PDR® NURSE'S DRUG HANDBOOK

2012 EDITION

Director, *Clinical Services:* Sylvia Nashed, PharmD
Manager, *Clinical Services:* Nermin Shenouda-Kerolous, PharmD
Senior *Drug Information Specialists:* Anila Patel, PharmD; Christine Sunwoo, PharmD
Drug *Information Specialists:* Pauline Lee, PharmD; Peter Leighton, PharmD;
  Kristine Mecca, PharmD; See-Won Seo, PharmD
Managing Editor: J. Harris Fleming, Jr.
Project Manager: Gary Lew
Manager, Art Department: Livio Udina
Senior Director, Operations & Client Services: Stephanie Struble
Associate Director, Manufacturing & Distribution: Thomas Westburgh

PDR NETWORK, LLC

CEO: Edward Fotsch, MD
President: David Tanzer
Chief Medical Officer: Christine Côté, MD
Chief Technology Officer: David Cheng
Chief Financial Officer: Dawn Carfora
Senior Vice President, Publishing & Operations: Valerie Berger
Senior Vice President, Corporate Development, Product Sales & General Counsel:
  Andrew Gelman
Senior Vice President, Sales: John Loucks
Senior Vice President, Product Management: Lucian Taylor

ISBN: 978-1-56363-790-2

Printed in Canada

W9-BDX-194

Contents

Contents

FOREWORD

Nursing professionals are at the forefront when it comes to safe medication administration and patient education, and they play an especially crucial role in the new era of healthcare reform. As noted in the 2011 Institute of Medicine report on the future of nursing,[1] nurses must now more than ever practice at the fullest extent of their practice scope. Nurses are central to the goals of ensuring the quality of healthcare and reducing costs in healthcare. To accomplish these goals in the arena of pharmacotherapy and medication administration, nurses must decipher the constantly changing information regarding medications, new therapies, and interactions, and rapidly assess patient responses to multiple variables that are important to medication administration. To do this, it is vital for each nurse to have a reference that provides accurate and easily accessible drug information. The *PDR® Nurse's Drug Handbook, 2012 Edition* is this reference.

Physicians' Desk Reference® is a well-known and trusted resource for medication information—and *PDR Nurse's Drug Handbook* follows this tradition. This important reference is specifically designed for nurses, with each entry providing the following when applicable: therapeutic class, indications, dosage, how the medication is supplied, contraindications, relevant warnings and precautions, key adverse reactions, interactions, pregnancy category, mechanism of action, pharmacokinetics, and nursing considerations—a special section that includes content specific to assessing, monitoring, and counseling patients, as well as administering medications.

The *PDR Nurse's Drug Handbook* is organized to foster quick identification of key drug information. Medications can be identified by generic and brand names, as well as therapeutic class. Special sections provide important considerations when caring for women who are pregnant or breastfeeding, children, and older adults. Other useful resources include scores of charts and tables about medications for specific chronic problems such as hypertension, headache, HIV, hepatitis, and diabetes; immunizations; poison antidotes; lactose-, galactose-, and sugar-free products; cytochrome P450 enzyme inhibitors, substrates, and inducers; and a full-color visual identification guide. New in the 2012 edition are tables providing detailed information about FDA-approved treatments for lung cancer and primary immunodeficiency disorders. Additionally, the 2012 edition comes with a companion digital Herbal Medicine Tool Kit.

The *PDR® Nurse's Drug Handbook, 2012 Edition* is an essential reference for enhancing full-scope nursing practice and patient education efforts. Its convenient size and clear layout provide fast access to concise, authoritative drug information, making this book a trusted resource among nurses.

Ivy M. Alexander, PhD, APRN, ANP-BC, FAAN
Professor
Director–Adult, Family, Gerontological, and
  Women's Health Primary Care Specialty
Yale University School of Nursing

1. Committee on the Robert Wood Johnson Foundation Initiative on the Future of Nursing, at the Institute of Medicine. (2011). The Future of Nursing: Leading Change, Advancing Health. The National Academies Press; Washington, DC. Available at: *http://www.nap.edu/catalog.php?record_id=12956*.

How to Use This Book

The *PDR® Nurse's Drug Handbook, 2012 Edition* allows you to quickly locate important drug information so you can care for patients with confidence. The guide includes over 1,100 monographs providing current, organized information for more than 1,500 of the most commonly used drugs. This handy reference is the perfect companion for practicing nurses, nursing students, and other healthcare professionals.

This compact guide is divided into four discrete sections. The **first section** consists of **concise drug monographs** based on FDA-approved prescribing information. These monographs are organized alphabetically by brand name. When a brand is no longer available, the generic name is used. Monographs may include:

- Brand Name
- Generic Name
- Manufacturer
- FDA/DEA Schedule
- Boxed Warnings
- Therapeutic Class
- Indications
- Dosage (adults, pediatrics, special populations)
- How Supplied (dosage form/strength)
- Contraindications
- Warnings/Precautions
- Adverse Reactions
- Interactions
- Pregnancy Category/Breastfeeding Precautions
- Mechanism of Action
- Pharmacokinetics
- Nursing Considerations
    - —Assessment
    - —Monitoring
    - —Patient Counseling
    - —Administration and Storage

The **second section** comprises an extensive collection of **tables and key references** to help nurses assess drug therapy and patient safety. Tables provided include Rx and OTC drug comparisons; the most common abbreviations, acronyms, and symbols used by healthcare professionals; and professional associations for nurses. Within the drug comparison tables, drugs are organized alphabetically and by class for easy access. These tables and references may include, but are not limited to:

- Brand/Generic Name
- How Supplied (dosage form/strength)
- Indications
- Initial and Max Dosages
- Usual Dosage Range
- Most Common Side Effects

The **third section** contains two **indices**—one with drugs indexed by brand and generic name and the other organized by therapeutic class.

The **final section** contains a **Visual Identification Guide** featuring product images listed by brand name. This section helps you quickly verify the identity of a capsule, tablet, or other solid oral medication. Each product image contains both the generic and brand name, strength, and the name of its supplier. Other strengths and dosage forms may be available; please check FDA-approved prescribing information for a complete listing of all strengths and dosage forms.

Important Information About Product Labeling

Entries in the *PDR® Nurse's Drug Handbook, 2012 Edition* are drawn from FDA-approved product labeling as published in *Physicians' Desk Reference®* or supplied by the manufacturer. The entries are compiled and updated on a regular basis by a staff of experienced pharmacists. While diligent efforts have been made to ensure the accuracy of each entry, it is essential to bear in mind that the information presented here is merely a synopsis of key points in the official labeling, and that the complete labeling contains additional precautionary information that may be of significance in specific cases. Similarly, please remember that only common and dangerous adverse reactions and interactions are included here, and that numerous less-prevalent adverse effects may be reported in the complete labeling. If an entry leaves any question unanswered, be sure to consult *Physicians' Desk Reference* or ask the manufacturer for additional information.

The function of the Publisher is the compilation, organization, and distribution of this information. In organizing and presenting the material in the *PDR® Nurse's Drug Handbook, 2012 Edition*, the Publisher does not warrant or guarantee any of the products described, or perform any independent analysis in connection with any of the product information contained herein.

The Publisher assumes no obligation to obtain and include any information in these entries other than that provided by the manufacturer. The Publisher does not warrant, guarantee, or advocate the use of any product described herein. The Publisher and editors do not assume, and expressly disclaim, any liability for errors, omissions, or typographical errors in the information contained herein or for misuse of any of the products listed.

DRUG MONOGRAPH KEY[1,2]

BRAND NAME

FDA/DEA Class*

generic (Manufacturer)

> **Boxed Warning:** A brief description of the boxed warning(s) that appear in the beginning of the official FDA-approved labeling for the drug.

OTHER BRAND NAMES: Brand name drugs that have the same generic components as the monograph drug.

THERAPEUTIC CLASS: Based on the active ingredients and their mechanism of action.

INDICATIONS: Only includes FDA-approved indications.

DOSAGE: Dosages for adults, pediatrics, and/or special populations as indicated in the official FDA-approved labeling.

HOW SUPPLIED: Product description including strength, formulation, [package size], and scored tablet information.

CONTRAINDICATIONS: Details harmful conditions related to the use of the drug and disease states or patient populations in which use of the monograph drug should be avoided.

WARNINGS/PRECAUTIONS: Details harmful conditions related to the use of the drug and disease states or patient populations where caution is dictated.

ADVERSE REACTIONS: Denotes side effects and adverse reactions listed in the official FDA-approved labeling as occurring with greater frequency (generally at a rate of ≥3%) or deemed significant based on the clinical judgment of the editors. Other side effects may be included if deemed serious or life-threatening. For a complete list of adverse reactions, please refer to the official FDA-approved labeling.

INTERACTIONS: Includes the effects and implications of other drugs and food on the monograph drug based on official FDA-approved labeling.

PREGNANCY: Indicated pregnancy and breastfeeding precautions and, when available, the FDA pregnancy rating system category.[†]

MECHANISM OF ACTION: Includes pharmacologic drug class and a brief description, or proposed mechanism, of how the drug produces its therapeutic effect.

PHARMACOKINETICS: Brief description of the important parameters described in the FDA-approved labeling related to the absorption, distribution, metabolism, and elimination of the drug. The majority of parameters included are an average or the approximate values provided in the FDA-approved labeling. Only a select group of parameters are included. Refer to the full prescribing information for more detailed pharmacokinetics information.

- **Absorption:** The process by which the drug enters the bloodstream and becomes bioavailable. Absorption parameters may include time to peak plasma concentration (T_{max}), area under the curve (AUC), peak plasma concentration (C_{max}), and absolute bioavailability.
- **Distribution:** Parameters related to the dispersion and dissemination of the monograph drug through bodily fluids and tissues. Distribution parameters may include plasma protein binding and volume of distribution (V_d).
- **Metabolism:** Summary of the biotransformation or detoxification of the parent compound into metabolites. Associated enzymes and active metabolites are included if applicable.
- **Elimination:** The parameters associated with the removal of the drug from the body. Elimination parameters may include elimination/terminal half-life ($T_{1/2}$) and percentage eliminated through urine or feces.

NURSING CONSIDERATIONS

Assessment: Contains specific parameters and laboratory tests that the patient must be assessed for or undergo prior to starting treatment with the drug.

Monitoring: Information used for monitoring patients currently treated with the drug. Monitoring points may include specific lab tests and drug-related or condition-specific information.

Patient Counseling: A compilation of important treatment information to discuss with the patient.

Administration: Guidelines for preparing the monograph drug for administration, rate of administration, proper administration technique, and/or compatibility. Please see the Dosage section. For more details on the step-by-step administration process, refer to the full prescribing information for the drug.

Storage: Instructions for safe storage and disposal of the monograph drug.

---

[1] Drug monographs contain concise information. Not all fields described in the Drug Monograph Key are included in every monograph. For more detailed information, please see the full FDA-approved labeling information for the drug.

[2] To identify abbreviated terms used within monographs, refer to the Abbreviations, Acronyms, and Symbols table in the appendix on page A1.

---

*FDA/DEA CLASS

OTC:	Available over-the-counter.
RX:	Requires a prescription.
CII:	Controlled substance; high potential for abuse.
CIII:	Controlled substance; some potential for abuse.
CIV:	Controlled substance; low potential for abuse.
CV:	Controlled substance; subject to state and local regulation.

---

†FDA USE-IN-PREGNANCY RATINGS

The FDA use-in-pregnancy rating system weighs the degree to which available information has ruled out risk to the fetus against the drug's potential benefit to the patient. The ratings, and the interpretation, are as follows:

CATEGORY	INTERPRETATION
A	**CONTROLLED STUDIES SHOW NO RISK.** Adequate, well-controlled studies in pregnant women have failed to demonstrate a risk to the fetus in any trimester of pregnancy.
B	**NO EVIDENCE OF RISK IN HUMANS.** Adequate, well-controlled studies in pregnant women have not shown increased risk of fetal abnormalities despite adverse findings in animals, or, in the absence of adequate human studies, animal studies show no fetal risk. The chance of fetal harm is remote, but remains a possibility.
C	**RISK CANNOT BE RULED OUT.** Adequate, well-controlled human studies are lacking, and animal studies have shown a risk to the fetus or are lacking as well. There is a chance of fetal harm if the drug is administered during pregnancy; but the potential benefits may outweigh the potential risk.
D	**POSITIVE EVIDENCE OF RISK.** Studies in humans, or investigational or post-marketing data, have demonstrated fetal risk. Nevertheless, potential benefits from the use of the drug may outweigh the potential risk. For example, the drug may be acceptable if needed in a life-threatening situation or serious disease for which safer drugs cannot be used or are ineffective.
X	**CONTRAINDICATED IN PREGNANCY.** Studies in animals or humans, or investigational or post-marketing reports, have demonstrated positive evidence of fetal abnormalities or risk which clearly outweighs any possible benefit to the patient.

Concise Drug Monographs

ABELCET
amphotericin B lipid complex (Enzon)

THERAPEUTIC CLASS: Polyene antifungal

INDICATIONS: Treatment of invasive fungal infections in patients refractory to or intolerant of conventional amphotericin B therapy.

DOSAGE: *Adults:* 5mg/kg given as a single IV infusion at 2.5mg/kg/hr. *Pediatrics:* ≥16 yrs: 5mg/kg given as a single IV infusion at 2.5mg/kg/hr.

HOW SUPPLIED: Inj: 5mg/mL

WARNINGS/PRECAUTIONS: Anaphylaxis reported. D/C if respiratory distress occurs. Monitor SrCr frequently during therapy. Monitor LFTs, serum electrolytes (particularly Mg^{2+} and K^+) and CBC.

ADVERSE REACTIONS: Chills, fever, increased SrCr, multi-organ failure, N/V, hypotension, respiratory failure, dyspnea, sepsis, diarrhea, headache, heart arrest, HTN, hypokalemia, infection.

INTERACTIONS: Concurrent use of antineoplastic agents may potentiate renal toxicity, bronchospasm, hypotension. Corticosteroids and corticotropin may potentiate hypokalemia. May induce hypokalemia and potentiate digitalis toxicity with digitalis glycosides. May increase flucytosine toxicity. Acute pulmonary toxicity reported with leukocyte transfusions. Nephrotoxic drugs (eg, aminoglycosides, pentamidine) enhance potential for renal toxicity. Initiation with cyclosporine within several days of bone marrow ablation associated with nephrotoxicity. May enhance curariform effect of skeletal muscle relaxants due to hypokalemia. Caution with imidazoles (eg, ketoconazole, miconazole, clotrimazole, fluconazole). Monitor renal and hematologic function with zidovudine.

PREGNANCY: Category B, not for use in nursing.

MECHANISM OF ACTION: Antifungal agent; acts by binding to sterols in cell membrane of susceptible fungi, with resultant change in membrane permeability.

PHARMACOKINETICS: Absorption: C_{max}=1.7mcg/mL, AUC=14mcg•hr/mL. **Distribution:** V_d=131L/kg. **Elimination:** $T_{1/2}$=173.4 hrs.

NURSING CONSIDERATIONS

Assessment: Assess for hypersensitivity, previous amphotericin B use, hepatic/renal impairment, pregnancy/nursing status and possible drug interactions. Obtain baseline SrCr, LFTs, serum electrolytes (Mg^{2+}, K^+) and CBC.

Monitoring: Monitor for anaphylactic reactions and infusion reactions (eg, fever, chills, hypotension, bronchospasm, arrhythmias, shock), Monitor SrCr, LFTs, serum electrolytes (Mg^{2+}, K^+) and CBC.

Patient Counseling: Advise to seek medical attention if symptoms of acute reaction occur (eg, fevers, chills). Instruct patient to report all medications being used.

Administration: IV infusion. Shake the infusion bag q2h if the infusion time exceeds 2 hrs. Refer to PI for preparation of admixture for infusion. Do not dilute with saline solution or mix with other drugs or electrolytes. Do not use in-line filter. **Storage:** 2-8°C (36-46°F); admixture stable for 48 hrs at 2-8°C (36-46°F) and additional 6 hrs at room temperature. Avoid light exposure and freezing.

ABILIFY

RX

aripiprazole (Bristol-Myers Squibb/Otsuka America)

> Elderly patients with dementia-related psychosis treated with antipsychotic drugs are at an increased risk of death; most deaths appeared to be cardiovascular (CV) (eg, heart failure, sudden death) or infectious (eg, pneumonia) in nature. Not approved for the treatment of patients with dementia-related psychosis. Antidepressants increased the risk of suicidal thinking and behavior (suicidality) in short-term studies in children, adolescents, and young adults with major depressive disorder (MDD) and other psychiatric disorders. Monitor and observe closely for clinical worsening, suicidality, or unusual changes in behavior in patients who are started on antidepressant therapy. Not approved for use in pediatric patients with depression.

OTHER BRAND NAMES: Abilify Discmelt (Bristol-Myers Squibb/Otsuka America)

THERAPEUTIC CLASS: Partial $D_2/5HT_{1A}$ agonist/$5HT_{2A}$ antagonist

INDICATIONS: (PO) Treatment of schizophrenia in adults and adolescents (13-17 yrs). Acute treatment of manic and mixed episodes associated with bipolar I disorder in adults and pediatrics (10-17 yrs). Maintenance treatment of bipolar I disorder, both as monotherapy and adjunct to lithium or valproate in adults. Adjunctive therapy to antidepressants for treatment of MDD in adults. Treatment of irritability associated with autistic disorder in pediatric patients (6-17 yrs). (Inj) Acute treatment of agitation associated with schizophrenia or bipolar disorder, manic or mixed, in adults.

DOSAGE: *Adults:* (PO) Schizophrenia: Initial/Target: 10mg or 15mg qd. Titrate: Should not increase before 2 weeks. Usual: 10-30mg/day. Bipolar Disorder (Monotherapy): Initial/Target: 15mg qd. (Adjunct to Lithium or Valproate): Initial: 10-15mg qd. Target: 15mg qd. Titrate: May increase to 30mg/day based on clinical response. Max: 30mg/day. MDD Adjunct: Initial: 2-5mg/day. Titrate: May adjust dose at increments up to 5mg/day at intervals ≥1 week. Usual: 2-15mg/day. Periodically reassess need for maintenance therapy. Oral Sol: May give on mg-per-mg basis up to 25mg. Patients receiving 30mg tabs should receive 25mg of oral sol. (Inj) Schizophrenia or Bipolar Mania: 9.75mg IM. Usual: 5.25-15mg IM. Max: 30mg/day IM or not more frequent than q2h. If clinically indicated, may replace with PO at 10-30mg/day. Refer to PI for dose adjustments with concomitant CYP3A4/CYP2D6 inhibitors, CYP3A4 inducers, and in CYP2D6 poor metabolizers.
Pediatrics: Schizophrenia (13-17 yrs)/Bipolar Disorder (Monotherapy or Adjunct) (10-17 yrs): Initial: 2mg/day. Titrate: May increase to 5mg/day after 2 days to a target dose of 10mg/day after 2 additional days. Subsequent dose increases should be administered in 5mg increments. Schizophrenia (13-17 yrs): Usual: 10-30mg/day. Irritability Associated with Autistic Disorder (6-17 yrs): Individualize dose. Initial: 2mg/day. Titrate: Increase to 5mg/day. May increase to 10 or 15mg/day if necessary. Dose adjustments of up to 5mg/day should occur gradually at intervals ≥1 week. Usual: 5-15mg/day. Periodically reassess need for maintenance therapy. Oral Sol: May give on mg-per-mg basis up to 25mg. Patients receiving 30mg tabs should receive 25mg of oral sol. Refer to PI for dose adjustments with concomitant CYP3A4/CYP2D6 inhibitors, CYP3A4 inducers, and in CYP2D6 poor metabolizers.

HOW SUPPLIED: Tab, Disintegrating: (Discmelt) 10mg, 15mg; Tab: 2mg, 5mg, 10mg, 15mg, 20mg, 30mg; Sol: 1mg/mL [150mL]; Inj: 7.5mg/mL

WARNINGS/PRECAUTIONS: Neuroleptic malignant syndrome (NMS) reported. May develop tardive dyskinesia (TD); consider d/c therapy. Hyperglycemia reported; monitor for worsening blood glucose control in diabetes mellitus (DM) patients and fasting blood glucose (FBG) levels in patients with diabetes risk. May cause orthostatic hypotension; caution with CV disease, cerebrovascular disease, or conditions that predispose to hypotension (eg, dehydration, hypovolemia). Leukopenia, neutropenia, and agranulocytosis reported; d/c if severe neutropenia (absolute neutrophil count [ANC] <1000/mm³) occurs. Seizures/convulsions reported; caution with history of seizures or with conditions that lower seizure threshold (eg, Alzheimer's dementia). May impair physical/mental abilities. May disrupt body's ability to reduce core body temperature. Esophageal dysmotility and aspiration may occur; caution in patients at risk for aspiration pneumonia.

ADVERSE REACTIONS: Headache, blurred vision, fatigue, tremor, anxiety, insomnia, N/V, somnolence, constipation, akathisia, extrapyramidal disorder, nasopharyngitis, dizziness, restlessness.

INTERACTIONS: May potentiate effect of antihypertensives. Caution with anticholinergic medications, and other centrally acting drugs. Avoid alcohol. CYP3A4 inducers (eg, carbamazepine) may lower blood levels. CYP3A4 inhibitors (eg, ketoconazole, itraconazole) or 2D6 inhibitors (eg, quinidine, fluoxetine, paroxetine) may increase blood levels. (Inj) Greater intensity of sedation and greater orthostatic hypotension with lorazepam inj; monitor for excessive sedation and orthostatic hypotension with parenteral benzodiazepines.

PREGNANCY: Category C, not for use in nursing.

MECHANISM OF ACTION: Partial $D_2/5HT_{1A}$ agonist/$5HT_{2A}$ antagonist; not established.

PHARMACOKINETICS: Absorption: Absolute bioavailability 87% (Tab), 100% (IM); T_{max}=3-5 hrs (Tab), 1-3 hrs (IM). **Distribution:** V_d=404L or 4.9L/kg (IV); plasma protein binding >99% (IV). **Metabolism:** Hepatic via dehydrogenation (CYP2D6 and CYP3A4), hydroxylation (CYP2D6 and CYP3A4), and N-dealkylation (CYP3A4). Dehydro-aripiprazole (active metabolite). **Elimination:** Urine (25%, <1% unchanged), feces (55%, 18% unchanged); $T_{1/2}$=75 hrs (extensive metabolizers) and 146 hrs (PMs).

NURSING CONSIDERATIONS

Assessment: Assess for history of suicidal behavior in children, DM or risk factors for DM, conditions that predispose to hypotension, seizures etc. Assess for any other conditions where treatment is cautioned or contraindicated. Assess baseline FBG levels in patients at risk for hyperglycemia.

Monitoring: Monitor for clinical worsening, suicidality, unusual changes in behavior, NMS, TD, hyperglycemia, orthostatic hypotension, leukopenia, neutropenia, akathisia, agranulocytosis, seizures/convulsions, cognitive/motor impairment, body temperature disruption, esophageal dysmotility, and aspiration. Measure FBG levels if hyperglycemic symptoms develop. Periodically evaluate serum glucose levels in patients at risk for DM. Monitor CBC frequently during the 1st few months of therapy. Periodically reassess for continued need for maintenance treatment.

Patient Counseling: Instruct caregivers and patients to contact physician if signs of agitation, anxiety, panic attacks, insomnia, hostility, aggressiveness, impulsivity, akathisia, hypomania, mania, irritability, worsening of depression, changes in behavior, or suicidal ideation develop. Use caution when operating hazardous machinery. Avoid alcohol use while on therapy. Counsel to avoid overheating and dehydration. Notify physician if become pregnant or intend to become pregnant during therapy and if taking or planning to take any prescription or over-the-counter drugs. Do not to breastfeed during therapy. ODT: Inform phenylketonurics that product contains phenylalanine. Instruct not to open blister until ready to administer. Do not split tab and to take without liquid, if possible. Sol: Inform that sol contains sucrose and fructose.

Administration: Oral/IM route. **Storage:** 25°C (77°F); excursions permitted to 15-30°C (59-86°F). Oral Sol: May be used for ≤6 months after opening, not beyond expiration date. Inj: Store in original container; protect from light.

ABRAXANE

RX

paclitaxel protein-bound particles (Abraxis)

Should not be administered to patients with metastatic breast cancer who have baseline neutrophil counts of <1,500 cells/mm³. Recommended that frequent peripheral blood cell counts be performed on all patients to monitor for the occurrence of bone marrow suppression, primarily neutropenia. Should be administered under the supervision of a physician experienced in the use of cancer chemotherapeutic agents. Do not substitute for or use with other paclitaxel formulations.

ABRAXANE

THERAPEUTIC CLASS: Antimicrotubule agent

INDICATIONS: Treatment of breast cancer after failure of combination chemotherapy for metastatic disease or relapse within 6 months of adjuvant chemotherapy. Prior therapy should have included an anthracycline unless clinically contraindicated.

DOSAGE: *Adults:* 260mg/m^2 IV over 30 min every 3 weeks. Severe Neutropenia (neutrophil <500 cells/mm^3 for week or longer) or Severe Sensory Neuropathy During Therapy: Reduce dose to 220mg/m^2 for subsequent courses. For recurrence of severe neutropenia or severe sensory neuropathy, additional dose reduction should be made to 180mg/m^2. For grade 3 sensory neuropathy, hold treatment until resolution to grade 1 or 2, followed by a dose reduction for all subsequent courses. Moderate Hepatic Impairment (AST<10XULN, Bilirubin 1.26-2.0XULN): 200mg/m^2. Severe Hepatic Impairment (AST<10XULN, Bilirubin 2.01-5.0XULN): 130mg/m^2. Do not give if AST>10xULN or Bilirubin>5.0xULN.

HOW SUPPLIED: Inj: 100mg

CONTRAINDICATIONS: Patients with baseline neutrophil counts of <1,500 cells/mm^3.

WARNINGS/PRECAUTIONS: Bone marrow suppression is dose dependent and a dose-limiting toxicity; do not re-treat until neutrophils recover to >1,500 cells/mm^3 and platelets recover to >100,000 cells/mm^3. Use has not been studied in patients with renal dysfunction. May cause fetal harm. Men should be advised not to father a child while receiving treatment. Remote risk for transmission of viral diseases; theoretical risk for transmission of Creutzfeldt-Jakob disease (CJD). Sensory neuropathy occurs frequently. Injection-site reactions reported. Caution with hepatic impairment. May affect ability to drive and use machines.

ADVERSE REACTIONS: Neutropenia, infections, anemia, ECG abnormalities, dyspnea, fluid retention/edema, sensory neuropathy, ocular/visual disturbances, arthralgia/myalgia, N/V, asthenia, diarrhea, alopecia, alkaline phosphatase elevations, AST elevations.

INTERACTIONS: Caution with concomitant use of medications known to inhibit (eg, ketoconazole and other imidazole antifungals, erythromycin, fluoxetine, gemfibrozil, cimetidine, ritonavir, saquinavir, indinavir, nelfinavir) or induce (eg, rifampicin, carbamazepine, phenytoin, efavirenz, nevirapine) either CYP2C8 or CYP3A4; pharmacokinetics of drug may be altered by interactions with substrates, inducers or inhibitors of CYP2C8 and/or CYP3A4. Concomitant or previous use with neurotoxic agents may influence the frequency or severity of neurological manifestations.

PREGNANCY: Category D, not for use in nursing.

MECHANISM OF ACTION: Antimicrotubule agent; promotes assembly of microtubules from tubulin dimers and stabilizes microtubules by preventing depolymerization. This stability results in inhibition of the normal dynamic reorganization of the microtubule network that is essential for vital interphase and mitotic cellular functions.

PHARMACOKINETICS: Absorption: C_{max}=18,741ng/mL. **Distribution:** V_d=632L/m^2, plasma protein binding (89-98%). **Metabolism:** Liver, via CYP2C8 (6α-hydroxypaclitaxel, major metabolite) and CYP3A4 (3'-p-hydroxypaclitaxel and 6α, 3'-p-dihydroxypaclitaxel, minor metabolites). **Elimination:** Urine (4% unchanged, <1% metabolite), feces (approximately 20%), $T_{1/2}$=27 hrs.

NURSING CONSIDERATIONS

Assessment: Assess for history of heart disease, hepatic/renal impairment, pregnancy/nursing status, and for possible drug interactions. Assess that baseline neutrophil count is ≥1,500 cells/mm^3.

Monitoring: Monitor for signs/symptoms of bone marrow suppression, viral infections, sensory neuropathy, and injection-site reactions. Perform frequent peripheral blood cell counts.

Patient Counseling: Inform of risks and benefits of therapy. Advise women of childbearing potential to avoid becoming pregnant and men not to father a child while on therapy. Counsel to immediately report any signs of fever or other signs of infection. Avoid contact with skin; if contact occurs wash skin immediately and thoroughly with soap and water. Inform that may affect ability to drive or use machines.

Administration: IV route. See PI for reconstitution instructions. **Storage:** Store vials in original cartons at 20-25°C (68-77°F). Retain in original package to protect from light.

ACANYA
clindamycin phosphate - benzoyl peroxide (Valeant)

RX

THERAPEUTIC CLASS: Antibacterial/keratolytic

INDICATIONS: Topical treatment of acne vulgaris in patients ≥12 yrs.

DOSAGE: *Adults:* Apply pea-sized amount to face qd.
Pediatrics: ≥12 yrs: Apply pea-sized amount to face qd.

HOW SUPPLIED: Gel: (Clindamycin Phosphate-Benzoyl Peroxide) 1.2%-2.5% [50g]

CONTRAINDICATIONS: History of regional enteritis, ulcerative colitis, or antibiotic-associated colitis.

WARNINGS/PRECAUTIONS: Diarrhea, bloody diarrhea, and colitis (including pseudomembranous colitis) reported; d/c if significant diarrhea occurs. Minimize sun exposure following application. Not for oral, ophthalmic, or intravaginal use.

ADVERSE REACTIONS: Erythema, scaling, itching, burning, stinging.

INTERACTIONS: Avoid with topical or oral erythromycin-containing products. *In vitro* antagonism with erythromycin reported. Caution with concomitant topical acne therapy (eg, peeling, desquamating, or abrasive agents) due to potential cumulative irritancy effects. May potentiate neuromuscular blockers. Antiperistaltic agents (eg, opiates, diphenoxylate with atropine) may prolong and/or worsen severe colitis.

PREGNANCY: Category C, not for use in nursing.

MECHANISM OF ACTION: Clindamycin phosphate: Antibacterial; binds to 50S ribosomal subunits of susceptible bacteria and prevents elongation of peptide chains, thereby suppressing bacterial protein synthesis. Benzoyl peroxide: Oxidizing agent; bacteriocidal and keratolytic effects.

PHARMACOKINETICS: Absorption: Benzoyl peroxide: Skin. **Distribution:** Orally and parenterally administered clindamycin is found in breast milk. **Metabolism:** Benzoyl peroxide: Benzoic acid (metabolite).

NURSING CONSIDERATIONS

Assessment: Assess for history of regional enteritis, ulcerative colitis, or antibiotic-associated colitis, diarrhea, bloody diarrhea, and active colitis, pregnancy/nursing status, and for possible drug interactions.

Monitoring: Monitor for erythema, scaling, itching, burning, stinging, allergic reactions, diarrhea, bloody diarrhea, and colitis.

Patient Counseling: Instruct to apply medication as directed and avoid other topical acne products unless directed by physician. Avoid direct contact with mouth, eyes, inside the nose, and all mucous membranes, applying on cuts or open wounds, and washing of face more than 2-3 times a day. Wash hands with soap and water after application. Notify physician if any signs or symptoms of local skin irritation develop. Minimize exposure to natural and avoid artificial sunlight. Instruct that may bleach hair or colored fabric. Advise to d/c and notify physician if severe diarrhea, GI discomfort, or allergic reaction occurs.

Administration: Topical route. Wash gently with mild soap and pat dry affected areas prior to application. Refer to PI for admixing instructions. **Storage:** 25°C (77°F) for 2 months. Do not freeze. Keep jar tightly closed.

ACCOLATE

RX

zafirlukast (AstraZeneca)

THERAPEUTIC CLASS: Leukotriene receptor antagonist

INDICATIONS: Prophylaxis and chronic treatment of asthma in patients ≥5 yrs.

DOSAGE: *Adults:* 20mg bid. Administer 1 hr ac or 2 hrs pc.
Pediatrics: ≥12 yrs: 20mg bid. 5-11 yrs: 10mg bid. Administer 1 hr ac or 2 hrs pc.

HOW SUPPLIED: Tab: 10mg, 20mg

WARNINGS/PRECAUTIONS: Cases of life-threatening hepatic failure reported. Monitor for signs and symptoms of liver dysfunction (eg, right upper quadrant abdominal pain, nausea, fatigue, lethargy, pruritus, jaundice, flu-like symptoms, anorexia, enlarged liver); d/c if liver dysfunction suspected. Monitor LFTs periodically or if hepatic dysfunction is suspected. Not for reversal of bronchospasm in acute asthma attacks including status asthmaticus. Therapy can be continued during acute exacerbations of asthma. Systemic eosinophilia, eosinophilic pneumonia, and vasculitis consistent with Churg-Strauss syndrome reported rarely. Neuropsychiatric events (eg, insomnia and depression) reported; carefully evaluate risks and benefits of continuing therapy if such events occur.

ADVERSE REACTIONS: Headache, infection, nausea.

INTERACTIONS: Coadministration with warfarin increases PT time; monitor closely and adjust anticoagulant dose accordingly. Caution with drugs metabolized by CYP2C9 (eg, tolbutamide, phenytoin, carbamazepine) or CYP3A4 (eg, dihydropyridine calcium channel blockers, cyclosporine, cisapride). Increased levels with ASA. Decreased levels with erythromycin, theophylline. May increase theophylline levels. May cause infections with inhaled corticosteroids.

PREGNANCY: Category B, not for use in nursing.

MECHANISM OF ACTION: Leukotriene receptor antagonist; selective and competitive receptor antagonist of leukotriene D_4 and E_4 (LTD_4 and LTE_4), components of slow-reacting substance of anaphylaxis (SRSA); inhibits bronchoconstriction.

PHARMACOKINETICS: Absorption: Rapid. (Adult) C_{max}=326ng/mL; T_{max}=2 hrs; AUC=1137ng•h/mL. (7-11 yrs) C_{max}=601ng/mL; T_{max}=2.5 hrs; AUC=2027ng•h/mL. (5-6 yrs) C_{max}=756ng/mL; T_{max}=2.1 hrs; AUC=2458ng•h/mL. **Distribution:** V_d=approximately 70L; plasma protein binding (>99%). Found in breast milk. **Metabolism:** Liver, hydroxylation via CYP2C9. **Elimination:** Urine (10%); feces. (Adult) $T_{1/2}$=13.3 hrs.

NURSING CONSIDERATIONS

Assessment: Assess for hepatic dysfunction, bronchospasm, pregnancy/nursing status, and for possible drug interactions. Obtain baseline LFTs.

Monitoring: Monitor for signs/symptoms of hepatotoxicity, systemic eosinophilia, eosinophilic pneumonia, vasculitic rash, worsening pulmonary symptoms, cardiac complications, neuropathy, and for neuropsychiatric events (eg, insomnia, depression). Monitor LFTs and PT.

Patient Counseling: Counsel to take drug at least 1 hr before or 2 hrs after meals. Advise to take regularly as prescribed even during symptom-free periods. Inform that medication is not a bronchodilator and should not be used to treat acute episodes of asthma. Instruct not to decrease dose or stop taking other anti-asthma medications unless instructed by a physician. Instruct to seek medical attention if symptoms of liver dysfunction (eg, right upper quadrant abdominal pain, nausea, fatigue, lethargy, pruritus, jaundice, flu-like symptoms, anorexia) or neuropsychiatric events occur. Instruct to notify physician if pregnant, planning to become pregnant, or are nursing.

Administration: Oral route. **Storage:** 20-25°C (68-77°F). Protect from light and moisture.

ACCRETROPIN

RX

somatropin (Cangene)

THERAPEUTIC CLASS: Recombinant human growth hormone

INDICATIONS: Treatment of pediatric patients who have growth failure due to inadequate secretion of normal endogenous growth hormone. Treatment of short stature associated with Turner syndrome (TS) in patients whose epiphyses are not closed.

DOSAGE: *Pediatrics:* Individualize dose. Divide into equal daily doses given 6 or 7X/week SQ. Growth Hormone Deficiency: 0.18mg/kg body weight/week to 0.3 mg/kg (0.90 IU/kg) body weight/week. TS: 0.36mg/kg body weight/week.

HOW SUPPLIED: Inj: 5mg/mL (15 IU/mL)

CONTRAINDICATIONS: Closed epiphyses; proliferative or preproliferative diabetic retinopathy; active malignancy (eg, pituitary tumor, progression or recurrence of an underlying intracranial tumor); acute critical illness due to complications following open heart surgery, abdominal surgery, or multiple accidental trauma, or acute respiratory failure; patients with Prader-Willi syndrome (PWS) who are severely obese or have severe respiratory impairment.

WARNINGS/PRECAUTIONS: Increased mortality reported with acute critical illness due to complications following open heart or abdominal surgery, multiple accidental trauma, or with acute respiratory failure; weigh benefits vs risks of continuing therapy in patients who develop acute critical illnesses. Fatalities reported in children with PWS who had severe obesity, history of upper airway obstruction or sleep apnea, or unidentified respiratory tract infection; interrupt treatment if signs develop. Monitor for signs of respiratory infection and weight control with PWS. Not indicated for long-term treatment of growth failure due to genetically confirmed PWS. May decrease insulin sensitivity which may unmask undiagnosed impaired glucose tolerance and overt diabetes mellitus (DM); monitor glucose levels. Monitor for progression or recurrence of underlying disease process in patients with pre-existing tumors or growth hormone deficiency secondary to an intracranial lesion. Intracranial HTN with papilledema, visual changes, headache, N/V reported; perform funduscopic exam before and periodically during treatment; d/c if papilledema occurs. Monitor standard hormonal replacement therapy in patients with hypopituitarism (multiple hormone deficiencies). Undiagnosed/untreated hypothyroidism may prevent optimal response; perform periodic thyroid function tests. Monitor for any malignant transformation of skin lesions. Tissue atrophy may occur if administered at same site over long period; rotate injection site. Slipped capital femoral epiphyses may occur; evaluate carefully with the onset of a limp or complaints of hip or knee pain. Monitor for scoliosis progression. Increased risk of otitis media or other ear disorders in patients with TS. Monitor for CV disorders in patients with TS. Allergic reactions may occur.

ADVERSE REACTIONS: Injection site reactions (eg, bruising, erythema, hemorrhage, edema, pain, pruritus, rash, swelling), nausea, headache, fatigue, scoliosis.

INTERACTIONS: May impact cortisol and cortisone metabolism; glucocorticoid replacement therapy may be required for previously undiagnosed, unmasked central (secondary) hypoadrenalism. Use of glucocorticoid replacement therapy for previously diagnosed hypoadrenalism, especially cortisone acetate or prednisone, may require an increase in maintenance or stress doses. Excessive glucocorticoid therapy may attenuate growth- promoting effects; adjust dosage carefully. May alter clearance of compounds metabolized by CYP450 (eg, corticosteroids, sex steroids, anticonvulsants, cyclosporine). May require dosage adjustment of insulin and/or oral hypoglycemic agents. Thyroid replacement therapy may require dosage adjustment.

PREGNANCY: Category C, caution in nursing.

MECHANISM OF ACTION: Human growth hormone; stimulates linear growth in pediatrics. Also demonstrated to stimulate skeletal growth in children, increase the size and number of skeletal muscle cells, increase cellular protein synthesis, modulate carbohydrate metabolism, mobilize lipids, reduce body fat stores, increase plasma fatty acids, and cause Na$^+$, K$^+$, and phosphorus retention.

PHARMACOKINETICS: Absorption: Absolute Bioavailability (70%), AUC$_{(0-t)}$=238.09ng•h/mL, AUC$_{(0-inf)}$=255.31ng•h/mL, C$_{max}$=29.49ng/mL, T$_{max}$=3.5 hrs. **Metabolism:** Liver, kidneys. **Excretion:** T$_{1/2}$=3.63 hrs.

NURSING CONSIDERATIONS

Assessment: Assess for other causes of poor growth (eg, under-nutrition, advanced bone age, hypothyroidism), closed epiphyses, proliferative or pre-proliferative diabetic retinopathy, active malignancy, DM or impaired glucose tolerance, pregnancy/nursing status, and for possible drug interactions. Assess for pre-existing papilledema by performing funduscopic examination. In patients with TS, assess for presence of otitis media or other ear disorders and for CV disorders.

Monitoring: Monitor for growth/clinical response, malignant transformation of skin lesions, symptoms of slipped capital femoral epiphysis, progression of pre-existing scoliosis, tissue atrophy at the injection site, and for allergic reactions. Monitor glucose levels. Perform thyroid function test and funduscopic examination periodically. In patients with TS, monitor for signs/symptoms of ear disorders (eg, otitis media) and CV disorders. In patients with hypopituitarism (multiple hormone deficiencies), monitor standard hormonal therapy. In patients with PWS, monitor weight and for signs/symptoms of upper airway obstruction or apnea and for respiratory infections. In patients with pre-existing tumors or GH deficiency secondary to an intracranial lesion, monitor for progression or recurrence of underlying disease process.

Patient Counseling: Inform of the potential benefits/risks of therapy. Instruct on proper administration. Advise to seek medical attention if symptoms of an allergic reaction, slipped capital femoral epiphysis (eg, onset of limp, hip or knee pain), or any other adverse reaction occurs.

Administration: SQ route. Do not inject IV. Rotate injection site. Refer to PI for further administration instructions. **Storage:** Unopened Vial: 2-8°C (36-46°F). Avoid freezing and shaking. Opened Vial: 2-8°C (36-46°F); stable up to 14 days. Discard 14 days after first use. Protect from light.

ACCUNEB   RX
albuterol sulfate (Dey)

THERAPEUTIC CLASS: Beta$_2$-agonist

INDICATIONS: Relief of bronchospasm with asthma (reversible obstructive airway disease) in patients 2-12 yrs.

DOSAGE: *Pediatrics:* 2-12 yrs: Initial: 0.63mg or 1.25mg tid-qid PRN via nebulizer over 5-15 min. Patients 6-12 yrs with more severe asthma, weight >40kg, or patients 11-12 yrs old may achieve better intial response with 1.25mg dose.

HOW SUPPLIED: Sol, Inhalation: 1.25mg/3mL, 0.63mg/3mL [3mL, 25^s]

WARNINGS/PRECAUTIONS: Can produce paradoxical bronchospasm; d/c if occurs. Consider adding anti-inflammatory agents (eg, corticosteroids) to adequately control asthma. Re-evaluate patient and treatment regimen if deterioration of asthma observed. Can produce clinically significant cardiovascular (CV) effect (eg, ECG changes); caution with CV disorders (eg, coronary insufficiency, cardiac arrhythmias, HTN). Immediate hypersensitivity reactions reported. Aggravation of pre-existing diabetes mellitus (DM) and ketoacidosis reported with large doses of IV albuterol. May cause hypokalemia. Has not been studied with acute attacks of bronchospasm.

ADVERSE REACTIONS: Asthma exacerbation, otitis media, allergic reaction, gastroenteritis, cold symptoms.

INTERACTIONS: Avoid other short-acting sympathomimetic aerosol bronchodilators and epinephrine. Extreme caution with MAOIs or TCAs, or within 2 weeks of d/c of such agents. Monitor digoxin levels; mean decreases in digoxin levels observed. May worsen ECG changes and/or hypokalemia caused by non-K+ sparing diuretics (eg, loop/thiazide); caution is advised. Pulmonary effect blocked by β-blockers; caution with cardioselective β-blockers.

PREGNANCY: Category C, not for use in nursing.

MECHANISM OF ACTION: β_2-adrenergic agonist; stimulates adenyl cyclase, the enzyme which catalyzes formation of cyclic AMP from ATP.

PHARMACOKINETICS: Absorption: Bioavailability (<20%); (Inh) C_{max}=2.1ng/mL, T_{max}=0.5 hrs. **Elimination:** Urine; (PO) $T_{1/2}$=5-6 hrs.

NURSING CONSIDERATIONS

Assessment: Assess for previous hypersensitivity to the drug, CV disorders, HTN, DM, pregnancy/nursing status, and for possible drug interactions.

Monitoring: Monitor for signs/symptoms of CV effects (measured by pulse rate and BP), worsening of symptoms, paradoxical bronchospasm, deterioration of asthma, hypokalemia, and hypersensitivity reactions.

Patient Counseling: Instruct not to use more frequently than recommended. Advise not to increase dose or frequency without consulting physician. Seek medical attention if symptoms worsen, if therapy becomes less effective, or if need to use more frequently than usual. Inform of the common effects (eg, palpitations, chest pain, rapid HR, tremor, nervousness). Do not to use if vial changes color or becomes cloudy. Inform that drug compatibility, clinical efficacy, and safety, when mixed with other drugs in nebulizer, have not been established.

Administration: Inhalation route. Refer to PI for proper administration.
Storage: 2-25°C (36-77°F). Protect from light and excessive heat. Store in protective foil pouch at all times. Once removed, use within 1 week. Discard if solution not colorless.

ACCUPRIL RX
quinapril HCl (Parke-Davis)

> ACE inhibitors can cause death/injury to the fetus during 2nd and 3rd trimesters. D/C if pregnancy is detected.

THERAPEUTIC CLASS: ACE inhibitor

INDICATIONS: Treatment of hypertension alone or in combination with thiazide diuretics. Management of heart failure with diuretics and/or digitalis as adjunct therapy.

DOSAGE: *Adults:* HTN: If possible, d/c diuretic 2-3 days prior to therapy. Initial: 10mg or 20mg qd; 5mg qd with concomitant diuretic. Titrate: May adjust dosage based on BP response at intervals of at least 2 weeks. Usual: 20-80mg/day given qd-bid. CrCl >60mL/min: Initial: 10mg/day. CrCl 30-60mL/min: Initial: 5mg/day. CrCl 10-30mL/min: Initial: 2.5mg/day. Elderly: Initial: 10mg qd. Titrate: Increase to the optimal response. Heart Failure: Initial: 5mg bid. Titrate: May adjust dosage at weekly intervals. Usual: 20-40mg/day given bid. CrCl >30mL/min: Initial: 5mg/day. CrCl 10-30mL/min: Initial: 2.5mg/day. If inital dose is well tolerated, succeeding days may be given bid. Titrate dose at weekly intervals based on clinical and hemodynamic response. Elderly: Start at low end of dosing range.

HOW SUPPLIED: Tab: 5mg*, 10mg, 20mg, 40mg *scored

CONTRAINDICATIONS: History of ACE inhibitor-associated angioedema.

WARNINGS/PRECAUTIONS: D/C if angioedema, jaundice, or marked LFT elevation occurs. Risk of hyperkalemia with DM, renal dysfunction. Persistent nonproductive cough reported. Monitor WBCs in renal or collagen vascular disease. Anaphylactoid reactions reported. Monitor for hypotension in high-risk patients (heart failure, surgery/anesthesia, hyponatremia, high-dose diuretic therapy, recent intensive diuresis, dialysis, or severe volume and/or salt depletion). Caution with CHF, renal dysfunction, and renal artery stenosis. Less effective on BP in blacks and higher rates of angioedema than nonblacks. Caution in elderly.

ADVERSE REACTIONS: Headache, dizziness, cough.

INTERACTIONS: Decreases tetracycline absorption (possibly due to magnesium content in quinapril); consider interaction with drugs that interact with magnesium. May increase lithium levels and risk of toxicity. Hypotension risk with diuretics. Increased risk of hyperkalemia with K^+-sparing diuretics, K^+ supplements, or K^+-containing salt substitutes. May attenuate K^+ loss with thiazide diuretics. Nitritoid reactions reported (eg, facial flushing, N/V, hypotension) rarely with injectable gold (eg, sodium aurothiomalate).

PREGNANCY: Category C (1st trimester) and D (2nd and 3rd trimesters), caution in nursing.

MECHANISM OF ACTION: Angiotensin-converting enzyme inhibitor; inhibits ACE activity, reducing angiotensin II formation.

PHARMACOKINETICS: Absorption: T_{max}=1 hr. (Quinaprilat) T_{max}=2 hrs. **Distribution:** Plasma protein binding (97%); found in breast milk. **Metabolism:** De-esterification. Quinaprilat (active metabolite). **Elimination:** (Quinaprilat) Renal; $T_{1/2}$=2 hrs.

NURSING CONSIDERATIONS

Assessment: Assess for volume/salt depletion, collagen vascular disease, CHF, DM, possible drug interactions, ischemic heart disease, cerebrovascular disease, renal function, pregnancy/nursing status, and possible drug interactions.

Monitoring: Monitor renal function for 1st few weeks, WBC periodically in patients with collagen vascular disease. Monitor for signs/symptoms of hypotension, anaphylactoid or hypersensitivity reactions, head/neck and intestinal angioedema, agranulocytosis, hyperkalemia, and renal dysfunction.

Patient Counseling: Inform of pregnancy risks; d/c therapy if pregnancy detected. Instruct that inadequate fluid intake or fluid loss may lead to drop in BP resulting in lightheadedness or syncope; avoid K^+ supplements or salt substitutes. Seek medical attention if symptoms of hypotension (syncope), anaphylactoid or hypersensitivity reactions, angioedema (head/neck; abdominal pain with/without N/V), infection (sore throat, fever), or hyperkalemia occur.

Administration: Oral route. **Storage:** 15-30°C (59-86°F). Protect from light.

ACCURETIC   RX
quinapril HCl - hydrochlorothiazide (Parke-Davis)

> ACE inhibitors can cause death/injury to developing fetus during 2nd and 3rd trimesters. D/C therapy if pregnancy detected.

THERAPEUTIC CLASS: ACE inhibitor/thiazide diuretic

INDICATIONS: Treatment of hypertension.

DOSAGE: *Adults:* Initial (if not controlled on quinapril monotherapy): 10mg-12.5mg or 20mg-12.5mg tab qd. Titrate: May increase after 2-3 weeks based on clinical response. Initial (if controlled on HCTZ 25mg/day but significant K^+ loss): 10mg-12.5mg or 20mg-12.5mg tab qd. If previously treated with 20mg quinapril and 25mg HCTZ, may switch to 20mg-25mg tab qd. Elderly: Start at low end of dosing range.

HOW SUPPLIED: Tab: (Quinapril-HCTZ) 10mg-12.5mg*, 20mg-12.5mg*, 20mg-25mg *scored

CONTRAINDICATIONS: History of ACE inhibitor-associated angioedema, anuria, sulfonamide hypersensitivity.

WARNINGS/PRECAUTIONS: D/C if angioedema, jaundice, or marked LFT elevation occurs. Risk of hyperkalemia with DM, renal dysfunction. Persistent nonproductive cough reported. Monitor WBCs in renal or collagen vascular disease. Anaphylactoid reactions reported. Monitor for hypotension in high-risk patients (eg, heart failure, surgery/anesthesia, hyponatremia, severe volume/salt depletion, etc.). Caution with CHF, renal or hepatic dysfunction, and renal artery stenosis. Less effective on BP in blacks and more reports of angioedema than nonblacks. May exacerbate or activate systemic lupus erythematosus (SLE). Monitor serum electrolytes. Avoid if CrCl ≤30mL/min/1.73m². May increase cholesterol, TG, magnesium, calcium, and uric acid levels. May decrease glucose tolerance, serum protein-bound iodine levels without signs of thyroid disturbance. D/C for a few days before parathyroid function tests. Not for initial therapy. Caution in elderly.

ADVERSE REACTIONS: Dizziness, headache, cough, increases in serum creatinine and BUN levels.

INTERACTIONS: Quinapril: Decreases tetracycline absorption (possibly due to magnesium content in quinapril); consider interaction with drugs that interact with magnesium. Increased risk of hyperkalemia with K⁺-sparing diuretics, K⁺ supplements, or K⁺-containing salt substitutes. May increase lithium levels and risk of toxicity. Nitritoid reactions reported (eg, facial flushing, N/V, hypotension) rarely with injectable gold (eg, sodium aurothiomalate). HCTZ: Potentiates orthostatic hypotension with alcohol, barbiturates, and narcotics. Adjust antidiabetic drugs. Impaired absorption with cholestyramine, colestipol. Corticosteroids and ACTH deplete electrolytes. May decrease response to pressor amines. Potentiates other antihypertensives. May increase responsiveness to non-depolarizing skeletal muscle relaxants. Risk of lithium toxicity. NSAIDs decrease diuretic, natriuretic, and antihypertensive effects.

PREGNANCY: Category C (1st trimester) and D (2nd and 3rd trimesters), not for use in nursing.

MECHANISM OF ACTION: Quinapril: Angiotensin-converting enzyme inhibitor; inhibits ACE activity, reducing angiotensin II formation. HCTZ: Thiazide diuretic; affects renal tubular mechanism of electrolyte reabsorption directly increasing excretion of Na^+ and Cl^-, and indirectly reducing plasma volume.

PHARMACOKINETICS: Absorption: Quinapril: T_{max}=1 hr. (Quinaprilat) T_{max}=2 hrs. **Distribution:** Quinapril: Plasma protein binding (97%). HCTZ: V_d=3.6-7.8L/kg; plasma protein binding (67.9%); crosses placenta; found in breast milk. **Metabolism:** Quinapril: De-esterification. Quinaprilat (metabolite). **Elimination:** Quinaprilat: Renal; $T_{1/2}$=2 hrs. HCTZ: Kidney (61%, unchanged); $T_{1/2}$=4-15 hrs.

NURSING CONSIDERATIONS

Assessment: Assess for volume/salt depletion, collagen vascular disease (SLE, scleroderma), CHF, DM, ischemic heart disease, cerebrovascular disease, anuria, sulfonamide hypersensitivity, renal/hepatic function, pregnancy/nursing status, and possible drug interactions.

Monitoring: Monitor renal function for 1st few weeks; WBC periodically in patients with collagen vascular disease. Monitor cholesterol, TG, magnesium, calcium and uric acid levels. Monitor for signs/symptoms of hypotension, anaphylactoid or hypersensitivity reactions, head/neck and intestinal angioedema, agranulocytosis, hyperkalemia, electrolyte imbalance, exacerbation or activation of SLE, precipitation of gout, hyperglycemia, renal/hepatic dysfunction.

Patient Counseling: Inform of pregnancy risks. Advise that inadequate fluid intake or loss of fluids may lead to drop in BP resulting in lightheadedness or syncope. Seek medical attention if symptoms of angioedema (head/neck; abdominal pain with/without N/V), infection (sore throat, fever), hypotension (syncope), hypersensitivity reactions, hyperkalemia, or electrolyte imbalance (dry mouth, thirst, weakness) occurs.

Administration: Oral route. **Storage:** 20-25°C (68-77°F).

ACEON
perindopril erbumine (Abbott)

RX

> ACE inhibitors can cause death/injury to developing fetus. D/C therapy if pregnancy detected.

THERAPEUTIC CLASS: ACE inhibitor

INDICATIONS: Treatment of HTN as monotherapy or with other antihypertensives, especially thiazide diuretics. Treatment of stable coronary artery disease (CAD) to reduce risk of cardiovascular mortality or nonfatal myocardial infarction (MI); may be used with conventional treatment for CAD (eg, antiplatelet, antihypertensive, or lipid-lowering therapy).

DOSAGE: *Adults:* HTN: Initial: 4mg qd. May be titrated PRN to max of 16mg qd. Maint: 4-8mg qd or in 2 divided doses. Elderly: Initial: 4mg qd or in 2 divided dose. Monitor BP and titrate carefully with doses >8mg. Use with diuretics: Reduce diuretic dose prior to start of treatment. Stable CAD: Initial: 4mg qd for 2 weeks. Maint: 8mg qd. Elderly (>70 yrs): Initial: 2mg qd for 1 week, then 4mg qd for Week 2. Maint: 8mg qd. Renal Impairment: CrCl ≥30mL/min: Initial: 2mg/day. Max: 8mg/day.

HOW SUPPLIED: Tab: 2mg*, 4mg*, 8mg* *scored

CONTRAINDICATIONS: Hereditary or idiopathic angioedema.

WARNINGS/PRECAUTIONS: Angioedema of the face, extremities, lips, tongue, glottis, and/or larynx reported; d/c if occur. Intestinal angioedema reported; monitor for abdominal pain (with or without N/V). May cause symptomatic hypotension; caution with volume/salt depletion, ischemic heart disease (IHD), or cerebrovascular disease. May cause agranulocytosis and bone marrow depression. May cause changes in renal function; caution with severe congestive heart failure (CHF) and hypertensive patients with renal artery stenosis. Increase BUN or SrCr may occur. May cause hyperkalemia; caution in patients with diabetes mellitus (DM) and renal dysfunction. Persistent nonproductive cough reported. Rarely, a syndrome of cholestatic jaundice, fulminant necrosis and sometimes death occurs; d/c if jaundice or marked elevations of hepatic enzymes develop.

ADVERSE REACTIONS: Cough, drug intolerance, asthenia, dizziness, hypotension, back pain.

INTERACTIONS: May increase lithium levels. Hypotension risk with diuretics, and anesthetics. Increased risk of hyperkalemia with K⁺-sparing diuretics (eg, spironolactone, amiloride, triamterene), drugs that increase serum K⁺ (eg, indomethacin, heparin, cyclosporine), or K⁺ supplements. Nitritoid reactions (eg, facial flushing, N/V, hypotension) reported rarely with injectable gold. Caution with digoxin.

PREGNANCY: Category D, caution in nursing.

MECHANISM OF ACTION: Angiotensin-converting enzyme inhibitor; inhibits ACE activity resulting in decreased plasma angiotensin II, leading to decreased vasoconstriction, increased plasma renin activity, and decreased aldosterone secretion.

PHARMACOKINETICS: Absorption: Rapid; absolute bioavailability (75%, perindopril), (25%, perindoprilat); T_{max}=(1 hr, perindopril), (3-7 hrs, perindoprilat). **Distribution:** Plasma protein binding (60%, perindopril), (10-20%, perindoprilat); crosses the placenta. **Metabolism:** Hepatic (extensive); hydrolysis, glucuronidation, cyclization. Perindoprilat (active metabolite). **Elimination:** Urine (4-12%, unchanged); $T_{1/2}$=(0.8-1 hr, perindopril), (3-10 hrs, perindoprilat).

NURSING CONSIDERATIONS

Assessment: Assess for hereditary or idiopathic angioedema, volume and/or salt depletion, CHF, renal artery stenosis, IHD, cerebrovascular disease, pregnancy/nursing status, hepatic/renal impairment, risk factors for developing hyperkalemia (eg, DM, renal insufficiency), previous hypersensitivity, and possible drug interactions.

Monitoring: Monitor for signs/symptoms of anaphylactoid reactions, head/neck/intestinal angioedema, hypotension, agranulocytosis, hepatic failure, hyperkalemia, persistent nonproductive cough, and hypersensitivity reactions. Monitor hepatic/renal function.

Patient Counseling: Instruct to immediately report to physician any signs/symptoms of angioedema (eg, swelling of the face, extremities, eyes, lips, tongue, hoarseness or difficulty swallowing or breathing) and to take no more drug before consulting healthcare provider. Instruct to contact physician if lightheadedness occurs and d/c therapy if fainting occurs. Advise to avoid K⁺ supplements or salt substitutes unless physician has been notified. Counsel to report indication of infection (eg, sore throat, fever) which could be a sign of neutropenia. Inform of potential risks if used during pregnancy. Keep out of reach of children.

Administration: Oral route. **Storage:** 20-25°C (68-77°F).

ACETADOTE   RX
acetylcysteine (Cumberland)

THERAPEUTIC CLASS: Acetaminophen antidote

INDICATIONS: Prevent or lessen hepatic injury within 8-10 hrs after ingestion of potentially hepatotoxic dose of acetaminophen (APAP).

DOSAGE: *Adults:* Total Dose: 300mg/kg over 21 hrs. ≥40kg: LD: 150mg/kg IV in 200mL of diluent over 60 min. Second Dose: 50mg/kg in 500mL of diluent over 4 hrs. Third Dose: 100mg/kg in 1000mL of diluent over 16 hrs. >20kg-<40kg: LD: 150mg/kg IV in 100mL of diluent over 60 min. Second Dose: 50mg/kg in 250mL of diluent over 4 hrs. Third Dose: 100mg/kg in 500mL of diluent over 16 hrs. ≤20kg: LD: 150mg/kg IV in 3mL/kg of body weight of diluent over 60 min. Second Dose: 50mg/kg in 7mL/kg of body weight of diluent over 4 hrs. Third Dose: 100mg/kg in 14mL/kg of body weight of diluent over 16 hrs.
Pediatrics: <16 yrs: Total Dose: 300mg/kg over 21 hrs. ≥40kg: LD: 150mg/kg IV in 200mL of diluent over 60 min. Second Dose: 50mg/kg in 500mL of diluent over 4 hrs. Third Dose: 100mg/kg in 1000mL of diluent over 16 hrs. >20kg-<40kg: LD: 150mg/kg IV in 100mL of diluent over 60 min. Second Dose: 50mg/kg in 250mL of diluent over 4 hrs. Third Dose: 100mg/kg in 500mL of diluent over 16 hrs. ≤20kg: LD: 150mg/kg IV in 3mL/kg of body weight of diluent over 60 min. Second Dose: 50mg/kg in 7mL/kg of body weight of diluent over 4 hrs. Third Dose: 100mg/kg in 14mL/kg of body weight of diluent over 16 hrs.

HOW SUPPLIED: Inj: 200mg/mL [30mL]

WARNINGS/PRECAUTIONS: Serious anaphylactoid reactions (eg, rash, hypotension, wheezing, and SOB) reported; interrupt and carefully restart therapy if occur; d/c and consider alternative management if anaphylactoid reaction returns upon reinitiation of treatment or increases in severity. Acute flushing and erythema of skin may occur. Caution with asthma or history of bronchospasm. Adjust total volume administered in patients <40kg and for those requiring fluid restriction to avoid fluid overload. May increase plasma levels with hepatic cirrhosis.

ADVERSE REACTIONS: Anaphylactoid reactions, rash, urticaria, pruritus, N/V, tachycardia, facial flushing.

PREGNANCY: Category B, caution in nursing.

MECHANISM OF ACTION: Acetaminophen antidote; protects liver by maintaining or restoring glutathione levels. Also acts as an alternate substrate for conjugation with, and thus detoxification of, the reactive metabolite.

PHARMACOKINETICS: Distribution: V_d=0.47L/kg; plasma protein binding (83%); crosses the placenta. **Metabolism:** May form cysteine, disulfides and conjugates. **Elimination:** $T_{1/2}$=5.6 hrs (adults), 11 hrs (newborns).

NURSING CONSIDERATIONS

Assessment: Assess for previous hypersensitivity to drug, asthma, history of bronchospasm, hepatic impairment, and pregnancy/nursing status. Obtain baseline serum APAP levels, ALT, AST, bilirubin, PT, BUN, blood glucose levels and electrolytes. Determine time of APAP ingestion.

Monitoring: Monitor for anaphylactoid reactions, acute flushing, erythema, fluid overload, hepatic/renal dysfunction, and electrolyte imbalance.

Patient Counseling: Advise to report to the physician any history of sensitivity to the product or any history of asthma.

Administration: IV route. **Storage:** 20-25°C (68-77°F).

ACIPHEX
rabeprazole sodium (Eisai/PRICARA)

RX

THERAPEUTIC CLASS: Proton pump inhibitor

INDICATIONS: Short-term treatment in the healing and symptomatic relief of erosive or ulcerative gastroesophageal reflux disease (GERD). Maintenance of healing and reduction in relapse rates of heartburn symptoms in patients with erosive or ulcerative GERD. Treatment of daytime and nighttime heartburn and other symptoms associated with GERD. Short-term treatment in the healing and symptomatic relief of duodenal ulcers (DU). In combination with amoxicillin and clarithromycin as a 3-drug regimen for the treatment of patients with *H.pylori* infection and DU disease (active or history within the past 5 yrs) to eradicate *H.pylori* and reduce the risk of DU recurrence. Long-term treatment of pathological hypersecretory conditions, including Zollinger-Ellison syndrome.

DOSAGE: *Adults:* Erosive/Ulcerative GERD: Healing: 20mg qd for 4-8 weeks. May repeat for 8 weeks if needed. Maint: 20mg qd. Symptomatic Gastroesophageal Reflux Disease (GERD): 20mg qd for 4 weeks. May repeat for 4 weeks if needed. Duodenal Ulcer: 20mg qd after am meal for up to 4 weeks. May need additional therapy. *H.pylori* Triple Therapy: 20mg + clarithromycin 500mg + amoxicillin 1g, all bid (qam and qpm) with food for 7 days. Pathological Hypersecretory Conditions: Initial: 60mg qd. Titrate: Adjust according to need. Maint: Up to 100mg qd or 60mg bid. May treat up to 1 yr. *Pediatrics:* ≥12 yrs: Symptomatic GERD: 20mg qd for up to 8 weeks.

HOW SUPPLIED: Tab, Delayed-Release: 20mg

WARNINGS/PRECAUTIONS: Symptomatic response does not preclude the presence of gastric malignancy. Caution with severe hepatic impairment. May increase risk of osteoporosis-related fractures of the hips, wrist, or spine with high doses and long-term proton pump inhibitors (PPIs) therapy.

ADVERSE REACTIONS: Headache, flatulence, pain, pharyngitis, diarrhea, N/V, abdominal pain.

INTERACTIONS: May alter absorption of pH-dependent drugs (eg, ketoconazole, digoxin). May inhibit cyclosporine metabolism. May increase digoxin plasma levels and decrease ketoconazole levels. Concomitant use with warfarin increases the INR and PT time; monitor PT/INR. When used with clarithromycin, the levels of both drugs may be increased. May reduce plasma levels of atazanavir.

PREGNANCY: Category B, not for use in nursing.

MECHANISM OF ACTION: Proton pump inhibitor; suppresses gastric acid secretion by inhibiting the gastric (H^+, K^+)-ATPase enzyme at the secretory surface of the gastric parietal cell. Blocks the final step of gastric acid secretion.

PHARMACOKINETICS: Absorption: T_{max}=2-5 hrs; absolute bioavailability (52%). **Distribution:** Plasma protein binding (96.3%). **Metabolism:** Extensive. Liver via CYP3A4 to sulphone (primary metabolite) and CYP2C19 to desmethyl rabeprazole (primary metabolite). **Elimination:** Urine (90%), feces; $T_{1/2}$=1-2 hrs.

NURSING CONSIDERATIONS

Assessment: Assess for hypersensitivity to other PPIs, presence of gastric malignancy, osteoporosis-related fractures, severe hepatic impairment, pregnancy/nursing status, and possible drug interactions.

Monitoring: Monitor for hypersensitivity reactions, clinical improvement, and pathological changes in gastric mucosa. If on concomitant therapy with antibacterial agents, monitor for signs/symptoms of *C. difficile*. Monitor PT/INR when given with warfarin.

Patient Counseling: Inform about the risks and benefits of therapy. Instruct to swallow tablet whole with water; do not chew, crush, or split tablet. May take with/without food. Inform if dose is missed, take drug as soon as possible. If almost time for the next dose, skip missed dose and go back to normal schedule; do not take 2 doses at same time. Contact physician if signs of hypersensitivity reaction (rash, face swelling, throat tightness, difficulty breathing) occur.

Administration: Oral route. Swallow tabs whole; do not chew, crush, or split.

Storage: 25°C (77°F); excursions permitted to 15-30°C (59-86°F). Protect from moisture.

ACLOVATE   RX
alclometasone dipropionate (GlaxoSmithKline)

THERAPEUTIC CLASS: Corticosteroid

INDICATIONS: Relief of the inflammatory and pruritic manifestations of corticosteroid-responsive dermatoses.

DOSAGE: *Adults:* Apply a thin film to affected areas, bid-tid; massage gently until it disappears. D/C when control is achieved; reassess if no improvement after 2 weeks.
Pediatrics: ≥1 yr: Apply a thin film to affected areas bid-tid; massage gently until it disappears. D/C when control is achieved; reassess if no improvement after 2 weeks.

HOW SUPPLIED: Cre, Oint: 0.05% [15g, 60g]

WARNINGS/PRECAUTIONS: May produce reversible hypothalamic-pituitary-adrenal (HPA) axis suppression, manifestations of Cushing's syndrome, hyperglycemia, and glucosuria. Evaluate for HPA axis suppression when applied to large surface area or to areas under occlusion; monitor by using ACTH stimulation, A.M. plasma cortisol and urinary free cortisol test. If HPA axis suppression noted, d/c or reduce frequency of application or substitute a less potent steroid. Steroid withdrawal may occur upon d/c. Use appropriate antifungal or antibacterial agent with dermatological infections; d/c if infection does not clear or if irritation occurs. Pediatric patients may be more susceptible to systemic toxicity; chronic therapy may interfere with growth and development. Allergic contact dermatitis reported.

ADVERSE REACTIONS: Itching, burning, erythema, dryness, irritation, papular rash, folliculitis, acneiform eruptions, hypopigmentation, perioral dermatitis, allergic contact dermatitis, secondary infection, skin atrophy, striae.

PREGNANCY: Category C, caution in nursing.

MECHANISM OF ACTION: Corticosteroid; has anti-inflammatory, antipruritic, and vasoconstrictive properties. Anti-inflammatory mechanism not established. Suspected to act by the induction of phospholipase A_2 inhibitory proteins (lipocortins)which may inhibit the release arachidonic acid.

PHARMACOKINETICS: Absorption: Percutaneous; occlusion, inflammation, and other disease states may increase absorption. **Distribution:** Systemically administered corticosteroids are found in breast milk.

NURSING CONSIDERATIONS

Assessment: Assess for hypersensitivity, dermatological infection, and pregnancy/nursing status.

Monitoring: Monitor for development of skin irritation, if present d/c medication. Monitor response to treatment, HPA axis suppression, Cushing's syndrome and other adverse effects if used for long term treatment.

Patient Counseling: Instruct to use externally and as directed. Avoid contact with eyes and that treated skin area should not be bandaged. Do not to use medication on face, underarms, or groin areas unless directed by a physician. Notify physician if any signs of improvement do not occur within 2 weeks of starting medication. Advise not to bandage, otherwise covered or wrapped, unless otherwise directed. Inform not to use in treatment of diaper dermatitis; should not be applied in diaper areas as diapers or plastic pants may constitute occlusive dressing.

Administration: Topical route. **Storage**: 2-30°C (36-86°F).

ACTEMRA   RX
tocilizumab (Genentech)

> Increased risk for developing serious infections (eg, active tuberculosis [TB], invasive fungal infections, bacterial/viral infections due to opportunistic pathogens) that may lead to hospitalization or death. Most patients who developed these infections were taking concomitant immunosuppressants (eg, methotrexate [MTX], corticosteroids). If serious infections develop, interrupt treatment until infection is controlled. Test for latent TB prior to and during therapy; initiate latent TB treatment prior to therapy. Consider risks and benefits prior to initiating therapy with chronic or recurrent infections. Monitor for development of signs and symptoms of infection during and after treatment.

THERAPEUTIC CLASS: Interleukin-6 receptor antagonist

INDICATIONS: Treatment of moderate to severe active rheumatoid arthritis in adults who have had inadequate response to one or more tumor necrosis factor (TNF) antagonist therapies.

DOSAGE: *Adults:* Monotherapy/With MTX or Other Disease-Modifying Antirheumatic Drugs (DMARD): Initial: 4mg/kg once q4 weeks as 60-min IV infusion. Titrate: Increase to 8mg/kg based on clinical response. Max: 800mg/infusion. Refer to PI for dose modifications based on liver enzyme abnormalities, absolute neutrophil count (ANC), and platelet count. Do not initiate treatment if ANC <2,000/mm³, platelets <100,000/mm³, or ALT/AST >1.5X ULN. Reduce dose from 8mg/kg to 4mg/kg for management of dose-related laboratory changes (eg, elevated liver enzymes, neutropenia, and thrombocytopenia).

HOW SUPPLIED: Inj: 20mg/mL [80mg/4mL, 200mg/10mL, 400mg/20mL]

WARNINGS/PRECAUTIONS: Avoid with active infection, including localized infections. Caution in patients with chronic/recurrent infections who have been exposed to TB, with history of serious/opportunistic infection, who reside or traveled in areas of endemic TB/mycoses, or with underlying conditions that may predispose them to infection. D/C if serious/opportunistic infection or sepsis develops. Viral reactivation and herpes zoster exacerbation observed. GI perforation reported; caution in patients at risk for GI perforation. Neutropenia, thrombocytopenia, elevation of liver enzymes, and increase in lipid parameters reported; monitor with appropriate tests q4-8 weeks. Severe hypersensitivity reactions (eg, anaphylaxis) reported. May increase risk of malignancies. Multiple sclerosis (MS) and chronic inflammatory demyelinating polyneuropathy reported rarely; caution with pre-existing or recent onset demyelinating disorders. Avoid with active hepatic disease or hepatic impairment. Caution in elderly. D/C if ALT or AST >5X ULN, ANC <500/mm³, or platelets <50,000/mm³.

ADVERSE REACTIONS: Infections, upper respiratory tract infections, nasopharyngitis, headache, HTN, increased ALT, dizziness, bronchitis.

INTERACTIONS: See Boxed Warning. Avoid with live vaccines. Caution with CYP450 substrates (eg, CYP1A2, CYP2B6, CYP2C9, CYP2C19, CYP2D6, CYP3A4); may increase metabolism of CYP450 substrates and be especially relevant in those drugs with narrow therapeutic index where the dose is individually adjusted. Upon initiation or d/c of tocilizumab, therapeutic monitoring of effect (eg, warfarin) or drug concentration (eg, cyclosporine, theophylline) should be performed and dosing adjustments should be made as needed. Caution when coadministered with CYP3A4 substrates (eg, oral contraceptives, lovastatin, atorvastatin) where decrease in effectiveness is undesired. May decrease dextromethorphan levels. Avoid with biological DMARDs (eg, TNF antagonists, IL-1R antagonists, anti-CD20 monoclonal antibodies, and selective costimulation modulators) due to increased immunosuppression. GI perforation may develop with NSAIDs, corticosteroids, MTX. Increased frequency and magnitude of transaminase elevations with hepatotoxic drugs (eg, MTX). Decreased exposure with simvastatin and omeprazole.

PREGNANCY: Category C, not for use in nursing.

MECHANISM OF ACTION: Interleukin-6 (IL-6) receptor antagonist; binds specifically to both soluble and membrane-bound IL-6 receptors (sIL-6R and mIL-6R) and inhibits IL-6 mediated signaling through these receptors.

PHARMACOKINETICS: Absorption: (4mg/kg) C_{max}=88.3mcg/mL; AUC=13,000mcg•h/mL, (8mg/kg) C_{max}=183mcg/mL; AUC=35,000mcg•h/mL. (≥100kg) C_{max}=269mcg/mL; AUC=55,500mcg•h/mL. **Distribution:** V_d=6.4L. **Elimination:** (4mg/kg) $T_{1/2}$=11 days, (8mg/kg) $T_{1/2}$=13 days.

NURSING CONSIDERATIONS

Assessment: Assess for infections (eg, bacteria, fungi, or viruses), including latent TB. Assess for demyelinating disorders, risk of GI perforation, active hepatic disease or impairment, pregnancy/nursing status, and for possible drug interactions. Obtain baseline lipid levels, platelet and neutrophil counts.

Monitoring: Monitor for signs/symptoms of TB and infections. Monitor for hypersensitivity reactions, GI perforation, malignancies, and demyelinating disorders (eg, MS, chronic inflammatory demyelinating polyneuropathy). Monitor neutrophil and platelet counts, LFTs, and lipid levels q4-8 weeks.

Patient Counseling: Advise of the potential risks/benefits of therapy. Inform that therapy may lower resistance to infections and may develop serious GI side effects while on therapy; instruct to contact physician if symptoms of infection or severe, persistent abdominal pain appears. Inform physician of travel history, especially in places that are endemic for TB/mycoses.

Administration: IV route. See PI for proper administration technique. Do not administer as an IV bolus or push. Inspect for particulate matter and discoloration. **Storage:** 2-8°C (36-46°F). Do not freeze. Protect vials from light by storing in original package until time of use. May store fully diluted solutions at room temperature for ≤24 hrs.

ACTIGALL   RX
ursodiol (Watson)

THERAPEUTIC CLASS: Bile acid

INDICATIONS: Indicated for patients with radiolucent, noncalcified gallbladder stones <20mm in diameter in whom elective cholecystectomy would be undertaken if not for the presence of increased surgical risk or for patients who refuse surgery. Prevention of gallstone formation in obese patients experiencing rapid weight loss.

DOSAGE: *Adults:* Gallstone Dissolution: 8-10mg/kg/day given bid-tid. Obtain ultrasound at 6- month intervals for 1 yr. Continue therapy after stones have dissolved and confirm with repeat ultrasound within 1-3 months. Gallstone Prevention: 600mg/day (300mg bid).

HOW SUPPLIED: Cap: 300mg

CONTRAINDICATIONS: Calcified cholesterol stones, radiopaque stones, compelling reasons for cholecystectomy (radiolucent bile pigment stones, unremitting acute cholecystitis, cholangitis, biliary obstruction, gallstone pancreatitis, biliary-gastrointestinal fistula).

WARNINGS/PRECAUTIONS: Therapy is not associated with liver damage. Monitor SGOT (AST) and SGPT (ALT) at the initiation of therapy and periodically thereafter. Caution in elderly.

ADVERSE REACTIONS: Abdominal pain, constipation, diarrhea, dyspepsia, flatulence, N/V, arthralgia, coughing, viral infection, bronchitis, pharyngitis, back pain, myalgia, headache, sinusitis.

INTERACTIONS: Decreased absorption with bile acid sequestrants and aluminum-based antacids. Estrogens, oral contraceptives, and clofibrate (and perhaps other lipid-lowering drugs) may increase hepatic cholesterol secretion and encourage cholesterol gallstone formation.

PREGNANCY: Category B, caution in nursing.

MECHANISM OF ACTION: Bile acid; suppresses hepatic synthesis, cholesterol secretion, and inhibits intestinal cholesterol absorption; actions combine to change bile from cholesterol-precipitating to cholesterol-solubilizing, resulting in bile conducive to cholesterol stone dissolution.

PHARMACOKINETICS: Absorption: Small bowel (90%). **Metabolism:** Liver (1st pass, conjugation). **Elimination:** Feces.

NURSING CONSIDERATIONS

Assessment: Assess for type of bile pigment stones (calcified cholesterol, radiopaque, radiolucent), unremitting acute cholecystitis, cholangitis, biliary obstruction, gallstone pancreatitis, biliary GI fistula, nursing status, and possible drug interactions. Obtain baseline SGOT (AST) and SGPT (ALT).

Monitoring: Ultrasound should be taken in 6-month intervals for first year. If appear dissolved, continue therapy and confirm on repeat ultrasound within 1-3 months. If partial dissolution not seen by 12 months, success is greatly reduced. Monitor SGOT (AST) and SGPT (ALT) periodically. Signs/symptoms of hypersensitivity reactions.

Patient Counseling: Seek medical attention if symptoms of hypersensitivity or allergic reactions occur. Advise patient that gallbladder stone dissolution requires months of therapy.

Administration: Oral route. **Storage:** 25°C (77°F); excursions permitted to 15-30°C (59-86°F). Dispense in tight container.

ACTIQ
fentanyl citrate (Cephalon) **CII**

> Serious adverse events, including deaths, reported. May cause life-threatening respiratory depression in opioid non-tolerant patients. Contains fentanyl, with abuse liability similar to other opioid analgesics. Use only in the care of cancer patients and only by oncologists and pain specialists who are skilled/knowledgeable in the use of Schedule II opioids to treat cancer pain. Contraindicated in the management of acute or postoperative pain including headache/migraine. Do not convert on a mcg-per-mcg basis to Actiq from other fentanyl products. Do not substitute for other fentanyl products; may result in fatal overdose. Use special care when dosing. Keep out of reach of children and discard properly. Concomitant use with moderate and strong CYP3A4 inhibitors may cause fatal respiratory depression.

THERAPEUTIC CLASS: Opioid analgesic

INDICATIONS: Management of breakthrough cancer pain in patients ≥16 yrs with malignancies who are already receiving and are tolerant to around-the-clock opioid therapy.

DOSAGE: *Adults:* ≥16 yrs: Initial: 200mcg (consume over 15 min). Titrate: Redose 15 min after previous dose is completed if breakthrough pain episode not relieved; take only 1 additional dose of the same strength. Max: Two doses per breakthrough pain episode. Wait 4 hrs before treating another episode of breakthrough pain. May increase to next highest available strength if several breakthrough episodes require >1 unit per pain episode. Repeat titration for each new dose. Prescribe an initial titration supply of six units. Maint: Once titrated to an effective dose, use only 1 unit of the appropriate strength per breakthrough pain episode. If >4 breakthrough pain episodes per day are experienced, re-evaluate maint dose. Upon d/c, gradually titrate dose downward.

HOW SUPPLIED: Loz: 200mcg, 400mcg, 600mcg, 800mcg, 1200mcg, 1600mcg

CONTRAINDICATIONS: Opioid non-tolerant patients and management of acute or postoperative pain, including headache/migraine.

WARNINGS/PRECAUTIONS: Caution with chronic obstructive pulmonary disease (COPD), pre-existing medical conditions predisposing to respiratory depression. Extreme caution with evidence of increased intracranial pressure (ICP) or impaired consciousness. May obscure clinical course of head injuries. Caution with bradyarrhythmias. May impair mental and/or physical abilities. Anaphylaxis and hypersensitivity reported. Caution with hepatic or renal dysfunction, and in the elderly.

ADVERSE REACTIONS: Respiratory depression, circulatory depression, hypotension, shock, N/V, headache, constipation, dizziness, dyspnea, anxiety, somnolence, asthenia, confusion, depression.

INTERACTIONS: See Boxed Warning. Respiratory depression may occur more readily when given with other agents that depress respiration. Concomitant use with other CNS depressants, including opioids, sedatives, hypnotics, general anesthetics, phenothiazines, tranquilizers, skeletal muscle relaxants, sedating antihistamines, strong inhibitors of CYP3A4 (eg, ketoconazole, itraconazole, ritonavir, troleandomycin, clarithromycin, nelfinavir and nefazodone) or moderate inhibitors (eg, amprenavir, aprepitant, diltiazem, erythromycin, fluconazole, fosamprenavir, and verapamil) and alcohol may result in increased plasma concentrations resulting in increased depressant effect; adjust dose if warranted. Avoid grapefruit and grapefruit juice. CYP3A4 inducers may have the opposite effect. Not recommended with or within 14 days of d/c of MAOIs.

PREGNANCY: Category C, not for use in nursing.

MECHANISM OF ACTION: Opioid analgesic: μ-opioid receptor agonist. Exact mechanism not established. Specific CNS opioid receptors for endogenous compounds have been identified throughout brain and spinal cord and play a role in analgesic effects.

PHARMACOKINETICS: Absorption: Rapidly absorbed from buccal mucosa; more prolonged absorption of swallowed fentanyl from GI tract. Absolute bioavailability (50%); (200mcg) C_{max} = 0.39ng/mL, AUC= 102ng/mL•min, T_{max} = 40 min; (400mcg) C_{max} = 0.75ng/mL, AUC= 243ng/mL•min, T_{max} =25 min; (800mcg) C_{max} =1.55ng/mL, AUC= 573ng/mL•min, T_{max} =25 min; (1600mcg) C_{max} = 2.51ng/mL, AUC= 1026ng/mL•min, T_{max} =20 min. **Distribution:** V_{ss} =4L/kg; plasma protein binding (80-85%). Readily crosses placenta; found in breast milk. **Metabolism:** Liver and intestinal mucosa via CYP3A4; norfentanyl (metabolite). **Elimination:** Urine (<7%, unchanged) (major), feces (1%, unchanged); $T_{1/2}$ = 193 min (200mcg), 386 min (400mcg), 381 min (800mcg), 358 min (1600mcg).

NURSING CONSIDERATIONS

Assessment: Assess for degree of opioid tolerance, previous opioid dose, level of pain intensity, type of pain, patient's general condition and medical status, emotional status, or any other conditions where treatment is contraindicated or cautioned. Assess for history of hypersensitivity, pregnancy/nursing status, renal/hepatic function, and possible drug interactions.

Monitoring: Monitor for signs/symptoms of respiratory and CNS depression, bradycardia, circulatory depression, hypotension, shock, impairment of mental/physical abilities, abuse/addiction, dental decay, and hypersensitivity reactions. Monitor glucose levels with DM.

Patient Counseling: Inform that medication must be kept out of reach of children; may be fatal to child. Seek immediate help if child accidentally consumes medication. Instruct to properly discard partially used units; not to take medication for acute or postoperative pain, pain from injuries, headache, migraine, or any other short-term pain; not to take medication if not taking an opioid medication on a scheduled basis (around-the-clock). Counsel about breakthrough pain episodes and advise to notify physician if breakthrough pain is not alleviated or worsens. Inform that medication has potential for abuse. Use may impair mental/physical abilities; use caution if performing hazardous tasks (eg, operating machinery/driving). Notify physician of all concurrently used medications or before taking any other medications. Avoid consumption of grapefruit juice and alcohol. Maintain proper dental hygiene during therapy. Advise diabetics that medication contains approximately 2g sugar/unit. Avoid abrupt withdrawal and instruct not to share medication as it could result in death due to overdose. Counsel on proper administration and disposal. Instruct female patients to notify physician if pregnant or planning to become pregnant.

Administration: Oral route. The lozenge should be sucked, not chewed, and consumed over 15 min. Refer to PI for proper administration. **Storage:** 20-25°C (68-77°F); excursions permitted between 15-30°C (59-86°F). Protect from freezing and moisture. Do not use if blister package has been opened.

ACTIVASE

RX

alteplase (Genentech)

THERAPEUTIC CLASS: Thrombolytic agent

INDICATIONS: Management of acute myocardial infarction (AMI) for the improvement of ventricular function following AMI, the reduction of incidence of congestive heart failure (CHF) and reduction of mortality with AMI. Management of acute ischemic stroke and acute massive pulmonary embolism (PE).

DOSAGE: *Adults:* AMI: Accelerated Infusion: >67kg: 15mg IV bolus, then 50mg over next 30 min, and then 35mg over next 60 min. ≤67kg: 15mg IV bolus, then 0.75mg/kg (max 50mg) over next 30 min, then 0.50mg/kg (max 35mg) over next 60 min. Max: 100mg total dose. 3-hr Infusion: ≥65kg: 60mg in 1st hr (give 6-10mg as IV bolus), then 20mg over 2nd hr, and 20mg over 3rd hr. <65kg: 1.25mg/kg over 3 hrs as described above. Acute Ischemic Stroke: 0.9mg/kg IV over 1 hr (max 90mg total dose). Administer 10% of total dose as IV bolus over 1 min. PE: 100mg IV over 2 hrs. Start heparin at end or immediately after infusion when PTT or thrombin time ≤2x normal.

HOW SUPPLIED: Inj: 50mg, 100mg

CONTRAINDICATIONS: (AMI, PE) Active internal bleeding, history of cerebrovascular accident (CVA), recent intracranial/intraspinal surgery or trauma, intracranial neoplasm, arteriovenous (AV) malformation, aneurysm, bleeding diathesis, severe uncontrolled HTN. (Acute Ischemic Stroke) Active internal bleeding, AV malformation, intracranial neoplasm, history or evidence of intracranial hemorrhage, aneurysm, bleeding diathesis, uncontrolled HTN, subarachnoid hemorrhage, seizure at stroke onset. Recent (within 3 months) intracranial or intraspinal surgery, serious head trauma, previous stroke.

WARNINGS/PRECAUTIONS: Weigh benefits/risks with recent major surgery, cerebrovascular disease, recent GI or genitourinary (GU) bleeding, recent trauma, HTN (systolic BP ≥175mmHg and/or diastolic BP >110mmHg), left heart thrombus, acute pericarditis, subacute bacterial endocarditis, hemostatic defects, severe hepatic dysfunction, pregnancy, diabetic hemorrhagic retinopathy or other hemorrhagic ophthalmic conditions, septic thrombophlebitis or occluded AV cannula at a seriously infected site, advanced age or elderly, any other bleeding condition that is difficult to manage. For stroke, also weigh benefits/risks with severe neurological deficit or major early infarct signs on CT. Cholesterol embolism and internal/superficial bleeding reported. Arrhythmias may occur with reperfusion. Avoid IM injection, noncompressible arterial puncture, and internal jugular or subclavian venous puncture. Caution with readministration. D/C therapy if anaphylactoid reaction occurs.

ADVERSE REACTIONS: Bleeding, orolingual angioedema.

INTERACTIONS: Increased risk of bleeding with warfarin, heparin, vitamin K antagonists, drugs that alter platelets (eg, ASA, dipyridamole, abciximab) given before, during, or after alteplase therapy. Orolingual angioedema with ACE inhibitors.

PREGNANCY: Category C, caution in nursing.

MECHANISM OF ACTION: Tissue plasminogen activator (t-PA); serine protease enzyme that has property of fibrin-enhanced conversion of plasminogen to plasmin. Produces limited conversion of plasminogen in absence of fibrin. Binds to fibrin in thrombus and converts entrapped plasminogen to plasmin. Initiates local fibrinolysis with limited systemic proteolysis.

PHARMACOKINETICS: Metabolism: Liver. **Elimination:** $T_{1/2}$=<5 min (initial).

NURSING CONSIDERATIONS

Assessment: In patients with acute MI or PE, assess for presence of active internal bleeding, history of cerebrovascular accident, trauma, aneurysm, known bleeding diathesis, and severe uncontrolled HTN. In patients with acute ischemic stroke, assess for presence or history of hemorrhage, surgery, serious head trauma, previous stroke, uncontrolled HTN, and possible drug interactions.

Monitoring: Monitor for signs/symptoms of bleeding (eg, internal, superficial, surface bleeding), cholesterol embolism (eg, livedo reticularis, "purple toe" syndrome, acute renal failure, gangrenous digits), and for allergic reactions (eg, anaphylactoid reaction, laryngeal edema, orolingual angioedema, rash, urticaria). Monitor BP frequently and arrhythmias with acute MI.

Patient Counseling: Inform about risk of bleeding with medication. Instruct to notify physician if any type of allergic reaction develops during therapy.

Administration: IV route. Reconstitute using appropriate volume of SWFI (without preservatives) to vial. Do not use Bacteriostatic Water for Inj, USP. Reconstitute to a final concentration of 1mg/mL. Reconstitute just prior to use. May further dilute using an equal volume of 0.9% NS or D5W to yield concentration of 0.5mg/mL. Do not add any other medication to infusion solutions containing drug. Discard any unused infusion solution. Do not use if vacuum is not present in 50mg vials. **Storage:** Lyophilized: Controlled room temperature not to exceed 30°C (86°F), or under refrigeration 2-8°C (36-46°F). Protect from excessive exposure to light. Reconstituted: 2-30°C (36-86°F); use within 8 hrs.

ACTIVELLA   RX
norethindrone acetate - estradiol (Novo Nordisk)

> Estrogens and progestins should not be used for the prevention of cardiovascular disease or dementia. Increased risk of MI, stroke, invasive breast cancer, pulmonary embosim (PE), and deep vein thrombosis (DVT) in postmenopausal women (50-79 yrs of age) reported. Increased risk of developing probable dementia in postmenopausal women ≥65 yrs of age reported.

THERAPEUTIC CLASS: Estrogen/progestogen combination

INDICATIONS: For women with intact uterus, treatment of moderate to severe vasomotor symptoms associated with menopause, vulvar/vaginal atrophy and prevention of postmenopausal osteoporosis.

DOSAGE: *Adults:* 1 tab qd.

HOW SUPPLIED: Tab: (Estradiol-Norethindrone) 1mg-0.5mg, 0.5mg-0.1mg

CONTRAINDICATIONS: Pregnancy, breast cancer, abnormal genital bleeding, estrogen-dependent neoplasia, DVT, thromboembolic disorders, stroke, liver dysfunction or disease.

WARNINGS/PRECAUTIONS: Risk of gallbladder disease, endometrial and breast cancer, fetal congenital reproductive tract disorder, elevated BP, and hypercalcemia with breast cancer or bone metastases. Possible risk of cardiovascular disease. Increased risk of DVT, stroke, and PE; increased risk of endometrial, breast, and ovarian cancer with prolonged use. Risk of probable dementia-unknown risk in postmenopausal women under 65 years of age. Monitor for fluid retention with asthma, epilepsy, migraine, and cardiac/renal dysfunction. Avoid in post-menopausal women without a uterus. D/C if vision disturbances or thrombotic disorders occur. Caution with depression, diabetes mellitus (DM), severe hypocalcemia. Acceleration of PT, PTT and hypercoagulability effects observed. Impaired glucose tolerance, increased triglycerides, fibrin/fibrinogen, and plasmin/plasminogen activity.

ADVERSE REACTIONS: Back pain, headache, nasopharyngitis, sinusitis, insomnia, upper respiratory tract infection, breast pain, postmenopausal bleeding/vaginal hemorrhage, endometrial thickening, uterine fibroid, pain in extremities, nausea, and diarrhea.

INTERACTIONS: CYP3A4 inducers (eg, St. John's wort, phenobarbital, carbamazepine, rifampin) may reduce estrogen levels. CYP3A4 inhibitors (eg, erythromycin, clarithromycin, ketoconazole, itraconazole, ritonavir, grapefruit juice) may increase estrogen levels.

PREGNANCY: Category X, caution in nursing.

MECHANISM OF ACTION: Estrogen/progestogen combination. Estradiol: Binds to nuclear receptors in estrogen-responsive tissues and modulating pituitary secretion of gonadotropins, luteinizing hormone (LH) and follicle-stimulating hormone (FSH), through negative-feedback mechanism.

Norethindrone: Exerts effect in target cells by binding to specific progesterone receptors that interact with progesterone-response elements in target genes. Enhances cellular differentiation and opposing actions of estrogens by decreasing estrogen receptor levels, increasing local metabolism of estrogens to less active metabolites, and inducing gene products that blunt cellular responses to estrogen.

PHARMACOKINETICS: Absorption: Estradiol (E_2): Well-absorbed, T_{max}=5-8 hrs. Norethindrone (NET): Rapid. **Distribution:** Estrogens found in breast milk. E_2: Sex-hormone-binding globulin (37%); albumin (61%); unbound (1-2%). NET: Sex-hormone-binding globulin (36%); albumin (61%). **Metabolism:** E_2: Liver to estrone, E_1 (metabolite); estriol (major urinary metabolite); enterohepatic recirculation via sulfate and glucuronide conjugation; biliary secretion of conjugates into the intestine, and hydrolysis in intestine; CYP3A4 (partial). NET: 5α-dihydro-norethindrone and tetrahydro-norethindrone (metabolites). **Elimination:** E_2: Urine; $T_{1/2}$=12-14 hrs. E_1: Urine; $T_{1/2}$=12-14 hrs. NET: $T_{1/2}$=8-11 hrs.

NURSING CONSIDERATIONS

Assessment: Assess for abnormal genital bleeding, presence or history of breast cancer, estrogen-dependent neoplasias, DVT, PE, active or recent (within past yr) and any other conditions where treatment may be contraindicated or cautioned. Assess use in women ≥65 yrs, nursing patients, and those with DM, asthma, epilepsy, migraines or porphyria, SLE, and hepatic hemangiomas. Assess for possible drug and lab test interactions.

Monitoring: Monitor for signs/symptoms of CV disorders (eg, MI, stroke, venous thrombosis, PE), malignant neoplasms (eg, breast, endometrial, ovarian cancer), dementia, gallbladder disease, hypercalcemia, visual abnormalities (eg, retinal vascular thrombosis), increased BP, hypertriglyceridemia, hypothyroidism, fluid retention, cholestatic jaundice, exacerbation of endometriosis and other conditions. Perform annual mammography and periodic monitoring of BP. Monitor thyroid function if patient on thyroid hormone replacement therapy. In cases of undiagnosed, persistent, or recurrent vaginal bleeding in women with uterus, perform adequate diagnostic measures (eg, endometrial sampling) to rule out malignancies.

Patient Counseling: Inform that estrogens may increase risk for uterine and breast cancer, heart attack, stroke, blood clots, and dementia. Report any unusual vaginal bleeding, breast lumps, dizziness or faintness, changes in speech, severe headaches, chest pain, SOB, leg pain, changes in vision, or vomiting. Advise to perform monthly self breast exam, and have annual gynecologic exam (breast exam, mammography).

Administration: Oral route. **Storage:** Store in dry place; protect from light. Store at room temperature, 25°C (77°F), excursions permitted to 15-30°C (59-86°F).

ACTONEL   RX
risedronate sodium (Warner Chilcott)

THERAPEUTIC CLASS: Bisphosphonate

INDICATIONS: Treatment and prevention of osteoporosis in postmenopausal women and glucocorticoid-induced osteoporosis in men and women who are either initiating or continuing systemic glucocorticosteroids. Treatment to increase bone mass in men with osteoporosis. Treatment of Paget's disease of bone in men and women.

DOSAGE: *Adults:* Postmenopausal Osteoporosis Prevention/Treatment: 5mg qd, or 35mg once weekly, or 150mg once a month. Glucocorticoid-Induced Osteoporosis Prevention/Treatment: 5mg qd. To Increase Bone Mass in Men with Osteoporosis: 35mg once weekly. Paget's Disease: 30mg qd for 2 months. May retreat after 2 months if relapse occurs, or if treatment fails to normalize serum alkaline phosphatase. Take ≥30 min before 1st food or drink of the day other than water. Swallow tab in upright position with full glass of plain water (6-8 oz). Do not lie down for 30 min after dose.

HOW SUPPLIED: Tab: 5mg, 30mg, 35mg, 150mg

CONTRAINDICATIONS: Hypocalcemia, inability to stand or sit upright for ≥30 min, abnormalities of the esophagus which delay esophageal emptying (eg, stricture or achalasia).

WARNINGS/PRECAUTIONS: May cause local irritation of upper GI mucosa; caution with upper GI problems (eg, Barrett's esophagus, dysphagia, other esophageal diseases, gastritis, duodenitis, or ulcers). D/C if dysphagia, odynophagia, retrosternal pain, or new/worsening heartburn occurs. Gastric and duodenal ulcers reported. Treat hypocalcemia and other disturbances of bone and mineral metabolism before therapy. Osteonecrosis of the jaw (ONJ) reported; d/c for patients requiring invasive dental procedures or consider d/c if ONJ develops. Severe, incapacitating bone, joint, and/or muscle pain reported; d/c if severe symptoms develop. Atypical, low-energy, or low trauma fractures of the femoral shaft reported; consider interrupting therapy. Ascertain sex steroid hormonal status and consider replacement before initiating therapy for the treatment/prevention of glucocorticoid-induced osteoporosis. Avoid with severe renal impairment (CrCl <30mL/min).

ADVERSE REACTIONS: Back pain, arthralgia, abdominal pain, dyspepsia, acute phase reaction, allergic reaction, arthritis, diarrhea, headache, infection, urinary tract infection, bronchitis, HTN, nausea, rash.

INTERACTIONS: Calcium supplements, antacids, or oral medications containing divalent cations (aluminum, magnesium) may interfere with absorption. Risk of ONJ with concomitant corticosteroid or chemotherapy. May interfere with the use of bone-imaging agents. May increase risk of atypical femur fractures with glucocorticoids (eg, prednisone).

PREGNANCY: Category C, not for use in nursing.

MECHANISM OF ACTION: Bisphosphonate; has an affinity for hydroxyapatite crystals in bone and acts as an antiresorptive agent. Inhibits osteoclasts.

PHARMACOKINETICS: Absorption: Upper GI tract; T_{max}=1 hr; absolute bioavailability (0.63%). **Distribution**: V_d=13.8L/kg; plasma protein binding (24%). **Elimination**: Urine (50%), feces (unabsorbed dose); $T_{1/2}$=561 hrs.

NURSING CONSIDERATIONS

Assessment: Assess for hypocalcemia, esophageal abnormalities, upper GI problems or any other conditions where treatment is contraindicated or cautioned, drug hypersensitivity, pregnancy/nursing status and possible drug interactions. Assess sex steroid hormonal status if treatment is for glucocorticoid-induced osteoporosis.

Monitoring: Monitor for signs/symptoms of upper GI disorders (eg, dysphagia, esophagitis, esophageal or gastric ulcers), ONJ, hypersensitivity reactions, and musculoskeletal pain.

Patient Counseling: Instruct to take ≥30 min before 1st food or drink of the day other than water; take in an upright position (while sitting or standing) with a full glass of plain water (6-8 oz.), not to lie down for 30 min after taking medication, and to avoid chewing or sucking tablet. Contact physician if symptoms of esophageal disease develop. Take supplemental calcium and vitamin D if dietary intake is inadequate; take supplement and calcium-, aluminum-, and magnesium-containing medications at a different time of the day than risedronate. Refer to PI for instructions on missed doses.

Administration: Oral route. **Storage**: 20-25°C (68-77°F).

ACTOPLUS MET   RX
pioglitazone HCl - metformin HCl (Takeda)

> **Thiozolidinediones may cause or exacerbate congestive heart failure (CHF) in some patients. After initiation/dose increase, observe for signs/symptoms of heart failure (HF) and manage accordingly; consider d/c or dose reduction. Not recommended in patients with symptomatic HF. Contraindicated with established NYHA Class III or IV HF. Lactic acidosis may occur due to metformin accumulation; d/c if suspected.**

OTHER BRAND NAMES: Actoplus Met XR (Takeda)

ACTOPLUS MET

THERAPEUTIC CLASS: Thiazolidinedione/biguanide

INDICATIONS: Adjunct to diet and exercise to improve glycemic control in adults with type 2 diabetes mellitus (DM) who are already treated with pioglitazone and metformin or who have inadequate glycemic control on pioglitazone or metformin alone.

DOSAGE: *Adults:* Individualize dose. Prior Pioglitazone/Metformin: Base on current regimen. Actoplus Met: Initial: 15mg-500mg or 15mg-850mg qd or bid with food. Max: 45mg-2550mg/day in divided doses with meals. Actoplus Met XR: Initial: 15mg-1000mg or 30mg-1000mg qpm with meal. Max: 45mg-2000mg qpm with a meal. Elderly/Debilitated/Malnourished: Initiate conservative dosing; do not titrate to max dose. Actoplus Met XR must be swallowed whole; do not chew, cut or crush. Titrate gradually based on response.

HOW SUPPLIED: Tab: (Pioglitazone-Metformin) 15mg-500mg, 15mg-850mg; Tab, Extended-Release: (Pioglitazone-Metformin) 15mg-1000mg, 30mg-1000mg

CONTRAINDICATIONS: NYHA Class III or IV HF, renal disease/dysfunction (eg, SrCr ≥1.5mg/dL [males], ≥1.4mg/dL [females], or abnormal CrCl), and acute or chronic metabolic acidosis, including diabetic ketoacidosis. Temporarily d/c in patients undergoing radiologic studies involving intravascular iodinated contrast materials.

WARNINGS/PRECAUTIONS: (Metformin) Increased risk of lactic acidosis with renal dysfunction, increased age, DM, CHF, and other conditions with risk of hypoperfusion and hypoxemia. Avoid in patients ≥80 yrs unless renal function is normal. Monitor renal function, ketoacidosis, and metabolic acidosis. Avoid in renal/hepatic impairment. D/C in hypoxic states (eg, CHF, shock, acute MI), loss of blood glucose control due to stress (give insulin), acidosis, dehydration, sepsis. Caution against excessive alcohol intake. Temporarily d/c prior to surgery. May decrease serum vitamin B_{12} levels; perform routine serum vitamin B_{12} measurements at 2-3 yr intervals. Increased risk of hypoglycemia in elderly, in debilitated/malnourished, with adrenal or pituitary insufficiency, or with alcohol intoxication. Withhold therapy during states of stress (eg, fever, trauma, infection); temporary loss of glycemic control may occur. (Pioglitazone) Use lowest approved dose with type 2 DM and systolic HF (NYHA Class II). Not for use in type 1 diabetes or for diabetic ketoacidosis treatment. May cause hypoglycemia, edema, dose-related weight gain and decrease in Hgb and Hct. Ovulation in premenopausal anovulatory patients may occur; risk of pregnancy with inadequate contraception. Avoid with active liver disease and in ALT levels >2.5X ULN; monitor liver enzymes periodically. D/C if jaundice occurs or ALT >3X ULN on therapy. Macular edema reported; perform regular eye exams. Increased risk of fractures in female patients.

ADVERSE REACTIONS: Upper respiratory tract infection, diarrhea, nausea, headache, urinary tract infection, sinusitis, dizziness, edema of lower limb, weight increased.

INTERACTIONS: (Metformin) Furosemide, nifedipine, cimetidine, cationic drugs (eg, digoxin, amiloride, procainamide, quinidine, quinine, ranitidine, trimethoprim, vancomycin, triamterene, morphine) may increase metformin levels. Thiazides, other diuretics, corticosteroids, phenothiazines, thyroid products, estrogens, oral contraceptives, phenytoin, nicotinic acid, sympathomimetics, CCBs, or isoniazid may cause hyperglycemia. Risk of hypoglycemia with alcohol; excess alcohol may increase potential for lactic acidosis. May decrease glyburide and furosemide levels. (Pioglitazone) Possible loss of contraception with ethinyl estradiol and norethindrone; caution when coadministering. Risk of hypoglycemia with insulin or oral hypoglycemic agents. May cause reduction of midazolam levels. CYP2C8 inhibitors (eg, gemfibrozil) may significantly increase AUC of pioglitazone. CYP2C8 inducers (eg, rifampin) may significantly decrease AUC of pioglitazone.

PREGNANCY: Category C, not for use in nursing.

MECHANISM OF ACTION: Pioglitazone: Thiazolidinedione; insulin sensitizing agent, enhances peripheral glucose utilization, decreases insulin resistance in periphery and liver resulting in increased insulin-dependent glucose disposal and decreased hepatic glucose output. Metformin: Biguanide; decreases endogenous hepatic glucose production, also decreases intestinal absorption of glucose and improves insulin sensitivity by increasing peripheral glucose uptake and utilization.

PHARMACOKINETICS: Absorption: Variable doses of Actoplus Met and Actoplus Met XR resulted in different pharmacokinetic parameters. Refer to PI. **Distribution:** Pioglitazone: V_d =0.63L/kg, plasma protein binding (>99%). Metformin: V_d =654L. **Metabolism:** Pioglitazone: Hydroxylation and oxidation (extensive) via CYP450 (2C8, 3A4, 1A1); M-II and M-IV [hydroxy derivatives], M-III [keto derivative] (active metabolites). **Elimination:** Refer to PI for $T_{1/2}$ values. Pioglitazone: Urine (15-30%), bile/feces. Metformin: Urine (90%).

NURSING CONSIDERATIONS

Assessment: Assess for HF, lactic acidosis and conditions that increase risk for lactic acidosis (eg, increased age, tissue hypoperfusion/hypoxemia, sepsis, dehydration, excessive alcohol intake). Assess for hepatic insufficiency and renal function, secondary causes of poor glycemic control prior to initiation or escalation of therapy and any other conditions where treatment is cautioned or contraindicated. Before initiation of therapy and at least annually thereafter, renal function should be assessed and verified as normal. Obtain baseline LFTs, CBC.

Monitoring: Monitor FPG and HbA1c periodically for glycemic control and therapeutic response. Perform LFTs, hematologic parameters (eg, Hgb/Hct, RBC indices), renal function (eg, SrCr), and eye exams periodically. Measure blood lactate levels, blood pH, serum electrolytes and lactate/pyruvate ratio. Perform Vitamin B_{12} measurements. Monitor for signs/symptoms of heart HF (excessive, rapid weight gain, dyspnea, and/or edema), lactic acidosis, diabetic ketoacidosis, fractures, and non-specific symptoms such as malaise, myalgia, respiratory distress, somnolence and abdominal distress.

Patient Counseling: Instruct to adhere to diet, exercise program, and testing of blood glucose and HbA1c. Advise to seek medical attention during periods of stress (eg, fever, trauma, infection, or surgery). Explain risks of lactic acidosis; inform to d/c therapy immediately and notify physician if unexplained hyperventilation, myalgia, malaise, unusual somnolence or other symptoms occur. Counsel to report unexplained GI symptoms, rapid increase in weight or edema, SOB, N/V, abdominal pain, fatigue, anorexia, or dark urine. Inform to avoid excessive alcohol intake. Counsel females about use of reliable contraception. Explain risks of hypoglycemia, its symptoms and treatment, and conditions that predispose to its development. Advise on importance of regular follow-up visits. If dose is missed, inform patient to take the next dose as prescribed. Inform that Actoplus Met XR must be swallowed whole and not chewed, cut, or crushed, and that the inactive ingredients may occasionally be eliminated in the feces as a soft mass that may resemble the original tablet.

Administration: Oral route. **Storage:** 25°C (77°F); excursions permitted to 15-30°C (59-86°F). Keep container tightly closed. Protect from moisture and humidity. Dispense Actoplus Met XR in light-resistant container.

ACTOS RX
pioglitazone HCl (Takeda)

> Thiazolidinediones may cause or exacerbate congestive heart failure (CHF) in some patients. After initiation and dose increases, monitor carefully for signs and symptoms of heart failure (HF) and manage accordingly; consider d/c or dose reduction. Not recommended in patients with symptomatic HF. Contraindicated with established NYHA Class III or IV HF.

THERAPEUTIC CLASS: Thiazolidinedione

INDICATIONS: Adjunct to diet and exercise to improve glycemic control in adults with type 2 diabetes mellitus.

DOSAGE: *Adults:* Without CHF: Initial: 15mg or 30mg qd. With CHF (NHYA Class I or II): Initial: 15mg qd. Titrate: In increments of 15mg. Max: 45mg qd. With Insulin Secretagogue: Reduce dose of insulin secretagogue if hypoglycemia occurs. With Insulin: Decrease insulin dose by 10-25% if hypoglycemia occurs. With Strong CYP2C8 Inhibitor: Max: 15mg qd.

ACULAR

HOW SUPPLIED: Tab: 15mg, 30mg, 45mg

CONTRAINDICATIONS: Established NYHA Class III or IV HF.

WARNINGS/PRECAUTIONS: New onset or worsening of edema reported; caution with edema and patients at risk for CHF. Fatal and non-fatal hepatic failure reported. Obtain LFTs prior to initiation; caution with liver disease/abnormal LFTs. D/C if ALT >3X ULN and do not restart if cause of abnormal LFTs not established or if total bilirubin >2X ULN without alternative etiologies. Increased incidence of bone fractures noted in females. Macular edema reported; refer to an ophthalmologist if visual symptoms develop. Ovulation in premenopausal anovulatory patients may occur; use adequate contraception.

ADVERSE REACTIONS: Upper respiratory tract infection, hypoglycemia, edema, headache, cardiac failure, pain in extremity, sinusitis, back pain, myalgia, pharyngitis, chest pain.

INTERACTIONS: Increased exposure and $T_{1/2}$ with CYP2C8 inhibitors (eg, gemfibrozil). Decreased exposure with CYP2C8 inducers (eg, rifampin). Additive effect on glycemic control with a sulfonylurea, metformin or insulin. Risk of fluid retention and hypoglycemia with insulin and other antidiabetic medications (eg, insulin secretagogues such as sulfonylureas). Increased exposure of digoxin, norethindrone, fexofenadine, ranitidine, theophylline. Decreased exposure of warfarin, ethinyl estradiol, glipizide, metformin, midazolam, nifedipine ER, atorvastatin calcium. Increased exposure with ketoconazole, fexofenadine, nifedipine ER. Decreased exposure with ranitidine, atorvastatin calcium, theophylline.

PREGNANCY: Category C, not for use in nursing.

MECHANISM OF ACTION: Thiazolidinedione; decreases insulin resistance in the periphery and liver resulting in increased insulin-dependent glucose disposal and decreased hepatic glucose output.

PHARMACOKINETICS: Absorption: T_{max}=Within 2 hrs, 3-4 hrs (with food). **Distribution:** V_d=0.63L/kg; plasma protein binding (>99%). **Metabolism:** Hydroxylation and oxidation; M-III and M-IV (active metabolites). **Elimination:** Urine (15-30%), bile and feces; $T_{1/2}$=3-7 hrs (pioglitazone), 16-24 hrs (metabolites).

NURSING CONSIDERATIONS

Assessment: Assess for previous hypersensitivity, NYHA Class III or IV HF, CHF, edema, risk factors for developing HF, liver disease, bone health, pregnancy/nursing status, and possible drug interactions. Obtain baseline LFTs.

Monitoring: Monitor for signs and symptoms of HF, exacerbation of CHF, edema, weight gain, hematological changes (eg, decreases in Hgb, Hct), liver injury, macular edema, visual disturbances, and bone fractures. Perform periodic measurements of FPG, HbA1c and LFTs. Perform periodic eye exams.

Patient Counseling: Advise to adhere to dietary instructions, to regularly test blood glucose and HbA1c levels, to seek medical advice promptly during periods of stress (eg, fever, trauma, infection, or surgery) and to report SOB, rapid increase in weight or edema, or other symptoms of HF to physician. Instruct to d/c and consult physician if unexplained N/V, abdominal pain, anorexia, fatigue, and darkening of urine occurs. Advise to take qd with/without meals; if dose is missed, advise to not double dose the following day. Inform about the risk of hypoglycemia when using with insulin or other antidiabetic medications. Inform about the increased risk for pregnancy while on therapy; recommend adequate contraception for all premenopausal women.

Administration: Oral route. **Storage:** 25°C (77°F); excursions permitted to 15-30°C (59-86°F). Keep container tightly closed. Protect from light, moisture and humidity.

ACULAR   RX
ketorolac tromethamine (Allergan)

THERAPEUTIC CLASS: NSAID

INDICATIONS: Ocular itching due to seasonal allergic conjunctivitis. Postoperative inflammation in cataract extraction.

DOSAGE: *Adults:* 1 drop qid. Post-op Inflammation: Begin 24 hrs post-op and continue for 2 weeks.
Pediatrics: ≥3 yrs: 1 drop qid. Post-op Inflammation: Begin 24 hrs post-op and continue for 2 weeks.

HOW SUPPLIED: Sol: 0.5% [3mL, 5mL, 10mL]

WARNINGS/PRECAUTIONS: Potential for cross-sensitivity to acetylsalicylic acid, phenylacetic acid derivatives, and other NSAIDs. May increase ocular tissue bleeding in conjunction with ocular surgery. Avoid use with contact lenses. D/C if corneal epithelium breakdown occurs. Caution in known bleeding tendencies, complicated ocular surgeries, corneal denervation, corneal epithelial defects, diabetes mellitus (DM), ocular surface diseases (eg, dry eye syndrome), rheumatoid arthritis, or repeat ocular surgeries within a short period of time. Caution if used >24 hrs prior to surgery and use beyond 14 days post-surgery.

ADVERSE REACTIONS: Transient stinging/burning, superficial keratitis or infections, allergic reactions, ocular inflammation, corneal edema, iritis.

INTERACTIONS: Caution with agents that may prolong bleeding time. Increased potential for healing problems with topical steroids.

PREGNANCY: Category C, caution in nursing.

MECHANISM OF ACTION: NSAID; inhibits prostaglandin biosynthesis.

PHARMACOKINETICS: Absorption: C_{max}=95ng/mL; T_{max}=12hrs.

NURSING CONSIDERATIONS

Assessment: Assess for drug hypersensitivity, cross-sensitivity reactions, bleeding tendencies, complicated ocular surgeries, corneal denervation, corneal epithelial defects, DM, ocular surface disease (dry eye syndrome), rheumatoid arthritis, possible drug interactions.

Monitoring: Monitor for bleeding of ocular tissues (hyphema), healing problems, keratitis, epithelial breakdown, corneal thinning/erosion/ulceration/perforation.

Patient Counseling: Advise not to use while wearing contact lenses. Caution during nursing/late pregnancy.

Administration: Intraocular route. **Storage:** 15-25°C (59-77°F), protect from light.

ACULAR LS   RX
ketorolac tromethamine (Allergan)

OTHER BRAND NAMES: Acular PF (Allergan)

THERAPEUTIC CLASS: NSAID

INDICATIONS: (Acular PF) Reduction of ocular pain and photophobia after incisional refractive surgery. (Acular LS) Reduction of ocular pain and burning/stinging following corneal refractive surgery.

DOSAGE: *Adults:* 1 drop qid post-op PRN for up to 3 days (Acular PF) or 4 days (Acular LS).
Pediatrics: ≥3 yrs: 1 drop qid post-op PRN for up to 3 days (Acular PF) or 4 days (Acular LS).

HOW SUPPLIED: Sol: (Acular PF) 0.5% [0.4mL, 12s] (PF is preservative free); (Acular LS) 0.4% [5mL]

WARNINGS/PRECAUTIONS: Avoid use with contact lenses. Potential cross-sensitivity to acetylsalicylic acid, phenylacetic acid derivatives, and other NSAIDs. May increase bleeding of ocular tissue (including hyphemas) in conjunction with ocular surgery. May slow or delay healing. D/C if corneal epithelium breakdown occurs. Caution in known bleeding tendencies, complicated ocular surgeries, corneal denervation, corneal epithelial defects, diabetes mellitus (DM), ocular surface diseases (eg, dry eye syndrome), rheumatoid arthritis, or repeated ocular surgeries within a short period of time. Caution if used >24 hrs prior to surgery and use beyond 14 days post-surgery.

ADVERSE REACTIONS: Transient stinging/burning, allergic reactions, corneal edema, iritis, ocular inflammation/irritation/pain, superficial keratitis, superficial ocular infections.

INTERACTIONS: Concomitant use of topical NSAIDs and topical steroids may increase potential for healing problems. Caution with other medications which may prolong bleeding time.

PREGNANCY: Category C, caution in nursing.

MECHANISM OF ACTION: NSAID; inhibits prostaglandin biosynthesis.

PHARMACOKINETICS: Absorption: C_{max}=960ng/mL.

NURSING CONSIDERATIONS

Assessment: Assess for drug hypersensitivity, cross-sensitivity reactions, bleeding tendencies, complicated ocular surgeries, corneal denervation, corneal epithelial defects, DM, ocular surface disease (dry eye syndrome), rheumatoid arthritis, possible drug interactions.

Monitoring: Monitor for bleeding of ocular tissues (hyphema), healing problems, keratitis, corneal epithelial breakdown, corneal thinning/erosion/ulceration/perforation.

Patient Counseling: Advise not to use while wearing contact lenses. Caution during nursing/late pregnancy. Solution from one Acular PF single-use vial should be used immediately after opening and the remaining contents should be discarded immediately after administration. Avoid physical contact between tip of vial and any other surface.

Intraocular route. Storage: (Acular PF) 15-30°C (59-86°F), protect from light. (Acular LS) 15-25°C (59-77°F).

ADALAT CC

RX

nifedipine (Bayer Healthcare)

OTHER BRAND NAMES: Nifediac CC (Teva) - Afeditab CR (Watson)

THERAPEUTIC CLASS: Calcium channel blocker (dihydropyridine)

INDICATIONS: Treatment of HTN alone or in combination with other antihypertensive agents.

DOSAGE: *Adults:* Initial: 30mg qd. Titrate: Over 7-14 days. Base upward titration on therapeutic efficacy and safety. Usual: 30-60mg qd. Max: 90mg qd. Elderly: Start at low end of dosing range.

HOW SUPPLIED: Tab, Extended-Release: (Adalat CC) 30mg, 60mg, 90mg, (Afeditab CR) 30mg, 60mg, (Nifediac CC) 30mg, 60mg, 90mg

CONTRAINDICATIONS: (Adalat CC) Concomitant use with strong P450 inducers (eg, rifampin); cardiogenic shock.

WARNINGS/PRECAUTIONS: May cause hypotension; monitor BP initially or with titration. May increase frequency, duration, and/or severity of angina or acute myocardial infarction (MI) with severe obstructive coronary artery disease (CAD) upon starting or at time of dosage increases. May increase risk of congestive heart failure (CHF), especially with tight aortic stenosis or β-blockers. Peripheral edema may occur; rule out peripheral edema caused by left ventricular dysfunction if HTN is complicated by CHF. Transient elevated liver enzymes, cholestasis with or without jaundice, and allergic hepatitis reported (rare). Positive direct Coomb's test reported. Elevated BUN and SrCr reported with chronic renal insufficiency. Caution with renal/hepatic impairment and in elderly. (Adalat CC) Reduced clearance in cirrhosis. Careful monitoring and dose reduction may be necessary; initiate lowest dose possible. Contains lactose; avoid with hereditary galactose intolerance problems, Lapp lactase deficiency, and glucose-galactose malabsorption. (Nifediac CC [90mg]) Contains tartrazine; may cause allergic type reactions, including bronchial asthma, frequently seen in patients with aspirin hypersensitivity.

ADVERSE REACTIONS: Peripheral edema, headache, flushing, heat sensation, dizziness, fatigue, asthenia, nausea, constipation.

INTERACTIONS: See Contraindications. Impacts exposure with drugs known to either inhibit or induce CYP450 3A4 system. β-blockers may increase risk of CHF, severe hypotension, or angina exacerbation; avoid abrupt β-blocker withdrawal. Caution in patients already taking drugs that are known to lower blood pressure. Possible hypotension with fentanyl. Enhanced hypotensive effect with benazepril and timolol. Increased exposure with CYP3A inhibitors (eg, ketoconazole, erythromycin, grapefruit, nefazodone, fluoxetine, verapamil, amprenavir); monitor BP and consider dose adjustment. Increased exposure with valproic acid; monitor BP and consider dose adjustment. Increased levels with quinidine and diltiazem. Avoid use with strong CYP3A inducers (eg, rifampin, rifabutin, phenobarbital, phenytoin, carbamazepine, St. John's wort). Avoid with grapefruit juice; stop intake ≥3 days prior to therapy. Monitor blood glucose level and consider dose adjustment with acarbose. May increase PT with coumarin anticoagulants. May increase plasma levels of digoxin. Increased plasma levels and absorption of metformin. May increase exposure of tacrolimus; monitor blood levels and consider dose reduction. May decrease doxazosin levels; monitor BP and reduce dose. Increased levels with cimetidine, quinupristin/dalfopristin; monitor BP and reduce dose. Increased plasma concentrations with cisapride. (Adalat CC) May increase the BP-lowering effects of diuretics, PDE5 inhibitors, and α-methyldopa. Coadministration with IV magnesium sulfate in pregnant women may cause excessive fall in BP.

PREGNANCY: Category C, not for use in nursing.

MECHANISM OF ACTION: Calcium channel blocker; inhibits the transmembrane influx of calcium ions into vascular smooth muscle and cardiac muscle. Involves peripheral arterial vasodilation and reduction in peripheral vascular resistance, resulting in reduced arterial blood pressure.

PHARMACOKINETICS: Absorption: Complete; absolute bioavailability (84-89%); C_{max}=115ng/mL (90mg); T_{max}=2.5-5 hrs. **Distribution:** Plasma protein binding (92-98%); found in breast milk. **Metabolism:** Liver via CYP3A4. **Elimination:** Urine (60-80%, metabolite), (<0.1%, unchanged); feces (metabolite); $T_{1/2}$=7 hrs.

NURSING CONSIDERATIONS

Assessment: Assess for severity of HTN, CHF, hepatic/renal impairment, pregnancy/nursing status, drug hypersensitivity, or any other conditions where treatment is contraindicated or cautioned and for possible drug interactions.

Monitoring: Monitor for CHF, hypotension, cholestasis with/without jaundice, allergic hepatitis, peripheral edema, angina, MI, hemolytic anemia, allergic reactions and bronchial asthma. Monitor patients with cirrhosis. Carefully monitor vital signs during initial administration and titration. Monitor LFTs. Monitor BUN and SrCr in patients with chronic renal insufficiency.

Patient Counseling: Inform about potential benefits/risks of therapy. Swallow whole; do not chew, crush, or divide.Take on empty stomach. Do not take with grapefruit juice. Notify physician if pregnant/nursing and if any adverse reactions occur. (Afeditab CR) Advise patients that empty matrix "ghost" (tab) may pass in the stool and that this is not a cause for concern.

Administration: Oral route. Swallow whole, not bitten or divided. Take on empty stomach. **Storage:** <30°C (86°F). (Nifediac CC): 25°C (77°F); excursions permitted to 15-30°C (59-86°F). Protect from light and moisture.

ADCIRCA RX
tadalafil (Lilly)

THERAPEUTIC CLASS: Phosphodiesterase type 5 inhibitor

INDICATIONS: Treatment of pulmonary arterial hypertension (PAH) (WHO Group I) to improve exercise ability.

DOSAGE: *Adults:* 40mg qd. Mild (CrCl 51-80mL/min) or Moderate (CrCl 31-50mL/min) Renal Impairment/Coadministration in Patients on Ritonavir for ≥1 Week: Initial: 20mg qd. Titrate: May increase to 40mg qd. Mild or Moderate Hepatic Impairment (Child Pugh Class A or B): Initial: 20mg qd. Coadministration of Ritonavir in Patients on Tadalafil: Stop tadalafil ≥24 hrs before ritonavir initiation. After ≥1 week following ritonavir initiation, resume tadalafil at 20mg qd. Titrate: May increase to 40mg qd.

HOW SUPPLIED: Tab: 20mg

CONTRAINDICATIONS: Regular or intermittent use with any form of organic nitrate.

WARNINGS/PRECAUTIONS: Seek immediate medical attention if anginal chest pain, sudden vision loss, decreased or loss of hearing, or erection >4 hrs occurs following use. Transient decrease in BP reported; caution with underlying cardiovascular disease (CVD). Patients with severely impaired autonomic control of BP or left ventricular outflow obstruction may be more sensitive to vasodilatory effects. May worsen cardiovascular (CV) status with pulmonary veno-occlusive disease (PVOD); not recommended with veno-occlusive disease. Avoid use in severe renal impairment (CrCl <30mL/min and on hemodialysis) and hepatic impairment (Child-Pugh Class C). Not recommended with hereditary degenerative retinal disorders (eg, retinal pigmentosa). Non-arteritic anterior ischemic optic neuropathy (NAION) reported. Rare reports of prolonged erections (>4 hrs) and priapism; caution in conditions predisposing to priapism (eg, sickle cell anemia, multiple myeloma, leukemia) or with anatomical deformation of the penis (eg, angulation, cavernosal fibrosis, Peyronie's disease). Assess risk/benefit with bleeding disorders or significant active peptic ulceration.

ADVERSE REACTIONS: Headache, myalgia, nasopharyngitis, flushing, respiratory tract infection, pain in extremity, nausea, back pain, dyspepsia, nasal congestion.

INTERACTIONS: See Contraindications. Additive hypotensive effects with alcohol, α-adrenergic blockers (eg, doxazosin, alfuzosin, tamsulosin), vasodilators, and antihypertensives (eg, amlodipine, angiotensin II receptor blockers, bendroflumethiazide, enalapril, metoprolol). Increased exposure with ritonavir, other HIV protease inhibitors, ketoconazole, and other CYP3A inhibitors. Decreased exposure with rifampin, bosentan, and other CYP3A inducers. Avoid use during initiation of ritonavir. Avoid use with potent CYP3A inhibitors (eg, ketoconazole, itraconazole) and chronic potent CYP3A inducers (eg, rifampin). Increased exposure and levels of ethinyl estradiol. Reduced rate of absorption with antacids (magnesium hydroxide/aluminum hydroxide). Avoid use with Cialis or other PDE5 inhibitors. A small increase in HR seen with theophylline. May increase risk of NAION with smoking.

PREGNANCY: Category B, caution in nursing.

MECHANISM OF ACTION: Phosphodiesterase type 5 (PDE5) inhibitor; increases the concentrations of cGMP, resulting in relaxation of pulmonary vascular smooth muscle cells and vasodilation of the pulmonary vascular bed.

PHARMACOKINETICS: Absorption: T_{max}=2-8 hrs. **Distribution:** V_d=77L; plasma protein binding (94%). **Metabolism:** Via CYP3A to catechol metabolite, which undergoes extensive methylation and glucuronidation; methylcatechol glucuronide (major metabolite). **Elimination:** Feces (61%), Urine (36%); $T_{1/2}$=35 hrs.

NURSING CONSIDERATIONS

Assessment: Assess for CVD, BP, renal/hepatic function, hereditary degenerative retinal disorders, conditions that may predispose to priapism, bleeding disorders, active peptic ulceration, hypersensitivity to drug, nitrite use, pregnancy/nursing status, and possible drug interactions.

Monitoring: Monitor for signs/symptoms of anginal chest pain, vision or hearing loss, pulmonary edema, NAION, prolonged erections >4 hrs, and priapism. Monitor BP.

Patient Counseling: Inform that any use of organic nitrates is contraindicated, may take drug with or without food, and that drug is also marketed as Cialis for erectile dysfunction; instruct to avoid taking Cialis or other PDE5 inhibitors. Advise to seek immediate medical attention if sudden loss of vision in one or both eyes and sudden decrease or loss of hearing develop, or if erection lasts for >4 hrs.

Administration: Oral route. Dividing dose over the course of the day is not recommended. **Storage:** 25°C (77°F); excursions permitted to 15-30°C (59-86°F).

ADDERALL CII
amphetamine salt combo (Shire)

> High potential for abuse; avoid prolonged use. Misuse of amphetamine may cause sudden death and serious cardiovascular adverse events.

THERAPEUTIC CLASS: Sympathomimetic amine

INDICATIONS: Treatment of attention-deficit disorder with hyperactivity (ADHD) and narcolepsy.

DOSAGE: *Adults:* Narcolepsy: Initial: 10mg/day. Titrate: May increase by 10mg/day every week. Usual: 5-60mg/day. Give 1st dose upon awakening, and additional doses q4-6h.
Pediatrics: ADHD: 3-5 yrs: Initial: 2.5mg qd. Titrate: May increase by 2.5mg weekly. ≥6 yrs: 5mg qd-bid. May increase by 5mg weekly. Max (usual): 40mg/day. Narcolepsy: 6-12 yrs: Initial: 5mg/day. May increase by 5mg weekly. ≥12 yrs: Initial: 10mg/day. Titrate: May increase by 10mg/day every week. Usual: 5-60mg/day. Give 1st dose upon awakening, and additional doses q4-6h.

HOW SUPPLIED: Tab: 5mg*, 7.5mg*, 10mg*, 12.5mg*, 15mg*, 20mg*, 30mg*
*scored

CONTRAINDICATIONS: Advanced arteriosclerosis, symptomatic cardiovascular disease, moderate to severe HTN, hyperthyroidism, glaucoma, agitated states, history of drug abuse, during or within 14 days of MAOI use.

WARNINGS/PRECAUTIONS: May exacerbate symptoms of behavior disturbance and thought disorder in psychotic patients. Caution when using stimulants to treat patients with comorbid bipolar disorder because of concern for possible induction of mixed/manic episode in such patients. Stimulants at usual doses can cause treatment emergent psychotic or manic symptoms (eg, hallucinations, delusional thinking, mania) in children and adolescents without prior history of psychotic illness. Aggressive behavior or hostility reported in clinical trials and the postmarketing experience of some medications indicated for the treatment of ADHD. Monitor growth in children. May lower convulsive threshold; d/c in presence of seizures. Visual disturbances reported with stimulant treatment. May exacerbate Tourette's syndrome and phonic or motor tics. Caution with HTN and monitor BP. Interrupt occasionally to determine if patient requires continued therapy. Sudden death reported in children with structural cardiac abnormalities; avoid with known structural cardiac abnormalities or other serious cardiac problems.

ADVERSE REACTIONS: HTN, tachycardia, palpitations, CNS overstimulation, dry mouth, GI disorders, anorexia, impotence, urticaria, rash, angioedema, anaphylaxis, Stevens-Johnson syndrome.

INTERACTIONS: GI acidifying agents (eg, guanethidine, reserpine, glutamic acid, etc.) and urinary acidifying agents (eg, ammonium chloride, etc.) decrease efficacy. MAOIs may cause hypertensive crisis. Potentiated by GI and urinary alkalinizers, propoxyphene overdose. Potentiated effects of both agents with TCAs. May delay absorption of phenytoin, ethosuximide, phenobarbital. Potentiates meperidine, norepinephrine, phenobarbital, phenytoin. Antagonized by haloperidol, chlorpromazine, lithium. Antagonizes adrenergic blockers, antihistamines, antihypertensives, veratrum alkaloids (antihypertensive). Avoid coadministration with alkalinizing agents (eg, antacids).

PREGNANCY: Category C, not for use in nursing.

MECHANISM OF ACTION: CNS stimulant; thought to block reuptake of norepinephrine and dopamine into presynaptic neuron and increase release of these monoamines into extraneuronal space.

PHARMACOKINETICS: Absorption: T_{max}=approximately 3 hrs (fasted). **Metabolism**: CYP2D6 (oxidation): 4-hydroxy-amphetamine and norephedrine. **Elimination**: Urine, $T_{1/2}$=9.77-11 hrs (d-amphetamine), 11.5-13.8 hrs (l-amphetamine).

NURSING CONSIDERATIONS

Assessment: Assess for agitation, glaucoma, tics, family history of Tourette's syndrome, cardiovascular conditions (eg, severe HTN, angina pectoris, cardiac abnormalities, arrhythmias, heart failure, recent MI), hyperthyroidism or thyrotoxicosis, bipolar illness, history of drug dependence or alcoholism.

Monitoring: Monitor for cardiac abnormalities, exacerbations of behavior disturbances and thought disorder, bipolar illness, aggression, seizures, and visual disturbances. Periodic monitoring of CBC, differential and platelet count, LFTs. Monitor height and weight in children.

Patient Counseling: Inform about risks of treatment, appropriate use, drug abuse/dependence. Caution while operating machinery/driving.

Administration: Oral route. **Storage**: 20-25°C (68-77°F).

ADDERALL XR
amphetamine salt combo (Shire)

> High potential for abuse. Prolonged use may lead to drug dependence. Misuse may cause sudden death and serious cardiovascular adverse reactions.

THERAPEUTIC CLASS: Sympathomimetic amine

INDICATIONS: Treatment of attention deficit hyperactivity disorder (ADHD).

DOSAGE: *Adults:* Individualize dose. Amphetamine-Naive/Switching from Another Medication: 20mg qam. Currently on Amphetamine (immediate-release): Switch to ER at the same total daily dose, taken once daily. Titrate at weekly intervals as needed. Swallow cap whole or open cap and sprinkle contents on applesauce; do not chew beads.
Pediatrics: Individualize dose. Currently on Amphetamine (immediate-release): Switch to ER at the same total daily dose, taken once daily. Titrate at weekly intervals as needed. 13-17 yrs: Amphetamine-Naive/Switching from Another Medication: Initial: 10mg/day. Titrate: May increase to 20mg/day after one week if symptoms not controlled. 6-12 yrs: Amphetamine-Naive/Switching from Another Medication: 10mg qam or 5mg qam when lower initial dose is appropriate. Titrate: Adjust daily dosage in increments of 5mg or 10mg at weekly intervals. Max: 30mg/day. Swallow cap whole or open cap and sprinkle contents on applesauce; do not chew beads.

HOW SUPPLIED: Cap, Extended-Release: 5mg, 10mg, 15mg, 20mg, 25mg, 30mg

CONTRAINDICATIONS: Advanced arteriosclerosis, symptomatic cardiovascular disease, moderate to severe HTN, hyperthyroidism, glaucoma, agitated states, history of drug abuse, during or within 14 days of MAOI use.

WARNINGS/PRECAUTIONS: Avoid with known serious structural cardiac abnormalities, cardiomyopathy, serious heart rhythm abnormalities, coronary artery disease, or other serious cardiac problems; sudden death reported in children and adolescents with structural cardiac abnormalities or other serious heart problems. Sudden death, stroke, and myocardial infarction (MI) reported in adults. May cause modest increase in HR and BP; caution with HTN, heart failure, recent MI, or ventricular arrhythmia. Prior to treatment perform a physical exam and medical history (including assessment for family history of sudden death or ventricular arrhythmia). Promptly evaluate if symptoms of cardiac disease develop during treatment. May exacerbate symptoms of behavior disturbance and thought disorder with pre-existing psychotic disorder. Caution in patients with comorbid bipolar disorder; may cause induction of mixed/manic episode. May cause treatment-emergent psychotic or manic symptoms (eg, hallucinations, delusional thinking, mania) in children and adolescents without prior history of psychotic illness or mania at usual doses; d/c may be appropriate. Aggressive behavior or hostility reported in children and adolescents with ADHD. Suppression of growth reported with long-term use in pediatrics; monitor height and weight. May lower convulsive threshold; d/c in presence of seizures. Difficulties in accommodation and blurred vision reported. Prescribe or dispense least amount feasible to minimize overdosage possibility. Reported to exacerbate motor and phonic tics and Tourette's syndrome.

ADVERSE REACTIONS: Loss of appetite, dry mouth, insomnia, headache, abdominal pain, weight loss, emotional lability, agitation, anxiety, N/V, dizziness, tachycardia, nervousness.

INTERACTIONS: See Contraindications. GI acidifying agents (eg, guanethidine, reserpine, glutamic acid HCl, ascorbic acid) and urinary acidifying agents (eg, ammonium chloride, sodium acid phosphate, methenamine salts) may decrease efficacy. GI alkalinizing agents (eg, sodium bicarbonate) may potentiate effects; avoid concomitant use. Urinary alkalinizing agents (eg, acetazolamide, some thiazides) may potentiate effects. Use in cases of propoxyphene overdose may potentiate CNS stimulation and cause fatal convulsions. May enhance activity of TCAs or sympathomimetic agents. May delay absorption of phenytoin, ethosuximide, phenobarbital. May potentiate effects of meperidine. Chlorpromazine and haloperidol may inhibit central stimulant effects. Lithium carbonate may inhibit anorectic and stimulatory effects. May antagonize effect of antihypertensives. May enhance the adrenergic effect of norepinephrine. May inhibit hypotensive effect of veratrum alkaloids. May counteract sedative effects of antihistamines. May reduce cardiovascular effects of adrenergic blockers. Monitor for changes in clinical effect with proton pump inhibitors (PPI).

PREGNANCY: Category C, not for use in nursing.

MECHANISM OF ACTION: Sympathomimetic amine; mechanism unknown. Thought to block reuptake of norepinephrine and dopamine into presynaptic neuron and increase release of these monoamines into extraneuronal space.

PHARMACOKINETICS: Absorption: T_{max}=7 hrs. **Distribution:** Found in breast milk. **Metabolism**: CYP2D6 (oxidation): 4-hydroxy-amphetamine and norephedrine (metabolites). **Elimination**: Urine (30-40%). (Cap, ER 20mg single dose) D-amphetamine: $T_{1/2}$=10 hrs (adults), 11 hrs (adolescents aged 13-17 years), 9 hrs (6-12 years). l-amphetamine: $T_{1/2}$=13 hrs (adults), 13-14 hrs (adolescents aged 13-17), 11 hrs (6-12 yrs).

NURSING CONSIDERATIONS

Assessment: Assess for pre-existing psychotic disorder, history of seizures, history of drug abuse, pregnancy/nursing status, and for possible drug interactions. Assess for structural cardiac abnormalities, cardiomyopathy, heart rhythm abnormalities, coronary artery disease, HTN, or other serious cardiac problems.

Monitoring: Monitor for exacerbations of behavior disturbances and thought disorder, psychotic or manic symptoms, aggressive behavior, hostility, seizures, visual disturbances, exacerbation of Tourette's syndrome, and for phonic or motor tics exacerbation. Monitor BP and HR. Monitor height and weight in children.

Patient Counseling: Inform about benefits and risks of treatment and counsel on appropriate use. Advise to store in a safe place to prevent misuse/abuse. Advise of serious cardiovascular risk (including sudden death, MI, stroke and HTN). Inform that psychotic or manic symptoms may occur. Advise parents or guardians of pediatric patients that growth will need to be monitored during treatment. Instruct to notify physician if pregnant, planning become pregnant, or if nursing. Advise that therapy may impair the ability to engage in hazardous activities and therefore caution should be used while operating machinery or vehicles.

Administration: Oral route. **Storage:** 25°C (77°F); excursion permitted to 15-30°C (59-86°F).

ADENOCARD

RX

adenosine (Astellas)

THERAPEUTIC CLASS: Endogenous nucleoside

INDICATIONS: Conversion to sinus rhythm (SR) of paroxysmal supraventricular tachycardia (PSVT), including that associated with accesory bypass tracts (Wolff-Parkinson-White syndrome).

DOSAGE: *Adults:* 6mg rapid IV bolus over 1-2 sec. If not converted to SR within 1-2 min, give 12mg rapid IV bolus; may give 2nd 12mg dose if needed. Max: 12mg/dose.
Pediatrics: <50kg: 0.05-0.1mg/kg rapid IV bolus. If not converted to SR within 1-2 min, give additional bolus doses, incrementally increasing amount by 0.05-0.1mg/kg. Follow each bolus with a saline flush. Continue process until SR or a maximum single dose of 0.3mg/kg is used. ≥50kg: 6mg rapid IV bolus over 1-2 sec. If not converted to SR within 1-2 min, give 12mg rapid IV bolus; may give second 12mg dose if needed. Max: 12mg/dose.

HOW SUPPLIED: Inj: 3mg/mL [2mL, 4mL]

CONTRAINDICATIONS: 2nd- or 3rd-degree AV block (except with pacemaker), sinus node disease such as sick sinus syndrome or symptomatic bradycardia (except with pacemaker).

WARNINGS/PRECAUTIONS: May produce short-lasting 1st-, 2nd-, 3rd-degree heart block; institute appropriate therapy as needed. Transient or prolonged asystole, respiratory alkalosis, ventricular fibrillation reported. Caution with obstructive lung disease not associated with bronchoconstriction (eg, emphysema, bronchitis). Avoid with bronchoconstriction/bronchospasm (eg, asthma). D/C if severe respiratory difficulties develop. Resuscitative measures should be available. New arrhythmias may appear on ECG at time of conversion. Caution in elderly.

ADVERSE REACTIONS: Arrhythmias, facial flushing, dyspnea/SOB, chest pressure, nausea.

INTERACTIONS: Antagonized by methylxanthines (eg, theophylline, caffeine); may need larger dose. Potentiated by nucleoside transport inhibitors (eg, dipyridamole); use lower dose. Caution with digoxin, digoxin/verapamil combination, digitalis; ventricular fibrillation (rare) reported and potential for additive/synergistic depressant effects on SA and AV nodes. Possible higher degrees of heart block with carbamazepine.

PREGNANCY: Category C, safety in nursing not known.

MECHANISM OF ACTION: Endogenous nucleoside; slows conduction time through AV node, can interrupt reentry pathways through the AV node, and can restore normal sinus rhythm in patients with PSVT, including PSVT associated with Wolff-Parkinson-White syndrome.

PHARMACOKINETICS: Metabolism: Rapid (intracellular), through phosphorylation and deamination. **Elimination:** $T_{1/2}=$ <10 seconds.

NURSING CONSIDERATIONS

Assessment: Assess for AV block, presence of functioning pacemaker, sinus node disease, ventricular fibrillation, arrhythmias at time of conversion (eg, premature ventricular/atrial contractions, sinus bradycardia/tachycardia, skipped beats) obstructive lung disease, bronchoconstriction/bronchospasm (eg, asthma), previous hypersensitivity, pregnancy status, and possible drug interactions. Obtain baseline ECG and vital signs.

Monitoring: Monitor for AV block, bradycardia, ventricular fibrillation, prolonged asystole, and arrythmias at time of conversion. Monitor for signs of respiratory stimulation/alkalosis/ difficulties, or hypersensitivity reactions. Monitor ECG and vital signs.

Patient Counseling: Inform about benefits/risks of therapy. Advise to promptly report any adverse reactions to physician.

Administration: IV route. **Storage:** 15-30°C (59-86°F). Do not refrigerate. Dissolve crystals by warming to room temperature if crystallization occurs.

Discard unused portion. Needles should not be recapped, purposely bent or broken by hand.

ADRENACLICK
RX
epinephrine (Sciele)

THERAPEUTIC CLASS: Sympathomimetic catecholamine

INDICATIONS: Emergency treatment of severe allergic reactions (Type 1) including anaphylaxis to stinging insects (eg, order *Hymenoptera*, which includes bees, wasps, hornets, yellow jackets and fire ants), and biting insects (eg, triatoma, mosquitos), allergen immunotherapy, foods, drugs, diagnostic testing substances (eg, radiocontrast media), and other allergens, as well as anaphylaxis to unknown substances (idiopathic anaphylaxis) or exercise-induced anaphylaxis. For immediate administration with history of anaphylactic reactions.

DOSAGE: *Adults:* 15-30kg: Inject 0.15mg IM/SQ into the anterolateral aspect of the thigh. ≥30kg: Inject 0.3mg IM/SQ into the anterolateral aspect of the thigh.
Pediatrics: 15-30kg: Inject 0.15mg IM/SQ into the anterolateral aspect of the thigh. ≥30kg: Inject 0.3mg IM/SQ into the anterolateral aspect of the thigh.

HOW SUPPLIED: Inj: 1mg/mL [0.15mg, 0.3mg]

WARNINGS/PRECAUTIONS: Avoid injecting into the hands, feet, or buttocks; may result in loss of blood flow if accidentally injected into these areas. Avoid IV use; may result in cerebral hemorrhage due to sharp rise in BP if accidentally injected. Caution with cardiac arrhythmias, coronary artery or heart disease, or HTN. May precipitate/aggravate angina pectoris and produce ventricular arrhythmias in patients with coronary insufficiency or ischemic heart disease. High risk of developing adverse reactions with hyperthyroidism, CV disease, HTN, DM, elderly, and pregnant women. Contains sodium bisulfite; may cause allergic-type reactions including anaphylactic symptoms or life-threatening asthmatic episodes in certain susceptible persons.

ADVERSE REACTIONS: Anxiety, apprehensiveness, restlessness, tremor, weakness, dizziness, sweating, palpitations, pallor, N/V, headache, respiratory difficulties.

INTERACTIONS: Monitor for cardiac arrhythmias with anti-arrhythmics, cardiac glycosides and diuretics. Effects may be potentiated by tricyclic antidepressants, MAOIs, sodium levothyroxine, and certain antihistamines (eg, chlorpheniramine, tripelennamine, diphenhydramine). Cardiostimulating and bronchodilating effects antagonized by β-adrenergic blockers (eg, propranolol). Vasoconstricting and hypertensive effects antagonized by α-adrenergic blockers (eg, phentolamine). Ergot alkaloids and phenothiazines may reverse pressor effects.

PREGNANCY: Category C, caution in nursing.

MECHANISM OF ACTION: Sympathomimetic catecholamine; acts on α-adrenergic receptors by lessening the vasodilation and increasing vascular permeability that occurs during anaphylactic reaction. Acts on β-adrenergic receptors causing bronchial smooth muscle relaxation that helps alleviate bronchospasm, wheezing, and dyspnea that may occur during anaphylaxis.

NURSING CONSIDERATIONS

Assessment: Assess for arrhythmias, coronary artery or organic heart disease, HTN, hyperthyroidism, CV disease, DM, Parkinson's disease, pregnancy/nursing status, and possible drug interactions.

Monitoring: Monitor BP, HR, blood glucose, signs of cerebral hemorrhage, ventricular arrhythmia, HTN, anginal pain, and other adverse reactions.

Patient Counseling: Inform about side effects of therapy (eg, increased pulse rate, sensation of a more forceful heartbeat, palpitations, throbbing headache, pallor, feelings of overstimulation, anxiety, weakness, shakiness, dizziness, or nausea). Side effects may subside rapidly, especially with rest, quiet, and recumbency. Avoid injecting into the hands, feet, or buttocks and to avoid IV route. Inform physician if accidental injection occur into these areas. Inspect the solution for particulate matter and discoloration. Inform that patients may develop more severe/persistent effects if with HTN/hyperthyroidism; could experience angina if with coronary artery disease; may increase blood glucose if with diabetes; and may worsen symptoms of Parkinson's disease.

Administration: SQ or IM route. Inject only at the anterolateral aspect of the thigh. **Storage:** 20°-25°C (68°-77°F); excursions permitted to 15°-30°C (59°-86°F). Light sensitive; store in the carrying case provided. Protect from light and freezing. Do not refrigerate. Discard if discolored, cloudy, or has particulate matter. The remaining volume left after the fixed dose should not be further administered and should be discarded.

ADVAIR   RX
fluticasone propionate - salmeterol (GlaxoSmithKline)

> Long-acting β₂-adrenergic agonists (LABA), such as salmeterol, increase the risk of asthma-related death. LABAs may increase the risk of asthma-related hospitalization in pediatric and adolescent patients. Should only be prescribed for patients not adequately controlled on a long-term asthma control medication or whose disease severity clearly warrants initiation of treatment with both an inhaled corticosteroid and a LABA. Do not use in patients whose asthma is adequately controlled on low- or medium-dose inhaled corticosteroids.

THERAPEUTIC CLASS: Corticosteroid/beta₂ agonist

INDICATIONS: Treatment of asthma in patients ≥4 yrs. (250/50) Maintenance treatment of airflow obstruction in patients with chronic obstructive pulmonary disease (COPD), including chronic bronchitis and/or emphysema, and to reduce exacerbations of COPD in patients with history of exacerbations.

DOSAGE: *Adults:* Asthma: Initial: Based upon asthma severity. Usual: 1 inh bid (am/pm q12h). Max: 500/50 bid. Increase to higher strength if response to initial dose is inadequate after 2 weeks. COPD: (250/50): 1 inh bid (am/pm q12h). If asthma symptoms or SOB occurs between doses, use short-acting β₂-agonist for immediate relief.
Pediatrics: ≥12 yrs: Asthma: Initial: Based upon asthma severity. Usual: 1 inh bid (am/pm q12h). Max: 500/50 bid. Increase to higher strength if response to initial dose is inadequate after 2 weeks. If asthma symptoms arise between doses, use short-acting β₂-agonist for immediate relief. 4-11 yrs: (100/50): Not Controlled on Inhaled Corticosteroid: 1 inh bid (am/pm q12h).

HOW SUPPLIED: Disk: (Fluticasone Propionate-Salmeterol) (100/50) 100mcg-50mcg/inh, (250/50) 250mcg-50mcg/inh, (500/50) 500mcg-50mcg/inh

CONTRAINDICATIONS: Primary treatment of status asthmaticus or other acute episodes of asthma or COPD where intensive measures are required; severe hypersensitivity to milk proteins.

WARNINGS/PRECAUTIONS: Do not use more often or at higher doses than recommended; cardiovascular (CV) effects and fatalities reported. Localized infections of the mouth and pharynx with *Candida albicans* reported; consider d/c when necessary. Lower respiratory tract infections (eg, pneumonia) reported in patients with COPD. Increased susceptibility to infections; avoid exposure to chickenpox or measles. Caution with active or quiescent tuberculosis (TB) infections of the respiratory tract, untreated systemic infections, or ocular herpes simplex. Deaths due to adrenal insufficiency have occurred with transfer from a systemic to inhaled corticosteroids. Wean slowly from systemic corticosteroid therapy. Transfer from systemic to inhaled corticosteroid therapy may unmask conditions previously suppressed (eg, rhinitis). May produce systemic corticosteroid effects; reduce dose slowly if such effects develop. May produce paradoxical bronchospasm; d/c immediately, treat, and institute alternative therapy. Upper airway symptoms reported. Immediate hypersensitivity reactions may occur. Caution in patients with CV disorders. Long-term use may result in decreases in bone mineral density (BMD), glaucoma, increased intraocular pressure (IOP), and cataracts. May reduce growth velocity in pediatric patients. Rare cases of eosinophilic conditions (eg, Churg-Strauss syndrome) observed. Caution in elderly and patients with convulsive disorders, thyrotoxicosis, hepatic disease, if unusually responsive to sympathomimetic amines, diabetes mellitus (DM) and ketoacidosis. May cause changes in blood glucose and serum K^+ levels.

ADVERSE REACTIONS: Upper respiratory tract infection/inflammation, pharyngitis, dysphonia, oral candidiasis, bronchitis, cough, headache, N/V, pneumonia, throat irritation, viral respiratory infection, musculoskeletal pain.

INTERACTIONS: Extreme caution with TCAs or MAOIs, or within 2 weeks of d/c such products. May produce severe bronchospasm in patients with reversible obstructive airway disease with β-blockers. May increase salmeterol levels, increase heart rate, and prolong QTc interval with erythromycin. Avoid with strong CYP3A4 inhibitors (eg, ritonavir, atazanavir, clarithromycin, indinavir, itraconazole, nefazodone, nelfinavir, saquinavir, ketoconazole, telithromycin). Avoid use with other medications containing LABAs. Caution with cardioselective β-blockers, non-K^+-sparing diuretics (eg, loop or thiazide diuretics), tobacco and chronic use of drugs that can reduce bone mass (eg, anticonvulsants, oral corticosteroids). Increased fluticasone propionate exposure and reduced cortisol levels with ritonavir and ketoconazole. Increased exposure of salmeterol with ketoconazole; combination may be associated with QTc prolongation. D/C regular use of oral/inhaled short-acting β$_2$-agonists at initiation of therapy.

PREGNANCY: Category C, not for use in nursing.

MECHANISM OF ACTION: Fluticasone: Corticosteroid with anti-inflammatory activity. Asthma: inhibits multiple cell types (eg, mast cells, eosinophils, basophils, lymphocytes, macrophages, neutrophils) and mediator production or secretion (eg, histamine, eicosanoids, leukotrienes, cytokines) involved in the asthmatic response. COPD: Not well defined. Salmeterol: Selective LABA; stimulates intracellular adenyl cyclase, which catalyzes conversion of ATP to cAMP, producing relaxation of bronchial smooth muscle and inhibits mediator release of immediate hypersensitivity from cells, especially from mast cells.

PHARMACOKINETICS: Absorption: Administration in healthy, asthmatic, and COPD patients resulted in different pharmacokinetic parameters. **Distribution:** Fluticasone: V_d=4.2L/kg; plasma protein binding (91%). Salmeterol: Plasma protein binding (96%). **Metabolism:** Fluticasone: Liver via CYP3A4; 17 β-carboxylic acid derivative (metabolite). Salmeterol: Liver, via CYP3A4 to α-hydroxysalmeterol (metabolite). **Elimination:** Fluticasone: (PO) Urine (<5%); (Inh) $T_{1/2}$=5.6 hrs. Salmeterol (PO): Urine (25%), feces (60%); $T_{1/2}$=5.5 hrs.

NURSING CONSIDERATIONS

Assessment: Assess for hypersensitivity to milk proteins, acute asthma/COPD episodes, rapidly deteriorating asthma or COPD, risk factors for decreased bone mineral content, CV disease, convulsive disorder, thyrotoxicosis, DM, history of increased IOP, glaucoma, cataracts, active or quiescent pulmonary TB, ocular herpes simplex, untreated systemic infections, hepatic disease, pregnancy/nursing status, and for possible drug interactions. Obtain baseline BMD, eye exam, and lung function prior to therapy.

Monitoring: Monitor for localized oral *Candida albicans* infections, upper airway symptoms, worsening or acutely deteriorating asthma, development of glaucoma, increased IOP, CV effects, CNS effects, cataracts, hypercorticism, adrenal suppression, paradoxical bronchospasm, eosinophilic conditions, hypokalemia, hyperglycemia, and for hypersensitivity reactions. Monitor BMD and lung function periodically. Perform periodic eye exams. Monitor growth in pediatric patients. Monitor for lower respiratory tract infections (eg, pneumonia) in patients with COPD.

Patient Counseling: Inform that salmeterol, a component of Advair, increases the risk of asthma-related death. Advise that medication is not for the relief of acute asthma symptoms or exacerbations of COPD and extra doses should not be used for this purpose. Inform not to d/c unless directed by physician and on administration instructions. Advise to rinse mouth after inhalation and to spit water out; do not swallow water. Inform that medication may cause reduction in growth velocity (pediatric) and may also unmask conditions. Instruct to avoid exposure to chickenpox or measles and to seek medical attention if exposed to chickenpox or measles, if existing TB infections or ocular herpes simplex symptoms do not improve or worsen, during periods of stress or severe asthmatic attack, or if adrenal insufficiency, paradoxical bronchospasm, or hypersensitivity reactions occur.

Administration: Oral inhalation. Rinse mouth with water without swallowing after inhalation. Refer to PI for further administration instructions. **Storage:** 20-25°C (68-77°F). Keep in a dry place, away from direct heat or sunlight. Discard 1 month after removal from pouch or when indicator reads "0," whichever comes 1st.

ADVAIR HFA   RX
fluticasone propionate - salmeterol (GlaxoSmithKline)

> Long-acting β_2-adrenergic agonists (LABA), such as salmeterol, increase the risk of asthma-related death. LABA may increase the risk of asthma-related hospitalization in pediatric and adolescent patients. Should only be prescribed for patients not adequately controlled on a long-term asthma control medication or whose disease severity clearly warrants initiation of treatment with both an inhaled corticosteroid and a LABA. Do not use in patients whose asthma is adequately controlled on low- or medium-dose inhaled corticosteroids.

THERAPEUTIC CLASS: Corticosteroid/beta$_2$ agonist

INDICATIONS: Treatment of asthma in patients ≥12 yrs.

DOSAGE: *Adults:* Initial: Based upon patient's current asthma therapy. Usual: 2 inh bid (am/pm q12h). Increase to higher strength if response to initial dose inadequate after 2 weeks. Max: 2 inh of 230/21 bid. If symptoms arise between doses, use an inhaled short-acting β_2-agonist for immediate relief.
Pediatrics: ≥12 yrs: Initial: Based upon patient's current asthma therapy. Usual: 2 inh bid (am/pm q12h). Increase to higher strength if response to initial dose inadequate after 2 weeks. Max: 2 inh of 230/21 bid. If symptoms arise between doses, use an inhaled short-acting β_2-agonist for immediate relief.

HOW SUPPLIED: MDI: (Fluticasone Propionate-Salmeterol) (45/21) 45mcg-21mcg/inh, (115/21) 115mcg-21mcg/inh, (230/21) 230mcg-21mcg/inh [60 inhalations, 120 inhalations]

CONTRAINDICATIONS: Primary treatment of status asthmaticus or other acute episodes of asthma where intensive measures are required.

WARNINGS/PRECAUTIONS: Do not use more often or at higher doses than recommended; fatalities and prolonged QTc interval reported. Deaths due to adrenal insufficiency have occurred during and after transfer from systemic to inhaled corticosteroids. During periods of stress or a severe asthma attack, resume oral corticosteroids in patients who have withdrawn from systemic corticosteroids, and immediately contact physician. Can produce paradoxical bronchospasm; d/c immediately, treat and institute alternative therapy. Immediate hypersensitivity reactions may occur. Upper airway symptoms reported. Cardiovascular (CV) effects may occur; caution with CV disorders. Transferring from systemic corticosteroid therapy may unmask conditions previously suppressed (eg, rhinitis). Increased susceptibility to infections; avoid exposure to chickenpox or measles. Caution with active or quiescent tuberculosis (TB) infection, untreated systemic infections, or ocular herpes simplex. Caution in elderly, patients with convulsive disorder or thyrotoxicosis, hepatic problems, and in those unusually responsive to sympathomimetic amines, diabetes mellitus (DM), and ketoacidosis. Systemic corticosteroid effects may occur; reduce dose slowly if such effects develop. May cause reduction in growth velocity in pediatrics. Long-term use may result in decrease of bone mineral density (BMD), glaucoma, increased intraocular pressure (IOP), and cataracts. Lower respiratory tract infections (eg, pneumonia) reported. Localized *Candida albicans* infection of the pharynx may occur. Significant changes in systolic and/or diastolic BP and pulse rate reported. May cause changes in blood glucose and serum K$^+$ levels. Rare cases of eosinophilic conditions (eg, Churg-Strauss) observed.

ADVERSE REACTIONS: Upper respiratory tract infection, headache, throat irritation, musculoskeletal pain, N/V, menstruation symptoms, muscle pain, dizziness, viral GI infections, hoarseness, GI signs and symptoms, pain, intoxication hangover.

INTERACTIONS: Extreme caution with TCAs or MAOIs, or within 2 weeks of d/c such products. May produce severe bronchospasm in patients with asthma with β-blockers. Caution with cardioselective β-blockers. May increase salmeterol levels, increase heart rate, and prolong QTc interval with erythromycin. Avoid strong CYP3A4 inhibitors (eg, ketoconazole, ritonavir, atazanavir, clarithromycin, indinavir, itraconazole, nefazodone, nelfinavir, saquinavir, telithromycin). Caution with non-K$^+$ sparing diuretics (eg, loop or thiazide diuretics); ECG changes, hypokalemia may result. Do not use any additional inhaled LABAs. Increased risk of decreased BMD with tobacco and chronic use of drugs which can reduce bone mass (eg, anticonvulsants, corticosteroids). D/C regular use of oral/inhaled short-acting β$_2$ agonists at initiation of therapy.

PREGNANCY: Category C, not for use in nursing.

MECHANISM OF ACTION: Fluticasone: Corticosteroid with anti-inflammatory activity; inhibits multiple cell types (eg, mast cells, eosinophils, basophils, lymphocytes, macrophages, neutrophils) and mediator production or secretion (eg, histamine, eicosanoids, leukotrienes, cytokines) involved in the asthmatic response. Salmeterol: LABA; stimulates intracellular adenyl cyclase, which catalyzes conversion of adenosine triphosphate (ATP) to cyclic AMP, producing relaxation of bronchial smooth muscle and inhibits mediator release of immediate hypersensitivity from cells, especially mast cells.

PHARMACOKINETICS: Absorption: Fluticasone: Absolute Bioavailability (5.3%); Salmeterol: C_{max}=150pg/mL. **Distribution:** Fluticasone: V_d=4.2L/kg; plasma protein binding (99%). Salmeterol: Plasma protein binding (96%). **Metabolism:** Fluticasone: Liver, via CYP3A4. Salmeterol: Extensive by hydroxylation. **Elimination:** Fluticasone: Feces (major), urine (<5%); $T_{1/2}$=7.8 hrs. Salmeterol: Feces (60%), urine (25%); $T_{1/2}$=5.5 hrs.

NURSING CONSIDERATIONS

Assessment: Assess for previous hypersensitivity, acute asthma episode, severe asthma, risk factors for decreased bone mineral content, recent trauma or surgery, CVD, convulsive disorder, thyrotoxicosis, DM, history of increased IOP, glaucoma, cataracts, status asthmaticus, active or quiescent pulmonary TB, ocular herpes simplex, untreated systemic infections, hepatic impairment, pregnancy/nursing status, and possible drug interactions. Obtain baseline BMD, eye exam, and lung function prior to therapy.

Monitoring: Monitor for *Candida albicans* infections, upper airway symptoms, worsening or acutely deteriorating asthma, CV effects, development of glaucoma, increased IOP, cataracts, hypercorticism, adrenal suppression, paradoxical bronchospasm, eosinophilic conditions, hypokalemia, hyperglycemia, and for hypersensitivity reactions. Monitor BMD and lung function periodically. Perform periodic eye exams. Monitor growth in pediatric patients.

Patient Counseling: Inform that salmeterol, a component of Advair HFA, increases the risk of asthma-related death. Advise that medication is not for the relief of acute asthma symptoms and extra doses should not be used for this purpose. Inform not to d/c unless directed by physician and on administration instructions. Inform that medication may cause reduction in growth velocity (pediatric) and may also unmask conditions. Instruct to avoid exposure to chickenpox or measles and to seek medical attention if exposed to chickenpox or measles, if existing TB infections or ocular herpes simplex symptoms do not improve or worsen, during periods of stress or severe asthmatic attack, or if adrenal insufficiency, paradoxical bronchospasm, or hypersensitivity reactions occur. Advise to read Medication Guide.

Administration: Oral inhalation. Prime inhaler before 1st use by releasing 4 test sprays into air, away from face, shaking well for 5 sec before each spray. If not used for 4 weeks or dropped, reprime by releasing 2 test sprays into air, away from face, shaking well before each spray. **Storage:** 25°C (77°F); excursions permitted to 15-30°C (59-86°F). Store with mouthpiece down. May cause bursting when exposed to >120°F. Do not puncture, use or store near heat or open flame, or throw container into fire/incinerator.

Advicor   RX
lovastatin - niacin (Abbott)

THERAPEUTIC CLASS: HMG-CoA reductase inhibitor/Nicotinic acid

INDICATIONS: As an adjunct to diet, for the treatment of hypercholesterolemia when use of both Niaspan (niacin ER) and lovastatin is appropriate. (Niacin ER) As adjunct to diet for the treatment of primary hypercholesterolemia and mixed dyslipidemia, as an adjunct for the treatment of hypertriglyceridemia, and for the secondary prevention of cardiovascular events. (Lovastatin) Adjunct to diet for the treatment of primary hypercholesterolemia, and for primary and secondary prevention of cardiovascular events. See individual labeling for further details.

DOSAGE: *Adults:* Place on a standard cholesterol-lowering diet before treatment. Individualize dose based on targeted goals for cholesterol, TG, and on patients response. Not Currently on Niaspan: Initial: 500mg-20mg qhs. Titrate: Increase by no more than 500mg of niacin every 4 weeks. Max: 2000mg-40mg qd. Concomitant Cyclosporine/Danazol: Initial: 10mg/day of lovastatin. Max Lovastatin: 20mg/day. Concomitant Amiodarone/Verapamil: Max Lovastatin: 40mg/day. CrCl <30mL/min: Caution with dosage increases >20mg/day of lovastatin. May pretreat with aspirin (ASA) 30 min prior to treatment (up to 325mg) to reduce flushing. If d/c for an extended period of time (>7 days), reinstitute at the lowest dose. Refer to PI for further dosing information.

HOW SUPPLIED: Tab, Extended Release: (Niacin-Lovastatin) 500mg-20mg, 750mg-20mg, 1000mg-20mg, 1000mg-40mg

CONTRAINDICATIONS: Active liver disease or unexplained persistent elevations in serum transaminases, active peptic ulcer disease (PUD), arterial bleeding, pregnancy, nursing mothers.

WARNINGS/PRECAUTIONS: Do not substitute for equivalent dose of immediate-release niacin; severe hepatic toxicity may occur. Myopathy and rhabdomyolysis reported. Caution with history of liver disease or jaundice, hepatobiliary disease, history of peptic ulcer, diabetes, unstable angina, acute phase of myocardial infarction (MI), renal dysfunction. Monitor LFTs prior to therapy, every 6-12 weeks for first 6 months, and periodically thereafter; d/c if transaminase progression rise to 3 times ULN or if associated with nausea, fever, and/or malaise. May increase PT; caution in patients undergoing surgery. Elevated uric acid levels reported; caution in patients predisposed to gout. Lovastatin may elevate creatine phosphokinase (CPK). D/C if myopathy diagnosed or suspected and a few days before surgery. May cause CNS toxicity. May reduce platelet count and phosphorous levels. May cause endocrine dysfunction.

ADVERSE REACTIONS: Flushing, asthenia, flu syndrome, headache, infection, pain, back pain, diarrhea, N/V, hyperglycemia, myalgia, pruritus, rash, abdominal pain, dyspepsia.

INTERACTIONS: May potentiate ganglionic blockers, vasoactive drugs. Decreased niacin clearance by ASA. Separate bile acid sequestrants (eg, cholestyramine, colestipol) by 4-6 hrs. Avoid concomitant alcohol and hot drinks; may increase flushing and pruritus. Antidiabetic agents may need adjustment. Caution with vitamins or other nutritional supplements containing large doses of niacin or related compounds (eg, nicotinamide). Increased risk of skeletal muscle disorders with potent CYP3A4 inhibitors (eg, cyclosporine, itraconazole, clarithromycin, telithromycin, danazol, HIV protease inhibitors, nefazodone, >1 quart/day of grapefruit juice), fibrates (eg, gemfibrozil). Caution with drugs that diminish levels or activity of steroid hormones (eg, ketoconazole, spironolactone, cimetidine). Caution with vasoactive drugs (eg, nitrates, calcium channel blockers (CCBs), adrenergic blockers) and CYP3A4 substrates. Monitor PT before initiating therapy and during early treatment in patients on anticoagulants (eg, warfarin).

PREGNANCY: Category X, not for use in nursing.

MECHANISM OF ACTION: Niacin: Nicotinic acid; mechanism not established. May partially inhibit release of free fatty acids from adipose tissue and increase lipoprotein lipase activity. Decreases hepatic synthesis rate of VLDL-C and LDL-C. Lovastatin: HMG-CoA reductase inhibitor. Inhibits conversion of HMG-CoA to mevalonate. Has LDL-lowering effect by involving both reduction of VLDL-C concentration and induction of the LDL receptor, leading to reduction of production and/or increased catabolism of LDL-C.

PHARMACOKINETICS: Absorption: Niacin: C_{max}=18mcg/mL, T_{max}=5 hrs. Lovastatin: Incomplete, C_{max}=11ng/mL, T_{max}=2 hrs. **Distribution:** Niacin: Plasma protein binding (<20%), found in breast milk. Lovastatin: Plasma protein binding (>95%). **Metabolism:** Niacin: Rapid and extensive. Liver to nicotinamide adenine dinucleotide (NAD) metabolite and other metabolites; conjugation to nicotinuric acid (NUA) (metabolite). Lovastatin: Liver (extensive) via CYP3A4. Lovastatin acid, 6'-hydroxy (active metabolites). **Elimination:** Niacin: Urine (60%), (12%, unchanged); $T_{1/2}$=20-48 min. Lovastatin: Urine (10%), feces (83%), bile; $T_{1/2}$=4.5 hrs.

NURSING CONSIDERATIONS

Assessment: Assess for any conditions where treatment is contraindicated or cautioned, pregnancy/nursing status, and for possible drug interactions. Perform LFTs and lipid profile prior to therapy. Attempt to control dyslipidemia with appropriate diet, exercise, and weight reduction in obese patients and treat other underlying medical problems before instituting therapy.

Monitoring: Monitor for signs and symptoms of hepatotoxicity, myopathy (eg, muscle pain, tenderness, weakness), rhabdomyolysis with or without acute renal failure, endocrine dysfunction, CNS toxicity, and for laboratory test interactions. Perform periodic determinations of CK levels, phosphorus levels, glucose levels, uric acid levels, platelet count, and PT. Monitor LFTs every 6-12 weeks during the first 6 months of therapy and periodically thereafter. Perform lipid profile at intervals no less than 4 weeks.

Patient Counseling: Counsel to take at bedtime after a low-fat snack. Instruct to take as prescribed. Inform about risks/benefits of therapy. Advise to avoid alcohol, hot drinks and spicy foods around time of drug administration to minimize flushing. Counsel to avoid administration with grapefruit juice. Instruct to notify physician if pregnant/nursing or if dizziness occurs. Inform that flushing may occur but should subside after several weeks of therapy and that taking aspirin or another NSAID (eg, ibuprofen) 30 min before administration may minimize it. Advise not to break, crush, or chew, and to swallow whole. Instruct to contact physician if dosing is interrupted for any length of time, taking vitamins or other nutritional supplements, or if unexplained muscle pain, tenderness or weakness, or dizziness occurs. Instruct diabetic patients to contact physician if changes in blood glucose levels occur.

Administration: Oral route. Take drug whole at bedtime with a low-fat snack; do not break, crush or chew. Do not take on empty stomach or with grapefruit juice, alcohol, or hot drinks. **Storage:** 20-25°C (68-77°F).

AFINITOR   RX
everolimus (Novartis)

THERAPEUTIC CLASS: Kinase inhibitor

INDICATIONS: Treatment of advanced renal cell carcinoma (RCC) after failure of treatment with sunitinib or sorafenib. Treatment of patients with subependymal giant cell astrocytoma (SEGA) associated with tuberous sclerosis (TS) who require therapeutic intervention but are not candidates for curative surgical resection.

DOSAGE: *Adults:* Administer qd at the same time every day. Advanced RCC: 10mg qd. Dose Modifications: Severe and/or Intolerable Adverse Reactions/ Moderate Hepatic Impairment (Child-Pugh B): 5mg qd. SEGA: Initial dose based on body surface area (BSA). BSA: 0.5-1.2m²: 2.5mg qd. 1.3-2.1m²: 5mg qd. ≥2.2m²: 7.5mg qd. Refer to PI for dose modifications with moderate/strong CYP3A or PgP inhibitors, and for therapeutic drug monitoring.
Pediatrics: ≥3 yrs: ≥0.58m²: SEGA: Initial dose based on BSA. BSA: 0.5-1.2m²: 2.5mg qd. 1.3-2.1m²: 5mg qd. ≥2.2m²: 7.5mg qd. Refer to PI for dose

modifications with moderate/strong CYP3A or PgP inihibitors, and for thera-peutic drug monitoring.

HOW SUPPLIED: Tab: 2.5mg, 5mg, 10mg

WARNINGS/PRECAUTIONS: Non-infectious pneumonitis reported; for mod-erate symptoms, consider stopping therapy until symptoms resolve and con-sider corticosteroid use. D/C if symptoms are severe; consider corticosteroid use until symptoms resolve. Immunosuppressive properties may predispose patients to infections, including infections with opportunistic pathogens. Localized and systemic infections (eg, pneumonia, other bacterial infections, invasive fungal infections, viral infections including reactivation of hepatitis B virus) have occurred. Monitor for infection and institute appropriate treat-ment; d/c if invasive systemic fungal infection occurs. Mouth ulcers, stomati-tis, and oral mucositis reported. Elevated SrCr, hyperglycemia, hyperlipidemia, hypertriglyceridemia; decreased Hgb, lymphocytes, neutrophils, and platelets reported. Avoid with severe hepatic impairment (Child-Pugh Class C). Fetal harm may occur in pregnant woman.

ADVERSE REACTIONS: Stomatitis, infections, asthenia, fatigue, cough, diar-rhea, upper respiratory tract infection, sinusitis, otitis media, pyrexia, dyspnea, dehydration, pneumonitis, abdominal pain, anemia.

INTERACTIONS: Reduce dose and use with caution in combination with mod-erate CYP3A4 and/or PgP inhibitors (eg, amprenavir, fluconazole, verapamil, diltiazem). Avoid concomitant strong inhibitors of CYP3A4 (eg, ketoconazole, itraconazole, clarithromycin, atazanavir) may significantly increase levels. Strong CYP3A4 inducers (eg, phenytoin, carbamazepine, rifampin, rifapentine, phenobarbital, St. John's wort) may decrease levels; avoid and if combination cannot be avoided, increase dose of everolimus. Avoid concomitant use with grapefruit, grapefruit juice and other foods that are known to inhibit cyto-chrome P450 and PgP activity; may increase everolimus exposures. Avoid live vaccines and close contact with those who have received live vaccines.

PREGNANCY: Category D, not for use in nursing.

MECHANISM OF ACTION: Kinase inhibitor; binds to an intracellular protein, FKBP-12, resulting in an inhibitory complex formation and leading to inhibition of mTOR (mammalian target of rapamycin) kinase activity. In addition, inhibits the expression of hypoxia-inducible factor and reduces the expression of vas-cular endothelial growth factor. Reduces cell proliferation, angiogenesis, and glucose uptake in in vitro and/or in vivo studies.

PHARMACOKINETICS: Absorption: T_{max}=1-2 hrs. **Distribution:** Plasma protein binding (74%). **Metabolism:** Via CYP3A4 and PgP. **Excretion:** Urine (5%), feces (80%); $T_{1/2}$=30 hrs.

NURSING CONSIDERATIONS

Assessment: Assess for hypersensitivity reactions, active infections especially pre-existing fungal infections, hepatic impairment, pregnancy/nursing status, and possible drug interactions. Obtain baseline BUN, SrCr, FPG, lipid profile and CBC. Consider timing of routine vaccinations in pediatric patients with SEGA prior to therapy.

Monitoring: Monitor for signs/symptoms of hypersensitivity reactions, non-infectious pneumonitis, infections, reactivation of hepatitis B, mouth ulcers, stomatitis, and oral mucositis. Monitor CBC, blood chemistry, renal function including BUN or SrCr, serum glucose, and lipid profile periodically. For SEGA, evaluate SEGA volume 3 months after initiation and periodically thereafter. Routine therapeutic drug monitoring is recommended.

Patient Counseling: Instruct to swallow whole with a glass of water; if un-able to swallow, instruct to disperse completely in a glass of water by gently stirring, immediately prior to drinking. Inform patients that non-infectious pneumonitis or infections may develop; advise to report new or worsening respiratory symptoms or any signs or symptoms of infection. May develop mouth ulcers, stomatitis, oral mucositis, and hepatitis B reactivation. Use topi-cal treatments and mouthwashes (without alcohol or peroxide) if oral ulcer-ation develops. Inform of need to monitor blood chemistry and hematology before therapy and periodically thereafter. Notify healthcare providers of all concomitant medications, including OTC and dietary supplements. Avoid use of live vaccines and close contact with those who have received live vaccines. Advise of risk of fetal harm and to use an effective method of contraception during, and for 8 weeks after, therapy. If dose is missed, may take dose up to 6 hrs after the time the dose is normally taken; if >6 hrs have elapsed, skip the dose for that day and take it at the usual time on the next day. Do not take 2 doses to make up for the missed dose.

Administration: Oral route. Swallow whole with a glass of water. Do not chew or crush. Disperse completely in a glass of water if unable to swallow; see PI. Take either consistently with food or consistently without food. **Storage:** 25°C (77°F); excursions permitted between 15-30°C (59-86°F). Protect from light and moisture.

AFLURIA   RX
influenza virus vaccine (Merck)

THERAPEUTIC CLASS: Vaccine

INDICATIONS: Active immunization of individuals ≥6 months against influenza disease caused by influenza virus subtypes A and type B present in the vaccine.

DOSAGE: *Adults*: 0.5mL IM as single dose.
Pediatrics: ≥9 yrs: 0.5mL IM. ≥36 months-8 yrs: Unvaccinated/Previously vaccinated once with 1 dose last season: Give 2 doses of 0.5mL, 1 on day 1 followed by another 4 weeks later. Previously vaccinated with 2 doses last season or 1 dose ≥2 yrs ago: Give 1 dose of 0.5mL. ≥6 months-35 months: Unvaccinated/Previously vaccinated once with 1 dose last season: Give 2 doses of 0.25mL IM, 1 on day 1 followed by another 4 weeks later. Previously vaccinated with 2 doses last season or 1 dose ≥2 yrs ago: Give 1 dose of 0.25mL IM.

HOW SUPPLIED: Inj: 0.5mL [single-dose prefilled syringe], 5mL [multi-dose vial]

CONTRAINDICATIONS: Hypersensitivity to eggs, neomycin or polymyxin.

WARNINGS/PRECAUTIONS: Caution if Guillain-Barre syndrome (GBS) has occurred within 6 weeks of previous influenza vaccination. Immunosuppressed patients may have lower immune system. Medical treatment and supervision must be available to manage possible anaphylactic reaction. Influenza virus vaccine may not protect all individuals. Fever and febrile seizures reported in children <5 yrs.

ADVERSE REACTIONS: Local site reactions, headache, malaise, muscle aches, N/V, chills/shivering, fever, cough, loss of appetite, diarrhea, irritability, rhinitis, sore throat.

INTERACTIONS: Do not mix with any other vaccine in the same syringe or vial; administer other vaccine at different injection site if to be given at the same time. May diminish immune response with corticosteroids and immunosuppressive therapies.

PREGNANCY: Category C, caution in nursing.

MECHANISM OF ACTION: Vaccine; stimulates the immune system to elicit an immune response that produces antibodies that may protect against influenza virus subtypes A and type B.

NURSING CONSIDERATIONS

Assessment: Assess for age of patient, hypersensitivity to eggs, neomycin, polymyxin, any previous reactions to influenza vaccine, immunization history, immunosuppression, pregnancy/nursing status, and possible drug interactions.

Monitoring: Monitor for hypersensitivity reactions, injection-site any previous reactions to influenza vaccine. Assess for, immunization history, fever, headache, myalgia, irritability, insomnia, neurological complications (GBS), anaphylactic shock, and other adverse events that may occur.

AGGRASTAT

Patient Counseling: Inform about risk and benefits of immunization. Inform that cannot cause influenza but produce antibodies that protect against influenza. Inform that effect is achieved approximately 3 weeks after vaccination; advise annual revaccination. Instruct to in inform physician if any severe or unusual adverse reactions occur.

Administration: IM route. Inspect visually for particulate matter and discoloration; do not use if present. Do not use if frozen or suspected of being frozen. 1) Administer in deltoid muscle of upper arm for adults, toddlers, and young children and in the anterolateral aspect of the thigh in infants. 2) When using preservative-free, single-dose syringe, shake syringe and administer immediately. 3) When using multi-dose vial, shake vial before withdrawing each dose and administer immediately. **Storage:** 2-8°C (36-46°F). Do not freeze. Protect from light. Once stopper has been pierced, discard vial within 28 days.

AGGRASTAT   RX
tirofiban HCl (Medicure)

THERAPEUTIC CLASS: Glycoprotein IIb/IIIa inhibitor

INDICATIONS: In combination with heparin, for treatment of acute coronary syndrome, in patients being medically managed or undergoing percutaneous transluminal coronary angioplasty (PTCA) or atherectomy.

DOSAGE: *Adults:* Initial: 0.4mcg/kg/min IV for 30 min. Maint: 0.1mcg/kg/min IV. Continue through angiography and for 12-24 hrs after angioplasty or atherectomy. CrCl <30mL/min: Administer at half of usual rate of infusion.

HOW SUPPLIED: Inj: 0.05mg/mL

CONTRAINDICATIONS: Active internal bleeding, acute pericarditis, severe HTN, concomitant parenteral GP IIb/IIIa inhibitor, hemorrhagic stroke, aortic dissection, thrombocytopenia with prior exposure. Bleeding diathesis, stroke, major surgical procedure, or severe physical trauma within past 30 days. History of intracranial hemorrhage or neoplasm, arteriovenous malformation, aneurysm.

WARNINGS/PRECAUTIONS: Bleeding reported. Monitor platelets, Hgb, Hct before treatment, within 6 hrs after loading infusion, and daily during therapy. Monitor platelets earlier if previous GP IIb/IIIa inhibitor use. Determine activated partial thromboplastin time (APTT) before and during therapy with heparin. Caution with platelets <150,000/mm³, hemorrhagic retinopathy, chronic hemodialysis patients, femoral access site in percutaneous coronary intervention. When obtaining intravenous access, non-compressible sites (eg, subclavian or jugular veins) should be avoided. Minimize vascular and other trauma. D/C if thrombocytopenia confirmed or if bleeding cannot be controlled by pressure.

ADVERSE REACTIONS: Bleeding, nausea, fever, headache, edema, anaphylaxis.

INTERACTIONS: See contraindications. Increased bleeding with heparin and ASA. Caution with other drugs that affect hemostasis (eg, warfarin). Increased clearance with levothyroxine, omeprazole.

PREGNANCY: Category B, not for use in nursing.

MECHANISM OF ACTION: Glycoprotein IIB/IIIa inhibitor; reversible antagonist of fibrinogen binding to the GP IIb/IIIa receptor, the major platelet surface receptor involved in platelet aggregation. Inhibits platelet aggregation.

PHARMACOKINETICS: Distribution: V_d=22-42L; plasma protein binding (not highly bound). **Metabolism:** Limited. **Elimination**: Urine (65%), feces (25%); $T_{1/2}$=2 hrs.

NURSING CONSIDERATIONS

Assessment: Assess for presence or history (within previous 30 days) of internal bleeding; history of intracranial hemorrhage/neoplasm, arteriovenous malformation, or aneurysm; history of thrombocytopenia following previous exposure to the medication; history of any stroke; major recent surgical procedure or severe trauma; history, symptoms, or findings of aortic dissection;

severe HTN; concomitant use of another parenteral GP IIb/IIIa inhibitor; and acute pericarditis. Assess use in patients with platelet counts <150,000/mm³, presence of hemorrhagic retinopathy, and those on chronic hemodialysis. Assess for drug interactions. Obtain baseline platelet counts, Hgb, Hct, and APTT.

Monitoring: Monitor for signs/symptoms of bleeding, allergic reactions (eg, anaphylaxis), and thrombocytopenia. Monitor platelet counts, Hgb, and Hct within 6 hours of loading infusion, and at least daily thereafter. Monitor APTT for anticoagulant effects of heparin.

Patient Counseling: Counsel to notify physician if allergic reaction (eg, anaphylaxis) or bleeding occurs.

Administration: IV route. Dilute. 1) If using 500mL of 0.9% NS or D5W, withdraw and discard 100mL from bag and replace this volume with 100mL of drug injection from two 50mL vials. 2) If using 250mL of 0.9% NS or D5W, withdraw and discard 50mL from bag and replace this volume with 50mL of drug injection from one 50mL vial. Mix well prior to administration. Refer to PI for proper administration. Any unused solution should be discarded. Do not administer in same line as diazepam. **Storage:** 25°C (77°F) with excursions permitted between 15-30°C (59-86°F). Protect from light. Do not freeze.

AGGRENOX   RX

dipyridamole - aspirin (Boehringer Ingelheim)

THERAPEUTIC CLASS: Platelet aggregation inhibitor

INDICATIONS: Reduce risk of stroke in patients who have had transient ischemia of the brain or completed ischemic stroke due to thrombosis.

DOSAGE: *Adults:* Usual: 1 cap bid (am and pm). Intolerable Headaches: 1 cap qhs and low-dose ASA qam. Return to usual regimen as soon as possible (≤1 week). Swallow caps whole without chewing.

HOW SUPPLIED: Cap: (ASA-Dipyridamole Extended-Release) 25mg-200mg

CONTRAINDICATIONS: NSAID allergy, children or teenagers with viral infections, syndrome of asthma, rhinitis, nasal polyps.

WARNINGS/PRECAUTIONS: Risk of intracranial hemorrhage. Risk of GI side effects (eg, stomach pain, heartburn, N/V, gross GI bleeding, dyspepsia); monitor for signs of ulceration and bleeding. May increase bleeding time, elevations of hepatic enzymes, hepatic failure and exacerbation of hypotension. Caution with chronic heavy alcohol users (≥3 alcoholic drinks/day), inherited or acquired (liver disease or vitamin K deficiency) bleeding disorders, and hypotension. Avoid with history of peptic ulcer disease, severe hepatic insufficiency, and severe renal failure (GFR <10mL/min). Caution in coronary artery disease; may precipitate/aggravate chest pain. Aspirin in this product may not provide adequate treatment for cardiac indications for stroke/TIA patients for whom aspirin is indicated to prevent recurrent MI or angina pectoris. Not interchangeable with individual components of ASA and dipyridamole tabs. May cause fetal harm; avoid in 3rd trimester of pregnancy.

ADVERSE REACTIONS: Headache, dyspepsia, abdominal pain, N/V, diarrhea, fatigue, arthralgia, pain, hemorrhage, back pain.

INTERACTIONS: May decrease effects of ACE inhibitors, cholinesterase inhibitors, phenytoin, β-blockers. Potentiates adenosine, acetazolamide, methotrexate, oral hypoglycemics, valproic acid. Increased risk of bleeding with anticoagulants (heparin and warfarin) and chronic alcohol use (≥3 alcoholic drinks/day). Decreased effects of diuretics in renal or CV disease. NSAIDs may increase risk of bleeding or decrease renal function. May antagonize uricosuric agents (probenecid and sulfinpyrazone).

PREGNANCY: Category D, caution in nursing.

MECHANISM OF ACTION: Dipyridamole: Platelet aggregation inhibitor. Inhibits uptake of adenosine into platelets, endothelial cells, and erythrocytes. ASA: Platelet aggregation inhibitor. Irreversibly inhibits platelet cyclooxygenase and thus inhibits the generation of thromboxane A_2, a powerful inducer of platelet aggregation and vasoconstriction.

AGRIFLU

PHARMACOKINETICS: Absorption: Dipyridamole: C_{max}=1.98mcg/mL; T_{max}=2 hrs. ASA: C_{max}=319ng/mL; T_{max}=0.63 hrs. **Distribution:** Dipyridamole/ASA: Found in breast milk. Dipyridamole: V_d=92L; plasma protein binding (99%). ASA: V_d=10L; plasma protein binding (concentration-dependent); **Metabolism:** Dipyridamole: Liver (conjugation); into monoglucuronide (primary metabolite). ASA: Plasma (hydrolysis) into salicylic acid (metabolite) then liver (conjugation). **Elimination:** Dipyridamole: Feces (95%), Urine; $T_{1/2}$=13.6 hrs. ASA: Urine; $T_{1/2}$=0.33 hrs, $T_{1/2}$=1.71 hrs (salicylic acid).

NURSING CONSIDERATIONS

Assessment: Assess for hypersensitivity to NSAIDs, asthma, rhinitis, nasal polyps, renal/hepatic function, inherited or acquired bleeding disorders (eg, liver disease, vitamin K deficiency), alcohol use, history of active peptic ulcer disease, presence of severe coronary artery disease (eg, unstable angina or recently sustained MI), hypotension, pregnancy/nursing status, and for possible drug interactions.

Monitoring: Monitor for signs/symptoms of allergic reactions (eg, urticaria, angioedema, bronchospasm), GI effects (eg, stomach pain, heartburn, N/V), elevated hepatic enzymes, hepatic failure, and for bleeding (eg, GI, intracranial hemorrhage). Monitor platelet function (eg, bleeding time), BP, and hepatic enzymes.

Patient Counseling: Counsel patients who consume ≥3 alcoholic drinks daily about the risk for bleeding. Contact physician if any signs of abnormal bleeding or allergic reactions occur. Inform about signs and symptoms of GI side effects and what steps to take if they occur. Swallow medication whole, and not to chew or crush. If dose is missed, advise to take next dose on regular schedule and not take a double dose. Inform that transient headache may occur; notify physician if intolerable headache develops. Inform of risks to fetus if used during pregnancy; notify physician if pregnant or if become pregnant. Inform patients to protect drug from moisture.

Administration: Oral route. Swallow caps whole without chewing. **Storage:** 25°C (77°F); excursions permitted to 15-30°C (59-86°F). Protect from excessive moisture.

AGRIFLU   RX
influenza virus vaccine (Novartis)

THERAPEUTIC CLASS: Vaccine

INDICATIONS: Active immunization of persons ≥18 yrs for prevention of disease caused by influenza virus subtypes A and type B contained in the vaccine.

DOSAGE: *Adults:* 0.5mL IM as a single dose, preferably in the deltoid muscle of the upper arm.

HOW SUPPLIED: Inj: 0.5mL

CONTRAINDICATIONS: Hypersensitivity reactions to egg proteins (eggs or egg products), kanamycin, neomycin or life-threatening reaction to previous administration of any influenza vaccine.

WARNINGS/PRECAUTIONS: Do not inject in gluteal area or areas with major nerve trunk. Caution if Guillain-Barre syndrome has occured within 6 weeks of receipt of prior influenza vaccine. May not obtain expected immune response in immunocompromised persons. Have appropriate medical treatment available to manage possible anaphylactic reactions. May not protect all recipients.

ADVERSE REACTIONS: Local reaction (pain, induration, swelling, erythema), headache, myalgia, malaise, anaphylactic shock, fatigue, chills, arthralgia, sweating, fever, influenza-like illness.

INTERACTIONS: Immunosuppressive therapies (including corticosteroids) may reduce effectiveness.

PREGNANCY: Category B, caution in nursing.

MECHANISM OF ACTION: Vaccine; elicits the formation of antibodies that may protect against influenza virus subtypes A and B.

NURSING CONSIDERATIONS

Assessment: Assess immunity and current health status, hypersensitivity to egg proteins, immunization history, pregnancy/nursing status, and possible drug interactions. Assess potential benefits and risks if Guillain-Barre syndrome occurred with previous influenza vaccination.

Monitoring: Monitor hypersensitivity reactions, local injection-site reactions (eg, pain, induration, swelling, erythema), systemic adverse events (eg, headache, myalgia, malaise) and serious allergic reactions (eg, anaphylactic shock).

Patient Counseling: Inform of potential benefits and risks of immunization. Inform that vaccine contains noninfectious particles and cannot cause influenza. Advise that vaccine is intended to provide protection against illness due to influenza viruses only and cannot protect against other respiratory illnesses. Instruct to report any adverse reaction to healthcare provider. Inform that annual vaccination is recommended.

Administration: IM route. Inject into deltoid muscle of upper arm; should not be injected in gluteal region or areas where there may be a major nerve trunk. Allow to reach room temperature and shake before use. **Storage:** 2-8°C (35-46°F). Do not freeze. Protect from light.

ALACORT RX
hydrocortisone acetate (Crown Laboratories)

OTHER BRAND NAMES: U-cort (Taro)

THERAPEUTIC CLASS: Corticosteroid

INDICATIONS: Relief of the inflammatory and pruritic manifestations of corticosteroid-responsive dermatoses.

DOSAGE: *Adults:* Apply a thin film to affected area(s) bid-qid depending on the severity of the condition.
Pediatrics: Apply a thin film to affected area(s) bid-qid depending on the severity of the condition.

HOW SUPPLIED: Cre: (Alacort) 1% [28.4g, 85.2g]; (U-cort) 1% [28.35g, 85g, 123g]

WARNINGS/PRECAUTIONS: Reversible hypothalamic-pituitary-adrenal (HPA) axis suppression, Cushing's syndrome, hyperglycemia and glucosuria reported with systemic absorption. Application of more potent steroids, use over large areas and with occlusive dressings augment systemic absorption; monitor for HPA axis suppression, d/c, reduce frequency, or substitute less potent steroid if occurs. Signs and symptoms of steroid withdrawal may occur infrequently; may require supplemental systemic corticosteroids. D/C if irritation develops. Use appropriate antifungal or antibacterial agent with dermatological infections. Pediatric patients may be more susceptible to systemic toxicity; Cushing's syndrome, intracranial HTN (eg, bulging fontanelles, headaches, and bilateral papilledema), adrenal suppression, (eg, linear growth retardation, delayed weight gain, low plasma cortisol levels and absence of response to adrenocorticotrophic hormone (ACTH) stimulation). Chronic corticosteroid therapy may interfere with growth and development of children. (Alacort) Not for ophthalmic use. (U-cort) Contains sodium bisulfite; may cause allergic-type reactions in susceptible people; caution with asthmatics. Atrophy of skin and SQ tissues may occur with prolonged use and even with short-term use when used on intertriginous or flexor areas, or on the face.

ADVERSE REACTIONS: HPA suppression, Cushing's syndrome, burning/itching/irritation/dryness at application site, growth retardation, skin atrophy, allergic contact dermatitis, hypertrichosis, maceration of the skin, miliaria, striae, hypopigmentation, folliculitis.

PREGNANCY: Category C, caution in nursing

MECHANISM OF ACTION: Corticosteroid; possesses anti-inflammatory, antipruritic and vasoconstrictive properties. Mechanism of anti-inflammatory effects has not established.

PHARMACOKINETICS: Absorption: Extent of percutaneous absorption depends on skin integrity, vehicle and use of occlusive dressing. Inflammation and/or other disease processes in the skin increase absorption. **Metabolism:** Liver. **Elimination:** Urine, bile.

NURSING CONSIDERATIONS

Assessment: Assess for dermatological infections, hypersensitivity, surface area, pregnancy/nursing status and possible drug interactions.

Monitoring: Monitor for signs/symptoms of glucocorticoid insufficiency, hyperglycemia, glucosuria, skin irritation, and skin infections (eg, fungal, bacterial). Monitor for HPA-axis suppression by using periodic ACTH stimulation and urinary free cortisol tests in patients applying medication to large surface areas or using occlusive dressings. Monitor for signs/symptoms of systemic toxicity in pediatric patients.

Patient Counseling: Instruct patient to use medication as directed by the physician; to avoid contact with the eyes. Advise not to use medication for any disorder other than for which it was prescribed. Do not wrap, cover, or bandage treated skin unless directed by physician. Instruct patients to report adverse reactions. Advise not to use tight-fitting diapers or plastic pants on a child being treated in the diaper area.

Administration: Topical route. Occlusive dressings may be used for psoriasis or recalcitrant conditions; d/c if infection develops. **Storage:** (U-cort) 15-30°C (59-86°F). Protect from freezing. Dispense in tight container.

ALAMAST   RX
pemirolast potassium (Vistakon)

THERAPEUTIC CLASS: Mast cell stabilizer

INDICATIONS: Prevention of ocular itching due to allergic conjunctivitis.

DOSAGE: *Adults:* 1-2 drops in affected eye qid.
Pediatrics: ≥3 yrs: 1-2 drops in affected eye qid.

HOW SUPPLIED: Sol: 0.1% [10mL]

WARNINGS/PRECAUTIONS: May reinsert soft contact lens after 10 min if eyes are not red. Contains lauralkonium chloride; may be absorbed by soft contact lens.

ADVERSE REACTIONS: Headache, rhinitis, cold/flu symptoms, ocular burning/discomfort, dry eye, foreign body sensation.

PREGNANCY: Category C, caution in nursing.

MECHANISM OF ACTION: Mast cell stabilizer; inhibits type I immediate hypersensitivity reaction, antigen-induced release of inflammatory mediators (eg, histamine, leukotriene C_4, D_4, E_4) from human mast cell; also inhibits the chemotaxis of eosinophils into ocular tissue, blocks the release of mediators from human eosinophils, and prevents calcium influx into mast cells upon antigen stimulation (not established).

PHARMACOKINETICS: Absorption: C_{max}=4.7ng/mL, T_{max}=0.42 hrs. **Elimination:** Urine (10-15% unchanged); $T_{1/2}$=4.5 hrs.

NURSING CONSIDERATIONS

Assessment: Assess for known drug hypersensitivity.

Monitoring: Monitor for anaphylaxis and adverse reactions.

Patient Counseling: Counsel not to touch dropper tip to eyelid or surrounding areas and not to wear contact lenses if eye is red.

Administration: Intraocular route. **Storage:** 15-25°C (59-77°F).

ALBUTEROL   RX
albuterol sulfate (Various)

THERAPEUTIC CLASS: Beta$_2$-agonist

INDICATIONS: (Aerosol) Prevention and treatment of bronchospasm with reversible obstructive airway disease. Prevention of Exercise-Induced Bronchospasm (EIB). (Sol) Relief of bronchospasm with reversible obstructive airway disease and acute attacks of bronchospasm in patients ≥2 yrs. (Tab; Tab, Extended-Release) Relief of bronchospasm with reversible obstructive airway disease in patients ≥6 yrs. (Syrup) Relief of bronchospasm in patients ≥2 yrs with reversible obstructive airway disease.

DOSAGE: *Adults:* Bronchospasm: (Aerosol) 2 inh q4-6h or 1 inh q4h. (Repetabs) Initial: 4-8mg q12h. Max: 32mg/day. (Sol) 2.5mg tid-qid by nebulizer. (Syrup, Tabs) 2-4mg tid-qid. Max: 32mg/day (8mg qid). Elderly/β-Adrenergic Sensitivity: (Syrup, Tabs) Initial: 2mg tid-qid. Max: (Tabs) 8mg tid-qid. EIB: (Aerosol) 2 inh 15 min before activity.
Pediatrics: Bronchospasm: >14 yrs: (Syrup) Initial: 2-4mg tid-qid. Max: 8mg qid. ≥12 yrs: (Aerosol) 2 inh q4-6h or 1 inh q4h. (Tabs) Initial: 2-4mg tid-qid. Max: 8mg qid. >12 yrs: (Repetabs) Initial: 4-8mg q12h. Max: 32mg/day. 6-14 yrs: (Syrup) Initial: 2mg tid-qid. Max: 24mg/day. 6-12 yrs: (Repetabs) Initial: 4mg q12h. Max: 24mg/day. (Tabs) Initial: 2mg tid-qid. Max: 24mg/day. 2-12 yrs: ≥15 kg: (Sol) 2.5mg tid-qid by nebulizer. <15 kg: Use 0.5% sol if require <2.5mg/dose. 2-6 yrs: (Syrup) Initial: 0.1mg/kg tid (not to exceed 2mg tid). Titrate: May increase to 0.2mg/kg/day. Max: 4mg tid. EIB: ≥12 yrs: (Aerosol) 2 inh 15 min before activity.

HOW SUPPLIED: MDI: 0.09mg/inh [17g]; Sol (neb): 0.083% [3mL, 25^s], 0.5% [20mL]; Syrup: 2mg/5mL; Tab: 2mg*, 4mg*; Tab, Extended-Release (Repetabs): 4mg *scored

WARNINGS/PRECAUTIONS: Hypersensitivity reactions reported. Monitor for worsening asthma. Fatalities reported with excessive use. Caution with cardiovascular disorders, especially coronary insufficiency, arrhythmias and HTN. May need concomitant corticosteroids. Can produce paradoxical bronchospasm. Caution with DM, hyperthyroidism, seizures. May cause transient hypokalemia.

ADVERSE REACTIONS: Tachycardia, increased BP, tremor, nervousness, dizziness, N/V, palpitations, paradoxical bronchospasm, heartburn, rhinitis, respiratory tract infection.

INTERACTIONS: Avoid other sympathomimetic agents. Extreme caution with MAOIs and TCAs. Monitor digoxin. May worsen ECG changes and/or hypokalemia with non-K$^+$-sparing diuretics. Antagonized by β-blockers.

PREGNANCY: Category C, not for use in nursing.

MECHANISM OF ACTION: β$_2$-adrenergic agonist; stimulates intracellular adenyl cyclase, which catalyzes conversion of ATP to cAMP to produce relaxation of bronchial smooth muscle and inhibition of release of mediators of immediate hypersensitivity from cells (mast cells).

PHARMACOKINETICS: Absorption: (Aerosol) T$_{max}$=2-4 hrs. (Syrup, Tab) Rapid. C$_{max}$=18ng/mL; T$_{max}$=2 hrs. **Elimination:** (Aerosol) Urine (28%); T$_{1/2}$=3.8 hrs. (Syrup, Tab) T$_{1/2}$=5 hrs.

NURSING CONSIDERATIONS

Assessment: Assess for CVD (coronary insufficiency, cardiac arrhythmias, HTN), convulsive disorder, hyperthyroidism, DM, and possible drug interactions.

Monitoring: Monitor for signs/symptoms of CV effects (increased BP, palpitations), worsening of symptoms, destabilization of asthma, paradoxical bronchospasm, and hypersensitivity reactions (anaphylactic, urticaria, angioedema, rash, bronchospasm).

Patient Counseling: Seek medical attention if worsening of symptoms, therapy becomes less effective, need more inhalation from short-acting β$_2$-agonist than usual, paradoxical bronchospams, and hypersensitivity (anaphylactic, urticaria, angioedema, rash, bronchospasm) occur.

Administration: Oral inhalation, oral route. (Aerosol) 1) Shake well. 2) Breathe out fully through mouth. 3) While breathing in deeply and slowly through mouth, depress the top of metal canister. 4) Hold breath as long as possible. 5) Cleanse inhaler thoroughly and frequently. 6) Recommend "test spray" into air before using for first time. **Storage:** (Inhalation) 2-25°C (36-77°F). Protect from light. Store in pouch until time of use. (Aerosol) 15-30°C (59-86°F). Shake well before using. (Tab) 20-25°C (36-77°F). Protect from light. Dispense in tight, light-resistant container. (Syrup) 15-30°C (59-86°F). Dispense in tight, light-resistant container.

ALCORTIN
iodoquinol - hydrocortisone (Primus)
RX

THERAPEUTIC CLASS: Corticosteroid/Anti-infective

INDICATIONS: "Possibly" Effective: Contact or atopic dermatitis, impetiginized eczema, nummular eczema, endogenous chronic infectious dermatitis, stasis dermatitis, pyoderma, nuchal eczema and chronic eczematoid otitis externa, acne urticata, localized or disseminated neurodermatitis, lichen simplex chronicus, anogenital pruritus (vulvae, scroti, ani), folliculitis, bacterial dermatoses, mycotic dermatoses such as tinea (capitis, cruris, corporis, pedis), monliasis, intertrigo.

DOSAGE: *Adults:* Apply to affected area(s) tid-qid.
Pediatrics: ≥12 yrs: Apply to affected area(s) tid-qid.

HOW SUPPLIED: Gel: (Hydrocortisone-Iodoquinol) 2%-1% [2g]

WARNINGS/PRECAUTIONS: For external use only. Avoid eyes. D/C if irritation develops. May stain skin, hair, or fabrics. Risk of systemic absorption with treatment of extensive areas or use of occlusive dressings. Increased risk of systemic absorption in children. Iodoquinol may interfere with thyroid tests. False-positive phenylketonuria test reported. Prolonged use may result in overgrowth of nonsusceptible organisms.

ADVERSE REACTIONS: Burning, itching, irritation, dryness, folliculitis, hypertrichosis, acneiform eruptions, hypopigmentation, perioral dermatitis, allergic dermatitis, skin maceration, secondary infection, skin atrophy, striae, miliaria.

PREGNANCY: Category C, caution in nursing.

MECHANISM OF ACTION: Corticosteroid/Anti-infective. Hydrocortisone: Corticosteroid; possesses anti-inflammatory, antipruritic, and vasoconstrictive properties. Anti-inflammatory effect unclear; however, there is a recognizable correlation between vasoconstrictor potency and therapeutic efficacy. Iodoquinol: Anti-infective; possesses both antifungal and antibacterial properties.

PHARMACOKINETICS: Absorption: Hydrocortisone: Absorbed from normal intact skin. Inflammation of skin increases absorption. **Metabolism:** Hydrocortisone: Liver and most body tissues. Tetrahydrocortisone and tetrahydrocortisol (metabolites). **Elimination:** Hydrocortisone: Urine (unchanged and glucuronides). Iodoquinol: Urine (3-5% glucuronide).

NURSING CONSIDERATIONS

Assessment: Assess for known hypersensitivity to aloe vera, glycine, histidine, lysine, or palmitic acid. Assess use in pregnant/nursing females.

Monitoring: Monitor for development of systemic toxicity in children if large areas of body are treated or if occlusive dressings used (eg, diapers, plastic pants) on treated areas. With prolonged therapy, monitor for occurrence of overgrowth of non-susceptible bacteria. Monitor for lab test interactions (eg, thyroid function tests, ferric chloride tests for phenylketonuria [PKU]). If necessary, perform thyroid function tests 1 month after therapy end.

Patient Counseling: Instruct parents of pediatric patients not to use tight-fitting diapers or plastic pants on child being treated in diaper area. Counsel to keep medication away from eyes. If contact occurs and irritation develops, counsel to d/c medication and apply appropriate therapy. Inform that medication may cause staining of skin, hair, or fabrics and burning, itching, irritation, or dryness.

Administration: Topical route; external use only. **Storage:** Store at room temperature, 15-30°C (59-86°F). Keep out of reach of children. Keep tightly closed.

ALDACTAZIDE RX
hydrochlorothiazide - spironolactone (Pharmacia & Upjohn)

> Tumorigenic in chronic toxicity animal studies; avoid unnecessary use. Not for initial therapy.

THERAPEUTIC CLASS: K+-sparing diuretic/thiazide diuretic

INDICATIONS: Management of edematous conditions (congestive heart failure (CHF), hepatic cirrhosis with edema/ascites, nephrotic syndrome) and hypertension.

DOSAGE: *Adults:* Edema: 100mg/day per component qd or in divided doses. Maint: 25-200mg/day per component. HTN: 50-100mg/day per component qd or in divided doses.

HOW SUPPLIED: Tab: (Spironolactone-HCTZ) 25mg-25mg, 50mg-50mg* *scored

CONTRAINDICATIONS: Acute renal impairment, significantly impaired renal excretory function, hyperkalemia, acute or severe hepatic dysfunction, anuria, sulfonamide hypersensitivity.

WARNINGS/PRECAUTIONS: Monitor for fluid/electrolyte imbalance. Caution with renal and hepatic dysfunction. Hyperchloremic metabolic acidosis reported with decompensated hepatic cirrhosis. Mild acidosis, gynecomastia, transient BUN elevation, hypercalcemia, hyperglycemia, hyperuricemia, hypomagnesemia, and sensitivity reactions may occur. D/C if hyperkalemia occurs. Risk of dilutional hyponatremia. Enhanced effects in post-sympathetectomy patient. May increase cholesterol and TG levels. May manifest latent DM.

ADVERSE REACTIONS: Gastric bleeding, ulceration, gynecomastia, impotence, agranulocytosis, fever, urticaria, confusion, ataxia, renal dysfunction, blood dyscrasias, electrolyte disturbances, weakness, irregular menses, amenorrhea.

INTERACTIONS: Risk of hyperkalemia with K+-sparing diuretics, K+ supplements, NSAIDs, ACE inhibitors. Alcohol, barbiturates, or narcotics potentiate orthostatic hypotension. Corticosteroids, adrenocorticotrophic hormone (ACTH) may intensify electrolyte depletion. Reduced vascular response to norepinephrine. Increased response to nondepolarizing skeletal muscle relaxants. Risk of digoxin, lithium toxicity. NSAIDs may reduce effects. Antidiabetic agents may need adjustment.

PREGNANCY: Category C, not for use in nursing.

MECHANISM OF ACTION: Spironolactone: Aldosterone antagonist; competitively binds to receptors at aldosterone-dependent sodium-potassium exchange site. HCTZ: Thiazide diuretic; promotes excretion of sodium and water by inhibiting reabsorption.

PHARMACOKINETICS: Absorption: Spironolactone: C_{max}=80ng/mL; T_{max}=2.6 hrs. HCTZ: Rapid; T_{max}=1-2 hrs. **Distribution:** Spironolactone: Plasma protein binding (90%). **Elimination:** Spironolactone: Urine (major), bile (minor). HCTZ: Urine.

NURSING CONSIDERATIONS

Assessment: Assess for renal/hepatic function, hyperkalemia, pregnancy status, possible drug interactions, SLE, DM, sulfonamide hypersensitivity, history of allergy or bronchial asthma.

Monitoring: Monitor serum electrolytes, serum K+, and renal function periodically. Monitor for signs/symptoms of electrolyte imbalance, hyperkalemia, gynecomastia, hyperglycemia, exacerbation or activation of SLE, hyperuricemia or precipitation of gout, hypersensitivity reactions, hepatic/renal impairment.

Patient Counseling: Instruct to avoid K⁺ supplements and foods containing high levels of K⁺. Inform of pregnancy risks. Advise to seek medical attention if symptoms of electrolyte imbalance (dry mouth, thirst, weakness), hyperkalemia (paresthesia, fatigue, muscle weakness), or hypersensitivity reactions occur.

Administration: Oral route. **Storage:** Below 25°C (77°F).

ALDACTONE   RX

spironolactone (G.D. Searle)

> Tumorigenic in chronic toxicity animal studies; avoid unnecessary use.

THERAPEUTIC CLASS: Aldosterone blocker

INDICATIONS: Management of primary hyperaldosteronism (diagnosis, short-term preoperative and long-term maintenance treatment), edematous conditions (CHF, hepatic cirrhosis with edema/ascites, nephrotic syndrome, pathological causes of edema in pregnancy), essential hypertension. Treatment and prophylaxis of hypokalemia. In addition to standard therapy in severe heart failure (NYHA Class III-IV).

DOSAGE: *Adults:* Primary Hyperaldosteronism: (Diagnostic) 400mg/day for 3-4 weeks or 400mg/day for 4 days. (Preoperative) 100-400mg/day. (Unsuitable for Surgery) Maint: Lowest effective dose. Edema: Initial: 100mg/day given qd or in divided doses for at least 5 days. Maint: 25-200mg/day given qd-bid. HTN: Initial: 50-100mg/day given qd or in divided doses. Titrate: Adjust at 2-week intervals. Diuretic-Induced Hypokalemia: 25-100mg/day. Severe Heart Failure (SrK⁺ ≤5.0mEq/L, SrCr ≤2.5mg/dL): Initial: 25mg qd. May increase to 50mg qd if tolerated or reduce to 25mg every other day if not tolerated.

HOW SUPPLIED: Tab: 25mg, 50mg*, 100mg* *scored

CONTRAINDICATIONS: Anuria, acute renal insufficiency, significantly impaired renal excretory function, hyperkalemia.

WARNINGS/PRECAUTIONS: Monitor for fluid/electrolyte imbalance. Caution with renal and hepatic dysfunction. Hyperchloremic metabolic acidosis reported with decompensated hepatic cirrhosis. Mild acidosis, gynecomastia, transient BUN elevation may occur. D/C and monitor ECG and K⁺ levels if hyperkalemia occurs. May cause/aggravate dilutional hyponatremia.

ADVERSE REACTIONS: Gastric bleeding, ulceration, gynecomastia, agranulocytosis, fever, urticaria, confusion, ataxia, renal dysfunction, irregular menses, postmenopausal bleeding.

INTERACTIONS: Risk of hyperkalemia with K⁺-sparing diuretics, K⁺ supplements, NSAIDs (eg, indomethacin), ACE inhibitors. Alcohol, barbiturates, or narcotics potentiate orthostatic hypotension. Corticosteroids, ACTH may intensify electrolyte depletion, particularly hypokalemia. Reduced vascular response to norepinephrine; caution in patients subjected to regional or general anesthesia. Increased response to nondepolarizing skeletal muscle relaxants (eg, tubocurarine). Risk of digoxin, lithium toxicity. NSAIDs may reduce effects.

PREGNANCY: Category C, not for use in nursing.

MECHANISM OF ACTION: Aldosterone antagonist; competitively binds to receptors at aldosterone-dependent Na⁺-K⁺ exchange site in distal convoluted renal tubule, causing increased Na⁺ and water excretion and K⁺ retention.

PHARMACOKINETICS: Absorption: C_{max}=80ng/mL; T_{max}=2.6 hrs. **Distribution:** Plasma protein binding (>90%). **Elimination:** Urine (major), bile (minor).

NURSING CONSIDERATIONS

Assessment: Assess for renal/hepatic function, hyperkalemia, pregnancy/nursing status and possible drug interactions.

Monitoring: Monitor serum K⁺, electrolytes, ECG and renal function (eg, BUN, creatinine) periodically. Monitor for signs/symptoms of fluid/electrolyte imbalance, dilutional hyponatremia, hyperkalemia, acidosis, gynecomastia, hypersensitivity reactions, renal/hepatic dysfunction.

Patient Counseling: Instruct to avoid K⁺ supplements and foods containing high levels of K⁺, including salt substitutes. Advise to seek medical attention if symptoms of electrolyte imbalance (dry mouth, thirst, weakness), hyperkalemia (paresthesia, fatigue, muscle weakness) or hypersensitivity reactions occur.

Administration: Oral route. **Storage:** <25°C (77°F).

ALDARA
imiquimod (Graceway)

RX

THERAPEUTIC CLASS: Immune response modifier

INDICATIONS: Topical treatment of nonhyperkeratotic, nonhypertrophic actinic keratoses on face or scalp and biopsy-confirmed, primary superficial basal cell carcinoma (sBCC), with a maximum tumor diameter of 2cm, located on trunk (excluding anogenital skin), neck, or extremities (excluding hands and feet), only when surgical methods are medically less appropriate and follow-up can be assured in immunocompetent adults. Treatment of external genital and perianal warts/condyloma acuminata in patients ≥12 yrs.

DOSAGE: *Adults:* Apply before hs and rub in until no longer visible. Actinic Keratosis: Usual: Apply 2x/week for a full 16 weeks to defined area on face or scalp (but not both concurrently). Wash off after 8 hrs with soap and water. Max: 36 pkts for 16 weeks. External Genital and Perianal Warts/Condyloma: Usual: Apply 3x/week. Use until warts are totally cleared. Wash off after 6-10 hrs with soap and water. May suspend use for several days to manage local reactions. Max: 16 weeks. Do not occlude treatment area. Superficial Basal Cell Carcinoma (sBCC): Apply 5x/week for a full 6 weeks. If tumor diameter is 0.5 to <1cm, use 4mm (10mg) of cre. If tumor is ≥1 to <1.5cm, use 5mm (25mg) of cre. If tumor is ≥1.5 to 2cm, use 7mm (40mg) of cre. Max diameter of tumor: 2cm. Treatment area should include a 1cm margin of skin around the tumor. Wash off after 8 hrs with soap and water. Max: 36 pkts for 6 weeks.
Pediatrics: ≥12 yrs: External Genital and Perianal Warts/Condyloma: Usual: Apply 3x/week before hs. Rub in until no longer visible. Use until warts are totally cleared. Wash off after 6-10 hrs with soap and water. May suspend use for several days to manage local reactions. Max: 16 weeks. Do not occlude treatment area.

HOW SUPPLIED: Cre: 5% [250mg]

WARNINGS/PRECAUTIONS: Not for oral, ophthalmic, or intravaginal use. Not for urethral, intravaginal, cervical, rectal, or intra-anal human papilloma viral disease. Not for repeated use in treatment of actinic keratosis in same area; not for treatment of actinic keratosis on areas of skin >25cm². Not recommended from any previous drug or surgical treatment or with sunburn until fully recovered. Not recommended for treatment of basal cell carcinoma (BCC) subtypes, other than sBCC. Avoid or minimize exposure to sunlight. Avoid contact with eyes, lips, nostrils. Caution with inherent sensitivity to sunlight and patients who may have considerable sun exposure. May exacerbate inflammatory skin conditions. Interruption of dosing should be considered, if systemic reactions (eg, flu-like signs/symptoms) or local inflammatory reactions occur. Not effective in pediatrics 2-12 yrs with molluscum contagiosum.

ADVERSE REACTIONS: Application-site reactions, upper respiratory tract infection, sinusitis, headache, squamous cell carcinoma, diarrhea, back pain, rhinitis, lymphadenopathy, influenza-like symptoms.

PREGNANCY: Category C, caution in nursing.

MECHANISM OF ACTION: Immune response modifier; mechanism has not been established. In basal cell carcinoma, suspected to increase infiltration of lymphocytes, dendritic cells, and macrophages into the tumor lesion. In external genital warts, suspected to induce mRNA encoding cytokines, including interferon-α at the treatment site.

PHARMACOKINETICS: Absorption: C_{max}=0.1ng/mL (12.5mg face), 0.2ng/mL (25mg scalp), 3.5ng/mL (75mg hands/arms), 0.4ng/mL (4.6mg average dose). **Elimination:** Urine (0.11% in males, 2.41% in females with 4.6mg average dose), (0.08% in males, 0.15% in females with 75mg dose).

NURSING CONSIDERATIONS

Assessment: Assess for age, pre-existing autoimmune conditions, immuno-suppression, human papilloma viral disease, basal cell nevus syndrome or xeroderma pigmentosum. For treatment of superficial basal cell carcinoma, assess proper diagnosis (eg, biopsy). Assess use in patients with inherent sensitivity to sunlight, current sunburn, and in pregnancy/nursing.

Monitoring: Monitor for signs/symptoms of local inflammatory reactions (eg, weeping or erosion) and for systemic reactions (eg, flu-like symptoms: malaise, fever, nausea, myalgias, rigors). Monitor for clinical signs of improvement.

Patient Counseling: Inform to wash hands before and after applying cream. Before applying, wash treatment area with mild soap and water and allow area to dry thoroughly. Avoid contact with eyes, lips, and nostrils and exposure to sunlight (including sunlamps) and to use protective clothing (eg, hat) or sunscreen when using medication. May experience local skin reactions and flu-like systemic signs and symptoms during therapy. Advise patients with sunburns not to use the cream until fully recovered. Advise female patients to take special care when applying the cream at the vaginal opening because of local skin reactions on the delicate moist surfaces, which may result in pain or swelling and may cause difficulty in passing urine. When using for the treatment of actinic keratosis or superficial basal cell carcinoma, wash the treatment area with mild soap and water 8 hrs following application of the cream. When using for the treatment of external genital warts, wash treatment area with mild soap and water 6-10 hrs following application of cream. Inform that new warts may develop during therapy. May weaken condoms and vaginal diaphragms; concurrent use not recommended.

Administration: Topical route. **Storage:** 4-25°C (39-77°F). Do not freeze.

ALFENTANIL
alfentanil HCl (Various)   CII

OTHER BRAND NAMES: Alfenta (Akorn)

THERAPEUTIC CLASS: Opioid analgesic

INDICATIONS: As an analgesic adjunct given in incremental doses in the maintenance of anesthesia with barbiturate/nitrous oxide/oxygen. As an analgesic administered by continuous infusion with nitrous oxide/oxygen in the maintenance of general anesthesia. As a primary anesthetic agent for the induction of anesthesia in patients undergoing general surgery in which endo-tracheal intubation and mechanical ventilation are required. As the analgesic component for monitored anesthesia care (MAC).

DOSAGE: *Adults:* Individualize dose. Spontaneous Breathing/Assisted Ventilation: Induction: 8-20mcg/kg. Maint: 3-5mcg/kg q 5-20 min or 0.5-1mcg/kg/min. Total: 8-40mcg/kg. Assisted or Controlled Ventilation: Incremental Injection: Induction: 20-50mcg/kg. Maint: 5-15mcg/kg q5-20 min. Total: Up to 75mcg/kg. Continuous Infusion: Induction: 50-75mcg/kg. Maint: 0.5-3mcg/kg/min (average rate 1-1.5mcg/kg/min). Total: Dependent on duration of procedure. Anesthetic Induction: Induction: 130-245 mcg/kg. Maint: 0.5-1.5mcg/kg/min or general anesthetic. Total: dependent on duration of procedure. Monitored Anesthesia Care (MAC): Induction: 3-8mcg/kg. Maint: 3-5 mcg/kg q 5-20 min or 0.25-1mcg/kg/min. Total: 3-40mcg/kg.

HOW SUPPLIED: Inj: 500mcg/mL

WARNINGS/PRECAUTIONS: May cause delayed respiratory depression, respiratory arrest, bradycardia, asystole, arrhythmias, and hypotension; an opioid antagonist, resuscitative and intubation equipment and oxygen should be readily available. Use in caution with patients with head injury, increased intracranial pressure, pulmonary disease, and liver or kidney dysfunction.

Initial dose of alfentanil should be appropriately reduced in elderly and debilitated patients.

ADVERSE REACTIONS: Respiratory depression, skeletal muscle rigidity, N/V, HTN, hypotension, bradycardia, tachycardia, dizziness, skeletal muscle movements, apnea, chest wall rigidity.

INTERACTIONS: Coadministration with CNS depressants such as barbituates, tranquilizers, opioids, or inhalation general anesthetics may enhance CNS effects and postoperative respiratory depression. Erythromycin may significantly inhibit alfentanil clearance and increase the risk of prolonged or delayed respiratory depression. Cimetidine reduces clearance of alfentanil and may extend duration of action.

PREGNANCY: Category C, caution in nursing

MECHANISM OF ACTION: Opioid analgesic; attenuates the catecholamine response with more rapid recovery and reduced need for postoperative analgesics.

PHARMACOKINETICS: Distribution: V_d=0.4-1L/kg, plasma protein binding (approximately 92%). **Metabolism:** Liver **Elimination:** Urine (1% unchanged, drug); $T_{1/2}$=90-111 min.

NURSING CONSIDERATIONS

Assessment: Assess for pulmonary disease, decreased respiratory reserve, hepatic/renal function, bradycardia, arrhythmias, head injury, and possible drug interactions

Monitoring: Monitor for cardiovascular depression (bradycardia and hypotension), respiratory depression, muscle rigidity of neck and extremities, N/V, chills, arrhythmias, chest wall rigidity. Monitor vital signs routinely. Appropriate postoperative monitoring should ensure that adequate spontaneous breathing is established and maintained prior to discharging.

Patient Counseling: Counsel about side effects and abuse potential.

Administration: IV route. **Storage:** 15-25°C (59-77°F). Protect from light.

ALIMTA   RX
pemetrexed disodium (Lilly)

THERAPEUTIC CLASS: Antifolate

INDICATIONS: In combination with cisplatin for the initial treatment of locally advanced or metastatic nonsquamous non-small cell lung cancer (NSCLC). Maintenance treatment in patients with locally advanced or metastatic nonsquamous NSCLC whose disease has not progressed after 4 cycles of platinum-based first-line chemotherapy. Single agent for the treatment of patients with locally advanced or metastatic nonsquamous NSCLC after prior chemotherapy. In combination with cisplatin for the treatment of patients with malignant pleural mesothelioma whose disease is unresectable or who are otherwise not candidates for curative surgery.

DOSAGE: *Adults:* Premedication: Dexamethasone (or equivalent) 4mg PO bid day before, day of, and day after administration. Give at least five daily doses of folic acid (350-1000mcg) PO during the 7 days prior to first dose. Continue throughout therapy and for 21 days after last dose. Give vitamin B_{12} 1000mcg IM once during week preceding first dose and every three cycles thereafter. Combination with Cisplatin: Nonsquamous NSCLC/ Mesothelioma: 500mg/m² IV infused over 10 min on Day 1 of each 21-day cycle. Give cisplatin 75mg/m² infused over 2 hrs beginning 30 min after the end of administration. Patient should receive appropriate hydration prior to and/or after receiving cisplatin. Single Agent: Nonsquamous NSCLC: 500mg/m² IV infused over 10 min on Day 1 of each 21-day cycle. Refer to PI for dose adjustments for hematologic, nonhematologic, and neurotoxicities.

HOW SUPPLIED: Inj: 100mg, 500mg

WARNINGS/PRECAUTIONS: Premedicate with folic acid and vitamin B_{12} to reduce hematologic and GI toxicity and with dexamethasone or its equivalent to reduce the incidence and severity of cutaneous reactions. Bone marrow suppression may occur; myelosuppression is usually the dose-limiting toxicity. Caution with renal/hepatic dysfunction and the elderly. Avoid in patients with CrCl <45mL/min. D/C if hematologic or ≥Grade 3 nonhematologic toxicities experienced after two dose reductions or with ≥Grade 3 neurotoxicity. Do not start new cycle unless CrCl ≥45mL/min, absolute neutrophil count (ANC) ≥1500 cells/mm³, platelet count ≥100,000 cells/mm³. May cause fetal harm; use effective contraception to prevent pregnancy. In patients with clinically significant third space fluid, consider draining the effusion prior to therapy.

ADVERSE REACTIONS: Anemia, anorexia, fatigue, leukopenia, N/V, stomatitis, neutropenia, rash/desquamation, thrombocytopenia, constipation, pharyngitis, diarrhea.

INTERACTIONS: Delayed clearance with nephrotoxic or tubularly secreted drugs (eg, probenecid). Reduced clearance with ibuprofen; caution with concomitant use of ibuprofen in patients with mild-moderate renal insufficiency (CrCl from 45-79mL/min). In mild-moderate renal insufficiency, avoid NSAIDs with short elimination half-lives for a period of 2 days before, the day of, and 2 days following therapy. Interrupt dosing of NSAIDs with longer half-lives for at least 5 days before, the day of, and 2 days following therapy.

PREGNANCY: Category D, not for use in nursing.

MECHANISM OF ACTION: Antifolate; disrupts folate-dependent metabolic processes essential for cell replication. Inhibits thymidylate synthase, dihydrofolate reductase and glycinamide ribonucleotide formyltransferase.

PHARMACOKINETICS: Distribution: V_d=16.1L. Plasma protein binding (81%). **Elimination:** Urine (70-90% unchanged); $T_{1/2}$=3.5 hrs (normal renal function).

NURSING CONSIDERATIONS

Assessment: Assess for renal/hepatic functon, pregnancy/nursing status, history of hypersensitivity reaction to the drug, significant third space fluid (eg, ascites, pleural effusion) and possible drug interactions. Obtain baseline vital signs, ANC, CBC with platelets, renal function (CrCl), LFTs.

Monitoring: Monitor for signs and symptoms of hematologic/nonhematologic toxicities, bone marrow suppression (eg, neutropenia, thrombocytopenia, anemia), GI toxicity (eg, diarrhea, mucositis), neurotoxicity, cutaneous reactions (eg, rash), hypersensitivity reactions, and other adverse events that may occur. Monitor vital signs, CBC with platelets, renal function (CrCl), LFTs.

Patient Counseling: Inform about benefits and risks of therapy. Instruct to take folic acid and vitamin B_{12} as prophylactic measures to reduce treatment-related hematological and GI toxicities. Inform about risks of low blood counts. Instruct to contact physician if any sign of infection (eg, fever), bleeding, anemia, vomiting, diarrhea, dehydration, and if other adverse events occur. Inform physician if taking any concomitant prescription or over-the-counter (OTC) medications (eg, NSAID). Inform that drug may cause fetal harm; advise women of childbearing potential to avoid becoming pregnant and to use effective contraceptive measures to prevent pregnancy during treatment.

Administration: IV route. Refer to PI for further details on preparation and administration. Reconstitution and further dilution is only recommended with 0.9% NaCl injection (preservative free). Physically incompatible with calcium-containing diluents (eg, Lactated Ringer's). **Storage:** 25°C (77°F); excursions permitted to 15-30°C (59-86°F). Reconstituted and infusion solution can be used up to 24 hrs following initial reconstitution, when refrigerated, 2-8°C (36-46°F) or at 25°C (77°F); excursions permitted to 15-30°C (59-86°F). Discard unused portion.

ALINIA   RX
nitazoxanide (Romark)

THERAPEUTIC CLASS: Antiprotozoal agent

INDICATIONS: Treatment of diarrhea caused by *Cryptosporidium parvum* and *Giardia lamblia* in patients ≥1 yr (Sus) and ≥12 yrs (Tab).

DOSAGE: *Adults:* Give for 3 days. (Sus) 25mL q12h; (Tab) 1 tab q12h. Take with food.
Pediatrics: Give for 3 days. 1-3 yrs: 5mL (100mg) q12h. 4-11 yrs: 10mL (200mg) q12h. ≥12 yrs: (Sus) 25mL q12h. (Tab) 1 tab q12h. Take with food.

HOW SUPPLIED: Sus: 100mg/5mL [60mL]; Tab: 500mg.

WARNINGS/PRECAUTIONS: Caution with hepatic and biliary disease, renal disease, and combined renal and hepatic disease. Oral suspension contains 1.48g sucrose/5mL.

ADVERSE REACTIONS: Abdominal pain, diarrhea, headache, nausea (tab), vomiting (sus).

INTERACTIONS: Caution with other highly plasma protein-bound drugs with narrow therapeutic indices, as competition for binding sites may occur (eg, warfarin).

PREGNANCY: Category B; caution in nursing.

MECHANISM OF ACTION: Antiprotozoal agent; interferes with the pyruvate: ferredoxin oxidoreductase (PFOR) enzyme-dependent electron transfer reaction, which is essential to anaerobic energy metabolism.

PHARMACOKINETICS: Absorption: (Tab) (500mg) Tizoxanide: 12-17 yrs: C_{max}=9.1mcg/mL, T_{max}=2 hrs, AUC=39.5mcg•hr/mL; ≥18 yrs: C_{max}=10.6mcg/mL, T_{max}=3 hrs, AUC=41.9mcg•hr/mL. (Sus) Bioavailability (70%); Tizoxanide: 1-3 yrs: (100mg) C_{max}=3.11mcg/mL, T_{max}=3.5 hrs, AUC=11.7mcg•hr/mL; 4-11 yrs: (200mg) C_{max}=3mcg/mL, T_{max}=2 hrs, AUC=13.5mcg•hr/mL; ≥18 yrs: (500mg) C_{max}=5.49mcg/mL, T_{max}=2.5 hrs, AUC= 30.2mcg•hr/mL. ≥18 yrs: (500mg) C_{max}=3.21mcg/mL, T_{max}=4 hrs, AUC= 22.8mcg•hr/mL. **Distribution:** Tizoxanide: Plasma protein binding (>99%). **Metabolism:** Tizoxanide, tizoxanide glucuronide (active metabolites). Conjugation, primarily by glucuronidation. **Elimination:** Nitazoxanide: urine (1/3 of dose), bile and feces (2/3 of the dose). Tizoxanide glucuronide: urine, bile. Tizoxanide: urine, bile, feces. Refer to PI for parameters for active metabolite.

NURSING CONSIDERATIONS

Assessment: Assess for hepatic, renal/biliary impairment, HIV infection, DM, pregnancy/nursing status, and possible drug interactions.

Monitoring: Monitor for abdominal pain, diarrhea, N/V, headache, LFTs, and CBC.

Patient Counseling: Counsel to take exactly as directed. Shake sus well prior to administration. Instruct to report any adverse effects. Inform patient that it should be taken with food. Advise diabetic patients oral sus contains 1.48g of sucrose/5mL.

Administration: Oral route. Take with food. Reconstitute sus with 48mL of water and keep tightly closed. Shake well before administration. **Storage:** 25°C (77°F); excursions permitted to 15-30°C (59-86°F). Reconstituted sus may be stored for 7 days, after which unused portion should be discarded.

ALLEGRA   RX
fexofenadine HCl (Sanofi-Aventis)

THERAPEUTIC CLASS: H_1-antagonist

INDICATIONS: Relief of symptoms associated with seasonal allergic rhinitis in adults and children ≥2 years of age. Treatment of uncomplicated skin manifestations of chronic idiopathic urticaria in adults and children ≥6 months of age.

DOSAGE: *Adults:* Tab: Rhinitis/Urticaria: 60mg bid or 180mg qd. Renal Dysfunction: Initial: 60mg qd.
Pediatrics: Tab: ≥12 yrs: Rhinitis/Urticaria: 60mg bid or 180mg qd. Renal Dysfunction: Initial: 60mg qd. 6-11 yrs: Rhinitis/Urticaria: 30mg bid. Renal Dysfunction: Initial: 30mg qd. ODT: Rhinitis/Urticaria: 6-11 yrs: 30mg bid. Renal Dysfunction: 30mg qd. Sus: Rhinitis: 2-11 yrs: 30mg (5mL) bid. Renal Dysfunction: 30mg (5mL) qd. Urticaria: 2-11 yrs: 30mg (5mL) bid. Renal

Dysfunction: 30mg (5mL) qd. 6 months to <2 yrs: 15mg (2.5mL) bid. Renal
Dysfunction: 15mg (2.5mL) qd.

HOW SUPPLIED: Tab: 30mg, 60mg, 180mg; Tab, Disintegrating: 30mg; Sus:
30mg/5mL

WARNINGS/PRECAUTIONS: Oral disintegrating tablet contains phenylalanine, a component of aspartame. Hypersensitivity reactions reported. Caution
in elderly.

ADVERSE REACTIONS: Vomiting, headache, cough, diarrhea.

INTERACTIONS: Increased plasma levels with erythromycin or ketoconazole.
Avoid concomitant aluminum- and magnesium-containing antacids. Fruit
juices (eg, grapefruit, orange, and apple) may decrease levels.

PREGNANCY: Category C, caution in nursing.

MECHANISM OF ACTION: Antihistamine with selective peripheral H_1-receptor
antagonist activity; prevents antigen-induced bronchospasm and histamine
release from peritoneal mast cells.

PHARMACOKINETICS: Absorption: Rapid; (Cap, 120mg) T_{max} =2.6 hrs;
(Cap, 60mg) C_{max} =131ng/mL; (Tab, 60mg) C_{max} =142ng/mL; (Tab, 180mg)
C_{max} =494ng/mL; (Sus, 30mg) C_{max} =118.0ng/mL, T_{max} =1.0 hrs. **Distribution:**
Plasma protein binding (60%). **Metabolism:** Liver (5%). **Elimination:** Urine
(80%), feces (11%); $T_{1/2}$ =14.4 hrs.

NURSING CONSIDERATIONS

Assessment: Assess for hepatic/renal impairment, pregnancy/nursing status,
and possible drug interactions.

Monitoring: Monitor for side effects and treatment efficacy.

Patient Counseling: Advise to take as prescribed and not to exceed recommended dose. D/C and consult physician if adverse effects occur. Advise not
to take with fruit juices.

Administration: Oral route. Take with water. Oral disintegrating tablet can
be taken with or without water and on an empty stomach. Shake suspension
bottle before use. **Storage:** 20-25°C (68-77°F).

ALLEGRA-D   RX
fexofenadine HCl - pseudoephedrine HCl (Sanofi-Aventis)

THERAPEUTIC CLASS: H_1-antagonist/sympathomimetic amine

INDICATIONS: Relief of symptoms of seasonal allergic rhinitis in adults and
children ≥12 yrs.

DOSAGE: *Adults:* 60mg-120mg tab bid or 180mg-240mg tab qd without food.
Renal Dysfunction: Initial: 60mg-120mg tab qd; avoid 180mg-240mg tab.
Swallow whole; do not crush or chew. Take with water.
Pediatrics: ≥12 yrs: 60mg-120mg tab bid or 180mg-240mg tab qd without
food. Renal Dysfunction: Initial: 60mg-120mg tab qd; avoid 180mg-240mg
tab. Swallow whole; do not crush or chew. Take with water.

HOW SUPPLIED: Tab, Extended-Release: (Fexofenadine-Pseudoephedrine)
(12-Hour) 60mg-120mg, (24-Hour) 180mg-240mg

CONTRAINDICATIONS: Narrow-angle glaucoma, urinary retention, severe
HTN, severe coronary artery disease (CAD), MAOI therapy or within 14 days
of d/c.

WARNINGS/PRECAUTIONS: Caution with HTN, diabetes mellitus (DM),
ischemic heart disease, increased intraocular pressure (IOP), hyperthyroidism,
renal impairment, or prostatic hypertrophy. May produce CNS stimulation with
convulsions or cardiovascular collapse with accompanying hypotension. Avoid
use or lower initial dose with decreased renal function/insufficiency. Caution
in elderly.

ADVERSE REACTIONS: Headache, upper respiratory infection (URI), back
pain, insomnia, nausea, dry mouth, arrhythmia, angioedema, cardiovascular
collapse, convulsions, chest tightness, dyspnea, hypotension, dizziness.

INTERACTIONS: See Contraindications. Increased plasma levels with erythromycin or ketoconazole. Increased ectopic pacemaker activity with digitalis. Caution with other sympathomimetic amines, combined effects on cardiovascular system may be harmful. Reduced effects of antihypertensive drugs which interfere with sympathetic activity (eg, methyldopa, mecamylamine, reserpine). Decrease plasma concentrations with aluminum- and magnesium-containing antacid (Maalox).

PREGNANCY: Category C, caution in nursing.

MECHANISM OF ACTION: Fexofenadine: Selective peripheral H_1-receptor antagonist; inhibits antigen-induced bronchospasm and histamine release from peritoneal mast cells. Pseudoephedrine: Orally active sympathomimetic amine; exerts a decongestant action on the nasal mucosa.

PHARMACOKINETICS: Absorption: Fexofenadine: Rapidly absorbed; (12 Hour) C_{max}=191ng/mL (single dose), 255ng/mL (multiple doses); T_{max}=2 hrs. (24 Hour) C_{max}=634ng/mL (single dose), 674ng/mL (multiple doses); T_{max}=1.8 hrs. Pseudoephedrine: (12 Hour) C_{max}=206ng/mL (single dose), 411ng/mL (multiple doses); T_{max}=6 hrs (single dose), 5 hrs (multiple dose). (24 Hour) C_{max}=394ng/mL (single dose), 495ng/mL (multiple doses); T_{max}=12 hrs. **Distribution:** Fexofenadine: Plasma protein binding (60-70%). Pseudoephedrine: V_d=2.6-3.5L/kg. Found in breast milk. **Metabolism:** Hepatic (5% of fexofenadine; <1% of pseudoephedrine). **Elimination:** Fexofenadine: Feces (80%), urine (11%); $T_{1/2}$=14.4 hrs (12 Hour), 14.6 hrs (24 Hour). Pseudoephedrine: Urine (43-96%, unchanged); $T_{1/2}$=4-6 hrs, 7 hrs (24 Hour).

NURSING CONSIDERATIONS

Assessment: Assess for hepatic/renal function, severity of symptoms, history of HTN, DM, and any other conditions where treatment is cautioned or contraindicated.

Monitoring: Monitor for signs/symptoms of hypotension, renal function, dizziness, nervousness, or sleepiness, and other adverse reactions.

Patient Counseling: Instruct to take on empty stomach with water. Swallow tab whole; do not break or chew. Instruct to take as prescribed; do not exceed recommended dose. Counsel to d/c and contact physician if nervousness, dizziness, or sleeplessness occurs. Avoid concurrent use with OTC antihistamines and decongestants. Instruct patient that inactive ingredient resembling original tablet may be eliminated in the feces occasionally. Counsel of pregnancy/nursing risks. Instruct not to use in patient with narrow-angle glaucoma, urinary retention, HTN, CAD, or by patients receiving MAO inhibitors.

Administration: Oral route. Swallow whole; do not crush or chew. Take on an empty stomach with water. **Storage:** 20-25°C (68-77°F). Store in tightly-closed container in a cool, dry place, away from children.

ALOPRIM   RX
allopurinol sodium (Bioniche)

THERAPEUTIC CLASS: Xanthine oxidase inhibitor

INDICATIONS: Management of elevated serum and urinary uric acid levels in patients with leukemia, lymphoma, and solid tumor malignancies receiving cancer therapy when oral therapy is not tolerated.

DOSAGE: *Adults:* Usual: 200-400mg/m²/day IV infusion qd or in equally divided infusions every 6, 8, or 12 hrs. Max: 600mg/day. CrCl 10-20mL/min: 200mg/day. CrCl 3-10mL/min: 100mg/day. CrCl <3mL/min: 100mg/day at extended intervals. Elderly: Start at lower end of dosing range.
Pediatrics: Usual: 200mg/m²/day IV qd or in divided doses every 6, 8, or 12 hrs.

HOW SUPPLIED: Inj: 500mg

WARNINGS/PRECAUTIONS: D/C at first appearance of hypersensitivity (eg, skin rash or other signs which indicate an allergic reaction); increased risk in patients with decreased renal function. Caution with renal/hepatic impairment or concurrent illnesses affecting renal function such as HTN and diabetes mellitus (DM). Hepatotoxicity may occur; monitor LFTs during early stages of therapy if with pre-existing liver disease. Monitor renal function and uric acid levels; adjust dose if needed. Maintain sufficient fluid intake to yield a daily urinary output ≥2L and maintain neutral/slightly alkaline urine. May impair mental/physical abilities. Drowsiness and bone marrow suppression reported. Caution in elderly.

ADVERSE REACTIONS: Skin rash, eosinophilia, local injection-site reaction, N/V, diarrhea, renal failure/insufficiency.

INTERACTIONS: Inhibits oxidation of mercaptopurine and azathioprine; reduce mercaptopurine and azathioprine dose to 1/3-1/4 of usual dose. Increased frequency of skin rash with ampicillin and amoxicillin. Increased toxicity and risk of hypersensitivity in patients with renal dysfunction with concomitant thiazide diuretics; monitor renal function. Increased risk of hypoglycemia in the presence of renal insufficiency with concomitant chlorpropamide. Enhanced bone marrow suppression when used with cyclophosphamide and other cytotoxic agents among patients with neoplastic disease, except leukemia. May increase cyclosporine levels; monitor cyclosporine levels and dose ajust as required. Decreased inhibition of xanthine oxidase by oxypurinol and increased urinary excretion of uric acid with uricosuric agents. Prolongs half-life of dicumarol; monitor PT with concomitant use.

PREGNANCY: Category C, caution in nursing.

MECHANISM OF ACTION: Xanthine oxidase inhibitor; reduces production of uric acid by inhibiting the biochemical reactions immediately preceding its formation.

PHARMACOKINETICS: Absorption: Absolute bioavailability (100%); C_{max}=1.58µg/mL (100mg), 5.12µg/mL (300mg); T_{max}=0.5 hrs; AUC=1.99 hr•µg/mL (100mg), 7.1 hr•µg/mL (300mg). **Distribution:** V_d=0.84L/kg (100mg), 0.87L/kg (300mg); found in breast milk. **Metabolism:** Oxidative; oxypurinol (active metabolite). **Elimination:** Urine (12% unchanged, 76% as oxypurinol); $T_{1/2}$=(100mg) 1 hr (parent), 24.1 hrs (oxypurinol), (300mg) 1.21 hrs (parent), 23.5 hrs (oxypurinol).

NURSING CONSIDERATIONS

Assessment: Assess for renal/hepatic function, concurrent illnesses affecting renal function (eg, HTN, DM), hypersensitivity reactions (eg, skin rash, Stevens-Johnson syndrome [SJS]), pregnancy/nursing status and possible drug interactions. Obtain serum uric acid to provide correct dosage and schedule.

Monitoring: Monitor for allergic reactions, severe hypersensitivity reactions (eg, exfoliative, urticarial, purpuric lesions, SJS), generalized vasculitis, hepatotoxicity, drowsiness, bone marrow suppression and fluid intake. Monitor LFTs, serum uric acid, BUN and SrCr.

Patient Counseling: Inform about benefits/risks of therapy. Inform may impair mental/physical abilities. Advise to take sufficient fluid to yield a daily urinary output of at least 2L in adults and the need to maintain a neutral or preferably slightly alkaline urine. Advise to report any adverse events to physician.

Administration: IV infusion. Refer to PI for reconstitution and dilution. Rate of infusion depends on the volume of infusate. Whenever possible, initiate therapy 24-48 hrs before the start of chemotherapy known to cause tumor cell lysis (including adrenocorticosteroids). Do not mix or administer through the same IV port with agents which are incompatible in solution (refer to PI). Begin administration within 10 hrs after reconstitution. **Storage:** 25°C (77°F); excursions permitted to 15-30°C (59-86°F). After dilution, store solution at 20-25°C (68-77°F). Do not refrigerate the reconstituted and/or diluted product.

ALOXI   RX
palonosetron HCl (Eisai)

THERAPEUTIC CLASS: 5-HT$_3$ receptor antagonist

INDICATIONS: Prevention of acute and delayed N/V associated with initial and repeat courses of moderately emetogenic cancer chemotherapy and prevention of acute N/V associated with initial and repeat courses of highly emetogenic cancer chemotherapy. Prevention of postoperative nausea and vomiting (PONV) for up to 24 hrs following surgery.

DOSAGE: *Adults:* Prevention of Chemotherapy-Induced N/V: 0.25mg IV single dose over 30 sec. Dosing should occur approximately 30 min before the start of chemotherapy. PONV: 0.075mg IV single dose over 10 sec immediately before induction of anesthesia.

HOW SUPPLIED: Inj: 0.25mg/5mL, 0.075mg/1.5mL

WARNINGS/PRECAUTIONS: Hypersensitivity reactions may occur in patients who have exhibited hypersensitivity to other 5-HT$_3$ receptor antagonists. Routine prophylaxis is not recommended in patients in whom there is little expectation that N/V will occur postoperatively. In patients where N/V must be avoided during the postoperative period, prophylaxis is recommended even when the incidence of PONV is low.

ADVERSE REACTIONS: Headache, constipation, QT prolongation, bradycardia.

PREGNANCY: Category B, not for use in nursing.

MECHANISM OF ACTION: 5-HT$_3$ receptor antagonist; antiemetic and antinauseant.

PHARMACOKINETICS: Absorption: (IV, 3mcg/kg) C_{max}=5.6ng/mL, AUC=35.8ng•hr/mL. **Distribution:** V_d=8.3L/kg; plasma protein binding (62%). **Metabolism:** 50% metabolized via CYP2D6, CYP3A4, CYP1A2; N-oxide-palonosetron and 6-S-hydroxy-palonosetron (primary metabolites). **Elimination:** Urine (80% of dose, 40% palonosetron); $T_{1/2}$=40 hrs.

NURSING CONSIDERATIONS

Assessment: Assess for previous hypersensitivity to other 5-HT$_3$ receptor antagonists and for pregnancy/nursing status. Obtain baseline vital signs and ECG.

Monitoring: Monitor for hypersensitivity reactions and other adverse events that may occur. Monitor vital signs and ECG for QT interval prolongation.

Patient Counseling: Instruct to read patient insert. Advise to report to physician of all medical conditions and infusion-site reactions (eg, pain, redness, swelling).

Administration: IV route. Flush infusion line with normal saline before and after administration. Do not mix with other drugs. Inspect visually for particulate matter and discoloration before administration. **Storage:** 20-25°C (68-77°F); excursions permitted to 15-30°C (59-86°F). Protect from light and freezing.

ALPHAGAN P   RX
brimonidine tartrate (Allergan)

THERAPEUTIC CLASS: Selective alpha$_2$ agonist

INDICATIONS: Lowering of intraocular pressure (IOP) in patients with open-angle glaucoma or ocular hypertension.

DOSAGE: *Adults:* 1 drop in the affected eye(s) tid (approx. 8 hrs apart). Space dosing of other topical ophthalmics that lower IOP at least 5 min apart. *Pediatrics:* ≥2 yrs: 1 drop in the affected eye(s) tid (approx. 8 hrs apart). Space dosing of other topical ophthalmics that lower IOP at least 5 min apart.

HOW SUPPLIED: Sol: 0.1%, 0.15% [5mL, 10mL, 15mL]

CONTRAINDICATIONS: Concomitant MAOI therapy.

WARNINGS/PRECAUTIONS: Caution with severe cardiovascular disease (CVD), hepatic or renal dysfunction, depression, cerebral or coronary insufficiency, Raynaud's phenomenon, orthostatic hypotension, thromboangiitis obliterans.

ADVERSE REACTIONS: Allergic conjunctivitis, conjunctival hyperemia, eye pruritus, burning sensation, conjunctival folliculosis, HTN, oral dryness, ocular allergic reaction, visual disturbance, somnolence, decreased alertness.

INTERACTIONS: See Contraindications. May potentiate effect with CNS depressants (alcohol, barbiturates, opiates, sedatives, anesthetics). Caution with antihypertensives, cardiac glycosides, and TCAs.

PREGNANCY: Category B, not for use in nursing.

MECHANISM OF ACTION: Selective α_2 agonist; reduces aqueous humor production and increases uveoscleral outflow.

PHARMACOKINETICS: Absorption: T_{max}=0.5-2.5 hrs. **Metabolism:** Liver (extensive). **Elimination:** Urine (74%); $T_{1/2}$=2 hrs.

NURSING CONSIDERATIONS

Assessment: Assess for hypersensitivity, history of CVD, depression, orthostatic hypotension. Assess renal/hepatic function prior to therapy, possible drug interactions, and pregnancy/nursing status.

Monitoring: Perform routine monitoring of IOP while on therapy. Monitor pulse rate and BP while on medication.

Patient Counseling: Advise that drug may cause fatigue and/or drowsiness. Use caution during hazardous activities that require mental alertness. Advise that if more than one topical ophthalmic product is being used, the administration of the products should be at least 5 min apart.

Administration: Ocular route. **Storage:** 15-25°C (59-77°F).

ALREX   RX
loteprednol etabonate (Bausch & Lomb)

THERAPEUTIC CLASS: Corticosteroid

INDICATIONS: Relief of signs and symptoms of seasonal allergic conjunctivitis.

DOSAGE: *Adults:* 1 drop qid.

HOW SUPPLIED: Sus: 0.2% [5mL, 10mL]

CONTRAINDICATIONS: Viral diseases of the cornea and conjunctiva, including epithelial herpes simplex keratitis, vaccinia, and varicella. Mycobacterial infection and fungal diseases of the eye.

WARNINGS/PRECAUTIONS: Caution with glaucoma, herpes simplex, diseases causing thinning of cornea/sclera and other ocular viral infections. Prolonged use can cause glaucoma or secondary ocular infections (eg, fungal). Monitor IOP beyond 10 days of therapy. Wait 10 min after instillation before inserting soft contact lenses. Re-evaluate if no response after 2 days.

ADVERSE REACTIONS: Elevated IOP, foreign body sensation, itching, chemosis, epiphora, blurred vision, burning on instillation, discharge, dry eyes, photophobia.

PREGNANCY: Category C, caution in nursing.

MECHANISM OF ACTION: Corticosteroid; anti-inflammatory agent, not established. Inhibits edema, fibrin deposition, capillary dilation, leukocyte migration, fibroblast proliferation, deposition of collagen, and scar formation associated with inflammation by induction of phospholipase A_2 inhibitory protein lipocortin.

PHARMACOKINETICS: Absorption: C_{max}<1ng/mL.

NURSING CONSIDERATIONS

Assessment: Assess for viral diseases of the cornea and conjunctiva (eg, epithelial herpes simplex, keratitis (dendritic keratitis), vaccinia and varicella, mycobacterial infection of the eye and fungal diseases of ocular structure, known hypersensitivity to drug components, glaucoma, and possible drug interactions.

Monitoring: Monitor for secondary ocular infections, fungal infections, masking or enhancement of existing infections, thinning of the cornea or sclera, perforation, damage to optic nerve, defects in visual acuity, and posterior subcapsular cataract formation.

Patient Counseling: Avoid touching dropper tip to eyes, fingers, or any surface. Notify physician if symptoms persist or worsen. Do not wear contact lenses if eyes are red or irritated.

Administration: Intraocular route. **Storage:** 15-25°C (59-77°F). Do not freeze.

ALSUMA   RX
sumatriptan (King)

THERAPEUTIC CLASS: 5-HT$_{1B/1D}$ agonist

INDICATIONS: Acute treatment of migraine attacks, with or without aura. Acute treatment of cluster headache episodes.

DOSAGE: *Adults:* ≥18 yrs: Usual: 6mg SQ. Max: Two 6-mg doses/24 hrs. Separate doses by at least 1 hr.

HOW SUPPLIED: Inj: 6mg/0.5mL

CONTRAINDICATIONS: IV administration. Ischemic heart disease (eg, angina pectoris, MI, or silent ischemia), or symptoms/findings consistent with ischemic heart disease, coronary vasospasm (eg, Prinzmetal's variant angina), or other significant underlying cardiovascular (CV) disease, cerebrovascular syndromes (eg, stroke, transient ischemic attack [TIA]), peripheral vascular disease (eg, ischemic bowel disease), uncontrolled HTN, or hemiplegic or basilar migraine, administration of any ergotamine-containing or ergot-type agents (eg, dihydroergotamine or methysergide) or other 5-HT$_1$ agonists (eg, triptan) within 24 hrs.

WARNINGS/PRECAUTIONS: Serious adverse cardiac events (eg, acute myocardial infarction [MI], life-threatening arrhythmias), cerebrovascular events, vasospastic reactions and hypersensitivity (anaphylaxis/anaphylactoid) reactions reported. Evaluate for coronary artery disease (CAD) and its risk factors; administer 1st dose under medical supervision and consider an ECG following administration. Sensations of tightness, pain, pressure and heaviness in the chest, throat, neck, and jaw may occur and should be evaluated for CAD or predisposition to Prinzmetal's variant angina before receiving additional doses; monitor ECG if symptoms persist. Seizures reported; caution with history of epilepsy or lowered seizure threshold. Serotonin syndrome may occur; symptoms may include mental status changes, autonomic instability, neuromuscular aberrations, and GI symptoms. Caution with controlled HTN. BP elevation, including hypertensive crisis reported rarely. Corneal opacities may occur. Signs or symptoms suggestive of decreased arterial flow should be evaluated for atherosclerosis or predisposition to vasospasm.

ADVERSE REACTIONS: Injection-site reactions, tingling, warm/hot sensation, burning sensation, feeling of heaviness, pressure sensation, feeling of tightness, flushing, numbness, tightness in chest, chest discomfort, dizziness/vertigo, drowsiness/sedation, N/V, weakness, neck pain/stiffness.

INTERACTIONS: See Contraindications. Use with an MAO-A inhibitor increases levels and is not recommended; if clinically warranted, suitable dose adjustment is advised. Serotonin syndrome reported with combined use of an SSRI or SNRI.

PREGNANCY: Category C, caution in nursing.

MECHANISM OF ACTION: Selective 5-HT$_{1B/1D}$ agonist; binds to vascular 5-HT$_1$-type receptors in cranial arteries, basilar artery, and vasculature of isolated dura mater, which causes vasoconstriction.

PHARMACOKINETICS: Absorption: Bioavailability (97%); (Deltoid) C$_{max}$=74ng/mL; T$_{max}$=12 min. (Thigh) Manual: C$_{max}$=61ng/mL. Auto-Injector: C$_{max}$=52ng/mL. **Distribution:** V$_d$=50L; plasma protein binding (14%-21%). **Metabolism:** Indole acetic acid (38%, metabolite). **Elimination:** Urine, (22%, unchanged); T$_{1/2}$=115 min.

NURSING CONSIDERATIONS

Assessment: Assess for presence/history of ischemic heart disease, CAD and its risk factors (eg, hypercholesterolemia, smoking, obesity, diabetes mellitus), cerebrovascular/peripheral vascular disease, uncontrolled HTN, hemiplegic/basilar migraine, history of epilepsy, pregnancy/nursing status, and possible drug interactions. Establish proper diagnosis of migraine or cluster headache; exclude other potentially serious neurological conditions. Obtain baseline vital signs, weight, CV function, ECG, LFTs.

Monitoring: Monitor for cardiac ischemia; give 1st dose in physician's office or medical facility and obtain ECG after administration for those with CAD risk factors. Monitor for signs/symptoms of cardiac events (eg, MI, cardiac arrhythmias, peripheral vascular ischemia, hypertensive crisis, chest tightness), colonic ischemia, bloody diarrhea, serotonin syndrome (eg, mental status changes, autonomic instability, neuromuscular aberrations, and/or GI symptoms), hypersensitivity reactions, chest/throat/jaw/neck tightness, seizures, headache, increased BP, ophthalmic changes (eg, corneal opacities). For long-term therapy or with CAD risk factors, perform periodic monitoring of CV function. Monitor vital signs and weight, LFTs.

Patient Counseling: Inform about risks and benefits of therapy, proper use, importance of follow-up, and possible drug interactions. Inform to notify physician if any symptoms such as chest pain, SOB, weakness, or slurring of speech occur, or if pregnant or nursing. Advise on the proper administration techniques and appropriate sites of injection (eg, lateral thigh or upper arms).

Administration: SQ route. **Storage:** 25°C (77°F); excursions permitted 15-30°C (59-86°F). Protect from light. Do not refrigerate.

ALTABAX   RX
retapamulin (GlaxoSmithKline)

THERAPEUTIC CLASS: Pleuromutilin antibacterial

INDICATIONS: Topical treatment of impetigo due to *Staphylococcus aureus* (methicillin-susceptible isolates only) or *Streptococcus pyogenes,* in patients ≥9 months.

DOSAGE: *Adults*: Apply thin layer to the affected area (up to 100 cm² in total area) bid for 5 days. May cover with sterile bandage or gauze.
Pediatrics: ≥9 mos: Apply thin layer to the affected area (up to 2% total BSA) bid for 5 days. May cover with sterile bandage or gauze.

HOW SUPPLIED: Oint: 1% [5g, 10g, 15g, 30g]

WARNINGS/PRECAUTIONS: D/C if sensitization or severe local irritation occurs; use appropriate alternative therapy. Not intended for oral, intranasal, ophthalmic or intravaginal use. Not evaluated for use on mucosal surfaces. May cause superinfection during therapy.

ADVERSE REACTIONS: Application-site reactions, headache, diarrhea, nausea, nasopharyngitis, pruritus, fever, eczema.

INTERACTIONS: Coadministration with ketoconazole may increase levels.

PREGNANCY: Category B, caution in nursing.

MECHANISM OF ACTION: Pleuromutilin antibacterial; selectively inhibits bacterial protein synthesis by interacting at a site on the 50S subunit of the bacterial ribosome. The binding site involves ribosomal protein L3 and is in the region of the ribosomal P site and peptidyl transferase center. By binding to this site, peptidyl transfer is inhibited, P-site interactions are blocked, and the formation of normal active 50S ribosomal subunits is prevented.

PHARMACOKINETICS: Absorption: Low systemic exposure. Following application to 800cm² of intact skin: C_{max}=3.5ng/mL (multiple doses). Following application to 200cm² of abraded skin: C_{max}=11.7ng/mL (single dose), 9.0ng/mL (multiple doses). **Distribution:** Plasma protein binding (94%). **Metabolism:** Liver (extensive) via CYP3A4 (mono-oxygenation, N-demethylation).

NURSING CONSIDERATIONS

Assessment: Assess for proper diagnosis of bacterial organisms, pregnancy/nursing status, and possible drug interactions with other topical agents.

Monitoring: Monitor for signs/symptoms of sensitization reactions or severe local irritation, and for the development of overgrowth of nonsusceptible organisms (superinfection).

Patient Counseling: Counsel that drug is for external use only; avoid contact with eyes, mouth or lips, inside the nose, or inside the female genital area. Inform that the treated area may be covered by sterile bandage or gauze dressing after applying ointment. Instruct to wash hands following application (if hands are not the treatment area). Instruct to take the medication for the full recommended time and to notify physician if symptoms do not improve within 3-4 days after starting treatment. Notify physician if irritation, redness, itching, burning, blistering, oozing at treatment site develop.

Administration: Topical route. Do not use in eyes, mouth, lips, or inside the nose. **Storage:** Store at 25°C (77°F); excursions permitted to 15-30°C (59-86°F).

ALTACE CAPSULES   RX
ramipril (King)

> ACE inhibitors can cause death/injury to developing fetus during 2nd and 3rd trimesters. D/C if pregnancy is detected.

OTHER BRAND NAMES: Altace Tablets (King)

THERAPEUTIC CLASS: ACE inhibitor

INDICATIONS: To reduce risk of myocardial infarction (MI), stroke, and death from cardiovascular (CV) causes in patients ≥55 yrs who are at high risk due to history of coronary artery disease, stroke, peripheral vascular disease, or diabetes with at least one other CV risk factor. Treatment of HTN, alone or with thiazide diuretics. To reduce risk of CV death, heart failure related hospitalization, and progression to severe/resistant heart failure in stable post-MI patients who show signs of congestive heart failure (CHF).

DOSAGE: *Adults:* Risk Reduction of MI, Stroke, CV Death: Initial: 2.5mg qd for 1 week. Titrate: Increase to 5mg qd for next 3 weeks, and then increase as tolerated. Maint: 10mg qd. Give as divided dose if hypertensive or recently post MI. HTN: Initial: 2.5mg qd. Adjust dosage according to BP. Maint: 2.5-20mg/day given qd or in 2 equally divided doses. Add diuretic if BP not controlled. CrCl <40mL/min: Initial: 1.25mg qd. May be titrated upward until BP is controlled. Max: 5mg/day. CHF Post-MI: Initial: 2.5mg bid, or switch to 1.25mg bid if hypotensive. Titrate: May increase up to 5mg bid at 3 week intervals after 1 week of initial dose. CrCl <40mL/min: Initial: 1.25mg qd. Titrate: May increase to 1.25mg bid up to 2.5mg bid depending on response and tolerability. Max: 2.5mg bid. With Volume Depletion/Renal Artery Stenosis: Initial: 1.25mg qd. Adjust according to BP response.

HOW SUPPLIED: Cap: 1.25mg, 2.5mg, 5mg, 10mg; Tab: 1.25mg, 2.5mg, 5mg, 10mg

CONTRAINDICATIONS: History of ACE inhibitor-associated angioedema.

WARNINGS/PRECAUTIONS: May increase risk of angioedema in patients with history of angioedema unrelated to ACE inhibitor therapy. Angioedema of the face, extremities, lips, tongue, glottis, and larynx reported; d/c and administer appropriate therapy if this occurs. Intestinal angioedema reported; monitor for abdominal pain (with or without N/V). More reports of angioedema in blacks than nonblacks. Anaphylactoid reactions reported during desensitization with hymenoptera venom and with dialysis with high-flux membranes and LDL apheresis with dextran sulfate absorption. May cause symptomatic hypotension; caution with volume and/or salt depletion (eg, diuretic therapy, dietary salt restriction, dialysis, diarrhea, vomiting). Correct volume and/or salt depletion prior to therapy. Caution with CHF; excessive hypotension associated with oliguria, azotemia, acute renal failure (ARF) or death may occur. Monitor patients during first 2 weeks of therapy and whenever dose is increased. Caution with unilateral/bilateral renal artery stenosis; may increase SrCr and BUN. Rarely, a syndrome of cholestatic jaundice, fulminant hepatic necrosis and sometimes death occurs; d/c if jaundice or marked elevations of hepatic enzymes develops. Agranulocytosis, pancytopenia, bone marrow depression, reduction in RBC, Hgb content, WBC or platelet count may develop. Hematologic reactions are more likely to occur with collagen vascular disease (eg, systemic lupus erythematosus [SLE], scleroderma) and renal impairment; monitor WBC count. Risk of hyperkalemia with diabetes mellitus (DM) and renal dysfunction. Persistent nonproductive cough reported. Caution with severe liver cirrhosis and/or ascites.

ADVERSE REACTIONS: Hypotension, cough increased, dizziness, angina pectoris, headache.

INTERACTIONS: May increase lithium levels; monitor levels and symptoms of lithium toxicity. Hypotension risk with diuretics. Increased risk of hyperkalemia with K+-sparing diuretics, K+ supplements, or K+-containing salt substitutes; monitor serum K+ frequently. NSAIDs may worsen renal failure and increase serum K+ Nitritoid reactions (eg, facial flushing, N/V, hypotension) reported rarely with injectable gold (sodium aurothiomalate). Hypotension reported with anesthesia agents. Hypoglycemia reported with oral hypoglycemic agents or insulin. May attenuate K+ loss caused by thiazide diuretics. Avoid use with telmisartan. May increase BUN and SrCr levels in patients with no apparent pre-existing renal vascular disease when given concomitantly with a diuretic.

PREGNANCY: Category C (1st trimester) and D (2nd and 3rd trimesters), not for use in nursing.

MECHANISM OF ACTION: ACE inhibitor; inhibition of ACE results in decreased plasma angiotensin II, which leads to decreased vasopressor activity and to decreased aldosterone secretion.

PHARMACOKINETICS: Absorption: Absolute bioavailability (28%); T_{max}=1 hr. (ramiprilat) Absolute bioavailability (44%); T_{max}=2-4 hrs. **Distribution:** Plasma protein binding (73%), (56% ramiprilat); crosses the placenta; found in breast milk. **Metabolism:** Cleavage of ester group; ramiprilat (active metabolite). **Elimination:** Urine (60%; <2% unchanged); Feces (40%). (ramiprilat) $T_{1/2}$= >50 hrs (terminal $T_{1/2}$), 13-17 hrs (multiple-dose).

NURSING CONSIDERATIONS

Assessment: Assess for hypersensitivity, history of angioedema, volume/salt depletion (diuretic therapy, dietary salt restriction, dialysis, diarrhea, vomiting), DM, collagen vascular disease (SLE, scleroderma), CHF, unilateral/bilateral renal stenosis, liver cirrhosis, ascites, hepatic/renal impairment, pregnancy/nursing status, and possible drug interactions. Obtain baseline BP, BUN, SrCr, renal function and RBC, WBC and platelet count.

Monitoring: Monitor renal function periodically. Monitor patients during first 2 weeks of therapy and whenever dose is increased. Monitor for signs/symptoms of hypotension, anaphylactoid or hypersensitivity reactions, abdominal pain, infection, cholestatic jaundice, fulminant hepatic necrosis, neutropenia, agranulocytosis, and bone marrow depression. Monitor BP, WBC, RBC and platelet count, BUN, SrCr levels, K+ and LFT levels.

Patient Counseling: Inform of pregnancy risks and advise to report pregnancy to physician as soon as possible. Instruct that inadequate fluid intake or excessive perspiration, diarrhea, or vomiting may lead to drop in BP resulting in lightheadedness or syncope. Advise to seek medical attention if signs and symptoms of angioedema (swelling of face, eyes, lips, or tongue, or difficulty in breathing), infection (sore throat, fever), syncope, or hypersensitivity reactions occur. Advise not to use salt substitutes containing K+ and other drugs without consulting prescribing physician.

Administration: Oral route. Swallow whole. (Cap) May sprinkle contents on a small amount (about 4 oz.) of applesauce or mixed in 4 oz. of water or apple juice. Consume mixture in its entirety. **Storage:** (Cap) 15-30°C (59-86°F). May store pre-prepared mixture for up to 24 hrs at room temperature or up to 48 hrs under refrigeration. (Tab) 20-25°C (68-77°F); excursion permitted between 15-30°C (59-86°F).

ALTOPREV   RX
lovastatin (Sciele)

THERAPEUTIC CLASS: HMG-CoA reductase inhibitor

INDICATIONS: Adjunct to diet, to slow progression of coronary atherosclerosis in coronary heart disease. Adjunct to diet, for reduction of elevated total cholesterol (total-C), LDL-C, Apo B, and TG, and to increase HDL-C in patients with primary hypercholesterolemia (heterozygous familial and non-familial) and mixed dyslipidemia (Fredrickson types IIa and IIb). To reduce risk of MI, unstable angina, and coronary revascularization procedures in patients without symptomatic cardiovascular disease, average to moderately elevated Total-C and LDL-C, and below average HDL-C.

DOSAGE: *Adults:* Individualize dosing. Initial: 20, 40, or 60mg qhs. Range: 20-60mg/day. Consider immediate-release lovastatin in patients requiring smaller reductions. May adjust at intervals of ≥4 weeks. Elderly (>65 yrs)/ Renal Insufficiency/Diabetes Mellitus: Initial: 20mg qhs. Severe Renal Insufficiency (CrCl <30mL/min): Consider dose increase of >20mg/day carefully and implement cautiously. Concomitant Fibrates/Niacin (≥1g/day): Try to avoid. Max: 20mg/day. Concomitant Amiodarone/Verapamil: Max: 20mg/day. Swallow whole; do not chew, crush or cut.

HOW SUPPLIED: Tab: Extended-Release: 20mg, 40mg, 60mg

CONTRAINDICATIONS: Active liver disease, unexplained persistent elevations of serum transaminases, pregnancy, nursing mothers.

WARNINGS/PRECAUTIONS: Myopathy and rhabdomyolysis with or without acute renal failure secondary to myoglobinuria reported. May increase serum transaminases and CPK levels; consider in differential diagnosis of chest pain. D/C if AST or ALT ≥3X ULN persists, if myopathy diagnosed or suspected, and a few days before major surgery. Monitor LFTs prior to therapy, at 6 weeks and 12 weeks after initiation of therapy or elevation of dose, and then periodically thereafter. Caution with heavy alcohol use and/or history of hepatic disease. Caution with dose escalation in renal insufficiency. May cause endocrine dysfunction and CNS toxicity. Lovastatin immediate-release found to be less effective with homozygous familial hypercholesterolemia.

ADVERSE REACTIONS: Nausea, abdominal pain, insomnia, dyspepsia, headache, asthenia, myalgia, diarrhea, back pain, flu syndrome, infection, arthralgia, sinusitis.

INTERACTIONS: Due to increased risk of myopathy, suspend lovastatin if itraconazole, ketoconazole, erythromycin, or clarithromycin must be used. Avoid other CYP3A4 inhibitors unless benefits outweigh the risk (eg, HIV protease inhibitors, nefazodone, >1 quart/day grapefruit juice). Avoid use with cyclosporine. Avoid use with gemfibrozil, other fibrates, or lipid lowering doses of (>1g/day) of niacin; if necessary, lovastatin dose should not exceed 20mg/day. Avoid lovastatin doses >20mg/day if used with amiodarone or verapamil. Monitor PT in patients taking anticoagulants (eg, warfarin) before starting lovastatin and following initiation of therapy. Caution with drugs that may decrease the levels or activity of endogenous steroid hormones (eg, ketoconazole, spironolactone, cimetidine).

PREGNANCY: Category X, not for use in nursing.

MECHANISM OF ACTION: HMG-CoA reductase inhibitor; inhibits the conversion of HMG-CoA to mevalonate which is an early step in the biosynthetic pathway for cholesterol. Reduces LDL-C and total-C.

PHARMACOKINETICS: Absorption: Lovastatin: C_{max}=5.5ng/mL, T_{max}=14.2 hrs, AUC=77ng•hr/mL. Lovastatin acid: C_{max}=5.8ng/mL, T_{max}=11.8 hr, AUC=87ng•hr/mL. **Distribution:** Plasma protein binding (>95%). Crosses blood brain/placental barriers. **Metabolism:** Liver (extensive), β-hydroxy acid, 6'-hydroxy derivative, and two additional metabolites (major active metabolites). **Elimination:** Urine, bile.

NURSING CONSIDERATIONS

Assessment: Assess for active or history of iver disease or unexplained persistent elevations in serum transaminases, pregnancy/nursing status, renal insufficiency, homozygous familial hypercholesterolemia, alcohol use, and for possible drug interactions. Assess LFTs prior to therapy.

Monitoring: Monitor for signs/symptoms of myopathy/rhabdomyolysis (eg, pain, tenderness, or weakness), increases in serum transaminases, CNS toxicity, and endocrine dysfunction. Monitor creatine kinase levels. Monitor LFTs at 6 and 12 weeks after initiation of therapy or dose elevations, and periodically thereafter.

Patient Counseling: Inform about risks/benefits of therapy. Instruct to promptly report unexplained muscle pain, tenderness, or weakness. Advise to avoid grapefruit juice. Instruct to swallow tablet whole and to not chew, crush, or cut tablet. Counsel to inform physician of all medical conditions and medicines being taken.

Administration: Oral route. Take drug whole; do not crush, chew or cut.
Storage: 20-25°C (68-77°F); excursions permitted to 15-30°C (59-86°F). Avoid excessive heat and humidity.

Alvesco   RX
ciclesonide (Sunovion)

THERAPEUTIC CLASS: Non-halogenated glucocorticoid

INDICATIONS: Maintenance treatment of asthma as prophylactic therapy in adults and adolescents ≥12 yrs.

DOSAGE: *Adults:* Previous Bronchodilator Alone: Initial: 80mcg bid. Max: 160mcg bid. Previous Inhaled Corticosteroid: Initial: 80mcg bid. Max: 320mcg bid. Previous Oral Corticosteroid: Initial: 320mcg bid. Max: 320mcg bid. Elderly: Start at low end of dosing range. Titrate to the lowest effective dosage after asthma is stable. If inadequate response to initial dose after 4 weeks, may use higher doses.
Pediatrics: ≥12 yrs: Previous Bronchodilator Alone: Initial: 80mcg bid. Max: 160mcg bid. Previous Inhaled Corticosteroid: Initial: 80mcg bid. Max: 320mcg bid. Previous Oral Corticosteroid: Initial: 320mcg bid. Max: 320mcg bid. Titrate to the lowest effective dosage after asthma is stable. If inadequate response to initial dose after 4 weeks, may use higher doses.

HOW SUPPLIED: MDI: 80mcg/actuation, 160mcg/actuation [60 actuations]

CONTRAINDICATIONS: Primary treatment of status asthmaticus or other acute episodes of asthma where intensive measures are required.

WARNINGS/PRECAUTIONS: Localized *Candida albicans* infections of mouth and pharynx may occur; treat accordingly. Not indicated for rapid relief of bronchospasm. Increased susceptibility to infections (eg, chickenpox, measles); avoid exposure in patients who have not had the disease or been properly immunized. Caution with active or quiescent tuberculosis (TB) infections, untreated systemic bacterial, fungal, viral, parasitic infections, or ocular herpes simplex. Caution in patients transferred from systemic to inhaled corticosteroids; deaths due to adrenal insufficiency have occurred and may unmask allergic conditions. Hypercorticism and adrenal suppression may appear with more than recommended doses over prolonged periods of time. May decrease bone mineral density (BMD) with prolonged treatment; monitor those with major risk factors and treat accordingly. May reduce growth velocity in pediatrics. Glaucoma, increased intraocular pressure (IOP) and cataracts reported; monitor closely in patients with change in vision, history of IOP, glaucoma, and/or cataracts. Bronchospasm may occur; d/c use and institute alternative treatment if occur. Caution in elderly.

ADVERSE REACTIONS: Headache, nasopharyngitis, sinusitis, pharyngolaryngeal pain, upper respiratory infection, arthralgia, nasal congestion, pain in extremity, back pain.

INTERACTIONS: Oral ketoconazole may increase levels of the pharmacologically active metabolite des-ciclesonide. Caution with chronic use of drugs that can reduce bone mass (eg, anticonvulsants, oral corticosteroids).

PREGNANCY: Category C, caution in nursing.

MECHANISM OF ACTION: Non-halogenated glucocorticoid; not established. Exerts anti-inflammatory actions with affinity to glucocorticoid receptor that inhibits activities of multiple cell types (mast cells, eosinophils, basophils, lymphocytes, macrophages, and neutrophils) and mediators (histamine, eicosanoids, leukotrienes, and cytokines) involved in asthmatic response.

PHARMACOKINETICS: Absorption: Ciclesonide: Absolute bioavailability (22%). Des-ciclesonide: AUC=2.18ng•hr/mL (multiple dose), C_{max}=1.02ng/mL (single dose), 0.369ng/mL (multiple dose); T_{max}=1.04 hrs. **Distribution:** (IV) V_d=2.9L/kg (ciclesonide), 12.1L/kg (des-ciclesonide); plasma protein binding (≥99%). **Metabolism:** Liver, via CYP3A4, CYP2D6; des-ciclesonide (active metabolite). **Elimination:** (IV) Feces (66%), urine (≤20% des-ciclesonide). $T_{1/2}$=0.71 hrs (ciclesonide), 6-7 hrs (des-ciclesonide).

NURSING CONSIDERATIONS

Assessment: Assess for status asthmaticus, acute episodes of asthma, previous corticosteroid use, risk for decreased bone mineral content, history of glaucoma, increased IOP, and/or cataracts, pregnancy/nursing status and possible drug interactions.

Monitoring: Monitor for glaucoma, increased IOP, cataracts, visual changes, growth in children, localized infections with Candida albicans, hypercorticism, adrenal insufficiency, bronchospasm, hypersensitivity, and other adverse events that may occur. Monitor lung function and BMD.

Patient Counseling: Inform patient of the benefits and risks of the treatment. Advise that drug is not a bronchodilator or a rescue medication. Contact physician immediately if deterioration of asthma occurs. Advise to rinse mouth after inhalation. Instruct to use at regular intervals. Inform that maximum benefit may not be seen for ≥4 weeks after starting treatment. Report if symptoms do not improve or if condition worsens; do not increase prescribed dosage. Instruct not to d/c abruptly. Avoid exposure to chickenpox or measles; notify physician immediately if exposed. Inform that drug may worsen existing TB, fungal, bacterial, viral, or parasitic infections, or ocular herpes simplex, and may cause decrease in BMD and growth velocity in children. Instruct to prime drug before using for the 1st time or when not used for >10 days. Instruct on proper administration.

Administration: Inhalation route. Prime pump by actuating 3 times. Refer to PI for further administration instructions. **Storage:** 25°C (77°F); excursions permitted to 15-30°C (59-86°F). Contents under pressure. Do not puncture. Exposure to >49°C (120°F) may cause bursting. Never throw into fire or incinerator.

AMANTADINE RX
amantadine HCl (Endo)

THERAPEUTIC CLASS: Dopamine receptor agonist

INDICATIONS: Prophylaxis and treatment of uncomplicated influenza A infections. Treatment of parkinsonism and drug-induced extrapyramidal reactions.

DOSAGE: *Adults:* Influenza A Virus Prophylaxis/Treatment: 200mg qd given as a single dose of two 100mg tabs (or 4 tsp of syrup). May give 100mg (or 2 tsp) bid if CNS effects develop. Elderly: ≥65 yrs: 100mg qd. Parkinsonism: Initial: 100mg bid if used alone. Serious Associated Illness/Concomitant High-Dose Antiparkinson Agent: Initial: 100mg qd. Titrate: May increase to 100mg bid after 1 to several weeks. Max: 400mg/day. Drug-Induced Extrapyramidal Reactions: 100mg bid. Titrate: May increase to 300mg/day in divided doses. CrCl 30-50mL/min: 200mg on Day 1, then 100mg qd. CrCl 15-29mL/min: 200mg on Day 1, then 100mg every other day. CrCl <15mL/min/Hemodialysis: 200mg every 7 days.

Pediatrics: Influenza A Virus Prophylaxis/Treatment: 9-12 yrs: 100mg (or 2 tsp of syrup) bid. 1-9 yrs: 4.4-8.8mg/kg/day. Max: 150mg/day.

HOW SUPPLIED: Cap: 100mg; Syrup: 50mg/5mL; Tab: 100mg

WARNINGS/PRECAUTIONS: Deaths reported from overdose. Suicide attempts, neuroleptic malignant syndrome (NMS) reported. May exacerbate mental illness in patients with history of psychotropic disorder or substance abuse. Caution with CHF, peripheral edema, orthostatic hypotension, renal or hepatic dysfunction, recurrent eczematoid rash, uncontrolled psychosis or severe psychoneurosis. Avoid in untreated angle-closure glaucoma. Do not d/c abruptly in Parkinson's disease. May increase seizure activity. Increased risk of melanoma with Parkinson's disease; monitor periodically. May impair mental/physical abilities. Compulsive behaviors (eg, intense urges to gamble, increased sexual urges) reported.

ADVERSE REACTIONS: Nausea, dizziness, insomnia, depression, anxiety, hallucinations, confusion, anorexia, dry mouth, constipation, ataxia, livedo reticularis, peripheral edema, orthostatic hypotension, irritability, headache.

INTERACTIONS: Caution with CNS stimulants. Alcohol may potentiate CNS effects (eg, dizziness, confusion, orthostatic hypotension). Anticholinergic agents may potentiate the anticholinergic side effects. Increased tremor in elderly Parkinson's patients with thioridazine. Increased plasma levels with quinine or quinidine, triamterene/hydrochlorothiazide. Avoid use of attenuated influenza vaccine within 2 weeks before or 48 hours after.

PREGNANCY: Category C, not for use in nursing.

MECHANISM OF ACTION: Antiviral; appears to prevent release of infectious viral nucleic acid into host cell by interfering with function of transmembrane domain of viral M2 protein, preventing virus assembly during replication. Parkinson's disease; may have direct/indirect effect on dopamine neurons and is a weak, noncompetitive NMDA receptor antagonist.

PHARMACOKINETICS: Absorption: Well absorbed; (Tab) C_{max}=0.51mcg/mL, T_{max}=2-4 hrs. (Syrup) C_{max}=0.24mcg/mL, T_{max}=2-4 hrs. **Distribution:** (IV) V_d=3-8L/kg; plasma protein binding (67%); excreted in breast milk. **Metabolism:** N-acetylation; acetylamantadine (metabolite). **Elimination:** Urine; excreted unchanged; $T_{1/2}$=16 hrs.

NURSING CONSIDERATIONS

Assessment: Assess for history of CHF, peripheral edema, epilepsy or other "seizures", recurrent eczematoid rash, psychiatric illness, untreated angle-closure glaucoma, pregnancy/nursing status, possible drug interactions, renal/hepatic impairment, and hypersensitivity.

Monitoring: Monitor for signs/symptoms of CHF, peripheral edema, epilepsy or other "seizures", recurrent eczematoid rash, psychiatric illness, untreated angle-closure glaucoma, NMS (eg, fever, muscle rigidity, altered mental status), renal/hepatic impairment, melanoma, compulsive behaviors (eg, pathological gambling, hypersexuality), and hypersensitivity reactions. Monitor lab tests such as CPK, WBC, serum myoglobin, BUN, SrCr, alkaline phosphatase, LDH, bilirubin, GGT, SGOT and SGPT.

Patient Counseling: Advise blurry vision and impaired mental acuity may occur. Avoid excessive alcohol use, getting up suddenly from sitting or lying position, and abrupt d/c. Notify physician if no improvement in a few days or appears less effective after a few weeks. Seek medical attention if experience symptoms of CHF (eg, lightheadedness, SOB), peripheral edema, epilepsy or other "seizures", recurrent eczematoid rash, psychiatric illness (eg, suicidal ideation, mood changes), untreated angle-closure glaucoma, hypersensitivity reaction, NMS (eg, fever, muscle rigidity, altered mental status), renal/hepatic impairment. Consult a physician before discontinuing medication. Caution against driving/working where alertness and adequate motor coordination are important. Notify physician if new or increased gambling urges, increased sexual urges or other intense urges occur.

Administration: Oral route. Influenza A: Treatment: should be started within 24-48 hrs after onset and after disappearance of signs and symptoms; continue for at least 10 days after known exposure. Prophylaxis: Administer for 2-4 weeks after vaccine is given. If vaccine unavailable, continue for entire duration of exposure in community. **Storage:** 25°C (77°F); excursions permitted to 15-30°C (59-86°F). Dispense in tight container.

AMARYL RX
glimepiride (Sanofi-Aventis)

THERAPEUTIC CLASS: Sulfonylurea (2nd generation)

INDICATIONS: Adjunct to diet and exercise, to improve glycemic control in type 2 diabetes mellitus. May use in combination with metformin or insulin.

DOSAGE: *Adults:* Initial: 1-2mg qd with breakfast or 1st main meal. Titrate: After 2mg, may increase by up to 2mg every 1-2 weeks. Maint: 1-4mg qd. Max: 8mg qd. Amaryl/Metformin: Add Metformin to 8mg qd for better glucose control. Amaryl/Insulin Therapy: If FBG >150mg/dL on 8mg qd, add low-dose insulin; increase insulin weekly as needed. Renal Insufficiency: Initial: 1mg qd. Elderly/Debilitated/Malnourished/Hepatic Insufficiency: Dose conservatively to avoid hypoglycemia.

HOW SUPPLIED: Tab: 1mg, 2mg, 4mg

CONTRAINDICATIONS: Diabetic ketoacidosis with or without coma.

WARNINGS/PRECAUTIONS: Increased cardiovascular (CV) mortality. Hypoglycemia risk if debilitated, malnourished, or with adrenal, pituitary, renal or hepatic insufficiency. Hypoglycemia may be masked in elderly and patients with autonomic neuropathy. May lose blood glucose control with stress (eg, fever, trauma, infection, or surgery). Secondary failure may occur. Risk of hemolytic anemia reported with G6PD deficiency; use with caution and consider alternative therapy. Allergic reaction may develop if allergic to other sulfonamide derivatives.

ADVERSE REACTIONS: Dizziness, nausea, asthenia, headache, hypoglycemia.

INTERACTIONS: Potentiates hypoglycemia with alcohol, NSAIDs, insulin, metformin, highly protein-bound drugs, such as salicylates, sulfonamides, chloramphenicol, coumarin, probenecid, MAOIs, miconazole, β-blockers, disopyramide, fluoxetine, quinolones, and clarithromycin. Risk of hyperglycemia with diuretics, corticosteroids, phenothiazines, thyroid products, estrogens, oral contraceptives, phenytoin, nicotinic acid, sympathomimetics, and isoniazid. Monitor for hypoglycemia when switching from long-acting sulfonylurea, and with combination therapy with insulin and metformin. Hypoglycemia may be masked with β-blockers or other sympatholytic agents.

PREGNANCY: Category C, not for use in nursing.

MECHANISM OF ACTION: Sulfonylurea; lowers blood glucose by stimulating insulin release from functioning pancreatic β cells.

PHARMACOKINETICS: Absorption: Administration of variable doses resulted in different parameters. Complete (GI tract, 100%); T_{max}=2-3 hrs; **Distribution:** (IV) V_d=8.8L; plasma protein binding (99.5%). **Metabolism:** Complete (liver); CYP2C9; major metabolites: M1 & M2. **Elimination:** Urine (60%), feces (40%).

NURSING CONSIDERATIONS

Assessment: Assess for signs/symptoms of hypoglycemia, loss of glucose control (fever, trauma, infection), risk of CV mortality, G6PD deficiency, pregnancy/nursing status, and potential drug interactions.

Monitoring: Monitor fasting blood glucose and glycosylated hemoglobin (every 3-6 months) to determine response to therapy and glycemic control.

Patient Counseling: Instruct to have a proper diet and exercise and regularly test blood glucose. Inform about risks of hypoglycemia (symptoms, treatment) and conditions that predispose to development. Inform risks, advantages, and alternative modes of therapy.

Administration: Oral route. **Storage:** 15-30°C (59-86°F). Dispense in tightly closed container.

AMBIEN
zolpidem tartrate (Sanofi-Aventis)

THERAPEUTIC CLASS: Imidazopyridine hypnotic

INDICATIONS: Short-term treatment of insomnia characterized by difficulties with sleep initiation.

DOSAGE: *Adults:* Individualize dose. 10mg qhs. Max: 10mg/day. Elderly/Debilitated/Hepatic Insufficiency: 5mg qhs. Adjust dose with other CNS depressants.

HOW SUPPLIED: Tab: 5mg, 10mg

WARNINGS/PRECAUTIONS: Initiate only after careful evaluation; failure of insomnia to remit after 7-10 days of treatment may indicate presence of psychiatric and/or medical illness. Severe anaphylactic/anaphylactoid reactions reported. Abnormal thinking, behavior changes, visual/auditory hallucinations, and complex behaviors (eg, sleep-driving) reported. Worsening of depression, including suicidal thoughts and actions have been reported in depressed patients. Withdrawal symptoms may occur with rapid dose reduction or abrupt d/c. Potential impairment of performance of activities requiring complete mental alertness (eg, operating machinery or driving a motor vehicle) may occur the day following ingestion. Monitor elderly and debilitated patients for impaired motor/cognitive performance and for unusual sensitivity. Caution with hepatic impairment, compromised respiratory function or sleep apnea syndrome, myasthenia gravis, depression, and conditions that could affect metabolism or hemodynamic responses. Closely monitor patients with renal impairment.

ADVERSE REACTIONS: Drowsiness, dizziness, headache, diarrhea, drugged feeling, lethargy, dry mouth, back pain, pharyngitis, sinusitis, allergic reactions.

INTERACTIONS: Consider pharmacology of any CNS-active drug to be used concomitantly. CNS depressants may potentially enhance effects. Avoid use with alcohol. Decreased alertness observed in combination with imipramine/chlorpromazine. Increased $T_{1/2}$ with fluoxetine in females. Increased C_{max} and decreased T_{max} with sertraline in females. Increased exposure with CYP3A inhibitors (itraconazole, ketoconazole). Caution with ketoconazole. Decreased levels with rifampin.

PREGNANCY: Category C, caution in nursing.

MECHANISM OF ACTION: Imidazopyridine, non-benzodiazepine hypnotic; interacts with a GABA-BZ receptor complex and binds the BZ_1 receptor preferentially with a high affinity ratio of the α_1/α_5 subunits.

PHARMACOKINETICS: Absorption: Rapid from GI tract. C_{max} =59ng/mL (5mg), 121ng/mL (10mg). T_{max} =1.6 hrs (5mg, 10mg). **Distribution:** Plasma protein binding (92.5%); found in breast milk. **Elimination**: Renal; $T_{1/2}$ =2.6 hrs (5mg), 2.5 hrs (10mg).

NURSING CONSIDERATIONS

Assessment: Assess for primary psychiatric and/or medical illness, myasthenia gravis, pre-existing respiratory impairment (sleep apnea syndrome), diseases/conditions that could affect metabolism or hemodynamic responses, depression, hypersensitivity to drug, hepatic/renal impairment, pregnancy/nursing status, possible drug interactions, and history of drug or alcohol addiction or abuse.

Monitoring: Monitor for anaphylactic/anaphylactoid reactions, withdrawal effects, motor/cognitive impairment, abnormal thinking, behavioral changes, complex behaviors, and visual/auditory hallucinations. Monitor patients with hepatic/renal impairment and history of drug or alcohol addiction or abuse.

Patient Counseling: Inform about risks/benefits of use. Instruct to read Medication Guide. Advise to seek medical attention immediately if anaphylactic/anaphylactoid reactions occur. Counsel to take just before bedtime and only when they are able to stay in bed a full night (7-8 hrs) before being active again. Advise not to take with or immediately after a meal. Caution against hazardous tasks (eg, operating machinery/driving); immediately report events such as sleep-driving and other complex behaviors. Advise to report all concomitant medications to the prescriber. Counsel on tolerance, dependence, and withdrawal signs/symptoms. Do not take with alcohol.

Administration: Oral route. **Storage:** 20-25°C (68-77°F).

AMBIEN CR   CIV
zolpidem tartrate (Sanofi-Aventis)

THERAPEUTIC CLASS: Imidazopyridine hypnotic

INDICATIONS: Treatment of insomnia characterized by difficulties with sleep onset and/or sleep maintenance.

DOSAGE: *Adults:* Individualize dose. 12.5mg qhs. Max: 12.5mg/day. Elderly/ Debilitated/Hepatic Insufficiency: 6.25mg qhs. Adjust dose with other CNS depressants.

HOW SUPPLIED: Tab, Extended-Release: 6.25mg, 12.5mg

WARNINGS/PRECAUTIONS: Initiate only after careful evaluation; failure of insomnia to remit after 7-10 days of treatment may indicate presence of psychiatric and/or medical illness. Severe anaphylactic/anaphylactoid reactions reported. Abnormal thinking, behavior changes, visual/auditory hallucinations, and complex behaviors (eg, sleep-driving) reported. Worsening of depression, including suicidal thoughts and actions have been reported in depressed patients. Withdrawal symptoms may occur with rapid dose reduction or abrupt d/c. Potential impairment of performance of activities requiring complete mental alertness (eg, operating machinery or driving a motor vehicle) may occur the day following ingestion. Monitor elderly and debilitated patients for impaired motor/cognitive performance and for unusual sensitivity. Caution with hepatic impairment, compromised respiratory function or sleep apnea syndrome, myasthenia gravis, depression, and conditions that could affect metabolism or hemodynamic responses. Closely monitor patients with renal impairment.

ADVERSE REACTIONS: Headache, somnolence, dizziness, anxiety, nausea, influenza, hallucinations, back pain, myalgia, fatigue, disorientation, memory disorder, visual disturbance, nasopharyngitis.

INTERACTIONS: Consider pharmacology of any CNS-active drug to be used concomitantly. CNS depressants may potentially enhance effects. Avoid use with alcohol. Decreased alertness observed in combination with imipramine/ chlorpromazine. Increased $T_{1/2}$ with fluoxetine in females. Increased C_{max} and decreased T_{max} with sertraline in females. Increased exposure with CYP3A inhibitors (itraconazole, ketoconazole). Caution with ketoconazole. Decreased levels with rifampin.

PREGNANCY: Category C, caution in nursing.

MECHANISM OF ACTION: Imidazopyridine, non-benzodiazepine hypnotic; interacts with a GABA-BZ receptor complex and binds the BZ_1 receptor preferentially with a high affinity ratio of the α_1/α_5 subunits.

PHARMACOKINETICS: Absorption: Biphasic, rapid from GI tract, then extended; C_{max}=134ng/mL, T_{max}=1.5 hrs, AUC=740ng•hr/mL. **Distribution:** Plasma protein binding (92.5%); found in breast milk. **Elimination:** Renal; $T_{1/2}$=2.8 hrs.

NURSING CONSIDERATIONS

Assessment: Assess for primary psychiatric and/or medical illness, myasthenia gravis, pre-existing respiratory impairment (sleep apnea syndrome), diseases/conditions that could affect metabolism or hemodynamic responses, depression, hypersensitivity to drug, hepatic/renal impairment, pregnancy/ nursing status, possible drug interactions, and history of drug or alcohol addiction or abuse.

Monitoring: Monitor for anaphylactic/anaphylactoid reactions, withdrawal effects, motor/cognitive impairment, abnormal thinking, behavioral changes, complex behaviors, and visual/auditory hallucinations. Monitor patients with hepatic/renal impairment and history of drug or alcohol addiction or abuse.

Patient Counseling: Instruct to read Medication Guide. Counsel to take just before bedtime and only when able to stay in bed a full night (7-8 hrs) before being active again. Advise not to take with or immediately after a meal; do not crush, divide, or chew, and do not take when drinking alcohol. Advise to seek medical attention immediately if any anaphylactic/anaphylactoid reactions occur. Caution against hazardous tasks (eg, driving/operating machines); immediately report events such as sleep-driving and other complex behaviors. Advise to report all concomitant medications to the prescriber. Inform about risks/benefits of use. Counsel on tolerance, dependence, and withdrawal signs/symptoms.

Administration: Oral route. Swallow whole; do not divide, crush, or chew.
Storage: 15-25°C (59-77°F); excursions permissible ≤30°C (86°F).

AmBisome RX
amphotericin B liposome (Astellas)

THERAPEUTIC CLASS: Polyene antifungal

INDICATIONS: Empirical therapy for presumed fungal infection in febrile, neutropenic patients. Treatment of *Aspergillus, Candida,* or *Cryptococcus* infections refractory to amphotericin B deoxycholate or where renal impairment or unacceptable toxicity precludes its use. Treatment of cryptococcal meningitis in HIV-infected patients. Treatment of visceral leishmaniasis.

DOSAGE: *Adults:* Empirical Therapy: 3mg/kg/day IV. Systemic Infections (*Aspergillus, Candida, Cryptococcus*): 3-5mg/kg/day IV. Cryptococcal Meningitis in HIV: 6mg/kg/day IV. Visceral Leishmaniasis: Immunocompetent: 3mg/kg/day IV on Days 1-5, 14, 21. May repeat course if needed. Immunocompromised: 4mg/kg/day IV on Days 1-5, 10, 17, 24, 31, 38. Infuse over 120 min but may be reduced to 60 min if tolerated.
Pediatrics: 1 month-16 yrs: Empirical Therapy: 3mg/kg/day IV. Systemic Infections (*Aspergillus, Candida, Cryptococcus*): 3-5mg/kg/day IV. Cryptococcal Meningitis in HIV: 6mg/kg/day IV. Visceral Leishmaniasis: Immunocompetent: 3mg/kg/day IV on Days 1-5, 14, 21. May repeat course if needed. Immunocompromised: 4mg/kg/day IV on Days 1-5, 10, 17, 24, 31, 38. Infuse over 120 min but may be reduced to 60 min if tolerated.

HOW SUPPLIED: Inj: 50mg/vial

WARNINGS/PRECAUTIONS: Anaphylaxis reported, d/c all further infusions if severe anaphylactic reaction occurs. Significantly less toxic than amphotericin B deoxycholate.

ADVERSE REACTIONS: Hypokalemia, chills/rigors, SrCr elevation, anemia, N/V, diarrhea, hypomagnesemia, rash, dyspnea, bilirubinemia, BUN increased, headache, abdominal pain.

INTERACTIONS: Concurrent use of antineoplastic agents may potentiate renal toxicity, bronchospasm, hypotension. Corticosteroids and corticotropin may potentiate hypokalemia. May induce hypokalemia and potentiate digitalis toxicity with digitalis glycosides. May increase flucytosine toxicity. Acute pulmonary toxicity reported with leukocyte transfusions. Nephrotoxic drugs enhance potential for renal toxicity. May enhance curariform effect of skeletal muscle relaxants due to hypokalemia. Imidazoles (eg, ketoconazole, miconazole, clotrimazole, fluconazole) may induce fungal resistance; caution with combination therapy, especially in immunocompromised patients.

PREGNANCY: Category B, not for use in nursing.

MECHANISM OF ACTION: Antifungal agent; acts by binding to the sterol component of the cell membrane leading to changes in cell permeability and cell death in susceptible fungi. Also binds to the cholesterol component of the mammalian cell, leading to cytotoxicity.

PHARMACOKINETICS: Absorption: IV administration of variable doses resulted from different pharmacokinetic parameters. **Elimination:** (24-hr dosing interval) $T_{1/2}$=7-10 hrs. (49 days after dosing) $T_{1/2}$=100-153 hrs.

NURSING CONSIDERATIONS

Assessment: Assess hypersensitivity, health status (eg, immunocompetent, immunocompromised), cultures, renal function, pregnancy/nursing status and possible drug interactions.

Monitoring: Monitor for anaphylaxis/severe allergic reaction, infusion reactions (eg, chills, hypotension, hypoxia, rash), renal, hepatic and hematopoietic function, and serum electrolytes (particularly Mg^{2+} and K^+).

Patient Counseling: Advise to seek medical attention if symptoms of acute reaction occur (eg, fevers, chills, respiratory symptoms). Instruct patient to report all medications being used. Inform that potential risks are involved when used during pregnancy and nursing.

Administration: IV infusion. Infuse over 120 min but may be reduced to 60 min if tolerated. An in-line membrane filter may be used provided the mean pore diameter of the filter is not <1.0 micron. Refer to PI for directions for reconstitution, filtration and dilution. Do not reconstitute with saline or add saline to the reconstituted concentration, or mix with other drugs. Discard partially used vials. **Storage:** Unopened vials: 25°C (77°F). Reconstituted: 2-8°C (36-46°F) up to 24 hrs. Diluted Product: Injection should commence within 6 hrs of dilution with 5% Dextrose Injection.

AMERGE   RX
naratriptan HCl (GlaxoSmithKline)

THERAPEUTIC CLASS: 5-HT$_{1B/1D}$ agonist

INDICATIONS: Acute treatment of migraine with or without aura.

DOSAGE: *Adults:* ≥18 yrs: 1mg or 2.5mg taken with fluids; may repeat dose once after 4 hrs. Max: 5mg/24 hrs. Mild-Moderate Renal/Hepatic Impairment: Initial: Lower dose. Max: 2.5mg/24 hrs. Safety of treating >4 headaches/30 days not known.

HOW SUPPLIED: Tab: 1mg, 2.5mg

CONTRAINDICATIONS: Uncontrolled HTN, ischemic cardiac disease, cerebrovascular or peripheral vascular syndromes, other significant cardiovascular disease (CVD), severe renal or hepatic impairment, basilar or hemiplegic migraine, within 24 hrs of another 5-HT$_1$ agonist, ergotamine-containing or ergot-type drugs (eg, dihydroergotamine, methysergide).

WARNINGS/PRECAUTIONS: Confirm diagnosis. Potential to cause coronary artery vasospasm; do not give with documented ischemic/vasospastic coronary artery disease (CAD). Not for patients in whom unrecognized CAD is predicted by presence of risk factors (eg, HTN, hypercholesterolemia, smoker, obesity, diabetes, CAD family history, menopause, males >40 yrs.) unless with a satisfactory cardiovascular evaluation; administer 1st dose under medical supervision; obtain ECG to assess presence of cardiac ischemia. Monitor cardiovascular function with long-term intermittent use. May cause vasospastic reactions or cerebrovascular events. Serotonin syndrome may occur; symptoms may include mental status changes, autonomic instability, neuromuscular aberrations, and GI symptoms. HTN and hypertensive crisis reported rarely. Caution with renal or hepatic dysfunction. Avoid in elderly.

ADVERSE REACTIONS: Paresthesias, dizziness, drowsiness, malaise/fatigue, throat and neck symptoms, pain/pressure sensation, N/V.

INTERACTIONS: See Contraindications. Serotonin syndrome reported with combined use of an SSRI or serotonin norepinephrine reuptake inhibitor (SNRI). Oral contraceptives elevate concentrations of naratriptan. Smoking increased the clearance by 30%.

PREGNANCY: Category C, caution in nursing.

MECHANISM OF ACTION: Selective 5-HT$_1$ receptor agonist; binds with high affinity to 5-HT$_{1D/1B}$ receptors. Suspected to perform its action by (1) activation of 5-HT$_{1D/1B}$ receptors located on intracranial blood vessels, including those on arteriovenous anastomoses, leads to vasoconstriction that correlates with relief of migraine, or (2) activation of 5-HT$_{1D/1B}$ receptors in the trigeminal system results in inhibition of pro-inflammatory neuropeptide release.

PHARMACOKINETICS: Absorption: Well-absorbed; bioavailability (70%); T$_{max}$=2-3 hrs. **Distribution:** V$_d$=170L, plasma protein binding (28-31%). **Metabolism:** Via CYP450 isoenzymes. **Elimination:** Urine (50% unchanged, 30% metabolites); T$_{1/2}$=6 hrs.

NURSING CONSIDERATIONS

Assessment: Confirm diagnosis of migraine before therapy. Assess for ischemic heart disease, HTN, hemiplegic/basilar migraine, presence of risk factors (eg, hypercholesterolemia, smoking, obesity, DM, strong family history of CAD, female with surgical/physiological menopause, or male >40 yrs), ECG changes, hepatic/renal function, pregnancy/nursing status, and possible drug interactions.

Monitoring: Administration of 1st dose should be in physician's office or medically staffed and equipped facility as cardiac ischemia may occur in absence of clinical symptoms; ECG should be obtained immediately during interval in those with risk factors. Monitor for signs/symptoms of cardiac events (eg, coronary vasospasm, acute MI, arrhythmia, ECG changes, follow-up coronary angiography), cerebrovascular events (eg, hemorrhage, stroke, TIAs), peripheral vascular ischemia, colonic ischemia with bloody diarrhea and abdominal pain, serotonin syndrome (eg, mental status changes, autonomic instability, neuromuscular aberrations and/or GI symptoms), ophthalmic effects, increased BP, and anaphylaxis/anaphylactoid reactions.

Patient Counseling: Inform about potential risks of therapy (eg, symptoms of serotonin syndrome such as confusion, hallucinations, fast heartbeat, fever, sweating, muscle spasms, and diarrhea), especially if taken with SSRIs or SNRIs. Instruct to report adverse reactions to physician. Take exactly as directed. Notify if pregnant/nursing or planning to become pregnant.

Administration: Oral route. **Storage:** 20-25°C (68-77°F).

AMEVIVE   RX
alefacept (Astellas)

THERAPEUTIC CLASS: Immunosuppressive agent

INDICATIONS: Treatment of moderate to severe chronic plaque psoriasis for candidates of systemic therapy or phototherapy.

DOSAGE: *Adults:* 15mg IM once weekly for 12 weeks. May initiate retreatment with an additional 12-week course if CD4+ T-lymphocyte counts are within normal range and a 12-week minimum interval has passed since the previous course of treatment. If CD4+ T-Lymphocyte Counts <250 cells/μL, withhold dose. D/C if counts remain below 250 cells/μL for 1 month.

HOW SUPPLIED: Inj: 15mg

CONTRAINDICATIONS: HIV.

WARNINGS/PRECAUTIONS: Dose-dependent reductions in circulating CD4+ and CD8+ T-lymphocyte counts reported. Do not initiate with CD4+ T-lymphocyte counts below normal; monitor every 2 weeks. May increase risk of malignancies; do not administer to patients with history of systemic malignancy, caution in patients at high risk for malignancy. May increase risk of infection or reactivate latent, chronic infections; avoid with clinically important infections, caution with chronic infection or history of recurrent infections; d/c if serious infection develops. Hypersensitivity reactions (eg, urticaria, angioedema) reported; d/c if anaphylactic or serious allergic reactions occur. Liver injury (fatty infiltration, hepatitis) reported; d/c if significant clinical signs of liver injury develop. Caution in elderly. Avoid concurrent phototherapy.

ADVERSE REACTIONS: Lymphopenia, malignancies, serious infections, hypersensitivity reactions, pharyngitis, dizziness, increased cough, nausea, pruritus, myalgia, chills, injection-site reactions, immunogenecity.

INTERACTIONS: Avoid with other immunosuppressive agents.

PREGNANCY: Category B, not for use in nursing.

MECHANISM OF ACTION: Immunosuppressive agent; interferes with lymphocyte activation by specifically binding to the lymphocyte antigen CD2, and inhibiting LFA-2/CD2 interaction. Reduces subsets of CD2+ T lymphocytes (primarily CD45RO+), presumably by bridging between CD2 on target lymphocytes and immunoglobulin Fc receptors on cytotoxic cells, such as natural killer cells, which results in reduction of circulating total CD4+ and CD8+ T-lymphocyte counts.

PHARMACOKINETICS: Absorption: Bioavailability (63%). **Distribution:** V_d=94mL/kg. **Elimination:** $T_{1/2}$=270 hrs.

NURSING CONSIDERATIONS

Assessment: Assess for HIV infection, history of systemic malignancy or risk of malignancy, chronic infections or history of recurrent infection, immunosuppressants or phototherapy, immunization status, hepatic impairment, pregnancy/nursing status, and possible drug interactions. Prior to initiation or subsequent course of therapy, patient should have normal CD4+ T lymphocytes.

Monitoring: Requires monitoring of CD4+ T lymphocyte counts every 2 weeks throughout the course of the 12-week dosing regimen. Monitor for signs/ symptoms of infection during or after a course of therapy. Monitor for new infections, malignancies, hypersensitivity reactions (urticaria, angioedema, anaphylactic reactions, or serious allergic reaction), signs/symptoms of hepatic injury, and WBCs.

Patient Counseling: Inform about potential risks/benefits of therapy and to report any signs/symptoms of infections, malignancy, or liver injury (eg, N/V, fatigue, jaundice, dark urine) to physician. Notify physician if pregnant/ nursing or planning to become pregnant (or within 8 weeks of d/c). Inform of the need for regular monitoring of WBC counts. Inform that therapy reduces lymphocyte counts increasing the chances of infection or malignancy.

Administration: IM route. Use only under supervision of a physician. **Storage:** 2-8°C (36-46°F). Protect from light, retain in drug/diluent pack until time of use.

AMICAR   RX
aminocaproic acid (Xanodyne)

THERAPEUTIC CLASS: Monoamino carboxylic acid anti-fibrinolytic

INDICATIONS: To enhance hemostasis when fibrinolysis contributes to bleeding.

DOSAGE: *Adults:* IV: 16-20mL (4-5g) in 250mL diluent during 1st hr, then 4mL/hr (1g) in 50mL of diluent. PO: 5g during 1st hr, then 5mL (syr) or 1g (tabs) per hr. Continue therapy for 8 hrs or until bleeding is controlled.

HOW SUPPLIED: Inj: 250mg/mL [20mL]; Syrup: 1.25g/5mL; Tab: 500mg*, 1000mg* *scored

CONTRAINDICATIONS: Active intravascular clotting process, disseminated intravascular coagulation without concomitant heparin.

WARNINGS/PRECAUTIONS: Avoid in hematuria of upper urinary tract origin due to risk of intrarenal obstruction from glomerular capillary thrombosis or clots in renal pelvis and ureters. Skeletal muscle weakness with necrosis of muscle fibers reported after prolonged therapy. Consider cardiac muscle damage with skeletal myopathy. Avoid rapid IV infusion. Thrombophlebitis may occur. Contains benzyl alcohol; do not administer to neonates due to risk of fatal "gasping syndrome." Do not administer without a definite diagnosis of hyperfibrinolysis.

ADVERSE REACTIONS: Edema, headache, anaphylactoid reactions, injection-site reactions, pain, bradycardia, hypotension, abdominal pain, diarrhea, N/V, agranulocytosis, increased CPK, confusion, dyspnea, pruritus, tinnitus.

INTERACTIONS: Increased risk of thrombosis with Factor IX complex concentrates, anti-inhibitor coagulant concentrates.

PREGNANCY: Category C, caution in nursing.

MECHANISM OF ACTION: Monoamino carboxylic acid anti-fibrinolytic; fibrinolysis inhibitory effects are exerted principally by inhibition of plasminogen activators and, to a lesser extent, through antiplasmin activity.

PHARMACOKINETICS: Absorption: (PO) C_{max}=164mcg/mL; T_{max}=1.2 hrs. **Distribution:** (PO) V_d=23.1L; (IV) V_d=30L. **Metabolism:** Adipic acid (metabolite). **Elimination:** Renal: Urine (65% unchanged), (11% metabolite); $T_{1/2}$=2 hrs.

NURSING CONSIDERATIONS

Assessment: Assess for evidence of active intravascular clotting, proper diagnosis of hyperfibrinolysis (hyperplasminemia), pregnancy/nursing status, and possible drug interactions. Assess use in presence of hematuria of the upper urinary tract origin.

Monitoring: Monitor for signs/symptoms of subendocardial hemorrhages, fatty degeneration of the myocardium, skeletal muscle weakness with necrosis of muscle fibers (rhabdomyolysis, myoglobinuria, acute renal failure), cardiac muscle damage, thrombophlebitis, and neurological deficits (eg, hydrocephalus, cerebral ischemia, cerebral vasospasm). In patients with upper urinary tract bleeding, monitor for signs/symptoms of intrarenal obstruction (eg, glomerular capillary thrombosis, clots in renal pelvis and ureters). If used in pediatrics, monitor for "gasping syndrome" in neonates. Monitor CPK levels in patients on long-term therapy. Perform periodic monitoring to determine amount of fibrinolysis present.

Patient Counseling: Advise not to administer without definite diagnosis (laboratory finding indicative of hyperfibrinolysis). Instruct to contact physician if unusual muscle weakness or pain develops.

Administration: IV or Oral routes. IV: Use compatible intravenous vehicles (eg, Sterile Water for Injection, Sodium Chloride for Injection, 5% Dextrose or Ringer's Injection). Rapid IV administration may induce hypotension, bradycardia, and/or arrhythmias. **Storage:** 15-30°C (59-86°F).

AMIKACIN   RX
amikacin sulfate (Various)

> Potential for ototoxicity/nephrotoxicity; reduce dose or d/c on evidence of ototoxicity/nephrotoxicity. Neurotoxicity (eg, vestibular and permanent bilateral auditory ototoxicity) can occur with preexisting renal damage and normal renal function treated at higher doses and/or longer treatment periods than recommended. Neuromuscular blockade, respiratory paralysis reported. Monitor renal and 8th-nerve function and serum amikacin concentration. Increased risk of neuromuscular blockade and respiratory paralysis with anesthetics, neuromuscular blockers (eg, tubocurarine, succinylcholine, decamethonium) or massive transfusions of citrate-anticoagulated blood. Avoid potent diuretics (eg, ethacrynic acid, furosemide) and other neurotoxic, nephrotoxic drugs (eg, bacitracin, cisplatin, amphotericin B, cephaloridine, paromomycin, viomycin, polymyxin B, colistin, vancomycin, aminoglycosides). Safety not established with treatment >14 days.

THERAPEUTIC CLASS: Aminoglycoside

INDICATIONS: Short-term treatment of serious infections due to susceptible strains of gram-negative bacteria. Shown to be effective in bacterial septicemia; respiratory tract, bone/joint, CNS (including meningitis), skin and soft tissue, and intra-abdominal infections; burns and postoperative infections; complicated and recurrent urinary tract infections (UTI) due to susceptible strains of microorganisms; infections caused by gentamicin-and/or tobramycin-resistant strains of Gram-negative organisms; staphylococcal infectons; severe infections such as neonatal sepsis in combination with a penicillin-type drug.

DOSAGE: *Adults:* IM/IV: 15mg/kg/day given q8h or q12h. Max: 15mg/kg/day. Heavier Wt Patients: Max: 1.5g/day. Recurrent Uncomplicated UTI: 250mg bid. Usual Duration: 7-10 days. Renal Impairment: Reduce dose.

Pediatrics: IM/IV: 15mg/kg/day given q8h or q12h. Newborns: LD: 10mg/kg. Maint: 7.5mg/kg q12h. Usual Duration: 7-10 days. D/C therapy if no response after 3-5 days. Renal Impairment: Reduce dose.

HOW SUPPLIED: Inj: 50mg/mL, 250mg/mL

WARNINGS/PRECAUTIONS: May cause fetal harm. Contains sodium metabisulfite; allergic reactions may occur especially in asthmatics. Maintain adequate hydration. Assess kidney function before therapy, then daily. Reduce dose with decreased creatinine clearance and urine specific gravity, increased BUN, creatinine and oliguria. D/C therapy if azotemia increases or if progressive decrease in urinary output occurs. Caution with muscular disorders (eg, myasthenia gravis, parkinsonism); may aggravate muscle weakness.

ADVERSE REACTIONS: Ototoxicity, neuromuscular blockage, nephrotoxicity, skin rash, drug fever, headache, paresthesia, tremor, N/V, arthralgia, anemia, hypotension.

INTERACTIONS: See Boxed Warning. Increased nephrotoxicity with aminoglycosides, antibiotics, cephalosporins. Should not be given concurrently with potent diuretics. Significant mutual inactivation may occur with β-lactams (eg, penicillin, cephalosporins). Cross-allergenicity between aminoglycosides.

PREGNANCY: Category D, not for use in nursing.

MECHANISM OF ACTION: Semisynthetic aminoglycoside antibiotic derived from kanamycin.

PHARMACOKINETICS: Absorption: (IM) Rapid. (IV) C_{max}=38mcg/mL. **Distribution:** V_d=24L; plasma protein binding (0-11%); crosses placenta. **Elimination:** Urine (IM, 91.9-98.2%), (IV, 84-94%); $T_{1/2}$>2 hrs.

NURSING CONSIDERATIONS

Assessment: Assess for pregnancy/nursing status, renal impairment, eighth cranial nerve function, muscular disorders (eg, myasthenia gravis, parkinsonism) and for possible drug interactions. Assess renal function tests prior to and throughout therapy.

Monitoring: Periodic monitoring of urea, creatinine, CrCl, audiometric testing changes, eigth cranial nerve function, serum concentrations of the drug and urine (specific gravity, proteins, presence of cells/casts). Monitor for signs/symptoms of nephrotoxicity, neurotoxicity (vestibular and permanent bilateral auditory ototoxicity, vertigo, numbness, skin tingling, muscle twitches, and convulsions), cochlear damage, neuromuscular blockade, and respiratory paralysis.

Patient Counseling: Inform about potential risks/benefits of therapy and to report signs of ototoxicity (eg, dizziness, vertigo, tinnitus, roaring in the ears, and hearing loss). Notify physician if pregnant/nursing or planning to become pregnant. Inform that drug treats bacterial infections only. Take as prescribed.

Administration: IV, IM route. Obtain pretreatment body weight to calculate correct dosage. Do not physically premix with other drugs; administer separately. **Storage:** 15-30°C (59-86°F).

AMIODARONE IV   RX
amiodarone HCl (Various)

THERAPEUTIC CLASS: Class III antiarrhythmic

INDICATIONS: Initiation of treatment and prophylaxis of frequently recurring ventricular fibrillation (VF) and hemodynamically unstable ventricular tachycardia (VT) refractory to other therapies. Treatment of patients with VT/VF for whom oral amiodarone is indicated, but who are unable to take oral medication.

DOSAGE: *Adults:* LD: 150mg over 1st 10 min (15mg/min), then 360mg over next 6 hrs (1mg/min), then 540mg over remaining 18 hrs (0.5mg/min). Maint: 0.5mg/min (720mg/24 hrs) for 2-3 weeks. Increase rate to achieve arrhythmia suppression. Do not exceed an initial infusion rate of 30mg/min. Breakthrough Episodes of Ventricular Fibrillation/Hemodynamically Unstable Ventricular

AMIODARONE IV

Tachycardia: 150mg supplemental infusion mixed in 100mL D$_5$W over 10 min. Switching to Oral Amiodarone (Assuming a 720mg/day IV infusion): <1 week of IV infusion: 800mg-1600mg/day; 1-3 weeks of IV infusion: 600mg-800mg/day; >3 weeks of IV infusion: 400mg/day. Elderly: Start at lower end of dosing range.

HOW SUPPLIED: Inj: 50mg/mL [3mL]

CONTRAINDICATIONS: Cardiogenic shock, marked sinus bradycardia, 2nd- or 3rd-degree atrioventricular (AV) block (unless a functioning pacemaker is available).

WARNINGS/PRECAUTIONS: Hypotension reported; do not exceed the recommended rate of infusion. Treat hypotension initially by slowing the infusion; additional standard therapy may be needed (eg, vasopressor drugs, positive inotropic agents, and volume expansion). Bradycardia and AV block reported; ensure availability of temporary pacemaker in patients with known predisposition. Elevations of hepatic enzymes reported. Acute centrolobular confluent hepatocellular necrosis leading to hepatic coma and acute renal failure may occur at a much higher LD concentration and much faster rate of infusion than recommended. Consider d/c or reducing rate of administration with evidence of progressive hepatic injury. May worsen or precipitate a new arrhythmia. Proarrhythmia, primarily torsades de pointes (TdP), has been associated with QTc prolongation; monitor during infusion. Reserve use with other antiarrhythmics for life-threatening ventricular arrhythmias incompletely responsive to a single agent. Acute-onset pulmonary injury/pulmonary toxicity and adult respiratory distress syndrome (ARDS) reported. Optic neuropathy/neuritis may occur; perform ophthalmic examination if symptoms of visual impairment appear. May induce hyperthyroidism leading to thyrotoxicosis and/or the possibility of arrhythmia breakthrough or aggravation; consider d/c or dose reduction. When aggressive treatment has failed or amiodarone cannot be d/c, surgical management may be an option. Experience with this form of therapy is limited; thyroidectomy could induce thyroid storm. May cause potential hazard to the fetus (eg, congenital goiter/hypothyroidism, hyperthyroidism). Thyroid abnormalities (eg, thyroid nodules, thyroid cancer) reported; caution in patients with history of thyroid nodules, goiter, or other thyroid dysfunction. Corneal refractive laser surgery devices contraindicated in patients taking amiodarone. Correct hypokalemia or hypomagnesemia before therapy to prevent exaggeration of QTc prolongation and potential for TdP. Contains benzyl alcohol; gasping syndrome reported in neonates. Caution in elderly.

ADVERSE REACTIONS: Elevated liver enzymes, hypotension, injection-site reactions, bradycardia, AV block, hypothyroidism, nausea.

INTERACTIONS: Potential for drug interactions may persist after d/c due to long half-life. May increase levels with CYP2C8/CYP3A4 inhibitors (eg, protease inhibitors, loratadine, cimetidine, trazodone, grapefruit juice). QT prolongation and TdP with loratadine and trazodone reported. Increases QT prolongation leading to arrhythmia when used with disopyramide. QTc prolongation, with or without TdP, when used with fluoroquinolones, macrolide antibiotics, or azoles. May increases levels of CYP1A2/CYP2C9/CYP2D6/CYP3A4 and p-glycoprotein substrates. May elevate levels of cyclosporine leading to increased creatinine. Myopathy/rhabdomyolysis reported when used with simvastatin. May elevate levels of digoxin and flecainide. May elevate levels of quinidine and procainamide; reduce dose by 1/3 when coadministered. If used with other antiarrhythmic agents, initial dose of antiarrhythmics should be half of the usual recommended dose. Caution in patients receiving β-receptor blocking agents (eg, propranolol) or calcium channel antagonists (eg, verapamil, diltiazem); possible potentiation of bradycardia, sinus arrest, and AV block may occur. Potentiation of warfarin-type anticoagulant response, which may lead to serious or fatal bleeding with concomitant use. Monitor PT and reduce anticoagulant dose by 1/3 to 1/2. Ineffective inhibition of platelet aggregation reported with clopidogrel. May decrease levels with CYP3A4 inducers. Decreased levels with phenytoin, rifampin, St. John's wort and cholestyramine. Hypotension, bradycardia, and decreased cardiac output may occur when used with fentanyl. Seizure and sinus bradycardia reported with concomitant lidocaine. Hemodynamic and electrophysiologic interactions observed with concomitant use of propranolol, diltiazem, and verapamil. May impair metabolism of phenytoin, dextromethorphan and MTX. Action of antithyroid drugs may be especially delayed in amiodarone-induced thyrotoxicosis. Radioactive iodine therapy is contraindicated with amiodarone-induced hyperthyroidism. Monitor electrolyte and acid-base balance when receiving concomitant diuretics. Increased sensitivity to myocardial depressant and conduction defects of halogenated inhalational anesthetics.

PREGNANCY: Category D, not for use in nursing.

MECHANISM OF ACTION: Class III antiarrhythmic; blocks sodium, calcium, and potassium channels; exerts noncompetitive antisympathetic action, and negative chronotropic and dromotropic effects; lengthens cardiac action potential, decreases cardiac workload and myocardial oxygen consumption.

PHARMACOKINETICS: Absorption: (single 5mg/kg 15-minute IV infusion, healthy subjects) C_{max}=5-41mg/L, (150mg 10-minute IV infusion, VF/VT patients) C_{max}=7-26mg/L. **Distribution:** Plasma protein binding (>96%); crosses the placenta, found in breast milk. **Metabolism:** CYP3A4, 2C8; N-desethylamiodarone (major active metabolite). **Elimination:** Urine, bile; (Amiodarone) $T_{1/2}$=9-36 days, (N-desethylamiodarone) $T_{1/2}$=9-30 days.

NURSING CONSIDERATIONS

Assessment: Assess for cardiogenic shock, marked sinus bradycardia, 2nd- or 3rd-degree AV block, functioning pacemaker, pre-existing arrhythmia, history of thyroid dysfunction, hypersensitivity reactions, pregnancy/nursing status, and possible drug interactions. Prior to initiation, hypokalemia and hypomagnesemia should be corrected with special attention to electrolyte and acid-base balance in patients experiencing severe/prolonged diarrhea.

Monitoring: Monitor initial rate of infusion closely. Monitor for hypotension, bradycardia, AV block, acute centrolobular confluent hepatocellular necrosis, hepatic coma, hepatic injury, acute renal failure, worsening of existing or precipitation of new arrhythmia, ARDS, acute onset pulmonary injury/toxicity, pulmonary fibrosis, optic neuropathy/neuritis, visual impairment, hypo/hyperthyroidism, thyrotoxicosis, and congenital goiter/hypothyroidism/hyperthyroidism in infants. Monitor LFTs and thyroid function. Monitor when switching to oral therapy, especially for elderly. Perform regular ophthalmic examination (eg, fundoscopy, slit-lamp examination) during administration.

Patient Counseling: Inform about benefits and risks of therapy. Advise that corneal refractive laser surgery devices are contraindicated with concurrent use. Advise female patients to d/c nursing while on therapy. Instruct to avoid grapefruit juice, cough medicines (which may contain dextromethorphan), and St. John's wort. Discuss the symptoms of hypo/hyperthyroidism, particularly if switching to oral amiodarone. Advise to take as directed. Advise to report any adverse reactions promptly to physician.

Administration: IV route. Use of drop counter infusion set may lead to underdosage; deliver via volumetric infusion pump. Infusions >1 hr should not exceed 2mg/mL unless a central venous catheter is used. Administer infusions >2 hrs in a glass or polyolefin bottle containing D_5W. Amiodarone leaches out plasticizers (eg, DEHP from IV tubing) especially at higher infusion concentrations, and lower flow rates than recommended. Inspect for particulate matter and discoloration prior to administration. **Storage:** 20-25°C (68-77°F). Protect from light. Avoid excessive heat. Do not freeze. Use carton to protect contents from light until used.

AMITIZA RX
lubiprostone (Sucampo/Takeda)

THERAPEUTIC CLASS: Chloride channel activator

INDICATIONS: Treatment of chronic idiopathic constipation in adults. Treatment of irritable bowel syndrome with constipation (IBS-C) in women ≥18 yrs.

DOSAGE: *Adults:* Chronic Idiopathic Constipation: 24mcg bid with food and water. Hepatic Dysfunction: Moderate (Child-Pugh Class B): 16mcg bid. Severe (Child-Pugh Class C): 8mcg bid. If dose is tolerated but adequate response not obtained, escalate to full dose with appropriate monitoring. IBS-C: 8mcg bid with food and water. Severe Hepatic Dysfunction (Child-Pugh Class C): 8mcg qd. If dose is tolerated but adequate response not obtained, escalate to full dose with appropriate monitoring.

HOW SUPPLIED: Cap: 8mcg, 24mcg

CONTRAINDICATIONS: Known or suspected mechanical GI obstruction.

WARNINGS/PRECAUTIONS: Use only during pregnancy if benefit justifies the risk to fetus; confirm a negative pregnancy test prior to initiation of therapy and advise effective contraceptive measures. May cause nausea and diarrhea; may administer with food to reduce symptoms of nausea. Avoid with severe diarrhea. Dyspnea reported; resolves within a few hours after dose but may recur with subsequent doses. Confirm absence of mechanical GI obstruction prior to initiating therapy.

ADVERSE REACTIONS: Diarrhea, N/V, abdominal distention/pain/discomfort, flatulence, loose stools, dyspnea, headache, dizziness, edema.

PREGNANCY: Category C, not for use in nursing.

MECHANISM OF ACTION: Chloride channel activator; enhances chloride-rich intestinal fluid secretion, increasing motility in the intestine, thereby facilitating the passage of stool.

PHARMACOKINETICS: Absorption: (M3) C_{max}=41.5pg/mL, T_{max}=1.1 hrs, AUC_{0-t}=57.1pg•hr/mL. **Distribution:** Plasma protein binding (94%). **Metabolism:** Rapid and extensive via carbonyl reductase; M3 (active metabolite). **Elimination:** Urine (60%), feces (30%); (M3) $T_{1/2}$=0.9-1.4 hrs.

NURSING CONSIDERATIONS

Assessment: Assess for known or suspected mechanical GI obstruction, severe diarrhea, pregnancy/nursing status and possible drug interactions. Perform pregnancy test and thorough evaluation to confirm absence of obstruction (if symptoms suggestive of mechanical obstruction) prior to therapy.

Monitoring: Monitor for symptoms of allergic reactions, nausea, dyspnea, severe diarrhea, and other adverse reactions. Assess the need for continued therapy.

Patient Counseling: Advise to take with food and water to reduce symptoms of nausea. Report severe nausea, diarrhea, or dyspnea to physician. Advise that the capsule should be swallowed whole, should not be broken or chewed, and should be taken once in the morning and once in the evening as prescribed.

Administration: Oral route. **Storage:** 25°C (77°F); excursions permitted to 15-30°C (59-86°F). Protect from extreme temperatures.

AMITRIPTYLINE   RX
amitriptyline HCl (Mylan)

> Antidepressants increased the risk of suicidal thinking and behavior (suicidality) in short-term studies in children, adolescents, and young adults with major depressive disorder (MDD) and other psychiatric disorders. Monitor and observe closely for clinical worsening, suicidality, or unusual changes in behavior in patients who are started on antidepressant therapy. Amitriptyline is not approved for use in pediatric patients.

THERAPEUTIC CLASS: Tricyclic antidepressant

INDICATIONS: Relief of symptoms of depression, especially endogenous depression.

DOSAGE: *Adults:* PO: Initial: (Outpatient) 75mg/day in divided doses or 50-100mg qhs. (Inpatient) 100mg/day. Titrate: (Outpatient) Increase by 25-50mg qhs. (Inpatient) Increase to 200mg/day. Increases are made preferably in the late afternoon and/or bedtime doses. Maint: 50-100mg qhs. Max: (Outpatient) 150mg/day. (Inpatient) 300mg/day. Elderly: 10mg tid and 20mg qhs. *Pediatrics:* >12 yrs: Adolescents: 10mg tid and 20mg qhs.

HOW SUPPLIED: Tab: 10mg, 25mg, 50mg, 75mg, 100mg, 150mg

CONTRAINDICATIONS: MAOI use or within 14 days; acute recovery period following MI; concurrent cisapride.

WARNINGS/PRECAUTIONS: Screen for risk for bipolar disorder. Caution with history of seizures, urinary retention, angle-closure glaucoma, increased IOP, hyperthyroidism, cardiovascular disorders, liver dysfunction. Increases symptoms with schizophrenia and bipolar disorder. D/C several weeks before elective surgery. May alter blood glucose levels. May impair physical/mental abilities. Caution in elderly.

ADVERSE REACTIONS: MI, stroke, seizure, paralytic ileus, urinary retention, constipation, blurred vision, dry mouth, hyperpyrexia, rash, bone marrow depression, testicular swelling, gynecomastia (male), breast enlargement (female), alopecia, edema.

INTERACTIONS: See Contraindications. May block antihypertensive effects of guanethidine. Potentiates other CNS depressants, alcohol, barbiturates. Increased levels with CYP2D6 inhibitors (eg, quinidine, cimetidine, SSRIs). Avoid within 5 weeks of fluoxetine use. Caution with thyroid drugs. Delirium reported with disulfiram and ethchlorvynol. Paralytic ileus and hyperpyrexia with anticholinergics. Monitor with sympathomimetics and neuroleptics. Increased plasma levels with cimetidine. Very rare cases of serotonin syndrome (SS) have been reported with other drugs that have a recognized association with SS.

PREGNANCY: Category C, not for use in nursing.

MECHANISM OF ACTION: Dibenzocycloheptadiene derivative; suspected to inhibit the membrane pump mechanism responsible for uptake of norepinephrine and serotonin in adrenergic and serotonergic neurons.

PHARMACOKINETICS: Absorption: Rapid. **Distribution:** Excreted in breast milk; crosses the placenta. **Metabolism:** N-demethylation and hydroxylation.

NURSING CONSIDERATIONS

Assessment: Assess if acute recovery period after MI, for bipolar disorder risk, history of mania, paranoia, seizures, unrecognized/history of schizophrenia, CVD, hyperthyroidism, IOP, narrow-angle glaucoma, urinary retention, hepatic impairment, hypersensitivity, pregnancy/nursing status, and possible drug interactions.

Monitoring: Periodically monitor LFTs, thyroid function tests, blood glucose, and CBC. Monitor for signs/symptoms of clinical worsening (suicidality, unusual changes in behavior), mania, cardiovascular events, increasing psychosis or paranoia, mydriasis, hypo/hyperglycemia, seizures, hepatic dysfunction, cognitive/motor impairment, and hypersensitivity reactions.

Patient Counseling: Advise to avoid alcohol. Seek medical attention for symptoms of mania, clinical worsening (suicidal ideation, unusual changes in behavior), cardiovascular events, increasing psychosis or paranoia, mydriasis, hypo/hyperglycemia, seizures, and discontinuation symptoms (irritability, agitation, dizziness, anxiety, headache, insomnia). Caution in engaging hazardous tasks (eg, driving automobile).

Administration: Oral route. **Storage:** 20-25°C (68-77°F). Dispense in tight, light-resistant container. Keep out the reach of children

AMNESTEEM

RX

isotretinoin (Genpharm)

Not for use by females who are or may become pregnant, or if breastfeeding. Birth defects have been documented. Increased risk of spontaneous abortion, and premature births reported. D/C if pregnancy does occur during treatment and refer to an obstetrician-gynecologist experienced in reproductive toxicity for evaluation and counseling. Approved for marketing only under special restricted distribution program called iPLEDGE™. Must have 2 negative pregnancy tests. Repeat pregnancy test monthly. Use 2 forms of contraception at least 1 month prior, during, and 1 month following discontinuation. Must fill written prescriptions within 7 days; refills require new prescriptions. Prescriber, dispensing pharmacy, and patient must be registered with iPLEDGE.

OTHER BRAND NAMES: Claravis (Barr) - Sotret (Ranbaxy)

THERAPEUTIC CLASS: Retinoid

INDICATIONS: Severe recalcitrant nodular acne unresponsive to conventional therapy, including systemic antibiotics in female patients who are not pregnant.

DOSAGE: *Adults:* Initial/Usual: 0.5-1mg/kg/day given bid for 15-20 weeks. Max: 2mg/kg/day (for very severe disease with scarring or primary trunk manifestation). Adjust for side effects and disease response. May d/c if nodule count reduced by >70% prior to completion. Repeat only if necessary after 2 months off drug. Take with food.
Pediatrics: ≥12 yrs: Initial/Usual: 0.5-1mg/kg/day given bid for 15-20 weeks. Max: 2mg/kg/day (for very severe disease with scarring or primary trunk manifestation). Adjust for side effects and disease response. May d/c if nodule count reduced by >70% prior to completion. Repeat only if necessary after 2 months off drug. Take with food.

HOW SUPPLIED: Cap: 10mg, 20mg, 40mg, (Claravis, Sortret) 30mg

CONTRAINDICATIONS: Pregnancy, paraben sensitivity (preservative in gelatin cap).

WARNINGS/PRECAUTIONS: Acute pancreatitis, impaired hearing, inflammatory bowel disease, elevated TG and LFTs, hepatotoxicity, premature epiphyseal closure, and hyperostosis reported. May cause depression, psychosis, aggressive and/or violent behaviors, rarely suicidal ideation/attempts and suicide; may need further evaluation after d/c. May cause decreased night vision, and corneal opacities. Associated with pseudotumor cerebri. Check lipids before therapy, and then at intervals until response established (within 4 weeks). D/C if significant decrease in WBC, hearing or visual impairment, abdominal pain, rectal bleeding, or severe diarrhea occurs. May develop musculoskeletal symptoms. Caution with genetic predisposition for age-related osteoporosis, history of childhood osteoporosis, osteomalacia, other bone metabolism disorders (eg, anorexia nervosa). Spontaneous osteoporosis, osteopenia, bone fractures, and delayed fracture healing reported; caution in sports with repetitive impact.

ADVERSE REACTIONS: Cheilitis, dry skin and mucous membranes, conjunctivitis, blood dyscrasias, epistaxis, decreased HDL, elevated cholesterol and TG, elevated blood sugar, arthralgias, back pain, hearing/vision impairment, rash, photosensitivity reactions, psychiatric disorders, abnormal menses, cardiovascular disorders.

INTERACTIONS: Avoid vitamin A. Limit alcohol consumption. Avoid use with tetracyclines; increased incidence of pseudotumor cerebri. Pregnancy reported with oral and injectable/implantable contraceptives. Avoid St. John's wort; may cause breakthrough bleeding with oral contraceptives. Caution with drugs that cause drug-induced osteoporosis/osteomalacia and affect vitamin D metabolism (eg, corticosteroids, phenytoin).

PREGNANCY: Category X, not for use in nursing.

MECHANISM OF ACTION: Retinoid; not established. Suspected to inhibit sebaceous gland function and keratinization.

PHARMACOKINETICS: Absorption: C_{max}=862ng/mL (fed), 301ng/mL (fasted); T_{max}=5.3 hrs (fed), 3.2 hrs (fasted); AUC=10,004ng•hr/mL (fed), 3703ng•hr/mL (fasted). **Distribution:** Plasma protein binding (99.9%). **Metabolism:** Liver via CYP2C8, 2C9, 3A4, and 2B6; 4-*oxo*-isotretinoin, retinoic acid, and 4-*oxo*-retinoic acid (active metabolites). **Elimination:** Urine, feces; $T_{1/2}$=21 hrs (isotretinoin), 24 hrs (4-*oxo*-isotretinoin).

NURSING CONSIDERATIONS

Assessment: Assess that females have had 2 negative pregnancy tests separated by at least 19 days, and are on 2 forms of effective contraception: A primary form (eg, tubal sterilization, partner's vasectomy, intrauterine device, or hormonal) and a secondary form (barrier, vaginal sponge) for at least 1 month prior to administration. Assess for hypersensitivity to parabens, history of psychiatric disorder, depression, risk of hyperlipidemia (eg, DM, obesity, increased alcohol intake, lipid metabolism disorder or family history of such disorder) possible drug interactions and nursing status. Obtain lipid levels profile and LFTs.

Monitoring: Monitor for signs/symptoms of psychiatric disorders (eg, depression, mood disturbances, psychosis, aggression, suicidal ideation), pseudotumor cerebri (eg, papilledema, headache, N/V, visual disturbances), hyperlipidemias (eg, elevated serum TG), acute pancreatitis, hearing impairment, hepatotoxicity, inflammatory bowel disease (regional ileitis), decreased bone mineral density, hyperostosis, premature epiphyseal closure, musculoskeletal symptoms (eg, arthralgia), neutropenia, agranulocytosis, hypersensitivity reactions, visual impairments, corneal opacities, and decreased night vision. Monitor lipid levels and LFTs (weekly or biweekly), glucose levels, and creatine phosphokinase levels until response to drug is established. Monitor that females remain on 2 forms of contraception during therapy and for 1 month following discontinuation.

Patient Counseling: Instruct to read the guidelines (Medication Guide/iPledge) and sign the Patient Information/Informed Consent form. For females of childbearing potential, instruct that 2 forms of contraception are required starting 1 month prior to initiation, during treatment, and for 1 month following discontinuation. Inform that monthly pregnancy tests are required before new prescription is issued. Counsel not to share drug with anyone and not to donate blood during therapy and 1 month following discontinuation. Instruct to take with a meal and swallow capsule with a full glass of liquid. Inform that transient flare of acne may occur when initiating treatment. Notify physician if signs of depression, mood disturbances, psychosis, or aggression occur. Avoid wax epilation and skin resurfacing procedures during therapy and for 6 months following; avoid prolonged exposure to UV rays or sunlight. Inform that decreased tolerance to contact lenses during and after therapy may occur. Inform that musculoskeletal symptoms, transient pain in chest, back pain in pediatrics, arthralgias, neutropenia, agranulocytosis, anaphylactic reactions, allergic vasculitis, purpura or extremities and extraneous involvement may occur.

Administration: Oral route. **Storage:** (Amnesteem) 15-30°C (59-86°F). (Claravis, Sortret) 20-25°C (68-77°F). Protect from light. Keep out of reach of children.

AMOXIL RX
amoxicillin (GlaxoSmithKline)

THERAPEUTIC CLASS: Semisynthetic ampicillin derivative

INDICATIONS: Treatment of infections of the ear, nose, throat, genitourinary tract (GU), skin and skin structure (SSSI), lower respiratory tract (LRTI); acute, uncomplicated gonorrhea due to susceptible (β-lactamase negative) strains of microorganisms. Combination therapy for *H.pylori* eradication to reduce the risk of duodenal ulcer recurrence.

DOSAGE: *Adults:* Ear/Nose/Throat/SSSI/GU: (Mild/Moderate) 500mg q12h or 250mg q8h. (Severe) 875mg q12h or 500mg q8h. LRTI: 875mg q12h or 500mg q8h. Continue for a minimum of 48 to 72 hrs beyond the time that patient becomes asymptomatic or evidence of bacterial eradication has been obtained. *Streptococcus pyogenes* infections: ≥10 days. Gonorrhea/Uncomplicated Anogenital/Urethral Infections: 3g as single dose. *H.pylori:* (Dual Therapy) 1g + 30mg lansoprazole, both tid x 14 days. (Triple Therapy) 1g + 30mg lansoprazole + 500mg clarithromycin, all q12h x 14 days. (Amoxicillin) GFR 10-30mL/min: 250-500mg q12h. GFR<10mL/min: 250-500mg q24h. Hemodialysis: 250-500mg q24h, additional dose during and at end of dialysis. Refer to PI for more information.

Pediatrics: Neonates: ≤12 weeks: Max: 30mg/kg/day divided q12h. >3 months: Ear/Nose/Throat/SSSI/GU: (Mild/Moderate) 25mg/kg/day given in divided doses q12h or 20mg/kg/day given in divided doses q8h. (Severe): 45mg/kg/day given in divided doses q12h or 40mg/kg/day given in divided doses q8h. LRTI: 45mg/kg/day given in divided doses q12h or 40mg/kg/day given in divided doses q8h. Continue for a minimum of 48 to 72 hrs beyond the time that patient becomes asymptomatic or evidence of bacterial eradication has been obtained. *Streptococcus pyogenes* infections: ≥10 days. Gonorrhea/Uncomplicated Anogenital/Urethral Infections: (Prepubertal) 50mg/kg with 25mg/kg probenecid as single dose (not for <2 yrs). >40kg: Dose as adult.

HOW SUPPLIED: (Amoxil) Cap: 500mg; Sus: 50mg/mL [30mL], 250mg/5mL [100mL, 150mL], 400mg/5mL [100mL]. (Generic) Cap: 250mg, 500mg; Sus: 125mg/5mL [80mL, 100mL, 150mL], 200mg/5mL [50mL, 75mL, 100mL], 250mg/5mL [80mL, 100mL, 150mL], 400mg/5mL [50mL, 75mL, 100mL]; Tab: 500mg, 875mg; Tab, Chewable: 125mg, 200mg, 250mg, 400mg

WARNINGS/PRECAUTIONS: Serious, fatal, hypersensitivity reactions reported with penicillin (PCN) therapy; d/c and treat accordingly. *Clostridium difficile*-associated diarrhea (CDAD) ranging from mild diarrhea to fatal colitis reported; d/c and treat accordingly. May develop superinfection with mycotic or bacterial pathogens; d/c if superinfection occurs. Erythematosus rash may develop; avoid use in patients with mononucleosis. Increases risk of the development of drug-resistant bacteria when used prophylactically or in the absence of bacterial infection. Perform periodic assessment of renal, hepatic, and hematopoietic function with prolonged use. Perform a serologic test for syphilis in all patients with gonorrhea at time of diagnosis, and a follow-up serologic test 3 months after therapy. High urine concentrations of amoxicillin may result in false-positive urinary glucose tests; glucose-tests based on enzymatic glucose oxidase reactions may be used. May cause a transient decrease in plasma concentrations of total conjugated estriol, estriol-glucuronide, conjugated estrone, and estradiol in pregnancy. Caution in elderly. The 200mg and 400mg chewable tabs contain phenylalanine.

ADVERSE REACTIONS: N/V, diarrhea, black hairy tongue, pseudomembranous colitis, hypersensitivity reactions, blood dyscrasias, hepatic dysfunction, tooth discoloration.

INTERACTIONS: Probenecid decreases renal tubular secretion of amoxicillin. Increased and prolonged levels with probenecid. Abnormal prolongation of PT may occur when used concomitantly with oral anticoagulants; monitor PT and adjust dose appropriately. May reduce efficacy of combined oral estrogen/progesterone contraceptives. Chloramphenicol, macrolides, sulfonamides, tetracyclines may interfere with bactericidal effects.

PREGNANCY: Category B, caution in nursing.

MECHANISM OF ACTION: Ampicillin analog; has broad-spectrum bactericidal activity against susceptible organisms during active multiplication; acts through inhibition of biosynthesis of cell-wall mucopeptide.

PHARMACOKINETICS: Absorption: Rapid. Cap (250mg): T_{max}=1-2 hrs. C_{max}=3.5-5mcg/mL. Cap (500mg): T_{max}=1-2 hrs. C_{max}=5.5-7.5mcg/mL. Tab (875mg): C_{max}=13.8mcg/mL, AUC=35.4mcg•hr/mL. Oral suspension (400mg): C_{max}=5.92mcg/mL, AUC=17.1mcg•hr/mL. Chewable tab (400mg): C_{max}=5.18mcg/mL, AUC=17.9mcg•hr/mL. Oral suspension (125mg): T_{max}=1-2 hrs. C_{max}=1.5-3mcg/mL. Oral Suspension (250mg) T_{max}=1-2 hrs, C_{max}=3.5-5mcg/mL. **Distribution:** Plasma protein binding (20%). Found in breast milk. **Elimination:** Urine (60%, unchanged); $T_{1/2}$=61.3 min.

NURSING CONSIDERATIONS

Assessment: Assess for history of allergic reaction to PCNs, cephalosporins, or other allergens, infectious mononucleosis, phenylketonurics, pregnancy/nursing status, renal/hepatic function, hematopoietic function, and for possible drug interactions.

Monitoring: Monitor for serious anaphylactic reactions, erythematous skin rash, development of drug resistance or superinfection with mycotic or bacterial pathogen, signs/symptoms of CDAD (may range from mild diarrhea to fatal colitis). In patients on prolonged therapy, periodically monitor renal, hepatic, and hematopoietic function. Perform serologic test for syphilis at diagnosis of gonorrhea and after 3 months of treatment.

Patient Counseling: Inform drug treats bacterial, not viral, infections. Instruct to take exactly as directed; skipping doses or not completing full course may decrease effectiveness and increase likelihood that bacteria will develop resistance. Inform about potential benefits/risks; notify physician if watery/bloody diarrhea (with/without stomach cramps and fever) develop (may occur as late as 2 months after treatment). Notify if pregnant/nursing.

Administration: Oral route. Sus can be added to formula, milk, fruit juice, water, ginger ale or cold drinks; should be taken immediately. **Storage:** ≤20°C (68°F) for caps and (250mg) unreconstituted powder; ≤25°C (77°F) for un-reconstituted powder (200-400mg), chewable tabs, and tabs. Store in tight container. (Generic) Store at 20-25°C (68-77°F). Dispense in a tight, light-resistant container with a child-resistant closure.

AMPHOTEC   RX
amphotericin B cholesteryl sulfate (InterMune)

THERAPEUTIC CLASS: Polyene antifungal

INDICATIONS: Treatment of invasive aspergillosis in patients with renal impairment, unacceptable toxicity, or previous failure to amphotericin deoxycholate.

DOSAGE: *Adults:* Test Dose: Infuse small amount over 15-30 min. Treatment: 3-4mg/kg/day IV at 1mg/kg/hr.
Pediatrics: Test Dose: Infuse small amount over 15-30 min. Treatment: 3-4mg/kg/day IV at 1mg/kg/hr.

HOW SUPPLIED: Inj: 50mg, 100mg

WARNINGS/PRECAUTIONS: Anaphylaxis may occur. D/C if severe respiratory distress occurs. Acute reactions (eg, fever, shaking chills, hypotension, nausea, tachypnea) 1-3 hrs after starting infusion. Monitor renal/hepatic function, electrolytes, CBC, PT during therapy.

ADVERSE REACTIONS: Chills, fever, headache, hypotension, tachycardia, HTN, N/V, thrombocytopenia, increased creatinine, hypokalemia, dyspnea, hypoxia.

INTERACTIONS: Antineoplastics may potentiate renal toxicity, broncho-spasm, hypotension. Corticosteroids and corticotropin may potentiate hypokalemia. May increase flucytosine toxicity. Caution with imidazoles (eg, ketoconazole, clotrimazole, miconazole, fluconazole). Increased risk of renal toxicity with nephrotoxic drugs (eg, aminoglycosides, cyclosporine, pentamidine). May enhance curariform effect of skeletal muscle relaxants (eg, tubocurarine) or digitalis toxicity with hypokalemia.

PREGNANCY: Category B, not for use in nursing.

MECHANISM OF ACTION: Polyene antibiotic; binds to sterols (primarily ergosterol) in cell membranes of sensitive fungi, with subsequent leakage of intracellular contents and cell death. Also binds to cholesterol in mammalian cell membranes, which may account for human toxicity.

PHARMACOKINETICS: Administration: Variable doses resulted in altered parameters. **Absorption:** (3mg/kg/day) AUC=29µg/mL•hr, C_{max}=2.6µg/mL. (4mg/kg/day) AUC=36µg/mL•hr, C_{max}=2.9µg/mL. **Distribution:** (3mg/kg/day) V_d=3.8L/kg. (4mg/kg/day) V_d=4.1L/kg. **Metabolism:** Unknown. **Elimination:** (3mg/kg/day) $T_{1/2}$=27.5 hrs. (4mg/kg/day) $T_{1/2}$=28.2 hrs.

NURSING CONSIDERATIONS

Assessment: Assess cultures, renal function, and possible drug interactions.

Monitoring: Monitor for acute infusion reactions (fevers, chills, hypoxia, hypotension), hepatic function, serum electrolytes, CBC, PT, and possible drug interactions.

Patient Counseling: Seek medical attention if symptoms of acute reaction occur (fever, chills, respiratory symptoms).

Administration: IV route. Refer to PI for proper reconstitution and administration. **Storage:** Unopened Vial: 15-30°C (59-86°F). Store in unopened carton. Reconstituted: Refrigerate 2-8°C (36-46°F). Use within 24 hrs, do not freeze. Further diluted with 5% Dextrose: Refrigerate 2-8°C. Use within 24 hrs.

AMPHOTERICIN B

RX

amphotericin B (Various)

> Treatment primarily for progressive and potentially life-threatening fungal infections. Not for noninvasive fungal disease (eg, oral thrush, vaginal and esophageal candidiasis) in patients with normal neutrophil counts. Exercise caution to prevent inadvertent overdosage; verify product name and dose especially if dose >1.5mg/kg.

OTHER BRAND NAMES: Fungizone (Geneva)

THERAPEUTIC CLASS: Polyene antifungal

INDICATIONS: Treatment of progressive, potentially life-threatening fungal infections including aspergillosis, cryptococcosis, North American blastomycosis, systemic candidiasis, coccidioido-mycosis, histoplasmosis, zygomycosis including mucormycosis due to susceptible species of the genera (*Absidia, Mucor* and *Rhizopus*), sporotrichosis, and infections due to susceptible species of *Conidiobolus* and *Basidiobolus*. May be useful for treatment of American mucocutaneous leishmaniasis.

DOSAGE: *Adults:* Administer by slow IV infusion. Test Dose: 1mg in 20mL of D5W over 20-30 min. Treatment: Initial: 0.25mg/kg. Severe or Rapidly Progressive Infection: Initial: 0.3mg/kg. Give smaller initial dose if impaired cardio-renal function or severe reaction to test dose. Titrate: May increase by 5-10mg/day, depending on cardio-renal status, up to 0.5-0.7mg/kg/day. Max: 1mg/kg/day or 1.5mg/kg/day when given on alternate days. Sporotrichosis: Therapy has ranged up to 9 months with total dose up to 2.5g. Aspergillosis: Total dose up to 3.6g for 11 months. Rhinocerebral Phycomycosis: Cumulative dose of at least 3g is recommended. Whenever therapy is interrupted for >7 days, resume with lowest dose.

HOW SUPPLIED: Inj: 50mg

WARNINGS/PRECAUTIONS: Acute reactions (eg, fever, shaking chills, hypotension, anorexia, N/V, headache, tachypnea) 1-3 hrs after starting infusion may occur. Avoid rapid IV infusion; may cause hypotension, hypokalemia, arrhythmias and shock. Caution with renal impairment. Reduced risk of nephrotoxicity with hydration and sodium repletion before drug administration. Leukoencephalopathy reported.

ADVERSE REACTIONS: Fever, malaise, weight loss, hypotension, tachypnea, anorexia, N/V, diarrhea, dyspepsia, normochromic normocytic anemia, injection site pain, renal dysfunction, phlebitis, headache, azotemia.

INTERACTIONS: Antineoplastics (eg, nitrogen mustard) may potentiate renal toxicity, bronchospasm, hypotension; caution when coadministering. Corticosteroids and corticotropin may potentiate hypokalemia; monitor serum electrolytes and cardiac function during coadministration. May increase flucytosine toxicity. Caution with imidazoles (eg, ketoconazole, clotrimazole, miconazole, fluconazole), especially in immunocompromised patients. Increased risk of renal toxicity with nephrotoxic drugs (eg, aminoglycosides, cyclosporine, pentamidine). May enhance curariform effect of skeletal muscle relaxants (eg, tubocurarine) or digitalis toxicity with amphotericin B-induced hypokalemia. Acute pulmonary reactions reported with leukocyte transfusions; separate infusions and monitor pulmonary function.

PREGNANCY: Category B, not for use in nursing.

MECHANISM OF ACTION: Fungistatic or fungicidal; binds to sterols in cell membranes of susceptible fungi, resulting in change in membrane permeability, allowing leakage of intracellular components.

PHARMACOKINETICS: Absorption: C_{max} = approximately 0.5-2mcg/mL. **Distribution:** Plasma protein binding (>90%). **Elimination:** Renal excretion. Urine (approximately 40%); $T_{1/2}$= approximately 15 days.

NURSING CONSIDERATIONS

Assessment: Assess cultures, renal function, hematological effects (normocytic anemia), hepatic function, nursing status and possible drug interactions.

Monitoring: Monitor for signs/symptoms of acute reaction (fever, shaking, chills, hypotension, tachypnea), serum electrolytes (Mg^{2+}, K^+), liver function, frequent renal function tests, Hgb, CBC, pulmonary function. Monitor temperature, pulse, respiration, and BP every 30 min for 2-4 hrs after initial (test) dose.

Patient Counseling: Advise to seek medical attention if symptoms of acute reactions (fever, shaking, chills, respiratory symptoms) occur. Maintain adequate hydration.

Administration: IV route. Observe aseptic technique strictly in all handling. 1) Reconstitute (add 10mL of Sterile Water for Inj, USP into vial). 2) Shake vial until sol is clear. 3) Dilute using 5% Dextrose Inj, USP. **Storage:** Refrigerate; protect against exposure to light. The concentrate may be stored in dark, at room temperature for 24 hrs or refrigerator for 1 week with minimal loss of potency and clarity. Discard unused material. Protect from light during administration.

AMPICILLIN INJECTION   RX

ampicillin sodium (Various)

THERAPEUTIC CLASS: Semisynthetic penicillin derivative

INDICATIONS: Treatment of respiratory tract, urinary tract, and GI infections, bacterial meningitis, septicemia, and endocarditis caused by susceptible strains of microorganisms.

DOSAGE: *Adults:* IM/IV: Respiratory Tract/Soft Tissues: ≥40kg: 250-500mg q6h. <40kg: 25-50mg/kg/day given q6-8h. GI/GU Tract Infections: ≥40kg: 500mg q6h. <40kg: 50mg/kg/day given q6-8h. Urethritis (Caused by *N.gonorrhoeae* in Males): 500mg q8-12h for 2 doses; may retreat if needed. Bacterial Meningitis: 150-200mg/kg/day given q3-4h. Septicemia: 150-200mg/kg/day IV for 3 days, continue with IM q3-4h. Treatment of all infections should be continued for a minimum of 48-72 hrs after becoming asymptomatic or evidence of bacterial eradication has been obtained. Treatment recommended for a minimum of 10 days for Group A β-hemolytic streptococci.
Pediatrics: Bacterial Meningitis: 150-200mg/kg/day given q3-4h. Septicemia: 150-200mg/kg/day IV for 3 days, continue with IM q3-4h. Treatment of all infections should be continued for a minimum of 48-72 hrs after becoming asymptomatic or evidence of bacterial eradication has been obtained. Treatment recommended for a minimum of 10 days for Group A β-hemolytic streptococci.

HOW SUPPLIED: Inj: 125mg, 250mg, 500mg, 1g, 2g, 10g

WARNINGS/PRECAUTIONS: Serious, sometimes fatal, hypersensitivity reactions reported; d/c if occurs. Prior to therapy, assess for previous hypesensitivity reactions to penicillins, cephalosporins, and other allergens. *Clostridium difficile*-associated diarrhea (CDAD) reported and may range from mild diarrhea to fatal colitis. D/C if superinfection develops. Avoid in infectious mononucleosis; skin rash reported. May increase risk of development of drug-resistant bacteria in the absence of proven or strongly suspected bacterial infection or a prophylactic indication. False-positive glucose reactions reported with Clinitest, Benedict's solution, or Fehling's solution. Perform periodic assessment of renal, hepatic, and hematopoietic function during prolonged therapy. Rapid direct IV administration may result in convulsive seizures.

ADVERSE REACTIONS: Skin rashes, urticaria, glossitis, N/V, diarrhea, stomatitis, enterocolitis, anemia, thrombocytopenia, eosinophilia, leukopenia, agranulocytosis.

INTERACTIONS: May delay excretion with probenecid. Increased incidence of skin rash with allopurinol.

PREGNANCY: Category B, caution in nursing.

MECHANISM OF ACTION: Penicillin derivative; bactericidal against penicillin-susceptible gram-positive organisms and many common gram-negative pathogens.

PHARMACOKINETICS: Distribution: Plasma protein binding (20%), found in breast milk. Penetrates to CSF and brain only if meninges are inflamed. **Elimination:** Urine (unchanged).

NURSING CONSIDERATIONS

Assessment: Assess for proper diagnosis, hypersensitivity to penicillins/cephalosporins or other allergens, infectious mononucleosis, pregnancy/nursing status, and for possible drug interactions.

Monitoring: Monitor for signs/symptoms of hypersensitivity reactions, CDAD, superinfection, and for skin rash. Perform periodic monitoring of renal, hepatic and hematopoietic function.

Patient Counseling: Inform that drug treats bacterial, not viral, infections. Instruct to take exactly as directed to prevent drug resistance. Instruct to notify physician if pregnant/nursing. Advise to contact physician if watery and bloody stools developed even after 2 or more months after therapy.

Administration: IM/IV routes. Administer within 1 hr after preparation. Administer IV slowly, over at least 10-15 min to avoid convulsive seizures. Refer to PI for information regarding dilution and storage instructions.

AMPICILLIN ORAL   RX
ampicillin (Various)

THERAPEUTIC CLASS: Semisynthetic penicillin derivative

INDICATIONS: Treatment of meningitis, and infections of genitourinary tract (GU) (including gonorrhea), respiratory tract, and GI tract caused by susceptible strains of microorganisms.

DOSAGE: *Adults:* GI/GU: 500mg qid in equally spaced doses. Gonorrhea: 3.5g single dose with 1g probenecid. Respiratory: 250mg qid in equally spaced doses. May need larger doses in chronic or severe infections. Treat hemolytic strains of streptococci for ≥10 days. Except for gonorrhea, continue therapy for a minimum of 48-72 hrs after patient becomes asymptomatic or evidence of bacterial eradication has been obtained.
Pediatrics: >20kg: GI/GU: 500mg qid in equally spaced doses. Gonorrhea: 3.5g single dose with 1g probenecid. Respiratory: 250mg qid in equally spaced doses. ≤20kg: GI/GU: 100mg/kg/day total qid, in equally divided and spaced doses. Respiratory: 50mg/kg/day total tid-qid, in equally divided and spaced doses. Do not exceed adult doses. May need larger doses in chronic or severe infections. Treat hemolytic strains of streptococci for ≥10 days. Except for gonorrhea, continue therapy for a minimum of 48-72 hrs after patient becomes asymptomatic or evidence of bacterial eradication has been obtained.

HOW SUPPLIED: Cap: 250mg, 500mg; Sus: 125mg/5mL, 250mg/5mL [100mL, 200mL]

CONTRAINDICATIONS: Infections caused by penicillinase-producing organisms.

WARNINGS/PRECAUTIONS: Serious and fatal hypersensitivity reactions reported with penicillin therapy; anaphylactoid reactions require immediate treatment with epinephrine, oxygen, IV steroids and airway management. Possible cross-sensitivity with cephalosporins. Pseudomembranous colitis reported; initiate therapeutic measures if diagnosed and consider d/c of treatment. Increased risk of developing drug-resistant bacteria in absence of proven/strongly suspected infection. Prolonged use may promote overgrowth of nonsusceptible organisms, including fungi. May develop superinfection; take appropriate measures. Give additional parenteral penicillin in patients with gonorrhea who also have syphilis. Treatment does not preclude the need for surgical procedures, particularly in staphylococcal infections. May cause false-positive reaction for urinary glucose using copper sulfate tests.

ADVERSE REACTIONS: Stomatitis, N/V, diarrhea, rash, SGOT elevation, agranulocytosis, anemia, eosinophilia, leukopenia, thrombocytopenia, thrombocytopenic purpura, hypersensitivity reactions.

INTERACTIONS: Increased risk of rash with allopurinol. Bacteriostatic antibiotics (eg, chloramphenicol, erythromycins, sulfonamides, or tetracyclines) may interfere with bactericidal activity. May increase breakthrough bleeding with oral contraceptives and decrease oral contraceptive effectiveness. Increased blood levels with probenecid.

PREGNANCY: Category B, not for use in nursing.

MECHANISM OF ACTION: Penicillin derivative; bactericidal against non-penicillinase-producing gram-positive and gram-negative organisms.

PHARMACOKINETICS: Absorption: Well-absorbed; (500mg Cap) C_{max}=3mcg/mL; (250mg Sus) C_{max}=2.3mcg/mL. **Distribution:** Plasma protein binding (20%); found in breast milk. **Elimination:** Urine (unchanged).

NURSING CONSIDERATIONS

Assessment: Assess for previous hypersensitivity reactions to penicillins, cephalosporins, or other allergens; a history of allergy, asthma, hay fever, or urticaria; pregnancy/nursing status, and possible drug interactions. Conduct susceptibility testing as guide to therapy. Assess for syphilis.

Monitoring: Monitor for hypersensitivity reactions, pseudomembranous colitis, and overgrowth of nonsusceptible organisms. Evaluate renal/hepatic/hematopoietic systems periodically with prolonged therapy. Upon completion, obtain cultures to determine organism eradication. Monitor for masked syphilis; perform follow-up serologic test for each month for 4 months for syphilis in patients without suspected lesions of syphilis.

Patient Counseling: Instruct to notify physician of history of hypersensitivity to penicillins, cephalosporins, or other allergens. Inform diabetics to consult with physician prior to changing diet or dosage of diabetic medication. Inform to take exactly as directed; skipping doses or not completing full course decreases effectiveness and increases bacterial resistance. D/C and notify physician if side effects occur. Inform that therapy only treats bacterial and not viral infections.

Administration: Oral route. Take at least 1/2 hr before or 2 hrs after meals with a full glass of water. Add water to suspension bottle in two portions and shake well after each addition. Refer to PI for directions for reconstitution. **Storage:** 20-25°C (68-77°F). Store reconstituted suspension in a refrigerator; discard unused portion after 14 days.

AMPYRA

RX

dalfampridine (Acorda)

THERAPEUTIC CLASS: Potassium channel blocker

INDICATIONS: Treatment to improve walking in patients with multiple sclerosis (MS).

DOSAGE: *Adults:* 10mg bid (approximately 12 hrs apart). Max recommended dose of 10mg bid should not be exceeded. Do not double dose or take extra if a dose is missed. Take whole; do not divide, crush, chew, or dissolve.

HOW SUPPLIED: Tab, Extended Release: 10mg

CONTRAINDICATIONS: History of seizure, and moderate or severe renal impairment.

WARNINGS/PRECAUTIONS: Increased incidence of seizures has been observed. D/C and do not restart if experience seizure while on treatment. The risk for seizures with mild renal impairment (CrCl 51-80mL/min) is unknown but dalfampridine plasma levels in these patients may approach those seen with 15mg bid, a dose that may increase the risk of seizures. CrCl should be estimated prior to initiating treatment.

ADVERSE REACTIONS: Seizures, urinary tract infection, insomnia, dizziness, headache, nausea, asthenia, multiple sclerosis relapse, paresthesia.

INTERACTIONS: Avoid use with other forms of 4-aminopyridine.

PREGNANCY: Category C, not use for nursing.

MECHANISM OF ACTION: Broad spectrum potassium channel blocker; therapeutic effect has not been fully elucidated. In animal studies it has been shown to increase conduction of action potentials in demyelinated axons through inhibition of potassium channels.

PHARMACOKINETICS: Absorption: Rapid and complete; relative bioavailability (96%); (Tab) C_{max}=17.3-21.6ng/mL (fasted) T_{max}=3-4 hrs (fasted). **Distribution:** V_d=2.6L/kg. **Metabolism:** CYP2E1 (major). **Elimination:** Urine (95.9%); feces (0.5%); $T_{1/2}$=5.2-6.5 hrs.

NURSING CONSIDERATIONS

Assessment: Assess for history of seizures, renal function, concomitant use of 4-aminopyridine, pregnancy/nursing status, and possible drug interactions. Obtain baseline CrCl.

Monitoring: Monitor for seizures, urinary tract infection, headache, dizziness and relapse of multiple sclerosis.

Patient Counseling: Inform patients that medication may cause seizures in a dose-dependent fashion, and that they must d/c use if experience a seizure. Instruct patients to take medication exactly as prescribed. Instruct to take tablet whole; do not crush, chew, or dissolve. Instruct not to take >2 tablets in a 24-hour period and to make sure that there is a 12-hour interval between doses.

Administration: Oral route. **Storage:** 25°C (77°F). Excursions permitted 15-30°C (59-86°F).

AMRIX   RX
cyclobenzaprine HCl (Cephalon)

THERAPEUTIC CLASS: Skeletal muscle relaxant (central acting)

INDICATIONS: Adjunct to rest and physical therapy to relieve muscle spasm associated with acute, painful musculoskeletal conditions. Use for only short periods of time (up to 2-3 weeks).

DOSAGE: *Adults:* Usual: 15mg qd. Titrate: May increase to 30mg qd if needed. Use for longer than 2-3 weeks not recommended.

HOW SUPPLIED: Cap, Extended-Release: 15mg, 30mg

CONTRAINDICATIONS: MAOI use during or within 14 days. Hyperpyretic crisis seizures and deaths associated with concomitant use of cyclobenzaprine (or drugs structurally similar to TCAs) and MAOIs reported. Acute recovery phase of myocardial infarction (MI), arrhythmias, heart block conduction disturbances, CHF, hyperthyroidism.

WARNINGS/PRECAUTIONS: Avoid in hepatic impairment and elderly patients. Caution with history of urinary retention, angle-closure glaucoma, increased intraocular pressure (IOP), and use of anticholinergic medication. May impair mental and/or physical performance.

ADVERSE REACTIONS: Drowsiness, dry mouth, dizziness, somnolence, headache.

INTERACTIONS: Contraindicated with MAOIs. Enhances effects of alcohol, barbiturates and other CNS depressants. TCAs may block antihypertensive action of guanethidine and similar compounds and may enhance seizure risk with tramadol.

PREGNANCY: Category B, caution in nursing.

MECHANISM OF ACTION: Skeletal muscle relaxant; acts primarily within the CNS at brain stem as opposed to spinal cord level, although overlapping action on the latter may contribute to its overall skeletal muscle relaxant activity; suggested to reduce tonic somatic motor activity influencing both gamma and α motor systems.

PHARMACOKINETICS: Absorption: C_{max}=8.3ng/mL, T_{max}=8.1 hrs, AUC=354.1ng•h/mL; see Full PI for more detailed information. **Metabolism:** Extensive; via CYP3A4, 1A2, and 2D6 through N-demethylation pathway. **Elimination:** Urine (glucuronides); $T_{1/2}$=33.4 hrs.

NURSING CONSIDERATIONS

Assessment: Assess for hepatic function, history of seizures, hyperthyroidism, urinary retention, angle-closure glaucoma, IOP, recent MI, arrhythmias, heart block, CHF, alcohol intake, pregnancy/nursing status, and possible drug interactions.

Monitoring: Monitor for cardiac arrhythmias, sinus tachycardia, MI, stroke, IOP, CBC, and LFTs.

Patient Counseling: Caution against performing hazardous tasks (eg, operating machinery/driving); avoid alcohol and other CNS depressants. Notify if pregnant/nursing.

Administration: Oral route; take at same time each day. **Storage:** 25°C (77°F); excursions permitted to 15-30°C (59-86°F); in tight, light-resistant container. Keep out of reach of children.

ANAGRELIDE HCl   RX
anagrelide HCl (Various)

OTHER BRAND NAMES: Agrylin (Shire)

THERAPEUTIC CLASS: Platelet-reducing agent

INDICATIONS: Treatment of thrombocythemia, secondary to myeloproliferative disorders, to reduce the elevated platelet count and the risk of thrombosis and to ameliorate associated symptoms (eg, thrombo-hemorrhagic events).

DOSAGE: *Adults:* Initial: 0.5mg qid or 1mg bid for ≥1 week. Moderate Hepatic Impairment: Initial: 0.5mg qd for ≥1 week. Titrate: Increase by no more than 0.5mg/day in any 1 week. Max: 10mg/day or 2.5mg/dose. Adjust to lowest effective dose to reduce and maintain platelets <600,000/μL. Monitor platelet counts q2 days during 1st week, then weekly thereafter until maintenance dose reached.
Pediatrics: Initial: 0.5mg qd-0.5mg qid. Titrate: Increase by no more than 0.5mg/day in any 1 week. Max: 10mg/day or 2.5mg/dose. Adjust to lowest effective dose to reduce and maintain platelets <600,000/μL. Monitor platelet counts q2 days during 1st week, then weekly thereafter until maintenance dose reached.

HOW SUPPLIED: Cap: 0.5mg, 1mg, (Agrylin) 0.5mg

CONTRAINDICATIONS: Severe hepatic impairment.

WARNINGS/PRECAUTIONS: Caution with known/suspected heart disease; may cause cardiovascular (CV) effects (eg, vasodilation, tachycardia, palpitations, and congestive heart failure [CHF]). Perform pretreatment CV exam and monitor during treatment. Caution with hepatic dysfunction; reduce dose in moderate hepatic impairment and monitor CV effects. Interstitial lung diseases reported. Monitor blood counts (Hgb, WBC) and renal function (SrCr, BUN). Cases of hepatotoxicity (eg, symptomatic ALT and AST elevations and elevation >3x ULN) reported; measure LFTs prior to and during therapy. Fall in standing BP accompanied by dizziness reported. Interruption of treatment may be followed by an increase in platelet count.

ADVERSE REACTIONS: Headache, palpitations, diarrhea, asthenia, edema, N/V, abdominal pain, dizziness, pain, dyspnea, flatulence, fever, peripheral edema, rash (including urticaria).

INTERACTIONS: Sucralfate may interfere with absorption. Exacerbated effects of products that inhibit cyclic adenosine monophosphate (AMP) phosphodiesterase (PDEIII) (eg, inotropes: milrinone, enoximone, amrinone, olprinone, cilostazol). Assess the potential risks and benefits of concomitant use with aspirin prior to coadministration, particularly in patients with a high risk profile for hemorrhage. Fluvoxamine and theophylline may adversely influence the clearance of drug.

PREGNANCY: Category C, not for use in nursing.

MECHANISM OF ACTION: Platelet-reducing agent; not established. Suspected to reduce platelet production resulting from a decrease in megakaryocyte hypermaturation. Inhibits cyclic AMP PDEIII. PDEIII inhibitors can also inhibit platelet aggregation.

PHARMACOKINETICS: Metabolism: RL603 and 3-hydroxy anagrelide (major metabolites). **Elimination:** Urine (>70%); $T_{1/2}$=1.3 hrs.

NURSING CONSIDERATIONS

Assessment: Assess cardiac/hepatic/renal function, pregnancy/nursing status, and for possible drug interactions. Assess for known/suspected heart disease. Measure blood count and BP prior to therapy.

Monitoring: Monitor for signs/symptoms of CV effects, thrombocytopenia, and interstitial lung diseases. Monitor platelet counts q2 days during 1st week of treatment and at least weekly thereafter until maint is reached. Periodically monitor blood counts, BP, cardiac/hepatic/renal function.

Patient Counseling: Instruct to notify physician if any CV effects develop. Advise that periodic laboratory tests will need to be performed while on therapy. Inform that platelet counts begin to respond within 7-14 days of therapy at the proper dosage. Instruct women of childbearing potential to avoid pregnancy and use contraception during therapy.

Administration: Oral route. **Storage:** 20-25°C (68-77°F). (Agrylin) 25°C (77°F); excursions permitted to 15-30°C (59-86°F). Store in light-resistant container.

ANAPROX DS

RX

naproxen sodium (Roche Labs)

> NSAIDs may cause an increased risk of serious cardiovascular thrombotic events, myocardial infarction (MI), stroke, and serious GI adverse events including bleeding, ulceration, and perforation of the stomach or intestines. Contraindicated for the treatment of perioperative pain in the setting of coronary artery bypass graft (CABG) surgery.

OTHER BRAND NAMES: Anaprox (Roche Labs)

THERAPEUTIC CLASS: NSAID

INDICATIONS: Relieves signs and symptoms of rheumatoid arthritis (RA), osteoarthritis (OA), ankylosing spondylitis (AS), juvenile arthritis (JA), tendinitis, bursitis, and acute gout. Management of pain and primary dysmenorrhea.

DOSAGE: *Adults:* RA/OA/AS: 275mg bid or 550mg bid. Acute Gout: 825mg followed by 275mg q8h. Pain/Dysmenorrhea/Tendinitis/Bursitis: 550mg followed by 550mg q12h or 275mg q6-8h prn. Max: 1375mg on Day 1, then 1100mg/day.

HOW SUPPLIED: (Anaprox) Tab: 275mg; (Anaprox DS) Tab: 550mg* *scored

CONTRAINDICATIONS: Asthma, urticaria, or other allergic-type reactions with aspirin (ASA) or other NSAIDs. Treatment of perioperative pain in the setting of CABG surgery.

WARNINGS/PRECAUTIONS: May lead to onset of new HTN or worsening of pre-existing HTN; monitor BP closely. Fluid retention, edema, and peripheral edema reported; caution with fluid retention, HTN, or heart failure. Renal papillary necrosis and other renal injury reported after long-term use. Not recommended for use with advanced renal disease; if therapy must be initiated, monitor renal function closely. Anaphylactoid reactions may occur. May cause serious skin adverse events (eg, exfoliative dermatitis, Stevens-Johnson syndrome, toxic epidermal necrolysis). Avoid in late pregnancy; may cause premature closure of ductus arteriosus. Not a substitute for corticosteroid or to treat corticosteroid insufficiency. Monitor for visual changes or disturbances. May cause elevations of LFTs; d/c if liver disease develops or systemic manifestations occur. Caution with high doses in chronic alcoholic liver disease and elderly. Anemia may occur with long-term use; monitor Hgb/Hct if signs or symptoms of anemia develop or if initial Hgb ≤10g. May inhibit platelet aggregation and prolong bleeding time; monitor with coagulation disorders. Caution with asthma and avoid with ASA-sensitive asthma.

ADVERSE REACTIONS: Edema, drowsiness, dizziness, constipation, heartburn, abdominal pain, nausea, headache, tinnitus, dyspnea, pruritus, skin eruptions, ecchymoses.

INTERACTIONS: Avoid other products containing naproxen. Potential for increased adverse effects with ASA. May reduce tubular secretion of methotrexate; monitor for toxicity. May diminish antihypertensive effect and potentiate renal disease with ACE inhibitors. May reduce natriuretic effect of furosemide and thiazides. May increase lithium levels; monitor for toxicity. Increase risk of GI bleeding with SSRIs, oral corticosteroids, and anticoagulants. Synergistic effects on GI bleeding with warfarin. Observe for dose adjustment with hydantoins, sulfonamides, or sulfonylureas. May reduce antihypertensive effects of propranolol and other β-blockers. Probenecid increases half-life significantly. Antacids (magnesium oxide or aluminum hydroxide) and sucralfate may delay absorption. May impair response of thiazides or loop diuretics.

PREGNANCY: Category C, not for use in nursing.

MECHANISM OF ACTION: NSAID; unknown, related to prostaglandin synthetase inhibition.

PHARMACOKINETICS: Absorption: Rapid and complete. Bioavailability (95%). T_{max}=1-2 hrs. **Distribution:** V_d=0.16 L/kg; plasma protein binding (>99%). **Metabolism:** Hepatic, metabolite (6-O-desmethyl naproxen). **Elimination:** Urine (95%), feces (≤3%), $T_{1/2}$=12-17 hrs.

NURSING CONSIDERATIONS

Assessment: Assess for history of asthma, CV disease (pre-existing HTN, CHF) or risk factors for disease, fluid retention, edema, CV thrombotic events, MI, stroke, CABG surgery, pregnancy status, risk factors for GI events (bleeding, ulceration, perforation), possible drug interactions, renal/hepatic dysfunction.

Monitoring: Monitor BP, CBC, LFTs, renal function, and chemistries periodically. Monitor for signs/symptoms of GI events (bleeding, ulceration, perforation), CV thrombotic events, CHF, HTN, anemia, salt depletion, renal/liver dysfunction.

Patient Counseling: Seek medical attention if symptoms of hepatotoxicity (eg, nausea, fatigue, pruritus), anaphylactic reaction (eg, difficulty breathing, swelling of face/throat), hypersensitivity reaction (eg, rash), CV events (eg, chest pain, SOB, weakness, slurring of speech), GI ulceration and bleeding (eg, epigastric pain, dyspepsia, melena, hematemesis), weight gain, or edema occur. Inform of pregnancy risks. Caution if drowsiness, dizziness, vertigo, or depression is experienced during therapy.

Administration: Oral route. **Storage:** 15-30°C (59-86°F) in well-closed containers.

ANCOBON RX
flucytosine (Valeant)

Extreme caution with renal dysfunction. Monitor hematologic, renal, and hepatic status closely.

THERAPEUTIC CLASS: 5-fluorocytosine antifungal

INDICATIONS: Treatment of septicemia, endocarditis, and urinary tract infections caused by *Candida*. Treatment of meningitis and pulmonary infection caused by *Cryptococcus*.

DOSAGE: *Adults:* 50-150mg/kg/day given q6h. Renal Impairment: Reduce initial dose. Take a few caps over 15 min to reduce N/V.

HOW SUPPLIED: Cap: 250mg, 500mg

WARNINGS/PRECAUTIONS: Caution with renal dysfunction and bone marrow depression. Bone marrow depression can be irreversible and fatal.

ADVERSE REACTIONS: Myocardial toxicity, chest pain, dyspnea, rash, pruritus, urticaria, photosensitivity, N/V, jaundice, renal failure, pyrexia, crystalluria, anemia, leukopenia, eosinophilia, thrombocytopenia, ataxia, hearing loss, neuropathy.

INTERACTIONS: Antagonized by cytosine. Drugs that impair glomerular filtration may prolong half-life. Antifungal synergism with polyene antibiotics (eg, amphotericin B).

PREGNANCY: Category C, not for use in nursing.

MECHANISM OF ACTION: Antifungal agent not established; metabolized to 5-fluorouracil by entering the fungal organism via cytosine permease. The 5-fluorouracil is then incorporated into the fungal RNA where it inhibits synthesis of both RNA and DNA, inhibiting fungal growth, leading to fungal death.

PHARMACOKINETICS: Administration: Absolute bioavailability (78%-89%); C_{max}=30-40µg/mL; T_{max}=2 hrs. **Distribution:** Penetrates blood-brain barrier. Clinically significant amounts found in CSF. **Metabolism:** α-fluoro-β-ureido-propionic acid (metabolite). **Elimination:** Renal; Urine (90%), feces (small amount); $T_{1/2}$=2.4-4.8 hrs.

NURSING CONSIDERATIONS

Assessment: Assess use with impaired renal function, history of bone marrow depression, or hematologic disease. Assess serum electrolytes and hematologic and renal function prior to treatment.

Monitoring: Monitor blood concentrations of drug in patients with renal impairment. Monitor hematologic (leukocyte and thrombocyte count) function, renal function (Jaffe reaction), and hepatic (alkaline phosphatase, SGOT, and SGPT) status.

Patient Counseling: Counsel to notify physician of all other medications being taken. Counsel females to avoid nursing. If N/V develops, divide dosage and administer over a 15-min period.

Administration: PO. **Storage:** 25°C (77°F); excursions permitted to 15-30°C (59-86°F).

ANDRODERM `CIII`
testosterone (Watson)

THERAPEUTIC CLASS: Androgen

INDICATIONS: Testosterone replacement therapy in men for conditions associated with a deficiency or absence of endogenous testosterone (eg, primary or secondary hypogonadism).

DOSAGE: *Adults:* Initial: 5mg/day. Maint: 2.5mg-7.5mg/day. Apply patch nightly to intact skin of back, abdomen, upper arm, or thigh. Rotate sites; avoid same site for 7 days. Do not apply to scrotum or oily, damaged, irritated areas. May apply two patches at same time.
Pediatrics: ≥15 yrs: Initial: 5mg/day. Maint: 2.5mg-7.5mg/day. Apply patch nightly to intact skin of back, abdomen, upper arm, or thigh. Rotate sites; avoid same site for 7 days. Do not apply to scrotum or oily, damaged, irritated areas. May apply two patches at same time.

HOW SUPPLIED: Patch: 2.5mg/24 hrs [60ˢ], 5mg/24 hrs [30ˢ]

CONTRAINDICATIONS: Breast or known or suspected prostate cancer in men. Women.

WARNINGS/PRECAUTIONS: Prolonged use or high doses of orally active androgens are associated with serious hepatic effects (eg, peliosis hepatis, cholestatic jaundice, hepatic neoplasms). Increased risk for prostatic hyperplasia/carcinoma in elderly. Risk of edema with pre-existing cardiac, renal, or hepatic disease; d/c if edema occurs and may require diuretic therapy. Gynecomastia may develop. Risk of virilization, changes in body hair distribution, and increase in acne reported in female sexual partner. Monitor LFTs, Hgb, Hct, prostate specific antigen (PSA), cholesterol, lipids. May decrease thyroxine-binding globulin leading to changes in T_3 and T_4 levels. Skin burns reported at patch site during magnetic resonance imaging (MRI) scan; prior removal of patch is recommended.

ADVERSE REACTIONS: Gynecomastia, pruritus/erythema/vesicles/blister/burning/induration at application site, prostate abnormalities, headache, depression.

INTERACTIONS: Decrease oral anticoagulant requirement with concomitant use. Coadministration may elevate serum levels of oxyphenbutazole. May decrease blood glucose and, therefore, insulin requirements in diabetics. Pretreatment with ointment formulations (eg, 0.1% triamcinolone acetonide) may reduce testosterone absorption.

PREGNANCY: Category X, not for use in nursing.

MECHANISM OF ACTION: Endogenous androgen; delivers physiologic amounts of testosterone producing circulating testosterone concentrations that approximate the normal circadian rhythm.

PHARMACOKINETICS: Absorption: C_{max}=753ng/dL; T_{max}=7.9 hrs. **Distribution:** Sex hormone-binding globulin and albumin binding. **Metabolism:** Liver; estradiol and dihydrotestosterone (major active metabolites). **Elimination:** (IM) Urine (90% glucuronide and sulfate conjugates), feces (6% unconjugated); $T_{1/2}$=71 min.

NURSING CONSIDERATIONS

Assessment: Assess for history of breast or prostate carcinoma, cardiac or renal/hepatic disease, hypersensitivity to components, pregnancy/nursing status of female partner, and possible drug interactions.

Monitoring: Periodically monitor Hgb, Hct, LFTs, PSA, cholesterol and HDL, and serum testosterone levels after initiation of therapy. Monitor for signs/symptoms of hypersensitivity reactions, edema with/without congestive heart failure, gynecomastia, prostatic hyperplasia/carcinoma in geriatrics.

Patient Counseling: Advise not to apply to the scrotum or over a bony prominence or any part of the body that could be subject to prolonged pressure during sleep or sitting. Instruct to contact physician if changes in body hair distribution, increase in acne, or other signs of virilization of female partner, too frequent or persistent erections, changes in skin color, ankle swelling, unexplained N/V, or hypersensitivity reactions occur. Instruct to use over-the-counter topical hydrocortisone cream after system removal in order to ameliorate mild skin irritation. Applying small amount of 0.1% triamcinolone acetonide cream to skin under the central drug reservoir of patch may reduce incidence and severity of skin irritation; ointment formulations should not be used. Counsel to remove patch before undergoing an MRI.

Administration: Transdermal patch system. Apply adhesive side of the system to a clean, dry area of the skin on the back, abdomen, upper arms, or thighs. Rotate application site with an interval of 7 days between applications to the same site. **Storage:** 25° (77°F); excursions permitted to 15-30°C (59-86°F). Do not store outside pouch provided.

ANDROGEL

CIII

testosterone (Abbott)

> Virilization reported in children secondarily exposed to testosterone gel. Children should avoid contact with unwashed or unclothed application sites in men using testosterone gel. Advise patients to strictly adhere to recommended use instructions.

THERAPEUTIC CLASS: Androgen

INDICATIONS: Replacement therapy in adult males for conditions associated with a deficiency or absence of endogenous testosterone (congenital/acquired primary hypogonadism or hypogonadotropic hypogonadism).

DOSAGE: *Adults:* Initial: Apply 5g qd, preferably in AM, to clean, dry, intact skin of shoulders and upper arms and/or abdomen. Titrate: May increase to 7.5g qd, then 10g qd if serum testosterone is below normal range. May decrease daily dose if serum testosterone exceeds normal range. D/C therapy if serum testosterone consistently exceeds the normal range at a daily dose of 5g.

HOW SUPPLIED: Gel: 1% [2.5g, 5g pkts; 75g pump]

CONTRAINDICATIONS: Known/suspected prostate carcinoma or breast carcinoma in men, women who are or may become pregnant, or nursing mothers. Hypersensitivity to alcohol or soy products.

WARNINGS/PRECAUTIONS: Patients with benign prostatic hyperplasia (BPH) may be at increased risk for worsening of signs/symptoms of BPH. May increase risk for prostate cancer; evaluate for prostate cancer prior to and during therapy. May increase prostate specific antigen (PSA) levels. May cause fetal harm. Suppression of spermatogenesis may occur at large doses. Rare reports of hepatocellular carcinoma with long-term therapy in high doses observed. Risk of edema with or without congestive heart failure (CHF) with pre-existing cardiac, renal, or hepatic disease. Gynecomastia may develop and may persist. May potentiate sleep apnea especially with obesity or chronic lung diseases. Increases in Hct and red blood cell mass may increase risk for thromboembolic events. Changes in serum lipid profile reported; adjust dose or d/c therapy if necessary. Caution in cancer patients at risk of hypercalcemia and associated hypercalciuria. Not indicated for use in women. Gel is flammable; avoid fire, flame, or smoking until the gel has dried.

ADVERSE REACTIONS: PSA increase, acne, application-site reactions, prostatic/urinary/testicular disorders, abnormal lab tests, headache, emotional lability, gynecomastia, HTN, nervousness, breast pain, asthenia, decreased libido.

INTERACTIONS: May decrease blood glucose and insulin requirements. May increase fluid retention with adrenocorticotropic hormone or corticosteroids. Changes in anticoagulant activity may occur; frequently monitor INR and PT in patients taking anticoagulants.

PREGNANCY: Category X, not for use in nursing.

MECHANISM OF ACTION: Androgen; responsible for normal growth and development of male sex organs and for maintenance of secondary sex characteristics.

PHARMACOKINETICS: Absorption: Systemic (10%). **Distribution:** Sex hormone-binding globulin (SHBG) binding (40%), albumin and plasma protein-binding (58%), unbound (2%). **Metabolism:** Estradiol and DHT (active metabolites). **Elimination:** (IM) Urine (90% glucuronic and sulfuric acid conjugates), feces (6% unconjugated); $T_{1/2}$=10-100 min.

NURSING CONSIDERATIONS

Assessment: Assess for conditions where treatment is contraindicated, BPH, cardiac or renal/hepatic disease, obesity, chronic lung disease, and for possible drug interactions.

Monitoring: Monitor for signs/symptoms of prostate carcinoma, edema with or without CHF, gynecomastia, sleep apnea, hepatocellular carcinoma, virilization, prostate cancer and worsening of BPH. Monitor Hct, Hgb, PSA, serum lipid profile, LFTs, and serum testosterone levels periodically. In cancer patients at risk for hypercalcemia, regularly monitor serum calcium levels.

Patient Counseling: Inform that men with known or suspected prostate/breast cancer should not use androgen therapy. Advise to report signs and symptoms of secondary exposure in children and women to the physician. Instruct to avoid contact with unwashed or unclothed application sites of men. Instruct to apply as directed; wash hands with soap and water after application, cover application site with clothing after gel dries, and wash application site with soap and water prior to direct skin-to-skin contact with others. Inform about possible adverse reactions. Advise to read Medication Guide before therapy and reread each time the prescription is renewed. Inform that drug is flammable. Keep out of reach of children. Inform about importance of adhering to all the recommended monitoring, to report changes in their state of health, and to wait 5 hrs before showering or swimming.

Administration: Topical route. Do not apply to genitals. Allow application site to dry prior to dressing. Wash hands with soap and water after application. Refer to PI for administration details and specific dosing guidelines using the multi-dose pump. **Storage:** 25°C (77°F); excursions permitted to 15-30°C (59-86°F).

ANGELIQ
drospirenone - estradiol (Bayer Healthcare)

RX

> Estrogens and progestins should not be used for prevention of cardiovascular disease or dementia. Increased risk of myocardial infarction (MI), stroke, invasive breast cancer, pulmonary embolism (PE), and deep vein thrombosis (DVT) in postmenopausal women (50-79 yrs of age) reported. Increased risk of developing probable dementia in postmenopausal women ≥65 yrs of age reported.

THERAPEUTIC CLASS: Estrogen/progestogen combination

INDICATIONS: Treatment of moderate to severe vasomotor symptoms and/or vulvar/vaginal atrophy associated with menopause.

DOSAGE: *Adults:* 1 tab qd. Re-evaluate after 3-6 months.

HOW SUPPLIED: Tab: (Drospirenone-Estradiol) 0.5mg-1mg

CONTRAINDICATIONS: Pregnancy, undiagnosed abnormal genital bleeding, breast cancer, estrogen-dependent neoplasia, DVT/PE, active or recent (eg, within past year) arterial thromboembolic disease (eg, stroke, MI), liver dysfunction or disease, renal insufficiency, adrenal insufficiency.

WARNINGS/PRECAUTIONS: Not for use in renal insufficiency, hepatic dysfunction, and adrenal insufficiency due to increased risk of hyperkalemia. May increase risk of cardiovascular events (eg, MI, stroke), venous thrombosis, and PE; d/c immediately if any of these events occur or are suspected. May increase risk of breast/endometrial cancer, and gallbladder disease. May lead to severe hypercalcemia with breast cancer and bone metastases; monitor and d/c if hypercalcemia occurs. Retinal vascular thrombosis reported; monitor and d/c if papilledema or retinal vascular lesions occur. May elevate BP; monitor at regular intervals. May cause elevations of plasma triglycerides with pre-existing hypertriglyceridemia. Caution with history of cholestatic jaundice associated with past estrogen use or with pregnancy; d/c with recurrence. May lead to increased thyroid-binding globulin levels; monitor thyroid function. May cause fluid retention; caution with cardiac/renal dysfunction. Caution with severe hypocalcemia. May increase risk of ovarian cancer. May exacerbate endometriosis, asthma, diabetes mellitus (DM), epilepsy, migraine, porphyria, systemic lupus erythematosus (SLE), and hepatic hemangiomas; use with caution.

ADVERSE REACTIONS: Abdominal pain, pain in extremity, back pain, flu syndrome, enlarged abdomen, headache, upper respiratory infection, sinusitis, breast pain, vaginal hemorrhage.

INTERACTIONS: CYP3A4 inducers (eg, St. John's wort, phenobarbital, carbamazepine, rifampin) may decrease levels which may decrease therapeutic effects and/or change uterine bleeding profile. CYP3A4 inhibitors (eg, erythromycin, clarithromycin, ketoconazole, itraconazole, ritonavir, grapefruit juice) may increase levels which may result in side effects. Increased risk of hyperkalemia with ACE inhibitors, angiotensin receptor blockers, NSAIDs, potassium-sparing diuretics, potassium supplements, and heparin.

PREGNANCY: Contraindicated in pregnancy, caution in nursing.

MECHANISM OF ACTION: Estrogen/progestogen combination. Estradiol: Binds to nuclear receptors in estrogen-responsive tissues. Modulates pituitary secretion of gonadotropins, leuteinizing hormone (LH) and follicle stimulating hormone (FSH), through negative feedback mechanism. Drospirenone (DRSP): Synthetic progestin and spironolactone analog with antimineralocorticoid activity. Possesses anti-androgenic activity. Counters estrogenic effects by decreasing number of nuclear estradiol receptors and suppressing epithelial DNA synthesis in endometrial tissue.

PHARMACOKINETICS: **Absorption:** DRSP: C_{max} =18.3ng/mL; T_{max} =1.0 hr; AUC_{0-24hr} =208ng•hr/mL. Absolute bioavailability (76-85%) Estradiol; C_{max} =43.8pg/mL; T_{max} =2.5 hrs; $AUC_{0-24 hr}$ =665pg•hr/mL. Estrone (metabolite): C_{max} =245pg/mL; T_{max} =4 hrs; $AUC_{(0-24 hr}$ =3814pg•hr/mL. **Distribution:** Estrogens and DRSP found in breast milk. DRSP: V_d =4.2L/kg, serum protein binding (97%). Estradiol: Sex hormone binding globulin (SHBG) (37%); albumin binding (61%). **Metabolism:** DRSP: Extensive; CYP3A4 (minor). Estradiol: Liver to estrone (metabolite); estriol (major urinary metabolite); enterohepatic recirculation via sulfate and glucuronide conjugation in the liver; biliary secretion of conjugates in the intestine; hydrolysis in the gut; reabsorption. **Elimination:** DRSP: Urine (38-47%, glucuronide and sulfate conjugates), feces (17-20%, glucuronide and sulfate conjugates); T$_{1/2}$=36-42 hrs. Estradiol: Urine. Estrone: Urine; T$_{1/2}$=23 hrs.

NURSING CONSIDERATIONS

Assessment: Assess for presence or history of breast cancer, estrogen dependent neoplasia, abnormal genital bleeding, active liver disease, and known/suspected pregnancy or any other conditions where treatment is cautioned or contraindicated. Assess use in patients undergoing surgeries associated with risk of thromboembolism, with prolonged immobilization, ≥65 yrs old, presence of hypothyroidism or hypocalcemia, and in nursing females. Assess for drug or lab interactions.

Monitoring: Monitor for signs/symptoms of CV disorders (eg, MI, stroke, venous thrombosis, PE), malignant neoplasms (eg, endometrial, breast, or ovarian cancer), dementia, gallbladder disease, cholestatic jaundice, hypercalcemia, visual abnormalities (eg, retinal vascular thrombosis), increased BP levels, fluid retention, hyponatremia, hypertriglyceridemia, hypothyroidism, exacerbation of endometriosis, and exacerbation of other conditions (eg, asthma, DM, epilepsy, migraines, porphyria, SLE, and hepatic hemangiomas). Periodically monitor BP levels, thyroid function in patients on thyroid hormone replacement therapy, serum potassium levels during first cycle of therapy in patients at risk for hyperkalemia. Perform proper diagnostic testing (eg, endometrial sampling) in patients with undiagnosed, persistent, or recurring vaginal bleeding. Perform annual breast exam (eg, mammography). Monitor use of therapy every 3-6 months.

Patient Counseling: Inform drug may increase risk for heart attack, stroke, breast cancer, blood clots, and dementia. Report any breast lumps, unusual vaginal bleeding, dizziness and faintness, changes in speech, severe headaches, chest pain, SOB, leg pains, changes in vision, or vomiting. Instruct to perform monthly breast exam.

Administration: Oral route. **Storage:** 25°C (77°F); excursions permitted to 15-30°C (59-86°F). Do not store above 30°C (86°F).

ANGIOMAX   RX
bivalirudin (The Medicines Company)

THERAPEUTIC CLASS: Thrombin inhibitor

INDICATIONS: Adjunct to aspirin for anticoagulation in patients with unstable angina undergoing percutaneous transluminal coronary angioplasty (PTCA) or percutaneous coronary intervention (PCI). Patients with, or at risk of, heparin-induced thrombocytopenia and thrombosis syndrome undergoing PCI.

DOSAGE: *Adults:* Initial: 0.75mg/kg IV bolus, then 1.75mg/kg/hr for duration of PCI procedure. Additional bolus of 0.3mg/kg can be given if needed based on ACT. Continuation of infusion for up to 4 hrs post-procedure is optional. After 4 hrs, if needed, an additional 0.2mg/kg/hr IV for up to 20 hrs may be initiated. Renal Impairment: CrCl <30mL/min: 1mg/kg/hr infusion. Hemodialysis: 0.25mg/kg/hr infusion. Reduction in bolus dose not necessary; monitor anticoagulation.

HOW SUPPLIED: Inj: 250mg

CONTRAINDICATIONS: Active major bleeding.

WARNINGS/PRECAUTIONS: Not for IM administration. Hemorrhage can occur at any site. D/C with unexplained symptoms, fall in BP or Hct. There is no known antidote to treatment, but can be hemodialyzable. Caution when used during brachytherapy procedures.

ADVERSE REACTIONS: Bleeding, back pain, pain, N/V, headache, hypotension, HTN, bradycardia, dyspepsia, urinary retention, insomnia, anxiety, abdominal pain, fever, nervousness.

INTERACTIONS: Increased risk of major bleed with heparin, warfarin, thrombolytics, glycoprotein IIb/IIIa inhibitors.

PREGNANCY: Category B, caution in nursing.

MECHANISM OF ACTION: Reversible direct thrombin inhibitor; inhibits thrombin by specifically binding to catalytic site and to anion-binding exosite of circulating and clot-bound thrombin.

PHARMACOKINETICS: Metabolism: Renal mechanisms and proteolytic cleavage. **Elimination:** Urine; $T_{1/2}$=25 min.

NURSING CONSIDERATIONS

Assessment: Assess for active major bleeding, renal impairment, and drug interactions. Assess use in patients with disease states associated with increased risk of bleeding.

Monitoring: Monitor for signs/symptoms of hemorrhage (eg, decreases in BP or Hct), and thrombus formation. For patients with renal impairment, monitor anticoagulant status.

Patient Counseling: Advise about increased risk of bleeding events and instruct to contact physician if any occur.

Administration: IV route. Not for IM administration. Reconstitute: 1) To each 250mg vial, add 5mL of sterile water for injection. 2) Gently swirl until all material is dissolved. Further dilute: 3) Use 500mL D5W or 0.9% NaCl for injection to yield a final concentration of 0.5mg/mL. 4) Infusion rate to be administered is adjusted according to patient's weight. During brachytherapy, maintain meticulous catheter technique (eg, frequent aspiration and flushing). **Storage:** 20-25°C (68-77°F); excursion permitted to 15-30°C. Do not freeze. Reconstituted: May be stored at 2-8°C for up to 24 hrs. Diluted preparation is stable at room temperature for up to 24 hrs.

ANSAID RX
flurbiprofen (Pharmacia & Upjohn)

> NSAIDs may cause an increased risk of serious cardiovascular (CV) thrombotic events, myocardial infarction (MI), stroke, and serious GI adverse events including bleeding, ulceration, and perforation of the stomach or intestines, which can be fatal. Contraindicated for the treatment of perioperative pain in the setting of coronary artery bypass graft (CABG) surgery.

THERAPEUTIC CLASS: NSAID

INDICATIONS: Relief of the signs and symptoms of rheumatoid arthritis (RA) or osteoarthritis (OA).

DOSAGE: *Adults:* Individualize dose. Initial: 200-300mg/day given bid, tid or qid. Max: 300mg/day or 100mg/dose.

HOW SUPPLIED: Tab: 50mg, 100mg

CONTRAINDICATIONS: ASA or other NSAID allergy that precipitates asthma, urticaria, or allergic reactions. Treatment of perioperative pain in the setting of CABG surgery.

WARNINGS/PRECAUTIONS: May lead to onset of new HTN or worsening of pre-existing HTN; monitor BP closely. Fluid retention and edema reported; caution with fluid retention or heart failure. Renal toxicity such as renal papillary necrosis and other renal injury reported after long-term use; caution with impaired renal function, heart failure, liver dysfunction, and the elderly. Not recommended for use with advanced renal disease; if therapy must be initiated, monitor renal function. Anaphylactoid reactions may occur; avoid with patients with the aspirin triad (symptom complex of rhinitis with or without nasal polyps and bronchospasm after taking ASA or other NSAIDs). Avoid in late pregnancy; may cause premature closure of ductus arteriosus. Not a substitute for corticosteroids or for the treatment of corticosteroid insufficiency. May cause elevations of LFTs; d/c if liver disease develops or systemic manifestations occur. Anemia may occur; monitor Hgb/Hct with long-term use. May inhibit platelet aggregation and prolong bleeding time; monitor with coagulation disorders. Caution with asthma and avoid with ASA-sensitive asthma. Visual changes reported. May cause serious skin adverse events (eg, exfoliative dermatitis, Stevens-Johnson syndrome [SJS], toxic epidermal necrolysis [TEN]). Caution in elderly. Use lowest effective dose for the shortest duration.

ADVERSE REACTIONS: Cardiovascular thrombotic events, GI adverse events, dyspepsia, diarrhea, abdominal pain, constipation, headache, nausea, edema, elevation of LFTs.

INTERACTIONS: May diminish antihypertensive effect of ACE inhibitors. Increased risk of GI bleeding with anticoagulants (eg, warfarin), smoking, alcohol and oral corticosteroid. Concomitant ASA is not recommended due to increased adverse effects. May decrease hypotensive effects of β-blockers (eg, propranolol). May decrease natriuretic effects of furosemide and thiazides diuretics; may interfere with effects of K$^+$-sparing diuretics. May elevate plasma lithium levels; observe for signs of lithium toxicity. Could enhance the toxicity of methotrexate. Impaired response to thiazides and loop diuretics. ACE inhibitors and diuretics may increase the risk of overt renal decompensation. Reduced rate of absorption with antacids in geriatrics. Increased levels with cimetidine. Slightly reduced blood sugar concentrations with hypoglycemic agents.

PREGNANCY: Category C, not for use in nursing.

MECHANISM OF ACTION: NSAID; has not been established, related to prostaglandin synthetase inhibition and exerts anti-inflammatory, analgesic, and antipyretic actions.

PHARMACOKINETICS: Absorption: Rapid; bioavailability (96%); T_{max}=2 hrs, C_{max}=14Tg/mL, AUC=83Tg•h/mL. **Distribution:** V_d=0.12L/kg; plasma protein binding (>99%); found in breast milk. **Metabolism:** CYP2C9. 4'-hydroxy-flurbiprofen (major metabolite). **Elimination:** Urine (<3% unchanged) (70% parent drug and metabolites); $T_{1/2}$=4.7 hrs (R-flurbiprofen), 5.7 hrs (S-flurbiprofen).

NURSING CONSIDERATIONS

Assessment: Assess BP, CBC, and coagulation profile. Assess for pre-existing HTN, CHF, CVD, history of ulcer disease or GI bleeding, smoking, alcohol use, renal/hepatic impairment, fluid retention, pre-existing asthma, coagulation disorders, pregnancy/nursing status, and possible drug interactions. Assess use in elderly, debilitated, and poor CYP2C9 metabolizers. Assess for contraindications.

Monitoring: Monitor for signs/symptoms of CV thrombotic events, BP, new onset or worsening of pre-existing HTN, GI events (eg, inflammation, bleeding, ulceration, perforation), fluid retention and edema, renal effects (eg, renal papillary necrosis), hepatic effects (eg, jaundice, liver necrosis, liver failure), anaphylactoid reactions, skin reactions (eg, exfoliative dermatitis, SJS, TEN), hematological effects (eg, anemia, prolongation of bleeding time), visual changes, and for bronchospasm. Perform periodic monitoring of CBC, chemistry profile, renal function, and LFTs. Perform ophthalmologic exams if patient has eye complaints.

Patient Counseling: Counsel about risks and benefits of therapy. Counsel that therapy may cause CV (eg, MI or stroke), GI (ulcers, bleeding), and skin side effects (eg, exfoliative dermatitis, SJS, TEN); counsel patient of the signs/symptoms and advise to seek medical attention if any occur. Advise to report any signs/symptoms of unexplained weight gain or edema to physician. Inform about the warning signs/symptoms of hepatotoxicity (eg, nausea, fatigue, lethargy, pruritus, jaundice, right upper quadrant tenderness, flu-like symptoms) and anaphylactoid reactions (eg, difficulty breathing, swelling of face/throat); seek immediate medical therapy. Advise to take as prescribed. Advise pregnant women to avoid medication especially late in pregnancy.

Administration: Oral route. **Storage:** 20-25°C (68-77°F).

ANTARA   RX
fenofibrate (Oscient)

THERAPEUTIC CLASS: Fibric acid derivative

INDICATIONS: Adjunct to diet, to reduce elevated LDL-C, Total-C, TG, Apo B, and to increase HDL-C in adult patients with primary hypercholesterolemia or mixed dyslipidemia (Fredrickson Types IIa and IIb). Adjunct to diet, for treatment of hypertriglyceridemia (Fredrickson Types IV and V hyperlipidemia) in adult patients.

DOSAGE: *Adults:* Hypercholesterolemia/Mixed Hyperlipidemia: Initial: 130mg qd. Hypertriglyceridemia: Initial: 43-130mg/day. Titrate: Adjust if needed after repeat lipid levels at 4-8 week intervals. Max: 130mg/day. Renal Dysfunction/Elderly: Initial: 43mg/day. Take without regard to meals.

HOW SUPPLIED: Cap: 43mg, 130mg

CONTRAINDICATIONS: Hepatic or severe renal dysfunction (including primary biliary cirrhosis), unexplained persistent hepatic function abnormality, pre-existing gallbladder disease.

WARNINGS/PRECAUTIONS: Hepatocellular, chronic active, and cholestatic hepatitis and cirrhosis (rare) reported. Increases in serum transaminases reported; monitor LFTs regularly; d/c if >3X ULN. May cause cholelithiasis; d/c if gallstones found. May cause myositis, myopathy, or rhabdomyolysis; d/c if myopathy/myositis is suspected or diagnosed or if markedly elevated CPK levels occur. Acute hypersensitivity reactions (rare) and pancreatitis reported. Pulmonary embolus (PE) and deep vein thrombosis (DVT) were observed. Decreased Hgb, Hct, WBCs, thrombocytopenia, and agranulocytosis reported; monitor CBC during first 12 months of therapy. Minimize dose in severe renal impairment. Caution in elderly. Prior to therapy, attempt to control lipid levels with appropriate diet, exercise, and weight loss in obese patients and attempt to control any medical problems (eg, diabetes mellitus [DM]), hypothyroidism) that are contributing to lipid abnormalities. Measure lipid levels prior to therapy and during initial treatment; d/c use if inadequate response after 2 months on maximum recommended dose of 130mg/day.

ADVERSE REACTIONS: Abdominal pain, back pain, headache, abnormal LFTs, respiratory disorder, increased AST,ALT, and creatinine phosphokinase.

INTERACTIONS: Caution with anticoagulants because may potentiate coumarin anticoagulants; reduce anticoagulant dose to maintain desirable INR and PT. Avoid HMG-CoA reductase inhibitors unless benefits outweigh risks. Bile acid sequestrants may impede absorption; take at least 1 hr before or 4-6 hrs after bile acid binding resin. Evaluate benefits/risks with immunosuppressants (eg, cyclosporine) and other nephrotoxic agents. Prior to therapy, d/c or change if possible, medications known to exacerbate hypertriglyceridemia (eg, beta-blockers, thiazides, estrogens). Caution with drugs that are substrates of CYP2C19, CYP2A6, or CYP2C9.

PREGNANCY: Category C, not for use in nursing.

MECHANISM OF ACTION: Fibric acid derivative; activates peroxisome proliferator activated receptor α (PPARα), increasing lipolysis and elimination of triglyceride-rich particles from plasma by activating lipoprotein lipase and reducing production of apoprotein C-III. Decreased triglycerides produces an alteration in the size and composition of LDL particles. LDL particles then have a greater affinity for cholesterol receptors and are catabolized rapidly. Activation of PPARα also induces an increase in the synthesis of apoproteins A-I, A-II, and HDL cholesterol. Also reduces serum acid uric levels in hyperuricemic and normal individuals by increasing the urinary excretion of uric acid.

PHARMACOKINETICS: Absorption: Well absorbed; T_{max}=4-8 hrs. **Distribution:** Plasma protein binding (99%). **Metabolism:** Rapid, via hydrolysis by esterases to fenofibric acid (active metabolite), conjugation. **Elimination:** Urine (60%), feces (25%); $T_{1/2}$=23 hrs.

NURSING CONSIDERATIONS

Assessment: Assess for renal/hepatic function or primary biliary cirrhosis, pre-existing gallbladder disease, pregnancy/nursing status, and for possible drug interactions. Prior to therapy, attempt to control serum lipids with appropriate diet, exercise, and weight loss in obese patients and attempt to control medical problems (eg, DM, hypothyroidism) that are contributing to lipid abnormalities. Measure lipid levels and LFTs prior to therapy.

Monitoring: Monitor for signs/symptoms of myositis, myopathy, and rhabdomyolysis; measure CPK levels if myopathy is suspected. Monitor for signs/symptoms of increases in serum transaminase levels, hepatocellular, chronic active and cholestatic hepatitis; perform periodic monitoring of LFTs. Monitor for signs/symptoms of venothromboembolic disease (eg, PE, DVT), pancreatitis, and for hypersensitivity reactions (eg, severe skin rashes). Monitor for hematological changes (eg, thrombocytopenia, agranulocytosis); perform periodic monitoring of blood counts. Monitor for signs/symptoms of cholelithiasis; perform gallbladder studies if cholelithiasis is suspected. Perform periodic monitoring of lipid levels.

Patient Counseling: Inform about risks/benefits of therapy. Counsel need to be on a lipid-lowering diet while on therapy. Inform that may be taken without regard to meals. Instruct to promptly report to physician any signs of myopathy (eg, unexplained muscle pain, weakness, or tenderness) particularly if accompanied by malaise and fever. Inform to notify physician if pregnant or nursing.

Administration: Oral route. **Storage:** 25°C (77°F); excursions permitted to 15-30°C (59-86°F).

ANZEMET   RX
dolasetron mesylate (Sanofi-Aventis)

THERAPEUTIC CLASS: 5-HT$_3$ receptor antagonist

INDICATIONS: (Inj) Prevention and treatment of postoperative nausea and/or vomiting (PONV) ≥2 yrs. (Tab) Prevention of N/V associated with moderately emetogenic cancer chemotherapy, including initial and repeat courses, and PONV ≥2 yrs.

DOSAGE: *Adults:* Prevention of Cancer Chemotherapy-Induced N/V: (Tab) 100mg PO within 1 hr before chemotherapy. Prevention/Treatment of PONV: (IV) 12.5mg as a single dose 15 min before cessation of anesthesia (prevention) or as soon as N/V presents (treatment). (Tab) 100mg PO within 2 hrs before surgery. Elderly: Start at low end of dosing range.
Pediatrics: 2-16 yrs: Prevention of Cancer Chemotherapy-Induced N/V: (Tab) 1.8mg/kg PO within 1 hr before chemotherapy. Max: 100mg. Prevention/Treatment of PONV: (IV) 0.35mg/kg as a single dose 15 min before cessation of anesthesia or as soon as N/V presents. Max: 12.5mg. May mix 1.2mg/kg inj in apple or apple-grape juice and administer orally within 2 hrs before surgery. Max: 100mg. (Tab) 1.2mg/kg PO within 2 hrs before surgery. Max: 100mg.

HOW SUPPLIED: Inj: 20mg/mL [12.5mg/0.625mL, 100mg/5mL, 500mg/25mL]; Tab: 50mg, 100mg

CONTRAINDICATIONS: (Inj) Prevention of N/V associated with initial and repeat courses of emetogenic cancer chemotherapy due to dose dependant QT prolongation in adults and pediatrics.

WARNINGS/PRECAUTIONS: May cause PR, QT, and QRS interval prolongation, 2nd and 3rd degree atrioventricular (AV) block, cardiac arrest, and serious ventricular arrhythmias; avoid in patients who have or may develop prolongation of cardiac conduction intervals, particularly QTc, including congenital long QT syndrome, hypokalemia, and hypomagnesemia, with complete heart block or those at risk and use caution with underlying structural heart disease, pre-existing conduction system abnormalities, sick sinus syndrome, atrial fibrillation (A-fib) with slow ventricular response, myocardial ischemia, and in elderly. Correct hypokalemia and hypomagnesemia prior to therapy. Caution in elderly.

ADVERSE REACTIONS: Headache, dizziness, pain. (Inj) Drowsiness, urinary retention. (Tab) Tachycardia, pruritus, bradycardia, hypotension, fatigue, diarrhea, dyspepsia, fever.

INTERACTIONS: Increased risk of prolongation of cardiac conduction intervals with diuretics having potential for inducing electrolyte abnormalities, antiarrhythmics or other QT, PR (eg, verapamil), and QRS (eg, flecainide, quinidine) interval prolonging drugs, and cumulative high-dose anthracycline therapy. Caution with drugs causing hypokalemia or hypomagnesemia. (Tab)

Increased levels with cimetidine. Decreased levels with rifampin. Caution with drugs used in chemotherapy and surgery. (IV) Decreased clearance with atenolol.

PREGNANCY: Category B, caution in nursing.

MECHANISM OF ACTION: 5-HT$_3$ receptor antagonist; releases serotonin from the enterochromaffin cells of the small intestine to activate 5-HT$_3$ receptors located on vagal efferents to initiate the vomiting reflex.

PHARMACOKINETICS: Absorption: (Inj) T$_{max}$=0.6 hr (metabolite). (Tab) Well-absorbed; absolute bioavailability (75%); T$_{max}$=1 hr (metabolite). **Distribution:** V$_d$=5.8L/kg (metabolite); plasma protein binding (69-77%) (metabolite). **Metabolism:** Complete. Reduction via carbonyl reductase to hydrodolasetron (major metabolite); CYP2D6 (hydroxylation); N-oxidation of hydrodolasetron via CYP3A and flavin monooxygenase. **Elimination:** (Inj) Urine (53%, unchanged hydrodolasetron), feces; T$_{1/2}$=<10 min, 7.3 hrs (metabolite). (Tab) Urine (61%, unchanged hydrodolasetron), feces; T$_{1/2}$=8.1 hrs (metabolite). Refer to PI for pharmacokinetic values (hydrodolasetron) in special and targeted patient population.

NURSING CONSIDERATIONS

Assessment: Assess for possibility of cardiac conduction interval prolongation, hypersensitivity to drug, pregnancy/nursing status, and possible drug interactions.

Monitoring: Monitor ECG changes especially with congestive heart failure (CHF), bradycardia, elderly and renally impaired patients. Monitor for Torsades de Pointes, heart block, ventricular arrhythmias, and cardiac arrest. Monitor serum electrolytes (K$^+$, Mg^{+2}).

Patient Counseling: Instruct to not exceed the recommended dose. Inform that drug may cause serious cardiac arrhythmias; avoid in patients having higher chances of developing QT prolongation and Torsades de Pointes or heart block. Instruct to contact physician immediately if patients perceive HR change, lightheadedness occur, or if they have syncopal episode.

Administration: IV/Oral route. (Inj) Infuse as rapidly as 30 sec or dilute in a compatible IV sol to 50mL and infuse over ≤15 min. Do not mix with other drugs. Flush the infusion line before and after administration. **Storage:** (Tab) 20-25°C (68-77°F). Protect from light. (Inj) 20-25°C (68-77°F); excursions permitted to 15-30°C (59-86°F). Diluted product may be kept for 24 hrs at room temperature or under refrigeration for 48 hrs. Diluted product with apple or apple-grape juice may be kept ≤2 hrs at room temperature before use. Protect from light.

APIDRA

insulin glulisine, rdna (Sanofi-Aventis)

RX

OTHER BRAND NAMES: Apidra Solostar (Sanofi-Aventis)

THERAPEUTIC CLASS: Insulin

INDICATIONS: Indicated to improve glycemic control in adults and children with diabetes mellitus (DM).

DOSAGE: *Adults:* Individualize dose. Usual requirement: 0.5-1 unit/kg/day. Inject SQ within 15 min before a meal or within 20 min after starting a meal. Rotate inj site (abdomen, thigh, or deltoid). May be administered IV under medical supervision. Use concentration of 0.05-1 U/mL in infusion systems using polyvinyl chloride (PVC) bags.
Pediatrics: ≥4 yrs: Individualize dose. Usual requirement: 0.5-1 unit/kg/day. Inject SQ within 15 min before a meal or within 20 min after starting a meal. Rotate inj site (abdomen, thigh, or deltoid). May be administered IV under medical supervision. Use concentration of 0.05-1 U/mL in infusion systems using polyvinyl chloride (PVC) bags.

HOW SUPPLIED: Inj: (Apidra) 100 U/mL [10mL vial, 3mL cartridge]; Pre-filled: (Apidra-Solostar) 100 U/mL [3mL pen]

CONTRAINDICATIONS: Episodes of hypoglycemia.

WARNINGS/PRECAUTIONS: Hypoglycemia and hypokalemia may occur; monitor glucose and potassium levels frequently. Rapid onset and short duration of action; follow dosage directions. Adjust dose if change in physical activity or usual meal plan. Whether using an external pump for SQ infusion or administering intravenously, do not dilute or mix with any other insulin. Caution when changing insulin strength, manufacturer, type, or species. Concomitant antidiabetic therapy may need adjustment. Severe, generalized allergy including anaphylaxis may occur.

ADVERSE REACTIONS: Allergic reactions, injection-site reactions, lipodystrophy, pruritus, rash, hypoglycemia, influenza, nasopharyngitis, urinary tract infection, arthralgia, HTN, headache, peripheral edema.

INTERACTIONS: Decreased effect with corticosteroids, danazol, niacin, diuretics, sympathomimetic agents (eg, epinephrine, albuterol, terbutaline), glucagon, isoniazid, phenothiazine derivatives, somatropin, thyroid hormones, estrogens, progestogens (eg, in oral contraceptives), protease inhibitors, and atypical antipsychotic medications (eg, olanzapine and clozapine). Increased effect with ACE inhibitors, MAOIs, oral antidiabetics, disopyramide, fibrates, fluoxetine, pentoxifylline, propoxyphene, salicylates, sulfonamide antibiotics, somatostatin analogs and pramlintide. Decreased or increased effect with β-blockers, clonidine, lithium salts, and alcohol. Pentamidine may cause hypoglycemia followed by hyperglycemia. β-blockers, clonidine, guanethidine, and reserpine may reduce or mask signs of hypoglycemia.

PREGNANCY: Category C, caution in nursing.

MECHANISM OF ACTION: Insulin glulisine (rDNA origin); lowers blood glucose by stimulating peripheral glucose uptake by skeletal muscle and fat and by inhibiting hepatic glucose production.

PHARMACOKINETICS: Absorption: C_{max}=83, 84μU/mL (0.15, 0.2 IU/kg); T_{max}=60, 100 min (0.15, 0.2 IU/kg); Absolute bioavailability, 70% (SQ). **Distribution:** V_d=13L. **Elimination:** Rapidly eliminated; $T_{1/2}$=42 min.

NURSING CONSIDERATIONS

Assessment: Assess FPG, HbA1c, renal function, LFTs, episodes of hyperglycemia, infections, alcohol consumption, exercise routines, pregnancy/nursing status, and possible drug interactions.

Monitoring: Monitor glucose and potassium levels, FPG, HbA$_{1c}$, hypokalemia, renal function, diabetic ketoacidosis, vision changes, lipodystrophy, allergic reactions. Monitor for signs of hypoglycemia (sweating, palpitations, seizures, disorientation, tremors).

Patient Counseling: Use only if the solution is clear and colorless with no visible particles. Do not dilute or mix with other insulins or solutions. Counsel about signs/symptoms of hypoglycemia, hyperglycemia, diabetic ketoacidosis, the importance of frequent monitoring of blood glucose levels, and the need for eating a balanced diet and exercising regularly. Advise to avoid excessive alcohol use. During periods of stress (eg, trauma, infection, surgery), insulin requirements may be changed; advise patients to seek prompt medical advice. Counsel on proper administration techniques.

Administration: SQ/ IV route. Refer to Full Prescribing Information for administration techniques. **Storage:** Unopened vial/cartridge/prefilled pen: 2-8°C (36-46°F). Open (in-use): 25°C (77°F). Discard after 28 days. Protect from light. Insulin exposed to temperatures >37°C (98°F) should be discarded.

APLENZIN   RX
buproprion hydrobromide (Sanofi-Aventis)

> Antidepressants increased the risk of suicidal thinking and behavior (suicidality) in short-term studies in children, adolescents, and young adults with major depressive disorder (MDD) and other psychiatric disorders. Monitor and observe closely for clinical worsening, suicidality, or unusual changes in behavior in patients who are started on antidepressant therapy. Bupropion is not approved for use in pediatric patients.

THERAPEUTIC CLASS: Aminoketone

INDICATIONS: Treatment of major depressive disorder (MDD).

DOSAGE: *Adults:* ≥18 yrs: Initial: 174mg qam. Titrate: May increase to 348mg qd on Day 4 if tolerated. Max: 522mg/day given as single dose if no clinical improvement after several weeks. Switching from Wellbutrin, Wellbutrin SR, or Wellbutrin XL: Give equivalent dose. 522mg bupropion HBr = 450mg bupropion HCl, 348mg bupropion HBr = 300mg bupropion HCl, 174mg bupropion HBr = 150mg bupropion HCl. Mild-Moderate Hepatic Cirrhosis/Renal Impairment: Reduce frequency and/or dose. Severe Hepatic Cirrhosis: Max: 174mg every other day.

HOW SUPPLIED: Tab, Extended-Release: 174mg, 348mg, 522mg

CONTRAINDICATIONS: Seizure disorder, bulimia or anorexia nervosa, within 14 days of MAOIs, other forms of bupropion, abrupt d/c of alcohol or sedatives (including benzodiazepines).

WARNINGS/PRECAUTIONS: May worsen depression and/or emergence of suicidal ideation and behavior; monitor closely. May precipitate manic episodes in bipolar disorder. Dose-related risk of seizures; d/c and do not restart if seizures occur. Extreme caution with history of seizures, cranial trauma, severe hepatic cirrhosis, concomitant medications that lower seizure threshold. Agitation, insomnia, psychosis, confusion and other neuropsychiatric signs reported. Caution with hepatic impairment (including mild to moderate hepatic cirrhosis). Anorexia/weight loss may occur. HTN reported; caution with recent history of myocardial infarction (MI) or unstable heart disease. Anaphylactoid/anaphylactic reactions reported; d/c if any occur.

ADVERSE REACTIONS: Dry mouth, nausea, insomnia, dizziness, pharyngitis, abdominal pain, agitation, anxiety, tremor, palpitation, tremor, sweating, tinnitus, myalgia.

INTERACTIONS: See Contraindications. Extreme caution with drugs that lower seizure threshold (eg, antidepressants, antipsychotics, theophylline, systemic steroids). Increased seizure risk with opioids, cocaine, or stimulant addiction, OTC stimulants or anorectics, oral hypoglycemics, insulin, excessive use or abrupt d/c of alcohol or sedatives. Caution with levodopa, amantadine, and drugs that are metabolized by CYP2D6 (eg, SSRIs, TCAs, antipsychotics, β-blockers, Class 1C antiarrhythmics); use low initial dose and gradually titrate. Monitor HTN with transdermal nicotine. Caution with CYP2B6 substrates or inhibitors (eg, orphenadrine, cyclophosphamide, thiotepa). Carbamazepine, phenytoin, cimetidine, and phenobarbital may induce metabolism of bupropion. Infrequently associated with hemorrhagic or thrombotic complications when used with warfarin. Minimize or avoid alcohol.

PREGNANCY: Category C, not for use in nursing.

MECHANISM OF ACTION: Aminoketone antidepressant; mechanism of action not established, presumed that action is mediated by noradrenergic and/or dopaminergic mechanisms.

PHARMACOKINETICS: Absorption: T_{max}=5 hrs. **Distribution:** Plasma protein binding (84%). **Metabolism:** Extensive to hydroxybupropion (CYP2B6) via hydroxylation; threohydrobupropion, erythrohydrobupropion via reduction of carbonyl group. **Elimination:** Urine (87%), feces (10%), (0.5% unchanged). $T_{1/2}$= 21 hrs, 24 hrs, 31 hrs, 50 hrs (bupropion, hydroxybupropion, erythrohydrobupropion, threohydrobupropion respectively).

NURSING CONSIDERATIONS

Assessment: Assess for history of seizures, bulimia/anorexia nervosa, LFTs, renal function tests, DM, head trauma, use of alcohol, opiate sedatives, history of MI or unstable heart disease, psychosis, mixed/manic eposodes. Note other diseases/conditions and drug therapies especially other bupropion products.

Monitoring: Monitor for clinical worsening, suicidality, or unusual changes in behavior, seizures, increased restlessness, agitation, anxiety, insomnia, neuropsychiatric signs/symptoms (eg, delusions, hallucinations, psychosis, concentration disturbances, paranoia, and confusion), weight loss, loss of appetite, arthralgia, myalgia, HTN, and fever with rash.

Patient Counseling: Advise families and caregivers of need for close observation of clinical worsening and suicidal risks. Avoid alcohol, sedatives, and

OTC drugs. Exercise caution while driving or operating machinery. Advise not to use in combination with other medications that contains the same active ingredient. Advise that something that looks like a tablet may appear in the stool; this is the non-absorbable empty shell that is eliminated from the body. D/C and do not restart if seizures are experienced while on treatment.

Administration: Oral route. Swallow whole; do not chew, divide or crush tablets. **Storage**: 25°C (77°F); excursions permitted to 15-30°C (59-86°F).

APOKYN RX
apomorphine HCl (Ipsen/Tercica)

THERAPEUTIC CLASS: Non-ergoline dopamine agonist

INDICATIONS: Acute, intermittent treatment of hypomobility, "off" episodes ("end-of-dose wearing off" and unpredictable "on/off" episodes) associated with advanced Parkinson's disease.

DOSAGE: Trimethobenzamide (300mg tid PO) should be started 3 days prior to the initial dose and continued at least during the first 2 months of therapy. *Adults:* Test Dose: 0.2mL (2mg) SQ to patients in an "off" state; closely monitor BP. If 0.2mL is tolerated but ineffective, give a 0.4mL (4mg) test dose at the next "off" period (no sooner than 2 hrs after the first test dose). If 0.4mL (4mg) is tolerated, initiate with a starting dose of 0.3mL (3mg) prn. If 0.4mL (4mg) is not tolerated, administer a 0.3mL (3mg) test dose at the next "off" period (no sooner than 2 hrs after the prior test dose). If 0.3mL (3mg) is tolerated, initiate with a starting dose of 0.2mL (2mg) prn. Titrate: Increase by 0.1mL (1mg) every few days, if needed; assess efficacy/tolerability. Do not give a second dose for an "off" period if the first was ineffective. Usual: 0.3-0.6mL (3-6mg) tid. Max: 0.6mL (6mg)/dose. Renal Impairment: Test Dose/Initial: 0.1mL SQ.

HOW SUPPLIED: Inj: 10mg/mL [3mL]

CONTRAINDICATIONS: Concomitant use with 5HT$_3$ antagonists (eg, ondansetron, granisetron, dolasetron, palonosetron, alosetron).

WARNINGS/PRECAUTIONS: Avoid IV administration; serious adverse events reported (thrombus formation and pulmonary embolism). Nausea, vomiting, syncope, symptomatic hypotension, falls, hallucinations, falling asleep during activities of daily living, coronary events (eg, angina, myocardial infarction (MI), cardiac arrest, sudden death) reported. May prolong QT interval; potential proarrhythmic effects; caution with drugs that prolong QT/QTc interval. May cause or worsen dyskinesias. Withdrawal-emergent hyperpyrexia and confusion reported with rapid dose reduction/withdrawal/changes in therapy. Fibrotic complications (eg, retroperitoneal fibrosis, pulmonary infiltrates, pleural effusion/thickening, cardiac valvulopathy) reported with ergot-derived dopaminergic agents. May cause priapism. Caution with hepatic/renal impairment, sulfite sensitivity, known cardiovascular and cerebrovascular disease. Compulsive behaviors (eg, intense urges to gamble, increased sexual urges) reported.

ADVERSE REACTIONS: Yawning, somnolence, dizziness, rhinorrhea, edema, chest pain, increased sweating, flushing, pallor, dyskinesia, postural hypotension, hallucination, N/V, confusion.

INTERACTIONS: See Contraindications. Antihypertensives and vasodilators may increase risk of hypotension, MI, serious pneumonia, falls, bone and joint injuries. Dopamine antagonists such as neuroleptics (eg, phenothiazines, butyrophenones, thioxanthenes) and metoclopramide may diminish effectiveness.

PREGNANCY: Category C, not for use in nursing.

MECHANISM OF ACTION: Non-ergoline dopamine agonist; not established, suspected to stimulate post-synaptic dopamine D$_2$-type receptors within the caudate-putamen in the brain.

PHARMACOKINETICS: Absorption: Rapid; T$_{max}$=10-60 min. **Distribution:** V$_d$=218L. **Metabolism:** Sulfation, N-demethylation, glucuronidation and oxidation. **Elimination:** T$_{1/2}$=40 min.

NURSING CONSIDERATIONS

Assessment: Assess for asthma, history of psychotic disorders, dyskinesia, sulfite, sensitivity, pregnancy/nursing status. Note other diseases/conditions and drug therapy. Obtain baseline BP (supine and standing), liver/renal function parameters.

Monitoring: Monitor for coronary or cerebral ischemia, QT/QTc interval, hypotension, syncope, hallucinations, dyskinesia (or exacerbation), hepatic/renal impairment, fibrotic complications, drug abuse, and compulsive behaviors (eg, pathological gambling, hypersexuality). Perform periodic skin examinations to monitor for melanomas.

Patient Counseling: Inform that medication is intended only for SQ and not IV use. Instruct to take as prescribed; advise patients and caregivers to read attached PI for detailed instructions on proper use. Instruct to rotate the injection site and observe proper aseptic technique. Inform of the potential for hallucination, psychotic-like behavior, sedating effects including somnolence, and the possibility of falling asleep. Advise not to drive a car or engage in any other potentially dangerous activities while on treatment. Instruct to notify physician if become pregnant or intend to become pregnant or breastfeed. Advise to avoid alcohol and exercise caution with concomitant antihypertensive medications and/or vasodilators and sedating medications.

Administration: SQ. **Storage:** Store at 25°C (77°F); excursions permitted to 15-30°C (59-86°F).

APRISO   RX
mesalamine (Salix)

THERAPEUTIC CLASS: 5-Aminosalicylic acid derivative

INDICATIONS: Maintenance of remission of ulcerative colitis in patients ≥18 yrs.

DOSAGE: *Adults:* 1.5g (4 caps) qam. Take with or without food.

HOW SUPPLIED: Cap, Extended Release: 0.375g

WARNINGS/PRECAUTIONS: Renal impairment, including minimal change nephropathy, acute and chronic interstitial nephritis, renal failure (rare), reported. Evaluate renal function prior to initiation of therapy and periodically while on therapy. Caution in patients with known renal dysfunction or a history of renal disease. D/C if acute intolerance syndrome occurs (eg, acute abdominal pain, cramping, bloody diarrhea). Caution with sulfasalazine hypersensitivity, in patients with liver disease, and in the elderly.

ADVERSE REACTIONS: Headache, diarrhea, upper abdominal pain, nausea, nasopharyngitis, influenza/influenza-like illness, sinusitis.

INTERACTIONS: Avoid coadministration with antacids.

PREGNANCY: Category B, caution in nursing.

MECHANISM OF ACTION: Anti-inflammatory agent; Has not been established. Suspected that 5-ASA diminishes inflammation by blocking production of arachidonic acid metabolites.

PHARMACOKINETICS: Absorption: T_{max}=4 hrs, C_{max}=2.1μg/mL, AUC_{0-24}=11μg*h/mL. AUC_{0-inf}= 14 μg*h/mL. **Distribution:** Plasma protein binding (43%). **Metabolism:** Liver and intestinal mucosa via N-acetyltransferase activity; N-acetyl-5-aminosalicylic acid (major metabolite). **Elimination:** $T_{1/2}$=9-10 hrs. Urine (2%, unchanged).

NURSING CONSIDERATIONS

Assessment: Assess for pre-existing renal/liver disease, hepatic/renal impairment, obtain baseline LFTs, creatinine, and blood cell counts.

Monitoring: Monitor LFTs, CrCl, and blood cell counts periodically. Monitor for acute intolerance syndrome, hypersensitivity, and allergic reactions.

Patient Counseling: Instruct not to take with antacids. Advise to seek medical consultation if ulcerative colitis symptoms worsen. Advise patients with phenylketonuria that each capsule contains aspartame.

Administration: Oral route. **Storage:** Store at 20-25°C (68-77°F); excursions permitted between 15-30°C (59-86°F).

APTIVUS   RX

tipranavir (Boehringer Ingelheim)

> Both fatal and nonfatal intracranial hemorrhage reported. Clinical hepatitis and hepatic decompensation, including some fatalities, have been reported. Extra vigilance needed in patients with chronic hepatitis B or hepatitis C coinfection due to increased risk of hepatotoxicity.

THERAPEUTIC CLASS: Protease inhibitor

INDICATIONS: Coadministered with ritonavir for combination antiretroviral treatment of HIV-1-infected patients who are treatment-experienced and have HIV-1 strains resistant to more than one protease inhibitor (PI).

DOSAGE: *Adults:* 500mg (two 250mg or 5mL) with 200mg ritonavir bid with or without food.
Pediatrics: 2-18 yrs: 14mg/kg with 6mg/kg ritonavir (or 375mg/m² with ritonavir 150mg/m²) bid. Max: 500mg with 200mg ritonavir bid. Intolerance or Toxicity: Decrease dose to 12mg/kg with 5mg/kg ritonavir (or 290mg/m² with ritonavir 115mg/m²) bid. May switch to oral solution if unable to swallow caps.

HOW SUPPLIED: Cap: 250mg; Sol: 100mg/mL

CONTRAINDICATIONS: Moderate or severe (Child-Pugh Class B and C) hepatic impairment. Coadministration with drugs that are highly dependent on CYP3A for clearance or are potent CYP3A inducers. Concomitant administration with amiodarone, bepridil, flecainide, propafenone, quinidine, rifampin, dihydroergotamine, ergonovine, ergotamine, methylergonovine, cisapride, St. John's wort, lovastatin, simvastatin, pimozide, oral midazolam, triazolam, alfuzosin, and sildenafil (for treatment of pulmonary arterial HTN).

WARNINGS/PRECAUTIONS: Must be coadministered with ritonavir. Not recommended for use in treatment-naive patients. Caution with mild hepatic impairment (Child-Pugh Class A) and/or with chronic hepatitis B or C coinfection; monitor LFTs prior to therapy and during therapy. D/C if signs and symptoms of clinical hepatitis develop. D/C if asymptomatic elevations in AST or ALT >10X the ULN or if asymptomatic elevations in AST or ALT between 5-10X the ULN and increases in total bilirubin >2.5X the ULN occur. Caution in patients at risk of increased bleeding from trauma, surgery, or other medical conditions. Reports of new-onset diabetes mellitus (DM), exacerbation of pre-existing DM, diabetic ketoacidosis, and hyperglycemia reported. Spontaneous bleeding may occur in patients with hemophilia type A and B and additional factor VIII may be required. Rash (eg, urticarial/maculopapular) and possible photosensitivity accompanied with joint pain/stiffness, throat tightness, generalized pruritus reported; d/c with severe rash. Increased total cholesterol and triglycerides (TG) reported; assess lipid levels prior to and during therapy. Caution with known sulfonamide allergy. Possible redistribution/accumulation of body fat. Immune reconstitution syndrome reported with combination therapy. Caution in elderly.

ADVERSE REACTIONS: Diarrhea, N/V, abdominal pain, pyrexia, fatigue, headache, cough, rash, anemia, weight loss, hypertriglyceridemia, bleeding, elevated transaminases.

INTERACTIONS: See Contraindications. Combination therapy with other PIs not recommended. Decreased levels of abacavir, atazanavir, didanosine, zidovudine, amprenavir, lopinavir, saquinavir, valproic acid, methadone, meperidine and omeprazole. Increased levels of fluoxetine, paroxetine, sertraline, atorvastatin, rosuvastatin, tadalafil, trazodone, desipramine, colchicine, bosentan, and salmeterol. Weigh risks/benefits with fluticasone; coadministration not recommended. Decreased levels with buprenorphine, naloxone, carbamazepine, phenobarbital, and phenytoin. Increased levels with fluconazole and enfuvirtide. Caution with itraconazole, ketoconazole, voriconazole, diltiazem, felodipine, nicardipine, nisoldipine, verapamil, disulfiram/metronidazole, fluticasone, cyclosporine, sirolimus, and tacrolimus. Starting dose of sildenafil should not exceed 25mg within 48 hours, tadalafil 10mg every

72 hours, and vardenafil 2.5mg every 72 hours. Decreased levels of ethinyl estradiol; use alternative forms of birth control. Dosage reduction needed for clarithromycin by 50% if CrCl 30-60mL/min and 75% if <30mL/min; concomitant rifabutin by 75%. Dose reduction and concentration monitoring for desipramine. Monitor glucose with glimepiride, glipizide, glyburide, pioglitazone, repaglinide, or tolbutamine. Caution with antiplatelet and anticoagulants; may increase risk of bleeding. Monitor INR with warfarin. Caution with parenteral midazolam; monitor for respiratory depression/prolonged sedation and consider dose adjustments. Caution with supplemental high doses of vitamin E; avoid with oral solution. See Prescribing Information for detailed information.

PREGNANCY: Category C, not for use in nursing.

MECHANISM OF ACTION: Protease inhibitor; inhibits processing of Gag and Gag-Pol polyproteins, preventing formation of mature virions.

PHARMACOKINETICS: Absorption: Tipranavir/Ritonavir: (female) C_{max}=94.8µM, T_{max}=2.9 hrs, AUC=851µM•h. (male) C_{max}=77.6µM, T_{max}=3.0 hrs, AUC=710µM•h. **Distribution:** Plasma protein binding (>99.9%). **Metabolism:** Liver via CYP3A4. **Elimination:** Feces (82.3%), urine (4.4%). Tipranavir/Ritonavir: (healthy) $T_{1/2}$=4.8 hrs. (HIV-infected) $T_{1/2}$=6.0 hrs. Refer to prescribing information for pediatric parameters by age.

NURSING CONSIDERATIONS

Assessment: Assess for hepatitis B or C infection, hepatic impairment, hemophilia, sulfonamide allergy, DM, pregnancy/nursing status, and possible drug interactions. Determine baseline LFTs and lipid levels.

Monitoring: Monitor for signs and symptoms of clinical hepatitis, severe skin reaction, DM, and bleeding. LFTs and lipid levels should be monitored periodically during treatment. Enroll patients in the Antiretroviral Pregnancy Registry if they become pregnant while on treatment.

Patient Counseling: Inform that therapy is not cure for HIV, does not reduce risk of transmission of HIV, and that opportunistic infections may develop. Instruct to notify physician if pregnant, planning to become pregnant, or if nursing. Advise to seek medical attention for symptoms of hepatitis (eg, fatigue, malaise, anorexia, nausea), bleeding, severe skin reaction, infections, and hyperglycemia. Advise to inform healthcare provider about all medications, including prescription or nonprescription medications (eg, St. John's wort) before initiating therapy. Report any history of sulfonamide allergy. Avoid vitamin E supplements. Instruct to use additional or alternative contraceptive measures for patients taking estrogen-based hormonal contraceptives. Inform that if a dose is missed, take dose as soon as possible and then return to normal schedule. Instruct not to double the next dose.

Administration: Oral route. **Storage:** Must be used within 60 days of opening. (Cap) 2-8°C (36-46°F) prior to opening the bottle. After opening store at 25°C (77°F); excursions permitted to 15-30°C (59-86°F). (Sol) 25°C (77°F); excursions permitted to 15-30°C (59-86°F); do not refrigerate or freeze.

ARANESP   RX
darbepoetin alfa (Amgen)

> Increased mortality, serious cardiovascular (CV) events and stroke in chronic renal failure (CRF) patients when administered to target Hgb levels of ≥13g/dL. Individualize dosing to achieve and maintain Hgb levels within range of 10-12g/dL. Shortened overall survival and/or increased risk of tumor progression or recurrence in patients with breast, non-small cell lung, head and neck, lymphoid, and cervical cancers. Use lowest dose needed to avoid RBC transfusions. Prescribers and hospitals must enroll in and comply with the ESA APPRISE Oncology Program to prescribe and/or dispense to patients with cancer. Use only for treatment of anemia due to concomitant myelosuppressive chemotherapy. Not indicated for patients receiving myelosuppressive therapy when anticipated outcome is cure. D/C following completion of chemotherapy course.

THERAPEUTIC CLASS: Erythropoiesis stimulator

INDICATIONS: Treatment of anemia associated with CRF, including patients on dialysis and patients not on dialysis. Treatment of anemia due to the effect of concomitantly administered chemotherapy in patients with metastatic, non-myeloid malignancies.

DOSAGE: *Adults:* CRF: Individualize dose. Initial: 0.45mcg/kg IV/SQ weekly or 0.75mcg/kg SQ once q2 weeks for patient not on dialysis. Titrate: Adjust to target Hgb 10-12g/dL. If Hgb increases >1g/dL in a 2-week period or is approaching 12g/dL, reduce dose by 25%. If Hgb continues to increase, hold dose until Hgb begins to decrease, and reinitiate at 25% below previous dose. Do not increase more than once monthly. If Hgb increases <1g/dL over 4 weeks, with adequate iron stores, increase dose by 25% of the previous dose. If Hgb of 10-12g/dL is not attained in 12 weeks, do not give higher dose and use the lowest dose to maintain Hgb at levels sufficient to avoid transfusion, evaluate for other causes of anemia, and monitor Hgb thereafter. Conversion from Epoetin Alfa: Base dose on weekly epoetin dose. Administer less frequently than Epoetin alfa. Refer to PI for further details. Malignancy: Initial: 2.25mcg/kg SQ weekly or 500mcg SQ once q3 weeks. Do not initiate therapy if Hgb ≥10g/dL. Titrate: If Hgb increases by >1g/dL in a 2-week period or if Hgb reaches a level to avoid tranfusion, decrease dose by 40% of the previous dose. If Hgb exceeds a level needed to avoid transfusion, hold dose until Hgb approaches a level where transfusions may be required. Reinitiate at 40% below previous dose. If given weekly and <1g/dL Hgb increase after 6 weeks, may increase up to 4.5mcg/kg. D/C after 8 weeks if no response or if transfusions are still required. D/C if chemotherapy course is completed. *Pediatrics:* ≥1 year: CRF: Conversion from Epoetin Alfa: Base dose on weekly epoetin dose. Administer less frequently than Epoetin alfa. Refer to PI for further details.

HOW SUPPLIED: Inj: Autoinjector/Prefilled Syringe: 25mcg/0.42mL, 40mcg/0.4mL, 60mcg/0.3mL, 100mcg/0.5mL, 150mcg/0.3mL, 200mcg/0.4mL, 300mcg/0.6mL, 500mcg/mL; SDV: 25mcg/mL, 40mcg/mL, 60mcg/mL, 100mcg/mL, 150mcg/0.75mL, 200mcg/mL, 300mcg/mL, 500mcg/mL.

CONTRAINDICATIONS: Uncontrolled HTN.

WARNINGS/PRECAUTIONS: May increase BP; monitor and control BP during therapy. Hypertensive encephalopathy and seizures reported in patients with CRF. Pure red cell aplasia and severe anemia (with or without other cytopenias), associated with neutralizing antibodies to erythropoietin reported; evaluate etiology if lack/loss of response with or without severe anemia and low reticulocyte count occur; test for presence of antibodies to erythropoietin; d/c permanently if antibody-mediated anemia develops. Rare reports of allergic reactions; permanently d/c if serious allergic or anaphylactic reaction occurs. Formulation with albumin may carry risk for transmission of viral diseases. Safety and efficacy not established in patients with underlying hematologic disease (eg, hemolytic anemia, sickle cell anemia, thalassemia, porphyria). May cause allergic reaction in latex sensitive individuals. Evaluate for causative factors if there is a lack of response or failure to maintain a Hgb response with doses given within the recommended dosing range; exclude or correct deficiencies of folic acid, iron, or vitamin B12. May need interval of 2-6 weeks between dose adjustment and response. CRF patients not on dialysis may be more responsive to the drug. Monitor BP and Hgb especially in CRF patients not on dialysis and during transitioning to dialysis. May reduce dialysis efficiency; may require adjustment in dialysis prescription. Monitor Hgb weekly until stabilized and maint dose established, and for at least 4 weeks after dose adjustment. Supplemental iron is recommended if ferritin is <100mcg/L or serum transferrin saturation is <20%.

ADVERSE REACTIONS: Infection, abdominal pain, muscle spasm, HTN, hypotension, headache, diarrhea, fatigue, edema, N/V, fever, constipation, cardiac arrhythmias, dizziness.

PREGNANCY: Category C, caution in nursing.

MECHANISM OF ACTION: Erythropoiesis stimulating protein; stimulates erythropoiesis (same mechanism as endogenous erythropoietin) in response to hypoxia. Erythropoietin interacts with progenitor stem cells to increase RBC production.

PHARMACOKINETICS: Absorption: Adults with CRF: (SQ) Slow. T_{max}=48 hrs. Adult with cancer: (6.75mcg/kg) T_{max}=71 hrs; (2.25mcg/kg) T_{max}=90 hrs. **Elimination:** (IV) $T_{1/2}$=21 hrs. (SQ): $T_{1/2}$=74 hrs.

NURSING CONSIDERATIONS

Assessment: Assess for uncontrolled HTN, latex allergy, underlying hematologic disease (eg, hemolytic anemia, sickle cell anemia, thalassemia, porphyria), and pregnancy/nursing status. Obtain baseline iron status.

Monitoring: Monitor for signs/symptoms of an allergic reactions especially in latex-sensitive patients, CV events, thromboembolic events, stroke, premonitory neurologic symptoms, pure red cell aplasia, severe anemia and iron status. In cancer patients, monitor for progression and recurrence of tumor. Monitor response to therapy; if lack/loss of response, exclude or correct folic acid, iron and Vitamin B12 deficiencies and evaluate for presence of antibodies. Monitor Hgb, BP, and iron status. In CRF, monitor renal function, electrolyte and fluid balance. In patient on dialysis, monitor dialysis efficiency.

Patient Counseling: Inform of increased risks of mortality, serious CV events, thromboembolic events and increased risk of tumor progression/recurrence. Advise of possible side effects of therapy. Counsel on importance of compliance with treatment, dietary and dialysis prescriptions and the importance of judicious monitoring of BP and Hgb concentrations.

Administration: Syringe/SDV: IV route, SQ route. Prefilled Autoinjector: SQ route. In patients on hemodialysis IV route is recommended. Autoinjectors are designed to administer full content and should be used only for patients who need full dose. Do not dilute. Do not use vial, prefilled syringe and autoinjector more than one time. Do not administer in conjunction with other solutions. **Storage:** 2-8°C (36-46°F). Do not freeze or shake. Protect from light.

ARAVA RX
leflunomide (Sanofi-Aventis)

> Avoid pregnancy during treatment or before completion of drug elimination procedure after treatment. Severe liver injury, including fatal liver failure, reported; not for use with pre-existing acute or chronic liver disease, or those with serum ALT >2X ULN before initiating treatment. Caution with other potentially hepatotoxic drugs. Monitor ALT levels at least monthly for 6 months after starting therapy, and thereafter q6-8 weeks. Interrupt therapy if ALT elevation >3X ULN; if leflunomide-induced, start cholestyramine washout and monitor liver tests weekly until normalized. If not leflunomide-induced, resume therapy.

THERAPEUTIC CLASS: Pyrimidine synthesis inhibitor

INDICATIONS: Treatment of active rheumatoid arthritis (RA) to reduce signs/symptoms, inhibit structural damage as evidenced by x-ray erosions and joint space narrowing, or to improve physical function in adults.

DOSAGE: *Adults:* LD: 100mg qd for 3 days. Maint: 20mg qd. If not tolerated, reduce to 10mg qd. Max: 20mg/day.

HOW SUPPLIED: Tab: 10mg, 20mg, 100mg

CONTRAINDICATIONS: Women who are or may become pregnant.

WARNINGS/PRECAUTIONS: May cause immunosuppression. Avoid with severe immunodeficiency, bone marrow dysplasia, severe, uncontrolled infections. May cause increased susceptibility to infections especially *Pneumocystis jiroveci* pneumonia (PCP), tuberculosis (TB), aspergillosis. Rare cases of pancytopenia, agranulocytosis, thrombocytopenia, Stevens-Johnson syndrome (SJS), and toxic epidermal necrolysis (TEN) reported. D/C if SJS or TEN occurs. Monitor WBCs, platelets, Hgb, Hct, LFTs (especially ALT) at baseline then monthly for 6 months, and q6-8 weeks thereafter. D/C with evidence of bone marrow suppression. Monitor for hematologic toxicity if switching to another anti-rheumatic agent with a known potential for hematologic suppression. May need drug elimination if serious toxicity (eg, hypersensitivity), serious infection, SJS, or TEN occurs. Interstitial lung disease reported. New onset or worsening pulmonary symptoms (eg, cough, dyspnea) with or without associated fever, may be a reason for d/c; consider wash-out procedures if d/c is necessary. Screen for latent TB infection with a tuberculin skin test prior to initiating therapy. Caution with renal impairment. Monitor for BP before start of therapy and periodically thereafter.

ADVERSE REACTIONS: Severe liver injury, diarrhea, respiratory infections, alopecia, headache, nausea, rash, HTN, abnormal liver enzymes, dyspepsia, bronchitis, abdominal/back/GI pain, joint disorder, dizziness.

INTERACTIONS: See Boxed Warning. Decreased levels with cholestyramine or activated charcoal. Increased levels with rifampin; caution with concomitant use. May increase levels of diclofenac, ibuprofen, or tolbutamide. Possible interaction with other NSAIDs. Increased risk of hepatotoxicity with concomitant methotrexate. Avoid vaccination with live vaccines. Increased INR when coadministered with warfarin (rare). Increased susceptibility to infections and increased risk of malignancy with concomitant immunosuppressant therapy.

PREGNANCY: Category X, not for use in nursing.

MECHANISM OF ACTION: Pyrimidine synthesis inhibitor; isoxazole immuno-modulatory agent. Inhibits dihydroorotate dehydrogenase and has antiproliferative activity.

PHARMACOKINETICS: Absorption: A77 1726 (M1) (major active metabolite): T_{max}=6-12 hrs. Oral administration of various doses led to different parameters. **Distribution:** (M1) V_{ss}=0.13L/kg; plasma protein binding (>99.3%). **Metabolism:** M1 (major active) and many minor metabolites. **Elimination:** Urine (43%), feces (48%). (M1) $T_{1/2}$=2 weeks.

NURSING CONSIDERATIONS

Assessment: Assess for severe immunodeficiency, bone marrow dysplasia, severe uncontrolled infections, hepatic/renal function, comorbid illnesses, latent TB infection, drug hypersensitivity, pregnancy/nursing status, and possible drug interactions. Obtain baseline BP, platelet, WBC count, Hgb, Hct, and ALT levels.

Monitoring: Monitor for signs/symptoms of immunosuppression and opportunistic infections (eg, PCP, TB, aspergillosis), sepsis, bone marrow suppression, pancytopenia, agranulocytosis, thrombocytopenia, severe liver injury, skin reactions (eg, SJS, TEN), interstitial lung disease, malignancy, new onset or worsening pulmonary symptoms, hypersensitivity. Monitor BP, platelets, WBC count, Hgb/Hct, and ALT levels monthly for 6 months and q6-8 weeks thereafter. Monitor for hematologic toxicity when switching to another antirheumatic agent with known potential for hematologic suppression. Monitor for bone marrow suppression monthly if used concomitantly with immunosuppressants.

Patient Counseling: Advise women of increased risks of having a child with birth defects if taking medication while pregnant or if become pregnant when medication has not been completely eliminated from body. Instruct women of childbearing potential to use reliable form of contraception while on therapy. Promptly inform physician if there is any possibility of pregnancy. Contact physician if develop any type of skin rash or mucous membrane lesions, hepatotoxicity (eg, unusual tiredness, abdominal pain or jaundice), pancytopenia (eg, easy bruising, bleeding, recurrent infections), and interstitial lung disease.

Administration: Oral route. **Storage:** 25°C (77°F); excursions permitted to 15-30°C (59-86°F). Protect from light.

ARCALYST   RX
rilonacept (Regeneron)

THERAPEUTIC CLASS: Interleukin-1 receptor antagonist

INDICATIONS: Treatment of Cryopyrin-Associated Periodic Syndromes (CAPS), including Familial Cold Autoinflammatory Syndrome (FCAS) and Muckle-Wells Syndrome (MWS) in adults and children ≥12 yrs.

DOSAGE: *Adults:* ≥18 yrs: LD: 320mg (two 160mg) SQ on same day at two different sites. Maint: 160mg SQ per week. Do not give more than once weekly. *Pediatrics:* 12-17 yrs: LD: 4.4mg/kg SQ. Max: 320mg as 1 or 2 SQ injections with max volume of 2mL. If initial dose is given as 2 injections, give on same day at two different sites. Maint: 2.2mg/kg/week. Max: 160mg. Do not give more than once weekly.

HOW SUPPLIED: Inj (powder): 220mg

WARNINGS/PRECAUTIONS: Increased risk of infection reported; d/c if serious infection develops. Do not initiate with active or chronic infection. Tuberculosis (TB) reactivation may occur. May increase risk of malignancies. Monitor for changes in lipid profiles. D/C if hypersensitivity reactions develop. Concomitant use of other Interleukin-1 blockers is not recommended due to potential for pharmacologic interactions.

ADVERSE REACTIONS: Injection site reactions, infection, upper respiratory tract infection, sinusitis, cough, hypoesthesia, nausea, diarrhea, stomach discomfort, urinary tract infection.

INTERACTIONS: Avoid live vaccines. Increased risk of serious infections with TNF inhibitors; concomitant use is not recommended. Caution when given with CYP450 substrates (eg, warfarin); may need dose adjustment.

PREGNANCY: Category C, caution in nursing.

MECHANISM OF ACTION: Interleukin-1 blocker; acts as a soluble decoy receptor by binding IL-1β and prevents its interaction with cell surface receptors.

NURSING CONSIDERATIONS

Assessment: Assess for active and chronic infection, hypersensitivity reactions, vaccination history, latent TB, infections, pregnancy/nursing status, and possible drug interactions.

Monitoring: Monitor for signs/symptoms of serious infection, changes in lipid profile, injection site reactions, malignancies and hypersensitivity reactions.

Patient Counseling: 1st injection should be performed under supervision of qualified healthcare professional. Instruct on aseptic reconstitution and injection technique and to reconstitute with preservative-free Sterile Water for Injection. Use puncture-resistant container to dispose of vials, needles and syringes; use properly and do not reuse. Inform that injection site reactions may occur; inform physician if persistent. Advise not to inject at swollen or red area. Advise to rotate injection sites. D/C if serious infections occur; contact healthcare professional if infections develop; do not initiate treatment if with chronic or active infections. Instruct not to take IL-1 blocking drug if taking drugs that blocks TNF. Concomitant use of IL-1 blockers (eg, anakinra) is not recommended. Inform physician of vaccination history .

Administration: SQ route. Refer to PI for reconstitution procedures. **Storage:** 2-8°C (36-46°F). Store inside original carton to protect from light. After reconstitution, may keep at room temperature, protect from light and use within 3 hrs of reconstitution. Discard unused portions and vial after single withdrawal of drug.

AREDIA   RX
pamidronate disodium (Novartis)

THERAPEUTIC CLASS: Bisphosphonate

INDICATIONS: Treatment of moderate to severe hypercalcemia of malignancy, with or without bone metastasis. Treatment of moderate to severe Paget's disease of the bone. Adjunct to standard antineoplastic therapy for treatment of osteolytic bone metastases of breast cancer and osteolytic lesions of multiple myeloma.

DOSAGE: *Adults:* Moderate Hypercalcemia: 60-90mg IV single dose over 2-24 hrs. Severe Hypercalcemia: 90mg IV single dose over 2-24 hrs. Retreatment: Minimum of 7 days should elapse before retreatment to allow for full response to initial dose. Paget's Disease: 30mg IV over 4 hrs for 3 consecutive days. Retreatment: When indicated, retreat at the dose of initial therapy. Osteolytic Bone Lesions of Multiple Myeloma: 90mg IV over 4 hrs once a month. Osteolytic Bone Metastases of Breast Cancer: 90mg IV over 2 hrs every 3-4 weeks. Max: 90mg/single dose for all indications. Give oral calcium and vitamin D supplementation to minimize hypocalcemia. Renal Dysfunction With Bone Metastases: Withhold dose if SrCr increases by 0.5mg/dL (normal baseline) or by 1mg/dL (abnormal baseline). Resume when SrCr returns to within 10% of baseline. Elderly: Start at low end of dosing range.

HOW SUPPLIED: Inj: 30mg, 90mg

WARNINGS/PRECAUTIONS: Associated with renal toxicity; assess SrCr prior to each treatment. Focal segmental glomerulosclerosis with or without nephrotic syndrome reported. Do not use during pregnancy; may cause fetal harm. Asymptomatic cases of hypophosphatemia, hypokalemia, hypomagnesemia, and hypocalcemia reported. Rare cases of symptomatic hypocalcemia (including tetany) reported. Increased risk of hypocalcemia in patients with previous thyroid surgery and hypoparathyroidism. Monitor serum calcium, electrolytes, phosphate, magnesium, CBC with differential, Hct/Hgb closely. Monitor for 2 weeks post-treatment if pre-existing anemia, leukopenia, or thrombocytopenia exists. Increased risk of renal adverse reactions with renal impairment. Avoid treatment of bone metastases in severe renal impairment. Osteonecrosis of the jaw (ONJ) reported in cancer patients; avoid invasive dental procedures. Severe and occasionally incapacitating bone, joint/and or muscle pain is reported. Do not mix with calcium-containing infusion solutions (eg, Ringer's solution); should be given in a single IV solution in line separate from all other drugs. Caution in elderly.

ADVERSE REACTIONS: Fever, infusion-site reaction, anorexia, constipation, dyspepsia, N/V, upper respiratory tract infection, leukopenia, uremia, hypocalcemia, hypokalemia, hypomagnesemia, hypophosphatemia, rhinitis, atrial fibrillation.

INTERACTIONS: Concurrent use with thalidomide increases risk of renal dysfunction in multiple myeloma. Caution with other potential nephrotoxic drugs.

PREGNANCY: Category D, caution in nursing.

MECHANISM OF ACTION: Bone resorption inhibitor; mechanism of antiresorptive action not established. Adsorbs to calcium phosphate crystals in bone and may directly block dissolution of this mineral component of bone. Inhibition of osteoclast activity contributes to inhibition of bone resorption.

PHARMACOKINETICS: Elimination: Urine (46% unchanged); $T_{1/2}$=28 hrs.

NURSING CONSIDERATIONS

Assessment: Assess for renal impairment, history of thyroid surgery, pregnancy/nursing status, and for possible drug interactions. Assess SrCr prior to each treatment. In cancer patients, obtain dental exam with preventive dentistry prior to treatment.

Monitoring: Monitor for signs/symptoms of hypocalcemia, hypophosphatemia, hypokalemia, hypomagnesemia, renal toxicity, osteonecrosis of the jaw, and for musculoskeletal pain. Monitor serum calcium, electrolytes, phosphate, magnesium, and CBC, differential, and Hct/Hgb.

Patient Counseling: Instruct women of child bearing potential, to avoid pregnancy during therapy. Inform cancer patients to maintain good oral hygiene and avoid invasive dental procedures during therapy. Inform that periodic laboratory monitoring is required during treatment.

Administration: IV route. Reconstitute. 1) Add 10mL of Sterile Water for Injection to each vial resulting in a solution of 30mg/10mL or 90mg/10mL. Do not mix with calcium-containing infusion solutions (eg, Ringer's solution); administer in single IV sol and line separate from all other drugs. **Storage**: Vial: Do not store above 30°C (86°F). Reconstituted: Refrigerate at 2-8°C (36-46°F) for up to 24 hrs.

ARGATROBAN   RX
argatroban (GlaxoSmithKline)

THERAPEUTIC CLASS: Direct thrombin inhibitor

INDICATIONS: Prophylaxis or treatment of thrombosis in heparin-induced thrombocytopenia (HIT). As an anticoagulant in patients with or at risk for HIT undergoing percutaneous coronary intervention (PCI).

DOSAGE: *Adults:* Thrombosis: D/C heparin and obtain baseline activated partial thromboplastintime (aPTT). Initial: 2mcg/kg/min IV. Check aPTT after 2 hrs. Titrate: Increase dose until aPTT is 1.5-3x initial baseline. Max: 10mcg/kg/min. Moderate Hepatic Impairment: Initial: 0.5mcg/kg/min. PCI: Initial: 350mcg/kg bolus with 25mcg/kg/min IV. Check activated clotting time (ACT) 5-10 min after bolus. Proceed with PCI if ACT >300 sec. If ACT <300 sec, give additional 150mcg/kg bolus and increase infusion to 30mcg/kg/min. Check ACT 5-10 min later. If ACT >450 sec, decrease to 15mcg/kg/min and check ACT 5-10 min later. Continue infusion dose at therapeutic ACT (300-450 sec) during procedure. May give additional 150mcg/kg bolus and increase infusion to 40mcg/kg/min if dissection, impending abrupt closure, thrombus formation, or inability to achieve/maintain ACT >300 sec. After PCI, may use lower infusion rate if anticoagulation is needed.

HOW SUPPLIED: Inj: 100mg/mL

CONTRAINDICATIONS: Overt major bleeding.

WARNINGS/PRECAUTIONS: D/C all parenteral anticoagulants before administering. Extreme caution in conditions associated with an increased danger of hemorrhage (eg, severe HTN, immediately following lumbar puncture, bleeding disorder, GI lesions, spinal anesthesia, major surgery, etc). Caution in hepatic impairment. Avoid high doses in PCI patients with significant hepatic disease or AST/ALT ≥3X ULN. Monitor aPTT. For PCI, obtain ACT before dose, 5-10 min after bolus and infusion rate change, at the end of PCI, and every 20-30 min during prolonged procedures.

ADVERSE REACTIONS: GI bleed, GU bleed, Hct/Hgb decrease, hypotension, fever, diarrhea, sepsis, cardiac arrest, N/V, ventricular tachycardia, allergic reactions, chest pain (in PCI).

INTERACTIONS: Initiate after cessation of heparin therapy; allow time for heparin's effect on the aPTT to decrease. Prolongation of PT/INR with warfarin. Antiplatelets, thrombolytics, and other anticoagulants may increase risk of bleeding. D/C all anticoagulants before administration.

PREGNANCY: Category B, not for use in nursing.

MECHANISM OF ACTION: Direct thrombin inhibitor; reversibly binds to thrombin active site. Exerts anticoagulant effects by inhibiting thrombin-catalyzed or thrombin-induced reactions, including fibrin formation; activation of coagulation factors V, VIII, XIII; activation of protein C; and platelet aggregation. Capable of inhibiting both free and clot-associated thrombin.

PHARMACOKINETICS: Distribution: V_d=174mL/Kg; plasma protein binding (54%). **Metabolism:** Liver, via hydroxylation and aromatization; CYP3A4/5; M1 (primary metabolite). **Elimination:** Feces (primary), urine; $T_{1/2}$=39-51 min.

NURSING CONSIDERATIONS

Assessment: Assess for hepatic impairment, overt major bleeding, and for drug interactions. Assess use in patients with disease states at risk for a hemorrhagic event (eg, severe HTN). Obtain baseline aPTT and activated clotting time (ACT).

Monitoring: Monitor for signs/symptoms of hemorrhagic events (eg, unexplained fall in Hct, decrease in BP) and for allergic reactions. Monitor aPTT 2 hrs after initiation of therapy to confirm desired therapeutic range. Monitor ACT 5-10 min after bolus dosing, after changes in infusion rate, and at end of PCI procedure.

Patient Counseling: Inform about risk of hemorrhagic events. Instruct to contact physician if unusual bleeding or allergic reactions occur.

Administration: IV route. Do not mix with other drugs prior to dilution. 2.5 mL vial: 1) Dilute (0.9% NS, D5W, or LR) to a final concentration of 1 mg/mL. Each 2.5mL vial should be diluted 100-fold by mixing with 250mL of diluent. 2) Mix repeatedly by inversion for 1 min. **Storage:** Vial: 25°C (77°F); excursions permitted to 15-30°C. Retain in original carton to protect from light. Prepared Solution: 25°C (77°F); excursions permitted to 15-30° (59-86°F) in ambient indoor light for 24 hrs. Stable for 96 hrs when protected from light and stored at controlled room temperature, 20-25°C (68-77°F) or refrigerated, 5°C ± 3°C (41°F ± 5°F).

ARICEPT

RX

donepezil HCl (Eisai/Pfizer)

OTHER BRAND NAMES: Aricept ODT (Eisai/Pfizer)

THERAPEUTIC CLASS: Acetylcholinesterase inhibitor

INDICATIONS: Treatment of dementia of the Alzheimer's type.

DOSAGE: *Adults:* Mild to Moderate Alzheimer's Disease: Initial: 5mg qd. Usual: 5-10mg qd. Titrate: May increase to 10mg after 4-6 weeks. Moderate to Severe Alzheimer's Disease: Initial: 5mg qd. Usual: 10-23mg qd. Titrate: May increase to 10mg after 4-6 weeks, then to 23mg after ≥3 mth.

HOW SUPPLIED: Tab: 5mg, 10mg, 23mg; Tab, Disintegrating: (ODT) 5mg, 10mg

WARNINGS/PRECAUTIONS: May exaggerate succinylcholine-type muscle relaxation during anesthesia. May have vagotonic effects on sinoatrial and atrioventricular nodes, manifesting as bradycardia or heart block. Syncopal episodes reported. May produce diarrhea, N/V; observe closely at initiation of treatment and after dose increases. May increase gastric acid secretion; monitor for active or occult GI bleeding. Caution with increased risk for developing ulcers (eg, history of ulcer disease). May cause weight loss, generalized convulsions, and bladder outflow obstruction. Caution with asthma or obstructive pulmonary disease. .

ADVERSE REACTIONS: N/V, diarrhea, insomnia, muscle cramps, fatigue, anorexia, dizziness, insomnia, weight decrease, infection, HTN, back pain, abnormal dreams, ecchymosis.

INTERACTIONS: Synergistic effect with neuromuscular blocking agents (eg, succinylcholine) and cholinergic agonists (eg, bethanechol). May interfere with activity of anticholinergic medications. CYP2D6 and CYP3A4 inducers (eg, phenytoin, carbamazepine, dexamethasone, rifampin, phenobarbital) may increase elimination rate. Ketoconazole and quinidine, inhibitors of CYP3A4 and CYP2D6, respectively, inhibit donepezil metabolism in vitro. Monitor closely for GI bleeding with concurrent NSAID use.

PREGNANCY: Category C, caution in nursing.

MECHANISM OF ACTION: Acetylcholinesterase (AChE) inhibitor; may exert effect by increasing acetylcholine concentrations through reversible inhibition of its hydrolysis by AChE.

PHARMACOKINETICS: Absorption: T_{max}=3-8 hrs. **Distribution:** V_d: 12-16L/kg; plasma protein binding (96%). **Metabolism:** Hepatic (glucuronidation) via CYP2D6 and CYP3A4. **Elimination:** Urine (57%), feces (15%); $T_{1/2}$=70 hrs.

NURSING CONSIDERATIONS

Assessment: Assess for hypersensitivity, history of cardiovascular conditions, ulcer disease, NSAID use, GI bleeding (active/occult), seizures, asthma, obstructive pulmonary disease, possible drug interactions and pregnancy/nursing status.

Monitoring: Monitor for vagotonic effects on sinoatrial and atrioventricular nodes (eg, bradycardia, heart block), syncopal episodes, diarrhea, GI bleeding, N/V, and generalized convulsions.

Patient Counseling: Take qhs without regard to meals. Do not crush or chew tab. Swallow tab whole. For ODT, dissolve on tongue and follow with water. Caution with NSAID use. Advise that may cause N/V, diarrhea, insomnia, muscle cramps, fatigue, and decreased appetite.

Administration: Oral route. **Storage:** 15-30°C (59-86°F).

ARIMIDEX
anastrozole (AstraZeneca)

RX

THERAPEUTIC CLASS: Nonsteroidal aromatase inhibitor

INDICATIONS: Adjuvant treatment of postmenopausal women with hormone receptor-positive early breast cancer. First-line treatment of postmenopausal women with hormone receptor positive or hormone receptor-unknown locally advanced or metastatic breast cancer. Treatment of advanced breast cancer in postmenopausal women with disease progression following tamoxifen therapy.

DOSAGE: *Adults:* 1mg qd. Continue until tumor progression with advanced breast cancer.

HOW SUPPLIED: Tab: 1mg

CONTRAINDICATIONS: Pregnancy and premenopausal women.

WARNINGS/PRECAUTIONS: Increased incidence of ischemic cardiovascular events in patients with pre-existing ischemic heart disease reported. May cause reduction in bone mineral density. May elevate serum cholesterol.

ADVERSE REACTIONS: Hot flashes, asthenia, arthritis, pain, pharyngitis, HTN, depression, N/V, rash, osteoporosis, fractures, headache, bone pain, peripheral edema, dyspnea, pharyngitis.

INTERACTIONS: Concurrent use with tamoxifen decreases plasma levels. Avoid with estrogen-containing therapies.

PREGNANCY: Category X, not for use in nursing.

MECHANISM OF ACTION: Nonsteroidal aromatase inhibitor; lowers estradiol concentrations and has no detectable effect on formation of adrenal corticosteroids or aldosterone.

PHARMACOKINETICS: Absorption: Rapid, T_{max}=2 hrs. **Distribution:** Plasma protein binding (40%). **Metabolism:** Liver via N-dealkylation, hydroxylation, and glucuronidation. **Elimination**: Hepatic (85%), renal (10%); $T_{1/2}$=50 hrs.

NURSING CONSIDERATIONS

Assessment: Assess for hypersensitivity reactions, pre-existing ischemic cardiac disease, baseline bone mineral density, pregnancy/nursing status, menopausal status, hepatic/renal impairment and possible drug interactions.

Monitoring: Monitor bone mineral density, LFTs and cholesterol levels. Monitor for serious side effects.

Patient Counseling: Advise to take exactly as prescribed. Report to physician if serious allergic reactions (angioedema) occur. Inform patients with pre-existing ischemic heart disease that increased incidence of cardiovascular events has been observed. Inform that drug may lower the level of estrogen which may lead to a loss of the mineral content of bones, and might decrease the bone strength. Instruct to notify physician if pregnant/nursing or intend to become pregnant.

Administration: Oral route. **Storage:** 20-25°C (68-77°F).

ARIXTRA
fondaparinux sodium (GlaxoSmithKline)

RX

Epidural or spinal hematomas resulting in long-term or permanent paralysis may occur in patients anticoagulated with low molecular weight heparins, heparinoids, or fondaparinux sodium and who are receiving neuraxial anesthesia or undergoing spinal puncture. Increased risk of developing epidural or spinal hematomas in patients using indwelling epidural catheters, concomitant use of other drugs that affect hemostasis (eg, NSAIDs, platelet inhibitors, other anticoagulants), history of traumatic or repeated epidural or spinal puncture, or a history of spinal deformity or spinal surgery. Monitor frequently for signs/symptoms of neurologic impairment; if neurologic compromise noted, urgent treatment is necessary. Consider benefit and risks before neuraxial intervention in patients anticoagulated or to be anticoagulated for thromboprophylaxis.

THERAPEUTIC CLASS: Specific factor Xa inhibitor

INDICATIONS: Prophylaxis of deep vein thrombosis (DVT) in patients undergoing hip fracture surgery, including extended prophylaxis; hip replacement surgery; knee replacement surgery; abdominal surgery who are at risk of thromboembolic complications. Treatment of acute DVT when administered in conjunction with warfarin sodium. Treatment of acute pulmonary embolism (PE) when administered in conjunction with warfarin sodium when initial therapy is administered in the hospital.

DOSAGE: *Adults:* DVT Prophylaxis: 2.5mg SQ qd. Administer no earlier than 6-8 hrs post-op for 5-9 days. Hip Fracture Surgery Prophylaxis: Extended prophylaxis up to 24 additional days is recommended. DVT/PE Treatment: <50kg: 5mg SQ qd. 50-100kg: 7.5mg SQ qd. >100kg: 10mg SQ qd. Initiate concomitant treatment with warfarin as soon as possible, usually within 72 hrs. Continue treatment with fondaparinux for ≥5 days and until therapeutic oral anticoagulant effect is established (INR=2-3).

HOW SUPPLIED: Inj: 2.5mg/0.5mL, 5mg/0.4mL, 7.5mg/0.6mL, 10mg/0.8mL

CONTRAINDICATIONS: Severe renal impairment (CrCl <30mL/min), active major bleeding, bacterial endocarditis, thrombocytopenia associated with a positive *in vitro* test for anti-platelet antibody in the presence of fondaparinux sodium, body weight <50kg (for venous thromboembolism [VTE] prophylaxis only).

WARNINGS/PRECAUTIONS: Not for IM injection. Extreme caution in conditions with an increased risk of hemorrhage (eg, congenital or acquired bleeding disorders, active ulcerative and angiodysplastic GI disease, hemorrhagic stroke, uncontrolled arterial HTN, diabetic retinopathy, shortly after brain, spinal, or ophthalmological surgery). Isolated cases of elevated activated partial thromboplastintime temporally associated with bleeding events have been reported. Do not administer earlier than 6-8 hrs after surgery; increases risk of major bleeding. Risk of bleeding increases with renal impairment; monitor renal function periodically and d/c if severe renal impairment develops. Do not use for VTE prophylaxis and treatment if CrCl <30mL/min. Caution with CrCl 30-50mL/min. Avoid use as prophylactic therapy in hip fracture, hip replacement, knee replacement and abdominal surgery. Thrombocytopenia reported; monitor closely. D/C if platelet count <100,000/mm³. D/C if unexpected changes in coagulation parameters or major bleeding occurs during therapy. Perform routine CBC (including platelet count), SrCr, and stool occult blood tests during treatment. Packaging (needle guard) may cause allergic reaction in latex-sensitive individuals. Caution with hepatic impairment and in the elderly.

ADVERSE REACTIONS: Bleeding complications, thrombocytopenia, local reactions (eg, rash, pruritus), anemia, insomnia, increased wound drainage, hypokalemia, dizziness, purpura, hypotension, confusion, bullous eruption, hematoma

INTERACTIONS: See Boxed Warning. Agents that may enhance the risk of hemorrhage should be d/c prior to initiation of therapy unless these agents are essential; if coadministration is necessary, monitor closely for hemorrhage.

PREGNANCY: Category B, caution in nursing.

MECHANISM OF ACTION: Specific factor Xa inhibitor; selectively binds to antithrombin III (ATIII) and potentiates the innate neutralization of Factor Xa by ATIII thereby interrupting the blood coagulation cascade and inhibiting thrombin formation and thrombus development.

PHARMACOKINETICS: Absorption: Rapid, complete; absolute bioavailability (100%); C_{max}=0.39-0.50mg/L (2.5mg qd), 1.2-1.26mg/L (5mg, 7.5mg, 10mg qd); T_{max}=3 hrs (2.5mg qd). **Distribution:** V_d=7-11L; bound to ATIII (94%). **Elimination:** Urine (up to 77%, unchanged); $T_{1/2}$=17-21 hrs.

NURSING CONSIDERATIONS

Assessment: Assess for renal/hepatic function, presence of active major bleeding, conditions that increase the risk of hemorrhage or any other conditions where treatment is cautioned or contraindicated, latex sensitivity, PE, DVT, nursing/pregnancy status, and for possible drug interactions. Obtain weight and baseline CrCl, aPTT, PT, CBC, SrCr, and stool occult blood test.

Monitoring: Monitor for signs/symptoms of bleeding and thrombocytopenia. In patients undergoing neuraxial anesthesia or spinal puncture, monitor for epidural or spinal hematomas and neurologic impairment. Periodically monitor CBC (including platelet count), SrCr, stool occult blood tests, aPTT, CrCl and PT.

Patient Counseling: Instruct on proper administration technique. Counsel on signs and symptoms of possible bleeding. Inform that it may take longer than usual to stop bleeding and may bruise and/or bleed more easily while on therapy. Instruct to report any unusual bleeding, bruising, or signs of thrombocytopenia (eg, rash of dark red spots under the skin). Notify physician or dentist of all prescription and nonprescription medications currently taking. Instruct to watch for signs and symptoms of spinal or epidural hematomas such as tingling, numbness and muscular weakness; contact physician immediately if symptoms occur.

Administration: SQ route. Instructions for Use. Do not inject IM. Do not mix with other injections or infusions. Do not expel air bubble from prefilled syringe. Administer in fatty tissue, alternating injection sites. Refer to PI for further instructions on administration and preparation. **Storage:** 25°C (77°F); excursions permitted to 15-30°C (59-86°F).

ARMOUR THYROID   RX
thyroid (Forest)

THERAPEUTIC CLASS: Thyroid replacement hormone

INDICATIONS: Treatment of hypothyroidism. As a pituitary TSH suppressant in the treatment or prevention of various types of euthyroid goiters. Diagnostic agent in suppression tests to differentiate suspected mild hyperthyroidism or thyroid gland autonomy. Management of thyroid cancer.

DOSAGE: *Adults:* Hypothyroidism: Initial: 30mg qd. Titrate: Increase by 15mg q2-3 weeks. Myxedema with Cardiovascular Disorder: 15mg qd. Maint: 60-120mg/day. Thyroid Cancer: Higher doses than replacement therapy are required. Myxedema Coma: 400mcg IV levothyroxine sodium (100mcg/mL rapidly) followed by 100-200mcg/day IV. Switch to PO when stable. Thyroid Suppression: 1.56mg/kg/day for 7-10 days. Elderly: Initial: Use lower dose (eg, 15-30mg qd).
Pediatrics: Hypothyroidism: >12 yrs: 1.2-1.8mg/kg/day. 6-12 yrs: 2.4-3mg/kg/day. 1-5 yrs: 3-3.6mg/kg/day. 6-12 months: 3.6-4.8mg/kg/day. 0-6 months: 4.8-6mg/kg/day.

HOW SUPPLIED: Tab: 15mg, 30mg, 60mg, 90mg, 120mg, 180mg*, 240mg, 300mg* *scored

CONTRAINDICATIONS: Untreated thyrotoxicosis; uncorrected adrenal cortical insufficiency.

WARNINGS/PRECAUTIONS: Do not use in the treatment of obesity; larger doses in euthyroid patients can cause serious or even life-threatening toxicity. Caution with cardiovascular disease, diabetes mellitus (DM), diabetes insipidus, elderly, and adrenal cortical insufficiency.

INTERACTIONS: May increase insulin or oral hypoglycemic requirements. Reduced absorption with cholestyramine and colestipol; space dosing by 4-5 hrs. Altered effect of oral anticoagulants; monitor PT/INR. Estrogens increase thyroxine-binding globulin; increase in thyroid dose may be needed. Serious or life-threatening side effects can occur with sympathomimetic amines. Androgens, corticosteroids, estrogens, iodine-containing preparations, and salicylates may interfere with thyroid lab tests.

PREGNANCY: Category A, caution in nursing.

MECHANISM OF ACTION: Thyroid hormone; not established, suspected to enhance oxygen consumption by most body tissues, increase the basal metabolic rate and metabolism of carbohydrates, lipids, and proteins.

PHARMACOKINETICS: Abosrption: (T_3) Completely absorbed; T_{max} =4 hrs; (T_4) partially absorbed. **Distribution:** Plasma protein binding (>99%), found in breast milk. **Metabolism:** Deiodination in liver, kidneys, other tissues.

NURSING CONSIDERATIONS

Assessment: Assess for diagnosed but uncorrected adrenal cortical insufficiency, untreated thyrotoxicosis, hypersensitivity to any of its active or extraneous constituents, cardiovascular system, angina, DM, myxedema coma, and possible drug and test interactions.

Monitoring: Monitor urinary glucose levels in patients with DM, PT in patients receiving anticoagulants, and periodic assessment of thyroid status (TSH suppression test, serum T_4 levels, free T_4; if TSH is normal, total T_4 is low), free T_3, T_4, signs/symptoms of thyroid hormone toxicity (chest pain, increased pulse rate, palpitations, excessive sweating, heat intolerance, and nervousness), partial hair loss in children.

Patient Counseling: Inform that replacement therapy is to be taken essentially for life, with the exception of cases of transient hypothyroidism, which associated with thyroiditis, and those patients receiving a therapeutical trial of the drug. Report immediately any signs/symptoms of thyroid toxicity.

Administration: Oral route. **Storage:** Store at 15-30°C (59-86°F).

AROMASIN   RX
exemestane (Pharmacia & Upjohn)

THERAPEUTIC CLASS: Aromatase inactivator

INDICATIONS: In postmenopausal women, treatment of advanced breast cancer that has progressed after tamoxifen therapy. Adjuvant treatment of postmenopausal women with estrogen-receptor positive early breast cancer who have received 2-3 yrs of tamoxifen and are switched to exemestane for a total completion of 5 consecutive yrs to adjuvant hormonal therapy.

DOSAGE: *Adults:* Early/Advanced: 25mg qd after a meal. Continue in the absence of recurrence of contralateral breast cancer until completion of 5 yrs of adjuvant endocrine therapy in postmenopausal women with early breast cancer treated with 2-3 yrs of tamoxifen. Continue until tumor progression is evident. Concomitant Potent CYP3A4 Inducers (eg, rifampicin, phenytoin): 50mg qd after a meal.

HOW SUPPLIED: Tab: 25mg

WARNINGS/PRECAUTIONS: Fetal harm in pregnancy. Avoid in premenopausal women.

ADVERSE REACTIONS: Fatigue, N/V, hot flashes, pain, depression, insomnia, anxiety, dyspnea, dizziness, headache, increased sweating, edema, HTN, anorexia.

INTERACTIONS: Avoid coadministration with estrogen-containing agents. Potent CYP3A4 inducers (eg, rifampin, phenytoin, carbamazepine, phenobarbital, St. John's wort) may decrease plasma levels.

PREGNANCY: Category D, caution in nursing.

MECHANISM OF ACTION: Irreversible steroidal aromatase inactivator; acts as false substrate for aromatase enzyme; processed to intermediate that binds irreversibly to active site of enzyme, causing inactivation.

PHARMACOKINETICS: Absorption: Rapid. (Breast cancer) T_{max}=1.2 hrs; AUC=75.4ng•hr/mL. **Distribution:** Plasma protein binding (90%). **Metabolism:** Oxidation via CYP3A4; reduction. **Elimination:** Urine (<1%), $T_{1/2}$=24 hrs.

NURSING CONSIDERATIONS

Assessment: Assess for possible drug interactions, pregnancy/nursing status, and renal/hepatic function.

Monitoring: Monitor for hematological abnormalities, LFTs, creatinine, and bone mineral density.

Patient Counseling: Inform of pregnancy risks. Advise to take after meal.

Administration: Oral route. **Storage:** 25°C (77°F); excursions permitted to 15-30°C (59-86°F).

ARTHROTEC

RX

diclofenac sodium - misoprostol (G.D. Searle)

> Misoprostol can cause abortion, premature birth or birth defects. Uterine rupture reported when used to induce labor or induce abortion beyond 8th week of pregnancy. Patients must be advised of the abortifacient property and warned not to give the drug to others. Use only in women of childbearing age if at high risk for GI ulcers or complications with NSAID therapy; must have had a negative serum pregnancy test within 2 weeks before therapy, is capable of complying with effective contraceptive measures, has received both oral and written warnings, and will begin therapy on 2nd or 3rd day of menstrual period. NSAIDs may cause an increased risk of serious cardiovascular (CV) thrombotic events, myocardial infarction, stroke, and serious GI adverse events including bleeding, ulceration, and perforation of the stomach or intestines. Contraindicated for the treatment of perioperative pain in the setting of coronary artery bypass graft (CABG) surgery.

THERAPEUTIC CLASS: NSAID/prostaglandin E, analogue

INDICATIONS: Treatment of the signs and symptoms of osteoarthritis (OA) or rheumatoid arthritis (RA) in patients at high risk of developing NSAID-induced gastric and duodenal ulcers and their complications.

DOSAGE: *Adults:* OA: 50mg/200mcg tid. RA: 50mg/200mcg tid or qid. OA/RA: If intolerable, may give 50mg/200mcg or 75mg/200mcg bid. May adjust dose and frequency according to individual needs after observing response to initial therapy. Refer to PI for special dosing considerations.

HOW SUPPLIED: Tab: (Diclofenac-Misoprostol) 50mg-200mcg, 75mg-200mcg

CONTRAINDICATIONS: Pregnancy, patients who experienced asthma, urticaria or other allergic type reactions to ASA or other NSAIDs. Treatment of peri-operative pain in the setting of CABG.

WARNINGS/PRECAUTIONS: May lead to onset of new or worsening HTN. Caution in patients with HTN; monitor BP. Fluid retention and edema reported; caution in patients with fluid retention or heart failure (HF). Caution with history of ulcer disease or GI bleeding. May increase risk of GI bleeding with smoking, older age, debilitation and poor general health status. D/C if a serious GI event occurs. Renal papillary necrosis and other renal injury reported after long-term use. Renal toxicity reported in patients in whom renal prostaglandins have a compensatory role in the maintenance of renal perfusion; caution with impaired renal function, HF, liver dysfunction. Not recommended for use with advanced renal disease. May cause elevation of transaminases and hepatotoxicity; monitor transaminases prior to therapy and periodically thereafter. Anaphylactic reactions may occur. May cause serious skin adverse events [eg, exfoliative dermatitis, Stevens-Johnson syndrome (SJS), toxic epidermal necrolysis (TEN)]; d/c if skin rash or hypersensitivity occurs. May cause premature closure of ductus arteriosus if used late in pregnancy. Not a substitute for corticosteroids or for the treatment of corticosteroid insufficiency. Anemia may occur; monitor Hgb/Hct if signs/symptoms of anemia develop. May prolong bleeding time; monitor with coagulation disorders. Caution with preexisting asthma. Aseptic meningitis with fever and coma reported. Avoid with hepatic porphyria. Caution in elderly.

ADVERSE REACTIONS: Abdominal pain, diarrhea, dyspepsia, nausea, flatulence.

INTERACTIONS: May diminish the antihypertensive effect of ACE inhibitors and increase the risk of renal toxicity. May reduce the bioavailability of misoprostol acid and delay the absorption of diclofenac Na with antacids. Avoid with magnesium-containing antacids; misoprostol-associated diarrhea may be exacerbated when used concomitantly. May increase the risk of renal toxicity with diuretics; may reduce the natriuretic effect of furosemide and thiazides. Increased serum potassium with K+-sparing diuretics. Loop diuretics and thiazides may have impaired response when given concomitantly with NSAIDs. Synergistic GI bleeding effects when used concomitantly with warfarin. May increase risk of serious GI bleeding when used concomitantly with oral corticosteroids, anticoagulants, or alcohol. May alter response to insulin or oral hypoglycemics. Monitor for digoxin, methotrexate, cyclosporine, phenobarbital, and lithium toxicities. Caution with drugs that are known to be potentially hepatotoxic (eg, antibiotics, anti-epileptics). Avoid with ASA. Voriconazole may increase diclofenac Na levels Diclofenac Na may minimally interfere with protein binding of prednisolone.

PREGNANCY: Category X, caution in nursing.

MECHANISM OF ACTION: Diclofenac: NSAID; not established. May be related to prostaglandin synthetase inhibition. Possesses anti-inflammatory, analgesic, and antipyretic properties. Misoprostol: Prostaglandin E_1 analog with gastric antisecretory and mucosal protective properties.

PHARMACOKINETICS: Absorption: Oral administration of a single dose or multiple doses of medication is similar to pharmacokinetics of two individual components. Refer to PI for further information. **Distribution:** Found in breast milk. Diclofenac: V_d=550mL/kg; plasma protein binding (>99%). Misoprostol: Plasma protein binding (<90%). **Metabolism:** Diclofenac: Glucuronide and sulfate conjugation via CYP2C8, 2C9, 3A4; 4'-hydroxy diclofenac (major metabolite). Misoprostol: Rapid; misoprostol acid (active metabolite). **Elimination:** Diclofenac: Urine (65%), bile (35%); $T_{1/2}$=2 hrs. Misoprostol: Urine (70%); $T_{1/2}$=30 min.

NURSING CONSIDERATIONS

Assessment: Assess for history of hypersensitivity to ASA or other NSAIDs, or to misoprostol or other prostaglandins; history of asthma; presence of or risk factors for CV disease; HTN; HF; fluid retention; history of ulcer disease or GI bleeding; risk factors for a GI event; conditions affected by platelet function alterations; hepatic porphyria; underlying chronic disease; pregnancy/nursing status; and for possible drug interactions. Assess use of effective contraceptive measures. Obtain pregnancy test 2 weeks prior to therapy, and baseline BP, renal/hepatic function.

Monitoring: Monitor for CV thrombotic events, new onset or worsening of HTN, fluid retention, GI bleeding and ulceration, renal papillary necrosis or other renal injury/toxicity, hepatotoxicity, systemic manifestations, anaphylactic or skin reactions, anemia, prolonged bleeding time, bronchospasm, aseptic meningitis, and porphyria. Monitor BP; renal function if with renal disease; Hgb/Hct if anemia is suspected. Monitor transaminases within 4-8 weeks after initiating therapy. Periodically monitor CBC and chemistry profile for long-term use. Monitor use of effective contraception.

Patient Counseling: Advise of pregnancy risks; inform women of childbearing potential that they must not be pregnant when therapy is initiated and must use an effective contraception during treatment. Inform that therapy should not be taken by nursing mothers. Instruct not to give medication to other individuals. Instruct to contact physician if signs/symptoms of CV effects (eg, chest pain, SOB, weakness, slurring of speech), GI effects (eg, epigastric pain, dyspepsia, melena, hematemesis), or unexplained weight gain and edema occur. Instruct to contact physician and d/c if signs of skin reactions (eg, rash, blisters, fever, itching) or hepatotoxicity (eg, nausea, fatigue, jaundice) occur. Instruct to seek immediate medical attention if an anaphylactic reaction occurs (eg, breathing difficulty, facial or throat swelling). Instruct to take with meals and avoid the use of magnesium containing antacids. Instruct to swallow tab whole; do not chew, crush or dissolve.

Administration: Oral route. **Storage:** ≤25°C (77°F), in a dry area.

ARZERRA   RX
ofatumumab (GlaxoSmithKline)

THERAPEUTIC CLASS: Monoclonal antibody/CD20-blocker

INDICATIONS: Treatment of patients with chronic lymphocytic leukemia (CLL) refractory to fludarabine and alemtuzumab.

DOSAGE: *Adults:* Premedicate. 300mg (Dose 1), followed 1 week later by 2,000mg weekly for 7 doses (Doses 2 through 8), followed 4 weeks later by 2,000mg every 4 weeks for 4 doses (Doses 9 through 12). Refer to PI for detailed information on infusion rates and dose modifications.

HOW SUPPLIED: Inj: 20mg/mL [5mL]

WARNINGS/PRECAUTIONS: Do not administer as IV push or bolus. May cause serious infusion reactions (eg, bronchospasm, dyspnea, pulmonary/laryngeal edema, flushing, HTN, hypotension, syncope, cardiac ischemia/infarction, back pain, abdominal pain, pyrexia, rash, urticaria, angioedema); interrupt infusion if reaction develops. Premedicate with PO acetaminophen 1,000mg (or equivalent), PO/IV antihistamine (cetirizine 10mg or equivalent), and IV corticosteroid (prednisolone 100mg or equivalent). Avoid with moderate to severe COPD; bronchospasm may develop. Prolonged (≥1 week) severe neutropenia and thrombocytopenia may occur. Progressive multifocal leukoencephalopathy (PML) may occur; d/c if PML is suspected and initiate evaluation for PML. Hepatitis B virus (HBV) infection or reactivation, including fulminant hepatitis and death, may occur; screen patients at high risk of HBV infection before initiating therapy. Closely monitor carriers of HBV for clinical and laboratory signs of active HBV infection during treatment and for 6-12 months following last infusion. D/C if viral hepatitis or reactivation of viral hepatitis develops. Obstruction of small intestine may occur; perform diagnostic evaluation if suspected.

ADVERSE REACTIONS: Neutropenia, anemia, pneumonia, pyrexia, cough, diarrhea, fatigue, dyspnea, rash, nausea, bronchitis, sepsis, infusion reactions, chills, infections.

INTERACTIONS: Do not administer live viral vaccines to patients who have recently received ofatumumab.

PREGNANCY: Category C, caution in nursing.

MECHANISM OF ACTION: IgG$_1$kappa human monoclonal antibody; binds specifically to extracellular loops of CD20 molecule expressed on normal B lymphocytes and on B-cell CLL. The Fab domain of ofatumumab binds to the CD20 molecule and the Fc domain mediates immune effector functions to result in B-cell lysis in vitro.

PHARMACOKINETICS: Distribution: V$_d$= 1.7-5.1L. **Elimination**: T$_{1/2}$=14 days (mean between the 4th and 12th infusions).

NURSING CONSIDERATIONS

Assessment: Assess for HBV, COPD, pre-existing neurological signs or symptoms, pregnancy/nursing status, and possible drug interactions. Prior to therapy, assess that patient was premedicated with appropriate medications.

Monitoring: Monitor for signs/symptoms of infusion reactions, neutropenia, thrombocytopenia, PML, intestinal obstruction and other possible adverse reactions. Monitor CBC and platelet counts at regular intervals during therapy. Monitor carriers of HBV for clinical and laboratory signs of active infection during treatment and for 6-12 months following last infusion.

Patient Counseling: Contact physician if signs/symptoms of an infusion reaction (eg, fever, chills, rash, breathing problems), cytopenias (eg, bleeding, easy bruising, petechiae, pallor, worsening weakness, or fatigue), infection (eg, fever, cough), new neurological symptoms (eg, confusion, dizziness, difficulty talking or walking, vision problems), or hepatitis (eg, yellow discoloration of eyes or skin, worsening fatigue) are experienced or if new or worsening abdominal pain or nausea develops. Notify physician if pregnant or nursing. Advise that periodic monitoring of blood counts during therapy is required. Avoid vaccinations with live viral vaccines.

Administration: IV route. Refer to PI for preparation and administration instructions. Do not use if discoloration or if foreign particulate matter is present. Do not shake. **Storage:** 2-8°C (36-46°F). Do not freeze. Protect from light.

ASACOL   RX
mesalamine (Warner Chilcott)

OTHER BRAND NAMES: Asacol HD (Warner Chilcott)

THERAPEUTIC CLASS: 5-Aminosalicylic acid derivative

INDICATIONS: (Asacol): Treatment of mildly to moderately active ulcerative colitis and for the maintenance of remission of ulcerative colitis. (Asacol HD): Treatment of moderately active ulcerative colitis.

DOSAGE: *Adults:* (Asacol): Mild-Moderately Active Ulcerative Colitis: Usual: 2 tabs of 400mg tid for 6 weeks. Maintenance of Remission of Ulcerative Colitis: 1.6g/day in divided doses. (Asacol HD): Moderately Active Ulcerative Colitis: Usual: 2 tabs of 800mg tid for 6 weeks. One Asacol HD 800mg tab has not been shown to be bioequivalent to two Asacol 400mg tabs.

HOW SUPPLIED: Tab, Delayed-Release: 400mg (Asacol), 800mg (Asacol HD).

WARNINGS/PRECAUTIONS: Caution in patients with pyloric stenosis, may prolong gastric retention which could delay mesalamine release in the colon. Exacerbation of symptoms of colitis (eg, cramping, abdominal pain, bloody diarrhea) reported; symptoms abate with d/c. Caution with sulfasalazine hypersensitivity. Renal impairment, including minimal change nephropathy, acute and chronic interstitial nephritis, and rarely renal failure reported; caution with renal dysfunction or history of renal disease. Evaluate renal function prior to therapy and periodically thereafter. Caution in elderly. Reports of hepatic failure in patients with pre-existing liver disease; caution in patients with liver disease.

ADVERSE REACTIONS: Headache (Asacol): Abdominal pain, eructation, pain, nausea, pharyngitis, dizziness, asthenia, diarrhea, back pain, fever, rash, dyspepsia.

PREGNANCY: (Asacol) Category C; (Asacol HD) Category B; caution in nursing.

MECHANISM OF ACTION: 5-Aminosalicylic acid derivative; anti-inflammatory agent; mechanism unknown. Possibly diminishes inflammation by blocking cyclooxygenase and inhibiting prostaglandin production in the colon.

PHARMACOKINETICS: Absorption: (400 mg) T_{max}=4-12 hrs. (800mg): T_{max}=10-16 hrs, C_{max}=5mcg/mL, AUC_{tau}=20mcg• h/mL. **Distribution:** (400mg, 800mg): Found in breast milk; crosses placental barrier. **Metabolism:** Gut mucosal wall and liver via rapid acetylation. Metabolite (N-acetyl-5-aminosalicylic acid). **Elimination:** Renally excreted as metabolite. (400mg): $T_{1/2}$=2-15 hrs. (800mg) $T_{1/2}$=12.6 hrs.

NURSING CONSIDERATIONS

Assessment: Assess for hypersensitivity to sulfasalazine or salicylates, renal function or history of renal/liver disease, pyloric stenosis, and pregnancy/nursing status. Obtain baseline renal function.

Monitoring: Monitor for signs and symptoms of renal impairment including nephropathy, acute and chronic interstitial nephritis, and renal failure. Monitor for signs and symptoms of a colitis exacerbation (eg, cramping, abdominal pain, bloody diarrhea) and for hypersensitivity reactions. If pyloric stenosis exists, monitor for prolonged gastric retention. If pre-existing liver disease exists, monitor for signs and symptoms of hepatic failure. Perform periodic monitoring of renal function and blood cell counts.

Patient Counseling: Instruct to swallow whole and not to break, cut, or chew tabs. Inform physician if intact, partially intact and/or tablet shells are seen in stool repeatedly. Inform that ulcerative colitis rarely remits completely; risk of relapse can be substantially reduced by continued administration of medication. Seek medical attention if an exacerbation of colitis (cramping, abdominal pain, bloody diarrhea) occurs or if a hypersensitivity reaction develops. Inform that Asacol cannot be substituted with Asacol HD. (Asacol HD) Advise to d/c previous oral mesalamine therapy and follow dosing instructions for Asacol HD if switching therapy. Advise pregnant and breastfeeding women, or women of childbearing potential that drug contains dibutyl phthalate, which could possibly cause fetal malformations.

Administration: Oral route. Swallow whole without cutting, breaking, or chewing. **Storage:** 20-25°C (68-77°F). Protect tablets from moisture, close container tightly, and leave desiccant pouches present in bottle.

ASCLERA
polidocanol (BioForm Medical)

RX

THERAPEUTIC CLASS: Sclerosing Agent

INDICATIONS: To sclerose uncomplicated spider veins (varicose veins ≤1 mm in diameter) and uncomplicated reticular veins (varicose veins 1-3 mm in diameter) in the lower extremity.

DOSAGE: *Adults:* Spider Veins (Varicose Veins ≤1mm in Diameter): 0.5% IV. Reticular Veins (Varicose Veins 1-3mm in Diameter): 1% IV. Use 0.1-0.3mL/injection. Max: 10mL/session. Maintain compression 2-3 days after treatment for spider veins and 5-7 days for reticular veins. Extensive Varicosities: Longer compression treatment with compression bandages/gradient compression stocking of a higher compression class recommended. Repeat treatment if varicose veins requires >10mL; treatment should be separated by 1-2 weeks.

HOW SUPPLIED: Inj: 0.5%, 1% [2mL]

CONTRAINDICATIONS: Acute thromboembolic diseases.

WARNINGS/PRECAUTIONS: Severe allergic reactions, including anaphylactic reactions reported with use of larger volumes (>3mL); minimize dose. Tissue necrosis may occur following extravasation; care should be taken in IV placement and dosing. Apply compression with stocking/bandage after injection session is completed; have the patient walk for 15-20 mins. Avoid intra-arterial and perivascular injection.

ADVERSE REACTIONS: Injection-site reactions (hematoma, irritation, discoloration, pain, pruritus, warmth, thrombosis), neovascularisation.

PREGNANCY: Category C, not for use in nursing.

MECHANISM OF ACTION: Sclerosing agent. Locally damages the endothelium of blood vessels.

PHARMACOKINETICS: Elimination: $T_{1/2}$ = 1.5 hrs.

NURSING CONSIDERATIONS

Assessment: Assess for history of allergic reactions to product and pregnancy/nursing status.

Monitoring: Monitor for allergic reactions (including anaphylactic reactions), extravasation, and injection-site reactions.

Patient Counseling: Advise to wear thigh/knee high compression stockings/support hose on treated legs continuously for 2-3 days and for 2-3 weeks during daytime. Advise to walk for 15-20 mins immediately after procedure and daily for the next few days. Advise to avoid heavy exercise, sunbathing, long flights, and hot baths or sauna for 2-3 days after treatment.

Administration: IV route. Use a syringe (glass/plastic) with a fine needle (26- or 30- gauge). Insert tangentially into the vein and inject solution slowly. Apply gentle pressure during injection and compression (stocking/bandage) after the needle is removed. **Storage:** 15-30°C (59-86°F).

ASMANEX
mometasone furoate (Schering)

RX

THERAPEUTIC CLASS: Corticosteroid

INDICATIONS: Maintenance treatment of asthma as prophylactic therapy in patients ≥4 yrs.

DOSAGE: *Adults:* Previous Therapy with Bronchodilators Alone or Inhaled Corticosteroids: Initial: 220mcg qpm. Max: 440mcg qpm or 220mcg bid. Previous Therapy with Oral Corticosteroids: Initial: 440mcg bid. Max: 880mcg/day. Titrate: May need higher dose if inadequate response after 2 weeks. Adjust to lowest effective dose once asthma stability is achieved. *Pediatrics:* ≥12 yrs: Previous Therapy with Bronchodilators Alone or Inhaled Corticosteroids: Initial: 220mcg qpm. Max: 440mcg qpm or 220mcg bid.

Previous Therapy with Oral Corticosteroids: Initial: 440mcg bid. Max: 880mcg/day. Titrate: May need higher dose if inadequate response after 2 weeks. 4-11 yrs: Initial/Max: 110mcg qpm regardless of prior therapy. Adjust to lowest effective dose once asthma stability is achieved.

HOW SUPPLIED: Twisthaler: 110mcg/actuation, 220mcg/actuation

CONTRAINDICATIONS: Primary treatment of status asthmaticus or other acute episodes of asthma where intensive measures are required. Hypersensitivity to milk proteins.

WARNINGS/PRECAUTIONS: Localized *Candida albicans* infections of the mouth and pharynx reported; treat accordingly. D/C if hypersensitivity reactions occur. Contains small amount of lactose which contains milk proteins; anaphylactic reactions with milk protein allergy reported. Increased susceptibility to infections. Avoid exposure to chickenpox and measles. Caution with active or quiescent tuberculosis (TB) infection, untreated systemic fungal, bacterial, viral, or parasitic infections, or ocular herpes simplex. Deaths due to adrenal insufficiency have occurred with transfer from systemic to inhaled corticosteroids. Wean slowly from systemic corticosteroid therapy. Resume oral corticosteroids during stress or severe asthma attack. Transferring from oral to inhalation therapy may unmask allergic conditions (eg, rhinitis, conjunctivitis, eczema). Monitor for systemic corticosteroid effects such as hypercorticism and adrenal suppression. Prolonged use may result in decrease of bone mineral density (BMD). May cause reduction in growth velocity in pediatrics; monitor growth routinely. Glaucoma, increased intraocular pressure (IOP), and cataracts reported. D/C and institute alternative therapy if bronchospasm occurs after dosing.

ADVERSE REACTIONS: Headache, allergic rhinitis, pharyngitis, upper respiratory tract infection, sinusitis, oral candidiasis, dysmenorrhea, musculoskeletal pain, back pain, dyspepsia, myalgia, abdominal pain, nausea.

INTERACTIONS: Ketoconazole may increase plasma levels. Caution with drugs that reduce bone mass (eg, anticonvulsants and corticosteroids).

PREGNANCY: Category C, caution in nursing.

MECHANISM OF ACTION: Corticosteroid; not established. Shown to have inhibitory effects on multiple cell types (eg, mast cells, eosinophils, neutrophils, macrophages, and lymphocytes) and mediators (eg, histamine, eicosanoids, leukotrienes, and cytokines), involved in inflammatory and asthmatic response.

PHARMACOKINETICS: Absorption: Absolute bioavailability (<1%); C_{max}=94-114pcg/mL; T_{max}=1-2.5 hrs. **Distribution:** (IV) V_d=152L; plasma protein binding (98-99%). **Metabolism:** Liver via CYP3A4. **Elimination:** Feces (74%), urine (8%); $T_{1/2}$=5 hrs.

NURSING CONSIDERATIONS

Assessment: Assess for status asthmaticus, acute asthma episodes, bronchospasm, known hypersensitivity to milk proteins or to any drug component. Assess for risk factors for decreased BMD, history of increased IOP, glaucoma, cataracts, active or quiescent pulmonary TB, ocular herpes simplex, untreated systemic infections, chickenpox, measles, pregnancy/nursing status, and possible drug interactions.

Monitoring: Monitor for localized infections of mouth and pharynx with *Candida albicans*, decreased BMD, chickenpox, measles, asthma instability, growth in pediatrics, development of glaucoma, increased IOP, cataracts, hypercorticism, signs and symptoms of adrenal insufficiency, paradoxical bronchospasm, hypersensitivity reactions, and immunosuppression. Monitor for lung function, β-agonist use, and asthma symptoms during withdrawal of oral corticosteroids.

Patient Counseling: Advise that localized infection with *Candida albicans* may occur in mouth and pharynx; rinse mouth after inhalation. Inform that therapy should not be used to treat status asthmaticus or to relieve acute asthma symptoms. Counsel to d/c if hypersensitivity reactions (eg, rash, pruritus, angioedema, and anaphylactic reactions) occur. Advise to avoid exposure to chickenpox or measles and to seek medical attention if exposed. Inform of potential worsening of existing TB, other infections, or ocular herpes, and drug may cause systemic corticosteroid effects of hypercorticism and adrenal suppression, may reduce BMD, and may cause reduction in growth rate (pediatrics). Advise to take as directed, to use medication at regular intervals, and to contact physician if symptoms do not improve or if condition worsens. Instruct on proper administration procedures and on when to discard inhaler.

Administration: Oral inhalation. Inhale rapidly and deeply. Rinse mouth after inhalation. Refer to PI for further administration instructions. **Storage:** 25°C (77°F); excursions permitted to 15-30°C (59-86°F). Store in dry place. Discard inhaler 45 days after opening foil pouch or when dose counter reads "00," whichever comes 1st.

ASTELIN   RX
azelastine HCl (Meda)

THERAPEUTIC CLASS: Antihistamine

INDICATIONS: Treatment of the symptoms of seasonal allergic rhinitis and vasomotor rhinitis.

DOSAGE: *Adults:* 2 sprays per nostril bid.
Pediatrics: Seasonal Allergic/Vasomotor Rhinitis: ≥12 yrs: 2 sprays per nostril bid. Seasonal Allergic Rhinitis: 5-11 yrs: 1 spray per nostril bid.

HOW SUPPLIED: Spray: 137mcg/spray [30mL]

ADVERSE REACTIONS: Bitter taste, somnolence, weight increase, headache, nasal burning, pharyngitis, paroxysmal sneezing, dry mouth, nausea, atrial fibrillation, palpitations.

INTERACTIONS: Avoid alcohol or other CNS depressants; additive CNS impairment may occur. Increased azelastine levels with cimetidine.

PREGNANCY: Category C, caution in nursing.

MECHANISM OF ACTION: Phthalazinone derivative; inhibits histamine H_1 receptor activity.

PHARMACOKINETICS: Absorption: T_{max}=2-3 hrs. **Distribution:** Azelastine: plasma protein binding (88%). Desmethylazelastine: V_d=14.5L/kg; plasma protein binding (97%).

NURSING CONSIDERATIONS

Assessment: Assess for liver/renal functions, alcohol intake, and possible drug interactions.

Monitoring: Monitor for somnolence.

Patient Counseling: Caution against hazardous activities (eg, operating machinery/driving). Avoid concomitant use of drugs (eg, other antihistamines, CNS depressants) or alcohol. Avoid spraying in eyes. Consult physician if pregnant/nursing or planning to become pregnant.

Administration: Intranasal route. **Storage:** 20-25°C (68-77F°). Protect from freezing. Store bottle upright with pump tightly closed.

ASTEPRO   RX
azelastine HCl (Meda)

THERAPEUTIC CLASS: H_1-antagonist

INDICATIONS: Relief of symptoms of seasonal and perennial allergic rhinitis in patients ≥12 yrs.

DOSAGE: *Adults:* Seasonal allergic rhinitis: (0.1%, 0.15%): 1 or 2 sprays per nostril bid. (0.15%): May be administered as 2 sprays per nostril qd. Perennial allergic rhinitis: (0.15%): 2 sprays per nostril bid. Elderly: Start at the low end of dosing range.
Pediatrics: ≥12 yrs: Seasonal allergic rhinitis: (0.1%, 0.15%): 1 or 2 sprays per nostril bid. (0.15%): May be administered as 2 sprays per nostril qd. Perennial allergic rhinitis: (0.15%): 2 sprays per nostril bid.

ASTRAMORPH PF

HOW SUPPLIED: Spray: (0.1%) 137mcg; (0.15%) 205.5mcg

WARNINGS/PRECAUTIONS: Somnolence reported. May impair physical/mental abilities. Administer by intranasal route only. Caution in elderly.

ADVERSE REACTIONS: Bitter taste, somnolence, epistaxis, headache, nasal discomfort, fatigue, sneezing.

INTERACTIONS: Avoid concurrent use with alcohol or other CNS depressants; additional reductions in alertness and impairment of CNS performance may occur. Increased levels with cimetidine.

PREGNANCY: Category C, caution in nursing.

MECHANISM OF ACTION: H_1-receptor antagonist; phthalazinone derivative, which exhibits histamine H_1-receptor activity in isolated tissues, animal models, and humans; desmethylazelastine (major metabolite) also possesses H_1-receptor antagonist activity.

PHARMACOKINETICS: Absorption: Bioavailability (40%); (0.1%) C_{max}=200pg/mL; T_{max}=3 hrs; AUC =5122 pg•hr/mL. (0.15%) C_{max}=409pg/mL; T_{max}=4 hrs; AUC=9312pg•hr/mL. Desmethylazelastine: (0.1%) C_{max}=23pg/mL; T_{max}=24 hrs; AUC =2131 pg•hr/mL. (0.15%) C_{max}=38pg/mL; T_{max}=24 hrs; AUC=3824pg•hr/mL. **Distribution:** Plasma protein binding (azelastine, desmethylazelastine [major metabolite]): (88%, 97% respectively). V_d=14.5L/kg. **Metabolism:** Oxidation via CYP450 enzyme system. Desmethylazelastine (major metabolite). **Elimination:** Azelastine: Feces (75%, <10% unchanged); $T_{1/2}$=22-25 hrs. Desmethylazelastine: $T_{1/2}$=52-57 hrs.

NURSING CONSIDERATIONS

Assessment: Assess for hepatic/renal functions, alcohol intake, and possible drug interactions. Assess pregnancy/nursing status.

Monitoring: Monitor for somnolence, bitter taste, epistaxis, headache, nasal discomfort, fatigue, and sneezing.

Patient Counseling: Instruct to use exactly as prescribed. Instruct to use caution while engaging in hazardous activities (eg, operating machinery/driving) that require complete mental alertness and motor coordination. Advise to avoid alcohol or other CNS depressants. Must notify physician if pregnant/nursing or planning to become pregnant. Advise to prime medication before intial spray by releasing 6 sprays or until a fine mist appears. When medication has not been used for ≥3 days, counsel to reprime with 2 sprays or until a fine mist appears. Avoid spraying into eyes. Keep out of the reach of children.

Administration: Intranasal route. **Storage:** 20°-25°C (68°-77°F). Protect from freezing.

ASTRAMORPH PF   `CII`
morphine sulfate (APP Pharmaceuticals)

THERAPEUTIC CLASS: Opioid analgesic

INDICATIONS: Management of pain unresponsive to non-narcotic analgesics.

DOSAGE: *Adults:* IV: Initial: 2-10mg/70kg of body weight. Epidural Injection: Initial: 5mg in lumbar region. Titrate: If inadequate pain relief within 1 hr, increase by 1-2mg at intervals sufficient to assess effectiveness. Max: 10mg/24 hrs. Continuous Epidural: Initial: 2-4mg/24 hrs. Give additional 1-2mg if needed. Intrathecal: 0.2-1mg single dose, do not repeat; may follow with 0.6mg/hr naloxone IV infusion to reduce incidence of side effects. Consider alternative routes of administration if pain recurs. Elderly: Administer with extreme caution.

HOW SUPPLIED: Inj: 0.5mg/mL [2mL, 10mL], 1mg/mL [2mL, 10mL]

CONTRAINDICATIONS: Acute bronchial asthma, upper airway obstruction.

WARNINGS/PRECAUTIONS: Have resuscitation equipment, trained personnel and narcotic antagonists available; severe respiratory depression may occur. Avoid rapid administration. May be habit-forming. Caution with head injury, increased intracranial pressure, decreased respiratory reserve (eg, emphysema, severe obesity, kyphoscoliosis, or phrenic nerve paralysis), hepatic/

renal dysfunction, elderly. High doses may cause seizures. Smooth muscle hypertonicity secondary to morphine entering systemic circulation after neuraxial administration may cause biliary colic, urinary difficulty or retention. Orthostatic hypotension may occur with hypovolemia or myocardial dysfunction. Limit epidural/intrathecal route to lumbar area, and use epidural over intrathecal route whenever possible. Evaluate benefit versus risk of epidural/intrathecal administration in patients with infection of the injection site, bleeding diathesis, or on anticoagulant therapy.

ADVERSE REACTIONS: Respiratory depression, hypotension, pruritus, urinary retention, N/V, constipation, anxiety, cough reflex depression, oliguria.

INTERACTIONS: CNS depressants (eg, alcohol, sedatives, antihistamines, psychotropics) potentiate depressive effects. Neuroleptics may increase respiratory depression. May cause severe hypotension with general anesthesia and phenothiazines, and orthostatic hypotension with sympatholytic drugs.

PREGNANCY: Category C, safety in nursing not known.

MECHANISM OF ACTION: Opioid analgesic. Analgesic effect involves 3 areas of CNS; periaqueductal periventricular gray matter, ventromedial medulla, and spinal cord. Interacts predominantly with the μ-receptor to produce analgesic effects; μ-binding sites are found in the brain, spinal cord, and in the trigeminal nerve.

PHARMACOKINETICS: Absorption: (Epidural) C_{max}=33-40ng/mL; (intrathecal) C_{max}≤1-7.8ng/mL; (epidural, intrathecal) T_{max}=5-10 min. **Distribution:** (IV) V_d= 1-4.7L/kg; (intrathecal) V_d=22 mL. Plasma protein binding (36%), muscle tissue binding (54%). **Metabolism:** Hepatic glucuronidation. Found in breast milk. **Elimination:** Urine (major), feces (10%). (IV) $T_{1/2}$=1.5-2 hrs; (Epidural) $T_{1/2}$=30-249 min.

NURSING CONSIDERATIONS

Assessment: Assess for degree of opioid tolerance, previous opioid dose, level of pain intensity, type of pain, patient's general condition and medical status, emotional status or any other conditions where treatment is contraindicated or cautioned. Assess for history of hypersensitivity, pregnancy/nursing status, renal/hepatic function, and possible drug interactions.

Monitoring: Monitor for signs/symptoms of respiratory depression, hypotension, myoclonic-like spasms, seizures, urinary retention, and drug dependence. If administered via epidural and intrathecal route, monitor patients for 24 hrs for signs of respiratory depression.

Patient Counseling: Instruct to report if any signs/symptoms of respiratory depression (eg, difficulty breathing) occur. Inform physician of all medications currently taking. Advise to avoid alcohol or other CNS depressants. Inform drug may be habit forming. Avoid abrupt withdrawal.

Administration: IV, epidural, or intrathecal route. Administer in a setting where proper monitoring and resuscitative equipment are available. For epidural administration, proper placement of the needle or catheter in the epidural space should be verified before medication is injected. **Storage:** Store in carton at 20-25°C (68-77°F). Protect from light. Do not freeze. Discard any unused portion. Do not heat-sterilize.

ATACAND

RX

candesartan cilexetil (AstraZeneca)

> Can cause injury/death to developing fetus during 2nd and 3rd trimesters. D/C therapy if pregnancy is detected.

THERAPEUTIC CLASS: Angiotensin II receptor antagonist

INDICATIONS: Treatment of HTN, alone or with other antihypertensives, in adults or children 1-<17 yrs. Treatment of heart failure (HF) (NYHA Class II-IV) in adults with left ventricular systolic dysfunction (ejection fraction ≤40%) to reduce risk of death and HF hospitalizations; has an added effect when used with an ACE inhibitor.

DOSAGE: *Adults:* Individualize dose. HTN: Monotherapy Without Volume Depletion: Initial: 16mg qd. Usual: 8-32mg/day given qd-bid. Maximal effects attained within 4-6 weeks. May add diuretic if BP not controlled. Intravascular Volume Depletion/Moderate Hepatic Impairment: Lower initial dose. Heart Failure: Initial: 4mg qd. Titrate: Double dose every 2 weeks, as tolerated, to target dose of 32mg qd.
Pediatrics: HTN: 6-<17 yrs: <50kg: Initial: 4-8mg. Usual: 2-16mg/day. >50kg: Initial: 8-16mg. Usual: 4-32mg/day. 1-<6 yrs: Initial: 0.20mg/kg. Usual: 0.05-0.4mg/kg/day. Adjust according to BP response. Intravascular Volume Depletion: Initiate at a lower dose. Administer qd or divided into 2 equal doses. Full effect attained within 4 weeks. For children who cannot swallow tablets, oral suspension may be substituted. Refer to PI for preparation of oral suspension.

HOW SUPPLIED: Tab: 4mg*, 8mg*, 16mg*, 32mg* *scored

WARNINGS/PRECAUTIONS: Oligohydramnios reported; d/c unless it is considered life-saving for the mother. Avoid use in children <1 yr; may affect the development of immature kidneys. May cause symptomatic hypotension in volume- or salt-depleted patients; correct conditions before therapy or monitor closely. Hypotension may occur during major surgery and anesthesia. Caution initiating therapy with HF. May cause hyperkalemia and increase SrCr in patients with HF; monitor serum K⁺, SrCr, and BP during dose escalation and periodically thereafter. Changes in renal function may occur. Avoid in all pediatric patients with a glomerular filtration rate <30mL/min/1.73m². Consider low initial dose in patients with moderate hepatic impairment.

ADVERSE REACTIONS: Back pain, dizziness, URI, hyperkalemia, hypotension, abnormal renal function.

INTERACTIONS: May increase lithium levels when coadministered; monitor serum lithium levels carefully. Hypotension may occur with anesthesia. Increased risk of hyperkalemia with ACE inhibitors and potassium-sparing diuretics such as spirinolactone.

PREGNANCY: Category C (1st trimester) and D (2nd and 3rd trimesters), not for use in nursing.

MECHANISM OF ACTION: Angiotensin II receptor antagonist; blocks the vasoconstrictor and aldosterone-secreting effects of angiotensin II by selectively blocking the binding of angiotensin II to the AT_1 receptor in many tissues, such as vascular smooth muscle and adrenal gland.

PHARMACOKINETICS: Absorption: Rapid, complete; absolute bioavailability (15%); T_{max}=3-4 hrs. **Distribution:** V_d=0.13L/kg; plasma protein binding (>99%). **Metabolism:** GIT via ester hydrolysis, liver via O-deethylation (minor); candesartan (metabolite). **Elimination:** Feces (67%), urine (33%; 26%, unchanged); $T_{1/2}$=9 hrs.

NURSING CONSIDERATIONS

Assessment: Assess for hypersensitivity, hepatic/renal function, volume or salt depletion, HF, renal artery stenosis, pregnancy/nursing status, and possible drug interactions.

Monitoring: Monitor serum K⁺, SrCr, BUN, and BP periodically especially in patients with HF. Monitor for signs/symptoms of hypotension, hypersensitivity reactions, changes in renal function and oligohydramnios in pregnant women. Monitor infants with histories of *in utero* exposure for hypotension, oliguria and hyperkalemia.

Patient Counseling: Inform patient of pregnancy/nursing risks. Ask to report pregnancies as soon as possible. Regularly question post-menarche adolescents on changes in menstrual pattern and the possibility of pregnancy. Advise to seek medical attention if experience symptoms of hypotension, CV events, or hypersensitivity reactions. Take without regard to food.

Administration: Oral route. **Storage:** 25°C (77°F); excursions permitted to 15-30°C (59-86°F). Keep container tightly closed.

ATACAND HCT

RX

candesartan cilexetil - hydrochlorothiazide (AstraZeneca)

> Can cause injury/death to developing fetus during 2nd and 3rd trimesters. D/C therapy if pregnancy detected.

THERAPEUTIC CLASS: Angiotensin II receptor antagonist/thiazide diuretic

INDICATIONS: Treatment of HTN.

DOSAGE: *Adults:* Initial: If BP Not Controlled on HCTZ 25mg/day or Controlled But Serum K⁺ Decreased: 16mg-12.5mg tab qd. If BP not controlled on 32mg candesartan/day, give 32mg-12.5mg qd; may increase to 32mg-25mg qd. Replacement Therapy: Combination may be substituted for titrated components.

HOW SUPPLIED: Tab: (Candesartan-HCTZ) 16mg-12.5mg*, 32mg-12.5mg*, 32mg-25mg* *scored

CONTRAINDICATIONS: Anuria, hypersensitivity to sulfonamide-derived drugs.

WARNINGS/PRECAUTIONS: Not for initial therapy. Not recommended for initial titration with moderate hepatic impairment. Correct volume or salt depletion before therapy. Avoid with severe renal impairment. Candesartan: Caution with renal artery stenosis, and severe congestive heart failure. Risk of hypotension during major surgery. HCTZ: May cause idiosyncratic reaction, resulting in acute transient myopia and acute angle-closure glaucoma; d/c as rapidly as possible. Caution with hepatic impairment, progressive liver disease, and severe renal disease. Hypersensitivity reactions may occur. May exacerbate or activate systemic lupus erythematosus (SLE). Hyperuricemia, hyperglycemia, hypokalemia, hypomagnesemia, hyponatremia, hypochloremic alkalosis, hypercalcemia may occur. Enhanced effects in post-sympathectomy patient. D/C or withhold therapy if progressive renal impairment becomes evident. May increase cholesterol and TG levels.

ADVERSE REACTIONS: Fetal injury, upper respiratory tract infection, back pain.

INTERACTIONS: Symptomatic hypotension may occur in intravascular volume-depleted patients (eg, patients treated with diuretics). Candesartan: Increases lithium levels; monitor lithium levels during concomitant use. Hypotension may occur during anesthesia. HCTZ: Potentiates orthostatic hypotension with alcohol, barbiturates, and narcotics. Adjust dosage of insulin or oral hypoglycemic agents. Impaired absorption with cholestyramine, colestipol. Corticosteroids and adrenocorticotropic hormone may intensify electrolyte depletion. May decrease response to pressor amines (eg, norepinephrine). Potentiates other antihypertensives. May increase responsiveness to nondepolarizing skeletal muscle relaxants (eg, tubocurarine). Risk of lithium toxicity; avoid use. NSAIDs may reduce diuretic, natriuretic, and hypertensive effects. May cause hypokalemia, which may lead to cardiac arrhythmia and sensitize or exaggerate the response of the heart to the toxic effects of digitalis.

PREGNANCY: Category C (1st trimester) and D (2nd and 3rd trimesters), not for use in nursing.

MECHANISM OF ACTION: Candesartan: Angiotensin II receptor antagonist; blocks vasoconstrictor and aldosterone-secreting effects of angiotensin II by blocking binding of angiotensin II to AT_1 receptors. HCTZ: Thiazide diuretic; affects renal tubular mechanism of electrolyte reabsorption, directly increasing excretion of Na⁺ and Cl⁻, and indirectly reducing plasma volume.

PHARMACOKINETICS: Absorption: Candesartan: Rapid and complete; absolute bioavailability (15%); T_{max}=3-4 hrs. **Distribution:** Candesartan: Plasma protein binding (>99%); V_d=0.13L/kg. HCTZ: Crosses placenta; found in breast milk. **Metabolism:** Candesartan: Ester hydrolysis, liver via O-deethylation (minor); candesartan (active metabolite). **Elimination:** Candesartan: Biliary, feces (unchanged); urine (26% unchanged); $T_{1/2}$=9 hrs. HCTZ: Urine (61% unchanged); $T_{1/2}$=5.6-14.8 hrs.

NURSING CONSIDERATIONS

Assessment: Assess for volume/salt depletion, SLE, diabetes mellitus (DM), anuria, hypersensitivity to sulfonamide, hepatic/renal function, pregnancy/nursing status, and possible drug interactions.

Monitoring: Monitor serum electrolytes periodically. Monitor for signs/symptoms of fluid/electrolyte imbalance, exacerbation or activation of SLE, hypotension, hyperglycemia, hyperuricemia or precipitation of gout, hypersensitivity reactions, renal/hepatic dysfunction.

Patient Counseling: Inform of pregnancy risks. Counsel that lightheadedness may occur especially during the 1st days of therapy. Instruct to d/c therapy if syncope occurs. Advise that inadequate fluid intake, excessive perspiration, diarrhea, or vomiting may result in drop of BP, leading to lightheadedness or syncope. Instruct not to use K$^+$ supplements or salt substitutes containing K$^+$ without consulting physician.

Administration: Oral route. **Storage:** 25°C (77°F); excursions permitted to 15-30°C (59-86°F).

ATELVIA   RX
risedronate sodium (Warner Chilcott)

THERAPEUTIC CLASS: Bisphosphonate

INDICATIONS: Treatment of osteoporosis in postmenopausal women.

DOSAGE: *Adults:* 35mg once weekly. Take in am immediately following breakfast. Swallow tab whole in upright position and with at least 4 oz. of plain water. Do not lie down for 30 min after dose. Do not crush, cut, or chew tab.

HOW SUPPLIED: Tab, Delayed-Release: 35mg

CONTRAINDICATIONS: Hypocalcemia, inability to stand or sit upright for at least 30 min, abnormalities of the esophagus which delay esophageal emptying (eg, stricture or achalasia).

WARNINGS/PRECAUTIONS: Should not be given in patients treated with Actonel; contains the same active ingredient. May cause local irritation of the upper GI mucosa. Esophageal and GI adverse events reported; caution with active upper GI problems (eg, Barrett's esophagus, dysphagia, other esophageal diseases, gastritis, duodenitis or ulcers). D/C if signs and symptoms of esophageal reactions occur. Treat hypocalcemia and other disturbances of bone and mineral metabolism before therapy. Osteonecrosis of the jaw (ONJ) reported. Severe and occasionally incapacitating bone, joint, and/or muscle pain reported; d/c use if severe symptoms develop. Atypical femur fractures reported; evaluate patients with new thigh or groin pain to rule out femoral fracture. Avoid with severe renal impairment (CrCl <30mL/min). Caution in use with bone-imaging agents. Not for use in pediatrics.

ADVERSE REACTIONS: Diarrhea, abdominal pain, constipation, N/V, dyspepsia, influenza, bronchitis, upper respiratory tract infection, arthralgia, back pain, pain in extremity.

INTERACTIONS: Calcium supplements, antacids, magnesium-based supplements or laxatives, and iron preparations may reduce bioavailability of risedronate and should not be taken together. Reduced absorption with calcium/vitamin D supplement. Drugs that raise stomach pH (eg, H$_2$ blockers, proton pump inhibitors [PPIs], or antacids) may affect enteric coating and thereby reduce bioavailability of risedronate; should not be taken at the same time with antacids; not recommended with H$_2$ blockers and PPIs. Upper GI reactions with concomitant NSAID. Risk of ONJ with concomitant corticosteroid or chemotherapy. May interfere with the use of bone-imaging agents. May increase risk of atypical femur fractures with glucocorticoids (eg, prednisone).

PREGNANCY: Category C, not for use in nursing.

MECHANISM OF ACTION: Bisphosphonate; has an affinity for hydroxyapatite crystals in bone and acts as an antiresorptive agent. At the cellular level, it inhibits osteoclasts.

PHARMACOKINETICS: Absorption: T_{max}=3 hrs; (immediate release) absolute bioavailability (0.63%). **Distribution:** V_d=13.8L/kg; plasma protein binding (24%). **Elimination:** Urine (85% IV dose), feces (unabsorbed dose, unchanged); $T_{1/2}$=561 hrs.

NURSING CONSIDERATIONS

Assessment: Assess for hypocalcemia and other bone disturbances or problems with mineral metabolism. Assess for ability to stand or sit upright for 30 min, any mental disability, esophageal abnormalities, active upper GI problems, severe renal impairment (CrCl <30mL/min), risk factors for developing ONJ, known hypersensitivity to any drug component, pregnancy/nursing status, and possible drug interactions. Assess for history of bisphosphonate exposure with thigh or groin pain.

Monitoring: Monitor for signs/symptoms of upper GI disorders (eg, dysphagia, esophagitis, esophageal or gastric ulcers), ONJ, atypical femur fracture (unusual hip, groin, or thigh pain), musculoskeletal pain.

Patient Counseling: Instruct to take in am, while in an upright position (sitting or standing), with at least 4 oz. of plain water, immediately following breakfast. Advise to swallow tab whole and not to crush, cut or chew tab. Instruct not to lie down for 30 min after taking medication. Contact physician if symptoms of esophageal disease develop. Advise to take supplemental calcium and vitamin D if dietary intake is inadequate; take supplement at a different time of the day than risedronate. Advise to consider weight-bearing exercises and appropriate lifestyle modifications. Inform not to take with Actonel. Counsel about possible adverse reactions. Counsel about possible adverse reactions. Instruct if they miss a dose to take 1 tab on the morning after; return to original schedule and not to take 2 tabs on the same day. Instruct to read the Medication Guide before starting therapy and re-read it each time the prescription is renewed.

Administration: Oral route. **Storage:** 20-25°C (68-77°F).

ATIVAN

lorazepam (Biovail)

THERAPEUTIC CLASS: Benzodiazepine

INDICATIONS: Management of anxiety disorders or for short-term relief of the symptoms of anxiety or anxiety associated with depressive symptoms.

DOSAGE: *Adults:* Initial: 2-3mg/day given bid-tid. Usual: 2-6mg/day in divided doses. Insomnia: 2-4mg qhs. Elderly/Debilitated: 1-2mg/day in divided doses. *Pediatrics:* >12 yrs: Initial: 2-3mg/day given bid-tid. Usual: 2-6mg/day in divided doses. Insomnia: 2-4mg qhs.

HOW SUPPLIED: Tab: 0.5mg, 1mg*, 2mg* *scored

CONTRAINDICATIONS: Acute narrow-angle glaucoma.

WARNINGS/PRECAUTIONS: Avoid with primary depression or psychosis. Withdrawal symptoms with abrupt d/c. Careful supervision if addiction-prone. Caution in patients with compromised respiratory function. Caution with elderly, and renal or hepatic dysfunction. Monitor for GI disease with prolonged therapy. Periodic blood counts and LFTs with long-term therapy.

ADVERSE REACTIONS: Sedation, dizziness, weakness, unsteadiness, transient amnesia, memory impairment, visual disturbance, depression, respiratory depression, constipation, vertigo, change in appetite, headache.

INTERACTIONS: CNS-depressant effects with barbiturates, alcohol. Diminished tolerance to alcohol and other CNS depressants. Increased plasma levels with valproate and probenecid, decrease dose by 50%.

PREGNANCY: Not for use in pregnancy or nursing.

MECHANISM OF ACTION: Benzodiazepine; antianxiety agent, interacts with GABA-benzodiazepine receptor complex.

PHARMACOKINETICS: Absorption: Absolute bioavailability (90%); C_{max}=20ng/mL (2mg PO); T_{max}=2 hrs. **Distribution:** Plasma protein binding (85%). **Metabolism:** Glucuronidation. **Elimination:** Urine; $T_{1/2}$=12 hrs.

NURSING CONSIDERATIONS

Assessment: Assess for acute narrow-angle glaucoma, pre-existing depression and/or psychosis, compromised respiratory function, impaired renal/hepatic function, and possible drug interactions. Assess addiction-prone individuals (eg, drug addicts, alcoholics).

Monitoring: Monitor worsening of depression and/or suicidal thinking, physical/psychological dependence, paradoxical reactions, CNS depression, lab tests (CBC, LFTs, lactate dehydrogenase).

Patient Counseling: Inform that psychological/physical dependence may result; consult physician before increasing dose or abruptly d/c drug. Caution with hazardous tasks (eg, operating machinery/driving); do not drink alcohol or take other CNS depressants concomitantly.

Administration: Oral route. **Storage:** 20-25°C (68-77°F). Keep tightly closed.

ATIVAN INJECTION   CIV
lorazepam (Baxter)

THERAPEUTIC CLASS: Benzodiazepine

INDICATIONS: Treatment of status epilepticus and preanesthetic medication in adults.

DOSAGE: *Adults:* ≥18 yrs: Status Epilepticus: 4mg IV (given slowly at 2mg/min); may repeat 1 dose after 10-15 min if seizures recur or fail to cease. Preanesthetic Sedation: Usual: (IM) 0.05mg/kg given at least 2 hrs prior to operation; (IV) 2mg or 0.044mg/kg IV (whichever is smaller) 15-20 min prior to procedure. Max: 4mg IM/IV. Elderly: Start at the low end of the dosing range.

HOW SUPPLIED: Inj: 2mg/mL, 4mg/mL [1mL, 10mL]

CONTRAINDICATIONS: Acute narrow-angle glaucoma, sleep apnea syndrome, severe respiratory insufficiency. Not for intra-arterial injection.

WARNINGS/PRECAUTIONS: May produce heavy sedation; airway obstruction and respiratory depression may occur; ensure airway patency and monitor respiration. May impair mental/physical abilities. Avoid intra-arterial administration. Avoid in patients with hepatic and/or renal failure; caution in patients with hepatic and/or renal impairment. May cause fetal damage during pregnancy. When used for peroral endoscopic procedures; adequate topical/regional anesthesia is recommended to minimize reflex activity. Extreme caution when administering injections to elderly, very ill, or to patients with limited pulmonary reserve as hypoventilation and/or hypoxic cardiac arrest may occur. Paradoxical reaction, propylene glycol toxicity (eg, lactic acidosis, hyperosmolality, hypotension) and polyethylene glycol toxicity (eg, acute tubular necrosis) reported; premature and low birth weight infants as well pediatric patients receiving high-doses may be at higher risk. Pediatric patients may exhibit sensitivity to benzyl alcohol; "gasping syndrome" associated with administration of IV solutions containing benzyl alcohol in neonates. Repeated doses over a prolonged period of time may result in physical and psychological dependence and withdrawal symptoms following abrupt d/c.

ADVERSE REACTIONS: Respiratory depression/failure, somnolence, headache, hypoventilation, injection-site reactions (eg, pain, burning, redness), paradoxical excitement.

INTERACTIONS: Additive CNS depression with other CNS depressants (eg, ethyl alcohol, phenothiazines, barbiturates, MAOIs, antidepressants). Increased sedation, hallucinations and irrational behavior with scopolamine. Reduce dose by 50% when given in combination with valproate or probenecid due to decreased clearance. Increased clearance with oral contraceptives. Severe adverse effects with clozapine, loxapine, and haloperidol reported. Prolonged and profound effect with concomitant sedatives, tranquilizers, narcotic analgesics.

PREGNANCY: Category D, not for use in nursing.

MECHANISM OF ACTION: Benzodiazepine; antianxiety, sedative and anti-convulsant effects. Interacts with GABA-benzodiazepine receptor complex in human brain. Exhibits relatively high and specific affinity for its recognition site but does not displace GABA. Attachment to the specific binding site enhances the affinity of GABA for its receptor site on the same receptor complex.

PHARMACOKINETICS: Absorption: Complete, rapid; (IM) C_{max}=48ng/mL, T_{max}=within 3 hrs. **Distribution:** V_d=1.3L/kg, plasma protein binding (91%), crosses blood brain barrier. **Metabolism:** Liver. **Elimination:** Urine (88%), feces (7%), (0.3% unchanged); $T_{1/2}$=14 hrs.

NURSING CONSIDERATIONS

Assessment: Comprehensive review of benefits/risks in status epilepticus. Assess for hypersensitivity to benzodiazepine or its vehicle, acute-angle glaucoma, pre-existing respiratory impairment, hepatic/renal impairment, pregnancy/nursing status, and possible drug interactions.

Monitoring: Monitor for respiratory depression, airway obstruction, heavy sedation, drowsiness, excessive sleepiness, hypoglycemia and hyponatremia in status epilepticus, seizures, myoclonus, somnolence, injection-site reactions (eg, pain, burning sensation, and redness), and paradoxical reactions (eg, mania, agitation, psychosis). Signs of toxicity to the vehicle's components (eg, lactic acidosis, hyperosmolarity, hypotension, and acute tubular necrosis). Monitor for hypersensitivity reactions.

Patient Counseling: Inform of risks/benefits. Caution with hazardous tasks (eg, operating machinery/driving). Do not get out of bed unassisted. Avoid alcoholic beverages for at least 24-48 hrs after receiving drug. Advise about potential for physical/psychological dependence and withdrawal symptoms.

Administration: IM/IV route. **Storage:** Refrigerate; protect from light.

ATRALIN   RX
tretinoin (DPT Laboratories)

THERAPEUTIC CLASS: Retinoid

INDICATIONS: Topical treatment of acne vulgaris.

DOSAGE: *Adults:* Cleanse area(s) thoroughly, then apply thin layer qd before bedtime.
Pediatrics: ≥10 yrs: Cleanse area(s) thoroughly, then apply thin layer qd before bedtime.

HOW SUPPLIED: Gel: 0.05% [45g]

WARNINGS/PRECAUTIONS: Avoid eyes, mouth, paranasal creases, and mucous membranes. Skin may become dry, red, or exfoliated. If degree of irritation warrants, temporarily reduce amount/frequency, or d/c use temporarily or altogether. May cause mild to moderate dryness; use appropriate moisturizer. Caution with eczematous or sunburned skin, with high levels of exposure to sun, wind, or cold, or with known sensitivity to fish allergy.

ADVERSE REACTIONS: Dry skin, peeling, scaling, flaking skin, burning sensation, erythema.

INTERACTIONS: Caution with topical medications, medicated or abrasive soaps and cleansers, products with strong drying effects, high concentrations of alcohol, astringents, spices, or lime. Caution with benzoyl peroxide, sulfur, resorcinol, or salicylic acid; allow effects of these agents to subside before use.

PREGNANCY: Category C, caution in nursing.

MECHANISM OF ACTION: Retinoic acid derivative; binds with high affinity to three specific retinoic acid nuclear receptors (RARα, RARβ, and RAR$_γ$) which are located in both the cytosol and nucleus. Acts to modify gene expression, subsequent protein synthesis, and epithelial cell growth and differentiation. Decreases the cohesiveness of follicular epithelial cells with decreased microcomedo formation. Stimulates mitotic activity and increases turnover of follicular epithelial cells causing extrusion of the comedones.

PHARMACOKINETICS: Absorption: Tretinoin: Baseline plasma concentrations=0.68ng/mL; Day 14 plasma concentrations=0.69-2.88ng/mL. **Metabolism:** Major metabolites: 13-cis-retinoic acid and 4-oxo-13-cis-retinoic acid.

NURSING CONSIDERATIONS

Assessment: Assess use in patients with presence of eczematous or sunburned skin, known sensitivity or allergy to fish, inherent sensitivity to sun, and in pregnant/nursing females. Assess for possible drug interactions.

Monitoring: Monitor for development of dry, red, or exfoliated skin while on medication.

Patient Counseling: Advise to avoid unprotected exposure to sunlight/ sunlamps due to potential for increased photosensitization. Instruct to use sunscreen of, at least SPF 15, and wear protective clothing during sunlight exposure. Inform that weather extremes such as wind or cold may cause irritation. Instruct to use a moisturizer if mild-to-moderate skin dryness develops. Advise to continue using medication if these effects are tolerable. Instruct to remove any cosmetics and clean affected area thoroughly prior to administration. Instruct to avoid applying medication around the eyes, mouth, paranasal creases, and mucus membranes.

Administration: Topical. **Storage:** 20-25°C (68-77°F), excursions permitted to 15-30°C (59-86°F). Protect from freezing. Keep out of reach of children.

ATRIPLA   RX

tenofovir disoproxil fumarate - emtricitabine - efavirenz (Bristol-Myers Squibb/ Gilead Sciences)

> Lactic acidosis and severe hepatomegaly with steatosis, including fatal cases, have been reported with the use of nucleoside analogs in combination with other antiretrovirals. Not approved for the treatment of chronic hepatitis B virus (HBV) infection. Severe acute exacerbations of HBV have been reported in patients upon d/c of emtricitabine or tenofovir. Hepatic function should be monitored closely for at least several months after d/c of therapy in patients coinfected with HIV-1 and HBV. Initiation of anti-hepatitis B therapy may be warranted.

THERAPEUTIC CLASS: Non-nucleoside reverse transcriptase inhibitor/nucleoside analog combination

INDICATIONS: For use alone as a complete regimen or in combination with other antiretroviral agents for the treatment of HIV-1 infection in adults.

DOSAGE: *Adults:* ≥18 yrs: 1 tab qd on empty stomach, hs dosing may improve tolerability of nervous system symptoms.

HOW SUPPLIED: Tab: (Efavirenz-Emtricitabine-Tenofovir DF) 600mg-200mg-300mg

CONTRAINDICATIONS: Concomitant use with voriconazole, dihydroergotamine, ergonovine, ergotamine, methylergonovine, midazolam, triazolam, bepridil, cisapride, pimozide, St. John's wort.

WARNINGS/PRECAUTIONS: Caution with known risk factors for hepatic disease; suspend treatment if clinical or laboratory findings are suggestive of lactic acidosis or pronounced hepatotoxicity. Test for presence of chronic HBV prior to treatment. Monitor LFTs before or during treatment. Serious psychiatric adverse events (eg, severe depression, suicidal ideation, nonfatal suicide attempts, aggressive behavior, paranoid and manic reactions) and CNS symptoms reported; may impair mental/physical abilities. Renal impairment, including cases of acute renal failure and Fanconi syndrome reported; avoid in patients with CrCl <50mL/min; may cause fetal harm during 1st trimester; avoid pregnancy. Use adequate contraceptive measures for 12 weeks after d/c. Skin rash reported; d/c if severe rash associated with blistering, desquamation, mucosal involvement, or fever develops. Monitor bone mineral density (BMD) in patients with history of pathologic bone fracture or are at risk for osteopenia. Cases of osteomalacia reported. Caution in patients with history of seizures; convulsions reported. Immune reconstitution syndrome reported. May cause redistribution/accumulation of body fat.

ADVERSE REACTIONS: Diarrhea, nausea, fatigue, depression, dizziness, rash, headache, insomnia, abnormal dreams, laboratory abnormalities, lactic acidosis, severe hepatomegaly with steatosis.

INTERACTIONS: See Contraindications. Should not be use with adefovir dipivoxil. Avoid with concurrent or recent use of nephrotoxic agents. Avoid concomitant use with drugs with the same active components. Should not be coadministered with drugs containing lamivudine. May cause additive CNS effects when used with alcohol or psychoactive drugs. Coadministration with atazanavir is not recommended. Additional 100mg/day of ritonavir needed when concomitantly used with fosamprenavir/ritonavir once daily. Monitor LFTs when coadministered with ritonavir and other medications associated with liver toxicity. Coadministration with didanosine may increase didanosine concentrations. May decrease plasma concentrations of rifabutin. May decrease the levels of etonogestrel and the active metabolites of norgestimate. Efavirenz: May alter plasma concentrations of drugs metabolized by 2C9, 2C19, and 3A4. Drugs that induce CYP3A activity (eg, phenobarbital, rifampin, rifabutin) may increase clearance resulting in lowered plasma concentrations. May decrease levels of indinavir, lopinavir, maraviroc and saquinavir. May decrease the plasma levels of the anticonvulsants phenytoin, carbamazepine, and phenobarbital. May decrease levels of sertraline, ketoconazole, itraconazole, clarithromycin, calcium channel blockers that are CYP3A substrates and HMG-CoA reductase inhibitors. Avoid with posaconazole. May decrease methadone concentrations. Concomitant use with rifampin may decrease efavirenz concentrations. May increase or decrease warfarin concentrations. Emtricitabine (FTC) and Tenofovir DF (TDF): Coadministration with drugs that reduce renal function or compete for active tubular secretion (eg, acyclovir, adefovir dipivoxil, cidofovir, ganciclovir, valacyclovir, valganciclovir) may increase concentrations of FTC, TDF, and/or the coadministered drug. Concomitant use with lopinavir/ritonavir may increase TDF concentrations and may potentiate TDF-associated adverse events. May decrease the levels of cyclosporine, tacrolimus, sirolimus, and other immunosuppressants metabolized by CYP3A. Refer to PI for detailed information.

PREGNANCY: Category D, not for use in nursing.

MECHANISM OF ACTION: Efavirenz: Non-nucleoside reverse transcriptase inhibitor; noncompetitive inhibition of HIV-1 reverse transcriptase (RT). Emtricitabine: Nucleoside analog of cytidine; inhibits activity of HIV-1 RT by competing with natural substrate deoxycytidine 5'-triphosphate and incorporating into nascent viral DNA, resulting in chain termination. Tenofovir DF: Acyclic nucleoside phosphonate diester analog of adenosine monophosphate; inhibits activity of HIV-1 RT by competing with the natural substrate deoxyadenosine 5'-triphosphate and, after incorporation into the DNA, by DNA chain termination.

PHARMACOKINETICS: Absorption: Efavirenz: C_{max}=12.9μM, T_{max}=3-5 hrs, AUC=184μM•hr. Emtricitabine: Rapid; absolute bioavailability (93%), C_{max}=1.8μg/mL, T_{max}=1-2 hrs, AUC=10μg•hr/mL. Tenofovir DF: C_{max}=296ng/mL, T_{max}=1 hr, AUC=2287ng•hr/mL. **Distribution:** Efavirenz: Plasma protein binding (99.5-99.75%). Emtricitabine: Plasma protein binding (<4%). Tenofovir DF: Plasma protein binding (<0.7%). **Metabolism:** Efavirenz: Via CYP3A and CYP2B6. **Elimination:** Efavirenz: Urine (14-34%, <1% unchanged), feces (16-61%); $T_{1/2}$=52-76 hrs (single dose), 40-55 hrs (multiple doses). Emtricitabine: Urine (86%); $T_{1/2}$=10 hrs. Tenofovir DF: Urine (70-80% unchanged), IV; $T_{1/2}$=17 hrs.

NURSING CONSIDERATIONS

Assessment: Assess for obesity, prolonged nucleoside exposure, liver dysfunction or risk factors for liver disease, renal impairment, HBV or HCV infection, psychiatric history, history of injection drug use, history of seizures, hypersensitivity, pregnancy/nursing status, and possible drug interactions. Assess BMD in patients with a history of pathological bone fracture or those at risk for osteopenia. Obtain baseline LFTs, CrCl, serum phosphorus levels, total cholesterol and TG levels.

Monitoring: Monitor for signs/symptoms of lactic acidosis, severe hepatomegaly with steatosis, psychiatric symptoms (eg, severe depression, suicidal ideations, aggressive behavior) nervous system symptoms (eg, dizziness, insomnia, impaired concentration), new onset or worsening renal impairment, skin rash, decreases in BMD, convulsions, immune reconstitution syndrome, and for fat redistribution/accumulation. Monitor clinical and laboratory follow-up for acute exacerbations of hepatitis B in patients with HBV and HIV-1 upon d/c of therapy. Monitor CD4+ cell count, HIV-1 RNA levels, LFTs, CrCl, serum phosphorus, total cholesterol and TG levels. Monitor fetal outcomes, didanosine-associated adverse effects, anticonvulsants and immunosuppressant levels.

Patient Counseling: Inform that therapy is not a cure for HIV-1, does not reduce transmission of HIV-1, and illnesses associated with HIV-1 may still be experienced. Advise to continue to practice safer sex, use latex or polyurethane condoms, and never to reuse or share needles. Instruct to take on an empty stomach and to take on a regular dosing schedule. Instruct to contact physician if symptoms of lactic acidosis or severe hepatomegaly with steatosis (eg, nausea, vomiting, unusual stomach discomfort, weakness), new onset or worsening renal impairment, psychiatric symptoms (eg, aggressive behavior, depression, suicide attempts, delusions, paranoia), CNS symptoms (eg, dizziness, insomnia, impaired concentration, drowsiness, abnormal dreams), or skin rash develops. Advise that fat redistribution/accumulation and decreases in bone mineral density may occur. Counsel to avoid pregnancy while on therapy; instruct that barrier contraception must always be used in combination with other methods of contraception. Advise to avoid potentially hazardous tasks (eg, driving, operating machinery) if experiencing CNS or psychiatric symptoms. Advise that severe acute exacerbation of hepatitis B may occur if coinfected. Advise to report use of any prescription, nonprescription medication, or herbal products, particularly St. John's wort.

Administration: Oral route. Take on an empty stomach. **Storage:** 25°C (77°F); excursions permitted to 15-30°C (59-86°F). Keep container tightly closed. Dispense only in original container. Do not use if seal over bottle opening is broken or missing.

ATROVENT HFA   RX
ipratropium bromide (Boehringer Ingelheim)

THERAPEUTIC CLASS: Anticholinergic bronchodilator

INDICATIONS: Maintenance treatment of bronchospasm associated with chronic obstructive pulmonary disease (COPD), including chronic bronchitis and emphysema.

DOSAGE: *Adults:* Initial: 2 inh qid. Max: 12 inh/24 hrs.

HOW SUPPLIED: MDI: 17mcg/inh [12.9g]

CONTRAINDICATIONS: Hypersensitivity to atropine or its derivatives.

WARNINGS/PRECAUTIONS: Not for acute episodes. Immediate hypersensitivity reactions reported. Can produce paradoxical bronchospasm. Caution with narrow-angle glaucoma, prostatic hyperplasia or bladder-neck obstruction.

ADVERSE REACTIONS: Back pain, bronchitis, dyspnea, dizziness, headache, nausea, blurred vision, dry mouth, exacerbation of symptoms.

INTERACTIONS: Avoid coadministration with other anticholinergic-containing drugs.

PREGNANCY: Category B, caution in nursing.

MECHANISM OF ACTION: Anticholinergic; inhibits vagally mediated reflexes by antagonizing the action of acetylcholine.

PHARMACOKINETICS: Absorption: (4 inh) C_{max} =59pg/mL. **Distribution:** Plasma protein binding (0-9%). **Metabolism:** Partial. **Elimination:** $T_{1/2}$=2 hrs.

NURSING CONSIDERATIONS

Assessment: Assess for hypersensitivity to atropine or its derivatives, narrow-angle glaucoma, prostatic hyperplasia, bladder-neck obstruction, pregnancy/nursing status, and possible drug interactions.

Monitoring: Monitor for urinary retention, mydriasis, GI distress (diarrhea, N/V), paradoxical bronchospasm, and allergic type-reaction (pruritus, angioedema of tongue, lips and face, urticaria, laryngospasm, anaphylaxis).

Patient Counseling: Remind patients to read the Patient Instructions for Use. Advise not to increase the dose or frequency. Not for acute episodes of bronchospasm. Avoid spraying in the eyes. Inform patient that paradoxical bronchospasm, which can be life-threatening, can occur; if occurs d/c use. Seek medical attention if symptoms of precipitation or worsening of narrow-angle glaucoma, mydriasis, increased intraocular pressure, acute eye pain/discomfort, blurring of vision, visual halos or colored images with red eyes from conjunctival and corneal congestion, or allergic/hypersensitivity reactions occur. Contact physician if difficulty in urinating occurs. Instruct patient that priming the medication is essential to ensure proper dosing.

Administration: Oral inhalation. Prime medication before first use with 2 sprays. If not used for >3 days, reprime with 2 sprays. **Storage:** 25°C (77°F); excursions permitted to 15-30°C (59-86°F). Do not puncture, use or store near heat or open flame.

ATROVENT NASAL   RX
ipratropium bromide (Boehringer Ingelheim)

THERAPEUTIC CLASS: Anticholinergic

INDICATIONS: (0.03%) Symptomatic relief of rhinorrhea associated with allergic and nonallergic perennial rhinitis in adults and children ≥6 yrs. (0.06%) Symptomatic relief of rhinorrhea associated with the common cold or seasonal allergic rhinitis in adults and children ≥5 yrs.

DOSAGE: *Adults:* (0.03%) Rhinorrhea with Allergic/Nonallergic Perennial Rhinitis: 2 sprays/nostril bid-tid. (0.06%) Rhinorrhea Associated with Common Cold: 2 sprays/nostril tid-qid for ≤4 days. Rhinorrhea Associated with Seasonal Allergic Rhinitis: 2 sprays/nostril qid for ≤3 weeks.
Pediatrics: (0.03%) ≥6 yrs: Rhinorrhea with Allergic/Nonallergic Perennial Rhinitis: 2 sprays/nostril bid-tid. (0.06%) Rhinorrhea Associated with Common Cold: ≥12 yrs: 2 sprays/nostril tid-qid for ≤4 days. 5-11 yrs: 2 sprays/nostril tid for ≤4 days. ≥5 yrs: Rhinorrhea Associated with Seasonal Allergic Rhinitis: 2 sprays/nostril qid for ≤3 weeks.

HOW SUPPLIED: Spray: (0.03%) 21mcg/spray [31.1g], (0.06%) 42mcg/spray [16.6g]

CONTRAINDICATIONS: Hypersensitivity to atropine or its derivatives.

WARNINGS/PRECAUTIONS: Immediate hypersensitivity reactions reported; d/c once and consider alternative treatment. Caution with narrow-angle glaucoma, prostatic hyperplasia, or bladder-neck obstruction. Caution in patients with hepatic or renal insufficiency.

ADVERSE REACTIONS: Epistaxis, pharyngitis, upper respiratory tract infection, nasal dryness, dry mouth/throat, headache, taste perversion.

INTERACTIONS: May produce additive effects with other anticholinergic agents.

PREGNANCY: Category B, caution in nursing.

MECHANISM OF ACTION: Anticholinergic; inhibits vagally-mediated reflexes by antagonizing action of acetylcholine at the cholinergic receptor. Inhibits secretions from serous and seromucous glands lining the nasal mucosa.

PHARMACOKINETICS: Absorption: Bioavailability (<20%). **Distribution:** Plasma protein binding (0-9%). **Metabolism:** Partial; ester hydrolysis products, tropic acid, tropane. **Elimination:** Urine (unchanged). (IV) $T_{1/2}$=1.6 hrs.

NURSING CONSIDERATIONS

Assessment: Assess for hypersensitivity to atropine or its derivatives, narrow-angle glaucoma, prostatic hyperplasia, bladder-neck obstruction, hepatic/renal insufficiency, pregnancy/nursing status, and possible drug interactions.

Monitoring: Monitor for signs and symptoms of hypersensitivity reactions (eg, urticaria, angioedema, rash, bronchospasm, anaphylaxis, oropharyngeal edema). Monitor visual changes and nasal symptoms.

Patient Counseling: Advise not to alter size of nasal spray opening. Instruct to avoid spraying medication into the eyes. Inform that temporary blurring of vision, precipitation or worsening of narrow-angle glaucoma, mydriasis, increased intraocular pressure (IOP), acute eye pain or discomfort, visual halos or colored images in association with red eyes from conjunctival and corneal congestion may occur if medication comes into direct contact with the eyes. Instruct to contact physician if eye pain, blurred vision, excessive nasal dryness, or episodes of nasal bleeding occurs. Caution about engaging in activities requiring balance and visual acuity (eg, driving or operating machines).

Administration: Intranasal route. Prime the nasal spray pump and blow nose to clear nostrils before first use. Refer to PI for proper administration. **Storage:** 25°C (77°F); excursions permitted to 15-30°C (59-86°F). Avoid freezing.

AUGMENTIN   RX
clavulanate potassium - amoxicillin (GlaxoSmithKline)

THERAPEUTIC CLASS: Aminopenicillin/beta lactamase inhibitor

INDICATIONS: Treatment of lower respiratory tract (LRTI), skin and skin structure (SSSI), and urinary tract infections (UTI), otitis media (OM), sinusitis caused by susceptible strains of microorganisms.

DOSAGE: *Adults:* (Dose based on amoxicillin) 500mg q12h or 250mg q8h. Severe Infections/RTI: 875mg q12h or 500mg q8h. May use 125mg/5mL or 250mg/5mL sus in place of 500mg tab and 200mg/5mL sus or 400mg/5mL sus in place of 875mg tab. CrCl <30mL/min: Do not give 875mg tab. CrCl 10-30mL/min: 250-500mg q12h. CrCl <10mL/min: 250-500mg q24h. Hemodialysis: 250-500mg q24h, give additional dose during and at end of dialysis.
Pediatrics: (Dose based on amoxicillin) ≥40kg: Use adult dose. ≥12 Weeks: Sinusitis/OM/LRTI/Severe Infections: (Sus/Tab, Chewable) 45mg/kg/day given q12h or 40mg/kg/day given q8h. Treat OM for 10 days. Less Severe Infections: 25mg/kg/day given q12h or 20mg/kg/day given q8h. <12 Weeks: 15mg/kg q12h (use 125mg/5mL sus).

HOW SUPPLIED: (Amoxicillin-Clavulanate) Sus: 125-31.25mg/5mL [75mL, 100mL, 150mL], 200-28.5mg/5mL [50mL, 75mL, 100mL], 250-62.5mg/5mL [75mL, 100mL, 150mL], 400-57mg/5mL [50mL, 75mL, 100mL]; Tab: 250-125mg, 500-125mg, 875-125mg*; Tab, Chewable: 125-31.25mg, 200-28.5mg, 250-62.5mg, 400-57mg *scored

CONTRAINDICATIONS: History of penicillin (PCN) allergy or amoxicillin clavulanate-associated cholestatic jaundice/hepatic dysfunction.

WARNINGS/PRECAUTIONS: Serious, sometimes fatal, hypersensitivity reactions reported with PCN therapy. *Clostridium difficile*-associated diarrhea (CDAD) reported. Possibility of superinfection. Caution with hepatic dysfunction. Monitor renal, hepatic, and hematopoietic functions with prolonged use. Avoid with mononucleosis. Take with food to reduce GI upset. The 200mg and 400mg chewable tabs and 200mg/5mL and 400mg/5mL sus contain phenylalanine. The 250mg tab and chewable tab are not interchangeable due to unequal clavulanic acid amounts. Only use 250mg tab in pediatrics ≥40kg. False (+) for urine glucose with Clinitest and Benedict's or Fehling's solution.

ADVERSE REACTIONS: Diarrhea/loose stools, nausea, skin rashes, urticaria, pruritus, angioedema, hepatitis, cholestatic jaundice, serum sickness-like reactions, erythema multiforme, acute generalized exanthematous pustulosis, hypersensitivity vasculitis, exfoliative dermatitis.

INTERACTIONS: Increased and prolonged plasma levels with probenecid. May reduce effects of oral contraceptives. Allopurinol may increase incidence of rash. May increase PT with anticoagulant therapy.

PREGNANCY: Category B, caution in nursing.

MECHANISM OF ACTION: Amoxicillin: Semisynthetic antibiotic with broad-spectrum of bactericidal activity against gram-positive and gram-negative organisms. Clavulanate: β-lactamase inhibitor; possesses ability to inactivate a wide range of β-lactamase enzymes commonly found in microorganisms resistant to PCN and cephalosporins.

PHARMACOKINETICS: Absorption: Well absorbed from GI tract. C_{max} and AUC varied according to dose and regimen; see full PI for more information. (Tab, Sol) T_{max} =1.5 hrs, 1 hr. **Distribution:** Found in breast milk. Amoxicillin: Diffuses readily in body tissues and fluids. Clavulanic acid: Well distributed in body tissues. Plasma protein binding: Amoxicillin (18%), clavulanic acid (25%). **Elimination:** Urine, (amoxicillin) (50-70% unchanged), (clavulanic acid) (25-40% unchanged); $T_{1/2}$ =1.3 hrs (amoxicillin), 1 hr (clavulanic acid).

NURSING CONSIDERATIONS

Assessment: Assess for history of allergic reactions to penicillins or cephalosporins or other allergens, hepatic or renal or hematopoietic function, pregnancy/nursing status, and possible drug interactions.

Monitoring: Periodically monitor renal, hepatic, and hematopoietic functions. Monitor for anaphylactic reactions, hepatic toxicity, cholestatic jaundice, superinfection with mycotic or bacterial pathogen, drug resistance, and pseudomembranous colitis/CDAD.

Patient Counseling: Inform drug only treats bacterial, not viral, infections. Instruct to take as directed; skipping doses or not completing full course may decrease effectiveness and increase resistance. Inform about potential benefits/risks of therapy. Advise to d/c therapy and consult physician if allergic reactions or watery/bloody diarrhea (with/without stomach cramps) occur (may occur up to 2 months after therapy). Advise to notify physician if pregnant/nursing.

Administration: Oral route. Take at start of meals or snacks. Shake well before using. **Storage:** Tabs/Dry Powder at or below 25°C (77°F); store in original containers. Refrigerate reconstituted sus; discard after 10 days.

AUGMENTIN ES-600   RX
clavulanate potassium - amoxicillin (GlaxoSmithKline)

THERAPEUTIC CLASS: Aminopenicillin/beta lactamase inhibitor

INDICATIONS: Treatment of pediatric patients with recurrent or persistent acute otitis media due to susceptible strains of microorganisms.

DOSAGE: *Pediatrics:* ≥3 months: <40kg: (Dose based on amoxicillin content) 45mg/kg q12h for 10 days.

HOW SUPPLIED: Sus: (Amoxicillin-Clavulanate) 600mg-42.9mg/5mL [75mL, 125mL, 200mL]

CONTRAINDICATIONS: History of penicillin (PCN) allergy or amoxicillin-clavulanate associated cholestatic jaundice/hepatic dysfunction.

WARNINGS/PRECAUTIONS: Serious, sometimes fatal, hypersensitivity reactions reported with PCN therapy. *Clostridium difficile*-associated diarrhea (CDAD) reported. Possibility of superinfection with mycotic or bacterial pathogens. Caution with hepatic dysfunction. Avoid with mononucleosis.

ADVERSE REACTIONS: Diaper rash, coughing, vomiting, fever, upper respiratory infection, skin rashes, pruritus, urticaria, angioedema, serum sickness-like reactions, erythema multiforme, hypersensitivity vasculitis, exfoliative dermatitis.

INTERACTIONS: Increased and prolonged plasma levels with probenecid. Avoid with probenecid. May reduce effects of oral contraceptives. May increase PT with anticoagulant agents.

AUGMENTIN XR

PREGNANCY: Category B, caution in nursing.

MECHANISM OF ACTION: Amoxicillin: Semisynthetic antibiotic with broad spectrum of bactericidal activity against gram-positive and gram-negative organisms. Clavulanate: β-lactamase inhibitor. Possesses ability to inactivate a wide range of β-lactamase enzymes commonly found in microorganisms resistant to PCN and cephalosporins.

PHARMACOKINETICS: Absorption: Amoxicillin: C_{max}=15.7mcg/mL; T_{max}=2.0 hrs; AUC=59.8mcg•hr/mL. Clavulanic acid: C_{max}=1.7mcg/mL; T_{max}=1.1 hr; AUC=4.0mcg•hr/mL. **Distribution:** Plasma protein binding 18% (amoxicillin), 25% (clavulanic acid). Well distributed in bodily tissues except brain and spinal fluid. **Elimination:** Urine (unchanged) amoxicillin (50-70%); clavulanic acid (25-40%).

NURSING CONSIDERATIONS

Assessment: Assess for history of allergic reactions to PCNs, cephalosporins or other allergens, cholestatic jaundice, hepatic dysfunction, infectious mononucleosis, phenylketonuria, pregnancy/nursing status, and possible drug interactions.

Monitoring: Periodically monitor renal, hepatic and hematopoietic organ functions. Monitor for anaphylactic reactions, hepatic toxicity, cholestatic jaundice, development of superinfection with mycotic or bacterial pathogen, development of drug resistance, skin rash, diarrhea, pseudomembranous colitis/CDAD, false-positive reaction of urinary glucose if Benedict's or Fehling's solution or Clinitest are used, and for transient decrease in plasma concentration of total conjugated estriol, estriol-glucuronide, conjugated estrone and estradiol if given to pregnant women.

Patient Counseling: Inform drug only treats bacterial, not viral, infections. Instruct to take as directed; skipping doses or not completing full course may decrease effectiveness and increase resistance. Inform about potential benefits/risks of therapy. Advise to d/c therapy and consult physician if allergic reactions or watery/bloody diarrhea (with or without stomach cramps) occur (may occur up to 2 months or more after treatment). Advise to notify physician if pregnant/nursing.

Administration: Oral route. Take at start of meals or snacks to prevent gastric upset. Shake well before using. **Storage:** Store dry powder at or below 25°C (77°F); original container. Refrigerate reconstituted sus; discard after 10 days.

AUGMENTIN XR   RX
clavulanate potassium - amoxicillin (GlaxoSmithKline)

THERAPEUTIC CLASS: Aminopenicillin/beta lactamase inhibitor

INDICATIONS: Treatment of community-acquired pneumonia (CAP) or acute bacterial sinusitis due to confirmed or suspected β-lactamase-producing pathogens and *S.pneumoniae* with reduced susceptibility to penicillin (PCN).

DOSAGE: *Adults:* Sinusitis: 2 tabs q12h for 10 days. CAP: 2 tabs q12h for 7-10 days. Take at the start of a meal.
Pediatrics: ≥40kg: Sinusitis: 2 tabs q12h for 10 days. CAP: 2 tabs q12h for 7-10 days. Take at the start of a meal.

HOW SUPPLIED: Tab, Extended-Release: (Amoxicillin-Clavulanate) 1000mg-62.5mg* *scored

CONTRAINDICATIONS: History of penicillin (PCN) allergy. History of cholestatic jaundice/hepatic dysfunction associated with amoxicillin/clavulanate potassium, severe renal impairment (CrCl <30mL/min), hemodialysis.

WARNINGS/PRECAUTIONS: Serious, sometimes fatal, hypersensitivity reactions reported with PCN therapy. *Clostridium difficile*-associated diarrhea (CDAD) reported. Possibility of superinfection. Caution with hepatic dysfunction. Monitor renal, hepatic, and hematopoietic functions with prolonged use. Avoid with mononucleosis. False (+) for urine glucose with Clinitest and Benedict's or Fehling's solution. Prescribing in the absence of a proven or strongly suspected bacterial infection or for prophylaxis is unlikely to provide benefit and increases the risk of development of drug-resistant bacteria.

ADVERSE REACTIONS: Diarrhea, vaginal mycosis, N/V, loose stools.

INTERACTIONS: Increased and prolonged plasma levels with probenecid. May reduce effects of oral contraceptives. Allopurinol may increase incidence of rash. May increase PT/INR with anticoagulant therapy.

PREGNANCY: Category B, caution in nursing.

MECHANISM OF ACTION: Amoxicillin: Aminopenicillin; semisynthetic antibiotic with broad spectrum of bactericidal activity against gram-positive and gram-negative organisms. Clavulanate: β-lactamase inhibitor; possesses ability to inactivate a wide range of β-lactamase enzymes commonly found in microorganisms resistant to PCN and cephalosporins.

PHARMACOKINETICS: Absorption: Well-absorbed. Refer to PI for complete absorption parameters in adults and pediatrics. **Distribution:** Amoxicillin: Plasma protein binding (18%). Clavulanate Potassium: Plasma protein binding (25%). Found in breast milk. **Elimination:** Amoxicillin: Urine (60-80% unchanged); $T_{1/2}$=1.3 hrs. Clavulanate Potassium: Urine (30-50% unchanged); $T_{1/2}$=1.0 hrs.

NURSING CONSIDERATIONS

Assessment: Assess for history of allergic reactions to PCNs, cephalosporins or other allergens, cholestatic jaundice, hepatic/renal impairment, infectious mononucleosis, pregnancy/nursing status, and possible drug interactions.

Monitoring: Periodically monitor renal, hepatic and hematopoietic organ functions with prolonged use. Monitor for anaphylactic reactions, hepatic toxicity, cholestatic jaundice, development of superinfection, skin rash, diarrhea, pseudomembranous colitis/CDAD. Monitor for transient decrease in plasma concentration of total conjugated estriol, estriol-glucuronide, conjugated estrone and estradiol if given to pregnant women.

Patient Counseling: Instruct to take as directed; skipping doses or not completing the full course may decrease effectiveness and increase resistance. Inform about potential benefits/risks of therapy. Advise to d/c and consult physician if allergic reactions or watery/bloody diarrhea (with/without stomach cramps) occurs (may occur up to 2 months or more after treatment). Advise to notify physician if pregnant/nursing. Instruct to discard any unused medicine.

Administration: Oral route. Take at start of meals. **Storage:** ≤ 25°C (77°F).

AVALIDE   RX
irbesartan - hydrochlorothiazide (Bristol-Myers Squibb/Sanofi-Aventis)

> Can cause death/injury to developing fetus during 2nd and 3rd trimesters. Stop therapy if pregnancy detected.

THERAPEUTIC CLASS: Angiotensin II receptor antagonist/thiazide diuretic

INDICATIONS: Treatment of hypertension. May be used in patients not adequately controlled with monotherapy. May be used as initial therapy in patients likely to need multiple drugs to achieve BP goals.

DOSAGE: *Adults:* Initial: 150mg/12.5mg qd. Titrate: May increase after 1-2 weeks to a max dose of 300mg/25mg qd. Not Controlled with Monotherapy: Recommended doses in order of increasing mean effect are 150mg/12.5 mg, 300mg/12.5 mg, and 300mg/25 mg. Replacement Therapy: May substitute for titrated components. Avoid with CrCl <30mL/min.

HOW SUPPLIED: Tab: (Irbesartan-HCTZ) 150mg-12.5mg, 300mg-12.5mg, 300mg-25mg

CONTRAINDICATIONS: Anuria, sulfonamide hypersensitivity.

WARNINGS/PRECAUTIONS: Correct volume or salt depletion before therapy; risk of hypotension exists. Avoid if CrCl <30mL/min. Irbesartan may cause changes in renal function. If unilateral or bilateral renal artery stenosis is present, may increase SrCr and BUN. Use HCTZ with caution in severe renal disease, impaired hepatic function or progressive liver disease; may precipitate hepatic coma or azotemia. D/C or withhold diuretic therapy if progressive renal impairment becomes evident. Hypersensitivity reactions may occur; caution with history of allergy or bronchial asthma. May exacerbate or activate systemic lupus erythematosus (SLE). Monitor serum electrolytes. Hypokalemia, hyponatremia, hypochloremic alkalosis, hyperuricemia (or frank gout), hyperglycemia, hypomagnesemia, hypercholesterolemia, and hypercalcemia may occur. Enhanced effects may occur in the post-sympathectomy patient.

ADVERSE REACTIONS: Dizziness, hypokalemia, fatigue, musculoskeletal pain, influenza, edema, N/V.

INTERACTIONS: Potentiation of orthostatic hypotension may occur with alcohol, barbiturates, and narcotics. Dosage adjustment of insulin or oral hypoglycemic agents may be required. Impaired absorption with cholestyramine or colestipol resins. Intensified electrolyte depletion, particularly hypokalemia, with corticosteroids and adrenocorticotropic hormone (ACTH). May decrease response to pressor amines (eg, norepinephrine). Potentiation/additive effect with other antihypertensives. May increase responsiveness to nondepolarizing skeletal muscle relaxants (eg, tubocurarine). Increased risk of lithium toxicity; avoid concomitant use. NSAIDs may reduce diuretic, natriuretic, and antihypertensive effects. May cause symptomatic hypotension in patients on diuretic therapy. May sensitize or exaggerate the response of the heart to the toxic effects of digitalis.

PREGNANCY: Category D, not for use in nursing.

MECHANISM OF ACTION: Irbesartan: Angiotensin II receptor antagonist; blocks the vasoconstrictor and aldosterone-secreting effects of angiotensin II by selectively blocking binding to the AT_1angiotensin II receptor. HCTZ: Thiazide diuretic; antihypertensive effect not fully understood. Believed to affect renal tubular mechanisms of electrolyte reabsorption, directly increasing Na^+ and Cl^- excretion in approximately equivalent amounts, and indirectly reducing plasma volume.

PHARMACOKINETICS: Absorption: Irbesartan: Rapid, complete; absolute bioavailability (60-80%); T_{max}=1.5-2 hrs. **Distribution:** Irbesartan: V_d=53-93L; plasma protein binding (90%). HCTZ: Crosses placenta, excreted in breast milk. **Metabolism:** Irbesartan: CYP2C9 (oxidation), glucuronide conjugation. **Elimination:** Irbesartan: Biliary, kidney (20%); $T_{1/2}$=11-15 hrs. HCTZ: Kidney (61%, unchanged); $T_{1/2}$=5.6-14.8 hrs.

NURSING CONSIDERATIONS

Assessment: Assess for anuria, sulfonamide hypersensitivity, pregnancy/nursing status, intravascular volume/salt depletion (eg, dialysis), history of allergy or bronchial asthma, post-sympathectomy, congestive heart failure, renal artery stenosis, hepatic impairment or progressive liver disease, SLE, renal impairment, and possible drug interactions. Obtain baseline BP, renal function, CrCl, LFTs.

Monitoring: Monitor for signs/symptoms of electrolyte imbalance (hyponatremia, hypochloremic alkalosis, hypokalemia), exacerbation or activation of SLE, hypotension, hyperglycemia, hyperuricemia or precipitation of gout, hypersensitivity reactions, hepatic/renal dysfunction.

Patient Counseling: Inform of pregnancy risks; instruct to notify physician if pregnancy occurs during therapy. Inform patients that they may feel lightheaded during first days of use; d/c use if fainting occurs and notify healthcare provider. Inform that becoming dehydrated while on therapy can lower BP too much and lead to lightheadedness and possibly fainting. Inform that dehydration may occur with excessive sweating, diarrhea, vomiting, and not drinking enough liquids.

Administration: Oral route. **Storage:** 25°C (77°F); excursions permitted to 15-30°C (59-86°F).

AVANDAMET

RX

metformin HCl - rosiglitazone maleate (GlaxoSmithKline)

> Thiazolidinediones cause or exacerbate congestive heart failure (CHF) in some patients. After initiation and dose increases, observe for signs and symptoms of heart failure (HF) and manage accordingly; consider d/c or dose reduction. Not recommended in patients with symptomatic HF. Contraindicated with established NYHA Class III or IV HF. Meta-analysis showed association with increased risk of myocardial infarction (MI). Lactic acidosis reported due to metformin accumulation (rare); d/c if suspected.

THERAPEUTIC CLASS: Thiazolidinedione/biguanide

INDICATIONS: Adjunct to diet and exercise to improve glycemic control when treatment with both rosiglitazone and metformin is appropriate in adults with type 2 diabetes mellitus (DM) already taking rosiglitazone, or not taking rosiglitazone and unable to achieve glycemic control on other diabetes medication and have decided not to take pioglitazone or pioglitazone-containing products upon consultation.

DOSAGE: *Adults:* Take in divided doses with meals. Initial: Take rosiglitazone component at lowest recommended dose. Switching Prior Metformin Therapy of 1000mg/day: Initial: 2mg-500mg tab bid. Prior Metformin Therapy of 2000mg/day: Initial: 2mg-1000mg tab bid. Prior Rosiglitazone Therapy of 4mg/day: Initial: 2mg-500mg tab bid. Prior Rosiglitazone Therapy of 8mg/day: 4mg-500mg tab bid. Titrate: May increase by increments of 4mg rosiglitazone and/or 500mg metformin. After increasing metformin, titrate if inadequate after 1-2 weeks. After increasing rosiglitazone, titrate if inadequate after 8-12 weeks. Max: 8mg-2000mg/day. Elderly: Conservative dosing. Elderly/Debilitated/Malnourished: Do not titrate to max dose.

HOW SUPPLIED: Tab: (Rosiglitazone-Metformin) 2mg-500mg, 4mg-500mg, 2mg-1000mg, 4mg-1000mg

CONTRAINDICATIONS: Established NYHA Class III or IV HF, renal disease/dysfunction (SrCr ≥1.5mg/dL [males], ≥1.4mg/dL [females], or abnormal CrCl), acute or chronic metabolic acidosis (eg, diabetic ketoacidosis with or without coma). Temporarily d/c if undergoing radiologic studies involving IV administration of iodinated contrast materials.

WARNINGS/PRECAUTIONS: Initiation with patients experiencing acute coronary event is not recommended; consider d/c during the acute phase. Caution with edema and patients at risk for HF. Avoid with active liver disease or if ALT levels >2.5X ULN. May start or continue therapy with caution if ALT levels ≤2.5X ULN; monitor LFTs periodically. D/C if ALT levels remain >3X ULN or if jaundice occurs. Check LFTs if hepatic dysfunction symptoms occur. May lose glycemic control with stress; withhold therapy and temporarily administer insulin. Review benefits of continued therapy if menstrual dysfunction occurs. Avoid use during pregnancy. Caution in elderly. (Metformin) Avoid use in patients ≥80 yrs unless renal function is normal. Elderly, debilitated/malnourished, adrenal/pituitary insufficiency, or alcohol intoxication may have increased susceptibility to hypoglycemia. (Rosiglitazone) Increased risk of cardiovascular (CV) events with CHF NYHA Class I and II. Dose-related edema and weight gain reported. Macular edema reported; refer to an ophthalmologist if visual symptoms develop. Increased incidence of bone fracture; risk appears higher in females than males. May decrease Hgb and Hct. Decreased serum vitamin B_{12} levels reported. Ovulation in premenopausal anovulatory patients may occur, resulting in an increased risk of pregnancy; adequate contraception should be recommended.

ADVERSE REACTIONS: CHF, lactic acidosis, upper respiratory tract infection, headache, back pain, fatigue, sinusitis, diarrhea, viral infection, arthralgia, anemia.

INTERACTIONS: See Contraindications. Use with insulin is not recommended. Metformin: Alcohol may potentiate effect on lactate metabolism. Caution with drugs that may affect renal function or result in significant hemodynamic change or may interfere with the disposition of metformin (eg, cationic drugs eliminated by renal tubular secretion). Hypoglycemia may occur with concomitant use of hypoglycemic agents (eg, sulfonylureas, insulin) or ethanol. May be difficult to recognize hypoglycemia with concomitant use of β-adrenergic blocking drugs. Furosemide, nifedipine, cimetidine, and cationic drugs (eg, digoxin, amiloride, procainamide, quinidine etc.) may increase levels. Observe for loss of glycemic control with thiazides and other diuretics, corticosteroids, phenothiazines, thyroid products, estrogens, oral contraceptives, phenytoin, nicotinic acid, sympathomimetics, calcium channel blockers, and isoniazid. May decrease furosemide levels. Rosiglitazone: Higher incidence of MI with ramipril. Dose-related weight gain and risk of hypoglycemia with other hypoglycemic agents. Increased levels with CYP2C8 inhibitors (eg, gemfibrozil). Decreased levels with CYP2C8 inducers (eg, rifampin).

PREGNANCY: Category C, not for use in nursing.

MECHANISM OF ACTION: Rosiglitazone: Thiazolidinedione; insulin-sensitizing agent that acts by enhancing peripheral glucose utilization. Metformin: Biguanide; decreases hepatic glucose production, decreases intestinal absorption of glucose, and increases peripheral glucose uptake and utilization.

PHARMACOKINETICS: Absorption: Rosiglitazone: Absolute bioavailability (99%). (4mg) AUC_{0-inf}=1442ng•hr/mL; C_{max}=242ng/mL; T_{max}=0.95 hr. Metformin: (500mg) Absolute bioavailability (50-60%) (fasted); AUC_{0-inf}=7116ng•hr/mL; C_{max}=1106ng/mL; T_{max}=2.97 hrs. **Distribution:** Rosiglitazone: V_d=17.6L; plasma protein binding (99.8%); crosses the placenta. Metformin: (850mg) V_d=654L. **Metabolism:** Rosiglitazone: Extensive by N-demethylation and hydroxylation, then conjugation with sulfate and glucuronic acid; CYP2C8 (major), 2C9 (minor). **Elimination:** Rosiglitazone: Urine (64%), feces (23%); $T_{1/2}$=3-4 hrs. Metformin: (PO) Urine (90%), (IV) Urine (unchanged); (PO) $T_{1/2}$=6.2 hrs (plasma), 17.6 hrs (blood).

NURSING CONSIDERATIONS

Assessment: Assess for renal/hepatic function, CHF, hypoxemia, dehydration, active liver disease, acute coronary event, edema, risk factors for HF, pregnancy/nursing status, and possible drug interactions. Obtain baseline FPG, HbA1c, renal function, LFTs, and hematological parameters.

Monitoring: Monitor for signs/symptoms of lactic acidosis, HF, MI, acute coronary event, edema, weight gain, hepatic function, macular edema, bone fractures, hematologic changes, hypoglycemia, menstrual function. Monitor renal function, especially in elderly, at least annually. Monitor vitamin B-12 levels in patients predisposed to develop subnormal vitamin B-12 levels. Periodically monitor LFTs, FPG, HbA1c, CBC, bone health, and hematologic parameters. Perform periodic eye exams in DM.

Patient Counseling: Inform about benefits and risks of therapy and on importance of adherence to dietary instructions and regular testing of blood glucose, HbA1c, renal function, and hematologic parameters. Advise to d/c and notify physician if unexplained hyperventilation, myalgia, malaise, unusual somnolence, or nonspecific symptoms occur. Report rapid increase in weight or edema, or SOB to physician and to avoid excessive alcohol intake. Inform that the drug is not recommended with symptomatic heart failure and patients taking insulin.

Administration: Oral route. **Storage:** 25°C (77°F); excursions permitted to 15-30°C (59-86°F).

AVANDARYL   RX
rosiglitazone maleate - glimepiride (GlaxoSmithKline)

> Thiazolidinediones cause or exacerbate congestive heart failure (CHF) in some patients. After initiation and dose increases, observe for signs and symptoms of heart failure (HF) and manage accordingly; consider d/c or dose reduction. Not recommended in patients with symptomatic HF. Contraindicated with established NYHA Class III or IV HF. Meta-analysis has shown to be associated with increased risk of myocardial infarction (MI).

THERAPEUTIC CLASS: Thiazolidinedione/sulfonylurea

INDICATIONS: Adjunct to diet and exercise to improve glycemic control when treatment with both rosiglitazone and glimepiride is appropriate in adults with type 2 diabetes mellitus (DM) already taking rosiglitazone or not taking rosiglitazone and unable to achieve glycemic control on other diabetes medication and have decided not to take pioglitazone or pioglitazone-containing products upon consultation.

DOSAGE: *Adults:* Initial: 4mg-1mg qd with 1st meal of day. Already Treated with Sulfonylurea or Rosiglitazone: Initial: 4mg-2mg qd. Switching from Prior Combination Therapy as Separate Tab: Start with dose of each component already being taken. Switching from Current Rosiglitazone Monotherapy: Increase glimepiride component in no >2mg increments if inadequately controlled after 1-2 weeks. After an increase in glimepiride component, titrate Avandaryl if inadequately controlled after 1-2 weeks. Switching from Current Sulfonylurea Monotherapy: Titrate rosiglitazone component if inadequately controlled after 8-12 weeks. After an increase in rosiglitazone component, titrate Avandaryl if inadequately controlled after 2-3 months. Max: 8mg-4mg/day. Elderly/Debilitated/Malnourished/Renal, Hepatic, or Adrenal Insufficiency: Initial: 4mg-1mg qd. Titrate carefully. Consider dose reduction of glimepiride component if hypoglycemia occurs during up-titration or maintenance.

HOW SUPPLIED: Tab: (Rosiglitazone-Glimepiride) 4mg-1mg, 4mg-2mg, 4mg-4mg, 8mg-2mg, 8mg-4mg

CONTRAINDICATIONS: Established NYHA Class III or IV HF.

WARNINGS/PRECAUTIONS: Avoid with active liver disease or if ALT levels >2.5X ULN. Caution if liver enzymes mildly elevated (ALT levels ≤2.5X ULN). D/C if ALT levels remain >3X ULN on therapy or if jaundice occurs. Check LFTs if hepatic dysfunction symptoms occur. May lose glycemic control with stress; withhold therapy and temporarily administer insulin. (Rosiglitazone) Increased risk of cardiovascular (CV) events with CHF NYHA Class I and II. Initiation with patients experiencing acute coronary event is not recommended; consider d/c during the acute phase. Caution with edema and patients at risk for HF. Edema and weight gain reported. Macular edema reported; refer to an ophthalmologist if visual symptoms develop. Increased incidence of bone fracture; risk appears higher in females than in males. May decrease Hgb and Hct. Ovulation in premenopausal anovulatory patients may occur, resulting in an increased risk of pregnancy; adequate contraception should be recommended. Review benefits of continued therapy if menstrual dysfunction occurs. (Glimepiride) Increased risk of CV mortality. Hypoglycemia may be masked in elderly; risk in debilitated, malnourished, or with adrenal, pituitary, renal or hepatic insufficiency. May elevate liver enzyme levels in rare cases. Hemolytic anemia reported; caution with G6PD deficiency.

ADVERSE REACTIONS: Headache, hypoglycemia, anemia. (Rosiglitazone) CHF, upper respiratory tract infection, nasopharyngitis, HTN, back pain, arthralgia. (Glimepiride) Dizziness, asthenia, nausea.

INTERACTIONS: Severe hypoglycemia with oral miconazole. Use with insulin is not recommended. Glimepiride: Hypoglycemia may be masked with β-blockers and other sympatholytic agents. Increased hypoglycemia risk with alcohol and use of >1 glucose-lowering drug. Observe for loss of glycemic control with thiazides and other diuretics, corticosteroids, phenothiazines, thyroid products, estrogens, oral contraceptives, phenytoin, nicotinic acid, sympathomimetics, and isoniazid (INH). Hypoglycemic action may be potentiated by certain drugs, including NSAIDs and other drugs that are highly protein bound (eg, salicylates, sulfonamides, chloramphenicol, coumarins, probenecid, MAOIs, and β-blockers). Potential interactions with inhibitors (eg, fluconazole), inducers (eg, rifampicin), other drugs metabolized by CYP2C9 (eg, phenytoin, diclofenac, ibuprofen, naproxen, mefenamic acid). Changes in levels with aspirin (ASA) and propranolol. Decrease in the pharmacodynamic response to warfarin. Rosiglitazone: Dose-related weight gain with other hypoglycemic agents. Higher incidence of MI with ramipril. Increased levels with CYP2C8 inhibitors (eg, gemfibrozil). Decreased levels with CYP2C8 inducers (eg, rifampin). Decreased glyburide levels in Caucasians and increased in Japanese.

PREGNANCY: Category C, not for use in nursing.

MECHANISM OF ACTION: Glimepiride: Sulfonylurea; stimulates insulin release from functional pancreatic β cells. Rosiglitazone: Thiazolidinedione; insulin-sensitizing agent that acts by enhancing peripheral glucose utilization.

PHARMACOKINETICS: Absorption: Glimepiride: Complete; T_{max} =2-3 hrs; (4mg) C_{max} =151ng/mL; $AUC_{(0\text{-inf, }0\text{-t})}$ =1052ng•hr/mL, 944ng•hr/mL. Rosiglitazone: Absolute bioavailability (99%); T_{max} =1 hr; (4mg) C_{max} =257ng/mL; $AUC_{(0\text{-inf, }0\text{-t})}$ =1259ng•hr/mL, 1231ng•hr/mL. **Distribution:** Glimepiride: (IV) V_d =8.8L; protein binding (>99.5%). Rosiglitazone: V_d =17.6L; plasma protein binding (99.8%); crosses the placenta. **Metabolism:** Glimepiride: Liver (complete) via oxidative biotransformation; cyclohexyl hydroxy methyl (M1) and carboxyl (M2) derivative (major metabolites); CYP2C9. Rosiglitazone: Liver (extensive) via N-demethylation and hydroxylation followed by conjugation; CYP2C8 (major), 2C9 (minor). **Elimination:** Glimepiride: (PO) Urine (60%, 80-90% major metabolites), feces (40%, 70% major metabolites). Rosiglitazone: Urine (64%), feces (23%); $T_{1/2}$ =3-4 hrs.

NURSING CONSIDERATIONS

Assessment: Assess for HF, active liver disease, acute coronary event, edema, G6PD deficiency, premenopausal anovulation, risk factors for HF, pregnancy/nursing status, and possible drug interactions. Assess baseline renal function, LFTs, CBC, and bone health.

Monitoring: Monitor for adverse events related to fluid retention during dose increases. Periodically monitor LFTs, fasting blood glucose, HbA1c, CBC, and bone health. Monitor for signs and symptoms of HF, MI, acute coronary event, edema, weight gain, hepatic function, macular edema, bone fractures, hematologic changes, hypoglycemia, hypersensitivity reactions, ovulation in premenopausal anovulatory women, and menstrual function. Perform periodic eye exams. Monitor renal function in elderly.

Patient Counseling: Inform about benefits and risks of therapy. Inform about importance of caloric restrictions, weight loss, exercise, and regular testing of blood glucose levels. Advise to immediately report unexplained N/V, anorexia, abdominal pain, fatigue, dark urine, unusual rapid increase in weight or edema, SOB, or other symptoms of HF to physician. Instruct to take drug with 1st meal of the day. Explain to patients and their family members the risks, symptoms, treatment, and conditions that predispose to the development of hypoglycemia.

Administration: Oral route. **Storage:** 25°C (77°F); excursions permitted to 15-30°C (59-86°F).

AVANDIA   RX
rosiglitazone maleate (GlaxoSmithKline)

> Thiazolidinediones, including rosiglitazone, cause or exacerbate congestive heart failure (CHF) in some patients. After initiation and dose increases, observe for signs and symptoms of heart failure (HF) and manage accordingly; consider d/c or dose reduction. Not recommended in patients with symptomatic HF. Contraindicated with established NYHA Class III or IV HF. Meta-analysis has shown to be associated with increased risk of myocardial infarction (MI).

THERAPEUTIC CLASS: Thiazolidinedione

INDICATIONS: Adjunct to diet and exercise to improve glycemic control in adults with type 2 diabetes mellitus (DM) who either are already taking rosiglitazone or not already taking rosiglitazone and have inadequate glycemic control on other diabetes medications and have decided not to take pioglitazone upon consultation.

DOSAGE: *Adults:* Initial: 4mg as qd dose or in 2 divided doses. Titrate: May increase to 8mg/day after 8-12 weeks if response to treatment is inadequate. Max: 8mg/day.

HOW SUPPLIED: Tab: 2mg, 4mg, 8mg

CONTRAINDICATIONS: Established NYHA Class III or IV HF.

WARNINGS/PRECAUTIONS: Increased risk of cardiovascular (CV) events with CHF NYHA Class I and II. Initiation not recommended if experiencing an acute coronary event; consider d/c therapy during the acute phase. Caution with edema and patients at risk for HF. Edema and weight gain reported. Monitor LFTs prior to initiation of therapy and during therapy. Avoid with active liver disease or if ALT levels >2.5X ULN. Caution if liver enzymes are mildly elevated (ALT levels ≤2.5X ULN). D/C if ALT levels remain 3X ULN while on therapy or if jaundice occurs. Check LFTs if hepatic dysfunction symptoms occur. Macular edema reported; refer to an ophthalmologist if visual symptoms develop. Increased incidence of bone fracture; risk appears higher in females than in males. Decreases in Hgb and Hct reported. Perform periodic measurements of FPG and HbA1c to monitor therapeutic response. May cause ovulation in premenopausal anovulatory patients resulting in an increased risk of pregnancy. Review benefits of continued therapy if menstrual dysfunction occurs.

ADVERSE REACTIONS: Upper respiratory tract infection, headache, back pain, hyperglycemia, fatigue, sinusitis, edema.

INTERACTIONS: Risk of hypoglycemia when used with other hypoglycemic agents. May increase levels with CYP2C8 inhibitors (eg, gemfibrozil). May decrease levels with CYP2C8 inducers (eg, rifampin). Coadministration with insulin is not recommended; may increase risk of CHF and MI. Higher incidence of MI reported with ramipril.

PREGNANCY: Category C, not for use in nursing.

MECHANISM OF ACTION: Thiazolidinedione; improves insulin sensitivity.

PHARMACOKINETICS: Absorption: Administration of variable doses resulted in different parameters. Absolute bioavailability (99%); T_{max}=1 hr. **Distribution:** V_d=17.6L; plasma protein binding (99.8%); crosses the placenta. **Metabolism:** N-demethylation and hydroxylation followed by conjugation (extensive); CYP2C8 (major), 2C9 (minor). **Elimination**: Urine (64%), feces (23%); $T_{1/2}$=3-4 hrs.

NURSING CONSIDERATIONS

Assessment: Assess for HF or risk factors for HF, presence of an acute coronary event, hepatic dysfunction, and edema. Assess baseline LFTs, CBC, and bone health.

Monitoring: Monitor for signs/symptoms of HF, MI, edema, weight gain, hepatic dysfunction, macular edema, bone fractures, hematologic changes, ovulation in premenopausal anovulatory women, and menstrual dysfunction. Perform periodic eye exams. Periodically monitor LFTs, fasting blood glucose, HbA1c, CBC and bone health.

Patient Counseling: Advise of risks and benefits of therapy. Inform that drug may be taken with or without food. Inform about importance of caloric restriction, weight loss, exercise, and regular testing of blood glucose levels. Instruct to immediately report to physician any symptoms of HF (eg, rapid increase in weight or edema, SOB) or hepatic dysfunction (eg, anorexia, N/V, dark urine, abdominal pain, fatigue). Inform about risk of hypoglycemia, its symptoms and treatment, and conditions that predispose to its development. Advise that ovulation may occur in some premenopausal anovulatory women and adequate contraception should be used.

Administration: Oral route. **Storage:** 25°C (77°F); excursions permitted to 15-30°C (59-86°F).

AVAPRO

RX

irbesartan (Bristol-Myers Squibb/Sanofi-Aventis)

> May cause death/injury to developing fetus during 2nd and 3rd trimesters. D/C if pregnancy detected.

THERAPEUTIC CLASS: Angiotensin II receptor antagonist

INDICATIONS: Treatment of HTN alone or in combination with other antihypertensives. Treatment of diabetic nephropathy with an elevated serum creatinine and proteinuria (>300mg/day) in patients with type 2 diabetes and hypertension.

DOSAGE: *Adults:* HTN: Initial: 150mg qd. Titrate: May increase to 300mg qd. A low-dose diuretic may be added if BP is not controlled. Intravascular Volume/Salt Depletion: Initial: 75mg qd. Nephropathy: Maint: 300mg qd.
Pediatrics: HTN: ≥17 yrs: Initial: 150mg qd. Titrate: May increase to 300mg qd. Intravascular Volume/Salt Depletion: Initial: 75mg qd.

HOW SUPPLIED: Tab: 75mg, 150mg, 300mg

WARNINGS/PRECAUTIONS: Symptomatic hypotension may occur in volume and/or salt depleted patients; correct volume depletion prior to therapy and monitor closely. Changes in renal function may occur; caution with renal artery stenosis, severe CHF. Increases in SrCr or BUN reported with renal artery stenosis.

ADVERSE REACTIONS: Diarrhea, fatigue, orthostatic hypotension, dizziness.

PREGNANCY: Category C (1st trimester) and D (2nd and 3rd trimesters), not for use in nursing.

MECHANISM OF ACTION: Angiotensin II receptor antagonist; blocks vasoconstrictor and aldosterone-secreting effects of angiotensin II by selectively binding to AT_1 angiotensin II receptor.

PHARMACOKINETICS: Absorption: Rapid and complete, absolute bioavailability (60-80%); T_{max}=1.5-2 hrs. **Distribution:** V_d=53-93L; plasma protein binding (90%); crosses placenta; excreted in breast milk. **Metabolism:** CYP2C9 (oxidation), glucuronide conjugation. **Elimination:** Urine, feces; $T_{1/2}$=11-15 hrs.

NURSING CONSIDERATIONS

Assessment: Assess for pregnancy/nursing status, renal impairment, and volume/salt depletion.

Monitoring: Monitor renal function periodically. Monitor for signs/symptoms of hypotension, hypersensitivity reactions, hyperkalemia, and renal dysfunction.

Patient Counseling: Inform of pregnancy risks. Advise to seek medical attention if symptoms of hypotension or hypersensitivity reactions occur. Inform that drug may be taken with/without food.

Administration: Oral route. **Storage:** 25°C (77°F); excursions permitted to 15-30°C (59-86°F).

AVASTIN   RX
bevacizumab (Genentech)

> Incidences of wound healing and surgical complications; d/c at least 28 days prior to elective surgery. Do not initiate for at least 28 days after surgery and until the surgical wound is fully healed. Severe or fatal hemorrhage including hemoptysis, GI bleeding, CNS hemorrhage, epistaxis, and vaginal bleeding have occurred; avoid with serious hemorrhage or recent hemoptysis. D/C if GI perforation or wound dehiscence develops.

THERAPEUTIC CLASS: Vascular endothelial growth factor (VEGF) inhibitor

INDICATIONS: 1st- or 2nd-line treatment of metastatic colorectal cancer (mCRC), in combination with 5-fluorouracil (5-FU)-based chemotherapy. 1st-line treatment of unresectable, locally advanced, recurrent or metastatic non-squamous non-small cell lung cancer (NSCLC), in combination with carboplatin and paclitaxel. Treatment of patients who have not received chemotherapy for metastatic HER2-negative breast cancer (mBC), in combination with paclitaxel. Treatment of glioblastoma with progressive disease following prior therapy as a single agent. Treatment of metastatic renal cell carcinoma (mRCC), in combination with interferon alfa.

DOSAGE: *Adults:* mCRC: 5mg/kg or 10mg/kg q2 weeks (in combination with 5-FU). 5mg/kg q2 weeks (in combination with bolus IFL). 10mg/kg q2 weeks (in combination with FOLFOX4). NSCLC: 15mg/kg q3 weeks (in combination with carboplatin/paclitaxel). mBC: 10mg/kg q2 weeks (in combination with paclitaxel). Glioblastoma: 10mg/kg q2 weeks. mRCC: 10mg/kg q2 weeks (in combination with interferon alfa).

HOW SUPPLIED: Inj: 100mg/4mL, 400mg/16mL

WARNINGS/PRECAUTIONS: Serious and fatal non-GI fistula formation (eg, in tracheo-esophageal, bronchopleural, biliary, vaginal, renal, and bladder sites), hemorrhage (eg, hemoptysis, GI, hematemesis, CNS, epistaxis, vaginal), arterial thromboembolic events (eg, cerebral infarction, transient ischemic attacks, MI, angina), nephrotic syndrome may occur; d/c use if any occur. Increased incidence of severe HTN; monitor BP every 2-3 weeks during therapy and treat with appropriate antihypertensive agents. D/C use with hypertensive crisis and hypertensive encephalopathy. Reversible posterior leukoencephalopathy syndrome reported. Increased incidence and severity of proteinuria; monitor by urine analysis. Suspend treatment for ≥2g proteinuria/24 hrs and resume when proteinuria is <2g/24 hrs. Infusion reactions (eg, HTN, hypertensive crisis with neurologic signs and symptoms, wheezing, oxygen desaturation, hypersensitivity) reported; stop infusion for severe cases and administer appropriate medical therapy.

ADVERSE REACTIONS: Epistaxis, headache, HTN, rhinitis, proteinuria, taste alteration, dry skin, rectal hemorrhage, lacrimation disorder, back pain, exfoliative dermatitis, polyserositis, pulmonary HTN, pancytopenia, dysphonia.

INTERACTIONS: Increased risk of arterial thromboembolic events when coadministered with chemotherapy. Serious or fatal pulmonary hemorrhage has occurred with chemotherapy in patients with NSCLC. May decrease paclitaxel exposure when coadministered.

PREGNANCY: Category C, not for use in nursing.

MECHANISM OF ACTION: VEGF inhibitor; binds VEGF and prevents interaction with receptors (Flt-1, KDR) on surface of endothelial cells, thereby inhibiting endothelial cell proliferation and new blood vessel formation.

PHARMACOKINETICS: Absorption: T_{max}=100 days. **Distribution:** V_d=3.25L (male) and 2.66L (female). **Elimination:** $T_{1/2}$=20 days.

NURSING CONSIDERATIONS

Assessment: Assess for history of hemoptysis, HTN, hepatic/renal dysfunction (proteinuria, nephrotic syndrome), baseline urinalysis, BP, CBC, pregnancy/nursing status, and possible drug interactions.

Monitoring: Monitor CBC, BP every 2-3 weeks, and perform serial urinalysis. Monitor for signs/symptoms of GI perforation, fistula formation, wound-healing complications, serious hemorrhage, arterial thromboembolic events, hypertensive events (eg, crisis, encephalopathy), reversible posterior leukoencephalopathy syndrome, neutropenia, proteinuria, nephrotic syndrome, severe infusion reactions, CHF, and hypersensitivity reactions.

Patient Counseling: Inform of pregnancy risks and need to continue contraception for 6 months after therapy. Inform of risk for adverse events and instruct to seek medical attention if symptoms of the following occur: GI perforation (abdominal pain, constipation, vomiting), fistula formation, wound-healing complications, serious hemorrhage, arterial thromboembolic events, hypertensive events, reversible posterior leukoencephalopathy syndrome (headache, seizures, lethargy, confusion, blindness), neutropenia (fever, infection), proteinuria, nephrotic syndrome, and hypersensitivity reactions. Advise patient to undergo BP monitoring and contact health care provider if BP is elevated.

Administration: IV route. Do not administer as an IV push or bolus. Give as IV infusion over 90 min; if 1st infusion is well tolerated, give 2nd infusion over 60 min and subsequent doses over 30 min. **Storage:** 2-8°C (36-46°F). (Diluted): 2-8°C (36-46°F) for up to 8 hrs. Protect from light. Do not freeze or shake.

AVELOX

moxifloxacin HCl (Merck)

RX

> Fluoroquinolones are associated with an increased risk of tendinitis and tendon rupture in all ages. Risk is further increased in patients >60 yrs, taking corticosteroids, and with kidney, heart, or lung transplants. May exacerbate muscle weakness with myasthenia gravis; avoid in patients with known history of myasthenia gravis.

THERAPEUTIC CLASS: Fluoroquinolone

INDICATIONS: Treatment of acute bacterial sinusitis, acute bacterial exacerbation of chronic bronchitis (ABECB), uncomplicated and complicated skin and skin structure infections (SSSI), community-acquired pneumonia (CAP), complicated intra-abdominal infections, including polymicrobial infections (eg, abscess), caused by susceptible strains of microorganisms in adults ≥18 yrs.

DOSAGE: *Adults:* Sinusitis: 400mg PO/IV q24h for 10 days. ABECB: 400mg PO/IV q24h for 5 days. Uncomplicated SSSI: 400mg PO/IV q24h for 7 days. Complicated SSSI: 400mg PO/IV q24h for 7-21 days. CAP: 400mg PO/IV q24h for 7-14 days. Complicated Intra-Abdominal Infections: 400mg PO/IV q24h for 5-14 days.

HOW SUPPLIED: Inj: 400mg/250mL; Tab: 400mg

WARNINGS/PRECAUTIONS: D/C if experience pain, swelling, inflammation, or rupture of tendon. May prolong QT interval; avoid with QT interval prolongation or uncorrected hypokalemia. Caution with ongoing proarrhythmic conditions (eg, significant bradycardia, acute myocardial ischemia) and liver cirrhosis. Serious anaphylactic and sometimes fatal reactions reported; d/c if skin rash, jaundice, or any other sign of hypersensitivity appears and institute appropriate therapy. Convulsions and CNS events may occur (eg, dizziness, confusion, hallucinations, depression); d/c if these events occur. Caution with CNS disorders (eg, severe cerebral arteriosclerosis, epilepsy) or risk factors that may predispose to seizures or lower seizure threshold. *Clostridium difficile*-associated diarrhea (CDAD) reported. Rare cases of sensory or sensorimotor axonal polyneuropathy, resulting in paresthesias, hypoesthesias, dysesthesias, and weakness reported. May cause photosensitivity/phototoxicity reactions; d/c if phototoxicity occurs. Avoid excessive exposure to sun/UV light. Caution in elderly and in patients with hepatic impairment. (Inj) Not for intra-arterial, IM, intrathecal, intraperitoneal, or SQ use.

ADVERSE REACTIONS: Tendinitis, tendon rupture, nausea, diarrhea, headache, dizziness.

INTERACTIONS: See Boxed Warning. Avoid Class IA (eg, quinidine, procainamide) or Class III (eg, amiodarone, sotalol) antiarrhythmics. Caution with drugs that prolong the QT interval (eg, cisapride, erythromycin, antipsychotics, TCAs). NSAIDs may increase risk of CNS stimulation and convulsions. May enhance anticoagulant effects with warfarin; monitor PT and INR with warfarin or its derivatives. Blood glucose levels slightly decreased with glyburide. Reduced C_{max} and prolonged T_{max} when coadministered with calcium. (Tab) Antacids containing aluminum or magnesium, with sucralfate, with metal cations such as iron, with multivitamins containing iron or zinc, or with formulations containing divalent and trivalent cations such as didanosine chewable/buffered tabs or the pediatric powder for oral sol, may substantially interfere with the absorption and lower systemic concentrations.

PREGNANCY: Category C, not for use in nursing.

MECHANISM OF ACTION: Fluoroquinolone; inhibits topoisomerase II (DNA gyrase) and topoisomerase IV, which are required for bacterial DNA replication, transcription, repair, and recombination.

PHARMACOKINETICS: Absorption: Well-absorbed (PO); absolute bioavailability (90%). Refer to PI for various parameters. **Distribution:** V_d=1.7-2.7L/kg; plasma protein binding (30-50%); found in breast milk. **Metabolism:** Glucuronide and sulfate conjugation. **Elimination:** Single dose: $T_{1/2}$=11.5-15.6 hrs (PO), 8.2-15.4 hrs (IV). Multiple dose: $T_{1/2}$=12.7 hrs (PO), 14.8 hrs (IV). 45% unchanged; urine (20%), feces (25%).

NURSING CONSIDERATIONS

Assessment: Assess for risk factors for developing tendinitis and tendon rupture, history of myasthenia gravis, drug hypersensitivity, QT interval prolongation, uncorrected hypokalemia, ongoing proarrhythmic conditions, liver cirrhosis, CNS disorders or risk factors that may predispose to seizures or lower seizure threshold, pregnancy/nursing status, and possible drug interactions.

Monitoring: Monitor for ECG changes, signs/symptoms of anaphylactic reactions, QT interval prolongation, ventricular arrhythmia/torsades de pointes, CNS events, drug resistance, CDAD, peripheral neuropathy, tendon rupture, tendinitis, and photosensitivity/phototoxicity reactions. Monitor for muscle weakness in patients with myasthenia gravis.

Patient Counseling: Instruct to take exactly as directed; skipping doses or not completing full course may decrease effectiveness and increase bacterial resistance. Inform to notify physician if experience pain, swelling, or inflammation of a tendon, or weakness or inability to move joints; rest and refrain from exercise and d/c therapy. Advise to notify physician of any personal or family history of QT prolongation, proarrhythmic conditions, and convulsions. Instruct to d/c and notify physician if an allergic reaction, skin rash, watery and bloody stools, or symptoms of peripheral neuropathy develop. Notify prescriber if worsening muscle weakness or breathing problems, palpitations or fainting spells, or sunburn-like reaction occurs, if pregnant/nursing, and all medications and supplements currently taking. Use caution while performing hazardous tasks (eg, operating machinery/driving). Avoid exposure to sunlight and artificial light. (Tab) Inform that may be taken with or without food, to drink fluids liberally, and that antacids, metal cations, and multivitamins should be taken ≥4 hrs before or 8 hrs after.

Administration: Oral, IV routes. (Tab) Administer ≥4 hrs before or 8 hrs after products containing magnesium, aluminum, iron or zinc, including antacids, sucralfate, multivitamins, and didanosine chewable/buffered tabs or the pediatric powder for oral sol. May take with or without food; drink fluids liberally. (Inj) Infuse over 60 min. Avoid rapid or bolus IV infusion. Do not add other IV substances, additives, or other medications to inj or infuse simultaneously through same IV line. Inspect for particulate matter and discoloration prior to administration. Refer to PI for preparation for administration. **Storage:** 25°C (77°F); excursions permitted to 15-30°C (59-86°F). (Tab) Avoid high humidity. (IV) Do not refrigerate.

AVIANE   RX
ethinyl estradiol - levonorgestrel (Duramed)

> Cigarette smoking increases the risk of serious cardiovascular (CV) side effects. Risk increases with age (>35 yrs) and with heavy smoking (≥15 cigarettes/day). Women who use oral contraceptives should be strongly advised not to smoke.

OTHER BRAND NAMES: Lessina (Barr)

THERAPEUTIC CLASS: Estrogen/progestogen combination

INDICATIONS: Prevention of pregnancy.

DOSAGE: *Adults:* 1 tab qd for 28 days, then repeat. Start 1st Sunday after menses begin or 1st day of menses.
Pediatrics: Postpubertal: 1 tab qd for 28 days, then repeat. Start first Sunday after menses begin or 1st day of menses.

HOW SUPPLIED: Tab: (Ethinyl Estradiol-Levonorgestrel) 0.02mg-0.1mg

CONTRAINDICATIONS: Thrombophlebitis, deep vein thrombosis, or thromboembolic disorders, pregnancy, cerebrovascular or coronary artery disease, undiagnosed abnormal genital bleeding, cholestatic jaundice of pregnancy or jaundice with prior pill use, hepatic adenomas or carcinomas, active liver disease (as long as liver function has not returned to normal), breast cancer or other estrogen-dependent neoplasia, thrombogenic valvulopathies, thrombogenic rhythm disorders, diabetes with vascular involvement, uncontrolled HTN.

WARNINGS/PRECAUTIONS: Cigarette smoking increases risk of serious cardiovascular side effects; risk increases with age (especially >35 yrs) and heavy smoking. Increased risk of myocardial infarction (MI), vascular disease, thromboembolism, stroke and gallbladder disease. Retinal thrombosis, hepatic neoplasia, carcinoma of breast and reproductive organs reported. May cause glucose intolerance. May increase BP, elevate LDL levels or cause other lipid changes, fluid retention, breakthrough bleeding, and spotting. May cause or exacerbate migraine. May develop visual changes with contact lens. Diarrhea and/or vomiting may reduce absorption. Increased risk of MI with HTN, hyperlipidemia, obesity, and diabetes. D/C if jaundice, significant depression or ophthalmic irregularities develop. Perform annual physical exam. Use before menarche is not indicated. May affect certain endocrine, LFTs and blood components.

ADVERSE REACTIONS: N/V, breakthrough bleeding, spotting, amenorrhea, migraine, depression, vaginal candidiasis, edema, weight changes.

INTERACTIONS: Reduced effects, increased breakthrough bleeding, and menstrual irregularities with rifampin, barbiturates, phenylbutazone, phenytoin, griseofulvin, topiramate, some protease inhibitors, modafinil, ampicillin, tetracyclines, and possibly with St. John's wort. Troleandomycin may increase risk of intrahepatic cholestasis. Ascorbic acid, APAP, CYP3A4 inhibitors (eg, indinavir, fluconazole, troleandomycin), atorvastatin may increase plasma levels. Increased plasma levels of cyclosporine, theophylline, and corticosteroids.

PREGNANCY: Category X, not for use in nursing.

MECHANISM OF ACTION: Oral contraceptive: Inhibits ovulation by suppression of gonadotropins. Causes changes in cervical mucus (increases difficulty of sperm entry into uterus) and in endometrium (reduces likelihood of implantation).

PHARMACOKINETICS: Absorption: Levonorgestrel: Rapid and complete, bioavailability (100%), C_{max}=2.8ng/mL (single dose), 6.0ng/mL (multiple doses), T_{max}=1.6 hrs (single dose), 1.5 hrs (multiple doses); Ethinyl Estradiol: Rapid, bioavailability; (38-48%); C_{max}=62 pg/mL (single dose), 77pg/mL (multiple doses), T_{max}=1.5 hrs (single dose), 1.3 hrs (multiple doses). **Distribution:** Levonorgestrel: Primarily bound to SHBG. Ethinyl estradiol: Plasma protein binding (97%). **Metabolism:** Levonorgestrel: Reduction, hydroxylation, and conjugation. Ethinyl Estradiol: Hepatic, via CYP3A4 (hydroxylation), methylation, and glucuronidation. **Elimination:** Levonorgestrel: Urine (40-68%), feces (16-48%); $T_{1/2}$=36 hrs. Ethinyl Estradiol: $T_{1/2}$=18 hrs.

NURSING CONSIDERATIONS

Assessment: Assess for presence or history of breast cancer, estrogen dependent neoplasia, abnormal genital bleeding, active liver disease, and known/suspected pregnancy or any other conditions where treatment is cautioned or contraindicated. Assess use in patients who are >35 yrs and heavy smokers (≥15 cigarettes/day). Assess use with HTN, hyperlipidemias, obesity, diabetes mellitus (DM), or in patients at increased risk for thrombosis. Assess for possible drug interactions.

Monitoring: Monitor bleeding irregularities, thromboembolic events, onset or exacerbation of headaches or migraines, and ectopic pregnancy. Monitor fasting blood glucose levels in DM and prediabetic patients, BP with history of HTN, lipid levels with a history of hyperlipidemia. Monitor for signs of liver dysfunction (eg, jaundice) and signs of depression with previous history. Refer patients with contact lenses to an ophthalmologist if visual changes occur. Perform annual history and physical exam.

Patient Counseling: Inform that drug does not protect against HIV infection and other sexually transmitted diseases. Instruct women who are initiating therapy to use additional method of protection during first 7 days of use. Take exactly as directed and at intervals not exceeding 24 hrs. Advise that if pill missed, take as soon as remembered; take next dose at regularly scheduled time. Inform may experience spotting, light bleeding, or stomach upset during first 1-3 packs of pills. Instruct to continue using therapy and to contact physician if symptoms persist. Counsel to avoid smoking while on medication.

Administration: Oral route. **Storage:** Store at controlled room temperature 20-25°C (68-77°F).

AVINZA

morphine sulfate (King)

> Swallow capsules whole or sprinkle contents on applesauce. Do not crush, chew, or dissolve capsule beads. Avoid alcohol and alcohol-containing medications; consumption of alcohol may result in the rapid release and absorption of potentially fatal dose of morphine.

THERAPEUTIC CLASS: Opioid analgesic

INDICATIONS: Relief of moderate to severe pain requiring continuous opioid therapy for an extended period of time.

DOSAGE: *Adults:* Individualize dose. Conversion from Other Oral Morphine Products: Give total daily dose as a single dose q24h. Conversion from Parenteral Morphine: Initial: Give about 3x the previous daily parenteral requirement. Conversion from Other Parenteral or Oral Non-Morphine Opioids: Initial: Give 1/2 of estimated daily requirement q24h. Supplement with immediate-release (IR) morphine or short-acting analgesics if needed. Titrate: Adjust dose as frequently as qod. Non-Opioid Tolerant: Initial: 30mg q24h. Titrate: Increase by increments ≤30mg every 4 days. The 45, 60, 75, 90, and 120mg caps are for opioid-tolerant patients. Max: 1,600mg/day. Doses >1,600mg/day contain a quantity of fumaric acid, which may cause renal toxicity. Elderly: Start at low end of dosing range.

HOW SUPPLIED: Cap, Extended-Release: 30mg, 45mg, 60mg, 75mg, 90mg, 120mg

CONTRAINDICATIONS: Respiratory depression in the absence of resuscitative equipment, acute or severe bronchial asthma, paralytic ileus.

WARNINGS/PRECAUTIONS: Abuse potential. Extreme caution with chronic obstructive pulmonary disease (COPD), cor pulmonale, decreased respiratory reserve (eg, severe kyphoscoliosis), hypoxia, hypercapnia, pre-existing respiratory depression. May obscure neurologic signs of increased intracranial pressure (ICP) with head injury. May cause orthostatic hypotension, syncope, severe hypotension with depleted blood volume. Caution with circulatory shock, biliary tract disease (eg, acute pancreatitis), severe renal/hepatic insufficiency, Addison's disease, hypothyroidism, prostatic hypertrophy, urethral stricture, elderly or debilitated; consider dose reduction. Caution with CNS depression, toxic psychosis, acute alcoholism, delirium tremens, seizure disorders. Avoid with GI obstruction. Avoid abrupt withdrawal. Tolerance and physical dependence may develop. Potential for severe constipation; use laxatives, stool softeners at onset of therapy. May impair mental/physical abilities. Not for use as a PRN or postoperative analgesic.

ADVERSE REACTIONS: Constipation, N/V, somnolence, dehydration, headache, peripheral edema, diarrhea, abdominal pain, infection, urinary tract infection (UTI), flu syndrome, back pain, rash, insomnia, depression.

INTERACTIONS: See Boxed Warning. Additive effects with alcohol, other opioids, illicit drugs that cause CNS depression. Reduce dose with other CNS depressants (eg, sedatives, hypnotics, general anesthetics, antiemetics, phenothiazines, tranquilizers, alcohol); caution when coadministering. May enhance neuromuscular blocking action of skeletal muscle relaxants and increase risk of respiratory depression. Avoid with mixed agonist/antagonists (eg, pentazocine, nalbuphine, butorphanol) and within 14 days of MAOI use. Risk of precipitating apnea, confusion, muscle twitching reported with cimetidine; monitor for respiratory and CNS depression.

PREGNANCY: Category C, not for use in nursing.

MECHANISM OF ACTION: Opioid analgesic; pure opioid agonist that is relatively selective for μ-receptor but may interact with other opioid receptors at higher doses. Mechanism of analgesic action is unknown. Specific CNS opiate receptors (eg, μ-receptors) and endogenous compounds with morphine-like activity are found throughout brain and spinal cord and are likely to play a role in analgesic effects.

PHARMACOKINETICS: Absorption: C_{max}=18.65ng/mL; AUC=273.25ng/mL•hr. **Distribution:** Plasma protein binding (20-35%), V_d=1-6L/kg, distributed to skeletal muscle, kidneys, liver, GI tract, lung, spleen, and brain. Small quantities cross the blood-brain barrier. Crosses the placenta and found in human breast milk. **Metabolism:** Hepatic conjugation; 3-glucuronide (M3G) (metabolite); 6-glucuronide (M6G) (active metabolite). **Elimination:** Urine (major M3G/ M6G, 10% unchanged), feces (7-10%), bile (small); $T_{1/2}$=15 hrs, PO

NURSING CONSIDERATIONS

Assessment: Assess for degree of opioid tolerance, previous opioid dose, level of pain intensity, type of pain, patient's general condition and medical status, emotional status or any other conditions where treatment is contraindicated or cautioned. Assess for history of hypersensitivity, pregnancy/nursing status, renal/hepatic function, and possible drug interactions.

Monitoring: Monitor for signs/symptoms of respiratory depression, orthostatic hypotension, syncope, drug dependence and tolerance, and withdrawal syndrome (eg, restlessness, lacrimation, rhinorrhea, myalgia, mydriasis). Monitor for signs of increased ICP with head injuries. Monitor for relief of pain and need for IR morphine.

Patient Counseling: Advise that medication should be taken once daily and that it may be taken with/without food. Instruct to swallow whole (not to chew, crush, or dissolve) or open and sprinkle onto small amount of applesauce. Instruct not to consume alcohol during therapy, including Rx/OTC drugs containing alcohol. Notify physician of all concurrent medications and avoid use of other CNS depressants. Caution when performing hazardous tasks (eg, operating machinery/driving). Do not adjust dose or abruptly d/c medication without consulting physician. Advise that medication has potential for abuse. Instruct to keep out of reach of children. Advise to dispose of any unused medication via toilet. Counsel about severe constipation; take appropriate laxatives or stool softeners at start of therapy.

Administration: Oral route. Swallow capsules whole or sprinkle contents on a small amount of applesauce. **Storage:** 25°C (77°F); excursions permitted to 15-30°C (59-86°F). Protect from light and moisture.

AVODART   RX
dutasteride (GlaxoSmithKline)

THERAPEUTIC CLASS: Type I and II 5 alpha-reductase inhibitor (2nd generation)

INDICATIONS: Treatment of symptomatic benign prostatic hyperplasia (BPH) in men with an enlarged prostate, either as monotherapy or in combination with the α-blocker tamsulosin.

DOSAGE: *Adults:* Monotherapy: 0.5mg qd. Combination Therapy with Tamsulosin: 0.5mg qd and tamsulosin 0.4mg qd. Swallow whole; do not chew or open.

HOW SUPPLIED: Cap: 0.5mg

CONTRAINDICATIONS: Pregnancy, women of childbearing potential, and pediatric patients.

WARNINGS/PRECAUTIONS: Risk to male fetus; should not be handled by pregnant women or women who may become pregnant. Rule out prostate cancer and other urological diseases prior to treatment and periodically thereafter. Monitor for obstructive uropathy in patients with a large residual urinary volume and/or severely diminished urinary flow; these patients may not be good candidates for therapy with dutasteride. Avoid donating blood until 6 months after last dose. May decrease serum prostate-specific antigen (PSA) levels by about 40-50%; obtain a new baseline PSA concentration after 3-6 months of treatment. To interpret an isolated PSA value in a man treated for ≥6 months, the PSA value should be doubled for comparison with normal values. Any confirmed increases in PSA from NADIR while on therapy may signal the presence of prostate cancer and should be carefully evaluated, even if values are still within normal range for men not taking 5α-reductase inhibitor. Contact with contents of drug may cause oropharyngeal mucosal irritation.

ADVERSE REACTIONS: Impotence, decreased libido, breast disorders, ejaculation disorders.

INTERACTIONS: Caution with potent CYP3A4 inhibitors (eg, ritonavir); may increase blood levels. Coadministration of verapamil or diltiazem decreases clearance and may increase exposure of dutasteride; no dose adjustment required.

PREGNANCY: Category X, not for use in nursing.

MECHANISM OF ACTION: Type I, II 5α-reductase inhibitor; inhibits conversion of testosterone to dihydrotestosterone (DHT), the androgen primarily responsible for development and enlargement of the prostate gland.

PHARMACOKINETICS: Absorption: Absolute bioavailability (60%); T_{max}=2-3 hrs. **Distribution:** V_d=300-500L; plasma protein binding (99%). **Metabolism:** Liver (extensive) via CYP3A4, CYP3A5. Major active metabolites: 4'-hydroxy-dutasteride, 1,2-dihydroxydutasteride, 6-hydroxydutasteride. **Elimination:** Feces (5% unchanged, 40% metabolites), urine (<1%); $T_{1/2}$=5 weeks.

NURSING CONSIDERATIONS

Assessment: Assess for hepatic impairment, large residual urinary volume or severely diminished urinary flow, and for possible drug interactions. Rule out prostate cancer and other urologic diseases prior to treatment and periodically thereafter.

Monitoring: Monitor for signs/symptoms of prostate cancer and other urological diseases (eg, obstructive uropathy) and for hepatic dysfunction. Obtain new baseline PSA after 3-6 months of treatment.

Patient Counseling: Advise not to donate blood for at least 6 months after d/c therapy. Inform females who are pregnant, or intend to become pregnant, not to handle drug due to potential risk to fetus; inform that if contact is made, wash area immediately with soap and water. Advise to take as prescribed and should swallow the capsule whole; do not crush, chew, or open. Contact with contents of drug may cause oropharyngeal mucosal irritation. Inform that may take with or without food.

Administration: Oral route. **Storage:** 25°C (77°F); excursions permitted to 15-30°C (59-86°F).

AXERT   RX
almotriptan malate (Ortho-Mcneil/Janssen)

THERAPEUTIC CLASS: 5-HT$_{1B/1D}$ agonist

INDICATIONS: Acute treatment of migraine attacks with a history of migraine with or without aura in adults. Acute treatment of migraine headache pain with a history of migraine attacks with or without aura usually lasting ≥4 hrs in adolescents 12-17 yrs.

DOSAGE: *Adults:* Initial: 6.25-12.5mg at onset of headache. May repeat after 2 hrs. Max: 25mg/day. Hepatic/Renal Impairment: 6.25mg at onset of headache. Max: 12.5mg/24 hrs. Elderly: Start at lower end of dosing range.
Pediatrics: 12-17 yrs: Initial: 6.25-12.5mg at onset of headache. May repeat after 2 hrs. Max: 25mg/day. Hepatic/Renal Impairment: 6.25mg at onset of headache. Max: 12.5mg/24 hrs.

HOW SUPPLIED: Tab: 6.25mg, 12.5mg

CONTRAINDICATIONS: Ischemic heart disease, coronary artery vasospasm, other significant cardiovascular disease, cerebrovascular syndromes (eg, stroke, transient ischemic attacks [TIA]), peripheral vascular disease (eg, ischemic bowel disease), uncontrolled HTN, hemiplegic or basilar migraine. Avoid use within 24 hrs of another 5-HT$_1$ agonist (eg, triptans) or ergotamine-containing or ergot-type medications (eg, dihydroergotamine, ergotamine tartrate, methysergide).

WARNINGS/PRECAUTIONS: Confirm diagnosis. Supervise first dose and monitor cardiac function in those at risk of coronary artery disease (CAD) (eg, HTN, hypercholesterolemia, smoker, obesity, diabetes, CAD family history, postmenopausal women, males >40 yrs). Monitor cardiovascular function with long-term intermittent use. May cause vasospastic reactions or cerebrovascular events. Serotonin syndrome symptoms (eg, mental status changes, autonomic instability, neuromuscular aberrations, and GI symptoms) reported. Sensations of tightness, pain, presure, and heaviness in the precordium, throat, neck, and jaw reported. May bind to melanin in the eye. Caution with renal or hepatic dysfunction. Caution with known hypersensitivity to sulfonamides. Caution in elderly.

ADVERSE REACTIONS: N/V, dizziness, somnolence, headache, paresthesia, coronary artery vasospasm, myocardial infarction (MI), ventricular tachycardia, ventricular fibrillation, transient myocardial ischemia, dry mouth.

INTERACTIONS: See Contraindications. Additive vasospastic reactions with ergotamines. Selective serotonin reuptake inhibitors (SSRIs) may cause weakness, hyperreflexia, and incoordination. Life-threatening serotonin syndrome reported with combined use of SSRIs or serotonin norepinephrine reuptake inhibitors (SNRIs). Clearance may be decreased by MAOIs. Increased levels possible with CYP3A4 inhibitors (eg, ketoconazole).

PREGNANCY: Category C, caution in nursing.

MECHANISM OF ACTION: Selective 5-HT$_{1B/1D}$ receptor agonist; binds with high affinity to 5-HT$_{1B/1D}$ receptors on extracerebral, intracranial blood vessels that become dilated during migraine attack and on nerve terminal in trigeminal system. Activation of these receptors results in cranial nerve constriction, inhibition of neuropeptide release, and reduced transmission in trigeminal pain pathways.

PHARMACOKINETICS: Absorption: Absolute bioavailability (70%); T_{max}=1-3 hrs. **Distribution:** V_d=180-200L; plasma protein binding (35%). **Metabolism:** Monoamine oxidase (MAO)-mediated oxidative deamination and CYP450-mediated oxidation (major pathways), flavin monooxygenase (minor pathway); indoleacetic acid, gamma-aminobutyric acid (inactive metabolites). **Elimination:** Urine (75%, 40% unchanged), feces (13%, unchanged and metabolite); $T_{1/2}$=3-4 hrs.

NURSING CONSIDERATIONS

Assessment: Confirm diagnosis of migraine before therapy. Assess for cluster headache, ischemic heart disease (eg, angina pectoris, Prinzmetal's variant angina, MI or documented silent MI), HTN, hemiplegic or basilar migraine, presence of risk factors (eg, hypercholesterolemia, smoking, obesity, diabetes mellitus), ECG changes, hepatic/renal impairment, hypersensitivity to the drug and to sulfonamides, pregnancy/nursing status, and possible drug interactions.

Monitoring: Administration of 1st dose should be in physician's office or medically staffed and equipped facility as cardiac ischemia may occur in absence of clinical symptoms; ECG should be obtained immediately during interval in those with risk factors. Monitor for signs/symptoms of cardiac events (eg, coronary vasospasm, acute MI, arrhythmia, ECG changes, follow-up coronary angiography), cerebrovascular events (eg, hemorrhage, stroke, TIAs), peripheral vascular ischemia, colonic ischemia with bloody diarrhea and abdominal pain, serotonin syndrome (eg, mental status changes, autonomic instability, neuromuscular aberrations and/or GI symptoms), ophthalmic effects, hypersensitivity reactions, and increased BP.

Patient Counseling: Inform about potential risks (eg, serotonin syndrome manifestations such as confusion, hallucinations, fast heartbeat, fever, sweating, muscle spasm, and diarrhea), especially if taken with SSRIs or SNRIs. Report adverse reactions to physician. Advise to take exactly as directed. Counsel to use caution during hazardous tasks (eg, driving/operating machinery). Notify if pregnant/nursing or planning to become pregnant.

Administration: Oral route. **Storage:** 25°C (77°F); excursions permitted to 15-30°C (59-86°F).

AXID

RX

nizatidine (GlaxoSmithKline)

OTHER BRAND NAMES: Axid Oral Solution (Braintree)

THERAPEUTIC CLASS: H_2-blocker

INDICATIONS: Short-term treatment of active duodenal ulcer (DU) and benign gastric ulcer (GU). Maintenance therapy for duodenal ulcers. Treatment of endoscopically diagnosed esophagitis, including erosive and ulcerative esophagitis, and heartburn due to gastroesophageal reflux disease (GERD).

DOSAGE: *Adults:* Active DU/Active Benign GU: Usual: 300mg qhs or 150mg bid up to 8 weeks. Healed DU: Maint: 150mg qhs, up to 1 year. GERD: 150mg bid up to 12 weeks. Renal Impairment: Treatment: CrCl 20-50mL/min: 150mg/day. CrCl <20mL/min: 150mg every other day. Maint: CrCl 20-50mL/min: 150mg every other day. CrCl <20mL/min: 150mg every 3 days.
Pediatrics: ≥12 yrs: (Sol) Erosive Esophagitis/GERD: 150mg bid up to 8 weeks. Max: 300mg/day. Renal Impairment: Treatment: CrCl 20-50mL/min: 150mg/day. CrCl <20mL/min: 150mg every other day. Maint: CrCl 20-50mL/min: 150mg every other day. CrCl <20mL/min: 150mg every 3 days.

HOW SUPPLIED: Cap: 150mg, 300mg; Sol: 15mg/mL

WARNINGS/PRECAUTIONS: Caution with renal dysfunction; reduce dose. Symptomatic response does not preclude the presence of gastric malignancy. False positive tests for urobilinogen with Multistix.

ADVERSE REACTIONS: Headache, abdominal pain, pain, asthenia, diarrhea, N/V, flatulence, dyspepsia, rhinitis, pharyngitis, dizziness.

INTERACTIONS: May elevate serum salicylate levels with high dose aspirin.

PREGNANCY: Category B, not for use in nursing.

MECHANISM OF ACTION: H_2 receptor antagonist; competitive, reversible inhibitor of histamine at the histamine H_2 receptors, particularly those in gastroparietal cells.

PHARMACOKINETICS: Absorption: Absolute bioavailability (>70%); (150mg, 300mg) C_{max}=700-1800mcg/L, 1400-3600mcg/L; T_{max}=0.5-3 hrs. (12-18 yrs, 150mg) C_{max}=1422.9ng/mL; T_{max}=1.3 hrs; AUC=3764ng•hr/mL. **Distribution:** (Adult) V_d=0.8-1.5L/kg; (12-18 yrs) V_d=71.4L. Plasma protein binding (35%); found in breast milk. **Metabolism:** N_2-monodesmethylnizatidine (major). **Excretion:** Urine (90%, 60% unchanged); feces (6%). (Adult) $T_{1/2}$=1-2 hrs; (12-18 yrs) $T_{1/2}$=1.2 hrs.

NURSING CONSIDERATIONS

Assessment: Assess for hypersensitivity to other H_2 receptor antagonists, renal dysfunction, presence of gastric malignancy, pregnancy/nursing status, and possible drug interactions.

Monitoring: Monitor for signs/symptoms of hepatocellular injury (eg, elevation in liver enzymes), hematological effects (eg, anemia), hypersensitivity reactions (eg, anaphylaxis), and for signs of clinical improvement. If treatment is for active duodenal ulcer, monitor for signs of healing after 4 weeks and for complete healing by 8 weeks.

Patient Counseling: Advise if taking single dosing, take at bedtime. Contact physician if hypersensitivity reaction develops. Notify pregnant/nursing females about risks of use.

Administration: Oral route. **Storage:** Dispense in tightly closed container. Cap: 20-25° (68-77°F). Sol: 25° (77°F); excursions permitted to 15-30°C (59-86°F).

AXIRON
testosterone (Lilly)

CIII

> Virilization reported in children secondarily exposed to topical testosterone. Children should avoid contact with unwashed or unclothed application sites in men using topical testosterone. Advise patients to strictly adhere to recommended instructions for use.

THERAPEUTIC CLASS: Androgen

INDICATIONS: Replacement therapy in males for conditions associated with a deficiency or absence of endogenous testosterone (eg, congenital or acquired primary hypogonadism or hypogonadotropic hypogonadism).

DOSAGE: *Adults:* Initial: Apply 60mg (1 pump actuation of 30mg to each axilla) qam, to clean, dry, intact skin of the axilla. May adjust dose based on serum testosterone concentration from a single blood draw 2-8 hrs after application and ≥14 days after starting treatment or following dose adjustment. Serum concentration <300ng/dL: May increase from 60mg to 90mg (3 pump actuations) or from 90mg to 120mg (4 pump actuations). Serum concentration >1050ng/dL: Decrease from 60mg (2 pump actuations) to 30mg (1 pump actuation). D/C if consistently >1050ng/dL at lowest qd dose of 30mg (1 pump actuation). Refer to PI for application techniques.

HOW SUPPLIED: Sol: 30mg [110mL]

CONTRAINDICATIONS: Prostate or breast carcinoma in men, women who are or may become pregnant or who are breastfeeding.

WARNINGS/PRECAUTIONS: Application site and dose are not interchangeable with other topical testosterone products. Patients with BPH may be at increased risk for worsening of signs/symptoms of BPH. May increase risk for prostate cancer; evaluate for prostate cancer prior to and during therapy. May increase prostate-specific antigen (PSA) levels. Risk of virilization in women (eg, changes in body hair distribution, significant increase in acne) and children due to secondary exposure to testosterone; d/c if occur. Increases in Hct and RBC mass may increase risk for thromboembolic events. Not indicated for use in women. Suppression of spermatogenesis may occur. Prolonged use may cause serious hepatic effects (eg, peliosis hepatitis, hepatic neoplasms, cholestatic hepatitis, jaundice). Risk of edema with or without coongestive heart failure (CHF) with pre-existing cardiac, renal, or hepatic disease. Gynecomastia may develop and persist. May potentiate sleep apnea especially with obesity or chronic lung disease. Changes in serum lipid profile reported. Caution in cancer patients at risk of hypercalcemia and associated hypercalciuria. May decrease concentrations of thyroxin-binding globulins, resulting in decreased total T4 and increased resin uptake of T3 and T4. Alcohol-based and flammable; avoid fire, flame, or smoking during use.

ADVERSE REACTIONS: PSA increase, application-site irritation, application-site erythema, diarrhea, headache, Hct increase, vomiting.

INTERACTIONS: May decrease blood glucose and insulin requirements. Concurrent use with adrenocorticotrophic hormone or corticosteroids may increase fluid retention; monitor cautiously with cardiac, renal or hepatic disease. Changes in anticoagulant activity may be seen with androgens; increase frequency of PT/INR monitoring.

PREGNANCY: Category X, not for use in nursing.

MECHANISM OF ACTION: Androgen; responsible for normal growth and development of male sex organs and for maintenance of secondary sex characteristics.

PHARMACOKINETICS: Absorption: Systemic. **Distribution:** Sex hormone-binding globulin (SHBG) (40%), albumin and plasma protein-binding (rest), unbound (2%). **Metabolism:** Estradiol and dihydrotestosterone (DHT) (active metabolites). **Elimination:** (IM) urine (90% glucuronic and sulfuric acid conjugates), feces (6% unconjugated); $T_{1/2}$=10-100 min.

NURSING CONSIDERATIONS

Assessment: Assess for breast or prostate carcinoma, BPH, cardiac/renal/ hepatic disease, obesity, chronic lung disease, pregnancy/nursing status of female partner, Hct, and possible drug interactions. Assess use in cancer patients at risk of hypercalcemia.

Monitoring: Monitor for signs/symptoms of prostate carcinoma (3-6 months after, then following screening practices), hepatic effects, edema with or without CHF, gynecomastia, and sleep apnea. In patients with BPH, monitor for signs/symptoms of worsening BPH. Perform periodic monitoring of Hgb, Hct, PSA, serum lipid profile, LFTs, thyroxine-binding globulin, and serum testosterone levels. In cancer patients at risk for hypercalcemia, regularly monitor serum calcium levels.

Patient Counseling: Inform children and women to avoid contact with application sites. Apply only to axilla, not to any other part of the body. Instruct to wash hands immediately with soap and water after application. Advise to cover application site with clothing after waiting 3 min for the solution to dry. Instruct to wash application site with soap and water prior to direct skin-to-skin contact with others. Wash with soap and water immediately if unwashed/ unclothed skin comes in direct contact with skin of another person. Contact physician if changes in body hair distribution, increase in acne, virilization of female partner or child occurs. Inform that treatment may lead to adverse reactions which include changes in urinary habits, breathing disturbances, frequent or persistent erections of the penis, N/V, changes in skin color, or ankle swelling. Advise to read Medication Guide before therapy. Keep out of reach of children.

Administration: Topical route. Refer to PI for administration instructions.
Storage: 25°C (77°F); excursions permitted to 15-30°C (59-86°F).

AYGESTIN   RX
norethindrone acetate (Duramed)

THERAPEUTIC CLASS: Progestogen

INDICATIONS: Treatment of secondary amenorrhea, endometriosis, and abnormal uterine bleeding due to hormonal imbalance in the absence of organic pathology.

DOSAGE: *Adults:* Assume interval between menses is 28 days. Secondary Amenorrhea/Abnormal Uterine Bleeding: 2.5-10mg qd for 5-10 days during second half of menstrual cycle. Endometriosis: Initial: 5mg qd for 2 weeks. Titrate: Increase by 2.5mg qd every 2 weeks until 15mg/day. Continue for 6-9 months or until breakthrough bleeding demands temporary termination.

HOW SUPPLIED: Tab: 5mg* *scored

CONTRAINDICATIONS: Pregnancy, thrombophlebitis, thromboembolic disorders, cerebral apoplexy, liver impairment, breast carcinoma, undiagnosed vaginal bleeding, missed abortion, use as a pregnancy diagnostic test.

WARNINGS/PRECAUTIONS: D/C with migraine, vision loss, proptosis, diplopia, papilledema, or retinal vascular lesions. May cause thrombophlebitis, pulmonary embolism (PE), and fluid retention. Caution with epilepsy, migraine, psychic depression, asthma, cardiac or renal dysfunction, depression, diabetes mellitus (DM), and hyperlipidemia. May mask onset of climacteric. Not for use during the first trimester of pregnancy; risk to the fetus.

ADVERSE REACTIONS: Breakthrough bleeding, spotting, change in menstrual flow, amenorrhea, edema, weight changes, cervical changes, cholestatic jaundice, rash, melasma, chloasma, depression.

PREGNANCY: Category X, safety in nursing is not known.

MECHANISM OF ACTION: Progestogen; induces secretory changes in estrogen-primed endometrium.

PHARMACOKINETICS: Absorption: Rapid; C_{max}=26.19ng/mL; T_{max}=1.83 hrs; AUC=166.9ng/mL•hr. **Distribution:** V_d=4L/kg; sex hormone binding globulin (SHBG) (36%); albumin binding (61%); found in breast milk. **Metabolism:**

Extensive, via reduction; sulfate and glucuronide conjugation. **Elimination:** Urine, feces (metabolites); $T_{1/2}$=9 hrs.

NURSING CONSIDERATIONS

Assessment: Assess for known/suspected pregnancy, vaginal bleeding, presence or history of breast cancer, deep vein thrombosis, PE, active or recent (within past yr) arterial thromboembolic disease (eg, stroke, myocardial infarction), and impaired renal/hepatic function. Assess use in nursing females, history of depression, and those at risk for arterial vascular disease (eg, presence of HTN, hypercholesterolemia, DM, obesity, tobacco use) and for possible lab interactions.

Monitoring: Monitor for signs/symptoms of cardiovascular disorders (eg, thromboembolic events), visual abnormalities (eg, loss of vision, proptosis, diplopia), fluid retention, and breakthrough bleeding. Monitor for signs of worsening depression in patients with previous history. Monitor with hyperlipidemias and DM for changes in lipid and carbohydrate metabolism.

Patient Counseling: Counsel to contact physician if breast lumps, dizziness or faintness, changes in speech, severe headaches, chest pain, SOB, leg pain, or changes in vision occur. Advise to have annual breast exam and mammography unless otherwise directed by physician. Counsel to avoid using tobacco.

Administration: Oral route. **Storage:** 20-25°C (68-77°F).

AZACTAM   RX
aztreonam (Bristol-Myers Squibb)

THERAPEUTIC CLASS: Monobactam

INDICATIONS: Treatment of septicemia and lower respiratory tract (eg, pneumonia, bronchitis) infections, skin and skin-structure infections (eg, postoperative wounds, ulcers, burns), complicated/uncomplicated urinary tract infections (UTI) including pyelonephritis and initial/recurrent cystitis, gynecologic infections (eg, endometritis, pelvic cellulitis), and intra-abdominal (eg, peritonitis) infections caused by susceptible gram-negative microorganisms. Adjunct therapy to surgery for management of infections caused by susceptible microorganisms (eg, abscesses, hollow viscus perforation infections, cutaneous infections, infections of serous surfaces).

DOSAGE: *Adults:* UTI: 500mg-1g IM/IV q8-12h. Moderately Severe Systemic Infections: 1-2g IM/IV q8-12h. Severe Systemic/Life-Threatening Infections/ *Pseudomonas aeruginosa:* 2g IV q6-8h. Max: 8g/day. CrCl 10-30mL/ min/1.73m²: Initial: LD: 1 or 2g. Maint: 50% of usual dose. CrCl <10mL/ min/1.73m²: Usual: 500mg, 1g or 2g. Maint: 25% of usual initial dose at usual intervals of 6, 8 or 12 hrs. Serious/Life-Threatening Infections: In addition to maint dose, give 1/8 initial dose after each hemodialysis session. IV route recommended for single doses >1g or for bacterial septicemia, localized parenchymal abscess (eg, intra-abdominal abscess), peritonitis, or other severe systemic or life-threatening infections. Continue for at least 48 hrs after patient is asymptomatic or evidence of bacterial eradication. Elderly: Creatinine clearance should be obtained and appropriate dosage modification made if necessary.
Pediatrics: 9 months-16 yrs: Mild-Moderate Infections: 30mg/kg IV q8h. Moderate-Severe Infections: 30mg/kg IV q6-8h. Max: 120mg/kg/day. In patients with cystic fibrosis, higher doses may be warranted.

HOW SUPPLIED: Inj: 1g, 2g, 1g/50mL, 2g/50mL

WARNINGS/PRECAUTIONS: Caution with hypersensitivity to other β-lactams (eg, penicillins, cephalosphorins, carbapenems) or allergens; d/c if occurs. *Clostridium difficile*-associated diarrhea (CDAD) reported. May promote overgrowth of nonsusceptible organisms; take appropriate measures if superinfection develops. Toxic epidermal necrolysis (TEN) reported (rarely) in bone marrow transplant with multiple risk factors including sepsis and radiation therapy. Increased risk of development of drug-resistant bacteria in the absence of a proven or strongly suspected bacterial infection or a prophylactic indication. Monitor patients with impaired renal or hepatic function. If using concomitantly with an aminoglycoside, renal function should be monitored. Caution in the elderly.

ADVERSE REACTIONS: ALT/AST elevation, rash, eosinophilia, neutropenia, pain at injection site, increased serum creatinine, thrombocytosis.

INTERACTIONS: TEN reported (rarely) in bone marrow transplant (BMT) patients who were receiving concomitant therapy with other drugs associated with TEN. Avoid concomitant use with beta-lactamase inducing antibiotics (eg, cefoxitin, imipinem). Potential nephrotoxicity and ototoxicity when given with aminoglycosides. Increase serum levels with probenecid or furosemide.

PREGNANCY: Category B, not for use in nursing.

MECHANISM OF ACTION: Monobactam: Synthetic bactericidal antibiotic; inhibits bacterial cell-wall synthesis due to high affinity of aztreonam for penicillin-binding protein 3 (PBP3).

PHARMACOKINETICS: Absorption: C_{max}=90mcg/mL (1g dose), 204mcg/mL (2g dose), 54mcg/mL (500mg dose); T_{max}=1 hr. **Distribution:** V_d=12.6L; crosses placenta; found in breast milk. **Metabolism:** Hydrolysis. **Elimination:** Urine (60-70%), feces (12%); $T_{1/2}$=1.7 hr.

NURSING CONSIDERATIONS

Assessment: Assess for proven/strongly suspected bacterial infection, drug hypersensitivity, hypersensitivity to any allergens, history of hypersensitivity to other beta-lactams (eg, penicillins, cephalosporins, carbapenems), hepatic/renal impairment, pregnancy/nursing status, and for possible drug interactions. Assess use in patients undergoing BMT with multiple risk factors (eg, sepsis, radiation therapy).

Monitoring: Monitor for signs/symptoms of hypersensitivity reactions, CDAD, overgrowth of non-susceptible organisms, development of drug resistance, superinfection, TEN in patients undergoing BMT and hepatic/renal function.

Patient Counseling: Inform about potential benefits/risks of therapy. Advise that drug treats bacterial, not viral, infections. Instruct to take exactly as directed; inform that skipping doses or not completing full course may decrease effectiveness and increase bacterial resistance. Instruct to d/c therapy and notify physician if allergic reactions, watery/bloody diarrhea (with/without stomach cramps) occur (may occur as late as 2 or more months after therapy).

Administration: IM/IV route. Refer to PI for preparation instructions and compatibility information. **Storage:** Prior to Reconstitution: Store at room temperature; avoid excessive heat. Refer to PI for storage information of reconstituted solution.

AZASITE RX
azithromycin (Inspire)

THERAPEUTIC CLASS: Macrolide

INDICATIONS: Treatment of bacterial conjunctivitis caused by susceptible strains of microorganisms.

DOSAGE: *Adults:* Initial: 1 drop bid, 8 to 12 hrs apart, for first 2 days. Maint: 1 drop qd for next 5 days.
Pediatrics: ≥1 yr: Initial: 1 drop bid, 8 to 12 hrs apart, for first 2 days. Maint: 1 drop qd for next 5 days.

HOW SUPPLIED: Sol: 1% [2.5mL]

WARNINGS/PRECAUTIONS: Not for injection; do not give systemically, inject subconjunctivally or into chamber of eye. Caution may cause hypersensitivity reactions. Growth of resistant organisms including fungi may occur with prolonged use. Avoid contact lens use.

ADVERSE REACTIONS: Eye irritation, burning, stinging and irritation upon instillation, contact dermatitis, corneal erosion, dry eye, dysgeusia, nasal congestion, ocular discharge, punctate keratitis, sinusitis.

PREGNANCY: Category B, caution in nursing.

MECHANISM OF ACTION: Macrolide; binds to the 50S ribosomal subunit of susceptible microorganisms and interferes with microbial protein synthesis.

PHARMACOKINETICS: Absorption: $C_{max} \leq 10$ng/mL.

NURSING CONSIDERATIONS

Assessment: Assess proper diagnosis of causative bacteria.

Monitoring: Monitor for signs/symptoms of anaphylaxis (angioedema, Stevens-Johnson syndrome), development of growth of resistant organisms, and eye irritation.

Patient Counseling: Advise patients with signs/symptoms of bacterial conjuctivitis to avoid wearing contact lenses. Instruct not to allow applicator tip to touch the eye, fingers, or other sources. Take exactly as directed. Advise if doses are skipped or medication is stopped early, treatment effectiveness will be decreased and bacteria may develop resistance. Direct to d/c and contact physician if signs of allergic reaction occur.

Administration: Ocular route. **Storage:** Store unopened bottle under refrigeration at 2-8°C (36-46°F). Once bottle is opened, store at 2-25°C (36-77°F) for up to 14 days. Discard after 14 days.

AZILECT   RX
rasagiline mesylate (Teva)

THERAPEUTIC CLASS: Monoamine oxidase inhibitor (Type B)

INDICATIONS: Treatment of signs and symptoms of idiopathic Parkinson's disease as initial monotherapy and adjunct therapy to levodopa.

DOSAGE: *Adults:* Monotherapy: 1mg qd. Adjunctive Therapy: Initial: 0.5mg qd. Titrate: May increase to 1mg qd. May reduce dose of levodopa with concomitant use. Concomitant Ciprofloxacin or Other CYP1A2 Inhibitors/Mild Hepatic Impairment: 0.5mg qd.

HOW SUPPLIED: Tab: 0.5mg, 1mg

CONTRAINDICATIONS: Concomitant use with meperidine, tramadol, methadone, propoxyphene, dextromethorphan, St. John's wort, cyclobenzaprine, during or within 14 days of other MAOI use.

WARNINGS/PRECAUTIONS: Avoid with moderate or severe hepatic impairment. Should not exceed recommended doses due to risks of hypertensive crisis. Avoid foods containing very large amounts of tyramine while on therapy; potential for large increases in BP. May increase risk of melanoma. Concomitant use with levodopa may potentiate dopaminergic side effects and exacerbate pre-existing dyskinesia. Postural hypotension and high blood pressure reported in combination with levodopa. Orthostatic hypotension reported. Symptom complex resembling neuroleptic malignant syndrome (NMS) reported with rapid dose reduction, withdrawal of, or changes in drugs that increase central dopaminergic tone. Hallucinations may develop. May cause or exacerbate psychotic-like behavior; caution with major psychotic disorder.

ADVERSE REACTIONS: Headache, arthralgia, dyspepsia, rash, fall, somnolence, dyskinesia, diarrhea, N/V, weight loss, constipation, postural hypotension, dry mouth, hallucinations.

INTERACTIONS: See Contraindications. Concomitant use with SSRIs, serotonin norepinephrine reuptake inhibitors, tricyclic, tetracyclic and triazolopyridine antidepressants is not recommended due to severe CNS toxicity. Increased plasma concentrations up to 2-fold with concomitant ciprofloxacin and other CYP1A2 inhibitors. Severe hypertensive reactions reported with concomitant use of sympathomimetics (eg, ephedrine, tetrahydrozoline); caution when using nasal, oral, and ophthalmic decongestants, cold remedies, and tyramine-containing food.

PREGNANCY: Category C, caution in nursing.

MECHANISM OF ACTION: MAO-B inhibitor; suspected to inhibit MAO type B, which causes an increase in extracellular dopamine levels in the striatum which subsequently increases dopaminergic activity.

PHARMACOKINETICS: Absorption: Rapid. Absolute bioavailability (36%); T_{max}=1 hr. **Distribution**: V_d=87 L; plasma protein binding (88-94%). **Metabolism**: Liver via N-dealkylation, hydroxylation; CYP1A2: 1-aminoindan (AI), 3-hydroxy-N-propargyl-1 aminoindan (3-OH-PAI) and 3-hydroxy-1-aminoindan (3-OH-AI). **Elimination**: Urine (62% over 7 days), (84% over 38 days), (<1% unchanged), feces (7% over 7 days); $T_{1/2}$=3 hrs.

NURSING CONSIDERATIONS

Assessment: Assess LFTs, renal function tests, dyskinesia and major psychotic disorder. Assess for pregnancy/nursing status and possible drug interactions.

Monitoring: Monitor LFTs, renal function test, BP, signs of melanoma, hallucinations, psychotic-like behavior, postural hypotension, HTN, dyskinesia.

Patient Counseling: Instruct to inform physician if taking or planning to take any prescription or over-the-counter (OTC) drugs, especially antidepressant, ciprofloxacin, and OTC cold meds. Advise to avoid foods containing very large amounts of tyramine (eg, aged cheese) and to monitor for melanomas. Inform of the possibility of developing hallucinations, dyskinesia with concomitant levodopa, and increases in BP; instruct to report if develop. Inform that postural (orthostatic) hypotension with or without symptoms such as dizziness, nausea, syncope, and sometimes sweating may occur; caution against standing up rapidly after sitting or lying down, especially if they have been doing so for prolonged periods, and at the initiation of treatment. Inform about the risks of therapy. Inform that it can be taken with/without food. Instruct to take as prescribed and not to double dose if a dose is missed. Instruct to report adverse side effects and contact healthprovider if they wish to d/c therapy. Inform physician if experience new or increased gambling urges, increased sexual urges, or other intense urges.

Administration: Oral route. **Storage**: 25°C (77°F); excursions permitted to 15-30°C (59-86°F).

AZMACORT   RX
triamcinolone acetonide (Abbott)

THERAPEUTIC CLASS: Corticosteroid

INDICATIONS: Maintenance treatment of asthma as prophylactic therapy in patients ≥6 yrs; to reduce or eliminate the need for oral corticosteroidal therapy.

DOSAGE: *Adults:* 2 inh (150mcg) tid-qid or 4 inh (300mcg) bid. Severe Asthma: Initial: 12-16 inh/day. Max: 16 inh/day (1200mcg). Rinse mouth after use.

Pediatrics: >12 yrs: 2 inh (150mcg) tid-qid or 4 inh (300mcg) bid. Severe Asthma: Initial: 12-16 inh/day. Max: 16 inh/day (1200mcg). 6-12 yrs: 1-2 inh (75-150mcg) tid-qid or 2-4 (150-300mcg) inh bid. Max: 12 inh/day (900mcg). Rinse mouth after use.

HOW SUPPLIED: MDI: 75mcg/inh [20g]

CONTRAINDICATIONS: Primary treatment of status asthmaticus or other acute asthma attacks.

WARNINGS/PRECAUTIONS: Deaths due to adrenal insufficiency have occurred with transfer from systemic corticosteroids to inhaled corticosteroids. Resume oral corticosteroids during stress or severe asthma attack. Observe for adrenal insufficiency, systemic corticosteroid withdrawal effects, hypercorticoidism and growth suppression (children). More susceptible to infections. Not for acute bronchospasm. D/C if bronchospasm occurs after dosing. Caution with tuberculosis (TB) of respiratory tract; untreated systemic fungal, bacterial, viral or parasitic infections; or ocular herpes simplex. *Candida* infection of mouth and pharynx reported.

ADVERSE REACTIONS: Pharyngitis, sinusitis, headache, flu syndrome.

INTERACTIONS: Caution with prednisone.

PREGNANCY: Category C, caution in nursing.

MECHANISM OF ACTION: Corticosteroid; not established. Inhaled route makes possible to provide local anti-inflammatory activity.

PHARMACOKINETICS: Absorption: T_{max}=1.5-2 hrs. **Distribution:** V_d=99.5L; plasma protein binding (68%). **Elimination:** Urine (40%), feces (60%); $T_{1/2}$=88 min.

NURSING CONSIDERATIONS

Assessment: Assess for concomitant diseases such as status asthmaticus, active or quiescent pulmonary TB, untreated systemic fungal, bacterial, parasitic or viral infections, and possible drug interactions.

Monitoring: Monitor for localized oral infections with *Candida albicans*, body height in children, adrenal insufficiency, paradoxical bronchospasm, and hypersensitivity reactions.

Patient Counseling: Inform not for relief of acute bronchospasm. Advise that drug may unmask allergies (rhinitis, conjunctivitis, eczema). Instruct to track use of drug and dispose canister after 240 actuations since reliable dose delivery not assured after 240 doses. Warn to avoid exposure to chickenpox or measles. Advise to seek medical attention if exposed to chickenpox or measles, symptoms do not improve or worsen, during periods of stress or severe asthmatic attack, paradoxical bronchospasm or hypersensitivity reaction occurs. Counsel to avoid spraying in eyes and shake well before each use.

Administration: Oral inhalation. **Storage:** 20-25°C (68-77°F). Do not puncture, use, or store near heat or open flame; do not freeze.

AZOPT   RX
brinzolamide (Alcon)

THERAPEUTIC CLASS: Carbonic anhydrase inhibitor

INDICATIONS: Treatment of elevated intraocular pressure (IOP) in patients with ocular HTN or open-angle glaucoma.

DOSAGE: *Adults:* 1 drop in the affected eye(s) tid. Space dosing with other topical ophthalmic drugs by at least 10 min.

HOW SUPPLIED: Sus: 1% [5mL, 10mL, 15mL]

WARNINGS/PRECAUTIONS: Systemically absorbed. Rare fatalities have occurred due to severe sulfonamide reactions, including Stevens-Johnson syndrome (SJS), toxic epidermal necrolysis (TEN), fulminant hepatic necrosis, agranulocytosis, aplastic anemia, and other blood dyscrasias. Sensitization may recur when re-administered. D/C if signs of serious reactions or hypersensitivity occur. Caution with low endothelial cell counts; increased potential for corneal edema. Avoid with severe renal impairment (CrCl <30mL/ min). The preservative used, benzalkonium chloride, may be absorbed by soft contact lenses; contact lenses should be removed during instillation and reinserted 15 min after instillation. Not studied in acute angle closure glaucoma.

ADVERSE REACTIONS: Blurred vision, taste disturbances, blepharitis, dermatitis, dry eye, foreign body sensation, headache, hyperemia, ocular discharge, ocular discomfort, ocular keratitis, ocular pain, ocular pruritus, rhinitis.

INTERACTIONS: Acid-base alterations reported with oral carbonic anhydrase inhibitors; caution with high-dose salicylates. Potential additive systemic effects with oral carbonic anhydrase inhibitors; coadministration is not recommended.

PREGNANCY: Category C, not for use in nursing.

MECHANISM OF ACTION: Carbonic anhydrase II inhibitor; inhibits aqueous humor formation and reduces elevated intraocular pressure.

PHARMACOKINETICS: Distribution: Plasma protein binding (60%). **Elimination:** Urine (unchanged).

NURSING CONSIDERATIONS

Assessment: Assess for sulfonamide hypersensitivity, low endothelial cell counts, acute angle-closure glaucoma, contact lens use, renal function, pregnancy/nursing status, and possible drug interactions.

Monitoring: Monitor for sulfonamide hypersensitivity reactions. If using chronically, monitor for ocular reactions (eg, conjunctivitis and lid reactions); d/c therapy and evaluate patient if such reactions occur. Monitor for bacterial keratitis if using multiple dose container. Monitor for choroidal detachment following filtration procedures.

Patient Counseling: Advise to d/c and contact physician if any serious or unusual ocular or systemic reactions or signs of hypersensitivity occur. Inform that temporary blurred vision may occur after dosing; caution with operating machinery or driving motor vehicle. Instruct to avoid touching container tip to the eye or any other surfaces. Instruct to contact physician about the continued use of present multidose container if having ocular surgery or if an intercurrent ocular condition (eg, trauma, infection) develops. Instruct to remove contact lenses during instillation and reinsert 15 min after instillation. Advise that if using >1 topical ophthalmic medication, separate administration by at least 10 min.

Administration: Ocular route. Shake well before use. **Storage:** 4-30°C (39-86°F).

AZOR   RX
amlodipine besylate - olmesartan medoxomil (Daiichi Sankyo)

> Can cause injury/death to developing fetus during 2nd and 3rd trimesters. D/C therapy if pregnancy is detected.

THERAPEUTIC CLASS: ARB/Calcium channel blocker (dihydropyridine)

INDICATIONS: Treatment of hypertension, alone or with other antihypertensive agents. Initial therapy in patients likely to need multiple antihypertensive agents to achieve their BP goals.

DOSAGE: *Adults:* Replacement Therapy: May substitute for individually titrated components for patients on amlodipine and olmesartan. When substituting for individual components, the dose of 1 or both components may be increased if needed. Add-On Therapy: May be used to provide additional BP lowering when not adequately controlled on amlodipine or olmesartan alone. Initial Therapy: Initiate at 5mg-20mg qd. Titrate: May increase dose after 1-2 weeks to maximum dose of 10mg-40mg qd as needed to control BP. Max: 10mg-40mg qd.

HOW SUPPLIED: Tab: (Amlodipine-Olmesartan) 5mg-20mg, 5mg-40mg, 10mg-20mg, 10mg-40mg

WARNINGS/PRECAUTIONS: Hypotension, especially in volume- or salt-depleted patients, may occur with treatment initiation; monitor closely. Caution with severe aortic stenosis and heart failure (HF). Increased risk of severe obstructive coronary artery disease (CAD), angina, or myocardial infarction (MI) with calcium channel blockers may occur with dosage initiation or increase. Changes in renal function, oliguria, progressive azotemia, or acute renal failure may occur. Avoid initial therapy in patients ≥75 yrs or in patients with hepatic impairment

ADVERSE REACTIONS: Edema, dizziness, headache, palpitations.

PREGNANCY: Category C (1st trimester) and D (2nd and 3rd trimester), not for use in nursing.

MECHANISM OF ACTION: Amlodipine: Calcium channel receptor blocker (dihydropyridine); inhibits transmembrane influx of calcium ions into vascular smooth muscle and cardiac muscle. Olmesartan: Angiotensin II receptor blocker; blocks vasoconstrictor effect of angiotensin II.

PHARMACOKINETICS: Absorption: Amlodipine: T_{max}=6-12 hrs, absolute bioavailability (64-90%). Olmesartan: Rapid and complete, absolute bioavailability (26%), T_{max}=1-2 hrs. **Distribution:** Amlodipine: Plasma protein binding (93%).

Olmesartan: V_d=17L, plasma protein binding (99%), crosses placental barrier; excreted in breast milk. **Metabolism:** Amlodipine: Liver. Olmesartan: Ester hydrolysis. **Elimination:** Amlodipine: Urine (60%); $T_{1/2}$=30-50 hrs. Olmesartan: Urine (35-50%), feces; $T_{1/2}$=13 hrs.

NURSING CONSIDERATIONS

Assessment: Assess for severe obstructive CAD, HF, severe aortic stenosis, volume/salt depletion, renal/hepatic function and pregnancy/nursing status.

Monitoring: Monitor for signs/symptoms of hypotension, hypersensitivity reactions, renal/hepatic dysfunction. Monitor for symptoms of severe obstructive CAD, angina or MI after dosage initiation or increase.

Patient Counseling: Inform of pregnancy risks. Notify physician if pregnant/intend to become pregnant, or if breastfeeding. Advise to seek medical attention if symptoms of hypotension or hypersensitivity reactions occur.

Administration: Oral route. **Storage:** 25°C (77°F); excursions permitted to 15-30°C (59-86°F).

AZULFIDINE   RX
sulfasalazine (Pharmacia & Upjohn)

THERAPEUTIC CLASS: 5-Aminosalicylic acid derivative/sulfapyridine

INDICATIONS: Treatment of mild to moderate ulcerative colitis. Adjunct therapy in severe ulcerative colitis. To prolong remission period between acute attacks of ulcerative colitis.

DOSAGE: *Adults:* Initial: 3-4g/day in evenly divided doses not >8-hr interval. May initiate at 1-2g/day to reduce GI intolerance. Maint: 2g/day. Response to therapy can be evaluated by clinical criteria (eg, presence of fever, weight changes, degree and frequency of diarrhea and bleeding, sigmoidoscopy, evaluation of biopsy samples). When endoscopic examination confirms satisfactory improvement, dosage should be reduced to maintenance level. If diarrhea recurs, dosage should be increased to previously effective levels. If symptoms of GI intolerance occur after 1st few doses, reduce dose in 1/2, then gradually increase. If GI intolerance persists, d/c for 5-7 days, then reintroduce at a lower dose.
Pediatrics: ≥6 yrs: 40-60mg/kg/day divided into 3-6 doses. Maint: 30mg/kg/day divided into 4 doses. Response to therapy can be evaluated by clinical criteria (eg, presence of fever, weight changes, degree and frequency of diarrhea and bleeding, sigmoidoscopy, evaluation of biopsy samples). When endoscopic examination confirms satisfactory improvement, dosage should be reduced to maintenance level. If diarrhea recurs, dosage should be increased to previously effective levels. If symptoms of GI intolerance occur after 1st few doses, reduce dose in 1/2, then gradually increase. If GI intolerance persists, d/c for 5-7 days, then reintroduce at a lower dose.

HOW SUPPLIED: Tab: 500mg* *scored

CONTRAINDICATIONS: Intestinal or urinary obstruction, porphyria.

WARNINGS/PRECAUTIONS: Caution with hepatic/renal impairment, blood dyscrasias, severe allergy, and bronchial asthma. Monitor patients with glucose 6-phosphate dehydrogenase deficiency for signs of hemolytic anemia. Deaths reported from hypersensitivity reactions, agraunulocytosis, aplastic anemia, other blood dyscrasias, renal and liver damage, irreversible neuromuscular and CNS changes, and fibrosing alveolitis. Presence of sore throat, fever, pallor, purpura, or jaundice may be the indications of serious blood disorder or hepatotoxicity. Monitor CBC including differential WBC, LFTs, at baseline, every 2nd week for 1st 3 months, monthly for next 3 months, and every 3 months thereafter. D/C while awaiting the results of blood tests. Monitor urinalysis and renal function periodically. Maintain adequate fluid intake to prevent crystalluria and stone formation. D/C if hypersensitivity or toxic reaction occurs. Oligospermia and infertility reported in males.

ADVERSE REACTIONS: Anorexia, headache, N/V, gastric distress, reversible oligospermia.

INTERACTIONS: Reduces absorption of folic acid, digoxin.

PREGNANCY: Category B, caution in nursing.

MECHANISM OF ACTION: 5-aminosalicylic acid (5-ASA) derivative/sulfapyridine (SP); not established, may be related to anti-inflammatory and/or immunomodulatory properties of sulfasalazine (SSZ) or its metabolites (5-ASA and SP), its affinity for connective tissue, and/or to relatively high concentration reached in serous fluids, the liver, and intestinal walls.

PHARMACOKINETICS: Absorption: SSZ: C_{max}=6µg/mL, T_{max}=6 hrs; Absolute bioavailability=<15%. 5-ASA, SP: T_{max} =10 hrs. SP: Well absorbed from colon. 5-ASA: Much less well absorbed from GI tract. **Distribution:** SSZ: V_d=7.5L; Plasma protein binding (>99.3%). SP: Plasma protein binding (70%). AcSP: Plasma protein binding (90%). **Metabolism:** Intestinal bacteria to 5-ASA and SP (metaolites); liver (acetylation). Found in breast milk. **Elimination:** Urine (37%), feces. SSZ: $T_{1/2}$=7.6 hrs (IV); SP: $T_{1/2}$=10.4 hrs (fast acetylators), 14.8 hrs (slow acetylators).

NURSING CONSIDERATIONS

Assessment: Assess for intestinal or urinary obstruction, porphyria, blood dyscrasias, renal/liver damage, severe allergy or bronchial asthma, glucose 6-phosphate dehydrogenase deficiency, pregnancy/nursing status, and for possible drug interactions. Obtain baseline CBC, including differential WBC, LFTs.

Monitoring: Monitor for signs/symptoms of hypersensitivity reactions, agranulocytosis, aplastic anemia or other blood dyscrasias, renal and liver damage, neuromuscular and CNS changes, and for fibrosing alveolitis. Monitor for signs of hemolytic anemia in patients with glucose-6 phosphate dehydrogenase deficiency. Perform CBC, including differential WBC, and LFTs before start of therapy, every 2 weeks during the first 3 months of therapy, every month for second 3 months of therapy, then every 3 months during treatment. Perform periodic monitoring of serum SP levels, urinalysis, and renal function.

Patient Counseling: Advise about the possibility of adverse reactions and of the need for careful medical supervision. Instruct to seek medical attention if develop sore throat, fever, pallor, purpura, or jaundice. Inform that ulcerative colitis rarely remits completely and that risk of relapse can be substantially reduced by continued administration at a maintenance dosage. Instruct to take in evenly divided doses, preferably after meals. Advise that orange-yellow discoloration of urine or skin may occur.

Administration: Oral route. **Storage:** 25°C (77°F); excursions permitted to 15-30°C (59-86°F).

AZULFIDINE EN   RX
sulfasalazine (Pharmacia & Upjohn)

THERAPEUTIC CLASS: 5-Aminosalicylic acid derivative/sulfapyridine

INDICATIONS: Treatment of mild to moderate ulcerative colitis. Adjunct treatment of severe ulcerative colitis. To prolong the remission period between acute attacks of ulcerative colitis. Treatment of rheumatoid arthritis and polyarticular-course juvenile rheumatoid arthritis that has responded inadequately to salicylates or other NSAIDs.

DOSAGE: *Adults:* Ulcerative Colitis: Initial: 3-4g/day in evenly divided doses at intervals not >8 hrs. May initiate at 1-2g/day to reduce GI intolerance. Maint: 2g/day. Rheumatoid Arthritis: Initial: 0.5-1g/day. Maint: 2g/day given bid. Swallow tabs whole after meals.
Pediatrics: ≥6 yrs: Ulcerative Colitis: Initial: 40-60mg/kg/day in 3-6 divided doses. Maint: 30mg/kg/day in 4 divided doses. Juvenile Rheumatoid Arthritis: 30-50mg/kg/day in 2 divided doses. To reduce GI effects give 1/4 to 1/3 initial dose; increase weekly for 1 month. Max: 2g/day. Swallow tabs whole after meals.

HOW SUPPLIED: Tab, Delayed-Release: 500mg

CONTRAINDICATIONS: Intestinal or urinary obstruction, porphyria.

WARNINGS/PRECAUTIONS: Caution with hepatic or renal impairment, blood dyscrasias, severe allergy, bronchial asthma, or glucose 6-phosphate dehydrogenase deficiency. Monitor CBC, WBC, and LFTs prior to therapy and every 2nd week for the 1st 3 months, once monthly for next 3 months, then every 3 months thereafter. D/C while awaiting the result of blood tests. Monitor urinalysis and renal function periodically. Maintain adequate fluid intake to prevent crystalluria and stone formation. D/C if tabs pass undisintegrated, or if hypersensitivity or toxic reactions occur. Oligospermia and infertility reported in males.

ADVERSE REACTIONS: Anorexia, headache, N/V, gastric distress, reversible oligospermia, rash, pruritus, fever, dyspepsia, abdominal pain, dizziness, stomatitis, abnormal LFT, leukopenia.

INTERACTIONS: Reduced absorption of folic acid and digoxin. Increased incidence of GI adverse events (nausea) with combination of sulfasalazine (2g/day) and methotrexate (7.5mg/week).

PREGNANCY: Category B, caution in nursing.

MECHANISM OF ACTION: 5-aminosalicylic acid (5-ASA) derivative/sulfapyridine (SP); not established, may be related to the anti-inflammatory and/or immunomodulatory properties, its affinity for connective tissue, and/or to the relatively high concentration reached in serous fluids, liver, and intestinal wall.

PHARMACOKINETICS: Absorption: SSZ: C_{max}=6µg/mL, T_{max}=6 hrs; Absolute bioavailability (≤15%). 5-ASA, SP: T_{max}=10 hrs. SP: Well absorbed from colon, estimated bioavailability (60%). 5-ASA: Much less well absorbed from GI tract, estimated bioavailability (10-30%). **Distribution:** SSZ: V_d=7.5L; plasma protein binding (≥99.3%). SP: Plasma protein binding (70%). AcSP: plasma protein binding (90%). **Metabolism:** Intestinal bacteria to 5-ASA and SP; liver (acetylation). Found in breast milk. **Elimination:** Urine (37%), feces. SSZ: $T_{1/2}$=7.6 hrs (IV), SP: $T_{1/2}$=10.4 hrs (fast acetylators), 14.8 hrs (slow acetylators).

NURSING CONSIDERATIONS

Assessment: Assess for intestinal or urinary obstruction, porphyria, blood dyscrasias, renal/liver damage, severe allergy or bronchial asthma, pregnancy/nursing status, glucose 6-phosphate dehydrogenase deficiency, and drug interactions. Obtain baseline CBC, WBC, LFTs.

Monitoring: Perform CBC, including differential WBC and LFTs before initiation, every 2 weeks during the first 3 months, every month for next 3 months, then every 3 months thereafter. Monitor serum SP levels, urinalysis and renal function tests periodically. Monitor for signs/symptoms of serious blood disorder (eg, sore throat, fever, pallor, purpura, jaundice), hypersensitivity/allergic reactions, renal/hepatic dysfunction.

Patient Counseling: Inform that ulcerative colitis rarely remits completely and that risk of relapse can be substantially reduced by continued administration at maintenance dosage. Inform patients that rheumatoid arthritis rarely remits and that patients should follow up with their physician to determine the need for continued therapy. Instruct to take in evenly divided doses after meals and to swallow tablet whole. Orange-yellow discoloration of urine or skin may occur. Inform to seek medical attention if sore throat, fever, pallor, purpura, or jaundice, allergic reactions, or hypersensitivity occur.

Administration: Oral route. **Storage:** 25°C (77°F); excursions permitted to 15-30°C (59-86°F).

BACTRIM   RX
sulfamethoxazole - trimethoprim (AR Scientific)

OTHER BRAND NAMES: Bactrim DS (AR Scientific)

THERAPEUTIC CLASS: Sulfonamide/tetrahydrofolic acid inhibitor

INDICATIONS: Treatment of urinary tract infection (UTI), acute otitis media in pediatric patients, acute exacerbations of chronic bronchitis (AECB) in adults, traveler's diarrhea in adults, and for enteritis caused by susceptible strains of microorganisms. Treatment and prophylaxis against *Pneumocystis carinii* pneumonia (PCP) in immunosuppressed and those at increased risk.

DOSAGE: *Adults:* UTI/Shigellosis: 800mg-160mg or 2 tabs of 400mg-80mg q12h for 10-14 days (UTI) or 5 days (Shigellosis). AECB: 800mg-160mg or 2 tabs of 400mg-80mg q12h for 14 days. Traveler's Diarrhea: 800mg-160mg or 2 tabs of 400mg-80mg q12h for 5 days. PCP Treatment: 75-100mg/kg SMX and 15-20mg/kg TMP per 24 hrs given in equally divided doses q6h for 14-21 days. PCP Prophylaxis: 800mg-160mg qd. Renal Impairment: CrCl 15-30mL/min: 1/2 of usual dose. CrCl <15mL/min: Not recommended.
Pediatrics: ≥2 months: UTI/Otitis Media/Shigellosis: 40mg/kg SMX and 8mg/kg TMP per 24 hrs given in 2 divided doses q12h for 10 days (UTI/Otitis Media) or 5 days (Shigellosis). PCP Treatment: 75-100mg/kg SMX and 15-20mg/kg TMP per 24 hrs given in equally divided doses q6h for 14-21 days. PCP Prophylaxis: Usual: 750mg/m²/day SMX and 150mg/m²/day TMP given in equally divided doses bid, on 3 consecutive days/week. Max: 1,600mg SMX and 320mg TMP/day. Renal Impairment: CrCl 15-30mL/min: 1/2 of usual dose. CrCl <15mL/min: Not recommended.

HOW SUPPLIED: (Sulfamethoxazole [SMX]-Trimethoprim [TMP]) Tab: 400mg-80mg*; Tab, DS: 800mg-160mg* *scored

CONTRAINDICATIONS: Megaloblastic anemia due to folate deficiency, history of drug-induced immune thrombocytopenia with TMP and/or sulfonamides, pregnancy, nursing, infants <2 months, marked hepatic damage, severe renal insufficiency when renal status cannot be monitored.

WARNINGS/PRECAUTIONS: Fatal reactions (eg, Stevens-Johnson syndrome [SJS], toxic epidermal necrolysis [TEN], fulminant hepatic necrosis, agranulocytosis, aplastic anemia and other blood dyscrasias) may occur; d/c at 1st appearance of skin rash or any sign of adverse reaction. *Clostridium difficile*-associated diarrhea (CDAD) reported. Cough, SOB, and pulmonary infiltrates are hypersensitivity reactions of the respiratory tract that have been reported. Thrombocytopenia reported; usually resolves within a week upon d/c. Monitor CBC frequently; d/c if with significant reduction in any formed blood element. Avoid use with group A β-hemolytic streptococcal infections. Hemolysis may occur in glucose-6-phosphate dehydrogenase (G6PD)-deficient patients. Cases of hypoglycemia in non-diabetic patients seen rarely; patients with renal dysfunction, liver disease, malnutrition, or those receiving high doses are at risk for hypoglycemia. Hematological changes indicative of folic acid deficiency may occur in elderly patients or in patients with pre-existing folic acid deficiency or kidney failure; reversible by folinic acid therapy. Caution with hepatic/renal impairment, possible folate deficiency (eg, elderly, chronic alcoholics, malabsorption syndrome, malnutrition), bronchial asthma and severe allergies. Increased incidence of adverse events (eg, hyperkalemia, mild intolerance, rash, fever, leukopenia, elevated transaminase values) reported in AIDS patients; re-evaluate therapy if develops skin rash or any sign of adverse reaction develops. Hyperkalemia reported; caution in patients receiving high doses of TMP, underlying disorders of K⁺ metabolism and renal insufficiency. Ensure adequate fluid intake and urinary output to prevent crystalluria. Slow acetylators more prone to idiosyncratic reactions to sulfonamides. Caution with porphyria or thyroid dysfunction. TMP may impair phenylalanine metabolism.

ADVERSE REACTIONS: N/V, anorexia, allergic skin reactions (eg, rash, urticaria), agranulocytosis, aplastic anemia, SJS, TEN, hepatitis, renal failure, hyperkalemia, aseptic meningitis, arthralgia, convulsions, cough.

INTERACTIONS: Increased incidence of thrombocytopenia with purpura in elderly patients with diuretics (primarily thiazides). May prolong PT with anticoagulant warfarin. May increase the effects of phenytoin and levels of methotrexate and digoxin. Marked but reversible nephrotoxicity reported with cyclosporine in renal transplant recipients. May develop megaloblastic anemia with pyrimethamine >25mg/week. Increased SMX levels with indomethacin. May decrease efficacy of TCAs. Single case of toxic delirium reported with amantadine. Potentiates effects of oral hypoglycemics. May cause hyperkalemia in elderly patients with ACE inhibitors.

PREGNANCY: Category C, not for use in nursing.

MECHANISM OF ACTION: SMX: Sulfonamide; inhibits bacterial synthesis of dyhydrofolic acid by competing with para-aminobenzoic acid (PABA). TMP: Tetrahydrofolic acid inhibitor; blocks the production of tetrahydrofolic acid from dihydrofolic acid by binding to and reversibly inhibiting the required enzyme, dihydrofolate reductase.

PHARMACOKINETICS: Absorption: Rapid; T_{max}=1-4 hrs. **Distribution:** Crosses placenta; found in breast milk. SMX: Plasma protein binding (70%); TMP: Plasma protein binding (44%). **Metabolism:** SMX: N_4-acetylation; TMP: 1- and 3-oxides, 3'- and 4'-hydroxy derivatives (principal metabolites). **Elimination:** Urine (84.5% total sulfonamide), (66.8%, free TMP); $T_{1/2}$=10 hrs (SMX), 8-10 hrs (TMP).

NURSING CONSIDERATIONS

Assessment: Assess for hypersensitivity reaction to drug components, history of drug-induced immune thrombocytopenia, documented megaloblastic anemia due to folate deficiency (eg, malabsorption syndrome, group A β-hemolytic streptococcal infections, chronic alcoholic, malnutrition status, elderly, receiving anticonvulsant therapy), hepatic/renal insufficiency, CDAD, severe allergies, bronchial asthma, G6PD deficiency, phenylketonurics, porphyria or thyroid dysfunction, underlying disorders of K+ metabolism, slow acetylators, pregnancy/nursing status, and for possible drug interactions. Obtain baseline CBC.

Monitoring: Monitor for severe allergic reactions (eg, SJS, TEN, fulminant hepatic necrosis, agranulocytosis, aplastic anemia and other blood dyscrasias), thrombocytopenia, CDAD (mild diarrhea to fatal colitis), development of drug resistance, overgrowth of nonsusceptible microorganisms, hypersensitivity reactions of the respiratory tract (eg, cough, SOB, pulmonary infiltrates), kernicterus, hypogylcemia, signs of bone marrow depression after chronic use. Periodically monitor CBC, renal function, LFTs and K+ levels, coagulation time, digoxin levels, and perform urinalysis with careful microscopic exam.

Patient Counseling: Inform about potential benefits/risks of therapy. Inform that drug only treats bacterial, not viral infections (eg, common colds). Instruct to take exactly as directed; skipping doses or not completing full course may decrease effectiveness and increase bacterial resistance. Instruct to notify physician if allergic reaction, watery/bloody diarrhea (with/without stomach cramps and fever) occur (may occur up to ≥2 months after treatment). Counsel to drink adequate fluids to prevent crystalluria and stone formation. Notify physician if pregnant/nursing or planning to become pregnant.

Administration: Oral route. **Storage:** 20-25°C (68-77°F).

BACTROBAN   RX
mupirocin (GlaxoSmithKline)

THERAPEUTIC CLASS: Bacterial protein synthesis inhibitor

INDICATIONS: (Oint) Topical treatment of impetigo due to *S. aureus* and *S. pyogenes*. (Cre) Treatment of secondarily infected traumatic skin lesions (up to 10cm in length or 100cm²) due to *S. aureus* and *S. pyogenes*.

DOSAGE: *Adults:* (Oint) Apply tid. (Cre) Apply tid for 10 days. May cover with gauze. Re-evaluate if no response within 3-5 days.
Pediatrics: (Oint) 2 months -16 yrs: Apply tid. (Cre) 3 months-16 yrs: Apply tid for 10 days. May cover with gauze. Re-evaluate if no response within 3-5 days.

HOW SUPPLIED: Cre: 2% [15g, 30g]; Oint: 2% [22g]

WARNINGS/PRECAUTIONS: Avoid eyes. D/C if sensitization or irritation occurs. May cause superinfection with prolonged use. Caution with oint in renal dysfunction. Avoid mucosal surfaces. Avoid open wounds or damaged skin with oint.

ADVERSE REACTIONS: Burning, pain, pruritus, headache, rash, nausea.

PREGNANCY: Category B, caution in nursing.

MECHANISM OF ACTION: Bacterial protein synthesis inhibitor; inhibits bacterial protein synthesis by reversibly and specifically binding to bacterial isoleucyl transfer-RNA synthetase. Active against a wide range of gram-positive bacteria including methicillin-resistant *Staphylococcus aureus* (MRSA). Also active against certain gram-negative bacteria.

PHARMACOKINETICS: Absorption: Minimal percutaneous absorption. **Metabolism:** Rapid. Monic acid (inactive metabolite). **Elimination:** Renal (metabolite).

NURSING CONSIDERATIONS

Assessment: Perform proper diagnosis of skin infection. Assess use in pregnant/nursing females.

Monitoring: Monitor for sensitization or severe local irritation of the skin. In patients on prolonged therapy, monitor for possible overgrowth of nonsusceptible microorganisms, including fungi.

Patient Counseling: Inform that medication is for external use only and to avoid contact of medication with the eyes. Counsel that treated area can be covered with a gauze dressing. Advise to contact physician and d/c medication if any signs of local adverse reactions (eg, irritation, severe itching, rash) develop. Notify if no clinical improvement is seen within 3-5 days.

Administration: Topical. **Storage:** Store at or below 25°C (77°F). Do not freeze.

BACTROBAN NASAL   RX
mupirocin calcium (GlaxoSmithKline)

THERAPEUTIC CLASS: Bacterial protein synthesis inhibitor

INDICATIONS: Eradication of nasal colonization of methicillin-resistant *staphylococcus aureus* (MRSA) in adults and healthcare workers in certain institutional settings during outbreaks of MRSA.

DOSAGE: *Adults:* Apply 1/2 of the single-use tube into each nostril bid for 5 days. Spread oint by pressing together and releasing the sides of the nose repetitively for 1 min. Do not re-use tube.
Pediatrics: ≥12 yrs: Apply 1/2 of the single-use tube into each nostril bid for 5 days. Spread oint by pressing together and releasing the sides of the nose repetitively for 1 min. Do not re-use tube.

HOW SUPPLIED: Oint: 2% [1g pkt]

WARNINGS/PRECAUTIONS: Avoid eyes. D/C if sensitization or irritation occur. May cause superinfection with prolonged use.

ADVERSE REACTIONS: Headache, rhinitis, respiratory disorder, pharyngitis, taste perversion.

INTERACTIONS: Avoid use with other intranasal products.

PREGNANCY: Category B, caution in nursing.

MECHANISM OF ACTION: Antibacterial agent; inhibits protein synthesis by reversibly and specifically binding to bacterial isoleucyl transfer-RNA synthetase.

PHARMACOKINETICS: Absorption: Significant in neonates and premature infants. **Elimination:** Urine.

NURSING CONSIDERATIONS

Assessment: Assess for drug hypersensitivity, high-risk healthcare workers during institutional outbreaks of methicillin-resistant *S.aureus,* possible drug interactions.

Monitoring: Monitor for sensitization, severe local irritation, tearing, and for overgrowth of nonsusceptible microorganisms (eg, fungi).

Patient Counseling: Avoid contact with eyes. Consult physician if sensitization or severe irritation occurs.

Administration: Intranasal route. Apply approximately half of ointment from single-use tube directly into 1 nostril and other half into other nostril; discard tube after using. Press sides of nose together and gently massage after

B

application to spread ointment throughout inside of nostril. **Storage:** 20-25°C (68-77°F); excursions permitted to 15-30°C (59-86°F). Do not refrigerate.

BANZEL   RX
rufinamide (Eisai)

THERAPEUTIC CLASS: Triazole derivative

INDICATIONS: Adjunctive treatment of seizures associated with Lennox-Gastaut syndrome in adults and children ≥4 yrs.

DOSAGE: *Adults:* Initial: 400-800mg/day in two equally divided doses. Titrate: May increase by 400-800mg/day every other day until reach max of 3200mg/day, given in two equally divided doses. Max: 3200mg/day. Take with food. May give as whole tabs, half-tabs, or crushed. Elderly: Start at the low end of the dosing range.
Pediatrics: ≥4 yrs: Initial: 10mg/kg/day in two equally divided doses. Titrate: May increase by 10mg/kg increments every other day to target dose of 45mg/kg/day or 3200mg/day, whichever is less, given in two equally divided doses. Take with food. May give as whole tabs, half-tabs, or crushed.

HOW SUPPLIED: Tab: 200mg*, 400mg* *scored

CONTRAINDICATIONS: Familial short QT syndrome.

WARNINGS/PRECAUTIONS: May increase risk of suicidal thoughts or behavior; monitor for emergence or worsening of depression, suicidal thoughts or behavior, and/or or any unusual changes in mood or behavior. Associated with CNS-related adverse effects (eg, somnolence/fatigue, coordination abnormalities, dizziness, gait disturbances, ataxia). QT interval shortening reported. Multi-organ hypersensitivity syndrome reported; d/c if suspected. Withdraw gradually to minimize risk of precipitating seizures, seizure exacerbation, or status epilepticus. Leukopenia reported. Avoid with severe hepatic impairment. Caution with mild to moderate hepatic impairment and elderly.

ADVERSE REACTIONS: Somnolence, N/V, headache, fatigue, dizziness, tremor, nystagmus, nasopharyngitis, rash, ataxia, diplopia, bronchitis, blurred vision.

INTERACTIONS: Potent CYP450 inducers (eg, carbamazepine, phenytoin, primodone, phenobarbital) may increase clearance of rufinamide. May increase phenytoin and phenobarbital levels. Valproate may reduce clearance and increase levels; initiate valproate at low dose and titrate to clinically effective dose. May decrease lamotrigine and carbamazepine levels. May decrease levels of hormonal contraceptives; additional forms of non-hormonal contraception are recommended during coadministration. May decrease levels of drugs that are substrates of CYP3A4 (eg, triazolam). May increase plasma levels of drugs that are substrates of CYP2E1 (eg, chlorzoxazone). Caution with other drugs that shorten QT interval. May increase clearance with carboxylesterase inducers. May decrease metabolism with carboxylesterase inhibitors. Other CNS-acting medications and alcohol may cause additive CNS effects.

PREGNANCY: Category C, not for use in nursing.

MECHANISM OF ACTION: Triazole derivative; mechanism not established. Suspected to modulate activity of sodium channels and, in particular, prolongation of the inactive state of the channel. Slows sodium channel recovery from inactivation after prolonged prepulse in cultured cortical neurons, and limited sustained repetitive firing of sodium-dependent action potentials.

PHARMACOKINETICS: Absorption: Well-absorbed, T_{max}=4-6 hrs. **Distribution:** Plasma protein binding (34%); V_d=50L (3200mg/day); likely found in breast milk. **Metabolism:** Extensive; via carboxylesterase mediated hydrolysis; CYP2E1 (weak inhibitor), CYP3A4 (weak inducer). **Elimination:** Urine (<2%, unchanged; 66%, acid metabolite CGP 47292); $T_{1/2}$=6-10 hrs.

NURSING CONSIDERATIONS

Assessment: Assess for familial short QT syndrome, presence or history of depression, hepatic/renal impairment, pregnancy/nursing status, and for possible drug interactions.

Monitoring: Monitor for emergence or worsening of depression, suicidal thoughts, changes in behavior, CNS reactions (eg, somnolence, fatigue, coordination abnormalities, dizziness, gait disturbances, ataxia), QT interval shortening, multi-organ hypersensitivity syndrome, and for leucopenia. Upon withdrawal of therapy, monitor for precipitation of seizures, exacerbation of seizures, and status epilepticus.

Patient Counseling: Inform patients, caregivers, and families of the high risk of suicidal thoughts and behavior and to be alert for emergence or worsening of signs/symptoms of depression, unusual changes in mood or behavior, suicidal thoughts and behavior, and thoughts of self-harm. Instruct to take only as prescribed and to avoid alcohol. Counsel about potential to develop somnolence or dizziness. Advise not to drive or operate machinery until gain sufficient experience to gauge whether therapy adversely affects mental and/or motor performance. Instruct to notify physician if pregnant or intend to become pregnant, and if breastfeeding or intend to breastfeed. If pregnant or intending to become pregnant, encourage to enroll in North American Antiepileptic Drug (NAAED) Pregnancy Registry. Instruct to take with food; inform that tabs may be taken whole, cut in half, or crushed. Instruct to contact physician if rash develops.

Administration: Oral route. **Storage:** 25°C (77°F); excursions permitted to 15-30°C (59-86°F). Protect from moisture.

BARACLUDE

entecavir (Bristol-Myers Squibb)

RX

> Lactic acidosis and severe hepatomegaly with steatosis, including fatal cases, have been reported alone or in combination with antiretrovirals. Severe acute exacerbations of hepatitis B upon d/c of therapy reported; monitor liver function for at least several months after d/c. If appropriate, may initiate anti-hepatitis B therapy. Limited clinical experience suggests there is a potential for the development of resistance to HIV nucleoside reverse transcriptase inhibitors if entecavir is used to treat chronic hepatitis B virus (HBV) infection in patients with untreated HIV infection. Not recommended for HIV/HBV coinfected patients not receiving highly active antiretroviral therapy (HAART).

THERAPEUTIC CLASS: Guanosine nucleoside analogue

INDICATIONS: Treatment of chronic HBV infection with active viral replication and persistent elevations in serum aminotransferases (ALT or AST) or histologically active disease.

DOSAGE: *Adults:* Compensated Liver Disease: Nucleoside-Treatment-Naive: 0.5mg qd. History of Hepatitis B Viremia While Receiving Lamivudine or Known Lamivudine/Telbivudine Resistant Mutations: 1mg qd. Decompensated Liver Disease: 1mg qd. Take on an empty stomach (≥2 hrs after and 2 hrs before a meal). Renal Impairment: Refer to PI for dose modifications.
Pediatrics: ≥16 yrs: Compensated Liver Disease: Nucleoside-Treatment-Naive: 0.5mg qd. History of Hepatitis B Viremia While Receiving Lamivudine or Known Lamivudine/Telbivudine Resistant Mutations: 1mg qd. Decompensated Liver Disease: 1mg qd. Take on an empty stomach (≥2 hrs after and 2 hrs before a meal). Renal Impairment: Refer to PI for dose modifications.

HOW SUPPLIED: Sol: 0.05mg/mL [210mL]; Tab: 0.5mg, 1mg

WARNINGS/PRECAUTIONS: Reduce dose in renal dysfunction (CrCl <50mL/min), including patients on hemodialysis or continuous ambulatory peritoneal dialysis (CAPD). Caution with known risk factors of liver disease. D/C if lactic acidosis or profound hepatotoxicity occurs. Careful with dose selection in elderly.

ADVERSE REACTIONS: Headache, fatigue, dizziness, nausea, ALT/lipase elevation, total bilirubin elevation, hyperglycemia, glycosuria, hematuria, hepatitis exacerbation, lactic acidosis, severe hepatomegaly with steatosis.

INTERACTIONS: See Boxed Warning. Serum concentrations of entecavir or coadministered drug may be increased if coadministered with drugs that reduce renal function or compete for active tubular secretion; closely monitor for adverse events.

B

PREGNANCY: Category C, not for use in nursing.

MECHANISM OF ACTION: Guanosine nucleoside analogue; inhibits base priming, reverse transcription of negative strand from pregenomic mRNA, and synthesis of positive strand of HBV DNA.

PHARMACOKINETICS: Absorption: C_{max}=4.2ng/mL (0.5mg), 8.2ng/mL (1.0mg); T_{max}=0.5-1.5 hrs. **Distribution:** Plasma protein binding (13%). **Metabolism:** Hepatic (minor). **Elimination:** Urine (62-73% unchanged); $T_{1/2}$=128-149 hrs.

NURSING CONSIDERATIONS

Assessment: Assess for hepatic/renal impairment, HIV antibody testing, pregnancy/nursing status, current medications, and possible drug interactions.

Monitoring: Periodic monitoring of hepatic/renal function is recommended during treatment and for those who d/c anti-hepatitis B therapy, monitor hepatic function for at least several months.

Patient Counseling: Advise to take on an empty stomach (≥2 hrs after and 2 hrs before a meal). Inform that treatment may lower the amount of HBV in the body, may lower the ability of HBV to multiply and infect new liver cells, and may improve the condition of the liver, but will not cure HBV. Inform that deterioration of liver disease may occur in some cases if treatment is d/c. Inform that treatment has not shown to reduce risk of transmission of HBV. Inform that it is not known whether treatment will reduce risk of liver cancer or cirrhosis. Advise to remain under care of physician; discuss new symptoms, changes in regimen, or concurrent medications. Offer HIV antibody testing before starting therapy. Inform that drug may increase the chance of HIV resistance to HIV medication if HIV infected and not receiving effective HIV treatment. Instruct to hold dosing spoon in a vertical position and fill gradually to the mark corresponding to prescribed dose for oral solution.

Administration: Oral route. **Storage:** 25°C (77°F); excursions permitted between 15-30°C (59-86°F). Protect oral solution from light.

BAYER ASPIRIN   OTC
aspirin (Bayer Healthcare)

OTHER BRAND NAMES: Bayer Aspirin Children's (Bayer Healthcare) - Bayer Aspirin Regimen with Calcium (Bayer Healthcare) - Bayer Aspirin Regimen (Bayer Healthcare) - Genuine Bayer Aspirin (Bayer Healthcare)

THERAPEUTIC CLASS: Salicylate

INDICATIONS: To reduce the risk of death and nonfatal stroke with previous ischemic stroke or transient ischemia of the brain. To reduce risk of vascular mortality with suspected acute myocardial infarction (MI). To reduce risk of death and nonfatal MI with previous MI or unstable angina. To reduce risk of MI and sudden death in chronic stable angina pectoris. For patients who have undergone revascularization procedures with a pre-existing condition for which ASA is indicated. Relief of signs of rheumatoid arthritis (RA), juvenile rheumatoid arthritis (JRA), osteoarthritis (OA), spondyloarthropathies, arthritis, and pleurisy associated with systemic lupus erythematosus (SLE). For minor aches and pains.

DOSAGE: *Adults:* Ischemic Stroke/TIA: 50-325mg qd. Suspected Acute MI: Initial: 160-162.5mg qd as soon as suspect MI. Maint: 160-162.5mg qd for 30 days post-infarction, consider further therapy for prevention/recurrent MI. Prevention or Recurrent MI/Unstable Angina/Chronic Stable Angina: 75-325mg qd. CABG: 325mg qd, start 6 hrs post-surgery. Continue for 1 yr. PTCA: Initial: 325mg, 2 hrs pre-surgery. Maint: 160-325mg qd. Carotid Endarterectomy: 80mg qd to 650mg bid, start pre-surgery. RA: Initial: 3g qd in divided doses. Increase for anti-inflammatory efficacy to 150-300mcg/mL plasma salicylate level. Spondyloarthropathies: Up to 4g/day in divided doses. OA: Up to 3g/day in divided doses. Arthritis/SLE Pleurisy: Initial: 3g/day in divided doses. Increase for anti-inflammatory efficacy to 150-300mcg/mL plasma salicylate level. Pain: 325-650mg q4-6h. Max: 4g/day.

Pediatrics: JRA: Initial: 90-130mg/kg/day in divided doses. Increase for anti-inflammatory efficacy to 150-300mcg/mL plasma salicylate level. Pain: ≥12 yrs: 325-650mg q4-6h. Max: 4g/day.

HOW SUPPLIED: Tab: (Genuine Bayer Aspirin) 325mg; Tab: (Bayer Aspirin Regimen with Calcium) 81mg; Tab, Chewable: (Bayer Aspirin Children's) 81mg; Tab, Delayed-Release: (Bayer Aspirin Regimen) 81mg, 325mg

CONTRAINDICATIONS: NSAID allergy, viral infections in children or teenagers, syndrome of asthma, rhinitis, and nasal polyps.

WARNINGS/PRECAUTIONS: Increased risk of bleeding with heavy alcohol use (≥3 drinks/day). May inhibit platelet function; can adversely affect inherited (hemophilia) or acquired (hepatic disease, vitamin K deficiency) bleeding disorders. Monitor for bleeding and ulceration. Avoid in history of active peptic ulcer, severe renal failure, severe hepatic insufficiency, and sodium restricted diets. Associated with elevated LFTs, BUN, and SrCr; hyperkalemia; proteinuria; and prolonged bleeding time. Avoid 1 week before and during labor.

ADVERSE REACTIONS: Fever, hypothermia, dysrhythmias, hypotension, agitation, cerebral edema, dehydration, hyperkalemia, dyspepsia, GI bleed, hearing loss, tinnitus, problems in pregnancy.

INTERACTIONS: Diminished hypotensive and hyponatremic effects of ACE inhibitors. May increase levels of acetazolamide, valproic acid. Increased bleeding risk with heparin, warfarin. Decreased levels of phenytoin. Decreased hypotensive effects of β-blockers. Decreased diuretic effects with renal or cardiovascular disease. Decreased methotrexate clearance; increased risk of bone marrow toxicity. Avoid NSAIDs. Increased effects of hypoglycemic agents. Antagonizes uricosuric agents.

PREGNANCY: Avoid in 3rd trimester of pregnancy and nursing.

MECHANISM OF ACTION: Provides temporary relief from arthritis pain and arthritis inflammation.

NURSING CONSIDERATIONS

Assessment: Assess for hypersensitivity, stomach problems, bleeding problems, ulcers, history of chickenpox or flu symptoms, and possible drug interactions.

Monitoring: Monitor for Reye's syndrome, allergic reactions include hives, facial swelling, asthma (wheezing) and shock.

Patient Counseling: Instruct to immediately report worsening of any adverse effects.

Administration: Oral route. **Storage:** Room temperature.

BECONASE AQ
RX

beclomethasone dipropionate (GlaxoSmithKline)

THERAPEUTIC CLASS: Corticosteroid

INDICATIONS: Relief of symptoms of seasonal or perennial allergic and nonallergic rhinitis. Prevention of nasal polyp recurrence following surgical removal.

DOSAGE: *Adults:* 1-2 sprays per nostril bid. Max: 2 sprays per nostril bid. *Pediatrics:* >12 years: 1-2 sprays per nostril bid. 6-12 yrs: Initial: 1 spray per nostril bid. Titrate: May increase to 2 sprays per nostril. Decrease to 1 spray per nostril bid once adequate control achieved. Max: 2 sprays per nostril bid.

HOW SUPPLIED: Spray: 42mcg/spray [25g]

WARNINGS/PRECAUTIONS: Risk of adrenal insufficiency and withdrawal symptoms when replacing systemic corticosteroids with topical corticosteroids. Caution with active or quiescent tuberculous (TB), ocular herpes simplex, or untreated bacterial, fungal and systemic viral or parasitic infections. Avoid with recent nasal trauma/surgery or septum ulcers. Risk for more severe/fatal course of infections (eg, chickenpox, measles) and for *Candida* infections of nose and pharynx. Potential for reduced growth velocity in pediatrics. Rare cases of nasal septum perforation, wheezing, cataracts, glaucoma, increased intraocular pressure reported. Hypersensitivity reactions may occur. D/C if nasopharyngeal irritation persists. Caution in elderly.

ADVERSE REACTIONS: Nasopharyngeal irritation, sneezing, headache, nausea, lightheadedness, irritated/dry nose and throat, unpleasant taste/smell.

INTERACTIONS: Concomitant systemic corticosteroids increase risk of hypercorticism and/or HPA axis suppression.

PREGNANCY: Category C, caution in nursing.

MECHANISM OF ACTION: Corticosteroid; mechanism not established; anti-inflammatory and vasoconstrictor effects.

PHARMACOKINETICS: Absorption: Absolute bioavailability (44%) (for the active metabolite B-17-MP). C_{max} <50pg/mL. **Distribution:** V_d=20L (parent drug); V_d=424L (B-17-MP). Plasma protein binding (87%). **Metabolism:** B-17-MP (active metabolite) via esterase enzymes. **Elimination:** Urine (12% metabolites), feces (60% metabolites). $T_{1/2}$=0.5 hrs (parent drug), 2.7 hrs (B-17-MP).

NURSING CONSIDERATIONS

Assessment: Assess for associated asthma with history of long-term therapy with systemic steroids, active or quiescent TB of upper respiratory tract, untreated local or systemic fungal or bacterial infections, systemic viral or parasitic infections, ocular herpes simplex, nasal polyps or recent nasal septal ulcers, nasal surgery/trauma, and possible drug interactions.

Monitoring: Monitor for reduced growth velocity (in pediatrics), nasal septum perforation, localized infection, *Candida* infection, exacerbation of infections, nasopharyngeal irritation, signs of adrenal insufficiency, and symptoms of hypercorticism.

Patient Counseling: Instruct to take as directed at regular intervals and to avoid exposure to chickenpox or measles. Consult physician immediately if exposed to infection or symptoms do not improve, if the condition worsens, or if sneezing or nasal irritation occurs. Advise to avoid spraying in the eyes.

Administration: Intranasal route. **Storage:** 15-30°C (59-86°F).

BENICAR   RX
olmesartan medoxomil (Daiichi Sankyo)

| Avoid use in pregnancy; may cause death/injury to developing fetus. |

THERAPEUTIC CLASS: Angiotensin II receptor antagonist

INDICATIONS: Treatment of hypertension alone or in combination with other antihypertensives.

DOSAGE: *Adults:* Individualized dosing. Monotherapy Without Volume Depletion: Initial: 20mg qd. Titrate: May increase to 40mg qd after 2 weeks if needed. May add diuretic if BP not controlled. Intravascular Volume Depletion (eg, with diuretics, impaired renal function): Lower initial dose; monitor closely.
Pediatrics: 6-16 yrs: Individualized dosing. 20-<35 kg: Usual: 10mg qd. Titrate: May increase to 20 mg qd after 2 weeks if needed. ≥35 kg: Usual: 20mg qd. Titrate: May increase to 40mg qd after 2 weeks if needed. If Cannot Swallow Tablets: Refer to PI for preparation of suspension; follow same dose as tablets.

HOW SUPPLIED: Tab: 5mg, 20mg, 40mg

WARNINGS/PRECAUTIONS: Symptomatic hypotension may occur in volume-and/or salt-depleted patients; correct volume depletion prior to therapy and monitor closely. Changes in renal function may occur; caution in renal artery stenosis and severe congestive heart failure. Increase in SrCr or BUN reported with renal artery stenosis.

ADVERSE REACTIONS: Dizziness.

PREGNANCY: Category C (1st trimester) and D (2nd and 3rd trimesters), not for use in nursing.

MECHANISM OF ACTION: Angiotensin II receptor antagonist; blocks vasoconstrictor effects of angiotensin II by selectively blocking binding of angiotensin II to AT$_1$ receptor in vascular smooth muscle.

PHARMACOKINETICS: Absorption: Rapid, complete. Absolute bioavailability (26%); T$_{max}$=1-2 hrs. **Distribution:** V$_d$=17L; plasma protein binding (99%). **Metabolism:** Ester hydrolysis. **Elimination:** Urine (35-50%), feces; T$_{1/2}$=13 hrs.

NURSING CONSIDERATIONS

Assessment: Assess for pregnancy/nursing status, volume/salt depletion, and renal/hepatic impairment.

Monitoring: Monitor LFTs and renal function periodically. Monitor for signs/symptoms of hypotension, renal/hepatic dysfunction.

Patient Counseling: Inform of pregnancy risks. Advise to seek medical attention if symptoms of hypotension occur. Inform that drug may be taken with/without food.

Administration: Oral route. **Storage:** 20-25°C (68-77°F).

BENICAR HCT   RX
olmesartan medoxomil - hydrochlorothiazide (Daiichi Sankyo)

> Can cause death/injury to developing fetus during 2nd and 3rd trimesters. Stop therapy if pregnancy detected.

THERAPEUTIC CLASS: Angiotensin II receptor antagonist/thiazide diuretic

INDICATIONS: Hypertension. Not for initial therapy.

DOSAGE: *Adults:* If BP not controlled with olmesartan alone: Add HCTZ 12.5mg qd. May titrate to 25mg qd if BP uncontrolled after 2-4 weeks. If BP not controlled with HCTZ alone: Add olmesartan 20mg qd. May titrate to 40mg qd if BP uncontrolled after 2-4 weeks. Intravascular Volume Depletion (eg, with diuretics, impaired renal function): Lower initial dose; monitor closely. Elderly: Start at lower end of dosing range.

HOW SUPPLIED: Tab: (Olmesartan-HCTZ) 20mg-12.5mg, 40mg-12.5mg, 40mg-25mg

CONTRAINDICATIONS: Sulfonamide hypersensitivity.

WARNINGS/PRECAUTIONS: Can cause fetal injury/death. Correct volume or salt depletion before therapy or monitor closely. Caution with hepatic or severe renal dysfunction, progressive liver disease, history of allergies or asthma, renal artery stenosis, severe congestive heart failure. Avoid if CrCl ≤30mL/min. May exacerbate or activate systemic lupus erythematosus (SLE). Monitor serum electrolytes. Hyperuricemia, hyperglycemia, hypercalcemia, hypomagnesemia may occur. May increase cholesterol and triglyceride levels.

ADVERSE REACTIONS: Dizziness, upper respiratory tract infection, hyperuricemia, N/V, asthenia, angioedema, hyperkalemia, rhabdomyolysis, ARF, alopecia, urticaria.

INTERACTIONS: Potentiates orthostatic hypotension with alcohol, barbiturates, or narcotics. May need to adjust antidiabetics. Potentiates other antihypertensives. Impaired absorption with cholestyramine, colestipol. Corticosteroids, adrenocorticotrophic hormone deplete electrolytes. May decrease response to pressor amines. May potentiate non-depolarizing skeletal muscle relaxants. Risk of lithium toxicity. NSAIDs decrease diuretic effects.

PREGNANCY: Category C (1st trimester) and D (2nd and 3rd trimesters), not for use in nursing.

MECHANISM OF ACTION: Olmesartan: Angiotensin II receptor antagonist; blocks vasoconstrictor effects of angiotensin II by selectively blocking binding of angiotensin II to AT$_1$ receptor in vascular smooth muscle. HCTZ: Thiazide diuretic; affects renal tubular mechanism of electrolyte reabsorption, directly increasing excretion of Na$^+$ and Cl$^-$ and indirectly reducing plasma volume.

PHARMACOKINETICS: Absorption: Olmesartan: Rapid, complete; absolute bioavailability (26%); T_{max}=1-2 hrs. **Distribution:** Olmesartan: V_d=17 L; plasma protein binding (99%). Crosses placenta; excreted in breast milk. HCTZ: Crosses placenta; excreted in breast milk. **Metabolism:** Olmesartan: Ester hydrolysis. **Elimination:** Olmesartan: Urine (35-50%), feces; $T_{1/2}$=13 hrs. HCTZ: Kidney (61%); $T_{1/2}$=5.6-14.8 hrs.

NURSING CONSIDERATIONS

Assessment: Assess for pregnancy status, possible drug interactions, volume/salt depletion, SLE, diabetes mellitus, anuria, sulfonamide hypersensitivity, history of allergy or bronchial asthma, hepatic/renal impairment.

Monitoring: Monitor serum electrolytes periodically. Monitor for signs/symptoms of electrolyte imbalance, exacerbation or activation of SLE, hypotension, hyperglycemia, hyperuricemia or precipitation of gout, hypersensitivity reactions, renal/hepatic dysfunction.

Patient Counseling: Inform of pregnancy risks. Advise that inadequate fluid intake or loss of fluids may result in drop of BP, leading to lightheadedness or syncope. Advise to seek medical attention if syncope, symptoms of electrolyte imbalance (dry mouth, thirst, weakness, lethargy), or hypersensitivity reactions occur.

Administration: Oral route. **Storage:** 20-25°C (68-77°F).

BENTYL   RX
dicyclomine HCl (Axcan Scandipharm)

THERAPEUTIC CLASS: Anticholinergic

INDICATIONS: Treatment of functional bowel/irritable bowel syndrome.

DOSAGE: *Adults:* (Tab/Syrup) Initial: 20mg qid. Usual: 40mg qid if tolerated. Discontinue if no improvement after 2 weeks or if doses ≥80mg/day are not tolerated. (Inj) 20mg IM qid for 1-2 days, followed by oral dicyclomine. Not for IV use.

HOW SUPPLIED: Cap: 10mg; Inj: 10mg/mL; Syrup: 10mg/5mL; Tab: 20mg

CONTRAINDICATIONS: GI tract obstruction, obstructive uropathy, severe ulcerative colitis, reflux esophagitis, glaucoma, myasthenia gravis, unstable cardiovascular status and in acute hemorrhage, nursing mothers, infants <6 months of age.

WARNINGS/PRECAUTIONS: Caution in autonomic neuropathy, hepatic/renal impairment, ulcerative colitis, hyperthyroidism, HTN, congestive heart failure, cardiac tachyarrhythmia, coronary heart disease, hiatal hernia, and prostatic hypertrophy. Heat prostration may occur in high environmental temperature. Monitor for diarrhea, may be the early symptom of intestinal obstruction. Psychosis reported. Serious respiratory symptoms, seizures, syncope and death reported in infants.

ADVERSE REACTIONS: Dry mouth, N/V, blurred vision, dizziness, drowsiness, nervousness, mental confusion/excitement (especially in the elderly), mydriasis, increased ocular tension, urinary retention, dyspnea, apnea, tachycardia, decreased sweating, lactation suppression, impotence.

INTERACTIONS: Potentiated by amantadine, Class I antiarrhythmics (eg, quinidine), antihistamines, antipsychotics (eg, phenothiazines), benzodiazepines, MAOIs, narcotic analgesics (eg, meperidine), nitrates/nitrites, sympathomimetics, TCAs. Antagonizes the effects of antiglaucoma agents; do not give with corticosteroid eye drops. Antagonizes the effect of metoclopramide. May effect the GI absorption of delayed release digoxin. Decreased absorption with antacids. Antagonized by drugs treating achlorhydria and those used to test gastric secretion.

PREGNANCY: Category B, contraindicated in nursing.

MECHANISM OF ACTION: Dicyclomine anticholinergic and antispasmodic agent; relieves smooth muscle spasm of the GI tract, and antagonizes bradykinin- and histamine-induced spasms.

PHARMACOKINETICS: Absorption: Rapidly absorbed; T_{max}=60-90 mins. **Distribution:** V_d=approximately 3.65L/Kg (extensive); excreted in breast milk **Elimination:** Urine (79.5%), feces (8.4%); $T_{1/2}$=1.8 hrs.

NURSING CONSIDERATIONS

Assessment: Assess for glaucoma, obstructive uropathy, obstructive disease of GI tract, paralytic ileus, ulcerative colitis, myasthenia gravis, hiatal hernia associated with reflux esophagitis, renal/hepatic dysfunction, hyperthyroidism, cardiac disorders.

Monitoring: Monitor for heat prostration, drowsiness, blurred vision, increased HR, constipation, diarrhea, urinary hesitancy/retention, hypersensitivity reactions.

Patient Counseling: Review side effects and report if any develop. Exercise caution while operating machinery/driving. Avoid high environmental temperatures.

Administration: PO, IM. IM form should not be used for more than 2 days. **Storage:** Cap/Tab/Syrup/Inj: Room temperature below 30°C (86°F). Syrup: Protect from excessive heat. Inj: Protect from freezing.

BENZACLIN   RX
clindamycin phosphate - benzoyl peroxide (Dermik)

OTHER BRAND NAMES: Clindamycin Phosphate and Benzoyl Peroxide Gel 1%/5% (Mylan)

THERAPEUTIC CLASS: Antibacterial/keratolytic

INDICATIONS: Topical treatment of acne vulgaris.

DOSAGE: *Adults:* Wash face and pat dry. Apply bid (am and pm) or ud. *Pediatrics:* ≥12 yrs: Wash face and pat dry. Apply bid (am and pm) or ud.

HOW SUPPLIED: Gel: (Clindamycin Phosphate-Benzoyl Peroxide) 10mg-50mg [25g, 35g, 50g]; (Generic) [50g]

CONTRAINDICATIONS: History of regional enteritis, ulcerative colitis (UC), or antibiotic-associated colitis. Hypersensitivity to lincomycin.

WARNINGS/PRECAUTIONS: Severe colitis reported with oral and parenteral clindamycin. Topical use of clindamycin may result in absorption of the antibiotic from the skin surface. Diarrhea, bloody diarrhea, and colitis (including pseudomembranous colitis) reported; d/c if significant diarrhea occurs. Avoid contact with eyes and mucous membranes. May cause an overgrowth of non-susceptible organisms, including fungi; d/c use and treat appropriately.

ADVERSE REACTIONS: Dry skin, application-site reactions.

INTERACTIONS: Antiperistaltic agents (eg, opiates, diphenoxylate with atropine) may prolong and/or worsen severe colitis. Caution with concomitant topical acne therapy (eg, peeling, desquamating, or abrasive agents) because of possible cumulative irritancy. Avoid erythromycin agents.

PREGNANCY: Category C, not for use in nursing.

MECHANISM OF ACTION: Antibacterial/keratolytic; acts against *Propionibacterium acnes* an organism associated with acne vulgaris.

PHARMACOKINETICS: Absorption: (Benzoyl peroxide) Skin. (Clindamycin Phosphate) Bioavailability (>1%). C_{max}=(1.47-2.77ng/mL, Day 1), (1.43-7.18ng/mL, Day 5). AUC=(2.74-12.86ng•h/mL, Day 1), (11.4-69.7ng•h/mL, Day 5). **Distribution:** Orally and parenterally administered clindamycin has been reported to appear in breast milk. **Metabolism:** (Benzoyl peroxide) Benzoic acid. **Elimination:** (Clindamycin Phosphate) Urine (0.03-0.08%).

NURSING CONSIDERATIONS

Assessment: Assess for hypersensitivity to lincomycin, history of regional enteritis, UC, antibiotic-associated colitis, pregnancy/nursing status and for possible drug interactions.

Monitoring: Monitor for signs/symptoms of diarrhea, bloody diarrhea and colitis (pseudomembranous colitis), overgrowth of nonsusceptible organisms (eg, fungi), local adverse reactions, and allergic reactions. Perform endoscopic exam to diagnose pseudomembranous colitis. Perform stool culture for *Clostridium difficile* and stool assay for *Clostridium difficile* toxin if diarrhea occurs. Perform large bowel endoscopy if severe diarrhea occurs.

Patient Counseling: Counsel to notify physician if diarrhea develops during therapy and up to several weeks after. Advise to use as directed, for external use only, to avoid contact with eyes, inside the nose, mouth, and mucous membranes. Advise not to use any other topical acne preparation unless otherwise directed by physician. Inform that drug may bleach hair or colored fabric. Advise to limit exposure to sunlight and to wear protective clothing. Instruct to contact physician if develop any signs of adverse reactions. Counsel to d/c use if severe allergic symptoms (eg, severe swelling, shortness of breath) develop. Instruct to wash gently, then rinse with warm water and pat dry prior to use. Keep out of reach of children.

Administration: Topical route. **Storage:** 25°C (77°F). Do not freeze. Keep tightly closed. Keep out of reach of children. Discard unused product after 3 months.

BENZTROPINE RX
benztropine mesylate (Various)

OTHER BRAND NAMES: Cogentin (Lundbeck)

THERAPEUTIC CLASS: Anticholinergic

INDICATIONS: Adjunct in all forms of parkinsonism. Control of drug-induced extrapyramidal disorders.

DOSAGE: *Adults:* Individualize dose. Titrate: May increase by 0.5mg/day q5-6d. Idiopathic Parkinsonism: Initial: 0.5-1mg qhs. Postencephalitic Parkinsonism: 2mg/day given in 1 or more doses. Extrapyramidal Disorders: 1-4mg/day given qd-bid. D/C and re-evaluate necessity after 1-2 weeks; may reinstitute if disorders recur. (Inj) Acute Dystonic Reactions: 1-2mg IM/IV. *Pediatrics:* >3 yrs: Individualize dose. Titrate: May increase by 0.5mg/day q5-6d. Idiopathic Parkinsonism: Initial: 0.5-1mg qhs. Postencephalitic Parkinsonism: 2mg/day given in 1 or more doses. Extrapyramidal Disorders: 1-4mg/day given qd-bid. D/C and re-evaluate necessity after 1-2 weeks; may reinstitute if disorders recur. (Inj) Acute Dystonic Reactions: 1-2mg IM/IV.

HOW SUPPLIED: Inj: 1mg/mL; Tab: 0.5mg*, 1mg*, 2mg* *scored

CONTRAINDICATIONS: Patients <3 yrs.

WARNINGS/PRECAUTIONS: May produce anhidrosis, caution in hot weather. Muscle weakness and dysuria may occur. Caution in pediatrics >3 years of age. Not recommended for tardive dyskinesia (TD). Avoid with angle-closure glaucoma. Caution with CNS disease, mental disorders, tachycardia, prostatic hypertrophy, alcoholics, chronically ill, those exposed to hot environments. May impair mental/physical abilities.

ADVERSE REACTIONS: Tachycardia, paralytic ileus, constipation, N/V, dry mouth, confusion, blurred vision, urinary retention, heat stroke, hyperthermia, fever.

INTERACTIONS: Paralytic ileus, hyperthermia and heat stroke reported with phenothiazines and TCAs. Caution with other atropine-like agents.

PREGNANCY: Safety in pregnancy and nursing not known.

MECHANISM OF ACTION: Anticholinergic agent; controls extrapyramidal symptoms in parkinsonism.

NURSING CONSIDERATIONS

Assessment: Assess for tachycardia, prostatic hypertrophy, anhidrosis, TD. Note other diseases/conditions and drug therapy.

Monitoring: Monitor for tachycardia, prostatic hypertrophy, anhidrosis, hyperthermia, constipation, urinary retention, paralytic ileus, toxic psychosis.

Patient Counseling: Caution during hot weather, especially when given concomitantly with other atropine-like drugs to the chronically ill, alcoholics, those who have CNS disease, and those who do manual labor in a hot environment. Caution while operating machinery/driving.

Administration: IV/IM, Oral route. **Storage:** 15-30°C. Dispense in tightly closed container.

BEPREVE   RX
bepotastine besilate (Ista)

THERAPEUTIC CLASS: H_1-antagonist

INDICATIONS: Treatment of itching associated with signs and symptoms of allergic conjunctivitis.

DOSAGE: *Adults:* 1 drop into the affected eye(s) bid.
Pediatrics: >2 yrs: 1 drop into the affected eye(s) bid.

HOW SUPPLIED: Sol: 1.5% [2.5mL, 5mL, 10mL]

WARNINGS/PRECAUTIONS: For topical ophthalmic use only. Not for treatment of contact lens-related irritation. Remove contact lenses prior to instillation and reinsert after 10 min. This product contains benzalkonium chloride.

ADVERSE REACTIONS: Mild taste, eye irritation, headache, and nasopharyngitis.

INTERACTIONS: Low potential for drug interaction via inhibition of CYP3A4, CYP2C9, and CYP2C19. May be absorbed by soft contact lenses because of benzalkonium chloride.

PREGNANCY: Category C, caution in nursing.

MECHANISM OF ACTION: H_1 antagonist; antagonizes H_1 receptor and inhibits release of histamine from mast cells.

PHARMACOKINETICS: Absorption: T_{max}=1-2 hrs. C_{max}=7.3 ng/mL. **Distribution:** Plasma protein binding (55%). **Metabolism:** Liver via CYP450 (minimal). **Excretion:** Urine (75-90%, unchanged).

NURSING CONSIDERATIONS

Assessment: Assess for contact lens usage, pregnancy/nursing status.

Monitoring: Monitor for relief of itching associated with signs and symptoms of allergic conjunctivitis.

Patient Counseling: Counsel the patient that therapy is not for the treatment of lens-related irritation and not to wear contact lenses if their eyes are red. Remove lens first prior to instillation and reinsert after 10 min. Advise that solution contains benzalkonium chloride, which may be absorbed by soft lenses. Advise not to touch the dropper's tip to any surface to maintain sterility. Inform that solution is for topical ophthalmic use only.

Administration: Ocular route. **Storage:** 15-25°C (59-77°F).

BERINERT   RX
cl inhibitor (human) (CSL Behring)

THERAPEUTIC CLASS: C1 inhibitor

INDICATIONS: Treatment of acute abdominal or facial attacks of hereditary angioedema (HAE) in adults and adolescents.

DOSAGE: *Adults:* 20 U/kg IV. Administer at a rate of 4mL/min.
Pediatrics: Adolescents: 20 U/kg IV. Administer at a rate of 4mL/min.

HOW SUPPLIED: Inj: 500 U

WARNINGS/PRECAUTIONS: Severe hypersensitivity reactions (eg, hives, generalized urticaria, chest tightness, wheezing, hypotension, and/or anaphylaxis) may occur; d/c therapy immediately and institute appropriate treatment; have epinephrine available. Thrombotic events at reported when used off-label and at higher than labeled doses. May contain infectious agents (eg, viruses, Creutzfeldt-Jakob [CJD] agent, acute hepatitis C) that can cause disease. Report all infections thought to be transmitted by the product to the manufacturer.

ADVERSE REACTIONS: Hereditary Angioedema (HAE) exacerbation, headache, N/V, abdominal pain, muscle spasms, dysgeusia, diarrhea, nasopharyngitis, pain.

PREGNANCY: Category C, caution in nursing.

MECHANISM OF ACTION: C1 esterase inhibitor; has inhibiting potential on several of the major cascade systems of the human body. Regulation is performed through formation of complexes between the proteinase and the inhibitor, resulting in inactivation of both and consumption of C1 esterase inhibitor.

PHARMACOKINETICS: Absorption: Adults: AUC =27.5hr•IU/mL (unadjusted for baseline), 12.8hr•IU/mL (adjusted for baseline); **Pediatrics:** 25.45hr•IU/mL (unadjusted for baseline), 9.78hr•IU/mL (adjusted for baseline). **Distribution: Adults:** V_{ss}=18.6mL/kg (unadjusted for baseline), 35.4mL/kg (adjusted for baseline); Pediatric: V_{ss}=19.8mL/kg (unadjusted for baseline), 38.8mL/kg (adjusted for baseline). **Elimination: Adults:** $T_{1/2}$=21.9hrs (unadjusted for baseline), 18.4hrs (adjusted for baseline); **Pediatrics:** 22.4hrs (unadjusted for baseline), 16.7hrs (adjusted for baseline).

NURSING CONSIDERATIONS

Assessment: Assess for signs and symptoms of hypersensitivity reactions, known risk factors for thrombotic events or a history of blood clotting problems, pregnancy/nursing status.

Monitoring: Monitor for hypersensitivity reactions (eg, hives, generalized urticaria, chest tightness, wheezing, hypotension, anaphylaxis during or after injection). Reactions may have symptoms similar to HAE attacks; treatment methods should be carefully considered. Monitor for thrombotic events.

Patient Counseling: Counsel about the risks and benefits of C1 inhibitor prior to treatment. Inform that medication is made from human plasma and may contain infectious agents that can cause disease (eg, viruses, CJD agent). Inform patients to immediately report signs and symptoms of allergic hypersensitivity reactions (eg, hives, urticaria, chest tightness, wheezing, hypotension, anaphylaxis), and thrombosis (eg, new onset swelling and pain in the limbs or abdomen, new onset of chest pain, shortness of breath, loss of sensation or motor power, altered consciousness, vision or speech). Advise female patients to inform their physician if pregnant or plan to become pregnant. Notify physician if breastfeeding or plan to breastfeed. Advise patients to consult with their healthcare provider prior to travel.

Administration: IV route. Refer to PI for preparation and handling/detailed reconstitution and administration information. **Storage:** 2°-25°C (36°-77°F); up to 30 months. Do not freeze. Protect from light.

BESIVANCE

RX

besifloxacin (Bausch & Lomb)

THERAPEUTIC CLASS: Fluoroquinolone

INDICATIONS: Treatment of bacterial conjunctivitis caused by susceptible microorganisms.

DOSAGE: *Adults:* Instill 1 drop in affected eye(s) tid, 4-12 hrs apart for 7 days. *Pediatrics:* >1 yr : Instill 1 drop in affected eye(s) tid, 4-12 hrs apart for 7 days.

HOW SUPPLIED: Sus (Ophthalmic): 0.6% [7.5mL]

WARNINGS/PRECAUTIONS: For topical ophthalmic use only; should not be injected subconjuctivally, nor should be introduced directly into the anterior chamber of the eye. May result in overgrowth of non-susceptible organisms (eg, fungi). D/C if superinfection occurs; institute alternative therapy. Avoid contact lenses if signs or symptoms of bacterial conjunctivitis occur, or during the course of therapy.

ADVERSE REACTIONS: Conjunctival redness, blurred vision, eye pain, eye irritation, eye pruritus and headache.

PREGNANCY: Category C, caution in nursing.

MECHANISM OF ACTION: Fluoroquinolone antibacterial; inhibits bacterial DNA gyrase and topoisomerase. May be active against pathogens that are resistant to aminoglycoside, macrolide, and β-lactam antibiotics.

PHARMACOKINETICS: Absorption: C_{max}=0.37ng/mL (Day 1), 0.43ng/mL (Day 6). **Elimination:** $T_{1/2}$=7 hrs.

NURSING CONSIDERATIONS

Assessment: Assess for bacterial conjunctivitis, pregnancy/nursing status.

Monitoring: Monitor for overgrowth of non-susceptible organisms (eg, fungi), superinfection, conjunctival redness, blurring of vision, eye pain, eye irritation, eye pruritus, headache, and hypersensitivity reactions.

Patient Counseling: Advise to avoid contaminating applicator tip with material from the eye, fingers, or other source. D/C if rash or allergic reaction occurs; notify physician immediately. Instruct to take medication exactly as directed. Advise to avoid wearing contact lenses if signs or symptoms of bacterial conjunctivitis occur during the course of therapy. Advise to wash hands thoroughly before use. Instruct to invert closed bottle and shake once before each use. Inform that skipping doses or not completing the therapy may decrease effectiveness and increase likelihood that bacteria may develop resistance.

Administration: Ocular route. Invert closed bottle and shake once before each use. tilt head back, and gently squeeze bottle to instill one drop into the affected eye. **Storage:** Store at 15-25°C (59-77°F). Protect from light.

BETAGAN   RX
levobunolol HCl (Allergan)

THERAPEUTIC CLASS: Nonselective beta-blocker

INDICATIONS: Treatment of elevated intraocular pressure (IOP) in chronic open-angle glaucoma and ocular hypertension.

DOSAGE: *Adults:* (0.5%) 1-2 drops qd; bid for more severe or uncontrolled glaucoma. (0.25%): 1-2 drops bid.

HOW SUPPLIED: Sol: 0.25% [5mL, 10mL], 0.5% [2mL, 5mL, 10mL, 15mL]

CONTRAINDICATIONS: Bronchial asthma, chronic obstructive pulmonary disease (COPD), overt cardiac failure, sinus bradycardia, 2nd- and 3rd-degree AV block, cardiogenic shock.

WARNINGS/PRECAUTIONS: Caution with cardiac failure, diabetes mellitus (DM), COPD, cerebral insufficiency, pulmonary disease, bronchospastic disease, surgery and hepatic impairment. May mask symptoms of hypoglycemia and thyrotoxicosis. Contains sodium metabisulfite. Follow with a miotic in angle-closure glaucoma. Potentiates muscle weakness (eg, diplopia, ptosis).

ADVERSE REACTIONS: Ocular burning, ocular stinging, decreased heart rate, decreased blood pressure.

INTERACTIONS: Mydriasis with epinephrine. Additive effects with catecholamine-depleting drugs (eg, reserpine) and systemic β-blockers. AV conduction disturbance with calcium antagonists and digitalis. Left ventricular failure and hypotension with calcium antagonists. Additive hypotensive effects with phenothiazine-related drugs. Risk of hypoglycemia with insulin and oral hypoglycemic agents.

PREGNANCY: Category C, caution in nursing.

MECHANISM OF ACTION: Noncardioselective β-adrenoceptor blocking agent; equipotent at both β_1 and β_2 receptors. Responsible for reducing cardiac output, increasing airway resistance, and lowering elevated as well as normal IOP. Presumed to lower IOP through decreasing production of aqueous humor.

PHARMACOKINETICS: Absorption: T_{max}=2 and 6 hrs.

B

NURSING CONSIDERATIONS

Assessment: Assess for conditions where treatment may be contraindicated or cautioned. Assess for possible sulfite allergy prior to therapy. Assess use in patients who have DM, hyperthyroidism, diminished pulmonary function, cerebrovascular insufficiencies, patients undergoing major elective surgery, and in pregnant/nursing females. Assess that patients with angle-closure glaucoma are not using this drug as monotherapy. Assess for possible drug interactions.

Monitoring: Monitor for signs/symptoms of muscle weakness (eg, diplopia, ptosis), severe respiratory and cardiac reactions, and anaphylactic reactions. Monitor for occurrence of a thyroid storm in patients who have thyrotoxicosis and withdraw abruptly from medication. Monitor for signs/symptoms of acute hypoglycemia with DM.

Patient Counseling: Counsel to notify physician immediately if any signs of anaphylactic reaction, cardiac or respiratory symptoms develop while on medication. Counsel patients with DM medication may mask symptoms of hypoglycemia.

Administration: Ocular route. **Storage:** 15-25°C (59-77°F), protect from light.

BETAPACE
sotalol HCl (Bayer Healthcare)

RX

> To minimize risk of arrhythmia, for a minimum of 3 days, place patients initiated or reinitiated on therapy in a facility that can provide cardiac resuscitation and continuous ECG monitoring. Obtain CrCl before therapy. Not approved for atrial fibrillation or atrial flutter; do not substitute for Betapace AF.

THERAPEUTIC CLASS: Beta-blocker (group II/III antiarrhythmic)

INDICATIONS: Treatment of documented life-threatening ventricular arrhythmias such as sustained ventricular tachycardia.

DOSAGE: *Adults:* Individualize dose. Initial: 80mg bid. Titrate: May increase to 120-160mg bid PRN. Adjust dose gradually, allowing 3 days between dosing increments. Usual: 160-320mg/day given bid-tid. Refractory Ventricular Arrhythmia Patients: 480-640mg/day; use this dose when benefit outweighs risk. Renal Impairment: CrCl 30-59mL/min: Dose q24h. CrCl 10-29mL/min: Dose q36-48h. CrCl <10mL/min: Individualize dose. May increase dose with renal impairment after ≥5-6 doses. Transfer to Betapace: Withdraw previous antiarrhythmic for a minimum of 2-3 plasma half-lives before start of Betapace. After d/c of amiodarone, do not initiate Betapace until QT interval is normalized.

Pediatrics: Individualize dose. ≥2 yrs: Initial: 30mg/m² tid. Titrate: Wait ≥36 hrs between dose increases. Guide dose by response, HR, and QTc. Max: 60mg/m². <2 yrs: See dosing chart in PI. Reduce dose or d/c if QTc >550msec. Renal Impairment: Reduce dose or increase interval. Transfer to Betapace: Withdraw previous antiarrhythmic for a minimum of 2-3 plasma half-lives before start of Betapace. After d/c of amiodarone, do not initiate Betapace until QT interval is normalized.

HOW SUPPLIED: Tab: 80mg*, 120mg*, 160mg* *scored

CONTRAINDICATIONS: Bronchial asthma, sinus bradycardia, 2nd- and 3rd-degree AV block (unless a functioning pacemaker is present), congenital or acquired long QT syndromes, cardiogenic shock, uncontrolled congestive heart failure (CHF).

WARNINGS/PRECAUTIONS: May provoke new or worsen existing ventricular arrhythmias. Torsades de pointes reported; incidence is dose-related and risk increases with prolongation of QT interval, HR reduction, serum K⁺ reduction, female gender, and history of cardiomegaly or CHF. Avoid with hypokalemia, hypomagnesemia, excessive QT interval prolongation (>550msec). Anticipate proarrhythmic events upon initiation and every upward dose adjustment. Correct electrolyte imbalances before therapy. Caution with heart failure controlled by digitalis and/or diuretics, left ventricular dysfunction, sick sinus syndrome, renal impairment, renal failure undergoing hemodialysis, and 2 weeks post-myocardial infarction (MI). Avoid abrupt withdrawal. Avoid in patients with bronchospastic diseases. May mask hypoglycemia, hyperthyroidism symptoms. Use in surgery is controversial.

ADVERSE REACTIONS: Torsades de pointes, dyspnea, fatigue, dizziness, bradycardia, chest pain, palpitation, asthenia, abnormal ECG, hypotension, headache, light-headedness, edema, N/V.

INTERACTIONS: Avoid with Class Ia (eg, disopyramide, quinidine and procainamide) and Class III (eg, amiodarone) antiarrhythmics; potential to prolong refractoriness. Additive Class II effects with β-blockers. Caution with drugs that prolong the QT interval (eg, Class I and III antiarrhythmics, phenothiazines, TCAs, astemizole, bepridil, certain quinolones and oral macrolides). Reduced levels with antacids containing aluminum oxide and magnesium hydroxide. Potentiates rebound HTN with clonidine withdrawal. May produce excessive reduction of resting sympathetic nervous tone with catecholamine-depleting drugs (eg, reserpine and guanethidine). Additive effects on AV conduction or ventricular function and BP with calcium-blocking agents. Insulin and antidiabetic agents may need dose adjustment. $β_2$-agonists (eg, salbutamol, terbutaline and isoprenaline) may need dose increase. Proarrhythmic events were more common with digoxin. Caution with diuretics/digitalis. Increase risk of bradycardia with digitalis glycosides. Severe hypotension and difficulty in restoring and maintaining normal cardiac rhythm after anesthesia reported in patients receiving β-blockers. May block epinephrine effects.

PREGNANCY: Category B, not for use in nursing.

MECHANISM OF ACTION: Antiarrhythmic drug (Class II and III properties); has both β-adrenoreceptor-blocking and cardiac action potential duration prolongation antiarrhythmic properties.

PHARMACOKINETICS: Absorption: Bioavailability (90-100%); T_{max}=2.5-4 hrs. **Distribution:** Crosses placenta; found in breast milk. **Elimination:** Urine (unchanged); $T_{1/2}$=12 hrs.

NURSING CONSIDERATIONS

Assessment: Establish CrCl prior to dosing. Assess for previous evidence of hypersensitivity to drug, bronchial asthma, sinus bradycardia, sick sinus syndrome, 2nd- and 3rd-degree AV block, pacemaker, long QT syndromes, cardiogenic shock, left ventricular dysfunction or uncontrolled CHF, recent MI, ischemic heart disease, hypokalemia or hypomagnesemia, bronchospastic disease, diabetes mellitus (DM), episodes of hypoglycemia, upcoming major surgery, hyperthyroidism, renal impairment, nursing status, and for possible drug interactions.

Monitoring: After initiation, ensure ≥3 days at facility for continuous ECG monitoring and resuscitation. Monitor ECG changes, proarrhythmia, HR, CrCl, asystole, new arrhythmias, signs/symptoms of depressed myocardial contractility and more severe HF, anaphylaxis, bronchospasm, MI, hypotension, masking of hypoglycemia, signs of electrolyte imbalance, and thyrotoxicosis.

Patient Counseling: Advise not to d/c without consulting physician. Inform of benefits/risks of drug. Report any adverse reactions to physician. Inform that drug is not for use by nursing women.

Administration: Oral route. Preparation of 5mg/mL Oral Sol: Refer to PI for preparation. **Storage:** 25°C (77°F); excursions permitted to 15-30°C (59-86°F). Sus: Stable for 3 months at controlled room temperature and ambient humidity.

BETAPACE AF   RX
sotalol HCl (Bayer Healthcare)

> To minimize risk of arrhythmia, for a minimum of 3 days, place patients initiated or reinitiated on therapy in a facility that can provide cardiac resuscitation, continuous ECG monitoring and calculations of CrCl. Do not substitute Betapace for Betapace AF.

THERAPEUTIC CLASS: Beta-blocker (group II/III antiarrhythmic)

INDICATIONS: Maintenance of normal sinus rhythm in patients with symptomatic atrial fibrillation/atrial flutter (AFIB/AFL) who are currently in sinus rhythm.

DOSAGE: *Adults:* Individualize dose. Start only if baseline QT interval is ≤450 msec (average of 5 beats). Initial: 80mg qd (CrCl 40-60mL/min) or bid (CrCl >60mL/min). Monitor QT 2-4 hrs after each dose. Reduce or d/c if QT ≥500msec. May discharge patient if QT <500msec after at least 3 days (after 5th or 6th dose if receiving qd dosing). Alternatively, may increase dose to 120mg bid during hospitalization, and follow for 3 days (follow for 5 or 6 doses if receiving qd doses). If 120mg is inadequate, may increase to 160mg qd or bid depending on CrCl. Maint: Reduce dose if QT interval is ≥520msec and d/c if maintained on 80mg. Max: 160mg bid (CrCl >60mL/min). Transfer to Betapace AF: Withdraw previous antiarrhythmic for a minimum of 2-3 plasma half-lives before start of Betapace AF. After d/c of amiodarone, do not initiate Betapace AF until QT interval is normalized.
Pediatrics: Individualize dose. ≥2 yrs: Initial: 30mg/m² tid. Titrate: Wait ≥36 hrs between dose increases. Guide dose by response, HR and QTc. Max: 60mg/m². <2 yrs: See dosing chart in PI. Reduce dose or d/c if QTc >550msec. Renal Impairment: Reduce dose or increase interval. Transfer to Betapace AF: Withdraw previous antiarrhythmic for a minimum of 2-3 plasma half-lives before start of Betapace AF. After d/c of amiodarone, do not initiate Betapace AF until QT interval is normalized.

HOW SUPPLIED: Tab: 80mg*, 120mg*, 160mg* *scored

CONTRAINDICATIONS: Sinus bradycardia (<50bpm during waking hrs), sick sinus syndrome or 2nd- or 3rd-degree AV block (unless a functioning pacemaker is present), congenital or acquired long QT syndromes, baseline QT interval >450msec, cardiogenic shock, uncontrolled heart failure (HF), hypokalemia (<4meq/L), CrCl <40mL/min, bronchial asthma.

WARNINGS/PRECAUTIONS: Can cause serious ventricular arrhythmias, primarily torsades de pointes; incidence is dose-related and risk increases with sustained ventricular tachycardia, prolongation of QT interval, history of cardiomegaly or congestive heart failure (CHF), reduced renal clearance and female gender. Avoid with hypokalemia, hypomagnesemia; correct electrolyte imbalances before therapy. Bradycardia reported. Caution with heart failure controlled by digitalis and/or diuretics, sick sinus syndrome, left ventricular dysfunction, renal dysfunction, post-myocardial infarction (MI). Avoid abrupt withdrawal. Avoid in patients with bronchospastic disease. May mask hypoglycemia, hyperthyroidism symptoms. Use in surgery is controversial.

ADVERSE REACTIONS: Bradycardia, dyspnea, fatigue, QT interval prolongation, abnormal ECG, chest pain, abdominal pain, disturbance rhythm subjective, diarrhea, N/V, hyperhidrosis, dizziness, headache.

INTERACTIONS: Avoid with Class 1a (eg, disopyramide, quinidine and procainamide) and Class III (eg, amiodarone) antiarrhythmics; potential to prolong refractoriness. Not recommended with drugs that prolong the QT interval (eg, many antiarrhythmics, phenothiazines, TCAs, bepridil, and oral macrolides). Reduced levels with antacids containing aluminum oxide and magnesium hydroxide. Potentiates rebound HTN with clonidine withdrawal. May produce excessive reduction of resting sympathetic nervous tone with catecholamine-depleting drugs (eg, reserpine and guanethidine). Additive effects on AV conduction or ventricular function or BP with calcium-blocking agents. Insulin and antidiabetic agents may need adjustment. β₂-agonists (eg, salbutamol, terbutaline and isoprenaline) may need dose increase. Proarrhythmic events more common with digoxin. Caution with diuretics and digitalis. Increased risk of bradycardia with digitalis glycosides. Severe hypotension and difficulty in restoring and maintaining normal cardiac rhythm after anesthesia have been reported in patients receiving β-blockers. May block epinephrine effects.

PREGNANCY: Category B, not for use in nursing.

MECHANISM OF ACTION: Antiarrhythmic drug (Class II and III properties); has both β-adrenoreceptor blocking and cardiac action potential duration prolongation antiarrhythmic properties.

PHARMACOKINETICS: Absorption: Bioavailability (90-100%); T_{max}=2.5-4 hrs. **Distribution:** Crosses placenta; found in breast milk. **Elimination:** Urine (unchanged); $T_{1/2}$=12 hrs.

NURSING CONSIDERATIONS

Assessment: Establish CrCl prior to dosing. Assess for sinus bradycardia, sick sinus syndrome, 2nd- and 3rd-degree AV block, pacemaker, long QT syndromes, cardiogenic shock, uncontrolled HF, bronchial asthma, previous evidence of hypersensitivity to drug, recent MI, ischemic heart disease, hypokalemia or hypomagnesemia, bronchospastic disease, diabetes mellitus, episodes of hypoglycemia, upcoming major surgery, hyperthyroidism, renal impairment, nursing status, and for possible drug interactions.

Monitoring: After initiation, ensure ≥3 days at facility for continuous ECG monitoring and resuscitation. Monitor ECG changes, proarrhythmia, HR, CrCl, asystole, new arrhythmias, signs/symptoms of depressed myocardial contractility and more severe HF, anaphylaxis, bronchospasm, MI, hypotension, masking of hypoglycemia, signs of electrolyte imbalance, and thyrotoxicosis.

Patient Counseling: Advise not to abruptly d/c therapy without consulting physician. Inform of benefits/risks of drug, to report signs of electrolyte balance (eg, diarrhea, vomiting), and if taking any other medications or over-the-counter drugs. Instruct the need for compliance with recommended dosing. Instruct if a dose is missed, do not double next dose; take next dose at the usual time.

Administration: Oral route. Preparation of 5mg/mL Oral Sol: Refer to PI. **Storage:** 25°C (77°F); excursions permitted to 15-30°C (59-86°F). Susp: Stable for 3 months at controlled room temperature and ambient humidity.

BETIMOL   RX
timolol (Vistakon)

THERAPEUTIC CLASS: Nonselective beta-blocker

INDICATIONS: Treatment of elevated intraocular pressure (IOP) in patients with open-angle glaucoma or ocular hypertension.

DOSAGE: *Adults:* Initial: 1 drop 0.25% bid. May increase to max of 1 drop 0.5% bid. Maint: If adequate control, may try 1 drop 0.25-0.5% qd.

HOW SUPPLIED: Sol: 0.25%, 0.5% [2.5mL, 5mL, 10mL, 15mL]

CONTRAINDICATIONS: Bronchial asthma, history of bronchial asthma, severe chronic obstructive pulmonary disease (COPD), sinus bradycardia, 2nd- or 3rd-degree AV block, overt cardiac failure, cardiogenic shock.

WARNINGS/PRECAUTIONS: Caution with cardiac failure, diabetes mellitus (DM), cerebrovascular insufficiency. Severe cardiac and respiratory reactions reported. May mask symptoms of hypoglycemia and hyperthyroidism. Bacterial keratitis reported with contaminated containers. May reinsert contacts 5 min after applying drops. Avoid with COPD, bronchospastic disease. Not for use alone in angle-closure glaucoma. May potentiate muscle weakness. D/C if cardiac failure develops. Withdrawal before surgery is controversial.

ADVERSE REACTIONS: Burning/stinging on instillation, dry eyes, itching, foreign body sensation, eye discomfort, eyelid erythema, conjunctival injection, headache.

INTERACTIONS: May potentiate systemic β-blockers and catecholamine-depleting drugs (eg, reserpine). Oral/IV calcium antagonists can cause AV conduction disturbances, left ventricular failure, or hypotension. Digitalis can cause additive effects in prolonging AV conduction time. May antagonize epinephrine.

PREGNANCY: Category C, not for use in nursing.

MECHANISM OF ACTION: Nonselective β-adrenergic antagonist; blocks both $β_1$- and $β_2$-adrenergic receptors. Thought to reduce IOP through reducing production of aqueous humor.

PHARMACOKINETICS: Elimination: Urine (metabolites); $T_{1/2}$=4 hrs

NURSING CONSIDERATIONS

Assessment: Assess for overt heart failure, cardiogenic shock, sinus brady-cardia, 2nd-or 3rd-degree AV block, active or history of bronchial asthma, and severe COPD. Assess use in patients with cerebrovascular insufficiencies, undergoing elective surgery, with diabetes mellitus (DM), with hyperthyroid-ism, and in pregnant/nursing females. Assess patients with angle-closure glaucoma are not on monotherapy with this drug. Assess for possible drug interactions.

Monitoring: Monitor for signs/symptoms of reduced cerebral blood flow, cardiac failure, muscle weakness, bacterial keratitis when using multi-dose container, severe anaphylactic reactions, and hypoglycemia in patients with DM. Monitor for occurrence of thyroid storm in patients who abruptly with-draw from medication and have thyrotoxicosis.

Patient Counseling: Counsel to immediately notify physician if signs of cardiac, respiratory, or anaphylactic symptoms develop while on medication. Instruct patients with DM that this medication may mask signs of hypogly-cemia. To avoid contaminating solution, avoid touching container tip to the eye or surrounding structures. Counsel that if taking concomitant topical ophthalmic medications, to separate dosing by at least 5 min. Instruct patients who wear soft contact lenses to wait at least 5 min after administration before reinserting.

Administration: Ocular route. **Storage:** 15-25°C (59-77°F). Do not freeze. Protect from light.

BETOPTIC S   RX
betaxolol HCl (Alcon)

THERAPEUTIC CLASS: Selective beta₁-blocker

INDICATIONS: Treatment of elevated intraocular pressure (IOP) in patients with chronic open-angle glaucoma or ocular HTN.

DOSAGE: *Adults:* Instill 1 drop in affected eyes bid.
Pediatrics: Instill 1 drop in affected eyes bid.

HOW SUPPLIED: Sus: 0.25% [2.5mL, 5mL, 10mL, 15mL]

CONTRAINDICATIONS: Sinus bradycardia, >1st-degree atrioventricular (AV) block, cardiogenic shock, overt cardiac failure.

WARNINGS/PRECAUTIONS: Do not use alone in treating angle-closure glau-coma. Absorbed systemically; severe respiratory/cardiac reactions reported. Caution with history of cardiac failure or heart block, diabetes mellitus (DM), and cerebrovascular insufficiency. D/C on 1st sign of cardiac failure. May mask signs/symptoms of acute hypoglycemia and hyperthyroidism. Avoid abrupt withdrawal; may precipitate thyroid storm. May potentiate muscle weakness consistent with certain myasthenic symptoms. Withdrawal prior to major sur-gery is controversial. Caution in glaucoma patients with excessive restriction of pulmonary function; asthmatic attacks and pulmonary distress reported. May be more reactive to repeated challenge with history of atopy or severe anaphylactic reaction to variety of allergens; may be unresponsive to usual doses of epinephrine. Bacterial keratitis and choroidal detachment may occur.

ADVERSE REACTIONS: Transient ocular discomfort, blurred vision, corneal punctuate keratitis, foreign body sensation, photophobia, tearing, itching, dryness of eye, erythema, inflammation, discharge, ocular pain, decreased visual acuity, crusty lashes.

INTERACTIONS: Potential additive effects with oral β-blockers and cate-cholamine-depleting drugs (eg, reserpine). May produce hypotension and/or bradycardia with catecholamine-depleting drugs. Caution with adrenergic psychotropics and in patients receiving insulin or oral hypoglycemic agents. May augment risk of general anesthesia.

PREGNANCY: Category C, caution with nursing.

MECHANISM OF ACTION: Cardioselective (β-1-adrenergic) receptor inhibitor; reduces IOP through a reduction of aqueous production.

NURSING CONSIDERATIONS

Assessment: Assess for conditions where treatment is contraindicated or cautioned, hypersensitivity to the drug, pregnancy/nursing status, and possible drug interactions.

Monitoring: Monitor for signs/symptoms of cardiac/respiratory reactions, cardiac failure, muscle weakness, reduced cerebral blood flow, choroidal detachment, and hypersensitivity reactions. Monitor for development of bacterial keratitis in patients who are using multidose containers.

Patient Counseling: Instruct to avoid allowing tip of dispensing container to contact eye(s) or surrounding structures. Ocular solutions may become contaminated by bacteria that may cause ocular infections. Seek physician's advice if having an ocular surgery or if ocular condition (eg, trauma or infection) develops. Administer ≥10 min apart when receiving concomitant ophthalmic medications.

Administration: Ocular route. May be used alone or in combination with other IOP lowering medications. Refer to PI for administration instructions. Shake well before use. **Storage:** 2-25°C (36-77°F). Store upright.

BEXXAR   RX
iodine I 131 tositumomab - tositumomab (GlaxoSmithKline)

> Hypersensitivity reactions, including anaphylaxis, and prolonged and severe cytopenias reported. Can cause fetal harm if given during pregnancy. Contains radioactive component.

THERAPEUTIC CLASS: Monoclonal antibody/CD20-blocker

INDICATIONS: Treatment of CD20-positive, follicular, non-Hodgkin's lymphoma (NHL), with and without transformation, in patients refractory to rituximab and who have relapsed following chemotherapy.

DOSAGE: *Adults:* Premedication: Day 1: Begin thyro-protective regimen of either SSKI (4 drops PO tid), Lugol's sol (20 drops PO tid), or potassium iodide (130mg PO qd). Continue until 14 days post-therapeutic dose. Day 0: APAP 650mg and diphenhydramine 50mg. Dosimetric Step: IV: 450mg tositumomab over 60 min followed by 5mCi Iodine I 131 tositumomab (35mg) over 20 min. Day 0 + Day 2, 3, or 4 + Day 6 or 7: Whole body dosimetry and biodistribution. Day 6 or 7: Calculation of patient-specific activity of iodine I 131 tositumomab to deliver 75cGy total body irradiation or 65cGy if platelets ≥100,000 but <150,000 platelets/mm³. Day 7 (up to Day 14): Premedicate with APAP and diphenhydramine. Therapeutic Step: IV: Do not administer if biodistribution is altered. 450mg tositumomab over 60 min followed by prescribed therapeutic dose of iodine I 131 tositumomab (35mg) over 20 min.

HOW SUPPLIED: Inj: For Dosimetric Dosing: Tositumomab: 225mg [2 single-use vials], 35mg [1 single-use vial]; Iodine I 131 Tositumomab: 1 single-use vial. For Therapeutic Dosing: Tositumomab: 225mg [2 single-use vials], 35mg [1 single-use vial]; Iodine I 131 Tositumomab: 1 or 2 single-use vials.

CONTRAINDICATIONS: Pregnant women.

WARNINGS/PRECAUTIONS: Obtain CBCs weekly for 10-12 weeks. Safety not established with >25% lymphoma marrow involvement, platelet <100,000 cells/mm³, or neutrophil count <1,500 cells/mm³. Secondary malignancies reported. May cause hypothyroidism; monitor TSH prior to initiation and then annually. Thyroid blocking agents must be used; initiate at least 24 hrs before dosimetric dose and continue until 14 days after therapeutic dose. Caution with impaired renal function. Effective contraceptive methods should be used during, and for 12 months following treatment. Increased risk of serious allergic reactions if positive for human anti-murine antibodies (HAMA).

ADVERSE REACTIONS: Neutropenia, thrombocytopenia, anemia, asthenia, fever, infection, cough, pain, chills, headache, GI effects, myalgia, arthralgia, pharyngitis, dyspnea.

INTERACTIONS: Weigh risks vs benefits of concomitant agents that interfere with platelet function and/or anticoagulation.

PREGNANCY: Category X, not for use in nursing.

MECHANISM OF ACTION: Monoclonal antibody; possibly induces apoptosis, complement-dependent cytotoxicity, antibody-dependent cellular cytotoxicity mediated by the antibody; cell death associated with ionizing radiation from radioisotope. Tositumomab; murine IgG2a lambda monoclonal antibody directed against CD20 antigen found on surface of B lymphocytes. Iodine I 131 tositumomab; radio-iodinated derivative of Tositumomab, covalently linked to Iodine-131.

PHARMACOKINETICS: Elimination: (Iodine-131): Decay (β and gamma emissions). Physical $T_{1/2}$=8.04 days. Excreted in urine; (Iodine I 131 Tositumomab): Urine; $T_{1/2}$=67 hrs.

NURSING CONSIDERATIONS

Assessment: Assess for known hypersensitivity to murine proteins, lymphoma marrow involvement, impaired bone marrow reserve, renal function, pregnancy/nursing status, use of thyroid-blocking agent. Screen for human anti-mouse antibody (prior murine protein use) and possible drug interactions. Obtain baseline CBC, SrCr, TSH, and platelet count

Monitoring: Monitor CBC weekly for 10-12 weeks. Monitor renal function (periodically) and TSH (annually). Monitor for signs/symptoms of thrombocytopenia, neutropenia, anemia, secondary malignancies, hypersensitivity reaction (bronchospasm and angioedema), and hypothyroidism.

Patient Counseling: Inform of pregnancy risks and to d/c nursing. Instruct to use effective contraceptive methods during treatment and for 12 months after completion. Advise of importance of compliance with thyroid-blocking agents and need for lifelong monitoring. Seek medical attention if symptoms of thrombocytopenia, neutropenia, anemia, secondary malignancies, hypersensitivity reaction (bronchospasm and angioedema), and hypothyroidism occur.

Administration: IV infusion. Do not administer therapeutic dose if biodistribution is altered. Same IV tubing set and filter must be used throughout all steps. Changes in filter can result in loss of drug. Refer to full PI for detailed administration. **Storage:** Tositumomab: 2-8°C (36-46°). Do not freeze or shake. Protect from strong light. (Diluted): Stable for 24 hrs if refrigerated 2-8°C (36-46°F); stable for 8 hrs at room temperature. Do not freeze. Iodine I 131 Tositumomab: Frozen in original lead pots at -20°C or below. (Thawed): Stable for 8 hrs at 2-8°C (36-46°), or room temperature. (Diluted): Refrigerate 2-8°C (36-46°).

BEYAZ   RX
levomefolate calcium - drospirenone - ethinyl estradiol (Bayer Healthcare)

> Cigarette smoking increases the risk of serious cardiovascular (CV) side effects from combination oral contraceptives (COC) use. Risk increases with age (>35 yrs) and with the number of cigarettes smoked. Should not be used by women who are >35 yrs and smoke.

THERAPEUTIC CLASS: Estrogen/progestogen combination

INDICATIONS: Prevention of pregnancy. Treatment of symptoms of premenstrual dysphoric disorder (PMDD). Treatment of moderate acne vulgaris in women ≥14 yrs who have achieved menarche and desire an oral contraceptive for birth control. To raise folate levels for the purpose of reducing the risk of neural tube defect in a pregnancy conceived while taking the product or shortly after d/c.

DOSAGE: *Adults:* ≥18 yrs: Start 1st Sunday after menses begins or 1st day of menses. 1 pink tab (active) qd for 24 consecutive days, followed by 1 light orange tab (folate) on Days 25-28. Should be taken at the same time each day, preferably pm pc or qhs. Begin next and all subsequent regimens on the same day of the week on which first regimen began. Postpartum women who do not breastfeed or after a second trimester abortion should start no earlier than

4 weeks postpartum. If vomiting occurs within 3-4 hrs after taking tab, this can be regarded as a missed tab.

Pediatrics: Postpubertal: ≥14 yrs (acne): Start 1st Sunday after menses begins or 1st day of menses. 1 pink tab (active) qd for 24 consecutive days, followed by 1 light orange tab (folate) on Days 25-28. Should be taken at the same time each day, preferably pm pc or qhs. Begin next and all subsequent regimens on the same day of the week on which first regimen began. Postpartum women who do not breastfeed or after a second trimester abortion should start no earlier than 4 weeks postpartum. If vomiting occurs within 3-4 hrs after taking tab, this can be regarded as a missed tab.

HOW SUPPLIED: Tab: (Ethinyl Estradiol-Drospirenone-Levomefolate calcium) 0.02mg-3mg-0.451mg; Tab: (Levomefolate calcium) 0.451mg

CONTRAINDICATIONS: Renal impairment, adrenal insufficiency, high risk of arterial/venous thrombotic disease (eg, smoking at >35 yrs, history/present deep vein thrombosis [DVT]/pulmonary embolism [PE], cerebrovascular disease [CVD], coronary artery disease [CAD], thrombogenic valvular or thrombogenic rhythm diseases of the heart [eg, subacute bacterial endocarditis with valvular disease, atrial fibrillation], inherited/acquired hypercoagulopathies, uncontrolled HTN, diabetes mellitus [DM] with vascular disease, headache with focal neurological symptoms, migraine with/without aura if >35 yrs), undiagnosed abnormal uterine bleeding, history/present breast/other estrogen-/progestin-sensitive cancer, benign/malignant liver tumors, liver disease, pregnancy.

WARNINGS/PRECAUTIONS: Increased risk of venous thromboembolism and arterial thromboses (eg, strokes, myocardial infarction [MI]). D/C if arterial or deep venous thrombotic events, unexplained loss of vision, proptosis, diplopia, papilledema, or retinal vascular lesions occur. D/C at least 4 weeks before and through 2 weeks after major surgery or other surgeries with an elevated risk of thromboembolism. May cause hyperkalemia in high-risk patients; avoid use in patients predisposed to hyperkalemia (eg, renal insufficiency, hepatic dysfunction, adrenal insufficiency). Monitor K⁺ levels during 1st cycle with conditions predisposing to hyperkalemia. May increase risk of cervical cancer or intraepithelial neoplasia and gallbladder disease. Hepatic adenoma and increased risk of hepatocellular carcinoma reported. D/C if jaundice develops. Cholestasis may occur with history of pregnancy-related cholestasis. Increased BP reported; for well-controlled HTN, monitor BP and d/c if BP rises significantly. May decrease glucose tolerance (dose-related); monitor prediabetic and diabetic women. Consider alternative contraception with uncontrolled dyslipidemias. Increased risk of pancreatitis with hypertriglyceridemia or family history thereof. May increase frequency or severity of migraine; d/c if new headaches are recurrent, persistent or severe. Unscheduled (breakthrough) bleeding and spotting may occur; if bleeding persists, check for causes (eg, pregnancy or malignancy). Should not be used to test for pregnancy. Caution with history of depression; d/c if depression recurs to serious degree. May change results of laboratory tests (eg, coagulation factors, lipids, glucose tolerance, binding proteins). Folate may mask vitamin B12 deficiency. Caution with hereditary angioedema. Chloasma may occur especially with history of chloasma gravidarum; avoid sun exposure or ultraviolet radiation.

ADVERSE REACTIONS: Menstrual irregularities, N/V, headache/migraine, breast pain/tenderness, fatigue, irritability, decreased libido, increased weight, affect lability.

INTERACTIONS: Reduced effectiveness or increased incidence of breakthrough bleeding with drugs or herbal products that induce enzymes (eg, CYP3A4) that metabolize contraceptive hormones (eg, barbiturates, bosentan, carbamazepine, felbamate, griseofulvin, oxcarbazepine, phenytoin, rifampicin, St. John's wort, topiramate). Significant changes (increase or decrease) in plasma levels with protease inhibitors or non-nucleoside reverse transcriptase inhibitors. Pregnancy reported with use of hormonal contraceptives and antibiotics. Increased levels with atorvastatin, ascorbic acid, APAP, and CYP3A4 inhibitors (eg, itraconazole, ketoconazole). Decreases levels of lamotrigine and may reduce seizure control; may require dosage adjustment of lamotrigine. May need to increase dose of thyroid hormone in patients on thyroid hormone replacement therapy due to increased thyroid binding globulin. Risk of hyperkalemia with ACE inhibitors, angiotensin-II receptor antagonists, K⁺-sparing diuretics, K⁺ supplementation, heparin, aldosterone antagonists, and NSAIDs; monitor K⁺ levels during 1st treatment cycle. Decrease pharmacological effect of antifolate drugs (eg, antiepileptics, methotrexate or pyrimethamine). Reduced folate levels reported with dihydrofolate reductase enzyme inhibitors (eg, methotrexate, sulfasalazine), by reducing folate absorption (eg, cholestyramine), or via unknown mechanism (eg, antiepileptics [eg, carbamazepine, phenytoin, phenobarbital, primidone, valproic acid]).

PREGNANCY: Contraindicated in pregnancy; not for use in nursing.

MECHANISM OF ACTION: Estrogen/progestogen oral contraceptive; primarily acts by suppressing ovulation. Also causes cervical mucus changes that inhibit sperm penetration and endometrial changes that reduce the likelihood of implantation.

PHARMACOKINETICS: Absorption: Drospirenone (DRSP): Absolute bioavailability (76%); (Cycle 1/Day 21) C_{max}=70.3ng/mL; T_{max}=1.5 hrs; AUC=763ng•h/mL. Ethinyl estradiol (EE): Absolute bioavailability (40%); (Cycle 1/Day 21) C_{max}=45.1pg/mL; T_{max}=1.5 hrs; AUC=220pg•h/mL. Levomefolate T_{max}=0.5-1.5 hrs. **Distribution:** DRSP: V_d=4L/kg; serum protein binding (97%). EE: V_d=4-5L/kg; serum albumin binding (98.5%). **Metabolism:** DRSP: Liver, via CYP3A4 (minor). EE: Hydroxylation (via CYP3A4), conjugation with glucuronide and sulfate. **Elimination:** DRSP: Urine, feces; $T_{1/2}$=30 hrs. EE: Urine, feces; $T_{1/2}$=24 hrs. Levomefolate (L-5-methyl-THF): Urine, feces; $T_{1/2}$=4-5 hrs.

NURSING CONSIDERATIONS

Assessment: Assess for presence or history of breast cancer, estrogen dependent neoplasia, abnormal genital bleeding, active liver disease, and known/suspected pregnancy or any other conditions where treatment is cautioned or contraindicated. Assess use in patients who are >35 yrs and heavy smokers (≥15 cigarettes/day). Assess use with HTN, hyperlipidemias, obesity, diabetes mellitus (DM), or in patients at increased risk for thrombosis. Assess for possible drug interactions.

Monitoring: Monitor bleeding irregularities, thromboembolic events, onset or exacerbation of headaches or migraines, and ectopic pregnancy. Monitor fasting blood glucose levels in DM and prediabetic patients, BP with history of HTN, lipid levels with a history of hyperlipidemia. Monitor for signs of liver dysfunction (eg, jaundice) and signs of depression with previous history. Perform annual history and physical exam. All women taking combined oral contraceptive (COC) should have yearly visit for BP check and other healthcare. Monitor K⁺ levels during first treatment cycle in patients at risk for hyperkalemia.

Patient Counseling: Inform that drug does not protect against HIV infection and other sexually transmitted diseases. Advise that cigarette smoking increases the risk of serious CV events from COC use, and that women who are >35 yrs and smoke should not use COCs. Counsel on warnings and precautions associated with COCs. Instruct to take at the same time everyday, what to do in the event pills are missed, and to use a backup or alternative method of contraception when enzyme inducers are used with COCs. Inform that COCs may reduce breast milk production if breastfeeding. Counsel any patient who starts COCs postpartum, and who has not yet had a period, to use an additional method of contraception until she has taken a pink tablet for 7 consecutive days. Also, counsel patients that if started later than the first day of the menstrual cycle, an additional non-hormonal contraceptive should be used during the first 7 days. Inform that amenorrhea may occur and pregnancy should be ruled out if amenorrhea occurs in two or more consecutive cycles. Counsel patients to report if they are taking folate supplements and to maintain folate supplementation if d/c Beyaz due to pregnancy.

Administration: Oral route. **Storage:** 25°C (77°F); excursions permitted to 15-30°C (59-86°F).

BIAXIN

RX   B

clarithromycin (Abbott)

THERAPEUTIC CLASS: Macrolide

INDICATIONS: Treatment of the following infections caused by susceptible strains of microorganisms: (Adults) Pharyngitis/tonsillitis, acute maxillary sinusitis, acute bacterial exacerbation of chronic bronchitis (ABECB), community-acquired pneumonia (CAP), uncomplicated skin and skin structure infections (SSSI), and disseminated mycobacterial infections. Mycobacterium avium complex (MAC) prophylaxis in advanced HIV. (Tab) Combination therapy for *H.pylori* infection with duodenal ulcers. (Pediatrics) Pharyngitis/tonsillitis, CAP, acute maxillary sinusitis, acute otitis media, uncomplicated SSSI, disseminated mycobacterial infections. MAC prophylaxis in advanced HIV.

DOSAGE: *Adults:* Pharyngitis/Tonsillitis: 250mg q12h for 10 days. Sinusitis: 500mg q12h for 14 days. ABECB: 250-500mg q12h for 7-14 days. SSSI/CAP: 250mg q12h for 7-14 days. MAC Prophylaxis/Treatment: 500mg bid. CrCl <30mL/min: Give 50% dose or double the dosing interval. *H.pylori:* Triple Therapy: 500mg + amoxicillin 1g + omeprazole 20mg, all q12h for 10 days (give additional omeprazole 20mg qd for 18 days with active ulcer); or 500mg + amoxicillin 1g + lansoprazole 30mg, all q12h for 10-14 days. Dual Therapy: 500mg q8h + omeprazole 40mg qd (qAM) for 14 days (give additional omeprazole 20mg qd for 14 days with active ulcer); or 500mg q8h or q12h + ranitidine bismuth citrate 400mg q12h for 14 days (give additional ranitidine bismuth citrate 400mg bid for 14 days with active ulcer). May be taken with or without food.
Pediatrics: ≥6 months: Usual: 15mg/kg/day q12h for 10 days. MAC Prophylaxis/Treatment: ≥20 months: 7.5mg/kg bid, up to 500mg bid. CrCl <30mL/min: Give 50% dose or double the dosing interval. May be taken with or without food. Refer to PI for further pediatric dosage guidelines.

HOW SUPPLIED: Sus: 125mg/5mL, 250mg/5mL [50mL, 100mL]; Tab: 250mg, 500mg

CONTRAINDICATIONS: Concomitant use with cisapride, pimozide, astemizole, terfenadine, ergotamine or dihydroergotamine.

WARNINGS/PRECAUTIONS: Avoid in pregnancy. *Clostridium difficile*-associated diarrhea (CDAD) reported and may range in severity from mild diarrhea to fatal colitis. Adjust dose with severe renal impairment. Use in the absence of a proven or strongly suspected bacterial infection or a prophylactic indication is unlikely to provide benefit and increases the risk of development of drug resistant bacteria. May exacerbate symptoms of myasthenia gravis; new onset of symptoms of myasthenic syndrome reported.

ADVERSE REACTIONS: Diarrhea, N/V, abnormal taste, abdominal pain, rash.

INTERACTIONS: See Contraindications. Increases serum levels of theophylline, carbamazepine, omeprazole, ranitidine bismuth citrate, digoxin, drugs metabolized by CYP3A, HMG-CoA reductase inhibitors, and tolterodine. Hypotension, bradyarrhythmias, and lactic acidosis observed with CCBs (eg, verapamil). Decreases zidovudine plasma levels. Potentiates oral anticoagulant effects. Increases AUC of midazolam; avoid coadministration of oral midazolam and monitor IV closely to allow dose adjustment. Caution with benzodiazepines that are metabolized by CYP3A (eg, triazolam, alprazolam). Somnolence and confusion may occur with concomitant use of triazolam; monitor for additive CNS effects. Concomitant use with strong inducers of CYP450 (eg, efavirenz, nevirapine, rifampicin, rifabutin, rifapentine) may decrease plasma levels of clarithromycin. Occurrence of torsades de pointes with antiarrhythmics (eg, quinidine, disopyramide) reported. Increased phosphodiesterase inhibitor exposure with sildenafil, tadalafil, or vardenafil. Avoid ranitidine bismuth citrate if CrCl <25mL/min or history of porphyria. Reduce dose with ritonavir if CrCl ≤60mL/min. Increased levels with fluconazole. Reduce dose with atazanavir if CrCl ≤60mL/min; doses of clarithromycin >1,000mg/day should not be coadministered with protease inhibitors. Concomitant use with colchicine may increase colchicine exposure; colchicine toxicity reported especially in elderly. Concomitant use with itraconazole may increase levels of itraconazole and clarithromycin. Rare cases of rhabdomyolysis reported with HMG-CoA reductase inhibitors (eg, lovastatin, simvastatin). Interaction may occur when concomitantly used with cyclosporine, tacrolimus, alfentanil, methylprednisolone, cilostazol, bromocriptine, vinblastine, hexobarbital, phenytoin, or valproate. Rare reports of hypoglycemia with oral hypoglycemic agents or insulin.

PREGNANCY: Category C, caution in nursing.

MECHANISM OF ACTION: Semisynthetic macrolide antibiotic; exerts antibacterial action by binding to the 50S ribosomal subunit of susceptible microorganisms, resulting in inhibition of protein synthesis. Active against aerobic and anaerobic gram-positive and gram-negative microorganisms.

PHARMACOKINETICS: Absorption: Rapid; (250mg tab) Absolute bioavailability (50%); C_{max}=1-2µcg/mL (250mg tab), 3-4µcg/mL (500mg tab), 2µcg/mL (sus); T_{max}=2-3 hrs. **Distribution:** Body tissues, fluids. **Metabolism:** 14-OH clarithromycin (active metabolite). **Elimination:** Urine: 20% (250mg tab), 30% (500mg tab), 40% (250mg sus), 10-15% (14-OH). Parent drug; $T_{1/2}$=3-4 hrs (250mg tab, sus), 5-7 hrs (500mg tab). 14-OH: $T_{1/2}$=5-6 hrs (250mg tab, sus), 7-9 hrs (500mg tab).

NURSING CONSIDERATIONS

Assessment: Assess for renal impairment, myasthenia gravis, pregnancy/nursing status, a history of acute porphyria, and for possible drug interactions.

Monitoring: Monitor for anaphylactic reactions, development of drug-resistant bacteria, CDAD ranging from mild diarrhea to fatal colitis, overgrowth of nonsusceptible microorganisms. Monitor for exacerbation of myasthenia gravis. Monitor for colchicine toxicity if taken concurrently with colchicine, especially in elderly, and changes in LFTs, CBC, PT, and renal function.

Patient Counseling: Inform about potential benefits/risks of therapy. Counsel that drug only treats bacterial, not viral infections. Instruct to take exactly as directed; inform that skipping doses or not completing full course may decrease effectiveness and increase antibiotic resistance. Advise that may take with or without food. Notify physician if watery/bloody diarrhea (with/without stomach cramps) develop; inform that may occur up to 2 or more months after treatment. Notify physician if pregnant/nursing and all medications currently taking. Do not refrigerate suspension.

Administration: Oral route. **Storage:** (250 mg tab) 15-30°C (59-86°F). Protect from light. (500 mg tab) 20-25°C (68-77°F). (Sus) 15-30°C (59-86°F). Do not refrigerate.

BIAXIN XL

RX

clarithromycin (Abbott)

THERAPEUTIC CLASS: Macrolide

INDICATIONS: Treatment of acute maxillary sinusitis, community-acquired pneumonia (CAP), and acute bacterial exacerbation of chronic bronchitis (ABECB) in adults.

DOSAGE: *Adults:* Sinusitis: 1000mg qd for 14 days. ABECB/CAP: 1000mg qd for 7 days. CrCl <30mL/min: Give 50% dose or double the dosing interval. Swallow whole; do not chew, break, or crush. Take with food.

HOW SUPPLIED: Tab, Extended-Release: 500mg [PAC 14ˢ]

CONTRAINDICATIONS: Concomitant use with cisapride, pimozide, astemizole, terfenadine, ergotamine or dihydroergotamine.

WARNINGS/PRECAUTIONS: Avoid in pregnancy. *Clostridium difficile*-associated diarrhea (CDAD) reported and may range in severity from mild diarrhea to fatal colitis. Adjust dose with severe renal impairment. Use in the absence of a proven or strongly suspected bacterial infection or a prophylactic indication is unlikely to provide benefit and increases the risk of development of drug-resistant bacteria. May exacerbate symptoms of myasthenia gravis; new onset of symptoms of myasthenic syndrome reported.

ADVERSE REACTIONS: Diarrhea, abnormal taste, nausea.

INTERACTIONS: See Contraindications. Increases serum levels of theophylline, carbamazepine, omeprazole, ranitidine bismuth citrate, digoxin, drugs metabolized by CYP3A, HMG-CoA reductase inhibitors, and tolterodine. Hypotension, bradyarrhythmias, and lactic acidosis observed with calcium channel blockers (eg, verapamil). Concomitant use with itraconazole may increase levels of itraconazole and clarithromycin. Decreases zidovudine plasma levels. Potentiates oral anticoagulant effects. Increases AUC of midazolam; avoid coadministration of oral midazolam and monitor IV closely to allow dose adjustment. Caution with benzodiazepines that are metabolized by CYP3A (eg, triazolam, alprazolam). Somnolence and confusion may occur with concomitant use of triazolam; monitor for additive CNS effects. Concomitant use with strong inducers of CPY450 (eg, efavirenz, nevirapine, rifampicin, rifabutin, rifapentine) may decrease plasma levels of clarithromycin. Occurrence of torsades de pointes with antiarrhythmics (eg, quinidine, disopyramide) reported. Increased phosphodiesterase inhibitor exposure with sildenafil, tadalafil, or vardenafil. Avoid ranitidine bismuth citrate if CrCl <25 mL/min or history of acute porphyria. Reduce dose with ritonavir if CrCl ≤60mL/min. Increased levels with fluconazole. Concomitant use with colchicine may increase colchicine exposure; colchicine toxicity reported especially in elderly. Reduce dose with atazanavir if CrCl ≤60ml/min; doses of clarithromycin >1,000mg/day should not be coadministered with protease inhibitors. Rare cases of rhabdomyolysis reported with HMG-CoA reductase inhibitors (eg, lovastatin, simvastatin). Interaction may occur when concomitantly used with cyclosporine, tacrolimus, alfentanil, methylprednisolone, cilostazol, bromocriptine, vinblastine, hexobarbital, phenytoin, or valproate. Rare reports of hypoglycemia with oral hypoglycemic agents or insulin.

PREGNANCY: Category C, caution in nursing.

MECHANISM OF ACTION: Semisynthetic macrolide antibiotic; exerts antibacterial action by binding to the 50S ribosomal subunit of susceptible microorganisms resulting in inhibition of protein synthesis. Active against aerobic and anaerobic gram-positive and gram-negative microorganisms.

PHARMACOKINETICS: Absorption: Rapid. (2 x 500mg dose): (Parent drug) C_{max}=2-3μcg/mL, T_{max}=5-8 hrs.(14-OH) C_{max}=0.8μcg/mL, T_{max}=6-9 hrs. (1 x 500mg dose): (Parent drug) C_{max}=1-2μcg/mL, T_{max}=5-6 hr; (14-OH) C_{max}=0.6μcg/mL, T_{max}=6 hrs. **Distribution:** Body tissues, fluids. **Metabolism:** 14-OH clarithromycin (active metabolite). **Elimination:** Urine (30%).

NURSING CONSIDERATIONS

Assessment: Assess for renal impairment, myasthenia gravis, pregnancy/nursing status, a history of acute porphyria, and for possible drug interactions.

Monitoring: Monitor for anaphylactic reactions, development of drug-resistant bacteria, CDAD ranging from mild diarrhea to fatal colitis, overgrowth of nonsusceptible microorganisms. Monitor for exacerbation of myasthenia gravis and new onset of symptoms of myasthenic syndrome. Monitor for colchicine toxicity if taken concurrently with colchicine, and changes in LFTs, CBC, PT, and renal function.

Patient Counseling: Inform about potential benefits/risks of therapy. Counsel that drug only treats bacterial, not viral, infections. Instruct to take exactly as directed; inform that skipping doses or not completing full course may decrease effectiveness and increase antibiotic resistance. Instruct to swallow tab whole; do not chew, break, or crush. Advise to take with food. Notify physician if watery/bloody diarrhea (with/without stomach cramps) develops; inform that may occur as late as 2 or more months after treatment. Notify physician if pregnant/nursing and all medications currently taking.

Administration: Oral route. Swallow whole with food; do not chew, crush, or break. **Storage:** 20-25°C (68-77°F); excursions permitted 15-30°C (59-86°F).

Boniva   RX
ibandronate sodium (Genentech)

THERAPEUTIC CLASS: Bisphosphonate

INDICATIONS: (Inj) Treatment of osteoporosis in postmenopausal women. (PO) Treatment and prevention of postmenopausal osteoporosis.

DOSAGE: *Adults:* Inj: 3mg IV over 15-30 sec q3 months. PO: 150mg once monthly on the same date each month. Swallow whole with 6-8 oz. water. Do not lie down for 60 min after dose. Take ≥60 min before 1st food, drink (other than water), medication, or supplementation. Must not take 2 tabs within the same week.

HOW SUPPLIED: Inj: 3mg/3mL; Tab: 150mg

CONTRAINDICATIONS: Hypocalcemia. (PO) Inability to stand or sit upright for ≥60 min and abnormalities of the esophagus that delay esophageal emptying (eg, stricture or achalasia).

WARNINGS/PRECAUTIONS: Not recommended in severe renal impairment (CrCl <30mL/min). Osteonecrosis, primarily in the jaw reported; weigh benefit/risk. Caution with risk factors for osteonecrosis of the jaw (ONJ) including dental procedures, cancer diagnosis, and comorbid disorders (eg, anemia, coagulopathy, infection, and pre-existing dental disease). Severe, incapacitating bone, joint, and/or muscle pain reported; consider d/c if severe symptoms develop. Treat hypocalcemia and other bone and mineral disturbances prior to therapy; hypocalcemia reported. Atypical, low-energy, or low-trauma fractures of the femoral shaft reported; consider interrupting therapy. (PO) May cause local irritation of upper GI mucosa. Caution with upper GI problems (eg, Barrett's esophagus, dysphagia, esophageal diseases, gastritis, duodenitis or ulcer). D/C if dysphagia, odynophagia, retrosternal pain or new or worsening heartburn develops. Gastric and duodenal ulcers reported. (Inj) Avoid intra-arterial or paravenous inj.

ADVERSE REACTIONS: Acute phase reaction, arthralgia, abdominal pain, headache, dyspepsia, back pain. (Inj) Influenza, nasopharyngitis, constipation, HTN. (PO) Extremity pain, diarrhea.

INTERACTIONS: Caution with risk factors for osteonecrosis (eg, chemotherapy, radiotherapy, corticosteroids). May increase risk of atypical femur fractures with glucocorticoids (eg, prednisone). May interfere with bone-imaging agents. (PO) Products containing calcium and other multivalent cations (eg, aluminum, magnesium, iron) may interfere with absorption. Should be taken ≥60 min before any oral medication. Caution when used concomitantly with NSAIDs or aspirin due to GI irritation. Increased bioavailability with ranitidine.

PREGNANCY: Category C, caution in nursing.

MECHANISM OF ACTION: Bisphosphonate; has affinity for hydroxyapatite, a component of the mineral matrix of the bone. Inhibits osteoclast activity and reduces bone resorption and turnover. In postmenopausal women, it reduces the elevated rate of bone turnover, leading to, on average, net gain in bone mass.

PHARMACOKINETICS: Absorption: (PO) Upper GI tract; T_{max}=0.5-2 hrs. **Distribution:** V_d= ≥90L; Plasma protein binding: PO (90.9-99.5%); IV (86%). **Elimination:** (IV/PO) Kidney (50-60%); (PO) Feces (unabsorbed dose); (PO) (150mg): $T_{1/2}$=37-157 hrs; (IV, 2mg): $T_{1/2}$=4.6-15.3 hrs; (IV, 4mg): $T_{1/2}$=5-25.5 hrs.

NURSING CONSIDERATIONS

Assessment: Assess for any other conditions where treatment is contraindicated or cautioned, pregnancy/nursing status, and possible drug interactions. Obtain baseline serum calcium, CrCl.

Monitoring: Monitor for signs/symptoms of ONJ, musculoskeletal pain, hypocalcemia, atypical femur fracture, and renal function. PO: Monitor for signs/symptoms of upper GI disorders (eg, dysphagia, esophageal disease or ulcer).

Patient Counseling: (PO) Counsel to take ≥60 min before 1st food or drink (other than water) and before taking other oral medication or supplementation. Instruct to swallow whole with full glass of plain water (6-8 oz) while standing or sitting in upright position; avoid lying down for ≥60 min. Inform not to chew or suck medication. Advise to take supplemental calcium and vitamin D if dietary intake is inadequate. Counsel to take tab on the same date each month. If dose is missed and next scheduled dose is >7 days away, instruct to take one tab in the morning following the date it is remembered. If next dose is 1-7 days away, instruct to wait for next scheduled day to take tab. Instruct to d/c treatment and seek medical attention if signs of esophageal irritation develop during therapy. (Inj) Advise patients to take supplemental calcium and vitamin D.

Administration: Oral or IV route. (Inj) Do not mix with calcium-containing solutions or other IV drugs. Inspect visually for particulate matter and discoloration before administration. **Storage:** 25°C (77°F); excursions permitted to 15-30°C (59-86°F).

BOOSTRIX   RX
pertussis vaccine, acellular - diphtheria toxoid - tetanus toxoid
(GlaxoSmithKline)

THERAPEUTIC CLASS: Vaccine/toxoid combination

INDICATIONS: Active booster immunization against tetanus, diphtheria, and pertussis as a single dose in individuals 10-64 yrs of age.

DOSAGE: *Adults:* ≤64 yrs: 0.5mL IM into the deltoid muscle of the upper arm. Wound Management: May be given as a tetanus prophylaxis if no previous dose of any Tetanus Toxoid, Reduced Diphtheria Toxoid and Acellular Pertussis Vaccine, Adsorbed (Tdap) has been administered.
Pediatrics: ≥10 yrs: 0.5mL IM into the deltoid muscle of the upper arm. Wound Management: May be given as a tetanus prophylaxis if no previous dose of any Tdap has been administered.

HOW SUPPLIED: Inj: 0.5mL [vial, prefilled syringe]

CONTRAINDICATIONS: Encephalopathy (eg, coma, decreased level of consciousness, prolonged seizures) within 7 days of administration of a previous pertussis antigen-containing vaccine that is not attributable to another identifiable cause.

WARNINGS/PRECAUTIONS: Not for IV, intradermal, or SQ administration. Administer 5 yrs after last dose of recommended series of Diphtheria and Tetanus Toxoids and Acellular Pertussis Vaccine Adsorbed (DTaP) and/or Tetanus and Diphtheria Toxoids Adsorbed for Adult Use (Td) vaccine. May cause allergic reactions in latex-sensitive patients. May increased risk of Guillain-Barre syndrome following a subsequent dose of tetanus toxoid-containing vaccine if Guillain-Barre syndrome occurs within 6 weeks of receipt of a prior tetanus toxoid-containing vaccine. Defer vaccination in cases of progressive/unstable neurologic conditions (eg, cerebrovascular events, acute encephalopathic conditions). Avoid if previously experienced an Arthus-type hypersensitivity reaction following a prior dose of tetanus toxoid-containing vaccine unless ≥10 yrs have elapsed since last dose of tetanus toxoid-containing vaccine. Expected immune response may not be obtained in immunosuppressed persons. Have epinephrine and other appropriate agents used for the control of immediate allergic reactions available for anaphylactic reactions.

ADVERSE REACTIONS: Local: pain, redness, swelling, increased arm circumference (>5mm). Systemic: headache, fatigue, fever, GI symptoms.

INTERACTIONS: Concomitant use of meningococcal conjugate vaccine lowers post-vaccination geometric mean antibody concentrations (GMCs) to pertactin.Concomitant use with influenza virus vaccine lowers GMCs for antibodies to the pertussis antigens filamentous hemagglutinin and pertactin. Immunosuppressive therapies, including irradiation, antimetabolites, alkylating agents, cytotoxic drugs, and corticosteroids (used in greater than physiological doses), may reduce the immune response to vaccines.

PREGNANCY: Category C, caution in nursing.

MECHANISM OF ACTION: Vaccine/toxoid combination; produces neutralizing antibodies that may protect against tetanus, diphtheria, and pertussis.

NURSING CONSIDERATIONS

Assessment: Assess immunization history and current health/medical status (eg, immunosuppression). Assess for latex hypersensitivity, progressive/unstable neurologic conditions, history of seizures, pregnancy/nursing status, and for possible drug interactions.

Monitoring: Monitor for signs and symptoms of Guillain-Barre syndrome, brachial neuritis, and for allergic reactions (eg, anaphylaxis).

Patient Counseling: Inform about benefits/risks of immunization. Inform about the potential for adverse reactions and instruct to report any adverse events to physician. Inform that safety and efficacy have not been established in pregnant women. Advise patient, parent or guardian to acquire vaccine information statements prior to immunization.

Administration: IM route. Prior to administration, shake vial vigorously to obtain homogeneous, turbid, white suspension. Do not use if resuspension does not occur with vigorous shaking. Inspect visually for particulate matter and discoloration; if any of these conditions exist, do not administer. Do not mix with any other vaccine in the same syringe or vial. **Storage:** 2-8°C (36-46°F). Do not freeze. Discard if frozen.

BOTOX   RX
onabotulinumtoxinA (Allergan)

> Distant spread of toxin effects hours to weeks after injection reported (eg, asthenia, generalized muscle weakness, diplopia, ptosis, dysphagia, dysphonia, dysarthria, urinary incontinence, breathing difficulties). Swallowing and breathing difficulties can be life threatening and there have been reports of death. Risk of symptoms is greater in children treated for spasticity than in adults. In unapproved uses and approved indications, cases of spread of effect have occurred at doses comparable to those used to treat cervical dystonia and at lower doses.

THERAPEUTIC CLASS: Purified neurotoxin complex

INDICATIONS: Prophylaxis of headaches in adults with chronic migraine (≥15 days/month with headache lasting ≥4 hrs/day. Treatment of strabismus and blepharospasm associated with dystonia, including benign essential blepharospasm or VII nerve disorders in patients ≥12 yrs. Treatment of upper limb spasticity in adults, to decrease the severity of increased muscle tone in elbow flexors (biceps), wrist flexors (flexor carpi radialis and flexor carpi ulnaris) and finger flexors (flexor digitorum profundus and flexor digitorum sublimis). Treatment of adults with cervical dystonia, to reduce severity of abnormal head position and neck pain associated with cervical dystonia. Treatment of severe primary axillary hyperhidrosis that is inadequately managed with topical agents.

DOSAGE: *Adults:* Chronic Migraine: Usual: 155 U IM as 0.1mL (5 U)/site. Should be divided across 7 specific head/neck muscle areas. Refer to PI for recommended injection sites and recommended dose (number of sites). Re-treatment schedule: Every 12 weeks. Upper Limb Spasticity: Individualize dose. Range: 75-360 U divided among selected muscles. Biceps Brachii: 100-200 U divided in 4 sites. Flexor Carpi Radialis/Flexor Carpi Ulnaris: 12.5-50 U in 1 site. Flexor Digitorum Profundus/Flexor Digitorum Sublimis: 30-50 U in 1 site. Max: 50 U/site. May repeat no sooner than 12 weeks after previous injection. Cervical Dystonia: Individualize dose. Average Dose: 236 U divided among affected muscles. Max: 50 U/site. Primary Axillary Hyperhidrosis: 50 U/axilla intradermally (ID). Repeat injections when clinical effect of previous injection diminishes. Blepharospasm: Initial: 1.25-2.5 U into medial and lateral pre-tarsal orbicularis oculi of the upper lid and into the lateral pre-tarsal orbicularis oculi of the lower lid. May increase up to 2-fold if initial treatment response is insufficient. Max: 200 U/30 days. Strabismus: Initial: Vertical Muscle and Horizontal Strabismus <20 Prism Diopters: 1.25-2.5 U in any one muscle. Horizontal Strabismus of 20-50 Prism Diopters: 2.5-5 U in any one muscle. Persistent VI Nerve Palsy ≥1 Month: 1.25-2.5 U into medial rectus muscle. Max: 25 U/muscle. Dose may be increased by up to 2-fold if previous dose resulted in incomplete paralysis of target muscle. Reassess 7-14 days after each injection. Instill several drops of a local anesthetic and an ocular decongestant

several minutes prior to injection. ≥1 Indications: Max Cumulative Dose: 360 U, in a 3 month interval. Elderly: Start at low end of dosing range.
Pediatrics: ≥16 yrs: Cervical Dystonia: Individualize dose. Average Dose: 236 U divided among affected muscles. Max: 50 U/site. ≥12 yrs: Blepharospasm: Initial: 1.25-2.5 U into medial and lateral pre-tarsal orbicularis oculi of the upper lid and into the lateral pre-tarsal orbicularis oculi of the lower lid. May increase up to 2-fold if initial treatment response is insufficient. Max: 200 U/30 days. Strabismus: Initial: Vertical Muscle and Horizontal Strabismus <20 Prism Diopters: 1.25-2.5 U in any one muscle. Horizontal Strabismus of 20-50 Prism Diopters: 2.5-5 U in any one muscle. Persistent VI Nerve Palsy ≥1 Month: 1.25-2.5 U into the medial rectus muscle. Max: 25 U/muscle. Dose may be increased by up to 2-fold if previous dose resulted in incomplete paralysis of target muscle. Reassess 7-14 days after each injection. Instill several drops of a local anesthetic and an ocular decongestant several minutes prior to injection.

HOW SUPPLIED: Inj: 100 U, 200 U

CONTRAINDICATIONS: Presence of infection at proposed injection site(s).

WARNINGS/PRECAUTIONS: Units of onabotulinumtoxinA are specific to the preparation and assay method utilized and are not interchangeable with other botulinum toxin products and cannot be compared or converted into units of any other botulinum toxin products. Hypersensitivity reactions (eg, anaphylaxis, serum sickness, urticaria, soft tissue edema, dyspnea) reported; d/c and institute appropriate therapy. Caution in patients whose swallowing or respiratory function is already compromised; aspiration resulting from severe dysphagia may occur. Serious breathing difficulties, including respiratory failure reported in patients with cervical dystonia. Increased risk of dysphagia in patients with smaller neck muscle mass and those who require bilateral injections into sternocleidomastoid muscle; limit dose injected into sternocleidomastoid muscle. Injection in levator scapulae may increase risk of upper respiratory infection and dysphagia. May require immediate medical attention if swallowing, speech or respiratory disorders occur. Caution with peripheral motor neuropathic diseases, amyotrophic lateral sclerosis (ALS), or neuromuscular junction disorders (eg, myasthenia gravis, Lambert-Eaton syndrome). Closely monitor patients being treated for spasticity with compromised respiratory status. Reduced blinking from injection of orbicularis muscle may lead to corneal exposure, persistent epithelial defect, and corneal ulceration especially with VII nerve disorders; vigorously treat any epithelial defect. Retrobulbar hemorrhages compromising retinal circulation reported. Bronchitis and upper respiratory tract infections (URI) reported in patients being treated for spasticity. Contains albumin; risk for viral disease and Creutzfeldt-Jakob disease (CJD) transmission. Potential for immunogenicity. Not intended to substitute for usual standard of care rehabilitation regimens. Weakness of hand muscles and blepharoptosis may occur in patients treated for palmar hyperhidrosis and facial hyperhidrosis. Caution with inflammation at injection site or when excessive weakness or atrophy is present in target muscle. Caution in elderly.

ADVERSE REACTIONS: Asthenia, muscle weakness, diplopia, ptosis, dysphonia, dysarthria, urinary incontinence, dysphagia, dyspnea, upper respiratory tract infection, headache, neck pain, musculoskeletal stiffness, myalgia, fatigue.

INTERACTIONS: Toxin effects may be potentiated with coadministration of aminoglycosides or other agents interfering with neuromuscular transmission (eg, curare-like compounds). Excessive neuromuscular weakness may be exacerbated if another botulinum toxin is administered before effects resolve from the previous botulinum toxin injection administration. Excessive weakness may also be exaggerated by administration of a muscle relaxant before or after administration. Use of anticholinergic drugs after administration may potentiate systemic anticholinergic effects.

PREGNANCY: Category C, caution in nursing.

MECHANISM OF ACTION: Purified neurotoxin complex; blocks neuromuscular transmission by binding to acceptor sites on motor or sympathetic nerve terminals, entering the nerve terminals, and inhibiting release of acetylcholine.

NURSING CONSIDERATIONS

Assessment: Assess for infection or inflammation at proposed injection site, weakness/atrophy in target muscle, pre-existing breathing or swallowing difficulties, compromised swallowing or respiratory function, peripheral motor neuropathic diseases, ALS, neuromuscular junction disorders (eg, myasthenia gravis or Lambert-Eaton syndrome), increased risk for dysphagia (eg, small neck muscle mass, patients requiring bilateral injections into sternocleidomastoid muscle), VII nerve disorders, potential causes of secondary hyperhidrosis (eg, hyperthyroidism), hypersensitivity to any botulinum toxin preparation or other components of the drug, pregnancy/nursing status, and for possible drug interactions.

Monitoring: Monitor for distant spread of toxin effect (eg, asthenia, generalized muscle weakness, diplopia, ptosis, dysphagia, dysphonia, dysarthria, urinary incontinence, breathing difficulties), hypersensitivity reactions, aspiration due to severe dysphagia, URI, bronchitis, respiratory failure, transmission of viral diseases and CJD. Monitor for corneal exposure, persistent epithelial defect, and corneal ulceration when given for blepharospasm. Closely monitor patients with compromised respiratory status. In patients with strabismus, monitor for retrobulbar hemorrhage during administration, and for effects of dose by re-examining 7-14 days after injection.

Patient Counseling: Provide a copy and review the contents of the Medication Guide with the patient. Advise to seek immediate medical attention if swallowing, speech, or breathing difficulties arise, or if any existing symptom worsens. Counsel to avoid driving a car or engaging in other potentially hazardous activities if loss of strength, muscle weakness, impaired vision, or drooping eyelids occurs.

Administration: ID or IM routes. Refer to PI for preparation, dilution technique and administration. **Storage:** 2-8°C; up to 24 months (200 U) or 36 months (100 U). Reconstituted Sol: Refrigerate (2-8°C) and use within 24 hrs.

BOTOX COSMETIC   RX
onabotulinumtoxinA (Allergan)

> Distant spread of toxin effects hours to weeks after injection reported (eg, asthenia, generalized muscle weakness, diplopia, blurred vision, ptosis, dysphagia, dysphonia, dysarthria, urinary incontinence, breathing difficulties). Swallowing and breathing difficulties can be life-threatening and there have been reports of death. Risk of symptoms is greater in children treated for spasticity than in adults. In unapproved uses and approved indications, cases of spread of effect have occurred at doses comparable to those used to treat cervical dystonia and at lower doses.

THERAPEUTIC CLASS: Purified neurotoxin complex

INDICATIONS: For temporary improvement in appearance of moderate to severe glabellar lines associated with corrugator and/or procerus muscle activity in adults ≤65 years of age.

DOSAGE: *Adults:* ≤65 yrs: Inject a dose of 0.1mL IM into each of five sites, two in each corrugator muscle and one in the procerus muscle for a total dose of 20 U. Intervals should be no more frequent than every 3 months.

HOW SUPPLIED: Inj: 50 U, 100 U

CONTRAINDICATIONS: Infection at proposed injection sites.

WARNINGS/PRECAUTIONS: Not interchangeable with other botulinum toxin products and cannot be compared or converted to other products. Do not exceed dosing recommendations. Caution with peripheral motor neuropathic diseases, amyotrophic lateral sclerosis (ALS), neuromuscular junctional disorders (eg, myasthenia gravis, Lambert-Eaton syndrome); increased risk of dysphagia and respiratory compromise. Hypersensitivity reactions (eg, anaphylaxis, urticaria, soft tissue edema, and dyspnea) reported. Contains albumin; possible risk of transmission of (eg, viruses, Creutzfeldt-Jakob disease). Caution with inflammation at injection sites, excessive weakness or atrophy in target muscles. Injection of the orbicularis muscle may reduce blinking, especially with VII nerve disorders. Reduced blinking can lead to corneal exposure, persistent epithelial defect, and corneal ulceration. Carefully test corneal sensation in eyes previously operated upon, avoid injection into lower lid area to avoid ectropion, and vigorously treat any epithelial defect. Inducing paralysis in one or more extraocular muscles may produce spatial disorientation, double vision, or past pointing; covering affected eye may alleviate symptoms. Caution with inflammatory skin problems at the injection site, marked facial asymmetry, ptosis, excessive dermatochalasis, deep dermal scarring, thick sebaceous skin, or inability to substantially lessen glabellar lines by physically spreading them apart. Cardiovascular system adverse events including arrhythmia and myocardial infarction reported; caution with pre-existing cardiovascular disease (CVD). Needle-related pain and/or anxiety may result in vasovagal responses.

ADVERSE REACTIONS: Asthenia, generalized muscle weakness, diplopia, blurred vision, ptosis, dysphagia, dysphonia, dysarthria, urinary incontinence, breathing difficulties, headache, respiratory infection, flu syndrome, blepharoptosis, nausea.

INTERACTIONS: May be potentiated with aminoglycosides, and agents interfering with neuromuscular transmission (eg, curare-like nondepolarizing blockers, lincosamides, polymyxins, quinidine, magnesium sulfate, anticholinesterases, succinylcholine chloride). Excessive neuromuscular weakness may be exacerbated if another botulinum toxin is administered before effects resolve from the previous botulinum toxin injection.

PREGNANCY: Category C, caution in nursing.

MECHANISM OF ACTION: Purified neurotoxin complex; blocks neuromuscular transmission by binding to acceptor sites on motor nerve terminals, entering the nerve terminals, and inhibiting the release of acetylcholine. Produces partial chemical denervation of the muscle resulting in a localized reduction in muscle activity if injected IM.

NURSING CONSIDERATIONS

Assessment: Assess for breathing or swallowing difficulties, infection at proposed injection site or weakness/atrophy in target muscle, and other conditions where treatment is contraindicated or cautioned. Assess for pregnancy/nursing status and possible drug interactions.

Monitoring: Monitor for spread of toxin effect, breathing difficulties, injection site reactions, and other severe side effects.

Patient Counseling: Provide a copy and review the contents of the FDA-approved Patient Medication Guide with the patient. Advise to inform doctor or pharmacist if they develop any unusual symptoms (including difficulty with swallowing, speaking, or breathing), or if any existing symptom worsens. Counsel to avoid driving a car or engaging in other potentially hazardous activities if loss of strength, muscle weakness, or impaired vision occur.

Administration: IM route. Refer to PI for proper dilution and injection technique. **Storage:** Refrigerate (2-8°C) for up to 36 months for 100 U vial (unopened) or up to 24 months for 50 U vial (unopened). Refrigerate (2-8°C) reconstituted solution and administer within 24 hrs.

BREVIBLOC   RX
esmolol HCl (Baxter)

THERAPEUTIC CLASS: Selective beta₁-blocker

INDICATIONS: For rapid control of ventricular rate in atrial fibrillation or atrial flutter in perioperative, postoperative, or other emergent circumstances. For noncompensatory sinus tachycardia. Treatment of tachycardia and hypertension that occur during induction and tracheal intubation, during surgery, on emergence from anesthesia, and in the postoperative period.

DOSAGE: *Adults:* Supraventricular Tachycardia: Titrate dose based on ventricular rate. Initial Load: 0.5mg/kg over 1 min. Maint: 0.05mg/kg/min for next 4 min. May increase by 0.05mg/kg/min or increased step-wise at intervals of 4 min or more up to 0.2mg/kg/min depending upon the desired response. Rapid slowing of ventricular response: Repeat 0.5mg/kg load over 1 min, then

0.1mg/kg/min for 4 min. If needed, another (final) load of 0.5mg/kg over 1 min, then 0.15mg/kg/min for 4 min up to 0.2mg/kg/min. May continue infusions for as long as 24 hrs. Intraoperative/Postoperative Tachycardia and/or HTN: Immediate Control: Initial: 80mg (approx 1mg/kg) bolus over 30 sec followed by 0.15mg/kg/min prn. May titrate up to 0.3mg/kg/min to maintain desired heart rate and BP. Gradual Control: Initial: 0.5mg/kg over 1 min followed by maintenance infusion of 0.05mg/kg/min for 4 min. Then, may repeat load and follow maintenance infusion increased to 0.1mg/kg/min prn.

HOW SUPPLIED: Inj: 10mg/mL [10mL, 250mL], 20mg/mL [5mL, 100mL]

CONTRAINDICATIONS: Sinus bradycardia, heart block greater than first degree, cardiogenic shock or overt heart failure.

WARNINGS/PRECAUTIONS: Hypotension may occur; monitor BP and reduce dose or d/c if needed. May cause cardiac failure; withdraw at 1st sign of impending cardiac failure. Caution with supraventricular arrhythmias when patient is compromised hemodynamically. Not for HTN associated with hypothermia. Caution in bronchospastic diseases; titrate to lowest possible effective dose and terminate immediately in the event of bronchospasm. Caution in diabetics; may mask tachycardia occuring with hypoglycemia. Caution with renal impairment. Local infusion site reaction may develop; use alternate infusion site; caution should be taken to prevent extravasation. Avoid use of butterfly needles. Use caution when abruptly discontinuing infusions in coronary artery disease patients.

ADVERSE REACTIONS: Hypotension, dizziness, diaphoresis, somnolence, confusion, headache, agitation, bronchospasm, nausea, infusion-site reactions.

INTERACTIONS: Additive effects with catecholamine-depleting agents (eg, reserpine); monitor for evidence of hypotension or marked bradycardia. Levels increased by warfarin or morphine; titrate with caution. May increase digoxin levels; titrate with caution. May prolong effects of succinylcholine; titrate with caution. Caution when using with verapamil in depressed myocardial function; fatal cardiac arrest may occur. Do not use to control supraventricular tachycardia with vasoconstrictive and inotropic agents (eg, dopamine, epinephrine, norepinephrine) because of the danger of blocking cardiac contractility when systemic vascular resistance is high. Patients with a history of severe anaphylactic reaction may be more reactive to repeated challenge and unresponsive to the usual doses of epinephrine used to treat allergic reaction. Caution with supraventricular arrhythmias when patient is taking other drugs that decrease peripheral resistance, myocardial filling/contractility, and/or electrical impulse propagation in the myocardium.

PREGNANCY: Category C, caution in nursing.

MECHANISM OF ACTION: Selective β_1 blocker; inhibits β_1 receptors located chiefly in cardiac muscle, and at higher doses begins to inhibit β_2 receptors located chiefly in the bronchial and vascular musculature.

PHARMACOKINETICS: Distribution: Plasma protein binding (55%). **Metabolism:** Rapid. Through hydrolysis of the ester linkage in red blood cells to methanol and free acid. **Elimination:** Urine (73-88%, <2% unchanged); $T_{1/2}$=9 min (esmolol HCl), 3.7 hrs (acid metabolites).

NURSING CONSIDERATIONS

Assessment: Assess for sinus bradycardia, heart block greater than first degree, cardiogenic shock or overt heart failure, hypotension, HTN associated with hypothermia, bronchospastic disease, diabetes mellitus, renal impairment, and possible drug interactions.

Monitoring: Monitor BP, HR. Monitor for signs/symptoms of impending cardiac failure, hypotension (eg, diaphoresis or dizziness), postoperative tachycardia/HTN, bronchospasm, and masking signs of tachycardia occuring with hypoglycemia.

Patient Counseling: Inform about benefits/risks. Report any adverse reactions to physician.

Administration: IV route. Refer to PI for Directions for Use of Premixed Bag and Ready-to- Use Vials. Prediluted to provide ready-to-use vials. Do not introduce additives to premixed injections. **Storage:** 25°C (77°F); excursions permitted to 15-30°C (59-86°F). Protect from freezing. Avoid excessive heat.

BROMDAY

bromfenac (Ista)

RX

THERAPEUTIC CLASS: NSAID

INDICATIONS: Treatment of postoperative inflammation and reduction of ocular pain after cataract surgery.

DOSAGE: *Adults:* 1 drop qd in affected eye(s), start 1 day prior to surgery, the day of surgery and continue for 2 weeks post surgery.

HOW SUPPLIED: Sol: 0.09% [1.7mL]

WARNINGS/PRECAUTIONS: Contains sodium sulfite; may cause allergic-type reactions (eg, anaphylactic symptoms, asthmatic episodes). Sulfite sensitivity is seen more frequently in asthmatics. May slow or delay healing. Potential cross-sensitivity to acetylsalicylic acid, phenylacetic acid derivatives, and other NSAIDs. Caution when treating individuals who previously exhibited sensitivity to these drugs. May increase bleeding of ocular tissues (eg, hyphemas) in conjunction with ocular surgery. Caution in patients with known bleeding tendencies. May result in keratitis. Continued use may lead to sight-threatening epithelial breakdown, corneal thinning, corneal erosion, corneal ulceration, or corneal perforation; d/c if corneal epithelium breakdown occurs. Caution in patients with complicated ocular surgeries, corneal denervation, corneal epithelial defects, diabetes mellitus (DM), ocular surface diseases (eg, dry eye syndrome), rheumatoid arthritis (RA), or repeat ocular surgeries within a short period of time. Increased risk for occurrence and severity of corneal adverse events if used >24 hrs prior to surgery or use beyond 14 days post-surgery. Avoid use with contact lenses. Avoid use during late pregnancy because of the known effects on the fetal cardiovascular system (closure of ductus arteriosus).

ADVERSE REACTIONS: Abnormal sensation in eye, conjunctival hyperemia, eye irritation (burning/stinging), eye pain, eye pruritus, eye redness, headache, iritis.

INTERACTIONS: Concomitant use of topical NSAIDs and topical steroids may increase potential for healing problems. Caution with other medications which may prolong bleeding time.

PREGNANCY: Category C, caution in nursing.

MECHANISM OF ACTION: NSAID; thought to block prostaglandin synthesis by inhibiting cyclooxygenase 1 and 2.

NURSING CONSIDERATIONS

Assessment: Assess for hypersensitivity (eg, sodium sulfite) or cross-sensitivity (eg, ASA) reactions, history of complicated or repeated ocular surgeries, corneal denervation, corneal epithelial defects, DM, ocular surface diseases (eg, dry eye syndrome), RA, bleeding tendencies, pregnancy/nursing status, and possible drug interactions.

Monitoring: Monitor for anaphylactic symptoms, severe asthma attacks, wound-healing problems, keratitis, corneal epithelial breakdown, corneal thinning/erosion/ulceration/perforation, increased bleeding time, and bleeding of ocular tissues (hyphemas) in conjunction with ocular surgery.

Patient Counseling: Advise not to wear contact lenses during therapy. Advise patients of the possibility of slow or delayed healing which may occur while using this product. Advise not to touch the dropper tip to any surface, as this may contaminate the contents. If >1 topical ophthalmic medication is used, instruct to administer 5 min apart.

Administration: Ocular route. May be used in conjunction with other topical ophthalmic medications (eg, α-agonists, β-blockers, carbonic anhydrase inhibitors, cycloplegics, mydriatics). Administer at least 5 min apart. **Storage:** 15-25°C (59-77°F).

B

BROVANA
RX
arformoterol tartrate (Sunovion)

> Long-acting β_2-adrenergic agonists (LABA) may increase the risk of asthma-related death. All LABA, including arformoterol tartrate, are contraindicated in patients with asthma without use of a long-term asthma control medication.

THERAPEUTIC CLASS: Beta$_2$-agonist

INDICATIONS: Long-term maintenance treatment of bronchoconstriction in patients with chronic obstructive pulmonary disease (COPD), including chronic bronchitis and emphysema.

DOSAGE: *Adults:* Usual: 15mcg bid (am and pm) by nebulization. Max: 30mcg/day.

HOW SUPPLIED: Sol, Inhalation: 15mcg/2mL [30^s, 60^s]

CONTRAINDICATIONS: Patients with asthma without use of a long-term asthma control medication.

WARNINGS/PRECAUTIONS: Not indicated for treatment of acute episodes of bronchospasm (rescue therapy). COPD may deteriorate acutely over a period of hrs or chronically over several days or longer; re-evaluate and institute COPD treatment regimen. May produce life-threatening paradoxical bronchospasm; d/c immediately and institute alternative therapy. Caution in patients with convulsive disorders or thyrotoxicosis, cardiovascular disorders (CVD) especially coronary insufficiency, cardiac arrhythmias and HTN, and who are unusually responsive to sympathomimetic amines. May produce significant hypokalemia and cardiovascular (CV) effects. Changes in blood glucose and/or serum K$^+$ reported during long-term use at recommended dose. Immediate hypersensitivity reactions (eg, anaphylactic reaction, urticaria, angioedema, rash, and bronchospasm) may occur. Fatalities reported with excessive use. Should not be initiated in patients with acutely deteriorating COPD. D/C regular intake of inhaled, short-acting β2-agonists upon initiation of therapy; use only for symptomatic relief of acute respiratory symptoms. Caution with hepatic impairment. For use by nebulization only.

ADVERSE REACTIONS: Pain, chest/back pain, diarrhea, sinusitis, leg cramps, dyspnea, rash, flu syndrome, peripheral edema.

INTERACTIONS: Caution with concomitant use of additional adrenergic agonists; sympathetic effects may be potentiated. Concomitant use with methylxanthines (aminophylline, theophylline), steroids, or diuretics may potentiate hypokalemia. Caution with coadministration with non-K$^+$ sparing diuretics (eg, loop, thiazide diuretics); ECG changes and/or hypokalemia may be acutely worsened. Use extreme caution with MAOIs, TCAs, or any drugs known to prolong the QT$_c$ interval. Caution with β-blockers. Avoid use with other LABAs.

PREGNANCY: Category C, caution in nursing.

MECHANISM OF ACTION: Selective LABA; stimulates intracellular adenyl cyclase, which catalyzes conversion of adenosine triphosphate (ATP) to cyclic-3',5'-adenosine monophosphate (cAMP) to produce relaxation of bronchial smooth muscle and inhibition of release of mediators of immediate hypersensitivity from cells, especially in mast cells.

PHARMACOKINETICS: Absorption: C$_{max}$=4.3pg/mL, T$_{max}$=30 min, AUC$_{0-12h}$=34.5pg•hr/mL. **Distribution:** Plasma protein binding (52-65%). **Metabolism:** Glucuronidation (major) via uridine diphosphoglucuronosyltransferase (UGT) isoenzymes, O-demethylation (minor) via CYP2D6, CYP2C19. **Elimination:** Urine (1% unchanged); feces; T$_{1/2}$=26 hrs.

NURSING CONSIDERATIONS

Assessment: Assess for acute episodes of bronchospasm/symptoms of COPD, conditions where treatment is contraindicated or cautioned, pregnancy/nursing status, and possible drug interactions. Assess if using inhaled, short-acting β_2-agonists on regular basis before therapy.

Monitoring: Monitor pulse rate, BP, ECG changes, serum K$^+$ and glucose levels. Monitor for acute deteriorating COPD, CV effects, paradoxical bronchospasm, immediate hypersensitivity reactions, hypokalemia, and other adverse reactions. Monitor patients with hepatic impairment.

Patient Counseling: Inform about risks and benefits of therapy. Instruct to use by nebulizer only and not to inject or swallow. Advise to contact physician if pregnant/nursing. Instruct on the correct use of drug; read Medication Guide. Inform that treatment may lead to adverse events including palpitations, chest pain, rapid HR, tremor, or nervousness. Inform that drug compatibility, efficacy and safety when mixed with other drugs in a nebulizer have not been established. Inform that the drug is not for use in asthma without use of long-term asthma control medication and not indicated to relieve acute respiratory symptoms. Instruct to seek medical attention if symptoms worsen, treatment becomes less effective, or inhalations of a short-acting β_2-agonist are needed more than usual.

Administration: Oral inhalation route. Administer via a standard jet nebulizer connected to an air compressor. Refer to PI for proper administration and use.
Storage: Store in the protective foil pouch at 2-8°C (36-46°F) or at 20-25°C (68-77°F) for ≤6 weeks. Use opened ready-to-use vial immediately; discard if sol is not colorless. Protect from light and excessive heat.

BUMETANIDE   RX
bumetanide (Various)

Can lead to profound water and electrolyte depletion with excessive use.

THERAPEUTIC CLASS: Loop diuretic

INDICATIONS: Treatment of edema associated with congestive heart failure (CHF), hepatic disease, and renal disease including nephrotic syndrome.

DOSAGE: *Adults:* ≥18 yrs: PO: Usual: 0.5-2mg qd. Maint: May give every other day or every 3-4 days. Max: 10mg/day. IV/IM: Initial: 0.5-1mg over 1-2 min, may repeat every 2-3 hrs for 2-3 doses. Max: 10mg/day. Elderly: Start at low end of dosing range.

HOW SUPPLIED: Inj: 0.25mg/mL; Tab: 0.5mg*, 1mg*, 2mg* *scored

CONTRAINDICATIONS: Anuria, hepatic coma, severe electrolyte depletion.

WARNINGS/PRECAUTIONS: Monitor for volume/electrolyte depletion, hypokalemia, blood dyscrasias, hepatic damage. Elderly are prone to volume/electrolyte depletion. Caution in elderly, hepatic cirrhosis and ascites. Associated with ototoxicity, hypocalcemia, thrombocytopenia, hypomagnesemia, hypokalemia, and hyperuricemia. Hypersensitivity with sulfonamide allergy. D/C if marked increase in BUN or creatinine or if develop oliguria with progressive renal disease.

ADVERSE REACTIONS: Muscle cramps, dizziness, hypotension, headache, nausea, hyperuricemia, hypokalemia, hyponatremia, hyperglycemia, azotemia, increased serum creatinine.

INTERACTIONS: Avoid aminoglycosides, ototoxic and nephrotoxic drugs, indomethacin. Lithium toxicity. Probenecid reduces effects. Potentiates antihypertensives.

PREGNANCY: Category C, not for use in nursing.

MECHANISM OF ACTION: Loop diuretic; inhibits sodium reabsorption in ascending loop of Henle.

PHARMACOKINETICS: Absorption: (IV) T_{max}=15-30 min. (Tab) T_{max}=1-2 hrs. **Distribution:** Plasma protein binding (94-96%). **Metabolism:** Oxidation. **Elimination:** Urine, bile (2%); $T_{1/2}$=1-1.5 hrs.

NURSING CONSIDERATIONS

Assessment: Assess for progressive renal disease, severe electrolyte depletion, anuria, oliguria, risk for vetricular arrhythmia, possible drug interactions, DM, impaired GI absorption, CHF, sulfonamide allergy, and liver disease (hepatic coma).

Monitoring: Periodically monitor serum potassium, serum electrolytes, CBC, blood glucose, and renal function. Monitor for signs/symptoms of ototoxicity, hypersensitivity reactions, hyperuricemia, oliguria, and thrombocytopenia.

Patient Counseling: Advise to seek medical attention if symptoms of ototoxicity, oliguria, hypersensitivity reactions, or thrombocytopenia occur.

Administration: Oral route. **Storage:** IV: 20-25°C (68-77°F). Protect from light. Tab: 15-30°C (59-86°F).

BUPHENYL   RX
sodium phenylbutyrate (Ucyclyd Pharma)

THERAPEUTIC CLASS: Urea cycle disorder agent

INDICATIONS: Adjunctive therapy in chronic management of urea cycle disorders involving deficiencies of carbamylphosphate synthetase (CPS), ornithine transcarbamylase (OTC), or argininosuccinic acid synthetase (AS), neonatal-onset deficiency (complete enzymatic deficiency presenting within the first 28 days of life), and late-onset disease (partial enzymatic deficiency, presenting after the first month of life) in patients who have a history of hyperammonemic encephalopathy.

DOSAGE: *Adults:* <20kg: 450-600mg/kg/day. >20kg: 9.9-13g/m²/day. Take in equally divided amounts with each meal or feeding (eg, 3-6 times a day). Powder is for oral use via mouth, gastronomy, or nasogastric tube only. Mix powder with food (solid or liquid) for immediate use.
Pediatrics: <20kg: 450-600mg/kg/day. >20kg: 9.9-13m²/day. Take in equally divided amounts with meal or feeding (eg, 3-6 times a day). Powder is for oral use via mouth, gastronomy, or nasogastric tube only. Mix powder with food (solid or liquid) for immediate use.

HOW SUPPLIED: Powder: 250g; Tab: 500mg

CONTRAINDICATIONS: Acute hyperammonemia.

WARNINGS/PRECAUTIONS: Caution with congestive heart failure (CHF), hepatic/renal insufficiency, inborn errors of beta oxidation, and sodium retention with edema. Maintain plasma glutamine <1,000µmol/L. Monitor serum phenylbutyrate and its metabolites, phenylacetate, and phenylacetylglutamine periodically. Use of tablets for neonates, infants, and children <20kg is not recommended.

ADVERSE REACTIONS: Amenorrhea/menstrual dysfunction, decreased appetite, body odor, bad taste/taste aversion, hypoalbuminemia, metabolic acidosis/alkalosis, anemia, hyperchloremia, hypophosphatemia, decreased total protein, increased alkaline phosphatase, increased liver transaminase, leukopenia/leukocytosis, thrombocytopenia.

INTERACTIONS: Probenecid may affect renal excretion of conjugated product of sodium phenylbutyrate, including metabolite. Reports of hyperammonemia being induced by haloperidol and valproic acid. Use of corticosteroids may cause the breakdown of body protein and increase plasma ammonia levels.

PREGNANCY: Category C, caution in nursing.

MECHANISM OF ACTION: Prodrug of phenylacetate; decreases elevated plasma ammonia glutamine levels and increases waste nitrogen excretion in the form of phenylacetylglutamine.

PHARMACOKINETICS: Absorption: (Powder/tab) T_{max} =1 hr; C_{max}=195mcg/mL (powder) and 218mcg/mL (tab). Phenylbutyrate: T_{max}= 1.35 hrs; C_{max}=218mcg/mL. Phenylacetate: T_{max}=3.74 hrs; C_{max}=48.5mcg/mL. **Metabolism:** Hepatic and renal. **Elimination:** Renal (80-100%, phenylacetylglutamine). (Powder) $T_{1/2}$=0.76 hrs; (Tab) $T_{1/2}$=0.77 hrs.

NURSING CONSIDERATIONS

Assessment: Assess for acute hyperammonemia, CHF, hepatic/renal insufficiency, inborn errors of beta oxidation, sodium retention with edema, hypersensitivity to drug, pregnancy/nursing status, and possible drug interactions.

Assess for plasma levels of ammonia, arginine, branched-chain amino acids, serum proteins, glutamine.

Monitoring: Monitor for adverse reactions and hypersensitivity reactions. Monitor periodically serum phenylbutyrate and its metabolites, phenylacetate and phenylacetylglutamine levels. Monitor urinalysis, blood chemistry profiles, and hematologic tests.

Patient Counseling: Instruct to take drug exactly as prescribed and follow the prescribed diet. If a dose is missed, take as soon as possible that same day. Total daily dose should be taken in equally divided amounts with meals. Inform the physician of other medications being taken and when symptoms of sleepiness and lightheadedness occur.

Administration: Oral route, nasogastric or gastrostomy tube. Powder should be mixed with food (solid or liquid); however, when dissolved in water, it is stable for 1 week at room temperature or refrigerated. **Storage:** 15-30°C (59-86°F). Keep bottle tightly closed.

BUPRENEX CIII
buprenorphine HCl (Reckitt Benckiser)

THERAPEUTIC CLASS: Opioid analgesic

INDICATIONS: Relief of moderate to severe pain.

DOSAGE: *Adults:* 0.3mg IM/IV q6h prn. Repeat if needed, 30-60 min after initial dose and then prn. High Risk Patients/Concomitant CNS depressants: Reduce dose by approximately 50%. May use single doses ≤0.6mg IM if not at high risk.
Pediatrics: ≥13 yrs: 0.3mg IM/IV q6h prn. Repeat if needed, 30-60 min after initial dose and then prn. High Risk Patients/Concomitant CNS depressants: Reduce dose by approximately 50%. May use single doses ≤0.6mg IM if not at high risk. 2-12 yrs: 2-6mcg/kg IM/IV q4-6h.

HOW SUPPLIED: Inj: 0.3mg/mL

WARNINGS/PRECAUTIONS: Significant respiratory depression reported; caution with compromised respiratory function. May increase cerebrospinal fluid (CSF) pressure; caution with head injury, intracranial lesions. Caution with debilitated, BPH, biliary tract dysfunction, myxedema, hypothyroidism, urethral stricture, acute alcoholism, Addison's disease, CNS disease, coma, toxic psychoses, delirium tremens, elderly, pediatrics, kyphoscoliosis or hepatic/renal/pulmonary impairment. May impair mental or physical abilities. May precipitate withdrawal in narcotic-dependence. May lead to psychological dependence.

ADVERSE REACTIONS: Sedation, N/V, dizziness, sweating, hypotension, headache, miosis, hypoventilation.

INTERACTIONS: Caution with MAOIs, CNS and respiratory depressants. Respiratory and cardiovascular collapse reported with diazepam. Increased CNS depression with other narcotic analgesics, general anesthetics, anti-histamines, benzodiazepines, phenothiazines, other tranquilizers, sedative-hypnotics. Decreased clearance with CYP3A4 inhibitors (eg, macrolides, azole antifungals, protease inhibitors). Increased clearance with CYP3A4 inducers (eg, rifampin, carbamazepine, phenytoin).

PREGNANCY: Category C, not for use in nursing.

MECHANISM OF ACTION: Opioid analgesic; high affinity binding to μ-opiate receptors in CNS. Possesses slow rate of dissociation from its receptor. Also possesses narcotic antagonist activity.

PHARMACOKINETICS: Absorption: T_{max}=1 hr. **Distribution:** Found in breast milk. **Metabolism:** Liver. **Elimination:** $T_{1/2}$=1.2-7.2 hrs.

NURSING CONSIDERATIONS

Assessment: Assess for compromised respiratory function (eg, COPD, hypoxia), head injury, intracranial lesions, age of patient, hepatic/renal function, myxedema or hypothyroidism, adrenal cortical insufficiencies (eg, Addison's disease), CNS depression or coma, toxic psychosis, prostatic hypertrophy or urethral stricture, acute alcoholism, delirium tremens, kyphoscoliosis, biliary tract dysfunction, pregnancy/nursing, and possible drug interactions.

Monitoring: Monitor for signs/symptoms of respiratory depression, CNS depression, elevation of CSF pressure, increased intracholedochal pressure, drug dependence, and withdrawal effects.

Patient Counseling: Inform that medication may impair mental/physicial abilities; use caution when performing dangerous tasks (eg, operating machinery/driving). Advise to notify physician of all medications currently taken. Instruct to avoid use of other CNS depressants and alcohol during therapy. Advise that medication may lead to dependence. Counsel to not exceed prescribed dosage. Advise to avoid abruptly discontinuing medication. Counsel to contact physician if signs/symptoms of respiratory depression develop.

Administration: Deep IM or slow IV route. **Storage:** Avoid excessive heat (over 40°C or 104°F). Protect from prolonged exposure to light.

BuSpar   RX
buspirone HCl (Bristol-Myers Squibb)

THERAPEUTIC CLASS: Atypical anxiolytic

INDICATIONS: Management of anxiety disorders, short-term relief of anxiety symptoms.

DOSAGE: *Adults:* Usual: 7.5mg bid. Titrate: May increase by 5mg/day every 2-3 days. Usual: 20-30mg/day. Max: 60mg/day. Use low dose with potent CYP3A4 inhibitors (eg, 2.5mg qd with nefazodone). Take consistently with or without food; bioavailability increased with food.

HOW SUPPLIED: Tab: 5mg*, 10mg*, 15mg*, 30mg* *scored

WARNINGS/PRECAUTIONS: Avoid with hepatic or renal impairment.

ADVERSE REACTIONS: Dizziness, nausea, headache, nervousness, lightheadedness, excitement, dystonia, fatigue, parkinsonism, akathisia, restless legs syndrome, restlessness.

INTERACTIONS: Avoid MAOIs and alcohol. Withdraw other CNS depressants gradually before therapy. Caution with psychotropics. Elevated liver transaminases reported with trazodone. Increases haloperidol levels. Verapamil, diltiazem, grapefruit juice, nefazodone, itraconazole, cimetidine, erythromycin increase plasma levels. May increase levels of both drugs with nefazodone; decrease dose of buspirone. Decreased plasma levels and effects with rifampin; may need to adjust buspirone dose. CYP3A4 inhibitors may increase plasma levels and CYP3A4 inducers may increase metabolism of buspirone; may need dose adjustment. Presystemic clearance may be decreased with food. May displace digoxin.

PREGNANCY: Category B, not for use in nursing.

MECHANISM OF ACTION: Atypical antianxiety agent; not fully established. Binds with high affinity to serotonin receptors (5-HT$_{1A}$) and moderate affinity to dopamine receptors (D$_2$); may have indirect effects on other neurotransmitter systems.

PHARMACOKINETICS: Absorption: Rapid; C$_{max}$=1-6ng/mL; T$_{max}$=40-90 min. **Distribution:** Plasma protein binding (86%). **Metabolism:** CYP3A4; oxidation and hyroxylation; 1-pyrimidinylpiperazine (active metabolite). **Elimination:** Urine (29-63%), feces (18-38%); T$_{1/2}$=2-3 hrs.

NURSING CONSIDERATIONS

Assessment: Assess for hypersensitivity, hepatic/renal functions, and possible drug interactions (eg, MAOIs).

Monitoring: Monitor BP, CNS disturbances, withdrawal symptoms (eg, irritability, anxiety, agitation, insomnia, tremor, abdominal cramps/muscle cramps, vomiting, sweating, flu-like symptoms w/o fever, and seizures), pseudo-parkinsonism, akathisia, tardive dyskinesia, dystonia.

Patient Counseling: Counsel to avoid hazardous tasks (eg, operating machinery/driving), ingesting large amounts of grapefruit juice. Advise to notify physician of current medications, alcohol use, and pregnancy status.

Administration: Oral route. **Storage:** 25°C (77°F); excursions permitted to 15-30°C (59-86°F). Dispense in tight, light-resistant container.

BUTORPHANOL SPRAY   CIV
butorphanol tartrate (Various)

THERAPEUTIC CLASS: Opioid agonist-antagonist analgesic

INDICATIONS: Management of pain when the use of an opioid analgesic is appropriate.

DOSAGE: *Adults:* Initial: 1 spray (1mg) in 1 nostril, may repeat after 60-90 min (after 90-120 min in elderly or renal/hepatic disease) and may repeat in 3-4 hrs after 2nd dose; or may use 1 spray in each nostril, may repeat after 3-4 hrs. Renal/Hepatic Disease: Increase dose interval to no less than 6 hrs.

HOW SUPPLIED: Nasal Spray: 10mg/mL [2.5mL]

CONTRAINDICATIONS: Hypersensitivity to benzethonium chloride.

WARNINGS/PRECAUTIONS: Not for use in narcotic-dependent patients. May result in physical dependence or tolerance. Avoid abrupt cessation. D/C if severe HTN occurs. Caution with hepatic or renal disease, acute myocardial infarction (MI), ventricular dysfunction, or coronary insufficiency. May impair ability to operate machinery. Increased respiratory depression with CNS disease or respiratory impairment. Severe risks with head injury.

ADVERSE REACTIONS: Somnolence, dizziness, N/V, nasal congestion, insomnia.

INTERACTIONS: Increased CNS depression and respiratory depression with alcohol, barbiturates, tranquilizers, and antihistamines. May be potentiated by erythromycin, theophylline and other drugs that affect hepatic metabolism. Decreased absorption rate with nasal vasoconstrictors (eg, oxymetazoline). Diminished analgesic effect if administered shortly after sumatriptan nasal spray.

PREGNANCY: Category C, caution in nursing.

MECHANISM OF ACTION: Opioid agonist-antagonist analgesic; has activity at receptors of mu-opioid type, and agonist at kappa-opioid receptors.

PHARMACOKINETICS: Absorption: Absolute bioavailability (60-70%); C_{max}=0.9-1.04ng/mL; T_{max}=30-60 mins. **Distribution:** V_d=305-901L; plasma protein binding (80%); crosses placenta, found in breast milk. **Metabolism:** Liver. Hydroxybutorphanol (major metabolite). **Elimination:** Urine (5%), feces. Hydroxybutorphanol: Urine (49%); $T_{1/2}$=18 hrs.

NURSING CONSIDERATIONS

Assessment: Assess for benzethonium chloride hypersensitivity; acute MI; ventricular dysfunction; coronary insufficiency; narcotic dependence; head injury; possible drug interactions; respiratory, renal, and hepatic impairment.

Monitoring: Monitor for hypotension, respiratory depression, increased ICP, withdrawal symptoms, and hypersensitivity reactions.

Patient Counseling: May impair physical/mental abilities. Advise to seek medical attention if symptoms of hypotension (syncope), respiratory depression, increased intracranial pressure, withdrawal symptoms, or hypersensitivity reactions occur.

Administration: Intranasal route. **Storage:** 25°C (77°F).

B

BUTRANS

buprenorphine (Purdue Pharmaceutical)

CIII

> Potential for abuse; assess for clinical risks for opioid abuse or addiction prior to prescribing opioids. Monitor all patients receiving opioids for signs of misuse, abuse and addiction. Do not exceed a dose of one 20-mcg/hr buprenorphine transdermal system due to the risk of QTc interval prolongation. Avoid exposing application site and surrounding area to direct external heat sources. Temperature-dependent increases in buprenorphine release from the system may result in a possible overdose and death.

THERAPEUTIC CLASS: Opioid Analgesics

INDICATIONS: Management of moderate to severe chronic pain in patients requiring a continuous, around-the-clock opioid anaglesic for an extended period of time.

DOSAGE: *Adults*: Individualize dose. Determine dose based on opioid tolerance, previous analgesic requirements, and general condition and medical status of the patient. Conversion from Other Opioids: Refer to PI. Opioid-Naive: Initial: 5mcg/hr. Titrate: Dose may be titrated to the next higher level after a minimum of 72 hrs. Max: 20mcg/hr. Maint: Continue therapy at individualized dose for as long as pain management is necessary. During chronic therapy, periodically reassess the continued need for around-the-clock therapy. Patch is intended to be worn for 7 days. Mild to Moderate Hepatic Impairment: Initial: 5mcg/hr. Titrate: Increase to level that provides adequate analgesia and tolerable side effects.

HOW SUPPLIED: Patch: 5mcg/hr, 10mcg/hr, 20mcg/hr

CONTRAINDICATIONS: Management of acute pain or opioid analgesia for a short period of time, postoperative pain, mild/intermittent pain. Known or suspected paralytic ileus, severe bronchial asthma or significant respiratory depression.

WARNINGS/PRECAUTIONS: May cause respiratory depression; caution with significant chronic obstructive pulmonary disease or cor pulmonale, other risks of substantially decreased respiratory reserve (eg, asthma, severe obesity, sleep apnea, myxedema, clinically significant kyphoscoliosis, CNS depression), hypoxia, hypercapnia, and pre-existing respiratory depression. May cause CNS depression. May increase cerebrospinal fluid (CSF) pressure; caution with head injury, intracranial lesions, or other sources of pre-existing increased intracranial pressure (ICP). May obscure neurological signs associated with increased ICP with head injuries. May prolong QTc interval; caution with hypokalemia or clinically unstable cardiac disease. Avoid use with history of long QT syndrome or if an immediate family member has this condition. May cause severe hypotension; caution in circulatory shock. May cause hepatic abnormalities; obtain baseline and periodic LFTs in patients at increased risk of hepatotoxicity. D/C if severe application-site reaction develops. Acute and chronic hypersensitivity reactions reported. If fever develops, monitor for side effects and adjust dose if necessary. May impair mental and physical abilities. Not approved for management of addictive disorders. Caution with history of a seizure disorder, alcoholism, delirium tremens, debilitation, adrenocortical insufficiency, kyphoscoliosis associated with respiratory compromise, myxedema or hypothyroidism, prostatic hypertrophy or urethral stricture, toxic psychosis, biliary tract dysfunction, or severe impairment of hepatic, pulmonary, or renal function. May cause spasm of the spincter of Oddi; caution with biliary tract disease. May increase serum amylase. May obscure diagnosis or clinical course of patients with acute abdominal conditions; caution in patients at risk of developing ileus.

ADVERSE REACTIONS: Nausea, headache, application-site pruritus, irritation, erythema or rash, dizziness, constipation, somnolence, vomiting, dry mouth, peripheral edema, fatigue, hyperhidrosis, falling.

INTERACTIONS: Concomitant use with other CNS depressants (eg, alcohol, sedatives, anxiolytics, hypnotics, neuroleptics, muscle relaxants, other opioids) may cause respiratory depression, hypotension, profound sedation, or coma. Avoid use within 14 days of MAOIs. Avoid use with Class IA antiarrhythmics (eg, quinidine, procainamide, disopyramide) or Class III antiarrhythmics (eg, sotalol, amiodarone, dofetilide). Concurrent use with phenothiazines or other agents may cause hypotensive effects. Concomitant use with certain protease inhibitors (eg, atazanavir, atazanavir/ritonavir) may elevate levels. May interact with CYP3A4 inhibitors depending on route of administration as well as specificity of enzyme inhibition. May reduce efficacy if coadministered with CYP3A4 inducers (eg, phenobarbital, carbamazepine, phenytoin, rifampin). Caution with benzodiazepines. Concomitant use with skeletal muscle relaxants may enhance neuromuscular blocking action.

PREGNANCY: Category C, not for use in nursing.

MECHANISM OF ACTION: Opioid analgesic; clinical action results from binding to opioid receptors.

PHARMACOKINETICS: Absorption: Absolute bioavailability (15%). (5mcg/hr) C_{max}=176pg/mL, AUC=12087pg•h/mL. (10mcg/hr) C_{max}=191pg/mL, AUC=27035pg•h/mL. (20mcg/hr) C_{max}=471pg/mL, AUC=54294pg•h/mL. **Distribution:** Plasma protein binding (96%); Found in breast milk; readily crosses placenta. (IV) V_d=430L. **Metabolism:** Liver. N-dealkylation by CYP3A4 to norbuprenorphine (major metabolite). Glucuronidation by UGT isoenzymes (mainly UGT1A1 and 2B7) to buprenorphine 3-O-glucuronide. **Elimination:** Feces (70%), urine (27%).

NURSING CONSIDERATIONS

Assessment: Assess for opioid tolerance, level of pain intensity, type of pain, clinical risk for opioid abuse or addiction, patient's general condition and medical status such as compromised respiratory function, hepatic/renal function, debilitation, hypothyroidism, prostatic hypertrophy, seizures, toxic psychosis, biliary tract dysfunction, fever, pregnancy/nursing status, and for possible drug interactions.

Monitoring: Monitor for signs/symptoms of respiratory depression, CNS depression, elevation of CSF pressure, QTc prolongation, hypotension, hepatotoxicity, seizures, spasm of the spincter of Oddi, drug addiction, and level of pain intensity. Monitor LFTs and serum amylase levels.

Patient Counseling: Advise that patch is intended to be worn for 7 days. Apply to upper outer arms, upper chest, upper back, or the side of the chest. Rotate application site with a minimum of 3 weeks between applications to a previously used site. Apply patch to a hairless or nearly hairless skin site. Avoid exposing application site to external heat sources. If patch falls off during use, a new patch should be applied to a different skin site. Medication may impair mental/physicial abilities; use caution when performing dangerous tasks (eg, operating machinery/driving). Notify physician of all medications currently taking and avoid use of other CNS depressants and alcohol during therapy. Advise that medication may lead to dependence and to not exceed prescribed dosage. Advise to avoid abruptly d/c medication. Contact physician if signs/symptoms of respiratory depression develop.

Administration: Transdermal patch. Apply immediately after removal from individually sealed pouch. Do not use if the pouch seal is broken, cut, damaged, or changed in any way. Next patch should be applied to a different site. Apply to intact skin on upper outer arm, upper chest, upper back, or the side of the chest. **Storage:** 25°C (77°F); excursions permitted to 15-30°C (59-86°F).

BYETTA
exenatide (Amylin/Lilly)

RX

THERAPEUTIC CLASS: Incretin mimetic

INDICATIONS: Adjunct to diet and exercise to improve glycemic control in adults with type 2 diabetes mellitus (DM).

DOSAGE: *Adults:* Initial: 5mcg SQ bid, at anytime within 60 mins before am & pm meals (or before the two main meals of day approx. 6 hrs or more apart). Titrate: May increase to 10mcg bid after 1 month. CrCl 30-50mL/min: Caution when initiating or escalating doses from 5mcg to 10mcg. Reduction of sulfonylurea dose may be considered to reduce risk of hypoglycemia.

HOW SUPPLIED: Inj: 5mcg/dose, 10mcg/dose [60-dose prefilled pen]

WARNINGS/PRECAUTIONS: Not a substitute for insulin. Should not be used in patients with type 1 diabetes or for the treatment of diabetic ketoacidosis. Acute pancreatitis reported; d/c if suspected. Increased SrCr, renal impairment, worsened chronic renal failure, and acute renal failure reported; avoid with severe renal impairment (CrCl <30mL/min) or end stage renal disease (ESRD). Avoid with severe GI disease or a history of pancreatitis. Caution with renal transplantation. May develop immunogenicity; consider alternative antidiabetic therapy if there is worsening glycemic control or failure to achieve targeted glycemic control. Hypersensitivity reactions reported; d/c if hypersensitivity reaction occurs. Caution in elderly.

ADVERSE REACTIONS: N/V, immunogenicity, diarrhea, feeling jittery, dizziness, headache, dyspepsia, asthenia, gastroesophageal reflux disease, hyperhidrosis, hypoglycemia.

INTERACTIONS: Caution with oral medications with narrow therapeutic indexes or require rapid GI absorption. Drugs dependent on threshold concentrations for efficacy (eg, contraceptives, antibiotics) should be taken 1 hr before. Concomitant use of warfarin may increase INR; monitor PT more frequently. Increased risk of hypoglycemia when used in combination with sulfonylureas and with other glucose-independent insulin secretagogues (eg, meglitinides). May decrease concentrations of acetaminophen, digoxin, lovastatin. Concurrent use with insulin has not been studied and cannot be recommended.

PREGNANCY: Category C, not for use in nursing.

MECHANISM OF ACTION: Incretin-mimetic agent, GLP-1 receptor agonist; enhances glucose-dependent insulin secretion by the pancreatic β-cell, suppresses inappropriately elevated glucagon secretion, and slows gastric emptying.

PHARMACOKINETICS: Absorption: (SQ) C_{max}=211pg/mL, AUC=1036pg•h/mL, T_{max}=2.1 hrs. **Distribution:** V_d=28.3L. **Elimination:** $T_{1/2}$=2.4 hrs.

NURSING CONSIDERATIONS

Assessment: Assess for type 1 diabetes, diabetic ketoacidosis, history of pancreatitis, renal impairment, severe GI disease, pregnancy/nursing status, and for possible drug interactions. Assess glucose and HbA1c levels.

Monitoring: Monitor for signs/symptoms of acute pancreatitis (eg, severe abdominal pain, vomiting), hypoglycemia, GI events (eg, N/V, diarrhea), immunogenicity, and for hypersensitivity reactions. Monitor renal function, glucose levels, and HbA1c levels.

Patient Counseling: Advise of the potential risks and benefits of therapy. Never share injection pen with another patient. Inform about self-management practices (eg, proper storage of drug, injection technique, timing of dosage and concomitant oral drugs, adherence to meal planning, regular physical activity). Administer within 60-min period before morning and evening meals. Advise to not administer after a meal. Inform that if a dose is missed, treatment regimen should be resumed as prescribed with the next scheduled dose. Inform physician if pregnant or intend to become pregnant. Contact physician if signs/symptoms suggestive of acute pancreatitis (eg, severe abdominal pain), renal dysfunction, or hypersensitivity develop.

Administration: SQ route. Inject into thigh, abdomen, or upper arm. Refer to PI for further information on administration and preparation. **Storage:** Prior to first use, keep at 2-8°C (36-46°F). After first use, can be kept at ≤77°F (25°C). Do not freeze. Protect from light. Discard pen 30 days after the first use, even if some drug remains.

BYSTOLIC   RX
nebivolol (Forest)

THERAPEUTIC CLASS: Selective beta₁-blocker

INDICATIONS: Treatment of HTN alone or in combination with other antihypertensive agents.

DOSAGE: *Adults:* Individualize dose. Initial: 5mg qd, as monotherapy or in combination with other agents. Titrate: May increase dose at 2-week intervals. Max: 40mg. Moderate Hepatic/Severe Renal Impairment (CrCl <30mL/min): Initial: 2.5mg qd; titrate up slowly if needed.

HOW SUPPLIED: Tab: 2.5mg, 5mg, 10mg, 20mg

CONTRAINDICATIONS: Severe bradycardia, heart block >1st degree, cardiogenic shock, decompensated cardiac failure, sick sinus syndrome (unless permanent pacemaker in place), severe hepatic impairment (Child-Pugh >B).

WARNINGS/PRECAUTIONS: Severe exacerbation of angina, myocardial infarction, and ventricular arrhythmias reported in patients with coronary artery disease (CAD) following abrupt d/c; taper over 1-2 weeks when possible. Avoid with bronchospastic disease. May precipitate/aggravate symptoms of arterial insufficiency in patients with peripheral vascular disease (PVD). Caution with severe renal/moderate hepatic impairment. May mask signs/symptoms of hypoglycemia or hyperthyroidism. Abrupt withdrawal may also exacerbate symptoms of hyperthyroidism or precipitate a thyroid storm. Caution with history of severe anaphylactic reactions. Patients with known/suspected pheochromocytoma should initially receive an α-blocker prior to use of any β-blocker.

ADVERSE REACTIONS: Headache, fatigue, dizziness, diarrhea, nausea.

INTERACTIONS: Increased levels with CYP2D6 inhibitors (eg, quinidine, propafenone, paroxetine, fluoxetine) and cimetidine. Decreases AUC and C_{max} of sildenafil. Monitor closely with anesthetic agents which depress myocardial function (eg, ether, cyclopropane, trichloroethylene). May potentiate hypoglycemic effect of glucose-lowering agents (eg, insulin, oral hypoglycemic agents). Can exacerbate the effects of myocardial depressants/inhibitors of AV conduction, such as certain calcium antagonists (particularly verapamil and diltiazem type) or antiarrhythmic agents (eg, disopyramide). Excessive reduction of sympathetic activity may occur with catecholamine-depleting drugs (eg, reserpine, guanethidine). D/C for several days before gradually tapering clonidine. Increased risk of bradycardia with digitalis glycosides. Monitor closely and adjust dose with CYP2D6 inducers. Avoid with other β-blockers. Additional antihypertensive effects with up to two other antihypertensive agents (ACE inhibitors, angiotensin II antagonists, thiazide diuretics).

PREGNANCY: Category C, not for use in nursing.

MECHANISM OF ACTION: β-adrenergic receptor blocking agent; mechanism has not been established. Possible factors include decreased HR and myocardial contractility, diminution of tonic sympathetic outflow to the periphery from cerebral vasomotor centers, suppression of renin activity, vasodilation, and decreased peripheral vascular resistance.

PHARMACOKINETICS: Absorption: T_{max}=1.5-4 hrs. **Distribution:** Plasma protein binding (98%). **Metabolism**: Glucuronidation and hydroxylation via CYP2D6. **Elimination**: Urine (38% extensive metabolizers [EM]), (67% poor metabolizers [PM]); feces (44% EM), (13% PM); $T_{1/2}$=12 hrs (CYP2D6 EM), 19 hrs (PM).

NURSING CONSIDERATIONS

Assessment: Assess for hypersensitivity, severe bradycardia, heart block, cardiogenic shock, cardiac failure, sick sinus syndrome, CAD, bronchospastic disease, hepatic/renal impairment, PVD, history of severe anaphylactic reactions, pheochromocytoma, diabetes, hyperthyroidism, pregnancy/nursing status, and possible drug interactions. Obtain baseline LFTs, renal function and blood glucose.

Monitoring: Monitor vital signs, serum glucose level, ECG, hepatic/renal function. Monitor for signs/symptoms of cardiac failure, thyrotoxicosis, precipitation or aggravation of arterial insufficiency, hypotension, and hypersensitivity reactions. Monitor closely when therapy is continued perioperatively.

Patient Counseling: Advise patients to take nebivolol regularly and continuously, as directed. Inform that drug can be taken with/without food and if a dose is missed, take the next scheduled dose only. Advise to consult a physician if any difficulty in breathing occurs or signs and symptoms of worsening congestive heart failure (CHF) (eg, weight gain, increased SOB, excessive bradycardia) develop. Caution about operating automobiles, using machinery, or engaging in tasks requiring alertness. Instruct not to interrupt or d/c therapy without consulting physician. Caution about possible drug interactions. Caution diabetic patients receiving insulin or PO hypoglycemic agents of masking of the manifestations of hypoglycemia, particularly tachycardia.

Administration: Oral route. **Storage:** 20-25°C (68-77°F). Dispense in a tight, light-resistant container.

CADUET   RX
atorvastatin calcium - amlodipine besylate (Pfizer)

THERAPEUTIC CLASS: Calcium channel blocker/HMG-CoA reductase inhibitor

INDICATIONS: (Amlodipine) Treatment of HTN, chronic stable or vasospastic angina (Prinzmetal's or Variant Angina) alone or in combination with other antihypertensives/antianginals. To reduce the risks of hospitalization due to angina and to reduce risk of coronary revascularization procedure in patients with recently documented coronary artery disease (CAD) by angiography and without heart failure (ejection fraction <40%). (Atorvastatin) To reduce the risk of myocardial infarction (MI), stroke, revascularization procedures, and angina in adults without clinically evident coronary heart disease (CHD) but with multiple risk factors for CHD. To reduce the risk of MI and stroke in patients with type 2 diabetes mellitus, and without clinically evident CHD, but with multiple risk factors for CHD. To reduce the risk of non-fatal MI, fatal and non-fatal stroke, revascularization procedures, hospitalization for congestive heart failure (CHF), and angina in patients with clinically evident CHD. Adjunct to diet to reduce total cholesterol (total-C), LDL-C, TG, and Apo B levels, and to increase HDL-C in primary hypercholesterolemia (heterozygous familial and nonfamilial) and mixed dyslipidemia (Types IIa and IIb). Treatment of primary dysbetalipoproteinemia (Type III) inadequately responding to diet. Adjunct to other lipid-lowering treatments or if treatments are unavailable, to reduce total-C and LDL-C in homozygous familial hypercholesterolemia. Adjunct to diet to lower total-C, LDL-C, and Apo B in boys and postmenarchal girls, 10-17 yrs of age, with heterozygous familial hypercholesterolemia.

DOSAGE: *Adults:* Individualize dosing. (Amlodipine): HTN: Initial: 5mg qd. Titrate over 7-14 days according to patient's need. Max: 10mg qd. Elderly/Hepatic Dysfunction/Concomitant Antihypertensive Therapy: Initial: 2.5mg qd. Angina/CAD: 5-10mg qd. Elderly/Hepatic Dysfunction: 5mg qd. (Atorvastatin): Hypercholesterolemia/Mixed Dyslipidemia: Initial: 10-20mg qd (or 40mg qd for LDL-C reduction >45%). Titrate: Adjust dose if needed at 2-4 week intervals. Usual: 10-80mg qd. Homozygous Familial Hypercholesterolemia: 10-80mg qd. Concomitant with Cyclosporine: 10mg qd. Concomitant with Clarithromycin/Itraconazole/Ritonavir plus Saquinavir or Lopinavir: 20mg qd. Replacement Therapy: May substitute for individually titrated components.
Pediatrics: 6-17 yrs: (Amlodipine): HTN: 2.5-5mg qd. Max: 5mg/day. 10-17 yrs (Postmenarchal): (Atorvastatin): Heterozygous Familial Hypercholesterolemia: Initial: 10mg/day. Titrate: Adjust dose if needed at intervals of ≥4 weeks. Max: 20mg/day.

HOW SUPPLIED: Tab: (Amlodipine-Atorvastatin) 2.5mg-10mg, 2.5mg-20mg, 2.5mg-40mg, 5mg-10mg, 5mg-20mg, 5mg-40mg, 5mg-80mg, 10mg-10mg, 10mg-20mg, 10mg-40mg, 10mg-80mg

CONTRAINDICATIONS: Active liver disease, unexplained persistent elevations of serum transaminases, pregnancy, nursing mothers.

WARNINGS/PRECAUTIONS: Rare cases of rhabdomyolysis with acute renal failure secondary to myoglobinuria reported. Increased risk of rhabdomyolysis in patients with history of renal impairment. D/C if markedly elevated CPK levels occur, if myopathy is diagnosed or suspected, or if predisposition to renal failure secondary to rhabdomyolysis develop. May cause biochemical abnormalities of liver function; monitor LFTs prior to therapy, at 12 weeks after initiation, with dose elevation, and periodically thereafter. Reduce dose or d/c if AST or ALT >3X ULN persists. Symptomatic hypotension may occur. May cause worsening angina and acute MI after starting or increasing the dose. Increased risk of hemorrhagic stroke in patients with recent stroke or transient ischemic attack (TIA). Caution in the elderly.

ADVERSE REACTIONS: Headache, edema, palpitations, dizziness, fatigue, infection, diarrhea, rash, arthralgia, asthenia, abdominal pain, pain in extremities, urinary tract infection, dyspepsia, myalgia.

INTERACTIONS: (Atorvastatin) May increase levels with strong CYP3A4 inhibitors and grapefruit juice (>1.2L/day). Inhibitors of OATP1B1 (eg, cyclosporine) may increase bioavailability. Decreased levels with inducers of CYP3A4. Coadministration with digoxin may increase digoxin levels. Coadministration with oral contraceptives increases AUC of norethindrone and ethinyl estradiol. Increased risk of myopathy with immunosuppressive drugs, strong CYP3A4 inhibitors, cyclosporine, fibric acid derivatives, erythromycin, clarithromycin, combination of ritonavir plus saquinavir or lopinavir plus ritonavir, niacin, and azole antifungals. Caution with drugs that decrease levels and activity of endogenous steroid hormones (eg, ketoconazole, spironolactone, cimetidine). Refer to PI for detailed pharmacokinetic changes with co-administered drugs.

PREGNANCY: Category X, not for use in nursing

MECHANISM OF ACTION: Amlodipine: Dihydropyridine calcium channel blocker; inhibits transmembrane influx of Ca^{2+} ions into vascular smooth muscle and cardiac muscle. Atorvastatin: HMG-CoA reductase inhibitor; inhibits conversion of HMG-CoA to mevalonate (precursor of sterols, including cholesterol).

PHARMACOKINETICS: Absorption: Amlodipine: Absolute bioavailability (64-90%); T_{max}=6-12 hrs. Atorvastatin: Rapid; absolute bioavailability (14%); T_{max}=1-2 hrs; **Distribution:** Amlodipine: Plasma protein binding (93%). Atorvastatin: V_d=381L; plasma protein binding (≥98%); found in breast milk. **Metabolism:** Amlodipine: (Extensive) Liver. Atorvastatin: (Extensive) CYP3A4; ortho- and parahydroxylated derivatives (active metabolites). **Elimination:** Amlodipine: Urine (10% unchanged; 60% metabolite); $T_{1/2}$=30-50 hrs. Atorvastatin: Bile (major), urine (<2%); $T_{1/2}$=14 hrs.

NURSING CONSIDERATIONS

Assessment: Assess for active or history of liver disease, unexplained and persistent elevations in serum transaminase levels, pregnancy/nursing status, alcohol intake, recent stroke or TIA, heart disease (eg, MI, severe aortic stenosis), severe obstructive CAD and for possible drug interactions. Perform LFTs prior to therapy.

Monitoring: Monitor LFTs at 12 weeks following initiation of therapy and any drug dose elevation, then periodically thereafter. Monitor for signs/symptoms of hypotension, rhabdomyolysis with acute renal failure, hypersensitivity reaction, angina, and myopathy. Monitor LFTs, creatine phosphokinase.

Patient Counseling: Inform about potential risks/benefits of therapy. Instruct to follow standard cholesterol-lowering diet and . Advise to seek medical attention if symptoms of hypotension, hypersensitivity reaction, angina, myopathy (eg, unexplained muscle pain, tenderness, fever, malaise) or other adverse reactions occur. Instruct to avoid alcohol consumption Instruct to notify physician if pregnant/nursing or planning to become pregnant.

Administration: Oral route. **Storage:** 25°C (77°F); excursions permitted to 15-30°C (59-86°F).

CALAN
RX

verapamil HCl (G.D. Searle)

THERAPEUTIC CLASS: Calcium channel blocker (nondihydropyridine)

INDICATIONS: Treatment of essential hypertension and vasospastic, unstable, and chronic stable angina. Control of ventricular rate at rest and during stress in patients with chronic atrial flutter and/or atrial fibrillation (A-Fib), in association with digitalis. Prophylaxis of repetitive paroxysmal supraventricular tachycardia (PSVT).

DOSAGE: *Adults:* HTN: Individualize dosing by titration. Initial: 80mg tid. Usual: 360-480mg qd. Elderly/Small Stature: Initial: 40mg tid. Upward titration should be based on therapeutic efficacy. Angina: Usual: 80-120mg tid. Patients with Increased Response to Verapamil (eg, Elderly, Decreased Hepatic Function): Initial: 40mg tid. Titrate: Increase daily or weekly. Upward titration should be based on therapeutic efficacy and safety evaluated approximately 8 hrs after the previous dose. A-Fib (Digitalized): Usual: 240-320mg qd given in divided doses tid-qid. PSVT Prophylaxis (Non-Digitalized): 240-480mg/day given in divided doses tid-qid. Max: 480mg qd. Severe Hepatic Dysfunction: Give 30% of normal dose.

HOW SUPPLIED: Tab: 40mg, 80mg*, 120mg* *scored

CONTRAINDICATIONS: Severe left ventricular dysfunction, hypotension and cardiogenic shock. Sick-sinus syndrome and 2nd- or 3rd-degree atrioventricular (AV) block (except with functioning ventricular pacemaker). A-Fib/Flutter with an accessory bypass tract (eg, Wolff-Parkinson-White, Lown-Ganong-Levine syndromes).

WARNINGS/PRECAUTIONS: Avoid with moderate to severe cardiac failure, and ventricular dysfunction if taking a β-blocker. May cause hypotension, congestive heart failure (CHF), pulmonary edema, AV block, transient bradycardia, PR interval prolongation. Elevated transaminases (eg, elevations in alkaline phosphatase, SGOT, SGPT and bilirubin) occurred; monitor LFTs periodically. Hepatocellular injury reported. Caution with impaired hepatic function; give 30% of normal dose with severe hepatic dysfunction. Caution with renal impairment; monitor for abnormal PR interval prolongation. May decrease neuromuscular transmission in patients with Duchenne's muscular dystrophy; reduce dose with decreased neuromuscular transmission. Sinus bradycardia, 2nd-degree AV block, pulmonary edema, hypotension, and sinus arrest reported in patients with hypertrophic cardiomyopathy. Ventricular fibrillation has occurred in patients with A-fib/flutter and an accessory bypass tract.

ADVERSE REACTIONS: Constipation, dizziness, sinus bradycardia, hypotension, 2nd-degree AV block.

INTERACTIONS: Additive effects on HR, AV conduction, and contractility with β-blockers. Potentiates other antihypertensives (eg, vasodilators, ACE inhibitors, diuretics). May increase digoxin, carbamazepine, theophylline, cyclosporine, and alcohol levels. Avoid disopyramide within 48 hrs before or 24 hrs after verapamil. May reduce clearance of digitoxin. Additive negative inotropic effects and AV conduction prolongation with flecainide. Avoid quinidine with hypertrophic cardiomyopathy. Increased sensitivity to effects of lithium when used concomitantly; monitor carefully. Increased clearance with phenobarbital. Rifampin may reduce oral bioavailability. May potentiate neuromuscular blockers (curare and depolarizing); both agents may need dose reduction. Careful titration is needed when concomitantly used with inhalation anesthetics to avoid excessive cardiovascular (CV) depression. Concurrent use with telithromycin may cause hypotension and bradyarrhythmias. May produce asymptomatic bradycardia with a wandering pacemaker with timolol eyedrops. Decrease metoprolol and propranolol clearance while variable effect with atenolol. Excessive reduction in BP with prazosin. Monitor HR with clonidine.

PREGNANCY: Category C, not for use in nursing.

MECHANISM OF ACTION: Calcium channel blocker (nondihydropyridine); modulates influx of ionic calcium across cell membrane of arterial smooth muscle, and in conductile and contractile myocardial cells.

PHARMACOKINETICS: Absorption: Bioavailability (20-35%), T_{max}=1-2 hrs. **Distribution:** Plasma protein binding (90%); found in CSF and breast milk, crosses blood-brain barrier and placenta. **Metabolism:** Liver (extensive); norverapamil (metabolite). **Elimination:** Urine (70%, metabolites) (3-4%, unchanged), feces (≥16%); $T_{1/2}$=2.8-7.4 hrs (single dose), 4.5-12 hrs (repetitive dose).

NURSING CONSIDERATIONS

Assessment: Assess for severe left ventricular dysfunction, Duchenne's muscular dystrophy, hypertrophic cardiomyopathy, cardiac failure, cardiogenic shock, hypotension, sick sinus syndrome, AV block, A-Fib/Flutter with accessory bypass tract (WPW), hepatic/renal impairment, hypersensitivity, pregnancy/nursing status, and possible drug interactions.

Monitoring: Monitor LFTs and renal function periodically. Monitor for abnormal PR interval prolongation for toxicity; signs/symptoms of hepatotoxicity, renal dysfunction, CV events (hypotension), and hypersensitivity reactions.

Patient Counseling: Advise to seek medical attention if symptoms of hepatotoxicity (malaise, fever, right upper quadrant pain), CV events (hypotension), or hypersensitivity reactions occur. Counsel not to breastfeed and to report immediately if pregnant.

Administration: Oral route. **Storage:** 15-25°C (59-77°F). Protect from light. Dispense in tight, light-resistant containers.

CALAN SR   RX
verapamil HCl (Pharmacia & Upjohn)

THERAPEUTIC CLASS: Calcium channel blocker (nondihydropyridine)

INDICATIONS: Management of essential hypertension.

DOSAGE: *Adults:* ≥18 yrs: Initial: 180mg qam. Titrate: If inadequate response, increase to 240mg qam, then 180mg bid; or 240mg qam plus 120mg qpm, then 240mg q12h. Elderly/Small Stature: Initial: 120mg qam. Take with food.

HOW SUPPLIED: Tab, Extended-Release: 120mg, 180mg*, 240mg* *scored

CONTRAINDICATIONS: Severe left ventricular dysfunction, hypotension, cardiogenic shock, sick sinus syndrome or 2nd- or 3rd-degree AV block (except with functioning ventricular pacemaker), atrial fibrillation/flutter (A-Fib/Flutter) with an accessory bypass tract (eg, Wolff-Parkinson-White, Lown-Ganong-Levine syndromes).

WARNINGS/PRECAUTIONS: Avoid with moderate to severe cardiac failure, and ventricular dysfunction if taking a β-blocker. May cause hypotension, congestive heart failure (CHF), pulmonary edema, AV block, transient bradycardia, PR interval prolongation. Monitor LFTs periodically; hepatocellular injury reported. Caution with hypertrophic cardiomyopathy, renal or hepatic dysfunction. Decrease dose with decreased neuromuscular transmission.

ADVERSE REACTIONS: Constipation, dizziness, nausea, hypotension, headache, edema, CHF, fatigue, elevated liver enzymes, bradycardia, AV block, heart failure.

INTERACTIONS: Additive effects on HR, AV conduction, and contractility with β-blockers. Potentiates other antihypertensives. May increase digoxin, carbamazepine, theophylline, cyclosporine, and alcohol levels. Avoid disopyramide within 48 hrs before or 24 hrs after verapamil. Additive negative inotropic effects and AV conduction prolongation with flecainide. Avoid quinidine with hypertrophic cardiomyopathy. Inceased sensitivity to effects of lithium; monitor carefully. Increased clearance with phenobarbital. Rifampin may reduce oral bioavailability. May potentiate neuromuscular blockers; both agents may need dose reduction. Careful titration is needed with inhalation anesthetics to avoid excessive cardiovascular (CV) depression. May produce asymptomatic bradycardia with timolol eyedrops. Decrease metoprolol and propranolol clearance.

PREGNANCY: Category C, not for use in nursing.

MECHANISM OF ACTION: Calcium channel blocker; modulates influx of ionic calcium across cell membrane of arterial smooth muscle and in conductile and contractile myocardial cells.

PHARMACOKINETICS: Absorption: Absolute bioavailability (20-35%); T_{max}=7.7 hrs; C_{max}=79ng/mL; AUC=841ng•h/mL. **Distribution:** Plasma protein binding (90%). **Metabolism:** Biotransformation; norverapamil (metabolite). **Elimination:** Urine (70%, metabolites), (3-4%, unchanged); feces (16%); $T_{1/2}$=4.5-12 hrs.

NURSING CONSIDERATIONS

Assessment: Assess for severe left ventricular dysfunction, Duchenne's muscular dystrophy, severe heart failure, hypotension, sick sinus syndrome, AV block, atrial flutter/fibrillation with accessory bypass tract (eg, Wolff-Parkinson-White), hypertrophic cardiomyopathy, hepatic/renal impairment, hypersensitivity, pregnancy/nursing status, and possible drug interactions.

Monitoring: Monitor LFTs and renal function periodically; abnormal PR-interval prolongation for toxicity. Monitor for signs/symptoms of hepatotoxicity, renal dysfunction, CV events (hypotension), and hypersensitivity reactions.

Patient Counseling: Advise to seek medical attention if symptoms of hepatotoxicity (malaise, fever, right upper quadrant pain), cardiovascular events (hypotension), or hypersensitivity reactions occur.

Administration: Oral route. **Storage:** 15-25°C (59-77°F). Protect from light and moisture. Dispense in tight, light-resistant containers.

CALDOLOR   RX

ibuprofen (Cumberland)

> NSAIDs increase risk of serious cardiovascular (CV) thrombotic events, myocardial infarction (MI), stroke, and serious GI adverse events including bleeding, ulceration, and perforation of the stomach and intestine. Contraindicated for the treatment of perioperative pain in the setting of coronary artery bypass graft (CABG) surgery.

THERAPEUTIC CLASS: NSAID

INDICATIONS: Management of mild to moderate pain and moderate to severe pain as an adjunct to opioid analgesics in adults. For reduction of fever in adults.

DOSAGE: *Adults:* Analgesia: 400-800mg IV q6h prn. Infusion time must be no less than 30 min. Antipyretic: 400mg IV followed by 400mg q4-6h or 100-200mg q4h prn. Infusion time must be no less than 30 min. Elderly: Start at lower end of dosing range.

HOW SUPPLIED: Inj: 100mg/mL

CONTRAINDICATIONS: Asthma, urticaria, or allergic-type reactions to aspirin or other NSAIDs. Treatment of perioperative pain in the setting of coronary artery bypass graft (CABG) surgery.

WARNINGS/PRECAUTIONS: Severe hepatic reactions (rare) reported (eg, jaundice, fulminant hepatitis, liver necrosis, and hepatic failure); d/c if signs/symptoms of liver disease develop or if systemic manifestations occur. May lead to onset of new HTN or worsening of pre-existing HTN; monitor BP closely. Fluid retention and edema reported; caution in patients with fluid retention or heart failure. Caution in patients with considerable dehydration. Renal papillary necrosis and other renal injury reported after long-term use. Caution with impaired renal function, heart failure, liver dysfunction, the elderly and those taking diuretics and ACE inhibitors. Anaphylactoid reactions may occur. May cause serious skin adverse events (eg, exfoliative dermatitis, Stevens-Johnson syndrome [SJS], and toxic epidermal necrolysis [TEN]). Avoid in late pregnancy; may cause premature closure of ductus arteriosus. May mask signs of inflammation and fever. Anemia may occur; with long-term use, monitor Hgb/Hct if signs or symptoms of anemia develop. May inhibit platelet aggregation and prolong bleeding time; monitor with coagulation disorders. Infusion of drug product without dilution may cause hemolysis. Caution with pre-existing asthma. Blurred or diminished vision, scotomata, and changes in color vision reported; d/c if such complaints develop. Aseptic meningitis with fever and coma reported in patients on oral ibuprofen therapy. Caution in elderly.

ADVERSE REACTIONS: N/V, flatulence, headache, hemorrhage, dizziness, urinary retention, peripheral edema, anemia, dyspepsia, eosinophilia, hypokalemia, hypoproteinemia, neutropenia.

INTERACTIONS: May increase adverse effects with ASA. Synergistic effects on GI bleeding with warfarin. May decrease natriuretic effect of furosemide and thiazides; monitor for renal failure. May impair therapeutic response to ACE inhibitors, thiazides or loop diuretics. Increase risk of renal effects with diuretics or ACE inhibitors. May increase lithium levels; monitor for toxicity. May enhance methotrexate toxicity; caution when coadministered. Increase GI bleeding with use of oral corticosteroids or anticoagulants and use of alcohol.

PREGNANCY: Category C (prior to 30 weeks' gestation); Category D (starting 30 weeks' gestation), not for use in nursing.

MECHANISM OF ACTION: NSAID; not established. May be related to prostaglandin synthetase inhibition. Possesses anti-inflammatory, analgesic, and antipyretic activity.

PHARMACOKINETICS: Absorption: (400mg) AUC=109.3mcg•h/mL, (800mg) AUC=192.8mcg•h/mL; (400mg) C_{max}=39.2mcg/mL, (800mg) C_{max}=72.6mcg/mL. **Distribution:** Plasma protein binding (>99%). **Elimination:** (400mg) $T_{1/2}$=2.22 hrs, (800mg) $T_{1/2}$= 2.44 hrs.

NURSING CONSIDERATIONS

Assessment: Assess LFTs, CBC and coagulation profile. Assess for history of asthma, urticaria or allergic-type reaction with previous use of NSAIDs, asthma, perioperative pain in setting of CABG surgery, cardiovascular disease (CVD) or risk factors for CVD, HTN, fluid retention or HF, ulcer disease or GI bleeding, coagulation disorders or anticoagulant therapy, renal/hepatic impairment, pregnancy/nursing status, possible drug interactions.

Monitoring: Monitor BP during initiation of therapy and thereafter. Monitor Hgb/Hct, coagulation profiles, LFTs, and renal function. Monitor signs/symptoms of anaphylactic/anaphylactoid reactions, adverse skin events (eg, exfoliative dermatitis, SJS, TEN), eosinophilia, rash, GI bleeding/ulceration and perforation, anemia, CV thrombotic events, MI, stroke, new or worsening HTN, renal toxicity, renal papillary necrosis and other renal injury, ophthalmological effects (blurred or diminished vision, scotomata and changes in color vision) and aseptic meningitis.

Patient Counseling: Counsel about potential CV, GI, hepatotoxic, and skin adverse events, as well as possible weight gain/edema. Inform of the signs of an anaphylactoid reaction; d/c and initiate medical therapy if this occurs. Inform pregnant women starting at 30 weeks' gestation to avoid use of the product. Counsel patients to be well hydrated prior to administration in order to reduce renal adverse reactions.

Administration: IV (infusion) route. Infusion time must be no less than 30 mins. Must be diluted prior to infusion. Refer to PI for preparation and administration. **Storage:** 20-25°C (68-77°F). Diluted solutions are stable for up to 24 hrs at ambient temperature (approximately 20-25°C) and room lighting.

CAMBIA   RX
diclofenac potassium (Kowa)

NSAIDs may cause an increased risk of serious cardiovascular (CV) thrombotic events, myocardial infarction (MI), stroke and serious GI adverse events including bleeding, ulceration, and perforation of the stomach or intestines. Contraindicated for the treatment of perioperative pain in the setting of coronary artery bypass graft (CABG) surgery.

THERAPEUTIC CLASS: NSAID

INDICATIONS: Acute treatment of migraine attacks with or without aura in adults ≥18 yrs.

DOSAGE: *Adults:* ≥18 yrs: Administer 1 packet (50mg) in 1-2 oz. (30-60mL) water. Mix well and drink immediately. Do not use liquids other than water.

HOW SUPPLIED: Powder: 50mg

CONTRAINDICATIONS: Asthma, urticaria, or allergic reactions after taking ASA or other NSAIDs. Treatment of peri-operative pain in the setting of CABG surgery.

WARNINGS/PRECAUTIONS: Not indicated for prophylactic therapy of migraine. Safety and effectiveness not established for cluster headache. May lead to new onset or worsening of pre-existing HTN; monitor BP regularly. Elevation of one or more liver tests reported. D/C if abnormal LFTs or renal tests persist or worsen, if clinical signs and/or symptoms consistent with liver disease develop, or if systemic manifestations occur (eg, eosinophilia, rash, abdominal pain, diarrhea, dark urine). Caution with hepatic impairment. Fluid retention and edema reported; caution with fluid retention or heart failure. Caution when initiating treatment with considerable dehydration. Renal papillary necrosis and other renal injury reported after long-term use. Caution with renal/liver dysfunction. Not recommended for use with advanced renal disease; if therapy must be initiated, closely monitor renal function. May cause anaphylactoid reactions, serious skin adverse events (eg, exfoliative dermatitis, Stevens-Johnson syndrome [SJS], and toxic epidermal necrolysis [TEN]). May cause premature closure of ductus arteriosus; avoid in pregnancy starting at 30 weeks' gestation. May mask symptoms of infection (eg, fever, inflammation). Anemia may occur; monitor Hgb/Hct with long-term use. May inhibit platelet aggregation and prolong bleeding time; monitor platelet function in patients with coagulation disorders. Caution with pre-existing asthma, phenylketonurics and in the elderly.

ADVERSE REACTIONS: Abdominal pain, constipation, diarrhea, dyspepsia, flatulence, anemia, edema, N/V, dizziness, headache, rashes, heartburn, pruritus, abnormal renal function.

INTERACTIONS: See Contraindications. Caution with concomitant use of potentially hepatotoxic drugs (eg, acetaminophen, certain antibiotics, antiepileptics). Increased adverse effects with ASA. Synergistic effects on GI bleeding with anticoagulants (eg, warfarin). May diminish antihypertensive effect of ACE inhibitors. May reduce natriuretic effect of furosemide and thiazides. May increase lithium levels. May enhance methotrexate toxicity. May increase nephrotoxicity of cyclosporine. May affect pharmacokinetics with CYP2C9 inhibitors.

PREGNANCY: Category C (prior to 30 weeks' gestation) and D (starting at 30 weeks' gestation); not for use in nursing.

MECHANISM OF ACTION: NSAID (benzeneacetic acid derivative); mechanism not completely understood but may be related to prostaglandin synthetase inhibition.

PHARMACOKINETICS: Absorption: Absolute bioavailability (50%). T_{max}=0.25 hr. **Distribution:** V_d=1.3 L/kg; plasma protein binding (>99%). **Metabolism:** Glucoronidation or sulfation via CYP2C8, 2C9, 3A4; 4'-hydroxydiclofenac (major metabolite), 5-hydroxy-, 3'-hydroxy-, 4',5-dihydroxy- and 3'-hydroxy-4'-methoxy diclofenac (minor metabolites). **Elimination:** Urine (65%), bile (35%); $T_{1/2}$=2 hrs.

NURSING CONSIDERATIONS

Assessment: Assess LFTs, renal function, CBC, platelet count and chemistry profile. Assess for asthma, urticaria or allergic-type reactions after taking aspirin or other NSAIDs, risk factors for cardiovascular (CV) disease, GI adverse events, history of ulcer disease, GI bleeding, smoking, alcohol use, health status, pre existing HTN, fluid retention, heart failure, dehydration, renal/liver dysfunction, coagulation disorders, pregnancy/nursing status, and possible drug interactions.

Monitoring: Monitor for signs/symptoms of CV thrombotic events, MI, stroke, GI adverse events (eg, inflammation, bleeding, ulceration, perforation), liver injury, anaphylactoid reactions, serious skin reactions (eg, exfoliative dermatitis, SJS, TEN). Periodic monitoring of BP, LFTs, renal function. CBC with differential and platelet count, coagulation parameters (especially if on anticoagulation therapy or with coagulation disorders).

Patient Counseling: Advise patients to be alert for signs/symptoms of chest pains, shortness of breath, weakness, slurring of speech, GI ulcerations, bleeding, epigastric pain, dyspepsia, melena, hematemesis, anaphylactoid reactions (eg, difficulty breathing, swelling of face or throat), skin rash and blisters, fever, other signs of hypersensitivity (eg, itching) during therapy. Inform about signs/symptoms of hepatotoxicity (eg, nausea, fatigue, lethargy, pruritus, jaundice, right upper quadrant tenderness and flulike symptoms); d/c therapy immediately if any of these occur. Notify healthcare professional if signs/symptoms of unexplained weight gain or edema occur. Advise women to avoid use in late pregnancy. Inform about the product contains aspartame equivalent to phenylalanine 25mg/packet.

Administration: Oral route. Mix packet well with 1-2 ounces of water and drink immediately. **Storage:** 25°C (77°F) Excursions permitted from 15-30°C (59-86°F).

CAMPATH
alemtuzumab (Genzyme)

RX

> Serious cytopenias including fatal pancytopenia/marrow hypoplasia, autoimmune idiopathic thrombocytopenia, and autoimmune hemolytic anemia may occur; avoid single doses >30mg or cumulative doses >90mg/week. Serious, including fatal, infusion reactions may occur; gradually escalate dose to prevent. Serious, including fatal, bacterial, viral, fungal, and protozoan infections can occur; administer prophylaxis against *Pneumocystis jirovecii* pneumonia (PCP) and herpes virus infections.

THERAPEUTIC CLASS: Monoclonal antibody/CD52-blocker

INDICATIONS: Treatment of B-cell chronic lymphocytic leukemia (B-CLL).

DOSAGE: *Adults:* Administer as IV infusion over 2 hrs. Initial: 3mg IV qd until tolerated, then increase to 10mg IV qd. Continue until tolerated, then increase to maint dose of 30mg (escalation to 30mg usually takes 3-7 days). Maint: 30mg/day IV 3x/week on alternate days up to 12 weeks. Max: 30mg single dose or 90mg/week. Refer to PI for recommended concomitant medications and dose modifications for neutropenia or thrombocytopenia.

HOW SUPPLIED: Inj: 30mg/mL.

WARNINGS/PRECAUTIONS: Premedicate with oral antihistamine, acetaminophen to avoid infusion reactions. Monitor BP, hypotensive symptoms in ischemic heart disease, with antihypertensives. If serious infection occurs, withhold treatment until infection resolves. Monitor CBC, platelets weekly during therapy and CD4 counts after therapy. D/C for autoimmune or severe hematologic adverse reactions. Severe, including fatal, autoimmune anemia and thrombocytopenia, and prolonged myelosuppression reported. Hemolytic anemia, pure red cell aplasia, bone marrow aplasia, and hypoplasia reported. D/C for autoimmune cytopenias. Severe and prolonged lymphopenias with increased incidence of opportunistic infections reported. Administer PCP and herpes viral prophylaxis for a minimum of 2 months after completion or until CD4+ count is ≥200 cells/μL and monitor for cytomegalovirus (CMV) infection during and for at least 2 months after completion of treatment. Administer only irradiated blood products to avoid transfusion-associated graft versus host disease (TAGVHD), unless emergent circumstances dictate immediate transfusion.

ADVERSE REACTIONS: Cytopenias, infusion reactions, CMV and other infections, immunosuppression, nausea, emesis, abdominal pain, insomnia, anxiety.

INTERACTIONS: Avoid live viral vaccines.

PREGNANCY: Category C, not for use in nursing.

C

MECHANISM OF ACTION: Monoclonal antibody/CD52-blocker; binds to CD52 on surfaces of B and T lymphocytes, monocytes, macrophages, NK cells, granulocytes and bone marrow cells, causing antibody-dependent cellular-mediated cell death.

PHARMACOKINETICS: Distribution: V_d=0.18L/kg. **Elimination:** (1st dose) $T_{1/2}$=11 hrs. (Last dose) $T_{1/2}$=6 days.

NURSING CONSIDERATIONS

Assessment: Assess pregnancy status. Obtain baseline CBC, CD4, and platelet count.

Monitoring: Monitor CBC and platelet counts weekly; CD4 count after therapy until recovery to >200 cells/mL; for CMV infections during therapy and 2 months following completion. Monitor for signs/symptoms of autoimmune anemia, thrombocytopenia, myelosuppression, hemolytic anemia, pure red cell aplasia, bone marrow aplasia, hypoplasia, infusion reactions (eg, pyrexia, chills/rigors, nausea, hypotension, urticaria, dyspnea, rash, emesis, bronchospasm), immunosuppression, and exacerbation of infection.

Patient Counseling: Instruct to administer only irradiated blood products to avoid TAGVHD, unless emergent circumstances dictate immediate transfusion. Use effective contraceptive methods during treatment and at least 6 months following therapy. Inform should not be immunized with live vaccines if recently treated. Counsel on importance of need to take premedications and prophylactic anti-infectives as prescribed. Advise to seek medical attention if symptoms of bleeding, easy bruising, petechiae/purpura, pallor, weakness, fatigue, infusion reactions, or infections occur.

Administration: IV infusion. Refer to PI for complete administration technique. **Storage:** 2-8°C (36-46°F). Do not freeze. If frozen, thaw at 2-8°C before administration. Protect from direct sunlight.

CAMPRAL   RX
acamprosate calcium (Forest)

THERAPEUTIC CLASS: GABA analog

INDICATIONS: Maintenance of abstinence from alcohol in patients with alcohol dependence who are abstinent at treatment initiation.

DOSAGE: *Adults:* 2 tabs tid. CrCl 30-50mL/min: 1 tab tid.

HOW SUPPLIED: Tab: 333mg

CONTRAINDICATIONS: Severe renal impairment (CrCl ≤30mL/min).

WARNINGS/PRECAUTIONS: Use does not eliminate or diminish withdrawal symptoms. Dose reduction required with renal impairment (CrCl ≤30-50mL/min). Suicidal events reported.

ADVERSE REACTIONS: Asthenia, pain, anorexia, diarrhea, flatulence, nausea, anxiety, depression, dizziness, dry mouth, insomnia, paresthesia, pruritus, sweating.

INTERACTIONS: Naltrexone may increase levels. Weight gain/weight loss may occur with antidepressants.

PREGNANCY: Category C, caution in nursing.

MECHANISM OF ACTION: GABA analogue; not completely understood; suspected to interact with glutamate and GABA neurotransmitter systems centrally, hypothesized that the drug restores this balance.

PHARMACOKINETICS: Absorption: Absolute bioavailability (11%); C_{max}=350ng/mL; T_{max}=3-8 hrs. **Distribution:** V_d=72-109L. **Elimination:** Urine; T$_{1/2}$=20-33 hrs.

NURSING CONSIDERATIONS

Assessment: Assess for renal impairment.

Monitoring: Monitor for emergence of symptoms of depression and suicidality.

Patient Counseling: Caution while performing hazardous tasks (operating machinery/driving). Notify if pregnant/nursing or planning to become pregnant. Alert families/caregivers to look for symptoms of suicidality or depression.

Administration: Oral route. **Storage:** 25°C (77°F); excursions permitted to 15-30°C (59-86°F).

CAMPTOSAR RX
irinotecan HCl (Pfizer)

> Administer under the supervision of a physician experienced in the use of cancer chemo agents. May induce early and/or late forms of diarrhea. Early diarrhea (occurring during or shortly after infusion) may be accompanied by cholinergic symptoms that can cause abdominal cramping; may be prevented or ameliorated by atropine. Late diarrhea (occurring >24 hrs after administration) can be life-threatening since it may be prolonged and may lead to dehydration, electrolyte imbalance, or sepsis; should be treated with loperamide. Monitor with diarrhea; give fluid/electrolyte replacement if dehydrated or give antibiotics if ileus, fever, or severe neutropenia develop. Interrupt and reduce subsequent doses if severe diarrhea occurs. Severe myelosuppression may occur.

THERAPEUTIC CLASS: Topoisomerase I inhibitor

INDICATIONS: First-line therapy in combination with 5-fluorouracil (5-FU) and leucovorin (LV) for metastatic carcinoma of the colon and rectum, and for patients with metastatic carcinoma of the colon or rectum whose disease has progressed or recurred following initial 5-FU therapy.

DOSAGE: *Adults:* Combination Therapy (with 5-FU/LV): Dose of LV should be administered immediately after irinotecan, then 5-FU after LV. Regimen 1 (6-week cycle with bolus 5-FU/LV): 125mg/m² IV over 90 min on Days 1, 8, 15, 22. Regimen 2 (6-week cycle with infusional 5-FU/LV): 180mg/m² IV over 90 min on Days 1, 15, and 29. Both regimens: Begin next cycle on Day 43. Refer to PI for dose of 5-FU/LV. Single Therapy: Weekly Regimen: 125mg/m² IV over 90 min on Days 1, 8, 15, 22 followed by 2-week rest. Titrate: Dose may be adjusted to as high as 150mg/m² or as low as 50mg/m² in 25-50mg/m² decrements depending upon individual tolerance. Once-Every-3-Week Regimen: 350mg/m² IV over 90 min once q3 weeks. Titrate: Dose may be adjusted as low as 200mg/m² in 50mg/m² decrements depending upon individual tolerance. Refer to PI for Dose Modifications for Combination and Single-agent schedules. All dose modifications should be based on worst preceding toxicity. Premedicate with antiemetics at least 30 min prior to therapy. Prophylactic or therapeutic administration of atropine should be considered in patients with cholinergic symptoms. Reduced UGT1A1 Activity: Reduce starting dose by at least one level. Subsequent dose modifications should be based on patient's tolerance; refer to PI.

HOW SUPPLIED: Inj: 20mg/mL [2mL, 5mL]

WARNINGS/PRECAUTIONS: If late diarrhea occurs, delay therapy until return of pretreatment bowel function for at least 24 hrs without antidiarrheals; decrease subsequent doses if late diarrhea is Grade 2, 3, or 4. Deaths due to sepsis following severe neutropenia reported; temporarily hold therapy if neutropenic fever occurs or if neutrophils <1000/mm³. Increased risk for neutropenia in patients homozygous for the UGT1A1*28 allele; consider reduced initial dose. Hypersensitivity reactions, colitis, renal impairment/failure and thromboembolic events reported. May cause fetal harm. Monitor for extravasation and inflammation at infusion site. Premedicate with antiemetics. Caution with hepatic dysfunction, deficient glucuronidation of bilirubin (eg, Gilbert's syndrome), elderly with comorbidities, previous pelvic/abdominal irradiation. Careful monitoring of WBC with differential, Hgb, and platelets is recommended before each dose. Avoid in severe bone marrow failure, fructose intolerant patients, or unresolved bowel obstruction. Interstitial pulmonary disease (IPD)-like events reported; d/c therapy if diagnosed and institute appropriate treatment if needed.

ADVERSE REACTIONS: N/V, diarrhea, abdominal pain, anemia, asthenia, mucositis, anorexia, alopecia, fever, pain, constipation, infection, dyspnea, increased bilirubin.

INTERACTIONS: Exacerbated myelosuppression and diarrhea with antineoplastic agents having similar adverse effects. Avoid concurrent irradiation therapy. Possible hyperglycemia and lymphocytopenia with dexamethasone. Greater incidence of akathisia reported with prochlorperazine. Laxatives may worsen diarrhea. Consider withholding diuretics with irinotecan therapy. Decreased levels with CYP3A4 inducing anticonvulsants, phenytoin, phenobarbital, carbamazepine and St. John's wort; d/c at least 2 weeks prior to first cycle. Consider substituting non-enzyme inducing anticonvulsants 2 weeks prior to and during treatment. Increased levels with ketoconazole; d/c ketoconazole at least 1 week prior to and during therapy. Increased systemic exposure of SN-38 with atazanavir sulfate. May prolong neuromuscular blocking effects of suxamethonium and the neuromuscular blockade of non-depolarizing drugs may be antagonized.

PREGNANCY: Category D, not for use in nursing.

MECHANISM OF ACTION: Topoisomerase I inhibitor; binds to topoisomerase I-DNA complex and prevents religation of single-strand breaks induced by the enzyme to relieve torsional strain in DNA.

PHARMACOKINETICS: Absorption: Irinotecan: (125mg/m²); C_{max}=1660ng/mL; AUC_{0-24}=10200ng•h/mL. (340mg/m²) C_{max}=3392ng/mL; AUC_{0-24}=20604ng•h/mL. SN-38: (125mg/m²) C_{max}=26.3ng/mL; AUC_{0-24}=229ng•h/mL. (340mg/m²) C_{max}=56ng/mL; AUC_{0-24}=474ng•h/mL. **Distribution:** Irinotecan: (125mg/m²) V_d=110L/m². (340mg/m²) V_d=234L/m². Plasma protein binding (30-68%). SN-38: Plasma protein binding (95%). **Metabolism:** Liver via carboxyl esterase. SN-38 (active metabolite). **Elimination:** Irinotecan: Urine (11-20%). (125mg/m²) $T_{1/2}$=5.8 hrs. (340mg/m²) $T_{1/2}$=11.7 hrs. SN-38: Urine (<1%). (125mg/m²) $T_{1/2}$=10.4 hrs. (340mg/m²) $T_{1/2}$=21 hrs.

NURSING CONSIDERATIONS

Assessment: Assess for severe bone marrow failure, unresolved bowel obstruction, hereditary fructose intolerance, reduced UDP-glucuronosyl transferase 1A1 activity, pregnancy/nursing status, diabetes mellitus, glucose intolerance, pelvic/abdominal radiation. Assess for deficient glucuronidation of bilirubin (Gilbert's syndrome), possible drug interactions, renal/hepatic function, underlying cardiac disease, pre-existing lung disease. Assess use in elderly patients with comorbid conditions. Obtain baseline CBC with platelets.

Monitoring: Monitor for diarrhea, signs/symptoms of neutropenia, neutropenic complications (eg, neutropenic fever), ileus, pulmonary symptoms, inflammation and/or extravasation of infusion site, dehydration, cholinergic symptoms (eg, rhinitis, increased salivation, miosis, lacrimation, diaphoresis) especially when receiving higher doses, infections and hypersensitivity reactions, For patients with diarrhea, monitor for signs/symptoms of dehydration, electrolyte imbalance, ileus, fever, or severe neutropenia. Monitor WBC with differential, Hgb, platelet count before each dose.

Patient Counseling: Instruct to avoid vaccinations with live vaccines. Inform of pregnancy risks, toxic effects (GI complications). Instruct to have loperamide readily available and to begin treatment of late diarrhea at 1st episode of poorly formed or loose stool or the earliest onset of bowel movement more frequent than normally expected. Seek medical attention if the following occur: diarrhea for first time during treatment; black or bloody stools; unexplained pulmonary symptoms (eg, dyspnea, cough, fever), dehydration (eg, lightheadedness, dizziness, faintness), inability to take fluids by mouth due to N/V, inability to get diarrhea under control within 24 hrs, fever, evidence of infection, toxicity, or anaphylactic reactions. Inform of the potential of dizziness or visual disturbances which may occur within 24 hrs and advise not to drive or operate machinery if these symptoms occur. Alert for the possibility of alopecia.

Administration: IV route. Administer as IV infusion over 90 min. Use gloves. If solution contacts the skin/mucous membranes, wash immediately and thoroughly. Inspect visually for particulates and discoloration. Dilute in 5%

dextrose or 0.9% NaCl to final concentration range of 0.12-2.8mg/mL. Other drugs should not be added to the infusion solution. **Storage:** 15-30°C (59-86°F). Protect from light. Keep in the carton until the time of use. Solution: Room temperature (25°C), stable for 24 hrs. Solutions diluted in 5% dextrose and store at 2-8°C and protected from light are stable for 48 hrs. Diluted in 0.9% NaCl: avoid refrigeration. Avoid freezing. Use admixtures prepared with 5% dextrose within 24 hours if refrigerated. Use admixture prepared with 5% dextrose/NaCl with 6 hrs if kept at room temperature 15-30°C (59-86°F).

CANASA RX
mesalamine (Axcan Scandipharm)

THERAPEUTIC CLASS: 5-Aminosalicylic acid derivative

INDICATIONS: Treatment of active ulcerative proctitis.

DOSAGE: *Adults:* 1000mg rectally qhs. Retain suppository for at least 1-3 hrs.

HOW SUPPLIED: Sup: 1000mg

CONTRAINDICATIONS: Hypersensitivity to suppository vehicle (eg, saturated vegetable fatty acid esters).

WARNINGS/PRECAUTIONS: D/C if acute intolerance syndrome develops (eg, cramping, bloody diarrhea, abdominal pain, headache); consider sulfasalazine hypersensitivity. If rechallenge is considered, perform under careful observation. Caution with sulfasalazine hypersensitivity. Carefully monitor with renal dysfunction. Pancolitis, pericarditis (rare) reported.

ADVERSE REACTIONS: Dizziness, rectal pain, fever, acne, colitis, rash, hair loss.

PREGNANCY: Category B, caution in nursing.

MECHANISM OF ACTION: Not fully established; anti-inflammatory drug appears to act topically rather than systemically. Postulated to have a role as free radical scavenger or inhibitor of tumor necrosis factor.

PHARMACOKINETICS: Absorption: Variable; C_{max}=361ng/mL. **Metabolism:** Extensively metabolized to N-acetyl-5-ASA. **Elimination:** Urine; $T_{1/2}$=7 hrs.

NURSING CONSIDERATIONS

Assessment: Assess for hypersensitivity to the suppository vehicle, sulfa allergy, pre-existing renal disease, history of pancreatitis, and pericarditis. Obtain baseline renal function (BUN, creatinine, urinalysis).

Monitoring: Monitor renal function (BUN, creatinine, urinalysis) periodically, signs/symptoms of pericarditis, pancreatitis, acute intolerance syndrome (cramping, abdominal pain, bloody diarrhea), renal dysfunction, hypersensitivity, and allergic reactions.

Patient Counseling: Inform may cause stains. Advise to empty rectum before use and not to handle too much. If miss dose, use as soon as possible, unless almost time for next dose. Do not use 2 doses at once. Seek medical attention if chest pain, SOB, cramping, abdominal pain, bloody diarrhea, hypersensitivity, and allergic reactions occur. Inform to d/c if rash or fever occur.

Administration: Rectal route. 1) Remove plastic wrapper. 2) Avoid excessive handling. 3) Insert completely into rectum. 4) Lubricant may be used to assist insertion. **Storage:** 25°C (77°F), do not freeze. Keep away from direct heat, light or humidity, and out of reach of children.

CANCIDAS RX
caspofungin acetate (Merck)

THERAPEUTIC CLASS: Glucan synthesis inhibitor

INDICATIONS: Empirical therapy for presumed fungal infections in febrile, neutropenic patients. Treatment of candidemia and the following *Candida* infections: intra-abdominal abscesses, peritonitis, and pleural space infections. Treatment of esophageal candidiasis. Treatment of invasive aspergillosis in

C

patients who are refractory to or intolerant of other therapies (eg, amphotericin B, lipid formulations of amphotericin B, itraconazole).

DOSAGE: *Adults:* Infuse slowly over approximately 1 hr. Usual: LD: 70mg IV on Day 1. Maint: 50mg IV qd. Empirical Therapy: LD: 70mg IV on Day 1, followed by 50mg qd thereafter. May be continued until resolution of neutropenia. If fungal infection found, treat for ≥14 days; continue for at least 7 days after both neutropenia and clinical symptoms resolve. Increase to 70mg if 50mg dose is well tolerated but does not provide adequate clinical response. Candidemia/*Candida* Infections (Intra-abdominal Abscesses, Peritonitis, and Pleural Space Infections): LD: 70mg IV on Day 1, followed by 50mg qd thereafter. Duration based on patient's clinical and microbiological response. In general, treat for ≥14 days after the last positive culture. Persistently neutropenic patients may require longer therapy. Esophageal Candidiasis: 50mg IV qd for 7-14 days after symptom resolution. Invasive Aspergillosis: LD: 70mg IV on Day 1, followed by 50mg qd thereafter. Duration of treatment based on severity of underlying disease, recovery from immunosuppression, and clinical response. Moderate Hepatic Insufficiency (Child-Pugh Score 7-9): LD: 70mg IV on Day 1 (where recommended). Usual: 35mg IV qd. Concomitant with Rifampin: 70mg IV qd. Concomitant with Nevirapine/Efavirenz/Carbamazepine/Dexamethasone/Phenytoin: May require an increase to 70mg IV qd. Max: 70mg/day.

Pediatrics: 3 months-17 yrs: For all indications: LD: 70mg/m² IV on Day 1, followed by 50mg/m² IV qd thereafter. Dose can be increased to 70mg/m² qd if 50mg/m² daily dose is well tolerated but does not provide an adequate clinical response. Dosing is based on the patient's BSA. Max: 70mg/day. Concomitant Rifampin/Nevirapine/Efavirenz/Carbamazepine/Dexamethasone/Phenytoin: 70mg/m² IV qd. Max: 70mg/day.

HOW SUPPLIED: Inj: 50mg, 70mg

WARNINGS/PRECAUTIONS: LFT abnormalities may be seen; if abnormal LFTs develop, monitor for worsening hepatic function and re-evaluate therapy. Do not mix or coinfuse with other medications. Do not use diluents containing dextrose.

ADVERSE REACTIONS: Fever, chills, hypokalemia, hypotension, diarrhea, N/V, abdominal pain, edema, headache, rash, pneumonia, respiratory failure, tachycardia, septic shock, infusion-site reactions.

INTERACTIONS: Reduces blood levels of tacrolimus. Inducers of drug clearance (eg, efavirenz, nevirapine, phenytoin, rifampin, dexamethasone, carbamazepine) may decrease levels. Increased levels with cyclosporine; use only when benefits outweigh risks.

PREGNANCY: Category C, caution in nursing.

MECHANISM OF ACTION: Glucan synthesis inhibitor; inhibits the synthesis of β (1, 3)-D-glucan, an essential component of the cell wall of susceptible *Aspergillus* and *Candida* species.

PHARMACOKINETICS: Absorption: Administration to different age groups resulted in different pharmacokinetic parameters. **Distribution:** Plasma protein binding (97%). **Metabolism:** Hydrolysis and N-acetylation (slowly). **Elimination:** Urine (41%, 1.4% unchanged), feces (35%).

NURSING CONSIDERATIONS

Assessment: Assess use in patients who are on concomitant therapy with cyclosporine. Assess hepatic function prior to therapy, hypersensitivity, pregnancy/nursing status and possible drug interactions.

Monitoring: Monitor for histamine-related and anaphylactic reactions (eg, rash, facial swelling, bronchospasm) when administering. Monitor LFTs and CBC while on therapy.

Patient Counseling: Inform that there have been isolated reports of serious hepatic effects, and that therapy can cause hypersensitivity reactions (eg, rash, facial swelling, pruritus, sensation of warmth, or bronchospasm).

Administration: IV route. Administer by slow IV infusion over approximately 1 hr. Not for IV bolus administration. Refer to PI for preparation instructions. **Storage:** 2-8°C (36-46°F). Reconstituted: ≤25°C (≤77°F) for 1 hr prior to preparation of infusion solution. Diluted product: ≤25°C (≤77°F) for 24 hrs or 2-8°C (36-46°F) for 48 hrs.

CAPOZIDE RX

hydrochlorothiazide - captopril (Par)

> ACE inhibitors can cause death/injury to developing fetus during 2nd and 3rd trimesters. Stop therapy if pregnancy detected.

THERAPEUTIC CLASS: ACE inhibitor/thiazide diuretic

INDICATIONS: Treatment of hypertension.

DOSAGE: *Adults:* Initial: 25mg-15mg tab qd. Titrate: Adjust dose at 6-week intervals. Max: 150mg captopril/50mg HCTZ per day. Replacement Therapy: Substitute combination for titrated components. Renal Impairment: Decrease dose or increase interval. Take 1 hr before meals.

HOW SUPPLIED: Tab: (Captopril-HCTZ) 25mg-15mg*, 25mg-25mg*, 50mg-15mg*, 50mg-25mg* *scored

CONTRAINDICATIONS: History of ACE inhibitor-associated angioedema, anuria, sulfonamide hypersensitivity.

WARNINGS/PRECAUTIONS: D/C if angioedema, jaundice, or marked LFT elevation occurs. Risk of hyperkalemia with diabetes mellitus (DM), renal dysfunction may occur. Monitor WBCs in renal or collagen vascular disease. Anaphylactoid reactions reported. Fetal/neonatal morbidity and death reported. Monitor for hypotension in high-risk patients (heart failure, surgery/anesthesia, severe volume/salt depletion, on dialysis, etc.) Caution with congestive heart failure (CHF), renal or hepatic dysfunction, and renal artery stenosis. May exacerbate or activate systemic lupus erythematosus (SLE). Monitor serum electrolytes. Hypercalcemia, hypomagnesemia, hyperuricemia may occur. Neutropenia with myeloid hypoplasia, persistent nonproductive cough, anaphylactoid reactions, proteinuria reported. Enhanced effects in post-sympathectomy. Avoid with severe renal impairment.

ADVERSE REACTIONS: Anaphylactoid reactions, tachycardia, chest pain, dysguesia, rash, pruritis, fever, arthralgia, eosinophilia.

INTERACTIONS: Increased risk of hyperkalemia with K⁺-sparing diuretics, K⁺ supplements, or K⁺-containing salt substitutes. Caution with agents affecting sympathetic activity. D/C vasodilators before therapy. Caution and decrease vasodilator dose if resumed during therapy. Potentiates orthostatic hypotension with alcohol, barbiturates, and narcotics. Adjust other antihypertensives, anticoagulants, antidiabetic, or antigout drugs. Reduced absorption with cholestyramine, colestipol. Amphotericin B, corticosteroids, adrenocorticotropic hormone deplete electrolytes. May decrease methenamine effects. May decrease response to pressor amines. May potentiate non-depolarizing skeletal muscle relaxants, anesthetics. Risk of lithium toxicity. NSAIDs (eg, indomethacin) reduce effects. Enhanced hypotensive effects with MAOIs. Probenecid, sulfinpyrazone may need dose increase. Diazoxide enhances hyperglycemic, hyperuricemic, and antihypertensive effects. Monitor serum calcium levels with calcium salts. Monitor potassium levels with cardiac glycosides.

PREGNANCY: Category C (1st trimester) and D (2nd and 3rd trimesters), not for use in nursing.

MECHANISM OF ACTION: Captopril: ACE inhibitor; not established. Effects appear to result from suppression of renin-angiotensin-aldosterone system. HCTZ: Thiazide diuretic. Affects renal tubular mechanism of electrolyte reabsorption.

PHARMACOKINETICS: Absorption: Captopril: Rapid; T_{max}=1 hr. **Distribution:** Captopril: Plasma protein binding (25-30%). **Elimination:** Captopril: Urine (40-50%); $T_{1/2}$≤2 hrs. HCTZ: Kidney; $T_{1/2}$=2.5 hrs.

NURSING CONSIDERATIONS

Assessment: Assess volume/salt depletion, SLE, DM, anuria, sulfonamide hypersensitivity, history of allergy, angioedema or bronchial asthma, collagen vascular disease, congestive heart failure, hepatic/renal impairment. Obtain baseline serum electrolytes, renal function, and WBC with differential (impaired renal function), pregnancy/nursing status and possible drug interactions.

Monitoring: Monitor serum electrolytes and renal function periodically. If impaired renal function or collagen vascular disease, monitor WBC with differential before therapy, at 2-week intervals for 3 months, and then periodically during therapy. Monitor for signs/symptoms of electrolyte imbalance, exacerbation or activation of SLE, hypotension, hyperuricemia or precipitation of gout, anaphylactoid or hypersensitivity reactions, head/neck and intestinal angioedema, infection and neutropenia/agranulocytosis.

Patient Counseling: Instruct to take 1 hr before meal. Inform of pregnancy risks. Advise that inadequate fluid intake or loss of fluids may lead to drop in BP, resulting in lightheadedness or syncope. Instruct not to interrupt or d/c therapy without consulting physician; may cause withdrawal symptoms (eg, angina). Advise to seek medical attention if symptoms of angioedema (head/neck; intestinal; abdominal pain with/without N/V), infection (eg, sore throat, fever), syncope, edema, hypersensitivity reactions, or electrolyte imbalance (eg, dry mouth, thirst, lethargy) occur.

Administration: Oral route. **Storage:** Below 30°C (86°F).

CAPTOPRIL   RX
captopril (Various)

> ACE inhibitors can cause death/injury to developing fetus during 2nd and 3rd trimesters. D/C if pregnancy detected.

OTHER BRAND NAMES: Capoten (Par)

THERAPEUTIC CLASS: ACE inhibitor

INDICATIONS: Treatment of hypertension alone or in combination with other antihypertensive agents (eg, thiazide-type diuretics) and congestive heart failure (CHF) in combination with diuretics and digitalis. To improve survival in stable post-myocardial infarction patients with left ventricular dysfunction and to reduce the incidence of overt heart failure or hospitalizations for CHF in these patients. Treatment of diabetic nephropathy (proteinuria >500mg/day) in patients with type I diabetes mellitus (DM) and retinopathy.

DOSAGE: *Adults:* Take 1 hr before meals. HTN: If possible, d/c recent antihypertensive drug for 1 week prior to therapy. Initial: 25mg bid-tid. Titrate: May increase to 50mg bid-tid after 1-2 weeks. With Concomitant Diuretic Therapy: Range: 25-150mg bid-tid. Max: 450mg qd. CHF: Initial: 25mg tid. Titrate: May increase to 50-100mg tid. With Risk of Hypotension or Salt/Volume Depletion: Initial: 6.25mg or 12.5mg tid. Max: 450mg qd. Left Ventricular Dysfunction Post-MI: Initial: 6.25mg single dose, then 12.5mg tid. Titrate: Increase to 25mg tid over next several days, then to 50mg tid over next several weeks. Usual: 50mg tid. Diabetic Nephropathy: 25mg tid. Significant Renal Dysfunction: Decrease initial dose and titrate slowly.

HOW SUPPLIED: Tab: 12.5mg*, 25mg*, 50mg*, 100mg* *scored

CONTRAINDICATIONS: History of ACE inhibitor-associated angioedema.

WARNINGS/PRECAUTIONS: Persistent nonproductive cough, anaphylactoid reactions, angioedema (face, tongue, larynx), and neutropenia/agranulocytosis with myeloid hypoplasia reported. D/C if jaundice or marked LFT elevation occurs. Risk of hyperkalemia with DM, renal dysfunction. Fetal/neonatal morbidity and death reported. Monitor for hypotension in high-risk patients (surgery/anesthesia, dialysis, heart failure, volume/salt depletion, etc). Caution with CHF, renal dysfunction, renal artery stenosis, collagen vascular disease (especially with renal dysfunction). Monitor WBC before therapy, then every

2 weeks for 3 months, then periodically. Less effective on BP and higher rates of angioedema reported in blacks than nonblacks.

ADVERSE REACTIONS: Rash, fever, arthralgia, eosinophilia, loss of taste.

INTERACTIONS: May increase lithium levels. NSAIDs (eg, aspirin) and indomethacin may decrease antihypertensive effects. Hypotension risk with diuretics. Increased risk of hyperkalemia with K^+-sparing diuretics, K^+-containing salt substitutes, or K^+ supplements. Caution with vasodilators or agents affecting sympathetic activity. Augmented effect by antihypertensives that cause renin release (eg, thiazides). Nitritoid reactions (eg, facial flushing, N/V, hypotension) reported rarely with injectable gold.

PREGNANCY: Category C (1st trimester) and D (2nd and 3rd trimesters), not for use in nursing.

MECHANISM OF ACTION: ACE inhibitor; not established. Effects appear to result from suppression of renin-angiotensin-aldosterone system.

PHARMACOKINETICS: Absorption: Rapid; T_{max}=1 hr. **Distribution:** Plasma protein binding (25-30%). **Elimination:** Urine (40-50%) unchanged; $T_{1/2}$=<2 hrs.

NURSING CONSIDERATIONS

Assessment: Assess for pregnancy status, possible drug interactions, volume/salt depletion, DM, collagen vascular disease, CHF, aortic stenosis, hepatic/renal impairment. Obtain baseline BP, renal function, and WBC with differential (impaired renal function).

Monitoring: Monitor renal function periodically and BP in first 2 weeks and whenever dosage changes. If renal function is impaired, monitor WBC with differential before therapy, at 2-week intervals for 3 months, and then periodically during therapy. Monitor for signs/symptoms of hypotension, anaphylactoid or hypersensitivity reactions, head/neck and intestinal angioedema, infection, and neutropenia/agranulocytosis.

Patient Counseling: Inform of pregnancy risks; inadequate fluid intake or loss of fluids may lead to drop in BP resulting in lightheadedness or syncope. Instruct not to interrupt or d/c therapy without consulting physician; may cause withdrawal symptoms (eg, angina). Advise to seek medical attention if symptoms of angioedema (eg, swelling of extremities, lips, face, tongue; difficulty swallowing or breathing; intestinal/abdominal pain with/without N/V), infection (eg, sore throat, fever), syncope, edema, or hypersensitivity reactions occur. Caution patients against excessive perspiration and dehydration to avoid excessive fall in BP.

Administration: Oral route. Take 1 hr before meals. **Storage:** 20-25°C (68-77°F). Protect from moisture. Keep bottles tightly closed.

CARBAGLU   RX
carglumic acid (R&D)

THERAPEUTIC CLASS: Carbamoyl Phosphate Synthetase 1

INDICATIONS: Adjunctive therapy for the treatment of acute hyperammonemia due to deficiency of the hepatic enzyme N-acetylglutamate synthase (NAGS). Maintenance therapy for chronic hyperammonemia due to deficiency of NAGS.

DOSAGE: *Adults:* Acute Hyperammonemia: Initial: 100-250mg/kg/day bid-qid ac. Titrate dose based on individual plasma ammonia levels and clinical symptoms. Chronic Hyperammonemia: Maint: Usual: <100mg/kg/day bid-qid. Titrate to target normal plasma ammonia by age. Disperse tablets in water immediately before use. Do not swallow whole or crush.
Pediatrics: Acute Hyperammonemia: Initial: 100-250mg/kg/day bid-qid ac. Titrate dose based on individual plasma ammonia levels and clinical symptoms. Chronic Hyperammonemia: Maint: Usual: <100mg/kg/day bid-qid. Titrate to target normal plasma ammonia by age. Disperse tablets in water immediately before use. Do not swallow whole or crush.

HOW SUPPLIED: Tab: 200* *scored

WARNINGS/PRECAUTIONS: Any episode of acute symptomatic hyperammonemia should be treated as a life-threatening emergency. Uncontrolled hyperammonemia can rapidly result in brain injury/damage or death. Monitor plasma ammonia levels, neurological status, laboratory tests and clinical responses during treatment. Maintain normal range of plasma ammonia levels for age via individual dose adjustment. Protein restriction and hypercaloric intake is recommended until plasma ammonia levels normalize, then aim for unrestricted protein intake.

ADVERSE REACTIONS: Infection, abdominal pain, anemia, ear infection, diarrhea, vomiting, pyrexia, tonsilitis, headache, nasopharyngitis.

PREGNANCY: Category C, not for use in nursing.

MECHANISM OF ACTION: Carbamoyl phosphate synthetase 1 activator; synthetic analog of NAG which converts ammonia into urea.

PHARMACOKINETICS: Absorption: T_{max} =3 hrs. **Distribution:** V_d =2657L. **Elimination:** $T_{1/2}$ =5.6 hrs; Urine (9%, unchanged), feces (up to 60%, unchanged).

NURSING CONSIDERATIONS

Assessment: Assess for hyperammonemia, plasma ammonia levels, pregnancy/nursing status.

Monitoring: Monitor plasma ammonia levels, neurological status, laboratory tests and clinical responses.

Patient Counseling: Inform that tablets should not be swallowed whole or crushed; disperse in a minimum of 2.5mL of water. Advise that dietary protein may be increased when plasma ammonia levels have normalized. Inform of the most common adverse reactions.

Administration: Oral route. Refer to PI to Oral and Nasogastric Tube Administration. **Storage:** 2°-8°C (36°-46°F). After opening the container do not store above 30°C (86°F). Discard after 1 month after first opening. Protect from moisture.

CARBATROL   RX
carbamazepine (Shire)

> Serious and fatal dermatologic reactions, including toxic epidermal necrolysis (TEN) and Stevens-Johnson syndrome (SJS) reported; increased risk with presence of HLA-B*1502 allele; screen prior to initiation of therapy. Aplastic anemia and agranulocytosis reported. Obtain complete pretreatment hematological testing as a baseline. Consider d/c if evidence of bone marrow depression develops.

THERAPEUTIC CLASS: Carboxamide

INDICATIONS: Treatment of partial seizures with complex symptomatology (psychomotor, temporal lobe), generalized tonic-clonic seizures (grand mal), and mixed seizure patterns of these, or other partial or generalized seizures. Treatment of pain associated with true trigeminal or glossopharyngeal neuralgia.

DOSAGE: *Adults:* Epilepsy: Initial: 200mg bid. Titrate: Increase weekly by ≤200mg/day. Maint: Adjust to minimum effective level, usually 800-1200mg/day. Max: 1600mg/day. Combination Therapy: When added to existing anticonvulsant therapy, may be added gradually while other anticonvulsants are maintained or gradually decreased, except phenytoin, which may be increased. Trigeminal Neuralgia: Initial (Day 1): 200mg qd. Titrate: May increase by ≤200mg/day q12h PRN. Maint: Usual: 400-800mg/day. Attempts to reduce dose to minimum effective level or even to d/c therapy is at least once q3 months. Max: 1200mg/day.
Pediatrics: Epilepsy: >12 yrs: Initial: 200mg bid. Titrate: Increase weekly by ≤200mg/day. Maint: Adjust to minimum effective level, usually 800-1200mg/day. >15 yrs: Max: 1200mg/day. 12-15 yrs: Max: 1000mg/day. <12 yrs: May convert immediate-release dose ≥400mg/day to equal daily dose using bid regimen. Usual: <35mg/kg/day. Max: ≤35mg/kg/day.

HOW SUPPLIED: Cap, Extended-Release: 100mg, 200mg, 300mg

CONTRAINDICATIONS: History of bone marrow depression, MAOI use within 14 days, sensitivity to TCAs (eg, amitriptyline, desipramine, imipramine, protriptyline, nortriptyline), coadministration with nefazodone.

WARNINGS/PRECAUTIONS: Increased risk of suicidal thoughts or behavior reported. May cause fetal harm with pregnancy. Avoid abrupt d/c in patients with seizure disorder; may precipitate status epilepticus. Caution in patients with history of cardiac, hepatic, or renal damage; adverse hematologic reactions to other drugs; interrupted courses of therapy with carbamazepine; increased intraocular pressure (IOP); and mixed seizure disorder. May cause activation of latent psychosis and, in the elderly, confusion or agitation. Caution with history of liver disease; d/c immediately in cases of aggravated liver dysfunction or active liver disease. Hyponatremia, interference with some pregnancy tests, decreased values of thyroid function tests, renal dysfunction, eye changes, increased total cholesterol, LDL, and HDL reported.

ADVERSE REACTIONS: Dizziness, drowsiness, unsteadiness, N/V, bone marrow depression, congestive heart failure (CHF), aplastic anemia, agranulocytosis, SJS, TEN.

INTERACTIONS: See Contraindications. CYP3A4 and/or epoxide hydrolase inhibitors (eg, azole antifungals, cimetidine, erythromycin, protease inhibitors) may increase plasma level. CYP3A4 inducers (eg, cisplatin, doxorubicin, rifampin) may decrease plasma level. May decrease plasma levels of CYP1A2 and CYP3A4 substrates (eg, acetaminophen, oral contraceptives, trazodone, warfarin). Breakthrough bleeding reported with oral contraceptives. May reduce warfarin's anticoagulant effect. May increase plasma levels of clomipramine HCl and primidone. May increase or decrease plasma level of phenytoin. Increased risk of neurotoxic side effects with lithium. Antimalarial drugs (eg, chloroquine, mefloquine) may antagonize activity. Caution with other centrally acting drugs and alcohol. Coadministration with delavirdine may lead to loss of virologic response and possible resistance to non-nucleoside reverse transcriptase inhibitors (NNRTIs). Hyponatremia and a case of meningitis reported in combination with other drugs. Isolated cases of neuroleptic malignant syndrome reported with psychotropic drugs.

PREGNANCY: Category D, not for use in nursing.

MECHANISM OF ACTION: Anticonvulsant: Reduces polysynaptic response and blocks post-tetanic potentiation. Neuralgia: Depresses thalamic potential and bulbar and polysynaptic reflexes.

PHARMACOKINETICS: Absorption: (Single 200mg dose) C_{max}=1.9μg/mL, 0.11 μg/mL (CBZ-E); T_{max}=19 hrs, 36 hrs (CBZ-E). (Multiple 800mg dose) C_{max}=11μg/mL, 2.2μg/mL (CBZ-E); T_{max}=5.9 hrs, 14 hrs (CBZ-E). **Distribution:** Plasma protein binding (76%), (50% CBZ-E); crosses the placenta; found in breast milk. **Metabolism:** Liver via CYP3A4; carbamazepine-10,11-epoxide (CBZ-E) (active metabolite). **Elimination:** Urine (72%, 3% unchanged), feces (28%); $T_{1/2}$=35-40 hrs (single dose), 12-17 hrs (multiple doses), 34 hrs (CBZ-E).

NURSING CONSIDERATIONS

Assessment: Assess for conditions where treatment is contraindicated or cautioned, pregnancy/nursing status, and possible drug interactions. Perform detailed history and physical exam prior to treatment. Screen for HLA-B*1502 allele in suspected population. Obtain baseline CBC with platelet and reticulocyte counts, serum iron, LFTs, urinalysis, BUN, lipid profile, and eye exam.

Monitoring: Monitor for signs/symptoms of dermatologic reactions, aplastic anemia, agranulocytosis, signs of bone marrow depression, emergence or worsening of depression, suicidal thoughts or behavior, unusual changes in mood or behavior, and liver dysfunction aggravation or active liver disease. Periodically monitor WBC, platelet count, LFTs, urinalysis, BUN, lipid profile, and serum drug levels. Perform periodic eye exams, including slit-lamp exam, funduscopy, and tonometry.

Patient Counseling: Instruct to read Medication Guide prior to taking drug. Report toxic signs/symptoms of potential hematologic problems (eg, fever, sore throat, rash, ulcers in mouth, easy bruising, petechial or purpuric hemorrhage), and emergence of suicidal thoughts or behavior. Use caution while operating machinery/driving. Inform that caps can be opened and contents sprinkled over food (eg, teaspoon of applesauce) if necessary; do not crush or chew. Notify physician if pregnant or intend to become pregnant, and to report the use of any other prescription or nonprescription medication or herbal products. Encourage patients to enroll in North American Antiepileptic Drug (NAAED) Pregnancy Registry by calling 1-888-233-2334 or go to www. aedpregnancyregistry.org.

Administration: Oral route. **Storage:** 25°C (77°F); excursions permitted to 15-30°C (59-86°F). Protect from light and moisture.

CARDENE IV
nicardipine HCl (EKR)
RX

THERAPEUTIC CLASS: Calcium channel blocker (dihydropyridine)

INDICATIONS: Short-term treatment of HTN when PO therapy is not feasible or not desirable.

DOSAGE: *Adults:* Individualize dose. Patients Not Receiving PO Nicardipine: Initial: 5mg/hr IV infusion. Titrate: May increase by 2.5mg/hr q5 min (for rapid titration) to 15 min (for gradual titration). Max: 15mg/hr. Decrease rate to 3mg/hr after BP goal achieved with rapid titration. Equivalent PO Dose to IV Dose: 20mg q8h=0.5mg/hr; 30mg q8h=1.2mg/hr; 40mg q8h=2.2mg/hr. Transition to PO Nicardipine: Give 1st dose 1 hr prior to d/c of infusion. Hepatic Impairment/Reduced Hepatic Blood Flow: Consider lower dosages. Renal Impairment: Titrate gradually. Elderly: Start at low end of dosing range. (Cardene Premixed) Impending Hypotension/Tachycardia: D/C when restart at 3-5mg/hr when BP has stabilized and adjust to maintain desired BP.

HOW SUPPLIED: Inj: 2.5mg/mL [10mL], 0.1mg/mL [200mL], 0.2mg/mL [200mL]

CONTRAINDICATIONS: Advanced aortic stenosis.

WARNINGS/PRECAUTIONS: May induce or exacerbate angina in coronary artery disease (CAD) patients. Caution with heart failure (HF) or significant left ventricular dysfunction. To reduce possibility of venous thrombosis, phlebitis, local irritation, swelling, extravasation, and occurrence of vascular impairment, administer through large peripheral or central veins. Change IV site q12h to minimize risk of peripheral venous irritation. May occasionally produce symptomatic hypotension or tachycardia. Avoid systemic hypotension when administering in sustained acute cerebral infarction or hemorrhage. Caution in hepatic/renal impairment, reduced hepatic blood flow, and elderly.

ADVERSE REACTIONS: Headache, hypotension, tachycardia, N/V.

INTERACTIONS: Titrate slowly with β-blockers in HF or significant left ventricular dysfunction due to possible negative inotropic effects. Increased nicardipine levels when PO nicardipine is given with cimetidine. Elevated cyclosporine levels reported with PO nicardipine; closely monitor cyclosporine levels and reduce its dose accordingly.

PREGNANCY: Category C, not for use in nursing.

MECHANISM OF ACTION: Calcium channel blocker (dihydropyridine); inhibits transmembrane influx of calcium ions into cardiac muscle and smooth muscles without changing serum calcium concentration.

PHARMACOKINETICS: Distribution: V_d=8.3L/kg; plasma protein binding (>95%); found in breast milk. **Metabolism:** Liver (extensive). **Elimination:** Urine (49%), feces (43%); $T_{1/2}$=14.4 hrs.

NURSING CONSIDERATIONS

Assessment: Assess for advanced aortic stenosis, HF, CAD, left ventricular dysfunction, sustained acute cerebral infarction or hemorrhage, hepatic/renal impairment, pregnancy/nursing status, and possible drug interactions.

Monitoring: Monitor BP and HR during administration. Monitor for symptomatic hypotension, tachycardia, induction or exacerbation of angina, and hepatic/renal function.

Patient Counseling: Advise to seek medical attention if adverse reactions occur.

Administration: IV route. Refer to PI for preparation and administration instructions. Cardene IV: Dilute before infusion. Cardene Premixed: No further dilution required. **Storage:** 20-25°C (68-77°F). Avoid elevated temperatures. Protect from light. Store in carton until ready to use. Diluted Sol: Stable at room temperature for 24 hrs. Premixed: Protect from freezing.

CARDENE SR   RX
nicardipine HCl (PDL BioPharma)

THERAPEUTIC CLASS: Calcium channel blocker (dihydropyridine)

INDICATIONS: Treatment of hypertension.

DOSAGE: *Adults:* Initial: 30mg bid. Usual: 30-60mg bid. Adjust according to BP response.

HOW SUPPLIED: Cap, Sustained-Release: 30mg, 45mg, 60mg

CONTRAINDICATIONS: Advanced aortic stenosis.

WARNINGS/PRECAUTIONS: Increased angina reported in patients with angina. Caution with congestive heart failure (CHF) when titrating dose. Caution in hepatic/renal impairment, or reduced hepatic blood flow. May cause symptomatic hypotension. Monitor BP during initial administration and dose titration.

ADVERSE REACTIONS: Headache, pedal edema, vasodilation, palpitations, N/V, dizziness, asthenia, postural hypotension, increased urinary frequency, pain, rash, increased sweating.

INTERACTIONS: Increased levels with cimetidine. Elevates cyclosporine levels. With β-blocker withdrawal, gradually reduce over 8-10 days. Monitor digoxin levels. Severe hypotension reported with fentanyl anesthesia.

PREGNANCY: Category C, not for use in nursing.

MECHANISM OF ACTION: Ca^{2+} channel blocker; inhibits transmembrane influx of Ca^{2+} ions into cardiac muscle and smooth muscle without changing serum Ca^{2+} concentration.

PHARMACOKINETICS: Absorption: Complete; bioavailability (35%); C_{max}=13.4ng/mL (30mg), 34.0ng/mL (45mg), 58.4ng/mL (60mg); T_{max}=1-4 hrs. **Distribution:** Plasma protein binding (>95%). **Metabolism:** Liver. **Elimination:** Urine (<1%, intact), feces; $T_{1/2}$=8.6 hrs.

NURSING CONSIDERATIONS

Assessment: Assess for advanced aortic stenosis, CHF, acute cerebral infarction or hemorrhage, liver/renal impairment, pregnancy/nursing status, and possible drug interactions. Obtain baseline BP.

Monitoring: Monitor BP initially and during titration. Monitor for signs/symptoms of angina, hypersensitivity reactions, hypotension, liver/renal dysfunction.

Patient Counseling: Advise to seek medical attention if symptoms of hypotension, angina, or hypersensitivity reactions occur.

Administration: Oral route. **Storage:** 15-30°C (59-86°F); keep in light-resistant container.

CARDIZEM   RX
diltiazem HCl (Biovail)

THERAPEUTIC CLASS: Calcium channel blocker (nondihydropyridine)

INDICATIONS: Management of chronic stable angina and angina due to coronary artery spasm.

DOSAGE: *Adults:* Initial: 30mg qid (before meals and hs). Titrate: Increase gradually (given in divided doses tid-qid) at 1-2 day intervals until optimum response obtained. Usual: 180-360mg/day. Elderly: Start at lower end of dosing range.

HOW SUPPLIED: Tab: 30mg, 60mg*, 90mg*, 120mg* *scored

CONTRAINDICATIONS: Sick sinus syndrome and 2nd- or 3rd-degree AV block (except with functioning ventricular pacemaker); hypotension (<90mmHg systolic); acute myocardial infarction (MI) and pulmonary congestion documented by x-ray on admission.

WARNINGS/PRECAUTIONS: May cause abnormally slow heart rates, particularly in patients with sick sinus syndrome. May cause second- or third-degree AV block. Periods of asystole reported in patient with Prinzmetal's angina. Caution in renal, hepatic, or ventricular dysfunction. Symptomatic hypotension may occur. Elevations in enzymes (eg, alkaline phosphatase, lactate dehydrogenase [LDH], AST, ALT) and other phenomena consistent with acute hepatic injury reported; reversible upon d/c. Monitor LFTs and renal function. Dermatologic reactions (eg, erythema multiforme, exfoliative dermatitis) may occur; d/c if a dermatologic reaction persists. Caution in elderly.

ADVERSE REACTIONS: Edema, headache, nausea, dizziness, rash, asthenia.

INTERACTIONS: May increase levels of propranolol, carbamazepine, quinidine, midazolam, triazolam, lovastatin, simvastatin; monitor closely. Increased levels with cimetidine. Monitor digoxin and cyclosporine levels if used concomitantly. Potentiates depression of cardiac contractility, conductivity, automaticity and vascular dilation with anesthetics. Additive cardiac conduction effects with digitalis or β-blockers. Potential additive effects with agents known to affect cardiac contractility and/or conduction; caution and careful titration warranted. May have significant impact on efficacy and side effect profile with CYP450 3A4 substrates, inducers, and inhibitors. Avoid with CYP3A4 inducers (eg, rifampin). May enhance the effects and increase the toxicity of buspirone. Concomitant use with statins metabolized by CYP3A4 may increase the risk of myopathy and rhabdomyolysis. Sinus bradycardia resulting in hospitalization and pacemaker insertion reported with clonidine; monitor heart rate.

PREGNANCY: Category C, not for use in nursing.

MECHANISM OF ACTION: Calcium channel blocker; inhibits cellular influx of calcium ions during membrane depolarization of cardiac and vascular smooth muscle. Angina Due to Coronary Artery Spasm: A potent dilator of coronary arteries both epicardial and subendocardial; inhibits spontaneous and ergonovine-induced coronary artery spasm. Exertional Angina: Produces increases in exercise tolerance by its ability to reduce myocardial oxygen demand; accomplished via reduction in heart rate and systemic BP.

PHARMACOKINETICS: Absorption: Well absorbed; Absolute bioavailability (40%); T_{max}=2-4 hrs. **Distribution:** Plasma protein binding (70-80%); found in breast milk. **Metabolism:** Liver (extensive). **Elimination:** Urine (2-4%, unchanged), bile. $T_{1/2}$=3-4.5 hrs.

NURSING CONSIDERATIONS

Assessment: Assess for sick sinus syndrome, 2nd- or 3rd-degree AV block, hypotension, acute MI, pulmonary congestion, congestive heart failure (CHF), ventricular dysfunction, hepatic/renal impairment, pregnancy/nursing status, and for possible drug interactions.

Monitoring: Monitor for slow HR, second- or third-degree AV block, hypotension, hepatic injury (eg, increased alkaline phosphatase, increased LDH, increased AST, increased ALT) and for dermatologic events (eg, skin eruptions progressing to erythema multiforme and/or exfoliative dermatitis). Monitor liver and renal function regularly.

Patient Counseling: Inform about benefits/risks of therapy. Counsel to report any adverse reactions to physician and to notify physician if pregnant or nursing.

Administration: Oral route. **Storage:** 25°C (77°F); excursions permitted to 15-30°C (59-86°F). Avoid excessive humidity.

CARDIZEM CD

RX

diltiazem HCl (Biovail)

OTHER BRAND NAMES: Cardizem LA (Abbott) - Cartia XT (Watson)

THERAPEUTIC CLASS: Calcium channel blocker (nondihydropyridine)

INDICATIONS: Treatment of hypertension used alone or in combination with other antihypertensive medications. Management of chronic stable angina and (CD, Cartia XT) angina due to coronary artery spasm.

DOSAGE: *Adults:* Individualize dose. HTN: (CD, Cartia XT) Initial (monotherapy): 180-240mg qd. Titrate: Adjust to individual patient needs. Usual: 240-360mg qd. Max: 480mg qd. (LA) Initial (monotherapy): 180-240mg qd (am or hs). Titrate: Adjust to individual patient needs. Usual: 120-540mg qd. Max: 540mg qd. Angina: (CD, Cartia XT) Initial: 120-180mg qd. Titrate: Adjust at 1-2 week intervals. Max: 480mg qd. (LA) Initial: 180mg qd. Titrate: Increase at 1-2 week intervals. Max: 360mg. Elderly: Start at lower end of dosing range. Swallow tab whole. Do not chew or crush.

HOW SUPPLIED: Cap, Extended-Release: (Cardizem CD, Cartia XT) 120mg, 180mg, 240mg, 300mg, (Cardizem CD) 360mg; Tab, Extended-Release: (Cardizem LA) 120mg, 180mg, 240mg, 300mg, 360mg, 420mg

CONTRAINDICATIONS: Sick sinus syndrome and 2nd- or 3rd-degree AV block (except with functioning pacemaker); hypotension (<90mmHg systolic); acute myocardial infarction (MI) and pulmonary congestion documented by x-rays on admission.

WARNINGS/PRECAUTIONS: May cause abnormally slow heart rates, particularly in patients with sick sinus syndrome. May cause second- or third-degree heart block. Periods of asystole reported in patient with Prinzmetal's angina. Caution in renal, hepatic, or ventricular dysfunction. Symptomatic hypotension may occur. Elevations in enzymes (eg, alkaline phosphatase, lactate dehydrogenase [LDH], AST, ALT) and other phenomena consistent with acute hepatic injury reported; reversible upon d/c. Monitor LFTs and renal function. Dermatologic reactions (eg, erythema multiforme, exfoliative dermatitis) may occur; d/c if a dermatologic reaction persists. Caution in elderly.

ADVERSE REACTIONS: Headache, edema, dizziness, bradycardia, 1st-degree AV block (CD, Cartia XT). Edema lower limb, dizziness, fatigue, bradycardia, 1st-degree AV block (LA).

INTERACTIONS: May increase levels of propranolol, carbamazepine, quinidine, midazolam, triazolam, lovastatin, simvastatin. (CD, LA) Concomitant use with statins metabolized by CYP3A4 may increase the risk of myopathy and rhabdomyolysis; monitor closely. (CD, LA) Increased levels with cimetidine. Monitor digoxin and cyclosporine levels if used concomitantly. Potentiates depression of cardiac contractility, conductivity, automaticity and vascular dilation with anesthetics. Additive cardiac conduction effects with digitalis or β-blockers. Potential additive effects with agents known to affect cardiac contractility and/or conduction; caution and careful titration warranted. May have significant impact on efficacy and side effect profile with CYP450 3A4 substrates, inducers, and inhibitors. Avoid with CYP3A4 inducers (eg, rifampin). May enhance the effects and increase the toxicity of buspirone. Sinus bradycardia resulting in hospitalization and pacemaker insertion reported with clonidine; monitor heart rate (CD, LA).

PREGNANCY: Category C, not for use in nursing.

MECHANISM OF ACTION: Calcium channel blocker; inhibits cellular influx of calcium ions during membrane depolarization of cardiac and vascular smooth muscle. HTN: Relaxes vascular smooth muscle resulting in decreased peripheral vascular resistance. Angina: Produces increases in exercise tolerance by its ability to reduce myocardial oxygen demand; accomplished via reduction in heart rate and systemic BP.

PHARMACOKINETICS: Absorption: Well absorbed; Absolute bioavailability (40%). T_{max}=10-14 hrs (CD), 11-18 hrs (LA). **Distribution:** Plasma protein binding (70-80%); found in breast milk. **Metabolism:** Liver (extensive). **Elimination:** Urine (2-4%, unchanged), bile. $T_{1/2}$=5-8 hrs (CD), 6-9 hrs (LA).

NURSING CONSIDERATIONS

Assessment: Assess for sick sinus syndrome, 2nd- or 3rd-degree AV block, hypotension, acute MI, pulmonary congestion, congestive heart failure, ventricular dysfunction, hepatic/renal impairment, pregnancy/nursing status, and for possible drug interactions.

Monitoring: Monitor for slow HR, second- or third-degree AV block, hypotension, hepatic injury (eg, increased alkaline phosphatase, increased LDH, increased AST, increased ALT) and for dermatological events (eg, skin eruptions progressing to erythema multiforme and/or exfoliative dermatitis). Perform regular monitoring of liver and renal function regularly.

Patient Counseling: Inform about benefits/risks of therapy. Counsel to report any adverse reactions to physician and to notify physician if pregnant or nursing. Instruct to swallow tab whole; do not chew or crush.

Administration: Oral route. **Storage:** 25°C (77°F); excursions permitted to 15-30°C (59-86°F) (CD, LA); 20-25°C (68-77°F) (Cartia XT). Avoid excessive humidity and (LA) temperatures >30°C (86°F).

CARDURA   RX
doxazosin mesylate (Pfizer)

THERAPEUTIC CLASS: Alpha$_1$-blocker (quinazoline)

INDICATIONS: Treatment of hypertension and/or treatment of both the urinary outflow obstruction and obstructive and irritative symptoms associated with benign prostatic hyperplasia (BPH).

DOSAGE: *Adults:* HTN: Initial: 1mg qd. Monitor BP 2-6 hrs and 24 hrs after 1st dose. Titrate: Increase stepwise to 2mg, 4mg, 8mg, or 16mg qd based on patient's standing blood pressure response. BPH: Initial: 1mg qd (am or pm). Titrate: Increase stepwise to 2mg, 4mg, and 8mg in 1-2 week intervals based on patient's urodynamics and BPH symptomatology. Max: 8mg/day.

HOW SUPPLIED: Tab: 1mg*, 2mg*, 4mg*, 8mg* *scored

WARNINGS/PRECAUTIONS: Syncope and orthostatic hypotension (eg, dizziness, light-headedness, vertigo) can occur with 1st dose, dose increase and if interrupted for more than a few days. Caution with hepatic dysfunction. Rule out prostate cancer. Priapism (rare) and leukopenia/neutropenia reported. Intraoperative floppy iris syndrome observed during cataract surgery in some patients on, or previously treated with alpha blockers.

ADVERSE REACTIONS: Dizziness, headache, fatigue/malaise, somnolence, edema, nausea, rhinitis, vertigo.

INTERACTIONS: Caution with additional antihypertensive agents and drugs known to influence hepatic metabolism. Concomitant use with PDE-5 inhibitors may result in additive BP-lowering effects and symptomatic hypotension.

PREGNANCY: Category C, caution with nursing.

MECHANISM OF ACTION: Alpha$_1$-blocker; (BPH) antagonizes phenylephrine-induced contractions in prostate; (HTN) competitively antagonizes pressor effects of phenylephrine and systolic pressor effect of norepinephrine.

PHARMACOKINETICS: Absorption: Absolute bioavailability (65%); T_{max} =2-3 hrs. **Distribution:** Plasma protein binding (98%). **Metabolism:** Liver (extensive); O-demethylation or hydroxylation. **Elimination:** Feces (63%, 4.8% unchanged), urine (9%, trace amounts unchanged); $T_{1/2}$=22 hrs.

NURSING CONSIDERATIONS

Assessment: Assess for liver impairment, pregnancy/nursing status and possible drug interactions. Rule out prostate cancer.

Monitoring: Monitor BP periodically. Monitor for signs/symptoms of hypotension, priapism, liver dysfunction, and hypersensitivity reactions.

Patient Counseling: Inform of possibility of syncope and orthostatic symptoms, especially at initiation of therapy; urge to avoid driving or hazardous tasks for 24 hrs after first dose, dosage increase, and interruption of therapy when treatment is resumed. Caution to avoid situations where injury could result should syncope occur. Advise to sit or lie down when symptoms of low BP occur. Inform of possibility of priapism; advise to seek medical attention if priapism occurs. Instruct to inform ophthalmologist of drug use prior to cataract surgery.

Administration: Oral route. If drug use discontinued for several days, restart using the initial dosing regimen. **Storage:** 25°C (77°F); excursions permitted to 15-30°C (59-86°F).

CARDURA XL   RX
doxazosin mesylate (Pfizer)

THERAPEUTIC CLASS: Alpha$_1$-blocker (quinazoline)

INDICATIONS: Treatment of the signs and symptoms of benign prostatic hyperplasia (BPH).

DOSAGE: *Adults:* Initial: 4mg qd with breakfast. Titrate: May increase to 8mg after 3-4 weeks. Max: 8mg. If d/c for several days, restart using 4mg qd dose. Switching from Cardura to Cardura XL: Initial: 4mg qd. Final evening dose of Cardura should not be taken.

HOW SUPPLIED: Tab, Extended-Release: 4mg, 8mg

WARNINGS/PRECAUTIONS: Postural hypotension with or without symptoms (eg, dizziness) and syncope may develop; caution with symptomatic hypotension or patients who have hypotensive response to other medications. Rule out prostate cancer. Intraoperative floppy iris syndrome has been observed during cataract surgery in some patients on, or previously treated with, alpha$_1$ blockers. Caution with pre-existing severe GI narrowing (pathologic or iatrogenic). Caution with mild or moderate hepatic dysfunction; avoid with severe hepatic dysfunction. D/C with worsening of or new-onset angina pectoris symptoms.

ADVERSE REACTIONS: Dizziness, asthenia, headache, respiratory tract infection

INTERACTIONS: Caution with potent CYP3A4 inhibitors (eg, atazanavir, clarithromycin, indinavir, itraconazole, ketoconazole, nefazodone, nelfinavir, ritonavir, saquinavir, telithromycin, voriconazole). Caution with drugs known to influence hepatic metabolism. Increased systemic exposure with drugs that reduce GI motility (eg, anticholinergics). Additive blood pressure lowering effects and symptomatic hypotension with phosphodiesterase-5 (PDE-5) inhibitor.

PREGNANCY: Category C, not for use in nursing.

MECHANISM OF ACTION: Alpha$_1$-blocker; antagonizes α_1-agonist-induced contractions, decreasing urethral resistance, which may relieve BPH symptoms and improve urine flow.

PHARMACOKINETICS: Absorption: (4mg) C_{max}=10.1ng/mL, AUC=183ng•hr/mL, T_{max}=8 hrs. (8mg) C_{max}=25.8ng/mL, AUC=472ng•hr/mL, T_{max}=9 hrs. **Distribution:** Plasma protein binding (98%). **Metabolism:** Liver (extensive) via CYP3A4 (major) and CYP2D6, CYP2C19 (minor). **Elimination:** $T_{1/2}$=15-19 hrs.

NURSING CONSIDERATIONS

Assessment: Assess for hepatic impairment, symptomatic hypotension, history of hypotensive response to other medications, severe GI narrowing (chronic constipation), coronary insufficiency, and possible drug interactions. Rule out prostate cancer.

Monitoring: Monitor for signs/symptoms of postural hypotension and new onset or worsening of angina pectoris.

Patient Counseling: Instruct to take with breakfast; swallow whole; do not chew, divide, cut, or crush. Advise symptoms related to postural hypotension (eg, dizziness, syncope) may occur; caution about driving, operating machinery, and performing hazardous tasks. Avoid situations where injury could result if syncope occurs. Caution not to be alarmed if a tablet is noticed in the stool. Instruct to inform ophthalmologist of drug use prior to cataract surgery.

Admininistration: Oral route. Swallow whole; do not chew, divide, cut, or crush. **Storage:** 25°C (77°F); excursions permitted to 15-30°C (59-86°F).

CASODEX

RX

bicalutamide (AstraZeneca)

THERAPEUTIC CLASS: Nonsteroidal antiandrogen

INDICATIONS: Treatment of stage D_2 metastatic carcinoma of the prostate in combination with a luteinizing hormone-releasing hormone (LHRH) analogue.

DOSAGE: *Adults:* 50mg qd at same time. Initiate with LHRH analog therapy.

HOW SUPPLIED: Tab: 50mg

CONTRAINDICATIONS: Women, pregnancy.

WARNINGS/PRECAUTIONS: Not for use in women. Cases of death or hospitalization due to severe liver injury reported. Hepatitis and marked increases in liver enzymes leading to drug d/c have occurred. Measure serum transaminase levels prior to treatment, at regular intervals for first 4 months, then periodically. Hepatoxicity reported; d/c use if jaundice occurs or ALT >2X ULN. Caution with moderate-severe hepatic impairment; monitor LFTs periodically. Monitor prostate specific antigen (PSA) regularly to assess therapy. For patients who have objective progression of disease together with elevated PSA, a treatment-free period of antiandrogen, while continuing LHRH analogue, may be considered. Reduction in glucose tolerance (diabetes, loss of glycemic control) with pre-existing diabetes mellitus (DM) observed; monitor blood glucose.

ADVERSE REACTIONS: Hot flashes, HTN, constipation, nausea, diarrhea, anemia, peripheral edema, bone pain, dizziness, dyspnea, rash, nocturia, hematuria, urinary tract infection, gynecomastia.

INTERACTIONS: Can displace coumarin anticoagulants from binding sites; monitor PT and consider anticoagulant dose adjustment. Concomitant use of LHRH agonist may reduce glucose tolerance. Caution with CYP3A4 substrates (eg, midazolam).

PREGNANCY: Category X, not for use in nursing.

MECHANISM OF ACTION: Nonsteroidal antiandrogen; inhibits the action of androgens by binding to cytosol androgen receptors in target tissue.

PHARMACOKINETICS: Absorption: Well-absorbed, C_{max}=0.768mcg/mL, T_{max}=31.3 hrs. **Distribution:** Plasma protein binding (96%). **Metabolism:** Liver via oxidation and glucuronidation. **Elimination:** Urine, feces; $T_{1/2}$=5.8 days.

NURSING CONSIDERATIONS

Assessment: Assess for hypersensitivity, DM, and hepatic impairment. Note other diseases/conditions and drug therapies. Obtain baseline vital signs and weight, CBC, LFTs, and PSA levels.

Monitoring: Monitor for hot flashes, hypersensitivity reactions, hyperuricemia, and dyspnea. Monitor vital signs and weight, CBC, LFTs, PSA levels.

Patient Counseling: Inform about risks and benefits of therapy. Advise not to interrupt or d/c without consulting physician. Start treatment at the same time as LHRH analog. Inform that somnolence may occur; caution when driving or operating machinery. Counsel about the risks of DM or loss of glycemic control with pre-existing DM that may occur during therapy.

Administration: Oral route. May be taken in the morning or evening, with or without food. **Storage:** 20-25°C (68-77°F).

CATAFLAM
diclofenac potassium (Novartis)

RX

NSAIDs may cause an increased risk of serious cardiovascular (CV) thrombotic events, myocardial infarction (MI), stroke, and serious GI adverse events including bleeding, ulceration, and perforation of the stomach or intestines. Contraindicated for the treatment of perioperative pain in the setting of coronary artery bypass graft (CABG) surgery.

THERAPEUTIC CLASS: NSAID

INDICATIONS: Relief of signs and symptoms of osteoarthritis (OA) and rheumatoid arthritis (RA). Treatment of primary dysmenorrhea and relief of mild to moderate pain.

DOSAGE: *Adults:* OA: 100-150mg/day in divided doses, 50mg bid or tid. RA: 150-200mg/day in divided doses, 50mg tid or qid. Pain/Primary Dysmenorrhea: Initial: 50mg tid or 100mg on 1st dose, then 50mg on subsequent doses.

HOW SUPPLIED: Tab: 50mg

CONTRAINDICATIONS: ASA or other NSAID allergy that precipitates asthma, urticaria, or allergic reactions. Treatment of perioperative pain in the setting of CABG surgery.

WARNINGS/PRECAUTIONS: May lead to onset of new HTN or worsening of pre-existing HTN; monitor BP closely. Fluid retention and edema reported; caution in patients with fluid retention or heart failure. Caution with history of ulcer disease or GI bleeding. Caution in patients with considerable dehydration. Renal papillary necrosis and other renal injury reported after long-term use. Caution with impaired renal function, heart failure, liver dysfunction, and the elderly. Not recommended for use with advanced renal disease; if therapy must be initiated, monitor renal function. May cause elevations of LFTs; d/c if liver disease develops or systemic manifestations occur. Anaphylactoid reactions may occur. May cause serious skin adverse events (eg, exfoliative dermatitis, Stevens-Johnson syndrome, toxic epidermal necrolysis). Avoid in late pregnancy; may cause premature closure of ductus arteriosus. Not a substitute for corticosteroids or for the treatment of corticosteroid insufficiency. Anemia may occur; with long-term use, monitor Hgb/Hct if signs or symptoms of anemia develop. May inhibit platelet aggregation and prolong bleeding time; monitor with coagulation disorders. Caution with asthma and avoid with ASA-sensitive asthma.

ADVERSE REACTIONS: Dyspepsia, constipation, diarrhea, GI ulceration/perforation, N/V, flatulence, abnormal renal function, anemia, dizziness, edema, elevated liver enzymes, headache, increased bleeding time, rash, tinnitus.

INTERACTIONS: Avoid use with ASA. May enhance methotrexate toxicity; caution when co-administering. May increase nephrotoxicity of cyclosporine; caution when co-administering. May diminish antihypertensive effect of ACE-inhibitors. May reduce natriuretic effect of furosemide and thiazides; monitor for renal failure. May increase lithium levels; monitor for toxicity. Synergistic effects on GI bleeding with warfarin. Caution with hepatotoxic drugs (eg, antibiotics, anti-epileptics). Increase risk for GI bleeding with concomitant oral corticosteroids, anticoagulants, or alcohol. ACE inhibitors and diuretics may increase the risk of overt renal decompensation.

PREGNANCY: Category C, not for use in nursing.

MECHANISM OF ACTION: NSAID (benzeneacetic acid derivative); suspected to inhibit prostaglandin synthetase.

PHARMACOKINETICS: Absorption: Absolute bioavailabilty (55%), T_{max}=1 hr. **Distribution**: V_d=1.3L/kg; serum protein binding (>99%). **Metabolism**: Metabolites: 4'-hydroxy-, 5-hydroxy-, 3'-hydroxy-, 4',5-dihydroxy-, and 3'-hydroxy-4'-methoxy diclofenac. **Elimination:** Urine (65%), bile (35%); $T_{1/2}$=2 hrs.

NURSING CONSIDERATIONS

Assessment: Assess for history of a hypersensitivity reaction to aspirin or other NSAIDS, asthma, cardiovascular disease (eg, pre-existing HTN, congestive heart failure) or risk factors for CVD, risk factors for a GI event (eg, prior history of ulcer disease or GI disease, smoking), fluid retention, renal/hepatic dysfunction, coagulation disorders, pregnancy/nursing status, and for possible drug interactions. Assess baseline LFTs, renal function, and CBC.

Monitoring: Monitor for signs/symptoms of CV thrombotic events, new onset or worsening of pre-existing HTN, GI events (eg, inflammation, bleeding, ulceration, perforation), fluid retention and edema, renal effects (eg, renal papillary necrosis), hepatic effects (eg, jaundice, liver necrosis, liver failure), anaphylactoid reactions, skin reactions (eg, exfoliative dermatitis, Stevens-Johnson syndrome, toxic epidermal necrolysis), hematological effects (eg, anemia, prolongation of bleeding time), and for bronchospasm. Monitor BP. Perform periodic monitoring of CBC, renal function, and LFTs.

Patient Counseling: Instruct to seek medical attention for symptoms of hepatotoxicity (eg, nausea, fatigue, jaundice), anaphylactic reactions (eg, difficulty breathing, swelling of the face/throat), rash, CV events (eg, chest pain, SOB, weakness, slurring of speech), or if unexplained weight gain or edema occur. Inform of risks if used during pregnancy.

Administration: Oral route. **Storage:** Do not store above 30°C (86°F). Dispense in tight container.

CATAPRES   RX
clonidine HCl (Boehringer Ingelheim)

OTHER BRAND NAMES: Catapres-TTS (Boehringer Ingelheim)

THERAPEUTIC CLASS: Alpha-adrenergic agonist

INDICATIONS: Treatment of hypertension, alone or with other antihypertensives.

DOSAGE: *Adults:* (Patch) Apply to hairless, intact area of upper outer arm or chest once every 7 days. Each new patch should be applied on different skin site from previous location. Initial: Adjust according to individual therapeutic requirements, starting with TTS-1/Generic 0.1mg/day. Titrate: If inadequate reduction in BP after 1-2 weeks, increase dosage by adding another TTS-1/Generic 0.1mg/day or changing to a larger system. Renal Impairment: Adjust according to the degree of impairment. (Tab) Adjust dose according to patient's individual BP response. Initial: 0.1mg bid (am and hs). Maint: May increase by 0.1mg/day at weekly intervals if necessary until desired response is achieved. Usual: 0.2-0.6mg/day in divided doses. Max Dose: 2.4mg/day. Renal Impairment: Adjust according to the degree of impairment. Elderly: May benefit from lower end of dosing.

HOW SUPPLIED: Patch, Extended-Release (TTS): (TTS-1) 0.1mg, (TTS-2) 0.2mg, (TTS-3) 0.3mg; (Generic): 0.1mg, 0.2mg, 0.3mg. Tab: 0.1mg, 0.2mg, 0.3mg

WARNINGS/PRECAUTIONS: Avoid abrupt d/c; reduce dose gradually over 2 to 4 days to avoid withdrawal symptomatology. Rare instances of hypertensive encephalopathy, cerebrovascular accidents (CVA) and death reported after withdrawal. Caution with severe coronary insufficiency, conduction disturbances, recent myocardial infarction (MI), cerebrovascular disease, or chronic renal failure. Substitution from clonidine transdermal system to PO clonidine may elicit an allergic reaction (eg, generalized rash, urticaria, angioedema) if a localized contact sensitization or an allergic reaction to clonidine transdermal system previously occurred. Monitor BP during surgery; additional measures to control BP should be available. (Tab) Continue to within 4 hrs of surgery and resume as soon as possible thereafter. (Patch) Do not remove during surgery. (Patch) Remove before defibrillation or cardioconversion due to the potential risk of altered electrical conductivity and remove before undergoing an MRI or due to the occurrence of skin burns.

ADVERSE REACTIONS: Dry mouth, drowsiness, sedation. (Tab) Dizziness, constipation. (Patch) Fatigue, headache, lethargy, erythema, pruritus, allergic contact sensitization, localized vesiculation, hyperpigmentation, edema, excoriation.

INTERACTIONS: May potentiate CNS depression with alcohol, barbiturates, or other sedating drugs. Hypotensive effect reduced by TCAs. Monitor HR with agents that affect sinus node function or AV nodal conduction (eg, digitalis, calcium channel blockers, β-blockers). D/C β-blockers several days before the gradual withdrawal of clonidine in patients taking both. Catapres Tab, TTS: Sinus bradycardia reported with diltiazem or verapamil.

PREGNANCY: Category C, caution in nursing.

MECHANISM OF ACTION: Central acting α-agonist; stimulates α-adrenoreceptors in brain stem, reducing sympathetic outflow from CNS and decreasing HR, BP, peripheral resistance and renal vascular resistance.

PHARMACOKINETICS: Absorption: (Tab) T_{max}=3-5 hrs. **Distribution:** Found in breast milk. **Metabolism:** Liver. **Elimination:** Urine (40-60%, unchanged); (Tab) $T_{1/2}$=12-16 hrs; (Patch) $T_{1/2}$=12.7 hrs.

NURSING CONSIDERATIONS

Assessment: Assess for severe coronary insufficiency, conduction disturbances, recent MI, cerebrovascular disease, renal impairment, allergic reactions/contact sensitization, pregnancy/nursing status, and for possible drug interactions.

Monitoring: Monitor BP and renal function periodically. Monitor for withdrawal signs/symptoms (eg, hypertensive encephalopathy, CVA), presence of generalized skin rash and allergic reactions.

Patient Counseling: Caution against interruption of therapy without physician's advice. May impair mental/physical abilities. Inform that sedative effect may be increased by concomitant use of alcohol, barbiturates, or other sedating drugs. Inform that medication may cause dryness of eyes; caution with contact lenses. (Patch) Instruct to consult a physician promptly about possible need to remove patch due to adverse skin reactions. Inform that if patch begins to loosen, place adhesive cover directly over the patch to ensure adhesion for 7 days total. Advise to keep used and unused patch out of reach of children; fold in half with adhesive sides together and discard.

Administration: Oral route; transdermal route. **Storage:** (Tab) 25°C (77°F); excursions permitted to 15-30°C (59-86°F). Dispense in tight, light-resistant container. (Patch) TTS: Below 30°C (86°F). Generic: 20-25°C (68-77°F).

CAYSTON   RX
aztreonam (Gilead Sciences)

THERAPEUTIC CLASS: Monobactam

INDICATIONS: To improve respiratory symptoms in cystic fibrosis patients with *Pseudomonas aeruginosa.*

DOSAGE: *Adults:* 75mg tid administered via inhalation using an Altera Nebulizer System for 28 days followed by 28 days off therapy. Doses should be taken at least 4 hrs apart. Use bronchodilator before administration. Short-acting Bronchodilator: Give 15 min-4 hrs prior to each dose. Long-acting Bronchodilator: Give 30 min-12 hrs prior to each dose. Order of Administration if Taking Multiple Inhaled Therapies: Bronchodilator, mucolytics, aztreonam. *Pediatrics:* ≥7 yrs: 75mg tid via inhalation using an Altera Nebulizer System for 28 days followed by 28 days off therapy. Doses should be taken at least 4 hrs apart. Use bronchodilator before administration. Short-acting Bronchodilator: Give 15 min-4 hrs prior to each dose. Long-acting Bronchodilator: Give 30 min-12 hrs prior to each dose. Order of Administration if Taking Multiple Inhaled Therapies: Bronchodilator, mucolytics, aztreonam.

HOW SUPPLIED: Sol: 75mg/mL

WARNINGS/PRECAUTIONS: Not for IV or IM administration. Severe allergic reactions reported; d/c if an allergic reaction occurs (eg, facial rash, facial swelling, throat tightness). Caution with beta-lactam allergy (eg, penicillins, cephalosporins, carbapenems), cross-reactivity may occur. Bronchospasm reported. Decreases in FEV_1 reported after 28-day treatment cycle; consider baseline FEV_1 prior to therapy and presence of other symptoms when

C

evaluating whether post-treatment changes in FEV$_1$ are caused by a pulmonary exacerbation. May increase the risk of development of drug-resistant bacteria if given in the absence of known *P. aeruginosa* infection.

ADVERSE REACTIONS: Cough, nasal congestion, wheezing, pharyngolaryngeal pain, pyrexia, chest discomfort, abdominal pain, vomiting, bronchospasm.

PREGNANCY: Category B, safe in nursing.

MECHANISM-OF ACTION: Monobactam; binds to penicillin-binding proteins of susceptible bacteria, which leads to inhibition of bacterial cell wall synthesis and death of the cell.

PHARMACOKINETICS: Absorption: C$_{max}$=0.55mcg/mL, 0.67mcg/mL, 0.65mcg/mL (Days 0, 14, and 28, respectively). **Distribution:** Plasma protein binding (56%); found in breastmilk; crosses the placenta. **Elimination:** Urine (10%, unchanged), feces (12%), T$_{1/2}$=2.1 hrs.

NURSING CONSIDERATIONS

Assessment: Assess for history of beta-lactam allergy and pregnancy/nursing status. Assess baseline FEV$_1$.

Monitoring: Monitor for signs/symptoms of an allergic reaction (eg, facial rash, facial swelling, throat tightness). Monitor for pulmonary exacerbations following the 28-day treatment cycle. Measure FEV$_1$.

Patient Counseling: Advise that therapy is for inhalation use only and therapy should only be administered using the Altera Nebulizer System. Reconstitute only with the diluent provided and not mix with other drugs in the nebulizer. Complete full 28-day course of therapy and take as directed, even if feeling better. Inform that if dose is missed, all 3 daily doses should be taken, as long as the doses are at least 4 hrs apart. Advise to use bronchodilator prior to administration and instruct to take medications in the following order: bronchodilator, mucolytics, aztreonam. Contact physician if an allergic reaction develops, new symptoms develop, or if symptoms worsen. Counsel that it should only be used to treat bacterial, not viral infections. Counsel that skipping dose and not completing therapy may decrease effectiveness of the treatment and may increase the likelihood that bacteria will develop resistance to the drug.

Administration: Inhalation route via Altera Nebulizer System. Do not administer with any other nebulizer and do not mix with any other drugs in the nebulizer. Administer immediately after reconstitution. See PI for reconstitution and administration details. **Storage:** 2-8°C (36-46°F). Once removed from refrigerator, store at 25°C (77°F) for up to 28 days. Protect from light.

CEFACLOR   RX
cefaclor (Various)

THERAPEUTIC CLASS: Cephalosporin (2nd generation)

INDICATIONS: Treatment of otitis media, pharyngitis, tonsillitis, lower respiratory tract, urinary tract, and skin and skin structure infections caused by susceptible strains of microorganisms.

DOSAGE: *Adults:* Usual: 250mg q8h. Severe Infections/Pneumonia: 500mg q8h. Treat β-hemolytic strep for 10 days.
Pediatrics: ≥1 month: Usual: 20mg/kg/day given q8h. Otitis Media/Serious Infections/Infections Caused by Less Susceptible Organisms: 40mg/kg/day. Max: 1g/day. May administer q12h for otitis media and pharyngitis. Treat β-hemolytic strep for 10 days.

HOW SUPPLIED: Cap: 250mg, 500mg; Sus: 125mg/5mL [75mL, 150mL], 250mg/5mL [75mL, 150mL], 375mg/5mL [50mL, 100mL]

WARNINGS/PRECAUTIONS: Cross-sensitivity to penicillins (PCNs) and other cephalosporins may occur. *Clostridium difficile*-associated diarrhea (CDAD) reported. Positive direct Coombs' test reported. Caution with markedly impaired renal function, history of GI disease. False (+) for urine glucose with Benedict's and Fehling's solution, and Clinitest tabs.

ADVERSE REACTIONS: Hypersensitivity reactions, diarrhea, eosinophilia, genital pruritus and vaginitis, serum-sickness-like reactions.

INTERACTIONS: Renal excretion inhibited by probenecid. May potentiate warfarin and other anticoagulants; monitor PT/INR.

PREGNANCY: Category B, caution in nursing.

MECHANISM OF ACTION: Cephalosporin; bactericidal agent, inhibits cell-wall synthesis.

PHARMACOKINETICS: Absorption: Well-absorbed; (Fasting): C_{max}=7mcg/mL (250mg), 13mcg (500mg), 23mcg (1g); T_{max}=30-60 min. **Elimination:** Urine (60-85% unchanged); $T_{1/2}$= 0.6-0.9 hrs.

NURSING CONSIDERATIONS

Assessment: Assess for hypersensitivity reactions to cephalosporins, PCNs and other drugs; pregnancy/nursing status; renal function; and possible drug interactions.

Monitoring: Monitor for anaphylactic reactions, CDAD, superinfection, drug resistance, positive Coombs' test, increased anticoagulant effect when used concomitantly with anticoagulants, false (+) reaction for urinary glucose when using Benedict's and Fehling's solutions, and Clinitest tablets.

Patient Counseling: Inform drug only treats bacterial, not viral, infections. Take exactly as directed; skipping doses or not completing full course may decrease effectiveness and increase resistance. Inform about potential benefits/risks. D/C and notify physician if experience allergic reaction or watery/bloody diarrhea (with/without muscle cramps and fever) as late as 2 months after treatment end. Notify if pregnant/nursing.

Administration: Oral route. **Storage:** 20-25°C (68-77°F).

CEFACLOR ER   RX
cefaclor (Various)

> Used only to treat or prevent infections that are proven or strongly suspected to be caused by bacteria to reduce the development of drug-resistant bacteria and maintain effectiveness of antibacterial drugs.

THERAPEUTIC CLASS: Cephalosporin (2nd generation)

INDICATIONS: Treatment of acute bacterial exacerbations of chronic bronchitis (ABECB), secondary bacterial infections of acute bronchitis, pharyngitis, tonsillitis, and uncomplicated skin and skin structure infections (SSSI) caused by susceptible strains of microorganisms.

DOSAGE: *Adults:* ABECB/Acute Bronchitis: 500mg q12h for 7 days. Pharyngitis/Tonsillitis: 375mg q12h for 10 days. SSSI: 375mg q12h for 7-10 days. Take with meals. Do not crush, cut, or chew tab.
Pediatrics: ≥16 yrs: ABECB/Acute Bronchitis: 500mg q12h for 7 days. Pharyngitis/Tonsillitis: 375mg q12h for 10 days. SSSI: 375mg q12h for 7-10 days. Take with meals. Do not crush, cut, or chew tab.

HOW SUPPLIED: Tab, Extended-Release: 500mg

WARNINGS/PRECAUTIONS: Cross-sensitivity among beta-lactam antibiotics reported; d/c if allergic reaction occurs. *Clostridium difficile*-associated diarrhea (CDAD) reported; if suspected/confirmed, d/c and institute appropriate therapy. Prolonged use may result in overgrowth of nonsusceptible bacteria; take appropriate measures if superinfection occurs. Positive direct Coombs' test reported.

ADVERSE REACTIONS: Headache, rhinitis, diarrhea, nausea.

INTERACTIONS: Decreased absorption with aluminum or magnesium hydroxide-containing antacids; take within 1 hr of administration. Renal excretion inhibited by probenecid. Concomitant use with warfarin may increase PT.

PREGNANCY: Category B, caution in nursing.

MECHANISM OF ACTION: Cephalosporin; bactericidal, inhibits cell-wall synthesis.

PHARMACOKINETICS: Absorption: Fed: (375mg) C_{max}=3.7mcg/mL, T_{max}=2.7 hr, AUC=9.9mcg•hr/mL. (500mg) C_{max}=8.2mcg/mL, T_{max}=2.5 hr, AUC=18.1mcg•hr/mL. Fasting: C_{max}=5.4, T_{max}=1.5 hrs, AUC=14.8mcg•hr/mL. **Elimination:** $T_{1/2}$= approximately 1 hr.

NURSING CONSIDERATIONS

Assessment: Assess for hypersensitivity reactions to cephalosporins, penicillins, and other drugs, pregnancy/nursing status, and possible drug interactions. Document indications for therapy, culture, and susceptibility testing.

Monitoring: Monitor for anaphylactic reactions, pseudomembranous colitis, CDAD, superinfection, and drug resistance. Monitor CBC, LFTs, renal function tests, and blood chemistry.

Patient Counseling: Inform that drug only treats bacterial, not viral infections. Take exactly as directed; skipping doses or not completing full course may decrease effectiveness and increase resistance. Inform about benefits/risks. Inform that diarrhea may occur; d/c and notify physician if with watery and bloody stools (with/without abdominal cramps and fever) even as late as ≥2 months after taking last dose of therapy. Notify if pregnant/nursing and if allergic reactions occur.

Administration: Oral route. Take with meals. Do not crush, cut, or chew tab.
Storage: 20-25°C (68-77°F). Dispense in tight, light-resistant container, and with child-resistant closure.

CEFADROXIL   RX
cefadroxil monohydrate (Various)

THERAPEUTIC CLASS: Cephalosporin (1st generation)

INDICATIONS: Treatment of skin and skin structure (SSSI) and urinary tract infections (UTI), pharyngitis, and tonsillitis caused by susceptible strains of microorganisms.

DOSAGE: *Adults:* Uncomplicated Lower UTI: 1-2g/day given qd or bid. Other UTI: 2g in divided doses (bid). SSSI: 1g qd or 500mg bid. Group A β-hemolytic Strep Pharyngitis/Tonsillitis: 1g qd or 500mg bid for 10 days. CrCl ≤50mL/min: Initial: 1g. Maint: CrCl 25-50mL/min: 500mg q12h; CrCl 10-25mL/min: 500mg q24h; CrCl 0-10mL/min: 500mg q36h.
Pediatrics: UTI/SSSI: 15mg/kg q12h. Pharyngitis/Tonsillitis/Impetigo: 30mg/kg qd or 15mg/kg q12h. Treat β-hemolytic strep infections for at least 10 days.

HOW SUPPLIED: Cap: 500mg; Sus: 250mg/5mL [100mL], 500mg/5mL [75mL, 100mL]; Tab: 1g

WARNINGS/PRECAUTIONS: Caution in patients with penicillin (PCN) allergy; cross-sensitivity among β-lactam antibiotics may occur. D/C if an allergic reaction occurs. *Clostridium difficile*-associated diarrhea (CDAD) reported. Caution with renal impairment (CrCl <50mL/min/1.73 m²); careful observation and appropriate laboratory studies should be made prior to and during therapy in patients with known or suspected renal impairment. If superinfection occurs; appropriate measure should be taken. Caution with history of colitis or other GI diseases. Positive Coombs' test reported.

ADVERSE REACTIONS: Diarrhea, hypersensitivity reactions, hepatic dysfunction, genital moniliasis, vaginitis, fever, superinfection (prolonged use).

PREGNANCY: Category B, caution in nursing.

MECHANISM OF ACTION: Cephalosporin; bactericidal due to inhibition of cell-wall synthesis.

PHARMACOKINETICS: Absorption: Rapid; C_{max}(500, 1000mg)=16mcg/mL, 28mcg/mL. **Elimination:** Urine (90% unchanged).

NURSING CONSIDERATIONS

Assessment: Assess for history of hypersensitivity to PCNs, renal impairment, history of GI disease, and pregnancy/nursing status. Document indications for therapy, culture, and susceptibility testing.

Monitoring: Monitor for signs/symptoms of a hypersensitivity reaction, CDAD, and for superinfection. Monitor renal function and perform culture and susceptibility tests during therapy.

Patient Counseling: Inform drug only treats bacterial, not viral infections. Instruct to take exactly as directed; skipping doses or not completing full course may decrease effectiveness and increase resistance. Advise that may develop diarrhea during therapy; instruct to contact physician if watery/bloody stools, superinfection, or hypersensitivity reactions occur.

Administration: Oral route. **Storage:** 20-25°C (68-77°F). (Sus): Following reconstitution: Store in refrigerator; discard after 14 days. Shake well before use. Keep container tightly closed.

CEFAZOLIN   RX
cefazolin sodium (Various)

THERAPEUTIC CLASS: Cephalosporin (1st generation)

INDICATIONS: Treatment of respiratory tract, urinary tract (UTI), skin and skin structure, biliary tract, bone and joint, and genital infections, septicemia, and endocarditis caused by susceptible strains of microorganisms. Perioperative prophylaxis for surgical procedures classified as contaminated or potentially contaminated.

DOSAGE: *Adults:* Moderate-Severe Infections: 500mg-1g q6-8h. Mild Gram-Positive Cocci Infection: 250-500mg q8h. Acute, Uncomplicated UTI: 1g q12h. Pneumococcal Pneumonia: 500mg q12h. Severe Life-Threatening Infection (eg, Endocarditis, Septicemia): 1-1.5g q6h; Max: 12g/day (rare). Perioperative Prophylaxis: 1g IV 0.5-1 hr before surgery. For Procedures ≥2 hrs: 500mg-1g IV during surgery. Maint: 500mg-1g IV q6-8h for 24 hrs post-op. Continue for 3-5 days post-op for devastating procedures (eg, open-heart surgery, prosthetic arthroplasty). Renal Impairment: CrCl 35-54mL/min or SrCr of 1.6-3mg/dL: Full dose q8h. CrCl 11-34mL/min or SrCr of 3.1-4.5mg/dL: 1/2 usual dose q12h. CrCl ≤10mL/min or SrCr of ≥4.6mg/dL: 1/2 usual dose q18-24h. Apply reduced dosage recommendations after initial LD is given.
Pediatrics: Mild to Moderately Severe Infections: 25-50mg/kg/day, given tid or qid. Titrate: May increase to 100mg/kg/day for severe infections. Renal Impairment: CrCl 40-70mL/min: 60% of normal daily dose given in equally divided doses every 12 hrs. CrCl 20-40mL/min: 25% of normal daily dose given in equally divided doses every 12 hrs. CrCl 5-20mL/min: 10% of normal daily dose every 24 hrs. Apply reduced dosage recommendations after initial LD is given.

HOW SUPPLIED: Inj: 500mg, 1g, 10g, 20g

WARNINGS/PRECAUTIONS: Caution with penicillin (PCN) allergy; possible cross-hypersensitivity among β-lactam antibiotics. D/C if an allergic reaction develops. *C.difficile*-associated diarrhea (CDAD) reported. Prolonged use may result in overgrowth of nonsusceptible organisms. Lower doses are required in patients with low urinary output due to renal impairment; seizures may occur if inappropriate high doses are administered to patients with renal impairment. Caution with history of colitis or other GI diseases. Safety in premature infants and neonates not established. Positive Coombs' tests reported. False positive reaction for glucose in the urine may occur with Benedict's solution, Fehling's solution, or with Clinitest tabs. May cause a fall in prothrombin activity; caution in patients with renal/hepatic impairment, patients on protracted course of antimicrobial therapy, and in patients previously stabilized on anticoagulant therapy; monitor PT and administer vitamin K as indicated.

ADVERSE REACTIONS: Diarrhea, oral candidiasis, N/V, stomach cramps, anorexia, allergic reactions, blood dyscrasias, renal failure, transient rise in AST/ALT/BUN/SrCr/alkaline phosphatase, genital and anal pruritus.

INTERACTIONS: Decreased renal tubular secretion with probenecid.

PREGNANCY: Category B, caution in nursing.

MECHANISM OF ACTION: Cephalosporin; inhibits cell wall synthesis.

PHARMACOKINETICS: Absorption: C_{max}=185mcg/mL. **Distribution:** Crosses placenta; found in breast milk. **Elimination:** Urine (unchanged); $T_{1/2}$=1.8 hrs.

NURSING CONSIDERATIONS

Assessment: Assess for hypersensitivity to PCN, renal/hepatic impairment, history of GI disease (eg, colitis), nutritional status, pregnancy/nursing status, and possible drug interactions.

Monitoring: Monitor for signs/symptoms of a hypersensitivity reaction, CDAD, drug resistance or superinfection. Monitor PT in patients at risk of a fall in prothrombin activity. Monitor for seizures in patients with renal dysfunction.

Patient Counseling: Inform drug only treats bacterial, not viral, infections. Instruct to take as directed; skipping doses or not completing full course may decrease effectiveness and increase resistance. Advise to d/c therapy and notify physician if an allergic reaction or diarrhea occurs. Instruct to notify if pregnant/nursing.

Administration: IV route. **Storage:** -20°C (-4°F). Do not force thaw by immersion in water baths or by microwave irridiation. Thawed solution is stable for 30 days under refrigeration 5°C (41°F) and for 48 hrs at 25°C (77°F). Do not refreeze thawed antibiotics.

CEFDINIR   RX
cefdinir (Various)

THERAPEUTIC CLASS: Cephalosporin (3rd generation)

INDICATIONS: Community-acquired pneumonia (CAP), acute exacerbations of chronic bronchitis (AECB), acute maxillary sinusitis, pharyngitis/tonsillitis, and uncomplicated skin and skin structure infections (SSSIs) in adult and adolescent patients. Acute bacterial otitis media, pharyngitis/tonsillitis, and uncomplicated SSSIs in pediatric patients.

DOSAGE: *Adults:* (Cap) SSSI/CAP: 300mg q12h for 10 days. AECB/ Pharyngitis/Tonsillitis: 300mg q12h for 5-10 days or 600mg q24h for 10 days. Sinusitis: 300mg q12h or 600mg q24h for 10 days. CrCl <30mL/min: 300mg qd. Hemodialysis: Initial: 300mg or 7mg/kg qod. 300mg or 7mg/kg should be given at end of each hemodialysis session. Usual: 300mg or 7mg/kg qod. *Pediatrics:* (Sus) ≥43 kg: Max dose: 600mg/day. 6 months-12 yrs: Otitis Media/ Pharyngitis/Tonsillitis: 7mg/kg q12h for 5-10 days or 14mg/kg q24h for 10 days. Sinusitis: 7mg/kg q12h or 14mg/kg q24h for 10 days. SSSI: 7mg/kg q12h for 10 days. (Cap) ≥13 yrs: CAP/SSSI: 300mg q12h for 10 days. AECB/ Pharyngitis/Tonsillitis: 300mg q12h for 5-10 days or 600mg q24h for 10 days. Sinusitis: 300mg q12h or 600mg q24h for 10 days. CrCl <30mL/min/1.73m²: 7mg/kg qd. Max: 300mg qd.

HOW SUPPLIED: Cap: 300mg; Sus: 125mg/5mL, 250mg/5mL [60mL, 100mL]

WARNINGS/PRECAUTIONS: Cross-sensitivity to penicillins (PCNs) and other cephalosporins may occur. D/C use if an allergic reaction occurs. *Clostridium difficile*-associated diarrhea (CDAD) has been reported. Use in the absence of a proven or strongly suspected bacterial infection or prophylactic indication is unlikely to provide benefit and increases risk of development of drug-resistant bacteria. Prolonged treatment may result in emergence and overgrowth of resistant organisms; administer appropriate alternate therapy if superinfection develops. Reduce dose in patients with transient or persistent renal insufficiency (CrCl <30mL/min). Caution in patients with a history of colitis. Sus contains sucrose; caution in diabetes. Positive direct Coombs' tests may occur as well as false (+) for urine glucose with Clinitest and Benedict's or Fehling's solution. A false (+) reaction for ketones in the urine may occur with tests using nitroprusside.

ADVERSE REACTIONS: Diarrhea, vaginal moniliasis, nausea.

INTERACTIONS: Iron-fortified foods, iron supplements, and aluminum- or magnesium-containing antacids reduce absorption; separate doses by 2 hrs. Probenecid inhibits the renal excretion. Reddish stools reported with iron-containing products. Possible interaction between cefdinir and diclofenac.

PREGNANCY: Category B, safe in nursing.

MECHANISM OF ACTION: Extended-spectrum cephalosporin; bactericidal activity from inhibition of cell-wall synthesis.

PHARMACOKINETICS: Absorption: Cap: (300mg) C_{max}=1.6mcg/mL, T_{max}=2.9 hrs, AUC=7.05mcg•hr/mL. (600mg) C_{max}=2.87mcg/mL, T_{max}=3 hrs, AUC=11.1mcg•hr/mL. Sus: (7mg/kg) C_{max}=2.3mcg/mL, T_{max}=2.2 hrs, AUC=8.31mcg•hr/mL. (14mg/kg) C_{max}=3.86mcg/mL, T_{max}=1.8 hrs, AUC=13.4mcg•hr/mL. **Distribution:** V_d=0.35L/kg (adults), 0.67L/kg (pediatrics); plasma protein binding (60-70%). **Elimination:** (300mg) Urine (18.4% unchanged); (600mg) Urine (11.6% unchanged); $T_{1/2}$=1.7 hrs.

NURSING CONSIDERATIONS

Assessment: Assess for allergy to other cephalosporins, PCN, or to other drugs, history of colitis, renal impairment, and for possible drug interactions. Assess for diabetes if planning to use sus formulation. Assess proper diagnosis of causative organisms.

Monitoring: Monitor for signs/symptoms of hypersensitivity reactions, CDAD, and for development of a superinfection.

Patient Counseling: Treats bacterial, not viral, infections. Take as directed; skipping doses or not completing full course may decrease effectiveness and increase bacterial resistance. Take 2 hrs before or after antacid or iron supplements. Inform diabetics that sus contains sucrose. Diarrhea may occur; notify physician if watery/bloody stools, superinfection, or hypersensitivity reactions occur.

Administration: Oral route. **Storage:** Cap/Unsuspended Powder: 25°C (77°F); excursions permitted to 15-30°C (59-86°F). Reconstituted Sus: Can be stored at controlled room temperature for 10 days.

CEFOXITIN
cefoxitin sodium (Various)

RX

THERAPEUTIC CLASS: Cephalosporin (2nd generation)

INDICATIONS: Treatment of lower respiratory tract/urinary tract/intra-abdominal/gynecological/skin and skin structure/bone and joint infections and septicemia caused by susceptible strains of microorganisms. Prophylaxis in patients undergoing uncontaminated GI surgery, abdominal/vaginal hysterectomy, or cesarean section (CS).

DOSAGE: *Adults:* Usual: 1-2g IV q6-8h. Uncomplicated Infections: 1g IV q6-8h. Moderate-Severe Infections: 1g IV q4h or 2g IV q6-8h. Gas Gangrene/Other Infections Requiring Higher Dose: 2g IV q4h or 3g IV q6h. Renal Insufficiency: LD: 1-2g IV. Maint: CrCl 30-50mL/min: 1-2g IV q8-12h. CrCl 10-29mL/min: 1-2g IV q12-24h. CrCl 5-9mL/min: 0.5-1g IV q12-24h. CrCl <5mL/min: 0.5-1g IV q24-48h. Hemodialysis: LD: 1-2g IV after dialysis. Maint: See renal insufficiency doses above. Group A β-Hemolytic Streptococcal Infection: Maintain therapy ≥10 days. Prophylaxis: Uncontaminated GI Surgery/Hysterectomy: 2g IV prior to surgery (1/2-1 hr before initial incision), then 2g IV q6h after 1st dose ≤24 hrs. CS: 2g IV single dose as soon as umbilical cord is clamped, or 2g IV as soon as umbilical cord is clamped, followed by 2g IV at 4 and 8 hrs after initial dose.
Pediatrics: ≥3 months: 80-160mg/kg/day divided into 4-6 equal doses. Max: 12g/day. Renal Insufficiency: Modify dosage and frequency of dosage consistent with recommendations for adults. Prophylaxis: Uncontaminated GI Surgery/Hysterectomy: 30-40mg/kg IV prior to surgery (1/2-1 hr before initial incision), then 30-40mg/kg IV q6h after 1st dose ≤24 hrs.

HOW SUPPLIED: Inj: 1g, 2g. Also available as a Duplex and Pharmacy Bulk Package; refer to individual PI.

WARNINGS/PRECAUTIONS: Caution with previous hypersensitivity to cephalosporins, penicillins (PCNs), or other drugs. D/C if allergic reaction occurs. *Clostridium difficile*-associated diarrhea (CDAD) reported; d/c if suspected/confirmed and institute appropriate fluid and electrolyte management, protein supplementation, antibiotic treatment of *C. difficile*, and surgical evaluation. Use in absence of a proven bacterial infection or a prophylactic indication is unlikely to provide benefit and increases the risk of drug-resistant bacteria. Caution with GI disease, particularly colitis. Prolonged use may result in overgrowth of nonsusceptible organisms. May interfere with lab test measurements of serum/urinary creatinine levels by Jaffe reaction and urinary 17-hydroxy-corticosteroid by Porter-Silber reaction at high concentrations, and false (+) reaction for urinary glucose using Clinitest.

ADVERSE REACTIONS: Thrombophlebitis, rash, pseudomembranous colitis, pruritus, fever, dyspnea, hypotension, diarrhea, blood dyscrasias, elevated LFTs, changes in renal function tests, exacerbation of myasthenia gravis.

INTERACTIONS: Increased nephrotoxicity with aminoglycoside antibiotics.

PREGNANCY: Category B, caution in nursing.

MECHANISM OF ACTION: 2nd-generation cephalosporin; inhibits bacterial cell-wall synthesis.

PHARMACOKINETICS: Distribution: Passes pleural and joint fluids; found in breast milk. **Elimination:** Urine (85% unchanged); $T_{1/2}$=41-59 min.

NURSING CONSIDERATIONS

Assessment: Assess for previous hypersensitivity reactions to cephalosporins, PCNs, or other drugs, renal/hepatic function, GI disease, pregnancy/nursing status, and possible drug interactions. Perform appropriate culture and susceptibility studies to determine susceptible causative organisms.

Monitoring: Periodically monitor renal/hepatic/hematopoietic functions, especially with prolonged therapy. Monitor for CDAD (may range from mild diarrhea to fatal colitis), development of superinfections or drug resistance, allergic reactions (eg, toxic epidermal necrolysis or exfoliative dermatitis), and other adverse reactions. Monitor LFTs.

Patient Counseling: Inform that drug only treats bacterial, not viral infections. Instruct to take exactly as directed; skipping doses or not completing full course may decrease effectiveness and increase resistance. Inform about potential benefits/risks. Advise to notify physician if watery/bloody stools (with/without muscle cramps or fever) occurs even ≥2 months after therapy. Notify if pregnant/nursing.

Administration: IV route. Inspect for particulate matter and discoloration prior to use. Refer to PI for preparation, administration, and compatibility and stability instructions. **Storage:** Dry state at 2-25°C (36-77°F). Avoid >50°C.

CEFPODOXIME RX
cefpodoxime proxetil (Various)

THERAPEUTIC CLASS: Cephalosporin (3rd generation)

INDICATIONS: Treatment of mild to moderate infections (acute otitis media, pharyngitis/tonsillitis, community-acquired pneumonia [CAP], acute bacterial exacerbation of chronic bronchitis [ABECB], acute uncomplicated urethral and cervical gonorrhea, acute uncomplicated anorectal infections in women, uncomplicated skin and skin structure infections [SSSI], acute maxillary sinusitis, and uncomplicated urinary tract infections [cystitis]) caused by susceptible strains of microorganisms.

DOSAGE: *Adults:* Pharyngitis/Tonsillitis: 100mg q12h for 5-10 days. CAP: 200mg q12h for 14 days. ABECB: 200mg q12h for 10 days. Uncomplicated Gonorrhea (Men/Women)/Rectal Gonococcal Infections (Women): 200mg single dose. SSSI: 400mg q12h for 7-14 days. Sinusitis: 200mg q12h for 10 days. Cystitis: 100mg q12h for 7 days. CrCl <30mL/min: Increase interval to q24h. Hemodialysis: Dose 3 times weekly after dialysis. Take with food. *Pediatrics:* ≥12 yrs: (Susp/Tabs): Pharyngitis/Tonsillitis: 100mg q12h for 5-10 days. CAP: 200mg q12h for 14 days. Uncomplicated Gonorrhea (Men/Women)/Rectal Gonococcal Infections (Women): 200mg single dose. SSSI: 400mg q12h for 7-14 days. Sinusitis: 200mg q12h for 10 days. Cystitis: 100mg q12h for 7 days. (Tabs) ABECB: 200mg q12h for 10 days. 2 months to 12 yrs:

(Susp): Otitis media: 5mg/kg (Max 200mg/dose) q12h for 5 days. Pharyngitis/Tonsillitis: 5mg/kg/dose (Max 100mg/dose) q12h for 5-10 days. Sinusitis: 5mg/kg (Max 200mg/dose) for 10 days. CrCl <30mL/min: Increase interval to q24h. Hemodialysis: Dose 3 times weekly after dialysis. Take with food.

HOW SUPPLIED: Sus: 50mg/5mL, 100mg/5mL; Tab: 100mg, 200mg

WARNINGS/PRECAUTIONS: Caution with penicillin (PCN)-sensitive patients; cross hypersensitivity reaction may occur; d/c if an allergic reaction occurs. *Clostridium difficile*-associated diarrhea (CDAD) reported. Pseudomembranous colitis reported. Positive direct Coombs' tests reported. Caution with renal impairment; dose reduction may be needed. May result in overgrowth of nonsusceptible organisms with prolonged use; take appropriate measures if superinfection develops. Use in the absence of a proven or strongly suspected bacterial infection or prophylactic indication is unlikely to provide benefit and increases the risk of development of drug-resistant bacteria. Oral sus may contain phenylalanine. Tabs may contain tartrazine which may cause an allergic reaction in susceptible individuals.

ADVERSE REACTIONS: Diarrhea, nausea.

INTERACTIONS: Decreased plasma levels and extent of absorption with antacids and H_2-blockers. Delayed peak plasma levels with oral anticholinergics. Probenecid inhibits renal excretion. Closely monitor renal function with nephrotoxic agents. Caution with potent diuretics.

PREGNANCY: Category B, not for use in nursing.

MECHANISM OF ACTION: Cephalosporin; inhibits cell-wall synthesis.

PHARMACOKINETICS: Absorption: C_{max}(100mg)=1.4mcg/mL, (200mg)=2.3mcg/mL, (400mg)=3.9mcg/mL; T_{max}=2-3 hrs. **Distribution:** Plasma protein binding (21-29%), found in breast milk. **Metabolism:** Via desterification; cefpodoxime (active metabolite). **Elimination:** Urine; $T_{1/2}$= 2.09-2.84 hrs.

NURSING CONSIDERATIONS

Assessment: Assess for history of hypersensitivity to cephalosporins/PCNs, renal impairment, pregnancy/nursing status, and for possible drug interactions. Document indications for therapy, culture, and susceptibility testing.

Monitoring: Monitor for signs/symptoms of hypersensitivity reactions, CDAD, pseudomembranous colitis, and for superinfection. Monitor renal function.

Patient Counseling: Inform that drug only treats bacterial, not viral infections. Instruct to take as directed; inform that skipping doses or not completing full course of therapy may decrease effectiveness of immediate treatment and increase resistance to drug. Inform that may experience diarrhea; instruct to contact physician if watery/bloody stools develop.

Administration: Oral route. **Storage:** Sus (Prior to reconstitution)/Tab: 20-25°C (68-77°F). Sus (Following reconstitution) 2-8°C (36-46°F) Shake well before using. Keep tightly closed. May be used for 14 days; discard unused portion after 14 days. (Tab) Protect from excessive moisture.

CEFPROZIL   RX
cefprozil (Various)

THERAPEUTIC CLASS: Cephalosporin (2nd generation)

INDICATIONS: Treatment of mild to moderate pharyngitis/tonsillitis, otitis media, acute sinusitis, secondary bacterial infection of acute bronchitis, acute bacterial exacerbation of chronic bronchitis (ABECB), and uncomplicated skin and skin structure infections (SSSI) caused by susceptible strains of microorganisms.

DOSAGE: *Adults:* Pharyngitis/Tonsillitis: 500mg q24h for 10 days. Acute Sinusitis: 250-500mg q12h for 10 days. ABECB/Acute Bronchitis: 500mg q12h for 10 days. SSSI: 250-500mg q12h or 500mg q24h for 10 days. CrCl <30mL/min: 50% of standard dose.
Pediatrics: ≥13 yrs: Use adult dose. 2-12 yrs: Pharyngitis/Tonsillitis: 7.5mg/kg

q12h for 10 days. SSSI: 20mg/kg q24h for 10 days. 6 months-12 yrs: Otitis Media: 15mg/kg q12h for 10 days. Acute Sinusitis: 7.5-15mg/kg q12h for 10 days. Do not exceed adult dose. CrCl <30mL/min: 50% of standard dose.

HOW SUPPLIED: Sus: 125mg/5mL, 250mg/5mL [50mL, 75mL, 100mL]; Tab: 250mg, 500mg

WARNINGS/PRECAUTIONS: Caution with previous hypersensitivity to cephalosporins, penicillins (PCNs), or other drugs; cross-sensitivity may occur with history of PCN allergy. D/C if allergic reaction occurs. *Clostridium difficile*-associated diarrhea (CDAD) reported. Prolonged use may result in overgrowth of nonsusceptible organisms; take appropriate measures if superinfection occurs. Caution with GI disease, particularly colitis. Positive direct Coombs' tests reported with cephalosporin. Caution with renal impairment and elderly. May produce false (+) reaction for urine glucose with Benedict's, Fehling's solution, and Clinitest tabs. False (-) ferricyanide test for blood glucose may occur.

ADVERSE REACTIONS: Diarrhea, N/V, ALT/AST elevation, eosinophilia, genital pruritus, vaginitis, superinfection, diaper rash, dizziness, abdominal pain.

INTERACTIONS: Nephrotoxicity with aminoglycosides reported. Probenecid may increase plasma levels. Caution with potent diuretics.

PREGNANCY: Category B, caution in nursing.

MECHANISM OF ACTION: 2nd-generation cephalosporin; inhibits bacterial cell-wall synthesis.

PHARMACOKINETICS: Absorption: C_{max}=6.1mcg/mL (250mg), 10.5mcg/mL (500mg), 18.3mcg/mL (1g); T_{max}=1.5 hrs (adults), 1-2 hrs (peds). Plasma concentration (peds) at 7.5, 15, and 30mg/kg doses similar to those observed within same time frame in normal adults at 250, 500, and 1000mg doses, respectively. **Distribution:** V_d=0.23L/kg; plasma protein binding (36%); found in breast milk. **Elimination:** Urine (60%); $T_{1/2}$=1.3 hrs (adults), 1.5 hrs (peds).

NURSING CONSIDERATIONS

Assessment: Assess for previous hypersensitivity reactions to PCNs/cephalosporins or other drugs, renal/hepatic function, GI disease, pregnancy/nursing status, and possible drug interactions. Perform appropriate culture and susceptibility studies to determine susceptible causative organisms.

Monitoring: Periodically monitor renal/hepatic/hematopoietic functions. Monitor for CDAD (may range from mild diarrhea to fatal colitis), development of superinfections or drug resistance, allergic reactions, and other adverse reactions.

Patient Counseling: Inform that the oral sus contains phenylalanine. Inform that drug only treats bacterial, not viral infections. Instruct to take exactly as directed; skipping doses or not completing full course may decrease effectiveness and increase resistance. Inform about potential benefits/risks. Notify physician if watery/bloody stools (with/without stomach cramps/fever) occur even ≥2 months after therapy. Notify if pregnant/nursing.

Administration: Oral route. Shake sus well before use. Refer to PI for reconstitution direction. **Storage:** Tab/Dry Powder: 20-25°C (68-77°F). Reconstituted Sus: Refrigerate after mixing and discard unused portion after 14 days.

CEFTAZIDIME   RX
ceftazidime (Various)

THERAPEUTIC CLASS: Cephalosporin (3rd generation)

INDICATIONS: Treatment of lower respiratory tract (eg, pneumonia), skin and skin structure (SSSI), bone and joint, gynecologic, CNS (eg, meningitis), intra-abdominal, and urinary tract infections (UTI), and septicemia caused by susceptible strains of microorganisms. For use in sepsis.

DOSAGE: *Adults:* Usual: 1g IM/IV q8-12h. Uncomplicated UTI: 250mg IM/IV q12h. Complicated UTI: 500mg IM/IV q8-12h. Bone and Joint Infection: 2g IV q12h. Uncomplicated Pneumonia/SSSI: 500mg-1g IM/IV q8h. Gynecological/Intra-Abdominal/Meningitis/Severe Life-Threatening Infection: 2g IV q8h.

Lung Infection caused by *Pseudomonas* spp. in Cystic Fibrosis (normal renal function): 30-50mg/kg IV q8h. Max: 6g/day. CrCl 31-50mL/min: 1g q12h. CrCl 16-30mL/min: 1g q24h. CrCl 6-15mL/min: 500mg q24h. CrCl <5mL/min: 500mg q48h. For severe infections (6g/day), increase renal impairment dose by 50% or increase dosing interval. Apply reduced dosage recommendations after initial 1g LD is given. Hemodialysis: Give 1g before then 1g after each hemodialysis. Intra-Peritoneal Dialysis/Continuous Ambulatory Peritoneal Dialysis: Give 1g followed by 500mg q24h.

Pediatrics: ≥12 yrs: Usual: 1g IM/IV q8-12h. Uncomplicated UTI: 250mg IM/IV q12h. Complicated UTI: 500mg IM/IV q8-12h. Bone and Joint Infection: 2g IV q12h. Uncomplicated Pneumonia/SSSI: 500mg-1g IM/IV q8h. Gynecological/Intra-Abdominal/Meningitis/Severe Life-Threatening Infection: 2g IV q8h. Lung Infection caused by *Pseudomonas* spp. in Cystic Fibrosis (normal renal function): 30-50mg/kg IV q8h. Max: 6g/day. CrCl 31-50mL/min: 1g q12h. CrCl 16-30mL/min: 1g q24h. CrCl 6-15mL/min: 500mg q24h. CrCl <5mL/min: 500mg q48h. For severe infections (6g/day), increase renal impairment dose by 50% or increase dosing interval. Apply reduced dosage recommendations after initial 1g LD is given. Hemodialysis: Give 1g before then 1g after each hemodialysis. Intra-Peritoneal Dialysis/Continuous Ambulatory Peritoneal Dialysis: Give 1g followed by 500mg q24h.

HOW SUPPLIED: Inj: 1g, 2g, 6g

WARNINGS/PRECAUTIONS: Monitor renal function; potential for nephrotoxicity. Prolonged use may result in overgrowth of nonsusceptible organisms. Possible cross-sensitivity between penicillins (PCNs), cephalosporins, and other β-lactam antibiotics. Pseudomembranous colitis and CDAD reported. Elevated levels with renal insufficiency can lead to seizures, encephalopathy, asterixis, coma, and neuromuscular excitability. Possible decrease in PT; caution with renal or hepatic impairment, poor nutritional state; monitor PT and give vitamin K if needed. Caution with colitis and other GI diseases. Distal necrosis can occur after inadvertent intra-arterial administration. Continue therapy for 2 days after the signs and symptoms of infection have disappeared, but in complicated infections longer therapy may be required. False (+) for urine glucose with Benedict's, Fehling's solution, and Clinitest tabs.

ADVERSE REACTIONS: Phlebitis and inflammation at injection site, pruritus, rash, fever, diarrhea.

INTERACTIONS: Nephrotoxicity reported with aminoglycosides or potent diuretics (eg, furosemide). Avoid with chloramphenicol; may decrease effect of β-lactam antibiotics.

PREGNANCY: Category B, not for use in nursing.

MECHANISM OF ACTION: Broad spectrum, β-lactam antibiotic; exerts effects by inhibiting enzymes responsible for cell-wall synthesis.

PHARMACOKINETICS: Absorption: (IV) C_{max}=45mcg/mL (500mg), 90mcg/mL (1g). (IM) C_{max}=17mcg/mL (500mg), 39mcg/mL (1g), T_{max}=1 hr. **Distribution:** Plasma protein binding (<10%); found in breast milk. **Elimination:** Urine, (80-90% unchanged). $T_{1/2}$=1.9 hrs (IV), 2 hrs (IM).

NURSING CONSIDERATIONS

Assessment: Assess for previous hypersensitivity to cephalosporins/PCNs or other drugs, renal/hepatic insufficiency, nutritional status, history of GI disease, pregnancy/nursing status, and possible drug interactions.

Monitoring: Periodically monitor PT, with vitamin K administration if indicated. Monitor for allergic reactions (eg, Stevens-Johnson syndrome), signs/symptoms of pseudomembranous colitis or CDAD, seizures, encephalopathy, coma, asterixis, neuromuscular excitability, and myoclonia, development of superinfection or drug resistance, renal function tests/urine output for daily dosage, LFTs, hematopoietic function, and lab test interactions.

Patient Counseling: Inform that drug only treats bacterial, not viral, infections. Take exactly as directed; skipping doses or not completing full course may decrease effectiveness and increase resistance. Inform about potential benefits/risks. D/C and notify physician if allergic reactions, watery/bloody diarrhea (with/without muscle cramps), or fever occurs. Notify if pregnant/nursing.

C

Administration: IV/IM routes. Do not use plastic containers for series connections to avoid development of air embolism. **Storage:** Dry state at 15-30°C (59-86°F); protect from light. As premixed solution not >-20°C; do not force thaw by immersion in water baths or by microwave irradiation; store thawed solutions for up to 24 hrs at room temperature or for 7 days in a refrigerator. Do not refreeze thawed solution.

CEFTIN   RX
cefuroxime axetil (GlaxoSmithKline)

THERAPEUTIC CLASS: Cephalosporin (2nd generation)

INDICATIONS: Treatment of the following infections caused by susceptible strains of microorganisms: (Sus/Tab) Pharyngitis/tonsillitis and acute otitis media. (Sus) Impetigo. (Tab) Uncomplicated skin and skin structure infections (SSSI), uncomplicated urinary tract infections (UTI), uncomplicated gonorrhea, early Lyme disease, acute bacterial maxillary sinusitis, acute bacterial exacerbations of chronic bronchitis (ABECB), and secondary bacterial infections of acute bronchitis.

DOSAGE: *Adults:* (Tab) Pharyngitis/Tonsillitis/Sinusitis: 250mg bid for 10 days. ABECB/SSSI: 250-500mg bid for 10 days. Acute Bronchitis: 250-500mg bid for 5-10 days. UTI: 250mg bid for 7-10 days. Gonorrhea: 1000mg single dose. Lyme Disease: 500mg bid for 20 days.
Pediatrics: ≥13 yrs: (Tab) Pharyngitis/Tonsillitis/Sinusitis: 250mg bid for 10 days. ABECB/SSSI: 250-500mg bid for 10 days. Acute Bronchitis: 250-500mg bid for 5-10 days. UTI: 250mg bid for 7-10 days. Gonorrhea: 1000mg single dose. Lyme Disease: 500mg bid for 20 days. 3 months-12 yrs: (Sus) Pharyngitis/Tonsillitis: 20mg/kg/day divided bid for 10 days. Max: 500mg/day. Otitis Media/Sinusitis/Impetigo: 30mg/kg/day divided bid for 10 days. Max: 1000mg/day. (Tab-if can swallow whole) Otitis Media/Sinusitis: 250mg bid for 10 days.

HOW SUPPLIED: Sus: 125mg/5mL [100mL], 250mg/5mL [50mL, 100mL]; Tab: 250mg, 500mg

WARNINGS/PRECAUTIONS: Tabs are not bioequivalent to sus. Caution in patients with previous hypersensitivity to penicillins (PCNs) or other drugs; cross-sensitivity may occur in patients with a history of PCN allergy. D/C if an allergic reaction occurs. Watery, bloody stools (with or without stomach cramps and fever) may develop after starting treatment. *Clostridium difficile*-associated diarrhea (CDAD) reported and may range in severity from mild diarrhea to fatal colitis. Caution with a history of colitis. Prolonged administration may result in overgrowth of nonsusceptible organisms; take appropriate measures if superinfection occurs. Safety and efficacy not established in patients with GI malabsorption. May cause fall in PT; those at risk include patients previously stable on anticoagulants, patients receiving protracted course of antibiotics, patients with renal/hepatic impairment, and in patients with a poor nutritional state. Monitor PT and give vitamin K as needed. Use in the absence of a proven or strongly suspected bacterial infection or a prophylactic indication may increase the risk of the development of drug-resistant bacteria. Safety and efficacy not established in patients with renal failure. False (+) for urine glucose with Benedict's, Fehling's solution, and Clinitest tabs. False (-) results may occur in ferricyanide test. (Sus) Contains phenylalanine.

ADVERSE REACTIONS: Diarrhea, N/V, vaginitis, (suspension) dislike of taste, diaper rash.

INTERACTIONS: Probenecid increases plasma levels. Lower bioavailability with drugs that lower gastric acidity. Caution with agents causing adverse effects on renal function (diuretics). May lower estrogen reabsorption and reduce the efficacy of combined oral estrogen/progesterone contraceptives.

PREGNANCY: Category B, not for use in nursing.

MECHANISM OF ACTION: 2nd-generation cephalosporin; binds to essential target proteins and the resultant inhibition of cell-wall synthesis.

PHARMACOKINETICS: Absorption: Absolute bioavailability (37% before food), (52% after food). PO administration of variable doses resulted in different parameters. **Distribution:** Plasma protein binding (50%); found in breast milk. **Metabolism:** Rapid hydrolysis, via nonspecific esterases in the intestinal mucosa and blood. **Elimination:** Urine (50% unchanged).

NURSING CONSIDERATIONS

Assessment: Assess for previous hypersensitivity reactions to cephalosporins/PCNs or other drugs, renal/hepatic impairment, nutritional state, history of colitis, GI malabsorption, pregnancy/nursing status, and for possible drug interactions. For patients planning on using sus formulation, assess for phenylketonuria.

Monitoring: Monitor signs/symptoms of an allergic reaction, CDAD, superinfection, and lab test interactions. Monitor PT and renal function.

Patient Counseling: Advise of potential benefits/risks of therapy. Inform that drug only treats bacterial, not viral infections. Instruct to take exactly as directed; skipping doses or not completing full course may decrease effectiveness and increase resistance. Counsel to d/c and notify physician if an allergic reaction or if watery/bloody diarrhea (with/without stomach cramps or fever) develop. Instruct to notify physician if pregnant/nursing. Inform caregivers of pediatric patients that if cannot swallow tab whole, should receive oral sus. Advise that crushed tab, has a strong/persistent bitter taste. Inform that tab may be administered without regard to meals but oral sus must be administered with food.

Administration: Oral route. Tab and sus not bioequivalent and not substitutable on mg-per-mg basis. Refer to PI for reconstitution instructions for sus. Shake sus well before use. **Storage:** Tab: Store at 15-30°C (59-86°F). Sus Powder: Store at 2-30°C (36-86°F). Reconstituted Sus: Store at 2-8°C (36-46°F) in a refrigerator; discard after 10 days.

CEFTRIAXONE   RX
ceftriaxone sodium (Various)

OTHER BRAND NAMES: Rocephin (Roche)

THERAPEUTIC CLASS: Cephalosporin (3rd generation)

INDICATIONS: Treatment of lower respiratory tract infections, skin and skin structure infections (SSSI), bone and joint infections, intra-abdominal infections, urinary tract infections, acute bacterial otitis media, uncomplicated gonorrhea, pelvic inflammatory disease, bacterial septicemia, and meningitis caused by susceptible strains of microorganisms. Surgical prophylaxis during surgical procedures classified as contaminated or potentially contaminated.

DOSAGE: *Adults:* Usual: 1-2g/day IV/IM given qd or bid in equally divided doses depending on the type and severity of infection. Max: 4g/day. Gonorrhea: 250mg IM single dose. Surgical Prophylaxis: 1g IV 1/2-2 hrs before surgery. Continue therapy for ≥2 days after signs and symptoms of infection disappear. Usual duration: 4-14 days; complicated infections may require longer therapy. *S. pyogenes* Infections: Continue therapy for ≥10 days.
Pediatrics: SSSI: 50-75mg/kg/day IV/IM given qd or in equally divided doses bid. Max: 2g/day. Otitis Media: 50mg/kg (up to 1g) IM single dose. Serious Infections: 50-75mg/kg IV/IM given q12h. Max: 2g/day. Meningitis: Initial: 100mg/kg (up to 4g) IV/IM, then 100mg/kg/day IV/IM given qd or in equally divided doses q12h for 7-14 days. Max: 4g/day.

HOW SUPPLIED: Inj: (Rocephin) 500mg, 1g; (Generic) 250mg, 500mg, 1g, 2g. Also available as a Pharmacy Bulk Package. Refer to individual package insert for more information

CONTRAINDICATIONS: Hyperbilirubinemic neonates (≤28 days), especially if premature; concurrent use of calcium-containing IV solutions used in neonates.

WARNINGS/PRECAUTIONS: Caution in penicillin-sensitive patients and in patients who have demonstrated any form of an allergy, particularly to drugs.

Serious acute hypersensitvity reactions may require the use of SQ epinephrine and other emergency measures. Anaphylactic reactions reported. *Clostridium difficile*-associated diarrhea (CDAD) reported; if suspected/confirmed, d/c and institute appropriate therapy. Severe cases of hemolytic anemia reported; d/c until cause is determined. Increased risk of drug-resistant bacteria if used in the absence of a proven or strongly suspected bacterial infection or a prophylactic indication. Transient BUN and SrCr elevations may occur. Caution in patients with both hepatic and significant renal disease, Max: 2g/day. Alterations in PT may occur; monitor with impaired vitamin K synthesis or low vitamin K stores during treatment. Prolonged use may result in overgrowth of nonsusceptible organisms; take appropriate measures if superinfection develops. Caution with history of GI disease, especially colitis. Gallbladder sonographic abnormalities reported; d/c if gallbladder disease develops. Pancreatitis reported rarely.

ADVERSE REACTIONS: Injection-site reactions (eg, warmth, tightness, induration), eosinophilia, thrombocytosis, AST elevation, ALT elevation.

INTERACTIONS: See Contraindications.

PREGNANCY: Category B, caution in nursing.

MECHANISM OF ACTION: 3rd-generation cephalosporin; bactericidal activity results from inhibition of cell-wall synthesis.

PHARMACOKINETICS: Absorption: (Adults IM) Complete; T_{max}=2-3 hrs. (Pediatrics) Bacterial meningitis: C_{max}=216mcg/mL (50mg/kg IV), 275mcg/mL (75mg/kg IV). Middle ear fluid: C_{max}=35mcg/mL; T_{max}=24 hrs. **Distribution:** Found in breast milk and crosses blood placenta barrier; plasma protein binding (95%) (<25mcg/mL), (85%) (300mcg/mL); (Adults) V_d=5.78-13.5L. (Pediatrics) Bacterial meningitis: V_d=338mL/kg (50mg/kg IV), 373mL/kg (75mg/kg IV). **Elimination:** Urine (33-67%, unchanged), feces. (Adults) $T_{1/2}$=5.8-8.7 hrs. (Pediatrics) Bacterial meningitis: $T_{1/2}$=4.6 hrs (50mg/kg IV), 4.3 hrs (75mg/kg IV); Middle ear fluid: $T_{1/2}$=25 hrs.

NURSING CONSIDERATIONS

Assessment: Assess for hyperbilirubinemic neonates, especially if premature, hypersensitivity to penicillins or other drugs, presence of both hepatic dysfunction and significant renal disease, impaired vitamin K synthesis or low vitamin K stores, history of GI disease (eg, colitis), pregnancy/nursing status, and for possible drug interactions.

Monitoring: Monitor for signs/symptoms of hypersensitivity reactions, CDAD, overgrowth of nonsusceptible organisms (eg, superinfection), gallbladder disease, and pancreatitis. Periodically monitor BUN and SrCr levels. Monitor PT levels in patients with low impaired vitamin K synthesis or in patients with low vitamin K stores (eg, chronic hepatic disease, malnutrition).

Patient Counseling: Inform that therapy only treats bacterial, not viral, infections (eg, common cold). Instruct to take as directed; skipping doses or not completing full course may decrease drug effectiveness and increase risk of bacteria developing resistance. Inform that diarrhea (watery/bloody stools) may be experienced as late as 2 months or more after last dose; contact a physician as soon as possible if this occur.

Administration: IV/IM route. Incompatible with vancomycin, amsacrine, aminoglycosides, and fluconazole; when administered concomitantly by intermittent IV infusion, give sequentially, with thorough flushing of the intravenous lines between administrations. Avoid physically mixing with or piggybacking with solutions containing antimicrobial drugs. IV infusion should be administered over a period of 30 min. Refer to PI for reconstitution directions. **Storage:** ≤25°C (77°F). Protect from light. Do not refreeze unused portions.

CELEBREX

RX

celecoxib (G.D. Searle)

> NSAIDs may cause an increased risk of serious cardiovascular (CV) thrombotic events, myocardial infarction (MI), stroke and serious GI adverse events (eg, bleeding, ulceration, and perforation of the stomach or intestines), which can be fatal. These events can occur at any time during use without warning symptoms. Contraindicated for the treatment of perioperative pain in the setting of coronary artery bypass graft (CABG) surgery. Elderly patients are at greater risk for serious GI events.

THERAPEUTIC CLASS: COX-2 inhibitor

INDICATIONS: Relief of signs and symptoms of rheumatoid arthritis (RA), osteoarthritis (OA), and ankylosing spondylitis (AS). Management of acute pain in adults. Treatment of primary dysmenorrhea. Relief of signs and symptoms of juvenile rheumatoid arthritis (JRA) in patients ≥2 yrs.

DOSAGE: *Adults:* OA: 200mg qd or 100mg bid. RA: 100-200mg bid. AS: 200mg qd or divided (bid) doses. Titrate: May increase to 400mg/day after 6 weeks if no effect. Acute Pain/Primary Dysmenorrhea: Day 1: 400mg, then 200mg if needed. Maint: 200mg bid prn. Moderate Hepatic Impairment: Reduce daily dose by 50%. Poor Metabolizers of CYP2C9 Substrates: Half the lowest recommended dose. Elderly: <50kg: Initial: Lowest recommended dose.
Pediatrics: JRA: ≥2 yrs: 10-25kg: 50mg bid. >25kg: 100mg bid.

HOW SUPPLIED: Cap: 50mg, 100mg, 200mg, 400mg

CONTRAINDICATIONS: Asthma, urticaria, or allergic-type reactions after aspirin (ASA), NSAID, or sulfonamide use. Treatment of perioperative pain in the setting of CABG surgery.

WARNINGS/PRECAUTIONS: May lead to onset of new HTN or worsening of pre-existing HTN; caution with HTN and monitor BP closely during initiation of therapy. Fluid retention and edema reported; caution with fluid retention or heart failure. Rare cases of severe hepatic reactions (eg, jaundice, fatal fulminant hepatitis, liver necrosis, hepatic failure) reported. May cause elevations of LFTs; d/c if liver disease develops or systemic manifestations occur (eg, eosinophilia, rash). Renal papillary necrosis and other renal injury reported after long-term use. Anaphylactoid reactions may occur; ask emergency help. Do not give with ASA-triad. May cause serious skin adverse events (eg, exfoliative dermatitis, Stevens-Johnson syndrome [SJS], and toxic epidermal necrolysis [TEN]); d/c at first appearance of skin rash or any other sign of hypersensitivity. Avoid in late pregnancy; may cause premature closure of ductus arteriosus. Not a substitute for corticosteroid. Anemia may occur; monitor Hgb/Hct with long-term use. Caution in pediatrics with systemic onset JRA due to risk of disseminated intravascular coagulation (DIC), in poor CYP2C9 metabolizers, in elderly and debilitated and with asthma. D/C if abnormal liver/renal tests persist or worsen. May diminish utility of diagnostic signs in detecting infectious complications of presumed noninfectious, painful conditions. Not recommended with severe hepatic impairment and severe renal insufficiency.

ADVERSE REACTIONS: CV thrombotic events, GI adverse events, headache, HTN, diarrhea, fever, dyspepsia, upper respiratory infection, abdominal pain, N/V, cough, arthralgia, nasopharyngitis, sinusitis.

INTERACTIONS: Monitor anticoagulant activity with warfarin or similar agents; reports of serious bleeding, some fatal. May increase lithium plasma levels; monitor closely. Decreased effects of thiazides and loop diuretics. May diminish antihypertensive effects of ACE-inhibitors and angiotensin II antagonists. May reduce the natriuretic effect of furosemide and thiazides. Increased risk of renal toxicity with diuretics, ACE-inhibitors, angiotensin II antagonists. Increased levels with fluconazole. Caution with CYP2C9 inhibitors. Potential interaction with drugs metabolized by CYP2D6. ASA may increase GI complications. Avoid with non-aspirin NSAID. Increased risk of GI bleeding with concomitant use of oral corticosteroids, anticoagulants, smoking and alcohol. Reduced plasma concentrations with aluminum- and magnesium-containing antacids.

PREGNANCY: Category C and D (≥30 weeks gestation), caution in nursing.

MECHANISM OF ACTION: NSAID; inhibits prostaglandin synthesis primarily via inhibition of cyclooxygenase-2 (COX-2).

PHARMACOKINETICS: Absorption: C_{max}=705ng/mL, T_{max}=2.8 hrs (fasted, 200mg). **Distribution:** V_d=429L (fasted); plasma protein binding (97%); found in breast milk. **Metabolism:** CYP2C9. Primary alcohol, carboxylic acid, glucuronide conjugate (metabolites). **Elimination:** Urine (27%), feces (57%); $T_{1/2}$=11.2 hrs (fasted, 200mg).

NURSING CONSIDERATIONS

Assessment: Assess for CV disease or risk factors, CABG surgery, renal/hepatic insufficiency, HTN, fluid retention, heart failure, history of peptic ulcer disease and/or GI bleeding, ASA triad, systemic onset of JRA in pediatrics, pre-existing asthma, and hypersensitivity. Assess for pregnancy/nursing status and possible drug interactions.

Monitoring: Monitor renal function, LFTs, chemistries, and CBC periodically. Monitor for signs and symptoms of CV thrombotic events, GI events, HTN, fluid retention, edema, anaphylactoid/hypersensitivity reactions, renal/hepatic dysfunction, and abnormal coagulation in systemic onset JRA.

Patient Counseling: Instruct to read Medication Guide before use. Inform of risk for CV side effects (eg, MI, stroke) and GI adverse reactions (eg, ulcers, bleeding). Inform of serious skin side effects (eg, exfoliative dermatitis, SJS, TEN); d/c and report immediately if rash develops. Inform not to take if allergic to sulfa. Advise to seek medical attention if symptoms of GI ulceration/bleeding, skin rash/hypersensitivity (eg, itching), unexplained weight gain or edema, anaphylactoid reactions (eg, difficulty breathing, swelling of face or throat), hepatotoxicity (eg, nausea, fatigue, lethargy, pruritus, jaundice, right upper quadrant tenderness, "flu-like" symptoms), or worsening of asthma occur. Inform that drug can lead to onset of new HTN or worsening of preexisting HTN and may impair response of some antihypertensive agents; instruct on proper follow up for BP monitoring. Inform of pregnancy risks. Instruct to tell physician if they have history of asthma or ASA-sensitive asthma; not for ASA-sensitive.

Administration: Oral route. For patients with difficulty swallowing, contents may be added to applesauce and ingested with water. **Storage:** 25°C (77°F); excursions permitted to 15-30°C (59-86°F). Sprinkled contents on applesauce are stable for up to 6 hrs under 2-8°C (35-45°F).

CELEXA   RX
citalopram hbr (Forest)

> Antidepressants increased the risk of suicidal thinking and behavior (suicidality) in short-term studies in children, adolescents, and young adults with major depressive disorder (MDD) and other psychiatric disorders. Monitor and observe closely for clinical worsening, suicidality, or unusual changes in behavior in patients who are started on antidepressant therapy. Citalopram is not approved for use in pediatric patients.

THERAPEUTIC CLASS: Selective serotonin reuptake inhibitor

INDICATIONS: Treatment of depression.

DOSAGE: *Adults:* Initial: 20mg qd, in the am or pm. Titrate: Increase by 20mg at intervals of no less than 1 week. Max: 40mg/day (non-responders may require 60mg/day). Elderly/Hepatic Impairment: 20mg/day. Titrate: Increase to 40mg/day in nonresponders.

HOW SUPPLIED: Sol: 10mg/5mL [240mL]; Tab: 10mg, 20mg*, 40mg* *scored

CONTRAINDICATIONS: Concomitant use of MAOI or pimozide.

WARNINGS/PRECAUTIONS: Avoid abrupt withdrawal. May increase risk of bleeding events. Activation of mania/hypomania, syndrome of inappropriate antidiuretic hormone secretion, hyponatremia reported. Caution with history of mania or seizures, hepatic impairment, severe renal impairment, conditions that alter metabolism or hemodynamic responses. May impair judgment, thinking, or motor skills. Serotonin syndrome or neuroleptic malignant syndrome (NMS)-like reactions may occur. Monitor for clinical worsening and/or suicidality, especially at initiation of therapy or dose changes.

ADVERSE REACTIONS: N/V, dyspepsia, diarrhea, dry mouth, somnolence, insomnia, increased sweating, ejaculation disorder, rhinitis, anxiety, anorexia, tremor, agitation.

INTERACTIONS: See Contraindications. Avoid alcohol, tryptophan. Caution with other centrally acting drugs, SSRIs, SNRIs, TCAs, lithium, carbamazepine, cimetidine. Increased risk of bleeding with warfarin, ASA, NSAIDs. Rare reports of weakness, hyperreflexia, incoordination with SSRIs and sumatriptan. Clearance may be decreased with potent CYP3A4 (eg, ketoconazole, itraconazole, fluconazole, erythromycin) and CYP2C19 (eg, omeprazole) inhibitors. May increase metoprolol levels, which leads to decreased cardioselectivity. Concomitant use of serotonergic drugs and with drugs that impair metabolism of serotonin may cause serotonin syndrome. Caution with other agents that may affect serotonergic neurotransmitter systems (eg, triptans, linezolid, tramadol, or St. John's wort).

PREGNANCY: Category C, not for use in nursing.

MECHANISM OF ACTION: SSRI; inhibits CNS neuronal reuptake of serotonin.

PHARMACOKINETICS: Absorption: Absolute bioavailability (80%); T_{max}=4 hrs. **Distribution:** V_d=12L/kg. **Metabolism:** Hepatic (biotransformation: N-demethylation) via CYP3A4 and CYP2C19. **Elimination:** Urine (10%); $T_{1/2}$=35 hrs.

NURSING CONSIDERATIONS

Assessment: Assess for risk for bipolar disorder, history of mania, history of seizures, disease/condition that alters metabolism or hemodynamic response, hepatic/renal impairment, pregnancy/nursing status, and possible drug interactions.

Monitoring: Monitor for signs/symptoms of clinical worsening (suicidality, unusual changes in behavior), serotonin syndrome/NMS-like reactions, abnormal bleeding, hyponatremia, seizures, cognitive and motor impairment, and hepatic/renal dysfunction. If therapy is abruptly d/c, monitor for symptoms of dysphoric mood, irritability, agitation, dizziness, sensory disturbances, anxiety, confusion, headache, lethargy, emotional lability, insomnia, and hypomania.

Patient Counseling: Advise to avoid alcohol. Seek medical attention for symptoms of serotonin syndrome (mental status changes, tachycardia, hyperthermia, N/V, diarrhea, incoordination), abnormal bleeding (particularly if using NSAID or ASA), hyponatremia, activation of mania, seizures, clinical worsening (suicidal ideation, unusual changes in behavior) and discontinuation of symptoms (irritability, agitation, dizziness, anxiety, headache, insomnia). Caution against hazardous tasks (eg, operating machinery and driving). May notice improvement in 1-4 weeks; continue therapy as directed. Notify physician if pregnant/intend to become pregnant, or breastfeeding. Counsel about benefits and risks of therapy. Inform physician if taking, or plan to take any over-the-counter prescriptions.

Administration: Oral route. **Storage:** 25°C (77°F); excursions permitted to 15-30°C (59-86°F).

CELLCEPT   RX
mycophenolate mofetil (Genentech)

> Immunosuppression may lead to increased susceptibility to infection and possible development of lymphoma. Only physicians experienced in immunosuppressive therapy and management of renal, cardiac or hepatic transplant patients should use mycophenolate mofetil. Women of child-bearing potential must use contraception; use during pregnancy is associated with increased risk of pregnancy loss and congenital malformations.

THERAPEUTIC CLASS: Inosine monophosphate dehydrogenase inhibitor

INDICATIONS: Prophylaxis of organ rejection in allogeneic renal, cardiac, or hepatic transplants; used concomitantly with cyclosporine and corticosteroids.

DOSAGE: *Adults:* Renal Transplant: 1g IV/PO bid. Cardiac Transplant: 1.5g IV/PO bid. Hepatic Transplant: 1g IV bid or 1.5g PO bid. Start PO as soon as possible after transplant. Start IV within 24 hrs after transplant; can continue for up to 14 days. IV infusion should be administered over at least 2 hrs. Switch to oral when tolerated. Give on an empty stomach.
Pediatrics: 3 months-18 yrs: Renal Transplant: (Sus) 600mg/m² PO bid. Max: 2g/10mL/day. (Cap) BSA 1.25m² to 1.5m²: 750mg PO bid. (Cap/Tab) BSA >1.5m²: 1g PO bid.

HOW SUPPLIED: Cap: 250mg; Tab: 500mg; Inj: 500mg/20mL; Sus: 200mg/mL

CONTRAINDICATIONS: (Inj) Hypersensitivity to Polysorbate 80 (TWEEN).

WARNINGS/PRECAUTIONS: Do not administer by rapid or bolus IV injection. Risk of lymphomas and other malignancies, especially of the skin. Limit exposure to sunlight to decrease risk of skin cancer. May cause fetal harm; must have negative serum/urine pregnancy test within 1 week before therapy. Two reliable forms of contraception required before and during therapy, and 6 weeks following d/c. Severe neutropenia reported; if ANC <1.3 x 10³/µL, d/c or reduce dose. Monitor for bone marrow suppression. Risk of GI ulceration, hemorrhage, and perforation; caution with active digestive system disease. Caution with delayed renal graft function post-transplant. Oral suspension contains phenylalanine; caution with phenylketonurics. Monitor CBC weekly during the 1st month, twice monthly for the 2nd and 3rd months, and then monthly through 1st year. Avoid with rare hereditary deficiency of hypoxanthine-guanine phosphoribosyl-transferase (eg, Lesch-Nyhan and Kelley-Seegmiller syndromes). Increased susceptibility to infections/sepsis. Cases of pure red cell aplasia reported when used with other immunosuppressive agents. Activation of latent viral infections, including progressive multifocal leukoencephalopathy (PML) and BK virus-associated nephropathy (BKVAN), reported; reduce dose in patients who develop evidence of BKVAN or PML. Caution in elderly.

ADVERSE REACTIONS: Infections, diarrhea, leukopenia, sepsis, N/V, HTN, peripheral edema, constipation, pain, abdominal pain, fever, headache, asthenia, insomnia, anemia.

INTERACTIONS: Additive bone marrow suppression with azathioprine; avoid use. Reduced efficacy with drugs that interfere with enterohepatic recirculation (eg, cholestyramine); avoid concomitant use. Avoid live attenuated vaccines. Increased levels of both drugs with acyclovir, ganciclovir. Decreased levels with sevelamer and other calcium-free phosphate binders, magnesium- and aluminum-containing antacids; space dosing. Decreased levels of oral contraceptives; caution and consider additional birth control. Decreased exposure with rifampin; concomitant use not recommended unless benefit outweighs risk. May decrease levels with ciprofloxacin or amoxicillin plus clavulanic acid. Decreased exposure with combination of norfloxacin and metronidazole; avoid concomitant use. Other drugs that compete for renal tubular secretion may raise levels of both drugs.

PREGNANCY: Category D, not for use in nursing.

MECHANISM OF ACTION: Inosine monophosphate dehydrogenase inhibitor; inhibits the de novo pathway of guanosine nucleotide synthesis without incorporation into DNA.

PHARMACOKINETICS: Absorption: Oral: Rapid and complete, absolute bioavailability (94%). **Distribution:** V_d=3.6L/kg (IV), 4L/kg (oral); plasma protein binding of MPA (97%), MPAG (82%). **Metabolism:** MPA (active metabolite) metabolized by glucuronyl transferase to MPAG, which is converted to MPA via enterohepatic recirculation. **Elimination:** Oral: Urine (93%), feces (6%). Urine: MPA (<1%) and MPAG (87%). MPA: (Oral) $T_{1/2}$=17.9 hrs. (IV) $T_{1/2}$=16.6 hrs. **Pediatrics:** Oral administration in different age groups ranging between 1-18 years results in different pharmacokinetics.

NURSING CONSIDERATIONS

Assessment: Assess for drug hypersensitivity, hepatic/renal impairment, phenylketonuria, hereditary deficiency of hypoxanthin-guanine phosphoribosyl tranferase such as Lesch-Nyhan and Kelley-Seegmiller syndromes, and active digestive disease. Assess vaccination history, pregnancy/nursing status, and possible drug interactions.

Monitoring: Monitor for signs of delayed graft rejection (eg, anemia, thrombocytopenia, and hyperkalemia), neutropenia, lymphomas, skin cancer, GI bleeding/perforation/ulceration, infections (including opportunistic infections, latent viral infections, herpes, sepsis), unexpected bruising, bleeding, or any signs of bone marrow suppression. Monitor CBC weekly during the 1st month, twice monthly for the 2nd and 3rd months, and then monthly through the 1st year. Monitor pregnancy status and enroll patient in the National Transplantation Pregnancy Registry if patient becomes pregnant while on medication.

Patient Counseling: Counsel on importance of following dosage instructions and having periodic laboratory tests. Inform about increased risk of malignancies and infection, and reduced efficacy of concurrent vaccines; notify physician for any signs of infection, bruising, and/or bleeding. Advise to avoid prolonged exposure to sunlight. Not for use in pregnant/nursing women or those planning to become pregnant; inform of need for highly effective contraception before, during, and after therapy. Take on an empty stomach.

Administration: Oral route and slow IV infusion route. Administration of the infusion solution should be within 4 hrs from reconstitution and dilution.
Storage: 25°C (77°F); excursions permitted to 15-30°C (59-86°F). Constituted Sus: Stable up to 60 days and may be refrigerated at 2-8°C (36-46°F). Do not freeze.

CEPHALEXIN   RX
cephalexin (Various)

OTHER BRAND NAMES: Keflex (Middlebrook)

THERAPEUTIC CLASS: Cephalosporin (1st generation)

INDICATIONS: Treatment of otitis media and skin and skin structure (SSSI), bone, genitourinary tract, and respiratory tract infections caused by susceptible strains of microorganisms.

DOSAGE: *Adults:* Usual: 250mg q6h. Streptococcal Pharyngitis/SSSI/ Uncomplicated Cystitis (>15yrs): 500mg q12h. Treat cystitis for 7-14 days. Max: 4g/day.
Pediatrics: Usual: 25-50mg/kg/day in divided doses. Streptococcal Pharyngitis (>1 yr)/SSSI: May divide dose and give q12h. Otitis Media: 75-100mg/kg/day in 4 divided doses. Administer for at least 10 days in β-hemolytic streptococcal infections. In severe infections, the dosage may be doubled.

HOW SUPPLIED: (Keflex) Cap: 250mg, 500mg, 750mg; (Generic) Cap: 250mg, 500mg; Tab: 250mg, 500mg; Sus: 125mg/5mL [60mL, 100mL, 200mL], 250mg/5mL [100mL, 200mL]

WARNINGS/PRECAUTIONS: Caution in penicillin (PCN) sensitive patients, cross-hypersensivity reactions may occur. Caution in patients with any type of allergy. D/C use if an allergic reaction occurs. *Clostridium difficile*-associated diarrhea (CDAD) reported. Use in the absence of a proven or strongly suspected bacterial infection or prophylactic indication is unlikely to provide benefit and increases the risk of the development of drug-resistant bacteria. Prolonged use may result in overgrowth of nonsusceptible bacteria; take appropriate measures if superinfection occurs. Indicated surgical procedures should be performed in conjunction with antibiotic therapy. Caution in patients with markedly impaired renal function, history of GI disease. Positive direct Coombs' tests reported. False (+) for urine glucose with Benedict's, Fehling's solution, and Clinitest tabs. May cause a fall in PT; monitor PT in pa-

C

tients at risk (eg, hepatic/renal impairment, protracted course of antimicrobial therapy) and administer vitamin K as indicated.

ADVERSE REACTIONS: Diarrhea, allergic reactions, dyspepsia, gastritis, abdominal pain.

INTERACTIONS: Probenecid inhibits excretion. Concomitant use with metformin may increase concentrations of metformin and produce adverse effects; monitor patient closely and adjust dose of metformin accordingly. Patients previously stabilized on anticoagulants may be at risk for a fall in PT; monitor PT and administer vitamin K as indicated.

PREGNANCY: Category B, caution in nursing.

MECHANISM OF ACTION: Cephalosporin; bactericidal due to inhibition of cell-wall synthesis.

PHARMACOKINETICS: Absorption: Rapid; oral administration of variable doses resulted in different parameters. T_{max}=1 hr. **Distribution:** Found in breast milk. **Elimination:** Urine (90% unchanged).

NURSING CONSIDERATIONS

Assessment: Assess for history of hypersensitivity to cephalosporins/PCNs, pregnancy/nursing status, renal impairment, history of GI disease, and for possible drug interactions. Document indications for therapy, culture and susceptibility testing. Perform indicated surgical procedures in conjunction with antibiotic therapy when indicated.

Monitoring: Monitor for signs/symptoms of hypersensitivity reactions (eg, anaphylaxis), CDAD, superinfection, seizures, and aplastic anemia. Monitor renal function, and LDH. Monitor PT in patients at risk for a decrease in PT (eg, hepatic/renal impairement, poor nutritional state, protracted course of antimicrobial therapy).

Patient Counseling: Inform drug only treats bacterial, not viral, infections. Instruct to take exactly as directed; skipping doses or not completing full course may decrease effectiveness and increase bacterial resistance. Inform patient may experience diarrhea. Instruct to contact physician if watery/bloody stools, superinfection, or hypersensitivity reactions occur.

Administration: Oral route. Sus: Refer to label for reconstitution instructions. Shake well before use. **Storage:** 20°-25°C (68°-77°F). Store sus in refrigerator after mixing.

CEREBYX   RX
fosphenytoin sodium (Parke-Davis)

THERAPEUTIC CLASS: Hydantoin

INDICATIONS: Short-term (up to 5 days) parenteral administration when other means of phenytoin administration are unavailable, inappropriate, or less advantageous, including to control general convulsive status epilepticus, prevent or treat seizures during neurosurgery, or as a short-term substitute for oral phenytoin.

DOSAGE: *Adults:* Doses, concentration in dosing solutions, and infusion rates are expressed as phenytoin sodium equivalents (PE). Status Epilepticus: LD: 15-20 PE/kg IV at 100-150mg PE/min then switch to maintenance dose. Non-Emergent Cases: LD: 10-20mg PE/kg IV (max 150mg PE/min) or IM. Maint: Initial: 4-6mg PE/kg/day. May substitute for oral phenytoin sodium at the same total daily dose. Elderly: Lower and less frequent dosing required.

HOW SUPPLIED: Inj: 50mg PE/mL (2mL, 10mL)

CONTRAINDICATIONS: Sinus bradycardia, sino-atrial block, 2nd- and 3rd-degree AV block, Adams-Stokes syndrome.

WARNINGS/PRECAUTIONS: Avoid abrupt d/c. Not for use in absence seizures. Hypotension and severe cardiovascular reactions and fatalities reported especially after IV administration at high doses and rates; continuously monitor ECG, BP, and respiration during and for at least 20 min after IV infusion and monitor phenytoin levels at least 2 hrs after IV infusion or 4 hrs after

IM injection. Caution with severe myocardial insufficiency, porphyria, hepatic/renal dysfunction, hypoalbuminemia, elderly, and diabetes. Acute hepatotoxicity, lymphadenopathy, hemopoietic complications, hyperglycemia reported. D/C if rash or acute hepatotoxicity occurs. Severe sensory disturbances (eg, burning, itching, paresthesia) reported. Neonatal postpartum bleeding disorder, congenital malformations, and increased seizure frequency reported with use during pregnancy. Avoid use with seizures caused by hypoglycemia or other metabolic causes. Caution with phosphate restriction because of phosphate load (0.0037mmol phosphate/mg PE).

ADVERSE REACTIONS: Nystagmus, dizziness, pruritus, paresthesia, headache, somnolence, ataxia, tinnitus, stupor, nausea, hypotension, vasodilation, tremor, incoordination, dry mouth.

INTERACTIONS: Increased levels with acute alcohol intake, amiodarone, chloramphenicol, chlordiazepoxide, cimetidine, diazepam, dicumarol, disulfiram, estrogens, ethosuximide, fluoxetine, H_2-antagonists, halothane, isoniazid, methylphenidate, phenothiazines, phenylbutazone, salicylates, succinimides, sulfonamides, tolbutamide, trazodone. Decreased levels with carbamazepine, chronic alcohol abuse, reserpine. Decreases efficacy of anticoagulants, corticosteroids, coumarin, digitoxin, doxycycline, estrogens, furosemide, oral contraceptives, rifampin, quinidine, theophylline, vitamin D. Variable effects (increased or decreased levels) with phenobarbital, valproic acid, and sodium valproate. Caution with drugs highly bound to serum albumin. TCAs may precipitate seizures. May lower folate levels.

PREGNANCY: Category D, not for use in nursing.

MECHANISM OF ACTION: Anticonvulsant; prodrug of phenytoin. Modulates voltage-dependent sodium and calcium channels of neurons, inhibits calcium flux across neuronal membranes, and enhances sodium-potassium ATPase activity of neurons and glial cells.

PHARMACOKINETICS: Absorption: Fosphenytoin is completely converted to phenytoin. (IM) T_{max}=30 min. **Distribution:** Plasma protein binding (95-99%); V_d=4.3-10.8L. **Metabolism:** Phosphatases (conversion to phenytoin); liver (phenytoin metabolism). **Elimination:** Urine (1-5% phenytoin and metabolites); $T_{1/2}$=15 min (fosphenytoin), 12-28.9 hrs (phenytoin).

NURSING CONSIDERATIONS

Assessment: Assess LFTs, renal function, CBC with platelets and differential, hypoalbuminemia, porphyria, cardiac conduction defects, pregnancy status, and phosphate levels. Note other diseases/conditions and drug therapies.

Monitoring: Careful cardiac monitoring is needed when administering IV loading doses. Monitor LFTs, renal function, CBC with differential and platelets, hypersensitivity reactions, myasthenia, pneumonia, and hypokalemia.

Patient Counseling: Instruct patient to call a physician if skin rash develops. Inform patient about the importance of adhering strictly to prescribed dosage regimen and not to abruptly d/c medication. Advise patient of possible risk to fetus during pregnancy. Encourage patients to enroll in North American Antiepileptic Drug (NAAED) Pregnancy Registry by calling 888-233-2334 or go to www.aedpregnancyregistry.org.

Administration: IM/IV route. Should be prescribed in phenytoin sodium equivalent units (PE). Rate of IV administration should not exceed 150mg PE/min. **Storage:** Refrigerate at 2-8°C (36-46°F). Do not store at room temperature for more than 48 hours.

CERVARIX   RX
human papillomavirus recombinant vaccine, bivalent (GlaxoSmithKline)

THERAPEUTIC CLASS: Vaccine

INDICATIONS: Prevention of the following diseases caused by oncogenic human papillomavirus (HPV) types 16 and 18 in females 10-25 yrs: cervical cancer, cervical intraepithelial neoplasia (CIN) grade 2 or worse and adenocarcinoma *in situ*, and CIN grade 1.

DOSAGE: *Adults:* ≤25 yrs: Give 3 separate doses of 0.5mL IM in deltoid region of the upper arm at 0, 1, and 6 months.
Pediatrics: ≥10 yrs: Give 3 separate doses of 0.5mL IM in deltoid region of the upper arm at 0, 1, and 6 months.

HOW SUPPLIED: Inj: 0.5mL [vial, prefilled syringe]

WARNINGS/PRECAUTIONS: Does not provide protection against disease due to all HPV types or from vaccine/non-vaccine HPV types to which a woman has previously been exposed through sexual activity. May not result in protection in all vaccine recipients. Continue adherence to recommended cervical cancer screening procedures. Syncope may occur, sometimes resulting in falling with injury and may be associated with tonic-clonic movements and other seizure-like activity; observe for 15 min after administration. Tip cap and rubber plunger of needleless prefilled syringes contain dry natural latex; may cause allergic reactions in latex-sensitive individuals. Immune response to vaccine may be diminished in immunocompromised individuals. Appropriate medical treatment and supervision should be readily available in case of anaphylactic reaction following administration.

ADVERSE REACTIONS: Local-site reactions (eg, pain, redness, swelling), fatigue, headache, myalgia, GI symptoms, arthralgia, fever, rash, urticaria, nasopharyngitis, influenza.

INTERACTIONS: Immunosuppressive therapies, including irradiation, antimetabolites, alkylating agents, cytotoxic drugs, and corticosteroids (used in greater than physiologic doses), may reduce the immune response.

PREGNANCY: Category B, caution in nursing.

MECHANISM OF ACTION: Vaccine; may be mediated by the development of IgG-neutralizing antibodies directed against HPV-L1 capsid proteins generated as a result of vaccination.

NURSING CONSIDERATIONS

Assessment: Assess immunization history and current health/medical status (eg, immunosuppression), age of patient, latex hypersensitivity, pregnancy/nursing status, and for possible drug interactions.

Monitoring: Monitor for signs/symptoms of syncope, tonic-clonic movements, seizure-like activity, and for anaphylactic reactions.

Patient Counseling: Instruct to acquire Vaccine Information Statements prior to immunization. Advise of potential benefits and risks of immunization. Inform that vaccine does not substitute for routine cervical cancer screening and should continue to undergo cervical screening per standard of care. Counsel that vaccine does not protect against disease from HPV types to which a woman has previously been exposed through sexual activity. Inform that syncope may develop following vaccination; instruct to observe for 15 min after administration is recommended. Advise to report any adverse events to healthcare provider. Inform that vaccine is not recommended during pregnancy. Advise to enroll pregnant women who are on therapy in the pregnancy registry to monitor maternal and fetal outcomes.

Administration: IM route. Shake well before withdrawal and use. Inspect for particulate matter and discoloration; do not administer if these conditions exist. Do not administer IV, intradermally, or SQ. **Storage:** 2-8°C (36-46°F). Do not freeze. Discard if frozen.

CESAMET   CII
nabilone (Meda)

THERAPEUTIC CLASS: Cannabinoid

INDICATIONS: Treatment of N/V associated with cancer chemotherapy in patients who have failed to respond adequately to conventional antiemetic treatments.

DOSAGE: *Adults:* Usual: 1 or 2mg bid. Day of Chemotherapy: Initial: Administer 1-3 hrs before giving the chemotherapeutic agent. Start with lower dose and increase as necessary. 1 or 2mg the night before may be useful to minimize side effects. May be given bid or tid during the chemotherapy cycle and, if needed, for 48 hrs after the last dose of each cycle. Max: 6mg/day given in divided doses tid. Elderly: Start at the low end of dosing range.

HOW SUPPLIED: Cap: 1mg

WARNINGS/PRECAUTIONS: Patients should remain under the supervision during treatment, especially during initial use and dose adjustments due to individual variation in response and tolerance to the effects of the drug. Caution with HTN, heart disease, elderly, current or previous psychiatric disorders (including manic depressive illness, depression, and schizophrenia) and with history of substance abuse. May impair mental/physical abilities. May cause dizziness, drowsiness, euphoria, ataxia, anxiety, disorientation, depression, hallucinations, psychosis, tachycardia and orthostatic hypotension. Caution in pregnant/nursing patients and pediatrics. Adverse psychiatric reactions can persist for 48-72 hrs following cessation of treatment. Not intended for use on prn basis or as first antiemetic product prescribed.

ADVERSE REACTIONS: Drowsiness, vertigo, dry mouth, euphoria, ataxia, headache, concentration difficulties, dysphoria, sleep/visual disturbance, asthenia, anorexia, depression, hypotension, sedation.

INTERACTIONS: Additive HTN, tachycardia, possibly cardiotoxicity may occur with amphetamines, cocaine, other sympathomimetics. Additive or super-additive tachycardia, drowsiness may occur with atropine, scopolamine, antihistamines, other anticholinergics. Additive tachycardia, HTN, drowsiness may occur with amitriptyline, amoxapine, desipramine and other TCAs. Additive drowsiness and CNS depression may occur with barbiturates, benzodiazepines, ethanol, lithium, opioids, buspirone, antihistamines, muscle relaxants, and other CNS depressants. Hypomanic reaction reported with disulfiram, fluoxetine. May decrease clearance of antipyrine, barbiturates. May increase metabolism of theophylline. Cross-tolerance and mutual potentiation with opioids. Effects may be enhanced by opioid receptor blockade of naltrexone. Alcohol may increase the positive subjective mood effects. Avoid with alcohol, sedatives, hypnotics, or other psychoactive drugs. Impaired psychomotor function with diazepam. Change in dosage requirements with highly protein-bound drugs.

PREGNANCY: Category C, not for use in nursing.

MECHANISM OF ACTION: Cannabinoid; interacts with the cannabinoid receptor system CB (1) receptor that has been discovered in neural tissues.

PHARMACOKINETICS: Absorption: Complete, C_{max}=2ng/mL, T_{max}=2.0 hrs. **Distribution:** V_d=12.5L/kg. **Metabolism:** Liver (extensive), via stereospecific enzymatic reduction, oxidation, and CYP450 enzymes. **Elimination:** Feces (60%), urine (24%); $T_{1/2}$=2 hrs, 35 hrs (metabolites).

NURSING CONSIDERATIONS

Assessment: Assess for heart disease, HTN, previous/current psychiatric disorders, alcohol intake or substance abuse, pregnancy/nursing status, and possible drug interactions.

Monitoring: Monitor for adverse psychiatric reactions or unmasking of symptoms of psychiatric disorders, signs/symptoms of CNS effects (eg, dizziness, drowsiness, euphoria, ataxia, anxiety, disorientation, depression, hallucinations and psychosis), postural hypotension. Monitor BP and HR. Monitor for signs of excessive use, abuse and misuse. Monitor for signs and symptoms of hypersensitivity reactions.

Patient Counseling: Caution against performing hazardous tasks such as driving or operating machinery, or engage in any hazardous activity. Instruct to avoid concomitant use of alcohol and other CNS depressants such as benzodiazepines and barbiturates. Inform of possible changes in mood and other adverse behavioral effects so as to avoid panic in the event of such manifestations. Instruct to remain under supervision of responsible adult during treatment.

Administration: Oral route. **Storage:** 25°C (77°F); excursions permitted to 15-30°C (59-86°F).

CHANTIX RX

varenicline (Pfizer)

> Serious neuropsychiatric events including, but not limited to, depression, suicidal ideation, and attempted/completed suicide reported. Some cases may be complicated by nicotine withdrawal symptoms. Monitor for symptoms including changes in behavior, hostility, agitation, depressed mood, and suicide-related events. Advise to d/c and contact a healthcare provider immediately if these symptoms are observed. Weigh risks against benefits of use.

THERAPEUTIC CLASS: Nicotinic Acetylcholine Receptor Agonist

INDICATIONS: Aid to smoking cessation treatment.

DOSAGE: *Adults:* Days 1-3: 0.5mg qd. Days 4-7: 0.5mg bid. Day 8-End of Treatment: 1mg bid. Treat for 12 weeks; additional 12 weeks recommended after successful completion to ensure long-term abstinence. Severe Renal Impairment (CrCl <30mL/min): Initial: 0.5mg qd. Titrate: May be titrated as needed to a max dose of 0.5mg bid. End-Stage Renal Disease with Hemodialysis: Max: 0.5mg qd if tolerated. Consider temporary/permanent dose reduction in patients unable to tolerate adverse effects. Elderly: Careful dose selection. Take pc and with a full glass of water.

HOW SUPPLIED: Tab: 0.5mg, 1mg

WARNINGS/PRECAUTIONS: Hypersensitivity reactions including angioedema reported. Rare but serious skin reactions (Stevens-Johnson syndrome [SJS] and erythema multiforme) reported. D/C and contact healthcare provider immediately at first appearance of skin rash with mucosal lesions or any other signs of hypersensitivity. May impair physical/mental abilities. Nausea, sometimes persistent over several months, reported; consider dose reduction for patients with intolerable nausea. Caution in elderly patients and those with impaired renal function.

ADVERSE REACTIONS: N/V, flatulence, headache, insomnia, abnormal dreams, dysgeusia, constipation, fatigue, malaise, dyspepsia, asthenia, sleep disorder, abdominal pain, dry mouth, upper respiratory tract disorder.

INTERACTIONS: Reduced renal clearance and increased exposure with cimetidine. Increased incidence of adverse events with nicotine replacement therapy (NRT). Physiological changes resulting from smoking cessation may alter pharmacokinetics or pharmacodynamics of some drugs (eg, theophylline, warfarin, insulin).

PREGNANCY: Category C, not for use in nursing.

MECHANISM OF ACTION: Nicotinic acetylcholine receptor agonist; binds with high affinity and selectivity at α4β2 neuronal nicotinic acetylcholine receptors, producing agonist activity while simultaneously preventing nicotine from binding to these receptors and stimulating the central nervous mesolimbic dopamine system.

PHARMACOKINETICS: Absorption: Complete; T_{max}=3-4 hrs. **Distribution:** Plasma protein binding (≤20%). **Metabolism:** Minimal. **Elimination:** Urine (92% unchanged); $T_{1/2}$=24 hrs.

NURSING CONSIDERATIONS

Assessment: Assess for pre-existing psychiatric illness and impaired renal function, history of hypersensitivity/skin reaction to the drug, pregnancy/nursing status and possible drug interactions.

Monitoring: Monitor for neuropsychiatric symptoms (eg, changes in behavior, agitation, depressed mood, suicidal ideation/behavior), worsening of pre-existing psychiatric illness, nausea, somnolence, dizziness, loss of consciousness, difficulty concentrating, insomnia, hypersensitivity and skin reactions (eg, SJS, angioedema). Monitor renal function especially in elderly.

Patient Counseling: Instruct to set a date to quit smoking and start treatment 1 week before the quit date. Encourage to continue attempt to quit even with early lapses after quit day. Advise to take pc, and with full glass of water. Instruct how to take the medication from Day 1 to end of treatment until additional course of treatment. Inform about side effects such as nausea and insomnia, and to notify physician if persistent. Provide with educational materials and necessary counseling to support attempt at quitting smoking. Advise to d/c treatment and notify healthcare provider immediately if neuropsychiatric symptoms occur. Encourage to reveal any history of psychiatric illness prior to treatment. Inform patients of serious skin reactions and reports of angioedema with swelling of face, mouth and neck; instruct to d/c and contact physician immediately if these occur. Inform that quitting smoking may be associated with nicotine withdrawal symptoms or exacerbation of pre-existing psychiatric illness. Caution about performing hazardous tasks (eg, driving/operating machinery). Inform that vivid, unusual or strange dreams may be experienced. Counsel pregnant/breastfeeding or planning to become pregnant patients on the risks of smoking and the benefits of smoking cessation.

Administration: Oral route. **Storage:** 25°C (77°F); excursions permitted to 15-30°C (59-86°F).

CHENODAL   RX
chenodiol (Manchester)

THERAPEUTIC CLASS: Bile acid

INDICATIONS: Patients with radiolucent stones in well-opacifying gallbladders, in whom selective surgery would be undertaken except for the presence of increased surgical risk due to systemic disease or age.

DOSAGE: *Adults:* Initial: 250mg bid the first two weeks. Titrate: Increase by 250mg/day each week thereafter until recommended or maximum tolerated dose is reached. Range: 13-16mg/kg/day in two divided doses, am and pm. 45-58kg: 3 tabs/day; 59-75kg: 4 tabs/day; 76-90kg: 5 tabs/day; 91-107kg: 6 tabs/day; 108-125kg: 7 tabs/day. Adjust dose temporarily if diarrhea occurs until symptoms abate. D/C if no response by 18 months.

HOW SUPPLIED: Tab: 250mg

CONTRAINDICATIONS: Presence of known hepatocyte dysfunction or bile ductal abnormalities (eg, intrahepatic cholestasis, primary biliary cirrhosis, sclerosing cholangitis), nonvisualizing gallbladder after two consecutive single doses of dye, radiopaque stones, gallstone complications or compelling reasons for gallbladder surgery including unremitting acute cholecystitis, cholangitis, biliary obstruction, gallstone pancreatitis, or biliary GI fistula.

WARNINGS/PRECAUTIONS: Has the potential to cause hepatotoxicity or may increase rate of a need for cholecystectomy. Treatment should be reserved for carefully selected patients and must be accompanied by systemic monitoring for liver function alterations. Will not dissolve radiolucent bile pigment stones. May cause serious hepatic disease and fetal harm. May contribute to colon cancer in susceptible individuals. Use in patient without pre-existing liver disease; monitor for serum aminotransferase to detect drug-induced liver toxicity. D/C if with aminotransferase elevations over 3X ULN, if cholesterol rises above acceptable age-adjusted limit and if there is confirmed dissolution. Caution in patients with history of jaundice. Stone recurrence may occur; maintenance of reduced weight recommended. Safety of use beyond 24 months not established.

ADVERSE REACTIONS: Aminotransferase elevations (mainly SGPT), intrahepatic cholestasis, diarrhea, gastrointestinal side effects, increase in serum total cholesterol and LDL, decrease in WBC count.

INTERACTIONS: May reduce absorption with bile acid sequestering agents (eg, cholestyramine, colestipol) and aluminum-based antacids. Estrogen, oral contraceptive and clofibrate (and perhaps other lipid-lowering drugs) may counteract the effectiveness of chenodiol. May cause unexpected prolongation of PT and hemorrhages with coumarin and its derivatives.

PREGNANCY: Category X, caution in nursing.

MECHANISM OF ACTION: Bile acid; suppresses hepatic synthesis of both cholesterol and cholic acid, gradually replacing the latter and its metabolite, deoxycholic acid in an expanded bile acid pool that contributes to biliary cholesterol desaturation and gradual dissolution of radiolucent cholesterol gallstone.

PHARMACOKINETICS: Absorption: Well absorbed. **Metabolism:** Liver, converted in the colon by bacterial action to lithocholic acid (metabolite). **Elimination:** Lithocholate: Feces (80%).

NURSING CONSIDERATIONS

Assessment: Assess for hepatocyte dysfunction or bile ductal abnormalities or any other diseases or conditions where treatment is contraindicated or cautioned. Assess for pregnancy/nursing status and possible drug interactions. Obtain LFTs (AST/ALT), serum cholesterol and TG levels.

Monitoring: Monitor for patient's weight, increased risk for cholecystectomy and for signs and symptoms of hepatotoxicity, colon cancer or other adverse reactions. Monitor liver function alterations. Monitor serum aminotransferase levels monthly for the first 3 months and every 3 months thereafter during medication. Monitor serum cholesterol at 6-month intervals. Monitor response and/or recurrence with cholecystograms or ultrasonograms at 6-9-month intervals.

Patient Counseling: Counsel on the importance of periodic visits for LFTs and oral cholecystograms (or ultrasonograms) for monitoring stone dissolution. Inform about the symptoms of gallstone complications and advise to notify physician immediately if occurs. Instruct ways to facilitate faithful compliance with the dosage regimen throughout the usual long term of therapy, and on temporary dose reduction if episodes of diarrhea occur. Advise to maintain reduced weight to forestall stone recurrence.

Administration: Oral route. **Storage:** 20-25°C (68-77°F). Dispense in tight container.

CIALIS RX
tadalafil (Lilly)

THERAPEUTIC CLASS: Phosphodiesterase type 5 inhibitor

INDICATIONS: Treatment of erectile dysfunction (ED).

DOSAGE: *Adults:* Prn Use: Initial: 10mg prior to sexual activity. May increase to 20mg or decrease to 5mg based on efficacy and tolerability. Renal Impairment: CrCl 31-50mL/min: Initial: 5mg. Max: 10mg/48 hrs. CrCl <30mL/min/Hemodialysis: Max: 5mg/72 hrs. Mild/Moderate Hepatic Impairment: Max: 10mg qd. With Alpha Blockers: Initial: Use lowest recommended dose. With Potent CYP3A4 Inhibitors (eg, ketoconazole, ritonavir): Max: 10mg/72 hrs. Once-Daily Use: Initial: 2.5mg qd, taken at the same time every day. Titrate: May increase to 5mg based on efficacy and tolerability. With Alpha Blockers: Initial: Use lowest recommended dose. With Potent CYP3A4 Inhibitors (eg, ketoconazole, ritonavir): Max: 2.5mg.

HOW SUPPLIED: Tab: 2.5mg, 5mg, 10mg, 20mg

CONTRAINDICATIONS: Any form of organic nitrate, either regularly and/or intermittently used.

WARNINGS/PRECAUTIONS: Avoid in men for whom sexual activity is inadvisable due to underlying cardiovascular (CV) status. Avoid with myocardial infarction (within last 90 days), unstable angina or angina occurring during sexual intercourse, NYHA Class 2 or greater heart failure (in the last 6 months), uncontrolled arrhythmias, hypotension (<90/50mmHg), or uncontrolled HTN (>170/100mmHg), and stroke within the last 6 months. May cause transient decrease in BP. Increased sensitivity to vasodilatory effect with left ventricular outflow obstruction and severely impaired autonomic control of BP. Rare reports of prolonged erections (>4 hrs) and priapism; caution in conditions predisposing to priapism (eg, sickle cell anemia, multiple myeloma, leukemia), anatomical deformation of the penis (eg, angulation, cavernosal fibrosis, Peyronie's disease). Non-arteritic anterior ischemic optic neuropathy (NAION) reported; d/c if sudden loss of vision is experienced in one or both eyes. Sudden decrease or loss of hearing reported with tinnitus and dizziness;

d/c if occurs. Avoid prn use in severe renal insuffiency (CrCl <30mL/min and on hemodialysis). Avoid use with hepatic impairment (Child-Pugh Class C), hereditary degenerative retinal disorders including retinal pigmentosa. Caution with mild to moderate hepatic insufficiency, bleeding disorders or significant peptic ulceration.

ADVERSE REACTIONS: Headache, dyspepsia, back pain, myalgia, nasal congestion, flushing, limb pain, nasopharyngitis, upper respiratory tract infection, gastroenteritis (viral), influenza, cough, gastroesophageal reflux disease, myalgia, HTN.

INTERACTIONS: See Contraindications. Avoid concomitant use with nitrates within 48 hrs. Additive hypotensive effects with alcohol, α-adrenergic blockers (eg, doxazosin, alfuzosin, tamsulosin), antihypertensives (eg, amlodipine, angiotensin II receptor blockers, bendrofluazide, enalapril, metoprolol). Increased tadalafil exposure with ritonavir and possibly other HIV protease inhibitors. CYP3A4 inhibitors (eg, ketoconazole, itraconazole, erythromycin, grapefruit juice) may result in increased exposure of tadalafil. CYP3A4 inducers (eg, rifampin, carbamazepine, phenytoin, phenobarbital) may result in decreased tadalafil exposure. Antacids (magnesium hydroxide/aluminum hydroxide) shown to reduce rate of absorption. Avoid concomitant use with Adcirca or other PDE5 inhibitors. A small increase in heart rate seen with theophylline.

PREGNANCY: Category B, not for use in nursing.

MECHANISM OF ACTION: Phosphodiesterase type 5 inhibitor; increases amount of cGMP that causes smooth muscle relaxation and increased blood flow into the corpus cavernosum.

PHARMACOKINETICS: Absorption: T_{max}=2hrs. **Distribution:** V_d=63L; plasma protein binding (94%). **Metabolism:** Via CYP3A4 to a catechol metabolite which undergoes extensive methylation and glucuronidation; methylcatechol glucuronide (major metabolite). **Elimination:** Urine (36%), feces (61%); $T_{1/2}$=17.5 hrs.

NURSING CONSIDERATIONS

Assessment: Assess for CV disease, long QT syndrome, retinitis pigmentosa, bleeding disorders, active peptic ulceration, anatomical deformation of the penis or presence of conditions that would predispose to priapism (eg, sickle cell anemia, multiple myeloma, leukemia), renal/hepatic impairment, contraindications for sexual activity. Assess for potential underlying causes of erectile dysfunction and for possible drug interactions.

Monitoring: Monitor for signs/symptoms of decreases in BP, prolonged erection, NAION, hearing loss, and for hypersensitivity reactions. Monitor therapeutic effect when used in combination with other drugs.

Patient Counseling: Instruct to seek medical assistance if erection persists >4 hrs. Advise of potential BP-lowering effect of α-blockers, other antihypertensive medications, alcohol, and cardiac risk of sexual activity. Counsel about the protective measures necessary to guard against STDs, including HIV. Inform about drug's contraindication with organic nitrates and potential interactions with other medications. Instruct to d/c and contact physician if sudden loss of vision or hearing occur. Counsel to take as prescribed.

Administration: Oral route. 1) For prn use, take at least 30 min before anticipated sexual activity. 2) For qd use, take one tablet at the same time of day. **Storage:** 25°C (77°F); excursions permitted to 15-30°C (59-86°F).

CILOXAN   RX
ciprofloxacin HCl (Alcon)

THERAPEUTIC CLASS: Fluoroquinolone

INDICATIONS: Bacterial conjunctivitis and corneal ulcers.

DOSAGE: *Adults:* Bacterial Conjunctivitis: (Sol) 1-2 drops q2h while awake for 2 days, then 1-2 drops q4h while awake for 5 days. (Oint) 1/2 inch tid for 2 days, then bid for 5 days. Corneal Ulcer: (Sol) 2 drops every 15 min for 1st

C

6 hrs, then 2 drops every 30 min for rest of Day 1, then 2 drops every hr on Day 2, then 2 drops q4h on Days 3-14. May continue if re-epithelialization has not occurred.

Pediatrics: Bacterial Conjunctivitis: ≥1 yr: (Sol) 1-2 drops q2h while awake for 2 days, then 1-2 drops q4h while awake for 5 days. ≥2 yrs: (Oint) 1/2 inch tid for 2 days, then bid for 5 days. Corneal Ulcer: (Sol) ≥1 yr: 2 drops every 15 min for 1st 6 hrs, then 2 drops every 30 min for rest of Day 1, then 2 drops every hr on Day 2, then 2 drops q4h on Days 3-14. May continue if re-epithelialization has not occurred.

HOW SUPPLIED: Oint: 0.3% [3.5g]; Sol: 0.3% [2.5mL, 5mL, 10mL]

WARNINGS/PRECAUTIONS: Not for injection into eye. Superinfection may result with prolonged use. Fatal hypersensitivity reactions reported after 1st dose of systemic quinolone therapy. Avoid allowing tip of container to contact eye or surrounding structures. Avoid contact lenses with conjunctivitis. Risk of crystalline precipitate in cornea. Ointment may slow corneal healing and cause visual blurring.

ADVERSE REACTIONS: Local burning, white crystalline precipitants, lid margin crusting, crystals/scales, foreign body sensation, itching, conjunctival hyperemia, bad taste.

INTERACTIONS: Systemic quinolone therapy may increase theophylline levels, interfere with caffeine metabolism, enhance warfarin effects, and elevate serum creatinine with cyclosporine.

PREGNANCY: Category C, caution in nursing.

MECHANISM OF ACTION: Fluoroquinolone antibacterial agent; bactericidal, interferes with the enzyme DNA gyrase which is needed for synthesis of bacterial DNA.

PHARMACOKINETICS: Absorption: C_{max}≤5ng/mL.

NURSING CONSIDERATIONS

Assessment: Assess for proper diagnosis of causative organisms and for hypersensitivity to other quinolones. Assess for possible drug interactions.

Monitoring: During prolonged use, monitor for overgrowth (eg, superinfection) of nonsusceptible organisms, including fungi. Monitor for signs of hypersensitivity or anaphylactic reaction (eg, cardiovascular collapse, loss of consciousness, pharyngeal or facial edema, dyspnea, and urticaria). Monitor for development of precipitate in the superficial portion of the corneal defect.

Patient Counseling: Instruct not to touch dropper tip to any surface; may contaminate solution. Advise to contact physician if any hypersensitivity reaction occurs (eg, rash). Instruct to remove contact lenses prior to therapy.

Administration: Ocular route. **Storage:** 2-25°C (36-77°F). Protect from light.

CIMZIA   RX
certolizumab pegol (UCB)

> Increased risk for developing serious infections (eg, tuberculosis (TB), TB reactivation, invasive fungal infection, bacterial/viral infection due to opportunistic pathogens) that may lead to hospitalization or death. Concomitant use of immunosuppressants (eg, methotrexate [MTX] or corticosteroids) may predispose to these infections. Evaluate for latent TB and treat prior to initiation of therapy. Empiric antifungal therapy should be considered in patients at risk for invasive fungal infection who develop severe systemic illness. Consider risks and benefits of treatment prior to initiating therapy with chronic or recurrent infections. Monitor for development of infection during and after treatment. D/C if serious infection or sepsis develops. Lymphoma and other malignancies reported in children and adolescents.

THERAPEUTIC CLASS: TNF-receptor blocker

INDICATIONS: Reducing signs and symptoms of Crohn's disease and maintaining clinical response in adults with moderately to severely active disease who have had an inadequate response to conventional therapy. Treatment of moderately to severely active rheumatoid arthritis (RA) in adults.

DOSAGE: *Adults:* Crohn's disease: Initial: 400mg (given as 2 SQ inj of 200mg) initially and at Weeks 2 and 4. Maint: 400mg SQ every 4 weeks. RA: Initial: 400mg (given as 2 SQ inj of 200mg) initially and at Weeks 2 and 4, followed by 200mg every other week. Maint: 400mg SQ every 4 weeks. Concomitant MTX: 200mg SQ every other week.

HOW SUPPLIED: Inj: 200mg/mL

WARNINGS/PRECAUTIONS: Avoid with active infection. Caution in patients with history of recurrent infections, underlying conditions predisposing to infections, and with exposure to TB or those who travel in areas where TB and mycoses are endemic. Malignancies reported, including Hodgkin's and non-Hodgkin's lymphoma. Patients with RA are at a higher risk for lymphoma and leukemia. Increased risk of hepatitis B virus (HBV) reactivation in carriers; if reactivation occurs, d/c and start antiviral therapy. Hypersensitivity reactions (eg, angioedema, dyspnea, hypotension, rash, serum sickness, urticaria) reported; d/c if severe reactions occur. Caution with pre-existing or recent onset CNS demyelinating disorders (eg, multiple sclerosis) or peripheral demyelinating disorders (Guillain-Barre syndrome). Rare cases of neurological disorders (eg, seizure disorder, optic neuritis, peripheral neuropathy). Pancytopenia, including aplastic anemia, and significant cytopenia reported; caution in patients who have ongoing or a history of significant hematologic abnormalities. Cases of worsening congestive heart failure observed. May result in autoantibody formation; d/c if lupus-like syndrome develops. Caution in elderly.

ADVERSE REACTIONS: Infections, upper respiratory infections (URI), rash, urinary tract infections (UTI), HTN, nasopharyngitis, fever.

INTERACTIONS: See Boxed Warning. Increased risk of infection with anakinra, abatacept, rituximab, natalizumab, and biological disease-modifying antirheumatic drugs (DMARDs); avoid combination. Do not give live/attenuated vaccines concurrently. Additive hypertensive effects with NSAIDs and corticosteroids. Do not use with other TNF blocker therapies.

PREGNANCY: Category B, not for use in nursing.

MECHANISM OF ACTION: TNF-blocker; binds to TNFα and selectively neutralizes and inhibits its central role in inflammatory processes.

PHARMACOKINETICS: Absorption: T_{max}=54-171 hrs; C_{max}=43-49mcg/mL; Bioavailability (80%). **Distribution:** V_d=6-8L. **Elimination:** $T_{1/2}$=14 days.

NURSING CONSIDERATIONS

Assessment: Assess for localized or chronic infections, heart disease, hematologic disorders, pre-existing or recurrent CNS demyelinating disorders, pregnancy/nursing status, and possible drug interactions. Assess for active and inactive/latent TB infection; perform TB skin test prior to therapy.

Monitoring: Monitor for signs/symptoms of serious infection (eg, sepsis, pneumonia, TB, invasive fungal infection, HBV infection, neurologic disorders (eg, seizures, optic neuritis, peripheral neuropathy), hematologic reactions (eg, aplastic anemia, pancytopenia, leukopenia, neutropenia, thrombocytopenia), hypersensitivity reactions (eg, angioedema, dyspnea, rash, serum sickness, urticaria), malignancies (eg, lymphoma), lupus-like syndrome, and injection-site reactions. In patients with heart failure, monitor for worsening of symptoms.

Patient Counseling: Inform about risks/benefits of therapy. Inform that drug may lower ability to fight infections; seek medical attention if any severe allergic reactions occur. Instruct to report any signs of new or worsening medical conditions such as heart disease; neurological or autoimmune disorders; bruising, bleeding, pallor, cough, persistent fever, or flu-like symptoms; or if any symptoms of TB, histoplasmosis, or HBV develop. Counsel about possible risk of lymphoma and other malignancies. Instruct not to use if cloudy or if foreign particulate matter is present and to discard unused portions of drug remaining in the syringe or vial.

Administration: SQ route. Rotate injection sites; avoid tender, bruised, red, or hard areas of the skin. Refer to PI for proper reconstitution and administration.
Storage: 2-8°C (36-46°F). Do not freeze. Protect from light. Reconstituted Vials: Up to 24 hrs at 2-8°C (36-46°F) prior to injection. Do not freeze.

CINRYZE
c1 inhibitor (human) (Viro Pharma)

RX

THERAPEUTIC CLASS: C1 inhibitor

INDICATIONS: Routine prophylaxis against angioedema attacks in adolescent and adult patients with hereditary angioedema (HAE).

DOSAGE: *Adults:* 1,000 U IV every 3 or 4 days. Infusion Rate: Initial/Maintenance: 1mL/min (10 min).
Pediatrics: Adolescents: 1,000 U IV every 3 or 4 days. Infusion Rate: Initial/Maintenance: 1mL/min (10 min).

HOW SUPPLIED: Inj: 500 U [vial]

WARNINGS/PRECAUTIONS: Severe hypersensitivity reactions (eg, hives, urticaria, chest tightness, wheezing, hypotension, and/or anaphylaxis) may occur; d/c therapy immediately. Epinephrine should be immediately available to treat hypersensitivity. Thrombotic events at high doses reported. Treatment may carry a risk of transmitting infectious agents [eg, viruses, Creutzfeldt-Jakob (CJD) agent].

ADVERSE REACTIONS: Upper respiratory tract infection, sinusitis, rash, headache, bronchitis, limb injury, back pain, pain in extremity, pruritus.

PREGNANCY: Category C, caution in nursing.

MECHANISM OF ACTION: C1 inhibitor; regulates the activation of the complement and intrinsic coagulation (contact system) pathway and regulates the fibrinolytic system; increases plasma levels of C1 inhibitor activity.

PHARMACOKINETICS: Absorption: C_{max}=0.68 U/mL (single dose), 0.85 U/mL (double dose); T_{max}=3.9 hrs (single dose), 2.7 hrs (double dose); $AUC_{(0-t)}$=74.5 U•hr/mL (single dose), 95.9 U•hr/mL (double dose). **Elimination:** $T_{1/2}$=56 hrs (single dose), 62 hrs (double dose).

NURSING CONSIDERATIONS

Assessment: Assess signs and symptoms of hypersensitivity reactions, known risk factors for thrombotic events, and pregnancy/nursing status.

Monitoring: Monitor for hypersensitivity reactions and thrombotic events.

Patient Counseling: Counsel about the risks and benefits of therapy prior to treatment. Inform that medication is made from human plasma and may contain infectious agents that can cause disease (eg, viruses, CJD agent). Advise to d/c use and contact physician if hypersensitivity occurs. Advise to consult with physician prior to travel.

Administration: IV route. Administer at room temperature within 3 hrs after reconstitution. See PI for detailed reconstitution information. **Storage:** 2-25°C (36-77°F). Do not freeze, mix with other materials, and/or use after expiration date. Protect from light prior to reconstitution.

CIPRO HC
ciprofloxacin HCl - hydrocortisone (Alcon)

RX

THERAPEUTIC CLASS: Antibacterial/corticosteroid combination

INDICATIONS: Acute otitis externa in adults and pediatric patients ≥1 year.

DOSAGE: *Adults:* 3 drops into affected ear bid for 7 days. Warm bottle in hand for 1-2 min to avoid dizziness. Shake well before use.
Pediatrics: ≥1 yr: 3 drops into affected ear bid for 7 days. Warm bottle in hand for 1-2 min to avoid dizziness. Shake well before use.

HOW SUPPLIED: Sus: (Ciprofloxacin-Hydrocortisone) 0.2%-1% [10mL]

CONTRAINDICATIONS: Perforated tympanic membrane, viral infections of external ear canal (eg, varicella and herpes simplex infections).

WARNINGS/PRECAUTIONS: D/C if hypersensitivity reaction occurs. Re-evaluate if no improvement after 1 week.

ADVERSE REACTIONS: Headache, pruritus.

PREGNANCY: Category C, not for use in nursing.

MECHANISM OF ACTION: Broad-spectrum anti-inflammatory antibiotic; exerts antimicrobial activity against gram-positive and gram-negative bacteria.

NURSING CONSIDERATIONS

Assessment: Assess for history of hypersensitivity to hydrocortisone or quinolones, perforated tympanic membrane, and viral infection of the external canal.

Monitoring: Monitor for possible occurrence of superinfection, ear pain, fungal dermatitis, headache, hypersensitivity reactions, and pruritus.

Patient Counseling: Inform that if rash or allergic reactions occur, d/c and contact physician immediately. Counsel to use as directed. Advise to avoid contact with eyes to avoid contaminating dropper. Protect from light, shake well before use, and discard unused portion after completion.

Administration: Otic route. **Storage:** Below 25°C (77°F). Avoid freezing. Protect from light.

CIPRO IV   RX
ciprofloxacin (Bayer/Schering)

> Fluoroquinolones are associated with an increased risk of tendinitis and tendon rupture in all ages. Risk is further increased in patients >60 yrs, patients taking corticosteroids, and patients with kidney, heart, or lung transplants. May exacerbate muscle weakness with myasthenia gravis; avoid in patients with known history of myasthenia gravis.

THERAPEUTIC CLASS: Fluoroquinolone

INDICATIONS: Treatment of skin and skin structure infections (SSSI), bone and joint infections, complicated intra-abdominal infections (in combination with metronidazole), lower respiratory tract infections (LRTI), acute exacerbations of chronic bronchitis, urinary tract infections (UTI), nosocomial pneumonia, acute sinusitis, chronic bacterial prostatitis, and empirical therapy for febrile neutropenia in adults. Treatment of complicated UTI and pyelonephritis in pediatrics 1-17 yrs. To reduce the incidence or progression of post-exposure inhalational anthrax in both adults and pediatrics.

DOSAGE: *Adults:* Infuse as IV over 60 min. UTI: Mild-Moderate: 200mg q12h for 7-14 days. Complicated/Severe: 400mg q12h for 7-14 days. LRTI/SSSI: Mild-Moderate: 400mg q12h for 7-14 days. Complicated/Severe: 400mg q8h for 7-14 days. Bone and Joint: Mild-Moderate: 400mg q12h for ≥4-6 weeks. Complicated/Severe: 400mg q8h for ≥4-6 weeks. Nosocomial Pneumonia: Mild/Moderate/Severe: 400mg q8h for 10-14 days. Complicated Intra-Abdominal (with metronidazole): 400mg q12h for 7-14 days. Acute Sinusitis: 400mg q12h for 10 days. Chronic Bacterial Prostatitis: Mild-Moderate: 400mg q12h for 28 days. Febrile Neutropenia (Empirical Therapy): 400mg q8h (with piperacillin 50mg/kg q4h; Max: 24g/day) for 7-14 days. Inhalational Anthrax (post-exposure): 400mg q12h for 60 days. CrCl 5-29mL/min: 200-400mg q18-24h. Elderly: Start at lower end of dosing range. Refer to PI for conversion of IV to PO dosing.
Pediatrics: Infuse as IV over 60 min. Inhalational Anthrax: 10mg/kg q12h for 60 days. Max: 400mg/dose. 1-17 yrs: Complicated UTI/Pyelonephritis: 6-10mg/kg q8h for 10-21 days. Max: 400mg/dose.

HOW SUPPLIED: Inj: (Vial) 200mg/20mL, 400mg/40mL; (Flexible container) 200mg/100mL (0.2%), 400mg/200mL (0.2%)

CONTRAINDICATIONS: Concomitant administration with tizanidine.

WARNINGS/PRECAUTIONS: D/C if experience pain, swelling, inflammation, or rupture of tendon. Convulsions, increased intracranial pressure (ICP), and toxic psychosis reported; d/c if CNS events (eg, dizziness, confusion, tremors, hallucinations, depression, suicidal thoughts/acts) occur. Caution with CNS disorders or other factors that may predispose to seizures or lower the seizure threshold. Serious and occasionally fatal hypersensitivity reactions reported; d/c immediately if signs of hypersensitivity appear. *Clostridium difficile*-associated diarrhea (CDAD) reported. Rare cases of sensory or sensorimotor axonal polyneuropathy reported; d/c if symptoms of neuropathy occur. Local site reactions reported. Crystalluria reported; maintain hydration and avoid alkalinity of urine. Photosensitivity/phototoxicity reactions may occur; d/c if phototoxicity occurs. Monitor renal, hepatic, and hematopoietic function with prolonged use. Caution with risk factors for torsades de pointes (eg, known QT prolongation, uncorrected hypokalemia). Caution in elderly and with hepatic/renal impairment.

ADVERSE REACTIONS: Tendinitis, tendon rupture, musculoskeletal symptoms, GI disorders, arthralgia, N/V, diarrhea, abdominal pain, neurological disability, rhinitis, abnormal LFTs, rash.

INTERACTIONS: See Boxed Warning and Contraindications. Coadministration with drugs primarily metabolized by CYP1A2 (eg, theophylline, methylxanthines, tizanidine) results in increased plasma concentrations of these drugs and could lead to adverse events of the coadministered drug. Increased levels of and serious and fatal reactions reported with theophylline; monitor theophylline level and adjust dose. Decreased caffeine clearance and inhibits formation of paraxanthine after caffeine administration. May alter serum levels of phenytoin. Severe hypoglycemia with glyburide (rare). Increased levels with probenecid. Transient SrCr elevations with cyclosporine. Enhances oral anticoagulant effects with warfarin or its derivatives; monitor PT or other coagulation tests. May increase risk of methotrexate toxic reactions due to inhibition of renal tubular transport. High-dose quinolones shown to provoke convulsions with NSAIDs (not aspirin [ASA]). Caution with drugs that can result in prolongation of the QT interval (eg, class IA or III antiarrhythmics). Caution with drugs that may lower seizure threshold. Mean serum concentration changes reported with piperacillin sodium 6-8 hrs after end of infusion.

PREGNANCY: Category C, not for use in nursing.

MECHANISM OF ACTION: Fluoroquinolone; inhibits topoisomerase II (DNA gyrase) and topoisomerase IV, which are required for bacterial DNA replication, transcription, repair, and recombination.

PHARMACOKINETICS: Absorption: Oral absolute bioavailability (70-80%). Administration of various doses resulted in different parameters. **Distribution:** Plasma protein binding (20-40%); found in breast milk. **Elimination:** Bile (<1%, unchanged), urine (50-70%, unchanged), feces (15%); $T_{1/2}$=5-6 hrs.

NURSING CONSIDERATIONS

Assessment: Assess for risk factors for developing tendinitis and tendon rupture, myasthenia gravis, drug hypersensitivity, renal/hepatic function, risk factors for torsades de pointes, CNS disorders or factors that may predispose to seizures or lower the seizure threshold, pregnancy/nursing status, and possible drug interactions. Obtain baseline culture and susceptibility test.

Monitoring: Monitor for tendinitis or tendon rupture, convulsions, increased ICP, toxic psychosis, CNS events, CDAD, peripheral neuropathy, photosensitivity reactions, hypersensitivity reactions and local site reactions. Periodically assess renal, hepatic and hematopoietic functions and repeat culture and susceptibility tests.

Patient Counseling: Instruct to take exactly as directed; skipping doses or not completing full course may decrease effectiveness and increase bacterial resistance. Inform to notify healthcare provider if experience pain, swelling, or inflammation of a tendon, or weakness or inability to move joints; rest and refrain from exercise and d/c therapy. Instruct to d/c and notify physician if an allergic reaction, skin rash, watery and bloody stools, or symptoms of peripheral neuropathy develop. Notify prescriber if worsening muscle weakness or breathing problems, or sunburn-like reaction occurs, if pregnant/nursing, and all medications currently taking. Avoid exposure to natural or artificial sunlight. Instruct to see how they react to therapy before engaging in activities that require mental alertness or coordination.

Administration: IV route. Refer to PI for preparation/administration. **Storage:** Vial: 5-30°C (41-86°F). Flexible container: 5-25°C (41-77°F). Protect from light and freezing. Avoid excessive heat.

CIPRO ORAL

RX

ciprofloxacin HCl - ciprofloxacin (Bayer/Schering)

> Fluoroquinolones are associated with an increased risk of tendinitis and tendon rupture in all ages. Risk is further increased in patients >60 yrs, patients taking corticosteroids, and with kidney, heart, or lung transplants. May exacerbate muscle weakness with myasthenia gravis; avoid in patients with known history of myasthenia gravis.

THERAPEUTIC CLASS: Fluoroquinolone

INDICATIONS: Treatment of lower respiratory tract infections (LRTI), complicated intra-abdominal infections (in combination with metronidazole), skin and skin structure infections (SSSI), bone and joint infections, urinary tract infections (UTI), acute exacerbations of chronic bronchitis, acute sinusitis, acute uncomplicated cystitis in females, chronic bacterial prostatitis, infectious diarrhea, typhoid fever, and uncomplicated cervical and urethral gonorrhea in adults. Treatment of complicated UTI and pyelonephritis in pediatrics 1-17 yrs. To reduce the incidence or progression of post-exposure inhalational anthrax in both adults and pediatrics.

DOSAGE: *Adults:* Acute Sinusitis/Typhoid Fever: 500mg q12h for 10 days. LRTI/SSSI: Mild-Moderate: 500mg q12h for 7-14 days. Severe/Complicated: 750mg q12h for 7-14 days. Acute Uncomplicated UTI: 250mg q12h for 3 days. Mild-Moderate UTI: 250mg q12h for 7-14 days. Severe/Complicated UTI: 500mg q12h for 7-14 days. Chronic Bacterial Prostatitis: 500mg q12h for 28 days. Intra-Abdominal (with metronidazole): 500mg q12h for 7-14 days. Bone and Joint: Mild-Moderate: 500mg q12h for ≥4-6 weeks. Severe/Complicated: 750mg q12h for ≥4-6 weeks. Infectious Diarrhea: 500mg q12h for 5-7 days. Uncomplicated Urethral/Cervical Gonococcal Infections: 250mg single dose. Inhalational Anthrax (Post-Exposure): 500mg q12h for 60 days. CrCl 30-50mL/min: 250-500mg q12h. CrCl 5-29mL/min: 250-500mg q18h. Hemodialysis/Peritoneal Dialysis: 250-500mg q24h (after dialysis). Elderly: Start at lower end of dosing range. Refer to PI for conversion of IV to PO dosing.
Pediatrics: Inhalational Anthrax (Post-Exposure): 15mg/kg q12h for 60 days. Max: 500mg/dose. 1-17 yrs: Complicated UTI/Pyelonephritis: 10-20mg/kg q12h for 10-21 days. Max: 750mg/dose.

HOW SUPPLIED: Sus: 250mg/5mL, 500mg/5mL [100mL]; Tab: 250mg, 500mg, 750mg

CONTRAINDICATIONS: Concomitant administration with tizanidine.

WARNINGS/PRECAUTIONS: D/C if experience pain, swelling, inflammation, or rupture of tendon. Convulsions, increased intracranial pressure (ICP), and toxic psychosis reported; d/c if CNS events (eg, dizziness, confusion, tremors, hallucinations, depression, suicidal thoughts/acts) occur. Caution with CNS disorders or other factors that may predispose to seizures or lower the seizure threshold. Serious and occasionally fatal hypersensitivity reactions reported; d/c immediately if signs of hypersensitivity appear. *Clostridium difficile*-associated diarrhea (CDAD) reported. Rare cases of sensory or sensorimotor axonal polyneuropathy reported; d/c if symptoms of neuropathy occur. May mask or delay symptoms of incubating syphilis. All patients should have a serologic test for syphilis; repeat after 3 months. Crystalluria reported; maintain hydration and avoid alkalinity of urine. Photosensitivity/phototoxicity reactions may occur; d/c if phototoxicity occurs. Monitor renal, hepatic, and hematopoietic function with prolonged use. Caution with risk factors for torsades de pointes (eg, known QT prolongation, uncorrected hypokalemia). Caution in elderly and with renal/hepatic impairment.

ADVERSE REACTIONS: Tendinitis, tendon rupture, musculoskeletal symptoms, GI disorders, arthralgia, N/V, diarrhea, abdominal pain, neurological disability, rhinitis, abnormal LFTs, rash.

INTERACTIONS: See Boxed Warning and Contraindications. Coadministration with drugs primarily metabolized by CYP1A2 (eg, theophylline, methylxanthines, tizanidine) results in increased plasma concentrations of these drugs and could lead to adverse events of the coadministered drug. Increased levels of and serious and fatal reactions reported with theophylline; monitor theophylline level and adjust dose. Decreased caffeine clearance and inhibits formation of paraxanthine after caffeine administration. Multivalent cation-containing products (eg, magnesium- or aluminum-containing antacids, sucralfate, didanosine chewable/buffered tab or pediatric powder, other highly buffered drugs, products containing calcium, iron, or zinc) decrease absorption, resulting in lower serum and urine levels; administer ≥2 hrs before or 6 hrs after these drugs. May alter serum levels of phenytoin. Severe hypo-glycemia with glyburide (rare). Increased levels with probenecid. Transient SrCr elevations with cyclosporine. Enhances oral anticoagulant effects with warfarin or its derivatives; monitor PT or other coagulation tests. May increase risk of methotrexate toxic reactions due to inhibition of renal tubular trans-port. Acceleration of absorption with metoclopramide. High-dose quinolones shown to provoke convulsions with NSAIDs (not aspirin [ASA]). Caution with drugs that can result in prolongation of the QT interval (eg, class IA or III anti-arrhythmics). Caution with drugs that may lower seizure threshold.

PREGNANCY: Category C, not for use in nursing.

MECHANISM OF ACTION: Fluoroquinolone; inhibits topoisomerase II (DNA gyrase) and topoisomerase IV, which are required for bacterial DNA replica-tion, transcription, repair, and recombination.

PHARMACOKINETICS: Absorption: Rapid, well absorbed; absolute bioavail-ability (70%); T_{max}=1-2 hrs. Administration of various doses resulted in different parameters. **Distribution:** Plasma protein binding (20-40%); found in breast milk. **Elimination:** Urine (40-50%, unchanged), feces (20-35%); $T_{1/2}$=4 hrs.

NURSING CONSIDERATIONS

Assessment: Assess for risk factors for developing tendinitis and tendon rupture, myasthenia gravis, drug hypersensitivity, renal/hepatic function, risk factors for torsades de pointes, CNS disorders or factors that may predispose to seizures or lower seizure threshold, pregnancy/nursing status, and possible drug interactions. Obtain baseline culture and susceptibility test and serologic test for syphilis.

Monitoring: Monitor for tendinitis or tendon rupture, convulsions, increased ICP, toxic psychosis, CNS events, CDAD, peripheral neuropathy, photosensitiv-ity reactions, and hypersensitivity reactions. Periodically assess renal, hepatic and hematopoietic functions and repeat culture and susceptibility tests. Perform follow-up serologic test for syphilis after 3 months.

Patient Counseling: Instruct to take exactly as directed; skipping doses or not completing full course may decrease effectiveness and increase bacterial resistance. Inform to notify healthcare provider if experience pain, swelling, or inflammation of a tendon, or weakness or inability to move joints; rest and refrain from exercise and d/c therapy. Instruct to d/c and notify physician if an allergic reaction, skin rash, watery and bloody stools, or symptoms of peripheral neuropathy. Notify prescriber if worsening muscle weakness or breathing problems, or sunburn-like reaction occurs, if pregnant/nursing, and all medications and supplements currently taking. Inform to take with or without food, and drink fluids liberally. Instruct to avoid concomitant use with dairy products or calcium-fortified juices alone. Avoid exposure to natural or artificial sunlight. Instruct to see how they react to therapy before engaging in activities that require mental alertness or coordination.

Administration: Oral route. Administer ≥2 hrs before or 6 hrs after magne-sium- or aluminum-containing antacids, sucralfate, didanosine chewable/buff-ered tab or pediatric powder, other highly buffered drugs, or other products containing calcium, iron, or zinc. **Storage:** Tab/Reconstituted Sol: <30°C (<86°F). Reconstituted Sol: Store for 14 days. Microcapsules and Diluent: <25°C (<77°F). Protect from freezing.

CIPRO XR

RX

ciprofloxacin (Bayer/Schering)

> Fluoroquinolones are associated with an increased risk of tendinitis and tendon rupture in all ages. Risk is further increased in patients >60 yrs, taking corticosteroids, and with kidney, heart, or lung transplants. May exacerbate muscle weakness with myasthenia gravis; avoid in patients with known history of myasthenia gravis.

THERAPEUTIC CLASS: Fluoroquinolone

INDICATIONS: Treatment of urinary tract infections (UTI), including uncomplicated (acute cystitis) and complicated UTI, and acute uncomplicated pyelonephritis caused by susceptible strains of microorganisms.

DOSAGE: *Adults:* Uncomplicated UTI: 500mg q24h for 3 days. Complicated UTI/Acute Uncomplicated Pyelonephritis: 1000mg q24h for 7-14 days. CrCl <30mL/min: 500mg qd. Dialysis: Give after procedure is completed. May switch from ciprofloxacin IV to extended release at discretion of physician.

HOW SUPPLIED: Tab, Extended-Release: 500mg, 1000mg

CONTRAINDICATIONS: Concomitant administration with tizanidine.

WARNINGS/PRECAUTIONS: D/C if experience pain, swelling, inflammation or rupture of a tendon. Convulsions, intracranial pressure (ICP), toxic psychosis, and other CNS events reported; d/c if CNS events occur. Caution with CNS disorders or risk factors that may predispose to seizures or lower seizure threshold. Serious and occasionally fatal hypersensitivity reactions reported; d/c immediately if signs of hypersensitivity appear. *Clostridium difficile*-associated diarrhea (CDAD) reported. Rare cases of sensory or sensorimotor axonal polyneuropathy reported; d/c if symptoms of neuropathy occur. Crystalluria reported; maintain hydration and avoid alkalinizing urine. Photosensitivity/phototoxicity reactions may occur; d/c if phototoxicity occurs. Avoid excessive sunlight and UV light. Not interchangeable with immediate-release tablets. Caution in elderly and with renal impairment.

ADVERSE REACTIONS: N/V, headache, diarrhea, dizziness, vaginal moniliasis, dyspepsia.

INTERACTIONS: See Boxed Warning and Contraindications. Increase in plasma concentration of drugs metabolized by CYP1A2 (eg, theophylline, methylxanthines, tizanidine) when coadministered. Serious and fatal reactions reported with theophylline; monitor theophylline level and adjust. May reduce clearance of caffeine. Concurrent administration with multivalent-containing products such as magnesium -or aluminum-containing antacids, sucralfate, didanosine chewable/buffered tablets or pediatric powder, other highly buffered drugs and products containing calcium, iron, or zinc may decrease serum and urine levels; administer ≥2 hrs before or 6 hrs after. Slightly diminished absorption with omeprazole. May alter serum levels of phenytoin. Severe hypoglycemia with glyburide (rare). Transient elevations in SrCr with cyclosporine. Enhances the oral anticoagulant effects of warfarin and its derivatives; monitor PT and other suitable coagulation tests closely. Increased levels with probenecid. Increases methotrexate levels and may increase risk of toxic reactions. Accelerated absorption with metoclopramide. Caution with drugs that lower seizure threshold. High-dose quinolones shown to provoke convulsions with NSAIDs (not aspirin [ASA]). Caution with drugs that can result in prolongation of the QT interval (eg, class IA or class III antiarrhythmics). Avoid concomitant administration with dairy products alone, or with calcium-fortified products.

PREGNANCY: Category C, not for use in nursing.

MECHANISM OF ACTION: Fluoroquinolone; inhibits topoisomerase II (DNA gyrase) and topoisomerase IV, which are required for bacterial DNA replication, transcription, repair, and recombination.

PHARMACOKINETICS: Absorption: (500mg): C_{max}=1.59mg/L; T_{max}=1.5 hrs; AUC_{0-24h}=7.97mg•h/L. (1000mg): C_{max}=3.11mg/L; T_{max}=2 hrs; AUC_{0-24h}=16.83mg•h/L. **Distribution:** (IV) V_d=2.1-2.7L/kg; plasma protein binding (20-40%); found in breast milk. **Metabolism:** Primary metabolites: oxociprofloxacin (M_3) and sulfociprofloxacin (M_2). **Elimination:** Urine (35%, unchanged).

NURSING CONSIDERATIONS

Assessment: Assess for risk factors for developing tendinitis and tendon rupture, myasthenia gravis, drug hypersensitivity, renal function, risk factors for torsades de pointes, CNS disorders or risk factors that may predispose to seizure or lower seizure threshold, pregnancy/nursing status, and for possible drug interactions.

Monitoring: Monitor for tendinitis, tendon rupture, convulsions, increased ICP, toxic psychosis, CNS events, CDAD, peripheral neuropathy, photosensitivity reactions, and hypersensitivity reactions. Assess renal function.

Patient Counseling: Instruct to take exactly as directed; skipping doses or not completing full course may decrease effectiveness and increase bacterial resistance. Inform to notify healthcare provider if experience pain, swelling, or inflammation of a tendon, or weakness or inability to move joints; rest and refrain from exercise and d/c therapy. Instruct to d/c and notify physician if an allergic reaction, skin rash, watery and bloody stools, or symptoms of peripheral neuropathy develop. Notify prescriber if worsening muscle weakness or breathing problems, or sunburn-like reaction occurs, if pregnant/nursing, and all medications and supplements currently taking. Inform to take with or without food, and drink fluids liberally. Instruct to avoid concomitant use with dairy products or calcium-fortified juices alone. Avoid exposure to natural or artificial sunlight. Instruct to see how they react to therapy before engaging in activities that require mental alertness or coordination. Advise not to take more than one tab/day, even if dose is missed.

Administration: Oral route. Swallow tab whole; do not split, crush, or chew. Administer ≥2 hrs before or 6 hrs after magnesium- or aluminum-containing antacids, sucralfate, didanosine chewable/buffered tablets or pediatric powder, metal cations (eg, iron), multivitamins with zinc. Space calcium intake (>800mg) by ≥2 hrs. **Storage:** 25°C (77°F), excursions permitted to 15-30°C (59-86°F).

CIPRODEX   RX
dexamethasone - ciprofloxacin (Alcon)

THERAPEUTIC CLASS: Antibacterial/corticosteroid combination

INDICATIONS: Acute otitis media in pediatric patients with tympanostomy tubes. Acute otitis externa.

DOSAGE: *Adults:* Acute Otitis Externa: 4 drops in affected ear(s) bid for 7 days. Warm bottle in hand for 1-2 min to avoid dizziness. Shake well before use.
Pediatrics: ≥6 months: 4 drops in affected ear(s) bid for 7 days. Warm bottle in hand for 1-2 min to avoid dizziness. Shake well before use.

HOW SUPPLIED: Sus: (Ciprofloxacin-Dexamethasone) 0.3%-0.1% [5mL, 7.5mL]

CONTRAINDICATIONS: Viral infections of external ear canal including herpes simplex infections.

WARNINGS/PRECAUTIONS: D/C if hypersensitivity reaction occurs. Re-evaluate if no improvement after one week.

ADVERSE REACTIONS: Ear pain/discomfort/pruritus.

PREGNANCY: Category C, not for use in nursing.

MECHANISM OF ACTION: Fluoroquinolone, corticosteroid; antibacterial/anti-inflammatory; bactericidal action results from interference with the enzyme (DNA gyrase), which is needed for the synthesis of bacterial DNA.

PHARMACOKINETICS: Absorption: Ciprofloxacin: C_{max} =1.39ng/mL; T_{max} =15 min-2 hrs. Dexamethasone: C_{max} =1.14ng/mL; T_{max} =15 min-2 hrs.

NURSING CONSIDERATIONS

Assessment: Assess for history of drug hypersensitivity and viral infection of the external canal, including herpes simplex virus infection.

Monitoring: Monitor for anaphylactic reactions, skin rash, overgrowth of non-susceptible organisms (eg, fungi and yeast) in large doses, lesions or erosions of cartilage in weight-bearing joints, and other signs of arthropathy.

Patient Counseling: Inform drug is for otic use only. Avoid touching dropper tip to ear material or any other surface. D/C if rash or allergic reaction occurs. Instruct to keep infected ear dry and clean. Take as prescribed.

Administration: Otic route. Warm suspension by holding bottle in hand for 1-2 min. Lie with affected ear up, then instill drops. Maintain position for 60 sec and repeat, if necessary, with opposite ear. **Storage:** Store at 15-30°C (59-86°F). Protect from light; avoid freezing.

CLARINEX   RX
desloratadine (Merck)

THERAPEUTIC CLASS: H_1-antagonist

INDICATIONS: Relief of nasal and non-nasal symptoms of seasonal allergic rhinitis in patients ≥2 yrs. Relief of nasal and non-nasal symptoms of perennial allergic rhinitis in patients ≥6 months. Symptomatic relief of pruritus and reduction in number and size of hives in patients ≥6 months with chronic idiopathic urticaria.

DOSAGE: *Adults:* 5mg or 10mL qd. Hepatic/Renal Impairment: Initial: 5mg tab qod.
Pediatrics: ≥12 yrs: 5mg or 10mL qd. 6-11 yrs: 2.5mg (RediTabs) or 5mL qd. 12 months-5 yrs: 2.5mL (1.25mg) qd. 6-11 months: 2mL (1mg) qd.

HOW SUPPLIED: Tab: 5mg; Tab, Disintegrating (RediTabs): 2.5mg, 5mg; Sol: 0.5mg/mL

WARNINGS/PRECAUTIONS: Hypersensitivity reactions (eg, rash, pruritus, urticaria, edema, dyspnea, anaphylaxis) reported; d/c therapy if such reaction occurs and consider alternative treatment. Caution in elderly.

ADVERSE REACTIONS: Pharyngitis. (Tab) Dry mouth, headache, nausea, fatigue, myalgia. (Sol) Fever, diarrhea, cough, upper respiratory tract infection, irritability, somnolence, bronchitis, otitis media, vomiting.

INTERACTIONS: Increased plasma concentrations with erythromycin, ketoconazole, azithromycin, fluoxetine, and cimetidine.

PREGNANCY: Category C, not for use in nursing.

MECHANISM OF ACTION: Long-acting tricyclic histamine antagonist with selective H_1-receptor histamine antagonist activity; inhibits histamine release from human mast cells.

PHARMACOKINETICS: Absorption: (5mg tab) T_{max}=3 hrs; C_{max}=4ng/mL, AUC=56.9ng•hr/mL. **Distribution:** Plasma protein binding (82-87%, desloratadine), (85-89%, 3-hydroxydesloratadine); found in breast milk. **Metabolism:** Extensive; 3-hydroxydesloratadine (active metabolite). **Elimination:** Urine and feces (87% metabolites); $T_{1/2}$=27 hrs.

NURSING CONSIDERATIONS

Assessment: Assess for hypersensitivity to drug, renal/hepatic function, pregnancy/nursing status, and possible drug interactions.

Monitoring: Monitor for hypersensitivity and other adverse reactions.

Patient Counseling: Instruct to take drug as directed; may be taken without regard to meals. Advise not to increase dose or dosing frequency. Inform that RediTabs contain phenylalanine.

Administration: Oral route. (RediTabs) Dissolve on tongue and allow to disintegrate before swallowing. Take immediately after opening the blister. Administer with or without water. (Sol) Administer age-appropriate dose of sol with a measuring dropper or syringe calibrated to deliver 2mL and 2.5mL.

Storage: 25°C (77°F); excursions permitted to 15-30°C (59-86°F). (Tab) Avoid exposure at ≥30°C (86°F). (Sol) Protect from light.

CLARINEX-D

RX

pseudoephedrine sulfate - desloratadine (Schering)

THERAPEUTIC CLASS: H_1-antagonist/sympathomimetic amine

INDICATIONS: Relief of nasal and non-nasal symptoms of seasonal allergic rhinitis, including nasal congestion in adults and adolescents ≥12 yrs.

DOSAGE: *Adults:* (12-hr) 1 tab bid or (24-hr) 1 tab qd w/ or w/o food. *Pediatrics:* ≥12 yrs: (12-hr) 1 tab bid or (24-hr) 1 tab qd w/ or w/o food.

HOW SUPPLIED: Tab, Extended-Release: (Desloratadine-Pseudoephedrine) (12-Hr) 2.5mg-120mg, (24-Hr) 5mg-240mg

CONTRAINDICATIONS: Narrow-angle glaucoma, urinary retention, MAOI therapy or within 14 days of d/c, severe HTN, severe coronary artery disease (CAD).

WARNINGS/PRECAUTIONS: Cardiovascular (eg, CV collapse with hypotension) and CNS (eg, CNS stimulation, convulsions, tremor, arrhythmias) effects reported; caution in patients with CV disorder and should not be used in severe HTN or severe CAD. Caution in patients with diabetes mellitus (DM) and hyperthyroidism. Caution in patients with prostatic hypertrophy or increased intraocular pressure (IOP); urinary retention and narrow angle glaucoma may occur. Hypersensitivity reactions reported; d/c if any occur. Avoid in patients with hepatic and/or renal impairment. Caution in elderly.

ADVERSE REACTIONS: Dry mouth, headache, insomnia, fatigue, pharyngitis, somnolence.

INTERACTIONS: See Contraindications. Antihypertensive effects of β-adrenergic blocking agents, methyldopa, and reserpine may be reduced by sympathomimetics (eg, pseudoephedrine). Increased ectopic pacemaker activity with digitalis. Increased plasma concentrations with CYP450 3A4 inhibitors (eg, ketoconazole, erythromycin, azithromycin), cimetidine and fluoxetine.

PREGNANCY: Category C, not for use in nursing.

MECHANISM OF ACTION: Desloratadine: H_1-receptor antagonist; inhibits histamine release from human mast cells *in vitro*. Pseudoephedrine: Sympathomimetic amine; exerts a decongestant action on nasal mucosa.

PHARMACOKINETICS: Absorption: Desloratadine: (24 hr) C_{max}=1.79ng/mL; T_{max}=6-7 hrs, AUC=61.1ng•hr/mL. (12 hr) C_{max}=1.09ng/mL; T_{max}=4-5 hrs, AUC=31.6ng•hr/mL. Pseudoephedrine: (24 hr) C_{max}=328ng/mL, T_{max}=8-9 hrs, AUC=6438ng•hr/mL. (12 hr) C_{max}=263ng/mL, T_{max}=6-7 hrs, AUC=4588ng•hr/mL. **Distribution:** Desloratadine: Found in breast milk, plasma protein binding (82-87%), 3-hydroxydesloratadine (85-89%). **Metabolism:** Desloratadine (major metabolite): extensive, 3-hydroxydesloratadine (active metabolite) and glucuronidation pathway. Pseudoephedrine: Liver (incomplete), through N-demethylation. **Elimination:** Desloratadine: (24 hr) $T_{1/2}$=24 hrs, (12 hr) $T_{1/2}$=27 hrs. Pseudoephedrine: Urine (55-96% unchanged). If urinary pH=5, ($T_{1/2}$=3-6 hrs); if urinary pH=8, ($T_{1/2}$=9-16 hrs).

NURSING CONSIDERATIONS

Assessment: Assess for drug hypersensitivity, hepatic/renal impairment, history of increased IOP, narrow-angle glaucoma, prostatic hypertrophy, urinary retention, HTN, CAD, DM, hyperthyroidism, pregnancy/nursing status and possible drug interactions (eg, MAOIs).

Monitoring: Monitor for CV and CNS effects (eg, insomnia, dizziness, weakness, tremor, arrhythmias), hypersensitivity reactions, BP, IOP, urinary retention in patients with prostatic hyperthrophy and hepatic/renal function.

Patient Counseling: Inform patients that CV or CNS effects such as insomnia, dizziness, tremor or arrhythmias may occur. Advise not to increase the dose or dosing frequency. Advise not to use other antihistamines or decongestants.

Instruct to inform physician of present illness such as severe HTN, severe CAD, narrow angle glaucoma, or urinary retention prior to treatment. Not to be taken during nursing/pregnancy.

Administration: Oral route. Do not break or chew, swallow tab whole.
Storage: 25°C (77°F); excursions permitted to 15-30°C (59-86°F). Heat sensitive. Avoid exposure at or above 30°C (86°F). Protect from excessive moisture. Protect from light.

CLARIPEL RX
hydroquinone (Stiefel)

THERAPEUTIC CLASS: Depigmentation agent

INDICATIONS: Gradual treatment of ultraviolet induced dyschromia and discoloration resulting from use of oral contraceptives, pregnancy, hormone replacement therapy, or skin trauma.

DOSAGE: *Adults:* Apply bid.
Pediatrics: ≥12 yrs: Apply bid.

HOW SUPPLIED: Cre: 4% [28g, 45g]

WARNINGS/PRECAUTIONS: Avoid sun exposure on bleached skin. Claripel contains sunscreen. May produce unwanted cosmetic effects if not used as directed. Test for skin sensitivity. D/C if no lightening effect after 2 months of therapy, if blue-black skin discoloration occurs, or if itching, vesicle formation, or excessive inflammatory reactions occur. Contains sodium metabisulfite; may cause serious allergic type reactions. Avoid contact with eyes.

ADVERSE REACTIONS: Cutaneous hypersensitivity (contact dermatitis).

PREGNANCY: Category C, caution in nursing.

MECHANISM OF ACTION: Produces a reversible depigmentation of the skin by inhibition of the enzymatic oxidation of tyrosine to 3-(3,4-dihydroxy-phenyl) alanine (dopa)[1] and suppression of other melanocyte metabolic processes.

NURSING CONSIDERATIONS

Assessment: Test for skin sensitivity prior to treatment.

Monitoring: Monitor allergic-type reactions including anaphylactic symptoms and life-threatening or severe asthmatic episodes in susceptible patients, itching, vesicles and gradual blue-darkening of the skin.

Patient Counseling: Take drug as prescribed and use sunscreen during therapy. D/C drug and contact physician if any signs of allergy occur. Avoid contact with eyes.

Administration: Topical route. **Storage:** 15-30°C (59-86°F).

CLEOCIN RX
clindamycin (Pharmacia & Upjohn)

Clostridium difficile-associated diarrhea (CDAD) reported and may range in severity from mild diarrhea to fatal colitis. Not for use with nonbacterial infections. CDAD must be considered in all patients with diarrhea following antibiotic use. If CDAD is suspected or confirmed, ongoing antibiotic use not directed against *C.difficile* may need to be d/c. Appropriate fluid and electrolyte management, protein supplementation, antibiotic treatment of *C.difficile* and surgical evaluation may be instituted as clinically indicated.

THERAPEUTIC CLASS: Lincomycin derivative

INDICATIONS: Treatment of serious infections caused by susceptible anaerobes, streptococci, pneumococci, and staphylococci.

DOSAGE: *Adults:* Serious Infection: 150-300mg PO q6h or 600-1200mg/day IM/IV given bid-qid. More Severe Infections: 300-450mg PO q6h or 1200-2700mg/day IM/IV given bid-qid. Life-Threatening Infections: Up to 4800mg/day IV. Max: 600mg per IM injection. Alternatively may administer as a single rapid infusion for the first dose followed by continuous IV infusion; see PI for dosing. Treat β-hemolytic strep for at least 10 days.

Pediatrics: PO: Serious Infections: (Cap) 8-16mg/kg/day given tid-qid or (Sol) 8-12mg/kg/day tid-qid. Severe Infection: (Sol) 13-16mg/kg/day tid-qid. More Severe Infections: (Cap) 16-20mg/kg/day given tid-qid or (Sol) 17-25mg/kg/day tid-qid. ≤10kg: 1/2 tsp (37.5mg) tid should be the minimum recommended dose. IM/IV: 1 month-16 yrs: 20-40mg/kg/day tid-qid; use the higher dose for more serious infections. Alternately may give 350mg/m²/day for serious infections and 450mg/m²/day for more serious infections. <1 month: 15-20mg/kg/day tid-qid. Treat β-hemolytic strep for at least 10 days.

HOW SUPPLIED: Cap: (HCl) 75mg, 150mg, 300mg; Inj: (Phosphate) 150mg/mL [2mL, 4mL, 6mL, 60mL] 300mg/50mL, 600mg/50mL, 900mg/50mL; Sol: (Palmitate) 75mg/5mL [100mL]

WARNINGS/PRECAUTIONS: Due to association with severe colitis, reserve use for serious infections where less toxic agents are inappropriate. Use in the absence of a proven or strongly suspected infection is unlikely to provide benefit and may increase the risk of development of drug-resistant bacteria. May cause overgrowth of nonsusceptible organisms. Not for treatment of meningitis. Caution with patients with liver disease; perform periodic liver enzyme determinations with severe liver disease. Caution with atopic patients, renal disease, history of GI disease (eg, colitis), and the elderly. Perform periodic monitoring of blood counts, hepatic and renal function with long-term use. Do not give injection undiluted as bolus. (75mg/150mg caps) Contain tartrazine, may cause allergic-type reactions. (Inj) Contains benzyl alcohol; associated with "gasping syndrome" in premature infants.

ADVERSE REACTIONS: Abdominal pain, colitis, esophagitis, N/V, diarrhea, maculopapular skin rash, jaundice, pruritus, vaginitis.

INTERACTIONS: Antagonism may occur with erythromycin. May potentiate neuromuscular blockers.

PREGNANCY: Category B, not for use in nursing.

MECHANISM OF ACTION: Lincomycin-derivative antibiotic; inhibits bacterial protein synthesis by binding to the 50s subunit of the ribosome.

PHARMACOKINETICS: Absorption: Cap: Rapid, complete; C_{max}=2.5mcg/mL, T_{max}=45 min. Inj: C_{max}=10.8mcg/mL (Adults, 600mg IV q8h), 9mcg/mL (Adults, 600 mg IM q12h), 10mcg/mL (Peds, 5-7mg/kg IV in 1 hr), 8mcg/mL (Peds, 5-7mg/kg IM); T_{max}=3 hrs (Adults, IM), 1 hr (Peds, IM). **Distribution:** Wide; body fluids, tissues, and bones; found in breast milk. **Elimination:** Cap: Urine (10% unchanged), feces (3.6% unchanged); $T_{1/2}$=2.4 hr. Inj: $T_{1/2}$=3 hrs (Adults), 2.5 hrs (Peds). Sol: $T_{1/2}$=2 hrs.

NURSING CONSIDERATIONS

Assessment: Assess for previous sensitivities to drugs and other allergens, history of GI disease (eg, colitis), renal/hepatic function, pregnancy/nursing status, presence of meningitis, upcoming surgical procedures, and for possible drug interactions. Assess use in atopic patients and in elderly patients with severe illness.

Monitoring: Monitor for CDAD, overgrowth of nonsusceptible organisms, and for anaphylactoid reactions. Monitor for changes in bowel frequency in older patients. When culture and susceptibility information is available, consider modifying antibacterial therapy. If on prolonged therapy, perform periodic liver and kidney function tests and blood counts. Perform periodic liver enzyme determinations in patients with severe liver disease.

Patient Counseling: Inform about potential benefits/risks of use. Inform that therapy only treats bacterial, not viral infections. Instruct to take exactly as directed; skipping doses or not completing full course may decrease effectiveness and increase antibiotic resistance. Instruct to contact physician if an allergic reaction develops. Advise that watery and bloody stools may occur as late as 2 months after therapy. Instruct to notify physician if pregnant/nursing.

Administration: Oral/IM/IV route. See PI for proper preparation and administration. **Storage:** 20-25°C (68-77°F). (Sol) Do not refrigerate the reconstituted solution; stable at room temperature for 2 weeks.

CLEVIPREX

clevidipine butyrate (The Medicines Company)

THERAPEUTIC CLASS: Calcium channel blocker (dihydropyridine)

INDICATIONS: Reduction of BP in patients when oral therapy is not desirable or feasible.

DOSAGE: *Adults:* IV use only: Individualize dose. Initial: 1-2mg/hr. Titrate: Double dose at 90-second intervals initially and then adjust dose less than double every 5-10 min. Maint: 4-6mg/hr. Max: 16mg/hr. Due to lipid load restrictions, no more than 1000mL or an average of 21mg/hr is recommended/24 hrs. Transition to Oral Therapy: D/C or titrate downward until oral therapy is established. Consider lag time of oral agent's effect and monitor BP until desired effect is reached.

HOW SUPPLIED: Inj: 0.5mg/mL [50mL, 100mL]

CONTRAINDICATIONS: Allergy to soybeans, soy products, eggs, or egg products. Severe aortic stenosis, defective lipid metabolism (eg, pathologic hyperlipidemia, lipoid nephrosis, or acute pancreatitis accompanied with hyperlipidemia).

WARNINGS/PRECAUTIONS: Discard unused portions, including product being infused, within 4 hrs of stopper puncture. Systemic hypotension and reflex tachycardia may occur; decrease dose. Lipid intake restrictions may be necessary with significant disorders of lipid metabolism. May produce negative inotropic effects and exacerbation of heart failure (HF); monitor HF patients. Does not lower HR and does not protect against effects of abrupt beta-blocker withdrawal. Monitor for rebound hypertension for at least 8 hrs after withdrawal.

ADVERSE REACTIONS: Headache, N/V, MI, cardiac arrest, syncope, dyspnea, hypotension, reflex tachycardia.

PREGNANCY: Category C, safety not known in nursing.

MECHANISM OF ACTION: Calcium channel blocker (dihydropyridine); mediates the influx of calcium in arterial smooth muscle and reduces mean arterial blood pressure by decreasing systemic vascular resistance; does not reduce preload.

PHARMACOKINETICS: Distribution: V_d=0.17L/kg; plasma protein binding (>99.5%). **Metabolism:** Hydrolysis, glucuronidation, oxidation; carboxylic acid and formaldehyde (primary metabolites). **Excretion:** $T_{1/2}$=15 min; urine (63-74%); feces (7-22%).

NURSING CONSIDERATIONS

Assessment: Assess BP and HR, history of allergy to soy and egg products, defective lipid metabolism disorders, history of beta-blocker usage, and pregnancy/nursing status. Obtain baseline parameters (eg, BP, lipid profile).

Monitoring: Monitor BP and HR, hypotension, reflex tachycardia, rebound HTN (at least 8 hrs after the last dose), and HF.

Patient Counseling: Advise that underlying HTN requires follow up and continuation of oral antihypertensive medications as prescribed. Report any signs of new hypertensive emergency such as neurological symptoms, visual changes, or heart failure to healthcare provider immediately.

Administration: IV route. Refer to PI for details on administration. **Storage:** 2-8°C (36-46°F). Do not freeze. May be transferred to 25°C (77°F) for a period not to exceed 2 months. Do not return to refrigerated storage after exposing to room temperature. Protect from light.

CLIMARA

RX

estradiol (Bayer Healthcare)

> Estrogens increase the risk of endometrial cancer. Estrogens, with or without progestins, should not be used for the prevention of cardiovascular disease or dementia. Increased risk of myocardial infarction (MI), stroke, invasive breast cancer, pulmonary embolism (PE), and deep vein thrombosis (DVT) in postmenopausal women (50-79 yrs of age) reported. Increased risk of developing probable dementia in postmenopausal women ≥65 yrs of age reported.

THERAPEUTIC CLASS: Estrogen

INDICATIONS: Treatment of moderate to severe vasomotor symptoms and/or vulvar/vaginal atrophy associated with menopause. Treatment of hypoestrogenism due to hypogonadism, castration, or primary ovarian failure. Prevention of postmenopausal osteoporosis.

DOSAGE: *Adults:* Apply 1 patch weekly to lower abdomen or upper area of buttocks (avoid breasts and waistline). Rotate application sites. Vasomotor Symptoms: Initial: 0.025mg/day patch once weekly. Titrate: Adjust dose as needed. Wait 1 week after withdrawal of oral therapy before initiating patch. D/C or taper at 3-6 month intervals. Osteoporosis Prevention: Minimum Effective Dose: 0.025mg/day once weekly.

HOW SUPPLIED: Patch: 0.025mg/day, 0.0375mg/day, 0.05mg/day, 0.06mg/day, 0.075mg/day, 0.1mg/day [4[s]]

CONTRAINDICATIONS: Pregnancy, undiagnosed abnormal genital bleeding, breast cancer (or history of), estrogen-dependent neoplasia, DVT (or history of), PE (or history of), active or recent (eg, within 1 year) arterial thromboembolic disease (eg, stroke, MI), liver dysfunction or disease.

WARNINGS/PRECAUTIONS: May increase risk of cardiovascular (CV) events (eg, MI, stroke), venous thrombosis, and PE; d/c immediately if any of these events occur or are suspected. May increase risk of breast/endometrial cancer, and gallbladder disease. Retinal vascular thrombosis reported; monitor and d/c if papilledema or retinal vascular lesions occur. May increase risk of dementia. May cause severe hypercalcemia in patients with breast cancer and bone metastases; d/c if severe hypercalcemia occurs. Consider addition of a progestin if no hysterectomy. May elevate BP; monitor at regular intervals. May cause elevations of plasma triglycerides with pre-existing hypertriglyceridemia. Caution with history of cholestatic jaundice associated with past estrogen use or with pregnancy; d/c with recurrence. May lead to increased thyroid-binding globulin levels; monitor thyroid function in patients dependent on thyroid replacement therapy. May cause fluid retention; caution with cardiac/renal dysfunction. May increase risk of ovarian cancer. May exacerbate endometriosis, asthma, diabetes mellitus (DM), epilepsy, migraine, porphyria, systemic lupus erythematosus (SLE), hepatic hemangiomas; use with caution.

ADVERSE REACTIONS: Headache, arthralgia, edema, abdominal pain, flatulence, depression, breast pain, leukorrhea, upper respiratory tract infection, sinusitis, rhinitis, pruritus.

INTERACTIONS: CYP3A4 inducers (eg, St. John's wort, phenobarbital, carbamazepine, rifampin) may decrease levels, which may decrease therapeutic effects and/or change uterine bleeding profile. CYP3A4 inhibitors (eg, erythromycin, clarithromycin, ketoconazole, itraconazole, ritonavir, grapefruit juice) may increase levels, which may result in side effects.

PREGNANCY: Contraindicated in pregnancy, caution in nursing.

MECHANISM OF ACTION: Estrogen; binds to nuclear receptors in estrogen-responsive tissues. Modulates pituitary secretion of gonadotropins, luteinizing hormone (LH), and follicle stimulating hormone (FSH), through negative feedback mechanism.

PHARMACOKINETICS: Absorption: Transdermal administration of different doses resulted in different parameters. **Distribution:** Estrogens are found in breast milk. Wide; largely bound to sex hormone binding globulin (SHBG) and albumin. **Metabolism:** Liver to estrone (metabolite); estriol (major urinary metabolite); enterohepatic recirculation via sulfate and glucuronide conjugation;

biliary secretion of conjugates into the intestine; hydrolysis in the gut; and reasborbtion. **Elimination:** Urine.

NURSING CONSIDERATIONS

Assessment: Assess for abnormal genital bleeding, presence or history of breast cancer, estrogen-dependent neoplasias, DVT, PE, active or recent (within past yr) and any other conditions where treatment may be contraindicated or cautioned. Assess use in women ≥65 yrs, nursing patients, and those with DM, asthma, epilepsy, migraines or porphyria, SLE, and hepatic hemangiomas. Assess for possible drug and lab test interactions.

Monitoring: Monitor for signs/symptoms of CV disorders (eg, MI, stroke, venous thrombosis, PE), malignant neoplasms (eg, breast, endometrial, ovarian cancer), dementia, gallbladder disease, hypercalcemia, visual abnormalities (eg, retinal vascular thrombosis), increased BP, hypertriglyceridemia, hypothyroidism, fluid retention, cholestatic jaundice, exacerbation of endometriosis and other conditions. Perform annual mammography and periodic monitoring of BP. Monitor thyroid function if patient on thyroid hormone replacement therapy. In cases of undiagnosed, persistent, or recurrent vaginal bleeding in women with uterus, perform adequate diagnostic measures (eg, endometrial sampling) to rule out malignancies.

Patient Counseling: Inform that medication increases risk for uterine cancer and may increase chances for heart attack, stroke, breast cancer, and blood clots. Advise to contact physician if breast lumps, unusual vaginal bleeding, dizziness or faintness, changes in speech, severe headaches, chest pain, SOB, leg pain, visual changes, or vomiting occur. Inform once in place, transdermal system should not be exposed to sun for prolonged periods of time. Removal of system should be done carefully and slowly to avoid skin irritation. If patch falls off during dosing interval, apply new patch for remainder of the 7-day period.

Administration: Transdermal application. Site of application should not be oily, damaged, or irritated. Apply patch after opening pouch and removing protective liner. Ensure patch sticks completely, especially around edges.

Storage: Do not store above 30°C (86°F). Do not store unpouched. Keep out of reach of children.

CLIMARA PRO RX
levonorgestrel - estradiol (Bayer Healthcare)

> Estrogens and progestins should not be used for the prevention of cardiovascular disease (CVD) or dementia. Increased risks of myocardial infarction (MI), stroke, invasive breast cancer, pulmonary embolism (PE), and deep vein thrombosis (DVT) in postmenopausal women (50-79 yrs of age) reported. Increased risk of developing probable dementia in postmenopausal women ≥65 yrs of age reported. Prescribe at the lowest effective dose for the shortest duration consistent with treatment goals and risks for the individual woman.

THERAPEUTIC CLASS: Estrogen/progestogen combination

INDICATIONS: Treatment of moderate to severe vasomotor symptoms associated with menopause. Prevention of postmenopausal osteoporosis.

DOSAGE: *Adults:* Apply 1 patch weekly to lower abdomen (avoid breasts and waistline). Rotate application site; allow 1 week between applications to same site. Re-evaluate periodically (3- to 6-month intervals). Women currently using continuous estrogen or combination estrogen/progestin therapy should complete the current cycle of therapy, before initiating treatment; women not currently using continuous estrogen or combination estrogen/progestin may start anytime.

HOW SUPPLIED: Patch: (Estradiol-Levonorgestrel): 0.045mg-0.015mg/day [4ˢ]

CONTRAINDICATIONS: Pregnancy, undiagnosed abnormal genital bleeding, known/suspected/history of breast cancer, known/suspected estrogen-dependent neoplasia, active/history of DVT/PE, active or recent (eg, within 1 yr) arterial thromboembolic disease (eg, stroke, MI), liver dysfunction or disease.

WARNINGS/PRECAUTIONS: D/C immediately if CV events (eg, MI, stroke, venous thrombosis or PE) occur or are suspected. If possible, d/c at least 4-6 weeks before surgery associated with an increased risk of thromboembolism or during periods of prolonged immobilization. Increase risk of coronary heart disease (CHD), breast cancer, ovarian cancer, and gallbladder disease. Unopposed estrogens in women with intact uteri has been associated with increased risk of endometrial cancer. Adding progestin to estrogen therapy has been shown to reduce the risk of endometrial hyperplasia, which may be a precursor to endometrial cancer. May lead to severe hypercalcemia with breast cancer and bone metastases; monitor and d/c if hypercalcemia occurs. Retinal vascular thrombosis reported; d/c pending an exam if sudden partial or complete loss of vision, or sudden onset of proptosis, diplopia, or migraine occur. D/C permanently if papilledema or retinal vascular lesions are found. May elevate BP; monitor at regular intervals. Oral estrogen therapy may cause elevations of plasma triglycerides, which may lead to pancreatitis in patients with pre-existing hypertriglyceridemia. Caution with history of cholestatic jaundice associated with past estrogen use or with pregnancy; d/c with recurrence. May lead to increased thyroid-binding globulin levels; monitor thyroid function for patients dependent on thyroid hormone replacement therapy. May cause fluid retention; caution with cardiac/renal dysfunction. Caution with severe hypocalcemia. May exacerbate endometriosis, asthma, diabetes mellitus (DM), epilepsy, migraine, porphyria, systemic lupus erythematosus (SLE) and hepatic hemangiomas; use with caution.

ADVERSE REACTIONS: Application-site reaction, vaginal bleeding, breast pain, upper respiratory tract infection (URI), back pain, headache, depression, arthralgia, flu syndrome, abdominal pain, HTN, flatulence, edema, bronchitis, sinusitis.

INTERACTIONS: CYP3A4 inducers (eg, St. John's wort, phenobarbital, carbamazepine, rifampin) may decrease levels, which may decrease therapeutic effects and/or change uterine bleeding profile. CYP3A4 inhibitors (eg, erythromycin, clarithromycin, ketoconazole, itraconazole, ritonavir, grapefruit juice) may increase levels, which may result in side effects. Inducers or inhibitors of CYP3A, CYP2E and CYP2C may either, respectively, decrease the therapeutic effects or result in side effects.

PREGNANCY: Contraindicated in pregnancy, caution in nursing.

MECHANISM OF ACTION: Estradiol: Estrogen. Binds to nuclear receptors in estrogen-responsive tissue. Modulates pituitary secretion of gonadotropins, luteinizing hormone (LH) and follicle stimulating hormone (FSH), through negative feedback mechanism. Levonorgestrel: Progestogen. Inhibits gonadotropin production resulting in retardation of follicular growth and inhibition of ovulation. Counteracts proliferative effects of estrogens in endometrium.

PHARMACOKINETICS: Absorption: (Single dose) Estradiol: C_{max}=54.3pg/mL, T_{max}=42 hrs, AUC=6340pg•hr/mL; Estrone (metabolite): C_{max}=43.9pg/mL, T_{max}=84 hrs, AUC=6890pg•hr/ mL; Levonorgestrel: C_{max}=138pg/mL, T_{max}=90 hrs, AUC=22900pg•hr/mL. **Distribution:** Estrogens and progestin found in breast milk. Estradiol: Widely distributed; largely bound to sex hormone binding globulin (SHBG) and albumin. Levonorgestrel: Bound to SHBG and albumin. **Metabolism:** Estradiol: Hepatic, to estrone (metabolite); estriol (major urinary metabolite); enterohepatic recirculation, via sulfate and glucuronide conjugation; biliary secretion of conjugates into intestine; hydrolysis in intestine, reabsorption. CYP3A4 (partial). Levonorgestrel: Reduction, hydroxylation, conjugation. **Elimination:** Estradiol, estrone, estriol: Urine. Estradiol: $T_{1/2}$=3 hrs. Levonorgestrel: Urine; $T_{1/2}$=28 hrs.

NURSING CONSIDERATIONS

Assessment: Assess for abnormal genital bleeding, presence or history of breast cancer, DVT/PE or history of, presence of estrogen-dependent neoplasia, active or recent (within past yr) arterial thromboembolic disease (eg, stroke, MI), liver dysfunction/disease, known/suspected pregnancy. Assess use in patients ≥65 yrs, nursing females, hypocalcemia, asthma, DM, epilepsy, migraine or porphyria, SLE, and hepatic hemangiomas. Assess for drug and lab interactions.

Monitoring: Monitor for signs/symptoms of CV events (eg, stroke, MI, venous thrombosis, PE), malignant neoplasms (eg, cancers of endometrium, breast, ovaries), dementia, gallbladder disease, hypercalcemia, visual abnormalities (eg, retinal vascular thrombosis), elevated BP, hypertriglyceridemia, fluid retention, exacerbation of endometriosis and other conditions (eg, asthma, DM, epilepsy, migraines or porphyria, SLE, and hepatic hemangiomas) and hypersensitivity reactions. Perform annual breast exam. Periodically monitor BP. Monitor thyroid function in patients on thyroid replacement therapy. Periodically reassess use of therapy (every 3-6 months). If abnormal genital bleeding occurs, perform proper diagnostic measures (eg, endometrial sampling) to rule out malignancy.

Patient Counseling: Inform that drug may increase risk for heart attack, stroke, breast cancer, blood clots, and dementia. Instruct to report breast lumps, unusual vaginal bleeding, dizziness/faintness, changes in speech, severe headaches, chest pain, SOB, leg pain, visual changes, or vomiting. Inform once transdermal system is in place, it should not be exposed to sun for prolonged periods of time. Counsel that if patch falls off, may reapply same patch or place new patch on different area. Remove patch carefully and slowly to avoid skin irritation. Instruct to read the patient information leaflet before use. Keep out of reach of children.

Administration: Transdermal route. Site of application should not be oily, damaged, or irritated. Apply patch immediately after opening pouch and removing protective liner. Ensure that patch sticks, especially around edges. **Storage:** 20-25°C (68-77°F); excursions permitted to 15-30°C (59-86°F). Do not store unpouched.

CLINDAGEL RX
clindamycin phosphate (Galderma)

THERAPEUTIC CLASS: Lincomycin derivative

INDICATIONS: Acne vulgaris.

DOSAGE: *Adults:* Apply thin film once daily.
Pediatrics: ≥12 yrs: Apply thin film once daily.

HOW SUPPLIED: Gel: 1% [40mL, 75mL]

CONTRAINDICATIONS: Hypersensitivity to lincomycin. History of regional enteritis, ulcerative colitis, or antibiotic-associated colitis.

WARNINGS/PRECAUTIONS: D/C if significant diarrhea occurs. Caution in atopic individuals.

ADVERSE REACTIONS: Peeling, pruritus, pseudomembranous colitis (rare).

INTERACTIONS: May potentiate neuromuscular blockers.

PREGNANCY: Category B, not for use in nursing.

MECHANISM OF ACTION: Lincomycin derivative; inhibits bacteria protein synthesis at ribosomal level by binding to the 50S ribosomal subunit and affecting the process of peptide chain initiation.

PHARMACOKINETICS: Absorption: C_{max} ≤5.5ng/mL. **Distribution:** Orally and parenterally administered clindamycin appears in breast milk. **Excretion:** Urine (<0.4% of total dose).

NURSING CONSIDERATIONS

Assessment: Assess for hypersensitivity to lincomycin, history of regional or ulcerative colitis, antibiotic-associated colitis, nursing status. Assess use in atopic individuals and for possible drug interactions.

Monitoring: Monitor for signs/symptoms of colitis (pseudomembranous colitis), diarrhea, and bloody diarrhea. In patients with diarrhea, consider stool culture for *C. difficile* and stool assay for *C. difficile* toxin. In patients with significant diarrhea, consider large bowel endoscopy.

Patient Counseling: Instruct to notify physician of significant diarrhea during therapy or up to several weeks following therapy end.

C

Administration: Topical application. **Storage:** Controlled room temperature, 20-25°C (68-77°F); excursions permitted to 15-30°C (59-86°F). Keep container tightly closed, out of direct sunlight.

CLINDESSE RX
clindamycin phosphate (KV Pharm)

THERAPEUTIC CLASS: Lincomycin derivative

INDICATIONS: Treatment of bacterial vaginosis in non-pregnant women.

DOSAGE: *Adults:* 1 applicatorful intravaginally qd at any time of day.
Pediatrics: Postmenarchal: 1 applicatorful intravaginally qd at any time of day.

HOW SUPPLIED: Cre: 2% [5g]

CONTRAINDICATIONS: Regional enteritis, ulcerative colitis, or history of *Clostridium difficile*-associated diarrhea (CDAD).

WARNINGS/PRECAUTIONS: Contains mineral oil that may weaken latex or rubber products; do not use condoms or vaginal contraceptive diaphragms concurrently or for 5 days following treatment. CDAD reported; d/c therapy if suspected or confirmed. Not for ophthalmic, dermal, or oral use.

ADVERSE REACTIONS: Fungal vaginosis, headache.

INTERACTIONS: May potentiate neuromuscular blockers.

PREGNANCY: Category B, not for use in nursing

MECHANISM OF ACTION: Lincosamide antibacterial drug; inhibits bacterial protein synthesis at the level of the bacterial ribosome by binding preferentially to the 50S ribosomal subunit and affecting the process of peptide chain initiation.

PHARMACOKINETICS: Absorption: C_{max}=6.6ng/mL, T_{max}=20 hrs, AUC=175ng/mL•hr.

NURSING CONSIDERATIONS

Assessment: Assess for regional enteritis, ulcerative colitis, history of CDAD, history of hypersensitivity, pregnancy/nursing status, and for possible drug interactions.

Monitoring: Monitor for CDAD (mild diarrhea to fatal colitis), hypersensitivity, overgrowth of nonsusceptible organisms in the vagina, and for any possible adverse reactions.

Patient Counseling: Instruct not to engage in vaginal intercourse or use other vaginal products (eg, tampons, douches) during treatment. Inform that medication may weaken latex or rubber products such as condoms or vaginal contraceptive diaphragms; instruct not to use such barrier contraceptives concurrently or for 5 days following treatment. Inform that vaginal fungal infection can occur. Inform that medication can cause burning and irritation of the eye. Instruct to rinse eye with copious amounts of cool tap water and consult physician if accidental eye contact occurs.

Administration: Intravaginal. Insert one prefilled applicator into vagina, push plunger to release cream and discard applicator. **Storage:** 20-25°C (68-77°F). Avoid heat above 30°C (86°F).

CLODERM RX
clocortolone pivalate (Healthpoint)

THERAPEUTIC CLASS: Corticosteroid

INDICATIONS: Corticosteroid-responsive dermatoses.

DOSAGE: *Adults:* Apply tid. Use with occlusive dressing for management of psoriasis or recalcitrant conditions.
Pediatrics: Apply TID. Use with occlusive dressing for management of psoriasis or recalcitrant conditions.

HOW SUPPLIED: Cre: 0.1% [15g, 45g, 90g]

WARNINGS/PRECAUTIONS: May produce reversible hypothalamic-pituitary-adrenal (HPA) axis suppression, manifestations of Cushing's syndrome, hyperglycemia, glucosuria. Caution when applied to large surface areas or under occlusive dressings. Use appropriate antifungal or antibacterial agent with dermatological infections. D/C if infection is not adequately controlled or if irritation develops.

ADVERSE REACTIONS: Burning, itching, irritation, dryness, folliculitis, hypertrichosis, acneiform eruptions, hypopigmentation, perioral/allergic contact dermatitis, secondary infection, skin atrophy.

PREGNANCY: Category C, caution in nursing.

MECHANISM OF ACTION: Topical corticosteroid; mechanism not established. Possesses anti-inflammatory, anti-pruritic, and vasoconstrictive actions.

PHARMACOKINETICS: Absorption: Percutaneous; occlusion, inflammation, and other skin diseases increase absorption. **Distribution:** Bound to plasma protein to varying degrees. Systemically administered corticosteroids found in breast milk. **Metabolism:** Liver. **Elimination:** Kidney and bile.

NURSING CONSIDERATIONS

Assessment: Assess use in pregnant/nursing females and in pediatric patients.

Monitoring: Monitor for signs/symptoms of HPA axis suppression, Cushing's syndrome, hyperglycemia, and glucosuria. In patients on large doses of medication or using occlusive dressings, perform periodic testing for HPA axis suppression by using the urinary free cortisol and adrenocorticotropic hormone stimulation tests. Monitor for systemic toxicity in pediatric patients. Monitor for signs of skin irritation, dermatological infections (eg, bacterial, fungal), and treat appropriately.

Patient Counseling: Counsel to use as directed; avoid contact with eyes. Advise not to bandage or wrap treated skin areas unless directed. Instruct to report any signs of local adverse reactions. Instruct caregivers of pediatric patients to avoid using tight-fitting diapers or plastic pants on treatment area.

Administration: Topical application. **Storage:** Store at 15-30°C (59-86°F). Avoid freezing.

CLORPRES   RX
clonidine HCl - chlorthalidone (Mylan)

THERAPEUTIC CLASS: Alpha-agonist/monosulfamyl diuretic

INDICATIONS: Treatment of hypertension. Not for initial therapy.

DOSAGE: *Adults:* Determine dose by individual titration. 0.1mg clonidine-15mg chlorthalidone tab qd-bid. Max: 0.6mg clonidine-30mg chlorthalidone/day.

HOW SUPPLIED: Tab: (Clonidine-Chlorthalidone) 0.1mg-15mg*, 0.2mg-15mg*, 0.3mg-15mg* *scored

CONTRAINDICATIONS: Anuria, sulfonamide hypersensitivity.

WARNINGS/PRECAUTIONS: Caution with severe renal disease, hepatic dysfunction, asthma, severe coronary insufficiency, recent myocardial infarction (MI), cerebrovascular disease. May develop allergic reaction to oral clonidine if sensitive to clonidine patch. Avoid abrupt withdrawal. Continue therapy to within 4 hrs of surgery and resume after. Monitor for fluid/electrolyte imbalance. Hyperuricemia, hypokalemia, hyponatremia, hypochloremic alkalosis, and hyperglycemia may occur.

ADVERSE REACTIONS: Drowsiness, dizziness, constipation, sedation, fatigue, dry mouth, N/V, orthostatic symptoms.

INTERACTIONS: Potentiates other antihypertensives. May increase response to tubocurarine. May decrease arterial response to norepinephrine. Antidiabetic agents may need adjustment. Risk of lithium toxicity. TCAs may reduce effects of clonidine. Amitriptyline may enhance ocular toxicity. Enhanced CNS-depressive effects of alcohol, barbiturates, or other sedatives. Orthostatic hypotension aggravated by alcohol, barbiturates, narcotics. D/C β-blockers several days before the gradual withdrawal of clonidine in patients taking both.

PREGNANCY: (Clonidine) Category C, caution in nursing. (Chlorthalidone) Category B, not for use in nursing.

MECHANISM OF ACTION: Clonidine: Imidazoline derivative; stimulates α-adrenoceptor in brain stem, resulting in reduced sympathetic outflow from CNS and decrease in peripheral resistance, renal vascular resistance, HR, and BP. Chlorthalidone: Monosulfamyl diuretic; increases excretion of Na⁺ and Cl⁻; decreases extracellular fluid volume, plasma volume, cardiac output, total exchangeable sodium, glomerular filtration rate, and renal plasma flow.

PHARMACOKINETICS: Absorption: Clonidine: T_{max}=3-5 hrs. **Distribution:** Chlorthalidone: Plasma protein binding (75%). **Metabolism:** Clonidine: Liver (50%). **Elimination:** Clonidine: Urine (40-60% unchanged); $T_{1/2}$=12-16 hrs; $T_{1/2}$ in severe renal impairment=41 hrs. Chlorthalidone: Urine (unchanged); $T_{1/2}$=40-60 hrs.

NURSING CONSIDERATIONS

Assessment: Assess for anuria, sulfonamide hypersensitivity, coronary insufficiency, recent MI, cerebrovascular disease, history of allergy or bronchial asthma, systemic lupus erythematosus (SLE), diabetes mellitus, renal/hepatic impairment, pregnancy/nursing status, and possible drug interactions. Perform and obtain serum and urine electrolytes.

Monitoring: Monitor blood pressure. Periodically monitor serum and urine electrolytes, serum PBI level, serum K⁺ levels, and renal function. Monitor for signs/symptoms of electrolyte imbalance, hypokalemia, possible exacerbation or activation of SLE, hyperglycemia, withdrawal symptoms, hyperuricemia or precipitation of gout, hypersensitivity reactions, renal/hepatic dysfunction.

Patient Counseling: Caution that drug may impair physical/mental abilities. Inform to avoid alcohol. Instruct not to interrupt or d/c therapy without consulting physician. Seek medical attention if symptoms of electrolyte imbalance (dry mouth, thirst, weakness), hypokalemia (thirst, tiredness, restlessness), withdrawal (nervousness, agitation, headaches), or hypersensitivity reactions occur.

Administration: Oral route. **Storage:** 15-30°C (59-86°F). Avoid excessive humidity.

CLOZAPINE
clozapine (Various)

RX

> Risk of potentially life-threatening agranulocytosis. Reserve use for severely ill patients with schizophrenia unresponsive to standard antipsychotic treatment or for patients with schizophrenia/schizoaffective disorder at risk for re-experiencing suicidal behavior. Obtain baseline WBC count and absolute neutrophil count (ANC) prior to therapy, regularly during treatment, and for ≥4 weeks after d/c. Seizures associated with use and with greater likelihood at higher doses; caution with history of seizures or other predisposing factors. Increased risk of fatal myocarditis, especially during 1st month of therapy; d/c if suspected. Orthostatic hypotension, with or without syncope can occur. Rare reports of profound collapse with respiratory and/or cardiac arrest in patients taking benzodiazepines or any other psychotropic drugs. Elderly patients with dementia-related psychosis treated with atypical antipsychotic drugs are at an increased risk for death. Not approved for the treatment of dementia-related psychosis.

OTHER BRAND NAMES: Clozaril (Novartis)

THERAPEUTIC CLASS: Dibenzapine derivative

INDICATIONS: Management of severely ill schizophrenic patients who fail to respond adequately to standard drug treatment for schizophrenia. Reduction of risk for recurrent suicidal behavior in patients with schizophrenia/schizoaffective disorder who are judged to be at chronic risk for re-experiencing suicidal behavior.

DOSAGE: *Adults:* Treatment-Resistant Schizophrenia: Initial: 12.5mg qd-bid. Titrate: Increase by 25-50mg/day, up to 300-450mg/day by end of 2 weeks, then increase once or twice weekly in increments ≤100mg. Usual: 300-

600mg/day on a divided basis. Titrate: May increase to 600-900mg/day. Max: 900mg/day. Maint: Lowest effective dose. To d/c, gradually reduce dose over 1-2 weeks. Re-initiation (even with brief interval off clozapine): Start with 12.5 mg qd-bid. May titrate more quickly if initial dosing tolerated. Do not restart if d/c for WBC <2000/mm³ or ANC <1000/mm³. Reduction of Risk of Suicidal Behavior in Schizophrenia/Schizoaffective Disorder: May follow dosing recommendations for treatment-resistant schizophrenia. Range: 12.5-900mg/day (mean 300mg). To reduce the risk of suicidal behavior in patients who otherwise responded to therapy with another antipsychotic, treat for ≥2 years and then re-evaluate. If risk for suicidal behavior is still present, continue treatment and revisit at regular intervals. If no longer at risk of suicidal behavior, d/c treatment. Elderly: Start at lower end of dosing range.

HOW SUPPLIED: Tab: (Generic) 25mg, 50mg,100mg, 200mg; (Clozaril) 25mg*, 100mg* *scored

CONTRAINDICATIONS: Myeloproliferative disorders, uncontrolled epilepsy, paralytic ileus, history of clozapine-induced agranulocytosis or severe granulocytopenia, severe CNS depression, comatose states. Concomitant use with agents having potential to cause agranulocytosis or suppress bone marrow function.

WARNINGS/PRECAUTIONS: Hyperglycemia, sometimes with ketoacidosis, hyperosmolar coma or death, reported. Monitor for worsening of glucose control with diabetes mellitus (DM) and fasting blood glucose (FBG) levels with diabetes risk or symptoms of hyperglycemia. Tachycardia and cardiomyopathy reported. D/C if cardiomyopathy is confirmed unless benefits outweigh risk. Neuroleptic malignant syndrome (NMS), tardive dyskinesia (TD), impaired intestinal peristalsis, deep vein thrombosis (DVT), pulmonary embolism (PE), and ECG changes reported. Fever reported; rule out infection or agranulocytosis. Consider NMS in the presence of high fever. Hepatitis reported. If N/V and/or anorexia develop, perform LFTs. D/C if symptoms of jaundice occur. Has potent anticholinergic effects; caution with prostatic enlargement and narrow-angle glaucoma. May impair mental/physical abilities. Caution with renal, cardiac, hepatic, or pulmonary disease. Increased risk of cerebrovascular adverse events; caution with risk factors for stroke. Obtain WBC and ANC at baseline, then weekly for 1st six months of therapy, then every 2 weeks for next 6 months, and then every 4 weeks thereafter if counts are acceptable (WBC ≥3500/mm³ or ANC ≥2000/mm³). Refer to PI for frequency of monitoring based on stage of therapy, WBC count and ANC. Avoid treatment if WBC <3500/mm³ or ANC <2000/mm³. D/C treatment and do not rechallenge if WBC <2000/mm³, ANC <1000/mm³. Interrupt therapy if eosinophilia (>4000/mm³) develops. Caution in elderly.

ADVERSE REACTIONS: Drowsiness, vertigo, headache, tremor, salivation, sweating, dry mouth, visual disturbances, tachycardia, hypotension, syncope, constipation, N/V, weight gain, fever.

INTERACTIONS: See Contraindications and Boxed Warning. Avoid using epinephrine to treat clozapine-induced hypotension. Use with carbamazepine is not recommended. Caution with CNS-active drugs, general anesthesia, alcohol, paroxetine, fluoxetine, fluvoxamine, sertraline, or inhibitors/inducers of CYP1A2, 2D6, 3A4. Consider reduced dose with paroxetine, fluoxetine, fluvoxamine, and sertraline. Dosage reduction may be needed with drugs metabolized by CYP2D6 (eg, antidepressants, phenothiazines, carbamazepine, Type 1C antiarrhythmics) or that inhibit this enzyme (eg, quinidine). May potentiate hypotensive effects of antihypertensives and anticholinergic effects of atropine-type drugs. CYP450 inducers (eg, phenytoin, tobacco smoke, carbamazepine, rifampin) may decrease plasma levels. CYP450 inhibitors (eg, cimetidine, caffeine, citalopram, ciprofloxacin, fluvoxamine, erythromycin) may increase plasma levels. NMS reported with lithium and other CNS-active drugs. Concurrent psychopharmaceuticals may affect plasma clozapine levels. May interact with other highly protein-bound drugs.

PREGNANCY: Category B, not for use in nursing.

MECHANISM OF ACTION: Tricyclic dibenzodiazepine derivative; atypical antipyschotic agent. Interferes with binding of dopamine at D_1, D_2, D_3, and D_5 receptors and has a high affinity for D_4 receptor. Also acts as an antagonist at the adrenergic, cholinergic, histaminergic, and serotonergic receptors.

PHARMACOKINETICS: Absorption: C_{max}=319ng/mL; T_{max}=2.5 hrs (100mg bid). **Distribution:** Plasma protein binding (97%). **Metabolism:** Demethylation, hydroxylation, N-oxidation. **Elimination:** Urine (50%), feces (30%); $T_{1/2}$=8 hrs (75mg single dose), $T_{1/2}$=12 hrs (100mg bid).

NURSING CONSIDERATIONS

Assessment: Assess previous course of standard therapy prior to treatment. Assess for myeloproliferative disorders, uncontrolled epilepsy, paralytic ileus, history of clozapine-induced agranulocytosis or severe granulocytopenia, and severe CNS depression or comatose states, history of seizures or other predisposing factors, other conditions where treatment is cautioned or contraindicated. Assess pregnancy/nursing status and possible drug interactions. Obtain baseline WBC count and ANC prior to therapy, and baseline FBG levels in patients at risk for hyperglycemia/DM.

Monitoring: Monitor for clinical response and need to continue treatment. Monitor for agranulocytosis, myocarditis, orthostatic hypotension, HF, tachycardia, severe respiratory effects, seizures, flu-like symptoms, infection (eg, pneumonia), eosinophilia, fever, DVT, PE, NMS, TD, impairment of intestinal peristalsis, impairment of mental/physical abilities, and signs/symptoms of hyperglycemia. Monitor WBC counts and ANC during and for ≥4 weeks following d/c or until WBC ≥3500/mm³ and ANC ≥2000/mm³. Check periodic FBG levels if at risk for hyperglycemia and for signs/symptoms of hepatitis while on therapy. Obtain LFTs if patient develops N/V and/or anorexia.

Patient Counseling: Inform that drug is available only through a program designed to ensure the required blood monitoring schedule. Counsel on risks of treatment (eg, agranulocytosis, seizures, orthostatic hypotension). Inform about signs/symptoms of agranulocytosis; advise to immediately report lethargy, weakness, fever, sore throat, malaise, mucous membrane ulceration, flulike complaints, or other possible signs of infection. Instruct to avoid potentially hazardous activities (eg, operating machinery, driving). Notify physician if intending to become pregnant, planning to take any prescription or over-the-counter drugs or alcohol. Advise females to avoid breastfeeding. Advise drug can be taken with/without food. If a dose is missed for >2 days, consult physician before restarting medication.

Administration: Oral route. **Storage:** (Clozapine) 20-25°C (68-77°F). (Clozaril) ≤30°C (86°F).

COARTEM   RX
lumefantrine - artemether (Novartis)

THERAPEUTIC CLASS: Artemisinin-based combination therapy

INDICATIONS: Treatment of acute, uncomplicated malaria infections due to *Plasmodium falciparum* in patients ≥5kg.

DOSAGE: *Adults:* >16 yrs: ≥35kg: Initial: 4 tabs as single dose. Maint: 4 tabs again after 8 hrs and then 4 tabs bid (am and pm) for the following 2 days. <35kg: See dosage in pediatric patients. Take with food. If unable to swallow tab, tab may be crushed and mixed with small amount of water (1-2 tsp). *Pediatrics:* 5-<15kg: Initial: 1 tab. Maint: 1 tab again after 8 hrs and then 1 tab bid (am and pm) for the following 2 days. 15-<25kg: Initial: 2 tabs. Maint: 2 tabs again after 8 hrs and then 2 tabs bid for the following 2 days. 25-<35kg: Initial: 3 tabs. Maint: 3 tabs again after 8 hrs and then 3 tabs bid for the following 2 days. ≥35kg: Initial: 4 tabs as single dose. Maint: 4 tabs again after 8 hrs and then 4 tabs bid for the following 2 days. Take with food. If unable to swallow tab, tab may be crushed and mixed with small amount of water (1-2 tsp).

HOW SUPPLIED: Tab: (Artemether-Lumefantrine) 20mg-120mg* *scored

WARNINGS/PRECAUTIONS: May prolong the QT interval; avoid with congenital prolongation of the QT interval (eg, long QT syndrome) or any other clinical conditions known to prolong the QTc interval (eg, history of symptomatic cardiac arrhythmias with bradycardia or with severe cardiac disease). Avoid with a family history of congenital prolongation of the QT interval or sudden death. Avoid with known disturbances of electrolyte balance (eg, hypokalemia, hypomagnesemia). Caution with severe renal/hepatic impairment. Not approved for prevention of malaria or for patients with severe or complicated *P. falciparum* malaria. Risk of recrudescence may be greater in patients who remain adverse to food during treatment.

ADVERSE REACTIONS: Headache, abdominal pain, anorexia, dizziness, asthenia, arthralgia, myalgia, pyrexia, cough, N/V, chills, fatigue, splenomegaly, hepatomegaly, sleep disorder.

INTERACTIONS: Avoid with other medications that prolong the QT interval such as class IA (eg, quinidine, procainamide, disopyramide) or class III (eg, amiodarone, sotalol) antiarrhythmic agents; antipsychotics (eg, pimozide, ziprasidone); antidepressants; certain antibiotics (eg, macrolide or fluroquinolone antibiotics, imidazole, and triazole antifungal agents); certain non-sedating antihistaminics (eg, terfenadine, astemizole), or cisapride. Avoid concurrent use with medications metabolized by CYP2D6, which also have cardiac effects (eg, flecainide, imipramine, amitriptyline, clomipramine). Avoid coadministration with halofantrine within 1 month of each other due to potential additive effects on the QT interval. Avoid with other antimalarials. May decrease efficacy with mefloquine. Concomitant use with CYP3A4 substrates may decrease substrate concentration and substrate efficacy. May increase levels and potentiate QT prolongation with CYP3A4 inhibitors (eg, ketoconazole, grapefruit juice). Coadministration with CYP3A4 inducers may decrease levels and antimalarial efficacy. May reduce hormonal contraceptives effectiveness. Caution with quinine. Caution with drugs that have a mixed effect on CYP3A4 (eg, antiretroviral drugs).

PREGNANCY: Category C, caution in nursing.

MECHANISM OF ACTION: Artemether: Artemisinin derivative; antimalarial activity attributed to endoperoxide moiety. Lumefantrine: Not established; suspected to inhibit the formation of β-hematin by forming a complex with hemin. Both artemether and lumefantrine inhibit nucleic acid and protein synthesis.

PHARMACOKINETICS: Absorption: T_{max} = 2 hrs (Artemether), 6-8 hrs (Lumefantrine). Refer to PI for additional absorption parameters. **Distribution:** Plasma protein binding (95.4% [Artemether], 47-76% [DHA], 99.7% [Lumefantrine]). **Metabolism:** Artemether: Liver via CYP3A4/5 (Major), CYP2B6, CYP2C9, CYP2C19 (minor); Dihydroartemisinin [DHA] (active metabolite). Lumefantrine: Liver via CYP3A4. **Elimination:** $T_{1/2}$=2 hrs (Artemether and DHA), 3-6 days (Lumefantrine).

NURSING CONSIDERATIONS

Assessment: Assess for severe/complicated *P. falciparum* malaria, hepatic/renal impairment, congenital prolongation of the QT interval (eg, long QT syndrome), symptomatic cardiac arrhythmias with clinically relevant bradycardia or severe cardiac disease, family history of congenital prolongation of the QT interval or sudden death, electrolyte disturbances (eg, hypokalemia, hypomagnesemia), pregnancy/nursing status, and for possible drug interactions. Obtain baseline ECG, serum electrolytes, LFTs, renal function.

Monitoring: Monitor for hepatic/renal impairment, ECG changes (eg, QT interval prolongation), electrolyte imbalance, and other adverse events that may occur. Monitor ECG, serum electrolytes, LFTs, renal function, and for recrudescence of malaria.

Patient Counseling: Inform about risks and benefits of therapy. Instruct to take with food. Inform that if unable to swallow tab, then tab may be crushed and mixed with a small amount of water (1-2 tsps). Inform that administration should be over 3 days for a total of six doses. Counsel about risk for recrudescence of malaria with inadequate food intake. Instruct to notify physician of any personal/family history of QT prolongation or proarrhythmic conditions (eg, hypokalemia, bradycardia or recent myocardial infarction), taking any other medications that may prolong the QT interval, and symptoms of prolongation of the QT interval (eg, prolonged heart palpitations, loss of consciousness). Advise childbearing patients to use an additional nonhormonal method of birth control. Instruct to d/c therapy if hypersensitivity reactions (eg, rash, hives, rapid heart beat, difficulty swallowing/breathing, any swelling suggesting angioedema) or other symptoms of an allergic reaction occur; advise to inform physician if these and other adverse events develop.

Administration: Oral route. Encourage to resume normal eating as soon as food can be tolerated. For patients unable to swallow (eg, infants/children), may crush tablets and mix with a small amount of water (eg, 1-2 tsp.) in a clean container prior to administration; crushed tablet preparation should be followed whenever possible by food/drink (eg, milk, formula, pudding, broth, and porridge). If vomiting occurs within 1-2 hrs of administration, repeat the dose. If vomiting continues, d/c and start alternative antimalarial treatment. **Storage:** 25°C (77°F); excursions permitted to 15-30°C (59-86°F).

COLAZAL   RX
balsalazide disodium (Salix)

THERAPEUTIC CLASS: 5-Aminosalicylic acid derivative

INDICATIONS: Treatment of mild-to-moderate active ulcerative colitis in patients ≥5 yrs.

DOSAGE: *Adults:* 3 caps tid for up to 8 weeks (or 12 weeks if needed). May open cap and sprinkle on applesauce.
Pediatrics: 5-17 yrs: 1 or 3 caps tid for 8 weeks. May open cap and sprinkle on applesauce.

HOW SUPPLIED: Cap: 750mg

WARNINGS/PRECAUTIONS: May exacerbate symptoms of colitis. Prolonged gastric retention with pyloric stenosis. Caution with renal dysfunction or history of renal disease.

ADVERSE REACTIONS: Headache, abdominal pain, diarrhea, N/V, respiratory problems, arthralgia, rhinitis, insomnia, fatigue, rectal bleeding, flatulence, fever, dyspepsia.

INTERACTIONS: Oral antibiotics may interfere with the release of mesalamine in the colon.

PREGNANCY: Category B, caution in nursing.

MECHANISM OF ACTION: Not established; a prodrug enzymatically cleaved in colon to produce mesalamine (5-ASA), an anti-inflammatory drug that acts locally to block production of arachidonic acid metabolites in the colon.

PHARMACOKINETICS: Absorption: Different dosing conditions (fasted, fed, sprinkled) resulted in variable parameters. **Distribution:** Plasma protein binding (≥99%). **Metabolism:** Key metabolites: 5-ASA and N-acetyl-5-ASA. **Elimination:** Urine, feces.

NURSING CONSIDERATIONS

Assessment: Assess for pyloric stenosis, possible drug interactions, history of renal/hepatic disease.

Monitoring: Monitor renal function, LFTs, and CBC, signs/symptoms of prolonged gastric retention with pyloric stenosis, worsening of colitis symptoms, and hypersensitivity.

Patient Counseling: Inform can take with/without food or sprinkle on applesauce. Teeth and/or tongue may get stained when using sprinkle form with food. Seek medical attention if diagnosed with pyloric stenosis or renal dysfunction, experience worsening of colitis symptoms or hypersensitivity (eg, anaphylaxis, bronchospasm, skin reaction).

Administration: Oral route. **Storage:** 20-25°C (68-77°F); excursions permitted to 15-30°C (59-86°F).

COLCHICINE/PROBENECID   RX
probenecid - colchicine (Various)

THERAPEUTIC CLASS: Uricosuric

INDICATIONS: Chronic gouty arthritis complicated by frequent, recurrent acute gout attacks.

DOSAGE: *Adults:* Initial: 1 tab qd for 1 week, then 1 tab bid. Titrate: May increase by 1 tab/day every 4 weeks. Max: 4 tabs/day. May reduce dose by 1 tab every 6 months if acute attacks have been absent ≥6 months. Decrease dose with gastric intolerance. Renal Impairment: May need to increase dose. May not be effective if CrCl ≤30mL/min.

HOW SUPPLIED: Tab: (Colchicine-Probenecid) 0.5mg-500mg

CONTRAINDICATIONS: Blood dyscrasias, uric acid kidney stones, children <2 yrs and pregnancy. Do not use in acute gout attack.

WARNINGS/PRECAUTIONS: Exacerbation of gout may occur. Use acetaminophen (APAP) if analgesic needed. Severe allergic reaction and anaphylaxis reported (rare). D/C if hypersensitivity occurs. Caution with peptic ulcer. Monitor for glycosuria. Determine benefit/risk ratio with long-term therapy. Maintain liberal fluid intake and alkalization of urine.

ADVERSE REACTIONS: Headache, dizziness, hepatic necrosis, N/V, anorexia, sore gums, uric acid stones, renal colic, anaphylaxis, fever, pruritus, blood dyscrasias, peripheral neuritis, muscular weakness, abdominal pain, diarrhea, alopecia, dermatitis.

INTERACTIONS: Probenecid increases plasma levels of penicillin and other β-lactams; psychic disturbances reported. Salicylates and pyrazinamide antagonize uricosuric effects. Increased plasma levels of methotrexate, sulfonamides, sulfonylureas, thiopental or ketamine-induced anesthesia, some NSAIDs (eg, indomethacin, naproxen), lorazepam, APAP, and rifampin. Possible false high plasma levels of theophylline.

PREGNANCY: Contraindicated in pregnancy; safety in nursing not known.

MECHANISM OF ACTION: Probenecid: Uricosuric/renal tubular blocking agent; inhibits tubular reabsorption of urate, increasing urinary excretion of uric acid and decreasing serum urate levels. Colchicine: Colchicum alkaloid; not been established, has prophylactic, suppressive effect helping to reduce incidence of acute attacks and relieve residual pain and mild discomfort.

NURSING CONSIDERATIONS

Assessment: Assess for known blood dyscrasias, uric acid kidney stones, acute vs chronic attack, history of peptic ulcer, and possible drug interactions.

Monitoring: Monitor for signs/symptoms of gout exacerbation, allergic reactions, hematuria, renal colic, costovertebral pain, and uric acid stone formation.

Patient Counseling: Instruct on importance of liberal fluid intake. Advise to seek medical attention if symptoms of allergic reaction, hematuria, renal colic, or costovertebral pain occur.

Administration: Oral route. **Storage:** 20-25°C (68-77°F). Protect from light.

COLCRYS   RX
colchicine (AR Scientific)

THERAPEUTIC CLASS: Miscellaneous gout agent

INDICATIONS: Treatment and prophylaxis of acute gout flares. Treatment of familial Mediterranean fever (FMF) in adults and children ≥4 yrs.

DOSAGE: *Adults:* Individualize dose. Gout Flares: Prophylaxis: 0.6mg qd or bid. Max: 1.2mg/day. Treatment: 1.2mg (2 tabs) at the first sign of the flare followed by 0.6mg (1 tab) 1 hr later. Max: 1.8mg over a 1-hr period. May be administered for treatment of a gout flare during prophylaxis; wait 12 hrs and then resume the prophylactic dose. FMF: Usual Range: 1.2-2.4mg/day in one or two divided doses. Titrate: Increase by 0.3mg/day as needed to control disease and as tolerated to maximum dose. Decrease by 0.3mg/day if with intolerable side effects. Gout Flares: Severe Renal Impairment: Prophylaxis: 0.3mg/day. May increase with adequate monitoring for colchicine adverse effects. Treatment: Do not repeat more than once every 2 weeks. Dialysis:

Prophylaxis: 0.3mg twice a week. Treatment: Reduce dose to 0.6mg (1 tab) single dose. Do not repeat more than once every 2 weeks. Severe Hepatic Impairment: Prophylaxis: Reduce dose. Treatment: Do not repeat course more than once every 2 weeks. Treatment of gout flare not recommended in patients with renal/hepatic impairment receiving prophylaxis. FMF: Mild (CrCl 50-80mL/min) to Moderate (30-50mL/min) Renal Impairment: Dose reduction may be necessary. Severe Renal Impairment (CrCl <30mL/min)/ Dialysis: Initial: 0.3 mg/day. May increase with adequate monitoring for adverse effects. Severe Hepatic Impairment: Prophylaxis: Reduce dose. Please refer to the PI for dose modifications with concomitant CYP3A4 strong / moderate inhibitors/P-gp Inhibitors and protease inhibitors.
Pediatrics: Gout Flares: >16 yrs: Prophylaxis: 0.6mg qd or bid. Max: 1.2mg/day. FMF: >12 yrs: 1.2-2.4mg/day in one or two divided doses. 6-12 yrs: 0.9-1.8mg/day in one or two divided doses. 4-6 yrs: 0.3-1.8mg/day in one or two divided doses. Please refer to the PI for dose modifications with concomitant CYP3A4 strong/moderate inhibitors/P-gp inhibitors and protease inhibitors.

HOW SUPPLIED: Tab: 0.6mg* *scored

CONTRAINDICATIONS: Concomitant use with P-glycoprotein (P-gp) or strong CYP3A4 inhibitors in patients with renal or hepatic impairment.

WARNINGS/PRECAUTIONS: Fatal overdoses (accidental/intentional), myelosuppression, leukopenia, granulocytopenia, thrombocytopenia, pancytopenia and aplastic anemia reported. Drug-induced neuromuscular toxicity and rhabdomyolysis reported with chronic treatment at therapeutic doses; caution in elderly and in patients with renal dysfunction. D/C if colchicine toxicity is suspected. Not intended to treat pain from other causes.

ADVERSE REACTIONS: Diarrhea, pharyngolaryngeal pain, cramping, abdominal pain, N/V, fatigue.

INTERACTIONS: See Contraindications. Significant increase in plasma levels with moderate (amprenavir, aprepitant, diltiazem, erythromycin, fluconazole, fosamprenavir, grapefruit juice, verapamil) and strong (atazanavir, clarithromycin, indinavir, itraconazole, ketoconazole, nefazodone, nelfinavir, ritonavir, saquinavir, telithromycin) CYP3A4 inhibitors, and P-gp inhibitors (cyclosporine, ranolazine). Fatal toxicity reported with clarithromycin and cyclosporine. Neuromuscular toxicity with diltiazem and verapamil. Potentiate the development of myopathy and rhabdomyolysis when used concomitantly with HMG-CoA reductase inhibitors (atorvastatin, simvastatin, pravastatin, fluvastatin), gemfibrozil and fibrates. Rhabdomyolysis reported with concomitant digitalis glycosides.

PREGNANCY: Category C, caution in nursing.

MECHANISM OF ACTION: Alkaloid; disrupts cytoskeletal functions through inhibition of β-tubulin polymerization into microtubules, consequently preventing the activation, degranulation, and migration of neutrophils thought to mediate some gout symptoms. May interfere with the intracellular assembly of the inflammasome complex in neutrophils and monocytes that mediates activation of interleukin-1β in patients with FMF.

PHARMACOKINETICS: Absorption: C_{max}=2.5ng/mL; T_{max}=1-2 hrs; absolute bioavailability (45%). Variable doses resulted in different parameters.
Distribution: Found in breast milk and crosses the placenta; V_d=5-8L/kg; plasma binding protein (39%). **Metabolism:** Demethylation; 2-O-methylcolchicine and 3-O-demethylcolchicine (primary metabolites). **Elimination:** Urine (40-65%, unchanged) $T_{1/2}$=26.6-31.2 hrs.

NURSING CONSIDERATIONS

Assessment: Assess for renal/hepatic impairment, pregnancy/nursing status, and possible drug interactions. Weigh potential benefits/risks when coadministered with other drugs. Note other diseases/conditions and drug therapies.

Monitoring: Monitor for rhabdomyolysis, signs and symptoms of toxicities (cramping, diarrhea, abdominal pain, N/V, vomiting). Monitor for blood dyscrasias (myelosupression, leukopenia, granulocytopenia, pancytopenia, agranulocytosis, aplastic anemia, thrombocytopenia).

Patient Counseling: Inform about benefits and risks of therapy. Advise patients to take as directed. Instruct that if a dose is missed, take the next dose as soon as possible but do not double the next dose. Advise not to consume grapefruit/grapefruit juice during treatment. Inform that bone marrow depression may occur with therapeutic doses and that toxicities may occur when taken with certain drugs. Advise to d/c drug and notify a physician if abdominal pain, N/V, diarrhea, muscle pain/weakness, and/or tingling/numbness of fingers/toes occur. Notify healthcare provider of all current medications being taken and before starting any new medications, particularly antibiotics.

Administration: Oral route. **Storage:** 20-25°C (68-77°F). Protect from light.

COLESTID   RX
colestipol HCl (Pharmacia & Upjohn)

THERAPEUTIC CLASS: Bile acid sequestrant

INDICATIONS: Adjunct to diet, to reduce elevated serum total and LDL-C in primary hypercholesterolemia.

DOSAGE: *Adults:* Initial: Tab: 2g qd-bid. Granules: 1 pkt or 1 scoopful qd-bid. Titrate: Tab: Increase by 2g qd or bid at 1- to 2-month intervals. Granules: May increase at an increment of one dose/day (1 pkt or level tsp of granules) at 1- to 2-month intervals. Usual: 2-16g/day (tab) or 1-6 pkts or scoopfuls (granules) qd or in divided doses. Always mix granules with liquid. Take 1 tab at a time and swallow tabs whole with plenty of liquid.

HOW SUPPLIED: Granules: 5g/pkt [30^s 90^s], 5g/scoopful [300g, 500g]; Tab: 1g

WARNINGS/PRECAUTIONS: Exclude secondary causes of hypercholesterolemia and obtain a lipid profile prior to therapy. May interfere with normal fat absorption. Chronic use may increase bleeding tendency due to vitamin K deficiency. Monitor cholesterol and TG based on National Cholesterol Education Program guidelines. May cause hypothyroidism. May produce or worsen constipation. Avoid constipation with symptomatic coronary artery disease. Constipation associated with colestipol may aggravate hemorrhoids. May produce hyperchloremic acidosis with prolonged use. (Granules) Flavored form contains phenylalanine. Always mix granules with water or other fluids before ingesting.

ADVERSE REACTIONS: Constipation, abdominal discomfort, indigestion, musculoskeletal pain, headache, AST elevation, ALT elevation, alkaline phosphatase elevation, headache, chest pain, rash, anorexia, fatigue, tachycardia, SOB.

INTERACTIONS: May interfere with absorption of folic acid, fat-soluble vitamins (eg, A, D, K), oral phosphate supplements, hydrocortisone. May delay or reduce absorption of concomitant oral medication; take other drugs 1 hr before or 4 hrs after colestipol. Reduces absorption of chlorothiazide, tetracycline, furosemide, penicillin G, HCTZ, and gemfibrozil. Caution with digitalis agents, propranolol.

PREGNANCY: Safety in pregnancy not known, caution in nursing.

MECHANISM OF ACTION: Bile acid sequestrant; binds bile acids in the intestine, forming a complex that is excreted in the feces, leading to increased fecal loss of bile acids and increased oxidation of cholesterol to bile acids, a decrease in β lipoprotein or LDL, and a decrease in serum cholesterol levels.

PHARMACOKINETICS: Elimination: Feces.

NURSING CONSIDERATIONS

Assessment: Assess for secondary causes of hypercholesterolemia (eg, hypothyroidism, diabetes mellitus, nephrotic syndrome, dysproteinemia, obstructive liver disease, alcoholism), pre-existing constipation, pregnancy/nursing status, and for possible drug interactions. Determine baseline lipid profile.

Monitoring: Monitor for signs/symptoms of vitamin K deficiency (eg, tendency for bleeding), constipation, hypothyroidism, and for hyperchloremic acidosis. Monitor serum cholesterol, lipoprotein and TG levels.

Patient Counseling: Instruct to take as prescribed. Advise to take other medications at least 1 hr before or 4 hrs after taking colestipol. Inform about benefits/risks of therapy. Instruct to report any adverse reactions to physician. (Tab) Instruct to take tab one at a time, with plenty of water. Counsel not to cut, crush, or chew tab. (Granules) Advise to mix with water or other fluids before ingesting.

Administration: Oral route. **Storage:** 20-25°C (68-77°F).

COMBIGAN

RX

timolol maleate - brimonidine tartrate (Allergan)

THERAPEUTIC CLASS: Alpha$_2$-agonist/beta-blocker

INDICATIONS: Reduction of elevated intraocular pressure (IOP) in patients with glaucoma or ocular hypertension who require adjunctive or replacement therapy due to inadequately controlled IOP.

DOSAGE: *Adults:* 1 drop in affected eye(s) bid approximately 12 hrs apart. Instill other topical ophthalmic products at least 5 min apart.
Pediatrics: ≥2 yrs: 1 drop in affected eye(s) bid approximately 12 hrs apart. Instill other topical ophthalmic products at least 5 min apart.

HOW SUPPLIED: Sol: (Brimonidine-Timolol) 2mg-5mg/mL

CONTRAINDICATIONS: Bronchial asthma, history of bronchial asthma, severe chronic obstructive pulmonary disease (COPD), sinus bradycardia, second- or third-degree AV block, overt cardiac failure, cardiogenic shock.

WARNINGS/PRECAUTIONS: Systemic absorption, leading to adverse reactions (including severe respiratory reactions) may occur. Caution with cardiac failure; d/c if cardiac failure develops. Avoid with bronchospastic disease and/or mild-to-moderate COPD. May potentiate syndromes associated with vascular insufficiency; caution with depression, cerebral or coronary insufficiency, Raynaud's phenomenon, orthostatic hypotension, or thromboangiitis obliterans. May increase reactivity to allergens. May potentiate muscle weakness consistent with certain myasthenic symptoms. May mask signs/symptoms of acute hypoglycemia; caution in patients subject to spontaneous hypoglycemia or diabetic patients receiving insulin or hypoglycemic agents. May mask signs of hyperthyroidism. Bacterial keratitis reported with use of multiple-dose containers of topical ophthalmic products. May need to gradually withdraw β-blocking agents in patients undergoing elective surgery.

ADVERSE REACTIONS: Allergic conjunctivitis, conjunctival folliculosis, conjunctival hyperemia, eye pruritus, ocular burning/stinging.

INTERACTIONS: May reduce BP; caution with antihypertensives and/or cardiac glycosides. Monitor with concomitant oral β-blockers; avoid concomitant use of 2 topical β-blocking agents. Caution with concomitant oral or IV calcium antagonists; avoid concomitant use with impaired cardiac function. Monitor closely with concomitant catecholamine-depleting drugs (eg, reserpine). Possibility of additive or potentiating effect with CNS depressants (eg, alcohol, barbiturates, opiates, sedatives, anesthetics). Concomitant use of β-blockers with digitalis and/or calcium antagonists may have additive effects in prolonging AV-conduction time. Potentiated systemic β-blockade reported with CYP2D6 inhibitors and timolol. Caution with TCAs and/or MAOIs.

PREGNANCY: Category C, not for use in nursing.

MECHANISM OF ACTION: Decreases elevated IOP. Brimonidine: Selective α-2 adrenergic receptor. Timolol: Nonselective β-blocker.

PHARMACOKINETICS: Absorption: Brimonidine: C_{max}=30pg/mL; T_{max}= 1-4 hrs. Timolol: C_{max}=400pg/mL; T_{max}=1-3 hrs. **Distribution:** Timolol: Plasma protein binding (60%). **Metabolism:** Brimonidine: Liver (extensive). Timolol: Liver (partial). **Elimination:** Brimonidine: Urine (74%); $T_{1/2}$=3 hrs. Timolol: Excreted mainly by kidney; $T_{1/2}$=7 hrs.

NURSING CONSIDERATIONS

Assessment: Assess for ocular infection; signs/symptoms of systemic absorption of β-adrenergic blockers (eg, potentiation of bronchial asthma, COPD, cerebral or coronary insufficiency, cardiac failure).

Monitoring: Monitor IOP, vital signs, renal function, LFTs, and adverse reactions (eg, allergic conjunctivitis, conjunctival folliculosis, conjunctival hyperemia, eye pruritis, ocular burning and stinging).

Patient Counseling: To avoid ocular infection, avoid contact of container tip to affected eye. If more than 1 ophthalmic drug is being used, administer at least 5 min apart. Remove contact lenses prior to administration; may be reinserted after 15 min.

Administration: Ocular route. **Storage:** 15-25°C (59-77°F). Protect from light.

COMBIPATCH   RX
norethindrone acetate - estradiol (Novartis)

> Estrogens and progestins should not be used for prevention of cardiovascular disease or dementia. Increased risks of myocardial infarction (MI), stroke, invasive breast cancer, pulmonary embolism (PE), and deep vein thrombosis (DVT) in postmenopausal women (50-79 yrs of age) reported. Increased risk of developing probable dementia in postmenopausal women ≥65 yrs of age reported.

THERAPEUTIC CLASS: Estrogen/progestogen combination

INDICATIONS: In women with an intact uterus, for the treatment of moderate to severe vasomotor symptoms associated with menopause, vulvar/vaginal atrophy. Treatment of hypoestrogenism due to hypogonadism, castration, or primary ovarian failure.

DOSAGE: *Adults:* Continuous Combined Regimen: Apply 0.05mg/0.14mg patch on lower abdomen (avoid breasts and waistline). Apply twice weekly during 28-day cycle. Continuous Sequential Regimen: Wear estradiol-only patch for 1st 14 days of 28-day cycle, replace twice weekly. Apply 0.05mg/0.14mg patch for remaining 14 days, replace twice weekly. For both regimens, use 0.05mg/0.25mg patch if additional progestin required. Re-evaluate at 3-6 month intervals. Rotate sites; allow 1 week between same site.

HOW SUPPLIED: Patch: (Estradiol-Norethindrone) 0.05-0.14mg/day, 0.05-0.25mg/day [8^s, 24^s]

CONTRAINDICATIONS: Undiagnosed abnormal genital bleeding, breast cancer, estrogen-dependent neoplasia, DVT, PE, arterial thromboembolic disorder (eg, stroke, MI), liver dysfunction or disease.

WARNINGS/PRECAUTIONS: May increase risk of cardiovascular events (eg, MI, stroke), venous thrombosis, and PE; d/c immediately if any of these events occur or are suspected. May increase risk of breast/endometrial cancer, and gallbladder disease. May lead to severe hypercalcemia with breast cancer and bone metastases; monitor and d/c if hypercalcemia occurs. Retinal vascular thrombosis reported; monitor and d/c if papilledema or retinal vascular lesions occur. May elevate BP; monitor at regular intervals. May cause elevations of plasma triglycerides with pre-existing hypertriglyceridemia. Caution with history of cholestatic jaundice associated with past estrogen use or with pregnancy; d/c with recurrence. May lead to increased thyroid-binding globulin levels; monitor thyroid function. May cause fluid retention; caution with cardiac/renal dysfunction. Caution with severe hypocalcemia. May increase risk of ovarian cancer. May exacerbate endometriosis, asthma, diabetes mellitus (DM), epilepsy, migraine, porphyria, systemic lupus erythematosus (SLE), and hepatic hemangiomas; use with caution.

ADVERSE REACTIONS: Abdominal pain, back pain, asthenia, flu syndrome, application site reaction, nausea, nervousness, pharyngitis, respiratory disorder, breast pain, dysmenorrhea, menstrual disorder, vaginitis.

INTERACTIONS: CYP3A4 inducers (eg, St. John's wort, phenobarbital, carbamazepine, rifampin) may decrease levels which may decrease therapeutic effects and/or change uterine bleeding profile. CYP3A4 inhibitors (eg, erythromycin, clarithromycin, ketoconazole, itraconazole, ritonavir, grapefruit juice) may increase levels which may result in side effects.

PREGNANCY: Contraindicated in pregnancy, caution in nursing.

MECHANISM OF ACTION: Estrogen/progestogen. Acts by binding to nuclear receptors in estrogen-responsive tissues. Modulates pituitary secretion of gonadotropins, luteinizing hormone and follicle stimulating hormone, through negative feedback mechanism.

PHARMACOKINETICS: Absorption: Estradiol: Well-absorbed. Administration of various doses led to altered parameters. Norethindrone: Well-absorbed. Administration of various doses led to altered parameters. **Distribution:** Estrogens and progestins found in breast milk. Estradiol: Largely bound to sex hormone binding globulin (SHBG) and albumin. Norethindrone: 90% to SHBG and albumin. **Metabolism:** Liver, to estrone (metabolite); estriol (major urinary metabolite); enterohepatic recirculation, via sulfate and glucuronide conjugation; biliary secretion of conjugates in the intestine; hydrolysis in gut; reabsorption; CYP 3A4 (partial). Norethindrone: Liver. **Elimination:** Estradiol, estrone, estriol: Urine; $T_{1/2}$=2-3 hrs. Norethindrone: $T_{1/2}$=6-8 hrs.

NURSING CONSIDERATIONS

Assessment: Assess for abnormal genital bleeding, presence or history of breast cancer, estrogen-dependent neoplasias, DVT, PE, active or recent (within past yr) and any other conditions where treatment may be contraindicated or cautioned. Assess use in women ≥65 yrs, nursing patients, and those with DM, asthma, epilepsy, migraines or porphyria, SLE, and hepatic hemangiomas. Assess for possible drug and lab test interactions.

Monitoring: Monitor for signs/symptoms of CV disorders (eg, MI, stroke, venous thrombosis, PE), malignant neoplasms (eg, breast, endometrial, ovarian cancer), dementia, gallbladder disease, hypercalcemia, visual abnormalities (eg, retinal vascular thrombosis), increased BP, hypertriglyceridemia, hypothyroidism, fluid retention, cholestatic jaundice, exacerbation of endometriosis and other conditions. Perform annual mammography and periodic monitoring of BP. Monitor thyroid function if patient on thyroid hormone replacement therapy. In cases of undiagnosed, persistent, or recurrent vaginal bleeding in women with uterus, perform adequate diagnostic measures (eg, endometrial sampling) to rule out malignancies.

Patient Counseling: Inform that drug may increase risk for heart attack, stroke, breast cancer, blood clots, and dementia. Report any breast lumps, unusual vaginal bleeding, dizziness or faintness, changes in speech, chest pain, SOB, leg pain, changes in vision, and vomiting. Counsel that if patch falls off, reapply same patch to different area of lower abdomen or use new patch.

Administration: Transdermal route. **Storage:** Prior to dispensing: Store refrigerated at 2-8°C (36-46°F). After dispensed: May be stored at room temperature below 25°C (77°F). Do not store in areas where extreme temperatures may occur.

COMBIVENT   RX
ipratropium bromide - albuterol sulfate (Boehringer Ingelheim)

THERAPEUTIC CLASS: Beta$_2$-agonist/anticholinergic

INDICATIONS: Treatment of patients with chronic obstructive pulmonary disease (COPD) on a regular aerosol bronchodilator who continue to have evidence of bronchospasm and who require a second bronchodilator.

DOSAGE: *Adults:* 2 inh qid. Max: 12 inh/24 hrs.

HOW SUPPLIED: MDI: (Albuterol-Ipratropium) 0.09mg-0.018mg/inh [14.7g]

CONTRAINDICATIONS: History of hypersensitivity to soya lecithin or related food products (eg, soybeans, peanuts).

WARNINGS/PRECAUTIONS: Paradoxical bronchospasm and rare occurrences of myocardial ischemia reported. Hypersensitivity reactions reported. Caution with coronary insufficiency, arrhythmias, narrow-angle glaucoma, prostatic hyperplasia, bladder-neck obstruction, HTN, diabetes mellitus (DM), hyperthyroidism, convulsive disorders, renal or hepatic insufficiency and in those unusually responsive to sympathomimetic amines. May produce transient hypokalemia. Fatalities reported with excessive use.

ADVERSE REACTIONS: Headache, cough, upper respiratory tract infection, dyspnea, bronchitis.

INTERACTIONS: Potential additive interactions with other anticholinergic drugs. Increased risk of adverse cardiovascular (CV) effects with other sympathomimetics. β-blockers and albuterol inhibit effects of each other. ECG changes and/or hypokalemia may occur with non-K$^+$-sparing diuretics. Action of albuterol on CV system maybe potentiated with MAOIs and TCAs or within 2 weeks of d/c of these drugs.

PREGNANCY: Category C, not for use in nursing.

MECHANISM OF ACTION: Ipratropium: Anticholinergic bronchodilator; inhibits vagally-mediated reflexes by antagonizing the action of acetylcholine. Albuterol: Selective β$_2$-adrenergic bronchodilator; activates β$_2$-receptors on airway smooth muscle, leading to activation of adenylyl cyclase and increase of intracellular cyclic adenosine monophosphate (AMP) concentrations. This leads to activation of protein kinase A, which inhibits phosphorylation of myosin and lowers intracellular ionic calcium concentrations, resulting in relaxation.

PHARMACOKINETICS: Absorption: Ipratropium: Not readily absorbed. Albuterol: Rapid, complete; C_{max}=492pg/mL; T_{max}=3 hrs. **Distribution:** Ipratropium: Plasma protein binding (0-9%). **Metabolism:** Ipratropium: Partial; ester hydrolysis. Albuterol: Conjugation; albuterol 4'-O-sulfate (metabolite). **Elimination:** Ipratropium: Urine (50% unchanged); $T_{1/2}$=2 hrs. Albuterol: Urine (unchanged); $T_{1/2}$=3.9 hrs.

NURSING CONSIDERATIONS

Assessment: Assess for known history of hypersensitivity to soya lecithin or related food products (eg, soybeans, peanuts). Assess for concomitant diseases (eg, narrow-angle glaucoma, prostatic hyperplasia, convulsive disorders, hyperthyroidism, DM, hepatic/renal insufficiency, cardiovascular disease). Assess pregnancy/nursing status, potassium levels and possible drug interactions.

Monitoring: Monitor for hypersensitivity reactions, paroxdonal bronchospasm, MI, CV effects such as flattening of the T wave, prolongation of the QT interval, and ST segment depression, unexpected development of severe acute asthmatic crisis and hypoxia.

Patient Counseling: Advise to avoid spraying into eyes, to not exceed recommended dose, and to shake canister vigorously for at least 10 seconds before use. Discard canister after labeled number of actuations have been used. Advise not to puncture, not to use or store near heat or open flame, and to never throw inhaler into fire or incinerator; exposure to temperature >120°C may cause bursting.

Administration: Inhalation route. 1) Insert metal canister into end of mouthpiece. 2) Remove orange dust cap and shake. Test spray into the air 3x before using for the first time or in cases when aerosol has not been used for 24 hrs. 3) Shake canister for 10 sec. 4) Inhale and exhale through mouth and at the same time spray product into mouth. 5) Hold breath for 10 sec and remove mouth piece. 6) Wait for 2 min before next spray. 7) Replace cap and keep mouthpiece clean. 8) Keep track of the number of sprays used and discard after 200 sprays. **Storage:** 25°C (77°F); excursions permitted to 15-30°C (59-86°F). Keep out of reach of children. Store the canister at room temperature before use and avoid excessive humidity. Do not store near heat or open flame.

COMBIVIR

RX

zidovudine - lamivudine (ViiV Healthcare)

> Zidovudine has been associated with hematologic toxicity (eg, neutropenia, anemia), especially with advanced HIV-1 disease. Symptomatic myopathy reported with prolonged use. Lactic acidosis and hepatomegaly with steatosis, including fatal cases, reported with nucleoside analogues; suspend treatment if lactic acidosis or pronounced hepatotoxicity occurs. Acute exacerbations of hepatitis B reported in patients coinfected with hepatitis B virus (HBV) and HIV-1 who discontinued lamivudine; monitor hepatic function closely for at least several months after d/c and initiate anti-hepatitis B therapy if needed.

THERAPEUTIC CLASS: Nucleoside analog combination

INDICATIONS: Treatment of HIV-1 infection in combination with other antiretrovirals.

DOSAGE: *Adults:* ≥30 kg: 1 tab bid.
Pediatrics: ≥30 kg: 1 tab bid.

HOW SUPPLIED: Tab: (Lamivudine-Zidovudine) 150mg-300mg* *scored

WARNINGS/PRECAUTIONS: Caution in patients with granulocyte count <1000cells/mm³ or Hgb <9.5g/dL; monitor blood counts frequently with advanced HIV-1 and periodically with other HIV-1 infected patients. Interrupt therapy if anemia or neutropenia develops. Caution in patients with history and known risk factors for liver disease. Lamivudine-resistant HBV reported. Caution in patient with history of pancreatitis or significant risk factors for the development of pancreatitis; d/c if pancreatitis occurs. Possible redistribution or accumulation of body fat. Immune reconstitution syndrome reported. Caution in elderly. Do not use in patients with reduced renal function (CrCl <50mL/min), pediatrics weighing <30 kg, with hepatic impairment, or patients experiencing dose-limiting adverse reactions.

ADVERSE REACTIONS: Headache, malaise, fatigue, fever, chills, N/V, diarrhea, anorexia, neuropathy, insomnia, dizziness, nasal signs and symptoms, cough, musculoskeletal pain.

INTERACTIONS: Should not be administered concomitantly with other lamivudine-, zidovudine- or, emtricitabine-containing products. Nelfinavir may increase the AUC of lamivudine and decrease the AUC of zidovudine. Lamivudine: Hepatic decompensation may occur in HIV/hepatitis C virus co-infected patients receiving combination antiretroviral therapy for HIV-1 and interferon alfa with or without ribavirin; monitor for treatment-associated toxicities. Trimethoprim/sulfamethoxazole may increase lamivudine concentrations. Avoid use with zalcitabine; may inhibit phosphorylation of lamuvidine. Zidovudine: Avoid with stavudine, doxorubin, and nucleoside analogues affecting DNA replication such as ribavirin. Coadministration of ganciclovir, interferon alfa, ribavirin, bone marrow suppressive or cytotoxic agents may increase the hematologic toxicity of zidovudine. Atovaquone, fluconazole, methadone, probenecid, and valproic acid may increase zidovudine AUC. Rifampin, clarithromycin, and ritonavir may decrease zidovudine AUC.

PREGNANCY: Category C, not for use in nursing.

MECHANISM OF ACTION: Nucleoside analog combination; inhibits reverse transcriptase via DNA chain termination after incorporation of the nucleotide analogue.

PHARMACOKINETICS: Absorption: Lamivudine: Rapid. Absolute bioavailability (86%). Zidovudine: Rapid. Absolute bioavailability (64%). **Distribution:** Lamivudine: V_d=1.3L/kg; plasma protein binding (<36%). Zidovudine: V_d=1.6L/kg; plasma protein binding (<38%). **Metabolism:** Zidovudine: Hepatic: 3'-azido-3'-deoxy-5'-O-β-D-glucopyranuronosylthymidine (major metabolite). **Elimination:** Lamivudine: Urine (70% unchanged); $T_{1/2}$=5-7 hrs. Zidovudine: Urine (14% unchanged, 74% metabolite); $T_{1/2}$=0.5-3 hrs.

NURSING CONSIDERATIONS

Assessment: Assess for advanced symptomatic HIV disease, bone marrow suppression, liver function and risk factors for liver disease, hepatitis B infection, history of pancreatitis and risk factors for its development, renal function, hypersensitivity to drug, pregnancy/nursing status, and possible drug interaction. Obtain baseline weight, CBC and renal/liver function test.

Monitoring: Monitor CBC, platelet counts, renal/liver function. Monitor signs/symptoms that suggest pancreatitis, lactic acidosis, or hepatotoxicity including hepatomegaly with steatosis, peripheral neuropathy, myopathy and myositis, exacerbations of hepatitis, immune reconstitution syndrome, and hypersensitivity reactions.

Patient Counseling: Advise patients that they may continue to experience illnesses associated with HIV-1 while on therapy and that risk of transmission to others is not reduced. Inform that deterioration of liver disease can occur when drug is discontinued. Advise of zidovudine-related toxicities, such as neutropenia and anemia. Instruct patients to have their blood counts followed closely while on therapy. Inform that redistribution/accumulation of fat that may occur. Inform about potential drug interactions including ganciclovir, interferon alfa, and ribavirin which may exacerbate toxicity of zidovudine. Advice to take exactly as prescribed and not to administer with other drugs containing lamivudine, zidovudine, or emtricitabine.

Administration: Oral route. Take w/ or w/o food. **Storage:** 2-30°C (36-86°F).

COMBUNOX   `CII`
oxycodone HCl - ibuprofen (Forest)

> NSAIDs may cause an increased risk of serious cardiovascular (CV) thrombotic events, myocardial infarction (MI), stroke, and serious GI adverse events including bleeding, ulceration, and perforation of the stomach or intestines. Contraindicated for the treatment of perioperative pain in the setting of coronary artery bypass graft (CABG) surgery.

THERAPEUTIC CLASS: Opioid analgesic

INDICATIONS: Short-term (≤7 days) management of acute, moderate to severe pain.

DOSAGE: *Adults:* 1 tab PO. Adjust dose and frequency based on the response to initial therapy. Max: 4 tabs/24 hrs. Do not exceed 7 days.
Pediatrics: ≥14 yrs: 1 tab PO. Adjust dose and frequency based on the response to initial therapy. Max: 4 tabs/24 hrs. Do not exceed 7 days.

HOW SUPPLIED: Tab: (Oxycodone-Ibuprofen) 5mg-400mg

CONTRAINDICATIONS: Significant respiratory depression, acute or severe bronchial asthma, hypercarbia, paralytic ileus, or in patients who have experienced asthma, urticaria, allergic-type reactions after taking ASA or NSAIDs. Treatment of perioperative pain in the setting of CABG surgery.

WARNINGS/PRECAUTIONS: Use lowest effective dose for the shortest duration to minimize the risk of CV or GI events. May lead to HTN or worsening of pre-existing HTN. Fluid retention and edema reported; caution with fluid retention or heart failure (HF). Extreme caution with history of ulcer disease, GI bleeding or with risk factors for GI bleeding (eg, smoking, use of alcohol, older age, poor general health). May cause drug dependence and tolerance; potential for abuse. Risk of respiratory depression is increased in elderly/debilitated patients or with large initial doses to opioid-intolerant patients. Extreme caution with chronic obstructive pulmonary disease, cor pulmonale, decreased respiratory drive, hypoxia, hypercapnia or pre-existing respiratory depression. May produce orthostatic hypotension and severe hypotension may occur with depleted blood volume. Caution with circulatory shock; may further reduce cardiac output and BP. Respiratory depressant effects and capacity to elevate cerebrospinal fluid (CSF) pressure may be exaggerated with head injury, intracranial lesions or pre-existing increase in intracranial pressure. May obscure diagnosis or clinical course with head injuries or acute abdominal conditions. Anaphylactoid reactions may occur; avoid in patients with history of angioedema or patients with the aspirin triad. Renal papillary necrosis and other renal injury reported after long-term NSAID use. Caution with renal/liver impairment and HF. Not recommended for use with advanced renal disease. May cause exfoliative dermatitis, Stevens-Johnson syndrome (SJS), and toxic epidermal necrolysis (TEN). Not a substitute for corticosteroids or for the treatment of corticosteroid insufficiency. Caution in elderly and debilitated or with pulmonary dysfunction, hypothyroidism, Addison's disease, acute alcoholism, convulsive disorders, CNS depression or coma, delirium tremens, kyphoscoliosis associated with respiratory depression, toxic psychosis, prostatic hypertrophy, urethral stricture. May cause spasm of sphincter of Oddi and increase serum amylase; caution with biliary tract disease and acute pancreatitis. May suppress the cough reflex; caution when used postoperatively and with pulmonary disease. May elevate LFTs; d/c if liver disease or systemic manifestations occur. May cause anemia with long-term use. May inhibit platelet aggregation and prolong bleeding time. Caution with pre-existing and ASA-sensitive asthma. Aseptic meningitis observed.

ADVERSE REACTIONS: N/V, somnolence, dizziness, asthenia, fever, headache, vasodilation, constipation, GI effects (bleeding, ulcer, perforation), cardiovascular thrombotic events, MI.

INTERACTIONS: Oxycodone: Additive CNS depression, respiratory depression, hypotension, profound sedation, or coma with other CNS depressants (eg, narcotics, tranquilizers, sedative-hypnotics, general anesthetics, alcohol). Concurrent use with anticholinergics may produce paralytic ileus. Mixed agonist/antagonist analgesics may reduce the analgesic effect and/or cause withdrawal. Do not use with or within 14 days of d/c MAOIs. May enhance skeletal muscle relaxant effects and increase respiratory depression. Risk of severe hypotension with phenothiazines or other agents that compromise vasomotor tone. Respiratory depression may occur when given in conjunction with other agents that depress respiration. Metabolism to oxymorphone may be blocked by variety of drugs (eg, antidepressants, cardiovascular drugs). Ibuprofen: May diminish antihypertensive effect of ACE inhibitors. Concomitant use with corticosteroids, anticoagulants and warfarin may increase risk of GI bleeding. May enhance methotrexate toxicity. May decrease natriuretic effect of furosemide and thiazides. Avoid with ASA. May increase plasma levels and decrease clearance of lithium; monitor for toxicity.

PREGNANCY: Category C <30 weeks gestation; Category D ≥30 weeks gestation, not for use in nursing.

MECHANISM OF ACTION: Oxycodone: Opioid analgesic; not established. Suspected to be related to binding to opiate receptors in the CNS; may produce sedation and respiratory depression. Ibuprofen: NSAID; not established. Possess analgesic and antipyretic activity; inhibits cyclooxygenase activity and prostaglandin synthesis.

PHARMACOKINETICS: Absorption: Oxycodone: Rapid; C_{max}=9.8-11.7ng/mL; T_{max}=1.3-2.1 hrs. Ibuprofen: Rapid; C_{max}=18.5-34.3mcg/mL; T_{max}=1.6-3.1 hrs. **Distribution:** Oxycodone: Plasma protein binding (45%); found in breastmilk. Ibuprofen: Plasma protein binding (99%). **Metabolism:** Oxycodone: Liver via CYP2D6 (N-demethylation, O-demethylation, 6-ketoreduction, glucuronidation); noroxycodone (major circulating metabolite), oxymorphone (active metabolite). Ibuprofen: Undergoes interconversion in plasma from R- to S-isomer: (+)-2-4'-(2-hydroxy-2-methyl-propyl) phenyl propionic acid, (+)-2-4'-(carboxypropyl) phenyl propionic acid (primary metabolites). **Elimination:** Oxycodone: Urine (4%, unchanged); $T_{1/2}$=3.1-3.7 hrs. Ibuprofen: Urine (≤0.2%, unchanged); $T_{1/2}$=1.8-2.6 hrs.

NURSING CONSIDERATIONS

Assessment: Assess for level of pain intensity, type of pain, patient's general condition and medical status, or any other conditions where treatment is contraindicated or cautioned. Assess for history of hypersensitivity, pregnancy/nursing status, renal/hepatic function, and possible drug interactions.Obtain baseline BP, CBC,and coagulation profile.

Monitoring: Monitor for signs/symptoms of CV thrombotic events, MI, stroke, new onset/worsening of HTN, fluid retention/edema, serious GI events (eg, ulceration, bleeding, perforation), physical dependence and tolerance, abuse or misuse of medication, respiratory depression, hypotension, CSF pressure elevation, anaphylactoid reactions, renal papillary necrosis, renal/liver impairment, skin reactions, anemia and aseptic meningitis. Monitor patients who may be adversely affected by platelet function changes. Monitor BP, renal function, chemistry profile including LFTs (eg, ALT, AST), CBC (eg, Hgb, Hct), platelet count and coagulation profile.

Patient Counseling: Inform that drug may impair mental/physical abilities; use caution when performing dangerous tasks (eg, operating machinery/driving). Advise to avoid other CNS depressants and alcohol during therapy. Counsel that medication has abuse potential; only take as prescribed. Instruct to notify physician if develop any serious CV effects (eg, chest pain, SOB), GI effects (eg, ulcers, bleeding), serious skin reactions (eg, exfoliative dermatitis, SJS), unexplained weight gain or edema, hepatotoxicity (eg, nausea, fatigue, jaundice), or anaphylactoid reactions (eg, difficulty breathing, facial swelling) develops. Advise pregnant women to avoid medication especially in late pregnancy.

Administration: Oral route. **Storage:** 25°C (77°F); excursions permitted to 15-30°C (59-86°F).

COMTAN   RX
entacapone (Novartis)

THERAPEUTIC CLASS: COMT inhibitor

INDICATIONS: Adjunct to levodopa/carbidopa to treat patients with idiopathic Parkinson's disease who experience the signs and symptoms of end-of-dose "wearing-off."

DOSAGE: *Adults:* 200mg with each levodopa/carbidopa dose. Max: 1600mg/day.

HOW SUPPLIED: Tab: 200mg

WARNINGS/PRECAUTIONS: Orthostatic hypotension/syncope and hallucinations reported. Diarrhea and colitis reported; d/c if prolonged diarrhea is suspected to be related to therapy and institute appropriate care. May cause and/or exacerbate pre-existing dyskinesia. Severe rhabdomyolysis and symptom complex resembling neuroleptic malignant syndrome (NMS) reported. Retroperitoneal fibrosis, pulmonary infiltrates, pleural effusion, and pleural thickening reported. May increase risk of developing melanoma; perform periodic skin exams. May increase risk of developing renal toxicity. Caution with hepatic impairment (eg, biliary obstruction). Avoid rapid withdrawal or abrupt dose reduction.

ADVERSE REACTIONS: Dyskinesia, hyperkinesia, hypokinesia, N/V, diarrhea, abdominal pain, urine discoloration, dizziness, constipation, dry mouth, fatigue, dyspnea, back pain.

INTERACTIONS: Avoid nonselective MAOIs (eg, phenelzine, tranylcypromine). Caution with drugs metabolized by catechol-O-methyltransferase (COMT) (eg, isoproterenol, epinephrine, norepinephrine, dopamine, dobutamine, α-methyldopa, apomorphine, isoetherine, bitolterol); increased HR, arrhythmias, and BP changes may occur. Caution with concomitant use of drugs known to interfere with biliary excretion, glucuronidation, and intestinal β-glucuronidase (eg, probenecid, cholestyramine, some antibiotics [eg, erythromycin, rifampicin, ampicillin, chloramphenicol]). May potentiate dopaminergic side effects of levodopa.

PREGNANCY: Category C, caution in nursing.

MECHANISM OF ACTION: COMT inhibitor; inhibits COMT and alters the plasma pharmacokinetics of levodopa.

PHARMACOKINETICS: Absorption: (PO) Rapid; absolute bioavailability (35%); C_{max}=1.2µg/mL; T_{max}=1 hr. **Distribution:** Plasma protein binding (98%); (IV) V_d=20L. **Metabolism:** Isomerization to *cis*-isomer, and direct glucuronidation. **Elimination:** Urine (10%, 0.2% unchanged), feces (90%); $T_{1/2\ (\beta\text{-phase})}$=0.4-0.7 hrs; $T_{1/2\ (\text{gamma-phase})}$=2.4 hrs.

NURSING CONSIDERATIONS

Assessment: Assess for dyskinesia, biliary obstruction, hepatic function, history of hypotension, hypersensitivity to drug, pregnancy/nursing status, and for possible drug interactions.

C

Monitoring: Monitor for signs/symptoms of orthostatic hypotension, diarrhea, hallucinations, dyskinesia, rhabdomyolysis, a symptom complex resembling NMS (eg, elevated temperature, muscular rigidity, altered consciousness), retroperitoneal fibrosis, pulmonary infiltrates, pleural effusion, pleural thickening, and for renal toxicity. Monitor for signs of melanoma; perform periodic skin examinations.

Patient Counseling: Instruct to take only as prescribed. Inform that postural hypotension, hallucinations, nausea, diarrhea, increased dyskinesia, and change in urine color may occur. Caution against rising rapidly after sitting or lying down, especially during initiation of treatment. Instruct to avoid driving a car or operating other complex machinery until aware of how medication affects mental and/or motor performance. Advise to inform physician if experiencing new or increased gambling urges, sexual urges, or other intense urges. Instruct to notify physician if intend to become or are pregnant/nursing.

Administration: Oral route. **Storage:** 25°C (77°F); excursions permitted to 15-30°C (59-86°F).

CONCERTA CII
methylphenidate HCl (Ortho-Mcneil/Janssen)

> Caution with history of drug dependence or alcoholism. Marked tolerance and psychological dependence with varying degrees of abnormal behavior may result from chronic abusive use. Frank psychotic episodes may occur. Careful supervision required for withdrawal from abusive use to avoid severe depression. Withdrawal following chronic use may unmask symptoms of underlying disorder that may require follow-up.

THERAPEUTIC CLASS: Sympathomimetic amine

INDICATIONS: Treatment of attention-deficit/hyperactivity disorder (ADHD) in patients ≥6-65 yrs.

DOSAGE: *Adults:* ≤65 yrs: Methylphenidate-Naive or Receiving Other Stimulant: Initial: 18mg or 36mg qam. Titrate: May increase by 18mg weekly if optimal response not achieved. Max: 72mg/day. Currently on Methylphenidate: Initial: 18mg qam if previous dose 10-15mg/day; 36mg qam if previous dose 20-30mg/day; 54mg qam if previous dose 30-45mg/day; 72mg qam if previous dose 40-60mg/day. Conversion should not exceed 72mg/day. Titrate: May increase by 18mg weekly if optimal response not achieved. Max: 72mg/day. Reduce dose or d/c if paradoxical aggravation of symptoms or other adverse effects occur. D/C if no improvement after appropriate dosage adjustments over 1 month. Swallow whole with liquids; do not crush, divide, or chew.
Pediatrics: ≥6 yrs: Methylphenidate-Naive or Receiving Other Stimulant: Initial: 18mg qam. Titrate: May increase by 18mg weekly if optimal response not achieved. Max: 6-12 yrs: 54mg/day; 13-17 yrs: 72mg/day not to exceed 2mg/kg/day. Currently on Methylphenidate: Initial: 18mg qam if previous dose 10-15mg/day; 36mg qam if previous dose 20-30mg/day; 54mg qam if previous dose 30-45mg/day; 72mg qam if previous dose 40-60mg/day. Conversion should not exceed 72mg/day. Titrate: May increase by 18mg weekly if optimal response not achieved. Max: 6-12 yrs: 54mg/day; 13-17 yrs: 72mg/day. Reduce dose or d/c if paradoxical aggravation of symptoms or other adverse effects occur. D/C if no improvement after appropriate dosage adjustments over 1 month. Swallow whole with liquids; do not crush, divide, or chew.

HOW SUPPLIED: Tab, Extended-Release: 18mg, 27mg, 36mg, 54mg

CONTRAINDICATIONS: Patients with marked anxiety, tension, agitation, glaucoma, motor tics or family history or diagnosis of Tourette's syndrome. Treatment with or within a minimum of 14 days following d/c of an MAOI.

WARNINGS/PRECAUTIONS: Sudden death, stroke, and MI reported; avoid with known structural cardiac abnormalities, cardiomyopathy, serious heart abnormalities, coronary artery disease or other serious cardiac problems. May increase BP and HR; caution with pre-existing HTN, heart failure, myocardial infarction, or ventricular arrhythmias. Promptly evaluate when symptoms suggestive of cardiac disease develop. May exacerbate symptoms of behavior disturbance and thought disorder in psychotic patients. May induce mixed/manic episode in patients with bipolar disorder. Use at usual doses can cause treatment-emergent psychotic or manic symptoms (eg, hallucinations, delusional thinking, mania) without prior history of psychotic illness. Aggressive behavior or hostility reported. May lower convulsive threshold; d/c if seizures develop. May cause long-term suppression of growth in children. Visual disturbances reported. Avoid with pre-existing severe GI narrowing (eg, esophageal motility disorders, small bowel inflammatory disease, "short gut" syndrome). Perform periodic monitoring of CBC, differential, and platelet counts during prolonged use.

ADVERSE REACTIONS: Decreased appetite, headache, dry mouth, nausea, insomnia, anxiety, dizziness, decreased weight, irritability, upper abdominal pain, hyperhidrosis, palpitations, tachycardia, depressed mood, nervousness.

INTERACTIONS: See Contraindications. Caution with vasopressor agents; increased blood pressure may result. May inhibit metabolism of coumarin anticoagulants, anticonvulsants (eg, phenobarbital, phenytoin, primidone), and some antidepressants (eg, TCAs, SSRIs).

PREGNANCY: Category C, caution in nursing.

MECHANISM OF ACTION: Sympathomimetic amine; not established. CNS stimulant, thought to block the reuptake of norepinephrine and dopamine into the presynaptic neuron and increase the release of these monoamines into the extraneuronal space.

PHARMACOKINETICS: Absorption: Readily absorbed; (18mg qd dose) C_{max}=3.7ng/mL, AUC=41.8ng•hr/mL; T_{max}=6.8 hrs. **Metabolism:** De-esterification. α-phenyl-piperidine acetic acid (metabolite). **Elimination:** Urine (90%); $T_{1/2}$=3.5 hrs.

NURSING CONSIDERATIONS

Assessment: Assess for history of drug dependence or alcoholism, presence of anxiety, tension, family history or diagnosis of Tourette's syndrome, underlying medical conditions that might be compromised by increased BP or HR, psychotic disorders, seizure disorder, severe GI narrowing, drug hypersensitivity, pregnancy/nursing status, and for possible drug interactions. Perform careful history and physical exam to assess for presence of cardiac disease and psychiatric history. Prior to treatment, adequately screen patients with depressive symptoms to determine risk for bipolar disorder. Obtain baseline CBC, differential and platelet counts. Obtain baseline height/weight in children.

Monitoring: Monitor for cardiac abnormalities, increased BP and HR, cardiac disease symptoms, behavioral disturbances, thought disorder, new psychotic or manic symptoms, aggression, hostility, seizures, and for visual disturbances. In patients suspected of chronic abuse, monitor for marked tolerance or psychological dependence. In patients with bipolar disorder, monitor for mixed/manic episode. Perform periodic monitoring of height and weight in children, CBC, differential and platelet counts.

Patient Counseling: Inform about benefits, risks, and appropriate use of therapy. Instruct to swallow tablet whole with the aid of liquids; do not crush, divide, or chew. Advise to read Medication Guide. Inform that therapy may impair mental/physical abilities; caution with hazardous tasks (eg, operating machinery, driving). Inform that medication contains a nonabsorbable shell and to not be concerned if something that looks like a tablet is seen in the stool.

Administration: Oral route. Administer qam. Swallow whole with liquids; do not crush, divide, or chew. **Storage:** 25°C (77°F); excursions permitted to 15-30°C (59-86°F). Protect from humidity.

COPAXONE   RX
glatiramer acetate (Teva Neuroscience)

THERAPEUTIC CLASS: Immunomodulatory agent

INDICATIONS: To reduce frequency of relapses in patients with relapsing-remitting multiple sclerosis (RRMS), including patients who have experienced a first clinical episode and have magnetic resonance imaging (MRI) features of MS.

DOSAGE: *Adults:* 20mg SQ qd.

HOW SUPPLIED: Inj: 20mg/mL

CONTRAINDICATIONS: Hypersensitivity to mannitol.

WARNINGS/PRECAUTIONS: Not for IV use. Immediate post-injection reaction (eg, flushing, palpitations, dyspnea, urticaria, anxiety, throat constriction), chest pain, lipoatrophy, skin necrosis (rare) reported. May interfere with normal functioning of immune system.

ADVERSE REACTIONS: Injection-site reactions, vasodilation, chest pain, dyspnea, rash, asthenia, infection, pain, nausea, arthralgia, anxiety, hypertonia, depression, tachycardia, tremor.

PREGNANCY: Category B, caution in nursing.

MECHANISM OF ACTION: Immunomodulatory agent; not fully established. Presumed to modify immune processes in multiple sclerosis (MS).

NURSING CONSIDERATIONS

Assessment: Assess for mannitol therapy, clinical episodes of MS, MRI.

Monitoring: Monitor for immediate post-injection reactions (eg, flushing, chest pain, palpitations, anxiety, dyspnea, constriction of throat, urticaria), hypersensitivity, pregnancy/nursing status.

Patient Counseling: Notify physician if pregnant/nursing or planning to become pregnant. Counsel about transient and self-limiting symptoms of adverse reactions (eg, flushing, chest pain, palpitations, anxiety, dyspnea, throat constriction, and urticaria). Inform to seek medical consultation if chest pain of unusual duration or intensity occurs. Instruct to follow proper injection technique and rotate injection sites on a daily basis. Use aseptic technique.

Administration: SQ route. **Storage:** 2-8°C (36-46°F); 15-30°C (59-86°F) for 1 month. Do not expose to high temperatures and intense light.

COPEGUS   RX
ribavirin (Genentech)

> Not for monotherapy treatment of chronic hepatitis C (CHC) virus infection. Primary toxicity is hemolytic anemia. Anemia associated with therapy may result in worsening of cardiac disease that may lead to fatal and nonfatal myocardial infarctions (MI). Avoid with significant or unstable cardiac disease. Contraindicated in pregnancy and male partners of pregnant women. Use ≥2 reliable forms of effective contraception during therapy and for 6 months after d/c.

THERAPEUTIC CLASS: Nucleoside analogue

INDICATIONS: Treatment of CHC virus infection in combination with Pegasys (peginterferon α-2a) in adults with compensated liver disease not previously treated with interferon α.

DOSAGE: *Adults:* CHC monoinfection: Individualize dose: 800-1200mg daily in 2 divided doses. Treat for 24-48 weeks with Pegasys 180mcg. Genotypes 1 and 4: <75kg: 1000mg/day for 48 weeks. ≥75kg: 1200mg/day for 48 weeks. Genotypes 2 and 3: 800mg/day for 24 weeks. CHC with HIV Coinfection: 800mg qd. Treat for 48 weeks with Pegasys 180mcg SQ once a week. Dose Modifications: Reduce to 600mg/day: Give 200mg qam and 400mg qpm if Hgb <10g/dL with no cardiac disease, or if Hgb decreases by ≥2g/dL during any 4-week period treatment with history of stable cardiac disease. D/C if Hgb <8.5g/dL with no cardiac history or if Hgb <12g/dL after 4 weeks of dose reduction with history of stable cardiac disease. After dose modification, may restart at 600mg/day, then may increase to 800mg/day but do not increase to original assigned dose (1000-1200mg). Take with food. D/C if patient fails to demonstrate at least a 2 $\log_{10}$ reduction from baseline in HCV RNA by 12 weeks of therapy, or undetectable HCV RNA levels after 24 weeks of therapy.

HOW SUPPLIED: Tab: 200mg

CONTRAINDICATIONS: Pregnancy, male partners of pregnant women, hemoglobinopathies (eg, thalassemia major, sickle cell anemia); autoimmune hepatitis and hepatic decompensation (Child-Pugh score >6; class B and C) in cirrhotic CHC monoinfected patients, and (Child-Pugh score ≥6) in cirrhotic CHC patients coinfected with HIV before treatment when used in combination with Pegasys; combination with didanosine.

WARNINGS/PRECAUTIONS: Combination therapy associated with significant adverse reactions (eg, severe depression, suicidal ideation, hemolytic anemia, suppression of bone marrow function, autoimmune/infectious/ophthalmologic/cerebrovascular disorders, pulmonary dysfunction, colitis, pancreatitis, diabetes). Do not start therapy unless negative for pregnancy. Caution with baseline risk of severe anemia (eg, spherocytosis, history of GI bleeding). D/C with hepatic decompensation, confirmed pancreatitis, severe acute hypersensitivity reactions and serious skin reactions. Pulmonary disorders (eg, dyspnea, pulmonary infiltrates, pneumonitis, pulmonary HTN, pneumonia, sarcoidosis/exacerbation of sarcoidosis, pulmonary function impairment) reported; monitor closely and if appropriate, d/c therapy. Caution with pre-existing cardiac disease; d/c if cardiovascular (CV) status deteriorates. Avoid if CrCl <50mL/min.

ADVERSE REACTIONS: Fatigue, asthenia, neutropenia, headache, pyrexia, myalgia, irritability, anxiety, nervousness, insomnia, alopecia, rigors, N/V, anorexia.

INTERACTIONS: See Contraindications. Hepatic decompensation can occur with concomitant use of nucleoside reverse transcriptase inhibitors (NRTIs). May reduce phosphorylation of lamivudine, stavudine and zidovudine in vitro. May induce severe pancytopenia and may increase the risk of azathioprine-related myelotoxicity with azathioprine.

PREGNANCY: Category X, not for use in nursing.

MECHANISM OF ACTION: Nucleoside analogue; not established. Has direct antiviral activity in tissue culture against many RNA viruses; increases mutation frequency in the genomes of several RNA viruses and ribavirin triphosphate inhibits HCV polymerase in a biochemical reaction.

PHARMACOKINETICS: Absorption: C_{max}=2748ng/mL; T_{max}=2 hrs; AUC_{0-12h}=25,361ng•hr/mL. **Elimination:** $T_{1/2}$=120-170 hrs.

NURSING CONSIDERATIONS

Assessment: Assess for history of hemoglobinopathies (eg, thalassemia major, sickle cell anemia), autoimmune hepatitis, hepatic decompensation, baseline risk of severe anemia (eg, spherocytosis, history of GI bleeding), history of drug abuse, history of significant or unstable cardiac disease, renal/hepatic/pulmonary function, pulmonary infiltrates, pancreatitis, hypersensitivity, pregnancy (including female partners of male patients), nursing status, and possible drug interactions. Obtain baseline hematological laboratory test (eg, CBC, Hgb, Hct), biochemical laboratory test, ECG with pre-existing cardiac abnormalities, thyroid function, pregnancy test, and CD4 count in HIV/AIDS patients. Confirm use of ≥2 forms of effective contraception.

Monitoring: Monitor CBC, LFTs, TSH and ECG periodically. Obtain Hct and Hgb (Weeks 2 and 4, more if needed) and biochemical tests at Week 4. Perform pregnancy testing monthly and for 6 months after d/c (including female partners of male patients). Monitor the use of effective contraception during therapy and for 6 months after d/c. Monitor for severe depression, suicidal ideation, hemolytic anemia, suppression of bone marrow function, autoimmune/infectious/ophthalmologic/cerebrovascular disorders, colitis, diabetes, pancreatitis, laboratory abnormalities, hemolytic anemia, worsening of cardiac disease, MI, hepatic decompensation, severe acute hypersensitivity reactions and skin reactions. Monitor clinical status and hepatic/renal/pulmonary function.

Patient Counseling: Counsel on risks/benefits associated with treatment. Inform of pregnancy risks; instruct to use 2 forms of effective contraception during therapy and 6 months after d/c of therapy (including female partners of male patients). Inquire about prior history of drug abuse before initiating therapy; relapse of drug addiction and drug overdoses reported with interferons. Advise not to drink alcohol; may exacerbate CHC infection. Inform to take missed doses as soon as possible during the same day; do not double next dose. Advise to call healthcare provider if they have questions. Inform that the effect of treatment of hepatitis C infection on transmission is not known, and that appropriate precautions to prevent HCV transmission should be taken. Caution to avoid driving/operating machinery if symptoms of dizziness, confusion, somnolence, or fatigue occurs. Counsel to take with food and to keep well-hydrated. Advise that laboratory evaluations are required prior to starting therapy and periodically thereafter.

Administration: Oral route. **Storage:** 25°C (77°F); excursions permitted between 15-30°C (59-86°F). Keep bottle tightly closed.

CORDARONE   RX
amiodarone HCl (Wyeth)

> Use only in patients with the indicated life-threatening arrhythmias because use is accompanied by potentially fatal toxicities, the most important of which is pulmonary toxicity (hypersensitivity pneumonitis or interstitial/alveolar pneumonitis). Liver injury is common, usually mild, and evidenced by abnormal liver enzymes. Overt liver disease may occur, and has been fatal in a few cases. May exacerbate arrhythmia. Significant heart block or sinus bradycardia reported. Patients must be hospitalized while loading dose is given, and a response generally requires at least 1 week, usually 2 or more. Maintenance dose selection is difficult and may require dosage decrease or d/c of treatment.

THERAPEUTIC CLASS: Class III antiarrhythmic

INDICATIONS: Treatment of documented, life-threatening recurrent ventricular fibrillation and recurrent hemodynamically unstable ventricular tachycardia when these have not responded to documented adequate doses of other available antiarrhythmics or when alternative agents could not be tolerated.

DOSAGE: *Adults:* Give LD in hospital. LD: 800-1600mg/day for 1-3 weeks. Give in divided doses with meals for total daily dose ≥1000mg or if GI intolerance occurs. After control is achieved or with prominent side effects, 600-800mg/day for 1 month. Maint: 400mg/day; up to 600mg/day if needed. May be administered as a single dose, or in patients with severe GI intolerance, as a bid dose. Use lowest effective dose. Take consistently with regard to meals. Elderly: Start at low end of dosing range.

HOW SUPPLIED: Tab: 200mg* *scored

CONTRAINDICATIONS: Cardiogenic shock, severe sinus-node dysfunction causing marked sinus bradycardia, 2nd- or 3rd-degree AV block, when episodes of bradycardia have caused syncope (except when used with a pacemaker).

WARNINGS/PRECAUTIONS: Pulmonary toxicities reported; d/c if hypersensitivity pneumonitis occurs and d/c or reduce dose if interstitial/alveolar pneumonitis occurs and institute appropriate treatment. In patients with implanted defibrillators or pacemakers, pacing and defibrillation thresholds should be assessed before and during treatment. Can cause either hypo- or hyperthyroidism. Amiodarone-induced hyperthyroidism may result in thyrotoxicosis and/or the possibility of arrhythmia breakthrough or aggravation. Liver injury is common but usually mild; d/c or reduce dose if LFTs are >3x normal or doubles in patients with elevated baseline; monitor LFTs regularly. Optic neuropathy and/or optic neuritis usually resulting in visual impairment reported. Fetal harm in pregnancy. May develop corneal microdeposits (eg, visual halos, blurred vision), photosensitivity, and peripheral neuropathy (rare). Adult respiratory distress syndrome (ARDS) reported with surgery. Rare occurrences of hypotension reported upon d/c of cardiopulmonary bypass during open-heart surgery. Correct K+ or magnesium deficiency before therapy. Caution in elderly.

ADVERSE REACTIONS: Pulmonary toxicity, malaise, fatigue, involuntary movements, abnormal gait, constipation, arrhythmia exacerbation, hepatic injury, tremor, poor coordination, paresthesia, N/V, anorexia, photosensitivity, CHF.

INTERACTIONS: Risk of interactions after d/c due to its long half-life. May increase sensitivity to myocardial depressant and conduction effects of halogenated inhalation anesthetics. D/C or reduce digoxin dose by 50%. Reduce warfarin dose by 1/3-1/2; monitor PTT closely. Avoid grapefruit juice. Hemodynamic and electrophysiologic interactions have been observed with propranolol, diltiazem, verapamil. Caution with β-blockers, calcium channel blockers. Sinus bradycardia reported with lidocaine; seizure associated with increased lidocaine reported with IV amiodarone. May increase levels of cyclosporine, methotrexate, dextromethorphan, quinidine, procainamide, phenytoin, flecainide. Initiate added antiarrhythmic drug at 50% of usual dose. Quinidine and procainamide doses should be reduced by 1/3 if coadministered. Caution with loratadine, trazodone, disopyramide, fluoroquinolones, macrolides, azoles; QT prolongation reported. Decreased levels with cholestyramine, rifampin, phenytoin, St. John's wort. Rhabdomyolysis/myopathy reported with HMG-CoA reductase inhibitors that are CYP3A4 substrates (eg, simvastatin, atorvastatin); consider lower starting or maintenance doses of these drugs. Ineffective inhibition of platelet aggregation with clopidogrel. Fentanyl may cause hypotension, bradycardia, and decreased cardiac output. Increased levels with protease inhibitors; monitor for toxicity. Inhibits P-glycoprotein, CYP1A2, CYP2C9, CYP2D6, CYP3A4 and may increase levels of their substrates. Interactions reported with CYP3A4 inducers. CYP2C8 and CYP3A4 (eg, cimetidine) inhibitors may increase amiodarone levels. Antithyroid drugs' action may be delayed in amiodarone-induced thyrotoxicosis. Radioactive iodine is contraindicated with amiodarone-induced hyperthyroidism. Caution with drugs which may induce hypokalemia and/or hypomagnesemia.

PREGNANCY: Category D, not for use in nursing.

MECHANISM OF ACTION: Class III antiarrhythmic; prolongs myocardial cell-action potential duration and refractory period, and causes noncompetitive α- and β-adrenergic inhibition.

PHARMACOKINETICS: Absorption: Slow and variable; T_{max}=3-7 hrs; bioavailability (35%-65%). **Distribution:** V_d=60L/kg; plasma protein binding (96%); crosses the placenta; found in breast milk. **Metabolism:** CYP3A4, 2C8; desethylamiodarone (major metabolite). **Elimination:** Bile, urine; $T_{1/2}$=58 days, 36 days (metabolite).

NURSING CONSIDERATIONS

Assessment: Assess for cardiogenic shock, severe sinus node dysfunction causing marked sinus bradycardia, 2nd or 3rd degree AV block, episodes of bradycardia causing syncope (except when used with a pacemaker), life-threatening arrhythmias, renal/hepatic impairment, thyroid function, pre-existing pulmonary disease, recent myocardial infarction, hypersensitivity to the drug including iodine, presence of implanted defibrillators or pacemakers, pregnancy/nursing status and possible drug interactions. Assess for failure of prior therapies. Correct hypokalemia and hypomagnesemia prior to initiation. Obtain chest x-ray, pulmonary function tests (including diffusion capacity), and physical exam.

Monitoring: Monitor for pulmonary toxicities and worsened arrhythmia. Perform history, physical exam, and chest x-ray every 3-6 months. Monitor for sinus bradycardia, sinus arrest, and heart block. Monitor for induced hyperthyroidism/thyrotoxicosis, hypothyroidism, hepatic failure, optic neuritis/neuropathy, corneal microdeposits, vision loss, fetal harm, peripheral neuropathy, photosensitivity. Monitor LFTs and thyroid function tests. Peri- and postoperative monitoring for hypotension and ARDS recommended. Monitor patients with severe left ventricular dysfunction. Perform regular ophthalmic examination including fundoscopy and slit-lamp examination.

Patient Counseling: Advise to notify physician if pregnant/nursing. Inform about benefits/risks, including possibility of vision impairment, thyroid abnormalities, peripheral neuropathy, photosensitivity, and skin discoloration. Advise to report any adverse reactions to physician. Counsel to take as directed and not to take with grapefruit juice. Advise to avoid prolonged sunlight exposure and to use sun-barrier creams or protective clothing. Advise that corneal refractive laser surgery is contraindicated with concurrent use.

Administration: Oral route. **Storage:** 20-25°C (68-77°F). Protect from light. Dispense in a tight, light-resistant container.

CORDRAN   RX
flurandrenolide (Watson)

OTHER BRAND NAMES: Cordran SP (Watson)

THERAPEUTIC CLASS: Corticosteroid

INDICATIONS: Treatment of corticosteroid-responsive dermatoses.

DOSAGE: *Adults:* (Cre, Lot) Apply qd-qid depending on severity. For moist lesions, apply cream bid-tid. Apply lotion bid-tid. (Tape) Clean and dry skin. Shave or clip hair. Apply tape q12-24h.
Pediatrics: (Cre, Lot) Apply qd-qid depending on severity. For moist lesions, apply cream bid-tid. Apply lotion bid-tid. (Tape) Clean and dry skin. Shave or clip hair. Apply tape q12-24h.

HOW SUPPLIED: Cre (SP): 0.05% [15g, 30g, 60g]; Lot: 0.05% [15mL, 60mL]; Tape: 4mcg/cm² [60cm x 7.5cm, 200cm x 7.5cm]

CONTRAINDICATIONS: (Tape) Not for lesions exuding serum or in intertriginous areas.

WARNINGS/PRECAUTIONS: Systemic absorption may produce reversible HPA axis suppression, manifestations of Cushing's syndrome, hyperglycemia, and glucosuria. Application of more potent steroids, use on large surfaces, prolonged use, or occlusive dressings may augment systemic absorption. Evaluate periodically for hypothalamic-pituitary-adrenal (HPA) suppression if large dose applied to large area or with occlusive dressings. Pediatrics are more susceptible to toxicity. D/C if irritation develops. May use occlusive dressing for psoriasis or recalcitrant conditions.

ADVERSE REACTIONS: Burning, itching, irritation, dryness, folliculitis, hypertrichosis, acneiform eruptions, hypopigmentation, dermatitis. Occlusive dressing may cause skin maceration, secondary infection, skin atrophy, miliaria.

PREGNANCY: Category C, caution in nursing.

MECHANISM OF ACTION: Corticosteroid; possesses anti-inflammatory, antipruritic, and vasoconstrictive properties. Suspected to stabilize cellular and lysosomal membranes, thereby preventing release of proteolytic enzymes, and consequently reducing inflammation.

PHARMACOKINETICS: Absorption: Extent of percutaneous absorption depends on integrity of skin, vehicle, and use of occlusive dressings. **Distribution:** Plasma protein binding (variable). **Metabolism:** Liver. **Elimination:** Kidney (major), bile.

NURSING CONSIDERATIONS

Assessment: Assess severity of dermatoses and pregnancy/nursing status.

Monitoring: Monitor for signs/symptoms of reversible HPA axis suppression, Cushing's syndrome, hyperglycemia, glucosuria, skin irritation, and for development of dermatological infections (eg, bacterial, fungal). In patients on large doses or using occlusive dressings, perform periodic testing for HPA-axis suppression by using urinary free cortisol, and ACTH stimulation tests. Following d/c of therapy, monitor for signs/symptoms of steroid withdrawal. In pediatric patients, monitor for systemic toxicity, HPA-axis suppression, Cushing's syndrome, and intracranial HTN.

Patient Counseling: Inform to use exactly as directed, externally. Avoid contact with eyes. Counsel not to bandage or wrap treated skin unless directed by physician. (Tape) Cleanse treatment area and allow it to dry for 1 hour prior to application. Report adverse reactions. Instruct parents of pediatric patients to avoid using tight-fitting diapers or plastic pants on children receiving treatment in diaper area.

Administration: Topical. Application of Tape: 1) Clean treatment area so that scales, crusts, dried exudates, and previously used ointments or creams are removed. Use germicidal soap or cleanser to prevent odor from developing under tape. Shave or clip hair in treatment area. If shower or tub bath is to be taken, complete before application of tape. Dry skin prior to application. 2) Apply tape, keeping skin smooth; press tape into place. **Storage:** 15-30°C (59-86°F).

COREG CR RX

carvedilol phosphate - carvedilol (GlaxoSmithKline)

OTHER BRAND NAMES: Coreg (GlaxoSmithKline)

THERAPEUTIC CLASS: Alpha₁/Beta-blocker

INDICATIONS: Treatment of mild to severe chronic heart failure (CHF) of ischemic or cardiomyopathic origin. Reduction of cardiovascular mortality in clinically stable patients who have survived the acute phase of a myocardial infarction (MI) and have a left ventricular ejection fraction of ≤40%. Management of essential HTN.

DOSAGE: *Adults:* Individualize dose. (Tab) CHF: Initial: 3.125mg bid for 2 weeks. Titrate: May double dose every ≥2 weeks up to 25mg bid as tolerated. Max: 50mg bid if >85kg. Reduce dose if HR <55 beats/min. HTN: Initial: 6.25mg bid for 7-14 days. Titrate: May double dose at 7-14 day intervals. Max: 50mg/day. LVD Post-MI: Initial: 6.25mg bid for 3-10 days. Titrate: May double dose q3-10 days. Target dose: 25mg bid. May begin with 3.125mg bid and/or slow up-titration rate if clinically indicated. (Cap, ER) CHF: Initial: 10mg qd for 2 weeks. Titrate: May double dose every ≥2 weeks up to 80mg qd as tolerated. Reduce dose if HR <55 beats/min. HTN: Initial: 20mg qd for 7-14 days. Titrate: May double dose q7-14 days as tolerated. Max: 80mg/day. LVD Post-MI: Initial: 20mg qd for 3-10 days. Titrate: May double dose q3-10 days. Target dose: 80mg qd. May begin with 10mg qd and/or slow up-titration if clinically indicated. Elderly: Start at lower end of dosing range when switching from higher doses of immediate release; may titrate after ≥2 weeks. Take caps in am. Monitor dose increases. Minimize fluid retention prior to initiation.

HOW SUPPLIED: Tab: 3.125mg, 6.25mg, 12.5mg, 25mg; Cap, Extended-Release: 10mg, 20mg, 40mg, 80mg

CONTRAINDICATIONS: Bronchial asthma or related bronchospastic conditions, 2nd- or 3rd-degree atrioventricular (AV) block, sick sinus syndrome, severe bradycardia (without permanent pacemaker), cardiogenic shock, decompensated heart failure requiring IV inotropic therapy, severe hepatic impairment.

WARNINGS/PRECAUTIONS: Severe exacerbation of angina, MI, and ventricular arrhythmias reported with abrupt d/c; whenever possible, d/c over 1-2 weeks. Bradycardia reported. Hypotension, postural hypotension, and syncope reported, most commonly during up-titration period; avoid driving or hazardous tasks. May mask signs of hypoglycemia and hyperthyroidism (eg, tachycardia). Monitor renal function during up-titration with low BP (systolic blood pressure [SBP] <100mmHg), ischemic heart disease, diffuse vascular disease, and/or renal insufficiency. Worsening heart failure or fluid retention may occur during up-titration. Caution in pheochromocytoma, peripheral vascular disease (PVD), Prinzmetal's variant angina, and bronchospastic disease. May be more reactive to repeated challenge with history of severe anaphylactic reaction to variety of allergens; may be unresponsive to usual doses of epinephrine. Intraoperative Floppy Iris Syndrome (IFIS) observed during cataract surgery. (Tab) Chronically administered β-blocking therapy should not be routinely withdrawn prior to major surgery.

ADVERSE REACTIONS: Bradycardia, fatigue, hypotension, dizziness, headache, diarrhea, N/V, hyperglycemia, weight increase, increased cough, asthenia, angina pectoris, syncope, edema.

INTERACTIONS: May increase levels with potent CYP2D6 inhibitors (eg, quinidine, fluoxetine, paroxetine, propafenone). Monitor for hypotension and bradycardia with catecholamine-depleting agents (eg, reserpine, MAOIs). BP- and HR-lowering effects potentiated with clonidine. Reduced plasma levels with rifampin. Increased AUC with cimetidine. Conduction disturbances seen with diltiazem; monitor ECG and BP with verapamil and diltiazem. May enhance blood glucose-reducing effect of insulin and oral hypoglycemics; monitor blood glucose. May increase concentration of cyclosporine. Monitor levels of cyclosporine and digoxin. Caution with anesthetic agents that may depress myocardial function (eg, ether, cyclopropane, trichloroethylene). Digitalis glycosides and β-blockers slow AV conduction and decrease HR; concomitant use can increase the risk of bradycardia. Amiodarone or other CYP2C9 inhibitors (eg, fluconazole) may enhance β-blocking properties resulting in further slowing of the HR or cardiac conduction. Additive effects and exaggerated orthostatic component with diuretics.

PREGNANCY: Category C, not for use in nursing.

MECHANISM OF ACTION: Nonselective β-adrenergic and $α_1$ blocker.

PHARMACOKINETICS: Absorption: (Tab) Rapid and extensive; absolute bio-availability (25-35%). (Cap, ER) T_{max}=5 hrs. **Distribution:** Plasma protein binding (>98%); V_d=115L. **Metabolism:** Extensive by oxidation and glucuronidation; CYP2D6, 2C9 (primary); CYP3A4, 2C19, 1A2, 2E1 (minor); 3 active metabolites. **Elimination:** Urine (<2% unchanged), feces; $T_{1/2}$=7-10 hrs.

NURSING CONSIDERATIONS

Assessment: Assess for bronchial asthma, bronchospastic disease, AV block, sick sinus syndrome, severe bradycardia, cardiogenic shock, decompensated heart failure requiring IV inotropic therapy, severe hepatic impairment, diabetes mellitus (DM), Prinzmetal's variant angina, coronary artery disease (CAD), hypotension, ischemic heart disease, diffuse vascular disease, pheochromocytoma, PVD, hyperthyroidism, renal impairment, pregnancy/nursing status, and possible drug interactions. Assess for history of serious hypersensitivity reaction. Obtain baseline blood glucose levels, LFTs, and renal function. Assess for any upcoming surgery.

Monitoring: Monitor blood glucose during initiation/dosage adjustments, and upon d/c of therapy. Monitor LFTs and renal function. Monitor for bradycardia, signs/symptoms of cardiac failure, hyperglycemia, masking of hypoglycemia/hyperthyroidism, withdrawal symptoms, precipitation or aggravation of arterial insufficiency, hypotension, and hypersensitivity reactions. Monitor for IFIS during cataract surgery.

Patient Counseling: Instruct not to d/c or interrupt therapy without consulting physician. Instruct patients with heart failure to consult physician if signs/symptoms of worsening heart failure (eg, weight gain, increasing SOB) occur. Inform that a drop in BP when standing, resulting in dizziness and, rarely, fainting, may be experienced; advise to sit or lie down. Advise to avoid driving or hazardous tasks if experiencing dizziness or fatigue and to notify physician if dizziness or faintness occurs. Inform contact lens wearers that decreased lacrimation may be experienced, diabetic patients to report any changes in blood sugar levels, and to take with food. (Cap, ER) Advise not to divide, chew, or crush.

Administration: Oral route. Take with food. (Cap, ER) Swallow caps whole or may open and sprinkle contents on applesauce. Do not chew, crush, or divide. **Storage:** (Tab) <30°C (86°F). Protect from moisture. (Cap, ER) 25°C (77°F); excursions permitted to 15-30°C (59-86°F).

CORTISPORIN-TC OTIC   RX

hydrocortisone acetate - thonzonium bromide - neomycin sulfate - colistin sulfate (JHP Pharmaceuticals, LLC)

THERAPEUTIC CLASS: Antibacterial/corticosteroid combination

INDICATIONS: Treatment of superficial bacterial infections of the external auditory canal and infections of mastoidectomy and fenestration cavities, caused by susceptible organisms.

DOSAGE: *Adults:* Instill 5 drops into affected ear tid or qid.
Pediatrics: ≥1 yr: Instill 4 drops into affected ear tid or qid.

HOW SUPPLIED: Sus: (Colistin-Hydrocortisone-Neomycin-Thonzonium bromide) 3mg-10mg-3.3mg-0.5mg/mL [10mL]

CONTRAINDICATIONS: External auditory disorder suspected or due to cutaneous viral infection (eg, herpes simplex virus, varicella zoster virus).

WARNINGS/PRECAUTIONS: Prolonged treatment may result in overgrowth of nonsusceptible organisms or fungi; verify causative organism with culture studies if infection does not improve after a week. Limit therapy to 10 days. Neomycin: Sensorineural hearing loss due to cochlear damage may occur; risk is greater with prolonged use. Caution in patients with perforated tympanic membranes. May cause cutaneous sensitization. Examine periodically for redness with swelling, dry scaling and itching, or failure to heal; d/c if observed. Allergic cross-reactions may occur. Hydrocortisone: Excessive systemic levels of hydrocortisone may reduce number of circulating eosinophils and urinary excretion of 17-hydroxycorticosteroids. D/C if sensitivity or irritation occurs. Do not heat above body temperature to avoid loss of potency.

ADVERSE REACTIONS: Skin sensitization, ototoxicity, allergic skin reactions, burning, itching, irritation, dryness, folliculitis, hypertrichosis, acneiform eruptions, hypopigmentation, perioral dermatitis, maceration of the skin.

PREGNANCY: Category C, caution in nursing.

MECHANISM OF ACTION: Colistin: Polypeptide antibiotic; penetrates into and disrupts bacterial cell membrane. Neomycin sulfate: Aminoglycoside antibiotic; inhibits protein synthesis, disrupting the normal cycle of ribosomal function. Hydrocortisone acetate: Corticosteroid hormone; regulates rate of protein synthesis, controls inflammation, inhibit the body's defense mechanism against infection. Thonzonium bromide: surface active agent; promotes tissue contact by dispersion and penetration of the cellular debris and exudate.

NURSING CONSIDERATIONS

Assessment: Assess for external auditory canal disease (viral/nonviral), perforated tympanic membrane, drug hypersensitivity and pregnancy/nursing status.

Monitoring: Monitor for sensorineural hearing loss, cutaneous sensitization or irritation (eg, redness with swelling, dry scaling, itching). Monitor for persistence of infection >1 week.

Patient Counseling: Instruct regarding proper use; avoid contaminating the dropper. D/C use and contact physician if sensitization or irritation occurs. Counsel on proper application; do not use in the eyes. Instruct to notify physician if pregnant, plan to become pregnant or breastfeeding.

Administration: Otic route. Clean and dry ear canal with sterile cotton before application. Lie down with affected ear upward, instill drops, and maintain position for 5 mins to ensure penetration into ear canal. If preferred, insert cotton wick saturated with suspension into canal; keep moist by adding further solution every 4 hrs and replace wick at least once every 24 hrs. Shake well before using. **Storage:** 20-25°C (68-77°F).

CORVERT   RX
ibutilide fumarate (Pharmacia & Upjohn)

Can cause potentially fatal arrhythmias, particularly sustained polymorphic ventricular tachycardia, usually in association with QT prolongation (torsades de pointes), but sometimes without documented QT prolongation. Administer in a setting of continuous ECG monitoring and by personnel trained in identification and treatment of acute ventricular arrhythmias. Patients with atrial fibrillation of more than 2 to 3 days' duration must be adequately anticoagulated, generally for at least 2 weeks. Patients should be carefully selected such that the expected benefits of maintaining sinus rhythm outweigh the immediate and maintenance therapy risks.

THERAPEUTIC CLASS: Class III antiarrhythmic

INDICATIONS: For rapid conversion of atrial fibrillation or flutter (A-Fib/Flutter) of recent onset to sinus rhythm.

DOSAGE: *Adults:* ≥60kg: 1mg over 10 min. <60kg: 0.01mg/kg over 10 min. If arrhythmia still present within 10 min after the end of the initial infusion, repeat infusion 10 min after completion of 1st infusion.

HOW SUPPLIED: Inj: 0.1mg/mL

WARNINGS/PRECAUTIONS: Proarrhythmic; can cause potentially fatal arrhythmias. Administer in setting with continuous ECG monitoring and person able to treat acute ventricular arrhythmia. Adequately anticoagulate if A-Fib >2-3 days. Correct hypokalemia and hypomagnesemia before therapy. Caution in elderly.

ADVERSE REACTIONS: Sustained and nonsustained polymorphic ventricular tachycardia, sustained and nonsustained monomorphic ventricular tachycardia, bundle branch and AV block, ventricular and supraventricular extrasystoles, hypotension, bradycardia.

INTERACTIONS: Avoid Class IA (eg, disopyramide, quinidine, procainamide) and other Class III (eg, amiodarone, sotalol) antiarrhythmics with or within 4 hrs postinfusion of ibutilide. Increase proarrhythmia potential with drugs that prolong the QT interval (eg, phenothiazines, TCAs). Supraventricular arrhythmias may mask cardiotoxicity associated with excessive digoxin levels.

PREGNANCY: Category C, not for use in nursing.

MECHANISM OF ACTION: Class III antiarrhythmic agent; prolongs atrial and ventricular action potential duration and refractoriness. Delays repolarization by activation of a slow, inward current, rather than blocking outward potassium currents.

PHARMACOKINETICS: Distribution: V_d=11 L/kg; plasma protein binding (40%). **Metabolism:** Omega-oxidation and β-oxidation; omega-hydroxy metabolite (active). **Elimination:** Urine 82% (7% unchanged), feces (19%); $T_{1/2}$=6 hrs.

NURSING CONSIDERATIONS

Assessment: Assess for arrhythmia, bradycardia, hypokalemia, renal/hepatic impairment, and possible drug interactions.

Monitoring: Monitor for worsening of induction of new ventricular arrhythmia, torsade de pointes (a polymorphic ventricular tachycardia), and HR.

Patient Counseling: Inform about benefits/risks. Report any adverse reactions to physician. Patients with chronic A-Fib of ≥2-3 days duration must be adequately anticoagulated for at least 2 weeks. May cause potentially fatal arrhythmia, particularly sustained polymorphic ventricular tachycardia.

Administration: IV route. **Storage:** 20-25°C (68-77°F).

COSOPT   RX
dorzolamide HCl - timolol maleate (Merck)

THERAPEUTIC CLASS: Carbonic anhydrase inhibitor/nonselective beta-blocker

INDICATIONS: Reduction of elevated intraocular pressure (IOP) in patients with ocular HTN or open-angle glaucoma who are insufficiently responsive to β-blockers.

DOSAGE: *Adults:* 1 drop bid. Space dosing of other ophthalmic drugs by 10 min.

HOW SUPPLIED: Sol: (Dorzolamide-Timolol) 2%-0.5% [10mL]

CONTRAINDICATIONS: Bronchial asthma, history of bronchial asthma, severe chronic obstructive pulmonary disease (COPD), sinus bradycardia, 2nd- or 3rd-degree AV block, overt cardiac failure, cardiogenic shock.

WARNINGS/PRECAUTIONS: Caution with sulfonamide allergy, cardiac failure, diabetic patients (especially those with labile diabetes), major surgery, hepatic impairment, and patients suspected of developing thyrotoxicosis. May mask symptoms of acute hypoglycemia and certain clinical signs of hyperthyroidism (eg, tachycardia). Bacterial keratitis reported with contaminated containers. Avoid in severe renal impairment (CrCl <30mL/min). D/C if hypersensitivity or ocular reactions occur. Choroidal detachment after filtration procedures reported. Potentiation of muscle weakness consistent with myasthenic symptoms (eg, diplopia, ptosis, and generalized weakness) reported. Caution in patients with low endothelial cell counts.

ADVERSE REACTIONS: Taste perversion, ocular burning/stinging, conjunctival hyperemia, blurred vision, superficial punctate keratitis, eye itching.

INTERACTIONS: Avoid oral carbonic anhydrase inhibitors, oral β-blockers, or topical β-blockers due to potential additive effects. Oral/IV calcium antagonists can cause atrioventricular (AV)-conduction disturbances, left ventricular failure or hypotension; avoid with impaired cardiac function. Potentiated systemic β-blockade with concomitant CYP2D6 inhibitors (eg, quinidine, SSRIs). Close observation of patients with catecholamine-depleting drugs (eg, reserpine). AV conduction time prolonged with digitalis. Increased risk of hypoglycemia with insulin or oral hypoglycemic agents. Caution with high dose salicylate therapy.

PREGNANCY: Category C, not for use in nursing.

MECHANISM OF ACTION: Dorzolamide: Carbonic anhydrase inhibitor; decreases aqueous humor secretion, presumably by slowing formation of bicarbonate ions with subsequent reduction in Na^+ and fluid transport. Timolol: β_1 and β_2 (non-selective) adrenergic receptor blocking agent; decreases elevated IOP by reducing aqueous humor secretion.

PHARMACOKINETICS: Absorption: Timolol: C_{max}=0.46ng/mL. **Distribution:** Dorzolamide: Plasma protein binding (33%). Timolol: Found in breast milk. **Elimination:** Dorzolamide: Urine (unchanged).

NURSING CONSIDERATIONS

Assessment: Assess for history of bronchial asthma, severe COPD, sinus bradycardia, 2nd- or 3rd-degree AV block, overt cardiac failure, and cardiogenic shock. Assess sulfonamide allergy, use in elective surgery, risk for hypoglycemia with diabetes mellitus, with hyperthyroidism, acute angle-closure glaucoma, severe renal impairment (CrCl <30mL/min), hepatic impairment, in pregnancy/nursing, and for possible drug interactions.

Monitoring: Monitor for improvement in IOP, ocular HTN, signs/symptoms of anaphylaxis, primary conjunctivitis and lid reactions with chronic therapy, and bacterial keratitis with use of multi-dose containers.

Patient Counseling: Contact physician immediately if any type of cardiac, respiratory, or anaphylactic reactions occur. Advise to d/c and report if ocular reactions (eg, conjunctivitis, lid reactions) occur. Instruct to handle solution properly. Instruct not to touch container tip to eye or surrounding structures; may become contaminated. Advise to immediately contact physician concerning use of present multidose container if undergoing ocular surgery or a concomitant ocular condition (eg, trauma, infection) develops. Remove contact lenses prior to administration; may be reinserted 15 min after. Administer at least 10 min apart if using other ophthalmic medications. Contains dorzolamide (a sulfonamide); advise to d/c use if serious/unusual reactions or hypersensitivity occurs.

Administration: Ocular route. 1) Tilt head back and pull lower eyelid down to form pocket between eyelid and eye. 2) Invert bottle and press lightly until single drop is released. **Storage:** 15-30°C (59-86°F). Protect from light.

COUMADIN   RX
warfarin sodium (Bristol-Myers Squibb)

> May cause major or fatal bleeding; monitor INR regularly. Patients should be instructed about prevention measures to minimize risk of bleeding and to report immediately if signs and symptoms of bleeding occur.

OTHER BRAND NAMES: Jantoven (Upsher-Smith)

THERAPEUTIC CLASS: Vitamin K-dependent coagulation factor inhibitor

INDICATIONS: Prophylaxis and treatment of venous thrombosis and its extension, pulmonary embolism (PE), and thromboembolic complications associated with atrial fibrillation (AF) and/or cardiac valve replacement. To reduce risk of death, recurrent myocardial infarction (MI), and thromboembolic events such as stroke or systemic embolization after MI.

C

DOSAGE: *Adults:* Individualize dose. Adjust dose based on PT/INR. Give IV as alternate to PO. Initial: 2-5mg qd. Maintenance: 2-10mg qd. Venous Thromboembolism (including deep vein thrombosis (DVT) and PE): Target INR 2.5 (INR Range, 2-3). Atrial Fibrillation: INR 2-3. Post-MI: INR 2.5-3.5. Mechanical/Bioprosthetic Heart Valve: St. Jude Medical Bileaflet Valve in the Aortic Position: Target INR: 2.5 (INR Range, 2-3). Tilting Disk Valves and Bileaflet Mechanical Valves in the Mitral Position: Target INR: 3 (INR Range, 2.5-3.5). Caged Ball or Caged Disk Valve: Target INR 3 (INR Range, 2.5-3.5) in combination with ASA, 75-100mg/day. Bioprosthetic Valves in the Mitral and Aortic Position: Target INR: 2.5 (INR Range, 2-3). Valvular Heart Disease Associated with Atrial Fibrillation/Mitral Stenosis/Recurrent Systemic Embolism of Unknown Etiology: INR 2-3. Elderly/Debilitated: Start at the low end of dosing range. Refer to PI for recommended durations.

HOW SUPPLIED: Inj: (Coumadin) 5mg; Tab: (Coumadin, Jantoven) 1mg*, 2mg*, 2.5mg*, 3mg*, 4mg*, 5mg*, 6mg*, 7.5mg*, 10mg* *scored

CONTRAINDICATIONS: Pregnancy. Hemorrhagic tendencies or blood dyscrasias. Recent or contemplated surgery of the central nervous system, eye, or traumatic surgery resulting in large open surfaces. Bleeding tendencies associated with active ulceration or overt bleeding of GI/genitourinary/respiratory tract, cerebrovascular hemorrhage, cerebral aneurysms, dissecting aorta, pericarditis and pericardial effusions, bacterial endocarditis. Threatened abortion, eclampsia, and preeclampsia. Inadequate laboratory facilities. Unsupervised patients with senility, alcoholism, or psychosis or other lack of patient cooperation. Spinal puncture and other diagnostic/therapeutic procedures with potential for uncontrollable bleeding. Major regional, lumbar block anesthesia, and malignant HTN.

WARNINGS/PRECAUTIONS: Monitor PT/INR; many endogenous and exogenous factors may affect PT/INR. Risk of hemorrhage, necrosis and/or gangrene of the skin and other tissues which may result in death or permanent disability; perform careful diagnosis to determine whether necrosis is caused by underlying disease or warfarin therapy. D/C if warfarin suspected to be the cause of necrosis. Individualize therapy. Caution in any predisposing condition where added risk of hemorrhage, necrosis, and/or gangrene is present. D/C if systemic cholesterol microembolization ("purple toes syndrome") occurs. Caution in patients with heparin-induced thrombocytopenia and DVT; cases of venous limb ischemia, necrosis, and gangrene reported when heparin d/c and warfarin started or continued. Weigh benefits/risks of therapy with lactation, severe to moderate hepatic or renal insufficiency, infectious diseases, disturbances of the intestinal flora, trauma which may result in internal bleeding, surgery or trauma resulting in large exposed raw surfaces, indwelling catheters, severe to moderate HTN, protein C deficiency, polycythemia vera, vasculitis, and severe diabetes. Caution in the elderly.

ADVERSE REACTIONS: Fatal or non-fatal hemorrhage from any tissue or organ, necrosis of the skin and other tissues, paralysis, paresthesia, headache, chest/abdomen/joint/muscle pain, dizziness, shortness of breath, difficulty breathing or swallowing, unexplained swelling, weakness, hypotension, unexplained shock.

INTERACTIONS: May interact with protein-bound drugs, hepatic enzyme inducers and inhibitors. Caution with drugs that may cause hemorrhage (eg, NSAIDs, ASA), botanicals. Some botanicals (eg, bromelains, danshen, garlic, gingko biloba, ginseng, cranberry products) may increase coumadin effects; others (eg, coenzyme Q$_{10}$, St. John's wort) may decrease effects. May potentiate hypoglycemic and anticonvulsant drugs. May interact with antihyperlipidemic drugs like ezetimibe, thrombolytics, and many other drug classes. Concomitant administration with ticlopidine may be associated with cholestatic hepatitis. Refer to PI for extensive list of drug interactions.

PREGNANCY: Category X, safety not known in nursing.

MECHANISM OF ACTION: Vitamin K-dependent coagulation factor inhibitor; interferes with clotting factor synthesis by inhibition of the C1 subunit of the vitamin K epoxide reductase enzyme complex, thereby reducing the regeneration of vitamin K$_1$ epoxide.

PHARMACOKINETICS: Absorption: (PO) Complete; T_{max}=4 hrs. **Distribution:** V_d=0.14L/kg; plasma protein binding (99%); crosses placenta, found in fetal plasma. **Metabolism:** Hepatic via CYP2C9, 2C19, 2C8, 2C18, 1A2, 3A4. **Elimination:** Urine (92%, metabolites), bile (metabolites); $T_{1/2}$=1 week.

NURSING CONSIDERATIONS

Assessment: Assess pregnancy status, presence of hemorrhagic tendencies or blood dyscrasias, bleeding tendencies and any other conditions where treatment is contraindicated or cautioned. Assess PT/INR, drug and drug-disease interactions.

Monitoring: Monitor for signs/symptoms of bleeding, necrosis of the skin and other organs, and systemic atheroemboli or cholesterol microemboli (eg, "purple toes syndrome," livedo reticularis, rash). Perform periodic monitor PT/INR testing.

Patient Counseling: Counsel to maintain strict adherence to dosing regimen. Advise not to start or stop other medication, including salicylates (eg, aspirin, topical analgesics), over-the-counter drugs, or herbal medications except on advice of physician. Avoid any activity or sport that may result in traumatic injury. Inform of pregnancy risks. Instruct that regular PT tests are required during therapy. Advice patient to carry ID card stating drug is being taken. Inform that vitamin K in diet may affect medication. Instruct to eat normal, balanced diet; avoid drastic changes in diet such as eating large amounts of leafy green vegetables. Avoid alcohol consumption, cranberry juice, and cranberry products. Contact physician if dose is missed and to take missed dose as soon as possible on the same day, but not to double dose the next day. Contact physician to report any illness, such as diarrhea, infection or fever. Advise to immediately report unusual bleeding (eg, pain, swelling or discomfort, prolonged bleeding from cuts, increased menstrual flow or vaginal bleeding, nosebleeds, bleeding of gums from brushing, unusual bleeding or bruising, red or dark brown urine, red or tar black stools, headache, dizziness, or weakness). If warfarin is d/c'd, anticoagulant effects may persist for about 2 to 5 days. Inform that all warfarin sodium products represent the same medication. Keep out of reach of children.

Administration: (Coumadin, Jantoven) Oral or (Coumadin) IV route. IV: Reconstitute with 2.7mL sterile water for inj to yield 2mg/mL. Administer as slow bolus injection over 1-2 mins into a peripheral vein. Not for IM use.

Storage: Tab: (Coumadin) 15-30°C (59-86°F). Dispense in tight, light-resistant container. (Jantoven) 20-25°C (68-77°F); excursions permitted 15-30°C (59-86°F). Keep tightly closed. Protect from light and moisture; dispense in tight, light-resistant container. Inj: (Coumadin) 15-30°C (59-86°F). Use within 4 hrs after reconstitution. Do not refrigerate. Discard any unused solution.

COVERA-HS   RX
verapamil HCl (G.D. Searle)

THERAPEUTIC CLASS: Calcium channel blocker (nondihydropyridine)

INDICATIONS: Management of hypertension and angina.

DOSAGE: *Adults:* Individualize by titration. Initial: 180mg qhs. Titrate: If inadequate response with 180mg, increase to 240mg qhs, then 360mg qhs, then 480mg qhs. Elderly: Start at the low end of the dosing range. Swallow whole; do not chew, break, or crush.

HOW SUPPLIED: Tab, Extended-Release: 180mg, 240mg

CONTRAINDICATIONS: Severe left ventricular dysfunction (LVD), hypotension (systolic pressure <90mm Hg), cardiogenic shock, sick sinus syndrome, 2nd- or 3rd-degree AV block (except with functioning artificial ventricular pacemaker), atrial fibrillation/flutter and an accessory bypass tract (eg, Wolff-Parkinson-White [WPW], Lown-Ganong-Levine syndromes).

WARNINGS/PRECAUTIONS: Congestive heart failure (CHF) or pulmonary edema may develop; avoid with severe LVD (eg, ejection fraction <30%) or moderate to severe symptoms of cardiac failure and any degree of ventricular dysfunction if taking β-blockers. Hypotension, AV block, transient bradycardia, PR interval prolongation may occur. Elevated transaminases (eg, elevations in alkaline phosphate, SGOT, SGPT, and bilirubin) have been reported; monitor LFTs periodically. Hepatocellular injury reported. Caution with impaired hepatic function; give 30% of normal dose with severe hepatic dysfunction. Caution with renal impairment; monitor for abnormal PR interval prolongation. Reduce dose with decreased neuromuscular transmission. Sinus bradycardia, 2nd-degree AV block, pulmonary edema, hypotension, and sinus arrest reported in patients with hypertrophic cardiomyopathy. Ventricular fibrillation occurred in patients with atrial fibrillation/flutter and an accessory bypass tract. May cause worsening of myasthenia gravis. Caution with severe GI narrowing and in elderly.

ADVERSE REACTIONS: Constipation, dizziness, headache, edema, fatigue, sinus bradycardia, 2nd-degree AV block, upper respiratory infection.

INTERACTIONS: Additive negative effects on HR, AV conduction, and/or cardiac contractility with β-blockers. Asymptomatic bradycardia (36 beats/min) with a wandering atrial pacemaker observed with timolol eyedrops. May decrease metoprolol and propranolol clearance. Variable effects with atenolol. Potentiates other oral antihypertensive agents (eg, vasodilators, ACE inhibitors, diuretics). May increase digoxin, carbamazepine, theophylline, cyclosporine, and alcohol levels. Avoid disopyramide within 48 hrs before or 24 hrs after administration. May reduce clearance of digitoxin. Additive negative inotropic effects and AV conduction prolongation with flecainide. Avoid quinidine with hypertrophic cardiomyopathy. Increased sensitivity to neurotoxic effects of lithium reported with concomitant use; monitor lithium levels. CYP3A4 inhibitors (eg, erythromycin, ritonavir) and grapefruit juice may increase levels. CYP3A4 inducers (eg, rifampin) may decrease levels. Increased bleeding time with aspirin reported. May potentiate neuromuscular blockers (curare-like and depolarizing); both agents may need dose reduction. Caution with inhalation anesthetics. Hypotension and bradyarrhythmias observed with telithromycin. Reduced or unchanged clearance with cimetidine. Sinus bradycardia resulting in hospitalization and pacemaker insertion has been reported with concurrent use with clonidine; monitor HR. Excessive reduction in BP with prazosin observed. Phenobarbital may increase clearance. Rifampin may reduce oral bioavailability. Prolonged recovery from neuromuscular blocking agent vecuronium.

PREGNANCY: Category C, not for use in nursing.

MECHANISM OF ACTION: Calcium channel blocker (nondihydropyridine); selectively inhibits transmembrane influx of calcium ions into arterial smooth muscle and conductile/contractile myocardial cells without altering serum calcium concentrations.

PHARMACOKINETICS: Absorption: T_{max}=11 hrs. Bioavailability (33-65%, R-verapamil), (13-34%, S-verapamil). Oral administration of variable doses resulted in different pharmacokinetic parameters. **Distribution:** Plasma protein binding (94% to albumin and 92% to α-1 acid glycoprotein, R-verapamil), (88% to albumin and 86% to α-1 acid glycoprotein, S-verapamil). Found breast milk; crosses placenta. **Metabolism:** Liver (extensive); norverapamil (active metabolite). **Elimination:** Urine (70%, metabolites), (3-4%, unchanged), feces (≥16%).

NURSING CONSIDERATIONS

Assessment: Assess for left ventricular dysfunction, hypotension, sick sinus syndrome, AV block, atrial flutter/fibrillation with accessory bypass tract (eg, WPW), hypertrophic cardiomyopathy, severe GI narrowing, hepatic/renal impairment, hypersensitivity to drug, pregnancy/nursing status, and possible drug interactions.

Monitoring: Monitor LFTs and renal function, abnormal PR interval prolongation (toxicity), hepatotoxicity, renal dysfunction, cardiovascular (CV) events (eg, hypotension), and hypersensitivity reactions.

Patient Counseling: Instruct to swallow tab whole; do not chew, break, or crush. Advise to seek medical attention if symptoms of hepatotoxicity (malaise, fever, right upper quadrant pain), CV events (hypotension), or hypersensitivity reactions occur. Inform that outer shell of tablet does not dissolve; may occasionally be observed in stool. Counsel not to breastfeed and to report immediately if pregnant.

Administration: Oral route. **Storage:** 20-25°C (68-77°F). Keep in tight, light-resistant container.

COZAAR

RX

losartan potassium (Merck)

> Can cause death/injury to developing fetus during 2nd and 3rd trimesters. D/C therapy if pregnancy detected.

THERAPEUTIC CLASS: Angiotensin II receptor antagonist

INDICATIONS: Treatment of HTN, alone or with other antihypertensives. Reduce the risk of stroke in patients with HTN and left ventricular hypertrophy (LVH) (may not apply to black patients). Treatment of diabetic nephropathy with an elevated SrCr and proteinuria (urinary albumin to creatinine ratio ≥300mg/g) in patients with type 2 diabetes and a history of HTN.

DOSAGE: *Adults:* HTN: Individualize dose. Initial: 50mg qd. Usual: 25-100mg/day given qd-bid. Intravascular Volume Depletion/Hepatic Impairment: Initial: 25mg qd. HTN with LVH: Initial: 50mg qd. Add hydrochlorothiazide (HCTZ) 12.5mg qd and/or increase losartan to 100mg qd, followed by an increase in HCTZ to 25mg qd based on BP response. Diabetic Nephropathy: Initial: 50 mg qd. Titrate: Increase to 100mg qd based on BP response.
Pediatrics: ≥6 yrs: HTN: Initial: 0.7mg/kg qd (up to 50mg total). Adjust dose according to BP response. Max: 1.4mg/kg qd (or 100mg qd).

HOW SUPPLIED: Tab: 25mg, 50mg, 100mg

WARNINGS/PRECAUTIONS: Symptomatic hypotension may occur in patients who are intravascularly volume-depleted; correct volume depletion before therapy or start therapy at a lower dose. Hypersensitivity including angioedema reported. Consider dose adjustment with hepatic dysfunction. Changes in renal function may occur. Caution with severe congestive heart failure (CHF). Oliguria, and/or progressive azotemia and rarely acute renal failure and/or death reported. Caution with unilateral or bilateral renal artery stenosis; may increase serum creatinine and BUN. Electrolyte imbalances may occur in patients with renal impairment, with or without diabetes. Caution in type 2 diabetics with proteinuria; hyperkalemia reported. Not recommended in pediatrics with GFR <30mL/min/1.73m^2 and <6 yrs.

ADVERSE REACTIONS: Fetal injury, dizziness, cough, upper respiratory infection, diarrhea, asthenia/fatigue, chest pain, anemia, hypoglycemia, back pain, sinusitis, nasal congestion, muscle cramp, leg pain.

INTERACTIONS: Concomitant use with K$^+$-sparing diuretics (eg, spironolactone, triamterene, amiloride), K$^+$ supplements, or K$^+$-containing salt substitutes may increase serum K$^+$. May reduce excretion of lithium; monitor lithium levels. Combination with NSAIDs, including cyclooxygenase-2 (COX-2) inhibitors, may lead to further deterioration of renal function and attenuate antihypertensive effect. Increased levels with cimetidine, fluconazole and erythromycin. Decreased levels with phenobarbital and rifampin. Symptomatic hypotension may occur with diuretics.

PREGNANCY: Category C (1st trimester) and D (2nd and 3rd trimesters), not for use in nursing.

MECHANISM OF ACTION: Angiotensin II receptor antagonist; blocks vasoconstrictor and aldosterone-secreting effects of angiontensin II by selectively blocking the binding of angiotensin II to AT$_1$ receptor in many tissues (eg, vascular smooth muscle, adrenal gland).

PHARMACOKINETICS: Absorption: Well-absorbed. Administration of variable doses resulted in different pharmacokinetic parameters. **Distribution:** Plasma protein binding (98.7%, 99.8% [metabolite]). V$_d$=34L, 12L (metabolite). **Metabolism:** Liver via CYP2C9, 3A4; carboxylic acid (active metabolite). **Elimination:** Urine (4% unchanged, 6% [metabolite]); T$_{1/2}$=2 hrs, 6-9 hrs (metabolite).

NURSING CONSIDERATIONS

Assessment: Assess for volume depletion (eg, diuretic therapy), CHF, diabetes mellitus, unilateral or bilateral renal artery stenosis, hepatic/renal impairment, history of hypersensitivity, pregnancy/nursing status and possible drug interactions. Obtain baseline SrCr, BUN and serum electrolytes.

Monitoring: Monitor BP, serum electrolytes and renal function periodically. Monitor for signs/symptoms of electrolyte imbalance, hypotension, hypersensitivity reactions (eg, angioedema), oliguria, azotemia, renal failure, hyperkalemia, renal/hepatic dysfunction. Perform serial ultrasound examinations and fetal testing to pregnant patients under therapy.

Patient Counseling: Inform of pregnancy risks and instruct to report pregnancy to their physician immediately. Instruct patients not to use K⁺ supplements or salt substitutes containing K⁺ without consulting prescribing physician. Advise to seek medical attention if symptoms of electrolyte imbalance, hypotension, or hypersensitivity reactions (eg, angioedema) occur.

Administration: Oral route. Refer to PI for preparation of suspension. **Storage:** Tab: 25°C (77°F); excursions permitted to 15-30°C (59-86°F). Protect from light. Sus: 2-8°C (36-46°F) for up to 4 weeks.

CREON   RX
pancrelipase (Solvay)

THERAPEUTIC CLASS: Pancreatic enzyme supplement

INDICATIONS: Treatment of exocrine pancreatic insufficiency due to cystic fibrosis, chronic pancreatitis, pancreatectomy or other conditions.

DOSAGE: *Adults:* Individualize dose. Initial: 500 lipase U/kg/meal. Titrate: May increase dose based on clinical symptoms, degree of steatorrhea present, and fat content of diet. Max: 2,500 U lipase/kg/meal (≤10,000 lipase U/kg/day) or <4,000 lipase U/g fat ingested/day. Approximately half the dose used for meals should be given with each snack. Swallow whole; do not crush or chew. *Pediatrics:* Individualize dose. ≥4 yrs: Initial: 500 lipase U/kg/meal. Max: 2,500 lipase U/kg/meal (≤10,000 lipase U/kg/day) or <4,000 lipase U/g fat ingested/day. Approximately half the dose used for meals should be given with each snack. >12 months-<4 yrs: Initial: 1,000 lipase U/kg/meal. Max: 2,500 lipase U/kg/meal (≤10,000 lipase U/kg/day) or <4,000 lipase U/g fat ingested/day. Titrate: May increase dose based on clinical symptoms, degree of steatorrhea present, and fat content of diet. Infants-12 months: 2,000-4,000 lipase U/120mL of formula or/breastfeeding.

HOW SUPPLIED: Cap, Delayed-Release: (Amylase-Lipase-Protease) (Creon 1206) 30,000 U-6,000 U-19,000 U; (Creon 1212) 60,000 U-12,000 U-38,000 U; (Creon 1224) 120,000 U-24,000 U-76,000 U

WARNINGS/PRECAUTIONS: Fibrosing colonopathy reported; monitor closely for progression to stricture formation. Caution in doses >2500 lipase U/kg/meal. When receiving doses >6,000 lipase U/kg/meal, examine patients either immediately decrease dose or titrate downward to a lower range. Caution with gout, renal impairment, or hyperuricemia. May increase blood uric acid levels. Should not be crushed or chewed, or mixed in foods with pH >4.5; may disrupt enteric coating of cap and cause early release of enzymes, cause irritation of the oral mucosa, and/or cause loss of enzyme activity; take care to ensure that no drug is retained in the mouth. Risk for transmission of viral disease, including diseases caused by novel or unidentified viruses. Caution with a known allergy to proteins of porcine origin. Severe allergic reactions including anaphylaxis, asthma, hives, and pruritus may occur. Do not interchange with any other pancrealipase products. May diminish efficacy if contents of cap are mixed directly into formula or breast milk.

ADVERSE REACTIONS: Vomiting, flatulence, abdominal pain, headache, cough, dizziness, frequent bowel movements, abnormal feces, hyperglycemia, hypoglycemia, nasopharyngitis, weight loss.

PREGNANCY: Category C, caution in nursing.

MECHANISM OF ACTION: Pancreatic enzyme supplement; catalyzes the hydrolysis of fats to monoglyceride, glycerol and free fatty acids, proteins into peptides and amino acids, and starch into dextrins and short-chain sugars.

NURSING CONSIDERATIONS

Assessment: Assess for allergy to porcine protein, gout, renal impairment, hyperuricemia, and pregnancy/nursing status.

Monitoring: Monitor for fibrosing colonopathy, colonic stricture, oral mucosa irritation, viral diseases, and for allergic reactions (eg, anaphylaxis, asthma, hives and pruritus). Monitor serum uric acid levels.

Patient Counseling: Instruct to take as prescribed. Counsel to take with food. Instruct to swallow cap whole; instruct not to crush or chew cap or cap contents. Inform that if unable to swallow intact cap, may sprinkle contents of cap on a small amount of acidic soft food (eg, applesauce). Inform that care should be taken to ensure that no drug is retained in the mouth to avoid oral mucosa irritation. Instruct not to mix directly with formula or breast milk. Counsel to contact healthcare professional immediately if an allergic reaction develops.

Administration: Oral route. Administer to infants immediately prior to each feeding. Contents should be administered directly to the mouth or with a small amount of applesauce; avoid mixing directly with formula or breast milk.

Storage: 25°C (77°F); excursions permitted between 25-40°C (77-104°F) for up to 30 days. Discard if exposed to higher temperature and moisture conditions higher than 70%. Keep tightly closed. Protect from moisture.

CRESTOR RX
rosuvastatin calcium (AstraZeneca)

THERAPEUTIC CLASS: HMG-CoA reductase inhibitor

INDICATIONS: Adjunct to diet in primary hyperlipidemia and mixed dyslipidemia to reduce elevated total cholesterol (total-C), LDL, apolipoprotein (ApoB), non-HDL, and TG levels and to increase HDL in adults. Adjunct to diet in adolescent boys and girls, 10-17 yrs old, who are ≥1 year post-menarche (girls) with heterozygous familial hypercholesterolemia to reduce total-C, LDL and ApoB levels. Adjunct to diet for the treatment of hypertriglyceridemia in adults. Adjunct to diet for the treatment of primary dysbetalipoproteinemia (Type III hyperlipoproteinemia). Adjunct to other lipid-lowering treatments (eg, LDL apheresis) or alone if such treatments are unavailable, to reduce LDL, total-C, and ApoB in adult patients with homozygous familial hypercholesterolemia. Adjunct to diet to slow the progression of atherosclerosis in adults as part of a treatment strategy to lower total-C and LDL to target levels. Reduces risk of myocardial infarction, stroke, and arterial revascularization procedures in patients without clinically evident coronary heart disease, but with multiple risk factors.

DOSAGE: *Adults:* General: Initial: 10-20mg qd. Titrate: Analyze lipid levels within 2-4 weeks and adjust dose accordingly. Dosing Range: 5-40mg qd. Use the 40mg dose only if LDL-C goal not achieved with 20mg. Homozygous Familial Hypercholesterolemia: Initial: 20mg qd. Asian Patients: Initial: 5mg qd. Concomitant Cyclosporine: Max: 5mg qd. Concomitant Lopinavir/Ritonavir or Atazanavir/Ritonavir: Max 10mg qd. Concomitant with Niacin/Fenofibrate: Reduce dose. Concomitant Gemfibrozil: Max: 10mg qd. Severe Renal Impairment: (CrCl <30mL/min/1.73m², not on hemodialysis): Initial: 5mg qd. Max: 10mg qd.
Pediatrics: 10-17 yrs: Heterozygous Familial Hypercholesterolemia: Individualize dose. Usual: 5-20mg qd. Titrate: Adjust dose at intervals of ≥4 weeks. Max: 20mg/day.

HOW SUPPLIED: Tab: 5mg, 10mg, 20mg, 40mg

CONTRAINDICATIONS: Active liver disease, including unexplained persistent elevations of hepatic transaminase levels, women who are pregnant or may become pregnant, nursing mothers.

C

WARNINGS/PRECAUTIONS: Cases of myopathy and rhabdomyolysis with acute renal failure secondary to myoglobinuria reported; increased risk at highest dose (40mg). Caution in patients with predisposing factors for myopathy (eg, ≥65 yrs old, inadequately treated hypothyroidism, renal impairment). D/C if markedly elevated creatinine kinase levels occur or myopathy diagnosed or suspected. Withhold with acute, serious condition predisposing to the development of renal failure secondary to rhabdomyolysis (eg, sepsis, hypotension, dehydration, major surgery, trauma, severe metabolic, endocrine and electrolyte disorders, uncontrolled seizures). Increases in serum transaminases (AST, ALT) reported; perform LFTs prior to and at 12 weeks following initiation of therapy and any dose elevation, and periodically thereafter. Reduce dose or d/c if AST/ALT >3X ULN persists. Caution with heavy alcohol use and/or history of chronic liver disease. Dipstick-positive proteinuria and microscopic hematuria observed; consider dose reduction with unexplained persistent proteinuria and/or hematuria. Increase in HbA1c and FPG levels reported. Caution in elderly, renal/hepatic impairment, Asian patients.

ADVERSE REACTIONS: Headache, myalgia, nausea, dizziness, arthralgia, constipation.

INTERACTIONS: Increased risk of myopathy with lipid-lowering therapies (fibrates or niacin), gemfibrozil, cyclosporine, certain protease inhibitors in combination with ritonavir (eg, lopinavir/ritonavir or atazanavir/ritonavir). Prolonged PT/INR with coumarin anticoagulants (eg, warfarin); monitor INR before and frequently during early therapy. Caution with drugs that decrease levels or activity of endogenous steroid hormones (eg, ketoconazole, spironolactone, cimetidine), heavy alcohol use. Decreased levels with aluminum and magnesium hydroxide antacid combo; administer 2 hrs apart.

PREGNANCY: Category X, not for use in nursing.

MECHANISM OF ACTION: HMG-CoA reductase inhibitor; selectively and competitively inhibits enzyme HMG-CoA reductase, hence inhibiting conversion of HMG-CoA to mevalonate, a precursor of cholesterol. Produces its effect by increasing the number of hepatic LDL receptors on the cell-surface to enhance uptake and catabolism of LDL and inhibiting hepatic synthesis of VLDL, which reduces the total number of VLDL and LDL particles

PHARMACOKINETICS: **Absorption:** Absolute bioavailability (20%). T_{max}=3-5 hrs. **Distribution:** V_d=134L, plasma protein binding (88%). **Metabolism:** CYP2C9; N-desmethyl rosuvastatin (major metabolite). **Elimination:** Feces (90%); $T_{1/2}$=19 hrs.

NURSING CONSIDERATIONS

Assessment: Assess for active liver disease, pregnancy/nursing status, and for possible drug interactions, with history of alcohol abuse or have a history of chronic liver disease and in patients with predisposing factors for myopathy (eg, ≥65 yrs, inadequately treated hypothyroidism, renal impairment). Assess LFTs prior to therapy. If taking coumarin type anticoagulant, assess INR prior to therapy.

Monitoring: Monitor for signs/symptoms of myopathy, rhabdomyolysis, increases in serum transaminase levels, and for proteinuria and hematuria (via urinalysis). Monitor creatinine kinase levels. Monitor LFTs 12 weeks after treatment initiation or any dose elevation and then periodically thereafter.

Patient Counseling: Inform about potential risks/benefits of therapy. Instruct to notify physician if pregnant/nursing or planning to become pregnant. Counsel females on appropriate contraceptive methods. Counsel to promptly report any signs of unexplained muscle pain, tenderness or weakness, particularly if accompanied by malaise or fever. Counsel to take at least 2 hrs after antacids containing aluminum and magnesium hydroxide.

Administration: Oral route. **Storage:** 20-25°C (68-77°F). Protect from moisture.

CRIXIVAN   RX
indinavir sulfate (Merck)

THERAPEUTIC CLASS: Protease inhibitor

INDICATIONS: Treatment of HIV infection in combination with other antiretrovirals.

DOSAGE: *Adults:* Usual: 800mg PO q8h. Take without food but with water 1 hr before or 2 hrs after meals. Maintain adequate hydration (1.5L fluid/24 hrs). Mild-Moderate Hepatic insufficiency/Concomitant Delavirdine, Itraconazole, Ketoconazole: Reduce to 600mg PO q8h. Concomitant Didanosine: Administer at least 1 hr apart. Concomitant Rifabutin: 1g PO q8h (reduce rifabutin dose by 1/2).

HOW SUPPLIED: Cap: 100mg, 200mg, 400mg

CONTRAINDICATIONS: Concomitant use with pimozide, cisapride, amiodarone, triazolam, oral midazolam, alprazolam, dihydroergotamine, ergonovine, ergotamine, methylergonovine, alfuzosin and sildenafil (for treatment of pulmonary arterial HTN).

WARNINGS/PRECAUTIONS: May cause nephrolithiasis/urolithiasis; temporary interrupt (eg, 1-3 days) or d/c if signs/symptoms occur. Maintain adequate hydration. Hemolytic anemia, including cases resulting in death reported; d/c once diagnosis is apparent. Hepatitis, hepatic failure and indirect hyperbilirubinemia reported. Reduce dose with hepatic insufficiency due to cirrhosis. Immune reconstitution syndrome reported. New onset/(exacerbation of diabetes mellitus (DM) and hyperglycemia reported. Tubulointerstitial nephritis with medullary calcification and cortical atrophy reported with asymptomatic severe leukocyturia; monitor frequently with urinalyses. Consider d/c with severe leukocyturia (>100 cells/high power field). Spontaneous bleeding may occur with hemophilia A and B. Possible redistribution/accumulation of body fat. Not recommended in HIV-infected pregnant patients. Caution in elderly.

ADVERSE REACTIONS: Nephrolithiasis/urolithiasis, hyperbilirubinemia, abdominal pain, headache, N/V, dizziness, pruritus, asthenia/fatigue, diarrhea, back pain.

INTERACTIONS: See Contraindications. Avoid coadministration with rifampin, St. John's wort, atazanavir, lovastatin, simvastatin, salmeterol and rosuvastatin. Substantially increases sildenafil, tadalafil, vardenafil plasma levels; increased risk of hypotension, visual changes, priapism. Caution with parenteral midazolam. Increased plasma concentration with delavirdine, ketoconazole and itraconazole; consider dose reduction. Decreased level with and increases levels of rifabutin; adjust dose of both drugs. Increased concentration of antiarrhythmic agents (bepridil, lidocaine, quinidine) and dihydropyridine calcium channel blockers (eg, felodipine, nifedipine, nicardipine); clinical monitoring recommended. Increased fluticasone concentration; consider alternatives. Decreased plasma concentrations with CYP3A4 inducers, efavirenz, nevirapine, anticonvulsants, and venlafaxine. Higher incidence of nephrolithiasis with ritonavir. Avoid with colchicine in patient with renal/hepatic impairment. Increased concentrations with CYP3A4 inhibitors, nelfinavir and clarithromycin. May increase plasma levels of drugs metabolized by CYP3A4, saquinavir, bosentan, immunosuppressants (cyclosporine, tacrolimus, sirolimus) and trazodone. Careful monitoring with pravastatin, fluvastatin and atorvastatin (use lowest dose). May need dose adjustments of insulin or oral hypoglycemic agents with DM.

PREGNANCY: Category C, not for use in nursing.

MECHANISM OF ACTION: Protease inhibitor; binds to protease active site and inhibits enzyme activity hence preventing cleavage of viral polyproteins resulting in the formation of immature noninfectious viral particles.

PHARMACOKINETICS: Absorption: Rapid; C_{max}=12617nM; T_{max}=0.8 hrs; AUC=30691nM•hr. **Distribution:** Plasma protein binding (60%). **Metabolism:** Hepatic via CYP3A4 (major). **Elimination:** Urine (<20%, unchanged); $T_{1/2}$=1.8 hrs.

NURSING CONSIDERATIONS

Assessment: Assess for asymptomatic severe leukocyturia, hemophilia, hepatic/renal dysfunction, DM, hypersensitivity reactions, pregnancy/nursing status, and possible drug interactions.

Monitoring: Monitor for possible indirect hyperbilirubinemia, increase in serum transaminase, immune reconstitution syndrome, signs and symptoms of nephrolithiasis/urolithiasis, hemolytic anemia, hepatitis, hyperglycemia and new onset/exacerbation of DM. Monitor urinalyses frequently with severe leukocyturia and for possible tubulointerstitial nephritis.

Patient Counseling: Inform that therapy is not cure for HIV, does not reduce risk of transmission of HIV and that opportunistic infections may develop. Advice to seek medical attention if symptoms of infection, nephrolithiasis/ urolithiasis (flank pain, with or without hematuria), anemia, hepatitis fat redistribution/accumulation and hyperglycemia occur. Instruct to notify physician any use of prescription, non-prescription/herbal medication, particularly St. John's wort. Instruct to take without food but with water, other liquid or a light meal. Instruct to keep well hydrated during therapy.

Administration: Oral route. **Storage:** 15-30°C (59-86°F). Store in a tightly-closed container; protect from moisture.

CUBICIN   RX
daptomycin (Cubist)

THERAPEUTIC CLASS: Cyclic lipopeptide

INDICATIONS: Susceptible complicated skin and skin structure infections (cSSSI) and *Staphylococcus aureus* bloodstream infections (bacteremia), including right-sided infective endocarditis.

DOSAGE: *Adults:* ≥18 yrs: Administer as IV inj over 2 min or infusion over a 30 min period. cSSSI: 4mg/kg once q24h for 7-14 days. *S. aureus* Bacteremia: 6mg/kg once q24h for 2-6 weeks. Limited safety data for use >28 days. Do not dose more frequently than qd. Renal impairment: CrCl <30mL/min, Hemodialysis, Continuous Ambulatory Peritoneal Dialysis: 4mg/kg (cSSSI) or 6mg/kg (*S. aureus* bacteremia) once q48h.

HOW SUPPLIED: Inj: 500mg [10mL]

WARNINGS/PRECAUTIONS: Anaphylaxis/hypersensitivity reactions reported; d/c and institute appropriate therapy if allergic reaction occurs. Myopathy, creatine phosphokinase (CPK) elevation and rhabdomyolysis with or without acute renal failure reported. D/C with unexplained signs and symptoms of myopathy and CPK elevations to levels >1,000 U/L (~5X ULN), or without symptoms and levels >2,000 U/L (≥10X ULN). Eosinophilic pneumonia reported; d/c therapy and treat with systemic steroids if fever, dyspnea with hypoxic respiratory insufficiency, and diffuse pulmonary infiltrates occur. Peripheral neuropathy reported. *Clostridium difficile*-associated diarrhea (CDAD) reported; d/c if CDAD is suspected or confirmed. May cause superinfections. Repeat blood cultures for persisting or relapsing *S. aureus* bacteremia/endocarditis or poor clinical response; appropriate surgical intervention and/or change in antibiotic regimen may be required. Not indicated for the treatment of pneumonia and left-sided infective endocarditis due to *S. aureus*. May cause false prolongation of PT and elevation of INR when certain recombinant thromboplastin reagents are utilized for the assay.

ADVERSE REACTIONS: Headache, diarrhea, insomnia, CPK increased, chest pain, abdominal pain, pharyngolaryngeal pain, rash, abnormal LFTs, sepsis, bacteremia, edema, pruritus, sweating increased, HTN.

INTERACTIONS: Concomitant tobramycin increased daptomycin levels and decreased tobramycin levels. Concomitant therapy with agents associated with rhabdomyolysis (eg, HMG-CoA reductase inhibitors) may increase CPK levels; consider temporary d/c.

PREGNANCY: Category B, caution in nursing.

MECHANISM OF ACTION: Cyclic lipopeptide; binds to bacterial membranes and causes a rapid depolarization of membrane potential, causing inhibition of DNA, RNA, and protein synthesis, which results in bacterial cell death.

PHARMACOKINETICS: Absorption: (4mg/kg) C_{max}=57.8µg/mL, AUC=494µg•h/mL (over 30 min); AUC=475µg•h/mL (over 2 min). (6mg/kg) C_{max}=93.9µg/mL, AUC=632µg•h/mL (over 30 min); AUC=701µg•h/mL (over 2 min). Refer to PI for pharmacokinetic parameters with various degrees of renal function. **Distribution:** Plasma protein binding (90-93%); V_d=0.1L/kg. **Elimination:** Urine (78%), feces (5.7%); (4mg/kg over 30 min) $T_{1/2}$=8.1 hrs; (6mg/kg over 30 min) $T_{1/2}$=7.9 hrs.

NURSING CONSIDERATIONS

Assessment: Assess renal function, hypersensitivity to the drug, pregnancy/nursing status and possible drug interactions. Obtain baseline CPK levels. Obtain specimens for microbiological examination to determine pathogen identity and susceptibility.

Monitoring: Monitor renal/hepatic function. Monitor for anaphylaxis or hypersensitivity reactions, eosinophilic pneumonia, CDAD, rhabdomyolysis, myopathy, muscle pain or weakness particularly of the distal extremities, peripheral neuropathy, and persisting or relapsing *S. aureus* infection or poor clinical response. Monitor CPK levels weekly, and more frequently in patients who received recent prior or concomitant therapy with an HMG-CoA reductase inhibitor or if CPK elevations occur during therapy. Monitor renal function and CPK levels more frequently than once weekly with renal impairment.

Patient Counseling: Instruct to report any previous allergic reactions to the drug. Inform that serious allergic reactions may occur and require immediate treatment. Instruct to report muscle pain or weakness, tingling, numbness, cough, breathlessness or fever. Instruct to notify physician immediately if watery/bloody diarrhea (with or without stomach cramps and fever) develops even as late as 2 months after therapy. Inform that drug is used to treat bacterial, not viral infections (eg, common cold). Administer exactly as directed; skipping doses or not completing full course of therapy may decrease effectiveness and increase likelihood of drug resistance. Notify physician if pregnant/nursing.

Administration: IV route. Refer to PI for instructions on reconstitution and administration. Not compatible with dextrose-containing diluents. Do not add with other IV substances, additives and other medications. **Storage:** 2-8°C (36-46°F). Avoid excessive heat. Reconstituted/Diluted Solution: Stable for 12 hrs at room temperature or ≤48 hrs if refrigerated.

CUTIVATE   RX
fluticasone propionate (PharmaDerm)

THERAPEUTIC CLASS: Corticosteroid

INDICATIONS: (Cre, Oint) Relief of the inflammatory and pruritic manifestations of corticosteroid-responsive dermatoses. Cream may be used with caution in pediatric patients ≥3 months of age. (Lot) Relief of the inflammatory and pruritic manifestations of atopic dermatitis in patients ≥1 yr of age.

DOSAGE: *Adults:* Atopic Dermatitis: (Cre) Apply a thin film to affected areas qd-bid. (Lot) Apply a thin film to affected areas qd. Other Corticosteroid-Responsive Dermatoses: (Cre) Apply a thin film to affected areas bid. (Oint) Apply a thin film to affected areas bid. (Cre, Lot, Oint) Avoid occlusive dressings and re-evaluate if no improvement within 2 weeks. Rub in gently. *Pediatrics:* ≥3 months: (Cre) Atopic Dermatitis: Apply a thin film to affected areas qd-bid. Other Corticosteroid-Responsive Dermatoses: Apply a thin film to affected areas bid. Avoid in diaper area. ≥1 yr: (Lot) Atopic Dermatitis: Apply a thin film to affected areas qd. Avoid in diaper area. (Cre, Lot): Avoid occlusive dressings and re-evaluate if no improvement within 2 weeks. Rub in gently.

HOW SUPPLIED: Cre: 0.05% [15g, 30g, 60g]; Lot: 0.05% [60mL]; Oint: 0.005% [15g, 30g, 60g]

WARNINGS/PRECAUTIONS: Caution with cream in pediatrics. May produce reversible hypothalamic-pituitary-adrenal (HPA) axis suppression, manifestations of Cushing's syndrome, hyperglycemia and glucosuria. Withdraw, reduce frequency, or substitute to a less potent steroid if adrenal suppression noted. Infrequently, glucocorticosteroid insufficiency may occur, requiring supplemental systemic steroids. Use appropriate antifungal or antibacterial agent with dermatological infection; d/c until infection controlled. May cause cutaneous local adverse reactions. D/C if irritation occurs. Pediatrics may be more susceptible to systemic toxicity. HPA axis suppression, Cushing's syndrome and intracranial HTN reported in pediatrics. Caution when applied to large surface areas or areas under occlusion. Avoid with pre-existing skin atrophy and presence of infection at treatment site. Not for use in rosacea or perioral dermatitis. Cre/Lot contains imidurea excipient which releases formaldehyde as a breakdown product; avoid with hypersensitivity to formaldehyde.

ADVERSE REACTIONS: (Cre) Pruritus, dryness, numbness of fingers, burning, facial telangiectasia. (Oint) Pruritus, burning, hypertrichosis, increased erythema, hives, irritation, light-headedness. (Lot) Common cold, upper respiratory tract infection, cough, fever, dry skin, stinging at application site.

PREGNANCY: Category C, caution in nursing.

MECHANISM OF ACTION: Corticosteroid; possesses anti-inflammatory, antipruritic, and vasoconstrictive properties. Anti-inflammatory activity not established; suspected to act by the induction of phospholipase A_2 inhibitory proteins (lipocortins). Lipocortins control biosynthesis of potent mediators of inflammation (eg, prostaglandins, leukotrienes) by inhibiting release of common precursor, arachidonic acid.

PHARMACOKINETICS: Absorption: Extent of percutaneous absorption depends on skin integrity, vehicle, and use of occlusive dressings. **Distribution:** (IV) V_d=4.2L/kg; plasma protein binding (91%). Systemically administered corticosteroids are found in breast milk. **Metabolism:** (Oral) Hydrolysis via CYP450 3A4. **Elimination:** (IV) $T_{1/2}$=7.2 hrs.

NURSING CONSIDERATIONS

Assessment: Assess for hypersensitivity, proper diagnosis, pre-existing skin atrophy, presence of skin infection at treatment site, rosacea and perioral dermatitis, pregnancy/nursing status. (Cre, Lot) Assess use in pediatrics.

Monitoring: Monitor for signs/symptoms of reversible HPA-axis suppression, presence of dermatological infections (eg, fungal, bacterial). Monitor for withdrawal symptoms following d/c of therapy. If applying high doses of medication to large surface area or if using occlusive dressings, monitor for HPA-axis suppression by using urinary free cortisol and adrenocorticotropic hormone stimulation tests. Monitor for signs/symptoms of systemic toxicity in pediatrics.

Patient Counseling: (Cre, Lot, Oint) Use as directed. Avoid contact with eyes; not to bandage, cover, or wrap treated skin. Avoid using on face, underarms or groin areas unless directed by physician. Contact physician if any signs of adverse reactions or no clinical improvement within 2 weeks of therapy occurs. Not for treatment of diaper dermatitis and not for application in diaper areas. (Cre, Lot) Report to physician if allergic to formaldehyde. (Lot) Counsel that should not be used longer than 4 weeks as safety has not been established past 4 weeks.

Administration: Topical route. **Storage**: (Cre, Oint) 2-30°C (36-86°F). (Lot) 15-30°C (59-86°F). Do not refrigerate. Keep container tightly sealed.

CYCLESSA   RX
desogestrel - ethinyl estradiol (Organon)

> Cigarette smoking increases the risk of serious cardiovascular (CV) side effects from oral contraceptive use. Risk increases with age (>35yrs) and with heavy smoking (≥15 cigarettes/day). Women who use oral contraceptives should be strongly advised not to smoke.

OTHER BRAND NAMES: Velivet (Barr) - Cesia (Prasco)

THERAPEUTIC CLASS: Estrogen/progestogen combination

INDICATIONS: Prevention of pregnancy.

DOSAGE: *Adults:* 1 tab qd for 28 days without interruption, then repeat. Start 1st Sunday after menses begin or 1st day of menses. Take sequentially following the arrows marked on the dispenser. Intervals between doses should not exceed 24 hrs. When initiating a Sunday-start regimen, use another method of contraception until after first 7 consecutive days of administration. Initiate 4-6 weeks postpartum in women who elect not to breastfeed.

Pediatrics: Postpubertal adolescents: 1 tab qd for 28 days without interruption, then repeat. Start 1st Sunday after menses begin or 1st day of menses. Take sequentially following the arrows marked on the dispenser. Intervals between doses should not exceed 24 hrs. When initiating a Sunday-start regimen, use another method of contraception until after first 7 consecutive days of administration. Initiate 4-6 weeks postpartum in women who elect not to breast-feed.

HOW SUPPLIED: Tab: (Ethinyl Estradiol-Desogestrel) 0.025mg-0.1mg, 0.025mg-0.125mg, 0.025mg-0.15mg

CONTRAINDICATIONS: Thrombophlebitis, thromboembolic disorders, history of deep vein thrombophlebitis (DVT) or thromboembolic disorders, current or history of cerebral vascular disease (CVD) or coronary artery disease (CAD), known or suspected breast carcinoma (or personal history), carcinoma of the endometrium or other known or suspected estrogen-dependent neoplasia, undiagnosed abnormal genital bleeding, cholestatic jaundice of pregnancy or jaundice with prior hormonal contraceptive use, hepatic tumors (benign or malignant), pregnancy. (Cesia, Cyclessa) Valvular heart disease with thrombogenic complications, severe HTN, diabetes with vascular involvement, headaches with focal neurological symptoms, major surgery with prolonged immobilization, active liver disease, heavy smoking (≥15 cigarettes/day) and >35 years.

WARNINGS/PRECAUTIONS: Increased risk of venous and arterial thrombotic and thromboembolic events (such as myocardial infarction (MI), thromboembolism, and stroke), vascular disease, hepatic neoplasia, gallbladder disease, and HTN. May increase risk of breast and cervical cancer. Benign hepatic adenomas and hepatocellular carcinoma reported (rare). Retinal thrombosis reported; d/c if unexplained partial or complete loss of vision, onset of proptosis or diplopia, papilledema, or retinal vascular lesions develop. Should not be used to induce withdrawal bleeding as a test for pregnancy, or to treat threatened or habitual abortion during pregnancy. May cause glucose intolerance; monitor prediabetic and diabetic patients. May cause fluid retention and increase BP; monitor closely with HTN and d/c if significant elevation of BP occurs. D/C with onset or exacerbation of migraine or development of headache with new pattern which is persistent, recurrent and severe. May cause breakthrough bleeding and spotting; if persistent or recurrent rule out malignancy or pregnancy. Ectopic and intrauterine pregnancies may occur with contraceptive failures. Perform annual physical exam. Monitor closely with hyperlipidemias; may elevate LDL and/or plasma triglycerides. Caution in patient with impaired liver function; d/c if jaundice develops. May cause depression; caution with history of depression and d/c if depression recurs to serious degree. Visual changes or changes in lens tolerance may develop with contact lens use. Use before menarche is not indicated. May affect certain endocrine tests, LFTs, and blood components. Does not protect against HIV infection (AIDS) and other sexually transmitted disease.

ADVERSE REACTIONS: N/V, breakthrough bleeding, spotting, amenorrhea, migraine headache, mood changes (including depression), vaginitis, including candidiasis, edema/fluid retention, weight or appetite changes, GI symptoms (such as abdominal pain, cramps and bloating), cholestatic jaundice, rash (allergic).

INTERACTIONS: Reduced contraceptive effectiveness leading to unintended pregnancy or breakthrough bleeding with some antibiotics, anticonvulsants, other drugs that increase the metabolism of contraceptive steroids (eg, barbiturates, rifampin, phenylbutazone, phenytoin, carbamazepine, felbamate, oxcarbazepine, topiramate, griseofulvin) and (Velivet) possibly with ampicillin and tetracyclines. Since desogestrel is mainly metabolized by CYP2C9 there is a possible interaction with CYP2C9 substrates or inhibitors. Anti-HIV protease inhibitors may increase or decrease levels. Effectiveness reduced with St. John's wort. Atorvastatin, ascorbic acid, acetaminophen, CYP3A4 inhibitors (eg, itraconazole, ketoconazole) may increase hormone levels. Increased plasma concentrations of cyclosporine, prednisolone, and theophylline. Decreased plasma concentrations of APAP and increased clearance of temazepam, salicylic acid, morphine, and clofibric acid.

PREGNANCY: Category X, not for use in nursing.

MECHANISM OF ACTION: Estrogen/progestogen combination; acts by suppression of gonadotropins and inhibition of ovulation. Also inhibits ovulation and causes changes in cervical mucus (increasing difficulty of sperm entry into uterus) and changes in endometrium (reducing likelihood of implantation).

PHARMACOKINETICS: Absorption: Desogestrel and ethinyl estradiol: Rapid and complete. Refer to PI for pharmacokinetic parameter during third cycle following multiple dose administration. **Distribution:** Etonogestrel: Plasma protein binding (98%); found in breast milk. **Metabolism:** Desogestrel: Liver (first pass effect) and hydroxylation in intestinal mucosa to etonogestrel (major active metabolite); further metabolism catalyze by CYP3A4. Ethinyl estradiol: gut and hepatic conjugation. **Elimination:** Urine, bile, feces. Etonogestrel: $T_{1/2}$=37.1 hrs. Ethinyl estradiol: $T_{1/2}$=28.2 hrs.

NURSING CONSIDERATIONS

Assessment: Assess for abnormal genital bleeding, presence or history of breast cancer, DVT/PE or history of, presence of estrogen-dependent neoplasia, active or recent (within past yr) arterial thromboembolic disease (eg, stroke, MI), liver dysfunction/disease, known/suspected pregnancy. Assess for drug and lab interactions. migraine (particularly migraine with aura), history of depression, pregnancy/nursing status and possible drug interactions. Assess use in heavy smokers and >35 years, morbidly obese and/or contact lens wearers.

Monitoring: Monitor for venous and arterial thrombotic and thromboembolic events (eg, MI, thromboembolism, stroke) hepatic neoplasia, gallbladder disease, HTN, vascular disease, carcinoma of the breast and reproductive organs, ocular lesions, fluid retention, bleeding irregularities, and onset or exacerbation of headaches or migraines, hypertriglyceridemia, jaundice, pancreatitis, worsening of depression, and pregnancy. Monitor BP in patients with HTN. Monitor lipid levels in patients with a history of hyperlipidemia. Monitor serum glucose levels in prediabetic and diabetic patients. Refer patients with contact lenses to ophthalmologist if ocular changes develop. Perform annual physical exam.

Patient Counseling: Counsel about possible side effects, and to avoid smoking while on therapy. Inform that medication does not protect against sexually transmitted diseases, and to use other forms of contraception to protect against such diseases. Advise to undergo annual physical exam while on medication. Inform may experience spotting or light bleeding, or may feel sick to stomach during first 1-3 packs of pills; advise this will usually subside and if not, to contact physician. Inform not to skip pills and to take at the same time everyday, and that there is a risk of pregnancy if pills are missed. If a dose is missed, take as soon as possible; take next dose at regular time, or may take two pills in one day. Counsel to use additional contraception for 7 days after a missed dose. Refer to PI for detailed instructions on administration regarding missed doses. Instruct to continue taking medication, even if irregular vaginal bleeding occurs; notify physician if bleeding occurs in more than one cycle or lasts for more than a few days.

Administration: Oral route. **Storage:** (Cyclessa, Cesia) 25°C (77°F); excursions permitted to 15-30°C (59-86°F). (Velivet) 20-25°C (68-77°F).

CYCLOSET RX
bromocriptine mesylate (VeroScience)

THERAPEUTIC CLASS: Dopamine receptor agonist

INDICATIONS: Adjunct to diet and exercise to improve glycemic control in adults with type 2 diabetes mellitus (DM).

DOSAGE: *Adults:* Initial: 1.6-4.8mg qd within 2 hrs after waking in am. Titrate: May increase by 1 tab (0.8mg)/week until maximum daily dose of 6 tabs (4.8mg) or until the maximal tolerated number of tablets between 2 and 6/day is reached. Max: 6 tabs. Take with food.

HOW SUPPLIED: Tab: 0.8mg

CONTRAINDICATIONS: Syncopal migraine, nursing women.

WARNINGS/PRECAUTIONS: Orthostatic hypotension may occur; assess orthostatic vital signs prior to therapy and monitor periodically. May exacerbate psychotic disorders or reduce the effectiveness of drugs to treat psychosis; avoid with severe psychotic disorders. Somnolence reported. May impair mental/physical abilities. Caution with renal/hepatic impairment.

ADVERSE REACTIONS: N/V, fatigue, dizziness, headache, asthenia, constipation, sinusitis, diarrhea, amblyopia, dyspepsia, vomiting, infection, anorexia, cold, rhinitis.

INTERACTIONS: Concomitant use with dopamine receptor agonists is not recommended. Decreased effects with dopamine receptor antagonists (eg, butyrophenones, phenothiazines, thioxanthenes, or metoclopramide); concomitant use not recommended. Caution with antihypertensives. May increase unbound fraction with highly protein-bound therapies (eg, salicylates, sulfonamides, chloramphenicol, and probenecid). Avoid concomitant use of ergot-related agents within 6 hrs. Caution with strong inhibitors, inducers, or substrates of CYP3A4 (eg, azole antimycotics, HIV protease inhibitors). HTN and tachycardia reported with sympathomimetic agents (eg, phenylpropanolamine, isometheptene) in postpartum women. Avoid concomitant use with sympathomimetic agents for >10 days and selective 5-hydroxytryptamine$_{1B}$ (5-HT$_{1B}$) agonists (eg, sumatriptan).

PREGNANCY: Category B, not for use in nursing.

MECHANISM OF ACTION: Dopamine receptor agonist; ergot derivative; mechanism not established. Improves glycemic control in patients with type 2 diabetes without increasing plasma insulin concentrations. Increases circulating levels of bromocriptine.

PHARMACOKINETICS: Absorption: Absolute bioavailability (65-95%), T_{max}=53 mins. **Distribution:** V_d=61L; plasma protein binding (90-96%). **Metabolism:** GI and liver (extensive) via CYP3A4; **Excretion:** Bile (major), Urine (2-6%); $T_{1/2}$=6 hrs.

NURSING CONSIDERATIONS

Assessment: Assess FPG, HbA1c, renal function, LFTs, CBCs. Assess for cardiovascular complications and hypoglycemia risk factors. Assess for renal/hepatic impairment, and DM complications, syncopal migraine, hypotension, psychotic disorders, orthostatic vital signs, pregnancy/nursing status, and possible drug interactions.

Monitoring: Monitor FPG, HBA1c, renal function (at baseline and annually), LFTs, orthostatic vital signs, and hematological parameters. Monitor for hypersensitivity reactions.

Patient Counseling: Inform that drug is an adjunct to diet and exercise and should be taken as prescribed with meals. Counsel about potential risks, benefits and alternative therapies. Stress importance of adherence to dietary instructions, regular exercise programs, and regular testing of blood glucose levels. Caution against operating heavy machinery if symptoms of somnolence occur. Notify physician if any unusual symptoms develop.

Administration: Oral route. **Storage:** 25°C (77°F).

CYMBALTA   RX
duloxetine HCl (Lilly)

> Antidepressants increased the risk of suicidal thinking and behavior (suicidality) in short-term studies in children, adolescents, and young adults with major depressive disorder (MDD) and other psychiatric disorders. Monitor and observe closely for clinical worsening, suicidality, or unusual changes in behavior in patients who are started on antidepressant therapy. Not approved for use in pediatric patients.

THERAPEUTIC CLASS: Serotonin and norepinephrine reuptake inhibitor

INDICATIONS: Treatment of major depressive disorder (MDD) and of generalized anxiety disorder (GAD) in adults. Management of neuropathic pain associated with diabetic peripheral neuropathy (DPNP). Management of fibromyalgia (FM). Management of chronic musculoskeletal pain in patients with chronic low back pain (CLBP) and chronic pain due to osteoarthritis.

DOSAGE: *Adults:* MDD: Initial: 40mg/day (given as 20mg bid) to 60mg/day (given qd or as 30mg bid) or 30mg qd for 1 week before increasing to 60mg qd. Maint: 60mg qd. Max: 120mg/day. Reassess periodically to determine need for maint therapy and appropriate dose. GAD: Initial: 60mg qd or 30mg qd for 1 week before increasing to 60mg qd. Dose increases above 60mg/day should be in increments of 30mg qd. Maint: 60-120mg qd. Max: 120mg/day. Reassess periodically to determine need for maint and appropriate dose. DPNP: Initial: 60mg qd. May lower starting dose if tolerability is a concern. Consider lower starting dose with gradual increase in renal impairment. Maint: Individualize dose. Treat for up to 12 weeks. Max: 60mg qd. FM: Initial: 60mg qd or 30mg qd for 1 week before increasing to 60mg qd. Max: 60mg qd. Maint: Based on patient's response. Chronic Musculoskeletal Pain: Initial: 60mg qd or 30mg qd for 1 week before increasing to 60mg qd. Maint: 60mg qd for up to 13 weeks. Swallow whole. Do not chew, crush, open, sprinkle on food or mix with liquids.

HOW SUPPLIED: Cap, Delayed-Release: 20mg, 30mg, 60mg

CONTRAINDICATIONS: Concomitant use with or within 14 days of MAOIs; uncontrolled narrow-angle glaucoma.

WARNINGS/PRECAUTIONS: Fatal hepatic failure and cholestatic jaundice with minimal elevation of serum transaminase reported; d/c if jaundice or other evidence of hepatic dysfunction occurs. Avoid with substantial alcohol use or evidence of chronic liver disease and/or hepatic insufficiency. Serotonin syndrome or neuroleptic malignant syndrome (NMS)-like reactions reported; monitor and d/c if signs/symptoms develop. Orthostatic hypotension and syncope reported; consider d/c if symptomatic hypotension and/or syncope develops. May increase risk of bleeding events. D/C should be gradual. Activation of mania reported in patients with MDD. Caution with history of mania and/or seizures. May increase BP; obtain baseline and monitor periodically throughout therapy. May cause hyponatremia; d/c if symptomatic hyponatremia occurs and institute appropriate management. Urinary hesitation and retention reported. Caution with conditions that may slow gastric emptying, controlled narrow-angle glaucoma, diabetes, and in the elderly. Avoid in end-stage renal disease/severe renal impairment (CrCl <30mL/min).

ADVERSE REACTIONS: N/V, dry mouth, constipation, diarrhea, decreased appetite, fatigue, dizziness, somnolence, hyperhidrosis, headache, insomnia.

INTERACTIONS: See Contraindications. Upon d/c, wait ≥5 days before starting MAOI therapy. Avoid thioridazine, CYP1A2 inhibitors (eg, fluvoxamine, cimetidine, some quinolone antibiotics), substantial alcohol use. Increased levels with potent CYP2D6 inhibitors (eg, paroxetine, fluoxetine, quinidine). Caution with drugs metabolized by CYP2D6 having a narrow therapeutic index (eg, TCAs, phenothiazines, type 1C antiarrhythmics), and CNS-acting drugs. May increase free concentration levels of highly protein-bound drugs. Potential for interaction with drugs that affect gastric acidity. Caution with serotonergic drugs (eg, triptans, tramadol, linezolid, lithium, or St. John's wort). Avoid with other SSRIs, serotonin norepinephrine reuptake inhibitors, or tryptophan. Caution with NSAIDs, ASA, or other drugs that affect coagulation. Greater risk of hypotension with concomitant use of medications that induce orthostatic hypotension (eg, antihypertensives) and potent CYP1A2 inhibitors. Increased risk of hyponatremia with diuretics.

PREGNANCY: Category C, not for use in nursing.

MECHANISM OF ACTION: Selective serotonin and norepinephrine reuptake inhibitor; not established. Believed to be related to potentiation of serotonergic and noradrenergic activity in the CNS.

PHARMACOKINETICS: Absorption: Well absorbed; T_{max}=6 hrs. **Distribution:** V_d=1640L; plasma protein binding (>90%); found in breast milk. **Metabolism:** Hepatic via CYP1A2, 2D6; oxidation and conjugation. **Elimination:** Urine (70% metabolites; <1% unchanged), feces (20%); $T_{1/2}$=12 hrs.

NURSING CONSIDERATIONS

Assessment: Assess for bipolar disorder risk, history of mania, chronic liver disease, substantial alcohol use, history of seizures, disease/condition that slows gastric emptying (eg, diabetes mellitus), narrow-angle glaucoma, risk factors for hyponatremia, history of urinary retention, hepatic/renal impairment, pregnancy/nursing status, and possible drug interactions. Assess baseline BP, LFTs, BUN, SrCr, and blood glucose.

Monitoring: Monitor for signs/symptoms of clinical worsening (suicidality, unusual changes in behavior), hepatotoxicity, serotonin syndrome or NMS-like reactions, abnormal bleeding, hyponatremia, seizures, orthostatic hypotension, decreased glycemic control, urinary hesitation/retention, mydriasis, and hepatic/renal dysfunction. If abruptly d/c, monitor for symptoms of dizziness, N/V, headache, paresthesia, fatigue, irritability, insomnia, diarrhea, anxiety, and hyperhidrosis. Periodically monitor BP, LFTs, SrCr, and BUN.

Patient Counseling: Inform patients, families, and caregivers about benefits/risks and to read Medication Guide. Counsel to swallow whole, and not to chew, crush, open, sprinkle on food or mix with liquid. Advise to avoid alcohol. Instruct to seek medical attention for clinical worsening (suicidal ideation, unusual changes in behavior) and symptoms of serotonin syndrome (with use of triptans, tramadol, or other serotonergic agents). Abnormal bleeding (with use of NSAIDs, ASA, warfarin, or other drugs that affect coagulation), hyponatremia, orthostatic hypotension, hepatotoxicity, urinary hesitation/retention, seizures, or d/c symptoms (irritability, agitation, dizziness, anxiety, headache, insomnia) may occur. Advise to inform if taking or planning to take any prescription or OTC medications, ir pregnant, intend to become pregnant or are breastfeeding. Register pregnant patients while on treatment by calling Cymbalta Pregnancy Registry at 1-866-814-6975 or visiting www.cymbaltapregnancy.com. Caution with operating hazardous machinery including automobiles; may impair judgement, thinking, or motor skills. May notice improvement within 1-4 weeks; instruct to continue therapy as directed.

Administration: Oral route. **Storage:** 25°C (77°F); excursions permitted to 15-30°C (59-86°F).

Cytomel   RX
liothyronine sodium (King)

THERAPEUTIC CLASS: Thyroid replacement hormone

INDICATIONS: As replacement or supplemental therapy in patients with hypothyroidism of any etiology, except transient hypothyroidism during the recovery phase of subacute thyroiditis. In the treatment or prevention of various types of euthyroid goiters, including thyroid nodules, and Hashimoto's and multinodular goiter. As diagnostic agent in suppression tests to differentiate mild hyperthyroidism or thyroid gland autonomy.

DOSAGE: *Adults:* Individualize dose. Mild Hypothyroidism: Initial: 25mcg qd. Titrate: May increase by up to 25mcg qd every 1-2 weeks. Maint: 25-75mcg qd. Myxedema: Initial: 5mcg qd. Titrate: May increase by 5-10mcg qd every 1-2 weeks up to 25mcg qd, then increase by 5-25mcg qd every 1-2 weeks until desired response. Maint: 50-100mcg/day. Simple (Non-Toxic) Goiter: Initial: 5mcg/day. Titrate: May increase by 5-10mcg qd every 1-2 weeks up to

25mcg qd, then by 12.5-25mcg qd every 1-2 weeks. Maint: 75mcg qd. Elderly/ Angina Pectoris/Coronary Artery Disease: Initial: 5mcg qd. Titrate: Increase by no more than 5mcg qd at 2-week intervals. Switch to Cytomel Tablets from Thyroid, L-Thyroxine or Thyroglobulin: D/C other medication and initiate Cytomel at low dose then increase gradually based on patient response. Thyroid Suppression Therapy: 75-100mcg qd for 7 days. Radioactive iodine uptake is determined before and after administration of the hormone. *Pediatrics:* Congenital Hypothyroidism: Initial: 5mcg qd. Titrate: Increase by 5mcg qd every 3-4 days until desired response achieved. Maint: >3 yrs: 25-75mcg/day. 1-3 yrs: 50mcg qd. <1 yr: 20mcg qd.

HOW SUPPLIED: Tab: 5mcg, 25mcg*, 50mcg* *scored

CONTRAINDICATIONS: Uncorrected adrenal cortical insufficiency and untreated thyrotoxicosis.

WARNINGS/PRECAUTIONS: Do not use in the treatment of obesity; larger doses in euthyroid patients can cause serious or life-threatening toxicity. Caution with cardiovascular (CV) disorders (eg, angina pectoris) and in the elderly; use lower doses. Not for the treatment of male or female infertility unless accompanied by hypothyroidism. Rule out morphological hypogonadism and nephrosis prior to therapy. If hypopituitarism present, adrenal insufficency must be corrected prior to starting therapy. Caution in myxedematous patients; start at very low dose and increase gradually. Severe and prolonged hypothyroidism can lead to adrenocortical insufficiency; supplement with adrenocortical steroids. May precipitate a hyperthyroid state or aggravate hyperthyroidism. Concurrent use with androgens, corticosteroids, estrogens, oral contraceptives containing estrogens, iodine-containing preparations, and salicylates may interfere with thyroid laboratory tests. May aggravate symptoms diabetes mellitus (DM) or insipidus (DI) or adrenal cortical insufficiency. Add glucocorticoids with myxedema coma. Excessive doses may cause craniosynostosis in infants.

ADVERSE REACTIONS: Allergic skin reactions (rare).

INTERACTIONS: Coadministration of larger doses with sympathomimetic amines such as those used for their anorectic effects may cause serious or even life-threatening toxicity. Hypothyroidism decreases and hyperthyroidism increases sensitivity to oral anticoagulants; monitor PT. May cause increases in insulin and oral hypoglycemics requirements. Impaired absorption with cholestyramine; space dosing by 4-5 hrs. Estrogens increase thyroxine-binding globulin; increase in thyroid dose may be needed. Increased effects of both agents with TCAs (eg, imipramine). HTN and tachycardia may occur with ketamine. May potentiate digitalis toxicity. Increased adrenergic effects of catecholamines (eg, epinephrine, norepinephrine); caution with coronary artery disease (CAD).

PREGNANCY: Category A, caution in nursing.

MECHANISM OF ACTION: Synthetic thyroid hormone; mechanism not established. Suspected to enhance oxygen consumption by tissues and increase the basal metabolic rate and metabolism of carbohydrates, lipids, and proteins.

PHARMACOKINETICS: Distribution: Minimal amount found in breast milk. **Elimination:** $T_{1/2}$=2.5 days.

NURSING CONSIDERATIONS

Assessment: Assess thyroid status, CV disease (eg, CAD, angina pectoris), DM/DI, adrenal cortical insufficiency, thyrotoxicosis, myxedema, hypogonadism, nephrosis, pregnancy/nursing status, and for possible drug interactions.

Monitoring: Monitor thyroid function periodically. Monitor PT on oral anticoagulants, urinary glucose with DM and renal function. Monitor for signs/symptoms of precipitation of adrenocortical insufficiency, aggravation of DM/DI, hypoglycemia, hyperthyroidism, toxicity, and hypersensitivity reactions.

Patient Counseling: Inform that replacement therapy is taken for life. Warn that partial hair loss may be seen in pediatrics in first few months of therapy. Instruct to seek medical attention if symptoms of toxicity (eg, chest pain, increased HR, palpitations, excessive sweating, heat intolerance, nervousness), hypoglycemia, aggravation of DM/DI, or hypersensitivity reactions occur.

Administration: Oral route. **Storage:** 15-30°C (59-86°F).

CYTOXAN   RX

cyclophosphamide (Bristol-Myers Squibb)

THERAPEUTIC CLASS: Nitrogen mustard alkylating agent

INDICATIONS: Treatment of malignant lymphomas, Hodgkin's disease, lymphocytic lymphoma, mixed-cell type or histiocytic lymphoma, Burkitt's lymphoma, multiple myeloma, chronic lymphocytic leukemia, chronic granulocytic leukemia, acute myelogenous and monocytic leukemia, acute lymphoblastic leukemia in children, mycosis fungoides, neuroblastoma, ovary adenocarcinoma, retinoblastoma, breast carcinoma. Treatment of biopsy proven "minimal change" nephrotic syndrome in children, but not as primary therapy.

DOSAGE: *Adults:* Malignant Diseases (Without Hematologic Deficiency): Monotherapy: Initial: 40-50mg/kg IV in divided doses over 2-5 days, or 10-15mg/kg IV given every 7-10 days, or 3-5mg/kg twice weekly. Oral Dosing: Initial/Maint: 1-5mg/kg/day PO. Adjust dose according to antitumor activity and/or leukopenia. May need to reduce dose when combined with other cytotoxic drugs.
Pediatrics: Malignant Diseases (Without Hematologic Deficiency): Monotherapy: Initial: 40-50mg/kg IV in divided doses over 2-5 days, or 10-15mg/kg IV given every 7-10 days, or 3-5mg/kg twice weekly. Oral Dosing: Initial/Maint: 1-5mg/kg/day PO. Adjust dose according to antitumor activity and/or leukopenia. May need to reduce dose when combined with other cytotoxic drugs. Nephrotic Syndrome: 2.5-3mg/kg/day PO for 60-90 days.

HOW SUPPLIED: Inj (Lyophilized): 500mg, 1g, 2g; Tab: 25mg, 50mg

CONTRAINDICATIONS: Severely depressed bone marrow function.

WARNINGS/PRECAUTIONS: Second malignancies, cardiac dysfunction, and hemorrhagic cystitis reported. May cause fetal harm in pregnancy. Serious, fatal infections may develop if severely immunosuppressed. Monitor for toxicity with leukopenia, thrombocytopenia, tumor cell infiltration of bone marrow, previous x-ray therapy or cytotoxic therapy, and impaired hepatic and/or renal function. Monitor hematologic profile for hematopoietic suppression. Examine urine for red blood cells. Anaphylactic reactions reported. Possible cross-sensitivity with other alkylating agents. May cause sterility. May interfere with normal wound healing. Consider dose adjustment with adrenalectomy.

ADVERSE REACTIONS: Impairment of fertility, amenorrhea, N/V, anorexia, abdominal discomfort, diarrhea, alopecia, leukopenia, thrombocytopenia, hemorrhagic ureteritis, interstitial pneumonitis, malaise, asthenia, renal tubular necrosis.

INTERACTIONS: Chronic, high doses of phenobarbital increase metabolism and leukopenic activity. Potentiates succinylcholine chloride effects and doxorubicin-induced cardiotoxicity. Alert anesthesiologist if treated within 10 days of general anesthesia.

PREGNANCY: Category D, not for use in nursing.

MECHANISM OF ACTION: Nitrogen mustard alkylating agent; exerts action by cross linking of tumor cell DNA.

PHARMACOKINETICS: Absorption: Well absorbed; bioavailability (≥75%). **Distribution:** Plasma protein binding (≥60% as metabolites). **Metabolism:** Liver; active metabolites. **Elimination:** Urine (5-25% unchanged); $T_{1/2}$=3-12 hrs.

NURSING CONSIDERATIONS

Assessment: Assess for bone marrow function, leukopenia, thrombocytopenia, tumor cell infiltration of bone marrow, previous X-ray therapy, previous therapy with other cytotoxic agents, hepatic/renal function.

Monitoring: Monitor for second malignancies, amenorrhea, sterility, ovarian fibrosis, oligospermia or azoospermia, hemorrhagic cystitis, cardiac dysfunction, infection, anaphylactic reactions, CBC with differential and platelets.

Patient Counseling: Counsel about possible side effects and required contraceptive methods while on therapy. Take in the morning and drink adequate fluids. Report adverse side effects.

Administration: Oral, IV, IM, intraperitoneal, intrapleural route. Inspect drug product visually for particulate matter and discoloration prior to parenteral administration. **Storage:** Vial: Below 25°C (77°F). Tab: Below 25°C (77°F); excursions permitted to 30°C (86°F); protect from temperatures above 30°C (86°F).

DACOGEN RX
decitabine (Eisai)

THERAPEUTIC CLASS: DNA methyltransferase inhibitor

INDICATIONS: Treatment of myelodysplastic syndromes (MDS).

DOSAGE: *Adults*: Patients should be treated for a minimum of 4 cycles. Treatment Option 1: 15mg/m² by continuous IV infusion over 3 hrs q8h for 3 days. Repeat cycle every 6 weeks. Adjust dose based on hematologic recovery and disease progression; see PI. May premedicate with antiemetic therapy. Treatment Option 2: 20mg/m² by continuous IV infusion over 1 hr qd for 5 days. Repeat cycle every 4 weeks. Myelosuppression: Delay susbsequent treatment cycles until hematologic recovery. May premedicate with antiemetic therapy.

HOW SUPPLIED: Inj: 50mg

WARNINGS/PRECAUTIONS: Neutropenia and thrombocytopenia may occur; monitor CBC and platelets periodically (at minimum, before each dosing cycle). May cause fetal harm. Avoid pregnancy in women of childbearing potential. Men should be advised not to father a child while receiving treatment and for 2 months following completion of treatment. Caution with renal and hepatic dysfunction. Avoid with SrCr ≥2mg/dL; serum glutamate pyruvate transaminase, total bilirubin ≥2 times ULN, and active or uncontrolled infection.

ADVERSE REACTIONS: Neutropenia, thrombocytopenia, anemia, fatigue, pyrexia, nausea, cough, petechiae, constipation, diarrhea, hyperglycemia, febrile neutropenia, leukopenia, headache, insomnia.

PREGNANCY: Category D, not for use in nursing.

MECHANISM OF ACTION: DNA methyltransferase inhibitor; inhibition of methyltransferase causes hypomethylation of DNA and cellular differentiation or apoptosis.

PHARMACOKINETICS: Absorption: (15mg/m²) C_{max} = 73.8ng/mL, AUC=163ng•h/mL; (20mg/m²) C_{max} =147ng/mL, AUC=115ng•h/mL. **Elimination:** Deamination in liver, granulocytes, intestinal epithelium, and blood; $T_{1/2}$=0.62 hrs (15mg/m²), 0.54 hrs (20mg/m²).

NURSING CONSIDERATIONS

Assessment: Assess CBC with platelets, renal/hepatic function, pregnancy status. Note other diseases/conditions and drug therapies.

Monitoring: Monitor for hypersensitivity reactions, CBC with platelets, renal/hepatic impairment, cardiac disorders, infections and infestations, intracranial hemorrhage, mental status change, cholecystitis, and hyperglycemia.

Patient Counseling: Advise women of childbearing potential to avoid becoming pregnant and for men not to father a child while on therapy; counsel about effective contraception. Advise to monitor and report any symptoms of neutropenia, thrombocytopenia or fever.

Administration: IV route (IV infusion). Reconstitute aseptically with 10mL of SWFI. Dilute with 0.9% NS, D5W, or LR to final concentration of 0.1-1.0mg/mL. Unless used within 15 min of reconstitution, diluted sol must be prepared using cold (2-8°C) infusion fluids. **Storage**: Vials: 25°C (77°F); excursions permitted to 15-30°C (59-86°F). Diluted solution: 2-8°C (36-46°F) for up to max of 7 hrs, until administration.

DANTRIUM

dantrolene sodium (JHP Pharmaceuticals, LLC)

Has potential for hepatotoxicity. Symptomatic/overt hepatitis, liver dysfunction reported. Risk of hepatic injury greater in females, patients >35 yrs, and patients taking other medications. Monitor hepatic function. D/C if no benefit after 45 days. Lowest possible effective dose should be prescribed.

THERAPEUTIC CLASS: Direct acting skeletal muscle relaxant

INDICATIONS: To control manifestations of clinical spasticity from upper motor neuron disorders (eg, spinal cord injury, stroke, cerebral palsy, multiple sclerosis). Preoperatively to prevent or attenuate development of malignant hyperthermia, and after a malignant hyperthermia crisis.

DOSAGE: *Adults:* Chronic Spasticity: Individualize dose. Initial: 25mg qd for 7 days. Titrate: Increase to 25mg tid for 7 days, then 50mg tid for 7 days, then 100mg tid. Max: 100mg qid. If no further benefit at next higher dose, decrease to previous lower dose. Malignant Hyperthermia: Pre-Op: 4-8mg/kg/day given tid-qid for 1-2 days before surgery, with last dose given 3-4 hrs before surgery with minimum of water. Adjust dose within recommended dose range to avoid incapacitation or excessive gastrointestinal irritation. Post-Op Following Malignant Hyperthermia Crisis: 4-8mg/kg/day given qid for 1-3 days. *Pediatrics:* ≥5 yrs: Chronic Spasticity: Individualize dose. Initial: 0.5mg/kg qd for 7 days. Titrate: Increase to 0.5mg/kg tid for 7 days, then 1mg/kg tid for 7 days, then 2mg/kg tid. Max: 100mg qid. If no further benefit at next higher dose, decrease to previous lower dose.

HOW SUPPLIED: Cap: 25mg, 50mg, 100mg

CONTRAINDICATIONS: Active hepatic disease (eg, hepatitis, cirrhosis), where spasticity is utilized to sustain upright posture and balance in locomotion, when spasticity is utilized to obtain or maintain increased function.

WARNINGS/PRECAUTIONS: Not for treatment of skeletal muscle spasms resulting from rheumatic disorder. Brief withdrawal for 2 to 4 days may exacerbate manifestations of spasticity. Liver disorders (eg, idiosyncratic or hypersensitivity type) may occur. Monitor LFTs at baseline, then periodically. D/C if LFT abnormalities or jaundice appear. Caution with pulmonary dysfunction (eg, obstructive pulmonary disease), severely impaired cardiac function due to myocardial disease, and history of liver disease/dysfunction. Photosensitivity reaction may occur; limit sunlight exposure.

ADVERSE REACTIONS: Drowsiness, dizziness, weakness, malaise, fatigue, diarrhea, hepatitis, tachycardia, aplastic anemia, thrombocytopenia, depression, seizure.

INTERACTIONS: Increased drowsiness with CNS depressants (eg, sedatives, tranquilizers). Caution with estrogens; risk of hepatotoxicity especially in women >35 yrs. Increased risk of hepatic injury in patients taking other medications. Avoid with calcium channel blockers; cardiovascular collapse with concomitant verapamil reported (rare). May potentiate vecuronium-induced neuromuscular block.

PREGNANCY: Category C, not for use in nursing.

MECHANISM OF ACTION: Direct-acting skeletal muscle relaxant; interferes with release of calcium ions from the sarcoplasmic reticulum.

PHARMACOKINETICS: Absorption: Incomplete/slow but consistent. **Metabolism:** Hepatic microsomal enzymes; 5-hydroxy and acetamido analog (major metabolites). **Elimination:** Urine; $T_{1/2}$=8.7 hrs.

NURSING CONSIDERATIONS

Assessment: Assess for active hepatic disease (eg, hepatitis and cirrhosis), history of liver disease/dysfunction, skeletal muscle spasm from rheumatic disorders, pulmonary dysfunction, impaired cardiac function due to myocardial disease, pregnancy/nursing status, and possible drug interactions. Perform baseline LFTs to establish pre-existing liver disease. Assess use in patients >35 yrs due to increased risk of drug-induced hepatocellular disease.

Monitoring: Monitor for liver disorders, photosensitivity reactions, and signs/symptoms of hepatitis. Monitor LFTs (eg, SGOT, SGPT) regularly.

Patient Counseling: Inform about risks and benefits of therapy. Caution against performing hazardous tasks (eg, operating machinery/driving), and avoid prolonged sunlight exposure. Inform about other medications being taken. Notify if pregnant/nursing.

Administration: Oral route. **Storage:** Avoid excessive heat, over 40°C (104°F).

DANTRIUM IV   RX
dantrolene sodium (Procter & Gamble Pharmaceuticals)

THERAPEUTIC CLASS: Direct acting skeletal muscle relaxant

INDICATIONS: Adjunct management of fulminant hypermetabolism of skeletal muscle characteristic of malignant hyperthermia crises. For pre- and post-operative use to prevent or attenuate development of malignant hyperthermia.

DOSAGE: *Adults:* Malignant Hyperthermia: Initial: Minimum 1mg/kg IV push. Continue until symptoms subside or max cumulative dose 10mg/kg. Pre-Op Malignant Hyperthermia Prophylaxis: 2.5mg/kg 1.25 hrs before anesthesia and infuse over 1 hr. May need additional therapy during anesthesia/surgery if symptoms arise. Post-Op Prophylaxis: Initial: 1mg/kg or more as clinical situation dictates.
Pediatrics: Malignant Hyperthermia: Initial: Minimum 1mg/kg IV push. Continue until symptoms subside or max cumulative dose 10mg/kg.

HOW SUPPLIED: Inj: 20mg

WARNINGS/PRECAUTIONS: Use with supportive therapies to treat malignant hyperthermia. Take steps to prevent extravasation. Fatal and non-fatal hepatic disorders reported. Do not operate automobile or engage hazardous activity for 48 hrs after therapy. Caution at meals on day of administration because difficulty in swallowing/choking reported. Monitor vital signs if receive pre-operatively.

ADVERSE REACTIONS: Loss of grip strength, weakness in legs, drowsiness, dizziness, pulmonary edema, thrombophlebitis, urticaria, erythema.

INTERACTIONS: Plasma protein-binding reduced by warfarin and clofibrate, and increased by tolbutamide. Avoid with calcium channel blockers (CCBs); possible risk of cardiovascular collapse. Caution with tranquilizers. Possible increased metabolism by drugs known to induce hepatic microsomal enzymes. May potentiate vecuronium-induced neuromuscular block.

PREGNANCY: Category C, safety in nursing not known.

MECHANISM OF ACTION: Direct acting skeletal muscle relaxant; interferes with release of calcium ions from sarcoplasmic reticulum.

PHARMACOKINETICS: Distribution: Found in breast milk. **Metabolism:** Hydrolysis and oxidation; 5-hydroxy dantrolene and acetylamino analog (major metabolites). **Elimination:** Urine; $T_{1/2}$=4-8 hrs.

NURSING CONSIDERATIONS

Assessment: Assess for active hepatic disease (hepatitis and cirrhosis), pregnancy/nursing status, and possible drug interactions.

Monitoring: Monitor for vital signs, tissue necrosis, LFTs. Monitor for cardiovascular collapse if given concomitantly with CCBs.

Patient Counseling: Caution against performing hazardous tasks (eg, operating machinery/driving). Inform that at meals, on administration day, choking and difficulty swallowing have been reported. Inform about postop muscle weakness, reduced grip strength, and lightheadedness. Notify if pregnant/nursing.

Administration: IV route. **Storage:** 15-30°C (59-86°F); avoid prolonged light exposure.

DAYPRO

RX

oxaprozin (G.D. Searle)

> NSAIDs may cause an increased risk of serious cardiovascular (CV) thrombotic events, myocardial infarction (MI), stroke and serious GI adverse events including bleeding, ulceration, and perforation of the stomach or intestines. Contraindicated for the treatment of perioperative pain in the setting of coronary artery bypass graft (CABG) surgery.

THERAPEUTIC CLASS: NSAID

INDICATIONS: Relief of signs and symptoms of osteoarthritis (OA), rheumatoid arthritis (RA), and juvenile rheumatoid arthritis (JRA).

DOSAGE: *Adults:* RA: 1200mg qd. Max: 1800mg/day in divided doses (not to exceed 26mg/kg/day). OA: 1200mg qd, give 600mg qd for low weight or milder disease. Max: 1800mg/day in divided doses (not to exceed 26mg/kg/day). Renal Dysfunction/Hemodialysis: Initial: 600mg qd. *Pediatrics:* 6-16yrs: JRA: ≥55kg: 1200mg qd. 32-54kg: 900mg qd. 22-31kg: 600mg qd.

HOW SUPPLIED: Tab: 600mg* *scored

CONTRAINDICATIONS: ASA or other NSAID allergy that precipitates asthma, urticaria, or allergic-type reactions. Treatment of perioperative pain in the setting of CABG surgery.

WARNINGS/PRECAUTIONS: May lead to onset of new HTN or worsening of pre-existing HTN; monitor BP during initiation and throughout the course of therapy. Fluid retention and edema reported; caution with fluid retention or heart failure. Renal papillary necrosis and other renal injury reported after long-term use. Not recommended for use with advanced renal disease; if therapy must be initiated, monitor renal function. Anaphylactoid reactions may occur. May cause serious skin adverse events (eg, exfoliative dermatitis, Stevens-Johnson syndrome (SJS), and toxic epidermal necrolysis). Avoid with patients with the aspirin triad (complex symptoms of rhinitis with or without nasal polyps and bronchospasm). Avoid in late pregnancy; may cause premature closure of ductus arteriosis. May cause elevations of LFTs; d/c if liver disease develop or systemic manifestations (eg, eosinophilia, rash) occur. Not a substitute for corticosteroids or for treatment of corticosteroid insufficiency. Caution in elderly. Anemia may occur; with long-term use, monitor Hgb/Hct if signs or symptoms of anemia develop. May inhibit platelet aggregation and prolong bleeding time; monitor with coagulation disorders. Caution with pre-existing asthma and avoid with ASA-sensitive asthma. Rash and/or mild photosensitivity reactions reported.

ADVERSE REACTIONS: Edema, abdominal pain/distress, anorexia, diarrhea, dyspepsia, GI ulcers (gastric/duodenal), gross bleeding/perforation, heartburn, liver enzyme elevations, N/V, rash, anemia, CNS inhibition (eg, depression, sedation, somnolence, or confusion), headache.

INTERACTIONS: Avoid use with ASA. May diminish antihypertensive effect of ACE inhibitors. May decrease natriuretic effects of furosemide and thiazide diuretics; monitor for renal failure. May elevate lithium plasma levels; observe for signs of lithium toxicity. May increase methotrexate toxicities. Increased risk of GI bleeding with anticoagulants (eg, warfarin), smoking, alcohol, and oral corticosteroids. Monitor blood glucose in the beginning phase of glyburide and oxaprozin co-therapy. Monitor BP levels when coadministered with β-blockers (eg, metoprolol). Concurrent use with H₂-receptor antagonists (eg, cimetidine or ranitidine) reduced total body clearance of oxaprozin.

PREGNANCY: Category C, not for use in nursing.

MECHANISM OF ACTION: NSAIDs; unknown, suspected to inhibit prostaglandin synthetase.

PHARMACOKINETICS: **Absorption:** 95% absorbed. **Distribution:** V_d/F=11-17L/70kg; plasma protein binding primarily albumin (99%). **Metabolism:** Liver via oxidation (65%) and glucuronic acid conjugation (35%). **Elimination:** Feces (35%), urine (5% unchanged, 65% as metabolite).

NURSING CONSIDERATIONS

Assessment: Assess for hypersensitivity reaction to ASA or other NSAIDs, history of asthma, CV disease (eg, pre-existing HTN, congestive heart failure) or risk factors for cardiovascular disease, fluid retention, edema, SJS, pregnancy status, risk factors for GI events (eg, prior history of ulcer disease or GI bleeding, ulceration, perforation, smoking), coagulation disorders, pregnancy/nursing status, possible drug interactions, and renal/hepatic dysfunction. Assess use in elderly and debilitated patients. Obtain baseline LFTs, renal function, BP, and CBC.

Monitoring: Monitor CBC, LFTs, renal function, blood glucose, and chemistries periodically. Monitor for signs/symptoms of serious skin side effects (exfoliative dermatitis, SJS, and toxic epidermal necrolysis), GI events (bleeding, ulceration, perforation), CV thrombotic events, MI, stroke, HTN, renal/liver dysfunction, and anaphylactoid reaction (difficulty breathing, swelling of face/throat), hematological effects (eg, anemia, prolongation of bleeding time), and bronchospasm.

Patient Counseling: Instruct to read medication guide. Seek medical attention for symptoms of hepatotoxicity (nausea, fatigue, pruritus), anaphylactic reactions (difficulty breathing, swelling of face/throat), hypersensitivity reaction (rash), CV events (chest pain, SOB, weakness, slurring of speech), GI ulceration and bleeding (epigastric pain, dyspepsia, melena, hematemesis), weight gain, and edema. Inform of risks in pregnancy.

Administration: Oral route. **Storage:** 25°C (77°F); excursions permitted to 15-30°C (59-86°F). Dispense in a tight, light-resistant container with a child-resistant closure. Protect from light.

DAYTRANA   `CII`
methylphenidate (Shire)

> Give cautiously to patients with history of drug dependence or alcoholism. Chronic abusive use may lead to marked tolerance and psychological dependence with varying degrees of abnormal behavior. Careful supervision required during withdrawal from abusive use to avoid severe depression. Withdrawal following chronic therapeutic use may unmask symptoms of the underlying disorder that may require follow-up.

THERAPEUTIC CLASS: Sympathomimetic amine

INDICATIONS: Treatment of attention-deficit/hyperactivity disorder (ADHD).

DOSAGE: *Adults:* Individualize dose. Apply to hip area 2 hrs before effect is needed and remove 9 hrs after application. Recommended Titration Schedule: Week 1: 10mg/9 hrs. Week 2: 15mg/9 hrs. Week 3: 20mg/9 hrs. Week 4: 30mg/9 hrs.
Pediatrics: ≥6 yrs: Individualize dose. Apply to hip area 2 hrs before effect is needed and remove 9 hrs after application. Recommended Titration Schedule: Week 1: 10mg/9 hrs. Week 2: 15mg/9 hrs. Week 3: 20mg/9 hrs. Week 4: 30mg/9 hrs.

HOW SUPPLIED: Patch: 10mg/9 hrs, 15mg/9 hrs, 20mg/9 hrs, 30mg/9 hrs [30⁵]

CONTRAINDICATIONS: Patients with marked anxiety, tension, agitation, glaucoma, motor tics or family history or diagnosis of Tourette's syndrome. Treatment with or within a minimum of 14 days following D/C of an MAOI.

WARNINGS/PRECAUTIONS: Sudden death, stroke, myocardial infarction (MI) reported; avoid with known structural cardiac abnormalities or other serious cardiac problems. May increase BP and heart rate; caution with underlying conditions that may be compromised by increased BP or HR (eg, pre-existing HTN, heart failure, recent myocardial infarction, ventricular arrhythmia). Perform history and physical exam prior to use to assess for cardiac disease; perform prompt cardiac evaluation if cardiac disease symptoms develop during treatment. May exacerbate symptoms of behavior disturbance and thought disorder in psychotic patients. Caution in treating patients with co-morbid bipolar disorder because of concern for possible induction of mixed/manic episode. May cause treatment-emergent psychotic or manic symptoms (eg, hallucinations, delusional thinking, mania) in children and adolescents without prior history of psychotic illness at usual doses. Aggressive behavior or hostility reported. May lower convulsive threshold; d/c in the presence of seizures. Monitor growth during treatment in children; consider interrupting treatment if expected height or weight gain does not occur. Difficulties with accommodation and blurred vision reported with stimulant treatment. May lead to contact sensitization; d/c if suspected. Avoid exposing application site to external heat sources (eg, heating pads, electric blankets, heated water beds, etc.). Caution with history of drug dependence or alcoholism.

ADVERSE REACTIONS: Decreased appetite, headache, insomnia, N/V, decreased weight, irritability, tics, affect lability, anorexia, abdominal pain, dizziness.

INTERACTIONS: See Contraindications. Caution with pressor agents. May decrease effectiveness of antihypertensive agents. May inhibit metabolism of coumarin anticoagulants, anticonvulsants (eg, phenobarbital, phenytoin, primidone), some tricyclic drugs (eg, imipramine, clomipramine, desipramine), and SSRIs. Monitor drug levels (or coagulation times with coumarin) and consider dose adjustments with concomitant use. Serious adverse events reported with concomitant clonidine use.

PREGNANCY: Category C, caution in nursing.

MECHANISM OF ACTION: Sympathomimetic amine; CNS stimulant. Suspected to block reuptake of norepinephrine and dopamine into presynaptic neuron and increase release of these monoamines into extraneuronal spaces.

PHARMACOKINETICS: Absorption: Different doses (single and repeated) resulted in different pharmacokinetic parameters. T_{max}=10 hrs (single dose); T_{max}=8 hrs (repeated patch application). **Metabolism:** De-esterification; ritalinic acid (metabolite). **Elimination:** $T_{1/2}$=4-5 hrs (d-methylphenidate); $T_{1/2}$=1.4-2.9 hrs (l-methylphenidate).

NURSING CONSIDERATIONS

Assessment: Assess for history of marked anxiety, tension, agitation, known hypersensitivity to methylphenidate, glaucoma, behavior disturbances, thought disorder, bipolar disorder, depression, family history of suicide, pre-existing structural cardiac abnormalities, psychiatric history, history of seizures or any other conditions where treatment is contraindicated. Assess for presence of cardiac disease and careful history (eg, family history of sudden death or ventricular arrhythmia); perform further cardiac evaluation if findings suggest such disease (eg, ECG). Assess for history of drug dependence or alcoholism.

Monitoring: Monitor periodically for long-term usefulness, possible drug interactions, BP, HR, contact sensitization evidenced by erythema, edema, papules, vesicles, psychotic or manic symptoms such as hallucinations, delusional thinking, mania, confused state, crying, tics, headaches, irritability, anorexia, insomnia, infectious mononucleosis, and viral infection. Monitor for appearance of or worsening aggressive behavior or hostility. Perform follow-up weight and height in children 7-10 yrs. Perform periodic CBC, differential, and platelet counts during prolonged therapy.

Patient Counseling: Counsel about drug abuse/dependence potential. Avoid exposing application site to direct external heat sources while wearing the patch. Apply intact patches only; do not cut patches. Apply patch to a clean, dry site on hip. Site of application must be alternated daily and patch should not be applied to waistline, where tight clothing may rub the patch. Encourage parent/caregiver to use administration chart to monitor application and removal time, and method of disposal. Patient/caregiver should avoid touching adhesive side of patch during application; if touched, wash hands after application. If any swelling or blistering occurs, remove patch and inform physician. Do not apply hydrocortisone or other solutions, creams, ointments, or emollients immediately prior to patch application. Inform of potential side effects (eg, heart-related problems, mental problems); notify physician if any occur. Caution in operating potentially hazardous machinery or vehicles.

Administration: Transdermal route. Apply patch immediately upon removal from protective pouch. If patch does not fully adhere to skin, or is partially or fully detached during wear time, discard patch and apply a new one. Inspect release liner to ensure no adhesive-containing medication has transferred to liner; if adhesive transfer has occurred, discard patch. If a patch is replaced, total recommended wear time for the day should remain 9 hrs. Peel patches off slowly. Patches should not be applied or re-applied with dressings, tape, or other common adhesives. May take patch off earlier if unacceptable duration of appetite loss or insomnia in the evening occurs. **Storage:** 25°C (77°F); excursions permitted to 15-30°C (59-86°F). Do not store patches unpouched; once sealed tray/outer pouch is opened, use within 2 months. Do not refrigerate or freeze patches.

DEMEROL INJECTION `CII`
meperidine HCl (Hospira)

THERAPEUTIC CLASS: Opioid analgesic

INDICATIONS: For relief of moderate to severe pain. For preoperative medication, anesthesia support, and obstetrical analgesia.

DOSAGE: *Adults:* Pain: Usual: 50-150mg IM/SQ q3-4h prn. Preoperative: Usual: 50-100mg IM/SQ 30-90 min before anesthesia. Anesthesia Support: Use repeated slow IV inj of fractional doses (eg, 10mg/mL) or continuous IV infusion of a more diluted solution (eg, 1mg/mL). Titrate as needed. Obstetrical Analgesia: Usual: 50-100mg IM/SQ when pain is regular, may repeat at 1- to 3-hr intervals. Elderly: Start at lower end of dosage range and observe. With Phenothiazines/Other Tranquilizers: Reduce dose by 25-50%. IM method preferred with repeated use. For IV injection: Reduce dose and administer slowly, preferably using diluted solution.
Pediatrics: Pain: Usual: 0.5-0.8mg/lb IM/SQ, up to 50-150mg, q3-4h prn. Preoperative: Usual: 0.5-1mg/lb IM/SQ, up to 50-100mg, 30-90 min before anesthesia. With Phenothiazines/Other Tranquilizers: Reduce dose by 25-50%. IM method preferred with repeated use. For IV injection: Reduce dose and administer slowly, preferably using diluted solution.

HOW SUPPLIED: Inj: 25mg/mL, 50mg/mL, 75mg/mL, 100mg/mL

CONTRAINDICATIONS: MAOIs during or within 14 days of use.

WARNINGS/PRECAUTIONS: May develop tolerance and dependence; abuse potential. Extreme caution with head injury, increased intracranial pressure, intracranial lesions, acute asthmatic attack, chronic obstructive pulmonary disease or cor pulmonale, decreased respiratory reserve, respiratory depression, hypoxia, and hypercapnia. Rapid IV infusion may result in increased adverse reactions. Caution with acute abdominal conditions, atrial flutter, supraventricular tachycardias. May aggravate convulsive disorders. Caution and reduce initial dose with elderly or debilitated, renal/hepatic impairment, hypothyroidism, Addison's disease, prostatic hypertrophy or urethral stricture. Severe hypotension may occur post-op or if depleted blood volume. Orthostatic hypotension may occur. May impair mental/physical abilities. Not for use in pregnancy prior to labor. May produce depression of respiration and psychophysiologic functions in newborns when used as an obstetrical analgesic.

ADVERSE REACTIONS: Lightheadedness, dizziness, sedation, N/V, sweating, respiratory/circulatory depression.

INTERACTIONS: See Contraindications. Caution and reduce dose with other CNS depressants (eg, narcotics, anesthetics, phenothiazines, tranquilizers, sedative-hypnotics, TCAs, alcohol).

PREGNANCY: Safety in pregnancy and nursing not known.

MECHANISM OF ACTION: Narcotic analgesic; produces actions similiar to morphine. Principal actions involve the CNS and organs composed of smooth muscle. Produces analgesic and sedative effects.

PHARMACOKINETICS: Distribution: Crosses placental barrier; found in breast milk.

NURSING CONSIDERATIONS

Assessment: Assess for pain intensity, or any other conditions where treatment is contraindicated or cautioned. Assess for pregnancy/nursing status, renal/hepatic function, and possible drug interactions.

Monitoring: Monitor for signs/symptoms of drug dependence (eg, psychic dependence, physical dependence), respiratory depression, circulatory depression (eg, hypotension), and convulsions.

Patient Counseling: Inform that medication may impair mental/physical abilities; use caution when performing hazardous tasks (eg, operating machinery/driving). Notify physician of all medications currently taking. Avoid using other CNS depressants and alcohol during medication. Advise about potential for dependence upon repeated administration.

Administration: SQ, IM, IV route. SQ route is suitable for occasional use, IM administration is preferred if repeated doses are required. IM injection should be injected well into the body of a large muscle. If IV route is required, dosage should be decreased and injection should be made very slowly, preferably using a diluted solution. Dosage should be adjusted according to severity of pain. **Storage:** 20-25°C (68-77°F).

DEMEROL ORAL CII
meperidine HCl (Sanofi-Aventis)

THERAPEUTIC CLASS: Opioid analgesic

INDICATIONS: Relief of moderate to severe pain.

DOSAGE: *Adults:* Usual: 50-150mg q3-4h prn. Concomitant Phenothiazines/Other Tranquilizers: Reduce dose by 25-50%.
Pediatrics: Usual: 1.1-1.8mg/kg, up to adult dose, q3-4h prn. Concomitant Phenothiazines/Other Tranquilizers: Reduce dose by 25-50%.

HOW SUPPLIED: Tab: 50mg*, 100mg* *scored

CONTRAINDICATIONS: During or within 14 days of MAOI use.

WARNINGS/PRECAUTIONS: May develop tolerance and dependence; abuse potential. Extreme caution with head injury, increased intracranial pressure, intracranial lesions, acute asthma attack, chronic obstructive pulmonary disease, cor pulmonale, decreased respiratory reserve, respiratory depression, hypoxia, and hypercapnia. Caution with sickle cell anemia, pheochromocytoma, acute alcoholism, Addison's disease, CNS depression or coma, delirium tremens, elderly or debilitated, kyphoscoliosis associated with respiratory depression, myxedema, hypothyroidism, acute abdominal conditions, epilepsy, atrial flutter and other supraventricular tachycardias, renal/hepatic impairment, prostatic hypertrophy, urethral stricture, drug dependencies, neonates, and young infants. Severe hypotension may occur post-op or if depleted blood volume. Orthostatic hypotension may occur. Not for use in pregnancy prior to labor. May impair mental/physical abilities.

ADVERSE REACTIONS: Lightheadedness, dizziness, sedation, N/V, sweating, respiratory depression.

INTERACTIONS: See Contraindications. Reduce dose with other CNS depressants (eg, narcotics, anesthetics, phenothiazines, tranquilizers, sedative-hypnotics, TCAs, alcohol). Mixed agonist/antagonist analgesics (eg, pentazocine, nalbuphine, butorphanol, buprenorphine) may reduce analgesic effects and/or precipitate withdrawal symptoms. Caution with acyclovir, cimetidine. Phenytoin may enhance hepatic metabolism. May enhance neuromuscular blocking action of skeletal muscle relaxants. Increased levels with ritonavir; avoid concomitant administration.

PREGNANCY: Category C, not for use in nursing.

MECHANISM OF ACTION: Narcotic analgesic; produces actions similiar to morphine. Principal actions involve the CNS and organs composed of smooth muscle. Produces analgesic and sedative effects.

PHARMACOKINETICS: Distribution: Crosses placental barrier; found in breast milk.

NURSING CONSIDERATIONS

Assessment: Assess for pain intensity, or any other conditions where treatment is contraindicated or cautioned. Assess for history of hypersensitivity, pregnancy/nursing status, renal/hepatic function, and possible drug interactions.

Monitoring: Monitor for signs/symptoms of tolerance or dependence, misuse or abuse, increase in CSF pressure, circulatory depression (eg, hypotension), respiratory depression, and convulsions.

Patient Counseling: Counsel to notify physician of all medications currently taking. Avoid with MAOI use within 14 days. Notify physician of any pain or adverse events during treatment. Do not adjust dosage or abruptly d/c therapy without consulting physician. Inform medication contains meperidine, a morphine-like substance that has potential for drug abuse; protect from theft and use by anyone other than the prescribed patient. Drug may impair mental/physical abilities; use caution when performing hazardous tasks (eg, operating machinery, driving). Avoid using other CNS depressants and alcohol. Inform pregnant women about effects of medication on pregnancy.

Administration: Oral route. **Storage:** 25°C (77°F); excursions permitted to 15-30°C (59-86°F).

DENAVIR   RX
penciclovir (Novartis)

THERAPEUTIC CLASS: Nucleoside analogue

INDICATIONS: Treatment of recurrent herpes labialis (cold sores) in adults and children ≥12 yrs.

DOSAGE: *Adults:* Apply q2h while awake for 4 days. Start with earliest sign or symptom.
Pediatrics: ≥12 yrs: Apply q2h while awake for 4 days. Start with earliest sign or symptom.

HOW SUPPLIED: Cre: 1% [1.5g]

WARNINGS/PRECAUTIONS: Only use on herpes labialis on the lips and face. Avoid mucous membranes or near the eyes. Effectiveness not established in immunocompromised patients.

ADVERSE REACTIONS: Headache, application-site reaction, local anesthesia, taste perversion, rash.

PREGNANCY: Category B, not for use in nursing.

MECHANISM OF ACTION: Antiviral agent; active against herpes simplex virus types 1 (HSV-1) and 2 (HSV-2). Inhibits HSV polymerase competitively with deoxyguanosine triphosphate. Consequently, herpes viral DNA synthesis and replication are selectively inhibited.

NURSING CONSIDERATIONS

Assessment: Assess for severity, signs and symptoms of cold sore, use in pregnancy/nursing.

Monitoring: Monitor lesions for clinical response. If lesions worsen or do not improve, monitor for secondary bacterial infection.

Patient Counseling: Counsel to avoid applying medication in or near eyes. Instruct to wash hands with soap and water after applying product. Advise females to notify physician if they become pregnant or are nursing.

Administration: Topical. **Storage:** 20-25°C (68-77°F).

DEPACON

RX

valproate sodium (Abbott)

> Fatal hepatic failure may occur, especially in children <2 yrs on multiple anticonvulsants, with congenital metabolic disorders, severe seizure disorders with mental retardation, and organic brain disease. Hepatotoxicity may be preceded by nonspecific symptoms such as malaise, weakness, lethargy, facial edema, anorexia, and vomiting, or loss of seizure control in patients with epilepsy. Monitor LFTs prior to therapy, frequently during 1st 6 months of treatment and at frequent intervals thereafter. Teratogenic effects (eg, neural tube defects), and life-threatening pancreatitis reported; d/c if pancreatitis diagnosed and initiate appropriate treatment.

THERAPEUTIC CLASS: Valproate compound

INDICATIONS: Alternative when oral administration of valproate products is temporarily not feasible in the following conditions: monotherapy and adjunctive therapy for treatment of simple and complex absence seizures, and complex partial seizures; adjunctive therapy for multiple seizure types that include absence seizures.

DOSAGE: *Adults:* Simple/Complex Absence Seizure: Initial: 15mg/kg/day. Titrate: Increase weekly by 5-10mg/kg/day until optimal response. Max: 60mg/kg/day. Complex Partial Seizure/Conversion to Monotherapy/ Adjunctive Therapy: Initial: 10-15mg/kg/day. Titrate: Increase weekly by 5-10mg/kg/day until optimal response. Max: 60mg/kg/day. Elderly: Reduce initial dose and titrate slowly. Replacement Therapy: Give equivalent total daily dose as that of oral valproate. Administer as 60 min IV infusion, not >20mg/min. If dose >250mg/day, give in divided doses. Not for use >14 days; switch to oral route as soon as clinically feasible. Decrease dose or d/c if decreased food or fluid intake or if excessive somnolence occurs.
Pediatrics: ≥2 yrs: Simple/Complex Absence Seizure: Initial: 15mg/kg/day. Titrate: Increase weekly by 5-10mg/kg/day until optimal response. Max: 60mg/kg/day. ≥10 yrs: Complex Partial Seizure/Conversion to Monotherapy/ Adjunctive Therapy: Initial: 10-15mg/kg/day. Titrate: Increase weekly by 5-10mg/kg/day until optimal response. Max: 60mg/kg/day. Replacement Therapy: Give equivalent total daily dose as that of oral valproate. Administer as 60 min IV infusion, not >20mg/min. If dose >250mg/day, give in divided doses. Not for use >14 days; switch to oral route as soon as clinically feasible. Decrease dose or d/c if decreased food or fluid intake or if excessive somnolence occurs.

HOW SUPPLIED: Inj: 100mg/mL [5mL]

CONTRAINDICATIONS: Hepatic disease, significant hepatic dysfunction, known urea cycle disorders (UCD).

WARNINGS/PRECAUTIONS: Caution in hepatic disease; d/c if hepatic dysfunction suspected or apparent. Hyperammonemic encephalopathy in UCD patients; d/c if this occurs. Prior to therapy, evaluate for UCD in high-risk patients (eg, history of unexplained encephalopathy, coma, etc). If unexplained lethargy, vomiting, or mental status changes occur, measure ammonia levels. Caution in the elderly; monitor for fluid/nutritional intake, dehydration, somnolence. Dose-related thrombocytopenia and elevated liver enzymes reported. Monitor platelet and coagulation tests prior to therapy, then periodically. Altered thyroid function tests and urine ketone test. Avoid abrupt d/c. Multi-organ hypersensitivity reactions reported. May impair mental/physical abilities. Not for prophylaxis of post-traumatic seizures in acute head trauma. May stimulate replication of HIV and cytomegalovirus.

ADVERSE REACTIONS: Dizziness, headache, N/V, elevated amylase, injection-site pain/reaction, somnolence, thrombocytopenia, ecchymosis.

INTERACTIONS: Drugs that affect the level of expression of hepatic enzymes (eg, phenytoin, carbamazepine, phenobarbital, primidone) may increase valproate clearance. Concomitant use with ASA decreases protein binding and metabolism of valproate. Carbapenem antibiotics (eg, meropenem, ertapenem, imipenem) may reduce serum valproic concentration to subtherapeutic levels. Rifampin increases oral clearance and may require valproate dosage adjustment. Concomitant use with felbamate leads to an increase in valproate C_{max}. Reduces the clearance of amitriptyline, nortriptyline, and lorazepam.

Induces metabolism of carbamazepine. Inhibits metabolism of diazepam, ethosuximide, phenobarbital and phenytoin; monitor drug serum concentrations and adjust dose appropriately. Breakthrough seizures reported with concomitant valproate and phenytoin use. Administration with clonazepam may induce absence status in patients with absence seizures. Increases $T_{1/2}$ of lamotrigine; serious skin reactions reported. Concomitant use with topiramate associated with hyperammonemia with or without encephalopathy. May displace protein-bound warfarin; monitor coagulation tests. Additive CNS depression with other CNS depressants (eg, alcohol). May decrease clearance of zidovudine in HIV-seropositive patients.

PREGNANCY: Category D, not for use in nursing.

MECHANISM OF ACTION: Anticonvulsant; has not been established. Proposed to increase GABA concentration in the brain.

PHARMACOKINETICS: Distribution: V_d=11L/1.73m²; plasma protein binding (81.5%-90%); found in breast milk, CSF. **Metabolism:** Liver; glucuronidation, mitochondrial β-oxidation. **Elimination:** Urine (<3% unchanged); $T_{1/2}$=16 hrs.

NURSING CONSIDERATIONS

Assessment: Assess LFTs, CBC with platelets, pancreatitis, plasma ammonia levels, other diseases/conditions, acute head injuries, pregnancy/nursing status, and possible drug interactions. Note other diseases/conditions and drug therapies.

Monitoring: Monitor LFTs, CBC with platelets, coagulation parameters, pancreatitis, hypersensitivity reactions, hyperammonemia, thyroid function tests.

Patient Counseling: Advise to avoid alcohol, sedatives, and other over-the-counter drugs. Advise not to engage in hazardous activities (eg, driving/operating machinery). Counsel about signs/symptoms of pancreatitis, hepatotoxicity, hyperammonemia; notify physician if any symptoms or adverse effects occur. Instruct that a fever associated with other organ system involvement (rash, lymphadenopathy, etc.) may be drug-related and should be reported to physician immediately. Notify physician if pregnant or intend to become pregnant. Encourage patients to enroll in North American Antiepileptic Drug (NAAED) Pregnancy Registry by calling 888-233-2334 or go to www.aed-pregnancyregistry.org.

Administration: IV route. Give as a 60-min infusion after diluting with at least 50mL of a compatible diluent. **Storage:** 15-30°C (59-86°F).

DEPAKENE   RX
valproic acid (Abbott)

> Fatal hepatic failure may occur, especially in children <2 yrs on multiple anticonvulsants, with congenital metabolic disorders, severe seizure disorders with mental retardation, or organic brain disease. Hepatotoxicity may be preceded by nonspecific symptoms such as malaise, weakness, lethargy, facial edema, anorexia, and vomiting, or loss of seizure control in patients with epilepsy. Monitor LFTs prior to therapy, frequently during 1st 6 months of treatment and at frequent intervals thereafter. Teratogenic effects (eg, neural tube defects), and life-threatening pancreatitis reported; d/c if pancreatitis diagnosed and initiate appropriate treatment.

THERAPEUTIC CLASS: Carboxylic acid derivative

INDICATIONS: Monotherapy and adjunctive therapy for treatment of simple and complex absence seizures, and complex partial seizures. Adjunctive therapy for multiple seizure types, including absence seizures.

DOSAGE: *Adults:* Simple/Complex Absence Seizures: Initial: 15mg/kg/day. Titrate: Increase weekly by 5-10mg/kg/day until optimal response. Max: 60mg/kg/day. If dose >250mg/day, give in divided doses. Complex Partial Seizures: Monotherapy/Conversion to Monotherapy/Adjunctive Therapy: Initial: 10-15mg/kg/day. Titrate: Increase weekly by 5-10mg/kg/week until optimal response. If clinical response has not been achieved, plasma levels should be measured to determine whether they are in usually accepted therapeutic range (50-100µg/mL). Max: 60mg/kg/day. Concomitant anti-epileptic drug (AED) dosage can ordinarily be reduced by approximately 25% q2 weeks starting at initiation of valproic acid or delayed 1-2 weeks if there is concern seizures are likely to occur. Elderly: Reduce initial dose and titrate slowly. Consider dose reduction or d/c in patients with decreased food or fluid intake and in patients with excessive somnolence. GI irritation: May benefit from administration of the drug with food or by slowly building up the dose from an initial low level.

Pediatrics: >2 yrs: Simple/Complex Absence Seizure: Initial: 15mg/kg/day. Titrate: Increase by 5-10mg/kg/day until optimal response. Max: 60 mg/kg/day. If dose >250mg/day, give in divided doses. ≥10 yrs: Complex Partial Seizure: Monotherapy/Conversion to Monotherapy/Adjunctive Therapy: Initial: 10-15mg/kg/day. Titrate: Increase weekly by 5-10mg/kg/week until optimal response. If clinical response has not been achieved, plasma levels should be measured to determine whether they are in usually accepted therapeutic range (50-100µg/mL). Max: 60mg/kg/day. Concomitant AED dosage can ordinarily be reduced by approximately 25% q2 weeks starting at initiation of valproic acid or delayed 1-2 weeks if there is a concern that seizures are likely to occur. GI irritation: May benefit from administration of the drug with food or by slowly building up the dose from an initial low level.

HOW SUPPLIED: Cap: 250mg; Sol: 250mg/5mL

CONTRAINDICATIONS: Hepatic disease, significant hepatic dysfunction, known urea cycle disorders (UCD).

WARNINGS/PRECAUTIONS: Increased risk of suicidal thoughts or behavior; monitor for emergence or worsening of depression. Hyperammonemic encephalopathy in UCD patients; d/c if this occurs. Prior to therapy, evaluate for UCD in high-risk patients (eg, history of unexplained encephalopathy, coma, etc.). Measure ammonia levels if develop unexplained lethargy, vomiting, or mental status changes. Caution in elderly; monitor for fluid/nutritional intake, dehydration, somnolence. Multi-organ hypersensitivity reactions and hypothermia, with or without hyperammonemia, reported. Monitor platelets and coagulation tests before therapy and periodically thereafter. Elevated liver enzymes and thrombocytopenia may be dose-related. May interfere with urine ketone and thyroid function tests. May impair mental/physical abilities. Caution with history of hepatic disease. May stimulate replication of HIV and CMV. Avoid abrupt d/c.

ADVERSE REACTIONS: Abdominal pain, amblyopia/blurred vision, alopecia, asthenia, diarrhea, diplopia, dizziness, headache, nystagmus, N/V, peripheral edema, somnolence, tremor, thrombocytopenia, weight gain.

INTERACTIONS: Carbapenem antibiotics may reduce serum valproic concentration to subtherapeutic levels, leading to loss of seizure control. Oral clearance increased by rifampin. Concomitant administration with clonazepam may induce absence status in patients with history thereof. Increases $T_{1/2}$ of lamotrigine; may result in serious skin reaction with lamotrigine. Reports of breakthrough seizures with the combination of valproate and phenytoin; monitor levels of both. Concomitant use with ASA decreases protein binding and metabolism of valproate. Reduces the clearance of amitriptyline, nortriptyline, zidovudine, and lorazepam. Induces metabolism of carbamazepine. Displaces protein-bound diazepam and decreases its V_d and clearance. Inhibits metabolism and decreases clearance of ethosuximide. Concomitant use with felbamate leads to an increase in valproate C_{max}. Inhibits the metabolism of phenobarbital. Monitor for neurological toxicity when used with barbiturates. Displaces protein-bound tolbutamide, and warfarin; monitor coagulation tests. Concomitant use with topiramate has been associated with hyperammonemia with or without encephalopathy and hypothermia. Drugs that affect the level of expression of hepatic enzymes (eg, phenytoin, carbamazepine, phenobarbital, primidone) may increase valproate clearance. Additive CNS depression with other CNS depressants (eg, alcohol). Increased plasma level with chlorpromazine.

PREGNANCY: Category D, not for use in nursing.

MECHANISM OF ACTION: Carboxylic acid derivative; has not been established. Activity in epilepsy is proposed to be related to increased GABA concentration in the brain.

PHARMACOKINETICS: Absorption: Depakote:(Tab) T_{max}=4 hrs (fasting), 8 hrs (fed); (Cap) T_{max}=3.3 hrs (fasting), 4.8 hrs (fed). **Distribution:** V_d=11L/1.73m^2; plasma protein binding (10%-18.5%). **Metabolism:** Liver; glucuronidation, mitochondrial β-oxidation. **Elimination:** Urine (<3% unchanged); $T_{1/2}$=9-16 hrs.

NURSING CONSIDERATIONS

Assessment: Assess LFTs, CBC with platelets, pancreatitis, plasma ammonia levels, hepatic dysfunction/disease, pregnancy/nursing status. Note other diseases/conditions and drug therapies. Prior to therapy, evaluate for UCD in high-risk patients (eg, history of unexplained encepalopathy, coma, etc.).

Monitoring: Monitor LFTs (at frequent intervals during first 6 months), CBC with platelets, coagulation parameters, pancreatitis, thyroid function tests, hypersensitivity reactions, hyperammonemia, ketone and thyroid function tests. Monitor for emergence of worsening of depression, suicidal thoughts or behavior, and/or unusual changes in mood or behavior.

Patient Counseling: Counsel to avoid alcohol, sedatives, over-the-counter drugs. Caution while operating machinery/driving. Counsel about signs/symptoms of hepatotoxicity, pancreatitis, and hyperammonemic encephalopathy; notify physician if symptoms or adverse effects occur. Instruct that a fever associated with other organ system involvement (eg, rash, lympadenopathy, etc.) may be drug-related and should be reported to physician immediately. Notify physician if suicidal thoughts, behavior, or thoughts about self-harm emerge. Advise patients to enroll in the North American Antiepilepetic Drug (NAAED) Pregnancy Registry if they become pregnant. To enroll, call 888-233-2334 or go to www.aedpregnancyregistry.org.

Administration: Oral route. Swallow caps whole; do not chew. **Storage:** Cap: 15-25°C (59-77°F). Sol: Below 30°C (86°F).

DEPAKOTE   RX

divalproex sodium (Abbott)

> Fatal hepatic failure may occur, especially in children <2 yrs on multiple anticonvulsants, with congenital metabolic disorders, severe seizure disorders with mental retardation, and organic brain disease. Hepatotoxicity may be preceded by nonspecific symptoms such as malaise, weakness, lethargy, facial edema, anorexia, and vomiting, or loss of seizure control in patients with epilepsy. Monitor LFTs prior to therapy, frequently during 1st 6 months of treatment and at frequent intervals thereafter. Teratogenic effects (eg, neural tube defects), and life-threatening pancreatitis reported; d/c if pancreatitis diagnosed and initiate appropriate treatment.

OTHER BRAND NAMES: Depakote Sprinkle Capsules (Abbott)

THERAPEUTIC CLASS: Valproate compound

INDICATIONS: (Tab, Cap) Management of simple and complex absence seizures, complex partial seizures, and adjunctively with multiple seizure types including absence seizures. (Tab) Treatment of mania associated with bipolar disorder and migraine prophylaxis.

DOSAGE: *Adults:* (Cap/Tab) Complex Partial Seizures: Initial: 10-15mg/kg/day. Titrate: Increase by 5-10mg/kg/week. Max: 60mg/kg/day. Absence Seizures: Initial: 15mg/kg/day. Titrate: Increase weekly by 5-10mg/kg/day. Max: 60mg/kg/day. Give in divided doses if >250mg/day. Sprinkle capsules may be swallowed whole or contents may be sprinkled on soft food. Drug food mixture should be swallowed immediately; avoid chewing. (Tab) Migraine: Initial: 250mg bid. Max: 1000mg/day. Mania: 750mg daily in divided doses. Titrate: Increase dose rapidly to clinical effect. Max: 60mg/kg/day. Elderly: Reduce initial dose and titrate slowly. Decrease dose or d/c if decreased food or fluid intake or if excessive somnolence occurs.
Pediatrics: ≥16 yrs: (Tab) Migraine: Initial: 250mg bid. Max: 1000mg/day. ≥10 yrs: (Cap/Tab) Complex Partial Seizures: Initial: 10-15mg/kg/day. Titrate: Increase by 5-10mg/kg/week. Max: 60mg/kg/day. Absence Seizures: Initial: 15mg/kg/day. Titrate: Increase weekly by 5-10mg/kg/day. Max: 60mg/kg/day. Give in divided doses if >250mg/day. Sprinkle capsules may be swallowed whole or contents may be sprinkled on soft food. Drug food mixture should be swallowed immediately; avoid chewing.

HOW SUPPLIED: Cap, Delayed-Release: (Sprinkle) 125mg; Tab, Delayed-Release: 125mg, 250mg, 500mg

CONTRAINDICATIONS: Hepatic disease, significant hepatic dysfunction, known urea cycle disorders (UCD).

WARNINGS/PRECAUTIONS: Increased risk of suicidal thoughts or behavior; monitor for the emergence of worsening, and/or any unusual changes in mood or behavior. Hyperammonemic encephalopathy in UCD patients; d/c if this occurs. Prior to therapy, evaluate for UCD in high-risk patients (eg, history of unexplained encephalopathy, coma, etc). If unexplained lethargy, vomiting, or mental status changes occur, measure ammonia levels. Caution with hepatic disease; d/c if significant hepatic dysfunction suspected or apparent. Caution in the elderly; monitor fluid/nutritional intake, dehydration, and somnolence. Dose-related thrombocytopenia and elevated liver enzymes reported. Monitor platelet and coagulation tests prior to therapy, then periodically. Altered thyroid function tests and urine ketone tests. May stimulate replication of HIV and cytomegalovirus. Avoid abrupt d/c. Multi-organ hypersensitivity reactions and hypothermia reported.

ADVERSE REACTIONS: Diarrhea, N/V, somnolence, dyspepsia, thrombocytopenia, asthenia, abdominal pain, tremor, headache, anorexia, diplopia, blurred vision, dizziness, weight gain, rash.

INTERACTIONS: Drugs that affect the level of expression of hepatic enzymes (eg, phenytoin, carbamazepine, phenobarbital, primidone) may increase valproate clearance. Concomitant use with ASA decreases protein binding and metabolism of valproate. Carbapenem antibiotics (eg, ertapenem, imipenem, meropenem) may reduce serum valproic concentration to subtherapeutic levels, resulting in loss of seizure control. Rifampin increases oral clearance and may requre valproate dosage adjustment. Concomitant use with felbamate leads to an increase in valproate C_{max}. Reduces the clearance of amitriptyline, nortriptyline, and lorazepam. Induces metabolism of carbamazepine. Inhibits metabolism of diazepam, ethosuximide, phenobarbital and phenytoin; monitor drug serum concentrations and adjust dose appropriately. Breakthrough seizures reported with concomitant valproate and phenytoin use. Administration with clonazepam may induce absence status in patients with absence seizures. Increases $T_{1/2}$ of lamotrigine; serious skin reactions reported. Concomitant use with topiramate associated with hyperammonemia, with or without encephalopathy, and hypothermia. May displace protein-bound warfarin; monitor coagulation tests. Additive CNS depression with other CNS depressants (eg, alcohol). May decrease clearance of zidovudine in HIV-seropositive patients.

PREGNANCY: Category D, not for use in nursing.

MECHANISM OF ACTION: Anticonvulsant; has not been established. Proposed to increases GABA concentrations in the brain.

PHARMACOKINETICS: Absorption: T_{max}=4-8 hrs (tab), T_{max}=3.3-4.8 hrs (cap). **Distribution:** Plasma protein binding (10%-18.5%). Found in breast milk. **Metabolism:** Liver; glucuronidation, mitochondrial β-oxidation. **Elimination:** Urine (<3% unchanged); $T_{1/2}$=9-16 hrs.

NURSING CONSIDERATIONS

Assessment: Assess LFTs, CBC with platelets, pancreatitis, plasma ammonia levels, pregnancy status. Note other diseases/conditions and drug therapies.

Monitoring: Monitor LFTs, CBC with platelets, coagulation parameters, pancreatitis, hypersensitivity reactions, hyperammonemia, thyroid function tests.

Patient Counseling: Counsel to avoid alcohol, sedatives, OTC agents. Advise not to engage in hazardous activities (eg, driving/operating machinery). Counsel about signs/symptoms of pancreatitis, hepatotoxicity, hyperammonemia; notify physician if any symptoms or adverse effects occur. Instruct that a fever associated with other organ system involvement (eg, rash, lymphadenopathy, etc.) may be drug-related and should be reported to physician immediately. Notify physician if suicidal thoughts, behavior, or thoughts about self-harm emerge. Notify physician if pregnant or intend to become pregnant. Encourage patients to enroll in North American Antiepileptic

Drug (NAAED) Pregnancy Registry by calling 888-233-2334 or go to www.aedpregnancyregistry.org.

Administration: Oral route. **Storage:** Store below 30°C (86°F).

DEPAKOTE ER

RX

divalproex sodium (Abbott)

> Fatal hepatic failure may occur, especially in children <2 yrs on multiple anticonvulsants, with congenital metabolic disorders, severe seizure disorders with mental retardation, and organic brain disease. These incidents usually have occurred during the first 6 months of treatment. Hepatotoxicity may be preceded by nonspecific symptoms such as malaise, weakness, lethargy, facial edema, anorexia, vomiting, or loss of seizure control in patients with epilepsy. Monitor LFTs prior to therapy, especially during the first 6 months of treatment and at frequent intervals thereafter. Teratogenic effects (eg, neural tube defects) reported, including developmental delay, autism and/or autism spectrum disorder; use only if benefits of therapy outweigh risk. Life-threatening pancreatitis reported. Some cases have been described as hemorrhagic with rapid progression from initial symptoms to death. D/C if pancreatitis diagnosed and initiate appropriate treatment.

THERAPEUTIC CLASS: Valproate compound

INDICATIONS: Migraine prophylaxis. Acute manic or mixed episodes associated with bipolar disorder, with or without psychotic features. In adults and children ≥10 years, monotherapy and adjunctive therapy of complex partial seizures, and simple and complex absence seizures; an adjunct for multiple seizure types that include absence seizures.

DOSAGE: *Adults:* Individualize dose. Migraine: Initial: 500mg qd for 1 week. Titrate: Increase to 1000mg qd. Mania: Initial: 25mg/kg/day given qd. Titrate: Increase dose rapidly to achieve clinical effect. Max: 60mg/kg/day. Complex Partial Seizures: Monotherapy/Conversion to Monotherapy/Adjunctive Therapy: Initial: 10-15mg/kg/day. Titrate: Increase weekly by 5-10mg/kg/week until optimal response. Max: 60mg/kg/day. When converting to monotherapy, reduce concomitant antiepilepsy drug by 25% every 2 weeks starting at initiation or delay 1-2 weeks after start of therapy. Simple/Complex Absence Seizures: Initial: 15mg/kg/day. Titrate: Increase weekly by 5-10mg/kg/day until optimal response. Max: 60mg/kg/day. Conversion from Depakote: Administer dose 8-20% higher than total daily dose of Depakote. Refer to PI for dose conversion. If dose cannot be directly converted, consider increasing to next higher Depakote total daily dose before converting to appropriate total daily Depakote ER dose. Elderly: Reduce initial dose and titrate slowly. Decrease dose or d/c if decreased food or fluid intake or if excessive somnolence occurs.

Pediatrics: ≥10 yrs: Complex Partial Seizures: Monotherapy/Conversion to Monotherapy/Adjunctive Therapy: Initial: 10-15mg/kg/day. Titrate: Increase weekly by 5-10mg/kg/week until optimal response. Max: 60mg/kg/day. When converting to monotherapy, reduce concomitant antiepilepsy drug by 25% every 2 weeks starting at initiation or delay 1-2 weeks after start of therapy. Simple/Complex Absence Seizures: Initial: 15mg/kg/day. Titrate: Increase weekly by 5-10mg/kg/day until optimal response. Max: 60mg/kg/day. Conversion from Depakote: Administer dose 8-20% higher than total daily dose of Depakote. Refer to PI for dose conversion. If dose cannot be directly converted, consider increasing to next higher Depakote total daily dose before converting to appropriate total daily Depakote ER dose.

HOW SUPPLIED: Tab, Extended-Release: 250mg, 500mg

CONTRAINDICATIONS: Hepatic disease, significant hepatic dysfunction, known urea cycle disorders (UCD).

WARNINGS/PRECAUTIONS: Increased risk of suicidal thoughts or behavior; monitor for the emergence of worsening of depression, suicidal thoughts or behavior, and/or any unusual changes in mood or behavior. Hyperammonemic encephalopathy in UCD patients; d/c and initiate treatment if symptoms develop. Prior to therapy, evaluate for UCD in high-risk patients (eg, history of unexplained encephalopathy, coma, etc). Measure ammonia levels if unexplained lethargy, vomiting, or mental status changes occur. Caution in the elderly; monitor fluid/nutritional intake, and for dehydration and somnolence. Dose-related thrombocytopenia and elevated liver enzymes reported. Monitor platelet and coagulation tests prior to therapy, then periodically. Altered thyroid function tests and urine ketone tests. May stimulate replication of HIV and cytomegalovirus. May impair mental/physical abilities. Multi-organ hypersensitivity reactions and hypothermia reported.

ADVERSE REACTIONS: N/V, dyspepsia, diarrhea, abdominal pain, asthenia, somnolence, headache, fever, anorexia, infection, dizziness, hepatotoxicity, neural tube defects, pancreatitis.

INTERACTIONS: Drugs that affect the level of expression of hepatic enzymes (eg, phenytoin, carbamazepine, phenobarbital, primidone) may increase valproate clearance. Concomitant use with ASA decreases protein binding and metabolism. Carbapenem antibiotics (eg, ertapenem, imipenem, meropenem) may reduce serum concentration to subtherapeutic levels, resulting in loss of seizure control. Rifampin increases oral clearance and may require valproate dosage adjustment. Concomitant use with felbamate leads to an increase in valproate C_{max}. Reduces the clearance of amitriptylline, nortriptyline, and lorazepam. Induces metabolism of carbamazepine. Inhibits metabolism of diazepam, ethosuximide, phenobarbital and phenytoin; monitor drug serum concentrations and adjust dose appropriately. Breakthrough seizures reported with concomitant use with phenytoin. Administration with clonazepam may induce absence status in patients with absence seizures. Increases $T_{1/2}$ of lamotrigine; serious skin reactions reported. Concomitant use with topiramate associated with hyperammonemia, with or without encephalopathy, and hypothermia. May displace protein-bound warfarin; monitor coagulation tests. Additive CNS depression with other CNS depressants (eg, alcohol). May decrease clearance of zidovudine in HIV-seropositive patients. May increase concentrations of tolbutamide.

PREGNANCY: Category D, not for use in nursing.

MECHANISM OF ACTION: Anticonvulsant; mechanism not established. Proposed to increase GABA concentrations in the brain.

PHARMACOKINETICS: Absorption: Bioavailability (90%); T_{max}=4-17 hrs. **Distribution:** Plasma protein binding (10-18.5%). Found in breast milk, CSF. (Free valproate) V_d = 92 L/1.73m^2. (Total valproate) V_d = 11 L/1.73m^2. **Metabolism:** Liver; glucuronidation, mitochondrial β-oxidation. **Elimination:** Urine (<3% unchanged); $T_{1/2}$=9-16 hrs.

NURSING CONSIDERATIONS

Assessment: Assess hepatic dysfunction, UCD, pancreatitis, plasma ammonia levels, platelets, coagulation tests, history of hypersensitivity, pregnancy/nursing status. Note other diseases/conditions and possible drug interactions.

Monitoring: Monitor LFTs, CBC with platelets, coagulation parameters, pancreatitis, hypersensitivity reactions, hyperammonemia, thyroid function tests. Monitor for emergence/worsening of depression, suicidality, unusual changes in behavior.

Patient Counseling: Counsel to avoid alcohol, sedatives, over-the-counter drugs. Advise not to engage in hazardous activities (eg, driving/operating machinery). Counsel about signs/symptoms of pancreatitis, hepatotoxicity, hyperammonemia; notify physician if any symptoms or adverse effects occur. Instruct that a fever associated with other organ system involvement (eg, rash, lymphadenopathy, etc.) may be drug-related and should be reported to physician immediately. Notify physician if suicidal thoughts, behavior, or thoughts about self-harm emerge. Inform to take as prescribed and if dose is missed take as soon as possible; do not skip or double the dose. Notify physician if pregnant or intend to become pregnant. Encourage patients to enroll in North American Antiepileptic Drug (NAAED) Pregnancy Registry by calling 888-233-2334 or go to aedpregnancyregistry.org

Administration: Oral route. Swallow whole. Do not crush or chew. **Storage:** 25°C (77°F); excursions permitted to 15-30°C (59-86°F).

DEPO-MEDROL

RX

methylprednisolone acetate (Pharmacia & Upjohn)

D

THERAPEUTIC CLASS: Glucocorticoid

INDICATIONS: Steroid-responsive disorders.

DOSAGE: *Adults:* Local Effect: Rheumatoid/Osteoarthritis: Large Joint: 20-80mg. Medium Joint: 10-40mg. Small Joint: 4-10mg. Administer intra-articularly into synovial space q1-5 weeks or more depending on relief. Ganglion/Tendinitis/Epicondylitis: 4-30mg into cyst/area of greatest tenderness. May repeat if necessary. Dermatologic Conditions: Inject 20-60mg into lesion. Distribute 20-40mg dose by repeated injections into large lesions. Usual: 1-4 injections. Systemic Effect: Substitute for Oral Therapy: IM dose should equal total daily PO methylprednisolone dose q24 h. Prolonged Therapy: Administer weekly PO dose as single IM injection. Androgenital Syndrome: 40mg IM q2 weeks. Rheumatoid Arthritis: 40-120mg IM weekly. Dermatologic Lesions: 40-120mg IM weekly for 1-4 weeks. Acute Severe Dermatitis (Poison Ivy): 80-120mg IM single dose. Chronic Contact Dermatitis: May repeat injections q5-10 days. Seborrheic Dermatitis: 80mg IM weekly. Multiple Sclerosis: 160mg/day methylprednisolone for 1 week, then 64mg qod for 1 month. Asthma/Allergic Rhinitis: 80-120mg IM. Elderly: Start at lower end of dosing.
Pediatrics: Initial: 0.11-1.6mg/kg/day. Individualize dose depending on the severity of disease and response.

HOW SUPPLIED: Inj: 20mg/mL, 40mg/mL, 80mg/mL

CONTRAINDICATIONS: Idiopathic thrombocytopenic purpura (IM preparations), intrathecal administration, premature infants, systemic fungal infections except as an intra-articular injection for localized joint conditions.

WARNINGS/PRECAUTIONS: Contains benzyl alcohol, which is potentially toxic to neural tissue. Excessive amounts of benzyl alcohol have been associated with toxicity, particularly in neonates, and an increased incidence of kernicterus, particularly in small preterm infants. Injection may result in dermal/subdermal changes forming depressions in the skin at the injection site; do not exceed recommended doses. Avoid injection into deltoid muscle or into an infected site or a previously infected joint. Rare instances of anaphylactoid reactions reported. Do not use to treat traumatic brain injury. May cause elevation of BP, salt and water retention, and increased excretion of K^+ and Ca^{2+}; dietary salt restriction and K^+ supplementation may be necessary. Caution with recent myocardial infarction. HPA axis suppression, Cushing's syndrome, and hyperglycemia reported; monitor prolonged use. Possible increased susceptibility to infections (eg, viral, fungal, protozoan, or helminthic). May exacerbate systemic fungal infections. Latent disease due to certain pathogens may be activated or intercurrent infections exacerbated. Assess for latent or active amebiasis prior to therapy. Caution with known or suspected *Strongyloides*, active or latent tuberculosis (TB), HTN, congestive heart failure (CHF), renal insufficiency, active ocular herpes simplex, osteoporosis, active or latent peptic ulcer, diverticulitis, fresh intestinal anastomoses, and nonspecific ulcerative colitis. Not for use in cerebral malaria and optic neuritis. May produce posterior subscapular cataracts, glaucoma with possible damage to optic nerves, and enhance the establishment of secondary ocular infections due to bacteria, fungi, or viruses. May elevate intraocular pressure (IOP). Kaposi's sarcoma reported. Chickenpox and measles may have more serious or fatal course in pediatric and adult patients. Metabolic clearance is decreased in hypothyroidism and increased in hyperthyroidism. May decrease bone formation and increase bone resorption. Acute myopathy reported with high doses. May elevate creatine kinase levels. Psychic derangements may appear during therapy (eg, euphoria, insomnia, mood swings, personality changes, and severe depression to frank psychotic manifestations).

ADVERSE REACTIONS: Anaphylactoid reaction, bradycardia, cardiac arrhythmias, cardiac enlargement, acne, erythema, sodium retention, abdominal distention, decreased carbohydrate and glucose tolerance, glycosuria, hirsutism, fluid retention, convulsions, depression.

INTERACTIONS: Administration of live or live, attenuated vaccines is contandicated in patients receiving immunosuppressive doses. Killed or inactivated vaccines may be administered, though response can not be predicted. Use with aminoglutethimide may lead to a loss of corticosteroid-induced adrenal supression. May develop hypokalemia with K⁺-depleting agents (eg, ampothericin-B, diuretics). Case reports of cardiac enlargement and CHF reported when coadministered with amphotericin-B. Macrolide antibiotics decrease clearance. Anticholinesterase agents may produce severe weakness in patients with myasthenia gravis. Serum concentrations of isoniazid may be decreased. Cholestyramine may increase clearance. Coadministration of digitalis glycosides increases risk of arrhythmias due to hypokalemia. Estrogens (eg, oral contraceptives) may decrease hepatic metabolism leading to increased effects. Hepatic enzyme inducers (eg, barbiturates, phenytoin, carbamazepine, and rifampin) enhance metabolism. Hepatic enzyme inhibitors (eg, ketoconazole, macrolide antibiotics such as erythromycin and troleandomycin) may increase plasma concentrations. Concomitant use with ASA or other NSAIDs increases risks of GI side effects. The clearance of salicylates may be increased. Coadministration with warfarin usually results in inhibition of response to warfarin. Antidiabetic agents may require dosage adjustment. Increased activity of both cyclosporine and corticosteroids when used concomitantly; convulsions reported. Ketoconazole decreases metabolism leading to increased risk of side effects. Acute myopathy observed in patients receiving concomitant therapy with neuromuscular blocking drugs (eg, pancuronium).

PREGNANCY: Category C, not for use in nursing.

MECHANISM OF ACTION: Glucocorticoid; causes profound and varied metabolic effects and modifies the body's immune responses to diverse stimuli.

NURSING CONSIDERATIONS

Assessment: Assess for hypersensitivity to drug, unusual stress, systemic fungal infections, current infections, active TB, vaccination history, ulcerative colitis, renal/hepatic insufficiency, septic arthritis/unstable joint, HTN, osteoporosis, myasthenia gravis, thyroid status, psychotic tendencies, and possible drug interactions.

Monitoring: Monitor for anaphylactoid reactions, Cushing's syndrome, hyperglycemia, adrenocortical insufficiency, occurrence of infections, psychic derangement, cataracts, acute myopathy, Kaposi's sarcoma, fluid retention, measurement of serum electrolytes, creatine kinase, thyroid-stimulating hormone, LFTs, IOP, BP, and HR. Monitor urinalysis, blood sugar, weight, ECG for cardiac arrhythmias and bradycardia, chest X-ray, and upper GI X-ray (if ulcer history) regularly during prolonged therapy. Monitor linear growth in pediatrics.

Patient Counseling: Inform that susceptibility to infections may increase. Advise that exposure to chicken pox and measles must be reported immediately. Advise not to d/c abruptly or without medical supervision. Instruct to seek medical advice once fever or signs of infection develops. Warn not to d/c abruptly or without medical supervision.

Administration: IM, intra-articular, or intralesional. **Storage:** 20-25°C (68-77°F).

DEPO-PROVERA RX
medroxyprogesterone acetate (Pharmacia & Upjohn)

THERAPEUTIC CLASS: Progestogen

INDICATIONS: Adjunct and palliative treatment of inoperable, recurrent, and metastatic endometrial or renal carcinoma.

DOSAGE: *Adults:* Initial: 400-1000mg IM weekly. Maint: 400mg/month if disease stabilizes and/or improves within a few weeks or months.

HOW SUPPLIED: Inj: 400mg/mL [2.5mL]

CONTRAINDICATIONS: Pregnancy, undiagnosed vaginal bleeding, breast malignancy, thrombophlebitis, thromboembolic disorders, cerebral vascular disease, liver dysfunction.

WARNINGS/PRECAUTIONS: Avoid during first 4 months of pregnancy; risk of genital abnormalities in fetuses with exposure. May cause thromboembolic disorders, ocular disorders, fluid retention. Caution with history of depression; d/c if depression recurs to serious degree. Caution with family history of breast cancer or patients with breast nodules. Annual physical exam for all patients, with attention to BP, breasts, abdomen and pelvic organs. May mask the onset of climacteric.

ADVERSE REACTIONS: Menstrual irregularities, nervousness, dizziness, edema, weight and cervical changes, cholestatic jaundice, breast tenderness, galactorrhea, rash, acne, alopecia, hirsutism, depression, pyrexia, fatigue, insomnia, nausea.

INTERACTIONS: Aminoglutethimide may decrease serum levels.

PREGNANCY: Not recommended in pregnancy, caution in nursing.

MECHANISM OF ACTION: Progestogen; inhibits secretion of gonadotropins, preventing follicular maturation and ovulation, resulting in endometrial thinning and producing a contraceptive effect.

PHARMACOKINETICS: Absorption: C_{max}=1-7ng/mL; T_{max}=3 weeks. **Distribution:** Found in breast milk. **Elimination:** $T_{1/2}$=50 days.

NURSING CONSIDERATIONS

Assessment: Physical exam of BP, breast, abdominal, pelvic exam, including cervical cytology and relevant lab tests, with assessment of pregnancy status, vaginal bleeding, history of breast cancer, thromboembolic disorders/active thrombophlebitis and/or cerebrovascular disease, drug hypersensitivity, diabetes mellitus, mental depression, hepatic/renal impairment, and possible drug/lab test interactions.

Monitoring: Monitor for amenorrhea, menstrual irregularity, breast cancer risk, manifestations of thrombotic disorders (eg, thrombophlebitis, pulmonary embolism, cerebrovascular disorders, retinal thrombosis), ocular disorders (eg, partial/complete vision loss, proptosis, diplopia, migraine), anaphylaxis/anaphylactoid reaction, manifestations of fluid retentions, epilepsy, abdominal pain, weight changes. Lab monitoring of plasma/urinary steroid levels, gonadotropin level, sex hormone-binding globulin level, LFTs, glucose, lipid profile, and coagulation tests.

Patient Counseling: Counsel on risk/benefits. Notify if pregnant/nursing.

Administration: IM route. **Storage:** 20-25°C (68-77°F).

DEPO-PROVERA CONTRACEPTIVE   RX
medroxyprogesterone acetate (Pharmacia & Upjohn)

> May lose significant bone mineral density (BMD); greater with increasing duration of use and may not be completely reversible. Unknown if use during adolescence or early adulthood will reduce peak bone mass and increase risk of osteoporotic fractures in later life. Should not be used as long-term birth control (>2 yrs) unless other birth control methods are considered inadequate.

THERAPEUTIC CLASS: Progestogen

INDICATIONS: Prevention of pregnancy.

DOSAGE: *Adults:* 150mg IM every 3 months (13 weeks) in gluteal or deltoid muscle. Give 1st injection during 1st 5 days of menses; within 1st 5 days postpartum if not nursing; or at 6th postpartum week if exclusively nursing. If >13 weeks between injections, physician should determine that the patient is not pregnant before administering the drug.
Pediatrics: Postpubertal Adolescents: 150mg IM every 3 months (13 weeks) in gluteal or deltoid muscle. Give 1st injection during 1st 5 days of menses; within 1st 5 days postpartum if not nursing; or at 6th postpartum week if exclusively nursing. If >13 weeks between injections, physician should determine that the patient is not pregnant before administering the drug.

D

HOW SUPPLIED: Inj: 150mg/mL

CONTRAINDICATIONS: Known or suspected pregnancy or as a diagnostic test for pregnancy; undiagnosed vaginal bleeding; known or suspected malignancy of breast; active thrombophlebitis, current or past history of thromboembolic disorders or cerebral vascular disease; significant liver disease.

WARNINGS/PRECAUTIONS: Caution in patients with osteoporosis risk factors (eg, metabolic bone disease, anorexia nervosa, family history of osteoporosis); consider other birth control methods. Serious thrombotic events reported; d/c if thrombosis develops while on therapy. Do not readminister pending examination if with sudden partial or complete loss of vision; sudden onset of proptosis, diplopia, or migraine; or if examination reveals papilledema or retinal vascular lesions. May carry cancer risk (breast and cervix). Monitor women with family history of breast cancer or with breast nodules carefully. Be alert to the possibility of ectopic pregnancy. Anaphylaxis and anaphylactoid reaction reported. D/C if jaundice or acute or chronic disturbances of liver function develop. Convulsion reported. Monitor patients who have a history of depression; do not readminister if depression recurs. May cause disruption of menstrual bleeding patterns (eg, amenorrhea, irregular or unpredictable bleeding/spotting, prolonged spotting/bleeding, heavy bleeding). Rule out organic pathology if abnormal bleeding persists or is severe. May cause weight gain and decrease glucose tolerance; monitor diabetic patients. Detectable amounts have been identified in breast milk. May cause fluid retention; caution with epilepsy, migraine, asthma, and cardiac/renal dysfunction. Return to fertility after stopping therapy may be delayed. Does not protect against HIV infection and other sexually transmitted diseases (STDs). Annual physical exam recommended for a BP check and for other indicated healthcare. May change the results of some laboratory tests (eg, coagulation factors, lipids, glucose tolerance, binding proteins).

ADVERSE REACTIONS: Menstrual irregularities, weight gain, abdominal pain/discomfort, dizziness, headache, asthenia/fatigue, nervousness, decreased libido, nausea, leg cramps.

INTERACTIONS: May decrease effectiveness with drugs or herbal products that induce enzymes, including CYP3A4, (eg, barbiturates, bosentan, carbamazepine, felbamate, griseofulvin, oxcarbazepine, phenytoin, rifampin, St. John's wort, topiramate) that metabolize contraceptive hormones. Significant changes (increase or decrease) in plasma levels with protease inhibitors or non-nucleoside reverse transcriptase inhibitors. Pregnancy reported with use of antibiotics. Aminoglutethimide may decrease serum levels. May cause a significant loss of BMD; additional risk with risk factors for osteoporosis (eg, chronic alcohol and/or tobacco use, chronic use of drugs that can reduce bone mass, such as anticonvulsants or corticosteroids).

PREGNANCY: Contraindicated in pregnancy; safety in nursing not known.

MECHANISM OF ACTION: Progestogen; inhibits secretion of gonadotropins which, in turn, prevents follicular maturation and ovulation, resulting in endometrial thinning.

PHARMACOKINETICS: Absorption: C_{max}=1-7ng/mL; T_{max}=3 weeks. **Distribution:** Plasma protein binding (86%); found in breast milk. **Metabolism:** Liver (extensive) by P450 enzymes; reduction, loss of the acetyl group and hydroxylation. **Elimination:** Urine; $T_{1/2}$=50 days.

NURSING CONSIDERATIONS

Assessment: Assess for active thrombophlebitis, current/past history of thromboembolic disorders or cerebral vascular disease, malignancy of breast, hypersensitivity reactions, significant liver disease, vaginal bleeding, breast nodules, history of depression, diabetes mellitus (DM), pregnancy/nursing status and possible drug interactions. Assess use in patients with known osteoporosis risk factors (metabolic bone disease, anorexia nervosa, chronic alcohol and/or tobacco use, strong family history of osteoporosis), strong history of breast cancer, epilepsy, migraine, asthma and cardiac/renal dysfunction.

Monitoring: Monitor for thrombosis, loss of vision, proptosis, diplopia, migraine, papilledema, retinal vascular lesions, severe abdominal pain, anaphylaxis or anaphylactoid reactions, jaundice, disturbances in liver function, convulsions, fluid retention, and disruption of menstrual bleeding patterns (eg, amenorrhea, irregular or unpredictable bleeding/spotting, prolonged spotting/bleeding, heavy bleeding). Monitor patients with DM. Monitor for recurrence of depression with previous history. Monitor BP and BMD and perform annual physical exam while on therapy. Monitor carefully in women with a strong family history of breast cancer or who have breast nodules.

Patient Counseling: Counsel about risk/benefits of drug. Inform that drug does not protect against HIV infection and other sexually transmitted diseases. Advise at the beginning of treatment that their menstrual cycle may be disrupted and that irregular and unpredictable bleeding or spotting results, and that this usually decreases to the point of amenorrhea. Advise to take adequate calcium and vitamin D.

Administration: IM route. Shake vigorously before use. Administer by deep IM injection in the gluteal or deltoid muscle. **Storage:** 20-25°C (68-77°F). Must be stored upright.

DEPO-TESTOSTERONE

CIII

testosterone cypionate (Pharmacia & Upjohn)

THERAPEUTIC CLASS: Androgen

INDICATIONS: Testosterone replacement in males with primary hypogonadism and hypogonadotropic hypogonadism.

DOSAGE: *Adults:* Male Hypogonadism: 50-400mg IM every 2-4 weeks. Dose based on age, sex, and diagnosis. Adjust dose according to response and adverse reactions.
Pediatrics: ≥12 yrs: Male Hypogonadism: 50-400mg IM every 2-4 weeks. Dose based on age, sex, and diagnosis. Adjust dose according to response and adverse reactions.

HOW SUPPLIED: Inj: 100mg/mL, 200mg/mL

CONTRAINDICATIONS: Severe renal, hepatic and cardiac disease. Males with carcinoma of the breast or prostate gland. Pregnancy.

WARNINGS/PRECAUTIONS: May accelerate bone maturation without linear growth; monitor bone growth every 6 months. Risk of hepatic damage with long-term use. D/C if hypercalcemia occurs in immobilized patients. D/C with acute urethral obstruction, priapism, excessive sexual stimulation, or oligospermia; restart at lower doses. Risk of edema; caution with pre-existing cardiac, renal or hepatic disease. Caution in the elderly; increased risk of prostatic hypertrophy and prostatic carcinoma. Caution with BPH. Should not be used for enhancement of athletic performance. Do not administer IV. Monitor Hct, Hgb, cholesterol periodically.

ADVERSE REACTIONS: Gynecomastia, excessive frequency/duration of penile erections, male pattern baldness, increased/decreased libido, oligospermia, hirsutism, acne, fluid and electrolyte disturbances, nausea, hypercholesterolemia, clotting factor suppression, polycythemia, altered LFTs, priapism, anxiety, depression.

INTERACTIONS: May potentiate oral anticoagulants (eg, warfarin) and oxyphenbutazone. May decrease blood glucose and insulin requirements in diabetics.

PREGNANCY: Category X, not for use in nursing.

MECHANISM OF ACTION: Endogenous androgen; responsible for normal growth and development of male sex organs and for maintenance of secondary sex characteristics.

PHARMACOKINETICS: Distribution: Plasma protein binding (98%). **Elimination:** Urine (90%), feces (6%); $T_{1/2}$=8 days.

NURSING CONSIDERATIONS

Assessment: Assess for known hypersensitivity to drug, males with carcinoma of the breast, males with known or suspected carcinoma of the prostate gland, hepatic/renal disease, delayed puberty, and benign prostatic hypertrophy.

Monitoring: Periodically monitor Hgb, Hct, LFTs, prostate-specific antigen, cholesterol and HDL, serum testosterone levels, serum calcium after initiation of therapy. Monitor for signs/symptoms of hypersensitivity reactions, edema with/without congestive heart failure, gynecomastia, prostatic hyperplasia/carcinoma, hepatocellular carcinoma. Assess bone development every 6 months in male adolescents.

Patient Counseling: Inform to contact physician if notice changes in body hair distribution, increase in acne, virilization, too frequent or persistent erections, changes in skin color, ankle swelling, unexplained N/V, hypersensitivity reactions.

Administration: IM route, preferably gluteal muscle. **Storage:** Controlled temperature, 20-25°C (68-77°F). Protect from light.

DESOXYN
methamphetamine HCl (Lundbeck)

CII

> High potential for abuse. Administration for prolonged periods of time in obesity may lead to drug dependence and must be avoided. Misuse may cause sudden death and serious cardiovascular adverse events.

THERAPEUTIC CLASS: Sympathomimetic amine

INDICATIONS: Attention deficit disorder with hyperactivity (ADHD). Short-term adjunct to treat exogenous obesity.

DOSAGE: *Adults:* Obesity: 5mg, 1/2 hr before each meal. Do not exceed a few weeks of treatment.
Pediatrics: ADHD: ≥6 yrs: Initial: 5mg qd-bid. Titrate: May be raised in increments of 5mg at weekly intervals until optimum response is achieved. Usual: 20-25mg/day. Total daily dose may be given in two divided doses daily. Obesity: ≥12 yrs: 5mg, 1/2 hr before each meal. Do not exceed a few weeks of treatment.

HOW SUPPLIED: Tab: 5mg

CONTRAINDICATIONS: Advanced arteriosclerosis, symptomatic cardiovascular (CV) disease, moderate to severe HTN, hyperthyroidism, glaucoma, agitated states, history of drug abuse, during or within 14 days of monoamine oxidase inhibitor (MAOI) use.

WARNINGS/PRECAUTIONS: Tolerance to anorectic effect develop within a few weeks; do not exceed recommended dose to increase effect. Sudden death reported in children and adolescents with structural cardiac abnormalities or other serious heart problems. Sudden death, stroke, and myocardial infarction (MI) reported in adults. Avoid use with serious structural abnormalities, cardiomyopathy, serious heart rhythm abnormalities, coronary artery disease, or other serious cardiac problems. May increase BP and HR; caution with underlying medical conditions that might be compromised by increases in BP/HR (eg, preexisting HTN, heart failure, recent MI, ventricular arrhythmia). Patients with symptoms suggestive of cardiac disease (eg, exertional chest pain, unexplained syncope) should undergo prompt cardiac evaluation. May exacerbate behavior disturbance and thought disorder in psychotic patients. Treatment-emergent psychotic or manic symptoms may occur. Aggressive behavior or hostility reported in patients treated for ADHD. May cause growth suppression; monitor growth in children; interrupt therapy if not growing or gaining height/weight. Caution in patients with comorbid bipolar disorder. May lower convulsive threshold and cause blurring of vision and difficulty with accommodation. Do not use to combat fatigue or replace rest. Exacerbation of motor and phonic tics and Tourette's syndrome reported. Prescription should be limited to the smallest feasible amount to minimize overdosage. May cause significant elevation of plasma corticosteroids.

ADVERSE REACTIONS: BP elevation, tachycardia, palpitations, dizziness, dysphoria, overstimulation, insomnia, tremor, diarrhea, constipation, dry mouth, urticaria, impotence, changes in libido, growth suppression in children.

INTERACTIONS: See Contraindications. May alter insulin requirements. May decrease hypotensive effect of guanethidine. Caution with TCAs. Antagonized by phenothiazines.

PREGNANCY: Category C, not for use in nursing.

MECHANISM OF ACTION: Sympathomimetic amine; CNS stimulant: peripheral actions involve elevation of BP, weak bronchodilation, and respiratory stimulant actions. Anorectics/anorexigenics: mechanism not established; suspected to suppress appetite.

PHARMACOKINETICS: Absorption: Rapid. **Metabolism:** Liver; aromatic hydroxylation, N-dealkylation and deamination. **Elimination:** Urine (62%); $T_{1/2}$=4-5 hrs.

NURSING CONSIDERATIONS

Assessment: Assess for glaucoma, agitation, CV conditions, hyperthyroidism, history of drug abuse. Screen for comorbid depressive symptoms, psychiatric history (including family history of suicide, bipolar disorder, depression, psychotic disorder, mania). Assess for history of motor and phonic tics and Tourette's syndrome. Assess pregnancy/nursing status and for possible drug interactions. Assess for history of seizures, diabetes.

Monitoring: Monitor BP and HR. Monitor for cardiac abnormalities, exacerbations of behavior disturbances and thought disorders, aggression or hostility, psychotic or manic symptoms, seizures, and visual disturbances. Monitor growth (height and weight) in children. Interrupt occasionally to determine if patient requires continued therapy.

Patient Counseling: Inform about risks and benefits of treatment, appropriate use, drug abuse/dependence. Advise not to engage in hazardous activities (eg, operating machinery/driving). Avoid late evening doses; insomnia may result. Instruct not to increase dosage unless advised by physician.

Administration: Oral route. **Storage**: Store below 30°C (86°F). Dispense in a tight, light-resistant container.

DETROL LA   RX
tolterodine tartrate (Pharmacia & Upjohn)

OTHER BRAND NAMES: Detrol (Pharmacia & Upjohn)

THERAPEUTIC CLASS: Muscarinic antagonist

INDICATIONS: Treatment of overactive bladder with symptoms of urinary frequency, urgency, or urge incontinence.

DOSAGE: *Adults:* (LA Cap) Usual: 4mg qd may lower to 2mg. (Tab) Initial: 2mg bid, may lower to 1mg bid. Titrate based on individual response and tolerability. Significant Hepatic/Renal Dysfunction/Concomitant Potent CYP3A4 Inhibitors: (Tab) 1mg bid, (LA Cap) 2mg qd.

HOW SUPPLIED: Cap, Extended-Release: 2mg, 4mg; Tab: 1mg, 2mg

CONTRAINDICATIONS: Urinary retention, gastric retention, uncontrolled narrow-angle glaucoma.

WARNINGS/PRECAUTIONS: Risk of urinary retention with clinically significant bladder outflow obstruction and risk of gastric retention with GI obstructive disorders. Caution with narrow-angle glaucoma, decreased GI motility (eg, intestinal atony), myasthenia gravis, known history of QT prolongation and hepatic/renal dysfunction. Not recommended in patients with severe hepatic impairment (Child-Pugh Class C) and CrCl <10mL/min.

ADVERSE REACTIONS: Dry mouth, dizziness, headache, abdominal pain, constipation, diarrhea, dyspepsia, fatigue, somnolence.

INTERACTIONS: May increase concentration with fluoxetine (potent CYP2D6 inhibitors) and ketoconazole (potent CYP3A4 inhibitor). Reduce dose with concomitant potent CYP3A4 inhibitors (eg, clarithromycin, ketoconazole, itraconazole, miconazole). May increase anticholinergic effects with concomitant anticholinergic agents. Caution with Class IA (eg, quinidine, procainamide) or Class III (eg, amiodarone, sotalol) antiarrhythmics and cholinesterase inhibitors.

PREGNANCY: Category C, not for use in nursing.

MECHANISM OF ACTION: Muscarinic receptor antagonist; competitive antagonist of acetylcholine at postganglionic muscarinic receptors mediating urinary bladder contraction and salivation.

PHARMACOKINETICS: Absorption: (Tab) Extensive metabolizers (EM): Multiple Dose: C_{max}=2.6mcg/L ; T_{max}=1.2 hrs; Single Dose: C_{max}=1.6mcg/L ; T_{max}=1.6 hrs. Poor metabolizers (PM): Multiple Dose: C_{max}=19mcg/L; T_{max}=1.9 hrs; Single Dose: C_{max}=10mcg/L; T_{max}=1.4 hrs.(Cap, Extended-Release) EM: Multiple Dose: C_{max}=3.4mcg/L; T_{max}=4 hrs; Single Dose: C_{max}=1.3mcg/L; T_{max}=4 hrs. PM: C_{max}=19mcg/L; T_{max}=4 hrs. **Distribution:** (IV) V_d=113L; high plasma protein binding. **Metabolism:** EM: CYP2D6 (oxidation); 5-hydroxymethyl (active metabolite). PM: CYP3A4 (dealkylation). **Elimination:** Urine (77% unchanged), feces (17% unchanged). (Tab) EM: $T_{1/2}$=2.2 hrs; PM: $T_{1/2}$=9.6 hrs. (Cap, Extended-Release) EM: $T_{1/2}$=6.9 hrs; PM: $T_{1/2}$=18 hrs.

NURSING CONSIDERATIONS

Assessment: Assess for bladder outflow obstruction (urinary retention), GI obstructive disorder (gastric retention), narrow-angle glaucoma, myasthenia gravis, history of QT prolongation, hepatic/renal impairment, pregnancy/nursing status and possible drug interactions.

Monitoring: Monitor for signs/symptoms of urinary retention, gastric retention and hypersensitivity reactions. Monitor renal/hepatic function, QT prolongation and HR.

Patient Counseling: Inform may produce blurred vision, dizziness or drowsiness. Caution against potentially dangerous activities until drug effects have been determined. Notify physician if pregnant/nursing or planning to become pregnant. Do not change dose unless instructed by physician. Take capsule with water, tell your physician if difficulty swallowing. Can be taken with or without food. Do not take 2 doses at the same time. If miss a dose, take again the next day. Call your physician or poison control center if taken more than the prescribed dose.

Administration: Oral route. (Cap, extended release) Take with liquids and swallow whole. **Storage:** Tab: 25°C (77°F). Cap: 20-25°C (68-77°F); excursions permitted to 15-30°C (59-86°F). Protect from light.

DEXAMETHASONE RX
dexamethasone (Various)

THERAPEUTIC CLASS: Glucocorticoid

INDICATIONS: (PO) Treatment of steroid-responsive disorders. (Inj) Treatment of steroid-responsive disorders when oral therapy not feasible.

DOSAGE: *Adults:* Individualize for disease and patient response. Withdraw gradually. (Tab) Initial: 0.75-9mg/day PO. Maint: Decrease in small amounts to lowest effective dose. Cushing's Syndrome Test: 1mg PO at 11pm; draw blood at 8am next morning. Or, 0.5mg PO q6h for 48 hrs; or 2mg (to distinguish if excess pituitary adrenocorticotropic hormone [ACTH] or other causes) PO q6h for 48 hrs; obtain 24-hr urine collections. (Inj) Initial: 0.5-9mg/day IV/IM. Cerebral Edema: Initial: 10mg IV, then 4mg IM q6h until edema subsides. Reduce dose after 2-4 days and gradually d/c over 5-7 days. Palliative Management of Recurrent/Inoperable Brain Tumors: Maint: 2mg IV/PO bid-tid. Acute Allergic Disorders: 4-8mg IM on 1st day, then 1.5mg PO bid for 2 days, then 0.75mg PO bid for 1 day, then 0.75mg PO qd for 2 days. (Inj) Usual: 0.2-9mg. Maint: Decrease in small amounts to lowest effective dose. Intra-Articular/Intralesional/Soft Tissue Injection: Usual: 0.2-6mg once every 3-5 days to once every 2-3 weeks. See PI for Shock Treatment. Take tabs and oral Sol with meals and antacids to prevent peptic ulcer.

Pediatrics: Individualize for disease and patient response. Withdraw gradually. (Tab) Initial: 0.75-9mg/day PO. Maint: Decrease in small amounts to lowest effective dose. Cushing's Syndrome Test: 1mg PO at 11pm; draw blood at 8am next morning. Or, 0.5mg PO q6h for 48 hrs; or 2mg (to distinguish if excess pituitary ATCH or other causes) PO q6h for 48 hrs; obtain 24-hr urine collections. (Inj) Initial: 0.5-9mg/day IV/IM. Cerebral Edema: Initial: 10mg IV, then 4mg IM q6h until edema subsides. Reduce dose after 2-4 days and gradually d/c over 5-7 days. Palliative Management of Recurrent/Inoperable Brain Tumors: Maint: 2mg IV/PO bid-tid. Acute Allergic Disorders: 4-8mg IM on 1st day, then 1.5mg PO bid for 2 days, then 0.75mg PO bid for 1 day, then 0.75mg PO qd for 2 days. (Inj) Usual: 0.2-9mg. Maint: Decrease in small amounts to lowest effective dose. Intra-Articular/Intralesional/Soft Tissue Injection: Usual: 0.2-6mg once every 3-5 days to once every 2-3 weeks. See PI for shock treatment. Take tabs and oral Sol with meals and antacids to prevent peptic ulcer.

HOW SUPPLIED: Inj: (Dexamethasone Sodium Phosphate) 4mg/mL, 10mg/mL; Sol: (Dexamethasone) 0.5mg/5mL, 1mg/mL; Tab: (Dexamethasone) 0.5mg*, 0.75mg*, 1mg*, 1.5mg*, 2mg*, 4mg*, 6mg* *scored

CONTRAINDICATIONS: Systemic fungal infections.

WARNINGS/PRECAUTIONS: Increase dose before, during, and after stressful situations. Avoid abrupt withdrawal. May mask signs of infection, activate latent amebiasis, elevate BP, cause salt/water retention, increase excretion of potassium and calcium. Prolonged use may produce cataracts, glaucoma, secondary ocular infections. Caution with recent myocardial infarction (MI), ocular herpes simplex, emotional instability, nonspecific ulcerative colitis, diverticulitis, peptic ulcer, renal insufficiency, HTN, osteoporosis, myasthenia gravis, threadworm infection, active tuberculosis (TB). Enhanced effect with hypothyroidism, cirrhosis. Consider prophylactic therapy if exposed to measles or chickenpox. Risk of glaucoma, cataracts, and eye infections. False negative dexamethasone suppression test with indomethacin.

ADVERSE REACTIONS: Fluid/electrolyte disturbances, muscle weakness, osteoporosis, peptic ulcer, pancreatitis, ulcerative esophagitis, impaired wound healing, headache, psychic disturbances, growth suppression (pediatrics), glaucoma, hyperglycemia, weight gain, nausea, malaise.

INTERACTIONS: Caution with ASA. Inducers of CYP3A4 (eg, phenytoin, phenobarbital, carbamazepine, rifampin) and ephedrine enhance clearance; increase steroid dose. Inhibitors of CYP3A4 (ketoconazole, macrolides) may increase plasma levels. Drugs that affect metabolism may interfere with dexamethasone suppression tests. Increased clearance of drugs metabolized by CYP3A4 (eg, indinavir, erythromycin). May increase or decrease phenytoin levels. Ketoconazole may inhibit adrenal corticosteroid synthesis and cause adrenal insufficiency during corticosteroid withdrawal. Antagonizes or potentiates coumarins. Hypokalemia with potassium-depleting diuretics. Live virus vaccines are contraindicated with immunosuppressive doses.

PREGNANCY: Category C, not for use in nursing.

MECHANISM OF ACTION: Adrenocortical steroid; produces anti-inflammatory effects.

PHARMACOKINETICS: Distribution: Found in breast milk. **Metabolism:** Liver; CYP3A4.

NURSING CONSIDERATIONS

Assessment: Assess for hypersensitivity to drug, systemic fungal or current infections, active TB, vaccination, unusual stress, hypothyroidism, hepatic/renal impairment, ulcerative colitis, diverticulitis, peptic ulcer with/without impending perforation, fresh intestinal anastomoses, HTN, recent MI, osteoporosis, myasthenia gravis, unstable joints, septic arthritis, existing psychotic tendencies, and for possible drug interactions (eg, indomethacin).

Monitoring: Monitor for anaphylactoid reactions, appearance/exacerbation of infections, cataracts, fluid retention, psychic derangement. Monitor infants for hypoadrenalism and growth development. Monitor for fat embolism, adrenocortical insufficiency, LFTs, thyroid stimulating hormone, PT, glucose with intraocular pressure, BP, and ECG.

Patient Counseling: Inform that susceptibility to infection may increase. Avoid exposure to chickenpox or measles; report immediately if exposed. Advise to restrict dietary sodium and potassium supplements. Counsel not to overuse joint after intra-articular injection, and not to d/c abruptly without medical supervision.

Administration: Oral route. Parenteral: IM, IV, intra-articular, intralesional, and soft-tissue injection. **Storage:** Inj: 20-25°C (68-77°F); excursions permitted to 15-30°C (59-86°F).

DEXEDRINE SPANSULES   CII
dextroamphetamine sulfate (GlaxoSmithKline)

> High potential for abuse. Prolonged use may lead to drug dependence and must be avoided. Misuse may cause sudden death and serious cardiovascular adverse events.

THERAPEUTIC CLASS: Sympathomimetic amine

INDICATIONS: Treatment of attention deficit disorder with hyperactivity (ADHD) in patients 6-16 yrs and narcolepsy.

DOSAGE: *Adults:* Individualize dose. Administer at lowest effective dose. Narcolepsy: Initial: 10mg/day. Titrate: May increase by 10mg/day at weekly intervals until optimal response is obtained. Usual: 5-60mg/day in divided doses. May give once daily. Avoid late-evening doses.
Pediatrics: Individualize dose. Administer at lowest effective dose. Narcolepsy: 6-12 yrs: Initial: 5mg qd. Titrate: May increase weekly by 5mg/day until optimal response is obtained. ≥12 yrs: Initial: 10mg qd. Titrate: May increase by 10mg/day at weekly intervals until optimal response is obtained. Usual: 5-60mg/day in divided doses. ADHD: ≥6 yrs: Initial: 5mg qd-bid. Titrate: May increase 5mg/day at weekly intervals until optimal response is obtained. Only in rare cases will it be necessary to exceed a total of 40mg/day. May give once daily. Avoid late-evening doses.

HOW SUPPLIED: Cap, Sustained-Release: (Spansules) 5mg, 10mg, 15mg

CONTRAINDICATIONS: Advanced arteriosclerosis, symptomatic cardiovascular disease (CVD), moderate to severe HTN, hyperthyroidism, glaucoma, agitated states, history of drug abuse, during or within 14 days of MAOI use.

WARNINGS/PRECAUTIONS: Sudden death reported in children and adolescents with structural cardiac abnormalities or other serious heart problems. Sudden death, stroke, myocardial infarction (MI) reported in adults. Avoid use with serious structural cardiac abnormalities, cardiomyopathy, serious heart rhythm abnormalities, coronary artery disease (CAD), or other serious cardiac problems. Caution with HTN. Prior to treatment, obtain a careful history and perform physical exam to assess for cardiac disease. May exacerbate symptoms of behavior disturbance and thought disorder in psychotic patients. May induce mixed/manic episode in patients with bipolar disorder. Use at usual doses can cause treatment-emergent psychotic or manic symptoms (eg, hallucinations, delusional thinking, mania) in children and adolescents without prior history of psychotic illness. Monitor for appearance of, or worsening of, aggressive behavior or hostility in patients being treated for ADHD. May cause long-term suppression of growth in children; monitor growth during treatment. May lower seizure threshold; d/c if seizures develop. Visual disturbances (eg, difficulties with accommodation, blurring of vision) reported. May exacerbate motor and phonic tics and Tourette's syndrome.

ADVERSE REACTIONS: Palpitations, tachycardia, BP elevation, CNS overstimulation, restlessness, insomnia, dry mouth, GI disturbances, anorexia, urticaria, impotence.

INTERACTIONS: See Contraindications. GI acidifying agents (eg, guanethidine, reserpine, glutamic acid HCl, ascorbic acid, fruit juices) and urinary acidifying agents (eg, ammonium chloride, sodium acid, phosphate) lower blood levels and efficacy. Increased blood levels and potentiated by GI alkalinizing agents (eg, sodium bicarbonate) and urinary alkalinizing agents (eg, acetazolamide, some thiazides). Potentiates CNS stimulation and fatal convulsions may occur with propoxyphene overdosage. Urinary excretion

D

of amphetamines is increased and efficacy is reduced by acidifying agents used in methenamine therapy. Potentiated effects of both agents with TCAs (eg, desipramine, protriptyline). May delay intestinal absorption of phenytoin, ethosuximide, phenobarbital. Enhanced effect with sympathomimetic agents. Inhibits adrenergic blockers. Counteracts the sedative effect of antihistamines. Antagonizes the hypotensive effect of antihypertensives. Inhibits the central stimulant effect by chlorpromazine, haloperidol, and lithium carbonate. Potentiates the analgesic effect of meperidine. Enhances the adrenergic effect of norepinephrine. Inhibits the hypotensive effect of veratrum alkaloids. Increases plasma levels of corticosteroids.

PREGNANCY: Category C, not for use in nursing.

MECHANISM OF ACTION: Amphetamine; noncatecholamine sympathomimetic amine with CNS stimulant activity. Peripheral actions include elevation of BP, weak bronchodilation, and respiratory stimulant action.

PHARMACOKINETICS: Absorption: (15mg cap) C_{max}=23.5ng/mL; T_{max}=8 hrs. **Distribution:** Found in breast milk. **Elimination:** $T_{1/2}$=12 hrs.

NURSING CONSIDERATIONS

Assessment: Assess for cardiovascular conditions (eg, advanced arteriosclerosis, moderate to severe HTN, cardiac structural abnormalities, cardiomyopathy, arrhythmias, heart failure, recent MI, symptomatic CVD), hyperthyroidism, agitation, glaucoma, history of drug abuse, pre-existing psychosis, bipolar disorder, prior history of seizures, pregnancy/nursing status, and possible drug interactions. Assess for presence or family history of Tourette's syndrome.

Monitoring: Monitor for cardiac abnormalities, exacerbations of behavior disturbances and thought disorders, new psychotic or manic symptoms (eg, hallucinations, delusional thinking, mania), seizures, and visual disturbances. Monitor for signs/symptoms of mixed/manic episodes in patients with bipolar disorder. Monitor HR and BP. Monitor for appearance/worsening of aggressive behavior or hostility. Monitor growth in pediatrics.

Patient Counseling: Inform of benefits and risks of treatment. Advise on appropriate use of medication. Instruct that therapy may impair the ability to engage in potentially hazardous activities (eg, operating machinery or vehicles). Inform that late-evening doses should be avoided due to the risk of insomnia. Instruct to read and understand the medication guide. Instruct to notify physician of present or family history of any health conditions.

Administration: Oral route. **Storage:** 20-25°C (68-77°F).

DEXILANT   RX
dexlansoprazole (Takeda)

THERAPEUTIC CLASS: Proton pump inhibitor

INDICATIONS: Healing of all grades of erosive esophagitis (EE) for up to 8 weeks. Maintain healing of EE for up to 6 months. Treatment of heartburn associated with symptomatic non-erosive gastroesophageal reflux disease (GERD) for 4 weeks.

DOSAGE: *Adults*: Healing of EE: 60mg qd for up to 8 weeks. Maint: 30mg qd for up to 6 months. Symptomatic Non-Erosive GERD: 30mg qd for 4 weeks. Moderate Hepatic Impairment (Child-Pugh Class B): Max: 30mg qd.

HOW SUPPLIED: Cap, Delayed-Release: 30mg, 60mg

WARNINGS/PRECAUTIONS: Symptomatic response does not preclude the presence of gastric malignancy. May increase risk of osteoporosis-related fractures of the hip, wrist or spine; use lowest dose and shortest duration of PPI therapy needed.

ADVERSE REACTIONS: Diarrhea, abdominal pain.

INTERACTIONS: May reduce plasma levels of atazanavir; avoid concurrent use. May interfere with the absorption of other drugs where gastric pH is an important determinant of oral bioavailability (eg, ampicillin esters, digoxin, iron salts, ketoconazole). Concomitant use with warfarin may increase INR and PT. Concomitant use with tacrolimus may increase whole blood levels of tacrolimus.

PREGNANCY: Category B, not for use in nursing.

MECHANISM OF ACTION: Proton pump inhibitor; suppresses gastric acid secretion by specific inhibition of the (H^+, K^+) -ATPase in the gastric parietal cell. Blocks the final step of acid production.

PHARMACOKINETICS: Absorption: T_{max}=4-5 hrs; different doses resulted in variable parameters. **Distribution:** V_d=40.3L; Plasma Protein binding (96.1%-98.8%). **Metabolism:** Liver (extensive) via CYP3A4 and CYP2C19. **Elimination:** Urine (50.7%), feces (47.6%); $T_{1/2}$=1-2 hrs.

NURSING CONSIDERATIONS

Assessment: Assess for presence of gastric malignancy, osteoporosis-related fractures, hepatic impairment, hypersensitivity, pregnancy/nursing status, and possible drug interactions.

Monitoring: Monitor for signs and symptoms of hypersensitivity (anaphylaxis) and osteoporosis-related fractures of the hip, wrist or spine.

Patient Counseling: Instruct to swallow caps whole or may open caps and sprinkle intact granules on 1 tbsp of applesauce and swallow immediately without chewing. Inform that drug may be taken without regard to food. Inform to watch for signs of allergic reactions as these could be serious and may require d/c. Instruct to notify physician if pregnant or intend to become pregnant, breastfeeding, or have liver problems. Counsel about potential drug interactions.

Administration: Oral route. Swallow whole, do not chew. **Storage:** 25°C (77°F); excursions permitted to 15-30°C (59-86°F).

DIABETA   RX
glyburide (Sanofi-Aventis)

THERAPEUTIC CLASS: Sulfonylurea (2nd generation)

INDICATIONS: Adjunct to diet and exercise, to improve glycemic control in adults with type 2 diabetes mellitus (DM).

DOSAGE: *Adults:* Initial: 2.5-5mg qd with breakfast or first main meal; give 1.25mg if sensitive to hypoglycemia. Titrate: Increase by no more than 2.5mg/day at weekly intervals. Maint: 1.25-20mg given qd or in divided doses. May give bid with doses >10mg/day. Max: 20mg/day. Transfer From Other Oral Antidiabetic Agents: Initial: 2.5-5mg/day. Transfer From Maximum Dose of Other Sulfonylureas: Initial: 5mg qd. Switch From Insulin: If <20 U/day: 2.5-5mg qd. If 20-40 U/day: 5mg qd. If >40 U/day: Decrease insulin dose by 50% and give 5mg qd. Titrate: Progressive withdrawal of insulin and increase by 1.25-2.5mg/day every 2-10 days. Elderly/Debilitated/Malnourished/Renal or Hepatic Impairment/Adrenal or Pituitary Insufficiency: Initial: 1.25mg qd. Dose conservatively.

HOW SUPPLIED: Tab: 1.25mg*, 2.5mg*, 5mg* *scored

CONTRAINDICATIONS: Diabetic ketoacidosis with or without coma, treatment with bosentan.

WARNINGS/PRECAUTIONS: Increased risk of cardiovascular (CV) mortality. Risk of hypoglycemia, especially with renal and hepatic disease; elderly, debilitated, or malnourished patients; and those with adrenal or pituitary insufficiency. May need to d/c and give insulin with stress (eg, fever, trauma). Secondary failure may occur. Hemolytic anemia may occur in patients with G6PD deficiency; caution during administration.

ADVERSE REACTIONS: Hypoglycemia, cholestatic jaundice, hepatitis, nausea, epigastric fullness, heartburn, allergic skin reactions (eg, pruritus, erythema, urticaria, morbilliform), disulfiram-like reactions (rarely), hyponatremia, LFT abnormalities, photosensitivity reactions, hematologic reactions (eg, leukopenia, agranulocytosis, thrombocytopenia), porphyria, cutanea tarda, blurred vision.

D

INTERACTIONS: See Contraindications. Potentiate hypoglycemia with alcohol, NSAIDs, miconazole, fluoroquinolones, highly protein-bound drugs, salicylates, sulfonamides, chloramphenicol, probenecid, MAOIs, β-blockers, ACE inhibitors, disopyramide, fluoxetine, and clarithromycin. Risk of hyperglycemia and loss of glucose control with thiazides and other diuretics, corticosteroids, phenothiazines, thyroid products, estrogens, oral contraceptives, phenytoin, nicotinic acid, sympathomimetics, calcium channel blockers, and isoniazid. Increased or decreased coumarin effects. Disulfiram-like reactions (rarely) with alcohol. Elevated liver enzymes reported with bosentan. May increase cyclosporine plasma levels and toxicity. May worsen glucose control with rifampin. β-blockers may mask signs of hyperglycemia.

PREGNANCY: Category C, not for use in nursing.

MECHANISM OF ACTION: Sulfonylurea; acts by stimulating the release of insulin from functioning β-cells in the pancreas.

PHARMACOKINETICS: Absorption: T_{max}=4 hrs. **Distribution:** Plasma protein binding (extensive). **Metabolism**: Hydroxylation. **Elimination:** Bile (50%), urine (50%); $T_{1/2}$=10 hrs.

NURSING CONSIDERATIONS

Assessment: Assess for fasting blood glucose levels, glycosylated hemoglobin, type 1 DM, CV complications, hypoglycemia risk factors, renal/hepatic impairment, G6PD deficiency, pregnancy/nursing status, and possible drug interactions.

Monitoring: Monitor fasting blood glucose levels regularly and glycosylated hemoglobin periodically. Monitor GI, dermatologic, hematologic, metabolic, DM complications (eg, diabetic ketoacidosis), hypersensitivity reactions, and blurring of vision.

Patient Counseling: Stress importance of adherence to dietary instructions, regular exercise programs, and regular testing of blood glucose levels. Advise to take with breakfast or first meal. Inform patients for potential risks, advantages, and alternative modes of therapy. Counsel about the risks, symptoms, treatment, and conditions of hypoglycemia.

Administration: Oral route. **Storage:** 25°C (77°F); excursions permitted to 15-30°C (59-86°F).

DIABINESE   RX
chlorpropamide (Pfizer)

THERAPEUTIC CLASS: Sulfonylurea (1st generation)

INDICATIONS: Adjunct to diet and exercise to improve glycemic control in adults with type 2 diabetes mellitus.

DOSAGE: *Adults:* Take with breakfast. Divide dose with GI intolerance. Initial: 250mg qd. Titrate: After 5-7 days, adjust dose by 50-125mg/day every 3-5 days. Usual: 100-500mg qd. Max: 750mg/day. Switch From Insulin: If ≤40 U/day: D/C insulin; start 250mg qd. If >40 U/day: Reduce insulin dose by 50%; begin 250mg qd. Further insulin reductions depend on response. Elderly/Debilitated/Malnourished/Renal or Hepatic Impairment: Initial: 100-125mg qd. Dose conservatively.

HOW SUPPLIED: Tab: 100mg, 250mg

CONTRAINDICATIONS: Type 1 diabetes mellitus (DM), diabetic ketoacidosis with or without coma.

WARNINGS/PRECAUTIONS: Increased risk of hypoglycemia with the elderly, debilitated, malnourished, renal and hepatic disease, adrenal or pituitary insufficiency. Increased risk of cardiovascular mortality reported. Loss of blood glucose control when exposed to stress (eg, fever, trauma, infection, or surgery); d/c therapy and start insulin. Secondary failure can occur over period of time. Treatment of patients with glucose 6-phosphate dehydrogenase (G6PD) deficiency with sulfonylurea agents can lead to hemolytic anemia. Caution in patients with G6PD deficiency and consider a non-sulfonylurea alternative. Hemolytic anemia reported in patients without G6PD deficiency. Caution in Elderly.

ADVERSE REACTIONS: Hypoglycemia, cholestatic jaundice, pruritus, photosensitivity reactions, skin eruptions, hepatic porphyria, disulfiram-like reactions, leukopenia, agranulocytosis, thrombocytopenia, hemolytic anemia, SIADH.

INTERACTIONS: Hypoglycemic effects potentiated by alcohol, NSAIDs, other highly protein-bound drugs, salicylates, sulfonamides, chloramphenicol, probenecid, coumarins, MAOIs, and β-blockers. Severe hypoglycemia reported with oral hypolycemics and oral miconazole. Alcohol may produce disulfiram-like reaction. Certain drugs have a tendency to cause hyperglycemia and may lead to loss of glycemic control including thiazides and other diuretics, corticosteroids, phenothiazines, thyroid products, estrogens, oral contraceptives, phenytoin, nicotinic acid, sympathomimetics, calcium channel blockers, and isoniazid. β-blockers may mask signs of hypoglycemia. May prolong the effects of barbiturates; use with caution.

PREGNANCY: Category C, not for use in nursing.

MECHANISM OF ACTION: Sulfonylurea; lowers blood glucose acutely by stimulating the release of insulin from the pancreas.

PHARMACOKINETICS: Absorption: Rapid; T_{max}=2-4 hrs. **Elimination:** Urine (80-90%); $T_{1/2}$=36 hrs.

NURSING CONSIDERATIONS

Assessment: Assess cardiovascular risk factors prior to therapy. Assess for signs/symptoms of hyperglycemia, drug hypersensitivity, diabetic ketoacidosis with/without coma, type 1 DM, adrenal or pituitary insufficiency, pregnancy/nursing status and possible drug interactions.

Monitoring: Monitor blood glucose and HbA1c levels regularly. Monitor for hypoglycemia and other possible side effects.

Patient Counseling: Inform of importance of caloric restriction, weight loss, and regular exercise. Discuss primary and secondary therapy failure with patients. Counsel on signs/symptoms of cardiovascular mortality and hypoglycemia and its management. Instruct to take therapy once daily with breakfast. Promptly notify physician if symptoms of hypoglycemia or other adverse reactions occur.

Administration: Oral route. **Storage:** Below 30°C (86°F).

DIAZEPAM INJECTION   CIV
diazepam (Various)

THERAPEUTIC CLASS: Benzodiazepine

INDICATIONS: Management of anxiety disorders and short-term relief of anxiety symptoms. Symptomatic relief of acute alcohol withdrawal. Adjunct prior to endoscopic procedures, surgical procedures and cardioversion. Adjunct therapy in skeletal muscle spasm (eg, tetanus, etc), status epilepticus and severe recurrent convulsive disorders.

DOSAGE: *Adults:* Anxiety (moderate): 2-5mg IM/IV, may repeat in 3-4 hrs. Anxiety (severe): 5-10mg IM/IV, may repeat in 3-4 hrs. Alcohol Withdrawal (acute): 10mg IM/IV, then 5-10mg in 3-4 hrs if needed. Endoscopic Procedures: Usual: ≤10mg IV (up to 20mg) or 5-10mg IM 30 min prior to procedure. Muscle Spasm: 5-10mg IM/IV, then 5-10mg in 3-4 hrs if needed. Status Epilepticus/Severe Seizures: Initial: 5-10mg IV. Maint: May repeat at 10-15 min intervals. Max: 30mg. Preoperative: 10mg IM. Cardioversion: 5-15mg IV, 5-10 min prior to procedure. Elderly/Debilitated: Usual: 2-5mg.
Pediatrics: Tetanus: 30 days-5 yrs: 1-2mg IM/IV (slowly), may repeat every 3-4 hrs prn. ≥5 yrs: 5-10mg IM/IV, may repeat every 3-4 hrs. Status Epilepticus/Severe Seizures: 30 days-5 yrs: 0.2-0.5mg IV (slowly) every 2-5 min up to 5mg. ≥5 yrs: 1mg IV (slowly) every 2-5 min up to 10mg, may repeat in 2-4 hrs.

HOW SUPPLIED: Inj: 5mg/mL

CONTRAINDICATIONS: Acute narrow-angle glaucoma, untreated open-angle glaucoma.

WARNINGS/PRECAUTIONS: Inject slowly and avoid small veins with IV. Do not mix or dilute with other products in syringe or infusion flask. Extreme caution in elderly, severely ill and those with limited pulmonary reserve. Avoid if in shock, coma or acute alcohol intoxication with depressed vital signs. May impair mental/physical abilities. Increase in grand mal seizures reported. Caution with kidney or hepatic dysfunction. Not for obstetrical use. Withdrawal symptoms may occur. Hypotension and muscular weakness reported. Monitor blood counts and LFTs. Not for maintenance of seizures once controlled.

ADVERSE REACTIONS: Drowsiness, fatigue, ataxia, venous thrombosis and phlebitis (injection site).

INTERACTIONS: Phenothiazines, narcotics, barbiturates, MAOIs, and other antidepressants may potentiate effects. Delayed clearance with cimetidine. Reduce narcotic dose by at least one-third. Risk of apnea with concomitant barbiturates, alcohol, or other CNS depressants.

PREGNANCY: Not for use during pregnancy, safety in nursing unknown.

MECHANISM OF ACTION: Benzodiazepine/hypnotic agent; induces calming effect on parts of the limbic system, thalamus, and hypothalamus (animal study).

NURSING CONSIDERATIONS

Assessment: Assess for acute narrow-angle glaucoma, open-angle glaucoma, acute alcoholic intoxication, shock, coma, cardiac arrest, apnea, hypotension, hypersensitivity, and for possible drug interactions.

Monitoring: Monitor injection site for thrombosis and phlebitis, tonic status epilepticus, drowsiness, fatigue, ataxia, CNS depression, and for habituation and dependence.

Patient Counseling: Caution against hazardous tasks (operating machinery/driving).

Administration: IV, IM route. **Storage:** 20-25°C (6°-77°F). Protect from light.

DICLOXACILLIN
diclocacillin sodium (Various)   **RX**

THERAPEUTIC CLASS: Penicillin (penicillinase-resistant)

INDICATIONS: Infections caused by penicillinase-producing staphylococci.

DOSAGE: *Adults:* Mild-Moderate Infection: 125mg q6h. Severe Infection: 250mg q6h for at least 14 days.
Pediatrics: <40kg: Mild-Moderate Infection: 12.5mg/kg/day in divided doses q6h. Severe Infection: 25mg/kg/day in divided doses q6h for at least 14 days.

HOW SUPPLIED: Cap: 250mg, 500mg

WARNINGS/PRECAUTIONS: Serious, fatal hypersensitivity reactions reported. Pseudomembranous colitis has been reported. Caution with history of allergy and/or asthma. Monitor renal, hepatic, and hematopoietic function with prolonged use. Not for use as initial therapy with serious, life-threatening infections, or with N/V, gastric dilation, cardiospasm, or intestinal hypermotility.

ADVERSE REACTIONS: Allergic reactions, N/V, diarrhea, stomatitis, black or hairy tongue, superinfection (prolonged use), hepatotoxicity.

INTERACTIONS: Tetracycline may antagonize the bactericidal effects. Potentiated by probenecid.

PREGNANCY: Category B, caution in nursing.

MECHANISM OF ACTION: Penicillin (penicillinase-resistant); bactericidal against penicillin-susceptible microorganisms during state of active multiplication. Inhibits biosynthesis of bacterial cell wall.

PHARMACOKINETICS: Absorption: Rapid, incomplete; C_{max}=1-1.5 hrs; T_{max}=10-17mcg/mL. **Distribution:** Serum protein binding (95%-99%); found in breast milk. **Elimination:** Urine (unchanged); $T_{1/2}$=0.7 hrs.

NURSING CONSIDERATIONS

Assessment: Assess for comprehensive drug/allergy history, presence of severe illness or with N/V, gastric dilation, cardiospasm and intestinal hyper-motility, pregnancy/nursing status, renal/hepatic function and possible drug interactions. Perform blood cultures, WBC with differential prior to therapy and weekly thereafter.

Monitoring: Monitor for anaphylactic shock with collapse, pseudomembra-nous colitis or *C.difficle*-associated diarrhea (can range from mild diarrhea to fatal colitis), development of drug resistance, overgrowth of nonsusceptible organisms and lab monitoring for urine analysis, BUN, creatinine, SGOT, SGPT during therapy with dosage alteration if values elevated. Evaluate renal, he-patic, and hematopoietic functions during prolonged therapy.

Patient Counseling: Advise not to take drug if previous allergic reaction oc-curred. Take 1 hr before or 2 hrs after meal. Take exactly as prescribed to avoid developing drug resistance and to maintain effectiveness. Notify physician if pregnant/nursing or experience SOB, wheezing, skin rash, mouth irritation, black tongue, sore throat, N/V, diarrhea, fever, swollen joints, or any unusual bleeding or bruising. Notify if taking additional medications. Counsel that drug only treats bacterial, not viral, infections.

Administration: Oral route. **Storage:** 20-25°C (68-77°F).

DIDRONEL   RX
etidronate disodium (Warner Chilcott)

THERAPEUTIC CLASS: Bisphosphonate

INDICATIONS: Treatment of symptomatic Paget's disease of bone. Treatment and prevention of heterotopic ossification following total hip replacement or due to spinal cord injury.

DOSAGE: *Adults:* Paget's Disease: Initial: 5-10mg/kg/day ≤6 months or 11-20mg/kg/day ≤3 months. Retreatment only after a drug-free period of 90 days and if evidence of active disease process. Heterotopic Ossification: Total Hip Replacement: 20mg/kg/day 1 month before and 3 months after surgery. Spinal Cord Injury: 20mg/kg/day for 2 weeks, followed by 10mg/kg/day for 10 weeks.

HOW SUPPLIED: Tab: 400mg* *scored

CONTRAINDICATIONS: Overt osteomalacia, abnormalities of the esophagus which delay esophageal emptying (eg, stricture or achalasia).

WARNINGS/PRECAUTIONS: Therapy response in Paget's disease may be of slow onset and continue for months after d/c. Maintain adequate dietary intake of calcium and vitamin D. Therapy may need to be withheld in patients with enterocolitis due to diarrhea. Monitor with renal impairment; may reduce dose with decreased GFR. Esophageal and GI adverse events reported; cau-tion with active upper GI problems, d/c if symptoms of esophageal reactions occur. Caution in elderly. Reports of severe bone, joint, and/or muscle pain recorded. Osteonecrosis of the jaw reported. Caution in pregnant/nursing women.

ADVERSE REACTIONS: Diarrhea, nausea, bone pain, alopecia, arthropathy, esophagitis, hypersensitivity reactions, osteomalacia, amnesia, confusion.

INTERACTIONS: Food, especially food high in calcium, vitamins with mineral supplements or antacids that contain calcium, iron, aluminum, or magnesium may reduce absorption. Coadministration with warfarin may increase PT.

PREGNANCY: Category C, caution with nursing.

MECHANISM OF ACTION: Bone metabolism regulator; inhibits the forma-tion, growth, and dissolution of hydroxyapatite crystals and their amorphous precursors by chemisorption to calcium phosphate surfaces.

PHARMACOKINETICS: Absorption: Absolute bioavailability (3%). **Elimination:** Urine (50%, unchanged), feces; $T_{1/2}$=1-6 hrs.

D

NURSING CONSIDERATIONS

Assessment: Assess for clinically overt osteomalacia, abnormalities of the esophagus (eg, stricture, achalasia), GI problem (eg, Barrett's esophagus, dysphagia, other esophageal diseases, gastritis, duodenitis or ulcers), renal impairment, enterocolitis, presence of fractures, upcoming dental procedures, pregnancy/nursing status, and possible drug interactions.

Monitoring: Monitor for signs/symptoms of osteonecrosis (eg, jaw), musculo-skeletal pain, osteomalacia and fractures, diarrhea, esophageal adverse experiences (eg, esophagitis, esophageal ulcers, esophageal erosions, followed by esophageal stricture or perforation), and hyperphosphatemia. Monitor renal function in patients with renal impairment. In patients with lytic lesions, monitor radiographically and biochemically to determine if responsive to therapy.

Patient Counseling: Counsel to maintain adequate nutritional status, particularly adequate intake of calcium and vitamin D. Advise food high in calcium, vitamins with mineral supplements, or antacids which are high in metals (eg, calcium, iron, magnesium, aluminum) should be separated from dose administration by 2 hrs. Advise dose may be divided if GI discomfort occurs. Instruct to drink with full glass (6-8 oz) of water, and to avoid lying down after taking oral bisphosphonates.

Administration: Oral route. **Storage:** 25°C (77°F); excursions permitted to 15-30°C (59-86°F).

DIFFERIN   RX
adapalene (Galderma)

THERAPEUTIC CLASS: Naphthoic acid derivative (retinoid-like)

INDICATIONS: Topical treatment of acne vulgaris in patients ≥12 yrs.

DOSAGE: *Adults:* (Cre/Gel) Apply to entire face or affected area qhs after washing. (Lot) Apply to entire face (3-4 actuations of pump) or affected areas qd after washing.
Pediatrics: ≥12 yrs: (Cre/Gel) Apply to entire face or affected area qhs after washing. (Lot) Apply to entire face (3-4 actuations of pump) or affected areas qd after washing.

HOW SUPPLIED: Cre: 0.1% [45g]; Gel: 0.1%, 0.3% [45g, 75g]; Lot: 0.1% [59mL, 118mL]

WARNINGS/PRECAUTIONS: May cause irritation (eg, erythema, scaling, dryness, stinging/burning). Patient may apply moisturizer; depending on severity, reduce application frequency or d/c use. Avoid sun exposure; use sunscreen products/protective apparel if exposure cannot be avoided. Extreme weather (eg, wind, cold) may cause irritation. Avoid application to cuts, abrasions, eczematous or sunburned skin, to areas around eyes, lips, and mucous membranes. Avoid waxing.

ADVERSE REACTIONS: Skin erythema, scaling, dryness, burning/stinging sensation, (Gel) skin discomfort, (Cre) pruritus.

INTERACTIONS: Avoid peeling, desquamating, or abrasive agents, and other topicals with strong drying effects, high concentration of alcohol, astringents, spices, or lime. Caution with sulfur, resorcinol, or salicylic acid; possible cumulative irritancy effect may occur.

PREGNANCY: Category C, caution in nursing.

MECHANISM OF ACTION: Naphthoic acid derivative; not established. Binds to specific retinoic acid nuclear receptors and modulates cellular differentiation, keratinization and inflammatory processes. (Cre/Gel) Suspected to normalize differentiation of follicular epithelial cells resulting in decreased microcomedone formation.

PHARMACOKINETICS: Absorption: (Cre/Gel) Low. **Elimination:** (Cre/Gel) Bile.

NURSING CONSIDERATIONS

Assessment: Assess for sunburn or eczematous skin. Assess use in pregnant/nursing patients and for possible drug interactions.

Monitoring: Monitor for sensitivity or chemical irritation, cutaneous signs/symptoms (eg, erythema, dryness, scaling, burning, or pruritus).

Patient Counseling: Instruct to avoid exposure to sunlight and sunlamps; use sunscreen and protective clothing over treated areas when exposed. May cause skin irritation when exposed to wind or cold. Avoid contact with eyes, lips, angles of the nose, and mucous membranes. Do not apply medication to cuts, abrasions, eczematous or sunburned skin. Avoid use of waxing as depilatory method. Instruct to use moisturizers if necessary; however avoid products that contain α-hydroxyl or glycolic acid. Instruct to use as directed by physician.

Administration: Topical application. **Storage:** 20-25°C (68-77°F), excursions permitted to 15-30°C (59-86°F). Protect from freezing/light. Do not refrigerate. Keep away from heat. Keep bottle tightly closed.

DIFLUCAN   RX
fluconazole (Pfizer)

THERAPEUTIC CLASS: Azole antifungal

INDICATIONS: Treatment of vaginal, oropharyngeal, and esophageal candidiasis; systemic *Candida* infections (eg, candidemia, disseminated candidiasis, pneumonia); peritonitis and urinary tract infection (UTI) caused by *Candida*; and cryptococcal meningitis. Prophylaxis in patients undergoing bone marrow transplantation who receive cytotoxic chemotherapy and/or radiation therapy.

DOSAGE: *Adults:* Vaginal Candidiasis: 150mg PO single dose. IV/PO: Oropharyngeal Candidiasis: 200mg on first day, then 100mg qd for at least 2 weeks. Esophageal Candidiasis: 200mg on first day, then 100mg qd for at least 3 weeks and for at least 2 weeks following resolution of symptoms. Max: 400mg/day. Systemic *Candida* Infections: Up to 400mg/day. UTI/Peritonitis: 50-200mg/day. Cryptococcal Meningitis: 400mg on first day, then 200mg qd for 10-12 weeks after negative CSF culture. Suppression of Cryptococcal Meningitis Relapse in AIDS: 200mg qd. Prophylaxis in Bone Marrow Transplant: 400mg qd. Renal Impairment (Multiple Doses) CrCl ≤50mL/min (No Dialysis): Initial: LD 50-400mg. Maint: Give 50% of recommended dose. Dialysis: Give 100% of dose after each dialysis.
Pediatrics: IV/PO: Oropharyngeal Candidiasis: 6mg/kg on first day, then 3mg/kg/day for at least 2 weeks. Esophageal Candidiasis: 6mg/kg on first day, then 3mg/kg/day for at least 3 weeks and for at least 2 weeks following resolution of symptoms. Max: 12mg/kg/day. Systemic *Candida* Infections: 6-12mg/kg/day. Cryptococcal Meningitis: 12mg/kg first day, then 6mg/kg/day for 10-12 weeks after negative CSF culture. Suppression of Cryptococcal Meningitis Relapse in AIDS: 6mg/kg qd. Renal Impairment: CrCl ≤50mL/min (No Dialysis): Initial: LD: 50-400mg. Maint: Give 50% of recommended dose. Dialysis: Give 100% of dose after each dialysis.

HOW SUPPLIED: Inj: 200mg/100mL, 400mg/200mL; Sus: 50mg/5mL, 200mg/5mL [35ml]; Tab: 50mg, 100mg, 150mg, 200mg

CONTRAINDICATIONS: Coadministration with terfenadine (with multiple doses ≥400mg of fluconazole) and cisapride.

WARNINGS/PRECAUTIONS: Rarely associated with serious hepatic toxicity; monitor LFTs. D/C if signs and symptoms of liver disease develop. Rare exfoliative skin disorders reported; monitor for rash and d/c if lesions progress. Anaphylaxis reported. Rare cases of QT prolongation and torsades de pointes reported; caution with potentially proarrhythmic conditions. Consider risk vs. benefits of single PO tab dose vs. intravaginal agent therapy for the treatment of vaginal yeast infections. Caution in elderly.

ADVERSE REACTIONS: Headache, N/V, abdominal pain, diarrhea, serious hepatic reactions, anaphylaxis, rash.

INTERACTIONS: See Contraindications. Severe hypoglycemia with oral hypoglycemics. May increase PT with coumarin-type drugs (eg, warfarin). Increases levels of phenytoin, cyclosporine, zidovudine, rifabutin, tacrolimus, terfenadine, cisapride, glipizide, glyburide, tolbutamide, theophylline, astemizole, and other drugs metabolized by the CYP450 system. Rifampin enhances metabolism of fluconazole. Increases levels and psychomotor effects of midazolam; consider dose reduction of short-acting benzodiazepines. Decreased levels with cimetidine. Increased levels with HCTZ. May increase levels of ethinyl estradiol-, levonorgestrel-, and norethindrone-containing oral contraceptives. Greater incidence of abnormally elevated serum transaminases with one or more of the following medications: rifampin, phenytoin, isoniazid, valproic acid, or oral sulfonylureas. Uveitis reported with rifabutin. Nephrotoxicity reported with tacrolimus. Cardiac events reported with cisapride.

PREGNANCY: Category C, not for use in nursing.

MECHANISM OF ACTION: Triazole antifungal; inhibits fungal CYP450 dependent enzyme lanosterol 14-α-demethylase, which converts lanosterol to ergosterol. Subsequent loss of normal sterol correlates with accumulation of 14-α-methyl sterols in fungi and may be responsible for its fungistatic activity.

PHARMACOKINETICS: Absorption: Oral: C_{max}=6.72μg/mL (50-400mg), T_{max}=1-2 hrs (fasted). **Distribution:** Plasma protein binding (11-12%); found in breast milk. **Elimination:** Urine (80% unchanged, 11% metabolites); Oral: $T_{1/2}$=30 hrs. Refer to PI for pediatric and elderly pharmacokinetic parameters.

NURSING CONSIDERATIONS

Assessment: Assess for clinical diagnosis of fungal infection, AIDS, malignancies, renal impairment, potentially proarrhythmic conditions, hypersensitivity, pregnancy/nursing status, and possible drug interactions.

Monitoring: Monitor for signs/symptoms of anaphylaxis, hepatotoxicity, exfoliative skin disorders, QT prolongation, torsades de pointes. Monitor LFTs, renal function, and ECG.

Patient Counseling: Instruct to contact physician if signs of hepatotoxicity, anaphylaxis, or rash develop. Counsel to d/c if skin lesions progress. Advise to notify physician if pregnant/nursing and inform of all medications currently taking.

Administration: IV infusion, Oral route. IV infusion max rate is 200mg/hr. **Storage:** Tab: Below 30°C (86°F). Sus: Dry Powder: Below 30°C (86°F). Reconstituted: 5-30°C (41-86°F); discard unused portion after 2 weeks. Protect from freezing. Inj in Glass Bottles: 5-30°C (41-86°F). Protect from freezing. Inj in Viaflex Plus Plastic Container: 5-25°C (41-77°F). Brief exposure up to 40°C (104°F) does not adversely affect the product. Protect from freezing.

DIGIBIND   RX
digoxin immune fab (ovine) (GlaxoSmithKline)

THERAPEUTIC CLASS: Antidote, digoxin toxicity

INDICATIONS: Treatment of life-threatening digoxin intoxication. Also has been successfully used to treat digitoxin overdose.

DOSAGE: *Adults:* Acute Ingestion of Unknown Amount: Usual: Administer 10 vials, observe response, then additional 10 vials if clinically indicated. Calculation: # vials = total digitalis body load (mg)/0.5mg of digitalis bound per vial. 1 vial will bind approximately 0.5mg of digoxin (or digitoxin). Steady-State Serum Digoxin Concentrations: # of vials = (serum dig conc in ng/mL) x (wt in kg)/100. Steady-State Digitoxin Concentrations: # of vials = (serum digitoxin conc in ng/mL) x (wt in kg)/1000. If toxicity not adequately reversed after several hrs or appears to recur, may need readministration. See PI for details.

Pediatrics: Acute Ingestion of Unknown Amount: Usual: Administer 10 vials, observe response, then additional 10 vials if clinically indicated. Calculation: # vials = total digitalis body load (mg)/0.5mg of digitalis bound per vial. 1 vial will bind approximately 0.5mg of digoxin (or digitoxin). Steady-State Serum Digoxin Concentrations: Dose (mg) = (# vials) (38mg/vial). Steady-State Digitoxin Concentrations: # of vials = (serum digitoxin conc in ng/mL) x (wt in kg)/1000. If toxicity not adequately reversed after several hrs or appears to recur, may need readministration. See PI for details.

HOW SUPPLIED: Inj: 38mg

WARNINGS/PRECAUTIONS: Obtain digoxin level before initiation. Do not overlook possibility of multiple drug overdose. Risk of hypersensitivity is greater with allergies to papain, chymopapain, or other papaya extracts; skin testing may be appropriate for high-risk individuals. K⁺ levels may drop rapidly after administration; monitor closely. Digitalis toxicity may recur with renal dysfunction; caution and monitor closely. Caution with cardiac dysfunction, further deterioration may occur from digoxin withdrawal. Consider additional support with inotropes or vasodilators. Monitor for volume overload in children. D/C if anaphylactoid reaction occurs and treat appropriately.

ADVERSE REACTIONS: Allergic reactions, exacerbation of low cardiac output, congestive heart failure, hypokalemia.

PREGNANCY: Category C, caution in nursing.

MECHANISM OF ACTION: Antidote; digoxin toxicity. Binds to molecules of digoxin, making them unavailable for binding at their site of action on cells.

PHARMACOKINETICS: Elimination: Urine; $T_{1/2}$=15-20 hrs.

NURSING CONSIDERATIONS

Assessment: Assess for serum digoxin or digitoxin concentration, serum electrolytes, hypoxia, acid base disturbances, cardiovascular disease, and renal functions. Note other diseases/conditions and drug therapies.

Monitoring: Monitor for serum potassium concentration, arrhythmias, and renal function.

Patient Counseling: Counsel about adverse effects.

Administration: IV route. Refer to PI for further information. **Storage:** 2-8°C (36-46°F). Unreconstituted vials can be stored at up to 30°C (86°F) for 30 days.

DILACOR XR   RX
diltiazem HCl (Watson)

OTHER BRAND NAMES: Diltia XT (Watson)

THERAPEUTIC CLASS: Calcium channel blocker (nondihydropyridine)

INDICATIONS: Treatment of hypertension alone or in combination with other antihypertensives. Management of chronic stable angina.

DOSAGE: *Adults:* Individualize dose. HTN: Initial: 180-240mg qd. Usual: 180-480mg qd. ≥60 yrs: Initial: 120mg qd. Max: 540mg qd. Angina: Initial: 120mg qd. Titrate: May titrate to a dose of up to 480mg qd over a 7-14 day period. Take in am on an empty stomach. Swallow caps whole; do not open, crush, or chew.

HOW SUPPLIED: Cap, Extended-Release: 120mg, 180mg, 240mg

CONTRAINDICATIONS: Sick sinus syndrome, 2nd- or 3rd-degree AV block (except with functioning ventricular pacemaker), hypotension (<90mmHg systolic), acute myocardial infarction (MI), pulmonary congestion documented by x-ray.

WARNINGS/PRECAUTIONS: Prolongs AV node refractory periods. May develop asystole with Prinzmetal's angina. Caution in patients with pre-existing ventricular dysfunction; congestive heart failure (CHF) worsening reported. Mild elevations of transaminases (eg, alkaline phosphatase, bilirubin, LDH, SGOT, SGPT) and acute hepatic injury reported. Symptomatic hypotension may occur. Caution in renal, hepatic, and preexisting GI narrowing (pathologic or iatrogenic). Monitor LFTs and renal function with prolonged use. D/C if persistent dermatologic reactions (eg, skin eruptions progressing to erythema multiforme and/or exfoliative dermatitis) occur.

ADVERSE REACTIONS: Rhinitis, pharyngitis, increased cough, asthenia, headache, constipation.

INTERACTIONS: Increase levels of propranolol and carbamazepine. Increase levels with cimetidine and ranitidine. Potentiates depression of cardiac contractility, conductivity, and automaticity as well as vascular dilation with anesthetics. Additive cardiac conduction effects with digitalis or β-blockers. Monitor digoxin levels. Sinus bradycardia reported with clonidine. Potential additive effects with agents known to affect cardiac contractility and/or conduction. Competitive inhibition of metabolism with agents that undergo biotransformation by CYP450 mixed function oxidase. Additive antihypertensive effect when used concomitantly with other antihypertensive agents.

PREGNANCY: Category C, not for use in nursing.

MECHANISM OF ACTION: Calcium channel blocker; inhibits influx of calcium ions during membrane depolarization of cardiac and vascular smooth muscles. HTN: Relaxation of vascular smooth muscle with resultant decrease in peripheral vascular resistance. Angina: Reduces myocardial oxygen demand via reductions in heart rate and systemic blood pressure at submaximal and maximal work loads.

PHARMACOKINETICS: Absorption: Well absorbed; absolute bioavailability (41%); T_{max}=4-6 hrs. **Distribution:** Plasma protein binding (70-80%); found in breast milk. **Metabolism:** Liver (extensive). Desacetyldiltiazem (major metabolite). **Elimination:** Urine (2-4%, unchanged); $T_{1/2}$=5-10 hrs.

NURSING CONSIDERATIONS

Assessment: Assess for other conditions where treatment is contraindicated or cautioned, pre-existing impairment of ventricular function, preexisting GI narrowing, renal/hepatic impairment, hypersensitivity to drug, pregnancy/nursing status, and possible drug interactions.

Monitoring: Monitor renal/hepatic function and LFTs (eg, alkaline phosphatase, bilirubin, LDH, SGOT, SGPT), HR, ECG abnormalities. Monitor for signs/symptoms of worsening of CHF, hypotension, obstruction from strictures. Monitor for signs/symptoms of angina, dermatological reactions (eg, skin eruptions progressing to erythema multiforme and/or exfoliative dermatitis).

Patient Counseling: Instruct to take on empty stomach, not to open capsule and swallow whole; do not chew or crush.

Administration: Oral route. Take in am on an empty stomach. Swallow caps whole; do not open, crush or chew. **Storage:** 20-25°C (68-77°F).

DILANTIN   RX
phenytoin sodium (Parke-Davis)

OTHER BRAND NAMES: Dilantin Kapseals (Parke-Davis) - Dilantin-125 (Parke-Davis) - Dilantin Infatabs (Parke-Davis)

THERAPEUTIC CLASS: Hydantoin

INDICATIONS: (CER, CTB) Control of generalized tonic-clonic (grand mal) and complex partial (psychomotor, temporal lobe) seizures. Prevention and treatment of seizures during or following neurosurgery. (Sus) Control of tonic-clonic (grand mal) and psychomotor (temporal lobe) seizures.

DOSAGE: *Adults:* Individualize dose. (CER) Initial: 100mg tid. Titrate: May increase at 7- to 10-day intervals. Maint: 100mg tid-qid. Max: 200mg tid. May give 300mg qd if seizure is controlled on divided doses of three 100mg cap daily. LD (Clinic/Hospital): 1g in 3 divided doses (400mg, 300mg, 300mg) given 2 hrs apart. Start maintenance dose 24 hrs after LD. (CTB) Initial: 100mg tid. Titrate: May increase at 7- to 10-day intervals. Maint: 300-400mg/day. Max: 600mg/day. May chew or swallow tab whole. Not for qd dosing. (Sus) Initial: 125mg tid. Titrate: May increase to 5 tsp (625mg) daily if necessary. Determine serum level for optimal dosage adjustment.
Pediatrics: (CER, CTB, Sus) Individualize dose. Initial: 5mg/kg/day bid-tid in

equally divided doses. Maint: 4-8mg/kg/day. Max: 300mg/day. >6 yrs: May require the minimum adult dose (300mg/day).

HOW SUPPLIED: Cap, Extended-Release (CER): 30mg, 100mg, [Kapseals] 30mg; Sus: 125mg/5mL; Tab, Chewable (CTB) [Infatabs]: 50mg* *scored

WARNINGS/PRECAUTIONS: Caution in switching patient from a product formulated with the free acid (eg, Suspension, Infatabs) to a product formulated with the sodium salt (eg, Kapseals) and vice versa; Infatabs/Suspension yield higher plasma levels than Kapseals in equal doses; dose adjustments and serum level monitoring may be necessary. Avoid abrupt d/c; may precipitate status epilepticus. Increased risk of suicidal thoughts or behavior reported; monitor for worsening of depression and any unusual changes in mood or behavior. Lymphadenopathy (eg, lymph node hyperplasia, pseudolymphoma, lymphoma, Hodgkin's disease) reported; d/c and use alternative antiepileptic drugs. Caution with porphyria, hepatic dysfunction, and in elderly, gravely ill, diabetes. Caution in pregnancy; may increase seizure frequency during pregnancy, congenital malformation and malignancies, osteomalacia. Bleeding disorder in newborns may occur; give vitamin K to mother before delivery and to neonate after birth. Can cause serious skin adverse events (eg, exfoliative dermatitis, Stevens-Johnson syndrome [SJS], toxic epidermal necrolysis [TEN]); d/c if rash occurs. Anticonvulsant hypersensitivity syndrome (AHS), hyperglycemia, osteomalacia reported. May produce confusional states (eg, delirium, psychosis, encephalopathy, or cerebral dysfunction) at levels above optimal range; reduce dose or d/c if symptoms persist. Avoid use for seizures due to hypoglycemia or other metabolic causes. Not effective for absence (petit mal) seizures.

ADVERSE REACTIONS: Nystagmus, ataxia, slurred speech, decreased coordination, confusion, dizziness, insomnia, transient nervousness, motor twitching, headaches, N/V, constipation, rash, hypersensitivity reactions.

INTERACTIONS: Increased levels with acute alcohol intake, amiodarone, chloramphenicol, chlordiazepoxide, cimetidine, diazepam, dicumarol, disulfiram, estrogens, ethosuximide, fluoxetine, H2-antagonists, halothane, isoniazid, methylphenidate, phenothiazines, phenylbutazone, salicylates, succinimides, sulfonamides, ticlopidine, tolbutamide, trazodone. Decreased levels with chronic alcohol abuse, carbamazepine, reserpine, sucralfate. Decreases effects of corticosteroids, coumarin anticoagulants, digitoxin, doxycycline, estrogens, furosemide, oral contraceptives, paroxetine, quinidine, rifampin, theophylline, vitamin D. Phenobarbital, sodium valproate, valproic acid may increase or decrease levels. May increase or decrease levels of phenobarbital, sodium valproate, valproic acid. Calcium antacids decrease absorption; space dosing. Moban® brand molindone contains calcium ions that interfere with absorption. TCAs may precipitate seizures. Caution with barbiturates, succinimides, oxazolidinediones in patients with phenytoin hypersensitivity. Avoid with enteral feeding preparations and/or nutritional supplements.

PREGNANCY: Pregnancy D, not for use in nursing.

MECHANISM OF ACTION: Hydantoin; inhibits seizure activity by promoting sodium efflux from neurons, stabilizing threshold against hyperexcitability caused by excessive stimulation of environmental changes capable of reducing membrane sodium gradient. Reduces the maximal activity of the brain stem centers responsible for the tonic phase of the tonic-clonic (grand mal) seizures.

PHARMACOKINETICS: Absorption: (CTB, Sus) T_{max}=1.5-3 hrs; (CER) T_{max}=4-12 hrs. **Distribution:** Highly protein bound; found in breast milk. **Metabolism:** Liver (hydroxylation). **Elimination:** Bile, urine; $T_{1/2}$=22 hrs.

NURSING CONSIDERATIONS

Assessment: Assess that seizure is not due to hypoglycemia or other metabolic causes and that seizure is not an absence seizure. Assess for previous hypersensitivity, family history of AHS, immunosuppression, presence of grave illness, impaired hepatic function, porphyria, pregnancy/nursing status, and possible drug interactions.

Monitoring: Monitor for signs/symptoms of skin rash (eg, SJS, TEN), lymphadenopathy, and hyperglycemia in diabetic patients. Monitor for occurrence of confused states (eg, delirium, psychosis, encephalopathy), osteomalacia, and serum levels in pregnant women. Monitor for emergence/worsening of depression, suicidal thoughts, and/or any unusual changes in mood/behavior.

Patient Counseling: Inform of the importance of strictly adhering to prescribed dosage regimen. Caution on use of other drugs or alcoholic beverages without consulting physician. Instruct to immediately contact physician if skin rash develops. Instruct to maintain proper dental hygiene while on medication to minimize risk of gingival hyperplasia. Instruct to notify physician if suicidal thoughts or mood/behavior changes emerge. Advise females about dangers of using medication during pregnancy and apprise of the potential harm to fetus. Advise that Infatabs can either be chewed thoroughly before swallowing or swallowed whole. Encourage pregnant patients to enroll in the North American Antiepileptic Drug (NAAED) Pregnancy Registry by calling 888-233-2334 or go to www.aedpregnancyregistry.org.

Administration: Oral route. **Storage:** (CTB) 15-30°C (59-86°F). (CER/Sus) 20-25°C (68-77°F). (CER/CTB) Protect from moisture. (CER) Preserve in tight, light-resistant containers. (Sus) Protect from freezing and light.

DILAUDID

CII

hydromorphone HCl (Purdue Pharma)

> Highest potential for abuse and risk of respiratory depression exists. HP formulation is a more concentrated solution of hydromorphone and for use only in opioid-tolerant patients; do not confuse with standard parenteral formulations of hydromorphone or other opioids as overdose and death could result. Alcohol, other opioids and CNS depressants potentiate respiratory depressant effects, increasing the risk of respiratory depression that may result in death.

OTHER BRAND NAMES: Dilaudid-HP (Purdue Pharma)

THERAPEUTIC CLASS: Opioid analgesic

INDICATIONS: Management of pain where use of an opioid analgesic is appropriate. (HP) Relief of moderate to severe pain in opioid-tolerant patients who require larger than usual doses of opioids to provide adequate pain relief.

DOSAGE: *Adults:* Individualize dose. (Inj) Initial: 1-2mg SQ/IM q4-6h prn. If IV is necessary, give IV slowly, over at least 2-3 min depending on dose. Titrate: Adjust dose based on response. (HP) If switching from regular Dilaudid to Dilaudid-HP, similar doses should be used. If substituting for a different opioid, see PI. Adjust dose based on response. (Sol) Usual: 2.5-10mg PO q3-6h ud. (Tab) Initial: 2-4mg PO q4-6h. Titrate: May require gradual increase in dose if analgesia is inadequate, as tolerance develops, or pain severity increases. If substituting for a different opioid: See PI. Elderly/Hepatic/Renal Impairment: Start at lower end of dosing range.

HOW SUPPLIED: Inj: 1mg/mL, 2mg/mL, 4mg/mL, (HP) 10mg/mL, 50mg/5mL, 500mg/50mL, 250mg; Sol: 1mg/mL; Tab: 2mg, 4mg, 8mg* *scored.

CONTRAINDICATIONS: Respiratory depression in the absence of resuscitative equipment; status asthmaticus; obstetrical analgesia (labor and delivery); (HP) patients not already receiving large amounts of opioids.

WARNINGS/PRECAUTIONS: May cause respiratory depression; use extreme caution with chronic obstructive pulmonary disease (COPD) or cor pulmonale, decreased respiratory reserve, hypoxia, hypercapnia, or with pre-existing respiratory depression. May cause neonatal withdrawal syndrome. May exaggerate respiratory depression in the presence of head injuries, intracranial lesions, or a pre-existing increase in intracranial pressure (ICP). May obscure clinical course and neurologic signs of increases in ICP with head injury. May cause severe hypotension; caution with circulatory shock. Contains sodium metabisulfite; may cause allergic-type reactions including anaphylactic symptoms and life-threatening or less severe asthmatic episodes. Caution with elderly, debilitated, severe impairment of hepatic, pulmonary or renal function, myxedema, hypothyroidism, adrenocortical insufficiency (eg, Addison's disease), CNS depression or coma, toxic psychoses, prostatic hypertrophy, urethral stricture, (PO) gallbladder disease, acute alcoholism, delirium tremens, kyphoscoliosis or (PO) following GI surgery; reduce initial dose. May obscure the diagnosis or clinical course in patients with acute abdominal condition. May aggravate pre-existing convulsions. Mild to severe seizures and myoclonus reported in severely compromised patients. May impair mental/physical abilities. May cause spasm of the sphincter of Oddi; (PO) caution with upcoming biliary tract surgery. Physical dependence and tolerance are common during chronic therapy. Avoid abrupt d/c. Use Dilaudid-HP only in patients already receiving large doses of opioids and if required amount can be delivered accurately. (Inj) Diminishes propulsive peristaltic wave in the GI tract and may prolong obstruction; not for use with GI obstruction especially paralytic ileus. May diminish biliary/pancreatic secretions; caution with biliary tract disease including acute pancreatitis. Caution in alcoholism and other drug dependencies.

ADVERSE REACTIONS: Respiratory depression, apnea, cardiac arrest, light-headedness, dizziness, sedation, N/V, sweating, flushing, dysphoria, euphoria, dry mouth, pruritus.

INTERACTIONS: See Boxed Warning. Additive depressant effects with general anesthetics, phenothiazines, tranquilizers, sedatives or hypnotics, or (Inj) skeletal muscle relaxants. May enhance action of neuromuscular blocking agents. Mixed agonist/antagonist analgesics (ie, pentazocine, nalbuphine, butorphanol, buprenorphine) may reduce analgesia and/or may precipitate withdrawal symptoms; use with caution.

PREGNANCY: Category C, not for use in nursing.

MECHANISM OF ACTION: Opioid analgesic; mechanism not established. Suspected to bind to specific CNS opiate receptors to produce analgesia.

PHARMACOKINETICS: Absorption: (PO) Rapid; (Tab) bioavailability (24%); C_{max}=5.5ng, T_{max}=0.74 hrs, AUC=23.7ng•hr/mL. (Sol) C_{max}=5.7ng, T_{max}=0.73 hrs, AUC=24.6ng•hr/mL. **Distribution:** Plasma protein binding (8-19%); (IV Bolus) V_d=302.9 L; crosses placenta, found in breast milk. **Metabolism:** Liver (extensive) via glucuronidation; hydromorphone-3-glucuronide (metabolite). **Elimination:** Urine; (IV) $T_{1/2}$=2.3 hrs. (Tab) $T_{1/2}$=2.6 hrs. (Sol) $T_{1/2}$=2.8 hrs.

NURSING CONSIDERATIONS

Assessment: Assess for pain intensity or any other conditions where treatment is contraindicated or cautioned. Asses for pregnancy/nursing status, renal/hepatic function, and possible drug interactions.

Monitoring: Monitor for signs/symptoms of respiratory depression, increasing airway resistance, apnea, circulatory shock (eg, hypotension), misuse or abuse, addiction, tolerance or dependence, allergic/anaphylactic reactions, asthmatic episodes, hypersensitivity, seizures, myoclonus, and for alleviation of pain. Monitor BP and cardiac output.

Patient Counseling: Inform that medication may cause serious adverse effects (eg, respiratory depression) if not taken as directed. Report pain and any adverse effects experienced. Do not adjust dosage without prescriber's consent. May impair mental/physical abilities; use caution when performing hazardous tasks (eg, operating machinery/driving). Avoid using other CNS depressants and alcohol. Inform pregnant women and women who plan to become pregnant about effects of analgesics and other drug use on pregnancy. Avoid abrupt withdrawal; dosage should be tapered. Educate that medication has abuse potential. Advise to keep secure and to dispose of unused tablets and injections down the toilet.

Administration: Oral, SQ, IM, IV routes. (Inj) Inspect visually for particulate matter and discoloration before use. If needed, give as IV slowly over 2-3 min, depending on dose. (Dilaudid HP) Reconstitute 250mg single dose vial immediately prior to use with 25mL of sterile water for injection to provide a sterile solution containing 10mg/mL. **Storage:** Oral: 25°C (77°F), Inj: 20-25°C (68-77°F). Excursions permitted to 15-30° (59-86°F); protect from light.

DILTIAZEM INJECTION

RX

diltiazem HCl (Various)

THERAPEUTIC CLASS: Calcium channel blocker (nondihydropyridine)

INDICATIONS: Temporary control of rapid ventricular rate in atrial fibrillation/flutter (A-Fib/Flutter). Rapid conversion of paroxysmal supraventricular tachycardia (PSVT) to sinus rhythm.

DOSAGE: *Adults:* Bolus: 0.25mg/kg IV over 2 min. If no response after 15 min, may give 2nd dose of 0.35mg/kg over 2 min. Continuous Infusion: 0.25-0.35mg/kg IV bolus, then 10mg/hr. Titrate: Increase by 5mg/hr. Max: 15mg/hr and duration up to 24 hrs.

HOW SUPPLIED: Inj: 5mg/mL

CONTRAINDICATIONS: Sick sinus syndrome and 2nd- or 3rd-degree AV block (except with functioning pacemaker), severe hypotension, cardiogenic shock, concomitant IV β-blockers or within a few hrs of use, A-Fib/Flutter associated with accessory bypass tract (eg, Wolff-Parkinson-White syndrome, short PR syndrome), ventricular tachycardia.

WARNINGS/PRECAUTIONS: Initiate in setting with resuscitation capabilities. Caution if hemodynamically compromised, and renal, hepatic, or ventricular dysfunction. Monitor ECG continuously and BP frequently. Symptomatic hypotension, acute hepatic injury reported. D/C if high-degree AV block occurs in sinus rhythm or if persistent rash occurs. Ventricular premature beats may be present on conversion of PSVT to sinus rhythm.

ADVERSE REACTIONS: Hypotension, injection-site reactions (eg, itching, burning), vasodilation (flushing), arrhythmias.

INTERACTIONS: Caution with drugs that decrease peripheral resistance, intravascular volume, myocardial contractility or conduction. Increased AUC of midazolam, triazolam, buspirone, quinidine, and lovastatin, which may require a dose adjustment due to increased clinical effects or increased adverse events. Elevates carbamazepine levels, which may result in toxicity. Cyclosporine may need dose adjustment. Potentiates the depression of cardiac contractility, conductivity, automaticity, and vascular dilation with anesthetics. Possible bradycardia, AV block, and contractility depression with oral β-blockers. Possible competitive inhibition of metabolism with drugs metabolized by CYP450. Avoid IV β-blockers and rifampin. Monitor for excessive slowing of HR and/or AV block with digoxin. Cimetidine increases peak diltiazem plasma levels and AUC.

PREGNANCY: Category C, not for use in nursing.

MECHANISM OF ACTION: Calcium channel blocker; inhibits influx of Ca^{2+} ions during membrane depolarization of cardiac and vascular smooth muscle. Has ability to slow AV nodal conduction time and prolong AV nodal refractoriness, which has therapeutic benefits on supraventricular tachycardia. Decreases peripheral resistance, resulting in decreased systolic and diastolic BP.

PHARMACOKINETICS: Distribution: V_d=305-391L; plasma protein binding (70-80%); found in breast milk. **Metabolism:** Liver (extensive) via CYP450; deacetylation, N-demethylation, O-demethylation, and conjugation; N-monodesmethyldiltiazem and desacetyldiltiazem (major metabolites). **Elimination:** Urine and bile; $T_{1/2}$=3.4 hrs (single IV inj), 4.1-4.9 hrs (constant IV infusion).

NURSING CONSIDERATIONS

Assessment: Assess for sick sinus syndrome and 2nd- or 3rd-degree AV block, presence of functioning pacemaker, severe hypotension, cardiogenic shock, A-fib or atrial flutter associated with accessory bypass tract (eg, Wolff-Parkinson-White syndrome, short PR syndrome), ventricular tachycardia, wide complex tachycardia, AMI, CHF, pulmonary congestion documented by X-ray, hypertrophic cardiomyopathy, renal/hepatic impairment, pregnancy/nursing status, and possible drug interactions.

Monitoring: Initiation of therapy should be done in setting with monitoring and resuscitation capabilities, including DC cardioversion/defibrillation.

Monitor BP, HR, LFTs, and ECG. Monitor for hemodynamic deterioration, ventricular fibrillation, cardiac conduction abnormalities (eg, 2nd- or 3rd-degree AV block), hypotension, bradycardia, ventricular premature beats, dermatologic events (erythema multiforme/exfoliative dermatitis), and acute hepatic injury.

Patient Counseling: Initiation of therapy should be done in a setting with monitoring and resuscitation capabilities, including DC cardioversion/defibrillation. Inform risks/benefits; report adverse reactions. Notify if pregnant/nursing.

Administration: IV. **Storage:** 2-8°C (36-46°F). Do not freeze. Room temperature for up to 1 month. Destroy after 1 month.

DIOVAN RX
valsartan (Novartis)

> When used in pregnancy, drugs that act directly on the renin-angiotensin system can cause injury and even death to the developing fetus. D/C therapy when pregnancy is detected.

THERAPEUTIC CLASS: Angiotensin II receptor antagonist

INDICATIONS: Treatment of hypertension alone or in combination with other antihypertensives. Treatment of heart failure (NYHA Class II-IV). Reduction of cardiovascular mortality in clinically stable patients with left ventricular failure or dysfunction following MI.

DOSAGE: *Adults:* HTN: Monotherapy Without Volume Depletion: Initial: 80mg or 160mg qd. Titrate: May increase up to 320mg or add diuretic (greater effect than increasing dose >80mg). Max: 320mg/day. Heart Failure: Initial: 40mg bid. Titrate: May increase to 80mg or 160mg bid (use highest dose tolerated). Max: 320mg/day in divided doses. Post-MI: Initial: 20mg bid as early as 12 hrs after MI. Titrate: May increase to 40mg bid within 7 days, with subsequent titrations up to 160mg bid as tolerated. Maint: 160mg bid. May be given with other standard post-MI treatments including thrombolytics, aspirin, β-blockers, statins.
Pediatrics: 6-16 yrs: HTN: Initial: 1.3mg/kg qd (up to 40mg total). Adjust dose according to BP response. Max: 2.7mg/kg (up to 160mg) qd. Adjust dose accordingly when switching dosage forms.

HOW SUPPLIED: Tab: 40mg*, 80mg, 160mg, 320mg *scored

WARNINGS/PRECAUTIONS: Risk of hypotension; place patient in supine position and consider giving IV infusion of normal saline if excessive hypotension occurs; caution when initiating therapy in heart failure or post-MI. Caution with mild-moderate hepatic impairment (including biliary obstructive disorders). Changes in renal function may occur; caution with severe renal disease. Consider dose reduction and/or d/c of therapy with renal dysfunction. Use of a suspension recommended for children who cannot swallow tabs, or children for whom calculated dosage (mg/kg) does not correspond to available tab strengths. Avoid use in pediatric patients with GFR <30mL/min/1.73m².

ADVERSE REACTIONS: Fetal injury, cough, dizziness, hypotension, diarrhea, arthralgia, fatigue, viral infection, back pain.

INTERACTIONS: Coadministration of inhibitors of the hepatic uptake transporter OATP1B1 (eg, rifampin, cyclosporine) or efflux transporter MRP2 (eg, ritonavir) may increase systemic exposure. Concomitant use of K⁺-sparing diuretics (eg, spironolactone, triamterene, amiloride), K⁺ supplements, or salt substitutes containing K⁺ may increase serum K⁺ levels, and in heart failure patients may increase in SrCr. Symptomatic hypotension may occur in volume and/or salt-depleted patients receiving high doses of diuretics. Antihypertensive effect potentiated with atenolol. Concomitant use of ACE inhibitors may increase SrCr or K⁺ levels.

PREGNANCY: Category D, not for use in nursing.

MECHANISM OF ACTION: Angiotensin II receptor antagonist; blocks vasoconstrictor and aldosterone-secreting effects of angiotensin II by selectively blocking the binding of angiotensin II to the AT₁ receptor in many tissues, such as vascular smooth muscle and the adrenal gland.

PHARMACOKINETICS: Absorption: Absolute bioavailability (25%); T_{max}=2-4 hrs. **Distribution:** (IV) V_d=17L; plasma protein binding (95%). **Metabolism:** Valeryl 4-hydroxy valsartan (primary metabolite). **Elimination:** (Sol) Feces (83%), urine (13%); (IV)$T_{1/2}$=6 hrs.

NURSING CONSIDERATIONS

Assessment: Assess for HTN, CHF, renal/hepatic impairment, obstructive biliary disorders, renal function, pregnancy/nursing status, and possible drug interactions. Assess for volume or salt depletion and correct before initiating therapy.

Monitoring: Monitor serum K^+, SrCr, and BUN periodically. Monitor for signs/symptoms of hypotension, and renal/hepatic dysfunction. Monitor BP, HR, CBC. Perform ultrasound and routine fetal testing in exposed pregnant patients.

Patient Counseling: Counsel women of childbearing potential about the risks of therapy. Inform that drug can cause serious problems in the fetus. Advise to d/c and notify physician when pregnancy is detected while on therapy. Advise to seek medical attention if symptoms of hypotension occur. Inform physician of all medical conditions and medicines being taken.

Administration: Oral route. Refer to PI for instructions on preparation of oral sus for children who cannot swallow tablets. Shake bottle well for at least 10 sec prior to administration. **Storage:** Tab: 25°C (77°F); excursions permitted to 15-30°C (59-86°F). Protect from moisture. Dispense in tight container. Sus: <30°C (<86°F) for up to 30 days or refrigerate 2-8°C (35-46°F) for up to 75 days.

DIOVAN HCT   RX
hydrochlorothiazide - valsartan (Novartis)

> When used in pregnancy, drugs that act directly on the renin-angiotensin system can cause injury and even death to the developing fetus. D/C therapy when pregnancy is detected.

THERAPEUTIC CLASS: Angiotensin II receptor antagonist/thiazide diuretic

INDICATIONS: Treatment of hypertension in patients whose BP is uncontrolled on monotherapy and as initial therapy in patients who are likely to need multiple drugs to achieve BP goals.

DOSAGE: *Adults:* Uncontrolled with Valsartan (or another ARB) or HCTZ Alone: Initial: May be switched to valsartan-HCTZ. If dose-limiting adverse reactions are experienced on either component alone, switch to valsartan-HCTZ containing a lower dose of that component in combination with the other to achieve similiar BP reductions. Titrate: May increase after 3-4 weeks of therapy. Max: 320mg-25mg. Replacement Therapy: Initial Therapy: 160mg-12.5mg qd. Titrate: May increase after 1-2 weeks of therapy. Max: 320mg-25mg qd. Hepatic Impairment: Start at low dose and titrate slowly.

HOW SUPPLIED: Tab: (Valsartan-HCTZ) 80mg-12.5mg, 160mg-12.5mg, 160mg-25mg, 320mg-12.5mg, 320mg-25mg

CONTRAINDICATIONS: Anuria, hypersensitivity to sulfonamides.

WARNINGS/PRECAUTIONS: Symptomatic hypotension may occur in volume- and/or salt-depleted patients; correct volume or salt depletion before therapy and monitor closely. Caution with hepatic dysfunction or progressive liver disease, renal dysfunction, biliary obstructive disorders, renal artery stenosis, severe congestive heart failure (CHF), history of allergies or bronchial asthma. May exacerbate or activate systemic lupus erythematosus (SLE). Avoid with severe renal impairment (CrCl ≤30mL/min). If progressive renal impairment becomes evident, consider withholding or d/c diuretic therapy. Hyponatremia, hypochloremic alkalosis, chloride deficit, hypokalemia, hypomagnesemia, hypercalcemia, hyperglycemia, and hyperuricemia may occur. Enhanced effects in post-sympathectomy patients. May increase cholesterol and triglyceride levels.

ADVERSE REACTIONS: Fetal death, fetal injury, headache, dizziness, hypokalemia.

INTERACTIONS: Alcohol, barbiturates, and narcotics may potentiate orthostatic hypotension. Insulin and oral antidiabetic agents may require dosage adjustment. May impair absorption of HCTZ with cholestyramine or colestipol. Corticosteroids and ACTH deplete electrolytes. May decrease response to pressor amines (eg, norepinephrine). Potentiates other antihypertensives. May increase responsiveness to nondepolarizing skeletal muscle relaxants (eg, tubocurarine). Risk of lithium toxicity; avoid concurrent use. NSAIDs may decrease diuretic effects; monitor closely. Coadministration with carbamazepine may lead to symptomatic hyponatremia. May sensitize or exaggerate response of heart to the toxic effects of digitalis. Coadministration of inhibitors of the hepatic uptake transporter OATP1B1 (eg, rifampin, cyclosporine) or efflux transporter MRP2 (eg, ritonavir) may increase systemic exposure. Symptomatic hypotension may occur in volume- and/or salt-depleted patients receiving high doses of diuretics. Antihypertensive effect potentiated with atenolol.

PREGNANCY: Category D, not for use in nursing.

MECHANISM OF ACTION: Valsartan: Angiotensin II receptor antagonist; blocks vasoconstrictor and aldosterone-secreting effects of angiotensin II by selectively blocking binding of angiotensin II to AT_1 receptor in many tissues, such as vascular smooth muscle and the adrenal gland. HCTZ: Thiazide diuretic; affects renal tubular mechanisms of electrolyte reabsorption, directly increasing excretion of sodium and chloride and indirectly reducing plasma volume.

PHARMACOKINETICS: Absorption: Valsartan: Absolute bioavailability (25%); T_{max}=2-4 hrs. **Distribution:** Valsartan: V_d=17L (IV); plasma protein binding (95%). HCTZ: Crosses placenta; found in breast milk. **Metabolism:** Valsartan: Valeryl 4-hydroxy valsartan (primary metabolite). **Elimination:** Valsartan: (PO) Feces (83%), urine (13%); $T_{1/2}$=6 hrs. HCTZ: Urine (61%); $T_{1/2}$=5.8-18.9 hrs.

NURSING CONSIDERATIONS

Assessment: Assess for volume/salt depletion, SLE, DM, anuria, hypersensitivity to sulfonamide or any component of the drug, history of allergies or bronchial asthma, hepatic/renal impairment, pregnancy/nursing status, and possible drug interactions.

Monitoring: Perform periodic measurements of serum electrolytes and renal function. Monitor for signs and symptoms of fluid or electrolyte imbalance, hypotension, hyperuricemia or precipitation of gout, exacerbation or activation of SLE, hypersensitivity reactions, hyperglycemia, increases in cholesterol and triglyceride levels, BP, HR, CBC, and renal/hepatic dysfunction. Perform ultrasound and routine fetal testing in exposed pregnant patients.

Patient Counseling: Counsel women of childbearing potential about risks of therapy. Inform that drug can cause serious problems in the fetus. Advise to d/c therapy and notify physician if pregnancy is detected. Counsel that lightheadedness may occur especially during the first days of therapy and to notify physician if this occurs. Advise to d/c if syncope occurs. Advise that inadequate fluid intake, excessive perspiration, diarrhea or vomiting may result in drop of BP. Advise to seek medical attention if symptoms of electrolyte imbalance (eg, dry mouth, thirst, weakness), or hypersensitivity reactions occur. Advise not to use potassium supplements or salt substitutes containing potassium without consulting the physician.

Administration: Oral route. **Storage:** 25°C (77°F); excursion permitted to 15-30°C (59-86°F). Protect from moisture. Dispense in tight container.

DIPHENHYDRAMINE HCL INJECTION   RX
diphenhydramine HCl (Various)

THERAPEUTIC CLASS: Antihistamine

INDICATIONS: Amelioration of allergic reactions to blood or plasma. Adjunct to epinephrine in anaphylaxis. For other uncomplicated immediate-type allergic conditions when oral therapy is contraindicated. Treatment of motion sickness. For parkinsonism when oral therapy is not possible or contraindicated.

DOSAGE: *Adults:* Usual: 10-50mg IV or up to 100mg IM if needed. Max: 400mg/day.
Pediatrics: Usual: 5mg/kg/24 hrs or 150mg/m²/24 hrs IV/IM in 4 divided doses. Max: 300mg/day.

HOW SUPPLIED: Inj: 50mg/mL

CONTRAINDICATIONS: Neonates, premature infants, nursing, as a local anesthetic.

WARNINGS/PRECAUTIONS: Caution with narrow-angle glaucoma, stenosing peptic ulcer, pyloroduodenal obstruction, symptomatic prostatic hypertrophy, or bladder-neck obstruction. May cause excitation in pediatrics. Increased risk of dizziness, sedation, and hypotension in elderly. Caution with lower respiratory diseases, bronchial asthma, increased IOP, hyperthyroidism, CV disease, or HTN. Local necrosis with SQ or intradermal use.

ADVERSE REACTIONS: Sedation, drowsiness, dizziness, disturbed coordination, epigastric distress, thickening of bronchial secretions.

INTERACTIONS: Additive effects with alcohol and CNS depressants. MAOIs prolong and intensify anticholinergic effects.

PREGNANCY: Category B, contraindicated in nursing.

MECHANISM OF ACTION: Antihistamine; competes with histamine for cell receptor sites on effector cells.

PHARMACOKINETICS: Metabolism: Liver. **Elimination:** Urine.

NURSING CONSIDERATIONS

Assessment: Assess for narrow-angle glaucoma, stenosing peptic ulcer, pyloroduodenal obstruction, prostatic hypertrophy, bladder-neck obstruction, history of bronchial asthma, increased IOP, hyperthyroidism, cardiovascular disease, lower respiratory disease, possible drug interactions, and nursing status.

Monitoring: Monitor for signs/symptoms of hypersensitivity reactions.

Patient Counseling: Caution may impair physical/mental abilities. Advise to seek medical attention if symptoms of hypersensitivity reactions occur.

Administration: IV, IM route **Storage:** 20-25°C (68-77°F). Protect from freezing and light.

DITROPAN XL   RX
oxybutynin chloride (Ortho-McNeil)

OTHER BRAND NAMES: Oxybutynin Chloride (Various) - Ditropan (Ortho-McNeil)

THERAPEUTIC CLASS: Anticholinergic

INDICATIONS: (All) Overactive bladder/bladder instability with symptoms of urge urinary incontinence, urgency, and frequency. (Tab, Extended-Release) Detrusor overactivity associated with a neurological condition in pediatrics ≥6 yrs.

DOSAGE: *Adults:* (Tab) Usual: 5mg bid-tid. Max: 5mg qid. Frail Elderly: 2.5mg bid-tid.(Tab, Extended-Release) Initial: 5 or 10mg qd. Titrate: May increase by 5mg weekly. Max: 30mg/day. Swallow XL whole with liquid; do not chew, divide, or crush tab.
Pediatrics: >5 yrs: (Tab) Usual: 5mg bid. Max: 5mg tid. ≥6 yrs: (Tab, Extended-Release) Initial: 5mg qd. Titrate: May increase by 5mg weekly. Max: 20mg/day. Swallow XL whole with liquid; do not chew, divide, or crush tab.

HOW SUPPLIED: Tab: 5mg*; Tab, Extended-Release: 5mg, 10mg, 15mg
*scored; Sol (generic): 5mg/5mL

CONTRAINDICATIONS: Urinary retention, gastric retention and other severe decreased GI motility conditions, uncontrolled narrow-angle glaucoma, and in patients at risk for these conditions.

WARNINGS/PRECAUTIONS: Caution with hepatic or renal impairment, bladder outflow obstruction, GI obstruction/narrowing, ulcerative colitis, intestinal atony, gastroesophageal reflux disorder, myasthenia gravis, and pre-existing dementia. May aggravate symptoms of hyperthyroidism, CHD, CHF, arrythmias, hiatal hernia, tachycardia, HTN, myasthenia gravis, and prostatic hypertrophy. Reduce dose or d/c if anticholinergic CNS effects occur. Caution in frail elderly.

ADVERSE REACTIONS: Dry mouth, constipation, somnolence, headache, diarrhea, nausea, blurred vision, dyspepsia, pain, dizziness, UTI, memory impairment, QT interval prolongation, rash, impotence.

INTERACTIONS: Increased adverse effects with other anticholinergics. Increased drowsiness with alcohol. May alter GI absorption of other drugs due to GI motility effects. Increased levels with ketoconazole; caution with CYP3A4 inhibitors (eg, antimycotics, macrolides). Caution with bisphosphonates or other drugs that may exacerbate esophagitis.

PREGNANCY: Category B, caution in nursing.

MECHANISM OF ACTION: Antispasmodic/anticholinergic agent; inhibits muscarinic action of acetylcholine on smooth muscle exerting direct antispasmodic effect; relaxes smooth muscle of bladder.

PHARMACOKINETICS: Absorption: (Tab) Rapid; absolute bioavailability (6%). Refer to PI for pediatric, isomer, and metabolite parameters. **Distribution:** V_d=193L. **Metabolism:** Liver via CYP3A4; desethyloxybutynin (active metabolite). **Elimination:** Urine (<0.1% unchanged); $T_{1/2}$=2-3 hrs.

NURSING CONSIDERATIONS

Assessment: Assess for bladder outflow obstruction (urinary retention), GI obstructive disorders (gastric retention), decreased GI motility conditions (UC, intestinal atony), GERD, GI narrowing, narrow-angle glaucoma, myasthenia gravis, hyperthyroidism, CAD, CHF, arrhythmias, hiatal hernia, HTN, prostatic hypertrophy, preexisting dementia, pregnancy/nursing status, possible drug interactions, and hepatic/renal impairment.

Monitoring: Monitor for aggravation of myasthenia gravis, hyperthyroidism, CAD, CHF, arrhythmias, hiatal hernia, HTN, prostatic hypertrophy symptoms, signs/symptoms of hypersensitivity reactions, GI narrowing (strictures), aggravation of dementia, and hepatic/renal impairment.

Patient Counseling: Inform heat prostration (fever, heat stroke due to decreased sweating), drowsiness, and blurred vision may occur. Instruct to avoid with alcohol. Swallow tab whole with liquid; do not chew, divide, or crush. Take approximately same time each day, with/without food. (Tab, Extended-Release) Inform that tablet shell may be excreted in the stool, and patient should not be concerned.

Administration: Oral route. **Storage:** (Tab): 15-30°C (59-86°F). (Tab, Extended-Release): 25°C (77°F); excursions permitted to 15-30°C (59-86°F). Protect from moisture and humidity.

DIVIGEL   RX
estradiol (Upsher-Smith)

> Estrogens increase the risk of endometrial cancer. Estrogens, with or without progestins, should not be used for the prevention of CVD or dementia. Increased risks of MI, stroke, invasive breast cancer, PE, and DVT in postmenopausal women (50-79 yrs of age) reported. Increased risk of developing probable dementia in postmenopausal women ≥65 yrs of age reported.

THERAPEUTIC CLASS: Estrogen

INDICATIONS: Treatment of moderate to severe vasomotor symptoms associated with menopause.

D

DOSAGE: *Adults:* Initial: 0.25g qd applied on skin of right or left upper thigh. Re-evaluate periodically. Adjust dose based on individual response.

HOW SUPPLIED: Gel: 0.1% (0.25g, 0.5g, and 1g single-dose foil pkts containing 0.25mg, 0.5mg, and 1mg estradiol, respectively)

CONTRAINDICATIONS: Undiagnosed abnormal genital bleeding, breast cancer, estrogen-dependent neoplasia, DVT/PE, active or recent (within past year) arterial thromboembolic disease (eg, stroke, MI), liver dysfunction or disease, pregnancy.

WARNINGS/PRECAUTIONS: May increase risk of cardiovascular events (eg, MI, stroke), venous thrombosis, and PE; d/c immediately if any occur or are suspected. May increase risk of breast/endometrial cancer, dementia and gallbladder disease. May lead to severe hypercalcemia with breast cancer and bone metastases; monitor and d/c if hypercalcemia occurs. Retinal vascular thrombosis reported; monitor and d/c if papilledema or retinal vascular lesions occur. Consider addition of a progestin if no hysterectomy. May elevate BP; monitor at regular intervals. May cause elevations of plasma triglycerides with pre-existing hypertriglyceridemia. Caution with history of cholestatic jaundice associated with past estrogen use or with pregnancy; d/c with recurrence. May lead to increased TBG levels; monitor thyroid function. May cause fluid retention; caution with cardiac/renal dysfunction. Caution with severe hypocalcemia. May increase risk of ovarian cancer. May exacerbate endometriosis, asthma, DM, epilepsy, migraine, porphyria, SLE, and hepatic hemangiomas; use with caution. Alcohol-based gels are flammable; avoid fire, flame, or smoking until gel has dried.

ADVERSE REACTIONS: Nasopharyngitis, upper respiratory tract infection, vaginal mycosis, breast tenderness, metrorrhagia, headache, nausea, pruritus, abdominal cramps.

INTERACTIONS: May increase prothombin time, partial thromboplastin time, and platelet aggregation time. May require higher doses of thyroid hormone. May elevate binding proteins and decrease free hormone concentration. May increase plasma HDL concentration, reduce LDL concentration and increased triglyceride levels. Impaired glucose tolerance. Reduced response to metyrapone test.

PREGNANCY: Contraindicated in pregnancy, caution in nursing.

MECHANISM OF ACTION: Estrogen; binds to nuclear receptors in estrogen-responsive tissues. Circulating estrogens modulate pituitary secretion of gonadotropins, luteinizing hormone and follicle stimulating hormone, through negative feedback mechanism. Acts to reduce elevated levels of these hormones seen in postmenopausal women.

PHARMACOKINETICS: Absorption: Administration of variable doses led to altered parameters. **Distribution:** Largely bound to sex hormone binding globulin and albumin; found in breast milk. **Metabolism:** Liver to estrone (metabolite), estriol (major urinary metabolite), sulfate and glucuronide conjugation (liver), intestinal hydrolysis; CYP3A4 (partial metabolism). **Elimination:** Urine (parent compound and metabolites); $T_{1/2}$=10 hrs.

NURSING CONSIDERATIONS

Assessment: Assess for undiagnosed abnormal genital bleeding, presence or history of breast cancer, estrogen-dependent neoplasia, DVT, PE, active or recent (within past yr) arterial thromboembolic disease (eg, stroke, MI), liver dysfunction, history of cholestatic jaundice, pregnancy/nursing status, (≥65) yrs), hypertriglyceridemia, hypothyroidism, hypocalcemia, renal dysfunction, asthma, DM, epilepsy, migraines or porphyria, SLE, and possible drug interactions. Assess need for progestin in women who have not had a hysterectomy.

Monitoring: Monitor for signs/symptoms of CV disorders (eg, stroke, coronary heart disease, VTE), malignant neoplasms (endometrial, breast, or ovarian cancer), dementia, gallbladder disease, hypercalcemia, visual abnormalities (eg, retinal vascular thrombosis), BP elevations, elevations in plasma triglycerides and development of pancreatitis, hypothyroidism, fluid retention, exacerbation of endometriosis or other conditions (eg, asthma, DM, epilepsy, migraine or porphyria, SLE, hepatic hemangiomas). Monitor thyroid function in patients on thyroid replacement therapy. If undiagnosed, persistent, or recurring abnormal vaginal bleeding occurs, perform endometrial sampling to rule out malignancy. Monitor BP levels. Perform annual breast exam and periodic monitoring (every 3-6 months) to determine therapy need.

Patient Counseling: Inform that medication increases risk for uterine cancer. Instruct to contact physician for signs/symptoms of breast lumps, unusual vaginal bleeding, dizziness or faintness, changes in speech or vision, severe headaches, chest pain, SOB, leg pains, or vomiting. Instruct to notify physician if planning surgery or prolonged immobilization. Counsel to have annual gynecological exam and perform self-breast exams. Apply medication to left or right upper thigh and allow to dry before dressing; do not apply to face, breast, irritated skin, or area around vagina. Instruct to keep area dry as long as possible following application and to rotate between left and right upper thigh to prevent skin irritation. Wash hands before and following application. Others should avoid contact of skin area for at least 1 hr following administration. Medication should be applied by patient, if others need to apply, a disposable plastic glove should be used. Inform that medication contains alcohol; avoid fire, flame, or smoking until dry. Instruct that if missed a dose and next dosing is <12 hrs away, wait to apply regular dose at normal time; if dosing is >12 hrs away, apply missed dose and resume normal dosing schedule.

Administration: Topical route. **Storage:** 20-25°C (68°-77°F); excursions permitted to 15-30°C (59-86°F). Keep out of reach of children.

DOBUTAMINE   RX
dobutamine (Various)

THERAPEUTIC CLASS: Inotropic agent

INDICATIONS: Short-term treatment of cardiac decompensation due to depressed contractility resulting from organic heart disease or from cardiac surgical procedures.

DOSAGE: *Adults:* Initial: 0.5-1mcg/kg/min. Usual: 2-20mcg/kg/min. Max: 40mcg/kg/min (rare). Adjust rate and duration based on BP, urine flow, ectopic activity, HR, and when possible, cardiac output, central venous pressure, and/or pulmonary capillary wedge pressure.
Pediatrics: Initial: 0.5-1mcg/kg/min. Usual: 2-20mcg/kg/min. Max: 40mcg/kg/min (rare). Adjust rate and duration based on BP, urine flow, ectopic activity, HR, and when possible, cardiac output, central venous pressure, and/or pulmonary capillary wedge pressure.

HOW SUPPLIED: Inj: 12.5mg/mL

CONTRAINDICATIONS: Idiopathic hypertrophic subaortic stenosis (IHSS).

WARNINGS/PRECAUTIONS: May increase HR or BP, especially systolic pressure; caution with atrial fibrillation and HTN. May precipitate or exacerbate ventricular ectopic activity. Hypersensitivity reactions (eg, skin rash, fever, eosinophilia, bronchospasm) reported. Contains sulfites; caution in asthmatics. Monitor EKG, BP, pulmonary wedge pressure, and cardiac output. Correct hypovolemia prior to infusion. Caution in elderly. May decrease serum K⁺ levels. Improvement may not be observed with marked mechanical obstruction (eg, severe valvular aortic stenosis).

ADVERSE REACTIONS: Increased HR, BP and ventricular ectopic activity, hypotension, infusion-site reactions, nausea, headache, anginal pain, palpitations, shortness of breath, decreased K⁺ levels, nonspecific chest pain, phlebitis.

INTERACTIONS: Recent administration of β-blockers may reduce effectiveness and increase peripheral vascular resistance. Increased cardiac output and lower pulmonary wedge pressure with nitroprusside.

PREGNANCY: Category B, caution in nursing.

MECHANISM OF ACTION: Direct-acting inotropic agent; stimulates β-receptors of the heart while producing comparatively mild chronotropic, hypertensive, arrhythmogenic, and vasodilative effects.

PHARMACOKINETICS: Metabolism: Methylation of the catechol and conjugation. **Elimination**: Urine (the conjugates of dobutamine and 3-O-methyl dobutamine; inactive metabolite).

NURSING CONSIDERATIONS

Assessment: Assess for IHSS, mechanical obstruction (eg, valvular aortic stenosis), HTN, atrial fibrillation, drug or sulfite hypersensitivity and pregnancy/nursing status. Prior to treatment, correct hypovolemia if present.

Monitoring: Continuous monitoring of ECG, BP, pulmonary wedge pressure, cardiac output. Monitor for HR and BP, hypersensitivity reactions (eg, skin rash, fever, eosinophilia, and bronchospasm), allergic-type reactions, including anaphylactic symptoms and life-threatening or less severe asthmatic episodes, ectopic activity or ventricular tachycardia, and serum potassium.

Patient Counseling: Inform that drug may increase HR and BP. Report if experience any reactions at infusion site, palpitations, or SOB.

Administration: IV route. Observe for particulate matter prior to administration. **Storage:** 15-30°C (59-86°F).

DOLOPHINE
methadone HCI (Roxane)

> Only approved hospitals and pharmacies can dispense oral methadone for the treatment of narcotic addiction. Deaths, cardiac and respiratory, have been reported during initiation and conversion of pain in patients to methadone treatment from treatment with other opioid agonists. Respiratory depression is the main hazard associated with administration. QT interval prolongation and serious arrhythmias have been observed during treatment. Initiate treatment for analgesia in patients with acute or chronic pain only if benefits outweigh the risks.

OTHER BRAND NAMES: Methadone (Various)

THERAPEUTIC CLASS: Opioid analgesic

INDICATIONS: Detoxification and maintenance treatment of opioid addiction (heroin or other morphine-like drugs). Treatment of moderate to severe pain not responsive to non-narcotic analgesics.

DOSAGE: *Adults:* Detoxification: Initial: 20-30mg single dose. Max: 30mg. Evaluate after 2-4 hrs. Give 5-10mg if withdrawal symptoms reappear. Total daily dose on 1st day of treatment should not exceed 40mg. Short-term Detoxification: Titrate to a total daily dose of 40mg in divided doses. Stabilize for 2-3 days, then may decrease every 1-2 days depending on symptoms. Maint: Titrate to a dose at which opioid symptoms are prevented for 24 hrs. Usual range: 80-120mg/day. Withdrawal after Maintenance Treatment: Reduce dose <10% of established tolerance q10-14 days. Pain (Opioid Non-Tolerant): Usual: 2.5-10mg q8-12h slowly titrated to effect. Conversion from Parenteral to Oral Methadone: Use 1:2 dose ratio initially. See PI for switching to methadone from other chronic opioids.

HOW SUPPLIED: Tab: 5mg, 10mg

CONTRAINDICATIONS: Acute bronchial asthma or hypercarbia, respiratory depression, with suspicion of a paralytic ileus.

WARNINGS/PRECAUTIONS: Extreme caution if narcotic antagonists used in patients physically dependent on narcotics. Incomplete cross-tolerance and iatrogenic overdose may occur. Can cause CSF pressure elevation. Caution with head injuries, acute asthma attacks, COPD, cor pulmonale, decreased respiratory reserve, pre-existing respiratory depression, hypoxia, or hypercapnia. Reduce initial dose in elderly, debilitated, severe hepatic or renal impairment, hypothyroidism, Addison's disease, prostatic hypertrophy, or urethral stricture. Drug tolerance, dependence, and abuse may occur. Infants born to opioid-dependent mothers may exhibit respiratory difficulties and withdrawal symptoms. Impairs physical and mental abilities. Ineffective in relieving anxiety. May mask symptoms and clinical course of acute abdominal conditions and head injuries. May produce hypotension. Incomplete cross-tolerance and iatrogenic overdose may occur.

ADVERSE REACTIONS: Lightheadedness, dizziness, sedation, sweating, N/V, asthenia, cardiomyopathy, ECG abnormalities, abdominal pain, agitation, seizures, confusion, hallucinations, respiratory depression.

INTERACTIONS: Concomitant use with other opioid analgesics, general anesthesia, phenothiazines, sedatives, hypnotics, and other CNS depressants (including alcohol) may experience respiratory depression, hypotension, profound sedation, or coma. Concomitant use with phenytoin, rifampin, opioid antagonists, mixed agonists/antagonists, and partial agonists may precipitate withdrawal symptoms. Decreased plasma levels with antiretrovirals. Increased AUC of zidovudine. Decreased AUC and peak levels of didanosine and stavu- dine. May precipitate severe reactions with MAOIs. Increased levels of desi- pramine. Caution with drugs known to prolong QT interval. Pharmacodynamic interaction may occur with Class I and III antiarrhythmics, some neurolep- tics, tricyclic antidepressants (TCAs), and calcium channel blockers (CCBs). Caution with drugs capable of inducing electrolyte imbalance (eg, diuretics, laxatives, mineralocorticoids). Decreased effects with CYP450 inducers while CYP450 inhibitors (eg, azole antifungals, macrolide antibiotics, SSRIs) may potentiate effects.

PREGNANCY: Category C, not for use in nursing.

MECHANISM OF ACTION: Opioid analgesic; μ-agonist. Produces many actions similiar to morphine. Acts prominently in the CNS and in organs composed of smooth muscle. Also acts as an antagonist at the N-methyl-D-aspartate (NMDA) receptor.

PHARMACOKINETICS: Absorption: Bioavailability (36-100%); C_{max}=124- 1255ng/mL; T_{max}=1-7.5 hrs. **Distribution:** V_d=1.0-8.0L/kg; plasma protein binding (85-90%); found in saliva, breast milk, amniotic fluid, and umbilical cord plasma. **Metabolism:** Liver (N-demethylation) via CYP450 enzymes: 3A4 (primary), 2B6 (primary), 2C19 (primary); 2C9; 2D6. **Elimination:** Urine, feces; $T_{1/2}$=8-59 hrs.

NURSING CONSIDERATIONS

Assessment: Assess for pain intensity or any other conditions where treat- ment is contraindicated or cautioned. Assess for pregnancy/nursing status, renal/hepatic function, and possible drug interactions.

Monitoring: Monitor for signs/symptoms of respiratory depression, QT prolongation and arrhythmia (eg, torsades de pointes), elevations in CSF pressure, hypotension, misuse or abuse and tolerance or dependence, and hypersensitivity reactions.

Patient Counseling: Inform that drug may impair mental/physical abilities; use caution when performing hazardous tasks (eg, operating machinery/driv- ing). Avoid use of other CNS depressants and alcohol during therapy. Notify physician if symptoms suggestive of arrhythmia (eg, palpitations, dizziness, lightheadedness, syncope) develop. Medication may produce orthostatic hypotension. Avoid abrupt withdrawal from medication. Instruct that if using for treatment of opioid dependence, discontinuation may lead to relapse of illicit drug use.

Administration: Oral route. **Storage:** 25°C (77°F); excursions permitted to 15- 30°C (59-86°F). Dispense in tight, light-resistant container.

DONNATAL   RX

hyoscyamine sulfate - atropine sulfate - scopolamine hydrobromide - phenobarbital (PBM Pharmaceuticals)

OTHER BRAND NAMES: Donnatal Extentabs (PBM Pharmaceuticals)

THERAPEUTIC CLASS: Anticholinergic/barbiturate

INDICATIONS: Adjunct therapy for irritable bowel syndrome (irritable colon, spastic colon, mucous colitis), acute enterocolitis, and duodenal ulcers.

DOSAGE: *Adults:* (Elixir/Tab) 1-2 tabs or 5-10mL tid-qid. (Extentabs) 1 tab q8- q12h. Hepatic Disease: Use lower doses.

Pediatrics: (Elixir) 4.5kg: 0.5mL q4h or 0.75mL q6h. 9.1kg: 1mL q4h or 1.5mL q6h. 13.6kg: 1.5mL q4h or 2mL q6h. 22.7kg: 2.5mL q4h or 3.75mL q6h. 34kg: 3.75mL q4h or 5mL q6h. 45.4kg: 5mL q4h or 7.5mL q6h. Hepatic Disease: Use lower doses.

HOW SUPPLIED: (Atropine-Hyoscyamine-Phenobarbital-Scopolamine) Elixir: 0.0194mg-0.1037mg-16.2mg-0.0065mg/5mL; Tab: 0.0194mg-0.1037mg-16.2mg-0.0065mg; Tab, Extended-Release: (Extentabs) 0.0582mg-0.3111mg-48.6mg-0.0195mg

CONTRAINDICATIONS: Glaucoma, obstructive uropathy (eg, bladder neck obstruction due to prostatic hypertrophy), obstructive GI disease (achalasia, pyloroduodenal stenosis, etc.), paralytic ileus, intestinal atony in elderly or debilitated, unstable cardiovascular status in acute hemorrhage, severe ulcerative colitis especially if complicated by toxic megacolon, myasthenia gravis, hiatal hernia associated with reflux esophagitis, acute intermittent porphyria, and for patients in whom phenobarbital produces restlessness and/or excitement.

WARNINGS/PRECAUTIONS: Inconclusive whether anticholinergic/antispasmodic drugs aid in duodenal ulcer healing, decrease recurrence rate, or prevent complications. Heat prostration can occur with high environmental temperatures. May be habit forming; caution with history of physical and/or psychological drug dependence. Exercise caution while operating machinery/driving. Use with caution and lower dosage in patients with hepatic dysfunction. Caution with hepatic/renal disease, autonomic neuropathy, hyperthyroidism, coronary heart disease, congestive heart failure (CHF), arrhythmias, tachycardia, HTN. May delay gastric emptying. Diarrhea may be an early symptom of incomplete intestinal obstruction, especially with ileostomy or colostomy; treatment would be inappropriate. Avoid abrupt withdrawal in patients habituated to barbiturates.

ADVERSE REACTIONS: Xerostomia, urinary hesitancy/retention, blurred vision, tachycardia, mydriasis, cycloplegia, increased ocular tension, loss of taste, headache, nervousness, drowsiness, weakness, dizziness, insomnia, N/V.

INTERACTIONS: Phenobarbital may decrease anticoagulant effects; adjust dose.

PREGNANCY: Category C, caution in nursing.

MECHANISM OF ACTION: Anticholinergic/barbiturate; provides natural belladonna alkaloids in a specific, fixed ratio combined with phenobarbital to provide peripheral anticholinergic/antispasmodic action and mild sedation.

NURSING CONSIDERATIONS

Assessment: Assess for glaucoma, obstructive uropathy (eg, bladder neck obstruction due to prostatic hypertrophy) obstructive disease of the GIT (achalasia, pyloroduodenal stenosis, etc.) paralytic ileus, intestinal atony, coronary heart disease, CHF, cardiac arrhythmias, tachycardia, HTN, hypersensitivity and for any other conditions where treatment is contraindicated or cautioned. Assess pregnancy/nursing status and possible drug interactions.

Monitoring: Monitor occurrence of heat prostration, drowsiness, blurred vision, HR, constipation, diarrhea, urinary hesitancy/retention, and hypersensitivity reactions.

Patient Counseling: Counsel about possible side effects and to report to a healthcare provider if any occur. Counsel about drug abuse/dependence. Advise not to engage in activities requiring mental alertness, such as operating a motor vehicle or other machinery, and not to perform hazardous work. Advise to avoid high environmental temperatures.

Administration: Oral route. **Storage:** 20-25°C (68-77°F). Protect from light and moisture.

DOPAMINE
dopamine HCl (Various)

RX

OTHER BRAND NAMES: Dopamine HCl and 5% Dextrose (Baxter)

THERAPEUTIC CLASS: Inotropic agent

INDICATIONS: For correction of hemodynamic imbalances present in shock due to MI, trauma, endotoxic septicemia, open-heart surgery, renal failure, and chronic cardiac decompensation. (Dextrose); Hypotension due to inadequate cardiac output.

DOSAGE: *Adults:* Initial: 2-5mcg/kg/min. Use 5mcg/kg/min in seriously ill. Increase in 5-10mcg/kg/min increments, up to 20-50mcg/kg/min. (Dextrose): Avoid bolus administration. Elderly: Start at low end of dosing range. Drug additives should not be made.
Pediatrics: (Dextrose): Initial: 1-5mcg/kg/min. Max: 15-20mcg/kg/min, occasional ≥50mcg/kg/min.

HOW SUPPLIED: Inj: 40mg/mL, 80mg/mL, 160mg/mL, (Dopamine HCl and Dextrose) 800mcg/mL, 1600mcg/mL, 3200mcg/mL

CONTRAINDICATIONS: Pheochromocytoma, uncorrected tachyarrhythmias or ventricular fibrillation. (Dextrose); Allergy to corn or corn products.

WARNINGS/PRECAUTIONS: Contains sulfites. Monitor BP, urine flow, cardiac output and pulmonary wedge pressure. Correct hypovolemia, hypoxia, hypercapnia, and acidosis prior to use. Reduce infusion rate with increase in diastolic BP/marked decrease in pulse pressure; increase rate if hypotension occurs. D/C if hypotension persists. Reduce dose if increased ectopic beats occurs. Caution with history of occlusive vascular disease (eg, atherosclerosis, arterial embolism, Raynaud's disease, cold injury, diabetic endarteritis, and Buerger's disease); monitor for changes in skin color or temperature. Administer phentolamine if extravasation noted. Avoid abrupt withdrawal. (Dextrose): Do not add to any alkaline diluent solution. Do not administer at the same set as blood; pseudoagglutination or hemolysis may result. May cause fluid overloading. Caution in children and elderly. Avoid bolus administration.

ADVERSE REACTIONS: Tachycardia, palpitation, ventricular arrhythmia (high doses), dyspnea, N/V, headache, anxiety, bradycardia, hypotension, HTN, vasoconstriction.

INTERACTIONS: If treated with MAOIs within 2-3 weeks prior to administration of dopamine, reduce initial dose of dopamine to not greater than 1/10th of usual dose. Potential additive or potentiating effects on urine flow with diuretics. TCAs may potentiate cardiovascular effects of adrenergic agents. Cardiac effects antagonized by β-blockers. Peripheral vasoconstriction antagonized by α-blockers. Butyrophenones (eg, haloperidol) and phenothiazines may suppress renal and mesenteric vasodilation. Extreme caution with cyclopropane or halogenated hydrocarbon anesthetics. Concomitant use with vasopressors, vasoconstricting agents (eg, ergonovine), some oxytocic drugs, and local anesthetics may result in severe HTN. Hypotension and bradycardia reported with phenytoin; consider alternatives.

PREGNANCY: Category C, caution in nursing.

MECHANISM OF ACTION: Catecholamine; produces positive chronotropic and inotropic effects on the myocardium, resulting in increased heart rate and cardiac contractility. Acts directly by exerting an agonist action on β-adrenoreceptor and indirectly by causing release of norepinephrine from storage sites in sympathetic nerve endings.

PHARMACOKINETICS: Metabolism: Liver, kidneys, and plasma via MAO and catechol-O-methyltransferase. **Elimination:** Urine (80%) as homovanillic acid and 3,4-dihydroxyphenylacetic acid.

NURSING CONSIDERATIONS

Assessment: Assess for sulfite hypersensitivity, pheochromocytoma, uncorrected tachyarrhythmias/ventricular fibrillation, history of occlusive vascular disease (eg, atherosclerosis, arterial embolism, Raynaud's disease, cold injury, diabetic endarteritis, and Buerger's disease), pregnancy status, and possible

D

drug interactions. Assess and correct prior to, or concurrently with, administration of therapy for hypovolemia, hypoxia, acidosis, and hypercapnia. Assess pregnancy/nursing status.

Monitoring: Close monitoring of urine flow, cardiac output, BP, and central venous pressure. Monitor for ventricular arrhythmias, decreased pulse pressure, hypotension, extravasation/peripheral ischemia; sloughing and necrosis of the surrounding tissue and allergic-type reactions, including anaphylactic symptoms and life-threatening or less severe asthmatic episodes. In occlusive vascular disease, monitor for changes in color or temperature of skin in extremities.

Patient Counseling: Inform about benefits/risks of therapy.

Administration: IV infusion route. Not for direct IV injection; drug must be diluted before administration to patient. Avoid injection to sodium bicarbonate or other alkaline and/or amphotericin B solutions. **Storage:** 15-30°C (59-86°F). (Dopamine HCl and Dextrose): 25-40°C. Avoid excessive heat. Protect from freezing.

Doribax RX
doripenem (Ortho-McNeil)

THERAPEUTIC CLASS: Carbapenem

INDICATIONS: Treatment of complicated intra-abdominal and urinary tract infections, including pyelonephritis, caused by susceptible microorganisms.

DOSAGE: Adults: ≥18 yrs: 500mg IV q8h for 5-14 days (intra-abdominal) or 10 days (UTI). Infuse over 1 hour. Renal Impairment: CrCl: >50mL/min: No dose adjustment. CrCl 30-50mL/min: 250mg IV q8h. CrCl >10 to <30mL/min: 250mg IV q12h.

HOW SUPPLIED: Inj: 500mg

CONTRAINDICATIONS: Anaphylactic reactions to β-lactams.

WARNINGS/PRECAUTIONS: Serious hypersensitivity (anaphylactic) reactions reported. *Clostridium difficile*-associated diarrhea (CDAD) reported (ranging from mild diarrhea to fatal colitis); evaluate if diarrhea occurs. Consider alternative antibacterial therapies in patients receiving valproic acid or sodium valproate due to increased risk of breakthrough seizures. Increased risk of development of drug-resistant bacteria in the absence of proven or strongly suspected bacterial infection. Do not administer via inhalation.

ADVERSE REACTIONS: Headache, nausea, diarrhea, rash, phlebitis, anemia, pruritus, anaphylaxis, neutropenia, leukopenia.

INTERACTIONS: May reduce serum valproic acid levels, which may increase risk of breakthrough seizures. Probenecid may increase levels; avoid coadministration.

PREGNANCY: Category B, caution in nursing.

MECHANISM OF ACTION: Broad-spectrum carbapenem; exerts bactericidal activity by inhibiting cell wall biosynthesis, resulting in cell death.

PHARMACOKINETICS: Absorption: C_{max}=23mcg/mL, AUC=36.3mcg•hr/mL. **Distribution:** V_d=16.8L; plasma protein binding (8.1%). **Metabolism:** Via dehydropeptidase-1. **Elimination:** Urine (70% unchanged and 15% metabolites), feces (<1%); $T_{1/2}$=1 hr.

NURSING CONSIDERATIONS

Assessment: Assess for previous hypersensitivity reactions to other carbapenems, cephalosporins, PCNs, or other allergens. Assess for renal impairment and possible drug interactions. Document indications for therapy and culture and susceptibility testing.

Monitoring: Monitor for signs/symptoms of anaphylactoid/hypersensitivity reactions, CDAD, superinfection, seizures, anemia, phlebitis, rash.

Patient Counseling: Inform drug only treats bacterial, not viral, infections. Take exactly as directed; skipping doses or not completing full course may decrease effectiveness and increase resistance. May experience diarrhea; notify physician if taking valproic acid or if watery/bloody stools, hypersensitivity reactions, infection, or seizures occur.

Administration: IV route. **Storage:** Store at 25°C (77°F); excursions permitted to 15-30°C (59-86°F).

DORYX

RX D

doxycycline hyclate (Warner Chilcott)

THERAPEUTIC CLASS: Tetracycline derivative

INDICATIONS: Treatment of the following infections: upper respiratory tract, respiratory tract, urinary tract, lymphogranuloma venereum, psittacosis, trachoma, uncomplicated urethral/endocervical/rectal, nongonococcal urethritis, relapsing fever, Rocky Mountain spotted fever, typhus fever and the typhus group, Q fever, rickettsialpox, tick fevers, inclusion conjunctivitis, tularemia, *Campylobacter* fetus infections, bartonellosis, granuloma inguinale, plague, cholera, brucellosis, anthrax (including inhalational anthrax, post-exposure). When penicillin is contraindicated, treatment of syphilis, yaws, Vincent's infection, actinomycosis, and infections caused by *Clostridium* species. Adjunct therapy for acute intestinal amebiasis and severe acne. Prophylaxis of malaria due to *Plasmodium falciparum* in short-term travelers (<4 months) to areas with chloroquine and/or pyrimethamine-sulfadoxine resistant strains.

DOSAGE: *Adults:* Usual: 100mg q12h on 1st day, followed by 100mg/day (single dose or as 50mg q12h) or 100mg q12h for more severe infections (eg, chronic UTIs). *Streptococcus* Infection: Treat for 10 days. Uncomplicated Urethral, Endocervical, or Rectal Infection/ Nongonococcal Urethritis: 100mg bid for 7 days. Syphilis (Early): 100mg bid for 14 days. Syphilis (>1 yr): 100mg bid for 28 days. Acute Epididymo-orchitis: 100mg bid for ≥10 days. Inhalational Anthrax (post-exposure): 100mg bid for 60 days. Malaria Prophylaxis: 100mg qd, beginning 1-2 days before travel, continuing daily during travel and for 28 days after departure from malarious area. Elderly: Start at lower end of dosing range.
Pediatrics: >8 yrs: >100 lbs: Usual: 100mg q12h on 1st day, followed by 100mg/day (single dose or as 50mg q12h) or 100mg q12h for more severe infections (eg, chronic UTIs). *Streptococcus* Infection: Treat for 10 days. Inhalational Anthrax (post-exposure): 100mg bid for 60 days. Malaria Prophylaxis: 100mg qd, beginning 1-2 days before travel, continuing daily during travel and for 28 days after departure from malarious area. ≤100 lbs: Usual: 2mg/lb divided into 2 doses on 1st day, followed by 1mg/lb/day or up to 2mg/lb/day (single dose or divided into 2 doses) for more severe infections thereafter. *Streptococcus* Infection: Treat for 10 days. Inhalational Anthrax (post-exposure): 1mg/lb bid for 60 days. Malaria Prophylaxis: 2mg/kg qd, beginning 1-2 days before travel, continuing daily during travel and for 28 days after departure from malarious area. Max: 100mg/day

HOW SUPPLIED: Tab, Delayed-Release: 75mg*, 100mg*, 150mg* *scored

WARNINGS/PRECAUTIONS: *Clostridium difficile*-associated diarrhea (CDAD) reported. May decrease bone growth in premature infants, and cause fetal harm during pregnancy. May cause permanent discoloration of the teeth or enamel hypoplasia if used in last half of pregnancy, infancy or <8 yrs. Photosensitivity, increased BUN, false elevations of urinary catecholamines, and superinfection may occur. Bulging fontanels in infants and benign intracranial HTN in adults reported. Incision and drainage or other surgical procedures should be performed in conjunction when indicated. Those using doxycycline as a prophylaxis for malaria may transmit the infection to mosquitoes outside endemic areas. Use in the absence of the proper indication increases the risk of drug-resistance. When coexistent syphilis is suspected, perform dark-field examination before treatment and blood serology repeatedly monthly for at least 4 months. Caution in elderly.

ADVERSE REACTIONS: Anorexia, N/V, diarrhea, dysphagia, enterocolitis, rash, inflammatory lesions in the anogenital area, exfoliative dermatitis, renal toxicity, hemolytic anemia, hypersensitivity reactions.

INTERACTIONS: May depress plasma PT, adjust anticoagulant dose with concomitant use. May interfere with bactericidal action of penicillin; avoid concurrent use when possible. Impaired absorption with bismuth subsalicylate and antacids containing aluminum, calcium or magnesium and iron-containing preparations. Decreased $T_{1/2}$ with barbiturates, carbamazepine and phenytoin. Fatal renal toxicity with methoxyflurane. May render oral contraceptives less effective.

PREGNANCY: Category D, not for use in nursing.

MECHANISM OF ACTION: Tetracycline; exert bacteriostatic effect by the inhibition of protein synthesis.

PHARMACOKINETICS: Absorption: Complete; C_{max}=2.6 mcg/mL; T_{max}=2 hrs. **Distribution:** Found in breast milk. **Metabolism:** Liver. **Elimination:** Urine and feces. $T_{1/2}$=18-22 hrs.

NURSING CONSIDERATIONS

Assessment: Assess for hypersensitivity reactions, renal impairment, pregnancy/nursing status and possible drug interactions. Document indications for therapy, culture and susceptibility testing. Perform incision and drainage in conjunction with antibiotic therapy when indicated. When coexistent syphilis is suspected, perform dark-field examination before treatment and blood serology repeatedly monthly for at least 4 months.

Monitoring: Monitor for hypersensitivity reactions, photosensitivity, superinfection, CDAD, benign intracranial HTN. Monitor LFTs, hematopoietic values and renal function in long term therapy. When coexistent syphilis is suspected, perform blood serology repeatedly monthly for at least 4 months.

Patient Counseling: Inform of pregnancy risks and to avoid pregnancy. Counsel about photosensitivity reactions and to d/c at first sign of skin erythema. Avoid excessive sunlight/UV light and wear sunscreen or sunblock. Take exactly as directed, skipping doses or not completing full course may decrease effectiveness and increase resistance. Avoid foods with calcium and drink fluids liberally to reduce risk of esophageal irritation or ulceration. May increase the incidence of vaginal candidiasis. Inform that drug only treats bacterial, not viral, infections. Diarrhea may occur; contact physician if watery/bloody stools, hypersensitivity reactions, superinfections, photosensitivity or benign intracranial HTN occurs. Counsel on malaria prophylaxis to begin therapy 2 days before travel; continue while in the malarious area and for 4 weeks after return. Therapy should not exceed 4 months. Counsel on appropriate way to take medicine, eg, take with adequate amount of fluid, take with food or milk if gastric irritation occurs, and may sprinkle contents on a spoonful of applesauce to be swallowed without chewing followed by a glass of water.

Administration: Oral route. **Storage:** 25°C (77°F); excursions permitted to 15-30°C (59-86°F). Dispense in tight, light-resistant container.

DOVONEX   RX
calcipotriene (Warner Chilcott)

THERAPEUTIC CLASS: Vitamin D_3 derivative

INDICATIONS: Treatment of plaque psoriasis.

DOSAGE: *Adults:* Apply thin layer to affected skin bid and rub in gently and completely for up to 8 weeks. Wash hands after application.

HOW SUPPLIED: Cre: 0.005% [60g, 120g]

CONTRAINDICATIONS: Hypercalcemia, vitamin D toxicity.

WARNINGS/PRECAUTIONS: Avoid contact with face and eyes. Transient irritation may occur; d/c if develops. D/C if hypercalcemia occurs; may continue once calcium levels are normal. Avoid excessive exposure to either natural or artificial sunlight. Pediatric patients are at greater risk than adults of systemic adverse effects when they are treated with topical medication. For external use only; not for ophthalmic, oral or intravaginal use.

ADVERSE REACTIONS: Skin irritation, rash, pruritus, dermatitis, worsening of psoriasis.

PREGNANCY: Category C, caution in nursing.

MECHANISM OF ACTION: Vitamin D$_3$ derivative.

PHARMACOKINETICS: Metabolism: Liver. **Elimination:** Bile.

NURSING CONSIDERATIONS

Assessment: Assess for drug hypersensitivity reactions, hypercalcemia, evidence of vitamin D toxicity, pregnancy/nursing status.

Monitoring: Monitor for serum calcium concentration, irritation of lesions and surrounding uninvolved skin.

Patient Counseling: Advise to use drug as directed. Instruct to report signs of adverse reactions. Counsel to avoid excessive exposure to natural or artificial sunlight (eg, tanning booths, sun lamps) after application. For external use only; avoid contact with eyes or face. Advise to wash hands after application. Counsel that drug should not to be used for any disorder other than which is prescribed. Instruct to keep out of the reach of children.

Administration: Topical route. Wash hands thoroughly after use. **Storage:** 15-25°C (59-77°F). Do not freeze.

DOVONEX SCALP   RX
calcipotriene (Warner Chilcott)

THERAPEUTIC CLASS: Vitamin D$_3$ derivative

INDICATIONS: Topical treatment of chronic, moderately severe psoriasis of the scalp.

DOSAGE: *Adults:* Comb hair to remove scaly debris. After parting hair, apply and rub into affected area(s) bid for up to 8 weeks. Wash hands after application.

HOW SUPPLIED: Sol: 0.005% [60mL]

CONTRAINDICATIONS: Acute psoriatic eruptions, hypercalcemia, vitamin D toxicity.

WARNINGS/PRECAUTIONS: Avoid contact with mucous membranes and eyes. Transient irritation and sensitivity reaction may occur; d/c if develops. D/C if hypercalcemia occurs; may continue once calcium levels are normal. Avoid excessive exposure to either natural or artificial sunlight. Pediatric patients are greater risk than adults of systemic adverse effects when they are treated with topical medication. For external use only; not for ophthalmic, oral or intravaginal use.

ADVERSE REACTIONS: Transient burning, stinging, tingling, rash, dry skin, irritation and worsening of psoriasis.

PREGNANCY: Category C, caution in nursing.

MECHANISM OF ACTION: Vitamin D$_3$ derivative; has not been established. It is roughly equipotent to the natural vitamin in its effects on proliferation and differentiation of a variety of cell types.

PHARMACOKINETICS: Metabolism: Liver. **Elimination:** Bile.

NURSING CONSIDERATIONS

Assessment: Assess for drug hypersensitivity, acute psoriatic eruptions, hypercalcemia, evidence of vitamin D toxicity, pregnancy/nursing status.

Monitoring: Monitor for irritation of both lesions and surrounding uninvolved skin, hypersensitivity reactions and serum calcium concentration.

Patient Counseling: Advise to use as directed; d/c and contact physician if any adverse reactions occur. Avoid excessive exposure to natural or artificial sunlight (eg, tanning booths, sun lamps) after application. Counsel that drug is for external use only; avoid contact with face or eyes. Keep away from open flame. Counsel that drug should not be used for any disorder other than which is prescribed. Keep away from children. Counsel to avoid application of the solution to uninvolved scalp margins. Advise to wash hands after application.

Administration: Topical route. Wash hands thoroughly after use. **Storage:** 15-25°C (59-77°F). Do not freeze. Avoid sunlight. Keep away from open flame.

DOXIL

RX

doxorubicin HCl liposome (Centocor Ortho Biotech)

> May lead to cardiac toxicity; consider prior use of anthracyclines or anthracenediones in cumulative dose calculations. Myocardial damage may lead to congestive heart failure (CHF) when cumulative dose approaches 550mg/m². Cardiac toxicity may occur at lower cumulative doses with prior mediastinal irradiation or cyclophosphamide therapy. Acute infusion-associated reactions reported. Severe myelosuppression may occur. Reduce dose with impaired hepatic function. Severe side effects reported with accidental substitution for doxorubicin HCl; do not substitute on mg-per-mg basis.

THERAPEUTIC CLASS: Anthracycline

INDICATIONS: Treatment of ovarian cancer which has progressed or recurred after platinum-based chemotherapy. Treatment of AIDS-related Kaposi's sarcoma (KS) in patients after failure of prior systemic chemotherapy or intolerance to such therapy. In combination with bortezomib for the treatment of multiple myeloma (MM) in patients who have not previously received bortezomib and have received ≥1 prior therapy.

DOSAGE: *Adults:* Administer as IV infusion at initial rate of 1mg/min to minimize risk of infusion-related reactions; if no reactions, may increase rate to complete infusion over 1 hr. Ovarian Cancer: 50mg/m² IV q4 weeks for a minimum of 4 courses. Pretreatment with or concomitant use of antiemetics may be considered. KS: 20mg/m² IV q3 weeks for as long as responding satisfactorily and tolerating treatment. MM: Give bortezomib 1.3mg/m² IV bolus on Days 1, 4, 8 and 11, q3 weeks. Give doxorubicin 30mg/m² IV as a 1-hr IV infusion on Day 4 following bortezomib. May treat for ≤8 cycles until disease progression or occurrence of unacceptable toxicity. Hepatic Dysfunction: If serum bilirubin 1.2-3mg/dL, give 50% of normal dose. If serum bilirubin >3mg/dL, give 25% of normal dose. Adjust or delay dose based on toxicities; refer to PI for recommended dose modification guidelines.

HOW SUPPLIED: Inj: 2mg/mL

CONTRAINDICATIONS: Nursing mothers.

WARNINGS/PRECAUTIONS: Monitor cardiac function. Administer only when benefits outweigh the risks in patients with a history of cardiovascular disease (CVD). Perform hematological monitoring during use, including WBC, neutrophil, and platelet count, and Hgb/Hct. If hematologic toxicity occurs, dose reduction, delay of therapy, or suspension of therapy may be required. Evaluate hepatic function before therapy. Hand-foot syndrome reported. Recall reaction reported after radiotherapy. May cause fetal harm. Avoid extravasation.

ADVERSE REACTIONS: Neutropenia, severe myelosuppression, anemia, thrombocytopenia, stomatitis, fever, anorexia, fatigue, N/V, asthenia, rash, acute infusion-related reactions, diarrhea, constipation, hand-foot syndrome.

INTERACTIONS: See Boxed Warning. May potentiate toxicity of other anti-cancer therapies. May exacerbate cyclophosphamide-induced hemorrhagic cystitis. May enhance hepatotoxicity of 6-mercaptopurine. May increase radiation-induced toxicity of the myocardium, mucosa, skin, and liver. Hematological toxicity may be more severe with agents that cause bone-marrow suppression.

PREGNANCY: Category D, not for use in nursing.

MECHANISM OF ACTION: Anthracycline topoisomerase inhibitor; suspected to bind DNA and inhibit nucleic acid synthesis.

PHARMACOKINETICS: Absorption: (10mg/m²) C_{max}=4.12μg/mL, AUC=277μg/mL•h. (20mg/m²) C_{max}=8.34μg/mL, AUC=590μg/mL•h. **Distribution:** (10mg/m²) V_d=2.83L/m²; (20mg/m²) V_d=2.72L/m². **Metabolism:** Doxorubicinol (metabolite). **Elimination:** 1st Phase: $T_{1/2}$=4.7 hrs (10mg/m²); 5.2 hrs (20mg/m²). 2nd Phase: $T_{1/2}$=52.3 hrs (10mg/m²); 55 hrs (20mg/m²).

NURSING CONSIDERATIONS

Assessment: Assess for history of CVD, hepatic dysfunction, hypersensitivity, pregnancy/nursing status, history of radiotherapy use, and for possible drug interactions. Obtain baseline WBC, neutrophil and platelet counts, Hgb/Hct, hepatic function, and cardiac function.

Monitoring: Monitor signs/symptoms of cardiotoxicity, infusion reactions, myelosuppression, radiation recall reaction, extravasation, hand-foot syndrome, hypersensitivity reactions. Periodically monitor CBC including WBC, neutrophil, and platelet count, Hgb/Hct, hepatic function, and cardiac function (endomyocardial biopsy, ECG, multigated radionuclide scan).

Patient Counseling: Inform that reddish-orange color may appear in urine and other bodily fluids may occur. Advise of pregnancy risks. Instruct to seek medical attention if symptoms of an infusion reaction (eg, flushing, tightness in chest or throat), hand-foot syndrome (eg, tingling, burning, redness, flaking, bothersome swelling, small blisters), fever 100.5°F or higher, N/V, tiredness, weakness, rash, mild hair loss, or stomatitis occur.

Administration: IV route. Administer diluted preparation ≤24 hrs. Do not administer as bolus injection or undiluted solution. Do not use with any diluent except 5% Dextrose inj. Do not use any bacteriostatic agent (eg, benzyl alcohol). Do not mix with other drugs. Refer to PI for further instruction on handling, preparation, administration, and disposal. **Storage:** 2-8°C (36-46°F). Avoid freezing.

DOXYCYCLINE IV RX
doxycycline hyclate (Bedford)

THERAPEUTIC CLASS: Tetracycline derivative

INDICATIONS: Treatment of rickettsiae, *Mycoplasma pneumoniae*, psittacosis, ornithosis, lymphogranuloma venereum, granuloma inguinale, relapsing fever, chancroid, *Pasteurella pestis*, *Pasturella tularensis*, *Bartonella bacilliformis*, *Bacteroides* species, *Vibrio comma*, *Vibrio fetus*, *Brucella* species, *E.coli*, *Enterobacter aerogenes*, *Shigella* species, *Mima* species, *Herellea* species, *Haemophilus influenzae*, *Klebsiella* species, *Streptococcus* species, *Diplococcus pneumoniae*, *Staphylococcus aureus*, anthrax, and trachoma. When PCN is contraindicated; treatment of *Neisseria gonorrhoeae*, *N.meningitis*, syphilis, yaws, *Listeria monocytogenes*, *Clostridium* species, *Fusobacterium fusiforme*, and *Actinomyces* species. Adjunct therapy for amebiasis.

DOSAGE: *Adults:* Usual: 200mg IV divided qd-bid on Day 1 then 100-200mg/day IV depending on severity, with 200mg administered in 1 or 2 infusions. Primary/Secondary Syphilis: 300mg/day IV for at least 10 days. Inhalational Anthrax (post-exposure): 100mg IV bid. Institute oral therapy as soon as possible and continue therapy for a total of 60 days.
Pediatrics: >8 yrs: >100 lbs: Usual: 200mg IV divided qd-bid on Day 1 then 100-200mg/day IV depending on severity, with 200mg administered in 1 or 2 infusions. ≤100 lbs: 2mg/lb IV qd-bid on Day 1 then 1-2mg/lb/day IV divided qd-bid depending on severity. Inhalational Anthrax (post-exposure): <100 lbs: 1 mg/lb IV bid. Institute oral therapy as soon as possible and continue therapy for total of 60 days.

HOW SUPPLIED: Inj: 100mg

WARNINGS/PRECAUTIONS: *Clostridium difficile*-associated diarrhea (CDAD) reported. May cause fetal harm during pregnancy. Permanent tooth discoloration during tooth development (last half of pregnancy and children <8 yrs) reported; avoid use in this age group except for anthrax treatment. Decreased bone growth in premature infants reported. May increase BUN. Photosensitivity, enamel hypoplasia reported. Superinfection with prolonged use. Monitor hematopoietic, renal and hepatic values periodically with long term therapy. Bulging fontanels in infants and benign intracranial HTN in adults reported.

ADVERSE REACTIONS: GI effects, increased BUN, rash, hypersensitivity reactions, hemolytic anemia, thrombocytopenia.

INTERACTIONS: May decrease PT; adjust anticoagulants. Avoid use with bactericidal agents (eg, penicillin).

PREGNANCY: Safety in pregnancy not known; not for use in nursing.

MECHANISM OF ACTION: Tetracycline derivative; thought to inhibit protein synthesis.

PHARMACOKINETICS: Absorption: Readily absorbed; C_{max}=2.5mcg/mL. **Elimination:** $T_{1/2}$=18-22 hrs.

NURSING CONSIDERATIONS

Assessment: Assess pregnancy status, possible drug interactions, and renal impairment. Document indications for therapy, culture, and susceptibility testing. Perform incision and drainage in conjunction with antibiotic therapy when indicated.

Monitoring: Monitor for signs/symptoms of hypersensitivity reactions, photosensitivity, superinfection, *C.difficile*-associated diarrhea, vaginal candidiasis, benign intracranial HTN, LFTs, renal function, and hematological manifestations. In venereal disease with suspected coexistent syphilis, perform dark field exam before treatment; repeat monthly for 4 months.

Patient Counseling: Inform of pregnancy risks and photosensitivity reactions (d/c at 1st sign of skin erythema). Advise to avoid excessive sunlight/UV light; wear sunscreen or sunblock. Take as directed; skipping doses or not completing full course may decrease effectiveness and increase resistance. Inform may experience diarrhea; contact physician if watery or bloody stools, hypersensitivity reactions, superinfections, photosensitivity, or benign intracranial HTN occurs.

Administration: IV route. **Storage:** Solutions after reconstitution are stable for 8 weeks when stored at -20°C. If product warmed, care should be taken to avoid heating after thawing is complete.

DUETACT   RX
pioglitazone HCl - glimepiride (Takeda)

> Thiazolidinediones, including pioglitazone, may cause or exacerbate congestive heart failure (CHF) in some patients. After initiation, observe for signs/symptoms of heart failure (HF) and manage accordingly or consider d/c therapy. Not recommended in patients with symptomatic HF. Initiation with NYHA Class III or IV HF is contraindicated.

THERAPEUTIC CLASS: Thiazolidinedione/sulfonylurea

INDICATIONS: Adjunct to diet and exercise to improve glycemic control in adults with type 2 diabetes already being treated with a thiazolidinedione and a sulfonylurea or who have inadequate glycemic control on a thiazolidinedione alone or sulfonylurea alone.

DOSAGE: *Adults:* Individualize dose. Base recommended starting dose on current regimen of pioglitazone and/or sulfonylurea. Give with 1st main meal of day. Current Glimepiride Monotherapy or Switching from Combination Therapy of Pioglitazone plus Glimepiride as Separate Tablets: Initial: 30mg-2mg or 30mg-4mg qd. Current Pioglitazone or Different Sulfonylurea Monotherapy or Switching from Combination Therapy of Pioglitazone plus a Different Sulfonylurea: Initial: 30mg-2mg qd. Elderly/Debilitated/Malnourished/Renal or Hepatic Insufficiency (ALT ≤2.5X ULN): Initial: 1mg glimepiride prior to prescribing Duetact. Systolic Dysfunction: Initial: 15-30mg of pioglitazone; titrate carefully to lowest Duetact dose. Max: Not given more than once daily at any tablet strength.

HOW SUPPLIED: Tab: (Pioglitazone-Glimepiride) 30mg-2mg, 30mg-4mg

CONTRAINDICATIONS: Established NYHA Class III or IV heart failure; diabetic ketoacidosis with or without coma.

WARNINGS/PRECAUTIONS: Glimepiride: Increased CV mortality. May produce severe hypoglycemia; risk may be increased if debilitated, malnourished;

with adrenal, pituitary, renal, or hepatic insufficiency; and after severe or prolonged exercise. Hypoglycemia may be masked in elderly patients and in patients taking β-adrenergic blocking drugs or other sympatholytic agents. May lose blood glucose control with stress. Hemolytic anemia reported; use caution in patient with glucose-6-phosphate dehydrogenase (G6PD) deficiency and consider alternate non-sulfonylurea treatment. Pioglitazone: May cause fluid retention and exacerbation/initiation of heart failure; consider dose reduction or d/c therapy. Not indicated if NYHA Class III or IV cardiac status. Not for use in type 1 DM or diabetic ketoacidosis treatment. Caution with edema. Dose-related weight gain reported. Ovulation in premenopausal anovulatory patient may occur; risk of pregnancy with inadequate contraception. May decrease Hgb and Hct. Hepatitis and hepatic enzyme elevations >3X or more ULN reported and rarely hepatic failure reported. Avoid with active liver disease or if ALT levels >2.5X ULN. Check LFTs if hepatic dysfunction symptoms occur. D/C if ALT >3X ULN on therapy or if jaundice occurs. Macular edema reported; refer patients who develop any type of visual symptoms to an ophthalmologist. Increased incidence of bone fractures reported in female patients. Perform periodic measurements of FPG and A_{1c} measurements to monitor glycemic control and therapeutic response. Measure LFTs prior to therapy and periodically thereafter.

ADVERSE REACTIONS: Hypoglycemia, upper respiratory tract infection, edema/peripheral edema, increased weight, lower limb pain, headache, UTI, diarrhea, nausea.

INTERACTIONS: Pioglitazone: May be at risk for hypoglycemia if used concomitantly with insulin or oral hypoglycemic agents; may require dose reduction of concomitant agent. May be a weak inducer of CYP3A4 substrates. CYP2C8 inhibitors (eg, gemfibrozil) may significantly increase the AUC levels of pioglitazone. CYP2C8 inducers (eg, rifampin) may significantly decrease the AUC levels of pioglitazone. May decrease levels of midazolam and ethinyl estradiol levels. Glimepiride: Combined use with insulin, metformin, or when more than one glucose agent is used may increase the potential for hypoglycemia. Hypoglycemia more likely to occur when alcohol is ingested. Hypoglycemia may be potentiated with NSAIDs and other drugs that are highly protein bound (eg, salicylates, sulfonamides, chloramphenicol, coumarins, probenecid, MAOIs, β-blockers). Risk of severe hypoglycemia with oral miconazole. Risk of hyperglycemia with thiazides and other diuretics, corticosteroids, phenothiazines, thyroid products, estrogens, oral contraceptives, phenytoin, nicotinic acid, sympathomimetics, and isoniazid. Concomitant use with aspirin may decrease glimepiride concentrations. Concomitant use with propranolol may increase C_{max}, AUC and $T_{1/2}$ of glimepiride. May interact with inhibitors (eg, fluconazole) and inducers (eg, rifampicin) of CYP2C9.

PREGNANCY: Category C, not for use in nursing.

MECHANISM OF ACTION: Pioglitazone: Thiazolidinedione; insulin-sensitizing agent acts by enhancing peripheral glucose utilization. Glimepiride: Sulfonylurea; stimulates release of insulin from functional pancreatic β-cells.

PHARMACOKINETICS: Absorption: Administration of variable doses resulted in different parameters. Glimepiride: Complete. T_{max}=2-3 hrs. Pioglitazone: T_{max}=2 hrs. **Distribution:** Pioglitazone: V_d=0.63L/kg, plasma protein binding (>99%). Glimepiride: (IV) V_d=8.8L, plasma protein binding (>99.5%). **Metabolism:** Pioglitazone: Extensive (hydroxylation & oxidation) via CYP2C8, CYP3A4, CYP1A1. M-II and M-IV (hydroxy derivatives) and M-III (keto derivatives) (active metabolites). Glimepiride: Complete. Oxidative biotransformation via CYP2C9. Cyclohexyl hydroxy methyl derivative (M1), carboxyl derivative (M2) (major metabolites). **Elimination:** Pioglitazone: Urine (15-30%), bile (unchanged), feces (metabolites); $T_{1/2}$=3-7 hrs (pioglitazone), 16-24 hrs (total pioglitazone). Glimepiride: Urine (60%), feces (40%).

NURSING CONSIDERATIONS

Assessment: Assess for diabetic ketoacidosis, heart failure, macular edema, risk factors for developing heart failure, active liver disease, renal insufficiency, G6PD deficiency, pregnancy/nursing status, and for possible drug interactions. Assess LFTs and obtain CBC prior to therapy.

Monitoring: Monitor for signs and symptoms of heart failure, edema, hypoglycemia, weight gain, hematological changes (eg, decreases in Hgb and Hct), hepatic dysfunction (eg, N/V, abdominal pain, anorexia, dark urine, jaundice), macular edema, bone fractures and for hemolytic anemia. Perform periodic monitoring of LFTs, FBG and A1c. Perform periodic eye exams.

Patient Counseling: Counsel to report unexplained GI symptoms, rapid increase in weight or edema, SOB, N/V, abdominal pain, fatigue, anorexia or dark urine. Advise to avoid excessive alcohol intake. Counsel females about use of reliable contraception. Inform about importance of adherence to meal planning, regular physical activity, regular blood glucose monitoring, periodic HbA1c testing, recognition and management of hypo- and hyperglycemia, and periodic assessment for diabetes complications. Inform that during periods of stress (eg, trauma, infection, surgery), medication requirements may change; seek prompt medical advice.

Administration: Oral route. **Storage:** 25°C (77°F); excursions permitted to 15-30°C (59-86°F). Keep container tightly closed. Protect from moisture and humidity.

DULERA RX

mometasone furoate - formoterol fumarate dihydrate (Schering)

> Long-acting β₂-adrenergic agonists (LABA), such as formoterol, increase the risk of asthma-related death. LABA may increase the risk of asthma-related hospitalization in pediatric and adolescent patients. Use only for patients not adequately controlled on a long-term asthma control medication, such as an inhaled corticosteroid, or whose disease severity clearly requires initiation of treatment with both an inhaled corticosteroid and LABA. Do not use for patients whose asthma is adequately controlled on low- or medium- dose inhaled corticosteroids.

THERAPEUTIC CLASS: Corticosteroid/beta₂ agonist

INDICATIONS: Treatment of asthma in patients ≥12 yrs.

DOSAGE: *Adults:* 2 inh bid (am/pm). Previous Corticosteroid Therapy: Inhaled Medium-Dose Corticosteroids: Initial: 2 inh bid of 100mcg-5mcg. Max: 400mcg-20mcg daily. Inhaled High-Dose Corticosteroids: Initial: 2 inh bid of 200mcg-5mcg. Max: 800mcg-20mcg daily. Do not use more than 2 inh bid of the prescribed strength. If symptoms arise between doses, use an inhaled short-acting β₂-agonist (SABA) for immediate relief. May need higher strength in patients who do not respond adequately after 2 weeks of therapy. Rinse mouth after use.
Pediatrics: ≥12 yrs: 2 inh bid (am/pm). Previous Corticosteroid Therapy: Inhaled Medium-Dose Corticosteroids: Initial: 2 inh bid of 100mcg-5mcg. Max: 400mcg-20mcg daily. Inhaled High-Dose Corticosteroids: Initial: 2 inh bid of 200mcg-5mcg. Max: 800mcg-20mcg daily. Do not use more than 2 inh bid of the prescribed strength. If symptoms arise between doses, use an inhaled SABA for immediate relief. May need higher strength in patients who do not respond adequately after 2 weeks of therapy. Rinse mouth after use.

HOW SUPPLIED: MDI: (Mometasone furoate-Formoterol fumarate dihydrate) 100mcg-5mcg, 200mcg-5mcg.

CONTRAINDICATIONS: Primary treatment of status asthmaticus or acute episodes of asthma requiring intensive measures.

WARNINGS/PRECAUTIONS: Not indicated for the relief of acute symptoms; use a SABA. Do not initiate during rapidly deteriorating or potentially life-threatening episodes of asthma. Increased use of an inhaled SABA is a marker of deteriorating asthma; re-evaluate and reassess treatment regimen. At treatment initiation, regular use of an oral or inhaled SABA should be d/c. Should not be used more often or at higher doses than recommended; cardiovascular (CV) effects and fatalities reported. Do not use any additional inhaled LABAs for prevention of exercise-induced bronchospasm or the treatment of asthma. Localized *Candida albicans* infections of the mouth and pharynx may occur; if one develops treat accordingly. Increased susceptibility to infections. Avoid exposure to chickenpox and measles. Caution in patients with active or quiescent TB infection, untreated systemic fungal, bacterial, viral, or parasitic infections, or ocular herpes simplex. Deaths due to adrenal insufficiency have occurred with transfer from systemic to inhaled corticosteroids. Resume oral corticosteroids during stress or severe asthma attack. Transferring from oral to inhalation therapy may unmask allergic conditions (eg, rhinitis, conjunctivitis, eczema). Monitor for systemic corticosteroid effects such as hypercorticism and adrenal suppression; if effects occur reduce dose slowly. May produce paradoxical bronchospasm and upper airway symptoms; d/c immediately, treat, and institute alternative therapy. Immediate hypersensitivity reactions (eg, urticaria, flushing, allegic dermatitis) reported. CV effects may occur; caution in patients with CV disorders, especially coronary insufficiency, arrhythmia, HTN. May cause ECG changes (eg, flattened T-wave, QTc interval prolongation, ST segment depression). Prolonged use may result in decrease of bone mineral density, glaucoma, increased IOP, and cataracts. May cause reduction in growth velocity in pediatrics; monitor growth routinely. Caution in elderly, patients with convulsive disorders, thyrotoxicosis, diabetes, and in those unusually responsive to sympathomimetic amines. Hypokalemia and hyperglycemia may occur.

ADVERSE REACTIONS: Nasopharyngitis, sinusitis, headache.

INTERACTIONS: Oral ketoconazole increases plasma levels. Strong CYP3A4 inhibitors (eg, ritonavir, atazanavir, clarithromycin, indinavir, itraconazole, nefazodone, nelfinavir, saquinavir, telithromycin) may inhibit metabolism and increase systemic corticosteroid effects. Caution with additional adrenergic drugs, xanthine derivatives and non-K⁺-sparing diuretics (eg, loop or thiazide diuretics), β-blockers. Extreme caution within 14 days of using MAOIs or TCAs. Drugs known to prolong QTc interval may increase risk of ventricular arrhythmias.

PREGNANCY: Category C, not for use in nursing.

MECHANISM OF ACTION: Mometasone furoate: Corticosteroid; shown to have inhibitory effects on multiple cell types (eg, mast cells, eosinophils, neutrophils, macrophages, and lymphocytes) and mediators (eg, histamine, eicosanoids, leukotrienes, and cytokines) involved in inflammatory and asthmatic response. Formoterol: β₂-adrenergic agonist; stimulates intracellular adenyl cyclase, which catalyzes conversion of ATP to cAMP, to produce relaxation of bronchial smooth muscle and inhibition of release of mediators of immediate hypersensitivity from cells (especially mast cells).

PHARMACOKINETICS: Absorption: Mometasone: (Asthma) C_{max}=20pg/mL; AUC=170pg•hr/mL; T_{max}=1-2 hrs. Formoterol: (Asthma) C_{max}=22pmol/L; AUC=125pmol•h/L; T_{max}=0.58-1.97 hrs. **Distribution**: Mometasone: V_d=152L; plasma protein binding (98-99%). Formoterol: Plasma protein binding (61-64%). **Metabolism**: Mometasone: Liver (extensive) via CYP3A4. Formoterol: Liver (direct glucuronidation and O-demethylation) via CYP2D6, CYP2C19, CYP2C9, CYP2A6. **Elimination**: Mometasone: $T_{1/2}$=5 hrs; urine (8%), feces (74%). Formoterol: (R,R enantiomers) $T_{1/2}$=13 hrs; urine (37%); (S,S enantiomers) $T_{1/2}$=9.5 hrs; urine (63%).

NURSING CONSIDERATIONS

Assessment: Assess if asthma controlled by inhaled corticosteroids and occasional use of a SABA. Assess for risk factors for decreased bone mineral content, history of CVD, convulsive disorder, thyrotoxicosis, diabetes, concomitant diseases such as status asthmaticus, immunosupression, immunization history (eg, chickenpox, measles), active or quiescent pulmonary TB or any other condition where treatment is contraindicated or cautioned. Assess pregnancy/nursing status, and possible drug interactions. Obtain baseline bone mineral density and lung function prior to therapy.

Monitoring: Monitor bone mineral density and lung function, BP, PR, ECG, serum K⁺ and glucose levels periodically. Perform regular eye exams. Monitor for localized oral infections with *Candida albicans*, decreased bone mass, upper airway symptoms, worsening or acutely deteriorating asthma (increased use of an inhaled SABA, decreased lung function), growth in children, visual changes, development of glaucoma, increased IOP, posterior cataracts, hypercorticism, adrenal insufficiency (eg, fatigue, weakness, N/V and hypotension), rhinitis, conjunctivitis, eczema, arthritis, eosinophilic conditions, paradoxical bronchospasm, and hypersensitivity reactions (eg, urticaria, flushing, allergic dermatitis), ECG changes (eg, flattened T-wave, QTc interval prolongation, ST segment depression).

Patient Counseling: Instruct to avoid spraying in eyes. Advise to rinse mouth after inhalation. Do not d/c therapy unless directed by a physician. Therapy should not be used for sudden symptoms of SOB or acute bronchospasm. Inform that therapy may cause reduction in growth rate in pediatric patients. Counsel that may unmask allergies (eg, rhinitis, conjunctivitis, eczema, arthritis). Avoid exposure to chickenpox or measles; advise to seek medical attention if exposed to chickenpox or measles, or if experience worsening of existing TB, other infections or ocular herpes simplex, symptoms do not improve or worsen, during periods of stress or severe asthmatic attack, adrenal insufficiency (fatigue, weakness, N/V, and hypotension), paradoxical bronchospasm, or hypersensitivity reactions.

Administration: Inhalational route. See PI for proper administration. **Storage**: 20-25°C (68-77°F); excursions permitted to 15-30°C (59-86°F). Do not puncture. Do not use or store near heat or open flame.

DUONEB   RX
ipratropium bromide - albuterol sulfate (Dey)

THERAPEUTIC CLASS: Beta$_2$-agonist/anticholinergic

INDICATIONS: Treatment of bronchospasm in COPD in patients requiring more than one bronchodilator.

DOSAGE: *Adults:* 3mL qid via nebulizer. May give 2 additional doses/day.

HOW SUPPLIED: Sol, Inhalation: (Albuterol-Ipratropium) 3mg-0.5mg/3mL [3mL, 30^s 60^s]

CONTRAINDICATIONS: Hypersensitivity to atropine and its derivatives.

WARNINGS/PRECAUTIONS: Paradoxical bronchospasm and hypersensitivity reactions reported. Caution with cardiovascular disorders, convulsive disorders, hyperthyroidism, DM, narrow-angle glaucoma, prostatic hypertrophy, and bladder-neck obstruction.

ADVERSE REACTIONS: Pain, chest pain, diarrhea, dyspepsia, nausea, leg cramps, bronchitis, lung disease, pharyngitis, pneumonia, UTI.

INTERACTIONS: Additive interactions with anticholinergic agents. Increased risk of cardiovascular side effects with sympathomimetics. Use β_1-selective blockers with hyper-reactive airways. Caution within 2 weeks of discontinuation of MAOIs or TCAs.

PREGNANCY: Category C (albuterol) and B (ipratropium), not for use in nursing.

MECHANISM OF ACTION: Albuterol: β_2-adrenergic bronchodilator; stimulates adenyl cylase, enzyme that catalyzes formation of cAMP from ATP. Increased cAMP levels are associated with relaxation of bronchial smooth muscle and inhibition of release of mediators of immediate hypersensitivity. Ipratropium: Anticholinergic bronchodilator; blocks muscarinic receptors of acetylcholine. Prevents the increase in intracellular concentration of cGMP, resulting from interaction of acetylcholine with the muscarinic receptors of bronchial smooth muscle.

PHARMACOKINETICS: Absorption: Albuterol: C_{max}=4.65mg/mL; T_{max}=0.8 hrs; AUC=24.2ng•h/mL. **Distribution:** Ipratropium: Plasma protein binding (0-9%). **Metabolism:** Albuterol: Conjugation. Ipratropium: Ester hydrolysis. **Elimination:** Albuterol: Urine (8.4% unchanged). Ipratropium: Urine (3.9% unchanged); $T_{1/2}$=6.7 hrs.

NURSING CONSIDERATIONS

Assessment: Assess for history of hypersensitivity to atropine or its derivatives. Assess for concomitant diseases such as narrow-angle glaucoma, prostatic hyperplasia, convulsive disorders, hyperthyroidism, DM, hepatic/renal insufficiency, CVD, and possible drug interactions.

Monitoring: Monitor serum potassium, pulse rate and BP, hypersensitivity reactions, paradoxical brochospasm, cardiovascular effects such as flattening of the T wave, prolongation of QT interval, and ST segment depression, severe acute asthmatic crisis, hypoxia, and adverse effects (eg, headache, cough, respiratory disorders, pain, dyspnea, and bronchitis). Monitor for anticholinergic effects.

Patient Counseling: Caution to avoid spraying aerosol into eyes; may cause precipitation or worsening of narrow-angle glaucoma, mydriasis, increased IOP, acute eye pain or discomfort, temporary blurring vision, visual halos or colored images. Advise not to exceed recommended dose. Report lack of response and adverse side effects.

Administration: Oral inhalation. 1) Remove vial and squeeze contents into nebulizer reservoir. 2) Connect nebulizer to mouthpiece and compressor. 3) Place mouthpiece in mouth or put on face mask and turn on compressor. 4) Breathe as calmly as possible through mouth until no more mist is formed (5-15 min). 5) Clean nebulizer. **Storage:** 2-30°C (36-86°F). Protect from light.

DURAGESIC   CII
fentanyl (Ortho-McNeil)

> Life-threatening hypoventilation can occur. May be a target for abuse/diversion. Monitor for signs of misuse, abuse, or addiction. Avoid in patients <2 yrs. Only for use in patients who are already receiving opioid therapy, opioid-tolerant patients, and those who require a total dose at least equivalent to 25mcg/hr. Use in nonopioid-tolerant patients may lead to fatal respiratory depression. Overestimating the fentanyl transdermal dose when converting patients from another opioid medication can result in fatal overdose with the first dose. Concomitant use with CYP3A4 inhibitors may increase plasma concentrations and cause fatal respiratory depression. For transdermal use only. Avoid exposing application site to direct external heat source (eg, heating pads, tanning lamps). Monitor patient with fever or exercise-induced increase in core body temperature for side effects and adjust dose if necessary.

OTHER BRAND NAMES: Fentanyl Transdermal System (Mylan)

THERAPEUTIC CLASS: Opioid analgesic

INDICATIONS: Management of persistent, moderate to severe chronic pain in opioid-tolerant patients that requires continuous, around-the-clock opioid administration for an extended period of time, and cannot be managed by other means such as nonsteroidal analgesics, opioid combination products, or immediate-release opioids.

DOSAGE: *Adults:* Individualize dose. Determine dose based on opioid tolerance, previous analgesic requirement, and general condition and medical status of the patient. Minimum Initial Dose: 25mcg/hr for 72 hrs. Titrate: Initial dose may be increased after 3 days; further increase in dosage should be made after the higher dose is worn through two applications. Dosage increments may be based on the daily dose of supplementary opioids using the ratio of 45mg/24 hrs of oral morphine to a 12.5mcg/hr increase in dose. Some patients may not achieve adequate analgesia and may require systems to be applied q48h rather than q72h; an increase in dose should first be evaluated prior to changing the interval. Refer to PI for Dose Conversion Guidelines. Elderly/Debilitated/Cachectic/Renal/Hepatic Impairment: Reduce dose. *Pediatrics:* ≥2 yrs: Individualize dose. Determine dose based on opioid tolerance, previous analgesic requirement, and general condition and medical status of the patient. Minimum Initial Dose: 25mcg/hr for 72 hrs. Titrate: Initial dose may be increased after 3 days; further increase in dosage should be made after the higher dose is worn through two applications. Dosage increments may be based on the daily dose of supplementary opioids using the ratio of 45mg/24 hrs of oral morphine to a 12.5mcg/hr increase in dose. Refer to PI for Dose Conversion Guidelines.

HOW SUPPLIED: Patch: 12mcg/hr (2.1mg), 25mcg/hr (4.2mg), 50mcg/hr (8.4mg), 75mcg/hr (12.6mg), 100mcg/hr (16.8mg). (Generic) 12mcg/hr (1.28mg), 25mcg/hr (2.55mg), 50mcg/hr (5.10mg), 75mcg/hr (7.65mg), 100mcg/hr (10.20mg) [5*].

CONTRAINDICATIONS: Opioid non-tolerant patients, management of acute pain or in patients who require opioid analgesia for a short period of time, post-operative pain, mild/intermittent pain. Diagnosis or suspicion of paralytic ileus, acute or severe bronchial asthma, significant respiratory depression especially in unmonitored settings where there is a lack of resuscitative equipment.

WARNINGS/PRECAUTIONS: Do not use if seal is broken or patch is cut, damaged, or changed. Monitor patients with serious adverse events for at least 24 hrs after removal. Death and other serious medical problems have occurred from accidental exposure to fentanyl (eg, transfer from adult's body to a child while hugging, accidentally sitting on a patch). Respiratory depression may occur; caution with elderly, cachectic or debilitated patients, chronic pulmonary diseases or cor pulmonale, decreased respiratory reserve, hypoxia, hypercapnia, or pre-existing respiratory depression. May cause bradycardia; caution with bradyarrhythmias. Caution with brain tumors and renal/hepatic impairment. May cause spasm of the sphincter of Oddi; caution with biliary tract disease (eg, acute pancreatitis). May cause increases in serum amylase concentrations. Avoid with increased intracranial pressure, impaired consciousness, or coma. May obscure clinical course of head injury. Tolerance and physical dependence may occur. May impair mental/physical abilities. Withdrawal symptoms may occur; gradual downward titration recommended.

ADVERSE REACTIONS: Hypoventilation, headache, fever, N/V, constipation, dry mouth, somnolence, confusion, asthenia, sweating, nervousness, pruritus, apnea, dyspnea.

INTERACTIONS: See Boxed Warning. Concomitant use with CNS depressants (eg, opioids, sedatives, hypnotics, tranquilizers, general anesthetics, phenothiazines, skeletal muscle relaxants, alcohol) may cause respiratory depression, hypotension, profound sedation, or potentially coma. Coadministration with CYP3A4 inducers may lead to reduced efficacy of fentanyl. Avoid use within 14 days of an MAOI. Concomitant use with CNS-active drugs requires special patient care and observation.

PREGNANCY: Category C, not for use in nursing.

MECHANISM OF ACTION: Opioid analgesic; interacts predominantly with the opioid µ-receptor in the brain, spinal cord and other tissues. Exerts principal pharmacological actions on CNS.

PHARMACOKINETICS: Absorption: T_{max} = 20-72 hrs. Transdermal administration of variable doses resulted in different parameters. **Distribution:** V_d=6L/kg; found in breast milk; readily crosses placenta. **Metabolism**: Liver via CYP3A4; oxidative N-dealkylation to norfentanyl and other inactive metabolites. **Elimination**: Urine (75%, <10% unchanged), feces (9%); $T_{1/2}$= 20-27 hrs.

NURSING CONSIDERATIONS

Assessment: Assess for degree of opioid tolerance, previous opioid dose, level of pain intensity, type of pain, patient's general condition and medical status, emotional status or any other conditions where treatment is contraindicated or cautioned. Assess for history of hypersensitivity, pregnancy/nursing status, renal/hepatic function, and possible drug interactions.

Monitoring: Monitor for signs/symptoms of respiratory depression; bradycardia; increases in serum amylase levels; abuse or misuse, addiction, and tolerance or physical dependence. Monitor for signs and symptoms of overdose especially when converting patient from another opioid. Monitor development of fever/increase in core body temperature.

Patient Counseling: Advise that patch contains fentanyl, an opioid pain medicine similar to morphine, hydromorphone, methadone, oxycodone, and oxymorphone. Wear patch continuously for 72 hrs, and apply patch to different area of intact, nonirritated, and nonirradiated skin on a flat surface (eg, chest, back, flank, upper arm) following removal of previous patch. Following use, advise to fold patch and flush down the toilet. Apply immediately upon removal from sealed package and after removal of protective liner. Do not use a broken, cut or damaged patch. Never adjust the dose or the number of patches applied to the skin without instruction from the healthcare professional. In pediatric or cognitively impaired patients, advise to place on upper back to decrease chance of removal. Clean with water and dry skin prior to application; avoid soaps, oils, lotions, or any skin irritants. Avoid exposing patch to direct external heat sources. Contact physician if fever develops. Use caution if performing hazardous tasks (eg, driving, operating machinery). Notify physician of all medications currently taking and to avoid using other CNS depressants and alcohol. Inform that constipation may develop during therapy. Instruct to avoid abrupt withdrawal of medication; taper dose. Inform that medication has high potential for abuse and to keep in secure place; keep patches (new and used) out of reach of children. Instruct that if patch sticks to a person other than the patient, remove patch and wash exposed area with water, and contact physician. Advise that if gel from the drug reservoir accidentally contacts the skin, the area should be washed clean with water. Advise that if patch falls off before 72 hours, a new patch should be applied to a different skin site.

Administration: Transdermal patch. Apply immediately after removal from individually sealed pouch. Do not use if the pouch seal is broken. The next patch should be applied to a different site. Apply to intact, nonirritated, and nonirradiated skin on flat surface such as the chest, back, flank or upper arm. In pediatric or cognitively impaired patients the upper back is the preferred site. Refer to PI for further details on proper application. **Storage:** Store up to 25°C (77°F). Excursions permitted to 15-30°C (59-86°F). (Generic): 20-25°C (68-77°F). Store in original unopened pouch.

DURAMORPH
morphine sulfate (Baxter)

CII

> Risk of severe adverse reactions; patient must be observed in an equipped and staffed environment for at least 24 hrs after initial dose.

THERAPEUTIC CLASS: Opioid analgesic

INDICATIONS: Management of pain unresponsive to non-narcotic analgesics.

DOSAGE: *Adults:* IV: Initial: 2-10mg/70kg. Epidural Injection: Initial: 5mg in lumbar region. Titrate: If inadequate pain relief within 1 hr, increase by 1-2mg. Max: 10mg/24 hrs. Continuous Epidural: Initial: 2-4mg/24 hrs. Give additional 1-2mg if needed. Intrathecal: 0.2-1mg single dose, do not repeat; may follow with 0.6mg/hr naloxone infusion to reduce incidence of side effects.

HOW SUPPLIED: Inj: 0.5mg/mL, 1mg/mL

CONTRAINDICATIONS: Allergy to opiates, acute bronchial asthma, upper airway obstruction. Severe hypotension may occur in volume-depleted patients or with concurrent administration of phenothiazines or general anesthetics.

WARNINGS/PRECAUTIONS: Have resuscitation equipment, oxygen, and antidote (eg, naloxone) available; severe respiratory depression may occur. Avoid rapid administration. May be habit-forming. Caution with head injury, increased intracranial/intraocular pressure, decreased respiratory reserve, hepatic/renal dysfunction, elderly, debilitated. High doses may cause seizures. Smooth muscle hypertonicity may cause biliary colic, urinary difficulty or retention. Orthostatic hypotension may occur with hypovolemia or myocardial dysfunction. Acute respiratory failure reported with COPD or acute asthmatic attack. Limit epidural/intrathecal route to lumbar area.

ADVERSE REACTIONS: Respiratory depression, convulsions, dysphoric reactions, pruritus, urinary retention, constipation, lumbar puncture-type headache, toxic psychoses.

INTERACTIONS: CNS depressants (eg, alcohol, sedatives, antihistamines) and psychotropics potentiate CNS depression. Neuroleptics may increase respiratory depression.

PREGNANCY: Category C, safety in nursing not known.

MECHANISM OF ACTION: Opioid analgesic; analgesic effects are produced via at least 3 areas of the CNS: the periaqueductal-periventricular gray matter, the ventromedial medulla, and the spinal cord. Interacts predominantly with μ-receptors which are found distributed in the brain, spinal cord, and in the trigeminal nerve.

PHARMACOKINETICS: Absorption: (Epidural): Rapid absorption; C_{max}=33-40ng/mL; T_{max}=10-15 min; (Intrathecal): C_{max}<1-7.8ng/mL; T_{max}=5-10 min. **Distribution:** Plasma protein binding (36%); Muscle tissue binding (54%). Readily passes into fetal circulation, found in breast milk. (IV): V_d=1.0-4.7L/kg. **Metabolism:** Hepatic glucuronidation. **Elimination:** Kidneys (major), urine (2-12% unchanged), feces (10%); (IV, IM) $T_{1/2}$=1.5-4.5 hrs; (epidural) $T_{1/2}$=39-249 min.

NURSING CONSIDERATIONS

Assessment: Assess for pain intensity or any other conditions where treatment is contraindicated or cautioned. Assess for history of hypersensitivity, pregnancy/nursing status, renal/hepatic function, and possible drug interactions.

Monitoring: Monitor for signs/symptoms of respiratory depression and/or respiratory arrest, myoclonic events, seizures, dysphoric reactions, toxic psychoses, biliary colic, urinary retention, drug abuse, and drug dependence. If administered intrathecally or via epidural, monitor closely for 24 hrs for signs/symptoms of respiratory depression.

Patient Counseling: Counsel to notify physician immediately if develop signs/symptoms of respiratory depression. Avoid using other CNS depressants and alcohol during therapy. Inform that medication has potential for abuse and dependence. Avoid abrupt withdrawal of medication; withdrawal symptoms may occur. If accidental skin contact occurs, wash affected area with water.

Administration: IV, epidural, or intrathecal route. Proper placement of needle or catheter should be verified before epidural injection. **Storage:** 20-25°C (68-77°F); excursions permitted to 15-30°C (59-86°F). Protect from light. Do not freeze.

DUREZOL   RX
difluprednate (Alcon)

THERAPEUTIC CLASS: Corticosteroid

INDICATIONS: Treatment of inflammation and pain associated with ocular surgery.

DOSAGE: *Adults:* 1 drop into affected conjunctival sac of affected eye(s) qid beginning 24 hrs after ocular surgery and continue throughout the first 2 weeks post-op, followed by bid for a week and then taper based on response.

HOW SUPPLIED: Emulsion: 0.05% [5mL]

CONTRAINDICATIONS: Active viral diseases of the cornea and conjunctiva including epithelial herpes simplex keratitis, vaccinia, varicella, mycobacterial infection of the eye, and fungal disease of ocular structures.

WARNINGS/PRECAUTIONS: Prolonged use may result in glaucoma with optic nerve damage, visual acuity and visual field defects. Caution with glaucoma. Monitor intraocular pressure (IOP) if used ≥10 days. May cause posterior subcapsular cataract formation. Use in cataract surgery may delay healing and increase incidence of bleb formation. Caution with diseases causing thinning of the cornea or sclera; perforations may occur. Perform eye exam (eg, slit lamp biomicroscopy, fluorescein staining) prior to therapy and renewal of medication order >28 days. Prolonged use may suppress host response and increase risk of secondary ocular infections. May mask or enhance existing infection in acute purulent conditions; re-evaluate if fail to improve after 2 days. May prolong the course or exacerbate severity of many viral infections; caution with herpes simplex. Fungal infections of the cornea may develop with long-term use; consider fungal invasion in any persistent corneal ulceration. Not for intraocular administration.

ADVERSE REACTIONS: Corneal edema, ciliary and conjunctival hyperemia, eye pain, photophobia, posterior capsular opacification, anterior chamber cells and flare, conjunctival edema, blepharitis, reduced visual acuity, punctate keratitis, eye inflammation, and iritis.

PREGNANCY: Category C, caution in nursing.

MECHANISM OF ACTION: Corticosteroid; Not established. Suspected to induce phospholipase A_2 inhibitory proteins which control the biosynthesis of potent mediators of inflammation such as prostaglandins and leukotrienes.

PHARMACOKINETICS: Absorption: Limited. **Metabolism**: Deacetylation; 6α, 9-difluoroprednisolone 17-butyrate (active metabolite).

NURSING CONSIDERATIONS

Assessment: Assess for active viral diseases of the cornea and conjunctiva, epithelial herpes simplex keratitis, vaccinia, varicella, mycobacterial infection of the eye, fungal disease of ocular structures, glaucoma, optic nerve damage, visual acuity and visual field defects, diseases causing thinning of sclera or cornea, acute purulent conditions and pregnancy/nursing status. Perform eye exam (eg, slit lamp biomicroscopy, fluorescein staining) prior to therapy in certain patients.

Monitoring: Monitor for signs and symptoms of glaucoma, optic nerve damage, visual acuity and visual field defects, subcapsular cataract, ocular/corneal perforations, acute purulent conditions, bacterial, viral, fungal infections. Monitor post-operative cataract patients (eg, delayed healing, bleb formation) and increased risk for secondary ocular infections. Monitor IOP and perform eye exams.

Patient Counseling: Advise not to touch dropper tip to any surface; may contaminate drug. Advise to consult physician when pain develops or if redness, itching, or inflammation becomes aggravated. Instruct not to wear contact lenses during therapy.

Administration: Ocular route. **Storage**: 15-25°C (59-77°F). Do not freeze. Protect from light. Keep bottles in the protective carton when not in use.

DYAZIDE   RX
triamterene - hydrochlorothiazide (GlaxoSmithKline)

> Abnormal elevation of serum K+ levels (≥5.5mEq/L) may occur with all K+-sparing diuretic combinations. Hyperkalemia is more likely to occur with renal impairment and diabetes (even without evidence of renal impairment), and in elderly or severely ill; monitor serum K+ levels at frequent intervals.

THERAPEUTIC CLASS: K+-sparing diuretic/thiazide diuretic

INDICATIONS: Treatment of HTN or edema if hypokalemia occur on HCTZ alone, or when a thiazide diuretic is required and cannot risk hypokalemia. May be used alone or as an adjunct to other antihypertensives, such as β-blockers.

DOSAGE: *Adults:* 1-2 caps PO qd.

HOW SUPPLIED: Cap: (HCTZ-Triamterene) 25mg-37.5mg

CONTRAINDICATIONS: Anuria, acute and chronic renal insufficiency or significant renal impairment, sulfonamide hypersensitivity, pre-existing elevated serum K+ (hyperkalemia), K+-sparing agents (eg, spironolactone, amiloride, or other formulations containing triamterene), K+ salt substitutes, K+ supplements (except with severe hypokalemia).

WARNINGS/PRECAUTIONS: Avoid in severely ill in whom respiratory or metabolic acidosis may occur; if used, frequent evaluations of acid/base balance and serum electrolytes are necessary. May cause idiosyncratic reaction, resulting in acute transient myopia and acute angle-closure glaucoma; d/c as rapidly as possible. Caution with diabetes; may cause hyperglycemia and glycosuria. May manifest diabetes mellitus (DM). Caution with hepatic impairment; may precipitate hepatic coma with severe liver disease. Corrective measures must be taken if hypokalemia develops; d/c and initiate potassium chloride (KCl) supplementation if serious hypokalemia develops (serum K+<3.0 mEq/L). May potentiate electrolyte imbalance with heart failure, renal disease, or cirrhosis of the liver. May cause hypochloremia. Dilutional hyponatremia may occur in edematous patients in hot weather. Caution with history of renal stones. May increase BUN and SrCr. May decrease serum PBI levels. Decreased calcium excretion reported. Changes in parathyroid glands with hypercalcemia and hypophosphatemia reported during prolonged therapy. May interfere with the fluorescent measurement of quinidine.

ADVERSE REACTIONS: Muscle cramps, N/V, pancreatitis, weakness, arrhythmia, impotence, dry mouth, jaundice, paresthesia, renal stones, anaphylaxis, acute renal failure, hyperkalemia, hyponatremia.

INTERACTIONS: See Contraindications. Increased risk of hyperkalemia with ACE inhibitors, blood from blood bank, and low-salt milk. Increased risk of severe hyponatremia with chlorpropamide. Possible interaction resulting in acute renal failure with indomethacin; caution with NSAIDs. Avoid with lithium due to risk of lithium toxicity. Decreased arterial responsiveness to norepinephrine. Amphotericin B, corticosteroids, and corticotropin (ACTH) may intensify electrolyte imbalance, particularly hypokalemia. Adjust dose of antigout drugs to control hyperuricemia and gout. May decrease effect of oral anticoagulants. May alter insulin requirements. Increased paralyzing effects of nondepolarizing muscle relaxants (eg, tubocurarine). Reduced K⁺ levels with chronic or overuse of laxatives or use of exchange resins (eg, sodium polystyrene sulfonate). May reduce effectiveness of methenamine. Potentiated action of other antihypertensive drugs (eg, β-blockers).

PREGNANCY: Category C, not for use in nursing.

MECHANISM OF ACTION: Triamterene: K⁺-sparing diuretic; exerts diuretic effect on distal renal tubules to inhibit the reabsorption of Na in exchange for K⁺ and hydrogen ions. HCTZ: thiazide diuretic; blocks reabsorption of Na and chloride ions and thereby increases the quantity of Na transversing the distal tubule and the volume of water excreted.

PHARMACOKINETICS: Absorption: Well absorbed. Triamterene: C_{max}=46.4ng/mL; T_{max}=1.1 hrs; AUC=148.7ng•hrs/mL. HCTZ: C_{max}=135.1ng/mL; T_{max}=2 hrs; AUC=834ng•hrs/mL. **Distribution:** Crosses placenta; found in breast milk.

NURSING CONSIDERATIONS

Assessment: Assess for anuria, renal/hepatic impairment, sulfonamide hypersensitivity, hyperkalemia, diabetes, history of renal stones, pregnancy/nursing status, and for possible drug interactions. Obtain baseline BUN, SrCr, and serum electrolytes.

Monitoring: Monitor for signs/symptoms of hyperkalemia, hypokalemia, hyperglycemia, hypochloremia, renal stones, and for electrolyte imbalance. Monitor for hepatic coma in patients with severe liver disease. Monitor serum K⁺ levels, BUN, SrCr, and serum electrolytes.

Patient Counseling: Inform about risks/benefits of therapy. Advise to seek medical attention if symptoms of hyperkalemia (eg, paresthesias, muscular weakness, fatigue), hypokalemia, hyperglycemia, renal stones, electrolyte imbalance (eg, dry mouth, thirst, weakness), or hypersensitivity reactions occur.

Administration: Oral route. **Storage:** 20-25°C (68-77°F); excursions permitted to 15-30°C (59-86°F). Protect from light. Dispense in a tight, light-resistant container.

DYNACIN   RX
minocycline HCl (Medicis)

THERAPEUTIC CLASS: Tetracycline derivative

INDICATIONS: Treatment of rocky mountain spotted fever, typhus fever and the typhus group, Q fever, rickettsialpox, tick fevers, respiratory tract infections, lymphogranuloma venereum, psittacosis, trachoma, inclusion conjunctivitis, non-gonococcal urethritis, endocervical or rectal infections in adults, relapsing fever, chancroid, plague, tularemia, cholera, campylobacter fetus infections, brucellosis, bartonellosis and granuloma inguinale caused by susceptible strains of microorganisms. Treatment of infections caused by gram-negative microorganisms when bacteriologic testing indicates appropriate susceptibility to the drug (eg, respiratory tract and urinary tract infections) and gram-positive microorganisms (eg, upper respiratory tract, skin and skin structure infections). Alternative treatment in certain other infections (eg, uncomplicated urethritis in men, gonococcal infections, syphilis, yaws, listeriosis, anthrax, Vincent's infection, actinomycosis). Adjunctive therapy in acute intestinal amebiasis and severe acne. Treatment of *Mycobacterium marinum* and asymptomatic carriers of *Neisseria meningitidis*.

DOSAGE: *Adults:* Usual: 200mg initially, then 100mg q12h; alternative is 100-200mg initially, then 50mg qid. Uncomplicated Gonococcal Infection (Men, other than urethritis and anorectal infections): 200mg initially, then 100mg q12h for minimum 4 days, with post therapy cultures within 2-3 days. Uncomplicated Gonococcal Urethritis (Men): 100mg q12h for 5 days. Syphilis: Administer usual dose for 10-15 days. Meningococcal Carrier State: 100mg q12h for 5 days. *Mycobacterium marinum:* 100mg q12h for 6-8 weeks. Uncomplicated urethral, endocervical, or rectal infection: 100mg q12h for at least 7 days. Renal Dysfunction: Reduce dose and/or extend dose intervals. Take with plenty of fluids. Take 1 hr before or 2 hrs after meals.
Pediatrics: >8 yrs: 4mg/kg initially followed by 2mg/kg q12h. Take with plenty of fluids. Taken 1 hr before or 2 hrs after meals.

HOW SUPPLIED: Tab: 50mg, 75mg, 100mg

WARNINGS/PRECAUTIONS: May cause fetal harm during pregnancy. Use during tooth development (eg, last half of pregnancy, infancy, ≤8 yrs) may cause permanent discoloration of the teeth or enamel hypoplasia; avoid use during this period. Bulging fontanels in infants have been associated with use. May decrease bone growth in premature infants. Renal toxicity, hepatotoxicity, photosensitivity, increased BUN, superinfection, pseudotumor cerebri may occur; perform hematopoietic, renal and hepatic monitoring. May impair mental/physical abilities. Not for treatment of meningococcal infections.

ADVERSE REACTIONS: Anorexia, N/V, diarrhea, dysphagia, enterocolitis, pancreatitis, increased liver enzymes, maculopapular/erythematous rash, exfoliative dermatitis, Stevens-Johnson syndrome, skin and mucous membrane pigmentation, hemolytic anemia, headache.

INTERACTIONS: May require downward adjustments of anticoagulant dosage with concomitant use. May interfere with bactericidal action of penicillin; avoid concurrent use when possible. May decrease efficacy of oral contraceptives. Impaired absorption with antacids containing aluminum, calcium or magnesium and iron-containing products. Fatal renal toxicity with methoxyflurane has been reported.

PREGNANCY: Category D, not for use in nursing.

MECHANISM OF ACTION: Tetracycline derivative; bacteriostatic. Thought to inhibit protein synthesis.

PHARMACOKINETICS: Absorption: Rapid; C_{max}= 758.29ng/mL; T_{max}= 1.71 hrs. **Distribution:** Found in breast milk. **Elimination:** Urine and feces; $T_{1/2}$= 17.03 hrs, (hepatic dysfunction) 11-16 hrs, (renal dysfunction) 18-69 hrs.

NURSING CONSIDERATIONS

Assessment: Assess for renal impairment, meningococcal infection, pregnancy/nursing status and possible drug interactions. Document indications for therapy, culture and susceptibility testing. Perform incision and drainage in conjunction with antibiotic therapy when indicated.

Monitoring: Monitor for signs/symptoms of hypersensitivity reactions, photosensitivity, superinfection, benign intracranial HTN, LFTs, renal function, CBC with platelet and differential count. In venereal disease with coexistent syphilis, conduct serologic test before treatment and after 3 months.

Patient Counseling: Inform of pregnancy risks and photosensitivity reactions (d/c at 1st sign of skin erythema). Avoid excessive sunlight/UV light and wear sunscreen/sunblock. Inform therapy treats bacterial, not viral, infections. Take as directed; skipping doses or not completing full course may decrease effectiveness and increase resistance. Notify physician if hypersensitivity reactions, superinfections, photosensitivity or benign intracranial HTN occur. Inform that concomitant use of tetracyclines may render oral contraceptives less effective.

Administration: Oral route. **Storage:** Store at 20-25°C (68-77°F). Protect from light, moisture and excessive heat.

DynaCirc CR

isradipine (Reliant)

RX

THERAPEUTIC CLASS: Calcium channel blocker (dihydropyridine)

INDICATIONS: Management of hypertension alone or in combination with thiazide diuretics.

DOSAGE: *Adults:* Individualized dosing. Initial: 5mg qd alone or with a thiazide diuretic. Titrate: May adjust by 5mg/day at 2-4 week intervals. Max: 20mg/day. Swallow whole; do not bite or divide.

HOW SUPPLIED: Tab, Controlled-Release: 5mg, 10mg

WARNINGS/PRECAUTIONS: May produce symptomatic hypotension. Caution in patients with congestive heart failure (CHF), especially with concomitant β-blockers. Caution with pre-existing severe GI narrowing; obstructive symptoms reported. Dose-related, mild to moderate peripheral edema reported. Caution in elderly.

ADVERSE REACTIONS: Headache, edema, dizziness, constipation, fatigue, flushing, abdominal discomfort.

INTERACTIONS: Severe hypotension possible with fentanyl anesthesia and β-blockers; increased volume of circulating fluid might be required if such interaction occurred. May increases AUC and C_{max}, and may decrease T_{max} of propranolol.

PREGNANCY: Category C, not for use in nursing.

MECHANISM OF ACTION: Dihydropyridine calcium channel blocker; binds to calcium channels with high infinity and specificity, and inhibits calcium flux into cardiac and smooth muscle.

PHARMACOKINETICS: Absorption: Bioavailability (15-24%); (10mg) C_{max}=3-4ng/mL; AUC=62-73ng•h/mL. **Distribution:** Plasma protein binding (95%). **Metabolism:** Oxidation, ester cleavage; CYP3A4. **Elimination:** Urine (60-65%), feces (25-30%).

NURSING CONSIDERATIONS

Assessment: Assess for hypersensitivity, HTN, symptomatic hypotension, renal/hepatic impairment, CHF, pre-existing GI narrowing, ingestion of GITS products, pregnancy/nursing status, and possible drug interactions.

Monitoring: Monitor for signs/symptoms of hypotension (eg, syncope and dizziness), peripheral edema, obstruction from strictures, and hypersensitivity reactions.

Patient Counseling: Instruct to swallow tablet whole; do not bite or divide. Inform that tablet shell may be seen in stool.

Administration: Oral route. Swallow whole; do not bite or divide. **Storage:** Below 30°C (86°F). Store in a tight container, protected from moisture and humidity.

Dyrenium

triamterene (WellSpring)

RX

> Abnormal elevation of serum K⁺ levels (≥5.5mEq/L) can occur with all K⁺-sparing agents, including triamterene. Hyperkalemia is more likely to occur with renal impairment and diabetes (even without evidence of renal impairment), and in the elderly, or severely ill. Monitor serum K⁺ at frequent intervals.

THERAPEUTIC CLASS: K⁺-sparing diuretic

INDICATIONS: Treatment of edema associated with congestive heart failure, liver cirrhosis, and nephrotic syndrome. Treatment of steroid induced edema, idiopathic edema, and edema due to secondary hyperaldosteronism.

DOSAGE: *Adults:* Initial: 100mg bid pc. Max: 300mg/day. Titrate dose to the needs of the individual patient.

HOW SUPPLIED: Cap: 50mg, 100mg

CONTRAINDICATIONS: Anuria, severe or progressive kidney disease or dysfunction (except with nephrosis), severe hepatic disease, hyperkalemia, K^+ supplements, K^+ salts or K^+ containing salt substitutes, K^+-sparing agents (eg, spironolactone, amiloride hydrochloride).

WARNINGS/PRECAUTIONS: Check ECG if hyperkalemia occurs. Isolated reports of hypersensitivity reactions; monitor for possible occurrence of blood dyscrasias, liver damage, or other idiosyncratic reactions. In cirrhotics with splenomegaly, may contribute to megaloblastosis in cases where folic stores have been depleted; perform periodic blood studies and observe for exacerbation of liver disease. Monitor BUN periodically. Caution with gouty arthritis; may elevate uric acid levels. May aggravate or cause electrolyte imbalances in CHF, renal disease, or cirrhosis. Caution with history of renal stones.

ADVERSE REACTIONS: Hypersensitivity reactions, hyper- or hypokalemia, azotemia, renal stones, jaundice, thrombocytopenia, megaloblastic anemia, N/V, diarrhea, weakness, dizziness.

INTERACTIONS: See Contraindications. Increased risk of hyperkalemia with ACE inhibitors. Indomethacin may cause renal failure; caution with NSAIDs. Risk of lithium toxicity. Hyperkalemia may occur when used concomitantly with blood from blood bank, low-salt milk, or potassium containing medications (eg, parenteral penicillin G potassium). May cause hyperglycemia; adjust antidiabetic agents. Chlorpropamide may increase risk of severe hyponatremia. May potentiate nondepolarizing muscle relaxants, antihypertensives, other diuretics, preanesthetics, and anesthetics.

PREGNANCY: Category C, not for use in nursing.

MECHANISM OF ACTION: K^+ sparing diuretic; inhibits reabsorption of Na^+ ions in exchange for K^+ and H^+ ions at segment of distal tubule under control of adrenal mineralocorticoids.

PHARMACOKINETICS: Absorption: Rapid; C_{max}=30ng/mL, T_{max}=3 hrs. **Distribution:** Plasma protein binding (67%); crosses placental barrier. **Metabolism:** Hydroxytriamterene (metabolite). **Elimination:** Urine (21%).

NURSING CONSIDERATIONS

Assessment: Assess for anuria, CHF, DM, gout, hyperkalemia, history of kidney stones, liver/renal impairment, pregnancy/nursing status, and for possible drug interactions.

Monitoring: Monitor for signs/symptoms of electrolyte imbalance, exacerbation of gout, hypersensitivity reactions (eg, blood dyscrasias, liver damage), and for liver/renal dysfunction. Monitor for signs/symptoms of hyperkalemia and perform ECG if suspected. Monitor BUN, serum K^+ levels, and CBC periodically.

Patient Counseling: Advise to take after meals to avoid stomach upset. Inform that if single dose is prescribed, it may be preferable to take in a.m. to minimize frequency of urination during nighttime sleep. Instruct not to take more than prescribed dose at next dosing interval if dose missed. Seek medical attention if symptoms of hyperkalemia, electrolyte imbalance, or hypersensitivity reactions occur.

Administration: Oral route. **Storage:** 25°C (77°F); excursions permitted to 15-30°C (59-86°F). Dispense in tight, light-resistant container.

DYSPORT

abobotulinumtoxina (Ipsen)

> Spread of toxin effects hours to weeks after injection reported (eg, asthenia, generalized muscle weakness, diplopia, blurred vision, ptosis, dysphagia, dysphonia, dysarthria, urinary incontinence and breathing difficulties). Swallowing and breathing difficulties can be life threatening and there have been reports of death. Risk of symptoms is greater in children treated for spasticity than in adults. In unapproved uses and approved indications, effects have spread at doses comparable to those used to treat cervical dystonia and at lower doses.

THERAPEUTIC CLASS: Purified neurotoxin complex

INDICATIONS: Treatment of adults with cervical dystonia to reduce the severity of abnormal head position and neck pain in both toxin-naive and previously treated patients. Temporary improvement in the appearance of moderate to severe glabellar lines associated with procerus and corrugator muscle activity in adults <65 yrs.

DOSAGE: *Adults:* Initial: Cervical Dystonia: 500 U IM as a divided dose among affected muscles. Titrate: 250 U steps according to response; retreat q12 weeks or longer prn based on return of clinical symptoms. Max: 250-1000 U. Do not retreat in intervals of <12 weeks. Glabellar Lines: 50 U IM in 5 equal aliquots of 10 U each. Do not administer more frequently than q3 mth.

HOW SUPPLIED: Inj: 300 U, 500 U

CONTRAINDICATIONS: Allergy to cow's milk protein and infection at the proposed site(s).

WARNINGS/PRECAUTIONS: Not interchangeable with other botulinum toxin products; cannot be compared or converted into units of any other botulinum toxin products. Swallowing or breathing difficulties reported. May weaken neck muscles that serve as accessory muscles of ventilation. Respiratory failure reported in patients with cervical dystonia Deaths due to severe dysphagia reported. May require immediate medical attention if swallowing, speech or respiratory disorders occur. Caution with surgical alterations to face, excessive weakness or atrophy in the target muscle(s), marked facial asymmetry, inflammation at the injection site(s), ptosis, excessive dermatochalasis, deep dermal scarring, thick sebaceous skin, or the inability to substantially lessen glabellar lines by physically spreading them apart. Increased incidence of eyelid ptosis with higher doses. Monitor patients with peripheral motor neuropathic diseases, amyotrophic lateral sclerosis, neuromuscular junction disorders (eg, myasthenia gravis or Lambert-Eaton syndrome); may increase risk of clinically significant effects including severe dysphagia and respiratory compromise from typical doses. Contains albumin; may carry risk of transmitting viral disease (eg, Creutzfeldt-Jakob disease). Potential for immunogenicity.

ADVERSE REACTIONS: Asthenia, generalized muscle weakness, diplopia, blurred vision, ptosis, dysphagia, dysarthria, dysphonia, urinary incontinence, breathing difficulties, discomfort at injection site, dysphonia, eye disorder, dry mouth, headache.

INTERACTIONS: May potentiate systemic anticholinergic effects (eg, blurred vision) when used concomitantly with anticholinergic drugs. Effects may be potentiated with aminoglycosides or agents interfering with neuromuscular transmission (eg, curare-like agents). Excessive weakness may be exacerbated by another administration of botulinum toxin or a muscle relaxant prior to resolution of effects from prior botulinum toxin.

PREGNANCY: Category C, safety not known in nursing.

MECHANISM OF ACTION: Purified neurotoxin type A complex; inhibits release of acetylcholine from peripheral cholinergic nerve endings; produces chemical denervation of the muscle resulting in a localized reduction in muscle activity.

NURSING CONSIDERATIONS

Assessment: Assess for pre-existing breathing and swallowing difficulties, allergy to cow's milk, infection at proposed injection site, surgical facial alterations, excessive weakness or atrophy in the target muscle(s), marked facial asymmetry, inflammation at injection site(s), deep dermal scarring, ptosis, excessive dermatochalasis, thick sebaceous skin, inability to substantially lessen glabellar lines by physically spreading them apart, pre-existing neuromuscular disorders, hypersensitivity, pregnancy/nursing status and for possible drug interactions.

Monitoring: Monitor for spread of the toxin effects (eg, asthenia, generalized muscle weakness, diplopia, blurred vision, ptosis, dysphagia, dysphonia, dysarthria, urinary incontinence and breathing difficulties), swallowing difficulty, weakening of neck muscles, development of speech, swallowing or respiratory disorders. Monitor patients with peripheral motor neuropathic diseases, amyotrophic lateral sclerosis, neuromuscular junction disorders (eg, myasthenia gravis or Lambert-Eaton syndrome).

Patient Counseling: Notify healthcare professional if any unusual symptoms develop (eg, difficulty with swallowing, speaking or breathing) or if any known symptom persists or worsens. Instruct to avoid driving or engaging in potentially hazardous activities if loss of strength, muscle weakness, blurred vision, or drooping eyelids occurs.

Administration: IM route. Use within 4 hrs of reconstitution. Refer to PI for instructions for preparation and administration techniques. **Storage:** 2-8°C (36-46°F). Protect from light. Do not freeze after reconstitution.

EDARBI   RX
azilsartan medoxomil (Takeda)

> Drugs that act directly on the renin-angiotensin system can cause injury and death to the developing fetus. D/C therapy when pregnancy is detected.

THERAPEUTIC CLASS: Angiotensin II receptor antagonist

INDICATIONS: Treatment of HTN, alone or in combination with other antihypertensives.

DOSAGE: *Adults:* Usual: 80mg qd. With High Dose Diuretics: Initial: 40mg qd. Take with other antihypertensives if BP is not controlled with drug alone.

HOW SUPPLIED: Tab: 40mg, 80mg

WARNINGS/PRECAUTIONS: Symptomatic hypotension may occur in volume-and/or salt-depleted patients; correct volume/salt depletion prior to therapy. Changes in renal function may occur; caution with severe congestive heart failure (CHF), renal artery stenosis, or volume depletion. May increase SrCr or BUN in patients with renal artery stenosis.

ADVERSE REACTIONS: Fetal injury, dizziness, postural dizziness, diarrhea, nausea, asthenia, fatigue, muscle spasm, cough.

INTERACTIONS: May result in deterioration of renal function, including possible renal failure, when coadministered with NSAIDs, including selective COX-2 inhibitors in elderly, volume-depleted, or patients have compromised renal function; monitor renal function periodically. Antihypertensive effect may be attenuated by NSAIDs, including selective COX-2 inhibitors. May cause symptomatic hypotension with high doses of diuretics.

PREGNANCY: Category C (1st trimester) and D (2nd and 3rd trimesters), not for use in nursing.

MECHANISM OF ACTION: Angiotensin II receptor antagonist; blocks vasoconstrictor and aldosterone-secreting effects of angiotensin II by selectively blocking binding of angiotensin II to AT_1 receptor in many tissues, such as vascular smooth muscle and the adrenal gland.

PHARMACOKINETICS: Absorption: Absolute bioavailability (60%); T_{max}=1.5-3 hrs. **Distribution:** V_d=16L; plasma protein binding (>99%). **Metabolism:** GI tract via hydrolysis to azilsartan (active metabolite). Azilsartan: Liver via CYP2C9. **Elimination:** Urine (42%) (15% azilsartan), feces (55%); $T_{1/2}$=11 hrs.

NURSING CONSIDERATIONS

Assessment: Assess for pregnancy/nursing status, volume/salt depletion, renal function, history of CHF, renal artery stenosis, and possible drug
interactions.

Monitoring: Monitor for signs/symptoms of hypotension, SrCr, and BUN.
Monitor renal function periodically when coadministered with NSAIDs, including selective COX-2 inhibitors, especially in patients who are elderly, volume-
depleted, or have compromised renal function.

Patient Counseling: Inform of pregnancy risks. Notify physician if pregnant
or become pregnant. Seek medical attention if symptoms of hypotension or
other adverse events occur. Inform that drug may be taken with/without food.

Administration: Oral route. **Storage:** 25°C (77°F); excursions permitted to
15-30° (59-86°).

EDLUAR   CIV
zolpidem tartrate (Meda)

THERAPEUTIC CLASS: Imidazopyridine hypnotic

INDICATIONS: Short-term treatment of insomnia, characterized by difficulties
with sleep initiation.

DOSAGE: *Adults:* Individualize dose. 10mg SL qhs. Max: 10mg/day. Elderly/
Debilitated Patients: 5mg SL qhs. Concomitant Use with CNS-Depressant
Drugs: Require dose adjustment.

HOW SUPPLIED: Tab, Sublingual: 5mg, 10mg

WARNINGS/PRECAUTIONS: Evaluate for primary psychiatric and/or medical
illness if insomnia fails to remit after 7-10 days of treatment. Severe anaphylactic and anaphylactoid reactions reported; do not rechallenge if patient
develops reactions. Visual/auditory hallucinations, complex behavior (eg,
sleep-driving), abnormal thinking and behavior changes reported. Worsening
of depression, including suicidal thoughts and actions have been reported in
depressed patients. May impair mental/physical abilities. Caution with conditions that could affect metabolism or hemodynamic responses, sleep apnea,
myasthenia gravis, and worsening depression. Signs and symptoms of withdrawal reported with abrupt d/c of sedative/hypnotics. Monitor elderly and
debilitated patients for impaired motor and/or cognitive performance.

ADVERSE REACTIONS: Drowsiness, dizziness, diarrhea, headache, drugged
feeling, dry mouth, back pain, allergy, sinusitis, pharyngitis.

INTERACTIONS: CNS-active drugs may potentially enhance effects.
Additive effects on psychomotor performance with alcohol/chlorpromazine.
Decreased alertness observed with imipramine/chlorpromazine. Ketoconazole
may enhance sedative effects. May decrease effects with rifampin.

PREGNANCY: Category C, caution in nursing.

MECHANISM OF ACTION: Imidazopyridine, non-benzodiazepine hypnotic;
binds to GABA-BZ receptor complex at the α1/α5 subunits.

PHARMACOKINETICS: Absorption: Rapid; C_{max}=106ng/mL; T_{max}=82 min.
Distribution: Plasma protein binding (92.5%). **Elimination:** Renal; (5mg)
$T_{1/2}$=2.85 hrs, (10mg) $T_{1/2}$=2.65 hrs.

NURSING CONSIDERATIONS

Assessment: Assess for primary psychiatric and/or medical illness, pre-existing respiratory impairment (eg, sleep apnea syndrome), myasthenia gravis,
hypersensitivity reactions, hepatic impairment, history of alcohol, pregnancy/
nursing status, and possible drug interactions.

Monitoring: Monitor for anaphylactic/anaphylactoid reactions, abnormal
thinking, behavioral changes, complex behavior (eg, sleep-driving), hepatic
impairment, and those on long-term treatment for drug abuse/dependence.

Patient Counseling: Instruct not to swallow or take with water. Tablet should
be placed under the tongue. Should not to be given with or immediately after
a meal. Inform to take just before bedtime. Advise not to take with alcohol.

Caution against hazardous tasks (eg, driving/operating machinery). Counsel about risks/benefits of use. Seek medical attention if severe anaphylactic and anaphylactoid reactions occur. Notify physician of all concomitant medications and any episodes of sleep-driving or complex behaviors.

Administration: Oral route. Tablet should be placed under the tongue.
Storage: 20-25°C (68-77°F). Protect from light and moisture.

EFFEXOR   RX
venlafaxine HCl (Wyeth)

> Antidepressants increased the risk of suicidal thinking and behavior (suicidality) in children, adolescents, and young adults in short-term studies of major depressive disorder (MDD) and other psychiatric disorders. Monitor and observe closely for clinical worsening, suicidality, or unusual changes in behavior. Not approved for use in pediatric patients.

THERAPEUTIC CLASS: Serotonin and norepinephrine reuptake inhibitor

INDICATIONS: Treatment of major depressive disorder (MDD).

DOSAGE: *Adults:* Initial: 75mg/day given bid-tid with food. Titrate: Increase by 75mg/day at no less than 4-day intervals. Max: 375mg/day given tid. Hepatic Impairment (mild to moderate): Reduce dose by 50%. Renal Impairment (mild to moderate): Reduce dose by 25%. Hemodialysis: Reduce dose by 50%.

HOW SUPPLIED: Tab: 25mg*, 37.5mg*, 50mg*, 75mg*, 100mg* *scored

CONTRAINDICATIONS: Concomitant use of MAOI or within 14 days of stopping an MAOI.

WARNINGS/PRECAUTIONS: Avoid abrupt withdrawal; monitor for new symptoms when d/c treatment and re-evaluate periodically. Assess bipolar disorder risk before initiating therapy. Serotonin syndrome or neuroleptic malignant syndrome (NMS)-like reactions reported; d/c immediately and monitor. May cause sustained increases in BP; pre-existing hypertension should be controlled before initiation of therapy. Mydriasis reported; monitor patients with increase of intraocular pressure (IOP) or risk of acute narrow-angle glaucoma. May increase risk of bleeding events. Treatment-emergent anxiety, nervousness, insomnia, weight loss, anorexia, and activation of mania/hypomania reported. May cause hyponatremia; d/c if with symptomatic hyponatremia and institute appropriate intervention. Caution with history of mania or seizures and conditions affecting hemodynamic responses or metabolism; d/c if seizures occur. Elevation of cholesterol levels reported; monitor periodically. Caution with hyperthyroidism, heart failure, recent MI, renal or hepatic impairment. Interstitial lung disease and eosinophilic pneumonia reported rarely. Caution in elderly.

ADVERSE REACTIONS: Asthenia, sweating, N/V, headache, diarrhea, constipation, anorexia, insomnia, somnolence, dry mouth, dizziness, nervousness, anxiety, abnormal ejaculation/orgasm, impotence in men.

INTERACTIONS: See Contraindications. Avoid alcohol, tryptophan. Increased risk of bleeding with ASA, NSAIDs, warfarin, and other anticoagulants. Caution with cimetidine in elderly, HTN, hepatic dysfunction. Altered coagulation effects with warfarin. Decreases clearance of haloperidol. Increases risperidone and desipramine plasma levels. Increased levels with ketoconazole. Caution with metoprolol, potent inhibitors of CYP3A4 and CYP2D6, CNS-active drugs, and serotonergic drugs (eg, triptans, SSRIs, other SNRIs, linezolid, lithium, tramadol, or St. John's wort). Dose-dependent weight loss reported; coadministration with weight-loss agents not recommended. Coadministration with tryptophan supplements is not recommended.

PREGNANCY: Category C, not for use in nursing.

MECHANISM OF ACTION: Serotonin and norepinephrine reuptake inhibitor; potentiates neurotransmitter activity of CNS activity by inhibiting neuronal serotonin and norephinephrine reuptake.

PHARMACOKINETICS: Absorption: Well absorbed; relative bioavailability (100%). **Distribution:** Venlafaxine: V_d=7.5L/kg; plasma protein binding (27%). ODV: V_d=5.7L/kg; plasma protein binding (30%). Found in breastmilk. **Metabolism:** Hepatic; metabolite: O-desmethylvenlafaxine (ODV). **Elimination:** Venlafaxine: Urine, unchanged (5%); $T_{1/2}$=5 hrs. ODV: Urine: un-conjugated (29%), conjugated (26%); $T_{1/2}$=11 hrs.

NURSING CONSIDERATIONS

Assessment: Assess for bipolar disorder risk, history of mania and drug abuse, hyperthyroidism, heart failure, recent MI, history of glaucoma, increased IOP, risk factors for acute-narrow angle glaucoma, pre-existing HTN, history of seizures, disease/condition that alters metabolism or hemodynamic response, cholesterol levels, hepatic/renal impairment, pregnancy/nursing status, and possible drug interactions.

Monitoring: Monitor HR, BP, LFTs, renal function, cholesterol, triglycerides (TG) and ECG changes, height and weight. Monitor for signs/symptoms of clinical worsening (suicidality, unusual changes in behavior), serotonin syndrome or NMS-like reactions, mydriasis, severe HTN, lung disease (progressive dyspnea, cough, chest discomfort), abnormal bleeding, allergic reactions (rash, hives), hyponatremia (headache, weakness, unsteadiness), seizures, cognitive/motor impairment, and hepatic/renal dysfunction. If abruptly d/c, monitor for symptoms of dysphoric mood, irritability, agitation, dizziness, sensory disturbances, anxiety, confusion, headache, lethargy, emotional lability, insomnia, and hypomania.

Patient Counseling: Advise to avoid alcohol. Inform about the risks and benefits associated with treatment. Instruct to read the Medication Guide. Advise to inform physician if taking, or plan to take, any prescription or OTC drugs, including herbal preparations and nutritional supplements, since there is a potential for interactions. Seek medical attention for symptoms of serotonin syndrome (mental status changes, tachycardia, hyperthermia, N/V, diarrhea, incoordination), abnormal bleeding (particularly if using NSAIDs or ASA), hyponatremia (headache, weakness, unsteadiness), mydriasis, severe HTN, lung disease (progressive dyspnea, cough, chest discomfort), activation of mania, seizures, clinical worsening (suicidal ideation, unusual changes in behavior), or discontinuation symptoms (irritability, agitation, dizziness, anxiety, headache, insomnia). Notify physician if pregnant or breastfeeding, if rash, hives, or related allergic phenomenon develop. Notify healthcare provider of glaucoma history or an increase in IOP.

Administration: Oral route. **Storage:** 20-25°C (68-77°F) in a dry place.

Effexor XR   RX
venlafaxine HCl (Wyeth)

> Antidepressants increased the risk of suicidal thinking and behavior (suicidality) in children, adolescents, and young adults in short-term studies of major depressive disorder (MDD) and other psychiatric disorders. Monitor and observe closely for clinical worsening, suicidality, or unusual changes in behavior in patients who are started on antidepressant therapy. Not approved for use in pediatric patients.

THERAPEUTIC CLASS: Serotonin and norepinephrine reuptake inhibitor

INDICATIONS: Treatment of major depressive disorder (MDD), generalized anxiety disorder (GAD), social anxiety disorder (SAD), and panic disorder (PD).

DOSAGE: *Adults:* Give qd, either in the qam or qpm. MDD/GAD/SAD: Initial: 75mg qd, or 37.5mg qd increase to 75mg qd after 4-7 days. Titrate: May increase by increments of up to 75mg/day at no less than 4-day intervals. Max: 225mg/day. PD: Initial: 37.5mg qd for 7 days. Titrate: May increase by increments of up to 75mg/day at no less than 7 day intervals. Max: 225mg/day. Switching from Effexor IR Tablets: Give the nearest equivalent dose (mg/day) qd. Individual dose adjustments may be necessary. Hepatic Impairment (Mild-Moderate): Reduce initial dose by 50%. Renal Impairment: Reduce total daily dose by 25-50%. Hemodialysis: Reduce total daily dose by 50%.

HOW SUPPLIED: Cap, Extended-Release: 37.5mg, 75mg, 150mg

CONTRAINDICATIONS: Concomitant use of MAOIs.

WARNINGS/PRECAUTIONS: Avoid abrupt withdrawal. Re-evaluate periodically. Monitor for clinical worsening, suicidality, and/or unusual behavioral changes, especially at initiation of therapy or dose changes. Serotonin syndrome or neuroleptic malignant syndrome (NMS)-like reactions reported; d/c immediately and monitor. May cause sustained increases in BP. Activation of mania/hypomania, mydriasis, hyponatremia, SIADH, altered platelet function, treatment-emergent nervousness, insomnia, and anorexia reported. Caution with history of mania or seizures, conditions affecting hemodynamic responses or metabolism; d/c if seizures occur. Monitor increase of intraocular pressure (IOP) or risk of acute narrow-angle glaucoma. May increase risk of bleeding events. Elevation of cholesterol levels reported; monitor periodically. Caution with hyperthyroidism, heart failure, recent MI, renal or hepatic impairment. Interstitial lung disease and eosinophilic pneumonia reported rarely. Caution in elderly.

ADVERSE REACTIONS: Asthenia, sweating, headache, N/V, constipation, anorexia, dry mouth, dizziness, insomnia, nervousness, somnolence, abnormal ejaculation, abnormal dreams, pharyngitis.

INTERACTIONS: See Contraindications. Avoid alcohol, tryptophan. Increased risk of bleeding with ASA, NSAIDs, warfarin, and other anticoagulants. Caution with cimetidine in elderly, HTN, hepatic dysfunction. Altered coagulation effects with warfarin. Decreases clearance of haloperidol. Increases risperidone and desipramine plasma levels. Increase levels with ketoconazole. Caution with metoprolol, potent inhibitors of CYP3A4 and CYP2D6, CNS-active drugs, and serotonergic drugs (eg, triptans, SSRIs, other SNRIs, linezolid, lithium, tramadol, or St. John's wort). Coadministration with tryptophan supplements and weight-loss agents are not recommended.

PREGNANCY: Category C, not for use in nursing.

MECHANISM OF ACTION: 5-HT and NE reuptake inhibitor; potentiates neurotransmitter activity of CNS by inhibiting neuronal serotonin and norepinephrine reuptake.

PHARMACOKINETICS: Absorption: Venlafaxine: Absolute bioavailability (45%), C_{max}=150ng/mL, T_{max}=5.5 hrs. ODV (metabolite): C_{max}=260ng/mL, T_{max}=9 hrs. **Distribution:** Venlafaxine: V_d=7.5L/kg; plasma protein binding (27%). ODV: V_d=5.7L/kg; plasma protein binding (30%). **Metabolism:** Hepatic via CYP2D6; Active metabolite: O-desmethylvenlafaxine (ODV). Found in breast milk. **Elimination:** Urine (5% unchanged). Venlafaxine: $T_{1/2}$=5 hrs. ODV: $T_{1/2}$=11 hrs.

NURSING CONSIDERATIONS

Assessment: Assess for bipolar disorder risk, history of mania, hyperthyroidism, HF, recent MI, acute narrow-angle glaucoma, elevated IOP, HTN, seizures, hypersensitivity, concomitant use of MAOIs, serotonin syndrome, disease/condition that alters metabolism or hemodynamic response, cholesterol levels, hepatic/renal impairment, pregnancy/nursing status, and possible drug interactions.

Monitoring: Monitor HR, BP, LFTs, renal function, cholesterol, TG and ECG changes, signs/symptoms of clinical worsening (suicidality, unusual behavior), serotonin syndrome or NMS-like reactions (agitation, hallucinations, coma, uncoordination, tachycardia, hyperthermia, labile BP, N/V, diarrhea), mydriasis, severe HTN, lung disease (progressive dyspnea, cough, chest discomfort), abnormal bleeding, allergic reactions (rash, hives), hyponatremia (headache, weakness, unsteadiness), seizures, cognitive/motor impairment, and hepatic/renal dysfunction. If abruptly d/c, monitor for dizziness, sensory disturbances, anxiety, confusion, headache, lethargy, emotional lability, insomnia, and hypomania.

Patient Counseling: Advise to avoid alcohol; may impair physical/mental abilities. Seek medical attention for symptoms of serotonin syndrome (mental status changes, tachycardia, hyperthermia, N/V, diarrhea, incoordination), abnormal bleeding (particularly if using NSAIDs or ASA), hyponatremia (headache, weakness, unsteadiness), mydriasis, severe HTN, lung disease (progressive dyspnea, cough, chest discomfort), activation of mania, allergic reaction (rash, hives), seizures, clinical worsening (suicidal ideation, unusual changes in behavior), or discontinuation symptoms (irritability, agitation, dizziness, anxiety, headache, insomnia). Caution that medication may impair physical/mental abilities. Notify a physician if a rash, hives, or related allergic phenomenon develop.

Administration: Oral route. Take with food; swallow whole without chewing or open cap and sprinkle on spoonful of applesauce followed with water.
Storage: 20-25°C (68-77°F).

EFFIENT

prasugrel (Daiichi Sankyo/Eli Lilly)

RX

> May cause significant, sometimes fatal, bleeding; risk factors include <60kg body weight, propensity to bleed, and concomitant use of medications that may increase bleeding (eg, warfarin, heparin, fibrinolytic therapy, chronic use of NSAIDs). Do not use in patients with active pathological bleeding or history of transient ischemic attacks (TIA) or stroke. Not recommended in patients ≥75 yrs due to increased risk of fatal intracranial bleeding and uncertain benefits, except in diabetes or history of prior myocardial infarction (MI). Do not start in patients likely to undergo urgent coronary artery bypass graft surgery (CABG); d/c at least 7 days prior to surgery. Suspect bleeding in any patient who is hypotensive and has recently undergone coronary angiography, percutaneous coronary intervention (PCI), CABG, or other surgical procedures; if possible, manage bleeding without d/c. D/C in the first few weeks after ACS increases the risk of subsequent cardiovascular (CV) events.

THERAPEUTIC CLASS: Platelet aggregation inhibitor

INDICATIONS: Reduction of thrombotic CV events (eg, stent thrombosis) in patients with acute coronary syndrome (ACS) (eg, unstable angina, non-ST-elevation MI, ST-elevation MI) who are to be managed with percutaneous coronary intervention (PCI). Reduction of combined endpoint of CV death, nonfatal MI, or nonfatal stroke.

DOSAGE: *Adults:* LD: 60mg PO single dose. Maint: 10mg qd. <60 kg: Reduce to 5mg qd. Take with ASA 75-325mg qd.

HOW SUPPLIED: Tab: 5mg, 10mg

CONTRAINDICATIONS: Active pathological bleeding (eg, peptic ulcer, intracranial hemorrhage), history of prior TIA or stroke.

WARNINGS/PRECAUTIONS: Withholding a dose will not be useful in managing a bleeding event or the risk of bleeding associated with an invasive procedure. CABG-related bleeding may be treated with blood transfusion; platelet transfusion within 6 hrs of loading dose or 4 hrs of maintenance dose may be less effective. D/C if active bleeding, elective surgery, stroke or TIA occurs. Premature d/c of therapy will increase risk for cardiac events. Lapses in therapy should be avoided; if therapy is temporarily d/c because of adverse events, restart as soon as possible. Thrombotic thrombocytopenic purpura (TTP) reported, sometimes after brief exposure (<2 weeks) and may require treatment (eg, plasmapheresis).

ADVERSE REACTIONS: CABG and Non-CABG-related bleeding, HTN, hypercholesterolemia/hyperlipidemia, headache, back pain, dyspnea, nausea, dizziness, cough, hypotension, fatigue, non-cardiac chest pain.

INTERACTIONS: See Boxed Warning. Coadministration of ranitidine or lansoprazole decreased C_{max} of prasugrel active metabolite. Decreased C_{max} of ketoconazole. Increased bleeding time when coadministered with aspirin 150mg.

PREGNANCY: Category B, caution in nursing.

MECHANISM OF ACTION: Platelet aggregation inhibitor (thienopyridine class); inhibits platelet activation and aggregation through irreversible binding of its active metabolite to the $P2Y_{12}$ class of ADP receptors on platelets.

PHARMACOKINETICS: Absorption: (Prodrug) Rapid (≥79%); T_{max}=30 min. **Distribution:** Serum albumin (98%); V_d=44-68L (active metabolite). **Metabolism:** Hydrolysis via CYP3A4 and CYP2B6 and to a lesser extent by CYP2C9 and CYP2C19 in the intestine to thiolactone. **Elimination:** Urine (68%), feces (27%); $T_{1/2}$=7 hrs (active metabolite).

NURSING CONSIDERATIONS

Assessment: Assess for presence of active bleeding (recent or recurrent GI bleeding, active peptic ulcer disease, intracranial hemorrhage), history of prior TIA or stroke, ACS, concomitant use of medications that may increase bleeding, recent trauma, recent surgery, hepatic function, age, weight, nursing/pregnancy status, and possible drug interactions. Obtain baseline hematologic parameters, including PT/PTT.

Monitoring: Monitor for signs/symptoms of hypotension, TTP (eg, thrombocytopenia) and active bleeding. Monitor for cardiac events in patients who require premature d/c.

Patient Counseling: Counsel about benefits/risks of therapy. Counsel to take as prescribed and encourage not to d/c therapy without consulting prescribing physician. Inform that they will bleed and bruise more easily and take longer to stop bleeding. Advise to report any unanticipated, prolonged, or excessive bleeding, or blood in urine or stool. Inform patients about signs and symptoms requiring medical attention such as TTP. Instruct to get prompt medical attention if fever, weakness, extreme skin paleness, purple skin patches, yellowing of the skin or eyes, or neurological changes occur. Counsel to inform physicians and dentists of medication before any invasive procedure is scheduled. Instruct to notify physician of all concomitant prescription/OTC medications or dietary supplements.

Administration: Oral route. Take with or without meals. **Storage:** 25°C (77°F); excursions permitted to 15-30°C (59-86°F). Dispense and keep in original container. Keep container closed and do not remove desiccant from bottle. Do not break the tablet.

EGRIFTA   RX
tesamorelin (EMD Serono)

THERAPEUTIC CLASS: Growth hormone-releasing factor

INDICATIONS: Reduction of excess abdominal fat in HIV-infected patients with lipodystrophy.

DOSAGE: *Adults:* 2mg SQ in the abdomen qd.

HOW SUPPLIED: Inj (powder): 1mg

CONTRAINDICATIONS: Pregnancy, newly diagnosed or recurrent active malignancy, and disruption of hypothalamic-pituitary axis (HPA) due to hypophysectomy, hypopituitarism, pituitary tumor/surgery, head irradiation or head trauma.

WARNINGS/PRECAUTIONS: Carefully consider continuation of treatment in patients who do not show clear efficacy response. Not indicated for weight loss management. Caution with history of non-malignant neoplasms or treated and stable malignancies. Increases serum IGF-I; monitor IGF-I levels closely and consider d/c with persistent elevations. Fluid retention (eg, edema, arthralgia, carpal tunnel syndrome) may occur. May cause glucose intolerance and diabetes; evaluate glucose status prior to therapy then monitor periodically. May develop or worsen retinopathy in patients with diabetes. Hypersensitivity reactions may occur; d/c treatment immediately when reactions suspected. Rotate site of injection to different areas of abdomen to reduce injection-site reactions (eg, erythema, pruritus, pain, irritation, bruising). Consider d/c in critically ill patients; increased mortality reported in patients with acute critical illness after treatment with growth hormone (GH).

ADVERSE REACTIONS: Arthralgia, pain in extremity, myalgia, injection-site reactions (eg, erythema, pruritus, pain), peripheral edema, paresthesia, hypoesthesia, nausea, rash.

INTERACTIONS: GH may modulate CYP450 mediated antipyrine clearance; caution with CYP450 substrates (eg, corticosteroids, sex steroids, anticonvulsants, cyclosporine). May require an increase in maintenance or stress doses of glucocorticoids particularly in patients taking cortisone acetate and prednisone. Decreased absorption of simvastatin, simvastatin acid, and ritonavir.

PREGNANCY: Category X, not for use in nursing.

E

MECHANISM OF ACTION: Human Growth Hormone-Releasing Factor (GRF) synthetic analog; acts on pituitary somatotroph cells to stimulate the synthesis and pulsatile release of endogenous GH, which is both anabolic and lipolytic.

PHARMACOKINETICS: Absorption: Absolute bioavailability (<4%, healthy); AUC=634.6pg•h/mL (healthy), 852.8pg•h/mL (HIV-infected); C_{max}=2874.6pg/mL (healthy), 2822.3pg/mL (HIV-infected); T_{max}=0.15 hr (healthy, HIV infected). **Distribution:** V_d=9.4L/kg (healthy), 10.5L/kg (HIV-infected). **Elimination:** $T_{1/2}$=26 min (healthy), 38 min (HIV-infected).

NURSING CONSIDERATIONS

Assessment: Assess for active malignancy, hypersensitivity to tesamorelin and/or mannitol, HPA disruption due to hypophysectomy, hypopituitarism, pituitary tumor/surgery, head irritation or head trauma, history of non-malignant neoplasms or treated and stable malignancies, increased background risk of malignancies, glucose status, acute critical illness, pregnancy/nursing status, and possible drug interactions.

Monitoring: Monitor for response, IGF-I levels, HbA1c levels, changes in glucose metabolism, glucose intolerance, diabetes, worsening or development of retinopathy, and hypersensitivity reactions.

Patient Counseling: Advise that treatment may cause transient symptoms consistent with fluid retention (eg, edema, arthralgia, carpal tunnel syndrome) which resolve upon d/c. Seek medical attention and d/c therapy immediately when hypersensitivity reactions occur (eg, rash, urticaria). Advise to rotate the site of injection to different areas of abdomen to reduce incidence of injection site reactions (eg, erythema, pruritus, pain, irritation, bruising). Counsel not to share syringe with another person, even if the needle is changed. Advise women to d/c treatment if pregnant and not to breastfeed; apprise of the potential hazard to the fetus.

Administration: SQ route. Recommended site is the abdomen. Do not inject into scar tissue, bruises, or the navel. Refer to Instructions For Use leaflet for reconstitution procedures. **Storage:** Non-reconstituted: 2-8°C (36-46°F). Diluent/Syringes/Needles: 20-25°C (68-77°F). Protect from light. Keep in the original box until use.

ELDEPRYL RX
selegiline HCl (Somerset)

THERAPEUTIC CLASS: Monoamine oxidase inhibitor (Type B)

INDICATIONS: Adjunct in the management of Parkinsonian patients being treated with levodopa/carbidopa who exhibit deterioration in the quality of their response to this therapy.

DOSAGE: *Adults:* 10mg qd as divided doses of 5mg each taken at breakfast and lunch. Max: 10mg/day. May attempt to reduce levodopa/carbidopa after 2-3 days of therapy. Usual reduction of 10-30%; may reduce further with continued therapy.

HOW SUPPLIED: Cap: 5mg; (Generic) Tab: 5mg

CONTRAINDICATIONS: Concomitant meperidine, or other opioids.

WARNINGS/PRECAUTIONS: Selegiline should not be used at doses >10 mg/day due to risks associated with non-selective inhibition of MAO. Decrease levodopa/carbidopa by 10-30% to prevent exacerbation of levodopa-associated side effects. Patients with Parkinson's disease have higher risk of melanoma; monitor frequently for melanoma.

ADVERSE REACTIONS: Nausea, dizziness/lightheadedness/fainting, abdominal pain, confusion, hallucinations, dry mouth, vivid dreams, dyskinesias, headache.

INTERACTIONS: See Contraindications. Avoid SSRIs and TCAs; severe toxicity reported. Allow ≥2 weeks between d/c of selegiline and initiation of TCAs or SSRIs. Allow ≥5 weeks between d/c of fluoxetine and initiation of selegiline due to long half-lives of fluoxetine and its active metabolite. Caution with ephedrine and tyramine-containing foods; hypertensive crises/reactions reported.

PREGNANCY: Category C, not for use in nursing.

MECHANISM OF ACTION: Monoamine oxidase inhibitor (type B); mechanism not established. Irreversibly inhibits MAO type B (selectivity is dose-dependent) blocking the catabolism of dopamine. May also act through other mechanisms to increase dopaminergic activity.

PHARMACOKINETICS: Absorption: C_{max}=1ng/mL. **Metabolism:** Extensive via gut and liver. N-desmethylselegiline (active metabolite). **Elimination:** $T_{1/2}$=2 hrs (single-dose), 10 hrs (steady-state).

NURSING CONSIDERATIONS

Assessment: Assess pregnancy/nursing status, hypersensitivity and possible drug interactions.

Monitoring: Monitor for hypersensitivity reactions, adverse effects, hypertensive crisis, hallucinations, myoclonic jerks, intense urges to gamble and for increased sexual urges. Monitor frequently for melanoma. Periodic skin examinations should be performed by qualified individuals (eg, dermatologists).

Patient Counseling: Advise of the possible need to reduce levodopa dosage, not to exceed 10mg/day, and of the risk of using higher daily doses. Inform patients or their families about signs and symptoms of MAOI-induced hypertensive reactions; immediately report severe headache or other atypical/unusual symptoms. Report any intense urges to gamble, increased sexual urges and other intense urges and inability to control these urges. Avoid tyramine-containing foods (eg, cheese), and provide a description of the 'cheese reaction.'

Administration: Oral route. **Storage:** 20-25°C (68-77°F).

ELESTAT   RX
epinastine HCl (Inspire)

THERAPEUTIC CLASS: H_1-antagonist

INDICATIONS: Prevention of itching associated with allergic conjunctivitis.

DOSAGE: *Adults:* 1 drop in each eye bid.
Pediatrics: ≥3 yrs: 1 drop in each eye bid.

HOW SUPPLIED: Sol: 0.05% [5mL]

WARNINGS/PRECAUTIONS: Not for contact lens-related irritation. May reinsert contact lens 10 min after dosing if eye is not red.

ADVERSE REACTIONS: Burning sensation in the eye, folliculosis, hyperemia, pruritus, infection (cold symptoms and upper respiratory infections).

PREGNANCY: Category C, caution in nursing.

MECHANISM OF ACTION: H_1-receptor antagonist; inhibits histamine release from the mast cell; selective for the histamine H_1-receptor and has affinity for the histamine H_2-receptor and possesses affinity for the α_1-α_2 and 5-HT_2-receptors.

PHARMACOKINETICS: Absorption: C_{max}=0.04ng/ml; T_{max}=2 hrs. **Distribution:** Plasma protein binding (64%). **Metabolism:** Active tubular secretion. **Elimination:** Urine (55%, unchanged), feces (30%, unchanged); $T_{1/2}$=12 hrs.

NURSING CONSIDERATIONS

Assessment: Assess for drug hypersensitivity and severity of symptoms.

Monitoring: Monitor adverse events such as burning sensation in the eye, folliculosis, hyperemia, pruritus, and infection (cold symptoms and upper respiratory infections).

Patient Counseling: Counsel not to wear contact lenses if eye is red; remove prior to instillation. Inform that medication is not for treatment of contact lens-related irritation. Instruct to avoid touching tip of container to eye or any other surface to avoid contamination.

Administration: Ocular route. **Storage:** 15-25°C (59-77°F). Keep tightly closed.

ELIDEL
pimecrolimus (Novartis) RX

> Rare cases of malignancy (eg, skin and lymphoma) reported with topical calcineurin inhibitors including pimecrolimus, although causal relationship is not established. Avoid long-term use and application should be limited to areas of involvement with atopic dermatitis. Not indicated for children <2 yrs.

THERAPEUTIC CLASS: Macrolactam ascomycin derivative

INDICATIONS: Second-line therapy for the short-term and non-continuous chronic treatment of mild to moderate atopic dermatitis in non-immunocompromised patients ≥ 2 yrs who failed to respond adequately to other topical prescription treatments, or when those treatments are not advisable.

DOSAGE: *Adults:* Apply thin layer to the affected area(s) bid until signs and symptoms resolve. Re-evaluate if signs and symptoms persist beyond 6 weeks.
Pediatrics: ≥2 yrs: Apply thin layer to the affected area(s) bid until signs and symptoms resolve. Re-evaluate if signs and symptoms persist beyond 6 weeks.

HOW SUPPLIED: Cre: 1% [30g, 60g, 100g]

WARNINGS/PRECAUTIONS: Long-term safety, beyond 1 year of non-continuous use, has not been established. Avoid with malignant or pre-malignant skin conditions, Netherton's syndrome, or other skin diseases that may increase the potential for systemic absorption. Avoid in immunocompromised patients. May cause local symptoms such as skin burning (eg, burning sensation, stinging, soreness) or pruritus and may improve as the lesions resolve. Resolve bacterial or viral infections at treatment sites before starting treatment. Increased risk of varicella zoster infection, herpes simplex virus infection or eczema herpeticum. Skin papilloma/warts reported; consider d/c if skin papillomas worsen or are unresponsive to conventional treatment. Lymphadenopathy reported; d/c if lymphadenopathy of uncertain etiology or acute infectious mononucleosis occurs. Minimize or avoid natural or artificial sunlight exposure.

ADVERSE REACTIONS: Application-site burning, application-site reaction, upper respiratory tract infection, headache, nasopharyngitis, influenza, abdominal pain, diarrhea, sore throat, hypersensitivity, pyrexia, cough, rhinitis, N/V.

INTERACTIONS: Caution with CYP3A4 inhibitors (eg, erythromycin, itraconazole, ketoconazole, fluconazole, calcium channel blockers, cimetidine) in patients with widespread and/or erythrodermic disease. Skin flushing associated with concomitant alcohol use has been reported.

PREGNANCY: Category C, not for use in nursing.

MECHANISM OF ACTION: Macrolactam ascomycin derivative; not fully established. Suspected to bind with high affinity to macrophilin-12 (FKBP-12) and inhibit the calcium-dependent phosphatase, calcineurin. Consequently, this inhibits T cell activation by blocking the transcription of early cytokines. In particular, pimecrolimus inhibits at nanomolar concentrations Interleukin-2 and interferon gamma (Th1-type) and Interleukin-4 and Interleukin-10 (Th2-type) cytokine synthesis in human T cells. In addition, pimecrolimus prevents the release of inflammatory cytokines and mediators from mast cells in vitro after stimulation by antigen/IgE.

PHARMACOKINETICS: **Absorption:** C_{max}=1.4ng/mL (adults). **Distribution:** Plasma protein binding (99.5%). **Metabolism:** Liver via CYP3A. **Elimination:** Feces (78.4% metabolites, <1% unchanged).

NURSING CONSIDERATIONS

Assessment: Assess for malignant or pre-malignant skin conditions (eg, cutaneous-cell lymphoma), Netherton's syndrome or other skin diseases, viral or bacterial skin infections, generalized erythroderma, and possible drug interactions. Assess patient's age and pregnancy/nursing status.

Monitoring: Monitor for infections (eg, varicella virus infection, herpes simplex virus infection, eczema herpeticum), lymphomas, lymphadenopathy, skin malignancies, local symptoms such as skin burning (eg, burning sensation, stinging, soreness) or pruritus, and adverse reactions (eg, application-site reactions).

Patient Counseling: Inform not to use drug continuously for long periods of time and should be used only on areas of skin with eczema. Advise to d/c medication when signs/symptoms of eczema subside (eg, itching, rash, and redness). Contact physician if symptoms get worse, a skin infection develops, if burning on skin lasts >1 week or if symptoms do not improve after 6 weeks of treatment. Instruct to wash hands and dry skin before applying cream. Do not bathe, shower, or swim after applying cream. Avoid natural or artificial sunlight exposure while on therapy. Instruct not to cover treated skin area with bandages, dressings, or wraps. For external use only; avoid contact with eyes.

Administration: Topical route. **Storage:** 25°C (77°F); excursions permitted to 15-30°C (59-86°F). Do not freeze.

ELIGARD
leuprolide acetate (Sanofi-Aventis)

RX

THERAPEUTIC CLASS: Synthetic gonadotropin releasing hormone analog

INDICATIONS: Palliative treatment of advanced prostate cancer.

DOSAGE: *Adults:* 7.5mg SQ monthly or 22.5mg SQ q3 months or 30mg SQ q4 months or 45mg SQ q6 months.

HOW SUPPLIED: Inj: 7.5mg, 22.5mg, 30mg, 45mg

CONTRAINDICATIONS: Women who are or may become pregnant.

WARNINGS/PRECAUTIONS: Transient increase in serum concentration of testosterone and worsening of symptoms or onset of new signs/symptoms during 1st few weeks of therapy may occur. Closely monitor patients with metastatic vertebral lesions and/or urinary tract obstruction during 1st few weeks of therapy. Cases of ureteral obstruction and/or spinal cord compression reported; institute standard treatment if these complications occur. Suppression of pituitary-gonadal system reported. Hyperglycemia, increased risk of developing diabetes and myocardial infarction (MI), sudden cardiac death, and stroke reported in men.

ADVERSE REACTIONS: Hot flashes/sweats, injection site reactions (eg, pain, erythema, bruising), malaise/fatigue, testicular atrophy, weakness, gynecomastia, myalgia, dizziness, decreased libido, clamminess.

PREGNANCY: Category X, not for use in nursing.

MECHANISM OF ACTION: Synthetic gonadotropin releasing hormone analog; inhibits pituitary gonadotropin secretion and suppresses testicular and ovarian steroidogenesis when given continuously.

PHARMACOKINETICS: Absorption: (7.5mg dose; 1st inj) C_{max}=25.3ng/mL, T_{max}=5 hrs. (22.5mg dose; 1st inj, 2nd inj) C_{max}=127ng/mL, 107ng/mL, T_{max}=5 hrs. (30mg dose; 1st inj) C_{max}=150ng/mL, T_{max}=3.3 hrs. (45mg dose; 1st inj, 2nd inj): C_{max}=82ng/mL, 102ng/mL, T_{max}=4.5 hrs. **Distribution**: (IV bolus dose) V_d=27L; plasma protein binding (43-49%). **Metabolism**: Pentapeptide (M-1) metabolite (major metabolite). **Elimination**: (1mg IV bolus dose) $T_{1/2}$=3 hrs.

NURSING CONSIDERATIONS

Assessment: Assess for pregnancy, diabetes, cardiovascular disease (CVD) risk factors, severity of prostate cancer, hypersensitivity to the drug or its components, metastatic vertebral lesions, and urinary tract obstructions.

Monitoring: Periodically monitor pregnancy, blood glucose, HbA1c, and response by measuring serum concentrations of testosterone and prostate specific antigen (PSA). Monitor for worsening/onset of signs and symptoms (eg, bone pain, neuropathy, hematuria, bladder outlet obstruction), spinal cord compression, ureteral obstruction, anaphylactic reactions, suppression of pituitary-gonadal system, and signs/symptoms suggestive of CVD development.

Patient Counseling: Inform that hot flashes may be experienced. Inform that increased bone pain and difficulty in urinating, and onset or aggravation of weakness or paralysis may be experienced during the 1st few weeks of therapy. Notify a doctor if new or worsened symptoms after initial treatment develop. Inform about injection-site related adverse reactions (eg, transient burning/stinging, pain, bruising, and redness); inform the doctor if such reactions do not resolve. Contact physician immediately if an allergic reaction develops.

Administration: SQ route. Rotate inj sites. Specific inj location chosen should be an area with sufficient soft or loose SQ tissue; avoid brawny or fibrous SQ tissue or locations that can be rubbed or compressed. Refer to PI for mixing and administration procedures. Allow product to reach room temperature before using. **Storage:** 2-8°C (35.6-46.4°F). Once mixed, discard if not administered within 30 min.

ELLA RX
ulipristal acetate (Watson)

THERAPEUTIC CLASS: Emergency contraceptive kit

INDICATIONS: Emergency contraceptive for prevention of pregnancy following unprotected intercourse or a known or suspected contraceptive failure.

DOSAGE: *Adults:* Take 1 tab as soon as possible within 120 hrs (5 days) after unprotected intercourse or a known or suspected contraceptive failure. Consider repeating the dose if vomiting occurs within 3 hrs of intake. Take with or without food. Can be taken at any time during the menstrual cycle. *Pediatrics:* Postpubertal adolescent: Take 1 tab as soon as possible within 120 hrs (5 days) after unprotected intercourse or a known or suspected contraceptive failure. Consider repeating the dose if vomiting occurs within 3 hrs of intake. Take with or without food. Can be taken at any time during the menstrual cycle.

HOW SUPPLIED: Tab: 30mg

CONTRAINDICATIONS: Known or suspected pregnancy.

WARNINGS/PRECAUTIONS: Not indicated for termination of existing pregnancy. Exclude pregnancy prior to prescribing; perform pregnancy test if pregnancy cannot be excluded. History of ectopic pregnancy is not a contraindication to use. Consider possible ectopic pregnancy if lower abdominal pain or pregnancy occurs following use. For occasional use as emergency contraceptive only; should not replace regular method of contraception. Repeated use not recommended within the same menstrual cycle. Rapid return of fertility is likely following use; routine contraception should be continued or initiated as soon as possible following use. After intake, menses sometimes occur earlier or later than expected; rule out pregnancy if menses delayed >1 week. Intermenstrual bleeding reported. Does not protect against HIV infection (AIDS) or other sexually transmitted infections (STIs).

ADVERSE REACTIONS: Headache, abdominal/upper abdominal pain, nausea, dysmenorrhea, fatigue, dizziness.

INTERACTIONS: Concomitant use with drugs or herbal products that induce enzymes including CYP3A4, may decrease plasma concentrations and may decrease effectiveness (eg, barbiturates, bosentan, carbamazepine, felbamate, griseofulvin, oxcarbazepine, phenytoin, rifampin, St. John's wort, topiramate). CYP3A4 inhibitors (eg, itraconazole, ketoconazole) may increase plasma concentrations. May reduce contraceptive action of regular hormonal contraceptive methods.

PREGNANCY: Category X, not for use in nursing.

MECHANISM OF ACTION: Synthetic progesterone agonist/antagonist; postpones follicular rupture when taken immediately before ovulation. The likely primary mechanism of action for emergency contraception is inhibition or delay of ovulation; however, alterations to the endometrium that may affect implantation may also contribute to efficacy.

PHARMACOKINETICS: Absorption: C_{max}=176ng/mL; T_{max}=0.9 hr; AUC_{0-t}=548ng•hr/mL. (Monodemethyl-ulipristal acetate) C_{max}=69ng/mL; T_{max}=1 hr; AUC_{0-t}=240ng•hr/mL. **Distribution:** Plasma protein binding (>94%). **Metabolism:** CYP3A4. Monodemethyl-ulipristal acetate (active metabolite). **Elimination:** $T_{1/2}$=32.4 hrs. (Monodemethyl-ulipristal acetate) $T_{1/2}$=27 hrs.

NURSING CONSIDERATIONS

Assessment: Assess for pregnancy/nursing status and possible drug interactions.

Monitoring: Monitor for ectopic pregnancy (eg, lower abdominal pain) and effect on menstrual cycle.

Patient Counseling: Instruct to take as soon as possible and not >120 hrs after unprotected intercourse or a known or suspected contraceptive failure. Advise not to take if pregnancy is known or suspected; inform that therapy is not indicated for termination of an existing pregnancy. Advise to contact healthcare provider immediately if vomiting occurs within 3 hrs of taking the tablet or if menstration is delayed by more than a week, beyond the date that was expected. Instruct to seek medical attention if severe lower abdominal pain 3-5 weeks after taking medication is experienced. Advise not to use as routine contraception, or to use it repeatedly in the same menstrual cycle. Inform that therapy may reduce contraceptive action of regular hormonal contraceptive methods; instruct to use a reliable barrier method of contraception after using medication, for any subsequent acts of intercourse that occur in that same menstrual cycle. Inform that drug does not protect against HIV infection (AIDS) and other STDs. Advise not to use if breastfeeding.

Administration: Oral route. **Storage:** 20-25°C (68-77°F). Keep blister in the outer carton in order to protect from light.

ELLENCE   RX
epirubicin HCl (Pfizer)

> Severe local tissue necrosis with extravasation. Not for IM/SQ administration. Myocardial toxicity manifested by congestive heart failure may occur during therapy or months to years after. May increase risk of cardiac toxicity with concomitant radiotherapy to the mediastinal/pericardial area, previous therapy with other anthracyclines or anthracenediones, or concomitant use of other cardiotoxic drugs. Secondary acute myelogenous leukemia (AML) reported in breast cancer-treated patients. Occurrence of refractory secondary leukemia with DNA-damaging antineoplastics, heavy pretreatment with cytotoxic drugs, or escalated doses of anthracyclines. Reduce dose with hepatic dysfunction. Severe myelosuppression may occur. Administer only under supervision of a physician experienced in chemotherapeutic agents.

THERAPEUTIC CLASS: Anthracycline

INDICATIONS: Component of adjuvant therapy in patients with evidence of axillary node tumor involvement following resection of primary breast cancer.

DOSAGE: *Adults:* Initial: 100-120mg/m², repeat at 3- to 4-week cycles. May give total dose on Day 1 of each cycle or divide equally on Days 1 and 8. Bone Marrow Dysfunction: Initial: 75-90mg/m². Hepatic Dysfunction: Bilirubin 1.2-3mg/dL or AST 2-4X ULN: Give 1/2 of initial dose. Bilirubin >3mg/dL or AST >4X ULN: Give 1/4 of initial dose. Severe Renal Dysfunction: Serum Creatinine >5mg/dL: Lower dose. Give prophylactic therapy with SMZ-TMP or fluoro-quinolone with 120mg/m² regimen. Consider pretreatment with antiemetics. Adjust dose after first treatment cycle based on hematologic and nonhematologic toxicities; refer to PI for dosing. Administer by IV infusion.

HOW SUPPLIED: Inj: 2mg/mL [25mL, 100mL]

CONTRAINDICATIONS: Baseline neutrophils <1500 cells/mm³, severe myocardial insufficiency, recent MI, severe arrhythmias, previous anthracycline therapy with maximum cumulative dose, anthracenedione hypersensitivity, severe hepatic dysfunction.

WARNINGS/PRECAUTIONS: Increased risk of cardiotoxicity with active or dormant CV disease. Use extreme caution if exceeding cumulative dose of 900mg/m². Resolve acute toxicities from other cytotoxic agents prior to initiation. Monitor CBC, total bilirubin, AST, SrCr, and cardiac function before and during each cycle. May induce hyperuricemia. Potential for tumor lysis syndrome; monitor serum uric acid, potassium, calcium phosphate, and creatinine immediately after initial therapy. Thrombophlebitis, thromboembolic phenomena reported. Excessive rapid administration may cause facial flushing as well as local erythematous streaking along the vein.

ADVERSE REACTIONS: AML, tissue necrosis, myocardial toxicity, myelosuppression, hematologic abnormalities, amenorrhea, hot flashes, lethargy, fever, GI disturbances, infection, conjunctivitis/keratitis, alopecia, local toxicity, rash/itch.

INTERACTIONS: See Boxed Warning. Additive toxicity with other cytotoxic drugs. Cyclophosphamide and fluorouracil may cause severe leukopenia, neutropenia, thrombocytopenia, and anemia. Monitor closely with cardioactive compounds that could cause heart failure (eg, CCBs). Caution with agents that cause changes in hepatic function. AUC increased with cimetidine; d/c cimetidine during therapy. Previous radiation therapy may induce inflammatory recall reaction at irradiation site. Administration of paclitaxel prior to therapy increases AUC levels.

PREGNANCY: Category D, not for use in nursing.

MECHANISM OF ACTION: Anthracycline; complexes with DNA by intercalating its planar rings between nucleotide base pairs, inhibiting nucleic acid (DNA and RNA) and protein synthesis, triggering DNA cleavage by topoisomerase II, inhibits DNA helicase activity, and generates free radicals.

PHARMACOKINETICS: Absorption: IV administration of variable doses resulted in different parameters. **Distribution:** Plasma protein binding (77%). **Metabolism:** Liver (extensive and rapid); reduction, conjugation, hydrolytic, and redox process. Epirubicinol (metabolite). **Elimination:** Biliary (major), urine (minor).

NURSING CONSIDERATIONS

Assessment: Assess for baseline neutrophil count >1500 cells/mm³, CVD (insufficiency, MI, arrhythmias), acute toxicities (prior therapy), hepatic/renal dysfunction, risk factors for cardiac toxicities, pregnancy status, and possible drug interactions. Obtain baseline CBC, total bilirubin, AST, creatinine, and cardiac function (LVEF). Assess need for antiemetics.

Monitoring: Monitor total and differential WBC, RBC, platelet count, AST, total bilirubin, and cardiac function (MUGA, ECHO) before and during each cycle. Monitor for hypersensitivity reaction, CHF, liver dysfunction, myelosuppression, hyperuricemia (tumor lysis syndrome), extravasation, facial flushing or local erythematous streaking, and recall reaction (prior radiation).

Patient Counseling: Advise to seek medical attention if vomiting, dehydration, fever, evidence of infection, symptoms of CHF, or injection-site pain occur. Inform alopecia will develop and urine may appear red for 1-2 days after administration. Inform of risk of irreversible myocardial damage. Instruct men to use effective contraceptive methods. Inform females about risk of premature menopause.

Administration: IV route. Administer by IV infusion; see PI for administration technique. **Storage:** Refrigerate; 2-8°C (36-46°F). Do not freeze. Protect from light.

ELOCON   RX
mometasone furoate (Schering)

THERAPEUTIC CLASS: Corticosteroid

INDICATIONS: Relief of inflammatory and pruritic manifestations of corticosteroid-responsive dermatoses.

DOSAGE: *Adults:* (Cre, Oint) Apply qd. (Lot) Apply a few drops qd. Re-assess if no improvement seen within 2 weeks.
Pediatrics: (Cre, Oint) ≥12 yrs: Apply qd. (Lot) ≥2yrs: Apply a few drops qd. Re-assess if no improvement seen within 2 weeks.

HOW SUPPLIED: Cre, Oint: 0.1% [15g, 45g]; Lot: 0.1% [30mL, 60mL]

WARNINGS/PRECAUTIONS: Systemic absorption may produce reversible hypothalamic-pituitary-adrenal (HPA) axis suppression, manifestations of Cushing's syndrome, hyperglycemia, and glucosuria. D/C if irritation occurs. Use appropriate antifungal or antibacterial agent with dermatological infections. Pediatric patients may be more susceptible to systemic toxicity. Lotion not recommended in children <12 yrs old. Caution when applied to large surface areas or with occlusive dressings.

ADVERSE REACTIONS: Burning, pruritus, skin atrophy, rosacea, acneiform reaction, tingling, stinging, furunculosis, folliculitis, hypertrichosis, hypopigmentation, perioral dermatitis, allergic contact dermatitis, striae, miliaria.

PREGNANCY: Category C, caution in nursing.

MECHANISM OF ACTION: Corticosteroid; possesses anti-inflammatory, antipruritic, and vasconstrictive properties. Suspected to induce phospholipase A_2 inhibitory proteins, lipocortins. Lipocortins control biosynthesis of potent mediators of inflammation (eg, prostaglandins and leukotrienes) by inhibiting release of their precursor, arachidonic acid.

PHARMACOKINETICS: Absorption: Extent of absorption depends on skin integrity, vehicle, and use of occlusive dressing.

NURSING CONSIDERATIONS

Assessment: Assess for hypersensitivity and use in pregnant/nursing patients.

Monitoring: Monitor for signs/symptoms of HPA axis suppression, glucocorticoid insufficiency, Cushing's syndrome, hyperglycemia, glucosuria, skin irritation, allergic contact dermatitis (eg, failure to heal), and skin infections. In patients applying medication to large surface areas or using occlusive dressings, perform periodic monitoring for HPA-axis suppression by using ACTH stimulation, AM plasma cortisol, and urinary free cortisol tests. In pediatric patients, monitor for systemic toxicity, HPA-axis suppression, Cushing's syndrome, linear growth retardation, delayed weight gain, and intracranial HTN.

Patient Counseling: Avoid contact with eyes, face, underarms, and groin. Do not wrap, cover, or bandage treated skin unless directed by physician. Instruct patients to report adverse reactions. Do not apply medication in diaper area. Contact physician if no improvement within 2 weeks. Notify physician before using other corticosteroid therapies.

Administration: Topical route. **Storage:** 25°C (77°F); excursions permitted to 15-30°C (59-86°F).

ELOXATIN   RX
oxaliplatin (Sanofi-Aventis)

> Anaphylactic-like reactions may occur within minutes of administration.

THERAPEUTIC CLASS: Organoplatinum complex

INDICATIONS: Treatment of advanced metastatic carcinoma of colon or rectum and adjuvant treatment of Stage III colon cancer patients who have undergone complete resection of the primary tumor in combination with infusional 5-fluorouracil (5-FU) and leucovorin (LV).

DOSAGE: *Adults:* Advanced Colorectal Cancer: Day 1: 85mg/m² IV with LV 200mg/m²; give over 120 min in separate bags using a Y-line; followed by 5-FU 400mg/m² bolus over 2-4 min, then 5-FU 600mg/m² as a 22-hr infusion. Day 2: LV 200mg/m² over 120 min; followed by 5-FU 400mg/m² bolus over 2-4 min, then 5-FU 600mg/m² as a 22-hr infusion. Repeat cycle every 2 weeks. Persistent Grade 2 Neurosensory Events: Reduce oxaliplatin to 65mg/m². Grade 3 Neurosensory Events: Consider d/c. After Recovery From Grade 3/4 GI or Grade 4 Hematologic Toxicity: Reduce oxaliplatin to 65mg/m² and 5-FU by 20%. Adjuvant Therapy Stage III Colon Cancer: Recommended cycle every 2 weeks for 6 months. Persistent Grade 2 Neurosensory Events: Reduce oxaliplatin to 75mg/m². Persistent Grade 3 Neurosensory Events: Consider d/c. After Recovery From Grade 3/4 GI or Grade 3/4 Hematologic Toxicity: Reduce oxaliplatin to 75mg/m² and 5-FU to 300mg/m² bolus and 500mg/m² 22-hr infusion.

HOW SUPPLIED: Inj: 50mg, 100mg, 200mg

WARNINGS/PRECAUTIONS: Acute and persistent neuropathy reported. Cold may exacerbate acute neurological symptoms; avoid ice for mucositis prophylaxis. Potentially fatal pulmonary fibrosis reported. If unexplained respiratory symptoms develop, d/c until interstitial lung disease or pulmonary fibrosis is ruled out. Monitor WBC with differential, Hgb, platelets, and blood chemistries (including ALT, AST, bilirubin, creatinine) before each cycle. Caution with pre-existing renal impairment.

ADVERSE REACTIONS: Peripheral sensory neuropathy, fatigue, nausea, neutropenia, emesis, diarrhea, thrombocytopenia, anemia, increase in transaminases and alkaline phosphatase, stomatitis, transient vision loss, and interstitial or other lung diseases.

INTERACTIONS: Increased 5-FU plasma levels with doses of 130mg/m² oxaliplatin dosed every 3 weeks; clearance may be decreased with nephrotoxic agents.

PREGNANCY: Category D, not for use in nursing.

MECHANISM OF ACTION: Organoplatinum complex; inhibits DNA replication and transcription.

PHARMACOKINETICS: Absorption: C_{max}=0.814mcg/mL. **Distribution**: V_d=440L; plasma protein binding (>90%). **Metabolism**: Rapid, nonenzymatic biotransformation. **Elimination**: Urine (54%), feces (2%).

NURSING CONSIDERATIONS

Assessment: Assess for pre-existing hepatic/renal impairment, pregnancy status, hypersensitivity to platinum compounds, and possible drug interactions.

Monitoring: Monitor LFTs, WBC with differential, Hgb, platelet count, bilirubin, and creatinine periodically and before each dose. Monitor for signs/symptoms of anaphylactic reactions, neuropathy, neurosensory toxicity, portal HTN, liver/renal dysfunction, and pulmonary toxicity.

Patient Counseling: Inform of pregnancy risks and of neurologic effects and persistent neurosensory toxicity that may be precipitated by exposure to cold or cold objects. Avoid cold drinks and ice, cover exposed skin prior to exposure to cold temperature or cold objects. Advise to seek medical attention if persistent vomiting, diarrhea, fever, signs of dehydration or infection, cough, breathing difficulties, and allergic reactions (eg, rash, urticaria, erythema, pruritus, bronchospasm, and hypotension) occur. Vision abnormalities may impair ability to drive and use machinery; promptly report any vision problems to physician.

Administration: IV route. Infusion line should be flushed with D5W prior to administration of any concomitant medication. **Storage**: 25°C (77°F); excursions permitted to 15-30°C (59-86°F). Protect from light and do not freeze.

EMEND   RX
aprepitant (Merck)

THERAPEUTIC CLASS: Substance P/neurokinin 1 receptor antagonist

INDICATIONS: For prevention of acute and delayed N/V, in combination with other antiemetics, associated with initial and repeat courses of highly emetogenic cancer chemotherapy including high-dose cisplatin or moderately emetogenic cancer chemotherapy. Prevention of postoperative nausea and vomiting (PONV).

DOSAGE: *Adults:* Prevention of Chemo-Induced N/V: Day 1: 125mg 1 hr prior to chemotherapy. Days 2 and 3: 80mg qam. Regimen should include a corticosteroid and a 5-HT$_3$ antagonist. Refer to PI for dosing with corticosteroid (dexamethasone) and 5-HT$_3$ antagonist (ondansetron). Prevention of PONV: 40mg within 3 hrs prior to induction of anesthesia.

HOW SUPPLIED: Cap: 40mg, 80mg, 125mg; TriPack: (one 125mg & two 80mg caps)

CONTRAINDICATIONS: Concurrent treatment with pimozide, terfenadine, astemizole, or cisapride.

WARNINGS/PRECAUTIONS: Not recommended for chronic continuous use. Caution with severe hepatic impairment (Child-Pugh score >9).

ADVERSE REACTIONS: Asthenia/fatigue, N/V, constipation, diarrhea, hiccups, anorexia, headache, dehydration, pruritus, dizziness, alopecia, hypotension, pyrexia.

INTERACTIONS: See Contraindications. May increase levels of drugs metabolized by CYP3A4, including chemotherapeutic agents (eg, docetaxel, paclitaxel, etoposide, irinotecan, ifosfamide, imatinib, vinorelbine, vinblastine, and vincristine), and certain benzodiazepines (eg, midazolam, alprazolam, triazolam). Reduce dose of dexamethasone or methylprednisolone. May reduce efficacy of oral contraceptives; use alternative or back-up contraception during treatment and for 1 month after last dose. May decrease levels of warfarin, tolbutamide, phenytoin, or other drugs metabolized by CYP2C9. May increase plasma concentration with CYP3A4 inhibitors. Caution when used with strong/moderate inhibitors of CYP3A4 (eg, ketoconazole, itraconazole, nefazodone, troleandomycin, clarithromycin, ritonavir, nelfinavir, diltiazem). Decreased efficacy with strong CYP3A4 inducers (eg, rifampin, carbamazepine, phenytoin). Concomitant paroxetine may decrease levels of both drugs. Coadministration with warfarin may result in a clinically significant decrease in INR of prothrombin time.

PREGNANCY: Category B, not for use in nursing.

MECHANISM OF ACTION: Substance P/neurokinin 1 receptor antagonist; augments the antiemetic activity of the 5-HT$_3$ receptor antagonist ondansetron and the corticosteroid dexamethasone and inhibits both the acute and delayed phases of cisplatin-induced emesis.

PHARMACOKINETICS: Absorption: (40mg) AUC=7.8mcg•hr/mL, C$_{max}$=0.7mcg/mL, T$_{max}$=3 hrs. Refer to PI for detailed information. **Distribution:** V$_d$=70L; plasma protein binding (>95%); crosses blood-brain barrier. **Metabolism:** Liver (extensive via CYP3A4 (major), 1A2 (minor), 2C19 (minor). Oxidation. **Elimination:** Urine (57%), feces (45%); T$_{1/2}$=9-13 hrs.

NURSING CONSIDERATIONS

Assessment: Assess for history of hypersensitivity reactions to the drug and its components, hepatic impairment, pregnancy/nursing status and possible drug interactions (eg, drugs metabolized, primarily by CYP3A4).

Monitoring: Monitor INR in 2-week period following therapy (especially at 7-10 days if on chronic warfarin therapy). Monitor for hypersensitivity reactions.

Patient Counseling: Instruct to take drug as prescribed. Instruct to d/c medication and to inform physician immediately if allergic reactions (eg, hives, rash, itching, and difficulty in breathing or swallowing) occur. Patients on chronic warfarin therapy should have clotting status closely monitored. Notify physician if using other prescription, OTC, or herbal products. Advise patient using hormonal contraceptives to use alternative or backup methods of contraception during therapy and for 1 month after the last dose of the medication.

Administration: Oral route. **Storage:** 20-25°C (68-77°F).

EMEND FOR INJECTION   RX
fosaprepitant dimeglumine (Merck)

THERAPEUTIC CLASS: Substance P/neurokinin 1 receptor antagonist

INDICATIONS: Prevention of acute and delayed N/V associated with initial and repeat courses of highly emetogenic cancer chemotherapy (HEC) including high-dose cisplatin or moderately emetogenic cancer chemotherapy (MEC) in adults in combination with other antiemetics.

DOSAGE: *Adults:* N/V Associated with HEC: 150mg IV infusion over 20-30 min. N/V Associated with HEC/MEC: 115mg IV infusion over 15 min. Give 30 min prior to chemotherapy on Day 1 only of a single or 3-day dosing regimen. Regimen should include a corticosteroid and a 5-HT$_3$ antagonist. Refer to PI for dosing with corticosteroid (dexamethasone) and 5-HT$_3$ antagonist (ondansetron).

HOW SUPPLIED: Inj (powder): 115mg, 150mg

CONTRAINDICATIONS: Concurrent use with pimozide or cisapride.

WARNINGS/PRECAUTIONS: Has not been studied for treatment of established N/V. Hypersensitivity reactions reported; avoid reinitiating infusion if hypersensitivity occurs during 1st-time use. Not recommended for chronic continuous use. Caution with severe hepatic insufficiency (Child-Pugh score >9).

ADVERSE REACTIONS: Infusion-site reactions (erythema, pruritus, pain, induration), erythema, BP increased, thrombophlebitis.

INTERACTIONS: See Contraindications. May increase levels of drugs metabolized by CYP3A4, including chemotherapeutic agents (eg, docetaxel, paclitaxel, etoposide, irinotecan, ifosfamide, imatinib, vinorelbine, vinblastine, vincristine), and certain benzodiazepines (eg, midazolam, alprazolam, triazolam). May increase levels of dexamethasone and methylprednisolone; reduce dose of PO dexamethasone/methylprednisolone by 50% and IV methylprednisolone by 25% when given with 115mg fosaprepitant followed by aprepitant. May reduce efficacy of hormonal contraceptives (eg, ethinyl estradiol, norethindrone); use alternative or back-up contraception during treatment and for 1 month after last dose. May decrease levels of warfarin, tolbutamide. May increase levels with CYP3A4 inhibitors; caution with strong/moderate inhibitors of CYP3A4 (eg, ketoconazole, itraconazole, nefazodone, troleandomycin, clarithromycin, ritonavir, nelfinavir, diltiazem). May increase levels of diltiazem resulting in further max decrease in BP. Decreased levels and efficacy with strong CYP3A4 inducers (eg, rifampin, carbamazepine, phenytoin). Concomitant paroxetine may decrease levels of both drugs. Coadministration with warfarin may result in a clinically significant decrease in INR of PT.

PREGNANCY: Category B, not for use in nursing.

MECHANISM OF ACTION: Substance P/neurokinin 1 receptor antagonist; prodrug of aprepitant. Augments the antiemetic activity of the 5-HT$_3$ receptor antagonist ondansetron and the corticosteroid dexamethasone and inhibits both the acute and delayed phases of cisplatin-induced emesis.

PHARMACOKINETICS: Absorption: (Aprepitant, given as 150mg IV fosaprepitant) AUC=37.38mcg•hr/mL, C_{max}=4.15mcg/mL; (Given as 115mg IV fosaprepitant) AUC=31.7mcg•hr/mL, C_{max}=3.27mcg/mL. **Distribution:** (Aprepitant) V_d=70L; plasma protein binding (>95%). **Metabolism:** Rapidly converted to aprepitant by liver and extrahepatic tissues. Aprepitant by CYP3A4 (major), 1A2 and 2C19 (minor) via oxidation. **Elimination:** (100mg IV fosaprepitant) Urine (57%), feces (45%); (Aprepitant) $T_{1/2}$=9-13 hrs.

NURSING CONSIDERATIONS

Assessment: Assess for history of hypersensitivity to drug and its components, hepatic function, pregnancy/nursing status, and possible drug interactions.

Monitoring: Monitor INR in the 2-week period following therapy, especially at 7-10 days if taking chronic warfarin therapy. Monitor for hypersensitivity reactions and other adverse reactions.

Patient Counseling: Instruct to d/c medication and to inform physician immediately if allergic reactions (eg, hives, rash, itching, red face/skin, difficulty in breathing or swallowing) occur. Advise patients on chronic warfarin therapy should have clotting status closely monitored particularly 7-10 days following initiation with each chemotherapy cycle. Counsel patients how to care for local reactions and when to seek further evaluation. Notify physician if using other prescription, OTC, or herbal products. Instruct patient using hormonal contraceptives to use alternative or back-up methods of contraception during therapy and for 1 month after the last dose.

Administration: IV route. Refer to PI for compatibility and preparation.
Storage: 2-8°C (36-46°F). Reconstituted Sol: Stable for 24 hrs ≤25°C.

EMLA
RX

prilocaine - lidocaine (APP Pharmaceuticals)

THERAPEUTIC CLASS: Acetamide local anesthetic

INDICATIONS: Topical anesthetic for use on normal intact skin. Topical anesthetic for genital mucous membranes for superficial minor surgery and as pretreatment for infiltration anesthesia.

DOSAGE: *Adults:* Apply thick layer of cream to intact skin and cover with occlusive dressing. Minor Dermal Procedure: Apply 2.5g over 20-25cm^2 of skin surface for at least 1 hr. Major Dermal Procedure: Apply 2g/10cm^2 of skin for 2 hrs. Adult Male Genital Skin: Apply 1g/10cm^2 of skin surface for 15 min. Female External Genitalia: Apply 5-10g for 5-10 min.
Pediatrics: 7-12 yrs and >20kg: Max: 20g/200cm^2 for up to 4 hrs. 1-6 yrs and >10 kg: Max:10g/100cm^2 for up to 4 hrs. 3-12 months and >5 kg: Max: 2g/20cm^2 for up to 4 hrs. 0-3 months or <5kg: Max: 1g/10cm^2 for up to 1 hr. If >3 months and does not meet minimum weight requirement, max dose restricted to corresponding weight.

HOW SUPPLIED: Cre: (Lidocaine-Prilocaine) 2.5%-2.5%

WARNINGS/PRECAUTIONS: Application to larger areas or for longer than recommended times, may result in serious adverse effects. Should not be used where penetration or migration beyond the tympanic membrane into the middle ear is possible. Avoid with congenital or idiopathic methemoglobinemia and infants <12 months receiving treatment with methemoglobin-inducing agents. Very young or patients with glucose-6-phosphate dehydrogenase (G6PD) deficiency are more susceptible to methemoglobinemia. Reports of methemoglobinemia in infants and children following excessive applications. Monitor neonates and infants up to 3 months for Met-Hb levels before, during, and after application. Repeated doses may increase blood levels; caution in patients who may be more susceptible to systemic effects (eg, acutely ill, debilitated, elderly). Avoid eye contact and application to open wounds. Has been shown to inhibit viral and bacterial growth. Caution with severe hepatic disease and in patients with drug sensitivities.

ADVERSE REACTIONS: Erythema, edema, abnormal sensations, paleness (pallor or blanching), altered temperature sensations, burning sensation, itching, rash.

INTERACTIONS: Additive and potentially synergistic toxic effects with Class I antiarrhythmic drugs (eg, tocainide, mexiletine). May have additive cardiac effects with Class III antiarrhythmic drugs (eg, amiodarone, bretylium, sotalol, dofetilide). Avoid drugs associated with drug-induced methemoglobinemia (eg, sulfonamides, acetaminophen, acetanilid, aniline dyes, benzocaine, chloroquine, dapsone, naphthalene, nitrates/nitrites, nitrofurantoin, nitroglycerin, nitroprusside, phenobarbital, phenytoin, primaquine, pamaquine, para-aminosalicylic acid, phenacetin, quinine). Caution with other products containing lidocaine/prilocaine; consider the amount absorbed from all formulations.

PREGNANCY: Category B, caution in nursing.

MECHANISM OF ACTION: Amide-type local anesthetics; stabilizes neuronal membranes by inhibiting ionic fluxes required for initiation and conduction impulses, thereby effecting local anesthetic action.

PHARMACOKINETICS: Absorption: Lidocaine: (3 hrs 400cm^2) C_{max}=0.12mcg/mL, T_{max}=4 hrs; (24 hrs 400cm^2) C_{max}=0.28mcg/mL, T_{max}=10 hrs. Prilocaine: (3 hrs 400cm^2) C_{max}=0.07mcg/mL, T_{max}=4 hrs; (24 hrs 400 cm^2) C_{max}=0.14mcg/mL, T_{max}=10 hrs. **Distribution:** (IV) V_d=1.5L/kg (lidocaine), 2.6L/kg (prilocaine); (Cre) plasma protein binding 70% (lidocaine), 55% (prilocaine).

Crosses placental and blood-brain barrier; found in breast milk. **Metabolism:** Lidocaine: Liver (rapid); monoethylglycinexylidide and glycinexylidide (active metabolites). Prilocaine: Liver and kidneys by amidases; ortho-toluidine and N-n-propylalanine (metabolites). **Elimination:** (IV) Lidocaine: Urine (>98%); $T_{1/2}$=110 min. Prilocaine: $T_{1/2}$=70 min.

NURSING CONSIDERATIONS

Assessment: Assess for congenital or idiopathic methemoglobinemia, G6PD deficiency, hepatic disease, open wounds, presence of acute illness, presence of debilitation, history of drug sensitivities, pregnancy/nursing status, and for possible drug interactions. In neonates and infants ≤3 months, obtain Met-Hb levels prior to application.

Monitoring: Monitor for signs/symptoms of methemoglobinemia, ototoxicity, local skin reactions and for allergic/anaphylactoid reactions. Monitor Met-Hb levels in neonates and infants ≤3 months during and after application.

Patient Counseling: Inform about potential risks/benefits of drug. Advise to avoid inadvertent trauma to treated area. Instruct not to apply near eyes or on open wounds. Apply as directed by physician. Advise to notify physician if pregnant/nursing or planning to become pregnant. Instruct to remove cream and consult physician if child becomes very dizzy, excessively sleepy, or develops duskiness on the face or lips after application.

Administration: Topical route. Not for ophthalmic use. **Storage:** 20-25°C (68-77°F). Keep tightly closed.

EMSAM   RX
selegiline (Dey)

> Antidepressants increased the risk of suicidal thinking and behavior (suicidality) in short-term studies in children, adolescents, and young adults with major depressive disorder (MDD) and other psychiatric disorders. Monitor and observe closely for clinical worsening, suicidality, or unusual changes in behavior in patients who are started on antidepressant therapy. Not approved for use in pediatric patients.

THERAPEUTIC CLASS: Monoamine oxidase inhibitor (Type B)

INDICATIONS: Treatment of major depressive disorder.

DOSAGE: *Adults:* Initial/Target Dose: 6mg/24 hrs. Titrate: May increase in increments of 3mg/24 hrs at intervals no less than 2 weeks. Max: 12mg/24 hrs. Elderly: 6mg/24 hrs. Increase dose cautiously and monitor closely.

HOW SUPPLIED: Patch: 6mg/24 hrs, 9mg/24 hrs, 12mg/24 hrs [30ˢ]

CONTRAINDICATIONS: Pheochromocytoma. Concomitant SSRIs (eg, fluoxetine, sertraline, paroxetine), dual serotonin and norepinephrine reuptake inhibitors (eg, venlafaxine, duloxetine), TCAs (eg, imipramine, amitriptyline), bupropion, buspirone, meperidine, analgesic agents (eg, tramadol, methadone, and propoxyphene), dextromethorphan, St. John's wort, mirtazapine, cyclobenzaprine, carbamazepine, oxcarbazepine, sympathetic amines (including amphetamines), cold products and weight-reducing preparations that contain vasoconstrictors (eg, pseudoephedrine, phenylephrine, phenylpropanolamine, ephedrine), oral selegiline, other MAOIs (eg, isocarboxazid, phenelzine, tranylcypromine), general anesthesia agents, cocaine, or local anesthesia-containing sympathomimetic vasoconstrictors. Dietary modifications required with 9mg/24 hrs and 12mg/24 hrs systems.

WARNINGS/PRECAUTIONS: Monitor for clinical worsening of depression, suicidality, and unusual changes in behavior, especially during the initial few months of therapy or at times of dose changes. Hypertensive crisis may occur with ingestion of foods with a high concentration of tyramine. Postural hypotension may occur; consider dosage adjustment with orthostatic symptoms. Activation of mania/hypomania may occur; caution with history of mania. Caution with disorders or conditions that can produce altered metabolism or hemodynamic responses. Avoid elective surgery requiring general anesthesia.

ADVERSE REACTIONS: Headache, diarrhea, dyspepsia, insomnia, dry mouth, pharyngitis, sinusitis, application-site reaction, rash, low systolic BP, orthostatic hypotension, weight change.

INTERACTIONS: See Contraindications. Avoid alcohol.

PREGNANCY: Category C, caution in nursing.

MECHANISM OF ACTION: MAOI: Mechanism of action as antidepressant not established; presumed to be linked to potentiation of monoamine neurotransmitter activity in the central nervous system (CNS) resulting from its inhibition of MAO activity.

PHARMACOKINETICS: Absorption: AUC=46.2ng•hr/mL. **Distribution**: Plasma protein binding (90%). **Metabolism**: Hepatic (N-dealkylation, N-depropargylation) via CYP2B6, 2C9, 3A4/5 (major), CYP2A6 (minor); N-desmethylselegiline, methamphetamine, amphetamine (metabolites). **Elimination**: Urine (10%), feces (2%); $T_{1/2}$=18-25 hrs.

NURSING CONSIDERATIONS

Assessment: Assess for risk of bipolar disorder, history of mania, pre-existing orthostasis, and disease/condition that alters metabolism or hemodynamic response, pregnancy/nursing status, and possible drug interactions.

Monitoring: Monitor for signs/symptoms of clinical worsening (suicidality, unusual changes in behavior), hypertensive crises (occipital headaches, neck stiffness, N/V, sweating), postural hypotension, and cognitive and motor impairment.

Patient Counseling: Avoid concomitant use of alcohol, tyramine-containing foods/supplements/beverages (during and 2 weeks following d/c), and cough medicine containing dextromethorphan. Instruct to use only one patch at a time; do not cut patch into smaller portions. Seek medical attention for symptoms of hypertensive crises (occipital headaches, neck stiffness, N/V, sweating), postural hypotension, mania, and clinical worsening (suicidal ideation, unusual changes in behavior). May impair physical/mental abilities. Instruct to continue therapy as directed despite improvement. Avoid exposing application site to external sources of direct heat (heating pads, hot tubs). Advise to change position gradually if lightheaded, faint, or dizzy.

Administration: Transdermal route. Apply to dry, intact skin on the upper torso, upper thigh, or outer surface of upper arm once every 24 hrs. **Storage**: 20-25°C (68-77°F). Do not store outside sealed pouch.

EMTRIVA   RX
emtricitabine (Gilead)

> Lactic acidosis and severe hepatomegaly with steatosis, including fatal cases, reported with nucleoside analogs alone or with concomitant antiretrovirals. Not indicated for the treatment of chronic hepatitis B virus (HBV) infection. Severe acute exacerbations of hepatitis B reported in patients coinfected with HBV and HIV-1 upon discontinuation. Monitor hepatic function closely for at least several months. If appropriate, initiation of anti-HBV therapy may be warranted.

THERAPEUTIC CLASS: Nucleoside analogue

INDICATIONS: Treatment of HIV-1 infection in combination with other antiretroviral agents.

DOSAGE: *Adults:* ≥18 yrs: Cap: 200mg qd. CrCl 30-49mL/min: 200mg q48h. CrCl 15-29mL/min: 200mg q72h. CrCl <15mL/min (including hemodialysis): 200mg q96h. Sol: 240mg (24mL) qd. CrCl 30-49mL/min: 120mg (12mL) qd. CrCl 15-29mL/min: 80mg (8mL) qd. CrCl <15mL/min (including hemodialysis): 60mg (6mL) qd.
Pediatrics: 3 months-17 yrs: Cap: >33kg: 200mg qd. Sol: 6mg/kg qd. Max: 240mg (24mL). 0-3 months: Sol: 3mg/kg qd.

HOW SUPPLIED: Cap: 200mg; Sol: 10mg/mL [170mL]

WARNINGS/PRECAUTIONS: Obesity and prolonged nucleoside exposure may be risk factors for lactic acidosis and severe hepatomegaly with steatosis. Caution with known risk factors for hepatic disease. D/C if findings suggestive of lactic acidosis or pronounced hepatotoxicity (hepatomegaly and steatosis) even in the absence of marked transaminase elevations) develop. Prior to treatment, all patients with HIV-1 should be tested for the presence of chronic HBV. Reduce dose with impaired renal function. Fat redistribution/accumulation including central obesity, dorsocervical fat enlargement, peripheral wasting, facial wasting, breast enlargement, and "cushingoid appearance" may develop. Immune reconstitution syndrome reported. Caution in elderly.

ADVERSE REACTIONS: Headache, diarrhea, nausea, fatigue, dizziness, depression, insomnia, abnormal dreams, rash, abdominal pain, asthenia, increased cough, rhinitis.

INTERACTIONS: Avoid coadministration with Atripla, Truvada, or lamivudine-containing products.

PREGNANCY: Category B, not for use in nursing.

MECHANISM OF ACTION: Nucleoside analog of cytidine; inhibits the activity of HIV-1 reverse transcriptase by competing with the natural substrate deoxycytidine 5'-triphosphate and incorporating into nascent viral DNA, resulting in chain termination.

PHARMACOKINETICS: Absorption: Rapid and extensive. T_{max}=1-2 hrs. (Cap) Absolute bioavailability (93%). C_{max}=1.8mcg/mL, AUC=10.0mcg•hr/mL. (Sol) Absolute bioavailability (75%). **Distribution:** Plasma protein binding (<4%). **Metabolism:** Hepatic (conjugation and oxidation). Metabolites: 3'-sulfoxide diastereomers and 2'-O-glucuronide. **Elimination:** Urine (86%), feces (14%); $T_{1/2}$=10 hrs.

NURSING CONSIDERATIONS

Assessment: Assess for risk factors for lactic acidosis, chronic HBV infection, hypersensitivity, renal impairment, risk factors for liver disease, obesity, prolonged nucleoside exposure, pregnancy/nursing status, and for possible drug interactions. Prior to therapy, assess CrCl in all patients. In HIV-1 patients, perform testing for presence of chronic HBV.

Monitoring: Monitor for signs/symptoms of lactic acidosis, hepatotoxicity (hepatomegaly and steatosis) exacerbations of hepatitis (liver decompensation, liver failure), immune reconstitution syndrome, redistribution/accumulation of body fat including central obesity, dorsocervical fat enlargement, peripheral wasting, facial wasting, breast enlargement, and cushingoid appearance. Closely monitor hepatic and renal function. Perform renal function test (CrCl).

Patient Counseling: Advise patients that therapy is not a cure for HIV-1 infection and they may continue to experience illnesses associated with HIV-1 including opportunistic infections. Inform that therapy has not been shown to reduce risk of transmission of HIV-1 to others through sexual contact or blood contamination. Advise to seek medical attention if symptoms of lactic acidosis, hepatotoxicity (including N/V, unusual or unexpected stomach discomfort, and weakness) occur. Advise that HIV-1 patients should be tested for HBV prior to therapy. Inform that severe acute exacerbations of hepatitis B may occur. Inform that it should not be coadministered with other drugs containing lamivudine. Inform that it is for oral ingestion only and to take with combination therapy on a regular dosing schedule to avoid missing doses.

Administration: Oral route. **Storage:** (Cap): 25°C (77F°); excursions permitted to 15-30°C (59-86°F). (Sol): Refrigerated 2-8°C (36-46°F); if stored at 25°C (77°), use within 3 months; excursions permitted to 15-30°C (59-86°F).

ENABLEX   RX
darifenacin (Warner Chilcott)

THERAPEUTIC CLASS: Muscarinic antagonist

INDICATIONS: Treatment of overactive bladder with symptoms of urge urinary incontinence, urgency and frequency.

DOSAGE: *Adults:* Initial: 7.5mg qd. Titrate: May increase to 15mg qd as early as 2 weeks after starting therapy. Moderate Hepatic Impairment (Child-Pugh

B)/Concomitant Potent CYP3A4 Inhibitors (eg, ketoconazole, itraconazole, ritonavir, nelfinavir, clarithromycin, nefazodone): Max: 7.5mg/day.

HOW SUPPLIED: Tab, Extended-Release: 7.5mg, 15mg

CONTRAINDICATIONS: Urinary retention, gastric retention, uncontrolled narrow-angle glaucoma, and in patients at risk for these conditions.

WARNINGS/PRECAUTIONS: Angioedema of the face, lips, tongue, and/or larynx reported. Angioedema with upper airway swelling may be life-threatening; d/c and institute appropriate therapy if involvement of the tongue, hypopharynx, or larynx occur. Risk of urinary retention; caution with significant bladder outflow obstruction. Risk of gastric retention; caution with GI obstructive disorders. May decrease GI motility; caution with severe constipation, ulcerative colitis, and myasthenia gravis. Caution with moderate hepatic impairment and in patients being treated for narrow-angle glaucoma. Avoid use with severe hepatic impairment.

ADVERSE REACTIONS: Dry mouth, constipation, dyspepsia, abdominal pain, nausea, urinary tract infection, headache, flu syndrome.

INTERACTIONS: CYP3A4 inducers and CYP2D6 and CYP3A4 inhibitors may alter darifenacin pharmacokinetics. Do not exceed 7.5mg/day when given concomitantly with potent CYP3A4 inhibitors (eg, ketoconazole, itraconazole, ritonavir, nelfinavir, clarithromycin, nefazodone). Caution with medications metabolized by CYP2D6 and which have a narrow therapeutic window (eg, flecainide, thioridazine, tricyclic antidepressants). Concomitant use with other anticholinergic agents may increase the frequency and/or severity of anticholinergic pharmacologic effects. May increase concentrations with concomitant use of cimetidine or ketoconazole. May increase imipramine concentrations. Monitor PT with concomitant use of warfarin. Perform routine therapeutic drug monitoring for digoxin. May increase midazolam exposure.

PREGNANCY: Category C, caution in nursing.

MECHANISM OF ACTION: Muscarinic receptor antagonist; inhibits cholinergic muscarinic receptors, which mediate contractions of urinary bladder smooth muscle, and stimulation of salivary secretions.

PHARMACOKINETICS: Absorption: Variable doses resulted in different pharmacokinetic parameters in extensive metabolizers and poor metabolizers of CYP2D6. **Distribution:** V_d=163L; plasma protein binding (98%). **Metabolism:** CYP2D6, 3A4 (monohydroxylation, ring opening, N-dealkylation). **Elimination:** Urine (60%); Feces (40%); unchanged, 3%. $T_{1/2}$=13-19 hrs.

NURSING CONSIDERATIONS

Assessment: Assess for urinary retention, gastric retention, uncontrolled narrow-angle glaucoma and risk for these conditions, bladder outflow obstruction, GI obstructive disorders, severe constipation, ulcerative colitis, myasthenia gravis, hepatic impairment, pregnancy/nursing status, and for possible drug interactions.

Monitoring: Monitor for symptoms of urinary retention, gastric retention, decreased GI motility, hepatic impairment, and for angioedema (face, lips, tongue, hypopharynx, larynx).

Patient Counseling: Advise that dizziness or blurred vision may occur; instruct to use caution when engaging in potentially dangerous activities. Instruct take once daily with liquid, with/without food. Instruct to swallow whole; advise to not chew, divide, or crush. Inform that symptoms of constipation, retention, heat prostration (due to decreased sweating), or angioedema may occur. Advise to d/c therapy if edema of the tongue or laryngopharynx, or difficulty breathing occurs.

Administration: Oral route. Take with liquid, with or without food. Swallow whole; do not chew, divide, or crush. **Storage:** 25°C (77°F); excursions permitted to 15-30°C (59-86°). Protect from light.

ENALAPRIL/HCTZ

RX

enalapril maleate - hydrochlorothiazide (Various)

> ACE inhibitors can cause death/injury to developing fetus during 2nd and 3rd trimesters. D/C therapy if pregnancy detected.

OTHER BRAND NAMES: Vaseretic (Biovail)

THERAPEUTIC CLASS: ACE inhibitor/thiazide diuretic

INDICATIONS: Treatment of HTN.

DOSAGE: *Adults:* Not Controlled with either Enalapril/HCTZ Monotherapy: Initial: 5mg-12.5mg (generic) or 10mg-25mg qd. Titrate: May increase HCTZ dose after 2-3 weeks. Max: 20mg-50mg qd. Replacement Therapy: Substitute combination for titrated individual components. Elderly: Start at lower end of dosing range.

HOW SUPPLIED: Tab: (Enalapril-HCTZ) (generic) 5mg-12.5mg, 10-25mg, (Vaseretic) 10mg-25mg* *scored

CONTRAINDICATIONS: History of ACE inhibitor-associated angioedema, hereditary or idiopathic angioedema, anuria, hypersensitivity to other sulfonamide-derived drugs.

WARNINGS/PRECAUTIONS: Not for initial therapy of HTN. Angioedema of the face, extremities, lips, tongue, glottis, and/or larynx reported; d/c and administer appropriate therapy if this occurs. Intestinal angioedema reported. Anaphylactoid reactions reported during desensitization with hymenoptera venom, with dialysis with high-flux membranes, and LDL apheresis with dextran sulfate absorption. Excessive hypotension reported. Neutropenia or agranulocytosis, and bone marrow depression reported; monitor WBCs in patients with renal disease and collagen vascular disease. D/C if jaundice or marked elevation of hepatic enzymes occur. Caution with severe renal disease, hepatic dysfunction, left ventricular outflow obstruction, renal artery stenosis, and in elderly. May exacerbate or activate systemic lupus erythematosus (SLE). Risk of hyperkalemia with diabetes mellitus (DM) and renal insufficiency. Persistent nonproductive cough reported. Sensitivity reactions may occur in patients with/without history of allergy or bronchial asthma. Not recommended in patients with severe renal impairment (CrCl <30mL/min). May increase cholesterol and TG. May cause idiosyncratic reaction, resulting in acute transient myopia and acute angle-closure glaucoma. Fluid/electrolyte imbalance, hypercalcemia, hyperglycemia, hyperuricemia, and hypomagnesemia may occur. Enhanced effects with postsympathectomy patients.

ADVERSE REACTIONS: Dizziness, cough, fatigue, headache.

INTERACTIONS: Enalapril: Hypotension risk with diuretics. Hypotension may occur during anesthesia. Antihypertensive effect augmented by antihypertensive agents that cause renin release (eg, diuretics). May cause further deterioration of renal function in patients with compromised renal function taking NSAIDs. Increased risk of hyperkalemia with K$^+$-sparing diuretics, K$^+$ supplements, or K$^+$-containing salt substitutes; use with caution. Lithium toxicity reported; monitor serum lithium levels frequently. Nitritoid reactions with injectable gold reported. HCTZ: Potentiation of orthostatic hypotension with alcohol, barbiturates, and narcotics. Dose adjustment of insulin or oral hypoglycemic agents may be required. Potentiation or additive effects with other antihypertensives. Reduced absorption with cholestyramine or colestipol. Increased risk of electrolyte depletion (eg, hypokalemia) with corticosteroids and adrenocorticotropic hormone (ACTH). May decrease response to pressor amines (eg, norepinephrine). May increase responsiveness to nondepolarizing skeletal muscle relaxants (eg, tubocurarine). Increased risk of lithium toxicity; avoid with lithium. NSAIDs may reduce diuretic, natriuretic, and antihypertensive effects. May cause hypokalemia, which may lead to cardiac arrhythmia and sensitize or exaggerate the response of the heart to the toxic effects of digitalis.

PREGNANCY: Category C (1st trimester) and D (2nd and 3rd trimesters), not for use in nursing.

MECHANISM OF ACTION: Enalapril: ACE inhibitor; inhibition results in decreased plasma angiotensin II, which leads to decreased vasopressor activity and decreased aldosterone secretion. HCTZ: Thiazide diuretic; not established. Affects distal renal tubular mechanism of electrolyte reabsorption. Increases excretion of Na^+ and Cl^-.

PHARMACOKINETICS: Absorption: T_{max} (enalapril, enalaprilat)=1 hr, 3-4 hrs. **Distribution:** Crosses placenta; found in breast milk. **Metabolism:** Via hydrolysis; enalaprilat (metabolite). **Elimination:** Enalapril: Urine and feces (94% enalaprilat or enalapril); $T_{1/2}$ (enalaprilat)=11 hrs. HCTZ: Kidneys (≥61% unchanged); $T_{1/2}$=5.6-14.8 hrs.

NURSING CONSIDERATIONS

Assessment: Assess for CHF, renal artery stenosis, SLE, collagen vascular disease, risk factors for hyperkalemia, histories of angioedema, allergy or bronchial asthma, and any other conditions where treatment is contraindicated or cautioned. Assess for hypersensitivity to drug, renal/hepatic function, pregnancy/nursing status, and possible drug interactions.

Monitoring: Monitor BP, LFTs, renal function, (BUN, SrCr), and cholesterol/TG. Monitor for angioedema, anaphylactoid reactions, hypotension, jaundice, SLE, hyperuricemia, hyperglycemia, and sensitivity reactions. Periodically monitor serum electrolytes, and WBCs in patients with collagen vascular and renal diseases.

Patient Counseling: Inform about fetal risks if taken during pregnancy; report pregnancies to physicians as soon as possible. Advise to use caution with excessive perspiration, dehydration, and other causes of volume depletion (eg, diarrhea, vomiting); may lead to fall in BP. Instruct to report lightheadedness, to d/c therapy if actual syncope occurs, not to use K^+ supplements or salt substitutes containing K^+ without consulting physician, and to report immediately any signs/symptoms of neutropenia (eg, fever, sore throat, infection), and angioedema (eg, swelling of face, extremities, eyes, lips, tongue, difficulty swallowing or breathing).

Administration: Oral route. **Storage:** 25°C (77°F); excursions permitted to 15-30°C (59-86°F).

ENBREL   RX
etanercept (Amgen)

Increased risk for developing serious infections (eg, tuberculosis [TB], TB reactivation, invasive fungal infection, bacterial/viral and other infections due to opportunistic pathogens) that may lead to hospitalization or death. Most patients who developed these infections were taking concomitant immunosuppressants (eg, methotrexate [MTX] or corticosteroids). Evaluate for latent TB and treat prior to and during therapy, and treat latent TB prior to initiation of therapy. Consider empiric antifungal therapy in patients at risk for invasive fungal infection who develop severe systemic illness. Monitor for development of signs and symptoms of infection during and after treatment. Consider risks and benefits prior to therapy with chronic and recurrent infection. D/C if serious infection or sepsis develops. Lymphoma and other malignancies reported in children and adolescents.

THERAPEUTIC CLASS: TNF-receptor blocker

INDICATIONS: Reduce signs/symptoms, induce major clinical response, inhibit progression of structural damage, and improve physical function in moderate to severe active rheumatoid arthritis (RA), alone or in combination with MTX. Reduce signs/symptoms, inhibit progression of structural damage of active arthritis, and improve physical function in psoriatic arthritis (PsA), alone or in combination with MTX. Reduce signs/symptoms of moderate to severe active polyarticular juvenile idiopathic arthritis (JIA) in patients ≥2 yrs. Reduce signs/symptoms of active ankylosing spondylitis (AS). Treatment of adults ≥18 yrs with chronic moderate to severe plaque psoriasis (PsO) who are candidates for systemic therapy or phototherapy.

DOSAGE: *Adults*: RA/AS/PsA: 50mg SQ once weekly. May continue MTX, glucocorticoids, salicylates, NSAIDs, or analgesics. Max: 50mg/week. PsO: Initial: 50mg SQ twice weekly for 3 months. May begin with 25-50mg/week. Maint:

50mg once weekly.

Pediatrics: ≥2 yrs: JIA: <63kg: 0.8mg/kg SQ weekly. ≥63kg: 50mg SQ weekly. May continue glucocorticoids, NSAIDs or analgesics.

HOW SUPPLIED: Inj: (MDV) 25mg, (Prefilled Syringe) 25mg, 50mg

CONTRAINDICATIONS: Sepsis.

WARNINGS/PRECAUTIONS: Do not use with an active infection. New onset or exacerbation of CNS demyelinating disorders, transverse myelitis, optic neuritis, multiple sclerosis, Guillain-Barre syndromes, other peripheral demyelinating neuropathies, and new onset or exacerbation of seizure disorders, reported; caution with pre-existing or recent onset CNS or peripheral nervous system demyelinating disorders. Cases of acute and chronic leukemia reported. Non-melanoma skin cancer (NMSC) reported; perform periodic skin exams for patients at increased risk. New onset or worsening of pre-existing heart failure (HF) reported; caution with HF and monitor closely. Rare cases of pancytopenia and aplastic anemia reported. Caution with previous history of significant hematologic abnormalities; seek medical attention if blood dyscrasias/ infection develop, and d/c if significant hematologic abnormalities occur. May reactivate hepatitis B virus (HBV) in chronic HBV carriers. Allergic reactions reported; d/c if anaphylaxis or other serious allergic reaction occurs. Needle cap on prefilled syringe and autoinjector contains dry natural rubber; caution with latex allergy. Pediatric patients should be brought up-to-date with current immunization guidelines prior to therapy. May result in auto-antibodies formation; d/c if lupus-like syndrome or autoimmune hepatitis develops. May affect host defenses against infections. Caution with moderate to severe alcoholic hepatitis and in elderly.

ADVERSE REACTIONS: Infections, sepsis, upper respiratory infections, non-upper respiratory infections, injection site reactions, diarrhea, rash, pruritus, lymphoma, other malignancies.

INTERACTIONS: See Boxed Warning. Do not give live vaccines. May cause neutropenia and increased rate of infection with anakinra. May increase rate of serious adverse events (eg, infections) with abatacept. Use with antidiabetic agents may cause hypoglycemia. Mild decrease in mean neutrophil count reported with sulfasalazine. Avoid with immunosuppressive agents (eg, cyclophosphamide) in patients with Wegener's granulomatosis. Concomitant immunosuppressants may contribute to HBV reactivation.

PREGNANCY: Category B, not for use in nursing.

MECHANISM OF ACTION: TNF-receptor blocker; inhibits binding of TNF-α and TNF-β (lymphotoxin alpha [LT-α]) to cell surface TNF-receptors, rendering TNF biologically inactive.

PHARMACOKINETICS: Absorption: Various doses resulted in different parameters. **Elimination:** (25mg) $T_{1/2}$ =102 hrs.

NURSING CONSIDERATIONS

Assessment: Assess for sepsis, active/localized/chronic/recurrent infection, TB exposure, recent travel in areas of endemic TB/mycoses, predisposition to infection (eg, diabetes), CNS/peripheral nervous system demyelinating disorders, seizure disorder, HF, hematological abnormalities, HBV infection, latex allergy, alcoholic hepatitis, Wegener's granulomatosis, pregnancy/nursing status and possible drug interactions. Assess for immunization history in pediatric patients. Test for latent TB infection, HBV infection prior to therapy.

Monitoring: Monitor for serious infections, sepsis, lymphoma, other malignancies, NMSC, CNS/peripheral nervous system demyelinating disorders, transverse myelitis, optic neuritis, multiple sclerosis, Guillain-Barre syndrome, seizure disorders, leukemia, HF, pancytopenia, aplastic anemia, blood dyscrasias, hematological abnormalities, allergic/anaphylactic reactions, lupus-like syndrome and autoimmune hepatitis. Evaluate for latent infection periodically. Perform periodic skin examination with increased risk for NMSC. Monitor for active HBV infection during and for several months after therapy.

Patient Counseling: Inform about risks/benefits of therapy. Advise to contact physician if symptoms of infection, TB or reactivation of HBV, severe allergic reactions, any signs of new or worsening medical conditions, or symptoms suggestive of pancytopenia develop. Inform that needle cap on prefilled syringe and on autoinjector contains dry natural rubber; caution if there is sensitivity to latex. Instruct patient or caregiver of proper injection techniques, accurate measurement/administration of correct dose, proper syringe/needle disposal.

Administration: SQ route. Refer to PI for preparation and administration.
Storage: Refrigerate at 2-8°C (36-46°F). Do not freeze. Pre-filled Syringe: Keep in original carton; protect from light. Do not shake. Reconstituted Sol: May store for ≤14 days. Discard after 14 days.

ENGERIX-B

RX

hepatitis B (recombinant) (GlaxoSmithKline)

THERAPEUTIC CLASS: Vaccine

INDICATIONS: Immunization against infection caused by all known hepatitis B virus (HBV) subtypes.

DOSAGE: *Adults:* ≥20 yrs: 1mL IM at 0, 1, 6 months. Booster: 1mL IM. Hemodialysis: 2mL IM at 0, 1, 2, 6 months. Booster: 2mL IM, given when antibody levels <10 mIU/mL. Alternate Schedule: ≥20 yrs: 1mL IM at 0, 1, 2, 12 months. Additional hepatitis B immune globulin (HBIG) should be given with known or presumed exposure to HBV.
Pediatrics: ≤19 yrs/Infants Born of HBsAg-Positive/Negative Mothers: 0.5mL IM at 0, 1, 6 months. Booster: 11-19 yrs: 1mL IM. ≤10 yrs: 0.5mL IM. Alternate Schedule: 11-19 yrs: 1mL IM at 0, 1, 6 months/0, 1, 2, 12 months. 5-16 yrs: 0.5mL IM at 0, 12, 24 months. ≤10 yrs/Infants Born of HBsAg-Positive Mothers: 0.5mL IM at 0, 1, 2, 12 months. Additional HBIG should be given with known or presumed exposure to HBV.

HOW SUPPLIED: Inj: 10mcg/0.5mL, 20mcg/mL [prefilled syringes, vial]

CONTRAINDICATIONS: Yeast hypersensitivity.

WARNINGS/PRECAUTIONS: May cause allergic reactions in latex-sensitive individuals. May not prevent hepatitis B infection in individuals who had unrecognized hepatitis B infection at time of vaccine administration. May not prevent infection in individuals who do not achieve protective antibody titers. Postpone vaccination with moderate/severe acute illness unless at immediate risk of hepatitis B infection. Diminished immune response with immunocompromised persons. Medical and immunization history should be reviewed prior to vaccination. Epinephrine and other appropriate agents must be immediately available if an acute anaphylactic reaction occurs. May exacerbate multiple sclerosis (rare). Apnea in premature infants following IM administration observed; decisions about when to administer vaccine should be based on consideration of potential benefits, medical status, and possible risks. Defer for infants weighing <2000g if mother is documented to be HBsAg negative at the time of infant's birth.

ADVERSE REACTIONS: Inj site soreness/erythema/swelling/induration, fatigue, fever, headache, dizziness.

INTERACTIONS: Diminished immune response with immunosuppressant therapy.

PREGNANCY: Category C, caution in nursing.

MECHANISM OF ACTION: Vaccine; may produce immune response for protection against infection caused by all known subtypes of hepatitis B virus.

NURSING CONSIDERATIONS

Assessment: Assess hypersensitivity to yeast/latex, presence of moderate/severe acute illness and medical history, immunocompromised status, immunization history, previous vaccine-related adverse reactions, multiple sclerosis, weight of infants, pregnancy/nursing status, and possible drug interactions.

Monitoring: Monitor for hypersensitivity reactions, inj site reactions (eg, induration, erythema, swelling, soreness), and general reactions (eg, fever, headache, dizziness). Perform annual antibody testing in hemodialysis patients to assess the need for booster doses.

Patient Counseling: Inform of potential benefits/risks of immunization. Instruct to report any adverse reactions to healthcare provider. Advise that vaccine cannot cause hepatitis B infection. Give vaccine recipients and parents or guardians the Vaccine Information Statements, which are required to be given prior to immunization.

Administration: IM route. Do not administer in the gluteal region. Administer in the anterolateral aspect of thigh (<1 yr) and deltoid muscle (>1 yr). May give SQ if at risk of hemorrhage (eg, hemophiliacs). Shake well before use. Do not dilute to administer. Inspect for particulate matter and discoloration; if either of these exists do not use. Concomitant administration of other vaccines or immune globulin should be given at different inj sites; do not mix with any other vaccine or product in the same syringe or vial. **Storage:** 2-8°C (36-46°F). Do not freeze; discard if frozen.

ENJUVIA   RX
conjugated estrogens (Teva)

> Estrogens increase the risk of endometrial cancer. Estrogens and progestins should not be used for the prevention of cardiovascular disease or dementia. Increased risks of MI, stroke, invasive breast cancer, PE, and DVT in postmenopausal women (50 to 79 yrs) reported. Increased risk of developing probable dementia in postmenopausal women ≥65 yrs reported.

THERAPEUTIC CLASS: Estrogen

INDICATIONS: Treatment of moderate-severe vasomotor symptoms associated with menopause. Treatment of symptoms of vulvar and vaginal atrophy associated with menopause. Treatment of moderate-severe vaginal dryness and pain with intercourse; if used solely for this purpose, topical vaginal products should be considered.

DOSAGE: *Adults:* Individualize dosing. Initial: 0.3mg qd. Adjust dose based on response.

HOW SUPPLIED: Tab: 0.3mg, 0.45mg, 0.625mg, 0.9mg, 1.25mg

CONTRAINDICATIONS: Pregnancy, undiagnosed abnormal genital bleeding, breast cancer, estrogen-dependent neoplasia, DVT/PE, arterial thromboembolic disease (eg, stroke, MI), liver dysfunction.

WARNINGS/PRECAUTIONS: Increased risk of retinal vascular thrombosis, severe hypercalcemia in patients with breast cancer and bone metastases, gallbladder disease and breast and ovarian cancers. Elevated BP reported; monitor BP at regular intervals. May elevate plasma triglycerides resulting in pancreatitis. Caution in patients with impaired liver function or history of cholestatic jaundice. May increase TBG; monitor thyroid function of patients dependent on thyroid hormone replacement therapy and adjust dosage if needed. May cause fluid retention; caution with cardiac or renal dysfunction. Caution in individuals with severe hypocalcemia. May cause exacerbation of asthma, diabetes mellitus, epilepsy, migraine or porphyria, systemic lupus erythematosus, and hepatic hemangiomas.

ADVERSE REACTIONS: Abdominal pain, accidental injury, flu syndrome, headache, pain, flatulence, nausea, dizziness, paresthesia, bronchitis, rhinitis, sinusitis, breast pain, dysmenorrhea, vaginitis.

INTERACTIONS: CYP3A4 inducers (eg, St. John's wort, phenobarbital, carbamazepine, rifampin) may decrease levels, which may decrease therapeutic effects and/or uterine bleeding profile. CYP3A4 inhibitors (eg, erythromycin, clarithromycin, ketoconazole, itraconazole, ritonavir, grapefruit juice) may increase levels, which may result in side effects.

PREGNANCY: Category X, caution in nursing.

MECHANISM OF ACTION: Estrogen; binds to nuclear receptors in estrogen-responsive tissues. Circulating estrogens modulate pituitary secretion of the gonadotropins, luteinizing hormone and follicle stimulating hormone, through negative feedback mechanism. Reduces elevated levels of these hormones in postmenopausal women.

PHARMACOKINETICS: Absorption: Refer to package insert for conjugated and unconjugated estrogen parameters. **Distribution:** Largely bound to sex hormone binding globulin and albumin; found in breast milk. **Metabolism:** Liver to estrone (metabolite), estriol (major urinary metabolite); sulfate and glucuronide conjugation (liver); intestinal hydrolysis; CYP 3A4 (partial metabolism). **Elimination:** Urine (parent compound and metabolites); Conjugated estrone: $T_{1/2}$=14 hrs; Conjugated equilin: $T_{1/2}$=11 hrs.

NURSING CONSIDERATIONS

Assessment: Assess for undiagnosed abnormal genital bleeding, presence or history of breast cancer, DVT, PE, estrogen-dependent neoplasia, liver dysfunction, history of cholestatic jaundice, pregnancy/nursing status, age of patient (≥65 yrs), hypertriglyceridemia, hypothyroidism, hypocalcemia, asthma, DM, epilepsy, migraine, porphyria, SLE, and possible drug interactions. Assess need for progestin therapy in patients who have not had a hysterectomy.

Monitoring: Monitor for signs/symptoms of CV disorders (eg, stroke, coronary heart disease, venous thromboembolism), malignant neoplasms (eg, endometrial, breast, or ovarian cancer), dementia, gallbladder disease, hypercalcemia, visual abnormalities, elevations in BP, fluid retention, elevations in serum triglycerides, pancreatitis, hypothyroidism, hypocalcemia, exacerbation of endometriosis and other conditions (eg, asthma, DM, epilepsy, migraine, SLE). Monitor BP levels. Monitor thyroid function in patients on thyroid replacement therapy. If undiagnosed, persistent, or recurring abnormal vaginal bleeding occurs, perform proper diagnostic testing (eg, endometrial sampling) to rule out malignancy. Perform annual breast exam. Perform periodic monitoring (every 3-6 months) to determine therapy need.

Patient Counseling: Inform medication increases risk for uterine cancer. Report breast lumps, unusual vaginal bleeding, dizziness or faintness, changes in speech, severe headaches, chest pain, SOB, leg pains, changes in vision, or vomiting. Inform physician if planning surgery or prolonged immobilization. Perform monthly breast self-exams. Take with/without food. If a dose is missed, take as soon as possible; if almost time for next dose, skip missed dose and return to normal dosing schedule.

Administration: Oral route. **Storage:** 20-25°C (68-77°F). Dispense in tight container with child-resistant closure.

ENTEREG   RX

alvimopan (GlaxoSmithKline)

> Available only for short-term (15 doses) use in hospitalized patients. Only hospitals that have registered and met requirements for the Entereg Access Support and Education (E.A.S.E.) program may use drug.

THERAPEUTIC CLASS: Opioid antagonist

INDICATIONS: To accelerate time to upper and lower GI recovery following partial large or small bowel resection surgery with primary anastomosis.

DOSAGE: *Adults:* ≥18 yrs: 12mg given 30 min to 5 hrs prior to surgery followed by 12mg bid beginning day after surgery for maximum of 7 days or until discharge. Max: 15 doses.

HOW SUPPLIED: Cap: 12mg

CONTRAINDICATIONS: Therapeutic doses of opioids for >7 consecutive days immediately prior to therapy.

WARNINGS/PRECAUTIONS: Recent exposure to opioids may increase sensitivity to adverse reactions, mainly GI (eg, abdominal pain, N/V, diarrhea) associated with alvimopan; caution in patients receiving >3 doses of opioids within the week prior to surgery. Avoid using in severe hepatic impairment (Child-Pugh Class C), end-stage renal disease (ESRD), surgery for correction of complete bowel obstruction. Myocardial Infarction (MI) reported in patients treated with opioids for chronic pain. Caution in Japanese patients.

ADVERSE REACTIONS: Anemia, constipation, dyspepsia, flatulence, hypokalemia, back pain, urinary retention.

INTERACTIONS: See Contraindications.

PREGNANCY: Category B, caution in nursing.

MECHANISM OF ACTION: Selective antagonist of μ-opioid receptor; antagonizes the peripheral effects of opioids on GI motility and secretion by competitively binding to GI tract μ-opioid receptors.

PHARMACOKINETICS: Absorption: Absolute bioavailability (6%); T_{max}=2 hrs; C_{max}=10.98ng/mL; AUC_{0-12h}=40.2ng•h/mL; (Metabolite): T_{max}=36 hrs; C_{max}=35.73ng/mL. **Distribution:** V_d=30L. Plasma protein binding (80%, alvimopan; 94%, metabolite). **Elimination:** Renal excretion (35% of total clearance); Biliary (primary pathway); $T_{1/2}$=10-17 hrs; (Metabolite): $T_{1/2}$=10-18 hrs.

NURSING CONSIDERATIONS

Assessment: Assess for hepatic/renal impairment, bowel obstruction, history of opioid use, and pregnancy/nursing status, and for possible drug interactions.

Monitoring: Monitor for signs/symptoms of possible side effects when recently exposed to opioids (eg, abdominal pain, N/V, diarrhea) and for MI. Monitor hepatic and renal function.

Patient Counseling: Instruct to disclose long-term or intermittent opioid pain therapy, including any use of opioids in the week prior to receiving therapy. Inform that recent use of opioids may cause adverse reactions primarily those limited to the GI tract (eg, abdominal pain, N/V, diarrhea). Advise that therapy must be administered in a hospital setting for no more than 7 days after bowel resection surgery. Inform that constipation, dyspepsia, and flatulence may occur.

Administration: Oral route. **Storage:** 25°C (77°F); excursions permitted to 15-30°C (59-86°F).

ENTOCORT EC   RX
budesonide (Prometheus)

THERAPEUTIC CLASS: Corticosteroid

INDICATIONS: Treatment of mild to moderate active Crohn's disease of the ileum and/or ascending colon. Maintenance of clinical remission of mild to moderate Crohn's disease of the ileum and/or ascending colon for up to 3 months.

DOSAGE: *Adults:* Usual: 9mg qd, in the am for up to 8 weeks. Recurring Episodes: Repeat therapy for 8 weeks. Maint: 6mg qd for 3 months, then taper to complete cessation. Moderate to Severe Hepatic Insufficiency/Concomitant CYP3A4 Inhibitors: Reduce dose. Swallow whole; do not chew or break.

HOW SUPPLIED: Cap, Delayed-Release: 3mg

WARNINGS/PRECAUTIONS: May reduce response of HPA axis to stress. Supplement with systemic glucocorticosteroids if undergoing surgery or other stressful situations. Increased risk of infection; avoid exposure to varicella/varicella zoster and measles. Caution with TB, HTN, DM, osteoporosis, peptic ulcer, glaucoma, cirrhosis, cataracts, family history of DM or glaucoma. Replacement of systemic glucocorticosteroids may unmask allergies. Chronic use may cause hypercorticism and adrenal suppression.

ADVERSE REACTIONS: Headache, respiratory infection, N/V, back pain, dyspepsia, dizziness, abdominal pain, diarrhea, flatulence, sinusitis, viral infection, arthralgia, benign intracranial HTN, signs/symptoms of hypercorticism.

INTERACTIONS: Ketoconazole caused an eight-fold increase of systemic exposure to oral budesonide. Increased levels with CYP3A4 inhibitors (eg, ketoconazole, itraconazole, saquinavir, erythromycin, grapefruit, grapefruit juice); monitor for increased signs and symptoms of hypercorticism and reduce budesonide dose if coadministered.

PREGNANCY: Category C, not for use in nursing.

MECHANISM OF ACTION: Glucocorticosteroid.

PHARMACOKINETICS: Absorption: C_{max}=5nmol/L; T_{max}=30-600 min; AUC=30nmol•hr/L. Bioavailability=9-21%. **Distribution:** V_d=2.2-3.9L/kg; plasma protein binding (85-90%). **Metabolism:** Liver; CYP3A4. **Elimination:** Urine (60%); $T_{1/2}$=2-3.6 hrs.

NURSING CONSIDERATIONS

Assessment: Assess for liver disease, history of chickenpox or measles, TB, HTN, osteoporosis, peptic ulcers, cataracts, history and/or family history of DM or glaucoma and possible drug interactions. Obtain baseline LFTs.

Monitoring: Monitor LFTs periodically and for signs/symptoms of hypercorticism and hypersensitivity reactions.

Patient Counseling: Advise to swallow whole; do not chew or break. Avoid consumption of grapefruit and grapefruit juice during therapy. Take particular care to avoid exposure to chickenpox or measles.

Administration: Oral route. **Storage:** 25° (77°F); excursions permitted to 15-30°C (59-86°F). Keep container tightly closed.

EPIDUO   RX
benzoyl peroxide - adapalene (Galderma)

THERAPEUTIC CLASS: Antibacterial/keratolytic

INDICATIONS: Topical treatment of acne vulgaris in patients ≥12 yrs.

DOSAGE: *Adults:* Apply a pea-sized amount to the affected areas of the face and/or trunk qd after washing.
Pediatrics: ≥12 yrs: Apply a pea-sized amount to the affected areas of the face and/or trunk once qd after washing.

HOW SUPPLIED: Gel: (Adapalene-Benzoyl Peroxide) 0.1%-2.5% [45g]

WARNINGS/PRECAUTIONS: Not for oral, ophthalmic, or intravaginal use. Minimize exposure to sunlight and sunlamps. Extreme weather may increase skin irritation. Avoid contact with eyes, lips, mucous membranes, cuts, abrasions, eczematous or sunburned skin. Local cutaneous reactions or irritant and allergic dermatitis may occur; may apply moisturizer, reduce frequency of application, or d/c use. Avoid "waxing" as depilatory method on the treated skin.

ADVERSE REACTIONS: Local cutaneous reactions (eg, erythema, scaling, stinging/burning, dryness), contact dermatitis, skin irritation.

INTERACTIONS: Caution with topical acne therapy, especially with peeling, desquamating, or abrasive agents. Avoid with other potentially irritating topical products (medicated or abrasive soaps and cleansers, soaps and cosmetics that have strong skin-drying effect, and products with high concentrations of alcohol, astringents, spices, or limes).

PREGNANCY: Category C, caution in nursing.

MECHANISM OF ACTION: Adapalene: Naphthoic acid derivative; not established. Binds to specific retinoic acid nuclear receptors. Benzoyl peroxide: Oxidizing agent with bactericidal and keratolytic effects.

PHARMACOKINETICS: Absorption: (Adapalene) C_{max}=0.21ng/mL; AUC_{0-24h}=1.99ng•h/mL. **Excretion:** (Adapalene) Bile. (Benzoyl peroxide) Urine.

NURSING CONSIDERATIONS

Assessment: Assess for sunburned skin, eczema, abrasion, skin cuts, use in pregnancy/nursing and possible drug interactions.

Monitoring: Monitor for sensitivity or irritation, cutaneous signs/symptoms (eg, erythema, dryness, scaling, burning, stinging, contact dermatitis).

Patient Counseling: Advise to cleanse area with mild or soapless cleanser; pat dry. Avoid contact with eyes, lips, and mucous membranes. Do not use more than the recommended amount. May cause irritation and bleach hair and colored fabric. Minimize exposure to sunlight and sunlamps; use sunscreen and protective clothing.

Administration: Topical route. **Storage:** 25°C; excursions permitted to 15-30°C (59-86°F). Protect from light. Keep away from heat. Keep tube tightly closed.

EPIFOAM

RX

pramoxine HCl - hydrocortisone acetate (Alaven)

THERAPEUTIC CLASS: Corticosteroid/anesthetic

INDICATIONS: Relief of the inflammatory and pruritic manifestations of corticosteroid-responsive dermatoses.

DOSAGE: *Adults:* Apply tid-qid. May use occlusive dressings for management of psoriasis or recalcitrant conditions. D/C occlusive dressing if infection develops.
Pediatrics: Apply tid-qid. May use occlusive dressings for management of psoriasis or recalcitrant conditions. D/C occlusive dressing if infection develops. Use the least amount compatible with an effective therapeutic regimen.

HOW SUPPLIED: Foam: (Hydrocortisone-Pramoxine) 1%-1% [10g]

WARNINGS/PRECAUTIONS: Avoid prolonged use. D/C use if redness, pain, irritation or swelling persists. Systemic absorption may produce reversible HPA axis suppression, manifestations of Cushing's syndrome, hyperglycemia and glucosuria. Pediatric patients are more susceptible to systemic toxicity. Chronic therapy may interfere with growth and development of pediatric patients. D/C if irritations develop. If HPA axis suppression noted, d/c or reduce frequency of application or substitute a less potent steroid. Steroid withdrawal may occur upon discontinuation. In the presence of dermatological infections, the use of appropriate antifungal or antibacterial agent should be instituted. Do not burn or puncture aerosol container. If no favorable response, d/c corticosteroid until infection has been controlled. Avoid contact with eyes.

ADVERSE REACTIONS: Burning, itching, irritation, dryness, folliculitis, hypertrichosis, acneiform eruptions, hypopigmentation, perioral dermatitis, allergic contact dermatitis, maceration, secondary infection, skin atrophy, striae, miliaria.

PREGNANCY: Category C, caution in nursing.

MECHANISM OF ACTION: Hydrocortisone: Corticosteroid; possesses anti-inflammatory, antipruritic, and vasoconstrictive properties. Anti-inflammatory activity not established. Pramoxine: Local anesthetic.

PHARMACOKINETICS: Absorption: Percutaneous; inflammation, other disease states, and use of occlusive dressings may increase absorption. **Distribution:** Systemically administered corticosteroids are found in breast milk. **Metabolism:** Liver. **Elimination:** Kidneys, bile.

NURSING CONSIDERATIONS

Assessment: Assess for hypersensitivity, dermatological infections, and pregnancy/nursing status.

Monitoring: Monitor for signs/symptoms of reversible HPA-axis suppression, Cushing's syndrome, hyperglycemia, glucosuria, treatment-site irritation, and development of dermatological infections. If applying high doses to large surface area or using occlusive dressings, monitor for HPA-axis suppression by using urinary free cortisol and ACTH stimulation tests. In pediatric patients, monitor for signs/symptoms of systemic toxicity, HPA-axis suppression (eg, linear growth retardation, delayed weight gain), and intracranial HTN.

Patient Counseling: Instruct to use externally and exactly as directed; avoid contact with eyes. Advise not to bandage or wrap treatment area as to be occlusive, unless directed by physician. Instruct to report signs of local adverse events. Inform caregivers of pediatric patients to avoid using tight fitting diapers or plastic pants in treatment area.

Administration: Topical route. **Storage:** 20-25°C (68-77°F). Do not store at temperature ≥120°F (49°C). Do not refrigerate. Keep out of the reach of children.

EPIPEN
epinephrine (Dey)

OTHER BRAND NAMES: EpiPen Jr. (Dey)

THERAPEUTIC CLASS: Sympathomimetic catecholamine

INDICATIONS: Immediate self-administered, emergency treatment of allergic reactions (Type I) including anaphylaxis to stinging insects (eg, order Hymenoptera, which includes bees, wasps, hornets, yellow jackets and fire ants) or biting insect (eg, triatoma, mosquitoes), allergen immunotherapy, foods, drugs, diagnostic testing substances (eg, radiocontrast media), and other allergens, as well as idiopathic or exercise-induced anaphylaxis.

DOSAGE: *Adults:* 15-30kg: 0.15mg (Epipen Jr) IM/SQ into anterolateral aspect of thigh. May repeat with severe anaphylaxis. ≥30 kg: 0.3mg (Epipen) IM/SQ into anterolateral aspect of thigh. May repeat with severe anaphylaxis. *Pediatrics:* 15-30kg: 0.15mg (Epipen Jr) IM/SQ into anterolateral aspect of thigh. May repeat with severe anaphylaxis. ≥30 kg: 0.3mg (Epipen) IM/SQ into anterolateral aspect of thigh. May repeat with severe anaphylaxis.

HOW SUPPLIED: Inj: (Epipen Jr) 0.5mg/mL, (Epipen) 1mg/mL

WARNINGS/PRECAUTIONS: Not intended as a substitute for immediate medical care. Do not inject into buttock; may not provide effective treatment of anaphylaxis. May result in loss of blood flow to the affected areas if accidentally injected into digits, hands or feet. Not for IV use; may cause cerebral hemorrhage due to sharp rise in BP if accidentally injected IV. Contains sodium metabisulfite; sulfite-sensitivity is not a contraindication in serious allergic or emergency situations. Caution with heart disease, including cardiac arrhythmias, coronary artery or organic heart disease, or hypertension. High risk of developing adverse reactions with hyperthyroidism, CVD, HTN, and DM, and in elderly, pregnant women, pediatrics <30kg using Epipen and pediatrics <15kg using Epipen Jr.

ADVERSE REACTIONS: Palpitations, sweating, N/V, respiratory difficulty, pallor, dizziness, weakness, tremor, headache, apprehensiveness, anxiety, restlessness, arrhythmias (including fatal ventricular fibrillation), angina, cerebral hemorrhage.

INTERACTIONS: Can counteract the marked pressor effects of epinephrine with rapidly acting vasodilators. Drugs that sensitize the heart to arrhythmias (eg, digitalis, diuretics, quinidine, or anti-arrhythmias) may precipitate or aggravate angina pectoris as well as produce ventricular arrhythmias. Co-administration with TCAs, MAOIs, levothyroxine sodium, and certain antihistamines, including chlorpheniramine, tripelennamine and diphenhydramine, may lead to potentiation of epinephrine effects. Antagonized cardiostimulating and bronchodilating effects with beta-adrenergic blocking drugs, such as propranolol. Antagonized vasoconstricting and hypertensive effects with alpha-adrenergic blocking drugs such as phentoloamine. Ergot alkaloids may reverse pressor effects.

PREGNANCY: Category C, safety not known in nursing.

MECHANISM OF ACTION: Sympathomimetic catecholamine; acts on α receptors to lessen the vasodilation and increased vascular permeability that occurs during anaphylaxis, which can lead to loss of intravascular fluid volume and hypotension. Acts on β receptors to cause bronchial smooth muscle relaxation that helps alleviate bronchospasm, wheezing and dyspnea that may occur during anaphylaxis.

NURSING CONSIDERATIONS

Assessment: Assess for anaphylaxis severity, sulfite sensitivity.

Monitoring: Monitor for anginal pain, arrhythmia, BP, and cerebral hemorrhage (particularly in overdosage or inadvertent intravascular injection).

Patient Counseling: Inform about the signs and symptoms produced by the drug. Advise to go to nearest emergency room if accidentally injected into hands or feet; may result in loss of blood flow to affected area. Never inject into buttock or by IV route. Advise that epinephrine is not intended as a substitute for immediate medical care.

Administration: IM or SQ route. **Storage:** 25°C (77°F); excursions permitted to 15-30°C (59-86°F). Light sensitive; store in the tube provided. Do not refrigerate.

EPIQUIN MICRO   RX
hydroquinone (SkinMedica)

THERAPEUTIC CLASS: Depigmentation agent

INDICATIONS: Gradual treatment of ultraviolet induced dyschromia and discoloration resulting from the use of oral contraceptives, pregnancy, hormone replacement therapy, or skin trauma.

DOSAGE: *Adults/Pediatrics:* ≥12yrs: Apply bid (am and hs). Use sunscreen.

HOW SUPPLIED: Cre: 4% [30g]

WARNINGS/PRECAUTIONS: Avoid sun exposure on bleached skin. Use sunscreen. May produce unwanted cosmetic effects if not used as directed. Test for skin sensitivity. D/C if no lightening effect after 2 months of therapy, if blue-black darkening of the skin occurs, or if itching, vesicle formation, or excessive inflammatory reactions occur. Contains sodium metabisulfite; may cause serious allergic type reactions. Avoid contact with eyes.

ADVERSE REACTIONS: Cutaneous hypersensitivity (contact dermatitis).

PREGNANCY: Category C, caution in nursing.

MECHANISM OF ACTION: Produces a reversible depigmentation of the skin by inhibition of the enzymatic oxidation of tyrosine to 3-(3,4-dihydroxyphenyl) alanine (dopa)[2] and suppresses the melanocyte metabolic processes.

NURSING CONSIDERATIONS

Assessment: Assess for skin sensitivity by skin test, drug and sulfite hypersensitivity, and pregnancy/nursing status.

Monitoring: Monitor for allergic reactions (eg, hives, itching, wheezing, anaphylaxis and severe asthma attack), blue-black darkening of the skin, and unwanted cosmetic effects.

Patient Counseling: Avoid prolonged sun exposure. Instruct to d/c drug if no lightening effect noted after 2 months of therapy or apperance of blue-black darkening of skin. Take as directed. Not to be taken by pregnant/nursing women or children ≤12 yrs. Avoid contact with eyes.

Administration: Topical route. **Storage:** 25°C (77°F); excursions permitted to 15-30°C (59-86°F).

EPIVIR®   RX
lamivudine (ViiV Healthcare)

> Lactic acidosis and severe hepatomegaly with steatosis, including fatal cases, reported; suspend treatment if lactic acidosis or pronounced hepatotoxicity occur. Severe acute exacerbations of hepatitis B (HBV) reported in patients coinfected with HBV and HIV-1 and who d/c therapy. Monitor hepatic function closely for at least several months after d/c and initiate antihepatitis B therapy if needed. Epivir tabs and sol, used to treat HIV-1 infection, contain higher dose of lamivudine than Epivir-HBV tabs and sol, used to treat chronic HBV infection; only use appropriate dosing forms for HIV-1 treatment.

THERAPEUTIC CLASS: Nucleoside analogue

INDICATIONS: Treatment of HIV-1 infection in combination with other antiretrovirals.

DOSAGE: *Adults:* 150mg bid or 300mg qd, concomitantly with other antiretrovirals. Renal Impairment (≥ 30 kg): CrCl 30-49mL/min: 150mg qd. CrCl 15-29mL/min: 150mg first dose, then 100mg qd. CrCl 5-14mL/min: 150mg first dose, then 50mg qd. CrCl <5mL/min: 50mg first dose, then 25mg qd.

Pediatrics: ≥16 yrs: 150mg bid or 300mg qd, concomitantly with other antiretrovirals. 3 months-16 yrs: (Sol) 4mg/kg bid, concomitantly with other antiretrovirals. Max: 150mg bid. (Tab, scored) 14-21kg: 1/2 tab (75mg) in am and 1/2 tab (75mg) in pm. >21-<30kg: 1/2 tab (75mg) in am and 1 tab (150mg) in pm. ≥30kg: 1 tab (150mg) in am and 1 tab (150mg) in pm. Renal Impairment (≥ 30kg): CrCl 30-49mL/min: 150mg qd. CrCl 15-29mL/min: 150mg first dose, then 100mg qd. CrCl 5-14mL/min: 150mg first dose, then 50mg qd. CrCl <5mL/min: 50mg first dose, then 25mg qd.

HOW SUPPLIED: Sol: 10mg/mL [240mL]; Tab: 150mg*, 300mg *scored

WARNINGS/PRECAUTIONS: Caution in pediatric patients with history of prior antiretroviral nucleoside exposure, history of pancreatitis, or other significant risk factors for development of pancreatitis; d/c if pancreatitis develops. May cause redistribution or accumulation of body fat. Immune reconstitution syndrome reported. Reduce dose in renal dysfunction. Caution in elderly.

ADVERSE REACTIONS: Lactic acidosis, severe hepatomegaly with steatosis, severe acute exacerbations of hepatitis B, headache, malaise, fatigue, N/V, diarrhea, nasal signs/symptoms, neuropathy, insomnia/sleep disorders, musculoskeletal pain, cough, fever, chills.

INTERACTIONS: Hepatic decompensation occurred when used with interferon-α, with or without ribavirin. Avoid use with zalcitabine; may inhibit intracellular phosphorylation of drug. Avoid use with other lamivudine-containing products such as Epivir-HBV and fixed-dose combinations of abacavir, lamivudine, and zidovudine. Also avoid use with emtricitabine and fixed-dose combinations of emtricitabine, efavirenz, and tenofovir. Trimethoprim/ Sulfamethoxazole may increase lamivudine levels. Possible interaction with drugs that are secreted via the organic cationic transport system.

PREGNANCY: Category C, not for use in nursing.

MECHANISM OF ACTION: Nucleoside analogue; inhibits HIV-1 reverse transcriptase (RT) via DNA chain termination after incorporation of the nucleotide analogue into viral DNA.

PHARMACOKINETICS: Absorption: Rapid; Absolute bioavailability (tab 86%, sol 87%); C_{max}=1.5mcg/mL (HIV); T_{max}=0.9 hrs (fasting), 3.2 hrs (fed); administration with varying degrees of renal function resulted in different pharmacokinetic parameters. **Distribution:** V_d=1.3L/kg (IV); plasma protein binding (<36%); found in breast milk. **Metabolism:** Trans-sulfoxide (metabolite). **Elimination:** Urine (unchanged); $T_{1/2}$=5-7 hrs.

NURSING CONSIDERATIONS

Assessment: Assess for impaired hepatic/renal function, risk factors for liver disease, history of pancreatitis, risk factors for pancreatitis, HIV-1 and HBV coinfection, previous hypersensitivity, pregnancy/nursing status and possible drug interactions. Assess for obesity, prolonged nucleoside exposure, and use in women.

Monitoring: Monitor for signs/symptoms of pancreatitis, immune reconstitution syndrome, fat redistribution, lactic acidosis, severe hepatomegaly with steatosis, hepatitis B exacerbation, hepatic/renal dysfunction. Monitor hepatic function closely for several months in patients with HIV/HBV coinfection who d/c therapy.

Patient Counseling: Instruct to take with combination therapy on regular dosing schedule; avoid missing doses. Inform that drug is not a cure for HIV-1 infection and that patients may continue to experience illnesses associated with HIV-1 infection, including opportunistic infections. Counsel that therapy does not reduce risk of HIV transmission through sexual contact or blood contamination. Inform that redistribution or accumulation of body fat may occur. Instruct not to take concomitantly with emtricitabine-containing or other lamivudine-containing products. Inform of liver disease deterioration when treatment is d/c. Advise to monitor pediatrics for signs and symptoms of pancreatitis. Advise that each 15-mL dose of solution contains 3g of sucrose. Counsel about the differences in the formulations of Epivir.

Administration: Oral route. **Storage:** (Tab) 25°C (77°F); excursions permitted to 15-30°C (59-86°F). (Sol) 25°C (77°F). Store in tightly closed bottles.

EPIVIR-HBV

lamivudine (GlaxoSmithKline)

RX

Lactic acidosis and severe hepatomegaly with steatosis, including fatal cases reported with nucleoside analogues alone or in combination with other antiretrovirals. Epivir-HBV contains a lower dose of lamivudine than Epivir used to treat HIV; perform HIV counseling and testing to all patients prior to therapy and periodically thereafter. Rapid emergence of HIV resistance is likely if prescribed for unrecognized/untreated HIV infection. Severe acute exacerbations of hepatitis B reported upon d/c of therapy; monitor hepatic function closely for at least several months after d/c and initiate anti-hepatitis B therapy if needed.

THERAPEUTIC CLASS: Nucleoside analogue

INDICATIONS: Treatment of chronic hepatitis B (HBV) associated with evidence of viral replication and active liver inflammation.

DOSAGE: *Adults:* CrCl ≥50mL/min: 100mg qd. CrCl 30-49mL/min: 100mg 1st dose, then 50mg qd. CrCl 15-29mL/min: 100mg 1st dose, then 25mg qd. CrCl 5-14mL/min: 35mg 1st dose, then 15mg qd. CrCl <5mL/min: 35mg 1st dose, then 10mg qd. Elderly: Start at lower end of dosing range. Safety and efficacy of treatment >1 yr, and optimum duration of treatment not known. *Pediatrics:* 2-17 yrs: 3mg/kg qd. Max: 100mg/day. Renal Impairment: Dose reduction should be considered. Safety and efficacy of treatment >1 yr, and optimum duration of treatment not known.

HOW SUPPLIED: Sol: 5mg/mL [240mL]; Tab: 100mg

WARNINGS/PRECAUTIONS: Should only be used when alternative antiviral agent with a higher genetic barrier to resistance is not available/appropriate. Not established with decompensated liver disease/organ transplants. Not appropriate for patients dually infected with HBV and HCV, hepatitis delta, or HIV. Use appropriate infant immunizations to prevent neonatal acquisition of HBV. Caution with obesity, prolonged nucleoside exposure and known risk factors for liver disease; d/c therapy if lactic acidosis or pronounced hepatotoxicity occur. Pancreatitis reported, especially in HIV-infected pediatrics with prior nucleoside exposure. Emergence of resistance-associated HBV mutations reported; monitor ALT and HBV DNA levels during treatment. Caution in elderly.

ADVERSE REACTIONS: Lactic acidosis, severe hepatomegaly with steatosis, exacerbations of hepatitis, pancreatitis, fatigue, ear/nose/throat infections, myalgia, abdominal discomfort/pain, diarrhea, headache, N/V.

INTERACTIONS: Concomitant use with zalcitabine is not recommended. Possibility of interaction with other drugs whose main route of elimination is active renal secretion via the organic cationic transport system should be considered. May increase AUC when given with trimethoprim/sulfamethoxazole. Caution with other lamivudine-containing products (eg, Epivir, Combivir, Epzicom or Trivizir).

PREGNANCY: Category C, not for use in nursing.

MECHANISM OF ACTION: Nucleoside analogue; phosphorylated to active 5'-triphosphate metabolite intracellularly; incorporation of monophosphate form into viral DNA by HBV reverse transcriptase results in DNA termination.

PHARMACOKINETICS: Absorption: Rapid; C_{max}=1.28mcg/mL (HBV), C_{max}=1.05mcg/mL (healthy); T_{max}=0.5-2.0 hrs; AUC=4.3mcg•hr/mL (HBV), AUC=4.7mcg•hr/mL (healthy). Absolute bioavailability: Tab: (86%). Sol: (87%). Refer to PI for pharmacokinetic parameters in patients with impaired renal/hepatic function. **Distribution:** Plasma protein binding (<36%); V_d=1.3L/kg (IV); found in breast milk. **Metabolism:** Hepatic (minor); trans-sulfoxide (metabolite). **Elimination:** Urine (unchanged); $T_{1/2}$=5-7 hrs.

NURSING CONSIDERATIONS

Assessment: Assess weight, hepatic/renal function. Assess for nucleoside exposure, risk factors for liver disease, HIV infection, history of pancreatitis, drug hypersensitivity, pregnancy/nursing status and possible drug interactions. Perform HIV counseling and testing to all patients prior to therapy and periodically thereafter.

Monitoring: Monitor renal/hepatic function, therapeutic response. Monitor for signs/symptoms of pancreatitis, lactic acidosis, hepatomegaly with steatosis, emergence of resistant HIV, exacerbations of hepatitis. Monitor maternal-fetal outcomes by enrolling patients in the Antiretroviral Pregnancy Registry. Monitor ALT and HBV DNA levels if emergence of viral mutants is suspected. Monitor patients during and for at least several months after d/c therapy.

Patient Counseling: Advise to discuss any new symptoms or concurrent medications with physician. Inform that drug is not a cure for HBV; long-term benefits and relationship of initial treatment response are unknown. Inform that liver disease deterioration may occur upon d/c. Advise to discuss any changes in regimen with physician. Counsel on importance of HIV testing to avoid inappropriate therapy and development of resistant HIV. Instruct not to take concurrently with other lamivudine-containing products such as Epivir, Combivir, Epzicom or Trivizir. Inform that therapy does not reduce risk of HBV transmission through sexual contact/blood contamination. Inform diabetics that each 20mL of oral sol contains 4g of sucrose.

Administration: Oral route. **Storage:** Tab: 25°C (77°F); excursions permitted to 15-30°C (59-86°F). Sol: 20-25°C (68-77°F); store in tightly closed bottles.

EPOGEN   RX
epoetin alfa (Amgen)

> Increased mortality, serious cardiovascular (CV) events and stroke in CRF patients when administered to target Hgb levels of ≥13g/dL. Individualize dosing to achieve and maintain Hgb levels within range of 10-12g/dL. Shortened overall survival and/or increased risk of tumor progression or recurrence in patients with breast, non-small cell lung, head and neck, lymphoid, and cervical cancers. To decrease these risks, as well as risk of serious cardio- and thrombovascular events, use lowest dose needed to avoid RBC transfusions. Because of these risks, prescribers and hospitals must enroll in and comply with the ESA APPRISE Oncology Program to prescribe and/or dispense to patients with cancer. Use only for treatment of anemia due to concomitant myelosuppressive chemotherapy. Not indicated for patients receiving myelosuppressive therapy when anticipated outcome is cure. D/C following completion of chemotherapy course. Increased the rate of deep venous thromboses (DVT) in patients not receiving prophylactic anticoagulation during surgery. Consider DVT prophylaxis.

THERAPEUTIC CLASS: Erythropoiesis stimulator

INDICATIONS: Treatment of anemia of chronic renal failure (CRF); anemia related to therapy with zidovudine in HIV-infected patients; anemic patients (Hgb >10-≤13g/dL) who are at high risk for perioperative blood loss to reduce the need for allogeneic blood transfusions; anemia due to the effect of concomitantly administered chemotherapy based on studies that have shown a reduction in the need for RBC transfusions in patients with metastatic, non-myeloid malignancies receiving chemotherapy for minimum of 2 months.

DOSAGE: *Adults:* CRF: (IV/SQ) Individualize dose. Initial: 50-100 U/kg TIW. IV route recommended in hemodialysis patients. See PI for dose adjustments based on Hgb levels. Maint: Individually titrate for each patient on dialysis; Hgb levels between 10-12g/dL. Median Maint: (Hemodialysis) 75 U/kg TIW with the range of 12.5-525 U/kg TIW. Zidovudine-Treated HIV Patients: If serum erythropoietin ≤500 mU/mL and zidovudine ≤4200mg/week give 100 U/kg IV/SQ TIW for 8 weeks. Titrate: Increase by 50-100 U/kg TIW after 8 weeks if necessary. Max: 300 U/kg TIW. Maint: If Hgb >12g/dL, d/c until Hgb <11g/dL, then reduce dose by 25% when therapy is resumed. Surgery Patients: Initial: (Hgb >10-≤13g/dL) 300 U/kg/day SQ for 10 days before, on day of, and for 4 days after surgery; or 600 U/kg SQ once weekly on 21, 14, and 7 days before surgery. Cancer Patients on Chemotherapy: 150 U/kg SQ TIW or 40,000 U SQ weekly. Titrate: (TIW dosing) Increase to 300 U/kg TIW if response not satisfactory after 4 weeks to avoid need for RBC transfusion or (Weekly dosing) 60,000 U SQ weekly if Hgb is not increased by ≥1g/dL after 4 weeks. See PI for dose adjustments based on Hgb levels.
Pediatrics: CRF: (IV/SQ) Individualize dose. Initial: 50 U/kg TIW. See PI for dose adjustments based on Hgb levels. Median Maint (Hemodialysis and Peritoneal dialysis): 167 U/kg/week (49-447 U/kg/week) and 76 U/kg/week (24-323 U/kg/week) in divided doses (TIW or BIW). If transferrin saturation is

>20%, dose may be increased. Maintain Hgb levels between 10-12g/dL; 75-150 U/kg/week maintains the Hct of 36%-38% for 6 months. Cancer Patients on Chemotherapy: 600 U/kg IV weekly. Titrate: If Hgb is not increased by ≥1g/dL after 4 weeks increase to 900 U/kg IV weekly. See PI for dose adjustments based on Hgb levels. Max: 60,000 U

HOW SUPPLIED: Inj: 2000 U/mL, 3000 U/mL, 4000 U/mL, 10,000 U/mL, 20,000 U/mL, 40,000 U/mL [1mL single dose]; 10,000 U/mL [2mL multidose]; 20,000 [1mL multidose]

CONTRAINDICATIONS: Uncontrolled HTN. Hypersensitivity to mammalian cell-derived products and albumin (human).

WARNINGS/PRECAUTIONS: Contains benzyl alcohol; increased incidence of neurological and other complications in premature infants reported. Pure red cell aplasia and severe anemia (with or without other cytopenias) may occur. Evaluate etiology if lack/loss of response occurs; test for presence of antibodies to erythropoietin; if present d/c permanently. Should not be switched to other ESAs as antibodies may cross-react. Formulation with albumin may carry risk for transmission of viral diseases. Do not use in patients with uncontrolled HTN. Closely monitor and aggressively control BP in those treated and adjust dose in CRF patients on dialysis with clinically evident ischemic heart disease or CHF. Seizures reported; presence of premonitory neurologic symptoms should be monitored. Avoid potentially hazardous activities such as driving or operating heavy machinery. Exacerbation of porphyria observed; caution in patients with known porphyria. Transient rashes occasionally observed. ESAs resulted in decreased locoregional control/progression-free survival and/or overall survival in patients with advanced head and neck cancer receiving radiation therapy, in patients receiving chemotherapy for metastatic breast cancer or lymphoid malignancy, and in patients with non-small cell lung cancer or various malignancies who were not receiving chemotherapy or radiotherapy. Functional iron deficiency may develop; evaluate iron stores prior to and during therapy. Monitor Hct, BP, iron levels, serum chemistry, and CBC. Menses may resume.

ADVERSE REACTIONS: HTN, headache, fatigue, arthralgias, N/V, diarrhea, edema, rash, pyrexia, clotted vascular access, respiratory congestion, dyspnea, asthenia, dizziness, seizures, thrombotic events.

INTERACTIONS: Adjust anticoagulant dose in dialysis patients.

PREGNANCY: Category C, caution in nursing.

MECHANISM OF ACTION: Erythropoiesis stimulator.

PHARMACOKINETICS: Absorption: (SC) T_{max}=5-24 hrs. **Elimination:** (IV) $T_{1/2}$=4-13 hrs.

NURSING CONSIDERATIONS

Assessment: Assess for uncontrolled HTN, porphyria, history of HTN, CVD (ischemic heart disease, CHF), renal failure, cancer, pure red cell aplasia, seizure, pregnancy/nursing status, possible drug interactions, hypersensitivity to mammalian cell-derived products and albumin. Obtain baseline BP measurements and iron status (transferrin saturation, serum ferritin).

Monitoring: Monitor BP, Hct, CBC with differential and platelet count, iron status (transferrin saturation, serum ferritin) regularly. CRF: Serum chemistries (BUN, uric acid, creatinine, phosphorus, K⁺) regularly, Hgb twice weekly. HIV and cancer: Hgb once weekly. Monitor for signs/symptoms of CV events (MI, stroke, CHF), pure red cell aplasia, severe anemia, viral diseases, seizures, lack/loss of response to therapy, and hypersensitivity reactions.

Patient Counseling: Inform may impair physical/mental abilities. Seek medical attention if symptoms of CV events, anemia, infections, seizures, or hypersensitivity reactions occur. Inform that it can increase the risk of having serious CV events, thromboembolic events and tumor progression or recurrence. Instruct for the proper dosage and administration. Inform about the proper disposal and caution against the reuse of needles, syringes or drug product. A puncture-resistant container should be available for disposal of used syringes and needles.

Administration: IV, SQ route. **Storage:** 2-8°C (36-46°F). Do not freeze or shake. Protect from light.

EPZICOM

RX

abacavir sulfate - lamivudine (ViiV Healthcare)

THERAPEUTIC CLASS: Nucleoside analog combination

INDICATIONS: Treatment of HIV-1 infection in combination with other antiretrovirals.

DOSAGE: *Adults:* CrCl ≥50mL/min: 1 tab qd.

HOW SUPPLIED: Tab: (Abacavir Sulfate-Lamivudine) 600mg-300mg

CONTRAINDICATIONS: Hepatic impairment.

WARNINGS/PRECAUTIONS: Caution with obesity and prolonged nucleoside exposure; d/c therapy if lactic acidosis or pronounced hepatotoxicity occurs. Caution with history or known risk factors for liver disease. Lamivudine-resistant HBV reported. Immune reconstitution syndrome reported. Redistribution/accumulation of body fat observed. Increased risk of myocardial infarction (MI) reported; consider the underlying risk of coronary heart disease. Cross-resistance potential with nucleoside reverse transcriptase inhibitors (NRTIs) reported. Avoid use with impaired renal function (CrCl <50mL/min). Caution in elderly.

ADVERSE REACTIONS: Hypersensitivity, insomnia, depression, headache, fatigue/malaise, dizziness/vertigo, nausea, diarrhea, rash, pyrexia, abdominal pain/gastritis, abnormal dreams, anxiety.

INTERACTIONS: Hepatic decompensation reported in HIV-1/HCV co-infected patients receiving combination antiretroviral therapy for HIV and interferon α, with or without ribavirin; d/c Epzicom as medically appropriate and reduce or d/c interferon alfa, ribavirin, or both. May increase methadone clearance. Decreased elimination with ethanol. TMP/SMX and/or nelfinavir may increase lamivudine exposure. Avoid any other abacavir- and lamivudine-containing (eg, Ziagen, Epivir, Combivir, Trizivir) or emtricitabine-containing products (Atripla, Emtriva, Truvada).

PREGNANCY: Category C, not for use in nursing.

MECHANISM OF ACTION: Abacavir: Carbocyclic nucleoside analogue; inhibits HIV-1 reverse transcriptase (RT) activity by competing with natural substrate dGTP and incorporating into viral DNA. Lamivudine: Nucleoside analogue; inhibits RT via DNA chain termination after incorporation of the nucleotide analogue.

PHARMACOKINETICS: Absorption: Abacavir: Rapid. Bioavailability (86%); C_{max}=4.26mcg/mL, AUC=11.95mcg•hr/mL. Lamivudine: Rapid. Bioavailability (86%); C_{max}=2.04mcg/mL, AUC=8.87mcg•hr/mL. **Distribution:** Abacavir: V_d=0.86L/kg, plasma protein binding (50%). Lamivudine: V_d=1.3L/kg; found in breast milk. **Metabolism:** Abacavir: Via alcohol dehydrogenase and glucuronyl transferase; 5'-carboxylic acid, 5'-glucuronide (metabolites). Lamivudine: Trans-sulfoxide (metabolite). **Elimination:** Abacavir: $T_{1/2}$=1.45 hrs. Lamivudine: (IV) Urine (70%, unchanged); $T_{1/2}$=5-7 hrs.

NURSING CONSIDERATIONS

Assessment: Assess medical history and prior exposure to any abacavir-containing product. Assess for HBV infection, history of hypersensitivity reactions, HLA-B*5701 allele carriers, hepatic/renal impairment, obesity, prolonged nucleoside use, risk factors for CHD, pregnancy/nursing status, and possible drug interactions.

Monitoring: Monitor for signs/symptoms of hypersensitivity, lactic acidosis, hepatomegaly, HBV exacerbation, immune reconstitution syndrome, fat redistribution, MI. Monitor hepatic/renal function. Follow-up LFTs for several months after d/c therapy. May enroll patients in the Antiretroviral Pregnancy Registry if they become pregnant while on treatment.

Patient Counseling: Counsel regarding hypersensitivity reactions; call doctor right away if suspected. Do not restart or replace with any drug containing abacavir following hypersensitivity reaction. Liver disease may worsen if therapy is d/c in patients co-infected with HIV and HBV. Lactic acidosis with liver enlargement and fat redistribution may occur. Instruct not to take with other abacavir- or lamivudine-containing agents. Counsel to take on regular dosing schedule and to avoid missing doses. Advise patients that they may continue to experience illnesses associated with HIV-1 while on therapy and that risk of transmission to others is not reduced.

Administration: Oral route. Take with or without food. **Storage:** 25°C (77°F); excursions permitted to 15-30°C (59-86°F).

EQUETRO

RX

carbamazepine (Validus)

> Serious and sometimes fatal dermatologic reactions, including toxic epidermal necrolysis (TEN) and Stevens-Johnson syndrome (SJS) reported; increased risk with presence of HLA-B*1502 allele. Patients with ancestry in genetically at-risk populations should be screened for presence of HLA-B*1502 prior to initiating treatment. Aplastic anemia and agranulocytosis reported. Obtain complete pretreatment hematological testing as baseline. D/C if evidence of bone marrow depression develops.

THERAPEUTIC CLASS: Carboxamide

INDICATIONS: Treatment of acute manic and mixed episodes associated with Bipolar I Disorder.

DOSAGE: *Adults:* Initial: 400mg/day, given in divided doses, bid. Titrate: Adjust in increments of 200mg/day. Max: 1600mg/day.

HOW SUPPLIED: Cap, Extended-Release: 100mg, 200mg, 300mg

CONTRAINDICATIONS: History of previous bone marrow depression, hypersensitivity to TCAs (eg, amitriptyline, desipramine, imipramine, protriptyline, and nortriptyline), MAOI use within 14 days, coadministration with nefazodone.

WARNINGS/PRECAUTIONS: D/C at first sign of rash, unless rash is clearly not drug-related. Increased risk of suicidal thoughts or behavior; monitor for emergence or worsening of depression, suicidal thoughts and behavior, and/or any unusual changes in mood or behavior. May cause fetal harm if administered to a pregnant woman. In patients with seizure disorder, avoid abrupt d/c; may precipitate status epilepticus. Mild anticholinergic activity may occur; observe closely with increased intraocular pressure (IOP). Caution in patients with a history of cardiac, hepatic, or renal damage, or interrupted courses of therapy with carbamazepine. Previous adverse hematologic reaction to other drugs may increase risk of bone marrow depression. May activate latent psychosis. May cause confusion/agitation in elderly. May impair physical/mental abilities. Before initiating therapy, obtain a detailed history and perform physical exam.

ADVERSE REACTIONS: Dizziness, somnolence, N/V, agranulocytosis, headache, infection, pain, rash, diarrhea, dyspepsia, asthenia, aplastic anemia, amnesia, TEN, SJS.

INTERACTIONS: See Contraindications. CYP3A4 and/or epoxide hydrolase inhibitors (eg, acetazolamide, azole antifungals, cimetidine, clarithromycin, protease inhibitors) may increase plasma levels. CYP3A4 inducers (eg, cisplatin, phenobarbital, phenytoin) may decrease plasma levels. May lower plasma levels of CYP1A2 substrates and CYP3A4 substrates (eg, acetaminophen, bupropion, clonazepam, doxycycline, oral contraceptives, warfarin). May decrease effectiveness and increase incidence of breakthrough bleeding with oral contraceptives. May increase or decrease plasma levels of phenytoin;

monitor phenytoin levels. May reduce warfarin's anticoagulant effect. May increase plasma levels of clomipramine and primidone. May increase the risk of neurotoxic side effects with lithium. May decrease levels of trazodone. Antimalarial drugs (eg, chloroquine, mefloquine) may antagonize the activity of carbamazepine. Caution with other centrally acting drugs and alcohol. Coadministration with delavirdine may lead to loss of virologic response and possible resistance to NNRTIs.

PREGNANCY: Category D, not for use in nursing.

MECHANISM OF ACTION: Carboxamide; mechanism has not been established. Suspected to modulate sodium and calcium ion channels, receptor-mediated neurotransmitters, and intracellular signaling pathways.

PHARMACOKINETICS: Absorption: C_{max}=1.9mcg/mL (single 200mg dose), 11mcg/mL (multiple 800mg dose); T_{max}=19 (single 200mg dose), 5.9 hrs (multiple 800mg dose). **Distribution:** Plasma protein binding (76%); found in breast milk, crosses the placenta. **Metabolism:** Liver via CYP3A4; carbamazepine-10,11-epoxide (metabolite). **Elimination:** Urine (72%; 3% unchanged), feces (28%); $T_{1/2}$=35-40 hrs (single dose), 12-17 hrs (multiple doses).

NURSING CONSIDERATIONS

Assessment: Assess use in patients with history of cardiac, hepatic or renal damage. Assess use in patients who have had a history of interrupted courses of therapy with carbamazepine and in patients who had a previous hematological reaction to other medications. Assess for history of bone marrow depression, sensitivity to any tricyclic compounds, presence of a seizure disorder, presence of increased IOP, pregnancy/nursing status, and for possible drug interactions. Assess for HLA-B*1502 allele in suspected patient populations. Prior to initiating therapy, obtain a detailed history and perform physical exam. Obtain baseline CBC, including reticulocyte count, serum iron levels, LFTs, urinalysis, BUN, and eye exam.

Monitoring: Monitor for signs/symptoms of dermatological reactions (eg, TEN, SJS), aplastic anemia, agranulocytosis, suicidal behavior or ideation, worsening of depression, mood changes, activation of latent psychosis, development of bone marrow depression, and for increased IOP. In elderly patients, monitor for signs/symptoms of agitation. Perform periodic monitoring of CBC including reticulocytes, serum iron levels, liver function, urinalysis, BUN, total cholesterol levels, LDL levels, HDL levels, thyroid function tests, and serum drug levels. Perform periodic eye exams, including slit-lamp examination, funduscopy, and tonometry.

Patient Counseling: Instruct to immediately report signs/symptoms of hematologic disorders (eg, fever, sore throat, rash, ulcers in the mouth, easy bruising, petechial or purpuric hemorrhage). Inform that therapy may increase the risk of suicidal thoughts and behaviors; instruct to contact physician if symptoms of worsening depression develop or unusual changes in behavior or mood develop. Advise that dizziness or drowsiness may occur; caution against performing hazardous tasks (eg, operating machinery/driving). Inform that, if necessary, caps may be opened and contents sprinkled over food; instruct not to crush or chew caps. Advise to notify physician of all prescription, OTC, and herbal products currently taking. Instruct to notify physician if pregnant or planning to get pregnant.

Administration: Oral route; do not crush or chew. **Storage:** 25°C (77°F); excursions permitted to 15-30°C (59-86°F). Protect from light and moisture.

ERAXIS   RX
anidulafungin (Pfizer)

THERAPEUTIC CLASS: Echinocandin

INDICATIONS: Treatment of esophageal candidiasis, candidemia, and other forms of *Candida* infections (intra-abdominal abscess and peritonitis).

DOSAGE: *Adults:* Duration of treatment based on patient's clinical response. Candidemia/*Candida* Infections: LD: 200mg on Day 1. Follow with 100mg qd

E

thereafter. Continue therapy for at least 14 days after last positive culture. Esophageal Candidiasis: LD: 100mg on Day 1 followed by 50mg qd thereafter. Treat for minimum of 14 days and for at least 7 days after symptoms resolve. Consider suppressive antifungal therapy for esophageal candidiasis in patients with HIV infections due to risk of relapse.

HOW SUPPLIED: Inj: 50mg, 100mg

WARNINGS/PRECAUTIONS: Laboratory abnormalities in LFTs reported; monitor hepatic function and evaluate risk/benefit of continuing therapy if abnormal LFTs develop during therapy.

ADVERSE REACTIONS: Diarrhea, hypokalemia.

INTERACTIONS: Hepatic abnormalities may occur with multiple concomitant medications in patients with serious underlying medical conditions. Slightly increased levels with cyclosporine.

PREGNANCY: Category C, caution in nursing.

MECHANISM OF ACTION: Echinocandin; inhibits glucan synthase which results in the inhibition of the synthesis of 1, 3-β-D-glucan, an essential component of fungal cell walls.

PHARMACOKINETICS: Absorption: IV infusion of variable doses resulted in different parameters. **Distribution:** V_d=30-50L; plasma protein binding (>99%). **Elimination:** Urine (<1%), feces (30%; <10% intact drug); $T_{1/2}$=40-50 hrs.

NURSING CONSIDERATIONS

Assessment: Obtain cultures and perform other laboratory studies prior to therapy to properly identify causative organisms. Assess for infections, intra-abdominal abscess, peritonitis, liver function, underlying medical conditions, hypersensitivity, pregnancy/nursing status and other possible drug interactions.

Monitoring: Monitor LFTs for possible hepatic dysfunction, hepatitis or hepatic failure. Monitor for histamine-mediated symptoms, serum electrolytes (K⁺), and other adverse reactions.

Patient Counseling: Counsel about risks/benefits of therapy. Inform of possible histamine-mediated symptoms including rash, urticaria, flushing, pruritus, dyspnea, and hypotension. Notify about signs/symptoms of hepatic dysfunction.

Administration: IV route. Refer to PI for preparation for administration. Rate of infusion should not exceed 1.1mg/min (equivalent to 1.4mL/min or 84mL/hr when reconstituted and diluted per instructions). Visually inspect for particulate matter and discoloration prior to administration. **Storage:** (Unreconstituted/Reconstituted vials/Infusion solution) 2-8°C (36-46°F). (Reconstituted vials) Stable for up to 1 hr. (Infusion solution) Administer within 24 hrs. Do not freeze.

ERBITUX   RX

cetuximab (Bristol-Myers Squibb)

> Serious infusion reactions reported; immediately interrupt and permanently d/c infusion if these reactions occur. Cardiopulmonary arrest and/or sudden death have occurred with squamous cell carcinoma of the head and neck (SCCHN) treated with radiation therapy and cetuximab; closely monitor serum electrolytes during and after therapy.

THERAPEUTIC CLASS: Epidermal growth factor receptor (EGFR) antagonist

INDICATIONS: In combination with radiation therapy for the initial treatment of locally or regionally advanced SCCHN. As monotherapy with recurrent or metastatic SCCHN for whom prior platinum-based therapy has failed and for treatment of epidermal growth factor receptor (EGFR)-expressing metastatic colorectal cancer in patients who are intolerant to irinotecan-based regimens or after failure of both irinotecan- and oxaliplatin-based regimens. In combination with irinotecan for the treatment of EGFR-expressing metastatic colorectal cancer in patients who are refractory to irinotecan-based chemotherapy.

DOSAGE: *Adults:* Premedication: H₁ antagonist (eg, 50mg diphenhydramine) IV 30-60 min prior to 1st dose. SCCHN: Combination with Radiation Therapy: Initial: 400mg/m² IV over 120 min, 1 week prior to initiation of a course of radiation therapy. Maint: 250mg/m² over 60 min weekly for duration of radiation therapy (6-7 weeks). Complete administration 1 hr prior to radiation therapy. Monotherapy: Initial: 400mg/m² IV over 120 min. Maint: 250mg/m² over 60 min weekly until disease progression or unacceptable toxicity. Max Infusion Rate: 10mg/min. Colorectal Cancer as Monotherapy/In Combination with Irinotecan: Initial: 400mg/m² IV over 120 min. Maint: 250mg/m² over 60 min weekly until disease progression or unacceptable toxicity. Dose Modifications: Refer to PI for dose modifications for infusion or dermatologic toxicities.

HOW SUPPLIED: Inj: 2mg/mL [50mL, 100mL]

WARNINGS/PRECAUTIONS: Not recommended for colorectal cancer treatment with KRAS mutations in codon 12 or 13. Caution when used in combination with radiation therapy in head and neck cancer with history of coronary artery disease (CAD), congestive heart failure (CHF), or arrhythmias. Interstitial lung disease (ILD) reported; interrupt for acute onset or worsening of pulmonary symptoms and d/c if ILD confirmed. Dermatologic toxicities (eg, acneform rash, skin drying/fissuring, paronychial inflammation, infectious sequelae) and hypertrichosis may occur; limit sun exposure during therapy. Hypomagnesemia and electrolyte abnormalities may occur; replete electrolytes as necessary.

ADVERSE REACTIONS: Cutaneous reactions (eg, rash, pruritus, nail changes), headache, diarrhea, infection, infusion reactions, cardiopulmonary arrest, dermatologic toxicity, radiation dermatitis, sepsis, renal failure, ILD, pulmonary embolus.

INTERACTIONS: Serious cardiotoxicity and death observed with radiation therapy and cisplatin with locally advanced SCCHN.

PREGNANCY: Category C, not for use in nursing.

MECHANISM OF ACTION: Epidermal growth factor receptor antagonist; binds specifically to EGFR on normal and tumor cells and inhibits binding of epidermal growth factor and other ligands, such as transforming growth factor-α.

PHARMACOKINETICS: Absorption: C_{max}=168-235mcg/mL. **Distribution:** V_d=2-3L/m²; crosses the placenta. **Elimination:** $T_{1/2}$=112 hrs.

NURSING CONSIDERATIONS

Assessment: Assess for SCCHN, history of CAD, CHF, arrhythmias, pulmonary disorders, and colorectal cancer with mutations. Assess pregnancy/nursing status and possible drug interactions. Obtain baseline serum electrolyte levels (Mg^{2+}, K^+, Ca^{2+}).

Monitoring: Periodically monitor electrolytes (Mg^{2+}, K^+, Ca^{2+}) during and 8 weeks after drug administration. Monitor for signs/symptoms of hypomagnesemia, hypocalcemia, hypokalemia, acute onset or worsening of pulmonary symptoms, infusion reactions, dermatologic toxicities, and infectious sequelae. Monitor patients for 1 hr after infusion, and for a longer period to confirm resolution of the event in patients requiring treatment for infusion reactions.

Patient Counseling: Inform of pregnancy/nursing risks; advise to use effective contraceptive methods during and 6 months after therapy for both sexes. Inform that nursing is not recommended during and for 2 months following therapy. Instruct to limit sun exposure (eg, use of sunscreen) during and for 2 months after therapy. Seek medical attention if symptoms of infusion reaction (eg, fever, chills, breathing problems) occur.

Administration: IV route. Do not administer as IV push or bolus. Administer through low protein binding 0.22-μm in-line filter. Inspect visually for particulate matter and discoloration prior to administration. Do not shake or dilute.

Storage: Vials: 2-8°C (36-46°F). Do not freeze. Infusion Containers: Stable for 12 hrs at 2-8°C (36-46°F) and up to 8 hrs at 20-25°C (68-77°F). Discard unused portion of vial.

ERTACZO   RX
sertaconazole nitrate (Ortho Neutrogena)

THERAPEUTIC CLASS: Azole antifungal

INDICATIONS: Treatment of interdigital tinea pedis in immunocompetent patients ≥12 yrs caused by *Trichophyton rubrum*, *Trichophyton mentagrophytes* and *Epidermophyton floccosum*.

DOSAGE: *Adults:* Apply bid to affected areas between toes and adjacent areas for 4 weeks. Re-evaluate if no clinical improvement is seen 2 weeks after the treatment period.
Pediatrics: ≥12 yrs: Apply bid to affected areas between toes and adjacent areas for 4 weeks. Re-evaluate if no clinical improvement is seen 2 weeks after the treatment period.

HOW SUPPLIED: Cre: 2% [30g, 60g]

WARNINGS/PRECAUTIONS: Not for ophthalmic, oral or intravaginal use. D/C if irritation or sensitivity occurs. Caution in patients sensitive to other imidazole antifungals; cross-reactivity may occur. Confirm diagnosis by direct microscopic examination or culture.

ADVERSE REACTIONS: Application-site reaction, hyperpigmentation, vesiculation, desquamation.

PREGNANCY: Category C, caution in nursing.

MECHANISM OF ACTION: Azole antifungal agent; not established. Suspected to act primarily by inhibiting CYP450-dependent synthesis of ergosterol, a key component of fungi cell membranes. Lack of ergosterol leads to fungal cell injury through leakage of key constituents in cytoplasm from cell.

NURSING CONSIDERATIONS

Assessment: Assess for hypersensitivity to imidazoles and for proper diagnosis of the disease (eg, direct microscopic exam, culture). Assess pregnancy/nursing status.

Monitoring: Monitor for signs/symptoms of skin irritation or sensitivity. Monitor for signs of clinical response. If no clinical improvement seen 2 weeks after the treatment period, reassess diagnosis.

Patient Counseling: Instruct to dry affected area before application and to avoid contact with eyes, mouth, or other mucous membranes. Advise to wash hands after applying medication and avoid occlusive dressings on treated site unless directed. Use medication for fully prescribed treatment time, even if symptoms improve. Advise to contact physician if no clinical improvement or if condition worsens or if signs of irritation, itching, burning, blistering, swelling, or oozing develop from application site.

Administration: Topical route. **Storage:** 25°C (77°F); excursions permitted to 15-30°C (59-86°F).

ERY-TAB   RX
erythromycin (Abbott)

THERAPEUTIC CLASS: Macrolide

INDICATIONS: Treatment of mild to moderate upper/lower respiratory tract and skin and skin structure infections, listeriosis, pertussis, diphtheria, erythrasma, intestinal amebiasis, acute pelvic inflammatory disease (PID) (*N.gonorrhoeae*), primary syphilis (if PCN allergy), Legionnaires' disease, chlamydial infections (eg, newborn conjunctivitis, pneumonia of infancy, urogenital infections during pregnancy, or urethral, endocervical, or rectal infections when tetracyclines are contraindicated or not tolerated), and nongonococcal urethritis caused by susceptible strains of microorganisms. Prophylaxis of initial and recurrent attacks of rheumatic fever if PCN allergy.

DOSAGE: *Adults:* Usual: 250mg qid, 333mg q8h or 500mg q12h. Max: 4g/day. Do not take bid when dose is >1g/day. Treat strep infections for at least 10

days. Streptococcal Infection Long-Term Prophylaxis with Rheumatic Fever: 250mg bid. Chlamydial Urogenital Infection During Pregnancy: 500mg qid or 666mg q8h for at least 7 days, or 500mg q12h, 333mg q8h or 250mg qid for at least 14 days. Urethral/Endocervical/Rectal Chlamydial Infections and Nongonococcal Urethritis: 500mg qid or 666mg q8h for at least 7 days. Primary Syphilis: 30-40g in divided doses for 10-15 days. Acute PID: 500mg (erythromycin lactobionate) IV q6h for 3 days, then 500mg PO q12h or 333mg q8h for 7 days. Intestinal Amebiasis: 500mg q12h, 333mg q8h or 250mg q6h for 10-14 days. Pertussis: 40-50mg/kg/day in divided doses for 5-14 days. Legionnaires' Disease: 1-4g/day in divided doses.
Pediatrics: Usual: 30-50mg/kg/day in divided doses. Severe Infections: May double dose. Max: 4g/day. Treat strep infections for at least 10 days. Streptococcal Infection Long-Term Prophylaxis with Rheumatic Fever: 250mg bid. Chlamydial Conjunctivitis of Newborns/Chlamydial Pneumonia in Infancy: 12.5mg/kg qid for 2 weeks and 3 weeks, respectively. Intestinal Amebiasis: 30-50mg/kg/day in divided doses for 10-14 days.

HOW SUPPLIED: Tab, Delayed-Release: 250mg, 333mg, 500mg

CONTRAINDICATIONS: Concomitant terfenadine, astemizole, pimozide, or cisapride.

WARNINGS/PRECAUTIONS: Pseudomembranous colitis, hepatic dysfunction reported. Caution with impaired hepatic function. May aggravate weakness of patients with myasthenia gravis. Erythromycin does not reach adequate concentrations in fetus to prevent congenital syphilis.

ADVERSE REACTIONS: N/V, abdominal pain, diarrhea, anorexia, abnormal LFTs, allergic reactions, superinfection (prolonged use).

INTERACTIONS: See Contraindications. Rhabdomyolysis reported with lovastatin. May increase levels of theophylline, digoxin, drugs metabolized by CYP450 (eg, carbamazepine, cyclosporine, phenytoin, alfentanil, disopy-ramide, lovastatin, bromocriptine, valproate, etc). Increases effects of oral anticoagulants, triazolam, midazolam. Risk of acute ergot toxicity with ergot-amine or dihydroergotamine. May increase AUC of sildenafil; consider dose reduction of sildenafil.

PREGNANCY: Category B, caution in nursing.

MECHANISM OF ACTION: Macrolide antibiotic; inhibits protein synthesis by binding 50S ribosomal subunits of susceptible organisms.

PHARMACOKINETICS: Absorption: (PO) Readily absorbed. **Distribution:** Largely bound to plasma proteins. Crosses blood-brain barrier, placenta, and breast milk. Diffuses into most bodily fluids. **Elimination:** Biliary and urinary excretion (<5%).

NURSING CONSIDERATIONS

Assessment: Assess age of patient, conditions such as myasthenia gravis, arrhythmias and hepatic/renal function. Note other diseases/conditions and drug therapies.

Monitoring: Monitor LFTs, renal function, CDAD, pancreatitis, arrhythmias, and hypersensitivity reactions.

Patient Counseling: Inform to take exactly as directed and to complete entire course of therapy. Instruct to take on empty stomach. Advise to report any adverse effects, lack of response, and prolonged/persistent diarrhea.

Administration: Oral route. **Storage:** 30°C (86°F).

ERYTHROMYCIN BASE   RX
erythromycin (Various)

THERAPEUTIC CLASS: Macrolide

INDICATIONS: Treatment of mild to moderate upper/lower respiratory tract and skin/skin structure infections, listeriosis, pertussis, diphtheria, erythrasma, intestinal amebiasis, acute pelvic inflammatory disease (PID) (*N.gonorrhoeae*), primary syphilis (if PCN allergy), Legionnaires' disease, chlamydial infections (eg, newborn conjunctivitis, pneumonia of infancy, urogenital infections during pregnancy or urethral, endocervical, or rectal infections when tetracyclines are contraindicated or not tolerated), and nongonococcal urethritis caused by susceptible strains of microorganisms. Prophylaxis of initial and recurrent attacks of rheumatic fever if PCN allergy.

DOSAGE: *Adults:* Usual: 250mg qid or 500mg q12h without food. Max: 4g/day. Treat strep infections for at least 10 days. Streptococcal Infection Long-Term Prophylaxis of Rheumatic Fever: 250mg bid. Chlamydial Urogenital Infection During Pregnancy: 500mg qid for at least 7 days or 500mg q12h or 250mg qid for at least 14 days. Urethral/Endocervical/Rectal Chlamydial Infections and Nongonococcal Urethritis: 500mg qid for at least 7 days. Primary Syphilis: 30-40g in divided doses over 10-15 days. Acute PID: 500mg (erythromycin lactobionate) IV q6h for 3 days, then 500mg PO q12h for 7 days. Intestinal Amebiasis: 500mg q12h or 250mg q6h for 10-14 days. Pertussis: 40-50mg/kg/day in divided doses for 5-14 days. Legionnaires' Disease: 1-4g/day in divided doses.
Pediatrics: Usual: 30-50mg/kg/day in divided doses without food. Severe Infections: May double dose. Max: 4g/day. Treat strep infections for at least 10 days. Streptococcal Infection Long-Term Prophylaxis of Rheumatic Fever: 250mg bid. Chlamydial Conjunctivitis of Newborns/Chlamydial Pneumonia in Infancy: (Sus) 12.5mg/kg qid for 2 weeks and 3 weeks, respectively. Intestinal Amebiasis: 30-50mg/kg/day in divided doses for 10-14 days.

HOW SUPPLIED: Tab: 250mg, 500mg

CONTRAINDICATIONS: Concomitant terfenadine, astemizole, pimozide, or cisapride.

WARNINGS/PRECAUTIONS: Pseudomembranous colitis, hepatic dysfunction reported. Caution with impaired hepatic function. May aggravate weakness of patients with myasthenia gravis.

ADVERSE REACTIONS: Abdominal pain, N/V, diarrhea, anorexia, abnormal LFTs, allergic reactions, superinfection (prolonged use).

INTERACTIONS: See Contraindications. Rhabdomyolysis reported with lovastatin. May increase levels of theophylline, digoxin, drugs metabolized by CYP450 (eg, carbamazepine, cyclosporine, phenytoin, etc). Increases effects of oral anticoagulants, triazolam. Risk of acute ergot toxicity with ergotamine or dihydroergotamine. May increase AUC of sildenafil; consider dose reduction of sildenafil.

PREGNANCY: Category B, caution in nursing.

MECHANISM OF ACTION: Macrolide; inhibits protein synthesis by binding 50S ribosomal subunits of susceptible organisms.

PHARMACOKINETICS: Absorption: (PO) Readily absorbed. **Distribution:** Largely bound to plasma proteins. Crosses blood-brain barrier, placenta, breast milk. Diffuses into most body fluids. **Elimination:** Bile, urine (<5% unchanged).

NURSING CONSIDERATIONS

Assessment: Assess age of patient, conditions such as myasthenia gravis, arrhythmias, and hepatic/renal function. Note other diseases/conditions and drug therapies.

Monitoring: Monitor LFTs, renal function tests, *C.difficile*-associated diarrhea, pancreatitis, arrhythmias, and hypersensitivity reactions.

Patient Counseling: Inform that therapy only treats bacterial infections. Instruct to take exactly as directed and to report any adverse effects, lack of response, or prolonged/persistent diarrhea.

Administration: Oral route. **Storage:** Below 30°C (86°F). Keep tightly closed.

ERYTHROMYCIN DELAYED-RELEASE RX
erythromycin (Various)

THERAPEUTIC CLASS: Macrolide

INDICATIONS: Treatment of mild to moderate upper/lower respiratory tract and skin/skin structure infections, listeriosis, pertussis, diphtheria, erythrasma, intestinal amebiasis, acute pelvic inflammatory disease (PID) (*N.gonorrhoeae*), primary syphilis (if PCN allergy), Legionnaires' disease, chlamydial infections (eg, newborn conjunctivitis, pneumonia of infancy, urogenital infections during pregnancy, or urethral, endocervical, or rectal infections when tetracyclines are contraindicated or not tolerated), and nongonococcal urethritis caused by susceptible strains of micro-organisms. Prophylaxis of initial and recurrent attacks of rheumatic fever if PCN allergy.

DOSAGE: *Adults:* Usual: 250mg q6h or 500mg q12h without food. Max: 4g/day. Treat strep infections for 10 days. Streptococcal Infection Prophylaxis with Rheumatic Heart Disease: 250mg bid. Primary Syphilis: 30-40g in divided doses over 10-15 days. Intestinal Amebiasis: 250mg q6h for 10-14 days. Legionnaires' Disease: 1-4g/day in divided doses. Chlamydial Urogenital Infection During Pregnancy: 500mg qid for 7 days or 250mg qid for 14 days. Urethral/Endocervical/Rectal Chlamydial Infections and Nongonococcal Urethritis: 500mg qid for at least 7 days. Pertussis: 40-50mg/kg/day in divided doses for 5-14 days. Acute PID: 500mg (erythromycin lactobionate) IV q6h for 3 days, then 250mg PO q6h for 7 days.
Pediatrics: Usual: 30-50mg/kg/day in divided doses without food. Severe Infections: May double dose. Max: 4g/day. Treat strep infections for 10 days. Streptococcal Infection Prophylaxis with Rheumatic Heart Disease: 250mg bid. Intestinal Amebiasis: 30-50mg/kg/day in divided doses for 10-14 days.

HOW SUPPLIED: Cap, Delayed-Release: 250mg

CONTRAINDICATIONS: Concomitant terfenadine, astemizole, pimozide, or cisapride.

WARNINGS/PRECAUTIONS: Hepatic dysfunction and pseudomembranous colitis reported. May aggravate weakness of patients with myasthenia gravis.

ADVERSE REACTIONS: Abdominal pain, N/V, diarrhea, anorexia, hepatic dysfunction, abnormal LFTs, superinfection (prolonged use).

INTERACTIONS: See Contraindications. Rhabdomyolysis reported with lovastatin. May increase levels of theophylline, digoxin, drugs metabolized by CYP450 (eg, carbamazepine, cyclosporine, phenytoin, etc). Increases effects of oral anticoagulants, triazolam. Risk of acute ergot toxicity with ergotamine or dihydroergotamine. Extreme caution with terfenadine.

PREGNANCY: Category B, caution in nursing.

MECHANISM OF ACTION: Macrolide; inhibits protein synthesis by binding 50S ribosomal subunits of susceptible organisms.

PHARMACOKINETICS: Absorption: (PO) Readily absorbed; C_{max}=1.13-1.68mcg/mL; T_{max}=3 hrs. **Distribution:** Largely bound to plasma proteins; diffuses into most bodily fluids; crosses blood-brain barrier, placenta, and breast milk. **Elimination:** Bile, urine (<5% unchanged).

NURSING CONSIDERATIONS

Assessment: Assess age of patient, conditions such as myasthenia gravis, arrhythmias and hepatic/renal function. Note other diseases/conditions and drug therapies.

Monitoring: Monitor LFTs, renal function, *C.difficile* associated diarrhea, pancreatitis, arrhythmias, and hypersensitivity reactions.

Patient Counseling: Inform therapy treats bacterial, not viral, infections. Take exactly as directed; complete entire course of therapy. Take medication on empty stomach and report adverse effects, lack of response, and prolonged/persistent diarrhea.

Administration: Oral route. **Storage:** Below 30°C (86°F). Protect from moisture and excessive heat.

ESTRACE

RX

estradiol (Warner Chilcott)

> Estrogens increase the risk of endometrial cancer. Perform adequate diagnostic measures, including endometrial sampling, to rule out malignancy in all cases of undiagnosed persistent or recurring abnormal vaginal bleeding. Estrogens, with or without progestins, should not be used for the prevention of CV disease. Increased risks of myocardial infarction (MI), stroke, invasive breast cancer, pulmonary embolism (PE), and deep vein thrombosis (DVT) in postmenopausal women (50-79 yrs of age) reported. Increased risk of developing probable dementia in post-menopausal women ≥65 yrs of age reported. Estrogens, with or without progestins, should be prescribed at the lowest effective dose and for the shortest duration consistent with treatment goals and risks for the individual women.

THERAPEUTIC CLASS: Estrogen

INDICATIONS: (Cre/Tab) Treatment of vulval and vaginal atrophy. (Tab) Treatment of moderate to severe vasomotor symptoms associated with menopause. Treatment of hypoestrogenism due to hypogonadism, castration, or primary ovarian failure. Palliative treatment of metastatic breast cancer and advanced androgen-dependent prostate carcinoma. Prevention of osteoporosis.

DOSAGE: *Adults:* (Cre) Vulval/Vaginal Atrophy: Initial: 2-4g/day for 1-2 weeks, then decrease to 1-2g/day for 1-2 weeks. Maint: 1g, 1-3x/week. D/C or taper at 3- to 6-month intervals. (Tab) Vasomotor Symptoms/Vulval/Vaginal Atrophy: Initial: 1-2mg/day (3 weeks on, 1 week off). Maint: Minimum effective dose. D/C or taper at 3- to 6-month intervals. Hypoestrogenism: Initial: 1-2mg/day. Maint: minimum effective dose. Metastatic Breast Cancer: 10mg tid for at least 3 months. Prostate Carcinoma: 1-2mg tid. Osteoporosis Prevention: 0.5mg qd cyclically (23 days on and 5 days off).

HOW SUPPLIED: Cre, Vaginal: 0.1mg/g [42.5g]; Tab: 0.5mg*, 1mg*, 2mg*
*scored

CONTRAINDICATIONS: Pregnancy, undiagnosed abnormal genital bleeding, known, suspected or history of breast cancer unless being treated for meta-static disease, estrogen-dependent neoplasia, active or history of DVT, active or history of pulmonary embolism, active or recent arterial thromboembolic disease (eg, stroke, MI), liver dysfunction or disease.

WARNINGS/PRECAUTIONS: May increase risk of CV events (eg, MI, stroke), venous thrombosis, PE; d/c immediately if any of these events occur or are suspected. May increase risk of breast/endometrial cancer, and gallbladder disease. Retinal vascular thrombosis reported; d/c if papilledema or retinal vascular lesions occur. May cause severe hypercalcemia in patients with breast cancer and bone metastases; d/c if occurs. Consider addition of a progestin if no hysterectomy. May elevate BP; monitor at regular intervals. May cause elevation of triglycerides leading to pancreatitis in patients with pre-existing hypertriglyceridemia. Caution with history of cholestatic jaundice associated with past estrogen use or with pregnancy; d/c with recurrence. May lead to increased thyroid-binding globulin levels; monitor thyroid function in patients dependent on thyroid replacement therapy. May cause fluid retention; caution with cardiac/renal dysfunction. Caution with severe hypocalcemia. May increase risk of ovarian cancer. May exacerbate endometriosis, asthma, DM, epilepsy, migraine, porphyria, systemic lupus erythematosus (SLE), hepatic hemangiomas; use with caution. Acceleration of PT, PTT. Hypercoagulability effects. Impaired glucose tolerance.

ADVERSE REACTIONS: Altered vaginal bleeding, vaginal candidiasis, breast tenderness/enlargement, galactorrhea, N/V, thrombophlebitis, melasma, abdominal cramps, headache, mental depression, weight changes, edema, altered libido.

INTERACTIONS: CYP3A4 inducers (eg, St. John's wort, phenobarbital, carbamazepine, rifampin) may decrease levels, which may decrease therapeutic effects and/or change uterine bleeding profile. CYP3A4 inhibitors (eg, erythromycin, clarithromycin, ketoconazole, itraconazole, ritonavir, grapefruit juice) may increase levels, which may result in side effects. Patients on thyroid replacement therapy may require higher dose of thyroid hormones.

PREGNANCY: Contraindicated in pregnancy. (Tab) Category X. Caution in nursing.

MECHANISM OF ACTION: Estrogen; binds to nuclear receptors in estrogen-responsive tissue. Circulating estrogens modulate pituitary secretion of gonadotropins, luteinizing hormone (LH), and follicle stimulating hormone (FSH) through a negative feedback mechanism. Reduces elevated levels of these hormones in postmenopausal women.

PHARMACOKINETICS: Absorption: (Cre) Absorbed through skin, mucous membranes, and GI tract. **Distribution**: Largely bound to sex hormone-binding globulin and albumin; found in breast milk. **Metabolism**: Liver to estrone (metabolite), estriol (major urinary metabolite); sulfate and glucuronide conjugation (liver); gut hydrolysis followed by reabsorption. **Elimination**: Urine.

NURSING CONSIDERATIONS

Assessment: Assess for abnormal genital bleeding, presence or history of breast cancer, DVT/PE or history of, presence of estrogen-dependent neoplasia, active or recent (within past yr) arterial thromboembolic disease (eg, stroke, MI), liver dysfunction/disease, known/suspected pregnancy. Assess use in patients ≥65 yrs, nursing females, hypocalcemia, asthma, DM, epilepsy, migraine or porphyria, SLE, and hepatic hemangiomas. Assess for drug and lab interactions. pregnancy/nursing status, and possible drug interactions. Assess need for progestin therapy in women who have not had a hysterectomy.

Monitoring: Monitor for signs/symptoms of CV disorders (eg, MI, stroke, venous thrombosis, PE), malignant neoplasms (eg, endometrial, breast, ovarian cancer), dementia, gallbladder disease, hypercalcemia, visual abnormalities (eg, retinal vascular thrombosis), elevations in BP, elevations in plasma triglycerides, pancreatitis, hypothyroidism, fluid retention, exacerbation of endometriosis and other conditions (eg, asthma, DM, epilepsy, migraine, SLE). For cream formulation, monitor for hypersensitivity reactions. Monitor thyroid function in patients on thyroid replacement therapy. Monitor BP at regular intervals. If undiagnosed, persistent, or recurring abnormal vaginal bleeding occurs, perform proper diagnostic measures (eg, endometrial sampling) to rule out malignancy. Perform periodic monitoring (eg, every 3-6 months) to determine if treatment still required.

Patient Counseling: Inform medication increases chances of uterine cancer. Instruct to notify physician of upcoming surgery or need for prolonged bed rest. Advise to contact physician if breast lumps, unusual vaginal bleeding, dizziness and faintness, changes in speech, severe headaches, chest pain, SOB, leg pains, changes in vision, or vomiting occur. Instruct to notify physician if pregnant or nursing. Advise to perform monthly self breast exams.

Administration: Cre: Intravaginal route. Tab: Oral route. **Storage**: Cre: Store at room temperature; protect from temperatures >40°C (104°F). Keep out of reach of children. Tab: 15-30°C (59-86°F); dispense tight, light-resistant container.

ESTRADERM RX
estradiol (Novartis)

> Estrogens increase the risk of endometrial cancer. Estrogens, with or without progestins, should not be used for the prevention of CV disease or dementia. Increased risks of MI, stroke, invasive breast cancer, PE, and DVT in postmenopausal women (50-79 yrs of age) reported. Increased risk of developing probable dementia in postmenopausal women ≥65 yrs of age reported.

THERAPEUTIC CLASS: Estrogen

INDICATIONS: Treatment of moderate-to-severe vasomotor symptoms and/or vulvar/vaginal atrophy associated with menopause. Treatment of hypoestrogenism due to hypogonadism, castration, or primary ovarian failure. Prevention of postmenopausal osteoporosis.

DOSAGE: *Adults:* Apply to clean, dry area on trunk of body. Do not apply to breast or waistline. Replace twice weekly. Rotate application sites. May give continuously without intact uterus. May give cyclically (3 weeks on, 1 week off) with intact uterus. Vasomotor Symptoms/Vulvar/Vaginal Atrophy: Initial: Apply 0.05mg/day twice weekly. Discontinue/Taper at 3-6 month intervals. Start 1 week after discontinuing oral hormone therapy. Osteoporosis Prevention: Initial: 0.05mg/day.

HOW SUPPLIED: Patch: 0.05mg/24 hrs, 0.1mg/24 hrs [8^s, 24^s]

CONTRAINDICATIONS: Pregnancy, undiagnosed abnormal genital bleeding, breast cancer unless being treated for metastatic disease, estrogen-dependent neoplasia, DVT/PE, active or recent (eg, within past year) arterial thromboembolic disease (eg, stroke, MI), liver dysfunction or disease.

WARNINGS/PRECAUTIONS: May increase risk of cardiovascular events (eg, MI, stroke), venous thrombosis, and PE; d/c immediately if any of these events occur or are suspected. May increase risk of breast/endometrial cancer, and gallbladder disease. May lead to severe hypercalcemia with breast cancer and bone metastases; monitor and d/c if hypercalcemia occurs. Retinal vascular thrombosis reported; monitor and d/c if papilledema or retinal vascular lesions occur. Consider addition of a progestin if no hysterectomy. May elevate BP; monitor at regular intervals. May cause elevations of plasma triglycerides with pre-existing hypertriglyceridemia. Caution with history of cholestatic jaundice associated with past estrogen use or with pregnancy; d/c with recurrence. May lead to increased thyroid-binding globulin levels; monitor thyroid function. May cause fluid retention; caution with cardiac/renal dysfunction. Caution with severe hypocalcemia. May increase risk of ovarian cancer. May exacerbate endometriosis, asthma, DM, epilepsy, migraine, porphyria, SLE, and hepatic hemangiomas; use with caution.

ADVERSE REACTIONS: Redness/irritation at application site, altered vaginal bleeding, vaginal candidiasis, breast tenderness/enlargement, GI effects, melasma, CNS effects, retinal vascular thrombosis, weight changes, edema, altered libido.

INTERACTIONS: CYP3A4 inducers (eg, St. John's wort, phenobarbital, carbamazepine, rifampin) may decrease levels resulting in decreased therapeutic effects and/or changes in uterine bleeding profile. CYP3A4 inhibitors (eg, erythromycin, clarithromycin, ketoconazole, itraconazole, ritonavir, grapefruit juice) may increase levels and result in side effects.

PREGNANCY: Category X, caution in nursing.

MECHANISM OF ACTION: Estrogen; binds to nuclear receptors in estrogen-responsive tissues. Modulates pituitary secretion of gonadotropins, luteinizing hormone and follicle stimulating hormone, through negative feedback mechanism. Reduces elevated levels of these hormones in postmenopausal women,

PHARMACOKINETICS: Distribution: Largely bound to sex hormone binding globulin and albumin; found in breast milk. **Metabolism**: Liver to estrone (metabolite) and estriol (major urinary metabolite); sulfate and glucuronide conjugation (liver), gut hydrolysis; CYP3A4 (partial metabolism). **Elimination**: Urine (parent compound and metabolites); $T_{1/2}$=1 hr.

NURSING CONSIDERATIONS

Assessment: Assess for abnormal genital bleeding, presence or history of breast cancer, DVT/PE or history of, presence of estrogen-dependent neoplasia, active or recent (within past yr) arterial thromboembolic disease (eg, stroke, MI), liver dysfunction/disease, known/suspected pregnancy. Assess use in patients ≥65 yrs, nursing females, hypocalcemia, asthma, DM, epilepsy, migraine or porphyria, SLE, and hepatic hemangiomas. Assess for drug and lab interactions. Assess need for progestin therapy in women who have not had a hysterectomy.

Monitoring: Monitor for signs/symptoms of cardiovascular events (eg, MI, stroke, venous thrombosis, PE), malignant neoplasms (eg, endometrial, breast, ovarian cancer), dementia, gallbladder disease, hypercalcemia, visual disorders (eg, retinal vascular thrombosis), elevations in BP, elevations in plasma triglycerides, pancreatitis, hypothyroidism, fluid retention, exacerbation of endometriosis and other conditions (eg, asthma, DM, epilepsy, migraines, SLE). Monitor thyroid function in patients on thyroid replacement therapy. Perform regular monitoring of BP levels, annual breast exam, and periodic evelation (every 3-6 months) to determine need for therapy. If undiagnosed, persistent, or recurring bleeding occurs, perform proper diagnostic testing (eg, endometrial sampling) to rule out malignancy.

Patient Counseling: Inform drug increases risk for uterine cancer. Report breast lumps, unusual vaginal bleeding, dizziness or faintness, changes in speech, severe headaches, chest pain, SOB, leg pains, changes in vision, or vomiting. Instruct to place medication system on clean, dry skin on the trunk (including buttocks and abdomen); site should not be exposed to sunlight; area should not be oily, damaged, or irritated; do not apply to breasts. Rotate application sites. Apply immediately after opening pouch. If medication system falls off, reapply same system; if not able to, apply new system; continue with original treatment schedule. Notify physician if planning surgery or prolonged immobilization. Advise to perform monthly self breast exams.

Administration: Transdermal route. **Storage**: Do not store above 30°C (86°F). Do not store unpouched.

ESTRASORB

RX

estradiol (Graceway)

> Estrogens increase the risk of endometrial cancer. Estrogens, with or without progestins, should not be used for the prevention of cardiovascular (CV) disease or dementia. Increased risks of MI, stroke, invasive breast cancer, pulmonary emboli (PE), and deep vein thrombosis (DVT) in post-menopausal women (50-79 yrs of age) reported. Increased risk of developing probable dementia in postmenopausal women ≥65 yrs of age reported.

THERAPEUTIC CLASS: Estrogen

INDICATIONS: Treatment of moderate to severe vasomotor symptoms associated with menopause.

DOSAGE: *Adults:* Apply 2 pouches qam. Apply one pouch to each leg from the upper thigh to the calf. Rub in for 3 min until thoroughly absorbed.

HOW SUPPLIED: Emulsion, Topical: 4.35mg/1.74g (pouch)

CONTRAINDICATIONS: Undiagnosed abnormal genital bleeding, known/suspected/history of breast cancer, known/suspected history of estrogen-dependent neoplasia, DVT/PE, active or recent arterial thromboembolic disease (eg, stroke, MI), liver dysfunction or disease, pregnancy.

WARNINGS/PRECAUTIONS: Limit use to the shortest duration consistent with goals and risks; re-evaluate periodically. Increased risk of CV events (eg, MI, stroke, venous thromboembolism, PE), gallbladder disease, breast and endometrial cancer. D/C 4-6 weeks before surgery associated with an increased risk of thromboembolism or during prolonged immobilization. Possible increased risk of ovarian cancer. May lead to severe hypercalcemia in patients with breast cancer and bone metastases; monitor and d/c if hypercalcemia occurs. Consider adding progestin in patients with intact uterus to avoid endometrial hyperplasia. Increased thyroid-binding globulin levels (may need higher doses of thyroid hormone). May cause fluid retention; caution in cardiac or renal dysfunction. Retinal vascular thrombosis and elevated BP reported. May exacerbate endometriosis, asthma, diabetes mellitus (DM), epilepsy, migraine, porphyria, systemic lupus erythematosus (SLE), or hepatic hemangiomas; use with caution. Avoid use in close proximity to sunscreen application; may increase absorption. Potential for estradiol transfer through physical contact; wash application site 8 hrs post-application. May cause elevations of plasma triglycerides with pre-existing hypertriglyceridemia. Caution with history of cholestatic jaundice associated with past estrogen use or with pregnancy; d/c with recurrence.

ADVERSE REACTIONS: Headache, infection, sinusitis, pruritus, breast pain, endometrial disorder.

INTERACTIONS: CYP3A4 inducers (eg, St. John's wort, phenobarbital, carbamazepine, rifampin) may decrease levels, which may decrease therapeutic effects and/or change uterine bleeding profile. CYP3A4 inhibitors (eg, erythromycin, clarithromycin, ketoconazole, itraconazole, ritonavir, grapefruit juice) may increase levels, which may result in side effects. Increased abnormal mammogram results reported with estrogen plus progestin that requires further evaluation.

PREGNANCY: Contraindicated in pregnancy, caution in nursing.

MECHANISM OF ACTION: Estrogen; binds to nuclear receptors in estrogen-responsive tissues. Circulating estrogens modulate pituitary secretion of gonadotropins, LH and FSH, through negative feedback mechanism. Reduces elevated levels of these hormones in postmenopausal women.

PHARMACOKINETICS: Distribution: Largely bound to sex hormone binding globulin (SHBG) and albumin. **Metabolism:** Liver to estrone (metabolite), estriol (major urinary metabolite); sulfate and glucuronide conjugation (liver), gut hydrolysis; CYP 3A4 (partial metabolism). **Excretion:** Urine (parent compound and metabolites).

NURSING CONSIDERATIONS

Assessment: Assess for undiagnosed abnormal genital bleeding, presence or history of breast cancer, DVT, PE, estrogen-dependent neoplasia, active or recent arterial thromboembolic disease (eg, MI, stroke), liver dysfunction, pregnancy/nursing status, familial hyperlipoproteinemia, age (≥65 yrs), hypothyroidism, hypocalcemia, asthma, DM, epilepsy, migraine, porphyria, SLE, and possible drug interactions. Assess need for progestin therapy in women who have not had a hysterectomy.

Monitoring: Monitor for signs/symptoms of CV events (eg, MI, stroke, venous thrombosis, PE), malignant neoplasms (eg, endometrial, breast, ovarian cancer), dementia, gallbladder disease, hypercalcemia, visual abnormalities (retinal vascular thrombosis), elevations in BP, elevations in plasma triglycerides, pancreatitis, hypothyroidism, fluid retention, exacerbation of endometriosis, and exacerbation of other conditions (eg, asthma, DM, epilepsy, migraines, SLE). Perform annual breast exam. Monitor thyroid function in patients on thyroid replacement therapy. Monitor BP levels at regular intervals. Perform proper diagnostic testing (eg, endometrial sampling) for abnormal, undiagnosed, persistent or recurring vaginal bleeding to rule out malignancy. Perform periodic evaluation (every 3-6 months) to determine need for therapy.

Patient Counseling: Inform that estrogens increase chances of developing uterine cancer. Contact physician if breast lumps, unusual vaginal bleeding, dizziness or faintness, changes in speech, severe headaches, chest pain, SOB, leg pains, changes in vision, or vomiting occur. Advise to open medication pouches just prior to use. Apply in the morning to clean, dry skin of both thighs and calves. Avoid applying medication to irritated or red skin. Sunscreen should not be applied to treatment area at same time; may interact with medication. Advise patients to have yearly breast examinations conducted by a healthcare provider and to perform monthly breast self-examinations.

Administration: Topical route. Refer to PI for proper application. **Storage:** 20-25°C (68-77°F); excursions permitted to 15-30°C (59-86°F).

ESTROSTEP FE   RX
norethindrone acetate - ferrous fumarate - ethinyl estradiol (Warner Chilcott)

> Cigarette smoking increases the risk of serious cardiovascular (CV) side effects. Risk increases with age (>35 years) and with heavy smoking (≥15 cigarettes/day). Women who use oral contraceptives should be strongly advised not to smoke.

THERAPEUTIC CLASS: Estrogen/progestogen combination

INDICATIONS: Prevention of pregnancy. Treatment of moderate acne vulgaris in females ≥15 yrs who want contraception (for at least 6 months), have achieved menarche, and are unresponsive to topical acne agents.

DOSAGE: *Adults:* Contraception/Acne: 1 tab qd for 28 days, then repeat. Start 1st Sunday after menses begins or the 1st day of menses.
Pediatrics: ≥15 yrs: Contraception (Postpubertal Adolescents)/Acne: 1 tab qd for 28 days, then repeat. Start 1st Sunday after menses begins or the 1st day of menses.

HOW SUPPLIED: Tab: (Ethinyl Estradiol-Norethindrone) 0.035mg-1mg, 0.030mg-1mg, 0.020mg-1mg; Tab: (Ferrous Fumarate) 75mg

CONTRAINDICATIONS: Thrombophlebitis, thromboembolic disorders, history of deep vein thrombophlebitis or thromboembolic disorders, pregnancy, cerebrovascular disease, CAD, undiagnosed abnormal genital bleeding, cholestatic jaundice of pregnancy, jaundice with prior pill use, hepatic adenoma or carcinoma, breast carcinoma, carcinoma of the endometrium or other estrogen-dependent neoplasia.

WARNINGS/PRECAUTIONS: Increased risk of MI, vascular disease, thromboembolism, stroke, hepatic neoplasia and gallbladder disease. May increase risk of breast and cervical cancer. Benign hepatic adenomas and hepatocellular carcinoma reported; d/c if jaundice develops. Retinal thrombosis reported; d/c if unexplained partial or complete loss of vision, onset of proptosis or diplopia, papilledema, or retinal vascular lesions develops. Should not be used to induce withdrawal bleeding as a test for pregnancy, or to treat threatened or habitual abortion during pregnancy. May cause glucose intolerance; monitor prediabetic and diabetic patients. May cause fluid retention and increase BP; monitor closely with HTN and d/c if significant elevation of BP occurs. May elevate LDL levels or cause other lipid changes. May cause/exacerbate migraine or may develop headache with new pattern. Breakthrough bleeding and spotting reported; rule out malignancy or pregnancy. Perform annual physical exam. Monitor closely with depression and d/c if depression recurs to serious degree. Use before menarche is not indicated. May affect certain endocrine tests, LFTs, and blood components. Does not protect against HIV infection (AIDS) and other sexually transmitted disease.

ADVERSE REACTIONS: Thrombophlebitis, arterial thromboembolism, pulmonary embolism, MI, cerebral hemorrhage, cerebral thrombosis, HTN, gallbladder disease, Hepatic adenomas, benign liver tumors, N/V, breakthrough bleeding, spotting, amenorrhea.

INTERACTIONS: Reduced effects, increased breakthrough bleeding, and menstrual irregularities with rifampin, phenylbutazone and St. John's wort. Increased plasma levels with atorvastatin, ascorbic acid and APAP. Decreased plasma levels of APAP. Increased clearance of temazepam, salicylic acid, morphine, and clofibric acid. Increased plasma levels of cyclosporine, prednisolone, and theophylline. Pregnancy reported when administered with antimicrobials such as ampicillin, tetracycline and griseofulvin. Reduced effects when used with anticonvulsants such as phenobarbital, phenytoin, and carbamazepine.

PREGNANCY: Category X, not for use in nursing.

MECHANISM OF ACTION: Estrogen/progestogen oral contraceptive; acts by suppressing gonadotropins, inhibiting ovulation, and causing other alterations, including changes in the cervical mucus (increasing difficulty of sperm entry into uterus) and the endometrium (reducing likelihood of implantation). Acne: not established; increases sex hormone binding globulin and decreases free testosterone (reducing androgen stimulation of sebum production).

PHARMACOKINETICS: Absorption: Rapid and complete. Absolute bioavailability: Norethindrone (64%), ethinyl estradiol (43%); T_{max}=1-2 hrs. Refer to PI for dose specific parameters. **Distribution:** V_d=2-4L/kg; plasma protein binding (>95%). Excreted in breast milk. **Metabolism:** Norethindrone: Extensive; reduction, sulfate/glucuronide conjugation. Ethinyl estradiol: Extensive; oxidation via CYP3A4 and conjugation; 2-hydroxy ethinyl estradiol (major metabolite) **Elimination:** Urine, feces. Norethindrone: $T_{1/2}$=13 hrs. Ethinyl estradiol: $T_{1/2}$=19 hrs.

NURSING CONSIDERATIONS

Assessment: Assess for current or history of thrombophlebitis or thromboembolic disorders, cerebrovascular or coronary artery disease, known or suspected carcinoma of the breast, endometrium or other known or suspected estrogen-dependent neoplasia, undiagnosed abnormal genital bleeding, history of cholestatic jaundice of pregnancy or jaundice with previous pill use, hepatic adenomas or carcinomas, known or suspected pregnancy. Assess use in patients >35 who smoke ≥15 cigarettes/day. Assess use in patients with HTN, hyperlipidemias, DM and obesity. Assess for conditions that might be aggravated by fluid retention, nursing status and for possible drug interactions.

Monitoring: Monitor for venous and arterial thrombotic and thromboembolic events (eg, MI, stroke), hepatic neoplasia, gallbladder disease, ocular lesions, HTN, fluid retention, bleeding irregularities, and onset or exacerbation of headaches or migraines. Monitor blood glucose levels with history of DM or in prediabetic patients, BP with history of HTN, lipid levels with a history of hyperlipidemia. Monitor for signs/symptoms of liver toxicity (eg, jaundice), GI upset (eg, diarrhea, vomiting), and signs of worsening depression with previous history. Refer patients with contact lenses to ophthalmologist if ocular changes develop. Perform annual physical exam.

Patient Counseling: Counsel about possible side effects. Inform that medication does not protect against HIV and other STDs. Counsel to avoid smoking while on medication. Advise if spotting, light bleeding, or nausea develops during first 1-3 packs of pills, to continue taking medication, and to notify physician if symptoms do not subside. If N/V or diarrhea occurs, instruct use of backup birth control method until physician is contacted. Counsel to go for an annual physical. Counsel on the appropriate way to use the pack and when to start. Advise to take at the same time every day; if a dose is missed, take as soon as possible, then take next dose at regular time. See PI for detailed notes on administration regarding missed doses.

Administration: Oral route. **Storage:** Do not store above 25°C (77°F). Protect from light. Store tablets inside pouch when not in use.

ETODOLAC RX
etodolac (Various)

> NSAIDs may cause an increased risk of serious cardiovascular thrombotic events, MI, stroke and serious GI adverse events including bleeding, ulceration, and perforation of the stomach or intestines. Contraindicated for the treatment of perioperative pain in the setting of coronary artery bypass graft (CABG) surgery.

THERAPEUTIC CLASS: NSAID

INDICATIONS: Management of osteoarthritis (OA), rheumatoid arthritis (RA), and acute pain.

DOSAGE: *Adults:* ≥18 yrs: Acute Pain: Usual: 200-400mg q6-8h. Max: 1000mg/day. OA/RA: Initial: 300mg bid-tid, or 400-500mg bid. May give 600mg/day for long-term use. Titrate: Lowest effective dose. Max: 1000mg/day.

HOW SUPPLIED: Cap: 200mg, 300mg; Tab: 400mg, 500mg

CONTRAINDICATIONS: ASA or other NSAID allergy that precipitates asthma, urticaria or other allergic type reactions. Treatment of perioperative pain in the setting of CABG surgery.

WARNINGS/PRECAUTIONS: May lead to onset of new HTN or worsening of pre-existing HTN; monitor BP closely. Fluid retention and edema reported; caution with fluid retention or heart failure. Renal papillary necrosis and other renal injury reported after long-term use. Not recommended for use with advanced renal disease; if therapy must be initiated, monitor renal function. Anaphylactoid reactions may occur. May cause serious skin adverse events (eg, exfoliative dermatitis, Stevens-Johnson syndrome, and toxic epidermal necrolysis). Avoid in late pregnancy; may cause premature closure of ductus arteriosis. May cause elevations of LFTs; d/c if liver disease develops or systemic manifestations occur. Caution in elderly. Anemia may occur; with long-term use, monitor Hgb/Hct if signs or symptoms of anemia develop. May inhibit platelet aggregation and prolong bleeding time; monitor with coagulation disorders. Caution with asthma and avoid with ASA-sensitive asthma. Risk of GI ulceration, bleeding, and perforation.

ADVERSE REACTIONS: Dyspepsia, abdominal pain, diarrhea, flatulence, nausea, constipation, gastritis, asthenia, malaise, dizziness, increased bleeding time, GI ulcers, GI bleeding/perforation, heartburn, abnormal renal function.

INTERACTIONS: May elevate digoxin, lithium, and methotrexate serum levels. May enhance nephrotoxicity associated with cyclosporine. Avoid with phenylbutazone and ASA. Increased adverse effect potential with ASA. Caution with warfarin. Diuretics may increase risk of renal toxicity. May diminish antihypertensive effects of ACE inhibitors.

PREGNANCY: Category C, not for use in nursing.

MECHANISM OF ACTION: NSAID; suspected to inhibit prostaglandin synthetase, exerts anti-inflammatory, analgesic, and antipyretic actions.

PHARMACOKINETICS: Absorption: Well absorbed. Bioavailability (100%); C_{max}=14-37mcg/mL, T_{max}=80 min. **Distribution:** V_d=390mL/kg; plasma protein binding (99%). **Elimination:** Urine, feces; $T_{1/2}$=6.4 hrs.

NURSING CONSIDERATIONS

Assessment: Assess LFTs, renal function, CBC and coagulation profile. Assess for history of CABG surgery, asthma and allergic reactions to aspirin or other NSAIDs, active ulceration or chronic inflammation of GI tract, CVD, asthma, pregnancy status. Note other diseases/conditions and drug therapies.

Monitoring: Monitor for hypersensitivity reactions, cardiac complications, stroke, GI bleeding, asthma, skin side effects. Monitor BP, LFTs, renal function, CBC with differential and platelet count, coagulation profile, ocular effects and Reye's syndrome.

Patient Counseling: Counsel about side effects; seek medical attention if any occur. Tablet should be swallowed; not chewed or crushed. Advise to take as prescribed. Caution women against using medication late in pregnancy.

Administration: Oral route. **Storage:** 25-30°C (68-77°F). Protect from excessive heat and humidity.

ETOPOPHOS   RX
etoposide phosphate (Bristol-Myers Squibb)

> Administer under the supervision of a qualified physician experienced in use of cancer chemotherapeutic agents. Severe myelosuppression with resulting infection or bleeding may occur.

THERAPEUTIC CLASS: Podophyllotoxin derivative

INDICATIONS: Adjunct therapy for management of refractory testicular tumors. First-line combination therapy for management of small cell lung cancer (SCLC).

DOSAGE: *Adults:* Testicular Cancer: Usual: 50-100mg/m²/day IV on Days 1-5 to 100mg/m²/day on Days 1, 3, and 5. SCLC: 35mg/m²/day IV for 4 days to 50mg/m²/day for 5 days. Administer at infusion rates 5-210 min. After adequate recovery from any toxicity, repeat course for either therapy at 3-4 week intervals. CrCl 15-50mL/min: 75% of dose.

HOW SUPPLIED: Inj: 100mg

WARNINGS/PRECAUTIONS: Observe for myelosuppression during and after therapy. Withhold therapy if platelet count <50,000/mm³ or if absolute neutrophil count (ANC) <500/mm³. Risk of anaphylactic reaction, manifested by chills, fever, tachycardia, bronchospasm, dyspnea, and hypotension reported. Inj site reactions may occur; monitor infusion site for possible infiltration during administration. May be carcinogenic in humans; acute leukemia with or without a preleukemic phase may occur. Caution with low serum albumin; increased risk of toxicity. May cause fetal harm in pregnancy. D/C or reduce dose if severe reactions occur. Dosage may be modified to account for other myelosuppressive drugs or the effects of prior x-ray or chemotherapy, which may have compromised bone marrow reserve. Do not give by bolus IV inj. Caution in elderly.

ADVERSE REACTIONS: Leukopenia, neutropenia, thrombocytopenia, anemia, constipation, diarrhea, leukopenia, dizziness, alopecia, N/V, mucositis, asthenia/malaise, chills, fever, anorexia.

INTERACTIONS: Caution with drugs known to inhibit phosphatase activities (eg, levamisole hydrochloride). High-dose cyclosporin A reduces clearance and increases exposure of oral etoposide. Prior use of cisplatin may decrease etoposide total body clearance in children. Displaced from protein binding sites by phenylbutazone, sodium salicylate, and aspirin.

PREGNANCY: Category D, not for use in nursing.

MECHANISM OF ACTION: Podophyllotoxin derivative; induces DNA strand breaks by interacting with DNA-topoisomerase II or formation of free radicals.

PHARMACOKINETICS: Absorption: Rapid, complete; Etopophos 150mg/m^2: AUC=168.3µg•hr/mL, C_{max}=20µg/mL. Refer to PI for pharmacokinetic parameters for VePesid, which is similar to Etoposide.

NURSING CONSIDERATIONS

Assessment: Assess for renal function, low serum albumin, pregnancy/nursing status, and possible drug interactions. Obtain platelet, Hgb, and WBC with differential at start of therapy.

Monitoring: Monitor for signs/symptoms of anaphylactic reaction, severe myelosuppression, severe reactions, and renal dysfunction. Monitor for infusion site reactions. Perform periodic CBC prior to each cycle of therapy and at appropriate intervals during and after therapy.

Patient Counseling: Inform of pregnancy risks; avoid pregnancy. Advise to seek medical attention if experience symptoms of severe myelosuppression (infection or bleeding) or anaphylactic reaction (chills, fever, tachycardia, bronchospasm, dyspnea, hypotension).

Administration: IV (infusion) route. Refer to PI for preparation and administration. **Storage:** 2-8°C (36-46°F); protect from light. Reconstituted and diluted vials stable for 7 days at 2-8°C (36-46°F) or 24 hrs at 20-25°C (68-77°F).

EUFLEXXA   RX
sodium hyaluronate (Ferring)

THERAPEUTIC CLASS: Hyaluronan

INDICATIONS: Treatment of pain in osteoarthritis of the knee in patients who have failed to respond adequately to conservative non-pharmacologic therapy and simple analgesics (eg, APAP).

DOSAGE: *Adults:* Inject 2mL intra-articularly into affected knee at weekly intervals for 3 weeks, for a total of 3 injections. Use strict aseptic injection procedures.

HOW SUPPLIED: Inj: 1% [2mL]

CONTRAINDICATIONS: Avoid with knee joint infections, infections or skin diseases in area of injection site.

WARNINGS/PRECAUTIONS: Avoid mixing with quaternary ammonium salts (eg, benzalkonium chloride); may result in formation of a precipitate. Avoid injecting intravascularly. Patients having repeated exposure have the potential for an immune response. Safety and effectiveness in joints other than the knee or in conjunction with other intra-articular injectables have not been established. Remove any joint effusion before injecting. Transient pain and/or swelling of the injected joint may occur. Avoid any strenuous activities or prolonged (eg, more than 1 hr) weight-bearing activities within 48 hrs following injection. Safety and effectiveness have not been demonstrated in children.

ADVERSE REACTIONS: Arthralgia, nausea, back pain, rhinitis, BP increase, joint effusion/swelling, tendonitis, knee pain, skin irritation, headache, paresthesia.

PREGNANCY: Safety in pregnancy and nursing not known.

NURSING CONSIDERATIONS

Assessment: Assess for knee joint infections, skin infections, or disease in the injection-site area.

Monitoring: Monitor for knee pain or swelling of joint.

Patient Counseling: Inform that drug may cause transient pain/swelling of injected joint. Avoid strenuous activities or prolonged weight-bearing activities (jogging, tennis) within 48 hrs following injection.

Administration: Intra-articular injection. **Storage:** 2-25°C (36-77°F). Protect from light. Remove from refrigeration at least 20-30 min before use. Do not freeze.

EVAMIST   RX
estradiol (Ther-Rx)

Estrogens increase the risk of endometrial cancer in women with a uterus; undertake diagnostic measures, including endometrial sampling when indicated, to rule out malignancy in all cases of undiagnosed persistent or recurring abnormal vaginal bleeding. Estrogens, with or without progestins, should not be used for the prevention of cardiovascular disease or dementia. Increased risks of myocardial infarction (MI), stroke, invasive breast cancer, pulmonary embolism (PE), and deep-vein thrombosis (DVT) in postmenopausal women (50-79 yrs of age) reported. Increased risk of developing probable dementia in postmenopausal women ≥65 yrs of age reported. Prescribe at the lowest effective dose for the shortest duration consistent with treatment goals and risks for the individual woman.

THERAPEUTIC CLASS: Estrogen

INDICATIONS: Treatment of moderate to severe vasomotor symptoms due to menopause.

DOSAGE: *Adults:* Initial: 1 spray qd. Adjust dose based on response. Usual: 1-3 sprays qam to adjacent, non-overlapping areas on the inner surface of the forearam near the elbow. Use lowest effective dose for shortest duration consistent to treatment goals; re-evaluate need periodically.

HOW SUPPLIED: Spray: 1.53mg/spray [8.1mL]

CONTRAINDICATIONS: Undiagnosed abnormal genital bleeding, known, suspected or history of breast cancer, known or suspected estrogen-dependent neoplasia, active or history of DVT or PE, active or recent (within past year) arterial thromboembolic disease (eg, stroke, MI), liver dysfunction or disease, pregnancy.

WARNINGS/PRECAUTIONS: May increase risk of gallbladder disease. May lead to severe hypercalcemia with breast cancer and bone metastases; monitor and d/c if hypercalcemia occurs. Retinal vascular thrombosis reported; d/c pending an exam if sudden partial or complete loss of vision, or sudden onset of proptosis, diplopia, or migraine occur. D/C permanently if papilledema or retinal vascular lesions are found. Consider addition of progestin if no hysterectomy; may reduce risk of endometrial cancer. May elevate BP; monitor at regular intervals. May cause elevations of plasma triglycerides with pre-existing hypertriglyceridemia. May be poorly metabolized in patients with impaired liver function. Caution with history of cholestatic jaundice associated with past estrogen use or with pregnancy; d/c with recurrence. May lead to increased thyroid-binding globulin levels; monitor thyroid function. May cause fluid retention; caution with cardiac/renal dysfunction. Caution with severe hypocalcemia. May increase risk of ovarian cancer. May exacerbate endometriosis, asthma, diabetes mellitus, epilepsy, migraine, porphyria, systemic lupus erythematosus and hepatic hemangiomas. Avoid fire, flame or smoking until spray has dried.

ADVERSE REACTIONS: Breast tenderness, nipple pain, nausea, nasopharyngitis, back pain, arthralgia, headache.

INTERACTIONS: CYP3A4 inducers (eg, St. John's wort, phenobarbital, carbamazepine, rifampin) may reduce plasma concentrations, possibly resulting in a decrease therapeutic effects and/or change uterine bleeding profile. CYP3A4 inhibitors (eg, erythromycin, clarithromycin, ketoconazole, itraconazole, ritonavir, grapefruit juice) may increase levels which may result in side effects. Patients dependent on thyroid replacement therapy may require increased doses of their thyroid replacement therapy; estrogen leads to increased thyroid-binding globulin (TBG) levels. Decreased absorption with sunscreen applied 1 hr after estradiol application.

PREGNANCY: Contraindicated in pregnancy, not for use in nursing.

MECHANISM OF ACTION: Estrogen; binds to nuclear receptors in estrogen-responsive tissues. Circulating estrogens modulate pituitary secretion of the gonadotrophins, luteinizing hormone and follicle stimulating hormone, through negative feedback mechanism. Reduces elevated levels of these hormones in postmenopausal women.

PHARMACOKINETICS: Absorption: Administration of various doses resulted in different parameters. **Distribution:** Found in breast milk. Largely bound to sex hormone binding globulin (SHBG) and albumin. **Metabolism:** Liver; converted to estrone and/or estriol (major metabolite). Enterohepatic recirculation via sulfate and glucuronide conjugation (liver). **Elimination:** Urine (parent compound and metabolites).

NURSING CONSIDERATIONS

Assessment: Assess for abnormal genital bleeding, presence or history of breast cancer, estrogen-dependent neoplasias, DVT, PE, active or recent (within past yr) and any other conditions where treatment may be contraindicated or cautioned. Assess use in women ≥65 yrs, nursing patients, and those with DM, asthma, epilepsy, migraines or porphyria, SLE, and hepatic hemangiomas. Assess for possible drug and lab test interactions. Assess need for progestin in women who have not had a hysterectomy.

Monitoring: Monitor for signs/symptoms of CV disorders (eg, stroke, coronary heart disease, VTE), malignant neoplasms (eg, endometrial, breast, or ovarian cancer), dementia, gallbladder disease, hypercalcemia, visual abnormalities (eg, retinal vascular thrombosis), elevations in plasma triglycerides and pancreatitis, fluid retention, exacerbation of endometriosis or other conditions (eg, asthma, DM, epilepsy, migraines, SLE, hepatic hemangiomas). If undiagnosed, persistent, or recurring abnormal vaginal bleeding occurs, perform adequate diagnostic measures (eg, endometrial sampling) to rule out malignancy. Perform annual breast exam. Monitor BP levels at regular intervals and thyroid function in patients on thyroid hormone replacement therapy. Perform periodic evaluation (every 3-6 months) to determine therapy need.

Patient Counseling: Inform of the importance of reporting vaginal bleeding to their healthcare provider as soon as possible. Inform of the possible side effects of therapy (eg, headache, breast pain and tenderness, nausea and vomiting). Inform that if using medication for first time, container must be primed by fully depressing applicator 3 times. Apply medication at same time daily. Apply to clean, dry, unbroken skin, on inside of forearm between elbow and wrist; do not apply directly to breast or around vagina. Inform medication contains alcohol; avoid fire, flame, or smoking until medication is dry. Inform if dose missed and next scheduled dose is <12 hrs away, wait and apply normal dose; if >12 hrs away, apply missed dose and return to normal dosing schedule. Advise to perform monthly self-breast exams.

Administration: Topical route. Apply to adjacent, non-overlapping areas on the inner surface of the forearm, starting near the elbow. Allow to dry for 2 mins; do not wash site for 30 min. Should not be applied to skin surfaces other than the forearm. **Storage:** 25°C (77°F); excursions permitted to 15-30°C (59-86°F). Do not freeze.

EVISTA   RX
raloxifene HCl (Lilly)

> Increased risk of deep vein thrombosis (DVT) and pulmonary embolism (PE) reported. Avoid use in women with active or past history of venous thromboembolism. Increased risk of death due to stroke in postmenopausal women with documented coronary heart disease or at increased risk for major coronary events; consider risk-benefit balance in women at risk for stroke.

THERAPEUTIC CLASS: Selective estrogen receptor modulator

INDICATIONS: Treatment and prevention of osteoporosis in postmenopausal women. Reduction in risk of invasive breast cancer in postmenopausal women with osteoporosis and in postmenopausal women at high risk for invasive breast cancer.

DOSAGE: *Adults:* 60mg qd. May be given at any time of day without regard to meals. Refer to PI for recommendations regarding calcium and vitamin D supplementation.

HOW SUPPLIED: Tab: 60mg

CONTRAINDICATIONS: Nursing, pregnancy, women who may become pregnant, active/past history of venous thromboembolism (VTE) (eg, DVT, PE, retinal vein thrombosis).

WARNINGS/PRECAUTIONS: Venous thromboembolism events including superficial venous thrombophlebitis reported; d/c at least 72 hrs prior to and during prolonged immobilization (eg, post-surgical recovery, prolonged bed rest); therapy should only be resumed after fully ambulatory. Caution in women at risk of thromboembolic disease. Should not be used for primary or secondary prevention of cardiovascular disease. Avoid in premenopausal women. Use not adequately studied in women with a history of breast cancer. Not recommended for use in men. May increase levels of triglycerides with pre-existing hypertriglyceridemia; monitor serum triglyceride levels in women with history of hypertriglyceridemia. Caution with hepatic impairment or with moderate or severe renal impairment. Monitor for unexplained uterine bleeding and breast abnormalites.

ADVERSE REACTIONS: DVT, pulmonary embolism, vaginal bleeding, hot flashes, leg cramps, arthralgia, infection, flu syndrome, headache, nausea, weight gain, sinusitis, rhinitis, cough increased, peripheral edema.

INTERACTIONS: Cholestyramine may decrease absorption; avoid concomitant administration with cholestyramine and other anion exchange resins. Monitor PT with warfarin and other warfarin derivatives. Caution with other highly protein-bound drugs (eg, diazepam, diazoxide, lidocaine). Avoid concomitant use with systemic estrogens.

PREGNANCY: Category X, contraindicated in nursing.

MECHANISM OF ACTION: Selective estrogen receptor modulator; binds to estrogen receptors. Binding results in activation of estrogenic pathways in some tissues and blockade of estrogenic pathways in others depending on extent of recruitment of coactivators and corepressors to estrogen receptor target gene promotors. Acts as an estrogen agonist in bone. Decreases bone resorption and bone turnover, increases bone mineral density, and decreases fracture incidence.

PHARMACOKINETICS: Absorption: Rapid; Absolute bioavailability (2%); Single dose: C_{max}=0.5(ng/mL)/(mg/kg); AUC=27.2(ng•hr/mL)/(mg/kg). Multiple doses: C_{max}=1.36(ng/mL)/(mg/kg); AUC=24.2(ng•hr/mL)/(mg/kg). **Distribution:** V_d=2348L/kg. Plasma protein binding (95%). **Metabolism:** Extensive; glucuronidation; raloxifene-4'-glucuronide, raloxifene-6-glucuronide, raloxifene-6',4'-diglucuronide (metabolites). **Elimination:** Feces (primary), urine (<0.2% unchanged); $T_{1/2}$=27.7 hrs (single dose); $T_{1/2}$=32.5 hrs (multiple doses).

NURSING CONSIDERATIONS

Assessment: Assess for active or history of VTE (eg, DVT, PE, retinal vein thrombosis), CVD, risk factors for stroke, history of breast cancer, history of hypertriglyceridemia, prolonged immobilization, renal/hepatic impairment, pregnancy/nursing status, and for possible drug interactions.

Monitoring: Monitor for VTE (eg, DVT, PE, retinal vein thrombosis), stroke, unexplained uterine bleeding, and breast abnormalities. Monitor serum TG with history of hypertriglyceridemia.

Patient Counseling: For osteoporosis treatment/prevention, instruct to take supplemental calcium and/or vitamin D if intake is inadequate. Consider weight-bearing exercise and behavioral modification factors (eg, smoking, excessive alcohol consumption) for osteoporosis treatment/prevention. Advise to d/c therapy at least 72 hrs prior to and during prolonged immobilization. Avoid prolonged restrictions of movement during travel. Counsel that therapy may increase incidence of hot flashes or hot flashes may occur upon initiation of therapy. Inform that regular breast exams and mammography should be done before initiation of therapy and should continue during therapy. Instruct to read the medication guide before starting therapy.

Administration: Oral route. **Storage:** 20-25°C (68-77°F); excursions permitted to 15-30°C (59-86°F).

EVOCLIN

RX

clindamycin phosphate (Stiefel)

THERAPEUTIC CLASS: Lincomycin derivative

INDICATIONS: Treatment of acne vulgaris in patients ≥12 yrs.

DOSAGE: *Adults*: Apply to affected area qd. Use enough to cover the entire affected area.
Pediatrics: ≥12 yrs: Apply to affected area qd. Use enough to cover the entire affected area.

HOW SUPPLIED: Foam: 1% [50g, 100g]

CONTRAINDICATIONS: History of regional enteritis, ulcerative colitis, or antibiotic-associated colitis.

WARNINGS/PRECAUTIONS: Diarrhea, bloody diarrhea, and colitis (including pseudomembranous colitis) reported; d/c if significant diarrhea occurs. May cause irritation. Avoid contact with eyes; rinse eyes thoroughly with water if contact occurs. Caution in atopic individuals. Use caution when applying to the chest during lactation to avoid accidental ingestion by the infant.

ADVERSE REACTIONS: Diarrhea, bloody diarrhea, colitis, headache, application-site burning.

INTERACTIONS: May enhance the action of other neuromuscular blockers; caution with concomitant use. Possible antagonism with topical/oral erythromycin-containing products; avoid concomitant use.

PREGNANCY: Category B, not for use in nursing.

MECHANISM OF ACTION: Lincomycin derivative; not established. Shown to have activity against *Propionibacterium acnes*, which is associated with acne vulgaris.

PHARMACOKINETICS: Distribution: Orally and parenterally administered clindamycin found in breast milk. **Elimination:** Urine (<0.024% unchanged).

NURSING CONSIDERATIONS

Assessment: Assess for history of regional enteritis/ulcerative colitis or antibiotic-associated colitis, pregnancy/nursing status and possible drug interactions. Assess use in atopic individuals.

Monitoring: Monitor for colitis, including pseudomembranous colitis, and irritation. For colitis, perform stool culture and assay for *C.difficile* toxin.

Patient Counseling: Advise to wash skin with mild soap and allow drying before application. Instruct to dispense foam directly into cap or onto cool surface, then apply enough to cover the face. Instruct to wash hands after application. Advise that drug may cause irritation (eg, erythema, scaling, itching, burning, stinging). Instruct to avoid contact with eyes; rinse eyes thoroughly with water if contact occurs. Instruct to d/c and contact physician if severe diarrhea or GI discomfort develops. Instruct that medication is flammable; avoid smoking or contact with fire during and immediately following application.

Administration: Topical route. Not for oral, ophthalmic, or intravaginal use. Wash skin with mild soap and dry prior to administration. **Storage:** 20-25°C (68-77°F). Do not expose to heat or store >49°C (120°F). Contents under pressure; do not puncture or incinerate.

EXALGO
hydromorphone HCl (Mallinckrodt)

`CII`

THERAPEUTIC CLASS: Opioid Analgesics

INDICATIONS: Management of moderate to severe pain in opioid-tolerant patients requiring continuous, around-the-clock opioid analgesia for an extended period of time.

DOSAGE: *Adults:* >17 yrs: Individualize dose. Dose range: 8-64mg. Administer once q24h. Titrate: Not more often than 3-4 days. Increase 25-50% of the current daily dose for each titration step. Titrate dose upward, if >2 doses of rescue medication are needed within 24 hr period for 2 consecutive days. Conversion from intermediate-release hydromorphone: Starting dose equivalent to the patient's total daily oral hydromorphone dose taken qd. Conversion from other oral opioids: Refer to published relative potency information. Administer 50% of the calculated total daily dose every 24 hrs. Conversion from Transdermal Fentanyl: Administer 12mg q24h for each 25mcg/hr of transdermal fentanyl after 18 hrs following the removal of fentanyl transdermal patch. Moderate/Severe Hepatic and Moderate Renal Impairment: Reduce dose; closely monitor during dose titration. Severe Renal Impairment: Consider alternate analgesic. Elderly: Reduce initial dose. Maintenance: Assess the continued need for around-the-clock opioid therapy periodically, particularly with high-dose formulations. Discontinuation: Taper dose gradually, 25-50% every 2 or 3 days down to a dose of 8mg. Refer to PI for standard conversion of total daily (24-hr) dose of previous opioid therapy and for dosing recommendations.

HOW SUPPLIED: Tab, Extended-Release: 8mg, 12mg, 16mg

CONTRAINDICATIONS: Opiod non-tolerant patients. Significant respiratory depression, especially in the absence of resuscitative equipment or in unmonitored settings. Acute or severe bronchial asthma or hypercarbia, known or suspected paralytic ileus, previous surgical procedures and/or underlying disease that would result in narrowed or obstructed GI tract or presence of "blind loops" of the GI tract or GI obstruction.

WARNINGS/PRECAUTIONS: Do not use as a first opioid. May cause respiratory depression; caution with conditions accompanied by hypoxia, hypercapnia, or decreased respiratory reserve such as asthma, COPD or cor pulmonale, severe obesity, sleep apnea, myxedema, kyphoscoliosis, or CNS depression. Avoid with head injury, intracranial lesions, or pre-existing elevated intracranial pressure (ICP). May obscure neurologic signs of further increases in ICP in patients with head injury. May cause severe hypotension; caution in patients with circulatory shock. May obscure the diagnosis or clinical course in patients with acute abdominal condition. Contains sodium metabisulfite; may cause allergic-type reactions including anaphylactic symptoms and life-threatening or less severe asthmatic episodes. Caution with adrenocortical insufficiency, delirium tremens, hypothyroidism, prostatic hypertrophy or urethral stricture, and toxic psychosis. May aggravate convulsions in patients with convulsive disorders. May increase biliary tract pressure; caution with inflammatory or obstructive bowel disorder, acute pancreatitis secondary to biliary tract disease, and in biliary surgery. May cause mental/physical impairment. Avoid abrupt withdrawal. Tolerance and physical dependence may occur. Caution with elderly/debilitated.

ADVERSE REACTIONS: Constipation, N/V, somnolence, headache, asthenia, dizziness, diarrhea, insomnia, back pain, pruritus, anorexia, peripheral edema, hyperhidrosis, respiratory depression, hypotension, arthralgia, weight loss.

INTERACTIONS: Concomitant use with CNS depressants (eg, other opioids, illicit drugs, sedatives, hypnotics, tranquilizers, general anesthetics, phenothiazines, muscle relaxants, alcohol) may cause respiratory depression, hypotension, profound sedation, or potentially coma. Avoid concomitant use with alcohol. May cause CNS excitation or depression, hypotension, or HTN with MAOIs. Mixed agonist/antagonist analgesics (eg, buprenorphine, nalbuphine, pentazocine, butorphanol) may reduce analgesic effect and/or may precipitate withdrawal symptoms. May increase risk of urinary retention and/or severe constipation, leading to paralytic ileus with anticholinergics or other medications with anticholinergic activity.

PREGNANCY: Category C, not for use in nursing.

MECHANISM OF ACTION: Opioid analgesic; not established. Mediated through opioid-specific receptors located in central nervous system (CNS) to produce analgesia.

PHARMACOKINETICS: Absorption: Single dose: (8mg) T_{max}=12 hrs, C_{max}=0.93ng/mL. Refer to PI for pharmacokinetic parameters for different dosage forms. **Distribution:** Plasma protein binding (27%); (IV) V_d=2.9 L/kg; crosses placenta, found in breast milk. **Metabolism:** Liver; glucuronidation (extensive); hydromorphone-3-glucuronide (metabolite). **Elimination:** Urine (75%), (7% unchanged); Feces (1% unchanged); $T_{1/2}$=11 hrs.

NURSING CONSIDERATIONS

Assessment: Assess for degree of opioid tolerance; level of pain intensity; previous opioid dose; patient's general condition, age, and medical status; risk factors for abuse; or any other conditions where treatment is contraindicated or cautioned. Assess for history of hypersensitivity, pregnancy/nursing status, renal/hepatic function, and possible drug interactions.

Monitoring: Monitor for signs/symptoms of respiratory depression, circulatory depression (eg, hypotension), misuse or abuse, addiction, tolerance or dependence, hypersensitivity, seizures, and for alleviation of pain.

Patient Counseling: Advise to take as directed; swallow whole. Advise that drug is for use only in patients who are already receiving opioid pain medicine. Advise not to change the dose without consulting a healthcare provider. Report episodes of breakthrough pain and adverse experiences occurring during therapy. Advise that certain stomach or intestinal problems such as narrowing of the intestines or previous surgery may be at higher risk of developing a blockage. Contact healthcare provider if GI obstruction symptoms develop such as abdominal pain/distention, severe constipation, or vomiting. May impair mental and/or physical abilities. Advise not to combine other pain medications, sleep aids, or tranquilizers. Avoid abrupt withdrawal. Educate that medication has the potential for abuse. Advise to keep reach out of children and to dispose unused tablets down the toilet.

Administration: Oral route. **Storage:** 25°C (77°F); excursions permitted to 15-30°C (59-86°F).

EXELON   RX
rivastigmine tartrate (Novartis)

THERAPEUTIC CLASS: Acetylcholinesterase inhibitor

INDICATIONS: Treatment of mild to moderate dementia of the Alzheimer's type and mild to moderate dementia associated with Parkinson's disease.

DOSAGE: *Adults:* Alzheimer's Dementia: Initial: 1.5mg bid. Titrate: May increase by 1.5mg bid every 2 weeks. Max: 12mg/day. If not tolerating, suspend therapy for several doses and restart at same or next lower dose. If interrupted longer than several days, reinitiate with lowest daily dose and titrate as above. Dementia Associated with Parkinson's Disease: Initial: 1.5mg bid. Titrate: May increase by 1.5mg every 4 weeks. Max: 12mg/day. Take with food in am and pm. May mix solution with water, cold fruit juice, or soda. Patch: Alzheimer's Dementia/Dementia Associated with Parkinson's Disease: Initial: Apply 4.6mg/24 hrs patch qd to clean, dry, hairless, intact skin. Maint: Increase dose after 4 weeks. Max: 9.5mg/24 hrs if well tolerated. Switching from Capsules/Oral Sol: Total Oral Daily Dose <6mg: Switch to 4.6mg/24 hrs patch. Total Oral Daily Dose 6-12mg: Switch to 9.5mg/24 hrs patch. Apply 1st patch on day following last oral dose.

HOW SUPPLIED: Cap: 1.5mg, 3mg, 4.5mg, 6mg; Patch: 4.6mg/24 hrs, 9.5mg/24 hrs [30s]; Sol: 2mg/mL [120mL]

CONTRAINDICATIONS: Hypersensitivity to carbamate derivatives.

WARNINGS/PRECAUTIONS: Significant GI intolerance (eg, N/V, diarrhea, anorexia, weight loss); always follow dosing guidelines. Vagotonic effect on HR (bradycardia), especially in "sick sinus syndrome" or supraventricular conduction abnormalities. May cause urinary obstruction and seizures. Monitor for peptic ulcers/GI bleeds. Caution in asthma and COPD. May exacerbate or induce extrapyramidal symptoms. (Patch) May impair mental/physical abilities. Caution with low body weight (<50kg).

ADVERSE REACTIONS: N/V, abdominal pain, dyspepsia, constipation, somnolence, anorexia, asthenia, headache, dizziness, fatigue, diarrhea, tremor, depression.

INTERACTIONS: May block effects of anticholinergics. May be synergistic with succinylcholine, similar neuromuscular blockers, or cholinergic agonists (eg, bethanechol). May exaggerate succinylcholine-type muscle relaxation during anesthesia. Nicotine may increase oral clearance.

PREGNANCY: Category B, not for use in nursing.

MECHANISM OF ACTION: Reversible cholinesterase inhibitor; not fully established, suspected to enhance cholinergic function by increasing concentration of acetylcholine through reversible inhibition of cholinesterase.

PHARMACOKINETICS: Absorption: Patch: T_{max}=8-16 hrs. Cap, Sol: Rapid, complete; absolute bioavailability (36%); T_{max}=1 hr. **Distribution:** V_d=1.8-2.7L/kg; plasma protein binding (40%). **Metabolism:** Cholinesterase-mediated hydrolysis. **Elimination:** Cap, Sol: Urine (97%), feces (0.4%); $T_{1/2}$=1.5 hrs. Patch: Urine (>90%), feces (<1%); $T_{1/2}$=3 hrs.

NURSING CONSIDERATIONS

Assessment: Assess for history of ulcer disease, sick sinus syndrome, conduction defects, asthma or COPD, urinary obstruction, body weight, seizures, and possible drug interactions.

Monitoring: Monitor body weight and mental status; signs/symptoms of active or occult GI bleeding, extrapyramidal symptoms (EPS), and hypersensitivity reactions.

Patient Counseling: Inform to monitor for loss of weight or appetite, N/V, anorexia, or diarrhea; may exacerbate or induce EPS. (Sol) Instruct to use provided syringe to withdraw prescribed amount. (Patch) Instruct to wash hands after application, and avoid contact with eyes; do not rub in or apply to area that is red, irritated, cut or to areas where cream, lotion, powder has recently been applied; replace every 24 hrs and consistent time of day; do not apply new patch to same spot for at least 14 days; can be used while bathing but avoid exposure to external heat sources (eg, excess sunlight, saunas, solariums). If dose is missed, instruct apply new patch immediately, then continue scheduled dosage; do not apply 2 patches at once. Advise not to take capsule or oral solution or other drugs with cholinergic effect while wearing patch.

Administration: Oral, transdermal route. (Sol) Swallow directly from syringe or mix with small glass of water, juice or soda; stir before drinking. (Patch) Apply at upper or lower back. **Storage:** 25°C (77°F); excursions permitted to 15-30°C (59-86°F). Sol: Store in upright position and protect from freezing. Patch: Keep in sealed pouch until use. Cap: Store in a tight container.

EXFORGE   RX
amlodipine besylate - valsartan (Novartis)

> D/C therapy when pregnancy is detected. Drugs that act directly on the renin-angiotensin system can cause injury and even death to the developing fetus.

THERAPEUTIC CLASS: ARB/Calcium channel blocker (dihydropyridine)

INDICATIONS: Treatment of hypertension. May be used in patients whose BP is not adequately controlled on either monotherapy. May also be used as initial therapy in patients likely to need multiple drugs to achieve their BP goals.

DOSAGE: *Adults:* Initial Therapy: 5mg-160mg qd. Add-On/Replacement Therapy: May be substituted for titrated components. Titrate: If inadequate control, may increase after 1-2 weeks of therapy. Max: 10mg-320mg qd. Elderly: Initial: 2.5mg amlodipine.

HOW SUPPLIED: Tab: (Amlodipine-Valsartan) 5mg-160mg, 10mg-160mg, 5mg-320mg, 10mg-320mg

WARNINGS/PRECAUTIONS: May cause fetal harm, fetal/neonatal morbidity and mortality when taken by pregnant women. May cause excessive hypotension. May increase risk of angina and MI in patients with severe obstructive CAD. Caution with CHF, severe hepatic impairment, renal dysfunction, renal artery stenosis, and in the elderly.

ADVERSE REACTIONS: Peripheral edema, vertigo, nasopharyngitis, upper respiratory tract infection, dizziness.

INTERACTIONS: K^+ supplements, K^+-sparing diuretics (eg, spironolactone, triamterene, amiloride), or salt substitutes containing K^+ may increase serum K^+ and SrCr in heart failure patients. Concomitant use with atenolol may potentiate antihypertensive effects.

PREGNANCY: Category D, not for use in nursing.

MECHANISM OF ACTION: Amlodipine: Calcium channel blocker (dihydropyridine); inhibits transmembrane influx of calcium ions into vascular smooth muscle and cardiac muscle. Valsartan: Angiotensin II receptor blocker; blocks vasoconstrictor and aldosterone-secreting effects of angiotensin II by selectively blocking binding of angiotensin II to AT_1 receptor.

PHARMACOKINETICS: Absorption: Amlodipine: Absolute bioavailability (64-90%); T_{max}=6-12 hrs. Valsartan: Absolute bioavailability (25%); T_{max}=2-4 hrs. **Distribution:** Amlodipine: V_d=21L; plasma protein binding (93%). Valsartan: V_d=17L (IV); plasma protein binding (95%). **Metabolism:** Amlodipine: Liver (90%). Valsartan: Valeryl 4-hydroxy valsartan (metabolite). **Elimination:** Amlodipine: Urine (10%); $T_{1/2}$=30-50 hrs. Valsartan: Feces, urine; $T_{1/2}$=6 hrs.

NURSING CONSIDERATIONS

Assessment: Assess severe obstructive CAD, CHF, recent MI, severe aortic stenosis, pregnancy status, possible drug interactions, renal/hepatic impairment.

Monitoring: Monitor for signs/symptoms of hypotension, hypersensitivity reactions, renal/hepatic dysfunction, symptoms of angina or MI after dosage initiation or increase.

Patient Counseling: Inform of pregnancy risks. Advise to seek medical attention if symptoms of hypotension or hypersensitivity reactions occur.

Administration: Oral route. **Storage:** 25°C (77°F); excursions permitted to 15-30°C (59-86°F). Protect from moisture.

EXFORGE HCT   RX
amlodipine besylate - hydrochlorothiazide - valsartan (Novartis)

> D/C when pregnancy is detected. Drugs that act directly on the renin-angiotensin system can cause injury or even death to the developing fetus.

THERAPEUTIC CLASS: ARB/Calcium channel blocker (dihydropyridine)/Thiazide diuretic

INDICATIONS: Treatment of hypertension.

DOSAGE: *Adults:* CrCl >30mL/min: 1 tab qd. Titrate: May increase after 2 weeks of therapy. Max: 10mg-25mg-320mg qd. Add-on/Switch Therapy: May be used if not adequately controlled on any two of the following antihypertensive classes: calcium channel blockers, angiotensin receptor blockers, and diuretics. A patient who experiences dose-limiting adverse reactions to individual component while on any dual combination of the components of Exforge HCT may be switched to Exforge HCT containing a lower dose of that component. Replacement Therapy: May be substituted for the individually titrated components.

HOW SUPPLIED: Tab: (Amlodipine-HCTZ-Valsartan) 5mg-12.5mg-160mg, 5mg-25mg-160mg, 10mg-12.5mg-160mg, 10mg-25mg-160mg, 10mg-25mg-320mg

CONTRAINDICATIONS: Patients with anuria.

WARNINGS/PRECAUTIONS: Excessive hypotension, including orthostatic hypotension, reported; place patient in supine position and consider IV infusion of normal saline. Avoid in patients with aortic or mitral stenosis or obstructive hypertrophic cardiomyopathy. May rarely increase frequency, duration or severity of angina or acute MI in patients with severe obstructive coronary artery disease (CAD). Avoid with severe hepatic impairment. Monitor for worsening of hepatic or renal function in patients with mild-moderate hepatic impairment and biliary obstructive disorders. May precipitate azotemia with renal disease. Avoid in patients with severe renal disease (CrCl ≤30mL/min). Hypokalemia and hyperkalemia reported. (Amlodipine) Monitor fluid status, electrolytes, renal function, and BP in patients with heart failure. (Valsartan) May increase blood urea nitrogen (BUN), SrCr, and K^+ levels. Hypersensitivity reactions may occur in patients with or without a history of allergy or bronchial asthma. May cause exacerbation or activation of systemic lupus erythematosus. (HCTZ) Observe for signs of fluid or electrolyte imbalance (eg, hyponatremia, hypochloremic alkalosis, hypokalemia); may cause hyperuricemia or precipitation of frank gout, hyperglycemia, hypomagnesemia, hypercalcemia, hypercholesterolemia and hypertriglyceridemia.

ADVERSE REACTIONS: Dizziness, edema, headache, increase BUN, hyperkalemia, hypokalemia.

INTERACTIONS: (HCTZ) Potentiation of orthostatic hypotension with alcohol, barbiturates, or narcotics. Dosage adjustment of antidiabetic drugs (eg, oral agents and insulin) may be required during coadministration. Additive effect or potentiation with other antihypertensive drugs. Anionic exchange resins may impair absorption (eg, cholestyramine, colestipol). Hypokalemia reported with corticosteroid, ACTH. Decreased response to pressor amines. Increased responsiveness to nondepolarizing skeletal muscle relaxants (eg, tubocurarine). Avoid with lithium. NSAIDS may reduce diuretic, natriuretic, and antihypertensive effects of loop, potassium-sparing and thiazide diuretics. May lead to symptomatic hyponatremia with carbamazepine. May exaggerate the response of the heart to toxic effects of digitalis. (Valsartan) K^+ supplements, K^+-sparing diuretics (eg, spironolactone, triamterene, amiloride), or salt substitutes containing K^+ may increase serum K^+ and SrCr in heart failure patients. Potentiated antihypertensive effect with atenolol. Symptomatic hypotension may occur with volume- or salt-depleted patients receiving high doses of diuretics.

PREGNANCY: Category D, not for use in nursing.

MECHANISM OF ACTION: Amlodipine: Calcium channel blocker (dihydropyridine); inhibits transmembrane influx of calcium ions into vascular smooth muscle and cardiac muscle. HCTZ: Thiazide diuretic; antihypertensive effect unknown. Valsartan: Angiotensin II receptor blocker; blocks vasoconstrictor and aldosterone-secreting effects of angiotensin II by selectively blocking binding of angiotensin II to AT_1 receptor.

PHARMACOKINETICS: Absorption: Amlodipine: Absolute bioavailability (64-90%); T_{max} =6-12 hrs. Valsartan: Absolute bioavailability (25%); T_{max} =2-4 hrs. **Distribution:** Amlodipine: V_d=21 L; plasma protein binding (93%). HCTZ: Crosses the placental barrier and found in breast milk. Valsartan: V_d=17 L (IV); plasma protein binding (95%). **Metabolism:** Amlodipine: Liver. HCTZ: found in breast milk. Valsartan: CYP2C9; valeryl-4-hydroxy valsartan (metabolite). **Elimination:** Amlodipine: Urine (10%, parent; 60%, metabolites); $T_{1/2}$=30-50 hrs. HCTZ: Urine (61%, unchanged); $T_{1/2}$=5.8-18.9 hrs. Valsartan: Feces (83%), urine (13%); $T_{1/2}$=6 hrs.

NURSING CONSIDERATIONS

Assessment: Assess for LFTs, renal/hepatic function, biliary obstructive disorders, progressive liver disease, severe obstructive CAD, CHF, recent MI, aortic or mitral stenosis, obstructive hypertrophic cardiomyopathy, activated renin-angiotensin system, history of bronchial asthma, electrolyte imbalances, postsympathectomy patient, latent diabetes mellitus, pregnancy/nursing status and possible drug interactions.

Monitoring: Monitor for signs/symptoms of hypotension, hypersensitivity reactions, renal/hepatic impairment, worsening of hepatic or renal function and adverse reactions, symptoms of angina or MI after dosage initiation or increase. Monitor BP, fluid and electrolyte status, BUN, SrCr, CrCl levels.

Patient Counseling: Inform of pregnancy risks and serious fetal problems (eg, low BP, poor skull bone development, kidney problems, and death) may occur. Notify physician if pregnant/planning to become pregnant or breastfeeding. Caution about lightheadedness, especially during the first days of therapy, and advise to report to physician. Instruct to d/c if syncope occurs. Caution inadequate fluid intake, excessive perspiration, diarrhea, or vomiting may lead to an excessive fall in BP, that resulting in lightheadedness and possibly syncope. Instruct to avoid K⁺ supplements or salt substitutes containing K⁺ without consulting a physician.

Administration: Oral route. **Storage:** 25°C (77°F); excursions permitted to 15-30°C (59-86°F). Protect from moisture.

EXTAVIA   RX
interferon beta-1b (Novartis)

THERAPEUTIC CLASS: Biological response modifier

INDICATIONS: Treatment in patients who have experienced a first clinical episode and have MRI features consistent with multiple sclerosis (MS). To reduce frequency of clinical exacerbations in patients with relapsing-remitting MS.

DOSAGE: *Adults:* Initial: 0.0625mg SQ every other day. Titrate: Increase over 6 weeks to 0.25mg SQ every other day. Refer to PI for Dose Titration schedule.

HOW SUPPLIED: Inj: 0.3mg/3mL [vial]

CONTRAINDICATIONS: Hypersensitivity to human albumin.

WARNINGS/PRECAUTIONS: Caution with depression; increased frequency of depression and suicide reported; d/c if develops. Injection-site reactions (eg, inflammation, pain, hypersensitivity, mass, edema, and necrosis) reported; d/c if multiple leisions occur. Monitor for signs and symptoms of anaphylaxis/allergic reactions (eg, dyspnea, bronchospasm, tongue edema, skin rash, and urticaria). Flu-like symptoms, leukopenia, and LFTs elevation (SGPT, SGOT) reported. Perform CBC, differential WBC, LFTs, and platelet count before therapy and periodically thereafter. Contains albumin; risk of viral disease transmission.

ADVERSE REACTIONS: Injection-site reactions/necrosis, flu-like symptoms, headache, lymphopenia, hypertonia, asthenia, pain, fever, chills, rash, insomnia, myalgia, abdominal pain, incoordination, urinary urgency.

PREGNANCY: Category C, not for use in nursing.

MECHANISM OF ACTION: Interferon β-1b: Not established; believed that interferon β-1b receptor binding induces expression of proteins that are responsible for pleiotropic bioactivities. Immunomodulatory effects include the enhancement of suppressor T cell activity, reduction of pro-inflammatory cytokine production, down-regulation of antigen presentation, and inhibition of lymphocyte trafficking into the CNS.

PHARMACOKINETICS: **Absorption:** T_{max}=1-8 hrs, C_{max}=40 IU/mL. **Distribution:** V_d=0.25-2.88L/kg. **Elimination:** $T_{1/2}$=8 min-4.3 hrs.

NURSING CONSIDERATIONS

Assessment: Assess for hypersensitivity, depression, leukopenia, myelosuppression, liver function, thyroid function, myelosupression, and pregnancy/nursing status.

Monitoring: Monitor for anaphylaxis, depression, suicidal ideation, injection-site reactions, injection-site necrosis, flu-like symptoms, and periodically monitor CBC, WBC, LFTs, thyroid function.

Patient Counseling: Inform about potential benefits/risks of drug. Advise not to change dose or schedule of administration. Inform that depression and suicidal ideation, injection-site reactions, injection-site necrosis at 1 or multiple sites, symptoms of allergic reactions and anaphylaxis may occur; d/c and notify physician if symptoms is experienced. Inform patients to take antipyretics and analgesics if with flu-like symptoms. Advise patients not to use the drug during pregnancy unless the potential benefit justifies the potential risk to the fetus.

Administration: SC; rotate injection sites. Do not take in 2 consecutive days. Refer to PI for reconstitution. **Storage:** 25°C (77°F); excursions permitted to 15-30°C (59-86°F). After reconstitution, if not used immediately, refrigerate and use within 3 hrs. Avoid freezing.

EXTINA
ketoconazole (Stiefel)

RX

THERAPEUTIC CLASS: Azole antifungal

INDICATIONS: Topical treatment of seborrheic dermatitis in immunocompetent patients ≥12 yrs of age.

DOSAGE: *Adults:* Apply to affected area(s) bid (am and pm) for 4 weeks. *Pediatrics:* ≥12 yrs: Apply to affected area(s) bid (am and pm) for 4 weeks.

HOW SUPPLIED: Foam: 2% [50g, 100g]

WARNINGS/PRECAUTIONS: May cause contact sensitization, including photoallergenicity. Contents are flammable; avoid fire, flame, and/or smoking during and immediately following applications. Hepatitis, lowered testoterone, and ACTH-induced corticosteroid serum levels reported with orally administered ketoconazole; not seen with topical ketoconazole.

ADVERSE REACTIONS: Application-site burning, application-site reactions (eg, dryness, erythema, irritation, paresthesia, pruritus, rash, warmth), photoallergenicity, contact sensitization.

PREGNANCY: Category C, caution in nursing.

MECHANISM OF ACTION: Azole antifungal; inhibits the synthesis of ergosterol, a key sterol in the cell membrane of *Malassezia furfur*. Mechanism not established in the treatment of seborrheic dermatitis.

PHARMACOKINETICS: Absorption: C_{max}=11ng/mL.

NURSING CONSIDERATIONS

Assessment: Assess pregnancy/nursing status.

Monitoring: Monitor for contact sensitization reactions, including photoallergenicity, improvement/worsening of symptoms.

Patient Counseling: Counsel to notify physician if any type of skin irritation or contact sensitization reaction develops; or if no improvement after 4 weeks of treatment. Inform medication is flammable; do not administer near fire, open flame, or direct heat. Instruct to wash hands well following administration. Advise on the proper way to apply the foam. Keep out of reach of children.

Administration: Topical application. 1.) Hold the can at an upright angle. 2.) Push the button to spray foam directly into the cap of the can or other cool surface. Spray only the amount that will be needed to cover the affected area. Do not spray directly onto the affected skin or into hands because the foam will begin to melt right away when it touches the skin. 3.) If fingers are warm, rinse them in cold water first. Be sure to dry them well before handling the foam. If the can seems warm or the foam seems runny, place the can under cool running water for a few minutes. 4.) Using fingertips, gently massage foam into the affected areas until the foam disappears. 5.) If treating skin with hair such as the scalp, move any hair away so that the foam can be applied to the affected skin. 6.) Do not get foam in eyes, mouth or vagina; rinse areas well with water if contact occurs. **Storage:** 20-25°C (68-77°F). Do not store under refrigerated conditions or in direct sunlight. Do not expose containers to heat or store at temperatures above 49°C (120°F). Contents are flammable and under pressure. Do not puncture and/or incinerate container.

FACTIVE   RX
gemifloxacin mesylate (Cornerstone)

> Fluoroquinolones are associated with an increased risk of tendinitis and tendon rupture in all ages. Risk is further increased in patients >60 yrs, taking corticosteroids, with kidney, heart, or lung transplants. May exacerbate muscle weakness with myasthenia gravis; avoid in patients with known history of myasthenia gravis.

THERAPEUTIC CLASS: Fluoroquinolone

INDICATIONS: Treatment of community-acquired pneumonia (CAP), including multi-drug resistant *Streptococcus pneumoniae* (MDRSP), and acute bacterial exacerbation of chronic bronchitis (ABECB) caused by susceptible strains of microorganisms.

DOSAGE: *Adults:* ≥18 yrs: ABECB: 320mg qd for 5 days. CAP: 320mg qd for 5 days (*S. pneumoniae, H. influenzae, M. pneumoniae,* or *C. pneumoniae*) or 7 days (MDRSP, *K. pneumoniae,* or *M. catarrhalis*). CrCl ≤40mL/min or Dialysis: 160mg q24h. Take with fluids.

HOW SUPPLIED: Tab: 320mg

WARNINGS/PRECAUTIONS: May prolong QT interval; avoid in patients with history of prolonged QTc interval, uncontrolled electrolyte disorders, and risk factors for torsades de pointes. Caution with proarrhythmic conditions and CNS diseases (eg, epilepsy or patients predisposed to convulsions). D/C at 1st appearance of skin rash, jaundice, or any other sign of hypersensitivity, and if CNS stimulation, phototoxicity, and pain, swelling, inflammation, or rupture of a tendon occur. Peripheral neuropathy, CNS effects, photosensitivity and hypersensitivity (eg, rash) reactions, liver enzyme elevations, *Clostridium difficile*-associated diarrhea (CDAD), Achilles and other tendon ruptures reported. Caution in elderly and with renal impairment. Avoid excessive exposure to sunlight and UV light. Maintain hydration. Increased risk of development of drug-resistant bacteria if used in the absence of a strongly suspected bacterial infection.

ADVERSE REACTIONS: Diarrhea, rash, N/V, headache, abdominal pain, dizziness.

INTERACTIONS: See Boxed Warning. Avoid magnesium- or aluminum-containing antacids, ferrous sulfate (iron), didanosine chewable/buffered tab or pediatric powder for oral sol, and multivitamin preparations containing zinc or other metal cations within 3 hrs before or 2 hrs after therapy and sucralfate within 2 hrs of therapy. Decreased exposure with calcium carbonate after simultaneous administration. Reduced levels with oral estrogen/progesterone contraceptive product. Increased levels with cimetidine and omeprazole. Increased exposure with probenecid. Avoid Class IA (eg, quinidine, procainamide) or III (eg, amiodarone, sotalol) antiarrhythmics. Caution with drugs that prolong the QTc interval (eg, erythromycin, antipsychotics, TCAs). Increased INR or PT, and/or clinical episodes of bleeding with warfarin or its derivatives.

PREGNANCY: Category C, not for use in nursing.

MECHANISM OF ACTION: Fluoroquinolone; inhibits DNA synthesis through inhibition of both DNA gyrase and topoisomerase IV, which are essential for bacterial growth.

PHARMACOKINETICS: Absorption: Rapid; absolute bioavailability (71%); T_{max}=0.5-2 hrs, C_{max}=1.61µg/mL, AUC=8.36µg•hr/mL (respiratory and urinary tract infection [UTI]). **Distribution:** V_d=4.18L/kg; plasma protein binding (55-73%). **Metabolism:** Liver. **Elimination:** Feces (61%), urine (36%); $T_{1/2}$=7 hrs.

NURSING CONSIDERATIONS

Assessment: Assess for hypersensitivity to drug, factors that increase the risk of tendon rupture, history of myasthenia gravis and prolonged QTc interval, uncontrolled electrolyte disorders, proarrhythmic conditions, CNS disease, pregnancy/nursing status, and possible drug interactions. Obtain baseline renal function and LFTs.

Monitoring: Monitor for signs/symptoms of tendinitis or tendon rupture, muscle weakness exacerbation, hypersensitivity and photosensitivity/phototoxicity reactions, peripheral neuropathy, CNS effects, and CDAD. Monitor renal function and LFTs.

Patient Counseling: Notify healthcare provider if pain, swelling, or inflammation of a tendon, or weakness or inability to move joints occur; rest and refrain from exercise and d/c therapy. Inform that drug may worsen myasthenia gravis symptoms; immediately contact physician if worsening muscle weakness or breathing problems occur. Inform that drug treats bacterial, not viral, infections. Instruct to take exactly as directed and not to skip doses. Instruct to take with or without food, and drink fluids liberally. D/C and notify physician if rash or other allergic reaction develops. Notify physician for watery and bloody stools, palpitations, sunburn-like reaction, or skin eruption. Inform that drug may cause dizziness; caution in activities requiring mental alertness and coordination. Advise to avoid sun exposure. Instruct to swallow tab whole. Notify physician about medications taken concurrently.

Administration: Oral route. **Storage:** 25°C (77°F); excursions permitted to 15-30°C (59-86°F). Protect from light.

FAMOTIDINE   RX
famotidine (Various)

OTHER BRAND NAMES: Pepcid Tablet (Merck) - Pepcid Oral Suspension (Salix)

THERAPEUTIC CLASS: H_2-blocker

INDICATIONS: Short-term treatment of active duodenal ulcer (DU), active benign gastric ulcer (GU), gastroesophageal reflux disease (GERD), and esophagitis due to GERD including erosive or ulcerative disease. Maintenance therapy for DU patients at reduced dosage after the healing of an active ulcer. Treatment of pathological hypersecretory conditions (eg, Zollinger-Ellison syndrome, multiple endocrine adenomas). (Inj) Indicated in some hospitalized patients with pathological hypersecretory conditions or intractable ulcers, or as an alternative to oral dosage forms for short term use in patients who are unable to take oral medication.

DOSAGE: *Adults:* (PO) DU: Usual: 40mg qhs or 20mg bid for 4-8 weeks. Maint: 20mg qhs. Benign GU: Usual: 40mg qhs. (Inj) Intractable Ulcer: Usual: 20mg IV q12h. (PO) GERD: Usual: 20mg bid for ≤6 weeks. (PO) GERD with Esophagitis: 20-40mg bid for ≤12 weeks. Hypersecretory Conditions: Initial: (PO) 20mg q6h. Max: 160mg q6h. (Inj) Usual: 20mg IV q12h; higher starting dose may be required in some patients. Adjust dose according to individual patient needs and continue as long as indicated. Moderate (CrCl <50mL/min) or Severe (CrCl <10mL/min) Renal Impairment: Reduce to 1/2 dose, or increase dosing interval to q36-48h.
Pediatrics: 1-16 yrs: Peptic Ulcer: Usual: (PO) 0.5mg/kg/day qhs or divided bid. Max: 40mg/day. (Inj) 0.25mg/kg IV over not <2 min or as 15-min infusion q12h. Max: 40mg/day. Individualized based on clinical response, gastric pH determination, and endoscopy. GERD with or without Esophagitis: (PO) 1mg/kg/day divided bid. Max: 40mg bid. (Inj) 0.25mg/kg IV over not <2 min or as 15-min infusion q12h. Max: 40mg/day. Individualized based on clinical response, gastric pH determination, and endoscopy. 3 months-<1 yr: (PO) GERD: 0.5mg/kg bid for ≤8 weeks. <3 months: (PO) GERD: 0.5mg/kg qd for

≤8 weeks. Moderate (CrCl <50mL/min) or Severe (CrCl <10mL/min) Renal Impairment: Reduce to 1/2 dose, or increase dosing interval to q36-48h.

HOW SUPPLIED: Inj: (Generic) 10mg/mL [2mL, 4mL, 20mL], 20mg/50mL [50mL]; Sus: (Pepcid) 40mg/5mL; Tab: (Pepcid) 20mg, 40mg

WARNINGS/PRECAUTIONS: Symptomatic response to therapy does not preclude presence of gastric malignancy. CNS adverse effects reported with moderate to severe renal insufficiency; may need to prolong dosing intervals or reduce dose. (Inj) For IV use only. Inj from multiple dose vials contains benzyl alcohol; avoid in neonates and pregnant women.

ADVERSE REACTIONS: Headache, dizziness, constipation, diarrhea, agitation.

INTERACTIONS: (PO) Bioavailability may be slightly decreased by antacids.

PREGNANCY: Category B, not for use in nursing.

MECHANISM OF ACTION: Histamine H_2-receptor antagonist; inhibits both acid concentration and volume of gastric secretion.

PHARMACOKINETICS: Absorption: (PO) Incompletely absorbed; bioavailability (40-45%); T_{max}=1-3 hrs. **Distribution:** Plasma protein binding (15-20%); found in breast milk. **Metabolism:** Minimal first-pass metabolism; S-oxide (metabolite). **Elimination:** Renal (65-70%; 25-30% unchanged [PO], 65-70% unchanged [IV]); Metabolic (30-35%); $T_{1/2}$=2.5-3.5 hrs. Refer to PI for pediatric parameters.

NURSING CONSIDERATIONS

Assessment: Assess for hypersensitivity to drug and to other H_2-receptor antagonists, renal function, pregnancy/nursing status, and possible drug interactions.

Monitoring: Monitor for renal function, signs/symptoms of hypersensitivity reactions, and other adverse reactions.

Patient Counseling: Inform risks/benefits of therapy. Instruct to contact physician if hypersensitivity or other adverse reactions develop. Inform that antacids may be taken concomitantly. Advise to avoid nursing while on medication. Instruct to shake oral sus vigorously for 5-10 sec prior to each use. Instruct to discard unused constituted sus after 30 days.

Administration: IV and Oral route. May be given with antacids if needed. Refer to PI for directions for preparing oral sus and preparation/stability of inj/premixed inj. **Storage:** Inj: 2-8°C (36-46°). Bring to room temperature and solubilize if sol freezes. Diluted sol should be refrigerated and used within 48 hrs. Premixed Inj: Room temperature (25°C [77°F]); avoid exposure to excessive heat; brief exposure to temperatures ≤35°C (95°F) does not adversely affect product. Tab: Controlled room temperature; preserve in well-closed, light-resistant container. Sus: 25°C (77°F); excursions permitted to 15-30°C (59-86°F). Protect from freezing. Discard unused sus after 30 days.

FAMVIR   RX
famciclovir (Novartis)

THERAPEUTIC CLASS: Nucleoside analogue

INDICATIONS: Treatment of herpes zoster (shingles), herpes labialis (cold sores), treatment or suppression of recurrent genital herpes. Treatment of recurrent episodes of orolabial/genital herpes in HIV-infected adults.

DOSAGE: *Adults:* Immunocompetent Patients: Herpes Labialis: 1500mg as a single dose; initiate at the 1st sign/symptoms (eg, tingling, itching, burning, pain, or lesion). Genital Herpes: Recurrent Episodes: 1000mg bid for 1 day; initiate at the 1st sign/symptoms. Suppressive Therapy: 250mg bid. Herpes Zoster (shingles): 500mg q8h for 7 days; initiate as soon as herpes zoster is diagnosed. HIV-Infected Patients: Recurrent Orolabial/Genital Herpes: 500mg bid for 7 days; initiate at the first sign/symptoms. Elderly: Start at the low end of dosing range. Refer to PI for dosage recommendations for renal impairment.

HOW SUPPLIED: Tab: 125mg, 250mg, 500mg

WARNINGS/PRECAUTIONS: Acute renal failure reported; dose adjustment in renal disease recommended. Caution in elderly.

ADVERSE REACTIONS: Headache, N/V, diarrhea, elevated lipase, ALT elevation, fatigue, flatulence, pruritus, rash, neutropenia, abdominal pain, dysmenorrhea, migraine.

INTERACTIONS: Increased plasma concentration with probenecid and other drugs significantly eliminated by active renal tubular secretion. Potential interaction with drugs metabolized and/or inhibited by aldehyde oxidase. Raloxifene could decrease formation of penciclovir in vitro.

PREGNANCY: Category B, not for use in nursing.

MECHANISM OF ACTION: Nucleoside analogue; inhibits HSV-2 DNA polymerase competitively with deoxyguanosine triphosphate, inhibiting herpes viral DNA synthesis and replication.

PHARMACOKINETICS: Absorption: Penciclovir: Absolute bioavailability (77%); parameters varied for different doses. **Distribution:** Penciclovir (IV) V_d=1.08L/kg; plasma protein binding (<20%) **Metabolism**: Deacetylation and oxidation; famciclovir (prodrug) converted to penciclovir. **Elimination:** Urine (73%), feces (27%). Penciclovir: Urine (94%); $T_{1/2}$=2-3 hrs.

NURSING CONSIDERATIONS

Assessment: Assess for renal dysfunction, hypersensitivity to drug, pregnancy/nursing status, and possible drug interactions.

Monitoring: Monitor for acute renal failure and hypersensitivity reactions. Monitor CrCl and maternal-fetal outcomes of pregnant women exposed to the drug.

Patient Counseling: Inform to take exactly as directed. Advise to initiate treatment at the earliest signs/symptoms of recurrence of cold sores (eg, tingling, itching, burning, pain, or lesion), and genital herpes. Instruct that treatment for cold sores should not exceed 1 dose, that drug is not a cure for cold sores or genital herpes, and to avoid contact with lesions or intercourse when lesions and/or symptoms are present to avoid infecting partners. Counsel to use safer sex practices. Inform that if episodic therapy for recurrent genital herpes is indicated, advise to initiate therapy at the 1st sign or symptom of an episode. Instruct to refrain from driving or operating machinery if dizziness, somnolence, or confusion, or other CNS disturbances is experienced and to initiate as soon as possible once diagnosed with herpes zoster. Inform that contains lactose; advise to discuss with healthcare provider if with rare hereditary problems of galactose intolerance, severe lactase deficiency or glucose-galactose malabsorption.

Administration: Oral route. **Storage:** 25°C (77°F); excursions permitted to 15-30°C (59-86°F).

FANAPT   RX
iloperidone (Vanda)

Elderly patients with dementia-related psychosis treated with antipsychotic drugs are at an increased risk of death; most deaths appeared to be cardiovascular (eg, heart failure, sudden death) or infectious (eg, pneumonia) in nature. Iloperidone is not approved for treatment of patients with dementia-related psychosis.

THERAPEUTIC CLASS: Benzisoxazole derivative

INDICATIONS: Acute treatment of adults with schizophrenia.

DOSAGE: *Adults:* Initial: 1mg bid. Titrate: Titrate slowly from low starting dose. Day 2: 2mg bid. Day 3: 4mg bid. Day 4: 6mg bid. Day 5: 8mg bid. Day 6: 10mg bid. Day 7: 12mg bid. Range: 6-12mg bid. Max: 12mg bid (24mg/day). Concomitant Strong CYP2D6/CYP3A4 Inhibitors: Reduce dose by 50%. Increase to previous iloperidone dose upon withdrawal of CYP2D6/CYP3A4 inhibitors. Poor CYP2D6 Metabolizers: Reduce dose by 50%. Maint: Responding patients may continue beyond acute response; periodically reassess need for maintenance treatment. Reinitiation of Treatment: Follow initial titration schedule if have had an interval off for >3 days. Switching From Other Antipsychotics: Minimize overlapping period of antipsychotics.

HOW SUPPLIED: Tab: 1mg, 2mg, 4mg, 6mg, 8mg, 10mg, 12mg

WARNINGS/PRECAUTIONS: Avoid with hepatic impairment. QT prolongation reported; avoid with congenital long QT syndrome, history of cardiac arrhythmias, or with history of significant cardiovascular illnesses. Risk of torsades de pointes and/or sudden death may be increased by bradycardia, hypokalemia or hypomagnesemia, presence of congenital prolongation of the QT interval, recent acute MI, and/or uncompensated heart failure. Obtain baseline measurements and periodically monitor during treatment K+ and Mg levels in patients at risk of electrolyte disturbances. D/C if persistent QTc measurements >500 ms occur. Neuroleptic malignant syndrome (NMS) and tardive dyskinesia reported. Hyperglycemia reported; monitor for worsening blood glucose control in diabetes mellitus (DM) patients and fasting blood glucose (FBG) levels in patients with diabetes risk. Weight gain reported. Caution with history of seizures or conditions that lower seizure threshold. May induce orthostatic hypotension; caution with CVD, cerebrovascular disease or conditions that predispose to hypotension. Leukopenia, neutropenia and agranulocytosis reported; d/c in cases of severe neutropenia (ANC <1000/mm³). May elevate prolactin levels. May disrupt body's ability to reduce core body temperature; caution in conditions that may elevate body core temperature. Esophageal dysmotility and aspiration reported; caution in patients at risk of aspiration pneumonia. Closely supervise high-risk patients for suicide attempt. Priapism reported. May impair mental/physical abilities.

ADVERSE REACTIONS: Dizziness, somnolence, tachycardia, nausea, dry mouth, weight gain, nasal congestion, diarrhea, fatigue, extrapyramidal disorder, orthostatic hypotension, nasopharyngitis, arthralgia, tremor.

INTERACTIONS: May increase levels with concomitant use of CYP3A4 (eg, ketoconazole) or CYP2D6 (eg, fluoxetine, paroxetine) inhibitors. May increase total exposure of dextromethorphan with concomitant use. Avoid with Class IA (eg, quinidine, procainamide) or Class III (eg, amiodarone, sotalol) antiarrhythmics, antipsychotics (eg, chlorpromazine, thioridazine), antibiotics (eg, gatifloxacin, moxifloxacin), or other drugs known to prolong QTc interval (eg, pentamidine, levomethadyl acetate, methadone). Caution with other centrally acting drugs and alcohol. May potentiate effects of antihypertensive agents. Concomitant use with medications with anticholinergic activity may contribute to an elevation in core body temperature.

PREGNANCY: Category C, not for use in nursing.

MECHANISM OF ACTION: Piperidinyl-benzisoxazole derivative; has not been established. Proposed to be mediated through a combination of dopamine type 2 (D_2) and serotonin type 2 (5-HT_2) antagonisms.

PHARMACOKINETICS: Absorption: Well absorbed; T_{max}=2-4 hrs. **Distribution:** V_d=1340-2800L; plasma protein binding (95%). **Metabolism:** Liver via carbonyl reduction, hydroxylation (CYP2D6), O-demethylation (CYP3A4); P88, P95 (predominant metabolites). **Elimination:** Urine (58.2% in extensive metabolizers [EM], 45.1% in poor metabolizers [PM]); feces [19.9% (EM), 22.1% (PM)]. Refer to PI for $T_{1/2}$ in CYP2D6 EM and PM.

NURSING CONSIDERATIONS

Assessment: Assess for dementia-related psychosis, DM, risk factors for DM (eg, obesity, family history of DM), CVD, cerebrovascular disease, conditions that predispose to hypotension, history of clinically significant low WBCs or drug-induced leukopenia/neutropenia, history of seizures, risk for aspiration pneumonia, risk for suicide, pregnancy/nursing status, and possible drug interactions. Obtain baseline FBG in patients with DM and risk factors for DM. Perform baseline CBC, orthostatic vital signs, serum K+ and Mg levels.

Monitoring: Monitor for TD, NMS, priapism, extrapyramidal symptoms, cerebrovascular events, CVD, esophageal dysmotility, aspiration, orthostatic hypotension, body temperature lability, seizures, QT prolongation, suicidal attempts, and cognitive/motor impairment. Monitor for signs of hyperglycemia; perform periodic monitoring of FBG levels in patients with DM or at risk for DM. Monitor for signs/symptoms of leukopenia, neutropenia, and agranulocytosis; perform frequent monitoring of CBC in patients with risk factors for leukopenia/neutropenia. Monitor serum K+ and Mg, prolactin levels, and orthostatic vital signs.

Patient Counseling: Advise to inform physician immediately if feeling faint, lose consciousness or have heart palpitations. Counsel to avoid drugs that cause QT interval prolongation and inform physician if taking or planning to take any drug. Advise of the risk of NMS and orthostatic hypotension. Inform that therapy may impair judgment, thinking, or motor skills; caution against driving or operating hazardous machinery. Instruct to notify physician if pregnant or intend to become pregnant. Advise not to breastfeed. Instruct to avoid alcohol. Counsel about appropriate care to avoid dehydration.

Administration: Oral route. **Storage:** 25°C (77°F); excursions permitted to 15-30°C (59-86°F). Protect from light and moisture.

FASLODEX

fulvestrant (AstraZeneca)

RX

THERAPEUTIC CLASS: Estrogen receptor antagonist

INDICATIONS: Treatment of hormone receptor positive metastatic breast cancer in postmenopausal women with disease progression following antiestrogen therapy.

DOSAGE: *Adults:* 500mg IM into buttocks slowly (1-2 min/inj) as two 5-mL inj, one in each buttock. Moderate Hepatic Impairment (Child-Pugh Class B): 250mg IM into buttock slowly (1-2 min) as one 5-mL inj. Administer on Days 1, 15, 29, and once monthly thereafter.

HOW SUPPLIED: Inj: 50mg/mL [5mL]

WARNINGS/PRECAUTIONS: Caution with bleeding diatheses and thrombocytopenia. Not studied in severe hepatic impairment (Child-Pugh Class C). May cause fetal harm during pregnancy.

ADVERSE REACTIONS: Inj-site pain, headache, back pain, diarrhea, N/V, bone pain, fatigue, pain in extremity, asthenia, hot flash, anorexia, musculoskeletal pain, cough, dyspnea.

INTERACTIONS: Caution with anticoagulant use.

PREGNANCY: Category D, not for use in nursing.

MECHANISM OF ACTION: Estrogen receptor antagonist; binds to estrogen receptor (ER) and downregulates ER protein in human breast cancer cells.

PHARMACOKINETICS: Absorption: (Single dose) C_{max}=25.1ng/mL; AUC=11400ng•hr/mL. (Multiple dose) C_{max}=28ng/mL; AUC=13100ng•hr/mL. **Distribution:** V_d=3-5L/kg; plasma protein binding (99%). **Metabolism:** CYP3A4 (oxidation), aromatic hydroxylation, conjugation. **Elimination:** Feces (90%), urine (<1%); $T_{1/2}$=40 days.

NURSING CONSIDERATIONS

Assessment: Assess for hypersensitivity to drug, bleeding diatheses, thrombocytopenia, hepatic impairment, pregnancy/nursing status, and possible drug interactions.

Monitoring: Monitor for inj-site reactions, hepatic impairment, and other adverse reactions. Monitor use in women of childbearing potential.

Patient Counseling: Advise women of childbearing potential not to become pregnant. Instruct to notify physician if pregnant, nursing, or planning to become pregnant, or if have a bleeding disorder, thrombocytopenia, or taking anticoagulants.

Administration: IM route. Refer to PI for further administration instructions. **Storage:** 2-8°C (36-46°F). Protect from light. Store in original carton until time of use.

FAZACLO RX

clozapine (Azur)

> Risk of potentially life-threatening agranulocytosis. Reserve use for severely ill patients with schizophrenia unresponsive to standard antipsychotic treatment or for patients with schizophrenia/schizoaffective disorder at risk for re-experiencing suicidal behavior. Obtain baseline WBC count and absolute neutrophil count (ANC) prior to therapy, regularly during treatment, and for ≥4 weeks after d/c. Seizures associated with use and with greater likelihood at higher doses; caution with history of seizures or other predisposing factors. Increased risk of fatal myocarditis, especially during 1st month of therapy; d/c if suspected. Orthostatic hypotension, with or without syncope can occur. Rare reports of profound collapse with respiratory and/or cardiac arrest in patients taking benzodiazepines or any other psychotropic drugs. Elderly patients with dementia-related psychosis treated with atypical antipsychotic drugs are at an increased risk for death. Not approved for the treatment of dementia-related psychosis.

THERAPEUTIC CLASS: Dibenzapine derivative

INDICATIONS: Management of severely ill schizophrenic patients who fail to respond adequately to standard drug treatment for schizophrenia. Reduction of risk for recurrent suicidal behavior in patients with schizophrenia/schizo-affective disorder who are judged to be at chronic risk for re-experiencing suicidal behavior.

DOSAGE: *Adults:* Treatment-Resistant Schizophrenia: Initial: 12.5mg qd-bid. Titrate: Increase by 25-50mg/day, up to 300-450mg/day by end of 2 weeks; then increase once or twice weekly in increments of ≤100mg. Usual: 300-600mg/day given on a divided basis. Titrate: May increase to 600-900mg/day. Max: 900mg/day. Maint: Continue at lowest level needed to maintain remission. To d/c, gradually reduce dose over 1-2 weeks. Monitor for psychotic and cholinergic rebound symptoms if abrupt d/c warranted (eg, leukopenia). Re-initiation (even with brief interval off clozapine): Start with 12.5mg qd-bid; may titrate more quickly if initial dosing tolerated. Retitrate with extreme caution in those who experienced cardiac or respiratory arrest with initial dosing but was then successfully titrated to therapeutic dose. Do not restart in patients d/c for WBC <2000/mm³ or ANC <1000/mm³. Reduction of Risk of Suicidal Behavior in Schizophrenia/Schizoaffective Disorder: May follow dosing recommendations for treatment-resistant schizophrenia. Range: 12.5-900mg/day (mean 300mg). To reduce the risk of suicidal behavior in patients who otherwise responded to therapy with another antipsychotic, treat for ≥2 years and then re-evaluate. If risk for suicidal behavior is still present, continue treatment and revisit at regular intervals. If no longer at risk of suicidal behavior, d/c treatment. Elderly: Start at lower end of dosing range.

HOW SUPPLIED: Tab, Disintegrating: 12.5mg, 25mg, 100mg, 150mg, 200mg

CONTRAINDICATIONS: Myeloproliferative disorders, uncontrolled epilepsy, paralytic ileus, history of clozapine-induced agranulocytosis or severe granulocytopenia, severe CNS depression, comatose states. Concomitant use with agents with potential to cause agranulocytosis or suppress bone marrow function.

WARNINGS/PRECAUTIONS: Hyperglycemia, sometimes with ketoacidosis, hyperosmolar coma or death, reported. Monitor for worsening of glucose control with diabetes mellitus (DM) and fasting blood glucose (FBG) levels with diabetes risk or symptoms of hyperglycemia. Tachycardia and cardiomyopathy reported. D/C if cardiomyopathy is confirmed unless benefits outweigh risk. Neuroleptic malignant syndrome (NMS), tardive dyskinesia (TD), impaired intestinal peristalsis, deep-vein thrombosis, pulmonary embolism, and ECG changes reported. Fever reported; rule out infection or agranulocytosis. Consider NMS in the presence of high fever. Hepatitis reported. If N/V and/or anorexia develop, perform LFTs. D/C if symptoms of jaundice occur. Has potent anticholinergic effects; caution with prostatic enlargement and narrow-angle glaucoma. May impair mental/physical abilities. Caution with renal, cardiac, hepatic, or pulmonary disease. Increased risk of cerebrovascular adverse events; caution with risk factors for stroke. Obtain WBC and ANC at baseline, then weekly for 1st six months of therapy, then every 2 weeks for next 6 months, and then every 4 weeks thereafter if counts are acceptable

(WBC ≥3500/mm³ or ANC ≥2000/mm³). Refer to PI for frequency of monitoring based on stage of therapy, WBC count and ANC. Avoid treatment if WBC <3500/mm³ or ANC <2000/mm³. D/C treatment and do not rechallenge if WBC <2000/mm³, ANC <1000/mm³. Interrupt therapy if eosinophilia (>4000/mm³) develops. Contains aspartame (of which phenylalanine is a component); caution with phenylketonurics. Not for use in infants. Caution in elderly.

ADVERSE REACTIONS: Agranulocytosis, seizure, myocarditis, orthostatic hypotension, drowsiness/sedation, salivation, somnolence, tachycardia, dizziness/vertigo, constipation, insomnia, N/V, dyspepsia.

INTERACTIONS: See Contraindications and Boxed Warning. Avoid using epinephrine to treat clozapine-induced hypotension. Use with carbamazepine is not recommended. Caution with CNS-active drugs, general anesthesia, alcohol, paroxetine, fluoxetine, fluvoxamine, sertraline, or inhibitors/inducers of CYP1A2, 2D6, 3A4. Consider reduced dose with paroxetine, fluoxetine, fluvoxamine, and sertraline. Dosage reduction may be needed with drugs metabolized by CYP2D6 (eg, antidepressants, phenothiazines, carbamazepine, Type 1C antiarrhythmics) or that inhibit this enzyme (eg, quinidine). May potentiate hypotensive effects of antihypertensives and anticholinergic effects of atropine-type drugs. CYP450 inducers (eg, phenytoin, tobacco smoke, carbamazepine, rifampin) may decrease plasma levels. CYP450 inhibitors (eg, cimetidine, caffeine, citalopram, ciprofloxacin, fluvoxamine, erythromycin) may increase plasma levels. NMS reported with lithium and other CNS-active drugs. Concurrent psychopharmaceuticals may affect plasma clozapine levels. May interact with other highly protein-bound drugs.

PREGNANCY: Category B, not for use in nursing.

MECHANISM OF ACTION: Tricyclic dibenzodiazepine derivative; atypical antipsychotic agent. Interferes with the binding of dopamine specifically at the D_1, D_2, D_3, and D_5 receptors, and has a high affinity for D_4 receptor. Also acts as an antagonist at the adrenergic, cholinergic, histaminergic, and serotonergic receptors.

PHARMACOKINETICS: Absorption: C_{max}=413ng/mL, T_{max}=2.3 hrs (100mg bid). **Distribution:** Plasma protein binding (97%). **Metabolism:** Demethylation, hydroxylation, N-oxidation. Norclozapine (active metabolite). **Elimination:** Urine (50%), feces (30%); $T_{1/2}$=8 hrs (Single 75mg dose), 12 hrs (100mg bid).

NURSING CONSIDERATIONS

Assessment: Assess previous course of standard therapy prior to treatment. Assess for myeloproliferative disorders, uncontrolled epilepsy, paralytic ileus, history of clozapine-induced agranulocytosis or severe granulocytopenia, and severe CNS depression or comatose states, history of seizures or other predisposing factors, other conditions where treatment is cautioned or contraindicated. Assess pregnancy/nursing status and possible drug interactions. Obtain baseline WBC count and ANC prior to therapy, and baseline FBG levels in patients at risk for hyperglycemia/DM.

Monitoring: Monitor for clinical response and need to continue treatment. Monitor for agranulocytosis, myocarditis, orthostatic hypotension, HF, tachycardia, respiratory effects, seizures, flu-like symptoms, infection (eg, pneumonia), eosinophilia, fever, DVT, PE, NMS, TD, impairment of intestinal peristalsis, impairment of mental/physical abilities, and signs/symptoms of hyperglycemia. Monitor WBC counts and ANC during and for ≥4 weeks following d/c or until WBC ≥3500/mm³ and ANC ≥2000/mm³. Check periodic FBG levels if at risk for hyperglycemia and for signs/symptoms of hepatitis while on therapy. Obtain LFTs if patient develops N/V and/or anorexia.

Patient Counseling: Inform that drug is available only through a program designed to ensure the required blood monitoring schedule. Counsel on risks of treatment (eg, agranulocytosis, seizures, orthostatic hypotension). Inform about signs/symptoms of agranulocytosis; advise to immediately report lethargy, weakness, fever, sore throat, malaise, mucous membrane ulceration, flu-like complaints, or other possible signs of infection. Inform phenylketonuric patients that drug contains phenylalanine. Avoid potentially hazardous activities (eg, operating machinery, driving). Notify physician if intending to become pregnant, planning to take any prescription or OTC drugs or alcohol.

Advise females to avoid breastfeeding. Advise drug can be taken with/without food. If a dose is missed for >2 days, consult physician before restarting medication. Tablets should remain in the original package until immediately prior to use.

Administration: Oral route. Allow to disintegrate in mouth and swallow with saliva or chew if desired. No water needed. **Storage:** 25°C (77°F); excursions permitted to 15-30°C (59-86°F). Protect from moisture.

FELBATOL   RX
felbamate (Meda)

> Associated with increased incidence of aplastic anemia; d/c if any evidence of bone marrow depression occurs. Acute liver failure reported; d/c if AST or ALT increased ≥2x ULN or if clinical signs and symptoms suggest liver failure. Monitor blood count and LFTs routinely. Avoid with history of hepatic dysfunction.

THERAPEUTIC CLASS: Dicarbamate anticonvulsant

INDICATIONS: Monotherapy or adjunctive therapy in partial seizures, with and without generalization, in adults with epilepsy. Adjunctive therapy for partial and generalized seizures with Lennox-Gastaut syndrome in children.

DOSAGE: *Adults:* Initial Monotherapy: 300mg qid or 400mg tid. Titrate: Increase by 600mg every 2 weeks to 2.4g/day. Max: 3.6g/day. Initial Monotherapy Conversion/Adjunct Therapy: 300mg qid or 400mg tid while reducing present antiepileptic drugs (AED) (refer to PI). Titrate: Monotherapy Conversion: Increase at Week 2 to 2.4g/day, at Week 3 up to 3.6g/day. Adjunct Therapy: Increase by 1.2g/day every week up to 3.6mg/day. Renal Impairment: Initial/Maint: Reduce by one-half. Adjunct Therapy: May need further dose reductions. Elderly: Start at lower end of dosing range. *Pediatrics:* ≥14 yrs: Initial Monotherapy: 300mg qid or 400mg tid. Titrate: Increase by 600mg every 2 weeks to 2.4g/day. Max: 3.6g/day. Initial Monotherapy Conversion/Adjunct Therapy: 300mg qid or 400mg tid while reducing present AED (refer to PI). Titrate: Monotherapy Conversion: Increase at Week 2 to 2.4g/day, at Week 3 up to 3.6g/day. Adjunct Therapy: Increase by 1.2g/day every week up to 3.6mg/day. Renal Impairment: Initial/Maint: Reduce by one-half. Adjunct therapy: May need further dose reductions. 2-14 yrs: Lennox-Gastaut Adjunct Therapy: Initial: 15mg/kg/day in 3-4 divided doses while reducing present AEDs by 20%. Titrate: Increase by 15mg/kg/day every week to 45mg/kg/day.

HOW SUPPLIED: Sus: 600mg/5mL [8 oz, 32 oz]; Tab: 400mg*, 600mg* *scored

CONTRAINDICATIONS: History of blood dyscrasias or hepatic dysfunction.

WARNINGS/PRECAUTIONS: Not for first-line therapy. Avoid abrupt d/c. Increased risk of suicidal thoughts or behavior; monitor for emergence or worsening of depression, suicidal thoughts/behavior and any unusual changes in mood or behavior. Obtain full hematologic evaluations (eg, blood counts including platelets and reticulocytes) and LFTs before, during and after d/c. Caution with renal dysfunction. Caution in elderly.

ADVERSE REACTIONS: Anorexia, N/V, insomnia, headache, somnolence, dizziness, dyspepsia, constipation, fatigue, upper respiratory tract infection, diplopia, nervousness.

INTERACTIONS: Increases plasma concentrations of phenytoin, valproate, carbamazepine epoxide and phenobarbital. Decreases carbamazepine concentration. Decreased felbamate levels with phenytoin, carbamazepine and phenobarbital. Caution with oral contraceptives.

PREGNANCY: Category C, safety in nursing not known.

MECHANISM OF ACTION: Anticonvulsant; has not been established. Weak inhibitory effects on GABA-receptor binding and benzodiazepine receptor binding. Acts as an antagonist at the strychnine-insensitive glycine recognition site of the NMDA receptor-ionophore complex.

PHARMACOKINETICS: Absorption: Well-absorbed. **Distribution:** V_d=756mL/kg; plasma protein binding (22-25%); found in breast milk. **Metabolism:** Parahydroxyfelbamate, 2-hydroxyfelbamate, felbamatemonocarbamate (metabolites). **Elimination:** Urine (90%, 40-50% unchanged); $T_{1/2}$=20-23 hrs.

NURSING CONSIDERATIONS

Assessment: Assess for history of blood dyscrasias or hepatic dysfunction, depression and suicidal thoughts/behavior. Assess renal function and pregnancy/nursing status prior to therapy. Obtain baseline CBC (reticulocytes, platelets) and LFTs.

Monitoring: Monitor for signs/symptoms of hepatic failure, aplastic anemia (signs of infection, bleeding, anemia), bone marrow depression and seizures. Monitor for emergence or worsening of depression, suicidal thoughts/behavior and any unusual changes in mood or behavior. Monitor renal function. Monitor LFTs and CBC (platelets, reticulocytes) while on therapy and following treatment.

Patient Counseling: If signs of aplastic anemia (infection, bleeding, anemia) or liver dysfunction (jaundice, anorexia, GI complaints, and malaise) occur, advise to contact physician immediately. Advise not to abruptly d/c medication. Inform of risk for hematological/hepatic complications following d/c; continued monitoring of CBC and LFTs required. Notify physician if emergence or worsening of depression, suicidal thoughts/behavior and any unusual changes in mood or behavior occur. If pregnant, encourage to enroll in the North American Antiepileptic Drug (NAAED) Pregnancy Registry. Call 888-233-2334 or go to aedpregnancyregistry.org. Inform of the need to obtain written, informed consent prior to therapy.

Administration: Oral route. Shake oral suspension well before using. **Storage:** 20-25°C (68-77°F). Dispense in tight container.

FELODIPINE   RX
felodipine (Various)

THERAPEUTIC CLASS: Calcium channel blocker (dihydropyridine)

INDICATIONS: Treatment of hypertension alone or concomitantly with other antihypertensive agents.

DOSAGE: *Adults:* Initial: 5mg qd. Titrate: May increase to 10mg qd or decrease to 2.5mg qd at intervals not <2 weeks depending on patient's response. Range: 2.5-10mg qd. Hepatic dysfunction/Elderly: Initial: 2.5mg qd. Take without food or with a light meal. Swallow whole; do not crush or chew.

HOW SUPPLIED: Tab, Extended-Release: 2.5mg, 5mg, 10mg

WARNINGS/PRECAUTIONS: May cause hypotension and syncope (rare). May lead to reflex tachycardia, which may precipitate angina pectoris. Caution with heart failure or compromised ventricular function. Monitor BP during dose adjustment with hepatic impairment or elderly. Peripheral edema reported. Caution in elderly.

ADVERSE REACTIONS: Peripheral edema, headache, flushing, dizziness, asthenia, dyspepsia, upper respiratory infection.

INTERACTIONS: CYP3A4 inhibitors (eg, itraconazole, ketoconazole, erythromycin, grapefruit juice, cimetidine) may increase plasma levels. Decreased levels with long-term anticonvulsant therapy (eg, phenytoin, carbamazepine, phenobarbital). May increase metoprolol and tacrolimus levels. Caution with β-blockers in patients with heart failure or compromised ventricular function.

PREGNANCY: Category C, not for use in nursing.

MECHANISM OF ACTION: Calcium channel blocker: reversibly competes with nitredipine and/or other calcium channel blockers for dihydropyridine binding sites and blocks voltage-dependent Ca^{++} currents in vascular smooth muscle.

PHARMACOKINETICS: Absorption: (PO) Complete, systemic bioavailability (20%); T_{max}=2.5-5 hrs. **Distribution:** V_d=10L/kg; plasma protein binding (99%). **Elimination:** Urine (70%), feces (10%); $T_{1/2}$=11-16 hrs (immediate-release).

NURSING CONSIDERATIONS

Assessment: Assess for heart failure, compromised ventricular function, hepatic dysfunction, age, pregnancy/nursing status, and possible drug interactions. Obtain baseline LFTs.

Monitoring: Monitor BP, syncope, angina pectoris, and peripheral edema.

Patient Counseling: Instruct to take tab whole; do not crush or chew. Counsel about adverse side effects; notify physician if any develop. Inform that mild gingival hyperplasia (gum swelling) has been reported; maintain good dental hygiene.

Administration: Oral route. **Storage:** <30°C (86°F). Protect from light.

FEMARA   RX
letrozole (Novartis)

THERAPEUTIC CLASS: Nonsteroidal aromatase inhibitor

INDICATIONS: Adjuvant treatment of postmenopausal women with hormone-receptor positive early breast cancer. Extended adjuvant treatment of early breast cancer in postmenopausal women who have received 5 yrs of adjuvant tamoxifen therapy. First-line treatment of postmenopausal women with hormone receptor positive or unknown locally advanced or metastatic breast cancer. Treatment of advanced breast cancer with disease progression following antiestrogen therapy in postmenopausal women.

DOSAGE: *Adults:* 2.5mg qd. Adjuvant Early Breast Cancer: D/C at tumor relapse. Advanced Breast Cancer: Continue until tumor progression is evident. Cirrhosis/Severe Hepatic Dysfunction: Usual: 2.5mg qod.

HOW SUPPLIED: Tab: 2.5mg

CONTRAINDICATIONS: Premenopausal women with breast cancer, pregnant women.

WARNINGS/PRECAUTIONS: May decrease bone mineral density (BMD); bone fractures and osteoporosis reported; consider monitoring BMD. Hypercholesterolemia reported; consider monitoring serum cholesterol levels. Reduce dose by 50% with cirrhosis and severe hepatic dysfunction. May cause fatigue, dizziness and somnolence; caution when driving or using machinery. Decreased lymphocyte counts and thrombocytopenia reported.

ADVERSE REACTIONS: Hypercholesterolemia, hot flushes, asthenia, edema, arthralgia/arthritis, myalgia, headache, dizziness, night sweats, constipation, nausea, sweating increased, bone fractures, weight increased, fatigue.

INTERACTIONS: Reduced plasma levels with tamoxifen.

PREGNANCY: Category X, not for use in nursing.

MECHANISM OF ACTION: Nonsteroidal aromatase inhibitor; inhibits conversion of androgens to estrogens. Inhibits the aromatase enzyme by competitively binding to the heme of cytochrome P450 subunit of the enzyme, resulting in a reduction of estrogen biosynthesis in all tissues.

PHARMACOKINETICS: Absorption: Rapid and complete. **Distribution:** V_d=1.9L/kg. **Metabolism:** Liver via CYP3A4, CYP2A6. **Elimination:** Urine (75% glucuronide of carbinol metabolite, 9% unidentified metabolites, 6% unchanged); $T_{1/2}$=2 days.

NURSING CONSIDERATIONS

Assessment: Assess for premenopausal endocrine status, cirrhosis or hepatic impairment, pregnancy/nursing status, and for possible drug interactions. Obtain baseline BMD.

Monitoring: Monitor for bone fractures, osteoporosis, fatigue, dizziness, somnolence, decreased lymphocytes, and for thrombocytopenia. Monitor LFTs, bone mineral density, and serum cholesterol levels.

Patient Counseling: Inform that the drug is contraindicated in pregnant women and women of premenopausal endocrine status. Counsel perimenopausal and recently menopausal women to use contraception until postmenopausal status is clinically established. Advise about possible fatigue, dizziness, and somnolence; caution against operating machinery/driving. Advise that bone mineral density may be monitored while on therapy. Counsel about side effects; instruct to seek medical attention if any develop.

Administration: Oral route. **Storage:** 25°C (77°F); excursions permitted to 15-30°C (59-86°F).

FEMCON FE RX

ethinyl estradiol - ferrous fumarate - norethindrone (Warner Chilcott)

> Cigarette smoking increases the risk of serious CV side effects from oral contraceptive use. Risk increases with age (>35 yrs) and with heavy smoking (≥15 cigarettes/day). Women who use oral contraceptives should be strongly advised not to smoke.

THERAPEUTIC CLASS: Estrogen/progestogen combination

INDICATIONS: Prevention of pregnancy.

DOSAGE: *Adults:* Take 1 white tab qd for 21 days, followed by 1 brown tab qd for 7 days. Begin next and all subsequent courses of tablets on the same day of the week first course began. Intervals between doses should not exceed 24 hrs. Start first Sunday after menses begin or the first day of menses. Take at the same time each day. Initiate no earlier than Day 28 postpartum in nonlactating mother.
Pediatrics: Postpubertal: Take 1 white tab qd for 21 days, followed by 1 brown tab qd for 7 days. Begin next and all subsequent courses of tablets on the same day of the week first course began. Intervals between doses should not exceeding 24 hrs. Start first Sunday after menses begin or the first day of menses. Take at the same time each day. Initiate no earlier than Day 28 postpartum in nonlactating mother.

HOW SUPPLIED: Tab, Chewable: (Ethinyl Estradiol-Norethindrone) 0.035mg-0.4mg, Tab: (Ferrous Fumarate) 75mg

CONTRAINDICATIONS: Thrombophlebitis, current or history of thromboembolic disorders, history of deep vein thrombophlebitis (DVT), current or history of cerebral vascular disease (CVD) or coronary artery disease (CAD), valvular heart disease with thrombogenic complications, uncontrolled HTN, diabetes with vascular involvement, headaches with focal neurological symptoms such as aura, major surgery with prolonged immobilization, known or suspected breast carcinoma (or personal history), carcinoma of the endometrium or other known or suspected estrogen-dependent neoplasia, undiagnosed abnormal genital bleeding, cholestatic jaundice of pregnancy or jaundice with prior hormonal contraceptive use, hepatic adenomas or carcinoma or active liver disease, and known or suspected pregnancy.

WARNINGS/PRECAUTIONS: Increased risk of venous and arterial thrombotic and thromboembolic events (such as MI, thromboembolism, and stroke), vascular disease, hepatic neoplasia, gallbladder disease, and HTN. May increase risk of breast and cervical cancer. Benign hepatic adenomas and hepatocellular carcinoma reported (rare). Retinal thrombosis reported; d/c if unexplained partial or complete loss of vision, onset of proptosis or diplopia, papilledema, or retinal vascular lesions develop. Should not be used to induce withdrawal bleeding as a test for pregnancy, or to treat threatened or habitual abortion during pregnancy. May cause glucose intolerance; monitor prediabetic and diabetic patients. May cause fluid retention and increase BP; monitor closely with HTN and d/c if significant elevation of BP occurs. D/C with onset or exacerbation of migraine or development of headache with new pattern which is persistent, recurrent, and severe. May cause breakthrough bleeding and spotting; if persistent or recurrent rule out malignancy or pregnancy. Ectopic and intrauterine pregnancies may occur with contraceptive failures. Perform annual physical exam. Monitor closely with hyperlipidemias; may elevate LDL and/or plasma TG. Caution with impaired liver function; d/c if jaundice develops. May cause depression; caution with history of depression and d/c if it recurs to serious degree. Visual changes or changes in lens tolerance may develop with contact lens use. Use before menarche is not indicated. May affect certain endocrine tests, LFTs, and blood components. Does not protect AIDS and other sexually transmitted disease.

ADVERSE REACTIONS: N/V, breakthrough bleeding, spotting, amenorrhea, migraine, depression, vaginal candidiasis, edema, weight changes.

INTERACTIONS: Reduced contraceptive effectiveness leading to unintended pregnancy or breakthrough bleeding with some anticonvulsants, other drugs that increase the metabolism of contraceptive steroids (eg, barbiturates, rifampin, phenylbutazone, phenytoin, carbamazepine, felbamate, oxcarbazepine, topiramate, griseofulvin). Contraceptive failure and breakthrough bleeding reported with antibiotics such as ampicillin and tetracyclines. Anti-HIV protease inhibitors may increase or decrease levels. Reduced effectiveness with St. John's wort. Atorvastatin, ascorbic acid, acetaminophen, CYP3A4 inhibitors (eg, itraconazole, ketoconazole) may increase hormone levels. Increased plasma concentrations of cyclosporine, prednisolone, and theophylline. Decreased plasma concentrations of APAP and increased clearance of temazepam, salicylic acid, morphine, and clofibric acid.

PREGNANCY: Category X, not for use in nursing.

MECHANISM OF ACTION: Estrogen/progestogen combination oral contraceptive; acts by suppressing gonadotropins. Primarily inhibits ovulation. Also causes changes in cervical mucus (increases difficulty of sperm entry into uterus) and endometrium (reduces likelihood of implantation).

PHARMACOKINETICS: Absorption: Rapid. Norethindrone: Absolute bioavailability (65%), C_{max}=4210.6pg/mL, T_{max}=1.24 hr, AUC=18034.9pg•h/mL. Ethinyl estradiol: Absolute bioavailability (43%), C_{max}=131.4pg/mL, T_{max}=1.44 hrs, AUC=1065.8pg•h/mL. **Distribution:** V_d=2-4L/kg; Norethindone: Sex hormone-binding globulin binding (36%), albumin binding (61%). Ethinyl estradiol: Albumin binding (98.5%). **Metabolism:** Norethindone: Reduction, sulfate, glucuronide conjugation. Ethinyl estradiol: CYP3A4, via oxidation (conjugation with sulfate and glucuronide), 2-hydroxy-ethinyl estradiol (primary oxidative metabolite). **Elimination:** Norethindrone: Urine (>50%), feces (20-40%); $T_{1/2}$=8.6 hrs. Ethinyl Estradiol: Urine, feces; $T_{1/2}$=17.1 hrs.

NURSING CONSIDERATIONS

Assessment: Assess for presence or history of breast cancer, estrogen dependent neoplasia, abnormal genital bleeding, active liver disease, and known/suspected pregnancy or any other conditions where treatment is cautioned or contraindicated. Assess use in patients who are >35 yrs and heavy smokers (≥15 cigarettes/day). Assess use with HTN, hyperlipidemias, obesity, DM, or in patients at increased risk for thrombosis and for possible drug interactions.

Monitoring: Monitor bleeding irregularities, thromboembolic events, onset or exacerbation of headaches or migraines, and ectopic pregnancy. Monitor fasting blood glucose levels in DM and prediabetic patients, BP with history of HTN, lipid levels with a history of hyperlipidemia. Monitor for signs of liver dysfunction (eg, jaundice) and signs of depression with previous history. Refer patients with contact lenses to an ophthalmologist if visual changes occur. Perform annual history and physical exam.

Patient Counseling: Advise about possible serious CV and respiratory effects. Inform that medication does not protect against HIV infection (AIDS) and other STDs. Avoid smoking while on medication. Instruct to take medication at same time each day. Instruct if dose missed, take as soon as possible; take next pill at regularly scheduled time. If patient misses more than one dose, instruct to ask a pharmacist, physician, or refer to PI and to use back up contraception. Inform may have spotting, light bleeding, or stomach upset during first 1-3 packs of pills; advise not to d/c medication and if symptoms persist, notify physician. Vomiting, diarrhea, or concomitant medications may alter efficacy; use backup forms of contraception. Perform regular physical exams.

Administration: Oral route. **Storage:** 25° (77°F); excursions permitted to 15-30°C (59-86°F).

FENTORA

CII

fentanyl citrate (Cephalon)

> Serious adverse events, including deaths, reported. Substitution for any other fentanyl product may result in fatal overdose. Not indicated for opioid non-tolerant patients. Contraindicated in the management of acute or post-operative pain including headache/migraine. Life-threatening respiratory depression may occur in opioid non-tolerant patients. Do not convert on a mcg-per-mcg basis from Actiq to Fentora. Do not substitute for other fentanyl products; may result in fatal overdose. Use special care when dosing. Contains fentanyl with abuse potential similiar to other opioid analgesics. Must be kept out of the reach of children. Use only by healthcare professionals knowledgeable and skilled in the use of Schedule II opioids to treat cancer pain. Concomitant use with strong and moderate P450 3A4 inhibitors may cause potentially fatal respiratory depression.

THERAPEUTIC CLASS: Opioid analgesic

INDICATIONS: Management of breakthrough pain in patients with cancer who are already receiving and tolerant to around-the-clock opioid therapy for their underlying persistent cancer pain.

DOSAGE: *Adults*: Initial: Breakthrough Pain: 100mcg. Max: 2 doses per breakthrough pain episode. Titration Above 100mcg: Use two 100-mcg tabs (one on each side of mouth in the buccal cavity) with next breakthrough pain episode. If unsuccessful, use two 100-mcg tabs on each side of mouth in the buccal cavity (total of four 100-mcg tabs). Titration Above 400mcg: Use 200-mcg increments. Max: Not more than 4 tabs simultaneously. Maint: Once titrated to an effective dose, use only one tab of the appropriate strength per breakthrough pain episode. If breakthrough pain not relieved after 30 min, may take only one additional dose of the same strength. Wait at least 4 hrs before treating another breakthrough pain episode. Re-evaluate maintenance (around the clock) opioid dose if >4 episodes of breakthrough pain per day. Refer to PI for information on conversion of dosing from Actiq to Fentora. Hepatic/Renal impairment/With CYP3A4 Inhibitors: Use lowest possible dose.

HOW SUPPLIED: Tab, Buccal: 100mcg, 200mcg, 300mcg, 400mcg, 600mcg, 800mcg

CONTRAINDICATIONS: Opioid non-tolerant patients and management of acute or postoperative pain including headache/migraine.

WARNINGS/PRECAUTIONS: Caution in patients who have higher risk of substance abuse, including patients with bipolar disorder and/or schizophrenia; monitor for signs of abuse and addiction. Appropriate measures should be taken to limit the incidence of abuse (eg, proper assessment of patient, proper prescribing practices, periodic re-evaluation of therapy, proper dispensing, and storage). May cause physical dependence, which results in withdrawal symptoms when abruptly d/c therapy. May cause respiratory depression; caution with underlying respiratory disorders (eg, COPD), elderly, debilitated patients, patients predisposed to respiratory depression or when using large initial doses in opioid non-tolerant patients. May impair physical or mental abilities. Extreme caution in patients who may be susceptible to the intracranial effects of CO_2 retention (eg, evidence of increased intracranial pressure or impaired consciousness). May obscure clinical course of a head injury. Application-site reactions (eg, paresthesia, ulceration, bleeding) reported. Caution in patients with renal/hepatic impairment, bradyarrhythmias, and those at risk for suicide.

ADVERSE REACTIONS: Application-site reactions (eg, pain, ulcer, irritation), headache, N/V, constipation, dizziness, dyspnea, somnolence, fatigue, anemia, neutropenia, asthenia, abdominal pain, dehydration, peripheral edema, diarrhea.

INTERACTIONS: See Boxed Warning. Respiratory depression may occur more readily when given with other agents that depress respiration. Avoid concomitant use with grapefruit or grapefruit juice. CYP3A4 inducers may produce the opposite effects of CYP3A4 inhibitors. Concomitant use with other CNS depressants, including other opioids, sedatives, hypnotics, general anesthetics, phenothiazines, tranquilizers, skeletal muscle relaxants, sedating antihistamines, potent inhibitors of CYP450 4A isoform (eg, erythromycin,

ketoconazole, certain protease inhibitors), and alcoholic beverages may produce increased depressant effects. Avoid use within 14 days of MAOIs.

PREGNANCY: Category C, not for use in nursing.

MECHANISM OF ACTION: Opioid agonist; produces analgesia. Precise analgesic action not established; known to be μ-opioid receptor agonist. Specific
CNS opioid receptors with opioid-like activity are found throughout the brain
and spinal cord and play a role in producing analgesic effects.

PHARMACOKINETICS: Absorption: Readily absorbed. Absolute bioavailability (65%); (400mcg) C_{max}=1.02ng/mL, T_{max}=46.8 min, AUC_{0-inf}=6.48ng•hr/
mL. **Distribution:** V_d=25.4 L/kg; plasma protein binding (80-85%); found in
breast milk, readily passes across the placenta. **Metabolism:** Liver and intestinal mucosa via CYP3A4; norfentanyl (metabolite). **Elimination:** Urine (<7%
unchanged), feces (1% unchanged); $T_{1/2}$=2.63 hrs (100mcg, healthy subjects),
11.70 hrs (800mcg, healthy subjects).

NURSING CONSIDERATIONS

Assessment: Assess for degree of opioid tolerance, previous opioid dose,
level of pain intensity, type of pain, patient's general condition and medical
status, emotional status or any other conditions where treatment is contraindicated or cautioned. Assess for history of hypersensitivity, pregnancy/nurs-
ing status, renal/hepatic function, and possible drug interactions.

Monitoring: Monitor for signs/symptoms of respiratory depression, abuse,
tolerance, physical dependence, application-site reactions, bradycardia, and
for suicidality.

Patient Counseling: Advise to notify physician if signs/symptoms of respiratory depression develop. Medication must be kept out of reach of children;
may be fatal to child. Do not take for acute pain, postoperative pain, pain
from injuries, headache, migraine or any other short-term pain. Instruct if
not taking an opioid medication on scheduled basis (around the clock), they
should not take fentanyl citrate and to not take more than one tablet per dose
(unless instructed to titrate to achieve a desired dose). Contact physician if
breakthrough pain is not alleviated or worsens. Instruct not to chew, suck,
swallow, or split tablet; immediately place entire tablet in the buccal cavity.
Take exactly as prescribed and do not take more than prescribed. May cause
mental/physical impairment; instruct to use caution during hazardous tasks
(eg, operating machinery/driving). Notify physician if pregnant, planning to
become pregnant or if nursing. Avoid using concomitant therapy with other
CNS depressants including alcohol and avoid abrupt withdrawal. Medication
has potential for abuse. Dispose of unused medication down the toilet. Do not
share medication with anyone else; sharing may result in other individual's
death due to overdose. Counsel on proper administration.

Administration: Oral route. Do not open blister package until ready for
use. Do not attempt to push tablet through blister card. 1) Place tablet in
buccal cavity (above a rear molar, between the upper cheek and gum).
Do not attempt to split tablet. 2) Do not suck, chew or swallow. 3) Leave
tablet between cheek and gum until disintegrated. 4) After 30 min, swallow
remnants with glass of water. Alternate sides of the mouth when administering subsequent doses. **Storage:** 20-25°C (68-77°F); excursions permitted to
15-30°C (59-86°F). Protect from freezing and moisture. Should not be stored
once it has been removed from blister package. Do not use if blister package
has been tampered with. Keep out of reach of children.

FERRLECIT   RX
sodium ferric gluconate complex (Sanofi-Aventis)

THERAPEUTIC CLASS: Hematinic

INDICATIONS: Treatment of iron deficiency anemia in patients ≥6 yrs undergoing chronic hemodialysis and receiving supplemental epoetin therapy.

DOSAGE: *Adults:* 10mL (125mg) diluted in 100mL of 0.9% NaCl IV infusion over 1 hr or undiluted at a rate of up to 12.5mg/min. Most patients will

require a minimum cumulative dose of 1g of elemental iron administered over 8 sessions at sequential dialysis sessions to achieve a favorable Hgb or Hct response. Elderly: Start at the low end of dosing range.

Pediatrics: ≥6 yrs: 0.12mL/kg (1.5mg/kg) diluted in 25mL 0.9% NaCl IV infusion over 1 hr at 8 sequential dialysis sessions. Max: 125mg/dose.

HOW SUPPLIED: Inj: 62.5mg elemental iron/5mL

CONTRAINDICATIONS: Anemia not associated with iron deficiency. Evidence of iron overload.

WARNINGS/PRECAUTIONS: Hypersensitivity reactions and hypotension reported. Iron overload is more common in patients with hemoglobinopathies and other refractory anemias; avoid in patients with iron overload. May cause hypotension; usually resolved with 1 to 2 hrs. Contains benzyl alcohol; avoid in neonates. Do not mix with other medications or add parenteral nutritional solutions for IV infusion. Caution in elderly.

ADVERSE REACTIONS: Injection-site reactions, chest pain, pain, asthenia, headache, abdominal pain, cramps, dizziness, dyspnea, hypotension, HTN, N/V, diarrhea, pruritus, abnormal erythrocytes.

INTERACTIONS: May reduce absorption of concomitantly administered oral iron. Concomitant use with ACE inhibitors may increase the incidence of drug intolerance and suspected allergic events.

PREGNANCY: Category B, caution in nursing.

MECHANISM OF ACTION: Hematinic; used to replete the total body content of iron, which is critical for normal Hgb synthesis to maintain oxygen transport.

PHARMACOKINETICS: Absorption: Adults: Parameters varied by different dosage. (62.5mg) AUC=17.5mg-h/L; (125mg) C_{max}=19mg/L; T_{max}=7 min; AUC=35.6mg-h/L. **Pediatrics:** (1.5mg/kg) C_{max}=12.9mg/L; AUC=95mg•h/L. (3mg/kg) C_{max}=22.8mg/L; AUC=170.9mg•h/L. **Distribution:** V_d=6L. **Elimination: Adults:** $T_{1/2}$=1 hr. **Pediatrics:** (1.5mg/kg) $T_{1/2}$=2 hrs; (3mg/kg) $T_{1/2}$=2.5 hrs.

NURSING CONSIDERATIONS

Assessment: Assess for evidence of iron overload, type of anemia, hypersensity, pregnancy/nursing status, and for possible drug interactions.

Monitoring: Monitor for signs/symptoms of hypersensitivity reactions, iatrogenic hemosiderosis, and hypotension.

Patient Counseling: Advise to seek medical attention if symptoms of a hypersensitivity reaction, hypotension (light-headedness, malaise, fatigue, weakness), or if hemosiderosis occur.

Administration: IV route. Do not mix with other medications or add to parenteral nutrition solutions. If diluted in saline, use immediately after dilution. **Storage:** 20-25°C (68-77°F); excursions permitted to 15-30° (59-86°F). Do not freeze.

FIBRICOR   RX
fenofibric acid (AR Scientific)

THERAPEUTIC CLASS: Fibric acid derivative

INDICATIONS: Adjunctive therapy to diet for treatment of severe hypertriglyceridemia (≥500mg/dL). Adjunctive therapy to diet to reduce elevated LDL-C, Total-C, TG, and Apo B, and to increase HDL-C in patients with primary hypercholesterolemia or mixed dyslipidemia.

DOSAGE: *Adults:* Severe Hypertriglyceridemia: Individualize dose. Initial: 35-105mg/day. Titrate: May adjust dose if necessary following repeat lipid determinations at 4-8 week intervals. Max: 105mg/day. Primary Hyperlipidemia or Mixed Dyslipidemia: 105mg/day. Max: 105mg/day. Mild-to-Moderate Renal Impairment: Initial: 35mg/day. Titrate: May increase dose after evaluation of effects on renal function and lipid levels. Elderly: Base dose selection on renal function. Monitor serum lipids periodically during initiation to establish lowest effective dose. Reduce dose if lipid levels significantly falls below target range. D/C if no adequate response after 2 months of treatment at max dose.

HOW SUPPLIED: Tab: 35mg, 105mg

CONTRAINDICATIONS: Severe renal impairment (including dialysis), active liver disease (including primary biliary cirrhosis and unexplained persistent liver function abnormalities), pre-existing gallbladder disease, and nursing mothers.

WARNINGS/PRECAUTIONS: May cause increases in serum transaminases (eg, AST, ALT); chronic active hepatocellular and cholestatic hepatitis reported; monitor LFTs, and d/c therapy if enzyme levels >3X ULN. May cause cholelithiasis; d/c if gallstones found. Increased risk of myopathy and associated rhabdomyolysis in elderly, diabetes, renal failure, or hypothyroidism; d/c therapy if myopathy or marked CPK elevation occurs. Elevation of serum creatinine reported; monitor renal function in patients with renal impairment and those at risk for renal insuffiency (eg, elderly, diabetes). Acute hypersensitivity reactions (including Stevens-Johnson syndrome [SJS], toxic epidermal necrolysis [TEN]) and pancreatitis reported. Decreased Hgb, Hct, WBCs, thrombocytopenia, and agranulocytosis reported. Pulmonary embolus (PE) and deep vein thrombosis (DVT) observed. Caution in elderly. Ascertain lipid abnormality before therapy. Place patients on lipid-lowering diet prior to and during therapy.

ADVERSE REACTIONS: Abdominal pain, back pain, headache, abnormal liver tests, increased ALT, increased creatinine phosphokinase, increased AST, respiratory disorder.

INTERACTIONS: May potentiate anticoagulant effects of coumarin anticoagulants; monitor PT/INR. Bile acid binding resins may bind other drugs given concurrently; take at least 1 hr before or 4-6 hrs after the resin. May impair renal function with immunosuppressants (eg, cyclosporine, tacrolimus) and other potentially nephrotoxic agents; use lowest effective dose and monitor renal function. Increased risk of rhabdomyolysis with HMG-CoA reductase inhibitors (statins). May decrease levels with atorvastatin, pravastatin, fluvastatin, simvastatin, glimepiride, metformin. May increase levels with ezetimibe and rosiglitazone. May decrease levels of atorvastatin, simvastatin, rosiglitazone, efavirenz. May increase levels of pravastatin, fluvastatin, ezetimibe, glimepiride, metformin. D/C medications known to exacerbate hypertriglyceridemia (β-blockers, estrogens, thiazides) prior to therapy.

PREGNANCY: Category C, not for use in nursing.

MECHANISM OF ACTION: Fibric acid derivative; activates peroxisome proliferator activated receptor α (PPARα). This causes an increase in lipolysis and elimination of triglyceride-rich particles from plasma by activating lipoprotein lipase and reducing production of apoprotein C-III (an inhibitor of lipoprotein lipase activity). Activation of PPARα also induces an increase in the synthesis of apoproteins A-I, A-II, and HDL cholesterol.

PHARMACOKINETICS: Absorption: T_{max}=2.5 hrs. **Distribution:** Plasma protein binding (99%). **Metabolism:** Conjugation with glucuronic acid. **Elimination:** Urine; $T_{1/2}$=20 hrs.

NURSING CONSIDERATIONS

Assessment: Assess for severe renal impairment, active liver disease (eg, primary biliary cirrhosis, unexplained liver function abnormality), diabetes, hypothyroidism, pre-existing gallbladder disease, pregnancy/nursing status, and possible drug interactions. Obtain baseline LFTs (including ALT/AST), renal function, and lipid levels.

Monitoring: Monitor for signs/symptoms of active liver disease, cholelithiasis, pancreatitis, hypersensitivity reactions (eg, SJS, TEN), hematological changes (eg, agranulocytosis, thrombocytopenia), PE, DVT, myopathies, rhabdomyolysis, PE, DVT. Perform periodic monitoring of liver function (including ALT/AST) and blood counts. Perform periodic monitoring of serum lipid levels. If myopathy suspected, obtain CPK levels.

Patient Counseling: Inform of the potential benefits and risks of the drug and medications that should not be taken in combination with the drug. Instruct that it may be taken once daily, with/without food, at the prescribed dose.

Recommend to continue/follow an appropriate lipid-modifying diet during therapy. Instruct to notify physician of all medications, supplements, and herbal preparations taken and any changes in medical conditions. Instruct to notify physician of any muscle pain, tenderness, or weakness, onset of abdominal pain or if any other new symptoms develop.

Administration: Oral route. **Storage:** 20-25°C (68-77°F).

FIORICET RX
acetaminophen - caffeine - butalbital (Watson)

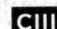

THERAPEUTIC CLASS: Barbiturate/analgesic

INDICATIONS: Tension or muscle contraction headaches.

DOSAGE: *Adults:* 1-2 tabs q4h prn. Max: 6 tabs/day. Not for extended use. *Pediatrics:* ≥12 yrs: 1-2 tabs q4h prn. Max: 6 tabs/day. Not for extended use.

HOW SUPPLIED: Tab: (Butalbital-APAP-Caffeine) 50mg-325mg-40mg

CONTRAINDICATIONS: Porphyria.

WARNINGS/PRECAUTIONS: May be habit-forming. Not for long-term use. Caution in elderly, debilitated, severe renal or hepatic impairment, acute abdominal conditions. Caution in mentally depressed and those with suicidal tendencies, history of drug abuse.

ADVERSE REACTIONS: Drowsiness, lightheadedness, dizziness, sedation, SOB, N/V, abdominal pain, intoxicated feeling.

INTERACTIONS: Enhanced CNS effects with MAOIs. May enhance CNS depressant effects of other narcotic analgesics, alcohol, general anesthetics, tranquilizers, sedative hypnotics, or other CNS depressants.

PREGNANCY: Category C, not for use in nursing.

MECHANISM OF ACTION: Butalbital: Short- to intermediate-acting barbiturate. APAP: Nonopiate, nonsalicylate analgesic, antipyretic. Caffeine: CNS stimulant.

PHARMACOKINETICS: Absorption: Well absorbed (butalbital), rapid (APAP, caffeine). **Distribution:** Butalbital: Plasma protein binding (45%); found in breast milk; crosses placenta. Caffeine: Found in CNS, placenta, and breast milk. **Metabolism:** APAP: Liver (conjugation). Caffeine: Hepatic; 1-methylxanthine, 1-methyluric acid. **Elimination:** Butalbital: Urine (59-88% unchanged or metabolite); $T_{1/2}$=35 hrs. APAP: Urine (85% metabolite, unchanged); $T_{1/2}$=1.25-3 hrs. Caffeine: Urine 70% (3% unchanged); $T_{1/2}$=3 hrs.

NURSING CONSIDERATIONS

Assessment: Assess for porphyria, elderly/debilitated patients, renal/hepatic impairment, acute abdominal condition, alcohol intake, and possible drug interactions (eg, MAOIs).

Monitoring: Monitor for drug abuse/dependence. Monitor LFTs , renal function, false (+) test for urinary 5-hydroxyindoleacetic acid.

Patient Counseling: Advise to use caution during hazardous tasks (eg, operating machinery/driving). Instruct not to take with alcohol/other CNS depressants. Advise to take as directed. Inform drug may be habit-forming. Instruct to notify physician if pregnant/nursing.

Administration: Oral route. **Storage:** 30°C (86°F); tight container.

FIORICET WITH CODEINE CIII
codeine phosphate - acetaminophen - caffeine - butalbital (Watson)

THERAPEUTIC CLASS: Barbiturate/analgesic

INDICATIONS: Tension or muscle contraction headaches.

DOSAGE: *Adults:* 1-2 caps q4h prn. Max: 6 caps/day. Not for extended use.

HOW SUPPLIED: Cap: (Butalbital-APAP-Caffeine-Codeine) 50mg-325mg-40mg-30mg

CONTRAINDICATIONS: Porphyria.

WARNINGS/PRECAUTIONS: May be habit-forming. Not for extended use. Respiratory depression and CSF pressure enhanced with head injury or intracranial lesions. Caution in elderly, debilitated, severe renal or hepatic impairment, hypothyroidism, urethral stricture, Addison's disease, BPH, and history of drug abuse. May mask signs of acute abdominal conditions.

ADVERSE REACTIONS: Drowsiness, lightheadedness, dizziness, sedation, SOB, N/V, abdominal pain, intoxicated feeling.

INTERACTIONS: Enhanced CNS effects with MAOIs. May enhance CNS depressant effects of other narcotic analgesics, alcohol, general anesthetics, tranquilizers, sedative hypnotics, or other CNS depressants.

PREGNANCY: Category C, not for use in nursing.

MECHANISM OF ACTION: Codeine: Narcotic analgesic and antitussive. Butalbital: Short- to intermediate-acting barbiturate. Caffeine: CNS stimulant. APAP: Nonopiate, nonsalicylate analgesic and antipyretic. The role each component plays in relief of complex of symptoms, known as tension headache, is incompletely understood.

PHARMACOKINETICS: Absorption: Butalbital: Well absorbed. Codeine, caffeine, acetaminophen: Rapid. **Distribution:** Codeine: Crosses blood-brain barrier, found in fetal tissue, breast milk. Butalbital: Plasma protein binding (45%); found in breast milk; crosses placental barrier. Caffeine: Found in fetal tissue, CNS, breast milk. **Metabolism:** Caffeine: Hepatic biotransformation to 1-methylxanthine, 1-methyluric acid. APAP: Liver (conjugation). **Elimination:** Codeine: Urine (90%), feces; $T_{1/2}$=2.9 hrs. Butalbital: Urine (59-88% unchanged or metabolites); $T_{1/2}$=35 hrs. Caffeine: Urine (70%, only 3% unchanged); $T_{1/2}$=3 hrs. APAP: Urine (85% unchanged, conjugates); $T_{1/2}$=1.25-3 hrs.

NURSING CONSIDERATIONS

Assessment: Assess for severity of headache, previous hypersensitivity to drug, renal/hepatic fucntion, or any other conditions where treatment is cautioned or contraindicated. Assess for pregnancy/nursing status, for possible drug interactions, and alcohol intake.

Monitoring: Serial monitoring of LFTs, renal function, improvement in symptoms. Monitor serum amylase levels, false (+) test results for urinary 5-hydroxyindoleacetic acid, drug abuse/dependence, CSF, and signs of CNS depression (eg, drowsiness, confusion, or shallow breathing).

Patient Counseling: Advise to use caution during hazardous tasks (eg, driving/operating machinery). Instruct not to take with other CNS depressants or alcohol. Advise to take as prescribed. Notify physician if pregnant/nursing or planning to become pregnant. Counsel that drug may be habit-forming.

Administration: Oral route. **Storage:** 30°C (86°F); tight container.

FIORINAL   CIII
caffeine - aspirin - butalbital (Watson)

THERAPEUTIC CLASS: Barbiturate/analgesic

INDICATIONS: Tension or muscle contraction headache.

DOSAGE: *Adults:* 1-2 caps q4h prn. Max: 6 caps/day. Not for extended use.

HOW SUPPLIED: Cap: (Butalbital-ASA-Caffeine) 50mg-325mg-40mg

CONTRAINDICATIONS: Porphyria, peptic ulcer disease, serious GI lesions, hemorrhagic diathesis. Syndrome of nasal polyps, angioedema, and bronchospastic reactivity to ASA or NSAIDs.

WARNINGS/PRECAUTIONS: May be habit-forming. Not for extended use. Caution in elderly, debilitated, severe renal or hepatic impairment, hypothyroidism, urethral stricture, head injuries, elevated ICP, acute abdominal conditions, Addison's disease, prostatic hypertrophy, peptic ulcer, coagulation disorders. Avoid with ASA allergy. Risk of ASA hypersensitivity with nasal polyps and asthma. Caution in children with chickenpox or flu. Preoperative ASA may prolong bleeding time.

ADVERSE REACTIONS: Drowsiness, lightheadedness, dizziness, sedation, N/V, flatulence.

INTERACTIONS: CNS effects enhanced by MAOIs. Additive CNS depression with alcohol, other narcotic analgesics, general anesthetics, tranquilizers (eg, chloral hydrate), sedatives/hypnotics, other CNS depressants. May enhance effects of anticoagulants. May cause hypoglycemia with oral antidiabetic agents and insulin. May cause bone marrow toxicity and blood dyscrasias with 6-MP and methotrexate. Increased risk of peptic ulceration and bleeding with NSAIDs. Decreased effects of uricosuric agents (eg, probenecid, sulfinpyrazone). Withdrawal of corticosteroids may cause salicylism with chronic ASA use.

PREGNANCY: Category C, not for use in nursing.

MECHANISM OF ACTION: Combines analgesic properties of ASA with anxiolytic and muscle relaxant properties of butalbital.

PHARMACOKINETICS: Absorption: ASA: T_{max}=40 min, C_{max}=8.8mcg/mL. Butalbital: Well-absorbed; C_{max}=202ng/mL, T_{max}=1.5 hrs. Caffeine: Rapid; C_{max}=1660ng/mL, T_{max} ≤1 hr. **Distribution:** ASA: Found in fetal tissue, breast milk, CNS; Plasma protein binding (50-80%). Butalbital: Crosses placenta, found in breast milk; Plasma protein binding (45%). Caffeine: Found in placenta, breast milk, CNS. **Metabolism:** ASA: Liver; salicyluric acid, phenolic/acyl glucuronides of salicylate, and gentisic and gentisuric acid (major metabolites). Caffeine: Liver; 1-methylxanthine and 1-methyluric acid (metabolites). **Elimination:** ASA: Urine; $T_{1/2}$=12 min (ASA), 3 hrs (salicylic acid/total salicylates). Butalbital: Urine (59-88%); $T_{1/2}$=35 hrs. Caffeine: Urine 70% (3% unchanged); $T_{1/2}$=3 hrs.

NURSING CONSIDERATIONS

Assessment: Assess for severity of headache, previous hypersensitivity to drug, renal/hepatic fucntion, or any other conditions where treatment is cautioned or contraindicated. Assess for pregnancy/nursing status and for possible drug interactions.

Monitoring: Serial monitoring of LFTs and renal function. Monitor for anaphylactoid reactions, drug abuse/dependence, bleeding, prolongation of bleeding time, PT, urinary (glucose, 5-hydroxyindoleactic acid, Gerhardt ketone, VMA, uric acid, diacetic acid, spectrophotometric detection of barbiturates), Reye's syndrome, serum amylase, FBG, cholesterol, protein, and uric acid.

Patient Counseling: Advise not to take with ASA allergy. Instruct to take exactly as prescribed; do not take with alcohol or other CNS depressants. Advise to use caution during hazardous tasks (eg, operating machinery/driving). Counsel that drug may be habit-forming. Advise to notify physician if pregnant, nursing, or planning to become pregnant.

Administration: Oral route. **Storage:** 77°F (25°C); tight container.

FIORINAL WITH CODEINE   `CIII`
codeine phosphate - caffeine - aspirin - butalbital (Watson)

OTHER BRAND NAMES: Ascomp with Codeine (Breckenridge)

THERAPEUTIC CLASS: Barbiturate/analgesic

INDICATIONS: Relief of the symptom complex of tension or muscle contraction headache.

DOSAGE: *Adults:* 1-2 caps q4h prn. Max: 6 caps/day. Not for extended use. Elderly: Start at low end of dosing range.

HOW SUPPLIED: Cap: (Butalbital-ASA-Caffeine-Codeine) 50mg-325mg-40mg-30mg

CONTRAINDICATIONS: Porphyria, peptic ulcer disease, serious GI lesions, hemorrhagic diathesis (eg, hemophilia, hypoprothrombinemia, von Willbrand's disease, thrombocytopenias, thromboasthenia and other ill-defined hereditary platelet dysfunctions, severe vitamin K deficiency and severe liver damage). Syndrome of nasal polyps, angioedema and bronchospastic reactivity to ASA or NSAIDs.

WARNINGS/PRECAUTIONS: May cause anaphylactic shock and other severe allergic reactions. Caution with peptic ulcer, GI lesions and bleeding disorders; significant bleeding may result. Aspirin administered pre-operatively may prolong bleeding time. May be habit-forming and potentially abusable. Not for extended use. Respiratory depression and CSF pressure may be enhanced with head injury or intracranial lesions. Caution in elderly, debilitated, severe renal or hepatic impairment, hypothyroidism, urethral stricture, elevated ICP, acute abdominal conditions, Addison's disease, prostatic hypertrophy. Caution in children with chickenpox or flu. Avoid with ASA allergy. Risk of ASA hypersensitivity with nasal polyps and asthma. Ultra-rapid metabolizers may experience overdose symptoms (eg, extreme sleepiness, confusion, or shallow breathing). May impair physical/mental ability.

ADVERSE REACTIONS: Drowsiness, lightheadedness, dizziness, sedation, SOB, N/V, abdominal pain, intoxicated feeling.

INTERACTIONS: CNS effects enhanced by MAOIs. Additive CNS depression with alcohol, other narcotic analgesics, general anesthetics, tranquilizers (eg, chlordiazepoxide), sedatives/hypnotics, other CNS depressants. May enhance effects of anticoagulants. May cause hypoglycemia with oral antidiabetic agents, insulin. May cause bone marrow toxicity, blood dyscrasias with 6-MP and methotrexate. Increased risk of peptic ulceration, bleeding with NSAIDs. Decreased effects of uricosuric agents (eg, probenecid, sulfinpyrazone). Withdrawal of corticosteroids may cause salicylism with chronic ASA use.

PREGNANCY: Category C, not for use in nursing.

MECHANISM OF ACTION: Butalbital: Short to intermediate acting barbiturate. ASA: Analgesic, antipyretic, and anti-inflammatory. Caffeine: Stimulates CNS. Codeine: Narcotic analgesic and antitussive. Role each component plays in relief of complex of symptoms known as tension headache is incompletely understood.

PHARMACOKINETICS: Absorption: ASA: C_{max}=8.8mcg/mL, T_{max}=40 mins; Codeine: Readily absorbed; C_{max}=198ng/mL, T_{max}=1 hr. Butalbital: Well-absorbed; C_{max}=2020ng/mL, T_{max}=1.5 hrs. Caffeine: Rapid; C_{max}=1660ng/mL, T_{max}<1 hr. **Distribution:** ASA: Plasma protein binding (50-80%); found in breast milk. Codeine: Found in breast milk. Butalbital: Plasma protein binding (45%); crosses placenta; found in breast milk. Caffeine: Found in breast milk. **Metabolism:** ASA: Liver; salicyluric acid, phenolic/acyl glucuronides of salicylate, and gentisic and gentisuric acid (major metabolites). Codeine: Glucuronidation. Caffeine: Liver; 1-methylxanthine and 1-methyluric acid. **Elimination:** ASA: Urine; $T_{1/2}$=12 min (ASA), 3 hrs (salicylic acid/total salicylate). Codeine: Urine (90%), feces; $T_{1/2}$=2.9 hrs. Butalbital: Urine (59-88%); $T_{1/2}$=35 hrs. Caffeine: Urine 70% (3% unchanged); $T_{1/2}$=3 hrs.

NURSING CONSIDERATIONS

Assessment: Assess for severity of headache, previous hypersensitivity to drug, renal/hepatic fucntion, or any other conditions where treatment is cautioned or contraindicated. Assess for pregnancy/nursing status, history of drug abuse, and for possible drug interactions.

Monitoring: Serial monitoring of LFTs, renal function tests. Monitor for anaphylactoid reactions, symptoms of CNS depression (eg, drowsiness, confusion, shallow breathing), drug abuse/dependence, bleeding, prolonged bleeding time, PT, urinary (glucose, 5-hydroxyindoleactic acid, Gerhardt ketone, VMA, uric acid, diacetic acid, spectrophotometric detection of barbiturates), Reye's syndrome, serum amylase, FBG, cholesterol, SGOT, protein, and uric acid. Monitor mother-infant pairs and notify doctor about the use of codeine during breastfeeding.

Patient Counseling: Advise not to take if patient has aspirin allergy. Take as prescribed; do not take with alcohol or other CNS depressants. Caution during hazardous tasks (eg, operating machinery/driving). Potential psychological dependence and abuse. Notify if pregnant/nursing or planning to become pregnant. Inform about risks/benefits and to report any adverse reactions to physician.

Administration: Oral route. **Storage:** <25°C (77°F); tight container. Protect form moisture.

FLAGYL

metronidazole (G.D. Searle)

> Shown to be carcinogenic in mice and rats. Avoid unnecessary use. Use should be reserved for conditions for which it is indicated.

THERAPEUTIC CLASS: Nitroimidazole

INDICATIONS: Treatment of symptomatic/asymptomatic trichomoniasis, asymptomatic consorts, acute intestinal amebiasis, amebic liver abscess, and anaerobic bacterial infections (following IV metronidazole therapy for serious infections) caused by susceptible strains of microorganisms. Treatment of intra-abdominal, skin and skin structure, bone/joint, CNS, lower respiratory tract, and gynecologic infections, bacterial septicemia, and endocarditis caused by susceptible strains of microorganisms.

DOSAGE: *Adults:* Trichomoniasis (Female/Male): Individualize dose. Seven-Day Treatment: (Cap) 375mg bid or (Tab) 250mg tid for 7 days. One-Day Treatment: (Tab) 2g as single dose or in two divided doses of 1g each given in the same day. If repeat course needed, reconfirm diagnosis and allow 4-6 weeks between courses. Acute Intestinal Amebiasis: 750mg tid for 5-10 days. Amebic Liver Abscess: (Tab) 500mg or (Cap, Tab) 750mg tid for 5-10 days. Anaerobic Bacterial Infection: Usually IV therapy administered initially if serious. Usual: 7.5mg/kg q6h for 7-10 days or longer. Approximately 500mg for a 70-kg adult. Max: 4g/24 hrs. Elderly: Adjust dose based on serum levels. Severe Hepatic Disease: Give lower dose cautiously; monitor levels for toxicity. *Pediatrics:* Amebiasis: 35-50mg/kg/24 hrs in 3 divided doses for 10 days.

HOW SUPPLIED: Cap: 375mg; Tab: 250mg, 500mg

CONTRAINDICATIONS: 1st trimester of pregnancy in patients with trichomoniasis.

WARNINGS/PRECAUTIONS: Convulsive seizures, encephalopathy, aseptic meningitis, optic and peripheral neuropathy; d/c if abnormal neurological signs occur. Caution with Crohn's disease, severe hepatic disease, evidence or history of blood dyscrasias, CNS disease, and with the elderly. Mild leukopenia reported; monitor total and differential leukocyte counts before and after treatment for trichomoniasis and amebiasis. Use in the absence of proven or strongly suspected bacterial infection or prophylactic indication is unlikely to provide benefit and increases the risk of drug-resistant bacteria. Candidiasis may present with more prominent symptoms; treat with candidacidal agents. May interfere with serum chemistry values (eg, AST, ALT, LDH, triglycerides, hexokinase glucose).

ADVERSE REACTIONS: Convulsive seizures, encephalopathy, aseptic meningitis, optic and peripheral neuropathy, N/V, headache, anorexia, unpleasant metallic taste, reversible neutropenia.

INTERACTIONS: Avoid alcohol during and for at least 1 day (Tab) or 3 days (Cap) afterward. Should not be given within 2 weeks of disulfiram; psychotic reactions reported in alcoholic patients who are concurrently using disulfiram. May potentiate anticoagulant effects of warfarin and other oral coumarin anticoagulants; monitor PT. Increased elimination with microsomal liver enzyme inducers (eg, phenytoin, phenobarbital). May impair phenytoin clearance. Half-life increased and clearance decreased by microsomal liver enzyme inhibitors (eg, cimetidine). May increase serum lithium levels.

PREGNANCY: Category B, not for use in nursing.

MECHANISM OF ACTION: Antibacterial and antiprotozoal nitroimidazole; exerts effect in anaerobic environment. Possesses bactericidal, amoebicidal, and trichomonacidal activity.

PHARMACOKINETICS: Absorption: Well absorbed. (Tab) T_{max}=1-2 hrs, C_{max}=(250mg) 6mcg/mL, (500mg) 12mcg/mL, (2000mg) 40mcg/mL. (750mg, Cap) C_{max}=21.4mcg/mL, T_{max}=1.6 hrs, AUC=223mcg•hr/mL. **Distribution:** Plasma protein binding (<20%); found in breast milk; crosses the placenta. **Metabolism:** Liver, via side-chain oxidation and glucuronide conjugation; 1-(β-hydroxyethyl)-2-hydroxymethyl-5-nitroimidazole and 2-methyl-5-nitroimidazole-1-yl-acetic acid (metabolites). **Elimination:** Urine (60-80%), feces (6-15%); $T_{1/2}$=8 hrs.

NURSING CONSIDERATIONS

Assessment: Assess for hepatic impairment, alcohol use, evidence/history of blood dyscrasias, CNS disease, candidiasis infections, Crohn's disease, pregnancy/nursing status, and for possible drug interactions. Obtain LFTs, and total and differential leukocyte count.

Monitoring: Monitor for symptoms of alcohol use (eg, abdominal distress, N/V, flushing, headache), neurologic symptoms (eg, convulsive seizures, encephalopathy, aseptic meningitis, optic and peripheral neuropathy), candidiasis infections, leukopenia and hypersensitivity reactions. Monitor LFTs, and total and differential leukocyte counts.

Patient Counseling: Instruct to avoid alcohol during and for at least 1 day (Tab) or 3 days (Cap) after therapy. Inform that drug treats bacterial, not viral infections. Instruct to take exactly as directed; inform that skipping doses or not completing full course may decrease effectiveness and increase resistance.

Administration: Oral route. **Storage:** Cap: 15-25°C (59-77°F). Dispense in well-closed container with child-resistant closure. Tab: Below 25°C (77°F). Protect from light.

FLAGYL ER   RX
metronidazole (G.D. Searle)

> Shown to be carcinogenic in mice and rats. Avoid unnecessary use. Use should be reserved for treatment of women with bacterial vaginosis (BV).

THERAPEUTIC CLASS: Nitroimidazole

INDICATIONS: Treatment of bacterial vaginosis.

DOSAGE: *Adults:* 750mg qd for 7 days. Take ≥1 hr before or ≥2 hrs after meals. Severe Hepatic Disease: Give lower dose cautiously; monitor levels. Elderly: Adjust dose based on serum levels.

HOW SUPPLIED: Tab, Extended-Release: 750mg

CONTRAINDICATIONS: Treatment during 1st trimester of pregnancy.

WARNINGS/PRECAUTIONS: Convulsive seizures, encephalopathy, aseptic meningitis, optic and peripheral neuropathy reported; d/c if abnormal neurological signs occur. Caution with Crohn's disease, severe hepatic disease, evidence or history of blood dyscrasias, CNS diseases, and with the elderly. Mild leukopenia reported; monitor total and differential leukocyte counts before and after re-treatment. Use in the absence of proven or strongly suspected bacterial infection or prophylactic indication is unlikely to provide benefit and increases the risk of drug-resistant bacteria. May interfere with serum chemistry values (eg, AST, ALT, LDH, triglycerides, hexokinase glucose). Candidiasis may present with more prominent symptoms and require treatment with a candidacidal agent.

ADVERSE REACTIONS: Headache, vaginitis, nausea, metallic taste, bacterial infection, influenza-like symptoms, genital pruritus, abdominal pain, dizziness, diarrhea, upper respiratory tract infection, rhinitis, sinusitis, pharyngitis, dysmenorrhea.

INTERACTIONS: Avoid alcohol during and for at least 3 days afterward. Should not be given within 2 weeks of disulfiram; psychotic reactions reported in alcoholic patients who are concurrently using disulfiram. Potentiates anticoagulant effects of warfarin and other oral coumarin anticoagulants; monitor PT. Increased elimination with microsomal liver enzyme inducers (eg, phenytoin, phenobarbital). May impair phenytoin clearance. Decreased elimination with microsomal liver enzyme inhibitors (eg, cimetidine). May increase lithium levels.

PREGNANCY: Category B, not for use in nursing.

MECHANISM OF ACTION: Antibacterial and antiprotozoal nitroimidazole; exerts effect in anaerobic environment. Upon entering the organism, drug is reduced by intracellular electron transport proteins. Because of this alteration, a concentration gradient is maintained which promotes the drug 's intracellular transport. Presumably, free radicals are formed which, in turn, react with cellular components resulting in death of the microorganism.

PHARMACOKINETICS: **Absorption:** C_{max}=19.4µg/mL (fed), 12.5µg/mL (fasting); T_{max}=4.6 hrs (fed), 6.8 hrs (fasting); AUC=211µg•hr/mL (fed), 198µg•hr/mL (fasting). **Distribution:** Found in breast milk; crosses the placental barrier. **Metabolism:** Liver, via side-chain oxidation and glucuronide conjugation; 1-(β-hydroxyethyl)-2-hydroxymethyl-5-nitroimidazole and 2-methyl-5-nitroimidazole-1-yl-acetic acid (metabolites). **Elimination:** Urine (60-80%), feces (6-15%); $T_{1/2}$=8 hrs.

NURSING CONSIDERATIONS

Assessment: Assess for hepatic impairment, alcohol use, evidence/history of blood dyscrasias, CNS diseases, candidiasis infections, Crohn's disease, pregnancy/nursing status, and for possible drug interactions. Obtain LFTs and total and differential leukocyte count.

Monitoring: Monitor for convulsive seizures, encephalopathy, aseptic meningitis, optic and peripheral neuropathy, candidiasis infections, and leukopenia. Monitor LFTs, and total/differential leukocyte counts.

Patient Counseling: Instruct to avoid alcohol during therapy and for at least 3 days afterward. Inform that drug only treats bacterial, not viral infections. Counsel to take exactly as directed; inform that skipping doses or not completing full course may decrease effectiveness and increase resistance.

Administration: Oral route. **Storage:** 25°C (77°F); excursions permitted to 15-30°C (59-86°F). Store in a dry place. Dispense in a well-closed container with a child-resistant closure.

FLAGYL IV

RX

metronidazole (Baxter)

> Shown to be carcinogenic in mice and rats. Use should be reserved only for conditions for which it is indicated.

THERAPEUTIC CLASS: Nitroimidazole

INDICATIONS: Treatment of serious infections caused by susceptible anaerobic bacteria. Treatment of intra-abdominal, skin and skin structure, gynecologic, bone and joint, CNS, and lower respiratory tract infections caused by susceptible microorganisms; also treatment of bacterial septicemia and endocarditis caused by susceptible microorganisms. Prophylaxis of postoperative infection in contaminated or potentially contaminated colorectal surgery. Effective against *B. fragilis* infections resistant to clindamycin, chloramphenicol, and PCN.

DOSAGE: *Adults:* Anaerobic Infections: LD: 15mg/kg IV (infused over 1 hr). Maint: 7.5mg/kg IV (infused over 1 hr) q6h, starting 6 hrs after LD. Usual duration: 7-10 days, or longer. Max: 4g/24 hrs. Surgical Prophylaxis: 15mg/kg IV (infused over 30-60 min) given 1 hr before surgery, then 7.5mg/kg IV (infused over 30-60 min) given 6 hrs and 12 hrs after initial dose. Whole of initial infusion must be completed, approximately 1 hr before surgery.

HOW SUPPLIED: Inj: 500mg [100mL]

WARNINGS/PRECAUTIONS: Encephalopathy (associated with cerebellar toxicity and CNS lesions on MRI), peripheral neuropathy, convulsive seizures, aseptic meningitis reported; evaluate benefit/risk ratio of therapy if abnormal neurologic signs/symptoms occur. Caution with severe hepatic impairment, presence or history of blood dyscrasias, and in patients predisposed to edema. Sodium retention may occur due to Na⁺ in solution. Monitor leukocytes before and after therapy. Candidiasis may present with more prominent symptoms; treat with candicidal agents. May interfere with serum chemistry values (eg, AST, ALT, LDH, triglycerides, hexokinase glucose). Do not use in absence of proven or strongly suspected infection due to susceptible organisms.

ADVERSE REACTIONS: Convulsive seizures, encephalopathy, aseptic meningitis, optic neuropathy, peripheral neuropathy (characterized by numbness/paresthesia of an extremity), N/V, diarrhea, leukopenia, erythematous rash, pruritus, fever, headache, syncope, Stevens-Johnson syndrome, thrombophlebitis.

INTERACTIONS: Avoid alcoholic beverages during therapy. Avoid within 2 weeks of disulfiram; increased possibility of psychotic reactions. Potentiates warfarin and other oral coumarin anticoagulants. Increased elimination with microsomal liver enzyme inducers (eg, phenytoin, phenobarbital). May impair phenytoin clearance. May prolong the half-life and decrease plasma clearance with microsomal liver enzyme inhibitors (eg, cimetidine). Caution with corticosteroids.

PREGNANCY: Category B, not for use in nursing.

MECHANISM OF ACTION: Nitroimidazole antibacterial; exerts effect in anaerobic environment. Possess bactericidal, amebicidal, and trichomonacidal activity.

PHARMACOKINETICS: Distribution: Plasma protein binding (<20%); found in CSF, saliva and breast milk. **Metabolism:** Liver, via side-chain oxidation and glucuronide conjugation; 1-(β-hydroxyethyl)-2-hydroxymethyl-5-nitroimidazole and 2-methyl-5-nitroimidazole-1-yl-acetic acid (metabolites). **Elimination:** Urine (60-80%), feces (6-15%); $T_{1/2}$=8 hrs.

NURSING CONSIDERATIONS

Assessment: Assess for evidence or history of a blood dyscrasia, hepatic impairment, predisposition to edema, pregnancy/nursing status, and for possible drug interactons. Obtain baseline LFTs and leukocyte count.

Monitoring: Monitor for signs/symptoms of encephalopathy, peripheral neuropathy, convulsive seizures, aseptic meningitis, and for candidiasis. Monitor LFTs and leukocyte counts.

Patient Counseling: Inform that drug treats bacterial infections, not viral infections. Instruct to take as directed and to not skip doses. Advise to report any symptoms of CNS toxicity or other adverse side effects.

Administration: IV route; via slow infusion. **Storage:** 15-30°C (59-86°F). Protect from light. Do not remove unit from overwrap until ready for use.

FLECTOR   RX
diclofenac epolamine (King)

> NSAIDs may cause an increased risk of serious cardiovascular thrombotic events, myocardial infarction (MI), stroke and serious GI adverse events including bleeding, ulceration, and perforation of the stomach or intestines, which can be fatal. Patients with cardiovascular disease (CVD) or risk factors for CVD may be at greater risk. Elderly patients are at a greater risk for GI events. Contraindicated in the perioperative setting of coronary artery bypass graft (CABG) surgery.

THERAPEUTIC CLASS: NSAID

INDICATIONS: Topical treatment of acute pain due to minor strains, sprains, and contusions.

DOSAGE: *Adults:* Apply 1 patch to most painful area bid.

HOW SUPPLIED: Patch: 180mg (1.3%) [5ˢ]

CONTRAINDICATIONS: Patients who experienced asthma, urticaria or other allergic type reactions to aspirin (ASA) or other NSAIDs. Treatment of perioperative pain in the setting of coronary artery bypass graft (CABG) surgery. Use on non-intact or damaged skin.

WARNINGS/PRECAUTIONS: May lead to new-onset or worsening of preexisting HTN; caution with HTN and monitor BP closely. Fluid retention and edema reported; caution with fluid retention or heart failure. May cause elevations of LFTs; monitor LFTs periodically and d/c if abnormal LFTs persist or worsen, liver disease develops, or systemic manifestations occur. Cases of severe hepatic reactions (eg, fulminant hepatitis with and without jaundice, liver necrosis, hepatic failure) reported. Caution when initiating treatment in patients with dehydration. Renal papillary necrosis and other renal injury reported after long-term use. Not recommended for use with advanced renal disease; if therapy must be initiated, monitor renal function. Anaphylactic reactions may occur. May cause serious skin adverse events (eg, exfoliative dermatitis, Stevens-Johnson syndrome [SJS], toxic epidermal necrolysis [TEN]); d/c at 1st appearance of skin rash or any other signs of hypersensitivity. Avoid at the start of 30 weeks gestation; may cause premature closure of ductus arteriosus. Cannot replace corticosteroid or treat corticosteroid insufficiency. May diminish the utility of diagnostic signs in detecting complications of presumed noninfectious, painful conditions. Anemia may occur; monitor Hgb/Hct if signs or symptoms of anemia develop with long-term use. May inhibit platelet aggregation and prolong bleeding time; carefully monitor patients with coagulation disorders. Caution with pre-existing asthma. Avoid contact with eyes and mucosa. Prescribe with extreme caution in history of ulcer disease or GI bleeding. Caution in elderly and debilitated patients. Use lowest effective dose for shortest possible duration.

ADVERSE REACTIONS: Application site reaction, pruritus, GI bleeding/perforation/ulceration, nausea.

INTERACTIONS: May diminish the antihypertensive effect of ACE inhibitors. Increased adverse effects with ASA; avoid use. May reduce natriuretic effect of furosemide and thiazides; monitor for renal failure. May impair response to ACE inhibitors, thiazides or loop diuretics. Greater risk of renal toxicity with diuretics and ACE inhibitors. May enhance lithium and methotrexate toxicity; caution when coadministering. Caution with drugs known to be potentially hepatotoxic (eg, acetaminophen, certain antibiotics, anti-epileptics). May result in higher rate of hemorrhage, more frequent abnormal creatinine, urea and Hgb with oral NSAIDs; avoid combination unless benefit outweighs risk. Increased risk of GI bleeding with oral corticosteroids, anticoagulants (eg, warfarin), smoking and alcohol. May increase cyclosporine's nephrotoxicity.

PREGNANCY: Category C (<30 weeks gestation) and D (≥30 weeks gestation), not for use in nursing.

MECHANISM OF ACTION: NSAID; mechanism not established. Suspected to involve inhibition of prostaglandin synthesis.

PHARMACOKINETICS: Absorption: C_{max}=0.7-6ng/mL, T_{max}=10-20 hrs. **Distribution:** Plasma protein binding (>99%). **Metabolism:** 4'hydroxy-diclofenac (major) via CYP2C9. See PI. **Elimination:** Urine (65%), bile (35%); $T_{1/2}$=12 hrs.

NURSING CONSIDERATIONS

Assessment: Assess for hypersensitivity to drug, conditions where treatment is cautioned or contraindicated, pregnancy/nursing status, and possible drug interactions.

Monitoring: Monitor BP and renal function. Periodically monitor CBC, LFTs, and chemistry profile. Monitor for signs/symptoms of GI events, CV thrombotic events, liver disease, edema, HTN, anaphylactic reactions, skin rash or other signs of hypersensitivity, and hematologic effects.

Patient Counseling: Instruct only to use on intact skin. Instruct to wash hands after applying, handling or removing the patch. Instruct not to wear patch during bathing or showering. Instruct to avoid contact with eyes and mucosa; advise to wash out the eye with water or saline immediately and consult physician if irritation persists for >1 hr. Advise to seek medical attention if experience symptoms of hepatotoxicity (nausea, fatigue, lethargy, pruritus, jaundice, right upper quadrant tenderness, "flu-like" symptoms), anaphylactic reaction (difficulty breathing, swelling of face/throat), skin and hypersensitivity reactions (rash, blisters, fever, itching), CV events (chest pain, SOB, weakness, slurring of speech), GI ulceration and bleeding (epigastric pain, dyspepsia, melena, hematemesis), bronchospasm (wheezing, SOB), weight gain or edema. Inform of pregnancy risks. Inform not to use with ASA-sensitive asthma.

Instruct to tape down edges of patch if it begins to peel-off. Instruct to keep out of the reach of children and pets.

Administration: Transdermal route. **Storage:** 25°C (77°F); excursions permitted to 15-30°C (59-86°F). Keep sealed at all times when not in use.

FLEXERIL RX
cyclobenzaprine HCl (McNeil Consumer)

THERAPEUTIC CLASS: Skeletal muscle relaxant (central-acting)

INDICATIONS: Relief of muscle spasm associated with acute, painful musculoskeletal conditions.

DOSAGE: *Adults:* Usual: 5mg tid. Titrate: May increase to 10mg tid. Mild Hepatic Dysfunction/Elderly: Initial: 5mg qd, then slowly increase. Moderate/Severe Hepatic Dysfunction: Avoid use. Treatment should not exceed 2-3 weeks.
Pediatrics: ≥15 yrs: Usual: 5mg tid. Titrate: May increase to 10mg tid. Mild Hepatic Dysfunction/Elderly: Initial: 5mg qd, then slowly increase. Moderate/Severe Hepatic Dysfunction: Avoid use. Treatment should not exceed 2-3 weeks.

HOW SUPPLIED: Tab: 5mg, 10mg

CONTRAINDICATIONS: Acute recovery phase of MI, arrhythmias, heart block or conduction disturbances, CHF, hyperthyroidism, MAOI use during or within 14 days.

WARNINGS/PRECAUTIONS: Caution with history of urinary retention, angle-closure glaucoma, increased IOP, hepatic dysfunction. Caution in elderly due to increased risk of CNS effects. May produce arrhythmias, sinus tachycardia and conduction time prolongation. May impair mental/physical abilities.

ADVERSE REACTIONS: Drowsiness, dry mouth, headache, fatigue.

INTERACTIONS: See Contraindications. Enhances effects of alcohol, barbiturates, and other CNS depressants. May block antihypertensive action of guanethidine and similar compounds. May enhance seizure risk with tramadol. Caution with anticholinergic medication.

PREGNANCY: Category B, caution in nursing.

MECHANISM OF ACTION: Centrally acting skeletal muscle relaxant; relieves skeletal muscle spasm of local origin without interfering with muscle function; reduces tonic somatic motor activity by influencing both gamma and α motor systems.

PHARMACOKINETICS: Absorption: Oral bioavailability (33-55%); C_{max}=25.9ng/mL; AUC=177ng•hr/mL. **Metabolism:** Extensive; through N-demethylation pathway. Via CYP3A4, 1A2, and 2D6. **Elimination:** Urine (glucuronides); $T_{1/2}$=18 hrs.

NURSING CONSIDERATIONS

Assessment: Assess for hepatic impairment, seizures, hyperthyroidism, urinary retention, angle-closure glaucoma, IOP, recent MI, arrhythmias, heart block, CHF, alcohol intake, pregnancy/nursing status, and possible drug interactions (eg, MAOIs if concomitant use or within 14 days after d/c, and anticholinergic medications).

Monitoring: Monitor for cardiac arrhythmias, sinus tachycardia, MI, increased seizure risk, stroke, IOP, CBC, and LFTs.

Patient Counseling: Caution while performing hazardous tasks (eg, operating machinery/driving). Avoid alcohol or other CNS depressants. Notify if pregnant/nursing.

Administration: Oral route. **Storage:** 25°C (77°F); excursions permitted to 15-30°C (59-86°F).

FLOMAX   RX

tamsulosin HCl (Boehringer Ingelheim/Astellas Pharma)

THERAPEUTIC CLASS: Alpha₁-antagonist

INDICATIONS: Treatment of signs and symptoms of benign prostatic hyperplasia (BPH).

DOSAGE: *Adults:* Initial: 0.4mg qd, 30 min after same meal each day. Titrate: May increase to 0.8mg qd after 2-4 weeks. If therapy is interrupted, restart with 0.4mg qd.

HOW SUPPLIED: Cap: 0.4mg

WARNINGS/PRECAUTIONS: Screen for presence of prostate cancer prior to treatment and at regular intervals afterward. Orthostasis/syncope may occur. May cause priapism (rare). Intraoperative floppy iris syndrome (IFIS) has been observed during cataract surgery. Use with caution if sulfa allergy present. Not for use in treatment of HTN.

ADVERSE REACTIONS: Headache, dizziness, somnolence, diarrhea, asthenia, back pain, pharyngitis, rhinitis, abnormal ejaculation, chest pain, cough increased.

INTERACTIONS: Avoid use with other α-adrenergic blockers. Decreased clearance with cimetidine; caution with concomitant use, especially with doses higher than 0.4mg. Caution with warfarin. Avoid doses >0.4mg in combination with strong inhibitors of CYP3A4 (eg, ketoconazole); may increase plasma exposure. Caution in combination with moderate inhibitors of CYP3A4 (eg, erythromycin) in combination with strong (eg, paroxetine) or moderate (eg, terbinafine) inhibitors of CYP2D6 and known poor metabolizers of CYP2D6; avoid use with doses higher than 0.4mg. Caution with PDE5 inhibitors; may cause symptomatic hypotension.

PREGNANCY: Category B, not for use in nursing.

MECHANISM OF ACTION: α₁ₐ antagonist; selective blockade of α₁ receptors in the prostate result in relaxation of the smooth muscles of the bladder neck and prostate.

PHARMACOKINETICS: Absorption: Complete. (0.4mg) (light breakfast) C_{max}=10.1ng/mL, T_{max}=6 hrs, AUC=151ng•hr/mL; (fasting) C_{max}=17.1ng/mL, T_{max}=4 hrs, AUC=199ng•hr/mL . (0.8mg) (light breakfast) C_{max}=29.8ng/mL, T_{max}=7 hrs, AUC=440ng•hr/mL; (high-fat meal) C_{max}=29.1ng/mL, T_{max}=6.6 hrs, AUC=449ng•hr/mL; (fasting) C_{max}=41.6ng/mL, T_{max}=5 hrs, AUC=557ng•hr/mL. **Distribution:** (IV) V_d=16L, plasma protein binding (94-99%). **Metabolism:** Liver; CYP3A4, CYP2D6. **Elimination:** Urine (76%;<10% unchanged), feces (21%); $T_{1/2}$=9-13 hrs (healthy), 14-15 hrs.

NURSING CONSIDERATIONS

Assessment: Assess for BPH, sulfa allergy, pregnancy/nursing status, and possible drug interactions. Rule out prostate cancer.

Monitoring: Monitor for signs/symptoms of orthostasis, priapism, IFIS, and allergic reactions.

Patient Counseling: Advise about possible occurrence of symptoms related to postural hypotension; caution may impair physical/mental abilities. Avoid situations where injury could result if syncope occurs. Take as prescribed. Do not crush, chew, or open capsule. Advise if considering cataract surgery to inform ophthalmologist of drug use. Advise about the possibility of priapism and to seek immediate medical attention if this occurs.

Administration: Oral route. **Storage:** 25°C (77°F); excursions permitted to 15-30°C (59-86°F).

FLONASE   RX

fluticasone propionate (GlaxoSmithKline)

THERAPEUTIC CLASS: Corticosteroid

INDICATIONS: Management of the nasal symptoms of seasonal and perennial allergic and nonallergic rhinitis in adults and pediatrics ≥4 yrs.

DOSAGE: *Adults:* Initial: 2 sprays per nostril qd or 1 spray per nostril bid. Maint: 1 spray per nostril qd. May dose as 2 sprays per nostril qd prn for seasonal allergic rhinitis.
Pediatrics: ≥4 yrs: Initial: 1 spray per nostril qd. If inadequate response, may increase to 2 sprays per nostril. Maint: 1 spray per nostril qd. Max: 2 sprays per nostril/day. ≥12 yrs: May dose as 2 sprays per nostril qd prn for seasonal allergic rhinitis.

HOW SUPPLIED: Spray: 50mcg/spray [16g]

WARNINGS/PRECAUTIONS: Caution with active or quiescent tuberculosis (TB), ocular herpes simplex, or untreated bacterial, fungal, and systemic viral or parasitic infections. Avoid with recent nasal trauma, surgery or septal ulcers. Risk for more severe/fatal course of infections (eg, chickenpox, measles); avoid exposure in patients who have not had disease or not have been properly immunized. *Candida albicans* infection of nose and pharynx reported (rare). Potential for reduced growth velocity in pediatrics. Hypercorticism and adrenal suppression may appear when used at higher than recommended doses or in susceptible individuals at recommended doses; d/c slowly if such changes occur. Rare hypersensitivity reactions or contact dermatitis may occur. Rare instances of wheezing, nasal septum perforation, cataracts, glaucoma, and increased intraocular pressure (IOP) reported. Avoid spraying in eyes.

ADVERSE REACTIONS: Headache, pharyngitis, epistaxis, nasal burning/irritation, asthma symptoms, N/V, cough.

INTERACTIONS: Levels increased with ketoconazole or other potent CYP3A4 inhibitors. Concomitant inhaled corticosteroids increase risk of hypercorticism and/or HPA axis suppression. Increased levels with ritonavir; avoid use unless benefit outweighs risk.

PREGNANCY: Category C, caution in nursing.

MECHANISM OF ACTION: Synthetic trifluorinated corticosteroid; not established. Anti-inflammatory agent with wide range of effects on multiple cell types (eg, mast cells, eosinophils, macrophages, and lymphocytes) and mediators (eg, histamine, eicosanoids, leukotrienes, and cytokines) involved in inflammation.

PHARMACOKINETICS: Absorption: Absolute bioavailability (<2%), C_{max}=50pg/mL. **Distribution:** (IV) Plasma protein binding (91%); V_d=4.2L/kg. **Metabolism:** CYP3A4. **Elimination:** (IV) Urine (<5%, metabolite), feces (parent drug, metabolite); $T_{1/2}$=7.8 hrs.

NURSING CONSIDERATIONS

Assessment: Assess for hypersensitivity, TB, infections, ocular herpes simplex, history of recent nasal septal ulcers, nasal surgery/trauma, immunization status, pregnancy/nursing status and possible drug interactions. May give prophylaxis with varicella zoster immune globulin (VZIG) if exposed to chickenpox, or with pooled IM immunogobulin (IG) if exposed to measles.

Monitoring: Monitor for acute adrenal insufficiency, withdrawal symptoms, hypercorticism and/or HPA axis suppression, infections, chickenpox and measles, nasal or pharyngeal *Candida albicans* infections, hypersensitivity or contact dermatitis, wheezing, nasal septum perforation, cataracts, glaucoma, and increased IOP. Monitor growth of pediatric patients routinely.

Patient Counseling: Take as directed at regular intervals and do not increase prescribed dosage. Avoid exposure to chickenpox or measles; consult physician immediately if exposed. Do not spray into eyes. Contact physician if symptoms do not improve or worsen.

Administration: Intranasal route. **Storage:** 4-30°C (39-86°F).

FLOVENT DISKUS   RX
fluticasone propionate (GlaxoSmithKline)

THERAPEUTIC CLASS: Corticosteroid

INDICATIONS: Maintenance treatment of asthma as prophylactic therapy in patients ≥4 yrs and for patients requiring oral corticosteroid therapy for asthma.

DOSAGE: *Adults:* Previous Bronchodilator Only: Initial: 100mcg bid. Max: 500mcg bid. Previous Inhaled Corticosteroid: Initial: 100-250mcg bid. Max: 500mcg bid. Previous Oral Corticosteroid: Initial: 500-1000mcg bid. Max: 1000mcg bid. Starting dosages >100mcg bid may be considered for patients with poorer asthma control or previous high-dose inhaled corticosteroid requirement. Reduce PO prednisone no faster than 2.5 to 5mg/day weekly, beginning at least 1 week after starting fluticasone. Reduce to the lowest effective dose once prednisone reduction is complete.
Pediatrics: ≥12 yrs: Previous Bronchodilator Only: Initial: 100mcg bid. Max: 500mcg bid. Previous Inhaled Corticosteroid: Initial: 100-250mcg bid. Max: 500mcg bid. Previous Oral Corticosteroid: Initial: 500-1000mcg bid. Max: 1000mcg bid. 4-11 yrs: Previous Therapy: Initial: 50mcg bid. Max: 100mcg bid. Starting dosages >100mcg bid may be considered for adolescent patients and >50mcg for patients 4-11 yrs with poorer asthma control or previous high-dose inhaled corticosteroid requirement. Reduce PO prednisone no faster than 2.5 to 5mg/day weekly, beginning at least 1 week after starting fluticasone. Reduce to the lowest effective dose once prednisone reduction is complete.

HOW SUPPLIED: Disk: 50mcg/inh, 100mcg/inh, 250mcg/inh [60 blisters]

CONTRAINDICATIONS: Primary treatment of status asthmaticus or other acute episodes of asthma where intensive measures are required. Severe hypersensitivity to milk proteins.

WARNINGS/PRECAUTIONS: Deaths may occur due to adrenal insufficiency with transfer from systemic corticosteroids to inhaled corticosteroid. Resume oral corticosteroids during stress or severe asthma attack. Wean slowly from systemic corticosteroid therapy. Transfer from systemic corticosteroid therapy may unmask conditions previously suppressed (eg, rhinitis, conjunctivitis, eczema, arthritis, eosinophilic conditions). Observe for signs and symptoms of adrenal insufficiency (eg, fatigue, lassitude, weakness, N/V, hypotension). Monitor for systemic corticosteroid effects such as hypercorticism and adrenal suppression; if effects occur reduce dose slowly. May cause reduction in growth velocity in pediatric patients. Hypersensitivity reactions, including anaphylaxis, angioedema, urticaria, and bronchospasm may occur. Long-term use may result in loss of bone mineral density, glaucoma, increased intraocular pressure (IOP), and cataracts. Avoid exposure to chickenpox or measles; more serious or even fatal course may occur. May produce paradoxical bronchospasm; treat immediately with an inhaled, fast-acting bronchodilator, d/c and institute alternative therapy. Caution with active or quiescent tuberculosis (TB) infections of the respiratory tract, untreated systemic fungal, bacterial, viral, or parasitic infections, or ocular herpes simplex. Localized infections of the mouth and pharynx with *Candida albicans* reported; treat accordingly and interrupt therapy if needed. Rare cases of eosinophilic conditions observed.

ADVERSE REACTIONS: Upper respiratory tract infection, throat irritation, headache, sinusitis/sinus infection, N/V, rhinitis, cough, muscle pain, oral candidiasis, arthralgia, articular rheumatism, fatigue, nasal congestion/blockage, malaise.

INTERACTIONS: May increase levels and reduce serum cortisol levels with ritonavir and ketoconazole; avoid concomitant use. Concurrent use with strong CYP3A4 inhibitors (eg, ritonavir, atazanavir, clarithromycin, indinavir, itraconazole, nefazodone, nelfinavir, saquinavir, telithromycin) may increase occurrence of systemic corticosteroid adverse effects.

PREGNANCY: Category C, caution in nursing.

MECHANISM OF ACTION: Corticosteroid; potent anti-inflammatory activity, inhibits multiple cell types and mediator production or secretion involved in asthmatic response.

PHARMACOKINETICS: Absorption: Acts locally in lung, absolute bioavailability (7.8%); C_{max} =110pg/mL (500mcg bid). **Distribution:** (IV) V_d=4.2 L/kg; plasma protein binding (99%). **Metabolism:** Liver via CYP3A4. **Elimination:** (IV) Feces, urine (<5%); $T_{1/2}$=7.8 hrs.

NURSING CONSIDERATIONS

Assessment: Assess for hypersensitivity to milk proteins, acute asthma episodes, rapidly deteriorating asthma, risk factors for decreased bone mineral content, CV disease, convulsive disorder, thyrotoxicosis, DM, history of increased IOP, glaucoma, cataracts, active or quiescent pulmonary TB, ocular herpes simplex, untreated systemic infections, hepatic disease, pregnancy/nursing status, and for possible drug interactions. Obtain baseline BMD, eye exam, and lung function prior to therapy.

Monitoring: Monitor respiratory status and lung sounds, airflow changes, signs and symptoms of asthma and adrenal insufficiency, systemic corticosteroid effects, growth rate in pediatric patients (via stadiometry), development of infections, hypersensitivity reactions, withdrawal symptoms (eg, joint/muscular pain, lassitude, depression) during withdrawal from systemic corticosteroids, changes in vision, serum and urine glucose concentrations, adrenal function tests to assess degree of hypothalamic-pituitary-adrenal axis suppression in chronic therapy, eosinophilic conditions, and hepatic disease.

Patient Counseling: Advise that localized infections with *Candida albicans* may occur in the mouth and pharynx in some patients; treat with appropriate local or systemic (ie, oral antifungal) therapy while still continuing therapy if oropharyngeal candidiasis develops. Advise to rinse mouth after inhalation. Advise that product is not intended as a rescue medication for acute asthma exacerbations; contact physician immediately if deterioration of asthma occurs. Counsel of risks of decreased bone mineral density (BMD) and reduced growth velocity in children. Instruct to taper slowly from systemic corticosteroids if transferring to oral inhalation and not to stop use abruptly. Instruct to avoid exposure to chickenpox or measles. Seek medical attention if exposed to chickenpox or measles, if existing TB infections, fungal/bacterial/viral/parasitic infections or ocular herpes simplex symptoms do not improve or worsen, or if adrenal insufficiency, paradoxal bronchospasm or hypersensitivity reactions occur. Instruct to get regular eye examinations. Use drugs at regular intervals as directed. Inform not to exceed recommended dose. Instruct not to use with a spacer device. Notify physician if pregnant or intend to become pregnant, or nursing. Instruct to carry a warning card indicating the need for supplementary systemic corticosteroids during periods of stress or a severe asthma attack.

Administration: Oral inhalation. Rinse mouth after inhalation. **Storage:** 20-25°C (68-77°F). Store in a dry place away from direct heat or sunlight. Device is not reusable. Discard in 6 weeks (50mcg) or 2 months (100mcg and 250mcg) after removal from pouch or when the indicator reads "0," whichever comes first.

FLOVENT HFA   RX
fluticasone propionate (GlaxoSmithKline)

THERAPEUTIC CLASS: Corticosteroid

INDICATIONS: Maintenance treatment of asthma as prophylactic therapy in patients ≥4 years, and for patients requiring oral corticosteroid therapy for asthma.

DOSAGE: *Adults:* Previous Bronchodilator Only: Initial: 88mcg bid. Max: 440mcg bid. Previous Inhaled Corticosteroids: Initial: 88-220mcg bid. Max: 440mcg bid. Previous Oral Corticosteroids: Initial: 440mcg bid. Max: 880mcg bid. May consider starting dose >88 mcg bid with poorer asthma control or previous high-dose inhaled corticosteroid requirement. For patients currently receiving chronic oral corticosteroid, reduce PO prednisone no faster than 2.5 to 5mg/day on a weekly basis, beginning ≥1 week after starting fluticasone. Titrate: Lowest effective dose. Increase to higher strength if response to initial dose inadequate after 2 weeks.
Pediatrics: ≥12 yrs: Previous Bronchodilator Only: Initial: 88mcg bid. Max: 440mcg bid. Previous Inhaled Corticosteroids: Initial: 88-220mcg bid. Max: 440mcg bid. Previous Oral Corticosteroids: Initial: 440mcg bid. Max: 880mcg bid. 4-11 yrs: Initial/Max: 88mcg bid. May consider starting dose >88 mcg

bid with poorer asthma control or previous high-dose inhaled corticosteroid requirement. For patients currently receiving chronic oral corticosteroid therapy, reduce PO prednisone no faster than 2.5 to 5mg/day on a weekly basis, beginning ≥1 week after starting fluticasone. Titrate: Lowest effective dose. Increase to higher strength if response to initial dose inadequate after 2 weeks.

HOW SUPPLIED: MDI: 44mcg/inh [10.6g], 110mcg/inh [12g], 220mcg/inh [12g]

CONTRAINDICATIONS: Primary treatment of status asthmaticus or other acute episodes of asthma where intensive measures are required.

WARNINGS/PRECAUTIONS: Localized *Candida albicans* infections of the mouth and pharynx reported. Increased susceptibility to infections; avoid exposure to chickenpox and measles. Caution in patients with active/quiescent tuberculosis (TB), untreated systemic infections, or ocular herpes simplex. Deaths due to adrenal insufficiency may occur with transfer from systemic to inhaled corticosteroid. Wean slowly from systemic corticosteroid therapy. Resume oral corticosteroids during periods of stress or a severe asthma attack if patient previously withdrawn from systemic corticosteroids and immediately contact physician. Transfer from systemic corticosteroid therapy may unmask conditions previously suppressed (eg, rhinitis). Monitor for systemic corticosteroid effects particularly in postoperative patients and during periods of stress. Hypercorticism and adrenal suppression/crisis may occur; reduce dose slowly if such effects occur. Hypersensitivity reactions may occur. Long-term use may result in loss of bone mineral density (BMD), glaucoma, increased intraocular pressure (IOP), and cataracts. May cause reduction in growth velocity in pediatric patients. May produce paradoxical bronchospasm; d/c immediately, treat, with and institute alternative therapy. Rare cases of systemic eosinophilic conditions observed; monitor for eosinophilia, vasculitic rash, worsening pulmonary symptoms, cardiac complications, and/or neuropathy.

ADVERSE REACTIONS: Upper respiratory tract infection, upper respiratory tract inflammation, throat irritation, sinusitis, dysphonia, candidiasis, cough, bronchitis, headache.

INTERACTIONS: May increase levels with ritonavir and ketoconazole; avoid concomitant use. Concomitant use with strong CYP3A4 inhibitors (eg, ritonavir, atazanavir, clarithromycin, indinavir, itraconazole, nefazodone, nelfinavir, saquinavir, ketoconazole, telithromycin) is not recommended because increased systemic corticosteroid adverse effects may occur. Increased risk of BMD with tobacco use and drugs that reduce bone mass (eg, anticonvulsants, oral corticosteroids).

PREGNANCY: Category C, caution in nursing.

MECHANISM OF ACTION: Corticosteroid; possesses potent anti-inflammatory activity. Inhibits multiple cell types and mediator production or secretion involved in the asthmatic response.

PHARMACOKINETICS: Absorption: Acts locally in lung. **Distribution:** (IV) V_d=4.2 L/kg; plasma protein binding (99%). **Metabolism:** via CYP3A4; 17β-carboxylic acid (metabolite). **Elimination:** (PO) Feces, urine (<5%); (IV) $T_{1/2}$=7.8 hrs.

NURSING CONSIDERATIONS

Assessment: Assess for status asthmaticus, acute asthma episode, acute bronchospasm, active or quiescent TB, ocular herpes simplex; untreated systemic infections, risk factors for decreased bone mineral content, history of increased IOP, glaucoma or cataracts, vision changes, hepatic disease, drug hypersensitivity, pregnancy/nursing status, and for possible drug interactions. Obtain baseline BMD and eye exam. In pediatric patients, obtain baseline height.

Monitoring: Monitor for signs of infection, immunosuppression, systemic corticosteroid effects, adrenal insufficiency, hypersensitivity reactions, decreased BMD, glaucoma, increased IOP, cataracts, bronchospasm, eosinophilic conditions, asthma instability and adrenal insufficiency. Monitor growth in pediatric patients. Monitor lung function (FEV1) or morning peak expiratory flow, β-agonist use, and asthma symptoms during oral corticosteroid with-drawal. Monitor patients with hepatic disease.

Patient Counseling: Advise that localized infections with *Candida albicans* may occur in the mouth and pharynx; advise to rinse mouth after use. Inform that product is not intended for acute asthma exacerbations; instruct to con-tact physician immediately if deterioration of asthma occurs. Counsel on risks of decreased BMD and reduced growth velocity in children, to avoid exposure to chickenpox or measles, that long-term use may increase risk of some eye problems, and that systemic corticosteroid effects and adrenal suppres-sion may occur. Instruct to d/c therapy if a hypersensitivity reaction occurs. Instruct to use at regular intervals as directed and not to stop use abruptly. Full benefit may not be achieved for 1-2 weeks or longer after starting treat-ment. Instruct to contact physician immediately if drug is d/c.

Administration: Oral inhalation. Rinse mouth after inhalation. Prime inhaler before using for 1st time by releasing 4 test sprays into air, away from face, shaking well for 5 sec before each spray. If not used for >7 days, or when dropped, prime inhaler again by shaking well before each spray and releasing 1 test spray into air. **Storage:** 25°C (77°F); excursions permitted to 15-30°C (59-86°F). Store inhaler with mouthpiece down. Inhaler should be at room temperature before use. Discard when the counter reads 000.

FLUARIX   RX
influenza virus vaccine (GlaxoSmithKline)

THERAPEUTIC CLASS: Vaccine

INDICATIONS: Active immunization in persons ≥3 yrs for prevention of disease caused by influenza virus subtypes A and type B contained in the vaccine.

DOSAGE: *Adults:* 0.5mL IM as a single dose.
Pediatrics: 3-<9 yrs: Unvaccinated or vaccinated for first time last season with only 1 dose: Two 0.5mL IM doses, each 0.5mL dose should be administered at least 4 weeks apart. Vaccinated with 2 doses: 0.5mL IM as 1 dose. ≥9 yrs: 0.5mL IM as 1 dose.

HOW SUPPLIED: Inj: (Syringe) 0.5mL

CONTRAINDICATIONS: Hypersenstivity reactions to egg proteins or life-threatening reaction to previous administration of any influenza vaccine.

WARNINGS/PRECAUTIONS: Not for intradermal, IV or SQ administration. Do not inject in gluteal area or areas with major nerve trunk. Caution if Guillain-Barre syndrome has occurred within 6 weeks of receipt of prior influenza vaccine. Caution in patients with bleeding disorders (eg, hemophilia). Tip caps contain latex; may cause allergic reactions in latex-sensitive individuals. Immunosuppressed patients may have a lower immune response. Medical treatment and supervision must be available to manage possible anaphylactic reactions. May not protect all susceptible individuals.

ADVERSE REACTIONS: Local reactions (pain, redness, swelling), muscle aches, fatigue, headache, arthralgia, shivering, irritability, loss of appetite, drowsiness, fever, cough, upper respiratory tract infection, vomiting.

INTERACTIONS: Caution with anticoagulants. Immunosuppressive therapies (eg, irradiation, antimetabolites, alkylating agents, cytotoxic drugs, corti-costeroids [used in greater than physiological doses]) may reduce immune response to influenza virus vaccine.

PREGNANCY: Category B, caution in nursing.

MECHANISM OF ACTION: Vaccine; elicits the formation of antibodies that may protect against influenza virus subtypes A and B.

NURSING CONSIDERATIONS

Assessment: Assess for hypersensitivity to egg proteins or latex, presence of immunosuppression, immunization history, bleeding disorders (eg, hemo-philia), pregnancy/nursing status, and for possible drug interactions. Assess potential benefits and risks if Guillain-Barre syndrome occurred with previous influenza vaccination.

Monitoring: Monitor for allergic reactions, local injection-site reactions (eg, pain, redness, swelling), and for general adverse events (eg, headache, fatigue, muscle aches, arthralgia, fever).

Patient Counseling: Inform of potential benefits and risks of immunization. Educate about potential adverse reactions. Inform that vaccine contains noninfectious killed viruses and cannot cause influenza. Advise that vaccine is intended to provide protection against illness due to influenza viruses only and cannot provide protection against all respiratory illnesses. Instruct to report any adverse events to healthcare provider. Inform that annual revaccination is recommended.

Administration: IM route. Inject into deltoid muscle of upper arm. **Storage:** 2-8°C (36-46°F). Do not freeze. Discard if frozen. Store in original container and protect from light.

FLUDROCORTISONE   RX
fludrocortisone acetate (Various)

THERAPEUTIC CLASS: Corticosteroid

INDICATIONS: Partial replacement therapy for primary & secondary adrenocortical insufficiency in Addison's disease. Treatment of salt-losing adrenogenital syndrome.

DOSAGE: *Adults:* Addison's Disease: Usual: 0.1mg/day with concomitant cortisone 10-37.5mg/day or hydrocortisone 10-30mg/day in divided doses. Dose Range: 0.1mg 3 times weekly to 0.2mg/day. If HTN develops, reduce to 0.05mg/day. Salt-Losing Adrenogenital Syndrome: 0.1-0.2mg/day.

HOW SUPPLIED: Tab: 0.1mg* *scored

CONTRAINDICATIONS: Systemic fungal infections.

WARNINGS/PRECAUTIONS: Treatment of conditions other than those indicated is not advised. May mask signs of infection, and new infections may appear; may decrease resistance and inability to localize infection. Prolonged use may produce posterior subcapsular cataracts, glaucoma with possible optic nerve damage, and may enhance the establishment of secondary ocular infection due to fungi or viruses. Can cause HTN, salt and water retention, and hypokalemia; monitor carefully for the dosage and salt intake. Serum electrolyte monitoring is advised with prolonged use; salt restriction diet and K⁺ supplementation may be necessary. May increase calcium excretion. Reactivation of TB may occur. Caution with hypothyroidism, cirrhosis, ocular herpes simplex, HTN, ulcerative colitis, diverticulitis, intestinal anastomosis, peptic ulcer, renal insufficiency, osteoporosis and myasthenia gravis. Avoid exposure to chickenpox or measles. Psychic derangements may appear. Adverse reactions produced if large doses used or upon rapid withdrawal. May affect the nitrobluetetrazolium test for bacterial infections and produce false-negative results.

ADVERSE REACTIONS: HTN, CHF, edema, cardiac enlargement, hypokalemia, hypokalemic alkalosis.

INTERACTIONS: Decreases pharmacologic effect of aspirin; monitor salicylate levels or therapeutic effect of aspirin. Enhanced hypokalemia with amphotericin B and potassium-depleting diuretics (eg, furosemide, ethacrynic acid). Increased risk of digitalis toxicity and arrhythmias with hypokalemia when given with digitalis glycosides. Decreased effects with rifampin, barbiturates, and phenytoin. Decrease PT with oral anticoagulants; monitor for PT. Diminish effects of oral hypoglycemics and insulin. Enhanced edema with other anabolic steroids (eg, oxymethalone, norethandrolone). Adjust dose with initiation or termination of estrogen. Avoid live virus vaccines (including smallpox) and other immunizations.

PREGNANCY: Category C, caution in nursing.

MECHANISM OF ACTION: Synthetic adrenocortical steroid; acts on electrolyte balance and carbohydrate metabolism and on distal tubules of kidney to enhance reabsorption of sodium ions from tubular fluid into the plasma. Increases urinary excretion of both K⁺ and hydrogen ions.

PHARMACOKINETICS: Distribution: Found in breast milk. **Elimination**: $T_{1/2}$=3.5 hrs (Plasma), 18-36 hr (Biological).

NURSING CONSIDERATIONS

Assessment: Assess for hypersensitivity reactions to drug, systemic fungal infections, other current infections, active TB, vaccination, HTN, heart disease, renal/hepatic impairment, unusual stress, psychotic tendencies, thyroid function, hypoprothrombinemia, osteoporosis, myasthenia gravis, peptic ulcers with/without impending perforation, fresh intestinal anastomosis, diverticulitis/ulcerative colitis, possible drug/lab test interactions (eg, nitrobluetetrazolium test for bacterial infection) and pregnancy/nursing status.

Monitoring: Monitor for occurrence of infections, edema, weight gain, psychic derangement, cataracts, and frequent measuring of serum electrolytes, TSH, LFTs, glucose, IOP, and BP.

Patient Counseling: Inform drug increases susceptibility to infections. Instruct to avoid exposure to chickenpox or measles. Counsel to carry supply of medication for emergency use. Advise on the importance of regular follow-up visits and to use medication exactly as directed. Advise to notify physician of dizziness, severe or continuing headaches, swelling of feet or lower legs, or unusual weight gain. Advise to report any medical history of heart disease, HTN, kidney or liver disease, and to report current use of any medicines. Inform patient to keep medication out of reach of children.

Administration: Oral route. **Storage**: 15-30°C (59-86°F). Avoid excessive heat. Dispense in a tightly-closed, light-resistant container.

FLUZONE   RX
influenza virus vaccine (Sanofi Pasteur)

OTHER BRAND NAMES: Fluzone HD (Sanofi Pasteur)

THERAPEUTIC CLASS: Vaccine

INDICATIONS: Active immunization against influenza disease caused by influenza virus subtypes A and type B contained in the vaccine in persons (Fluzone) ≥6 months of age or (Fluzone HD) ≥65 yrs of age.

DOSAGE: *Adults:* (Fluzone): 0.5mL IM in deltoid muscle as 1 dose; (Fluzone HD) ≥65 yrs: 0.5mL IM in deltoid muscle as 1 dose.
Pediatrics: Previously Unvaccinated or Incompletely Vaccinated for first time last season with only 1 dose: 3-8 yrs: Two 0.5mL IM doses, each 0.5mL dose should be 1 month apart. 6-35 months: Two 0.25mL IM doses, each 0.25mL dose should be 1 month apart. Vaccinated 2 doses last season or one or more doses at any time before last season: 3-8 yrs: 0.5mL IM as 1 dose. 6-35 months: 0.25mL IM as 1 dose. ≥9 yrs: 0.5mL IM as 1 dose. Administer in deltoid muscle in children (1-17 years) or anterolateral aspect of thigh muscle in infants (6-12 months).

HOW SUPPLIED: Inj: (Fluzone) 0.25mL, 0.5mL [prefilled syringe], 0.5 mL [single-dose vial], 5mL [multi-dose vial]; (Fluzone HD) 0.5mL [prefilled syringe]

CONTRAINDICATIONS: Hypersensitivity to egg proteins.

WARNINGS/PRECAUTIONS: Caution if Guillain-Barre Syndrome (GBS) has occurred with 6 weeks of previous influenza vaccination. Immunosuppressed patients may have lower immune response. Medical treatment and supervision must be available to manage possible anaphylactic reactions. May not protect all susceptible individuals. Prefilled syringes may contain natural rubber latex which may cause allergic reactions in latex sensitive individuals.

ADVERSE REACTIONS: Injection-site reactions (pain, tenderness, erythema, swelling), myalgia, malaise, headache, fever, arm stiffness.

INTERACTIONS: Immunosuppressive therapies may reduce immune response.

PREGNANCY: Category C, caution in nursing.

MECHANISM OF ACTION: Vaccine; stimulates the immune system to produce antibodies that may protect against influenza virus subtypes A and B.

NURSING CONSIDERATIONS

Assessment: Assess age, immunization and health/medical status, immuno-suppression, previous hypersensitivity to egg proteins or any of its components and rubber latex, or vaccination events (Guillain-Barre syndrome), pregnancy/nursing status, and possible drug interactions.

Monitoring: Monitor for hypersensitivity reactions, injection-site reactions (eg, swelling, pain, tenderness, erythema), fever, headache, myalgia, malaise, arm stiffness, and other adverse events that may occur.

Patient Counseling: Inform patients or caregivers of benefits/risks ratio. Inform that injection site reactions (eg, swelling, pain, tenderness, erythema), fever, headache, myalgia, malaise, arm stiffness may occur; advise to inform physician if these and other adverse events occur. Inform patient or guardian that vaccine contains killed viruses and cannot cause influenza. Advise that vaccine do not prevent other respiratory infections. Advise to inform physician if pregnant or nursing.

Administration: IM route. Administer in deltoid muscle in children (1-17 yrs) or anterolateral aspect of thigh muscle in infants (6-12 months). Administer at separate injection sites if to be given at the same time as another injectable vaccine(s). Do not inject into gluteal region or areas where there may be a major nerve trunk. Inspect visually for particulate matter and/or discoloration prior to administration. Shake the syringe or single-dose vial before administering and the multi-dose vial each time before withdrawing a dose. **Storage:** 2-8°C (35-46°F). Do not freeze; discard if frozen. Between uses, return the multi-dose vial to recommended condition, 2-8°C (35-46°F).

FML   RX
fluorometholone (Allergan)

OTHER BRAND NAMES: FML Forte (Allergan)

THERAPEUTIC CLASS: Corticosteroid

INDICATIONS: Treatment of inflammation of the palpebral and bulbar conjunctiva, cornea, and anterior segment of the globe.

DOSAGE: *Adults:* (Sus) 1 drop bid-qid or (Oint) apply 1/2 inch qd-tid. May give 0.1% q4h during initial 24-48 hrs. Re-evaluate after 2 days if no improvement. *Pediatrics:* ≥2 yrs: (Sus) 1 drop bid-qid or (Oint) apply 1/2 inch qd-tid. May give 0.1% q4h during initial 24-48 hrs. Re-evaluate after 2 days if no improvement.

HOW SUPPLIED: Oint: (S.O.P.) 0.1% [3.5g]; Sus: 0.1% [5mL, 10mL, 15mL]; (Forte) 0.25% [2mL, 5mL, 10mL, 15mL]

CONTRAINDICATIONS: Viral diseases of the cornea and conjunctiva including epithelial herpes simplex keratitis, vaccinia, and varicella. Mycobacterial infection and fungal diseases of the eye.

WARNINGS/PRECAUTIONS: Caution with glaucoma, herpes simplex, diseases causing thinning of cornea/sclera and other ocular viral infections. Prolonged use can cause glaucoma or secondary ocular infections (eg, fungal). Monitor IOP after 10 days of therapy. Re-evaluate if no response after 2 days. Ointment may retard corneal healing. May delay healing and increase incidence of bleb formation after cataract surgery. Avoid abrupt withdrawal with chronic use.

ADVERSE REACTIONS: Elevation of IOP, glaucoma, infrequent optic nerve damage, posterior subcapsular cataract formation, delayed wound healing, burning/stinging upon instillation, ocular irritation, taste perversion, visual disturbance.

PREGNANCY: Category C, not for use in nursing.

MECHANISM OF ACTION: Corticosteroid; suspected to act by induction of phospholipase A_2 inhibitory proteins called lipocortins, which control the biosynthesis of potent inflammation mediators (eg, prostaglandins, leukotrienes) by inhibiting release of their precursor, arachidonic acid.

NURSING CONSIDERATIONS

Assessment: Assess for viral diseases of cornea and conjunctiva, dendritic keratitis, vaccinia, varicella, mycobacterial infection of eye, fungal disease of ocular structures, glaucoma, mustard gas keratitis, Sjogren's keratoconjuctivitis, thinning of corneal/scleral epithelium, hypersensitivity, and for cataract surgery.

Monitoring: Frequent measuring of IOP and slit lamp microscopy exam when appropriate, fluorescein staining for monitoring of glaucoma with damage to the optic nerve (with defects in visual acuity and fields of vision), posterior subcapsular cataract, delayed corneal healing, thinning of cornea and sclera, ulceration, perforation, and secondary ocular infections or masking of existing infections.

Patient Counseling: Advise to d/c and notify physician if symptoms persist or worsen. Instruct to wait 15 min after instillation to wear soft contact lenses. Counsel to avoid touching bottle tip to eyelids or any other surface.

Administration: Ocular route. **Storage:** Store between 2-25°C (36-77°F); protect from freezing.

FOCALIN
dexmethylphenidate HCl (Novartis)

> Caution with history of drug dependence or alcoholism. Marked tolerance and psychological dependence with varying degrees of abnormal behavior may occur with chronic abusive use. Frank psychotic episodes may occur. Careful supervision is necessary during withdrawal from abusive use, since severe depression may occur. Withdrawal after chronic use may unmask symptoms of underlying disorder that may require follow-up.

THERAPEUTIC CLASS: Sympathomimetic amine

INDICATIONS: Treatment of attention deficit hyperactivity disorder (ADHD).

DOSAGE: *Adults:* Take bid at least 4 hrs apart. Methylphenidate-Naive: Initial: 5mg/day (2.5mg bid). Titrate: May increase weekly by 2.5-5mg/day. Max: 20mg/day (10mg bid). Currently on Methylphenidate: Initial: Take 1/2 of methylphenidate dose. Max: 20mg/day (10mg bid). Reduce or d/c if paradoxical aggravation of symptoms occur. D/C if no improvement after appropriate dosage adjustments over 1 month.
Pediatrics: ≥6 yrs: Take bid at least 4 hrs apart. Methylphenidate-Naive: Initial: 5mg/day (2.5mg bid). Titrate: May increase weekly by 2.5-5mg/day. Max: 20mg/day (10mg bid). Currently on Methylphenidate: Initial: Take 1/2 of methylphenidate dose. Max: 20mg/day (10mg bid). Reduce or d/c if paradoxical aggravation of symptoms occur. D/C if no improvement after appropriate dosage adjustments over 1 month.

HOW SUPPLIED: Tab: 2.5mg, 5mg, 10mg

CONTRAINDICATIONS: Marked anxiety, tension, agitation; glaucoma, motor tics or family history or diagnosis of Tourette's syndrome. Treatment with or within 14 days of monoamine oxidase inhibitor (MAOI) use.

WARNINGS/PRECAUTIONS: Avoid with known serious structural cardiac abnormalities, cardiomyopathy, serious heart rhythm abnormalities, or other serious cardiac problems; sudden death reported in children and adolescents with structural cardiac abnormalities or other serious heart problems. Sudden death, stroke, myocardial infarction (MI) reported in adults. May cause modest increase in HR and BP; caution with HTN, heart failure, recent MI or ventricular arrhythmia. Prior to treatment, perform a physical exam and medical history (including assessment for family history of sudden death or ventricular arrhythmia). Promptly evaluate if symptoms of cardiac disease develop during treatment. May exacerbate symptoms of behavior disturbance and thought disorder with pre-existing psychotic disorder. Caution in patients with comorbid bipolar disorder; may cause induction of mixed/manic episodes. May cause treatment-emergent psychotic or manic symptoms (eg, hallucinations, delusional thinking, mania) in children and adolescents without prior history of psychotic illness or mania at usual doses; d/c may be appropriate. Aggressive behavior or hostility reported in children with ADHD. Suppression of growth reported with long-term use; monitor height and weight. May lower convulsive threshold; d/c in the presence of seizures. Difficulties with accommodation and blurred vision reported. Monitor CBC, differential, and platelets with prolonged therapy. Not for use in pediatrics <6 yrs.

ADVERSE REACTIONS: Abdominal pain, fever, anorexia, nausea, nervousness, insomnia. (Pediatrics) Loss of appetite, weight loss, tachycardia.

INTERACTIONS: See Contraindications. May decrease the effectiveness of drugs used to treat HTN. Caution with pressor agents. May inhibit metabolism of coumarin anticoagulants, anticonvulsants (eg, phenobarbital, phenytoin, primidone) and some antidepressants (eg, TCAs, SSRIs); adjust dose. May possibly interact with venlafaxine.

PREGNANCY: Category C, caution in nursing.

MECHANISM OF ACTION: Sympathomimetic amine; CNS stimulant. Mechanism in ADHD has not been established; suspected to block the reuptake of norepinephrine and dopamine into the presynaptic neuron and increase release of these monoamines into extraneuronal space.

PHARMACOKINETICS: Absorption: Readily absorbed; T_{max}=2.9 hrs (fed), 1.5 hrs (fasted). **Metabolism:** Via de-esterification (d-ritalinic acid; primary metabolite). **Elimination:** Urine (90%); $T_{1/2}$=2.2 hrs.

NURSING CONSIDERATIONS

Assessment: Assess for marked anxiety, agitation, tension, glaucoma, tics, family history of or diagnosis of Tourette's syndrome, pre-existing psychotic disorders, seizure disorder, bipolar disorder, history of drug dependence or alcoholism, pregnancy/nursing status and for possible drug interactions. Assess for medical conditions that might be compromised by increases in BP and HR (eg, HTN, heart failure, recent MI, ventricular arrhythmia), structural cardiac abnormalities, cardiomyopathy, serious heart rhythm abnormalities, or other serious cardiac problems. Perform physical exam and obtain a medical history prior to therapy.

Monitoring: Monitor for symptoms of cardiac disease (eg, exertional chest pain, unexplained syncope, MI, stroke, exacerbations of behavioral disturbances and thought disorders, bipolar disorder, worsening of aggressive behavior or hostility, emergent psychotic or manic symptoms (eg, hallucinations, delusional thinking, mania), seizures, and for visual disturbances. During prolonged use, perform periodic monitoring of CBC, differential and platelet counts. In pediatric patients, monitor height and weight. Monitor BP and HR.

Patient Counseling: Inform about risks and benefits of treatment. Advise that may take with or without food. Advise to notify physician of all medications currently taking and if any adverse events develop.

Administration: Oral route. **Storage:** 25°C (77°F); excursions permitted to 15-30°C (59-86°F). Protect from light and moisture.

FOCALIN XR   `CII`
dexmethylphenidate HCl (Novartis)

> Caution with history of drug dependence or alcoholism. Marked tolerance and psychological dependence with varying degrees of abnormal behavior may occur with chronic abusive use. Frank psychotic episodes may occur. Careful supervision is necessary during withdrawal from abusive use, since severe depression may occur. Withdrawal after chronic use may unmask symptoms of underlying disorder that may require follow-up.

THERAPEUTIC CLASS: Sympathomimetic amine

INDICATIONS: Treatment of attention deficit hyperactivity disorder (ADHD) in patients ≥6 yrs.

DOSAGE: *Adults:* Individualize dose. Methylphenidate-Naive: Initial: 10mg/day qam. Titrate: May adjust weekly in 10mg increments. Max: 40mg/day. Currently on Methylphenidate: Initial: Take 1/2 of methylphenidate total daily dose. Currently on Dexmethylphenidate Immediate-Release: Switch to same daily dose of XR. Reduce or d/c if paradoxical aggravation of symptoms occurs. D/C if no improvement after appropriate dosage adjustments over 1 month.

Pediatrics: ≥6 yrs: Individualize dose. Methylphenidate-Naive: Initial: 5mg/day qam. Titrate: May adjust weekly in 5mg increments. Max: 30mg/day. Currently on Methylphenidate: Initial: Take 1/2 of methylphenidate total daily dose. Currently on Dexmethylphenidate Immediate-Release: Switch to same daily dose of XR. Reduce or d/c if paradoxical aggravation of symptoms occurs. D/C if no improvement after appropriate dosage adjustments over 1 month.

HOW SUPPLIED: Cap, Extended-Release: 5mg, 10mg, 15mg, 20mg, 30mg, 40mg

CONTRAINDICATIONS: Marked anxiety, tension, agitation, glaucoma, motor tics or family history or diagnosis of Tourette's syndrome. Treatment with or within a minimum of 14 days following d/c of a monoamine oxidase inhibitor (MAOI).

WARNINGS/PRECAUTIONS: Avoid with known serious structural cardiac abnormalities, cardiomyopathy, serious heart rhythm abnormalities, or other serious cardiac problems; sudden death reported in children and adolescents with structural cardiac abnormalities or other serious heart problems. Sudden death, stroke, myocardial infarction (MI) reported in adults. May cause modest increase in BP and HR; caution with HTN, heart failure, recent MI, or ventricular arrhythmia. Prior to treatment, perform a physical exam and medical history (including assessment for family history of sudden death or ventricular arrhythmia). Promptly evaluate if symptoms of cardiac disease develop during treatment. May exacerbate symptoms of behavior disturbance and thought disorder with pre-existing psychotic disorder. Caution in patients with comorbid bipolar disorder; may cause induction of mixed/manic episodes. May cause treatment-emergent psychotic or manic symptoms (eg, hallucinations, delusional thinking, mania) in children and adolescents without prior history of psychotic illness or mania at usual doses; d/c may be appropriate. Aggressive behavior or hostility reported in children with ADHD. Suppression of growth reported with long-term use in pediatric patients; monitor height and weight. May lower convulsive threshold; d/c in the presence of seizures. Difficulties in accommodation and blurring of vision reported. Monitor CBC, differential, and platelets with prolonged therapy.

ADVERSE REACTIONS: Dyspepsia, headache, anxiety. (Adults) Dry mouth, pharyngolaryngeal pain, feeling jittery, dizziness. (Pediatrics) Decreased appetite, insomnia, depression, vomiting, anorexia, irritability, nasal congestion, pruritus.

INTERACTIONS: See Contraindications. May decrease the effectiveness of drugs used to treat HTN. Caution with pressor agents. May inhibit metabolism of coumarin anticoagulants, anticonvulsants (eg, phenobarbital, phenytoin, primidone), and tricyclic drugs (eg, imipramine, clomipramine, desipramine); adjust dose. Coadministration with antacids or acid suppressants could alter the release of dexmethylphenidate. May possibly interact with venlafaxine.

PREGNANCY: Category C, caution in nursing.

MECHANISM OF ACTION: Sympathomimetic amine; CNS stimulant. Mechanism in ADHD has not been established; suspected to block reuptake of norepinephrine and dopamine into the presynaptic neuron and increase release of these monoamines into extraneuronal space.

PHARMACOKINETICS: Absorption: Absolute bioavailability (22-25%). T_{max}=1.5 hrs (first peak), 6.5 hrs (second peak). **Distribution:** Plasma protein binding (12-15%, racemic methylphenidate); V_d=2.65L/kg. **Metabolism:** De-esterification; d-ritalinic acid (metabolite). **Elimination:** Urine (90%, racemic methylphenidate); $T_{1/2}$=2-4.5 hrs (adults), 2-3 hrs (children).

NURSING CONSIDERATIONS

Assessment: Assess for marked anxiety, agitation, tension, glaucoma, tics, family history of or diagnosis of Tourette's syndrome, pre-existing psychotic disorders, seizure disorder, bipolar disorder, history of drug dependence or alcoholism, pregnancy/nursing status and for possible drug interactions. Assess for medical conditions that might be compromised by increases in BP and HR (eg, HTN, heart failure, recent MI, ventricular arrhythmia), structural cardiac abnormalities, cardiomyopathy, serious heart rhythm abnormalities, or other serious cardiac problems. Perform physical exam and obtain a medical history prior to therapy.

Monitoring: Monitor for symptoms of cardiac disease (eg, exertional chest pain, unexplained syncope), MI, stroke, exacerbations of behavioral disturbances and thought disorders, bipolar disorder, worsening of aggressive behavior or hostility, emergent psychotic or manic symptoms (eg, hallucinations, delusional thinking, mania), seizures, and for visual disturbances. During prolonged use, perform periodic monitoring of CBC, differential and platelet counts. In pediatric patients, monitor height and weight. Monitor BP and HR.

Patient Counseling: Inform about risks/benefits of therapy. Instruct to take once daily in am. Counsel to swallow capsule whole; never crush or chew. If unable to swallow, instruct to sprinkle over spoonful of applesauce and swallow without chewing. Advise to notify physician of all medications currently taking and if any adverse events develop. Instruct to read Medication Guide.

Administration: Oral route. Swallow whole or sprinkle contents on applesauce. Do not crush, chew or divide. **Storage:** 25°C (77°F), excursions permitted to 15-30°C (59-86°F).

FOLGARD RX 2.2   RX
vitamin B12 - vitamin B6 - folic acid (Upsher-Smith)

THERAPEUTIC CLASS: Folic acid/vitamin combination

INDICATIONS: For nutritional support and folic acid supplementation.

DOSAGE: *Adults:* 1 tab qd.

HOW SUPPLIED: Tab: Folic Acid 2.2mg-Vitamin B_6 25mg-Vitamin B_{12} 0.5mg*
*scored

WARNINGS/PRECAUTIONS: Folic acid >0.1mg/day may obscure pernicious anemia.

ADVERSE REACTIONS: Allergic sensitization.

PREGNANCY: Safety in pregnancy and nursing is not known.

MECHANISM OF ACTION: Folic acid/vitamin combination.

NURSING CONSIDERATIONS

Assessment: Assess for pernicious anemia.

Monitoring: Monitor hematological parameters and for hypersensitivity reactions.

Patient Counseling: Report hypersensitivity reactions.

Administration: Oral route. **Storage:** 15-30°C (59-86°F). Protect from light and moisture. Dispense in tight container with child-resistant closure.

FOLIC ACID   RX
folic acid (Various)

THERAPEUTIC CLASS: Erythropoiesis agent

INDICATIONS: Treatment of megaloblastic anemia due to folic acid deficiency and in anemias of nutritional origin, pregnancy, infancy or childhood.

DOSAGE: *Adults:* Usual: Up to 1mg/day. Maint: 0.4mg qd. Pregnancy/Nursing: Maint: 0.8mg qd. Max: 1mg/day. Increase maintenance dose with alcoholism, hemolytic anemia, anticonvulsant therapy, chronic infection.
Pediatrics: Usual: Up to 1mg/day. Maint: Infants: 0.1mg qd. <4 yrs: 0.3mg qd. ≥4 yrs: 0.4mg qd.

HOW SUPPLIED: Inj: 5mg/mL; Tab: (OTC) 0.4mg, 0.8mg, (RX) 1mg

WARNINGS/PRECAUTIONS: Not for monotherapy in pernicious anemia and other megaloblastic anemias with B_{12} deficiency. May obscure pernicious anemia in dosage >0.1mg/day. Decreased B_{12} serum levels with prolonged therapy.

F

ADVERSE REACTIONS: Allergic sensitization.

INTERACTIONS: Antagonizes phenytoin effects. Methotrexate, phenytoin, primidone, barbiturates, alcohol, alcoholic cirrhosis, nitrofurantoin, and pyrimethamine increase loss of folate. Increased seizures with phenytoin, primidone and phenobarbital reported. Tetracycline may cause false low serum and red cell folate due to suppression of *Lactobacillus casei*.

PREGNANCY: Category A, requirement increases during nursing.

MECHANISM OF ACTION: Acts as cofactor for transformylation reactions in biosynthesis of purines and thymidylates of nucleic acids; acts on megaloblastic bone marrow to produce normoblastic marrow; required for nucleoprotein synthesis and maintenance of normal erythropoiesis.

PHARMACOKINETICS: Absorption: Rapid (small intestine); T_{max}=1 hr. **Distribution:** Found in breast milk. **Metabolism:** Liver via reduced diphosphopyridine nucleotide and folate reductase. **Elimination:** Urine, feces.

NURSING CONSIDERATIONS

Assessment: Assess for alcoholism, chronic infection, and pernicious, megaloblastic, and hemolytic anemias, and for possible drug interactions.

Monitoring: Monitor for allergic/hypersensitivity reactions.

Patient Counseling: Advise to seek medical attention if symptoms of allergic/hypersensitivity reaction occurs.

Administration: Oral route. **Storage**: 20-25°C (68-77°F).

FOLOTYN RX
pralatrexate (Allos Therapeutics, Inc.)

THERAPEUTIC CLASS: Dihydrofolic acid reductase inhibitor

INDICATIONS: Treatment of patients with relapsed or refractory peripheral T-cell lymphoma (PTCL).

DOSAGE: *Adults:* Usual: 30mg/m² IV push over 3-5 min once weekly for 6 weeks in 7-week cycles until progressive disease or unacceptable toxicity. Vitamin Supplementation: Start low-dose (1.0-1.25mg) oral folic acid daily 10 days prior to 1st dose and continue during the full course of therapy and for 30 days after the last dose. Give vitamin B₁₂ (1mg) IM injection ≤10 weeks prior to 1st dose and q8-10 weeks thereafter. Subsequent vitamin B₁₂ injections may be given the same day as treatment with pralatrexate. Refer to PI for dose modifications following mucositis and hematologic/treatment-related toxicities.

HOW SUPPLIED: Inj: 20mg/mL [1mL, 2mL]

WARNINGS/PRECAUTIONS: May suppress bone marrow function, manifested by thrombocytopenia, neutropenia, and anemia. May cause mucositis; omit dose if ≥Grade 2 mucositis occurs. Dermatologic reactions reported; monitor closely and if severe, withhold or d/c therapy. Tumor lysis syndrome reported; monitor and treat for complications. Supplement with folic acid and vitamin B₁₂ to reduce treatment-related hematological toxicity and mucositis. May cause fetal harm. Caution with moderate to severe renal impairment; monitor for renal function and systemic toxicity. LFT abnormalities reported; monitor liver function.

ADVERSE REACTIONS: Mucositis, thrombocytopenia, N/V, fatigue, pyrexia, sepsis, febrile neutropenia, dehydration, dyspnea, anemia, constipation, edema, cough, epistaxis.

INTERACTIONS: Delayed clearance with increasing doses of probenecid. May delay clearance with drugs that are subject to substantial renal clearance (eg, NSAIDs, trimethoprim/sulfamethoxazole).

PREGNANCY: Category D, not for use in nursing.

MECHANISM OF ACTION: Folate analog metabolic inhibitor; competitively inhibits dihydrofolate reductase. Also a competitive inhibitor for polyglutamylation by the enzyme folylpolyglutamyl synthetase.

PHARMACOKINETICS: Distribution: V_d=105L (*S*-diastereomer), 37L (*R*-diastereomer); plasma protein binding (67%). **Elimination:** Urine (31% *S*-diastereomer, 38% *R*-diastereomer); $T_{1/2}$=12-18 hrs.

NURSING CONSIDERATIONS

Assessment: Assess renal/hepatic function, for dermatologic reactions, pregnancy/nursing status, and for possible drug interactions.

Monitoring: Monitor renal function, CBC, severity of mucositis, and LFTs. Monitor for systemic toxicity, thrombocytopenia, neutropenia, anemia, tumor lysis syndrome, and dermatologic reactions.

Patient Counseling: Instruct to take folic acid and vitamin B_{12} as a prophylactic measure to reduce possible side effects. Discuss signs and symptoms of mucositis, ways to reduce the risk of development, ways to maintain nutrition and control discomfort from mucositis if it occurs. Inform of the risk of low blood cell counts; instruct to contact physician if signs of infection, bleeding or symptoms of anemia occur. Discuss signs and symptoms of tumor lysis syndrome and instruct to notify physician if symptoms occur. Advise to inform physician if taking any concomitant medications, including prescription and OTC drugs. Inform physician if pregnant, planning to become pregnant, or if nursing. Notify physician if any untoward skin reactions occur.

Administration: IV route. Refer to PI for preparation and administration procedures. **Storage:** 2-8°C (36-46°F) in original carton to protect from light. Discard unused portion.

FOLTX   RX
vitamin B12 - vitamin B6 - folic acid (PamLab)

THERAPEUTIC CLASS: Folic acid/vitamin combination

INDICATIONS: To supply nutritional requirements for those with end stage renal failure, dialysis, hyperhomocysteinemia, homocystinuria, nutrient malabsorption.

DOSAGE: *Adults:* 1-2 tabs qd.

HOW SUPPLIED: Tab: Folic Acid 2.5mg-Vitamin B_6 25mg-Vitamin B_{12} 2mg

WARNINGS/PRECAUTIONS: Folic acid >0.1mg/day may obscure pernicious anemia (may be alleviated by B_{12} component).

ADVERSE REACTIONS: Allergic sensitization, paresthesia, somnolence, mild diarrhea, polycythemia vera, peripheral vascular thrombosis, itching, transitory exanthema, feeling of body swelling.

INTERACTIONS: Pyridoxine may antagonize levodopa; avoid concomitant use. May be used with carbidopa/levodopa. Decreases effect of phenytoin.

MECHANISM OF ACTION: Folic acid/vitamin combination.

NURSING CONSIDERATIONS

Assessment: Assess for Leber's optic atrophy, pernicious anemia, and hyperhomocysteinemia. Note other diseases/conditions and drug therapies.

Monitoring: Monitor for polycythemia vera, headache, paresthesia, and hypersensitivity reactions.

Patient Counseling: Counsel about adverse effects; immediately report if any occur. Take as directed by physician.

Administration: Oral route. **Storage:** Room temperature, 15-30°C (59-86°F). Protect from light and moisture. Dispense in original light-resistant container with child-resistant closure.

FORADIL

RX

formoterol fumarate (Schering)

Long-acting β₂-agonists (LABA), such as formoterol fumarate, may increase the risk of asthma-related death. Use for asthma without concomitant use of a long-term asthma control medication, such as an inhaled corticosteroid, is contraindicated. Do not use for patients whose asthma is adequately controlled on low- or medium-dose inhaled corticosteroids. LABAs may increase the risk of asthma-related hospitalization in pediatric and adolescent patients. For pediatric and adolescent patients with asthma who require addition of a LABA to an inhaled corticosteroid, a fixed-dose combination product containing both an inhaled corticosteroid and LABAs should be used to ensure adherence with both drugs.

THERAPEUTIC CLASS: Beta₂-agonist

INDICATIONS: Treatment of asthma and prevention of bronchospasm only as concomitant therapy with long-term asthma control medication (eg, inhaled corticosteroid) in adults and children ≥5 yrs with reversible obstructive airway disease, including nocturnal asthma. As PRN in acute prevention of exercise-induced bronchospasm (EIB) in adults and children ≥5 yrs. Long-term maintenance treatment of bronchoconstriction in chronic obstructive pulmonary disease (COPD), including chronic bronchitis and emphysema.

DOSAGE: *Adults:* Do not swallow cap; give only by inhalation with Aerolizer Inhaler. Asthma/COPD: 12mcg q12h. Max: 24mcg/day. EIB: 12mcg 15 min before exercise PRN; do not give additional doses for 12 hrs after administration or if already on q12h dose. Re-evaluate regimen if previously effective dose fails to provide usual response.
Pediatrics: ≥5 yrs: Do not swallow cap; give only by inhalation with Aerolizer Inhaler. Asthma: 12mcg q12h. Max: 24mcg/day. EIB: 12mcg 15 min before exercise PRN; do not give additional doses for 12 hrs after administration or if already on q12h dose. Re-evaluate regimen if previously effective dose fails to provide usual response.

HOW SUPPLIED: Cap, Inhalation: 12mcg [12ˢ, 60ˢ]

CONTRAINDICATIONS: Use for treatment of asthma without concomitant use of long-term asthma control medication (eg, inhaled corticosteroids).

WARNINGS/PRECAUTIONS: Has no anti-inflammatory effect and is not a substitute for corticosteroids; do not d/c or reduce inhaled corticosteroids. D/C regular use of short-acting β₂-agonist (SABA) inhaler and use only for relief of acute symptoms. D/C if paradoxical bronchospasm occurs. Deterioration of asthma may occur; monitor for signs of worsening asthma (eg, increased use of SABA, decrease in peak expiratory flow or lung function). May produce significant CV effects and ECG changes. Caution with CV disorders (eg, coronary insufficiency, HTN, arrhythmias), thyrotoxicosis, convulsive disorders, and in patients unusually responsive to sympathomimetic amines. Immediate hypersensitivity reactions (eg, anaphylactic reactions, urticaria, angioedema, rash, bronchospasm) may occur. Fatalities reported with excessive use. Not for use in acute asthmatic conditions. May cause hypokalemia and changes in blood glucose. Do not initiate in patients with significantly worsening/acutely deteriorating asthma. Contains lactose, which contains trace levels of milk protein; allergic reactions may occur in patients with severe milk protein allergy.

ADVERSE REACTIONS: Skeletal muscle tremor and cramps, insomnia, tachycardia, hypokalemia, hyperglycemia, viral infection, upper respiratory tract infection, asthma exacerbations, CV events, bronchitis, back pain, chest pain, pharyngitis, headache.

INTERACTIONS: Avoid with other LABAs. Potentiated sympathetic effects with additional adrenergic drugs. Hypokalemia potentiated with xanthine derivatives, steroids, and diuretics. Worsening of ECG changes and hypokalemia with non-potassium sparing diuretics (eg, loop, thiazide diuretics). Extreme caution with MAOIs, TCAs, and drugs known to prolong QT interval. Antagonized effect with β-blockers.

PREGNANCY: Category C, caution in nursing.

MECHANISM OF ACTION: LABA; acts as a bronchodilator, stimulates adenyl cyclase, which increases the intracellular concentration of cyclic AMP. Increased cyclic AMP levels cause relaxation of bronchial smooth muscle and inhibition of release of mediators of immediate hypersensitivity from cells, especially from mast cells.

PHARMACOKINETICS: Absorption: Rapid; C_{max}=92pg/mL, T_{max}=5 min. **Distribution:** Plasma protein binding (61-64%). **Metabolism:** Glucuronidation, O-demethylation via CYP2D6, 2C19, 2C9, 2A6. **Elimination:** With Asthma: Urine (10%, unchanged;15-18%, conjugates); COPD: Urine (7%, unchanged; 6-9%, conjugates). $T_{1/2}$=10 hrs.

NURSING CONSIDERATIONS

Assessment: Assess for CV disorders (eg, coronary insufficiency, HTN, arrhythmias), thyrotoxicosis, convulsive disorders, response to sympathomimetic amines, worsening or acutely deteriorating asthma, milk protein allergy, pregnancy/nursing status and possible drug interactions.

Monitoring: Monitor pulse rate, BP, and ECG changes, and for paradoxical bronchospasm and hypokalemia, glucose levels, hypersensitivity reactions, deterioration of asthma (eg, increased use of SABA, decrease in peak expiratory flow or lung function).

Patient Counseling: Inform that long-acting β_2-agonist may increase risk of asthma related death or hospitalization. Instruct to use with concomitant long-term asthma control medication (eg, inhaled corticosteroids) and not to use to relieve acute asthma symptoms. Seek medical attention if symptoms worsen, if treatment becomes less effective, or if they need more inhalations of SABA than usual. Do not increase dose or frequency without consulting physician and not to d/c or reduce concomitant asthma therapy without medical advice. Instruct to take 15 min before exercise for prevention of EIB. Inform that treatment may lead to palpitations, chest pain, rapid heart rate, tremor or nervousness. Inform not to use with a spacer and never to exhale into the device. Avoid exposing caps to moisture and to handle with dry hands. Advise to always use new Aerolizer Inhaler that comes with each refill. Report to physician if pregnant or nursing. Remove cap from blister immediately before use and pierce caps only once.

Administration: Oral inhalation route. 1) Pull off aerolizer inhaler cover. 2) Twist mouthpiece in the direction of the arrow to open. 3) Make sure four pins can be seen in the capsule well. 4) Place capsule in capsule chamber and twist mouthpiece back to closed position. 5) Hold mouthpiece of inhaler upright and press both buttons at the same time. Only press once. A click should be heard as the capsule is being pierced. 6) Release the button. 7) Exhale fully. 8) Place the mouthpiece in mouth and breathe in quickly and deeply. 9) Remove inhaler from mouth and hold breath as long as possible and then exhale. 10) Open the inhaler to see if any powder is still in the capsule. If drug remains, repeat steps 7-9. 11) After use, open the inhaler, remove and discard the empty capsule. Close the mouthpiece and replace the cover. **Storage:** Prior to dispensing: 2-8°C (36-46°F). After dispensing: 20-25°C (68-77°F). Protect from heat and moisture. Capsule should always be stored in blister and only removed from blister before use.

FORTAMET   RX
metformin HCl (Sciele)

THERAPEUTIC CLASS: Biguanide

INDICATIONS: Adjunct to diet and exercise, to improve glycemic control in type 2 diabetes mellitus.

DOSAGE: *Adults:* ≥17 yrs: Take with evening meal. Initial: 500-1000mg qd. With Insulin: Initial: 500mg qd. Titrate: May increase by 500mg/week. Max: 2500mg/day. Decrease insulin dose by 10-25% if FPG <120mg/dL. Elderly/Debilitated/Malnourished: Conservative dosing; do not titrate to max.

HOW SUPPLIED: Tab, Extended-Release: 500mg, 1000mg

CONTRAINDICATIONS: Renal disease/dysfunction (SrCr ≥1.5mg/dL [males], ≥1.4mg/dL [females], or abnormal CrCl), acute or chronic metabolic acidosis, including diabetic ketoacidosis. D/C temporarily (48 hrs) for radiologic studies with intravascular iodinated contrast materials.

WARNINGS/PRECAUTIONS: Lactic acidosis (rare) reported; may occur with pathophysiologic conditions, including DM, hypoperfusion, and hypoxemia. Increased risk with renal insufficiency (both intrinsic renal disease and renal hypoperfusion), CHF, and patient's age. Avoid use in patients ≥80 yrs unless renal function is not reduced. Should be promptly withheld with hypoxemia, dehydration, or sepsis. Caution against excessive alcohol intake. Lactic acidosis may be suspected in diabetic patient with metabolic acidosis lacking evidence of ketoacidosis (ketonuria and ketonemia). Immediately d/c with lactic acidosis; prompt hemodialysis is recommended to correct the acidosis and remove the accumulated metformin. Caution using concomitant medications that may affect renal function, or result in significant hemodynamic change, or interfere with the disposition of metformin (eg, cationic drugs eliminated by renal tubular secretion). Temporarily d/c prior to surgery (due to restricted food intake) and procedures requiring intravascular iodinated contrast materials. D/C in hypoxic states (eg, shock, CHF, acute MI). Avoid in patients with hepatic impairment. May decrease vitamin B_{12} levels. Increased risk of hypoglycemia in elderly, debilitated/malnourished, adrenal or pituitary insufficiency, or alcohol intoxication. If loss of glycemic control occurs due to stress, temporarily withhold metformin and administer insulin. Reinstitute metformin after acute episode is resolved.

ADVERSE REACTIONS: Infection, diarrhea, nausea, accidental injury, headache, dyspepsia, rhinitis.

INTERACTIONS: Furosemide, nifedipine, cimetidine, cationic drugs (eg, digoxin, amiloride, procainamide, quinidine, quinine, ranitidine, trimethoprim, vancomycin, triamterene, morphine) may increase metformin levels. Thiazides, other diuretics, corticosteroids, phenothiazines, thyroid products, estrogens, oral contraceptives, phenytoin, nicotinic acid, sympathomimetics, CCBs, and isoniazid may cause hyperglycemia. Risk of hypoglycemia with alcohol. Excess alcohol may increase potential for lactic acidosis. May decrease furosemide levels.

PREGNANCY: Category B, not for use in pregnancy or nursing.

MECHANISM OF ACTION: Biguanide; decreases hepatic glucose production, decreases intestinal absorption of glucose, and improves insulin sensitivity by increasing peripheral glucose uptake and utilization.

PHARMACOKINETICS: Absorption: C_{max}=2849ng/mL, T_{max}=6 hrs, AUC=26811ng•hr/mL. **Elimination:** Urine (90%); $T_{1/2}$=6.2 hrs (plasma), 17.6 hrs (blood).

NURSING CONSIDERATIONS

Assessment: Assess for renal FPG, HbA1c, renal function, LFTs, and CBC. Assess for CHF, septicemia, acute or chronic metabolic acidosis, adrenal or pituitary insufficiency, alcoholism, pregnancy status. Evaluate for other medical/surgical conditions and for possible drug interactions.

Monitoring: Monitor for infection, diarrhea, nausea, accidental injury, headache, dyspepsia, and rhinitis.

Patient Counseling: Inform of the potential risks and benefits and of alternative modes of therapy. Inform drug is adjunct to diet and exercise, and necessity of regular testing of blood glucose, glycosylated hemoglobin, renal function, and hematologic parameters. Temporarily d/c therapy prior to intravascular radiocontrast study or surgery. Report unexplained hyperventilation, myalgia, malaise, unusual somnolence, or other nonspecific symptoms. Counsel patient to avoid excessive alcohol intake, either acute or chronic. Drug alone does not cause hypoglycemia but can occur in conjunction with oral sulfonylureas and insulin. Instruct drug must be swallowed whole with a full glass of water and should not be chewed, cut, or crushed. Inactive ingredients may be eliminated in the feces as a soft mass.

Administration: Oral route. Must swallow whole with a full glass of water; do not crush or chew. **Storage:** 20-25°C (68-77°F); excursions permitted to 15-30°C (59-86°F). Keep tightly closed. Protect from light.

FORTAZ

RX

ceftazidime (GlaxoSmithKline)

THERAPEUTIC CLASS: Cephalosporin (3rd generation)

INDICATIONS: Treatment of lower respiratory tract (eg, pneumonia), skin and skin structure (SSSI), bone/joint, gynecologic, CNS (eg, meningitis), intra-abdominal, and urinary tract infections (UTI); and septicemia caused by susceptible strains of microorganisms. Treatment of sepsis.

DOSAGE: *Adults:* Usual: 1g IM/IV q8-12h. Uncomplicated UTI: 250mg IM/IV q12h. Complicated UTI: 500mg IM/IV q8-12h. Bone and Joint Infection: 2g IV q12h. Uncomplicated Pneumonia/SSSI: 500mg-1g IM/IV q8h. Gynecological/Intra-Abdominal/Meningitis/Severe Life-Threatening Infection: 2g IV q8h. Lung Infection Caused by *Pseudomonas* spp. in Cystic Fibrosis (Normal Renal Function): 30-50mg/kg IV q8h. Max: 6g/day. CrCl 31-50mL/min: 1g q12h. CrCl 16-30mL/min: 1g q24h. CrCl 6-15mL/min: 500mg q24h. CrCl <5mL/min: 500mg q48h. For severe infections (6g/day), increase renal impairment dose by 50% or increase dosing interval. Apply reduced dosage recommendations after initial 1g LD is given. Hemodialysis: Give 1g before, then 1g after each hemodialysis. Intra-Peritoneal Dialysis/Continuous Ambulatory Peritoneal Dialysis: Give 1g followed by 500mg q24h, or add to fluid at 250mg/2L. *Pediatrics:* 1 month-12 yrs: 30-50mg/kg IV q8h. Max: 6g/day. Neonates (0-4 weeks): 30mg/kg IV q12h. Higher doses for cystic fibrosis or meningitis. CrCl 31-50mL/min: 1g q12h. CrCl 16-30mL/min: 1g q24h. CrCl 6-15mL/min: 500mg q24h. CrCl <5mL/min: 500mg q48h. For severe infections (6g/day), increase renal impairment dose by 50% or increase dosing interval. Apply reduced dosage recommendations after initial 1g LD is given. Hemodialysis: Give 1g before, then 1g after each hemodialysis. Intra-Peritoneal Dialysis/Continuous Ambulatory Peritoneal Dialysis: Give 1g followed by 500mg q24h, or add to fluid at 250mg/2L.

HOW SUPPLIED: Inj: 500mg, 1g, 1g/50mL, 2g, 2g/50mL, 6g

WARNINGS/PRECAUTIONS: Monitor renal function; potential for nephrotoxicity. Prolonged use may result in overgrowth of nonsusceptible organisms. Possible cross-sensitivity between PCNs, cephalosporins, and other β-lactam antibiotics. *Clostridium difficile*-associated diarrhea (CDAD) reported and may range in severity from mild diarrhea to fatal colitis. Elevated levels with renal insufficiency can lead to seizures, encephalopathy, coma, asterixis, and neuromuscular excitability. Possible decrease in PT; caution with renal/hepatic impairment, poor nutritional state; monitor PT and give vitamin K if needed. Caution with colitis, other GI diseases, and elderly. Distal necrosis may occur after inadvertent intra-arterial administration. Continue therapy for 2 days after the signs and symptoms of infection have disappeared, but in complicated infections longer therapy may be required. False (+) for urine glucose with Benedict's solution, Fehling's solution, and Clinitest tabs.

ADVERSE REACTIONS: Phlebitis and inflammation at injection site, pruritus, rash, fever, diarrhea.

INTERACTIONS: Nephrotoxicity reported with aminoglycosides or potent diuretics (eg, furosemide). Avoid with chloramphenicol; may decrease effect of β-lactam antibiotics. Possible decrease in PT; caution with a protracted course of antimicrobial therapy; monitor PT and give vitamin K if needed. May reduce efficacy of oral contraceptives.

PREGNANCY: Category B, caution in nursing.

MECHANISM OF ACTION: 3rd-generation cephalosporin; bactericidal, inhibits cell-wall synthesis.

PHARMACOKINETICS: Absorption: (IV) Administration of variable doses resulted in different parameters. **Distribution:** Plasma protein binding (≤10%). **Elimination:** Urine (unchanged, 80-90%).

NURSING CONSIDERATIONS

Assessment: Assess for history of hypersensitivity to cephalosporins/PCNs, pregnancy status, possible drug interactions, renal impairment. Document indications for therapy, culture and susceptibility testing. Incision and drainage should be performed in conjunction with antibiotic therapy when indicated.

Monitoring: Monitor for signs and symptoms of hypersensitivity reactions (anaphylaxis), CDAD, seizures, LDH, LFTs, renal function, PT, hemolytic anemia, superinfection.

Patient Counseling: Inform therapy only treats bacterial, not viral, infections. Take exactly as directed; skipping doses or not completing full course may decrease effectiveness and increase resistance. May experience diarrhea; notify physician if watery/bloody stools, superinfection, or hypersensitivity reactions occur.

Administration: IM/IV route. For direct intermittent IV administration, slowly inject into vein over period of 3-5 min or give through tubing of administration set while patient also receives compatible IV fluid. **Storage:** In dry state, store between 15-30°C (59-86°F) and protect from light. Frozen as premixed solution should not be stored above -20°C.

FORTEO   RX
teriparatide (Lilly)

> Only prescribe when benefits outweigh risks. Not for those at increased baseline risk for osteosarcoma, including Paget's disease, unexplained alkaline phosphatase elevations, open epiphyses (pediatric and young adults), or prior external beam or implant radiation therapy involving the skeleton.

THERAPEUTIC CLASS: Recombinant human parathyroid hormone

INDICATIONS: Treatment of postmenopausal women with osteoporosis at high risk for fracture. To increase bone mass in men with primary or hypogonadal osteoporosis at high risk for fracture. Treatment of men and women with glucocorticoid-induced osteoporosis at high risk for fracture.

DOSAGE: *Adults:* 20mcg qd SQ into thigh or abdominal wall. Administer initially under circumstances where patient can sit or lie down if symptoms of orthostatic hypotension occur.

HOW SUPPLIED: Inj: 250mcg/mL [2.4mL, 3mL] [prefilled pen]

WARNINGS/PRECAUTIONS: Avoid in patient with bone metastases or history of skeletal malignancies, metabolic bone diseases other than osteoporosis, or pre-existing hypercalcemia (eg, primary hyperparathyroidism). Potential exacerbation of active or recent urolithiasis. Caution with active urolithiasis or pre-existing hypercalciuria; consider measuring urinary calcium excretion. May transiently increase serum calcium levels. Transient episodes of symptomatic orthostatic hypotension reported within 1st few doses. Use for >2 years is not recommended.

ADVERSE REACTIONS: Pain, arthralgia, asthenia, N/V, rhinitis, dizziness, headache, HTN, increased cough, pharyngitis, constipation, diarrhea, dyspepsia, gastritis, insomnia.

INTERACTIONS: Hypercalcemia may predispose to digitalis toxicity; caution with concomitant use of digoxin. Coadministration of IV furosemide (20-100mg) resulted in small increases in serum calcium (2%) and 24-hr urine calcium (37%).

PREGNANCY: Category C, not for use in nursing.

MECHANISM OF ACTION: Recombinant human parathyroid hormone; binds to specific high-affinity cell-surface receptors. Stimulates new bone formation on trabecular and cortical bone surfaces by preferential stimulation of osteoblastic activity over osteoclastic activity. Produces an increase in skeletal mass, markers of bone formation and resorption, and bone strength.

PHARMACOKINETICS: Absorption: Rapid; absolute bioavailability (95%); T_{max}=30 min. **Distribution:** (IV) V_d=0.12L/kg. **Metabolism:** Liver (nonspecific enzymatic mechanism). **Elimination:** Kidney. (IV) $T_{1/2}$=5 min; (SQ) $T_{1/2}$=1 hr.

NURSING CONSIDERATIONS

Assessment: Assess for risk factors for developing osteosarcoma (eg, Paget's disease of bone, unexplained alkaline phosphatase elevations, age of patient and open epiphyses, prior external beam or implant radiation therapy), bone metastases or history of skeletal malignancies, metabolic bone disease other than osteoporosis, pre-existing hypercalcemia or presence of hypercalcemic disorder (eg, primary hyperparathyroidism), pre-existing hypercalciuria, active or recent urolithiasis, hypersensitivity, pregnancy/nursing status, and for possible drug interactions. If active urolithiasis or hypercalciuria is present, measure urinary calcium excretion.

Monitoring: Monitor for signs/symptoms of osteosarcoma, orthostatic hypotension, hypercalcemia (eg, N/V, constipation, muscle weakness) and other adverse events that may occur.

Patient Counseling: Inform about benefits and risks of therapy. Counsel to sit or lie down if lightheadedness or palpitations following injection develop; if symptoms persist or worsen, advise to contact physician before continuing treatment. Inform physician if signs of hypercalcemia (eg, N/V, constipation, lethargy, muscle weakness) occur. Instruct on proper use of device, proper disposal of needles, not to share injection pens, and to discard pen after 28 days of use. Counsel on roles of supplemental calcium and/or vitamin D, weight-bearing exercise, and behavior modification factors (eg, smoking/alcohol use). Encourage to enroll in the voluntary Forteo patient registry and read medication guide and injection pen user manual before starting therapy and each time the prescription is renewed.

Administration: SQ route. Inject into thigh or abdominal wall. Inspect for particulate matter and discoloration. Avoid use if particles seen or if cloudy or colored. **Storage:** 2-8°C (36-46°F). Recap pen when not in use. Minimize time out of refrigerator. Do not freeze; do not use if frozen.

FORTESTA GEL `CIII`
testosterone (Endo)

> Virilization reported in children secondarily exposed to testosterone gel. Children should avoid contact with unwashed or unclothed application sites in men using testosterone gel. Advise patients to strictly adhere to recommended instructions for use.

THERAPEUTIC CLASS: Androgen

INDICATIONS: Replacement therapy in males for conditions associated with a deficiency or absence of endogenous testosterone (congenital or acquired primary hypogonadism or hypogonadotropic hypogonadism).

DOSAGE: *Adults:* Initial: Apply 40mg (4 pump actuations) qam to intact skin of the thighs. May adjust between 10-70mg based on serum testosterone concentration from a single blood draw 2 hrs after application, 14 days, and 35 days after starting treatment or following dose adjustment. Max: 70mg. Total Serum Testosterone Concentration: ≥2500ng/dL: Decrease daily dose by 20mg (2 pump actuations). ≥1250-<2500ng/dL: Decrease daily dose by 10mg (1 pump actuation). ≥500-<1250ng/dL: Continue on current dose. <500ng/dL: Increase daily dose by 10mg (1 pump actuation).

HOW SUPPLIED: Gel: 10mg/actuation [60g]

CONTRAINDICATIONS: Prostate or breast carcinoma in men, women who are or may become pregnant, or nursing mothers.

WARNINGS/PRECAUTIONS: Application site and dose are not interchangeable with other topical testosterone products. Patients with BPH may be at increased risk for worsening of signs/symptoms of BPH. May increase risk for prostate cancer; evaluate for prostate cancer prior to and during therapy. Risk of virilization in women and children due to secondary exposure; d/c until cause of virilization is identified. Increases in Hct and red blood cell mass may increase risk for thromboembolic events; may require reduction or d/c of drug. Suppression of spermatogenesis may occur. Prolonged use may cause serious hepatic effects (eg, peliosis hepatis, hepatic neoplasms, cholestatic hepatitis, jaundice). Risk of edema with or without CHF with pre-existing cardiac, renal, or hepatic disease. Gynecomastia may develop and persist. May potentiate sleep apnea, especially with obesity or chronic lung diseases. Changes in serum lipid profile reported. Caution in cancer patients at risk of hypercalcemia and associated hypercalciuria. May decrease concentrations of thyroxin-binding globulins, resulting in decreased total T4 serum concentrations and increased resin uptake of T3 and T4. Gel is flammable; avoid fire, flame, or smoking until dry.

ADVERSE REACTIONS: Application-site reactions, prostatic-specific antigen (PSA) increased, abnormal dreams.

INTERACTIONS: Changes in insulin sensitivity or glycemic control reported. Concurrent use with adrenocorticotrophic hormone (ACTH) or corticosteroids may increase fluid retention. Changes in anticoagulant activity may occur; frequently monitor INR and PT in patients taking anticoagulants.

PREGNANCY: Category X, contraindicated in nursing.

MECHANISM OF ACTION: Androgen; responsible for normal growth and development of male sex organs and for maintenance of secondary sex characteristics.

PHARMACOKINETICS: Metabolism: Estradiol and DHT (active metabolites). **Elimination:** (IM) Urine (90% glucuronic and sulfuric acid conjugates), feces (6% unconjugated); $T_{1/2}$=10-100 min.

NURSING CONSIDERATIONS

Assessment: Assess for conditions where treatment is contraindicated, BPH, cardiac/renal/hepatic disease, obesity, chronic lung disease, and for possible drug interactions. Assess use in cancer patients at risk of hypercalcemia. Obtain baseline Hct.

Monitoring: Monitor for prostate carcinoma, hepatic toxicity, edema with or without CHF, gynecomastia, and sleep apnea. In patients with BPH, monitor for signs/symptoms of worsening BPH. Perform periodic monitoring of Hgb, Hct, PSA, serum lipid profile, LFTs, and serum testosterone levels. In cancer patients at risk for hypercalcemia, regularly monitor serum Ca^{2+} levels.

Patient Counseling: Inform that men with known or suspected prostate/breast cancer should not use androgen therapy. Report signs/symptoms of secondary exposure in children (eg, penis/clitoris enlargement, premature development of pubic hair, increased erections) and in women (eg, changes in hair distribution, increase in acne). Advise family members to avoid contact with unwashed or unclothed application site of men. Apply product as directed: wash hands with soap and water after application, cover application site with clothing after gel dries, and wash application site with soap and water prior to direct skin-to-skin contact with others. Inform about possible adverse reactions. Advise to read the Medication Guide prior to therapy and reread each time prescription is renewed. Inform that drug is flammable until dry. Keep out of reach of children.

Administration: Topical route. Prime the canister pump in upright position, slowly and fully depress the actuator eight times. Refer to PI for administration details. **Storage:** 20-25°C (68-77°F); excursions permitted to 15-30°C (59-86°F). Do not freeze.

FORTICAL   RX
calcitonin-salmon (rdna origin) (Upsher-Smith)

THERAPEUTIC CLASS: Hormonal bone resorption inhibitor

INDICATIONS: Treatment of postmenopausal osteoporosis in women >5 yrs postmenopause with low bone mass relative to healthy postmenopausal women; recommended in conjunction with an adequate calcium and vitamin D intake.

DOSAGE: *Adults:* 200 IU qd intranasally. Alternate nostrils daily.

HOW SUPPLIED: Nasal Spray: 200 IU/activation

WARNINGS/PRECAUTIONS: Possibility of systemic allergic reactions (eg, anaphylaxis, anaphylactic shock). Allergic reactions should be differentiated from generalized flushing and hypotension. Consider skin testing if sensitivity suspected. Development of mucosal alterations or transient nasal conditions reported; perform periodic nasal exams. Rhinitis, epistaxis, sinusitis most commonly reported in postmenopausal patients. D/C if severe ulceration of nasal mucosa occurs (indicated by ulcers >1.5mm diameter or penetrating below mucosa, or associated with heavy bleeding). Incidence of rhinitis, irritation, erythema, and excoriation higher in geriatric patients.

ADVERSE REACTIONS: Rhinitis, nasal symptoms, back pain, arthralgia, epistaxis, headache, influenza-like symptoms, fatigue, erythematous rash, arthrosis, myalgia, sinusitis, bronchospasm, HTN, constipation.

INTERACTIONS: May reduce lithium levels; dose of lithium may need to be adjusted. Prior diphosphonate use appears to reduce the anti-resorptive response to calcitonin-salmon nasal spray in patients with Paget's disease.

PREGNANCY: Category C, not for use in nursing.

MECHANISM OF ACTION: Hormonal bone resorption inhibitor; actions on bone not fully established. Calcitonin receptors have been found in osteoclasts and osteoblasts. Initially causes a marked transient inhibition of the ongoing bone resorptive process. Prolonged use causes a smaller decrease in the rate of bone resorption. Associated with inhibition of osteoclast function and increased osteoblastic activity.

PHARMACOKINETICS: Absorption: T_{max}=13 min; Bioavailability (3%). **Elimination:** $T_{1/2}$=18 min.

NURSING CONSIDERATIONS

Assessment: Assess for previous allergy to calcitonin-salmon; perform skin testing if sensitivity suspected. Assess for pregnancy/nursing status and for possible drug interactions. Perform nasal and bone mineral density examination prior to treatment. Assess patient's intake of calcium and vitamin D and recommend adequate intake (at least 1000mg/day elemental calcium and 400 IU/day vitamin D) to retard progressive loss of bone mass.

Monitoring: Monitor for signs/symptoms of allergic reaction (eg, anaphylactic shock, anaphylaxis), nasal mucosal alterations, rhinitis, epistaxis, and sinusitis. Perform periodic nasal exams of nasal mucosa, turbinates, septum, and mucosal blood vessels. Perform periodic monitoring of urine sediment. Measure lumbar vertebral bone mass periodically to monitor for efficacy.

Patient Counseling: Counsel to notify physician of significant nasal irritation. Advise to seek emergency help if serious allergic reaction occurs (eg, troubled breathing, swelling of face, throat or tongue, rapid heartbeat, chest pain, feeling faint or dizzy). Advise to store new, unassembled medication in refrigerator away from light, and not to freeze. Instruct that before priming pump and using new medication, allow to reach room temperature. Inform that after opening, store at room temperature, in upright position; discard unused medication 30 days after 1st use. Recommend adequate intake of calcium and vitamin D.

Administration: Intranasal route. To prime pump, hold bottle upright and depress the 2 white side arms of pump toward the bottle at least 5X until a full spray is produced. To administer, carefully place the nozzle into the nostril with the head in upright position and pump firmly depressed toward the bottle. Do not prime pump before each daily use. **Storage:** Unopened: 2-8°C (36-46°F). Protect from freezing. Opened: 20-25°C (68-77°F); excursions permitted to 15-30°C (59-86°F). Store in upright position. Discard 30 days after 1st use.

FOSAMAX   RX
alendronate sodium (Merck)

THERAPEUTIC CLASS: Bisphosphonate

INDICATIONS: Treatment and prevention of osteoporosis in postmenopausal women. Treatment to increase bone mass in men with osteoporosis. Treatment of glucocorticoid-induced osteoporosis. Treatment of Paget's disease.

DOSAGE: *Adults:* Osteoporosis: Treatment: 70mg once weekly or 10mg qd. Prevention: 35mg once weekly or 5mg qd. Glucocorticoid-Induced: 5mg qd; 10mg qd for postmenopausal women not on estrogen. Paget's Disease: 40mg qd for 6 months. Take ≥30 min before the 1st food, beverage (other than plain water), or other medication. Take tabs with 6-8 oz. of plain water. Follow oral sol with 2 oz. of plain water. Do not lie down for ≥30 minutes and until after 1st food of the day.

HOW SUPPLIED: Sol: 70mg [75mL]; Tab: 5mg, 10mg, 35mg, 40mg, 70mg

CONTRAINDICATIONS: Esophageal abnormalities that delay esophageal emptying (eg, stricture or achalasia); inability to stand or sit upright for ≥30 min; hypocalcemia. Patients at increased risk of aspiration (oral sol).

WARNINGS/PRECAUTIONS: Not recommended with severe renal insufficiency (CrCl <35mL/min). May cause local irritation of the upper GI mucosa; caution with active upper GI problems (eg, Barrett's esophagus, dysphagia, esophageal diseases, gastritis, duodenitis, ulcers). Esophageal adverse events and gastric and duodenal ulcers reported. D/C if dysphagia, odynophagia, retrosternal pain, new or worsening heartburn develops. Supervise therapy in those who cannot comply with dosing instructions due to mental disability. Treat hypocalcemia or other mineral metabolism disorders prior to therapy; hypocalcemia reported; ensure adequate calcium and vitamin D intake. Severe, incapacitating bone, joint, and/or muscle pain reported; d/c if severe symptoms develop. Osteonecrosis of the jaw (ONJ) reported; d/c to reduce risk of ONJ in patients requiring invasive dental procedures. Atypical, low-energy, or low trauma fractures of the femoral shaft reported; consider interrupting therapy. In patients with glucocorticoid-induced osteoporosis, ascertain hormonal status and consider replacement therapy; measure bone mineral density (BMD) at initiation and repeat after 6-12 months after combined alendronate and glucocorticoid treatment.

ADVERSE REACTIONS: Nausea, abdominal pain, musculoskeletal pain (bone, muscle, or joint), acid regurgitation, flatulence, dyspepsia, constipation, diarrhea, dyspepsia.

INTERACTIONS: Calcium supplements and other multivalent cations, antacids, and some oral medications will interfere with absorption; take ≥1/2 hour after alendronate. Increased GI irritation with aspirin-containing products and alendronate >10mg. Caution with NSAID use due to associated GI irritation. Concomitant use with IV ranitidine may double bioavailability of oral alendronate. Concomitant use with hormone replacement therapy (eg, estrogen ± progestin) may lead to a greater degree of suppression of bone turnover. Increased oral bioavailability with oral prednisone. May increase risk of atypical femur fractures with glucocorticoids (eg, prednisone). Caution with risk factors for ONJ (eg, chemotherapy, corticosteroids). Reduced bioavailability with concomitant coffee or orange juice.

PREGNANCY: Category C, caution in nursing.

MECHANISM OF ACTION: Bisphosphonate; binds to hydroxyapatite found in bone, specifically inhibits the osteoclast-mediated bone resorption.

PHARMACOKINETICS: Absorption: Absolute bioavailability: Women (0.64%), men (0.59%). **Distribution:** V_d=28L; plasma protein binding (78%). **Elimination:** (IV) Urine (50%), feces (little or none); $T_{1/2}$>10 yrs.

NURSING CONSIDERATIONS

Assessment: Assess for esophageal abnormalities, ability to stand or sit upright for ≥30 min, hypocalcemia, active upper GI problems, mineral metabolism disorders, risk factors (invasive dental procedures, diagnosed cancer, chemotherapy, corticosteroids, poor oral hygiene, co-morbid disorders) of ONJ, renal impairment (eg, CrCl <35mL/min), hypersensitivity, pregnancy/nursing status, and possible drug interactions. Obtain BMD if taking glucocorticoids. Assess for risk of aspiration if using oral sol.

Monitoring: Monitor for signs/symptoms of ONJ, atypical fracture, esophageal reactions, musculoskeletal pain, hypocalcemia, mineral metabolism disorders. Monitor serum alkaline phosphatase especially in patients with Paget's disease and BMD q6-12 months if taking glucocorticoids.

Patient Counseling: Inform about risks and benefits of therapy and to read Medication Guide. Instruct to take supplemental calcium and vitamin D if dietary intake is inadequate. Counsel to consider weight-bearing exercise, modifying behavioral factors (eg, cigarette smoking, excessive alcohol use), to take medication with plain water in the am ≥30 min before the 1st food, beverage, or medication, and to swallow each tab with a full glass of water (6-8 oz.). If taking oral sol, advise to take ≥2 oz. of water after administration. Instruct to avoid chewing or sucking on tab, taking at hs or before arising for the day, and lying down for ≥30 min following administration and until after 1st food of the day. Advise to d/c and contact physician if symptoms of esophageal disease develop. Instruct to take the following am if dose is missed and return to taking dose on regularly scheduled day; avoid taking 2 doses at the same time.

Administration: Oral route. Refer to PI for proper administration. **Storage:** Tab: 15-30°C (59-86°F). Store in a well-closed container. Oral sol: 25°C (77°F); excursions permitted to 15-30°C (59-86°F). Do not freeze.

FOSAMAX PLUS D   RX
alendronate sodium - cholecalciferol (Merck)

THERAPEUTIC CLASS: Bisphosphonate/vitamin D analog.

INDICATIONS: Treatment of osteoporosis in postmenopausal women. Treatment to increase bone mass in men with osteoporosis.

DOSAGE: *Adults:* 1 tab (70mg/5600 IU or 70mg/2800 IU) once weekly. Usual: 70mg/5600 IU once weekly. Take with 6-8 oz. of plain water ≥30 min before the 1st food, beverage, or other medication. Do not lie down for ≥30 min and until after 1st food of the day.

HOW SUPPLIED: Tab: (Alendronate Sodium-Cholecalciferol) 70mg-2800 IU, 70mg-5600 IU

CONTRAINDICATIONS: Esophageal abnormalities that delay esophageal emptying (eg, stricture or achalasia), inability to stand or sit upright for ≥30 min, hypocalcemia.

WARNINGS/PRECAUTIONS: Not recommended with severe renal insufficiency (CrCl <35mL/min). May cause local irritation of the upper GI mucosa; caution with upper GI problems (eg, Barrett's esophagus, dysphagia, esophageal diseases, gastritis, duodenitis, ulcers). Esophageal adverse events and gastric and duodenal ulcers reported. D/C if dysphagia, odynophagia, retrosternal pain, new or worsening heartburn develops. Supervise therapy in those who cannot comply with dosing instructions due to mental disability. Treat hypocalcemia or other mineral metabolism disorders prior to therapy; hypocalcemia reported. Should not be used to treat vitamin D deficiency alone. Vitamin D_3 supplementation may worsen hypercalcemia and/or hypercalciuria in patients with disease associated with unregulated overproduction of 1,25-dihydroxyvitamin D (eg, leukemia, lymphoma, sarcoidosis); monitor urine and serum calcium. Severe, incapacitating bone, joint, and/or muscle pain reported; d/c if severe symptoms develop. Osteonecrosis of the jaw (ONJ) reported; d/c to reduce risk of ONJ in patients requiring invasive dental procedures. Atypical, low-energy, or low trauma fractures of the femoral shaft reported; consider interrupting therapy.

ADVERSE REACTIONS: Nausea, abdominal pain, musculoskeletal pain (bone, muscle, or joint), acid regurgitation, flatulence, dyspepsia, constipation, diarrhea, dyspepsia.

INTERACTIONS: Alendronate: Calcium supplements and other multivalent cations, antacids, other oral medications may interfere with absorption; take ≥1/2 hour after alendronate. Increased GI irritation with aspirin-containing products and alendronate >10mg. Caution with NSAID use due to associated GI irritation. Concomitant use with IV ranitidine may double bioavailability of oral alendronate. May increase oral bioavailability with oral prednisone.

May increase risk of atypical femur fractures with glucocorticoids (eg, prednisone). Caution with risk factors for ONJ (eg, chemotherapy, corticosteroids). Reduced bioavailability with concomitant coffee or orange juice. Cholecalciferol: Olestra, mineral oils, orlistat, bile acid sequestrants (eg, cholestyramine, colestipol) may impair absorption of vitamin D; consider additional supplementation. Anticonvulsants, cimetidine, and thiazides may increase catabolism of vitamin D; consider additional supplementation.

PREGNANCY: Category C, caution in nursing.

MECHANISM OF ACTION: Alendronate: Bisphosphonate; binds to bone hydroxyapatite, specifically inhibits the osteoclast-mediated bone resorption. Cholecalciferol: Vitamin D analog; increases intestinal absorption of calcium and phosphate. Regulates excretion of serum calcium, renal calcium and phosphate, bone formation, and bone resorption.

PHARMACOKINETICS: Absorption: Alendronate: Absolute bioavailability: women (0.64%), men (0.59%). Cholecalciferol: C_{max}=4.0ng/mL; T_{max}=10.6 hrs; AUC=120.7ng•hr/mL. **Distribution:** Alendronate: V_d= ≥28L; plasma protein binding (78%). Cholecalciferol: Found in breast milk. **Metabolism:** Cholecalciferol: Liver (rapid) via hydroxylation to 25-hydroxyvitamin D_3; subsequently metabolized in kidney to 1,25-dihydroxyvitamin D_3 (active metabolite). **Elimination:** Alendronate (IV): Urine (50%), feces (little or none); $T_{1/2}$=>10 yrs. Cholecalciferol (IV): Urine (2.4%), feces (4.9%); $T_{1/2}$=14 hrs.

NURSING CONSIDERATIONS

Assessment: Assess for esophageal abnormalities, ability to stand or sit upright for ≥30 min, hypocalcemia, active upper GI problems, mineral metabolism disorders, risk factors (invasive dental procedures, diagnosed cancer, chemotherapy, corticosteroids, poor oral hygiene, co-morbid disorders) of ONJ, renal impairment (eg, CrCl <35mL/min), hypersensitivity, pregnancy/nursing status, and possible drug interactions.

Monitoring: Monitor for signs/symptoms of ONJ, atypical fracture, esophageal reactions, musculoskeletal pain, hypocalcemia, mineral metabolism disorders, and diseases associated with unregulated overproduction of 1,25 dihydroxyvitamin D. Monitor urinalysis, serum calcium, and renal function.

Patient Counseling: Inform about risks and benefits of therapy and to read Medication Guide. Instruct to take supplemental calcium and vitamin D if dietary intake is inadequate. Counsel to consider weight-bearing exercise, modifying behavioral factors (eg, cigarette smoking, excessive alcohol use), to take medication with plain water in the am ≥30 min before the 1st food, beverage, or medication, and to swallow each tab with a full glass of water (6-8 oz.). Instruct to avoid chewing or sucking on tab, taking at hs or before arising for the day, and lying down for ≥30 min following administration and until after 1st food of the day. Advise to d/c and contact physician if symptoms of esophageal disease develop. Instruct to take the following am if dose is missed and return to taking dose on regularly scheduled day; avoid taking 2 doses at the same time.

Administration: Oral route. **Storage:** 20-25°C (68-77°F); excursions permitted to 15-30°C (59-86°F). Protect from moisture and light. Store in original package until use.

FOSINOPRIL/HCTZ RX

fosinopril sodium - hydrochlorothiazide (Various)

> ACE inhibitors can cause injury/death to developing fetus during 2nd and 3rd trimesters. D/C therapy if pregnancy detected.

THERAPEUTIC CLASS: ACE inhibitor/thiazide diuretic

INDICATIONS: Treatment of hypertension.

DOSAGE: *Adults:* Not Controlled with Fosinopril/HCTZ monotherapy: 10mg-12.5mg tab or 20mg-12.5mg tab qd.

HOW SUPPLIED: Tab: (Fosinopril-HCTZ) 10mg-12.5mg, 20mg-12.5mg

CONTRAINDICATIONS: Anuric patients and hypersensitivity to other sulfon-amide-derived drugs.

WARNINGS/PRECAUTIONS: Angioedema involving the face, extremities, lips, tongue, glottis, larynx and intestines reported; d/c if laryngeal stridor or angioedema of the face, tongue or glottis occur. Anaphylactoid reactions during desensitization and during membrane exposure reported. Can cause symptomatic hypotension; most likely to occur in volume- and/or salt-depleted patients and patients undergoing surgery or during anesthesia with agents that produce hypotension. Correct volume and/or salt depletion prior to therapy. Enhanced effects with postsympathectomy patients. May cause changes in renal function (eg, increase SrCr, BUN, azotemia); caution in patients with severe congestive heart failure (CHF), severe renal disease, renal artery stenosis, or pre-existing renal impairment. Associated with neutropenia/agranulocytosis; monitor WBC in patients with collagen-vascular disease and impaired renal function. Rarely, associated with syndrome that starts with cholestatic jaundice and progresses to fulminant necrosis and sometimes death; d/c if experience jaundice or marked elevations of hepatic enzymes. Caution in patients with impaired hepatic function or progressive liver disease. May exacerbate or activate systemic lupus erythematosus (SLE). Monitor electrolytes to detect possible electrolyte imbalance. Dilutional hyponatremia may occur in edematous patients. May cause hypercalcemia, hypophosphatemia, hypomagnesemia, reduce glucose tolerance and raise serum levels of cholesterol, TG and uric acid. Persistent nonproductive cough reported. Avoid if CrCl ≤30mL/min/1.73m^2.

ADVERSE REACTIONS: Headache, cough, fatigue, dizziness.

INTERACTIONS: Caution with other antihypertensives. May alter insulin requirements. Nitritoid reactions (eg, facial flushing, N/V, hypotension) reported rarely with injectable gold. Increased risk of lithium toxicity. Fosinopril: Increased risk of hyperkalemia with K$^+$-sparing diuretics, K$^+$supplements, or K$^+$-containing salt substitutes. Antacids may impair absorption; separate dose by 2 hrs. HCTZ: Potentiate effects of ganglionic or peripheral adrenergic-blocking agents. May decrease effects of methenamine. May increase responsiveness to tubocurarine. May decrease arterial responsiveness to norepinephrine. NSAIDs decrease diuretic, natriuretic, and antihypertensive effects. Potentiates orthostatic hypotension with alcohol, barbiturates, and narcotics. Reduced absorption with cholestyramine, colestipol. Increase risk of hypokalemia with corticosteroids and ACTH.

PREGNANCY: Category C (1st trimester) and D (2nd and 3rd trimesters), not for use in nursing.

MECHANISM OF ACTION: Fosinopril: ACE inhibitor; inhibition results in decreased plasma angiotensin II, which leads to decreased vasopressor activity and decreased aldosterone secretion. HCTZ: Thiazide diuretic; affects renal tubular mechanism of electrolyte reabsorption directly increasing excretion of Na$^+$ and Cl$^-$.

PHARMACOKINETICS: Absorption: Fosinoprilat: T_{max}=3 hrs; HCTZ: T_{max}=1-2.5 hrs. **Distribution:** Fosinopril: Found in breast milk. Fosinoprilat: Plasma protein binding (95%). HCTZ: V_d=3.6-7.8L/kg; plasma protein binding (67.9%), crosses placenta. **Metabolism:** Fosinopril: Hepatic, glucuronidation; fosinoprilat (active metabolite). **Elimination:** Fosinoprilat: Urine, feces, $T_{1/2}$=11.5 hrs. HCTZ: Renal; $T_{1/2}$=5-15 hrs.

NURSING CONSIDERATIONS

Assessment: Assess for anuria, history of allergy to sulfonamides, salt- and/or volume-depletion due to prolonged diuretic therapy, dietary salt restriction, diarrhea, vomiting, pre-existing CHF, renal disease, collagen-vascular disease, SLE, impaired hepatic function or progressive liver disease, severe renal disease, renal artery stenosis, and pre-existing renal vascular disease, pregnancy/nursing status and for possible drug interactions. Obtain baseline electrolytes (eg, K$^+$, Ca^{2+}, Mg^{2+}), SrCr and BUN.

Monitoring: Monitor for laryngeal stridor, angioedema of the face, tongue, or glottis, abdominal pain, anaphylactoid reactions especially during desensitization or membrane exposure, symptomatic hypotension, jaundice, infections

F

and marked elevation of hepatic enzymes. Monitor BP, serum electrolytes, serum uric acid, and glucose tolerance. Monitor WBC in patients with collagen-vascular disease.

Patient Counseling: Inform about fetal risks if taken during pregnancy. Caution that inadequate fluid intake, excessive perspiration, diarrhea, or vomiting can lead to excessive fall in BP, with the same consequences of light-headedness and possible syncope. Advise not to use salt or K+ supplements. Counsel about signs/symptoms of neutropenia (infections), angioedema, electrolyte imbalance (thirst, weakness, lethargy), and other adverse effects; advise to seek prompt medical attention.

Administration: Oral route. **Storage:** 20-25°C (68-77°F); excursions permitted to 15-30°C (59-86°F). Protect from moisture.

FOSRENOL   RX
lanthanum carbonate (Shire)

THERAPEUTIC CLASS: Phosphate binder

INDICATIONS: Reduction of serum phosphate in patients with end-stage renal disease.

DOSAGE: *Adults:* Initial: 750-1500mg/day in divided doses. Titrate: Every 2-3 weeks in increments of 750mg/day until acceptable serum phosphate level is reached. Take with meals and chew tablets completely before swallowing. Usual range: 1500-3000mg/day. Usual max: 3750mg/day.

HOW SUPPLIED: Tab, Chewable: 250mg, 500mg, 750mg, 1000mg

WARNINGS/PRECAUTIONS: Caution with acute peptic ulcer, ulcerative colitis, Crohn's disease or bowel obstruction.

ADVERSE REACTIONS: N/V, dialysis graft occlusion, abdominal pain.

INTERACTIONS: Should not be taken within 2 hrs of antacids.

PREGNANCY: Category C, caution in nursing.

MECHANISM OF ACTION: Inhibits absorption of phosphate by forming highly insoluble lanthanum phosphate complexes, consequently reducing both serum phosphate and calcium product.

PHARMACOKINETICS: Absorption: C_{max}=1.0ng/mL. **Distribution:** Plasma protein binding (>99%). **Metabolism:** Not metabolized. **Elimination:** $T_{1/2}$=53 hrs, ($T_{1/2}$=2-3.6 yrs, from bone).

NURSING CONSIDERATIONS

Assessment: Assess for acute peptic ulcer, ulcerative colitis, Crohn's disease, bowel obstruction, and pregnancy/nursing status.

Monitoring: Monitor for GI events and NV. Drug may appear as imaging agent in abdominal x-rays.

Patient Counseling: Take with or immediately after meals. Chew completely before swallowing. Do not swallow intact tablets.

Administration: Oral route. **Storage:** 25°C (77°F); excursions permitted to 15-30°C (59-86°F).

FRAGMIN

RX

dalteparin sodium (Eisai)

> Epidural or spinal hematomas resulting in long-term or permanent paralysis may occur in patients anticoagulated with low molecular weight heparins or heparinoids and who are receiving neuraxial anesthesia or undergoing spinal puncture. Increased risk with indwelling epidural catheters, concomitant use of other drugs that affect hemostasis (eg, NSAIDs, platelet inhibitors, other anticoagulants), history of traumatic or repeated epidural or spinal puncture, or a history of spinal deformity or spinal surgery. Monitor frequently for signs/symptoms of neurologic impairment; if neurological compromise noted, urgent treatment is necessary. Consider benefits and risks before neuraxial intervention in patients anticoagulated or to be anticoagulated for thromboprophylaxis.

THERAPEUTIC CLASS: Low molecular weight heparin

INDICATIONS: Prophylaxis of ischemic complications in unstable angina and non-Q-wave myocardial infarction (MI) in conjunction with ASA therapy. Prophylaxis of deep vein thrombosis (DVT) in hip replacement surgery, abdominal surgery in patients who are at risk for thromboembolic complications, and for those at risk for thromboembolic complications due to severely restricted mobility during acute illness. Extended treatment of symptomatic venous thromboembolism (VTE) (proximal DVT and/or pulmonary embolism(PE)) to reduce the recurrence of VTE in patients with cancer.

DOSAGE: _Adults:_ Administer SQ. Prophylaxis of Ischemic Complications in Unstable Angina/Non-Q-Wave MI: 120 IU/kg q12h w/ ASA (75-165mg/day) until patient is clinically stabilized (usual 5-8 days). Max: 10,000 IU q12h. Prophylaxis of VTE in Hip Replacement Surgery: Post-Op Start: Usual: 2500 IU 4-8 hrs after surgery (or later, if hemostasis has not been achieved). Maint: 5000 IU qd for 5-10 days (up to 14 days); start at least 6 hrs after post-op dose. Pre-Op (starting day of surgery): Usual: 2500 IU within 2 hrs before surgery followed by 2500 IU 4-8 hrs after surgery (or later, if hemostasis has not been achieved). Maint: 5000 IU qd for 5-10 days (up to 14 days); start at least 6 hrs after post-op dose. Pre-Op (starting evening prior to surgery): Allow approximately 24 hrs between doses. Usual: 5000 IU 10-14 hrs before surgery followed by 5000 IU 4-8 hrs after surgery (or later, if hemostasis has not been achieved). Maint: 5000 IU qd for 5-10 days (up to 14 days). Abdominal Surgery: 2500 IU 1-2 hrs pre-op then qd for 5-10 days post-op. High Thromboembolic Risk: 5000 IU evening before surgery then qd for 5-10 days post-op. Alternatively, in Patients with Malignancy: 2500 IU 1-2 hrs pre-op, 2500 IU 12 hrs later then 5000 IU qd for 5-10 days post-op. Severely Restricted Mobility During Acute Illness: 5000 IU qd for 12-14 days. Treatment of Symptomatic VTE in Cancer Patients: 200 IU/kg qd for first 30 days, then 150 IU/kg qd for months 2-6. Max: 18,000 IU/day. Platelet Count 50,000-100,000/mm³: Reduce dose by 2500 IU until platelet count ≥100,000/mm³. Platelet Count <50,000/mm³: D/C therapy until platelet count >50,000/mm³. Renal Impairment (CrCl <30mL/min): Monitor anti-Xa levels to determine appropriate dose.

HOW SUPPLIED: Inj: (Syringe) 2500 IU/0.2mL, 5000 IU/0.2mL, 7500 IU/0.3mL, 10,000 IU/0.4mL, 10,000 IU/1mL, 12,500 IU/0.5mL, 15,000 IU/0.6mL, 18,000 IU/0.72mL; (MDV) 95,000 IU/3.8mL, 95,000 IU/9.5 mL

CONTRAINDICATIONS: Active major bleeding and history of heparin-induced thrombocytopenia or heparin-induced thrombocytopenia with thrombosis, patients undergoing epidural/neuraxial anesthesia, as treatment for unstable angina and non-Q wave MI, for prolonged VTE prophylaxis, hypersensitivity to pork products.

WARNINGS/PRECAUTIONS: Not for IM injection. May cause heparin-induced thrombocytopenia with or without thrombosis; d/c or reduce dose if platelet count <100,000/mm³. Multi-dose vials contain benzyl alcohol; caution in pregnant women. In premature infants, benzyl alcohol has been reported to be associated with a fatal "gasping syndrome". Caution in elderly with low body weight (<45kg) and decreased renal function.

ADVERSE REACTIONS: Bleeding, thrombocytopenia, injection-site pain, elevation of serum transaminase (ALT, AST), hematoma at injection site.

INTERACTIONS: See Boxed Warning & Contraindications. Caution with oral anticoagulants, platelet inhibitors, and thrombolytic agents due to increased risk of bleeding.

PREGNANCY: Category B, caution in nursing.

MECHANISM OF ACTION: Low molecular weight heparin; enhances inhibition of Factor Xa and thrombin by antithrombin, while only slightly affecting the activated partial thromboplastin time (APTT).

PHARMACOKINETICS: Absorption: Absolute bioavailability (87%); (2500 IU) C_{max} =0.19 IU/mL. (5000 IU) C_{max} = 0.41 IU/mL; (10,000 IU) C_{max} =0.82 IU/mL; T_{max}=4 hrs. **Distribution:** V_d=40-60mL/kg; found in breast milk. **Elimination:** (40 IU/kg) (IV) $T_{1/2}$=2.1 hrs. (60 IU/kg) (IV) $T_{1/2}$=2.3 hrs; (SQ) $T_{1/2}$=3-5 hrs. (Chronic Renal Insufficiency Requiring Hemodialysis) (5000 IU) (IV) $T_{1/2}$=5.7 hrs.

NURSING CONSIDERATIONS

Assessment: Assess for active major bleeding, history of heparin-induced thrombocytopenia with or without thrombosis, patients undergoing epidural/neuraxial anesthesia, as treatment for unstable angina and non-Q wave MI, for prolonged VTE prophylaxis, pregnancy/nursing status, known hypersensitivity to heparin or pork products, and possible drug interactions. Assess use in patients with severe renal insufficiency.

Monitoring: Monitor for signs/symptoms of hemorrhage, thrombocytopenia, and allergic reactions. Monitor for signs/symptoms of spinal or epidural hematomas in patients receiving neuraxial anesthesia or undergoing spinal puncture. Perform periodic CBC with platelet count, blood chemistry, and stool occult blood tests. Monitor anti-Xa levels.

Patient Counseling: If patients have had neuraxial anesthesia or spinal puncture, and particularly, if they are taking concomitant NSAIDs, platelet inhibitors, or other anticoagulants, inform to watch for signs and symptoms of spinal or epidural hematoma (eg, tingling, numbness, muscular weakness) and notify physician immediately. Inform that the use of ASA and other NSAIDs may enhance the risk of hemorrhage. Instruct to contact physician if any unusual bleeding, bruising or signs of thrombocytopenia (eg, rash of dark red spots under skin). Advise that it will take longer than usual to stop bleeding; may bruise and/or bleed more easily when treated with dalteparin. Inform that periodic lab monitoring is required during medication. If pregnant, instruct to use preservative-free formulation. Instruct on proper administration technique. Advise to inform health practitioners when taking medications known to affect bleeding before any surgery is scheduled or any new drug is taken.

Administration: SQ route. Do not mix with other injections or infusions unless compatible. Patient should be sitting or lying down. May be administered in U-shaped area around navel, upper outer side of thigh, or upper outer quadrangle of buttock. Vary injection site daily. Inspect visually for particulates and discoloration prior to administration. Refer to PI for further details. **Storage:** 20-25°C (68-77°F). After first penetration of the rubber stopper, store the multiple dose vials at room temperature for up to 2 weeks. Discard any unused solution after 2 weeks.

FROVA   RX
frovatriptan succinate (Endo)

THERAPEUTIC CLASS: 5-HT$_{1B/1D}$ agonist

INDICATIONS: Acute treatment of migraine with or without aura.

DOSAGE: *Adults:* 2.5mg with fluids. If headache recurs after initial relief, may repeat after 2 hrs. Max: 7.5mg/day. Safety of treating >4 migraines/30 days not known.

HOW SUPPLIED: Tab: 2.5mg

CONTRAINDICATIONS: Ischemic heart disease (eg, angina pectoris, history of MI, or documented silent ischemia), or patients who have symptoms or findings consistent with ischemic heart disease, coronary artery vasospasm (eg, Prinzmetal's angina), significant cardiovascular disease (CVD), cerebro-vascular syndromes including strokes of any type as well as transient ischemic attacks (TIA), peripheral vascular disease including ischemic bowel disease, uncontrolled HTN, hemiplegic or basilar migraine, use within 24 hrs of treatment with another 5-HT1 agonist, an ergotamine containing or ergot-type medications.

WARNINGS/PRECAUTIONS: Confirm diagnosis. Potential to cause coronary artery vasospasm. Not for patients in whom unrecognized CAD is predicted by presence of risk factors (eg, HTN, hypercholesterolemia, smoker, obesity, diabetes, CAD family history, menopause, males >40 yrs.) unless a cardio-vascular evaluation provides evidence that the patient is free of underlying cardiovascular diseases. In these patients, administer 1st dose under medical supervision and obtain ECG to assess presence of cardiac ischemia; monitor cardiovascular function with long-term intermittent use. Serious adverse cardiac events, cerebrovascular events, vasospastic reactions and HTN reported. Serotonin syndrome symptoms (eg, mental status changes, autonomic instability, neuromuscular aberrations, and GI symptoms) reported. May bind to melanin in the eye, which may lead to toxicity with long-term use.

ADVERSE REACTIONS: Dizziness, headache, paresthesia, dry mouth, fatigue, hot or cold sensation, skeletal pain, flushing, N/V, coronary vasospasm, myocardial ischemia.

INTERACTIONS: See Contraindications. Prolonged vasospastic reactions with ergot-type agents and other 5-HT$_1$ agonists. Increased plasma levels with propranolol and oral contraceptives. Decreased levels with ergotamine tartrate. Serotonin syndrome reported when combined use with an SSRI or SNRI.

PREGNANCY: Category C, caution in nursing.

MECHANISM OF ACTION: 5-HT$_{1B/1D}$ agonist; binds with high affinity to 5-HT$_{1B/1D}$ receptors. Believed to act on extracerebral, intracranial arteries and to inhibit excessive dilation of these vessels in migraine.

PHARMACOKINETICS: Absorption: Absolute bioavailability: (20%) male, (30%) female; T$_{max}$=2-4 hrs. **Distribution:** V$_d$=4.2L/kg (male), 3L/kg (female); plasma protein binding (15%). **Metabolism:** via CYP1A2. Desmethyl frovatropin (active metabolite). **Elimination:** Feces (62%), urine (32%); T$_{1/2}$=26 hrs.

NURSING CONSIDERATIONS

Assessment: Confirm diagnosis of migraine before initiating therapy. Assess for ischemic heart disease or symptoms or findings consistent with ischemic heart disease, coronary artery vasospasm (eg, Prinzmetal's angina), CAD risk, hemiplegic or basilar migraine, hepatic/renal impairment, pregnancy/nursing status, ECG changes, any other conditions where treatment is contraindicated or cautioned and possible drug interactions.

Monitoring: In patients with risk factors predictive of CAD, administration of 1st dose should be in physician's office or medically staffed and equipped facility as cardiac ischemia may occur in absence of clinical symptoms; ECG should be obtained immediately during interval in those with risk factors. Monitor for signs/symptoms of cardiac events (eg, coronary vasospasm, acute MI, arrhythmia, ECG changes), cerebrovascular events (eg, hemorrhage, stroke, TIAs), peripheral vascular ischemia, colonic ischemia with bloody diarrhea and abdominal pain, serotonin syndrome (eg, mental status changes, autonomic instability, neuromuscular aberrations and/or GI symptoms), ophthalmic effects, and increased BP.

Patient Counseling: Instruct to read PI before use. Inform about potential risks (eg, serotonin syndrome manifestations), especially if taken with SSRIs or SNRIs. Report adverse reactions to physician. Advise to take as directed. Notify physician if pregnant/nursing or planning to become pregnant.

Administration: Oral route. **Storage:** 25°C (77°F); excursions permitted to 15-30°C (59-86°F). Protect from moisture.

FUROSEMIDE

RX

furosemide (Various)

> May lead to profound diuresis with excessive amounts; medical supervision required and dose and dose schedule must be adjusted to individual patient's needs.

OTHER BRAND NAMES: Lasix (Sanofi-Aventis)

THERAPEUTIC CLASS: Loop diuretic

INDICATIONS: (Inj, PO) Treatment of edema associated with congestive heart failure, liver cirrhosis, and renal disease including nephrotic syndrome in adults and pediatrics. (PO) Treatment of hypertension alone or in combination with other antihypertensive agents in adults. (Inj) Adjunct therapy for acute pulmonary edema.

DOSAGE: *Adults:* (PO): Individualize dose. HTN: Initial: 40mg bid. Concomitant Antihypertensives: Reduce dose of other agents by 50%. Edema: Initial: 20-80mg. May repeat or increase by 20-40mg after 6-8 hrs. Give individually determined single dose qd or bid. Max: 600mg/day. Dose on 2-4 consecutive days each week. Closely monitor if on >80mg/day. Geriatrics: Start at the low end of dosing range. (Inj) Individualize dose. Edema: Initial: 20-40mg IV/IM. May repeat or increase by 20mg after 2 hrs. Give individually determined single dose qd or bid. Acute Pulmonary Edema: Initial: 40mg IV. May increase to 80mg IV after 1 hr.
Pediatrics: Edema: (PO) Initial: 2mg/kg single dose. May increase by 1-2mg/kg after 6-8 hrs. Max: 6mg/kg. (Inj) Initial: 1mg/kg IV/IM. May increase by 1mg/kg IV/IM after 2 hrs. Max: 6mg/kg. Premature Infants: Max: 1mg/kg/day.

HOW SUPPLIED: (Generic) Inj: 10mg/mL; Sol: 10mg/mL, 40mg/5mL; (Generic, Lasix) Tab: 20mg, 40mg*, 80mg *scored

CONTRAINDICATIONS: Anuria.

WARNINGS/PRECAUTIONS: Monitor for fluid/electrolyte imbalance (eg, hypokalemia), renal or hepatic dysfunction. Initiate in hospital with hepatic cirrhosis and ascites. Tinnitus, hearing impairment, deafness reported. Ototoxicity associated with rapid injection, severe renal impairment, higher than recommended doses, or hypoproteinema; control IV infusion rate. Excessive diuresis may cause dehydration, blood volume reduction with circulatory collapse, vascular thrombosis and embolism; caution particularly in elderly. Hyperglycemia and precipitation of diabetes mellitus (DM) reported. Can cause acute urinary retention, asymptomatic hyperuricemia, and precipitation of gout. May activate/exacerbate systemic lupus erythematosus (SLE). Cross-sensitivity with sulfonamide allergy. (Inj) May increase risk of patent ductus arteriosus (PDA) in premature neonates with respiratory distress syndrome. May cause hearing loss in neonates.

ADVERSE REACTIONS: Pancreatitis, jaundice, anorexia, paresthesias, ototoxicity, blood dyscrasias, dizziness, rash, urticaria, photosensitivity, fever, thrombophlebitis, restlessness.

INTERACTIONS: Ototoxicity with aminoglycosides, ethacrynic acid, cisplatin or other ototoxic drugs. Avoid with aminoglycosides and ethacrynic acid. Caution with high-dose salicylates; risk of salicylate toxicity. Lithium toxicity. Antagonizes tubocurarine. Potentiates antihypertensives, succinylcholine, ganglionic or peripheral adrenergic blockers. Severe hypotension and renal function deterioration with ACE inhibitors or angiotensin II receptor blockers. Decreases arterial response to norepinephrine. Reduced natriuretic and antihypertensive effect with sucralfate and indomethacin. Separate by at least 2 hrs with sucralfate. Hypokalemia with ACTH, corticosteroids, licorice in large amounts, or prolonged use of laxatives. Digitalis may exacerbate metabolic effects of hypokalemia. Renal changes with NSAIDs. Orthostatic hypotension may be aggravated by alcohol, barbiturates, or narcotics. Avoid with chloral hydrate. Intestinal absorption decreased with phenytoin. Reduced effect with methotrexate and other drugs that undergo significant renal tubular secretion; conversely may increase serum levels of these drugs and potentiate toxicity of these drugs and furosemide. May increase risk of cephalosporin-induced nephrotoxicity, gouty arthritis with cyclosporine, nephrotoxicity with other nephrotoxic drugs. Higher risk of renal deterioration with radiocontrast.

PREGNANCY: Category C, caution in nursing.

MECHANISM OF ACTION: Loop diuretic; primarily inhibits reabsorption of Na^+ and Cl^- in proximal and distal tubules and in loop of Henle.

PHARMACOKINETICS: Distribution: Plasma protein binding (91-99%), found in breast milk. **Metabolism:** Biotransformation. Furosemide glucuronide (major metabolite). **Elimination:** Urine; $T_{1/2}$=2 hrs.

NURSING CONSIDERATIONS

Assessment: Assess for anuria, sulfonamide hypersensitivity, DM, SLE, possible drug interactions, hepatic/renal impairment, and pregnancy/nursing status. Obtain baseline serum electrolytes, renal function, urine, and blood glucose.

Monitoring: Monitor serum electrolytes, CO_2, creatinine and BUN frequently in first few months, then periodically; renal and hepatic function, urine, and blood glucose periodically. Monitor for signs/symptoms of electrolyte imbalance, blood dyscrasias, hyperglycemia, hyperuricemia or precipitation of gout, hypotension, ototoxicity, persistent PDA, and hypersensitivity reactions. Monitor renal function and consider renal ultrasonography in pediatrics.

Patient Counseling: Advise to seek medical attention if symptoms of electrolyte imbalance (eg, dry mouth, thirst, weakness), hypotension, ototoxicity (tinnitus, hearing impairment), or hypersensitivity reactions occur. Advise that postural hypotension can be managed by getting up slowly. K+ supplements/dietary measures may be needed to control or avoid hypokalemia. Advise diabetics that may increase blood glucose levels and thereby affect urine glucose tests. Inform that the skin may be more sensitive to the effects of sunlight. Inform to avoid medications that may increase blood pressure, including OTC products for appetite suppression and cold symptoms.

Administration: Oral, IV/IM route. See PI for high dose parenteral therapy.
Storage: Tab, Sol: 25°C (77°F); excursions permitted to 15-30°C (59-86°F). Protect sol from light and moisture. IV: 20-25°C (68-77°F). Protect from light.

FUSILEV   RX
levoleucovorin calcium (Spectrum)

THERAPEUTIC CLASS: Cytoprotective agent

INDICATIONS: Rescue therapy after high-dose methotrexate (MTX) therapy in osteosarcoma. To diminish the toxicity and counteract the effects of impaired MTX elimination and of inadvertent overdosage of folic acid antagonists.

DOSAGE: *Adults:* Levoleucovorin Rescue: 7.5mg (5mg/m²) IV q6h for 10 doses starting 24 hrs after beginning of MTX infusion. Continue therapy, hydration and urinary alkalinization until MTX level is <5x10⁻⁸M (0.05 micromolar). Refer to PI for guidelines on dosage adjustment and rescue extensions. Inadvertent MTX Overdosage: 7.5mg (5mg/m²) IV q6h until serum MTX is <10⁻⁸M. Titrate: Increase to 50mg/m² IV q3h if 24-hr SrCr is 50% over baseline, or if 24-hr MTX level is >5x10⁻⁶M, or 48-hr level is >9x10⁻⁷M. Employ concurrent hydration (3L/day) and urinary alkalinization with Na bicarbonate; adjust bicarbonate dose to maintain urine pH at ≥7. Start rescue therapy as soon as possible after overdose and within 24 hrs of MTX with delayed excretion. Do not infuse >16mL/min.

HOW SUPPLIED: Inj: 50mg

WARNINGS/PRECAUTIONS: Do not infuse >16mL/min. For IV use only; do not administer intrathecally. Not approved for pernicious anemia and megaloblastic anemias secondary to the lack of vitamin B_{12}; improper use may cause a hematologic remission while neurologic manifestations continue to progress.

ADVERSE REACTIONS: Stomatitis, N/V, diarrhea, dyspepsia, typhlitis, dyspnea, dermatitis, confusion, neuropathy, abnormal renal function, taste perversion.

INTERACTIONS: May reduce the antiepileptic effects of phenobarbital, phenytoin, and primidone, and increase seizure frequency in children; caution with concurrent anticonvulsant use. May enhance 5-FU toxicity. Increased treatment failure and morbidity rates with concurrent use of trimethoprim-sulfamethoxazole for treatment of PCP in HIV patients.

PREGNANCY: Category C, caution use in nursing.

MECHANISM OF ACTION: Folate analog; counteracts the therapeutic and toxic effects of folic acid antagonists, which act by inhibiting dihydrofolate reductase.

PHARMACOKINETICS: Absorption: (Total-THF) C_{max}=1722ng/mL; (5-methyl-THF) C_{max}=275ng/mL, T_{max}=0.9 hrs. **Metabolism:** 5-methyl-THF (active metabolite). **Elimination:** $T_{1/2}$=5.1 hrs (Total-THF), 6.8 hrs (5-methyl-THF).

NURSING CONSIDERATIONS

Assessment: Assess for third-space fluid accumulation (eg, ascites, pleural effusion), renal impairment, dehydration, pregnancy/nursing status and for possible drug interactions.

Monitoring: Monitor signs/symptoms of ascites, pleural effusion, renal impairment, and hypersensitivity reactions. Monitor fluid and electrolytes in patients with abnormalities in methotrexate excretion. Monitor creatinine and MTX levels daily while on therapy.

Patient Counseling: Inform about risks and benefits of therapy. Advise to notify physician if any adverse reaction occurs. Instruct to inform physician if pregnant/nursing.

Administration: IV route. Reconstitute with 5.3mL of 0.9% NaCl Injection to yield a levoleucovorin concentration of 10mg/mL. May further dilute to concentrations of 0.5mg/mL to 5mg/mL in 0.9% NaCl Injection or 5% Dextrose Injection. Do not administer >16mL/min. Refer to PI for further administration instructions. **Storage:** 25°C (77°F); excursions permitted from 15-30°C (59-86°F). Protect from light. Reconstitution/Dilution with 0.9% NaCl: Room temperature for 12 hrs max. Dilution with 5% Dextrose: Room temperature for 4 hrs max.

FUZEON   RX
enfuvirtide (Roche Labs)

THERAPEUTIC CLASS: Fusion inhibitor

INDICATIONS: In combination with other antiretroviral agents for the treatment of HIV-1 infection in treatment-experienced patients with evidence of HIV-1 replication despite ongoing antiretroviral therapy.

DOSAGE: *Adults:* 90mg SQ bid. Inject into upper arm, anterior thigh, or abdomen.
Pediatrics: 6-16 yrs: 2mg/kg SQ bid. Max: 90mg SQ bid. Refer to PI for weight-based dosing chart. Inject into upper arm, anterior thigh, or abdomen.

HOW SUPPLIED: Inj: 90mg/mL

WARNINGS/PRECAUTIONS: Local injection-site reactions (eg, pain, discomfort, erythema, nodules and cysts, pruritus, ecchymosis) reported; monitor for signs/symptoms of cellulitis or local infection. Administration with Biojector 2000 may result in neuralgia and/or paresthesia, bruising and hematomas. Patients with hemophilia or other coagulation disorders may have a higher risk of post-injection bleeding. May cause bacterial pneumonia; monitor for signs/symptoms of pneumonia, especially, those predisposed to pneumonia (eg, low initial CD4 cell count, high initial viral load, IV drug use, smoking, and prior history of lung disease). Associated with systemic hypersensitivity reactions; d/c immediately if signs/symptoms of systemic hypersensitivity develop. Use in noninfected HIV patients may lead to anti-enfuvirtide antibody production, which cross reacts with HIV gp41 and could result in false-positive HIV test with an ELISA assay. Immune reconstitution syndrome reported.

ADVERSE REACTIONS: Diarrhea, local injection-site reactions, fatigue, nausea, decreased weight, sinusitis, abdominal pain, cough, herpes simplex, decreased appetite, pancreatitis.

INTERACTIONS: Concomitant use with anticoagulants may result in a higher risk of post-injection bleeding.

PREGNANCY: Category B, not for use in nursing.

MECHANISM OF ACTION: Fusion inhibitor; interferes with the entry of HIV-1 into cells by inhibiting fusion of viral and cellular membranes; binds to the first heptad-repeat (HR1) in the gp41 subunit of the viral envelope glycoprotein and prevents the conformational changes required for the fusion of viral and cellular membranes.

PHARMACOKINETICS: Absorption: C_{max}=4.59mcg/mL; T_{max}=8 hrs; AUC=55.8mcg•hr/mL. Absolute bioavailabilty (84.3%). **Distribution:** V_d=5.5L; plasma protein binding (92%). **Metabolism:** Liver via hydrolysis; M_3 (metabolite). **Elimination:** $T_{1/2}$=3.8 hrs.

NURSING CONSIDERATIONS

Assessment: Assess for risk factors for pneumonia (eg, history of lung disease, decreased $CD4^+$ cell count, increased viral load, IV drug use, smoking), infections, hemophilia, history of coagulation disorders, pregnancy/nursing status, and for possible drug interactions.

Monitoring: Monitor for signs/symptoms of cellulitis or local injection-site reactions, immune reconstitution syndrome, post-injection bleeding, nerve pain/paresthesia, and hypersensitivity reactions. Monitor for signs/symptoms of pneumonia (eg, cough with fever, rapid breathing, SOB).

Patient Counseling: Inform of risk of developing injection-site reactions. Advise to seek medical attention if experience symptoms of pneumonia, systemic hypersensitivity (eg, rash, fever, N/V, chills, rigors, hypotension), post-injection bleeding, cellulitis, or nerve pain (paresthesia). Inform that may continue to contract illnesses associated with HIV-1 infection and may still transmit the infection through sexual contact or blood contamination. Advise that the drug must be taken as a part of a combination antiretroviral regimen. Instruct not to change dosage or schedule, or to stop drug without consulting physician. Instruct not to breastfeed. Advise to practice aseptic technique upon administration in order to avoid injection-site infections.

Administration: SQ route. Refer to PI for proper administration. Do not inject into moles, scar tissue, bruises, navel, surgical scars, tattoos, burn sites, directly over a blood vessel, or areas where large nerves course close to the skin, preceding site or on current injection-site reaction from an earlier dose. **Storage:** 25°C (77°F); excursions permitted to 15-30°C (59-86°F). Reconstituted Solution: 2-8°C (36-46°F). Use within 24 hrs.

GABITRIL   RX
tiagabine HCl (Cephalon)

THERAPEUTIC CLASS: Nipecotic acid derivative

INDICATIONS: Adjunctive therapy in adults and pediatrics ≥12 yrs in the treatment of partial seizures.

DOSAGE: *Adults:* Induced (patients already taking enzyme-inducing antiepilepsy drugs [AEDs]): Initial: 4mg qd. Titrate: May increase weekly by 4-8mg until clinical response achieved, or up to 56mg/day. Refer to PI for typical dosing titration. Usual: 32-56mg/day given bid-qid. Max: 56mg/day. Non-induced: Requires lower dose and may require slower titration. Hepatic Impairment: May require lower initial/maint doses and longer dosing intervals.
Pediatrics: 12-18 yrs: Induced: Initial: 4mg qd. Titrate: May increase by 4mg qd at beginning of Week 2, then increase weekly by 4-8mg until clinical response achieved, or up to 32mg/day. Refer to PI for typical dosing titration. Max: 32mg/day. Non-induced: Requires lower dose and may require slower titration. Hepatic Impairment: May require lower initial/maint doses and longer dosing intervals.

HOW SUPPLIED: Tab: 2mg, 4mg, 12mg, 16mg

WARNINGS/PRECAUTIONS: New-onset seizures and status epilepticus in patients without epilepsy reported; d/c therapy and evaluate for underlying seizure disorder. Increased risk of suicidal thoughts or behavior may occur; monitor for emergence or worsening of depression, suicidal thoughts/behavior, and any unusual changes in mood or behavior. Avoid abrupt d/c; may increase seizure frequency. May affect thought processes (eg, impaired concentration, speech or language problems, confusion) and level of consciousness (eg, somnolence, fatigue). May exacerbate EEG abnormalities; caution with history of spike and wave discharges on EEG and adjust dosage. Sudden unexpected death in epilepsy (SUDEP), incapacitating generalized weakness, and serious skin rash reported. Use in non-induced patients requires lower doses. There may be a possibility of long-term ophthalmologic effects. Caution with hepatic impairment.

ADVERSE REACTIONS: Dizziness, asthenia, tremor, somnolence, N/V, nervousness, abdominal pain, insomnia, depression, confusion, pharyngitis, rash, diarrhea.

INTERACTIONS: May reduce valproate concentrations. Clearance affected by hepatic AEDs; increased clearance with carbamazepine, phenytoin, and phenobarbital (primidone). Additive effects with alcohol, triazolam, and CNS depressants. Reports of new-onset seizures and status epilepticus in patients without epilepsy with concomitant drugs that lower the seizure threshold (antidepressants, antipsychotics, stimulants, narcotics). Potential interactions with drugs that induce or inhibit hepatic metabolizing enzymes. Use with highly protein bound drugs may lead to higher free fractions of tiagabine or competing drugs.

PREGNANCY: Category C, caution in nursing.

MECHANISM OF ACTION: Nipecotic acid derivative; not established. May enhance activity of gamma aminobutyric acid (GABA), the major inhibitory neurotransmitter in the CNS. Binds to recognition sites associated with the GABA uptake carrier, thereby blocking GABA uptake into presynaptic neurons, permitting more GABA to be available for receptor binding on the surfaces of postsynaptic cells.

PHARMACOKINETICS: Absorption: Rapid; absolute bioavailability (90%). T_{max}=2.5 hrs (fed), T_{max}=45 min (fasting). **Distribution:** Plasma protein binding (96%). **Metabolism:** Liver via CYP3A; oxidation and glucuronidation. **Elimination:** Urine (25%; 2% unchanged), feces (63%); $T_{1/2}$=7-9 hrs (non-induced), 2-5 hrs (induced).

NURSING CONSIDERATIONS

Assessment: Assess for underlying seizure disorder, history of status epilepticus and spike and wave discharges on EEG, depression, suicidal thoughts/behavior, history of hypersensitivity reactions, hepatic impairment, pregnancy/nursing status, and possible drug interactions.

Monitoring: Monitor for occurrence of new-onset seizures and status epilepticus in patients without a previous history of epilepsy, withdrawal seizures, cognitive and neuropsychiatric events, EEG changes, rash, emergence or worsening of depression, suicidal thoughts/behavior, unusual changes in mood or behavior, generalized weakness, and possible long-term ophthalmologic changes.

Patient Counseling: Instruct to read Medication Guide prior to therapy. Inform patients, caregivers, and families about increased risk of suicidal thoughts and behavior and to notify physician immediately if suicidal thoughts or behaviors emerge. Inform of possible drowsiness or dizziness; avoid operating machinery/driving until adjusted to effects. Advise to contact physician if signs of rash develop. Instruct to take with food and not to abruptly d/c medication. If multiple doses are missed, contact physician before restarting. Notify physician if pregnant, intend to become pregnant, if breastfeeding or intend to breastfeed. Encourage pregnant patients to enroll in North American Antiepileptic Drug (NAAED) Pregnancy Registry by calling 888-233-2334 or go to aedpregnancyregistry.org.

Administration: Oral route. Take with food. **Storage:** 20-25°C (68-77°F). Protect from light and moisture.

GANCICLOVIR   RX
ganciclovir sodium (Various)

> Risk of granulocytopenia, anemia, and thrombocytopenia. (Cap) Use only for prevention of cytomegalovirus (CMV) disease in patients with advanced HIV infection at risk for CMV disease and in solid organ transplant recipients. For maintenance treatment of CMV retinitis immunocompromised patients. Risk of more rapid rate of CMV retinitis progression with caps; only use as maintenance treatment when the risk is balanced by the benefit of avoiding daily IV infusions. (IV) Use only for the treatment of CMV retinitis in immunocompromised patients and for the prevention of CMV disease in transplant patients at risk for CMV disease.

OTHER BRAND NAMES: Cytovene IV (Genentech)

THERAPEUTIC CLASS: Synthetic guanine derivative nucleoside analogue

INDICATIONS: (Caps) Prevention of CMV in solid organ-transplant recipients and in advanced HIV patients at risk for CMV disease. Alternative to IV for maintenance treatment of CMV retinitis in immunocompromised patients, including patients with acquired immunodeficiency syndrome (AIDS) in whom retinitis is stable following appropriate induction therapy and for whom the risk of more rapid progression is balanced by the benefit associated with avoiding daily IV infusions. (IV) Treatment of CMV retinitis in immunocompromised patients, including patients with AIDS. Prevention of CMV disease in transplant recipients at risk for CMV disease.

DOSAGE: *Adults:* CMV Retinitis Treatment: Initial: 5mg/kg IV q12h for 14-21 days. Maint: 5mg/kg IV infusion qd for 7 days/week or 6mg/kg IV qd for 5 days/week or 1000mg PO tid or 500mg PO 6 times daily q3h, while awake. Progression of CMV Retinitis while on Therapy: Reinduction recommended. CMV Retinitis Prevention in HIV Patients: 1000mg PO tid. CMV Retinitis Prevention in Transplant Patients: Initial: 5mg/kg IV q12h for 7-14 days, followed by 5mg/kg IV qd for 7 days/week or 6mg/kg IV qd for 5 days/week or 1000mg PO tid. Renal Impairment: Refer to PI for Dosing. (PO) Take caps with food. (IV) Administer at constant rate over 1 hr.

HOW SUPPLIED: Cap: 250mg, 500mg; Inj: 500mg

WARNINGS/PRECAUTIONS: Avoid if ANC <500 cells/µL or platelets <25,000 cells/µL. Caution in pre-existing cytopenias or history of cytopenic reactions to other drugs, chemicals, or irradiation. Caution with renal impairment; adjust dose. May cause temporary or permanent inhibition of spermatogenesis and may suppress fertility in women. Mutagenic and teratogenic potential; women of childbearing potential should use effective contraception during treatment and men should practice barrier contraception during and for at least 90 days after therapy. Caution in elderly. (IV): Larger doses and more rapid infusions increase toxicity. Administration should be accompanied by adequate hydration. Phlebitis and/or pain may occur at infusion site. Administer into veins with adequate blood flow. May result in severe tissue irritation due to high pH of reconstituted solution with IM or SQ injection. Do not administer by rapid or bolus IV injection. Use extreme caution in pediatrics; administer only if potential benefits outweigh risks.

ADVERSE REACTIONS: Fever, diarrhea, anorexia, vomiting, leukopenia, anemia, sweating, infection, chills, thrombocytopenia, neutropenia, anemia, catheter infection, sepsis, hypokalemia.

INTERACTIONS: Concomitant use with zidovudine may increase AUC of zidovudine, decrease the AUC of ganciclovir, and increase the risk of neutropenia and anemia. Avoid imipenem-cilastatin; generalized seizures reported. Drugs that inhibit rapidly dividing cell populations such as bone marrow, spermatogonia and germinal layers of skin and GI mucosa (eg, dapsone, pentamidine, flucytosine, vincristine, vinblastine, adriamycin, amphotericin B, trimethoprim/sulfamethoxazole combinations, other nucleoside analogues) may have additive toxicity and should be administered only if benefits outweigh the risks. Concomitant use with probenecid may increase the AUC of ganciclovir and decrease the renal clearance of ganciclovir. (IV) Use with didanosine may increase the AUC and Cmax of didanosine. High frequency of impaired renal function in transplant patients and increases in SrCr when used concomitantly with amphotericin B or cyclosporine; monitor renal function when concomitantly using nephrotoxic drugs. (PO) Use with didanosine may increase the AUC of didanosine. A decrease in the AUC of ganciclovir may occur when didanosine is administered 2 hrs before ganciclovir.

PREGNANCY: Category C, not for use in nursing.

MECHANISM OF ACTION: Guanine derivative; believed to inhibit viral DNA synthesis by competitively inhibiting viral DNA polymerases and incorporating into viral DNA, resulting in eventual termination of viral DNA elongation.

PHARMACOKINETICS: Absorption: (PO): Absolute bioavailability (5%) (fasted), (6-9%) (fed state); AUC_{0-24}=15.9µg•hr/mL, C_{max}=1.02µg/mL (500mg q3h, 6 times daily, fed state), AUC_{0-24}=15.4µg•hr/mL, C_{max}=1.18µg/mL (1000mg tid, fed state). (IV): (1-hr infusion of 5mg/kg) C_{max}=8.27-9µg/mL; AUC=22.1-26.8µg•hr/mL. **Distribution:** Plasma protein binding (1-2%); (IV): V_d=0.74L/kg. **Elimination:** (IV): Urine (91.3%), $T_{1/2}$=3.5 hrs; (PO): $T_{1/2}$= 4.8 hrs.

NURSING CONSIDERATIONS

Assessment: Assess for hypersensitivity to acyclovir, pregnancy/nursing status, renal impairment, and for possible drug interactions. Assess for pre-existing cytopenias or a history of cytopenic reactions to other drugs, chemicals, or irradiation. Assess baseline renal function, absolute neutrophil count (≥500 cells/µL), and platelet count (≥25,000/µL).

Monitoring: Monitor for signs/symptoms of granulocytopenia, anemia, thrombocytopenia, and infertility. Perform frequent monitoring of CBC and platelet counts. Monitor SrCr or CrCl periodically. Ophthalmologic follow-up examinations in HIV patients. (IV) Monitor for infusion-site reactions (eg, pain, phlebitis).

Patient Counseling: Inform that the major toxicities of therapy are granulocytopenia (neutropenia), anemia, and thrombocytopenia. Advise that medication may increase SrCr levels. Inform that medication may decrease sperm production and cause infertility in men and women. Advise women of childbearing potential that medication should not be used during pregnancy and that effective contraception should be used. Inform men that barrier contraception should be used during therapy and for at least 90 days following treatment. Inform that therapy may be a potential carcinogen. Advise immunocompromised patients with CMV retinitis that medication is not a cure for CMV retinitis and that progression of retinitis may continue to occur during and after treatment; instruct to have ophthalmologic follow-up examinations at a minimum of every 4-6 weeks during treatment. (PO): Instruct to take with food. (IV) Inform to keep well hydrated during therapy.

Administration: IV/Oral route. Refer to PI for preparation of IV solution, handling and disposal. **Storage:** (IV) 25°C (77°F); excursions permitted to 15-30°C (59-86°F); (Cap): 20-25° (68-77°F); excursions permitted between 15-30°C (59-86°F).

GARDASIL   RX
human papillomavirus recombinant vaccine, quadrivalent (Merck)

THERAPEUTIC CLASS: Vaccine

INDICATIONS: Vaccination of girls and women 9-26 yrs of age for the prevention of cervical, vulvar, vaginal, and anal cancer caused by human papillomavirus (HPV) types 16 and 18, genital warts (condyloma acuminata) caused by HPV types 6 and 11, cervical intraepithelial neoplasia (CIN) Grade 2/3 and cervical adenocarcinoma in situ (AIS), CIN Grade 1, vulvar intraepithelial neoplasia (VIN) Grades 2 and 3, vaginal intraepithelial neoplasia (VaIN) Grades 2 and 3, and anal intraepithelial neoplasia (AIN) Grades 1, 2 and 3 caused by HPV types 6, 11, 16, and 18. Vaccination of boys and men 9-26 yrs of age for the prevention of anal cancer caused by HPV types 16 and 18, genital warts (condyloma acuminata) caused by HPV types 6 and 11, and AIN Grades 1, 2 and 3 caused by HPV types 6, 11, 16, and 18.

DOSAGE: *Adults:* ≤26 yrs: 0.5mL IM in the deltoid region of the upper arm or in the higher anterolateral area of the thigh at the following schedule: 0, 2 months, 6 months.
Pediatrics: ≥9 yrs: 0.5mL IM in the deltoid region of the upper arm or in the higher anterolateral area of the thigh at the following schedule: 0, 2 months, 6 months.

HOW SUPPLIED: Inj: 0.5mL

CONTRAINDICATIONS: Severe hypersensitivity reaction to yeast.

WARNINGS/PRECAUTIONS: Syncope may occur; observe for 15 min after administration. Appropriate medical treatment and supervision should be readily available if an anaphylactic reaction occurs. Response may be diminished in immunocompromised individuals. Does not protect against disease from vaccine and non-vaccine HPV types to which a person has previously been exposed through sexual activity. Not intended for treatment of active external genital lesions; cervical, vulvar, vaginal, and anal cancers; CIN; VIN; VaIN; AIN. Does not protect against diseases due to HPV types not contained in the vaccine and genital diseases not caused by HPV. Vaccination may not result in protection in all vaccine recipients. Patients should continue to undergo cervical and/or anal cancer screening.

ADVERSE REACTIONS: Local site reactions (eg, pain, swelling, erythema, pruritus, bruising), fever, nausea, dizziness, diarrhea, headache.

INTERACTIONS: Immunosuppressive therapies, including irradiation, antimetabolites, alkylating agents, cytotoxic drugs, and corticosteroids (used in greater than physiologic doses), may reduce the immune responses to vaccines.

PREGNANCY: Category B, caution in nursing.

MECHANISM OF ACTION: Vaccine; exact mechanism not established. Suspected to develop humoral immune response.

NURSING CONSIDERATIONS

Assessment: Assess current health and immune status, age of patient, pregnancy/nursing status, and for possible drug interactions. Assess for hypersensitivity to drug and yeast.

Monitoring: Monitor for signs/symptoms of anaphylactic reactions, syncope, tonic-clonic movements, and for seizure-like activity.

Patient Counseling: Inform about benefits and risks associated with vaccine. Advise to continue to undergo cervical and/or anal cancer screening. Advise that vaccine does not provide protection against disease from vaccine and non-vaccine HPV types to which a person has previously been exposed through sexual activity. Inform that syncope may occur following vaccination. Inform about importance of completing immunization series unless contraindicated. Advise that vaccine is not recommended during pregnancy. Instruct to contact physician if adverse events develop.

Administration: IM route. Shake well before use. Do not dilute or mix with other vaccines. Inspect for particulate matter and discoloration; do not use if these conditions exist. Refer to PI for instructions for using prefilled single-dose syringes. **Storage:** 2-8°C (36-46°F). Do not freeze. Protect from light. Administer as soon as possible after being removed from refrigeration; can be out of refrigeration (≤25°C/77°F) for ≤72 hrs.

GELNIQUE
RX
oxybutynin chloride (Watson)

THERAPEUTIC CLASS: Muscarinic antagonist

INDICATIONS: Treatment of overactive bladder with symptoms of urge urinary incontinence, urgency, and frequency.

DOSAGE: *Adults:* Apply contents of 1 sachet to dry, intact skin on the abdomen, upper arms/shoulders, or thighs qd. Rotate sites.

HOW SUPPLIED: Gel: 100mg/g (10%) [30s]

CONTRAINDICATIONS: Urinary retention, gastric retention, and uncontrolled narrow-angle glaucoma.

WARNINGS/PRECAUTIONS: For topical application only. Gel preparation is flammable; avoid open fire or smoking until gel has dried. Caution with bladder outflow obstruction, GI obstructive disorders, gastroesophageal reflux, and myasthenia gravis. May decrease gastrointestinal motility; caution with ulcerative colitis or intestinal atony. Skin hypersensitivity may occur; d/c if hypersensitivity develops. D/C and provide appropriate treatment in the event of angioedema. Skin transference may occur; cover application site with clothing after gel has dried.

ADVERSE REACTIONS: Dry mouth, application-site reactions, urinary tract/upper respiratory tract infections.

INTERACTIONS: Caution with bisphosphonates or other drugs that may cause or exacerbate esophagitis. Concomitant use with other anticholinergic (antimuscarinic) agents may increase the frequency and/or severity of dry mouth, constipation, blurred vision, somnolence, and pharmacological effects.

PREGNANCY: Category B, caution in nursing.

MECHANISM OF ACTION: Antispasmodic, antimuscarinic agent; acts as competitive antagonist of acetylcholine at postganglionic muscarinic receptors, resulting in relaxation of bladder smooth muscle.

PHARMACOKINETICS: Absorption: Abdomen: C_{max}=6.8ng/mL; AUC_{0-24}=112.7ng•hr/mL. Upper Arm/Shoulder: C_{max}=8.3ng/mL; AUC_{0-24}=133.8ng•hr/mL. Thigh: C_{max}=7ng/mL; AUC_{0-24}=125.1ng•hr/mL. **Distribution:** (IV) V_d=193L. **Metabolism:** CYP3A4, N-desethyloxybutynin (active metabolite). **Elimination:** Urine (<0.1% unchanged); (IV) $T_{1/2}$=2 hrs.

NURSING CONSIDERATIONS

Assessment: Assess for urinary retention, gastric retention, uncontrolled narrow-angle glaucoma, bladder outflow obstruction, GI obstructive disorders, ulcerative colitis or intestinal atony, gastroesophageal reflux, myasthenia gravis, pregnancy/nursing status, and for possible drug interactions.

Monitoring: Monitor for signs/symptoms of urinary retention, gastric retention, esophagitis, angioedema, and for skin hypersensitivity reactions.

Patient Counseling: Advise that therapy is for topical application only and not to be ingested. Instruct not to apply to recently shaved skin surfaces. Instruct to wash hands immediately after product application. Advise to avoid showering or water immersion for 1 hr after product application. Counsel to cover treated sites with clothing if close skin-to-skin contact is anticipated. Instruct to avoid open fire or smoking until gel is dried. Inform that the drug may produce significant adverse reactions related to anticholinergic pharmacological activity (eg, constipation, urinary retention, and blurred vision). Advise to exercise caution in engaging in potentially dangerous activities until effects have been determined. Inform that heat prostration may occur in hot environment. Inform that alcohol may enhance drowsiness.

Administration: Topical route. **Storage:** 25°C (77°F); excursions permitted to 15-30°C (59-86°F). Protect from moisture and humidity. Apply immediately after the sachets are opened and contents expelled. Discard used sachets in a manner that prevents accidental application or ingestion by children, pets, or others.

GEMZAR RX
gemcitabine (Lilly)

THERAPEUTIC CLASS: Nucleoside analogue antimetabolite

INDICATIONS: Combination with carboplatin for treatment of advanced ovarian cancer that has relapsed for ≥6 months after completion of platinum-based therapy. Combination with paclitaxel for 1st-line treatment of metastatic breast cancer after failure of prior anthracycline-containing adjuvant chemotherapy, unless anthracyclines were clinically contraindicated. Combination with cisplatin for 1st-line treatment of inoperable, locally advanced (Stage IIIA or IIIB), or metastatic (Stage IV) non-small cell lung cancer. First-line treatment of locally advanced (nonresectable Stage II or Stage III) or metastatic (Stage IV) adenocarcinoma of the pancreas in patients previously treated with 5-fluorouracil (5-FU).

DOSAGE: *Adults:* Refer to PI for dose modifications guideline for each indication. Ovarian Cancer: 1000mg/m² IV over 30 min on Days 1 and 8 of each 21-day cycle. Give carboplatin AUC 4 IV on Day 1 after gemcitabine. Breast Cancer: 1250mg/m² IV over 30 min on Days 1 and 8 of each 21-day cycle. Give paclitaxel 175mg/m² on Day 1 as 3-hr IV infusion before gemcitabine. Non-Small Cell Lung Cancer: 4-Week Cycle: 1000mg/m² IV over 30 min on Days 1, 8, and 15 of each 28-day cycle. Or 3-Week Cycle: 1250mg/m² IV over 30 min on Days 1 and 8 of each 21-day cycle. Then give cisplatin 100mg/m² IV on Day 1 after gemcitabine infusion. Pancreatic Cancer: 1000mg/m² IV over 30 min once weekly for ≤7 weeks (or until toxicity necessitates reducing or holding a dose), then 1 week off. Give subsequent cycles as once a week infusions for 3 consecutive weeks out of every 4 weeks.

HOW SUPPLIED: Inj: 200mg, 1g

WARNINGS/PRECAUTIONS: Increased toxicity with infusion time >60 min and more frequent than weekly dosing. Myelosuppression is a dose-limiting toxicity; bone marrow suppression (eg, leukopenia, thrombocytopenia, anemia) may occur. Pulmonary toxicity reported; d/c if severe lung toxicity occurs and institute appropriate supportive care measures. Hemolytic Uremic Syndrome (HUS), renal failure, and serious hepatotoxicity reported; caution with pre-existing renal impairment and hepatic insufficiency. Concurrent use with liver metastases or pre-existing history of hepatitis, alcoholism, or liver cirrhosis; may cause exacerbation of underlying hepatic insufficiency. May cause fetal harm.

ADVERSE REACTIONS: Myelosuppression, N/V, anemia, leukopenia, neutropenia, thrombocytopenia, elevated serum transaminases/alkaline phosphatases, proteinuria, fever, rash, hematuria, dyspnea.

INTERACTIONS: Serious hepatotoxicity reported with other potentially hepatotoxic drugs. Higher incidence of myelosuppression and SrCr toxicity with cisplatin. Has radiosensitizing activity; radiation toxicity reported with radiotherapy.

PREGNANCY: Category D, not for use in nursing.

MECHANISM OF ACTION: Nucleoside analogue antimetabolite; exhibits cell cycle specificity, primarily killing cells undergoing DNA synthesis (S-phase); also blocks progression of cells through the G1/S-phase boundary.

PHARMACOKINETICS: Distribution: V_d=50L/m² (infusion <70 min), 370L/m² (infusion 70-285 min). **Metabolism:** Intracellular by nucleoside kinases to the active diphosphate (dFdCDP) and triphosphate (dFdCTP) nucleosides. **Elimination:** Urine (92-98%); $T_{1/2}$=42-94 min (infusion <70 min), 245-638 min (infusion 70-285 min).

NURSING CONSIDERATIONS

Assessment: Assess for history of hepatitis, alcoholism or liver cirrhosis, liver metastases, previous hypersensitivity to drug, pre-existing hepatic/renal impairment, pregnancy/nursing status, and possible drug interactions. Obtain CBC, including differential and platelet count, prior to each dose. Obtain baseline renal and hepatic function.

Monitoring: Monitor for signs/symptoms of myelosuppression, pulmonary toxicity, HUS, renal failure, hepatotoxicity, and other adverse events/toxicities that may occur. Perform periodic monitoring of LFTs and renal function. Monitor SrCr, K⁺, Ca, and Mg when using concomitantly with cisplatin.

Patient Counseling: Inform about benefits and risks of therapy. Instruct to contact physician if any signs/symptoms of infection (eg, fever), anemia, or bleeding occur. Inform that drug may cause fetal harm; instruct to notify physician if pregnant or nursing.

Administration: IV route. Refer to PI for proper preparation, reconstitution, and administration instructions. **Storage:** (Unopened vials) 20-25°C (68-

77°F); excursions permitted to 15-30°C (59-86°F). (Reconstituted) 20-25°C (68-77°F) for 24 hrs. Discard unused portion. Do not refrigerate.

GEODON

RX

ziprasidone HCl - ziprasidone mesylate (inj) (Pfizer)

> Elderly patients with dementia-related psychosis treated with antipsychotic drugs are at an increased risk of death; most deaths appeared to be cardiovascular (eg, heart failure, sudden death) or infectious (eg, pneumonia) in nature. Not approved for the treatment of dementia-related psychosis.

OTHER BRAND NAMES: Geodon for Injection (Pfizer)

THERAPEUTIC CLASS: Benzisoxazole derivative

INDICATIONS: (PO) Treatment of schizophrenia. Monotherapy for acute treatment of manic or mixed episodes associated with bipolar I disorder. Adjunct to lithium or valproate for maintenance treatment of bipolar I disorder. (IM) Treatment of acute agitation in schizophrenic patients who need IM antipsychotic medication for rapid control of agitation.

DOSAGE: *Adults:* Schizophrenia: (PO) Initial/Maint: 20mg bid. Titrate: May increase ≥80mg bid; adjust dose at intervals of not <2 days if indicated. Max: 80mg bid. Maint: No additional benefit for dose >20mg bid. Bipolar Disorder: (PO) Initial: 40mg bid. Titrate: May increase to 60 or 80mg bid on 2nd day, then adjust dose based on tolerance and efficacy within the range 40-80mg bid. Maint (as adjunct to lithium/valproate): 40-80mg bid. Take with food. Agitation: (IM) Usual: 10mg q2h-20mg q4h. Max: 40mg/day. Administration >3 consecutive days has not been studied. Elderly: Start at lower end of dosing range.

HOW SUPPLIED: Cap: (HCl) 20mg, 40mg, 60mg, 80mg; Inj: (Mesylate) 20mg/mL

CONTRAINDICATIONS: Concomitant dofetilide, sotalol, quinidine, Class Ia/III antiarrhythmics, mesoridazine, thioridazine, chlorpromazine, droperidol, pimozide, sparfloxacin, gatifloxacin, moxifloxacin, halofantrine, mefloquine, pentamidine, arsenic trioxide, levomethadyl acetate, dolasetron mesylate, probucol, tacrolimus and drugs that prolong QT interval. History of QT prolongation (including congenital long QT syndrome), recent acute myocardial infarction (MI) and uncompensated heart failure.

WARNINGS/PRECAUTIONS: D/C if persistent QTc measurements >500 msec. Hypokalemia and/or hypomagnesemia may increase risk of QT prolongation and arrhythmia. Initiate further evaluation if symptoms of torsade de pointes (eg, dizziness, palpitations or syncope) occur. Neuroleptic malignant syndrome (NMS) reported; d/c therapy, institute intensive treatment and medical monitoring, and treat any concomitant illness if it occurs. Tardive dyskinesia may occur; consider d/c therapy. Hyperglycemia and DM reported. Rash/urticaria reported; d/c therapy upon appearance of rash. Orthostatic hypotension reported; caution with cardiovascular disease (CVD), cerebrovascular disease or conditions that predispose to hypotension. Leukopenia, neutropenia and agranulocytosis reported; d/c with severe neutropenia (ANC <1000/mm³). Caution with history of seizures or conditions that may lower seizure threshold. Esophageal dysmotility and aspiration pneumonia may occur. May elevate prolactin levels. May impair physical/mental abilities. Priapism reported. May disrupt the body's ability to reduce core body temperature. Closely supervise high-risk patients for suicide attempt. Caution in elderly. Caution with renal dysfunction when administered IM. Concomitant use of IM and oral preparations in schizophrenic patients not recommended.

ADVERSE REACTIONS: Heart failure, pneumonia, asthenia, N/V, constipation, dyspepsia, diarrhea, dry mouth, extrapyramidal symptoms, somnolence, akathisia, dizziness, respiratory tract infection, rash.

INTERACTIONS: See Contraindications. Caution with centrally acting drugs. May enhance effects of antihypertensives. May antagonize effects of levodopa and dopamine agonists. Carbamazepine may decrease levels. CYP3A4 inhibitors (eg, ketoconazole) may increase levels. Serotonin syndrome may occur with serotonergic medicinal products. Periodically monitor serum K⁺ and magnesium (Mg^{2+}) with diuretics. Caution with medication with anticholinergic activity; may elevate core body temperature.

PREGNANCY: Category C, not for use in nursing.

MECHANISM OF ACTION: Psychotropic agent; not established. Actions are mediated through a combination of dopamine type 2 (D_2) and serotonin type 2 ($5HT_2$) antagonism.

PHARMACOKINETICS: Absorption: (PO) Well-absorbed; absolute bioavailability (60%); T_{max}=6-8 hrs. (IM) Absolute bioavailability (100%); T_{max}=60 min. **Distribution:** (PO) V_d=1.5L/kg; plasma protein binding (>99%). **Metabolism:** (PO) Liver (extensive) via aldehyde oxidase (major), CYP3A4 (minor); benzisothiazole (BITP) sulphoxide, BITP-sulphone, ziprasidone sulphoxide, and S-methyl-dihydroziprasidone (major metabolites). **Elimination:** (PO) Urine (20%, <1% unchanged) and feces (66%, <4% unchanged); $T_{1/2}$=7 hrs. (IM) $T_{1/2}$=2-5 hrs.

NURSING CONSIDERATIONS

Assessment: Assess for conditions where treatment is contraindicated or cautioned. Perform baseline CBC and serum electrolytes (K⁺, Mg^{2+}) in patients at risk for significant electrolyte disturbances. Obtain baseline fasting blood glucose (FBG) in patients with increased risk for DM. Replete serum electrolytes prior to treatment. Assess for drug hypersensitivity, pregnancy/nursing status and possible drug interactions.

Monitoring: Monitor for QT prolongation, torsades de pointes, NMS, TD, rash, orthostatic hypotension, seizures, esophageal dysmotility, aspiration pneumonia, suicidal ideation, and weight gain. Monitor renal function, prolactin levels, serum electrolytes (K⁺, Mg^{2+}) and CBC, especially for decline of WBC with signs/symptoms of infection. Monitor for symptoms of hyperglycemia. Monitor regularly for FBG and worsening of glucose control in DM patients. Careful monitoring during the initial dosing period for some elderly.

Patient Counseling: Inform regarding the risks and benefits of therapy. Inform that use may impair mental/physical abilities. Counsel to take with food, avoid alcohol and high temperatures or humidity; drug may interfere with body's ability to regulate temperature. Advise to inform healthcare providers of the following: history of QT prolongation, recent acute MI, uncompensated heart failure, taking other QT-prolonging drugs, risk for electrolyte abnormalities, and history of cardiac arrhythmia. Instruct to report conditions that increase risk for electrolyte disturbances (eg, hypokalemia, taking diuretics, prolonged diarrhea) and if dizziness, palpitations, or syncope occurs.

Administration: Oral, IM route. (IM) Refer to PI for preparation instructions. **Storage:** Cap: 25°C (77°F), excursions permitted to 15-30°C (59-86°F). Inj: Dry form: 25°C (77°F); excursions permitted to 15-30°C (59-86°F). Protect from light. Reconstituted: 15-30°C (59-86°F) ≥24 hrs when protected from light or refrigerated at 2-8°C (36-46°F) for ≥7 days.

GLEEVEC   RX
imatinib mesylate (Novartis)

THERAPEUTIC CLASS: Protein-tyrosine kinase inhibitor

INDICATIONS: (Adults) Treatment of newly diagnosed patients with Philadelphia chromosome positive (Ph+) chronic myeloid leukemia (CML) in chronic phase. Treatment of Ph+ CML in blast crisis, accelerated phase, or in chronic phase after failure of interferon-α therapy. Treatment of relapsed or refractory Ph+ acute lympoblastic leukemia (ALL). Treatment of myelo-dysplastic/myeloproliferative diseases (MDS/MPD) associated with platelet-derived growth factor receptor (PDGFR) gene rearrangements. Treatment of aggressive systemic mastocytosis (ASM) patients without the D816V c-Kit mutation or with unknown c-Kit mutational status. Treatment of hypereosinophilic syndrome (HES) and/or chronic eosinophilic leukemia (CEL) patients who have the FIP1L1-PDGFRα fusion kinase (mutational analysis or FISH demonstration of CHIC2 allele deletion) and for patients with HES and/or CEL who are FIP1L1-PDGFRα fusion kinase negative or unknown. Treatment of unresectable, recurrent, and/or metastatic dermatofibrosarcoma protuberans (DFSP). Treatment of patients with Kit (CD117) positive unresectable and/or metastatic malignant gastrointestinal stromal tumors (GIST). Adjuvant treatment of patients following complete gross resection of Kit (CD117) positive GIST. (Pediatrics) Treatment of patients with Ph+ CML in chronic phase who are newly diagnosed or whose disease has recurred after stem cell transplant or who are resistant to interferon-α therapy.

DOSAGE: *Adults:* CML: Chronic Phase: Usual: 400mg qd. Titrate: May increase to 600mg qd. Accelerated Phase/Blast Crisis: Usual: 600mg qd. Titrate: May increase to 400mg bid. Relapsed/Refractory Ph+ ALL: 600mg qd. MDS or MPD/ASM without D816V c-Kit mutation/HES and/or CEL: 400mg qd. ASM with Eosinophilia/HES or CEL with FIP1L1-PDGFRα: Initial: 100mg qd. Titrate: May increase to 400mg qd in the absence of adverse reactions and insufficient response. DFSP: 800mg qd (as 400mg bid). GIST: Unresectable or Metastatic/Malignant: 400mg qd. Titrate: May increase to 400mg bid if signs/symptoms of disease progression at a lower dose are clear and in the absence of adverse reactions. Adjuvant treatment after complete gross resection: 400mg qd. Severe Hepatic Impairment: Reduce dose by 25%. Coadministration with Strong CYP3A4 Inducers: Avoid concomitant use, if necessary, increase dose by at least 50% and monitor carefully. Hepatotoxicity/Non-Hematologic Adverse Reaction: If bilirubin >3X ULN or transaminases >5X ULN, hold drug until bilirubin <1.5X ULN and transaminases <2.5X ULN. Continue at reduced dose. Moderate Renal Impairment (CrCl 20-39mL/min): Reduce starting dose by 50%. Titrate: As tolerated. Doses >400mg are not recommended. Mild Renal Impairment (40-59mL/min): Doses >600mg are not recommended. Neutropenia/Thrombocytopenia: See PI for dosage adjustments. Take with food and plenty of water.
Pediatrics: ≥2 yrs: CML: Newly Diagnosed: 340mg/m² qd. Max: 600mg. Chronic Phase: 260mg/m² qd or split into 2 doses (am and pm). Severe Hepatic Impairment: Reduce dose by 25%. Coadministration with Strong CYP3A4 Inducers: Avoid concomitant use, if necessary, increase dose by at least 50% and monitor carefully. Hepatotoxicity/Non-Hematologic Adverse Reaction: If bilirubin >3X ULN or transaminases >5X ULN, hold drug until bilirubin <1.5X ULN and transaminases <2.5X ULN. Continue at reduced dose. Moderate Renal Impairment (CrCl 20-39mL/min): Reduce starting dose by 50%. Titrate: As tolerated. Doses >400mg are not recommended. Mild Renal Impairment (40-59mL/min): Doses >600mg are not recommended. Neutropenia/Thrombocytopenia: See PI for dosage adjustments. Take with food and plenty of water.

HOW SUPPLIED: Tab: 100mg*, 400mg* *scored

WARNINGS/PRECAUTIONS: Fluid retention/edema (eg, pleural effusion, pericardial effusion, pulmonary edema, ascites) reported; monitor weight. Anemia/neutropenia/thrombocytopenia reported; monitor CBC weekly during 1st month, biweekly during 2nd month, and periodically thereafter. In pediatric CML patients, the most frequent toxicities observed were grade 3 and 4 cytopenias. May be hepatotoxic; monitor LFTs at baseline, then monthly or as needed. Interrupt and/or reduce dose if laboratory abnormalities occur. Severe congestive heart failure (CHF) and left ventricular dysfunction reported; monitor patients with cardiac disease or risk factors for cardiac failure. Hemorrhages reported. May cause GI irritation; take with food and large glass of water. GI perforation reported rarely. In patients with hypereosinophilic syndrome and cardiac involvement, cardiogenic shock/left ventricular dysfunction reported; reversible with administration of systemic steroids, circulatory support measures, and temporary d/c of treatment. Perform echocardiogram and troponin test in patients with HES/CEL and MDS/MPD or ASM associated with high eosinophil levels; consider prophylactic use of systemic steroids (1-2mg/kg) for 1-2 weeks concomitantly at initiation of therapy if either is abnormal. Bullous dermatological reactions (eg, erythema multiforme, Stevens-Johnson syndrome [SJS]) reported. Hypothyroidism reported in thyroidectomy patients undergoing levothyroxine treatment; monitor TSH levels. Avoid becoming pregnant. Interrupt treatment if severe non-hematologic adverse reaction develops (eg, severe hepatotoxicity, severe fluid retention); resume if appropriate.

ADVERSE REACTIONS: N/V, edema, muscle cramps, musculoskeletal pain, diarrhea, rash, fatigue, asthenia, abdominal pain, lethargy, hemorrhage, malaise, neutropenia, desquamation.

INTERACTIONS: Increased levels with CYP3A4 inhibitors; caution with strong CYP3A4 inhibitors (eg, ketoconazole, atazanavir, indinavir, nefazodone, nelfinavir, ritonavir, saquinavir, telithromycin, voriconazole, clarithromycin, itraconazole). Grapefruit juice may increase levels and should be avoided. Decreased levels with St. John's wort, enzyme-inducing antiepileptic drugs (EIAED) (eg, oxcarbamazepine, fosphenytoin, primidone) and other strong CYP3A4 inducers (eg, dexamethasone, phenytoin, carbamazepine, rifampin, rifabutin, rifampicin, phenobarbital); avoid concomitant use or increase dose by at least 50% if necessary. Caution with CYP3A4 substrates that have narrow therapeutic windows (eg, alfentanil, cyclosporine, diergotamine, ergotamine, fentanyl, quinidine, sirolimus, tacrolimus, pimozide). Increases levels of simvastatin, metoprolol, and drugs metabolized by CYP3A4 (eg, dihydropyridine calcium channel blockers, triazolo-benzodiazepines, HMG-CoA reductase inhibitors). Switch patients on warfarin to low molecular weight or standard heparin. Systemic exposure to acetaminophen is expected to increase. Caution with CYP2D6 substrates that have narrow therapeutic windows. When concomitantly used with chemotherapy, liver toxicity reported; monitor hepatic function. Hypothyroidism reported in thyroidectomy patients undergoing levothyroxine replacement; closely monitor TSH levels.

PREGNANCY: Category D, not for use in nursing.

MECHANISM OF ACTION: Protein-tyrosine kinase inhibitor; inhibits the bcr-abl tyrosine kinase, the constitutive abnormal tyrosine kinase created by the Philadelphia chromosome abnormality in CML; inhibits proliferation and induces apoptosis in bcr-abl positive cell lines as well as fresh leukemic cells from Ph+ CML. Also an inhibitor of the receptor tyrosine kinases for platelet-derived growth factor (PDGF) and stem cell factor (SCF), c-kit, and inhibits PDGF- and SCF-mediated cellular events; in vitro inhibits proliferation and induces apoptosis in GIST cells, which express an activating c-kit mutation.

PHARMACOKINETICS: Absorption: Rapid and well-absorbed; absolute bioavailability (98%); T_{max}=2-4 hrs. **Distribution:** Plasma protein binding (95%); found in breast milk. **Metabolism:** Liver via CYP3A4 (major role), CYP1A2, CYP2D6, CYP2C9, CYP2C19 (minor roles); N-demethylated piperazine derivative (major active metabolite). **Elimination:** Urine, feces (predominant); $T_{1/2}$=18 hrs (imatinib), 40 hrs (active metabolite).

NURSING CONSIDERATIONS

Assessment: Assess for renal/hepatic impairment, cardiac disease, hypereosinophilic syndrome, advanced age, pregnancy/nursing status, and for possible drug interactions. Assess liver function (transaminases, bilirubin, alkaline phosphatase) prior to therapy. Perform echocardiogram and troponin test in patients with HES/CEL and MDS/MPD or ASM associated with high eosinophil levels. Obtain baseline CBC, weight, LFTs, and renal function (CrCl).

Monitoring: Monitor for signs and symptoms of fluid retention (eg, unexpected rapid weight gain), edema, congestive heart failure, left ventricular dysfunction, hepatotoxicity, hemorrhage, GI disorders (eg, GI irritation, GI perforation), and for bullous dermatological reactions (eg, erythema multiforme, SJS). Monitor for signs and symptoms of anemia, neutropenia, and thrombocytopenia; perform CBC weekly for the first month of therapy, biweekly for the second month of therapy, and periodically thereafter. Monitor liver function (transaminases, bilirubin, alkaline phosphatase) monthly or as clinically indicated. In patients with hypereosinophilic syndrome and cardiac involvement, monitor for cardiogenic shock/left ventricular dysfunction. In thyroidectomy patients, monitor TSH levels.

Patient Counseling: Instruct to take exactly as prescribed with a meal and large glass of water. Advise to take the dose as soon as possible if missed; do not take if almost time for the next dose; never double the dose. Inform that it may cause fetal harm; instruct to notify physician if pregnant or nursing. Advise sexually active women to use adequate contraception while on therapy. Advise not to breastfeed while on therapy. Instruct to contact physician if any adverse effects (eg, fever, SOB, blood in stools, jaundice, sudden weight gain, symptoms of cardiac failure) develop while on therapy. Advise not to take any other medications (eg, acetaminophen, herbal products, warfarin, erythromycin, phenytoin) without consulting a pharmacist or doctor. Advise to notify physician if planning to take iron supplements. Advise to avoid grapefruit juice and other foods known to inhibit CYP3A4 while on therapy. Tablets should not be crushed; avoid direct contact of crushed tablets with skin or mucous membranes.

Administration: Oral route. If unable to swallow tablets, tablet may be dispersed in a glass of water or apple juice; required number of tablets should be placed in the appropriate volume of beverage (approximately 50mL for 100mg tablet and 200mL for a 400mg tablet); stir and administer suspension immediately after disintegration of tablets. **Storage:** 25°C (77°F); excursions permitted to 15-30°C (59-86°F). Protect from moisture. Dispense in a tight container.

G

GLUCAGON RX

glucagon (Lilly)

THERAPEUTIC CLASS: Glucagon

INDICATIONS: Treatment for severe hypoglycemia. Diagnostic aid for radiologic examination of the stomach, duodenum, small bowel, and colon when diminished intestinal motility would be advantageous.

DOSAGE: *Adults:* Severe Hypoglycemia: ≥20kg: 1mg (1 U) SQ/IM/IV. May give another dose after 15 min if patient does not respond, but IV glucose is a better alternative. Use immediately after reconstitution, discard unused portion. After patient responds, give supplemental carbohydrate. Diagnostic Aid: Stomach/Duodenum/Small Bowel: 0.25-0.5mg (0.25-0.5 U) IV, or 1mg (1 U) IM, or 2mg (2 U) IV/IM before procedure. Higher incidence of N/V with 2mg dose. Colon: 2mg (2 U) IM 10 min before procedure. Elderly: Start at low end of dosing range.
Pediatrics: Severe Hypoglycemia: ≥20kg: 1mg (1 U) SQ/IM/IV. <20kg: 0.5mg (0.5 U) or dose equivalent to 20-30mcg/kg. May give another dose after 15 min if patient does not respond, but IV glucose would be a better alternative. Use immediately after reconstitution; discard unused portion. After patient responds, give supplemental carbohydrate.

HOW SUPPLIED: Inj: 1mg

CONTRAINDICATIONS: Pheochromocytoma.

WARNINGS/PRECAUTIONS: Caution with history suggestive of insulinoma and/or pheochromocytoma. In patients with insulinoma, IV glucagon may produce an initial increase in blood glucose and then subsequently cause hypoglycemia. In the presence of pheochromocytoma, may cause the tumor to release catecholamines, which may result in a sudden and marked increase in BP. Generalized allergic reactions reported including urticaria, respiratory distress, and hypotension. Effective in treating hypoglycemia only if sufficient liver glycogen is present. Not effective in states of starvation, adrenal insufficiency, or chronic hypoglycemia; use glucose to treat.

ADVERSE REACTIONS: N/V, allergic reactions, urticaria, respiratory distress, hypotension.

INTERACTIONS: Addition of an anticholinergic during diagnostic study may increase side effects.

PREGNANCY: Category B, caution in nursing.

MECHANISM OF ACTION: Polypeptide hormone; increases blood glucose levels and relaxes smooth muscle of the GI tract.

PHARMACOKINETICS: Absorption: (SQ) C_{max}=7.9ng/mL, T_{max}=20 min; (IM) C_{max}=6.9ng/mL, T_{max}=13 min. **Distribution:** V_d=0.25L/kg. **Metabolism:** Extensively degraded in liver, kidneys, plasma. **Elimination:** Urine; $T_{1/2}$=8-18 min.

NURSING CONSIDERATIONS

Assessment: Assess for presence of pheochromocytoma, pregnancy/nursing status, and for possible drug interactions. Assess if patient is in a state of starvation, has adrenal insufficiencies, or has chronic hypoglycemia. Assess use in patients with a history suggestive of insulinoma and/or pheochromocytoma.

Monitoring: Monitor for occurrence of allergic reactions (eg, uticaria, respiratory distress, and hypotension). If pheochromocytoma, monitor for signs/ symptoms of HTN and treat accordingly. In patients with insulinoma, monitor for signs/symptoms of hypoglycemia. Monitor blood glucose levels in patients with hypoglycemia until asymptomatic.

Patient Counseling: Instruct patient and family members, in event of emergency, how to properly prepare and administer glucagon. Inform about measures to prevent hypoglycemia; includes following a uniform regimen on a regular basis, careful adjustment of insulin program, frequent testing of blood or urine for glucose, and routinely carrying hyperglycemic agents to quickly elevate blood glucose levels (eg, sugar, candy, readily absorbed carbohydrates). Inform about symptoms of hypoglycemia and how to treat it appropriately. Inform caregivers that if patient is hypoglycemic, patient should be kept alert and hypoglycemia should be treated as quickly as possible to prevent CNS damage. Advise to inform physician when hypoglycemia occurs.

Administration: IM/IV/SQ routes. Accompanying diluent should be used only for parental injection. Glucagon should not be used in concentrations ≥1mg/mL (1 U/mL). Use reconstituted solution immediately and discard any unused portion. Inspect for particulate matter and discoloration prior to administration. Severe hypoglycemia should be treated initially with IV glucose. If not available, then dissolve lyophilized glucagon using accompanying diluent solution. 1) Wipe rubber stopper on bottle. Do not remove plastic clip from syringe. 2) Swirl bottle gently until glucagon dissolves completely. Do not use unless solution is clear and water-like consistency. 3) Hold bottle upside down, making sure needle tip remains in solution, gently withdrawing solution. 4) Cleanse injection site. 5) Insert needle into loose tissue. Apply light pressure at injection site, and withdraw needle. Press alcohol swab against injection site. **Storage:** Before reconstitution: 20-25°C (68-77°F); excursions allowed between 15-30°C (59-86°F). After reconstitution: Should be used immediately; discard any unused portion.

GLUCOPHAGE XR   RX
metformin HCl (Bristol-Myers Squibb)

> Lactic acidosis reported (rare); increased risk with increased age, diabetes mellitus (DM), renal dysfunction, congestive heart failure (CHF), and conditions with risk of hypoperfusion and hypoxemia. Avoid use in patients ≥80 yrs unless renal function is normal. Withhold therapy in the presence of any condition associated with hypoxemia, dehydration, or sepsis. Avoid in patients with clinical or laboratory evidence of hepatic disease. Caution against excessive alcohol intake; may potentiate the effects of metformin on lactate metabolism. Temporarily D/C prior to any IV radiocontrast study or surgical procedures. D/C use and institute appropriate therapy if lactic acidosis occurs.

OTHER BRAND NAMES: Glucophage (Bristol-Myers Squibb)

THERAPEUTIC CLASS: Biguanide

INDICATIONS: Adjunct to diet and exercise, to improve glycemic control in type 2 DM.

DOSAGE: *Adults:* (Tab) Individualize dose. Initial: 500mg bid or 850mg qd with meals. Titrate: Increase by 500mg/week or 850mg every 2 weeks, or may increase from 500mg bid to 850mg bid after 2 weeks. Max: 2550mg/day. Give in 3 divided doses with meals if dose is >2g/day. (Tab, Extended-Release) Initial: ≥17 yrs: 500mg qd with evening meal. Titrate: Increase by 500mg/ week. Max: 2000mg/day. With Insulin: Initial: 500mg qd. Titrate: Increase by 500mg/week. Max: 2500mg/day and 2000mg/day (XR). Decrease insulin dose by 10-25% when FPG <120mg/dL. Elderly/Debilitated/Malnourished: Conservative dosing; do not titrate to max.

Pediatrics: 10-16 yrs: (Tab) Individualize dose. Initial: 500mg bid with meals. Titrate: Increase by 500mg/week. Max: 2000mg/day, given in divided doses.

HOW SUPPLIED: Tab: 500mg, 850mg, 1000mg; Tab, Extended-Release: 500mg, 750mg

CONTRAINDICATIONS: Renal disease/dysfunction (eg, SrCr ≥1.5mg/dL [males], ≥1.4mg/dL [females], or abnormal CrCl), metabolic acidosis, diabetic ketoacidosis with or without coma. D/C temporarily (48 hrs) for radiologic studies with intravascular iodinated contrast materials.

WARNINGS/PRECAUTIONS: Monitor renal function, FPG, HbA1c, and hematological parameters (eg, Hgb, Hct, red blood cell indices). Monitor for ketoacidosis and metabolic acidosis. Avoid in renal/hepatic impairment. D/C therapy in the presence of hypoxemia (eg, acute CHF, acute MI, cardiovascular collapse), dehydration, sepsis, or if loss of blood glucose occurs due to stress (give insulin). Temporarily d/c therapy prior to any surgical procedure (except minor procedures not associated with restricted intake of food and fluids). May decrease serum vitamin B12 levels. Increased risk of hypoglycemia in elderly, debilitated/malnourished, adrenal or pituitary insufficiency, or alcohol intoxication.

ADVERSE REACTIONS: Lactic acidosis, diarrhea, N/V, flatulence, asthenia, abdominal discomfort, hypoglycemia, dizziness, dyspnea, taste disorder, chest discomfort, flu syndrome, palpitations, indigestion, headache.

INTERACTIONS: See Boxed Warning and Contraindications. Furosemide, nifedipine, cimetidine, cationic drugs (eg, digoxin, amiloride, procainamide, quinidine, quinine, ranitidine, trimethoprim, vancomycin, triamterene, morphine) may increase metformin levels. Thiazides, other diuretics, corticosteroids, phenothiazines, thyroid products, estrogens, oral contraceptives, phenytoin, nicotinic acid, sympathomimetics, CCBs, and isoniazid may cause hyperglycemia. May interact with highly protein-bound drugs (eg, salicylates, sulfonamides, chloramphenicol, probenecid). May decrease furosemide levels. Caution with drugs that may affect renal function or result in significant hemodynamic change or may interfere with the disposition of metformin. Hypoglycemia may occur with concomitant use of other glucose-lowering agents (eg, sulfonylureas, insulin).

PREGNANCY: Category B, not for use in nursing.

MECHANISM OF ACTION: Biguanide; decreases hepatic glucose production, decreases intestinal absorption of glucose, and improves insulin selectivity by increasing peripheral glucose uptake and utilization.

PHARMACOKINETICS: Absorption: Absolute bioavailability (50-60%); (Tab) T_{max}=2.5 hrs, (Tab, Extended-Release) T_{max}=7 hrs. **Distribution:** V_d=654L. **Elimination:** Urine (90%); $T_{1/2}$=6.2 hrs (plasma), 17.6 hrs (blood).

NURSING CONSIDERATIONS

Assessment: Assess for renal/hepatic impairment, acute or chronic metabolic acidosis, presence of a hypoxic state (eg, CHF, acute MI, cardiovascular collapse), dehydration, sepsis, alcoholism, nutritional status, adrenal or pituitary insufficiency, pregnancy/nursing status, and for possible drug interactions. Assess baseline renal function, FPG, HbA1c, and hematological parameters (Hct, Hgb, red blood cell indices).

Monitoring: Monitor for lactic acidosis, hypoglycemia, hypoxemia (eg, cardiovascular collapse, acute CHF, acute MI), prerenal azotemia, and for decreases in Vitamin B12 levels. Monitor FPG, HbA1c, renal function (eg, SrCr), and hematological parameters (eg, Hgb, Hct, red blood cell indices).

Patient Counseling: Inform about the importance of adherence to dietary instructions and a regular exercise program. Inform of the risk of developing lactic acidosis during therapy; advise to d/c therapy immediately and contact physician if unexplained hyperventilation, myalgia, malaise, unusual somnolence, or other nonspecific symptoms occur. Instruct to avoid excessive alcohol intake. Inform that regular follow up is needed. Counsel to take with meals. Instruct that if taking the extended-release tablet, that tablet must be swallowed whole and not crushed or chewed.

Administration: Oral route. **Storage:** (Tab; Tab, Extended-Release) 20-25°C (68-77°F); excursions permitted to 15-30°C (59-86°F). Dispense in light-resistant containers.

GLUCOTROL
glipizide (Pfizer)

RX

THERAPEUTIC CLASS: Sulfonylurea (2nd generation)

INDICATIONS: Adjunct to diet and exercise to improve glycemic control in adults with type 2 diabetes mellitus (DM).

DOSAGE: *Adults:* Take 30 min before meals. Initial: 5mg qd before breakfast; give 2.5mg if elderly or with liver disease. Titrate: Increase by 2.5-5mg; several days should elapse between titration. May divide dose if unsatisfactory response to single dose. Maint: Total daily doses >15mg/day should be divided and given with meals of adequate caloric content. May give total daily doses >30mg bid to long-term patients. Max: 15mg qd or 40mg/day. Switch From Insulin: If ≤20 U/day: D/C insulin and start at 5mg qd. If >20 U/day: Reduce insulin dose by 50% and begin at 5mg qd. Titration: Several days should elapse between titration. Switching from Other Oral Hypoglycemics: No transition period necessary. Elderly/Debilitated/Malnourished/Renal or Hepatic Impairment: Dose conservatively.

HOW SUPPLIED: Tab: 5mg*, 10mg* *scored

CONTRAINDICATIONS: Type 1 DM, diabetic ketoacidosis, with or without coma.

WARNINGS/PRECAUTIONS: Increased risk of cardiovascular (CV) mortality reported; inform patient of potential risks, advantages, and alternative therapy. May produce severe hypoglycemia; proper patient selection, dosage, and instructions are important. Increased risk of hypoglycemia with elderly, debilitated, malnourished, renal/hepatic disease, adrenal or pituitary insufficiency. Loss of blood glucose control may occur when exposed to stress (eg, fever, trauma, infection, or surgery); d/c therapy and administer insulin. Secondary failure may occur over period of time. May cause hemolytic anemia in patients with glucose 6-phosphate dehydrogenase (G6PD) deficiency; observe caution and consider a non-sulfonylurea alternative. Caution in elderly.

ADVERSE REACTIONS: Hypoglycemia, GI disturbances, allergic skin reactions, dizziness, drowsiness, headache, leukopenia, thrombocytopenia, hemolytic anemia.

INTERACTIONS: Hypoglycemic effects potentiated by NSAIDs, some azoles, other highly protein-bound drugs, salicylates, sulfonamides, chloramphenicol, probenecid, coumarins, MAOIs, and β-blockers. Severe hypoglycemia reported with oral miconazole. Increase levels with fluconazole. Hyperglycemia and possible loss of glycemic control with thiazides and other diuretics, corticosteroids, phenothiazines, thyroid products, estrogens, oral contraceptives, phenytoin, nicotinic acid, sympathomimetics, calcium channel blockers, and isoniazid. Increased likelihood of hypoglycemia with alcohol and use of >1 glucose lowering drug. Caution with salicylates or dicumarol.

PREGNANCY: Category C, not for use in nursing.

MECHANISM OF ACTION: Sulfonylurea; lowers blood glucose acutely by stimulating the insulin release from the pancreas.

PHARMACOKINETICS: Absorption: Rapid and complete; T_{max} =1-3 hrs. **Distribution:** Plasma protein binding (98-99%); (IV) V_d=11L. **Metabolism:** Extensive via liver. **Elimination:** Urine (<10% unchanged); $T_{1/2}$=2-4 hrs.

NURSING CONSIDERATIONS

Assessment: Assess previous hypersensitivity, FPG, HbA1c, renal/hepatic function, LFTs, type 1 DM, diabetic ketoacidosis, GI disease, age, debilitated or malnourished patients, adrenal or pituitary insufficiency, G6PD deficiency, pregnancy/nursing status and for possible drug interactions.

Monitoring: Monitor blood and urine glucose, HbA1c, renal and hepatic function, SGOT, LDH, alkaline phosphate, BUN, creatinine, signs/symptoms of hypoglycemia, endocrine/metabolic/hematologic reactions, and any adverse reactions.

Patient Counseling: Instruct to take 30 min before meals. Inform about importance of adhering to dietary instructions, a regular exercise program, and regular testing of urine/blood glucose. Educate on risks/benefits of therapy; signs/symptoms of hypoglycemia/hyperglycemia, predisposing conditions, and treatment of hypoglycemia; and primary and secondary failure. Emphasize that diet is the primary form of treatment for type 2 diabetic patients; caloric restriction and weight loss for obese diabetic patient. Inform that regular physical activity is important, and CV risk factors should be identified and managed.

Administration: Oral route. **Storage:** <30°C (86°F).

GLUCOTROL **XL**   RX
glipizide (Pfizer)

OTHER BRAND NAMES: Glipizide ER (Various)

THERAPEUTIC CLASS: Sulfonylurea (2nd generation)

INDICATIONS: Adjunct to diet and exercise, to improve glycemic control in adults with type 2 diabetes mellitus (DM).

DOSAGE: *Adults:* Initial: 5mg qd with breakfast; use lower doses if sensitive to hypoglycemics. Titrate: Based on lab measures of glycemic control. Maint: 5-10mg qd. Max: 20mg/day. Switch from Immediate-Release (IR) Glipizide: Give a qd dose at nearest equivalent total daily dose. If receiving IR formulation, may titrate to ER starting with 5mg qd. Combination Therapy: Initial: 5mg qd. Switch From Insulin: If ≤20 U/day: D/C insulin and start at 5mg qd. If >20 U/day: Reduce insulin dose by 50% and begin at 5mg qd. Titrate: Several days should elapse between titration. Switching from Other Oral Hypoglycemics: No transition period necessary. Elderly/Debilitated/Malnourished/Renal or Hepatic Impairment: Dose conservatively.

HOW SUPPLIED: Tab, Extended-Release: 2.5mg, 5mg, 10mg

CONTRAINDICATIONS: Type 1 DM, diabetic ketoacidosis, with or without coma.

WARNINGS/PRECAUTIONS: Increased risk of cardiovascular (CV) mortality reported; inform patient of potential risks, advantages, and alternative therapy. Markedly reduced GI retention times reported. May produce severe hypoglycemia; proper patient selection, dosage, and instructions are important. Increased risk of hypoglycemia with elderly, debilitated, malnourished, renal/hepatic disease, adrenal or pituitary insufficiency. Loss of blood glucose control may occur when exposed to stress (eg, fever, trauma, infection, or surgery); d/c therapy and administer insulin. Secondary failure may occur over period of time. May cause hemolytic anemia in patients with glucose 6-phosphate dehydrogenase (G6PD) deficiency; observe caution and consider a non-sulfonylurea alternative.

ADVERSE REACTIONS: Hypoglycemia, asthenia, headache, dizziness, diarrhea, nervousness, tremor, flatulence.

INTERACTIONS: Hypoglycemic effects potentiated by NSAIDs, other highly protein-bound drugs, salicylates, sulfonamides, chloramphenicol, probenecid, coumarins, MAOIs, and β-blockers. Severe hypoglycemia reported with oral miconazole. Increased levels with fluconazole. Hyperglycemia and possible loss of glycemic control with thiazides and other diuretics, corticosteroids, phenothiazines, thyroid products, estrogens, oral contraceptives, phenytoin, nicotinic acid, sympathomimetics, calcium channel blockers, and isoniazid. Increased likelihood of hypoglycemia with alcohol and use of >1 glucose lowering drug. Caution with salicylates or dicumarol.

PREGNANCY: Category C, not for use in nursing.

MECHANISM OF ACTION: Sulfonylurea; lowers blood glucose acutely by stimulating the release of insulin from the pancreas.

PHARMACOKINETICS: Absorption: Rapid and complete (IR); absolute bioavailability (100%); T_{max}=6-12 hrs. **Distribution:** V_d=10L; plasma protein binding (98-99%). **Metabolism:** Liver; aromatic hydroxylation products (major metabolites). **Elimination:** Urine (80%, <10% unchanged), feces (10%, <10% unchanged); $T_{1/2}$=2-5 hrs.

NURSING CONSIDERATIONS

Assessment: Assess previous hypersensitivity, FPG, HbA1c renal/hepatic function, LFTs, type 1 DM, ketoacidosis, GI disease, pre-existing severe GI narrowing, debilitated or malnourished patients, adrenal or pituitary insufficiency, G6PD deficiency, pregnancy/nursing status and for possible drug interactions.

Monitoring: Monitor blood and urine glucose, HbA1c q3 months, renal and hepatic function, LFTs, signs/symptoms of hypoglycemia, loss control of blood glucose, hemolytic anemia, endocrine/metabolic/hematologic reactions, and any adverse reactions.

Patient Counseling: Counsel to swallow whole with breakfast; do not chew, divide, or crush. Inform that patients may notice something that looks like a tablet in their stool and about importance of adhering to dietary instructions, a regular exercise program, and regular testing of urine/blood glucose. Educate on risks/benefits and of therapy; signs/symptoms of hypoglycemia/hyperglycemia, predisposing conditions and treatment of hypoglycemia; and primary and secondary failure.

Administration: Oral route. Swallow whole; do not chew, divide, or crush tab. **Storage:** 15-30°C (59°-86°F). Protect from moisture and humidity.

GLUCOVANCE RX
metformin HCl - glyburide (Bristol-Myers Squibb)

> Lactic acidosis reported (rare); increased risk with increased age, DM with renal insufficiency, congestive heart failure (CHF), and conditions with risk of hypoperfusion and hypoxemia. Avoid use in patients ≥80 yrs unless renal function is normal. Withhold therapy in the presence of any condition associated with hypoxemia, dehydration, or sepsis. Avoid in patients with clinical or laboratory evidence of hepatic disease. Caution against excessive alcohol intake, may potentiate the effects of metformin on lactate metabolism. Temporarily D/C prior to any IV radiocontrast study or surgical procedures. D/C use and institute appropriate therapy if lactic acidosis occur. Monitor renal function and for metabolic acidosis.

THERAPEUTIC CLASS: Sulfonylurea/biguanide

INDICATIONS: Adjunct to diet and exercise to improve glycemic control in adults with type 2 diabetes mellitus (DM).

DOSAGE: *Adults:* Individualize dose. Inadequate Glycemic Control on Diet/Exercise Alone: Initial: 1.25mg-250mg qd-bid with meals. If HbA1c >9% or fasting plasma glucose (FPG) >200mg/dL, give 1.25mg-250mg bid (with morning and evening meals). Titrate: Increase by 1.25mg-250mg/day every 2 weeks. Do not use 5mg-500mg for initial therapy. Inadequate Glycemic Control on a Sulfonylurea and/or Metformin: Initial: 2.5mg-500mg or 5mg-500mg bid with meals. Starting dose should not exceed daily doses of glyburide or metformin already being taken. Titrate: Increase by no more than 5mg-500mg/day. Max: 20mg-2000mg/day. With Concomitant Thiazolidinediones (TZDs): Initiate and titrate TZD as recommended. If hypoglycemia occurs, reduce glyburide component. Elderly/Debilitated/Malnourished: Do not titrate to maximum dose.

HOW SUPPLIED: Tab: (Glyburide-Metformin) 1.25mg-250mg, 2.5mg-500mg, 5mg-500mg

CONTRAINDICATIONS: Renal disease or dysfunction (SrCr ≥1.5mg/dL [males], ≥1.4mg/dL [females], or abnormal CrCl), metabolic acidosis, including diabetic ketoacidosis. D/C temporarily for radiologic studies involving intravascular iodinated contrast materials.

WARNINGS/PRECAUTIONS: Increased risk of cardiovascular (CV) mortality. Increased risk of hypoglycemia with deficient caloric intake, in elderly, debilitated, malnourished, adrenal/pituitary insufficiency or alcohol intoxication. Caution in patients with glucose-6-phosphate dehydrogenase (G6PD) deficiency; may lead to hemolytic anemia. D/C if CV collapse (shock), acute CHF, acute MI, or prerenal azotemia occur. Temporarily suspend therapy before any surgical procedure (except minor procedures not associated with restricted intake of foods and fluids), and do not restart until oral intake has resumed and renal function returns to normal. May decrease serum vitamin B_{12} levels; caution in those with inadequate vitamin B12 or calcium intake or absorption.

ADVERSE REACTIONS: Upper respiratory infection, N/V, abdominal pain, headache, dizziness, diarrhea.

INTERACTIONS: See Boxed Warning & Contraindications. Furosemide, nifedipine, and cimetidine may increase metformin levels. Hypoglycemia is potentiated by ciprofloxacin, miconazole, thiazolidinedione, salicylates, sulfonamides, chloramphenicol, probenecid, coumarins, MAOIs, NSAIDs, highly protein bound drugs, other glucose lowering agents, phenylbutazone, warfarin and β-blockers. Thiazides and other diuretics, corticosteroids, phenothiazines, thyroid products, estrogens, oral contraceptives, phenytoin, nicotinic acid, sympathomimetics, calcium channel blockers, and isoniazid may cause hyperglycemia. Monitor LFTs and weight gain with TZD and rosiglitazone. May compete for common renal tubular transport systems with cationic drugs (eg, amiloride, digoxin, morphine, procainamide, quinidine, ranitidine, triamterene, trimethoprim, or vancomycin).

PREGNANCY: Category B, not for use in nursing.

MECHANISM OF ACTION: Glyburide: Sulfonylurea; stimulates release of insulin from the pancreas. Metformin: Biguanide; decreases hepatic glucose production and intestinal absorption of glucose, and improves insulin sensitivity by increasing peripheral glucose uptake and utilization.

PHARMACOKINETICS: Absorption: Glyburide: T_{max}=4 hrs. Metformin: absolute bioavailability (50-60%). **Distribution:** Glyburide: plasma protein binding (extensive). Metformin: V_d=654L. **Metabolism:** Glyburide: metabolites: 4-trans-hydroxy (major) and 3-cis hydroxy derivative. **Elimination:** Glyburide: bile, urine (50% each route); $T_{1/2}$=10 hrs. Metformin: urine (90%); $T_{1/2}$=6.2 hrs (plasma), 17.6 hrs (blood).

NURSING CONSIDERATIONS

Assessment: Assess for renal disease/dysfunction, metabolic acidosis, diabetic ketoacidosis, patients who have undergone radiologic studies using intravascular iodinated contrast materials or surgical procedures, CHF, conditions with risk of hypoperfusion and hypoxemia, septicemia, hydration status, patient's age, hepatic disease, alcoholism, CV disease, caloric intake, adrenal/pituitary insufficiency, G6PD deficiency, vitamin B_{12} or calcium deficiency, hypersensitivity, pregnancy/nursing status and for possible drug interactions. Assess FPG, HbA1c levels, renal function (eg, CrCl), LFTs, hematologic parameters (eg, Hgb, Hct and RBC indices)

Monitoring: Monitor for hypoglycemia, lactic acidosis, prerenal azotemia, CHF, CV disease, shock, acute MI, metabolic acidosis and hypersensitivity reactions. Monitor FPG, HbA1c, renal function (eg, SrCr), LFTs, hematologic parameters (eg, Hgb/Hct, CBC). Evaluate serum electrolytes and ketones, blood glucose, blood pH, lactate, pyruvate and metformin levels in the evidence of ketoacidosis or lactic acidosis.

Patient Counseling: Inform about potential risks and benefits of drug and alternative modes of therapy. Inform that drug is adjunct to diet and exercise to control diabetes. Inform about importance of adherence to dietary instructions, regular exercise programs, and regular testing of blood glucose, glycosylated Hgb, renal function, and hematologic parameters. Report unexplained hyperventilation, myalgia, malaise, N/V, and somnolence. Explain risk of lactic acidosis, its signs/symptoms, and conditions that predispose its development. Explain risk of hypoglycemia. Counsel against excessive alcohol intake.

Administration: Oral route. **Storage:** 25°C (77°F). Dispense in light-resistant container.

GLUMETZA

RX

metformin HCl (Depomed)

THERAPEUTIC CLASS: Biguanide

INDICATIONS: Adjunct to diet and exercise to improve glycemic control in type 2 diabetes mellitus.

DOSAGE: *Adults:* ≥18 yrs: Individualize dose. Take with evening meal. Initial: 1000mg qd. With Insulin: Initial: 500mg qd. Titrate: May increase by 500mg/week. Max: 2000mg/day. Decrease insulin dose by 10-25% if FPG <120mg/dL. Elderly/Debilitated/Malnourished: Conservative dosing; do not titrate to max. Swallow whole; do not crush or chew.

HOW SUPPLIED: Tab, Extended-Release: 500mg, 1000mg

CONTRAINDICATIONS: Renal disease or dysfunction (SrCr ≥1.5mg/dL [males], ≥1.4mg/dL [females], or abnormal CrCl), acute or chronic metabolic acidosis, including diabetic ketoacidosis with or without coma.

WARNINGS/PRECAUTIONS: Lactic acidosis reported (rare); increased risk with renal dysfunction, increased age, DM, CHF, and other conditions with risk of hypoperfusion and hypoxemia. Avoid use in patients ≥80 yrs unless renal function is normal. Avoid in hepatic impairment. D/C in hypoxic states (eg, CHF, shock, acute MI), acidosis, dehydration, sepsis. Loss of blood glucose control due to stress; d/c therapy and temporarily administer insulin. Temporarily d/c prior to surgery (due to restricted food/fluid intake) or procedures requiring intravascular iodinated contrast materials. May decrease serum vitamin B_{12} levels. Increased risk of hypoglycemia in elderly, debilitated/malnourished, adrenal or pituitary insufficiency, or alcohol intoxication.

ADVERSE REACTIONS: Hypoglycemia, diarrhea, nausea.

INTERACTIONS: Furosemide, nifedipine, cimetidine, cationic drugs (eg, digoxin, amiloride, procainamide, quinidine, quinine, ranitidine, trimethoprim, vancomycin, triamterene, morphine) may increase metformin levels. Thiazides, other diuretics, corticosteroids, phenothiazines, thyroid products, estrogens, oral contraceptives, phenytoin, nicotinic acid, sympathomimetics, CCBs, isoniazid may cause hyperglycemia. Risk of hypoglycemia with alcohol. Excess alcohol may increase potential for lactic acidosis. May decrease furosemide levels. Radiocontrast dyes may alter renal function leading to lactic acidosis in patients taking metformin.

PREGNANCY: Category B, not for use in nursing.

MECHANISM OF ACTION: Biguanide; decreases hepatic glucose production, decreases intestinal absorption of glucose, and improves insulin selectivity by increasing peripheral glucose uptake and utilization.

PHARMACOKINETICS: Absorption: Administration of variable doses resulted in different absorption parameters. T_{max}=7-8 hrs (1000mg, single dose). **Distribution:** V_d=654L (850mg, single dose). **Elimination:** Urine (90%); $T_{1/2}$=6.2 hrs (plasma), 17.6 hrs (blood).

NURSING CONSIDERATIONS

Assessment: Assess FPG, HbA1c, renal function, serum electrolytes, ketones, LFTs, CBC and body weight. Assess for CHF, septicemia, acute or chronic metabolic acidosis, adrenal or pituitary insufficiency, alcoholism, pregnancy status. Evaluate for other medical/surgical conditions and for possible drug interactions.

Monitoring: Monitor for hypoglycemia, lactic acidosis, prerenal azotemia, CHF, CVD. Monitor FPG, HbA1c, renal function, LFTs, CBC.

Patient Counseling: Inform of the potential risks and benefits of the drug and of alternative modes of therapy. Counsel about the importance of adherence to dietary instructions, regular exercise program, regular testing of blood glucose, glycosylated hemoglobin, renal function, and hematologic parameters. Counsel on signs and symptoms of lactic acidosis and instruct to d/c metformin and notify physician if suspected. Counsel against excessive alcohol intake, either acute or chronic while on therapy. Instruct to swallow tablet whole, not to crush or chew. Inactive ingredients may occasionally as eliminated in the feces resembling the tablet.

Administration: Oral route. **Storage:** 20-25°C (68-77°F); excursions permitted to 15-30°C (59-86°F).

GLYNASE PRESTAB RX

glyburide (Pharmacia & Upjohn)

THERAPEUTIC CLASS: Sulfonylurea (2nd generation)

INDICATIONS: Adjunct to diet and exercise, to improve glycemic control in adults with type 2 diabetes mellitus (DM).

DOSAGE: *Adults:* Initial: 1.5-3mg qd with breakfast or 1st main meal; give 0.75mg if sensitive to hypoglycemic drugs. Titrate: Increase by increments of ≤1.5mg at weekly intervals based on patient's response. Maint: 0.75-12mg qd or in divided doses. Max: 12mg/day. Transfer from Other Oral Antidiabetic Agents: Initial: 1.5-3mg/day. Retitrate when transferring from other glyburide products or oral hypoglycemic agents. Exercise particular care during 1st 2 weeks when transferring patients from chlorpropamide. Switch From Insulin: If <20 U/day: 1.5-3mg qd. If 20-40 U/day: 3mg qd. If >40 U/day, decrease insulin dose by 50% and give 3mg qd. Titrate: Progressive withdrawal of insulin, and increase in increments of 0.75-1.5mg every 2-10 days. Concomitant Metformin: Add glyburide gradually to max dose of metformin monotherapy after 4 weeks if needed. Elderly/Debilitated/Malnourished/Renal or Hepatic Impairment: Conservative initial and maintenance dose.

HOW SUPPLIED: Tab: 1.5mg*, 3mg*, 6mg* *scored

CONTRAINDICATIONS: Diabetic ketoacidosis with or without coma, type I DM.

WARNINGS/PRECAUTIONS: Increased risk of cardiovascular mortality reported. Risk of hypoglycemia, especially with renal/hepatic and adrenal/pituitary insufficiency, elderly, debilitated, and malnourished. Loss of blood glucose control may occur when exposed to stress (eg, fever, trauma, infection, surgery); d/c therapy and start insulin. Secondary failure may occur over period of time. Caution with glucose 6-phosphate dehydrogenase (G6PD) deficiency; treatment may lead to hemolytic anemia; thus, consider a non-sulfonylurea alternative.

ADVERSE REACTIONS: Hypoglycemia, liver function abnormalities, GI disturbances, leukopenia, agranulocytosis, thrombocytopenia, hemolytic anemia, aplastic anemia, pancytopenia, hyponatremia, changes in accomodation, blurred vision, allergic reactions.

INTERACTIONS: Hypoglycemic effects may be potentiated by NSAIDs, other drugs that are highly protein bound, ciprofloxacin, salicylates, sulfonamides, chloramphenicol, probenecid, coumarins, MAOIs, alcohol, and β-adrenergic blocking agents. Severe hypoglycemia reported with oral hypolycemics and oral miconazole. Hypoglycemia may occur with >1 glucose lowering drug used. Certain drugs, including thiazides and other diuretics, corticosteroids, phenothiazines, thyroid products, estrogens, oral contraceptives, phenytoin, nicotinic acid, sympathomimetics, calcium channel blockers, and isoniazid, tend to cause hyperglycemia and may lead to loss of glycemic control. May overlap drug effects when transferred from chlorpropamide. May be displaced from protein binding sites by phenylbutazone, warfarin and salicylates. Possible interaction with ciprofloxacin. Decrease levels with metformin.

PREGNANCY: Category B, not for use in nursing.

MECHANISM OF ACTION: Sulfonylurea; lowers blood glucose acutely by stimulating the release of insulin from the pancreas.

PHARMACOKINETICS: Absorption: C_{max}=106ng/mL (3mg); AUC=568ng•hr/mL (3mg); T_{max}=2-3 hrs. **Distribution:** Plasma protein binding (extensive). **Metabolism:** 4-trans-hydroxy derivative (major metabolite). **Elimination:** Bile (50%), urine (50%); $T_{1/2}$=4 hrs.

NURSING CONSIDERATIONS

Assessment: Assess for diabetic ketoacidosis, type I DM, renal/hepatic function, presence of debilitation or malnourishment, adrenal/pituitary insufficiency, G6PD deficiency, pregnancy/nursing status, and for possible drug interactions. Assess FPG and HbA1c levels. Assess adherence to diet before classifying secondary failure.

Monitoring: Monitor for signs/symptoms of hypoglycemia, hemolytic anemia, therapeutic response to therapy, primary/secondary failure. Periodically monitor FPG, glycosylated Hgb, and urine glucose.

Patient Counseling: Inform of the potential risks and advantages of therapy and of alternative modes of therapy. Instruct to take with breakfast or first main meal. Advise about the importance of adhering to dietary instructions, a regular exercise program, and regular testing of urine and/or blood glucose. Inform of risks of hypoglycemia, symptoms and treatment, and conditions that predispose to its development. Counsel about primary/secondary failure.

Administration: Oral route. **Storage:** 20-25°C (68-77°F).

GLYSET

miglitol (Pharmacia & Upjohn)

RX

THERAPEUTIC CLASS: Alpha-glucosidase inhibitor

INDICATIONS: Adjunct to diet and exercise to improve glycemic control in adults with type 2 diabetes mellitus.

DOSAGE: *Adults:* Initial: 25mg tid. May give 25mg qd (to minimize GI side effects) and gradually increase to tid. Titrate: After 4-8 weeks, increase to 50mg tid for 3 months. Maint: 50mg tid. May increase to 100mg tid if needed. Max: 100mg tid. One hour postprandial plasma glucose may be used to determine minimum effective dose. Take with first bite of each main meal.

HOW SUPPLIED: Tab: 25mg, 50mg, 100mg

CONTRAINDICATIONS: Diabetic ketoacidosis, inflammatory bowel disease, colonic ulceration, partial intestinal obstruction or predisposal to intestinal obstruction. Chronic intestinal diseases associated with digestion or absorption disorders or conditions that may deteriorate with increased gas formation in the intestine.

WARNINGS/PRECAUTIONS: Use oral glucose (dextrose) not sucrose (cane sugar) to treat mild-moderate hypoglycemia. Temporary insulin therapy may be necessary at times of stress such as fever, trauma, infection, or surgery. Not recommended with significant renal dysfunction (SrCr >2mg/dL).

ADVERSE REACTIONS: Flatulence, diarrhea, abdominal pain, skin rash, low serum iron.

INTERACTIONS: Intestinal absorbents (eg, charcoal) and digestive enzyme preparations containing carbohydrate-splitting enzmes (eg, amylase, pancreatin) may reduce effects. May reduce bioavailability of ranitidine and propranolol. Levels may be lowered with glyburide, metformin, or digoxin.

PREGNANCY: Category B, not for use in nursing.

MECHANISM OF ACTION: α-glucosidase inhibitor; reversibly inhibits membrane-bound intestinal α-glucosidase hydrolase enzymes.

PHARMACOKINETICS: Absorption: Complete, T_{max}=2-3 hrs. **Distribution:** V_d=0.18 L/kg; plasma protein binding (<4.0%); found in breast milk. **Elimination**: Urine (95% unchanged); $T_{1/2}$=2 hrs.

NURSING CONSIDERATIONS

Assessment: Assess for diabetic ketoacidosis, inflammatory bowel disease, colonic ulceration, partial intestinal obstruction, chronic intestinal disease, renal function, pregnancy/nursing status, hypersensitivity and possible drug interactions.

Monitoring: Monitor for hypoglycemia, FPG, HbA1c, renal function, diabetic ketoacidosis, GI symptoms, skin rash, serum iron.

Patient Counseling: Inform that drug is adjunct to diet and exercise. Counsel that during periods of stress (fever, trauma, infection, or surgery), medication requirements may change; patients should seek medical advice promptly. Counsel about dose-related gastrointestinal effects (eg, flatulence, soft stools, diarrhea, or abdominal discomfort). Inform that if side effects occur, they usually develop during the first few weeks of therapy. Advise to continue to adhere to dietary instructions, regular exercise program and regular testing of urine and/or blood glucose. Advise to take with the first bite of each meal.

Administration: Oral route. **Storage:** 25°C (77°F); excursions permitted to 15-30°C (59-86°F).

GRIFULVIN V   RX
griseofulvin (Ortho Neutrogena)

THERAPEUTIC CLASS: *Penicillium*-derived antifungal

INDICATIONS: Management of tinea capitis, tinea corporis, tinea pedis, tinea unguium, tinea barbae, and tinea cruris. Inhibits the growth of fungi that commonly cause ringworm infections of hair, skin, and nails.

DOSAGE: *Adults:* T. capitis: 500mg qd for 4-6 weeks. T. corporis: 500mg qd for 2-4 weeks. T. pedis: 1g qd for 4-8 weeks. T. cruris: 500mg qd. T. unguium: 1g qd for at least 4 months (fingernail) or at least 6 months (toenails). *Pediatrics:* Usual: 5mg/lb/day. 30-50 lbs: 125-250mg qd. >50 lbs: 250-500mg qd. T. capitis: Treat for 4-6 weeks. T. corporis: Treat for 2-4 weeks. T. pedis: Treat for 4-8 weeks. T. unguium: Treat for at least 4 months (fingernail) or at least 6 months (toenails).

HOW SUPPLIED: Sus: 125mg/5mL [120mL]; Tab: 250mg, 500mg

CONTRAINDICATIONS: Porphyria, hepatocellular failure, pregnancy.

WARNINGS/PRECAUTIONS: Confirm diagnosis. Not for prophylactic use. Monitor renal, hepatic, and hematopoietic functions periodically with prolonged therapy. Cross-sensitivity with PCN may exist. Photosensitivity reported. D/C if granulocytopenia occurs.

ADVERSE REACTIONS: Rash, urticaria, oral thrush, N/V, epigastric distress, diarrhea, headache, dizziness, insomnia, mental confusion.

INTERACTIONS: Oral anticoagulants may need adjustment. Barbiturates decrease effects. Decreases effects of oral contraceptives; may increase incidence of breakthrough bleeding.

PREGNANCY: Not for use in pregnancy or nursing.

MECHANISM OF ACTION: Acts systemically to inhibit the growth of *Trichophyton*, *Microsporum*, and *Epidermophyton* genera of fungi. Fungistatic amounts deposit in keratin, which is gradually exfoliated and replaced by noninfected tissue.

PHARMACOKINETICS: Absorption: C_{max}=0.5g; T_{max}=4 hrs.

NURSING CONSIDERATIONS

Assessment: Assess for proper diagnosis of infecting fungi. Assess for possible drug interactions and drug allergies (possible PCN cross-sensitivity).

Monitoring: Monitor for photosensitivity reactions. Periodically monitor organ system function, including renal, hepatic, and hematopoietic. Monitor for signs/symptoms of lupus erythematosus.

Patient Counseling: Counsel females to use additional forms of contraception while taking medication and for 1 month following cessation of therapy. Counsel males to use contraception while on treatment and for 6 months following. Warn patients to avoid exposure to intense natural or artificial sunlight. Counsel females to avoid use during pregnancy.

Administration: Oral route. **Storage:** Store at room temperature.

GRIS-PEG

RX

griseofulvin (Pedinol)

THERAPEUTIC CLASS: *Penicillium*-derived antifungal

INDICATIONS: Treatment of the following ringworm infections: tinea corporis, tinea pedis, tinea cruris, tinea barbae, tinea capitis, and tinea unguium when caused by one or more species of *Microsporum*, *Epidermophyton*, and *Trichophyton*.

DOSAGE: *Adults:* T. corporis/T. cruris/T. capitis: 375mg/day in single or divided doses. T. corporis: Treat for 2-4 weeks. T. capitis: Treat for 4-6 weeks. Difficult Fungal Infections to Eradicate/ T. pedis/ T. unguium: 750mg/day, given in a divided dose. T. pedis: Concomitant topical agents required. Treat for 4-8 weeks. T. unguium: Treat for at least 4 months (fingernails) and at least 6 months (toenails), depending on rate of growth.
Pediatrics: >2 yrs: Usual: 3.3mg/lb/day. 35-60 lbs: 125-187.5mg/day. >60 lbs: 187.5-375mg/day. T. capitis: Treat for 4-6 weeks. T. corporis: Treat for 2-4 weeks. T. pedis: Treat for 4-8 weeks. T. unguium: Treat for at least 4 months (fingernail) and at least 6 months (toenails), depending on rate of growth.

HOW SUPPLIED: Tab: 125mg*, 250mg* *scored

CONTRAINDICATIONS: Porphyria, hepatocellular failure, pregnancy.

WARNINGS/PRECAUTIONS: Not for prophylactic use. Severe skin reactions (eg, Stevens-Johnson syndrome (SJS), toxic epidermal necrolysis) reported; d/c if these occur. Elevations in AST, ALT, bilirubin and jaundice reported; monitor for hepatic adverse events and d/c if warranted. Periodically organ system function including renal, hepatic, and hematopoietic functions if on prolonged therapy; d/c if granulocytopenia occurs. Cross-sensitivity with PCN may exist. Photosensitivity reported. Lupus erythematosus or lupus-like syndromes reported. Clinical relapse may occur if therapy not continued until infecting organism eradicated.

ADVERSE REACTIONS: Hypersensitivity reactions (eg, skin rashes, urticaria, erythema multiforme-like reactions), granulocytopenia, oral thrush, N/V, epigastric distress, diarrhea, headache, dizziness, insomnia, mental confusion.

INTERACTIONS: Anticoagulants (warfarin-type) may require dosage adjustment. Decreased effect with barbiturates. Possible interaction with oral contraceptives. Increased alcohol effect, producing tachycardia and flush.

PREGNANCY: Contraindicated in pregnancy, safety not known in nursing.

MECHANISM OF ACTION: *Penicillium*-derived antifungal; fungistatic with *in vitro* activity against various species of *Microsporum*, *Epidermophyton* and *Trichophyton*.

PHARMACOKINETICS: Absorption: (250mg unaltered tab) C_{max}=600.61ng/mL; T_{max}=4.04 hrs; AUC=8,618.89ng•hr/mL. (250mg physically altered tab [crushed and in applesauce]) C_{max}=672.61ng/mL; T_{max}=3.08 hrs; AUC=9,023.71ng•hr/mL.

NURSING CONSIDERATIONS

Assessment: Assess for identification of fungi responsible for infection (eg, cultures, microscopic exam). Assess for hepatocellular failure, porphyria, hypersensitivity to penicillin, pregnancy/nursing status, and for possible drug interactions.

Monitoring: Monitor for signs/symptoms of serious skin reactions (eg, SJS, erythema multiforme), hepatotoxicity, photosensitivity reactions, and for lupus erythematosus or lupus-like syndromes. Perform periodic monitoring of organ system function including renal, hepatic, and hematopoietic functions in patients on prolonged therapy.

Patient Counseling: Inform of the importance of compliance with full course of therapy. Counsel to avoid intense natural or artificial sunlight while on medication. Instruct to take proper hygienic precautions to prevent spread of infection. Advise females to avoid pregnancy while on therapy. Instruct to notify physician if any adverse reactions occur.

Administration: Oral route. Swallow whole or crushed and sprinkled onto 1 tbsp of applesauce and swallow immediately without chewing. **Storage:** 15-30°C (59-86°F). Store in tight, light-resistant container.

HALAVEN   RX
eribulin mesylate (Eisai)

THERAPEUTIC CLASS: Antimicrotubule agent

INDICATIONS: Treatment of metastatic breast cancer in patients who have previously received ≥2 chemotherapeutic regimens (should have included anthracycline and taxane) for the treatment of metastatic disease.

DOSAGE: *Adults:* Administer IV over 2-5 min on Days 1 and 8 of a 21-day cycle. Usual: 1.4mg/m². Mild Hepatic (Child-Pugh A)/Moderate Renal Impairment (CrCl 30-50 mL/min): 1.1mg/m². Moderate Hepatic Impairment (Child-Pugh B): 0.7mg/m². Refer to PI for dose modifications and for recommended dose reductions.

HOW SUPPLIED: Inj: 0.5mg/mL [2mL]

WARNINGS/PRECAUTIONS: Severe neutropenia (ANC <500/mm³) may occur. Monitor CBC prior to each dose; increase frequency of monitoring if Grade 3 or 4 cytopenias develop. Peripheral neuropathy reported. Monitor closely for signs of peripheral motor and sensory neuropathy. May cause fetal harm. Monitor ECG in patients with CHF, bradyarrhythmias and electrolyte abnormalities. Correct hypokalemia or hypomagnesemia prior to therapy and monitor periodically. Avoid with congenital long QT syndrome

ADVERSE REACTIONS: Neutropenia, anemia, peripheral neuropathy, headache, asthenia/fatigue, pyrexia, weight decrease, constipation, diarrhea, N/V, arthralgia, dyspnea, alopecia.

INTERACTIONS: Caution with drugs known to prolong the QT interval (eg, Class Ia and III antiarrhythmics).

PREGNANCY: Category D, not for use in nursing.

MECHANISM OF ACTION: Antimicrotubule agent; inhibits growth phase of microtubules via tubulin-based antimitotic mechanism leading to G2/M cell-cycle block, disruption of mitotic spindles, and apoptotic cell death after prolonged mitotic blockage.

PHARMACOKINETICS: Distribution: V_d=43-114L/m²; plasma protein binding at concentrations of 100-1000ng/mL (49-65%). **Metabolism:** Liver via CYP3A4 (negligible). **Elimination:** Urine (9%; 91% unchanged), feces (82%; 88% unchanged); $T_{1/2}$=40 hrs.

NURSING CONSIDERATIONS

Assessment: Assess for renal/hepatic function, CHF, bradyarrhythmias, congenital long QT syndrome, electrolyte abnormalities, pregnancy/nursing status and possible drug interactions. Assess for peripheral neuropathy and obtain CBC prior to each dose.

Monitoring: Monitor ECG and serum electrolytes periodically. Monitor for signs of neuropathy and neutropenia. Monitor for prolonged QT intervals in patients with CHF, bradyarrhythmias, taking drugs known to prolong the QT interval and electrolyte abnormalities. Monitor CBC prior to each dose.

Patient Counseling: Advise to contact healthcare provider for a fever of ≥100.5°F or other signs/symptoms of infection (eg, chills, cough, or burning or pain on urination). Advise women of childbearing potential to avoid pregnancy and use effective contraception during treatment.

Administration: IV route. Administer undiluted or diluted in 100 mL of 0.9% NaCl. Do not dilute in or administer through IV line containing sol with dextrose. Do not administer in same IV line with the other medicinal products. **Storage:** 25°C (77°F); excursions permitted to 15-30°C (59-86°F). Do not freeze. Undiluted/Diluted Sol: Up to 4 hrs at room temperature or for up to 24 hrs under refrigeration (4°C or 40°F).

HALCION
triazolam (Pharmacia & Upjohn)

> Federally controlled substance (C-IV) because of potential for abuse or dependence. Prevent misuse and abuse by keeping in safe place. Inform doctor of any history of drug or alcohol dependence.

THERAPEUTIC CLASS: Benzodiazepine

INDICATIONS: Short-term treatment of insomnia.

DOSAGE: *Adults:* 0.25mg qhs. Max: 0.5mg. Elderly/Debilitated: Initial: 0.125mg. Max: 0.25mg.

HOW SUPPLIED: Tab: 0.125mg, 0.25mg* *scored

CONTRAINDICATIONS: Pregnancy. With ketoconazole, itraconazole, nefazodone, medications that impair CYP3A.

WARNINGS/PRECAUTIONS: Worsening or failure of response after 7-10 days may indicate other medical conditions. Increased daytime anxiety, abnormal thinking, and behavioral changes have occurred. May impair mental/physical abilities. Anterograde amnesia reported with therapeutic doses. Caution with baseline depression, suicidal tendencies, history of drug dependence, elderly/debilitated, renal/hepatic impairment, chronic pulmonary insufficiency, and sleep apnea. Withdrawal symptoms after d/c; avoid abrupt withdrawal.

ADVERSE REACTIONS: Drowsiness, dizziness, lightheadedness, headache, N/V, coordination disorders, ataxia.

INTERACTIONS: See Contraindications. Avoid the concomitant use with CYP3A inhibitors (eg, ketoconazole, itraconazole, all azole-type antifungals, nefazodone). Potentiated by the coadministration of isoniazid, oral contraceptives, grapefruit juice, ranitidine. Caution with fluvoxamine, diltiazem, verapamil, cimetidine, ergotamine, cyclosporine, amiodarone, nicardipine, nifedipine, sertraline, paroxetine, macrolides. Additive CNS depression with psychotropics, anticonvulsants, antihistamines, and alcohol.

PREGNANCY: Category X, not for use in nursing.

MECHANISM OF ACTION: Triazolobenzodiazepine hypnotic agent.

PHARMACOKINETICS: Absorption: C_{max}=1-6ng/mL, T_{max}=2 hrs. **Metabolism:** Hydroxylation via CYP3A. **Elimination:** Urine (79.9%), $T_{1/2}$=1.5-5.5 hrs.

NURSING CONSIDERATIONS

Assessment: Assess for primary psychiatric and/or medical illness, chronic pulmonary insufficiency (sleep apnea, COPD), renal/hepatic function, and possible drug interactions.

Monitoring: Monitor worsening of insomnia, suicidality, severe sedation, complex behaviors (sleep-driving), abnormal thinking/behavioral changes (aggressiveness, hallucinations, and bizzare behavior), anterograde amnesia, paradoxical reactions.

Patient Counseling: Inform of benefits/risks of therapy and potential for physical/psychological dependence. Caution against hazardous tasks (operating machinery/driving). Do not increase dose or d/c before consulting physician. Avoid alcohol consumption. Notify if pregnant or planning to become pregnant.

Administration: Oral route. **Storage:** 20-25°C (68-77°F).

HALFLYTELY   RX
polyethylene glycol 3350 - sodium bicarbonate - potassium chloride - sodium chloride - bisacodyl (Braintree)

THERAPEUTIC CLASS: Bowel cleanser/stimulant laxative

INDICATIONS: Colon cleansing prior to colonoscopy.

DOSAGE: *Adults:* Consume only clear liquids on day of preparation. Take 1 bisacodyl tab with water. Do not crush or chew tab. After 1st bowel movement (or max of 6 hrs) drink sol, at a rate of 8 oz. q10 mins. Drink all sol. Drink each portion at longer intervals or d/c sol temporarily if abdominal distension/discomfort occurs until symptoms improve.

HOW SUPPLIED: Kit: Tab, Delayed-Release: (Bisacodyl) 5mg. Sol: (Polyethylene Glycol 3350-Potassium Chloride-Sodium Bicarbonate-Sodium Chloride) 210g-0.74g-2.86g-5.6g [2000mL].

CONTRAINDICATIONS: Ileus, GI obstruction, gastric retention, bowel perforation, toxic colitis, toxic megacolon.

WARNINGS/PRECAUTIONS: Serious arrhythmias reported rarely; caution in patients at increased risk of arrhythmias (eg, history of prolonged QT, uncontrolled arrhythmias, recent myocardial infarction [MI], unstable angina, congestive heart failure [CHF], or cardiomyopathy), and consider pre-dose and post-colonoscopy ECGs. Perform post-colonoscopy lab tests (electrolytes, creatinine, BUN) if patient develops vomiting or signs of dehydration. Hydrate patients adequately before, during, and after administration. Caution in patients with increased risk for seizure, renal impairment, and fluid and electrolyte disturbances. Correct electrolyte abnormalities prior to treatment. Caution in severe active ulcerative colitis (UC). Caution in patients with impaired gag reflex and patients prone to regurgitation/aspiration. Ischemic colitis reported; evaluate if severe abdominal pain or rectal bleeding develops. Generalized tonic-clonic seizures reported with the use of large volume (4L) polyethylene glycol-based colon preparation products; caution in patients with a history of seizures and patients at risk of seizure or with known or suspected hyponatremia. Monitor closely with impaired water handling. Do not add additional ingredients other than flavor packs provided.

ADVERSE REACTIONS: N/V, abdominal fullness, abdominal cramping, overall discomfort.

INTERACTIONS: Oral medications taken within 1 hr of start of administration may not be absorbed from GI tract. Avoid bisacodyl delayed release tablets within 1 hr of taking an antacid. Caution with drugs that lower the seizure threshold (eg, tricyclic antidepressants), in patients withdrawing from alcohol or benzodiazepines, drugs that increase the risk of electrolyte abnormalities (eg, diuretics); monitor baseline and post-colonoscopy laboratory tests (Na, K$^+$, calcium, creatinine, BUN). Caution with drugs that may increase the risk of adverse events of arrhythmias and prolonged QT with fluid and electrolyte abnormalities. Caution with drugs that may affect renal function (eg, diuretics, ACE inhibitors, ARBs, NSAIDs); consider baseline and post-colonoscopy labs (electrolytes, SrCr, BUN) in these patients.

PREGNANCY: Category C, caution in nursing.

MECHANISM OF ACTION: Polyethylene glycol-3350: Osmotic laxative; causes water to be retained within the GI tract. Bisacodyl: Simulant laxative; active metabolite acts directly on the colonic mucosa to produce colonic peristalsis. The stimulant laxative effect of bisacodyl, together with the osmotic effect of the unabsorbed PEG when ingested with a large volume of water, produces watery diarrhea.

PHARMACOKINETICS: Absorption: Polyethylene glycol-3350: Minimal. **Metabolism:** Bisacodyl: Hydrolysis by intestinal brush border enzymes and colonic bacteria to form bis-(p-hydroxyphenyl) pyridyl-2 methane (active metabolite).

NURSING CONSIDERATIONS

Assessment: Assess for GI obstruction, bowel perforation, electrolyte/fluid abnormalities, history of seizures, known or suspected hyponatremia, renal impairment, any other conditions where treatment is contraindicated or cautioned, hypersensitivity, pregnancy/nursing status, and possible drug interactions. Obtain baseline electrolytes, Na, K$^+$, Ca, SrCr, and BUN in patients at risk for seizures and patients with renal impairment. Perform baseline ECGs in patients at risk for arrhythmias.

Monitoring: Perform baseline and post-colonoscopy lab tests in patients with seizure risk (eg, known/suspected hyponatremia), and consider these tests in patients with impaired renal function. Monitor for hypersensitivity reactions, aspiration, cardiac arrhythmias, abdominal pain, rectal bleeding, ischemic colitis, and seizures.

Patient Counseling: Oral medication administered within 1 hr of start of administration of sol may be flushed from GI tract, hence not absorbed. Instruct to take exactly as directed. Advise not to take other laxatives while taking HalfLytely and Bisacodyl Tablet Bowel Prep Kit. Notify physician if they have trouble swallowing or prone to regurgitation or aspiration. Instruct to slow or temporarily d/c administration if severe bloating, distention or abdominal pain occurs until symptoms abate and notify physician. Advise to d/c administration and contact physician if hives, rashes, allergic reaction, signs and symptoms of dehydration develops.

Administration: Oral route. **Storage:** 20-25°C (68-77°F); excursions permitted to 15-30°C (59-86°F). Refrigerate reconstituted solution and use within 48 hrs.

HALOPERIDOL
haloperidol (Various)

RX

> Elderly patients with dementia-related psychosis treated with antipsychotic drugs are at an increased risk of death; most deaths appeared to be cardiovascular (CV) (eg, heart failure, sudden death) or infectious (eg, pneumonia) in nature. Not approved for the treatment of patients with dementia-related psychosis.

OTHER BRAND NAMES: Haldol (Ortho-McNeil)

THERAPEUTIC CLASS: Butyrophenone

INDICATIONS: (Inj) Treatment of schizophrenia. (Inj/Sol/Tab) Control of tics and vocal utterances of Tourette's disorder. (Sol/Tab) Management of psychotic disorders in children. Treatment of severe behavior problems in non-psychotic children or short-term treatment of hyperactive children with accompanying conduct disorders only after failed to response to psychotherapy or medications other than antipsychotics.

DOSAGE: *Adults:* Individualize dose. (PO) Moderate Symptoms/Elderly/Debilitated: 0.5-2mg bid-tid. Severe Symptoms/Chronic or Resistant Patients: 3-5mg bid-tid. Max: 100mg/day. Maint: Gradually reduce to the lowest effective maint dose. (Inj) Schizophrenia: 2-5mg IM q4-8h or hourly as needed thereafter for acute, moderately severe or very severe symptoms. Refer to PI for dosing recommendations and switchover procedure.
Pediatrics: 3-12 yrs: (15-40kg): (PO) Individualize dose. Psychotic Disorders: Initial: 0.05-0.15mg/kg/day given bid-tid. Nonpsychotic Behavior/Tourette's Disorder: 0.05-0.075mg/kg/day given bid-tid. May increase by an increment of 0.5mg at 5-7 day intervals until therapeutic effect is obtained. Max: 6mg/day. Maint: Gradually reduce to the lowest effective maint dose.

HOW SUPPLIED: Inj: (Lactate) 5mg/mL [Haldol]; Sol: (Lactate) 2mg/mL; Tab: 0.5mg*, 1mg*, 2mg*, 5mg*, 10mg*, 20mg* *scored

CONTRAINDICATIONS: Severe toxic CNS depression or comatose states, Parkinson's disease.

WARNINGS/PRECAUTIONS: Risk of tardive dyskinesia (TD), especially in elderly; consider d/c if signs/symptoms appear. Neuroleptic malignant syndrome (NMS), hyperpyrexia, heat stroke, bronchopneumonia reported. Use only during pregnancy if benefit justifies the risk to fetus. May develop lethargy and decreased sensation of thirst due to central inhibition, which may lead to dehydration, hemoconcentration, reduced pulmonary ventilation, especially in the elderly; institute remedial therapy promptly. Cutaneous and ocular changes may occur. Leukopenia, neutropenia and agranulocytosis reported; d/c in cases of severe neutropenia (ANC<1000/mm3). Hypotension, precipitation of anginal pain may occur; caution with severe CV disorders. May lower convulsive threshold; caution with history of seizures and EEG abnormalities. Severe neurotoxicity may occur with thyrotoxicosis. May elevate prolactin levels during chronic administration. May impair mental/physical abilities. (Inj/Tab) Sudden death, QT-prolongation, and torsades de pointes reported; caution with QT-prolonging conditions (eg, electrolyte imbalance), underlying cardiac abnormalities, hypothyroidism, familial long QT-syndrome. (Inj) Not approved for IV administration.

ADVERSE REACTIONS: Extrapyramidal symptoms (EPS), TD, dystonia, ECG changes, ventricular arrhythmias, tachycardia, hypotension, HTN, N/V, constipation, diarrhea, dry mouth, blurred vision, urinary retention.

INTERACTIONS: Monitor for neurological toxicity with lithium. Caution with rifampin, anticonvulsants, anticoagulants, anticholinergics (eg, antiparkinson agents), drugs known to prolong QT. May potentiate CNS depressants (eg, alcohol, opiates, anesthetics); avoid use with alcohol. Vasopressor activity may be blocked and paradoxical further lowering of BP may occur with epinephrine; avoid concomitant use.

PREGNANCY: Safety not known in pregnancy, not for use in nursing.

MECHANISM OF ACTION: Butyrophenone; mechanism not established.

NURSING CONSIDERATIONS

Assessment: Assess for history of dementia-related psychosis or any other conditions where treatment is cautioned or contraindicated. Assess for hypersensitivity to drug, pregnancy/nursing status, and possible drug interactions. Obtain baseline CBC, ECG, EEG, and serum electrolytes.

Monitoring: Monitor for signs/symptoms of NMS, EPS, TD, bronchopneumonia, hypersensitivity reactions, and signs and symptoms of infection. Monitor for neurotoxicity in patients with thyrotoxicosis. Monitor vital signs, CBC, ECG, EEG, serum electrolytes, and cholesterol levels.

Patient Counseling: Inform risks/benefits of therapy. Instruct to use caution in performing hazardous tasks (eg, operating machinery/driving). Instruct to avoid alcohol due to possible additive effects and hypotension.

Administration: Oral and IM route. (Inj) Inspect visually for particulate matter and discoloration prior to administration. **Storage:** (Tab/Sol) 20-25°C (68-77°F). (Inj) 15-30°C (59-86°F). (Inj/Sol) Do not freeze. Protect from light.

HAVRIX   RX
hepatitis A vaccine (GlaxoSmithKline)

THERAPEUTIC CLASS: Vaccine

INDICATIONS: Active immunization against disease caused by hepatitis A virus (HAV) in persons ≥12 months of age.

DOSAGE: *Adults:* 1mL IM, then 1mL IM booster anytime between 6-12 months later. Administer in the deltoid region.
Pediatrics: 1-18 yrs: 0.5mL IM, then 0.5mL IM booster anytime between 6-12 months later. Administer in the anterolateral aspect of the thigh in infants and young children or in the deltoid muscle of the upper arm in older children.

HOW SUPPLIED: Inj: 720 EL U/0.5mL, 1440 EL U/mL [vial, prefilled syringes]

CONTRAINDICATIONS: Severe allergic reaction to neomycin.

WARNINGS/PRECAUTIONS: May cause severe allergic reaction. May cause allergic reactions in latex-sensitive individuals. Appropriate treatment must be available for possible anaphylactic reactions. Immunocompromised persons may have a diminished immune response. May not prevent hepatitis A in patients who have an unrecognized hepatitis A infection at time of vaccination. May not prevent infection in individuals who do not achieve protective antibody titers. Administer primary immunization at least 2 weeks prior to expected exposure to HAV. Lower antibody response in patients with chronic liver disease.

ADVERSE REACTIONS: Injection-site reactions (eg, induration, soreness, redness, swelling, pain), headache, irritability, fever, fatigue, malaise, anorexia, nausea, loss of appetite, drowsiness.

INTERACTIONS: Immunosuppressive therapies including irradiation, antimetabolites, alkylating agents, cytotoxic drugs, and corticosteroids (used in greater than physiological doses) may reduce immune response. Increased incidence of drowsiness and loss of appetite with Infanrix and Hib conjugate vaccine.

PREGNANCY: Category C, caution in nursing.

MECHANISM OF ACTION: Vaccine; presence of antibodies confers protection against hepatitis A virus infection.

NURSING CONSIDERATIONS

Assessment: Assess for hypersensitivity to the drug and latex, presence of immunosuppression, immunization status/vaccination history, pregnancy/ nursing status, and possible drug interactions.

Monitoring: Monitor for signs/symptoms of an allergic reaction and for injection-site reactions (eg, pain, redness, swelling), immune response, or possible adverse events.

Patient Counseling: Inform of potential benefits/risks of immunization. Counsel about potential adverse reactions and that the medication contains non-infectious killed viruses and cannot cause hepatitis A infection. Instruct to report any adverse events to healthcare provider. Give vaccine recipients and parents or guardians the Vaccine Information Statement, which is required to be given prior to immunization.

Administration: IM route. Do not administer in the gluteal region. Shake well before withdrawal and use. Do not dilute to administer. Inspect visually for particulate matter or discoloration prior to administration; if these conditions exist, do not administer. Concomitant administration of other vaccines or immune globulin should be given at different injection site; do not mix with any other vaccine or product in the same syringe or vial. **Storage:** 2-8°C (36-46°F). Do not freeze; discard if frozen.

HELIDAC   RX
tetracycline HCl - bismuth subsalicylate - metronidazole (Prometheus)

> Metronidazole has been shown to be carcinogenic in mice and rats. Unnecessary use of the drug should be avoided. Its use may be reserved for the eradication of *H.pylori* for treatment of patients with *H.pylori* infection and duodenal ulcer disease.

THERAPEUTIC CLASS: *H.pylori* treatment combination

INDICATIONS: In combination with an H$_2$ antagonist for eradication of *H.pylori* for treatment of patients with *H.pylori* infection and duodenal ulcer disease (active or history of duodenal ulcer).

DOSAGE: *Adults:* (Bismuth) (2 tabs) 525mg + (Metronidazole) 250mg + (Tetracycline) 500mg, all qid for 14 days with an H$_2$ antagonist taken as directed. Missed Dose: Continue normal dosing schedule until medication is gone. Do not take double doses. If >4 doses missed, contact the prescriber. Take at meals and hs. Chew and swallow bismuth tablets. Take metronidazole and tetracycline with a full glass of water; swallow whole.

HOW SUPPLIED: Cap: (Tetracycline) 500mg; Tab: (Metronidazole) 250mg; Tab, Chewable: (Bismuth Subsalicylate) 262.4mg

CONTRAINDICATIONS: Pregnancy, nursing, pediatrics, renal/hepatic impairment, known allergy to aspirin (ASA).

WARNINGS/PRECAUTIONS: Use in the absence of a proven or strongly suspected bacterial infection or prophylactic indication is unlikely to provide benefit and increases the risk of development of drug-resistant bacteria. Caution in elderly. (Bismuth subsalicylate) Do not use to treat nausea and vomiting in children or teenagers who have or are recovering from chickenpox or flu. Rare reports of neurotoxicity with excessive doses. May cause temporary and harmless darkening of the tongue and/or black stool. (Metronidazole) Encephalopathy, peripheral neuropathy, convulsive seizures, aseptic meningitis reported; d/c if abnormal neurological signs develop. Caution in patients with CNS disease. May produce teratogenic effects. Mild leukopenia reported; caution with evidence of or history of blood dyscrasias. Known or previously unrecognized candidiasis may present more prominent symptoms. (Tetracycline) May cause permanent discoloration of the teeth during tooth development (Last half of pregnancy, infancy, and childhood up to 8 yrs). Enamel hypoplasia reported. May cause fetal harm. Photosensitivity manifested by an exaggerated sunburn reaction reported; d/c at first evidence of skin erythema. May increase BUN which may lead to azotemia, hyperphosphatemia, and acidosis in patients with significant renal impairment. May result in overgrowth of nonsusceptible organisms (eg, fungi); d/c if superinfection occurs. Pseudotumor cerebri (benign intracranial hypertension) in adults reported.

ADVERSE REACTIONS: Nausea, diarrhea, abdominal pain, melena.

INTERACTIONS: (Bismuth subsalicylate) Increases risk of bleeding when administered with anticoagulant therapy. May enhance hypoglycemic effect of antidiabetic agents. Caution with ASA, probenecid, and sulfinpyrazone. (Tetracycline) Depressed plasma prothrombin activity with anticoagulants. Impaired absorption with antacids containing aluminum, calcium, or magnesium; preparations containing iron, zinc, or sodium bicarbonate; or milk or dairy products. Possible reduced absorption with bismuth or calcium carbonate. May interfere with bactericidal action of penicillin; avoid concomitant use. May render oral contraceptives less effective; breakthrough bleeding reported. (Metronidazole) Potentiates anticoagulant effect of warfarin and other oral coumarin anticoagulants. May prolong the half-life and decrease the plasma clearance when used concomitantly with drugs that decrease microsomal liver enzyme activity (eg, cimetidine). Accelerated elimination leading to reduced plasma levels of metronidazole when used concomitantly with drugs that induce microsomal liver enzymes (eg, phenytoin, phenobarbital). May impair phenytoin clearance. May increase lithium levels which may lead to toxicity. Avoid alcohol during and at least 1 day after therapy. Psychotic reactions reported in alcoholics with concomitant disulfiram; metronidazole should not be given to patients who have taken disulfiram within the last 2 weeks.

PREGNANCY: Category D, not for use in nursing.

MECHANISM OF ACTION: Antimicrobial; combination therapy with activity against *H.pylori*.

PHARMACOKINETICS: Absorption: (Salicylic acid, 525mg) C_{max}=13.1mcg/mL. (Metronidazole, 250mg) Well-absorbed; C_{max}=6mcg/mL; T_{max}=1-2 hrs. (Tetracycline) Readily absorbed. **Distribution**: (Bismuth) Plasma protein binding (>90%). (Salicylic acid) V_d=170mL/kg; plasma protein binding (90%). (Metronidazole) Plasma protein binding (<20%), appears in the CSF, saliva, breast milk. (Tetracycline) Crosses placenta, found in fetal tissues, secreted in breast milk. **Metabolism**: (Salicyclic acid) Extensive. (Metronidazole) Side chain oxidation, glucuronide conjugation; 2-hydroxymethyl (metabolite). **Elimination:** (Bismuth) Urine, bile; $T_{1/2}$=21-72 days. (Salicylic, 525mg) Urine (10%, unchanged); $T_{1/2}$=2-5 hrs. (Metronidazole) Urine (60-80%), feces (6-15%); $T_{1/2}$=8 hrs. (Tetracycline) Urine, feces.

NURSING CONSIDERATIONS

Assessment: Assess for proper diagnosis, age of patient, renal/hepatic impairment, hypersensitivity to ASA or salicylates, chickenpox, flu, candidiasis, CNS diseases, presence or history of blood dyscrasias, pregnancy/nursing status, and for possible drug interactions.

Monitoring: Monitor for signs/symptoms of encephalopathy, peripheral neuropathy, convulsive seizures, aseptic meningitis, neurotoxicity, photosensitivity, darkening of the tongue or black stools, increases in BUN, leukopenia, candidiasis, overgrowth of nonsusceptible organisms, and for pseudotumor cerebri.

Patient Counseling: Instruct to take 4 times a day, at meal times and bedtime. Instruct to chew and swallow bismuth subsalicylate tabs. Instruct to swallow tetracycline cap and metronidazole tab whole, with a full glass of water. Advise to take tetracycline with an adequate amount of fluid, particularly at bedtime, to help prevent esophageal irritation and ulceration. Inform if a dose is missed, continue normal dosing until medication is done, do not double up doses. Counsel to continue therapy for full treatment period to prevent development of bacterial resistance. Inform that ringing in the ears may occur when taken with ASA; advise to consult prescriber regarding d/c ASA until treatment is complete. Inform that therapy may make oral contraceptives less effective; advise to use a different or an additional form of contraception. Instruct to contact physician if breakthrough bleeding occurs. Advise to notify prescriber if pregnancy occurs while on therapy. Instruct to avoid alcohol while on medication and for 1 day after d/c. Counsel to avoid exposure to sun/sun lamps. Inform may develop darkening of tongue or stool. Instruct to avoid pregnancy/nursing during therapy.

Administration: Oral route. **Storage**: 20-25°C (68-77°F).

HEPARIN SODIUM RX
heparin sodium (Various)

OTHER BRAND NAMES: Heparin Sodium in Dextrose 5% (Baxter)

THERAPEUTIC CLASS: Glycosaminoglycan

INDICATIONS: Prophylaxis and treatment of venous and arterial thrombosis and its extension, pulmonary embolism (PE) and peripheral arterial embolism; atrial fibrillation (A-fib) with embolization. Diagnosis and treatment of acute and chronic consumptive coagulopathies/disseminated intravascular coagulation (DIC). Prevention of clotting in arterial and cardiac surgery. (Heparin Sodium Inj) Prevention of postoperative deep vein thrombosis (DVT) and PE. May also be used as anticoagulant in blood transfusion, extracorporeal circulation, dialysis procedures and in blood samples for laboratory purposes.

DOSAGE: *Adults:* Based on 68kg: (Heparin Sodium Inj) Initial: 5000 U IV, then 10,000-20,000 U SQ. Maint: 8000-10,000 U q8h or 15,000-20,000 U q12h. Intermittent IV Injection: Initial: 10,000 U. Maint: 5000-10,000 U q4-6h. Continuous IV Infusion: Initial: 5000 U. Maint: 20,000-40,000 U/24 hrs. (Heparin Sodium in Dextrose 5%) Initial: 5000 U IV, then 20,000-40,000 U q24h. Adjust to coagulation test results. See PI for details in specific disease states.
Pediatrics: Initial: 50 U/kg IV. Maint: 100 U/kg IV q4h or 20,000 U/m²/24 hrs continuously.

HOW SUPPLIED: Inj: 1000 U/mL, 5000 U/mL, 10,000 U/mL, 20,000 U/mL (Heparin Sodium Inj). 20,000 U [500mL], 25,000 U [250mL, 500mL] (Heparin Sodium in Dextrose 5%).

CONTRAINDICATIONS: Severe thrombocytopenia, if blood coagulation tests cannot be performed at appropriate intervals (with full-dose heparin), uncontrollable active bleeding state (except in DIC).

WARNINGS/PRECAUTIONS: Hemorrhage can occur at any site; caution with increased danger of hemorrhage (eg, severe HTN, bacterial endocarditis, surgery, increased bleeding tendencies, ulcerative lesions, menstruation, liver disease with impaired hemostasis). Thrombocytopenia, heparin-induced thrombocytopenia and thrombosis (HIT/HITT) and hyperaminotransferasemia reported, even up to several weeks after d/c of therapy. D/C if platelets <100,000/mm³, recurrent thrombosis develops, coagulation tests unduly prolonged, or hemorrhage occurs. Increased heparin resistance with fever, thrombosis, thrombophlebitis, infections with thrombosing tendencies, myocardial infarction (MI), cancer, and post-op. Higher bleeding incidence in women >60 yrs. (Heparin Sodium Inj) Not for IM use. Fatal hemorrhage reported in pediatrics due to medication errors (eg, confused with "catheter lock flush" vials). (Heparin Sodium in Dextrose 5%) D/C if HIT/HITT diagnosed/suspected. Avoid future use especially within 3-6 months after diagnosis of HIT/HITT and while positive for HIT antibodies. Not to be administered simultaneously with blood through same administration set; pseudoagglutination or hemolysis may occur. Sulfite sensitivity may occur; caution especially in asthmatics. Caution with overt/subclinical diabetes mellitus (DM). Use of electric flow control device is recommended.

ADVERSE REACTIONS: Thrombocytopenia, hemorrhage, local irritation, erythema, mild pain, hematoma, chills, fever, urticaria, asthma, lacrimation, N/V, anaphylactoid reactions, HIT/HITT.

INTERACTIONS: Wait ≥5 hrs after last IV dose or 24 hrs after last SQ dose before measuring PT when taken with dicumarol or warfarin. Platelet inhibitors (eg, aspirin [ASA], dextran, phenylbutazone, ibuprofen, indomethacin, dipyridamole, hydroxychloroquine) may induce bleeding. Digitalis, tetracyclines, nicotine, or antihistamines may counteract anticoagulant action. Decreased PTT with IV nitroglycerin; monitor PTT and adjust heparin dose with concurrent use.

PREGNANCY: Category C, safe in nursing.

MECHANISM OF ACTION: Glycosaminoglycan; inhibits reactions that lead to blood clotting and the formation of fibrin clots. Acts at multiple sites in the normal coagulation system.

PHARMACOKINETICS: Absorption: (SQ) T_{max}=2-4 hrs. **Metabolism:** Liver and reticulo-endothelial system. **Elimination:** $T_{1/2}$=10 mins.

NURSING CONSIDERATIONS

Assessment: Assess for severe thrombocytopenia, pregnancy status, and possible drug interactions. Assess use in disease states at risk for hemorrhage and use in older patients (>60 yrs). Assess that suitable coagulation tests (eg, whole blood clotting time, partial thromboplastin time) can be performed at appropriate intervals in patients on full-dose heparin. Assess for thrombocytopenia, HIT and HITT. Assess for hypersensitivity, including corn and sulfite hypersensitivity, and overt/subclinical DM. Obtain baseline CBC including platelet counts.

Monitoring: Monitor for signs/symptoms of hemorrhage, thrombocytopenia, heparin resistance, hypersensitivity reactions and hyperaminotransferasemia. Perform periodic monitoring of platelet counts, Hct, and tests for occult blood in stool. If given therapeutically, perform frequent coagulation tests. If given by continuous IV infusion, monitor coagulation time every 4 hrs during early stages of treatment. If given intermittently by IV inj, monitor coagulation tests before each inj during the initial phase of treatment and then at appropriate intervals thereafter.

Patient Counseling: Counsel about increased risk of bleeding tendencies while on medication. Instruct to notify physician if any type of unusual bleeding or hypersensitivity reaction occurs. Advise that periodic lab monitoring is required during treatment.

Administration: IV/SQ routes. If added to infusion solution for continuous IV administration, container should be inverted 6 times to ensure adequate mixing and prevention of heparin pooling in the solution. Visually inspect for particulate matter and discoloration prior to administration. **Storage:** (Heparin Sodium Inj) 20-25°C (68-77°F). (Heparin Sodium in Dextrose 5%) 25°C; brief exposure up to 40°C does not adversely affect product. Avoid excessive heat.

HEPSERA   RX
adefovir dipivoxil (Gilead Sciences)

> D/C may result in severe acute exacerbations of hepatitis; monitor hepatic function closely with both clinical and laboratory follow-up for at least several months in patients who d/c therapy; resumption of therapy may be warranted if appropriate. Chronic use may result in nephrotoxicity in patients at risk of or having underlying renal dysfunction; monitor renal function; dose adjustment may be required. HIV resistance may occur with unrecognized or untreated HIV infection. Lactic acidosis and severe hepatomegaly with steatosis, including fatal cases reported with the use of nucleoside analogs alone or in combination with other antiretrovirals.

THERAPEUTIC CLASS: Acyclic nucleotide analog

INDICATIONS: Treatment of chronic hepatitis B in patients ≥12 yrs with evidence of active viral replication and either evidence of persistent elevations in serum aminotransferases (ALT or AST) or histologically active disease.

DOSAGE: *Adults:* 10mg qd. Renal Impairment: CrCl 30-49mL/min: 10mg q48h. CrCl 10-29mL/min: 10mg q72h. Hemodialysis Patients: 10mg every 7 days following dialysis.
Pediatrics: ≥12 yrs: 10mg qd.

HOW SUPPLIED: Tab: 10mg

WARNINGS/PRECAUTIONS: Caution with use in adolescents with underlying renal dysfunction and monitor renal function closely in these patients. May require HIV antibody testing prior to treatment. Caution with use in patients with known risk factors for liver disease. Suspend treatment if clinical or laboratory findings suggestive of lactic acidosis or pronounced hepatotoxicity develop (eg, hepatomegaly, steatosis, transaminase elevations). Resistance to the drug can result in viral load rebound which may result in exacerbation of hepatitis B, leading to liver decompensation and possible fatal outcome. To reduce risk of resistance in patients with lamivudine-resistant HBV, adefovir dipivoxil should be used in combination with lamivudine and not as monotherapy. In order to reduce the risk of resistance in all patients receiving monotherapy, a modification of treatment should be considered if serum HBV DNA remains above 1000 copies/mL with continued treatment. Caution in elderly.

ADVERSE REACTIONS: Nephrotoxicity, asthenia, headache, abdominal pain, nausea, flatulence, diarrhea, dyspepsia, increased creatinine.

INTERACTIONS: Coadministration with drugs that reduce renal function or compete for active tubular secretion may increase concentrations of adefovir or the coadministered drugs; monitor closely for adverse events when used concomitantly with drugs that are excreted renally or with other drugs known to affect renal function. Avoid concomitant administration with tenofovir disoproxil fumarate (TDF) or TDF-containing products, including emtricitabine-TDF combination, and efavirenz-emtricitabine-TDF combination.

PREGNANCY: Category C, not for use in nursing.

MECHANISM OF ACTION: Acyclic nucleotide analog; inhibits HBV DNA polymerase by competing with natural substrate deoxyadenosine triphosphate and by causing DNA chain termination after incorporation into viral DNA.

PHARMACOKINETICS: Absorption: C_{max}=18.4ng/mL; T_{max}=1.75 hrs; AUC=220ng•h/mL. CrCl 50-80mL/min: C_{max}=22.4ng/mL; AUC=266ng•h/mL. CrCl 30-49mL/min: C_{max}=28.5ng/mL; AUC=455ng•h/mL., CrCl 10-29mL/min: C_{max}=51.6ng/mL; AUC=1240ng•h/mL. **Pediatrics:** C_{max}=23.3ng/mL; AUC=248.8ng•h/mL. **Distribution:** V_d=392mL/kg (IV, 1mg/kg/day), 352mL/kg (IV, 3mg/kg/day); plasma protein binding (≤4%). **Elimination:** Urine (45%); $T_{1/2}$=7.48 hrs.

NURSING CONSIDERATIONS

Assessment: Assess for renal dysfunction, risk factors for liver disease (eg, obesity), pregnancy/nursing status, and for possible drug interactions. Perform HIV antibody testing prior to therapy and assess CrCl prior to therapy.

Monitoring: Monitor for signs/symptoms of nephrotoxicity; monitor renal function. Monitor for signs and symptoms of acute exacerbations of hepatitis following d/c of therapy. Monitor for signs/symptoms of lactic acidosis, hepatomegaly with steatosis, and for clinical resistance.

Patient Counseling: Inform of risks and benefits of therapy. Advise patients to follow a regular dosing schedule to avoid missing doses. Instruct to notify physician if develop unusual symptoms, or any symptom persists or worsens. Instruct to immediately report any severe abdominal pain, muscle pain, yellowing of eyes, dark urine, pale stools, and/or loss of appetite. Instruct to not d/c therapy without first informing physician. Advise that routine laboratory monitoring and follow-up is important during therapy. Must obtain HIV antibody testing prior to starting therapy. Inform childbearing women about risks during pregnancy; may cause harm to nursing infant. Notify physician if the patient becomes pregnant while on therapy; encourage enrollment in pregnancy registry program to monitor maternal and fetal outcome. Inform about possible drug interactions. Instruct lamivudine-resistant patients to use as combination therapy with lamivudine and not as monotherapy.

Administration: Oral route. **Storage:** 25°C (77°F); excursions permitted to 15-30°C (59-86°F). Do not use if seal over bottle opening is broken or missing.

HERCEPTIN

RX

trastuzumab (Genentech)

> Use may result in cardiac failure manifesting as congestive heart failure (CHF) and decreased left ventricular ejection fraction (LVEF). Increased incidence/severity of left ventricular cardiac dysfunction in combination with anthracycline-containing chemotherapy regimens. Evaluate LVEF prior to and during therapy; d/c with significant decrease in left ventricular function or cardiomyopathy. Serious infusion reactions and pulmonary toxicity may occur. Interrupt infusion if dyspnea or clinically significant hypotension develops. D/C if anaphylaxis, angioedema, interstitial pneumonitis, or acute respiratory distress syndrome occurs.

THERAPEUTIC CLASS: Monoclonal antibody/HER2-blocker

INDICATIONS: Adjuvant treatment of HER2-overexpressing node-positive or node-negative breast cancer. 1st-line treatment of HER2-overexpressing metastatic breast cancer in combination with paclitaxel. Single agent for treatment of HER2-overexpressing breast cancer in patients who received one or more chemotherapy regimens for metastatic disease.

DOSAGE: *Adults:* Adjuvant treatment: during and following paclitaxel, docetaxel, or docetaxel/carboplatin for 52 weeks total: Initial: 4mg/kg over 90 min. Maint: 2mg/kg weekly over 30 min for the first 12 weeks (paclitaxel or docetaxel) or 18 weeks (docetaxel/carboplatin). 1 week following the last weekly dose: 6mg/kg IV over 30-90 min q3 weeks. Following completion of multimodality, anthracycline-based regimens: Initial: 8mg/kg IV over 90 min. Maint: 6mg/kg over 30-90 min q3 weeks. Metastatic breast cancer: Alone or with paclitaxel: Initial: 4mg/kg over 90 min. Maint: 2mg/kg weekly over 30 min until disease progression. Cardiomyopathy: Assess LVEF and withhold for at least 4 weeks when there is ≥16% absolute decrease in LVEF from pretreatment values or LVEF below institutional limits of normal and ≥10% absolute decrease in LVEF from pretreatment values. Resume treatment within 4-8 weeks when LVEF returns to normal limits and the absolute decrease from baseline is ≤15%. D/C permanently for persistent (>8 weeks) LVEF decline or for suspension of dosing on >3 occasions for cardiomyopathy.

HOW SUPPLIED: Inj: 440mg

WARNINGS/PRECAUTIONS: May cause left ventricular cardiac dysfunction, arrhythmias, HTN, disabling cardiac failure, cardiomyopathy, and cardiac death. Obtain baseline cardiac assessment (eg, history, physical, LVEF). Monitor LVEF prior to initiation, every 3 months during, and every 6 months following completion for at least 2 yrs. Fatal pulmonary toxicity may occur. May exacerbate chemotherapy-induced neutropenia. Detection of HER2 protein overexpression is necessary for selection of patients appropriate for therapy as these are the only patients for whom benefit has been shown. May cause severe infusion reactions; interrupt infusion and intervene with medical therapy. May cause fetal harm when administered to pregnant women; increased risk of oligohydramnios during second and third trimesters.

ADVERSE REACTIONS: Fever, N/V, infusion reactions, diarrhea, infections, increased cough, headache, fatigue, dyspnea, rash, neutropenia, anemia, myalgia, headache, nasopharyngitis.

INTERACTIONS: See Boxed Warning. Paclitaxel may increase serum levels. Concomitant anthracycline-containing chemotherapy regimens may increase incidence/severity of cardiac dysfunction.

PREGNANCY: Category D, not for use in nursing.

MECHANISM OF ACTION: Monoclonal antibody/HER2 blocker; inhibits the proliferation of human tumor cells that overexpress HER2.

PHARMACOKINETICS: Absorption: C_{max}=337mcg/mL (500mg). **Distribution:** V_d=44mL/kg. **Elimination:** $T_{1/2}$=2 days (10mg), $T_{1/2}$=12 days (500mg).

NURSING CONSIDERATIONS

Assessment: Assess cardiac function including history and physical exam and baseline LVEF by echocardiogram or MUGA scan. Assess for HER2 overexpression and HER2 gene amplification. Assess CBC with differential and platelets, pregnancy/nursing status, and possible drug interactions.

Monitoring: Monitor for cardiac failure and CHF. LVEF must be measured every 3 months during and upon completion of therapy and every 6 months for 2 yrs following completion. Monitor for cardiomyopathy, infusion reactions, pulmonary reactions/toxicity, exacerbation of chemotherapy-induced neutropenia, and other serious adverse events.

Patient Counseling: Contact health care professional if there is new onset or worsening shortness of breath, cough, swelling of ankles/legs or face, palpitations, weight gain of more than 5 lbs in 24 hrs, dizziness, or loss of consciousness. Advise females to use effective contraceptive methods during and at least 6 months following therapy. May enroll patients who become pregnant while on treatment in the Herceptin Pregnancy Registry.

Administration: IV route. Do not administer as IV push or bolus. See PI for proper reconstitution. **Storage:** 2-8°C (34-46°F). Diluted infusion solution may be stored at 2-8°C (34-46°F) for no longer than 24 hrs prior to use. Do not freeze.

HUMALOG   RX
insulin lispro (Lilly)

THERAPEUTIC CLASS: Insulin

INDICATIONS: Treatment of diabetes mellitus for the control of hyperglycemia.

DOSAGE: *Adults:* Individualize dose. Inject SQ within 15 min before or immediately after a meal. May need to reduce/adjust dose with renal/hepatic impairment. May use with external insulin pump; do not dilute or mix with other insulins when used with pump.
Pediatrics: ≥3 yrs: Individualize dose. Inject SQ within 15 min before or immediately after a meal. May need to reduce/adjust dose with renal/hepatic impairment. May use with external insulin pump; do not dilute or mix with other insulins when used with pump.

HOW SUPPLIED: Cartridge: 100 U/mL [3mL]; Inj: 100 U/mL [3mL, 10mL]; Pen: 100 U/mL [3mL]

CONTRAINDICATIONS: During episodes of hypoglycemia.

WARNINGS/PRECAUTIONS: Any change in insulin should be made cautiously. Changes in strength, manufacturer, type or method of manufacture may result in the need for a change in dosage. Hypoglycemia, hypokalemia, lipodystrophy or hypersensitivity may occur. An infection or illness may alter insulin requirements. With type 1 DM a longer-acting insulin is usually required to maintain glucose control. Caution with patients who are fasting or having autonomic neuropathy. Monitor glucose levels and adjust dose with hepatic impairment. Hyperglycemia or ketosis may occur; prompt identification and correction of the cause is necessary. May be used in an external insulin pump. Reduce requirements with renal impairment. Antibody production reported. Not for IV use.

ADVERSE REACTIONS: Hypoglycemia, hypokalemia, allergic reactions, injection-site reactions, lipodystrophy, pruritus, rash.

INTERACTIONS: Increased insulin requirements with corticosteroids, isoniazid, niacin, estrogens, oral contraceptives, phenothiazines, thyroid replacement therapy. Decreased insulin requirements with oral antidiabetic drugs, salicylates, sulfa antibiotics, MAOIs, ACEIs, ARBs, β-blockers, octreotide, and alcohol. β-blockers may mask symptoms of hypoglycemia. Caution with potassium-lowering drugs or drugs sensitive to serum potassium levels.

PREGNANCY: Category B, caution in nursing.

MECHANISM OF ACTION: Insulin lispro (rDNA origin); regulates glucose metabolism.

PHARMACOKINETICS: Absorption: (0.1-0.2 U/kg dose) Absolute bioavailability (55-77%); (0.1-0.4 U/kg dose)T_{max}=30-90 min. **Distribution:** V_d=0.26-0.36L/kg. **Elimination:** $T_{1/2}$=1 hr.

NURSING CONSIDERATIONS

Assessment: Assess renal function, LFTs, FPG, HbA1c, hypokalemia, pregnancy status, autonomic neuropathy, and possible drug interactions.

Monitoring: Monitor blood glucose, potassium levels, and HbA1c levels regularly. Monitor for antibody production, allergic reactions (eg, redness, swelling, or itching at injection site), SOB, wheezing, reduction in BP, rapid pulse or sweating, anaphylactic reactions, pruritus, lipodystrophy.

Patient Counseling: Inform about the potential risks and advantages of the drug and alternative therapies. Instruct that infusion set (reservoir syringe, tubing, and catheter), Disetronic D-TRON or D-TRON plus cartridge adapter, and Humalog in the external insulin pump reservoir should be replaced and a new infusion site selected every 48 hrs or less. Inform of the importance of proper insulin storage, injecting techniques, timing of dosage, adherence to meal planning, regular physical activity, regular blood glucose monitoring, periodic HbA1c testing, recognition and management of hypo/hyperglycemia, and periodic assessment for diabetes complications. Infrom physician if pregnant or intend to become pregant. Instruct or train on how to use the device.

Administration: SQ route. **Storage:** Refrigerate at 2-8°C (36-46°F). Do not use if frozen. Unrefrigerated [below 30ºC (86°F)] must be used within 28 days or be discarded. Protect from direct heat and sunlight.

HUMALOG MIX 75/25 RX
insulin lispro protamine - insulin lispro (Lilly)

THERAPEUTIC CLASS: Insulin

INDICATIONS: Treatment of diabetes mellitus for the control of hyperglycemia.

DOSAGE: *Adults:* Individualize dose. Inject SQ within 15 min before a meal. May need to reduce/adjust dose with renal/hepatic impairment.

HOW SUPPLIED: (Insulin Lispro Protamine, Human-Insulin Lispro, Human) Inj: 75 U-25 U/mL [10mL]; Pen: 75 U-25 U/mL [3mL]

CONTRAINDICATIONS: During episodes of hypoglycemia.

WARNINGS/PRECAUTIONS: Any change in insulin should be made cautiously. Changes in strength, manufacturer, type or method of manufacture may result in the need for a change in dosage. Hypoglycemia, hypokalemia, lipodystrophy or hypersensitivity may occur. An infection or illness may alter insulin requirements. With type 1 DM a longer-acting insulin is usually required to maintain glucose control. Caution with patients who are fasting or having autonomic neuropathy. Monitor glucose levels and adjust dose with hepatic impairment. Reduced requirements with renal impairment. Antibody production reported. Not for IV use.

ADVERSE REACTIONS: Hypoglycemia, hypokalemia, allergic reactions, injection-site reactions, lipodystrophy, pruritus, rash.

INTERACTIONS: Increased insulin requirements with corticosteroids, isoniazid, niacin, estrogens, oral contraceptives, phenothiazines, thyroid replacement therapy. Decreased insulin requirements with oral antidiabetic drugs, salicylates, sulfa antibiotics, MAOIs, ACEIs, ARBs, β-blockers, octreotide, and alcohol. β-blockers may mask symptoms of hypoglycemia. Caution with potassium-lowering drugs or drugs sensitive to serum potassium levels.

PREGNANCY: Category B, caution in nursing.

MECHANISM OF ACTION: Insulin; regulates glucose metabolism

PHARMACOKINETICS: Absorption: (0.3 U/kg dose) T_{max} = 30-240 min, 60 min (median).

NURSING CONSIDERATIONS

Assessment: Assess renal function, LFTs, FPG, HbA1c, hypokalemia, pregnancy status, autonomic neuropathy, and possible drug interactions.

Monitoring: Monitor blood glucose, potassium levels, and HbA1c levels regularly. Monitor for antibody production, allergic reactions (eg, redness, swelling, or itching at injection site), SOB, wheezing, reduction in BP, rapid pulse or sweating, anaphylactic reactions, pruritus, lipodystrophy.

Patient Counseling: Inform about the potential risks and advantages of drugs and alternative therapies. Inform of the importance of proper insulin storage, injecting techniques, timing of dosage, adherence to meal planning, regular physical activity, regular blood glucose monitoring, periodic HbA1c testing, recognition and management of hypo/hyperglycemia, and periodic assessment for diabetes complications. Inform physician if pregnant or intend to become pregnant. Instruct how to use the device.

Administration: SQ route (15 min before meals). **Storage:** Refrigerate at 2-8°C (36-46°F). Do not use if frozen. Unrefrigerated [below 30°C (86°F)] must be used within 28 days (vials), within 10 days (pens and kwikpens) or be discarded. Protect from direct heat and light.

HUMATROPE RX
somatropin (Lilly)

THERAPEUTIC CLASS: Human growth hormone

INDICATIONS: Treatment of pediatrics with growth failure due to inadequate secretion of endogenous growth hormone (GH), short stature associated with Turner syndrome (TS), idiopathic short stature (ISS), short stature or growth failure with short stature homeobox-containing gene (SHOX) deficiency, and for growth failure in children born small for gestational age (SGA) who fail to demonstrate catch-up growth by 2-4 yrs. Replacement of endogenous GH in adults with adult-onset or childhood-onset growth hormone deficiency (GHD).

DOSAGE: *Adults:* GHD: Non-Weight Based: Initial: 0.2mg/day SQ (range, 0.15-0.30mg/day). Titrate: Increase gradually q1-2 months by 0.1-0.2mg/day based on response and insulin-like growth factor-I (IGF-I) concentrations. Weight Based: Initial: ≤0.006mg/kg/day (6mcg/kg/day) SQ. Titrate: Increase based on individual requirement. Max: 0.0125mg/kg/day (12.5mcg/kg/day). Elderly: Lower starting dose and smaller dose increments. Estrogen-replete women may need higher doses than men.
Pediatrics: Individualize dose. GHD: 0.026-0.043mg/kg/day SQ (0.18-0.30mg/kg/week). TS: ≤0.054mg/kg/day SQ (0.375mg/kg/week). ISS: ≤0.053mg/kg/day SQ (0.37mg/kg/week). SHOX Deficiency: 0.050mg/kg/day SQ (0.35mg/kg/week). SGA: ≤0.067mg/kg/day SQ (0.47mg/kg/week). Refer to PI for further details.

HOW SUPPLIED: Inj: 5mg (vial); 6mg, 12mg, 24mg (cartridge)

CONTRAINDICATIONS: Pediatrics with closed epiphyses. Active proliferative or severe non-proliferative diabetic retinopathy. Active malignancy. Acute critical illness due to complications following open heart or abdominal surgery, multiple accidental trauma, or acute respiratory failure (ARF). Prader-Willi syndrome (PWS) with severe obesity, with history of upper airway obstruction or sleep apnea, or with severe respiratory impairment.

WARNINGS/PRECAUTIONS: Avoid use of cartridge if allergic to metacresol or glycerin. Examine for progression/recurrence of underlying disease in those with pre-existing tumors or GHD secondary to intracranial lesion. Monitor for malignant transformation of skin lesions. May unmask undiagnosed impaired glucose tolerance and overt diabetes mellitus (DM); monitor glucose levels. New onset type 2 DM reported. Intracranial HTN with papilledema, visual changes, headache, N/V reported; perform funduscopic exam before initiation and during therapy; d/c if papilledema occurs. Monitor other hormonal replacement treatments in patients with hypopituitarism. Undiagnosed/untreated hypothyroidism may prevent optimal response. Hypothyroidism may worsen or develop; perform periodic thyroid function tests. Slipped capital femoral epiphysis, fluid retention, or systemic allergic reactions may occur. Progression of scoliosis may occur in pediatrics with rapid growth. Increased risk of ear/hearing disorders and cardiovascular (CV) disorders in patients with TS. Pancreatitis reported (rare). Tissue atrophy may occur when administered at the same site over a long period of time. Serum levels of inorganic phosphorus, alkaline phosphatase, parathyroid hormone and IGF-I may increase after therapy. Caution in the elderly.

ADVERSE REACTIONS: Ear disorder, arthrosis, pain, edema, arthralgia, myalgia, HTN, paraesthesias, glucose intolerance, scoliosis, otitis media, hyperlipidemia, rhinitis, flu syndrome, headache.

INTERACTIONS: Use with glucocorticoid therapy may attenuate growth-promoting effects in children; carefully adjust glucocorticoid replacement dosing in children. May inhibit 11β-hydroxysteroid dehydrogenase type 1 (11βHSD-1), resulting in reduced serum cortisol concentrations; may need glucocorticoid replacement or dose adjustments in glucocorticoid therapy. May increase clearance of antipyrine. May alter clearance of compounds metabolized by CYP450 liver enzymes (eg, corticosteroids, sex steroids, anticonvulsants, cyclosporine). May require larger dose with oral estrogen replacement. May need to adjust dose of insulin and/or oral hypoglycemic agents in diabetic patients and hormone replacement therapy in patients with thyroid dysfunction.

PREGNANCY: Category C, caution in nursing.

MECHANISM OF ACTION: Human growth hormone; GH binds to dimeric GH receptors located within the cell membranes of target tissue cells, resulting in intracellular signal transduction and subsequent induction of transcription and translation of GH-dependent proteins, including IGF-1, IGF BP-3, and acid labile subunit.

PHARMACOKINETICS: Absorption: Absolute bioavailabilty (75%); C_{max}=63.3ng/mL; AUC=585ng•hr/mL. **Distribution:** V_d=0.957L/kg. **Metabolism:** Liver and kidney (protein catabolism). **Elimination:** Urine. $T_{1/2}$=3.81 hrs.

NURSING CONSIDERATIONS

Assessment: Assess for causes of poor growth, hypersensitivity to either metacresol or glycerin, pregnancy/nursing status, possible drug interactions, or any other conditions where treatment is contraindicated or cautioned. Perform funduscopic exam. In patients with Turner syndrome, assess for otitis media, other ear disorders, and CV disorders.

Monitoring: Monitor for growth, clinical response, compliance, malignant transformation of skin lesions, symptoms of slipped capital femoral epiphysis, progression of pre-existing scoliosis in pediatric patients, pancreatitis, fluid retention, and allergic reactions. Monitor patients with hypopituitarism who are on other hormone replacement therapy. Perform thyroid function test and funduscopic exam periodically. In patients with TS, monitor for signs or symptoms of ear disorders (eg, otitis media) and CV disorders. In patients with pre-existing tumors or GH deficiency secondary to an intracranial lesion, monitor for progression or recurrence of underlying disease process.

Patient Counseling: Inform of the potential benefits and risks of therapy, proper administration, usage and disposal, and caution against any reuse of needles and syringes. Instruct to dispose used needles and syringes in a puncture-resistant container.

Administration: SQ route. Refer to PI for reconstitution, administration, and preparation. **Storage:** (Vial) 2-8°C (36-46°F). Reconstituted: 2-8°C (36-46°F); stable up to 14 days. Reconstituted with Sterile Water: 2-8°C (36-46°F); use within 24 hrs; use only one dose per vial and discard unused portion. (Cartridge) 2-8°C (36-46°F). Reconstituted: 2-8°C (36-46°F); stable for 28 days. Avoid freezing.

HUMIRA

RX

adalimumab (Abbott)

> Increased risk for developing serious infections (eg, tuberculosis [TB], TB reactivation, invasive fungal infections, bacterial/viral infections due to opportunistic pathogens) that may lead to hospitalization or death, mostly with concomitant use of immunosuppressants (eg, methotrexate [MTX] or corticosteroids). Evaluate for latent TB and treat prior to initiation of therapy. Consider empiric antifungal therapy in patients at risk for invasive fungal infections who develop severe systemic illness. Monitor for development of signs/symptoms of infection during and after treatment. Consider risks and benefits prior to therapy with chronic or recurrent infections. D/C if serious infection or sepsis develops. Lymphoma and other malignancies reported in children and adolescents.

THERAPEUTIC CLASS: Monoclonal antibody/TNF-blocker

INDICATIONS: Reduce signs/symptoms, induce major clinical response, inhibit structural damage progression, and improve physical function in adults with moderately to severely active rheumatoid arthritis (RA), alone or in combination with MTX or other disease-modifying anti-rheumatic drugs (DMARDs). Reduce signs/symptoms of moderately to severely active polyarticular juvenile idiopathic arthritis in patients ≥4 yrs, alone or in combination with MTX. Reduce signs/symptoms of active arthritis, inhibit structural damage progression, and improve physical function in psoriatic arthritis (PA), alone or in combination with DMARDs. Reduce signs/symptoms of active ankylosing spondylitis (AS). Reduce signs/symptoms and induce and maintain clinical remission in adults with moderately to severely active Crohn's disease who have had an inadequate response to conventional therapy, also in those who have lost response to or are intolerant to infliximab. Treatment in adults with moderate to severe chronic plaque psoriasis who are candidates for systemic therapy or phototherapy.

DOSAGE: *Adults:* RA/PA/AS: 40mg SQ every other week. Some patients with RA not taking concomitant MTX may derive additional benefit from increasing to 40mg every week. Crohn's Disease: Initial: 160mg SQ at Day 1 (given as 4 inj of 40mg in 1 day or as 2 inj of 40mg/day for 2 consecutive days); then 80mg after 2 weeks (Day 15). Maint: 40mg every other week beginning at Week 4 (Day 29). Plaque Psoriasis: Initial: 80mg SQ. Maint: 40mg every other week starting 1 week after initial dose.
Pediatrics: 4-17 yrs: Juvenile Idiopathic Arthritis: 15kg-<30kg: 20mg SQ every other week. ≥30kg: 40mg SQ every other week.

HOW SUPPLIED: Inj: 20mg/0.4mL, 40mg/0.8mL [Prefilled syringe]; 40mg/0.8mL [Prefilled pen]

WARNINGS/PRECAUTIONS: Do not initiate with an active infection. Anaphylaxis and angioneurotic edema reported; d/c immediately and initiate appropriate therapy if occurs. Caution with hepatitis B virus (HBV) carriers; may increase risk of HBV reactivation; d/c and start antiviral therapy if occurs. New onset or exacerbation of CNS demyelinating disease reported; caution with pre-existing or recent-onset CNS/peripheral nervous system demyelinating disorders. Rare reports of pancytopenia (eg, aplastic anemia) reported; seek medical attention if blood dyscrasias/infection develop and d/c if significant hematologic abnormalities occur. New onset or worsening of congestive heart failure (CHF) reported; caution with heart failure. May result in autoantibody formation; d/c if lupus-like syndrome develops. May affect host defenses against infections and malignancies. Caution in elderly.

ADVERSE REACTIONS: Upper respiratory tract infections, injection-site pain/reactions, headache, rash, sinusitis, nausea, urinary tract infections, flu syndrome, abdominal pain, hyperlipidemia, hypercholesterolemia, back pain, hematuria.

INTERACTIONS: See Boxed Warning. Avoid with live vaccines and anakinra. Reduced clearance with MTX.

PREGNANCY: Category B, not for use in nursing.

MECHANISM OF ACTION: Monoclonal antibody/TNF-blocker; binds specifically to TNF-α and blocks its interaction with p55 and p75 cell surface TNF receptors. Modulates biological responses that are induced or regulated by

TNF. In plaque psoriasis, therapy reduces the epidermal thickness and infiltration of inflammatory cells.

PHARMACOKINETICS: Absorption: (40mg SQ single dose) Absolute bioavailability (64%), C_{max}=4.7mcg/mL, T_{max}=131 hrs. **Distribution:** (0.25-10mg/kg IV dose) V_d=4.7-6L. **Elimination:** (0.25-10mg/kg IV dose) $T_{1/2}$=2 weeks.

NURSING CONSIDERATIONS

Assessment: Assess for active infection, history of chronic/recurrent infection, predisposition to infection, TB risk factors, HBV carrier status, demyelinating disease, CHF, hypersensitivity to drug, latex allergy, pregnancy/nursing status, and possible drug interactions. Assess for immunization history in pediatric patients. Test for latent TB.

Monitoring: Monitor for serious infections, malignancies (eg, lymphoma), hypersensitivity reactions, HBV reactivation, demyelinating disease, hematological reactions, worsening/new onset CHF, lupus-like syndrome, immunosuppression, and other adverse reactions.

Patient Counseling: Inform about benefits/risks of therapy. Inform that therapy may lower the ability of immune system to fight infection; instruct to contact physician if any symptoms of infection, including TB and reactivation of HBV, occur. Counsel about risk of lymphoma and other malignancies. Advise to seek immediate medical attention if any symptoms of severe allergic reactions develop. Advise latex-sensitive patients that the needle cap of prefilled syringe contains latex. Advise to report any new/worsening medical conditions (eg, heart/neurological disease, autoimmune disorder) or any symptoms suggestive of a cytopenia (eg, bleeding, bruising, or persistent fever). Counsel about proper injection technique, as well as proper syringe and needle disposal.

Administration: SQ route. Rotate inj sites; avoid in areas where skin is tender, bruised, red, or hard. Inject full amount in the syringe. Inspect for particulate matter and discoloration prior to SQ administration. **Storage:** 2-8°C (36-46°F). Do not freeze. Protect prefilled syringe from exposure to light. Store in original carton until time of administration.

HUMULIN 70/30   OTC
insulin human, rdna origin - insulin, human (isophane/regular) (Lilly)

THERAPEUTIC CLASS: Insulin

INDICATIONS: To control hyperglycemia in diabetes.

DOSAGE: *Adults:* Individualize dose.
Pediatrics: Individualize dose.

HOW SUPPLIED: Inj: (Isophane-Regular) 70 U-30 U/mL

WARNINGS/PRECAUTIONS: Human insulin differs from animal-source insulin. Any change of insulin should be made cautiously. Changes in strength, manufacturer, type, or method of manufacturing may result in the need for a change in dosage. In cases where patients may require a change in dosage from that used with other insulin, adjustment should be done with the first dose, or during the first several weeks or months. Hypoglycemia may occur with too much insulin, missing or delaying meals, exercising, or working more than usual. Illness/infection (especially with N/V), pregnancy, exercise and travel may change insulin requirements. SQ administration may result in lipoatrophy or lipohypertrophy. May cause local (redness, swelling, itching at inj site that usually clears up in a few days) or generalized (rash over the whole body, SOB, wheezing, BP reduction, fast pulse, sweating) allergy. Not for IM or IV use.

ADVERSE REACTIONS: Hypoglycemia.

INTERACTIONS: Increased insulin requirements with oral contraceptives, corticosteroids, or thyroid replacement therapy. Reduced insulin requirements with oral hypoglycemics, salicylates (eg, aspirin [ASA]), sulfa antibiotics, alcohol, certain antidepressants, and some kidney and BP medicines. Early warning symptoms of hypoglycemia may be different or less pronounced with β-blockers.

PREGNANCY: Safety in pregnancy/nursing not known.

MECHANISM OF ACTION: Insulin; regulates glucose metabolism.

NURSING CONSIDERATIONS

Assessment: Assess FPG, HbA1c, renal function, LFTs, infections, alcohol consumption, exercise routines, diet, work schedule, travel plans, adrenal or thyroid or pituitary diseases, pregnancy/nursing status, and for possible drug interactions.

Monitoring: Monitor FPG, HbA1c, renal function, LFTs, diabetic ketoacidosis, lipodystrophy, and allergic reactions. Monitor for signs and symptoms of hypoglycemia (eg, sweating, palpitation, seizures, disorientation, tremors).

Patient Counseling: Advise to never share needles or syringes. Instruct to use syringe marked for U-100 insulin. Instruct to use disposable syringes and needles only once and discard by placing the used needle in a puncture-resistant disposable container. Advise to always wash hands before preparing the dose. Instruct to carefully shake or rotate the bottle several times to completely mix the insulin (should look uniformly cloudy or milky before administration); do not use if there is anything unusual in its appearance. Instruct to always carry a quick source of sugar (hard candy or glucose tablets). Counsel about signs/symptoms of hypoglycemia, importance of frequent monitoring of blood glucose levels, and need for a balanced diet and exercising regularly. Advise to keep an extra/spare supply of syringes and needles on hand and to always wear diabetic identification.

Administration: SQ route (Usual sites: abdomen, thigh, arms). Refer to PI for proper preparation and administration. **Storage:** (Not in use): Refrigerate. Do not freeze. (In use): <30°C (86°F). Protect from heat and light.

HUMULIN N
OTC

insulin, nph - insulin human, rdna origin - insulin, human isophane (Lilly)

THERAPEUTIC CLASS: Insulin

INDICATIONS: To control hyperglycemia in diabetes.

DOSAGE: *Adults:* Individualize dose.
Pediatrics: Individualize dose.

HOW SUPPLIED: Inj: 100 U/mL

WARNINGS/PRECAUTIONS: Human insulin differs from animal-source insulin. Any change of insulin should be made cautiously. Changes in strength, manufacturer, type, or method of manufacturing may result in the need for a change in dosage. In cases where patients may require a change in dosage from that used with other insulin, adjustment should be done with the 1st dose, or during the 1st several weeks or months. Hypoglycemia may occur with too much insulin, missing or delaying meals, exercising, or working more than usual. Illness/infection (especially with N/V), pregnancy, exercise and travel may change insulin requirements. SQ administration may result in lipoatrophy or lipohypertrophy. May cause local (redness, swelling, itching at inj site that usually clears up in a few days) or generalized (rash over the whole body, SOB, wheezing, BP reduction, fast pulse, sweating) allergy. Not for IM or IV use.

ADVERSE REACTIONS: Hypoglycemia, injection-site/allergic reaction.

INTERACTIONS: Increased insulin requirements with oral contraceptives, corticosteroids, or thyroid replacement therapy. Reduced insulin requirements with oral hypoglycemics, salicylates (eg, aspirin [ASA]), sulfa antibiotics, alcohol, certain antidepressants, and some kidney and BP medicines. β-blockers may mask symptoms of hypoglycemia.

PREGNANCY: Safety in pregnancy/nursing not known.

MECHANISM OF ACTION: Insulin; regulates glucose metabolism.

NURSING CONSIDERATIONS

Assessment: Assess FPG, HbA1c, renal function, LFTs, infections, alcohol consumption, exercise routines, diet, work schedule, travel plans, adrenal or thyroid or pituitary diseases, pregnancy/nursing status, and for possible drug interactions.

Monitoring: Monitor FPG, HbA1c, renal function, LFTs, diabetic ketoacidosis, lipodystrophy, and allergic reactions. Monitor for signs and symptoms of hypoglycemia (eg, sweating, palpitation, seizures, disorientation, tremors).

Patient Counseling: Instruct not to use any other insulin except on doctor's advise and direction. Advise to never share needles or syringes, use the proper and correct syringe type and use disposable syringes and needles only once and discard by placing the used needle in a puncture-resistant disposable container. Instruct to carefully shake or rotate the bottle several times to completely mix the insulin (should look uniformly cloudy or milky before administration); do not use if there is anything unusual in its appearance. Inform of proper dose preparation, mixing instructions with other human insulin and injection instructions. Instruct to always carry a quick source of sugar (hard candy or glucose tablets). Counsel about signs/symptoms of hypoglycemia, importance of frequent monitoring of blood glucose levels, and need for eating a balanced diet and exercising regularly. Advise to keep extra/spare supply of syringes and needles on hand and always wear diabetic identification and inform physician about medications concurrently being taken. Notify physician if pregnant/nursing or planning to be pregnant.

Administration: SQ route (alternate sites: abdomen, thigh, and arms). Refer to PI for proper preparation and administration. **Storage:** (Not-in use) Refrigerate. Do not freeze. (In-use): <30°C (86°F). Protect from heat and light.

HUMULIN R   OTC
insulin human, rdna origin - insulin, human regular (Lilly)

THERAPEUTIC CLASS: Insulin

INDICATIONS: Adjunct to diet and exercise to improve glycemic control in adults and children with type 1 and 2 diabetes mellitus (DM).

DOSAGE: *Adults:* Individualize dose. (SQ) ≥3x daily before meals. Inj should be followed by a meal within 30 min. (IV) 0.1-1 U/mL in infusion systems with 0.9% NaCl. Renal/Hepatic Impairment: May require dose reduction.
Pediatrics: Individualize dose. (SQ) ≥3x daily before meals. Inj should be followed by a meal within 30 min. (IV) 0.1-1 U/mL in infusion systems with 0.9% NaCl. Renal/Hepatic Impairment: May require dose reduction.

HOW SUPPLIED: Inj: 100 U/mL [3mL, 10mL]

CONTRAINDICATIONS: Hypoglycemia.

WARNINGS/PRECAUTIONS: Any change in insulin should be made cautiously. Changes in strength, manufacturer, type, or method of administration may result in the need for a change in dosage. Caution in patients with hypoglycemia unawareness and those who may be predisposed to hypoglycemia (pediatrics, those who fast or have erratic food intake). May require dose adjustment if physical activity or usual meal plan is changed. Illness, emotional disturbances, or other stresses may alter insulin requirements. Hyperglycemia, diabetic ketoacidosis, or hyperosmolar coma may develop if the patient takes less of the drug than needed to control blood glucose levels. May cause hypokalemia. Severe, life-threatening, generalized allergy (eg, anaphylaxis) may occur. May be administered IV under proper medical supervision.

ADVERSE REACTIONS: Hypoglycemia, hypokalemia, lipodystrophy, allergic reaction, weight gain, peripheral edema.

INTERACTIONS: Oral antihyperglycemics, salicylates, sulfa antibiotics, certain antidepressants (MAOIs, SSRIs), pramlintide, disopyramide, fibrates, fluoxetine, propoxyphene, pentoxifylline, ACE inhibitors, angiotensin II receptor blocking agents, and inhibitors of pancreatic function (eg, octreotide) may increase blood glucose-lowering effect and susceptibility to hypoglycemia. Corticosteroids, isoniazid, certain lipid-lowering drugs (eg, niacin), estrogens, oral contraceptives, phenothiazines, danazol, diuretics, sympathomimetic agents, somatropin, atypical antipsychotics, glucagon, protease inhibitors, and thyroid replacement therapy may reduce blood glucose-lowering effect. β-adrenergic blockers, clonidine, lithium salts, and alcohol may increase or decrease blood glucose-lowering effect. Pentamidine may cause hypoglycemia which may sometimes be followed by hyperglycemia. β-adrenergic blockers, clonidine, guanethidine, and reserpine may mask the signs of hypoglycemia. Hyperglycemia, diabetic ketoacidosis, or hyperosmolar coma may develop with drugs that affect glucose metabolism or insulin sensitivity. Use caution in patients using K$^+$-lowering medications or those taking medications sensitive to serum K$^+$ concentrations.

PREGNANCY: Category B, caution in nursing.

MECHANISM OF ACTION: Insulin; regulates glucose metabolism.

NURSING CONSIDERATIONS

Assessment: Assess FPG, HbA1c, renal/hepatic function, for hypoglycemia, conditions where treatment is cautioned, pregnancy/nursing status, and possible drug interactions.

Monitoring: Monitor for signs and symptoms of hypoglycemia, hyperglycemia, diabetic ketoacidosis, hyperosmolar coma, and allergic reactions. Monitor K$^+$ levels when drug is administered IV. Frequent glucose monitoring may be required in patients with renal/hepatic impairment and in those who experience hypoglycemia without early warning symptoms. Monitor FPG and HbA$_{1c}$.

Patient Counseling: Instruct not to use any other insulin except on doctor's advice and direction. Never share needles or syringes. Use the proper and correct syringe type. Use disposable syringes and needles only once and discard by placing the used needle in a puncture-resistant disposable container. Medication should look clear and colorless. Inform of proper dose preparation, mixing instructions with other human insulins and injection instructions. Always carry a quick source of sugar (hard candy or glucose tablets). Counsel about signs/symptoms of hypoglycemia, importance of frequent monitoring of blood glucose levels, and need for eating a balanced diet and exercising regularly. Keep extra/spare supply of syringes and needles on hand and always wear diabetic identification. Inform physician about medications concurrently being taken and if pregnant/nursing or planning to become pregnant.

Administration: SQ/IV route (SQ: abdomen, thigh, and arms). Refer to PI for preparation and administration. **Storage:** 2-8°C (36-46°F). Do not freeze. Opened: <30°C (86°F). Protect from heat and light. Use within 31 days. Admixture: Refrigerate (2-8°C [36-46°F]) for 48 hrs, then may use at room temperature for up to an additional 48 hrs.

HYALGAN   RX
sodium hyaluronate (Sanofi-Aventis)

THERAPEUTIC CLASS: Hyaluronan

INDICATIONS: Treatment of pain in osteoarthritis of the knee in patients who have failed to respond adequately to conservative nonpharmacologic therapy, and to simple analgesics (eg, APAP).

DOSAGE: *Adults:* Administer 2mL by intra-articular injection once a week for a total of 5 injections. Some patients may experience benefit with 3 injections given at weekly intervals.

HOW SUPPLIED: Inj: 2mL

CONTRAINDICATIONS: Intra-articular injections are contraindicated in cases of infections or skin disease in the area of the injection site.

WARNINGS/PRECAUTIONS: Avoid disinfectants containing quaternary ammonium salts for skin preparation; hyaluronic acid can precipitate in their presence. Anaphylactoid and allergic reactions reported. Transient increases in inflammation in the injected knee in some patients with inflammatory arthritis such as rheumatoid arthritis or gouty arthritis have been reported. Safety and effectiveness in joints other than the knee or concomitantly with other intra-articular injectables have not been established. Caution in patients who are allergic to avian proteins, feathers, and egg products. Avoid any strenuous activities or prolonged (eg, >1 hr) weight-bearing activities within 48 hrs following the intra-articular injection. Remove any joint effusion before injecting. Safety and effectiveness have not been demonstrated in children.

ADVERSE REACTIONS: GI complaints, injection-site pain, headache, local skin reactions (rash, ecchymosis), local joint pain, pruritus (local), knee swelling/effusion.

PREGNANCY: Safety in pregnancy and nursing not known.

NURSING CONSIDERATIONS

Assessment: Assess for knee joint infection, skin infection, or disease around injection site.

Monitoring: Monitor for anaphylactic and allergic reactions, injection-site pain, local skin reaction, and joint swelling/effusion.

Patient Counseling: Inform that drug may cause transient pain/swelling of injected joint. Avoid strenuous activities or prolonged weight-bearing activities (jogging, tennis) within 48 hrs following injection.

Adminstration: Intra-articular injection. Use strict aseptic technique. Inject full 2mL in one knee only. If treatment is bilateral, a separate vial should be used for each knee. **Storage:** Below 25°C (77°F). Do not freeze. Discard any used portions.

HYDROCHLOROTHIAZIDE   RX
hydrochlorothiazide (Various)

THERAPEUTIC CLASS: Thiazide diuretic

INDICATIONS: Management of HTN. Tab: Adjunct therapy in edema associated with CHF, hepatic cirrhosis, corticosteroid and estrogen therapy, renal dysfunction.

DOSAGE: *Adults:* Cap: Initial: 12.5mg qd. Max: 50mg/day. Elderly: Start at the low end of dosing range. Tab: Edema: 25-100mg qd or in divided doses. May give every other day or 3-5 days/week. HTN: Initial: 25mg qd. Titrate: May increase to 50mg/day.
Pediatrics: Tab: Diuresis/HTN: 1-2mg/kg/day given qd-bid. Max: Infants up to 2 yrs: 37.5mg/day. 2-12 yrs: 100mg/day. <6 months: Up to 3mg/kg/day given bid may be required.

HOW SUPPLIED: Cap: 12.5mg; Tab: 12.5mg, 25mg*, 50mg* *scored

CONTRAINDICATIONS: Anuria, sulfonamide hypersensitivity.

WARNINGS/PRECAUTIONS: Caution in severe renal disease, liver dysfunction, electrolyte/fluid imbalance. Can precipitate hepatic coma with severe liver disease, and azotemia with renal dysfunction. Latent diabetes mellitus may become manifest. Monitor electrolytes. Hyperuricemia, hyperglycemia, hypokalemia, hyponatremia, hypomagnesemia, hypercalcemia, hypophosphatemia may occur. Increases in cholesterol and triglyceride levels reported. May exacerbate systemic lupus erythematosus (SLE). Sensitivity reactions reported. D/C prior to parathyroid test. Parathyroid pathology reported with prolonged use. Enhanced effects in post-sympathectomy patients.

ADVERSE REACTIONS: Weakness, hypotension (including orthostatic hypotension), pancreatitis, jaundice, diarrhea, vomiting, blood dyscrasias, rash, photosensitivity, electrolyte imbalance, impotence, renal dysfunction/failure, interstitial nephritis.

INTERACTIONS: May potentiate orthostatic hypotension with alcohol, barbiturates, narcotics. Adjust dose of concomitant antidiabetic drugs. Possible decreased response to pressor amines. Concomitant corticosteroids, ACTH increase electrolyte depletion. May potentiate nondepolarizing skeletal muscle relaxants, antihypertensives. Lithium toxicity possible; avoid concomitant use. NSAIDs decrease effects. Decreased PO absorption with cholestyramine, colestipol resins.

PREGNANCY: Category B, not for use in nursing.

MECHANISM OF ACTION: Thiazide diuretic; affects renal tubular mechanism of electrolyte reabsorption, increasing excretion of Na^+ and Cl^-.

PHARMACOKINETICS: Absorption: C_{max}=70-490ng/mL; T_{max}= 1-5 hrs. **Distribution:** Crosses placenta; found in breast milk; plasma protein binding (40%-68%). **Elimination:** Urine (55%-77%), unchanged (>95%); $T_{1/2}$(cap)=6-15 hrs, (tab)=5.6-14.8 hrs.

NURSING CONSIDERATIONS

Assessment: Assess for anuria, SLE, DM, sulfonamide hypersensitivity, history of allergy or bronchial asthma, possible drug interactions, hepatic/renal impairment. Assess for pregnancy/nursing status.

Monitoring: Monitor serum electrolytes periodically. Monitor for signs/symptoms of electrolyte imbalance, exacerbation or activation of SLE, hyperglycemia, hyperuricemia or precipitation of gout, hypersensitivity reactions, renal/hepatic dysfunction.

Patient Counseling: Advise to seek medical attention if symptoms of electrolyte imbalance (dry mouth, thirst, weakness) or hypersensitivity reactions occur. Advise to avoid taking with food.

Administration: Oral route. **Storage:** 20-25°C (68-77°F). Cap: Protect from light, moisture, freezing.

HYDROXYZINE HCL   RX
hydroxyzine HCl (Various)

THERAPEUTIC CLASS: Piperazine antihistamine

INDICATIONS: (PO) Symptomatic relief of anxiety and tension associated with psychoneurosis and as adjunct in organic disease states in which anxiety is manifest. As a sedative when used as premedication and following general anesthesia. Management of pruritus due to allergic conditions and histamine-mediated pruritus. (Inj) Management of anxiety, tension, and psychomotor agitation in conditions of emotional stress. Management of acutely disturbed or hysterical patients or acute/chronic alcoholics with anxiety withdrawal symptoms or delirium tremens. As pre-/postoperative and pre-/postpartum adjunctive medication to permit reduction in narcotic dosage, allay anxiety, and control emesis. To control nausea and vomiting, excluding pregnancy.

DOSAGE: *Adults:* PO: Anxiety: 50-100mg qid. Pruritus: 25mg tid-qid. Sedation: 50-100mg. IM: Nausea/Vomiting, Pre-/Postoperative and Pre-/Postpartum Adjunct: 25-100mg. Psychiatric/Emotional Emergencies: 50-100mg q4-6h prn.
Pediatrics: PO: Anxiety/Pruritus: ≥6 yrs: 50-100mg/day in divided doses. <6 yrs: 50mg/day in divided doses. Sedation: 0.6mg/kg. IM: Nausea/Vomiting, Pre-/Postoperative Adjunct: 0.5mg/lb.

HOW SUPPLIED: Inj: 25mg/mL [1mL], 50mg/mL [1mL, 2mL, 10mL]; Syrup: 10mg/5mL [118mL, 473mL, 3785mL]; Tab: 10mg, 25mg, 50mg

CONTRAINDICATIONS: Early pregnancy. Injection is intended only for IM administration and should not, under any circumstances, be injected subcutaneously, intra-arterially, or IV. (Inj) Inadvertent SQ injection may result in significant tissue damage.

WARNINGS/PRECAUTIONS: Caution in elderly. May impair mental/physical abilities. Effectiveness as an antianxiety agent for long-term use (>4 months) has not been established.

ADVERSE REACTIONS: Dry mouth, drowsiness, involuntary motor activity.

INTERACTIONS: Potentiates CNS depression with other CNS depressants (eg, narcotics, non-narcotic analgesics, barbiturates, alcohol); rare cases of cardiac arrest and death have been reported following the combined use of the injection and other CNS depressants. May increase alcohol effects. Counteracts pressor action of epinephrine.

PREGNANCY: Not safe in pregnancy.

MECHANISM OF ACTION: Piperazine antihistamines; believed to suppress activity in key regions of subcortical area of CNS; shown to have primary skeletal muscle relaxation, bronchodilator, antihistaminic, and analgesic effects.

PHARMACOKINETICS: Absorption: Rapid (GIT).

NURSING CONSIDERATIONS

Assessment: Assess pregnancy/nursing status and possible drug interactions. Obtain baseline renal function.

Monitoring: Monitor for hypersensitivity reactions and renal dysfunction.

Patient Counseling: Caution may impair physical/mental abilities. Advise to avoid alcohol and other CNS depressants.

Administration: Oral route. **Storage:** Tab: 20-25°C (68-77°F). Dispense in a tight container. Syrup: 15-30°C (59-86°F). Protect from freezing. Protect from light. Dispense in a tight, light-resistant container. (Inj) 15-30°C (59-86°F). Protect from light.

HYDROXYZINE PAMOATE   RX
hydroxyzine pamoate (Various)

OTHER BRAND NAMES: Vistaril (Pfizer)

THERAPEUTIC CLASS: Piperazine antihistamine

INDICATIONS: Relief of anxiety. Allergic pruritus. For sedation as premedication and following anesthesia.

DOSAGE: *Adults:* Anxiety: 50-100mg qid. Pruritus: 25mg tid-qid. Sedation: 50-100mg.
Pediatrics: Anxiety/Pruritus: >6 yrs: 50-100mg/day in divided doses. <6 yrs: 50mg/day in divided doses. Sedation: 0.6mg/kg.

HOW SUPPLIED: Cap: 25mg, 50mg, 100mg

CONTRAINDICATIONS: Early pregnancy.

WARNINGS/PRECAUTIONS: Caution in elderly. May impair mental/physical abilities. Effectiveness as an antianxiety agent for long-term use (>4 months) has not been established.

ADVERSE REACTIONS: Dry mouth, drowsiness, involuntary motor activity.

INTERACTIONS: Potentiated by CNS depressants (eg, narcotics, non-narcotic analgesics, barbiturates); reduce dose.

PREGNANCY: Safety unknown in pregnancy and is contraindicated in early pregnancy, not for use in nursing.

MECHANISM OF ACTION: Believed to suppress activity in key regions of subcortical area of CNS; shown to have primary skeletal muscle relaxation, bronchodilator, antihistaminic, and analgesic effects.

PHARMACOKINETICS: Absorption: Rapid.

NURSING CONSIDERATIONS

Assessment: Assess for pregnancy/nursing status and possible drug interactions. Obtain baseline renal function.

Monitoring: Monitor for hypersensitivity reactions and renal dysfunction.

Patient Counseling: Caution may impair physical/mental abilities. Advise to avoid alcohol and other CNS depressants; seek medical attention if hypersensitivity reactions occur.

Administration: Oral route. **Storage:** Cap: Below 30°C (86°F). Susp: Shake vigorously until resuspended.

HYZAAR

RX

losartan potassium - hydrochlorothiazide (Merck)

> Can cause death/injury to developing fetus during 2nd and 3rd trimesters. D/C if pregnancy detected.

THERAPEUTIC CLASS: Angiotensin II receptor antagonist/thiazide diuretic

INDICATIONS: Treatment of HTN. Reduction of risk of stroke in patients with HTN and left ventricular hypertrophy (may not apply to Black patients).

DOSAGE: *Adults:* Individualize dose. HTN/HTN With Renal Impairment (CrCl >30mL/min): Usual: 50mg-12.5mg qd. Max: 100mg-25mg qd. Uncontrolled BP on Losartan Monotherapy or HCTZ Alone/Uncontrolled BP on 25mg qd HCTZ/Controlled BP With Hypokalemia: Switch to 50mg-12.5mg qd. Uncontrolled BP on 100mg Losartan Monotherapy: Switch to 100mg-12.5mg qd. Titrate: If BP remains uncontrolled after 3 weeks, increase to 100mg-25mg qd. Severe HTN: Initial: 50mg-12.5mg qd. Titrate: If inadequate response after 2-4 weeks, increase to 100mg-25mg qd. Max: 100mg-25mg qd. HTN With Left Ventricular Hypertrophy: Initial: Losartan 50mg qd. If inadequate BP reduction, add 12.5mg HCTZ or substitute losartan/HCTZ 50mg-12.5mg. If additional BP reduction needed, substitute with losartan 100mg and HCTZ 12.5mg or losartan/HCTZ 100mg-12.5mg, followed by losartan 100mg and HCTZ 25mg or losartan/HCTZ 100mg-25mg. Replacement Therapy: Combination may be substituted for titrated components.

HOW SUPPLIED: Tab: (Losartan-HCTZ) 50mg-12.5mg, 100mg-12.5mg, 100mg-25mg

CONTRAINDICATIONS: Anuria, hypersensitivity to sulfonamide-derived drugs.

WARNINGS/PRECAUTIONS: Not indicated for initial therapy of HTN. Symptomatic hypotension may occur in intravascular volume-depleted patients; correct volume depletion before therapy. Not recommended with hepatic impairment requiring losartan titration. Not recommended if CrCl ≤30mL/min. Angioedema reported. HCTZ: Caution with hepatic dysfunction or progressive liver disease; may precipitate hepatic coma. Hypersensitivity reactions may occur. May exacerbate or activate systemic lupus erythematosus (SLE). Observe for signs of fluid or electrolyte imbalance (hyponatremia, hypochloremic alkalosis, and hypokalemia). Hypokalemia may develop with brisk diuresis, severe cirrhosis, or after prolonged therapy. Dilutional hyponatremia may occur in edematous patients in hot weather; appropriate therapy is water restriction. May precipitate hyperuricemia or gout. Hyperglycemia, hypomagnesemia, and hypercalcemia may occur. D/C before testing for parathyroid function. Enhanced effects in postsympathectomy patients. Increased cholesterol, TG levels reported. May precipitate azotemia with renal disease. Losartan: Caution in patients with severe congestive heart failure (CHF); may cause oliguria and/or progressive azotemia, with acute renal failure and/or death (rare). May increase BUN and SrCr levels with renal artery stenosis.

ADVERSE REACTIONS: Fetal injury, hypokalemia, dizziness, upper respiratory infection, abdominal pain, palpitations, back pain, sinusitis, rash, cough, edema/swelling.

INTERACTIONS: NSAIDs, including selective COX-2 inhibitors, may decrease effects of diuretics and angiotensin II receptor antagonists and may further deteriorate renal function. Symptomatic hypotension may occur in intravascular volume-depleted patients (eg, those treated with diuretics). HCTZ: May reduce renal clearance of lithium; monitor for toxicity. Potentiates orthostatic hypotension with alcohol, barbiturates, narcotics. Adjust dose of antidiabetic drugs (eg, oral agents and insulin). Cholestyramine and colestipol resins impair absorption. Corticosteroids, adrenocorticotropic hormone (ACTH), and glycyrrhizin (found in liquorice) may intensify electrolyte depletion. May decrease response to pressor amines (eg, norepinephrine). Potentiates other antihypertensives and nondepolarizing skeletal muscle relaxants (eg, tubocurarine). May cause hypokalemia, which may lead to cardiac arrhythmia and sensitize or exaggerate the response of the heart to the toxic effects of digitalis. Losartan: Decreased levels with rifampin and phenobarbital. Increased levels with fluconazole, cimetidine, and erythromycin. Increased serum K+ with K+-sparing diuretics (eg, spironolactone, triamterene, amiloride), K+ supplements, K+-containing salt substitutes.

PREGNANCY: Category C (1st trimester) and D (2nd and 3rd trimesters), not for use in nursing.

MECHANISM OF ACTION: Losartan: Angiotensin II receptor antagonist; inhibits vasoconstrictor and aldosterone-secreting effects of angiotensin II by selectively blocking binding of angiotensin II to AT1 receptor. HCTZ: Thiazide diuretic; affects renal tubular mechanism of electrolyte reabsorption, directly increasing excretion of Na+ and Cl- and indirectly reducing plasma volume.

PHARMACOKINETICS: Absorption: Losartan: Well absorbed; T_{max}=1 hr, 3-4 hrs (metabolite). **Distribution:** Losartan: V_d=34L, 12L (metabolite); plasma protein binding (98.7%, 99.8% [metabolite]). HCTZ: Crosses placenta; found in breast milk. **Metabolism:** Losartan: CYP2C9, 3A4; carboxylic acid metabolite (active metabolite). **Elimination:** Losartan: Urine (4% unchanged, 6% metabolite); $T_{1/2}$=2 hrs, 6-9 hrs (metabolite). HCTZ: Kidney (≥61% unchanged); $T_{1/2}$=5.6-14.8 hrs.

NURSING CONSIDERATIONS

Assessment: Assess for hypersensitivity to drugs and its components, anuria, sulfonamide hypersensitivity, volume/salt depletion, SLE, DM, CHF, hepatic/renal function, postsympathectomy status, cirrhosis, renal artery stenosis, pregnancy/nursing status, and possible drug interactions. Obtain baseline BP.

Monitoring: Monitor for signs/symptoms of fluid/electrolyte imbalance, exacerbation/activation of SLE, hypotension, latent DM, hyperglycemia, hypomagnesemia, hypercalcemia, hyperuricemia or precipitation of gout, hypersensitivity reactions, and other adverse reactions. Monitor BP, serum electrolytes, renal function, cholesterol, and TG levels periodically.

Patient Counseling: Inform of pregnancy risks. Counsel that lightheadedness may occur especially during the 1st days of therapy. Instruct to d/c therapy if syncope occurs. Advise that inadequate fluid intake, excessive perspiration, diarrhea, or vomiting may result in drop of BP, leading to lightheadedness or syncope. Instruct not to use K+ supplements or salt substitutes containing K+ without consulting physician.

Administration: Oral route. **Storage:** 25°C (77°F); excursions permitted to 15-30°C (59-86°F). Keep container tightly closed. Protect from light.

IMDUR   RX
isosorbide mononitrate (Schering)

THERAPEUTIC CLASS: Nitrate vasodilator

INDICATIONS: Prevention of angina pectoris. Not for acute attack.

DOSAGE: *Adults:* Initial: 30-60mg qd in am. Titrate: May increase after several days to 120mg/day. Swallow whole with fluids. Elderly: Start at lower end of dosing range.

HOW SUPPLIED: Tab, Extended-Release: 30mg*, 60mg*, 120mg *scored

WARNINGS/PRECAUTIONS: Not for use with acute MI or CHF. Severe hypotension may occur; caution with volume depletion and hypotension. Hypotension may increase angina pectoris. May aggravate angina caused by hypertrophic cardiomyopathy. Monitor for tolerance. May interfere with cholesterol test.

ADVERSE REACTIONS: Headache, dizziness, hypotension.

INTERACTIONS: Severe hypotension with sildenafil. Orthostatic hypotension with CCBs. Additive vasodilation with other vasodilators (eg, alcohol).

PREGNANCY: Category B, caution with nursing.

MECHANISM OF ACTION: Nitrate vasodilator; relaxes vascular smooth muscle, and consequent dilatation of peripheral arteries and veins, especially the latter. Dilatation of veins leads to reducing the left ventricular end dia-stolic pressure and pulmonary capillary wedge pressure (preload). Arteriolar relaxation reduces systemic vascular resistance, systolic arterial pressure, and mean arterial pressure (afterload). It also dilates the coronary artery.

PHARMACOKINETICS: Absorption: Imdur: (60mg) C_{max}=557-572ng/mL, T_{max}=2.9-4.2 hrs, AUC=6625-7555ng•hr/mL. (120mg) C_{max}=1151-1180ng/mL, T_{max}=3.1-3.2 hrs, AUC=14241-16800ng•hr/mL. Absolute bioavailability (100%). **Distribution:** V_d=0.6-0.7L/kg; plasma protein binding (5%). **Metabolism:** Liver. Cleared through denitration and glucuronidation pathways. **Elimination:** Urine (96%), feces (1%). (60mg) $T_{1/2}$=6.2-6.3 hrs. (120mg) $T_{1/2}$=6.2-6.4 hrs.

NURSING CONSIDERATIONS

Assessment: Assess for severe hypotension, volume-depleted patients, angina caused by hypertrophic cardiomyopathy, pregnancy status, alcohol intake, and possible drug interactions.

Monitoring: Careful clinical or hemodynamic monitoring for hypotension and tachycardia. Monitor for paradoxical bradycardia and increased angina pectoris, headaches and lightheadedness on standing, manifestation of true physical dependence (chest pain, acute MI). Monitor for the interference with Zlatkis-Zak color reaction, causing false low readings in cholesterol levels and for manifestations of methemoglobinemia.

Patient Counseling: Counsel to carefully follow dosing regimen. Inform about headaches (markers of drug activity) and lightheadedness on standing. Avoid alcohol consumption.

Administration: Oral route. Swallow tab with glass of water; do not crush or chew. **Storage:** 25°C (77°F); excursions permitted to 15-30°C (59-86°F).

IMITREX   RX
sumatriptan succinate - sumatriptan (GlaxoSmithKline)

THERAPEUTIC CLASS: 5-HT$_1$-agonist

INDICATIONS: (Inj, Spray, Tab) Acute treatment of migraine attacks with or without aura in adults. (Inj) Acute treatment of cluster headache episodes.

DOSAGE: *Adults:* ≥18 yrs: (Inj) Initial: 6mg SQ. Max: Two 6mg inj/24 hrs. Injections must be separated by at least 1 hr. (Spray) 5mg, 10mg, or 20mg single dose administered into 1 nostril; may repeat after 2 hrs. 10mg dose may be obtained by administering a single 5mg dose in each nostril. Max: 40mg/24 hrs. (Tab) Initial: 25mg, 50mg, or 100mg single dose; may repeat after 2 hrs. Max: 200mg/24 hrs. If headache returns after initial treatment with inj dose, may give additional single tabs, (up to 100mg/day), with an interval of at least 2 hrs between doses. Hepatic Disease: Max: 50mg/single dose. Safety of treating >4 headaches/30 days not known.

HOW SUPPLIED: Inj: 4mg/0.5mL, 6mg/0.5mL; Tab: 25mg, 50mg, 100mg [9⁵]; Nasal Spray: 5mg, 20mg [6⁵]

CONTRAINDICATIONS: (Inj, Spray, Tab) History, symptoms, or signs of ischemic cardiac syndromes (eg, angina pectoris, MI, silent myocardial ischemia), cerebrovascular syndromes (eg, strokes, transient ischemic attacks), and peripheral vascular disease (eg, ischemic bowel disease). Other significant CVD, uncontrolled HTN, hemiplegic or basilar migraine, severe hepatic impairment, within 24 hrs of ergotamine-containing or ergot-type medications, or other 5-HT$_1$ agonists. (Inj) IV administration. (Spray, Tab) Concurrent administration of MAO-A inhibitors or use within 2 weeks of d/c of an MAO-A inhibitor.

WARNINGS/PRECAUTIONS: Caution in patients with risk factors for coronary artery disease (CAD); evaluate CV status before use and administer first dose with supervision and subsequent ECG monitoring. Serious adverse cardiac events (eg, acute MI, life-threatening arrhythmias), cerebrovascular events (eg, cerebral hemorrhage, subarachnoid hemorrhage, stroke) and vasospastic reactions (eg, coronary vasospasm, peripheral vascular ischemia, colonic ischemia) reported. Serotonin syndrome, elevation in BP, including hypertensive crisis, and hypersensitivity may occur. Chest, jaw, and neck tightness reported. Avoid in elderly. Caution with diseases that may alter the absorption, metabolism, or excretion of drugs (eg, hepatic or renal impairment). Rare reports of seizures; caution in patients with a history of epilepsy or conditions associated with a lower seizure threshold. Caution in patients with brain lesions and in patients with controlled HTN. Possible long-term ophthalmic effects. Reconsider diagnosis before 2nd dose. (Inj) Should only be used when a clear diagnosis of migraine or cluster headache has been established. (Spray, Tab) Should only be used with a clear diagnosis of migraine headache has been established. (Spray) May cause irritation in the nose and throat.

ADVERSE REACTIONS: (Inj) Atypical sensations, flushing, chest discomfort, neck pain/stiffness, injection-site reaction. (Spray) Nasal cavity/sinuses disorder/discomfort; N/V, bad/unusual taste. (Tab) Atypical sensations, pain sensation, pressure sensation, malaise/fatigue, drowsiness, hyposalivation, dizziness/vertigo.

INTERACTIONS: (Inj, Spray, Tab) See Contraindications. Serotonin syndrome reported with combined use of an SSRI or SNRI. Use with an MAO-A is not recommended; if clinically warranted, suitable dose adjustment is advised.

PREGNANCY: Category C, caution in nursing.

MECHANISM OF ACTION: Selective 5-HT_1 receptor subtype agonist; activates vascular 5-HT_1 receptors, located on cranial arteries, basilar artery, and in the vasculature of human dura mater. Responsible for mediating vasoconstriction.

PHARMACOKINETICS: Absorption: Intranasal, 5mg: C_{max}=5ng/mL; intranasal, 20mg: C_{max}=16ng/mL; SQ, 6mg: (Deltoid) C_{max}=74ng/mL, T_{max}=12 min. (Thigh) C_{max}=52ng/mL; (PO, 25mg) C_{max}=18ng/mL; (PO, 100mg) C_{max}=51ng/mL. **Distribution:** (PO) V_d=2.4L/kg, (SQ) V_d=50L, (Nasal Spray) V_d = 2.7L; plasma protein binding (14-21%); found in breast milk following SQ administration. **Metabolism:** Via monoamine oxidase. **Elimination:** (SQ) Urine (22% unchanged and 38% as indole acetic acid), $T_{1/2}$=115 min; (Nasal Spray) Urine (3% unchanged and 42% as metabolites), $T_{1/2}$=2 hrs. (Oral) Urine (60%), feces (40%), $T_{1/2}$=2.5 hrs.

NURSING CONSIDERATIONS

Assessment: Assess for presence/history of cardiac ischemic syndrome, cerebrovascular syndrome, or peripheral vascular syndrome, uncontrolled HTN, presence of hemiplegic or basilar migraines, presence of diseases that may alter the absorption, metabolism or excretion of drugs (eg, hepatic or renal impairment), history of epilepsy or conditions which lower seizure threshold, pregnancy/nursing status, and for possible drug interactions. Assess proper diagnosis of migraine headaches.

Monitoring: Monitor for signs/symptoms of cardiac events (eg, MI, cardiac rhythm disturbances, peripheral vascular ischemia, hypertensive crisis, chest tightness), colonic ischemia, bloody diarrhea, serotonin syndrome (eg, mental status changes), hypersensitivity reactions, jaw/neck tightness, seizures, exacerbation of headache, ophthalmic changes (eg, corneal opacities), and clinical response. In patients on long-term therapy and in patients with CAD risk factors, perform periodic monitoring of cardiovascular function. If clinical response does not occur following administration of first dose, reassess diagnosis.

Patient Counseling: Inform about possible adverse events (eg, cardiovascular effects, serotonin syndrome); instruct to consult physician if symptoms of any adverse event occur (eg, chest tightness, abdominal pain, SOB, confusion, hallucinations, flushing). Advise to notify physician of all medications currently taking and if pregnant or nursing.

Administration: Oral, SQ, or nasal route. **Storage:** 2-30°C (36-86°F). Protect from light.

IMURAN
azathioprine (Prometheus)

RX

> Increased risk of neoplasia with chronic immunosuppression. Physician should be familiar with this risk as well as mutagenic potential and possible hematologic toxicities.

THERAPEUTIC CLASS: Purine antagonist antimetabolite

INDICATIONS: Adjunct for prevention of rejection in renal homotransplantation. Management of active rheumatoid arthritis (RA) to reduce signs and symptoms.

DOSAGE: *Adults:* Renal Homotransplantation: Individualize dose. Initial: 3-5mg/kg/day, start at time of transplant. Usually given as a single dose on the day of, and minority of cases 1-3 days before transplantation. Maint: 1-3mg/kg/day. Rheumatoid Arthritis: Initial: 1mg/kg/day given qd-bid. Titrate: Increase by 0.5mg/kg/day after 6-8 weeks, then at 4-week intervals. Max: 2.5mg/kg/day. Maint: Lowest effective dose. Decrease by 0.5mg/kg/day or 25mg/day every 4 weeks. If no response by Week 12, then consider refractory. Renal Dysfunction: Lower dose.

HOW SUPPLIED: Tab: 50mg* *scored; Inj (azathioprine sodium): 100mg/20mL

CONTRAINDICATIONS: Pregnancy in RA treatment. Patients with RA previously treated with alkylating agents (eg, cyclophosphamide, chlorambucil, melphalan) may increase risk of neoplasia.

WARNINGS/PRECAUTIONS: Severe leukopenia, thrombocytopenia, macrocytic anemia, pancytopenia, and severe bone marrow suppression may occur. Monitor CBCs, including platelets, weekly during the 1st month, twice monthly for the 2nd and 3rd months, then monthly or more frequently if dose/therapy changes. Serious infections including fungal, viral, bacterial, and protozoal may occur and may be fatal; reduce dose and/or consider use of other drugs. The risk of post-transplant lymphoma may be increased in patients who receive aggressive treatment with immunosuppressive drugs. May cause fetal harm. Gastrointestinal hypersensitivity reactions (severe N/V) associated with diarrhea, rash, fever, malaise, myalgias, elevated liver enzymes, and hypotension may develop.

ADVERSE REACTIONS: Leukopenia, thrombocytopenia, infections, N/V, hepatotoxicity, bone marrow suppression, GI hypersensitivity, skin rashes, alopecia, fever, arthralgia, diarrhea, steatorrhea, negative nitrogen balance, interstitial pneumonitis.

INTERACTIONS: Caution with concomitant aminosalicylates (eg, sulphasalazine, mesalazine, olsalazine); may inhibit TPMT. Reduce dose to approximately 1/3-1/4 of the usual dose with allopurinol. Drugs affecting leukocyte production (eg, co-trimoxazole) may exaggerate leukopenia. ACE inhibitors may induce anemia, severe leukopenia. Inhibits anticoagulant effects of warfarin.

PREGNANCY: Category D, not for use in nursing.

MECHANISM OF ACTION: Immunosuppressive antimetabolite; an imidazolyl derivative of 6-mercaptopurine (6-MP). In homograft survival, it suppresses hypersensitivities of the cell-mediated type and causes variable alterations in antibody production. Immuno-inflammatory response mechanisms not established; suppresses disease manifestation and underlying pathology in autoimmune disease.

PHARMACOKINETICS: Absorption: (PO) Well absorbed; T_{max}=1-2 hrs. **Distribution:** Plasma protein binding (30%); crosses placenta; found in breast milk. **Metabolism:** Liver and erythrocytes (extensive); 6-MP activated to 6-thioguanine nucleotides (major metabolites); inactivated via thiol methylation by thiopurine S-methyltransferase (TPMT) and oxidation by xanthine oxidase. **Elimination:** Urine; $T_{1/2}$=5 hrs.

NURSING CONSIDERATIONS

Assessment: Assess for renal/hepatic dysfunction, previous treatment of rheumatoid arthritis with alkylating agents, pregnancy/nursing status, and for possible drug interactions. Conduct TPMT genotyping/phenotyping to identify absent or reduced enzymatic activity. Obtain baseline CBC with platelets.

Monitoring: Monitor for signs/symptoms of bone marrow suppression, malignancies (eg, skin cancer, reticulum cell or lymphomatous tumors), serious infections (eg, fungal, viral, bacterial, protozoal), and for GI hypersensitivity reactions. Monitor CBC, including platelet counts.

Patient Counseling: Inform about necessity of periodic CBC while on therapy. Instruct to report any unusual bleeding or bruising or signs of infections. Inform about risk of malignancy. Educate about careful dosage instructions, especially with impaired renal function or concomitant use with allopurinol. Advise to notify physician if pregnant or nursing.

Administration: IV and oral routes. **Storage:** 15-25°C (59-77°F). Protect from light. Store tablets in a dry place.

INDERAL LA

propranolol HCl (Akrimax)

THERAPEUTIC CLASS: Nonselective beta-blocker

INDICATIONS: Management of hypertension, angina pectoris due to coronary atherosclerosis, and hypertrophic subaortic stenosis. Migraine prophylaxis.

DOSAGE: *Adults:* HTN: Initial: 80mg qd. Maint: 120-160mg qd. Angina: Initial: 80mg qd. Titrate: Increase gradually every 3-7 days. Maint: 160mg qd. Max: 320mg qd. Migraine: Initial: 80mg qd. Maint: 160-240mg qd. D/C gradually if unsatisfactory response within 4-6 weeks. Hypertrophic Subaortic Stenosis: Usual: 80-160mg qd.

HOW SUPPLIED: Cap, Extended-Release: 60mg, 80mg, 120mg, 160mg

CONTRAINDICATIONS: Cardiogenic shock, sinus bradycardia and >1st-degree block, bronchial asthma.

WARNINGS/PRECAUTIONS: Reports of angina exacerbation and myocardial infarction (MI) following abrupt d/c. Gradually reduce dose over at least a few weeks if d/c therapy. Hypersensitivity reactions, including anaphylactic/anaphylactoid reactions, reported. Caution with well-compensated cardiac failure, nonallergic bronchospasm, Wolff-Parkinson-White (WPW) syndrome, hepatic or renal dysfunction. Withdrawal before surgery is controversial. May mask hypoglycemia or hyperthyroidism symptoms. May reduce IOP. Can cause cardiac failure. Stevens-Johnson syndrome, toxic epidermal necrolysis, exfoliative dermatitis, erythema multiforme, and urticaria reported. Caution in elderly. Not indicated for treatment of hypertensive emergencies.

ADVERSE REACTIONS: Bradycardia, CHF, hypotension, lightheadedness, mental depression, N/V, allergic reactions, agranulocytosis, dry eyes, alopecia, SLE-like reactions, male impotence, Peyronie's disease.

INTERACTIONS: Increased propranolol levels/toxicity with CYP2D6 inhibitors (eg, amiodarone, cimetidine, fluoxetine, paroxetine, quinidine, ritonavir), CYP1A2 inhibitors (eg, imipramine, cimetidine, ciprofloxacin, fluvoxamine, isoniazid, ritonavir, theophylline, zileuton, zolmitriptan, rizatriptan), and CYP2C19 inhibitors (eg, fluconazole, cimetidine, fluoxetine, fluvoxamine, teniposide, tolbutamide). Decreased blood levels with hepatic enzyme inducers (eg, rifampin, ethanol, phenytoin, phenobarbital, cigarette smoking). Propafenone levels increased with concurrent administration. Lidocaine metabolism is inhibited with coadministration. Increased levels with concurrent nisoldipine and nicardipine. Nifedipine levels increased with coadministration. Zolmitriptan and rizatriptan concentrations increased with concurrent administration. Decreased theophylline clearance with concurrent administration. Increased concentrations of diazepam and its metabolites with coadministration. Increased thioridazine plasma concentrations with concurrent administration of doses ≥160mg/day. Increased plasma concentrations with chlorpromazine. Aluminum hydroxide gel may decrease plasma concentrations. Decreased plasma concentrations with coadministration of cholestyramine or colestipol. Propranolol given with lovastatin or pravastatin may decrease levels of both drugs. Concurrent administration increases warfarin levels and

PT. Caution with ACE inhibitors, clonidine, terasozin/doxazosin, reserpine, inotropic agents, dobutamine/isoproterenol, NSAIDs, MAO inhibitors/TCA, methoxyflurane/trichloroethylene, neuroleptic drugs, and thyroxine. Avoid alcohol intake.

PREGNANCY: Category C, caution in nursing.

MECHANISM OF ACTION: Nonselective β-adrenergic receptor blocker; not fully established. Proposed to decrease cardiac output, inhibit renin release, and lessen tonic sympathetic nerve outflow from vasomotor centers in the brain.

PHARMACOKINETICS: Absorption: Complete; T_{max}=6 hrs. **Distribution:** V_d=4L/kg; plasma protein binding (90%); crosses placenta, blood-brain barrier; found in breast milk. **Metabolism:** CYP2D6 (hydroxylation and oxidation), CYP1A2, 2D6 (oxidation), N-dealkylation, glucuronidation. Propranolol glucuronide, naphthyloxylactic acid, glucuronic acid, sulfate conjugates (major metabolites). **Elimination:** $T_{1/2}$=10 hrs.

NURSING CONSIDERATIONS

Assessment: Assess for sinus bradycardia, AV heart block, cardiogenic shock, overt CHF, bronchial asthma, bronchospastic disease, hyperthyroidism, DM, WPW syndrome, history of HF, possible drug interactions, hepatic/renal impairment.

Monitoring: Monitor for signs/symptoms of cardiac failure, hypoglycemia, decreased IOP, thyrotoxicosis, withdrawal symptoms (eg, angina, MI), and hypersensitivity reactions.

Patient Counseling: Instruct not to interrupt or d/c therapy without consulting physician. Inform drug may mask signs of thyrotoxicosis and hypoglycemia. Inform may interfere with glaucoma screening test. Advise to contact physician if symptoms of HF, withdrawal (eg, angina), or hypersensitivity reactions occur.

Administration: Oral route. **Storage:** 20-25°C (68-77°F); excursions permitted to 15-30°C (59-86°F). Protect from light, moisture, freezing, and excessive heat.

INDOMETHACIN   RX
indomethacin (Various)

> NSAIDs may cause an increased risk of serious cardiovascular thrombotic events, MI, stroke and serious GI adverse events including bleeding, ulceration, and perforation of the stomach or intestines. Contraindicated for the treatment of perioperative pain in the setting of coronary artery bypass graft (CABG) surgery.

OTHER BRAND NAMES: Indocin (Merck)

THERAPEUTIC CLASS: NSAID

INDICATIONS: Management of moderate to severe rheumatoid arthritis (RA), ankylosing spondylitis, osteoarthritis (OA), acute painful shoulder (bursitis and/or tendinitis) and/or acute gouty arthritis.

DOSAGE: *Adults:* RA/Ankylosing Spondylitis/OA: Initial: 25mg PO bid-tid. Titrate: May increase by 25-50mg/day at weekly intervals. Max: 200mg/day. Bursitis/Tendinitis: 75-150mg/day given tid-qid for 7-14 days. Acute Gouty Arthritis: 50mg PO tid until pain is tolerable, then d/c. Take with food. *Pediatrics:* ≥14 yrs: RA/Ankylosing Spondylitis/OA: Initial: 25mg PO bid-tid. Titrate: May increase by 25-50mg/day at weekly intervals. Max: 200mg/day. Bursitis/Tendinitis: 75-150mg/day given tid-qid for 7-14 days. Acute Gouty Arthritis: 50mg PO tid until pain is tolerable, then d/c. 2-14 yrs (safety and effectiveness not established): Initial: 1-2mg/kg/day in divided doses. Max: 3mg/kg/day or 150-200mg/day. Take with food.

HOW SUPPLIED: Cap: 25mg, 50mg; Sus: 25mg/5mL [237mL]

CONTRAINDICATIONS: ASA or other NSAID allergy that precipitates acute asthmatic attack, urticaria, or rhinitis. Do not give suppositories with history of proctitis or recent rectal bleeding. Treatment of perioperative pain in the setting of CABG surgery.

WARNINGS/PRECAUTIONS: May lead to onset of new HTN or worsening of pre-existing HTN; monitor BP closely. Fluid retention and edema reported; caution with fluid retention or heart failure. Renal papillary necrosis and other renal injury reported after long-term use. Not recommended for use with advanced renal disease; if therapy must be initiated, monitor renal function. Anaphylactoid reactions may occur. May cause serious skin adverse events (eg, exfoliative dermatitis, Stevens-Johnson syndrome, and toxic epidermal necrolysis). Avoid in late pregnancy; may cause premature closure of ductus arteriosus. May cause elevations of LFTs; d/c if liver disease develops or systemic manifestations occur. Caution in elderly. Anemia may occur; with long-term use, monitor Hgb/Hct if signs or symptoms of anemia develop. May inhibit platelet aggregation and prolong bleeding time; monitor with coagulation disorders. Caution with asthma and avoid with ASA-sensitive asthma. Corneal deposits and retinal disturbances reported with prolonged therapy; perform eye exams at periodic intervals during prolonged therapy. May aggravate depression or other psychiatric disturbances, epilepsy, and parkinsonism; use with caution. D/C if severe CNS adverse reactions develop. May impair mental/physical abilities.

ADVERSE REACTIONS: Headache, dizziness, N/V, dyspepsia, diarrhea, abdominal pain, constipation, vertigo, somnolence, depression, fatigue.

INTERACTIONS: Avoid salicylates, diflunisal, other NSAIDs, and triamterene. Potassium-sparing diuretics may cause hyperkalemia. Increase toxicity of methotrexate, cyclosporine, lithium, and digoxin. Probenecid increases levels. Caution with antihypertensives and anticoagulants. May decrease effects of diuretics, β-blockers, captopril.

PREGNANCY: Category C, not for use in nursing.

MECHANISM OF ACTION: NSAID; not established; exhibits antipyretic, analgesic, and anti-inflammatory properties. Potent inhibitor of prostaglandin synthesis; decreases prostaglandins in peripheral tissues, suppresses inflammation in RA, and diminishes basal and CO_2-stimulated cerebral blood flow.

PHARMACOKINETICS: Absorption: Readily absorbed. Bioavailability (100%); C_{max}=1-2mcg/mL; T_{max}=2 hrs. **Distribution:** Plasma protein binding (99%); crosses blood-brain barrier and placenta; found in breast milk. **Metabolism:** Desmethyl, desbenzoyl, desmethyldesbenzoyl (metabolites). **Elimination:** Urine (60% as drug/metabolites), feces (33% as drug); $T_{1/2}$=4.5 hrs.

NURSING CONSIDERATIONS

Assessment: Assess for history of asthma, urticaria or allergic-type reaction after previous use of NSAIDs, perioperative pain in setting of CABG surgery, CVD or risk factors for CVD, HTN, fluid retention or HF, hyponatremia, ulcer disease or GI bleeding, coagulation disorders or anticoagulant therapy, renal/hepatic impairment, rhinitis with or without nasal polyps, pregnancy/nursing status, depression or other psychiatric disturbances, epilepsy, parkinsonism, and possible drug interactions.

Monitoring: Monitor BP during initiation of therapy and thereafter. Monitor platelet function, CBCs, LFTs, dexamethasone suppression tests, renal function, and chemistry profile. Monitor signs/symptoms of anaphylactic/anaphylactoid reactions, adverse skin events (eg, exfoliative dermatitis, Stevens-Johnson syndrome, toxic epidermal necrolysis), eosinophilia, rash, corneal deposits and retinal disturbances with periodic ophthalmic exam, CNS effects, aggravation of depression or other psychiatric disturbances, GI bleeding/ulceration and perforation, anemia, CV thrombotic events, MI, stroke, new or worsening HTN, renal toxicity, renal papillary necrosis, other renal injury, and hyperkalemia.

Patient Counseling: Inform about potential serious side effects (eg, CV side effects such as MI or stroke); seek medical attention if signs/symptoms of chest pain, SOB, weakness, slurred speech, skin rash, blisters or fever, GI effects, bleeding, ulceration and perforation, signs of anaphylactic/anaphylactoid reaction, or hepatic toxicity occurs. Caution while performing hazardous tasks (eg, operating machinery/driving). Advise to notify physician if pregnant, nursing, planning to become pregnant, or if weight gain/edema occurs.

Administration: Oral route. **Storage:** 20-25°C (68-77°F); tight, light-resistant container.

INFERGEN RX
interferon alfacon-1 (Valeant)

> May cause or aggravate fatal or life-threatening neuropsychiatric, autoimmune, ischemic, and infectious disorders. Monitor closely with periodic clinical and laboratory evaluations. D/C with severe or worsening signs or symptoms of these conditions. Use with ribavirin may cause birth defects and death of unborn child; avoid in pregnancy and in female partners of male patients. Ribavirin may cause hemolytic anemia and is genotoxic and mutagenic.

THERAPEUTIC CLASS: Biological response modifier

INDICATIONS: Treatment of chronic hepatitis C in patients ≥18 yrs with compensated liver disease.

DOSAGE: *Adults:* 9mcg three times per week SQ for 24 weeks. Patients who tolerated previous interferon therapy but did not respond/relapsed: 15mcg three times per week for up to 48 weeks. Hold dose temporarily with severe adverse effects and reduce to 7.5mcg. Combination Treatment with Ribavirin: 15mcg SQ qd with weight-based ribavirin 1,000mg - 1,200mg (<75kg and ≥75kg) PO in two divided doses for up to 48 weeks. Take with food. Reduce dose from 15mcg to 9mcg & from 9mcg to 6mcg if serious adverse reactions occur. Refer to PI for dose modifications and d/c based on depression or laboratory parameters. D/C if persistent or recurrent adverse effects despite dose adjustment, failure to achieve at least a 2 $\log_{10}$ drop or have detectable HCV-RNA levels after 24 weeks.

HOW SUPPLIED: Inj: 9mcg/0.3mL, 15mcg/0.5mL

CONTRAINDICATIONS: Hepatic decompensation (Child-Pugh score >6 [class B and C]), autoimmune hepatitis. In combination with ribavirin: pregnancy, men whose female partners are pregnant, hemoglobinopathies (eg, thalassemia major, sickle cell anemia), CrCL <50mL/min.

WARNINGS/PRECAUTIONS: May cause severe psychiatric adverse events; caution with history of depression. If patients develop psychiatric problems, monitor during treatment and in the 6-month follow up period. D/C if psychiatric symptoms persist or worsen, or suicidal ideation or aggressive behavior toward others identified. Hypotension, arrhythmia, tachycardia, cardiomyopathy, angina pectoris, myocardial infarction (MI) reported; caution with cardiovascular disease (CVD). Monitor patients with history of MI and arrhythmia. Dyspnea, pulmonary infiltrates, pneumonia, bronchiolitis obliterans, interstitial pneumonitis, pulmonary HTN, and sarcoidosis, some resulting in potentially fatal respiratory failure may occur; d/c if persistent or unexplained pulmonary infiltrates or pulmonary function impairment develops. Risk of hepatic decompensation with chronic hepatitis C with cirrhosis; monitor clinical status/hepatic function & d/c if symptoms of hepatic decompensation occur. Increases in SrCr, including renal failure reported; monitor closely for signs/symptoms of toxicity. Causes bone marrow suppression, including severe cytopenias; d/c if decreases in neutrophil (<0.5x10⁹/L) or platelet counts (<25x10⁹/L). Caution with abnormally low peripheral blood cell counts, transplant patients or chronically immunosuppressed patients. Potentially fatal hemorrhagic/ischemic colitis and pancreatitis observed; d/c if signs/symptoms develop. D/C if hypersensitivity reactions (eg, urticaria, angioedema, bronchoconstriction, anaphylaxis) occur. Decrease/loss of vision, retinopathy, retinal hemorrhage, cotton wool spots, optic neuritis, papilledema and serious retinal detachment reported; d/c with new or worsening symptoms. Administer periodic visual exams in patients with pre-existing ophthalmologic disorders. Caution with history of endocrine disorders (eg, hyper- or hypothyroidism) or DM. Thyroid disorder, hyperglycemia and DM reported; d/c if uncontrollable. Neutropenia, thrombocytopenia, hypertriglyceridemia and thyroid disorders reported; monitor lab parameters closely. Caution in elderly.

ADVERSE REACTIONS: Limb pain, insomnia, pharyngitis, headache, fatigue, fever, myalgia, rigors, body pain, arthralgia, back pain, abdominal pain, nausea, diarrhea, nervousness.

INTERACTIONS: Peripheral neuropathy reported with telbivudine. Caution with agents that cause myelosuppression.

PREGNANCY: Category C (monotherapy) and X (combination therapy), not for use in nursing.

MECHANISM OF ACTION: Type-I interferon; binds to the interferon cell-surface receptor, leading to the production of several interferon-stimulated gene products.

NURSING CONSIDERATIONS

Assessment: Assess for neuropsychiatric, autoimmune, ischemic, and infectious disorders. Assess for hepatic impairment (eg, chronic hepatitis C, cirrhosis, hepatic decompression, autoimmune hepatitis), hypersensitivity reactions, myelosuppression (including concurrent use of myelosuppressive therapy), pre-existing cardiac disease (eg, MI, arrhythmias), renal impairment, pre-existing ophthalmic disorders, history of pulmonary disease, history of endocrine disorders, DM, pre-existing thyroid disease, pregnancy/nursing status and possible drug interactions. Obtain baseline CBC with platelet count, SrCr/CrCl, serum albumin, bilirubin, TSH/T$_4$ and eye exam. Assess use with transplant or chronically immunosuppressed patients.

Monitoring: Monitor for occurrence or aggravation of neuropsychiatric, autoimmune, ischemic, and infectious disorders. Monitor for depression, psychiatric symptoms, CV events, persistent or unexplained pulmonary infiltrates, pulmonary function impairment, signs/symptoms of hepatic decompensation, colitis, pancreatitis, hypersensitivity reactions, ocular symptoms, occurrence or aggravation of hyper- or hypothyroidism, DM, hyperglycemia, and hypertriglyceridemia. Monitor for signs/symptoms of interferon toxicity, including increases in SrCr in patients with impaired renal function. Perform periodic ophthalmologic exam in patients with pre-existing ophthalmologic disorder (eg, diabetic retinopathy or hypertensive retinopathy). Monitor periodically CBC with platelet count, SrCr/CrCl, serum albumin, bilirubin, TSH and T$_4$.

Patient Counseling: Inform about the benefits and risks associated with therapy. Instruct to avoid pregnancy during treatment with combination therapy; do not initiate therapy until a report of negative pregnancy test has been obtained. Inform that there is no data regarding whether therapy will prevent transmission of HCV infection to others. Advise to take at bedtime or by use of antipyretics to minimize flulike symptoms. Inform possible development of depression. Advise to report any sign or symptoms of depression and/or suicidal ideation. Seek medical attention for symptoms of depression (suicidal ideation), chest pain, ocular symptoms, pancreatitis, colitis, fever, worsening of liver disease/failure (jaundice), respiratory, hyperglycemia and hypersensitivity reactions. Keep well-hydrated.

Administration: SQ route. Do not use if particulates or discoloration observed. **Storage:** 2-8°C (36-46°F). Do not freeze; avoid vigorous shaking and exposure to direct sunlight. May allow to reach room temperature prior to injection.

INFUMORPH
morphine sulfate (Baxter)

`CII`

> Risk of severe adverse reactions; observe patient for 24 hrs following test dose, and for 1st several days after catheter implantation.

THERAPEUTIC CLASS: Opioid analgesic

INDICATIONS: Treatment of intractable chronic pain in microinfusion devices.

DOSAGE: *Adults:* Lumbar Intrathecal: Opioid Intolerant: 0.2-1mg/day. Opioid Tolerant: 1-10mg/day. Max: Must be individualized. Caution with >20mg/day. Epidural: Opioid Intolerant: 3.5-7.5mg/day. Opioid Tolerant: 4.5-10mg/day. May increase to 20-30mg/day. Max: Must be individualized. Starting dose must be based on in-hospital evaluation of response to serial single-dose intrathecal/epidural bolus injections of regular morphine sulfate.

HOW SUPPLIED: Inj: 10mg/mL (200mg), 25mg/mL (500mg)

CONTRAINDICATIONS: For neuraxial analgesia: Infection at injection site, anticoagulants, uncontrolled bleeding diathesis, any therapy or condition that may render intrathecal or epidural administration hazardous.

WARNINGS/PRECAUTIONS: Have resuscitation equipment, oxygen, and antidote (eg, naloxone) available; severe respiratory depression may occur. Use only if less invasive means of controlling pain fail. Not for single-dose IV, IM, or SQ administration. May be habit-forming. Caution with determining refill frequency. Make sure needle is properly placed in the filling port of device. Myoclonic-like spasm of the lower extremities reported if dose >20mg/day; may need detoxification. Caution with head injury, increased ICP, decreased respiratory reserve, hepatic/renal dysfunction (epidural injection), elderly. Avoid with chronic asthma, upper airway obstruction, other chronic pulmonary disorders. Biliary colic reported. May cause micturition disturbances especially with BPH. Increased risk of orthostatic hypotension with reduced circulating blood volume and impaired myocardial function. Avoid abrupt withdrawal. Risk of withdrawal in patients maintained on parenteral/oral narcotics. Not for routine use in obstetric labor/delivery.

ADVERSE REACTIONS: Respiratory depression, myoclonus convulsions, dysphoric reactions, pruritus, urinary retention, constipation, lumbar puncture-type headache, peripheral edema, orthostatic hypotension.

INTERACTIONS: Depressant effect may be potentiated by CNS depressants (eg, alcohol, sedatives, antihistamines, psychotropics). Increased risk of respiratory depression with neuroleptics. Contraindicated with anticoagulants. Risk of withdrawal with narcotic antagonists. Increased risk of orthostatic hypotension with sympatholytic drugs.

PREGNANCY: Category C, safety in nursing not known.

MECHANISM OF ACTION: Opioid analgesic; analgesic effects are produced via at least 3 areas of the CNS: the periaqueductal-periventricular gray matter, the ventromedial medulla, and the spinal cord. Interacts predominantly with μ-receptors which are found distributed in the brain, spinal cord, and in the trigeminal nerve.

PHARMACOKINETICS: Absorption: (Epidural): Rapid absorption; C_{max}=33-40ng/mL, T_{max}=10-15 min; (Intrathecal): C_{max}≤1-7.8ng/mL, T_{max}=5-10 min. **Distribution:** Plasma protein binding (36%); Muscle tissue binding (54%). Readily passes into fetal circulation, found in breast milk. (IV): V_d=1.0-4.7L/kg. **Metabolism:** Hepatic glucuronidation. **Elimination:** Kidneys (major), urine (2-12% unchanged), feces (10%); $T_{1/2}$=1.5-4.5 hrs.

NURSING CONSIDERATIONS

Assessment: Assess for level of pain intensity, patient's general condition, age, and medical status, or any other conditions where treatment is contraindicated or cautioned. Assess for history of hypersensitivity, pregnancy/nursing status, renal/hepatic function, and possible drug interactions.

Monitoring: Monitor for signs/symptoms of respiratory depression and/or respiratory arrest, myoclonic events, seizures, dysphoric reactions, toxic psychoses, biliary colic, urinary retention, drug abuse and dependence. If administered intrathecally or via epidural, closely monitor for 24 hrs for signs/symptoms of respiratory depression.

Patient Counseling: Counsel to notify physician immediately if develop signs/symptoms of respiratory depression. Avoid using other CNS depressants and alcohol during therapy. Medication has potential for abuse and dependence. Avoid abrupt withdrawal of medication; withdrawal symptoms may occur. Instruct that if accidental skin contact occurs, wash affected area with water.

Administration: IV, epidural, or intrathecal route. Proper placement of needle or catheter should be verified before epidural injection. **Storage:** 20-25°C (68-77°F); excursions permitted to 15-30°C (59-86°F). Protect from light. Do not freeze.

INNOHEP

RX

tinzaparin sodium (Leo Pharma)

> Epidural or spinal hematomas resulting in long-term or permanent paralysis may occur in patients anticoagulated with low molecular weight heparins, heparinoids, or fondaparinux sodium and who are receiving neuraxial anesthesia or undergoing spinal puncture. Increased risk with indwelling epidural catheters, concomitant use of other drugs that affect hemostasis (eg, NSAIDs, platelet inhibitors, other anticoagulants), history of traumatic or repeated epidural or spinal puncture, or a history of spinal deformity or spinal surgery. Monitor frequently for signs/symptoms of neurologic impairment; if neurologic compromise noted, urgent treatment is necessary. Consider benefit and risks before neuraxial intervention in patients anticoagulated or to be anticoagulated for thromboprophylaxis.

THERAPEUTIC CLASS: Low molecular weight heparin

INDICATIONS: Treatment of acute symptomatic deep vein thrombosis (DVT) with or without pulmonary embolism (PE) in conjunction with warfarin.

DOSAGE: *Adults:* 175 anti-Xa IU/kg SQ qd for at least 6 days and until anticoagulated with warfarin (INR ≥2 for 2 consecutive days). Begin warfarin within 1-3 days of therapy. Refer to PI for dosing chart.

HOW SUPPLIED: Inj: 20,000 anti-Xa IU/mL [2mL]

CONTRAINDICATIONS: Hypersensitivity to heparin, sulfite, benzyl alcohol, or pork. Active major bleeding, or in patients with history of heparin-induced thrombocytopenia (HIT).

WARNINGS/PRECAUTIONS: Not for IM/IV injection. Cannot use interchangeably unit for unit with heparin or other low molecular weight heparins. Increased risk for death in elderly patients with renal insufficiency; consider alternative therapy. Extreme caution in patients at increased risk of bleeding (severe uncontrolled HTN, bacterial endocarditis, congenital or acquired bleeding disorders, active or recent ulceration and angioplastic GI disease, hemorrhagic stroke, diabetic retinopathy, or shortly after brain, spinal or ophthalmological surgery). Bleeding and thrombocytopenia may occur during therapy. D/C if severe hemorrhage occurs or if platelets <100,000/mm³. Sulfite sensitivity, especially in asthmatic patients, reported. Priapism reported (rare). Contains benzyl alcohol; "Gasping syndrome" in premature infants reported; caution in pregnant women. Periodic CBC including platelets, Hct, Hgb and stool occult blood test recommended.

ADVERSE REACTIONS: Bleeding, injection-site hematoma, asymptomatic increase in AST and ALT, urinary tract infection.

INTERACTIONS: See Boxed Warning. Prior to initiation of therapy, d/c agents that may enhance the risk of hemorrhage (eg, anticoagulants, platelet inhibitors, thrombolytics) unless the agents are essential; if coadministration is necessary, monitor closely for hemorrhage.

PREGNANCY: Category B, caution use in nursing.

MECHANISM OF ACTION: Low molecular weight heparin; inhibits reactions that lead to blood clotting, including the formation of fibrin clots. Acts as a potent co-inhibitor of several activated coagulation factors, including Factors Xa and IIa (thrombin). Primary inhibitory activity mediated through plasma protease inhibitor, antithrombin.

PHARMACOKINETICS: Absorption: (4,500 IU, Single Dose) C_{max}=0.25 IU/mL, T_{max}=3.7 hrs, AUC=2.0 IU•hr/mL. (175 IU/kg, Day 1) C_{max}=0.87 IU/mL, T_{max}=4.4 hrs, AUC=9.0 IU•hr/mL. (175 IU/kg, Day 5) C_{max}=0.93 IU/mL, T_{max}=4.6 hrs, AUC=9.7 IU•hr/mL; absolute bioavailability (86.7%). **Distribution:** V_d=3.1-5.0L. **Metabolism:** Partially metabolized by desulphation and depolymerization. **Elimination:** Renal; $T_{1/2}$=3-4 hrs.

NURSING CONSIDERATIONS

Assessment: Assess for signs of active major bleeding; presence or history of HIT; severe renal impairment; hypersensitivity to heparin, sulfites, benzyl alcohol or pork products; pregnancy/nursing status, and possible drug interactions. Assess use in conditions with increased risk of hemorrhage.

Monitoring: Monitor for signs/symptoms of bleeding (eg, decreases in Hct, Hgb, BP), thrombocytopenia, hypersensitivity reactions, and priapism. If concomitant therapy with neuraxial anesthesia, monitor for epidural or spinal hematomas and for neurological impairment. Perform periodic monitoring of CBC including platelet count, Hgb, Hct, and stool test for occult blood.

Patient Counseling: Advise about increased risk of bleeding during therapy. Instruct to notify physician if unusual bleeding or hypersensitivity reaction occurs. During pregnancy, advise risk of "Gasping syndrome." Counsel on the proper way to administer: patients should be lying down or sitting when administering SQ Injection; alternate between left and right anterolateral and posterolateral abdominal wall; hold skin fold between thumb and forefinger; insert whole length of needle into skin; to minimize bruising, do not rub injection site after administration.

Administration: SQ route. Patients should be lying down or sitting when administering SQ injection. Alternate between left and right anterolateral and posterolateral abdominal wall. **Storage:** Store at 25°C (77°F); excursions permitted to 15-30°C (59-86°F).

INNOPRAN XL
RX

propranolol HCl (GlaxoSmithKline)

> Exacerbation of angina and myocardial infarction (MI) reported following abrupt d/c; reduce dose gradually over at least a few weeks prior to d/c. Caution against interruption or cessation of therapy without a physician's advice. Reinstitute if exacerbation of angina occurs; take other measures for management of angina pectoris. Coronary artery disease (CAD) may be unrecognized; follow the above advice in patients at risk of having atherosclerotic heart disease who are given propranolol for other indications.

THERAPEUTIC CLASS: Nonselective beta-blocker

INDICATIONS: Management of HTN.

DOSAGE: *Adults:* Individualize dose. Initial: 80mg qhs (approximately 10 pm) taken consistently, either on empty stomach or with food. May titrate to 120mg qhs. Elderly: Start at low end of dosing range.

HOW SUPPLIED: Cap, Extended-Release: 80mg, 120mg

CONTRAINDICATIONS: Cardiogenic shock, sinus bradycardia, sick sinus syndrome and >1st-degree heart block (unless a permanent pacemaker is in place), bronchial asthma.

WARNINGS/PRECAUTIONS: Caution with congestive heart failure (CHF); may precipitate more severe failure. Hypersensitivity reactions and cutaneous reactions (eg, Stevens-Johnson syndrome [SJS]) reported. Caution with bronchospastic lung disease, hepatic or renal impairment, prolonged physical exertion, labile insulin-dependent diabetics, underlying skeletal muscle disease, and Wolff-Parkinson-White (WPW) syndrome and tachycardia. Avoid routine withdrawal before surgery. Exacerbation of myopathy and myotonia reported. May mask acute hypoglycemia and hyperthyroidism signs/symptoms. Abrupt withdrawal may exacerbate hyperthyroidism, including thyroid storm. May reduce intraocular pressure (IOP); may interfere with glaucoma screening test. May be more reactive to repeated challenge with history of severe anaphylactic reaction to variety of allergens; may be unresponsive to usual doses of epinephrine. Elevated serum K^+, transaminases and alkaline phosphatase observed. Elevated BUN reported in severe heart failure. Not for treatment of hypertensive emergencies. Caution in elderly.

ADVERSE REACTIONS: Fatigue, dizziness, constipation.

INTERACTIONS: Administration with CYP450 (CYP2D6, 1A2, 2C19) substrates, inhibitors or inducers may lead to relevant drug interactions. Increased levels and/or toxicity with CYP2D6 substrates/inhibitors (eg, fluoxetine, paroxetine, quinidine, ritonavir), CYP1A2 substrates/inhibitors (eg, imipramine, ciprofloxacin, fluvoxamine, isoniazid, theophylline, zileuton, zolmitriptan, rizatriptan), CYP2C19 substrates/inhibitors (eg, fluconazole, fluoxetine, fluvoxamine, teniposide, tolbutamide). Caution with drugs that slow down AV conduction (eg, digitalis, lidocaine, calcium channel blockers [CCBs]).

Increased levels with nisoldipine, nicardipine, propafenone, cimetidine, and acute alcohol use. ACE inhibitors can cause hypotension. May antagonize clonidine effects; caution when withdrawing from clonidine. Potentiated by propafenone and amiodarone. Decreased levels with hepatic metabolism inducers (eg, rifampin, cigarette smoking). Decreased clearance of lidocaine, bupivacaine, mepivacaine, and theophylline. Caution with amide anesthetics. May prolong 1st dose hypotension with prazosin. Postural hypotension reported with terazosin, doxazosin, quinidine. May experience uncontrolled HTN with epinephrine. May reduce resting sympathetic nervous activity with catecholamine-depleting drugs (eg, reserpine). Methoxyflurane and trichloroethylene may depress myocardial contractility. Effects can be reversed by β-agonists (eg, dobutamine, isoproterenol). May exacerbate hypotensive effects of MAOIs or TCAs. Hypotension and cardiac arrest reported with haloperidol. May reduce efficacy with indomethacin and NSAIDs. May lower T_3 levels with thyroxine. Increased levels of nifedipine, diazepam, zolmitriptan, rizatriptan, and thioridazine. Decreased levels with aluminum hydroxide gel, cholestyramine, colestipol, chronic alcohol use. Coadministration with chlorpromazine may increase levels of both drugs. Increased warfarin levels and PT. Decreased levels of lovastatin and pravastatin. May augment risks of general anesthesia. May be more difficult to adjust insulin dosage.

PREGNANCY: Category C, caution in nursing.

MECHANISM OF ACTION: Nonselective β-adrenergic receptor blocker; not established. Proposed to decrease cardiac output, inhibit renin release by the kidneys, and diminish tonic sympathetic nerve outflow from vasomotor centers in the brain.

PHARMACOKINETICS: Absorption: Almost complete; T_{max}=12-14 hrs (fasted). **Distribution:** V_d=4L; plasma protein binding (90%); found in breast milk. **Metabolism:** Liver (extensive); CYP2D6 (aromatic hydroxylation), CYP1A2, 2D6 (oxidation), CYP2C19, Pgp, N-dealkylation, glucuronidation. Propranolol glucuronide, naphthyloxylactic acid, and glucuronic acid and sulfate conjugates of 4-hydroxy propranolol (major metabolites). **Elimination:** $T_{1/2}$=8 hrs.

NURSING CONSIDERATIONS

Assessment: Assess for atherosclerotic heart disease, cardiogenic shock, sinus bradycardia, sick sinus syndrome, AV heart block, presence of pacemaker, bronchial asthma, CHF, bronchospastic lung disease, hepatic or renal impairment, prolonged physical exertion, underlying skeletal muscle disease, hyperthyroidism, diabetes, WPW syndrome, history of anaphylactic reactions, possible drug interactions, and pregnancy/nursing status. Obtain baseline vital signs, serum K^+, transaminase, alkaline phosphatase, and thyroid function tests.

Monitoring: Monitor for signs/symptoms of cardiac failure, hypoglycemia, decreased IOP, thyrotoxicosis, myopathy, myotonia, withdrawal symptoms, hypersensitivity reactions, cutaneous reactions, and other adverse reactions. Monitor vital signs, serum K^+, transaminase, alkaline phosphatase, LFTs, and renal/thyroid function tests.

Patient Counseling: Inform about risks and benefits of therapy. Instruct not to interrupt or d/c therapy without consulting physician. Advise to contact physician if symptoms of heart failure, withdrawal (angina), or hypersensitivity reactions occur. May interfere with glaucoma screening test.

Administration: Oral route. **Storage:** 25°C (77°F); excursions permitted to 15-30°C (59-86°F). Keep tightly closed.

INSPRA   RX
eplerenone (Pfizer)

THERAPEUTIC CLASS: Aldosterone blocker

INDICATIONS: Improve survival of stable patients with left ventricular systolic dysfunction and congestive heart failure (CHF) post-MI. Treatment of hypertension, alone or with other antihypertensives.

DOSAGE: *Adults:* CHF Post-MI: Initial: 25mg qd. Titrate: Increase to 50mg qd within 4 weeks. Maint: 50mg qd. Adjust dose based on K+ level: See table in PI. HTN: Initial: 50mg qd. May increase to 50mg bid if effect on BP is inadequate. Max: 100mg/day. With Moderate CYP3A4 Inhibitors: Initial: 25mg qd.

HOW SUPPLIED: Tab: 25mg, 50mg

CONTRAINDICATIONS: All Indications: Serum K+ >5.5mgEq/L at initiation, CrCl ≤30mL/min, concomitant potent CYP3A4 inhibitors (eg, ketoconazole, itraconazole, nefazodone, troleandomycin, clarithromycin, ritonavir, nelfinavir). When treating HTN: Type 2 diabetes with microalbuminuria, SrCr >2mg/dL (males) or >1.8mg/dL (females), CrCl <50mg/min, concomitant K+ supplements or K+-sparing diuretics (eg, amiloride, spironolactone, triamterene).

WARNINGS/PRECAUTIONS: Minimize risk of hyperkalemia (>5.5mEq/L) with proper patient selection and monitoring. Patients with CHF post-MI, with SrCr >2mg/dL (males) or >1.8mg/dL (females), CrCl ≤50mL/min, or are diabetic (especially those with proteinuria) should be treated cautiously. Increased risk of hyperkalemia with decreased renal function.

ADVERSE REACTIONS: Headache, dizziness, hyperkalemia, increased SrCr/TG/GGT, angina/MI, hypokalemia, diarrhea, coughing, fatigue, flu-like symptoms.

INTERACTIONS: See Contraindications. Increased levels with other CYP3A4 inhibitors (eg, erythromycin, verapamil, saquinavir, fluconazole). In HTN, use caution with ACE inhibitors and angiotensin II receptor antagonists; increased risk of hyperkalemia, especially with diabetics with microalbuminuria. Monitor lithium levels. Monitor antihypertensive effect with NSAIDs.

PREGNANCY: Category B, not for use in nursing.

MECHANISM OF ACTION: Aldosterone blocker; binds to mineralocorticoid receptor and blocks binding of aldosterone.

PHARMACOKINETICS: Absorption: Absolute bioavailability (69%); T_{max}=1.5 hrs. **Distribution:** V_d=43-90L; plasma protein binding (50%). **Metabolism:** CYP3A4. **Elimination:** Urine (67%, <5% unchanged), feces (32%, <5% unchanged); $T_{1/2}$=4-6 hrs.

NURSING CONSIDERATIONS

Assessment: Assess serum K+, SrCr. Assess for type 2 DM with microalbuminuria, proteinuria, impaired renal function, pregnancy/nursing status, and possible drug interactions.

Monitoring: Monitor serum K+, BP, and renal function tests periodically. Monitor for signs/symptoms of hyperkalemia and hypersensitivity reactions.

Patient Counseling: Advise against use of K+ supplements or salt substitutes containing K+, and strong CYP3A4 inhibitors. Advise to seek medical attention if symptoms of hyperkalemia, dizziness, diarrhea, vomiting, rapid or irregular heartbeat, lower extremity edema, difficulty breathing, or hypersensitivity reactions occur.

Administration: Oral route. **Storage:** 25°C (77°F); excursions permitted to 15-30°C (59-86°F).

INTEGRILIN   RX
eptifibatide (Schering)

THERAPEUTIC CLASS: Glycoprotein IIb/IIIa inhibitor

INDICATIONS: Treatment of acute coronary syndrome (ACS) in patients being medically managed or undergoing percutaneous coronary intervention (PCI) including intracoronary stenting.

DOSAGE: *Adults:* ACS: 180mcg/kg IV bolus, then 2mcg/kg/min IV infusion until discharge or initiation of CABG, up to 72 hrs. If undergoing PCI, continue until discharge or 18-24 hrs post-PCI, whichever comes first, allowing up to 96 hrs of therapy. CrCl <50mL/min: 180mcg/kg IV bolus, then 1mcg/kg/min IV infusion. PCI: 180mcg/kg IV bolus immediately before PCI, then 2mcg/kg/min

IV infusion. Give 2nd bolus of 180mcg/kg 10 min after 1st bolus. Continue until discharge or 18-24 hrs post-PCI. Recommend a minimum of 12 hr infusion. CrCl <50mL/min: 180mcg/kg IV bolus immediately before PCI, then 1mcg/kg/min IV infusion. Give 2nd bolus of 180mcg/kg 10 min after 1st bolus. See PI for concomitant ASA and heparin doses.

HOW SUPPLIED: Inj: 20mg, 75mg, 200mg

CONTRAINDICATIONS: Active abnormal bleeding, history of bleeding diathesis, or stroke within past 30 days. Severe HTN uncontrolled not adequately controlled on antihypertensives, major surgery within preceding 6 weeks, history of hemorrhagic stroke, current or planned concomitant parenteral glycoprotein IIb/IIIa inhibitor, renal dialysis dependency.

WARNINGS/PRECAUTIONS: Bleeding reported; mostly from arterial access site for cardiac catheterization, GI tract, or GU tract. Caution with renal dysfunction, platelets <100,000/mm³, femoral access site in PCI. Minimize vascular and other trauma. D/C if thrombocytopenia occurs. Monitor Hct, Hgb, platelets, SrCr, and PT/aPTT before therapy (and activated clotting time before PCI). D/C before CABG surgery.

ADVERSE REACTIONS: Bleeding (eg, intracranial hemorrhage, hematuria, hematemsis), thrombocytopenia, hypotension.

INTERACTIONS: Caution with other drugs that affect hemostasis (eg, thrombolytics, anticoagulants, NSAIDs, dipyridamole). Avoid other GPIIb/IIIa inhibitors. Cerebral, pulmonary, GI hemorrhage reported with ASA and heparin.

PREGNANCY: Category B, caution in nursing.

MECHANISM OF ACTION: Glycoprotein IIb/IIIa inhibitor; reversibly inhibits platelet aggregation by preventing the binding of fibrinogen, von Willebrand factor, and other adhesive ligands to GP IIb/IIIa.

PHARMACOKINETICS: Absorption: T_{max}=4-6 hrs. **Metabolism:** Deaminated eptifibatide (polar metabolite). **Distribution:** Plasma protein binding (25%). **Elimination:** Urine (50%; unchanged, metabolites); $T_{1/2}$=2.5 hrs.

NURSING CONSIDERATIONS

Assessment: Assess for history of bleeding diathesis, evidence of bleeding within previous 30 days, severe HTN, major surgery within the previous 6 weeks, history of any stroke, concomitant use of another GP IIb/IIIa inhibitor, dependency on renal dialysis, and for drug interactions. Assess use if platelet count is <100,000/mm³. Obtain baseline Hgb, Hct, platelet count, SrCr, and PT/aPTT. In patients undergoing PCI, obtain activated clotting time (ACT). Assess pregnancy/nursing status and for possible drug interactions.

Monitoring: Monitor for signs/symptoms of bleeding (eg, intracranial bleeding), and thrombocytopenia (eg, platelet count <100,000/mm³). Periodically monitor aPTT and ACT. Monitor for hypersensitivity reactions.

Patient Counseling: Inform about bleeding tendency during therapy and instruct to contact physician if signs of unusual bleeding develop.

Administration: IV route. Do not administer in same line with furosemide. Refer to PI for proper administration. **Storage:** 2-8°C (36-46°F). May be stored at 25°C (77°F) for a period not exceeding 2 months with excursions permitted to 15-30°C (59-86°F) . Protect from light and discard any unused portion in the vial.

INTELENCE
etravirine (Tibotec)

RX

THERAPEUTIC CLASS: Non-nucleoside reverse transcriptase inhibitor

INDICATIONS: Treatment of HIV-1 infection, in combination with other antiretrovirals, for antiretroviral treatment-experienced adult patients who have evidence of viral replication and HIV-1 strains resistant to a non-nucleoside reverse transcriptase inhibitor (NNRTI) and other antiretrovirals.

DOSAGE: *Adults:* 200mg (one 200mg tab or two 100mg tabs) bid pc. Elderly: Start at lower end of dosing range.

HOW SUPPLIED: Tab: 100mg, 200mg

WARNINGS/PRECAUTIONS: Severe and life-threatening skin (eg, Stevens Johnson syndrome, toxic epidermal necrolysis, erythema multiforme) and hypersensitivity reactions reported; d/c use and treat accordingly if severe skin/ hypersensitivity reactions develop. May cause redistribution/accumulation of body fat. Immune reconstitution syndrome reported. Risks and benefits have not been established in treatment naive adult patients. Caution in elderly.

ADVERSE REACTIONS: Rash, peripheral neuropathy.

INTERACTIONS: May alter therapeutic effect and adverse reaction profile with drugs that induce, inhibit, or are substrates of CYP3A, CYP2C9 and CYP2C19, or are transported by P-glycoprotein. Avoid concomitant use with efavirenz, nevirapine, and delavirdine. Atazanavir (ATV), fosamprenavir (FPV), nelfinavir, indinavir administered without low-dose ritonavir (RTV) is not recommended. RTV 600mg bid decreases plasma levels and should not be coadministered. Do not administer with tipranavir/RTV, FPV/RTV, ATV/RTV. Caution with digoxin; use lowest dose initially. May decrease levels of amiodarone, bepridil, disopyramide, flecainide, lidocaine (systemic), mexiletine, propafenone, quinidine; caution when coadministered; monitor drug levels. May increase warfarin concentrations; monitor INR. Do not use in combination with carbamazepine, phenobarbital, phenytoin, rifampin, rifapentine, rifabutin. Caution with fluconazole and voriconazole. Adjust dose with itraconazole, ketoconazole, posaconazole. Consider alternatives to clarithromycin such as azithromycin for treatment of *Mycobacterium avium* complex. May decrease levels of atorvastatin, lovastatin and simvastatin. May increase levels of fluvastatin. Caution when used with systemic dexamethasone and consider alternative therapy. May increase levels of diazepam. Caution with immunosuppressants (eg, cyclosporine, sirolimus, tacrolimus). Monitor for withdrawal symptoms when coadministered with methadone. May need to alter sildenafil dose. Caution when coadministered with lopinavir/RTV. Avoid concomitant use with St. John's wort. Decrease levels with darunavir/ritonavir and saquinavir/ritonavir. May decrease maraviroc levels. Coadministration with maraviroc/ darunavir/ritonavir may increase maraviroc levels. Activation of clopidogrel to its active metabolite may be decreased. Refer to PI for complete information.

PREGNANCY: Category B, not for use in nursing.

MECHANISM OF ACTION: Non-nucleoside reverse transcriptase inhibitor of HIV-1; binds directly to reverse transcriptase and blocks the RNA-dependent and DNA-dependent DNA polymerase activities, disrupting the enzyme's catalytic site.

PHARMACOKINETICS: Absorption: T_{max}=2.5-4 hrs. **Distribution:** Plasma protein binding (99.9%). **Metabolism:** Liver via CYP3A, CYP2C9 and CYP2C19; (methyl hydroxylation). **Elimination:** Feces (93.7%); urine (1.2%); $T_{1/2}$=41 hrs.

NURSING CONSIDERATIONS

Assessment: Assess treatment history, pregnancy/nursing status, and possible drug interactions. Perform resistance testing where possible.

Monitoring: Monitor for signs/symptoms of severe skin/hypersensitivity reactions, body fat redistribution/accumulation, presence of infections, and clinical status including liver transaminases.

Patient Counseling: Counsel that medication does not cure HIV and opportunistic infections may continue to develop. Inform that therapy does not reduce risk of HIV transmission to others; take precaution to avoid transmission (eg, safe sex practices). Instruct to swallow tab whole with water; may disperse tab in water, stir well and drink immediately. Instruct to rinse glass several times, each rinse completely swallowed to ensure entire dose is consumed. Instruct to always use with other antiretrovirals, not to alter dose or d/c therapy without consultation. If a dose is missed within 6 hrs of time usually taken, take as soon as possible with a meal; if scheduled time exceeds 6 hrs, do not take missed dose; resume normal dosing schedule. Advise to notify physician of all concomitant medications and herbal products currently taking. Counsel to d/c and notify physician if severe rash develops. Advise that redistribution or accumulation of body fat may occur. Inform mothers to avoid nursing to reduce risk of transmission.

Administration: Oral route. Tabs may be dispersed in glass of water if unable to swallow tab whole. Stir and drink immediately once dispersed. Rinse glass several times and each rinse completely swallowed to ensure entire dose is consumed. **Storage:** 25°C (77°F); excursions permitted to 15-30° C (59-86°F). Store in the original bottle. Keep bottle tightly closed to protect from moisture.

INTRON A   RX
interferon alfa-2b (Schering)

> May cause or aggravate fatal or life-threatening neuropsychiatric, autoimmune, ischemic, and infectious disorders. Monitor closely with periodic clinical and laboratory evaluations. D/C with severe or worsening signs or symptoms of these conditions.

THERAPEUTIC CLASS: Biological response modifier

INDICATIONS: Treatment of hairy cell leukemia in patients ≥18 yrs. Adjuvant to surgical treatment in patients ≥18 yrs with malignant melanoma who are free of disease but at high risk for systemic recurrence, within 56 days of surgery. Initial treatment of clinically aggressive follicular Non-Hodgkin's lymphoma with anthracycline-containing combination chemotherapy in patients ≥18 yrs. Treatment of AIDS-Related Kaposi's sarcoma and intralesional treatment of condylomata acuminata involving external surfaces of the genital and perianal areas in selected patients ≥18 yrs. Treatment of chronic hepatitis C with compensated liver disease who have a history of blood or blood-product exposure and are/or HCV antibody positive in patients ≥18 yrs. Treatment of chronic hepatitis C with compensated liver disease in patients ≥3 yrs previously untreated with α-interferon therapy, and in patients ≥18 yrs who have relapsed following α-interferon therapy, in combination with ribavirin; refer to ribavirin PI. Treatment of chronic hepatitis B in patients ≥1 yr with compensated liver disease and those who are serum HBsAg positive for ≥6 months and have evidence of HBV replication with elevated serum ALT.

DOSAGE: *Adults:* ≥18 yrs: Hairy Cell Leukemia: 2 MIU/m² IM/SQ 3x/week up to 6 months. Reduce dose by 50% or stop therapy with severe reactions. Platelet counts <50,000/mm³: SQ administration. Malignant Melanoma: Initial: 20 MIU/m² IV, over 20 min, for 5 consecutive days/week for 4 weeks. Maint: 10 MIU/m² SQ 3x/week for 48 weeks. Follicular Lymphoma: 5 MIU SQ 3x/week up to 18 months. Condylomata Acuminata: 1 MIU/lesion 3x/week alternating days for 3 weeks. Max: 5 lesions/course. An additional course may be administered at 12-16 weeks. Kaposi's Sarcoma: 30 MIU/m² IM/SQ 3x/week until disease progression or maximal response has been achieved after 16 weeks of treatment. Hepatitis C: 3 MIU IM/SQ 3x/week for 18-24 months. Hepatitis B: 5 MIU IM/SQ qd or 10 MIU IM/SQ 3x/week for 16 weeks. Dose adjust according to severe adverse reactions and laboratory abnormalities (See PI for more information).
Pediatrics: ≥3 yrs: Hepatitis C: 3 MIU IM/SQ 3x/week for 18-24 months. ≥1 yr: Hepatitis B: 3 MIU/m² SQ 3x/week for 1 week, then 6 MIU/m² 3x/week for total therapy of 16-24 weeks. Max: 10 MIU/m² 3x/week. Reduce dose by 50% or stop therapy with severe reactions. Dose adjust according to severe adverse reactions and laboratory abnormalities (See PI for more information).

HOW SUPPLIED: Inj: 10 MIU, 18 MIU, 50 MIU [Powder], 3 MIU/0.2mL, 5 MIU/0.2mL, 10 MIU/0.2mL [Pen], 3 MIU/0.5mL, 5 MIU/0.5mL [Vial]

CONTRAINDICATIONS: Autoimmune hepatitis, decompensated liver disease. In combination with ribavirin: Pregnancy, men whose female partners are pregnant, hemoglobinopathies (eg, thalassemia major, sickle cell anemia), CrCl <50mL/min.

WARNINGS/PRECAUTIONS: Caution with coagulation disorders (eg, thrombophlebitis, pulmonary embolism), severe myelosuppression, debilitating conditions such as pulmonary disease (eg, chronic obstructive pulmonary disease [COPD]), or diabetes mellitus (DM) prone to ketoacidosis. Caution with history of cardiovascular disease (CVD) including history of myocardial infarction (MI)and/or previous or current arrhythmic disorder; monitor closely. Supraventricular arrhythmias reported; modify dose or d/c treatment but may require specific additional therapy. Ischemic and hemorrhagic cerebrovascular events may occur with few or no reported risk factors for stroke and in patients <45 yrs. Psychiatric problems may occur; carefully monitor during treatment and in the 6-month follow-up period. Avoid with pre-existing psychiatric condition, especially depression or history of severe psychiatric disorder. D/C if psychiatric symptoms persist or worsen, or suicidal ideation or aggressive behavior towards others occur. Obtundation, coma and encephalopathy may occur in elderly treated with higher doses. May suppress bone marrow function resulting in severe cytopenias including aplastic anemia; d/c if severe decreases in neutrophil or platelet counts occur. Pulmonary disorders may be induced or aggravated; obtain chest x-ray if respiratory symptoms develop. Hepatotoxicity, pulmonary disorders and autoimmune disorders reported, monitor or d/c therapy if appropriate. Conduct baseline eye exam in all patients and periodic exams with pre-existing ophthalmologic disorders (eg, diabetic or hypertensive retinopathy); d/c if new or worsening ophthalmologic disorders (eg, decrease/loss of vision, retinopathy, optic neuritis, papilledema and serous retinal detachment) occur. Thyroid abnormalities (hypothyroid or hyperthyroid) and DM may develop; d/c therapy if cannot be normalized by medication. Avoid with pre-existing thyroid abnormalities that cannot be maintained by medication. Should not be used with rapidly progressive visceral disease. Avoid in patients with history of autoimmune disease or immunosuppressed transplant recipients. Birth defects and/or death of unborn child and hemolytic anemia reported when used in combination with ribavirin. Acute hypersensitivity reactions may occur; d/c immediately if occurs. New onset or exacerbated psoriasis or sarcoidosis may develop. Hypertriglyceridemia may result in pancreatitis. D/C if persistently elevated TG associated with symptoms of potential pancreatitis (eg, abdominal pain, N/V) occur. The powder formulation contain albumin; carries an extremely remote risk for transmission of viral diseases and Creutzfeldt-Jakob disease (CJD). Do not interchange brands. Caution in elderly.

ADVERSE REACTIONS: Flu-like symptoms, fatigue, fever, neutropenia, abnormal granulocyte count, myalgia, anorexia, decreased WBC count, N/V, asthenia, increased AST, headache, chills, GI disorders.

INTERACTIONS: Increases theophylline levels by 100%. Caution with myelosuppressive agents (eg, zidovudine). Higher incidence of neutropenia with concomitant zidovudine. Peripheral neuropathy reported in combination with telbivudine.

PREGNANCY: Category C, Category X when used with ribavirin, not for use in nursing.

MECHANISM OF ACTION: α-interferon; binds to specific membrane receptors on cell surface initiating induction of enzymes, suppression of cell proliferation, immunomodulating activities, and inhibition of virus replication.

PHARMACOKINETICS: Absorption: (IM, SQ) C_{max}=18-116 IU/mL, T_{max}=3-12 hrs; (IV) C_{max}=135-273 IU/mL. **Elimination:** (IM, SQ) $T_{1/2}$=2-3 hrs; (IV) $T_{1/2}$=2 hrs.

NURSING CONSIDERATIONS

Assessment: Establish diagnosis of compensated liver disease. Assess for conditions where treatment is contraindicated or cautioned. Assess for drug hypersensitivity, pregnancy/nursing status, and possible drug interactions. Obtain baseline CBC (eg, Hgb, Hct, WBC, neutrophil and platelet counts, PT), bilirubin and albumin levels, LFTs, serum ALT, SrCr, electrolytes, serum TSH, ECG, TG, chest x-ray and eye exams. Perform liver biopsy and test for presence of HCV antibody.

Monitoring: Monitor for psychiatric problems, CVD, cerebrovascular events, bone marrow toxicity, ocular symptoms, pancreatitis, worsening of liver disease/failure, pulmonary disorders, autoimmune disorders, hypersensitivity reactions, psoriasis and sarcoidosis. Closely monitor patients with history of MI or arrhythmic disorder, liver function abnormalities, pulmonary function impairment, WBC in myelosuppressed patients. Monitor LFTs, SrCr, alkaline phosphatase, albumin and bilirubin levels periodically and at approximately 2-week intervals during ALT flare. Monitor serum TSH, TG, electrolytes, ECG, chest x-ray periodically. Repeat CBC and platelet count 1-2 weeks after initiation of therapy, and monthly thereafter. Evaluate serum ALT at approximately 3-month intervals. Repeat TSH testing at 3 and 6 months during therapy. Evaluate HBeAg, HBsAg, and ALT at the end of therapy, then at 3 and 6 months post-therapy. Perform periodic ophthalmologic exams with those who develop ocular symptoms and with pre-existing ophthalmologic disorders.

Patient Counseling: Inform of risks and benefits associated with treatment. Instruct on proper use of product. Advise to seek medical attention for symptoms of depression (eg, suicidal ideation), cardiovascular (eg, chest pain), ophthalmologic toxicity (eg, decreased/loss of vision), pancreatitis or colitis (eg, abdominal pain, N/V), and cytopenias (eg, high persistent fevers, bruising, dyspnea). Keep well hydrated. Inform that use of antipyretic may ameliorate some of the flu-like symptoms. Instruct self-administering patients on the proper disposal of needles and syringes and caution against reuse. In combination with Ribavirin: Inform of the risks to fetus; instruct female patients and female partners of male patients to use 2 forms of birth control during treatment and for 6 months after therapy is d/c. Instruct to brush teeth twice daily and have regular dental examinations and instruct to rinse mouth when vomiting occurs.

Administration: IM, SQ, IV, and intralesional route. Refer to Medication Guide for proper administration. **Storage:** 2-8°C (36-46°F). (Powder) After reconstitution use immediately, store ≤24 hrs. (Sol for Inj/Sol for Inj in Multidose Pens) Do not freeze. Keep away from heat.

INTUNIV

guanfacine (Shire)

THERAPEUTIC CLASS: Alpha$_2$-agonist

INDICATIONS: Treatment of attention deficit hyperactivity disorder (ADHD) as monotherapy and as adjunctive therapy to stimulant medications.

DOSAGE: *Pediatrics:* 6-17 yrs: Monotherapy/Adjunctive Therapy: Initial: 1mg/day. Titrate: Adjust in increments of ≤1mg/week. Maint: 1-4mg/day for 9 weeks based on clinical response and tolerability. Range: (Monotherapy) 0.05-0.08mg/kg qd; if well tolerated, doses up to 0.12mg/kg/d may provide additional benefit. Max: 4mg/day. (Adjunctive Therapy) 0.05-0.12mg/kg/day. Switching from Immediate-Release: D/C immediate-release, and titrate with extended-release according to the recommended schedule. D/C: Taper in decrements of ≤1mg q3-7 days. Refer to PI for dosage reinitiation and adjustment.

HOW SUPPLIED: Tab, Extended-Release: 1mg, 2mg, 3mg, 4mg

WARNINGS/PRECAUTIONS: Hypotension, bradycardia, syncope, somnolence, and sedation reported. Caution with history of hypotension, heart block, bradycardia, cardiovascular disease (CVD), and syncope or condition(s) that predispose to syncope (eg, orthostatic hypotension, dehydration). Not intended for use in patients who exhibit symptoms secondary to environmental factors and/or other primary psychiatric disorders, including psychosis.

ADVERSE REACTIONS: Hypotension, decreased appetite, somnolence/sedation, headache, fatigue, abdominal pain, nausea, lethargy, dizziness, irritability, dry mouth, constipation.

INTERACTIONS: CYP3A4 inducer (eg, rifampin) may decrease exposure. May increase valproic acid concentrations. Additive effects with antihypertensives and CNS depressants (eg, alcohol, sedative/hypnotics, benzodiazepines, barbiturates, phenothiazines, antipsychotics); caution during coadministration. High-fat meals may increase exposure. Caution with ketoconazole or other strong CYP3A4/5 inhibitors. Avoid with other guanfacine-containing products. Increased exposure and C_{max} with Vyvanse (lisdexamfetamine dimesylate).

PREGNANCY: Category B, caution in nursing.

MECHANISM OF ACTION: $α_{2A}$-adrenergic agonist; mechanism not established. Known as an antihypetensive agent. Reduces sympathetic nerve impulses from the vasomotor center to the heart and blood vessels, resulting in decreased peripheral vascular resistance and reduction in heart rate.

PHARMACOKINETICS: Absorption: Adults: C_{max}=1ng/mL; AUC=32ng•hr/mL; T_{max}=6 hrs. **Children (6-12 yrs):** C_{max}=10ng/mL; AUC=162ng•hr/mL. **Adolescents (13-17 yrs):** C_{max}=7ng/mL; AUC=116ng•hr/mL. **Pediatrics:** T_{max}=5 hrs. **Distribution:** Plasma protein binding (70%). **Metabolism:** CYP3A4. **Elimination:** $T_{1/2}$=18 hrs (adults).

NURSING CONSIDERATIONS

Assessment: Assess HR and BP. Assess for history of hypotension, bradycardia, heart block, CVD, syncope, history of hypersensitivity to drug, renal/hepatic impairment, pregnancy/nursing status, and possible drug interactions.

Monitoring: Monitor HR and BP following dose increases and periodically while on therapy. Monitor for orthostatic hypotension, syncope, somnolence, and sedation.

Patient Counseling: Instruct to swallow whole with water, milk, or other liquid; do not crush, chew, or break before swallowing. Inform that taking drug with high-fat meal raises blood levels. Instruct caregiver to supervise the child or adolescent during therapy. Inform of the adverse reactions that may occur. Caution against operating heavy equipment or driving. Advise to avoid becoming dehydrated or overheated, and to avoid use with alcohol.

Administration: Oral route. Do not crush, chew, or break tabs before swallowing. **Storage:** 25°C (77°F); excursions permitted to 15-30°C (59-86°F).

INVANZ   RX
ertapenem sodium (Merck)

THERAPEUTIC CLASS: Carbapenem

INDICATIONS: Treatment of complicated intra-abdominal infections, complicated skin and skin structure infections (cSSSI) including diabetic foot infections without osteomyelitis, community-acquired pneumonia (CAP), complicated urinary tract infections (UTI) including pyelonephritis, and acute pelvic infections (including postpartum endomyometritis, septic abortion, and postsurgical gynecologic infections) caused by susceptible strains of microorganisms. Prophylaxis of surgical-site infection following elective colorectal surgery.

DOSAGE: *Adults:* 1g IM/IV qd. Duration: Intra-Abdominal Infections: 5-14 days. cSSSI: 7-14 days. CAP/UTI: 10-14 days. Acute Pelvic Infections (postpartum endomyometritis, septic abortion, postsurgical gynecologic infections): 3-10 days. Max: IV: 14 days. IM: 7 days. Prophylaxis Following Colorectal Surgery: 1g IV as single dose given 1 hr prior to surgical incision. CrCl ≤30mL/min/1.73m²: 500mg IM/IV qd. Hemodialysis: Give 150mg IM/IV after dialysis only if 500mg dose was given within 6 hrs prior to dialysis.
Pediatrics: ≥13 yrs: 1g IM/IV qd. 3 months-12 yrs: 15mg/kg IM/IV bid. Max: 1g/day. Duration: Intra-Abdominal Infections: 5-14 days. cSSSI: 7-14 days. CAP/UTI: 10-14 days. Acute Pelvic Infections (postpartum endomyometritis, septic abortion, postsurgical gynecologic infections): 3-10 days. Max: IV: 14 days. IM: 7 days.

HOW SUPPLIED: Inj: 1g

CONTRAINDICATIONS: Hypersensitivity to local anesthetics of the amide type (due to lidocaine diluent) if administered IM.

WARNINGS/PRECAUTIONS: Serious and occasionally fatal hypersensitivity reactions reported. Careful inquiry should be made concerning previous reactions to penicillins, cephalosporins, other β-lactams, and other allergens; d/c if allergic reaction occurs. *Clostridium difficile*-associated diarrhea (CDAD) reported; may need to d/c if CDAD is suspected or confirmed; institute appropriate fluid and electrolyte management, protein supplement, antibiotic treatment and surgical evaluation. Seizures and CNS adverse events reported. Increased risk of seizures with CNS disorders and/or compromised renal function. Prolonged use may result in overgrowth of nonsusceptible organisms.

Caution with IM administration; avoid accidental injection into blood vessel. Not recommended for treatment of meningitis in pediatric patients.

ADVERSE REACTIONS: Diarrhea, infused vein complication, N/V, anemia, headache, edema/swelling, fever, abdominal pain, constipation, altered mental status, insomnia, wound infection, ALT and AST increase.

INTERACTIONS: Decreased clearance with probenecid. May decrease serum levels of valproic acid or divalproex sodium.

PREGNANCY: Category B, caution in nursing.

MECHANISM OF ACTION: Carbapenem; bactericidal activity results from inhibition of cell wall synthesis, mediated through binding to penicillin binding proteins.

PHARMACOKINETICS: Absorption: Administration of different doses resulted in different parameters. (IM): Absolute bioavailability (90%); T_{max}=2.3 hrs. **Distribution:** V_d=0.12L/kg (adult); 0.2L/kg (3 months-12 yrs); 0.16L/kg (13-17 yrs). Plasma protein binding (85%-95%); found in breast milk. **Metabolism:** Liver via hydrolysis of the β-lactam ring. **Elimination:** Kidney: (Adults, 13-17 yrs) $T_{1/2}$=4 hrs. (3 months-12 yrs) $T_{1/2}$=2.5 hrs; urine (80% [38% unchanged, 37% metabolite]), feces (10%).

NURSING CONSIDERATIONS

Assessment: Assess for penicillin, cephalosporin, β-lactam, or local anesthetics of the amide type hypersensitivity, history of seizure or brain lesions, meningitis in pediatrics, renal impairment, pregnancy/nursing status, and possible drug interactions. Periodic assessment of organ system function, including renal, hepatic, and hematopoietic.

Monitoring: Monitor for signs/symptoms of anaphylactoid or hypersensitivity reactions, CDAD, superinfections, CNS disorders, and seizures. Monitor renal, hepatic, hematopoietic functions.

Patient Counseling: Counsel to inform physician if taking valproic acid or divalproex sodium. Inform that drug only treats bacterial, not viral infections. Instruct to take as directed; skipping doses or not completing full course may decrease effectiveness and increase resistance. May experience diarrhea; notify physician if watery/bloody stools (w/ or w/o stomach cramps and fever) occur.

Administration: IV/IM routes. Refer to PI for reconstitution and administration instructions. **Storage:** Before reconstitution: ≤25°C (77°F). Reconstituted and infusion solutions: 25°C and use within 6 hrs, or store for 24 hrs under refrigeration (5°C) and use within 4 hrs after removal from refrigeration. Do not freeze.

INVEGA   RX
paliperidone (Ortho-Mcneil/Janssen)

> Elderly patients with dementia-related psychosis treated with antipsychotic drugs are at an increased risk of death; most deaths appeared to be cardiovascular (CV) (eg, heart failure, sudden death) or infectious (eg, pneumonia) in nature. Not approved for the treatment of patients with dementia-related psychosis.

THERAPEUTIC CLASS: Benzisoxazole derivative

INDICATIONS: Treatment of schizophrenia in adults and adolescents. Treatment of schizoaffective disorder as monotherapy or as an adjunct to mood stabilizers and/or antidepressant therapy in adults.

DOSAGE: *Adults:* Schizophrenia: 6mg qd. Titrate: Increase by 3mg/day at intervals >5 days. Usual: 3-12mg/day. Max: 12mg/day. Schizoaffective Disorder: 6mg qd. Titrate: Increase by 3mg/day at intervals >4 days. Usual: 3-12mg/day. Max: 12mg/day. Renal Impairment: Individualize dose. CrCl ≥50-<80mL/min: Initial: 3mg qd. Max: 6mg qd. CrCl ≥10-<50mL/min: Initial: 1.5mg qd. Max: 3mg qd. Elderly: Adjust dose according to renal function. *Pediatrics:* 12-17 yrs: Schizophrenia: 3mg qd. Titrate: Increase by 3mg/day at intervals >5 days.

HOW SUPPLIED: Tab, Extended-Release: 1.5mg, 3mg, 6mg, 9mg

WARNINGS/PRECAUTIONS: Neuroleptic malignant syndrome (NMS) and tardive dyskinesia (TD) reported. May increase QTc interval; avoid with congenital long QT syndrome and history of cardiac arrhythmias. Have been associated with metabolic changes (eg, hyperglycemia, dyslipidemia, and weight gain) that may increase CV and cerebrovascular risk; monitor for weight gain, worsening blood glucose control in diabetes mellitus (DM) patients, and fasting blood glucose (FBG) levels in patients with diabetes risk. May elevate prolactin levels. Do not administer in patients with pre-existing severe GI narrowing. May induce orthostatic hypotension and syncope; caution with cardiovascular disease (CVD), cerebrovascular disease, and conditions that predispose to hypotension. Leukopenia, neutropenia, and agranulocytosis reported; d/c in cases of severe neutropenia (absolute neutrophil count [ANC] <1000/mm³). May impair mental/physical abilities. Seizures reported; caution with history of seizures or conditions that lower the seizure threshold. Esophageal dysmotility and aspiration reported; caution with increased risk of aspiration pneumonia. Priapism reported. May disrupt body's ability to reduce core body temperature; caution in conditions that may contribute to an elevation in core body temperature. May produce antiemetic effect that may mask signs/symptoms of overdosage with certain drugs or certain conditions (eg, intestinal obstruction, Reye's syndrome, brain tumor). Increased sensitivity reported with Parkinson's disease or dementia with Lewy bodies. Caution with suicidal tendencies, renal impairment, and in elderly.

ADVERSE REACTIONS: Extrapyramidal symptoms, tachycardia, somnolence, akathisia, dyskinesia, dyspepsia, dizziness, nasopharyngitis, headache, nausea, hyperkinesia, constipation, weight gain, Parkinsonism, tremors.

INTERACTIONS: Caution with other centrally acting drugs and alcohol. May antagonize the effect of levodopa and other dopamine agonists. Additive effect observed when administered with other agents that cause orthostatic hypotension. Avoid concomitant use with other drugs known to prolong QTc interval, including Class 1A (eg, quinidine, procainamide) or Class III (eg, amiodarone, sotalol) antiarrhythmics, antipsychotics (eg, chlorpromazine, thioridazine), antibiotics (eg, gatifloxacin, moxifloxacin). Concomitant use with carbamazepine may decrease levels. Increased exposure with paroxetine (a potent CYP2D6 inhibitor) in CYP2D6 extensive metabolizers. Divalproex sodium may increase plasma levels. Consider dose adjustment when administered with valproate (reduce dose) and carbamazepine (increase dose). Additive exposure with risperidone. Caution with drugs with anticholinergic activity.

PREGNANCY: Category C, caution in nursing.

MECHANISM OF ACTION: Benzisoxazole derivative; not established. Proposed to be mediated through a combination of central dopamine Type 2 (D_2) and serotonin Type 2 ($5HT_{2A}$) receptor antagonism.

PHARMACOKINETICS: Absorption: Absolute bioavailability (28%); T_{max}=24 hrs. **Distribution:** Plasma protein binding (74%); V_d=487L; found in breast milk. **Metabolism:** CYP2D6, 3A4 (limited); (immediate-release) dealkylation, hydroxylation, dehydrogenation, and benzisoxazole scission. **Elimination:** (Immediate-release) Urine (80%; 59% unchanged), feces (11%); $T_{1/2}$=23 hrs.

NURSING CONSIDERATIONS

Assessment: Assess for dementia-related psychosis, DM, risk factors for DM (eg, obesity, family history of DM), CVD, congenital long QT syndrome, history of cardiac arrhythmias, previously detected breast cancer, conditions that predispose to hypotension, history of clinically significant low WBCs or drug-induced leukopenia/neutropenia, history of seizures, severe GI narrowing, risk for aspiration pneumonia, Parkinson's disease, dementia with Lewy Bodies, renal impairment, pregnancy/nursing status, and possible drug interactions. Obtain baseline FBG in patients at risk for DM.

Monitoring: Monitor for NMS, TD, cerebrovascular/CV adverse reactions, hyperprolactinemia, orthostatic hypotension, syncope, cognitive and motor impairment, seizures, esophageal dysmotility, aspiration, priapism, metabolic changes, and disruption of body temperature. Monitor for weight gain, worsening blood glucose control in diabetes mellitus (DM) patients, and fasting blood glucose (FBG) levels in patients with diabetes risk. Monitor for signs/ symptoms of leukopenia, neutropenia (eg, fever, infection), and agranulocytosis; perform frequent monitoring of CBC in patients with history of clinically significant low WBC or drug-induced leukopenia/neutropenia. Monitor renal function.

Patient Counseling: Advise of the risk of orthostatic hypotension, particularly during initiation/re-initiation of treatment or dose increases. Inform that therapy has the potential to impair judgment, thinking, or motor skills; advise to use caution when operating hazardous machinery (eg, automobiles). Advise to avoid concomitant use with alcohol. Instruct to notify physician of all prescription and nonprescription drugs currently taking. Advise to notify physician if pregnant, intending to become pregnant, or if breastfeeding. Counsel on appropriate care in avoiding overheating and dehydration. Inform that medication must be swallowed whole with liquids; advise not to chew, divide, or crush. Advise that tab shell, along with insoluble core components, may be found in stool.

Administration: Oral route. Swallow tabs whole with liquids; do not chew, divide, or chew. **Storage**: ≤25°C (77°F); excursions permitted to 15-30°C (59-86°F). Protect from moisture.

INVEGA SUSTENNA   RX
paliperidone palmitate (Ortho-Mcneil/Janssen)

> Elderly patients with dementia-related psychosis treated with antipsychotic drugs, are at an increased risk of death; most deaths appeared to be cardiovascular (eg, heart failure, sudden death) or infectious (eg, pneumonia) in nature. Not approved for the treatment of patients with dementia-related psychosis.

THERAPEUTIC CLASS: Benzisoxazole derivative

INDICATIONS: Acute and maintenance treatment of schizophrenia in adults.

DOSAGE: *Adults:* Initial: 234mg IM on Day 1 and 156mg after 1 week. Administer in the deltoid muscle. Maint: 117mg/month. Range: 39mg-234mg based on tolerability and/or efficacy. Adjust dose monthly. After 2nd dose, administer monthly maint in deltoid or gluteal muscle. Maint: Continue at lowest dose needed. Reassess periodically to determine need to continue. CrCl ≥50-<80mL/min/Elderly with Decreased Renal Function: Initial: 156mg on Day 1 and 117mg after 1 week IM in deltoid. Maint: 78mg IM/month in deltoid or gluteal muscle. Switching from Oral Antipsychotics: D/C oral antipsychotics when initiating IM therapy. See PI for conversion. Switching from Long-Acting Injectable Antipsychotics: Initiate treatment in place of the next scheduled inj and continue at monthly intervals. Re-evaluate periodically. Refer to PI for instructions on missed/avoidance of missed doses.

HOW SUPPLIED: Inj, Extended-Release: 39mg, 78mg, 117mg, 156mg, 234mg

WARNINGS/PRECAUTIONS: Neuroleptic malignant syndrome (NMS) and tardive dyskinesia (TD) reported; d/c therapy if occur. May increase QTc interval; avoid with congenital long QT syndrome and with a history of cardiac arrhythmias. Hyperglycemia, in some cases extreme and associated with ketoacidosis or hyperosmolar coma or death, reported; monitor for hyperglycemia and perform fasting blood glucose testing at the beginning of therapy and periodically in patients at risk for diabetes mellitus (DM). Weight gain reported. May elevate prolactin levels. Leukopenia, neutropenia and agranulocytosis reported. D/C in cases of severe neutropenia (ANC <1000/mm³). May impair mental/physical abilities. Seizures reported; caution with history of seizures or conditions that lower the seizure threshold. May cause esophageal dysmotility and aspiration; caution with increased risk of aspiration pneumonia. May induce priapism; severe cases may require surgical intervention. May disrupt ability to reduce core body temperature; caution with conditions that may contribute to an elevated core body temperature. May have antiemetic effects that may mask the signs and symptoms of overdosage with certain drugs, intestinal obstruction, Reye's syndrome, or brain tumor. Patients with Parkinson's disease or dementia with Lewy bodies may have increased sensitivity to therapy. Caution with known suicidal tendencies, cardiovascular disease (CVD), cerebrovascular disease, conditions which predispose to hypotension, elderly, and renal impairment. Avoid in patients with CrCl <50mL/min. Intended for IM inj; avoid inadvertent inj into a blood vessel.

ADVERSE REACTIONS: Upper abdominal pain, constipation, N/V, injection-site reactions, nasopharyngitis, weight gain, dizziness, extrapyramidal disorder, headache, somnolence/sedation, agitation, anxiety, insomnia, akathisia.

INTERACTIONS: Caution with other CNS drugs and alcohol. May antagonize the effect of levodopa and other dopamine agonists. An additive effect may be observed when administered with other agents that cause orthostatic hypotension. Avoid in combination with other drugs known to prolong QTc interval, including Class 1A (eg, quinidine, procainamide) or Class III (eg, amiodarone, sotalol) antiarrhythmics, antipsychotics (eg, chlorpromazine, thioridazine), antibiotics (eg, gatifloxacin, moxifloxacin). Concomitant use with carbamazepine may decrease levels. Additive exposure with concurrent oral paliperidone or oral or injectable risperidone. Caution with concurrent anticholinergics; may contribue to an elevated body temperature.

PREGNANCY: Category C, not for use in nursing.

MECHANISM OF ACTION: Benzisoxazole derivative; not established. Proposed to be mediated through a combination of central dopamine Type 2 (D_2) and serotonin Type 2 ($5HT_{2A}$) receptor antagonism.

PHARMACOKINETICS: Absorption: T_{max}=13 days. **Distribution:** V_d=391L; plasma protein binding (74%); found in breast milk. **Metabolism:** Dealkylation, hydroxylation, dehydrogenation, and benzisoxazole scission; CYP2D6, 3A4 (limited). **Elimination:** (1mg IR single PO dose) Urine (80%, 59% unchanged), feces (11%); (39-234mg IM single-dose) $T_{1/2}$=25-49 days (median).

NURSING CONSIDERATIONS

Assessment: Assess for drug hypersensitivity and hypersensitivity to risperidone, dementia-related psychosis, Parkinson's disease, dementia, pre-existing low WBC or history of drug-induced leukopenia/neutropenia, known CVD, cerebrovascular disease, or conditions that predispose to hypotension. Assess use in patients with history of seizures, renal function, fasting blood glucose levels in patients at risk for DM, pregnancy/nursing status, and possible drug interactions.

Monitoring: Monitor for CV adverse events in the elderly, extrapyramidal symptoms (EPS), signs/symptoms of NMS, QT prolongation, TD, hyperglycemia, hyperprolactinemia, orthostatic hypotension, seizures, attempted suicide, and priapism. Perform periodic monitoring of fasting blood glucose levels in patients at risk for DM or experience hyperglycemia. Monitor CBC periodically in patients at risk for leukopenia/neutropenia.

Patient Counseling: Advise patients on risk of orthostatic hypotension. Caution about operating machinery/driving. Avoid concomitant use of alcohol. Instruct to inform physician about any concomitant medications. Notify physician if they become or intend to become pregnant.

Administration: IM route. Inject slowly, deep into muscle. Avoid inadvertent inj into a blood vessel. Do not administer dose in divided inj. Refer to PI for proper instructions for use. **Storage:** 25°C (77°F); excursions permitted to 15-30°C (59-86°F).

INVIRASE   RX
saquinavir mesylate (Roche Labs)

THERAPEUTIC CLASS: Protease inhibitor

INDICATIONS: Treatment of HIV-1 infection in combination with ritonavir and other antiretroviral agents in patients >16 yrs.

DOSAGE: *Adults:* 1000mg bid with ritonavir 100mg bid. Take within 2 hrs after a full meal. Concomitant therapy with lopinavir/ritonavir: 1000mg bid. *Pediatrics:* >16 yrs: 1000mg bid with ritonavir 100mg bid. Take within 2 hrs after a full meal. Concomitant therapy with lopinavir/ritonavir: 1000mg bid.

HOW SUPPLIED: Cap: 200mg; Tab: 500mg

CONTRAINDICATIONS: Congenital long QT syndrome, refractory hypokalemia or hypomagnesemia, complete atrioventricular (AV) block without implanted pacemakers, or patients at high risk of complete AV block, and with drugs that both increase saquinavir plasma concentrations and prolong the QT interval. Concomitant use with amiodarone, bepridil, dofetilide, flecainide, lidocaine (systemic), propafenone, quinidine, trazodone, rifampin, dihydroergotamine, ergonovine, ergotamine, methylergonovine, pimozide, cisapride, triazolam, orally administered midazolam, lovastatin, simvastatin, sildenafil (for treatment of pulmonary arterial HTN), alfuzosin. Severe hepatic impairment when coadministered with ritonavir.

WARNINGS/PRECAUTIONS: May prolong PR interval and dose-dependent QT prolongation. 2nd or 3rd degree AV block and torsade de pointes reported, rarely. Monitor ECG with congestive heart failure (CHF), bradyarrhythmias, hepatic impairment, electrolyte abnormalities and in patients with increased risk for cardiac conduction abnormalities (eg, underlying structural heart disease, pre-existing conduction system abnormalities, cardiomyopathies and ischemic heart disease). Correct hypokalemia/hypomagnesemia prior to therapy and monitor periodically. New onset diabetes mellitus (DM), exacerbation of pre-existing DM, hyperglycemia or diabetic ketoacidosis may occur. Caution with underlying hepatitis B or C, cirrhosis, chronic alcoholism, and/or other underlying liver abnormalities; worsening liver disease reported. Caution with hepatic/renal impairment. Spontaneous bleeding may occur with hemophilia A and B; additional factor VIII may be required. Redistribution or accumulation of body fat observed. Elevated cholesterol and/or triglyceride (TG) levels observed; monitor levels prior to therapy and periodically thereafter. Interrupt therapy if serious or severe toxicity occurs. Immune reconstitution syndrome reported. May increase likelihood of cross-resistance with other protease inhibitors. Contains lactose in amounts that should not induce specific symptoms of intolerance.

ADVERSE REACTIONS: Diarrhea, abdominal pain, pruritus, fever, rash, N/V, fatigue, pneumonia, lipodystrophy.

INTERACTIONS: See Contraindications. Caution with drugs that prolong PR interval, particularly drugs metabolized by CYP3A; clinical monitoring is recommended. Use atorvastatin or rosuvastatin at lowest possible dose. Avoid garlic capsules, tipranavir, fluticasone, bosentan, salmeterol. Decreased plasma levels with efavirenz, nevirapine, dexamethasone, St. John's wort, CYP3A inducers (eg, phenobarbital, phenytoin, carbamazepine). Ritonavir increases adverse effects. Delavirdine, atazanavir, indinavir increases plasma levels. Increases digoxin levels; monitor digoxin serum concentration and reduce dose if needed. Increase levels of CYP3A substrates, maraviroc, warfarin, colchicine, ketoconazole, rifabutin, vardenafil, tadalafil. Caution with ibutilide, sotalol, erythromycin, halofantrine, pentamidine, clozapine, haloperidol, mesoridazine, phenothiazines, thioridazine, ziprasidone. Adjust dose with clarithromycin in patients with renal impairment. Caution and monitor with CCB and PPIs. Decrease levels of methadone, ethinyl estradiol. Monitor with tricyclic antidepressants.

PREGNANCY: Category B, not for use in nursing.

MECHANISM OF ACTION: HIV protease inhibitor; binds to the protease active site and inhibits activity of the enzyme, preventing cleavage of the viral polyproteins and resulting in formation of immature, noninfectious virus particles.

PHARMACOKINETICS: Absorption: Administration of variable doses and combinations resulted in different parameters. **Distribution:** Plasma protein binding (98%). (IV): V_d=700L. **Metabolism:** Hepatic via CYP3A4. **Elimination:** (PO): Urine (1%), feces (88%). (IV): Urine (3%), feces (81%).

NURSING CONSIDERATIONS

Assessment: Assess for congenital long QT syndrome, refractory hypokalemia or hypomagnesemia, complete atrioventricular (AV) block without implanted pacemakers or patients at high risk of complete AV block, hypersensitivity, underlying structural heart disease, pre-existing conduction system abnormalities, cardiomyopathies and ischemic heart disease, CHF, bradyarrhythmias, electrolyte abnormalities, renal/hepatic impairment, pre-existing DM, underlying hepatitis B or C, cirrhosis, alcoholism, other underlying liver abnormalities, hemophilia, marked hypertriglyceridemia, lipid disorders, pregnancy/nursing status and possible drug interactions. Perform clinical chemistry tests (eg, TG and cholesterol levels) and ECG prior to initiation of treatment.

Monitoring: Monitor ECG (eg, PR interval prolongation, QT interval prolongation). Periodically monitor serum potassium and magnesium levels, TG and cholesterol levels. Monitor for signs/symptoms of, 2nd or 3rd degree block, cardiac conduction abnormalities, torsades de pointes, worsening liver disease, pancreatitis, spontaneous bleeding, immune reconstitution syndrome, fat redistribution/accumulation, hyperglycemia, new onset DM, diabetic ketoacidosis, infections, hepatic/renal function.

Patient Counseling: Inform the drug is not a cure for HIV and may continue to acquire illness associated with advanced HIV infection, including opportunistic infections. Report use of other Rx, OTC, or herbal products (eg, St. John's wort). Inform that drug therapy has not been shown to reduce the risk of transmitting HIV to others through sexual contact or blood contamination; use in combination with ritonavir; redistribution or accumulation of body fat may occur and long-term effects of these conditions are not known at this time. Take drug within 2 hrs of meals; do not alter or d/c therapy without consulting physician. Take medication every day, as prescribed, to achieve maximum benefit. If dose is missed, take as soon as possible; do not double next dose. Informed that changes in the ECG (PR interval or QT interval prolongation) may occurs. Inform healthcare provider if experiencing symptoms such as dizziness, lightheadedness, or palpitations.

Administration: Oral route. **Storage:** 25°C (77°F); excursions permitted to 15-30°C (59-86°F). Dispense in tightly closed bottles.

ISENTRESS

RX

raltegravir (Merck)

THERAPEUTIC CLASS: HIV-integrase strand transfer inhibitor

INDICATIONS: Treatment of HIV-1 infection in adults in combination with other antiretroviral agents.

DOSAGE: *Adults:* 400mg PO bid. With Rifampin: 800mg PO bid. Take with or without food.

HOW SUPPLIED: Tab: 400mg

WARNINGS/PRECAUTIONS: May develop immune reconstitution syndrome, an inflammatory response to indolent or residual opportunistic infections (eg, *Mycobacterium avium* complex, cytomegalovirus, *Pneumocystis jiroveci* pneumonia, *Mycobacterium* tuberculosis, or reactivation of varicella zoster virus) during initial phase of treatment, which may necessitate further evaluation and treatment. Caution in elderly. Avoid dosing before dialysis session.

ADVERSE REACTIONS: Hyperglycemia, insomnia, headache, rash, myopathy, rhabdomyolysis, ALT/AST elevation, total serum bilirubin increase, serum lipase elevation, low ANC, creatine increase, pancreatic amylase increase.

INTERACTIONS: Reduced levels with rifampin; increase dose of raltegravir. Reduced levels with efavirenz, etravirine, and tipranavir/ritonavir. Increased levels with drugs that inhibit UDP-glucuronosyltransferase (UGT) 1A1 (eg, atazanavir, atazanavir/ritonavir) and drugs that increase gastric pH (eg, omeprazole). Caution with drugs that cause myopathy or rhabdomyolysis.

PREGNANCY: Category C, not for use in nursing.

MECHANISM OF ACTION: HIV-1 integrase strand transfer inhibitor; inhibits the catalytic activity of HIV-1 integrase (an HIV-1 encoded enzyme required for viral replication) thus preventing the formation of HIV-1 provirus resulting in the prevention of propagation of the viral infection.

PHARMACOKINETICS: Absorption: T_{max}=3 hrs (fasting); variable doses resulted in different parameters. **Distribution:** Plasma protein binding (83%). **Metabolism:** Glucuronidation via UGT1A1; raltegravir-glucuronide (metabolite). **Elimination:** Urine (32%), feces (51%); $T_{1/2}$=9 hrs.

NURSING CONSIDERATIONS

Assessment: Assess for indolent or residual opportunistic infections, pre-existing history of psychiatric illness, risk of myopathy and rhabdomyolysis, liver disease, pregnancy/nursing status, and possible drug interactions. Obtain baseline CBC with platelet count, FPG, LFTs.

Monitoring: Monitor for inflammatory response to indolent or residual opportunistic infections. Monitor maternal-fetal outcomes of pregnant patients by enrolling them in the Antiretroviral Pregnancy Registry. Monitor CBC with platelet count, FPG, LFTs.

Patient Counseling: Inform about risks and benefits of therapy. Inform that therapy is not cure for HIV or AIDS, does not reduce risk of transmission of HIV, and that opportunistic infections may develop. Advise to practice safe sex by using latex or polyurethane condoms, or other barrier methods. Advise to never re-use or share needles. If dose is missed, instruct to take as soon as remembered; if not remembered until next dose, instruct to skip missed dose and go back to regular schedule. Advise not to take 2 tab at the same time. Instruct patients to read the Patient Package Insert before and during therapy. Advise to report development of unusual or persisting/worsening symptoms. Advise to inform physician if pregnant, plan to become pregnant, or nursing.

Administration: Oral route. **Storage:** 20-25°C (68-77°F); excursions permitted to 15-30°C (59-86°F).

ISONIAZID　　　　　　　　　　　　　　RX
isoniazid (Various)

> Severe, fatal hepatitis may develop. Monitor LFTs monthly. D/C drug if signs and symptoms of hepatic damage occur. Patients with tuberculosis (TB) who have isoniazid-induced hepatits should have appropriate treatment with alternative drugs. Defer preventive treatment in persons with acute hepatic disease.

THERAPEUTIC CLASS: Isonicotinic acid hydrazide

INDICATIONS: Prevention and treatment of TB.

DOSAGE: *Adults:* Active TB: 5mg/kg as a single dose. Max: 300mg qd or 15mg/kg 2 to 3 times/week. Max: 900mg/day. Use with other antituberculosis agents. Prevention: 300mg qd single dose.
Pediatrics: Active TB: 10-15mg/kg as a single dose. Max: 300mg qd or 20-40mg/kg 2 to 3 times/week. Max: 900mg/day. Use with other antituberculosis agents. Prevention: 10mg/kg qd single dose. Max: 300mg qd.

HOW SUPPLIED: Inj: 100mg/mL; Syrup: 50mg/5mL; Tab: 100mg, 300mg

CONTRAINDICATIONS: Severe hypersensitivity reactions including drug-induced hepatitis, previous INH-associated hepatic injury, severe adverse effects (eg, drug fever, chills, arthritis), acute liver disease of any etiology.

WARNINGS/PRECAUTIONS: D/C if hypersensitivity occurs. Monitor closely with liver or renal disease, daily alcohol users, pregnancy, age >35, and concurrent chronic medications. Precaution with HIV seropositive patients. Take with vitamin B_6 in malnourished and those predisposed to neuropathy.

ADVERSE REACTIONS: Peripheral neuropathy, N/V, anorexia, epigastric distress, elevated serum transaminases, bilirubinemia, jaundice, hepatitis, skin eruptions, pyridoxine deficiency.

INTERACTIONS: Alcohol is associated with hepatitis. May increase phenytoin, theophylline, and valproate serum levels. Do not take with food. Severe acetaminophen toxicity reported. Decreases carbamazepine metabolism and AUC of ketoconazole. Avoid tyramine- and histamine-containing foods.

PREGNANCY: Category C, caution in nursing.

MECHANISM OF ACTION: Isonicotinic acid hydrazide; inhibits mycoloic acid synthesis and acts against actively growing tuberculosis bacilli.

PHARMACOKINETICS: Absorption: T_{max}: 1-2 hrs. **Distribution**: Crosses placenta, found in breast milk. **Metabolism**: Acetylation and dehydrazination. **Elimination**: Urine (50-70%).

NURSING CONSIDERATIONS

Assessment: Assess for previous isoniazid-associated hepatic injury, acute liver disease, HIV status, pregnancy status, age, and drug interactions. Document reasons for therapy, culture, and susceptibility.

Monitoring: Prior to therapy and periodically thereafter, measure hepatic enzymes (AST, ALT). D/C at first sign of hypersensitivity reaction. Monitor for peripheral neuropathy, convulsions, N/V, agranulocytosis, hemolytic anemia, SLE-like syndrome, metabolic and endocrine reactions (hyperglycemia, pyridoxine deficiency, pellagra).

Patient Counseling: Immediately report signs/symptoms consistent with liver damage or other adverse events (unexplained anorexia, N/V, dark urine, icterus, rash, persistent paresthesias of the hands and feet, persistent fatigue, weakness or fever of >3 days duration, and/or abdominal tenderness). Drug should not be taken with food. Take pyridoxine tablets if peripheral neuropathy develops.

Administration: Oral and IM route. **Storage:** Tab: 20-25°C (68-77°F). Syrup: 15-30°C (59-86°F). Protect from light and moisture. Dispense in tight, light-resistant container. Inj: 20-25°C (68-77°F). Protect from light. If vial contents crystallize, warm vial to room temperature to redissolve crystals before use.

ISOSORBIDE DINITRATE

isosorbide dinitrate (Various)

OTHER BRAND NAMES: Isordil Titradose (Biovail) - Isordil (Biovail)

THERAPEUTIC CLASS: Nitrate vasodilator

INDICATIONS: Prevention of angina pectoris due to coronary artery disease.

DOSAGE: *Adults:* Prevention: Initial: 5-20mg bid-tid. Maint: 10-40mg bid-tid. Allow a dose-free interval of at least 14 hrs for both formulations. Elderly: Start at low end of dosing range.

HOW SUPPLIED: Tab: 5mg*, 10mg*, 20mg*, 30mg*; Tab, Extended-Release: 40mg; Tab, Sublingual: 2.5mg *scored

WARNINGS/PRECAUTIONS: Not for use with acute MI or CHF. Severe hypotension may occur. May aggravate angina caused by hypertrophic cardiomyopathy. Caution with volume depletion, hypotension, elderly. Monitor for tolerance.

ADVERSE REACTIONS: Headache, lightheadedness, hypotension, syncope, rebound HTN.

INTERACTIONS: Severe hypotension with sildenafil. Additive vasodilation with other vasodilators (eg, alcohol).

PREGNANCY: Category C, caution in nursing.

MECHANISM OF ACTION: Nitrate vasodilator; relaxes vascular smooth muscle, dilates peripheral arteries and veins, especially the latter. Dilatation of veins reduces left ventricular end diastolic pressure and pulmonary capillary wedge pressure (preload). Arteriolar relaxation reduces systemic vascular resistance, systolic arterial pressure, and mean arterial pressure (afterload). It also dilates the coronary artery.

PHARMACOKINETICS: Absorption: T_{max}=1 hr. **Distribution:** V_d=2-4L/kg. **Metabolism:** Liver; extensive first-pass metabolism; 2-mononitrate, 5-mononitrate (active metabolites). **Elimination:** $T_{1/2}$=5 hrs (5-mononitrate), 2 hrs (2-mononitrate).

NURSING CONSIDERATIONS

Assessment: Assess for severe hypotension, volume-depleted patients, angina caused by hypertrophic cardiomyopathy, alcohol intake, and possible drug interactions.

Monitoring: Careful clinical or hemodynamic monitoring for hypotension and tachycardia. Monitor for paradoxical bradycardia, increased angina pectoris, hemodynamic rebound, decreased exercise tolerance, headaches, lightheadedness on standing, manifestation of true physical dependence (chest pain, acute MI) and methemoglobinemia.

Patient Counseling: Counsel carefully follow dosing regimen. Inform about headaches (markers of drug activity) and lightheadedness on standing. Avoid alcohol consumption.

Administration: Oral route. **Storage:** 25°C (77°F).

IXEMPRA RX

ixabepilone (Bristol-Myers Squibb)

> Contraindicated in combination with capecitabine in patients with AST/ALT >2.5X ULN or bilirubin >1X ULN due to increased toxicity and neutropenia-related death.

THERAPEUTIC CLASS: Antimicrotubule agent

INDICATIONS: In combination with capecitabine for treatment of patients with metastatic or locally advanced breast cancer resistant to treatment with an anthracycline and a taxane, or whose cancer is taxane resistant and for whom further anthracycline therapy is contraindicated. As monotherapy for treatment of metastatic or locally advanced breast cancer in patients whose tumors are resistant or refractory to anthracyclines, taxanes, and capecitabine.

DOSAGE: *Adults:* 40mg/m² IV infusion over 3 hrs every 3 weeks. Patients with BSA >2.2m² should be dosed based on 2.2m². Adjust dose based on toxicities (see PI). Patient should not begin a new cycle of treatment unless the neutrophil count is at least 1500 cells/min³, the platelet count is at least 100,000 cell/mm³, and nonhematologic toxicities have improved to grade 1 (mild) or resolved. If toxicities recur, an additional 20% dose reduction should be made. Hepatic Impairment: Combination Therapy: AST or ALT ≤2.5X ULN and Bilirubin ≤1X ULN: 40mg/m². Monotherapy: Mild: AST and ALT ≤2.5X ULN and Bilirubin ≤1X ULN: 40mg/m². AST or ALT ≤10X ULN and Bilirubin ≤1.5X ULN: 32mg/m². Moderate (AST and ALT ≤10X ULN and Bilirubin >1.5 to ≤3X ULN): 20-30mg/m². Strong CYP3A4 Inhibitors: Avoid or reduce dose to 20mg/m². If d/c, allow a washout period of approximately 1 week before adjusting dose to the indicated dose. Strong CYP3A4 Inducers: Avoid or gradually increase dose to 40-60mg/m² given as a 4 hr IV infusion. If d/c, return to dose used prior to initiation of strong inducer. Premedicate all patients with H₁-antagonist (eg, diphenhydramine 50mg PO) and H₂-antagonist (eg, ranitidine 150-300mg PO) approximately 1 hr before infusion. Premedicate with corticosteroids (eg, dexamethasone 20mg, IV 30 min before infusion or PO 60 min before infusion) if prior hypersensitivity reaction experienced.

HOW SUPPLIED: Inj: 15mg, 45mg

CONTRAINDICATIONS: Neutrophil count <1500 cells/mm³ or platelet count <100,000 cells/mm³. In combination with capecitabine patients with AST or ALT >2.5x ULN or bilirubin >1x ULN. History of severe (CTC Grade 3/4) hypersensitivity reaction to Cremophor EL or derivatives (eg, polyoxyethylated castor oil).

WARNINGS/PRECAUTIONS: Peripheral neuropathy may occur early during treatment; monitor for symptoms and manage by dose adjustment, dose delays or d/c. Caution with DM or pre-existing peripheral neuropathy. Myelosuppression, primarily neutropenia, may occur and is dose-dependent; monitor with frequent peripheral blood cell counts and adjust dose as needed. Premedicate all patients with H₁- and H₂-antagonists 1 hr before treatment; d/c and institute aggressive supportive treatment if hypersensitivity occurs. May cause fetal harm; avoid during pregnancy. Caution with history of cardiac disease. D/C if cardiac ischemia or impaired cardiac function develops. Avoid monotherapy if AST or ALT >10X ULN or bilirubin >3X ULN and use caution if AST or ALT >5X ULN. Potential cognitive impairment may occur from excipients (eg, dehydrated alcohol USP).

ADVERSE REACTIONS: Peripheral neuropathy, fatigue/asthenia, myalgia/arthralgia, alopecia, N/V, stomatitis/mucositis, diarrhea, musculoskeletal pain, palmar-plantar erythrodysesthesia (hand-foot) syndrome, anorexia, abdominal pain, hepatic toxicity, neutropenia.

INTERACTIONS: CYP3A4 inhibitors may increase levels; avoid or reduce dose with strong CYP3A4 inhibitors (eg, ketoconazole, clarithromycin, atazanavir, nefazodone, saquinavir, grapefruit juice); use caution with mild/moderate CYP3A4 inhibitors (eg, erythromycin, fluconazole, verapamil), and monitor all patients closely for acute toxicities. Strong CYP3A4 inducers (eg, dexamethasone, phenytoin, carbamazepine, rifampin, rifampicin, rifabutin, phenobarbital) may decrease levels; consider gradual dose adjustment or alternative agents. St. John's wort may decrease levels and should be avoided.

PREGNANCY: Category D, not for use in nursing.

MECHANISM OF ACTION: Microtubule inhibitor; binds directly to β-tubulin subunits on microtubules, leading to suppression of microtubule dynamics. Blocks the mitotic phase of cell division, leading to cell death.

PHARMACOKINETICS: Absorption: C_{max}=252ng/mL; T_{max}=3 hrs; AUC=2143ng•hr/mL. **Distribution:** V_d= >1000L. Plasma protein binding=67-77%. **Metabolism:** Liver (oxidation) via CYP3A4. **Elimination:** Urine (21%, 5.6% unchanged), feces (65%, 1.6% unchanged); $T_{1/2}$=52 hrs.

NURSING CONSIDERATIONS

Assessment: Assess for hypersensitivity to Cremophor EL or polyoxyethylated castor oil, DM, pre-existing peripheral neuropathy, history of cardiac disease, renal dysfunction, hepatic impairment, pregnancy/nursing status, and possible drug interactions. Obtain baseline LFTs and peripheral blood cell count.

Monitoring: Monitor LFTs and peripheral blood cell count periodically. Monitor for signs/symptoms of neuropathy, myelosuppression, fever/neutropenia, cardiac adverse reactions, hepatic toxicity, and hypersensitivity reactions.

Patient Counseling: Advise to seek medical attention if symptoms of peripheral neuropathy (eg, numbness, tingling in hands or feet), fever/neutropenia (eg, chills, cough, burning or pain urinating), hypersensitivity reaction (eg, urticaria, pruritus, rash, flushing, swelling, chest tightness, dyspnea), or cardiac events (eg, chest pain, difficulty breathing, palpitations, unusual weight gain) occur. Instruct to avoid grapefruit juice. Inform of pregnancy/nursing risks; advise to use effective contraceptive methods and not to nurse.

Administration: IV infusion. Refer to PI for proper instructions of preparation and administration. **Storage:** 2-8°C (36-46°F). Protect from light. (Constituted) Store for maximum 1 hr at room temperature and room light. (Diluted) Stable at room temperature and room light for maximum of 6 hrs.

JALYN   RX
tamsulosin HCl - dutasteride (GlaxoSmithKline)

THERAPEUTIC CLASS: 5-alpha reductase inhibitor/alpha antagonist

INDICATIONS: Treatment of symptomatic benign prostatic hyperplasia (BPH) in men with an enlarged prostate.

DOSAGE: *Adults:* Initial: 1 cap qd, 30 min after the same meal each day. Swallow whole; do not chew or open cap.

HOW SUPPLIED: Cap: (Dutasteride-Tamsulosin HCl) 0.5mg-0.4mg

CONTRAINDICATIONS: Pregnancy, women of childbearing potential, and pediatric patients.

WARNINGS/PRECAUTIONS: Orthostatic hypotension/syncope may occur; avoid situations where injury could result if syncope occurs. Risk to male fetus; capsules should not be handled by pregnant women or women who may become pregnant. Rule out prostate cancer and other urological diseases prior to treatment and periodically thereafter. Monitor for obstructive uropathy in patients with a large residual urinary volume and/or severely diminished urinary flow; these patients may not be good candidates for therapy. Dutasteride may decrease serum prostate specific antigen (PSA) levels by about 40-50%; obtain a new baseline PSA concentration after 3-6 months of treatment. To interpret an isolated PSA value in a man treated for ≥6 months, double the PSA value for comparison with normal values. Any confirmed increases in PSA from nadir while on therapy may signal the presence of prostate cancer and should be carefully evaluated, even if values are still within normal range for men not taking a 5α-reductase inhibitor. May cause priapism, which can lead to permanent impotence if not properly treated. Avoid blood donation until 6 months after last dose. Intraoperative floppy iris syndrome (IFIS) has been observed during cataract surgery. Use with caution if sulfa allergy present. Contact with contents of drug may cause oropharyngeal mucosal irritation.

ADVERSE REACTIONS: Ejaculation disorders, impotence, decreased libido.

INTERACTIONS: Avoid concomitant use with strong inhibitors of CYP3A4 (eg, ketoconazole); may decrease tamsulosin metabolism and increase tamsulosin exposure. Caution when coadministered with moderate inhibitors of CYP3A4 (eg, erythromycin), strong (eg, paroxetine) or moderate (eg, terbinafine) inhibitors of CYP2D6 and known poor metabolizers of CYP2D6; may significantly increase tamsulosin metabolism. Decreased tamsulosin clearance with cimetidine; use with caution. Caution with warfarin. Avoid use with other α-adrenergic antagonists. Caution with PDE5 inhibitors; may cause symptomatic hypotension.

PREGNANCY: Category X, not for use in nursing.

MECHANISM OF ACTION: Dutasteride: Type I, II 5α-reductase inhibitor; inhibits the conversion of testosterone to dihydrotestosterone (DHT), the androgen primarily responsible for the initial development and subsequent enlargement of the prostate gland. Tamsulosin: α_{1A} antagonist; selective blockade of α_1 receptors in the prostate result in relaxation of the smooth muscles of the bladder neck and prostate.

PHARMACOKINETICS: Absorption: Dutasteride: Absolute bioavailability (60%); C_{max}=2.14ng/mL, T_{max}=3 hrs, AUC=39.6ng•hr/mL; Tamsulosin: Complete. (>90%); C_{max}=11.3ng/mL, T_{max}=6 hrs, AUC=187.2ng•hr/mL. **Distribution:** Dutasteride: V_d=300-500L; plasma protein binding (99%); Tamsulosin: (IV) V_d=16L, plasma protein binding (94-99%). **Metabolism:** Dutasteride: CYP3A4, 3A5. Major active metabolites: 4'-hydroxydutasteride, 1,2-dihydroxydutasteride, 6-hydroxydutasteride; Tamsulosin: Liver (extensive); CYP3A4, CYP2D6. **Elimination:** Dutasteride: Urine (<1%), feces (5% unchanged, 40% metabolites); $T_{1/2}$=5 weeks; Tamsulosin: Urine (76%), feces (21%); $T_{1/2}$=14-15 hrs.

NURSING CONSIDERATIONS

Assessment: Assess for BPH, large residual urinary volume or severely diminished urinary flow, sulfa allergy, pregnancy/nursing status, and possible drug interactions. Rule out prostate cancer and other urological diseases.

Monitoring: Monitor for signs/symptoms of prostate cancer and other urological diseases. Obtain new baseline PSA after 3-6 months of treatment. Monitor for signs/symptoms of orthostatic hypotension, syncope, priapism, IFIS, and allergic reactions.

Patient Counseling: Inform females who are pregnant or intend to become pregnant not to handle drug due to potential risk to fetus; inform that if contact is made, to wash area immediately with soap and water. Inform about the possible occurrence of symptoms related to orthostatic hypotension (eg, dizziness and vertigo) and the potential risk of syncope; avoid situations where injury could result if syncope occurs. Capsule may become deformed and/or discolored if kept at high temperatures; avoid use if this occurs. Advise about the possibility of priapism (rare) that can lead to permanent erectile dysfunction if not brought to immediate medical attention. If considering cataract surgery, advise to inform ophthalmologist of therapy. Advise not to donate blood for at least 6 months after last dose.

Administration: Oral route. **Storage:** 25°C (77°F); excursions permitted to 15-30°C (59-86°F).

JANUMET   RX
metformin HCl - sitagliptin (Merck)

> Lactic acidosis may occur due to metformin accumulation; increased risk with conditions such as sepsis, dehydration, excess alcohol intake, hepatic insufficiency, renal impairment, and acute congestive heart failure (CHF). If acidosis is suspected, d/c and hospitalize patient immediately.

THERAPEUTIC CLASS: Dipeptidyl peptidase-4 inhibitor/biguanide

INDICATIONS: Adjunct to diet and exercise to improve glycemic control in adults with type 2 diabetes mellitus (DM).

DOSAGE: *Adults:* Individualize dosing. Patients Not Currently on Metformin: Initial: 50mg sitagliptin/500mg metformin bid. Patients on Metformin: Initial: 50mg bid (100mg/day) of sitagliptin and current metformin dose. Patients on Metformin 850mg bid: Initial: 50mg sitagliptin/1000mg metformin bid. Max: 100mg sitagliptin/2000mg metformin. Take with meals with gradual dose escalation to reduce GI side effects of metformin. With Insulin/Insulin Secretagogue (eg, Sulfonylurea): May require lower dose of insulin secretagogue or insulin.

HOW SUPPLIED: Tab: (Metformin-Sitagliptin) 500mg-50mg, 1000mg-50mg

CONTRAINDICATIONS: Renal disease or renal dysfunction; acute or chronic metabolic acidosis, including diabetic ketoacidosis, with or without coma. Temporarily d/c if undergoing radiologic studies involving intravascular administration of iodinated contrast materials.

WARNINGS/PRECAUTIONS: Acute pancreatitis reported; d/c if pancreatitis suspected. Has not been studied in patients with history of pancreatitis. Avoid with hepatic impairment. D/C with evidence of renal impairment. May decrease vitamin B_{12} levels; monitor hematologic parameters annually. Suspend temporarily for any surgical procedures (except minor procedures not associated with restricted food and fluid intake); restart when oral intake is resumed and renal function is normal. Evaluate for evidence of ketoacidosis or lactic acidosis with lab abnormalities or clinical illness (especially vague and poorly defined illness); d/c if either form occurs. D/C in hypoxic states (eg, CHF, shock, acute MI). Temporary loss of glycemic control may occur when exposed to stress (eg, fever, trauma, infection, surgery); withhold therapy and temporarily administer insulin. Serious hypersensitivity reactions (eg, anaphylaxis, angioedema, exfoliative skin conditions including Stevens-Johnson syndrome [SJS]) reported; d/c if occur and institute alternative treatment. Avoid in patients ≥80 yrs unless renal function is normal. Caution in elderly.

ADVERSE REACTIONS: Lactic acidosis, diarrhea, upper respiratory tract infection, headache, N/V, abdominal pain.

INTERACTIONS: See Contraindications. Increased levels of digoxin observed; monitor digoxin levels. (Metformin) Furosemide, nifedipine, and cationic drugs (eg, digoxin, amiloride, procainamide, quinidine, quinine, ranitidine, trimethoprim, vancomycin, triamterene, morphine, cimetidine) may increase levels. Observe for loss of glycemic control with thiazides and other diuretics, corticosteroids, phenothiazines, thyroid products, estrogens, oral contraceptives, phenytoin, nicotinic acid, sympathomimetics, calcium channel blockers, and isoniazid. Alcohol may potentiate effect on lactate metabolism. Caution with drugs that may affect renal function or result in significant hemodynamic change or may interfere with the disposition of metformin (eg, cationic drugs eliminated by renal tubular secretion). May decrease furosemide and glyburide levels. Hypoglycemia may occur with ethanol. May be difficult to recognize hypoglycemia with β-adrenergic blocking drugs. (Sitagliptin) Hypoglycemia may occur with other glucose-lowering agents (eg, sulfonylureas, insulin); may require lower doses of sulfonylurea or insulin. Increased levels with cyclosporine.

PREGNANCY: Category B, caution in nursing.

MECHANISM OF ACTION: Sitagliptin: Dipeptidyl peptidase-4 inhibitor; acts by slowing the inactivation of incretin hormones. Metformin: Biguanide; decreases hepatic glucose production, decreases intestinal absorption of glucose, and improves insulin sensitivity by increasing peripheral glucose uptake and utilization.

PHARMACOKINETICS: Absorption: Sitagliptin: Absolute bioavailability (87%). Metformin: Absolute bioavailability (50-60%) (fasted). **Distribution:** Sitagliptin: (IV) V_d=198L; plasma protein binding (38%). Metformin: V_d=654L. **Metabolism:** Sitagliptin: CYP3A4 and CYP2C8. **Elimination:** Sitagliptin: Feces (13%), urine (87%, 79% unchanged); $T_{1/2}$12.4 hrs. Metformin: Urine (90%); $T_{1/2}$=6.2 hrs (plasma), 17.6 hrs (blood).

NURSING CONSIDERATIONS

Assessment: Assess for metabolic acidosis, renal/hepatic function, hypersensitivity, pregnancy/nursing status, and possible drug interactions. Assess if patient is planning to undergo any surgical procedure or is under any form of stress. Obtain baseline FPG, HbA1c, CrCl, LFTs, and hematological parameters.

Monitoring: Monitor for lactic acidosis, hypoglycemia, pancreatitis, clinical illness, hypoxic states, and for hypersensitivity reactions. Monitor renal function, especially in elderly, at least annually. Monitor vitamin B_{12} levels in patients predisposed to develop subnormal vitamin B_{12} levels. Monitor FPG, HbA1c, renal/hepatic function, and hematologic parameters periodically.

Patient Counseling: Inform the risks, benefits, and alternative modes of therapy. Advise on importance of adherence to dietary instructions, regular physical activity, periodic blood glucose monitoring, HbA1c testing, recognition/management of hypoglycemia/hyperglycemia, and assessment of diabetic complications. Advise of the risk of lactic acidosis. Counsel against excessive alcohol intake. Inform that GI symptoms may occur; consult physician if unexplained symptoms develop. Inform that acute pancreatitis is reported; d/c and contact physician if severe abdominal pain occurs. Contact physician during periods of stress (eg, fever, trauma, infection, surgery). D/C and seek medical attention if symptoms of an allergic reaction, unexplained hyperventilation, myalgia, malaise, unusual somnolence, dizziness, slow or irregular heart beat, sensation of feeling cold (especially in the extremities), or other nonspecific symptoms occurs. Inform about the importance of regular testing of renal function and hematological parameters. Read Medication Guide prior to therapy and reread each time prescription is renewed. Inform physician if any unusual symptom develops or if any symptom persists or worsens.

Administration: Oral route. **Storage:** 20-25°C (68-77°F); excursions permitted to 15-30°C (59-86°F).

JANUVIA   RX
sitagliptin (Merck)

THERAPEUTIC CLASS: Dipeptidyl peptidase-4 inhibitor

INDICATIONS: Adjunct to diet and exercise to improve glycemic control in adults with type 2 diabetes mellitus (DM).

DOSAGE: *Adults:* 100mg qd. Renal Insufficiency: Moderate (CrCl ≥30 to <50mL/min): 50mg qd. Severe (CrCl <30mL/min)/End Stage Renal Disease (ESRD) Requiring Hemodialysis or Peritoneal Dialysis: 25mg qd. With Insulin/Insulin Secretagogue (eg, Sulfonylurea): May require lower dose of insulin secretagogue or insulin.

HOW SUPPLIED: Tab: 25mg, 50mg, 100mg

WARNINGS/PRECAUTIONS: Acute pancreatitis reported; d/c if pancreatitis suspected. Dosage adjustment recommended with moderate/severe renal insufficiency. Hypersensitivity reactions (eg, anaphylaxis, angioedema, exfoliative skin conditions including Stevens-Johnson syndrome [SJS]) reported; d/c if hypersensitivity reaction is suspected and institute alternative treatment. Caution in elderly.

ADVERSE REACTIONS: Nasopharyngitis, upper respiratory tract infection, headache.

INTERACTIONS: May slightly increase digoxin levels; monitor appropriately. Cyclosporine may modestly increase sitagliptin levels. May require lower dose of insulin secretagogue (eg, sulfonylurea) or insulin therapy to reduce risk of hypoglycemia.

PREGNANCY: Category B, caution in nursing.

MECHANISM OF ACTION: Dipeptidyl peptidase-4 inhibitor; suspected to exert action by slowing the inactivation of incretin hormones. By increasing and prolonging active incretin levels, sitagliptin increases insulin release and decreases glucagon levels in the circulation in a glucose-dependent manner.

PHARMACOKINETICS: Absorption: Rapid. Absolute bioavailability (87%); T_{max}=1-4 hrs; AUC=8.52µM•hr; C_{max}=950nM. **Distribution:** (IV) V_d=198L; plasma protein binding (38%). **Metabolism:** Via CYP3A4 and CYP2C8. **Elimination:** Feces (13%), urine (87%, 79% unchanged); $T_{1/2}$=12.4 hrs.

NURSING CONSIDERATIONS

Assessment: Assess renal function, for previous hypersensitivity to the drug, history of pancreatitis, pregnancy/nursing status, and possible drug interactions. Obtain baseline FPG, HbA1c, and CrCl.

Monitoring: Monitor for pancreatitis and hypersensitivity reactions. Monitor FPG, HbA1c, and renal function periodically.

Patient Counseling: Inform of risks, benefits, and alternative modes of therapy. Advise on the importance of adherence to dietary instructions, regular exercise, periodic blood glucose monitoring, HbA1c testing, recognition/management of hypoglycemia/hyperglycemia, and assessment of diabetic complications. Instruct to seek medical attention during periods of stress (eg, fever, trauma, infection, surgery) as medication needs may change. Notify physician and d/c use if signs and symptoms of pancreatitis (eg, persistent severe abdominal pain), or allergic reactions (eg, rash, hives, and swelling of the face, lips, tongue, and throat) occur. Read Medication Guide prior to therapy and to reread each time prescription is renewed. Notify physician or pharmacist if any unusual symptom develops, or if any known symptom persists or worsens.

Administration: Oral route. May be taken with or without food. **Storage:** 20-25°C (68-77°F); excursions permitted to 15-30°C (59-86°F).

JENLOGA   RX
clonidine HCl (Shionogi)

THERAPEUTIC CLASS: Alpha-adrenergic agonist

INDICATIONS: Treatment of hypertension, alone or with other antihypertensives.

DOSAGE: *Adults:* Individualize dose. Initial: 0.1mg hs. Titrate: If inadequate reduction in BP, may increase in increments of 0.1mg/day at weekly intervals. Doses >0.1mg/day should be divided and taken am and hs. If am and hs doses are not equal, hs dose should be the larger of the two. Usual: 0.2-0.6mg/day. Max: 0.6mg/day. Renal Impairment: Initial: 0.1mg/day. Increase dose slowly. Carefully monitor to prevent excessive blood pressure lowering or bradycardia.

HOW SUPPLIED: Tab: 0.1mg

WARNINGS/PRECAUTIONS: Avoid abrupt d/c; reduce dose gradually over 2 to 4 days. Rare instances of hypertensive encephalopathy, cerebrovascular accidents (CVA) and death reported after withdrawal. Caution with severe coronary insufficiency, conduction disturbances, recent myocardial infarction (MI), cerebrovascular disease, or chronic renal failure; uptitrate dose slowly. In patients who have developed localized contact sensitization to a clonidine transdermal system, substitution of PO clonidine may result in the development of a generalized skin rash. In patients who develop an allergic reaction from a clonidine transdermal system, substitution of oral clonidine may elicit an allergic reaction (eg, generalized rash, urticaria, angioedema). Monitor BP during surgery; additional measures to control BP should be available. Continue to within 4 hrs of surgery and resume as soon as possible thereafter.

ADVERSE REACTIONS: Dry mouth, fatigue, dizziness, headache, nausea, somnolence, insomnia.

INTERACTIONS: May potentiate CNS depression with alcohol, barbiturates, or other sedating drugs. Hypotensive effect may be reduced by tricyclic antidepressants. Monitor HR with agents that affect sinus node function or AV nodal conduction (eg, digitalis, calcium channel blockers, β-blockers). Sinus bradycardia reported with diltiazem or verapamil. D/C β-blockers several days before the gradual withdrawal of clonidine in patients taking both.

PREGNANCY: Category C, not for use in nursing.

MECHANISM OF ACTION: Centrally acting alpha-2 adrenergic agonist; stimulates α-adrenoreceptors in the brain stem, reducing sympathetic outflow from CNS and decreasing peripheral resistance, renal vascular resistance, HR, and BP.

PHARMACOKINETICS: Absorption: T_{max}=4-7 hrs. **Distribution:** Found in breast milk. **Metabolism:** Liver. **Elimination:** Urine (40-60%, unchanged); $T_{1/2}$=13 hrs.

NURSING CONSIDERATIONS

Assessment: Assess for severe coronary insufficiency, conduction disturbances, recent MI, cerebrovascular disease, renal impairment, pregnancy/nursing status, and for possible drug interactions.

Monitoring: Monitor BP and renal function periodically. Monitor for withdrawal signs/symptoms (eg, hypertensive encephalopathy, CVA), presence of generalized skin rash, and allergic reactions.

Patient Counseling: Caution against interruption of therapy without physician's advice. Caution in engaging in hazardous activities (eg, operating machinery or driving). Inform that sedative effect may be increased by concomitant use of alcohol, barbiturates, or other sedating drugs. Inform that medication may cause dryness of the eyes; caution with contact lenses.

Administration: Oral route. **Storage:** 20-25°C (68-77°F).

JEVTANA   RX
cabazitaxel (Sanofi-Aventis)

> Neutropenic deaths reported. Perform frequent blood cell counts to monitor for neutropenia. Do not give to patients with neutrophil counts of ≤1,500 cells/mm³. Severe hypersensitivity reactions reported; d/c immediately if this occurs and administer appropriate therapy. Patients should receive premedication. Contraindicated in patients with history of severe hypersensitivity reactions to this medication or drugs formulated with polysorbate 80.

THERAPEUTIC CLASS: Antimicrotubule agent

INDICATIONS: In combination with prednisone for the treatment of patients with hormone-refractory metastatic prostate cancer previously treated with a docetaxel-containing treatment regimen.

DOSAGE: *Adults*: Individualize dose based on BSA. Initial: 25mg/m² over 1-hr IV infusion q3 weeks in combination with oral prednisone 10mg qd. Reduce dose to 20mg/m² if patients experience: Prolonged Grade ≥3 neutropenia (>1 week) despite appropriate medications (including G-CSF), febrile neutropenia, or Grade ≥3 diarrhea or persisting diarrhea despite appropriate medication, fluid and electrolyte replacement. Delay treatment until improvement or resolution of febrile neutropenia, diarrhea, and until neutrophil count is >1,500 cells/mm³. Use G-CSF for secondary prophylaxis for neutropenia and febrile neutropenia. D/C treatment if patient continues to experience any of these reactions at 20mg/m². Premedicate at least 30 min prior to each dose with antihistamine (dexchlorpheniramine 5mg, diphenhydramine 25mg, or equivalent antihistamine), corticosteroid (dexamethasone 8mg or equivalent steroid), H₂ antagonist (ranitidine 50mg or equivalent H₂ antagonist). Also give antiemetics as prophylaxis (PO or IV) prn.

HOW SUPPLIED: Inj: 60mg/1.5mL

CONTRAINDICATIONS: See Boxed Warning. Neutrophil counts ≤1,500/mm³.

WARNINGS/PRECAUTIONS: May cause GI symptoms (N/V, severe diarrhea), and intensive treatment measures may be required; may need to delay treatment or reduce dose with Grade ≥3 diarrhea. Renal failure, including cases with fatal outcome, reported; identify cause and treat aggressively. Caution in patients with severe renal impairment (CrCl <30mL/min) and in patients with end-stage renal disease. Avoid in patients with hepatic impairment (total bilirubin ≥ULN, or AST and/or ALT ≥1.5X ULN). May cause fetal harm. Caution in elderly. Caution when handling or preparing sol.

ADVERSE REACTIONS: Hypersensitivity reactions, neutropenia, anemia, leukopenia, thrombocytopenia, diarrhea, fatigue, N/V, constipation, asthenia, abdominal pain, anorexia, back pain, hematuria.

INTERACTIONS: Avoid with strong CYP3A inhibitors (eg, ketoconazole, itraconazole, clarithromycin, atazanavir, indinavir, nefazodone, nelfinavir, ritonavir, saquinavir, telithromycin, voriconazole). Caution with concomitant use of moderate CYP3A inhibitors. Strong CYP3A inducers (eg, phenytoin, carbamazepine, rifampin, rifabutin, rifapentin, phenobarbital) may decrease levels; avoid coadministration. Avoid concomitant use of St. John's wort.

PREGNANCY: Category D, not for use in nursing.

MECHANISM OF ACTION: Antimicrotubule agent; binds to tubulin and promotes its assembly into microtubules while simultaneously inhibiting disassembly which results in the inhibition of mitotic and interphase cellular functions.

PHARMACOKINETICS: Absorption: C_{max}=226 ng/mL; AUC=991 ng•hr/mL; T_{max}=1 hr. **Distribution**: V_{ss}=4,864L; Plasma protein binding (89%-92%). **Metabolism**: Liver (extensive); mainly by CYP3A4/5, and to a lesser extent CYP2C8. **Elimination**: Urine (3.7%) (2.3%, unchanged), feces (76%); $T_{1/2}$= 95 hrs.

NURSING CONSIDERATIONS

Assessment: Assess for hypersensitivity to drugs formulated with polysorbate 80, hepatic impairment (total bilirubin ≥ULN, or AST and/or ALT ≥1.5x ULN), severe renal impairment (CrCl <30mL/min), pregnancy/nursing status, and possible drug interactions. Obtain baseline neutrophil count. Assess use in the elderly. Assess for high-risk clinical features that may predispose to increased neutropenia complications (eg, age >65 yrs, poor performance status, previous episodes of febrile neutropenia, extensive poor radiation ports, poor nutritional status, or other serious comorbidities).

Monitoring: Monitor CBC on weekly basis during Cycle 1 and before each treatment cycle thereafter. Monitor for signs and symptoms of severe neutropenia, febrile neutropenia, infections, severe diarrhea, dehydration, renal failure and hypersensitivity reactions.

Patient Counseling: Counsel about the risk of potential hypersensitivity; instruct to immediately report signs of hypersensitivity reactions. Advise on the importance of routine blood cell counts. Instruct to monitor temperature frequently; report any occurrence of fever immediately. Instruct to report if not compliant with oral corticosteroid regimen. Counsel about side effects associated with exposure such as severe and fatal infections, dehydration, and renal failure. Advise to report significant vomiting or diarrhea, decreased urinary output, and hematuria. Advise to inform physician before taking any other medications. Advise women of childbearing age not to become pregnant while taking this drug. Inform elderly patients that certain side effects may be more frequent or severe.

Administration: IV route; refer to PI for preparation and administration procedures. Do not use PVC infusion containers or polyurethane infusions sets. **Storage**: 25°C (77°F); excursions permitted to 15-30°C (59-86°F). Do not refrigerate.

KADIAN
morphine sulfate (Actavis)

> Contains morphine sulfate, an opioid agonist and Schedule II controlled substance, with an abuse liability similar to other opioid analgesics. Not for use as a prn analgesic. The 100mg and 200mg capsules are for use in opioid-tolerant patients only. Swallow capsules whole or sprinkle contents on applesauce. Do not crush, chew, or dissolve pellets in capsules.

THERAPEUTIC CLASS: Opioid analgesic

INDICATIONS: Management of moderate to severe pain when continuous around-the-clock opioid analgesia is needed.

DOSAGE: *Adults:* Individualize dose. Not for initial opioid analgesic; it is advisable to begin treatment using IR formulation. Conversion from Other Oral Morphine: Give 50% of daily oral morphine dose q12h or give 100% oral morphine dose q24h. Do not give more frequently than q12h. Conversion from Parenteral Morphine: Oral morphine 3x the daily parenteral morphine dose may be sufficient in chronic-use settings. Conversion from Other Parenteral or Oral Opioids: Initial: Give 50% of estimated daily morphine demand and supplement with IR morphine. 1st dose may be taken with the last dose of any IR morphine. Conversion from Other Non-Opioids and Intermittent Use of Moderate or Strong Opioids: Give 50% (of estimated total daily oral morphine dose) q12h or q24h. Titrate: No more frequently than qod to stabilize before escalating the dose. Breakthrough Pain: Give <20% of daily dose of short act-ing analgesic. Switch to bid dosing after excessive sedation to qd dosing or inadequate analgesia before next dose. Opioid Non-Tolerant: Should only be started on 10-20mg. Titrate: Increase not >20mg qod. May sprinkle contents on small amount of applesauce or in water for gastrostomy tube (see PI for complete instructions). Do not chew, crush or dissolve pellets. Do not adminis-ter through NG-tube. Elderly: Start at low end of dosing range.

HOW SUPPLIED: Cap, Extended-Release: 10mg, 20mg, 30mg, 50mg, 60mg, 80mg, 100mg, 200mg

CONTRAINDICATIONS: Respiratory depression in the absence of resuscita-tive equipment, acute or severe bronchial asthma or hypercarbia, paralytic ileus.

WARNINGS/PRECAUTIONS: Do not administer pre-op for the manage-ment of post-op pain in patients not previously taking the drug. Respiratory depression possible; caution in COPD, cor pulmonale, decreased respiratory reserve. May obscure neurologic signs in head injuries, intracranial lesions, or a pre-existing increase in ICP. May cause severe hypotension. Avoid with GI obstruction. Caution in biliary tract disease (including pancreatitis), elderly, debilitated, renal/hepatic insufficiency, Addison's disease, myxedema, hypothyroidism, prostatic hypertrophy, urethral stricture, CNS depression, toxic psychosis, acute alcoholism, delirium tremens, kyphoscoliosis, inability to swallow and convulsive disorders. May impair mental/physical abilities. Depresses cough reflex. Decreases gastric, biliary, and pancreatic secretions. D/C 24 hrs before procedure that interrupts pain transmission pathways (eg, cordotomy); give short-acting parenteral opioid.

ADVERSE REACTIONS: Drowsiness, dizziness, constipation, nausea, anxiety.

INTERACTIONS: Increased risk of respiratory depression, hypotension, profound sedation or coma with CNS depressants (eg, sedatives, hypnot-ics, general anesthetics, antiemetics, phenothiazines, tranquilizers, alcohol); reduce initial dose of one or both agents by 50%. May enhance neuromuscular blocking action of skeletal relaxants. Mixed agonist/antagonist analgesics may reduce analgesic effects or precipitate withdrawal symptoms. Avoid MAOIs during or within 14 days of use. May reduce diuretic effects. Avoid concomitant use with cimetidine; confusion and severe respiratory depression reported.

PREGNANCY: Category C, not for use in nursing.

MECHANISM OF ACTION: Opioid analgesic; principal actions are analgesia and sedation. Precise mechanism of analgesic effects not established. Acts as a pure agonist, binding with and activating opioid receptors at sites in the peri-aqueductal and periventricular gray matter, the ventromedial medulla, and the spinal cord to produce analgesia.

PHARMACOKINETICS: Absorption: Various doses resulted in different parameters. **Distribution:** V_d=3-4L/kg; plasma protein binding (30-35%); distributed to skeletal muscle, kidneys, liver, intestinal tract, lungs, spleen, brain; crosses the blood brain barrier (small amount); crosses placental membranes; found in breast milk. **Metabolism:** Liver (conjugation) to glucuronide metabolites; morphine-3-glucuronide, morphine-6-glucuronide. **Elimination:** Urine (10% unchanged); bile (small amount); feces (7-10%); $T_{1/2}$=2-4 hrs.

NURSING CONSIDERATIONS

Assessment: Assess for degree of opioid tolerance, previous opioid dose, level of pain intensity, type of pain, patient's general condition and medical status, or any other conditions where treatment is contraindicated or cautioned. Assess for history of hypersensitivity, pregnancy/nursing status, renal/hepatic function, and possible drug interactions.

Monitoring: Monitor for signs/symptoms of respiratory depression, hypotension, anaphylaxis, convulsions, tolerance and physical dependence (eg, withdrawal symptoms), and signs of medication misuse or abuse. Monitor serum amylase levels.

Patient Counseling: Swallow medication whole (do not chew, crush, or dissolve) or open and sprinkle contents of capsule on small amount of applesauce (at room temperature or cooler). Rinse mouth after taking dose to ensure all pellets have been swallowed. Capsule may be administered through a French 16 gastrostomy tube if there is difficulty swallowing. Do not adjust dosing without physician's consent. Drug may impair mental/physical abilities; use caution when performing hazardous tasks (eg, operating machinery/driving). Avoid alcohol and other CNS depressants. Do not abruptly d/c medication. May develop severe constipation during therapy; appropriate concomitant therapy should be given at start of treatment. Medication has potential for abuse. Instruct to keep out of reach of children. If treatment is complete, dispose unused capsules via toilet.

Administration: Oral route. **Storage:** 25°C (77°F); excursions permitted to 15-30°C (59-86°F). Protect from light and moisture. Dispense in a sealed tamper-evident, childproof, light-resistant container.

KALBITOR RX
ecallantide (Dyax Corp.)

> Anaphylaxis reported. Should only be administered by a healthcare professional with appropriate medical support. Healthcare professionals should be aware of the similarity of symptoms between hypersensitivity and HAE; monitor closely.

THERAPEUTIC CLASS: Plasma kallikrein inhibitor

INDICATIONS: Treatment of acute attacks of hereditary angioedema (HAE) in patients ≥16 yrs.

DOSAGE: *Adults:* Usual: Three 10 mg (1mL) injections SQ. If attack persists, additional 30mg may be administered within a 24hr period. Elderly: Start at low end of dosing range.
Pediatrics: ≥16 yrs: Usual: Three 10 mg (1mL) injections SQ. If attack persists, additional 30mg may be administered within a 24hr period.

HOW SUPPLIED: Inj: 10mg/mL

WARNINGS/PRECAUTIONS: Serious hypersensitivity reactions (eg, chest discomfort, flushing, pharyngeal edema, pruritus, rhinorrhea, sneezing, nasal congestion, throat irritation, urticaria, wheezing, and hypotension) including anaphylaxis may occur within the first hour after dosing. Caution in elderly.

ADVERSE REACTIONS: Anaphylaxis, headache, N/V, fatigue, diarrhea, upper respiratory tract infection, injection-site reactions, nasopharyngitis, pruritus, upper abdominal pain, pyrexia, immunogenicity.

PREGNANCY: Category C, caution in nursing.

MECHANISM OF ACTION: Plasma kallikrein inhibitor; binds to plasma kallikrein and blocks the binding site, inhibiting the conversion of HMW kininogen to bradykinin.

PHARMACOKINETICS: Absorption: C_{max}=586ng/mL; T_{max}=2-3 hrs; AUC=3017ng•hr/mL. **Distribution**: V_d= 26.4L. **Elimination:** $T_{1/2}$=2 hrs.

NURSING CONSIDERATIONS

Assessment: Assess HAE and hypersensitivity reactions, and pregnancy/nursing status.

Monitoring: Monitor for anaphylaxis and hypersensitivity reactions such as chest discomfort, flushing, pharyngeal edema, pruritus, rhinorrhea, sneezing, nasal congestion, throat irritation, urticaria, wheezing, and hypotension.

Patient Counseling: Advise that it may cause anaphylaxis and other hypersensitivity reactions and must be administered by a healthcare professional with appropriate medical support to manage the reactions. Instruct patients not to receive additional doses with known hypersensitivity to the drug. Advise to consult Medication Guide for additional information regarding the risk of anaphylaxis and other hypersensitivity reactions.

Administration: SQ route. Refer to PI for preparation and handling/detailed reconstitution and administration information. **Storage:** 2°-8°C (36°-46°F). Vials removed from refrigeration: store below 30°C (86°F) and use within 14 days or return to refrigeration until use. Protect from light.

KALETRA   RX
ritonavir - lopinavir (Abbott)

THERAPEUTIC CLASS: Protease inhibitor

INDICATIONS: Treatment of HIV-1 infection in combination with other antiretrovirals.

DOSAGE: *Adults:* Usual: 400/100mg (2 tabs 200/50mg or 5mL) bid; or 800/200mg (4 tabs 200/50mg or 10mL) qd in patients with <3 lopinavir resistance-associated substitutions. Concomitant Therapy with Efavirenz, Nevirapine, Amprenavir, Nelfinavir: Tabs: Usual: 500/125mg (2 tabs 200/50mg and 1 tab 100/25mg) bid; Oral Sol: 533/133mg (6.5mL) bid. *Pediatrics:* 14 days-6 months: Oral Sol: Usual: 16/4mg/kg or 300/75mg/m² bid. 6 months-18 yrs: Oral Sol: Usual: 230/57.5mg/m² bid. Max: 400/100mg (5mL) bid. <15kg: Usual: 12/3mg/kg bid. ≥15-40kg: Usual: 10/2.5mg/kg bid. Tab: 15-25kg: Usual: 200/50mg (2 tabs 100/25mg) bid. >25-35kg: Usual: 300/75mg (3 tabs 100/25mg) bid. >35kg: Usual: 400/100mg (4 tabs 100/25mg or 2 tabs 200/50mg) bid. Concomitant Therapy with Efavirenz, Nevirapine, Amprenavir, or Nelfinavir: Treatment-Naive and Treatment-Experienced: 6 months-18 yrs: Oral Sol: Usual: 300/75mg/m² bid. Max: 533/133mg (6.5mL) bid. <15kg: Usual: 13/3.25mg/kg bid. >15-45kg: Usual: 11/2.75mg/kg bid. Tab: 15-20kg: Usual: 200/50mg (2 tabs 100/25mg) bid. >20-30kg: Usual: 300/75mg (3 tabs 100/25mg) bid. >30-45kg: Usual: 400/100mg (4 tabs 100/25mg or 2 tabs 200/50mg) bid. >45kg: Usual: 500/125mg (5 tabs 100/25mg) bid. Use oral sol for children with BSA <0.6m² or those who are unable to reliably swallow a tab.

HOW SUPPLIED: Tab: (Lopinavir-Ritonavir) 100mg-25mg, 200mg-50mg; Sol: 80mg-20mg/mL [160mL]

CONTRAINDICATIONS: Coadmistration with drugs that are highly dependent on CYP3A for clearance and for which elevated plasma concentrations are associated with serious and/or life-threatening reactions. Coadmistration with potent CYP3A inducers where significantly reduced lopinavir levels may be associated with the potential for loss of virologic response and possible resistance and cross-resistance (eg, alfuzosin, rifampin, dihydroergotamine, ergonovine, ergotamine, methylergonovine, St. John's wort, cisapride, lovastatin, simvastatin, sildenafil [when used to treat pulmonary arterial HTN], pimozide, triazolam, orally administered midazolam).

WARNINGS/PRECAUTIONS: Pancreatitis reported; suspend therapy as clinically appropriate if signs/symptoms (N/V, abdominal pain) or laboratory abnormalities (increased serum lipase/amylase) exhibit and suggestive of pancreatitis occur. Caution with underlying hepatitis B or C or marked transaminase elevation; may increase risk for developing or worsening of transaminase elevations or hepatic decompensation. Perform appropriate laboratory testing prior to and during therapy. Monitor AST/ALT with underlying chronic hepatitis or cirrhosis, especially during 1st several months of therapy. Diabetes mellitus (DM), exacerbation of pre-existing DM, and hyperglycemia reported; initiation or dose adjustments of insulin or oral hypoglycemic may be required. May elevate TG and total cholesterol levels. May cause redistribution/accumulation of body fat. Increased bleeding may occur with hemophilia A and B. Prolonged PR and QT interval may occur; caution with underlying structural heart disease, pre-existing conduction system abnormalities, ischemic heart disease, or cardiomyopathies. Avoid use with congenital long QT syndrome and hypokalemia. Immune reconstitution syndrome reported with combination therapy. Once-daily regimen is not recommended for adults with ≥3 of the following lopinavir resistance associated substitutions: L10F/I/R/V, K20M/N/R, L24I, L33F, M36I, I47V, G48V, I54L/T/V, V82A/C/F/S/T, I84V, and in pediatric patients. Avoid oral sol in preterm neonates; may be at increased risk of propylene glycol-associated adverse events. Life-threatening cases of cardiac toxicity (including AV block, bradycardia, and cardiomyopathy), lactic acidosis, acute renal failure, CNS depression and respiratory complications leading to death reported. Caution with hepatic impairment and in elderly.

ADVERSE REACTIONS: Asthenia, diarrhea, N/V, dysgeusia, hepatotoxicity, pancreatitis, rash, abdominal pain, dyspepsia, headache, decreased weight, insomnia.

INTERACTIONS: See Contraindications. CYP3A inhibitors may increase lopinavir (LPV) levels. Caution with drugs that prolong PR interval (eg, calcium channel blockers [CCBs], β-blockers, digoxin, atazanavir), particularly those metabolized by CYP3A. Avoid drugs that prolong QT interval (eg, salmeterol), parenteral midazolam, high doses of ketoconazole/itraconazole (>200mg/day), and tipranavir. Coadministration of fluticasone propionate is not recommended. May increase plasma concentrations of drugs metabolized by CYP3A. May increase biotransformation of some drugs metabolized by CYP450 enzymes. May increase sildenafil, tadalafil, and vardenafil levels; reduce dose and monitor for adverse effects. Increased atorvastatin and rosuvastatin levels; use lowest dose or consider alternate HMG-CoA reductase inhibitors (eg, pravastatin, fluvastatin). May decrease levels of methadone and atovaquone; dose increase may be needed. May decrease ethinyl estradiol levels; alternative contraception is recommended. May increase levels of antiarrhythmics (eg, amiodarone, bepridil, systemic lidocaine, quinidine), dihydropyridine CCBs (eg, felodipine, nifedipine, nicardipine), immunosuppressants (eg, cyclosporine, tacrolimus, rapamycin), trazodone, and tenofovir; monitoring recommended. May increase rifabutin levels; reduce usual rifabutin dose by 75%. Increased rate of adverse reactions observed with fosamprenavir. May increase levels of clarithromycin; dose adjustment recommended in patients with renal impairment. Should not administer qd with carbamazepine, phenytoin, phenobarbital, efavirenz, nevirapine, amprenavir, and nelfinavir. Concentration with warfarin may be affected. Increased levels of anticancer agents (eg, vincristine, vinblastine); d/c if significant hematologic and GI side effects occur. Increased levels of nilotinib and dasatinib; dose reduction or dosing interval adjustment needed. Increased levels of maraviroc, saquinavir, and indinavir. Take didanosine on an empty stomach 1 hr prior or 2 hrs after sol. May increase colchicine levels; adjust dose and avoid with renal/hepatic impairment. May increase levels of bosentan; d/c ≥36 hrs prior to initiation and resume bosentan ≥10 days after initiation of lopinavir/ritonavir. May increase fentanyl levels; monitor for adverse effects. Decreased levels with rifampin, and dexamethasone. May increase levels with delavirdine, fosamprenavir, omeprazole, rifabutin. Oral sol contains alcohol; may produce disulfiram-like reactions with disulfiram, metronidazole. May decrease levels of bupropion, abacavir, zidovudine, voriconazole, norethindrone desipramine, nevirapine, pravastatin. See PI for complete information.

PREGNANCY: Category C, not for use in nursing.

MECHANISM OF ACTION: Lopinavir: HIV-1 protease inhibitor; prevents cleavage of the Gag-Pol polyprotein, resulting in the production of immature, non-infectious viral particles. Ritonavir: HIV-1 protease inhibitor; CYP3A inhibitor that inhibits metabolism of lopinavir, increasing its plasma levels.

PHARMACOKINETICS: Absorption: Lopinavir: (400/100mg bid) C_{max}=9.8μg/mL, T_{max}=4 hrs, AUC=92.6μg•h/mL; (800/200mg qd) C_{max}=11.8μg/mL, T_{max}=6 hrs, AUC=154.1μg•h/mL. Refer to PI for pediatric parameters. **Distribution:** Lopinavir: Plasma protein binding (98-99%). **Metabolism:** Lopinavir: Hepatic via CYP3A. Ritonavir: Induces own metabolism. **Elimination:** Unchanged lopinavir: Urine (2.2%), feces (19.8%).

NURSING CONSIDERATIONS

Assessment: Assess for history of hypersensitivity reactions (eg, toxic epidermal necrolysis, Stevens-Johnson syndrome, erythema multiforme), history of pancreatitis, hepatitis B or C, cirrhosis, DM or hyperglycemia, hyperlipidemia, hemophilia type A or B, structural heart disease, pre-existing conduction system abnormalities, ischemic heart disease or cardiomyopathies, congenital long QT syndrome, hypokalemia, renal/hepatic impairment, pregnancy/nursing status, and for possible drug interactions. Obtain baseline TG, serum transaminase, total cholesterol levels. Assess children for the ability to swallow intact tab.

Monitoring: Monitor for signs/symptoms of pancreatitis, hyperglycemia, hepatic dysfunction, infection, fat redistribution, hypersensitivity reactions, and other adverse reactions. Monitor infants for increase in serum osmolality, SrCr, and toxicity (eg, hyperosmolality, renal toxicity, CNS depression, seizures, hypotonia, cardiac arrhythmias, ECG changes, hemolysis) if benefit of using oral sol immediately after birth outweighs the potential risks. Monitor TG, total cholesterol levels, LFTs, lipid profile, glucose, total bilirubin, ECG changes, serum lipase, and serum amylase levels. Monitor INR with warfarin.

Patient Counseling: Instruct to take prescribed dose as directed. Instruct that sol should be taken with food. Instruct to inform healthcare provider if weight changes in children occurs. Instruct that if a dose is missed, take dose as soon as possible and return to normal schedule; do not double next dose. Advise that product is not a cure for HIV; opportunistic infections may still occur. Advise to seek medical attention if symptoms of worsening liver disease (eg, loss of appetite, abdominal pain, jaundice), hyperglycemia (eg, frequent urination, excessive thirst, extreme hunger), fat redistribution, rash, sustained penile erection (eg, >4 hrs), dizziness, abnormal heart rhythm, or loss of consciousness occur. Inform of greater chance of developing diarrhea with qd regimen. Instruct to notify physician if using other Rx/OTC or herbal products, particularly St. John's wort. When taking didanosine, advise to take tab at the same time without food or take 1 hr or 2 hrs after sol. Instruct to report any symptoms (eg, hypotension, visual changes, sustained erection) to physician if receiving sildenafil, tadalafil, or vardenafil.

Administration: Oral route. Swallow tab whole; do not crush, break, or chew. Take sol with food. **Storage:** (Tab) 20-25°C (68-77°F); excursions permitted to 15-30°C (59-86°F). (Sol) 2-8°C (36-46°F). Avoid exposure to excessive heat. If stored at room temperature up to 25°C (77°F), sol should be used within 2 months.

KAPVAY **ER**   RX
clonidine HCl (Shionogi)

THERAPEUTIC CLASS: Alpha$_2$-agonist

INDICATIONS: Treatment of attention deficit hyperactivity disorder (ADHD) as monotherapy and as adjunctive therapy to stimulant medications.

DOSAGE: *Pediatrics:* 6-17 yrs: Initial: 0.1mg hs. Titrate: Adjust in increments of 0.1mg/day at weekly intervals until desired response is achieved. Max: 0.4mg/day. D/C in in decrements of no more than 0.1 mg every 3 to 7 days. Refer to PI for further dosing information.

HOW SUPPLIED: Tab, Extended-Release: 0.1mg, 0.2mg

WARNINGS/PRECAUTIONS: May cause dose related decreases in BP and HR; measure HR and BP prior to initiation of therapy, following dose increases, and periodically while on therapy. Somnolence and sedation reported. May impair mental/physical abilities. Avoid abrupt d/c; sudden cessation may result in headache, tachycardia, nausea, flushing, warm feeling, light-headedness, tightness in chest, and anxiety. Caution with history of hypotension, heart block, bradycardia, CV disease, syncope, severe coronary insufficiency, conduction disturbances, recent myocardial infarction (MI), cerebrovascular disease, and chronic renal failure. May elicit allergic reactions (eg, generalized rash, urticaria, angioedema).

ADVERSE REACTIONS: Somnolence, fatigue, upper respiratory infection, nasal congestion, nightmares, throat pain, increased body temperature, insomnia, emotional disorder, constipation, dry mouth, ear pain.

INTERACTIONS: May potentiate the CNS-depressive effects of alcohol, barbiturates or other sedating drugs. Decreased hypotensive effects with TCAs. Caution with agents known to affect sinus node function or AV nodal conduction (eg, digitalis, calcium channel blockers, β-blockers). Additive pharmacodynamic effects with other antihypertensives. Avoid with other products containing clonidine.

PREGNANCY: Category C, caution in nursing.

MECHANISM OF ACTION: Centrally acting alpha$_2$-adrenergic agonist; not established. Stimulates alpha$_2$-adrenergic receptors in the brain.

PHARMACOKINETICS: Absorption: (Adults) (Fed) C_{max}=235pg/mL, AUC=6505hr•pg/mL, T_{max}=6.8 hrs; (fasted) C_{max}=258pg/mL, AUC=6729hr•pg/mL, T_{max}=6.5 hrs; Absolute bioavailability (89%). **Distribution:** Found in breast milk. **Elimination:** (Adults) $T_{1/2}$=12.67 hrs (fed), 12.65 hrs (fasted).

NURSING CONSIDERATIONS

Assessment: Assess for history of hypotension, heart block, bradycardia, CVD, syncope, HTN, severe coronary insufficiency, conduction disturbances, recent MI, cerebrovascular disease, chronic renal failure, pregnancy/nursing status, and for possible drug interactions. Obtain baseline HR and BP.

Monitoring: Monitor for somnolence, sedation, hypotension, bradycardia, allergic reactions (eg, generalized rash, urticaria, angioedema), and for the presence of other side effects. Perform periodic BP and HR monitoring while on therapy.

Patient Counseling: Inform about risks and benefits of therapy and counsel appropriately. Advise not to d/c abruptly. If total daily dose does not allow equal bid dosing, instruct to take higher of two doses at bedtime. Instruct to swallow tab whole and never crush, cut or chew. Advise to consult a physician if pregnant, nursing or thinking of becoming pregnant. Caution against operating heavy equipment or driving until treatment response has been evaluated.

Administration: Oral route. **Storage:** 20-25°C (68-77°F).

KAYEXALATE   RX
sodium polystyrene sulfonate (Sanofi-Aventis)

THERAPEUTIC CLASS: Cation-exchange resin

INDICATIONS: Treatment of hyperkalemia.

DOSAGE: *Adults:* PO: 15g qd-qid. Rectal Enema: 30-50g q6h.
Pediatrics: Use 1mEq of K⁺ per 1g of resin as basis of calculation. Avoid PO administration in neonates.

HOW SUPPLIED: Powder: 453.6g

CONTRAINDICATIONS: Hypokalemia, obstructive bowel disease, neonates with reduced gut motility (post-op or drug-induced), oral administration in neonates.

K-Dur

WARNINGS/PRECAUTIONS: Cases of intestinal necrosis and other serious GI adverse events (eg, bleeding, ischemic colitis, perforation) reported. Avoid use in patients who have not had a bowel movement post-surgery and in patients at risk for developing constipation or impaction. Hypokalemia may occur. May be insufficient for emergency correction of hyperkalemia; consider other definitive measures (eg, dialysis). Monitor for electrolyte disturbances. Caution if intolerant to Na⁺ increases (eg, severe CHF or HTN, marked edema). Follow full aspiration precautions during administration. Caution with premature infants or low birth weight infants. If clinically significant constipation occurs d/c until normal bowel movement is resumed.

ADVERSE REACTIONS: Anorexia, N/V, constipation, hypokalemia, hypocalcemia, Na⁺ retention, diarrhea, fecal impaction, gastric irritation, intestinal necrosis.

INTERACTIONS: Avoid nonabsorbable cation-donating antacids and laxatives (eg, magnesium hydroxide, aluminum carbonate); systemic alkalosis may occur. Hypokalemia exaggerates toxic effects of digitalis. Intestinal obstruction reported with aluminum hydroxide. May decrease absorption of lithium and thyroxine. Concomitant use with sorbitol has been implicated in cases of intestinal necrosis; avoid use.

PREGNANCY: Category C, caution in nursing.

MECHANISM OF ACTION: Cation exchange resin; partially releases Na⁺ ions and are replaced by K⁺ ions.

NURSING CONSIDERATIONS

Assessment: Assess for hypokalemia, obstructive bowel disease, CHF, HTN, marked edema, prematurity, history of intestinal disease or surgery, hypovolemia, bowel function, renal insufficiency and failure, pregnancy/nursing status, and for possible drug interactions. Assess neonates for reduced gut motility.

Monitoring: Monitor for signs/symptoms of intestinal necrosis or other GI events (eg, bleeding, ischemic colitis, perforation), hypokalemia, cardiac arrhythmias, electrolyte disturbances, and constipation. Monitor ECG and serum electrolytes.

Patient Counseling: Counsel about potential side effects and advise to seek medical attention if signs/symptoms develop.

Administration: Oral/Rectal routes. Refer to PI for further administration instructions. **Storage:** 25°C (77°F); excursions permitted to 15-30°C (59-86°F). Suspension should be freshly prepared and not stored beyond 24 hrs.

K-Dur   RX
potassium chloride (Schering)

THERAPEUTIC CLASS: K⁺ supplement

INDICATIONS: (For those unable to tolerate liquid or effervescent potassium preparations). Treatment and prevention of hypokalemia with or without metabolic alkalosis. Treatment of digitalis intoxication and hypokalemic familial periodic paralysis.

DOSAGE: *Adults:* Prevention: 20mEq/day. Hypokalemia: 40-100mEq/day. Divide dose if >20mEq. Take with meals and a full glass of water or liquid. Tab can be broken in half or dissolved in water.

HOW SUPPLIED: Tab, Extended-Release: 10mEq, 20mEq* *scored

CONTRAINDICATIONS: Hyperkalemia, esophageal ulceration, delay in GI passage (from structural, pathological, pharmacologic causes), cardiac patients with esophageal compression due to enlarged left atrium.

WARNINGS/PRECAUTIONS: Potentially fatal hyperkalemia may occur. Extreme caution with acidosis, cardiac and renal disease; monitor ECG and electrolytes. Hypokalemia with metabolic acidosis should be treated with an alkalinizing potassium salt (eg, potassium bicarbonate, potassium citrate). May produce ulcerative or stenotic GI lesions.

ADVERSE REACTIONS: Hyperkalemia, GI effects (obstruction, bleeding, ulceration), N/V, abdominal pain, flatulence, diarrhea.

INTERACTIONS: Risk of hyperkalemia with ACE inhibitors (eg, captopril, enalapril), K⁺-sparing diuretics and K⁺ supplements. Contraindicated with anticholinergic agents due to possible delay in tablet passage through GI tract.

PREGNANCY: Category C, safe for use in nursing.

MECHANISM OF ACTION: K⁺ supplement (electrolyte replenisher); potassium ions participate in maintenance of intracellular tonicity, transmission of nerve impulses, contraction of cardiac, skeletal, and smooth muscle, and maintenance of normal renal function.

NURSING CONSIDERATIONS

Assessment: Assess for chronic renal disease, conditions which impair K⁺ excretion, esophageal compression due to enlarged left atrium, structural/pathologic cause for arrest/delay in passing through GI (diabetic gastroparesis), and possible drug interactions. Obtain baseline serum K⁺ levels and renal function test.

Monitoring: Monitor serum K⁺ levels, renal function, ECG, and acid-base balance. Monitor for hyperkalemia, signs of acute metabolic acidosis, acute dehydration, GI ulcerations, and hypersensitivity reactions.

Patient Counseling: Instruct to report symptoms of GI bleeding (tarry stools), ulcerations/perforations (severe vomiting, abdominal pain, distention), trouble swallowing, or tablet sticking in throat. Take with meals and full glass of water; swallow whole, do not crush, chew, or suck. If difficulty swallowing whole tablet; break tablet in half. Take each half separately with glass of water or place whole tab in 1/2 glass of water and allow 2 min to disintegrate, stir for half min after disintegration, swirl suspension and drink content. Add another 1oz of water, swirl, and drink immediately and repeat once more.

Administration: Oral route. **Storage:** 25°C (77°F); excursions permitted to 15-30°C (59-86°F). Keep tightly closed.

KEPIVANCE   RX
palifermin (Amgen)

THERAPEUTIC CLASS: Keratinocyte growth factor

INDICATIONS: To decrease the incidence and duration of severe oral mucositis in patients with hematologic malignancies receiving myelotoxic therapy requiring hematopoietic stem cell support.

DOSAGE: *Adults:* 60mcg/kg/day IV bolus 3 consecutive days before and after myelotoxic therapy for a total of 6 doses.

HOW SUPPLIED: Inj: 6.25mg

CONTRAINDICATIONS: Known hypersensitivity to *E. Coli*-derived proteins.

WARNINGS/PRECAUTIONS: Potential for stimulation of tumor growth. Safety and efficacy have not been established in patients with nonhematologic malignancies.

ADVERSE REACTIONS: Rash, erythema, edema, fever, pruritus, dysesthesia, tongue discoloration, tongue thickening, alteration of taste, pain arthralgias.

INTERACTIONS: Do not administer 24 hrs before, during infusion, or 24 hrs after administration of myelotoxic chemotherapy due to risk of increased severity and duration of oral mucositis. May interact with unfractionated as well as low molecular weight heparins; if heparin is used to maintain IV line, use saline to rinse prior to and after administration.

PREGNANCY: Category C, caution in nursing.

MECHANISM OF ACTION: Keratinocyte growth factor; binds to the KGF receptor, which results in proliferation, differentiation, and migration of the epithelial cells.

PHARMACOKINETICS: Elimination: $T_{1/2}$=4.5 hrs.

NURSING CONSIDERATIONS

Assessment: Assess for hypersensitivity to *E. coli*-derived proteins, pregnancy/nursing status, and for possible drug interactions.

Monitoring: Monitor for signs and symptoms of tumor growth, hypersensitivity reactions, rash, erythema, edema, pruritus, dysesthesia, tongue discoloration or thickening, taste alterations, and arthralgias.

Patient Counseling: Counsel about possible adverse effects, including mucocutaneous adverse effects. Instruct to seek medical attention if rash, erythema, edema, pruritus, oral/perioral dysesthesia, tongue discoloration, tongue thickening, or if taste alterations develop. Inform that use may stimulate tumor growth.

Administration: IV bolus for 3 consecutive days before and after myelotoxic therapy. **Storage:** Powder: 2-8°C (36-46°F). Reconstituted Sol: 2-8°C (36-46°F) for up to 24 hrs. May be allowed to reach room temperature for a maximum of one hour. Do not freeze. Protect from light.

KEPPRA   RX
levetiracetam (UCB)

THERAPEUTIC CLASS: Pyrrolidine derivative

INDICATIONS: (PO) Adjunctive therapy for partial onset seizures in adults and children ≥4 yrs. Adjunctive therapy in the treatment of myoclonic seizures in adults and children ≥12 yrs with juvenile myoclonic epilepsy (JME). Adjunctive therapy in the treatment of primary generalized tonic-clonic (PGTC) seizures in adults and children ≥6 yrs with idiopathic generalized epilepsy. (Inj) Alternative for patients ≥16 yrs when oral administration is temporarily not feasable in the adjunctive therapy of partial onset seizures, myoclonic seizures with JME and PGTC with idiopathic generalized epilepsy.

DOSAGE: *Adults:* Inj/PO: Initial: 500mg bid. Titrate: Increase by 1000mg/day every 2 weeks. Max: 3000mg/day. Inj: Replacement Therapy: Initial total daily dosage and frequency should equal total daily dosage and frequency of oral therapy. Dilute injection in 100mL of compatible diluent and give as 15-min IV infusion. Switching to PO: switch at equivalent daily dosage and frequency of the IV administration. Individualize dose: CrCl >80mL/min: 500mg-1500mg q12h. CrCl 50-80mL/min: 500mg-1000mg q12h. CrCl 30-50mL/min: 250mg-750mg q12h. CrCl <30mL/min: 250mg-500mg q12h. ESRD with Dialysis: 500-1000mg q24h. A supplemental dose of 250mg-500mg after dialysis is recommended. Elderly: Start at lower end of dosing range.
Pediatrics: PO: Partial Onset Seizures/PGTC: ≥16 yrs or Myoclonic Seizures with JME: ≥12 yrs: Initial: 500mg bid. Titrate: Increase by 1000mg/day every 2 weeks. Max: 3000mg/day. Partial Onset Seizures: 4 to <16 yrs or PGTC: 6-16 yrs: Initial: 10mg/kg bid. Titrate: Increase by 20mg/kg/day every 2 weeks. Max: 60mg/kg/day. Use oral sol for patients ≤20kg. (Inj): Partial Onset Seizures/Myoclonic Seizures with JME/PGTC: ≥16 yrs: Initial: 500mg bid. Titrate: Increase by 1000mg/day every 2 weeks. Max: 3000mg/day. Replacement Therapy: Initial total daily dosage and frequency should equal total daily dosage and frequency of oral therapy. Dilute injection in 100mL of compatible diluent and give as 15-min IV infusion. Switching to PO: switch at equivalent daily dosage and frequency of the IV administration. Individualize dose: CrCl >80mL/min: 500mg-1500mg q12h. CrCl 50-80mL/min: 500mg-1000mg q12h. CrCl 30-50mL/min: 250mg-750mg q12h. CrCl <30mL/min: 250mg-500mg q12h. ESRD with Dialysis: 500-1000mg q24h. A supplemental dose of 250mg-500mg after dialysis is recommended.

HOW SUPPLIED: Inj: 500mg/5mL; Sol: 100mg/mL; Tab: 250mg*, 500mg*, 750mg*, 1000mg* *scored

WARNINGS/PRECAUTIONS: Increased risk of suicidal thoughts or behavior reported; monitor for emergence or worsening of depression, suicidal thoughts/behavior and any unusual changes in mood or behavior. Associated with somnolence, fatigue, coordination difficulties and behavioral abnormalities (eg, psychotic symptoms, suicidal ideation and other abnormalities). Avoid abrupt withdrawal. Hematologic abnormalities reported. May impair physical/mental abilities. Caution with moderate to severe renal impairment and hemodialysis. Caution in elderly.

ADVERSE REACTIONS: Somnolence, asthenia, headache, infection, pain, anorexia, dizziness, nervousness, vertigo, ataxia, pharyngitis, rhinitis, irritability, vomiting, diarrhea.

INTERACTIONS: (PO) Increased clearance with enzyme-inducing antiepileptic drugs in pediatrics.

PREGNANCY: Category C, not for use in nursing.

MECHANISM OF ACTION: Pyrrolidine derivative; not established. Proposed to inhibit burst firing without affecting normal neuronal excitability, suggesting that it may selectively prevent hypersynchronization of epileptiform burst firing and propagation of seizure activity.

PHARMACOKINETICS: Absorption: Rapid; absolute bioavailability (100%); T_{max}=1 hr. **Distribution:** Plasma protein binding (<10%); found in breast milk. **Metabolism:** Enzymatic hydrolysis (not extensive); ucbL057 (metabolite). **Elimination:** Urine (66%, unchanged); $T_{1/2}$=7 hrs.

NURSING CONSIDERATIONS

Assessment: Assess for renal impairment, depression, suicidal thoughts/behavior, pregnancy/nursing status and possible drug interactions prior to therapy.

Monitoring: Monitor for CNS adverse effects such as somnolence, fatigue, coordination difficulties (ataxia, incoordination), behavioral abnormalities (agitation, anger, emotional lability), suicide ideation, emergence or worsening of depression, suicidal thoughts/behavior and any unusual changes in mood or behavior. Monitor renal function and hematological changes (RBCs, WBCs).

Patient Counseling: Instruct to take drug exactly as directed. Advise not to drive or operate heavy machinery until accustomed to the effects of medication. Monitor for changes in behavior (eg, aggression, anxiety, apathy, depression, irritability), psychotic symptoms and/or suicidal ideation. Notify if pregnant or intend to become pregnant. Encourage patients to enroll in North American Antiepileptic Drug (NAAED) Pregnancy Registry by calling 888-233-2334 or at UCB AED Pregnancy Registry by calling 888-537-7734 or go to aedpregnancyregistry.org.

Administration: Oral/IV route. Injection must be diluted prior to administration. Dilute in 100mL of compatible diluent (see PI). **Storage:** 25°C (77°F); excursions permitted to 15-30°C (59-86°F). Following IV dilution: Stable for 24 hrs at controlled room temperature 15-30°C (59-86°F).

KEPPRA XR   RX
levetiracetam (UCB)

THERAPEUTIC CLASS: Pyrrolidine derivative

INDICATIONS: Adjunct therapy for treatment of partial onset seizures in patients ≥16 yrs with epilepsy.

DOSAGE: *Adults:* Individualize dose. Initial: 1000mg qd. Titrate: Adjust dose in increments of 1000mg every 2 weeks. Max: 3000mg/day. CrCl >80mL/min/1.73m²: 1000-3000mg q24h. CrCl 50-80mL/min/1.73m²: 1000-2000mg q24h. CrCl 30-50mL/min/1.73m²: 500-1500mg q24h. CrCl <30mL/min/1.73m²: 500-1000mg q24h. Swallow tab whole; do not chew, break, or crush.
Pediatrics: ≥16 yrs: Initial: 1000mg qd. Titrate: Adjust dose in increments of 1000mg every 2 weeks. Max: 3000mg/day. Swallow tab whole; do not chew, break, or crush.

HOW SUPPLIED: Tab, Extended-Release: 500mg, 750mg

WARNINGS/PRECAUTIONS: Increased risk of suicidal thoughts or behavior reported; monitor for emergence or worsening of depression, suicidal thoughts/behavior, and any unusual changes in mood or behavior. May cause somnolence, dizziness, fatigue, coordination difficulties, and behavioral abnormalities (eg, psychotic symptoms, suicidal ideation, and other abnormalities). Withdraw gradually to minimize the potential of increased seizure frequency. Hematologic abnormalities and changes in LFTs may occur. Caution in renal impairment, hemodialysis, and elderly.

ADVERSE REACTIONS: Somnolence, influenza, nasopharyngitis, irritability, dizziness, nausea.

INTERACTIONS: Decreased metabolite renal clearance with probenecid.

PREGNANCY: Category C, not for use in nursing.

MECHANISM OF ACTION: Pyrrolidine derivative; mechanism not established. Proposed to inhibit burst firing without affecting normal neuronal excitability, suggesting that it may selectively prevent hypersynchronization of epileptiform burst firing and propagation of seizure activity.

PHARMACOKINETICS: Absorption: Almost complete. T_{max}=4 hrs.
Distribution: Plasma protein binding (<10%); found in breast milk.
Metabolism: Enzymatic hydrolysis (not extensive); ucbL057 (metabolite).
Elimination: Urine (66%, unchanged); $T_{1/2}$=7 hrs.

NURSING CONSIDERATIONS

Assessment: Assess for seizures, renal impairment, depression, suicidal thoughts/behavior, unusual changes in mood/behavior, hematologic disorders, pregnancy/nursing status and possible drug interactions prior to therapy.

Monitoring: Monitor for CNS adverse effects such as somnolence, fatigue, coordination difficulties (ataxia, incoordination), behavioral abnormalities (agitation, anger, emotional lability), suicidal ideation. Monitor for hematological changes (RBC, WBC), changes in LFTs and renal function.

Patient Counseling: Instruct to take drug exactly as directed. Advise not to drive or operate heavy machinery until accustomed to the effects of medication as dizziness and somnolence may occur. Advise patient, family, and caregivers to be alert of signs of behavior changes (eg, agitation, anger, anxiety, apathy, depression, hostility, irritability, psychotic symptoms), suicidal ideation, worsening of depression, thoughts about self-harm; notify physician if these and other adverse reaction occur. Advise that product may cause irritability and aggression. Notify physician if pregnant or intend to become pregnant. Encourage patients to enroll in North American Antiepileptic Drug (NAAED) Pregnancy Registry by calling 888-233-2334 or go to aedpregnancyregistry.org.

Administration: Oral route. Swallow tab whole; do not chew, break, or crush.
Storage: 25°C (77°F); excursions permitted to 15-30°C (59-86°F).

KETEK   RX
telithromycin (Sanofi-Aventis)

> Contraindicated with myasthenia gravis. Fatal and life-threatening respiratory failure in patients with myasthenia gravis reported.

THERAPEUTIC CLASS: Ketolide antibiotic

INDICATIONS: Treatment of mild to moderate community-acquired pneumonia (CAP) due to susceptible strains of microorganisms for patients ≥18 yrs.

DOSAGE: *Adults:* 800mg qd for 7-10 days. Severe Renal Impairment (CrCl <30mL/min) including Patients Who Need Dialysis: 600mg qd. Hemodialysis: Give after dialysis session on dialysis days. Severe Renal Impairment (CrCl <30mL/min) with Hepatic Impairment: 400mg qd.

HOW SUPPLIED: Tab: 300mg, 400mg

CONTRAINDICATIONS: Myasthenia gravis, history of hepatitis and/or jaundice associated with use of telithromycin or any macrolide antibiotic, hypersensitivity to macrolide antibiotics, concomitant use with cisapride or pimozide, and concomitant use with colchicine in patients with renal or hepatic impairment.

WARNINGS/PRECAUTIONS: Acute hepatic failure and severe liver injury, including fulminant hepatitis and hepatic necrosis reported; monitor closely and d/c if any signs/symptoms of hepatitis occur. Permanently d/c if hepatitis or transaminase elevations combined with systemic symptoms occur. May prolong QTc interval leading to risk for ventricular arrhythmias including torsades de pointes; avoid in patients with congenital prolongation, ongoing proarrhythmic conditions (eg, uncorrected hypokalemia/hypomagnesemia), and significant bradycardia. Visual disturbances and loss of consciousness reported; minimize hazardous activities such as driving and operating heavy machinery. *Clostridium difficile*-associated diarrhea (CDAD) reported. Unlikely to provide benefit and increases risk of drug resistance if used in the absence of bacterial infection or for prophylactic indication.

ADVERSE REACTIONS: Diarrhea, nausea, headache, dizziness.

INTERACTIONS: See Contraindications. Increases levels of drugs metabolized by the CYP450 system (eg, carbamazepine, cyclosporine, tacrolimus, sirolimus, hexobarbital, phenytoin), especially CYP3A4. Avoid simvastatin, lovastatin, atorvastatin, rifampin, ergot alkaloid derivatives (eg, ergotamine, dihydroergotamine), Class IA (eg, quinidine, procainamide) or Class III (eg, dofetilide) antiarrhythmics. Increased risk of myopathy and rhabdomyolysis with HMG-CoA reductase inhibitors. Caution with benzodiazepines metabolized by CYP3A4 (eg, triazolam). Caution with metoprolol in patients with heart failure. Increased levels with itraconazole, ketoconazole. Monitor with midazolam, digoxin. Decreased effects with CYP3A4 inducers (eg, phenytoin, carbamazepine, phenobarbital). Decreased levels of sotalol. Increased levels of levonorgestrel. Space dosing of theophylline by 1 hr to reduce GI effects. Concomitant administration with oral anticoagulants may potentiate effects of the oral anticoagulants. May cause hypotension, bradyarrhythmia, and loss of consciousness with calcium channel blockers metabolized by CYP3A4 (eg, verapamil, amlodipine, diltiazem). May increase levels of substrates of OATP1 (B1, B3) family members.

PREGNANCY: Category C, caution in nursing.

MECHANISM OF ACTION: Ketolide antibiotic; blocks protein synthesis by binding to domains II and V of 23S rRNA of 50S ribosomal subunit and may also inhibit assembly of nascent ribosomal units.

PHARMACOKINETICS: Absorption: Absolute bioavailability (57%); C_{max}=1.9µg/mL (single dose), 2.27µg/mL (multiple dose); T_{max}=1 hr (single/multiple dose); $AUC_{(0-24)}$=8.25µg•hr/mL (single dose), 12.5µg•hr/mL (multiple dose). **Distribution:** V_d=2.9L/kg; plasma protein binding (60-70%). **Metabolism:** Via CYP3A4 dependent and independent pathways. **Elimination:** Urine (13% unchanged); feces (7% unchanged); $T_{1/2}$=7.16 hrs (single dose), 9.81 hrs (multiple dose).

NURSING CONSIDERATIONS

Assessment: Assess for myasthenia gravis, history of hepatitis and/or jaundice, previous hypersensitivity to telithromycin or macrolides, renal/hepatic impairment, LFTs, QTc prolongation risk (eg, congenital prolongation, proarrhythmic conditions, significant bradycardia), pregnancy/nursing status, and possible drug interactions. Document indications for therapy, culture, and susceptibility testing.

Monitoring: Monitor LFTs and ECG for QTc prolongation. Monitor for visual disturbances, hepatitis, loss of consciousness associated with vagal syndrome, renal impairment, CDAD, pancreatitis, and allergic reactions (eg, angioedema, anaphylaxis).

Patient Counseling: Inform that therapy treats bacterial, not viral, infections. Advise to take as directed; skipping doses or not completing full course may decrease effectiveness and increase antibiotic resistance. Advise that therapy is contraindicated with myasthenia gravis. Instruct to d/c and seek medical attention if signs and symptoms of liver injury develop (eg, nausea, fatigue, anorexia, jaundice, dark urine, light colored stools, pruritus, tender abdomen). Instruct to report any fainting during therapy and to inform physician of history of QTc prolongation, proarrhythmic conditions, or significant bradycardia. Advise to contact physician if diarrhea (watery/bloody stools) occurs. Advise against operating machinery or driving and to seek physician's advice if visual difficulties, loss of consciousness, confusion, or hallucination is experienced. Advise to inform physician of any other medications taken concurrently with telithromycin.

Administration: Oral route. Can be given with or without food. **Storage:** 25°C (77°F); excursions permitted to 15-30°C (59-86°F).

KETOROLAC RX
ketorolac tromethamine (Various)

> For short-term use only (≤5 days). Contraindicated with peptic ulcer disease, GI bleeding/perforation, perioperative pain in coronary artery bypass graft (CABG) surgery, advanced renal impairment, risk of renal failure due to volume depletion, cerebrovascular bleeding, hemorrhagic diathesis, incomplete hemostasis, high-risk of bleeding, intrathecal/epidural use, labor and delivery, nursing, and with concurrent ASA or NSAIDs. Greater risk of GI events with elderly patients. May cause an increased risk of cardiovascular (CV) thrombotic events (MI, stroke). Contraindicated in pediatric patients and for minor or chronic painful conditions.

THERAPEUTIC CLASS: NSAID

INDICATIONS: Short-term (≤5 days) management of moderately severe acute pain that requires analgesia at the opioid level.

DOSAGE: Adults: >16 yrs to <65 yrs: Single-Dose: 60mg IM or 30mg IV. Multiple-Dose: 30mg IM/IV q6h. Max: 120mg/day. Transition from IM/IV to PO: 20mg PO single dose, then 10mg PO q4-6h prn. Max: 40mg/24 hrs. ≥65 yrs/Renal Impairment/<50kg: Single-Dose: 30mg IM or 15mg IV. Multiple-Dose: 15mg IM/IV q6h. Max: 60mg/day. Transition from IM/IV to PO: 10mg PO q4-6h prn. Max: 40mg/24 hrs.

HOW SUPPLIED: Inj: 15mg/mL, 30mg/mL; Tab: 10mg

CONTRAINDICATIONS: History or currently active peptic ulcer, recent GI bleeding/perforation, treatment of perioperative pain in CABG surgery, advanced renal impairment or risk of renal failure due to volume depletion, labor/delivery, nursing mothers, ASA or NSAID allergy, use as prophylactic analgesia before surgery, cerebrovascular bleeding, hemorrhagic diathesis, incomplete hemostasis, high risk of bleeding, neuraxial (epidural or intrathecal) administration, and concomitant ASA, NSAIDs, probenecid, or pentoxifylline.

WARNINGS/PRECAUTIONS: Do not exceed 5 days of therapy. Risk of GI ulcerations, bleeding, and perforation. Caution with renal/hepatic dysfunction, dehydration, HTN, CHF, coagulation disorders, pre-existing asthma. Preoperative use prolongs bleeding. CV thrombotic events, fluid retention, edema, NaCl retention, oliguria, anaphylactic reactions, elevated BUN and SrCr, anemia reported. Correct hypovolemia before therapy. Caution in elderly.

ADVERSE REACTIONS: Nausea, dyspepsia, abdominal pain, diarrhea, edema, headache, drowsiness, dizziness.

INTERACTIONS: May increase risk of serious bleeding with anticoagulants. May reduce diuretic response to furosemide and thiazide diuretics. Increased serum levels with salicylates. Avoid ASA, NSAIDs, and probenecid. Increased lithium and methotrexate levels. May increase risk of renal impairment with ACE-inhibitors/angiotension receptor angtagonist. May increase seizures with phenytoin and carbamazepine. Hallucinations reported with fluoxetine, thiothixene, and alprazolam. May cause apnea with nondepolarizing muscle relaxants.

PREGNANCY: Category C, not for use in nursing.

MECHANISM OF ACTION: NSAID; suspected to inhibit prostaglandin synthetase; exerts anti-inflammatory, analgesic, and antipyretic actions.

PHARMACOKINETICS: Absorption: Absolute oral bioavailability (100%). **Distribution:** V_d=13L; plasma protein binding (99%); enters breast milk. **Metabolism:** Liver; hydroxylation, conjugation. **Elimination:** Urine (92%; 40% metabolites, 60% unchanged), feces (6%); $T_{1/2}$=5-6 hrs.

NURSING CONSIDERATIONS

Assessment: Assess LFTs, renal function, CBC, and coagulation profile. Assess for history of asthma and allergic reactions to aspirin or other NSAIDs, active ulceration or chronic inflammation of GI tract, CVD, pregnancy status. Note other diseases/conditions and drug therapies.

Monitoring: Monitor for hypersensitivity reactions, cardiac complications, stroke, GI bleeding, asthma, dermatological side effects. Monitor BP, LFTs, renal function, CBC with differential and platelet count, coagulation profile, and ophthalmic exams.

Patient Counseling: Counsel about side effects; seek medical attention if any occur. Avoid alcohol and smoking during treatment. Advise to take exactly as prescribed. Notify physician if signs of CV side effects (chest pain, SOB, weakness), GI bleeding (epigastric pain, dyspepsia), skin rash, unexplained weight gain, hepatotoxicity (nausea, fatigue) occur. Caution women against using late in pregnancy. Inform that drug is used as continuation treatment following IM or IV dosing and should not exceed 5 days.

Administration: IM/IV/Oral routes. **Storage:** 15-30°C (59-86°F).

KINERET RX
anakinra (Amgen)

THERAPEUTIC CLASS: Interleukin-1 receptor antagonist

INDICATIONS: Reduce the signs/symptoms and slow the progression of structural damage in moderately to severely active rheumatoid arthritis (RA), in patients 18 yrs of age or older who have failed 1 or more disease modifying antirheumatic drugs (DMARDs). Can be used alone or in combination with DMARDs other than TNF blocking agents.

DOSAGE: *Adults:* ≥18 yrs: 100mg SQ qd at approximately same time every day. CrCl <30mL/min: 100mg SQ qod.

HOW SUPPLIED: Inj: 100mg/0.67mL

CONTRAINDICATIONS: Hypersensitivity to *E.coli*-derived proteins.

WARNINGS/PRECAUTIONS: Increased incidence of serious infections alone and in combination with etanercept. D/C if serious infection or if a hypersensitivity reaction occurs. Do not initiate with active infection. Decrease in neutrophil count may be experienced; obtain neutrophil count before therapy, monthly for 3 months, and thereafter quarterly for up to 1 yr. Needle cover of prefilled syringe contains dry latex rubber; caution in patients who are sensitive to latex. Caution in elderly.

ADVERSE REACTIONS: Serious infections, neutropenia, injection-site reactions, headache, nausea, diarrhea, infections, malignancy, worsening RA, abdominal pain, sinusitis, arthralgia, flu-like symptoms, URI.

INTERACTIONS: Neutropenia and higher rate of infections reported with etanercept; use with Tumor Necrosis Factor (TNF) blocking agents is not recommended. Avoid concomitant use with live vaccines.

PREGNANCY: Category B, caution in nursing.

MECHANISM OF ACTION: Interleukin-1 receptor antagonist; blocks biologic activity of IL-1 by competitively inhibiting IL-1 binding to the interleukin-1 type I receptor (IL-1RI), which is expressed in a wide variety of tissues and organs.

PHARMACOKINETICS: Absorption: Absolute bioavailability (95%); T_{max}=3-7 hrs. **Elimination:** $T_{1/2}$=4-6 hrs.

NURSING CONSIDERATIONS

Assessment: Assess for known hypersensitivity to *E.coli*-derived proteins, active infection, immunosuppression, severe renal insufficiency or end-stage renal disease, pregnancy/nursing status, and possible drug interactions. Obtain neutrophil count.

Monitoring: Monitor for signs/symptoms of serious infections (eg, cellulitis, pneumonia, bone and joint infections), hypersensitivity reactions, neutropenia, and malignancies (eg, lymphomas). Monitor neutrophil count monthly for 3 months, and quarterly thereafter for up to a year.

Patient Counseling: Advise to avoid receiving live vaccines while on therapy. Counsel about proper dosage, administration, and disposal of medication; caution against reuse of needles, syringes, and drug product. Not to be taken in combination with TNF-blocking agents. Counsel about signs/symptoms of allergic and adverse drug reactions. If severe hypersensitivity reaction occurs, d/c medication and start appropriate therapy. Advise that needle cover of prefilled syringe contains dry natural rubber, which may cause allergic reactions in latex-sensitive individuals.

Administration: SQ route. **Storage:** 2-8°C (36-46°F). Do not freeze or shake. Protect from light.

KLONOPIN

clonazepam (Roche Labs)

OTHER BRAND NAMES: Clonazepam ODT (Barr)

THERAPEUTIC CLASS: Benzodiazepine

INDICATIONS: Adjunct or monotherapy in the treatment of Lennox-Gastaut syndrome, akinetic and myoclonic seizures. May be useful with absence seizures who have failed to respond to succinimides. Treatment of panic disorder with or without agoraphobia.

DOSAGE: *Adults:* Seizure Disorders: Initial: Not to exceed 1.5mg/day given tid. Titrate: May increase in increments of 0.5-1mg every 3 days until seizures are controlled or until side effects preclude any further increase. Max: 20mg/day. Elderly: Start at low end of dosing range. Panic Disorder: Initial: 0.25mg bid. Titrate: Increase to 1mg/day after 3 days, then may increase in increments of 0.125-0.25mg bid every 3 days until panic disorder is controlled or until side effects preclude any further increase. Max: 4mg/day. Elderly: Start at low end of dosing range.
Pediatrics: Seizure Disorders: ≤10 yrs or 30kg: Initial: 0.01-0.03mg/kg/day up to 0.05mg/kg/day given bid-tid. Titrate: May increase by no more than 0.25-0.5mg every 3 days until maintenance dose is reached, unless seizures are controlled or until side effects preclude any further increase. Maint: 0.1-0.2mg/kg/day.

HOW SUPPLIED: Tab: 0.5mg*, 1mg, 2mg; Tab, Disintegrating: (Generic) 0.125mg, (Generic) 0.25mg, 0.5mg, 1mg, 2mg *scored

CONTRAINDICATIONS: Significant liver disease, open-angle glaucoma untreated, acute narrow-angle glaucoma.

WARNINGS/PRECAUTIONS: May impair physical/mental abilities. May increase risk of suicidal thoughts or behavior; monitor for the emergence or worsening of depression, suicidal thoughts or behavior, and/or any unusual changes in mood or behavior. Caution with use in pregnancy and women of childbearing potential; may increase risk of congenital malformations. Caution with renal impairment. May increase incidence or precipitate the onset of generalized tonic-clonic seizures; addition of appropriate anticonvulsants or increase in their dosages may be required. Monitor blood counts and LFTs periodically with long-term therapy. May produce an increase in salivation; caution in patients with chronic respiratory diseases. Withdrawal symptoms reported after d/c of therapy. Avoid abrupt withdrawal; may precipitate status epilepticus. Caution with addiction-prone individals and in the elderly.

ADVERSE REACTIONS: Ataxia, drowsiness, coordination abnormal, depression, behavior problems, dizziness, upper respiratory tract infection, memory disturbance, dysmenorrhea, fatigue, influenza, nervousness, sinusitis.

INTERACTIONS: Decreased serum levels with CYP450 inducers (eg, phenytoin, carbamazepine, phenobarbital), and propantheline. Caution with CYP3A inhibitors (eg, oral antifungals). Alcohol, narcotics, barbiturates, nonbarbiturate hypnotics, antianxiety agents, phenothiazines, thioxanthene and butyrophenone antipsychotics, monoamine oxidase inhibitors (MAOIs), tricyclic antidepressants (TCAs), and other anticonvulsant drugs may potentiate CNS-depressant effects. Avoid alcohol. May produce absence status with valproic acid.

PREGNANCY: Category D, not for use in nursing.

MECHANISM OF ACTION: Benzodiazepine; not established. Suspected to enhance activity of gamma aminobutyric acid (GABA), the major inhibitory neurotransmitter in the CNS.

PHARMACOKINETICS: Absorption: Rapid and complete. Absolute bioavailability (90%); T_{max}=1-4 hrs. **Distribution:** Plasma protein binding (85%). **Metabolism:** Liver via CYP450, then acetylation, hydroxylation, and glucuronidation. **Elimination:** Urine (<2% unchanged); $T_{1/2}$=30-40 hrs.

NURSING CONSIDERATIONS

Assessment: Assess for acute narrow-angle glaucoma, untreated open angle glaucoma, renal impairment, hepatic impairment, mental depression, history of drug or alcohol addiction, chronic respiratory diseases, pregnancy/nursing status, and for possible drug interactions.

Monitoring: Monitor for CNS depression, emergence or worsening of depression, suicidal thoughts or behavior, unusual changes in mood or behavior, and for worsening of seizures. In patients on prolonged therapy, perform periodic blood counts and monitor LFTs. Upon withdrawal, monitor for withdrawal symptoms and monitor for status epilepticus with abrupt withdrawal.

Patient Counseling: Instruct to take medication only as prescribed. Advise to inform physician if taking, or planning to take any prescription or OTC drugs and to avoid alcohol while on therapy. Inform that therapy may impair judgement, thinking or motor skills; advise to use caution while operating hazardous machinery including automobiles. Inform that therapy may produce physical and psychological dependence; instruct to consult physician before either increasing the dose or abruptly discontinuing the drug. Advise not to breast-feed while on therapy. Counsel that drug may increase risk of suicidal thoughts/behavior and advise of need to be alert for the emergence/worsening of symptoms of depression, or any unusual changes in mood or behavior. Advise to notify physician if patient becomes pregnant or intends to become pregnant during therapy.

Administration: Oral route. Tab, Disintegrating: 1) Peel back foil on blister. Do not push tablet through foil. 2) Using dry hands, remove tablet and place it in mouth. **Storage:** 25°C (77°F); excursions permitted to 15-30°C (59-86°F). Tab, Disintegrating: (Generic) 20-25°C (68-77°F).

KLOR-CON M   RX

potassium chloride (Upsher-Smith)

OTHER BRAND NAMES: Klor-Con (Upsher-Smith)

THERAPEUTIC CLASS: K⁺ supplement

INDICATIONS: Treatment of hypokalemia with or without metabolic alkalosis, in digitalis intoxication, and in patients with hypokalemic familial periodic paralysis. Prevention of hypokalemia in patients at risk (eg, digitalized patients, cardiac arrhythmias).

DOSAGE: *Adults:* Individualize dose. Prevention: 20mEq/day. Hypokalemia: 40-100mEq/day. Divide dose if >20mEq. Elderly: Start at low end of dosing range. Take with meals and fluids. (Klor-Con Extended-Release Tab): Swallow tab whole; do not crush, chew, or suck. (Klor-Con M) May break Klor-Con M in half or mix with 4 ounces of water.

HOW SUPPLIED: (Klor-Con M) Tab, Extended-Release: 10mEq, 15mEq, 20mEq; (Klor-Con) Pow: 20mEq, 25mEq; Tab, Extended-Release: 8mEq, 10mEq

CONTRAINDICATIONS: (Tab, ER) Hyperkalemia, cardiac patients with esophageal compression due to an enlarged left atrium. Structural, pathological (eg, diabetic gastroparesis) or pharmacological (eg, use of anticholinergic agents or other agents with anticholinergic properties) cause for arrest or delay through the GI tract with all solid dosage forms. (Powder) Hyperkalemia.

WARNINGS/PRECAUTIONS: (Tab, Extended-Release; Powder) Potentially fatal hyperkalemia and cardiac arrest may occur; monitor serum K^+ levels and adjust dose appropriately. Extreme caution with acidosis and cardiac and renal disease; monitor ECG and electrolytes. Hypokalemia with metabolic acidosis should be treated with an alkalinizing K^+ salt (eg, K^+ bicarbonate, K^+ citrate, K^+ acetate, K^+ gluconate). (Tab, Extended-Release) Solid oral dosage forms may produce ulcerative and/or stenotic lesions of the GI tract; d/c use if severe vomiting, abdominal pain, distention or GI bleeding occurs. Reserve use of ER preparations for those who cannot tolerate, cannot comply, or refuse to take liquid or effervescent preparations. Caution in elderly.

ADVERSE REACTIONS: Hyperkalemia, GI effects (eg, obstruction, bleeding, ulceration), N/V, abdominal pain/discomfort, flatulence, diarrhea.

INTERACTIONS: (Tab, Extended-Release) See Contraindications. Risk of hyperkalemia with ACE inhibitors (eg, captopril, enalapril). (Tab, Extended-Release; Powder) Risk of hyperkalemia with K^+-sparing diuretics (eg, spironolactone, triamterene, amiloride).

PREGNANCY: Category C, (Tab, Extended-Release) Safe for use in nursing, (Powder) caution in nursing.

MECHANISM OF ACTION: K^+ supplement (electrolyte replenisher); participates in a number of essential physiological processes, including the maintenance of intracellular tonicity, the transmission of nerve impulses, the contraction of cardiac, skeletal, and smooth muscle, and the maintenance of normal renal function.

PHARMACOKINETICS: Absorption: (Klor-Con Extended-Release Tab) GI tract. **Elimination:** (Klor-Con Extended-Release Tab) Urine and feces.

NURSING CONSIDERATIONS

Assessment: Assess for hyperkalemia, chronic renal failure, systemic acidosis, cardiac patients, if patient cannot tolerate, refuses to take, or cannot comply with taking liquid or effervescent K+ preparations prior to administration of an ER tab formulation. Obtain baseline ECG, serum electrolyte levels, and renal function.

Monitoring: Monitor for signs/symptoms of hyperkalemia and other adverse events that may occur. In patients taking solid oral dosage forms, monitor for signs/symptoms of GI lesions. In patients with cardiac disease, acidosis, or renal disease, monitor acid-base balance and perform appropriate monitoring of serum electrolytes, ECG, renal function, and the clinical status of the patient.

Patient Counseling: Inform about benefits and risks of therapy. Report to physician if develop any type of GI symptoms (eg, tarry stools or other evidence of GI bleeding, vomiting, abdominal pain/distention) or if other adverse events occur. Instruct to contact physician if develop difficulty swallowing or if the tablets are sticking in the throat. (Klor-Con): Swallow tablets whole and to take with meals and full glass of water or other liquid. Follow the frequency and amount prescribed by the physician, especially if also taking diuretics and/or digitalis preparations. (Klor-Con M): Take each dose with meals and with full glass of water or other liquid. Inform that may break tablets in half or make an oral aqueous suspension with tablets and 4 oz. of water (see PI for proper preparation). Inform that aqueous suspension not taken immediately should be discarded and use of other liquids for suspending is not recommended.

Administration: Oral route. (Klor-Con M) Refer to PI for preparation of aqueous suspension. **Storage:** (Klor-Con): 15-30°C (59-86°F). (Klor-Con M): 20-25°C (68-77°F); excursions permitted to 15-30°C (59-86°F).

KOMBIGLYZE XR
RX

metformin HCl - saxagliptin (Bristol-Myers Squibb/ AstraZeneca)

> Lactic acidosis may occur due to metformin accumulation; risk increases with conditions such as sepsis, dehydration, excess alcohol intake, hepatic impairment, renal impairment, and acute congestive heart failure (CHF). If suspected, d/c and hospitalize patient immediately.

THERAPEUTIC CLASS: Dipeptidyl peptidase-4 inhibitor/biguanide

INDICATIONS: Adjunct to diet and exercise, to improve glycemic control in type 2 diabetes mellitus (DM) when treatment with both saxagliptin and metformin is appropriate.

DOSAGE: *Adults:* Individualize dose. Take qd with evening meal, with gradual dose escalation to reduce GI side effects of metformin. Patient Treated with Metformin: Dose should provide metformin at the dose already being taken, or the nearest therapeutically appropriate dose. If switched from metformin IR to ER; monitor glycemic control and dose adjust accordingly. Starting Dose in Patients who need 5mg of Saxagliptin and not Currently Treated with Metformin: 5mg saxagliptin-500mg metformin. Starting Dose in Patients who need 2.5mg of Saxagliptin in Combination with Metformin XR: 2.5mg saxagliptin-1000mg metformin. Use individual components if need 2.5mg saxagliptin and are either metformin naive or require a dose of metformin higher than 1000mg. Max: 5mg saxagliptin-2000mg metformin. Limit the saxagliptin dose to 2.5mg (2.5mg/1000mg) qd if coadministered with strong CYP3A4/5 inhibitors.

HOW SUPPLIED: Tab, Extended-Release: (Saxagliptin-Metformin) 5mg-500mg, 5mg-1000mg, 2.5-1000mg

CONTRAINDICATIONS: Renal impairment (eg, SrCr ≥1.5mg/dL [men], ≥1.4mg/dL [women], or abnormal CrCl), acute or chronic metabolic acidosis, including diabetic ketoacidosis. D/C temporarily in patients undergoing radiologic studies involving intravascular administration of iodinated contrast materials.

WARNINGS/PRECAUTIONS: Not for the treatment of type 1 DM or diabetic ketoacidosis. Risk of lactic acidosis increases with the degree of renal dysfunction, presence of CHF, and patient's age. Avoid use in patients ≥80 yrs unless renal function is not reduced. Monitor renal function. Lactic acidosis should be suspected in diabetic patients with metabolic acidosis lacking evidence of ketoacidosis (ketonuria and ketonemia). May decrease vitamin B_{12} levels; monitor hematological parameters annually. Caution against excessive alcohol intake. Temporarily d/c for any surgical procedure (except minor procedures not associated with restricted intake of foods and fluids); do not restart until oral intake has resumed and renal function has been evaluated as normal. D/C in hypoxic states (eg, shock, CHF, acute MI). Avoid in patients with hepatic impairment. Increased risk of hypoglycemia in elderly, debilitated/malnourished, adrenal or pituitary insufficiency, or alcohol intoxication.

ADVERSE REACTIONS: Lactic acidosis, diarrhea, N/V, upper respiratory tract infection, UTI, headache, nasopharyngitis.

INTERACTIONS: See Contraindications. (Metformin) Concomitant use with cationic drugs that are eliminated by renal tubular secretion (eg, cimetidine, digoxin, amiloride, procainamide, quinidine, quinine, ranitidine, trimethoprim, vancomycin, triamterene, morphine) may potentially produce an interaction; monitor and dose adjust if necessary. Thiazides and other diuretics, corticosteroids, phenothiazines, thyroid products, estrogens, oral contraceptives, phenytoin, nicotinic acid, sympathomimetics, calcium channel blockers, and isoniazid may predispose to hyperglycemia and may lead to loss of glycemic control. Alcohol potentiates the effect of metformin on lactate metabolism. Less likely to interact with highly protein-bound drugs such as salicylates, sulfonamides, chloramphenicol, and probenecid. Caution with drugs that may affect renal function or result in significant hemodynamic change or may interfere with the disposition of metformin. Hypoglycemia may occur with concomitant use of other glucose-lowering agents (eg, sulfonylureas, insulin). (Saxagliptin) Increased plasma concentrations with ketoconazole and other strong CYP3A4/5 inhibitors (eg, atazanavir, clarithromycin, indinavir, itraconazole, nefazodone, nelfinavir, ritonavir, saquinavir, and telithromycin); limit dose. Strong CYP3A4/5 inducers and inhibitors may alter pharmacokinetics of saxagliptin and its active metabolite. Lower dose of insulin secretagogues (eg, sulfonylureas) may be required to reduce the risk of hypoglycemia.

PREGNANCY: Category B, caution in nursing.

MECHANISM OF ACTION: Metformin: Biguanide; decreases hepatic glucose production, decreases intestinal absorption of glucose, and improves insulin sensitivity by increasing peripheral glucose uptake and utilization. **Saxagliptin:** Dipeptidyl peptidase-4 inhibitor; slows the inactivation of the incretin hormones and increases their bloodstream concentrations resulting in reduction of fasting and postprandial glucose concentrations in a glucose-dependent manner in type 2 DM.

PHARMACOKINETICS: Absorption: Saxagliptin: C_{max}= 24ng/mL; AUC=78ng•hr/mL; T_{max} = 2 hrs. 5-hydroxy saxagliptin: C_{max}=47ng/mL; AUC=214ng•hr/mL; T_{max} = 4 hrs. Metformin: T_{max}=7 hrs. **Distribution:** Metformin: V_d=654L. **Metabolism:** Saxagliptin: Hepatic via CYP3A4/5; 5-hydroxy saxagliptin (active metabolite). **Elimination:** Saxagliptin: Feces (22%), Urine (24% unchanged, 36% active metabolite); $T_{1/2}$= 2.5 hrs (saxagliptin), 3.1 hrs (active metabolite). Metformin: Urine (90%); $T_{1/2}$=6.2 hrs (plasma), 17.6 hrs (blood).

NURSING CONSIDERATIONS

Assessment: Assess for renal/hepatic impairment, type 1 DM, diabetic ketoacidosis, acute or chronic metabolic acidosis, presence of a hypoxic state (eg, CHF, acute MI, cardiovascular collapse), dehydration, sepsis, alcoholism, nutritional status, adrenal or pituitary insufficiency, pregnancy/nursing status, and for possible drug interactions. Assess baseline renal function, FPG, HbA1c, and hematological parameters. Evaluate for other medical/surgical conditions.

Monitoring: Monitor for lactic acidosis, hypoglycemia, and for decreases in Vitamin B_{12} levels. Monitor for prerenal azotemia in patients with hypoxic conditions. Monitor FPG, HbA1c, renal function (eg, SrCr), and hematological parameters.

Patient Counseling: Inform of the potential risks and benefits and of alternative modes of therapy. Inform about the importance of adherence to dietary instructions, regular physical activity, periodic blood glucose monitoring and A1C testing, regular testing of renal function and hematological parameters, recognition and management of hypoglycemia and hyperglycemia, and assessment of diabetes complications. Seek medical advice promptly during periods of stress (eg, fever, trauma, infection, or surgery, medication requirements). Inform of the risk of developing lactic acidosis during therapy; advise to d/c therapy immediately and contact physician if unexplained hyperventilation, myalgia, malaise, unusual somnolence, or other nonspecific symptoms occur. Counsel against excessive alcohol intake. Inform that incidence of hypoglycemia may be increased if insulin secretagogues (eg, sulfonylurea) are added. Swallow whole and do not chew, cut, or crush. Inactive ingredients may be eliminated in the feces as a soft mass.

Administration: Oral route. **Storage:** 20-25°C (68-77°F); excursions permitted to 15-30°C (59-86°F).

KRISTALOSE   RX
lactulose (Cumberland)

THERAPEUTIC CLASS: Osmotic laxative

INDICATIONS: Treatment of constipation.

DOSAGE: *Adults:* 10-20g/day. Max 40g/day. Dissolve pkt contents in 4oz. of water.

HOW SUPPLIED: Powder (crystals for suspension): 10g/pkt, 20g/pkt [1⁵, 30⁵]

CONTRAINDICATIONS: Patients who require a low galactose diet.

WARNINGS/PRECAUTIONS: Caution in DM due to galactose and lactose content. Monitor electrolytes periodically in elderly or debilitated if used for >6 months. Potential for explosive reaction with electrocautery procedures during proctoscopy or colonoscopy.

ADVERSE REACTIONS: Flatulence, intestinal cramps, diarrhea, N/V.

INTERACTIONS: Nonabsorbable antacids may decrease effects.

PREGNANCY: Category B, caution in nursing.

MECHANISM OF ACTION: Osmotic laxative; increases osmotic pressure and slight acidification of the colonic contents.

PHARMACOKINETICS: Absorption: Poorly absorbed from GI tract.
Elimination: Urine (≤3%).

NURSING CONSIDERATIONS

Assessment: Assess for DM, patients requiring a low-galactose diet.

Monitoring: Monitor serum electrolytes (potassium, sodium, chloride, carbon dioxide), diarrhea, vomiting.

Patient Counseling: May be diluted with fruit juice, water, or milk. Report any potential adverse effects.

Administration: Oral route. Dissolve contents of packet in 4 oz. of water.
Storage: Store 15-30°C (59-86°F).

KRYSTEXXA   RX
pegloticase (Savient)

> Anaphylaxis and infusion reactions reported during and after administration; generally mani-
> fests within 2 hrs of infusion. Delayed-type hypersensitivity reactions also reported. Closely
> monitor for an appropriate period of time for anaphylaxis after administration. Premedicate
> with antihistamines and corticosteroids. Monitor serum uric acid levels prior to infusions and
> consider d/c treatment if levels increase >6mg/dL, particularly when 2 consecutive levels
> >6mg/dL are observed.

THERAPEUTIC CLASS: Recombinant urate-oxidase enzyme

INDICATIONS: Treatment of chronic gout in adults refractory to conventional therapy.

DOSAGE: *Adults:* 8mg IV infusion q2 weeks. Do not administer as IV push or bolus.

HOW SUPPLIED: Inj: 8mg/mL

CONTRAINDICATIONS: Glucose-6-phosphate dehydrogenase (G6PD) deficiency.

WARNINGS/PRECAUTIONS: Not recommended for treatment of asymptomatic hyperuricemia. Gout flares may occur after initiation; gout flare prophylaxis with an NSAID or colchicine is recommended starting ≥1 week before initiation of therapy and lasting ≥6 months, unless medically contraindicated or not tolerated. Caution with congestive heart failure (CHF); monitor closely following infusion. May increase risk of anaphylaxis and infusion reactions in re-treated patients due to immunogenicity.

ADVERSE REACTIONS: Gout flare, infusion reaction, N/V, contusion/ecchymosis, nasopharyngitis, constipation, chest pain, anaphylaxis, delayed-type hypersensitivity reactions.

PREGNANCY: Category C, not for use in nursing.

MECHANISM OF ACTION: Recombinant urate-oxidase enzyme; catalyzes oxidation of uric acid to allantoin, thereby lowering serum uric acid.

NURSING CONSIDERATIONS

Assessment: Assess for G6PD deficiency, asymptomatic hyperuricemia, CHF, and pregnancy/nursing status. Obtain serum uric acid levels prior to infusion.

Monitoring: Monitor for signs/symptoms of anaphylaxis, infusion reactions, and gout flares. Monitor serum uric acid levels.

Patient Counseling: Inform to read Medication Guide, that anaphylaxis and infusion reactions can occur while on therapy, and about the importance of adherence to help prevent or lessen the severity of these reactions. Instruct to seek immediate medical attention if an allergic reaction occurs. Inform that gout flares may initially increase when starting therapy and that medications to help reduce flares may need to be taken regularly for the 1st few months after therapy is started. Instruct patients with G6PD deficiency not to take the drug.

Administration: IV route. Inspect for particulate matter and discoloration prior to administration. Do not mix or dilute with other drugs. Refer to PI for further preparation and administration instructions. **Storage:** 2-8°C (36-46°F). Protect from light. Do not shake or freeze. Diluted Sol: Stable for 4 hrs at 2-8°C (36-46°F) and at 20-25°C (68-77°F).

K-TAB
potassium chloride (Abbott)

RX

OTHER BRAND NAMES: Klotrix (Apothecon)

THERAPEUTIC CLASS: K+ supplement

INDICATIONS: (For those unable to tolerate liquid or effervescent potassium preparations). Treatment and prevention of hypokalemia with or without metabolic alkalosis. Treatment of digitalis intoxication and hypokalemic familial periodic paralysis.

DOSAGE: *Adults:* Prevention: 20mEq/day. Hypokalemia: 40-100mEq/day. Divide dose if >20mEq. Take with meals and full glass of water or liquid. Do not cut, crush or chew tab.

HOW SUPPLIED: Tab, Extended-Release: 10mEq

CONTRAINDICATIONS: Hyperkalemia, esophageal ulceration, delay in GI passage (from structural, pathological, pharmacologic causes), cardiac patients with esophageal compression due to enlarged left atrium.

WARNINGS/PRECAUTIONS: Potentially fatal hyperkalemia may occur. Extreme caution with acidosis, cardiac and renal disease; monitor ECG and electrolytes. Hypokalemia with metabolic acidosis should be treated with an alkalinizing potassium salt (eg, potassium bicarbonate, potassium citrate). May produce ulcerative or stenotic GI lesions. Use with caution in elderly due to decreased renal function, start dose at low end of dosing range.

ADVERSE REACTIONS: Hyperkalemia, GI effects (obstruction, bleeding, ulceration), nausea, vomiting, abdominal pain, flatulence, diarrhea.

INTERACTIONS: Risk of hyperkalemia with ACE inhibitors (eg, captopril, enalapril), potassium-sparing diuretics and potassium supplements. Contraindicated with anticholinergic agents due to possible delay in tablet passage through GI tract.

PREGNANCY: Category C, safe for use in nursing.

MECHANISM OF ACTION: K+ supplement (electrolyte replenisher). Slows release of K+, so likelihood of high localized concentrations of K+ within GI is reduced.

NURSING CONSIDERATIONS

Assessment: Assess for chronic renal disease, conditions that impair K+ excretion, esophageal compression due to enlarged left atrium, structural/pathologic cause for arrest/delay in passing through GI tract (eg, diabetic gastroparesis), and possible drug interactions. Obtain baseline serum K+ levels and renal function test.

Monitoring: Monitor serum K+ levels, renal function, ECG, and acid-base balance. Monitor for hyperkalemia, signs of acute metabolic acidosis, acute dehydration, GI ulcerations, and hypersensitivity reactions.

Patient Counseling: Instruct to report symptoms of GI bleeding (tarry stools), ulcerations/perforations (severe vomiting, abdominal pain, distention), trouble swallowing, or tablet sticking in throat. Take with meals and full glass of water. Swallow whole; do not crush, chew, or suck.

Administration: Oral route. **Storage:** Below 30°C (86°F).

KUVAN
sapropterin dihydrochloride (Biomarin)

RX

THERAPEUTIC CLASS: Synthetic tetrahydrobiopterin

INDICATIONS: To reduce blood phenylalanine (Phe) levels in patients with hyperphenylalaninemia (HPA) due to tetrahydrobiopterin-(BH4)-responsive phenylketonuria (PKU) in conjunction with a Phe-restricted diet.

DOSAGE: *Adults:* Initial: 10mg/kg/day qd. Titrate: Adjust dose within the range of 5-20mg/kg/day. Max: 20mg/kg/day. Take with food.

HOW SUPPLIED: Tab: 100mg

WARNINGS/PRECAUTIONS: Monitor blood Phe levels during treatment. Active management of dietary Phe intake is required to ensure Phe control and nutritional balance. Caution in patients with hepatic impairment. Monitor for allergic reactions.

ADVERSE REACTIONS: Headache, diarrhea, abdominal pain, upper respiratory tract infection, pharyngolaryngeal pain, N/V.

INTERACTIONS: Use with caution when coadministering with drugs that inhibit folate metabolism (eg, methotrexate). Use with caution when coadministered with PDE-5 inhibitors such as sildenafil and vardenafil; may induce vasorelaxation. May cause exacerbation of convulsions, overstimulation, or irritability when coadministered with levodopa.

PREGNANCY: Category C, caution in nursing.

MECHANISM OF ACTION: Synthetic tetrahydrobiopterin; activates residual phenylalanine hydroxylase (PAH) enzyme, improves the normal oxidative metabolism of phenylalanine, and decreases phenylalanine levels.

PHARMACOKINETICS: Elimination: $T_{1/2}$=6.7 hrs.

NURSING CONSIDERATIONS

Assessment: Assess for hepatic and renal impairment, pregnancy status, nursing status, and possible drug interactions. Obtain baseline blood phenylalanine levels.

Monitoring: Monitor for signs and symptoms of an allergic reaction. Monitor for response to treatment; blood phenylalanine levels should be checked one week after initiating treatment and periodically thereafter for up to one month. If no response at 20mg/kg/day after one month, d/c medication. Monitor dietary intake of phenylalanine. Monitor hepatic or renal function if impairment exists.

Patient Counseling: Inform that should be on a phenylalanine restricted diet. Instruct to take medication at the same time everyday with food. Dissolve tablet in 4-8 oz. (120-240mL) of water or apple juice; take within 15 min of dissolution. Instruct that if remnants still exist, add more water or apple juice to ensure that full dose is taken. Instruct that if miss a dose, take as soon as possible; do not take 2 doses on the same day. Notify physician of all medications currently taking or if pregnant. Contact physician if develop any signs of an allergic reaction.

Administration: Oral route. **Storage:** 20-25°C (68-77°F); excursions allowed between 15-30°(59-86°F). Keep container tightly closed. Protect from moisture.

KYTRIL   RX
granisetron HCl (Roche Labs)

THERAPEUTIC CLASS: 5-HT$_3$ receptor antagonist

INDICATIONS: (Inj, PO) Prevention of N/V associated with initial and repeated courses of emetogenic cancer therapy (eg, high-dose cisplatin). (Inj) Prevention and treatment of postoperative nausea and vomiting (PONV) in adults. (PO) Prevention of N/V associated with radiation (eg, total body irradiation and fractionated abdominal radiation).

DOSAGE: *Adults:* Emetogenic Chemotherapy: (PO) 2mg tab or 10mL sol qd up to 1 hr before chemotherapy or 1mg tab or 5mL sol bid up to 1 hr before chemotherapy and 12 hrs later. (IV) 10mcg/kg, undiluted over 30 sec or diluted (with 0.9% NaCl or 5% dextrose) over 5 min, within 30 min before chemotherapy. Prevention of N/V with Radiation: (PO) 2mg tab or 10mL sol qd within

1 hr of radiation. Prevention of PONV: (IV) 1mg undiluted over 30 sec before induction of anesthesia or immediately before anesthesia reversal. Treatment of PONV: (IV) 1mg undiluted over 30 sec.

Pediatrics: 2-16 yrs: Emetogenic Chemotherapy: 10mcg/kg IV within 30 min before chemotherapy.

HOW SUPPLIED: Inj: 0.1mg/mL [1mL single-use vial], 1mg/mL [1mL single-use vial, 4mL multi-use vial]; Sol: 2mg/10mL [30mL]; Tab: 1mg

WARNINGS/PRECAUTIONS: Does not stimulate gastric or intestinal peristalsis; do not use instead of nasogastric suction. May mask progressive ileus or gastric distension. Hypersensitivity reactions may occur in patients who exhibited hypersensitivity to other selective 5-HT$_3$ receptor antagonists. Granisetron 1mg/mL contains benzyl alcohol; neonatal adverse events (eg, gasping syndrome) reported. QT prolongation reported; caution if with pre-existing arrhythmias, cardiac conduction disorders, cardiac disease, or cardio-toxic chemotherapy and electrolyte abnormalities.

ADVERSE REACTIONS: Headache, asthenia, somnolence, diarrhea, constipation, abdominal pain, dizziness, insomnia, dyspepsia, anemia, fever, alopecia, increased hepatic enzymes, bradycardia, leukocytosis.

INTERACTIONS: Hepatic CYP450 enzyme inducers or inhibitors may alter clearance and $T_{1/2}$. Avoid use with drugs known to prolong QT interval and/or arrhythmogenic drugs.

PREGNANCY: Category B, caution in nursing.

MECHANISM OF ACTION: 5-HT$_3$ receptor antagonist; blocks serotonin stimulation and subsequent vomiting after emetogenic stimuli.

PHARMACOKINETICS: Absorption: C_{max}=63.8ng/mL (IV, 40mcg/kg), 5.99ng/mL (PO, 1mg bid). **Distribution:** Plasma protein binding (65%). V_d=3.07L/kg (IV, 40mcg/kg), 2.42L/kg (IV, 1mg bid). **Metabolism:** CYP3A4; N-demethylation, aromatic ring oxidation, conjugation. **Elimination:** (PO) Urine (11% unchanged, 48% metabolites), feces (38% metabolites). (IV) Urine (12% unchanged, 49% metabolites), feces (34% metabolites); $T_{1/2}$=8.95 hrs (IV, 40mcg/kg), 8.63 hrs (IV, 1mg).

NURSING CONSIDERATIONS

Assessment: Assess for N/V (chemotherapy-induced and post-operative), pre-existing arrhythmias, cardiac conduction disorders, cardiac disease, cardiotoxic chemotherapy, electrolyte abnormalities, hypersensitivity reactions, pregnancy/nursing status and possible drug interactions.

Monitoring: Monitor for progressive ileus, gastric distention, QT prolongation and hypersensitivity reactions.

Patient Counseling: Discuss risks and benefits of therapy. Advise patients to report any adverse events to their healthcare provider.

Administration: Oral, IV route. **Storage:** (Tab) 15-30°C (59-86°F). Keep container tightly closed. Protect from light. (Sol/Inj) 25°C (77°F); excursions permitted to 15-30°C (59-86°F). Protect from light. (Inj) Once the multi-use vial is penetrated, its contents should be used within 30 days. Do not freeze. (Sol) Keep bottle tightly closed in an upright position.

LABETALOL   RX
labetalol HCl (Various)

THERAPEUTIC CLASS: Nonselective beta-blocker/alpha$_1$ blocker

INDICATIONS: (Tab) Management of hypertension. (Inj) Management of severe hypertension.

DOSAGE: *Adults:* (Tab) HTN: Initial: 100mg bid. Titrate: 100mg bid every 2-3 days. Maint: 200-400mg bid. Severe HTN: 1200-2400mg/day given bid-tid. Increments should not exceed 200mg bid for titration. (Inj) Severe HTN: Administer in supine position. Repeated IV Infusion: Initial: 20mg over 2 min. Titrate: Give additional 40mg or 80mg at 10-min intervals if needed. Max: 300mg. Slow Continuous Infusion: 200mg at rate of 2mg/min. Usual Dose

Range: 50-200mg. Max: 300mg. May adjust dose according to BP. Switch to tabs when BP is stable while in hospital. Initial: 200mg, then 200-400mg 6-12 hrs later on Day 1. Titrate: May increase at 1-day interval.

HOW SUPPLIED: Inj: 5mg/mL; Tab: 100mg*, 200mg*, 300mg *scored

CONTRAINDICATIONS: Bronchial asthma, overt cardiac failure, >1st degree heart block, cardiogenic shock, severe bradycardia, other conditions associated with severe and prolonged hypotension, history of obstructive airway disease.

WARNINGS/PRECAUTIONS: Severe hepatocellular injury reported; caution with hepatic dysfunction. Monitor LFTs periodically; d/c at 1st sign of liver injury or jaundice. Caution in well-compensated patients with a history of heart failure; CHF may occur. Avoid abrupt withdrawal; may exacerbate ischemic heart disease. Avoid with bronchospastic disease and in overt cardiac failure. Caution with pheochromocytoma; paradoxical HTN reported. Caution with DM; may mask symptoms of hypoglycemia. Withdrawal before surgery is controversial. Several deaths reported during surgery. Caution when reducing severely elevated BP; cerebral infarction, optic nerve infarction, angina and ECG ischemic changes reported. Avoid injection with low cardiac indices and elevated systemic vascular resistance.

ADVERSE REACTIONS: Fatigue, dizziness, dyspepsia, N/V, nasal stuffiness, somnolence, ejaculation failure, postural hypotension, increased sweating, paresthesia.

INTERACTIONS: Increased tremors with TCAs. Potentiated by cimetidine; may need to reduce dose. Synergistic antihypertensive effects blunt the reflex tachycardia with nitroglycerin. Caution with calcium antagonists. May need to adjust dose of antidiabetic drugs. Antagonizes effects of β-agonists (bronchodilators). May block epinephrine effects. (Inj) Synergistic effects with halothane; do not use ≥3% halothane.

PREGNANCY: Category C, caution in nursing.

MECHANISM OF ACTION: α-1 and nonselective β-adrenergic receptor blocker; produces dose-related falls in BP without reflex tachycardia and significant reduction in heart rate.

PHARMACOKINETICS: Absorption: Complete; T_{max}=1-2 hrs. **Distribution**: Plasma protein binding (50%); found in breast milk; crosses placenta. **Metabolism**: Liver (conjugation and glucuronidation). **Elimination**: Urine (IV, 55%-60% unchanged), feces; (Tab) $T_{1/2}$=6-8 hrs, (IV) $T_{1/2}$=5.5 hrs.

NURSING CONSIDERATIONS

Assessment: Assess for bronchospastic disease, heart block, severe bradycardia, cardiogenic shock, overt cardiac failure, DM, pheochromocytoma, ischemic heart disease, severe or prolonged hypotension, hepatic impairment, history of heart failure, and possible drug interactions.

Monitoring: Monitor LFTs periodically. Monitor for signs/symptoms of cardiac failure, HTN, exacerbation of ischemia following abrupt withdrawal, bronchospastic disease, hypoglycemia, hypersensitivity reactions, and hepatic dysfunction.

Patient Counseling: Instruct to remain supine during and immediately following (for up to 3 hrs) injection; advise on how to proceed gradually to become ambulatory. Instruct not to interrupt or d/c therapy without consulting physician. Instruct to report signs/symptoms of cardiac failure or hepatic dysfunction (eg, pruritus, dark urine, persistent anorexia, jaundice, RUQ tenderness, or unexplained flu-like symptoms). Transient scalp itching may occur, usually when treatment with tabs is initiated.

Administration: Oral, IV route; refer to PI for administration technique. **Storage**: Tab: 15-30°C (59-86°F). IV: 20-25°C (68-77°F). Protect from light and freezing.

LACTULOSE

lactulose (Various)

RX

OTHER BRAND NAMES: Enulose (Alpharma) - Generlac (Morton Grove) - Constulose (Actavis)

THERAPEUTIC CLASS: Osmotic laxative

INDICATIONS: Treatment of constipation. Prevention and treatment of portal-systemic encephalopathy, including stages of hepatic pre-coma and coma.

DOSAGE: *Adults:* Constipation: 15-30mL qd. Max 60mL/day. May mix with fruit juice, water, or milk. Portal-Systemic Encephalopathy: 30-45mL tid-qid. Adjust dose every 1 or 2 days to produce 2-3 soft stools daily. Rectal Use: Reversal of Coma: Mix 300mL with 700mL of water or saline and retain for 30-60 min. May repeat q4-6h. Oral doses should be started before completely stopping enema.
Pediatrics: Portal-Systemic Encephalopathy: Older Children/Adolescents: 40-90mL/day divided tid-qid adjusted to produce 2-3 soft stools daily. *Infants:* 2.5-10mL in divided doses to produce 2-3 soft stools daily.

HOW SUPPLIED: Sol: 10g/15mL

CONTRAINDICATIONS: Patients who require a low galactose diet.

WARNINGS/PRECAUTIONS: Caution in DM due to galactose and lactose content. Monitor electrolytes periodically in elderly or debilitated if used >6 months. Potential for explosive reaction with electrocautery procedures during proctoscopy or colonoscopy.

ADVERSE REACTIONS: Flatulence, intestinal cramps, diarrhea, N/V.

INTERACTIONS: Decreased effect with nonabsorbable antacids.

PREGNANCY: Category B, caution in nursing.

MECHANISM OF ACTION: Synthetic disaccharide; broken down primarily to lactic acid, by the action of colonic bacteria, resulting in increased osmotic pressure and slight acidification of colonic content, causing an increase in stool water content and softens the stool. In portal-systemic encephalopathy, acidification of colonic contents results in retention of ammonia in colon as ammonium ion; ammonia then migrates from blood into colon to form ammonium ion, which traps and prevents absorption of ammonia; finally, laxative actions expels trapped ammonium ion from colon.

PHARMACOKINETICS: Absorption: Poor. **Elimination:** Urine (≤3%).

NURSING CONSIDERATIONS

Assessment: Assess for DM. Assess patients requiring a low-galactose diet and those requiring electrocautery procedures.

Monitoring: Monitor serum electrolytes (potassium, sodium, chloride, carbon dioxide) periodically, diarrhea, vomiting.

Patient Counseling: Drug may be diluted with fruit juice, water, or milk. Report potential adverse effects.

Administration: Oral route. **Storage:** 25°C (77°F); excursions permitted to 15-30°C (59-86°F). Dispense in tight, light-resistant container with child-resistant closure.

LAMICTAL

lamotrigine (GlaxoSmithKline)

RX

> Serious life-threatening rash, including Stevens-Johnson syndrome, toxic epidermal necrolysis, and/or rash-related death, reported. Serious rash occurs more often in pediatrics than in adults. D/C at first sign of rash. Potential increased risk with concomitant valproate (including valproic acid and divalproex sodium) or exceeding the recommended initial dose/dose escalation.

OTHER BRAND NAMES: Lamictal ODT (GlaxoSmithKline) - Lamictal CD (GlaxoSmithKline)

THERAPEUTIC CLASS: Phenyltriazine

INDICATIONS: Adjunctive therapy in patients (≥2 yrs) with partial seizures, primary generalized tonic-clonic (PGTC) seizures, and for generalized seizures of Lennox-Gastaut syndrome. For conversion to monotherapy in adults (≥16 yrs) with partial seizures receiving a single antiepileptic drug (AED) (carbamazepine, phenytoin, phenobarbital, primidone or valproate). Maintenance treatment of Bipolar I Disorder to delay the time to occurrence of mood episodes (depression, mania, hypomania, mixed episodes) in patients (≥18 yrs) treated for acute mood episodes with standard therapy.

DOSAGE: *Adults:* Epilepsy: Concomitant Valproate: Weeks 1 and 2: 25mg qod. Weeks 3 and 4: 25mg qd. Week 5 Onwards: Increase every 1-2 weeks by 25-50mg/day. Maint: 100-200mg/day with valproate alone or 100-400mg/day with valproate and other drugs inducing glucuronidation in 1 or 2 divided doses. Patients Not Taking These Enzyme-Inducing Antiepileptic Drugs (EIAEDs) (Carbamazepine, Phenytoin, Phenobarbital, Primidone) or Valproate: Weeks 1 and 2: 25mg qd. Weeks 3 and 4: 50mg qd. Week 5 Onwards: Increase every 1-2 weeks by 50mg/day. Maint: 225-375mg/day in 2 divided doses. Concomitant EIAEDs without Valproate: Weeks 1 and 2: 50mg/day. Weeks 3 and 4: 100mg/day in 2 divided doses. Week 5 Onwards: Increase every 1-2 weeks by 100mg/day. Maint: 300-500mg/day in 2 divided doses. Conversion to Monotherapy: See PI. Bipolar Disorder: Patients Not Taking EIAEDs or Valproate: Weeks 1 and 2: 25mg qd. Weeks 3 and 4: 50mg qd. Week 5: 100mg qd. Weeks 6 and 7: 200mg qd. Concomitant Valproate: Weeks 1 and 2: 25mg qod. Weeks 3 and 4: 25mg qd. Week 5: 50mg qd. Weeks 6 and 7: 100mg qd. Concomitant EIAEDs without Valproate: Weeks 1 and 2: 50mg qd. Weeks 3 and 4: 100mg qd. Week 5: 200mg qd. Week 6: 300mg qd. Week 7: Up to 400mg qd. Weeks 3-7: Take in divided daily doses. D/C of Psychotropic Drugs Excluding EIAEDs or Valproate: Maintain current dose. D/C of Valproate with Current Dose of Lamotrigine 100mg qd: Week 1: 150mg qd. Week 2 Onward: 200mg qd. D/C of EIAEDs with Current Dose of Lamotrigine 400mg qd: Week 1: 400mg qd. Week 2: 300mg qd. Week 3 Onward: 200mg qd. Concomitant/Starting/Stopping Estrogen-Containing Oral Contraceptives: See PI. Hepatic Impairment: Moderate and Severe: Reduce by 25%. Severe with Ascites: Reduce by 50%. Adjust maint and escalation doses based on clinical response. Elderly: Start at lower end of dosing range.

Pediatrics: Epilepsy: >12 yrs: Same as adults. 2-12 yrs: Give in 1-2 divided daily doses, rounded down to the nearest whole tablet. Concomitant Valproate: Weeks 1 and 2: 0.15mg/kg/day. Weeks 3 and 4: 0.3mg/kg/day. Week 5 Onwards: Increase every 1-2 weeks by 0.3mg/kg/day. Maint: 1-3mg/kg/day with valproate alone or 1-5mg/kg/day. Max: 200mg/day. Initial Weight-Based Dosing Guide (Weeks 1-4): See PI. Patients Not Taking EIAEDs or Valproate: Weeks 1 and 2: 0.3mg/kg/day. Weeks 3 and 4: 0.6mg/kg/day. Week 5 Onwards: Increase every 1-2 weeks by 0.6mg/kg/day. Maint: 4.5-7.5mg/kg/day. Max: 300mg/day. Concomitant EIAEDs without Valproate: Weeks 1 and 2: 0.6mg/kg/day. Weeks 3 and 4: 1.2 mg/kg/day. Week 5 Onwards: Increase every 1-2 weeks by 1.2mg/kg/day. Maint: 5-15mg/kg/day. Max: 400mg/day. <30kg: May increase maint dose by up to 50% based on clinical response. ≥16 yrs: Conversion to Monotherapy: See PI.

HOW SUPPLIED: Tab: 25mg*, 100mg*, 150mg*, 200mg*; Tab, Chewable: (CD) 2mg, 5mg, 25mg; Tab, Disintegrating: (ODT) 25mg, 50mg, 100mg, 200mg *scored

WARNINGS/PRECAUTIONS: Rashes leading to hospitalization and d/c (eg, Stevens-Johnson syndrome [SJS], toxic epidermal necrolysis [TEN], angioedema, and rash associated with systemic manifestations: fever, lymphadenopathy, facial swelling, and hematologic and hepatologic abnormalities) reported. Hypersensitivity reactions (eg, multiorgan failure/dysfunction, hepatic abnormalities, disseminated intravascular coagulation [DIC]) reported; d/c if alternative etiology cannot be established. Note early manifestations of hypersensitivity (eg, fever, lymphadenopathy) even in the absence of rash. Majority of deaths from multiorgan failure occurred in association with other serious medical events (eg, status epilepticus, overwhelming sepsis, hantavirus) making it difficult to identify initial cause. Blood dyscrasias (eg, neutropenia, leukopenia, anemia, thrombocytopenia, pancytopenia, aplastic anemia, pure red cell aplasia) reported. Increased risk of suicidal thoughts or behavior;

balance risk of suicidal thoughts or behavior with risk of untreated illness prior to therapy. Worsening of depressive symptoms and/or emergence of suicidal ideation and behaviors (suicidality) may be experienced in bipolar disorder; consider d/c. Write prescriptions for smallest quantity of tablets to reduce risk of overdose. Aseptic meningitis reported; in most cases, symptoms (eg, headache, fever, N/V, nuchal rigidity, rash, photophobia, myalgia, chills, altered consciousness, somnolence) resolved after d/c. Avoid abrupt withdrawal due to risk of withdrawal seizures; taper over a period of at least 2 weeks. Sudden unexplained death in epilepsy (SUDEP) reported. May cause toxicity of the eyes and other melanin-containing tissues due to melanin binding. Medication errors reported. Do not exceed recommended initial dose and dose escalations. Caution with renal/hepatic impairment and in elderly. Safety and effectiveness in acute treatment of mood episodes and in patients <18 yrs with mood disorders not established. May impair mental/physical abilities.

ADVERSE REACTIONS: Dizziness, diplopia, infection, headache, ataxia, blurred vision, N/V, somnolence, fever, pharyngitis, rhinitis, serious rash/rash, diarrhea, abdominal pain, insomnia.

INTERACTIONS: See Boxed Warning. Decreased levels with phenytoin, carbamazepine, phenobarbital, primidone, rifampin and estrogen-containing oral contraceptives. May decrease levels of levonorgestrel. Increased levels with valproate. May increase carbamazepine epoxide levels. Higher incidence of dizziness, diplopia, ataxia and blurred vision with carbamazepine. Higher incidence of headache, dizziness, nausea and somnolence with oxcarbazepine. Inhibits dihydrofolate reductase; prescribe other folate metabolism inhibitors with caution. May affect clearance with drugs known to induce or inhibit glucuronidation; may require adjustment. Reduced AUC and C_{max} with olanzapine. May increase concentrations of topiramate. Increased clearance with ethinyl estradiol. Multiorgan dysfunction and DIC reported in 3 patients receiving concomitant therapy with valproate, carbamazepine and clonazepam.

PREGNANCY: Category C, not for use in nursing.

MECHANISM OF ACTION: Phenyltriazine; mechanism not established. Suspected to inhibit voltage-sensitive sodium channels, thereby stabilizing neuronal membranes and consequently modulating presynaptic transmitter release of excitatory amino acids (eg, glutamate, aspartate).

PHARMACOKINETICS: Absorption: Rapid and complete; absolute bioavailability (98%). T_{max}=1.4-4.8 hrs. **Distribution:** V_d=0.9-1.3L/kg; plasma protein binding (55%); found in breast milk. **Metabolism:** Liver via glucuronic acid conjugation; 2-N-glucuronide conjugate (major metabolite, inactive). **Elimination:** Urine (94%; 10%, unchanged), feces (2%). $T_{1/2}$=See PI. Refer to PI for pediatric parameters.

NURSING CONSIDERATIONS

Assessment: If restarting after d/c, assess for initial dosing recommendations. Assess for history of allergy/rash to other AEDs, renal/hepatic impairment, Parkinson's disease, systemic lupus erythematosus (SLE), and other autoimmune diseases. Assess for hypersensitivity to drug, pregnancy/nursing status and possible drug interactions.

Monitoring: Monitor for signs/symptoms of rash (eg, SJS, TEN, angioedema, systemic manifestations: fever, lymphadenopathy, facial swelling, hematologic and hepatologic abnormalities), hypersensitivity reactions (eg, multiorgan failure/dysfunction, hepatic abnormalities, DIC), status epilepticus, overwhelming sepsis, hantavirus, blood dyscrasias, emergence or worsening of depression, suicidal thoughts or behavior (suicidality), unusual mood/behavior changes, overdosage, symptoms of aseptic meningitis, long-term ophthalmologic effects, and occurrence of seizures in patients who abruptly d/c medication. Monitor drug levels with concomitant medications or if dosage adjustments are being made. Monitor effectiveness of long-term use (>16 weeks).

Patient Counseling: Instruct to notify physician immediately if rash, signs/symptoms of hypersensitivity (eg, fever, lymphadenopathy), blood dyscrasias, multiorgan failure, or aseptic meningitis occur. Inform patients, their caregivers, and families about increased risk of suicidal thoughts and behavior and advise them to be alert if signs/symptoms of depression, any unusual changes in mood/behavior, suicidal thoughts/behavior, or thoughts about self-harm emerge or worsen; notify physician immediately. Notify physician if worsening of seizure control occurs. Visually inspect tablets and verify if correct, as well as formulation, each time prescription is filled. Inform that CNS depression may occur; avoid operating machinery/driving until adjusted to effects. Advise females to notify physician if they plan to start or stop oral contraceptives or other hormonal preparations. Report changes in menstrual patterns. Encourage patients to enroll in North American Antiepileptic Drug (NAAED) Pregnancy Registry if they become or intend to become pregnant. Do not abruptly d/c therapy; if therapy is stopped, notify physician before restarting.

Administration: Oral route. Round dose down to the nearest whole tab; chewable dispersible tablets may be swallowed whole, chewed, dispersed in water or diluted in fruit juice. If tablets are chewed, consume a small amount of water or diluted fruit juice to aid in swallowing. When dispersing in water or diluted fruit juice, add tablets to small amount of liquid (1 tsp or enough to cover tablets) and approximately 1 min later, swirl solution and consume entire quantity immediately. Orally disintegrating tablets may be placed onto the tongue and moved around in the mouth. May disintegrate rapidly, swallow with or without water and may be taken with or without food. **Storage:** (Tab/Tab, Chewable) 25°C (77°F); excursions permitted to 15-30°C (59-86°F). Store in a dry place. (Tab) Protect from light. (Tab, Disintegrating) 20-25°C (68-77°F); excursions permitted between 15-30°C (59-86°F).

LAMISIL   RX
terbinafine HCl (Novartis)

THERAPEUTIC CLASS: Allylamine antifungal

INDICATIONS: (Granules) Treatment of tinea capitis in patients ≥4 yrs. (Tabs) Treatment of onychomycosis of toenail or fingernail due to dermatophytes (tinea unguium).

DOSAGE: *Adults:* Tabs: Fingernail: 250mg qd for 6 weeks. Toenail: 250mg qd for 12 weeks. Granules: Take qd with food for 6 weeks. <25kg: 125mg/day. 25-35kg: 187.5mg/day. >35kg: 250mg/day.
Pediatrics: ≥4 yrs: Granules: Take qd with food for 6 weeks. <25kg: 125mg/day. 25-35kg: 187.5mg/day. >35kg: 250mg/day.

HOW SUPPLIED: Granules: 125mg/pkt, 187.5mg/pkt; Tab: 250mg

WARNINGS/PRECAUTIONS: Liver disease and serious skin reactions reported; d/c therapy if these develop. Avoid with liver disease or renal impairment (CrCl ≤50 mL/min). Check serum transaminases before therapy. Monitor CBC if immunocompromised and taking terbinafine >6 weeks. Severe neutropenia reported; d/c therapy if neutrophil count ≤1,000 cells/mm³. Changes in ocular lens and retina reported (unknown significance).

ADVERSE REACTIONS: (Granules) Nasopharyngitis, headache, pyrexia, cough, vomiting, upper respiratory tract infection, upper abdominal pain, diarrhea, liver enzyme abnormalities, rash. (Tabs) Headache, diarrhea, dyspepsia, abdominal pain, liver enzyme abnormalities, rash.

INTERACTIONS: Increased clearance of cyclosporine. May potentiate levels of drugs metabolized by CYP2D6 (eg, TCAs, β-blockers, SSRIs, MAOIs-type B). Decreased clearance of IV caffeine. Clearance increased by rifampin and decreased by cimetidine.

PREGNANCY: Category B, not for use in nursing.

MECHANISM OF ACTION: Allylamine antifungal; acts by inhibiting squalene epoxidase, thus blocking biosynthesis of ergosterol, an essential component of fungal-cell membranes.

PHARMACOKINETICS: Absorption: (Tab) Well-absorbed (>70%), absolute bioavailability (40%); (250mg) C_{max}=1mcg/mL; T_{max}=2 hrs; AUC =4.56mcg.h/mL. **Distribution:** Plasma protein binding (>99%). **Metabolism:** Extensive, CYP2D6. **Elimination:** Urine (70%); $T_{1/2}$=200-400 hrs.

NURSING CONSIDERATIONS

Assessment: Prior to treatment, conduct LFTs and obtain appropriate nail specimens for lab testing (KOH preparation, fungal culture, or nail biopsy) to diagnose onychomycosis. Assess for pre-existing liver disease.

Monitoring: Monitor for signs of hepatotoxicity, occurrence of progressive skin rash (Stevens-Johnson syndrome), and signs/symptoms of lupus erythematosus. Perform CBC, LFTs, and renal function tests (CrCl) during therapy.

Patient Counseling: Inform that taste disturbances may occur while on medication. Counsel females to avoid nursing.

Administration: Oral route. **Storage:** Below 25°C (77°F). Dispense in a tight, light-resistant container.

LANOXIN   RX
digoxin (GlaxoSmithKline)

OTHER BRAND NAMES: Digoxin oral solution (Various) - Digitek (Mylan Bertek)

THERAPEUTIC CLASS: Cardiac glycoside

INDICATIONS: Treatment of mild to moderate heart failure and to control ventricular response rate with chronic atrial fibrillation.

DOSAGE: *Adults:* Rapid Digitalization: LD: (Inj) 0.4-0.6mg IV or (Tab) 0.5-0.75mg PO; may give additional (Inj) 0.1-0.3mg or (Tab) 0.125-0.375mg at 6-8 hr intervals until clinical effect. Maint: (Tab) 0.125-0.5mg qd. (Inj/Tab) Refer to PI for dose based on weight and renal function. Usual: 0.25mg qd. Elderly (>70 yrs)/Renal Dysfunction: Initial: 0.125mg qd. Marked Renal Dysfunction: Initial: 0.0625mg qd. Titrate: Increase q2 weeks based on response. A-Fib: Titrate to minimum effective dose for desired response. (Sol) Initial: 3mcg/kg/day. Refer to PI for Usual Daily Maintenance Requirements (mcg) for estimated peak body stores of 10mcg/kg in adults and Daily Dose in mL. Elderly: Start at low end of dosing range.
Pediatrics: (Ped Inj) IV Digitalizing Dose: Premature Infants: 15-25mcg/kg. Full-Term Infants: 20-30mcg/kg. 1-24 months: 30-50mcg/kg. 2-5 yrs: 25-35mcg/kg. 5-10 yrs: 15-30mcg/kg. >10 yrs: 8-12mcg/kg. Maint: Individualize dose. Premature Infants: 20-30% of IV digitalizing dose/day. Full-Term Infants to >10 yrs: 25-35% of IV digitalizing dose/day. (Tab) Maint: 2-5 yrs: 10-15mcg/kg. 5-10 yrs: 7-10mcg/kg. >10 yrs: 3-5mcg/kg. A-Fib: Titrate to minimum effective dose for desired response. (Sol) Children >2 yrs and Prepubertal Children: Initial: 10mcg/kg/day. Renal Dysfunction: Start at the low end of dosing range.

HOW SUPPLIED: Inj: (Pediatric Inj) 0.1mg/mL, 0.25mg/mL; Sol: (Generic) 50mcg/mL [60mL]; Tab: 0.125mg*, 0.25mg* *scored

CONTRAINDICATIONS: Ventricular fibrillation.

WARNINGS/PRECAUTIONS: May cause severe sinus bradycardia or sinoatrial block with pre-existing sinus node disease. May cause advanced or complete heart block with pre-existing incomplete AV block. May cause very rapid ventricular response or ventricular fibrillation. Caution with thyroid disorders, AMI, hypermetabolic states, disorders involving heart failure associated with preserved left ventricular ejection fraction (LVEF), hypertrophic cardiomyopathy, elderly, Wolff-Parkinson-White (WPW) syndrome, and (Inj/Sol) beri beri heart disease. Caution with renal dysfunction; high risk for toxicity. Caution with hypokalemia, hypomagnesemia, or hypercalcemia; toxicity may occur. Hypocalcemia can nullify effects of digoxin. Monitor electrolytes and renal function periodically. Risk of ventricular arrhythmia with electrical cardioversion. Bioavailability is different between dosage forms. (Inj/Sol) Avoid with myocarditis; may precipitate vasoconstriction.

ADVERSE REACTIONS: Heart block, rhythm disturbances, anorexia, N/V, diarrhea, visual disturbances, headache, weakness, dizziness, mental disturbances.

INTERACTIONS: Risk of toxicity with K⁺-depleting corticosteroids and diuretics. Increased risk of arrhythmias with calcium, sympathomimetics, and succinylcholine. Increased serum levels with quinidine, verapamil, amiodarone, propafenone, indomethacin, itraconazole, alprazolam, and spironolactone; monitor for toxicity. Increased absorption with propantheline, diphenoxylate, macrolides, and tetracycline; monitor for toxicity. Decreased serum levels with rifampin. Increased digoxin dose requirement with thyroid supplements. Additive effects on AV node conduction with β-blockers or CCBs. Caution with drugs that deteriorate renal function. May interfere with digoxin absorption with antacids, kaolin-pectin, sulfasalazine, neomycin, cholestyramine, certain anticancer drugs, and metoclopramide. (Sol) May interfere with digoxin absorption with activated charcoal, meals high in bran, sucralfate, lansoprazole, esomeprazole, and omeprazole. Potential digoxin pharmacokinetics alteration with P-glycoprotein inducers/inhibitors. Monitor digoxin levels when initiating, adjusting, and discontinuing with diltiazem, nifedipine, nitrendipine, and telmisartan. Increased serum concentration with carvedilol, epoprostenol, diclofenac, ketoconazole, rabeprazole, azithromycin, erythromycin, tetracycline, gatifloxacin, and clarithromycin. Decreased serum concentration with acarbose, miglitol, cyclosporine, albuterol, salbutamol, and St. John's Wort. Colestipol bind digoxin. Digoxin toxicity reported with tramadol. May compete for common renal tubular transport systems with metformin. Higher rate of torsade de pointes with dofetilide. Increased PR interval and QRS duration with moricizine. Caution with teriparatide. Increased levels with captopril in severe congestive heart failure.

PREGNANCY: Category C, (Inj/Tab) caution in nursing. (Sol) Not for use in nursing.

MECHANISM OF ACTION: Cardiac glycoside; inhibits Na$^+$-K$^+$ ATPase, leading to increase in intracellular concentration of Ca^{2+}.

PHARMACOKINETICS: Absorption: (Tab) Absolute bioavailability (60-80%), T_{max}=1-3 hrs. (Sol) Absolute bioavailability (70-85%), T_{max}=30-90 min. (Inj) Absolute bioavailability (100%). **Distribution:** Plasma protein binding (25%), crosses placenta; found in breast milk. **Metabolism:** Hydrolysis, oxidation, and conjugation. **Elimination:** Urine (50-70%); $T_{1/2}$=1.5-2 days. Anuric patients (3.5-5 days). (Sol) $T_{1/2}$= Children (18-26 hrs), adults (36-48 hrs).

NURSING CONSIDERATIONS

Assessment: Assess for drug hypersensitivity, ventricular fibrillation, possible drug interactions, thyroid and electrolyte disorders, hypermetabolic states, sinus node disease, incomplete AV block, renal impairment, atrial fibrillation/flutter with accessory AV pathway (WPW syndrome), restrictive cardiomyopathy, constrictive pericarditis, amyloid heart disease, pregnancy/nursing status, and (Inj/Tab) myocarditis .

Monitoring: Monitor serum electrolytes and renal function periodically. Monitor for signs/symptoms of sinoatrial block, severe sinus bradycardia, complete AV block, electrolyte imbalance, and hypersensitivity reactions. Monitor serum digoxin levels.

Patient Counseling: Advise to seek medical attention if symptoms of hypersensitivity, electrolyte imbalance, or CV events occur.

Administration: Oral, IV route. **Storage:** 25°C (77°F); excursions permitted to 15-30°C (59-86°F). Protect from light. (Tab) Store in dry place.

LANTUS   RX
insulin glargine, human (Sanofi-Aventis)

THERAPEUTIC CLASS: Insulin

INDICATIONS: Treatment of adults and pediatrics with type 1 diabetes mellitus (DM). Treatment of adults with type 2 DM.

DOSAGE: *Adults:* Individualize dose. Administer SQ qd at same time each day. Type 1 DM: Initial: 1/3 of total daily insulin requirement. Type 2 DM Not Currently Treated With Insulin: Initial: 10 U (or 0.2 U/kg) qd. Adjust dose according to blood glucose requirements. Switching from qd NPH Insulin: Initial: Same as the dose of NPH that is being d/c. Switching from bid NPH Insulin:

Initial: 80% of the total NPH dose that is being d/c. Dose reduction required for renal and hepatic impaired patient.

Pediatrics: ≥6 yrs: Individualize dose. Administer SQ qd at same time each day. Type 1 DM: Initial: 1/3 of total daily insulin requirement. Type 2 DM Not Currently Treated With Insulin: Initial: 10 U (or 0.2 U/kg) qd. Adjust dose according to blood glucose requirements. Switching from qd NPH Insulin: Same as the dose of NPH that is being d/c. Switching from bid NPH Insulin: Initial: 80% of the total NPH dose that is being d/c. Dose reduction required for renal and hepatic impaired patient.

HOW SUPPLIED: Inj: 100 U/mL; OptiClik: 100 U/mL; SoloStar: 100 U/mL

WARNINGS/PRECAUTIONS: Not recommended for the treatment of diabetic ketoacidosis. Use in regimens with short-acting insulin with type 1 DM. Glucose monitoring is essential for all patients receiving insulin therapy. Any change of insulin should be made cautiously and only under medical supervision. Changes in strength, manufacturer, type, or method of manufacture may result in the need for a change in dosage. Not for IV use or via an insulin pump; may result in severe hypoglycemia if given IV. Do not share disposable or reusable insulin devices or needles between patients; may carry a risk for transmission of blood-borne pathogens. Increased risk of hypoglycemia with intensive glycemic control, food intake changes (eg, amount of food or timing of meals), exercise, and concomitant medications. Severe hypoglycemia can lead to unconsciousness or convulsions and may result in temporary or permanent impairment of brain function or death. Caution in patients with hypoglycemia unawareness, patients predisposed to hypoglycemia (pediatrics, patients with fast or have erratic food intake). Patient's ability to concentrate and react may be impaired as a result of hypoglycemia; caution when driving or operating machinery. Severe, life-threatening, generalized allergy, including anaphylaxis, can occur. Not recommended with rapidly declining renal or hepatic function. Caution in elderly.

ADVERSE REACTIONS: Hypoglycemia, upper respiratory infection, peripheral edema, hypertension, influenza, sinusitis, cataracts, bronchitis, arthralgia, infection, pain in extremities, back pain, cough, urinary tract infection, retinal vascular disorder.

INTERACTIONS: Increased glucose-lowering effects with ACE inhibitors, pramlintide, disopyramide, fibrates, fluoxetine, MAOIs, propoxyphene, pentoxifylline, salicylates, somatostatin analogs, sulfonamide antibiotics, and other oral antidiabetic agents. Decreased blood glucose lowering effects with corticosteroids, niacin danazol, diuretics, sympathomimetic agents (eg, epinephrine, albuterol, terbutaline), glucagon, isoniazid, phenothiazine derivatives, somatropin, thyroid hormones, estrogens, progestogens (eg, in oral contraceptives), protease inhibitors, and atypical antipsychotics (eg, olanzapine and clozapine). Pentamidine may cause hypoglycemia, followed by hyperglycemia. β-blockers, clonidine, lithium salts, and alcohol may potentiate or weaken glucose lowering effect. Signs of hypoglycemia may be reduced or absent with sympatholytic drugs such as β-blockers, clonidine, guanethidine, and reserpine. Do not dilute or mix with any other insulin or solution; may alter pharmacokinetic or pharmacodynamic profile (eg, onset of action, time to peak).

PREGNANCY: Category C, caution in nursing.

MECHANISM OF ACTION: Insulin glargine (rDNA origin); regulates glucose metabolism by stimulating peripheral glucose uptake by skeletal muscle and fat, inhibiting hepatic glucose production, lipolysis in the adipocyte, proteolysis, and enhancing protein synthesis.

PHARMACOKINETICS: Absorption: Slow, prolonged, and relatively constant. **Metabolism:** Partly metabolized into 2 active metabolites [M1 (21^A-Gly-insulin) and M2 (21^A-Gly-des-30^B-Thr-insulin)].

NURSING CONSIDERATIONS

Assessment: Assess for diabetic ketoacidosis, patients predisposed to hypoglycemia (pediatrics, patients with fast or have erratic food intake), hypersensitivity, renal/hepatic dysfunction, pregnancy/nursing status and possible drug interactions including other diabetic medications. Assess blood glucose levels including fasting blood glucose, HbA1c, renal/hepatic function, LFTs, alcohol consumption and exercise routines.

Monitoring: Monitor for signs and symptoms of hypoglycemia (unconsciousness, convulsions, impairment of brain function), concentration impairment, hypersensitivity reactions (eg, anaphylaxis), pregnancy/nursing status and possible drug interactions. Monitor for food intake changes (amount of food or timing of meals) and exercise routines. Monitor glucose in all patients receiving therapy. Monitor fasting blood glucose, HbA1c, renal/hepatic function.

Patient Counseling: Inform patient that changes to insulin regimens must be made cautiously and under medical supervision. Inform about potential side effects including lipodystrophy, weight gain, allergic reactions, and hypoglycemia. Inform patient that the ability to concentrate and react may be impaired, caution when driving or operating machinery. Patients should be instructed to always check the insulin label before each injection. Instruct patient to inspect solution for particles and discoloration before administration. Use only if the solution is clear and colorless, with no visible particles. Do not dilute or mix with other insulins or solutions. Advise not to share disposable or reusable insulin devices or needles with other patients. Instruct patients on self-management procedures including glucose-monitoring, proper injection technique, and management of hypoglycemia and hyperglycemia. Advise to inform physician if they are pregnant or are contemplating pregnancy.

Administration: SQ route only. Injection sites should be rotated within the same region (abdomen, thigh, or deltoid) from one injection to the next. **Storage:** Unopened vial: 2-8°C (36-46°F). Do not freeze. In-use vial: Below 30°C (86°F). Opened cartridge system OptiClik and Solostar should not be refrigerated; keep at room temperature (below 30°C [86°F]) away from direct heat and light. Discard after 28 days.

LASTACAFT RX
alcaftadine (Allergan)

THERAPEUTIC CLASS: H₁-antagonist

INDICATIONS: Prevention of itching associated with allergic conjunctivitis.

DOSAGE: *Adults:* 1 drop in each eye qd.
Pediatrics: ≥2 yrs: 1 drop in each eye qd.

HOW SUPPLIED: Sol: 0.25% [3mL]

WARNINGS/PRECAUTIONS: For topical ophthalmic use only. Caution not to touch the dropper tip to eyelids or surrounding areas to minimize contamination. Do not wear contact lens if the eye is red. Not for treatment of contact lens-related irritation. Do not instill while wearing contact lenses; reinsert lenses after 10 min following administration.

ADVERSE REACTIONS: Eye irritation, burning and/or stinging upon instillation, eye redness, eye pruritus.

PREGNANCY: Category B, caution in nursing.

MECHANISM OF ACTION: H₁-receptor antagonist; inhibits release of histamine from mast cells, decreases chemotaxis, and inhibits eosinophil activation.

PHARMACOKINETICS: Absorption: C_{max}=60pg/mL, 3ng/mL (active metabolite); T_{max}=15 min (median), 1 hr after dosing (active metabolite). **Distribution:** Plasma protein binding (39.2%), (62.7%, active metabolite). **Metabolism:** non-CYP450 cytosolic enzymes; carboxylic acid metabolite (active metabolite). **Excretion:** Urine (unchanged); $T_{1/2}$=2 hrs (active metabolite).

NURSING CONSIDERATIONS

Assessment: Assess for contact lens-related irritation and pregnancy/nursing status.

Monitoring: Monitor for possible adverse reactions.

Patient Counseling: Advise to avoid touching the tip of dropper to any surface to avoid contamination. Advise not to wear contact lenses if the eye is red. Advise not to use to treat contact lens-related irritation. Advise to remove contact lenses prior to instillation, then reinsert lenses after 10 min following administration. Inform that the drug is for topical ophthalmic administration only.

Administration: Ocular route. **Storage:** 15-25°C (59-77°F). Keep bottle tightly closed when not in use.

LATISSE   RX
bimatoprost (Allergan)

THERAPEUTIC CLASS: Prostaglandin analog

INDICATIONS: Treatment of hypotrichosis of the eyelashes.

DOSAGE: *Adults:* 1 drop qd hs. Apply evenly along the skin of the upper eyelid margin at the base of the eyelashes.

HOW SUPPLIED: Sol: 0.03% [3mL, 5mL]

WARNINGS/PRECAUTIONS: May lower intraocular pressure (IOP). Increased risk of permanent brown iris pigmentation. May cause pigment changes to periorbital pigmented tissues and eyelashes. May cause hair growth outside the treatment area. Use applicators on one eye and then discard; do not reuse to avoid contamination and infections. Caution with active intraocular inflammation, aphakic patients, pseudophakic patients with a torn posterior lens capsule, patients at risk of macular edema, and renal or hepatic impairment. Do not use with contact lenses; may be reinserted 15 min following its administration.

ADVERSE REACTIONS: Eye pruritus, conjunctival hyperemia, skin pigmentation, ocular irritation, dry eye, erythema of the eyelid.

INTERACTIONS: Concurrent use with other IOP-lowering prostaglandin analogs may decrease the IOP-lowering effect.

PREGNANCY: Category C, caution in nursing.

MECHANISM OF ACTION: Prostaglandin analog; not established; increases the percentage of hairs in, and the duration of the anagen or growth phase.

PHARMACOKINETICS: Absorption: C_{max}=0.08ng/mL; T_{max}=1.5 hrs; AUC=0.09ng•hr/mL. **Distribution:** V_d=0.67L/kg. **Metabolism:** Via oxidation, N-deethylation, and glucuronidation. **Elimination:** Urine (67%), feces (25%); $T_{1/2}$=45 min.

NURSING CONSIDERATIONS

Assessment: Assess use in aphakic patients, pseudophakic patients with a torn posterior lens capsule, patients at risk for macular edema, pregnant/nursing females, and patients with angle-closure, inflammatory, and neovascular glaucoma.

Monitoring: Monitor for increased iris pigmentation, changes in the periorbital tissue (eyelid), changes in eyelashes or growth of eyelashes, macular edema (eg, cystoid macular edema), and bacterial keratitis.

Patient Counseling: Instruct to apply medication every night using only sterile applicators; use only on one eye and then discard. Do not apply in your eye or to lower lid. Counsel medication may cause permanent increase in brown pigmentation of the iris, eyelid skin darkening, which may be reversible, and changes in the eyelashes. Instruct to avoid touching container tip to the eye, surrounding structures, fingers, or any other surface to avoid contamination. Counsel medication may lower IOP. Notify physician if an intercurrent ocular condition (eg, trauma or infection), any type of ocular reactions (eg, conjunctivitis, eyelid reaction) develop while on medication. Instruct to remove contact lenses prior to instillation; reinsert 15 mins after administration. Inform that if more than 1 topical ophthalmic medication is used, seperate administration by at least 5 min. Counsel that if any solution gets into the eye, it is not expected to cause harm; the eye should not be rinsed.

Administration: Ocular route. **Storage:** Store at 2-25°C (36-77°F).

LATUDA

RX

lurasidone HCl (Sunovion)

> Elderly patients with dementia-related psychosis treated with antipsychotic drugs are at an increased risk of death; most deaths appeared to be cardiovascular (eg, heart failure (HF), sudden death) or infectious (eg, pneumonia) in nature. Lurasidone HCl is not approved for the treatment of dementia-related psychosis.

THERAPEUTIC CLASS: Benzoisothiazol derivative

INDICATIONS: Treatment of schizophrenia.

DOSAGE: *Adults:* Initial: 40mg qd. Max: 80mg/day. Concomitant Use with Moderate CYP3A4 Inhibitors/Moderate and Severe Renal Impairment/ Moderate and Severe Hepatic Impairment: Max: 40mg/day. Take with food (≥350 calories).

HOW SUPPLIED: Tab: 40mg, 80mg

CONTRAINDICATIONS: Concomitant use with strong CYP3A4 inhibitors (eg, ketoconazole) and strong CYP3A4 inducers (eg, rifampin).

WARNINGS/PRECAUTIONS: Neuroleptic malignant syndrome (NMS) reported. Tardive dyskinesia (TD) may occur. Atypical antipsychotics have been associated with metabolic changes (hyperglycemia, dyslipidemia, and weight gain). Clinical monitoring of weight, glucose, and lipids is recommended. May elevate prolactin levels. Leukopenia, neutropenia and agranulocytosis have been reported with atypical antipsychotics; d/c in cases of severe neutropenia (ANC<1000/mm³). May cause orthostatic hypotension; caution with cardiovascular (CVD) disease, cerebrovascular disease, and conditions that predispose to hypotension. Caution with history of seizures or with conditions that lower the seizure threshold. May impair mental/physical abilities. May disrupt body temperature regulation; caution when exposed to conditions that may elevate core body temperature. Suicidal ideation reported. Esophageal dysmotility and aspiration reported with atypical antipsychotics; avoid use in patients at risk for aspiration pneumonia.

ADVERSE REACTIONS: Somnolence, akathisia, N/V, parkinsonism, agitation, dyspepsia, fatigue, back pain, dystonia, dizziness, insomnia, anxiety, restlessness.

INTERACTIONS: See Contraindications. Caution with other centrally acting drugs and alcohol. May slightly increase digoxin and midazolam levels; dose adjustments are not required. Slight level increases with lithium; dose adjustments are not required. Increased levels with diltiazem (moderate CYP3A4 inhibitor), do not exceed 40mg/day if coadministered.

PREGNANCY: Category B, caution in nursing.

MECHANISM OF ACTION: Atypical antipsychotic, benzoisothiazol derivative; mechanism not established. Suggested that the efficacy is mediated through a combination of dopamine Type 2 (D_2) and serotonin Type 2 ($5HT_{2A}$) receptor antagonism.

PHARMACOKINETICS: Absorption: T_{max}=1-3 hrs. **Distribution:** V_d= 6173L; plasma protein binding (99%). **Metabolism:** mainly via CYP3A4; oxidative *N*-dealkylation, hydroxylation of norbornane ring, and *S*-oxidation; ID-14283, ID-14326 (active metabolites). **Elimination:** Urine (9%), feces (80%); (40mg dose) $T_{1/2}$=18 hrs, clearance 3902mL/min.

NURSING CONSIDERATIONS

Assessment: Assess for dementia-related psychosis, pre-existing low WBCs or drug-induced leukopenia/neutropenia, conditions which predispose to hypotension, conditions that lower the seizure threshold, risk of aspiration pneumonia, hepatic/renal impairment, pregnancy/nursing status, and for possible drug interactions (strong inhibitors/inducers of CYP3A4). Assess for DM or risk factors for DM and obtain a baseline FPG in patients at risk for DM.

Monitoring: Monitor for signs/symptoms of NMS, hyperglycemia, weight gain, hyperlipidemia, TD, orthostatic hypotension, leukopenia, neutropenia, agranulocytosis, dysphagia, seizures, body temperature disruption, cognitive and motor impairment, and hyperprolactinemia. Perform periodic monitoring of FBG, lipid levels, and weight of patient. Perform frequent monitoring of CBC in patients with a history of clinically significant low WBC or drug-induced leukopenia/neutropenia. In patients with clinically significant neutropenia, monitor for fever or other symptoms or signs of infection. In high-risk patients, monitor closely for suicide attempt.

Patient Counseling: Advise that elderly patients with dementia-related psychoses treated with atypical antipsychotic drugs are at increased risk of death and that this therapy is not approved for dementia-related psychosis. Counsel about signs/symptoms of NMS (eg, hyperpyrexia, muscle rigidity, altered mental status, autonomic instability); instruct to contact physician if signs/symptoms of NMS develop. Inform about symptoms of hyperglycemia and DM. Advise of risk of orthostatic hypotension particularly at the time of initiating treatment, re-initiating treatment, or increasing the dose. Counsel to notify physician if taking any other medications and if intending to become pregnant or if become pregnant during therapy. Advise that medication may impair judgment, thinking, or motor skills; instruct to use caution when operating hazardous machinery. Advise appropriate care in avoiding overheating and dehydration.

Administration: Oral route. Take with food. **Storage:** 25°C (77°F); excursions permitted to 15-30°C (59-86°F).

Lescol XL   RX
fluvastatin sodium (Novartis)

OTHER BRAND NAMES: Lescol (Novartis)

THERAPEUTIC CLASS: HMG-CoA reductase inhibitor

INDICATIONS: Adjunct to diet, to reduce total cholesterol (total-C), LDL, TG, and apolipoprotein B (Apo B) levels, and to increase HDL in primary hypercholesterolemia and mixed dyslipidemia (Types IIa and IIb) when response to nonpharmacological measures is inadequate. To slow coronary atherosclerosis progression in coronary heart disease by lowering total-C and LDL. To reduce risk of undergoing coronary revascularization procedures in patients with coronary heart disease. Adjunct to diet, to reduce Total-C, LDL-C, and Apo B levels in adolescent boys and postmenarchal girls, 10-16 yrs of age, with heterozygous familial hypercholesterolemia when response to dietary restriction is inadequate and LDL-C remains ≥190mg/dL, or if LDL-C remains ≥160mg/dL and there is positive family history of premature CV disease or 2 or more other CV disease risk factors are present.

DOSAGE: *Adults:* ≥18 yrs: (For LDL-C reduction of ≥25%) Initial: 40mg cap qpm or 80mg XL tab at any time of day or 40mg cap bid. (For LDL-C reduction of <25%) Initial: 20mg cap qpm. Range: 20-80mg/day. Severe Renal Impairment: Caution with dose >40mg/day.
Pediatrics: 10-16 yrs (≥1 year post menarche): Heterozygous Familial Hypercholesterolemia: Initial: One 20mg cap. Titrate: Adjust dose at 6-week intervals. Max: 40mg cap bid or 80mg XL tab qd.

HOW SUPPLIED: Cap: (Lescol) 20mg, 40mg; Tab, Extended-Release: (Lescol XL) 80mg

CONTRAINDICATIONS: Active liver disease or unexplained, persistent elevations of serum transaminases, pregnancy, nursing mothers.

WARNINGS/PRECAUTIONS: Monitor LFTs prior to therapy, at 12 weeks, and with dose elevation. D/C if AST or ALT ≥3X ULN on 2 consecutive occasions. Risk of myopathy and/or rhabdomyolysis reported. D/C if markedly elevated CPK levels occur, if myopathy is diagnosed or suspected, or if predisposition to renal failure secondary to rhabdomyolysis. Less effective with homozygous familial hypercholesterolemia. Caution with heavy alcohol use and/or history of hepatic disease. Evaluate if endocrine dysfunction develops.

ADVERSE REACTIONS: Dyspepsia, abdominal pain, headache, sinusitis, nausea, diarrhea, myalgia, flu-like symptoms, abnormal LFTs.

INTERACTIONS: Increases levels of glyburide, diclofenac, and phenytoin. Rifampicin significantly decreases serum levels. Glyburide, phenytoin, cimetidine, ranitidine, omeprazole, fluconazole, cyclosporine and digoxin increase levels of fluvastatin. Caution with drugs that decrease levels of endogenous steroid hormones (eg, ketoconazole, spironolactone, cimetidine). Avoid fibrates. Cyclosporine, colchicine, gemfibrozil, erythromycin, or niacin may increase risk of myopathy/rhabdomyolysis. Immediate-release fluvastatin given within 4 hrs of cholestyramine leads to decreased serum levels of fluvastatin but has additive effects when given 4 hrs after cholestyramine. Monitor PT of patients on warfarin-type anticoagulants.

PREGNANCY: Category X, not for use in nursing.

MECHANISM OF ACTION: HMG-CoA reductase inhibitor; inhibits conversion of HMG-CoA to mevalonate (precursor of sterols, including cholesterol). Inhibition of cholesterol biosynthesis reduces cholesterol in hepatic cells, which stimulates the synthesis of LDL receptors, thereby increasing uptake of LDL particles, resulting in reduction of plasma cholesterol concentration.

PHARMACOKINETICS: Absorption: Oral administration of variable doses resulted in different parameters. Cap: Rapid and complete, absolute bioavailability (24%); T_{max}=<1 hr. Tab: relative bioavailability (relative to cap) (29%); T_{max}=3 hrs (fasting), 2.5 hrs (Low-fat meal), 6 hrs (High-fat meal). **Distribution:** V_d=0.35L/kg, plasma protein binding (98%). **Metabolism:** Liver via CYP2C9, 2C8 and 3A4 through hydroxylation, N-dealkylation, and β-oxidation pathways. **Elimination:** Feces (90% metabolites, <2% unchanged), urine (5%); Tab: $T_{1/2}$=9 hrs.

NURSING CONSIDERATIONS

Assessment: Assess for active liver disease or unexplained, persistent elevations in serum transaminase, pregnancy/nursing status, alcohol intake, homozygous familial hypercholestrolemia, renal impairment, DM, and possible drug interactions. Perform LFTs prior to therapy and at 12 weeks thereafter. Control hypercholesterolemia through appropriate diet, exercise, and weight reduction prior to therapy.

Monitoring: Monitor LFTs, CPK, thyroid functions. Monitor for signs/symptoms of myopathy (eg, diffuse muscle pain, tenderness or weakness, and fever or malaise), rhabdomyolysis, renal failure, endocrine dysfunction, and CNS toxicity or CNS vascular lesions (eg, hemorrhage and edema).

Patient Counseling: Inform about potential risks/benefits of therapy. Report promptly unexplained muscle pain, tenderness, or weakness, changes in urine or skin color, stomach pain, N/V, and malaise or fever. Notify physician if pregnant/nursing or planning to become pregnant.

Administration: Oral route. **Storage:** 25°C (77°F); excursions permitted to 15-30°C (15-86°F). Dispense in a tight container. Protect from light.

LETAIRIS   RX
ambrisentan (Gilead)

> Contraindicated in pregnancy. May cause serious birth defects if used by pregnant women; exclude pregnancy before treatment and prevent during treatment and for 1 month after stopping treatment by using 2 acceptable methods of contraception unless the patient has had tubal sterilization or chooses to use Copper T 380A IUD or LNg 20 IUS, in which case no additional contraception is needed. Obtain monthly pregnancy tests. Available only through the Letairis Education and Access Program (LEAP).

THERAPEUTIC CLASS: Endothelin receptor antagonist

INDICATIONS: Treatment of pulmonary arterial hypertension (PAH) (WHO Group 1) to improve exercise ability and delay clinical worsening.

DOSAGE: *Adults:* Initial: 5mg PO qd. Titrate: May increase to 10mg PO qd if 5mg is tolerated. Max: 10mg qd. May be taken with or without food.

HOW SUPPLIED: Tab: 5mg, 10mg

CONTRAINDICATIONS: Women who are or may become pregnant.

WARNINGS/PRECAUTIONS: Order and review tests for serum liver enzymes as clinically indicated since some members of this pharmacologic class are hepatotoxic. Not recommended with moderate or severe hepatic impairment. May cause peripheral edema; reported with greater frequency and severity in elderly patients. If clinically significant fluid retention develops, with or without weight gain, evaluate further to determine cause and possible need for treatment or d/c therapy. May decrease sperm count. May decrease Hgb and Hct; measure Hgb prior to initiation, at 1 month, then periodically thereafter. Avoid with clinically significant anemia. If acute pulmonary edema occurs during initiation of therapy, consider the possibility of pulmonary veno-occlusive disease; d/c if confirmed.

ADVERSE REACTIONS: Peripheral edema, Hgb decrease, nasal congestion, sinusitis, flushing, palpitations, nasopharyngitis, abdominal pain, constipation, dyspnea, headache.

INTERACTIONS: Increased levels with cyclosporine and rifampin; limit dose to 5mg qd when coadministered with cyclosporine.

PREGNANCY: Category X, not for use in nursing.

MECHANISM OF ACTION: Endothelin receptor antagonist; selective for endothelin type-A (ET$_A$) receptor, blocks the vasoconstriction and cell proliferation effects of Endothelin-1 (ET-1) in vascular smooth muscle and endothelium.

PHARMACOKINETICS: Absorption: T$_{max}$=2 hrs. **Distribution:** Plasma protein binding (99%). **Metabolism:** Via CYP3A, CYP2C19, and UGTs 1A9S, 2B7S, and 1A3S. **Elimination:** T$_{1/2}$=9 hrs.

NURSING CONSIDERATIONS

Assessment: Assess for anemia, hepatic impairment, pregnancy/nursing status, and possible drug interactions. Obtain baseline LFTs, Hgb, and Hct levels.

Monitoring: LFTs, Hgb, Hct, and pregnancy tests monthly. Monitor for signs/symptoms of hepatotoxicity, peripheral edema, pulmonary edema, pulmonary veno-occlusive disease, and hypersensitivity reactions. Monitor for improvements in WHO class symptoms and exercise capacity.

Patient Counseling: Advise to enroll in LEAP and re-enroll after the 1st 12 months of treatment and annually thereafter. Inform that drug may cause fetal harm and instruct to use 2 forms of contraception during and 1 month after therapy. If IUD or tubal sterilization is used, inform that additional contraception is not needed. Instruct to obtain a monthly pregnancy test and to notify healthcare professional if pregnancy is suspected. Inform of the importance of Hgb testing. Advise to seek medical attention if symptoms of liver injury (eg, anorexia, N/V, fever, malaise, fatigue, right upper quadrant abdominal discomfort, jaundice, dark urine, itching) occur. Advise not to split, crush, or chew tablets.

Administration: Oral route. Do not split, crush, or chew tablets. **Storage:** 25°C (77°F); excursions permitted to 15-30°C (59-86°F). Store in original packaging.

LEUKERAN **RX**
chlorambucil (GlaxoSmithKline)

> Risk of severe bone marrow suppression. Potentially carcinogenic, mutagenic, and teratogenic. Produces human infertility.

THERAPEUTIC CLASS: Nitrogen mustard alkylating agent

INDICATIONS: Treatment of chronic lymphatic (lymphocytic) leukemia (CLL), malignant lymphomas, and Hodgkin's disease.

DOSAGE: *Adults:* Usual: 0.1-0.2mg/kg qd for 3-6 weeks. Adjust according to response; reduce with abrupt WBC decline. Lymphocytic Infiltration of Bone Marrow/Hypoplastic Bone Marrow: Max: 0.1mg/kg/day. Caution within 4 weeks of full course of radiation or chemotherapy.

HOW SUPPLIED: Tab: 2mg

CONTRAINDICATIONS: Prior resistance to therapy.

WARNINGS/PRECAUTIONS: Convulsions, infertility, leukemia and secondary malignancies observed. Shown to cause chromatid or chromosome damage and sterility. Skin rash progressing to erythema multiforme, toxic epidermal necrolysis, or Stevens-Johnson syndrome reported. Avoid becoming pregnant. Lymphopenia reported, usually returns to normal upon completion. Monitor Hgb, leukocyte count and differential, platelet counts weekly. Avoid live vaccines in the immunocompromised.

ADVERSE REACTIONS: Bone marrow suppression, N/V, diarrhea, tremors, muscular twitching, confusion, agitation, ataxia, urticaria, angioneurotic syndrome, pulmonary fibrosis, hepatotoxicity, jaundice.

INTERACTIONS: Cross-hypersensitivity may occur with other alkylating agents.

PREGNANCY: Category D, not for use in nursing.

MECHANISM OF ACTION: Nitrogen mustard alkylating agent.

PHARMACOKINETICS: Absorption: Rapid and complete. (0.6-1.2 mg/kg) T_{max}=1 hr; (0.2mg/kg) C_{max}=492ng/mL, T_{max}=0.83 hrs, AUC=883ng•hr/mL; (Phenylacetic acid mustard) C_{max}=306ng/mL, T_{max}=1.9 hrs; AUC=1204ng•hr/mL. **Distribution:** Plasma protein binding (99%); crosses placenta. **Metabolism:** Liver (rapid). Phenylacetic acid mustard (major metabolite). **Elimination:** Low urinary excretion; $T_{1/2}$=1.5 hrs (0.6-1.2mg/kg); $T_{1/2}$=1.3 hrs (0.2mg/kg); $T_{1/2}$=1.8 hrs (phenylacetic acid mustard).

NURSING CONSIDERATIONS

Assessment: Assess for prior resistance, history of seizure disorder or head trauma, and possible drug interactions. Obtain baseline WBC and platelet count.

Monitoring: Monitor Hgb, WBC with differential and platelet count weekly. During first 3-6 weeks of therapy, obtain WBC levels 3 or 4 days after each weekly blood count. Monitor for signs/symptoms of myelosuppression, hypersensitivity reactions, secondary malignancies, and skin reactions.

Patient Counseling: Inform of pregnancy risks; avoid pregnancy. Advise to avoid vaccinations with live vaccines. Inform that major toxicities are related to hypersensitivity, drug fever, myelosuppression, hepatotoxicity, infertility, seizures, GI toxicity, and secondary malignancies. Instruct not to take without medical supervision; consult physician if skin rash, bleeding, fever, jaundice, persistent cough, seizures, or unusual lumps/masses occur.

Administration: Oral route. **Storage:** Refrigerate; 2-8°C (36-46°F).

LEVAQUIN   RX
levofloxacin (Ortho-Mcneil/Janssen)

> Fluoroquinolones are associated with an increased risk of tendinitis and tendon rupture in all ages. Risk is further increased with patients >60 yrs, taking corticosteroids, and with kidney, heart or lung transplants. May exacerbate muscle weakness with myasthenia gravis; avoid in patients with known history of myasthenia gravis.

THERAPEUTIC CLASS: Fluoroquinolone

INDICATIONS: Treatment of uncomplicated and complicated skin and skin structure infections (SSSI), uncomplicated and complicated urinary tract infections (UTI), acute bacterial sinusitis, acute bacterial exacerbation of chronic bronchitis (ABECB), community-acquired pneumonia (CAP) including multi-drug resistant Streptococcus pneumoniae, nosocomial pneumonia, chronic bacterial prostatitis (CBP), and acute pyelonephritis (AP) including cases with concurrent bacteremia caused by susceptible strains of microorganisms in adults ≥18 yrs. To reduce the incidence or progression of disease following anthrax exposure in adults and pediatrics.

DOSAGE: *Adults:* ≥18 yrs: IV/PO: CAP: 750mg qd for 5 days or 500mg qd for 7-14 days. Acute Bacterial Sinusitis: 750mg qd for 5 days or 500mg qd for 10-14 days. ABECB: 500mg qd for 7 days. Complicated SSSI/ Nosocomial Pneumonia: 750mg qd for 7-14 days. Uncomplicated SSSI: 500mg qd for

7-10 days. Chronic Bacterial Prostatitis: 500mg qd for 28 days. Complicated UTI/AP: 750mg qd for 5 days or 250mg qd for 10 days. Uncomplicated UTI: 250mg qd for 3 days. Inhalational Anthrax: 500mg qd for 60 days. Elderly: Start at lower end of dosing range. Refer to PI for Dose Adjustment with Renal Impairment (CrCl <50mL/min).

Pediatrics: ≥6 Months:IV/PO: Inhalational Anthrax: >50kg: 500mg q24h for 60 days. <50kg: 8mg/kg q12h for 60 days. Max: 250mg/dose.

HOW SUPPLIED: Inj: 25mg/mL [vial], 5mg/mL in 5% Dextrose [pre-mixed sol]; Sol: 25mg/mL; Tab: 250mg, 500mg, 750mg

WARNINGS/PRECAUTIONS: D/C if experience pain, swelling, inflammation or rupture of tendon. Serious anaphylactic sometimes fatal reactions reported; d/c if skin rash, jaundice, or any other sign of hypersensitivity appears and institute appropriate therapy. Convulsions and toxic psychosis reported. Increased intracranial pressure and central nervous system stimulation (which may lead to tremors, restlessness, anxiety, lightheadedness, confusion, halluncinations, paranoia, depression, nightmares, insomnia and suicidal thoughts or acts) may occur; d/c and institute appropriate measures if these reactions occur. Caution with CNS disorders (eg, severe cerebral arteriosclerosis, epilepsy) or risk factors that may predispose to seizures or lower seizure threshold. Severe hepatotoxicity including acute hepatitis and fatal events reported; d/c if signs and symptoms of hepatitis occur. *Clostridium difficile*-associated diarrhea (CDAD) reported. Rare cases of sensory or sensorimotor axonal polyneuropathy resulting in paresthesias, hypoesthesias, dysesthesias, and weakness reported. May prolong QT interval; avoid with QT interval prolongation or uncorrected hypokalemia, and patients receiving Class IA (quinidine, procainamide) or Class III (amiodarone, sotalol) antiarrhythmic agents. Increased incidence of musculoskeletal disorders (arthralgia, arthritis, tendonopathy, and gait abnormality) in pediatric patients. Blood glucose disturbances reported in diabetics; d/c if hypoglycemic reactions occur. May cause photosensitivity/phototoxicity reactions; d/c if phototoxicity occurs. Avoid excessive exposure to sun/UV light. Increased risk of development of drug-resistant bacteria if used in the absence of a strongly suspected bacterial infection. Crystalluria and cylinduria reported; maintain adequate hydration. May produce false-positive urine screening results for opiates using commercially available immunoassay kits. Caution with renal impairment and in elderly. (Inj) Not for IM, intrathecal, intraperitoneal, or SQ use. Avoid rapid or bolus IV infusion.

ADVERSE REACTIONS: Tendinitis, tendon rupture, nausea, diarrhea, constipation, headache, insomnia, dizziness.

INTERACTIONS: See Boxed Warning. Caution with drugs that may lower seizure threshold. Avoid with drugs that can prolong QT interval. Class IA (eg, quinidine, procainamide) and Class III (eg, amiodarone, sotalol) antiarrhythmics. Concomitant use with an antidiabetic agent may alter blood glucose levels. Increase seizure risk and CNS stimulation with NSAIDs. May increase theophylline levels and increase risk of theophylline-related adverse reactions; monitor theophylline levels closely. May enhance effects of warfarin; monitor PT and INR with warfarin. Reduced renal clearance with concomitant administration of either cimetidine or probenecid. (PO) Antacids containing aluminum or magnesium, with sucralfate, with metal cations such as iron, with multivitamins containing zinc, or with didanosine chewable/buffered tabs or the pediatric powder for oral sol, may substantially interfere with the absorption and lower systemic concentrations.

PREGNANCY: Category C, not for use in nursing.

MECHANISM OF ACTION: Fluoroquinolone; inhibits bacterial topoisomerase IV and DNA gyrase, which are enzymes required for bacterial DNA replication, transcription, repair, and recombination.

PHARMACOKINETICS: Absorption: Rapid and complete; absolute bioavailability (99%); administration of variable doses resulted in different parameters. **Distribution:** V_d=74-112L; plasma protein binding (approximately 24-38%); found in breast milk. **Metabolism:** Limited. **Elimination:** (Oral) Urine (87% unchanged, <5% desmethyl and N-oxide metabolites), feces (<4%); $T_{1/2}$=6-8 hrs.

NURSING CONSIDERATIONS

Assessment: Assess for risk factors for developing tendinitis and tendon rupture, history of myasthenia gravis, drug hypersensitivity, CNS disorders or risk factors that may predispose to seizures or lower seizure threshold, QT interval prolongation, uncorrected hypokalemia, renal/hepatic function, pregnancy/nursing status, and possible drug interactions. Perform appropriate culture and susceptibility tests prior to therapy for proper diagnosis of causative organisms.

Monitoring: Monitor for ECG changes, signs/symptoms of anaphylactic reaction, hepatotoxicity, prolongation of QT interval, CNS events, drug resistance, CDAD, peripheral neuropathy, musculoskeletal disorders (pediatrics), tendon rupture, tendinitis, photosensitivity/phototoxicity reactions. Monitor hydration, blood glucose levels, and renal function. Monitor for muscle weakness in patients with myasthenia gravis.

Patient Counseling: Inform that drug treats only bacterial, not viral, infections. Take as prescribed; skipping doses or not completing full course may decrease effectiveness and increase drug resistance. May take tab with or without food. Take oral sol 1 hr before or 2 hrs after eating. Take tab and sol at same time each day. Notify healthcare provider if symptoms of pain, swelling, or inflammation of a tendon, or weakness or inability to move joints develop. Notify physician of any history of convulsions, QT prolongation, or myasthenia gravis. Instruct to d/c use and notify physician if allergic reaction, skin rash, signs/symptoms of liver injury or peripheral neuropathy occur. Caution in activities requiring mental alertness and coordination. Instruct to contact physician immediately if watery and bloody diarrhea (with or without stomach cramps and fever) develop. Inform physician if child has tendon or joint-related problems prior to, during or after therapy. Advise to minimize or avoid exposure to natural or artificial sunlight. Instruct diabetic patients being treated with antidiabetic agents to d/c therapy and notify physician if hypoglycemia occurs. Inform physician if taking warfarin.

Administration: IV, Oral route. (PO) Administer ≥2 hrs before or 2 hrs after antacids containing magnesium, aluminum, as well as sucralfate, metal cations such as iron, and multivitamin preparations with zinc or didanosine chewable/buffered tab or pediatric powder for oral sol. (Sol) 1 hr before or 2 hrs after eating. (Inj) Infuse over 90 minutes q24h. Refer to PI for more information on administration, preparation and instructions for use. **Storage:** (Tab) 15-30°C (59-86°F), in well-closed containers. (Sol) 25°C (77°F), excursions permitted to 15-30°C (59-86°F). (Inj) Single-use vials: Controlled room temperature, and protected from light. Pre-mixed solution: ≤25°C (77°F); brief exposure ≤40°C (104°F). Avoid excessive heat and protect from freezing and light.

LEVBID   RX
hyoscyamine sulfate (Alaven)

OTHER BRAND NAMES: Levsinex (Alaven) - Levsin (Alaven)

THERAPEUTIC CLASS: Anticholinergic

INDICATIONS: Adjunct treatment of peptic ulcer, irritable bowel syndrome, neurogenic bladder, and neurogenic bowel disturbances. Management of functional intestinal disorders (eg, mild dysenteries, diverticulitis). To control gastric secretion, visceral spasm, and hypermotility in spastic colitis, spastic bladder, cystitis, pylorospasm, and associated abdominal cramps. Symptomatic relief of biliary and renal colic with concomitant morphine or other narcotics. Drying agent for symptomatic relief of acute rhinitis. To reduce rigidity and tremors of Parkinson's disease and control associated sialorrhea and hyperhidrosis. For anticholinesterase poisoning. To reduce pain and hypersecretion in pancreatitis. For certain cases of partial heart block associated with vagal activity. (Elixir, Drops) Treatment of infant colic. (Inj) Facilitates GI diagnostic procedures. Reduces pain and hypersecretion in pancreatitis, in cases of partial heart block associated with vagal activity, and as antidote for anticholinesterase poisoning. In anesthesia as a pre-op antimuscarinic. In urology to improve radiologic visibility of kidneys.

DOSAGE: *Adults:* May also chew or swallow SL tab. (Drops, Elixir, Tab, and Tab, SL) 0.125-0.25mg q4h or prn. Max: 1.5mg/24 hrs. (Cap and Tab, Extended-Release) 0.375-0.75mg q12h; or 1 cap q8h. Max: 1.5mg/24 hrs. Do not crush or chew. (Inj) GI Disorders: 0.25-0.5mg IM/IV/SQ as single dose or up to qid at 4-hr intervals. Diagnostic Procedures: 0.25-0.5mg IV 5-10 min before procedure. Anesthesia: 5mcg/kg IM/IV/SQ 30-60 min before anesthesia or with narcotic/sedative administration. GI Disorders: 0.25-0.5mg IM/IV/SQ as single dose; may require bid-qid administration at 4-hr intervals. Diagnostic Procedures: 0.25-0.5mg IV 5-10 min prior. Drug-Induced Bradycardia (Surgery): Increments of 0.25mL IV; repeat prn. Neuromuscular Blockade Reversal: 0.2mg for every 1mg neostigmine or equal dose of physostigmine or pyridostigmine.

Pediatrics: May also chew or swallow SL tab. ≥12 yrs: (Drops, Elixir, Tab, and Tab, SL) 0.125-0.25mg q4h or prn. Max: 1.5mg/24 hrs. (Cap and Tab, Extended-Release) 0.375-0.75mg q12h; or 1 cap may be given q8h. Max: 1.5mg/24 hrs. Do not crush or chew. 2 to <12 yrs: (Tab and Tab, SL) 0.0625-0.125mg q4h or prn. Max: 0.75mg/24 hrs. (Elixir) Give q4h or prn. 10kg: 1.25mL. 20kg: 2.5mL. 40kg: 3.75mL. 50kg: 5mL. Max: 30mL/24 hrs. (Drops) 0.25-1mL q4h or prn. Max: 6mL/24 hrs. <2 yrs: (Drops) Give q4h or prn. 3.4kg: 4 drops. Max: 24 drops/24 hrs. 5kg: 5 drops. Max: 30 drops/24 hrs. 7kg: 6 drops. Max: 36 drops/24 hrs. 10kg: 8 drops. Max: 48 drops/24 hrs. >2 yrs: Anesthesia: (Inj) 5mcg/kg IM/IV/SQ 30-60 min before anesthesia or with narcotic/sedative administration.

HOW SUPPLIED: (Levbid) Tab, Extended-Release: 0.375mg. (Levsin) Drops: 0.125mg/mL [15mL]; Elixir: 0.125mg/5mL [473mL]; Inj: 0.5mg/mL; Tab: 0.125mg*; Tab, SL: 0.125mg*. (Levsinex) Cap, Extended-Release: 0.375mg *scored

CONTRAINDICATIONS: Glaucoma, obstructive uropathy, GI tract obstruction, paralytic ileus; intestinal atony of elderly/debilitated, unstable CV status in acute hemorrhage, toxic megacolon complicating ulcerative colitis, myasthenia gravis.

WARNINGS/PRECAUTIONS: Risk of heat prostration with high environmental temperature. Avoid activities requiring mental alertness. Psychosis has been reported. Caution with diarrhea, autonomic neuropathy, hyperthyroidism, coronary heart disease, CHF, arrhythmias/tachycardia, HTN, renal disease, and hiatal hernia associated with reflux esophagitis. D/C if diarrhea occurs.

ADVERSE REACTIONS: Anticholinergic effects, drowsiness, headache, nervousness.

INTERACTIONS: Additive effects with other antimuscarinics, amantadine, haloperidol, phenothiazines, MAOIs, TCAs, and some antihistamines. Antacids interfere with absorption; take ac and antacids pc.

PREGNANCY: Category C, caution in nursing.

MECHANISM OF ACTION: Anticholinergic/antispasmodic; inhibits specifically the actions of acetylcholine on structures innervated by postganglionic cholinergic nerves and on smooth muscles that respond to acetylcholine but lack cholinergic innervation.

PHARMACOKINETICS: Absorption: Complete. **Distribution:** Crosses blood-brain barrier and placental barrier. **Metabolism:** Hydrolyzed partially to tropic acid. **Elimination:** Urine (unchanged); $T_{1/2}$=2-3.5 hrs.

NURSING CONSIDERATIONS

Assessment: Assess for glaucoma, obstructive uropathy, GI obstruction, paralytic ileus, intestinal atony, unstable CV status in acute hemorrhage, severe ulcerative colitis, toxic megacolon complicating ulcerative colitis, myasthenia gravis, and possible drug interactions.

Monitoring: Monitor for diarrhea, drowsiness, dizziness or blurred vision, psychosis, and CNS signs/symptoms including confusion, disorientation, short-term memory loss, hallucinations, dysarthria, ataxia, euphoria, anxiety, fatigue, insomnia, agitation, and unusual mannerisms.

Patient Counseling: Warn not to engage in activities requiring mental alertness (eg, operating a motor vehicle or other machinery), or to perform hazardous work while on treatment. Inform that decreased sweating resulting in heat prostration, fever or heat stroke may occur; caution if febrile, or exposed to high environmental temperatures. Counsel that extended-release tab/cap may not completely disintegrate and may be excreted.

Administration: Oral, IV, IM, SQ routes. **Storage:** 15-30°C (59-86°F).

LEVEMIR

RX

insulin detemir, rdna origin (Novo Nordisk)

THERAPEUTIC CLASS: Insulin

INDICATIONS: Once-or-twice-daily SQ administration for the treatment of adults and pediatrics with type 1 diabetes or adults with type 2 diabetes who require basal (long-acting) insulin for the control of hyperglycemia.

DOSAGE: *Adults:* Individualize dose. Administer SQ qd or bid. Once-Daily Dosing: Administer with evening meal or hs. Twice-Daily Dosing: Administer pm dose with evening meal, hs, or 12 hrs after am dose. Titrate: Adjust dose according to blood glucose measurements. Type 1/Type 2 Diabetes on Basal-Bolus Treatment or Patients Only on Basal Insulin: Change on a unit-to-unit basis. Insulin-Naive with Type 2 Diabetes Inadequately Controlled on Oral Antidiabetics: Initial: 0.1-0.2 U/kg qpm or 10 U qd or bid. Administer SQ in thigh, abdominal wall or upper arm. Rotate injection sites within same region. *Pediatrics:* Individualize dose. Administer SQ qd or bid. Once-Daily Dosing: Administer with evening meal or hs. Twice-Daily Dosing: Administer pm dose with evening meal, hs, or 12 hrs after am dose. Titrate: Adjust dose according to blood glucose measurements. Type 1 Diabetes on Basal-Bolus Treatment or Patients Only on Basal Insulin: Change on a unit-to-unit basis. Administer SQ in thigh, abdominal wall or upper arm. Rotate injection sites within same region.

HOW SUPPLIED: Inj: 100 U/mL; Innolet: 100 U/mL; Flexpen: 100 U/mL

WARNINGS/PRECAUTIONS: Not for IV or IM use. IV administration may result in severe hypoglycemia. Hypoglycemia may occur; glucose monitoring recommended. Not for use in an insulin infusion pump. Caution with any change in insulin dose. Changes in insulin strength, timing of dosing, manufacturer, type, species, or method of manufacture may result in the need for change in dosage. Inadequate dosing or d/c may lead to hyperglycemia. Lipodystrophy, hypersensitivity, sodium retention and edema reported. Change in physical activity or usual meal plan may require dosage adjustment. Dose adjustment may be needed in renal or hepatic impairment and during intercurrent conditions such as illness, emotional disturbances, or other stresses. Injection site reactions (eg, redness, pain, itching, hives, swelling, and inflammation) may occur; continuous rotation of the injection site may help reduce these reactions. Generalized allergy to insulin (rash over whole body, SOB, wheezing, BP reduction, rapid pulse, sweating) may occur; severe cases including anaphylactic reaction may be life-threatening. Caution in elderly.

ADVERSE REACTIONS: Allergic reactions, injection site reactions, lipodystrophy, pruritus, rash, hypoglycemia, weight gain.

INTERACTIONS: Avoid mixing with other insulins. Increased blood-glucose-lowering effects with ACE inhibitors, disopyramide, fibrates, fluoxetine, MAOIs, propoxyphene, salicylates, somatostatin analog (eg, ocreotide), sulfonamide antibiotics, and oral antidiabetic agents. Decreased blood-glucose-lowering effects with corticosteroids, danazol, diuretics, sympathomimetic agents (eg, epinephrine, albuterol, terbutaline), isoniazid, phenothiazine derivatives, somatotropin, thyroid hormones, estrogens, progestogens (eg, in oral contraceptives). Pentamidine may cause hypoglycemia, followed by hyperglycemia. β-blockers, clonidine, lithium salts, and alcohol may potentiate or weaken glucose-lowering effect. β-blockers, clonidine, guanethidine, and reserpine may reduce signs of hypoglycemia.

PREGNANCY: Category C, caution in nursing.

MECHANISM OF ACTION: Insulin detemir (rDNA origin); regulates glucose metabolism and lowers blood glucose by facilitating cellular uptake of glucose into skeletal muscle and fat and inhibiting glucose output from the liver.

Inhibits lipolysis in the adipocyte, inhibits proteolysis, and enhances protein synthesis.

PHARMACOKINETICS: Absorption: Slow, prolonged; absolute bioavailability (60%); T_{max}=6-8 hrs. **Distribution:** V_d=0.1L/kg; plasma protein binding (≥98%). **Elimination:** $T_{1/2}$=5-7 hrs.

NURSING CONSIDERATIONS

Assessment: Assess FPG, HbA1c, renal/hepatic function, LFTs, pregnancy/nursing status, infections, alcohol consumption, exercise routines, hypersensitivity and possible drug interactions.

Monitoring: Monitor FPG, HbA$_{1c}$, hypokalemia, hypoglycemia, hyperglycemia, renal/hepatic function, diabetic ketoacidosis, vision changes, lipodystrophy, allergic reactions and injection site reactions. Monitor for signs of hypoglycemia (sweating, palpitations, seizures, disorientation, tremors).

Patient Counseling: Advise to use only if the solution is clear and colorless with no visible particles. Inform about potential risks and benefits of the medication, including possible side effects. Do not dilute or mix with other insulins or solutions. Counsel about signs/symptoms of hypoglycemia, hyperglycemia, diabetic ketoacidosis, the importance of frequent monitoring of blood glucose levels, the need for eating a balanced diet, lifestyle management, timing of dosage, complication of insulin therapy, and exercising regularly. Advise to avoid excessive alcohol. During periods of stress (eg, trauma, infection, surgery), insulin requirements may be changed; advise patients to seek prompt medical advice. Counsel on proper administration techniques. Instruct how to handle special situations (eg, intercurrent conditions, inadequate or skipped insulin dose, inadvertent administration of an increased insulin dose, inadequate food intake, or skipped meals. Advise that ability to concentrate and/or react may be impaired. Notify physician if pregnant/contemplating to be pregnant.

Administration: SQ route. Administer on thigh, abdominal wall, or upper arm. Do not be mix or dilute with any other insulin preparations. **Storage:** Unused: 2-8°C (36-46°F). Do not freeze. Do not use if frozen. After use: Vial: Refrigerate, do not freeze. If refrigeration is not possible, store at room temperature <30°C (86°F) for 42 days. PenFill Cartridges/InnoLet/FlexPen: Store at room temperature <30°C (86°F) for 42 days. Keep away from direct heat and light.

LEVITRA   RX
vardenafil HCl (Merck)

THERAPEUTIC CLASS: Phosphodiesterase type 5 inhibitor

INDICATIONS: Treatment of erectile dysfunction (ED).

DOSAGE: *Adults:* Initial: 10mg 1 hr prior to sexual activity. Titrate: May decrease to 5mg or increase to max of 20mg based on response. Max: 1 tab/day. Elderly: ≥65 yrs: Initial: 5mg. Moderate Hepatic Impairment (Child-Pugh B): Initial: 5mg. Max: 10mg. Concomitant Ritonavir: Max: 2.5mg/72 hrs. Concomitant Indinavir/Saquinavir/Atazanavir/Clarithromycin/Ketoconazole 400mg daily/Itraconazole 400mg daily: Max: 2.5mg/24 hrs. Concomitant Ketoconazole 200mg daily/Itraconazole 200mg daily/Erythromycin: Max: 5mg/24 hrs. Concomitant Stable Alpha-blocker: Initial: 5mg; 2.5mg when used with certain CYP3A4 inhibitors.

HOW SUPPLIED: Tab: 2.5mg, 5mg, 10mg, 20mg

CONTRAINDICATIONS: Concomitant nitrates or nitric oxide donors.

WARNINGS/PRECAUTIONS: Avoid when sexual activity is inadvisable due to underlying cardiovascular (CV) status. Increased sensitivity to vasodilation effects with left ventricular outflow obstruction. Decrease in supine BP reported. Avoid with unstable angina, hypotension (resting SBP<90 mmHg), uncontrolled HTN (>170/110 mmHg), recent history of stroke, life-threatening arrhythmia, myocardial infarction (MI) within last 6 months, severe cardiac failure, severe hepatic impairment (Child-Pugh C), end-stage renal disease

(ESRD) requiring dialysis, hereditary degenerative retinal disorders including retinitis pigmentosa, congenital QT prolongation. Rare reports of prolonged erections >4 hrs and priapism. Caution with bleeding disorders, peptic ulcers, anatomical deformation of the penis or predisposition to priapism. Rare reports of non-arteritic anterior ischemic optic neuropathy (NAION) with phosphodiesterase type 5 (PDE5) inhibitors. Sudden decrease or loss of hearing accompanied by tinnitus and dizziness reported.

ADVERSE REACTIONS: Headache, flushing, rhinitis, dyspepsia, sinusitis, flu syndrome, dizziness, nausea.

INTERACTIONS: See Contraindications. Avoid use with Class IA (eg, quinidine, procainamide) or Class III (eg, amiodarone, sotalol) antiarrhythmics and other agents for ED. Caution with medications known to prolong QT interval. Increased levels with CYP3A4 inhibitors (eg, ritonavir, indinavir, saquinavir, atazanavir, ketoconazole, itraconazole, clarithromycin, erythromycin). Additive hypotensive effect, which may lead to symptomatic hypotension when used with α-blockers. Reduced clearance with CYP3A4/5 and CYP2C9 inhibitors.

PREGNANCY: Category B, not for use in nursing.

MECHANISM OF ACTION: PDE5 inhibitor; increases the amount of cGMP, which causes smooth muscle relaxation, allowing increased blood flow into the penis, resulting in erection.

PHARMACOKINETICS: Absorption: Rapid, absolute bioavailability (15%); T_{max}=30 min-2 hrs. **Distribution:** V_d=208L; plasma protein binding (95%). **Metabolism:** Via CYP3A4, CYP3A5, CYP2C. M1 (major metabolite). **Elimination:** Feces (91-95%), urine (2-6%); $T_{1/2}$=4-5 hrs.

NURSING CONSIDERATIONS

Assessment: Assess for CV disease, left ventricular outflow obstruction (eg, aortic stenosis, idiopathic hypertrophic subaortic stenosis), congenital QT prolongation, retinitis pigmentosa, bleeding disorders, active peptic ulceration, anatomical deformation of the penis or conditions that predispose to priapism (eg, sickle cell anemia, multiple myleoma, leukemia), and renal/hepatic impairment. Assess potential underlying causes of erectile dysfunction and for possible drug interactions.

Monitoring: Monitor potential for cardiac risk due to sexual activity, hypotension, color vision changes or other eye adverse events (eg, NAION), hypersensitivity reactions, and hearing impairment. Monitor for adverse events when used in combination with other drugs.

Patient Counseling: Discuss risks and benefits of therapy. Seek medical assistance if erection persists >4 hrs. Inform that postural hypotension may occur. Advise of potential BP-lowering effect of nitrates, α-blockers and antihypertensive medications, and cardiac risk of sexual activity. Counsel about protective measures necessary to guard against STDs, including HIV; drug does not protect against STDs. D/C and inform doctor if sudden loss of vision or hearing occur. Counsel to take as prescribed.

Administration: Oral route. **Storage:** 25°C (77°F); excursions permitted to 15-30°C (59-86°F).

LEVOPHED   RX
norepinephrine bitartrate (Hospira)

> Antidote for Extravasation Ischemia: To prevent sloughing and necrosis in area of extravasation, area should be infiltrated with 10-15mL saline solution containing 5-10mg phentolamine, an adrenergic blocking agent. Sympathetic blockade with phentolamine causes immediate and conspicuous local hyperemic changes if infiltrated within 12 hrs. Give phentolamine as soon as possible after the extravasation is noted.

THERAPEUTIC CLASS: Alpha-adrenergic agonist

INDICATIONS: For BP control in certain acute hypotensive states (eg, pheochromocytomectomy, sympathectomy, poliomyelitis, spinal anesthesia, myocardial infarction, septicemia, blood transfusion, and drug reactions). As an adjunct in the treatment of cardiac arrest and profound hypotension.

DOSAGE: *Adults:* (Average Dosage) Initial: 8-12mcg/min (2mL-3mL) as IV infusion until low normal BP (80-100mmHg systolic) is established and maintained by adjusting rate of flow. Maint: 2-4mcg/min (0.5mL-1mL). (High Dosage) Individualize dose (as high as 68mg/day). Elderly: Start at lower end of dosing range.

HOW SUPPLIED: Inj: 4mg/4mL

CONTRAINDICATIONS: Hypotension from blood volume deficits except as an emergency measure to maintain coronary and cerebral artery perfusion until blood volume replacement therapy can be completed, mesenteric or peripheral vascular thrombosis (unless administration is necessary as a life-saving procedure in the opinion of the attending physician), profound hypoxia or hypercarbia, and concomitant use of cyclopropane and halothane anesthetics.

WARNINGS/PRECAUTIONS: Contains sodium metabisulfite; may cause allergic-type reactions (eg, anaphylactic symptoms, life-threatening or less severe asthmatic episodes). May produce dangerously high BP with overdoses due to potency and varying response; monitor BP every 2 min from initial administration until desired BP is obtained, then every 5 min if administration is to be continued. Headache may be a symptom of HTN due to overdosage; monitor rate of flow constantly. Infusions should be given into a large vein, particularly an antecubital vein whenever possible. Avoid a catheter tie-in technique if possible. Occlusive vascular diseases (eg, atherosclerosis, arteriosclerosis, diabetic endarteritis, Buerger's disease) more likely to occur in the lower than in the upper extremity; avoid leg veins in elderly patients or in those suffering from such disorders. Gangrene in a lower extremity reported when given in an ankle vein. Check infusion site frequently for free flow. Avoid extravasation into the tissues; local necrosis might ensue. Blanching may occur; consider changing the infusion site at intervals to allow local effects of vasoconstriction to subside. Caution in elderly.

ADVERSE REACTIONS: Ischemic injury, bradycardia, arrhythmias, anxiety, headache, respiratory difficulty, extravasation necrosis at injection site, gangrene.

INTERACTIONS: See Contraindications. Caution with MAOI or triptyline/imipramine antidepressants; severe, prolonged HTN may result.

PREGNANCY: Category C, caution in nursing.

MECHANISM OF ACTION: Alpha-adrenergic agonist; peripheral vasoconstrictor (α-adrenergic action) and inotropic stimulator of the heart and dilator of coronary arteries (β-adrenergic action).

NURSING CONSIDERATIONS

Assessment: Assess hypotension and need for blood volume replacement. Assess use as emergency measure or life-saving procedure (eg, hypotension from blood volume deficits to maintain coronary and cerebral artery perfusion until blood volume replacement therapy can be completed, mesenteric or peripheral vascular thrombosis). Assess sulfite sensitivity, pregnancy/nursing status, and for possible drug interactions. Assess use in elderly and occlusive vascular diseases (eg, atherosclerosis, arteriosclerosis, diabetic endarteritis, Buerger's disease). Obtain baseline BP.

Monitoring: Monitor for HTN, headache, gangrene, extravasation, blanching, hypersensitivity/allergic reactions. Monitor rate of flow, BP, HR, central venous pressure, and appropriate fluid and electrolyte replacement.

Administration: IV route. Refer to PI for proper dilution and administration. Avoid contact with iron salts, alkalis, or oxidizing agents. **Storage:** 20-25°C (68-77°F); excursions permitted to 15-30° (59-86°F). Protect from light.

LEVOTHROID   RX
levothyroxine sodium (Forest)

THERAPEUTIC CLASS: Thyroid replacement hormone

INDICATIONS: Hypothyroidism. As a pituitary TSH suppressant for non-endemic goiter and for chronic lymphocytic thyroiditis. Diagnostic agent in suppression tests to differentiate mild hyperthyroidism or thyroid gland autonomy. Adjunct therapy with antithyroid drugs to treat thyrotoxicosis. Adjunct to surgery and radioiodine therapy for TSH-dependent thyroid cancer.

DOSAGE: *Adults:* Hypothyroidism: Usual: 100-200mcg/day. Endocrine/Cardiovascular Complications: Initial: 50mcg/day. Titrate: Increase by 50mcg/day every 2-4 weeks until euthyroid. Hypothyroid with Angina: Initial: 25mcg/day. Titrate: Increase by 25-50mcg every 2-4 weeks until euthyroid. *Pediatrics:* Hypothyroidism: >12 yrs: Usual: 100-200mcg/day. 6-12 yrs: 4-5mcg/kg/day. 1-5 yrs: 5-6mcg/kg/day. 6-12 months: 6-8mcg/kg/day. 0-6 months: 10-15mcg/kg/day. May crush tab and sprinkle over food (applesauce) or mix with 5-10mL water, formula (non-soy), or breast milk.

HOW SUPPLIED: Tab: 25mcg*, 50mcg*, 75mcg*, 88mcg*, 100mcg*, 112mcg*, 125mcg*, 137mcg*, 150mcg*, 175mcg*, 200mcg*, 300mcg* *scored

CONTRAINDICATIONS: Untreated thyrotoxicosis, acute MI, and uncorrected adrenal insufficiency.

WARNINGS/PRECAUTIONS: Do not use in the treatment of obesity; larger doses in euthyroid patients can cause serious or even life-threatening toxicity. Caution with cardiovascular disease, HTN. May aggravate diabetes mellitus or insipidus and adrenal cortical insufficiency. Excessive doses in infants may produce craniosynostosis. Add glucocorticoid with myxedema coma.

ADVERSE REACTIONS: Lactose hypersensitivity, transient partial hair loss in children.

INTERACTIONS: Monitor insulin and oral hypoglycemic requirements. May potentiate anticoagulant effects of warfarin; adjust warfarin dose and monitor PT/INR. Increased adrenergic effects of catecholamines; caution with CAD. Decreased absorption with cholestyramine and colestipol; space dosing by 4-5 hrs. Estrogens increase thyroxine-binding globulin; increase in thyroid dose may be needed. Large dose may cause life-threatening toxicities with sympathomimetic amines. Avoid mixing crushed tabs with foods/formula with large amounts of iron, soybean or fiber.

PREGNANCY: Category A, caution in nursing.

MECHANISM OF ACTION: Thyroid hormone; not understood, suspected to control DNA transcription and protein synthesis. Regulates multiple metabolic processes.

PHARMACOKINETICS: Distribution: Plasma protein binding (99%). **Metabolism:** Deiodination (major pathway), conjugation (minor pathway) in liver (mainly), kidneys, and other tissues. **Elimination:** Urine; T_4 (feces 20% unchanged); $T_{1/2}$=6-7 days; $T_{1/2}$≤2 days (T_3).

NURSING CONSIDERATIONS

Assessment: Assess for drug hypersensitivity, CV disease, angina pectoris, acute MI, suppressed serum TSH level with normal T_3 and T_4 levels, overt thyrotoxicosis, DM, clotting disorder, adrenal/pituitary gland problems, malabsorption, autoimmune polyglandular syndrome, undergoing surgery, and possible drug and test interactions. Assess infants with congenital hypothyroidism for other congenital anomalies.

Monitoring: Requires frequent lab tests and clinical evaluation of thyroid function by TSH levels, and also glucose/lipid metabolism, urinary glucose in diabetics, and clotting status. Monitor for CV signs such as arrhythmia and coronary insufficiency, growth/development, bone metabolism, cognitive function, emotional state, GI function, reproductive function, partial hair loss in children, and signs/symptoms of thyrotoxicosis.

Patient Counseling: Counsel to take 1 hr before breakfast, and not to to use as part of weight control regimen. Inform that replacement therapy is essential for life, except in cases of transient hypothyroidism. Advise to notify physician if pregnant/nursing or intend to become pregnant or if taking any other drugs. Counsel to not d/c or change dosage. Report signs/symptoms of thyroid toxicity.

Administration: Oral route. **Storage:** 25°C (77°F); excursions permitted to 15-30°C (59-86°F). Protect from light and moisture.

LEVOXYL

RX

levothyroxine sodium (King)

THERAPEUTIC CLASS: Thyroid replacement hormone

INDICATIONS: Replacement or supplemental therapy in congenital or acquired hypothyroidism of any etiology, except transient hypothyroidism during the recovery phase of subacute thyroiditis. Treatment or prevention of various types of euthyroid goiters, including thyroid nodules, subacute or chronic lymphocytic thyroiditis, multinodular goiter and as an adjunct to surgery and radioiodine therapy for thyrotropin-dependent well-differentiated thyroid cancer.

DOSAGE: *Adults:* Take in the AM at least one-half hour before food. Take at least 4 hrs apart from drugs that are known to interfere with absorption. Hypothyroidism: Usual: 1.7mcg/kg/day. Doses >200mcg/day seldom required. >50 yrs/<50 yrs with cardiac disease: Initial: 25-50mcg/day. Titrate: Increase by 12.5-25mcg/day every 6-8 weeks until euthyroid. Elderly with Cardiac Disease: Initial: 12.5-25mcg/day. Titrate: Increase by 12.5-25mcg/day every 4-6 weeks until euthyroid. Severe Hypothyroidism: Initial: 12.5-25mcg/day. Titrate: Increase by 25mcg/day every 2-4 weeks until euthyroid. Pregnancy: May increase dose requirements. Subclinical Hypothyroidism: Lower doses may be adequate to normalize the TSH level (eg, 1mcg/kg/day). TSH Suppression in Well-differentiated Thyroid Cancer and Thyroid Nodules: Individualize dose based on the specific disease and the patient being treated. Take with water. Refer to PI for further details.
Pediatrics: Take in the AM at least one-half hour before food. Take at least 4 hrs apart from drugs that are known to interfere with absorption. Hypothyroidism: 0-3 months: 10-15mcg/kg/day. 3-6 months: 8-10mcg/kg/day. 6-12 months: 6-8mcg/kg/day. 1-5 yrs: 5-6mcg/kg/day. 6-12 yrs: 4-5mcg/kg/day. >12 yrs: 2-3mcg/kg/day. Growth/Puberty Complete: 1.7mcg/kg/day. Infants at Risk for Cardiac Failure: Use lower dose (eg, 25mcg/day). Titrate: Increase dose every 4-6 weeks as needed based until euthyroid. Infants with Serum T_4 <5mcg/dL: Initial: 50mcg/day. Chronic/Severe Hypothyroidism: Children: Initial: 25mcg/day. Titrate: Increase by 25mcg/day every 2-4 weeks until desired effect is achieved. Minimize Hyperactivity in Older Children: Initial: Give 1/4 of full replacement dose. Titrate: Increase on a weekly basis by an amount equal to 1/4 the full recommended replacement dose until the full recommended replacement dose is reached. May crush tab and mix with 5-10mL of water.

HOW SUPPLIED: Tab: 25mcg, 50mcg, 75mcg, 88mcg, 100mcg, 112mcg, 125mcg, 137mcg, 150mcg, 175mcg, 200mcg

CONTRAINDICATIONS: Untreated subclinical or overt thyrotoxicosis of any etiology, acute myocardial infarction (MI), and uncorrected adrenal insufficiency.

WARNINGS/PRECAUTIONS: Do not use for the treatment of obesity or weight loss; larger doses in euthyroid patients may cause serious or even life-threatening toxicity. Should not be used in the treatment of male or female infertility unless associated with hypothyroidism. Caution with nontoxic diffuse goiter or nodular thyroid disease. Carefully titrate dose to avoid over or under treatment. May decrease bone mineral density (BMD) with long term use; give minimum dose necessary to achieve desired clinical and biochemical response. Caution with CV disorders and the elderly with risk of occult cardiac disease. If cardiac symptoms develop or worsen, reduce or withhold dose for 1 week and then restart at lower dose. May produce CV effects (eg, increase HR, increase in cardiac wall thickness, increase in cardiac contractility, precipitation of angina or arrhythmias). Monitor patients with coronary artery disease (CAD) closely during surgical procedures, may precipitate cardiac arrhythmias. Caution in patients with adrenal insufficiency, insulin-dependent diabetes mellitus (DM), or pernicious anemia.

ADVERSE REACTIONS: Fatigue, increased appetite, weight loss, heat intolerance, headache, hyperactivity, irritability, insomnia, palpitations, arrhythmias, dyspnea, hair loss, menstrual irregularities, pseudotumor cerebri (children), slipped capital femoral epiphysis (children).

INTERACTIONS: Sympathomimetics may increase risk of coronary insufficiency with CAD. Upward dose adjustments may be needed for insulin and oral hypoglycemic agents. May decrease absorption with soybean flour, cottonseed meal, walnuts, and dietary fiber. May potentiate oral anticoagulant effects; adjust dose and monitor PT. May decrease levels and effects of digitalis glycosides. Reduced TSH secretion with dopamine/dopamine agonists, glucocorticoids, octreotide. Decreased thyroid hormone secretion with amino-glutethimide, amiodarone, iodine (including iodine-containing radiographic contrast agents), lithium, methimazole, propylthiouracil (PTU), sulfonamides, tolbutamide. May increase thyroid hormone secretion with amiodarone and iodide. May decrease T4 absorption with antacids (aluminum & magnesium hydroxides), simethicone, bile acid sequestrants (cholestyramine, colestipol), calcium carbonate, cation exchange resins (kayexalate), ferrous sulfate, orlistat, and sucralfate. May increase serum thyroxine-binding globulin (TBG) concentration with clofibrate, estrogen-containing oral contraceptives, oral estrogens, heroin/methadone, 5-FU, mitotane, and tamoxifen. May decrease serum TBG concentration with androgens/anabolic steroids, asparaginase, glucocorticoids, and slow-release nicotinic acid. May cause protein-binding site displacement with furosemide (>80mg IV), heparin, hydantoins, NSAIDs (fenamates, phenylbutazone), and salicylates (>2g/day). May alter T4 and T3 metabolism with carbamazepine, hydantoins, phenobarbital, and rifampin. May decrease T4 5'-deiodinase activity with amiodarone, β-adrenergic antagonists (eg, propranolol >160mg/day), glucocorticoids (eg, dexamethasone >4mg/day), and PTU. Concurrent use with tri/tetracyclic antidepressants may increase the therapeutic and toxic effects of both drugs. Coadministration with sertraline in patients stabilized on levothyroxine may result in increased levothyroxine requirements. Interferon-α may cause development of anti-thyroid microsomal antibodies causing transient hypothyroidism, hyperthyroidism, or both. Interleukin-2 has been associated with transient painless thyroiditis. Excessive use with growth hormones (eg, somatropin, somatrem) may accelerate epiphyseal closure. Ketamine may produce marked HTN and tachycardia. May reduce uptake of iodine-containing radiographic contrast agents. Decreased theophylline clearance may occur in hypothyroid patients. Altered levels of thyroid hormone and/or TSH level with choral hydrate, diazepam, ethionamide, lovastatin, metoclopramide, 6-mercaptopurine, nitroprusside, para-aminosalicylate sodium, perphenazine, resorcinol (excessive topical use), and thiazide diuretics.

PREGNANCY: Category A, caution in nursing.

MECHANISM OF ACTION: Thyroid hormone; mechanism not established. Suspected that principal effects are exerted through control of DNA transcription and protein synthesis.

PHARMACOKINETICS: Distribution: Plasma protein binding (99%); found in breast milk. **Metabolism:** Deiodination and conjugation in liver (mainly), kidneys, and other tissues. **Elimination:** Urine, feces (20% unchanged); $T_{1/2}$=6-7days (T4), ≤2 days (T3).

NURSING CONSIDERATIONS

Assessment: Assess for untreated subclinical or overt thyrotoxicosis, presence of acute MI, uncorrected adrenal insufficiency, CV disorders, nontoxic diffuse goiter, nodular thyroid disease, DM, pregnancy/nursing status, and for possible drug interactions. In patients with secondary or tertiary hypothyroidism, assess for additional hypothalamic/pituitary hormone deficiencies. Assess that therapy is not for the treatment of obesity or for weight loss. In infants with congenital hypothyroidism, assess for other congenital anomalies.

Monitoring: Monitor for CV effects (eg, increase in HR, increase in cardiac wall thickness, angina, arrhythmias). In patients on long-term therapy, monitor for signs/symptoms of decreased BMD. In patients with nontoxic diffuse goiter or nodular thyroid disease, monitor for precipitation of thyrotoxicosis. In adults with primary hypothyroidism, perform periodic monitoring of serum TSH levels. In pediatric patients with congenital hypothyroidism, perform periodic monitoring of serum TSH levels and total or free T4 levels. In patients with secondary and tertiary hypothyroidism, perform periodic monitoring of serum free T4 levels.

Patient Counseling: Instruct to notify physician if allergic to any foods or medicines, pregnant or planning to become pregnant, breastfeeding or taking any other drugs, including prescriptions and over-the-counter preparations. Notify physician of any other medical conditions particularly heart disease, diabetes, clotting disorders, and adrenal or pituitary gland problems. Instruct not to stop or change dose unless directed by physician. Take on empty stomach, with a full glass of water, at least 1/2 hr before eating any food. Advise that partial hair loss may occur during the first few months of therapy, but is usually temporary. Notify physician or dentist prior to surgery, that taking levothyroxine. Inform that should not use as a primary or adjunctive therapy in a weight control program.

Administration: Oral route. Take with water. **Storage:** 20-25°C (68-77°F); excursions permitted to 15-30°C (59-86°F).

LEXAPRO   RX
escitalopram oxalate (Forest)

> Antidepressants increased the risk of suicidal thinking and behavior (suicidality) in short-term studies in children, adolescents, and young adults with MDD and other psychiatric disorders. Monitor and observe closely for clinical worsening, suicidality, or unusual changes in behavior in patients who are started on antidepressant therapy. Not approved for use in pediatric patients <12 yrs of age.

THERAPEUTIC CLASS: Selective serotonin reuptake inhibitor

INDICATIONS: Acute and maintenance treatment of major depressive disorder (MDD) in adults and adolescents 12-17 yrs. Acute treatment of generalized anxiety disorder (GAD) in adults.

DOSAGE: *Adults:* MDD: Initial: 10mg qd. Titrate: May increase to 20mg after ≥1 week. Max: 20mg qd. GAD: Initial: 10mg qd. Titrate: May increase to 20mg after ≥1 week. Efficacy >8 weeks not studied. Elderly/Hepatic Impairment: 10mg qd. Periodically assess the need for maintenance. Allow ≥14 days interval between d/c of MAOI and initiation of escitalopram, or vice versa.
Pediatrics: 12-17 yrs: MDD: Initial: 10mg qd. Titrate: May increase to 20mg after ≥3 weeks. Max: 20mg qd. Periodically assess the need for maintenance. Allow ≥14 days interval between d/c of MAOI and initiation of escitalopram, or vice versa.

HOW SUPPLIED: Sol: 5mg/5mL; Tab: 5mg, 10mg*, 20mg* *scored

CONTRAINDICATIONS: Concomitant use of MAOI or pimozide.

WARNINGS/PRECAUTIONS: Serotonin syndrome or neuroleptic malignant syndrome (NMS)-like reactions may occur. Avoid abrupt d/c; gradually decrease dose. Activation of mania/hypomania reported; caution with history of mania. May increase the risk of bleeding events. Hyponatremia may occur; caution in elderly and volume-depleted patients. D/C if symptomatic hyponatremia occurs and institute appropriate intervention. Convulsions reported. Caution with history of seizures, conditions that alter metabolism or hemodynamic responses, severe renal impairment. May impair mental/physical abilities.

ADVERSE REACTIONS: N/V, insomnia, ejaculation disorder, increased sweating, somnolence, fatigue, diarrhea, dry mouth, headache, constipation, indigestion, neck/shoulder pain, anorgasmia.

INTERACTIONS: See Contraindications. Increased risk of serotonin syndrome or NMS-like reactions with serotonergic drugs (including triptans), antipsychotics, dopamine antagonists, linezolid, lithium, tramadol, St. John's wort; use with caution. Use with other SSRIs, SNRIs, tryptophan, or alcohol is not recommended. Caution with other CNS drugs, and drugs metabolized by CYP2D6 (eg, desipramine). Increased risk of bleeding with NSAIDs, aspirin (ASA), warfarin, and other anticoagulants. Rare reports of weakness, hyperreflexia, incoordination with sumatriptan. May increase levels with cimetidine. May decrease levels of ketoconazole. May increase levels of metoprolol. May increase clearance with carbamazepine. Increased risk of hyponatremia with diuretics.

PREGNANCY: Category C, caution in nursing.

MECHANISM OF ACTION: SSRI; presumed to be linked to potentiation of serotonergic activity in the CNS resulting from its inhibition of CNS neuronal reuptake of serotonin (5-HT).

PHARMACOKINETICS: Absorption: T_{max}=5 hrs. **Distribution:** Plasma protein binding (56%); found in breast milk. **Metabolism:** Hepatic; N-demethylation via CYP3A4, 2C19. **Elimination:** Urine (8%); $T_{1/2}$=27-32 hrs.

NURSING CONSIDERATIONS

Assessment: Assess for risk of bipolar disorder, bleeding events, history of seizures, history of mania, volume depletion, disease/condition that alters metabolism or hemodynamic response, hepatic/renal impairment, drug hypersensitivity, pregnancy/nursing status, and possible drug interactions. Obtain detailed psychiatric history.

Monitoring: Monitor for signs/symptoms of clinical worsening, suicidality, unusual changes in behavior, serotonin syndrome, NMS-like reactions, abnormal bleeding, hyponatremia, seizures, cognitive and motor impairment, and hepatic/renal dysfunction. If therapy is abruptly d/c, monitor for symptoms of dysphoric mood, irritability, agitation, dizziness, sensory disturbances, anxiety, confusion, headache, lethargy, emotional lability, insomnia, and hypomania.

Patient Counseling: Advise to avoid alcohol. Seek medical attention for symptoms of serotonin syndrome (mental status changes, tachycardia, hyperthermia, N/V, diarrhea, incoordination), abnormal bleeding (particularly if using NSAIDs or ASA), activation of mania, seizures, clinical worsening (suicidal ideation, unusual changes in behavior), and d/c symptoms (irritability, agitation, anxiety, headache, insomnia). Caution against hazardous tasks (eg, operating machinery and driving). May notice improvement in 1-4 weeks; continue therapy as directed. Instruct to notify physician if taking or plan to take any prescribed or over-the-counter drugs. Advise to notify physician if they become pregnant, intend to become pregnant, or breastfeeding.

Administration: Oral route. Administer qd, in am or pm, with or without food. **Storage:** 25°C (77°F); excursions permitted to 15-30°C (59-86°F).

LIALDA   RX
mesalamine (Shire)

THERAPEUTIC CLASS: 5-Aminosalicylic acid derivative

INDICATIONS: Induction of remission in adult patients with active, mild to moderate ulcerative colitis.

DOSAGE: *Adults:* 2-4 tabs qd with meals for up to 8 weeks. Max: 2.4g - 4.8g/day.

HOW SUPPLIED: Tab, Delayed-Release: 1.2g

WARNINGS/PRECAUTIONS: Patients with pyloric stenosis may have prolonged gastric retention, which could delay mesalamine release in the colon. Caution with sulfasalazine allergy. May cause acute intolerance syndrome; if suspected prompt withdrawal is required. Cardiac hypersensitivity reactions (myocarditis, pericarditis) reported; caution in patients with conditions predisposing to the development of myocarditis or pericarditis. Renal impairment, including minimal change nephropathy, and acute or chronic interstitial nephritis reported; caution with known renal dysfunction or history of renal disease. Caution with hepatic impairment or pre-existing liver disease. Caution in nursing women.

ADVERSE REACTIONS: Headache, flatulence, acute intolerance syndrome.

INTERACTIONS: Concurrent use with nephrotoxic agents (eg, NSAIDs) may increase risk of renal reactions. Concurrent use with azathioprine or 6-mercaptopurine can increase potential for blood disorders.

PREGNANCY: Category B, caution in nursing.

MECHANISM OF ACTION: Anti-inflammatory agent; not established. Suspected to diminish inflammation by blocking cyclooxygenase and inhibiting prostaglandin production in colon.

PHARMACOKINETICS: Absorption: PO administration of variable doses resulted in different parameters. C_{max} = 1595-2154 ng/mL. AUC = 21084-44775 ng•hr/mL. **Distribution:** Plasma protein binding (43%). Found in breast milk; crosses placental barrier. **Metabolism:** Liver and intestinal mucosa (acetylation), N-acetyl-5-aminosalicylic acid (major metabolite). **Elimination:** Urine (<8% unchanged, >13% N-acetyl-5-aminosalicylic acid); (2.4g) $T_{1/2}$=7-9 hrs, (4.8g) $T_{1/2}$=8-12 hrs.

NURSING CONSIDERATIONS

Assessment: Assess for pyloric stenosis, sensitivity to sulfasalazine, renal dysfunction, hepatic impairment, conditions predisposing to development of myo- and pericarditis, pregnancy/nursing status, and possible drug interactions. Obtain baseline renal function, cardiac function and LFTs.

Monitoring: Monitor for signs/symptoms of acute intolerance syndrome (eg, cramping, acute abdominal pain, bloody diarrhea), prolonged gastric retention, cardiac hypersensitivity reactions, and renal impairment (eg, nephropathy, acute/chronic interstitial nephritis). Perform periodic renal function monitoring during therapy.

Patient Counseling: Instruct to swallow tablet whole, keeping outer coating intact. Seek medical attention if symptoms of acute intolerance syndrome, prolonged gastric retention, or hypersensitivity reactions occur. Inform physician if allergic to sulfasalazine or mesalamine. Inform physician if taking NSAIDs or other nephrotoxic agents, azathioprine or 6-mercaptopurine concomitantly. Alert physician if pregnant or intend to become pregnant or breastfeeding.

Administration: Oral route. **Storage:** 15-25°C (59-77°F); excursions permitted to 30°C (86°F).

LIBRAX
chlordiazepoxide HCl - clidinium bromide (Valeant) `CIV`

THERAPEUTIC CLASS: Benzodiazepine/anticholinergic

INDICATIONS: Adjunct treatment of irritable bowel syndrome (IBS), acute enterocolitis, and peptic ulcer.

DOSAGE: *Adults:* Usual/Maint: 1-2 caps tid-qid ac and hs. Elderly/Debilitated: Initial: 2 caps/day and increase gradually, if needed.

HOW SUPPLIED: Cap: (Chlordiazepoxide-Clidinium) 5mg-2.5mg

CONTRAINDICATIONS: Glaucoma, prostatic hypertrophy, benign bladder neck obstruction.

WARNINGS/PRECAUTIONS: Risk of congenital malformations during first trimester of pregnancy; avoid use. Avoid abrupt withdrawal. Paradoxical reactions reported in psychiatric patients. Caution with depression, renal or hepatic dysfunction, the elderly. Inhibition of lactation may occur.

ADVERSE REACTIONS: Drowsiness, ataxia, confusion, skin eruptions, extrapyramidal symptoms, dry mouth, nausea, constipation, altered libido, blood dyscrasias, jaundice, hepatic dysfunction.

INTERACTIONS: Avoid with other psychotropics; if combination is indicated, use caution especially with MAOIs and phenothiazines. Caution with alcohol, other CNS depressants. Altered coagulation effects with oral anticoagulants.

PREGNANCY: Not for use in pregnancy; safety in nursing is not known.

MECHANISM OF ACTION: Anticholinergic/spasmolytic and antianxiety agent.

NURSING CONSIDERATIONS

Assessment: Assess for glaucoma, prostatic hypertrophy, benign bladder neck obstruction, renal/hepatic dysfunction, alcohol intake, and for possible drug interactions (eg, MAOIs).

Monitoring: Monitor for ataxia, oversedation, confusion, paradoxical reactions (eg, excitement, stimulation, acute rage), and for possible physical and psychological dependence.

Patient Counseling: Inform that psychological and physical dependence may develop, to avoid performing hazardous tasks (eg, operating machinery/driving), and to consult physician before increasing dose or abruptly d/c.

Administration: Oral route.

LIBRIUM

CIV

chlordiazepoxide HCl (Valeant)

THERAPEUTIC CLASS: Benzodiazepine

INDICATIONS: Management of anxiety disorders and short-term relief of anxiety symptoms, withdrawal symptoms of acute alcoholism, and preoperative apprehension and anxiety.

DOSAGE: *Adults:* Mild-Moderate Anxiety: 5-10mg tid-qid. Severe Anxiety: 20-25mg tid-qid. Alcohol Withdrawal: 50-100mg; repeat until agitation controlled. Max: 300mg/day. Preoperative Anxiety: 5-10mg PO tid-qid on days prior to surgery. Elderly/Debilitated: 5mg bid-qid.
Pediatrics: ≥6 yrs: 5mg bid-qid. May increase to 10mg bid-tid.

HOW SUPPLIED: Cap: 5mg, 10mg, 25mg

WARNINGS/PRECAUTIONS: Avoid in pregnancy. Paradoxical reactions reported in psychiatric patients and in hyperactive aggressive pediatrics. Caution with porphyria, renal or hepatic dysfunction. Reduce dose in elderly, debilitated. Avoid abrupt withdrawal after extended therapy. May impair mental/physical abilities.

ADVERSE REACTIONS: Drowsiness, ataxia, confusion, skin eruptions, edema, nausea, constipation, extrapyramidal symptoms, libido changes, EEG changes.

INTERACTIONS: Additive effects with CNS depressants and alcohol. Avoid other psychotropic agents.

PREGNANCY: Not for use in pregnancy, safety in nursing not known.

MECHANISM OF ACTION: Not established; has antianxiety, sedative, appetite stimulating, and weak analgesic actions; suspected to block EEG arousal from stimulation of brain stem reticular formation.

PHARMACOKINETICS: Elimination: Urine (1-2% unchanged, 3-6% as conjugates); $T_{1/2}$=24-48 hrs.

NURSING CONSIDERATIONS

Assessment: Assess for pregnancy status, hepatic/renal function, and possible drug interactions.

Monitoring: Monitor geriatric patients for ataxia and oversedation, drowsiness, confusion; paradoxical reactions in psychiatric patients and in hyperactive aggressive pediatric patients. Periodic blood counts and LFTs are advisable when treatment is protracted.

Patient Counseling: Inform that psychological/physical dependence may result; consult physician before increasing dose or abruptly d/c drug. May impair mental/physical abilities; caution while operating machinery/driving. May impair mental alertness in children. Avoid alcohol and other CNS depressant drugs.

Administration: Oral route. **Storage:** 25°C (77°F); excursions permitted to 15-30°C (59-86°F).

LIDODERM PATCH

RX

lidocaine (Endo)

THERAPEUTIC CLASS: Acetamide local anesthetic

INDICATIONS: Relief of pain associated with post-herpetic neuralgia.

DOSAGE: *Adults:* Apply to intact skin, cover most painful area. Apply up to 3 patches, once for up to 12 hrs within 24-hr period. May cut patches into smaller sizes before removal of the release liner. Debilitated/Impaired Elimination: Treat smaller areas. Remove if irritation or burning occurs; may reapply when irritation subsides.

HOW SUPPLIED: Patch: 5% [30^s]

WARNINGS/PRECAUTIONS: Serious adverse events may occur in children or pets if ingested; keep out of reach. Increased risk of toxicity in severe hepatic disease. Increased risk of toxicity in severe hepatic disease. Avoid broken or inflamed skin, placement of external heat (eg, heating pads, electric blankets) and eye contact. Caution with history of drug sensitivities (eg, procaine, tetracaine, benzocaine), smaller patients and patients with impaired elimination.

ADVERSE REACTIONS: Application-site reactions (eg, erythema, edema, bruising, papules, vesicles, discoloration, depigmentation, burning sensation, pruritus, dermatitis, petechia, blisters, exfoliation, abnormal sensation, irritation).

INTERACTIONS: Additive toxic effects with concomitant Class I antiarrhythmics (eg, tocainide, mexiletine). Consider total amount absorbed from all formulations containing other local anesthetics.

PREGNANCY: Category B, caution in nursing.

MECHANISM OF ACTION: Amide-type local anesthetic; stabilizes neuronal membranes by inhibiting ionic fluxes required for initiation and conduction of impulses.

PHARMACOKINETICS: Absorption: C_{max}=0.13mcg/mL; T_{max}=11 hrs. **Distribution:** V_d=0.7-2.7L/kg (IV); Plasma protein binding (70%). Crosses placenta; found in breast milk. **Metabolism:** Liver (rapid); monoethylglycinexylidide, glycinexylidide (active metabolites). **Elimination:** Urine (<10%, unchanged); $T_{1/2}$=81-149 min (IV).

NURSING CONSIDERATIONS

Assessment: Assess for hepatic disease, pregnancy/nursing status, history of drug sensitivities to local anesthetics of the amide type and para-aminobenzoic acid derivatives. Assess for possible drug interactions.

Monitoring: Monitor for local skin reactions, allergic/anaphylactoid reactions, liver function, pain intensity and pain relief periodically.

Patient Counseling: Instruct to remove patch and not to reapply if irritation or burning sensation occurs during application until irritation subsides. If eye contact occurs, immediately wash with water or saline and protect eye until sensation returns. Counsel to avoid application to larger areas and for longer than recommended wearing time. Avoid applying to broken or inflamed skin. Instruct to wash hands after handling patch and to fold used patches so adhesive side sticks to itself. Keep out of reach of children and pets.

Administration: Transdermal route. Refer to PI for proper handling and disposal. **Storage:** Store at 25°C (77°F); excursions permitted to 15-30°C (59-86°F).

LIPITOR

RX

atorvastatin calcium (Parke-Davis/Pfizer)

THERAPEUTIC CLASS: HMG-CoA reductase inhibitor

INDICATIONS: Adjunct to diet, to reduce total cholesterol (total-C), LDL, TG, and apolipoprotein B (Apo B) levels, and to increase HDL in primary hypercholesterolemia (heterozygous familial and nonfamilial) and mixed dyslipidemia (Types IIa and IIb). Adjunct to diet for elevated serum TG levels (type IV). Treatment of primary dysbetalipoproteinemia (Type III) inadequately responding to diet. Adjunct to other lipid-lowering treatments or if treatments are unavailable, to reduce total-C and LDL in homozygous familial hypercholesterolemia. Adjunct to diet to lower total-C, LDL, and Apo B in boys and postmenarchal girls, 10 to 17 yrs of age, with heterozygous familial hypercholesterolemia. To reduce the risk of MI, stroke, revascularization procedures, and angina in adults without clinically evident CHD but with multiple risk factors for CHD. To reduce the risk of MI and stroke in patients with Type II DM, and without clinically evident CHD, but with multiple risk factors for CHD. In patients with clinically evident CHD to reduce the risk of non-fatal MI, fatal and non-fatal stroke, revascularization procedures, hospitalization for CHF, and angina.

DOSAGE: *Adults:* Hyperlipidemia (Heterozygous Familial and Nonfamilial)/ Mixed Dyslipidemia: Initial: 10-20mg qd (or 40mg qd for LDL reduction >45%). Titrate: Adjust dose if needed at 2-4 week intervals. Usual: 10-80mg qd. Homozygous Familial Hypercholesterolemia: 10-80mg qd. With Cyclosporine: 10mg qd. With Clarithromycin, Itraconazole, or Combination of Ritonavir Plus Saquinavir or Lopinavir Plus Ritonavir: Caution in doses >20mg qd; the lowest dose necessary should be used.
Pediatrics: 10-17 yrs: Heterozygous Familial Hypercholesterolemia: Initial: 10mg/day. Titrate: Adjust dose if needed at intervals of ≥4 weeks. Max: 20mg/day.

HOW SUPPLIED: Tab: 10mg, 20mg, 40mg, 80mg

CONTRAINDICATIONS: Active liver disease which may include unexplained persistent elevations of serum transaminases, pregnancy or nursing mothers.

WARNINGS/PRECAUTIONS: May cause biochemical abnormalities of liver function; monitor LFTs prior to therapy, at 12 weeks or with dose elevation, and periodically thereafter. Reduce dose or withdraw if AST or ALT ≥3x ULN persists. Caution with heavy alcohol use and/or history of hepatic disease. Rare cases of rhabdomyolysis with acute renal failure secondary to myoglobinuria reported. Monitor for skeletal muscle effects in patients with history of renal impairment. D/C if markedly elevated CPK levels occur, if myopathy is diagnosed or suspected, or if there are risk factors predisposing renal failure secondary to rhabdomyolysis. May affect endocrine function or cause CNS toxicity. Caution in patients with recent stroke or TIA. Caution in elderly.

ADVERSE REACTIONS: Nasopharyngitis, arthralgia, diarrhea, dyspepsia, nausea, pain in extremity, urinary tract infection, myalgia, muscle spasms, musculoskeletal pain, fatigue, hepatic enzyme elevation, rhabdomyolysis, myopathy, peripheral neuropathy.

INTERACTIONS: May increase levels when used with strong CYP3A4 inhibitors (eg, clarithromycin, HIV protease inhibitors, itraconazole), and grapefruit juice (>1.2L/day). Inhibitors of OATP1B1 (eg, cyclosporine) may increase bioavailability of atorvastatin. Coadministration with digoxin may increase digoxin levels; monitor appropriately. Inducers of CYP3A4 (eg, efavirenz, rifampin) may decrease atorvastatin levels. Coadministration with oral contraceptives increases AUC of norethindrone and ethinyl estradiol. Increased risk of myopathy with cyclosporine, fibric acid derivatives, erythromycin, clarithromycin, combination of ritonavir plus saquinavir or lopinavir plus ritonavir, niacin, and azole antifungals. Caution with drugs that decrease the levels or activity of endogenous steroid hormones (eg, ketoconazole, spironolactone, cimetidine). Diltiazem may increase the AUC of atorvastatin. Amlodipine may increase the AUC of atorvastatin and decrease the C_{max} of atorvastatin. Colestipol may decrease the C_{max} of atorvastatin. Maalox TC may decrease the AUC and C_{max} of atorvastatin. Coadministration with antipyrine may increase the AUC and decrease the C_{max} of antipyrine.

PREGNANCY: Category X, not for use in nursing.

MECHANISM OF ACTION: HMG-CoA reductase inhibitor; inhibits conversion of HMG-CoA to mevalonate (precursor of sterols, including cholesterol).

PHARMACOKINETICS: Absorption: Rapid; absolute bioavailability (14%); T_{max}=1-2 hrs. **Distribution:** V_d=381L; plasma protein binding (≥98%); found in breast milk. **Metabolism:** Extensive; via CYP3A4; ortho- and parahydroxylated derivatives and various β-oxidation products (metabolites). **Elimination:** Bile (drug, metabolites), urine (<2%); $T_{1/2}$=14 hrs.

NURSING CONSIDERATIONS

Assessment: Assess for active or history of liver disease, unexplained and persistent elevations in serum transaminase levels, pregnancy/nursing status, alcohol intake, renal impairment, recent stroke or TIA, and for possible drug interactions. Assess for risk factors predisposing to the development of renal failure secondary to rhabdomyolysis (eg, severe acute infection, hypotension, major surgery, trauma, uncontrolled seizures). Perform LFTs prior to therapy. Try to control hypercholesterolemia through appropriate diet, exercise, and weight reduction prior to therapy.

Monitoring: Monitor for signs/symptoms of rhabdomyolysis with acute renal failure, myopathy (eg, muscle aches, muscle weakness, CPK elevations), liver dysfunction, endocrine dysfunction, and CNS toxicity. Monitor LFTs 12 weeks following initiation of therapy, with any elevation of dose, and periodically (eg, semiannually) thereafter.

Patient Counseling: Inform about potential risks/benefits of therapy. Instruct to follow standard cholesterol-lowering diet and regular exercise program as appropriate. Counsel to promptly report any signs of myopathy (eg, un-explained muscle pain, tenderness, weakness). Instruct to notify physician if pregnant/nursing or planning to become pregnant.

Administration: Oral route. **Storage:** 20-25°C (68-77°F).

LIPOFEN   RX
fenofibrate (Kowa)

THERAPEUTIC CLASS: Fibric acid derivative

INDICATIONS: Treatment of hypertriglyceridemia (Types IV and V) as adjunct to diet. Reduction of elevated total cholesterol, LDL, Apo B, TG, and to increase HDL in primary hypercholesterolemia or mixed dyslipidemia (Types IIa and IIb) as adjunct to diet.

DOSAGE: *Adults:* Hypercholesterolemia/Mixed Dyslipidemia: Initial: 150mg qd. Hypertriglyceridemia: Initial : 50-150mg/day. Titrate: Adjust if needed after repeat lipid determinations at 4-8 week intervals. Max: 150mg/day. Renal Dysfuntion/Elderly: Initial: 50mg/day. Titrate: Adjust if needed after lipid determinations and evaluation of the effects on renal function.

HOW SUPPLIED: Cap: 50mg, 150mg

CONTRAINDICATIONS: Pre-existing gallbladder disease, unexplained persis-tent liver function abnormality, hepatic or severe renal dysfunction (including primary biliary cirrhosis).

WARNINGS/PRECAUTIONS: Monitor LFTs regularly; d/c if >3X ULN. May cause cholelithiasis; d/c if gallstones found. D/C if myopathy or marked CPK elevation occurs. Decreased Hgb, Hct, WBCs, thrombocytopenia, and agranu-locytosis reported; monitor CBC during first 12 months of therapy. Acute hypersensitivity reactions (rare) and pancreatitis reported. Minimize dose in severe renal impairment. Increased rate of pulmonary embolus (PE) and deep vein thrombosis (DVT) reported. Not indicated for patients with Type I hyperlipoproteinemia.

ADVERSE REACTIONS: Abdominal/back pain, headache, abnormal LFTs, respiratory disorder, increased creatinine phosphokinase, ALT/AST increase.

INTERACTIONS: Potentiates coumarin anticoagulants; reduce anticoagulant dose and monitor PT/INR. Avoid HMG-CoA reductase inhibitors unless ben-efits outweigh risks. Bile acid sequestrants may impede absorption; take at least 1 hr before or 4-6 hrs after the resin. Evaluate benefits/risks with immu-nosuppressants (eg, cyclosporine) and other nephrotoxic agents. Medication known to exacerbate hypertriglyceridemia (eg, β-blockers, thiazides, estro-gens) should be discontinued or changed if possible prior to initiating therapy.

PREGNANCY: Category C, not for use in nursing.

MECHANISM OF ACTION: Fibric acid derivative; activates peroxisome pro-liferator-activated receptor α (PPARα), increasing lipolysis and elimination of triglyceride-rich particles from plasma by activating lipoprotein lipase and re-ducing production of apoprotein C-III (lipoprotein lipase inhibitor). Activation of PPARα also induces an increase in synthesis of apoproteins A-I, A-II, and HDL-cholesterol. Reduces serum uric acid levels in hyperuricemic and healthy individuals by increasing the urinary excretion of uric acid.

PHARMACOKINETICS: Absorption: Well absorbed. **Distribution:** Plasma pro-tein binding (99%). **Metabolism:** Hydrolysis, glucuronidation; fenofibric acid (active metabolite). **Elimination:** Urine (60%), feces (25%); $T_{1/2}$=10-35 hrs.

NURSING CONSIDERATIONS

Assessment: Assess for hepatic/renal dysfunction, pre-existing gallbladder disease, pregnancy/nursing status, and drug interactions. Obtain baseline lipid levels.

Monitoring: Monitor for signs/symptoms of liver dysfunction, cholelithiasis, pancreatitis, hypersensitivity reactions, hematological changes (eg, thrombo-cytopenia, agranulocytosis), myopathies, rhabdomyolysis, PE, DVT, and eleva-tions in SrCr. Periodically monitor liver function (eg, ALT, AST), cholesterol levels, and blood counts. Evaluate CPK levels in patients suspected of having myopathies. Monitor for clinical response; if adequate response not seen after 2 months with maximum dose, d/c therapy.

Patient Counseling: Advise to immediately contact physician if unexplained muscle pain, tenderness, or weakness develop, particularly when accompa-nied by malaise or fever. Recommend appropriate lipid-lowering diet. Instruct to take with/without meals.

Administration: Oral route. **Storage:** 15°-30°C (59°-86°F). Keep out of reach of children. Protect from moisture.

L

LITHOBID RX
lithium carbonate (Noven)

> Lithium toxicity is related to serum levels, and can occur at doses close to therapeutic levels. Facilities for prompt and accurate serum lithium determinations should be available before initiating therapy.

THERAPEUTIC CLASS: Antimanic agent

INDICATIONS: Treatment of manic episodes of bipolar disorder. Maintenance treatment for bipolar disorder.

DOSAGE: *Adults:* Acute Mania: Initial: 900mg bid or 600mg tid to achieve effective serum levels of 1-1.5mEq/L; monitor levels twice weekly until sta-bilized. Maint: 900-1200mg/day, given bid-tid to maintain serum levels of 0.6-1.2mEq/L; monitor levels every 2 months. Elderly: Start at lower end of dosing range.
Pediatrics: ≥12 yrs: Acute Mania: Initial: 900mg bid or 600mg tid to achieve ef-fective serum levels of 1-1.5mEq/L; monitor levels twice weekly until stabilized. Maint: 900-1200mg/day, given bid-tid to maintain serum levels of 0.6-1.2 mEq/L; monitor levels every 2 months.

HOW SUPPLIED: Tab, Extended-Release: 300mg, (Generic) 450mg* *scored

WARNINGS/PRECAUTIONS: Avoid with significant renal or CV disease, severe debilitation, dehydration, or sodium depletion. Assess kidney func-tion prior to and during therapy. Risk of encephalopathic syndrome (eg, weakness, lethargy, fever, tremulousness, confusion, EPS); d/c therapy. May impair mental/physical abilities. Reduce dose or d/c with sweating, diarrhea, infection with elevated temperatures. Caution with hypothyroidism; may need supplemental therapy. Chronic therapy associated with diminution of renal concentrating ability, glomerular and interstitial fibrosis, and nephron atrophy. Transient syndrome of acute dystonia and hyperreflexia reported in a <15kg child who ingested 300mg. May cause sodium depletion; maintain normal diet, including salt, and adequate fluid intake. Caution in elderly.

ADVERSE REACTIONS: Fine hand tremor, polyuria, mild thirst, general discomfort, diarrhea, N/V, drowsiness, muscular weakness, lack of coordination, ataxia, giddiness, tinnitus, blurred vision, large output of diluted urine.

INTERACTIONS: Avoid diuretics and ACE inhibitors; risk of lithium toxicity due to reduced renal clearance. May prolong effects of neuromuscular blockers. Decreased levels with acetazolamide, urea, xanthine preparations, and alkalinizing agents. May produce hypothyroidism with iodide preparations. Increased plasma levels with indomethacin, piroxicam, other NSAIDs. Increased risk of neurotoxic effects with carbamazepine and CCBs. Reduced renal clearance with metronidazole. Fluoxetine may increase and/or decrease lithium levels. (Generic) May increase plasma levels with angiotensin-converting enzyme inhibitors, such as enalapril and captopril, and angiotensin II receptor antagonists, such as losartan; reduce dosage and monitor serum levels periodically. Diarrhea, confusion, tremor, dizziness, and agitation reported with selective serotonin reuptake inhibitors; caution when coadministering. May interact with methyldopa and phenytoin.

PREGNANCY: Category D, not for use in nursing.

MECHANISM OF ACTION: Antimanic agent; not established. Suspected to alter sodium transport in nerve and muscle cells and effects a shift toward intraneuronal metabolism of catecholamines.

PHARMACOKINETICS: Distribution: Found in breast milk. **Elimination:** Urine (primary), feces (insignificant). $T_{1/2}$=24 hrs.

NURSING CONSIDERATIONS

Assessment: Assess use with significant renal dysfunction, CV disease, severe debilitation, dehydration, sodium depletion, concomitant therapy with either ACE inhibitors or diuretics. Assess renal function (urinalysis, SrCr) prior to therapy. Assess thyroid function with history of thyroid disease, pregnancy/nursing status, and possible drug interactions.

Monitoring: Monitor for diminution of renal concentrating ability (eg, nephrogenic diabetes insipidus), glomerular and interstitial fibrosis, and nephron atrophy in patients on long-term therapy, encephalopathic syndrome, renal function while on therapy, thyroid function in patients with a history of hypothyroidism, serum lithium levels, signs of lithium toxicity (eg, diarrhea, vomiting, tremor).

Patient Counseling: Instruct to maintain a normal diet, including proper sodium and fluid intake (2500mL-3500mL). Instruct to notify physician if protracted sweating or diarrhea, or concomitant infection with elevated temperatures develops; may require dose adjustment. Counsel to d/c therapy and notify physician if clinical signs of lithium toxicity (eg, diarrhea, vomiting, tremor, muscular weakness) occur. Inform may impair mental/physical abilities; use caution with activities requiring alertness.

Administration: Oral route. **Storage:** 15-30°C (59-86°F). Protect from moisture. Dispense in tight, light- and child-resistant containers.

LIVALO   RX
pitavastatin (Kowa)

THERAPEUTIC CLASS: HMG-CoA reductase inhibitor

INDICATIONS: Adjunctive therapy to diet to reduce elevated total cholesterol (TC), low-density lipoprotein cholesterol (LDL-C), apolipoprotein B (Apo B), triglycerides (TG), and to increase high-density lipoprotein cholesterol (HDL-C) in adults with primary hyperlipidemia or mixed dyslipidemia.

DOSAGE: *Adults:* Initial: 2mg qd. Usual: 1-4mg qd. Max: 4mg qd. Individualize according to goals of therapy and response. Upon initiation/titration, analyze lipid levels after 4 weeks and adjust dosage accordingly. Moderate Renal Impairment (GFR: 30 to <60mL/min/1.73m²)/End-Stage Renal Disease Receiving Hemodialysis: Initial: 1mg qd. Max: 2mg qd. Concomitant Erythromycin: Max: 1mg qd. Concomitant Rifampin: Max: 2mg qd.

HOW SUPPLIED: Tab: 1mg, 2mg, 4mg

CONTRAINDICATIONS: Active liver disease including unexplained persistent elevations of hepatic transaminase levels, pregnancy/nursing mothers, and coadministration with cyclosporine.

WARNINGS/PRECAUTIONS: Myopathy and rhabdomyolysis with acute renal failure secondary to myoglobinuria reported. Caution with predisposing factors for myopathy including advanced age (>65 yrs), renal impairment, and inadequately treated hypothyroidism; d/c if elevated creatine kinase (CK) levels occur or myopathy is diagnosed or suspected. Temporarily withhold therapy if patient has an acute, serious condition suggestive of myopathy or predisposing to the development of renal failure secondary to rhabdomyolysis (eg, sepsis, major surgery). Transient increased serum transaminases reported; d/c or reduce dose if AST/ALT >3X ULN persists. Monitor LFTs before and at 12 weeks following both therapy initiation and dose elevation and periodically thereafter. Caution with heavy alcohol use, renal impairment, and history of liver disease. Medication should not be used in patients with severe renal impairment (GFR <30mL/min/1.73m^2) not yet on hemodialysis.

ADVERSE REACTIONS: Back pain, constipation, myalgia, diarrhea, pain in extremity, arthralgia, headache, influenza, nasopharyngitis.

INTERACTIONS: See Contraindications. Levels may be increased with protease inhibitors (eg, lopinavir/ritonavir); avoid concomitant use. Erythromycin and rifampin increased exposure; dose adjust and do not to exceed 1mg qd with concomitant erythromycin and 2mg qd with rifampin. Caution with fibrates; increased risk of myopathy. Consider dose reduction with niacin; enhanced risk of skeletal effects. Monitor PT and INR with warfarin coadministration.

PREGNANCY: Category X, not for use in nursing.

MECHANISM OF ACTION: HMG-CoA reductase inhibitor; inhibits cholesterol synthesis in the liver.

PHARMACOKINETICS: Absorption: T_{max}=1 hr; Absolute bioavailability (51%). **Distribution:** Plasma protein binding (>99%); V_d=148L. **Metabolism:** Conjugation; CYP2C9, 2C8; uridine 5'-diphosphate (UDP) glucuronosyltransferase (UGT1A3 and UGT2B7) (active metabolites). **Elimination:** Urine (15%), feces (79%); $T_{1/2}$=12 hrs.

NURSING CONSIDERATIONS

Assessment: Assess for active liver disease or unexplained elevations in serum transaminase levels, pregnancy/nursing status, renal impairment, inadequately treated hypothyroidism, and possible drug interactions. Obtain baseline lipid profile and LFTs prior to therapy. Assess use in patients who consume substantial quantities of alcohol and/or have a past history of liver disease.

Monitoring: Monitor signs/symptoms of myopathy, rhabdomyolysis, acute renal failure, and hypersensitivity reactions. Perform periodic monitoring of lipid profile, CK levels, and LFTs. Analyze lipid levels 4 weeks after initiation/titration. Perform LFTs before and at 12 weeks following initiation/dose elevation and periodically thereafter. Monitor PT and INR when using wafarin.

Patient Counseling: Advise to notify physician immediately if unexplained muscle pain, tenderness, or weakness occur. Notify physician of all concurrently taken medications, both prescription and over the counter. Counsel women of childbearing age to use effective method of birth control to prevent pregnancy during therapy. Notify physician if pregnant or breastfeeding.

Administration: Oral route. Take at any time of the day with or without food.
Storage: 15-30°C (59-86°F). Protect from light.

LO/OVRAL   RX
norgestrel - ethinyl estradiol (Wyeth)

> Cigarette smoking increases the risk of serious cardiovascular (CV) side effects. Risk increases with age (>35 yrs) and with heavy smoking (≥15 cigarettes/day). Women who use oral contraceptives should be strongly advised not to smoke.

OTHER BRAND NAMES: Low-Ogestrel (Watson) - Cryselle (Duramed)

THERAPEUTIC CLASS: Estrogen/progestogen combination

INDICATIONS: Prevention of pregnancy.

DOSAGE: *Adults:* Start 1st Sunday after menses begins or the 1st day of menses. First cycle use: 1 white tab qd for 21 days followed by 1 pink /peach (inert) tab qd for 7 consecutive days. After the first cycle use: Begin next and all subsequent courses after taking the last pink/peach tab. Follow same dosing schedule. (Lo/Ovral) Switching from 21-day regimen: Start 7 days after taking last dose. Switching from progestin-only pill: Start the next day after last dose. Switching from implant/injection: Start on the day of implant removal or the day the next injection would be due. Use after pregnancy/abortion/miscarriage: Start on day 28 postpartum in nonlactating mother or after a second-trimester abortion.
Pediatrics: Postpubertal adolescents: Start 1st Sunday after menses begins or the 1st day of menses. First cycle use: 1 white tab qd for 21 days followed by 1 pink/peach (inert) tab qd for 7 consecutive days. After the first cycle use: Begin next and all subsequent courses after taking the last pink/peach tab. Follow same dosing schedule. (Lo/Ovral) Switching from 21-day regimen: Start 7 days after taking last dose. Switching from progestin-only pill: Start the next day after last dose. Switching from implant/injection: Start on the day of implant removal or the day the next injection would be due. Use after pregnancy/abortion/miscarriage: Start on day 28 postpartum in nonlactating mother or after a second-trimester abortion.

HOW SUPPLIED: Tab: (Ethinyl Estradiol-Norgestrel) 0.03mg-0.3mg

CONTRAINDICATIONS: Thrombophlebitis, thromboembolic disorders, history of DVT or thromboembolic disorders, cerebrovascular or coronary artery disease (current or past history), known or suspected carcinoma of the breast or personal history of breast cancer, carcinoma of the endometrium or other known or suspected estrogen-dependent neoplasia, undiagnosed abnormal genital bleeding, cholestatic jaundice of pregnancy or jaundice with prior pill use, pregnancy, hepatic adenomas or carcinomas or benign liver tumors. (Lo/Ovral) Active liver disease, valvular heart disease with thrombogenic complications, thrombogenic rhythm disorders, hereditary or acquired thrombophilias, major surgery with prolonged immobilization, diabetes with vascular involvement, headaches with focal neurological symptoms, uncontrolled HTN.

WARNINGS/PRECAUTIONS: Increased risk of venous and arterial thrombotic and thromboembolic events (eg, MI, thromboembolism, stroke), hepatic neoplasia, gallbladder disease. Retinal thrombosis reported; d/c use if unexplained partial or complete loss of vision occurs, onset of proptosis or diplopia, papilledema, or retinal vascular lesions develop. May cause glucose intolerance; monitor prediabetic and diabetic patients. May cause fluid retention and increase BP; monitor closely with HTN and d/c if significant elevation of BP occurs. May cause onset or exacerbation of migraine or development of headaches with new pattern. Breakthrough bleeding and spotting reported; rule out malignancy or pregnancy. Ectopic and intrauterine pregnancy may occur in contraceptive failures. Monitor closely with hyperlipidemias; consider non-hormonal contraception with uncontrolled dyslipidemias. D/C if jaundice develops. Monitor closely with depression and d/c if depression recurs to significant degree. May develop visual changes or changes in lens tolerance with contact-lens wearers. Diarrhea and/or vomiting may reduce hormone absorption. Perform annual physical exam. Use before menarche is not indicated. Does not protect against HIV infection (AIDS) and other sexually transmitted diseases. May affect certain endocrine, LFTs and blood components. Should not be used to induce withdrawal bleeding as a test for pregnancy, or to treat threatened or habitual abortion during pregnancy.

ADVERSE REACTIONS: N/V, breakthrough bleeding, spotting, amenorrhea, migraine, depression, vaginal candidiasis, edema, weight changes, abdominal cramps/bloating, menstrual flow changes, cervical erosion and secretion.

INTERACTIONS: Reduced contraceptive effectiveness resulting in unintended pregnancy and breakthrough bleeding with antibiotics (eg, ampicillin, other penicillins, tetracyclines), anticonvulsants and other drugs that increase the metabolism of contraceptive steroids (eg rifampin, rifabutin, barbiturates, primidone, phenylbutazone, phenytoin, dexamethasone, carbamazepine, felbamate, oxcarbazepine, topiramate, griseofulvin, St. John's wort and modafinil). Significant changes (increase or decrease) in plasma levels with anti-HIV protease inhibitors; safety and efficacy may be affected. Increased levels with atorvastatin, ascorbic acid, acetaminophen and CYP3A4 inhibitors (eg, indinavir, itraconazole, ketoconazole, fluconazole, troleandomycin). Increased risk of intrahepatic cholestasis with troleandomycin. Increased plasma levels of cyclosporin, prednisolone and other corticosteroids, and theophylline. Decreased plasma concentrations of acetaminophen and increased clearance of temazepam, salicylic acid, morphine and clofibric acid.

PREGNANCY: Category X, not for use in nursing.

MECHANISM OF ACTION: Estrogen/progestogen combination oral contraceptive; acts by suppressing gonadotropins. Primarily acts by inhibiting ovulation. Also responsible for causing changes in cervical mucus (increases difficulty of sperm entry into uterus) and in endometrium (reduces likelihood of implantation).

PHARMACOKINETICS: Distribution: Found in breast milk.

NURSING CONSIDERATIONS

Assessment: Assess for presence or history of breast cancer, estrogen dependent neoplasia, abnormal genital bleeding, active liver disease, and known/suspected pregnancy or any other conditions where treatment is cautioned or contraindicated. Assess use in patients who are >35 yrs and heavy smokers (≥15 cigarettes/day). Assess use with HTN, hyperlipidemias, obesity, DM, or in patients at increased risk for thrombosis. Assess for possible drug interactions.

Monitoring: Monitor bleeding irregularities, thromboembolic events, onset or exacerbation of headaches or migraines, and ectopic pregnancy. Monitor fasting blood glucose levels in DM and prediabetic patients, BP with history of HTN, lipid levels with a history of hyperlipidemia. Monitor for signs of liver dysfunction (eg, jaundice) and signs of depression with previous history. Refer patients with contact lenses to an ophthalmologist if visual changes occur. Perform annual history and physical exam.

Patient Counseling: Counsel about possible adverse effects of drug. Advise to avoid smoking while on medication. Inform that drug does not protect against HIV infection and other STDs. Instruct women to use additional method of birth control until after first 7 days of administration in initial cycle. Instruct to take medication at same time every day and at intervals not exceeding 24 hrs. Inform that if dose missed, take next pill as soon as possible, then take next dose at regular time. If patient skips 2 or more doses, advise to use another method of contraception until patient has taken medication for 7 consecutive days. Counsel that if spotting or breakthrough bleeding occurs, continue taking medication; notify physician if bleeding is persistent or prolonged.

Administration: Oral route. **Storage:** 20-25°C (68-77°F). (Low-Ogestrel) 15-25°C (59-77°F).

LOCOID   RX
hydrocortisone butyrate (Ferndale)

THERAPEUTIC CLASS: Corticosteroid

INDICATIONS: (Cre, Oint) Corticosteroid-responsive dermatoses. (Sol) Seborrheic dermatitis.

DOSAGE: *Adults:* (Cre, Oint) Apply bid-tid. May use occlusive dressings for psoriasis or recalcitrant conditions. D/C dressings if infection develops. (Sol) Apply bid-tid.
Pediatrics: (Cre, Oint) Apply bid-tid. May use occlusive dressings for psoriasis or recalcitrant conditions. D/C dressings if infection develops. (Sol) Apply bid-tid. Use least amount effective for condition.

HOW SUPPLIED: Cre, Oint: 0.1% [15g, 45g]; Sol: 0.1% [20mL, 60mL]

WARNINGS/PRECAUTIONS: May produce reversible HPA axis suppression, manifestations of Cushing's syndrome, hyperglycemia, and glucosuria. D/C if irritation occurs. Use appropriate antifungal or antibacterial agent with dermatological infections. Pediatric patients may be more susceptible to systemic toxicity. Caution when applied to large surface areas. Avoid contact with eyes. Limit to smallest amount compatible with an effective therapeutic regimen. Chronic corticosteroid therapy may interfere with the growth and development of children, use least amount effective for condition.

ADVERSE REACTIONS: Burning, itching, irritation, dryness, folliculitis, hypertrichosis, acneiform eruptions, hypopigmentation, perioral dermatitis, allergic dermatitis, skin maceration, secondary infection, skin atrophy, striae, miliaria.

PREGNANCY: Category C, caution in nursing.

MECHANISM OF ACTION: Corticosteroid; possesses anti-inflammatory, anti-pruritic, and vasoconstrictive properties. Anti-inflammatory actions not established.

PHARMACOKINETICS: Absorption: Percutaneous; inflammation, other disease states, and occlusive dressings may increase absorption. **Distribution:** Bound to plasma proteins to varying degrees. Systemically administered corticosteroids found in breast milk. **Metabolism:** Liver. **Elimination:** Renal (major), bile.

NURSING CONSIDERATIONS

Assessment: Assess for severity of infection and use in pregnant/nursing patients.

Monitoring: Monitor for signs/symptoms dermatological infections (eg, fungal, bacterial). For patients on large doses or in patients using occlusive dressings, perform periodic monitoring for HPA-axis suppression using urinary free cortisol and ACTH stimulation tests. Monitor for signs/symptoms of systemic toxicity in pediatrics.

Patient Counseling: Counsel to use externally and exactly as directed; avoid contact with eyes. Report signs of adverse reactions; do not bandage, cover or wrap treated skin area. Inform caregivers of pediatric patients to avoid using tight-fitting diapers or plastic pants on treatment area.

Administration: Topical route. **Storage:** Cream: 15-25°C (59-77°F), Ointment: 2-30°C (36-86°F), Solution: 5-25°C (41-77°F).

LOESTRIN 21   RX
norethindrone acetate - ethinyl estradiol (Duramed)

> Cigarette smoking increases the risk of serious cardiovascular (CV) side effects. Risk increases with age (>35 yrs) and with heavy smoking (≥15 cigarettes/day). Women who use oral contraceptives should be strongly advised not to smoke.

OTHER BRAND NAMES: Junel 1.5/30 (Barr) - Junel 1/20 (Barr) - Microgestin 1/20 (Watson) - Microgestin 1.5/30 (Watson) - Loestrin 21 1.5/30 (Duramed) - Loestrin 21 1/20 (Duramed)

THERAPEUTIC CLASS: Estrogen/progestogen combination

INDICATIONS: Prevention of pregnancy.

DOSAGE: *Adults:* 1 tab qd for 21 days, stop 7 days, then repeat. Start 1st Sunday after menses begin or the 1st day of menses.
Pediatrics: Postpubertal: 1 tab qd for 21 days, stop 7 days, then repeat. Start 1st Sunday after menses begin or the 1st day of menses.

HOW SUPPLIED: Tab: (Ethinyl Estradiol-Norethindrone) (1/20) 20mcg-1mg, (1.5/30) 30mcg-1.5mg

CONTRAINDICATIONS: Thrombophlebitis, thromboembolic disorders, past history of deep vein thrombophlebitis or thromboembolic disorders, cerebral vascular or coronary artery disease (CAD), known or suspected carcinoma of the breast, carcinoma of the endometrium or other known or suspected estrogen-dependent neoplasia, undiagnosed abnormal genital bleeding, cholestatic jaundice of pregnancy or jaundice with prior pill use, hepatic adenomas or carcinomas, and pregnancy.

WARNINGS/PRECAUTIONS: Increased risk of myocardial infarction (MI), thromboembolism, stroke, hepatic neoplasia, gallbladder disease, and vascular disease. Increased risk of morbidity and mortality with HTN, hyperlipidemia, obesity, and diabetes. Caution in women with CV disease risk factors. Start use ≥4-6 weeks post-partum if not breastfeeding. May increase risk of breast cancer and cancer of the reproductive organs. Retinal thrombosis reported; d/c if unexplained partial or complete loss of vision occurs, onset of proptosis or diplopia, papilledema, or retinal vascular lesions develop. Should not be used to induce withdrawal bleeding as a test for pregnancy, or to treat threatened or habitual abortion during pregnancy. May cause glucose intolerance; monitor prediabetic and diabetic patients. May elevate BP; monitor closely and d/c use if significant BP elevation occurs. New onset/exacerbation of migraine, or recurrent, persistent, severe headache may develop; d/c therapy if these occur. Breakthrough bleeding and spotting reported; rule out malignancy or pregnancy. May cause serum TG or other lipid changes (eg, elevated LDL). May be poorly metabolized with impaired liver function; d/c if jaundice develops. May cause fluid retention; caution with conditions that aggravate fluid retention. Caution with history of depression; d/c if depression recurs to serious degree. May develop changes in vision or lens tolerance in contact lens wearers. Does not protect against HIV infection (AIDS) and other sexually transmitted diseases (STDs). Perform annual history and physical exam. Use before menarche is not indicated. May affect certain endocrine, LFTs, and blood components in laboratory tests.

ADVERSE REACTIONS: N/V, breakthrough bleeding, spotting, amenorrhea, migraine, mental depression, vaginal candidiasis, edema, weight changes, abdominal cramps/bloating, menstrual flow changes, melasma.

INTERACTIONS: Reduced effects, increased breakthrough bleeding, and menstrual irregularities with rifampin. Reduced effects and increased incidence of breakthrough bleeding with phenylbutazone. Increased metabolism and reduced contraceptive effectiveness with anticonvulsants (phenobarbital, phenytoin, carbamazepine). Pregnancy reported with antimicrobials (ampicillin, griseofulvin, and tetracyclines). Increased levels with atorvastatin, ascorbic acid, and acetaminophen (APAP). Increased plasma levels of cyclosporine, prednisolone, and theophylline. Decreased levels of APAP. Increased clearance of temazepam, salicylic acid, morphine, and clofibric acid. Reduced plasma levels with troglitazone resulting in reduced contraceptive effectiveness.

PREGNANCY: Category X, not for use in nursing.

MECHANISM OF ACTION: Estrogen/progestogen oral contraceptive; acts by suppressing gonadotropins, primarily inhibiting ovulation, and causing other alterations, including changes in cervical mucus (increases difficulty of sperm entry into uterus) and endometrium (reduces likelihood of implantation).

PHARMACOKINETICS: Absorption: Ethinyl Estradiol: Absolute bioavailability (43%). Norethindrone: Rapid and complete. Absolute bioavailability (64%). **Distribution:** V_d=2-4L/kg; plasma protein binding (>95%); found in breast milk. **Metabolism:** Ethinyl Estradiol: Extensive via CYP3A4; oxidation, sulfate/glucuronide conjugation; 2-hydroxy ethinyl estradiol (primary oxidative metabolite). Norethindrone: Extensive; reduction, sulfate/glucuronide conjugation. **Elimination:** Urine, feces.

NURSING CONSIDERATIONS

Assessment: Assess for presence or history of breast cancer, estrogen dependent neoplasia, abnormal genital bleeding, active liver disease, and known/suspected pregnancy or any other conditions where treatment is cautioned or contraindicated. Assess use in patients who are >35 yrs and heavy smokers (≥15 cigarettes/day). Assess use with HTN, hyperlipidemias, obesity, DM, or in patients at increased risk for thrombosis. Assess for possible drug interactions.

Monitoring: Monitor bleeding irregularities, thromboembolic events, onset or exacerbation of headaches or migraines, and ectopic pregnancy. Monitor fasting blood glucose levels in DM and prediabetic patients, BP with history of HTN, lipid levels with a history of hyperlipidemia. Monitor for signs of liver dysfunction (eg, jaundice) and signs of depression with previous history. Refer patients with contact lenses to an ophthalmologist if visual changes occur. Perform annual history and physical exam.

Patient Counseling: Counsel about potential adverse effects. Inform that drug does not protect against HIV infection and other STDs. Instruct to use additional method of protection until after the 1st week of administration in the initial cycle when utilizing the Sunday-Start Regimen. Instruct to take exactly as directed and at intervals not exceeding 24 hrs. Take drug regularly with meal or hs; if dose is missed, take as soon as remembered, then take next dose at regularly scheduled time; continue regimen if spotting or breakthrough bleeding occurs; notify physician if bleeding persists. Avoid smoking while on medication.

Administration: Oral route. Refer to PI for special notes on administration.
Storage: 20-25°C (68-77°F).

LOFIBRA   RX
fenofibrate (Gate)

THERAPEUTIC CLASS: Fibric acid derivative

INDICATIONS: Adjunct to diet, for treatment of adults with hypertriglyceridemia (Fredrickson Types IV and V hyperlipidemia). Adjunct to diet, for reduction of LDL-C, Total-C, TG, and Apo B in adults with primary hypercholesterolemia or mixed dyslipidemia (Fredrickson Types IIa and IIb). (Tab) Adjunct to diet, to increase HDL-C in adults with primary hypercholesterolemia or mixed dyslipidemia (Fredrickson Types IIa and IIb).

DOSAGE: *Adults:* Primary Hypercholesterolemia/Mixed Hyperlipidemia: Initial: Cap: 200mg qd. Tab: 160mg qd. Hypertriglyceridemia: Individualize dose. Initial: Cap: 67-200mg/day. Tab: 54-160mg qd. Titrate: Adjust if needed after repeat lipid levels at 4-8 week intervals. Max: Cap: 200mg/day. Tab: 160mg/day. Renal Dysfunction/Elderly: Initial: Cap: 67mg/day. Tab: 54mg/day. Take with meals.

HOW SUPPLIED: Cap: 67mg, 134mg, 200mg; Tab: 54mg, 160mg

CONTRAINDICATIONS: Hepatic or severe renal dysfunction (including primary biliary cirrhosis and unexplained persistent liver function abnormality), pre-existing gallbladder disease.

WARNINGS/PRECAUTIONS: Hepatocellular, chronic active and cholestatic hepatitis and cirrhosis (rare) reported. Increases in serum transaminases (AST or ALT) reported; monitor LFTs regularly and d/c if >3X ULN. May cause cholelithiasis; d/c if gallstones found. May cause myositis, myopathy, or rhabdomyolysis; d/c if myopathy/myositis or marked CPK elevation occurs. Prior to therapy attempt to control serum lipids with appropriate diet, exercise, and weight loss in obese patients and attempt to control any medical problems (eg, diabetes mellitus [DM]), hypothyroidism) that are contributing to lipid abnormalities. Measure lipid levels prior to therapy and during initial treatment; d/c if inadequate response after 2 months on maximum dose of 200mg/day (Cap) or 160 mg/day (Tab). Acute hypersensitivity reactions (rare) and pancreatitis reported. Decreased Hgb, Hct, and WBCs reported; Periodically monitor CBC during the first 12 months of therapy. Pulmonary embolus (PE), deep vein thrombosis (DVT), and elevated serum creatinine observed (Tab). Avoid with (Tab) or minimize dose (Cap) in severe renal impairment and reduce dose in mild/moderate renal impairment. Caution in renally impaired elderly.

ADVERSE REACTIONS: Abdominal/pain, headache, abnormal LFTs, increased creatine phosphokinase, increased ALT, increased AST, respiratory disorder.

INTERACTIONS: Caution with anticoagulants due to potentiatiation of coumarin anticoagulants; reduce anticoagulant dose to maintain desirable PT/INR. Avoid HMG-CoA reductase inhibitors unless benefits outweigh risks. Rhabdomyolysis, increased creatine kinase (CK), myoglobinuria, and acute renal failure reported. Bile acid sequestrants may impede absorption; take at least 1 hr before or 4-6 hrs after bile acid binding resin. Evaluate benefits/risks with immunosuppressants (eg, cyclosporine) and other nephrotoxic agents;

use lowest effective dose. Prior to therapy, d/c or change if possible, medications that are known to exacerbate hypertriglyceridemia (eg, beta-blockers, thiazides, estrogens). Pravastatin, glimepiride, ezetimibe and fluvastatin increase plasma concentration (Tab). Atovastatin decreases plasma concentration (Tab).

PREGNANCY: Category C, not for use in nursing.

MECHANISM OF ACTION: Fibric acid derivative; activates peroxisome proliferator activated receptor α (PPARα), increasing lipolysis and elimination of triglyceride-rich particles from plasma by activating lipoprotein lipase and reducing production of apoprotein C-III. Decreased triglycerides alter the size and composition of LDL particles, which then have a greater affinity for cholesterol receptors and are catabolized rapidly. Activation of PPARα also induces an increase in the synthesis of apoproteins A-I, A-II, and HDL.

PHARMACOKINETICS: Absorption: Well absorbed; T_{max}=6-8 hrs. **Distribution:** Plasma protein binding (99%). **Metabolism:** Rapid, via hydrolysis by esterases to fenofibric acid (active metabolite), conjugation. **Elimination:** Urine (60%), feces (25%); $T_{1/2}$=20 hrs.

NURSING CONSIDERATIONS

Assessment: Assess for hepatic impairment including primary biliary cirrhosis and unexplained persistent liver function abnormality, renal dysfunction, pre-existing gallbladder disease, severe hypertriglyceridemia, pregnancy/nursing status, and for possible drug interactions. Assess for body weight and alcohol intake. Prior to therapy, attempt to control serum lipids with appropriate diet, exercise, and weight loss in obese patients and attempt to control any medical problems (eg, DM, hypothyroidism) that are contributing to lipid abnormalities. Obtain baseline CPK, lipid levels and LFTs prior to therapy.

Monitoring: Monitor for signs/symptoms of myositis, myopathy, and rhabdomyolysis; measure serum creatine kinase levels if myopathy is suspected. Monitor for signs/symptoms of increases in serum transaminases, hepatitis, and cirrhosis; perform periodic monitoring of LFTs. Monitor for signs/symptoms of cholelithiasis; perform gallbladder studies if cholelithiasis is suspected. Monitor for signs/symptoms of pancreatitis, hypersensitivity reactions, (Tab) PE and DVT. Periodically monitor hematological changes (eg, hemoglobin, hematocrit, and WBC decreases) and lipid levels.

Patient Counseling: Inform of risks/benefits of therapy. Instruct to take with meals. Advise to immediately contact physician if unexplained muscle pain, tenderness, or weakness, with malaise or fever occur. Recommend appropriate lipid-lowering diet.

Administration: Oral route. **Storage:** 20-25°C (68-77°F). Protect from moisture.

LOMOTIL
diphenoxylate HCl - atropine sulfate (Pfizer)

OTHER BRAND NAMES: Lonox (Sandoz)

THERAPEUTIC CLASS: Opioid/anticholinergic

INDICATIONS: Adjunctive therapy for management of diarrhea.

DOSAGE: *Adults:* Initial: 2 tabs or 10mL qid. Titrate: Reduce dose after symptoms are controlled. Maint: 2 tabs or 10mL qd. Max: 20mg/day diphenoxylate. D/C if symptoms not controlled after 10 days at max dose of 20mg/day (diphenoxylate).
Pediatrics: 2-12 yrs: Initial: 0.3-0.4mg/kg/day of solution in four divided doses. 13-16 yrs: Initial: 2 tabs or 10mL tid. Titrate: Reduce dose after symptoms are controlled. Maint: May be as low as 25% of initial dose. D/C if no improvement within 48 hrs.

HOW SUPPLIED: (Diphenoxylate-Atropine) Sol: 2.5mg-0.025mg/5mL [60mL]; Tab: 2.5mg-0.025mg

CONTRAINDICATIONS: Obstructive jaundice, diarrhea associated with pseudomembranous enterocolitis or enterotoxin-producing bacteria.

WARNINGS/PRECAUTIONS: Avoid in children <2 yrs. Overdosage may result in severe respiratory depression and coma, leading to brain damage or death. Avoid use with severe dehydration or electrolyte imbalance until corrective therapy is initiated. May induce toxic megacolon with acute ulcerative colitis; d/c if abdominal distention occurs or untoward symptoms develop. May cause intestinal fluid retention. Avoid with diarrhea associated with organisms that penetrate the intestinal mucosa, and with pseudomembranous enterocolitis. Extreme caution with advanced hepatorenal disease and liver dysfunction. Caution in pediatrics, especially with Down's syndrome.

ADVERSE REACTIONS: Numbness of extremities, dizziness, anaphylaxis, drowsiness, toxic megacolon, N/V, urticaria, pruritus, anorexia, pancreatitis, paralytic ileus, euphoria, malaise/lethargy.

INTERACTIONS: MAOIs may precipitate hypertensive crisis. (Diphenoxylate) May potentiate barbiturates, tranquilizers and alcohol. Potential to prolong $t_{1/2}$ of drugs for which the rate of elimination is dependent on the microsomal drug metabolizing enzyme system.

PREGNANCY: Category C, caution in nursing.

MECHANISM OF ACTION: Diphenoxylate: Antidiarrheal. Atropine: Anticholinergic.

PHARMACOKINETICS: Absorption: (4 tabs) C_{max}=163ng/mL; T_{max}=2 hrs. **Metabolism:** Rapid and extensive metabolism through ester hydrolysis to diphenoxylic acid (major metabolite). **Elimination:** Urine (14%), feces (49%). $T_{1/2}$=12-14 hrs (diphenoxylic acid).

NURSING CONSIDERATIONS

Assessment: Assess for hypersensitivity, obstructive jaundice, diarrhea associated with pseudomembranous enterocolitis or enterotoxin-producing bacteria, severe dehydration, electrolyte imbalance, hepatic dysfunction, hepatorenal disease, ulcerative colitis, Down's syndrome, diarrhea (caused by *E. coli, Salmonella, Shigella*), pregnancy/nursing status, and possible drug interactions.

Monitoring: Monitor for severe dehydration, electrolyte imbalance, renal function, toxic megacolon in ulcerative colitis, abdominal distention, signs of atropinism, and other adverse reactions.

Patient Counseling: Instruct to take as directed and not to exceed the recommended dosage. Inform of consequences of overdosage, including severe respiratory depression and coma, possibly leading to permanent brain damage or death. Instruct to exercise caution while operating machinery/driving. Advise to avoid alcohol and other CNS depressants. Advise to keep medicines out of reach of children. Inform patient that drowsiness or dizziness may occur.

Administration: Oral route. Plastic dropper should be used when measuring liquid for administration to children. **Storage:** Dispense liquids in original container.

LOPID   RX
gemfibrozil (Parke-Davis)

THERAPEUTIC CLASS: Fibric acid derivative

INDICATIONS: Treatment of Types IV and V hyperlipidemia with risk of pancreatitis not responding to dietary management (usually TG >2000mg/dL). May consider therapy if TG 1000-2000mg/dL with history of pancreatitis or recurrent abdominal pain typical of pancreatitis. Risk reduction of CAD in Type IIb patients without history or symptoms of existing coronary heart disease inadequately responding to weight loss, dietary therapy, exercise, other pharmacologic agents; with triad of low HDL, and elevated LDL and TG levels.

DOSAGE: *Adults:* 600mg bid. Give 30 min before morning and evening meals.

HOW SUPPLIED: Tab: 600mg* *scored

CONTRAINDICATIONS: Hepatic or severe renal dysfunction including primary biliary cirrhosis, pre-existing gallbladder disease, combination therapy with repaglinide.

WARNINGS/PRECAUTIONS: Cholelithiasis reported. Associated with myositis. Abnormal LFTs reported; monitor periodically. D/C if myositis and gallstones suspected/diagnosed or if abnormal LFTs persist. Only use if indicated and d/c if significant lipid response not obtained. Severe anemia, leukopenia, thrombocytopenia, and bone marrow hypoplasia (rare) reported. Monitor blood counts periodically during first 12 months. May worsen renal insufficiency.

ADVERSE REACTIONS: Dyspepsia, abdominal pain, diarrhea, fatigue, bacterial and viral infections, musculoskeletal symptoms, abnormal LFTs, hematologic changes, hypesthesia, paresthesia, taste perversion.

INTERACTIONS: See Contraindications. Increased risk for severe hypoglycemia with repaglinide. Caution with anticoagulants; reduce dose and monitor PT. Increased risk of myopathy and rhabdomyolysis with HMG-CoA reductase inhibitors (statins). Benefit with concomitant statins does not outweigh risks. Reduced bioavailability with resin-granule drugs (eg, colestipol); spaced dosing required.

PREGNANCY: Category C, not for use in nursing.

MECHANISM OF ACTION: Fibric acid derivative; not established. Suspected to inhibit peripheral lipolysis, decrease hepatic extraction of free fatty acids, thus reducing hepatic TG production and inhibiting synthesis and increasing clearance of VLDL carrier apolipoprotein B, leading to decreased VLDL production.

PHARMACOKINETICS: Absorption: Complete; T_{max}=1-2 hrs. **Metabolism:** Oxidation to hydroxymethyl and carboxyl metabolites. **Elimination:** Urine (70% glucoronide conjugate) (<2% unchanged), feces (6%).

NURSING CONSIDERATIONS

Assessment: Assess for hepatic/renal dysfunction, primary biliary cirrhosis, persistent abnormal levels of lipids, gallbladder disease, DM, hypothyroidism, pregnancy/nursing status, coronary heart disease, hypersensitivity to drug, and possible drug interactions (eg, anticoagulants). Control serum lipids with appropriate diet, exercise, and weight loss in obese patients prior to therapy.

Monitoring: Monitor lipids periodically and for LFTs, CPK, CBC, creatinine, INR, PT. Monitor for signs of myopathy (eg, unexplained muscle pain, weakness, or tenderness with fever or malaise), hypersensitivity reactions, cholelithiasis, cataracts, malignancy, abdominal pain leading to appendectomy, and noncoronary mortality.

Patient Counseling: Inform about potential risks/benefits of therapy. Report signs of myopathy (eg, unexplained muscle pain, tenderness, or weakness with fever or malaise). Notify physician if pregnant/nursing or planning to become pregnant.

Administration: Oral route. **Storage:** 20-25°C (68-77°F). Protect from light and moisture.

LOPRESSOR   RX
metoprolol tartrate (Novartis)

THERAPEUTIC CLASS: Selective beta$_1$-blocker

INDICATIONS: (Tab) Treatment of hypertension alone or in combination with other anti-hypertensives. Long-term treatment of angina pectoris. (Tab/inj) To reduce cardiovascular mortality in hemodynamically stable patients with definite or suspected acute myocardial infarction.

DOSAGE: *Adults:* HTN: Individualize dosing. Take with meals. Initial: 100mg/day PO in single or divided doses given alone or with a diuretic. Titrate: May increase at weekly (or longer) intervals until optimum BP reduction is achieved. Usual: 100-450mg/day. Max: 450mg/day. Angina: Individualize dosing. Take with meals. Initial: 100mg/day PO in two divided doses. Titrate: Increase weekly until optimum clinical response is achieved or pronounced slowing of HR. Usual: 100-400mg/day. Max: 400mg/day. MI (Early Phase): 5mg IV every 2 min for 3 doses (monitor BP, HR, and ECG). If tolerated, give 50mg PO q6h for 48 hrs. Maint: 100mg bid. If not tolerated, give 25-50mg PO q6h. If severe intolerance d/c. Initiate PO dose 15 min after last IV dose. MI (Late Phase): 100mg bid for at least 3 months.

HOW SUPPLIED: Inj: 1mg/mL [5mL]; Tab: 50mg*, 100mg* *scored

CONTRAINDICATIONS: (HTN, Angina) Sinus bradycardia, >1st-degree heart block, cardiogenic shock, overt cardiac failure, sick sinus syndrome, severe peripheral arterial circulatory disorders. (MI) HR <45 beats/min, 2nd- and 3rd-degree heart block, significant 1st-degree heart block, systolic blood pressure (SBP) <100mmHg, moderate to severe cardiac failure.

WARNINGS/PRECAUTIONS: Caution with ischemic heart disease; avoid abrupt withdrawal, taper over 1-2 weeks. Caution in hypertensive and angina patients who have congestive heart failure (CHF) controlled by digitalis and diuretics. Continued myocardial depression may lead to cardiac failure; at first sign/symptom, digitalize and/or give diuretic. Avoid with bronchospastic diseases. Withdrawal prior to major surgery is controversial; difficulty in restarting and maintaining heart beat reported. May mask tachycardia occurring with hypoglycemia; caution in diabetics. May cause paradoxical increase in BP with pheochromocytoma if administered alone; always initiate an alpha blocker before starting therapy. May mask clinical signs of hyperthyroidism; if suspected to develop thyrotoxicosis, avoid abrupt withdrawal. May decrease sinus HR, slow AV conduction, produce significant heart block and hypotension (SBP ≤90mmHg); d/c if heart block and hypotension occur. Caution with impaired hepatic function and in elderly.

ADVERSE REACTIONS: Bradycardia, tiredness, dizziness, depression, SOB, diarrhea, pruritus, rash, heart block, heart failure, hypotension.

INTERACTIONS: Additive effects with catecholamine-depleting drugs (eg, reserpine). May block epinephrine effects. Caution with digitalis; both agents slow AV conduction and decrease HR. May enhance cardiodepressant effect with some inhalational anesthetics. Potent CYP2D6 inhibitors may increase levels; caution when coadministering. When given concomitantly with clonidine, d/c several days before clonidine is withdrawn.

PREGNANCY: Category C, caution in nursing.

MECHANISM OF ACTION: β-blocker; not established. Proposed to competitively antagonize catecholamines at peripheral adrenergic-neuronal sites, has central effect leading to reduced sympathetic outflow to periphery and suppression of renin activity.

PHARMACOKINETICS: Absorption: Rapid and complete. **Distribution:** Serum albumin binding (12%); found in breast milk. **Metabolism:** Liver via CYP2D6 (oxidation). **Elimination:** PO: Urine (<5%, unchanged), IV: Urine (10%, unchanged); $T_{1/2}$=2.8 hrs (extensive metabolizers); $T_{1/2}$=7.5 hrs (poor metabolizers).

NURSING CONSIDERATIONS

Assessment: Assess for sinus bradycardia, heart block, cardiogenic shock, history of or overt CHF, cardiac failure, ischemic heart disease, bronchospastic diseases, hyperthyroidism, DM, sick sinus syndrome, severe peripheral arterial circulatory disorders, pheochromocytoma, hepatic impairment, hypersensitivity, pregnancy/nursing status, and possible drug interactions. Perform baseline BP, heart rate, and ECG.

Monitoring: Monitor BP, HR, ECG and hemodynamic status periodically. Monitor for signs/symptoms of cardiac failure, hypoglycemia, thyrotoxicosis, withdrawal symptoms (angina, MI), hypotension, and hypersensitivity reactions.

Patient Counseling: Instruct to take regularly and continuously, as directed, with or immediately following meals. If dose is missed, take next dose at scheduled time (without doubling). Do not d/c without consulting physician. May impair physical/mental abilities. Advise to contact physician before any surgery or if symptoms of heart failure (difficulty breathing), withdrawal (angina) or hypersensitivity occur. Inform that signs of thyrotoxicosis and hypoglycemia may be masked.

Administration: Oral, IV route. **Storage:** 25°C (77°F); excursions permitted to 15-30°C (59-86°F). (Tab) Protect from moisture. (Inj) Protect from light.

LOPROX   RX
ciclopirox (Medicis)

OTHER BRAND NAMES: Loprox TS (Medicis)

THERAPEUTIC CLASS: Broad-spectrum antifungal

INDICATIONS: (Cre/Sus) Topical treatment of dermal infections of tinea pedis, tinea cruris, tinea corporis, cutaneous candidiasis and tinea versicolor. (Gel) Topical treatment of interdigital tinea pedis and tinea corporis. (Gel/Shampoo) Topical treatment of seborrheic dermatitis of the scalp.

DOSAGE: *Adults:* (Cre/Gel/Sus) Massage affected and surrounding areas bid (am and pm). (Shampoo) Apply about 5mL (up to 10mL for long hair) to wet scalp. Lather and rinse off after 3 min. Repeat twice weekly for 4 weeks, at least 3 days apart. If no improvement after 4 weeks reassess treatment. *Pediatrics:* ≥16 yrs: (Gel): ≥10 yrs: (Cre/Sus) Massage affected and surrounding areas bid (am and pm) up to 4 weeks. ≥16 yrs: (Shampoo) Apply about 5mL (up to 10mL for long hair) to wet scalp. Lather and rinse off after 3 min. Repeat twice weekly for 4 weeks, at least 3 days apart. If no improvement after 4 weeks reassess treatment.

HOW SUPPLIED: Cre: 0.77% [15g, 30g, 90g]; Gel: 0.77% [30g, 45g, 100g]; Shampoo: 1% [120mL]; Sus: (Loprox TS) 0.77% [30mL, 60mL]

WARNINGS/PRECAUTIONS: Not for ophthalmic, oral, or intravaginal use. D/C if sensitization or chemical irritation occurs. Avoid eyes; if contact occurs, rinse thoroughly with water. (Shampoo) Hair discoloration reported in patients with lighter hair color.

ADVERSE REACTIONS: Pruritus, burning. (Gel) Contact dermatitis. (Shampoo) Itching, erythema.

PREGNANCY: Pregnancy B, caution in nursing.

MECHANISM OF ACTION: Broad-spectrum antifungal; acts by chelation of polyvalent cations (Fe^{3+} or Al^{3+}) resulting in the inhibition of the metal-dependent enzymes that are responsible for degradation of peroxides in the fungal cell wall. Inhibits the growth of pathogenic dermatophytes, yeasts, and *Malassezia furfur.*

PHARMACOKINETICS: Absorption: (Cre) (5g) C_{max}=18.62ng/mL. (Gel) (5g) C_{max}=25.02ng/mL. (15g) C_{max}=100ng/mL. **Elimination:** (Cre/Sus) Urine (0.01%), feces; $T_{1/2}$=1.7 hrs. (Gel) Urine (3%), $T_{1/2}$=5.5 hrs. (Shampoo) Urine (0.5%).

NURSING CONSIDERATIONS

Assessment: Assess proper diagnosis of causative organisms. Assess for hypersensitivity and use in pregnant/nursing patients.

Monitoring: Monitor for signs/symptoms of sensitivity or chemical irritation reactions.

Patient Counseling: Instruct to use medication as directed by physician. Counsel to continue therapy for the full treatment time even if symptoms improve. Instruct to notify physician if there are no signs of improvement after 4 weeks of therapy or if signs of increased irritation (eg, redness, itching, blistering, oozing) develop at the application site. Instruct to avoid occlusive wrappings or dressings. Advise that burning or itching may occur when using the gel formulation on the scalp. Advise patients with lighter hair color that the shampoo formulation may discolor hair.

Administration: Topical route. (Sus) Shake vigorously before use. **Storage:** (Cre/Gel/Shampoo) 15-30°C (59-86°F). (Sus) 5-25°C (41-77°F).

LORCET

hydrocodone bitartrate - acetaminophen (Forest)

 CIII

OTHER BRAND NAMES: Lorcet 10/650 (Forest) - Lorcet Plus (Forest)

THERAPEUTIC CLASS: Opioid analgesic

INDICATIONS: Relief of moderate to moderately severe pain.

DOSAGE: *Adults:* (Plus, 10/650) Usual: 1 cap/tab q4-6h prn pain. Max: 6 tabs or caps/day.

HOW SUPPLIED: (Hydrocodone-APAP) Tab: (Plus) 7.5mg-650mg*, (10/650) 10mg-650mg* *scored

WARNINGS/PRECAUTIONS: May produce dose-related respiratory depression. May obscure acute abdominal conditions or head injuries. Caution in elderly, debilitated, severe hepatic or renal dysfunction, hypothyroidism, Addison's disease, prostatic hypertrophy, urethral stricture, pulmonary disease and postoperative use. May be habit-forming. Suppresses cough reflex.

ADVERSE REACTIONS: Dizziness, drowsiness, N/V, dysphoria, urinary retention, urethral spasm, dyspnea, SOB, rash.

INTERACTIONS: May potentiate CNS depression with narcotics, alcohol, antianxiety agents, antihistamines, antipsychotics, other CNS depressants. Increased effect of antidepressant or hydrocodone with MAOIs or TCAs.

PREGNANCY: Category C, not for use in nursing.

MECHANISM OF ACTION: Hydrocodone: Narcotic analgesic; not established. Suspected to be related to existence of opiate receptors in the CNS. APAP: Nonopiate, nonsalicylate analgesic and antipyretic. Mechanism of analgesia not established; involves peripheral influences. Antipyretic activity is mediated through hypothalamic heat regulating centers. Inhibits prostaglandin synthetase.

PHARMACOKINETICS: Absorption: Hydrocodone: C_{max}=23.6ng/mL; T_{max}=1.3 hrs. APAP: Rapid. **Distribution:** APAP: Found in breast milk. **Metabolism:** Hydrocodone: O-demethylation, N-demethylation, and 6-keto reduction. APAP: Liver (conjugation). **Elimination:** Hydrocodone: $T_{1/2}$=3.8 hrs. APAP: Urine (85%); $T_{1/2}$=1.25-3 hrs.

NURSING CONSIDERATIONS

Assessment: Assess for level of pain intensity, type of pain, patient's general condition and medical status, or any other conditions where treatment is contraindicated or cautioned. Assess for history of hypersensitivity, pregnancy/nursing status, renal/hepatic function, and possible drug interactions..

Monitoring: Monitor for signs/symptoms of respiratory depression, elevated CSF pressure, dependence on medication, and abuse. Monitor serial hepatic/renal function tests in with severe hepatic/renal disease.

Patient Counseling: Advise that medication may impair mental/physical abilities; use caution when performing hazardous tasks (eg, operating machinery/driving). Advise to avoid using alcohol and other CNS depressants during therapy. Inform that medication may be habit-forming; counsel to take only as long as prescribed, in amounts prescribed, and not more frequently than prescribed.

Administration: Oral route. **Storage:** 20-25°(68-77°); excursions permitted to 15-30°C (59-86°F). Dispense in tight, light-resistant container.

LORTAB

hydrocodone bitartrate - acetaminophen (UCB)

 CIII

OTHER BRAND NAMES: Hycet (Xanodyne)

THERAPEUTIC CLASS: Opioid analgesic

INDICATIONS: Relief of moderate to moderately severe pain.

DOSAGE: *Adults:* (2.5/500, 5/500) Usual: 1-2 tabs q4-6h prn. Max: 8 tabs/day. (7.5/500, 10/500) Usual: 1 tab q4-6h prn. Max: 6 tabs/day. (Sol) Usual: 1 tbsp (15mL) q4-6h prn. Max: 90mL/day.
Pediatrics: ≥2 yrs: (Sol) Give q4-6h prn. 12-15kg: 3.75mL. Max: 22.5mL/day. 16-22kg: 5mL. Max: 30mL/day. 23-31kg: 7.5mL. Max: 45mL/day. 32-45kg: 10mL. Max: 60mL/day. ≥46kg: 15mL. Max: 90mL/day.

HOW SUPPLIED: (Hydrocodone-APAP) Sol: (Hycet) 7.5mg-325mg/15mL, (Lortab) 7.5mg-500mg/15mL; Tab: (Lortab) 2.5mg-500mg*, 5mg-500mg*, 7.5mg-500mg*, 10mg-500mg* *scored

WARNINGS/PRECAUTIONS: May produce dose-related respiratory depression. Exaggerated respiratory depressant effect and elevated cerebrospinal fluid (CSF) pressure with head injury, other intracranial lesions, or pre-existing increase in intracranial pressure (ICP). May obscure diagnosis or clinical course of acute abdominal conditions or head injuries. Caution in elderly, debilitated, severe hepatic or renal dysfunction, hypothyroidism, Addison's disease, prostatic hypertrophy, urethral stricture, pulmonary disease, postoperative use. May be habit-forming; increased risk of misuse, abuse, diversion and dependence. Suppresses cough reflex. (Sol) Infants may have increased sensitivity to respiratory depression; use substantially reduced initial doses.

ADVERSE REACTIONS: Lightheadedness, dizziness, sedation, N/V.

INTERACTIONS: Additive CNS depression with other narcotics, antihistamines, antipsychotics, antianxiety agents, or other CNS depressants (including alcohol). Increased effect of antidepressant or hydrocodone with MAOIs or TCAs.

PREGNANCY: Category C, not for use in nursing.

MECHANISM OF ACTION: Hydrocodone: Narcotic analgesic and antitussive; not established. Suspected to be related to existence of opiate receptors in CNS. APAP: Nonopioid, nonsalicylate analgesic, and antipyretic; analgesic action involves peripheral influences. Specific mechanism not established. Antipyretic activity is mediated through hypothalamic heat-regulating centers. Inhibits prostaglandin synthetase.

PHARMACOKINETICS: Absorption: Hydrocodone C_{max}=23.6ng/mL; T_{max}=1.3 hrs. APAP: Rapid. **Distribution:** Hydrocodone: Crosses placental barrier. APAP: Found in breast milk. **Metabolism:** Hydrocodone: O-demethylation, N-demethylation and 6-keto reduction; 6-α-and 6-β-hydroxymetabolites. APAP: Liver (conjugation). **Elimination:** Hydrocodone: $T_{1/2}$=3.8 hrs; APAP: Urine (85%); $T_{1/2}$=1.25-3 hrs.

NURSING CONSIDERATIONS

Assessment: Assess for level of pain intensity, type of pain, patient's general condition and medical status, or any other conditions where treatment is contraindicated or cautioned. Assess for history of hypersensitivity, pregnancy/nursing status, renal/hepatic function, and possible drug interactions.

Monitoring: Monitor for signs/symptoms of respiratory depression, elevated CSF pressure, drug dependence, and drug abuse. Monitor serial hepatic/renal function tests in severe hepatic/renal disease. (Sol) Monitor infants closely for respiratory depression.

Patient Counseling: May impair mental/physical abilities; use caution when performing hazardous tasks (eg, operating machinery/driving). Avoid the use of alcohol and other CNS depressants while on medication. May be habit forming; instruct to take only as prescribed.

Administration: Oral route. **Storage:** (2.5mg/500mg): 15-30°C (59-86°F); (5mg/500mg, 10mg/500mg, 7.5mg/500mg, Sol): 20-25°C (68-77°F).

LOSEASONIQUE RX
ethinyl estradiol - levonorgestrel (Duramed)

> Cigarette smoking increases the risk of serious CV events from combination oral contraceptive (COC) use. This risk increases with age and with number of cigarettes smoked. Women who are >35 yrs and smoke should not use COCs.

THERAPEUTIC CLASS: Estrogen/progestogen combination

INDICATIONS: Prevention of pregnancy.

DOSAGE: *Adults:* 1 tablet qd for 91 days. Begin taking on first Sunday after the onset of menstruation. If menses begin on Sunday, start on that day. Use non-hormonal back-up method of contraception (eg, condoms, spermicide) until levonorgestrel-ethinyl estradiol tablet has been taken daily for 7 consecutive days. Begin next and all subsequent 91 day cycles without interruption on same day of week (Sunday) upon which first course began, following the same schedule. Postpartum women should start COC no earlier than 4-6 weeks postpartum.
Pediatrics: Postpubertal: 1 tablet qd for 91 days. Begin taking on first Sunday after the onset of menstruation. If menses begin on Sunday, start on that day. Use non-hormonal back-up method of contraception (eg, condoms, spermicide) until levonorgestrel-ethinyl estradiol tablet has been taken daily for 7 consecutive days. Begin next and all subsequent 91 day cycles without interruption on same day of week (Sunday) upon which first course began, following the same schedule. Postpartum women should start COC no earlier than 4-6 weeks postpartum.

HOW SUPPLIED: Tab: (Ethinyl Estradiol-Levonorgestrel) 0.02mg-0.1mg; Tab: (Ethinyl Estradiol) 0.01mg.

CONTRAINDICATIONS: Patients with high risk of arterial or venous thrombotic diseases (eg, women who smoke, if over age 35; presence or history of deep vein thrombosis or pulmonary embolism; cerebrovascular or coronary artery disease; thrombogenic valvular or thrombogenic rhythm diseases of the heart; hypercoagulopathies; uncontrolled hypertension; diabetes with vascular disease; headaches with focal neurological symptoms or migraine headaches with or without aura if over age 35), presence or history of breast cancer or other estrogen or progestin sensitive cancer, liver tumors (benign or malignant) or liver disease, and pregnancy.

WARNINGS/PRECAUTIONS: Increases the risk of venous thromboembolism, arterial thromboses (eg, stroke, MI); d/c if arterial or deep venous thrombotic event occurs. D/C if unexplained loss of vision, proptosis, diplopia, papilledema, or retinal vascular lesions occur; evaluate for retinal vein thrombosis. May increase risk of cervical cancer or intraepithelial neoplasia. D/C if jaundice develops. Increases risk of hepatic adenomas, hepatocellular carcinoma, and gallbladder disease. Oral contraceptive cholestasis may occur in women with history of pregnancy related cholestasis. May cause HTN; d/c if BP rises significantly in women with history of well controlled HTN. May decrease glucose tolerance; monitor prediabetic and diabetic women. May affect lipid levels; consider alternate therapy in patients with uncontrolled dyslipidemias. Breakthrough bleeding and spotting may occur, especially during the first 3 months; if bleeding persists, check for causes. Amenorrhea may occur during use; check for pregnancy. Amenorrhea or oligomenorrhea may occur after d/c therapy. May change the results of some laboratory tests (eg, coagulation factors, lipids, glucose tolerance, binding proteins). May need to increase dose of thyroid hormone in patients on thyroid hormone replacement therapy.

ADVERSE REACTIONS: Headaches, irregular and/or heavy uterine bleeding, dysmenorrhea, N/V, backpain, breast tenderness, mood changes, acne, weight gain.

INTERACTIONS: Use with drugs or herbal products that induce enzymes, including CYP3A4, that metabolize contraceptive hormones, may decrease the plasma concentrations of contraceptive hormones and may decrease the effectiveness of the hormonal contraceptive or cause breakthrough bleeding; counsel to use additional contraception or a different method of contraception. Barbiturates, bosentan, carbamazepine, felbamate, griseofulvin, oxcarbazepine, phenytoin, rifampin, St. John's wort, and topiramate may decrease contraceptive effectiveness. HIV protease inhibitors may increase or decrease levels. Reports of pregnancy with antibiotic use. Increased levels with atorvastatin, ascorbic acid, acetaminophen, and CYP3A4 inhibitors (eg, itraconazole, ketoconazole). Decreases levels of lamotrigine and may reduce seizure control; may require dosage adjustment of lamotrigine.

PREGNANCY: Safety not known in pregnancy, caution in nursing.

MECHANISM OF ACTION: Estrogen/progestogen combination oral contraceptive; primarily suppresses ovulation. Also responsible for causing changes in cervical mucus (increases difficulty in sperm entry into uterus) and endometrium (reduces likelihood of implantation).

PHARMACOKINETICS: Absorption: Rapid; Levonorgestrel: Absolute bioavailability (nearly 100%); T_{max}=1.6 hrs; C_{max} = 6.0ng/mL; AUC=76.5ng•hr/mL. Ethinyl estradiol: Absolute bioavailability (43%); T_{max}=1.8 hrs; C_{max}=122.8pg/mL; AUC=1335.8pg•hr/mL. **Distribution:** Found in breast milk; Levonorgestrel: V_d=1.8L/kg; plasma protein binding (97.5%-99%). Ethinyl estradiol: V_d=4.3L/kg; plasma protein binding (95%-97%). **Metabolism:** Levonorgestrel: Sulfate and glucuronide conjugates. Ethinyl estradiol: 1st past metabolism in gut wall, Hepatic, via CYP3A4 (hydroxylation), methylation, conjugation. **Elimination:** Levonorgestrel: Urine (45%), feces (32%); $T_{1/2}$=28.5 hrs. Ethinyl estradiol: Urine, feces; $T_{1/2}$=17.5 hrs.

NURSING CONSIDERATIONS

Assessment: Assess for presence or history of breast cancer, estrogen dependent neoplasia, abnormal genital bleeding, active liver disease, and known/suspected pregnancy or any other conditions where treatment is cautioned or contraindicated. Assess use in patients who are >35 yrs and heavy smokers (≥15 cigarettes/day). Assess use with HTN, hyperlipidemias, obesity, DM, or in patients at increased risk for thrombosis. Assess for possible drug interactions.

Monitoring: Monitor for signs/symptoms of venous thromboembolism, arterial thromboses (eg, stroke, MI), cervical cancer or intraepithelial neoplasia, retinal vein thrombosis (eg, loss of vision, proptosis, diplopia, papilledema, retinal vascular lesions), jaundice, hepatic adenomas, hepatocellular carcinoma, gallbladder disease, headaches, bleeding irregularities, and for interference with laboratory tests. Monitor glucose levels in DM or prediabetic patients. Monitor for HTN, cholestasis in women who have a history of pregnancy related cholestasis.

Patient Counseling: Inform that drug does not protect against HIV infection (AIDS) and other STDs. Advise not to smoke while on medication. Instruct to take medication by mouth at the same time everyday, and what to do in the event pills are missed. Counsel to use back-up or alternative method of contraception when enzyme inducers are used with COCs. Counsel COCs may reduce breast milk production. Counsel any patient who uses COCs postpartum, and have not yet had a period, to use an additional method of contraception until she has taken a levonorgestrel-ethinyl estradiol tablet for 7 consecutive days.

Administration: Oral route. **Storage:** 20-25°C (68-77°F).

LOTEMAX   RX
loteprednol etabonate (Bausch & Lomb)

THERAPEUTIC CLASS: Corticosteroid

INDICATIONS: Treatment of inflammation of the palpebral and bulbar conjunctiva, cornea and anterior segment of the globe. Management of postoperative inflammation.

DOSAGE: *Adults:* Steroid-Responsive Disease: 1-2 drops qid, may increase up to 1 drop every hr within the 1st week of treatment. Re-evaluate after 2 days if no improvement. Postoperative: 1-2 drops qid starting 24 hrs post-op and continue for 2 weeks.

HOW SUPPLIED: Sus: 0.5% [2.5mL, 5mL, 10mL, 15mL]

CONTRAINDICATIONS: Viral diseases of the cornea and conjunctiva including epithelial herpes simplex keratitis, vaccinia, and varicella. Mycobacterial infection and fungal diseases of the eye.

WARNINGS/PRECAUTIONS: Caution with glaucoma, history of herpes simplex, and diseases causing thinning of cornea/sclera. Prolonged use can cause glaucoma, optic nerve damage, defects in visual acuity and fields of vision, cataracts, or secondary ocular infections (eg, fungal). Monitor IOP after 10 days of therapy. Re-evaluate if no response after 2 days. May delay healing and increase incidence of bleb formation after cataract surgery. May mask or enhance existing infection in acute, purulent conditions.

ADVERSE REACTIONS: Elevated IOP, abnormal vision, chemosis, discharge, dry eyes, burning on instillation, epiphora, itching, photophobia, foreign body sensation, optic nerve damage, visual field defects.

PREGNANCY: Category C, caution in nursing.

MECHANISM OF ACTION: Glucocorticoid; anti-inflammatory agent, no accepted explanation for MOA; suspected to inhibit edema, fibrin deposition, capillary dilation and deposition of collagen and scar formation by the induction of phospholipase A_2 inhibitory proteins, lipocortins.

NURSING CONSIDERATIONS

Assessment: Assess for viral diseases of cornea and conjunctiva, dendritic keratitis, vaccinia, varicella, mycobacterial infection, fungal disease of ocular structures, glaucoma, thinning of corneal/scleral epithelium, hypersensitivity, cataract surgery.

Monitoring: Frequent measuring of IOP and slit lamp microscopy exam where appropriate, fluorescein staining for monitoring of glaucoma with damage to optic nerve with defects in visual acuity and fields of vision, posterior subscapsular cataract, delayed corneal healing, thinning of cornea and sclera, ulceration, perforation, secondary ocular infections or masking of existing infections.

Patient Counseling: Advise to d/c drug and notify physician if symptoms persist or worsen. Instruct to not wear soft contact lenses during treatment. Counsel to avoid touching bottle tip to eyelids or any other surface.

Administration: Ocular route. Shake vigorously before using. **Storage:** 15-25°C (59-77°F). Do not freeze.

LOTENSIN   RX
benazepril HCl (Novartis)

> When used in pregnancy, ACE inhibitors can cause injury and even death to the developing fetus. D/C therapy when pregnancy detected.

THERAPEUTIC CLASS: ACE inhibitor

INDICATIONS: Treatment of hypertension. May be used alone or in combination with thiazide diuretics.

DOSAGE: *Adults:* If possible, d/c diuretic 2-3 days prior to initiation of therapy. Initial: 10mg qd or 5mg with concomitant diuretic. Maint: 20-40mg/day given qd-bid. Resume diuretic if BP not controlled. Max: 80mg/day. CrCl <30mL/min/1.73m²: Initial: 5mg qd. Max: 40mg/day.
Pediatrics: ≥6 yrs: Initial: 0.2mg/kg qd. Max: 0.6mg/kg or 40mg/day.

HOW SUPPLIED: Tab: 5mg, 10mg, 20mg, 40mg

CONTRAINDICATIONS: History of angioedema.

WARNINGS/PRECAUTIONS: D/C if angioedema, jaundice or if marked LFT elevation occurs. Less effective on BP in blacks and more reports of angioedema than nonblacks. Risk of hyperkalemia with diabetes mellitus (DM), renal dysfunction. Persistent nonproductive cough reported. May cause agranulocytosis and bone marrow depression; monitor WBC in patients with renal and collagen vascular disease. May increase BUN and SrCr levels. Anaphylactoid reactions reported. Monitor for hypotension in high-risk patients (eg, surgery/anesthesia, prolonged diuretic therapy, heart failure, volume and/or salt depletion, dialysis, diarrhea, vomiting). Caution with congestive heart failure (CHF), renal dysfunction and renal artery stenosis.

ADVERSE REACTIONS: Cough, dizziness, headache, fatigue.

INTERACTIONS: May increase lithium levels; risk of lithium toxicity. Hypotension risk with diuretics. Increased risk of hyperkalemia with K⁺-sparing diuretics, K⁺-containing salt substitutes, or K⁺ supplements. Nitritoid reactions (eg, facial flushing, N/V, hypotension) reported when used concomitantly with injectable gold (sodium aurothiomalate). Hypoglycemia may develop with concomitant use with oral anti-diabetics or insulin in diabetics.

PREGNANCY: Category D, not for use in nursing.

MECHANISM OF ACTION: ACE inhibitor; effects appear to result from suppression of renin-angiotensin-aldosterone system. Inhibition results in decreased plasma angiotensin II, which leads to decreased vasopressor activity and to decreased aldosterone secretion.

PHARMACOKINETICS: Absorption: Benazepril: T_{max} = 0.5-1 hr; absolute bioavailability (37%). Benazeprilat: T_{max} =1-2 hrs (fasting), 2-4 hrs (nonfasting). **Distribution:** Plasma protein binding (96.7%, benazepril) (95.3%, benazeprilat); excreted in breast milk. **Metabolism:** Liver, cleavage of ester group; benazeprilat (active metabolite). **Elimination:** Benazepril: Urine (trace). Benazeprilat: Urine (20%), biliary (11-12%); $T_{1/2}$= 10-11 hrs (adults), 5 hrs (pediatrics).

NURSING CONSIDERATIONS

Assessment: Assess for pregnancy/nursing status, volume/salt depletion, collagen vascular disease (SLE, scleroderma), CHF, DM, renal/hepatic impairment, history of angioedema or hypersensitivity reactions, and possible drug interactions.

Monitoring: Monitor renal function for 1st few weeks, LFTs, WBC (collagen vascular disease) and serum electrolytes periodically. Monitor for signs/symptoms of hypotension, anaphylactoid or hypersensitivity reactions, head/neck and intestinal angioedema, jaundice, agranulocytosis, bone marrow depression, hyperkalemia and renal/hepatic dysfunction.

Patient Counseling: Inform of pregnancy risks. Inform that inadequate fluid intake or fluid loss may lead to drop in BP resulting in lightheadedness or syncope; avoid K⁺ supplements or salt substitutes. Advise to seek medical attention if symptoms of hypotension (syncope), anaphylactoid or hypersensitivity reactions, angioedema (head/neck; abdominal pain with/without N/V), infection (eg, sore throat, fever), hyperkalemia, or hepatic dysfunction occur.

Administration: Oral route. **Storage:** ≤30°C (86°F). Protect from moisture. Dispense in a tight container.

LOTENSIN HCT   RX
benazepril HCl - hydrochlorothiazide (Novartis)

> When used in pregnancy, ACE inhibitors can cause injury and even death to the developing fetus. D/C therapy if pregnancy detected.

THERAPEUTIC CLASS: ACE inhibitor/thiazide diuretic

INDICATIONS: Treatment of HTN.

DOSAGE: *Adults:* Initial (if not controlled on benazepril monotherapy): 10mg-12.5mg or 20mg-12.5mg. Titrate: May increase after 2-3 weeks. Initial (if controlled on 25mg HCTZ/day with hypokalemia): 5mg-6.25mg. Replacement Therapy: Substitute combination for titrated components. Elderly: Start at lower end of dosing range.

HOW SUPPLIED: Tab: (Benazepril-HCTZ) 5mg-6.25mg*, 10mg-12.5mg*, 20mg-12.5mg*, 20mg-25mg* *scored

CONTRAINDICATIONS: Anuria, hypersensitivity to other sulfonamide-derived drugs, history of angioedema.

WARNINGS/PRECAUTIONS: Not for initial therapy. Avoid use if CrCl ≤30mL/min. Angioedema of head and neck reported; d/c and administer appropriate therapy if this occurs. Intestinal angioedema reported. Anaphylactoid reactions during desensitization with hymenoptera venom, with dialysis with high-flux membranes, and LDL apheresis with dextran sulfate absorption. Correct volume and/or salt depletion prior to therapy. Caution with congestive heart failure (CHF); excessive hypotension may occur. Enhanced effects may occur in post-sympathectomy patients. May increase BUN and SrCr levels. Caution with severe renal dysfunction, renal artery stenosis, impaired hepatic function or liver disease. Agranulocytosis and bone marrow depression reported; monitor WBCs in patients with renal and collagen vascular disease. D/C if jaundice or marked elevations in hepatic enzymes develop. May cause idiosyncratic reaction, resulting in acute transient myopia and acute-angle glaucoma; d/c as rapidly as possible. May exacerbate or activate systemic lupus erythematosus (SLE). May cause hyperkalemia, hyponatremia, hypokalemia, hypochloremic alkalosis, hypercalcemia, hypophosphatemia and hypomagnesemia. May reduce glucose tolerance and increase cholesterol, TG and serum uric acid levels. Persistent, nonproductive cough reported.

ADVERSE REACTIONS: Dizziness/postural dizziness, headache, fatigue, cough, angioedema.

INTERACTIONS: Increased risk of hyperkalemia with K^+ supplements, K^+-sparing diuretics (eg, spironolactone, amiloride, triamterene), or K^+-containing salt substitutes. May increase lithium levels; risk of lithium toxicity. Nitritoid reactions reported with injectable gold (sodium aurothiomalate). May increase responsiveness to tubocurarine. NSAIDs reduce effects. Cholestyramine, colestipol decrease absorption. Insulin requirements in diabetics may need adjustment. May decrease arterial responsiveness to norepinephrine. May potentiate other antihypertensives, especially ganglionic or peripheral adrenergic-blocking drugs. Risk of hypokalemia with use, which may sensitize or exaggerate the response of the heart to the toxic effects of digitalis. Increased risk of hypokalemia when used concomitantly with corticosteroids or ACTH. Orthostatic hypotension may be potentiated by alcohol, barbiturates or narcotics. Symptomatic hypotension may occur in patients undergoing anesthesia. Absorption of HCTZ is increased by agents that reduce GI motility.

PREGNANCY: Category D, not for use in nursing.

MECHANISM OF ACTION: Benazepril: ACE inhibitor; decreases plasma angiotensin II, which leads to decreased vasopressor activity and decreased aldosterone secretion. HCTZ: Thiazide diuretic; affects renal tubular mechanisms of electrolyte reabsorption, directly increasing excretion of Na^+ and Cl^-. Antihypertensive mechanism not established.

PHARMACOKINETICS: Absorption: Benazepril: T_{max}= 0.5-1 hr; absolute bioavailability (37%). Benazeprilat: T_{max}=1-2 hrs (fasting), 2-4 hrs (nonfasting). HCTZ: T_{max}=1-2.5 hrs; absolute bioavailability (50-80%). **Distribution:** Found in breast milk. Benazepril: Plasma protein binding (96.7%). Benazeprilat: Plasma protein binding (95.3%). HCTZ: Plasma protein binding (67.9%); V_d= 3.6-7.8 L/kg; crosses placenta. **Metabolism**: Benazepril: Cleavage of ester group (primarily in liver); benazeprilat (active metabolite). **Elimination:** Benazepril: Urine (trace amounts). Benazeprilat: Urine (20%), biliary (11-12%); $T_{1/2}$= 10-11 hrs. HCTZ: Kidney; $T_{1/2}$= 5-15 hrs.

NURSING CONSIDERATIONS

Assessment: Assess for anuria, history of angioedema, or allergy or bronchial asthma, volume/salt depletion, CHF, SLE, and any other conditions where treatment is contraindicated or cautioned. Assess for hypersensitivity to drug or sulfonamides, renal/hepatic function, electrolyte levels, pregnancy/nursing status, and possible drug interactions.

Monitoring: Monitor for angioedema, anaphylactoid reactions, hypotension, jaundice, sensitivity reactions, SLE, idiosyncratic reaction, myopia, and angle-closure glaucoma. Periodically monitor WBCs in patients with collagen vascular and renal diseases. Monitor serum electrolytes, BP, LFTs, renal function (BUN, SrCr), and cholesterol/TG levels. Monitor patients closely for the 1st 2 weeks of therapy and during dose increases.

Patient Counseling: Inform of pregnancy risks. Inadequate fluid intake or fluid loss may lead to drop in BP, resulting in lightheadedness or syncope. D/C if syncope occurs. Avoid K^+ supplements or salt substitutes. Seek medical attention if symptoms of angioedema (eg, swelling of face, eyes, lips, tongue), hypotension (eg, syncope), or infection (eg, sore throat, fever) occur.

Administration: Oral route. **Storage**: ≤30°C (86°F). Protect from moisture and light.

LOTREL RX

benazepril HCl - amlodipine besylate (Sandoz)

> ACE inhibitors can cause death/injury to the developing fetus. D/C if pregnancy detected.

THERAPEUTIC CLASS: Calcium channel blocker (dihydropyridine)/ACE inhibitor

INDICATIONS: Treatment of hypertension not adequately controlled on monotherapy with either agent.

DOSAGE: *Adults:* Usual: 2.5-10mg amlodipine and 10-80mg benazepril qd. Titrate: Dosage must be guided by clinical response. Small/Elderly/Frail/ Hepatic Impairment: Initial: 2.5mg amlodipine. Not recommended in patients with severe renal impairment (CrCl <30mL/min/1.73m²). Replacement Therapy: May be substituted for individual components.

HOW SUPPLIED: Cap: (Amlodipine-Benazepril) 2.5mg-10mg, 5mg-10mg, 5mg-20mg, 5mg-40mg, 10mg-20mg, 10mg-40mg.

CONTRAINDICATIONS: History of angioedema, with or without previous ACE inhibitor treatment.

WARNINGS/PRECAUTIONS: Angioedema involving the face, extremities, lips, tongue, glottis, larynx and intestines reported; d/c if laryngeal stridor or angioedema of the face, tongue or glottis occur. Anaphylactoid reactions during desensitization and during membrane exposure reported. Increased angina/ MI with severe obstructive CAD reported. Monitor for hypotension in high-risk patients (eg, surgery/anesthesia, volume/salt depletion). Rarely associated with cholestatic jaundice that progresses to fulminant hepatic necrosis and sometimes death; d/c if jaundice or marked elevations of hepatic enzymes occur. May cause changes in renal function (eg, increase creatinine, BUN); caution in patients with severe CHF, renal artery stenosis, or pre-existing renal impairment. May cause hyperkalemia; caution in patients with risk factors for hyperkalemia (eg, DM, renal dysfunction). Persistent nonproductive cough reported. Avoid if CrCl <30mL/min. Caution in elderly.

ADVERSE REACTIONS: Cough, headache, dizziness, edema, angioedema.

INTERACTIONS: May increase lithium levels; if coadministered monitor lithium levels and signs/symptoms of toxicity. Hypotension risk with diuretics, anesthesia. Increased risk of hyperkalemia with K⁺-sparing diuretics, K⁺ supplements, or K⁺-containing salt substitutes. Nitritoid reactions (eg, facial flushing, N/V, hypotension) reported when used concomitantly with injectable gold (sodium aurothiomalate).

PREGNANCY: Category D, not for use in nursing.

MECHANISM OF ACTION: Amlodipine: Ca^{2+} channel blocker (dihydropyridine); inhibits transmembrane influx of Ca^{2+} ions into vascular smooth muscle and cardiac muscle. Benazepril: ACE inhibitor; decreases plasma angiotensin II, which leads to decreased vasopressor activity and to decreased aldosterone secretion.

PHARMACOKINETICS: Absorption: Amlodipine: Absolute bioavailability (64-90%); T_{max}=6-12 hrs. Benazepril: Absolute bioavailability (≥37%); T_{max}=0.5-2 hrs, 1.5-4 hrs (metabolite). **Distribution:** Amlodipine: V_d=21L/kg; plasma protein binding (93%). Benazepril: V_d=0.7L/kg; plasma protein bound; found in breast milk (minimal amounts). **Metabolism:** Amlodipine: Liver. Benazepril: Liver, cleavage of ester group; benazeprilat (active metabolite). **Elimination:** Amlodipine: Urine (10% parent compound, 60% metabolites); $T_{1/2}$=2 days. Benazepril: Urine (trace), biliary (11-12%). Benazeprilat: Urine (20%); $T_{1/2}$=10-11 hrs.

NURSING CONSIDERATIONS

Assessment: Assess for history of angioedema, severe aortic stenosis, CHF, severe obstructive CAD, volume/salt depletion, collagen vascular disease (lupus, scleroderma), DM, unilateral or bilateral renal artery stenosis, and hepatic/renal impairment. Check for hypersensitivity to other ACE inhibitors, pregnancy/nursing status and possible drug interactions.

Monitoring: Monitor renal function for the 1st few weeks in patients with renal artery stenosis. Monitor WBC, blood potassium level and serum electrolytes periodically. Monitor for signs/symptoms of hypotension, anaphylactoid or hypersensitivity reactions, head/neck and intestinal angioedema, agranulocytosis, hyperkalemia, renal/hepatic dysfunction. Monitor for signs/symptoms of angina or MI after dosage initiation or increase.

Patient Counseling: Inform of pregnancy risks. Advise to seek medical attention if symptoms of hypotension, anaphylactoid or hypersensitivity reactions, angioedema (head/neck, intestinal), infection, hyperkalemia, or hepatic dysfunction occur. Advise patient to take missed dose as soon as remembered; if more than 12 hrs, just take the next dose at regular time.

Administration: Oral route. **Storage:** 25°C (77°F); excursions permitted to 15-30°C (59-86°F). Protect from moisture. Dispense in tight container.

LOTRISONE   RX
betamethasone dipropionate - clotrimazole (Schering)

THERAPEUTIC CLASS: Corticosteroid/azole antifungal

INDICATIONS: Topical treatment of symptomatic inflammatory tinea pedis, tinea cruris, and tinea corporis caused by *Trichophyton rubrum*, *Trichophyton mentagrophytes*, and *Epidermophyton floccosum* in patients ≥17 yrs.

DOSAGE: *Adults:* ≥17 yrs: Massage sufficient amount into affected skin area(s) bid (am and pm). Do not use for >2 weeks for the treatment of tinea cruris and tinea corporis or for >4 weeks for the treatment of tinea pedis. Amounts of cream >45g/week or of lotion >45mL/week should not be used.

HOW SUPPLIED: (Betamethasone Dipropionate-Clotrimazole) Cre: 0.643mg/g-10mg/g [15g, 45g]; Lot: 0.643mg/g-10mg/g [30mL]

WARNINGS/PRECAUTIONS: Systemic absorption of corticosteroids may produce reversible HPA axis suppression, Cushing's syndrome, hyperglycemia, and glucosuria. Use over large surface areas, prolonged use, and use under occlusive dressings augment systemic absorption. Not for use with occlusive dressing. D/C if irritation develops. Pediatrics may be more susceptible to systemic toxicity. Not recommended for patients <17 yrs or patients with diaper dermatitis.

ADVERSE REACTIONS: Cre, Lot: Itching, irritation, folliculitis, hypertrichosis, acneiform eruptions, hypopigmentation. Cre: Paresthesia, rash, edema, secondary infection. Lot: Burning, dry skin, stinging.

PREGNANCY: Category C, caution in nursing.

MECHANISM OF ACTION: Corticosteroid/azole antifungal agent. Clotrimazole: Imidazole antifungal agent; inhibits 14-α-demethylation of lanosterol in fungi by binding to 1 of the CYP450 enzymes. Leads to accumulation of 14-α-methylsterols and reduced concentrations of ergosterol, a sterol essential for a normal fungal cytoplasmic membrane. The methylsterols may affect the electron transport system, thereby inhibiting growth of fungi. Betamethasone: Corticosteroid; has been shown to have topical systemic pharmacologic and metabolic effects characteristic of this class of drugs.

PHARMACOKINETICS: Metabolism: Liver. **Elimination:** Renal, biliary.

NURSING CONSIDERATIONS

Assessment: Assess for hypersensitivity to other corticosteroids or imidazoles. Assess use in pediatric patients. Assess pregnancy/nursing status.

Monitoring: Monitor for signs/symptoms of HPA-axis suppression, skin irritation. When used on large surface areas and/or with occlusive dressings, perform periodic monitoring for HPA-axis suppression using ACTH test, morning plasma cortisol test, and urinary free-cortisol level test. Monitor for systemic toxicity, HPA-axis suppression, Cushing's syndrome, delayed weight gain, and intracranial HTN in pediatrics.

Patient Counseling: Counsel to use exactly as directed for fully prescribed treatment period. Advise to avoid contact with eyes, mouth, or intravaginally.

Inform to contact physician if no improvement after 1 week of treatment for tinea cruris or tinea corporis, or 2 weeks for tinea pedis. Instruct to avoid using occlusive dressings or tight-fitting clothing on treated areas and not to use with other corticosteroids. Counsel the patient to use only for 2 weeks if the affected area is the groin and notify physician if condition persists after 2 weeks. Advise that the medication should be used only for the disorder for which it was prescribed. Counsel on adverse events.

Administration: Topical route. Shake lotion well before each use. **Storage:** 25C°(77°F), excursions permitted to 15-30°C (59-86°F). Store lotion in upright position.

LOTRONEX   RX
alosetron HCl (Prometheus)

> Serious GI adverse events (eg, ischemic colitis, serious constipation complications) reported. Only prescribers enrolled in Prometheus Prescribing Program should prescribe this medication. Patients must read and sign the Patient Acknowledge Form before receiving initial prescription. D/C immediately if constipation or symptoms of ischemic colitis develop; do not resume therapy in patients with ischemic colitis. Indicated only for women with severe diarrhea-predominant irritable bowel syndrome (IBS) who have not responded adequately to conventional therapy.

THERAPEUTIC CLASS: 5-HT$_3$ receptor antagonist

INDICATIONS: Treatment for women with severe diarrhea-predominant irritable bowel syndrome (IBS) who have chronic symptoms (≥6 months), exclusion of anatomic or biochemical abnormalities of GI tract, failure to respond to conventional therapy.

DOSAGE: *Adults:* Initial: 0.5mg bid for 4 weeks. D/C if constipation occurs, then restart at 0.5mg qd if constipation resolves. D/C if constipation recurs at lower dose. Titrate: If tolerated and IBS symptoms are not adequately controlled, may increase to up to 1mg bid. D/C after 4 weeks if symptoms are not controlled in 1mg bid.

HOW SUPPLIED: Tab: 0.5mg, 1mg

CONTRAINDICATIONS: Current constipation. History of chronic/severe constipation or sequelae from constipation, intestinal obstruction, stricture, toxic megacolon, GI perforation/adhesions, ischemic colitis, impaired intestinal circulation, thrombophlebitis or hypercoagulable state, Crohn's disease, ulcerative colitis, diverticulitis, severe hepatic impairment. Inability to understand/comply with Patient Acknowledgment Form. Concomitant administration with fluvoxamine.

WARNINGS/PRECAUTIONS: Caution in elderly and debilitated patients; may be at greater risk for complications of constipation. Caution with mild/moderate hepatic impairment.

ADVERSE REACTIONS: Constipation, ischemic colitis, abdominal discomfort/pain, nausea, GI discomfort/pain.

INTERACTIONS: See Contraindications. Increased risk of constipation with medications that decrease GI motility. Inducers and inhibitors of CYP1A2, with minor contributions from CYP3A4 and CYP2C9, drug-metabolizing enzymes may alter clearance. Avoid with quinolone antibiotics and cimetidine. Caution with strong CYP3A4 inhibitors (eg, ketoconazole, clarithromycin, telithromycin, protease inhibitors, voriconazole, itraconazole).

PREGNANCY: Category B, caution in nursing.

MECHANISM OF ACTION: 5-HT$_3$ receptor antagonist; inhibits activation of non-selective cation channels, which results in the modulation of the enteric nervous system.

PHARMACOKINETICS: Absorption: Rapidly absorbed, absolute bioavailability (50-60%), 9ng/mL (young women); T_{max}=1 hr. **Distribution:** V_d=65-95L, plasma protein binding (82%). **Metabolism:** via Liver (extensive). **Elimination:** Urine (74%, metabolites), feces (11%, <1% unchanged); $T_{1/2}$=1.5 hrs.

NURSING CONSIDERATIONS

Assessment: Assess history of chronic or severe constipation or sequelae from constipation, intestinal obstruction or stricture, toxic megacolon, GI perforation or adhesion, ischemic colitis, impaired intestinal circulation, thrombophlebitis or hypercoagulable state, Crohn's disease or ulcerative colitis, diverticulitis, severe hepatic impairment, pregnancy/nursing status and possible drug interactions.

Monitoring: Monitor LFTs, signs/symptoms of ischemic colitis and serious complications of constipation, perforation and other adverse reactions.

Patient Counseling: Counsel on the risk and benefits of the treatment. Review side effects and advise to report if any develop. Inform that tab may be taken with or without meals. Do not start if patient is constipated. D/C and contact prescriber if become constipated and have symptoms of ischemic colitis. Instruct to d/c treatment and contact prescriber if IBS symptoms are not controlled after 4 weeks of taking 1mg bid.

Administration: Oral route. **Storage:** 25°C (77°F); excursions permitted to 15-30°C (59-86°F).

LOVAZA RX
omega-3-acid ethyl esters (GlaxoSmithKline)

THERAPEUTIC CLASS: Lipid-regulating agent

INDICATIONS: Adjunct to diet to reduce triglyceride (TG) levels in adults with severe (≥500mg/dL) hypertriglyceridemia.

DOSAGE: *Adults:* 4g/day (4 caps qd or 2 caps bid).

HOW SUPPLIED: Cap: 1g

WARNINGS/PRECAUTIONS: Contains ethyl esters of omega-3 fatty acids (EPA and DHA) obtained from oil of several fish sources; unknown whether patients allergic to fish and/or shellfish are at an increased risk of an allergic reaction. Caution with known hypersensitivity to fish and/or shellfish. Increase in ALT levels without concurrent increase in AST levels reported. May increase LDL-C levels.

ADVERSE REACTIONS: Eructation, taste perversion, dyspepsia.

INTERACTIONS: Possible prolongation of bleeding time with concomitant anticoagulants or other drugs affecting coagulation (aspirin [ASA], NSAIDs, warfarin, coumarin); monitor periodically. D/C or change medications known to exacerbate hypertriglyceridemia (eg, β-blockers, thiazides, estrogens) prior to consideration of therapy.

PREGNANCY: Category C, caution in nursing.

MECHANISM OF ACTION: Lipid-regulating agent; not established. Inhibits acyl CoA:1,2-diacylglycerol acyltransferase, increases mitochondrial and peroxisomal β-oxidation in the liver, decreases lipogenesis in the liver, and increases plasma lipoprotein lipase activity. May reduce the synthesis of TG in the liver because EPA and DHA are poor substrates for the enzymes responsible for TG synthesis, and EPA and DHA inhibit esterification of other fatty acids.

NURSING CONSIDERATIONS

Assessment: Assess for persistent abnormal TG levels, hypersensitivity (eg, anaphylactic reaction), pregnancy/nursing status, other conditions which may affect treatment, and possible drug interactions. Attempt to control serum TG levels with appropriate diet, exercise, and weight loss in obese patients before instituting therapy.

Monitoring: Periodically monitor ALT/AST/LDL-C levels, coagulation parameters (during concomitant use with drugs affecting coagulation) and check for possible adverse effects.

Patient Counseling: Caution patients with known sensitivity or allergy to fish and/or shellfish. Advise that the use of lipid-regulating agents does not reduce the importance of adhering to diet. Capsules should be swallowed whole and not altered in any way.

Administration: Oral route. Swallow whole. Do not break open, crush, dissolve, or chew. **Storage:** 25°C (77°F); excursions permitted to 15-30°C (59-86°F). Do not freeze.

LOVENOX

RX

enoxaparin sodium (Sanofi-Aventis)

> Epidural or spinal hematomas resulting in long-term or permanent paralysis may occur in patients anticoagulated with low molecular weight heparins or heparinoids and are receiving neuraxial anesthesia or undergoing spinal puncture. Increased risk with indwelling epidural catheters, concomitant use of other drugs that affect hemostasis (eg, NSAIDs, platelet inhibitors, other anticoagulants), history of traumatic or repeated epidural or spinal puncture, or a history of spinal deformity or spinal surgery. Monitor frequently for signs/symptoms of neurologic impairment; if neurologic compromise noted, urgent treatment is necessary. Consider benefit and risks before neuraxial intervention in patients anticoagulated or to be anticoagulated for thromboprophylaxis.

THERAPEUTIC CLASS: Low molecular weight heparin

INDICATIONS: Prophylaxis of deep vein thrombosis (DVT) in patients undergoing abdominal surgery who are at risk for thromboembolic complications, in patients undergoing hip replacement surgery during and following hospitalization, in patients undergoing knee replacement surgery, or medical patients who are at risk for thromboembolic complications due to severely restricted mobility during acute illness. Inpatient treatment of acute DVT with or without pulmonary embolism (PE) in conjunction with warfarin. Outpatient treatment of acute DVT without PE in conjunction with warfarin. Prophylaxis of ischemic complications of unstable angina and non-Q-wave myocardial infarction (MI) when administered with aspirin (ASA). Treatment of acute ST-segment elevation MI when administered with ASA in patients receiving thrombolysis and being medically managed or with percutaneous coronary intervention (PCI).

DOSAGE: *Adults:* SQ: DVT Prophylaxis: Abdominal Surgery: 40mg qd with initial dose given 2 hrs pre-op for up to 12 days (usually 7-10 days). Knee Surgery: 30mg q12h with initial dose given 12-24 hrs post-op for up to 14 days (usually 7-10 days). Hip Surgery: 30mg q12h with initial dose given 12-24 hrs post-op for up to 14 days (usually 7-10 days) or 40mg qd with initial dose given 9-15 hrs pre-op for up to 3 weeks. Acute Medical Illness: 40mg qd for up to 14 days (usually 6-11 days). Acute DVT Treatment: Outpatient without PE: 1mg/kg q12h for up to 17 days (usually 7 days). Inpatient, with or without PE: 1mg/kg q12h, or 1.5mg/kg qd, up to 17 days (usually 7 days), administered at the same time daily. Initiate concomitant warfarin therapy as soon as possible, usually within 72 hrs. Unstable Angina/Non-Q-Wave MI: 1mg/kg q12h in conjunction with ASA therapy (100-325mg/day) for up to 12.5 days (usually 2-8 days). Treatment of Acute STEMI: <75 yrs: 30mg single IV bolus plus a 1mg/kg SQ dose, followed by 1mg/kg q12h SQ (max 100mg for the first 2 doses only, followed by 1mg/kg dosing for the remaining doses) for ≥8 days or until hospital discharge. ≥75 yrs: Do not use initial IV bolus. Initial: 0.75mg/kg SQ q12h (maximum 75mg for the first 2 doses only, followed by 0.75mg/kg dosing for the remaining doses) for ≥8 days or until hospital discharge. All patients should receive 75-325mg/d aspirin as soon as they are identified as having STEMI. In Conjunction with Thrombolytic Therapy: Give enoxaparin dose between 15 min before and 30 min after start of fibrinolytic therapy. Continue treatment for ≥8 days or until hospital discharge. PCI: If last dose is given <8 hrs before balloon inflation, no additional dosing is needed. If last dose is given >8 hrs before balloon inflation, give an IV bolus of 0.3mg/kg. Severe Renal Impairment (CrCl <30mL/min): Refer to PI.

HOW SUPPLIED: Inj: (MDV) 300mg/3mL; (Syringe) 30mg/0.3mL, 40mg/0.4mL, 60mg/0.6mL, 80mg/0.8mL, 100mg/mL, 120mg/0.8mL, 150mg/mL

CONTRAINDICATIONS: Active major bleeding, thrombocytopenia associated with a positive *in vitro* test for antiplatelet antibody in the presence of enoxaparin sodium, hypersensitivity to heparin or pork products, hypersensitivity to benzyl alcohol (only with the multi-dose formulation).

WARNINGS/PRECAUTIONS: Not for IM injection. Extreme caution in conditions with an increased risk of hemorrhage such as bacterial endocarditis, congenital or acquired bleeding disorders, active ulcerative and angiodysplastic GI disease, hemorrhagic stroke, or shortly after brain, spinal, or ophthalmological surgery. Major hemorrhages including retroperitoneal and intracranial bleeding reported. To minimize the risk of bleeding following vascular instrumentation during treatment of unstable angina, non-Q-wave MI, and acute STEMI, adhere precisely to the intervals recommended between doses. Observe for signs of bleeding or hematoma formation at the site of the procedure. Caution in patients with bleeding diathesis, uncontrolled arterial HTN or history of a recent GI ulceration, diabetic retinopathy, renal dysfunction and hemorrhage. Use with extreme caution in patients who have a history of heparin-induced thrombocytopenia. Thrombocytopenia reported; d/c if platelets <100,000/mm^3. Cannot be used interchangeably (unit for unit) with heparin or other low molecular weight heparins. Pregnant women with mechanical prosthetic heart valves may be at higher risk for thromboembolism and have a higher rate of fetal loss; monitor anti-Factor Xa levels, and adjust dosage if needed. Multi-dose vial contains benzyl alcohol which crosses the placenta and has been associated with fatal "gasping syndrome" in premature neonates; use only when clearly needed in pregnant women. Periodic CBC including platelet count and stool occult blood tests are recommended during course of treatment. Anti-Factor Xa may be used to monitor anticoagulant activity in patients with significant renal impairment or if abnormal coagulation parameters or bleeding occur.

ADVERSE REACTIONS: Hemorrhage, thrombocytopenia, local reactions (ecchymosis, erythema), anemia, dyspnea, nausea, elevations of serum aminotransferase.

INTERACTIONS: See Boxed Warning. D/C agents that may enhance the risk of hemorrhage prior to therapy. These include anticoagulants, platelet inhibitors such as acetylsalicylic acid, salicylates, NSAIDs (including ketorolac tromethamine), dipyridamole, or sulfinpyrazone. If coadministration is essential, conduct close monitoring. Increased risk of hyperkalemia with K$^+$-sparing drugs, and administration of K$^+$.

PREGNANCY: Category B, not for use in nursing.

MECHANISM OF ACTION: Low molecular-weight heparin; has antithrombotic properties.

PHARMACOKINETICS: Absorption: (SQ) Absolute bioavailability=100%. T_{max}=3-5 hrs. **Distribution:** (Anti-Factor Xa activity) V_d=4.3L. **Metabolism:** Liver; via desulfation and/or depolymerization. **Elimination:** Urine; $T_{1/2}$=4.5-7 hrs.

NURSING CONSIDERATIONS

Assessment: Assess for presence of active major bleeding, thrombocytopenia, hypersensitivity to heparin or pork products, hypersensitivity to benzyl alcohol, bacterial endocarditis, congenital or acquired bleeding disorders, active ulcerative and angiodysplastic GI disease, hemorrhagic stroke; brain, spinal, or ophthalmological surgery; bleeding diathesis, uncontrolled arterial HTN or history of a recent GI ulceration, diabetic retinopathy, renal dysfunction and hemorrhage, nursing/pregnancy status, and for possible drug interactions.

Monitoring: Monitor for signs/symptoms of hemorrhage and thrombocytopenia. Monitor for epidural or spinal hematomas, and for neurological impairment if used concomitantly with spinal/epidural anesthesia or spinal puncture. Monitor for signs/symptoms of hyperkalemia. Periodically monitor CBC including platelet count, stool occult blood tests. If bleeding occurs, monitor anti-factor Xa levels.

Patient Counseling: If patients have had neuraxial anesthesia or spinal puncture, particularly, if they are taking concomitant NSAIDs, platelet inhibitors, or other anticoagulants, inform to watch for signs and symptoms of spinal or epidural hematoma (tingling, numbness, muscular weakness); contact physician if these occur. Contact physician if any type of unusual bleeding, bruising, signs of thrombocytopenia, or allergic reactions develop. Advise that it will take longer than usual to stop bleeding; may bruise and/or bleed more easily when treated with enoxaparin. Inform of instructions for injecting if therapy is to continue after discharge: Lie down during administration; do not expel air bubble before injection; alternate administration sites between left and right anterolateral and posterolateral abdominal wall; the entire length of the needle should be introduced into skin fold held between thumb and forefinger; skin fold should be held throughout injection. To minimize bruising, do not rub injection site. Notify physicians and dentists of enoxaparin therapy prior to surgery or taking a new drug.

Administration: SC or IV (for multiple dose vial) route. Inspect visually for particulate matter and discoloration. Use tuberculin syringe or equivalent when using multiple dose vial. **Storage:** 25°C (77°F); excursions permitted to 15-30°C (59-86°F). Do not store multiple-dose vials for >28 days after first use.

LUCENTIS RX
ranibizumab (Genentech)

THERAPEUTIC CLASS: Monoclonal antibody/VEGF-A blocker

INDICATIONS: Treatment of patients with neovascular (Wet) age-related macular degeneration (AMD) and macular edema following retinal vein occlusion (RVO).

DOSAGE: *Adults:* AMD/RVO: Administer 0.5mg (0.05mL) by intravitreal injection once a month (approximately q28 days). AMD: May reduce to 1 injection every 3 months after the first 4 injections if monthly injections are not feasible.

HOW SUPPLIED: Inj: 10mg/mL

CONTRAINDICATIONS: Ocular or periocular infections.

WARNINGS/PRECAUTIONS: Intravitreal injections have been associated with endophthalmitis and retinal detachments; use proper aseptic injection technique. Increases in IOP have been noted within 60 min of intravitreal injection. Risk of arterial thromboembolic events (eg, nonfatal stroke, nonfatal myocardial infarction, vascular death).

ADVERSE REACTIONS: Conjunctival hemorrhage, eye pain, vitreous floaters, increased IOP, intraocular inflammation, cataract, nasopharyngitis, foreign body sensation in the eyes, eye irritation, lacrimation increased, visual disturbances/vision blurred, ocular hyperemia, dry eye, maculopathy, headache.

INTERACTIONS: May develop serious intraocular inflammation when used adjunctively with Verteporfin photodynamic therapy (PDT); incidence reported when drug was administered 7 days after Verteporfin PDT.

PREGNANCY: Category C, caution in nursing.

MECHANISM OF ACTION: Monoclonal antibody/human vascular endothelial growth factor A (VEGF-A) blocker; binds to receptor binding site of VEGF-A; prevents the interaction of VEGF-A with its receptors (VEGFR1 and VEGFR2) on the surface of endothelial cells, thereby reducing endothelial cell proliferation, vascular leakage, and new blood vessel formation.

PHARMACOKINETICS: Absorption: C_{max}=1.5ng/mL; T_{max}=1 day. **Elimination:** $T_{1/2}$=9 days.

NURSING CONSIDERATIONS

Assessment: Assess for ocular or periocular infections, hypersensitivity to drug, and pregnancy/nursing status.

Monitoring: Monitor for signs/symptoms of endophthalmitis, retinal detachments, cataracts, elevated IOP, arterial thromboembolic events, and hypersensitivity reactions. Monitor perfusion of the optic nerve head. Perform tonometry within 30 min following injection. Monitor during the week following the injection to permit early treatment should an infection occur.

Patient Counseling: Inform about risks of developing endophthalmitis, rheg-matogenous retinal detachments, or traumatic cataracts following administration of the injection. Instruct to seek immediate care from an ophthalmologist if the eye becomes red, sensitive to light, painful, or develops a change in vision.

Administration: Ophthalmic intravitreal injection. Refer to PI for preparation for administration. **Storage:** 2-8°C (36-46°F). Do not freeze. Protect from light and store in the original carton until time of use.

LUMIGAN

RX

bimatoprost (Allergan)

THERAPEUTIC CLASS: Prostaglandin analog

INDICATIONS: Reduction of elevated intraocular pressure (IOP) in open-angle glaucoma or ocular hypertension.

DOSAGE: *Adults:* Usual: 1 drop in affected eye(s) qd in pm. Max: Once-daily dosing. Space dosing with other ophthalmic drugs by at least 5 min.

HOW SUPPLIED: Sol: 0.03% [2.5mL, 5mL, 7.5mL]

WARNINGS/PRECAUTIONS: Changes to pigmented tissues, including increased pigmentation of iris (may be permanent), eyelids and eyelashes (may be reversible), and growth of eyelashes reported. Macular edema, including cystoid macular edema, reported. May change eye color. Caution with active intraocular inflammation (eg, uveitis), aphakic patients, pseudophakic patients with a torn posterior lens capsule, and patients at risk of macular edema. Not for the treatment of angle-closure, inflammatory, or neovascular glaucoma. Bacterial keratitis reported with multi-dose container. Contains benzalkonium chloride; remove contact lenses prior to use and reinsert 15 min after administration.

ADVERSE REACTIONS: Conjunctival hyperemia, ocular pruritus, growth of eyelashes, ocular dryness, visual disturbances, eye burning, foreign body sensation, eye pain, periocular skin pigmentation, blepharitis, cataracts, eyelid erythema, eyelash darkening, superficial punctate keratitis.

PREGNANCY: Category C, caution in nursing.

MECHANISM OF ACTION: Prostaglandin analog: selectively mimics the effects of naturally occurring substances, prostamides. Believed to lower IOP by increasing outflow of aqueous humor through both the trabecular meshwork and uveoscleral routes.

PHARMACOKINETICS: Absorption: C_{max}=0.08ng/mL; T_{max}=10 min; AUC=0.09ng•hr/mL. **Distribution:** V_d=0.67L/kg. **Metabolism:** Via oxidation, N-de-ethylation, and glucuronidation. **Elimination:** Urine (67%), feces (25%); $T_{1/2}$=45 min.

NURSING CONSIDERATIONS

Assessment: Assess use in aphakic patients, pseudophakic patients with a torn posterior lens capsule, patients at risk for macular edema, pregnancy/nursing status, and patients with angle-closure, inflammatory, or neovascular glaucoma.

Monitoring: Monitor for increased iris pigmentation, changes in the periorbital tissue (eyelid), changes in eyelashes or growth of eyelashes, macular edema (eg, cystoid macular edema), and bacterial keratitis.

Patient Counseling: Inform about risk of brown pigmentation of the iris, which may be permanent, darkening of eyelid skin, eyelashes and vellus hair changes. Instruct to avoid touching container tip to the eye, surrounding structures, fingers, or any other surface to avoid contamination. Inform to contact physician if an intercurrent ocular condition (eg, trauma or infection) or any type of ocular reaction (eg, conjunctivitis, eyelid reaction) develops while on medication. Instruct to remove contact lenses prior to instillation; reinsert 15 min after administration. Administer at least 5 min apart if using >1 topical ophthalmic drug.

Administration: Ocular route. **Storage:** Store in original container at 2-25°C (36-77°F).

LUNESTA
eszopiclone (Sunovion)

THERAPEUTIC CLASS: Nonbenzodiazepine hypnotic agent

INDICATIONS: Treatment of insomnia.

DOSAGE: Adults: Initial: 2mg immediately before hs. Titrate: May be initiated at or raised to 3mg, if clinically required. Elderly: Use lowest possible effective dose. Difficulty Falling Asleep: Initial: 1mg immediately before hs. Titrate: May be increased to 2mg, if clinically indicated. Difficulty Staying Asleep: 2mg immediately before hs. Severe Hepatic Impairment: Initial: 1mg. With Potent CYP3A4 Inhibitors: Initial: Max 1mg. Titrate: May be raised to 2mg, if needed.

HOW SUPPLIED: Tab: 1mg, 2mg, 3mg

WARNINGS/PRECAUTIONS: Abnormal thinking and behavioral changes reported. Complex behavior such as "sleep driving" has been reported; d/c if episode of "sleep driving" occurred. Amnesia and other neuropsychiatric symptoms may occur. Worsening of depression, including suicidal thoughts and actions, reported in primarily depressed patients. Evaluate carefully and immediately for the emergence of new behavioral sign and symptom. Avoid rapid dose decrease or abrupt d/c. Should only be taken immediately prior to bed or after going to bed and experiencing difficulty falling asleep. Rare cases of angioedema (involving tongue, glottis or larynx) reported; do not rechallenge with the drug. Taking medications while still up and about may result in short-term memory impairment, hallucinations, impaired coordination, dizziness and lightheadedness. Caution in conditions affecting metabolism or hemodynamic responses, and compromised respiratory function. Reduce dose with severe hepatic impairment. Caution with signs and symptoms of depression. May impair physical/mental ability.

ADVERSE REACTIONS: Headache, unpleasant taste, somnolence, dry mouth, dizziness, infection, rash, chest pain, N/V, peripheral edema, migraine.

INTERACTIONS: May produce additive CNS-depressant effects with other psychotropic medications, anticonvulsants, antihistamines, ethanol, and other drugs that produce CNS depression. Avoid with alcohol. Decreased exposure with rifampicin. Increased levels with ketoconazole and other strong CYP3A4 inhibitors (eg, itraconazole, clarithromycin, nefazodone, troleandomycin, ritonavir, nelfinavir). Decreased levels with and of lorazepam. Coadministration with olanzapine produced a decrease in Digit Symbol Substitution Test (DSST) score.

PREGNANCY: Category C, caution in nursing.

MECHANISM OF ACTION: Nonbenzodiazepine hypnotic agent; mechanism not established. Suspected to interact with GABA-receptor complexes at binding domains located close to or allosterically coupled to benzodiazepine receptor.

PHARMACOKINETICS: Absorption: Rapidly absorbed; T_{max}=1 hr. **Distribution:** Plasma protein binding (52-59%). **Metabolism:** Liver (extensive); oxidation and demethylation pathways via CYP3A4 and CYP2E1. Primary Metabolites: (S)-zopiclone-N-oxide and (S)-N-desmethyl zopiclone. **Elimination:** Urine (75% metabolite), (<10% parent drug); $T_{1/2}$=6 hrs, 9 hrs (elderly).

NURSING CONSIDERATIONS

Assessment: Assess for psychiatric or physical illness, diseases/conditions that could affect metabolism or hemodynamic response. Assess for depression, suicidal ideations, respiratory function, hepatic/renal impairment, hypersensitivity reactions, pregnancy/nursing status, and other possible drug interactions.

Monitoring: Monitor for anaphylactic/anaphylactoid reactions, insomnia, angioedema, severe sedation, memory disorders, coordination, dizziness, lightheadedness, abnormal thinking/behavioral changes (eg, aggressiveness or extraversion that seem out of character), complex/bizarre behavior, worsening of depression, physical/psychological dependence, respiratory depression, motor or cognitive performance in elderly, withdrawal-emergent anxiety, and rebound insomnia.

Patient Counseling: Inform about potential benefits/risks of drug and possibility of physical/psychological dependence. Instruct to take immediately before hs when patient can dedicate 8 hrs to sleep. Do not take with alcohol or other sedating drugs. Advise to consult physician if have history of depression, mental illness or suicidal thoughts, history of drug or alcohol abuse or have liver disease. Report to physician if "sleep driving" and other complex behavior occurred. Caution in performing hazardous tasks (eg, operating machinery, driving).

Administration: Oral route. **Storage:** 25°C (77°F), excursions permitted to 15-30°C (59-86°F).

LUPRON DEPOT (ONCOLOGY)   RX
leuprolide acetate (Abbott)

OTHER BRAND NAMES: Lupron Depot 7.5mg (Abbott) - Lupron Depot 3-Month 22.5 mg (Abbott) - Lupron Depot 4-Month 30 mg (Abbott)

THERAPEUTIC CLASS: Synthetic gonadotropin releasing hormone analog

INDICATIONS: Palliative treatment of advanced prostatic cancer.

DOSAGE: *Adults:* 7.5mg IM single dose monthly, 22.5mg IM single dose q3 months, or 30mg IM single dose q4 months. Rotate injection site.

HOW SUPPLIED: Inj: (1-month) 7.5mg, (3-month) 22.5mg, (4-month) 30mg

CONTRAINDICATIONS: Women who are or may become pregnant. (30mg) Women.

WARNINGS/PRECAUTIONS: May increase serum levels of testosterone during 1st week of treatment; transient worsening of or occurrence of additional signs/symptoms of prostate cancer may develop. For patients at risk, may initiate daily inj for 1st 2 weeks to facilitate withdrawal of treatment if needed. Closely monitor patients with metastatic vertebral lesions and/or urinary tract obstruction during 1st few weeks of therapy. Hyperglycemia, increased risk of developing diabetes/myocardial infarction (MI), sudden cardiac death, and stroke reported in men receiving GnRH agonists. May suppress pituitary-gonadal system. (7.5mg, 30mg) May experience temporary increase in bone pain. Ureteral obstruction and spinal cord compression reported; institute standard treatment if spinal cord compression/renal impairment develops.

ADVERSE REACTIONS: Injection-site reactions, general pain, headache, hot flashes, sweating, edema, urinary/respiratory disorders, asthenia, GI disorders, impotence, testicular atrophy.

PREGNANCY: Category X, safety in nursing not known.

MECHANISM OF ACTION: LH-RH agonist; acts as a potent inhibitor of gonadotropin secretion, resulting in suppression of testicular and ovarian steroidogenesis.

PHARMACOKINETICS: Absorption: (22.5mg) C_{max}=48.9ng/mL; T_{max}=4 hrs. **Distribution:** (IV) V_d=27L; plasma protein binding (43-49%). **Metabolism:** M-I (major metabolite). **Elimination:** (3.75mg) Urine (<5% parent and M-I); (IV) $T_{1/2}$=3 hrs.

NURSING CONSIDERATIONS

Assessment: Assess pregnancy status, metastatic vertebral lesions, urinary tract obstruction, previous hypersensitivity to drug, cardiovascular disease (CVD), diabetes mellitus (DM), and possible drug interactions. Obtain serum testosterone, prostate-specific antigen (PSA) levels, blood glucose levels, LFTs.

Monitoring: Monitor response to drug and for signs/symptoms of worsening prostate cancer, ureteral obstruction, spinal cord compression, renal impairment, signs/symptoms suggestive of development of CVD, and other adverse reactions. Periodically monitor serum testosterone, PSA levels, (30mg) prostatic acid phosphatase, blood glucose and/or HbA1c, bone mineral density, LFTs.

Patient Counseling: Inform risks/benefits of therapy. Advise to seek medical attention if adverse events occur.

Administration: IM route. Refer to PI for preparation and administration instructions. **Storage:** 25°C (77°F); excursions permitted to 15-30°C (59-86°F).

LUPRON DEPOT-PED   RX
leuprolide acetate (Abbott)

THERAPEUTIC CLASS: Synthetic gonadotropin releasing hormone analog

INDICATIONS: Treatment of children with central precocious puberty (CPP).

DOSAGE: *Pediatrics:* Individualize dose. Initial: 0.3mg/kg/4 weeks (minimum 7.5mg) as single IM dose. Starting Dose: ≤25kg: 7.5mg; >25-37.5kg: 11.25mg; >37.5kg: 15mg. Titrate: Increase in increments of 3.75mg IM q4 weeks if downregulation not achieved. Maint: Dose that produces adequate downregulation. Verify adequate downregulation with significant weight increase. Consider d/c before age 11 in females and age 12 in males.

HOW SUPPLIED: Inj: 7.5mg, 11.25mg, 15mg

CONTRAINDICATIONS: Pregnancy.

WARNINGS/PRECAUTIONS: Noncompliance or inadequate dosing may cause inadequate control of the pubertal process, which may lead to the return of pubertal signs (eg, menses, breast development, testicular growth). Monitor hormonal effects after 1-2 months of therapy. Measure bone age for advancement q6-12 months. Sex steroids may increase or rise above prepubertal levels with inadequate dose; gonadotropin and sex steroid levels may decline to prepubertal levels once therapeutic dose established. Increase in clinical signs and symptoms may occur in early phase due to rise in gonadotropins and sex steroids. Normal function of the pituitary-gonadal system is usually restored within 3 months after d/c; may mislead diagnostic tests of pituitary gonadotropic/gonadal functions conducted during treatment and ≤3 months after d/c.

ADVERSE REACTIONS: Injection-site reactions, pain, emotional lability, acne/seborrhea, rash, headache, vaginal bleeding/discharge, vaginitis.

PREGNANCY: Category X, not for use in nursing.

MECHANISM OF ACTION: GnRH agonist; acts as a potent inhibitor of gonadotropin secretion, resulting in suppression of testicular and ovarian steroidogenesis.

PHARMACOKINETICS: Absorption: (7.5mg in adults) C_{max} =20ng/mL; T_{max} =4 hrs. **Distribution:** (IV) V_d=27L, plasma protein binding (43-49%). **Metabolism:** M-I (major metabolite). **Elimination:** Urine (<5% parent and M-I); (IV) $T_{1/2}$=3 hrs.

NURSING CONSIDERATIONS

Assessment: Confirm diagnosis of CPP (refer to PI). Assess for height and weight measurements, sex/adrenal steroid level, β- human chorionic gonadotropin (HCG) level, hypersensitivity to drug and pregnancy/nursing status. Perform pelvic/adrenal/testicular ultrasound and CT of the head.

Monitoring: Monitor GnRH stimulation test, sex steroid levels, and Tanner staging 1-2 months following initiation of therapy or dose changes. Monitor measurements of bone age for advancement q6-12 months.

Patient Counseling: Counsel about importance of continuous therapy and adherence to drug administration schedule. Inform females that menses or spotting may occur during first 2 months of therapy; instruct to notify physician if bleeding continues beyond 2nd month of therapy. Instruct to immediately report to physician any irritation at injection site and any unusual signs/symptoms.

Administration: IM route. Refer to PI for administration techniques. **Storage:** 25°C (77°F); excursions permitted to 15-30°C (59-86°F).

LUSEDRA
fospropofol disodium (Eisai)

THERAPEUTIC CLASS: Anesthetic agent

INDICATIONS: For monitored anesthesia care (MAC) sedation in adult patients undergoing diagnostic or therapeutic procedures.

DOSAGE: *Adults:* Individualize dose. Standard Dosing Regimen: 18-<65 yrs who are Healthy or Patients With Mild Systemic Disease (ASA P1 or P2): Initial: 6.5mg/kg IV bolus. Supplemental: 1.6mg/kg IV as necessary. Max: 16.5mL (initial dose) and 4mL (supplemental dose). Modified Dosing Regimen: ≥65 yrs or Patients with Severe Systemic Disease (ASA P3 or P4): Initial/Supplemental: 75% of the standard dosing regimen. Give supplemental doses only when patients can demonstrate purposeful movement in response to verbal or light tactile stimulation and no more frequently than every 4 min. Refer to PI for specific information regarding standard and modified dosing regimens. Use supplemental oxygen in all patients undergoing sedation.

HOW SUPPLIED: Inj: 35mg/mL

WARNINGS/PRECAUTIONS: Only trained persons in general anesthesia administration and not involved in the conduct of the diagnostic or therapeutic procedure should administer fospropofol. Sedated patients should be continuously monitored and facilities for maintenance of patent airway, providing artificial ventilation, administration of supplemental oxygen, and instituting of cardiovascular resuscitation must be immediately available. Respiratory depression and hypoxemia reported. Hypotension reported; caution in patients with compromised myocardial function, reduced vascular tone, or reduced intravascular volume. May cause unresponsiveness or minimal responsiveness to vigorous tactile or painful stimulation. Caution in hepatic impairment.

ADVERSE REACTIONS: Paresthesia, pruritus, N/V, hypoxemia, hypotension.

INTERACTIONS: Concomitant use with other cardiorespiratory depressants (eg, benzodiazepines, sedative-hypnotics, narcotic analgesics) may produce additive cardio-respiratory effects.

PREGNANCY: Category B, not for use in nursing.

MECHANISM OF ACTION: Sedative-hypnotic agent. Prodrug of propofol; metabolized by alkaline phosphatases following IV injection.

PHARMACOKINETICS: Absorption: (Fospropofol) AUC=19mcg•h/mL. (Propofol) AUC=1.2mcg•h/mL **Distribution:** (Fospropofol) V_d=0.33L/kg. (Propofol) V_d=5.8L/kg; plasma protein binding (98%). Crosses placenta, found in breast milk. **Metabolism:** Complete via alkaline phosphatases to propofol, formaldehyde, and phosphate; further metabolized to propofol glucuronide, quinol-4-sulfate, quinol-1-glucuronide, quinol-4-glucuronide (major metabolites). **Elimination:** (Fospropofol) $T_{1/2}$=0.88 hrs. (Propofol) $T_{1/2}$=1.13 hrs.

NURSING CONSIDERATIONS

Assessment: Assess for respiratory depression, hypotension or risk of hypotension (eg, compromised myocardial function, reduced vascular tone, reduced intravascular volume), hepatic impairment, pregnancy/nursing status, and for possible drug interactions.

Monitoring: Monitor continuously during sedation and recovery process for early signs of hypotension, apnea, airway obstruction, and/or oxygen desaturation. Monitor responsiveness to vigorous tactile or painful stimulation.

Patient Counseling: Inform that paresthesias (including burning, tingling, stinging) and/or pruritus are frequently experienced during the 1st injection and are typically mild to moderate in intensity, last a short time, and require no treatment. Counsel that a patient escort may be required after procedure. Instruct to avoid engaging in activities requiring complete alertness, coordination and/or physical dexterity (eg, operating hazardous machinery, signing legal documents, driving a motor vehicle) until physician has approved of performing such tasks.

Administration: IV route. **Storage:** 25°C (77°F); excursions permitted 15-30°C (59-86°F).

LUVOX CR

RX

fluvoxamine maleate (Jazz Pharmaceuticals, Inc.)

> Antidepressants increased the risk of suicidal thinking and behavior (suicidality) in short-term studies in children, adolescents, and young adults with major depressive disorder (MDD) and other psychiatric disorders. Monitor and observe closely for clinical worsening, suicidality, or unusual changes in behavior in patients who are started on antidepressant therapy. Not approved for use in pediatric patients.

THERAPEUTIC CLASS: Selective serotonin reuptake inhibitor

INDICATIONS: Treatment of obsessive compulsive disorder (OCD) and social anxiety disorder (social phobia).

DOSAGE: *Adults:* Initial: 100mg qhs. Titrate: May increase by 50mg every week. Maint: 100-300mg/day. Max: 300mg/day. Maint/Continuation of Extended Treatment: Lowest effective dose. Periodically reassess need to continue. Switching to/from MAOI: Allow ≥14 days between d/c and initiation of therapy. Elderly/Hepatic Impairment: Titrate slowly. 3rd Trimester Pregnancy: Taper dose. Do not crush or chew.

HOW SUPPLIED: Cap, Extended-Release: 100mg, 150mg

CONTRAINDICATIONS: Concomitant use of alosetron, tizanidine, thioridazine, or pimozide. Use during or within 14 days of MAOI therapy.

WARNINGS/PRECAUTIONS: May precipitate mixed/manic episode in patients at risk for bipolar disorder. Screen for risk for bipolar disorder prior to initiating treatment. Serotonin syndrome or neuroleptic malignant syndrome (NMS)-like reactions reported. D/C should be gradual. May increase risk of bleeding events. Caution with history of convulsive disorders; d/c if seizures occur or if seizure frequency increases. Avoid with unstable epilepsy and monitor patients with controlled epilepsy. Caution with history of mania, hepatic dysfunction, conditions that alter metabolism or hemodynamic responses. Hyponatremia may occur; caution in elderly and d/c with symptomatic hyponatremia. Consider potential risks and benefits of treatment during 3rd trimester of pregnancy.

ADVERSE REACTIONS: Headache, asthenia, nausea, diarrhea, anorexia, dyspepsia, insomnia, somnolence, nervousness, dizziness, anxiety, dry mouth, tremor, abnormal ejaculation.

INTERACTIONS: See Contraindications. Avoid with diazepam, ramelteon, serotonin precursors such as tryptophan and with other SSRIs or SNRIs. Caution with metoprolol or propranolol; reduce the initial β-blocker dose and titrate cautiously. Serotonin syndrome or NMS-like reactions reported with concomitant use of serotonergic drugs (including triptans), drugs that impair metabolism of serotonin (including MAOIs), or with antipsychotics or other dopamine antagonists. Caution with other drugs that may affect serotonergic neurotransmitter systems (eg, triptans, linezolid, lithium, tramadol, St. John's wort). Rare reports of weakness, hyperreflexia, and incoordination with sumatriptan. Risk of bleeding with concomitant use of NSAIDs, aspirin, warfarin, or other drugs that affect coagulation. Monitor PT with concomitant oral anticoagulants; adjust anticoagulant dose accordingly. Monitor plasma levels closely if used concomitantly with drugs eliminated via oxidative metabolism and has a narrow therapeutic window (eg, warfarin, theophylline, certain benzodiazepines, phenytoin). If used with alprazolam, initial alprazolam dosage should be halved and titrated to the lowest effective dose. If used with theophylline, reduce theophylline dose to one-third of the usual daily maintenance dose and monitor plasma concentrations of theophylline. May reduce clearance of benzodiazepines; use with caution. Monitor serum mexiletine levels with concomitant use. Monitor closely when used with clozapine; elevated clozapine levels reported. Caution with TCAs; monitor plasma TCA concentrations and may need to reduce TCA dose. Smoking increases metabolism. Greater risk of hyponatremia with diuretics. May increase absorption of tacrine. May increase methadone and carbamazepine plasma levels. Risk of bradycardia with diltiazem. Caution with CYP2D6 inhibitors (eg, quinidine). Inhibits several CYP450 in vitro that are known to be involved in metabolism of other drugs such as: CYP1A2 (eg, warfarin, theophylline, propranolol, tizanidine), CYP2C9 (eg, warfarin), CYP3A4 (eg, alprazolam), and CYP2C19 (eg, omeprazole).

PREGNANCY: Category C, not for use in nursing.

MECHANISM OF ACTION: SSRI; inhibits neuronal uptake of serotonin.

PHARMACOKINETICS: Absorption: C_{max} (at doses 100mg, 200mg, 300mg) =47ng/mL, 161ng/mL, 319ng/mL. **Distribution:** V_d=25L/kg; plasma protein binding (80%); found in breast milk. **Metabolism:** Liver (extensive) via oxidative demethylation and deamination. **Elimination:** Urine (94%), $T_{1/2}$ =16.3 hrs.

NURSING CONSIDERATIONS

Assessment: Assess for MDD, risk for bipolar disorder, depressive symptoms, history of mania, history of seizures, disease/condition that alters metabolism or hemodynamic response, hepatic impairment, history of hypersensitivity to drug, pregnancy/nursing status and possible drug interactions. Obtain a detailed psychiatric history prior to therapy.

Monitoring: Monitor for signs/symptoms of clinical worsening (suicidality, unusual changes in behavior), serotonin syndrome, NMS-like reactions (muscle rigidity, hyperthermia, mental status changes), abnormal bleeding, hyponatremia, seizures, hepatic dysfunction, and other adverse reactions. If d/c therapy (particularly if abrupt), monitor for symptoms of dysphoric mood, irritability, agitation, dizziness, sensory disturbances, anxiety, confusion, headache, lethargy, emotional lability, insomnia, and hypomania.

Patient Counseling: Advise to avoid alcohol, tizanidine and alosteron. Caution on risk of serotonin syndrome with concomitant use of triptans, tramadol or other serotonergic agents. Seek medical attention for symptoms of serotonin syndrome (mental status changes, tachycardia, hyperthermia, N/V, diarrhea, incoordination), NMS, allergic reactions (rash, hives), abnormal bleeding (particularly if using NSAIDs or ASA), hyponatremia, activation of mania, seizures, clinical worsening (suicidal ideation, unusual changes in behavior) and discontinuation symptoms (eg, irritability, agitation, dizziness, anxiety, headache, insomnia). Instruct not to crush or chew; may be taken with or without food. Caution against hazardous tasks (eg, operating machinery and driving). Notify physician if pregnant, intend to become pregnant, or breastfeeding. Counsel about benefits and risks of therapy. Inform physician if taking or plan to take any OTC medications.

Administration: Oral route. **Storage:** Store at 25°C (77°F); excursions permitted to 15-30°C (59-86°F). Avoid exposure to >30°C (86°F). Protect from high humidity. Dispense in tight containers.

LUXIQ   RX
betamethasone valerate (Stiefel)

THERAPEUTIC CLASS: Corticosteroid

INDICATIONS: Relief of the inflammatory/pruritic manifestations of corticosteroid-responsive dermatoses of the scalp.

DOSAGE: *Adults:* Apply to affected scalp area bid (am and pm). Repeat until entire affected scalp area is treated.

HOW SUPPLIED: Foam: 0.12% [50g, 100g]

WARNINGS/PRECAUTIONS: May produce reversible hypothalamic-pituitary-adrenal (HPA) axis suppression, manifestations of Cushing's syndrome, hyperglycemia, and glucosuria; pediatric patients are at greater risk. Caution when applied to large surface areas, for prolonged use, or under occlusive dressings; may increase systemic absorption. Evaluate periodically for HPA suppression; d/c or reduce frequency of application or substitute a less potent steroid if noted. D/C if irritation develops. Use appropriate antifungal or antibacterial agent with dermatological infections; if infection does not clear, d/c until infection is controlled. Administration to children should be limited to smallest amount compatible with an effective therapeutic regimen; may interfere with growth and development. Flammable; avoid fire, flame, or smoking during and immediately after application.

ADVERSE REACTIONS: Burning, stinging, pruritus, paresthesia, acne, alopecia, conjunctivitis.

PREGNANCY: Category C, caution in nursing.

MECHANISM OF ACTION: Corticosteroid; possesses anti-inflammatory, antipruritic, and vasoconstrictive properties. Anti-inflammatory mechanism not established. Suspected to induce phospholipase A_2 inhibitory proteins, lipocortins. Lipocortins control biosynthesis of potent mediators of inflammation (eg, prostaglandins, leukotrienes) by inhibiting release of their precursor, arachidonic acid.

PHARMACOKINETICS: Absorption: Percutaneous; occlusion, inflammation, and other diseases may increase absorption. **Distribution:** Systemically administered corticosteroids are found in breast milk. **Metabolism:** Liver. **Elimination:** Renal (major), bile.

NURSING CONSIDERATIONS

Assessment: Assess for hypersensitivity to corticosteroids and pregnancy/nursing status.

Monitoring: Monitor for signs/symptoms of HPA-axis suppression, Cushing's syndrome, hyperglycemia, glucosuria, local skin irritation, allergic contact dermatitis (eg, failure to heal), and for the development of dermatological infections (eg, fungal, bacterial). Monitor for signs of glucocorticoid insufficiency following withdrawal from treatment. In patients on high doses or using occlusive dressings, perform periodic monitoring for HPA-axis suppression using adrenocorticotropic hormone (ACTH) stimulation, A.M. plasma cortisol, and urinary free cortisol tests. In pediatric patients, monitor for signs/symptoms of systemic toxicity, Cushing's syndrome, linear growth retardation, delayed weight gain, and intracranial HTN (bulging fontanelles, headache, bilateral papilledema).

Patient Counseling: Inform to use exactly as directed; avoid contact with eyes. Counsel on proper dispensing and application. Instruct not to bandage, cover, or wrap treated scalp area unless directed by physician. Contact physician if no improvement within 2 weeks of starting therapy or if adverse reactions develop. Avoid fire, flame, or smoking during and immediately following drug application. Advise patient to wash hands immediately after application. Keep out of reach of children.

Administration: Topical route. Invert can and dispense foam onto saucer or other cool surface first, then apply in small amounts to scalp. Gently massage into affected area until foam disappear. **Storage:** 20-25°C (68-77°F). Do not expose to heat or store at temperatures above 49°C (120°F). Do not puncture or incinerate container. Contents under pressure.

LYBREL   RX
ethinyl estradiol - levonorgestrel (Wyeth)

> Cigarette smoking increases the risk of serious cardiovascular (CV) side effects from oral contraceptive use. Risk increases with age (>35yrs) and with heavy smoking (≥15 cigarettes/day). Women who use oral contraceptives should be strongly advised not to smoke.

THERAPEUTIC CLASS: Estrogen/progestogen combination

INDICATIONS: Prevention of pregnancy.

DOSAGE: *Adults:* 1 tab qd. No Current Contraceptive Therapy: Start on Day 1 of menstrual cycle. Current 21- or 28-day Contraceptive Regimen: Start on Day 1 of withdrawal bleed (at the latest 7 days after last active tablet). Current Progestin-Only Pill Regimen: Start on the day after taking progestin-only pill. Current Implant Regimen: Start on the day of implant removal. Current Inj Regimen: Start on the day the next inj is due. Use nonhormonal back-up method of birth control for 1st 7 days of therapy when initiating after progestin-only pill, implant, or inj. Start no earlier than Day 28 postpartum in the nonlactating mother or after second trimester abortion.

Pediatrics: Postpubertal adolescents: 1 tab qd. No Current Contraceptive Therapy: Start on Day 1 of menstrual cycle. 21- or 28-day Regimen: Start on Day 1 of withdrawal bleed (at the latest 7 days after last active tablet). Progestin-Only Pill: Start on the day after taking progestin-only pill. Implant: Start on the day of implant removal. Inj: Start on the day the next inj is due. Use nonhormonal back-up method of birth control for 1st 7 days of therapy when initiating after progestin-only pill, implant, or inj. Start no earlier than Day 28 postpartum in the nonlactating mother or after second trimester abortion.

HOW SUPPLIED: Tab: (Ethinyl Estradiol-Levonorgestrel) 20mcg-90mcg

CONTRAINDICATIONS: Thrombophlebitis or history of deep vein thrombophlebitis (DVT), thromboembolic disorders or history of thromboembolic disorders, current or past history of cerebrovascular or coronary artery disease (CAD), valvular heart disease with thrombogenic complications, thrombogenic rhythm disorders, uncontrolled HTN, diabetes with vascular involvement, headaches with focal neurological symptoms such as aura, major surgery with prolonged immobilization, hereditary or acquired thrombophilia, known or suspected breast carcinoma or personal history of breast carcinoma, carcinoma of the endometrium or other known or suspected estrogen-dependent neoplasia, undiagnosed abnormal genital bleeding, cholestatic jaundice of pregnancy or jaundice with prior pill use, hepatic adenomas or carcinomas or active liver disease, known or suspected pregnancy.

WARNINGS/PRECAUTIONS: Increased risk of MI, vascular disease, venous thromboembolic and thrombotic disease, cerebrovascular disease (thrombotic and hemorrhagic stroke), transient ischemic attacks (TIA), hepatic neoplasia, and gallbladder disease. Increased risk of morbidity and mortality in patients with inherited or acquired thrombophilias, HTN, hyperlipidemia, obesity, diabetes mellitus (DM) and surgery or trauma with increased risk of thrombosis. May increase risk of breast and cervical cancer. Retinal thrombosis reported; d/c if unexplained partial or complete loss of vision, onset of proptosis or diplopia, papilledema, or retinal vascular lesions develops. Should not be used to induce withdrawal bleeding as a test for pregnancy, or to treat threatened or habitual abortion during pregnancy. May cause glucose intolerance; monitor prediabetic and diabetic patients. May cause fluid retention and increase BP; monitor closely with HTN and d/c if significant elevation of BP occurs. D/C with onset or exacerbation of migraine headache. May cause unscheduled breakthrough bleeding and spotting. Ectopic and intrauterine pregnancies may occur with contraceptive failures. Caution in patients with history of depression; d/c if significant depression develops. Monitor closely with hyperlipidemias; may elevate LDL and/or plasma triglycerides. D/C if jaundice develop. Visual changes or changes in lens tolerance may develop with contact lens use. Diarrhea and/or vomiting may reduce serum concentrations. Perform annual physical exam. May affect certain endocrine, LFTs, and blood components. Does not protect against HIV infection (AIDS) or other STDs. Use before menarche is not indicated.

ADVERSE REACTIONS: Acne, Budd-Chiari syndrome, change in cervical erosion and secretion, dizziness, edema/fluid retention, focal nodular hyperplasia, GI symptoms (eg, abdominal pain, cramps, and bloating), hirsutism, infertility, lactation, persistent melasma/chloasma, N/V, pancreatitis, rash (allergic), loss of scalp hair.

INTERACTIONS: Reduced contraceptive effectiveness leading to unintended pregnancy or unscheduled bleeding with antibiotics, anticonvulsants, and other drugs that increase the metabolism of contraceptive steroids (eg, rifampin, rifabutin, barbiturates, phenylbutazone, primidone, dexamethasone, phenytoin, carbamazepine, felbamate, oxcarbazepine, griseofulvin, topiramate, and modafinil). Contraceptive failures and unscheduled bleeding reported with ampicillins and other penicillins and tetracyclines. Decreased enterohepatic recirculation with substances that reduce gastric transit time. Anti-HIV protease inhibitors may increase or decrease levels. Reduce effectiveness with St. John's wort (*Hypericum perforatum*). Atorvastatin, ascorbic acid, acetaminophen, CYP3A4 inhibitors (eg, itraconazole, ketoconazole) may increase hormone levels. Troleandomycin may increase risk for intrahepatic cholestasis. May increase levels of cyclosporine, theophylline, prednisolone, and other corticosteroids. May decrease levels of acetaminophen and lamotrigine. Increases clearance of temazepam, salicylic acid, morphine, clofibric acid.

PREGNANCY: Category X, not for use in nursing.

MECHANISM OF ACTION: Estrogen/progesterone combination oral contraceptive. Acts by suppression of gonadotropins. Primarily inhibits ovulation. Also responsible for changes in cervical mucus (increasing difficulty of sperm entry into uterus) and in endometrium (reducing likelihood of implantation).

PHARMACOKINETICS: Absorption: Oral administration on variable days resulted in different parameters. Levonorgestrel: Rapid and completely absorbed, absolute bioavailability (100%); Ethinyl estradiol: Rapid and completely absorbed, absolute bioavailability (between 38% and 43%). **Distribution:** Levonorgestrel: Sex hormone-binding globulin (SHBG). Ethinyl Estradiol: Plasma protein binding (97%). **Metabolism:** Levonorgestrel: Reduction, hydroxylation and conjugation. Ethinyl Estradiol: Liver; hydroxylation via CYP3A4; methylation sulfation, glucuronidation. **Elimination:** Levonorgestrel: Urine (40-68%), feces (16-48%); $T_{1/2}$=36 hrs. Ethinyl Estradiol: Urine, feces; $T_{1/2}$=21 hrs.

NURSING CONSIDERATIONS

Assessment: Assess for presence or history of breast cancer, estrogen dependent neoplasia, abnormal genital bleeding, active liver disease, and known/suspected pregnancy or any other conditions where treatment is cautioned or contraindicated. Assess use in patients who are >35 yrs and heavy smokers (≥15 cigarettes/day). Assess use with HTN, hyperlipidemias, obesity, DM, or in patients at increased risk for thrombosis. Assess for possible drug interactions.

Monitoring: Monitor bleeding irregularities, thromboembolic events, onset or exacerbation of headaches or migraines, and ectopic pregnancy. Monitor fasting blood glucose levels in DM and prediabetic patients, BP with history of HTN, lipid levels with a history of hyperlipidemia. Monitor for signs of liver dysfunction (eg, jaundice) and signs of depression with previous history. Refer patients with contact lenses to an ophthalmologist if visual changes occur. Perform annual history and physical exam.

Patient Counseling: Instruct that medication does not protect against HIV infection (AIDS) and other STDs. Counsel about potential adverse effects. Inform may experience spotting/bleeding; continue therapy and notify physician if persists. Advise to avoid smoking. Instruct to take pill at same time every day. Inform that if 1 pill missed, take as soon as remembered; take next pill at next regular scheduled time. Advise that pregnancy can occur if patient has sexual intercourse during 7 days after restarting pills; use nonhormonal birth control method during that time.

Administration: Oral route. **Storage:** 25°C (77°F); excursions permitted to 15-30°C (59-86°F).

LYRICA   `CV`
pregabalin (Pfizer)

THERAPEUTIC CLASS: GABA analog

INDICATIONS: Management of neuropathic pain associated with diabetic peripheral neuropathy. Management of post-herpetic neuralgia. Adjunctive therapy for adult patients with partial onset seizures. Management of fibromyalgia.

DOSAGE: *Adults:* Neuropathic Pain (diabetes associated): Initial: 50mg tid. Titrate: May increase to 300mg/day within 1 week based on efficacy and tolerability. Max: 300mg/day (100mg tid). Postherpetic Neuralgia: Initial: 150mg/day divided bid or tid. Titrate: May increase to 300mg/day within 1 week based on efficacy and tolerability. If tolerated, may increase to up to 600mg/day divided bid or tid if patient does not experience sufficient pain relief following 2 to 4 weeks of treatment with 300mg/day. **Partial-Onset Seizures:** Initial: 150mg/day divided bid-tid. Titrate: May increase based on response and tolerability up to 600mg/day. Max: 600mg/day. **Fibromyalgia:** Initial: 75mg bid. Titrate: May increase to 300mg/day (150mg bid) within 1 week based on efficacy and tolerability. May further increase to 450mg/day (225mg bid) if needed. Max: 450mg/day. Refer to PI for Dosage Adjustment based on Renal Function. D/C: Taper over minimum of 1 week.

HOW SUPPLIED: Cap: 25mg, 50mg, 75mg, 100mg, 150mg, 200mg, 225mg, 300mg. Sol: 20mg/mL.

WARNINGS/PRECAUTIONS: Avoid abrupt withdrawal; gradually taper over 1 week. Increased risk of suicidal thoughts/behavior; monitor for emergence or worsening of depression, suicidal thought or behavior, and/or unusual changes in mood or behavior. May cause dizziness, somnolence and impair physical/mental abilities. May cause weight gain and peripheral edema; caution in congestive heart failure (CHF). Blurred vision, decreased acuity and visual field changes reported. Associated with creatine kinase (CK) elevations and rhabdomyolysis, d/c if myopathy or markedly elevated CK levels occur. May cause a decrease in platelet count and/or mild PR-interval prolongation. Life-threatening angioedema reported; D/C if symptoms observed & caution with patients who have previous episode of angioedema. Hypersensitivity reactions, including skin redness, blisters, hives, rash, dyspnea, and wheezing, reported; d/c if these symptoms occur. Caution in patients with renal impairment.

ADVERSE REACTIONS: Somnolence, dizziness, dry mouth, edema, blurred vision, weight gain, abnormal thinking (difficulty with concentration/attention), headache, constipation, asthenia, infection, neuropathy, ataxia.

INTERACTIONS: Increased risk of angioedema with other drugs associated with angioedema (eg, ACE inhibitors). Additive effects on cognitive and gross motor functioning with oxycodone, lorazepam, or ethanol. Caution with thiazolidinedione class of antidiabetic drugs.

PREGNANCY: Category C, not for use in nursing.

MECHANISM OF ACTION: Gamma-aminobutyric acid derivative; not fully established; binds to the $alpha_2$-delta site (an auxillary subunit of voltage-gated calcium channels) in CNS tissues. *In vitro*, shown to reduce calcium-dependent release of several neurotransmitters, possibly by modulation of calcium channel function.

PHARMACOKINETICS: Absorption: Well absorbed; T_{max}=1.5 hrs (fasting), 3 hrs (fed); bioavailability (≥90%). **Distribution:** V_d=0.5L/kg. **Metabolism:** Negligible metabolism. **Elimination:** Urine (90% unchanged); $T_{1/2}$=6.3 hrs.

NURSING CONSIDERATIONS

Assessment: Assess for known hypersensitivity reactions, impaired renal function, history of drug abuse, history of depression, seizure disorder, previous episode of angioedema, CHF, pregnancy/nursing status, and for possible drug interactions. Obtain baseline weight.

Monitoring: Monitor patient's response, therapy efficacy, degree of sedation, skin integrity, emergence or worsening of depression, suicidal thoughts or behavior, and/or unusual changes in mood or behavior. Monitor for symptoms of myopathy and ophthalmic changes, creatine kinase, weight, PR interval prolongation nd peripheral edema.

Patient Counseling: Inform that drug may cause physical/mental impairment; use with caution when operating machinery/driving. Instruct to report unexplained muscle pain, tenderness, or weakness, particularly if these symptoms are accompanied by malaise or fever. Avoid consuming alcohol. Take with/without food. Inform about signs/symptoms of angioedema, and not to abruptly d/c; taper dose over a week. Advise to be alert of the emergence or worsening of symptoms of depression, any unusual changes in mood or behavior, or the emergence of suicidal thoughts, behavior or thoughts about self-harm. Instruct to notify physician if pregnant, tend to become pregnant, breast feeding or intend to breast feed. Encourage to enroll in the North

American Antiepileptic Drug (NAAED) Pregnancy Registry. Inform men of risk of male-mediated teratogenicity. Advise patient that hypersensitivity reactions, edema, weight gain, and ophthalmological effects may occur. Instruct diabetic patients to watch for the development of skin ulcers. Inform that a Medication Guide is available and should be read before taking the drug.

Administration: Oral route. **Storage:** 25°C (77°F); excursions permitted to 15-30°C (59-86°F). (Sol) Use within 45 days of first opening the bottle.

LYSTEDA   RX
tranexamic acid (Xanodyne)

THERAPEUTIC CLASS: Antifibrinolytic agent

INDICATIONS: Treatment of cyclic heavy menstrual bleeding.

DOSAGE: *Adults:* 2 tabs tid for ≤5 days. Renal Impairment: SrCr >1.4-≤2.8mg/dL: 2 tabs bid for ≤5 days. SrCr >2.8-≤5.7mg/dL: 2 tabs qd for ≤5 days. SrCr >5.7mg/dL: 1 tab qd for ≤5 days. Swallow whole.

HOW SUPPLIED: Tab: 650mg

CONTRAINDICATIONS: Active thromboembolic disease (eg, DVT, pulmonary embolism, or cerebral thrombosis); history of thrombosis or thromboembolism (including retinal vein or artery occlusion) or intrinsic risk of thrombosis or thromboembolism (eg, thrombogenic valvular disease, thrombogenic cardiac rhythm disease, or hypercoagulopathy).

WARNINGS/PRECAUTIONS: Severe allergic reaction and anaphylactic shock reported. Retinal venous and arterial occlusion as well as ligneous conjunctivitis reported; d/c with ocular symptoms pending ophthalmologic evaluation. May cause cerebral edema and cerebral infarction in women with subarachnoid hemorrhage.

ADVERSE REACTIONS: Headache, nasal and sinus symptoms, back pain, abdominal pain, musculoskeletal pain, arthralgia, muscle cramps/spasms, migraine, anemia, fatigue.

INTERACTIONS: Concomitant use of hormonal contraceptives may further increase inherent thrombotic risk. May increase risk of thrombosis in women taking Factor IX complex concentrates or anti-inhibitor coagulant concentrates. May exacerbate procoagulant effect of all-trans retinoic acid in women with acute promyelocytic leukemia. Concomitant use with tissue plasminogen activators may decrease efficacy of both drugs.

PREGNANCY: Category B, caution in nursing.

MECHANISM OF ACTION: Antifibrinolytic; synthetic lysine amino acid derivative, which diminishes the dissolution of hemostatic fibrin by plasmin. Reversibly binds to the lysine receptor binding sites of plasmin for fibrin, preventing binding to fibrin monomers, thus preserving and stabilizing fibrin's matrix structure.

PHARMACOKINETICS: Absorption: Absolute bioavailability (45%); (single dose) AUC_{inf}=80.19mcg•h/mL, C_{max}=13.83mcg/mL, T_{max}=2.5 hrs. (multiple dose) C_{max}=6.41mcg/mL, T_{max}=2.5hrs. **Distribution:** V_d=0.18L/kg; V_{ss}=0.39L/kg; plasma protein bound (3%); crosses placenta; found in breast milk. **Elimination:** Urine (95%, unchanged); $T_{1/2}$=11 hrs.

NURSING CONSIDERATIONS

Assessment: Assess for active thromboembolic disease (eg, DVT, pulmonary embolism, or cerebral thrombosis), history of thrombosis or thromboembolism (including retinal vein or artery occlusion) or intrinsic risk for such conditions (eg, thrombogenic valvular disease, thrombogenic cardiac rhythm disease, or hypercoagulopathy), promyelocytic leukemia, renal impairment, pregnancy/nursing status, hypersensitivity and possible drug interactions.

Monitoring: Monitor for venous thromboembolism, arterial thromboses, severe allergic reactions and anaphylactic shock, retinal venous and arterial occlusion, ligneous conjunctivitis, cerebral edema and cerebral infarction.

Patient Counseling: Instruct patients to adhere to dosing regimen. Advise to swallow whole and not to break or chew tabs. Inform that headache, sinus and nasal symptoms, back pain, abdominal pain, musculoskeletal pain, joint pain, muscle cramps, migraine, anemia, and fatigue may occur. D/C and notify physician if eye symptoms or change in vision, allergic reactions (eg, SOB or throat tightening), and if menstrual bleeding persists or worsens.

Administration: Oral route. **Storage:** 25°C (77°F); excursions permitted to 15-30°C (59-86°F).

MACROBID   RX
nitrofurantoin monohydrate (Procter & Gamble)

THERAPEUTIC CLASS: Imidazolidinedione antibacterial

INDICATIONS: Treatment of acute uncomplicated urinary tract infections (acute cystitis).

DOSAGE: *Adults:* 100mg q12h for 7 days. Take with food.
Pediatrics: >12 yrs: 100mg q12h for 7 days. Take with food.

HOW SUPPLIED: Cap: 100mg

CONTRAINDICATIONS: Anuria, oliguria, CrCl <60mL/min, pregnancy at term (38-42 weeks gestation), labor and delivery, and neonates <1 month of age, and previous history of cholestatic jaundice or hepatic dysfunction.

WARNINGS/PRECAUTIONS: Acute, subacute, or chronic pulmonary reactions have occurred. Anemia, diabetes mellitus (DM), renal dysfunction, electrolyte imbalance, vitamin B deficiency, and debilitating disease may enhance occurrence of peripheral neuropathy. D/C with acute and chronic pulmonary reactions, hepatic disorders, hemolysis, or peripheral neuropathy. Monitor renal function, LFTs, and pulmonary function periodically during long-term therapy. Optic neuritis and hepatic reactions reported. *Clostridium difficile*-associated diarrhea (CDAD) has been reported.

ADVERSE REACTIONS: Pulmonary disorders, hepatic damage, peripheral neuropathy, nausea, headache, flatulence, diarrhea, dizziness, alopecia, exfoliative dermatitis, Stevens-Johnson syndrome, anaphylaxis, aplastic anemia.

INTERACTIONS: Antacids, especially magnesium trisilicate, decrease rate and extent of absorption. Uricosuric drugs (eg, probenecid and sulfinpyrazone) increase nitrofurantoin levels.

PREGNANCY: Category B, not for use in nursing.

MECHANISM OF ACTION: Imidazolidinedione antibacterial; inhibits protein synthesis, aerobic energy metabolism, DNA, RNA, and cell-wall synthesis.

PHARMACOKINETICS: Absorption: C_{max}≤1mcg/mL. **Elimination:** Urine (20-25% unchanged).

NURSING CONSIDERATIONS

Assessment: Assess for anuria, oliguria, renal impairment (CrCl <60mL/min or significant SrCr elevation), G6PD deficiency, DM, anemia, hypersensitivity, and drug interactions.

Monitoring: Monitor for acute/chronic pulmonary reactions (eg, diffuse interstitial pneumonitis, fibrosis), hepatic reactions (eg, hepatitis, cholestatic jaundice, chronic active hepatitis, and hepatic necrosis), peripheral neuropathy, optic neuritis, hematologic manifestations, CDAD, renal function, LFTs, benign intracranial HTN, Stevens-Johnson syndrome, cyanosis (methemoglobinemia).

Patient Counseling: Advise to take with food to enhance tolerance and improve drug absorption. Advise not to use antacids containing magnesium trisilicate and uricosuric drugs. Inform that therapy treats bacterial, not viral, infections. Take exactly as directed; skipping doses or not completing full course may decrease effectiveness and increase bacterial resistance. Inform may experience diarrhea; notify physician if watery/bloody stools, hypersensitivity reactions, or benign intracranial HTN develops.

Administration: Oral route. **Storage:** 15-30°C (59-86°F).

MACRODANTIN RX
nitrofurantoin macrocrystals (Procter & Gamble)

THERAPEUTIC CLASS: Imidazolidinedione antibacterial

INDICATIONS: Treatment of urinary tract infections.

DOSAGE: *Adults:* 50-100mg qid for 1 week or at least 3 days after sterility of the urine obtained. Long-term Suppressive Use: 50-100mg qhs. Take with food.
Pediatrics: ≥1 month: 5-7mg/kg/day given qid for 1 week or at least 3 days after sterility of the urine obtained. Long-term Suppressive Use: 1mg/kg/day given qd-bid. Take with food.

HOW SUPPLIED: Cap: 25mg, 50mg, 100mg

CONTRAINDICATIONS: Anuria, oliguria, CrCl <60mL/min, pregnancy at term (38-42 weeks' gestation), labor and delivery, neonates <1 month of age, and previous history of cholestatic jaundice or hepatic dysfunction associated with nitrofurantoin.

WARNINGS/PRECAUTIONS: Acute, subacute or chronic pulmonary reactions have occurred. Anemia, DM, renal dysfunction, electrolyte imbalance, vitamin B deficiency, and debilitating diseases enhance occurrence of peripheral neuropathy. Stop therapy with acute and chronic pulmonary reactions, hepatic disorders, hemolysis, or peripheral neuropathy. Monitor renal function, LFTs, and pulmonary function periodically during long-term therapy. Optic neuritis and hepatic reactions reported. False-positive reaction for glucose in urine may occur with Benedict's and Fehling's solution. *Clostridium difficile*-associated diarrhea (CDAD) has been reported. Hepatic reactions including hepatitis, cholestatic jaundice, chronic active hepatitis, and hepatic necrosis occur rarely.

ADVERSE REACTIONS: Pulmonary disorders, hepatic damage, malaise, dyspnea, peripheral neuropathy, nausea, emesis, anorexia, dizziness, headache, drowsiness, asthenia, vertigo, fever, nystagmus.

INTERACTIONS: Antacids containing magnesium trisilicate decrease rate and extent of absorption. Uricosuric drugs (eg, probenecid and sulfinpyrazone) increase nitrofurantoin levels.

PREGNANCY: Category B, not for use in nursing.

MECHANISM OF ACTION: Imidazolidinedione antibacterial; inhibits protein synthesis, aerobic energy metabolism, DNA, RNA, and cell-wall synthesis.

NURSING CONSIDERATIONS

Assessment: Assess for anuria, oliguria, renal impairment (CrCl <60mL/min, significant SrCr elevation), glucose 6 phosphate dehydrogenase deficiency, DM, anemia, hypersensitivity, pregnancy/nursing status, and possible drug interactions.

Monitoring: Monitor for acute/chronic pulmonary reactions (eg, diffuse interstitial pneumonitis or fibrosis), hepatic reactions (eg, hepatitis, cholestatic jaundice, chronic active hepatitis, and hepatic necrosis), peripheral neuropathy, optic neuritis, hematologic manifestations, CDAD, renal function, LFTs, benign intracranial HTN, Stevens-Johnson syndrome, and cyanosis (methemoglobinemia).

Patient Counseling: Take with food to enhance tolerance and improve drug absorption. Do not to use antacids containing magnesium trisilicate or uricosuric drugs. Therapy treats bacterial, not viral, infections. Take exactly as directed; skipping doses or not completing full course may decrease effectiveness and increase drug resistance. Notify physician if experience watery/bloody stools, hypersensitivity reactions, or benign intracranial HTN.

Administration: Oral route.

M

MACUGEN RX
pegaptanib sodium (Eyetech/Pfizer)

THERAPEUTIC CLASS: Vascular endothelial growth factor (VEGF) inhibitor

INDICATIONS: Treatment of neovascular (wet) age-related macular degeneration.

DOSAGE: *Adults*: 0.3mg by intravitreous injection once every 6 weeks.

HOW SUPPLIED: Inj: 0.3mg

CONTRAINDICATIONS: Ocular or periocular infections.

WARNINGS/PRECAUTIONS: Rare post-marketing cases of anaphylaxis/anaphylactoid reactions, including angioedema, reported. Endophthalmitis associated with intravitreous injections. Use proper aseptic injection technique. Monitor for increased IOP. For ophthalmic intravitreal injection only.

ADVERSE REACTIONS: Anterior chamber inflammation, blurred vision, cataract, conjunctival hemorrhage, corneal edema, eye discharge, eye irritation, eye pain, HTN, increased IOP, ocular discomfort, punctate keratitis, reduced visual acuity, visual disturbance, vitreous floaters, vitreous opacities.

PREGNANCY: Category B, caution in nursing.

MECHANISM OF ACTION: Selective vascular endothelial growth factor (VEGF) antagonist; inhibits VEGF, which is responsible for inducing angiogenesis, increasing vascular permeability and inflammation. VEGF has also been implicated in blood retinal barrier breakdown and pathological ocular neovascularization.

PHARMACOKINETICS: Absorption: Slowly into circulation from eye. C_{max}=80ng/mL. AUC=25mcg•hr/mL. **Distribution:** Vitreous fluid, retina, aqueous fluid. Metabolism: Via endo- and exonucleases. **Elimination:** Urine; $T_{1/2}$=10 days.

NURSING CONSIDERATIONS

Assessment: Prior to therapy, assess for ocular or periocular infections. Assess medical history for hypersensitivity reactions.

Monitoring: Monitor for signs/symptoms of elevated IOP, endophthalmitis, anaphylaxis reactions (eg, angioedema), retinal detachment, and iatrogenic traumatic cataract. Monitor perfusion of optic nerve immediately, perform tonometry within 30 min and biomicroscopy between 2 and 7 days following injection.

Patient Counseling: Advise about risk of developing endophthalmitis following administration. Instruct to seek immediate care with ophthalmologist if eye becomes red, sensitive to light, painful, or if change in vision develops.

Administration: Ophthalmic intravitreal injection. Injection procedure should be carried out under controlled aseptic conditions, including sterile gloves, sterile drape, and sterile eyelid speculum. Adequate anesthesia and a broad-spectrum microbicide should be given prior to injection. **Storage:** 2-8°C (36-46°F). Do not freeze or shake vigorously.

MALARONE RX
proguanil HCl - atovaquone (GlaxoSmithKline)

OTHER BRAND NAMES: Malarone Pediatric (GlaxoSmithKline)

THERAPEUTIC CLASS: Pyrimidine synthesis inhibitor

INDICATIONS: Prophylaxis or treatment of acute, uncomplicated malaria caused by *P. falciparum*.

DOSAGE: *Adults:* Prevention: Begin 1-2 days before entering malaria-endemic area, continue daily during stay and for 7 days after return. 250mg-100mg qd. Treatment: 1000mg-400mg qd for 3 days. Repeat dose in the event of vomiting within 1 hr after dosing. Take at the same time each day with meal or milky drink.

Pediatrics: Prevention: Begin 1-2 days before entering endemic area, continue during stay and for 7 days after return. 11-20kg: 62.5mg-25mg qd. 21-30kg: 125mg-50mg qd. 31-40kg: 187.5mg-75mg qd. >40kg: 250mg-100mg qd. Treatment: Treat for 3 consecutive days. 5-8kg: 125mg-50mg qd. 9-10kg: 187.5mg-75mg qd. 11-20kg: 250mg-100mg. 21-30kg: 500mg-200mg qd. 31-40kg: 750mg-300mg. >40kg: 1000mg-400mg qd. Repeat dose in the event of vomiting within 1 hr after dosing. Take at the same time each day with meal or milky drink. May crush and mix with condensed milk just prior to administration for children who may have difficulty swallowing tablets.

HOW SUPPLIED: Tab: (Atovaquone-Proguanil) 62.5mg-25mg, 250mg-100mg

CONTRAINDICATIONS: Prophylaxis in patients with severe renal impairment (CrCl <30mL/min).

WARNINGS/PRECAUTIONS: Not evaluated for treatment of cerebral malaria or other severe manifestations of complicated malaria, including hyperparasitemia, pulmonary edema, or renal failure. Patients with severe malaria are not candidates for PO therapy. Rare cases of hepatitis and elevated LFTs reported with prophylactic use. Diarrhea or vomiting may reduce absorption; monitor for parasitemia and consider use of an antiemetic in patients who are vomiting. Alternative therapy may be required with severe or persistent diarrhea or vomiting. Parasite relapse occured commonly when used as monotherapy to treat *P. vivax*. Caution for the treatment of malaria in patients with severe renal impairment. Treat with a different blood schizoticide in the event of recrudescent *P. falciparum* infections or failure of chemoprophylaxis.

ADVERSE REACTIONS: Abdominal pain, headache, N/V, pruritus, diarrhea, elevated LFTs, asthenia, anorexia, dizziness, gastritis.

INTERACTIONS: Concomitant use of rifampin, rifabutin, tetracycline may decrease levels. Reduced bioavailability with metoclopramide. Caution with indinavir; may decrease trough levels of indinavir. May potentiate anticoagulant effect of warfarin and similar anticoagulants; caution when initiating and withdrawing Malarone therapy.

PREGNANCY: Category C, caution in nursing.

MECHANISM OF ACTION: Pyramidine synthesis inhibitor. Atovaquone: Acts as a selective inhibitor of parasite mitochondrial electron transport. Proguanil: Acts via its metabolite, cycloguanil, which inhibits dihydrofolate reductase in the malaria parasite, disrupting of deoxythymidylate synthesis.

PHARMACOKINETICS: Absorption: Atovaquone: Absolute bioavailability (23% with food). Proguanil: Extensively absorbed. **Distribution:** Atovaquone: V_d=8.8L/kg; plasma protein binding (≥99%). Proguanil: V_d=1617-2502L (adult and pediatric patients >15 yrs with body weight 31-110kg), V_d=462-966L (pediatric patients ≤15 yrs with body weight 11-56kg). Plasma protein binding (75%). **Metabolism:** Proguanil: Cycloguanil (active metabolite) via CYP2C19. **Elimination:** Atovaquone: Feces (94 unchanged), urine (<0.6%). $T_{1/2}$=2-3 days (adult). Proguanil: Urine (40-60%); $T_{1/2}$=12-21 hrs (adult and pediatric patients).

NURSING CONSIDERATIONS

Assessment: Assess for uncomplicated *P.falciparum* malaria, renal impairment, cerebral malaria, hyperparasitemia, pulmonary edema, diarrhea, vomiting, decreased hepatic/renal function, pregnancy/nursing status, and possible drug interactions.

Monitoring: Monitor for parasitemia and parasite relapse to determine if antiemetic or alternative antimalarial therapy is needed. Monitor for adverse reactions.

Patient Counseling: Take tablet at the same time each day with food or a milky drink; repeat dose if vomiting occurs within 1 hr after dosing. If dose is missed, take as soon as possible and then return to normal dosing schedule. Do not double dose if dose is skipped. Consult physician for any febrile illness that occurs during or after return from a malaria-endemic area. Pregnant/nursing women anticipating travel to malarious areas should inform physician.

Administration: Oral route. Take with food or a milky drink. **Storage:** 25°C (77°F); excursions permitted to 15-30°C (59-86°F).

MARINOL
dronabinol (Solvay)

THERAPEUTIC CLASS: Cannabinoid

INDICATIONS: Treatment of anorexia associated with weight loss in AIDS patients and N/V associated with chemotherapy when conventional treatment has failed.

DOSAGE: *Adults:* Appetite Stimulation: Initial: 2.5mg bid before lunch and supper or 2.5mg qpm or qhs if 5mg/day is intolerable. Max: 20mg/day in divided doses. Antiemetic: Initial: 5mg/m² given 1-3 hrs before chemotherapy, then q2-4h after chemotherapy, up to 4-6 doses/day. Titrate: May increase by 2.5mg/m² increments. Max: 15mg/m²/dose.

HOW SUPPLIED: Cap: 2.5mg, 5mg, 10mg

CONTRAINDICATIONS: Allergy to sesame oil.

WARNINGS/PRECAUTIONS: Do not drive, operate machinery, or engage in any hazardous activity until ability to tolerate drug is established. Seizure and seizure-like activity reported; caution in patients with history of seizure disorders and d/c if seizures develop. Caution with cardiac disorders due to possible HTN, occasional hypotension, syncope, or tachycardia. Caution with history of substance abuse. Caution and psychiatric monitoring are needed in patients with mania, depression, and schizophrenia as illness may be exacerbated. Caution in elderly due to increased sensitivity to the psychoactive, neurological, and postural hypotensive effects.

ADVERSE REACTIONS: Euphoria, dizziness, paranoid reaction, somnolence, abnormal thinking, abdominal pain, N/V.

INTERACTIONS: Highly protein-bound drugs may require dosage changes. Additive effects with phenothiazines, alcohol, sedatives, hypnotics, or other psychoactive drugs. Additive HTN, tachycardia, and possible cardiotoxicity with amphetamines, cocaine, and sympathomimetics. Increased tachycardia, and drowsiness with anticholinergic agents (eg, atropine, scopolamine) and antihistamines. Potentiates effects of TCAs (eg, amitriptyline, amoxapine, desipramine) and CNS depressants (eg, benzodiazepines, barbiturates). Additive drowsiness and CNS depression with lithium, opioids, buspirone, and muscle relaxants. Coadministration with theophylline in patients who smoked marijuana/tobacco increased theophylline metabolism. Coadministration with disulfiram and fluoxetine in patients who smoked marijuana resulted to hypomanic reactions. Decreased clearance of antipyrine and barbiturates.

PREGNANCY: Category C, not for use in nursing.

MECHANISM OF ACTION: Cannabinoid; has complex effects on the CNS, including central sympathomimetic activity.

PHARMACOKINETICS: Absorption: Complete (90-95%); (2.5mg bid) C_{max}=1.32ng/mL, T_{max}=1 hr, AUC=2.88ng•hr/mL; (5mg bid) C_{max}=2.96ng/mL, T_{max}=2.5 hr, AUC=6.16ng•hr/mL; (10mg bid) C_{max}=7.88ng/mL, T_{max}=1.5 hr, AUC=15.2ng•hr/mL. **Distribution:** V_d=10L/kg; plasma protein binding (97%). Found in breast milk. **Metabolism:** Liver via microsomal hydroxylation; 11-OH-delta-9-THC (active metabolite). **Elimination:** Urine (10-15%), bile/feces (50%, <5% unchanged); $T_{1/2}$=25-36 hrs.

NURSING CONSIDERATIONS

Assessment: Assess for history of hypersensitivity, especially to sesame oil, seizure/cardiac disorders, history of substance abuse (including alcohol abuse/dependence), mania, depression, schizophrenia, pregnancy/nursing status, hepatic/renal impairment, and possible drug interactions.

Monitoring: Monitor for psychiatric illness exacerbation, abdominal pain, N/V, dizziness, euphoria, paranoid reaction, somnolence, abnormal thinking, hypotension or HTN, syncope, tachycardia, and for psychological and physiological dependence.

Patient Counseling: Do not drink alcohol or take other CNS depressants. Use caution while performing hazardous tasks (eg, operating machinery/driving) until well tolerated. Inform of mood changes and other behavioral effects that may occur during therapy. Advise that patients must be under constant supervision of a responsible adult during initial use. Instruct to immediately report any adverse effects to physician.

Adminisration: Oral route. **Storage:** 8-15°C (46-59°F). Protect from freezing.

MAVIK   RX
trandolapril (Abbott)

> ACE inhibitors can cause death/injury to developing fetus during 2nd and 3rd trimesters. D/C if pregnancy detected.

THERAPEUTIC CLASS: ACE inhibitor

INDICATIONS: Treatment of hypertension (HTN) alone or in combination with other antihypertensives. Treatment of congestive heart failure (CHF) or left-ventricular dysfunction post myocardial infarction (MI).

DOSAGE: *Adults:* HTN: D/C diuretic 2-3 days prior to therapy if possible. Initial: 1mg qd in non-black patients; 2mg qd in black patients; 0.5mg with concomitant diuretic. Titrate: Adjust at 1-week intervals according to blood pressure response. Usual: 2-4mg qd. May be treated with 4mg bid if inadequately treated with qd dosing. Resume diuretic if not controlled. Max: 8mg. Post-MI: Initial: 1mg qd. Titrate: Increase to target dose of 4mg qd as tolerated; if not tolerated, continue with the greatest tolerated dose. CrCl <30mL/min/Hepatic Cirrhosis for HTN or Post-MI: Initial: 0.5mg qd. Titrate to optimal response.

HOW SUPPLIED: Tab: 1mg*, 2mg, 4mg *scored

CONTRAINDICATIONS: History of ACE inhibitor-associated angioedema.

WARNINGS/PRECAUTIONS: Angioedema involving the face, extremities, lips, tongue, glottis, and/or larynx reported; d/c if occurs. Intestinal angioedema reported; monitor for abdominal pain (with or without N/V). More reports of angioedema in blacks than nonblacks. Risk of hyperkalemia with DM, renal dysfunction. Monitor WBCs in renal impairment and/or collagen vascular disease. Rarely, a syndrome of cholestatic jaundice, fulminant necrosis and sometimes death occurs; d/c if jaundice or marked elevations of hepatic enzymes develops. Fetal/neonatal morbidity and death reported. Monitor for hypotension in high-risk patients (heart failure, surgery/anesthesia, prolonged diuretic therapy, volume and/or salt depletion, etc). Persistent nonproductive cough reported. Caution with CHF, renal dysfunction, and renal artery stenosis. Minor increases in BUN or SrCr reported.

ADVERSE REACTIONS: Cough, dizziness, hypotension, elevated serum uric acid, elevated BUN, elevated creatinine, cardiogenic shock, syncope, hyperkalemia, dyspepsia, bradycardia, hypocalcemia, myalgia, gastritis, intermittent claudication.

INTERACTIONS: May increase lithium levels. Hypotension risk with diuretics. Increased risk of hyperkalemia with K^+-sparing diuretics, K^+-containing salt substitutes, or K^+ supplements. Nitritoid reactions (eg, facial flushing, N/V, hypotension) reported rarely with injectable gold. Reduced antihypertensive effect with NSAIDs. May enhance hypotensive effect of certain inhalation anesthetics.

PREGNANCY: Category C (1st trimester) and D (2nd and 3rd trimesters), not for use in nursing.

MECHANISM OF ACTION: ACE inhibitor; reduces angiotensin II formation, decreases vasoconstriction and aldosterone secretion, and increases plasma renin.

PHARMACOKINETICS: Absorption: Absolute bioavailability (10%, trandolapril), (70%, trandolaprilat); Tmax=(1 hr, trandolapril), (4-10 hrs, trandolaprilat). **Distribution:** V_d=18L; plasma protein binding (80% trandolapril), (65-94%, trandolaprilat). **Metabolism:** Cleavage of ester group; trandolaprilat (metabolite). **Elimination:** Urine (33%), feces (66%); $T_{1/2}$=(6 hrs, trandolapril), (22.5, trandolaprilat).

NURSING CONSIDERATIONS

Assessment: Assess for pregnancy status, volume/salt depletion, collagen vascular disease (SLE, scleroderma), CHF, DM, possible drug interactions, ischemic heart disease, aortic stenosis, cerebrovascular disease, renal/hepatic impairment.

Monitoring: Monitor renal function for 1st few weeks; WBC (collagen vascular disease) periodically. Monitor for nitritoid reactions, hypotension, anaphylactoid or hypersensitivity reactions, head/neck and intestinal angioedema, agranulocytosis, hyperkalemia, renal/hepatic dysfunction.

Patient Counseling: Counsel about fetal risks during pregnancy and signs/symptoms of angioedema (eg, laryngeal/tongue edema, abdominal pain); advise to seek prompt medical attention if symptoms develop. Inform that inadequate fluid intake or fluid loss may lead to drop in BP resulting in lightheadedness or syncope; avoid K⁺ supplements or salt substitutes. Inform about need for periodic monitoring of electrolytes and blood counts. Advise to seek medical attention if symptoms of hypotension (syncope), anaphylactoid or hypersensitivity reactions, infection (sore throat, fever), hyperkalemia, or hepatic dysfunction occur.

Administration: Oral route. **Storage:** 20-25°C (68-77°F).

MAXAIR   RX
pirbuterol acetate (Graceway)

THERAPEUTIC CLASS: Beta$_2$-agonist

INDICATIONS: Prevention and reversal of bronchospasm in patients ≥12 yrs with reversible bronchospasm including asthma as monotherapy or with theophylline and/or corticosteroids.

DOSAGE: *Adults:* 1-2 inh q4-6h. Max: 12 inh/day.
Pediatrics: ≥12 yrs: 1-2 inh q4-6h. Max: 12 inh/day.

HOW SUPPLIED: MDI: 200mcg/actuation [2.8g, 14g]

WARNINGS/PRECAUTIONS: D/C if cardiovascular (CV) effects occurred. ECG changes reported. Caution with CV disorders (eg, coronary insufficiency, ischemic heart disease, HTN, arrhythmias), hyperthyroidism, diabetes mellitus (DM), convulsive disorders, and patients who are unusually responsive to sympathomimetic amines. Can produce paradoxical bronchospasm; d/c immediately when develops and institute alternative therapy. Consider adding anti-inflammatory agents to therapy (eg, corticosteroids) to adequately control asthma. Re-evaluate patient and treatment regimen if deterioration of asthma observed. Changes in systolic and diastolic BP and hypokalemia may occur.

ADVERSE REACTIONS: Nervousness, tremor, headache, dizziness, palpitations, tachycardia, cough, nausea.

INTERACTIONS: Avoid with other short-acting aerosol β$_2$ agonists. May potentiate action on the vascular system with MAOIs or TCAs. May worsen the ECG changes and/or hypokalemia caused by non-K⁺ sparing diuretics (eg, loop or thiazide diuretics); caution with use. Pulmonary effect blocked by β-blockers. Caution with cardioselective β-blockers.

PREGNANCY: Category C, caution in nursing.

MECHANISM OF ACTION: β$_2$-adrenergic bronchodilator; stimulates the intracellular adenyl cyclase, the enzyme that converts adenosine triphosphate to cyclic adenosine monophosphate (cAMP). Increased cAMP levels are associated with relaxation of bronchial smooth muscle and inhibition of release of mediators of immediate hypersensitivity from cells.

PHARMACOKINETICS: Elimination: Urine (51%); T$_{1/2}$=2 hrs.

NURSING CONSIDERATIONS

Assessment: Assess for previous hypersensitivity to the drug, CV disorders, HTN, unusual response to sympathomimetic amines, convulsive disorders, hyperthyroidism, DM, pregnancy/nursing status, and possible drug interactions.

Monitoring: Monitor pulse rate, BP, ECG changes, for CV effects, paradoxical bronchospasm and hypokalemia, hypersensitivity reactions, and deterioration of asthma.

Patient Counseling: Instruct patient to take as directed. Seek medical attention if treatment becomes less effective, symptoms becomes worse, and/or more frequent use is needed. Contact physician if pregnant/nursing, and/or experiencing adverse reactions. Instruct not to use with any other inhalation aerosol canister or any other actuator. Advise to keep out of reach of children and avoid spraying in eyes. Advise to prime before use for the first time and if not used in 48 hrs.

Administration: Oral inhalation route. Shake well. Prime before use for the 1st time and if has not been used in 48 hrs. **Storage:** 15-30°C (59-86°F). Do not use or store near heat or open flame.

MAXALT RX
rizatriptan benzoate (Merck)

OTHER BRAND NAMES: Maxalt-MLT (Merck)

THERAPEUTIC CLASS: 5-HT$_{1B/1D}$ agonist

INDICATIONS: Acute treatment of migraine attacks with or without aura in adults.

DOSAGE: *Adults:* Individualize dose. Usual: 5-10mg single dose. Separate doses by ≥2 hrs. Max: 30mg/24 hrs. Concomitant Propranolol: Use 5mg dose. Max: 3 doses/24 hrs. (MLT) Dissolve on tongue and swallow with saliva.

HOW SUPPLIED: Tab: 5mg, 10mg; (MLT) Tab, Disintegrating: 5mg, 10mg

CONTRAINDICATIONS: Ischemic heart disease (IHD) (eg, angina pectoris, history of myocardial infarction [MI], or documented silent ischemia), symptoms or findings consistent with IHD, coronary artery vasospasm (eg, Prinzmetal's variant angina), other significant underlying cardiovascular disease (CVD), uncontrolled HTN, hemiplegic/basilar migraine, concurrent use of MAOIs or use within 2 weeks of d/c of MAOI therapy, concomitant use with another 5-HT1 agonist or an ergotamine-containing or ergot-type medication (eg, dihydroergotamine, methysergide) within 24 hrs.

WARNINGS/PRECAUTIONS: Safety and effectiveness not established for cluster headache. Not intended for prophylactic therapy. Use only when diagnosis is confirmed. May cause coronary vasospasm. Avoid with unrecognized coronary artery disease (CAD) predicted by presence of risk factors (eg, HTN, hypercholesterolemia, smoker, obesity, diabetes, strong family history of CAD, female with surgical/physiological menopause, males >40 yrs) unless with a satisfactory cardiovascular (CV) evaluation; administer 1st dose under medical supervision and obtain ECG to assess presence of cardiac ischemia. Perform periodic interval CV evaluation with intermittent long-term use. Serious adverse cardiac events, including acute MI, reported within few hours following administration. Cerebrovascular events (eg, cerebral/subarachnoid hemorrhage, stroke), vasospastic reactions (eg, peripheral vascular/colonic ischemia with abdominal pain and bloody diarrhea), BP elevation, and hypertensive crisis reported. Sensations of tightness, pain, pressure, and heaviness in precordium, throat, neck, and jaw not associated with arrhythmias or ischemic ECG changes reported. Serotonin syndrome may occur; symptoms may include mental status changes, autonomic instability, neuromuscular aberrations, and GI symptoms. Caution with renal dialysis, moderate hepatic insufficiency, and diseases that may alter absorption, metabolism, or excretion of drugs. May possibly cause long-term ophthalmologic effects. (MLT) Contains phenylalanine; caution with phenylketonuria.

ADVERSE REACTIONS: Paresthesia, dry mouth, nausea, dizziness, somnolence, asthenia/fatigue, pain/pressure sensation.

INTERACTIONS: See Contraindications. Increased plasma levels with propranolol. Serotonin syndrome reported with SSRIs or serotonin norepinephrine reuptake inhibitors (SNRIs).

PREGNANCY: Category C, caution in nursing.

M

MECHANISM OF ACTION: $5-HT_{1B/1D}$ receptor agonist; binds with high affinity to human cloned $5-HT_{1B/1D}$ receptors on extracerebral, intracranial blood vessels, and on trigeminal system nerve terminals resulting in cranial vessel constriction, neuropeptide release inhibition, and reduced transmission in trigeminal pain pathways.

PHARMACOKINETICS: Absorption: Complete; (Tab) absolute bioavailability (45%), T_{max}=1-1.5 hrs; (MLT) T_{max}=1.6-2.5 hrs. **Distribution:** V_d=140L (male), 110L (female); plasma protein binding (14%). **Metabolism:** Oxidative deamination via monoamine oxidase-A (MAO-A). N-monodesmethyl-rizatriptan (active metabolite). **Elimination:** Urine (82%), (14% unchanged, 51% indole acetic acid metabolite), feces (12%); $T_{1/2}$=2-3 hrs.

NURSING CONSIDERATIONS

Assessment: Confirm diagnosis before instituting therapy. Assess for IHD, coronary artery vasospasm, CVD, HTN, hemiplegic/basilar migraine, risk factors for CAD, hepatic/renal function, diseases that may alter absorption, metabolism, or excretion of drugs, phenylketonuria, pregnancy/nursing status, drug hypersensitivity, and possible drug interactions. Perform CV evaluation prior to therapy.

Monitoring: Monitor for signs/symptoms of coronary vasospasm, CV adverse events, cerebrovascular events, peripheral vascular ischemia, colonic ischemia with bloody diarrhea and abdominal pain, serotonin syndrome, ophthalmologic effects, increased BP, and other adverse reactions. Monitor ECG during the interval immediately following therapy in patients with CAD risk factors. Perform periodic interval CV evaluation with intermittent long-term use.

Patient Counseling: Inform that the drug may cause somnolence and dizziness; evaluate ability to perform complex tasks during attacks and after administration. Caution about the risk of serotonin syndrome, especially if combined with SSRIs or SNRIs. Instruct to read patient package insert before taking the drug. (MLT) Instruct not to remove blister from outer pouch until just prior to dosing; peel open with dry hands and place disintegrating tab on tongue.

Administration: Oral route. (MLT) Just prior to dosing, peel open with dry hands and place on tongue, where it will be dissolved and swallowed with saliva. **Storage:** 15-30°C (59-86°F).

MAXIPIME   RX
cefepime HCl (Elan)

THERAPEUTIC CLASS: Cephalosporin (4th generation)

INDICATIONS: Treatment of uncomplicated/complicated urinary tract (UTI) including pyelonephritis, uncomplicated skin and skin structure (SSSI), complicated intra-abdominal infections, and pneumonia caused by susceptible strains of microorganisms. Empiric therapy for febrile neutropenia.

DOSAGE: *Adults:* Moderate-Severe Pneumonia: 1-2g IV q12h for 10 days. Febrile Neutropenia Empiric Therapy: 2g IV q8h for 7 days or until neutropenia resolved. Mild-Moderate UTI: (Maxipime): 0.5-1g IM/IV q12h for 7-10 days; IM only indicated for mild to moderate UTI due to *E.coli* when IM route is more appropriate. (Generic): 0.5-1g IV q12h for 7-10 days. Severe UTI/Moderate-Severe SSSI: 2g IV q12h for 10 days. Complicated Intra-Abdominal Infections: 2g IV q12h for 7-10 days in combination with metronidazole. Renal Impairment (CrCl ≤60mL/min): Initial (except for hemodialysis): Normal dose. Maint: CrCl 30-60mL/min: 500mg-2g q24h or 2g q12h. CrCl 11-29mL/min: 500mg-2g q24h. CrCl <11mL/min: 250mg-1g q24h. CAPD: 500mg-2g q48h. Hemodialysis: 1g on Day 1, then 500mg q24h or 1g q24h.
Pediatrics: 2 months-16 yrs: ≤40kg: UTI/SSSI/Pneumonia: (Maxipime): 50mg/kg IM/IV q12h. IM injection only indicated for mild to moderate UTI due to *E.coli* when IM route is more appropriate. (Generic): 50mg/kg IV q12h. Febrile Neutropenia: 50mg/kg IV q8h. Give for the same duration as adults. Max: Do not exceed adult dose.

HOW SUPPLIED: Inj: 500mg; (Generic/Maxipime) 1g, 2g

CONTRAINDICATIONS: Hypersensitivity to penicillins (PCNs) or other β-lactam antibiotics.

WARNINGS/PRECAUTIONS: Caution with PCN sensitivity; cross hypersensitivity may occur. D/C use if an allergic reaction occurs. Caution with renal impairment (CrCl ≤60mL/min) or history of GI disease, especially colitis. Encephalopathy, myoclonus, and seizures reported; most cases reported in patients with renal impairment who exceeded recommended dosing schedule. *Clostridium difficile*-associated diarrhea (CDAD) reported. Use in the absence of a proven or strongly suspected bacterial infection or prophylactic indication is unlikely to provide benefit and may increase risk of drug-resistant bacteria. Prolonged use may result in overgrowth of nonsusceptible organisms. May alter glucose values or elevate serum K^+ levels. Associated with a fall in PT; monitor PT in patients with renal or hepatic impairment, or poor nutritional state, and in patients on a protracted course of antimicrobials; give vitamin K as indicated. Associated with (+) direct Coombs' test. False (+) for urine glucose with Clinitest tabs. Superinfection occur; appropriate measurement should be taken. Caution with meningeal seeding/meningitis.

ADVERSE REACTIONS: Local reactions (eg, phlebitis), rash, diarrhea, (+) Coombs' test (without hemolysis).

INTERACTIONS: Increased risk of nephrotoxicity and ototoxicity with aminoglycosides. Risk of nephrotoxicity with potent diuretics (eg, furosemide).

PREGNANCY: Category B, caution in nursing.

MECHANISM OF ACTION: 4th generation cephalosporin; bactericidal agent that acts by inhibiting cell wall synthesis.

PHARMACOKINETICS: Absorption: Complete (IM). Refer to PI for IM and IV parameters. **Distribution:** V_d=18L; plasma protein binding (20%); found in breast milk. **Metabolism:** Metabolized to N-methylpyrrolidine (NMP), which is rapidly converted to N-oxide (NMP-N-oxide). **Elimination:** Urine, (85% unchanged, <1% NMP, 6.8% NMP-N-oxide); $T_{1/2}$=2 hrs.

NURSING CONSIDERATIONS

Assessment: Assess for PCN allergy, pregnancy/nursing status, renal/hepatic impairment, nutritional status, history of GI disease, and for possible drug interactions. Document indications for therapy with culture and susceptibility testing. (Generic): Assess for allergy to corn or corn products.

Monitoring: Monitor for signs/symptoms of hypersensitivity reactions (anaphylaxis), CDAD, renal function, encephalopathy, myoclonus, seizures, superinfection, a fall in prothrombin activity, changes in glucose metabolism, and for elevations in serum K^+ levels. Monitor PT in patients at risk for a fall in prothrombin activity (eg, renal/hepatic impairment, poor nutritional state, protracted course of antimicrobial therapy).

Patient Counseling: Inform that therapy only treats bacterial, not viral infections (eg, common colds). Instruct to take as directed; skipping doses or not completing full course of therapy may decrease effectiveness and increase bacterial resistance. Advise that diarrhea may occur. Instruct to notify physician if watery/bloody stools (with/without stomach cramps and fever), hypersensitivity reactions, neurological signs/symptoms including encephalopathy (disturbance of consciousness including confusion, hallucinations, and coma), myoclonus, or seizures occur.

Administration: IV/IM routes; give IV over 30 min. Refer to PI for administration instructions. **Storage:** Dry State: 2-25°C (36-77°F). Protect from light. (Generic): -20°C (-4°F). Thawed solution: remains stable for 7 days under refrigeration 5°C (41°F) or 24 hrs at room temperature 25°C (77°F). Do not refreeze.

MAXITROL OINTMENT RX
polymyxin B sulfate - neomycin sulfate - dexamethasone (Alcon)

OTHER BRAND NAMES: Maxitrol suspension (Alcon)
THERAPEUTIC CLASS: Antibacterial/corticosteroid combination

INDICATIONS: For steroid-responsive inflammatory ocular conditions for which a corticosteroid is indicated and where bacterial infection or the risk of bacterial ocular infection exist.

DOSAGE: *Adults:* (Oint) Apply 1/2 inch in conjunctival sac(s) up to 3-4 times daily. Max: 8g for initial prescription. (Sus) Instill 1-2 drops in conjunctival sac(s) up to 4-6 times daily in mild disease and qh in severe disease. Taper to d/c as inflammation subsides. Max: 20mL for initial prescription.

HOW SUPPLIED: Oint: (Dexamethasone-Neomycin sulfate-Polymyxin sulfate) 0.1%-3.5mg-10,000 U/g [3.5g]; Sus: (Dexamethasone-Neomycin sulfate-Polymyxin sulfate) 0.1%-3.5mg-10,000 U/mL [5mL]

CONTRAINDICATIONS: Epithelial herpes simplex keratitis (dendritic keratitis), vaccinia, varicella, and other viral diseases of the cornea and conjunctiva, mycobacterial infection of the eye, fungal diseases of ocular structures.

WARNINGS/PRECAUTIONS: For topical ophthalmic use only; not for injection. Glaucoma with damage to the optic nerve, defects in visual acuity and fields of vision, and posterior subcapsular cataract formation may occur after prolonged use. May cause perforations when used with diseases causing thinning of cornea or sclera. May mask infection or enhance existing infection in acute purulent conditions of the eye. Monitor intraocular pressure (IOP) if used for ≥10 days. Prolonged use may suppress host response, increase risk of secondary ocular infections, or cause persistent fungal infections of the cornea. May cause cutaneous sensitization. Caution in the treatment of herpes simplex. Perform eye exam (eg, slit lamp biomicroscopy, fluorescein staining) prior to therapy and renewal of medication. (Sus) Usage after cataract surgery may delay healing and increase incidence of bleb formation. May prolong course and exacerbate severity of ocular viral infections (eg, herpes simplex). Do not inject subconjunctivally, nor directly introduce into anterior chamber of the eye. If no improvement is seen after 2 days, re-evaluate patient. Suspect fungal invasion in any persistent corneal ulceration during/after therapy; take fungal cultures when appropriate.

ADVERSE REACTIONS: Allergic sensitizations, elevated IOP, posterior subcapsular cataract formation, delayed wound healing, secondary infections.

PREGNANCY: Category C, caution in nursing.

MECHANISM OF ACTION: Antibacterial/Corticosteroid. Dexamethasone: Corticosteroid; suppresses the inflammatory response to a variety of agents. May inhibit the body's defense mechanism against infection.

PHARMACOKINETICS: (Systemically administered) found in breast milk.

NURSING CONSIDERATIONS

Assessment: Assess for active viral diseases of the cornea and conjunctiva, epithelial herpes simplex keratitis, vaccinia, varicella, mycobacterial infection of the eye, fungal disease of ocular structures, diseases causing thinning of sclera or cornea, acute purulent conditions, history of cataract surgery, hypersensitivity to the drug or its components, and pregnancy/nursing status. Perform eye exam (eg, slit lamp biomicroscopy, flourescein staining) prior to therapy.

Monitoring: Monitor for signs and symptoms of glaucoma, optic nerve damage, visual acuity and visual field defects, subcapsular cataract, ocular/corneal perforations, cutaneous sensitizations, bacterial, viral, fungal infections. Monitor for increased risk of secondary ocular infections. Monitor IOP and perform eye exams (eg, slit lamp biomicroscopy, flourescein staining) prior to renewal of medication. (Sus) Monitor use after cataract surgery. Perform fungal cultures when fungal invasion is suspected.

Patient Counseling: Advise not to touch dropper tip to any surface; may contaminate drug. Keep out of reach of children. Instruct to use medication as prescribed. Advise that medication is for topical ophthalmic use only. Inform physician if pregnant or breastfeeding. (Oint) Advise not to wear contact lenses if signs and syptoms of bacterial ocular infection are present. Instruct not to use product if the imprinted carton seals have been damaged or removed. (Sus) Advise to d/c and consult physician if inflammation or pain persists >48 hrs or becomes aggravated. Inform that use of the same bottle by more than one person may spread infection. Instruct to shake well before use and to keep bottle tightly closed when not in use.

Administration: Ocular route. (Oint) Tilt head back. Place finger on cheek just under the eye and gently pull down until a "V" pocket is formed between eyeball and lower lid. Place small amount of ointment in the "V" pocket. Look downward before closing the eye. **Storage:** Oint: 2-25°C (36-77°F). Sus: 8-27°C (46-80°F). Store upright.

MAXZIDE
RX
triamterene - hydrochlorothiazide (Mylan Bertek)

> Abnormal elevation of serum K⁺ levels (≥5.5mEq/L) may occur with all K⁺-sparing diuretic combinations. Hyperkalemia is more likely to occur with renal impairment and diabetes (even without evidence of renal impairment), and in elderly or severely ill; monitor serum K⁺ levels at frequent intervals.

OTHER BRAND NAMES: Maxzide-25 (Mylan Bertek)

THERAPEUTIC CLASS: K⁺-sparing diuretic/thiazide diuretic

INDICATIONS: Treatment of HTN or edema if hypokalemia occurs on HCTZ alone, or when a thiazide diuretic is required and cannot risk hypokalemia. May be used alone or as an adjunct to other antihypertensives, such as β-blockers.

DOSAGE: *Adults:* (Maxzide-25) 1-2 tabs qd, given as a single dose or (Maxzide) 1 tab qd.

HOW SUPPLIED: Tab: (Triamterene-HCTZ) (Maxzide) 75mg-50mg*, (Maxzide-25) 37.5mg-25mg* *scored

CONTRAINDICATIONS: Elevated serum K⁺ (≥5.5mEq/L), anuria, acute or chronic renal insufficiency or significant renal impairment, sulfonamide hypersensitivity, K⁺-sparing agents (eg, spironolactone, amiloride, or other formulations containing triamterene), K⁺ supplements, K⁺ salt substitutes, K⁺-enriched diets.

WARNINGS/PRECAUTIONS: Obtain ECG if hyperkalemia is suspected. Avoid in severely ill in whom respiratory or metabolic acidosis may occur; if used, frequent evaluations of acid/base balance and serum electrolytes are necessary. May cause idiosyncratic reaction, resulting in acute transient myopia and acute angle-closure glaucoma; d/c as rapidly as possible. Monitor for fluid/electrolyte imbalances. May manifest latent diabetes mellitus (DM). Caution with hepatic impairment or progressive liver disease; minor alterations in fluid and electrolyte balance may precipitate hepatic coma. May cause hypochloremia. Dilutional hyponatremia may occur in edematous patients in hot weather. Caution with history of renal lithiasis. May increase BUN and SrCr; d/c if azotemia increases. May contribute to megaloblastosis in folic acid deficiency. Hyperuricemia may occur or acute gout may be precipitated. May decrease serum PBI levels. Decreased calcium excretion reported. Changes in parathyroid glands with hypercalcemia and hypophosphatemia reported during prolonged use. Sensitivity reactions may occur. May exacerbate or activate systemic lupus erythematosus (SLE). May interfere with the fluorescent measurement of quinidine.

ADVERSE REACTIONS: Hyperkalemia, jaundice, pancreatitis, N/V, taste alteration, drowsiness, dry mouth, depression, anxiety, tachycardia, electrolyte/fluid imbalances.

INTERACTIONS: See Contraindications. Increased risk of hyperkalemia with ACE inhibitors. Hypokalemia may develop with corticosteroids, ACTH, or amphotericin B. Insulin requirements may be increased, decreased, or unchanged. May potentiate other antihypertensives (eg, β-blockers); dosage adjustments may be necessary. Avoid with lithium due to risk of lithium toxicity. Acute renal failure reported with indomethacin; caution with NSAIDs. May increase responsiveness to tubocurarine. May decrease arterial responsiveness to norepinephrine. Alcohol, barbiturates, or narcotics may aggravate orthostatic hypotension. May cause hypokalemia, which can sensitize or exag-

M

gerate the response of the heart to the toxic effects of digitalis (eg, increased ventricular irritability).

PREGNANCY: Category C, not for use in nursing.

MECHANISM OF ACTION: Triamterene: K⁺-sparing diuretic; exerts diuretic effect on distal renal tubule to inhibit the reabsorption of Na⁺ in exchange for K⁺ and H⁺. HCTZ: Thiazide diuretic; blocks renal tubular absorption of Na⁺ and Cl⁻ ions. This natriuresis and diuresis is accompanied by a secondary loss of K⁺ and bicarbonate.

PHARMACOKINETICS: Absorption: Well absorbed. HCTZ: T_{max}=2 hrs. Triamterene: Rapid, T_{max}=1 hr. **Distribution:** Crosses placenta; found in breast milk. **Metabolism:** Triamterene: Sulfate conjugation; hydroxytriamterene (metabolite). **Elimination:** HCTZ: Urine (unchanged).

NURSING CONSIDERATIONS

Assessment: Assess for conditions where treatment is contraindicated or cautioned, diabetes, risk for respiratory or metabolic acidosis, SLE, pregnancy/nursing status, and for possible drug interactions. Obtain baseline BUN, SrCr, and serum electrolytes.

Monitoring: Monitor for signs/symptoms of hyperkalemia, idiosyncratic reaction, hypokalemia, azotemia, renal stones, hepatic coma, and for fluid/electrolyte imbalances. Monitor serum K⁺ levels, BUN, SrCr, folic acid levels. Monitor serum and urine electrolytes if vomiting or receiving parenteral fluids.

Patient Counseling: Inform about risks/benefits of therapy. Advise to seek medical attention if symptoms of hyperkalemia (eg, paresthesias, muscular weakness, fatigue), hypokalemia, renal stones, electrolyte imbalance (eg, dry mouth, thirst, weakness), or hypersensitivity reactions occur. Notify physician if pregnant/nursing.

Administration: Oral route. **Storage:** 20-25°C (68-77°F). Protect from light.

MEDROL   RX
methylprednisolone (Pharmacia & Upjohn)

OTHER BRAND NAMES: Medrol Dosepak (Pharmacia & Upjohn)

THERAPEUTIC CLASS: Glucocorticoid

INDICATIONS: Steroid-responsive treatment for acute control of severe intractable allergic conditions, rheumatic, collagen, dermatologic, respiratory, acute regional enteritis and ulcerative colitis, allergic and edematous states, tuberculous meningitis with subarachnoid block when used with antituberculous chemotherapy, and trichinosis with neurologic/myocardial involvement. For the short-term adjunct treatment of synovitis, osteoarthritis (OA), rheumatoid arthritis (RA), bursitis, acute gouty arthritis, epicondylitis and acute nonspecific tenosynovitis.

DOSAGE: *Adults:* Initial: 4-48mg/day depending on disease and response. Maint: Decrease dose by small amounts to lowest effective dose. MS: Initial: 160mg/day for 1 week. Maint: 64mg every other day for 1 month. Alternate Day Therapy: Twice the usual dose qod for long-term therapy.

HOW SUPPLIED: Tab: 2mg, 4mg, 8mg, 16mg, 32mg; (Dosepak) 4mg [21ˢ]

CONTRAINDICATIONS: Systemic fungal infections.

WARNINGS/PRECAUTIONS: May need to increase dose before, during, and after stressful situations. May mask signs of infection or cause new infections. Prolonged use may produce glaucoma, optic nerve damage, secondary ocular infections. Increases BP, salt/water retention, potassium excretion. More severe/fatal course of infections reported with chickenpox, measles. Caution with strongyloides, latent TB, hypothyroidism, cirrhosis, ocular herpes simplex, HTN, diverticulitis, fresh intestinal anastomoses, ulcerative colitis, osteoporosis, myasthenia gravis, renal insufficiency, peptic ulcer disease. Kaposi's sarcoma reported. Growth and development of children on prolonged therapy should be monitored. Monitor for psychic disturbances. Avoid abrupt withdrawal.

ADVERSE REACTIONS: Fluid and electrolyte disturbances, HTN, osteoporosis, muscle weakness, cushingoid state, menstrual irregularities, nervousness, insomnia, impaired wound healing, DM, ulcerative esophagitis, excessive sweating, increased ICP, carbohydrate intolerance, glaucoma, cataracts, weight gain, nausea, malaise.

INTERACTIONS: Reduced efficacy with hepatic enzyme inducers (eg, phenobarbital, phenytoin, and rifampin). Increases clearance of chronic high-dose ASA. Caution with ASA in hypoprothrombinemia. Effects on oral anticoagulants are variable; monitor PT. Increased insulin and oral hypoglycemic requirements in DM. Avoid live vaccines with immunosuppressive doses. Possible decreased vaccine response with killed or inactivated vaccines with immunosuppressive doses. Mutual inhibition of metabolism with cyclosporine; convulsions reported. Potentiated by ketoconazole and troleandomycin.

PREGNANCY: Safety in pregnancy and nursing not known.

MECHANISM OF ACTION: Anti-inflammatory glucocorticoid; causes profound and varied metabolic effects and modifies the body's immune responses to diverse stimuli.

PHARMACOKINETICS: Absorption: Readily absorbed from GI tract.

NURSING CONSIDERATIONS

Assessment: Assess for systemic fungal infections, current infections, active TB, vaccination history, ulcerative colitis, diverticulitis, peptic ulcer with impending perforation, renal/hepatic insufficiency, septic arthritis/unstable joint, HTN, osteoporosis, myasthenia gravis, thyroid status, psychotic tendencies, and possible drug interactions.

Monitoring: Monitor for adrenocortical insufficiency, occurrence of infection, psychic derangement, cataracts, acute myopathy, Kaposi's sarcoma, fluid retention, measurement of serum electrolytes, TSH, LFTs, IOP, and BP. Monitor urinalysis, blood sugar, weight, chest x-ray, and upper GI x-ray (if ulcer history) regularly during prolonged therapy.

Patient Counseling: Inform that susceptibility to infections may increase. Avoid exposure to chickenpox or measles; report immediately if exposed. Dietary salt restriction and supplementation of K^+ is advised.

Administration: Oral route. **Storage:** 20-25°C (68-77°F).

MEFLOQUINE HCL   RX
mefloquine HCl (Various)

THERAPEUTIC CLASS: Quinolinemethanol derivative

INDICATIONS: Treatment and prophylaxis of mild to moderate acute malaria caused by *P.falciparum* or *P.vivax.*

DOSAGE: *Adults:* Treatment: 1250mg single dose. Take with at least 8 oz. (240 mL) of water. Prophylaxis: 250mg weekly. Start 1 week before arrival in endemic malarial area and continue weekly (always on the same day each week). Continue for 4 weeks after leaving the area.
Pediatrics: ≥20kg: Treatment: Usual: 20-25mg/kg, split in 2 doses. Take 6-8 hrs apart. If vomiting occurs <30 min after dose, give a 2nd full dose. If vomiting occurs 30-60 min after dose, give additional half-dose. If vomiting continues, start alternative treatment. Prophylaxis: 5mg/kg weekly. >45kg: 1 tab weekly. 30-45kg: 3/4 tab weekly. 20-30kg: 1/2 tab weekly.

HOW SUPPLIED: Tab: 250mg* *scored

CONTRAINDICATIONS: Use as prophylaxis in patients with active or recent history of depression, generalized anxiety disorder, psychosis, schizophrenia, or other major psychiatric disorders, or with a history of convulsions.

WARNINGS/PRECAUTIONS: In life-threatening malaria infection due to *P.falciparum*, use IV antimalarials. High risk of relapse seen with acute *P.vivax*; after initial treatment, subsequently treat with 8-aminoquinoline (eg, primaquine). May cause psychiatric symptoms. During prophylaxis, d/c if symptoms of acute anxiety, depression, restlessness, or confusion occur. In long-term therapy, monitor LFTs and perform ophthalmic exams. May impair mental/physical abilities. Increased risk of convulsions in epileptic patients. Caution with cardiac disease, psychiatric disturbances, hepatic dysfunction, and the elderly. Should not be administered with halofantrine or ketoconazole within 15 weeks of the last dose of mefloquine due to fatal QTc interval prolongation risk.

ADVERSE REACTIONS: N/V, myalgia, fever, dizziness, headache, syncope, sleep disorders, chills, diarrhea, abdominal pain, fatigue, tinnitus, pruritus, skin rash, vertigo.

INTERACTIONS: Avoid halofantrine and ketoconazole; may prolong QTc interval. Concomitant administration with other related compounds (eg, quinine, quinidine, chloroquine) may cause ECG abnormalities and increased risk of convulsions; delay mefloquine dose for 12 hrs after last dose of these drugs. Avoid propranolol; cardiopulmonary arrest reported. Drugs that may alter cardiac conduction (eg, anti-arrhythmic or β-blockers, CCBs, antihistamines, H_1-blockers, TCAs, and phenothiazines) may prolong QT_c interval. May lower plasma levels of anticonvulsants (eg, valproic acid, carbamazepine, phenobarbital, phenytoin); monitor blood levels and adjust dosage accordingly. Complete vaccinations with live, attenuated vaccines (eg, typhoid vaccine) at least 3 days before mefloquine therapy. Caution with anticoagulants, antidiabetic agents, rifampin. May increase/decrease mefloquine plasma concentration with CYP450 inhibitors or inducers.

PREGNANCY: Category C, not for use in nursing.

MECHANISM OF ACTION: Quinolinemethanol derivative; suspected to act as blood schizonticide. Exact mechanism of action is not established.

PHARMACOKINETICS: Absorption: C_{max}=1000-2000mcg/L; T_{max}=6-24 hrs. **Distribution:** V_d=20L/kg; plasma protein binding (98%); crosses placenta; found in breast milk. **Metabolism:** Extensive. Liver via CYP3A4. **Elimination:** Bile/feces, urine (9% unchanged, 4% metabolite); $T_{1/2}$=2-4 weeks.

NURSING CONSIDERATIONS

Assessment: Assess LFTs, ECG. Assess for history of depression, epilepsy, pregnancy status, and possible drug interactions. Note other diseases/conditions and drug therapies.

Monitoring: Monitor for psychiatric symptoms, convulsions, QTc interval prolongation, and for possible drug interactions. Monitor CBC, platelet count, LFTs, and ECG periodically. Monitor anticonvulsant blood level when taking antiseizure medications concomitantly. Periodic ophthalmic exams recommended.

Patient Counseling: Inform that malaria can be a life-threatening infection. Report any adverse reactions and seek medical attention for any febrile illness that occurs after return from a malarious area. Advise that no chemoprophylactic regimen is 100% effective; use of protective clothing, insect repellants, and bednets are important components of malaria prophylaxis. Advise females to use effective birth control during treatment. Caution with activities requiring alertness and fine motor coordination (eg, driving, piloting aircraft, operating machinery, and deep-sea diving). Advise that when used as prophylaxis, the first dose should be taken 1 week prior to arrival in an endemic area. Advise not to take on an empty stomach; administer with at least 8oz (240mL) of water.

Administration: Oral route. Tablets may be crushed and suspended in a small amount of water, milk or other beverages for those who are unable to swallow the tablet. **Storage:** 25°C (77°F); excursions permitted to 15-30°C (59-86°F).

MEGACE ES   RX
megestrol acetate (Par)

OTHER BRAND NAMES: Megace Suspension (Bristol-Myers Squibb)
THERAPEUTIC CLASS: Progesterone

INDICATIONS: Treatment of anorexia, cachexia, or unexplained significant weight loss in AIDS (acquired immunodeficiency syndrome) patients.

DOSAGE: *Adults:* Shake well before use. (Megace) Initial: 800mg/day (20mL/day). Usual: 400-800mg/day. Elderly: Start at lower end of dosing range. (Megace ES) Initial/Usual: 625mg/day (5mL/day).

HOW SUPPLIED: Sus: 40mg/mL [240mL], (ES) 125mg/mL [150mL]

CONTRAINDICATIONS: Pregnancy.

WARNINGS/PRECAUTIONS: Caution with history of thromboembolic disease. May cause fetal harm; avoid in pregnancy. New onset or exacerbation of diabetes mellitus (DM) or Cushing's syndrome reported. Adrenal insufficiency if taking or withdrawing from chronic therapy observed; laboratory evaluation for adrenal insufficiency and consideration of replacement or stress doses of a rapidly acting glucocorticoid are strongly recommended. Failure to recognize inhibition of the hypothalamic-pituitary adrenal (HPA) axis may result in death. Caution in elderly.

ADVERSE REACTIONS: Diarrhea, impotence, rash, flatulence, N/V, HTN, asthenia, insomnia, anemia, fever, decreased libido, dyspepsia, headache, hyperglycemia.

INTERACTIONS: Decreased exposure of indinavir; higher dose should be considered.

PREGNANCY: Category X, not for use in nursing.

MECHANISM OF ACTION: Progesterone; not established; has appetite-enhancing property.

PHARMACOKINETICS: Absorption:
(800mg/day) C_{max}=753ng/mL, AUC=10476ng•hr/mL, T_{max}=5 hrs. (750mg/day) C_{max}=490ng/mL, AUC=6779ng•hr/mL, T_{max}=3 hrs. **Elimination:** Urine (major, 66.4%), feces (19.8%); (ES) $T_{1/2}$=20-50 hrs.

NURSING CONSIDERATIONS

Assessment: Assess for pre-existing DM, Cushing's disease, history of thromboembolic disease, renal dysfunction, treatable causes of weight loss, hypersensitivity, pregnancy/nursing status, and possible drug interactions.

Monitoring: Monitor for adrenal insufficiency, hypoadrenalism (hypotension, N/V, dizziness, weakness), HPA axis inhibition, breakthrough bleeding, renal function, worsening or new DM, and hypersensitivity reactions. Monitor adrenocorticotropin (ACTH) stimulation test.

Patient Counseling: Inform about benefits and risks of therapy. Advise to use as directed by physician and to use contraception while on therapy if capable of becoming pregnant; notify physician if becomes pregnant. Seek medical attention if symptoms of adrenal insufficiency, hypoadrenalism (hypotension, N/V, dizziness, weakness) or if any adverse reactions occur.

Administration: Oral route. **Storage:** 15-25°C (59-77°F). Protect from heat.

MENVEO   RX
meningococcal (groups A,C, Y and W-135) oligosaccharide diphtheria crm 197 conugate (Novartis)

THERAPEUTIC CLASS: Vaccine

INDICATIONS: Active immunization to prevent invasive meningococcal disease caused by *Neisseria meningitidis* serogroups A, C, Y and W-135 for persons 2-55 yrs.

DOSAGE: *Adults:* ≤55 yrs: Single 0.5mL IM preferably into the deltoid muscle (upper arm).
Pediatrics: ≥2 yrs: Single 0.5mL IM preferably into the deltoid muscle (upper arm). 2-5 yrs (Continued High Risk): May administer 2nd dose 2 months after 1st dose.

HOW SUPPLIED: Inj: 0.5mL

WARNINGS/PRECAUTIONS: Appropriate medical treatment must be available should an allergic reaction occur. Syncope associated with seizure-like movements reported; observe for 15 min after administration. Expected immune response may not be obtained in immunocompromised persons. May increase risk of Guillain-Barre syndrome (GBS). Avoid with bleeding disorders unless potential benefit outweighs risk.

ADVERSE REACTIONS: Pain at injection site, local erythema, irritability, sleepiness, induration at injection site, headache, myalgia, malaise, N/V, rash, chills, arthralgia.

INTERACTIONS: Immunosuppressive therapies (eg, irradiation, antimetabolite medications, alkylating agents, cytotoxic drugs, and corticosteroids [when used in greater than physiologic doses]) may reduce immune response. Avoid with anticoagulants unless potential benefit outweighs risk. Lower geometric mean antibody concentrations (GMCs) for antibodies to the pertussis antigens filamentous hemagglutinin (FHA) and pertactin observed when coadministered with Boostrix and Gardasil as compared with Boostrix alone.

PREGNANCY: Category B, caution in nursing.

MECHANISM OF ACTION: Vaccine; leads to production of bactericidal antibodies directed against the capsular polysaccharides of meningococcal serogroups A, C, Y and W-135.

NURSING CONSIDERATIONS

Assessment: Assess for previous hypersensitivity to vaccine or other vaccines containing similar components, bleeding disorders, immune system status, *N. meningitidis* serogroup B infections, pregnancy/nursing status and possible drug interactions. Assess children 2-5 yrs for continued high risk of meningococcal disease.

Monitoring: Monitor for syncope, seizure-like activity, GBS, allergic reactions, and other adverse effects.

Patient Counseling: Inform of the potential benefits and risks of immunization. Advise about the potential adverse reactions temporally associated with the vaccine. Instruct to report any side effects to the healthcare provider. Inform about the Novartis pregnancy registry as appropriate (1-877-311-8972).

Administration: IM route. Not for IV, SQ, or intradermal use. Do not mix with any other vaccine or diluent in the same syringe or vial. Refer to PI for reconstitution instructions. **Storage:** 2-8°C (36-46°F); maintain at 36-46°F during transport. Do not freeze or use frozen/previously frozen product. Protect from light. Use reconstituted vaccine immediately, but may be held at ≤25°C (77°F) for ≤8 hrs.

MERREM   RX
meropenem (AstraZeneca)

THERAPEUTIC CLASS: Carbapenem

INDICATIONS: Treatment of complicated intra-abdominal infections, bacterial meningitis, and complicated skin and skin structure infections (cSSSI) caused by susceptible strains of microorganisms.

DOSAGE: *Adults:* IV: Intra-Abdominal Infections: CrCl ≥51mL/min: 1g q8h. CrCl 26-50mL/min: 1g q12h. CrCl 10-25mL/min: 500mg q12h. CrCl <10mL/min: 500mg q24h. cSSSI: CrCl ≥ 51mL/min: 500mg q8h. CrCl 26-50mL/min: 500mg q12h. CrCl 10-25mL/min: 250mg q12h. CrCl <10mL/min: 250mg q24h. Administer as infusion over 15-30 min; doses of 1g may also be administered as bolus injection (5-20mL) over 3-5 min.
Pediatrics: ≥3 months: IV: >50kg: Intra-Abdominal Infections: 1g q8h. Meningitis: 2g q8h. cSSSI: 500mg q8h. ≤50kg: Intra-Abdominal Infections: 20mg/kg q8h. Max: 1g q8h. Meningitis: 40mg/kg q8h. Max: 2g q8h. cSSSI: 10mg/kg q8h. Max: 500mg q8h. Administer as infusion over 15-30 min, or as bolus injection (5-20mL) over 3-5 min.

HOW SUPPLIED: Inj: 500mg, 1g

WARNINGS/PRECAUTIONS: Serious and fatal hypersensitivity reactions reported. Careful inquiry should be made concerning previous reactions to penicillins, cephalosporins, other β-lactams, and other allergens; d/c if allergic reaction occurs. *Clostridium difficile*-associated diarrhea (CDAD) reported; if CDAD is suspected, d/c therapy. Seizures and other CNS effects reported, particularly with history of seizures or CNS abnormality, concomitant medications with seizure potential, and compromised renal function. Thrombocytopenia reported with renal impairment. Prolonged use may result in superinfection; appropriate measures should be taken. Not for treatment of viral infections (eg, common cold).

ADVERSE REACTIONS: Diarrhea, N/V, rash, headache, constipation, anemia, pain.

INTERACTIONS: Probenecid inhibits renal excretion; avoid concomitant use. May reduce valproic acid or divalproex sodium levels, thereby increasing risk of breakthrough seizures; if concomitant administration is necessary, consider supplemental anticonvulsant therapy.

PREGNANCY: Category B, caution in nursing.

MECHANISM OF ACTION: Broad-spectrum carbapenem; penetrates bacterial cells and interferes with synthesis of vital cell wall components, resulting in cell death.

PHARMACOKINETICS: Absorption: 30-min infusion: C_{max}=23mcg/mL (500mg); 49mcg/mL (1g). 5-min bolus injection: C_{max}=45mcg/mL (500mg); 112mcg/mL (1g). **Distribution:** Plasma protein binding (2%). **Elimination:** Urine (70%, unchanged); $T_{1/2}$=1 hr (in patients ≥2 yrs), 1.5 hrs (in pediatrics [3 months-2 yrs]).

NURSING CONSIDERATIONS

Assessment: Assess for penicillin, cephalosporin, or other β-lactam hypersensitivity, history of seizure or brain lesions, bacterial meningitis, renal impairment, pregnancy/nursing status, and possible drug interactions. Assess organ system function (eg, renal, hepatic, and hematopoietic).

Monitoring: Monitor for signs/symptoms of anaphylactic/hypersensitivity reactions, CDAD, superinfections, and seizures. Monitor renal, hepatic, hematopoietic functions.

Patient Counseling: Inform that drug only treats bacterial, not viral, infections. Instruct to take as directed; skipping doses or not completing full course may decrease effectiveness and increase antibiotic resistance. Inform that diarrhea may occur; advise to contact physician if experience watery/bloody stools, hypersensitivity reactions, infection, or seizures. Counsel to inform physician if taking valproic acid or divalproex sodium.

Administration: IV route. Infusion over 15-30 min, or as bolus injection (5-20mL) over 3-5 min. Refer to PI for preparation of solution and stability parameters. **Storage:** 20-25°C (68-77°F).

METADATE CD   `CII`
methylphenidate HCl (UCB)

> Give cautiously to patients with a history of drug dependence or alcoholism. Chronic abusive use may lead to marked tolerance and psychological dependence with varying degrees of abnormal behavior. Careful supervision required during withdrawal from abusive use.

THERAPEUTIC CLASS: Sympathomimetic amine

INDICATIONS: Treatment of attention deficit hyperactivity disorder (ADHD).

DOSAGE: *Pediatrics:* ≥6 yrs: Individualize dosing based on patient needs and response. Initial: 20mg every am before breakfast. Titrate: May increase by increments of 10-20mg to a maximum of 60mg/day weekly based on tolerability/efficacy. Daily dosage above 60mg/day is not recommended. Reduce dose or d/c if paradoxical aggravation of symptoms occur. D/C if no improvement after appropriate dose adjustments over 1 month.

HOW SUPPLIED: Cap, Extended-Release: 10mg, 20mg, 30mg, 40mg, 50mg, 60mg

CONTRAINDICATIONS: Rare hereditary problems of fructose intolerance, glucose-galactose malabsorption or sucrase-isomaltase insufficiency, marked anxiety/tension/agitation, glaucoma, motor tics, family history or diagnosis of Tourette's syndrome, severe HTN, angina pectoris, cardiac arrhythmias, heart failure, recent myocardial infarction (MI), hyperthyroidism or thyrotoxicosis, during or within 14 days of MAOI use and on the day of surgery.

WARNINGS/PRECAUTIONS: Sudden death, stroke, and MI reported; avoid with known structural cardiac abnormalities, cardiomyopathy, serious heart abnormalities, coronary artery disease or other serious cardiac problems. May increase BP and HR; caution with pre-existing HTN, heart failure, MI, or ventricular arrhythmias. When symptoms suggestive of cardiac disease develop, prompt evaluation required. May exacerbate symptoms of behavior disturbance and thought disorder in patients with a pre-existing psychotic disorder. Caution with comorbid bipolar disorder; risk for induction of mixed/manic episode in such patients. May cause treatment-emergent psychotic or manic symptoms (eg, hallucinations, delusional thinking, mania) in children and adolescents without prior history of psychotic illness. Monitor for appearance and worsening of aggressive behavior or hostility during initial treatment. Monitor growth during therapy; interrupt if patient is not growing or gaining height or weight as expected. May lower seizure threshold, especially with prior history of seizures or with prior EEG abnormalities; d/c if seizures occur. Visual disturbances (eg, accommodation difficulties and blurring of vision) reported. Caution with emotionally unstable patients or prior history of drug dependence or alcoholism; chronic abusive use may lead to tolerance and psychological dependence; monitor during withdrawal since severe depression may occur. May react adversely with an element of agitation; d/c therapy if necessary. May produce positive results during drug testing. Not to be used in children <6 yrs.

ADVERSE REACTIONS: Headache, abdominal pain, anorexia, insomnia, nervousness, cardiac arrest, stroke, myocardial infarction (MI), aggressive behavior, toxic psychosis, neuroleptic malignant syndrome (NMS).

INTERACTIONS: See Contraindications. May inhibit metabolism of coumarin anticoagulants, anticonvulsants (eg, phenobarbital, phenytoin, primidone), phenylbutazone, and some antidepressants (eg, tricyclics and selective serotonin reuptake inhibitors). Caution with centrally acting α-2 agonists (eg, clonidine) and pressor agents. Clearance might be affected by urinary pH; either increased with acidifying agents or decreased with alkalinizing agents. Risk of sudden blood pressure increase with halogenated anesthetics during surgery.

PREGNANCY: Category C, caution in nursing.

MECHANISM OF ACTION: CNS stimulant; not established, thought to block reuptake of norepinephrine and dopamine into presynaptic neuron and increase release of these monoamines into extraneuronal space.

PHARMACOKINETICS: Absorption: Readily absorbed. Administration of variable doses resulted in different parameters. **Metabolism:** Via de-esterification. Metabolite: α-phenyl-piperidine acetic acid (ritalinic acid). **Elimination:** $T_{1/2}$=6.8 hrs.

NURSING CONSIDERATIONS

Assessment: Assess for agitation, anxiety, tension, glaucoma, tics, family history of Tourette's syndrome, cardiovascular conditions (eg, severe HTN, angina pectoris, arrhythmias, HF, recent MI), structural cardiac abnormalities, hyperthyroidism or thyrotoxicosis, bipolar illness, seizure disorder or history of seizures, history of drug dependence or alcoholism. Assess if undergoing surgery and hereditary problems of fructose intolerance, glucose-galactose malabsorption, or sucrase-isomaltase insufficiency. Assess pregnancy/nursing status and possible drug interactions.

Monitoring: Monitor for cardiac abnormalities, exacerbations of behavior disturbances and thought disorders, bipolar illness, aggression, seizures, and visual disturbances. Monitor for larger changes in HR and BP. Periodic monitoring of CBC, differential and platelet count, LFTs. Height and weight follow-up in children.

Patient Counseling: Inform about the benefits and risks of therapy, appropriate use, and drug abuse/dependence. Instruct to take 1 dose in the morning before breakfast. Instruct that capsule may be swallowed whole or opened and sprinkled in 1 tbsp applesauce followed by water; never crush or chew. Keep out of reach of children. Instruct patient, their families, and caregivers to read the Medication Guide.

Administration: Oral route. Swallow whole with liquids or open and sprinkle on 1 tbsp applesauce followed by water. **Storage:** 25°C (77°F); excursions permitted to 15-30°C (59-86°F). Protect from moisture.

METADATE ER
methylphenidate HCl (UCB)

CII

> Give cautiously to patients with a history of drug dependence or alcoholism. Chronic abusive use may lead to marked tolerance and psychological dependence with varying degrees of abnormal behavior. Careful supervision required during withdrawal from abusive use.

THERAPEUTIC CLASS: Sympathomimetic amine

INDICATIONS: Treatment of attention deficit disorder (ADHD) and narcolepsy.

DOSAGE: *Adults:* (Immediate-Release Methylphenidate) 10-60mg/day given bid-tid 30-45 min ac. Take last dose before 6 pm if insomnia occurs. (Tab, Extended-Release) May use in place of immediate-release tabs when the 8-hr dose corresponds to the titrated 8-hr immediate-release dose. Swallow whole; do not chew or crush.
Pediatrics: ≥6 yrs: (Immediate-Release Methylphenidate) Initial: 5mg bid before breakfast and lunch. Titrate: Increase gradually by 5-10mg weekly. Max: 60mg/day. (Tab, Extended-Release) May use in place of immediate-release tabs when the 8-hr dose corresponds to the titrated 8-hr immediate-release dose. Swallow whole; do not chew or crush. Reduce dose or d/c if paradoxical aggravation of symptoms occur. D/C if no improvement after appropriate dose adjustment over 1 month.

HOW SUPPLIED: Tab, Extended-Release: 10mg, 20mg

CONTRAINDICATIONS: Marked anxiety, tension, and agitation; glaucoma; motor tics or family history or diagnosis of Tourette's syndrome; during or within 14 days of MAOI use.

WARNINGS/PRECAUTIONS: Caution with comorbid bipolar disorder. Monitor growth in children. Not for severe depression or fatigue. May exacerbate symptoms of behavior disturbance and thought disorder in psychotic children. Treatment emergent psychotic/manic symptoms in children and adolescents may occur. Aggressive behavior or hostility observed. May lower seizure threshold, especially in known EEG abnormalities. Caution with HTN, emotionally unstable patients. Monitor during withdrawal. Visual disturbances may occur (rare). Monitor CBC, differential, and platelets with prolonged use. Periodically d/c to assess condition.

ADVERSE REACTIONS: Nervousness, insomnia, hypersensitivity reactions, anorexia, nausea, dizziness, palpitations, headache, dyskinesia, drowsiness, BP and pulse changes, tachycardia, angina, arrhythmia, abdominal pain.

INTERACTIONS: See Contraindications. May decrease hypotensive effect of guanethidine. Caution with pressor agents. Potentiates anticoagulants, anticonvulsants (eg, phenobarbital, phenytoin, primidone), phenylbutazone, TCAs (eg, imipramine, clomipramine, desipramine).

PREGNANCY: Category C, caution in nursing.

MECHANISM OF ACTION: Not established, suspected to have sympathomimetic activity in the brain stem arousal system and cortex.

PHARMACOKINETICS: Absorption: Slowly absorbed. T_{max}=1.3-8.2 hrs (sustained-release tab), 0.3-4.4 hrs (immediate release tab).

NURSING CONSIDERATIONS

Assessment: Assess for agitation, hereditary problems of galactose intolerance, Lapp lactase deficiency or glucose-galactose malabsorption, glaucoma, tics, family history of Tourette's syndrome, cardiovascular conditions (severe HTN, angina pectoris, cardiac arrhythmias, heart failure, recent MI), hyperthyroidism or thyrotoxicosis, bipolar illness, history of drug dependence or alcoholism.

Monitoring: Monitor for cardiac abnormalities, exacerbations of behavior disturbances and thought disorder, bipolar illness, aggression, seizures, and visual disturbances. Periodic monitoring of CBC, differential and platelet count, LFTs. Height and weight follow-up in children.

Patient Counseling: Inform about potential risks of therapy, appropriate use, drug dependence/abuse. Must swallow, never crush or chew. Take last dose before 6 pm to avoid insomnia.

Administration: Administer PO, preferably 30-45 min before meals. **Storage:** 20-25°C (77°F); excursions permitted to 15-30°C (59-86°F). Keep tightly closed. Protect from moisture.

METAGLIP RX
metformin HCl - glipizide (Bristol-Myers Squibb)

THERAPEUTIC CLASS: Sulfonylurea/biguanide

INDICATIONS: Adjunct to diet and exercise to improve glycemic control in adults with type 2 diabetes mellitus.

DOSAGE: *Adults:* Individualize dose. Inadequate glycemic control on diet/exercise alone: Initial: 2.5mg-250mg with a meal qd. If fasting plasma glucose (FPG) 280-320mg/dL, give 2.5mg-500mg bid. Titrate: Increase by 1 tab/day q2 weeks. Max: 10mg-1000mg/day or 10mg-2000mg/day in divided doses. Inadequate glycemic control on sulfonylurea or metformin: Initial: 2.5mg-500mg or 5mg-500mg bid (with morning and evening meals). Starting dose should not exceed daily dose of metformin or glipizide already being taken. Titrate: Increase by no more than 5mg-500mg/day. Max: 20mg-2000mg/day.

HOW SUPPLIED: Tab: (Glipizide-Metformin) 2.5mg-250mg, 2.5mg-500mg, 5mg-500mg

CONTRAINDICATIONS: Renal disease/dysfunction (SrCr ≥1.5mg/dL [males], ≥1.4mg/dL [females], abnormal CrCl), metabolic acidosis including diabetic ketoacidosis. D/C temporarily (48 hrs) for radiologic studies involving intravascular iodinated contrast materials.

WARNINGS/PRECAUTIONS: Lactic acidosis reported (rare); increased risk with increased age, DM with renal insufficiency, congestive heart failure (CHF), and other conditions with risk of hypoperfusion and hypoxemia. Avoid use in patients ≥80 yrs unless renal function is normal. Increased risk of cardiovascular mortality. Increased risk of hypoglycemia in elderly, debilitated, malnourished, adrenal or pituitary insufficiency, or alcohol intoxication. D/C in hypoxic states (eg, CHF, shock, acute MI) and prior to surgical procedures (due to restricted food intake). Avoid in renal/hepatic impairment. May decrease serum vitamin B_{12} levels. Impaired renal and/or hepatic function may slow excretion. Withhold with any condition associated with hypoxemia, dehydration, or sepsis. Monitor renal function. Caution in patients with glucose-6-phosphate dehydrogenase (G6PD) deficiency; may lead to hemolytic anemia. Hemolytic anemia reported in patients without G6PD deficiency.

ADVERSE REACTIONS: Upper respiratory tract infection, HTN, headache, diarrhea, dizziness, musculoskeletal pain, N/V, abdominal pain, hypoglycemia.

INTERACTIONS: Furosemide, nifedipine, cimetidine, and cationic drugs (eg, digoxin, procainamide, quinidine, quinine, ranitidine, trimethoprim, vancomycin, triamterene, morphine) may increase metformin levels. Temporarily d/c metformin before and for 48 hrs after intravascular contrast studies with iodinated materials. Hypoglycemia is potentiated by alcohol, NSAIDs, some azoles, and other highly protein-bound drugs, salicylates, sulfonamides, chloramphenicol, probenecid, coumarins, MAOIs, and β-blockers. Severe hypoglycemia reported with concomitant oral miconazole. Thiazides and other diuretics, corticosteroids, phenothiazines, thyroid products, estrogens, oral contraceptives, phenytoin, nicotinic acid, sympathomimetics, CCBs, and isoniazid may cause hyperglycemia. Alcohol potentiates the effect of metformin on lactate metabolism. May decrease furosemide levels.

PREGNANCY: Category C, not for use in nursing.

MECHANISM OF ACTION: Glipizide: Sulfonylurea; stimulates release of insulin from the pancreas. Metformin: Biguanide; decreases hepatic glucose production and intestinal absorption of glucose and improves insulin sensitivity by increasing peripheral glucose uptake and utilization.

PHARMACOKINETICS: Absorption: Glipizide: Rapid, complete; T_{max}=1-3 hrs. Metformin: Absolute bioavailability (50-60%). **Distribution:** Glipizide: Plasma protein binding (98-99%); V_d=11L (IV). Metformin: V_d=654L (PO). **Metabolism:** Glipizide: Liver (extensive). **Elimination:** Glipizide: Urine; $T_{1/2}$=2-4 hrs. Metformin: Urine (90% [PO], unchanged [IV]); $T_{1/2}$=6.2 hrs (plasma), 17.6 hrs (blood).

NURSING CONSIDERATIONS

Assessment: Assess FPG, HbA1c, renal function (eg, SrCr), LFTs, hematologic parameters (eg, Hgb/Hct, CBC). Assess for CHF, septicemia, acute or chronic metabolic acidosis, adrenal or pituitary insufficiency, alcoholism, other medical conditions, hypersensitivity, pregnancy/nursing status, and possible drug interactions.

Monitoring: Monitor for hypoglycemia, lactic acidosis, prerenal azotemia, CHF, cardiovascular disease, and hypersensitivity reactions. Monitor FPG, HbA1c, renal function (eg, SrCr), LFTs, hematologic parameters (eg, Hgb/Hct, CBC).

Patient Counseling: Inform about potential risks and benefits of drug and alternative modes of therapy. Inform that drug is adjunct to diet and exercise to control diabetes. Inform about importance of adherence to dietary instructions, regular excercise programs, and regular testing of blood glucose, glycosylated Hgb, renal function, and hematologic parameters. Report unexplained hyperventilation, myalgia, malaise, N/V, and somnolence. Explain risk of lactic acidosis, its signs/symptoms, and conditions that predispose to its development. Explain risk of hypoglycemia. Counsel against excessive alcohol intake.

Administration: Oral route. **Storage:** 20-25°C (68-77°F); excursions permitted to 15-30°C (59-86°F).

METHADOSE `CII`
methadone HCl (Mallinckrodt)

> Deaths due to cardiac and respiratory effects reported during initiation and conversion from other opioid agonists. Respiratory depression and QT prolongation observed. Only certified/approved opioid treatment programs can dispense oral methadone for treatment of narcotic addiction. Use as analgesic should be initiated only if benefits outweigh risks. (Powder): For oral administration only and must be used in the preparation of a liquid by dissolving powder in an appropriate vehicle. Preparation must not be injected.

THERAPEUTIC CLASS: Opioid analgesic

INDICATIONS: Detoxification and maintenance treatment of opioid addiction (heroin or other morphine-like drugs) in conjunction with appropriate social and medical services. Tab: Treatment of moderate to severe pain not responsive to non-narcotic analgesics.

DOSAGE: Adults: Detoxification: Initial/Induction: 20-30mg/day. Titrate: Give 5-10mg 2-4 hrs later if needed. Max: 40mg on first day. Adjust dose to control withdrawal symptoms over first week. Short-Term Detoxification: Titrate to 40mg/day given in divided doses to achieve adequate stabilizing level. Stabilization can continue for 2-3 days, then decrease dose every 1-2 days depending on symptoms. Maint: Titrate to a dose at which symptoms prevented for 24 hrs. Usual: 80-120mg/day. Medically Supervised Withdrawal After a Period of Maintenance Treatment: Dose reductions should be <10% of established tolerance or maintenance dose, and 10- to 14-day intervals should elapse between dose reductions. Pregnancy: May increase dose or decrease dosing interval. (Tab) Pain in Opioid Non-Tolerant: Initial: 2.5-10mg q8-12h, slowly titrated to effect. Conversion From Parenteral: Use a 1:2 dose ratio parenteral to oral. Switching From Other Chronic Opioids: Use caution; see PI for dosing details.

HOW SUPPLIED: Oral Concentrate: 10mg/mL; Powder: 50g, 100g, 500g, 1kg; Tab: 5mg*, 10mg*; Tab, Dispersible: 40mg *scored

CONTRAINDICATIONS: In any situation where opioids are contraindicated such as respiratory depression (in the absence of resuscitative equipment or in unmonitored settings), acute bronchial asthma or hypercarbia, and paralytic ileus.

WARNINGS/PRECAUTIONS: Can cause respiratory depression and elevate CSF pressure; caution with decreased respiratory reserve, hypoxia, hypercapnia, head injuries, other intracranial lesions or a pre-existing increase in intracranial pressure. Cases of QT interval prolongation and serious arrhythmia observed; caution in patients with risk of prolonged QT interval and evaluate for risk factors. Caution in elderly. Caution in patients with severe hepatic/renal impairment, hypothyroidism, Addison's disease, prostatic hypertrophy, or urethral stricture. Risk of tolerance, dependence, and abuse. May obscure the diagnosis or clinical course of acute abdominal conditions. May impair mental/physical abilities. Patients tolerant to other opioids may be incompletely tolerant to methadone. Infants born to opioid-dependent mothers may exhibit respiratory difficulties and withdrawal symptoms. May produce hypotension.

ADVERSE REACTIONS: Lightheadedness, dizziness, sedation, sweating, N/V.

INTERACTIONS: Inhibitors and inducers of CYP3A4, CYP2B6, CYP2C19, CYP2C9 and CYP2D6 may alter metabolism and effects. Opioid antagonists, mixed agonist/antagonists, and partial agonists may precipitate withdrawal symptoms. Concomitant use with other opioid analgesics, general anesthetics, phenothiazines, tranquilizers, sedative-hypnotics, or other CNS depressants may cause respiratory depression, hypotension, profound sedation, or coma. Deaths reported when abused in conjunction with benzodiazepines. Caution with drugs that may prolong QT interval. MAOIs may cause severe reactions. May increase levels of desipramine. Abacavir, amprenavir, efavirenz, nelfinavir, nevirapine, ritonavir, lopinavir + ritonavir (combination) may increase clearance or decrease levels. May decrease levels of didanosine and stavudine. May increase AUC of zidovudine.

PREGNANCY: Category C, not for use in nursing.

MECHANISM OF ACTION: Synthetic opioid analgesic; μ-agonist. Produces actions similar to morphine; acts on CNS and organs composed of smooth muscle. May also act as an N-methyl-D-aspartate (NMDA) receptor antagonist.

PHARMACOKINETICS: Absorption: Bioavailability (36-100%); C_{max}=124-1255ng/mL; T_{max}=1-7.5 hrs. **Distribution:** V_d=1-8L/kg; plasma protein binding (85-90%); found in breast milk and umbilical cord plasma. **Metabolism:** Hepatic N-demethylation; CYP3A4, 2B6, 2C19 (major); 2C9, 2D6 (minor). **Elimination:** Urine, feces; $T_{1/2}$=7-59 hrs; (Tab) $T_{1/2}$=8-59 hrs.

NURSING CONSIDERATIONS

Assessment: Assess for respiratory status, history of acute bronchial asthma or COPD, CNS depression, cardiac conduction abnormalities, increased ICP, acute abdominal conditions, volume depletion, hepatic/renal impairment, or any other conditions where treatment is contraindicated or cautioned. Assess hypersensitivity to drug, pregnancy/nursing status, and possible drug interactions.

Monitoring: Monitor for signs/symptoms of respiratory depression, QT prolongation and arrhythmias, misuse or abuse of medication, physical dependence and tolerance, withdrawal symptoms, elevations in CSF pressure, orthostatic hypotension, and hypersensitivity reactions.

Patient Counseling: Inform that medication may impair mental/physical abilities; use caution when performing hazardous tasks (eg, operating machinery/driving). Advise to avoid using alcohol and other CNS depressants. Instruct to seek immediate medical care if signs/symptoms of arrhythmia (eg, palpitations, dizziness, syncope) or difficulty in breathing develops. Orthostatic hypotension may occur. Instruct to keep out of reach of children. Advise to avoid abrupt withdrawal; taper dosing with medical supervision. Inform patients treated for opioid dependence that d/c may lead to relapse of illicit drug use. Educate about potential for abuse and to protect from theft. Reassure that dose of methadone will "hold" for longer periods of time as treatment progresses after initiation.

Administration: Oral route. **Storage:** 20-25°C (68-77°F).

METHOTREXATE   RX
methotrexate (Various)

> Should only be used by physicians with knowledge and experience in the use of antimetabolite therapy. Only for life-threatening neoplastic diseases, or psoriasis or rheumatoid arthritis patients with severe, recalcitrant, disabling disease not adequately responsive to other forms of therapy. Fetal death/congenital anomalies reported. Elimination reduced with impaired renal function, ascites, or pleural effusions; monitor carefully. Severe, sometimes fatal, bone marrow suppression and GI toxicity reported with concomitant NSAIDs. May cause hepatotoxicity, fibrosis, and cirrhosis (usually after prolonged use). Lung disease, malignant lymphomas, and potentially fatal opportunistic infections may occur. Interrupt therapy if diarrhea or ulcerative stomatitis occur. May induce tumor lysis syndrome. Severe, occasionally fatal, skin reactions reported. Concomitant radiotherapy may increase risk of soft tissue necrosis and osteonecrosis.

THERAPEUTIC CLASS: Dihydrofolic acid reductase inhibitor

INDICATIONS: (Inj/PO) Treatment of neoplastic diseases such as acute lymphocytic leukemia (prophylaxis of meningeal leukemia or maintenance therapy), gestational choriocarcinoma, chorioadenoma destruens, hydatidiform mole, breast cancer, epidermoid cancer of the head and neck, advanced mycosis fungoides, lung cancer, advanced stage non-Hodgkin's lymphomas. Prolonging relapse-free survival in non-metastatic osteosarcoma followed by leucovorin. Symptomatic control of severe, recalcitrant, disabling psoriasis. (PO) Management of severe, active rheumatoid arthritis (RA) or polyarticular-course juvenile rheumatoid arthritis (JRA) unresponsive to other therapies.

DOSAGE: *Adults:* Choriocarcinoma/Trophoblastic Disease: 15-30mg qd PO/IM for 5 days. May repeat 3-5 times as required with rest period of ≥1 week. Leukemia: Induction: 3.3mg/m² with prednisone 60mg/m² qd. Remission Maintenance: 15mg/m² PO/IM twice weekly or 2.5mg/kg IV every 14 days. Burkitt's Tumor: Stages I-II: 10-25mg/day PO for 4-8 days. Administer several courses with rest periods of 7-10 days in between. Lymphosarcoma: Stage III: 0.625-2.5mg/kg qd with other antitumor agents. Mycosis Fungoides: 5-50mg once weekly. If poor response, give 15-37.5mg twice weekly. Adjust dose based on response and hematologic monitoring. Osteosarcoma: Initial: 12g/m² IV, increase to 15g/m² if peak serum levels of 1000 micromolar not reached at end of infusion. Meningeal Leukemia: 12mg/m² intrathecally at 2-5 day intervals. Max: 15mg. Psoriasis: Initial: 10-25mg PO/IM/IV weekly until adequate response or use divided oral dose schedule, 2.5mg at 12 hr intervals for 3 doses. Titrate: Increase gradually until optimal response. Maint: Reduce to lowest effective dose. Max: 30mg/week. RA: Initial: 7.5mg PO once weekly, or 2.5mg q12h for 3 doses given as a course once weekly. Titrate: Gradual increase. Max: 20mg/wk. After response, reduce dose to lowest effective amount of drug. See PI for proper leucovorin rescue therapy.
Pediatrics: Meningeal Leukemia: <1 yr: 6mg. 1 yr: 8mg. 2 yrs: 10mg. ≥3yrs: 12mg. If dosing based on weight: 12mg/m². Max: 15mg. Give intrathecally at 2-5 day intervals. JRA: 2-16 yrs: Initial: 10mg/m² once weekly. Adjust dose gradually to achieve optimal response.

HOW SUPPLIED: Inj: 25mg/mL; Tab: 2.5mg* *scored

CONTRAINDICATIONS: Pregnant women with psoriasis or RA (should be used in treatment of pregnant women with neoplastic diseases only when potential benefit outweighs risk), nursing mothers. Psoriasis or RA patients with alcoholism, alcoholic liver disease, chronic liver disease, immunodeficiency syndromes, and pre-existing blood dyscrasias (eg, bone marrow hypoplasia, leukopenia, thrombocytopenia, significant anemia).

WARNINGS/PRECAUTIONS: Monitor closely; toxicity may be related to dose and frequency of administration. When reactions do occur, doses should be reduced or discontinued and corrective measures should be taken. Avoid pregnancy if either partner is receiving therapy. Avoid intrathecal administration or high-dose therapy with formulations or diluents containing preservatives. Caution in elderly.

ADVERSE REACTIONS: Ulcerative stomatitis, leukopenia, nausea, abdominal distress, malaise, fatigue, chills, fever, dizziness, decreased resistance to infection, anemia, thrombocytopenia, rash, pruritus, hepatotoxicity.

INTERACTIONS: See Boxed Warnings. Avoid NSAIDs with high doses. Caution with nephrotoxic agents (eg, cisplatin), NSAIDs, probenecid, and highly protein bound drugs (eg, sulfonamides, phenytoin, phenylbutazone, salicylates). May increase levels of mercaptopurine. Oral antibiotics (eg, tetracycline, chloramphenicol) may decrease absorption or interfere with enterohepatic circulation. Penicillins may decrease clearance. Closely monitor with hepatotoxins (eg, azathioprine, retinoids, sulfasalazine). Folic acid may decrease response to MTX. TMP/SMZ may increase bone marrow suppression. May decrease theophylline clearance.

PREGNANCY: Category X, not for use in nursing.

MECHANISM OF ACTION: Dihydrofolic acid reductase inhibitor; interferes with DNA synthesis, repair, and cellular replication. Mechanism in RA not established; may affect immune function.

PHARMACOKINETICS: Absorption: (PO, Healthy) T_{max}=1-2 hrs. (IM) T_{max}=30-60 min. Oral administration resulted in different parameters according to disease state and dosing; refer to PI for further information. **Distribution:** (IV, Initial) V_d=0.18L/kg; (Steady state) V_d=0.4-0.8L/kg; plasma protein binding (50%); found in breast milk. **Metabolism:** Hepatic and intracellular; 7-hydroxymethotrexate (metabolite). **Elimination:** Renal (primary route), bile (≤10%). (Psoriasis, RA, low-dose chemotherapy at <30mg/m² $T_{1/2}$=3-10 hrs; (High dose) $T_{1/2}$=8-15 hrs.

NURSING CONSIDERATIONS

Assessment: Assess pregnancy/nursing status, alcoholism, chronic liver disease, immunodeficiency, active infection, blood dyscrasias (eg, bone marrow hypoplasia, leukopenia, thrombocytopenia), impaired renal function, ascites, pleural effusions, debility, and possible drug interactions. Obtain baseline CBC with differential and platelet counts, hepatic enzymes, renal function tests, and chest x-ray.

Monitoring: Monitor for signs/symptoms of bone marrow suppression, hematological effects, GI toxicity (eg, vomiting, diarrhea, stomatitis), hepatotoxicity, fibrosis, cirrhosis, lung disease (eg, dry, nonproductive cough), malignant lymphomas, opportunistic infections, neurotoxicity (eg, seizures, leukoencephalopathy), nephrotoxicity, and skin reactions (eg, toxic epidermal necrolysis, Stevens-Johnson syndrome). Monitor for tumor lysis syndrome in patients with rapidly growing tumors. If given concomitantly with radiotherapy, monitor for soft-tissue necrosis and osteonecrosis. For psoriasis treatment, monitor CBC with differential and platelet counts monthly; renal/liver function every 1-2 months. Perform more frequent monitoring of lab parameters during antineoplastic therapy. If drug-induced lung disease is suspected, perform pulmonary function tests. For psoriatic patients on long-term therapy, perform periodic liver biopsies.

Patient Counseling: Counsel about risks/benefits of therapy, effects on reproduction in both males and females. Advise about early signs/symptoms of toxicity; contact physician immediately if any are experienced. Periodic laboratory tests and close follow up are necessary during therapy.

Administration: Oral, IM, IV, intra-arterial, or intrathecal route. **Storage:** Tab/Inj: 20-25°C (68-77°F).

METHYLIN

CII

methylphenidate HCl (Mallinckrodt)

OTHER BRAND NAMES: Methylin ER (Mallinckrodt)

THERAPEUTIC CLASS: Sympathomimetic amine

INDICATIONS: Treatment of attention deficit disorder (ADHD) and narcolepsy.

DOSAGE: *Adults:* (Sol/Tab/Tab, Chewable) 10-60mg/day given bid-tid 30-45 min ac. Take last dose before 6 pm if insomnia occurs. (Tab, Extended-Release) May used in place of immediate-release tabs when 8-hr dose corresponds to titrated 8-hr immediate release dose. Swallow whole; do not chew or crush.
Pediatrics: ≥6 yrs: (Sol/Tab/Tab, Chewable) Initial: 5mg bid before breakfast and lunch. Titrate: Increase gradually by 5-10mg weekly. Max: 60mg/day. (Tab, Extended-Release) May be used in place of immediate-release tabs when 8-hr dose corresponds to titrated 8-hr immediate release dose. Swallow whole; do not chew or crush. Reduce dose or d/c if paradoxical aggravation of symptoms occur. D/C if no improvement after appropriate dose adjustment over 1 month.

HOW SUPPLIED: Sol: 5mg/5mL [500mL], 10mg/5mL [500mL]; Tab: 5mg, 10mg, 20mg; Tab, Chewable: 2.5mg, 5mg, 10mg; Tab, Extended-Release: 10mg, 20mg

CONTRAINDICATIONS: Marked anxiety, tension, and agitation; glaucoma; motor tics or family history or diagnosis of Tourette's syndrome; during or within 14 days of MAOI use. (Methylin ER) Severe hypertension, angina pectoris, cardiac arrhythmias, heart failure, recent myocardial infarction (MI), hyperthyroidism, thyrotoxicosis.

WARNINGS/PRECAUTIONS: Give cautiously to patients with a history of drug dependence or alcoholism. Chronic abusive use may lead to marked tolerance and psychological dependence with varying degrees of abnormal behavior. Careful supervision required during withdrawal from abusive use. Monitor growth in children. Not for severe depression or fatigue. May exacerbate symptoms of behavior disturbance or thought disorder in psychotic children. Caution when using stimulants to treat patients with comorbid bipolar disorder because of concern for possible induction of mixed/manic episode in such patients. Stimulants at usual doses can cause treatment emergent psychotic or manic symptoms (eg, hallucinations, delusional thinking, mania) in children and adolescents without prior history of psychotic illness. Aggressive behavior or hostility has been reported in clinical trials and the postmarketing experience of some medications indicated for the treatment of ADHD. May lower seizure threshold, especially in known EEG abnormalities. Monitor during withdrawal. Visual disturbances may occur (rare). Monitor CBC, differential, and platelets with prolonged use. Periodically d/c to assess condition. Sudden death reported in association with CNS stimulant treatment in children and adolescents with pre-existing cardiac abnormalities or problems while sudden death, MI, and stroke are reported in adults. Monitor heart rate and BP. Assess cardiac status before initiating therapy. Avoid with serious structural abnormalities, cardiomyopathy or other serious cardiac problems.

ADVERSE REACTIONS: Nervousness, insomnia, hypersensitivity reactions, anorexia, nausea, dizziness, palpitations, headache, dyskinesia, drowsiness, BP and pulse changes, tachycardia, angina, arrhythmia, abdominal pain.

INTERACTIONS: See Contraindications. May decrease hypotensive effect of guanethidine. Caution with pressor agents. Potentiates anticoagulants, anticonvulsants (eg, phenobarbital, diphenylhydantoin, primidone), phenylbutazone, TCAs (eg, imipramine, clomipramine, desipramine). Caution with $α_2$-agonists (eg, clonidine); serious adverse reactions reported with concurrent use. May decrease the effectiveness of antihypertensives.

PREGNANCY: Category C, caution in nursing.

MECHANISM OF ACTION: CNS stimulant; activates the brain-stem arousal system and cortex to produce its stimulant effect. Blocks the reuptake of

M

norepinephrine and dopamine into the presynaptic neuron and increases release of monoamines into extraneuronal space.

PHARMACOKINETICS: Absorption: (20mg, Sol) C_{max}=9ng/mL, T_{max}=1-2 hrs. **Metabolism:** Deesterification to α-phenyl-piperidine acetic acid. **Elimination:** Urine (90%), $T_{1/2}$=2.7 hrs (sol), 3 hrs (chewable), 2.8 hrs (extended-release).

NURSING CONSIDERATIONS

Assessment: Assess for agitation, history of depression, glaucoma, tics, family history of Tourette's syndrome, cardiovascular status and conditions (eg, severe HTN, angina pectoris, cardiac arrhythmias, heart failure, recent MI), hyperthyroidism or thyrotoxicosis, bipolar illness, history of drug dependence or alcoholism.

Monitoring: Monitor BP, cardiac abnormalities, exacerbations of behavior disturbances and thought disorders, bipolar illness, aggression, seizures, and visual disturbances. Periodic monitoring of CBC, differential and platelet count, and LFTs. Height and weight follow-up in children.

Patient Counseling: Inform about risks of treatment, its appropriate use, drug abuse/dependence. Inform to take last dose before 6pm to avoid insomnia. Advise not to take chewable tablets if having difficulty swallowing. Seek medical attention if chest pain, vomiting, or difficulty swallowing or breathing occur. Swallow ER tablets whole; never crush or chew. Advise to notify physician if new or worsening mental symptoms or problems occur.

Administration: Oral route. **Storage:** 20-25°C (68-77°F).

METOPROLOL/HCTZ　　　　　RX
metoprolol tartrate - hydrochlorothiazide (Various)

> Exacerbation of angina and myocardial infarction (MI) reported following abrupt d/c. When d/c therapy, avoid abrupt withdrawal even without overt angina pectoris. Caution patients against d/c without a physician's advice.

OTHER BRAND NAMES: Lopressor HCT (Novartis)

THERAPEUTIC CLASS: Selective beta₁-blocker/thiazide diuretic

INDICATIONS: Management of HTN.

DOSAGE: *Adults:* Individualize dose. (Metoprolol) Initial: 100mg/day in single or divided doses. May increase gradually until optimum BP control is achieved. Range: 100-450mg/day. (HCTZ) Usual: 12.5-50mg/day. Max: 50mg/day. May add another antihypertensive gradually, beginning with 50% of the usual recommended starting dose when necessary. Refer to PI for Dosage Schedule. Elderly: Start at lower end of dosing range.

HOW SUPPLIED: Tab: (Metoprolol-HCTZ) 50mg-25mg*, 100mg-25mg* (Generic) 100mg-50mg* *scored

CONTRAINDICATIONS: Sinus bradycardia, >1st-degree heart block, cardiogenic shock, overt cardiac failure, sick-sinus syndrome, severe peripheral arterial circulatory disorders, anuria, sulfonamide hypersensitivity.

WARNINGS/PRECAUTIONS: Not for initial therapy. May depress myocardial contractility, leading to cardiac failure. Do not give in bronchospastic diseases. Withdrawal before surgery is not recommended. May mask hypoglycemia and hypothyroidism symptoms. May manifest latent diabetes mellitus (DM). Paradoxical BP increase reported with pheochromocytoma; give in combination with and only after initiating α-blocker therapy. Caution with severe renal disease; consider d/c with progressive renal impairment. Caution with hepatic dysfunction. Sensitivity reactions are more likely to occur with history of allergy or bronchial asthma. May exacerbate or activate systemic lupus erythematosus (SLE). May cause idiosyncratic reaction, resulting in acute transient myopia and acute-angle glaucoma; d/c as rapidly as possible. Fluid or electrolyte imbalances reported. May cause hyperuricemia and precipitation of frank gout. Enhanced effects in post-sympathectomy patient. Pathological changes in the parathyroid gland with hypercalcemia and hypophosphatemia observed. Elevated levels of serum transaminase, alkaline phosphatase, and lactate dehydrogenase reported. Caution in elderly.

ADVERSE REACTIONS: Fatigue, lethargy, dizziness, vertigo, flu syndrome, drowsiness, somnolence, hypokalemia, headache, bradycardia, lethargy, vertigo.

INTERACTIONS: (Metoprolol) Potent CYP2D6 inhibitors (eg, antidepressants, antipsychotics, antiarrhythmics, antiretrovirals, antihistamines, antimalarials, antifungals, stomach ulcer drugs) may increase drug levels. Additive effects with catecholamine-depleting drugs (eg, reserpine). May block epinephrine effects. May increase risk of bradycardia with digitalis glycosides. Caution with diuretics. Increased risk for rebound hypotension following clonidine withdrawal; stop metoprolol several days before clonidine d/c. Inhalational anesthetics may enhance cardiodepressant effects. (Generic) Effects can be reversed by β-agonists (eg, dobutamine or isoproterenol). (HCTZ) Hypokalemia can sensitize or exaggerate heart's response to the toxic effects of digitalis. Risk of hypokalemia with steroids or ACTH. Risk of lithium toxicity. NSAIDs may reduce diuretic effects. Insulin may need adjustment. Impaired absorption with cholestyramine, colestipol. May increase response to tubocurarine. May decrease arterial responsiveness to norepinephrine. Alcohol, barbiturates, and narcotics may potentiate orthostatic hypotension. Rare reports of hemolytic anemia with methyldopa. May potentiate other antihypertensive drugs (eg, ganglionic or peripheral adrenergic blocking drugs).

PREGNANCY: Category C, not for use in nursing.

MECHANISM OF ACTION: Metoprolol: β-adrenergic receptor blocker; not established. Proposed to competitively antagonize catecholamines at peripheral adrenergic-neuron sites, have central effect leading to reduced sympathetic outflow to periphery and suppresses renin activity. HCTZ: Thiazide diuretic; not established. Affects renal tubular mechanism of electrolyte reabsorption and increases excretion of Na^+ and Cl^-.

PHARMACOKINETICS: Absorption: Metoprolol: Rapid and complete. HCTZ: Rapid; T_{max}=1-2.5 hrs. **Distribution:** Found in breast milk. Metoprolol: Plasma protein binding (12%). HCTZ: V_d=3.6-7.8L/kg; plasma protein binding (67.9%); crosses the placenta. **Metabolism:** Metoprolol: Extensive; CYP2D6 (oxidation). **Elimination:** Metoprolol: Urine (<5%, unchanged); $T_{1/2}$=2.8 hrs (extensive metabolizers), 7.5 hrs (poor metabolizers). HCTZ: Urine (72-97%); $T_{1/2}$=10-17 hrs.

NURSING CONSIDERATIONS

Assessment: Assess for history of heart failure, SLE, hyperthyroidism, DM, pheochromocytoma, hepatic/renal impairment, pregnancy/nursing status, possible drug interactions, or any other conditions where treatment is contraindicated. Obtain baseline serum electrolytes, and thyroid function tests. Assess for history of sulfonamide allergy.

Monitoring: Monitor for signs/symptoms of cardiac failure, hypoglycemia, thyrotoxicosis, electrolyte imbalance, exacerbation or activation of SLE, hyperglycemia, hyperuricemia or precipitation of gout, hypersensitivity reactions, hepatic/renal dysfunction, skin reactions, idiosyncratic reaction, myopia, and angle-closure glaucoma. Monitor vital signs, serum and urine electrolytes, and thyroid function tests.

Patient Counseling: Instruct to take regularly, as directed, with or immediately following meals. If dose is missed, take next dose at scheduled time (without doubling); do not d/c without consulting physician. Avoid driving, operating machinery, or engaging in tasks requiring alertness until response to therapy is determined. Contact physician if difficulty in breathing or other adverse reactions occur and inform physician/dentist of drug therapy before undergoing any type of surgery.

Administration: Oral route. **Storage:** (Lopressor HCT) 25°C (77°F); excursions permitted to 15-30°C (59-86°F). (Generic) 20-25°C (68-77°F). Protect from moisture.

METROGEL

RX

metronidazole (Galderma)

OTHER BRAND NAMES: MetroLotion (Galderma) - MetroCream (Galderma)

THERAPEUTIC CLASS: Imidazole antibiotic

INDICATIONS: Treatment of inflammatory lesions of rosacea.

DOSAGE: *Adults:* (Cre, Gel 0.75%, Lot) Wash affected area(s) then apply bid, am and pm. (Gel 1%) Wash affected area(s) then apply qd.

HOW SUPPLIED: Cre: 0.75% [45g]; Gel: 0.75% [45g], 1% [60g]; Lot: 0.75% [59mL]

WARNINGS/PRECAUTIONS: Peripheral neuropathy (eg, numbness, paresthesia) reported; re-evaluate therapy immediately should abnormal neurologic signs appear. Caution with CNS diseases, blood dyscrasias. Irritant and allergic contact dermatitis reported; consider d/c if dermatitis occurs. May cause tearing of the eye; avoid contact with eyes. Not for oral, ophthalmic, or intravaginal use.

ADVERSE REACTIONS: Burning/stinging, skin irritation, dryness, scaling, pruritus, nasopharyngitis, peripheral neuropathy, contact dermatitis.

INTERACTIONS: May potentiate anticoagulants; caution when using concomitantly with coumarin or warfarin.

PREGNANCY: Category B, not for use in nursing.

MECHANISM OF ACTION: Imidazole antibiotic; not established.

PHARMACOKINETICS: Absorption: (1g of 1% Gel) C_{max}=32ng/mL; T_{max}=6-10 hrs; AUC_{0-24}=595ng•hr/mL. (1g of 0.75% Lot) C_{max}=96ng/mL; AUC_{0-24}=962ng•hr/mL.

NURSING CONSIDERATIONS

Assessment: Assess pregnancy/nursing status, evidence/history of blood dyscrasias, CNS disease, and for possible drug interactions.

Monitoring: Monitor for abnormal neurologic signs particularly peripheral neuropathy (numbness/paresthesia of extremeties). Monitor for irritant/allergic contact dermatitis.

Patient Counseling: Instruct to use medication exactly as directed (for external use only, not for oral, opthalmic,vaginal use). Avoid contact with eyes, and cleanse affected area(s) before applying. Advise to report adverse reactions, and use less frequently or d/c if local skin irritation develops. May use cosmetics following application.

Administration: Topical use. **Storage:** 20-25°C (68-77°F); excursions permitted between 15-30°C (59-86°F).

METROGEL-VAGINAL

RX

metronidazole (Graceway)

THERAPEUTIC CLASS: Imidazole antibiotic

INDICATIONS: Treatment of bacterial vaginosis.

DOSAGE: *Adults:* Insert 1 applicatorful intravaginally qd-bid for 5 days. For once daily dosing, administer hs.

HOW SUPPLIED: Gel: 0.75% [70g]

CONTRAINDICATIONS: Hypersensitivity to other nitroimidazole derivatives.

WARNINGS/PRECAUTIONS: Caution with CNS or severe hepatic disease. D/C if abnormal neurologic signs appear. Avoid vaginal intercourse during therapy. May develop *Candida* vaginitis. May interfere with lab tests (ALT, SGPT, AST, SGOT, LDH, triglycerides, and glucose hexokinase).

ADVERSE REACTIONS: *Candida* cervicitis/vaginitis, vaginal discharge, pelvic discomfort, nausea, vomiting, headache, vulva/vaginal irritation, GI discomfort, change in WBC count.

INTERACTIONS: May potentiate warfarin, other anticoagulants, and lithium. Cimetidine may potentiate metronidazole. Avoid alcohol; possible disulfiram-like reaction may occur. Do not administer gel within 2 weeks of discontinuing disulfiram therapy.

PREGNANCY: Category B, not for use in nursing.

MECHANISM OF ACTION: Antibacterial/antiprotozoal agent; not established, suspected that 5-nitro group of metronidazole is reduced by metabolically active anaerobes and the reduced form of the drug interacts with bacterial DNA.

PHARMACOKINETICS: Absorption: C_{max}=237ng/mL; T_{max}=6-12 hrs. **Distribution:** Found in breast milk and crosses placental barrier.

NURSING CONSIDERATIONS

Assessment: Assess for hypersensitivity to drug, hepatic impairment, CNS diseases, vaginal candidiasis, alcohol intake, for possible drug/lab test interactions (eg, disulfiram).

Monitoring: Monitor for convulsive seizures and peripheral neuropathy, psychotic reactions, disulfiram-like reaction, *Candida* vaginitis, lab tests for AST, ALT, LDH, TG, glucose hexokinase, and WBCs.

Patient Counseling: Instruct not to engage in vaginal intercourse or drink alcohol during treatment. Avoid contact with eyes; rinse with cool tap water if occurs.

Administration: Intravaginal route. Insert applicator into vagina, push plunger to deposit gel, and then withdraw applicator. **Storage:** 15-30°C (59-86°F). Protect from freezing.

MEVACOR RX
lovastatin (Merck)

THERAPEUTIC CLASS: HMG-CoA reductase inhibitor

INDICATIONS: To reduce risk of myocardial infarction (MI), unstable angina, and coronary revascularization procedures in patients without symptomatic cardiovascular disease (CVD), average to moderately elevated total cholesterol (total-C) and LDL-C, and below average HDL-C. To slow progression of coronary atherosclerosis in patients with coronary heart disease to lower total-C and LDL-C. Adjunct to diet to lower total-C and LDL-C in primary hypercholesterolemia (Types IIa and IIb) when the response to diet restricted in saturated fat and cholesterol and to other nonpharmacological measures alone has been inadequate. Adjunct to diet to reduce total-C, LDL-C, apolipoprotein B (Apo B) levels in adolescents who are ≥1 yr postmenarche, 10-17 yrs of age, with heterozygous familial hypercholesterolemia (HeFH) if after an adequate trial of diet therapy the following findings are present: LDL remains >189mg/dL; or LDL remains >160 mg/dL and there is positive family history of premature CVD or ≥2 CVD risk factors are present.

DOSAGE: *Adults:* Individualize dose. Initial: 20mg qd with the evening meal. Usual: 10-80mg/day in single or 2 divided doses. Max: 80mg/day. Requiring LDL-C Reduction of ≥20%: Initial: 20mg/day. May consider 10mg ifsmaller reductions required. Titrate: Adjust at ≥4-week intervals. Reduce dose if cholesterol levels fall significantly below the targeted range. Concomitant Cyclosporine/Danazol: Initial: 10mg/day. Max: 20mg/day. Concomitant Gemfibrozil/Fibrates/Niacin (≥1g/day): Max: 20mg/day. Concomitant Amiodarone/Verapamil: Max: 40mg/day. Severe Renal Insufficiency (CrCl <30mL/min): Caution with increasing doses >20mg/day. *Pediatrics:* 10-17 yrs: Individualize dose. Heterozygous Familial Hypercholesterolemia: Usual: 10-40mg/day. Max: 40mg/day. Requiring LDL-C Reduction of ≥20%: Initial: 20mg/day. May consider 10mg if smaller reductions required. Titrate: Adjust at ≥4-week intervals. Reduce dose if cholesterol levels fall significantly below the targeted range. Concomitant Cyclosporine/ Danazol: Initial: 10mg/day. Max: 20mg/day. Concomitant Gemfibrozil/ Fibrates/Niacin (≥1g/day): Max: 20mg/day. Concomitant Amiodarone/

Verapamil: Max: 40mg/day. Severe Renal Insufficiency (CrCl <30mL/min): Caution with increasing doses >20mg/day.

HOW SUPPLIED: Tab: 20mg, 40mg

CONTRAINDICATIONS: Active liver disease/unexplained persistent elevations of serum transaminases, pregnancy and lactation.

WARNINGS/PRECAUTIONS: May cause myopathy/rhabdomyolysis (dose-related); d/c if myopathy is diagnosed or suspected. D/C a few days before elective major surgery and when any major medical or surgical condition supervenes. Symptomatic liver disease reported (rarely). Elevation of serum transaminases reported; perform LFTs prior to initiation of therapy in patients with a history of liver disease, or when otherwise clinically indicated; d/c if AST or ALT ≥3X ULN persists. Caution in patients who have history of hepatic disease. May elevate creatine phosphokinase levels. Less effective in homozygous familial hypercholesterolemia. At the time of hospitalization for acute coronary event, may initiate therapy at discharge if LDL-C ≥130mg/L. Children treated in adolescence should be re-evaluated in adulthood.

ADVERSE REACTIONS: Headache, constipation, flatulence, myalgia, creatine kinase (CK) elevations.

INTERACTIONS: Increased risk of myopathy/rhabdomyolysis with potent CYP3A4 inhibitors (eg, itraconazole, ketoconazole, erythromycin, clarithromycin, telithromycin, HIV protease inhibitors, nefazodone, >1 quart/day of grapefruit juice), verapamil, amiodarone, other fibrates, gemfibrozil, cyclosporine, danazol, and ≥1g/day of niacin. Monitor PT with coumarin anticoagulants. Caution with drugs that may decrease the levels or activity of endogenous steroid hormones (eg, ketoconazole, spironolactone, cimetidine). Caution with substantial quantities of alcohol.

PREGNANCY: Category X, not for use in nursing.

MECHANISM OF ACTION: HMG-CoA reductase inhibitor; specific inhibitor of HMG-CoA reductase, the enzyme that catalyzes the conversion of HMG-CoA to mevalonate. The conversion of HMG-CoA to mevalonate is an early step in the biosynthetic pathway for cholesterol. LDL-C-lowering effect involves both reduction of VLDL-C concentration, and induction of the LDL receptor, leading to reduced production and/or increased catabolism of LDL-C.

PHARMACOKINETICS: Absorption: T_{max}=2 hrs (lovastatin), 2-4 hrs (β-hydroxyacid, 6'hydroxy derivative). **Distribution:** Lovastatin and β-hydroxyacid: Plasma protein binding (>95%). **Metabolism:** Liver (extensive) via CYP3A4. β-hydroxyacid, 6'-hydroxy derivative (major active metabolites). **Elimination:** Urine (10%), feces (83%).

NURSING CONSIDERATIONS

Assessment: Assess for secondary causes of hypercholesterolemia, presence of active liver disease or unexplained elevations of serum transaminases, drug hypersensitivity, pregnancy/nursing status, and possible drug interactions. Assess lipid profile (total-C, HDL-C, and TG) and LFTs prior to therapy. Assess use in presence of homozygous familial hypercholesterolemia or renal insufficiency.

Monitoring: Monitor for signs/symptoms of myopathy (eg, muscle pain, tenderness, weakness), rhabdomyolysis, liver dysfunction, and endocrine dysfunction. Perform periodic monitoring of cholesterol levels, CK levels, and LFTs (eg, ALT, AST).

Patient Counseling: Inform about possible interactions with other drugs and grapefruit juice. Advise to report any signs/symptoms of unexplained muscle pain, tenderness, or weakness immediately. Inform that periodic blood testing is required to evaluate cholesterol levels and liver function. Counsel females about risks of use during pregnancy/nursing. Counsel adolescent females on appropriate contraceptive methods while on therapy.

Administration: Oral route. Take with meals. **Storage:** 20-25°C (68-77°F). Protect from light and store in a well-closed, light-resistant container.

MIACALCIN

RX

calcitonin-salmon (Novartis)

THERAPEUTIC CLASS: Hormonal bone resorption inhibitor

INDICATIONS: (Inj) Treatment of Paget's disease of bone and hypercalcemia. (Inj/Spray) Treatment of postmenopausal osteoporosis in females >5 yrs postmenopause.

DOSAGE: *Adults:* (Inj) Paget's Disease: Usual: 100 IU IM/SQ qd. Maint: 50 IU IM/SQ qd or qod. Maintain higher dose with serious deformity and neurological involvement. Hypercalcemia: Initial: 4 IU/kg IM/SQ q12h. Titrate: May increase to 8 IU/kg q12h after 1-2 days, then to 8 IU/kg q6h after 2 days if unsatisfactory response. Postmenopausal Osteoporosis: (Inj) 100 IU IM/SQ qod. If >2mL, use IM injection. (Spray) 200 IU qd intranasally. Alternate nostrils daily. Take with supplemental calcium (1.5g calcium carbonate qd) and vitamin D (400 IU qd) for postmenopausal osteoporosis.

HOW SUPPLIED: Inj: 200 IU/mL; Nasal Spray: 200 IU/inh

WARNINGS/PRECAUTIONS: Serious allergic-type reactions (eg, bronchospasm, swelling of tongue or throat, anaphylactic shock) reported. May lead to hypocalcemic tetany; provisions for parenteral calcium should be available on the first several administration of calcitonin. Monitor urine sediment periodically with chronic use. (Spray) D/C if severe ulceration (ulcers >1.5mm diameter, penetrating below mucosa or if with heavy bleeding) of the nasal mucosa occurs. Perform periodic nasal exams.

ADVERSE REACTIONS: (Inj) N/V, injection-site inflammation, flushing of face or hands, nocturia, ear lobe pruritus, poor appetite, abdominal pain. (Spray) Nasal symptoms, rhinitis, back pain, headache, arthralgia, epistaxis.

INTERACTIONS: Concomitant use with lithium may lead to reduced plasma lithium; lithium dose may need to be adjusted. Prior diphosphonate use with Paget's disease may reduce antiresorptive response.

PREGNANCY: Category C, not for use in nursing.

MECHANISM OF ACTION: Hormonal bone resorption inhibitor; actions on bone not fully established. Calcitonin receptors have been found in osteoclasts and osteoblasts. Initially causes a marked transient inhibition of the ongoing bone resorptive process. Prolonged use causes a smaller decrease in the rate of bone resorption. Thought to be associated with decrease in number of osteoclasts as well as decrease in resorptive activity.

PHARMACOKINETICS: Absorption: (Intranasal): Bioavailability (3-5%), T_{max}=13 min; (Inj): Absolute bioavailability (66% IM), (71% SQ), T_{max}=23 min (SQ). **Distribution:** V_d=0.15-0.3L/kg. **Metabolism:** Kidney, blood, peripheral tissues. **Elimination:** Urine; (Intranasal): $T_{1/2}$=18 mins; (Inj): $T_{1/2}$=58 mins (IM), $T_{1/2}$=59-64 mins (SQ).

NURSING CONSIDERATIONS

Assessment: Assess for hypersensitivity to medication; consider skin testing. Assess pregnancy/nursing status. If using intranasal formulation, obtain baseline nasal exam (eg, visualization of the nasal mucosa, turbinates, septum, and mucosal blood vessel status). If using parenteral formulation and treating osteoporosis, obtain baseline measurement of bone resorption/turnover and bone mineral density.

Monitoring: Monitor for signs/symptoms of allergic reaction (eg, bronchospasm, swelling of tongue or throat, anaphylactic shock). Perform periodic exams of urine sediment. If using intranasal formulation, monitor for nasal mucosal alterations, transient nasal conditions, and ulceration of nasal mucosa; perform periodic nasal exams. For intranasal formulation, perform periodic measurements of lumbar vertebral bone. If using parenteral formulation, monitor for hypocalcemic tetany. For parenteral administration in treatment of Paget's disease, perform periodic measurement of serum alkaline phosphatase and 24-hr urinary hydroxyproline. For parenteral administration in treatment of osteoporosis, monitor biochemical markers of bone resorption/turnover and bone mineral density.

M

Patient Counseling: Intranasal formulation: Instruct how to assemble and prime pump, and introduce medication in the nasal passages. Advise to contact physician if allergic reaction or nasal irritation occur. Inform that new, unassembled bottles should be refrigerated and protected from freezing. Allow medication to reach room temperature before priming pump and using a new bottle. Store opened bottle upright at room temperature for up to 35 days. Parenteral formulation: Advise to use sterile injection technique.

Administration: Intranasal/IM/SQ routes. **Storage:** (Intranasal) Unopened: 2-8°C (36-46°F). Protect from freezing. Used: 15-30°C (59-86°F) in upright position for up to 35 days. (Inj) 2-8°C (36-46°F).

MICARDIS   RX
telmisartan (Boehringer Ingelheim)

> May cause death/injury to the developing fetus when used in pregnancy. D/C immediately if pregnancy is detected.

THERAPEUTIC CLASS: Angiotensin II receptor antagonist

INDICATIONS: Treatment of HTN, alone or with other antihypertensives. Reduction of risk of myocardial infarction (MI), stroke, or death from cardiovascular causes in patients ≥55 yrs who are unable to take ACE inhibitors.

DOSAGE: *Adults:* HTN: Individualize dose. Initial: 40mg qd. Usual: 20-80mg/day. May add diuretic if additional BP reduction is desired. Cardiovascular Risk Reduction: 80mg qd. Monitor BP and adjust dose of medications that lower BP if needed.

HOW SUPPLIED: Tab: 20mg, 40mg, 80mg

WARNINGS/PRECAUTIONS: Correct volume or salt depletion before therapy due to risk of symptomatic hypotension. Changes in renal function (including acute renal failure) may occur. May precipitate azotemia in patients with renal disease. Caution with biliary obstructive disorders, hepatic insufficiency and unilateral or bilateral renal artery stenosis. Hyperkalemia may occur; consider periodic monitoring of serum electrolytes to detect possible imbalances.

ADVERSE REACTIONS: Upper respiratory tract infection, back pain, sinusitis, diarrhea, intermittent claudication, skin ulcer.

INTERACTIONS: Dual blockade of the renin-angiotensin-aldosterone system, oliguria, and progressive azotemia with ACE inhibitors. Hyperkalemia may occur with K+ supplements, K+-sparing diuretics, K+-containing salt substitutes or other drugs that increase K+ levels. May increase digoxin levels; monitor digoxin levels. May increase lithium levels/toxicity; monitor lithium levels during concomitant use. Possible additive effects with ramipril; concomitant use not recommended. Possible inhibition of the metabolism of drugs metabolized by CYP2C19.

PREGNANCY: Category C (1st trimester) and D (2nd and 3rd trimesters), not for use in nursing.

MECHANISM OF ACTION: Angiotensin II receptor antagonist; blocks vasoconstrictor and aldosterone-secreting effects of angiotensin II by selectively blocking the binding of angiotensin II to the AT_1 receptor in many tissues, such as vascular smooth muscle and adrenal gland.

PHARMACOKINETICS: Absorption: Absolute bioavailability=42% (40mg), 58% (160mg); T_{max}=0.5-1 hr. **Distribution:** V_d=500L; plasma protein binding (>99.5%). **Metabolism:** Conjugation. **Elimination**: Feces (>97%, unchanged), urine (0.91% [IV administration]; 0.49% [oral administration]); $T_{1/2}$=24 hrs.

NURSING CONSIDERATIONS

Assessment: Assess BP, hepatic/renal function, pregnancy/nursing status, and possible drug interactions.

Monitoring: Monitor BP, ECG, hepatic/renal function, and serum electrolytes. Monitor for signs and symptoms of electrolyte imbalance and adverse reactions (eg, upper respiratory tract infection, back pain, sinusitis, diarrhea).

Patient Counseling: Counsel about signs/symptoms of adverse effects, and advise to seek prompt medical attention if any occur. Inform about fetal risks if taken during pregnancy; instruct to report pregnancy immediately if detected.

Administration: Oral route. **Storage:** 25°C (77°F); excursions permitted to 15-30°C (59-86°F). Do not remove tablets from blisters until immediately before administration.

MICARDIS HCT

RX

telmisartan - hydrochlorothiazide (Boehringer Ingelheim)

> Can cause death/injury to the fetus during 2nd and 3rd trimesters. D/C immediately if pregnancy is detected.

THERAPEUTIC CLASS: Angiotensin II receptor antagonist/thiazide diuretic

INDICATIONS: Treatment of hypertension. Not for initial therapy.

DOSAGE: *Adults:* Uncontrolled BP on 80mg Telmisartan, or Uncontrolled BP on 25mg/day of HCTZ, or Controlled BP on 25mg/day of HCTZ but with Decreased Serum K$^+$: Initial: 80mg-12.5mg tab qd. Alternative (For Those with Uncontrolled BP on 25mg/day of HCTZ): Initial: 80mg-25mg tab qd. Titrate/Max: Increase to 160mg-25mg if BP uncontrolled after 2-4 weeks. Biliary Obstruction/Hepatic Insufficiency: Initial: 40mg-12.5mg tab qd; monitor closely. Replacement Therapy: Substitute combination for titrated components.

HOW SUPPLIED: Tab: (Telmisartan-HCTZ) 40mg-12.5mg, 80mg-12.5mg, 80mg-25mg

CONTRAINDICATIONS: Anuria, sulfonamide hypersensitivity.

WARNINGS/PRECAUTIONS: Correct volume or salt depletion before therapy due to risk of hypotension. May precipitate azotemia in patients with renal disease. (HCTZ) Caution with impaired hepatic function, liver disease or progressive liver disease; may precipitate hepatic coma. May exacerbate or activate systemic lupus erythematosus (SLE). Hypersensitivity reactions may occur with history of allergy or bronchial asthma. Hyponatremia (including dilutional hyponatremia), hypokalemia, hypochloremic alkalosis, hyperuricemia, hyperglycemia, hypercalcemia, and hypomagnesemia may occur; monitor serum electrolytes. (Telmisartan) Caution with biliary obstructive disorders, hepatic insufficiency, and unilateral or bilateral renal artery stenosis. Changes in renal function (including acute renal failure) reported.

ADVERSE REACTIONS: Fatigue, influenza-like symptoms, dizziness, diarrhea, sinusitis, upper respiratory tract infection.

INTERACTIONS: (HCTZ) Potentiation of orthostatic hypotension with alcohol, barbiturates, or narcotics. Adjust dose of insulin and oral antidiabetic drugs. Additive effect or potentiation with other antihypertensive drugs. Impaired absorption with cholestyramine and colestipol resins. Intensified electrolyte depletion (particularly leading to hypokalemia) with corticosteroids and ACTH. Decreased response to pressor amines (eg, norepinephrine). Increased responsiveness to non-depolarizing skeletal muscle relaxants (eg, tubocurarine). Avoid lithium; risk of toxicity. Reduced diuretic, natriuretic, and antihypertensive effects of diuretics, with NSAIDs. Thiazide-induced hypokalemia may sensitize or exaggerate response of heart to toxic effects of digitalis. (Telmisartan) May increase digoxin levels; monitor digoxin levels. May increase lithium levels/toxicity; avoid concomitant use. Possible additive effects with ramipril and ramiprilat. May decrease warfarin levels. Dual blockade of the renin-angiotensin-aldosterone system with ACE inhibitors. Possible inhibition of the metabolism of drugs metabolized by CYP2C19.

PREGNANCY: Category C (1st trimester) and D (2nd and 3rd trimesters), not for use in nursing.

MECHANISM OF ACTION: Telmisartan: Angiotensin II receptor antagonist; blocks the vasoconstrictor and aldosterone-secreting effects of angiotensin II by selectively blocking the binding of angiotensin II to the AT$_1$ receptor in many tissues such as vascular smooth muscle and adrenal gland. HCTZ:

M

Thiazide diuretic; affects renal tubular mechanisms of electrolyte reabsorption, directly increasing excretion of Na+ and Cl- and indirectly reducing plasma volume.

PHARMACOKINETICS: Absorption: Telmisartan: T_{max}=0.5-1 hr; Absolute bioavailability=42% (40mg), 58% (160mg). **Distribution:** Telmisartan: Plasma protein binding (>99.5%); V_d= 500L. HCTZ: Crosses placenta; found in breast milk. **Metabolism:** Telmisartan: Conjugation. **Elimination:** Telmisartan: Feces (>97%), urine (0.91% [IV administration]; 0.49% [oral administration]); $T_{1/2}$=24 hrs. HCTZ: Kidney (61%, unchanged); $T_{1/2}$=5.6-14.8 hrs.

NURSING CONSIDERATIONS

Assessment: Assess SLE, DM, CHF, MI, cirrhosis, history of allergy or bronchial asthma, biliary obstructive disorder, history of *in utero* exposure to angiotensin II receptor antagonist, hypersensitivity to sulfonamide-derived drugs, anuria, pregnancy/nursing status, and possible drug interactions.

Monitoring: Monitor BP, ECG, hepatic/renal function, CBC with platelet and differential count, serum electrolytes, hyperuricemia, lipid profile. Monitor for signs and symptoms of electrolyte imbalance, exacerbation or activation of SLE, angioneurotic edema, hypersensitivity reactions, and adverse reactions (eg, upper respiratory tract infection, diarrhea, sinusitis, pancreatitis, Stevens-Johnson syndrome [SJS], xanthopsia).

Patient Counseling: Counsel about the signs and symptoms of potential adverse effects, and advise to seek prompt medical attention if any occur. Inform of pregnancy risks; instruct to report pregnancy immediately if detected. Instruct to inform physician if syncope occurs. Inform that inadequate fluid intake or loss of fluids may lead to fall of BP; instruct to seek medical attention if vomiting/diarrhea/excessive perspiration occur. Advise against use of K+ supplements/salt substitutes that contain potassium without consulting physician.

Administration: Oral route. **Storage:** 25°C (77°F); excursions permitted to 15-30°C (59-86°F). Do not remove tablets from blisters until immediately before administration.

MICRO-K   RX
potassium chloride (Ther-Rx)

THERAPEUTIC CLASS: K+ supplement

INDICATIONS: (For those unable to tolerate liquid or effervescent potassium preparations). Treatment and prevention of hypokalemia with or without metabolic alkalosis. Treatment of digitalis intoxication and hypokalemic familial periodic paralysis.

DOSAGE: *Adults:* Prevention: 20mEq/day. Hypokalemia: 40-100mEq/day. Divide dose if >20mEq. Take with meal and full glass of water or liquid. May sprinkle on soft food; swallow without chewing.

HOW SUPPLIED: Cap, Extended-Release: 8mEq, 10mEq

CONTRAINDICATIONS: Hyperkalemia, esophageal ulceration, delay in GI passage (from structural, pathological, pharmacologic causes), cardiac patients with esophageal compression due to enlarged left atrium.

WARNINGS/PRECAUTIONS: Potentially fatal hyperkalemia may occur. Extreme caution with acidosis, cardiac and renal disease; monitor ECG and electrolytes. Hypokalemia with metabolic acidosis should be treated with an alkalinizing potassium salt (eg, potassium bicarbonate, potassium citrate). May produce ulcerative or stenotic GI lesions.

ADVERSE REACTIONS: Hyperkalemia, GI effects (obstruction, bleeding, ulceration), N/V, abdominal pain, diarrhea.

INTERACTIONS: Risk of hyperkalemia with ACE inhibitors (eg, captopril, enalapril), K+-sparing diuretics, and K+ supplements. Contraindicated with anticholinergic agents due to possible delay in tablet passage through GI tract.

PREGNANCY: Category C, safe for use in nursing.

MECHANISM OF ACTION: K^+ supplement; helps in maintenance of intracellular tonicity, transmission of nerve impulses, contraction of cardiac, skeletal, and smooth muscle, and maintenance of normal renal function.

NURSING CONSIDERATIONS

Assessment: Assess for conditions that impair excretion of K^+, hyperkalemia, esophageal compression due to enlarged left atrium, conditions causing arrest or delay in passage through GI, renal insufficiency, DM, and possible drug interactions.

Monitoring: Monitor serum K^+ levels regularly; renal function, ECG, and acid-base balance. Monitor for GI ulceration/obstruction/perforation, hyperkalemia, renal dysfunction, and hypersensitivity reactions.

Patient Counseling: Instruct to take with meals; swallow with full glass of water or other suitable liquid. Do not crush, chew, or suck. Seek medical attention if symptoms of GI ulceration, obstruction, perforation (vomiting, abdominal pain, distention, GI bleeding), hyperkalemia, or hypersensitivity reactions occur.

Administration: Oral route. **Storage:** 20-25°C (68-77°F).

MICRONOR   RX
norethindrone (Ortho-McNeil)

OTHER BRAND NAMES: Camila (Barr) - Errin (Barr)

THERAPEUTIC CLASS: Progestogen

INDICATIONS: Prevention of pregnancy.

DOSAGE: *Adults:* 1 tab qd without interruption (continuous regimen) on 1st day of menstrual period. If fully nursing, start 6 weeks postpartum. If partially nursing, start 3 weeks postpartum.
Pediatrics: Postpubertal: 1 tab qd without interruption (continuous regimen) on 1st day of menstrual period. If fully nursing, start 6 weeks postpartum. If partially nursing, start 3 weeks postpartum.

HOW SUPPLIED: Tab: 0.35mg

CONTRAINDICATIONS: Pregnancy, breast carcinoma, undiagnosed abnormal genital bleeding, benign or malignant liver tumors, acute liver disease.

WARNINGS/PRECAUTIONS: Avoid smoking. Perform annual physical exam. Not for use before menarche. May affect certain endocrine tests (eg, sex hormone binding globulin, thyroxine binding globulin). Monitor glucose tolerance in prediabetics and diabetics. May alter lipid metabolism. May increase risk of breast cancer and hepatic adenomas. May cause irregular menstrual patterns. Delayed follicular atresia/ovarian cysts and ectopic pregnancy may occur. D/C with recurrent migraines or severe headaches.

ADVERSE REACTIONS: Menstrual irregularities, frequent or irregular bleeding, headache, breast tenderness, nausea, dizziness, androgenic effects (rare).

INTERACTIONS: Reduced efficacy with hepatic enzyme inducers (eg, rifampin, phenytoin, carbamazepine, barbiturates).

PREGNANCY: Not for use in pregnancy, caution in nursing.

MECHANISM OF ACTION: Progestogen oral contraceptive; suppresses ovulation. Thickens cervical mucus to inhibit sperm penetration, lowers midcycle LH and FSH peaks, slows movement of ovum through fallopian tubes, and alters endometrium.

PHARMACOKINETICS: Absorption: T_{max}=2 hrs. **Distribution:** Rapid.

NURSING CONSIDERATIONS

Assessment: Assess for pregnancy, carcinoma of breast, undiagnosed abnormal genital bleeding, benign/malignant liver tumor, and acute liver disease. Assess use in smokers and for possible drug interactions.

Monitoring: Monitor for ectopic pregnancy, delayed follicular atresia, ovarian cysts, irregular genital bleeding, and hepatic neoplasias. Perform annual physical exam while on medication. Monitor serum glucose levels with DM and prediabetic patients, lipid levels while on medication, and for onset or exacerbation of migraine or development of severe headaches.

Patient Counseling: Counsel about possible adverse effects. Inform that drug does not protect against HIV infection (AIDS) or other STDs. Advise to avoid smoking while on medication. Instruct to take at same time daily. Instruct that if dose missed or taken 3 hrs past scheduled time, use backup form of contraception for next 48 hrs.

Administration: Oral route. **Storage:** 25°C (77°F); excursions permitted to 15-30°C (59-86°F). Keep out of reach of children.

MICROZIDE   RX
hydrochlorothiazide (Watson)

THERAPEUTIC CLASS: Thiazide diuretic

INDICATIONS: Management of hypertension.

DOSAGE: *Adults:* Initial: 12.5mg qd. Max: 50mg/day.

HOW SUPPLIED: Cap: 12.5mg

CONTRAINDICATIONS: Anuria, sulfonamide hypersensitivity.

WARNINGS/PRECAUTIONS: Caution in severe renal disease, liver dysfunction, electrolyte/fluid imbalance. Monitor electrolytes. Hyperuricemia, hyperglycemia, hypokalemia, hyponatremia, hypomagnesemia, hypercalcemia may occur. Increases in cholesterol and triglyceride levels reported. May exacerbate SLE. Sensitivity reactions reported. D/C prior to parathyroid test. Enhanced effects in post-sympathectomy patient.

ADVERSE REACTIONS: Weakness, hypotension, pancreatitis, jaundice, diarrhea, vomiting, blood dyscrasias, rash, photosensitivity, electrolyte imbalance, impotence.

INTERACTIONS: May potentiate orthostatic hypotension with alcohol, barbiturates, narcotics. Adjust antidiabetic drugs. Possible decreased response to pressor amines. Corticosteroids, ACTH increase electrolyte depletion. May potentiate nondepolarizing skeletal muscle relaxants, antihypertensives. Lithium toxicity. NSAIDs decrease effects. Decreased PO absorption with cholestyramine, colestipol.

PREGNANCY: Category B, not for use in nursing.

MECHANISM OF ACTION: Thiazide diuretic; affects renal tubular mechanism of electrolyte reabsorption, directly increasing excretion of Na$^+$ and Cl$^-$.

PHARMACOKINETICS: Absorption: Well absorbed (65-75%); C_{max}=70-490ng/mL; T_{max}=1-5 hrs. **Distribution:** Plasma protein binding (40-68%). **Elimination:** Urine (unchanged), $T_{1/2}$=6-15 hrs.

NURSING CONSIDERATIONS

Assessment: Assess for anuria, known hypersensitivity to sulfonamide-derived drugs, DM, hypoglycemia, impaired renal/hepatic function, serum electrolytes, parathyroid disease, pregnancy status, and possible drug interactions.

Monitoring: Monitor BP, hyperuricemia or acute gout, signs/symptoms of electrolyte imbalance, serum glucose, lipid profile, pancreatitis, Stevens-Johnson syndrome, xanthopsia, impotence.

Patient Counseling: Counsel about signs/symptoms of electrolyte imbalance (dryness of mouth, thirst, weakness, lethargy, drowsiness, restlessness, muscle pains or cramps, muscular fatigue, hypotension, oliguria, tachycardia, and GI disturbance such as N/V) and advise to seek prompt medical attention.

Administration: Oral route. **Storage:** 20-25°C (68-77°F). Protect from light, moisture, freezing -20°C (-4°F). Keep container tightly closed.

MIDAZOLAM INJECTION
midazolam HCl (Various)

> Associated with respiratory depression and respiratory arrest especially when used for sedation in noncritical care settings. Use only in hospital or ambulatory care settings that provide continuous monitoring of respiratory and cardiac function. For deeply sedated pediatric patients, a dedicated individual, other than the practitioner performing the procedure should monitor the patient throughout the procedure. The initial IV dose for sedation in normal, healthy adults should not exceed 2.5mg. Lower doses are necessary for older (>60 yrs) patients or debilitated patients and in patients receiving concomitant narcotic or other CNS depressants. Initial and all subsequent doses should always be titrated slowly. Doses for pediatrics must be calculated on a mg/kg basis. Do not administer by rapid injection to neonates.

THERAPEUTIC CLASS: Benzodiazepine

INDICATIONS: For sedation, anxiolysis, and amnesia induction pre-op, prior to or during diagnostic, therapeutic, or endoscopic procedures, either alone or in combination with other CNS depressants. For induction of general anesthesia. For sedation of intubated and ventilated patients.

DOSAGE: *Adults:* Sedation/Anxiolysis/Amnesia Induction: <60 yrs: Initial: 1-2.5mg IV over 2 min. Titrate: In small increments at 2 min intervals if needed. Max: 5mg IV. Concomitant Narcotics/Other CNS Depressants: Reduce dose by 30%. ≥60 yrs/Debilitated/Chronically Ill: Initial: 1-1.5mg IV over 2 min. Titrate: In small increments at 2-min intervals if needed. Max: 3.5mg IV. Concomitant Narcotics/Other CNS Depressants: Reduce dose by 50%. Maint: 25% of sedation dose by slow titration. Preoperative Sedation/Anxiolysis/Amnesia: <60 yrs: 0.07-0.08mg/kg IM up to 1 hr before surgery. ≥60 yrs/Debilitated: 1-3mg IM. Anesthesia Induction: Unpremedicated: <55 yrs: Initially: 0.3-0.35mg/kg IV over 20-30 seconds. May give additional doses of 25% of initial dose to complete induction. ≥55 yrs: 0.3mg/kg IV. Debilitated: Initial: 0.15-0.25mg/kg IV. Premedicated: <55 yrs: Initial: 0.25mg/kg IV over 20-30 seconds. ≥55 yrs: Initial: 0.2mg/kg IV. Debilitated: 0.15mg/kg IV. Continuous Infusion: LD: 0.01-0.05mg/kg IV. May repeat dose at 10-15 min intervals until adequate sedation is achieved. Maint: 0.02-0.1mg/kg/hr. Infusion rate should be adjusted up or down by 25-50% of the initial infusion rate so as to assure adequate titration of sedation level. Infusion rate should be decreased 10-25% every few hrs to find minimum effective infusion rate.
Pediatrics: Sedation/Anxiolysis/Amnesia Induction: IV by Intermittent Inj: <6 months: Limited information; titrate with small increments and monitor. 6 months-5 yrs: Initial: 0.05-0.1mg/kg IV over 2-3 min, up to 0.6mg/kg IV if needed. Max: 6mg IV. 6-12 yrs: Initial: 0.025-0.05mg/kg IV over 2-3 min, up to 0.4mg/kg IV if needed. Max: 10mg IV. 12-16 yrs: Should be dosed as adults. Max: 10mg IV. Continuous Infusion for Sedation/Anxiolysis/Amnesia in Critical Care Settings: LD: 0.05-0.2mg/kg IV over 2-3 min. Maint: 0.06-0.12mg/kg/hr IV. May adjust dose by 25%. Continuous IV Infusion for Sedation in Critical Care: Neonatal Dose: <32 weeks: Initial: 0.03mg/kg/hr IV. >32 weeks: Initial: 0.06mg/kg/hr IV. Adjust to lowest effective dose. IM (Non-Neonatal) Preoperative Sedation/Anxiolysis/Amnesia: 0.1-0.15mg/kg IM, up to 0.5mg/kg IM if needed. Max: 10mg IM.

HOW SUPPLIED: Inj: 1mg/mL, 5mg/mL

CONTRAINDICATIONS: Acute narrow-angle glaucoma, untreated open-angle glaucoma, intrathecal or epidural use.

WARNINGS/PRECAUTIONS: Must never be used without individualization of dosage. Agitation, involuntary movements, hyperactivity, and combativeness reported. Caution with CHF, chronic renal failure, pulmonary disease, uncompensated acute illnesses (eg, severe fluid or electrolyte disturbances), and in elderly or debilitated. Pediatric and adult patients undergoing procedures involving the upper airway are particularly vulnerable to episodes of desaturation and hypoventilation. Avoid use with shock or coma, or in acute alcohol intoxication with depression of vital signs. Precautions against unintended intra-arterial injection should be taken. Administer IM or IV only. Should not operate hazardous machinery or a motor vehicle until effects of drug have subsided or until one full day after anesthesia or surgery, whichever

M

is longer. May increase risk of congenital malformations and cause withdrawal symptoms in infants if used during pregnancy. Neonates may be vulnerable to profound and/or prolonged respiratory effects. Contains benzyl alcohol. Does not protect against the increase in intracranial pressure or against the HR rise and/or BP rise associated with endotracheal intubation under light anesthesia.

ADVERSE REACTIONS: Decreased tidal volume and/or respiratory rate, BP/HR variations, desaturation, local effects at injection site, apnea, hiccoughs.

INTERACTIONS: Prolonged sedation with CYP3A4 inhibitors (eg, erythromycin, diltiazem, verapamil, ketoconazole, itraconazole, cimetidine). Increased sedative effects with morphine, meperidine, fentanyl, secobarbital, droperidol, or other CNS depressants. May require a moderate reduction in induction dosage requirements of thiopental when used concomitantly with IM midazolam. IV midazolam may decrease the minimum alveolar concentration (MAC) of halothane required for general anesthesia. May cause severe hypotension with concomitant use of fentanyl in neonates. Concomitant use of barbiturates, alcohol, or other CNS depressants may increase the risk of hypoventilation, airway obstruction, desaturation, or apnea and may contribute to profound and/or prolonged drug effect. Narcotic premedication depresses the ventilatory response to carbon dioxide stimulation.

PREGNANCY: Category D, caution in nursing.

MECHANISM OF ACTION: Benzodiazepine; short-acting CNS depressant.

PHARMACOKINETICS: Absorption: (IM) Absolute bioavailability (>90%), C_{max}=90ng/mL, T_{max}=0.5 hr. (1-hydroxy-midazolam) C_{max}=8 ng/ml, T_{max}=1 hr. **Distribution:** Crosses placenta, found in breast milk and CSF. V_d=1.0-3.1L/kg; plasma protein binding (97%). **Metabolism:** Liver via CYP450-3A4;1-hydroxy-midazolam (major metabolite). **Elimination:** Urine; (0.5% unchanged, 45%-57% as 4-hydroxy-midazolam); $T_{1/2}$ = 3 hrs.

NURSING CONSIDERATIONS

Assessment: Assess for acute narrow angle glaucoma, untreated open-angle glaucoma, COPD, renal/hepatic impairment, CHF, shock, presence of a comatose state, uncompensated acute illnesses (eg, fluid or electrolyte disturbances), pregnancy/nursing status, and for possible drug interactions.

Monitoring: Monitor for signs/symptoms of cardiorespiratory complications (eg, respiratory depression, airway obstruction, oxygen desaturation, apnea, respiratory arrest, cardiac arrest), hypotension, agitation, involuntary movements, hyperactivity, and for combativeness. Monitor vital signs.

Patient Counseling: Advise of possible effects that medication may produce including sedation and amnesia. Inform that patient must use caution when engaging in activities requiring mental alertness (eg, driving, operating heavy machinery). Instruct to inform physician about any alcohol consumption and all medications currently taking. Counsel to notify physician if pregnant, planning to become pregnant, or if nursing. Advise that if receiving therapy over an extended period of time, may experience symptoms of withdrawl if abruptly d/c therapy.

Administration: IM/IV route. **Storage:** 20-25°C (68-77°F); excursions permitted to 59°-86°F.

MIGRANAL   RX
dihydroergotamine mesylate (Valeant)

> Serious and life-threatening peripheral ischemia reported with potent CYP3A4 inhibitors (eg, protease inhibitors, macrolides). Elevated levels of dihydroergotamine increases risk of vasospasm leading to cerebral ischemia or ischemia of the extremities. Concomitant use with CYP3A4 inhibitors is contraindicated.

THERAPEUTIC CLASS: Ergot alkaloid

INDICATIONS: Acute treatment of migraine headache with or without aura.

DOSAGE: *Adults:* 1 spray per nostril, repeat in 15 min. Max: 6 sprays/24 hrs or 8 sprays/week.

HOW SUPPLIED: Nasal Spray: 0.5mg/spray [3.5mL]

CONTRAINDICATIONS: Ischemic heart disease (angina, history of MI, documented silent ischemia), coronary artery vasospasm (Prinzmetal's variant angina), uncontrolled HTN, known peripheral artery disease, sepsis, following vascular surgery, severe renal or hepatic dysfunction, hemiplegic or basilar migraine, pregnancy or nursing, with potent CYP3A4 inhibitors (eg, ritonavir, nelfinavir, indinavir, erythromycin, clarithromycin, troleandomycin, ketoconazole, itraconazole). Do not use with peripheral and central vasoconstrictors or within 24 hrs of 5-HT$_1$ agonists, ergot-type drugs, or methysergide.

WARNINGS/PRECAUTIONS: Confirm diagnosis. Monitor and consider ECG with 1st dose in patients with CAD risk factors (eg, HTN, hypercholesterolemia, smoker, obesity, DM, strong family history, postmenopausal women, men >40 yrs). Risk of elevated BP, MI, and other adverse cardiac or vasospastic effects. Monitor cardiovascular function with intermittent long-term use. Fibrotic complications (eg, pleural and retroperitoneal fibrosis) reported.

ADVERSE REACTIONS: Rhinitis, altered taste, application-site reactions, dizziness, N/V, pharyngitis, somnolence.

INTERACTIONS: Potentiated BP elevation with peripheral and central vasoconstrictors. Additive coronary vasospastic effect with sumatriptan; avoid within 24 hrs of each other. Propranolol and nicotine may potentiate the vasoconstrictive action. Increased plasma levels and peripheral vasoconstriction with macrolides. Contraindicated with CYP3A4 inhibitors (eg, macrolides, protease inhibitors). Caution with less potent CYP3A4 inhibitors (eg, saquinavir, nefazodone, fluconazole, grapefruit juice, fluoxetine, fluvoxamine, zileuton, clotrimazole).

PREGNANCY: Category X, not for use in nursing.

MECHANISM OF ACTION: Ergotamine; binds with high affinity to 5-HT$_{1D}$ receptors on intracranial blood vessels, causing vasoconstriction, or activates 5-HT$_{1D}$ receptors on sensory nerve endings of trigeminal system, inhibiting proinflammatory neuropeptide release.

PHARMACOKINETICS: Absorption: Bioavailability (32%). **Distribution:** V$_d$=800L; plasma protein binding (93%). **Metabolism:** 8-β-hydroxydihydroergotamine (major metabolite). **Elimination:** Bile (major), urine (2%).

NURSING CONSIDERATIONS

Assessment: Assess for ischemic heart disease (angina pectoris, MI, silent ischemia), coronary artery vasospasm, Prinzmetal's variant angina, CAD or risk factors, HTN, peripheral arterial disease, sepsis, s/p vascular surgery, possible drug interaction, hemiplegic or basilar migraine, renal/hepatic impairment. Obtain baseline cardiac evaluation.

Monitoring: Perform periodic cardiac evaluations. Monitor for signs/symptoms of vasospasm, vasoconstriction, CV effects, and hypersensitivity reactions.

Patient Counseling: Once applicator prepared, discard after 8 hrs. Advise to seek medical attention immediately if numbness or tingling in fingers and toes, muscle pain in arms and legs, weakness in legs, chest pain, speeding or slowing of HR, swelling, or itching occur.

Administration: Intranasal. Prime (squeeze 4 times) before use. Spray once into each nostril; do not tilt back or sniff through nose while spraying or immediately after; wait 15 min; spray once again into each nostril. **Storage:** Below 25°C (77°F). Do not refrigerate, freeze, or keep opened vial for more than 8 hrs. Keep away from heat and light.

MINIPRESS   RX
prazosin HCl (Pfizer)

THERAPEUTIC CLASS: Alpha$_1$-blocker (quinazoline)

INDICATIONS: Treatment of hypertension either alone or in combination with other antihypertensive drugs.

DOSAGE: *Adults:* Initial: 1mg bid-tid. Titrate: Slowly increase to 20mg/day in divided doses. Maint: 6-15mg qd in divided doses. Max: 40mg/day. Concomitant with Diuretic/Antihypertensive Agent: Reduce to 1-2mg tid, then retitrate.

HOW SUPPLIED: Cap: 1mg, 2mg, 5mg

WARNINGS/PRECAUTIONS: Syncope with sudden loss of consciousness may occur, usually after initial dose or dose increase; Patient should be placed in the recumbent position and treated with supportive care. Due to excessive postural hypotensive effect, caution to avoid situations where injury could result should syncope occur during initiation of therapy. Always start on 1mg cap. Possible adverse effects (eg, dizziness, lightheadedness) may occur. Intraoperative Floppy Iris Syndrome (IFIS) may occur during cataract surgery. False (+) for pheochromocytoma may occur. D/C with elevated urinary VMA levels and retest after 1 month.

ADVERSE REACTIONS: Dizziness, headache, drowsiness, lack of energy, weakness, palpitations, N/V, edema, orthostatic hypotension, dyspnea, syncope, depression, urinary frequency, diarrhea, and blurred vision.

INTERACTIONS: Additive hypotensive effects with diuretics, PDE5 inhibitors, β-blockers, or other antihypertensives. Dizziness or syncope may occur with alcohol.

PREGNANCY: Category C, caution in nursing.

MECHANISM OF ACTION: α_1 blocker, quinazoline derivative; not established. Blocks the postsynaptic α-adrenoreceptors resulting in vasodilation and reduction in total peripheral resistance.

PHARMACOKINETICS: Absorption: T_{max}=3 hrs. **Distribution:** Plasma protein binding (highly bound). Found in breast milk. **Metabolism:** Demethylation and conjugation. **Elimination:** Bile and feces; $T_{1/2}$=2-3 hrs.

NURSING CONSIDERATIONS

Assessment: Assess BP, LFTs, urinary VMA levels, hypersensitivity, pregnancy/nursing status, and for possible drug interactions.

Monitoring: Monitor BP, LFTs, HR, urinary VMA levels. Monitor for orthostatic hypotension, edema, epistaxis, lichen planus, angina pectoris and hypersensitivity reactions.

Patient Counseling: Inform that dizziness or drowsiness may occur after first dose; avoid driving or performing hazardous tasks for first 24 hrs. Dizziness, lightheadedness or fainting may occur; get up slowly when rising from a lying or sitting position. Instruct to be careful in the amount of alcohol taken. Counsel to use extra care during exercise or hot weather, or if standing for long periods.

Administration: Oral route. **Storage:** Below 30°C (86°F)

MINOCIN   RX
minocycline HCl (Triax)

THERAPEUTIC CLASS: Tetracycline derivative

INDICATIONS: Treatment of the following infections caused by susceptible microorganisms: Rocky Mountain spotted fever; typhus fever and the typhus group; Q fever; rickettsialpox; tick fevers; respiratory tract infections; lymphogranuloma venereum; psittacosis (ornithosis); trachoma; inclusion conjunctivitis; nongonococcal urethritis, endocervical, or rectal infections in adults; relapsing fever; chancroid (PO only); plague; tularemia; cholera; *Campylobacter fetus* infections; brucellosis; bartonellosis; granuloma inguinale. Treatment of infections caused by *Escherichia coli*, *Enterobacter aerogenes*, *Shigella* species, *Acinetobacter* spp. Respiratory tract infections caused by *Haemophilus influenzae*, respiratory tract and urinary tract infections caused by *Klebsiella* spp. Treatment of upper respiratory tract infections caused by *Streptococcus pneumoniae*, skin and skin structure infections caused by *Staphylococcus aureus*. When penicillin is contraindicated, treatment of the following infections caused by susceptible microorganisms:

uncomplicated urethritis is men due to *Neisseria gonorrhoeae* and for the treatment of other gonococcal infections (PO only), infections in women caused by *N. gonorrhoeae* (PO only), meningitis (IV only), syphilis, yaws, listeriosis, anthrax, Vincent's infection, actinomycosis, infections caused by *Clostridium* species. Adjunct in acute intestinal amebiasis. (PO) May be used to treat asymptomatic carriers of *N. meningitidis* to eliminate meningococci from the nasopharynx. Limited clinical data show that it has been used successfully in the treatment of infections caused by *Mycobacterium marinum*.

DOSAGE: *Adults:* Usual: 200mg initially, then 100mg q12 hrs. Max: (IV) 400mg/24 hrs. (Cap) Alternative: 100-200mg initially, then 50mg qid. Uncomplicated Gonococcal Infections (Men, Other Than Urethritis and Anorectal Infections)/(Sus) Gonorrhea in Patients Sensitive to Penicillin: 200mg initially, then 100mg q12 hrs for minimum 4 days, with post-therapy cultures within 2-3 days. (Cap/Sus) Uncomplicated Gonococcal Urethritis (Men): 100mg q12 hrs for 5 days. Syphilis: Administer usual dose for 10-15 days. Meningococcal Carrier State: 100mg q12 hrs for 5 days. *Mycobacterium marinum*: 100mg q12 hrs for 6-8 weeks. Uncomplicated Urethral, Endocervical, or Rectal Infection Caused by *Chlamydia trachomatis* or *Ureaplasma urealyticum*: 100mg q12 hrs for at least 7 days. Renal Dysfunction: Max: 200mg/24 hrs. (Cap) Take with plenty of fluids.
Pediatrics: >8 yrs: 4mg/kg initially followed by 2mg/kg q12 hrs, not to exceed adult dose. Renal Impairment (CrCl < 80mL/min): Max: 200mg/24 hrs. (PO) Take with plenty of fluids.

HOW SUPPLIED: Cap: 50mg, 100mg; Inj: 100mg; Sus: 50mg/5mL [60mL]

WARNINGS/PRECAUTIONS: May cause fetal harm during pregnancy. Do not use during tooth development (last half of pregnancy, infancy, ≤8 yrs); may cause permanent discoloration of the teeth or enamel hypoplasia. Decrease in fibula growth rate has been observed when given to premature infants given PO tetracycline (25mg/kg q6 hrs); reversible upon d/c. Drug Rash with Eosinophilia and Systemic Symptoms (DRESS) including fatal cases reported; d/c if this syndrome is recognized. Caution in renal impairment; may increase BUN and lead to azotemia, hyperphosphatemia, acidosis and possible hepatotoxicity. Photosensitivity reported. May impair mental/physical abilities. CNS effects (light-headedness, dizziness or vertigo) reported; symptoms may disappear during therapy and upon d/c. *C.difficile*-associated diarrhea (CDAD) reported; ranges from mild diarrhea to fatal colitis. Consider CDAD in all patients who present diarrhea after use (over 2 months after administration). If CDAD develops, d/c antibiotic not directed against *C. difficile* and initiate appropriate therapy. May cause superinfection; d/c and institute appropriate therapy. Pseudotumor cerebri (benign intracranial HTN) in adults associated with use. Clinical manifestations are headache and blurred vision. May cause bulging fontanels in infants. Hepatotoxicity reported; caution in hepatic dysfunction. Caution in elderly. False elevations of urinary catecholamine levels due to intolerance with fluorescence test may occur. (Sus) Safety use during pregnancy not established. Contains Na⁺ sulfite, may cause allergic-type reactions (eg, anaphylactic symptoms and life-threatening or less severe asthmatic episodes) in certain susceptible people.

ADVERSE REACTIONS: Neutropenia, agranulocytosis, hypersensitivity syndrome, lupus-like syndrome, serum sickness-like syndrome, fever, N/V, diarrhea, increased LFTs, renal toxicity, rash, exfoliative dermatitis, Stevens-Johnson syndrome, skin and mucous membrane pigmentation, headache, tooth discoloration.

INTERACTIONS: May require downward adjustments of anticoagulant dosage. May interfere with bactericidal action of penicillin; avoid concurrent use when possible. May decrease efficacy of oral contraceptives. Fatal renal toxicity with methoxyflurane reported. Avoid isotretinoin shortly before, during and after therapy; each drug alone is associated with pseudotumor cerebri. Caution with other hepatotoxic drugs. Increased risk of ergotism with ergot alkaloids. (PO) Impaired absorption with antacids containing aluminum or calcium or magnesium and iron-containing products.

PREGNANCY: Category D, not for use in nursing.

MECHANISM OF ACTION: Tetracycline; bacteriostatic, thought to inhibit protein synthesis.

M

PHARMACOKINETICS: Absorption: (Cap) C_{max}=3.5µg/mL; T_{max}=2.1 hrs (fasted). **Distribution:** Crosses placenta (IV). **Elimination:** (Cap/Sus) Urine, feces; $T_{1/2}$=15.5 hrs (Cap), 11-17 hrs (Sus), 15-23 hrs (IV), 11-16 hrs (hepatic dysfunction), 18-69 hrs (renal dysfunction).

NURSING CONSIDERATIONS

Assessment: Assess for age, bacterial infection, hepatic/renal impairment, gonorrhea, syphilis, hypersensitivity, pregnancy/nursing status, possible drug interactions. (Sus) Assess for sulfite sensitivity.

Monitoring: Monitor growth rate, syphilis, organ systems, including hematopoietic, renal (BUN and creatinine) and hepatic, periodically. Monitor for signs/symptoms of thyroid cancer, DRESS, hepatotoxicity, hypersensitivity syndrome, lupus-like syndrome, serum sickness-like syndrome, photosensitivity, CNS effects, superinfection, CDAD, bulging fontanels and pseudotumor cerebri. (Cap) When coexistent syphilis is suspected, monitor blood serology monthly for at least 4 months. (Sus, IV) Serologic test for syphilis after 3 months.

Patient Counseling: Inform that therapy treats bacterial, not viral (eg, common cold), infections. Take as directed; skipping doses or not completing full course may decrease effectiveness and increase bacterial resistance. May experience diarrhea. If watery/bloody stools, with or without cramps and fever occur, notify physician as soon as possible. Inform pregnant patients about the potential hazard to the fetus. (PO) Swallow whole and take with full glass of liquid. Advise that photosensitivity manifested by an exaggerated sunburn reaction can occur; d/c treatment at the 1st evidence of skin erythema. Caution in patients who experience CNS symptoms about driving vehicles or using hazardous machinery. May decrease efficacy of oral contraceptives. Discard by expiration date.

Administration: Oral and IV route. (IV) Avoid rapid administration. Refer to PI for further information. **Storage:** 20-25°C (68-77°F). (Cap) Protect from light, moisture, and excessive heat. (Sus) Do not freeze.

Minoxidil   RX

minoxidil (Mutual Pharmaceutical Co Inc)

> May cause pericardial effusion, occasionally progressing to tamponade, and may exacerbate angina pectoris. Only for nonresponders to maximum therapeutic doses of two other antihypertensives and a diuretic. Administer under supervision with a β-blocker and diuretic. Monitor in hospital for a decrease in BP in those receiving guanethidine with malignant hypertension.

THERAPEUTIC CLASS: Peripheral vasodilator

INDICATIONS: Treatment of hypertension that is symptomatic or associated with target organ damage and is not manageable with maximum therapeutic doses of diuretic plus 2 other antihypertensive drugs.

DOSAGE: *Adults:* Initial: 5mg qd. Titrate: Increase daily dose to 10mg, 20mg and then to 40mg in single or divided doses. Usual: 10-40mg/day. Max: 100mg/day. Frequency: Give qd if diastolic BP is reduced to <30mmHg and if reduced to >30mmHg give bid. Give with a diuretic (eg, HCTZ 50mg bid; chlorthalidone 50-100mg qd; furosemide 40mg bid) and a β-blocker (equivalent to propranolol 80-160mg/day) or methyldopa (250-750mg bid starting 24 hrs before therapy) or clonidine (0.1-0.2mg bid). Renal Failure/Dialysis: Reduce dose.
Pediatrics: >12 yrs: Initial: 5mg qd. Titrate: Increase daily dose to 10mg, 20mg and then to 40mg in single or divided doses. Usual: 10-40mg/day. Max: 100mg/day. Frequency: Give qd if diastolic BP is reduced to <30mmHg and if reduced to >30mmHg give bid. Give with a diuretic (eg, HCTZ 50mg bid; chlorthalidone 50-100mg qd; furosemide 40mg bid) and a β-blocker (equivalent to propranolol 80-160mg/day) or methyldopa (250-750mg bid starting 24 hrs before therapy) or clonidine (0.1-0.2mg bid). <12 yrs: 0.2mg/kg qd. Titrate: May increase by 50-100% increments. Usual: 0.25-1mg/kg/day. Max: 50mg/day. Renal Failure/Dialysis: Reduce dose.

HOW SUPPLIED: Tab: 2.5mg*, 10mg* *scored

CONTRAINDICATIONS: Pheochromocytoma.

WARNINGS/PRECAUTIONS: Refractory fluid retention may require d/c of therapy. Monitor for pericardial disorder and consider d/c of minoxidil if pericardial effusion persists. With renal failure or dialysis, reduce dose to prevent renal failure exacerbation and precipitation of cardiac failure. Avoid rapid control with severe HTN. Monitor body weight, fluid and electrolyte balance. Extreme caution with post-MI. Hypersensitivity reactions reported.

ADVERSE REACTIONS: Salt and water retention, pericarditis, pericardial effusion, tamponade, hypertrichosis.

INTERACTIONS: See Boxed Warning. Severe orthostatic hypotension with guanethidine.

PREGNANCY: Category C, not for use in nursing.

MECHANISM OF ACTION: Antihypertensive peripheral vasodilator; reduces systolic and diastolic BP by decreasing peripheral vascular resistance.

PHARMACOKINETICS: Absorption: Almost complete (90%); T_{max}=1 hr. **Distribution:** Found in breast milk. **Metabolism:** Glucuronide conjugation. **Elimination:** Urine; $T_{1/2}$=4.2 hrs.

NURSING CONSIDERATIONS

Assessment: Assess for hypersensitivity, pheochromocytoma, MI, CHF, BP, pregnancy/nursing status, renal dysfunction, and possible drug interactions.

Monitoring: Monitor fluid and electrolyte balance, body weight, HR, BP, pericarditis, cerebrovascular episodes, orthostatic effects, hypertrichosis, Stevens-Johnson syndrome, renal functions, ECG, EKG, chest x-ray, urinalysis, for thrombocytopenia, leukopenia, and N/V. Observe for signs/symptoms of pericardial disorder.

Patient Counseling: Instruct to take as directed; do not d/c without consulting physician. Do not skip doses. If dose is missed, wait until time for next dose and continue with regular schedule. Advise to immediately report any adverse effects (eg, N/V, rash, change in HR or body weight, headache, fatigue, breast tenderness, chest pain, dizziness, difficulty breathing). Inform that body hair may grow darker or longer on certain parts of the body within 3-6 weeks from start and will disappear within 1-6 months after completion.

Administration: Oral route. **Storage:** 20°-25°C (68°-77°F). Dispense in tight, child-resistant container.

M

MiraLax OTC
polyethylene glycol 3350 (Schering-Plough)

THERAPEUTIC CLASS: Osmotic laxative

INDICATIONS: Treatment of occasional constipation.

DOSAGE: *Adults:* Stir and dissolve 17g in 4-8 oz of beverage and drink qd. Use no more than 7 days.
Pediatrics: ≥17 yrs: Stir and dissolve 17g in 4-8 oz of beverage and drink qd. Use no more than 7 days.

HOW SUPPLIED: Powder: 17g/dose [119g, 238g]

WARNINGS/PRECAUTIONS: Avoid in kidney disease.

Mirapex RX
pramipexole dihydrochloride (Boehringer Ingelheim)

THERAPEUTIC CLASS: Non-ergot dopamine agonist

INDICATIONS: Treatment of signs and symptoms of idiopathic Parkinson's disease. Treatment of moderate-to-severe primary Restless Legs Syndrome (RLS).

DOSAGE: *Adults:* Parkinson's: Initial: 0.125mg tid. Titrate: May increase every 5-7 days (eg, Week 2: 0.25mg tid; Week 3: 0.5mg tid; Week 4: 0.75mg tid; Week 5: 1mg tid; Week 6: 1.25mg tid; Week 7: 1.5mg tid). Maint: 0.5-1.5mg tid. Max: 1.5mg tid. Renal Impairment: Mild: CrCl >60mL/min: Initial: 0.125mg tid. Max: 1.5mg tid. Moderate: CrCl 35-59mL/min: Initial: 0.125mg bid. Max: 1.5mg bid. Severe: CrCl 15-34mL/min: Initial: 0.125mg qd. Max: 1.5mg qd. Recommend to d/c over a period of 1 week. RLS: Initial: 0.125mg once daily, 2-3 hours before bedtime. Titrate: May double dose every 4-7 days up to 0.5mg/day. Moderate/Severe Renal Impairment (CrCl 20-60mL/min): Increase duration between titration steps to 14 days.

HOW SUPPLIED: Tab: 0.125mg, 0.25mg*, 0.5mg*, 0.75mg, 1mg*, 1.5mg* *scored

WARNINGS/PRECAUTIONS: Somnolence, symptomatic hypotension, hallucinations and rhabdomyolysis reported. May impair mental/physical abilities. Caution with renal insufficiency. May potentiate dyskinesia. May cause retinal pathology, fibrotic complications, withdrawal-emergent hyperpyrexia and confusion. Consider d/c if significant daytime sleepiness or sudden onset of sleep occurs during daily activities. Cases of pathological gambling, hypersexuality, and compulsive eating reported. Rebound and augmentation in RLS reported. Falling asleep during activities of daily living. Melanoma reported; monitor regularly.

ADVERSE REACTIONS: Nausea, dizziness, somnolence, insomnia, constipation, asthenia, hallucinations, vision abnormalities, peripheral edema, arthritis, dry mouth, postural hypotension, chest pain, malaise.

INTERACTIONS: May increase risk of drowsiness with concomitant sedating medications and medications that increase pramipexole plasma levels. Decreased oral clearance with drugs that are secreted by the cationic transport system (eg, cimetidine, ranitidine, diltiazem, triamterene, verapamil, quinidine, and quinine) and amantidine. May increase half-life of cimetidine. May increase peak plasma concentration of levodopa. Dopamine antagonists (eg, phenothiazines, butyrophenones, thioxanthenes, metoclopramide) may decrease effects.

PREGNANCY: Category C, not for use in nursing.

MECHANISM OF ACTION: Non-ergot dopamine agonist; not established. Suspected to stimulate dopamine receptors on the striatum.

PHARMACOKINETICS: Absorption: Rapid, absolute bioavailability (>90%), T_{max}=2 hrs. **Distribution:** V_d=500L; plasma protein binding (15%). **Elimination:** Urine (90% unchanged); $T_{1/2}$=8hrs (healthy); $T_{1/2}$=12hrs (elderly).

NURSING CONSIDERATIONS

Assessment: Assess for symptomatic hypotension, sleep disorders, renal function test, dyskinesia, retinal exam, pregnancy/nursing status, and possible drug interactions. Note other diseases/conditions and drug therapies.

Monitoring: Monitor BP, renal function test, signs/symptoms of rhabdomyolysis, NMS, melanomas, fibrotic complications, hallucinations, impulse control behaviors/compulsive behaviors.

Patient Counseling: Instruct to take with/without food. Caution while operating machinery/driving. Counsel about impulse control disorders/compulsive behaviors; avoid concomitant use of alcohol; report side effects. Advise to inform regarding concomitant medications being taken. Advise that may cause hallucination especially in the elderly with Parkinson's disease. Notify physician if intense urge to gamble, increased sexual urges, and other intense urges occur. Notify physician if pregnant or intend to be pregnant during therapy, or intend to breast-feed or are breast feeding an infant.

Administration: Oral route. **Storage:** 25°C (77°F); excursions permitted to 15-30°C (59-86°F). Protect from light.

MIRCETTE

RX

desogestrel - ethinyl estradiol (Duramed)

> Cigarette smoking increases risk of serious cardiovascular (CV) side effects. Risk increases with age (>35 yrs) and heavy smoking (≥15 cigarettes/day). Women who use oral contraceptives should be strongly advised not to smoke.

OTHER BRAND NAMES: Kariva (Barr)

THERAPEUTIC CLASS: Estrogen/progestogen combination

INDICATIONS: Prevention of pregnancy.

DOSAGE: *Adults:* Start 1st Sunday after menses begin or 1st day of menses. 28-day: 1 tab qd for 28 days, then repeat.
Pediatrics: Postpubertal: Start 1st Sunday after menses begin or 1st day of menses. 28-day: 1 tab qd for 28 days, then repeat

HOW SUPPLIED: Tab: (Ethinyl Estradiol-Desogestrel) 0.02mg-0.15mg and 0.01mg-NA

CONTRAINDICATIONS: Thrombophlebitis, DVT or thromboembolic disorders, pregnancy, cerebrovascular or coronary artery disease, undiagnosed abnormal genital bleeding, cholestatic jaundice of pregnancy or jaundice with prior pill use, hepatic adenomas or carcinomas, breast cancer or other estrogen-dependent neoplasia.

WARNINGS/PRECAUTIONS: Increased risk of MI, vascular disease, thromboembolism, stroke and gallbladder disease. Retinal thrombosis, hepatic neoplasia, carcinoma of breast and reproductive organs reported. May cause glucose intolerance. May increase BP, elevate LDL levels or cause other lipid changes, fluid retention, breakthrough bleeding, and spotting. May cause or exacerbate migraine. May develop visual changes with contact lens. Increased risk of MI with HTN, hyperlipidemia, obesity, and diabetes. D/C if jaundice, significant depression, or ophthalmic irregularities develop. Perform annual physical exam. Not indicated for use before menarche. May affect certain endocrine, LFTs and blood components.

ADVERSE REACTIONS: NV, breakthrough bleeding, spotting, amenorrhea, migraine, depression, vaginal candidiasis, edema, weight changes.

INTERACTIONS: Reduced effects, increased breakthrough bleeding, and menstrual irregularities with rifampin, barbiturates, phenylbutazone, phenytoin, carbamazepine, and possibly with griseofulvin, ampicillin, and tetracyclines.

PREGNANCY: Category X, not for use in nursing.

MECHANISM OF ACTION: Oral contraceptive combination; supresses gonadotropins, inhibits ovulation, increases difficulty of sperm entry into uterus, and reduces likelihood of implantation by producing changes in cervical mucus and endometrium, respectively.

PHARMACOKINETICS: Absorption: Desogestrel: Rapid, complete; relative bioavailability (100%). Ethinyl estradiol: Rapid, complete; absolute bioavailability (93-99%). **Distribution:** Desogestrel: Sex hormone-binding globulin (99%, metabolite). Ethinyl estradiol: Plasma protein binding (98.3%). **Metabolism:** Desogestrel: Hydroxylation in intestinal mucosa; etonogestrel (metabolite). Ethinyl estradiol: Conjugation. **Elimination:** Urine, bile, feces. Desogestrel: $T_{1/2}$=27.8 hrs (metabolite). Ethinyl estradiol: $T_{1/2}$=23.9 hrs.

NURSING CONSIDERATIONS

Assessment: Assess for history or recent DVT or thromboembolic disorders, thrombophlebitis, or any other conditions where treatment is contraindicated or cautioned. Assess for pregnancy/nursing status and possible drug interactions. Obtain complete medical history and physical exam with special reference to BP, breasts, abdomen and pelvic organs, cervical cytology, and relevant lab tests.

Monitoring: Monitor for thromboembolic disorders and other vascular problems, malignant neoplasms, MI, stroke, hepatic neoplasia, jaundice, emotional disorders, ocular lesions, gallbladder disease, carbohydrate and lipid metabolic effects, elevated BP, bleeding irregularities, migraine headaches, lipid profile (HDL, LDL, TG), LFTs, PT, TBG, T_3 and T_4, blood glucose, and serum folate levels.

Patient Counseling: Strongly advise not to smoke; increases risk of CV side effects. Instruct to take daily at same time. Counsel that light bleeding is possible. Drug does not protect against HIV infections/AIDS and other STDs. Caution that some drugs decrease efficacy, and to consult with physician before use to determine appropriate back-up contraceptive method. Immediately report sharp chest pains, coughing of blood, sudden SOB, pain in calf, severe headache and vomiting, dizziness or fainting, disturbances of vision or speech, severe pain or tenderness in stomach area, difficulty sleeping, weakness, changes in mood, and jaundice.

Administration: Oral route. **Storage:** 20-25°C (68-77°F).

Mirena RX
levonorgestrel (Bayer Healthcare)

THERAPEUTIC CLASS: Progestogen

INDICATIONS: Intrauterine contraception up to 5 yrs. Treatment of heavy menstrual bleeding in women who choose to use intrauterine contraception as their method of contraception. Recommended for women who had ≥1 child.

DOSAGE: *Adults:* Initial release rate is 20mcg/day. Rate decreases by 50% after 5 yrs. Replace every 5 yrs. Initial insertion into uterine cavity is recommended within 7 days of menstruation onset or immediately after 1st trimester abortion. May replace at any time during menstrual cycle. May insert 6 weeks postpartum or until uterine involution is complete. If involution is substantially delayed, consider waiting until 12 weeks postpartum.

HOW SUPPLIED: Intrauterine Insert: 52mg

CONTRAINDICATIONS: Pregnancy, congenital or acquired uterine anomaly, acute or history of pelvic inflammatory disease (PID) unless there has been a subsequent intrauterine pregnancy, postpartum endometritis, infected abortion in the past 3 months, uterine or cervical neoplasia or unresolved, abnormal Pap smear, genital bleeding of unknown etiology, untreated acute cervicitis or vaginitis including bacterial vaginosis or other lower genital tract infections until infections is controlled, acute liver disease, liver tumor (benign or malignant), conditions associated with increased susceptibility to pelvic infections, previously inserted intrauterine device (IUD) that is not removed, breast carcinoma.

WARNINGS/PRECAUTIONS: If pregnancy occurs while device is in place, evaluate for ectopic pregnancy and remove device; may increase the risk of septic abortion, congenital anomalies, premature labor/delivery, and miscarriage. Group A streptococcal sepsis (GAS) reported. Does not protect against sexually transmitted disease (STD). Associated with an increased risk of PID and actinomycosis; remove device and initiate antibiotic therapy. Can alter bleeding patterns and result in spotting, irregular bleeding, heavy bleeding, oligomenorrhea, and amenorrhea; if bleeding irregularities develop during prolonged treatment, rule out endometrial pathology. Perforation or penetration of the uterine wall or cervix or embedment in myometrium may occur; may result to pregnancy; remove when this occurs. May increase risk of perforation in fixed retroverted uteri, during lactation, and postpartum. Partial or complete expulsion may occur; replace within 7 days of menstrual period after pregnancy has been ruled out. May cause enlarged ovarian follicles. Breast cancer reported. May affect glucose tolerance. Caution with increased risk of infective endocarditis and/or have coagulopathies. Remove device if with: new onset menorrhagia and/or metrorrhagia producing anemia; STD; endometritis; jaundice (first time); intractable pelvic pain; severe dyspareunia; endometrial or cervical malignancy. Remove if the following occurs for the 1st time: migraine, focal migraine with asymmetrical visual loss or other symptoms indicating transient cerebral ischemia, exceptionally severe headache; marked BP increase; or severe arterial disease (eg, stroke or MI).

ADVERSE REACTIONS: Uterine/vaginal bleeding alterations, amenorrhea, intramenstrual bleeding, spotting, abdominal/pelvic pain, ovarian cysts, headache/migraine, acne, depressed/altered mood, menorrhagia, vaginal discharge, IUD expulsion, breast tenderness/pain.

INTERACTIONS: May decrease serum concentrations of progestins with drugs or herbal products that induce enzymes such as CYP3A4 (eg, barbiturates, bosentan, carbamazepine, felbamate, griseofulvin, oxcarbazepine, phenytoin, rifampin, St. John's wort, topiramate). Significant changes (increase or decrease) in serum concentrations of progestin with HIV protease inhibitors, non-nucleoside reverse transcriptase inhibitors. Caution if receiving anticoagulants.

PREGNANCY: Contraindicated in pregnancy. Not for use in nursing.

MECHANISM OF ACTION: Progestogen; not conclusively demonstrated. Thickens cervical mucus (preventing passage of sperm into uterus), inhibits sperm capacitation or survival, and alters endometrium.

PHARMACOKINETICS: Distribution: V_d=1.8L/kg, plasma protein binding (97.5-99%). Found in breast milk. **Metabolism:** Sulfate and glucuronide (lesser extent) conjugates (metabolites). **Excretion:** Urine (45%), feces (32%); $T_{1/2}$=17 hrs.

NURSING CONSIDERATIONS

Assessment: Perform complete medical and social history (including that of partner) and physical exam including a pelvic exam, Pap smear, breast exam and appropriate tests for any other forms of genital or other STDs. Assess for any conditions where treatment is contraindicated or cautioned. Assess for pregnancy/nursing status. Assess for risk factors for infective endocarditis, coagulopathy, migraine, focal migraine with asymmetrical visual loss or other symptoms indicating transient cerebral ischemia, exceptionally severe headache; marked BP increase; jaundice (first time) or with severe arterial disease (eg, stroke or MI) and possible drug interactions. Prior to insertion, determine degree of patency of the endocervical canal and internal os and the direction and depth of the uterine cavity.

Monitoring: Re-examine/evaluate 4-12 weeks after insertion and at least once a year. Monitor for pregnancy, ectopic pregnancy, intrauterine pregnancy, GAS, PID, and other adverse effects. Monitor blood glucose in diabetics and monitor for marked BP increase. During insertion, monitor for decrease pulse, perspiration, or pallor. See if thread is still visible and for length of thread.

Patient Counseling: Drug does not protect against HIV infection (AIDS) and other STDs. Inform of risks/benefits of the drug device. Immediately report any symptoms of PID (eg, unusual vaginal discharge, abdominal/pelvic pain/tenderness, chills) and if partner becomes HIV-positive or acquires an STD. Inform that some bleeding (eg, irregular or prolonged bleeding, spotting) may occur during 1st few weeks; contact healthcare provider if symptoms continue or become severe. Contact healthcare provider if experiencing stroke or heart attack, develops very severe or migraine headaches, unexplained fever, yellowing of skin or whites in the eyes, may be pregnant, pelvic pain or pain during sex, HIV positive, exposed to STDs, unusual vaginal discharge, genital sores, severe or prolonged vaginal bleeding, or cannot feel threads. Instruct how to check after menstrual period that threads still protrude from cervix and caution not to pull on threads and displace drug device. No contraceptive protection exists if device is displaced or expelled.

Administration: Placed in uterine cavity. Refer to PI for insertion instructions. Observe strict asepsis during insertion. Fundal positioning is important. **Storage:** 25°C (77°F); excursions permitted to 15-30°C (59-86°F).

M-M-R II   RX

rubella vaccine live - measles vaccine live - mumps vaccine live (Merck)

THERAPEUTIC CLASS: Vaccine

INDICATIONS: Vaccination against measles, mumps, and rubella in individuals ≥12 months.

DOSAGE: *Adults:* 0.5mL SQ into outer aspect of upper arm.
Pediatrics: 12-15 months: 0.5mL SQ into outer aspect of upper arm. Repeat before elementary school entry. If first vaccinated <12 months of age, repeat dose between 12-15 months and then revaccinate before elementary school entry.

HOW SUPPLIED: Inj: 0.5mL

CONTRAINDICATIONS: Pregnant females; avoid pregnancy for 3 months after vaccination. Anaphylactic/anaphylactoid reactions to neomycin, febrile respiratory illness or other active febrile infection, immunosuppressive therapy (except corticosteroids as replacement therapy), blood dyscrasias, leukemia, lymphoma of any type, malignant neoplasms affecting bone marrow or lymphatic system, primary and acquired immunodeficiency states (including immunosuppressed associated with AIDS, other clinical manifestation of HIV infection, cellular immune deficiencies, hypogammaglobulinemic and dysgammaglobulinemic states), and family history of congenital or hereditary immunodeficiency.

WARNINGS/PRECAUTIONS: Caution with history of cerebral injury, individual or family history of convulsions or any other condition in which stress due to fever should be avoided. Caution with history of anaphylactic/anaphylactoid, or other immediate reactions to egg ingestion; may increase risk of hypersensitivity reactions. Have epinephrine (1:1000) available should an anaphylactic/anaphylactoid reaction occur. May develop severe thrombocytopenia in individuals with current thrombocytopenia. Evaluate serologic status to determine need for additional doses. Ensure that injection does not enter a blood vessel. Excretion of small amounts of the live attenuated rubella virus from the nose or throat 7-28 days after vaccination reported. Avoid with active untreated tuberculosis.

ADVERSE REACTIONS: Atypical measles, fever, syncope, headache, dizziness, malaise, diarrhea, local reactions, N/V, arthralgia, arthritis, pneumonitis, sore throat, Stevens-Johnson syndrome.

INTERACTIONS: See Contraindications. Do not give with immune globulin; may interfere with expected immune response. May be given 1 month before or after administration of other live viral vaccines. Defer vaccination for ≥3 months following administration of immune globulin (human), blood or plasma transfusions. Do not give concurrently with diphtheria, tetanus, pertussis (DTP) and/or oral poliovirus vaccines (OPV). May result in temporary depression of tuberculin skin sensitivity if given individually; administer test either before or simultaneously.

PREGNANCY: Category C, caution in nursing.

MECHANISM OF ACTION: Live virus vaccine; may induce antibodies that protect against measles, mumps, and rubella.

PHARMACOKINETICS: Distribution: Found in breast milk (live attenuated rubella).

NURSING CONSIDERATIONS

Assessment: Assess for immune and current health/medical status, vaccination history, thrombocytopenia, active untreated tuberculosis, conditions where treatment is contraindicated or cautioned, nursing status, and possible drug interactions.

Monitoring: Monitor for anaphylactic/anaphylactoid reactions, thrombocytopenia, vaccine-preventable diseases in HIV patients, and other adverse reactions.

Patient Counseling: Inform of benefits/risks of vaccination. Instruct to report any serious adverse reactions. Inform that pregnancy should be avoided for 3 months after vaccination.

Administration: SQ route. Refer to PI for proper reconstitution and administration procedures. **Storage:** Unreconstituted: -50 to 8°C (-58 to 46°F). Protect from light. Before Reconstitution: 2-8°C (36-46°F). May refrigerate diluent or store separately at room temperature; do not freeze. Reconstituted: 2-8°C (36-46°F), store in a dark place; discard if not used within 8 hrs.

MOBIC

RX

meloxicam (Boehringer Ingelheim)

> NSAIDs may cause an increased risk of serious cardiovascular thrombotic events, myocardial infarction (MI), stroke and serious GI adverse events including bleeding, ulceration, and perforation of the stomach or intestines. Contraindicated for the treatment of perioperative pain in the setting of coronary artery bypass graft (CABG) surgery.

THERAPEUTIC CLASS: NSAID

INDICATIONS: Relief of signs and symptoms of osteoarthritis (OA) and rheumatoid arthritis (RA). Relief of the signs and symptoms of pauciarticular or polyarticular course juvenile rheumatoid arthritis (JRA) in patients ≥2 yrs.

DOSAGE: *Adults:* OA/RA: Initial/Maint: 7.5mg qd. Max: 15mg/day. Severe Renal Impairment/Hemodialysis: Max: 7.5mg qd.
Pediatrics: ≥2 yrs: JRA: 0.125mg/kg qd. Max: 7.5mg/day.

HOW SUPPLIED: Sus: 7.5mg/5mL; Tab: 7.5mg, 15mg

CONTRAINDICATIONS: Aspirin (ASA) or other NSAID allergy that precipitates asthma, urticaria, or allergic-type reactions. Treatment of perioperative pain in the setting of CABG surgery.

WARNINGS/PRECAUTIONS: May lead to onset of new HTN or worsening of pre-existing HTN; monitor BP closely. Fluid retention and edema reported; caution with fluid retention, HTN, or heart failure. Renal papillary necrosis, renal insufficiency, acute renal failure, and other renal injury reported after long-term use. Caution with pre-existing kidney disease, impaired renal function, heart failure, liver dysfunction, asthma, dehydrated patients, and the elderly. Not recommended for use with severe renal impairment (CrCl <20mL/min); if therapy must be initiated, monitor renal function. May cause anaphylactoid reactions and serious skin adverse events (eg, exfoliative dermatitis, Stevens-Johnson syndrome (SJS), toxic epidermal necrolysis (TEN)); d/c if rash or other evidence of hypersensitivity occurs. Avoid with patients with the ASA triad (complex symptom of rhinitis with or without nasal polyps and bronchospasm). Avoid starting at 30 weeks gestation; may cause premature closure of ductus arteriosis. May cause elevation of LFTs; d/c if liver disease develops, or systemic manifestations (eg, eosinophilia, rash) occur. Not a substitute for corticosteroids or for treatment of corticosteroid insufficiency. May mask signs of inflammation and fever. Anemia may occur; with long-term use, monitor Hgb/Hct if symptoms of anemia develop. May inhibit platelet aggregation and prolong bleeding time; monitor patients with coagulation disorders.

ADVERSE REACTIONS: Abdominal pain, diarrhea, dyspepsia, nausea, headache, anemia, arthralgia, insomnia, upper respiratory tract infection, urinary tract infection, dizziness, pain, pharyngitis, rash.

INTERACTIONS: Avoid use with ASA. May diminish antihypertensive effect of ACE inhibitors or angiotensin II antagonists and may cause further deterioration of renal function in patients with compromised renal function. May decrease natriuretic effects of furosemide and thiazides diuretics; monitor for renal failure. Impaired response to thiazides and loop diuretics. May elevate lithium plasma levels; observe for signs of lithium toxicity. May increase cyclosporine and methotrexate toxicities. Increased risk of GI bleeding with anticoagulants (eg, warfarin), smoking, alcohol, and oral corticosteroids.

PREGNANCY: Category C (<30 weeks gestation) and D (≥30 weeks gestation), not for use in nursing.

MECHANISM OF ACTION: NSAIDs; inhibits prostaglandin synthetase resulting in reduced formation of prostaglandins, thromboxanes, and prostacyclin.

PHARMACOKINETICS: Absorption: Absolute bioavailability (89%), C_{max}=1.05mcg/mL, T_{max}=4.9 hrs. **Distribution:** V_d=10L, plasma protein binding (99.4%). **Metabolism:** Liver (extensive); oxidation via CYP2C9 (major), CYP3A4 (minor); 5-carboxy meloxicam (metabolite). **Elimination:** Urine (0.2% unchanged), feces (1.6% unchanged); $T_{1/2}$=20.1 hrs.

M

NURSING CONSIDERATIONS

Assessment: Assess for history of a hypersensitivity reaction to ASA or other NSAIDs, renal/hepatic impairment, pregnancy/nursing status, possible drug interactions, and any other conditions where treatment is contraindicated or cautioned. Assess use in elderly and debilitated patients. Obtain baseline LFTs, renal function, BP, and CBC.

Monitoring: Monitor for signs/symptoms of CV thrombotic events, new onset or worsening pre-existing HTN, GI events (eg, inflammation, bleeding, ulceration, perforation), fluid retention and edema, renal effects (eg, renal papillary necrosis), hepatic effects (eg, jaundice, liver necrosis, liver failure), anaphylactic/anaphylactoid reactions, skin reactions (eg, exfoliative dermatitis, SJS, TEN), hematological effects (eg, anemia, prolongation of bleeding time), and bronchospasm. Monitor BP. Perform periodic monitoring of CBC, renal function, and LFTs.

Patient Counseling: Advise to seek medical attention if symptoms of hepatotoxicity (eg, nausea, fatigue, lethargy, pruritus, jaundice, right upper quadrant tenderness), anaphylactic reaction (eg, difficulty breathing, swelling of face/throat), skin rash, blisters, fever, hypersensitivity reaction (eg, itching), CV events (eg, chest pain, SOB, weakness, slurring of speech), GI ulceration and bleeding (eg, epigastric pain, dyspepsia, melena, hematemesis), weight gain, or edema occur. Avoid starting at 30 weeks gestation. Advise to keep out of reach of children.

Administration: Oral route. (Sus) Shake gently before using. **Storage:** (Tab; Sus): 25°C (77°F); excursions permitted to 15-30°C (59-86°F). Keep tablets in a dry place; dispense in tight container. Keep suspension container tightly closed.

MONODOX   RX
doxycycline monohydrate (Watson)

THERAPEUTIC CLASS: Tetracycline derivative

INDICATIONS: Treatment of Rocky Mountain spotted fever, typhus fever and the typhus group, Q fever, rickettsialpox, ticks fever, respiratory tract infections, urinary tract infections, skin and skin structure infections, inclusion conjunctivitis, uncomplicated urethral/endocervical/rectal infections caused by *C.trachomatis*, nongonococcal urethritis caused by *C.trachomatis* and *U.urealyticum*, relapsing fever, lymphogranuloma, psittacosis, trachoma, tularemia, *campylobacter fetus*, chancroid, plague, cholera, brucellosis, bartonellosis, granuloma inguinale, and anthrax. Treatment of infections caused by *E.coli, Enterobacter aerogenes, Shigella species*, and *Acinetobacter species*. Treatment of uncomplicated gonorrhea, syphilis, yaws, listeriosis, Vincent's infection, actinomycosis, and *Clostridium* species infections when PCN is contraindicated. Adjunct therapy for acute intestinal amebiasis and severe acne.

DOSAGE: *Adults:* Usual: 100mg q12h or 50mg q6h for 1 day, then 100mg/day. Severe Infection: 100mg q12h. Uncomplicated Gonococcal Infections (Except Anorectal Infections in Men): 100mg bid for 7 days or 300mg stat, then repeat in 1 hr. Acute Epididymo-Orchitis caused by *N.gonorrhoeae* or *C.trachomatis*: 100mg bid for at least 10 days. Primary/Secondary Syphilis: 300mg/day in divided doses for at least 10 days. Uncomplicated Urethral/Endocervical/Rectal Infection caused by *C.trachomatis*: 100mg bid for at least 7 days. Nongonococcal Urethritis caused by *C.trachomatis* and *U.urealyticum*: 100mg bid for at least 7 days. Inhalational Anthrax (Post-Exposure): 100mg bid for 60 days. Take with full glass of water. Take with food if GI upset occurs. *Pediatrics:* >8 yrs: ≤100 lbs: 2mg/lb divided in 2 doses for 1 day, then 1mg/lb daily in single or 2 divided doses. Severe Infection: ≤100 lbs: May use up to 2mg/lb/day. >100 lbs: Use usual adult dose. Inhalation Anthrax (Post-Exposure): <100 lbs: 1mg/lb bid for 60 days. ≥100 lbs: 100mg bid for 60 days. Take with full glass of water. Take with food if GI upset occurs.

HOW SUPPLIED: Cap: 50mg, 75mg, 100mg

WARNINGS/PRECAUTIONS: Avoid direct sunlight or UV light. May cause permanent tooth discoloration during tooth development (last half of pregnancy and children <8 years). Enamel hypoplasia reported. Monitor renal/hepatic function, and blood with long-term therapy. A decrease in fibula growth rate may occur if given to prematures. May cause fetal harm. May increase BUN. Photosensitivity, pseudotumor cerebri reported. D/C if superinfection occurs. Bulging fontanels in infants and intracranial HTN in adults reported. *Clostridium difficile*-associated diarrhea (CDAD) reported. Use in the absence of proven or strongly suspected bacterial infection is unlikely to provide benefit and increases the risk of drug resistant bacteria.

ADVERSE REACTIONS: GI effects, photosensitivity, rash, blood dyscrasias, hypersensitivity reactions.

INTERACTIONS: Carbamazepine, barbiturates, phenytoin decrease half-life of doxycycline. May decrease PT; adjust anticoagulants. Avoid concomitant use with PCN. May decrease effects of oral contraceptives. Aluminum-, calcium-, iron-, and magnesium-containing products and bismuth subsalicylate impair absorption. Fatal renal toxicity may occur with methoxyflurane.

PREGNANCY: Category D, not for use in nursing.

MECHANISM OF ACTION: Tetracycline; bacteriostatic, thought to inhibit protein synthesis.

PHARMACOKINETICS: Absorption: C_{max}=3.61mcg/mL; T_{max}=2.6 hrs. **Distribution:** Found in breast milk. **Elimination:** Urine, feces; $T_{1/2}$=16.33 hrs.

NURSING CONSIDERATIONS

Assessment: Assess for renal impairment, pregnancy/nursing status, and for possible drug interactions. In venereal disease, when coexistent syphilis is suspected, perform a dark field examination before treatment.

Monitoring: Monitor for signs/symptoms of hypersensitivity reactions, photosensitivity, superinfection, CDAD, vaginal candidiasis, and benign intracranial HTN. In long-term therapy, perform periodic laboratory evaluation of organ systems, including hematopoietic, renal, and hepatic studies. In venereal disease, when coexistent syphilis is suspected, repeat blood serology for at least four months.

Patient Counseling: Inform of pregnancy risks. Avoid excessive sunlight or artificial UV light and d/c therapy if phototoxicity (eg, skin eruptions) occurs. Wear sunscreen or sunblock. Drink fluids liberally to reduce risk of esophageal irritation or ulceration. Therapy treats bacterial, not viral, infections. Take as directed; skipping doses or not completing full course may decrease effectiveness and increase antibiotic resistance. May experience diarrhea. Notify physician if watery/bloody stools, hypersensitivity reactions, superinfections, or photosensitivity occur.

Administration: Oral route. **Storage**: 20-25°C (68-77°F).

MONOPRIL   RX
fosinopril sodium (Bristol-Myers Squibb)

> ACE inhibitors can cause death/injury to developing fetus during 2nd and 3rd trimesters. D/C therapy if pregnancy detected.

THERAPEUTIC CLASS: ACE inhibitor

INDICATIONS: Treatment of hypertension (HTN), may be used alone or with thiazide diuretics. Adjunct therapy for heart failure (HF).

DOSAGE: *Adults:* HTN: If possible, d/c diuretic 2-3 days before therapy. Initial: 10mg qd, monitor carefully if cannot d/c diuretic. Maint: 20-40mg qd. Resume diuretic if BP not controlled. Max: 80mg qd. HF: Initial: 10mg qd, 5mg with moderate to severe renal failure or vigorous diuresis. Titrate: Increase over several weeks. Maint: 20-40mg qd. Max: 40mg qd. Elderly: Start at low end of dosing range.
Pediatrics >50kg: HTN: 5-10mg qd.

HOW SUPPLIED: Tab: 10mg*, 20mg, 40mg *scored

CONTRAINDICATIONS: History of ACE inhibitor associated angioedema.

WARNINGS/PRECAUTIONS: Head, neck, and intestinal angioedema reported; d/c if laryngeal stridor or angioedema of the face, lips, mucous membranes, tongue, glottis, or extremities occur. Anaphylactoid reactions during desensitization and during membrane exposure reported. Monitor for hypotension in high-risk patients (eg, HF, volume and/or salt depletion, surgery/anesthesia). May cause agranulocytosis; consider monitoring WBCs in patients with collagen vascular disease, especially if associated with renal impairment. Fetal/ neonatal morbidity and death reported. Rarely associated with cholestatic jaundice that progresses to fulminant hepatic necrosis and sometimes death; d/c if jaundice or if marked elevations of hepatic enzymes occur. Caution in patients with impaired liver function. May cause changes in renal function; caution in patients with severe CHF, renal artery stenosis, and in patients with pre-existing renal impairment. May cause hyperkalemia; caution in patients with risk factors for hyperkalemia (eg, diabetes mellitus (DM), renal dysfunction). Persistent non-productive cough reported. Less effective on BP in blacks and more reports of angioedema than nonblacks. Caution in elderly.

ADVERSE REACTIONS: Dizziness, cough, hypotension, musculoskeletal pain, headache, fatigue, diarrhea, N/V.

INTERACTIONS: May increase lithium levels. Hypotension risk with diuretics. Increased risk of hyperkalemia with K+-sparing diuretics (eg, spironolactone, amiloride, triamterene), K+-containing salt substitutes, or K+ supplements. Decreased absorption with antacids; space dosing by 2 hrs. Nitritoid reactions (eg, facial flushing, N/V, hypotension) reported rarely with injectable gold.

PREGNANCY: Category C (1st trimester) and D (2nd and 3rd trimesters), not for use in nursing.

MECHANISM OF ACTION: ACE inhibitor; inhibition results in decreased plasma angiotensin II, which leads to decreased vasopressor activity and decreased aldosterone secretion.

PHARMACOKINETICS: Absorption: Slow; T_{max}=3 hrs. **Distribution:** Plasma protein binding (99.4%); found in breast milk. **Metabolism:** Hepatic; glucuronidation; fosinoprilat (active metabolite). **Elimination:** Urine, feces; (HTN) $T_{1/2}$=11.5 hrs. (HF) $T_{1/2}$=14 hrs.

NURSING CONSIDERATIONS

Assessment: Assess for history of ACE inhibitor associated angioedema. Assess for volume and/or salt depletion, renal artery stenosis, CHF, pregnancy/nursing status, renal/hepatic function, hypersensitivity to drug, and for possible drug interactions. Assess for risk factors for developing hyperkalemia (eg, DM).

Monitoring: Monitor for signs/symptoms of head/neck and intestinal angioedema, anaphylactoid reactions, hypotension, agranulocytosis, hepatic failure, renal impairment, hyperkalemia, and for persistent non-productive cough. Monitor renal function. In patients with collagen vascular disease, consider monitoring WBC count.

Patient Counseling: Inform that angioedema including laryngeal edema can occur; instruct to immediately report to physician and d/c therapy if any signs or symptoms of angioedema (eg, swelling of face, eyes, lips, tongue, extremities; difficulty swallowing or breathing) occur. Lightheadedness may occur, instruct to d/c therapy if syncope occurs until physician has been contacted. Inadequate fluid intake or excessive perspiration, diarrhea, or vomiting can lead to an excessive fall in BP. Avoid using K+ supplements or salt substitutes containing K+ unless physician has been notified. Counsel to report any signs of infection (eg, sore throat, fever). Inform of potential risks of therapy if used during pregnancy.

Administration: Oral route. **Storage:** 25°C (77°F); excursions permitted to 15-30°C (59-86°F). Protect from moisture; keep bottle tightly closed.

MORPHINE SULFATE
morphine sulfate (Various)

> Solution form (100mg/5mL concentration) is indicated for use in opioid-tolerant patients only. Use caution when prescribing, dispensing, and administering to avoid dosing errors due to confusion between different concentrations and between mg and mL, which could result in accidental overdose and death. Ensure the proper dose is communicated and dispensed. Keep out of reach of children. Seek medical help in case of accidental ingestion.

THERAPEUTIC CLASS: Opioid analgesic

INDICATIONS: (Sol/Tab) Relief of moderate to severe acute chronic pain where use of an opioid analgesic is appropriate. (Sol, 100mg/5mL) Relief of moderate to severe acute chronic pain in opioid-tolerant patients.

DOSAGE: *Adults:* Individualize dose. Initial: (Sol) 10-20mg q4h prn for pain. (Tab) 15-30mg q4h prn for pain. Titrate: Based upon the individual patient's response. Use 100mg/5mL only for patients who have already been titrated to a stable analgesic regimen using lower strengths and who can benefit from use of a smaller volume of oral sol; always use the enclosed calibrated oral syringe. Conversion from Parenteral to Oral Morphine Sulfate: Anywhere from 3-6mg to provide pain relief equivalent to 1mg of parenteral morphine. Conversion from Parenteral Oral Non-Morphine Opioids to Oral Morphine Sulfate/Oral Controlled-Release to Oral Morphine Sulfate: Refer to published relative potency information. Close observation and dose adjustment is recommended. Periodically reassess the continued need for opioid analgesic use. Taper dose gradually. Elderly: Start at the low end of dosing range.

HOW SUPPLIED: Sol: 10mg/5mL [5mL, 100mL, 200mL], 20mg/5mL [100mL, 500mL], 100mg/5mL [30mL, 120mL]; Tab: 15mg*, 30mg* *scored

CONTRAINDICATIONS: Diagnosis or suspicion of paralytic ileus, acute or severe bronchial asthma or hypercarbia, respiratory depression in absence or lack of resuscitative equipment.

WARNINGS/PRECAUTIONS: Increased risk of respiratory depression in elderly, debilitated patients, those suffering from conditions accompanied by hypoxia, hypercapnia, or upper airway obstruction. Morphine sulfate is a Schedule II controlled substance with an abuse liability similar to other opioids. Respiratory depression and potential to elevate CSF pressure may be markedly exaggerated in the presence of head injury, other intracranial lesions; may obscure signs of increased intracranial pressure. May cause orthostatic hypotension and syncope; increased risk of hypotension with compromised ability to maintain BP. Avoid in patients with GI obstruction, especially paralytic ileus; may obscure diagnosis of acute abdominal conditions. Caution in patients with biliary tract disease; may cause spasm of the sphincter of Oddi and diminish biliary/pancreatic secretions. Use with caution and in reduced dosages in patients with severe renal/hepatic impairment, Addison's disease, hypothyroidism, prostatic hypertrophy, or urethral stricture, elderly, CNS depression, toxic psychosis, acute alcoholism and delirium tremens; may aggravate or induce seizures. May impair mental/physical abilities.

ADVERSE REACTIONS: Respiratory depression, lightheadedness, dizziness, constipation, somnolence, N/V, sweating.

INTERACTIONS: Caution with CNS depressants (including sedatives, hypnotics, general anesthetics, antiemetics, phenothiazines, TCAs, other opioids, illicit drugs, alcohol); may increase the risk of respiratory depression, hypotension, profound sedation, or coma. May enhance the neuromuscular blocking action of skeletal muscle relaxants. Avoid with mixed agonist/antagonist analgesics (eg, pentazocine, nalbuphine, and butorphanol). Precipitates apnea, confusion, and muscle twitching with cimetidine. Potentiated by MAOIs; allow at least 14 days after stopping MAOIs before initiating treatment. May result in increased risk of urinary retention/severe constipation, which may lead to paralytic ileus with anticholinergics or other medications with anticholinergic activity. Caution with P-glycoprotein (PGP) inhibitors.

PREGNANCY: Category C, not for use in nursing.

M

MECHANISM OF ACTION: Opioid analgesic; precise mechanism unknown. Binds to CNS opiate receptors, producing analgesic effects. Also produces respiratory depression by direct action on brain stem respiratory centers, and depresses cough reflex by direct action on cough center in the medulla.

PHARMACOKINETICS: Absorption: Bioavailability (<40%); C_{max}=78ng/mL (Tab), 58ng/mL (Sol). **Distribution:** V_d=1-6L/kg; plama protein binding (20-35%); crosses placenta; found in breast milk. **Metabolism:** Liver via conjugation; 3- and 6- glucuronide (metabolite). **Elimination:** Urine (10% unchanged), feces (7-10%), bile; $T_{1/2}$=2-15 hrs (IV).

NURSING CONSIDERATIONS

Assessment: Assess for degree of opioid tolerance, level of pain intensity, type of pain, patient's general condition and medical status, or any other conditions where treatment is contraindicated or cautioned. Assess for history of hypersensitivity, pregnancy/nursing status, renal/hepatic function, and possible drug interactions.

Monitoring: Monitor for signs/symptoms of respiratory/CNS depression and development of psychological and physical dependence. Monitor for hypersensitivity reactions.

Patient Counseling: Advise to take only as directed and not to adjust dose without consulting a physician. Inform physician if pregnant, become pregnant, or planning to become pregnant prior to therapy. Taper dose upon d/c. Potential for severe constipation; appropriate laxatives/stool softeners should be initiated. Therapy may produce physical or psychological dependence. Caution against performing hazardous tasks (eg, operating machinery/driving). Avoid alcohol or CNS depressants during therapy. Keep in a secure place out of reach of children.

Administration: Oral route. **Storage:** 15-30°C (59-86°F). Protect from moisture.

MOTRIN RX
ibuprofen (McNeil Consumer)

> NSAIDs may cause an increased risk of serious cardiovascular thrombotic events, myocardial infarction (MI), stroke, and serious GI adverse events including bleeding, ulceration, and perforation of the stomach or intestines. Contraindicated for the treatment of perioperative pain in the setting of coronary artery bypass graft (CABG) surgery.

THERAPEUTIC CLASS: NSAID

INDICATIONS: (Sus, Tab) For the relief of the signs and symptoms of rheumatoid arthritis (RA) and osteoarthritis (OA) and for the treatment of primary dysmenorrhea in adults. (Sus) For the reduction of fever in patients aged 6 months up to 2 yrs of age. For the relief of mild to moderate pain in patients aged 6 months up to 2 yrs of age. For the relief of signs and symptoms of juvenile arthritis (JA) in pediatrics. (Tab) For the relief of mild to moderate pain in adults.

DOSAGE: *Adults:* Pain: 400mg q4-6h prn. Max: 3200mg/day. Dysmenorrhea: 400mg q4h prn. Max: 3200mg/day. RA/OA: 300mg qid or 400mg, 600mg, or 800mg tid or qid. Max: 3200mg/day. If GI complaints occur, take tab with meals or milk.
Pediatrics: Fever: 6 months-2 yrs: 5mg/kg for temp <102.5°F; 10mg/kg if temp ≥102.5°F q6-8h. Max: 40mg/kg/day. Pain: 6 months-2 yrs: 10mg/kg q6-8h. Max: 40mg/kg/day. JA: 30-40mg/kg/day divided into 3 or 4 doses. Milder disease may use 20mg/kg/day.

HOW SUPPLIED: Sus: 100mg/5mL; Tab: 400mg, 600mg, 800mg

CONTRAINDICATIONS: Treatment of perioperative pain in the setting of CABG surgery. Asthma, urticaria, or allergic-type reactions after taking aspirin (ASA) or other NSAIDs.

WARNINGS/PRECAUTIONS: May lead to onset of new HTN or worsening of pre-existing HTN; monitor BP closely. Fluid retention and edema reported; caution in patients with fluid retention or heart failure. Caution with history

. of ulcer disease or GI bleeding. Renal papillary necrosis and other renal injury reported after long-term use. Renal toxicity also reported in patients in whom renal prostaglandins have a compensatory role in the maintenance of renal perfusion; caution with impaired renal function, heart failure, liver dysfunction, and the elderly. Not recommended for use with advanced renal disease; if therapy must be initiated, monitor renal function. Anaphylactoid reactions may occur. May cause serious skin adverse events (eg, exfoliative dermatitis, Stevens-Johnson syndrome, toxic epidermal necrolysis). Avoid in late pregnancy; may cause premature closure of ductus arteriosis. Not a substitute for corticosteroids or for the treatment of corticosteroid insufficiency. May cause elevations of LFTs; d/c if liver disease develops or systemic manifestations occur. Anemia may occur; with long-term use, monitor Hgb/Hct if signs or symptoms of anemia develop. May inhibit platelet aggregation and prolong bleeding time; monitor with coagulation disorders. Caution with asthma and avoid with ASA-sensitive asthma. D/C if visual disturbances occur. Aseptic meningitis with fever and coma reported. Suspension contains sucrose and calories; caution with diabetic patients.

ADVERSE REACTIONS: Anemia, abnormal renal function, dizziness, edema, elevated liver enzymes, abdominal pain, bloating, constipation, diarrhea, dyspepsia, flatulence, heartburn, N/V, pruritus, rashes.

INTERACTIONS: May enhance methotrexate toxicity. May decrease natriuretic effect of furosemide and thiazides. Avoid use with ASA. May decrease lithium clearance; monitor for toxicity. Concomitant use with ACE inhibitors may diminish the antihypertensive effect of ACE inhibitors. Synergistic GI bleeding effects when used concomitantly with warfarin. May increase risk of serious GI bleeding when used concomitantly with oral corticosteroids, anticoagulants, or alcohol. ACE inhibitors and diuretic may increase risk of overt renal decompensation.

PREGNANCY: Category C, not for use in nursing.

MECHANISM OF ACTION: NSAID; suspected to inhibit prostaglandin synthetase.

PHARMACOKINETICS: Absorption: (Tab) Rapid; T_{max}=1-2 hrs. (Sus) **Adults:** C_{max}=19µg/mL; T_{max}=0.79 hrs; AUC=64µg•h/mL. Febrile children: C_{max}= 55µg/mL; T_{max}=0.97 hrs; AUC=155µg•h/mL. **Distribution:** (Sus): Plasma protein binding (>99%). **Adults:** V_d=0.12L/kg; febrile children: V_d=0.2L/kg. **Metabolism:** Hepatic. **Elimination:** Urine. (Tab): $T_{1/2}$=1.8-2 hrs. (Sus): $T_{1/2}$=2 hrs.

NURSING CONSIDERATIONS

Assessment: Assess for history of hypersensitivity reaction to ASA or other NSAIDs, connective tissue diseases, renal/hepatic dysfunction, coagulation disorders, pregnancy/nursing status, possible drug interactions, or any other condition where treatment is contraindicated or cautioned. Assess baseline LFTs, CBC, and renal function. If planning to use sus formulation, assess for DM.

Monitoring: Monitor for signs/symptoms of CV thrombotic events, new onset or worsening of pre-existing HTN, fluid retention and edema, GI events (eg, bleeding, ulceration, perforation), renal effects (eg, renal papillary necrosis), anaphylactoid reactions, skin reactions (eg, exfoliative dermatitis, Stevens-Johnson syndrome, toxic epidermal necrolysis), hepatic effects (eg, jaundice, liver necrosis, hepatic failure), hematological effects (eg, anemia, prolongation of bleeding time), bronchospasm, and for aseptic meningitis. Perform periodic monitoring of BP, CBC, LFTs, and renal function. If using sus formulation, monitor blood glucose levels in patients with DM.

Patient Counseling: Instruct to seek medical attention for symptoms of hepatotoxicity (eg, nausea, fatigue, jaundice), anaphylactic reactions (eg, difficulty breathing, swelling of face/throat), rash, CV events (eg, chest pain, SOB, weakness, slurring of speech), GI ulceration and bleeding (eg, epigastric pain, dyspepsia, melena, hematemesis), and unexplained weight gain or edema. Inform of risks if used during pregnancy.

Administration: Oral route. **Storage:** (Sus) 15-30°C (59-86°F). Shake before use. (Tab) 20-25°C (68-77°F).

MoviPrep

RX

ascorbic acid - sodium ascorbate - polyethylene glycol 3350 - potassium chloride - sodium chloride - sodium sulfate (Salix)

THERAPEUTIC CLASS: Bowel cleanser

INDICATIONS: Cleansing of the colon as a preparation for colonoscopy in adults ≥18 yrs.

DOSAGE: *Adults:* ≥18 yrs: Split-Dose Regimen: 1L over 1 hr (8 oz. q15min) followed by 0.5L of clear liquid the evening prior to colonoscopy, then 1L over 1 hr followed by 0.5L of clear liquid in the morning at least 1 hr prior to colonoscopy. Evening-Only Regimen: Around 6 pm, take 1L over 1 hr (8 oz. q15min), after 1.5 hrs, take 1L over 1 hr. Additionally, take 1L of clear liquid during the evening before colonoscopy.

HOW SUPPLIED: Sol (powder): (PEG 3350-Sodium Sulfate-Sodium Chloride-Potassium Chloride-Ascorbic Acid-Sodium Ascorbate) 100g-7.5g-2.691g-1.015g-4.7g-5.9g

WARNINGS/PRECAUTIONS: Caution with severe ulcerative colitis, ileus, GI obstruction or perforation, gastric retention, toxic colitis, or toxic megacolon. If GI obstruction or perforation is suspected, perform appropriate tests to rule out these conditions before administration. During administration, closely observe patients prone to regurgitation or aspiration or those with impaired gag reflex. D/C temporarily or slow administration if severe bloating, abdominal distention or abdominal pain occurs. Caution with phenylketonurics. Caution with glucose-6-phosphate dehydrogenase (G6PD) deficiency especially with an active infection or with history of hemolysis. Generalized tonic-clonic seizures associated with electrolyte abnormalities (eg, hyponatremia, hypokalemia) rarely reported. Caution with hyponatremia.

ADVERSE REACTIONS: Abdominal distension, anal discomfort, thirst, N/V, abdominal pain, sleep disorder, rigors, hunger, malaise, dizziness, dyspepsia.

INTERACTIONS: Oral medications given within 1 hr of administration may be flushed from GI and may not be absorbed. Caution in G-6-PD deficiency patients taking drugs known to precipitate hemolytic reactions. Caution with drugs that increase the risk of electrolyte abnormalities (eg, diuretics, angiotensin converting enzyme (ACE) inhibitors).

PREGNANCY: Category C, caution in nursing.

MECHANISM OF ACTION: Bowel cleanser; produces watery stool leading to cleansing of colon.

NURSING CONSIDERATIONS

Assessment: Assess for electrolyte abnormalities, seizures, ileus, GI obstruction or perforation, gastric retention, toxic colitis or toxic megacolon, severe ulcerative colitis, phenylketonuria, impaired gag reflex, regurgitation or aspiration tendencies, G6PD deficiency especially with active infection or history of hemolysis, or with concomitant medications which precipitate hemolytic reactions, pregnancy/nursing status, and for possible drug interactions.

Monitoring: Perform baseline and post-colonoscopy lab tests with known or suspected hyponatremia or in patients using concomitant medications that increase the risk of electrolyte abnormalities. Monitor for severe bloating, abdominal distention, or abdominal pain. Monitor for hypersensitivity reactions.

Patient Counseling: Advise to adequately hydrate before, during, and after use. Inform that clear soup and/or plain yogurt may be taken for dinner, finishing evening meal at least 1 hr prior to start of treatment and no solid food should be taken from start of treatment until after the colonoscopy. First bowel movement may occur approximately 1 hr after the start of drug administration, and abdominal bloating and distention may occur before the first bowel movement. Advise that if severe abdominal discomfort or distention occurs, stop drinking temporarily or drink at longer intervals until symptoms disappear.

Administration: Oral route. Empty 1 pouch of A and 1 pouch of B into a glass container. Add 1L of lukewarm water and mix the solution until completely dissolved. May be refrigerated prior to drinking. Do not add additional ingredients (eg, flavoring) to the solution. Repeat procedure for the second liter of the solution. **Storage**: 25°C (77°F); excursions permitted to 15-30°C (59-86°F). When reconstituted, store upright and keep refrigerated. Use within 24 hrs.

MOXEZA   RX
moxifloxacin HCl (Alcon)

THERAPEUTIC CLASS: Fluoroquinolone

INDICATIONS: Treatment of bacterial conjunctivitis caused by susceptible strains of organisms.

DOSAGE: *Adults:* 1 drop bid for 7 days in the affected eye(s).
Pediatrics: ≥4 months: 1 drop bid for 7 days in the affected eye(s).

HOW SUPPLIED: Sol: 0.5% [3mL]

WARNINGS/PRECAUTIONS: For topical ophthalmic use only. Serious and sometimes fatal hypersensitivity reactions reported; d/c and institute appropriate therapy if allergic reaction occurs. Prolonged use may cause overgrowth of nonsusceptible organisms. D/C use and consider alternative therapy if superinfection occurs. Avoid wearing contact lenses when signs/symptoms of bacterial conjunctivitis are present.

ADVERSE REACTIONS: Eye irritation, pyrexia, conjunctivitis.

PREGNANCY: Category C, caution in nursing.

MECHANISM OF ACTION: Fluoroquinolone antibiotic; inhibits topoisomerase II (DNA gyrase) and topoisomerase IV, which are enzymes involved in replication, transcription, repair of bacterial DNA or partitioning of chromosomal DNA during bacterial cell division.

PHARMACOKINETICS: Absorption: AUC=8.17ng•hr/mL. **Distribution:** Presumed to be excreted in breast milk.

NURSING CONSIDERATIONS

Assessment: Assess severity of infection, symptoms, and pregnancy/nursing status.

Monitoring: Monitor for signs/symptoms of hypersensitivity/anaphylactic reactions and other adverse reactions. Monitor for superinfection; examine with magnification (eg, slit lamp biomicroscopy) and fluorescein staining, where appropriate.

Patient Counseling: Advise to avoid touching dropper tip to any surface. D/C medication and contact physician if rash or allergic reaction occurs. Do not wear contact lenses if signs/symptoms of bacterial conjunctivitis are present.

Administration: Ocular route. Do not inject into eye. **Storage:** 2-25°C (36-77°F).

MOZOBIL   RX
plerixafor (Genzyme)

THERAPEUTIC CLASS: Hematopoetic stem cell mobilizer

INDICATIONS: In combination with granulocyte-colony stimulating factor (G-CSF) to mobilize hematopoietic stem cells to the peripheral blood for collection and subsequent autologous transplantation in patients with non-Hodgkin's lymphoma (NHL) and multiple myeloma (MM).

DOSAGE: *Adults:* Begin treatment after patient has received G-CSF qd for 4 days. Administer approximately 11 hrs prior to initiation of apheresis for up to 4 consecutive days. Recommended dose: 0.24mg/kg SQ. Max: 40mg/day. Concomitant G-CSF: Administer 10mcg/kg G-CSF qam for 4 days prior to 1st

M

pm dose of plerixafor and qd prior to apheresis. Moderate and Severe Renal Impairment (CrCl ≤50mL/min): Reduce dose to 0.16mg/kg. Max: 27mg/day.

HOW SUPPLIED: Inj: 20mg/mL [1.2mL]

WARNINGS/PRECAUTIONS: May cause tumor cell mobilization; not intended for use in patients with leukemia. Hematologic changes (eg, leukocytosis and thrombocytopenia) may occur; monitor WBCs and platelet count. Caution in patients with peripheral blood neutrophil counts above 50,000/mcL. May have potential for splenic enlargement; evaluate patients if left upper abdominal pain and/or scapular or shoulder pain reported. May cause fetal harm. Caution in elderly.

ADVERSE REACTIONS: Diarrhea, N/V, flatulence, injection-site reactions, fatigue, arthralgia, headache, dizziness, insomnia.

INTERACTIONS: Coadministration with drugs that reduce renal function or compete for active tubular secretion may increase serum concentrations of plerixafor or the coadministered drug.

PREGNANCY: Category D, not for use in nursing.

MECHANISM OF ACTION: CXCR4 chemokine receptor inhibitor; blocks binding of its cognate ligand, stromal cell-derived factor-1α (SDF-1α).

PHARMACOKINETICS: Absorption: T_{max}=30-60 min. **Distribution:** Plasma protein binding (58%); V_d=0.3L/kg. **Elimination:** Urine (70%); $T_{1/2}$=3-5 hrs.

NURSING CONSIDERATIONS

Assessment: Assess for renal impairment, pregnancy/nursing status and possible drug interactions. Obtain baseline WBC count, neutrophil/platelet count, Hgb/Hct and renal function.

Monitoring: Monitor for splenic enlargement, injection-site reactions, and other adverse reactions. Monitor renal function and hematologic changes (eg, leukocytosis and thrombocytopenia).

Patient Counseling: Counsel about signs/symptoms of potential systemic reactions (eg, urticaria, periorbital swelling, dyspnea, or hypoxia). Notify physician immediately if vasovagal reactions (eg, orthostatic hypotension or syncope), itching, rash or injection-site reaction occurs. Inform that drug may cause GI disorders (eg, diarrhea, N/V, flatulence, abdominal pain). Instruct on how to manage specific GI disorders and to inform healthcare professional if severe events occurs. Advise female patients with reproductive potential to use effective contraceptive methods during therapy. Advise not to become pregnant while on treatment. Notify physician if pregnant/intend to become pregnant and if nursing.

Administration: SQ route. **Storage:** 25°C (77°F); excursions permitted to 15-30°C (59-86°F). For single use only. Discard unused drug after injection.

MS CONTIN
morphine sulfate (Purdue Pharma)

CII

> Indicated for opioid-tolerant patients only. Contains morphine sulfate, a Schedule II controlled substance that has a high potential for abuse and is subject to misuse, addiction, and criminal diversion. 100mg and 200mg tabs are for use in opioid-tolerant patients only; these strengths may cause fatal respiratory depression in non-opioid tolerant patients. Not indicated for use in the management of acute or postoperative pain and is not intended for use as a prn analgesic. Swallow whole. Do not break, chew, dissolve, crush or inject tabs.

THERAPEUTIC CLASS: Opioid analgesic

INDICATIONS: Management of moderate to severe pain when a continuous, around-the-clock opioid analgesic is needed for an extended period of time. Postoperative use if the patient is already receiving the drug prior to surgery or if postoperative pain is expected to be moderate to severe and persist for an extended period of time.

DOSAGE: *Adults:* Individualize dose. Conversion from Immediate-Release Oral Morphine: Give 1/2 of patient's 24-hr requirement q12h or give 1/3 of daily requirement q8h. Conversion from Parenteral Morphine: Initial: Estimates of oral to parenteral potency vary. A dose of oral morphine only 3 times the daily parenteral morphine requirement may be sufficient in chronic settings. Reassess periodically for need of continued around-the-clock therapy. Swallow whole; do not crush, chew, break or dissolve. Elderly: Start at the low end of dosing range.

HOW SUPPLIED: Tab, Controlled-Release: 15mg, 30mg, 60mg, 100mg, 200mg

CONTRAINDICATIONS: Paralytic ileus, respiratory depression in the absence of resuscitative equipment, acute or severe bronchial asthma or hypercarbia.

WARNINGS/PRECAUTIONS: Do not use as a first opioid. May cause respiratory depression; caution with conditions accompanied by hypoxia, hypercapnia, or decreased respiratory reserve such as asthma, COPD or cor pulmonale, severe obesity, sleep apnea, myxedema, kyphoscoliosis, or CNS depression. Avoid with head injury, intracranial lesions, or pre-existing elevated intracranial pressure. May obscure neurologic signs if further increases in intracranial pressure in patients with head injury. May aggravate convulsions with convulsive disorders. May cause severe hypotension; caution in patients with circulatory shock. Caution with severe hepatic/renal dysfunction, adrenocortical insufficiency, coma, toxic psychosis, prostatic hypertrophy, urethral stricture, alcoholism, delirium tremens, and inability to swallow. May cause neonatal withdrawal syndrome. May increase biliary tract pressure; caution with inflammatory or obstructive bowel disorder, acute pancreatitis secondary to biliary tract disease, and in biliary surgery. May cause mental/physical impairment. Avoid abrupt withdrawal. Tolerance and physical dependence may occur. Rare cases of anaphylaxis reported. Does not release morphine continuously over the course of dosing interval. Caution with elderly/debilitated.

ADVERSE REACTIONS: Constipation, lightheadedness, dizziness, sedation, N/V, sweating, dysphoria, euphoria.

INTERACTIONS: Additive depressant effects with other CNS depressants (eg, sedatives, hypnotics, general anesthetics, phenothiazines, tranquilizers, alcohol). Enhances neuromuscular blocking effects and increases respiratory depression with skeletal muscle relaxants. Caution with agonist/antagonist analgesics (eg, pentazocine, nalbuphine, butorphanol, buprenorphine); may reduce analgesic effect or cause withdrawal symptoms. Risk of hypotension with phenothiazines or general anesthetics.

PREGNANCY: Category C, not for use in nursing.

MECHANISM OF ACTION: Opioid analgesic; principal actions are analgesia and sedation. Precise mechanism of analgesic effects not established. Binds to CNS opiate receptors, producing analgesic effects. Also produces respiratory depression by direct action on brain stem respiratory centers, and depresses cough reflex by direct action on cough center in the medulla.

PHARMACOKINETICS: Absorption: (Immediate-release) Bioavailability (50%). **Distribution:** V_d=4L/kg; crosses placental membranes; found in breast milk. **Metabolism:** Liver to glucuronide metabolites, M3G (major metabolite), M6G (active metabolite). **Elimination:** Renal (primary), bile; (IV) $T_{1/2}$=2-4 hrs.

NURSING CONSIDERATIONS

Assessment: Assess for degree of opioid tolerance, previous opioid dose, level of pain intensity, type of pain, patient's general condition and medical status, or any other conditions where treatment is contraindicated or cautioned. Assess for history of hypersensitivity, pregnancy/nursing status, renal/hepatic function, and possible drug interactions.

Monitoring: Monitor for signs/symptoms of respiratory depression, elevation in CSF pressure, hypotension, convulsions, tolerance and physical dependence, and misuse or abuse.

Patient Counseling: Advise that the drug contains morphine and should be taken only as directed. Do not change the dose without consulting physician. Drug is designed to work properly only if swallowed whole. Report episodes of breakthrough pain and adverse experiences. May impair mental and/or physical ability required to perform hazardous tasks (eg, operating machinery/driving). Avoid alcohol or other CNS depressants. Avoid abrupt withdrawal if on medication for more than a few weeks; taper dose. Special care must

M

be taken to avoid accidental ingestion or use by individuals other than the patient for whom it was originally prescribed. Advise to flush unused medication down toilet; has drug abuse potential; protect from theft. May pass empty matrix "ghosts" (tablets) via colostomy or in the stool. Inform physician if pregnant or planning to become pregnant.

Administration: Oral route. **Storage:** 25°C (77°F); excursions permitted between 15-30°C (59-86°F). Dispense in a tight, light-resistant container.

MULTAQ   RX
dronedarone (Sanofi-Aventis)

> Contraindicated in patients with NYHA Class IV heart failure (HF), or NYHA Class II-III HF with a recent decompensation requiring hospitalization or referral to a specialized HF clinic.

THERAPEUTIC CLASS: Class III antiarrhythmic

INDICATIONS: To reduce the risk of cardiovascular (CV) hospitalization in patients with paroxysmal or persistent atrial fibrillation (A-fib) or atrial flutter (A-flutter), with a recent episode of A-fib/A-flutter and associated CV risk factors (eg, age >70, HTN, diabetes, prior cerebrovascular accident, left atrial diameter ≥50mm or left ventricular ejection fraction [LVEF] <40%), who are in sinus rhythm or who will be cardioverted.

DOSAGE: *Adult:* 400mg bid. Take 1 tab with am meal and 1 tab with pm meal.

HOW SUPPLIED: Tab: 400mg

CONTRAINDICATIONS: NYHA Class IV HF or NYHA Class II-III HF with a recent decompensation requiring hospitalization or referral to a specialized HF clinic. 2nd- or 3rd-degree atrioventricular (AV) block or sick sinus syndrome (except when used with a functioning pacemaker), bradycardia <50 bpm, concomitant use of strong CYP3A inhibitors, drugs or herbal products that prolong the QT interval and might increase the risk of torsade de pointes (eg, phenothiazine anti-psychotics, TCAs, certain oral macrolide antibiotics, Class I and III antiarrhythmics), QTc Bazett interval ≥500 msec or PR interval >280 msec, severe hepatic impairment, pregnancy, nursing.

WARNINGS/PRECAUTIONS: Consider d/c or suspending therapy if HF develops or worsens. May induce moderate QTc (Bazett) prolongation; d/c if the QTc Bazett interval is ≥500 msec. Hepatocellular liver injury reported; d/c if suspected and test serum enzymes, AST, ALT, alkaline phosphatase and serum bilirubin. Do not restart therapy in patients without another explanation for the observed liver injury. Increased SrCr levels by about 0.1 mg/dL reported. Premenopausal women who have not undergone hysterectomy/oophorectomy must use effective contraception while on therapy.

ADVERSE REACTIONS: Diarrhea, N/V, abdominal pain, asthenia, bradycardia, rashes, pruritus, eczema, dermatitis, allergic dermatitis, QT prolongation, SrCr increase.

INTERACTIONS: See Contraindications. Hypokalemia/hypomagnesemia may occur with K+-depleting diuretics. Blood levels may be affected by CYP3A inhibitors and inducers. May potentiate electrophysiologic effects with digoxin; reduce digoxin dose by half and monitor levels closely. Calcium channel blockers (CCBs) (eg, verapamil, diltiazem) may potentiate conduction and increase dronedarone exposure. Bradycardia observed with β-blockers. Increased exposure and levels with ketoconazole. Avoid grapefruit juice, rifampin or other CYP3A inducers (eg, phenobarbital, carbamazepine, phenytoin, St. John's wort). May increase simvastatin/simvastatin acid, digoxin, other P-glycoprotein substrates, propranolol, metoprolol and other CYP2D6 substrates (eg, TCAs, SSRIs), and CCB exposure. Concomitant administration may result in a higher exposure to dabigatran. Increased plasma levels of tacrolimus, sirolimus, and other CYP3A substrates; monitor and adjust dosage appropriately. Clinically significant INR elevations with oral anticoagulant and increased S-warfarin exposure by 1.2-fold; monitor INR.

PREGNANCY: Category X, not for use in nursing.

MECHANISM OF ACTION: Benzofuran derivative; not established. Antiarrhythmic properties belong to all 4 Vaughan-Williams classes.

PHARMACOKINETICS: Absorption: Absolute bioavailability (4% no food, 15% with high fat meal); T_{max}=3-6 hrs. **Distribution:** Plasma protein binding (>98%); (IV) V_d=1400L. **Metabolism:** Extensive via CYP3A; N-debutylation, oxidative deamination and direct oxidation; N-debutyl metabolite (active). **Elimination:** Urine (6%, metabolites), feces (84%, metabolites); $T_{1/2}$=13-19 hrs.

NURSING CONSIDERATIONS

Assessment: Assess for recent decompensation, pregnancy/nursing status, possible drug interactions, and conditions where treatment is contraindicated or cautioned. Determine baseline serum K^+ levels.

Monitoring: Monitor for signs or symptoms of new/worsening HF, hepatic injury, bradycardia, and QT interval prolongation. Monitor serum K^+, bilirubin, and SrCr levels. Obtain periodic hepatic serum enzymes, especially during 1st 6 months of therapy.

Patient Counseling: Advise to take with meals and to avoid grapefruit juice. If a dose is missed, take next dose at the regularly scheduled time and do not double the dose. Consult physician if signs/symptoms of worsening HF (eg, acute weight gain, dependent edema, or increasing SOB) or hepatic injury (eg, anorexia, N/V, fever, malaise, fatigue, right upper quadrant pain, jaundice, dark urine, or itching) occurs, or of any history of HF, rhythm disturbance other than A-fib or A-flutter, or predisposing conditions such as uncorrected hypokalemia. Report use of any other prescription, non-prescription medication, or herbal products, particularly St. John's wort. Counsel women of childbearing potential about appropriate contraceptive choices while on therapy.

Administration: Oral route. **Storage:** 25°C (77°F); excursions permitted to 15-30°C (59-86°F).

MYCAMINE RX M

micafungin sodium (Astellas)

THERAPEUTIC CLASS: Glucan synthesis inhibitor

INDICATIONS: Treatment of candidemia, acute disseminated candidiasis, *Candida* peritonitis, abscesses, and esophageal candidiasis. Prophylaxis of *Candida* infections in patients undergoing hematopoietic stem cell transplantation (HSCT).

DOSAGE: *Adults:* Candidemia/Acute Disseminated Candidiasis/*Candida* Peritonitis/Abscesses: 100mg IV qd (usual range 10-47 days). Esophageal Candidiasis: 150mg IV qd (usual range 10-30 days). *Candida* Infection Prophylaxis in HSCT: 50mg IV qd (usual range 6-51 days). Do not mix or co-infuse with other drugs.

HOW SUPPLIED: Inj: 50mg, 100mg

WARNINGS/PRECAUTIONS: Reports of serious hypersensitivity reactions (eg, anaphylaxis, anaphylactoid reactions, shock); d/c drug and administer appropriate treatment. LFT abnormalities reported; monitor for worsening hepatic function. Reports of significant renal dysfunction, acute renal failure, and elevations in BUN and creatinine. Reports of acute intravascular hemolysis, hemolytic anemia and hemoglobinuria.

ADVERSE REACTIONS: Hyperbilirubinemia, neutropenia, headache, rash, phlebitis, N/V, diarrhea, pyrexia, hypokalemia, thrombocytopenia.

INTERACTIONS: Monitor for sirolimus, nifedipine, or itraconazole toxicity; reduce dose if toxicity occurs. May precipitate when mixed or co-infused with other drugs.

PREGNANCY: Category C, caution in nursing.

MECHANISM OF ACTION: Antifungal agent; inhibits the synthesis of 1,3-β-D-glucan, a component of fungal cell walls.

PHARMACOKINETICS: Absorption: IV infusion of variable doses resulted in different parameters. **Distribution:** V_d=0.39L/kg (terminal phase); plasma protein binding (≥99%). **Metabolism:** Metabolized to M-1 (catechol form) by arylsulfatase and further metabolized to M-2 (methoxy form) by catechol-O-methyltransferase. Catalyzed by CYP450 isoenzymes. **Elimination:** Urine and feces (major route).

NURSING CONSIDERATIONS

Assessment: Assess cultures and other diagnostic tests prior to therapy, pregnancy/nursing status, and for possible drug interactions.

Monitoring: Monitor for hypersensitivity and anaphylaxis reaction (shock), LFTs for possible hepatic dysfunction, hepatitis or hepatic failure, elevations in BUN and creatinine, and signs/symptoms of renal dysfunction or acute renal failure. Monitor for hematological effects (hemolysis, hemoglobinuria).

Patient Counseling: Instruct to notify physician if signs/symptoms of hypersensitivity or anaphylaxis reactions, hematological reactions, hepatic complications, or renal complications develop.

Administration: IV infusion. Refer to PI for proper preparation and administration. **Storage:** Unopened vial: 25°C (77°F); excursions permitted to 15-30°C (59-86°F). Reconstituted, diluted infusions: 25°C (77°F) for up to 24 hrs.

MYFORTIC   RX
mycophenolic acid (Novartis)

> Immunosuppression may lead to increased susceptibility to infection and possible development of lymphoma and other neoplasms. Only physicians experienced in immunosuppressive therapy and management of organ transplant recipients should use mycophenolic acid. Women of child-bearing potential must use contraception. Use during pregnancy is associated with increased risks of pregnancy loss and congenital malformations.

THERAPEUTIC CLASS: Inosine monophosphate dehydrogenase inhibitor

INDICATIONS: Prophylaxis of organ rejection in patients receiving allogeneic renal transplants, administered in combination with cyclosporine and corticosteroids.

DOSAGE: *Adults:* 720mg bid (1440mg total daily dose). Elderly: Max: 720mg bid. Take on empty stomach, 1 hr before or 2 hrs after food intake. Swallow tab whole; do not crush, chew, or cut.
Pediatrics: 400mg/m² bid. Max: 720mg bid. BSA 1.19-1.58m²: 1080mg daily dose (3 tabs 180mg or 1 tab 180mg and 1 tab 360mg bid). BSA >1.58m²: 1440mg daily dose (4 tabs 180mg or 2 tabs 360mg bid). BSA <1.19m²: Cannot be accurately administered with current formulations. Take on empty stomach, 1 hr before or 2 hrs after food intake. Swallow tab whole; do not crush, chew, or cut.

HOW SUPPLIED: Tab, Delayed-Release: 180mg, 360mg

WARNINGS/PRECAUTIONS: Risk of lymphomas and other malignancies, particularly of the skin. Avoid sunlight, wear protective clothing and use sunscreen to decrease risk of skin cancer. Increased susceptibility to infections including opportunistic infections (eg, polyomavirus), fatal infections, and sepsis. Polyomavirus infections may produce serious and fatal outcomes including progressive multifocal leukoencephalopathy (PML) and Polyomavirus associated nephropathy (PVAN). Pure red cell aplasia (PRCA) reported. Monitor for blood dyscrasias (eg, neutropenia or anemia); interrupt or reduce dose if blood dyscrasias occur (eg, neutropenia [ANC <1.3x10³/μL] or anemia). Intestinal perforations, GI hemorrhage, gastric ulcers, and duodenal ulcers rarely reported; caution with active serious digestive system disease. Caution in patients with delayed graft function (DGF). Avoid with rare hereditary deficiency of hypoxanthine-guanine phosphoribosyl-transferase (HGPRT) (eg, Lesch-Nyhan and Kelley-Seegmiller syndrome). May cause fetal harm. Must have negative serum/urine pregnancy test sensitivity of at least 25 mIU/mL within 1 week before therapy. Two reliable forms of contraception are required four weeks before therapy, during therapy, and 6 weeks following discontinuation. May have increased levels in patients with severe chronic renal impairment (GFR <25mL/min/1.73m²). Caution in elderly.

ADVERSE REACTIONS: Constipation, diarrhea, leukopenia, N/V, anemia, dyspepsia, CMV infection, urinary tract infection, insomnia, postoperative pain, herpes simplex, herpes zoster, candida.

INTERACTIONS: Avoid concomitant use with azathioprine and mycophenolate mofetil. Reduced efficacy with drugs that interfere with enterohepatic recirculation (eg, cholestyramine) and drugs that bind bile acids (eg, bile acid sequestrants, oral activated charcoal). Decreased effects of live attenuated vaccines; avoid concomitant use. Increased levels of both drugs with acyclovir/ganciclovir. Decreased levels with magnesium- and aluminum-containing antacids; do not administer simultaneously. Decreased effects of oral contraceptives. Cases of PRCA reported with other immunosuppressive agents.

PREGNANCY: Category D, not for use in nursing.

MECHANISM OF ACTION: Inosine monophosphate dehydrogenase inhibitor; inhibits the de novo pathway of guanosine nucleotide synthesis without incorporation to DNA.

PHARMACOKINETICS: Absorption: Absolute bioavailability (72%); T_{max}=1.5-2.75 hrs. **Distribution:** V_d=54L; plasma protein binding (>98%, MPA), (82%, MPAG). **Metabolism:** Glucuronyl transferase (mycophenolic acid glucuronide, major metabolite). **Elimination:** Urine (>60% MPAG, 3% unchanged MPA), bile; $T_{1/2}$=8-16 hrs (MPA), 13-17 hrs (MPAG).

NURSING CONSIDERATIONS

Assessment: Assess for hepatic/renal impairment, inherited deficiency of HGPRT (eg, Lesch-Nyhan and Kelley-Seegmiller syndromes), pregnancy/nursing status, and for possible drug interactions.

Monitoring: Monitor for signs of delayed graft rejection, lymphomas, skin cancer, GI bleeding/perforation, infections (eg, sepsis, PML), PVAN, and for blood dyscrasias (eg, neutropenia, anemia). Monitor CBC weekly during the 1st month, twice monthly for the 2nd and 3rd months, and then monthly through 1st year.

Patient Counseling: Counsel to take on an empty stomach (1 hr before or 2 hrs after food intake) and to swallow tab whole; do not crush, chew, or cut. Instruct to avoid prolonged exposure to sunlight and UV light by wearing protective clothing and using sunscreen. Inform that use in pregnancy is associated with an increased risk of 1st trimester pregnancy loss and birth defects; instruct to use effective contraception (two methods) 4 weeks prior, during therapy, and for 6 weeks after d/c. Advise that periodic laboratory tests need to be performed. Inform about increased risk for malignancies, lymphoproliferative disease, and infections.

Administration: Oral route. Swallow tab whole; do not crush, chew, or cut. **Storage:** 25°C (77°F); excursions permitted to 15-30°C (59-86°F). Protect from moisture.

MYLERAN   RX
busulfan (GlaxoSmithKline)

> Do not use unless CML diagnosis is established. May induce severe bone marrow hypoplasia; reduce dose or d/c if unusual depression of bone marrow function occurs.

THERAPEUTIC CLASS: Alkylating agent

INDICATIONS: Palliative treatment of chronic myelogenous leukemia (CML).

DOSAGE: *Adults:* 60mcg/kg/day or 1.8mg/m²/day. Reserve dose >4mg/day for the most compelling symptoms. Remission Induction: Range: 4-8mg/day. *Pediatrics:* 60mcg/kg/day or 1.8mg/m²/day. Reserve dose >4mg/day for the most compelling symptoms.

HOW SUPPLIED: Tab: 2mg

CONTRAINDICATIONS: Lack of definitive diagnosis of CML.

WARNINGS/PRECAUTIONS: Induction of bone marrow failure resulting in severe pancytopenia reported. Bronchopulmonary dysplasia with pulmonary fibrosis, cellular dysplasia, malignant tumors, acute leukemias, hepatic veno-occlusive disease reported. Ovarian suppression and amenorrhea with menopausal symptoms have occurred. Cardiac tamponade in patients with thalassemia and seizures reported. Caution with compromised bone marrow reserve from prior irradiation/chemotherapy. Seizures reported.

ADVERSE REACTIONS: Myelosuppression, pulmonary fibrosis, cardiac tamponade, hyperpigmentation, weakness, fatigue, weight loss, N/V, melanoderma, hyperuricemia, myasthenia gravis, hepatic veno-occlusive disease.

INTERACTIONS: Additive myelosuppression with myelosuppressive drugs. Additive pulmonary toxicity with cytotoxic drugs. Increased clearance of cyclophosphamide and busulfan with phenytoin pretreatment. Decreased clearance with concomitant cyclophosphamide alone. Reduced clearance with itraconazole; monitor for signs of toxicity. Concurrent thioguanine was associated with portal HTN and esophageal varices with abnormal LFTs; caution with long-term therapy.

PREGNANCY: Category D, not for use in nursing.

MECHANISM OF ACTION: Bifunctional alkylating agent.

PHARMACOKINETICS: Absorption: (IV, PO) Absolute bioavailability (adults 80%, children 68%); C_{max}(2mg, 4mg)=30ng/mL, 68ng/mL; T_{max}=0.9 hrs; AUC (4mg) =269ng•hr/mL **Distribution**: Plasma protein binding (32%); crosses blood-brain barrier. **Metabolism**: Liver (extensive); 3-hydroxytetrahydrothiophene-1, 1-dioxide (major metabolite). **Elimination**: Urine (>2% unchanged); $T_{1/2}$=2.69 hrs.

NURSING CONSIDERATIONS

Assessment: Assess for chronic myelogenous leukemia, history of seizure disorder, head trauma, if receiving other potentially epilepteogenic drugs, pregnancy/nursing status. Note other diseases/conditions and drug therapies.

Monitoring: Periodically measure serum transaminases, alkaline phosphatase, and bilirubin for early detection of hepatotoxicity, and evaluate weekly Hgb/Hct, total WBC count and differential, quantitative platelet count, and bone marrow exam for evaluation of marrow status. Monitor for signs/symptoms of busulfan toxicity and bronchopulmonary dysplasia with pulmonary fibrosis, secondary malignancies, chromosomal aberrations.

Patient Counseling: Counsel about need for periodic blood counts and to report unusual bleeding, fever, breathing difficulty, anorexia, weight loss, or melanoderma.

Administration: Oral route. **Storage**: 25°C (77°F); excursions permitted to 15-30°C (59-86°F).

NABI-HB

RX

hepatitis B immune globulin (Biotest)

THERAPEUTIC CLASS: Vaccine

INDICATIONS: Treatment for acute exposure to blood containg HBsAg, perinatal exposure of infants born to HBsAg-positive mothers, sexual exposure to HBsAg-positive persons, and household exposure to persons with acute HBV infection.

DOSAGE: *Adults:* Acute Exposure to Blood Containing HBsAg: 0.06mL/kg IM after exposure and within 24 hrs. Sexual Exposure to HBsAg-Positive Person(s): 0.06mL/kg IM (single dose) and start hepatitis B vaccine series within 14 days of the last sexual contact or if sexual contact with the infected person will continue. Refer to PI for recommendations for hepatitis B prophylaxis following percutaneous or permucosal exposure.
Pediatrics: Prophylaxis of Infant to HBsAg-Positive Mother: 0.5mL IM within 12 hrs. Prophylaxis of Infant (<12 months) Exposed to Mother or Caregiver with Acute HBV-Infection: 0.5mL IM. Refer to PI for recommended schedule of hepatitis B immunoprophylaxis to prevent perinatal transmission.

HOW SUPPLIED: Inj: >312 IU [1mL]; >1560 IU [5mL]

CONTRAINDICATIONS: Anaphylactic or severe systemic reaction to human globulin or IgA-deficiency disorder.

WARNINGS/PRECAUTIONS: Caution in patients with severe thrombocytopenia or coagulation disorder that contraindicate IM administration; give only if expected benefits outweigh the potential risks. Products made from human plasma may contain infectious agents and cause disease. Must be administered intramuscularly.

ADVERSE REACTIONS: Headache, erythema, myalgia, malaise, nausea, injection-site pain, elevated alkaline phosphatase levels.

INTERACTIONS: May interfere with live virus vaccines; defer until 3 months following the last dose of vaccine.

PREGNANCY: Category C, caution in nursing.

MECHANISM OF ACTION: Vaccine; passive immunization from HBV exposure resulting in reduction of HBV infection rate.

PHARMACOKINETICS: Absorption: T_{max}=6.5 days. **Distribution:** V_d=11.2L. **Excretion:** $T_{1/2}$=23.1 days.

NURSING CONSIDERATIONS

Assessment: Assess HBsAg/HBeAg, thrombocytopenia, coagulation disorder, IgA-deficiency, previous history of severe anaphylactic or systemic reaction to human globulin, live virus vaccination, and pregnancy/nursing status. Assess for acute exposure to blood of HBsAg-positive mothers, sexual contact with HBsAg-positive persons, and household persons with acute HBV infection.

Monitoring: Monitor for erythema, headache, myalgia, malaise, nausea, and elevated alkaline phosphatase levels.

Patient Counseling: Advise to avoid live virus vaccination for 3 months after hepatitis B immune globulin administration; revaccinate persons immediately after live virus administration.

Administration: IM administration only for post-exposure prophylaxis. Preferred sites are anterolateral aspect of the upper thigh and deltoid muscle. **Storage:** 2-8°C (36-46°F). Do not freeze. Use within 6 hrs once opened; do not reuse or save for future use and partially used vials should be discarded.

NABUMETONE   RX
nabumetone (Various)

> NSAIDs may cause an increased risk of serious cardiovascular (CV) thrombotic events, myocardial infarction (MI), stroke and serious GI adverse events including bleeding, ulceration, and perforation of the stomach or intestines. Contraindicated for the treatment of perioperative pain in the setting of coronary artery bypass graft (CABG) surgery.

THERAPEUTIC CLASS: NSAID

INDICATIONS: Relief of signs and symptoms of osteoarthritis and rheumatoid arthritis.

DOSAGE: *Adults:* Initial: 1000mg qd with or without food. Titrate: May give 1500-2000mg depending on clinical response to initial therapy. Max: 2000mg/day given qd-bid. Renal impairment: Moderate: Initial : ≤750mg qd. Severe: Initial: ≤500mg qd.

HOW SUPPLIED: Tab: 500mg, 750mg

CONTRAINDICATIONS: History of asthma, urticaria, or allergic-type reactions after taking aspirin (ASA) or other NSAIDs. Treatment of perioperative pain in the setting of CABG surgery.

WARNINGS/PRECAUTIONS: Use lowest effective dose for shortest duration possible to minimize risk for CV events and adverse GI events. May lead to onset of new HTN or worsening of pre-existing HTN; Caution with HTN and monitor BP closely. Fluid retention and edema reported; caution with fluid retention or heart failure. Renal papillary necrosis and other renal injury reported after long-term use. Not recommended for use with advanced renal disease; if therapy must be initiated, monitor renal function closely.

Anaphylactoid reactions may occur. Should not be given with ASA triad. May cause serious skin adverse events (eg, exfoliative dermatitis, Stevens-Johnson syndrome, and toxic epidermal necrolysis). Avoid in late pregnancy; may cause premature closure of ductus arteriosus. May cause elevations of LFTs; d/c if liver disease develops or systemic manifestations occur. Caution in elderly. Anemia may occur; with long-term use, monitor Hgb/Hct if signs or symptoms of anemia develop. May inhibit platelet aggregation and prolong bleeding time; monitor with coagulation disorders. Caution with asthma and avoid with ASA-sensitive asthma. May induce photosensitivity.

ADVERSE REACTIONS: Diarrhea, dyspepsia, abdominal pain, constipation, flatulence, N/V, positive stool guaiac, dizziness, headache, pruritus, rash, tinnitus, edema.

INTERACTIONS: Caution with warfarin and other protein bound drugs. May decrease natriuretic effect of furosemide and thiazides; possible renal failure risk. May elevate lithium and methotrexate levels. May diminish antihypertensive effect of ACE inhibitors. Avoid concomitant ASA. May increase risk of GI bleeding with concomitant use of oral corticosteroids, anticoagulants or alcohol.

PREGNANCY: Category C, not for use in nursing.

MECHANISM OF ACTION: NSAID (naphthylalkanone derivative); suspected to inhibit prostaglandin synthesis, exerts anti-inflammatory, analgesic, and antipyretic actions.

PHARMACOKINETICS: Absorption: Well-absorbed (GIT). PO administration of variable doses resulted in different parameters. **Distribution:** Plasma protein binding (>99%). **Metabolism:** Liver (extensive biotransformation), 6-methoxy-2-naphthylacetic acid (active metabolite). **Elimination:** Urine (approximately 80%), feces (9%); $T_{1/2}$=24 hrs.

NURSING CONSIDERATIONS

Assessment: Assess LFTs, renal function, CBC and coagulation profile. Assess for history of CABG surgery, asthma and allergic reactions to ASA or other NSAIDs, active ulceration or chronic inflammation of GI tract, CVD, asthma, alcohol intake, pregnancy/nursing status. Note other diseases/conditions and drug therapies.

Monitoring: Monitor for hypersensitivity reactions, CV thrombotic events, MI, stroke, GI bleeding, asthma, skin adverse effects. Monitor BP, LFTs, renal function, CBC with differential and platelet count, coagulation profile, ocular effects, photosensitivity.

Patient Counseling: Counsel about potential side effects; seek medical attention if any develop, especially serious CV events or adverse GI events. Counsel about possible drug interactions. Take as prescribed. Advise women not to use in late pregnancy.

Administration: Oral route. **Storage:** 20-25°C (68-77°F). Dispense in tight, light-resistant container.

NADOLOL   RX
nadolol (Various)

OTHER BRAND NAMES: Corgard (King)

THERAPEUTIC CLASS: Nonselective beta-blocker

INDICATIONS: Long-term management of angina pectoris. Management of hypertension; may be used alone or in combination with other antihypertensive agents, especially thiazide type diuretics.

DOSAGE: *Adults:* Angina Pectoris: Initial: 40mg qd. Titrate: Increase by 40-80mg q 3-7 days until optimum response achieved or slowing of HR occurs. Usual Maintenance Dose: 40 or 80mg qd. Max: 240mg/day. HTN: Initial: 40mg qd. Titrate: Increase in 40-80mg increments. Usual Maintenance Dose: 40 or 80mg qd. Max: 320mg/day. Renal Dysfunction: CrCl >50mL/min: Dose q24h. CrCl 31-50mL/min: Dose q24-36h. CrCl 10-30mL/min: Dose q24-48h. CrCl <10mL/min: Dose q40-60h.

HOW SUPPLIED: Tab: 20mg*, 40mg*, 80mg* *scored

CONTRAINDICATIONS: Bronchial asthma, sinus bradycardia and >1st-degree conduction block, cardiogenic shock, overt cardiac failure.

WARNINGS/PRECAUTIONS: May lead to incidence or worsening of cardiac failure. Exacerbation of angina, myocardial infarction reported upon abrupt discontinuation of therapy. Avoid in patients with bronchospastic disease. Impairs ability of heart to respond to β-adrenergically mediated stimuli and may increase the risk of general anesthesia and surgical procedures; therapy should be wtihdrawn several days prior to surgery. May prevent appearance of signs and symptoms of acute hypoglycemia (eg, tachycardia, and BP changes). May mask clinical signs of hyperthyroidism; may precipitate thyroid storm with abrupt withdrawal. Caution in elderly and patients with renal dysfunction.

ADVERSE REACTIONS: Dizziness, fatigue, nausea, diarrhea, anorexia, abdominal discomfort, rash, pruritus, weight gain, blurred vision, peripheral vascular insufficiency, cardiac failure, rhythm/conduction disturbances.

INTERACTIONS: Additive hypotension and/or bradycardia with catecholamine-depleting drugs (eg, reserpine) and digitalis glycoside. Reduces insulin release in response to hyperglycemia and may prevent premonitory signs/symptoms of acute hypoglycemia; adjust antidiabetic agents accordingly. General anesthetics may exaggerate hypotension. May reduce effects of epinephrine.

PREGNANCY: Category C, not for use in nursing.

MECHANISM OF ACTION: Nonselective β-blocker; has not been established. Suspected to competitively antagonize catecholamines at peripheral adrenergic neuron sites, leading to decreased cardiac output; a central effect leading to reduced sympathetic outflow to the periphery; and suppression of renin activity.

PHARMACOKINETICS: Absorption: T_{max}=3-4 hrs. **Distribution:** Plasma protein binding (30%). **Elimination:** Urine (unchanged); $T_{1/2}$=20-24 hrs.

NURSING CONSIDERATIONS

Assessment: Assess for bronchial asthma, sinus bradycardia, AV block, cardiogenic shock, CHF, bronchospastic disease, CAD, hyperthyroidism, DM, renal impairment, possible drug interactions, pregnancy/nursing status.

Monitoring: Monitor renal function periodically. Monitor for signs/symptoms of cardiac failure, hypoglycemia, thyrotoxicosis, withdrawal symptoms, renal dysfunction, and hypersensitivity reactions.

Patient Counseling: Warn against interruption or d/c of therapy without consulting physician. Inform drug may mask signs of thyrotoxicosis and hypoglycemia. Advise to seek medical attention if symptoms of heart failure, withdrawal (angina, tremulousness, sweating, headache) or hypersensitivity reactions occur.

Administration: Oral route. **Storage:** 20-25°C (68-77°F). Protect from light. Dispense in a tight, light-resistant container.

NAMENDA   RX
memantine HCl (Forest)

OTHER BRAND NAMES: Namenda XR (Forest)

THERAPEUTIC CLASS: NMDA receptor antagonist

INDICATIONS: Treatment of moderate to severe dementia of the Alzheimer's type.

DOSAGE: *Adults:* (Sol, Tab) Initial: 5mg qd. Titrate: Increase at intervals ≥1 week in 5mg increments to 10mg/day (5mg bid), 15mg/day (5mg and 10mg as separate doses), and 20mg/day (10mg bid). Severe Renal Impairment: (CrCl 5-29mL/min): Target Dose: 5mg bid. (Cap, ER) Initial: 7mg qd. Titrate: Increase at intervals ≥1 week in 7mg increments to 28mg qd. Max: 28mg qd. Severe Renal Impairment (CrCl 5-29mL/min): Target dose: 14mg/day. Switching from Tabs to ER, Caps: Switch from 10mg bid tabs to 28mg qd caps the day following last dose of 10 mg tab. Severe Renal Impairment: Switch from 5mg bid tabs to 14mg qd caps the day following last dose of 5mg tab. Swallow caps intact or may be opened, sprinkled on applesauce. Do not divide, chew or crush.

HOW SUPPLIED: Sol: 2mg/mL [360mL]; Tab: 5mg, 10mg; Titration-Pak: 5mg [28's], 10mg [21's]. Cap, Extended-Release: 7mg, 14mg, 21mg, 28mg.

WARNINGS/PRECAUTIONS: Use not evaluated with seizure disorders. Conditions that raise urine pH may decrease the urinary elimination resulting in increased plasma levels. Caution in patients with severe hepatic impairment. Consider dose reduction with severe renal impairment.

ADVERSE REACTIONS: Dizziness, headache, constipation, confusion, HTN, coughing, somnolence, hallucination, vomiting, back pain, pain, diarrhea.

INTERACTIONS: Caution with other NMDA antagonists (eg, amantadine, ketamine, dextromethorphan), urinary alkalinizers (eg, carbonic anhydrase inhibitors, sodium bicarbonate). Drugs eliminated via renal (cationic system) mechanism, including HCTZ, triamterene, metformin, cimetidine, ranitidine, quinidine, nicotine, may alter levels of both agents.

PREGNANCY: Category B, caution in nursing.

MECHANISM OF ACTION: NMDA receptor antagonist; postulated to exert its therapeutic effect through its action as a low to moderate affinity uncompetitive (open-channel) NMDA receptor antagonist which binds preferentially to the NMDA receptor-operated cation channels.

PHARMACOKINETICS: Absorption: (Sol, Tab) T_{max}=3-7 hrs. (Cap, ER) T_{max}=9-12 hrs. **Distribution**: V_d=9-11L/kg. Plasma protein binding (45%). **Metabolism**: Liver (partial); N-glucuronide conjugate, 6-hydroxy memantine, 1-nitroso-deaminated memantine (metabolites). **Elimination**: Urine (48%, unchanged); $T_{1/2}$=60-80 hrs.

NURSING CONSIDERATIONS

Assessment: Assess for conditions that raise urine pH, presence of a seizure disorder, renal/hepatic impairment, pregnancy/ nursing status, and for possible drug interactions.

Monitoring: Monitor renal/hepatic function and for adverse events.

Patient Counseling: (Cap, ER; Sol; Tab) Instruct to take as prescribed. Inform about possible side effects associated with therapy and instruct to notify physician if any develop. (Cap, ER) Instruct to swallow cap whole or inform that cap may be opened and sprinkled on applesauce and the entire contents should be consumed. Inform that caps should not be divided, chewed, or crushed and can be taken with/without food.

Administration: Oral route. Refer to PI for instructions for oral solution.
Storage: 25°C (77°F); excursions permitted to 15-30°C (59-86°F).

NAPRELAN   RX
naproxen sodium (Elan)

> NSAIDs may cause an increased risk of serious cardiovascular (CV) thrombotic events, myocardial infarction (MI), stroke, and serious GI adverse events including bleeding, ulceration, and perforation of the stomach or intestines. Contraindicated for the treatment of perioperative pain in the setting of coronary artery bypass graft (CABG) surgery.

THERAPEUTIC CLASS: NSAID

INDICATIONS: Treatment of rheumatoid arthritis (RA), osteoarthritis (OA), ankylosing spondylitis (AS), tendinitis, bursitis, primary dysmenorrhea, and acute gout. Relief of mild to moderate pain.

DOSAGE: *Adults:* RA/OA/AS: Initial: 750mg-1g qd. Max: 1.5g/day. Pain/ Primary Dysmenorrhea/Tendinitis/Bursitis: 1g/day or 1.5g for a limited period. Max: 1g/day thereafter. Acute Gout: Initial: 1-1.5g qd for 1 day, Maint: 1g qd until attack subsides. Elderly/Renal/Hepatic Impairment: Start at lower end of dosing range.

HOW SUPPLIED: Tab, Controlled-Release: 375mg, 500mg, 750mg

CONTRAINDICATIONS: History of asthma, urticaria, allergic/anaphylactic type reactions with aspirin (ASA), or other NSAIDs. Treatment of perioperative pain in the setting of CABG surgery.

WARNINGS/PRECAUTIONS: Patients with known CV disease or risk factors for CV disease may be at greatest risk for thrombotic events, MI, or stroke; use lowest effective dose for the shortest duration possible. May lead to onset of new HTN or worsening of pre-existing HTN; monitor BP closely. Caution in patients with fluid retention or heart failure. Renal papillary necrosis and other renal injury reported after long-term use. Not recommended for use with advanced renal disease; if therapy must be initiated, monitor renal function. Anaphylactoid reactions may occur. May cause serious skin adverse events (eg, exfoliative dermatitis, Stevens-Johnson syndrome (SJS), and toxic epidermal necrolysis (TEN)). Avoid in late pregnancy; may cause premature closure of ductus arteriosis. May cause elevations of LFTs; d/c if liver disease develops or systemic manifestations occur. Caution in elderly. Anemia may occur; monitor Hgb/Hct if signs or symptoms of anemia develop with long-term use. May inhibit platelet aggregation and prolong bleeding time; monitor with coagulation disorders. Caution with asthma and avoid with ASA-sensitive asthma. Not intended to substitute for corticosteroids or treat corticosteroid insufficiency.

ADVERSE REACTIONS: Headache, dyspepsia, flu syndrome, pain, infection, nausea, diarrhea, constipation, tinnitus, heartburn, drowsiness, edema, skin rash, ecchymoses, pharyngitis.

INTERACTIONS: Avoid concomitant use with other products containing naproxen and ASA. May inhibit natriuretic effect of furosemide and thiazides. May diminish antihypertensive effect of angiotensin converting enzyme (ACE) inhibitors. May increase lithium levels; monitor for lithium toxicity. May enhance methotrexate toxicity. Synergistic effect with warfarin.

PREGNANCY: Category C, not for use in nursing.

MECHANISM OF ACTION: NSAID; not fully established, suspected to inhibit prostaglandin synthetase.

PHARMACOKINETICS: Absorption: Rapid, complete; bioavailability (95%); C_{max}=94mcg/mL; T_{max}=5 hrs; AUC=1448mcg•hr/mL. **Distribution:** V_d=0.16L/kg; plasma protein binding (>99%). **Metabolism:** Hepatic; 6-O-desmethyl naproxen (metabolite). **Elimination:** Urine, feces (≤5%); $T_{1/2}$=15 hrs.

NURSING CONSIDERATIONS

Assessment: Assess for CVD (HTN, CHF) or risk factors for disease, history of ulcer disease, asthma, pregnancy/nursing status, risk factors for GI events (bleeding, ulceration, perforation), possible drug interactions, renal and hepatic dysfunction.

Monitoring: Monitor BP, CBC, LFTs, renal function, and blood chemistries periodically. Monitor for signs/symptoms of GI events (bleeding, ulceration, perforation), hypersensitivity reaction (eosinophilia, rash), renal/liver dysfunction.

Patient Counseling: Advise to seek medical attention if symptoms of hepatotoxicity (eg, nausea, fatigue, lethargy, pruritus, jaundice, right upper quadrant tenderness, and flu-like symptoms), anaphylactic reaction (difficulty breathing, swelling of face/throat), hypersensitivity reaction (eg, rash, blisters, itching), fever, exfoliative dermatitis, SJS, TEN, CV events (eg, MI, stroke, chest pain, SOB, weakness, slurring of speech), GI ulceration and bleeding (eg, epigastric pain, dyspepsia, melena, hematemesis), weight gain, or edema occur. Inform of pregnancy risks.

Administration: Oral route. **Storage:** 20-25°C (68-77°F).

NAPROSYN   RX
naproxen (Roche Labs)

> NSAIDs may cause an increased risk of serious cardiovascular thrombotic events, MI, stroke, and serious GI adverse events including bleeding, ulceration, and perforation of the stomach or intestines. Contraindicated for the treatment of perioperative pain in the setting of coronary artery bypass graft (CABG) surgery.

OTHER BRAND NAMES: EC-Naprosyn (Roche Labs)

THERAPEUTIC CLASS: NSAID

INDICATIONS: (Naprosyn, EC-Naprosyn) Relieves signs and symptoms of rheumatoid arthritis (RA), osteoarthritis (OA), ankylosing spondylitis, and juvenile arthritis (JA). (Naprosyn) Relieves signs and symptoms of tendinitis, bursitis, and acute gout. Management of pain and primary dysmenorrhea. EC-Naprosyn not recommended for initial treatment of acute pain.

DOSAGE: *Adults:* RA/OA/Ankylosing Spondylitis: Naprosyn: 250, 375, or 500mg bid; EC-Naprosyn: 375 or 500mg bid. Max: 1500mg/day. Acute Gout: Naprosyn: 750mg followed by 250mg q8h until attack subsides. Pain/Dysmenorrhea/Tendinitis/Bursitis: Naprosyn: 500mg followed by 500mg q12h or 250mg q6-8h prn. EC-Naprosyn should not be chewed, crushed, or broken.
Pediatrics: ≥2 yrs: JA: (Sus) 5mg/kg bid. Max: 10mg/kg/day.

HOW SUPPLIED: (Naprosyn) Sus: 25mg/mL; Tab: 250mg*, 375mg, 500mg*; (EC-Naprosyn) Tab, Delayed-Release: 375mg, 500mg *scored

CONTRAINDICATIONS: Asthma, urticaria, or other allergic-type reactions with aspirin (ASA) or other NSAIDs. Treatment of perioperative pain in the setting of CABG surgery.

WARNINGS/PRECAUTIONS: May lead to onset of new HTN or worsening of pre-existing HTN; monitor BP closely. Fluid retention, edema, and peripheral edema reported; caution with fluid retention, HTN, or heart failure. Renal papillary necrosis and other renal injury reported after long-term use. Not recommended for use with advanced renal disease; if therapy must be initiated, monitor renal function closely. Anaphylactoid reactions may occur. May cause serious skin adverse events (eg, exfoliative dermatitis, Stevens-Johnson syndrome, toxic epidermal necrolysis). Avoid in late pregnancy; may cause premature closure of ductus arteriosis. Monitor for visual changes or disturbances. May cause elevations of LFTs; d/c if liver disease develops or systemic manifestations occur. Caution with high doses in chronic alcoholic liver disease and elderly. Anemia may occur with long-term use; monitor Hgb/Hct if signs or symptoms of anemia develop or if initial Hgb ≤10g. May inhibit platelet aggregation and prolong bleeding time; monitor with coagulation disorders. Caution with asthma and avoid with ASA-sensitive asthma.

ADVERSE REACTIONS: Edema, drowsiness, dizziness, constipation, heartburn, abdominal pain, nausea, headache, tinnitus, dyspnea, pruritus, skin eruptions, ecchymoses.

INTERACTIONS: (Naprosyn, EC-Naprosyn) Avoid with other products containing naproxen. Potential for increased effects with ASA. May reduce tubular secretion of methotrexate; monitor for toxicity. May increase nephrotoxicity of cyclosporine; caution with coadministration. May diminish antihypertensive effect and potentiate renal disease with ACE inhibitors. May reduce natriuretic effect of furosemide and thiazides; monitor for renal failure. May increase lithium levels; monitor for toxicity. Increased risk of GI bleeding with SSRIs. Synergistic effects on GI bleeding with warfarin. Observe for dose adjustment with hydantoins, sulfonamides, or sulfonylureas. May reduce antihypertensive effects of propranolol and other β-blockers. Probenecid increases half-life significantly. (EC-Naprosyn) Avoid with H_2-blockers, sucralfate, or intensive antacid therapy.

PREGNANCY: Category C, not for use in nursing.

MECHANISM OF ACTION: NSAID; unknown, related to prostaglandin synthetase inhibition.

PHARMACOKINETICS: Absorption: Rapid and complete. Bioavailability (95%), C_{max}=97.4mcg/mL; T_{max}=2-4 hrs; AUC_{0-12h}=767mcg•hr/mL. (Tab, Delayed-Release) C_{max}=94.9mcg/mL; T_{max}=4 hrs; AUC_{0-12h}=845mcg•hr/mL. (Sus) T_{max}=1-4 hrs. **Distribution:** V_d=0.16L/kg; plasma protein binding (>99%). **Metabolism:** Hepatic. Metabolite (6-O-desmethyl naproxen). **Elimination:** Urine (95%), feces (≤3%); $T_{1/2}$=12-17 hrs.

NURSING CONSIDERATIONS

Assessment: Assess for history of asthma, CV thrombotic events, CABG surgery, stroke, MI, CV disease (pre-existing HTN, CHF) or risk factors for disease, fluid retention, edema, pregnancy/nursing status, risk factors for GI events (bleeding, ulceration, perforation), possible drug interactions, renal/hepatic dysfunction.

Monitoring: Monitor BP, CBC, LFTs, renal function, and chemistries periodically. Monitor for signs/symptoms of GI events (bleeding, ulceration, perforation), CV thrombotic events, CHF, HTN, anemia, salt depletion, renal/liver dysfunction.

Patient Counseling: Seek medical attention if symptoms of hepatotoxicity (nausea, fatigue, pruritus), anaphylactic reaction (difficulty breathing, swelling of face/throat), hypersensitivity reaction (rash), CV events (chest pain, SOB, weakness, slurring of speech), GI ulceration and bleeding (epigastric pain, dyspepsia, melena, hematemesis), weight gain, and edema occur. Inform of pregnancy risks. Caution should be exercised if drowsiness, dizziness, vertigo or depression is experienced during therapy.

Administration: PO. **Storage:** (Sus) 15-30°C (59-86°); avoid excessive heat, above 40°C (104°F). Dispense in light-resistant containers. Shake before use. (Tab, Delayed-Release) 15-30° (59-86°F) in tightly closed containers; dispense in light-resistant containers. (Tab) 15-30°C (59-86°F) in tightly closed containers.

NARDIL   RX
phenelzine sulfate (Parke-Davis)

Antidepressants increased the risk of suicidal thinking and behavior (suicidality) in short-term studies in children, adolescents, and young adults with major depressive disorder (MDD) and other psychiatric disorders. Monitor and observe closely for clinical worsening, suicidality, or unusual changes in behavior in patients who are started on antidepressant therapy. Phenelzine is not approved for use in pediatric patients.

THERAPEUTIC CLASS: Monoamine oxidase inhibitor

INDICATIONS: Treatment of atypical, nonendogenous or neurotic depression not responsive to other antidepressants.

DOSAGE: *Adults:* Initial: 15mg tid. Titrate: Increase to 60-90mg/day at a fairly rapid pace until maximum benefit. Maint: Reduce slowly over several weeks to 15mg qd or 15mg qod.

HOW SUPPLIED: Tab: 15mg

CONTRAINDICATIONS: Pheochromocytoma, CHF, history of liver disease, abnormal LFTs, severe renal impairment or renal disease, meperidine, MAOIs, dextromethorphan, CNS depressants, alcohol, certain narcotics, sympathomimetic drugs (eg, amphetamines, cocaine, methylphenidate, dopamine, epinephrine, norepinephrine), or related compounds (eg, methyldopa, L-dopa, L-tryptophan, L-tyrosine, phenylalanine), high tyramine-containing food (eg, cheese, pickled herring, beer, wine, yeast extract, salami, yogurt), excessive caffeine and chocolate, dextromethorphan, CNS depressants, buspirone, serotoninergic agents (eg, dexfenfluramine, fluoxetine, fluvoxamine, paroxetine, sertraline, venlafaxine), bupropion, guanethidine.

WARNINGS/PRECAUTIONS: Hypertensive crisis, postural hypotension reported; monitor BP frequently. Caution with epilepsy, asthma, DM, or psychosis. D/C if palpitations or headache occur. Excessive stimulation in schizophrenics. D/C 10 days prior to elective surgery. Avoid abrupt withdrawal.

ADVERSE REACTIONS: Dizziness, headache, drowsiness, sleep disturbances, constipation, dry mouth, GI disturbances, elevated serum transaminases, weight gain, edema, sexual disturbances.

INTERACTIONS: See Contraindications. Hypertensive crisis with other MAOIs, sympathomimetics, high tyramine-containing foods. Allow 10 days between starting another MAOI, or antidepressant or buspirone. Serious reactions reported with serotoninergic agents. Allow 5 weeks after d/c fluoxetine before starting therapy. Allow 2 weeks after d/c therapy before starting bupropion. Avoid cocaine and local, general, and spinal anesthesia. Reduce dose of barbiturates. Caution with rauwolfia alkaloids. Exaggerated hypotensive effects with antihypertensives. Excitation, seizures, delirium, hyperpyrexia, circulatory collapse, coma, and death have been reported with meperidine.

PREGNANCY: Safety in pregnancy and nursing not known.

MECHANISM OF ACTION: MAOI; inhibits MAO activity.

PHARMACOKINETICS: Absorption: (30mg) C_{max}=19.8ng/mL, T_{max}=43 mins. **Metabolism:** Oxidation via MAO. Acetylation (minor). **Elimination:** (30mg) $T_{1/2}$=11.6 hrs.

NURSING CONSIDERATIONS

Assessment: Assess for DM, pheochromocytoma, CHF, history of liver disease, possible drug interactions, risk for bipolar disorder, history of mania or seizures or schizophrenia, pregnancy/nursing status, severe renal/hepatic impairment.

Monitoring: Monitor BP, renal/hepatic function, for signs/symptoms of clinical worsening (suicidality, unusual changes in behavior), hypertensive crisis (occipital headaches, neck stiffness, N/V, sweating), seizures, liver dysfunction, postural hypotension, hypoglycemia, increased psychosis, and activation of mania.

Patient Counseling: Instruct to avoid concomitant use of alcohol, tyramine-containing foods/supplements/beverages (during and 2 weeks following d/c), and any cough medicine containing dextromethorphan. Seek medical attention for symptoms of hypertensive crisis (occipital headaches, neck stiffness, N/V, sweating), hypoglycemia, increased psychosis, seizures, postural hypotension, mania, clinical worsening (suicidal ideation, unusual changes in behavior), and liver dysfunction. Advise to change position gradually if lightheaded, faint, or dizzy. Counsel about pregnancy risks.

Administration: Oral route. **Storage:** 15-30°C (59-86°F).

NAROPIN RX
ropivacaine HCl (APP Pharmaceuticals)

THERAPEUTIC CLASS: Local anesthetic

INDICATIONS: Production of local or regional anesthesia for surgery and for acute pain management.

DOSAGE: *Adults:* Individualize dose. Dosage varies depending on procedure, area to be anesthetized, tissue vascularity, number of neuronal segments to be blocked, depth and duration of anesthesia, degree of muscle relaxation required, tolerance, and physical condition of the patient. Test dose: 3-5mL prior to complete block. Surgical Anesthesia: Lumbar Epidural: Surgery: 75-200mg in 15-30mL; Cesarean: 100-150mg in 15-30mL. Thoracic Epidural for Surgery: 25-113mg in 5-15mL. Major Nerve Block: 75-300mg in 10-50mL. Field Block: 5-200mg in 1-40mL. Labor: Lumbar Epidural: Initial: 20-40mg; Continuous Infusion: 12-28mg/hr; Incremental Injection: 20-30mg/hr. Postoperative: Lumbar/Thoracic Epidural: 12-28mg/hr. Infiltration: 2-200mg in 1-100mL. Refer to PI for detailed dosage recommendations.

HOW SUPPLIED: Inj: 2mg/mL [10mL, 20mL, 100mL, 200mL]; 5mg/mL [20mL, 30mL]; 7.5mg/mL [20mL]; 10mg/mL [10mL, 20mL]

WARNINGS/PRECAUTIONS: Should only be administered by clinicians trained in diagnosis and management of dose related toxicity and other acute emergencies. Acidosis, cardiac arrest, death reported from delay in toxicity management. Administer in incremental doses. Optimize patient's condition; should have an IV line prior to major blocks. Not for emergency situations where fast onset of surgical anesthesia is necessary. Not for IV injection, IV regional anesthesia, production of obstetrical paracervical block, retrobulbar block, or spinal anesthesia. Not for intraarticular infusions following arthroscopic and other surgical procedures; chondrolysis reported. Perform syringe aspiration to avoid intravascular or subarachnoid inj. Use lowest effective dose. Caution with debilitated, elderly, and acutely ill patients; reduce dose. Caution with hepatic disease or impaired cardiovascular function. Administer test dose with epidural anesthesia. Caution with use of 300mg dose for brachial plexus block. Increased risk of intravascular inj and/or rapid systemic absorption when used in major peripheral nerve block. Caution with use in head and neck area; confusion, convulsions, respiratory depression/arrest, and cardiovascular stimulation/depression reported. Not recommended for use in ophthalmic surgery.

ADVERSE REACTIONS: Hypotension, bradycardia, N/V, paresthesia, back pain, fever, postoperative complications, headache, pain, urinary retention, dizziness, pruritus, HTN, anemia.

INTERACTIONS: Caution with other local anesthetics, amide-type anesthetics; additive toxic effects may occur. Caution with class III antiarrhythmics (eg, amiodarone). Increased levels with inhibitors of CYP1A2 (eg, fluvoxamine) and CYP3A4 (eg, ketoconazole). Possible interaction with CYP1A2 substrates (eg, theophylline, imipramine). Beta-blockers may mask changes in HR.

PREGNANCY: Category B, caution in nursing.

MECHANISM OF ACTION: Local anesthetic; blocks the generation and conduction of nerve impulses, presumably by increasing the threshold for electrical excitation in the nerve, by slowing the propagation of the nerve impulse and by reducing the rate of rise of the action potential.

PHARMACOKINETICS: Absorption: Complete and biphasic absorption (epidural space). Systemic concentration of drug is dependent on total dose, concentration, and route of administration; refer to PI for more information. **Distribution:** V_d=41L (IV); plasma protein binding (94%); crosses placenta. **Metabolism:** Liver (extensive); aromatic hydroxylation via CYP1A to 3-hydroxy ropivacaine (major metabolite). **Elimination:** Urine: IV (86%), (1% unchanged); $T_{1/2}$(IV)=1.8 hrs; $T_{1/2}$(Epidural)=14 min (1st phase) and 4.2 hrs (2nd phase).

NURSING CONSIDERATIONS

Assessment: Assess for drug hypersensitivity, hepatic disease, impaired cardiovascular function, hypotension, hypovolemia, heart block, pregnancy/nursing status, and possible drug interactions.

Monitoring: Monitor for signs/symptoms of cardiotoxicity and CNS toxicity, and for unintended intrathecal administration. Perform careful and constant monitoring of cardiovascular and respiratory (adequacy of ventilation) vital signs and patient's state of consciousness following each injection.

Patient Counseling: Inform risks of therapy. May experience temporary loss of sensation and motor activity in the anesthetized part of the body and of other adverse reactions.

Administration: Epidural route, Infiltration route. **Storage:** 20-25°C (68-77°F). Keep from freezing. Protect from light.

NASACORT AQ   RX
triamcinolone acetonide (Sanofi-Aventis)

THERAPEUTIC CLASS: Corticosteroid

INDICATIONS: Treatment of nasal symptoms of seasonal and perennial allergic rhinitis in adults and children ≥2 yrs.

DOSAGE: *Adults:* Initial/Max: 2 sprays per nostril qd. With improvement, may reduce dose to 1 spray per nostril qd. Elderly: Start at lower end of dosing range.
Pediatrics: ≥12 yrs: Initial/Max: 2 sprays per nostril qd. With improvement, may reduce dose to 1 spray per nostril qd. 6-12 yrs: Initial: 1 spray per nostril qd. Max: 2 sprays per nostril qd. 2-5 yrs: Initial/Max: 1 spray per nostril qd.

HOW SUPPLIED: Spray: 55mcg/spray [16.5g]

WARNINGS/PRECAUTIONS: Local nasal effects (eg, epistaxis, *Candida* infections of the nose and pharynx, nasal septal perforation, impaired wound healing) may occur. Glaucoma and/or cataracts may develop; monitor closely in patients with change in vision, history of increased intraocular pressure (IOP), glaucoma, and/or cataracts. Risk for more severe/fatal course of infections (eg, chickenpox, measles); avoid with patients who have not had such diseases or have not been properly immunized. Caution with active or quiescent tuberculosis (TB), ocular herpes simplex, untreated bacterial, fungal and systemic viral or parasitic infections; potential for worsening. Hypercorticism and adrenal suppression may appear in higher recommended dose or in susceptible individuals at recommended dose; d/c slowly following accepted procedures of oral therapy discontinuation. Potential for reduced growth velocity in pediatrics. Caution in elderly.

ADVERSE REACTIONS: Pharyngitis, epistaxis, increased cough, flu syndrome, bronchitis, dyspepsia, tooth disorder, headache, pharyngolaryngeal pain, nasopharyngitis, upper abdominal pain, diarrhea, asthma, rash, excoriation.

PREGNANCY: Category C, caution in nursing.

MECHANISM OF ACTION: Corticosteroid; mechanism not established; wide range of action on multiple cell types (eg, mast cells, eosinophils, neutrophils, macrophages, lymphocytes) and mediators (eg, histamine, eicosanoids, leukotrienes, cytokines) involved in inflammation.

PHARMACOKINETICS: Absorption: C_{max}=0.5ng/mL; T_{max}=1.5 hrs; AUC (110mcg, 400mcg)=1.4ng•hr/mL, 4.7ng•hr/mL. **Distribution:** V_d=99.5L (IV). **Elimination:** $T_{1/2}$=3.1 hrs.

NURSING CONSIDERATIONS

Assessment: Assess for history of hypersensitivity, increased IOP, glaucoma and/or cataracts. Assess for recent nasal ulcers, surgery/trauma, active or quiescent TB, untreated local or systemic infections, ocular herpes simplex, suppressed immune system, asthma or other conditions requiring chronic systemic corticosteroid therapy, pregnancy/nursing status, and possible drug interactions.

Monitoring: Monitor for acute adrenal insufficiency and withdrawal symptoms when replacing systemic corticosteroid with topical corticosteroid. Monitor for hypercorticism and/or HPA-axis suppression, disseminated infections (eg, chickenpox and measles), nasal or pharyngeal Candida infections, hypoadrenalism in infants whose mothers received corticosteroids during pregnancy, suppression of growth velocity in children, nasal septal perforation, epistaxis, glaucoma, and cataracts.

Patient Counseling: Advise to take as directed at regular intervals. Counsel to avoid exposure to chickenpox or measles and immediately notify physician if exposed or if symptoms worsen or do not improve, or if sneezing or nasal irritation occurs. Avoid spraying into eyes. Keep out of reach of children.

Administration: Intranasal route. Refer to PI for proper administration and safe use. **Storage:** 20-25°C (68-77°F).

NASONEX   RX
mometasone furoate monohydrate (Schering Corporation)

THERAPEUTIC CLASS: Corticosteroid

INDICATIONS: Treatment of nasal symptoms of seasonal and perennial allergic rhinitis and relief of nasal congestion associated with seasonal allergic rhinitis in patients ≥2 yrs. Prophylaxis of nasal symptoms of seasonal allergic rhinitis in patients ≥12 yrs. Treatment of nasal polyps in patients ≥18 yrs.

DOSAGE: *Adults:* Treatment (Seasonal/Perennial Allergic Rhinitis)/Prophylaxis and Treatment of Nasal Congestion (Seasonal Allergic Rhinitis): 2 sprays/nostril qd. Prophylaxis may start 2-4 weeks before pollen season. Nasal Polyps: 2 sprays/nostril qd-bid.
Pediatrics: ≥12 yrs: Treatment (Seasonal/Perennial Allergic Rhinitis)/Prophylaxis and Treatment of Nasal Congestion (Seasonal Allergic Rhinitis): 2 sprays/nostril qd. Prophylaxis may start 2-4 weeks before pollen season. 2-11 yrs: Treatment (Seasonal/Perennial Allergic Rhinitis)/Nasal Congestion (Seasonal Allergic Rhinitis): 1 spray/nostril qd.

HOW SUPPLIED: Spray: 50mcg/spray [17g]

WARNINGS/PRECAUTIONS: Local nasal effects (eg, epistaxis, *Candida* infections of nose and pharynx, nasal septum perforation, impaired wound healing) may occur; d/c when infection occurs. Glaucoma and/or cataracts may develop; monitor closely in patients with change in vision, history of increased intraocular pressure (IOP), glaucoma, and/or cataracts. D/C if hypersensitivity reactions, including instances of wheezing, occur. May increase susceptibility to infections; caution with active/quiescent tuberculosis (TB), ocular herpes simplex, or untreated bacterial, fungal, and systemic viral infections. Hypercorticism and adrenal suppression may appear when used at higher than recommended doses or in susceptible individuals at recommended doses; d/c slowly if such changes occur. May reduce growth velocity of pediatrics; monitor growth routinely.

ADVERSE REACTIONS: Headache, viral infection, pharyngitis, epistaxis/blood-tinged mucus, cough, upper respiratory tract infection, dysmenorrhea, musculoskeletal pain, sinusitis, N/V.

INTERACTIONS: May increase plasma concentrations with ketoconazole.

PREGNANCY: Category C, caution with nursing.

MECHANISM OF ACTION: Corticosteroid; not established. Demonstrates anti-inflammatory properties and is shown to have wide range of effects on multiple cell types (eg, mast cells, eosinophils, neutrophils, macrophages, lymphocytes) and mediators (eg, histamine, eicosanoids, leukotrienes, cytokines) involved in inflammation.

PHARMACOKINETICS: Absorption: Bioavailability (<1%). **Distribution:** Plasma protein binding (98-99%). **Metabolism:** Liver (extensive) via CYP3A4. **Elimination:** Bile (as metabolites); urine (limited extent); (IV) $T_{1/2}$=5.8 hrs.

NURSING CONSIDERATIONS

Assessment: Assess for previous hypersensitivity, active/quiescent TB, infections, ocular herpes simplex, change in vision, history of IOP, glaucoma or cataracts, recent nasal septum ulcers, nasal surgery/trauma, pregnancy/nursing status, and possible drug interactions.

Monitoring: Monitor for acute adrenal insufficiency, hypercorticism, nasal or pharyngeal *Candida* infections, suppression of growth velocity in children, hypersensitivity reactions, wheezing, nasal septum perforation, changes in vision, glaucoma, cataracts, increased IOP, epistaxis, wound healing, worsening of infections, and other adverse reactions.

Patient Counseling: Advise to take as directed at regular intervals and not to increase prescribed dosage. Inform patients that treatment may be associated with adverse reactions (eg, epistaxis, nasal septum perforation, *Candida* infection). Inform that glaucoma and/or cataracts may develop. Counsel to avoid exposure to chickenpox or measles and to immediately consult a physician if exposed. Contact physician if symptoms worsen or do not improve. Supervise young children during administration. Advise patient to take missed dose as soon as remembered. Counsel on proper priming and administration techniques.

Administration: Intranasal route. Refer to PI for proper administration. **Storage:** 25°C (77°F); excursions permitted to 15-30°C (59-86°F). Protect from light.

NATACYN   RX
natamycin (Alcon)

THERAPEUTIC CLASS: Tetraene polyene antifungal

INDICATIONS: Treatment of fungal blepharitis, conjunctivitis, and keratitis caused by susceptible organisms. Effectiveness as a single agent in fungal endophthalmitis has not been established.

DOSAGE: *Adults:* Keratitis: 1 drop q1-2h for 3-4 days, then 1 drop 6-8 times daily for 14-21 days or until the resolution of infection. Reduce dose at 4-7 day intervals. Blepharitis/Conjunctivitis: 1 drop 4-6 times daily.

HOW SUPPLIED: Sus: 5% [15mL]

WARNINGS/PRECAUTIONS: For topical ophthalmic use only, not for injection. Failure of improvement of keratitis following 7-10 days of administration suggests that the infection may be caused by a microorganism not susceptible to natamycin. Continuation of therapy should be based on clinical re-evaluation and additional laboratory studies. Adherence of suspension to areas of epithelial ulceration or retention of the suspension in the fornices occurs regularly.

ADVERSE REACTIONS: Allergic reaction, change in vision, chest pain, corneal opacity, dyspnea, eye discomfort, eye edema, eye hyperemia, eye irritation, eye pain, foreign body sensation, paresthesia, tearing.

PREGNANCY: Category C, caution in nursing.

MECHANISM OF ACTION: Tetraene polyene antifungal; binds to sterol moiety of the fungal cell membrane. Polyenesterol complex alters permeability of membrane to produce depletion of essential cellular constituents.

PHARMACOKINETICS: Absorption: GI (poor).

NURSING CONSIDERATIONS

Assessment: Assess proper diagnosis through clinical and lab evaluation (eg, smear and culture of corneal scrapings). Assess use in pregnant/nursing females.

Monitoring: Monitor for clinical response. In patients with keratitis, reassess therapy if no response within 7 to 10 days.

Patient Counseling: Advise not to touch dropper tip to any surface to avoid contamination of suspension. Instruct not to wear contact lenses if have signs/symptoms of fungal blepharitis, conjunctivitis, and keratitis.

Administration: Ocular route. Shake well before use. **Storage:**2-24°C (36-75°F). Do not freeze. Avoid exposure to light and excessive heat.

NATAZIA   RX
estradiol valerate - dienogest (Bayer Healthcare)

> Cigarette smoking increases risk of serious cardiovascular events; risk increases with age (especially >35 yrs) and number of cigarettes smoked. Should not be used if >35 yrs and smoke.

THERAPEUTIC CLASS: Estrogen/progestogen combination

INDICATIONS: Prevention of pregnancy.

DOSAGE: *Adults:* 1 tab qd at the same time for 28 days, then repeat. Take in the order directed on the blister pack. Start on Day 1 of menses or not earlier than 4 weeks postpartum for postpartum women who do not breasfeed or after second trimester abortion. When starting therapy, use a nonhormonal back-up contraceptive method for first 9 days of therapy.
Pediatrics: Post-pubertal Adolescents: 1 tab qd at the same time for 28 days, then repeat. Take in the order directed on the blister pack. Start on Day 1 of menses or not earlier than 4 weeks postpartum for postpartum women who do not breasfeed or after second trimester abortion. When starting therapy, use a nonhormonal back-up contraceptive method for first 9 days of therapy.

HOW SUPPLIED: Tab: (Estradiol valerate, Estradiol valerate-Dienogest) 1mg, 3mg, 2mg-2mg, 2mg-3mg

CONTRAINDICATIONS: High risk of arterial or venous thrombotic diseases including smoking and >35 years old, current or history of DVT or pulmonary embolism, cerebrovascular disease, CAD, thrombogenic valvular or thrombogenic rhythm diseases of the heart, inherited or acquired hypercoagulopathies, uncontrolled HTN, DM with vascular disease, headache with focal neurological symptoms or migraine headaches with or without aura; undiagnosed abnormal genital bleeding, breast cancer or other estrogen- or progestin-sensitive cancer (current or past history), benign or malignant liver tumors or liver disease, and pregnancy.

WARNINGS/PRECAUTIONS: Increased risk of venous thromboembolism, arterial thrombosis (eg, stroke, MI), and cerebrovascular events (thrombotic and hemorrhagic strokes). D/C if arterial or deep venous thrombotic event occurs. D/C at least 4 weeks before and for 2 weeks after major surgery or other surgeries known to have an elevated risk of thromboembolism. Caution with CV disease risk factors. D/C if there is unexplained loss of vision, proptosis, diplopia, papilledema, or retinal vascular lesions; evaluate for retinal vein thrombosis immediately. May increase risk of breast or cervical cancer or intraepithelial neoplasia, and gallbladder disease. May cause hepatic adenomas, hepatocellular carcinoma, and OCP-related cholestasis; d/c if jaundice develops. May increase BP; monitor BP closely with HTN and d/c if significant elevation occurs. May decrease glucose tolerance. Consider alternative contraception with uncontrolled dyslipedemia. Caution with hypertriglyceridemia; may increase risk of pancreatitis. If new headaches develop that are recurrent, persistent, or severe, evaluate cause and d/c if indicated. May increase frequency or severity of migraines. May cause bleeding irregularities (eg, breakthrough bleeding, spotting, amenorrhea); rule out malignancy or pregnancy. Not for use as a test for pregnancy. Monitor closely with depression and d/c if depression recurs to serious degree. Not indicated for use before menarche. May affect certain laboratory tests (eg, coagulation factors, lipids, glucose tolerance, binding proteins). May lead to increased thyroid-binding globulin levels; monitor thyroid function in patients dependent on thyroid replacement therapy. Chloasma reported; avoid exposure to sun or ultraviolet radiation. May induce or exacerbate symptoms of angioedema.

ADVERSE REACTIONS: N/V, headache, migraine, irregular menstruation, metrorrhagia, breast pain, discomfort or tenderness, acne, increased weight.

INTERACTIONS: CYP3A4 inducers (eg, St. John's wort, carbamazepine, felbamate, rifampicin, phenytoin, barbiturates, bosentan, griseofulvin, oxcarbazepine, topiramate) may decrease levels and decrease contraceptive efficacy and/or increase breakthrough bleeding; avoid strong CYP3A4 inducers (eg, carbamazepine, phenytoin, rifampicin, St. John's wort). CYP3A4 inhibitors (eg, erythromycin, ketoconazole, azole antifungals, cimetidine, verapamil, macrolides, diltiazem, antidepressants, grapefruit juice) may increase levels. Significant changes (increase/decrease) in plasma estrogen and progestin levels may occur with some HIV protease inhibitors. Patients on thyroid replacement therapy may require higher dose of thyroid hormones. Caution with concomitant use of antibiotics. May decrease plasma concentrations of lamotrigine; may need dosage adjustment.

PREGNANCY: Category X, caution in nursing.

MECHANISM OF ACTION: Estrogen/progestin combination oral contraceptive; acts primarily by suppressing ovulation. Also causes cervical mucus changes that inhibit sperm penetration and endometrial changes that reduce the likelihood of implantation.

PHARMACOKINETICS: Absorption: Dienogest: C_{max}=91.7ng/mL, T_{max}=1 hrs, AUC(0-24 hr)=964ng/mL; Estradiol: C_{max}=73.3pg/mL, T_{max}=6 hrs, AUC(0-24 hr)=1301pg•hr/mL. **Distribution:** Estradiol: V_d=1.2L/kg (IV); bound to sex hormone-binding globulin (38%) and albumin (60%); found in breast milk. Dienogest: V_d=46L (IV); bound to albumin (90%). **Metabolism:** Dienogest: extensive (hydroxylation, conjugation), CYP3A4 (main); Estradiol: CYP3A, estrone and its sulfate or glucuronide conjugates (main metabolites). **Elimination:** Estradiol: Urine (Main), Feces (10%), $T_{1/2}$=14 hrs; Dienogest: Renal (Main); $T_{1/2}$=11 hrs.

NURSING CONSIDERATIONS

Assessment: Assess for risk factors of arterial or venous thrombotic diseases, current or history of DVT or pulmonary embolism, cerebrovascular disease, CAD, or any other condition where treatment is contraindicated or cautioned, pregnancy/nursing status, depression, thyroid function, and for possible drug interactions.

Monitoring: Monitor for signs/symptoms of CV disorders (eg, MI, stroke, venous thrombosis), breast cancer, liver tumors or liver disease (eg, jaundice), gallbladder disease, retinal vascular thrombosis, elevations in BP, headache, pancreatitis, migraine aggravation, depression, bleeding irregularities, amenorrhea. Monitor thyroid function in patients on thyroid replacement therapy. Monitor BP at regular intervals. Monitor liver function. Monitor glucose levels in prediabetic and diabetic women.

Patient Counseling: Counsel that cigarette smoking increases the risk of serious CV events and to avoid use in women who are >35 years old and smoke. Inform that therapy does not protect against HIV infection and other STDs. Advise to take one tablet daily by mouth at the same time every day in the exact order noted on the blister. Instruct what to do in the event pills are missed. Inform of possible drug interactions. Counsel to use a back-up or alternative method of contraception when weak or moderate enzyme inducers are concomitantly used. Inform patients who are breastfeeding or who desire to breastfeed that therapy may reduce breast-milk production. Counsel any patient who starts medication postpartum, and who has not yet had a period, to use an additional method of contraception until she has taken medication for 9 consecutive days. Inform that amenorrhea may occur. Avoid exposure to sun or ultraviolet radiation in women with tendency to chloasma. Notify physician if pregnant or nursing.

Administration: Oral route. **Storage:** 25°C (77°F); excursions permitted to 15-30°C (59-86°F).

NATRECOR

RX

nesiritide (Scios Inc.)

THERAPEUTIC CLASS: Human B-type natriuretic peptide

INDICATIONS: Treatment of acutely decompensated congestive heart failure with dyspnea at rest or with minimal activity.

DOSAGE: *Adults:* 2mcg/kg IV bolus over 60 seconds, then 0.01mcg/kg/min IV infusion.

HOW SUPPLIED: Inj: 1.5mg

CONTRAINDICATIONS: Primary therapy with cardiogenic shock or systolic BP <90mmHg.

WARNINGS/PRECAUTIONS: Avoid with low cardiac filling pressures. Use precautions for parenteral administration of protein pharmaceuticals or *E.coli*-derived products; may cause allergic or untoward reaction. Avoid when vasodilators are inappropriate (eg, significant valvular stenosis, restrictive/obstructive cardiomyopathy, constrictive pericarditis, pericardial tamponade, conditions where cardiac output is dependent on venous return). May affect renal function; azotemia reported. Hypotension reported; reduce dose or d/c. Caution with BP <100mmHg at baseline.

ADVERSE REACTIONS: Hypotension, ventricular tachycardia, ventricular extrasystoles, headache, back pain, dizziness, anxiety, nausea, abdominal pain, insomnia.

INTERACTIONS: Increased risk of hypotension with drugs that cause hypotension, such as oral ACE inhibitors.

PREGNANCY: Category C, caution in nursing.

MECHANISM OF ACTION: Human B-type natriuretic peptide; binds to the particulate guanylate cyclase receptor of vascular smooth muscle and endothelial cells, leading to increased intracellular concentrations of cGMP and smooth muscle relaxation.

PHARMACOKINETICS: Distribution: V_d=0.19L/kg. **Elimination:** Renal; $T_{1/2}$=18 min.

NURSING CONSIDERATIONS

Assessment: Assess for cardiogenic shock or SBP ≤90mmHg, significant valvular stenosis, restrictive or obstructive cardiomyopathy, constrictive pericarditis, pericardial tamponade, low cardiac filling pressure, pregnancy/nursing status, possible drug interactions, and known hypersensitivity to drug or any of its components.

Monitoring: Monitor renal function, HR, BP, cardiac index/status, and hemodynamic parameters. Monitor for hypotension, ventricular tachycardia, bradiacardia, and N/V.

Patient Counseling: Counsel about potential adverse effects of drug.

Administration: (IV) Infusion bag preparation: 1) Reconstitute one 1.5mg vial by adding 5mL of diluent. 2) Do not shake the bottle. Rock the vial gently so that all surfaces, including the stopper, are in contact with the diluent to ensure complete reconstitution. 3) Withdraw the entire contents of the reconstituted vial and add to the 250mL plastic IV bag. The IV bag should be inverted several times to ensure complete mixing. 4) Use reconstituted solution within 24 hrs and store at 2-25°C (36-77°F). **Storage:** Store below 25°C. Do not freeze. Protect from light.

NATROBA   RX
spinosad (ParaPRO/Pernix Therapeutics)

THERAPEUTIC CLASS: Pediculocide

INDICATIONS: Topical treatment of head lice infestation in patients ≥4 yrs.

DOSAGE: *Adults:* Apply ≤120mL to adequately cover dry scalp and hair. Leave on for 10 min, then thoroughly rinse off with warm water. Apply 2nd treatment if live lice seen 7 days after the 1st.
Pediatrics: ≥4 yrs: Apply ≤120mL to adequately cover dry scalp and hair. Leave on for 10 min, then thoroughly rinse off with warm water. Apply 2nd treatment if live lice seen 7 days after the 1st.

HOW SUPPLIED: Sus: 0.9% [120mL]

WARNINGS/PRECAUTIONS: Not for oral, ophthalmic, or intravaginal use. Contains benzyl alcohol; avoid in neonates and infants <6 months.

ADVERSE REACTIONS: Application site erythema, irritation, ocular erythema.

PREGNANCY: Category B, caution in nursing.

MECHANISM OF ACTION: Pediculocide; causes neuronal excitation in insects; lice become paralyzed and die after periods of hyperexcitation.

NURSING CONSIDERATIONS

Assessment: Assess pregnancy/nursing status.

Monitoring: Monitor for presence of live lice after 7 days of 1st treatment.

Patient Counseling: Advise to use only on dry scalp and hair. Instruct not to swallow. Instruct to rinse thoroughly with water if medication gets in or near the eyes. Advise to wash hands after application. Inform to use on children only under direct supervision of an adult. Consult physician if pregnant/breastfeeding.

Administration: Topical route. Shake well before use. Avoid contact with eyes. **Storage:** 25°C (77°F); excursions permitted between 15-30°C (59-86°F).

NAVANE   RX
thiothixene (Pfizer)

> Elderly patients with dementia-related psychosis treated with antipsychotic drugs are at an increased risk of death; most deaths appeared to be cardiovascular (eg, heart failure, sudden death) or infectious (eg, pneumonia) in nature. Thiothixene is not approved for the treatment of patients with dementia-related psychosis.

THERAPEUTIC CLASS: Thioxanthene

INDICATIONS: Management of schizophrenia.

DOSAGE: *Adults:* Individualize dose. Mild Condition: Initial: 2mg tid. Titrate: May increase to 15mg/day. Severe Condition: Initial: 5mg bid. Usual: 20-30mg/day. Max: 60mg/day.
Pediatrics: ≥12 yrs: Individualize dose. Mild Condition: Initial: 2mg tid. Titrate:

N

May increase to 15mg/day. Severe Condition: Initial: 5mg bid. Usual: 20-30mg/day. Max: 60mg/day.

HOW SUPPLIED: Cap: 1mg, 2mg, 5mg, 10mg, 20mg

CONTRAINDICATIONS: Circulatory collapse, comatose states, CNS depression, blood dyscrasias.

WARNINGS/PRECAUTIONS: May cause tardive dyskinesia (TD) and neuroleptic malignant syndrome (NMS); d/c if this develops. May impair mental/physical abilities. May mask signs of overdosage of toxic drugs and obscure conditions such as intestinal obstruction and brain tumor. Caution with history of convulsive disorders or in a state of alcohol withdrawal; may lower convulsive threshold. Monitor for pigmentary retinopathy and lenticular pigmentation. Caution with CV disease, extreme heat exposure, activities requiring alertness. May elevate prolactin levels. May cause leukopenia, neutropenia, and agranulocytosis; consider d/c at 1st sign of significant decline in WBC in absence of other causes, and d/c when absolute neutrophil count (ANC) is <1000/mm³. False positive pregnancy tests may occur. Risk for extrapyramidal symptoms (EPS) and/or withdrawal symptoms following delivery in neonates exposed during 3rd trimester of pregnancy.

ADVERSE REACTIONS: NMS, TD, tachycardia, hypotension, lightheadedness, syncope, drowsiness, restlessness, agitation, insomnia, EPS, cerebral edema, CSF abnormalities, allergic reactions, hematologic effects.

INTERACTIONS: Possible additive effects with hypotensive agents, CNS depressants, and alcohol. Increased clearance with hepatic microsomal enzyme inducers (eg, carbamazepine). Potentiates the actions of barbiturates. Caution with atropine or related drugs. Paradoxical effects (lowering of BP) with pressor agents (eg, epinephrine).

PREGNANCY: Safety is not known in pregnancy and nursing.

MECHANISM OF ACTION: Thioxanthene derivative; antipsychotic agent.

NURSING CONSIDERATIONS

Assessment: Assess for dementia-related psychosis in elderly, history of convulsive disorders, history of CV disorders, CNS depression, circulatory collapse, comatose state, blood dyscrasias, alcohol intake, infection, intestinal obstruction, brain tumor, possibility of extreme heat exposure, previous hypersensitivity to the drug, pregnancy/nursing status and possible drug interactions. Obtain baseline vital signs, CBC, LFTs, prolactin levels.

Monitoring: Monitor for hypersensitivity reactions, TD, NMS, CV effects, visual disturbances, and EPS. Monitor LFTs, bilirubin, CBC, prolactin, and blood glucose.

Patient Counseling: Inform about the risks of the treatment particularly about the possibility of developing TD. Advise about risk of chronic use of drug. Use caution when performing hazardous tasks (operating machinery/driving). Warn about possible additive effects (eg, hypotension) when drug is combined with hypotensive agents, CNS depressants and/or alcohol.

Administration: Oral route.

NEORAL

RX

cyclosporine (Novartis)

Should only be prescribed by physicians experienced in management of systemic immunosuppressive therapy for indicated diseases. Increased susceptibility to infection and development of neoplasia (eg, lymphoma) may result from immunosuppression. Not bioequivalent to Sandimmune and cannot be used interchangeably without physician supervision. Caution in switching from Sandimmune. Cyclosporine may be coadministered with other immunosuppressive agents in kidney, liver, and heart transplant patients. Monitor cyclosporine blood concentrations in transplant and rheumatoid arthritis (RA) patients to avoid toxicity. Dose adjustments should be made to minimize possible organ rejection in transplant patients. Increased risk of developing skin malignancies in psoriasis patients previously treated with PUVA, methotrexate (MTX) or other immunosuppressive agents, UVB, coal tar, or radiation therapy. Cyclosporine may cause systemic HTN and nephrotoxicity. Monitor renal function for renal dysfunction including, structural kidney damage, during therapy.

THERAPEUTIC CLASS: Cyclic polypeptide immunosuppressant

INDICATIONS: Prophylaxis of organ rejection in kidney, liver, and heart allogeneic transplants. Has been used in combination with azathioprine and corticosteroids. Treatment of severe, active RA where disease has not adequately responded to MTX. May be used in combination with MTX. Treatment of nonimmunocompromised adults with severe (eg, extensive and/or disabling), recalcitrant, plaque psoriasis who failed to respond to at least one systemic therapy (eg, PUVA, retinoids, MTX) or when other systemic therapies are contraindicated and cannot be tolerated.

DOSAGE: *Adults:* All daily doses bid. Administer on a consistent schedule with regard to time of day and relation to meals. Newly Transplanted Patients: Initial: May be given 4-12 hrs prior to transplantation or be given postoperatively. Dose varies depending on the transplanted organ and other immunosuppressive agents included in immunosuppressive protocol. Renal Transplant: 9±3mg/kg/day. Liver Transplant: 8±4mg/kg/day. Heart Transplant: 7±3mg/kg/day. Adjust subsequent dose to achieve a pre-defined blood concentration. Adjunct therapy with adrenal corticosteroid recommended. Conversion from Sandimmune: Start with same daily dose as was previously used with Sandimmune, (1:1 dose conversion). Adjust subsequent dose to attain a pre-conversion blood trough concentration. Monitor blood levels every 4-7 days while adjusting to trough levels. Transplant Patients with Poor Sandimmune Absorption: Caution when converting patients at doses >10mg/kg/day. Titrate dose individually based on trough concentrations, tolerability, and clinical response. Measure blood trough concentration at least 2x a week until stabilized within desired range. RA: Initial: 2.5mg/kg/day. Titrate: May be increased by 0.5-0.75mg/kg/day after 8 weeks and again after 12 weeks. Max: 4mg/kg/day. Combined with MTX (15mg/week): ≤3mg/kg/day. Psoriasis: Initial: 2.5mg/kg/day for 4 weeks. If no significant clinical improvement occurs, may increase dosage at 2-week interval. Titrate: May increase approximately 0.5mg/kg/day based on clinical response. Max: 4mg/kg/day. (RA/Psoriasis) Reduce dose by 25-50% if adverse events (eg, HTN) occur. D/C if reduction is not effective or if no clinical response after 16 weeks of therapy. Elderly: Start at lower end of dosing range.

HOW SUPPLIED: Cap: 25mg, 100mg; Sol: 100mg/mL [50mL]

CONTRAINDICATIONS: Abnormal renal function, uncontrolled HTN, malignancies in RA or psoriasis patients; concomitant PUVA or UVB therapy, MTX, other immunosuppressants, coal tar, or radiation therapy in psoriasis patients.

WARNINGS/PRECAUTIONS: Elevation of SrCr and BUN may occur and reflect a reduction in GFR. Elevations in SrCr and BUN levels do not necessarily indicate rejection; evaluate patient before dose adjustment. Increase in SrCr is generally reversible upon dose reduction and its d/c. May develop syndrome of thrombocytopenia and microangiopathic hemolytic anemia; may result in graft failure. Significant hyperkalemia and hyperuricemia reported. May cause hepatotoxicity. Increased risk for opportunistic infections, including activation of latent viral infection. BK virus-associated nephropathy reported; reduce immunosuppression if it develops. Encephalopathy and optic disc edema reported; reversible upon d/c. Avoid excessive sun exposure. Evaluate before and during treatment for the presence of malignant and pre-malignant lesions. SrCr, BUN, BP, CBC, uric acid, K+, lipids, and magnesium should be monitored every 2 weeks for the first 3 months of therapy and then monthly if the patient is stable or more frequently when dosage adjustments are made. Monitor CBC and LFTs monthly with MTX. Monitor SrCr after initiation or increases in NSAID dose for RA. Caution in elderly.

ADVERSE REACTIONS: Renal dysfunction, HTN, hirsutism/hypertrichosis, tremor, headache, gingival hyperplasia, diarrhea, N/V, paresthesia, dyspepsia, stomatitis, hypomagnesemia, BK virus-associated nephropathy.

INTERACTIONS: See Contraindications. Avoid with K+-sparing diuretics, caution with K+-sparing drugs (eg, ACE inhibitors, angiotensin II receptor antagonists), K+-containing drugs and K+-rich diet. Ciprofloxacin, gentamicin, tobramycin, vancomycin, SMZ/TMP, amphotericin B, ketoconazole, melphalan, cimetidine, ranitidine, tacrolimus, fibric acid derivatives (eg, bezafibrate, fenofibrate), methotrexate, azapropazon, colchicine, diclofenac, naproxen, sulindac and NSAIDs may potentiate renal dysfunction. Monitor levels and adjust dose with CYP3A4 and/or P-glycoprotein inducers and inhibitors. Avoid with orlistat. Diltiazem, nicardipine, verapamil, fluconazole, itraconazole, ketoconazole, voriconazole, azithromycin, clarithromycin, erythromycin, quinupristin/dalfopristin, methylprednisolone, allopurinol, bromocriptine, danazol, metoclopramide, colchicine, amiodarone, imatinib, nefazodone, oral contraceptives may increase levels. Avoid with grapefruit and grapefruit juice. Nafcillin, rifampin, carbamazepine, oxcarbazepine, phenobarbital, phenytoin, bosentan, octreotide, ticlopidine, orlistat, sulfinpyrazone, terbinafine, St. John's wort may decrease levels. Caution with rifabutin. May double diclofenac blood levels. Increases levels of CYP3A4 and/or P-glycoprotein subtrates. May reduce clearance of digoxin, colchicine, prednisolone, HMG-CoA reductase inhibitors (eg, statins) and eposides. Increased levels with sirolimus; give 4 hrs after cyclosporine administration. Vaccination maybe less effective; avoid live vaccines during therapy. Convulsions reported with high dose methylprednisolone. Frequent gingival hyperplasia with nifedipine. Caution with nephrotoxic drugs and HIV protease inhibitors. May increase levels of repaglinide and thereby increase risk of hypoglycemia.

PREGNANCY: Category C, not for use in nursing.

MECHANISM OF ACTION: Cyclic polypeptide immunosuppressant; results from specific and reversible inhibition of immunocompetent lymphocytes in the G_0- and G_1-phase of the cell cycle. T-lymphocytes are preferentially inhibited with T-helper cell as main target while also possibly suppressing T-suppressor cells. Also inhibits lymphokine production and release (eg, interleukin-2).

PHARMACOKINETICS: Absorption: Incomplete; T_{max}=1.5-2 hrs. Pharmacokinetic parameters varied with different indications (renal, liver, RA and/or psoriasis). **Distribution:** V_d=3-5L/kg (IV); plasma protein binding (90%); found in breast milk. **Metabolism:** (Extensive) Liver via CYP3A , to a lesser extent GI tract and kidneys. M1, M9, and M4N (major metabolites); oxidation and demethylation pathways. **Elimination:** Bile (primary), urine (6%, 0.1% unchanged); $T_{1/2}$=8.4 hrs.

NURSING CONSIDERATIONS

Assessment: Assess for hypersensitivity to the drug, abnormal renal function, uncontrolled HTN, presence of malignancies, pregnancy/nursing status and possible drug interactions. RA: Before initiating treatment, BP (on at least 2 occasions) and two creatinine levels should be taken. Psoriasis: Careful dermatological and physical examinations, including BP on at least two occasions, should be performed before initiating treatment. Evaluate for presence of occult infections and tumors. Atypical skin lesions should be biopsied. Obtain baseline SrCr (at least twice), BUN, LFTs, bilirubin, CBC, Mg+, K+, uric acid, and lipids.

Monitoring: Monitor for renal/hepatic impairment. Cyclosporine blood concentrations should be routinely monitored in transplant patients and periodically in RA patients. RA: Monitor SrCr after an increase of the dose of NSAIDs and after initiation: Always monitor BP when starting new NSAID therapy. If coadministered with MTX, CBC and LFTs are recommended monthly. BP and

SrCr should be evaluated every 2 weeks during initial 3 months, then monthly if patient is stable. Psoriasis: Presence of occult infections and tumors should be evaluated throughout treatment. SrCr, BUN, BP, CBC, uric acid, K⁺, lipids, and Mg⁺ should be evaluated every 2 weeks during first 3 months of treatment, then monthly if stable.

Patient Counseling: Instruct to contact a physician before changing formulations of cyclosporine, which may require dose changes. Inform patients that repeated tests are required while on medication. Counsel not to administer concurrently with UVB or other radiation therapy/immunosuppressive agents. Instruct to take exactly as directed. Advise regarding potential risks during pregnancy, increased risk of neoplasia, HTN, and renal dysfunction. Inform that vaccinations may be less effective and to avoid live vaccines during therapy. Advise to take the medication on a consistent schedule with regard to time and meals and to avoid grapefruit and grapefruit juice.

Administration: Oral route. (Dilute only with orange or apple juice, not grapefruit juice). **Storage:** Cap/Sol: 20-25°C (68-77°F). Sol: Do not refrigerate. Use within 2 months upon opening. At <20°C (68°F) may form gel, light flocculation, or formation of light sediment; warm at 25°C (77°C) to reverse changes.

NEULASTA   RX
pegfilgrastim (Amgen)

THERAPEUTIC CLASS: Granulocyte colony stimulating factor

INDICATIONS: To decrease the incidence of infection, as manifested by febrile neutropenia, in patients with nonmyeloid malignancies receiving myelosuppressive anticancer drugs associated with a clinically significant incidence of febrile neutropenia.

DOSAGE: *Adults:* 6mg SQ once per chemotherapy cycle. Do not administer in the period between 14 days before and 24 hrs after cytotoxic chemotherapy.

HOW SUPPLIED: Inj: 6mg/0.6mL

WARNINGS/PRECAUTIONS: May cause splenic rupture; evaluate patients with left upper abdominal and/or shoulder pain. May cause acute respiratory distress syndrome (ARDS); evaluate patients who develop fever and lung infiltrates or respiratory distress; d/c if ARDS develops. Serious allergic reactions (eg, anaphylaxis) reported; d/c permanently if it occurs. May cause fatal sickle cell crises in patients with sickle cell disorders. May act as a growth factor for any tumor type; not approved for myeloid malignancies and myelodysplasia. Needle cover on prefilled syringe contains latex; avoid use with latex allergy.

ADVERSE REACTIONS: Splenic rupture, ARDS, allergic reactions, bone pain, pain in extremity.

PREGNANCY: Category C, caution in nursing.

MECHANISM OF ACTION: Pegylated granulocyte colony stimulating factor; acts on hematopoietic cells by binding to specific cell surface receptors, thereby stimulating proliferation, differentiation, commitment, and end cell functional activation.

PHARMACOKINETICS: Elimination: (SQ) T$_{1/2}$=15-80 hrs.

NURSING CONSIDERATIONS

Assessment: Assess for myeloid malignancies, myelodysplasia, history of hypersensitivity to the drug, latex allergy, sickle cell disorders, and pregnancy/nursing status.

Monitoring: Monitor for signs/symptoms of an allergic reaction, splenic rupture, ARDS (eg, fever, lung infiltrates), and for tumor growth. Monitor for signs/symptoms of sickle cell crises in patients with sickle cell disorders.

Patient Counseling: Discuss signs/symptoms of an allergic drug reaction and advise appropriate actions. Counsel on importance of compliance with treatment. Caution patient and caregivers against reuse of needles, syringes, or drug product, and thoroughly instruct on their proper disposal. Advise to report if left upper abdominal or shoulder pain, SOB, signs/symptoms of sickle cell crisis or infection, flushing, dizziness, or rash occurs.

Administration: SQ route. Inspect for particulate matter and discoloration prior to administration. **Storage:** Refrigerate at 2-8°C (36-46°F) in the carton to protect from light. Do not shake. Discard syringes stored at room temperature for >48 hrs. Avoid freezing; if frozen, thaw in the refrigerator before administration. Discard if frozen more than once.

NEUMEGA   RX
oprelvekin (Wyeth)

> Allergic or hypersensitivity reactions, including anaphylaxis, reported; permanently d/c if this develops.

THERAPEUTIC CLASS: Thrombopoietic agent

INDICATIONS: Prevention of severe thrombocytopenia and reduction of the need for platelet transfusions following myelosuppressive chemotherapy in nonmyeloid malignancy patients at high risk.

DOSAGE: *Adults:* 50mcg/kg qd SQ. Severe renal impairment (CrCl <30mL/min): 25mcg/kg qd SQ. Initiate 6-24 hrs after chemotherapy completion. Monitor platelets to assess optimal duration of therapy. Continue therapy until post-nadir platelets ≥50,000 cells/mcL. D/C at least 2 days before next chemotherapy cycle. Max: 21 days of therapy.

HOW SUPPLIED: Inj: 5mg

WARNINGS/PRECAUTIONS: Fluid retention reported; caution in CHF and patients receiving aggressive hydration. Capillary leak syndrome, pleural/pericardial effusion, renal failure, visual disturbances, papilledema, stroke, and rash reported. Monitor fluid and electrolyte balance with chronic diuretic therapy. Permanently d/c if significant allergic reactions occur. Moderate decreases in Hgb, Hct, and RBCs reported. Caution with history of atrial arrhythmias. May develop antibodies to therapy. Obtain CBC before therapy, then regularly. Monitor platelets during expected nadir time and until adequate recovery.

ADVERSE REACTIONS: Edema, dyspnea, tachycardia, conjunctival injection, palpitations, atrial arrhythmias, pleural effusions, syncope, pneumonia, neutropenic fever, headache, N/V, fever, mucositis, diarrhea.

PREGNANCY: Category C, not for use in nursing.

MECHANISM OF ACTION: Thrombopoietic agent; stimulates megakaryocytopoiesis and thrombopoiesis.

PHARMACOKINETICS: Absorption: Absolute bioavailability (>80%); C_{max}=17.4ng/mL; T_{max}=3.2 hrs. **Elimination:** Kidneys (animal studies); $T_{1/2}$=6.9 hrs.

NURSING CONSIDERATIONS

Assessment: Assess for pregnancy/nursing status, bone marrow transplant, fluid retention or overload, capillary leak syndrome, pleural/pericardial effusion, CHF, aggressive hydration, history of papilledema or tumors of CNS, renal failure, prior myeloablative chemotherapy, history of atrial arrhythmias, and history of stroke or transient ischemic attack. Obtain baseline CBC including platelet count.

Monitoring: Periodically monitor CBC, fluid balance, fluid and electrolyte status (chronic diuretics). Monitor platelets during expected nadir time and until adequate recovery. Monitor for signs/symptoms of hypersensitivity reactions, papilledema, fluid retention, pleural/pericardial effusion, atrial arrhythmias, and anemia.

Patient Counseling: Inform of pregnancy risks. Advise to seek medical attention if symptoms of hypersensitivity reactions (edema, SOB, wheezing, chest pain, hypotension), worsening of dyspnea (CHF, pleural effusion), atrial arrhythmias, anemia, or papilledema (blurred vision, blindness) occur.

Administration: SQ route; thigh, abdomen, or hip (upper arm if not self-injecting). **Storage:** 2-8°C (36-46°F). Protect from light; do not freeze. Reconstituted: 2-8°C (36-46°F) or 25°C (77°F); stable for 3 hrs. Do not freeze or shake.

NEUPOGEN RX
filgrastim (Amgen)

THERAPEUTIC CLASS: Granulocyte colony stimulating factor

INDICATIONS: To decrease incidence of infection, as manifested by febrile neutropenia in patients with nonmyeloid malignancies receiving myelosuppressive anticancer drugs associated with significant incidence of severe neutropenia with fever. To reduce the time to neutrophil recovery and duration of fever, following consolidation chemotherapy treatment of adults with acute myeloid leukemia (AML). To reduce the duration of neutropenia and neutropenia-related clinical sequelae in patients with nonmyeloid malignancies undergoing myeloablative chemotherapy followed by marrow transplantation. For mobilization of hematopoietic progenitor cells into the peripheral blood for collection by leukapheresis. For chronic administration to reduce incidence and duration of sequelae of neutropenia in symptomatic patients with congenital neutropenia, cyclic neutropenia, or idiopathic neutropenia.

DOSAGE: *Adults:* Myelosuppressive Chemotherapy: Initial: 5mcg/kg qd SQ bolus, short IV infusion (15-30 min), or continuous SQ/IV infusion. Titrate: May increase in increments of 5mcg/kg for each chemotherapy cycle, according to duration and severity of ANC nadir. Should be administered no earlier than 24 hrs after the administration of cytotoxic chemotherapy. Should not be administered in the period 24 hrs before the administration of chemotherapy. Continue therapy after chemotherapy daily for up to 2 weeks, until the post nadir ANC =10,000/mm³ is reached. D/C if ANC surpasses 10,000/mm³ after the expected chemotherapy-induced neutrophil nadir. Bone Marrow Transplant: 10mcg/kg/day by IV infusion of 4 or 24 hrs or by continuous 24-hr SQ infusion. First dose at least 24 hrs after cytotoxic chemotherapy and at least 24 hrs after bone marrow infusion. Dose Adjustment: Adjust according to ANC; see PI. Peripheral Blood Progenitor Cell Collection: 10mcg/kg/day SQ, either as a bolus or continuous infusion. Should be given at least four days before the 1st leukapheresis procedure and continue until the last leukapheresis. Monitor neutrophils after 4 days and consider dose modification if WBC >100,000/mm³. Chronic Neutropenia: Congenital Neutropenia: Initial: 6mcg/kg SQ bid. Idiopathic or Cyclic Neutropenia: Initial: 5mcg/kg SQ qd. Adjust dose based on clinical course and ANC.

HOW SUPPLIED: Inj: 300mcg/0.5mL, 300mcg/mL, 480mcg/0.8mL, 480mcg/1.6mL

CONTRAINDICATIONS: Hypersensitivity to *E. coli*-derived proteins.

WARNINGS/PRECAUTIONS: Allergic-type reactions reported. Splenic rupture reported, some fatal. Evaluate for enlarged spleen or splenic rupture if complaints of left upper abdominal and/or shoulder tip pain. Acute respiratory distress syndrome reported; d/c until resolved. Alveolar hemorrhage manifesting as pulmonary infiltrates and hemoptysis requiring hospitalization reported. Severe sickle cell crises reported with sickle cell disorders. Take care to confirm diagnosis of severe chronic neutropenia prior to therapy. Avoid simultaneous use with chemotherapy and radiation therapy. CBC monitoring is recommended twice a week during therapy to avoid potential complications of excessive leukocytosis. Safety not established in patients with chronic myeloid leukemia (CML) and myelodysplasia. Potential for immunogenicity. Avoid premature d/c of therapy prior to time of recovery from expected neutrophil nadir. Cutaneous vasculitis reported; continue therapy at a reduced dose.

ADVERSE REACTIONS: N/V, skeletal pain, alopecia, diarrhea, neutropenic fever, mucositis, fatigue, anorexia, dyspnea, headache, cough, skin rash, splenomegaly, thrombocytopenia.

INTERACTIONS: Caution with drugs that may potentiate the release of neutrophils (eg, lithium). Transient positive bone imaging changes have been associated with increased hematopoietic activity of the bone marrow in response to growth factor therapy.

PREGNANCY: Category C, caution in nursing.

MECHANISM OF ACTION: Granulocyte colony-stimulating factor (G-CSF); acts on hematopoietic cells by binding to specific cell surface receptors. Stimulates proliferation, differentiation commitment, and some end-cell functional activation.

PHARMACOKINETICS: Absorption: (SQ, 3.45mcg/kg, 11.5mcg/kg): C_{max}=4ng/mL, 49ng/mL; T_{max}=2-8 hrs. **Distribution:** V_d=150mL/kg. **Elimination:** $T_{1/2}$=3.5 hrs, (IV) $T_{1/2}$=231 min (34.5mcg/kg), (SQ) $T_{1/2}$=210 min (3.45mcg/kg).

NURSING CONSIDERATIONS

Assessment: Obtain CBC with differential and platelet count. Assess for severe chronic neutropenia, history of chemotherapy/radiation therapy, history of hypersensitivity to *E. coli*-derived proteins, pregnancy/nursing status, and for possible drug interactions.

Monitoring: Monitor CBC with differential and platelet count 2-3 times a week. Perform annual bone marrow and cytogenetic evaluations throughout treatment for patients with congenital neutropenia. Monitor for hypersensitivity reactions, splenic rupture, ARDS, alveolar hemorrhage, hemoptysis, and sickle cell crises (in patients with sickle cell disease).

Patient Counseling: Counsel about potential adverse effects; seek medical attention if any develop. Report any left upper abdominal or shoulder tip pain. Refer patients to Information for Patients and Caregivers included with package insert in each dispensing pack.

Administration: SQ/IV route. Refer to PI for further detail. **Storage:** 2-8°C (36-46°F). Avoid shaking.

NEURONTIN   RX
gabapentin (Parke-Davis)

THERAPEUTIC CLASS: GABA analog

INDICATIONS: Adjunct therapy for partial seizures with or without secondary generalization in patients >12 yrs. Adjunct therapy for partial seizures in pediatrics 3-12 yrs with epilepsy. Management of postherpetic neuralgia (PHN) in adults.

DOSAGE: *Adults:* Epilepsy: Initial: 300mg tid. Titrate: Increase up to 1800mg/day. The maximum time between doses in the tid schedule should not exceed 12 hrs. Max: 3600mg/day. PHN: 300mg single dose on Day 1, then 300mg bid on Day 2, and 300mg tid on Day 3. Titrate: Increase prn for pain up to 600mg tid. Renal Impairment: CrCl ≥60mL/min: 900-3600mg/day. CrCl 30-59mL/min: 400-1400mg/day. CrCl >15-29mL/min: 200-700mg/day. CrCl 15mL/min: 100-300mg/day. CrCl <15mL/min: Reduce dose in proportion to CrCl. Hemodialysis: Maint: Base on CrCl. Give supplemental dose (125-350mg) after 4 hrs of hemodialysis. Refer to PI for dose adjustment. Elderly: Start at the low end of the dosing range.
Pediatrics: Epilepsy: >12 yrs: Initial: 300mg tid. Titrate: Increase up to 1800mg/day. Max: 3600mg/day. 3-12 yrs: Initial: 10-15mg/kg/day tid. Titrate: Increase over 3 days. Usual: ≥5 yrs: 25-35mg/kg/day tid. 3-4 yrs: 40mg/kg/day tid. The maximum time between doses in the tid schedule should not exceed 12 hrs. Max: 50mg/kg/day. Renal Impairment: ≥12 yrs: CrCl ≥60mL/min: 900-3600mg/day. CrCl >30-59mL/min: 400-1400mg/day. CrCl >15-29mL/min: 200-700mg/day. CrCl 15mL/min: 100-300mg/day. CrCl <15mL/min: Reduce dose in proportion to CrCl. Hemodialysis: Maint: Base on CrCl. Give supplemental dose (125-350mg) after 4 hrs of hemodialysis. Refer to PI for dose adjustment.

HOW SUPPLIED: Cap: 100mg, 300mg, 400mg; Sol: 250mg/5mL [470mL]; Tab: 600mg*, 800mg* *scored

WARNINGS/PRECAUTIONS: Avoid abrupt withdrawal; may increase seizure frequency. Increased risk of suicidal thoughts or behavior reported; monitor for emergence or worsening of depression, suicidal thought or behavior, and/or any unusual changes in mood and behavior. Sudden and unexplained deaths reported. Neuropsychiatric adverse events (eg, emotional lability, hostility, thought disorder, hyperkinesia) in pediatrics (3-12 yrs). Possible tumorigenic potential. Caution in elderly.

ADVERSE REACTIONS: Somnolence, dizziness, peripheral edema, ataxia, nystagmus, fatigue, tremor, rhinitis, N/V, infection, diarrhea, asthenia, dry mouth, constipation, headache.

INTERACTIONS: Decreased levels when taken with Maalox; take 2 hrs following antacid. Increased levels with controlled-release morphine, naproxen Na. Hydrocodone increases gabapentin AUC values while gabapentin decreases hydrocodone levels in dose-dependent manner.

PREGNANCY: Category C, caution in nursing.

MECHANISM OF ACTION: GABA analog; not established. Anticonvulsant activity: Suspected to bind to different areas of the brain including neocortex and hippocampus. Analgesic effects: Prevents allodynia and hyperalgesia.

PHARMACOKINETICS: Absorption: PO administration of variable doses resulted in different parameters. Refer to PI. **Distribution:** V_d=58L (150mg IV); plasma protein binding (<3%); found in breast milk. **Metabolism:** Not appreciably metabolized. **Elimination:** Renal (unchanged); $T_{1/2}$=5-7 hrs.

NURSING CONSIDERATIONS

Assessment: Assess renal function, hypersensitivity, pre-existing tumors, pregnancy/nursing status, and possible drug interactions.

Monitoring: Monitor for neuropsychiatric events (emotional lability, hostility, thought disorders, and hyperkinesia) in pediatric patients. Monitor for withdrawal-precipitated seizures, status epilepticus, emergence or worsening of depression, suicidal thoughts, changes in behavior, adverse reactions, development of new tumors, worsening of pre-existing tumors, renal function, and hypersensitivity reactions.

Patient Counseling: Instruct that medication may be taken with or without food and to take only as prescribed. Caution against operating machinery/driving until accustomed to effects of medication. Carefully observe for signs of CNS depression. Do not change the dose without talking to healthcare provider. Counsel that if taking Maalox, separate dosing by 2 hrs. Encourage patients to enroll in North American Antiepileptic Drug (NAAED) Pregnancy Registry if they become pregnant. Advise patients to be alert for and to contact physician if they have any increase of suicidal thoughts, worsening of depression, or any unusual changes in mood or behavior. Advise that scored tabs can be broken in half. The remaining half tab should be administered at next dose, or discard if unused after several days.

Administration: Oral route. **Storage:** Cap/Tab: 25°C (77°F); excursions permitted to 15-30°C (59-86°F). Sol: 2-8°C (36-46°F).

NEVANAC   RX
nepafenac (Alcon)

THERAPEUTIC CLASS: NSAID

INDICATIONS: Treatment of pain and inflammation associated with cataract surgery.

DOSAGE: *Adults:* 1 drop tid, start 24 hrs prior to surgery, continue up to 2 weeks post-op.

HOW SUPPLIED: Sus: 0.1% [3mL]

WARNINGS/PRECAUTIONS: Possible cross-sensitivity to acetylsalicylic acid, phenylacetic acid derivatives, and other NSAIDs. May cause increased bleeding of ocular tissue; slowed or delayed healing; keratitis. With continued use, may cause epithelial breakdown, corneal thinning, erosion, ulceration, perforation. Caution with bleeding tendencies and in complicated ocular surgeries, corneal denervation, corneal epithelial defects, diabetes mellitus, ocular surface diseases, rheumatoid arthritis, or repeat ocular surgeries.

ADVERSE REACTIONS: Capsular opacity, decreased visual acuity, foreign body sensation, increased IOP, sticky sensation.

PREGNANCY: Category C, caution in nursing.

MECHANISM OF ACTION: NSAID; inhibits cyclo-oxygenase that is essential for the biosynthesis of prostaglandins.

NURSING CONSIDERATIONS

Assessment: Assess for hypersensitivity or cross-sensitivity with some drugs (eg, acetylsalicylic acid), history of complicated or repeated ocular surgeries, corneal denervation, corneal epithelial defects, DM, ocular surface diseases (eg, dry eye syndrome), RA, bleeding tendencies, and history of concomitant use of medications that may prolong bleeding time or delay wound healing.

Monitoring: Monitor for hypersensitivity reactions, wound healing problems, keratitis, corneal thinning, corneal erosion, corneal ulceration or perforation, increased bleeding time, and bleeding of ocular tissues (hyphemas) in conjunction with ocular surgery.

Patient Counseling: Instruct not to administer suspension while wearing contact lenses.

Administration: Intraocular route. **Storage:** 2-25°C (36-77°F).

Nexavar   RX
sorafenib tosylate (Bayer/Onyx)

THERAPEUTIC CLASS: Multikinase inhibitor

INDICATIONS: Treatment of advanced renal cell carcinoma (RCC) or unresectable hepatocellular carcinoma (HCC).

DOSAGE: *Adults:* 400mg bid without food (1 hr before or 2 hrs after eating). Continue until no clinical benefit or unacceptable toxicity. Temporary interruption or dose reduction to 400mg qd or qod may be necessary if serious adverse events suspected. Refer to PI for dose modifications for skin toxicity.

HOW SUPPLIED: Tab: 200mg

CONTRAINDICATIONS: Squamous cell lung cancer, when given in combination with carboplatin and paclitaxel.

WARNINGS/PRECAUTIONS: Risk of cardiac ischemia and/or infarction reported; temporary or permanent d/c should be considered. Increased risk of bleeding may occur; consider d/c if bleeding necessitates medical intervention. HTN reported. Hand-foot skin reaction and rash may occur; may require topical treatment, temporary treatment interruption, and/or dose modification, or permanent d/c in severe cases. D/C if GI perforation occurs. Temporary interruption of therapy recommended when undergoing major surgical procedures. May cause fetal harm. Monitor fluid balance and electrolytes in patients at risk of renal dysfunction. Hepatic impairment may reduce plasma concentrations.

ADVERSE REACTIONS: HTN, fatigue, weight loss, rash/desquamation, hand-foot skin reaction, alopecia, pruritus, diarrhea, N/V, anorexia, constipation, hemorrhage, dyspnea, abdominal pain.

INTERACTIONS: See Contraindications. Caution with compounds metabolized/eliminated predominantly by the UGT1A1 pathway (eg, irinotecan); systemic exposure of substrates of UGT1A1 and UGT1A9 may increase with coadministration. May increase levels of docetaxel and doxorubicin; coadminister with caution. May alter level of fluorouracil; caution when coadministered with fluorouracil/leucovorin. Systemic exposure to substrates of CYP2B6 and CYP2C8 may increase with coadministration. May increase metabolism and decrease levels with CYP3A4 inducers (eg, St. John's wort, phenytoin, carbamazepine, phenobarbital, and dexamethasone). May increase INR; monitor with concomitant warfarin. Decrease levels with continuous administration of rifampicin. May increase concentrations of P-glycoprotein substrates. Decreased exposure with oral neomycin.

PREGNANCY: Category D, not for use in nursing.

MECHANISM OF ACTION: Multikinase inhibitor; inhibits multiple intracellular (CRAF, BRAF, and mutant BRAF) and cell surface kinases (KIT, FLT-3, RET, VEGFR-1, VEGFR-2, VEGFR-3, and PDGFR-β) which are thought to be involved in tumor cell signaling, angiogenesis, and apoptosis.

PHARMACOKINETICS: Absorption: Relative bioavailability (tab) (38-49%): T_{max}=3 hrs. **Distribution:** Plasma protein binding (99.5%). **Metabolism:** Liver via oxidation and glucuronidation; CYP3A4, UGT1A9; pyridine N-oxide (metabolite). **Elimination:** (100mg dose sol) Feces (77%, 51% unchanged), urine (19% as glucuronidated metabolites); $T_{1/2}$=25-48 hrs.

NURSING CONSIDERATIONS

Assessment: Assess for squamous cell lung cancer, bleeding problems, renal/hepatic dysfunction, major surgical procedures, drug hypersensitivity, pregnancy/nursing status and possible drug interactions. Note other diseases/conditions and drug therapies.

Monitoring: Monitor BP weekly during the first 6 weeks and periodically thereafter. Monitor for cardiac ischemia or infarction, hemorrhage, HTN, dermatologic toxicities, GI perforation, fluid balance and electrolytes in patients at risk of renal dysfunction. Monitor changes in PT, INR, or clinical bleeding episodes when given with warfarin.

Patient Counseling: Counsel about possible side effects; report any episodes of bleeding, cardiac ischemia/and or infarction, GI perforation. Advise of possible occurrence of hand-foot skin reaction and rash during therapy and appropriate countermeasures. Inform that HTN may develop especially during the first 6 weeks; advise that BP should be monitored regularly during therapy. Inform female patients that the drug may cause birth defects or fetal loss during pregnancy and that they should not become pregnant during therapy or for at least 2 weeks after stopping therapy; both males and females should use effective birth control during treatment to avoid conception. Advise against breastfeeding.

Administration: Oral route. Take without food (at least 1 hr before or 2 hrs after a meal). **Storage:** 25°C (77°F); excursions permitted to 15-30°C (59-86°F). Store in dry place.

NEXIUM RX
esomeprazole magnesium (AstraZeneca)

THERAPEUTIC CLASS: Proton pump inhibitor

INDICATIONS: Short-term treatment (4-8 weeks) and maintenance (up to 6 months) of the healing and symptomatic resolution of erosive esophagitis. Short-term treatment of heartburn and other symptoms associated with GERD in adults and children ≥1 yr. Reduction in occurrence of gastric ulcers associated with continuous NSAID therapy in patients at risk for developing gastric ulcers. In combination with amoxicillin and clarithromycin, for the treatment of *H. pylori* infection and duodenal ulcer disease (active or history of within the past 5 yrs). Long term-treatment of pathological hypersecretory conditions, including Zollinger-Ellison syndrome.

DOSAGE: *Adults:* Erosive Esophagitis: Healing: 20mg or 40mg qd for 4-8 weeks; may extend treatment for 4-8 weeks if not healed. Maint of healing: 20mg qd for up to 6 months. Symptomatic GERD: 20mg qd for 4 weeks; may extend treatment for 4 weeks if symptoms do not resolve. Risk Reduction of NSAID-Associated Gastric Ulcer: 20mg or 40mg qd for up to 6 months. *H. pylori* Eradication: Triple Therapy: 40mg qd + amoxicillin 1000mg bid + clarithromycin 500mg bid, all for 10 days. Pathological Hypersecretory Conditions (eg, Zollinger-Ellison Syndrome): 40mg bid. Adjust dose based on patient's needs. Doses up to 240mg qd have been administered. Severe Hepatic Dysfunction (Child-Pugh Class C): Max: 20mg/day. Take 1 hr before meals. (Cap) Swallow capsule whole. Contents may be mixed with applesauce or delivered through a nasogastric tube.

Pediatrics: GERD: 12-17 yrs: 20mg or 40mg qd for up to 8 weeks. 1-11 yrs: 10mg qd for up to 8 weeks. Healing of Erosive Esophagitis: 1-11 yrs: <20kg: 10mg qd for 8 weeks. ≥20kg: 10mg or 20mg qd for 8 weeks. Severe Hepatic Dysfunction (Child-Pugh Class C): Max: 20mg/day. Take 1 hr before meals. (Cap) Swallow capsule whole. Contents may be mixed with applesauce or delivered through a nasogastric tube.

HOW SUPPLIED: Cap, Delayed-Release: 20mg, 40mg; Sus, Delayed-Release: 10mg, 20mg, 40mg (granules/pkt).

WARNINGS/PRECAUTIONS: Atrophic gastritis reported with long-term use. Symptomatic response does not preclude the presence of gastric malignancy. May be associated with an increased risk for osteoporosis-related fractures of the hip, wrist or spine; use lowest dose and shortest duration of PPI therapy.

ADVERSE REACTIONS: Headache, diarrhea, abdominal pain, constipation, nausea, flatulence, dry mouth.

INTERACTIONS: Decreases clearance of diazepam. May interfere with absorption of gastric pH-dependent drugs (eg, ketoconazole, atazanavir, digoxin, iron salts). May reduce atazanavir and nelfinavir levels; use not recommended. May increase cilostazol levels; consider dose reduction. May increase saquinavir levels; monitor for possible toxicity and consider dose reduction. Increased levels with amoxicillin and clarithromycin. Monitor INR and prothrombin time with warfarin. May increase levels with combined inhibitors of CYP2C19 and 3A4 (eg, voriconazole). May inhibit metabolism of CYP2C19 substrates. May change absorption of antiretroviral drugs.

PREGNANCY: Category B, not for use in nursing.

MECHANISM OF ACTION: Proton pump inhibitor; suppresses gastric acid secretion by specific inhibition of the H^+/K^+-ATPase in the gastric parietal cell.

PHARMACOKINETICS: Absorption: (40mg) C_{max} =4.7µmol/L; T_{max} =1.6 hrs; AUC=12.6µmol•hr/L. (20mg) C_{max} =2.1µmol/L; T_{max} =1.6 hrs; AUC=4.2µmol•hr/L. **Distribution:** V_d =16L; plasma protein binding (97%). **Metabolism:** Liver (extensive) via CYP2C19, CYP3A4. **Elimination:** Inactive metabolites: Urine (80%), feces (remainder); (40mg) $T_{1/2}$ =1.5 hrs (20mg) $T_{1/2}$ =1.2 hrs. For pediatric parameters, refer to PI.

NURSING CONSIDERATIONS

Assessment: Assess for hypersensitivity to other proton pump inhibitors, presence of gastric malignancy, severe hepatic impairment, pregnancy/nursing status, and possible drug interactions.

Monitoring: Monitor for signs/symptoms of atrophic gastritis, osteoporosis-related fractures, GI symptoms, and hypersensitivity reactions (eg, anaphylaxis, angioedema). Monitor INR and PT when given with warfarin. Monitor LFTs.

Patient Counseling: Counsel to contact physician if signs/symptoms of hypersensitivity reaction or any adverse events occur. May take antacids while on therapy. Instruct to tell physician if taking or begin taking other medication and take 1 hr before meals. Swallow capsules whole; do not chew, crush, and mix with food, granules can only be mixed with applesauce. If difficulty swallowing, open capsules and empty granules into applesauce, which should not be warm. For oral suspension, empty packet of medication into container containing 1 tbsp of water (15mL); stir contents, let stand for 2-3 min to thicken; drink solution within 30 min. If contents of solution remain, add more water, stir, and drink immediately.

Administration: Oral route. Refer to PI for administration options and instructions. **Storage:** 25°C (77°F); excursions permitted to 15-30°C (59-86°F). Dispense in tightly closed container.

NEXIUM IV   RX

esomeprazole sodium (AstraZeneca)

THERAPEUTIC CLASS: Proton pump inhibitor

INDICATIONS: Short-term treatment (up to 10 days) of GERD with history of erosive esophagitis when oral therapy not possible or appropriate.

DOSAGE: *Adults:* 20mg or 40mg qd IV injection (no less than 3 min) or infusion (10-30 min) for up to 10 days. D/C as soon as patient is able to resume treatment with cap. Severe Liver Impairment (Child Pugh Class C): Max: 20mg/day.

HOW SUPPLIED: Inj: 20mg, 40mg

WARNINGS/PRECAUTIONS: Atrophic gastritis reported with long-term use. Symptomatic response does not preclude the presence of gastric malignancy. D/C and convert to oral therapy as soon as possible. May be associated with an increased risk for osteoporosis-related fractures of the hip, wrist or spine; use lowest dose and shortest duration of PPI therapy.

ADVERSE REACTIONS: Headache, flatulence, dyspepsia, nausea, abdominal pain, diarrhea, dry mouth.

INTERACTIONS: Decreases clearance of diazepam. May interfere with absorption of gastric pH-dependent drugs (eg, ketoconazole, iron salts, digoxin). Monitor INR and prothrombin time with warfarin. May reduce plasma levels of atazanavir and nelfinavir; use not recommended. May increase cilostazol levels; consider dose reduction. May increase saquinavir levels; monitor for possible toxicity and consider dose reduction. May increase levels with combined inhibitors of CYP2C19 and 3A4 (eg, voriconazole). May inhibit metabolism of CYP2C19 substrates. May change the absorption of antiretroviral drugs.

PREGNANCY: Category B, not for use in nursing.

MECHANISM OF ACTION: Proton pump inhibitor; suppresses gastric acid secretion by specific inhibition of the H^+/K^+-ATPase in the gastric parietal cell.

PHARMACOKINETICS: Absorption: (20mg) AUC=5.11µmol•hr/L; C_{max}=3.86µmol/L; (40mg) AUC=16.21µmol•hr/L; C_{max}=7.51µmol/L. **Distribution:** V_d=16L; plasma protein binding (97%). **Metabolism:** Liver (extensive) via CYP2C19, 3A4. **Elimination:** Urine (primary, <1% unchanged), feces; (20mg) $T_{1/2}$=1.05 hrs. (40mg) $T_{1/2}$=1.41 hrs.

NURSING CONSIDERATIONS

Assessment: Assess for hypersensitivity to other proton pump inhibitors, presence of gastric malignancy, severe hepatic insufficiency/liver impairment, pregnancy/nursing status, and possible drug interactions.

Monitoring: Monitor for signs/symptoms of atrophic gastritis, osteoporosis-related fractures, hypersensitivity reaction. Monitor INR and PT when given with warfarin. Monitor LFTs.

Patient Counseling: Instruct to contact physician if any adverse events develop.

Administration: IV route. Refer to PI for reconstitution instructions. Should not be administered concomitantly with any other medications through same IV site or tubing. Always flush IV line both prior to and after administration. Inspect visually for particulate matter and discoloration prior to administration. **Storage:** Vial: 25°C (77°F); excursions permitted to 15-30°C (59-86°F). Protect from light. Store in carton until time of use. Refer to PI for storage information of reconstituted products.

NEXTERONE   RX
amiodarone HCl (Prism)

THERAPEUTIC CLASS: Class III antiarrhythmic

INDICATIONS: Initiation of treatment and prophylaxis of frequently recurring ventricular fibrillation (VF) and hemodynamically unstable ventricular tachycardia (VT) refractory to other therapies. Treatment of patients with VT/VF for whom oral amiodarone is indicated, but who are unable to take oral medication.

DOSAGE: *Adults:* May individualize 1st-24 hr dose. Max Infusion Rate: 30mg/min (initial); 2mg/mL (longer than 1 hr, unless a central venous catheter is used). LD: 150mg IV over 1st 10 min (15mg/min), then 360mg IV over next 6 hrs (1mg/min). Maint: 540mg IV over remaining 18 hrs (0.5mg/min). After 1st 24 hrs, continue with 720mg/24 hrs (0.5mg/min) for 2-3 weeks; may increase rate to achieve suppression. Breakthrough VF/Unstable VT: Supplemental 150mg IV over 10 min. Switching to Oral Amiodarone (assuming a 720mg/day IV infusion): <1 week of IV infusion: 800-1600mg/day; 1-3 weeks of IV infusion: 600-800mg/day; >3 weeks of IV infusion: 400mg/day. Elderly: Start at low end of dosing range.

HOW SUPPLIED: Inj: 1.5mg/mL, 1.8mg/mL

CONTRAINDICATIONS: Cardiogenic shock, marked sinus bradycardia, 2nd- or 3rd-degree atrioventricular (AV) block unless a functioning pacemaker is available.

WARNINGS/PRECAUTIONS: Hypotension reported; treat initially by slowing infusion. Bradycardia reported; treat by slowing infusion or d/c. Elevated hepatic enzymes reported. Acute centrolobular confluent hepatocellular necrosis leading to hepatic coma and acute renal failure may occur at a much higher LD concentration and much faster rate of infusion than recommended. Consider d/c or reducing infusion rate with evidence of progressive hepatic injury. May worsen or precipitate a new arrhythmia; monitor for QTc prolongation. Pulmonary toxicity/fibrosis and adult respiratory distress syndrome (ARDS) reported. Optic neuropathy and neuritis reported. Hypo- and hyperthyroidism, thyroid nodules/cancer/dysfunction reported. Hyperthyroidism may result in thyrotoxicosis and arrhythmia breakthrough or aggravation. May cause fetal harm. Corneal refractive laser surgery may be contraindicated. Correct hypokalemia or hypomagnesemia before initiation to prevent exaggeration of QTc prolongation or increased potential for torsade de pointes. Caution in elderly.

ADVERSE REACTIONS: Hypotension, asystole, cardiac arrest, pulseless electrical activity (PEA), cardiogenic shock, congestive heart failure, bradycardia, abnormal LFTs, fever, nausea, VT.

INTERACTIONS: CYP3A inhibitors (eg, protease inhibitors, cimetidine, grapefruit juice) may increase levels. CYP2C8 inhibitors may decrease metabolism and increase levels. May increases levels of CYP1A2/CYP2C9/CYP2D6/CYP3A and p-glycoprotein substrates. QT prolongation and TdP may occur with loratadine and trazodone. May elevate plasma levels of cyclosporine, digoxin, quinidine, procainamide, phenytoin, flecainide. D/C or reduce digitalis dose by 50%. Reduce quinidine and procainamide doses by one-third. Myopathy/rhabdomyolysis reported with simvastatin. Risk of bradycardia, sinus arrest, and AV block with β-receptor blocking agents (eg, propranolol) or calcium channel blockers (eg, verapamil, diltiazem). May increase PT with warfarin. Concomitant use with clopidogrel may result in ineffective inhibition of platelet aggregation. CYP3A inducers (eg, rifampin, St. John's wort) may decrease levels. Concomitant use with fentanyl may cause hypotension, bradycardia, and decreased cardiac output. Cholestyramine may decrease levels and half-life. QTc prolongation with disopyramide, fluoroquinolones, macrolides, and azoles. Concomitant use with propranolol, diltiazem, verapamil may result in hemodynamic and electrophysiologic interactions. May be more sensitive to myocardial depressant and conduction defects of halogenated inhalational anesthetics. Seizures, associated with increased lidocaine concentrations, reported. Action of antithyroid drugs may be delayed in amiodarone-induced thyrotoxicosis. Radioactive therapy is contraindicated with amiodarone-induced hyperthyroidism. Give special attention to electrolyte and acid-base balance in patients receiving concomitant diuretics. Initiate any added antiarrhythmic drug at a lower than usual dose.

PREGNANCY: Category D, not for use in nursing.

MECHANISM OF ACTION: Class III antiarrhythmic; blocks sodium, calcium, and potassium channels; exerts noncompetitive antisympathetic action, and negative chronotropic and dromotropic effects; lengthens cardiac action potential, decreases cardiac workload and myocardial oxygen consumption.

PHARMACOKINETICS: Absorption: C_{max}=7-26mg/L (150mg IV). **Distribution:** Plasma protein binding (>96%); crosses the placenta, found in breast milk. **Metabolism:** CYP3A, 2C8; N-desethylamiodarone (major active metabolite). **Elimination:** Urine, bile; $T_{1/2}$=9-36 days (amiodarone); 9-30 days (N-desethylamiodarone).

NURSING CONSIDERATIONS

Assessment: Assess for cardiogenic shock, marked sinus bradycardia, 2nd- or 3rd-degree AV block, functioning pacemaker, thyroid dysfunction, hypersensitivity, pregnancy/nursing status, and possible drug interactions. Prior to initiation, correct hypokalemia and hypomagnesemia.

Monitoring: Monitor for hypotension, asystole/cardiac arrest/PEA, bradycardia, VT, CHF, hepatic injury, acute renal failure, worsening of existing or precipitation of new arrhythmia, QTc prolongation, ARDS, pulmonary fibrosis, optic neuropathy/neuritis, visual impairment. Monitor LFTs and thyroid function. Perioperative monitoring for patients undergoing general anesthesia recommended. Perform regular ophthalmic exams including fundoscopy and slit-lamp exams. Monitor initial rate of infusion closely and do not exceed the recommended dose.

Patient Counseling: Instruct to d/c nursing while on therapy. Advise that corneal refractive laser surgery may be contraindicated. Do not to take grapefruit juice, over-the-counter cough medicine (dextromethorphan), and St. John's wort during therapy. Inform of the symptoms of hypo- and hyperthyroidism, particularly if transitioned to oral therapy.

Administration: IV route. Do not use plastic containers in series connections. Caution with admixture incompatibility, refer to PI. **Storage:** 20-25°C (68-77°F); excursions permitted to 15-30°C (59-86°F). Protect from light, excessive heat, and freezing.

NIASPAN   RX
niacin (Abbott)

THERAPEUTIC CLASS: Nicotinic acid

INDICATIONS: To reduce elevated total cholesterol (TC), LDL-C, TG, and Apo B levels, and to increase HDL-C in primary hyperlipidemia and mixed dyslipidemia. With concomitant lovastatin or simvastatin, to treat primary hyperlipidemia and mixed dyslipidemia when treatment with monotherapy is inadequate. To reduce the risk of recurrent nonfatal myocardial infarction (MI) with history of MI and hyperlipidemia. With concomitant bile acid binding resin, to slow progression/promote regression of atherosclerotic disease in patients with history of CAD and hyperlipidemia, and to reduce elevated TC and LDL-C levels in adult patients with primary hyperlipidemia. Adjunct therapy for treatment of adult patients with severe hypertriglyceridemia with risk of pancreatitis and who do not respond adequately to diet.

DOSAGE: *Adults:* Take qhs after low-fat snack. Individualize dose. Initial: 500mg qhs. Titrate: Increase by 500mg every 4 weeks. After Week 8, titrate to patient response and tolerance. Do not increase daily dose by more than 500mg in any 4-week period. Maint: 1-2g qhs. Max: 2g/day. With Lovastatin/Simvastatin: Initial Lovastatin/Simvastatin: 20mg qd. Adjust dose at intervals of ≥4 weeks. Max: 2g niacin/40mg lovastatin/simvastatin qd. May take aspirin (up to 325mg) 30 min before administration to reduce flushing. Do not chew, crush, or break; swallow whole. Women may respond at lower doses than men. Do not interchange 3 of 500mg and 2 of 750mg tab. If d/c therapy for an extended period of time, reinstitution should include titration phase. *Pediatrics:* >16 yrs: Take qhs after low-fat snack. Individualize dose. Initial: 500mg qhs. Titrate: Increase by 500mg every 4 weeks. After week 8, titrate to patient response and tolerance. Do not increase daily dose by more than 500mg in any 4-week period. Maint: 1-2g qhs. Max: 2g/day. With Lovastatin/Simvastatin: Initial Lovastatin/Simvastatin: 20mg qd. Adjust dose at intervals of ≥4 weeks. Max: 2g niacin/40mg lovastatin/simvastatin qd. May take aspirin (up to 325mg) 30 min before administration to reduce flushing. Do not chew, crush, or break; swallow whole. Women may respond at lower doses than men. Do not interchange 3 of 500mg and 2 of 750mg tab. If d/c therapy for an extended period of time, reinstitution should include titration phase.

HOW SUPPLIED: Tab, Extended-Release: 500mg, 750mg, 1000mg

CONTRAINDICATIONS: Active liver disease or unexplained persistent elevations in hepatic transaminases, active peptic ulcer disease, arterial bleeding.

WARNINGS/PRECAUTIONS: Do not substitute with equivalent doses of immediate-release niacin; severe hepatic toxicity may occur. Caution with heavy alcohol use and/or past history of liver disease, renal impairment, unstable angina, and acute phase of MI. Observe closely with history of jaundice, hepatobiliary disease, or peptic ulcer. Myopathy and rhabdomyolysis reported. Associated with abnormal LFTs; d/c if transaminase levels progress (3X ULN and are persistent), or if associated with nausea, fever, and/or malaise. May increase FPG; caution in diabetic patients. May reduce platelet count and phosphorus levels. May increase PT; caution in patients undergoing surgery. Elevated uric acid levels reported; caution in patients predisposed to gout.

ADVERSE REACTIONS: Flushing, diarrhea, N/V, increased cough, pruritus, rash.

INTERACTIONS: Rhabdomyolysis/myopathy may occur with HMG-CoA reductase inhibitors; consider performing periodic monitoring of creatine phosphokinase (CPK) and K^+ levels. May potentiate effects of ganglionic blocking agents and vasoactive drugs resulting in postural hypotension. Separate dosing from bile acid binding resins (eg, colestipol, cholestyramine) by at least 4-6 hrs. Concomitant aspirin use may decrease metabolic clearance of nicotinic acid. Concurrent use with vitamins or other nutritional supplements containing large doses of niacin or related compounds (eg, nicotinamide) may potentiate adverse effects of niacin. Avoid ingestion of alcohol, hot drinks, or spicy foods around time of administration; may increase flushing and pruritus. Caution with anticoagulants; monitor platelet counts and PT. Caution with unstable angina or acute phase MI and vasoactive drugs (eg, nitrates, calcium channel blockers, adrenergic blockers). Adjustment of hypoglycemic therapy may be necessary.

PREGNANCY: Category C, not for use in nursing.

MECHANISM OF ACTION: Nicotinic acid; mechanism not established. May partially inhibit release of free fatty acids from adipose tissue, and increase lipoprotein lipase activity, which may increase the rate of chylomicron TG removal from plasma. Decreases the rate of hepatic synthesis of VLDL and LDL.

PHARMACOKINETICS: Absorption: T_{max}=5 hrs. **Distribution:** Found in breast milk. **Metabolism:** Liver rapid and extensive to nicotinamide adenine dinucleotide (NAD), to nicotinuric acid (NUA) via conjugation and other metabolites. **Elimination:** Urine (60-76%; 12%, unchanged).

NURSING CONSIDERATIONS

Assessment: Assess for presence or history of liver disease, history of jaundice, uncontrolled hypothyroidism, or any other conditions where treatment is contraindicated or cautioned. Assess for upcoming surgery, pregnancy/nursing status, and for possible drug interactions. Assess LFTs and lipid levels prior to therapy. Assess that patient is on cholesterol-lowering diet prior to therapy.

Monitoring: Monitor for signs/symptoms of hepatotoxicity (eg, fulminant hepatic necrosis), rhabdomyolysis, decreases in platelet counts, increases in PT, and for increased uric acid levels. Monitor phosphorus levels in patients at risk for hypophosphatemia. Monitor LFTs (eg, AST, ALT) every 6-12 weeks during first year and periodically thereafter. Monitor periodically serum CPK, K^+, and fasting lipid levels. Monitor glucose levels frequently.

Patient Counseling: Advise to adhere to recommended diet, a regular exercise program, and periodic testing of a fasting lipid panel. Counsel to take at hs, after a low-fat snack. Advise not to break, crush, or chew; swallow whole. Inform that flushing may occur but may subside after several weeks of therapy. Inform that taking aspirin 30 min before dosing may minimize flushing. Avoid ingestion of alcohol, spicy foods, or hot drinks with administration to prevent flushing. Get up slowly if awakened by flushing at night. Contact physician if dosing is interrupted for any length of time, taking vitamins or other nutritional supplements, or if unexplained muscle pain, tenderness or weakness, or dizziness occurs. Instruct diabetic patients to contact physician if changes in blood glucose levels occur. Advise to d/c use and contact physician if patient becomes pregnant or if patient is currently breastfeeding.

Administration: Oral route. **Storage:** 20-25°C (68-77°F).

NIFEDIPINE RX
nifedipine (Various)

OTHER BRAND NAMES: Procardia (Pfizer)

THERAPEUTIC CLASS: Calcium channel blocker (dihydropyridine)

INDICATIONS: Management of vasospastic angina and chronic stable angina.

DOSAGE: *Adults:* Initial: 10mg tid. Usual: 10-20mg tid or 20-30mg tid-qid with evidence of coronary artery spasm. Titrate: Over a 7-14 day period. If symptoms warrant (eg, activity level, attack frequency, SL nitroglycerin consumption) dose may be increased from 10mg tid to 20mg tid then 30mg tid over a 3-day period. Ischemic hospitalized patients may increase in 10mg increments over 4-6 hr periods. Doses above 120mg qd are rarely necessary. Max: 180mg qd. Swallow cap whole.

HOW SUPPLIED: Cap: 10mg, 20mg

WARNINGS/PRECAUTIONS: May cause hypotension; monitor BP initially or with titration. CHF risk, especially with aortic stenosis or β-blockers. Peripheral edema reported. Not for acute reduction of BP or essential HTN. May increase angina or MI with severe obstructive CAD. Avoid with acute coronary syndrome or within 1-2 weeks of MI. Caution in elderly.

ADVERSE REACTIONS: Dizziness, lightheadedness, giddiness, flushing, heat sensation, heartburn, muscle cramps, tremor, headache, weakness, nausea, peripheral edema, nervousness/mood changes, palpitation.

INTERACTIONS: β-blockers may increase risk of CHF, severe hypotension, or angina exacerbation. Possible hypotension with fentanyl. Potentiates digoxin. Increase plasma levels with cimetidine and grapefruit juice. Increased prothrombin time with coumarin. Decreased plasma levels of quinidine.

PREGNANCY: Category C, unknown use in nursing.

MECHANISM OF ACTION: Calcium channel blocker; inhibits the transmembrane influx of calcium ions into cardiac muscle and smooth muscle. Angina: MOA not fully determined; believed to act by relaxation and prevention of coronary artery spasm, and reduction of oxygen utilization.

PHARMACOKINETICS: Absorption: Rapid and fully absorbed; T_{max}=30 min. **Distribution:** Plasma protein binding (92-98%). **Metabolism:** Liver, extensive. **Elimination:** Urine (80%); $T_{1/2}$=2 hrs.

NURSING CONSIDERATIONS

Assessment: Assess for CHF, aortic stenosis, hepatic/renal impairment, essential HTN, recent MI, β-blocker withdrawal syndrome with increased angina, pregnancy/nursing status, and possible drug interactions.

Monitoring: Monitor for hypotension and/or increased fluid volume requirements, increased angina, and/or MI, HF, peripheral edema, allergic hepatitis, cholestasis with/without jaundice. Monitor BP, LFTs, BUN, SrCr, decreased platelet aggregation, increased bleeding time, positive direct Coombs' test with/without hemolytic anemia.

Patient Counseling: Inform not to use for acute reduction of BP or for control of essential HTN. Advise not to take with grapefruit juice. Inform about potential risks/benefits of drug.

Administration: Oral route. **Storage:** 15-25°C (59-77°F). Protect from light and moisture.

NILANDRON

RX

nilutamide (Sanofi-Aventis)

Interstitial pneumonitis reported. Rare postmarketing reports of interstitial changes including pulmonary fibrosis that led to hospitalization and death have been reported. Symptoms included exertional dyspnea, cough, chest pain, and fever. X-rays showed interstitial or alveolo-interstitial changes, and pulmonary function tests revealed a restrictive pattern with decreased DLco. Most cases occurred within the first 3 months of treatment, and reversed with discontinuation. A routine x-ray should be performed prior to initiating treatment. Baseline pulmonary function tests may be considered. Instruct patients to report any new or worsening shortness of breath during treatment. If symptoms occur, treatment should be discontinued until it can be determined if the symptoms are drug related.

THERAPEUTIC CLASS: Nonsteroidal antiandrogen

INDICATIONS: Treatment of metastatic prostatic cancer (Stage D_2) in combination with surgical castration.

DOSAGE: *Adults:* Initial: 300mg/day for 30 days beginning on the day of, or on the day after, surgical castration. Maint: 150mg qd.

HOW SUPPLIED: Tab: 150mg

CONTRAINDICATIONS: Severe hepatic impairment, respiratory insufficiency.

WARNINGS/PRECAUTIONS: Not for use in women. Hepatotoxicity reported; d/c if jaundice or ALT >2X ULN develop. May cause aplastic anemia. Patients whose disease progresses while on therapy may experience clinical improvement with discontinuation. Delayed adaptation to dark reported; wearing tinted glasses may alleviate effect.

ADVERSE REACTIONS: Hot flushes, decreased libido, abnormal vision, increased LFTs, dyspnea, dizziness, HTN, anemia, testicular atrophy, gynecomastia, pain, N/V, constipation.

INTERACTIONS: Inhibits CYP450 in vitro and may reduce the metabolism of their substrates. May, thus, potentiate vitamin K antagonists, phenytoin, and theophylline leading to toxicity. May cause intolerance to alcohol (eg, hypotension, malaise).

PREGNANCY: Category C, safety not known in nursing.

MECHANISM OF ACTION: Nonsteroidal antiandrogen; acts by blocking effects of testosterone at the androgen receptor sites.

PHARMACOKINETICS: Absorption: Rapid and complete. **Distribution:** Plasma protein binding (Moderate). **Metabolism:** Extensive, via oxidation. **Elimination**: Urine (62%, <2% unchanged), feces (1.4%-7%); $T_{1/2}$=38-59.1 hrs (100mg-300mg single dose).

NURSING CONSIDERATIONS

Assessment: Measure baseline hepatic enzymes, chest x-ray, and pulmonary function test. Assess comorbidities and possible drug interactions.

Monitoring: Prior to treatment and periodically thereafter, measure baseline hepatic enzymes, routine chest x-ray, and pulmonary function tests. Monitor for occurrence of interstitial pneumonitis, hepatotoxicity, hypersensitivity reactions.

Patient Counseling: Report new or worsening SOB, N/V, abdominal pain, or jaundice. Start on day of or day after surgical castration; do not interrupt or d/c dosing without consulting physician. Avoid taking with alcohol. Wear tinted glasses to alleviate the delayed adaptation to dark; caution about driving at night and through tunnels.

Administration: Oral route. **Storage**: 25°C (77°F); excursions permitted to 15-30°C (59-86°F). Protect from light.

NIRAVAM
alprazolam (Schwarz)

THERAPEUTIC CLASS: Benzodiazepine

INDICATIONS: Management of anxiety disorders and short-term relief of anxiety symptoms. Treatment of panic disorder with or without agoraphobia.

DOSAGE: *Adults:* Anxiety: Initial: 0.25-0.5mg tid. Titrate: May increase every 3-4 days. Max: 4mg/day. Panic Disorder: Initial: 0.5mg tid. Titrate: Increase by no more than 1mg/day every 3-4 days; slower titration if ≥4mg/day. Usual: 1-10mg/day. Decrease dose slowly (no more than 0.5mg every 3 days). Elderly/Advanced Liver Disease/Debilitated: Initial: 0.25mg bid-tid. Titrate: Increase gradually as tolerated.

HOW SUPPLIED: Tab, Disintegrating: 0.25mg*, 0.5mg*, 1mg*, 2mg* *scored

CONTRAINDICATIONS: Acute narrow-angle glaucoma, untreated open-angle glaucoma, concomitant ketoconazole or itraconazole.

WARNINGS/PRECAUTIONS: Risk of dependence. Withdrawal symptoms, including seizure, reported with dose reduction or abrupt d/c; avoid abrupt withdrawal. Risk of CNS depression and impaired performance. May cause fetal harm. Caution with impaired renal, hepatic, or pulmonary function, severe depression, obesity, elderly and debilitated. Hypomania/mania reported with depression. Weak uricosuric effect.

ADVERSE REACTIONS: Drowsiness, fatigue/tiredness, impaired coordination, irritability, memory impairment, cognitive disorder, dysarthria, decreased libido, confusional state, lightheadedness, dry mouth, hypotension, increased salivation.

INTERACTIONS: See Contraindications. Avoid with potent CYP3A inhibitors (eg, azole antifungals). Potentiated by nefazodone, fluvoxamine, cimetidine, fluoxetine, oral contraceptives. Decreased plasma levels with propoxyphene and carbamazepine. Caution with diltiazem, isoniazid, macrolides, grapefruit juice, sertraline, paroxetine, ergotamine, cyclosporine, amiodarone, nicardipine, nifedipine and other CYP3A inhibitors. Increases levels of imipramine and desipramine. Additive CNS depressant effects with psychotropic agents, anticonvulsants, antihistamines, ethanol.

PREGNANCY: Category D, not for use in nursing.

MECHANISM OF ACTION: Benzodiazepine; not established, CNS depressant, believed to exert its effects by binding at stereo specific receptor at several sites within the CNS.

PHARMACOKINETICS: Absorption: Readily absorbed; C_{max}=8-37ng/mL; T_{max}=1.5-2 hrs. **Distribution:** Plasma protein binding (80%). **Metabolism:** Metabolized (extensively), hydroxylation, 4-hydroxyalprazolam and α-hydroxyalprazolam (major metabolites). **Elimination:** Urine, $T_{1/2}$=12.5 hrs.

NURSING CONSIDERATIONS

Assessment: Assess for known sensitivity to drug, open-angle and acute-closed glaucoma, renal/hepatic impairment, pulmonary function insufficiency, and possible drug interactions. Assess for risk of dependence among panic disorder patients.

Monitoring: Monitor early morning anxiety and emergence of anxiety symptoms, CNS depression, physical/psychological dependence, suicidality, mania/hypomania, uricosuric effects, acute renal failure, seizures and status epilepticus. Monitor blood counts, urinalysis, and blood chemistry analysis.

Patient Counseling: Inform of benefits/risks and possibilty of physical/ psychological dependence. Caution against hazardous tasks (eg, operating machinery/driving). Avoid alcohol. Notify physician if pregnant or planning to become pregnant or before increasing dose or d/c the drug.

Administration: Oral route. Remove tablets from bottle just before dosing. Can be swallowed with/without water. **Storage:** 20-25°C (68-77°F); excursions permitted to 15-30°C (59-86°F). Protect from moisture.

NITRO-DUR

RX

nitroglycerin (Schering)

OTHER BRAND NAMES: Nitrek (Mylan Bertek) - Minitran (Graceway)

THERAPEUTIC CLASS: Nitrate vasodilator

INDICATIONS: Prevention of angina pectoris. Not for acute attack.

DOSAGE: *Adults:* Initial: 0.2-0.4mg/hr for 12-14 hrs. Remove for 10-12 hrs.

HOW SUPPLIED: Patch: (Minitran) 0.1mg/hr, 0.2mg/hr, 0.4mg/hr, 0.6mg/hr [30^s]; (Nitrek) 0.2mg/hr, 0.4mg/hr, 0.6mg/hr [30^s]; (Nitro-Dur) 0.1mg/hr, 0.2mg/hr, 0.3mg/hr, 0.4mg/hr, 0.6mg/hr, 0.8mg/hr [30^s]

CONTRAINDICATIONS: Allergy to adhesives in NTG patches.

WARNINGS/PRECAUTIONS: Severe hypotension may occur; caution with volume depletion or hypotension. May aggravate angina caused by hypertrophic cardiomyopathy. Tolerance to other nitrate forms may decrease effects. Monitor with acute MI or CHF. Do not discharge defibrillator/cardioverter through the patch.

ADVERSE REACTIONS: Headache, lightheadedness, hypotension, syncope.

INTERACTIONS: Additive vasodilating effects with other vasodilators (eg, alcohol). Marked orthostatic hypotension reported with CCBs. Vasodilatory effects with phosphodiesterase inhibitors (eg, sildenafil) can result in severe hypotension.

PREGNANCY: Category C, caution in nursing.

MECHANISM OF ACTION: Nitrate vasodilator; relaxes vascular smooth muscle, and consequent dilatation of peripheral arteries and veins, especially the latter. Dilatation of veins leads to reduced left ventricular end-diastolic pressure and pulmonary capillary wedge pressure (preload). Arteriolar relaxation reduces systemic vascular resistance, systolic arterial pressure, and mean arterial pressure (afterload). It also dilates the coronary artery.

PHARMACOKINETICS: Absorption: T_{max}=2 hrs. **Distribution:** V_d=3L/kg. **Metabolism:** Extrahepatic metabolism (RBC and vascular walls). Inorganic nitrate and the 1,2- and 1,3- dinitroglycerols. Dinitrates are metabolized to mononitrates and to glycerol and CO_2. **Elimination:** $T_{1/2}$=3 min.

NURSING CONSIDERATIONS

Assessment: Assess for severe hypotension or volume depleted patients, angina caused by hypertrophic cardiomyopathy, alcohol intake, pregnancy/nursing status, and possible drug interactions.

Monitoring: Careful clinical or hemodynamic monitoring for hypotension and tachycardia. Monitor for paradoxical bradycardia and increased angina pectoris, decreased exercise tolerance and hemodynamic rebound, headaches and lightheadedness on standing, manifestation of true physical dependence (chest pain, acute MI), and methemoglobinemia.

Patient Counseling: Counsel to carefully follow dosing regimen. Inform about headaches (markers of drug activity) and lightheadedness on standing. Avoid alcohol consumption.

Administration: Transdermal route. **Storage:** 15-30°C (59-86°F).

NITROLINGUAL SPRAY

RX

nitroglycerin (Various)

OTHER BRAND NAMES: NitroMist (Akrimax)

THERAPEUTIC CLASS: Nitrate vasodilator

INDICATIONS: For acute relief of an attack or prophylaxis of angina pectoris due to coronary artery disease.

DOSAGE: *Adults:* Acute: 1-2 sprays at onset of attack onto or under tongue. May be repeated every 3-5 mins prn. Max: 3 sprays/15 min. Prophylaxis: 1-2 sprays onto or under tongue 5-10 min before activity that may cause acute attack. The spray should not be inhaled. Do not expectorate medication or rinse mouth for 5-10 min after administration.

HOW SUPPLIED: Spray: 400mcg/spray

CONTRAINDICATIONS: Use with certain drugs for erectile dysfunction (phosphodiesterase inhibitors), as their concomitant use can cause severe hypotension.

WARNINGS/PRECAUTIONS: Severe hypotension may occur; caution with volume depletion or hypotension. May aggravate angina caused by hypertrophic cardiomyopathy. Tolerance and cross-tolerance to other nitrates/nitrites may occur. Monitor during early days of AMI. (Nitrolingual Spray) Physical dependence may occur.

ADVERSE REACTIONS: Headache, hypotension, flushing, dizziness, weakness, rash, exfoliative dermatitis.

INTERACTIONS: See Contraindications. Alcohol may cause hypotension. Decreased or increased effect with other agents that depend on vascular smooth muscle. Concomitant use with calcium channel blockers may cause orthostatic hypotension. (NitroMist) Increased hypotensive effects with β-adrenergic blockers (eg, labetalol). ASA may increase levels. May decrease anticoagulant effect of heparin. Avoid ergotamine. Caution with tissue-type plasminogen activator.

PREGNANCY: Category C, caution in nursing.

MECHANISM OF ACTION: Nitrate vasodilator; relaxation of vascular smooth muscle, producing a vasodilator effect on both peripheral arteries and veins with more prominent effects on the latter.

PHARMACOKINETICS: Absorption: (Nitrolingual Spray) C_{max}=1041pg/mL•min, T_{max}=7.5min, AUC=12769pg/mL•min. **Metabolism:** Rapid, liver via reductase enzyme to glycerol nitrate metabolites and inorganic nitrates; hydrolysis to 1,2- and 1,3-dinitroglycerols (active metabolites)

NURSING CONSIDERATIONS

Assessment: Assess for angina pectoris, hypotension, presence of volume-depletion, angina caused by hypertrophic cardiomyopathy, pregnancy/nursing status, and possible drug interactions.

Monitoring: Monitor for hypotension with paradoxical bradycardia and increased angina, tolerance development and physical dependence. Monitor for methemoglobinemia and signs of impaired oxygen delivery despite adequate arterial O_2.

Patient Counseling: Inform about side effects of the drug (eg, headache, lightheadedness). Inform to not take drug concomitantly with drugs used for erectile dysfunction. Instruct patient to use 5-10 minutes prior to engaging in activities which might provoke an acute attack. Do not open the bottle forcibly or use near open flame. Avoid alcohol consumption. Instruct how to prime device prior to use and if device has not been used within 6 weeks.

Administration: Spray on or under the tongue. **Storage:** 25°C (77°F); excursions permitted to 15-30°C (59-85°F).

NITROSTAT
nitroglycerin (Parke-Davis)

RX

THERAPEUTIC CLASS: Nitrate vasodilator

INDICATIONS: For acute relief of an attack or acute prophylaxis of angina pectoris due to coronary artery disease.

DOSAGE: *Adults:* Treatment: 1 tab SL or in buccal pouch at onset of attack. May repeat every 5 min until relief is obtained. If pain persists after a total of 3 tabs in 15 min or pain is different than typically experienced, prompt medical attention is recommended. Prophylaxis: Take 5-10 min before activity which may cause acute attack. Elderly: Start at low end of dosing range.

HOW SUPPLIED: Tab, SL: 0.3mg, 0.4mg, 0.6mg

CONTRAINDICATIONS: Early myocardial infarction (MI), severe anemia, increased intracranial pressure (ICP), patients who are using a phophodi-esterase-5 (PDE-5) inhibitor (eg, sildenafil citrate).

WARNINGS/PRECAUTIONS: Do not swallow tabs; intended for sublingual or buccal administration. Severe hypotension may occur; caution with volume depletion or in patients who are already hypotensive. Nitroglycerin induced hypotension may be accompanied by paradoxical bradycardia and increased angina pectoris. May aggravate angina caused by hypertrophic cardiomyopathy. D/C if blurred vision or dry mouth develops. Use smallest dose for effective relief of acute attack; excessive use may lead to tolerance. Excessive dosage may produce severe headaches. As tolerance to other forms of nitroglycerin develops, effects of sublingual nitroglycerin on exercise tolerance is blunted. Physical dependence may occur. Caution in elderly.

ADVERSE REACTIONS: Headache, vertigo, dizziness, weakness, palpitation, syncope, flushing, drug rash, exfoliative dermatitis.

INTERACTIONS: See contraindications. Additive hypotension may occur with antihypertensive drugs, β-blockers, or phenothiazines. Marked orthostatic hypotension reported with calcium channel blockers. Concomitant use with alcohol may cause hypotension. Avoid ergotamine and related drugs, sildenafil. Vasodilatory and hemodynamic effects potentiated by ASA. Caution with alteplase. IV nitroglycerin reduces anticoagulant effect of heparin; effect of sublingual nitroglycerin with heparin is unknown. TCAs (eg, amitriptyline, desipramine, doxepin) and anticholinergics may make sublingual dissolution difficult. Long-acting nitrates may decrease effects.

PREGNANCY: Category C, caution in nursing.

MECHANISM OF ACTION: Nitrate vasodilator; forms free radical nitric oxide (NO) which activates guanylate cyclase, resulting in an increase of guanosine 3'5' monophosphate (cyclic GMP) in smooth muscle and other tissues leading to dephosphorylation of myosin light chains resulting in vasodilatation.

PHARMACOKINETICS: Absorption: (SL) Rapid; absolute bioavailability (40%). (0.3mg x 2 doses) C_{max}=2.3ng/mL, T_{max}=6.4 min, AUC=14.9ng•mL/min; (0.6mg x 1 dose) C_{max}=2.1ng/mL, T_{max}=7.2 min, AUC=14.9ng•mL/min. **Distribution:** (IV) V_d=3.3 L/kg; plasma protein binding (60%). **Metabolism:** Liver via reductase, extrahepatic (RBC and vascular walls). 1,2- and 1,3-dinitroglycerin (major metabolites). **Elimination:** $T_{1/2}$=2.8 min (0.3mg x 2 doses), 2.6 min (0.6mg x 1 dose).

NURSING CONSIDERATIONS

Assessment: Assess for hypotension, volume depletion, severe anemia, angina caused by hypertrophic cardiomyopathy, early MI, severe anemia, increased ICP, pregnancy/nursing status, and for possible drug interactions.

Monitoring: Monitor for hypotension, paradoxical bradycardia, increased angina pectoris, tolerance, headache and lightheadedness on standing, manifestations of physical dependence (chest pain, acute MI), blurring of vision, and methemoglobinemia. In patients with an acute MI or congestive heart failure (CHF), perform careful clinical or hemodynamic monitoring for hypotension and tachycardia.

Patient Counseling: Instruct to take sublingually; inform that tab is not to be chewed, crushed, or swallowed. Instruct to sit down when taking the drug and to use caution when standing up. May be used prophylactically 5 to 10 min prior to engaging in activities which may precipitate an acute attack. Inform about side effects of drug (eg, headaches, lightheadedness on standing, burning or tingling sensation when administered SL). Avoid alcohol. Keep the medicine in the original glass container tightly capped.

Administration: Sublingual route. Administer in sitting position. **Storage:** 20-25°C (68-77°F).

NIZORAL

RX

ketoconazole (Janssen)

> Risk of fatal hepatotoxicity. Concomitant terfenadine, astemizole and cisapride are contraindicated due to serious cardiovascular adverse events.

THERAPEUTIC CLASS: Azole antifungal

INDICATIONS: Treatment of the following systemic fungal infections: candidiasis, chronic mucocutaneous candidiasis, oral thrush, candiduria, blastomycosis, coccidioidomycosis, histoplasmosis, chromomycosis, and paracoccidioidomycosis. Treatment of severe recalcitrant cutaneous dermatophyte infections not responsive to topical therapy or oral griseofulvin. Not for treatment of fungal meningitis.

DOSAGE: *Adults:* Initial: 200mg qd. Max: 400mg qd.
Pediatrics: >2 yrs: 3.3-6.6mg/kg/day.

HOW SUPPLIED: Tab: 200mg* *scored

CONTRAINDICATIONS: Concomitant terfenadine, astemizole, cisapride or oral triazolam.

WARNINGS/PRECAUTIONS: Hepatotoxicity reported. Monitor LFTs prior to therapy and periodically thereafter. Serum testosterone levels may be lowered. Hypersensitivity reactions reported. Tablets require acidity for dissolution. Not for use in children unless benefit outweighs risk.

ADVERSE REACTIONS: N/V, abdominal pain, pruritus.

INTERACTIONS: See Boxed Warning and Contraindications. Give antacids, anticholinergics, and H$_2$ blockers 2 hrs after ketoconazole. May potentiate midazolam, triazolam, oral hypoglycemics. May enhance anticoagulant effect of coumarin-like drugs. Avoid rifampin, isoniazid. Monitor digoxin, phenytoin. May alter metabolism of cyclosporine, tacrolimus, methylprednisolone and drugs metabolized by CYP3A4.

PREGNANCY: Category C, not for use in nursing.

MECHANISM OF ACTION: Azole antifungal; impairs synthesis of ergosterol, a vital component of fungal cell membranes.

PHARMACOKINETICS: Absorption: C_{max}=3.5mcg/mL; T_{max}=1-2 hrs.
Distribution: Plasma protein binding (99%). **Metabolism:** Via oxidation, degradation of imidazole and piperazine rings, oxidative dealkylation and aromatic hydroxylation. **Elimination:** Biphasic. $T_{1/2}$=2 hrs (during first 10 hrs); $T_{1/2}$=8 hrs (thereafter); bile (major), urine (13%).

NURSING CONSIDERATIONS

Assessment: Assess for lab, as well as clinical, documentation of infection, LFTs and possible drug interactions (eg, terfenadine, astemizole).

Monitoring: Monitor LFTs, signs/symptoms of hepatotoxicity and anaphylaxis. Monitor for CV events if using concomitant therapy with terfenadine or astemizole.

Patient Counseling: Counsel females to avoid nursing while on medication. Advise to report any signs/symptoms of liver dysfunction (eg, fatigue, anorexia, N/V, jaundice, dark urine, or pale stools). If concomitant antacids, anticholinergics and H$_2$-blockers are needed, give at least 2 hrs after administration of drug. Continue treatment until tests indicate infection subsided.

Administration: Oral route. In cases of achlorhydria, instruct to dissolve each tab in 4mL aqueous solution of 0.2 N HCl. Use drinking straw to avoid contact with teeth. Follow administration with cup of water. **Storage:** 15-25°C (59-77°F). Protect from moisture.

NORCO

CIII

hydrocodone bitartrate - acetaminophen (Watson)

OTHER BRAND NAMES: Maxidone (Watson)

THERAPEUTIC CLASS: Opioid analgesic

INDICATIONS: Relief of moderate to moderately severe pain.

DOSAGE: *Adults:* Usual: 1 tab q4-6h prn pain (or 2 tabs of 5-325mg). (Norco) Max: 6 tabs/day. (Maxidone) 5 tabs/day. Elderly: Start at lower end of dosing range.

HOW SUPPLIED: Tab: (Hydrocodone bitartrate-APAP): (Norco) 5mg-325mg*, 7.5mg-325mg*, 10mg-325mg*. (Maxidone) 10mg-750mg* *scored

WARNINGS/PRECAUTIONS: May produce dose-related respiratory depression. Respiratory depressant effects and elevation of CSF pressure may be exaggerated in the presence of head injury, intracranial lesions, or pre-existing increase in intracranial pressure. May obscure diagnosis or clinical course of acute abdominal conditions or head injuries. Caution in elderly, debilitated, severe hepatic or renal dysfunction, hypothyroidism, Addison's disease, prostatic hypertrophy, urethral stricture, pulmonary disease, and postoperative use. May be habit-forming. Suppresses cough reflex.

ADVERSE REACTIONS: Lightheadedness, dizziness, sedation, N/V, rash, drowsiness, thrombocytopenia, agranulocytosis, allergic reactions.

INTERACTIONS: Additive CNS depression with narcotics, antipsychotics, antihistamines, antianxiety agents, alcohol, or other CNS depressants. Increased effect of antidepressants or hydrocodone with MAOIs or TCAs.

PREGNANCY: Category C, not for use in nursing.

MECHANISM OF ACTION: Hydrocodone: Opioid analgesic; most effects involve the CNS and smooth muscles. Precise MOA not established; suspected to relate to existence of opiate receptors in the CNS. Acetaminophen (APAP): Nonopiate, nonsalicylate analgesic and antipyretic. Analgesic activity involves peripheral influences; mechanism not established. Antipyretic activity is mediated through hypothalmic heat regulating-centers; inhibits prostaglandin synthetase.

PHARMACOKINETICS: Absorption: Hydrocodone: C_{max}=23.6ng/mL; T_{max}=1.3 hrs. APAP: Rapid. **Distribution:** APAP: Excreted in breast milk. **Metabolism:** Hydrocodone: O-demethylation, N-demethylation, and 6-ketoreduction; APAP: Liver via conjugation. **Elimination:** Hydrocodone: $T_{1/2}$=3.8 hrs. APAP: Urine (85%, glucuronide conjugate); $T_{1/2}$=1.25-3 hrs.

NURSING CONSIDERATIONS

Assessment: Assess for head injury, intracranial lesions, elevations in intracranial pressure, acute abdominal conditions, presence of debilitation (eg, elderly), hepatic/renal impairment, hypothyroidism, Addison's disease, prostatic hypertrophy or urethral stricture, pulmonary disease, nursing/pregnancy status, and possible drug interactions.

Monitoring: Monitor for signs/symptoms of respiratory depression, elevations in CSF pressure, medication dependence or tolerance, and medication abuse or misuse. Monitor serial hepatic/renal function tests with severe hepatic/renal disease.

Patient Counseling: May impair mental/physical abilities; use caution if performing hazardous tasks (eg, operating machinery/driving). Avoid alcohol and other CNS depressants. May be habit-forming; only take for as long as prescribed, in amounts prescribed, and no more frequently than prescribed.

Administration: Oral route. **Storage:** 15-30°C (59-86°F). Store in tight, light-resistant container with child-resistant closure.

NORDITROPIN   RX
somatropin (Novo Nordisk)

OTHER BRAND NAMES: Norditropin FlexPro (Novo Nordisk) - Norditropin Nordiflex (Novo Nordisk)

THERAPEUTIC CLASS: Human growth hormone

INDICATIONS: (Adults) Replacement of endogenous growth hormone deficiency who meet either of the following criteria: (1) adult-onset patients with growth hormone deficiency (GHD), either alone or associated with multiple hormone deficiencies (hypopituitarism), as a result of pituitary disease, hypo-thalamic disease, surgery, radiation therapy, or trauma; or (2) childhood-onset patients who were growth hormone-deficient during childhood as a result of congenital, genetic, acquired, or idiopathic causes. (Pediatrics) Treatment for growth failure due to inadequate endogenous growth hormone secretion. Treatment for short stature associated with Noonan syndrome and Turner syndrome. Treatment for short stature born small for gestational age (SGA) with no catch-up growth by age 2-4 yrs.

DOSAGE: *Adults:* Individualize dose. Weight-based: Initial: No more than 0.004mg/kg/day. Increase to no more than 0.016mg/kg/day after 6 weeks. Titrate dose based on clinical response, side effects, and determination of age- and gender-adjusted serum insulin-like growth factor I (IGF-I) concentra-tions. Non-Weight based: Initial: 0.2mg/day (range, 0.15-0.30mg/day). May increase gradually every 1-2 months by increments of 0.1-0.2mg/day based on clinical response and serum IGF-I concentrations. Decrease dose as necessary based on adverse events and/or serum IGF-I concentrations above the age-and gender- specific normal range. Maint: May vary from person to person, and between male and female. Elderly: Start at the low end of dosing range. *Pediatrics:* Individualize dose. GHD: 0.024-0.034mg/kg/day 6-7x/week. Noonan Syndrome: Dose up to 0.066mg/kg/day. Turner Syndrome/SGA: Dose up to 0.067mg/kg/day. Carefully monitor growth response and adjust dose as necessary.

HOW SUPPLIED: Inj: 5mg/1.5mL, 15mg/1.5mL [cartridge]; (FlexPro) 5mg/1.5mL, 10mg/1.5mL, 15mg/1.5mL [prefilled pen]; (Nordiflex) 5mg/1.5mL, 10mg/1.5mL, 15mg/1.5mL, 30mg/3mL [prefilled pen].

CONTRAINDICATIONS: Acute critical illness due to complications following open heart surgery, abdominal surgery or multiple accidental trauma, or acute respiratory failure; Prader-Willi syndrome in children with severe obesity, a history of upper airway obstruction or sleep apnea, or severe respiratory impairment; presence of active malignancy; active proliferative or severe non-proliferative diabetic retinopathy; pediatrics with closed epiphyses.

WARNINGS/PRECAUTIONS: Increased mortality reported with acute critical illness; weigh against the potential risk for treatment continuation. Reports of fatalities in pediatrics after initiating therapy in Prader-Willi syndrome; evaluate Prader-Willi patients for signs of upper airway obstruction and sleep apnea before treatment and interrupt therapy if it occurs during treatment. Not indicated for the treatment of pediatric patients who have growth failure due to genetically confirmed Prader-Willi syndrome. In patients with pre-existing tumors or GHD secondary to an intracranial lesion, monitor for progression or recurrence of underlying disease. Monitor for potential malignant trans-formation of skin lesions. May decrease insulin sensitivity. Intracranial HTN reported. Fluid retention may occur. Undiagnosed/untreated hypothyroidism may prevent optimal response. Slipped capital femoral epiphysis may occur; evaluate any pediatrics with onset of a limp or complaints of hip or knee pain during therapy. Progression of scoliosis may occur in pediatrics with rapid growth. Increased occurrence of otitis media with Turner syndrome; monitor for CV disorders. Patients with epiphyseal closure who were treated in child-hood should be re-evaluated before continuation of therapy as adults. Tissue atrophy may occur when administered at the same site over a long period of time. Allergic reactions may occur.

ADVERSE REACTIONS: Glucose intolerance, infection, arthralgia, headache, increased sweating, leg edema, myalgia, bronchitis, flu-like symptoms, HTN, gastroenteritis, paresthesia, skeletal pain, laryngitis.

INTERACTIONS: May impact metabolism of cortisol and cortisone; use of glucocorticoid replacement therapy for previously undiagnosed hypoadrenal-ism may require an increase in maintenance or stress doses, especially with cortisone acetate or prednisone. Adjust glucocorticoid therapy in children to avoid both hypoadrenalism and inhibitory effect on growth. May alter the clearance of compounds metabolized by CYP450 liver enzymes (eg, corticos-teroids, sex steroids, anticonvulsants, cyclosporine). May require larger dose with concomitant oral estrogen replacement. May require dosage adjustment of insulin or oral hypoglycemic agents.

N

PREGNANCY: Category C, caution in nursing.

MECHANISM OF ACTION: Human growth hormone; binds to dimeric GH receptor in cell membrane of target cells, resulting in intracellular signal transduction and a host of pharmacodynamic effects.

PHARMACOKINETICS: Absorption: T_{max}=4-5 hrs; C_{max}=13.8ng/mL (4mg), 17.1ng/mL (8mg). **Elimination**: $T_{1/2}$=7-10 hrs, $T_{1/2}$=21.2 mins (IV)

NURSING CONSIDERATIONS

Assessment: Assess for any condition where treatment is contraindicated or cautioned. Assess for pregnancy/nursing status, and possible drug interactions. Assess for intracranial HTN; perform baseline funduscopic examination to identify pre-existing papilledema. Assess for hypothyroidism; perform baseline thyroid function tests. In Prader-Willi syndrome, assess for signs of upper airway obstruction and sleep apnea. In patients with Turner syndrome, evaluate for otitis media, other ear disorders, and CV disorders. In patients with epiphyseal closure who were treated with somatotropin replacement therapy in childhood, reevaluate before continuing therapy as adults. Rule out presence of a pituitary tumor (or other brain tumors) before initiating treatment.

Monitoring: Monitor for signs and symptoms of malignant transformation of skin lesions, fluid retention, slipped capital femoral epiphysis, progression of scoliosis, tissue atrophy at injection site, allergic reactions, and increases in serum levels of inorganic phosphorus, alkaline phosphatase, parathyroid hormone, and IGF-I. Monitor for intracranial HTN; perform periodic funduscopic examinations. Monitor for glucose intolerance; perform periodic measurements of glucose levels. Monitor for hypothyroidism; perform periodic thyroid function tests. In Prader-Willi syndrome patients, monitor for signs of upper airway obstruction, proper weight control, and for signs of respiratory infection. In patients with pre-existing tumors or GHD secondary to an intracranial lesion, monitor for progression of underlying disease process. In patients with Turner's syndrome, monitor for signs/symptoms of otitis media and for CV disorders.

Patient Counseling: Inform about benefit/risks of therapy. Instruct on proper usage and disposal, and caution against reuse of needles and syringes. Seek medical attention if symptoms of allergic reactions, slipped capital femoral epiphysis (onset of limp, hip or knee pain), respiratory infections (eg, otitis media or ear or CV disorders) and/or progression of scoliosis occur. Instruct to read instruction booklets or leaflets provided.

Administration: SQ route. **Storage**: Unused: 2-8°C (36-46°F); do not freeze; avoid direct light. In-use: 5mg, 10mg: 2-8°C (36-46°F) and use within 4 weeks or store up to 25°C (77°F) for up to 3 weeks. Discard unused portion. 15mg, 30 mg: 2-8°C (36-46°F) and use within 4 weeks; discard unused portion after 4 weeks.

NORINYL 1/50   RX
norethindrone - mestranol (Watson)

> Cigarette smoking increases the risk of serious CV side effects. Risk increases with age (>35 yrs) and with heavy smoking (≥15 cigarettes/day). Women who use oral contraceptives should be strongly advised not to smoke.

OTHER BRAND NAMES: Necon 1/50 (Watson)

THERAPEUTIC CLASS: Estrogen/progestogen combination

INDICATIONS: Prevention of pregnancy.

DOSAGE: *Adults:* 1 tab qd for 28 days, then repeat. Start 1st Sunday after menses begin or 1st day of menses.
Pediatrics: Postpubertal Adolescents: 1 tab qd for 28 days, then repeat. Start 1st Sunday after menses begin or 1st day of menses.

HOW SUPPLIED: Tab: (Mestranol-Norethindrone) 0.05mg-1mg

CONTRAINDICATIONS: Thrombophlebitis, thromboembolic disorders, history of deep vein thrombophlebitis (DVT) or thromboembolic disorders, cerebral vascular or coronary artery disease (CAD), carcinoma of the endometrium or other known or suspected estrogen-dependent neoplasia, undiagnosed abnormal genital bleeding, cholestatic jaundice of pregnancy or jaundice with prior pill use, hepatic adenomas or carcinomas, known or suspected carcinoma of the breast, and pregnancy. (Norinyl 1/50) Benign liver tumors.

WARNINGS/PRECAUTIONS: Increased risk of MI, vascular disease, thromboembolism, stroke, gallbladder disease, and hepatic neoplasia. Increased risk of morbidity and mortality in patients with HTN, hyperlipidemias, obesity and diabetes. May increase risk of breast cancer and cancer of the reproductive organs. Retinal thrombosis reported; d/c if unexplained partial or complete loss of vision occurs, onset of proptosis or diplopia, papilledema, or retinal vascular lesions develop. May cause glucose intolerance; monitor prediabetic and diabetic patients. May cause fluid retention and increase BP; monitor closely and d/c if significant elevation of BP occurs. Breakthrough bleeding and spotting reported; rule out malignancy or pregnancy. May cause onset or exacerbation of a migraine or development of a headache. May develop visual changes with contact lens. May elevate LDL levels or cause other lipid effects. D/C if jaundice develops. Caution with history of depression; d/c if depression recurs to serious degree. Not indicated for use before menarche. Does not protect against HIV infection (AIDS) and other sexually transmitted diseases (STDs). May affect certain endocrine, LFTs, and blood components in laboratory tests. Ectopic and intrauterine pregnancies may occur with contraceptive failures. Should not be used to induce withdrawal bleeding as a test for pregnancy, or to treat threatened or habitual abortion during pregnancy.

ADVERSE REACTIONS: N/V, breakthrough bleeding, spotting, amenorrhea, migraine, mental depression, vaginal candidiasis, edema, weight changes, abdominal cramps/bloating, menstrual flow changes, melasma.

INTERACTIONS: Reduced effects, increased breakthrough bleeding, and menstrual irregularities with rifampin, barbiturates, phenylbutazone, phenytoin Na$^+$, and possibly with griseofulvin, ampicillin, tetracyclines, and (Necon 1/50) carbamazepine.

PREGNANCY: Category X, not for use in nursing.

MECHANISM OF ACTION: Estrogen/progestogen oral contraceptive; suppresses gonadotropins. Primarily inhibits ovulation. Also causes changes in cervical mucus (increases difficulty of sperm entry into uterus) and endometrium (reduces likelihood of implantation).

PHARMACOKINETICS: Distribution: Found in breast milk.

NURSING CONSIDERATIONS

Assessment: Assess for thrombophlebitis, thromboembolic disorders, history of DVT or thromboembolic disorders, any other conditions where treatment is contraindicated or cautioned. Assess for pregnancy/nursing status, and for possible drug interactions. Assess use in patients with hyperlipidemia, HTN, obesity, diabetes, history of depression, and in patients >35 yrs who smoke ≥15 cigarettes/day. (Norinyl 1/50) Assess for benign liver tumors.

Monitoring: Monitor for MI, thromboembolism, stroke, and other adverse effects. Monitor glucose levels in diabetic or prediabetic patients, BP with history of HTN, and lipid levels with history of hyperlipidemia. Monitor for signs of liver dysfunction (eg, jaundice), and signs of worsening depression with previous history. Refer patients with contact lenses to ophthalmologist if ocular changes develop. Perform annual physical exam while on therapy.

Patient Counseling: Inform that therapy does not protect against HIV infection and other STDs. Inform of potential risks/benefits of oral contraceptives. When initiating treatment, instruct to use additional form of contraception until after 7 days on therapy. Take 1 pill at same time daily at intervals not exceeding 24 hrs. If dose is missed, take as soon as possible; take next dose at regularly scheduled time. Continue medication if spotting or breakthrough bleeding occur; notify physician if symptoms persist. Inform that missing a pill can cause spotting or light bleeding. Advise not to smoke while on therapy.

N

Administration: Oral route. **Storage:** 15-25°C (59-77°F) (Norinyl 1/50); 20-25°C (68-77°F) (Necon 1/50).

NOROXIN   RX
norfloxacin (Merck)

> Fluoroquinolones are associated with an increased risk of tendinitis and tendon rupture in all ages. Risk further increased in patients >60 yrs, taking corticosteroids, and with kidney, heart, or lung transplants. Avoid with history of myasthenia gravis; may exacerbate muscle weakness.

THERAPEUTIC CLASS: Fluoroquinolone

INDICATIONS: Treatment of complicated and uncomplicated urinary tract infection (UTI) including cystitis, uncomplicated urethral and cervical gonorrhea, and prostatitis caused by susceptible strains of designated microorganisms.

DOSAGE: *Adults:* Uncomplicated UTI due to *E. coli, K. pneumoniae, P. mirabilis:* 400mg q12h for 3 days. Uncomplicated UTIs due to Other Organisms: 400mg q12h for 7-10 days. Complicated UTIs: 400mg q12h for 10-21 days. CrCl ≤30mL/min: 400mg qd. Uncomplicated Gonorrhea: 800mg single dose. Acute/Chronic Prostatitis: 400mg q12h for 28 days.

HOW SUPPLIED: Tab: 400mg

CONTRAINDICATIONS: History of tendinitis or tendon rupture associated with use of quinolones.

WARNINGS/PRECAUTIONS: D/C if experience pain, swelling, inflammation, or rupture of tendon. Convulsions, increased intracranial pressure (ICP), and toxic psychoses reported. D/C and institute appropriate measures if CNS stimulation occurs; may lead to tremors, restlessness, lightheadedness, confusion, and hallucinations. Caution with known or suspected CNS disorders. Serious and occasionally fatal hypersensitivity (anaphylactic) reactions reported; d/c immediately if signs of hypersensitivity appear. *Clostridium difficile*-associated diarrhea (CDAD) reported. Rare cases of sensory or sensorimotor axonal polyneuropathy, resulting in paresthesias, hypoesthesias, dysesthesias, and weakness reported. D/C if symptoms of neuropathy or deficits in light touch, pain, temperature, position sense, vibratory sensation, and/or motor strength occur. May mask or delay the symptoms of incubating syphilis. All patients with gonorrhea should have a serologic test for syphilis; repeat after 3 months. Photosensitivity/phototoxicity reactions may occur; d/c if phototoxicity occurs. Avoid excessive exposure to sun/UV light. Hemolytic reactions reported with glucose-6-phosphate dehydrogenase (G6PD) deficiency. Caution in elderly and with renal impairment.

ADVERSE REACTIONS: Tendinitis, tendon rupture, dizziness, nausea, headache, abdominal cramping, asthenia, rash.

INTERACTIONS: See Boxed Warning. May increase theophylline and cyclosporine levels. May enhance effects of oral anticoagulants including warfarin or its derivative. Diminished urinary excretion with probenecid. Avoid with nitrofurantoin; may antagonize antibacterial effect in urinary tract. Multivitamins, or other products containing iron or zinc, antacids or sucralfate, and didanosine (chewable/buffered tabs, pediatric oral sol) may interfere with absorption; space dose by 2 hrs. May reduce clearance of caffeine. Coadministration with NSAIDs may increase risk of CNS stimulation and convulsive seizures. On rare occasions, may result in severe hypoglycemia if coadministered with glyburide (a sulfonylurea agent). Drugs metabolized by CYP1A2 (eg, caffeine, clozapine, ropinirole, tacrine, theophylline, tizanidine) may result in increased substrate drug concentrations when given usual doses. Caution with drugs that can result in prolongation of the QTc interval (eg, class IA or class III antiarrhythmics).

PREGNANCY: Category C, not for use in nursing.

MECHANISM OF ACTION: Fluoroquinolone; inhibits bacterial DNA synthesis, ATP-dependent DNA supercoiling reaction catalyzed by DNA gyrase, relaxation of supercoiled DNA, and promotes double-stranded DNA breakage.

PHARMACOKINETICS: Absorption: C_{max}=0.8µg/mL (200mg), 1.5µg/mL (400mg), 2.4µg/mL (800mg); T_{max}=1 hr. Refer to PI for different pharmacokinetic parameters of different age groups. **Distribution:** Plasma protein binding (10-15%). **Elimination:** Urine (26-32%, 5-8% active metabolites); feces (30%); $T_{1/2}$=3-4 hrs.

NURSING CONSIDERATIONS

Assessment: Assess for risk factors for developing tendinitis and tendon rupture, myasthenia gravis, drug hypersensitivity, CNS disorders (eg, severe cerebral arteriosclerosis, epilepsy, other factor that predispose to seizure), G6PD deficiency, renal function, pregnancy/nursing status, and possible drug interactions. Obtain baseline culture and susceptibility test, and serologic test for syphilis.

Monitoring: Monitor for tendonitis, tendon rupture, exacerbation of muscle weakness/myasthenia gravis, convulsions, increased ICP, psychoses, CNS stimulation, hypersensitivity or anaphylactic reactions, CDAD, colitis, and other adverse events. Repeat culture and susceptibility testing performed periodically. Perform follow-up serologic test for syphilis after 3 months

Patient Counseling: Notify healthcare provider if symptoms of pain, swelling, or inflammation of a tendon, or weakness or inability to move joints occur; rest and refrain from exercise and d/c therapy. Advise that it may cause changes in ECG (eg, QTc interval prolongation), dizziness, or lightheadedness. Notify physician of history of QTc prolongation or proarrhythmic conditions, or convulsions. Advise to d/c and contact physician if symptoms of peripheral neuropathies develop or at 1st sign of skin rash or other allergic reaction. Instruct to take ≥1 hr before or ≥2 hrs after meals or ingestion of dairy products. Inform to drink fluids liberally and to take exactly as directed; skipping doses or not completing full course may decrease effectiveness and increase resistance. Advise to contact physician if diarrhea occurs. Counsel that the drug treats bacterial, not viral infections. Instruct to avoid exposure to natural or artificial sunlight. Counsel on possible drug interactions. Inform that multivitamins or other products containing iron or zinc, antacids, or didanosine should not be taken 2 hrs before or within taking drug.

Administration: Oral route. Take ≥1 hr before or ≥2 hrs after a meal or ingestion of milk and/or other dairy products. **Storage:** 25°C (77°F); excursions permitted to 15-30°C (59-86°F). Keep tightly closed.

NORPACE   RX
disopyramide phosphate (Pharmacia & Upjohn)

> In a long-term clinical study in patients with asymptomatic non-life-threatening ventricular arrhythmias who had a myocardial infarction, an excessive mortality or non-fatal cardiac arrest rate was seen in patients treated with encainide or flecainide compared to placebo. Considering the known proarrhythmic properties of Norpace or Norpace CR and the lack of evidence of improved survival, its use should be reserved for patients with life-threatening ventricular arrhythmias.

OTHER BRAND NAMES: Norpace CR (Pharmacia & Upjohn)

THERAPEUTIC CLASS: Class I antiarrhythmic

INDICATIONS: Treatment of documented life-threatening ventricular arrhythmias.

DOSAGE: *Adults:* Usual: 400-800mg/day in divided dose. Recommended: 150mg q6h immediate-release (IR) or 300mg q12h extended-release (CR). Adjust dose with anticholinergic effects. Weight <110 lbs/Moderate Hepatic or Renal Insufficiency (CrCl >40mL/min): 100mg q6h IR or 200mg q12h CR. Severe Renal Insufficiency (with or without initial 150mg LD): CrCl 30-40mL/min: 100mg q8h IR. CrCl 15-30mL/min: 100mg q12h IR. CrCl <15mL/min: 100mg q24h IR. Rapid Control of Ventricular Arrhythmia: LD: 300mg IR (200mg if <110lbs). Follow with maint dose. Cardiomyopathy/Cardiac Decompensation: Initial: 100mg q6-8h IR. Adjust gradually. See PI if no response or toxicity occurs. Elderly: Start at low end of dosing range. *Pediatrics:* 12-18 yrs: 6-15mg/kg/day. 4-12 yrs: 10-15mg/kg/day. 1-4 yrs: 10-

20mg/kg/day. <1 yrs: 10-30mg/kg/day. Give in equally divided doses q6h. Hospitalize patient during initial therapy. Start dose titration at lower end of range.

HOW SUPPLIED: Cap: (Norpace) 100mg, 150mg; Cap, Extended-Release: (Norpace CR) 100mg, 150mg

CONTRAINDICATIONS: Cardiogenic shock, 2nd- or 3rd-degree AV block (if no pacemaker present), congenital QT prolongation.

WARNINGS/PRECAUTIONS: May cause or worsen CHF and produce hypotension due to negative inotropic properties. Reduce dose if 1st-degree heart block occurs. Avoid with urinary retention, glaucoma, and myasthenia gravis unless adequate overriding measures taken. Atrial flutter/fibrillation; digitalize first. Monitor closely or withdraw if QT prolongation >25% occurs and ectopy continues. D/C if QRS widening >25% occurs. Avoid LD with cardiomyopathy or cardiac decompensation. Correct K^+ abnormalities before therapy. Reduce dose with renal/hepatic dysfunction; monitor ECG. Avoid CR formulation with CrCl ≤40mL/min. Caution with sick sinus syndrome, Wolff-Parkinson-White syndrome, bundle branch block, or elderly. May significantly lower blood glucose.

ADVERSE REACTIONS: Dry mouth, urinary retention/frequency/urgency, constipation, blurred vision, GI effects, dizziness, fatigue, headache.

INTERACTIONS: Avoid type IA and IC antiarrhythmics, and propranolol except in unresponsive, life-threatening arrhythmias. Hepatic enzyme inducers may lower levels. Avoid within 48 hrs before or 24 hrs after verapamil. Possible fatal interactions with CYP3A4 inhibitors. Monitor blood glucose with β-blockers, alcohol.

PREGNANCY: Category C, not for use in nursing.

MECHANISM OF ACTION: Type I antiarrhythmic; decreases rate of diastolic depolarization in cells with augmented automaticity, decreases upstroke velocity, and increases action potential duration of normal cardiac cells. Decreases disparity in refractoriness between infracted and adjacent normally perfused myocardium and has no effect on α- or β-adrenergic receptors.

PHARMACOKINETICS: Absorption: Rapid and complete; C_{max}=2.22mcg/mL, T_{max}=4.5 hrs. **Distribution:** Plasma protein binding (50-65%). **Metabolism:** Liver. **Elimination:** Urine (50% unchanged), (20% mono-N-dealkylated metabolite), (10% other metabolite); $T_{1/2}$=11.65 hrs.

NURSING CONSIDERATIONS

Assessment: Prior to therapy, patients with atrial flutter or AF should be digitalized and K^+ abnormalities should be corrected. Assess for cardiogenic shock, pre-existing 2nd- or 3rd-degree heart block, presence of functioning pacemaker, sick sinus syndrome (bradycardia/tachycardia syndrome), Wolff-Parkinson-White syndrome, bundle branch block, congenital QT prolongation, MI, life-threatening arrhythmia, CHF, cardiomyopathy or myocarditis, chronic malnutrition, hepatic/renal impairment, alcohol intake, glaucoma, myasthenia gravis, urinary retention or BPH, pregnancy/nursing status, and possible drug interactions.

Monitoring: Monitor for hypotension, HF, PR interval prolongation, widening of QRS, hypoglycemia, heart block, urinary retention, and myasthenia crisis.

Patient Counseling: Inform about risks/benefits; report adverse reactions. Notify if pregnant/nursing.

Administration: Oral route. **Storage:** 25°C (77°F); excursions permitted to 15-30°C (59-86°F).

NORVASC   RX
amlodipine besylate (Pfizer)

THERAPEUTIC CLASS: Calcium channel blocker (dihydropyridine)

INDICATIONS: Treatment of hypertension (HTN) and coronary artery disease (CAD) including chronic stable or vasospastic angina (Prinzmetal's or variant angina) alone or in combination with other antihypertensives/antianginals. To reduce risks of hospitalization due to angina and to reduce risk of coronary revascularization procedure in patients with recently documented CAD by angiography and without heart failure (ejection fraction <40%).

DOSAGE: *Adults:* HTN: Initial: 5mg qd. Titrate over 7-14 days. Max: 10mg qd. Small, Fragile, or Elderly Individuals/Hepatic Dysfunction/Concomitant Antihypertensive: 2.5mg qd. Angina: Usual dose: 5-10mg qd. CAD: 5-10mg qd. *Pediatrics:* 6-17 yrs: HTN: Usual Range: 2.5-5mg qd. Max: 5mg qd.

HOW SUPPLIED: Tab: 2.5mg, 5mg, 10mg

WARNINGS/PRECAUTIONS: Symptomatic hypotension possible with severe aortic stenosis. May cause worsening angina and acute MI after starting or increasing the dose particularly with severe obstructive CAD. Caution with severe hepatic impairment and in elderly.

ADVERSE REACTIONS: Edema, palpitations, dizziness, headache, fatigue, somnolence, flushing, nausea.

PREGNANCY: Category C, not for use in nursing.

MECHANISM OF ACTION: Dihydropyridine calcium antagonist (calcium ion antagonist or slow-channel blocker): Inhibits transmembrane influx or calcium ions into vascular smooth muscle and cardiac muscle; binds to both dihydro-pyridine and nondihydropyridine binding sites resulting in peripheral arterial vasodilation and reduction in BP.

PHARMACOKINETICS: Absorption: Absolute bioavailability (64-90%); T_{max}=6-12 hrs. **Distribution:** Plasma protein binding (93%). **Metabolism:** Hepatic. **Elimination:** Urine (10% parent compound; 60% inactive metabolites), $T_{1/2}$=30-50 hrs.

NURSING CONSIDERATIONS

Assessment: Assess for BP, heart disease (CAD, severe aortic stenosis, MI), liver disease, LFTs, and pregnancy/nursing status.

Monitoring: Monitor BP, LFTs, and adverse events (eg, edema, flushing, palpitations, headache, fatigue, jaundice, MI).

Patient Counseling: Counsel about potential adverse effects; advise to seek medical attention if any develop. Instruct to take as prescribed.

Administration: Oral route. **Storage:** 15-30°C (59-86°F); store in tight, light-resistant container.

NORVIR
ritonavir (Abbott)

RX

> Coadministration with sedative hypnotics, antiarrhythmics, or ergot alkaloids may result in potentially serious and/or life-threatening adverse events.

THERAPEUTIC CLASS: Protease inhibitor

INDICATIONS: Treatment of HIV infection in combination with other antiretrovirals.

DOSAGE: *Adults:* Initial: 300mg bid. Titrate: Increase every 2-3 days by 100mg bid. Maint: 600mg bid. Max: 600mg bid. Elderly: Start at low end of dosing range. Take with meals.
Pediatrics: >1 month: Initial: 250mg/m² bid. Titrate: Increase every 2-3 days by 50mg/m². Maint: 350-400mg/m² bid or highest tolerated dose. Max: 600mg bid. Take with meals. Refer to PI for pediatric dosage guideline.

HOW SUPPLIED: Cap: 100mg; Sol: 80mg/mL [240mL]; Tab: 100mg

CONTRAINDICATIONS: Coadministration with drugs mediated by CYP3A inhibitors can result in serious and/or life-threatening events. Coadministration with alfuzosin HCl, amiodarone, bepridil, flecainide, propafenone, quinidine, voriconazole, ergot derivatives (dihydroergotamine, ergonovine, ergotamine, methylergonovine), St. John's wort, lovastatin, simvastatin, pimozide, sildenafil (only when used for treatment of pulmonary arterial hypertension), oral midazolam, triazolam, and cisapride.

N

WARNINGS/PRECAUTIONS: Allergic reaction (eg, urticaria, mild skin eruptions, bronchospasm, and angioedema) may occur. D/C if signs and symptoms of pancreatitis, anaphylaxis, Stevens-Johnson syndrome occur. New onset/exacerbation of pre-existing diabetes mellitus (DM), hyperglycemia, and immune reconstitution syndrome reported. Caution with pre-existing liver disease, impaired hepatic function, liver enzyme abnormalities, or hepatitis. Hepatic transaminase elevations, clinical hepatitis, and jaundice reported. Monitor LFTs, especially first 3 months. Prolonged PR interval may occur; caution with underlying structural heart disease, pre-existing conduction system abnormalities, ischemic heart disease, and cardiomyopathies. May elevate triglycerides (TG) and total cholesterol levels; monitor levels at baseline then periodically. Increased bleeding may occur with hemophilia A and B. Possible redistribution or accumulation of body fat have been observed. May increase likelihood of cross-resistance to other protease inhibitors. Caution in elderly.

ADVERSE REACTIONS: Diarrhea, anorexia, N/V, abdominal pain, asthenia, headache, malaise, vasodilation, constipation, dizziness, taste perversion, circumoral/peripheral paresthesia, insomnia, sweating.

INTERACTIONS: See Contraindications. Neurologic and cardiac events reported with disopyramide, mexiletine, nefazodone, fluoxetine, and β-blockers. May decrease ritonavir levels with rifampin; may lead to loss of virologic response. Concomitant use with tipranavir may cause hepatitis and hepatic decompensation. May increase levels of clarithromycin with renal impairment; reduce clarithromycin dose by 50% if CrCl 30-60mL/min and by 75% if CrCl<30mL/min. May increase ketoconazole/itraconazole levels; avoid ketoconazole/itraconazole doses >200mg/day. May increase tadalafil, vardenafil and sildenafil levels; monitor for adverse events. May increase levels of tramadol, propoxyphene, antiarrhythmics, carbamazepine, clonazepam, ethosuximide, antidepressants, dronabinol, quinine, metoprolol, timolol, diltiazem, nifedipine, verapamil, atorvastatin, rosuvastatin, immunosuppressants, perphenazine, risperidone, thioridazine, sedative/hypnotics, fluticasone, methamphetamine, maraviroc, vincristine, vinblastine, digoxin, salmeterol, saquinavir, atazanavir, darunavir, fosamprenavir, desipramine, indinavir, rifabutin and parenteral midazolam. Please refer to PI for detailed Drug Interactions info. Reduce dose with dexamethasone, prednisone. May increase levels of trazodone; use with caution and consider lowering trazodone dose. May increase levels with delavirdine. May decrease levels of phenytoin, divalproex, lamotrigine, bupropion, atovaquone, meperidine, theophylline, and methadone. Separate dosing with didanosine by 2.5 hrs. May increase plasma levels of drugs metabolized by CYP3A or CYP2D6. May decrease ethinyl estradiol levels; use alternative contraceptive measures. Decreases warfarin levels; monitor INR. Solution contains alcohol; may produce disulfiram-like reactions with disulfiram, metronidazole. May increase colchicine levels; should not be given with ritonavir in patients with renal or hepatic impairment. May increase bosentan level; d/c bosentan at least 36 hrs prior to initiation of ritonavir and resume bosentan after 10 days following initiation of ritonavir. Caution with CCBs, β-blockers, digoxin and atazanavir.

PREGNANCY: Category B, not for use in nursing.

MECHANISM OF ACTION: HIV protease inhibitor; antiviral; renders enzyme incapable of processing Gag-Pol polyprotein precursor, which leads to production of noninfectious immature HIV particles.

PHARMACOKINETICS: Absorption: C_{max} =11.2mcg/mL; T_{max} =2 hrs (fasting), 4 hrs (fed); AUC=121.7mcg•hr/mL (Cap), AUC=129mcg•hr/mL (Sol). **Distribution:** Plasma protein binding (98-99%). **Metabolism:** CYP3A, CYP2D6 (oxidation); isopropylthiazole (major metabolite). **Elimination:** Urine (11.3%, 3.5% unchanged), feces (86.4%, 33.8% unchanged); $T_{1/2}$ =3-5 hrs.

NURSING CONSIDERATIONS

Assessment: Assess for pre-existing liver disease or impairment (eg, enzyme abnormalities, hepatitis), DM, hemophilia A and B, underlying cardiac problems (eg, structural heart disease, ischemic heart disease, cardiomyopathies, conduction system abnormalities), pregnancy/nursing status, and possible drug interactions. Obtain baseline ECG, ALT, AST, GGT, CPK, uric acid, TG, and cholesterol levels.

Monitoring: Monitor LFTs periodically for first 3 months. Monitor for signs/symptoms of anaphylactoid/allergic reactions, new onset or exacerbation of DM, hyperglycemia, pancreatitis, immune reconstitution syndrome, fat redistribution or accumulation, and hepatic dysfunction. Monitor ECG, ALT, AST, GGT, CPK, uric acid, TG, and cholesterol levels. May enroll patients in the Antiretroviral Pregnancy Registry if they become pregnant while on treatment.

Patient Counseling: Discuss risks and benefits of therapy. Inform that drug does not cure HIV and that opportunistic infections may continue to develop. Does not reduce risk of transmitting HIV. Notify physician if using Rx/OTC or herbal products, particularly St. John's wort. Seek medical attention if experience symptoms of PR interval prolongation (dizziness, lightheadedness, abnormal heart rhythm, or loss of consciousness), allergic reactions, pancreatitis (N/V, abdominal pain), infections, or fat redistribution/accumulation. Women taking estrogen-based hormonal contraceptives should use an additional/alternative method of birth control while on therapy. Advise that taking PDE5 inhibitors for erectile dysfunction may increase risk of hypotension, visual changes, and sustained erection; report any symptoms.

Administration: Oral route. (Tab) Do not chew, crush or break; swallow whole. (Sol) May mix with chocolate milk within 1 hr of dosing. **Storage**: Cap: 2-8°C (36-46°F). Refrigeration is recommended but not required if used within 30 days and stored below 25°C (77°F). Protect from light. Avoid exposure to excessive heat. Sol: 20-25°C (68-77°F). Do not refrigerate. Shake well before use. Tab: 20-25°C (68-77°F); excursions permitted to 15-30°C (59-86°F).

NOVACORT   RX
pramoxine HCl - hydrocortisone acetate (Primus)

THERAPEUTIC CLASS: Corticosteroid/anesthetic

INDICATIONS: Relief of the inflammatory and pruritic manifestations of corticosteroid-responsive dermatoses.

DOSAGE: *Adults:* Apply to affected area(s) tid-qid. May use occlusive dressings for psoriasis or recalcitrant conditions. D/C dressings if infection develops.
Pediatrics: Apply to affected area(s) tid-qid. May use occlusive dressings for psoriasis or recalcitrant conditions. D/C dressings if infection develops. Use least amount effective for condition.

HOW SUPPLIED: Gel: (Hydrocortisone-Pramoxine) 2%-1% [29g]

WARNINGS/PRECAUTIONS: May produce reversible HPA axis suppression, manifestations of Cushing's syndrome, hyperglycemia, and glucosuria. Caution when applied to large surface areas, under occlusive dressings, or with prolonged use. Use appropriate antifungal or antibacterial agent with dermatological infections; d/c if infection does not clear. Pediatrics may be more susceptible to systemic toxicity. D/C if irritation develops. Avoid eyes.

ADVERSE REACTIONS: Burning, itching, irritation, dryness, folliculitis, hypertrichosis, acneiform eruptions, hypopigmentation, perioral dermatitis, allergic dermatitis, skin maceration, secondary infection, skin atrophy, striae, miliaria.

PREGNANCY: Category C, caution in nursing.

MECHANISM OF ACTION: Topical corticosteroid/anesthetic. Hydrocortisone: Possesses anti-inflammatory, anti-pruritic, and vasoconstrictive properties. Anti-inflammatory mechanism not established. Pramoxine: Stabilizes neuronal membrane of nerve endings with which it comes into contact.

PHARMACOKINETICS: Absorption: Percutaneous; occlusion, inflammation, other disease states may increase absorption. **Distribution:** Bound to plasma protein in varying degrees. Systemically administered corticosteroids found in breast milk. **Metabolism:** Liver. **Elimination:** Kidney (major), bile.

NURSING CONSIDERATIONS

Assessment: Assess for severity of dermatoses and use in pregnant/nursing patients.

Monitoring: Monitor for signs/symptoms of reversible HPA-axis suppression, Cushing's syndrome, hyperglycemia, glucosuria, skin irritation, and dermatological infections (eg, fungal, bacterial). In patients on large doses of therapy and in patients using occlusive dressings, perform frequent monitoring of HPA-axis suppression using urinary free cortisol and ACTH stimulation tests. Monitor for signs of steroid withdrawal following d/c of therapy. In pediatric patients, monitor for signs/symptoms of systemic toxicity, HPA-axis suppression, Cushing's syndrome, and intracranial HTN.

Patient Counseling: Instruct to use medication exactly as directed; avoid contact with eyes. Report adverse reactions. Do not bandage, cover, or wrap treated skin unless directed by physician to do so. Advise caregivers of pediatric patients to avoid tight-fitting diapers or plastic pants on treatment diaper area.

Administration: Topical. **Storage:** Store at 15-30°C (59-86°F). Keep tightly closed.

NOVOLIN OTC

insulin human, rdna origin - insulin, human isophane - insulin, human regular (Novo Nordisk)

OTHER BRAND NAMES: Novolin R (Novo Nordisk) - Novolin N (Novo Nordisk)

THERAPEUTIC CLASS: Insulin

INDICATIONS: To control hyperglycemia in diabetes.

DOSAGE: *Adults:* Individualize dose.
Pediatrics: Individualize dose.

HOW SUPPLIED: Inj: 100 U/mL (Novolin N, Novolin R)

WARNINGS/PRECAUTIONS: Human insulin differs from animal source insulin. Any change in insulin should be made cautiously. Changes in strength, manufacturer, type or method of manufacture may result in the need for a change in dosage. Hypoglycemia may occur with taking too much insulin, missing or delaying meals, exercising or working more than usual. An infection or illness (especially if accompanied by diarrhea or vomiting) may change insulin requirements. Administration of insulin SQ can result in lipoatrophy. Novolin R is not recommended for use in insulin pumps.

ADVERSE REACTIONS: Hypoglycemia, sweating, dizziness, palpitations, tremor, hunger, restlessness, lightheadedness, inability to concentrate, headache, injection-site reaction, allergic reaction.

INTERACTIONS: Increased insulin requirements with oral contraceptives, corticosteroids, or thyroid replacement therapy. Reduced insulin requirements with oral hypoglycemics, salicylates, sulfa antibiotics, and certain antidepressants. Alcoholic beverages may change insulin requirements. β-blockers may mask symptoms of hypoglycemia.

PREGNANCY: Safety not known in pregnancy/nursing.

MECHANISM OF ACTION: Insulin (rDNA origin); regulates glucose metabolism, lowers blood glucose by facilitating cellular uptake of glucose and simultaneously inhibiting the glucose output from the liver.

NURSING CONSIDERATIONS

Assessment: Assess FPG, HbA1c, renal function, LFTs, pregnancy/nursing status, infections, alcohol consumption, exercise routines, and for possible drug interactions.

Monitoring: Monitor FPG, HbA1c, and renal function. Monitor for signs of hypoglycemia, hypokalemia, diabetic ketoacidosis, vision changes, lipodystrophy, and allergic reactions.

Patient Counseling: Use only if solution is clear and colorless with no visible particles. Counsel about signs/symptoms of hypoglycemia, hyperglycemia, diabetic ketoacidosis, the importance of frequent monitoring of blood glucose levels, eating a balanced diet and exercising regularly. Advise to avoid excessive alcohol. During periods of stress (eg, trauma, infection, surgery), insulin requirements may be changed; advise patients to seek prompt medical advice. Counsel on proper administration techniques.

Administration: SQ route. Refer to labeling for administration techniques.
Storage: Below 30°C (86°F). Do not freeze. Protect from light.

NOVOLIN 70/30 OTC
insulin human, rdna origin - insulin, human (isophane/regular) (Novo Nordisk)

THERAPEUTIC CLASS: Insulin

INDICATIONS: To control hyperglycemia in diabetes.

DOSAGE: *Adults:* Individualize dose.
Pediatrics: Individualize dose.

HOW SUPPLIED: (Isophane/Regular) Inj: 70 U-30 U/mL

WARNINGS/PRECAUTIONS: Human insulin differs from animal source insulin. Any change of insulin should be made cautiously. Changes in strength, manufacturer, type or method of manufacture may result in the need for a change in dosage. Hypoglycemia may occur with taking too much insulin, missing or delaying meals, exercising or working more than usual. An infection or illness (especially with diarrhea or vomiting) may change insulin requirements. Caution with diseases of adrenal, pituitary, or thyroid glands, or progression of kidney or liver disease. Administration of insulin SQ can result in lipodystrophy.

ADVERSE REACTIONS: Hypoglycemia, sweating, dizziness, palpitations, tremor, hunger, restlessness, lightheadedness, inability to concentrate, headache, injection-site reaction, allergic reaction.

INTERACTIONS: Increased insulin requirements with oral contraceptives, corticosteroids, or thyroid replacement therapy. Reduced insulin requirements with oral hypoglycemics, salicylates, sulfa antibiotics, and certain antidepressants. Alcoholic beverages may change insulin requirements. β-blockers may mask symptoms of hypoglycemia.

PREGNANCY: Safety not known in pregnancy/nursing.

MECHANISM OF ACTION: Insulin (rDNA origin). Regulates glucose metabolism, lowers blood glucose by facilitating cellular uptake of glucose and simultaneously inhibiting the glucose output from the liver.

NURSING CONSIDERATIONS

Assessment: Assess FPG, HbA1c, renal function, LFTs, pregnancy/nursing status, infections, alcohol consumption, exercise routines, and for possible drug interactions.

Monitoring: Monitor FPG, HbA1c, and renal function. Monitor for signs of hypoglycemia, hypokalemia, diabetic ketoacidosis, vision changes, lipodystrophy, and allergic reactions.

Patient Counseling: Use only if the solution is clear and colorless with no visible particles. Counsel about signs/symptoms of hypoglycemia, hyperglycemia, diabetic ketoacidosis, the importance of frequent monitoring of blood glucose levels, the need for eating a balanced diet and exercising regularly. Advise to avoid excessive alcohol. During periods of stress (eg, trauma, infection, surgery) insulin requirements may be changed; advise patients to seek prompt medical advice. Counsel on proper administration techniques.

Administration: SQ route. Refer to labeling for administration techniques.
Storage: Below 30°C (86°F). Do not freeze. Protect from light.

NOVOLOG RX
insulin aspart (Novo Nordisk)

THERAPEUTIC CLASS: Insulin

INDICATIONS: To improve glycemic control in adults and children with diabetes mellitus (DM).

DOSAGE: *Adults:* Individualize dose. Usual Requirement: 0.5-1 unit/kg/day. Inject SQ immediately within 5-10 min before a meal. Continuous SQ Insulin Infusion (CSII) by External Pump: Infuse pre-meal boluses immediately (within 5-10 mins) before a meal. Initial: Based on the total daily insulin dose of the previous regimen. Usual: 50% of total dose given as meal-related boluses and the remainder given as basal infusion. Change the reservoir at least q6 days; change infusion sets and infusion set insertion site at least q3 days. Rotate inj site (abdomen, buttocks, thigh, or upper arm). May be administered via IV under medical supervision. Use concentration of 0.05-1 U/mL in infusion systems using polypropylene infusion bags. Renal/Hepatic Impairment: May need to reduce dose.
Pediatrics: ≥2 yrs: Individualize dose. Usual requirement: 0.5-1 unit/kg/day. Inject SQ immediately within 5-10 min before a meal. Continuous SQ Insulin Infusion (CSII) by External Pump: Infuse pre-meal boluses immediately (within 5-10 mins) before a meal. Initial: Based on the total daily insulin dose of the previous regimen. Usual: 50% of total dose given as meal-related boluses and the remainder given as basal infusion. Change the reservoir at least q6 days; change infusion sets and infusion set insertion site at least q3 days. Rotate inj site (abdomen, buttocks, thigh, or upper arm). Renal/Hepatic Impairment: May need to reduce dose.

HOW SUPPLIED: Inj: 100 U/mL [10mL]; FlexPen: 100 U/mL [3mL]; PenFill: 100 U/mL [3mL]

CONTRAINDICATIONS: Episodes of hypoglycemia.

WARNINGS/PRECAUTIONS: Hypoglycemia may occur; caution in hypoglycemia unawareness and in predisposal to hypoglycemia (eg, patients who are fasting or have erratic food intake). Hypokalemia may occur; caution in patients who may be at risk. Redness, swelling or itching at the injection site may occur. Adjust dose if change in physical activity or usual meal plan. Any change of insulin dose should be made cautiously and under medical supervision. Changing from one insulin product to another or changing the insulin strength may result in the need for a change in dosage. Dose adjustment may be needed during intercurrent conditions such as illness, emotional disturbances, or other stresses. Severe, generalized allergy including anaphylaxis may occur. Needles/FlexPen must not be shared. IV-administered insulin requires close monitoring for hypoglycemia. Increases in anti-insulin antibodies observed. Whether using an external pump for SQ infusion or administering intravenously, do not dilute or mix with any other insulin. May impair mental/physical abilities.

ADVERSE REACTIONS: Hypoglycemia, headache, nausea, diarrhea, hyporeflexia, onychomycosis, sensory disturbance, urinary tract infection, chest pain, lipodystrophy, hypersensitivity reaction, abdominal pain, skin disorder, injection-site reaction, sinusitis.

INTERACTIONS: Increased blood-glucose-lowering effects with pramlintide, ACE inhibitors, disopyramide, fibrates, fluoxetine, MAOIs, propoxyphene, salicylates, somatostatin analog (eg, octreotide), sulfonamide antibiotics, and oral antidiabetic agents. Decreased blood-glucose-lowering effects with corticosteroids, danazol, niacin, diuretics, sympathomimetic agents (eg, epinephrine, salbutamol, terbutaline), isoniazid, phenothiazine derivatives, somatotropin, thyroid hormones, estrogens, progestogens (eg, in oral contraceptives), atypical antipsychotics. Pentamidine may cause hypoglycemia, followed by hyperglycemia. β-blockers, clonidine, lithium salts, and alcohol may potentiate or weaken glucose-lowering effect. β-blockers, clonidine, guanethidine, and reserpine may reduce signs of hypoglycemia. Caution with K⁺-lowering drugs, drugs sensitive to serum K⁺ levels, and IV insulin.

PREGNANCY: Category B, caution in nursing.

MECHANISM OF ACTION: Insulin aspart (rDNA origin); regulates glucose metabolism, lowers blood glucose by facilitating cellular uptake of glucose and simultaneously inhibiting glucose output from the liver.

PHARMACOKINETICS: **Absorption:** C_{max}=82mU/L; T_{max}=40-50 min. **Distribution:** Plasma protein binding (<10%). **Elimination:** $T_{1/2}$=81 min.

NURSING CONSIDERATIONS

Assessment: Assess FPG, HbA1c, renal function, LFTs, episodes of hyperglycemia, exercise routines, pregnancy/nursing status, infections, alcohol consumption, hypersensitivity and for possible drug interactions.

Monitoring: Monitor FPG, HbA1c, and renal/hepatic function. Monitor for hypokalemia, diabetic ketoacidosis, vision changes, lipodystrophy, allergic reactions, hypoglycemia, hyperglycemia, and injection-site reactions.

Patient Counseling: Advise to use solution only if it is clear and colorless with no visible particles. Counsel about signs/symptoms of diabetic ketoacidosis, the need to eat a balanced diet, and regular exercise. Inform about potential risks and benefits of taking insulin and possible adverse reactions. Counsel on proper administration techniques, lifestyle management, regular glucose monitoring, periodic glycosylated hemoglobin technique, hemoglobin testing, recognition and management of hypo- and hyperglycemia, complications of insulin therapy, timing of dose, instruction in the use of injection or SQ infusion device, and proper storage of insulin. Caution when driving or operating machinery. Check carefully when administering insulin to avoid medication errors.

Administration: SQ/ IV route. Refer to PI for administration techniques.

Storage: 2-8°C (36-46°F). Do not freeze. Do not use if frozen. After use: Vial: Refrigerate or store at room temperature <30°C (86°F) for 28 days, do not freeze. PenFill Cartridges/FlexPen: Store at room temperature <30°C (86°F) for 28 days. Keep away from direct heat and light. Pump: Discard Novolog in pump reservoir at least q6 days of use or after exposure to >37°C (98.6°F). Diluted Novolog: <30°C (86°F) for 28 days. IV Infusion: Store at room temperature for 24 hours.

NovoLog Mix 70/30   RX
insulin aspart protamine - insulin aspart (Novo Nordisk)

THERAPEUTIC CLASS: Insulin

INDICATIONS: To improve glycemic control in patients with diabetes mellitus (DM).

DOSAGE: *Adults:* Individualize dose. Type 1 DM: Inject SQ bid within 15 min before meals. Type 2 DM: Inject SQ bid within 15 min before/after meals. Rotate inj site (abdomen, buttocks, thigh, or upper arm). Hepatic/Renal Impairment: May require dose reductions. Do not mix with other insulins or use in IV or in insulin pumps. Elderly: Start at low end of dosing range.

HOW SUPPLIED: (Insulin Aspart Protamine-Insulin Aspart) Inj: 70 U-30 U/mL [10mL]; FlexPen: 70 U-30 U/mL [3mL]

CONTRAINDICATIONS: Episodes of hypoglycemia.

WARNINGS/PRECAUTIONS: Administer with meals. Not for IV use or in infusion pumps. Any change of insulin should be made cautiously and only under medical supervision. Changing from one insulin product to another or changing the insulin strength may result in the need for a change in dosage. Dose adjustments may be needed during illness, emotional stress, or other physiologic stresses in addition to changes in meals and exercise. Hypoglycemia may occur; caution in hypoglycemia unawareness and in predisposal to hypoglycemia (eg, patients who are fasting or have erratic food intake). Hypokalemia may occur; caution in patients who may be at risk for hypokalemia. Insulin antibodies may develop during treatment. Caution in elderly. Erythema, swelling, and pruritus at the injection site observed. Severe, generalized allergy including anaphylaxis may occur. May impair mental/physical abilities.

ADVERSE REACTIONS: Hypoglycemia, headache, influenza-like illness, back pain, diarrhea, pharyngitis, skeletal pain, upper respiratory tract infection, dyspepsia, neuropathy, abdominal pain, rhinitis.

INTERACTIONS: Increased blood-glucose-lowering effects with pramlintide, ACE inhibitors, disopyramide, fibrates, fluoxetine, MAOIs, propoxyphene, salicylates, somatostatin analog (eg, octreotide), sulfonamide antibiotics, and oral antidiabetic agents. Decreased blood-glucose-lowering effects with corticosteroids, danazol, niacin, diuretics, sympathomimetic agents (eg, epinephrine, salbutamol, terbutaline), isoniazid, phenothiazine derivatives, somatotropin, thyroid hormones, estrogens, progestogens (eg, in oral contraceptives), atypical antipsychotics. Pentamidine may cause hypoglycemia, followed by hyperglycemia. β-blockers, clonidine, lithium salts, and alcohol may potentiate or weaken glucose-lowering effect. β-blockers, clonidine, guanethidine, and reserpine may reduce signs of hypoglycemia. Do not mix with other insulin products. Caution with K^+-lowering drugs or drugs sensitive to serum K^+.

PREGNANCY: Category B, caution in nursing.

MECHANISM OF ACTION: Insulin; regulates glucose metabolism. Lowers blood glucose by facilitating cellular uptake of glucose, simultaneously inhibiting output of glucose from liver.

PHARMACOKINETICS: Absorption: Rapid; (0.2 U/kg) C_{max}=23.4 mU/L, T_{max}=60 min; (0.3 U/kg) C_{max}= 61.3 mU/L, T_{max}=85 min. **Distribution:** Plasma protein binding (0-9%). **Elimination:** $T_{1/2}$=8-9 hrs.

NURSING CONSIDERATIONS

Assessment: Assess FPG, HbA1c, renal function, LFTs, pregnancy/nursing status, infections, alcohol consumption, exercise routines, hypersensitivity and for possible drug interactions.

Monitoring: Monitor FPG, HbA1c, and renal/hepatic function. Monitor for signs and symptoms of hypoglycemia, hypokalemia, diabetic ketoacidosis, vision changes, lipodystrophy, and allergic reactions.

Patient Counseling: Inform to use only if solution is clear and colorless with no visible particles, and not to dilute or mix with other insulins or solution. Counsel about the signs and symptoms of hypoglycemia, hyperglycemia, and diabetic ketoacidosis. Explain the importance of frequent monitoring of blood glucose levels, need for a balanced diet, and regular exercise. Avoid excessive alcohol. Counsel that during periods of stress (eg, trauma, infection, surgery), insulin requirements may be changed; advise to seek prompt medical attention. Educate on proper administration techniques. Hypoglycemia may impair ability to concentrate and react; caution when driving or operating machinery. Check carefully when administering insulin to avoid medication errors. Careful monitoring of glucose control is essential in pregnant patients with DM or history of DM during pregnancy. Notify physician if pregnant or plan to become pregnant. Avoid sharing of needles and Flexpen.

Administration: SQ route. Refer to PI for administration techniques.
Storage: 2-8°C (36-46°F). Do not freeze. Do not use if frozen. After use: Vial: Refrigerate or store at room temperature <30°C (86°F) for 28 days, do not freeze. Avoid excessive exposure to heat or sunlight. FlexPen: Store at room temperature <30°C (86°F) for 14 days. Keep away from direct heat and light.

NOXAFIL   RX
posaconazole (Schering)

THERAPEUTIC CLASS: Azole antifungal

INDICATIONS: Prophylaxis of invasive *Aspergillus* and *Candida* infections in patients ≥13 yrs, who are at high risk of developing these infections due to being severely immunocompromised. Treatment of oropharyngeal candidiasis, including oropharyngeal candidiasis refractory to itraconazole and/or fluconazole.

DOSAGE: *Adults:* Prophylaxis of Invasive Fungal Infections: 200mg (5mL) tid. Base duration of therapy on recovery from neutropenia or immunosuppression. Oropharyngeal Candidiasis: LD: 100mg (2.5mL) bid on 1st day, then 100mg qd for 13 days. Oropharyngeal Candidiasis Refractory to Itraconazole and/or Fluconazole: 400mg (10mL) bid. Base duration of therapy on severity of underlying disease and clinical response.
Pediatrics: ≥13 yrs: Prophylaxis of Invasive Fungal Infections: 200mg (5mL) tid. Base duration of therapy on recovery from neutropenia or

immunosuppression. Oropharyngeal Candidiasis: LD: 100mg (2.5mL) bid on 1st day, then 100mg qd for 13 days. Oropharyngeal Candidiasis Refractory to Itraconazole and/or Fluconazole: 400mg (10mL) bid. Base duration of therapy on severity of underlying disease and clinical response.

HOW SUPPLIED: Sus: 40mg/mL [105mL]

CONTRAINDICATIONS: Coadministration with sirolimus, CYP3A4 substrates that prolong the QT interval (eg, pimozide, quinidine), simvastatin, ergot alkaloids.

WARNINGS/PRECAUTIONS: Prolongation of QT interval and rare cases of torsades de pointes reported; caution with potentially proarrhythmic conditions. Hepatic reactions (eg, mild to moderate elevations in ALT, AST, alkaline phosphatase, total bilirubin, and/or clinical hepatitis) reported. Cholestasis or hepatic failure reported in patients with serious underlying medical conditions. D/C if signs/symptoms of liver disease develop that may be attributable to therapy. Monitor closely for breakthrough fungal infections with severe renal impairment.

ADVERSE REACTIONS: Fever, headache, rigors, anemia, neutropenia, diarrhea, N/V, abdominal pain, coughing, dyspnea, anorexia, fatigue, asthenia, pain.

INTERACTIONS: See Contraindications. Elevated cyclosporine and tacrolimus levels reported; frequently monitor levels and consider dose adjustment of cyclosporine or tacrolimus. Avoid with cimetidine, esomeprazole, rifabutin, phenytoin, and efavirenz unless benefits outweigh risks. If concomitant phenytoin is required, monitor closely and consider phenytoin dose reduction. If concomitant rifabutin is required, monitor CBC and adverse events. Monitor adverse events with benzodiazepines metabolized through CYP3A4 (eg, midazolam, alprazolam, triazolam). May increase levels of vinca alkaloids; consider dose adjustment of vinca alkaloid. Consider dose reduction of concomitant statins that are metabolized through CYP3A4. Monitor for adverse events and toxicity with calcium channel blockers (CCBs) (eg, verapamil, diltiazem, nifedipine, nicardipine, felodipine) and drugs that are metabolized through CYP3A4 (eg, atazanavir, ritonavir); dose reduction of these drugs may be needed. Decreased levels with cimetidine, esomeprazole, and metoclopramide; monitor for breakthrough fungal infections. Increased digoxin levels; monitor digoxin plasma concentrations. Inhibitors or inducers of UDP glucuronidation or P-glycoprotein (P-gp) may affect posaconazole concentrations. Monitor glucose concentration with glipizide.

PREGNANCY: Category C, not for use in nursing.

MECHANISM OF ACTION: Triazole antifungal agent; blocks synthesis of ergosterol, a key component of fungal cell membrane, through inhibition of the enzyme lanosterol 14α-demethylase and accumulation of methylated sterol precursors.

PHARMACOKINETICS: Administration: Administration of variable doses resulted in different parameters. **Distribution:** V_d=1774L; plasma protein binding (>98%). **Metabolism:** Via UDP glucuronidation; glucuronide conjugates (metabolites). **Elimination:** Feces (71%), urine (13%); $T_{1/2}$=35 hrs.

NURSING CONSIDERATIONS

Assessment: Assess for drug hypersensitivity, renal function, proarrhythmic conditions, LFTs, pregnancy/nursing status, and for possible drug interactions.

Monitoring: Monitor for signs/symptoms of hypersensitivity reactions, hepatic reactions, QT prolongation, torsades de pointes, and LFTs. In patients with severe renal impairment, monitor for breakthrough fungal infections.

Patient Counseling: Instruct to take medication with full meal; if cannot eat full meal, may take with liquid nutritional supplement or acidic carbonated beverage. Inform physician of all medications being taken. Inform physician if severe diarrhea or vomiting develops, have a heart or circulatory condition, are pregnant or plan to become pregnant, nursing, have liver disease, flu symptoms, experience itching, eyes/skin turn yellow, feel more tired than usual, or had an allergic reaction to other antifungal medications.

Administration: Oral route. **Storage**: 25°C (77°F); excursions permitted to 15-30°C (59-86°F). Do not freeze.

NPLATE   RX
romiplostim (Amgen)

THERAPEUTIC CLASS: Thrombopoietin receptor agonist

INDICATIONS: Treatment of thrombocytopenia in patients with chronic immune (idiopathic) thrombocytopenic purpura (ITP) who have had an insufficient response to corticosteroids, immunoglobulins, or splenectomy.

DOSAGE: *Adults:* Administer weekly. Initial: 1mcg/kg SQ based on actual body wt. Titrate: Adjust dose by increments of 1mcg/kg until platelet count is ≥50 x 10^9/L. Max: 10mcg/kg/week. If platelet count <50 x 10^9/L, increase dose by 1mcg/kg. If platelet count >200 x 10^9/L x 2 consecutive weeks, reduce dose by 1mcg/kg. If platelet count >400 x 10^9/L, do not dose; continue assessing platelet count weekly. After platelet count falls to <200 x 10^9/L, resume therapy at a dose reduced by 1mcg/kg. D/C if platelet count does not increase to a sufficient level after 4 weeks of therapy at the maximum weekly dose.

HOW SUPPLIED: Inj: 250mcg, 500mcg

WARNINGS/PRECAUTIONS: Should only be used in patients with ITP whose degree of thrombocytopenia and clinical condition increases the risk for bleeding. Should not be used in an attempt to normalize platelet counts. May increase risk for development or progression of reticulin fiber deposition within bone marrow. Development of marrow fibrosis with collagen reported. Examine peripheral blood smear closely to establish baseline level of cellular morphological abnormalities; d/c if new or worsening morphological abnormalities or cytopenia develop. D/C may worsen thrombocytopenia and increase risk of bleeding, particularly if taking anticoagulants or antiplatelet agents. Excessive doses may result in thrombotic/thromboembolic complications. If hyporesponsiveness or failure to maintain a platelet response occurs, search for causative factors (eg, neutralizing antibodies, bone marrow fibrosis). May increase risk for hematologic malignancies or cause malignancy progression. Not indicated for thrombocytopenia due to MDS or any cause other than chronic ITP. Monitor CBCs, including platelet counts, and peripheral blood smears prior to initiation, throughout, and following d/c of therapy. Caution in renal/hepatic impairment and elderly. Available only through restricted distribution program.

ADVERSE REACTIONS: Headache, arthralgia, dizziness, insomnia, myalgia, pain in extremity, development of antibodies, abdominal pain, shoulder pain, dyspepsia, paresthesia.

PREGNANCY: Category C, not for use in nursing.

MECHANISM OF ACTION: Thrombopoietin receptor agonist; increases platelet production through binding and activation of the TPO receptor.

PHARMACOKINETICS: Absorption: T_{max}=7-50 hrs. **Elimination:** $T_{1/2}$=1-34 days.

NURSING CONSIDERATIONS

Assessment: Assess for degree of thrombocytopenia, risk factors for thromboembolism, hematological malignancies, hepatic/renal impairment, and pregnancy/nursing status. Obtain baseline CBC, platelet count, peripheral blood smear, and peripheral blood differential count.

Monitoring: Monitor CBC, platelet count, peripheral blood smear weekly during dose adjustment phase, then monthly after establishment of a stable dose, and after d/c for at least 2 weeks. Monitor for bone marrow reticulin deposition, new or worsening morphological abnormalities or cytopenias, worsening thrombocytopenia, thrombotic/thromboembolic complications, and malignancies.

Patient Counseling: Inform of risks and benefits of therapy. Advise that the risks associated with prolonged treatment are not fully established and that patients must enroll in Nplate NEXUS (Network of Experts Understanding and Supporting Nplate and Patients) program for proper use. Advise to follow up for monitoring of platelet count and CBCs, including peripheral blood smears, weekly, until stable dose has been achieved; thereafter, platelet counts and CBCs, including peripheral blood smears during therapy and for 2 weeks after d/c. Counsel to avoid situations or medications that may increase risk for bleeding.

Administration: SQ route. Refer to PI for preparation/reconstitution and administration instructions. **Storage:** Keep refrigerated at 2-8°C (36-46°F). Do not freeze. Reconstituted: Keep at 25°C (77°F) or refrigerated for up to 24 hrs prior to administration. Protect from light.

NUCYNTA `CII`
tapentadol (Ortho-Mcneil/Janssen)

THERAPEUTIC CLASS: Central acting analgesic

INDICATIONS: Relief of moderate to severe acute pain in patients ≥18 yrs.

DOSAGE: *Adults:* Individualize dose. Usual: 50mg, 75mg, or 100mg q4-6h depending on pain intensity. Day 1: 2nd dose may be given 1 hr after 1st dose if pain relief is inadequate, then 50mg, 75mg, or 100mg q4-6h. Max: 700mg on Day 1, then 600mg/day thereafter. Severe Renal/Hepatic Impairment: Do not use. Moderate Hepatic Impairment: Initial: 50mg q8h or longer between doses. Max: 3 doses/24 hrs. Elderly: Start at low end of dosing range.

HOW SUPPLIED: Tab: 50mg, 75mg, 100mg

CONTRAINDICATIONS: Significant respiratory depression, acute/severe bronchial asthma, or hypercapnia (in unmonitored settings or the absence of resuscitative equipment); paralytic ileus; MAOI use during or within 14 days of treatment.

WARNINGS/PRECAUTIONS: May cause respiratory depression; occurs more frequently in elderly, debilitated, and patients with hypoxia, hypercapnia, or upper airway obstruction. Caution with asthma, chronic obstructive pulmonary disease (COPD), cor pulmonale, severe obesity, sleep apnea syndrome, myxedema, kyphoscoliosis, CNS depression, and coma. Can raise CSF pressure; avoid in those susceptible to such effects. Caution with head injury, intracranial lesions, or other sources of pre-existing increased intracranial pressure (ICP). May obscure clinical course of patients with head injury. May be abused in a manner similar to other opioids; carefully monitor for signs of abuse and addiction. May impair mental/physical abilities. Caution with history of seizure disorder, risk of seizures, and moderate hepatic impairment. Potentially life-threatening serotonin syndrome may occur. Withdrawal symptoms may occur upon abrupt d/c. May cause spasm of sphincter of Oddi; caution with biliary tract disease, including acute pancreatitis.

ADVERSE REACTIONS: N/V, dizziness, somnolence, constipation, pruritus, dry mouth, hyperhidrosis, fatigue.

INTERACTIONS: See Contraindications. May exhibit additive CNS depression with other opioid analgesics, general anesthetics, phenothiazines, antiemetics, other tranquilizers, sedatives, hypnotics, other CNS depressants (eg, alcohol); consider dose reduction. Serotonin syndrome may occur, particularly with serotonergic drugs (eg, SSRIs, SNRIs, TCAs, MAOIs and triptans) and drugs that may impair metabolism of serotonin.

PREGNANCY: Category C, not for use in nursing.

MECHANISM OF ACTION: Centrally-acting analgesic; not established. Suspected to be due to mu-opioid agonist activity and the inhibition of norepinephrine reuptake.

PHARMACOKINETICS: Absorption: T_{max}=1.25 hrs; absolute bioavailability (32%). **Distribution:** (IV) V_d=540L; plasma protein binding (20%). **Metabolism:** Conjugation (extensive); tapentadol-O-glucuronide (major metabolite). **Elimination:** Kidneys (99%); urine (3% unchanged, 70% conjugated); $T_{1/2}$=4 hrs.

NURSING CONSIDERATIONS

Assessment: Assess for pain intensity, pregnancy/nursing status, possible drug interactions, and conditions where treatment is contraindicated or cautioned.

Monitoring: Monitor for signs of respiratory depression especially high-risk patients (eg, asthma, COPD), increased CSF pressure in patients with head injury or pre-existing increased ICP, abuse or addiction, withdrawal symptoms, mental/physical impairment, and for serotonin syndrome. Monitor hepatic/renal function.

Patient Counseling: Instruct to report episodes of breakthrough pain and adverse experiences during therapy. Counsel to take only as directed; instruct to not adjust dose without consulting the physician. Advise that it may be appropriate to taper dosing when discontinuing as withdrawal symptoms may occur. Inform of potential for drug abuse and that judgment, thinking, and motor skills when performing hazardous tasks (eg, operating machinery, driving) may be impaired. Advise to notify physician if pregnant/planning to become pregnant. Avoid breastfeeding and alcohol use. Inform of risk of seizures and serotonin syndrome. Instruct to notify physician of any prescription or OTC drugs currently taking.

Administration: Oral route. **Storage:** 25°C (77°F); excursions permitted to 15-30°C (59-86°F). Protect from moisture.

NUEDEXTA RX

quinidine sulfate - dextromethorphan hydrobromide (Avanir)

THERAPEUTIC CLASS: NMDA receptor antagonist

INDICATIONS: Treatment of pseudobulbar affect (PBA).

DOSAGE: *Adults:* Initial: 1 cap PO qd for 7 days. On 8th day of therapy and thereafter, 1 cap q12h.

HOW SUPPLIED: Cap: (Dextromethorphan HBr-Quinidine sulfate) 20mg-10mg

CONTRAINDICATIONS: Drug-induced thrombocytopenia, hepatitis, bone marrow depression or lupus-like syndrome. Prolonged QT interval, congenital long QT syndrome or history suggestive to torsades de pointes and patients with heart failure. Complete atrioventricular (AV) block without implanted pacemakers, or patients with high risk of complete AV block. During or within 14 days of MAOI therapy. Concomitant use with quinidine, quinine, or mefloquine, drugs that both prolong QT interval and metabolized by CYP2D6 (eg, thioridazine and pimozide).

WARNINGS/PRECAUTIONS: Quinidine may cause immune-mediated thrombocytopenia; d/c immediately if this occurs. Quinidine has also been associated with lupus-like syndrome involving polyarthritis, rash, bronchospasm, lymphadenopathy, hemolytic anemia, vasculitis, uveitis, angioedema, agranulocytosis, sicca syndrome, myalgia, skeletal-muscle enzymes elevation and pneumonitis. Hepatitis, including granulomatous hepatitis, reported. Fever and other signs of hypersensitivity may occur. QT prolongation reported; may cause torsades de pointes-type ventricular tachycardia. ECG evaluation should be conducted at baseline and 3-4 hrs after first dose in patients with left ventricular hypertrophy (LVH), left ventricular dysfunction (LVD), those taking drugs that prolong the QT interval, and drugs that are strong or moderate CYP3A4 inhibitors. Reevaluate ECG if risk factors of arrhythmia change during therapy. Hypokalemia and hypomagnesemia should be corrected prior to therapy and monitor during treatment. D/C if cardiac arrhythmia (eg, syncope or palpitations) occurs. May cause dizziness; caution in patients with motor impairment affecting gait or with history of falls. May cause serotonin syndrome. Monitor for worsening clinical condition in myasthenia gravis and other conditions adversely affected by anticholinergic effects.

ADVERSE REACTIONS: Diarrhea, dizziness, cough, vomiting, asthenia, peripheral edema, urinary tract infection (UTI), influenza, increased gamma-glutamyltransferase, flatulence.

INTERACTIONS: See Contraindications. Recommend ECG when taking moderate or strong CYP3A4 inhibitors. Concomitant use with SSRIs or TCAs increases risk of serotonin syndrome. Adjust doses of desipramine and paroxetine if given together. Concomitant administration with digoxin may result in increased digoxin levels; monitor plasma digoxin concentration and reduce dose if necessary. Additive effect with memantine. Caution in combination with alcohol and other centrally acting drugs.

PREGNANCY: Category C, caution in nursing.

MECHANISM OF ACTION: (Dextromethorphan) NMDA receptor antagonist; mechanism has not been established; sigma-1 receptor and uncompetitive NMDA receptor antagonist. (Quinidine) increases plasma levels of dextromethorphan by competitively inhibiting cytochrome P450 2D6, which catalyzes a major biotransformation pathway for dextromethorphan.

PHARMACOKINETICS: Absorption: Quinidine; C_{max}=2-5mcg/mL, T_{max}=1-2 hrs; Dextromethorphan: T_{max}=3-4 hrs. **Distribution:** Dextromethorphan: Plasma protein binding (60-70%). Quinidine: 3-hydroxyquinidine (major metabolite), plasma protein binding (80-89%). **Metabolism:** Liver. Dextromethorphan: CYP2D6. Quinidine: CYP3A4. **Elimination:** Dextromethorphan: $T_{1/2}$=13 hrs. Quinidine: Urine (20%, unchanged), $T_{1/2}$=7 hrs.

NURSING CONSIDERATIONS

Assessment: Assess for drug hypersensitivity, history of drug-induced thrombocytopenia, chronic HTN, known CAD, history of stroke, electrolyte abnormality (eg, hypokalemia, hypomagnesemia), bradycardia, family history of QT abnormality, or any other condition where treatment is contraindicated or cautioned. Assess renal/hepatic function, pregnancy/nursing status and possible drug interactions. Obtain baseline ECG and genotyping.

Monitoring: Monitor for development of thrombocytopenia, lightheadedness, chills, fever, N/V, fatal hemorrhage, lupus-like syndrome, polyarthritis, rash, bronchospasm, lymphadenopathy, hemolytic anemia, vasculitis, uveitis, angioedema, agranulocytosis, sicca syndrome, myalgia, skeletal-muscle enzyme elevation, pneumonitis, hepatitis including granulomatous hepatitis, fever, hypersensitivity, QTc prolongation, torsades de pointes, ventricular tachycardia, cardiac arrhythmias, dizziness, serotonin syndrome, hypokalemia, hypomagnesemia and other possible adverse reactions. Monitor ECG 3-4 hrs after the first dose in patients at risk of QT prolongation and torsades de pointes, plasma digoxin levels, worsening of myasthenia gravis and other conditions that may be affected by anticholinergic effects. Reevaluate ECG if risk factors of arrhythmia change during therapy.

Patient Counseling: Inform about the risks and benefits of the treatment. Report any adverse effects to healthcare provider. Take medication as prescribed; do not take >2 caps in 24-hr period and make sure there is an approximate 12-hr interval between doses, and do not double dose after a missed dose. Inform healthcare provider about all medications they are taking and planning to take. Advise patients to seek immediate medical attention if hypersensitivity reactions, fainting or loss of consciousness occur. Inform healthcare providers if with personal or family history of QTc prolongation. Instruct not to share or give medication to others even if with the same symptoms. Contact healthcare providers if PBA persists or worsens. Advise to use precautions to reduce risk of falls as dizziness may occur. Keep all medications out of reach of children.

Administration: Oral route. **Storage:** 25°C (77°F); excursions permitted to 15-30°C (59-86°F).

NUTROPIN   RX
somatropin (Genentech)

OTHER BRAND NAMES: Nutropin AQ (Genentech)
THERAPEUTIC CLASS: Human growth hormone

INDICATIONS: (Adults) Replacement of endogenous growth hormone (GH) in GH deficiency (GHD). (Pediatrics) Long-term treatment of growth failure due to lack of adequate endogenous GH secretion, in short stature associated with Turner syndrome, and in idiopathic short stature (ISS). Treatment of growth failure associated with chronic renal insufficiency (CRI) up to the time of renal transplantation.

DOSAGE: *Adults:* GHD: Initial: Up to 0.006mg/kg/day SQ. Max: <35 yrs: 0.025mg/kg qd. ≥35 yrs: 0.0125mg/kg/day. Alternatively may use 0.2mg/day (range: 0.15-0.30mg/day). Increase every 1-2 months by increments of 0.1-0.2mg qd. Elderly: Start at low end of dosing range.
Pediatrics: GHD: Usual: 0.3mg/kg/week divided into daily SQ doses. Pubertal Patients: Up to 0.7mg/kg/week divided into daily SQ doses. CRI: 0.35mg/kg/week divided into daily SQ doses. Continue until renal transplantation. Hemodialysis: Give qhs or 3-4 hrs post-dialysis. Chronic Cycling Peritoneal Dialysis: Give in am after dialysis. Chronic Ambulatory Peritoneal Dialysis: Give qhs during overnight exchange. Turner Syndrome: Up to 0.375mg/kg/week SQ in divided doses 3-7x/week. ISS: 0.3mg/kg/week divided into daily SQ doses.

HOW SUPPLIED: Inj: 5mg, 10mg, (AQ) 10mg/2mL, 20mg/2mL, (AQ NuSpin) 5mg/2mL, 10mg/2mL, 20mg/2mL

CONTRAINDICATIONS: Acute critical illness after serious surgeries (eg, open heart or abdominal surgery, accidental trauma, acute respiratory failure), closed epiphyses in pediatrics, active proliferative or severe nonproliferative diabetic retinopathy, active neoplasia, evidence of recurrence or progression of an intracranial tumor. Prader-Willi syndrome (unless also diagnosed with GH deficiency) with severe obesity or respiratory impairment.

WARNINGS/PRECAUTIONS: Caution with epiphyseal closure in adults treated with GH-replacement therapy in childhood. Recurrence/progression reported with intracranial lesions. Renal osteodystrophy may occur with growth failure secondary to renal impairment. Scoliosis and slipped capital femoral epiphysis may develop in rapid growth. Caution with Turner syndrome and ISS. Intracranial HTN with papilledema, visual changes, headache, N/V has been reported. Monitor for malignant transformation of skin lesions. Injecting SQ in same site over long period of time may cause tissue atrophy. May decrease insulin sensitivity. Caution in elderly.

ADVERSE REACTIONS: Antibodies to the protein, leukemia, transient peripheral edema, arthralgia, carpal tunnel syndrome, malignant transformations, gynecomastia, pancreatitis.

INTERACTIONS: Decreased effects with glucocorticoids. May reduce insulin sensitivity; may need insulin adjustment. May need to increase dose in adult women on estrogen replacement.

PREGNANCY: Category C, caution in nursing.

MECHANISM OF ACTION: Human growth hormone; increases growth rate and serum insulin-like growth factor-I levels.

PHARMACOKINETICS: **Absorption:** (SQ) Absolute bioavailability (81%), C_{max}=71.1mcg/L, T_{max}=3.9 hrs, AUC=677 mcg•hr/L. **Distribution:** V_d=50mL/kg. **Metabolism:** Liver and kidneys. **Elimination:** (SQ) $T_{1/2}$=2.1 hrs. (IV) $T_{1/2}$=19.5 min.

NURSING CONSIDERATIONS

Assessment: Assess for any conditions where treatment is contraindicated or cautioned, pre-existing type 1 or type 2 DM or impaired glucose tolerance, history of scoliosis, pre-existing papilledema, hypothyroidism, diagnostic imaging (rule out pituitary or intracranial tumor), hypopituitarism and possible drug interactions. Obtain baseline funduscopic exam. Chronic renal insufficiency (pediatrics): Baseline x-ray of hips. Prader-Willi syndrome: Evaluate for signs of upper airway obstruction or sleep apnea before initiation. Turner syndrome: Evaluate for otitis media or other ear disorders, and for CV disorders before initiation.

Monitoring: Monitor FPG, and thyroid function tests periodically, periodic funduscopic exam, weight control (Prader-Willi), signs/symptoms of malignant transformation of skin lesions, intracranial HTN, renal osteodystrophy, slipped capital femoral epiphysis (onset of limp, hip or knee pain), hypersensitivity/allergic reactions, respiratory infections (Prader-Willi), otitis media or ear disorders, CV disorders (Turner syndrome), and progression of scoliosis.

Patient Counseling: Instruct thoroughly on proper usage, proper disposal, and caution against reuse of needles and syringes. Seek medical attention if symptoms of slipped capital femoral epiphysis (onset of limp, hip or knee pain), hypersensitivity/allergic reactions, respiratory infections (Prader-Willi), otitis media or ear disorders and CV disorders (Turner syndrome), and progression of scoliosis occur.

Administration: SQ route. Do not shake. Refer to PI for proper administration.
Storage: Before and after reconstitution: 2-8°C (36-46°F) (under refrigeration). Avoid freezing. AQ: Stable for 28 days after initial use. Protect from light. Nutropin: Stable 14 days after reconstitution.

NuvaRing RX
etonogestrel - ethinyl estradiol (Organon)

> Cigarette smoking increases risk of serious cardiovascular (CV) side effects. Risk increases with age (>35 yrs) and heavy smoking (≥15 cigarettes/day). Women who use combination hormonal contraception should be strongly advised not to smoke.

THERAPEUTIC CLASS: Estrogen/progestogen combination

INDICATIONS: Prevention of pregnancy.

DOSAGE: *Adults:* Insert ring vaginally. Ring is to remain in place continuously for 3 weeks. It should be removed for 1 week break and then a new ring should be inserted on same day of week as the last ring was removed. No Hormonal Contraceptive Use in the Preceding Cycle: Insert ring on Day 1-5 of menstrual bleeding. If inserted on days 2-5 of cycle, use an additional barrier method of contraception (eg, condom, spermicide) for 1st 7 days. Changing from Combined Hormonal Contraceptive: May switch any day, but at the latest on the day following the usual hormone-free interval. Changing from Progestin-Only Method (minipill, implant, or injection) or from Progestogen-Releasing Intrauterine System (IUS): May switch on any day from the minipill. May switch from an implant or IUS on the day of its removal and from an injectable on the day when the next injection is due. In all cases, additional barrier method (eg, condom, spermicide) should be use for the 1st 7 days.
Pediatrics: Postpubertal: Insert ring vaginally. Ring is to remain in place continuously for 3 weeks. It should be removed for 1 week break and then a new ring should be inserted on same day of week as the last ring was removed. No Hormonal Contraceptive Use in the Preceding Cycle: Insert ring on Day 1-5 of menstrual bleeding. If inserted on days 2-5 of cycle, use an additional barrier method of contraception (eg, condom, spermicide) for 1st 7 days. Changing from Combined Hormonal Contraceptive: May switch any day, but at the latest on the day following the usual hormone-free interval. Changing from Progestin-Only Method (minipill, implant, or injection) or from Progestogen-Releasing Intrauterine System (IUS): May switch on any day from the minipill. May switch from an implant or IUS on the day of its removal and from an injectable on the day when the next injection is due. In all cases, additional barrier method (eg, condom, spermicide) should be use for the 1st 7 days.

HOW SUPPLIED: Vaginal ring: (Ethinyl estradiol-Etonogestrel) 0.015mg-0.120mg/day

CONTRAINDICATIONS: Thrombophlebitis, history of deep vein thrombophlebitis, active or history of thromboembolic disorders, current or history of cerebral vascular disease, current or history of coronary artery disease, valvular heart disease with thrombogenic complications, severe HTN, diabetes with vascular involvement, headaches with focal neurological symptoms, major surgery with prolonged immobilization, breast carcinoma or history of breast carcinoma, carcinoma of the endometrium or other estrogen-dependent neoplasia, undiagnosed abnormal genital bleeding, cholestatic jaundice of pregnancy or jaundice with prior hormonal contraceptive use, hepatic tumors (benign or malignant) or active liver disease, pregnancy, heavy smoking (≥15 cigarettes per day) and >35 yrs.

WARNINGS/PRECAUTIONS: Increases risk of MI, thromboembolism, stroke, hepatic neoplasia, vascular disease, gallbladder disease, and HTN. Increased risk of morbidity and mortality in certain inherited thrombophilias, HTN, hyperlipidemias, obesity, and diabetes. May increase risk of breast cancer and cancer of the reproductive organs. Retinal thrombosis reported; d/c if unexplained partial or complete loss of vision, onset of proptosis or diplopia, papilledema, or retinal vascular lesions develop. May cause decreased glucose tolerance, fluid retention, breakthrough bleeding, and spotting. May increase BP; d/c if significant elevation in BP occurs. May elevate LDL levels or cause other lipid changes. May cause or exacerbate migraine headaches; d/c if severe or recurrent headache or migraine develops. D/C if jaundice or if significant depression develops. May develop visual changes with contact lens. May be expelled while removing tampons on rare occasions. Toxic shock syndrome reported. Older women who take hormonal contraceptive should take the lowest possible dose formulation that is effective. Ectopic as well as intrauterine pregnancy may occur in contraceptive failures. Does not protect against HIV infection (AIDS) and other STDs. Vaginal/cervical erosion or ulceration rarely reported. May affect certain endocrine, LFTs, and blood components in laboratory tests.

ADVERSE REACTIONS: Vaginitis, headache, upper respiratory tract infection, vaginal secretion, sinusitis, weight gain, nausea.

INTERACTIONS: May reduce contraceptive effectiveness when co-administered with some anti-fungals, anticonvulsants, and other drugs that increase the metabolism of contraceptive steroids (eg, barbiturates, griseofulvin, rifampin, phenylbutazone, phenytoin, carbamazepine, felbamate, oxycarbazepine, topiramate, modafinil); use additonal form of contraception when taking such medications. HIV protease inhibitors may increase or decrease estrogen and progestin levels. St. John's wort may reduce contraceptive effectiveness and may cause breakthrough bleeding. Atorvastatin, ascorbic acid, acetaminophen, CYP3A4 inhibitors (eg, itraconazole, ketoconazole), vaginal miconazole nitrate may increase plasma hormone levels. May increase levels of cyclosporine, prednisolone, and theophylline. May decrease levels of acetaminophen and increase clearance of temazepam, salicylic acid, morphine, and clofibric acid.

PREGNANCY: Category X, not for use in nursing.

MECHANISM OF ACTION: Estrogen/progestogen combination; suppresses gonadotropins, leading to inhibition of ovulation, and increases difficulty of sperm entry into uterus and reduces likelihood of implantation by producing changes in cervical mucus and endometrium, respectively.

PHARMACOKINETICS: Absorption: Etonorgestrel: Rapid; bioavailability (100%); C_{max}=1716pg/mL; T_{max}=200.3 hrs. Ethinyl estradiol: Rapid; absolute bioavailability (56%); C_{max}=34.7pg/mL; T_{max}=59.3 hrs. **Distribution:** Found in breast milk. Etonorgestrel: Serum albumin binding (66%), sex hormone-binding globulin (32%). Ethinyl estradiol: Serum albumin binding (98.5%). **Metabolism:** Hepatic via CYP3A4. **Elimination:** Urine, bile, feces; Etonorgestrel: $T_{1/2}$=29.3 hrs; Ethinyl estradiol: $T_{1/2}$=44.7 hrs.

NURSING CONSIDERATIONS

Assessment: Assess for conditions in which treatment is contraindicated or cautioned. Assess for pregnancy/nursing status, and for possible drug interactions. Assess if a heavy smoker and over the age of 35. Assess use in patients who have inherited thrombophilias, HTN, hyperlipidemias, obesity, or DM.

Monitoring: Monitor for signs and symptoms of MI, thromboembolism, stroke, and other adverse effects. Monitor lipid levels with history of hyperlipidemia; monitor BP if have history of HTN; monitor serum glucose levels in DM or prediabetic patients. Refer patients with contact lenses to an opthalmologist if visual changes or changes in lens tolerance occur. Perform annual physical exam.

Patient Counseling: Counsel that drug does not protect against HIV infection/AIDS or other STDs and to take as directed. Counsel about possibility of light spotting. Advise to avoid smoking to prevent cardiovascular side effects. Instruct to seek immediate medical attention if develop sharp chest pain, coughing blood, shortness of breath, pain in the calf, chest pain or chest heaviness, vision or speech abnormalities, severe headache, severe vomiting, severe dizziness, severe abdominal pain, sudden fever or sunburn rash, breast lumps, irregular vaginal bleeding or spotting, urination problems, swelling of fingers or ankles, or if develop sleeping disturbances or fatigue. Caution that some medications decrease efficacy and should not be used without physician instructions. Inform that if ring is accidentally expelled and left outside of the vagina for less than three hours, contraceptive efficacy is not reduced; ring can be rinsed with cool to lukewarm water and reinserted as soon as possible or a new ring can be inserted and the regimen should continue without alteration.

Administration: Intravaginal route. Refer to PI for specific instructions.
Storage: 2-8°C (36-46°F). After dispensing, store up to 4 months at 25°C (77°F); excursions permitted to 15-30°C (59-86°F). Avoid direct sunlight or above 30°C (86°F).

NUVIGIL
armodafinil (Cephalon)

THERAPEUTIC CLASS: Wakefulness-promoting agent

INDICATIONS: To improve wakefulness in patients with excessive sleepiness associated with narcolepsy, obstructive sleep apnea (OSA), and shift work disorder (SWD). As adjunct to standard treatment for underlying obstruction in OSA.

DOSAGE: *Adults:* ≥17 yrs: OSA/Narcolepsy: 150mg or 250mg qam. SWD: 150mg qd 1 hr prior to work shift. Elderly: Consider dose reduction.

HOW SUPPLIED: Tab: 50mg, 150mg, 250mg

WARNINGS/PRECAUTIONS: May cause severe or life-threatening rash, including Stevens-Johnson syndrome (SJS), toxic epidermal necrolysis (TEN), and drug rash with eosinophilia and systemic symptoms (DRESS); d/c treatment at first sign of rash. Angioedema, anaphylactoid reactions, multi-organ hypersensitivity and psychiatric adverse experiences reported; d/c treatment if symptoms develop. Caution with history of psychosis, depression, or mania. Caution if recent myocardial infarction (MI) or unstable angina. Avoid in patients with history of left ventricular hypertrophy or with mitral valve prolapse who have experienced mitral valve prolapse syndrome (eg, ischemic ECG changes, chest pain, arrhythmia) with CNS stimulants. May impair mental/physical abilities. Reduce dose with severe hepatic impairment. Use low dose in elderly.

ADVERSE REACTIONS: Headache, nausea, dizziness, insomnia, diarrhea, dry mouth, anxiety, depression, rash.

INTERACTIONS: Potent CYP3A4/5 inducers (eg, carbamazepine, phenobarbital, rifampin) or inhibitors (eg, ketoconazole, erythromycin) may alter plasma levels. Effectiveness of CYP3A substrates (eg, cyclosporine, ethinyl estradiol, midazolam, triazolam) may be reduced; consider dose adjustment. May cause moderate inhibition of CYP2C19 activity; dosage reduction may be required for some CYP2C19 substrates (eg, omeprazole, diazepam, phenytoin, propranolol, clomipramine). Weakly induces CYP1A2; may affect CYP1A2 substrates. Methylphenidate or dextroamphetamine may delay absorption. Caution with MAOIs. Monitor PT/INR with warfarin. Effectiveness of steroidal contraceptives may be reduced during and for 1 month after d/c of therapy; alternate or concomitant methods of contraception are recommended.

PREGNANCY: Category C, caution in nursing.

MECHANISM OF ACTION: Wakefulness-promoting agent; not established. Binds to the dopamine transporter and inhibits dopamine reuptake.

PHARMACOKINETICS: Absorption: Readily absorbed. T_{max}=2 hrs (fasted), delayed by 2-4 hrs (fed). **Distribution**: V_d=42L; plasma protein binding (60%, based on modafinil). **Metabolism**: Liver via hydrolytic deamidation, S-oxidation, aromatic ring hydroxylation, and glucuronide conjugation;

CYP3A4/5. **Elimination**: Feces (1%), urine (80%, <10% parent compound); $T_{1/2}$=15 hrs.

NURSING CONSIDERATIONS

Assessment: Assess for hypersensitivity, hepatic impairment, pregnancy/nursing status, possible drug interactions, and a history of psychosis, depression, mania, left ventricular hypertrophy, or mitral valve prolapse. Assess for a recent history of MI or unstable angina. Use only in patients who have had a complete evaluation of their excessive sleepiness, and in whom a diagnosis of either narcolepsy, OSA, and/or SWD has been made.

Monitoring: Monitor for serious rash, SJS, TEN, DRESS, angioedema, hypersensitivity, multi-organ hypersensitivity reactions, psychiatric adverse symptoms, and other adverse reactions. Monitor BP. If used adjunctively with continuous positive airway pressure (CPAP), monitor for CPAP compliance. Periodically re-evaluate long-term usefulness if prescribed for an extended time.

Patient Counseling: Advise that this is not a replacement for sleep. Inform that drug may improve but does not eliminate sleepiness. Advise to avoid taking alcohol during therapy. Caution against hazardous tasks (eg, driving, operating machinery) or performing other activities that require mental alertness. Advise to notify physician if pregnant or intend to become pregnant or if nursing during therapy. Caution about increased risk of pregnancy when using steroidal contraceptives and for 1 month after d/c therapy. Inform physician if taking or planning to take any prescribed or OTC drugs. Instruct to contact physician if rash, depression, anxiety, or signs of psychosis or mania develop. Inform of importance of continuing previously prescribed treatments. Advise to d/c and notify physician if rash, hives, mouth sores, blisters, peeling skin, trouble swallowing or breathing or other allergic reactions develop.

Administration: Oral route. **Storage:** 20-25°C (68-77°F).

NYSTATIN ORAL   RX
nystatin (Various)

THERAPEUTIC CLASS: Polyene antifungal

INDICATIONS: (Sus) Treatment of oral candidiasis. (Tab) Treatment of non-esophageal mucous membrane GI candidiasis.

DOSAGE: *Adults:* Oral Candidiasis: (Sus) 2-3mL in each side of mouth qid. Retain in mouth as long as possible before swallowing. Non-Esophageal GI Candidiasis: (Tab) 1-2 tab tid.
Pediatrics: Oral Candidiasis: (Sus) 2-3mL in each side of mouth qid. Infants: 1mL in each side of mouth qid. Retain in mouth as long as possible before swallowing. Avoid feeding for 5 to 10 min after.

HOW SUPPLIED: Sus: 100,000 U/mL [60mL, 480mL]; Tab: 500,000 U

WARNINGS/PRECAUTIONS: Not for systemic mycoses; d/c if sensitization/irritation occurs. Continue for at least 48 hrs after symptoms have disappeared to prevent relapse. Caution with renal insufficiency.

ADVERSE REACTIONS: Oral irritation, sensitization, diarrhea, N/V, GI disturbances, rash, urticaria, Stevens-Johnson syndrome.

PREGNANCY: Category C, caution in nursing.

MECHANISM OF ACTION: Polyene antifungal; fungistatic and fungicidal agent. Binds to sterols in the cell membrane of susceptible *Candida* species with a resultant change in membrane permeability, allowing leakage of intracellular components.

PHARMACOKINETICS: Elimination: Feces (unchanged).

NURSING CONSIDERATIONS

Assessment: Assess for proper diagnosis of oral/non-esophageal GI candidiasis, renal insufficiency and pregnancy/nursing status.

Monitoring: Monitor for possible adverse reactions including oral irritation, hypersensitivity, diarrhea, N/V, GI upset/disturbance, rash, Stevens-Johnson syndrome. Monitor renal function.

Patient Counseling: Discuss risks and benefits of therapy. Not for treatment of systemic mycoses. D/C if sensitization or irritation occurs. Notify physician for any adverse reactions. Shake sus well before use.

Administration: Oral route. **Storage:** (Sus) 20-25°C (68°-77°F); excursions permitted to 15-30°C (59-86°F). (Tab) 20°-25°C (68°-77°F).

NYSTOP   RX
nystatin (Paddock)

THERAPEUTIC CLASS: Polyene antifungal

INDICATIONS: Treatment of cutaneous and mucocutaneous mycotic infections caused by susceptible *Candida* species.

DOSAGE: *Adults:* Apply to lesions bid-tid until healing is complete. For fungal infections of the feet, dust powder on feet and also in shoes.
Pediatrics: Neonates and Older: Apply to lesions bid-tid until healing is complete. For fungal infections of the feet, dust powder on feet and also in shoes.

HOW SUPPLIED: Powder, Topical: 100,000 U/g [15g, 30g, 60g]

WARNINGS/PRECAUTIONS: D/C if irritation or sensitization occurs. Confirm diagnosis. Not for systemic, oral, intravaginal, or ophthalmic use.

ADVERSE REACTIONS: Allergic reactions, burning, itching, rash, eczema, pain at application site.

PREGNANCY: Category C, caution in nursing.

MECHANISM OF ACTION: Polyene antifungal; binds sterols in the cell membrane of susceptible species causing a change in membrane permeability and subsequent leakage of intracellular components. Fungistatic and fungicidal.

PHARMACOKINETICS: Absorption: Not absorbed from intact skin or mucous membranes.

NURSING CONSIDERATIONS

Assessment: Assess proper diagnosis of cutaneous or mucocutaneous candidiasis through use of KOH smears, cultures, or other diagnostic methods. Assess use in pregnancy/nursing.

Monitoring: Monitor for irritation or sensitization and therapeutic response. If no therapeutic response, reassess diagnosis (eg, KOH smears, cultures, other diagnostic methods).

Patient Counseling: Instruct to use exactly as directed and not to interrupt or d/c therapy even if symptom relief occurs within first few days of treatment. Notify physician if skin irritation develops.

Administration: Topical route. **Storage:** 15-30°C (59-86°F); avoid excessive heat 40°C (104°F).

OFIRMEV   RX
acetaminophen (Cadence)

THERAPEUTIC CLASS: Analgesic

INDICATIONS: Management of mild to moderate pain, management of moderate to severe pain with adjunctive opioid analgesics and for reduction of fever.

DOSAGE: *Adults:* ≥50kg: Usual: 1000mg q6h or 650mg q4h. Max Daily Dose: 4000mg/day. Max Single Dose:1000mg/dose. <50kg: 15mg/kg q6h or 12.5mg/kg q4h. Max Daily Dose: 75g/kg/day. Max Single Dose: 15mg/kg/dose. Dosing interval must be a minimum of 4 hrs.
Pediatrics: ≥13 yrs: ≥50kg: Usual: 1000mg q6h or 650mg q4h. Max Daily dose: 4000mg/day. Max Single Dose: 1000mg/dose. <50kg:

15mg/kg q6h or 12.5mg/kg q4h. Max Daily Dose: 75mg/kg/day. Max Single Dose:15mg/kg/dose. ≥2-12 yrs: 15mg/kg q6h or 12.5mg/kg q4h. Max Daily Dose: 75mg/kg/day (up to 3750mg). Max Single Dose: 15mg/kg/dose (up to 750mg). Dosing interval must be a minimum of 4 hrs.

HOW SUPPLIED: Inj: 10mg/mL

CONTRAINDICATIONS: Severe hepatic impairment or severe active liver disease.

WARNINGS/PRECAUTIONS: May result in hepatic injury (eg, severe hepatotoxicity, death) in doses higher than recommended; do not exceed maximum recommended daily dose. Caution with hepatic impairment or active hepatic disease, alcoholism, chronic malnutrition, severe hypovolemia, or severe renal impairment (CrCl ≤30mL/min). Hypersensitivity and anaphylaxis reported; d/c immediately if symptoms associated with allergy/hypersensitivity occur. Life-threatening anaphylaxis requiring emergent medical attention reported.

ADVERSE REACTIONS: N/V, headache, insomnia, constipation, pruritus, agitation, atelectasis.

INTERACTIONS: Altered metabolism and increased hepatotoxic potential with substances that induce or regulate CYP2E1. Excessive alcohol use may induce hepatic cytochromes. Ethanol may inhibit metabolism. Increased international normalized ratio (INR) in some patients stabilized on warfarin.

PREGNANCY: Category C, caution in nursing.

MECHANISM OF ACTION: Analgesic/antipyretic; not established. Thought to primarily involve central actions.

PHARMACOKINETICS: Absorption: Variable doses to different age groups resulted in different parameters; refer to PI. **Distribution:** Plasma protein binding (10-25%); widely distributed throughout body tissues except fat; (PO) found in breast milk. **Metabolism:** Liver; glucuronide and sulfate conjugation, and oxidation via CYP2E1; N-acetyl-p-benzoquinone imine (NAPQI) (metabolite). **Elimination:** Urine (<5% unconjugated, >90% within 24 hrs).

NURSING CONSIDERATIONS

Assessment: Assess for previous hypersensitivity, severe hepatic impairment or severe active liver disease, alcoholism, chronic malnutrition, severe hypovolemia, or severe renal impairment (CrCl ≤30mL/min). Assess for pregnancy/nursing status and possible drug interactions.

Monitoring: Monitor for signs and symptoms of hypersensitivity and anaphylaxis (eg, swelling of face, mouth, and throat, respiratory distress, urticaria, rash, and pruritus), and other adverse reactions.

Patient Counseling: Inform about the risks and benefits of therapy. Warn not to exceed the recommended dose. Notify physician if any adverse reactions occur or if pregnant/nursing or planning to become pregnant. Counsel about possible drug interactions.

Administration: IV route. Administer by IV infusion. Do not add other medications to the vial or infusion device. Refer to PI for administration technique. **Storage:** 20-25°C (68-77°F). Use within 6 hrs after opening. Do not refrigerate or freeze.

OFLOXACIN   RX
ofloxacin (Various)

> Fluoroquinolones are associated with an increased risk of tendinitis and tendon rupture in all ages. Risk is further increased in patients >60 yrs, taking corticosteroids, and with kidney, heart or lung transplants. May exacerbate muscle weakness with myasthenia gravis; avoid with known history of myasthenia gravis.

THERAPEUTIC CLASS: Fluoroquinolone

INDICATIONS: Treatment of complicated urinary tract infections (UTI), uncomplicated skin and skin structure infections (SSSI), acute bacterial exacerbation of chronic bronchitis (ABECB), community-acquired pneumonia (CAP), acute uncomplicated urethral and cervical gonorrhea, nongonococcal urethritis and cervicitis, mixed infections of urethra and cervix, acute pelvic inflammatory disease (PID), uncomplicated cystitis, and prostatitis caused by susceptible strains of microorganisms.

DOSAGE: *Adults:* ABECB/CAP/SSSI: 400mg q12h for 10 days. Cervicitis/ Urethritis: 300mg q12h for 7 days. Gonorrhea: 400mg single dose. PID: 400mg q12h for 10-14 days. Uncomplicated Cystitis: 200mg q12h for 3 days (*E.coli* or *K.pneumoniae*) or 7 days (other pathogens). Complicated UTI: 200mg q12h for 10 days. Prostatitis: (*E.coli*) 300mg q12h for 6 weeks. CrCl 20-50mL/min: After regular initial dose, give q24h. CrCl <20mL/min: After regular initial dose, give 50% of normal dose q24h. Severe Hepatic Impairment: Max: 400mg/day.

HOW SUPPLIED: Tab: 200mg, 300mg, 400mg

WARNINGS/PRECAUTIONS: Convulsions, increased ICP, toxic psychosis, CNS stimulation, and serious, sometimes fatal, hypersensitivity reactions reported; d/c if any occur. Rare cases of sensory or sensorimotor axonal polyneuropathy reported; d/c if symptoms of neuropathy occur. *Clostridium difficile*-associated diarrhea (CDAD) and ruptures of shoulder, hand, and Achilles' tendon reported. Not shown to be effective for syphilis. Maintain adequate hydration. Caution with renal or hepatic dysfunction, risk for seizures, CNS disorder with predisposition to seizures. Avoid excessive sunlight. Monitor blood, renal and hepatic function with prolonged therapy. D/C immediately at the first appearance of skin rash, jaundice, or any other sign of hypersensitivity and supportive measures instituted. Drug therapy should be d/c if photosensitivity/phototoxicity occurs. Avoid in patients with known prolongation of the QT interval, and with uncorrected hypokalemia. Caution in elderly taking corticosteroids.

ADVERSE REACTIONS: N/V, insomnia, headache, dizziness, diarrhea, external genital pruritus in women, vaginitis.

INTERACTIONS: See Boxed Warning. Decreased absorption with antacids, sucralfate, multivitamins, zinc, didanosine; separate dosing by 2 hrs. Cimetidine may interfere with elimination. Cyclosporine levels may be elevated. NSAIDs may increase risk of seizures. Probenecid may affect renal tubular secretion. Avoid in patients receiving Class IA (quinidine, procainamide), or Class III (amiodarone, sotalol) antiarrhythmic agents. May potentiate theophylline, warfarin. May potentiate insulin, oral hypoglycemics; d/c if hypoglycemia occurs. May increase half-life of drugs metabolized by CYP450.

PREGNANCY: Category C, not for use in nursing.

MECHANISM OF ACTION: Fluoroquinolone; synthetic broad-spectrum antimicrobial agent; inhibits topoisomerase II (DNA gyrase) and topoisomerase IV, which are required for bacterial DNA replication, transcription, repair, and recombination.

PHARMACOKINETICS: Absorption: Oral administration of variable doses resulted in different parameters; T_{max}=1-2 hrs; bioavailability (98%). **Distribution:** Plasma protein binding (32%), found in breast milk. **Elimination:** Biphasic ($T_{1/2}$=4-5 hrs, 20-25 hrs), renal.

NURSING CONSIDERATIONS

Assessment: Assess for risk factors for developing tendinitis and tendon rupture, myasthenia gravis, renal function, LFTs, pregnancy/nursing status, history of seizures, QTc prolongation, and possible drug interactions. Obtain baseline culture and susceptibility test and serologic test for syphilis.

Monitoring: Monitor for tendinitis or tendon rupture, convulsions, increased ICP, toxic psychosis, CNS events, CDAD, peripheral neuropathy, photosensitivity reactions, and hypersensitivity reactions. Assess renal function and perform follow-up serologic test for syphilis after 3 months.

Patient Counseling: Notify healthcare provider if experience symptoms of pain, swelling, or inflammation of a tendon, or weakness or inability to move joints; rest and refrain from exercise and d/c therapy. Call healthcare provider if muscle weakness or breathing problems worsen. Inform that drug treats bacterial, not viral, infections. Take exactly as directed; skipping doses or not completing full course may decrease effectiveness and increase resistance. Inform about potential benefits/risks. D/C and notify physician if experience skin rash, other allergic reaction, watery or bloody stools, or symptoms of peripheral neuropathy develop. Use caution in activities requiring mental alertness and coordination. Advise diabetic patients to use caution; hypoglycemia may develop during therapy. Inform to take with or without meals, and to drink fluids. Avoid sun exposure. Take full course as prescribed.

Administration: Oral route. **Storage:** 25°C (77°F), excursions permitted to 15-30°C (59-86°F).

OFLOXACIN OTIC SOLUTION 0.3% RX
ofloxacin (Various)

OTHER BRAND NAMES: Floxin Otic Singles Solution (Daiichi Sankyo)

THERAPEUTIC CLASS: Fluoroquinolone

INDICATIONS: Treatment of otitis externa in patients ≥6 months, chronic suppurative otitis media in patients ≥12 yrs with perforated tympanic membranes, and acute otitis media in patients ≥1 yr with tympanostomy tubes, caused by susceptible isolates of designated microorganisms.

DOSAGE: *Adults:* Otitis Externa: 10 drops (0.5mL) or 2 single-dispensing containers (SDCs) into affected ear qd for 7 days. Chronic Suppurative Otitis Media with Perforated Tympanic Membrane: 10 drops (0.5mL) or 2 SDCs bid into affected ear for 14 days. Pump tragus 4 times by pushing inward to facilitate penetration into the middle ear.
Pediatrics: Otitis Externa: ≥13 yrs: 10 drops (0.5mL) or 2 SDCs into affected ear qd for 7 days. 6 months-13 yrs: 5 drops (0.25mL) or 1 single-dispensing container (SDC) into affected ear qd for 7 days. Chronic Suppurative Otitis Media with Perforated Tympanic Membrane: ≥12 yrs: 10 drops (0.5mL) or 2 SDCs bid into affected ear for 14 days. Pump tragus 4 times by pushing inward to facilitate penetration into the middle ear. Acute Otitis Media with Tympanostomy Tubes: 1-12 yrs: 5 drops (0.25mL) or 1 SDC bid into affected ear for 10 days. Pump tragus 4 times by pushing inward to facilitate penetration into the middle ear.

HOW SUPPLIED: Sol: 0.3% [5mL, 10mL], (Singles) 0.3% [20ˢ]

WARNINGS/PRECAUTIONS: D/C if hypersensitivity reaction occurs. Prolonged use may result in overgrowth in nonsusceptible organisms; re-evaluate if no improvement after one week. If otorrhea persists after a full course, or if two or more episodes occur within six months, further evaluation is recommended. Not for injection and ophthalmic use.

ADVERSE REACTIONS: Pruritus, application site reaction, taste perversion.

PREGNANCY: Category C, not for use in nursing.

MECHANISM OF ACTION: Fluoroquinolone; exerts antibacterial activity by inhibiting DNA gyrase (a bacterial topoisomerase), an essential enzyme which controls DNA topology and assists in DNA replication, repair, deactivation, and transcription.

PHARMACOKINETICS: Absorption: (Perforated tympanic membrane) C_{max}=10ng/mL.

NURSING CONSIDERATIONS

Assessment: Assess for drug hypersensitivity, pre-existing cholesteatoma, foreign body or tumor, pregnancy/nursing status.

Monitoring: Monitor for anaphylactic reactions, cardiovascular collapse, loss of consciousness, angioedema, airway obstruction, dyspnea, urticaria and itching, overgrowth of nonsusceptible organisms (fungi), for improvement/persistence of otorrhea.

Patient Counseling: Counsel to avoid touching applicator tip to fingers or other surfaces to avoid contamination. D/C and instruct to contact physician if signs of allergy occur. Instruct patients to warm bottle by holding for 1-2 min, to avoid dizziness which may result from instillation of a cold solution. Instruct to lie with affected ear upward, before instilling the drops; maintain position for 5 min. Repeat if necessary, for opposite ear.

Administration: Otic route. **Storage:** 20-25°C (68-77°F). Protect from light.

OFORTA   RX
fluticasone phosphate (Sanofi-Aventis)

> Severe neurologic effects, including blindness, coma, and death reported when administered at high doses in patients with acute leukemia. Similiar severe CNS toxicity reported rarely in patients who received doses in the recommended range for CLL. Periodic neurological assessments are recommended. Life-threatening and sometimes fatal autoimmune hemolytic anemia reported; monitor closely for hemolysis. High incidence of fatal pulmonary toxicity reported when used in combination with pentostatin.

THERAPEUTIC CLASS: Antimetabolite

INDICATIONS: Single agent for the treatment of adults with B-cell chronic lymphocytic leukemia (CLL) whose disease has not responded to or has progressed during or after treatment with at least one standard alkylating-agent containing regimen.

DOSAGE: *Adults:* Usual: 40mg/m² qd for 5 days. Each 5-day course of treatment should commence every 28 days. Refer to PI for specific dosing information based on BSA. CrCl 30-70mL/min/1.73m²: Reduce dose by 20%. CrCl <30mL/min/1.73m²: Reduce dose by 50%. May decrease or delay dose based on hematologic or nonhematologic toxicity. Consider delaying dose or d/c therapy if neurotoxicity occurs.

HOW SUPPLIED: Tab: 10mg

WARNINGS/PRECAUTIONS: Consider delaying or d/c therapy if neurotoxicity develops. Severe bone marrow suppression (eg, anemia, thrombocytopenia, and neutropenia) reported; perform careful hematologic monitoring. Fatalities due to infection reported; monitor for signs and symptoms of infection. Tumor lysis syndrome reported with large tumor burdens. Transfusion associated graft vs host disease reported following transfusion of non-irradiated blood; consider using irradiated blood products if transfusion required. May cause fetal harm if used during pregnancy; women of childbearing potential and fertile males must take contraceptive measures during and for at least 6 months after cessation of therapy. Caution with renal impairment. Patients with advanced age, renal insufficiency, or bone marrow impairment may be predisposed to increased toxicity; monitor for excessive toxicity and modify dose accordingly.

ADVERSE REACTIONS: Myelosuppression (neutropenia, thrombocytopenia, and anemia), fever, chills, infections, N/V, malaise, fatigue, anorexia, weakness, pain, cough.

INTERACTIONS: See Boxed Warning.

PREGNANCY: Category D, not for use in nursing.

MECHANISM OF ACTION: Purine nucleotide antimetabolite; competes with deoxyadenosine triphosphate for incorporation into DNA. Once incorporated into DNA, functions as a DNA chain terminator, inhibits DNA polymerase alpha, gamma, and delta, and inhibits ribonucleoside diphosphate reductase. Also inhibits DNA primase and DNA ligase I.

PHARMACOKINETICS: Absorption: 2F-ara-A: Absolute bioavailability (50-65%); T_{max}=1-2 hrs. **Distribution:** 2F-ara-A: Plasma protein binding (19-29%). **Metabolism:** 2F-ara-A (active metabolite). **Elimination:** 2F-ara-A: $T_{1/2}$=20 hrs.

NURSING CONSIDERATIONS

Assessment: Assess age of patient, renal impairment, bone marrow impairment, pregnancy/nursing status, and possible drug interactions.

Monitoring: Monitor for signs and symptoms of severe neurologic effects (eg, blindness, coma); perform periodic neurological assessments. Monitor for signs and symptoms of bone marrow suppression including autoimmune hemolytic anemia; monitor for hemolysis and perform periodic assessment of peripheral blood counts. Monitor for signs and symptoms of infection, tumor lysis syndrome in patients with large tumor burdens, and for graft vs host disease in patients undergoing blood transfusions.

Patient Counseling: Contact physician if a dose is missed. May cause bone marrow suppression; periodic blood testing is required while on therapy. Notify physician if fever or other signs of infection (eg, chills, cough, burning pain on urination) or neurotoxicity (eg, vision disturbances, impaired consciousness) develop. Women of childbearing potential and fertile males must take contraceptive measures during therapy and for at least 6 months after the cessation of therapy.

Administration: Oral route. May take on an empty stomach or with food; swallow tablet whole with water; do not chew or break tablet. **Storage:** 25°C (77°F); excursions permitted to 15-30°C (59-86°F).

OLEPTRO   RX
trazodone HCl (Labopharm)

> Antidepressants increased the risk of suicidal thinking and behavior (suicidality) in children, adolescents and young adults in short-term studies of major depressive disorder (MDD) and other psychiatric disorders. Monitor and observe closely for clinical worsening, suicidality, or unusual changes in behavior in patients who are started on antidepressant therapy. Trazodone is not approved for use in pediatric patients.

THERAPEUTIC CLASS: Triazolopyridine derivative

INDICATIONS: Treatment of MDD.

DOSAGE: *Adults:* Initial: 150mg qd. Titrate: May increase by 75mg qd every 3 days. Max: 375mg qd. Once adequate response is achieved, reduce dose gradually, with subsequent adjustment depending on therapeutic response. Maintain on the lowest effective dose and periodically reassess to determine the continued need for maintenance treatment. Do not chew or crush.

HOW SUPPLIED: Tab, Extended Release: 150mg*, 300mg* *scored

WARNINGS/PRECAUTIONS: Monitor for withdrawal symptoms when treatment is stopped; reduce dose gradually whenever possible. Serotonin syndrome (eg, mental status changes, autonomic instability, neuromuscular aberrations, GI symptoms) or neuroleptic malignant syndrome (NMS)-like reactions may occur. Screen patients (including psychiatric history, family history) for bipolar disorder; not approved in treating bipolar depression. Caution in patients with cardiac disease (eg, myocardial infarction [MI]); may cause cardiac arrhythmias. May cause QT/QTc interval prolongation and GI bleeding. Priapism rarely reported; caution in men with sickle cell anemia, multiple myeloma, leukemia or in men with penile anatomical deformation (eg, angulation, cavernosal fibrosis, Peyronie's disease). Hyponatremia may occur; d/c and institute appropriate medical intervention. Orthostatic hypotension and syncope reported. May impair mental/physical abilities. Caution in hepatic/renal impairment and elderly.

ADVERSE REACTIONS: Somnolence, sedation, headache, dry mouth, dizziness, nausea, fatigue, diarrhea, constipation, back pain, blurred vision, sexual dysfunction.

INTERACTIONS: May cause serotonin syndrome or NMS-like reactions with other serotogenic drugs (SSRIs, SNRIs and triptans), MAOIs, other antipsychotics, or dopamine antagonists. Not recommended with serotonin precursors (eg, tryptophan). May enhance response to alcohol, barbiturates and other CNS depressants. Increase risk of cardiac arrhythmia with drugs that prolong QT interval or CYP3A4 inhibitors. CYP3A4 inhibitors (eg, ritonavir, ketoconazole, indinavir, itraconazole, nefazodone) may increase levels; consider lower dose. Carbamazepine decreases levels; monitor to determine if a dose increase of trazodone is required. Increased serum digoxin or phenytoin levels; monitor serum levels and adjust dose as needed. May affect PT time in patients on warfarin. Concomitant use with an antihypertensive may require reduction in the dose of the antihypertensive drug. Not for use in combination or within 14 days of d/c treatment with an MAOI. Monitor and use caution with NSAIDs, ASA, and other drugs that affect coagulation or bleeding. Increased risk of hyponatremia with diuretics.

PREGNANCY: Category C, caution in nursing.

MECHANISM OF ACTION: Triazolopyridine derivative; mechanism not established. Suspected to potentiate serotonergic activity in the CNS. Preclinical trials shows selective inhibition of neuronal reuptake of serotonin and activity as an antagonist at 5-HT-2A/2C serotonin receptors.

PHARMACOKINETICS: Absorption: Well absorbed; (100mg tid dose) AUC=33058ng•h/mL, C_{max}=3118ng/mL; (300mg qd dose) AUC=29131ng•h/mL, C_{max}=1812ng/mL. **Distribution:** Plasma protein binding (89-95%). **Metabolism:** Liver (extensive); CYP3A4 via oxidative cleavage; m-chlorophenylpiperazine (active metabolite). **Elimination:** Urine (70-75%). $T_{1/2}$=10 hrs.

NURSING CONSIDERATIONS

Assessment: Assess for psychiatric history (eg, suicide, depression, bipolar disorder), family history, cardiac disease (eg, MI), serotonin syndrome, bleeding events, sickle cell anemia, multiple myeloma, leukemia, penile anatomical deformation in men, syndrome of inappropriate antidiuretic hormone secretion (SIADH), arrhythmias, hepatic/renal impairment, pregnancy/nursing status, and for possible drug interactions. Obtain baseline vital signs, serum electrolytes, ECG, hepatic/renal function.

Monitoring: Monitor for signs/symptoms of clinical worsening, suicidality, unusual behavior changes or mental status changes, neuromuscular aberrations, GI symptoms, priapism, arrhythmias, hyponatremia (eg, headache, confusion, weakness), bleeding events, hepatic/renal impairment, hypotension, and withdrawal symptoms when d/c treatment. Monitor vital signs, serum electrolytes, ECG, hepatic/renal function.

Patient Counseling: Inform about the benefits and risks of therapy. Advise patients, families and caregivers of need to observe for signs/symptoms of clinical worsening and suicidality (eg, agitation, anxiety, panic attacks, mania, changes in behavior) and sleep disturbances; instruct to contact physician if these and other symptoms occur. Counsel to avoid alcohol, sedatives and other CNS depressants. Instruct males to d/c use and contact physician if prolonged or inappropriate penile erection develops. Inform that mental and/or physical ability required for performing potentially hazardous tasks (eg, operating machinery, driving) may be impaired. Instruct to notify physician if pregnant or intend to become pregnant and if nursing.

Administration: Oral route. Take at the same time everyday, preferably at bedtime, on empty stomach. **Storage:** 15-30°C. Keep in tight, light-resistant containers.

OLUX   RX
clobetasol propionate (Stiefel)

THERAPEUTIC CLASS: Corticosteroid

INDICATIONS: Short-term treatment of inflammatory and pruritic manifestations of moderate to severe corticosteroid-responsive dermatoses of the scalp. Short-term treatment of mild to moderate plaque-type psoriasis of non-scalp regions excluding the face and intertriginous areas.

DOSAGE: *Adults:* Apply to affected area bid (am and pm). No more than 1.5 capfuls/application. Limit to 2 consecutive weeks. Avoid with occlusive dressings unless directed. Max 50g/week.
Pediatrics: ≥12 yrs: Apply to affected area bid (am and pm). No more than 1.5 capfuls/application. Limit to 2 consecutive weeks. Avoid with occlusive dressings unless directed. Max 50g/week.

HOW SUPPLIED: Foam: 0.05% [50g, 100g]

WARNINGS/PRECAUTIONS: May produce reversible hypothalamic-pituitary-adrenal (HPA) axis suppression, manifestations of Cushing's syndrome, hyperglycemia, and glucosuria. Caution when applied to large surface areas or under occlusive dressings. Withdraw, reduce frequency, or substitute a less potent steroid if adrenal suppression noted. Use appropriate antifungal or antibacterial agent with dermatological infections; d/c until infection controlled. Pediatric patients may be more susceptible to systemic toxicity.

Striae, adrenal suppression (low plasma cortisol, no response to ACTH stimulation), Cushing's syndrome, linear growth retardation, delayed weight gain, and intracranial HTN (bulging fontanelle, headache, bilateral papilledema) reported in pediatrics. Avoid contact with eyes. D/C if irritation occurs. Avoid extensive or prolonged use in pregnant patients. Not recommended in pediatrics <12 yrs. Caution in elderly. Flammable; avoid fire, flame, or smoking during and immediately following application.

ADVERSE REACTIONS: Burning/stinging, pruritus, irritation, erythema, folliculitis, cracking/fissuring of skin, numbness of fingers, telangiectasia, skin atrophy, hypertrichosis, acneiform eruptions, hypopigmentation, maceration of the skin.

PREGNANCY: Category C, caution in nursing.

MECHANISM OF ACTION: Corticosteroid; possesses anti-inflammatory, antipruritic and vasoconstrictive properties. Anti-inflammatory effects not established; suspected to act by induction of phospholipase A_2 inhibitory proteins, lipocortins. Lipocortins control biosynthesis of inflammation mediators (eg, prostaglandins and leukotrienes) by inhibiting release of their common precursor, arachidonic acid.

PHARMACOKINETICS: Absorption: Percutaneous; occlusion, inflammation, and other disease states may increase absorption. **Distribution:** Systemically administered corticosteroids are found in breast milk. **Metabolism:** Liver. **Elimination:** Kidney (major), bile.

NURSING CONSIDERATIONS

Assessment: Assess for severity of dermatoses, hypersensitivity reactions, pregnancy/nursing status, and use in pediatric patients.

Monitoring: Monitor for development of skin irritation, if present d/c medication. Monitor response to treatment, HPA axis suppression, Cushing's syndrome and other adverse effects if used for long term treatment.

Patient Counseling: Counsel patient on the signs/symptoms of adverse reactions and to contact physician if any occur. Counsel to use exactly as directed, externally, and not for >2 weeks. Propellant in this foam is flammable; avoid fire, flame, or smoking during and immediately following application. Advise not to bandage or wrap treated skin area, unless directed by physician. Advise to avoid contact with eyes or other mucous membranes and wash hands following application. Avoid extensive or prolonged use in pregnant patients.

Administration: Topical route. 1) Place small amount of medication into cap of medication container, onto a saucer, other cool surface or directly onto affected skin area. Do not use more than 1 1/2 capfuls. Do not squirt medication directly into the hands (unless hands are the treatment area); medication will melt in contact with warm skin. If fingers are warm, rinse in cold water and dry prior to application. If can is warm, run under cold water prior to administration. 2) Using fingertips, massage medication into treatment area. **Storage:** 20-25°C (68-77°F). Do not puncture or incinerate container. Do not expose to heat or store above 49°C (120°F).

Olux-E   RX
clobetasol propionate (Stiefel)

THERAPEUTIC CLASS: Corticosteroid

INDICATIONS: Treatment of inflammatory and pruritic manifestations of corticosteroid-responsive dermatoses in patients ≥12 yrs.

DOSAGE: *Adults:* Apply a thin layer to affected area bid (am and pm). Limit to 2 consecutive weeks; d/c when control achieved. Max: 50g/week or 21 capfuls/week.
Pediatrics: ≥12 yrs: Apply a thin layer to affected area bid (am and pm). Limit to 2 consecutive weeks; d/c when control achieved. Max: 50g/week or 21 capfuls/week.

HOW SUPPLIED: Foam: 0.05% [50g, 100g]

WARNINGS/PRECAUTIONS: May produce reversible hypothalamic-pituitary-adrenal (HPA) axis suppression, Cushing's syndrome, hyperglycemia, and unmasking of latent diabetes mellitus (DM). Identify predisposing factors (eg, use of more potent steroids, over large surface areas, over prolonged periods, under occlusion, on an altered skin barrier, with liver failure) and periodically evaluate for HPA axis suppression. Withdraw, reduce frequency, or substitute a less potent steroid. Pediatric patients may be more susceptible to systemic toxicity. Striae, HPA axis suppression (low plasma cortisol, no response to ACTH stimulation), Cushing's syndrome, linear growth retardation, delayed weight gain, and intracranial HTN (eg, bulging fontanelles, headache, bilateral papilledema) reported in pediatrics. Use appropriate antimicrobial agent with skin infections; d/c until infection is treated. D/C if irritation occurs. Avoid eyes, face, groin, axillae, and area of skin atrophy. Flammable; avoid fire, flame, or smoking during and immediately following application.

ADVERSE REACTIONS: Application site reaction, application site atrophy, folliculitis, acneiform eruptions, hypopigmentation, perioral dermatitis, allergic contact dermatitis, secondary infection, irritation, striae, miliaria.

PREGNANCY: Category C, caution in nursing.

MECHANISM OF ACTION: Corticosteroid; plays a role in cellular signaling, immune function, inflammation, and protein regulation.

PHARMACOKINETICS: Absorption: Percutaneous; occlusion, inflammation, and other disease states may increase absorption. C_{max}=59pg/mL, T_{max}=5 hrs (post-dose on day 8). **Distribution:** Systemically administered corticosteroids are found in breast milk. **Metabolism:** Liver. **Elimination:** Kidneys, bile.

NURSING CONSIDERATIONS

Assessment: Assess for presence of concomitant skin infections, severity of dermatoses, pregnancy/nursing status, and use in pediatric patients.

Monitoring: Monitor for signs/symptoms of reversible HPA axis suppression, Cushing's syndrome, hyperglycemia, treatment-site irritation, allergic contact dermatitis (eg, failure to heal) and skin infections. If applying to large surface area or to occluded areas, monitor for HPA axis suppression using cosyntropin (ACTH) stimulation test. Following d/c of therapy, monitor for glucocorticosteroid insufficiency. Monitor for systemic toxicity, HPA axis suppression, Cushing's syndrome, linear growth retardation, delayed weight gain, and intracranial HTN in pediatrics. Monitor response to therapy.

Patient Counseling: Counsel to use externally and exactly as directed; avoid use on face, skin folds (eg, underarms, groin), contact with eyes or other mucous membranes. Wash hands after use. Instruct not to use for any disorder other than for which it was prescribed. Advise not to bandage or wrap treatment area, unless directed by physician. Counsel to contact physician if any local or systemic adverse reactions occur, if no improvement is seen after 2 weeks, or if surgery is contemplated. Propellant in foam is flammable; avoid fire, flame, or smoking during and immediately following application.

Administration: Topical route. Shake can, hold upside down, and depress the actuator. Dispense small amount and gently massage into affected area. **Storage:** 20-25°C (68-77°F). Do not puncture or incinerate container. Do not expose to heat or store above 49°C (120°F).

OMNARIS NASAL SPRAY   RX
ciclesonide (Sunovion)

THERAPEUTIC CLASS: Non-halogenated glucocorticoid

INDICATIONS: Treatment of nasal symptoms associated with seasonal allergic rhinitis in adults/children ≥6 yrs and with perennial allergic rhinitis in adults/adolescents ≥12 yrs.

DOSAGE: *Adults:* Seasonal/Perennial Allergic Rhinitis: 2 sprays/nostril qd. Max: 2 sprays/nostril/day (200mcg/day). Elderly: Start at low end of dosing range.
Pediatrics: Perennial Allergic Rhinitis: ≥12 yrs: 2 sprays/nostril qd. Max: 2

sprays/nostril/day (200mcg/day). Seasonal Allergic Rhinitis: ≥6 yrs: 2 sprays/nostril qd. Max: 2 sprays/nostril/day (200mcg/day).

HOW SUPPLIED: Spray: 50mcg/spray [12.5g]

WARNINGS/PRECAUTIONS: Epistaxis reported. *Candida albicans* infections of nose or pharynx may occur; examine periodically and treat accordingly. Caution with active or quiescent tuberculosis (TB) infections, untreated local/systemic fungal/bacterial infections, systemic viral or parasitic infections, or ocular herpes simplex. Risk for more severe/fatal course of infections (eg, chickenpox, measles); avoid exposure in patients who have not had these diseases or have not been properly immunized. Nasal septal perforation may occur; avoid spraying directly onto nasal septum. Risk of acute adrenal insufficiency and withdrawal symptoms when replacing systemic corticosteroids with topical corticosteroids; monitor closely. D/C slowly if symptoms of hypercorticism and adrenal suppression occur. May exacerbate symptoms of asthma and other conditions requiring long-term systemic corticosteroid use with rapid dose decrease. May cause reduced growth velocity in pediatrics. May impair wound healing; avoid in recent nasal septal ulcers, nasal surgery, or nasal trauma until healed. Glaucoma and/or cataracts may develop; caution with vision changes, history of increased intraocular pressure (IOP), glaucoma and/or cataracts. Caution in elderly.

ADVERSE REACTIONS: Headache, epistaxis, nasopharyngitis, back pain, pharyngolaryngeal pain, sinusitis, influenza, nasal discomfort, bronchitis, urinary tract infection, cough.

INTERACTIONS: Ketoconazole may increase levels of the active metabolite des-ciclesonide.

PREGNANCY: Category C, caution in nursing.

MECHANISM OF ACTION: Non-halogenated glucocorticoid; mechanism not established. Shown to have a wide range of effects on multiple cell types (eg, mast cells, eosinophils, neutrophils, macrophages, and lymphocytes) and mediators (eg, histamine, eicosanoids, leukotrienes, and cytokines) involved in allergic inflammation.

PHARMACOKINETICS: Absorption: Des-ciclesonide: C_{max}=<30pg/mL. **Distribution:** (IV) V_d=2.9L/kg (Ciclesonide), 12.1L/kg (des-ciclesonide); plasma protein binding (≥99%). **Metabolism:** Hydrolyzed to des-ciclesonide (active metabolite); further metabolism in liver, via CYP3A4, CYP2D6. **Elimination:** (IV) Feces (66%), urine (≤20%).

NURSING CONSIDERATIONS

Assessment: Assess patients who have not been immunized or exposed to infections such as measles or chickenpox. Assess for drug hypersensitivity, TB, any infections, ocular herpes simplex, history of increased IOP, glaucoma, cataracts, recent nasal septal ulcers, nasal surgery/trauma, use of other inhaled or systemic corticosteroids, pregnancy/nursing status, and possible drug interactions.

Monitoring: Monitor for hypercorticism, adrenal suppression, TB, infections, ocular herpes simplex, chickenpox, and measles. Monitor for epistaxis, nasal septal perforation, growth velocity in children, wound healing, visual changes, hypoadrenalism in infants born to mothers receiving corticosteroids during pregnancy, and hypersensitivity reactions. Monitor for adrenal insufficiency and withdrawal symptoms in the event of replacing systemic with topical corticosteroids.

Patient Counseling: Counsel on appropriate priming and administration of spray. Avoid spraying in eyes or directly onto nasal septum. Take as directed at regular intervals; do not exceed prescribed dosage. Contact physician if symptoms do not improve by a reasonable time (over 1-2 weeks in seasonal allergic rhinitis and 5 weeks in perennial allergic rhinitis) or if condition worsens. Counsel about risks of epistaxis, nasal ulceration, *Candida* infections, and other adverse reactions. Instruct to avoid exposure to chickenpox or measles and to consult physician if exposed to chickenpox or measles. Inform that worsening of existing TB infections, fungal/bacterial/viral/parasitic infections, or ocular herpes simplex may occur. Glaucoma and cataracts may develop; inform physician if change in vision occurs.

Administration: Intranasal route. Shake bottle gently and prime pump by actuating 8 times before use. Reprime with 1 spray if not used for 4 consecutive days. **Storage:** 25°C (77°F); excursions permitted to 15-30°C (59-86°F). Do not freeze. Discard after 4 months after removal from pouch or after 120 actuations following initial priming, whichever comes first.

OMNITROPE RX
somatropin (Sandoz)

THERAPEUTIC CLASS: Human growth hormone

INDICATIONS: Treatment of pediatric patients with growth failure due to an inadequate secretion of endogenous growth hormone (GH), pediatric patients who have growth failure due to Prader-Willi syndrome (PWS) and children born small for gestational age (SGA) who fail to manifest catch-up growth by age 2. Replacement therapy of endogenous GH in adults of either childhood- or adult-onset etiology.

DOSAGE: *Adults:* Individualize dose. GHD: Initial: ≤0.04mg/kg/week. May increase at 4- to 8-week intervals. Max: 0.08mg/kg/week. GHD: Non-Weight Based: Initial: 0.2mg/day (0.15-0.30mg/day). May increase gradually every 1-2 months by increments of 0.1-0.2mg/day based on clinical response and serum IGF-I concentrations. Divide weekly dose into 6-7 daily SQ injections (give preferably in the evening). Elderly: Start at lower dose and consider smaller dose increments.
Pediatrics: Individualize dose. GHD: 0.16-0.24mg/kg/week. PWS: 0.24mg/kg/week. SGA: Up to 0.48mg/kg/week. Divide dose into 6-7 daily SQ injections (give preferably in the evening).

HOW SUPPLIED: Inj: 1.5mg, 5.8mg; Cartridge: 5mg/1.5mL (15 IU), 10mg/1.5mL (30 IU)

CONTRAINDICATIONS: Acute critical illness due to complications following open heart surgery, abdominal surgery, multiple accidental trauma, or with acute respiratory failure. Patients with PWS who are severely obese, have a history of upper airway obstruction or sleep apnea, or have severe respiratory impairment. Active malignancy. Active proliferative or severe non-proliferative diabetic retinopathy. Pediatric patients with closed epiphyses. (5mg/1.5mL cartridge, 5.8mg/vial) Contains benzyl alcohol; must not be given to premature babies or neonates.

WARNINGS/PRECAUTIONS: Increased mortality reported with acute critical illness; weigh against the potential risk for treatment continuation. Reports of fatalities in pediatrics after initiating therapy in PWS; evaluate PWS patients for signs of upper airway obstruction and sleep apnea before treatment and interrupt therapy if this occurs during treatment. In patients with pre-existing tumors or GHD secondary to an intracranial lesion, monitor for progression or recurrence of underlying disease. Increased risk of second neoplasm reported in childhood cancer survivors. Monitor closely for any malignant transformation of skin lesions. May decrease insulin sensitivity; monitor blood sugar. Intracranial HTN reported; d/c if papilledema occurs. Caution in patient with hypopituitarism. Undiagnosed/untreated hypothyroidism may prevent optimal response; perform periodic thyroid function tests. Slipped capital femoral epiphysis may occur; evaluate any pediatrics with onset of a limp or complaints of hip or knee pain during therapy. Progression of scoliosis may occur in pediatrics with rapid growth. Patients with epiphyseal closure who were treated in childhood should be reevaluated before continuation of therapy as adults. Tissue atrophy may occur when administered at the same site over a long period of time. Allergic reactions and fluid retention may occur.

ADVERSE REACTIONS: Hypothyroidism, elevated HbA1c, eosinophilia, hematoma, headache, hypertriglyceridemia, leg pain.

INTERACTIONS: Use with glucocorticoid therapy may attenuate growth promoting effects of somatropin in children; glucocorticoid replacement dosing should be carefully adjusted in children during concomitant use. May inhibit 11β-hydroxysteroid dehydrogenase type 1 (11βHSD-1), resulting in reduced serum cortisol concentrations; glucocorticoid replacement therapy may be required or adjustments in glucocorticoid therapy doses may be required. May alter clearance of compounds metabolized by CYP450 liver enzymes (eg, corticosteroids, sex steroids, anticonvulsants, antipyrine, cyclosporine). May require larger dose with oral estrogen replacement. Adjust dose of insulin and/or oral hypoglycemic agents in diabetic patients.

PREGNANCY: Category B, caution in nursing.

MECHANISM OF ACTION: Human growth hormone; binds to dimeric GH receptor in cell membrane of target cells resulting in intracellular signal transduction.

PHARMACOKINETICS: Absorption: C_{max}=72-74mcg/mL, T_{max}=4 hrs. **Metabolism:** Liver and kidneys (proteolytic degradation). **Elimination:** $T_{1/2}$=2.5-2.8 hrs.

NURSING CONSIDERATIONS

Assessment: Assess for pre-existing type 1, type 2 DM or impaired glucose tolerance, history of scoliosis, hypothyroidism, hypopituitarism, pregnancy/nursing status, possible drug interactions, or any conditions where treatment is contraindicated or cautioned. Assess for pre-existing papille-dema; perform funduscopic examination prior to treatment. In patients with PWS, assess for the presence of severe obesity, history of upper airway obstruction or sleep apnea, or for the presence of severe respiratory impairment.

Monitoring: Monitor for drug response, malignant transformation of skin lesions, fluid retention, and allergic reactions. Monitor for signs/symptoms of slipped capital femoral epiphysis and for the progression of pre-existing scoliosis in pediatric patients. Monitor for signs symptoms of hypothyroidism; perform periodic monitoring of thyroid function tests. Monitor for glucose levels periodically especially in patients with known risk factors. In patients with PWS, monitor weight of the patient and monitor for signs/symptoms of upper airway obstruction and for respiratory infections. Perform periodic fun-duscopic examination. In patients with pre-existing tumors or GH deficiency secondary to an intracranial lesion, monitor for progression or recurrence of underlying disease process. In patients with hypopituitarism, monitor other hormonal replacement therapy during treatment. Monitor for increases in serum levels of inorganic phosphorus, alkaline phosphatase, parathyroid hor-mone, and insulin-like growth factor-I (IGF-I).

Patient Counseling: Inform about potential benefits and risks of therapy. Instruct thoroughly as to proper usage, proper disposal, and caution against any reuse of needles and syringes.

Administration: SQ route. (Inj) Once diluent is added, swirl gently; do not shake. Use only if it is clear and colorless. **Storage:** 2-8°C (36-46°F). Protect from light. Do not freeze. (Cartridge) After 1st injection: Refrigerate, maybe be stored for a maximum of 28 days. (Inj 1.5mg/vial) After reconstitution, may refrigerate up to 24 hrs. Use once and discard any remaining solution. (Inj 5.8mg/vial) After reconstitution, must be used within 3 weeks.

ONCASPAR   RX
pegaspargase (Enzon)

THERAPEUTIC CLASS: Protein synthesis inhibitor

INDICATIONS: First line treatment of patients with acute lymphoblastic leu-kemia (ALL) or treatment of patients with ALL and hypersensitivity to native forms of L-asparaginase as a component of a multi-agent chemotherapeutic regimen.

DOSAGE: *Adults:* Usual: 2500 IU/m² IM or IV no more frequently than every 14 days.
Pediatrics: Usual: 2500 IU/m² IM or IV no more frequently than every 14 days.

HOW SUPPLIED: Inj: 750 IU/mL [5mL]

CONTRAINDICATIONS: History of pancreatitis, significant hemorrhagic events, or serious thrombosis with prior L-asparaginase therapy.

WARNINGS/PRECAUTIONS: May be a contact irritant. Avoid inhalation or contact with skin or mucous membranes. Serious allergic reaction, pancreatitis, or glucose intolerance can occur. Increased prothrombin time, partial thromboplastin time, and hypofibrinogenemia can occur; monitor coagulation parameters. May predispose to infections, bleeding, thrombosis. D/C in patients with serious thrombotic events including sagittal sinus thrombosis.

ADVERSE REACTIONS: Allergic reactions (including anaphylaxis), CNS thrombosis, coagulopathy, elevated transaminases, hyperbilirubinemia, hyperglycemia, pancreatitis.

PREGNANCY: Category C, not for use in nursing.

MECHANISM OF ACTION: Protein synthesis inhibitor; selectively kills leukemic cells due to depletion of plasma asparagine.

PHARMACOKINETICS: Elimination: $T_{1/2}$=5.8 days.

NURSING CONSIDERATIONS

Assessment: Assess for history of serious allergic reactions to L-asparaginase, thrombosis, pancreatitis, serious hemorrhagic events, and pregnancy/nursing status.

Monitoring: Monitor coagulation parameters at baseline and periodically during and after treatment. Monitor for occurrence of anaphylaxis, thrombosis, pancreatitis, glucose intolerance, and coagulopathy.

Patient Counseling: Immediately report swelling, SOB, severe headache, chest pain, severe abdominal pain, excessive thirst, or any increase in volume or frequency of urination.

Administration: IM or IV route. When administered IM, the volume at a single injection site should be limited to 2mL. If the volume to be administered is greater than 2mL, multiple inj sites should be used. When administered IV, should be given over 1-2 hrs in 100mL of NaCl or dextrose inj 5%, through an already running infusion. **Storage:** Refrigerate at 2-8°C (36-46°F).

ONGLYZA   RX

saxagliptin (Bristol-Myers Squibb/ AstraZeneca)

THERAPEUTIC CLASS: Dipeptidyl peptidase-4 inhibitor

INDICATIONS: Adjunct to diet and exercise to improve glycemic control in adults with type 2 diabetes mellitus (DM).

DOSAGE: *Adults:* 2.5mg or 5mg qd. Moderate or Severe Renal Impairment/ Hemodialysis with ESRD (CrCl ≤50mL/min): 2.5mg qd. Concomitant Strong CYP3A4/5 Inhibitors: 2.5mg qd.

HOW SUPPLIED: Tab: 2.5mg, 5mg

WARNINGS/PRECAUTIONS: May be administered following hemodialysis with end-stage renal disease (ESRD) requiring hemodialysis. Caution in elderly.

ADVERSE REACTIONS: Upper respiratory tract infection (URI), urinary tract infection (UTI), headache, peripheral edema, hypoglycemia.

INTERACTIONS: May alter pharmacokinetics with strong CYP3A4/5 inducers. Lower dose of insulin secretagogues (eg, sulfonylureas) may be required to reduce the risk of hypoglycemia. Increased plasma concentrations with ketoconazole and other strong CYP3A4/5 inhibitors (eg, atazanavir, clarithromycin, indinavir, itraconazole, nefazodone, nelfinavir, ritonavir, saquinavir, and telithromycin); limit dose to 2.5mg. Refer to PI for complete drug-drug interactions.

PREGNANCY: Category B, caution in nursing.

MECHANISM OF ACTION: Dipeptidyl peptidase-4 inhibitor; slows the inactivation of the incretin hormones and increases their bloodstream concentrations, resulting in reduction of fasting and postprandial glucose concentrations in a glucose-dependent manner in type 2 DM.

PHARMACOKINETICS: Absorption: C_{max} = 24ng/mL; AUC=78ng•hr/mL; T_{max} = 2 hrs. **Metabolism:** CYP3A4/5; 5-hydroxy saxagliptin (active metabolite). **Elimination:** Feces (22%), urine (24% unchanged); $T_{1/2}$ = 2.5 hrs.

NURSING CONSIDERATIONS

Assessment: Assess renal function, pregnancy/nursing status, and for possible drug interactions.

Monitoring: Monitor blood glucose, HbA1c levels, and renal function periodically.

Patient Counseling: Inform on potential risk/benefits. Advise on the importance of adherence to dietary instructions, regular physical activity, periodic blood glucose monitoring and HbA1c testing, recognition/management of hypoglycemia/hyperglycemia, and assessment of diabetic complications. Seek medical advice during periods of stress (eg, fever, trauma, infection, surgery) and if unusual/existing symptom persists or worsens. Inform that response to therapy should be monitored by measurements of blood glucose and HbA1c and on potential need to adjust dose based on changes in renal function. Instruct to read the Patient Package Insert before starting therapy and renewing prescription.

Administration: Oral route. **Storage:** 20-25°C (68-77°F); excursions permitted to 15-30°C (59-86°F).

ONSOLIS

`CII`

fentanyl (Meda)

> Contains fentanyl with abuse liability similar to other opioid analgesics. Must be used only in opioid-tolerant patients. Contraindicated for use in opioid non-tolerant patients and management of acute or postoperative pain, including headache/migraine, dental pain, or use in the emergency room. Do not convert on a mcg-per-mcg basis to Onsolis from other transmucosal fentanyl products. Life-threatening respiratory depression in opioid non-tolerant patients reported. Do not substitute for any other fentanyl product; may result in fatal overdose. If breakthrough pain is not relieved, patients should wait at least 2 hrs for the next dose. Keep out of reach of children and dispose of unneeded films properly. Concomitant use with CYP3A4 inhibitors may cause fatal respiratory depression. Use only by knowledgeable/skilled Schedule II opioid specialists. Available only through restricted distribution program (FOCUS).

THERAPEUTIC CLASS: Opioid analgesic

INDICATIONS: Management of breakthrough pain in patients with cancer (≥18 yrs) who are already receiving and who are tolerant to opioid therapy for their underlying persistent cancer pain.

DOSAGE: *Adults:* Initial: 200mcg. Titrate: May titrate by using multiples of 200mcg (for doses of 400mcg, 600mcg, or 800mcg) if adequate pain relief is not achieved after initiation. Do not use more than 4 of 200mcg films simultaneously. If adequate pain relief is not achieved after 800mcg, and patient has tolerated the 800mcg dose, may treat next episode by using one 1200mcg film. Max: 1200mcg. Single doses should only be used once per episode, and should be separated by at least 2 hrs. If adequate pain relief is not achieved within 30 min, use rescue medication ud. Limit to ≤4 doses/day. If >4 breakthrough pain episodes a day, may increase around-the-clock opioid medicine used for persistent cancer pain. Switching From Another Oral Transmucosal Fentanyl: Initial: ≤200mcg. Do not switch on a mcg-per-mcg basis.

HOW SUPPLIED: Film, Buccal: 200mcg, 400mcg, 600mcg, 800mcg, 1200mcg

CONTRAINDICATIONS: Opioid non-tolerant patients and management of acute or postoperative pain including headache/migraine, dental pain, or use in the emergency room.

WARNINGS/PRECAUTIONS: Caution with COPD (chronic obstructive pulmonary disease), pre-existing medical conditions predisposing to hypoventilation, severe renal or hepatic disease and bradyarrhythmias. Extreme caution with evidence of increased intracranial pressure or impaired consciousness;

may obscure the clinical course of a patient with head injury. May impair physical/mental abilities. Caution in elderly.

ADVERSE REACTIONS: Respiratory depression, circulatory depression, hypotension, shock, constipation, asthenia, fatigue, anorexia, N/V, constipation, dehydration, dizziness, dyspnea, headache.

INTERACTIONS: See Boxed Warning. Increased depressant effects with other CNS depressants (eg, other opioids, sedatives or hypnotics, general anesthetics, phenothiazines, tranquilizers, sedating antihistamines, skeletal muscle relaxants, alcoholic beverages). CYP3A4 inducers (eg, barbiturates, carbamazepine, efavirenz, glucocorticoids, modafinil, nevirapine, oxcarbazepine, phenobarbital, phenytoin, pioglitazone, rifabutin, rifampin, St. John's wort, or troglitazone) decrease plasma concentration and may reduce efficacy. Avoid use within 14 days of MAOIs. Respiratory depression reported with other drugs that depress respiration.

PREGNANCY: Category C, not for use in nursing.

MECHANISM OF ACTION: Pure opioid agonist; produces analgesia. Precise analgesic action not established; known to be μ-opioid receptor agonist. Specific CNS opioid receptors for endogenous compounds with opioid-like activity are found throughout the brain and spinal cord and are involved in producing analgesic effects.

PHARMACOKINETICS: Absorption: Rapid (buccal mucosa) and prolonged (GI tract). Absolute bioavailability (71%); various doses resulted in different parameters. **Distribution:** V_d=4L/kg; plasma protein binding (80-85%). Crosses the placenta; found in breast milk. **Metabolism:** Liver and intestinal mucosa via CYP3A4; norfentanyl (metabolite). **Elimination:** Urine (<7% unchanged), feces (1% unchanged); $T_{1/2}$=14 hrs.

NURSING CONSIDERATIONS

Assessment: Assess for degree of opioid tolerance, previous opioid dose, level of pain intensity, type of pain, patient's general condition, age and medical status, or any other conditions where treatment is contraindicated or cautioned. Assess for history of hypersensitivity, pregnancy/nursing status, renal/hepatic function, and possible drug interactions.

Monitoring: Monitor for signs/symptoms of respiratory depression, drug abuse, physical dependence, bradycardia, opioid toxicity, hypersensitivity, anaphylaxis, signs of increased drug activity.

Patient Counseling: Notify physician if signs/symptoms of respiratory depression develop. Inform that film contains medicine in an amount that can be fatal in children, in individuals for whom it is not prescribed, and in those who are not opioid tolerant. Safely dispose any unneeded films remaining from a prescription as soon as possible by removing from foil package, and flushing the film down the toilet; do not flush the foil packages or cartons. Notify physician if breakthrough pain is not alleviated or worsens. Avoid using concomitant therapy with other CNS depressants and alcohol. May cause mental/physical impairment and has potential for abuse. Encourage patients to read the Medication Guide. Patients must enroll in FOCUS program by calling 1-877-466-7654 (1-877-4Onsolis) or visit online.

Administration: Oral (buccal) route. May be placed on both sides of the mouth not on top of each other when multiple films are used. Do not cut or tear prior to use. Refer to PI for proper administration. **Storage:** 20-25°C (68-77°F); excursions permitted between 15-30°C (59-86°F) until ready to use. Protect from freezing and moisture. Do not use if the foil package has been opened.

OPANA ER `CII`
oxymorphone HCl (Endo)

(Tab, Extended-Release) Increased risk of misuse, abuse, or diversion. For continuous analgesia only; not intended for PRN use. To be swallowed whole; not to be broken, chewed, dissolved, or crushed. Avoid with alcohol or medications containing alcohol.

OTHER BRAND NAMES: Opana (Endo)

THERAPEUTIC CLASS: Opioid analgesic

INDICATIONS: (Tab) Relief of moderate to severe acute pain. (Tab, ER) Relief of moderate to severe pain in patients requiring continuous, around-the-clock opioid treatment for extended period of time.

DOSAGE: *Adults:* Individualize dose. (Tab) Initial: Opioid-Naive: 10-20mg q4-6h. May start with 5mg (eg, for renal/hepatic impairment, geriatrics) if necessary. Max: 20mg. Conversion from Parenteral Oxymorphone: Give 10x total daily parenteral oxymorphone dose in 4 or 6 equally divided doses (eg, [IV dose x 10] divided by 4 or 6). Conversion from Other Oral Opioids: Give 50% of calculated total daily dose in 4-6 equally divided doses, q4-6h. Maint: Identify source of increased pain and adjust dose. (Tab, ER) Swallow whole; do not break, chew, crush, or dissolve. Opioid-Naive: Initial: 5mg q12h. Titrate: Increase dose individually at increments of 5-10mg q12h every 3-7 days. Conversion from Opana: Give half of total daily Opana dose as ER, q12h. Conversion from Parenteral Oxymorphone: Give 10x total daily parenteral oxymorphone dose in 2 equally divided doses (eg, [IV dose x 10] divided by 2). Conversion from Other Oral Opioids: Give 50% of calculated total daily dose (refer to PI for conversion ratios) in 2 divided doses, q12h. Gradually adjust initial dose until adequate pain relief and acceptable side effects are achieved. Maint: Titrate if necessary; follow the same method as Initial Therapy. (Tab/Tab, ER) Mild Hepatic/Renal Impairment (CrCl <50mL/min): Start with lowest dose and titrate slowly while carefully monitoring side effects. With CNS Depressants: Start at 1/3 to 1/2 of usual dose. Elderly: Start at lower end of dosing range and slowly titrate to adequate analgesia. Cessation Therapy: Taper gradually. Take on an empty stomach ≥1 hr prior to or 2 hrs after eating.

HOW SUPPLIED: Tab: 5mg, 10mg; Tab, Extended-Release (ER): 5mg, 7.5mg, 10mg, 15mg, 20mg, 30mg, 40mg

CONTRAINDICATIONS: Respiratory depression (Tab: except in monitored settings with resuscitative equipment), acute/severe bronchial asthma or hypercarbia, paralytic ileus, moderate/severe hepatic impairment.

WARNINGS/PRECAUTIONS: Schedule II controlled substance with abuse liability. Respiratory depression may occur; extreme caution in elderly or debilitated patients, with hypoxia, hypercapnia, or decreased respiratory reserve such as asthma, chronic obstructive pulmonary disease (COPD) or cor pulmonale, severe obesity, sleep apnea syndrome, myxedema, kyphoscoliosis, CNS depression, or coma. With head injury, intracranial lesions or a pre-existing increase in intracranial pressure (ICP), possible respiratory depressant effects and potential to elevate CSF pressure may be markedly exaggerated; effects on papillary response and consciousness may obscure neurologic signs of further increases in ICP with head injuries. May cause severe hypotension. Caution with increased ICP, impaired consciousness, circulatory shock, adrenocortical insufficiency (eg, Addison's disease), prostatic hypertrophy or urethral stricture, severe pulmonary impairment, moderate/severe renal dysfunction, mild hepatic impairment and toxic psychosis. May aggravate convulsions with convulsive disorders and may induce/aggravate seizures. May obscure diagnosis or clinical course in patients with acute abdominal conditions. May cause spasm of the sphincter of Oddi; caution with biliary tract disease (including acute pancreatitis). May impair physical/mental abilities. May produce tolerance and dependence. Avoid abrupt d/c; may cause abstinence syndrome in physically dependent patients. (Tab, ER) Not indicated for pre-emptive analgesia (administration pre-operatively for the management of post-operative pain). Only indicated for post-operative use if already receiving drug prior to surgery or if post-operative pain is expected to be moderate or severe and persist for an extended period of time.

ADVERSE REACTIONS: Constipation, N/V, pyrexia, somnolence, headache, dizziness, pruritus, increased sweating, xerostomia, sedation, confusion, anxiety.

INTERACTIONS: See Boxed Warning. Additive CNS depression with other CNS depressants (eg, sedatives, hypnotics, tranquilizers, general anesthetics, phenothiazines, other opioids, alcohol). Caution with MAOIs; avoid within 14 days of MAOIs use. Anticholinergics may increase risk of urinary retention and/or severe constipation, which may lead to paralytic ileus. CNS side effects (eg, confusion, disorientation, respiratory depression, apnea, seizures) reported with cimetidine. Reduced effect and/or precipitate withdrawal symptoms with mixed agonist/antagonist analgesics (eg, pentazocine, nalbuphine, butorphanol, buprenorphine). Severe hypotension with phenothiazines or other agents that compromise vasomotor tone.

PREGNANCY: Category C, caution with nursing.

MECHANISM OF ACTION: Opioid analgesic; pure opioid agonist. Has not been established. Suspected that specific CNS opiate receptors and endogenous compounds with morphine-like activity have been identified throughout the brain and spinal cord and are likely to play a role in the expression and perception of analgesic effects.

PHARMACOKINETICS: Absorption: Absolute bioavailability (10%). Administration of variable doses resulted in different pharmacokinetic parameters. Refer to PI. **Distribution:** Plasma protein binding (10-12%); crosses placenta. **Metabolism:** Liver (reduction or conjugation); oxymorphone-3-glucuronide, 6-OH-oxymorphone (major metabolites). **Elimination:** Urine (<1% unchanged, 33-38% oxymorphone-3-glucuronide, 0.25-0.62% 6-OH-oxymorphone), feces.

NURSING CONSIDERATIONS

Assessment: Assess for patient's prior analgesic treatment experience, degree of opioid tolerance, previous opioid dose, type and severity of pain, age, patient's general condition and medical status, history or risk factors for abuse and addiction, respiratory depression, paralytic ileus, acute/severe bronchial asthma or hypercarbia, or any other conditions where treatment is cautioned. Assess for drug hypersensitivity or hypersensitivity to morphine analogs, pregnancy/nursing status, renal/hepatic function, and possible drug interactions.

Monitoring: Monitor for signs/symptoms of respiratory depression, presence of elevated CSF pressure, hypotension, convulsions, spasms of sphincter of Oddi, physical dependence and tolerance, and abuse or misuse of medication. Monitor patients closely to evaluate for adequate analgesia and side effects. Monitor all patients closely when converting to ER tab from methadone to other opioid agonists. Monitor for decreased bowel motility in post-operative patients. Periodically reassess continued need for around-the-clock opioid therapy.

Patient Counseling: Instruct to take as directed. ER tab should be swallowed whole; do not break, chew, dissolve, or crush. Inform that if broken or chewed, contents of tab may release all at once and cause fatal overdose. Instruct to take on empty stomach, ≥1 hr prior to or 2 hrs after eating. Caution in performing hazardous tasks (eg, operating machinery/driving). Avoid alcohol, medications containing alcohol or other CNS depressants. Report episodes of breakthrough pain or adverse events. Contact physician if inadequate pain control and avoid adjusting dose without consulting physician. Inform that drug has potential for abuse and should be protected from theft. Counsel on the importance of safely tapering dose and abrupt d/c if receiving treatment for more than a few days to weeks. Advise of the potential for severe constipation. Advise women regarding effects in pregnancy and nursing. Instruct to keep out of reach of children and dispose any unused tablet by flushing down in the toilet as soon as they are no longer needed.

Administration: Oral route. **Storage**: 25°C (77°F); excursions permitted to 15-30°C (59-86°F). Dispense in tight container with child-resistant closure.

OPTIVAR   RX
azelastine HCl (Meda)

THERAPEUTIC CLASS: H$_1$-antagonist

INDICATIONS: Treatment of itching of the eye associated with allergic conjunctivitis.

DOSAGE: *Adults:* 1 drop bid.
Pediatrics: ≥3 yrs: 1 drop bid.

HOW SUPPLIED: Sol: 0.05% [6mL]

WARNINGS/PRECAUTIONS: Not for injection or oral use. Do not wear contact lens if the eye is red. Not for treatment of contact lens irritation. Wait 10 min after instilling drops to insert contact lens.

ADVERSE REACTIONS: Transient eye burning/stinging, headaches, asthma, conjunctivitis, dyspnea, eye pain, fatigue, influenza-like symptoms, pharyngitis, pruritus, rhinitis, temporary blurring.

PREGNANCY: Category C, caution in nursing.

MECHANISM OF ACTION: Antihistaminic agent; relatively selective H₁-receptor antagonist; inhibits release of histamine and other mediators from cells (eg, mast cells) involved in the allergic response and decreases chemotaxis and activation of eosinophils.

PHARMACOKINETICS: Metabolism: N-desmethylazelastine (principle metabolite).

NURSING CONSIDERATIONS

Assessment: Assess for drug hypersensitivity.

Monitoring: Monitor for transient burning/stinging, headaches, and bitter taste.

Patient Counseling: Counsel not to wear contact lenses if the eye is red. Avoid touching tip of dropper to eye or any other surface to avoid contamination. Wait 10 min after instillation to wear soft-contact lenses.

Administration: Ocular route. **Storage:** Store upright at 2-25°C (36-77°F).

ORACEA   RX

doxycycline (Galderma)

THERAPEUTIC CLASS: Tetracycline derivative

INDICATIONS: Treatment of only inflammatory lesions (papules and pustules) of rosacea in adult patients.

DOSAGE: *Adults:* 40mg qd in am. Take on empty stomach, preferably at least 1 hr prior or 2 hrs after meals.

HOW SUPPLIED: Cap: 40mg

WARNINGS/PRECAUTIONS: May cause fetal harm during pregnancy. Use during tooth development (eg, last half of pregnancy, infancy, ≤8 yrs) may cause permanent tooth discoloration or enamel hypoplasia. Pseudomembranous colitis reported, diarrhea may occur; initiate appropriate treatment. Photosensitivity reported. Autoimmune syndrome reported; monitor LFTs, ANA, CBC. Tissue hyperpigmentation reported. Superinfection reported; caution in patients with history of or predisposition to candidiasis overgrowth. Bacterial resistance may develop; use only as indicated. May increase BUN; caution in patients with renal impairment. Bulging fontanels in infants and pseudotumor cerebri (benign intracranial HTN) in adults reported.

ADVERSE REACTIONS: Nasopharyngitis, sinusitis, diarrhea, HTN.

INTERACTIONS: May require downward adjustment of anticoagulant dosage. May interfere with bactericidal action of penicillin; avoid concurrent use when possible. Concomitant use with methoxyflurane may result in fatal renal toxicity. Bismuth subsalicylate, proton pump inhibitors, antacids containing aluminum, calcium or magnesium and iron-containing preparations may impair absorption. May interfere with the effectiveness of oral contraceptives. Avoid concurrent use with oral retinoids (eg, isotretinoin, acitretin). Barbiturates, carbamazepine, and phenytoin decrease the half-life of doxycycline.

PREGNANCY: Category D, not for use in nursing.

MECHANISM OF ACTION: Tetracycline-derivative antibacterial agent; has not been established.

PHARMACOKINETICS: Absorption: Single dose: C_{max}=510ng/mL; T_{max}=3 hrs; AUC=9227ng•hr/mL. Steady-state: C_{max}=600ng/mL; T_{max}=2 hrs; AUC=7543ng•hr/mL. **Distribution:** Plasma protein binding (>90%); crosses the placenta, found in breast milk. **Elimination:** Urine (unchanged), feces (unchanged); $T_{1/2}$=21.2 hrs (single dose), 23.2 hrs (steady-state).

NURSING CONSIDERATIONS

Assessment: Assess pregnancy/nursing status, for renal impairment, history of or predisposition to candidiasis overgrowth, and those with gastric insufficiencies (eg, patients with gastrectomy, gastric bypass surgery, or in patients who are achlorhydric), visual disturbances prior to therapy, and possible drug interactions.

Monitoring: Monitor for signs/symptoms of pseudomembranous colitis, infection, autoimmune syndrome, bulging fontanels in infants, and benign intracranial HTN in adults. Routinely monitor for papilledema during therapy. Monitor BUN level, LFTs, ANA, CBC. Monitor for signs/symptoms of azotemia, hyperphosphatemia, and acidosis in patients with renal insufficiencies. Perform periodic monitoring of drug serum levels in patients with renal impairment.

Patient Counseling: Take medication as directed (1 hr before or 2 hrs after meals with fluid); exceeding recommended dosage may increase incidence of side effects including the development of resistant microorganisms. Medication is not for treatment or prevention of infections. Minimize/avoid exposure to natural or artificial sunlight (eg, tanning beds). Wear loose-fitting clothing to protect skin from sun exposure; d/c at first evidence of sunburn. Medication may cause autoimmune disorders; contact physician if arthralgia, fever, rash, or malaise develop. Drug may cause discoloration of skin, scars, teeth, or gums. Inform females drug may render oral contraceptives less effective, and to avoid if pregnant or nursing. Counsel males and females who are attempting to conceive a child not to use. Inform that diarrhea, headache, blurred vision may occur; seek medical help if symptoms develop.

Administration: Oral route. **Storage:** 15-30°C (59-86°F). Dispense in tight, light-resistant containers.

ORAMORPH SR   CII

morphine sulfate (Xanodyne)

> This is a sustained-release tablet. Swallow tab whole; do not break in half, crush or chew.

THERAPEUTIC CLASS: Opioid analgesic

INDICATIONS: Relief of pain in patients who require opioid analgesics for more than a few days.

DOSAGE: *Adults:* Conversion from Parenteral or Immediate Release Oral Morphine: Daily dose determined by daily requirement of immediate-release formulation. Single dose is 1/2 of daily requirement given q12h. Initial: 30mg is recommended if daily morphine requirement is ≤120mg. Use 15mg for low daily morphine requirements. Titrate: Increase to 60mg or 100mg after stable dose reached.

HOW SUPPLIED: Tab, Extended-Release: 15mg, 30mg, 60mg, 100mg

CONTRAINDICATIONS: Respiratory depression in the absence of resuscitative equipment, acute or severe bronchial asthma, paralytic ileus.

WARNINGS/PRECAUTIONS: Not for initial treatment. Caution with hepatic and renal dysfunction, increased ICP or with head injury, decreased respiratory reserve (eg, emphysema, severe obesity, kyphoscoliosis, or paralysis of the phrenic nerve), chronic asthma, upper airway obstruction, or in other chronic pulmonary disorders. Tolerance, psychological and physical dependence may develop. Avoid abrupt discontinuation. Not for pediatrics or use in women during or immediately before labor.

ADVERSE REACTIONS: Constipation, N/V, dizziness, sedation, dysphoria, euphoria, sweating, respiratory depression.

INTERACTIONS: Potentiated depressant effects with CNS depressants, alcohol, sedatives, antihistaminics, or psychotropics. Increased risk of respiratory depression, hypotension, sedation and coma with neuroleptics. Mixed agonist/antagonist opioid analgesics (eg, pentazocine, nalbuphine, butorphanol, or buprenorphine) may alter effect or precipitate withdrawal symptoms.

PREGNANCY: Category C, not for use in nursing.

MECHANISM OF ACTION: Opioid analgesic; interacts predominantly with μ-receptor. μ binding sites are found distributed in the brain, spinal cord, and in trigeminal nerve. Primary actions are analgesia and sedation.

PHARMACOKINETICS: Absorption: Absolute bioavailability (40%), oral administration of variable doses resulted in different parameters. **Distribution:** V_d=4L/kg; crosses placental membrane; found in breast milk. **Metabolism:** Liver to glucuronide metabolites; morphine-3-glucuronide (major metabolite), morphine-6-glucuronide (active metabolite). **Elimination:** Kidneys (major), feces (10%), bile (small amount); $T_{1/2}$=2-4 hrs.

NURSING CONSIDERATIONS

Assessment: Assess for respiratory depression, acute or severe bronchial asthma, COPD, presence of debilitation (eg, elderly), paralytic ileus, ICP or head injury, hepatic/renal dysfunction, pregnancy/nursing status, and possible drug interactions.

Monitoring: Monitor for signs/symptoms of respiratory depression, elevations in CSF pressure, medication dependence and abuse.

Patient Counseling: Swallow medication whole; do not break, chew, or crush. May cause psychological and/or physical dependence. Do not adjust dose without consulting physician. Avoid abrupt withdrawal of medication. Advise to avoid alcohol or other CNS depressants. May impair mental/physical abilities; use caution if performing hazardous tasks (eg, operating machinery/driving).

Administration: Oral route. **Storage:** 25°C (77°F); excursions permitted to 15-30°C (59-86°F).

ORAPRED   RX
prednisolone sodium phosphate (Sciele)

OTHER BRAND NAMES: Orapred ODT (Shionogi)

THERAPEUTIC CLASS: Glucocorticoid

INDICATIONS: Steroid-responsive disorders.

DOSAGE: *Adults:* Individualize dose. (Sol) Initial: 5-60mg/day depending on disease and response. (Tab) Initial: 10-60mg/day depending on disease and response. Maint: Decrease dose by small amounts to lowest effective dose at appropriate time intervals. (Sol/Tab) Multiple Sclerosis Exacerbations: 200mg qd for 1 week, then 80mg qod for 1 month. Elderly: Start at lower end of dosing range.
Pediatrics: Individualize dose. (Sol/Tab) Initial: 0.14-2mg/kg/day, depending on disease and response, given in 3 or 4 divided doses (4-60mg/m²/day). Nephrotic Syndrome >2 yrs: 60mg/m²/day in 3 divided doses for 4 weeks followed by 40mg/m²/day qod for 4 weeks. Uncontrolled Asthma: 1-2mg/kg/day in single or divided doses until peak expiratory flow rate of 80% is achieved (usually 3-10 days).

HOW SUPPLIED: Sol: 15mg/5mL [237mL]; Tab, Orally Disintegrating: 10mg, 15mg, 30mg

CONTRAINDICATIONS: (Sol) Systemic fungal infections

WARNINGS/PRECAUTIONS: May produce reversible hypothalamic-pituitary-adrenal (HPA) axis suppression with potential for glucocorticosteroid insufficiency following withdrawal. May impair mineralocorticoid secretion; administer salt and/or mineralocorticoid concurrently. Changes in thyroid status may necessitate dose adjustment. May mask signs of or increase risk of infections. Caution with latent tuberculosis (TB); give chemoprophylaxis. May activate latent amebiasis; rule out latent or active amebiasis before starting. Chickenpox/measles may be more severe. May exacerbate systemic fungal infections; avoid use unless needed to control drug reactions. Not for use in cerebral malaria, optic neuritis or active ocular herpes simplex. Increases BP, salt/water retention, K^+ and Ca^{2+} excretion may occur. Caution with recent myocardial infarction (MI); left ventricular free wall rupture associated with corticosteroid therapy. Caution with active or latent peptic ulcers, diverticulitis, fresh intestinal anastomoses and abscess or other pyogenic infections; may increase risk of perforation. CNS effects may appear and existing emotional instability or psychotic tendencies may be aggravated. May decrease bone formation and increase bone resorption. May produce posterior subcapsular cataracts, glaucoma with possible damage to the optic nerves, and enhance the establishment of secondary ocular infections due to fungi or viruses. May elevate intraocular pressure (IOP); monitor IOP if steroid therapy >6 weeks. Acute myopathy observed with high doses. May elevate creatinine kinase may occur. Kaposi's sarcoma reported. May cause negative effects on pediatric growth/development and fetal harm. Caution with Strongyloides infestation, congestive heart failure (CHF), HTN, renal insufficiency, and increased risk of osteoporosis. Avoid abrupt withdrawal. Caution in elderly.

ADVERSE REACTIONS: Fluid retention, increased BP, behavioral/mood changes, increased appetite, weight gain.

INTERACTIONS: Enhanced metabolism with inducers of hepatic microsomal enzyme (eg, barbiturates, phenytoin, ephedrine, rifampin). Use with cyclosporine may increase activity of both drugs; convulsions reported. Decreased metabolism with estrogens or ketoconazole. (Tab) Decreased metabolism with macrolide antibiotics. May inhibit response to warfarin. Increased risk of GI side effects with aspirin (ASA) or other NSAIDs. May increase clearance of salicylates. High doses or concurrent neuromuscular blocking drugs may cause acute myopathy. Enhanced risk of hypokalemia when given with K^+-depleting agents (ie, diuretics, amphotericin B). May produce severe weakness in myasthenia gravis patients on anticholinesterase agents. Avoid live vaccines with immunosuppressive doses. Possible diminished response with toxoids, killed or inactivated vaccines. (Tab) May increase blood glucose; adjust antidiabetic agents. May lead to loss of corticosteroid-induced adrenal suppression with aminoglutethimide. Increased risk of arrhythmias due to hypokalemia with digitalis glycosides. (Tab) Increased clearance with cholestyramine.

PREGNANCY: Category C (Sol), D (Tab), caution in nursing.

MECHANISM OF ACTION: Synthetic adrenocortical steroid; promotes gluconeogenesis, increases deposition of glycogen in the liver, inhibits glucose utilization, possesses anti-insulin activity, increases catabolism of protein and lipolysis, stimulates fat synthesis and storage, increases glomerular filtration that leads to increased urinary excretion of urate and calcium.

PHARMACOKINETICS: Absorption: (Sol) Rapid and well-absorbed. (30mg) AUC=2408.1ng•hr/mL, C_{max}=420.91ng•hr/mL. **Distribution:** V_d=0.22-0.7L/kg; plasma protein binding (70-90%), found in breast milk (5-25%). **Metabolism:** Liver. **Elimination:** Urine (as sulfate and glucuronide conjugates); (Sol) $T_{1/2}$=2-4 hrs, (Tab) $T_{1/2}$=2.6 hrs.

NURSING CONSIDERATIONS

Assessment: Assess for hypersensitivity to drug, active or latent peptic ulcer disease, active or latent TB, systemic fungal infection, cerebral malaria, Strongyloides infestation, other current infections, HTN, CHF, MI, GI disorders, renal insufficiency, active or latent amebiasis, ophthalmic diseases, risk of osteoporosis, neuromuscular transmission disorders (eg, myasthenia gravis), emotional instability, psychotic tendencies. Assess vaccination status, thyroid status, pregnancy/nursing status, and for possible drug interactions. Obtain baseline bone density, TSH, LFTs, glucose, BP, weight, height.

Monitoring: Monitor for anaphylactic reactions, HPA axis suppression, Cushing's syndrome, hyperglycemia, occurrence of infections, CNS effects, psychotic manifestations, GI perforation, cataracts, glaucoma, acute myopathy, Kaposi's sarcoma, fluid retention, pediatric growth and development. Periodically monitor bone density, serum electrolytes, TSH, LFTs, renal function, glucose, IOP, BP, weight, height.

Patient Counseling: Do not d/c abruptly or without medical supervision. Seek medical advice if fever or other signs of infection develop. Take exactly as prescribed and with food to avoid GI irritation. Advise to report recent or ongoing infections, vaccination, and concurrent medicines. Advise to avoid exposure to chickenpox or measles; report immediately if exposed. Inform that may cause fetal harm; instruct to notify physician if pregnant. Counsel about common adverse reactions (eg, fluid retention, altered glucose tolerance, elevated BP, behavioral and mood changes, increased appetite and weight gain). May swallow tab whole or place on tongue and allow to dissolve in mouth, with/without water. Inform to take missed dose as soon as remembered, except if it is almost time for next dose; never take an extra dose to make up for missed dose. Instruct not to remove the tab from the blister until just prior to dosing. Do not cut, split, or break tab. Do not use partial tab.

Administration: Oral route. **Storage:** (Sol) 2-8°C (36-46°F). Keep tightly closed; (Tab) 20-25°C (68-77°F); excursions permitted to 15-30°C (59-86°F). Protect from moisture.

ORAVIG   RX
miconazole (Strativa)

THERAPEUTIC CLASS: Azole antifungal

INDICATIONS: Local treatment of oropharyngeal candidiasis.

DOSAGE: *Adults:* ≥16 yrs: Apply 1 buccal tab to the upper gum region (canine fossa) qd for 14 consecutive days.

HOW SUPPLIED: Tab, Buccal: 50mg

CONTRAINDICATIONS: Hypersensitivity to milk protein concentrate.

WARNINGS/PRECAUTIONS: Allergic reactions, including anaphylactic reactions reported; d/c at 1st sign of hypersensitivity. Caution in patients with hepatic impairment.

ADVERSE REACTIONS: Oral pain/discomfort, tongue/mouth ulceration, loss of/altered taste, N/V, diarrhea, headache, gingival pruritus/swelling.

INTERACTIONS: Caution with warfarin; may enhance anticoagulant effects. Closely monitor PT/INR and for evidence of bleeding. May interact with drugs metabolized through CYP2C9 and CYP3A4 (eg, oral hypoglycemics, phenytoin, ergot alkaloids).

PREGNANCY: Category C, caution in nursing.

MECHANISM OF ACTION: Azole antifungal; inhibits 14α-demethylase, inhibiting ergosterol synthesis (an essential part of the fungal cell membrane) and affects the synthesis of triglycerides and fatty acids and inhibits oxidative/peroxidative enzymes.

PHARMACOKINETICS: Absorption: C_{max}=15.1mcg/mL; T_{max}=7 hrs; AUC=55.23mcg•hr/mL. **Metabolism:** Hepatic (major), no active metabolites. **Elimination:** $T_{1/2}$=24 hrs, urine (<1%, unchanged).

NURSING CONSIDERATIONS

Assessment: Assess for possible drug interactions, pregnancy/nursing status, hypersensitivity to milk protein concentrate, hepatic impairment.

Monitoring: Closely monitor PT/INR and evidence of bleeding with concomitant anticoagulants. Monitor for hypersensitivity reactions, signs and symptoms of hepatic impairment, and other adverse events.

Patient Counseling: Apply buccal tab in the morning, after brushing teeth and with dry hands. Place rounded side of tab against the upper gum just above the incisor tooth and hold in place for 30 sec to ensure adhesion. Subsequent applications should be made to alternate sides of mouth. Allow tab to dissolve slowly; food/drink can be taken; avoid chewing gum and situations that could interfere with the sticking of the tab (eg, touching tab, hitting tab when brushing teeth, rinsing mouth too vigorously, wearing upper denture). If tab does not adhere or falls off within 1st 6 hrs, inform that the same tab should be repositioned immediately. If tab still does not adhere, apply a new tab. If swallowed within 1st 6 hrs, drink a glass of water and apply a new tab only once. If tab falls off or is swallowed after in place for 6 hrs or more, do not apply a new tab until the next scheduled dose. Do not to crush, chew, or swallow. Report adverse events to physician.

Administration: Buccal route. **Storage:** 20-25°C (68-77°F); excursions between 15-30°C permitted at room temperature. Protect from moisture.

ORENCIA   RX
abatacept (Bristol-Myers Squibb)

THERAPEUTIC CLASS: Selective costimulation modulator

INDICATIONS: To reduce signs and symptoms, induce major clinical response, inhibit progression of structural damage, and improve physical function in adult patients with moderately to severely active rheumatoid arthritis (RA). May be used as monotherapy or concomitantly with disease-modifying antirheumatic drugs (DMARDs) other than TNF-antagonists. To reduce signs and symptoms in pediatric patients ≥6 yrs with moderately to severely active polyarticular juvenile idiopathic arthritis. May be used alone or in combination with methotrexate (MTX).

DOSAGE: *Adults:* Rheumatoid Arthritis: Initial: <60kg: 500mg; 60-100kg: 750mg; >100kg: 1g; infuse over 30 min. Maint: Give at 2 and 4 weeks after initial infusion, then every 4 weeks thereafter.
Pediatrics: 6-17 yrs: Juvenile Idiopathic Arthritis: ≥75 kg: Follow adult dosing regimen. Max: 1000mg. <75kg: Initial: 10mg/kg; infuse over 30 min. Maint: Give at 2 and 4 weeks after initial infusion, then every 4 weeks thereafter.

HOW SUPPLIED: Inj: 250mg/15mL

WARNINGS/PRECAUTIONS: Anaphylaxis or anaphylactoid reactions reported. Caution with history of recurrent infections, underlying conditions that may predispose to infections, and chronic, latent, localized infections; d/c if serious infections develop. Screen for latent tuberculosis (TB) and viral hepatitis prior to initiation of therapy. Caution with COPD; monitor for worsening of respiratory status. May affect host defenses against infections and malignancies. Juvenile idiopathic arthritis patients should be up to date with all immunizations prior to therapy. Caution in elderly.

ADVERSE REACTIONS: Headache, nasopharyngitis, dizziness, cough, back pain, HTN, dyspepsia, urinary tract infection, rash, pain in extremities, upper respiratory tract infection, nausea, sinusitis, influenza, bronchitis.

INTERACTIONS: Concomitant use with TNF-antagonist may increase risk of serious infections, and is not recommended. Concomitant use with other biologic RA therapy, such as anakinra, is not recommended. Do not use live vaccines concurrently or within 3 months of d/c.

PREGNANCY: Category C, not for use in nursing.

MECHANISM OF ACTION: Selective costimulation modulator; inhibits T cell activation by binding to CD80 and CD86, thereby blocking interaction with CD28.

PHARMACOKINETICS: Absorption: C_{max}=292mcg/mL (Healthy subjects); C_{max}=295mcg/mL (RA patients); C_{max}=217 mcg/mL (Juvenile Idiopathic Arthritis patients). **Distribution:** V_d=0.09L/kg (Healthy subjects); V_d=0.07L/kg (RA patients). **Elimination:** $T_{1/2}$=16.7 days (Healthy subjects); $T_{1/2}$=13.1 days (RA patients)

NURSING CONSIDERATIONS

Assessment: Assess for immunization history in pediatrics, history of recurrent infections, chronic/latent/localized infections, underlying conditions that may predispose to infection, and COPD. Screen for latent TB infection and viral hepatitis. Assess pregnancy/nursing status and for possible drug interactions.

Monitoring: Monitor for signs/symptoms of hypersensitivity, infection, immunosuppression, malignancies, and hepatitis B reactivation. If COPD present, monitor for exacerbation, cough, rhonchi, dyspnea and worsening of respiratory status. When monitoring blood glucose in diabetic patients, use methods not based on GDH-PQQ.

Patient Counseling: Inform not to use concomitantly with TNF-antagonist (eg, adalimumab, etanercept, and infliximab) and other biologic RA therapy (eg, anakinra). Ask about history of recurrent infection, chronic/latent/localized infections, conditions which may predispose to infection, active/positive skin test/exposure to TB infection. Instruct that patient may be tested for TB prior to therapy. Instruct to immediately contact physician if allergic reaction or infection occur. Instruct not to receive live vaccines during therapy or within 3 months following d/c. Instruct to inform doctor if pregnant/nursing or planning to become pregnant. Inform diabetic patients that the infusion contains maltose, which can give falsely elevated blood glucose readings on the day of administration; may need alternate monitoring method.

Administration: IV. Refer to PI for complete preparation instructions. Administer diluted solution over 30 min. **Storage:** 2-8°C (36-46°F). Protect from light; store in original package until time of use.

ORTHO EVRA RX
ethinyl estradiol - norelgestromin (Ortho-McNeil)

> Cigarette smoking increases risk of serious cardiovascular (CV) events. Risk increases with age (>35 yrs) and with the number of cigarettes smoked. Hormonal contraceptives should not be used by women who are >35 yrs of age and smoke. Has higher steady state concentrations and lower peak concentrations than oral contraceptives. May increase risk of venous thromboembolism for current users of Ortho Evra.

THERAPEUTIC CLASS: Estrogen/progestogen combination

INDICATIONS: Prevention of pregnancy.

DOSAGE: *Adults:* Start on either the 1st Sunday after menses begins or on the 1st day of menses. Apply patch every week on same day for 3 weeks. Week 4 is patch-free. There should not be more than a 7-day patch-free interval between cycles. Apply to clean, dry, intact skin on buttock, abdomen, upper outer arm, or upper torso. Only 1 patch should be worn at a time. Refer to PI for further dosing guidelines.
Pediatrics: Postpubertal Adolescents: Start on either the 1st Sunday after menses begins or on the 1st day of menses. Apply patch every week on same day for 3 weeks. Week 4 is patch-free. There should not be more than a 7-day patch-free interval between cycles. Apply to clean, dry, intact skin on buttock, abdomen, upper outer arm, or upper torso. Only 1 patch should be worn at a time. Refer to PI for further dosing guidelines.

HOW SUPPLIED: Patch: (Ethinyl Estradiol-Norelgestromin): 0.75mg-6mg [1^s, 3^s]

CONTRAINDICATIONS: Thrombophlebitis or history of deep vein thrombophlebitis, current or history of thromboembolic disorders, current or history of cerebrovascular or coronary artery disease (CAD), known or suspected carcinoma of the breast or personal history of breast cancer, known thrombophilic conditions, valvular heart disease with complications, persistent BP ≥160mmHg systolic or ≥100mmHg diastolic, diabetes with vascular involvement, headaches with focal neurological symptoms, major surgery with prolonged immobilization, carcinoma of the endometrium or other known or suspected estrogen-dependent neoplasia, undiagnosed abnormal genital bleeding, cholestatic jaundice of pregnancy or jaundice with prior hormonal contraceptive use, acute/chronic hepatocellular disease with abnormal liver function, hepatic adenomas or carcinomas, pregnancy.

WARNINGS/PRECAUTIONS: Increased risk of myocardial infarction (MI), vascular disease, thromboembolism, thrombotic disease, and stroke. May increase risk of benign hepatic adenomas and hepatocellular carcinoma. D/C if jaundice develops. May increase risk of breast cancer and cancer of the reproductive organs. Retinal thrombosis reported; d/c if unexplained partial or complete loss of vision, onset of proptosis or diplopia, papilledema, or retinal vascular lesions develops. Should not be used to induce withdrawal bleeding as a test for pregnancy, or to treat threatened or habitual abortion during pregnancy. May increase the risk of or worsen existing gallbladder disease. May cause glucose intolerance and elevations in LDL levels or other lipid level changes. May cause fluid retention and increase BP; d/c if persistent elevation of BP occurs (≥160mmHg systolic or ≥100mmHg diastolic). D/C with onset or exacerbation of migraine headache or development of a headache with a new pattern. May cause breakthrough bleeding and spotting. Ectopic and intrauterine pregnancies may occur with contraceptive failures. May be less effective in women ≥198 lbs. Caution in patients with history of depression; d/c if significant depression develops. Visual changes or changes in lens tolerance may develop with contact lens use. Not indicated for use before menarche. May affect certain endocrine and LFTs and blood components. Does not protect against HIV and other sexually transmitted diseases (STDs).

ADVERSE REACTIONS: Breast symptoms (eg, breast discomfort, engorgement, pain), irregular uterine bleeding, dysmenorrhea, emotional lability, diarrhea, headache, application-site disorder, N/V, abdominal pain.

INTERACTIONS: May reduce effectiveness or increase incidence of breakthrough bleeding with drugs that induce enzymes (eg, CYP3A4) that metabolize contraceptive hormones (eg, barbiturates, bosentan, carbamazepine, felbamate, griseofulvin, oxcarbazepine, phenytoin, rifampin, St. John's wort, topiramate); additional or a different method of contraception is needed. May increase or decrease levels with protease inhibitors and non-nucleoside reverse transcriptase inhibitors. Pregnancy reported with antibiotics. HMG-CoA reductase inhibitors (eg, atorvastatin, rosuvastatin), ascorbic acid, APAP, and CYP3A4 inhibitors (eg, itraconazole, ketoconazole, voriconazole, fluconazole, grapefruit juice) may increase ethinyl estradiol levels. May increase levels of cyclosporine, prednisolone, and theophylline. May decrease levels of APAP, clofibric acid, morphine, salicylic acid, and temazepam. May decrease lamotrigine levels; dosage adjustment of lamotrigine may be necessary.

PREGNANCY: Category X, not for use in nursing.

MECHANISM OF ACTION: Estrogen/progestin combination contraceptive; suppresses gonadotropins. Inhibits ovulation, promotes changes in cervical mucus (which increases difficulty of sperm entry into uterus) and in the endometrium (which reduces likelihood of implantation).

PHARMACOKINETICS: Absorption: Administration of doses during different dosing cycles led to altered parameters. **Distribution:** Found in breast milk. Ethinyl estradiol: Serum albumin binding (extensive). Norelgestromin: Serum protein binding (>97%). **Metabolism:** Ethinyl estradiol: Hydroxylated, glucuronide and sulfate conjugates (metabolites). Norelgestromin: Hepatic; hydroxylated and conjugated metabolites, norgestrel (metabolites). **Elimination:** Urine, feces; $T_{1/2}$=17 hrs (ethinyl estradiol), 28 hrs (norelgestromin).

NURSING CONSIDERATIONS

Assessment: Assess for current or history of thrombophlebitis or thromboembolic disorders, thrombophilic conditions, or any other conditions where treatment is contraindicated or cautioned. Assess for pregnancy/nursing status and possible drug interactions. Assess use in patients with HTN, hyperlipidemias, obesity, diabetes, and in patients >35 yrs who smoke.

Monitoring: Monitor for signs/symptoms of thromboembolism, MI, stroke, and other adverse effects. Monitor for signs of HTN; perform regular monitoring of BP throughout duration of therapy. Monitor for changes in lipid levels; measure lipid levels periodically. Monitor serum glucose levels in prediabetic and diabetic patients. Refer patients with contact lenses to an ophthalmologist if visual changes or changes in lens tolerance develop. Perform annual physical exam.

Patient Counseling: Inform that drug does not protect against HIV and other STDs. Advise to avoid smoking and inform about possible adverse effects. Instruct to have annual physical exam and medical evaluation while on therapy. Instruct to apply patch to clean, dry, intact healthy skin (on buttock, abdomen, upper outer arm, or upper torso) where it will not be rubbed by tight clothing. Inform not to place patch on red, irritated, or cut skin, or on the breasts. Advise that there may be spotting, light bleeding, breast tenderness, or nausea during use; instruct that if symptoms persist, notify physician. Counsel to apply only one patch at a time. Advise not to skip patches and to never have the patch off for >7 days in a row.

Administration: Transdermal route. Apply immediately upon removal from protective pouch. Apply each new patch to a new spot. **Storage:** 25°C (77°F); excursions permitted to 15-30°C (59-86°F). Store patches in their protective pouches. Do not store in refrigerator or freezer.

ORTHO TRI-CYCLEN   RX
ethinyl estradiol - norgestimate (Ortho-McNeil)

> Cigarette smoking increases risk of serious cardiovascular (CV) side effects. Risk increases with age (>35 yrs) and heavy smoking (≥15 cigarettes/day). Women who use oral contraceptives should be strongly advised not to smoke.

OTHER BRAND NAMES: Tri-Previfem (Teva) - Trinessa (Watson)

THERAPEUTIC CLASS: Estrogen/progestogen combination

INDICATIONS: Prevention of pregnancy. Treatment of moderate acne vulgaris in females ≥15 yrs who want contraception and have achieved menarche.

DOSAGE: *Adults:* Contraception/Acne: 1 tab qd for 28 days, then repeat. Start 1st Sunday after menses begin or 1st day of menses.
Pediatrics: ≥15 yrs: Contraception (postpubertal adolescents)/Acne: 1 tab qd for 28 days, then repeat. Start 1st Sunday after menses begin or 1st day of menses.

HOW SUPPLIED: Tab: (Ethinyl Estradiol-Norgestimate) 0.035mg-0.18mg, 0.035mg-0.215mg, 0.035mg-0.25mg

CONTRAINDICATIONS: Thrombophlebitis or thromboembolic disorders, past history of deep vein thrombophlebitis or thromboembolic disorders, cerebral vascular or coronary artery disease (CAD) (current or past history), valvular heart disease with complications, severe HTN, diabetes with vascular involvement, headaches with focal neurological symptoms, major surgery with prolonged immobilization, known or suspected carcinoma of the breast or personal history of, carcinoma of the endometrium or other known or suspected estrogen-dependent neoplasia, undiagnosed abnormal genital bleeding, cholestatic jaundice of pregnancy or jaundice with prior pill use, acute or chronic hepatocellular disease with abnormal liver function, hepatic adenomas or carcinomas, known or suspected pregnancy.

WARNINGS/PRECAUTIONS: Increased risk of myocardial infarction (MI), thromboembolism, cerebrovascular events, gallbladder disease, and hepatic neoplasia. May increase risk of breast cancer and cervical intraepithelial dysplasia. Retinal thrombosis reported; d/c if unexplained partial or complete loss of vision, onset of proptosis or diplopia, papilledema, or retinal vascular lesions develop. May cause glucose intolerance, hypertriglyceridemia, and changes in lipoprotein levels. May cause fluid retention and increase BP; d/c if significant elevations in BP occur. May cause or exacerbate migraine headaches. Breakthrough bleeding and spotting reported; rule out malignancy or pregnancy. Ectopic as well as intrauterine pregnancy may occur in contraceptive failures. Does not protect against HIV infection (AIDS) or other sexually transmitted diseases. D/C if jaundice or if significant depression develops. Contact lens wearers may develop visual changes or changes in lens tolerance. Not indicated for use before menarche. May affect certain endocrine, LFTs, and blood components in laboratory tests. Do not use to treat threatened or habitual abortion.

ADVERSE REACTIONS: N/V, breakthrough bleeding, GI symptoms (eg, abdominal cramps, bloating), spotting, menstrual flow changes, amenorrhea, migraine, depression, vaginal candidiasis, edema, weight changes, cervical erosion and secretion.

INTERACTIONS: Reduced effects resulting in breakthrough bleeding or unintended pregnancy may occur when coadministered with antibiotics, anticonvulsants and other drugs that increase the metabolism of contraceptive steroids (eg, rifampin, barbiturates, phenylbutazone, phenytoin, carbamazepine, felbamate, oxcarbazepine, griseofulvin, topiramate, bosentan, St. John's wort). HIV protease inhibitors may increase or decrease levels. Atorvastatin, ascorbic acid, acetaminophen (APAP), CYP3A4 inhibitors (eg, itraconazole, ketoconazole) may increase hormone levels. May increase levels of cyclosporine, prednisolone, and theophylline. May decrease levels of APAP. May increase the clearance of temazepam, salicylic acid, morphine, and clofibric acid. (Ortho Tri-Cyclen) May decrease plasma levels of lamotrigine which may reduce seizure control; dosage adjustment of lamotrigine may be necessary.

PREGNANCY: Category X, not for use in nursing.

MECHANISM OF ACTION: Estrogen/progestogen combination oral contraceptive; acts by suppressing gonadotropins. Primarily inhibits ovulation. Also produces other alterations including changes in the cervical mucus (increases difficulty of sperm entry into uterus) and endometrium (reduces likelihood of implantation).

PHARMACOKINETICS: Absorption: Rapidly absorbed. Oral administration on various days during dosing led to altered parameters. **Distribution:** Found in breast milk. Norgestimate: Serum protein binding (>97%). Ethinyl estradiol: Serum albumin binding (>97%). **Metabolism:** Norgestimate: GI tract and/or liver (1st pass mechanism). Norelgestromin (primary active metabolite): Hepatic, norgestrel (active metabolite). Ethinyl estradiol: Hydroxylated, glucuronide and sulfate conjugates. **Elimination:** Norgestimate: Urine (47%), feces (37%).

NURSING CONSIDERATIONS

Assessment: Assess for thrombophlebitis or past history of DVT, current or history of thromboembolic disorders, or any other conditions where treatment is contraindicated or cautioned. Assess use in patients >35 who smoke ≥15 cigarettes/day. Assess use in patients with HTN, hyperlipidemias, DM and obesity. Assess for conditions that might be aggravated by fluid retention, pregnancy/nursing status and for possible drug interactions.

Monitoring: Monitor for signs/symptoms of MI, thromboembolism/thrombotic disease, stroke, and other adverse effects. Monitor serum glucose levels in DM and prediabetic patients. Monitor serum triglycerides and lipoprotein levels. Monitor for jaundice, depression and visual changes or changes in lens tolerance in contact lens wearer. Monitor serum folate level in patient who becomes pregnant shortly after d/c. Perform annual physical exam.

Patient Counseling: Inform that drug does not protect against HIV infection (AIDS) and other STDs. Advise to avoid smoking while on medication. Counsel about potential adverse effects. Instruct to take exactly as directed at intervals not exceeding 24 hrs. Advise about risk of pregnancy if dose is missed. Instruct that if one dose missed, take as soon as possible; take next pill at regularly scheduled time. May experiece spotting, light bleeding, or stomach sickness during first 1-3 packs of pills; advise not to d/c medication and if symptoms persist, notify physician.

Administration: Oral route. **Storage:** 25°C (77°F); excursions permitted to 15-30°C (59-86°F). Protect from light.

ORTHO TRI-CYCLEN LO   RX
ethinyl estradiol - norgestimate (Ortho-McNeil)

> Cigarette smoking increases risk of serious cardiovascular (CV) side effects. Risk increases with age (>35 yrs) and heavy smoking (≥15 cigarettes/day). Women who use oral contraceptives should be strongly advised not to smoke.

THERAPEUTIC CLASS: Estrogen/progestogen combination

INDICATIONS: Prevention of pregnancy.

DOSAGE: *Adults:* 1 tab qd for 28 days, then repeat. Start 1st Sunday after menses begin or 1st day of menses.
Pediatrics: Postpubertal adolescents: 1 tab qd for 28 days, then repeat. Start 1st Sunday after menses begin or 1st day of menses.

HOW SUPPLIED: Tab: (Ethinyl Estradiol-Norgestimate) 0.025mg-0.18mg, 0.025mg-0.215mg, and 0.025mg-0.25mg

CONTRAINDICATIONS: Thrombophlebitis or history of deep vein thrombophlebitis, thromboembolic disorders (current or past history), pregnancy, cerebrovascular or coronary artery disease (CAD) (current or past history), valvular heart disease with complications, severe HTN, diabetes with vascular involvement, headaches with focal neurological symptoms, major surgery with prolonged immobilization, undiagnosed abnormal genital bleeding, cholestatic jaundice of pregnancy or jaundice with prior pill use, hepatic adenomas or carcinomas, breast carcinoma (current or past history), endometrial carcinoma or other known or suspected estrogen-dependent neoplasia.

WARNINGS/PRECAUTIONS: Increased risk of MI, vascular disease, thromboembolism, stroke, hepatic neoplasia, and gallbladder disease. May increase risk of breast cancer and cervical intraepithelial neoplasia. Retinal thrombosis reported; d/c if unexplained partial or complete loss of vision, onset of proptosis or diplopia, papilledema, or retinal vascular lesions develop. May cause glucose intolerance, fluid retention, breakthrough bleeding, and spotting. May increase BP; d/c if significant elevations in BP occur. May elevate LDL levels or cause other lipid changes. May cause or exacerbate migraine headaches. May develop visual changes with contact lens. Increased risk of morbidity and mortality with HTN, hyperlipidemia, obesity, and DM. D/C if jaundice or if significant depression develops. Does not protect against HIV infection (AIDS) and other sexually transmitted diseases (STDs). Ectopic and intrauterine pregnancy may occur with contraceptive failure. Not indicated for use before menarche. May affect certain endocrine, LFTs, and blood components in laboratory tests.

ADVERSE REACTIONS: N/V, breakthrough bleeding, spotting, amenorrhea, migraine, depression, vaginal candidiasis, edema, weight changes, melasma, breast changes, changes in cervical erosion and secretion, rash (allergic).

INTERACTIONS: Reduced effects resulting in pregnancy or breakthrough bleeding may occur when coadministered with antibiotics, anticonvulsants, and other drugs that increase the metabolism of contraceptive steroids (eg, rifampin, barbiturates, phenylbutazone, phenytoin, carbamazepine, felbamate, oxcarbazepine, griseofulvin, topiramate, ampicillin, tetracyclines, St. John's wort). Atorvastatin, ascorbic acid, acetaminophen (APAP), CYP3A4 inhibitors (eg, itraconazole, ketoconazole) may increase hormone levels. HIV protease inhibitors may increase or decrease levels. May increases levels of cyclosporine, prednisolone, theophylline. May decrease levels of APAP. May increase the clearance of temazepam, salicylic acid, morphine, and clofibric acid. May decrease plasma levels of lamotrigine, which may reduce seizure control; dosage adjustments of lamotrigine may be necessary.

PREGNANCY: Category X, not for use in nursing.

MECHANISM OF ACTION: Estrogen/progestogen oral contraceptive; acts by suppression of gonadotropins. Primarily inhibits ovulation. Also produces other alterations including changes in the cervical mucus (increases difficulty of sperm entry into uterus) and the endometrium (reduces likelihood of implantation).

PHARMACOKINETICS: Absorption: Rapidly absorbed. Oral administration on various days during dosing schedule led to altered parameters. **Distribution:** Found in breast milk. Norgestimate: Serum protein binding (>97%). Ethinyl estradiol: Serum albumin binding (>97%). **Metabolism:** Norgestimate: GI tract and/or liver, 1st pass mechanism. Norelgestromin (active major metabolite): Hepatic, norgestrel (active metabolite). Ethinyl Estradiol: Hydroxylated, glucuronide and sulfate conjugates. **Elimination:** Urine, feces; $T_{1/2}$=28.1 hrs (norelgestromin), 36.4 hrs (norgestrel), 17.7 hrs (ethinyl estradiol).

NURSING CONSIDERATIONS

Assessment: Assess for current or history of thrombophlebitis or thromboembolic disorders, or any other conditions where treatment is contraindicated or cautioned. Assess use in patients >35 yrs who smoke ≥15 cigarettes/day. Assess use in patients with HTN, hyperlipidemias, DM, and obesity. Assess pregnancy/nursing status and for possible drug interactions.

Monitoring: Monitor for signs/symptoms of MI, thromboembolism, stroke, and other adverse effects. Monitor BP if have history of HTN; monitor serum glucose levels in DM or prediabetic patients, lipid levels with history of hyperlipidemia, for signs/symptoms of liver dysfunction while on therapy (eg, jaundice). Monitor for signs of worsening depression with previous history. Refer patients with contact lenses to an ophthalmologist if ocular changes occur. Perform annual physical exam.

Patient Counseling: Inform that drug does not protect against HIV infection (AIDS) and other STDs. Advise to avoid smoking. Counsel about potential adverse effects. Instruct to take exactly as directed at intervals not exceeding 24 hrs. Advise about risk of pregancy if dose is missed. Instruct that if one dose missed, take as soon as possible; take next pill at regularly scheduled time. May experience spotting, light bleeding, or nausea during first 1-3 packs of pills; advise not to d/c medication and if symptoms persist, notify physician.

Administration: Oral route. **Storage:** (Ortho Tri-Cyclen Lo) 25°C (77°F); excursions permitted to 15-30°C (59-86°F). Protect from light.

ORTHO-CYCLEN

RX

ethinyl estradiol - norgestimate (Ortho-McNeil)

> Cigarette smoking increases risk of serious cardiovascular (CV) side effects. Risk increases with age (>35 yrs) and heavy smoking (≥15 cigarettes/day). Women who use oral contraceptives should be strongly advised not to smoke.

OTHER BRAND NAMES: Sprintec (Barr) - MonoNessa (Watson)

THERAPEUTIC CLASS: Estrogen/progestogen combination

INDICATIONS: Prevention of pregnancy.

DOSAGE: *Adults:* 1 tab qd for 28 days, then repeat. Start 1st Sunday after menses begin or 1st day of menses.
Pediatrics: Postpubertal Adolescents: 1 tab qd for 28 days, then repeat. Start 1st Sunday after menses begin or 1st day of menses.

HOW SUPPLIED: Tab: (Ethinyl Estradiol-Norgestimate) 0.035mg-0.25mg

CONTRAINDICATIONS: Thrombophlebitis or past history of deep vein thrombophlebitis, thromboembolic disorders (current or past history of), cerebral vascular or coronary artery disease (current or past history of), carcinoma of the breast (current or past history of), carcinoma of the endometrium or other known or suspected estrogen dependent neoplasia, undiagnosed abnormal genital bleeding, cholestatic jaundice of pregnancy or jaundice with prior pill use, hepatic adenomas or carcinomas, known or suspected pregnancy. (Mononessa, Ortho-Cyclen) Valvular heart disease with complications, severe HTN, diabetes with vascular involvement, headaches with focal neurological symptoms, major surgery with prolonged immobilization, acute or chronic hepatocellular disease with abnormal liver function.

WARNINGS/PRECAUTIONS: Increased risk of MI, vascular disease, thromboembolism, stroke, gallbladder disease, and hepatic neoplasia. May increase risk of breast cancer and cancer of the reproductive organs. Retinal thrombosis reported; d/c if unexplained partial or complete loss of vision, onset of proptosis or diplopia, papilledema, or retinal vascular lesions develop. May cause glucose intolerance, fluid retention, breakthrough bleeding, and spotting. May increase BP; d/c if significant elevations in BP occur. May elevate LDL levels or cause other lipid changes. May cause or exacerbate migraine headaches. May develop visual changes with contact lens. Increased risk of morbidity and mortality with HTN, hyperlipidemia, obesity, and DM. D/C if jaundice or if significant depression develops. Not indicated for use before menarche. Does not protect against HIV infection (AIDS) or other sexually transmitted diseases (STDs). May affect certain endocrine, LFTs, and blood components in laboratory tests.

ADVERSE REACTIONS: N/V, breakthrough bleeding, GI symptoms (such as abdominal cramps, bloating), spotting, menstrual flow changes, amenorrhea, migraine, depression, vaginal candidiasis, edema, weight changes, cervical erosion and secretion.

INTERACTIONS: Reduced effects resulting in breakthrough bleeding or unintended pregnancy may occur when coadministered with antibiotics, anticonvulsants, and other drugs that increase metabolism (eg, rifampin, barbiturates, phenylbutazone, phenytoin, carbamazepine, felbamate, oxcarbazepine, griseofulvin, ampicillin, tetracyclines, topiramate, bosentan, St. John's wort). (Mononessa, Ortho-Cyclen) Atorvastatin, ascorbic acid, acetaminophen, CYP3A4 inhibitors (eg, itraconazole, ketoconazole) may increase hormone levels. Increases levels of cyclosporine, prednisolone, and theophylline. Decreases levels of acetaminophen. Increases clearance of temazepam, salicylic acid, morphine, and clofibric acid. May significantly decrease plasma levels of lamotrigine; dosage adjustment of lamotrigine may be necessary. Anti-HIV protease inhibitors may significantly change (increase and decrease) hormone levels.

PREGNANCY: Category X, not for use in nursing.

MECHANISM OF ACTION: Estrogen/progestogen combination oral contraceptive; acts by suppression of gonadotropins. Inhibits ovulation and produces changes in cervical mucus (increases difficulty of sperm entry into uterus) and the endometrium (reduces likelihood of implantation).

PHARMACOKINETICS: Absorption: Rapid. Oral administration of various doses led to altered parameters. Refer to PI for specific parameters for norelgestromin, norgestrel, and ethinyl estradiol. **Distribution:** Found in breast milk. Norelgestromin and norgestrel: Albumin binding (>97%). Ethinyl estradiol: Albumin binding (>97%). **Metabolism:** Norgestimate: GI tract and/or liver (1st pass mechanism); norelgestromin (primary active metabolite), norgestrel (active metabolite). Ethinyl estradiol: Hydroxylated, glucuronide, sulfate conjugates. **Elimination:** Norgestimate: Urine (47%), feces (37%).

NURSING CONSIDERATIONS

Assessment: Assess for thrombophlebitis or past history of deep vein thrombophlebitis, current or history of thromboembolic disorders, or any other conditions where treatment is contraindicated or cautioned. Assess use in patients >35 yrs old who smoke ≥15 cigarettes/day. Assess use with history of HTN, hyperlipidemia, obesity, or DM. Assess pregnancy/nursing status and for possible drug interactions.

Monitoring: Monitor for signs/symptoms of MI, thromboembolism, stroke, hepatic neoplasia, and other adverse effects. Monitor serum glucose levels in DM and prediabetic patients. Monitor BP with history of HTN, lipid levels with history of hyperlipidemia, and for signs of worsening depression with previous history. Refer patients to an ophthalmologist if ocular changes develop. Perform annual physical exam while on therapy. Monitor liver function and for signs of liver toxicity (eg, jaundice).

Patient Counseling: Inform that drug does not protect against HIV infection (AIDS) and other STDs. Advise to avoid smoking while on medication. Counsel about potential adverse effects. Instruct to take exactly as directed at intervals not exceeding 24 hrs. Advise about risk of pregnancy if dose is missed. Instruct that if one dose missed, take as soon as possible; take next pill at regularly scheduled time; this means you may take 2 pills in 1 day. May experience spotting, light bleeding, or stomach sickness during first 1-3 packs of pills; advise not to d/c medication and if symptoms persist, notify physician.

Administration: Oral route. **Storage:** (Mononessa, Ortho-Cyclen) 25°C (77°F); excursions permitted to 15-30°C (59-86°F). Protect from light. (Sprintec) 20-25°C (68-77°F).

ORTHO-NOVUM 1/35

RX

ethinyl estradiol - norethindrone (Ortho-McNeil)

> Cigarette smoking increases the risk of serious CV side effects. Risk increases with age (>35 yrs) and with heavy smoking (≥15 cigarettes/day). Women who use oral contraceptives should be strongly advised not to smoke.

OTHER BRAND NAMES: Nortrel 1/35 (Barr) - Norinyl 1/35 (Watson) - Necon 1/35 (Watson)

THERAPEUTIC CLASS: Estrogen/progestogen combination

INDICATIONS: Prevention of pregnancy.

DOSAGE: *Adults:* 28 day regimen: 1 tab qd for 28 days, then repeat. Start 1st Sunday after menses begin or 1st day of menses. 21 day regimen: 1 tab qd for 21 days, then stop for 7 days, then repeat. Start 1st Sunday after menses begin or 1st day of menses.
Pediatrics: Postpubertal Adolescents: 28 day regimen: 1 tab qd for 28 days, then repeat. Start 1st Sunday after menses begin or 1st day of menses. 21 day regimen: 1 tab qd for 21 days, then stop for 7 days, then repeat. Start 1st Sunday after menses begin or 1st day of menses.

HOW SUPPLIED: Tab: (Ethinyl Estradiol-Norethindrone) 0.035mg-1mg

CONTRAINDICATIONS: Thrombophlebitis, thromboembolic disorders, history of deep vein thrombophlebitis (DVT) or thromboembolic disorders, cerebral vascular or coronary artery disease (CAD), carcinoma of the endometrium or other known or suspected estrogen-dependent neoplasia, undiagnosed abnormal genital bleeding, cholestatic jaundice of pregnancy or jaundice with prior pill use, hepatic adenomas or carcinomas, known or suspected carcinoma of the breast, and pregnancy. (Ortho-Novum 1/35) Valvular heart disease with complications, severe HTN, diabetes with vascular involvement, headaches with focal neurological symptoms, major surgery with prolonged immobilization, acute or chronic hepatocellular disease with abnormal liver function. (Norinyl 1/35) Benign liver tumors.

WARNINGS/PRECAUTIONS: Increased risk of MI, vascular disease, thromboembolism, stroke, gallbladder disease, and hepatic neoplasia. Increased risk of morbidity and mortality in patients with HTN, hyperlipidemias, obesity and diabetes. May increase risk of breast cancer and cancer of the reproductive organs. Retinal thrombosis reported; d/c if unexplained partial or complete loss of vision occurs, or if onset of proptosis or diplopia, papilledema, or retinal vascular lesions develops. May cause glucose intolerance. May cause fluid retention and increase BP; monitor closely and d/c if significant elevation of BP occurs. Breakthrough bleeding and spotting reported; rule out malignancy or pregnancy. May cause onset or exacerbation of a migraine or development of a headache. May develop visual changes with contact lenses. May elevate LDL levels or cause other lipid effects. D/C if jaundice develops. Caution with history of depression; d/c if depression recurs to serious degree. Not indicated for use before menarche. Does not protect against HIV infection (AIDS) and other sexually transmitted diseases (STDs). May affect certain endocrine, LFTs, and blood components in laboratory tests. Ectopic and intrauterine pregnancies may occur with contraceptive failures. Should not be used to induce withdrawal bleeding as a test for pregnancy, or to treat threatened or habitual abortion during pregnancy.

ADVERSE REACTIONS: N/V, breakthrough bleeding, spotting, amenorrhea, migraine, mental depression, vaginal candidiasis, edema, weight changes, abdominal cramps/bloating, menstrual flow changes, melasma.

INTERACTIONS: Reduced effects, increased breakthrough bleeding, and menstrual irregularities with rifampin, barbiturates, phenylbutazone, phenytoin Na⁺, and possibly with griseofulvin, ampicillin, tetracyclines and (Necon, Nortrel 1/35, Ortho-Novum 1/35) carbamazepine. (Ortho-Novum 1/35) Reduced effects resulting in unintended pregnancy or breakthrough bleeding may occur when coadministered with antibiotics, anticonvulsants, and other drugs that increase the metabolism of contraceptive steroids (eg, felbamate, oxcarbazepine, topiramate, bosentan), and St. John's wort. Significant changes in plasma levels of estrogen and progestin may occur with coadministration with anti-HIV protease inhibitors. Atorvastatin, ascorbic acid, and acetaminophen (APAP) may increase plasma estradiol levels. CYP3A4 inhibitors (eg, itraconazole, ketoconazole) may increase plasma hormone levels. Bosentan may decrease hormone levels. May increase plasma concentrations of cyclosporine, prednisolone, and theophylline. May decrease plasma concentrations of APAP and lamotrigine. May increase clearance of temazepam, salicylic acid, morphine, and clofibric acid.

PREGNANCY: Category X, not for use in nursing.

MECHANISM OF ACTION: Estrogen/progestogen oral contraceptive; suppresses gonadotropins. Primarily inhibits ovulation. Also causes changes in cervical mucus (increases difficulty of sperm entry into uterus) and endometrium (reduces likelihood of implantation).

PHARMACOKINETICS: Distribution: Found in breast milk.

NURSING CONSIDERATIONS

Assessment: Assess for thrombophlebitis, thromboembolic disorders, history of DVT or thromboembolic disorders, or any other conditions where treatment is contraindicated or cautioned, Assess pregnancy/nursing status, and for possible drug interactions. Assess use in patients >35 yrs who smoke ≥15 cigarettes/day. Assess use in patients with HTN, hyperlipidemia, obesity, or diabetes.

Monitoring: Monitor for MI, thromboembolism, stroke, and other adverse effects. Monitor BP, serum glucose levels in diabetic and prediabetic patients, lipid levels with history of hyperlipidemia, and for signs of worsening depression with previous history. Monitor LFTs and for signs of liver dysfunction (eg, jaundice). Refer patients with contact lenses to ophthalmologist if ocular changes develop. Perform annual history and physical exam.

Patient Counseling: Inform that therapy does not protect against HIV infection and other STDs. Inform of potential risks/benefits of oral contraceptives. Advise not to smoke while on therapy. Instruct to take 1 pill at same time daily at intervals not exceeding 24 hrs. Counsel if dose is missed, take as soon as possible; advise to take next dose at regularly scheduled time. Instruct to continue medication if spotting or breakthrough bleeding occur; notify physician if symptoms persist. Inform that missing a pill can cause spotting or light bleeding.

Administration: Oral route. **Storage:** (Ortho-Novum 1/35) 25°C (77°F); excursions permitted to 15-30°C (59-86°F). (Norinyl 1/35) 15-25°C (59-77°F). (Nortrel, Necon 1/35) 20-25°C (68-77°F).

OSMOPREP   RX

monobasic sodium phosphate - dibasic sodium phosphate - sodium phosphate (Salix)

> Rare, but serious reports of acute phosphate nephropathy. Some cases resulted in permanent renal impairment requiring long-term dialysis. Patients at increased risk may include those with increased age, hypovolemia, increased bowel transit time (eg, bowel obstruction), active colitis, baseline kidney disease, and using medicines that affect renal perfusion or function (eg, diuretics, angiotensin converting enzyme [ACE] inhibitors, angiotensin receptor blockers [ARBs], and possibly NSAIDs). Use the recommended dose and dosing regimen (pm/am split dose).

THERAPEUTIC CLASS: Bowel cleanser

INDICATIONS: For cleansing the colon in preparation for colonoscopy in adults ≥18 yrs of age.

DOSAGE: *Adults:* ≥18 yrs: Evening Before Colonoscopy Procedure: 4 tabs with 8 oz. of clear liquids q15min for a total of 20 tabs. Day of Colonoscopy Procedure: Starting 3-5 hrs before procedure, 4 tabs with 8 oz. of clear liquids q15min for a total of 12 tabs. Drink only clear liquids. Do not use within 7 days of previous administration. Do not take any additional enema or laxative, particularly one containing sodium phosphate.

HOW SUPPLIED: Tab: (Sodium Phosphate Monobasic Monohydrate-Sodium Phosphate Dibasic Anhydrous) 1.102g-0.398g

CONTRAINDICATIONS: Patients with biopsy-proven acute phosphate nephropathy.

WARNINGS/PRECAUTIONS: Fatalities reported due to significant fluid shifts, severe electrolyte abnormalities, and cardiac arrhythmias. Adequately hydrate before, during and after use. Inadequate fluid intake may lead to excessive fluid loss, hypovolemia and dehydration. Use with caution in elderly, impaired renal function, congestive heart failure (CHF), ascites, unstable angina, acute bowel obstruction, bowel perforation, toxic megacolon, gastric retention, ileus, pseudo-obstruction of the bowel, severe chronic constipation, acute colitis, gastric bypass, stapling surgery, hypomotility syndrome, history of acute phosphate nephropathy and known or suspected electrolyte disturbances. Correct electrolyte abnormalities before treatment. Rare reports of generalized tonic-clonic seizures and/or loss of consciousness. Caution in patients with history of seizures and in patients at higher risk of seizures (eg, patients withdrawing from alcohol or benzodiazepines, patients with known or suspected hyponatremia). Rare reports of serious arrhythmias; caution in patients with high risk of arrhythmias (eg, patients with prolonged QT, history of cardiomyopathy, history of uncontrolled arrhythmias, and recent history of myocardial infarction [MI]). Prolongation of QT interval reported. May induce colonic mucosal aphthous ulcerations and exacerbate inflammatory bowel disease (IBD).

ADVERSE REACTIONS: Abdominal bloating, abdominal pain, N/V, colonic mucosal aphthous ulcers, renal impairment, acute phosphate nephropathy.

INTERACTIONS: See Boxed Warning. Medications administered in close proximity to sodium phosphate tablets may not be absorbed from the GI tract. Caution if taking medications that may affect electrolyte levels (eg, diuretics), reduce seizure threshold (eg, tricyclic antidepressants), or prolong the QT interval.

PREGNANCY: Category C, safety not known in nursing.

MECHANISM OF ACTION: Purgative: Mechanism not established, primary mode of action thought to be through the osmotic effect of Na⁺, causing large amounts of water to be drawn into the colon, promoting evacuation.

NURSING CONSIDERATIONS

Assessment: Assess if at increased risk of developing acute phosphate nephropathy or biopsy-proven acute phosphate nephropathy. Assess use in patients with severe renal insufficiency or renal impairment, or in any other conditions where treatment is contraindicated or cautioned. Consider baseline labs (phosphate, calcium, K⁺, Na⁺, SrCr, BUN) in patients who may be at increased risk for serious adverse events. Consider pre-dose ECG in patients with known prolonged QT or in patients with serious risk of cardiac arrhythmias. Assess hypersensitivity, pregnancy/nursing status, and for possible drug interactions.

Monitoring: Monitor for signs and symptoms of acute phosphate nephropathy, fluid shifts, severe electrolyte abnormalities, cardiac arrhythmias, renal failure, nephrocalcinosis, generalized tonic-clonic seizures, loss of consciousness, QT prolongation and colonic mucosal aphthous ulcerations. Consider performing post-colonoscopy labs (phosphate, calcium, Na⁺, K⁺, SrCr, BUN) in patients at increased risk for adverse events or if develop vomiting or signs of dehydration. Consider post-colonoscopy ECG in patients with high risk of serious cardiac arrhythmias or in patients with known prolonged QT.

Patient Counseling: Stress importance of adequate hydration before, during and after use. Instruct to drink 8 oz. of clear liquid with each 4-tab dose. Instruct to contact physician if experience symptoms of dehydration. Instruct not to use within 7 days of previous administration and not to administer additional laxative or purgative agents, particularly additional sodium phosphate-based products. Instruct to contact physician if develop worsening of bloating, abdominal pain, N/V, or headache.

Administration: Oral route. **Storage:** 25°C (77°F); excursions permitted to 15-30°C (59-86°F). Discard any unused portion.

OVCON-35

RX

ethinyl estradiol - norethindrone (Warner Chilcott)

> Cigarette smoking increases the risk of serious cardiovascular (CV) side effects. Risk increases with age (>35 yrs) and with heavy smoking (≥15 cigarettes/day). Women who use oral contraceptives should be strongly advised not to smoke.

OTHER BRAND NAMES: Balziva (Barr) - Ovcon-50 (Warner Chilcott)

THERAPEUTIC CLASS: Estrogen/progestogen combination

INDICATIONS: Prevention of pregnancy.

DOSAGE: *Adults:* 1 tab qd for 28 days, then repeat regimen on the next day after the last tab. Start on the 1st day of menses or 1st Sunday after menses begin. For the 1st cycle of a Sunday start regimen, use back-up method if had intercourse before having taken the seven pills.
Pediatrics: Postpubertal Adolescents: 1 tab qd for 28 days, then repeat regimen on the next day after the last tab. Start on the 1st day of menses or 1st Sunday after menses begin. For the 1st cycle of a Sunday start regimen, use back-up method if had intercourse before having taken the seven pills.

HOW SUPPLIED: Tab: (Ethinyl Estradiol-Norethindrone) (Ovcon 35, Balziva) 0.035mg-0.4mg; (Ovcon 50) 0.05mg-1mg

CONTRAINDICATIONS: Thrombophlebitis, current or history of thromboembolic disorders, past history of deep vein thrombophlebitis, cerebrovascular or coronary artery disease (CAD), known or suspected carcinoma of the breast, endometrial carcinoma or other known or suspected estrogen-dependent neoplasia, undiagnosed abnormal genital bleeding, cholestatic jaundice of pregnancy or jaundice with prior pill use, hepatic adenomas or carcinomas, known or suspected pregnancy.

WARNINGS/PRECAUTIONS: Increased risk of myocardial infarction (MI), thromboembolism, cerebrovascular events, gallbladder disease, and hepatic neoplasia. May increase risk of breast cancer and cervical intraepithelial neoplasia. May cause benign hepatic adenomas. Retinal thrombosis reported; d/c if unexplained partial or complete loss of vision, onset of proptosis or diplopia, papilledema, or retinal vascular lesions develop. Increased risk of gallbladder surgery reported. May cause glucose intolerance; caution with prediabetic and diabetic patients. May cause fluid retention and increase BP; monitor closely with HTN and d/c if significant elevation of BP occurs. May cause migraine or development of headaches; d/c and evaluate the cause. Breakthrough bleeding and spotting reported; rule out malignancy or pregnancy. Does not protect against HIV infection (AIDS) or other sexually transmitted diseases (STD). D/C if jaundice develops. Monitor closely with depression and d/c if depression recurs to serious degree. May develop visual changes or changes in contact lense tolerance. Not indicated for use before menarche. Use back-up method of contraception with significant GI disturbance.

ADVERSE REACTIONS: N/V, breakthrough bleeding, GI symptoms (eg, abdominal cramps, bloating), spotting, menstrual flow changes, amenorrhea, migraine, depression, vaginal candidiasis, edema, weight changes, cervical ectropion and secretion changes.

INTERACTIONS: Reduced effects, increased breakthrough bleeding, and menstrual irregularities with rifampin, barbiturates, phenylbutazone, phenytoin sodium, and possibly with griseofulvin, ampicillin, and tetracyclines.

PREGNANCY: Category X, not for use in nursing.

MECHANISM OF ACTION: Estrogen/progestogen combination oral contraceptive; acts by suppressing gonadotropins. Primarily inhibits ovulation but also produces other alterations including changes in the cervical mucus (increases difficulty of sperm entry into uterus) and endometrium (reduces likelihood of implantation).

PHARMACOKINETICS: Distribution: Found in breast milk.

NURSING CONSIDERATIONS

Assessment: Assess for pregnancy/nursing status, possible drug interactions, and conditions where treatment is contraindicated or cautioned. Assess use in patients >35 yrs who smoke ≥15 cigarettes/day, and with HTN, hyperlipidemia, obesity, and DM.

Monitoring: Monitor for signs/symptoms of thromboembolism, stroke, MI, and other adverse effects. Monitor BP in patients with a history of HTN, HTN-related disease, or renal disease. Monitor for signs of depression in patients with a history of depression. Perform annual history and physical exam. Monitor serum glucose levels in prediabetic and diabetic patients. Monitor lipid levels in patients with a history of hyperlipidemia.

Patient Counseling: Inform that medication does not protect against HIV/AIDS and other STDs. Counsel about possible serious side effects. Advise to avoid smoking while on therapy. Instruct to take 1 pill at same time daily. If dose is missed, refer to PI for instructions. If spotting, light bleeding, or nausea occurs during first 1-3 packs of pills, advise not to d/c medication and if symptoms persist, notify physician. Inform if vomiting or diarrhea occurs or if taking other medications, efficacy may decrease; use backup method of contraception. Refer patients with contact lenses to an ophthalmologist if changes in vision or lens tolerance develop.

Administration: Oral route. Take 1 pill at the same time every day until the pack is empty. If on 28 day regimen, start the next pack the day after the last inactive tablet and do not wait any days between packs. **Storage:** (Ovcon 35, Balziva) 20-25°C (68-77°F). (Ovcon 50) Below 30°C (86°F).

OXYCODONE IMMEDIATE-RELEASE   CII
oxycodone HCl (Various)

THERAPEUTIC CLASS: Opioid analgesic

INDICATIONS: Moderate to moderately severe pain.

DOSAGE: *Adults:* Usual: 5mg q6h prn for pain.

HOW SUPPLIED: Cap: 5mg

CONTRAINDICATIONS: Respiratory depression, acute or severe bronchial asthma, hypercarbia, paralytic ileus, situations where opioids are contraindicated.

WARNINGS/PRECAUTIONS: Extreme caution with COPD, cor pulmonale, decreased respiratory reserve, hypoxia, hypercapnia, pre-existing respiratory depression. Caution with circulatory shock, delirium tremens, acute alcoholism, adrenocortical insufficiency, CNS depression, myxedema or hypothyroidism, BPH, severe hepatic/renal/pulmonary impairment, toxic psychosis, biliary tract disease, increased ICP, or head injury, elderly or debilitated. May cause severe hypotension. May produce drug dependence; caution in known drug abuse. May aggravate convulsive disorders and mask abdominal disorders. May impair mental/physical abilities.

ADVERSE REACTIONS: Lightheadedness, dizziness, N/V, sedation.

INTERACTIONS: Respiratory depression, hypotension and profound sedation with other CNS depressants (eg, sedatives, anesthetics, phenothiazines, alcohol). Mixed agonist/antagonist analgesics may reduce the analgesic effect and/or cause withdrawal. Risk of severe hypotension with phenothiazines, or other agents that compromise vasomotor tone. May enhance skeletal muscle relaxant effects and increase respiratory depression. May interact with CYP2D6 inhibitors (eg, amiodarone, quinidine, polycyclic antidepressants). Caution with MAOIs.

PREGNANCY: Category B, not for use in nursing.

MECHANISM OF ACTION: Opioid analgesic; pure agonist opioid whose principal therapeutic effect is analgesia. Precise action not established. However, specific CNS opioid receptors for endogenous compounds with opioid-like activity are found throughout the brain and spinal cord and play a role in analgesic effects.

PHARMACOKINETICS: Distribution: Found in breast milk. **Metabolism:** Via CYP2D6 to oxymorphone (metabolite).

NURSING CONSIDERATIONS

Assessment: Assess for adrenocortical insufficiency (eg, Addison's disease), kyphoscoliosis associated with respiratory depression, prostatic hypertrophy or urethral stricture, acute pancreatitis, or any other conditions where treatment is contraindicated or cautioned. Assess for pregnancy/nursing status and possible drug interactions.

Monitoring: Monitor for signs/symptoms of respiratory depression, hypotension, convulsions, medication dependence and tolerance, medication abuse, sphincter of Oddi spasms, elevations in CSF pressure, and elevations in serum amylase levels.

Patient Counseling: Advise not to adjust dosing without consulting physician. Inform that medication may impair mental/physical abilities required for performing hazardous tasks (eg, operating machinery/driving). Counsel to avoid alcohol and other CNS depressants. Inform medication has potential for abuse; protect from theft. Advise not to abruptly d/c medication if on therapy for a few weeks; taper dosing.

Administration: Oral route. **Storage:** 20-25°C (68-77°F); protect from moisture and dispense in tight, light-resistant container.

OxyContin

CII

oxycodone HCl (Purdue Pharma)

> Contains oxycodone, a Schedule II controlled substance with abuse liability similar to morphine. Not intended for use as a prn analgesic. 60mg and 80mg, a single dose >40mg, or a total daily dose >80mg are only for use in opioid-tolerant patients; may cause fatal respiratory depression with intolerant patients. Abuse potential; assess for risks of opioid abuse/addiction prior to therapy. Swallow tab whole; do not cut, break, chew, crush or dissolve. Concomitant use with CYP3A4 inhibitors (eg, macrolides, azole-antifungals, protease inhibitors) may cause fatal respiratory depression.

THERAPEUTIC CLASS: Opioid analgesic

INDICATIONS: Management of moderate to severe pain when a continuous, around-the-clock analgesic is needed for an extended period of time. For use in the immediate postoperative period in patients already receiving the drug before surgery or those expected to have moderate to severe postoperative pain for an extended period of time.

DOSAGE: *Adults:* Individualize dose. Opioid-Naive: 10mg q12h. Titrate: Determine dose that provides adequate analgesia and minimizes adverse reactions while maintaining q12h dosing regimen. May increase total daily dose by 25-50% of the current dose every 1-2 days. Opioid-Tolerant Patients: Refer to PI for conversion to oxycodone from other opioid analgesics. Hepatic Impairment/CNS Depressants/Debilitated, Opioid-Naive: Start at 1/3 or 1/2 the usual starting dose. Reassess continued need regularly (eg, every 6-12 months). Taper dose gradually upon d/c of therapy.

HOW SUPPLIED: Tab, Controlled-Release: 10mg, 15mg, 20mg, 30mg, 40mg, 60mg, 80mg

CONTRAINDICATIONS: Significant respiratory depression, acute or severe bronchial asthma, known or suspected paralytic ileus.

WARNINGS/PRECAUTIONS: Not to be used for pre-emptive analgesia, mild pain, pain not expected to persist for an extended period of time, or pain in immediate postoperative period. May cause CNS and respiratory depression. Risk of respiratory depression is increased in elderly/debilitated patients or with large initial doses given to opioid-intolerant patients. Extreme caution with chronic obstructive pulmonary disease (COPD), cor pulmonale, decreased respiratory reserve, hypoxia, hypercapnia, and pre-existing respiratory depression. May induce or aggravate convulsions/seizures; caution with history of seizure disorders. Respiratory depressant effects may be exaggerated in the presence of head injury, intracranial lesions, or other sources of pre-existing increased intracranial pressure (ICP). May cause severe hypotension; increased risk with depleted blood volume. Caution with circulatory shock, alcoholism, delirium tremens, adrenocortical insufficiency, CNS depression, debilitation, kyphoscoliosis associated with respiratory compromise, myxedema or hypothyroidism, BPH or urethral stricture, severe hepatic/renal/pulmonary impairment, and toxic psychosis. May cause spasm of sphincter of Oddi and increase in serum amylase; caution with biliary tract disease, pancreatitis, and in patients at risk of developing ileus. Gradually increase dose if tolerance develops. May impair mental and physical abilities. May produce orthostatic hypotension in ambulatory patients. May obscure diagnosis or clinical course of acute abdominal conditions.

ADVERSE REACTIONS: Respiratory depression, constipation, N/V, somnolence, dizziness, pruritus, headache, dry mouth, asthenia, sweating, apnea, respiratory arrest, circulatory depression, hypotension.

INTERACTIONS: See Box Warning. Respiratory depression, hypotension, and profound sedation or coma may occur with other CNS depressants (eg, sedatives, hypnotics, anxiolytics, neuroleptics, tranquilizers, centrally acting antiemetics, general anesthetics, phenothiazines, alcohol, other opioids). Mixed agonist/antagonist analgesics (eg, pentazocine, nalbuphine, butorphanol) may reduce analgesic effect and/or cause withdrawal. Risk of severe hypotension with phenothiazines or other agents that compromise vasomotor tone. May enhance neuromuscular blocking action of skeletal muscle relaxants (eg, pancuronium) and increase respiratory depression. Increased levels with voriconazole. Decreased levels with CYP3A4 inducers (eg, rifampin, carbamazepine, phenytoin). May interact with CYP2D6 inhibitors (eg, amiodarone, quinidine, polycyclic antidepressants). Caution with monoamine oxidase inhibitors (MAOIs). Antipsychotics, β-blockers, antidepressants block the formation of oxymorphone, a minor metabolite of oxycodone.

PREGNANCY: Category B, not for use in nursing.

MECHANISM OF ACTION: Opioid analgesic; pure μ-receptor opioid agonist. Precise analgesic action not established. However, specific CNS opioid receptors have been found throughout the brain and spinal cord and play a role in analgesic effect.

PHARMACOKINETICS: Absorption: Administration of variable doses resulted in different parameters. Absolute bioavailability (60-87%). **Distribution:** V_d=2.6L/kg; plasma protein binding (45%); found in breast milk; crosses the placenta. **Metabolism:** Extensively via CYP3A and CYP2D6 to noroxycodone, noroxymorphone (major metabolites) and oxymorphone. **Elimination:** Urine; $T_{1/2}$=4.5 hrs.

NURSING CONSIDERATIONS

Assessment: Assess for degree of opioid tolerance, previous opioid dose, level of pain intensity, type of pain, patient's general condition and medical status, emotional status or any other conditions where treatment is contraindicated or cautioned. Assess for pregnancy/nursing status, renal/hepatic function, and for possible drug interactions.

Monitoring: Monitor for signs/symptoms of respiratory depression, CNS depression, seizures/convulsions, elevations in CSF pressure, hypotension, spasm of sphincter of Oddi, tolerance and physical dependence. Monitor BP and serum amylase levels. Routinely monitor for signs of misuse, abuse and addiction.

Patient Counseling: Instruct to swallow medication whole; do not cut, break, chew, dissolve or crush tabs. Advise to report episodes of breakthrough pain or adverse events (eg, respiratory depression). Instruct to not adjust dosing without consulting physician. Mental/physical abilities may be impaired; avoid alcohol or other CNS depressants. Medication has potential for abuse; protect from theft. Inform that if taking medication for more than a few weeks, to avoid abrupt withdrawal; advise that dosing will need to be tapered. Counsel to not share or permit use by individuals other than the patient for whom it was prescribed. Inform physician if pregnant or planning to become pregnant. Dispose of any unused medication by flushing down the toilet.

Administration: Oral route. Take 1 tab at a time with enough water. **Storage:** 25°C (77°F); excursions permitted to 15-30°C (59-86°F). Dispense in tight, light-resistant container.

OXYTROL   RX
oxybutynin (Watson)

THERAPEUTIC CLASS: Anticholinergic

INDICATIONS: Treatment of overactive bladder with symptoms of urge urinary incontinence, urgency, and frequency.

DOSAGE: *Adults:* One 3.9mg/day system applied twice weekly (every 3-4 days) to dry, intact skin on the abdomen, hip or buttock. Avoid reapplication to same site within 7 days.

HOW SUPPLIED: Patch: 3.9mg/day [8°]

CONTRAINDICATIONS: Urinary retention, gastric retention, uncontrolled narrow-angle glaucoma, and in patients at risk for these conditions.

WARNINGS/PRECAUTIONS: Angioedema may occur; d/c and provide appropriate therapy. Caution with hepatic/renal impairment, bladder outflow obstruction, GI obstructive disorders, ulcerative colitis, intestinal atony, myasthenia gravis, and gastroesophageal reflux. May decrease GI motility.

ADVERSE REACTIONS: Application-site reactions (pruritus, erythema, vesicles, rash), dry mouth, diarrhea, constipation.

INTERACTIONS: Other anticholinergics and other agents that produce dry mouth, constipation, somnolence, and/or other anticholinergic-like effects may increase frequency and/or severity of anticholinergic effects. Caution with bisphosphonates or other drugs that may exacerbate esophagitis. May alter GI absorption of other drugs due to GI motility effects.

PREGNANCY: Category B, caution in nursing.

MECHANISM OF ACTION: Antispasmodic, anticholinergic agent; acts as competitive antagonist of acetylcholine at postganglionic muscarinic receptors, resulting in relaxation of bladder smooth muscle.

PHARMACOKINETICS: Absorption: Administration using variable dosing studies resulted in different parameters. **Distribution:** (IV) V_d=193L. **Metabolism:** Liver (extensive); CYP3A4, N-desethyloxybutynin (active metabolite). **Elimination:** Urine (<0.1% unchanged, <0.1% N-desethyloxybutynin); (IV) $T_{1/2}$=2 hrs.

NURSING CONSIDERATIONS

Assessment: Assess for bladder outflow obstruction, urinary/gastric retention, uncontrolled narrow-angle glaucoma, gastroesophageal reflux, GI obstructive disorder, ulcerative colitis, intestinal atony, esophagitis, myasthenia gravis, renal/hepatic impairment, pregnancy/nursing status, and possible drug interactions.

Monitoring: Monitor for signs/symptoms of angioedema, gastric retention, urinary retention, decreased gastric motility, renal/hepatic dysfunction, and for exacerbation of esophagitis.

Patient Counseling: Advise that heat prostration may occur in hot environment. Counsel that dizziness, drowsiness, and blurred vision may occur and alcohol may enhance drowsiness. Inform that angioedema has been reported and instruct to d/c therapy and seek medical attention when angioedema occurs. Instruct to apply to dry, intact skin on abdomen, hip, or buttock; advise to avoid reapplication to same site within 7 days.

Administration: Transdermal route. Apply immediately after removal from protective pouch. **Storage:** 25°C (77°F); excursions permitted to 15-30°C (59-86°F). Protect from moisture and humidity. Do not store outside the sealed pouch.

OZURDEX

RX

dexamethasone (Allergan)

THERAPEUTIC CLASS: Corticosteroid

INDICATIONS: Treatment of macular edema following branch retinal vein occlusion (BRVO) or central retinal vein occlusion (CRVO) and of non-infectious uveitis affecting the posterior segment of the eye.

DOSAGE: *Adults:* 0.7mg intravitreal injection via Novadur drug delivery system.

HOW SUPPLIED: Intravitreal Implant: 0.7mg

CONTRAINDICATIONS: Advanced glaucoma, active or suspected ocular or periocular infections including most viral diseases of the cornea and conjunctiva, including active epithelial herpes simplex keratitis (dendritic keratitis), vaccinia, varicella, mycobacterial infections and fungal diseases.

WARNINGS/PRECAUTIONS: Endophthalmitis, eye inflammation, increased intraocular pressure (IOP), and retinal detachments may occur. May produce posterior subcapsular cataracts, increased IOP, glaucoma and may enhance the establishment of secondary ocular infections due to bacteria, fungi, or viruses. Caution in patients with history of ocular herpes simplex.

ADVERSE REACTIONS: Increased IOP, conjunctival hemorrhage, eye pain, conjunctival hyperemia, ocular HTN, cataract, headache.

PREGNANCY: Category C, caution in nursing.

MECHANISM OF ACTION: Corticosteroid; suppresses inflammation by inhibiting multiple inflammatory cytokines resulting in decreased edema, fibrin deposition, capillary leakage and migration of inflammatory cells.

PHARMACOKINETICS: Absorption: C_{max}=94pg/mL.

NURSING CONSIDERATIONS

Assessment: Assess for glaucoma and for active or suspected ocular or periocular infections (eg, herpes simplex keratitis, vaccinia, varicella, mycobacterial infections or fungal diseases), pregnancy/nursing status, and for hypersensitivity to product components.

Monitoring: Monitor for elevated IOP and endophthalmitis by checking for perfusion of the optic nerve head immediately after injection, tonometry within 30 min of application, and biomicroscopy between 2 to 7 days of administration. Monitor for eye inflammation and retinal detachment, posterior subcapsular cataracts, glaucoma and secondary ocular infections, and other adverse events that may occur.

Patient Counseling: Instruct to report any symptoms of endophthalmitis and increased IOP. If the eye becomes red, sensitive to light, painful, or develops a change in vision, advise to consult an ophthalmologist. Temporary visual blurring may occur after receiving treatment; avoid driving/using machines until this has resolved.

Administration: Intravitreal route. Procedure should be carried out under controlled aseptic conditions. Adequate anesthesia and a broad-spectrum microbicide should be given prior to injection. Refer to PI for proper administration. **Storage:** 15-30°C (59-86°F).

PACLITAXEL

RX

paclitaxel (Various)

Administer under supervision of a physician experienced in the use of cancer chemotherapeutic agents. Anaphylaxis, severe hypersensitivity reactions reported. Pretreat with corticosteroids, diphenhydramine, and H_2 antagonists. Do not rechallenge if severe hypersensitivity reaction occurs. Not given to patients with solid tumors having baseline neutrophil counts of <1500 cells/mm³ and with AIDS-related Kaposi's sarcoma having baseline neutrophil count of <1000 cells/mm³. Monitor peripheral blood cell counts frequently.

THERAPEUTIC CLASS: Antimicrotubule agent

INDICATIONS: First-line (with cisplatin) and subsequent treatment of advanced ovarian carcinoma. Adjuvant treatment of node-positive breast cancer administered sequentially to doxorubicin-containing chemotherapy. Treatment of breast cancer after failure of combination chemotherapy for metastatic disease or relapse within 6 months of adjuvant chemotherapy. Second-line treatment of AIDS-related Kaposi's sarcoma. First-line treatment of non-small cell lung cancer (NSCLC) in combination with cisplatin in patients who are not candidates for potentially curative surgery and/or radiation therapy.

DOSAGE: *Adults:* IV: Ovarian Carcinoma: Previously Untreated: 175mg/m^2 over 3 hrs or 135mg/m^2 over 24 hrs q3 weeks followed by cisplatin. Previously Treated: 135mg/m^2 or 175mg/m^2 over 3 hrs q3 weeks. Breast Cancer (adjuvant treatment of node positive): 175mg/m^2 over 3 hrs q3 weeks for 4 courses given sequentially to doxorubicin chemo. Breast Cancer (failure of initial chemo for metastatic disease or relapse): 175mg/m^2 over 3 hrs q3 weeks. NSCLC: 135mg/m^2 over 24 hrs q3 weeks followed by cisplatin. Kaposi's Sarcoma: 135mg/m^2 over 3 hrs q3 weeks or 100mg/m^2 over 3 hrs q2 weeks. Reduce dose of subsequent courses by 20% if neutrophils <500 cells/mm^3 for ≥1 week or severe peripheral neuropathy occurs. Refer to PI for dosing in patients with hepatic impairment.

HOW SUPPLIED: Inj: 30mg/5mL, 100mg/16.7mL, 150mg/25mL, 300mg/50mL

CONTRAINDICATIONS: Hypersensitivity to drugs formulated in polyoxyl 35 castor oil, NF; solid tumor patients with baseline neutrophils <1500 cells/mm^3, or AIDS-related Kaposi's sarcoma patients with baseline neutrophils <1000 cells/mm^3.

WARNINGS/PRECAUTIONS: Severe conduction abnormalities documented; administer appropriate therapy and monitor continuously during subsequent therapy if this develops. Injection-site reactions, peripheral neuropathy reported. Bone marrow suppression is dose dependent and is the dose-limiting toxicity. Can cause fetal harm. Hypotension, bradycardia, and HTN may occur during administration. Contains dehydrated alcohol; CNS and other alcohol effects may occur. Caution in patients with bilirubin >2x ULN.

ADVERSE REACTIONS: Anaphylaxis, bone marrow suppression, infections, bleeding, abnormal ECG, hypotension, peripheral neuropathy, myalgia/arthralgia, N/V, diarrhea, mucositis, alopecia, injection-site reactions.

INTERACTIONS: May increase doxorubicin levels. Caution with CYP450 2C8 and 3A4 substrates and inducers (eg, rifampicin, carbamazepine, phenytoin, efavirenz, nevirapine) or inhibitors (eg, erythromycin, fluoxetine, gemfibrozil). Myelosuppression more profound when given after than before cisplatin.

PREGNANCY: Category D, not for use in nursing.

MECHANISM OF ACTION: Antimicrotubule agent; promotes assembly of microtubules from tubulin dimers and stabilizes microtubules by preventing depolymerization inhibiting microtubule network essential for vital interphase and mitotic cellular functions.

PHARMACOKINETICS: Absorption: IV administration of multiple doses resulted in different parameters. **Distribution:** V$_d$=227-688L/m^2; plasma protein binding (89-98%). **Metabolism:** CYP2C8 (major), CYP3A4 (minor). 6α-hydroxypaclitaxel (metabolite). **Elimination:** Urine (1.3-12.6%), feces (5%).

NURSING CONSIDERATIONS

Assessment: Assess for pregnancy/nursing status, possible drug interactions, neutrophil count (>1500 cells/mm^3 for solid tumors; >1000 cells/mm^3 for Kaposi's sarcoma), hypersensitivity to polyoxyl 35 castor oil, and hepatic impairment.

Monitoring: Monitor blood count frequently and vital signs frequently during 1st hr of infusion. Monitor for signs/symptoms of anaphylaxis/hypersensitivity reactions, injection-site reactions, conduction abnormalities, bone marrow suppression, infections, neutropenia, and hepatic dysfunction.

Patient Counseling: Inform of pregnancy risks. Advise to seek medical attention if symptoms of infection, anaphylaxis/hypersensitivity reactions (eg, dyspnea, hypotension, angioedema, urticaria), conduction abnormalities, or injection-site reactions (eg, erythema, tenderness, swelling, discoloration) occur.

Administration: IV route. **Storage:** 20-25°C (68-77°F). Protect from light.

PAMELOR   RX
nortriptyline HCl (Mallinckrodt)

> Antidepressants increased the risk of suicidal thinking and behavior (suicidality) in short-term studies in children, adolescents, and young adults with major depressive disorder (MDD) and other psychiatric disorders. Monitor and observe closely for clinical worsening, suicidality, or unusual changes in behavior in patients who are started on antidepressant therapy. Nortriptyline is not approved for use in pediatric patients.

THERAPEUTIC CLASS: Tricyclic antidepressant

INDICATIONS: Relief of symptoms of depression.

DOSAGE: *Adults;* 25mg tid-qid. Max: 150mg/day. Total daily dose may be given once a day. Monitor serum levels if dose >100mg/day. Elderly/Adolescents: 30-50mg/day in single or divided doses.

HOW SUPPLIED: Cap: 10mg, 25mg, 50mg, 75mg; Sol: 10mg/5mL

CONTRAINDICATIONS: MAOI use within 14 days, acute recovery period following MI.

WARNINGS/PRECAUTIONS: MI, arrhythmia, strokes have occurred. Caution with cardiovascular disease (CVD), glaucoma, history of urinary retention, hyperthyroidism. May lower seizure threshold, exacerbate psychosis or activate schizophrenia, cause symptoms of mania in bipolar disease, or alter glucose levels. D/C several days prior to elective surgery.

ADVERSE REACTIONS: Arrhythmias, hypotension, HTN, tachycardia, MI, heart block, stroke, confusion, hallucination, insomnia, tremors, ataxia, dry mouth, blurred vision, skin rash.

INTERACTIONS: See Contraindications. May block guanethidine effects. Arrhythmia risk with thyroid agents. Alcohol may potentiate effects. "Stimulating" effect with reserpine. Monitor with anticholinergic and sympathomimetic drugs. Increased plasma levels with cimetidine. Hypoglycemia reported with chlorpropamide. SSRIs, antidepressants, phenothiazines, propafenone, flecainide and CYP2D6 inhibitors (eg, quinidine) may potentiate effects. Decreased clearance with quinidine.

PREGNANCY: Safety during pregnancy and nursing not known.

MECHANISM OF ACTION: Tricyclic antidepressant; inhibits activity of histamine, 5-hydroxytryptamine, and acetylcholine; increases pressor effect of NE, blocks pressor response of phenethylamine, and interferes with transport, release, and storage of catecholamine.

NURSING CONSIDERATIONS

Assessment: Assess if acute recovery period after MI, for bipolar disorder risk, history of mania, unrecognized/history of schizophrenia, possible drug interactions, history of seizures, CVD, hyperthyroidism, DM, glaucoma, urinary retention, history of agitation or overactivity, and pregnancy/nursing status.

Monitoring: Periodically monitor blood glucose. Monitor for signs/symptoms of clinical worsening (suicidality, unusual changes in behavior), mania, cardiovascular events, increasing psychosis, increasing anxiety/agitation, mydriasis, hypo/hyperglycemia, seizures, cognitive/motor impairment.

Patient Counseling: Advise to avoid alcohol. Seek medical attention for symptoms of activation of mania, seizures, clinical worsening (suicidal ideation, unusual changes in behavior), cardiovascular events, increasing psychosis, increasing anxiety/agitation, mydriasis, and hypo/hyperglycemia. May impair physical/mental abilities.

Administration: Oral route. **Storage:** 20-25°C (68-77°F).

PANCREAZE   RX
pancrelipase (McNeil Pediatrics)

THERAPEUTIC CLASS: Pancreatic enzyme supplement

INDICATIONS: Treatment of exocrine pancreatic insufficiency due to cystic fibrosis or other conditions.

DOSAGE: *Adults:* Individualize dose based on clinical symptoms, degree of steatorrhea present, and fat content of diet. Initial: 500 U lipase/kg/meal. Max: 2,500 U lipase/kg/meal (≤10,000 U lipase/kg/day) or <4,000 U lipase/g fat ingested/day. Usual: Half of the dose used for meals should be given with each snack. Approximately 3 meals plus 2 or 3 snacks/day should reflect a total daily dose. Swallow whole with sufficient fluid; do not crush or chew. *Pediatrics:* Individualize dose based on clinical symptoms, degree of steatorrhea present, and fat content of diet. ≥4 yrs: Initial: 500 U lipase/kg/meal. Max: 2,500 U lipase/kg/meal (≤10,000 U lipase/kg/day) or <4,000 U lipase/g fat ingested/day. Usual: Half of the dose used for meals should be given with each snack. Approximately 3 meals plus 2 or 3 snacks/day should reflect a total daily dose. Swallow whole with sufficient fluid; do not crush or chew. >12 months-<4 yrs: Initial: 1,000 U lipase/kg/meal. Max: 2,500 U lipase/kg/meal (≤10,000 U lipase/kg/day) or <4,000 U lipase/g fat ingested/day. Infants: ≤12 months: 2,000-4,000 lipase units/120mL of formula or/breast milk. Do not mix capsule contents directly into formula or breast milk.

HOW SUPPLIED: Cap, Delayed-Release: (Amylase-Lipase-Protease) (MT4) 17,500 U-4,200 U-10,000 U, (MT10) 43,750 U-10,500 U-25,000 U, (MT 16) 70,000 U-16,800 U-40,000 U, (MT20) 61,000 U-21,000 U-37,000 U

WARNINGS/PRECAUTIONS: Fibrosing colonopathy reported; monitor closely for some may be at risk of progressing to stricture formation. Colonic strictures reported in children <12 yrs with doses exceeding 6,000 U lipase/kg/meal; assess and titrate dosage downward to a lower range. Caution in doses >2,500 U lipase/kg/meal. May irritate oral mucosa; care should be taken to ensure that no drug is retained in the mouth. Caution with gout, renal impairment, or hyperuricemia; may increase blood uric acid levels. Theoretical risk for transmission of viral disease, including diseases caused by novel or unidentified viruses. Caution with known allergy to porcine protein. Do not interchange with other pancrelipase products.

ADVERSE REACTIONS: Abdominal pain, flatulence.

INTERACTIONS: May diminish efficacy if contents are mixed directly into formula or breast milk.

PREGNANCY: Category C, caution in nursing.

MECHANISM OF ACTION: Pancreatic enzyme supplement; catalyzes the hydrolysis of fats to monoglycerides, glycerol and free fatty acids, proteins into peptides and amino acids, and starches into dextrins and short chain sugars such as maltose and maltriose in the duodenum and proximal small intestine, thereby acting like digestive enzymes physiologically secreted by the pancreas.

NURSING CONSIDERATIONS

Assessment: Assess for allergy to porcine protein, gout, renal impairment, hyperuricemia, pregnancy/nursing status.

Monitoring: Monitor for fibrosing colonopathy, colonic stricture, oral mucosa irritation, viral diseases, and for allergic reactions (eg, anaphylaxis, asthma, hives and pruritus). Monitor serum uric acid levels.

Patient Counseling: Instruct to take medication as prescribed and follow dosing instructions carefully. Inform that if a dose was missed, take the next dose with the next meal/snack as directed. Instruct not to take a double dose or increase dose on their own. Take with food. Swallow whole with adequate amounts of liquid; do not crush, chew, or mix directly with formula or breast milk. If cannot swallow intact cap, it may be opened carefully and the contents may be added or sprinkled onto a small amount of acidic food (pH <4.5) such as applesauce. Care should be taken to ensure that no drug is retained in the mouth to avoid oral mucosa irritation. Notify healthcare professional if pregnant/breastfeeding or thinking of becoming pregnant/breastfeeding during therapy. Advise to contact healthcare professional immediately if allergic reactions develop.

Administration: Oral route. Administer immediately to infants prior to each feeding. Avoid mixing directly into formula or breast milk. Contents may be administered directly in the mouth followed by breast milk or formula. Ensure that no drug is retained in the mouth. Contents may be sprinkled on small amounts of acidic soft food with a pH of <4.5 (eg, applesauce) and should be swallowed immediately with sufficient fluid or given to infant within 15 mins.
Storage: Do not store above 25ºC (77ºF). Avoid heat. Store in a dry place in original container. Protect from moisture.

PARCOPA   RX
levodopa - carbidopa (Schwarz)

THERAPEUTIC CLASS: Dopa-decarboxylase inhibitor/dopamine precursor

INDICATIONS: Treatment of symptoms of idiopathic Parkinson's disease, postencephalitic parkinsonism, and symptomatic parkinsonism.

DOSAGE: *Adults:* 25mg-100mg tab: Initial: 1 tab tid. Titrate: Increase by 1 tab qd or qod until 8 tabs/day. 10mg-100mg tab: Initial: 1 tab tid-qid. Titrate: Increase 1 tab qd or qod until 2 tabs qid. 70-100mg/day carbidopa required. Max: 200mg/day carbidopa. Levodopa must be d/c 12 hrs before starting carbidopa-levodopa.

HOW SUPPLIED: Tab, Disintegrating: (Carbidopa-Levodopa) 10mg-100mg*, 25mg-100mg*, 25mg-250mg* *scored

CONTRAINDICATIONS: MAOIs during or within 14 days of use; narrow-angle glaucoma; suspicious, undiagnosed skin lesions; history of melanoma.

WARNINGS/PRECAUTIONS: Dyskinesias and mental disturbances may occur. Caution with severe cardiovascular(CV) or pulmonary disease, bronchial asthma, renal or hepatic disease, endocrine disease, chronic wide-angle glaucoma, peptic ulcer, and MI with residual arrhythmias. Neuroleptic malignant syndrome (NMS) reported during dose reduction or withdrawal. Dark color may appear in saliva, urine, or sweat. May cause false (+) ketonuria or false (-) glucosuria (glucose-oxidase method).

ADVERSE REACTIONS: Dyskinesias, choreiform, dystonia and other involuntary movements, nausea.

INTERACTIONS: See Contraindications. Risk of postural hypotension with antihypertensives, selegiline. HTN and dyskinesia may occur with TCAs. Reduced effects with dopamine D_2 antagonists (eg, phenothiazines, butyrophenones, risperidone), isoniazid. Antagonized by phenytoin, papaverine, metoclopramide. Reduced bioavailability with iron salts, high-protein diets.

PREGNANCY: Category C, caution in nursing

MECHANISM OF ACTION: Carbidopa: Inhibits decarboxylation of peripheral levodopa. Levodopa: Crosses blood-brain barrier, converting into dopamine and thereby increasing concentrations in the brain.

PHARMACOKINETICS: Absorption: Carbidopa: Bioavailability (99%).
Elimination: Urine.

NURSING CONSIDERATIONS

Assessment: Assess for glaucoma, CV or pulmonary disease, melanoma, asthma, phenylketonuria, or any other conditions where treatment is contraindicated or cautioned. Assess LFTs, renal function, CBC, pregnancy/nursing status, and possible drug interactions.

Monitoring: Monitor for cardiac, hepatic/renal functions during initial dosage adjustment period, depression and suicidal ideation, worsening of dyskinesia, rhabdomyolysis, diarrhea, hallucinations, fibrotic complications, hyperpyrexia, melanomas, IOP, and hypersensitivity reactions.

P

Patient Counseling: Instruct to take as prescribed. Caution while operating machinery/driving. Discoloration of body fluids may occur. High-protein diet, excessive acidity, and iron salts reduce clinical effectiveness. Wearing-off effect may be seen at end of dosing interval. Report any adverse effects. Place tablet on tongue and dissolve with saliva.

Administration: Oral route. **Storage:** 20-25°C (68-77°F); excursions permitted to 15-30°C (59-86°F).

PARLODEL
bromocriptine mesylate (Novartis)

RX

THERAPEUTIC CLASS: Dopamine receptor agonist

INDICATIONS: Treatment of dysfunctions associated with hyperprolactinemia including amenorrhea with or without galactorrhea, infertility, or hypogonadism. Treatment of prolactin-secreting adenomas, acromegaly, and signs and symptoms of idiopathic or postencephalitic Parkinson's disease.

DOSAGE: *Adults:* Take with food. Parkinson's Disease: Initial: 1.25mg bid. Titrate: If needed, increase by 2.5mg/day every 2-4 weeks. Max: 100mg/day. Hyperprolactinemia: Initial: 1.25mg-2.5mg qd. Titrate: If needed, increase by 2.5mg every 2-7 days. Usual: 2.5-15mg/day. Acromegaly: Initial: 1.25-2.5mg qhs for 3 days. Titrate: Increase by 1.25-2.5mg every 3-7 days until optimal response achieved. Usual: 20-30mg/day. Max: 100mg/day. Withdraw for 4-8 weeks every year in patients treated with pituitary irradiation.
Pediatrics: Take with food. 11-15 yrs: Prolactin-Secreting Pituitary Adenomas: Initial: 1.25-2.5mg/day. Titrate: Increase as tolerated. Usual: 2.5-10mg/day.

HOW SUPPLIED: Cap: 5mg; Tab: 2.5mg* *scored

CONTRAINDICATIONS: Uncontrolled HTN, postpartum period in women with history of CAD and other severe CV conditions unless withdrawal is medically contraindicated, pregnancy if treating hyperprolactinemia. Hypertensive disorders of pregnancy if used to treat acromegaly, prolactinoma, or Parkinson's disease, unless withdrawal is medically contraindicated.

WARNINGS/PRECAUTIONS: Perform evaluation of the pituitary before treatment. Safety during pregnancy not established. May cause somnolence and sudden sleep onset; consider dose reduction or d/c. Symptomatic hypotension may occur. HTN, seizures, strokes, and MI reported in postpartum patients; not recommended for use in prevention of physiological lactation; monitor BP; if HTN, severe, progressive, or unremitting headache, or evidence of CNS toxicity develops, d/c and evaluate. Pleural and pericardial effusions, pleural and pulmonary fibrosis, and constrictive pericarditis reported; perform exam and consider d/c if pleuropulmonary disorders develop. Retroperitoneal fibrosis reported; d/c if fibrotic changes in the retroperitoneum are diagnosed or suspected. Caution with a history of psychosis or CVD. Avoid with galactose intolerance. Monitor visual fields in patients with macroprolactinoma; rapidly progressive visual field loss should be evaluated by a neurosurgeon. Contraceptive measures, other than oral contraceptives should be used if not seeking pregnancy or if have large adenomas. In patients with amenorrhea, perform pregnancy test every 4 weeks during amenorrheic period, and once menses are reinitiated, every time a menstrual period is missed; d/c if pregnancy established. Cerebrospinal rhinorrhea observed in patients with prolactin-secreting adenomas. Cold-sensitive digital vasospasm and possible tumor expansion reported in acromegalic patients. Severe GI bleeding from peptic ulcers reported in acromegalic patients. High doses may cause confusion and mental disturbances; caution with dementia. May cause hallucinations. Caution with history of MI who have residual atrial, nodal, or ventricular arrhythmia.

ADVERSE REACTIONS: N/V, headache, dizziness, constipation, abdominal cramps, orthostatic hypotension, fatigue, insomnia, hallucinations, abnormal involuntary movements, depression,

INTERACTIONS: Decreased effects with dopamine antagonists (eg, butyrophenones, haloperidol, phenothiazines, pimozide, metoclopramide). Increased plasma levels with macrolide antibiotics (eg, erythromycin) and octreotide. Concomitant use with levodopa may cause hallucinations. Caution with antihypertensives and drugs that are strong inhibitors and/or substrates of CYP3A4 (eg, azole antimycotics, HIV protease inhibitors). Alcohol may potentiate side effects. Concomitant use with other ergot alkaloids is not recommended.

PREGNANCY: Category B, not for use in nursing.

MECHANISM OF ACTION: Dopamine receptor agonist; activates post-synaptic dopamine receptors and modulates prolactin secretion from anterior pituitary by secreting prolactin inhibitory factor.

PHARMACOKINETICS: Absorption: GI tract (28%); C_{max} =0.465ng/mL (5mg); T_{max}=1-3 hrs. **Distribution:** Serum albumin binding (90-96%) (*in vitro*). **Metabolism:** Liver, via CYP3A and hydroxylation. **Elimination:** Liver and kidneys (6%); $T_{1/2}$=15 hrs.

NURSING CONSIDERATIONS

Assessment: Assess for HTN, history of CAD or other severe CV conditions, pituitary tumors, dementia, history of psychosis, history of peptic ulcer or GI bleeding, galactose intolerance, renal/hepatic disease, pregnancy/nursing status, and for possible drug interactions. Perform complete pituitary evaluation.

Monitoring: Monitor for GI bleeding, somnolence, sudden sleep onset, hypotension, HTN, seizures, stroke, MI, pleural and pericardial effusions, pleural and pulmonary fibrosis, constrictive pericarditis, retroperitoneal fibrosis, visual disturbances, cold sensitive digital vasospasm, peptic ulcers, confusion and mental disturbances. Monitor BP, CBC, prolactin levels, LFTs, and renal function. Monitor visual fields in patients with macroprolactinoma; rapidly progressive visual field loss should be evaluated by a neurosurgeon.

Patient Counseling: Advise to use caution while operating machinery/driving. Instruct to take exactly as prescribed with food. Counsel to report lack of response, if adverse effects develop, or if pregnant or nursing.

Administration: Oral route. **Storage:** Store below 25°C (77°F); tight, light-resistant container.

PARNATE RX
tranylcypromine sulfate (GlaxoSmithKline)

> Antidepressants increased the risk of suicidal thinking and behavior (suicidality) in short-term studies in children, adolescents, and young adults with major depressive disorder (MDD) and other psychiatric disorders. Monitor and observe closely for clinical worsening, suicidality, or unusual changes in behavior in patients who are started on antidepressant therapy. Tranylcypromine is not approved for use in pediatric patients.

THERAPEUTIC CLASS: Monoamine oxidase inhibitor

INDICATIONS: Treatment of major depressive episode without melancholia.

DOSAGE: *Adults:* Usual: 30mg qd in divided doses. Titrate: If no improvement after 2 weeks, may increase by 10mg/day increments every 1-3 weeks. Max: 60mg/day.

HOW SUPPLIED: Tab: 10mg

CONTRAINDICATIONS: Concomitant use with MAO inhibitors or dibenzazepine derivatives, sympathomimetics (eg, amphetamines) or OTC drugs such as cold, hay fever, weight-reducing products that contain vasoconstrictors, some CNS depressants (eg, narcotics and alcohol), antihypertensive agents, diuretics, antihistamine, sedative or anesthetic drugs, bupropion, buspirone, dextromethorphan, SSRIs (eg, fluoxetine, paroxetine, sertraline), meperidine, anesthetic agents, anti-parkinsonism drugs, cheese or other foods with a high tyramine content, or excessive quantities of caffeine. Cerebrovascular disorders, cardiovascular disease (CVD), HTN, history of headaches, pheochromocytoma, history of liver disease, abnormal LFTs. Elective surgery requiring general anesthesia.

WARNINGS/PRECAUTIONS: Anxiety, agitation, panic attacks, insomnia, irritability, hostility, aggressiveness, impulsivity, akathisia, hypomania, mania reported. D/C if hypertensive crisis (eg, occipital headache, neck stiffness or soreness, N/V, tachycardia, bradycardia), palpitations, and/or frequent headaches occur. Hypotension reported. Caution in epileptic patients; may lower seizure threshold. D/C at first sign of hepatic dysfunction or jaundice; monitor LFTs periodically. Caution in patients with renal dysfunction, hyperthyroidism, elderly and diabetics taking insulin or glycemic agents. Drug dependency possible in doses excessive of the therapeutic range. May suppress anginal pain in myocardial ischemia. May precipitate mixed/manic episode in patients at risk for bipolar disorder; adequately screen patients to determine risk prior to initiating treatment. May impair mental/physical abilities.

ADVERSE REACTIONS: Restlessness, insomnia, weakness, drowsiness, nausea, diarrhea, tachycardia, anorexia, edema, tinnitus, muscle spasm, overstimulation, dizziness, dry mouth.

INTERACTIONS: See Contraindications. Caution with disulfiram. Additive hypotensive effects with phenothiazines. Tryptophan may precipitate disorientation, memory impairment and other neurological and behavioral signs. Avoid metrizamide; d/c 48 hrs before myelography and may resume 24 hrs post-procedure. Concurrent use with guanethidine, methyldopa, reserpine, dopamine, levodopa may precipitate HTN, headache and related symptoms.

PREGNANCY: Safety in pregnancy and nursing not known.

MECHANISM OF ACTION: Non-hydrazine MAOI; inhibits monoamine oxidase, increasing concentration of epinephrine, norepinephrine, and serotonin in storage sites throughout the nervous system.

NURSING CONSIDERATIONS

Assessment: Assess for risk of bipolar disorder, history of CVD, HTN, history of headaches, cerebrovascular disease, pheochromocytoma, seizure disorder, hyperthyroidism, DM, history of hepatic impairment, severe renal impairment, suicidal thinking and behavior, pregnancy/nursing status, and possible drug interactions.

Monitoring: Monitor BP, HR, renal/hepatic function, for signs and symptoms of clinical worsening, hypertensive crisis, seizures in epileptic patients, postural hypotension, and hypoglycemia in diabetics.

Patient Counseling: Inform family and caregivers the need to monitor for emergence of agitation, irritability, unusual changes in behavior, suicidality; notify healthcare provider if symptoms occur. Report occurrences of headache or other unusual symptoms (eg, palpitations, tachycardia, severe constriction in the throat or chest, N/V). Advise to seek medical attention for symptoms of hypertensive crisis, hypoglycemia, or seizures. Inform of the possibility of hypotension, faintness, drowsiness. May impair performance of potentially hazardous tasks, such as driving a car or operating machinery. Advise to avoid concomitant intake of alcohol, foods with a high tyramine content (eg, cheese), dextromethorphan, excessive quantities of caffeine. Caution not to take concomitant prescription or OTC medications without advice of a physician.

Administration: Oral route. **Storage:** 15-30°C (59-86°F). Dispense in tight, light-resistant container.

PATANOL   RX
olopatadine HCl (Alcon)

THERAPEUTIC CLASS: H₁-antagonist and mast cell stabilizer
INDICATIONS: Allergic conjunctivitis.
DOSAGE: *Adults:* 1 drop bid, q6-8h.
Pediatrics: ≥3 yrs: 1 drop bid, q6-8h.
HOW SUPPLIED: Sol: 0.1% [5mL]
WARNINGS/PRECAUTIONS: May re-insert contact lens 10 min after dosing if eye is not red. Not for injection or oral use.

ADVERSE REACTIONS: Headache, asthenia, blurred vision, burning, stinging, cold syndrome, dry eye, foreign body sensation, hyperemia, hypersensitivity, keratitis, lid edema, nausea, pharyngitis, pruritus, rhinitis.

PREGNANCY: Category C, caution in nursing.

MECHANISM OF ACTION: Antihistaminic drug; relatively selective histamine H₁-antagonist; inhibits the type 1 immediate hypersensitivity reaction, including inhibition of histamine induced effects on human conjunctival epithelial cells.

PHARMACOKINETICS: Absorption: C_{max}=0.5-1.3ng/mL; T_{max}=2 hrs. **Metabolism:** Metabolites: Mono-desmethyl and N-oxide. **Elimination:** Urine (60-70% parent drug).

NURSING CONSIDERATIONS

Assessment: Assess for drug hypersensitivity.

Monitoring: Monitor for headache and other adverse reactions.

Patient Counseling: Counsel not to wear contact lenses if eye is red; wait at least 10 min after instillation to wear contact lenses. Instruct to avoid touching tip of container to eye or any other surface to avoid contamination.

Administration: Ocular route. **Storage:** 4-25°C (39-77°F). Keep bottle tightly closed.

PAXIL **RX**
paroxetine HCl (GlaxoSmithKline)

> Antidepressants increased the risk of suicidal thinking and behavior (suicidality) in short-term studies in children, adolescents, and young adults with major depressive disorder (MDD) and other psychiatric disorders. Monitor and observe closely for clinical worsening, suicidality, or unusual changes in behavior in patients who are started on antidepressant therapy. Paroxetine HCl is not approved for use in pediatric patients.

THERAPEUTIC CLASS: Selective serotonin reuptake inhibitor

INDICATIONS: Treatment of major depressive disorder (MDD), panic disorder with or without agoraphobia, obsessive compulsive disorder (OCD), social anxiety disorder (SAD), generalized anxiety disorder (GAD), and post-traumatic stress disorder (PTSD).

DOSAGE: *Adults:* Give qd, usually in the am. To titrate, may increase in 10mg/day increments at intervals of ≥1 week. Maintain on the lowest effective dose and reassess periodically to determine the need for continued treatment. MDD: Initial: 20mg/day. Max: 50mg/day. Maint: Efficacy is maintained for periods of up to 1 year with doses that averaged about 30mg. OCD: Initial: 20mg/day. Usual: 40mg qd. Max: 60mg/day. Panic Disorder: Initial: 10mg/day. Usual: 40mg/day. Max: 60mg/day. GAD: Initial/Usual: 20mg/day. Dose range: 20-50mg/day. SAD: Initial/Usual: 20mg/day. Dose range: 20-60mg/day. PTSD: Initial: 20mg/day. Dose range: 20-50mg/day. Elderly/Debilitated/Severe Renal/Hepatic Impairment: Initial: 10mg/day. Max: 40mg/day. 3ʳᵈ Trimester Pregnancy: Taper dose. Allow 14-day interval between d/c of monoamine oxidase inhibitor (MAOI) and start of paroxetine HCl and vice versa.

HOW SUPPLIED: Sus: 10mg/5mL [250mL]; Tab: 10mg*, 20mg*, 30mg, 40mg *scored

CONTRAINDICATIONS: Concomitant use with thioridazine, pimozide, and MAOIs including linezolid and methylthioninium chloride (methylene blue) or use within 2 weeks of stopping treatment with MAOIs.

WARNINGS/PRECAUTIONS: Not approved for treatment of bipolar depression. Potentially life-threatening serotonin syndrome (eg, mental status changes, autonomic instability, neuromuscular aberrations and/or GI symptoms) or neuroleptic malignant syndrome (NMS)-like reactions reported. Increased risk of congenital malformations, reported in infants exposed in 1st trimester of pregnancy. Neonatal complications requiring prolonged hospitalization, respiratory support, and tube feeding may develop in neonates exposed in the late third trimester. Activation of mania/hypomania reported; caution in patients

P

with a history of mania. Caution with history of seizures; d/c if seizures occur. Adverse reactions (eg, dysphoric mood, irritability) reported upon d/c; avoid abrupt withdrawal. Akathisia may develop. Hyponatremia reported; caution in elderly and volume-depleted patients. May increase risk of bleeding events. Bone fracture risk reported; consider pathological fracture in patients with unexplained bone pain, point tenderness, swelling or bruising. Caution with disease/conditions that could affect metabolism or hemodynamic responses, narrow-angle glaucoma, severe renal/hepatic impairment, and in elderly and debilitated patients. May impair mental/physical abilities.

ADVERSE REACTIONS: Suicidality, somnolence, headache, insomnia, nausea, asthenia, abnormal ejaculation, dry mouth, constipation, dizziness, diarrhea, decreased libido, sweating, decreased appetite, tremor.

INTERACTIONS: See Contraindications. Serotonin syndrome or NMS-like reactions reported when used alone and in combination with serotonergic drugs (eg, triptans, fentanyl, lithium, tramadol, or St. John's wort), drugs that impair serotonin metabolism, antipsychotics, and dopamine antagonists. Use with other SSRIs, SNRIs, or tryptophan is not recommended. Avoid alcohol. Concomitant use with ASA, NSAIDs, warfarin, and other anticoagulants may increase risk of bleeding events. Use with diuretics may increase risk of developing hyponatremia. Metabolism and pharmacokinetics of paroxetine may be affected by induction or inhibition of drug-metabolizing enzymes. Increased levels with cimetidine. Reduced levels with phenobarbital, phenytoin, fosamprenavir/ritonavir. Increased phenytoin level after 4 weeks of coadministration reported. Caution with drugs that are metabolized by CYP2D6 (eg, antidepressants, phenothiazines, risperidone, Type 1C antiarrhythmics) and with drugs that inhibit CYP2D6 (eg, quinidine). May increase levels of desipramine, risperidone, atomoxetine. May reduce efficacy of tamoxifen. May inhibit metabolism of TCAs; caution with concomitant use. May displace other highly protein-bound drugs. Caution with digoxin. May increase procyclidine levels; reduce dose if anticholinergic effects are seen. Severe hypotension reported when added to chronic metoprolol treatment. May elevate theophylline levels. Caution with lithium.

PREGNANCY: Category D, caution in nursing.

MECHANISM OF ACTION: SSRI; inhibits CNS neuronal reuptake of serotonin.

PHARMACOKINETICS: Absorption: Complete; Tab (30 mg): C_{max}=61.7ng/mL; T_{max}=5.2 hrs. **Distribution:** Plasma protein binding (93-95%); found in breast milk. **Metabolism:** Extensive; oxidation and methylation via CYP2D6. **Elimination:** Sol (30 mg): Urine (62%, metabolites; 2%, parent compound); feces (36%, metabolites; <1%, parent compound); Tab (30 mg): $T_{1/2}$=21 hrs.

NURSING CONSIDERATIONS

Assessment: Assess for history of seizures, history of mania, volume depletion, diseases/conditions that alter metabolism or hemodynamic responses, hepatic/renal impairment, narrow-angle glaucoma, previous hypersensitivity, pregnancy/nursing status, and for possible drug interactions. Assess use in the elderly or debilitated patients. Screen for bipolar disorder.

Monitoring: Monitor for signs/symptoms of clinical worsening, serotonin syndrome or NMS-like reactions, seizures, manic episodes, akathisia, bone fracture, hyponatremia especially in the elderly, and abnormal bleeding. Upon d/c, monitor for symptoms of dysphoric mood, irritability, agitation, dizziness, sensory disturbances, anxiety, confusion, headache, lethargy, emotional lability, insomnia, and hypomania. Periodically assess for need of therapy.

Patient Counseling: Instruct to swallow whole, not to chew or crush. Advise to avoid alcohol. Instruct to notify physician of all prescription, over-the-counter drugs currently taking or planning to take. Caution about the risk of serotonin syndrome with concomitant use of triptans, tramadol, or other serotonergic agents. Instruct the patient, families, and caregivers to report emergence of anxiety, agitation, panic attacks, insomnia, irritability, hostility, aggressiveness, impulsivity, akathisia, hypomania, mania, unusual changes in behavior, worsening of depression, and suicidal ideation, especially during drug initiation or dose adjustment. Caution against hazardous tasks (eg, operating machinery, driving). Inform that improvement may be noticed in 1-4 weeks;

continue therapy as directed. Advise to notify physician if pregnant/intend to become pregnant, or breastfeeding. Caution about concomitant use with NSAIDs, aspirin, warfarin or other drugs that affect coagulation. Counsel about benefits and risks of therapy.

Administration: Oral route. (Tab) Swallow whole; do not crush or chew. (Sus) Shake well before use. **Storage:** (Tab): 15-30°C (59-86°F). (Sus): ≤25°C (77°F).

PAXIL CR

RX

paroxetine HCl (GlaxoSmithKline)

> Antidepressants increased the risk of suicidal thinking and behavior (suicidality) in short-term studies in children, adolescents, and young adults with major depressive disorder (MDD) and other psychiatric disorders. Monitor and observe closely for clinical worsening, suicidality, or unusual changes in behavior in patients who are started on antidepressant therapy. Not approved for use in pediatric patients.

THERAPEUTIC CLASS: Selective serotonin reuptake inhibitor

INDICATIONS: Treatment of major depressive disorder (MDD), panic disorder with or without agoraphobia, social anxiety disorder (SAD), and premenstrual dysphoric disorder (PMDD).

DOSAGE: *Adults:* Give qd, usually in the am with/without food. MDD: Initial: 25mg/day. Titrate: May increase by 12.5mg/day at intervals of ≥1 week. Max: 62.5mg/day. Panic Disorder: Initial: 12.5mg/day. Titrate: May increase by 12.5mg/day at intervals of ≥1 week. Max: 75mg/day. Maint: Lowest effective dose. SAD: Initial: 12.5mg/day. Titrate: May increase by 12.5mg/day at intervals of ≥1 week. Max: 37.5mg/day. Maint: Lowest effective dose. PMDD: Initial: 12.5mg/day. Give either qd throughout menstrual cycle or limited to luteal phase. 25mg/day also shown to be effective. Titrate: Changes should occur at intervals of ≥1 week. Elderly/Debilitated/Severe Renal or Hepatic Impairment: Initial: 12.5mg/day. Max: 50mg/day. 3rd Trimester Pregnancy: Taper dose. Allow ≥14 days interval between d/c of monoamine oxidase inhibitor (MAOI) and start of paroxetine HCl and vice versa. Reduce dose gradually.

HOW SUPPLIED: Tab, Controlled-Release: 12.5mg, 25mg, 37.5mg; (Generic) Tab, Extended-Release: 12.5mg, 25mg

CONTRAINDICATIONS: Concomitant use with thioridazine, pimozide and MAOIs including linezolid or (Paxil CR) methylthioninium chloride (methylene blue) or use within 2 weeks of stopping treatment with MAOIs.

WARNINGS/PRECAUTIONS: Not approved to treat bipolar depression. Serotonin syndrome (eg, mental status changes, autonomic instability, neuromuscular aberrations and/or GI symptoms) or neuroleptic malignant syndrome (NMS)-like reactions reported. Increased risk of congenital malformations reported in 1st trimester of pregnancy. Neonatal complications requiring prolonged hospitalization, respiratory support, and tube feeding may develop in neonates exposed in the late third trimester. Activation of mania/hypomania may occur; caution with a history of mania. Caution with history of seizures; d/c if seizures occur. Adverse reactions upon d/c (eg, dysphoric mood, irritability) reported; avoid abrupt withdrawal. Akathisia may develop. Hyponatremia reported; caution in elderly and volume-depleted patients. May increase risk of bleeding events. Caution with disease/conditions that could affect metabolism or hemodynamic responses, narrow-angle glaucoma, severe renal/hepatic impairment, and in elderly and debilitated patients. May impair mental/physical abilities. (Paxil CR) Bone fracture risk reported; consider pathological fracture in patients with unexplained bone pain, point tenderness, swelling or bruising.

ADVERSE REACTIONS: Suicidality, somnolence, insomnia, nausea, asthenia, abnormal ejaculation, dry mouth, constipation, dizziness, diarrhea, decreased libido, sweating, abnormal vision, headache, tremor.

INTERACTIONS: See Contraindications. Serotonin syndrome or NMS-like reactions reported when used alone and in combination with serotonergic drugs (eg, triptans, fentanyl, lithium, tramadol, or St. John's wort), drugs that impair serotonin metabolism, antipsychotics, and dopamine antagonists. Use

P

with other SSRIs, SNRIs, or tryptophan is not recommended. Avoid alcohol. Concomitant use with ASA, NSAIDs, warfarin, and other drugs that may affect coagulation may increase risk of bleeding events. Use with diuretics may increase risk of developing hyponatremia. Metabolism and pharma-cokinetics may be affected by induction or inhibition of drug-metabolizing enzymes. Increased levels with cimetidine. Reduced levels with phenobarbital, phenytoin, fosamprenavir/ritonavir. Increased phenytoin level after 4 weeks of coadministration reported. Caution with drugs that are metabolized by CYP2D6 (eg, antidepressants, phenothiazines, risperidone, tamoxifen, Type 1C antiarrhythmics) and with drugs that inhibit CYP2D6 (eg, quinidine). May increase levels of desipramine, risperidone, atomoxetine. May reduce efficacy of tamoxifen. May inhibit metabolism of TCAs; caution with concomitant use. May displace or be displaced by other highly protein-bound drugs. Caution with digoxin; decreased levels seen. May increase procyclidine levels; reduce dose if anticholinergic effects are seen. Severe hypotension may occur when added to chronic metoprolol treatment. May elevate theophylline levels. Caution with lithium.

PREGNANCY: Category D, caution in nursing.

MECHANISM OF ACTION: SSRI; inhibits CNS neuronal reuptake of serotonin.

PHARMACOKINETICS: Absorption: Complete; administration of variable doses resulted in different parameters; T_{max}=6-10 hrs. **Distribution:** Plasma protein binding (93-95%); found in breast milk. **Metabolism:** Extensive; oxida-tion and methylation via CYP2D6. **Elimination:** Sol: Urine (62%, metabolites; 2%, parent); feces (36%, metabolites; <1%, parent). $T_{1/2}$=15-20 hrs.

NURSING CONSIDERATIONS

Assessment: Assess for history of seizures or mania, volume depletion, dis-eases/conditions that affect metabolism or hemodynamic response, hepatic/renal impairment, narrow-angle glaucoma, previous hypersensitivity, preg-nancy/nursing status, and for possible drug interactions. Assess use in the elderly or debilitated patients. Screen for bipolar disorder.

Monitoring: Monitor for signs/symptoms of clinical worsening, serotonin syndrome or NMS-like reactions, seizures, mania, akathisia, bone fracture, hyponatremia especially in the elderly, and abnormal bleeding. Upon d/c, monitor for symptoms of dysphoric mood, irritability, agitation, dizziness, sen-sory disturbances, anxiety, confusion, headache, lethargy, emotional lability, insomnia, and hypomania. Periodically assess for need of therapy.

Patient Counseling: Inform patient to swallow whole, not to chew or crush, and to avoid alcohol use. Notify physician of all prescription, over-the-counter drugs currently taking or planning to take. Caution on risk of serotonin syndrome with concomitant use of triptans, tramadol, or other serotonergic agents. Instruct patient, families, and caregivers to report emergence of anxi-ety, agitation, panic attacks, insomnia, irritability, hostility, aggressiveness, impulsivity, akathisia, hypomania, mania, unusual changes in behavior, wors-ening of depression, and suicidal ideation, especially during drug initiation or dose adjustment. Caution against hazardous tasks (eg, operating machinery, driving). Inform that improvement may be noticed in 1-4 weeks; continue therapy as directed. Notify physician if pregnant/intend to become pregnant, or breastfeeding. Caution on concomitant use with NSAIDs, aspirin, warfarin or other drugs that affect coagulation.

Administration: Oral route. Swallow whole; do not chew or crush. **Storage:** ≤25°C (77°F). (Generic) 20-25°C (68-77°F).

PEDIAPRED   RX
prednisolone sodium phosphate (Celltech)

THERAPEUTIC CLASS: Glucocorticoid

INDICATIONS: Steroid-responsive dermatoses.

DOSAGE: *Adults:* Initial: 5-60mg/day depending on disease and response. Maint: Decrease dose by small amounts to lowest effective dose. MS

Exacerbations: 200mg qd for 1 week, then 80mg qod for 1 month.
Pediatrics: Initial: 0.14-2mg/kg/day given tid-qid. Nephrotic Syndrome:
20mg/m² tid for 4 weeks, then 40mg/m² qod for 4 weeks. Uncontrolled
Asthma: 1-2mg/kg/day in single or divided doses until peak expiratory rate of
80% is achieved (usually 3-10 days).

HOW SUPPLIED: Sol: 5mg/5mL [120mL]

CONTRAINDICATIONS: Systemic fungal infections.

WARNINGS/PRECAUTIONS: May produce reversible HPA axis suppression.
Adjust dose during stress or change in thyroid status. May mask signs of
infection or cause new infections. May activate latent amebiasis. Avoid with
cerebral malaria. Avoid exposure to chickenpox or measles. Not for treatment
of optic neuritis or active ocular herpes simplex. May cause elevation of BP
or IOP, cataracts, glaucoma, optic nerve damage, Kaposi's sarcoma, psychic
derangements, salt/water retention, increased excretion of K^+ and/or calcium,
osteoporosis, growth suppression in children, secondary ocular infections.
Caution with strongyloides, CHF, diverticulitis, HTN, renal insufficiency,
fresh intestinal anastomoses, active or latent peptic ulcer, ulcerative colitis.
Enhanced effect in hypothyroidism or cirrhosis. Avoid abrupt withdrawal.
Caution in elderly, increased risk of corticosteroid-induced side effects; start
at low end of dosing range; monitor bone mineral density.

ADVERSE REACTIONS: Edema, fluid/electrolyte disturbances, osteoporosis,
muscle weakness, pancreatitis, peptic ulcer, impaired wound healing, increased intracranial pressure, cushingoid state, hirsutism, menstrual irregularities, growth suppression in children, glaucoma, nausea, weight gain.

INTERACTIONS: Enhanced metabolism with barbiturates, phenytoin, ephedrine, and rifampin. Use with cyclosporine may increase activity of both drugs;
convulsions reported with concomitant use. Decreased metabolism with estrogens or ketoconazole. May inhibit response to warfarin. Increased risk of GI
side effects with ASA or other NSAIDs. May increase clearance of salicylates.
High doses or concurrent neuromuscular drugs may cause acute myopathy.
Enhanced possibility of hypokalemia when given with K^+-depleting agents.
May produce severe weakness in myasthenia gravis patients on anticholinesterase agents. Avoid live vaccines with immunosuppressive doses. Possible
diminished response with killed or inactivated vaccines. May increase blood
glucose; adjust antidiabetic agents. May suppress reactions to skin tests.

PREGNANCY: Category C, caution in nursing.

MECHANISM OF ACTION: Synthetic adrenocorticoid steroid; promotes gluconeogenesis, increases deposition of glycogen in the liver, inhibits glucose
utilization, increases catabolism of protein, lipolysis, glomerular filtration that
leads to increased urinary excretion of urate and calcium.

PHARMACOKINETICS: Absorption: Rapidly absorbed from GI tract.
Distribution: Plasma protein binding (70-90%); found in breast milk.
Metabolism: Liver. **Elimination:** Urine (as sulfate and glucuronide congu-
gates); $T_{1/2}$=2-4 hrs.

NURSING CONSIDERATIONS

Assessment: Assess for systemic fungal/other infections, active TB, vaccination history, HTN, CHF, renal insufficiency, ophthalmic disease, osteoporosis,
thyroid status, hepatic impairment, nonspecific ulcerative colitis, ulcers, preg-
nancy/nursing status, and possible drug interactions.

Monitoring: Monitor for adrenocortical insufficiency, occurrence of infections,
psychic derangement, cataracts, acute myopathy, Kaposi's sarcoma, fluid
retention, and measurement of serum electrolytes, TSH, LFTs, glucose, IOP,
and BP.

Patient Counseling: Advise not to d/c therapy abruptly or without medical
supervision. Avoid exposure to chickenpox or measles; report immediately if
exposed. Dietary salt restriction and K^+ supplementation is advised.

Administration: Oral route. **Storage:** 4-25°C (39-77°F).

PEDIARIX RX

pertussis vaccine, acellular - hepatitis B (recombinant) - poliovirus vaccine, inactivated - diphtheria toxoid - tetanus toxoid (GlaxoSmithKline)

THERAPEUTIC CLASS: Vaccine/toxoid combination

INDICATIONS: Active immunization against diphtheria, tetanus, pertussis, all known subtypes of hepatitis B virus (HBV), and poliomyelitis in infants born of HBsAg-negative mothers, beginning as early as 6 weeks through 6 years (prior to 7th birthday).

DOSAGE: *Pediatrics:* ≥6 weeks - 6 yrs: 3 doses of 0.5mL IM at 2, 4, and 6 months (6-8 week intervals, preferably 8 weeks). May be used to complete the first 3 doses of DTaP series in children who have received 1 or 2 doses of Infanrix and are also scheduled to receive other vaccine components of Pediarix. May be used to complete the HBV vaccination series following 1 or 2 doses of another HBV vaccine including vaccines from other manufacturers in children born of HBsAg-negative mothers who are also scheduled to receive the other components of Pediarix. May be used to complete first 3 doses of the IPV series in children who have received 1 or 2 doses of IPV from other manufacturers and are scheduled to receive other components of Pediarix. May use Infanrix and Kinrix to complete DTaP and IPV series.

HOW SUPPLIED: Inj: 0.5mL [prefilled syringe, vial]

CONTRAINDICATIONS: Encephalopathy (eg, coma, decreased level of consciousness, prolonged seizures) within 7 days of administration of a previous pertussis-containing vaccine that is not attributable to another cause. Progressive neurologic disorder, including infantile spasms, uncontrolled epilepsy, or progressive encephalopathy. Hypersensitivity to yeast, neomycin, or polymyxin B.

WARNINGS/PRECAUTIONS: Caution with Guillain-Barre syndrome occurring within 6 weeks of receipt of prior vaccine containing tetanus toxoid. Risk of fever. Caution if any of the following occur in temporal relation to receipt of any pertussis-containing vaccine: temperature ≥40.5°C (105°F) within 48 hrs not due to another identifiable cause; collapse or shock-like state (hypotonic-hyporesponsive episode) occurring within 48 hrs; persistent, inconsolable crying lasting ≥3 hrs occurring within 48 hrs; or seizures (with or without fever) occurring within 3 days. For children with a higher risk for seizures, administer antipyretic at the time of vaccination. Tip cap and rubber plunger of prefilled syringe contain dry natural rubber latex; use of these syringes may cause allergic reactions in latex sensitive individuals. Epinephrine and other appropriate agents should be immediately available for the control of allergic reactions. Apnea following IM vaccine has been observed in premature infants.

ADVERSE REACTIONS: Local injection-site reactions (eg, pain, redness, swelling), fever, fussiness, irritability, drowsiness, loss of appetite.

INTERACTIONS: Immunosuppressive therapies including irradiation, antimetabolites, alkylating agents, cytotoxic drugs, and corticosteroids (used in greater than physiologic doses) may reduce immune response.

PREGNANCY: Category C, safety in nursing not known.

MECHANISM OF ACTION: Vaccine/toxoid combination; stimulates immune system to elicit immune response, which produces neutralizing antibodies that may protect against diphtheria toxin, tetanus toxin, pertussis, hepatitis B, and poliovirus infections.

NURSING CONSIDERATIONS

Assessment: Review current health status, immunization history for possible vaccine sensitivity and previous vaccination-related adverse reactions. Assess for progressive neurologic disorder, including infantile spasms, uncontrolled epilepsy or progressive encephalopathy, possible drug interactions, or any other conditions where treatment is contraindicated or cautioned. Assess use in premature infants.

Monitoring: Monitor for signs/symptoms of Guillain-Barre syndrome, collapse or shock-like state, hypotonic-hyporesponsive episode, persistent inconsolable crying, fever, seizures, hematoma, and allergic reactions. Monitor for apnea in premature infants.

Patient Counseling: Inform of potential benefits and risks of immunization, and of the importance of completing the immunization series. Counsel about potential adverse reactions and instruct to report any adverse events to their healthcare provider.

Administration: IM route. Shake vial vigorously to obtain homogeneous, turbid, white suspension before use. Do not use if resuspension does not occur with vigorous shaking. Inspect visually for particulate matter and discoloration prior to administration; if any of these conditions exist, do not administer. Preferred administration site of <1 yr of age is anterolateral aspect of thigh; in older children, may administer via deltoid muscle. Do not inject in gluteal area or areas where there may be a major nerve trunk. Do not administer IV, intradermally, or SQ. Do not mix with any other vaccine in the same syringe or vial. **Storage:** 2-8°C (36-46°F). Do not freeze. Discard if frozen.

PEGASYS   RX
peginterferon alfa-2a (Roche)

> May cause or aggravate fatal or life-threatening neuropsychiatric, autoimmune, ischemic, and infectious disorders. Monitor closely with periodic clinical and laboratory evaluations. D/C with persistently severe or worsening signs or symptoms of these conditions. May cause birth defects, fetal death, and hemolytic anemia when used with ribavirin, including Copegus. Refer to the individual PI for more information on ribavirin.

THERAPEUTIC CLASS: Pegylated virus proliferation inhibitor

INDICATIONS: Treatment of chronic hepatitis C (CHC), alone or in combination with Copegus, in adults with compensated liver disease not previously treated with interferon α. Treatment of HBeAg positive and HBeAg negative chronic hepatitis B (CHB) in adults with compensated liver disease, evidence of viral replication, and liver inflammation.

DOSAGE: *Adults:* Administer in abdomen or thigh. CHC: Monotherapy: 180mcg SQ once weekly for 48 weeks. Combination Therapy With Copegus: 180mcg SQ once weekly. Genotype 2 and 3: Treat for 24 weeks. Genotype 1 and 4: Treat for 48 weeks. CHC w/ HIV Coinfection: Monotherapy: 180mcg SQ once weekly for 48 weeks. Combination Therapy with Copegus: 180mcg SQ once weekly for 48 weeks, regardless of genotype. CHB: Monotherapy: 180mcg SQ once weekly for 48 weeks. Refer to PI for dose modification and discontinuation.

HOW SUPPLIED: Inj: 180mcg/0.5mL [prefilled syringe]; 180mcg/mL [single-dose vial]

CONTRAINDICATIONS: Autoimmune hepatitis, hepatic decompensation (Child-Pugh score >6 [class B and C]) in cirrhotic patients before treatment, hepatic decompensation with Child-Pugh score ≥6 in cirrhotic CHC patients coinfected with HIV before treatment, neonates and infants (contains benzyl alcohol). When used with Copegus, refer to PI for additional contraindications.

WARNINGS/PRECAUTIONS: Life-threatening neuropsychiatric reactions may occur; extreme caution with history of depression; d/c immediately in severe cases. Serious infections reported. Risk of bone marrow suppression and may result in severe cytopenias; obtain CBCs prior to initiation and routinely thereafter. Caution with pre-existing cardiac disease. Ischemic and hemorrhagic cerebrovascular events reported. CHC patients with cirrhosis may be at risk for hepatic decompensation and death. Exacerbation of hepatitis B reported. May cause or aggravate hypothyroidism or hyperthyroidism. Hypoglycemia, hyperglycemia, and diabetes mellitus (DM) reported. Caution with autoimmune disorders. May induce or aggravate pulmonary disorders. D/C if pulmonary infiltrates or pulmonary function impairment develops. Hypersensitivity reactions, ulcerative and hemorrhagic/ischemic colitis, and pancreatitis reported; d/c if any of these develop. D/C if new or worsening ophthalmologic disorders occur. Caution with CrCl <50mL/min and in elderly. Safety and efficacy not established in liver or other organ transplant recipients, those who failed other α interferon treatments, hepatitis B patients coinfected with hepatitis C virus (HCV) or HIV, or in HCV patients coinfected with hepatitis B virus (HBV) or coinfected with HIV with a CD4$^+$ count <100 cells/μL.

ADVERSE REACTIONS: Injection-site reactions, fatigue/asthenia, diarrhea, pyrexia, rigors, N/V, neutropenia, myalgia, headache, irritability/anxiety/nervousness, insomnia, depression.

INTERACTIONS: May inhibit CYP1A2 and increase theophylline AUC; monitor theophylline serum levels. Hepatic decompensation can occur with concomitant use of NRTIs and peginterferon alfa-2a/ribavirin; refer to PI for respective NRTIs for guidance regarding toxicity management. May increase methadone levels; monitor for methadone toxicity. Concomitant use of peginterferon alfa-2a/ribavirin with zidovudine may cause severe neutropenia and severe anemia. Peripheral neuropathy reported in combination with telbivudine.

PREGNANCY: Category C, Category X when used with ribavirin, not for use in nursing.

MECHANISM OF ACTION: alfa-2a interferon; binds to human type 1 interferon receptor leading to receptor dimerization which activates multiple intracellular signal transduction pathways initially mediated by the JAK/STAT pathway. Expected to have pleiotropic biological effects in the body.

PHARMACOKINETICS: Absorption: T_{max}=72-96 hrs. **Elimination:** $T_{1/2}$=160 hrs (chronic HCV).

NURSING CONSIDERATIONS

Assessment: Assess for neuropsychiatric, autoimmune, ischemic or infectious disorders, hepatic/renal impairment, risk of severe anemia, known hypersensitivity reactions, pregnancy/nursing status, possible drug interactions, or any other conditions where treatment is contraindicated or cautioned. Obtain baseline CBC, SrCr, TSH, LFTs, CD4$^+$ (HIV), Hgb, Hct, and eye exam. Obtain baseline pregnancy test in women of childbearing potential.

Monitoring: Monitor for neuropsychiatric, autoimmune, ischemic, infectious disorders, bone marrow toxicities, CV disorders, cerebrovascular disorders, or other adverse effects. Monitor hematological (Weeks 2 and 4), biochemical tests (Week 4), LFTs, TSH (q12 weeks). Perform periodic eye exams in patients with pre-existing ophthalmologic disorders. Perform monthly pregnancy tests if on combination therapy with Copegus and for 6 months after d/c. Monitor CBC, clinical status, and hepatic/renal function.

Patient Counseling: Counsel on risks and benefits of therapy. Women who are pregnant or men whose female partners are pregnant should not use combination therapy with Copegus; inform of the teratogenic/embryocidal risks and to use two forms of effective contraception during and for 6 months after therapy. Remain well hydrated. It is not known if therapy will prevent transmission of HCV or HBV infection to others. Avoid driving or operating machinery if dizziness, confusion, somnolence, or fatigue occurs. Avoid drinking alcohol. Do not switch to another brand of interferon without consulting healthcare provider. Inform on preparation, administration, and disposal; do not reuse any needles and syringes.

Administration: SQ route. **Storage:** Refrigerate at 2-8°C (36-46°F). Do not freeze or shake. Protect from light. Discard any unused portion.

PEG-Intron   RX
peginterferon alfa-2b (Schering)

> May cause or aggravate fatal or life-threatening neuropsychiatric, autoimmune, ischemic, and infectious disorders. Monitor closely with periodic clinical and laboratory evaluations. D/C with severe or worsening signs or symptoms of these conditions. Use with Ribavirin: ribavirin may cause birth defects, death of unborn child, and hemolytic anemia. Refer to individual PI for more information on ribavirin.

THERAPEUTIC CLASS: Pegylated virus proliferation inhibitor

INDICATIONS: Treatment of chronic hepatitis C (CHC) in combination with Rebetol (ribavirin) in patients ≥3 yrs with compensated liver disease. Treatment of CHC alone in patients ≥18 yrs with compensated liver disease previously untreated with interferon-alpha.

DOSAGE: *Adults:* ≥18 yrs: Monotherapy: 1mcg/kg/week SQ for 1 yr. Combination Therapy with Ribavirin: 1.5mcg/kg/week SQ with 800-1400mg ribavirin PO based on body weight. Interferon Alpha-naive Patients: Genotype 1: Treat for 48 weeks. Genotype 2 and 3: Treat for 24 weeks. Prior Treatment Failures: Re-treat for 48 weeks, regardless of HCV genotype. Refer to PI for dose recommendation or reduction based on body weight and dose modifications or discontinuations based on depression or laboratory parameters. Renal Impairment: CrCl 30-50mL/min: Reduce dose by 25%. Hemodialysis/CrCl 10-29mL/min: Reduce dose by 50%. D/C if renal function decreases, <2 log$_{10}$ drop or loss of HCV-RNA at 12 weeks, or HCV-RNA levels remain detectable after 24 weeks.
Pediatrics: 3-17 yrs: Combination Therapy with Ribavirin: 60mcg/m2/week SQ with 15mg/kg/day ribavirin PO in 2 divided doses. Remain on pediatric dosing regimen if 18th birthday was reached while receiving therapy. Genotype 1: Treat for 48 weeks. Genotype 2 and 3: Treat for 24 weeks. Refer to PI for dose recommendation or reduction based on body weight and dose modification or discontinuation based on depression or laboratory parameters. Renal Impairment: CrCl 30-50mL/min: Reduce dose by 25%. Hemodialysis/CrCl 10-29mL/min: Reduce dose by 50%. D/C if renal function decreases, HCV-RNA dropped <2 log$_{10}$ at 12 weeks, or HCV-RNA levels remain detectable after 24 weeks.

HOW SUPPLIED: Inj: 50mcg/0.5mL, 80mcg/0.5mL, 120mcg/0.5mL, 150mcg/0.5mL

CONTRAINDICATIONS: Autoimmune hepatitis, hepatic decompensation (Child-Pugh score >6 [class B and C]) in cirrhotic CHC patients. In combination with ribavirin: Pregnancy, women of child-bearing potential, men whose female partners are pregnant, hemoglobinopathies (eg, thalassemia major, sickle cell anemia), CrCl <50mL/min.

WARNINGS/PRECAUTIONS: Caution with history of psychiatric disorders. Monitor patients during treatment and in 6-month follow-up period if psychiatric problems develop; d/c therapy if symptoms persist or worsen. Cases of encephalopathy reported if given in high doses. Hypotension, arrhythmia, tachycardia, cardiomyopathy, angina pectoris, myocardial infarction (MI) reported; caution with cardiovascular disease (CVD). Monitor patients with history of MI and arrhythmia. May cause or aggravate hypothyroidism and hyperthyroidism. Hyperglycemia and diabetes mellitus (DM) reported. Conduct baseline eye exam in all patients and periodic exams with pre-existing ophthalmologic disorders (eg, diabetic or hypertensive retinopathy); d/c if new or worsening ophthalmologic disorders occur. Ischemic and hemorrhagic cerebrovascular events may occur in patients with few or no reported risk factors for stroke and in patients <45 yrs. May cause bone marrow suppression; d/c if severe neutropenia or thrombocytopenia develop. Rare cases of aplastic anemia reported. Caution with CrCl <50mL/min, autoimmune disorders and history of pulmonary disease (eg, chronic obstructive pulmonary disease [COPD]). D/C if serious, acute hypersensitivity (eg, urticaria, angioedema, bronchoconstriction, anaphylaxis) reaction and cutaneous eruptions (Steven-Johnson syndrome [SJS], toxic epidermal necrolysis [TEN]) occur, or if ulcerative or hemorrhagic/ischemic colitis or pancreatitis develop. Risk of hepatic decompensation and death in CHC patients with cirrhosis. Monitor patients with renal impairment for toxicity, including increases in SrCr levels. Elevated ALT and TG levels reported. Concomitant use of peginterferon alpha/ribavirin with zidovudine may cause severe neutropenia and severe anemia. Caution in elderly.

ADVERSE REACTIONS: Headache, fatigue/asthenia, rigors, N/V, abdominal pain, anorexia, emotional lability/irritability, myalgia, injection-site inflammation/erythema/reaction, fever, neutropenia.

INTERACTIONS: May increase methadone levels; monitor signs/symptoms of increased narcotic effect. May decrease therapeutic effects of medications metabolized by CYP2C8/9 (eg, warfarin, phenytoin, tolbutamide) or

P

CYP2D6 (eg, flecainide, dextromethorphan). Monitor treatment-associated toxicities (eg, hepatic decompensation, anemia) with ribavirin and nucleoside reverse transcriptase inhibitors (NRTIs). Peripheral neuropathy reported with telbivudine.

PREGNANCY: Category C, Category X when used with ribavirin, not for use in nursing.

MECHANISM OF ACTION: Pegylated virus proliferation inhibitor; binds to and activates the human type 1 interferon receptor. Upon binding, the receptor subunits dimerize and activate multiple intracellular signal transduction pathways.

PHARMACOKINETICS: Absorption: T_{max}=15-44 hrs. **Elimination:** $T_{1/2}$=40 hrs (HCV-infected).

NURSING CONSIDERATIONS

Assessment: Assess for history of psychiatric disorders, MI, arrhythmia, pulmonary disease, autoimmune and ophthalmologic disorders, CVD, age of patient, risk factors of stroke, hypersensitivity to drug, pregnancy/nursing status and possible drug interactions. Obtain baseline CBC, blood chemistry, LFTs, and renal function (SrCr). Perform eye exam.

Monitoring: Monitor periodically CBC, blood chemistry, LFTs, renal function (SrCr), TSH, bilirubin, uric acid, glucose and TG levels, HCV RNA, and complete eye exam. Monitor for signs/symptoms of autoimmune, ischemic, infectious, endocrine, pulmonary, ophthalmologic, and cerebrovascular disorders, neuropsychiatric events, encephalopathy, bone marrow toxicity, hepatic failure/decompensation, CV events, ulcerative or hemorrhagic/ischemic colitis, pancreatitis, hypersensitivity reactions, and cutaneous eruptions.

Patient Counseling: Inform about the benefits and risks associated with therapy. Instruct to avoid pregnancy during treatment with combination therapy; do not initiate therapy until a report of negative pregnancy test has been obtained. Inform that there are no data regarding whether therapy will prevent transmission of HCV infection to others. Advise to administer drug at bedtime or use antipyretics to minimize flu-like symptoms. Advise to brush teeth thoroughly twice a day and have regular dental examinations during combination treatment. Inform that chest x-ray or other tests may be needed if fever, cough, SOB, or other symptoms of lung problem develop. Keep well-hydrated.

Administration: SQ route. Refer to PI for preparation and instructions for use. Monotherapy: Administer on the same day of the week. Combination therapy with ribavirin: Take with food. **Storage:** (Redipen) 2-8°C (36-46°F). Do not reuse. (Vials) 25°C (77°F); excursions permitted to 15-30°C (59-86°F). After redipen/vial reconstitution, use sol immediately, but may store for ≤24 hrs at 2-8°C (36-46°F). Do not freeze. Keep away from heat.

PENICILLIN VK   RX
penicillin V potassium (Various)

OTHER BRAND NAMES: Veetids (Sandoz)

THERAPEUTIC CLASS: Penicillin

INDICATIONS: Treatment of mild to moderately severe bacterial infections including conditions of the respiratory tract, oropharynx, skin and soft tissue caused by susceptible strains of microorganisms. Prevention of recurrence following rheumatic fever and/or chorea. May be useful as prophylaxis against bacterial endocarditis in patients with congenital heart disease or rheumatic or other acquired valvular heart disease who are undergoing dental procedures and surgical procedures of the upper respiratory tract.

DOSAGE: *Adults:* Usual: Streptococcal Infections (Scarlet Fever/Erysipelas/Upper Respiratory Tract): 125-250mg q6-8h for 10 days. Pneumococcal Infections (Otitis Media/Respiratory Tract): 250-500mg q6h until afebrile for at least 2 days. Staphylococcus Infections (Skin/Soft Tissue): 250-500mg q6-8h. Fusospirochetosis (Oropharynx): 250-500mg q6-8h. Rheumatic Fever/

Chorea Prevention: 125-250mg bid. Bacterial Endocarditis Prophylaxis: 2g 1 hr before procedure; 1g after 6 hrs.

Pediatrics: ≥12 yrs: Usual: Streptococcal Infections (Scarlet Fever/Erysipelas/Upper Respiratory Tract): 125-250mg q6-8h for 10 days. Pneumococcal Infections (Otitis Media/Respiratory Tract): 250-500mg q6h until afebrile for at least 2 days. Staphylococcus Infections (Skin/Soft Tissue): 250-500mg q6-8h. Fusospirochetosis (Oropharynx): 250-500mg q6-8h. Rheumatic Fever/Chorea Prevention: 125-250mg bid. Bacterial Endocarditis Prophylaxis: 2g or 1g (<60 lbs) 1 hr before procedure; 1g or 500mg (<60 lbs) after 6 hrs.

HOW SUPPLIED: Sus: 125mg/5mL, 250mg/5mL [100mL, 200mL]; Tab: 250mg, 500mg

WARNINGS/PRECAUTIONS: Not for severe pneumonia, empyema, bacteremia, pericarditis, meningitis and arthritis during the acute stage. Serious, fatal anaphylactic reactions reported. *Clostridium difficile*-associated diarrhea (CDAD) reported. Oral administration may not be effective with severe illnesses, N/V, gastric dilatation, cardiospasm, or intestinal hypermotility. Cross-sensitivity with cephalosporins. Use in the absence of a proven or strongly suspected bacterial infection or prophylaxis indication, may increase risk of development of drug-resistant bacteria. Prolonged use may promote overgrowth of nonsusceptible organisms (eg, fungi); take appropriate measures if superinfection develops. Caution with history of significant asthma and allergies. In streptococcal infections, perform culture following completion of treatment.

ADVERSE REACTIONS: Epigastric distress, N/V, diarrhea, hypersensitivity reactions, black hairy tongue, anaphylaxis, superinfection (prolonged use).

PREGNANCY: Safety in pregnancy/nursing is not known.

MECHANISM OF ACTION: Penicillin; exerts a bactericidal action against penicillin-sensitive microorganisms during the stage of active multiplication. Acts through inhibition of biosynthesis of cell-wall mucopeptide.

PHARMACOKINETICS: Distribution: Plasma protein binding (80%). **Elimination:** Urine.

NURSING CONSIDERATIONS

Assessment: Assess for history of significant allergies or asthma, N/V, gastric dilatation, severe illness, cardiospasm, intestinal hypermotility, and pregnancy/nursing status. Obtain culture and sensitivity tests especially in suspected staphylococcal infections.

Monitoring: Monitor for signs/symptoms of hypersensitivity reactions, CDAD (mild diarrhea to fatal colitis), and for superinfections. Perform culture following completion of streptococcal treatment to ensure eradication.

Patient Counseling: Therapy only treats bacterial, not viral, infections. Take as directed; skipping doses or not completing full course of therapy may decrease effectiveness and increase resistance. May experience diarrhea; contact physician if watery and bloody stools or hypersensitivity reactions occur.

Administration: Oral route. **Storage:** 20-25°C (68-77°F). Keep tightly closed.

PENLAC   RX
ciclopirox (Dermik)

THERAPEUTIC CLASS: Broad-spectrum antifungal

INDICATIONS: Mild to moderate onychomycosis of fingernails or toenails without lunula involvement due to *Trichophyton rubrum* (in immunocompetent patients).

DOSAGE: *Adults:* Apply qhs or 8 hrs before washing to nail bed, hyponychium, and under surface when it is free of nail bed. Apply daily over previous coat and remove with alcohol every 7 days. Repeat cycle up to 48 weeks.

HOW SUPPLIED: Sol: 8% [6.6mL]

WARNINGS/PRECAUTIONS: Only for use on nails and adjacent skin. Caution with removal of infected nail in insulin-dependent DM or diabetic neuropathy.

ADVERSE REACTIONS: Periungual erythema, erythema of proximal nail fold, nail shape change, nail irritation, ingrown toenail, nail discoloration.

INTERACTIONS: Avoid nail polish or other nail cosmetics on treated nails.

PREGNANCY: Category B, caution in nursing.

MECHANISM OF ACTION: Broad spectrum antifungal; acts by chelation of polyvalent cations (Fe^{+3} or Al^{+3}), resulting in the inhibition of the metal-dependent enzymes responsible for degradation of peroxides within fungal cell.

PHARMACOKINETICS: Absorption: Serum levels range from 12-80ng/mL following topical administration. **Elimination:** Urine (<5% of applied topical dose).

NURSING CONSIDERATIONS

Assessment: Assess use with insulin-dependent DM, diabetic neuropathy, and in pregnant/nursing females. Assess medication is only being used on nails or immediately adjacent skin.

Monitoring: Monitor for signs/symptoms of sensitivity reactions and chemical irritation. Perform frequent (eg, monthly) removal of unattached infected nails, trimming of onycholic nails, and filing of any excess horny material.

Patient Counseling: Advise to avoid bringing medication in contact with eyes and mucous membranes. Apply medication evenly over entire nail plate and 5mm of surrounding skin. Notify physician if signs of increased irritation at the application site develop (eg, redness, itching, burning, oozing, blistering). File away (with emery board) loose nail material and trim nails as required. Do not use nail polish or other nail cosmetic products on the treated nails. Instruct not to use medication near open flame. Inform that it may take up to 48 weeks of daily application of the medication (including monthly professional removal of unattached infected nails) before a clear or almost clear nail is seen.

Administration: Topical route. **Storage:** 15-30°C (59-86°F). Flammable; keep away from heat and flame.

PENNSAID
diclofenac sodium (Mallinckrodt)

RX

> NSAIDs may cause an increased risk of serious cardiovascular thrombotic events, MI, stroke and serious GI adverse events including bleeding, ulceration, and perforation of the stomach or intestines. Contraindicated for the treatment of perioperative pain in the setting of coronary artery bypass graft (CABG) surgery.

THERAPEUTIC CLASS: NSAID

INDICATIONS: Treatment of signs and symptoms of osteoarthritis of the knee(s).

DOSAGE: *Adults:* Usual: 40 drops per knee qid. Apply to clean, dry skin. Dispense 10 drops into the hand, or directly onto the knee. Spread evenly around front, back and sides of the knee. Repeat the procedure until 40 drops have been applied and the knee is completely covered. To treat the other knee, repeat the procedure.

HOW SUPPLIED: Sol: (1.5%) 150mL

CONTRAINDICATIONS: Aspirin (ASA) or other NSAID allergy that precipitates asthma, urticaria, or allergic reactions. Setting of coronary artery bypass graft (CABG) surgery.

WARNINGS/PRECAUTIONS: Not evaluated for use on spine, hip, or shoulder. May lead to onset of new HTN or worsening of pre-existing HTN; monitor BP closely. Fluid retention and edema reported; caution with fluid retention or heart failure. Renal papillary necrosis and other renal injury reported after long-term use. Not recommended for use with advanced renal disease; if therapy must be initiated, monitor renal function. Anaphylactoid reactions may occur. May cause serious skin adverse events (eg, exfoliative dermatitis, Stevens-Johnson syndrome [SJS], and toxic epidermal necrolysis [TEN]). Avoid in late pregnancy; may cause premature closure of ductus arteriosus. May cause elevations of LFTs; d/c if liver disease develops or systemic manifestations occur. To minimize the potential for adverse liver-related events, use the lowest effective dose for the shortest duration possible. Caution in elderly. Anemia may occur; with long-term use, monitor Hgb/Hct if signs or symptoms of anemia develop. May inhibit platelet aggregation and prolong bleeding time; monitor with coagulation disorders. Caution with asthma and avoid with ASA-sensitive asthma. Patients should minimize or avoid exposure to natural or artificial sunlight on treated areas. Caution in patients with prior history of ulcer or GI bleeding; monitor for signs or symptoms of GI bleeding. May diminish utility of diagnostic signs (eg, inflammation, fever) in detecting infectious complications of presumed noninfectious, painful conditions.

ADVERSE REACTIONS: Dyspepsia, dry skin, rash, pharyngitis, abdominal pain, infection, contact dermatitis, flatulence, pruritus, diarrhea, nausea, constipation, edema, paresthesia.

INTERACTIONS: Increased adverse effects with ASA; avoid use. Synergistic effects of anticoagulants such as warfarin on GI bleeding. May reduce natriuretic effect of furosemide and thiazides; monitor for signs of renal failure. May increase levels of lithium. Caution with methotrexate. Increased nephrotoxicity with cyclosporine. Avoid use with oral NSAID. Caution with drugs that are potentially hepatotoxic (eg, acetaminophen, certain antibiotics, antiepileptics). May impair response to therapies with ACE inhibitors, thiazide or loop diuretics.

PREGNANCY: Category C (prior to 30 weeks gestation); Category D (starting 30 weeks gestation), not for use in nursing.

MECHANISM OF ACTION: NSAID; inhibits enzyme, cyclooxygenase (COX), resulting in the reduced formation of prostaglandins, thromboxanes, and prostacylin.

PHARMACOKINETICS: Absorption: (Single Dose) C_{max}=8.1ng/mL; T_{max}=11 hrs; AUC_{0-t}=177.5ng.h/mL, AUC_{0-inf}=196.3ng.h/mL. (Multiple Dose) C_{max}=19.4ng/mL; T_{max}=4 hrs; AUC_{0-t}=695.4ng.h/mL, AUC_{0-inf}=745.2ng.h/mL. **Distribution:** Plasma protein binding (99%). **Metabolism:** 4'-hydroxy-diclofenac (major metabolite); glucuronidation or sulfation and oxidation. **Elimination:** Bile and urine; $T_{1/2}$= 36.7 hrs (single dose), 79 hrs (multiple dose).

NURSING CONSIDERATIONS

Assessment: Assess for hypersensitivity to ASA or NSAIDs, history of ulcer or GI bleeding, HTN, fluid retention, CHF, asthma, cardiovascular disease (or risk factors), renal/hepatic impairment, pregnancy/nursing status and possible drug interactions. Obtain baseline BP.

Monitoring: Monitor BP, LFTs, and renal function periodically. Monitor for signs/symptoms of cardiovascular events, GI events (eg, ulcerations, bleeding), hepatotoxicity, renal dysfunction, HTN, skin reactions, anemia, blood loss and hypersensitivity reactions.

Patient Counseling: Inform about the possible effects of the drug (eg, cardiovascular effects, GI effects, hepatotoxicity, weight gain/edema, anaphylactoid reactions, effects during pregnancy). Avoid contact with eyes and mucosa. Do not apply to open skin wounds, infections, inflammations or exfoliative dermatitis. Avoid exposure on treated knees to natural or artificial sunlight. Avoid showering/bathing for at least 30 min after application. Wash and dry hands after use. Do not apply external heat and/or occlusive dressings to treated area. Avoid wearing clothing or applying other topical products until treated knee is dry.

Administration: Topical route. **Storage:** 25°C (77°F); excursions permitted to 15°-30°C (50°-86°F).

PENTASA   RX
mesalamine (Shire)

THERAPEUTIC CLASS: 5-Aminosalicylic acid derivative

INDICATIONS: Induction of remission and for treatment of mild to moderate active ulcerative colitis.

DOSAGE: *Adults:* 1g qid. Can be given up to 8 weeks.

HOW SUPPLIED: Cap, Extended-Release: 250mg, 500mg

WARNINGS/PRECAUTIONS: Caution with hepatic and renal dysfunction; monitor closely. D/C if acute intolerance syndrome develops (eg, cramping, bloody diarrhea, abdominal pain, headache). If rechallenge is considered, perform under careful observation.

ADVERSE REACTIONS: Diarrhea, headache, nausea, abdominal pain.

PREGNANCY: Category B, caution in nursing.

MECHANISM OF ACTION: Unknown, suspected to act as anti-inflammatory agent for blocking cyclooxygenase and inhibiting prostaglandin in gastrointestinal use.

PHARMACOKINETICS: Absorption: C_{max}=1mcg/mL, T_{max}=3 hrs. (N-acetylmesalamine) C_{max}=1.8mcg/mL, T_{max}=3 hrs. **Metabolism:** N-acetylmesalamine (Metabolite). **Elimination:** Feces, N-acetylmesalamine: Urine (19-30%).

NURSING CONSIDERATIONS

Assessment: Assess for pre-existing renal disease, hepatic/renal impairment. Obtain baseline LFTs, BUN, creatinine, and urinalysis (protein).

Monitoring: Monitor LFTs, BUN, creatinine, and urinalysis (protein) periodically. Monitor signs/symptoms of hepatotoxicity, acute intolerance syndrome (cramping, acute abdominal pain, bloody diarrhea), hypersensitivity, and allergic reactions.

Patient Counseling: Seek medical attention if symptoms of hepatotoxicity, acute intolerance syndrome (cramping, acute abdominal pain, bloody diarrhea), hypersensitivity and allergic reactions occur.

Administration: Oral route. **Storage:** 25°C (77°F); excursions permitted to 15-30°C (59-86°F).

Percocet   `CII`

oxycodone HCl - acetaminophen (Endo)

OTHER BRAND NAMES: Endocet (Endo)

THERAPEUTIC CLASS: Opioid analgesic

INDICATIONS: Relief of moderate to moderately severe pain.

DOSAGE: *Adults:* (325mg-2.5mg): 1-2 tabs q6h prn. Max: 12 tabs/day. (325mg-5mg): 1 tab q6h prn. Max: 12 tabs/day. (500mg-7.5mg): 1 tab q6h prn. Max: 8 tabs/day. (650mg-10mg) 1 tab q6h prn. Max: 6 tabs/day. (325mg-7.5mg): 1 tab q6h prn. Max: 8 tabs/day. (325mg-10mg): 1 tab q6h prn. Max: 6 tabs/day. Do not exceed APAP 4g/day.

HOW SUPPLIED: Tab: (APAP-Oxycodone) 325mg-2.5mg, 325mg-5mg, 325mg-7.5mg, 325mg-10mg, 500mg-7.5mg, 650mg-10mg

CONTRAINDICATIONS: Oxycodone: Significant respiratory depression (in unmonitored settings or absence of resuscitative equipment), acute or severe bronchial asthma or hypercarbia, paralytic ileus.

WARNINGS/PRECAUTIONS: May cause physical dependence and tolerance; d/c gradually to avoid withdrawal symptoms. Potential for misuse, abuse or diversion; monitor for prevention or early detection. May induce or aggravate convulsions/seizures, produce severe hypotension in compromised patients and orthostatic hypotension in ambulatory patients. Risk of respiratory depression. May decrease bowel motility; monitor for ileus in postoperative patients. Capacity to elevate CSF pressure may be exaggerated with head injury, other intracranial lesions or a pre-existing increase in intracranial pressure (ICP). May obscure the diagnosis or clinical course with head injuries or acute abdominal conditions. May cause spasms of the Sphincter of Oddi. Caution with circulatory shock, acute asthma, chronic obstructive pulmonary disorder (COPD), cor pulmonale, or pre-existing respiratory impairment, CNS depression, severe hepatic/renal/pulmonary impairment, hypothyroidism, liver disease, Addison's disease, prostatic hypertrophy, urethral stricture, the elderly or debilitated, acute alcoholism, delirium tremens, kyphoscoliosis with respiratory depression, myxedema, toxic psychosis, biliary tract disease (eg, acute pancreatitis). May increase serum amylase levels. Anaphylactic reactions reported.

ADVERSE REACTIONS: Lightheadedness, dizziness, drowsiness, N/V, sedation, respiratory depression, apnea, respiratory arrest, circulatory depression, hypotension, shock.

INTERACTIONS: Oxycodone: May enhance neuromuscular-blocking action of skeletal muscle relaxants and produce an increase in the degree of respiratory depression. Additive CNS depression with other opioid analgesics, general anesthetics, centrally acting anti-emetics, phenothiazines, tranquilizers, sedatives-hypnotics, and other CNS depressants (eg, alcohol); reduce dose of one or both agents. Caution with concurrent agonist/antagonist analgesics (eg, pentazocine, nalbuphine and butorphanol) use; may reduce analgesic effect of oxycodone and/or may precipitate withdrawal symptoms. May produce paralytic ileus with anticholinergics. APAP: Increase in glucuronidation, plasma clearance and decreased half-life with oral contraceptives. Increase in pharmacologic effects with propranolol and probenecid. Decrease effects of loop diuretics, lamotrigine, and zidovudine effects.

PREGNANCY: Category C, not for use in nursing.

MECHANISM OF ACTION: Oxycodone: Opioid analgesic; semisynthetic pure opioid agonist whose principal therapeutic action is analgesia. Effects mediated by CNS receptors (eg, μ and kappa) for endogenous opioid-like compounds (eg, endorphins, enkephalins). APAP: Nonopiate, nonsalicyclic analgesic, and antipyretic. Site and mechanism of analgesic effect not established. Antipyretic effect produced through inhibition of endogenous pyrogen action on the hypothalamic heat-regulating centers.

PHARMACOKINETICS: Absorption: APAP: Rapid absorption. Oxycodone: Absolute bioavailability (87%). **Distribution:** Oxycodone: Plasma protein binding (45%); (IV): V_d=211.9L; found in breast milk; crosses the placenta. **Metabolism:** Acetaminophen: Liver via CYP450 (glucuronidation), NAPQI (toxic metabolite). Oxycodone: N-dealkylation to noroxycodone (metabolite); CYP2D6 (O-demethylation) to oxymorphone (metabolite). **Elimination:** APAP: Urine (90-100%). Oxycodone: Urine (parent compound and metabolites); $T_{1/2}$=3.51 hrs.

NURSING CONSIDERATIONS

Assessment: Assess for level of pain intensity, type of pain, patient's general condition and medical status, or any other conditions where treatment is contraindicated or cautioned. Assess for history of hypersensitivity, pregnancy/nursing status, renal/hepatic function, and possible drug interactions.

Monitoring: Monitor for signs/symptoms of respiratory depression, elevations in CSF pressure, hypotension, hepatotoxicity, convulsions, anaphylactic reactions, decreased bowel motility in postoperative patients, sphincter of Oddi spasms, increased serum amylase levels, tolerance and physical dependence, and medication abuse.

Patient Counseling: If accidental ingestion occurs, seek emergency medical care. Advise to flush unused medication down toilet. Do not adjust dose without consulting physician. Inform drug may impair mental/physical abilities required to perform hazardous tasks (eg, operating machinery/driving). Avoid alcohol or other CNS depressants. Do not abruptly d/c if on for few weeks; taper dosing. Has potential for abuse; protect from theft. Notify physician if pregnant or planning to become pregnant.

Administration: Oral route. **Storage:** 20-25°C (68-77°F).

P

PERCODAN

CII

oxycodone HCl - aspirin (Endo)

OTHER BRAND NAMES: Endodan (Endo)

THERAPEUTIC CLASS: Opioid analgesic

INDICATIONS: Management of moderate to moderately severe pain.

DOSAGE: *Adults:* Usual: 1 tab q6h prn for pain. Max: (ASA) Should not exceed 4g/day or 12 tabs/day. Dosage should be adjusted according to severity of pain and patient response.

HOW SUPPLIED: Tab: (Aspirin [ASA]-Oxycodone HCl) 325mg-4.8355mg* *scored

CONTRAINDICATIONS: ASA: Hemophilia, viral infection in children/teens with or w/o fever, syndrome of asthma, rhinitis, and nasal polyps. Oxycodone: Significant respiratory depression (in unmonitored settings or absence of resuscitative equipment), acute/severe bronchial asthma or hypercarbia, known/suspected paralytic ileus.

WARNINGS/PRECAUTIONS: May cause drug dependence and tolerance; potential for abuse. May cause respiratory depression; caution in elderly/ debilitated patients, acute asthma, chronic obstructive pulmonary disease (COPD), cor pulmonale, or pre-existing respiratory impairment. Respiratory depressant effects (eg, carbon dioxide retention, secondary elevation of CSF pressure) may be markedly exaggerated in the presence of head injury, intracranial lesions, or pre-existing increased intracranial pressure. May cause severe hypotension and orthostatic hypotension; caution in patients in circulatory shock and/or depleted blood volume. May inhibit platelet function and cause gastric mucosal irritation and bleeding; caution with peptic ulcer or coagulation abnormalities. Caution with acute alcoholism, hypothyroidism, Addison's disease, prostatic hypertrophy, urethral stricture, delirium tremens, kyphoscoliosis with respiratory depression, myxedema, toxic psychosis, and biliary disease. Monitor for decreased bowel motility in postoperative patients. May cause spasm of the sphincter of Oddi; caution with biliary tract disease (including acute pancreatitis). May aggravate convulsions and seizures. May cause elevated hepatic enzymes, BUN, creatinine, and amylase, hyperkalemia, proteinuria, and prolonged bleeding time. Avoid in pregnancy, especially during the 3rd trimester and during labor and delivery, severe renal failure (GFR <10mL/min), and severe hepatic insufficiency. Avoid abrupt d/c; may cause the precipitation of withdrawal symptoms.

ADVERSE REACTIONS: Respiratory depression, apnea, respiratory arrest, circulatory depression, hypotension, shock.

INTERACTIONS: ASA: May lead to high serum concentrations of acetazolamide. May diminish hyponatremic and hypotensive effects of ACE inhibitors. Increased risk for bleeding with anticoagulants (eg, warfarin, heparin) and chronic, heavy alcohol use. May decrease the total concentration of phenytoin and increase serum valproic acid levels. May diminish hypotensive effects of β-blockers. May diminish effectiveness of diuretics. Avoid NSAIDs; may increase bleeding or lead to decreased renal function. May enhance the serious side effects and toxicity of ketorolac and methotrexate. Antagonizes the uricosuric action of probenecid or sulfinpyrazone. May increase the serum glucose-lowering action of insulin and sulfonylureas leading to hypoglycemia. Oxycodone: May enhance neuromuscular-blocking action of skeletal muscle relaxants. Additive CNS depression with other opioid analgesics, general anesthetics, centrally acting anti-emetics, phenothiazines, tranquilizers, sedatives-hypnotics, and other CNS depressants (eg, alcohol); reduce dose of one or both agents. May cause severe hypotension with drugs which compromise vasomotor tone (eg, phenothiazines). Agonist/antagonist analgesics (eg, pentazocine, nalbuphine, naltrexone and butorphanol) may reduce analgesic effect and/or may precipitate withdrawal symptoms; administer with caution. Decreased clearance with CYP3A4 inhibitors [eg, macrolide antibiotics (eg, erythromycin), azole-antifungals (eg, ketoconazole), protease inhibitors (eg, ritonavir)]; caution when initiating therapy. Decreased plasma concentration with CYP450 inducers (eg, rifampin, carbamazepine, phenytoin); caution when initiating therapy.

PREGNANCY: Category B (Oxycodone) and D (ASA), not for use in nursing.

MECHANISM OF ACTION: ASA: Acetylsalicylic acid; inhibits prostaglandin production, including those involved in inflammation. In CNS, works on hypothalamus heat-regulating center to reduce fever. Oxycodone: Semisynthetic pure opioid agonist; principal therapeutic effect is analgesia. Other effects include anxiolysis, euphoria, and feelings of relaxation. Effects mediated by CNS receptors (eg, μ, kappa) for endogenous opioid-like compounds (eg, endorphins, enkephalins).

PHARMACOKINETICS: Absorption: ASA: Rapidly absorbed. Oxycodone: Absolute bioavailability (87%). **Distribution:** ASA: Found in most body tissues, fluids (eg, fetal tissues, breast milk, CNS, liver, kidneys); variable serum protein binding. Oxycodone: Plasma protein binding (45%); found in breast milk; (IV) V_d=211.9L. **Metabolism:** ASA: Liver, hydrolysis to salicylate, salicyluric acid, salicyl phenolic glucuronide, salicyl acyl glucuronide, gentisic acid, gentisuric acid (major metabolites). Oxycodone: CYP3A (N-demethylation) to noroxycodone (metabolite); CYP2D6 (O-demethylation) to oxymorphone (metabolite). **Elimination:** ASA: Urine (80%-100%; 10% unchanged salicylates, 90% metabolites). $T_{1/2}$=15 min (ASA), 2-3 hrs (salicylates). Oxycodone: Urine (parent compound and metabolites).

NURSING CONSIDERATIONS

Assessment: Assess for drug hypersensitivity, pregnancy/nursing status, drug abuse potential, possible drug interactions, or any other conditions where treatment is contraindicated or cautioned.

Monitoring: Monitor for signs/symptoms of respiratory depression, presence of elevated CSF pressure, GI ulceration and/or bleeding, anaphylactic reactions, decreased bowel motility in post-op patients, spasms of sphincter of Oddi, physical dependence and tolerance, abuse or misuse of medication, hypersensitivity reactions, and withdrawal syndrome during d/c.

Patient Counseling: Instruct if accidental ingestion occurs, seek medical attention. Dispose of unused drug via toilet. Advise to consult physician before adjusting dosing. May impair mental/physical abilities required for performing hazardous tasks (eg, operating machinery/driving). Avoid alcohol and other CNS depressants. Do not abruptly d/c if on medication for more than few weeks; taper dosing. Instruct to report adverse events (eg, respiratory depression). Has potential for abuse; protect from theft and do not give to anyone. Consult physician before taking the product if pregnant, planning to become pregnant, and nursing. May cause or worsen constipation.

Administration: Oral route. **Storage:** 25°C (77°F); excursions permitted to 15-30°C (59-86°F). Dispense in a tight, light-resistant container.

PERFOROMIST   RX
formoterol fumarate (Dey)

| Long-acting β₂-agonists may increase risk of asthma-related death. |

THERAPEUTIC CLASS: Beta₂-agonist

INDICATIONS: Long-term maintenance treatment of bronchoconstriction in patients with chronic obstructive pulmonary disease (COPD), including chronic bronchitis and emphysema.

DOSAGE: *Adults:* 20mcg q12h by nebulization. Max: 40mcg/day.

HOW SUPPLIED: Sol, Inhalation: 20mcg/2mL

WARNINGS/PRECAUTIONS: Only use short-acting β₂-agonist inhalers for acute symptoms. Should not be used with other long acting β₂-agonist medications. D/C if paradoxical bronchospasm occurs. D/C if ECG changes, QT interval increases, or ST depression occurs. Caution with cardiovascular (CV) disorders (eg, coronary insufficiency, arrhythmias, and HTN), convulsive disorders, thyrotoxicosis, and DM. May cause hypokalemia and hyperglycemia.

ADVERSE REACTIONS: Diarrhea, nausea, nasopharyngitis, dry mouth, angina, HTN, hypotension, tachycardia, arrhythmias, nervousness, headache, tremor, muscle cramps, palpitations, dizziness.

INTERACTIONS: Adrenergic drugs may potentiate effects. Xanthine derivatives, steroids, diuretics, or non-potassium sparing diuretics may potentiate hypokalemia or ECG changes; use with caution. MAOIs, TCAs, and drugs known to prolong QTc interval may potentiate effect on CV system; use with extreme caution. β-blockers may decrease effectiveness; use with caution.

PREGNANCY: Category C, caution in nursing.

MECHANISM OF ACTION: β_2-agonist; acts as bronchodilator, stimulates intracellular adenyl cyclase, the enzyme that catalyzes the conversion of ATP to cAMP. Increased cAMP levels cause relaxation of bronchial smooth muscle and inhibition of release of mediators of immediated hypersensitivity from cells such as mast cells.

PHARMACOKINETICS: Absorption: C_{max}=72pg/mL; T_{max}=12 min. **Distribution:** Plasma protein binding (61-64%). **Metabolism:** Glucuronidation, O-demethylation; CYP2D6, 2C19, 2A6. **Elimination:** Urine (unchanged); $T_{1/2}$=7 hrs.

NURSING CONSIDERATIONS

Assessment: Assess for acute COPD, asthma, acute bronchospasm, CV disease (coronary insufficiency, cardiac arrhythmias, HTN), convulsive disorders, thyrotoxicosis, K+ levels, DM, ketoacidosis, pregnancy/nursing status, and possible drug interactions.

Monitoring: Monitor for serious asthma exacerbations, paradoxical bronchospasm, CV effects, hypokalemia, hyperglycemia, aggravation of DM, ketoacidosis, pulse rate, BP, and ECG changes (T-wave flattening, prolongation of QTc interval, ST segment depression).

Patient Counseling: Do not inhale more than prescribed. Excessive use may increase likelihood of CV side effects. Maximum daily dose is 1 vial twice daily. Use other inhaler (albuterol) for acute symptoms, and consult with physician about use of other inhalers. Immediately report any side effects to physician (chest pain, rapid heart rate, headache, nervousness, dry mouth, muscle cramps, nausea, dizziness, fatigue, malaise, and BP changes). Always keep in foil pack; only remove for use and discard container and top right after use.

Administration: Oral inhalation. Only administered via a standard jet nebulizer connected to an air compressor with adequate airflow and equipped with a facemask or mouthpiece. **Storage:** Prior to dispensing: 2-8°C (36-46°F). After dispensing: 2-25°C (36-77°F) for up to 3 months. Protect from heat.

PEXEVA   RX
paroxetine mesylate (Noven)

> Antidepressants increased the risk of suicidal thinking and behavior (suicidality) in short-term studies in children, adolescents, and young adults with major depressive disorder (MDD) and other psychiatric disorders. Monitor and observe closely for clinical worsening, suicidality or unusual changes in behavior in patients who are started on antidepressant therapy. Paroxetine is not approved for use in pediatric patients.

THERAPEUTIC CLASS: Selective serotonin reuptake inhibitor

INDICATIONS: Treatment of MDD, obsessive compulsive disorder (OCD), panic disorder with or without agoraphobia, and generalized anxiety disorder (GAD).

DOSAGE: *Adults:* Give qd, usually in the am. To titrate, may increase weekly by 10mg/day. MDD: Initial: 20mg/day. Max: 50mg/day. OCD: Initial: 20mg/day. Usual: 40mg/day. Max: 60mg/day. Panic Disorder: Initial: 10mg/day. Usual: 40mg/day. Max: 60mg/day. GAD: Initial: 20mg/day. Usual: 20-50mg/day. Elderly/Debilitated/Severe Renal or Hepatic Impairment: Initial: 10mg/day. Max: 40mg/day.

HOW SUPPLIED: Tab: 10mg, 20mg*, 30mg, 40mg *scored

CONTRAINDICATIONS: Concomitant use of MAOIs, thioridazine, and pimozide.

WARNINGS/PRECAUTIONS: Avoid use in bipolar depression. Potentially life-threatening serotonin syndrome and neuroleptic malignant syndrome (NMS)-like reactions reported. Increased risk of congenital malformations reported in infants. Activation of mania/hypomania reported; caution in patients with a history of mania. Caution with history of seizures; d/c if seizures occur. Akathisia may develop. Hyponatremia reported, caution in elderly and volume-depleted patients. May increase risk of bleeding events. Caution with conditions that affect metabolism or hemodynamic responses, narrow-angle glaucoma and hepatic/renal impairment. May impair mental/physical abilities. Dysphoric mood, irritability, agitation, dizziness, sensory disturbances, anxiety, confusion, headache, lethargy, emotional lability, insomnia, and hypomania reported upon d/c; avoid abrupt withdrawal.

ADVERSE REACTIONS: Asthenia, sweating, nausea, decreased appetite, somnolence, dizziness, insomnia, tremor, nervousness, abnormal ejaculation, dry mouth, constipation, decreased libido, impotence, headache.

INTERACTIONS: See Contraindications. Serotonin syndrome or NMS-like reactions reported when used alone and in combination with serotonergic drugs (eg, triptans, linezolid, lithium, tramadol, or St. John's wort), drugs that impair serotonin metabolism, antipsychotics, and dopamine antagonists. Use with other SSRIs, SNRIs, or tryptophan is not recommended. Caution with warfarin, phenobarbital, phenytoin, lithium, and digoxin. Avoid alcohol. Concomitant use with ASA, NSAIDs, warfarin, and other anticoagulants may increase risk of bleeding events. Use with diuretics may increase risk of developing hyponatremia. Metabolism and pharmacokinetics of paroxetine may be affected by induction or inhibition of drug-metabolizing enzymes. Increased levels with cimetidine. Caution with drugs that are metabolized by CYP2D6 (eg, antidepressants, phenothiazines, risperidone, Type 1C antiarrhythmics) and with drugs that inhibit CYP2D6 (eg, quinidine). May increase levels of risperidone. May increase levels of atomoxetine; may require dose adjustments. May impair metabolism of TCAs, caution with concomitant use. May shift concentrations when concomitantly used with highly protein-bound drugs. May increase procyclidine and theophylline levels. Severe hypotension reported when added to chronic metoprolol treatment. Decreased level with fosamprenavir/ritonavir.

PREGNANCY: Category D, caution in nursing.

MECHANISM OF ACTION: SSRI; inhibits CNS neuronal reuptake of serotonin.

PHARMACOKINETICS: Absorption: Complete; C_{max}=81.3ng/mL; T_{max}=8.1 hr. **Distribution:** Plasma protein binding (95%); found in breast milk. **Metabolism:** Extensive; oxidation and methylation via CYP2D6. **Elimination:** Urine (62% metabolites; 2% parent compound); feces (36% metabolites; <1% parent compound); $T_{1/2}$=33.2 hrs.

NURSING CONSIDERATIONS

Assessment: Assess for bipolar disorder risk, history of seizures, history of mania, volume depletion, diseases/conditions that alter metabolism or hemodynamic responses, hepatic/renal impairment, narrow-angle glaucoma, pregnancy/nursing status, and for possible drug interactions. Assess use in the elderly.

Monitoring: Monitor for signs/symptoms of clinical worsening (eg, suicidality, unusual changes in behavior), serotonin syndrome or NMS-like reactions, seizures, and hyponatremia. Upon d/c, monitor for symptoms of dysphoric mood, irritability, agitation, dizziness, sensory disturbances, anxiety, confusion, headache, lethargy, emotional lability, insomnia, and hypomania.

Patient Counseling: Instruct to swallow whole, not to chew or crush. Advise to avoid alcohol. Seek medical attention for symptoms of serotonin syndrome, abnormal bleeding (particularly if using NSAIDs, ASA, warfarin), akathisia, hyponatremia, mydriasis, activation of mania, seizures, clinical worsening, or d/c symptoms (irritability, agitation, dizziness, anxiety, headache, insomnia). Caution against hazardous tasks (eg, operating machinery and driving). Inform may notice improvement in 1-4 weeks; continue therapy as directed. Notify physician if pregnant, intend to become pregnant, or are breastfeeding.

- Counsel about benefits and risks of therapy. Inform physician if taking, or plan to take, any prescription or OTC drugs.

Administration: Oral route. **Storage:** 25°C (77°F); excursions permitted to 15-30°C (59-86°F). Protect from humidity.

PHENERGAN INJECTION

RX

promethazine HCl (Baxter)

> Do not use in pediatric patients <2 yrs because of potential for fatal respiratory depression. Caution when used in pediatrics ≥2 yrs. Injection may cause severe chemical irritation and damage to tissue regardless of the route of administration. Irritation and damage may result from perivascular extravasation, unintentional intra-arterial injection, or intraneuronal/perineuronal infiltration; surgical intervention may be required. Preferred route of administration is deep IM injection.

THERAPEUTIC CLASS: Phenothiazine derivative

INDICATIONS: Amelioration of allergic reactions to blood or plasma. In anaphylaxis as an adjunct to epinephrine and other standard measures after acute symptoms have been controlled. For other uncomplicated allergic conditions of the immediate type when oral therapy is not possible or contraindicated. For sedation and relief of apprehension to produce light sleep. Active treatment of motion sickness. Prevention and control of N/V associated with certain types of anesthesia and surgery. Adjunct to analgesics for the control of postoperative pain. Preoperative, postoperative, and obstetric (during labor) sedation. IV in special surgical situations such as repeated bronchoscopy, ophthalmic surgery, and poor-risk patients, with reduced amounts of meperidine or other narcotic analgesic as adjunct to anesthesia and analgesia.

DOSAGE: *Adults:* (IM/IV) IM route is preferred. Allergy: Initial: 25mg, may repeat within 2 hrs. Adjust to the smallest adequate amount to relieve symptoms. For continued therapy, oral route preferred. Sedation: 25-50mg qhs in hospitalized patients. N/V: Usual: 12.5-25mg, not to be repeated more frequently than q4h. Preoperative/Postoperative Adjunct: 25-50mg. May be combined with appropriately reduced doses of analgesics and atropine-like drugs. Obstetrics: 50mg in early stages of labor, 25-75mg in established labor may be given with an appropriately reduced dose of any desired narcotic, may repeat once or twice q4h in normal labor. Max: 100mg/24 hrs of labor. Do not give IV administration >25mg/mL and at a rate >25mg/min. Elderly: Start at lower end of dosing range.
Pediatrics: ≥2 yrs: Dose should not exceed half of suggested adult dose. Premedication Adjunct: Usual: 1.1 mg/kg body weight in combination with an appropriately reduced dose of narcotic or barbiturate and appropriate dose of an atropine-like drug. Do not give IV administration >25mg/mL and at a rate >25mg/min.

HOW SUPPLIED: Inj: 25mg/mL, 50mg/mL

CONTRAINDICATIONS: Children <2 yrs, comatose states, intra-arterial or SQ injection.

WARNINGS/PRECAUTIONS: Not recommended for uncomplicated vomiting in pediatrics. May impair physical/mental ability. Fatal respiratory depression reported; avoid with compromised respiratory function or patients at risk of respiratory failure (eg, COPD, sleep apnea). May lower seizure threshold. Caution with bone marrow depression; leukopenia and agranulocytosis reported. Neuroleptic malignant syndrome (NMS) reported. Sulfite sensitivity may occur; caution especially in asthmatics. Avoid in pediatrics with Reye's syndrome or other hepatic diseases. Hallucinations and convulsions may occur in pediatrics. Increased susceptibility to dystonias in acutely ill pediatric patients with dehydration. May inhibit platelet aggregation in the newborn when used in pregnant women within two weeks of delivery. Caution with narrow-angle glaucoma, prostatic hypertrophy, stenosing peptic ulcer, bladder-neck or pyloroduodenal obstruction, cardiovascular (CV) disease, hepatic dysfunction. Cholestatic jaundice reported. May cause false interpretations of diagnostic pregnancy tests and may increase blood glucose. Caution in elderly.

ADVERSE REACTIONS: Respiratory depression, severe tissue injury, drowsiness, dizziness, tinnitus, blurred vision, dry mouth, increased or decreased BP, urticaria, N/V, blood dyscrasia, gangrene.

INTERACTIONS: Concomitant use with respiratory depressants in pediatric patients may result in death. May increase, prolong, or intensify sedation when used concomitantly with CNS depressants (eg, alcohol, sedative/hypnotics [including barbiturates], general anesthetics, narcotics, TCAs, tranquilizers); avoid concomitant use or reduce dose. Reduce dose of barbiturates by at least 50% if given concomitantly. Reduce dose of narcotics by 25-50% if given concomitantly. Caution with drugs that alter seizure threshold (eg, narcotics, local anesthetics). Leukopenia and agranulocytosis reported when used with other known marrow-toxic agents. Do not use epinephrine for promethazine injection overdose. Caution with anticholinergics. Possible adverse reactions with MAOIs. NMS reported alone and in combination with antipsychotics.

PREGNANCY: Category C, not for use in nursing.

MECHANISM OF ACTION: Phenothiazine derivative/H$_1$ receptor antagonist; possesses antihistamine (does not block release of histamine), sedative, anti-motion sickness, antiemetic, and anticholinergic effects.

PHARMACOKINETICS: Metabolism: Liver; sulfoxides, N-desmethylpromethazine (metabolites). **Elimination:** Urine; T$_{1/2}$=9-16 hrs (IV), 9.8 hrs (IM).

NURSING CONSIDERATIONS

Assessment: Assess for history of seizure disorder, compromised respiratory function or risk of respiratory failure (eg, COPD, sleep apnea), bone marrow depression, sulfite hypersensitivity, asthma, narrow-angle glaucoma, prostatic hypertrophy, stenosing peptic ulcer, pyloroduodenal obstruction, bladder-neck obstruction, CV disease, hepatic impairment, pregnancy/nursing status, and for possible drug interactions. Assess age of patient and presence of a comatose state. In pediatrics, assess for Reye's syndrome or presence of acute illness with dehydration.

Monitoring: Monitor for signs/symptoms of respiratory depression, seizures, leukopenia, agranulocytosis, NMS, cholestatic jaundice, injection-site reactions, and for hypersensitivity reactions. Monitor for hallucinations, convulsions, extrapyramidal symptoms and dystonia in pediatrics. In newborns, monitor platelet count, when used in pregnant women within 2 weeks of delivery.

Patient Counseling: Advise regarding risk of respiratory depression and risk of tissue injury. May impair physical/mental abilities. Seek medical attention if symptoms of respiratory depression, seizures, infections, NMS (hyperpyrexia, muscle rigidity, autonomic instability), injection site reactions (burning, pain, erythema), or hypersensitivity reactions occur. Avoid alcohol, certain other medications with possible interactions, and prolonged sun exposure.

Administration: IV, IM route. If pain occurs during IV injection, stop immediately and evaluate for possible arterial injection or perivascular extravasation. Inspect before use and discard if either color or particulate is observed. **Storage:** 20-25°C (68-77°F). Protect from light.

PHENOBARBITAL `CIV`
phenobarbital (Various)

THERAPEUTIC CLASS: Barbiturate

INDICATIONS: Treatment of generalized, tonic-clonic and cortical focal seizures. For relief of anxiety, tension and apprehension. Short-term treatment of insomnia.

DOSAGE: *Adults:* Sedation: 30-120mg/day given bid-tid. Max: 400mg/24h. Hypnotic: 100-200mg. Seizures: 60-200mg/day. Elderly/Debilitated/Renal or Hepatic Dysfunction: Reduce dosage.
Pediatrics: Seizures: 3-6mg/kg/day.

HOW SUPPLIED: Elixir: 20mg/5mL; Tab: 15mg, 30mg, 32.4mg, 60mg, 64.8mg, 100mg

CONTRAINDICATIONS: Respiratory disease with dyspnea or obstruction, porphyria, severe liver dysfunction. Large doses with nephritic patients.

WARNINGS/PRECAUTIONS: May be habit-forming. Avoid abrupt withdrawal. Caution with acute or chronic pain; may mask symptoms or paradoxical excitement may occur. Cognitive deficits reported in children with febrile seizures. May cause excitement in children; excitement, depression or confusion in elderly, debilitated. Caution with hepatic dysfunction, borderline hypoadrenal function, depression.

ADVERSE REACTIONS: Drowsiness, residual sedation, lethargy, vertigo, somnolence, respiratory depression, hypersensitivity reactions, N/V, headache.

INTERACTIONS: May be potentiated by MAOIs, antihistamines, alcohol, tranquilizers, sedative/hypnotics, other CNS depressants. Decreases effects of oral anticoagulants and oral contraceptives. Increases corticosteroid metabolism. Decreases absorption of griseofulvin. Decreases half-life of doxycycline. May alter phenytoin metabolism. Increased levels with sodium valproate and valproic acid.

PREGNANCY: Category D, caution in nursing.

MECHANISM OF ACTION: Barbiturate; nonselective CNS depressant. Capable of producing all levels of CNS mood alteration. Responsible for depressing the sensory cortex, decreasing motor activity, altering cerebellar function, causing sedation and hypnosis.

PHARMACOKINETICS: Distribution: Distributed to all tissues and fluids. High concentrations found in the brain, liver, and kidneys. Found in breast milk. **Metabolism:** Hepatic. **Elimination:** Urine (primary), feces; $T_{1/2}$=79 hrs (adults), 110 hrs (children and newborns less than 48 hrs old).

NURSING CONSIDERATIONS

Assessment: Assess for history of manifest or latent porphyria, hepatic impairment, or respiratory disease with evidence of dyspnea or obstruction. Assess use in children, pregnant/nursing women, history of drug abuse, elderly or debilitated patients, acute or chronic pain, borderline hypoadrenal function, and history of depression or suicidal tendencies. Assess for possible drug interactions.

Monitoring: For patients on prolonged therapy, perform periodic evaluations of hematopoietic, renal/hepatic function. Monitor for signs of psychological/physical dependence, cognitive deficits in children, signs/symptoms of CNS depression, acute intoxication of medication (eg, unsteady gait, slurred speech), signs of chronic intoxication (eg, confusion, insomnia), and for exfoliative dermatitis (eg, Stevens-Johnson syndrome, toxic epidermal necrosis). Monitor for withdrawal symptoms (eg, anxiety, muscle twitching, weakness, convulsions, delirium) after d/c medication.

Patient Counseling: Inform psychological/physical dependence may result. Instruct not to increase dosage without consulting physician. Inform medication may impair mental/physical abilities; use caution when performing hazardous tasks. Avoid alcohol or other CNS depressants while on medication. Notify physician if any type of rash develops.

Administration: Oral route. **Storage:** 15-30°C (59-86°F).

PHENYTEK   RX
phenytoin sodium (Mylan)

THERAPEUTIC CLASS: Hydantoin

INDICATIONS: Control of generalized tonic-clonic (grand mal) and complex partial (psychomotor, temporal lobe) seizures. Prevention and treatment of seizures occurring during or following neurosurgery.

DOSAGE: *Adults:* Individualize dose. No Previous Treatment: Initial: 100mg tid. Titrate: May increase at 7- to 10-day intervals. Maint: 100mg tid-qid. May increase up to 200mg tid. QD Dosing: May consider 300mg qd if controlled with divided doses of three 100mg caps daily. LD (clinic/hospital): 1g in 3 divided doses (400mg, 300mg, 300mg) given 2 hrs apart. Start maint dose 24 hrs later. Avoid LD with renal and hepatic disease.

Pediatrics: Individualize dose. Initial: 5mg/kg/day given in 2 or 3 equally divided doses. Titrate: May increase at 7- to 10-day intervals. Maint: 4-8mg/kg/day. Max: 300mg/day. >6 yrs: May require minimum adult dose (300mg/day).

HOW SUPPLIED: Cap, Extended-Release: 200mg, 300mg

WARNINGS/PRECAUTIONS: Avoid abrupt withdrawal; may precipitate status epilepticus. May increase risk of suicidal thoughts/behavior; monitor for worsening of depression and any unusual changes in mood or behavior, or thoughts of self-harm. Lymphadenopathy (benign lymph node hyperplasia, pseudolymphoma, lymphoma, and Hodgkin's disease) with or without serum sickness-like reactions reported; observe for an extended period and use alternative antiepileptic drugs. May exacerbate porphyria; use with caution. Caution in pregnancy; increased seizure frequency in mothers, congenital malformations (orofacial clefts, cardiac defects, dysmorphic facial features, nail and digit hypoplasia, growth abnormalities and mental deficiency), and malignancies (eg, neuroblastoma) observed. Life-threatening bleeding disorder may occur in newborns exposed to phenytoin in utero; give vitamin K to mother before delivery and to neonate after birth. Caution with hepatic impairment, elderly or if gravely ill; may show early signs of toxicity. D/C if rash (exfoliative, purpuric, bullous, lupus erythematosus, Stevens-Johnson syndrome [SJS], toxic epidermal necrolysis [TEN]) occurs. For milder types of rash (measles-like or scarlatiniform), may resume therapy after rash has completely disappeared. If rash recurs after reinstitution, further phenytoin medication is contraindicated. Hyperglycemia and osteomalacia reported. Avoid use for seizures due to hypoglycemia or other metabolic causes. Not effective for absence (petit mal) seizures. Confused states referred to as delirium, psychosis, encephalopathy, or irreversible cerebellar dysfunction reported with increased levels; reduce dose or d/c if symptoms persist. May increase serum glucose, alkaline phosphatase, gamma glutamyl transpeptidase (GGT) levels, interfere with dexamethasone and metyrapone tests, and decrease T_4 concentration. Avoid with enteral feeding preparation.

ADVERSE REACTIONS: Nystagmus, ataxia, slurred speech, decreased coordination, confusion.

INTERACTIONS: Increased levels with acute alcohol intake, amiodarone, chloramphenicol, chlordiazepoxide, cimetidine, diazepam, dicumarol, disulfiram, estrogens, ethosuximide, fluoxetine, H_2-antagonists, halothane, isoniazid, methylphenidate, phenothiazines, phenylbutazone, salicylates, succinamides, sulfonamides, ticlopidine, tolbutamide, trazodone. Decreased levels with chronic alcohol use, carbamazepine, reserpine, sucralfate. Impaired efficacy of corticosteroids, coumarin anticoagulants, digitoxin, doxycycline, estrogens, furosemide, oral contraceptives, paroxetine, quinidine, rifampin, theophylline, vitamin D. May increase or decrease levels with phenobarbital, sodium valproate, valproic acid. Calcium antacids decrease absorption; space dosing. Moban° (molindone) contains calcium ions that interfere with absorption. TCAs may precipitate seizures; may need to adjust phenytoin dose.

PREGNANCY: Category D, not for use in nursing.

MECHANISM OF ACTION: Hydantoin; inhibits seizure activity by promoting Na efflux from neurons, stabilizing the threshold against hyperexcitability caused by excessive stimulation or environmental changes capable of reducing membrane sodium gradient. Reduces the post-tetanic potentiation at synapses, which prevents cortical seizure foci from detonating adjacent cortical areas.

PHARMACOKINETICS: Absorption: Slow and extended. T_{max}=4-12 hrs. **Distribution:** Protein binding (high). **Metabolism:** Hepatic via hydroxylation. **Elimination:** Bile (inactive metabolite) and urine; $T_{1/2}$=22 hrs.

NURSING CONSIDERATIONS

Assessment: Assess for alcohol use, impaired liver function, grave illness, porphyria, seizures due to hypoglycemic or other metabolic causes, absence (petit mal) seizures, pregnancy/nursing status, possible drug interactions, and hypersensitivity reactions. Obtain baseline serum phenytoin levels.

Monitoring: Monitor alcohol use, alkaline phosphatase, GGT, phenytoin levels and serum concentrations of T_4. Monitor for signs and symptoms of status epilepticus, skin rash, hyperglycemia, osteomalacia, phenytoin toxicity (eg, delirium, psychosis, encephalopathy or irreversible cerebellar dysfunction), development of lymphadenopathy, serum sickness-like reactions, increased seizure frequency in pregnancy, and hypersensitivity reactions. Monitor for worsening of depression, suicidal thoughts/behavior, unusual change in mood/behavior, or thoughts of self-harm.

Patient Counseling: Advise of importance of strictly adhering to prescribed dosage regimen, and of informing physician of any clinical condition in which it is not possible to take the drug orally as prescribed (eg, surgery). Caution with the use of other drugs or alcohol while on medication. Notify physician if skin rash develops. Stress good dental hygiene to minimize development of gingival hyperplasia and its complications. May increase risk of suicidal thoughts and behavior; advise to report to healthcare provider immediately if emergence/worsening of depression, unusual change in mood/behavior, suicidal thoughts/behavior occurs. Notify physician if pregnant or intend to become pregnant. Encourage patients to enroll in North American Antiepileptic Drug (NAAED) Pregnancy Registry by calling 888-233-2334 or go to www.aedpregnancyregistry.org.

Administration: Oral route. **Storage:** 20-25°C (68-77°F). Protect from light and moisture.

PHOSLO   RX
calcium acetate (Fresenius)

THERAPEUTIC CLASS: Phosphate binder

INDICATIONS: Control of hyperphosphatemia in end stage renal failure (ESRF). Does not promote aluminum absorption.

DOSAGE: *Adults:* Initial: 2 caps/tabs with each meal. Titrate: Increase gradually until serum phosphate <6mg/dL, as long as hypercalcemia does not develop. Maint: 3-4 caps/tabs with each meal.

HOW SUPPLIED: Cap, Tab: 667mg

CONTRAINDICATIONS: Hypercalcemia.

WARNINGS/PRECAUTIONS: Increased risk of hypercalcemia when calcium given with meals in ESRF. Monitor serum calcium twice weekly during early dose adjustment period. If hypercalcemia develops, reduce dose or d/c depending on severity. Caution with arrhythmias.

ADVERSE REACTIONS: Hypercalcemia, constipation, anorexia, N/V, confusion, delirium, stupor, coma.

INTERACTIONS: Decreased bioavailability of tetracyclines. Hypercalcemia may precipitate arrhythmia; avoid digitalis. Avoid other calcium supplements.

PREGNANCY: Category C, safety in nursing not known.

MECHANISM OF ACTION: Phosphate binder; combines with dietary phosphate to form insoluble calcium phosphate, which is excreted in the feces.

NURSING CONSIDERATIONS

Assessment: Assess for hypercalcemia, patients taking digitalis, pregnancy status, and possible drug interaction.

Monitoring: Monitor serum calcium level twice weekly: (CaXP) product ≤66. X-ray suspect anatomical region to detect soft tissue calcification. Monitor for cardiac arrhythmia and vascular calcification.

Patient Counseling: Inform about compliance with dosage and diet instructions. Avoid use of nonprescription antacids. Inform about symptoms of hypercalcemia.

Administration: Oral route, taken with meal. **Storage:** 25°C (77°F); excursions permitted to 15-30°C (59-86°F).

PINDOLOL

RX

pindolol (Various)

THERAPEUTIC CLASS: Nonselective beta-blocker

INDICATIONS: Management of HTN.

DOSAGE: *Adults:* Initial: 5mg bid. Titrate: May increase by 10mg/day after 3-4 weeks. Max: 60mg/day.

HOW SUPPLIED: Tab: 5mg, 10mg

CONTRAINDICATIONS: Bronchial asthma, overt cardiac failure, cardiogenic shock, 2nd- and 3rd-degree heart block, severe bradycardia.

WARNINGS/PRECAUTIONS: Caution with well-compensated heart failure, nonallergic bronchospasm, renal or hepatic impairment. Can cause cardiac failure. Avoid abrupt withdrawal. Withdrawal before surgery is controversial. May mask hypoglycemia or hyperthyroidism symptoms.

ADVERSE REACTIONS: Dizziness, fatigue, insomnia, nervousness, dyspnea, edema, joint pain, muscle cramps/pain.

INTERACTIONS: Additive hypotension and/or bradycardia with catecholamine-depleting drugs. Both thioridazine and pindolol levels may increase when used concomitantly.

PREGNANCY: Category B, not for use in nursing.

MECHANISM OF ACTION: Nonselective β-blocker; inhibits β-adrenergic receptor with intrinsic sympathomimetic activity.

PHARMACOKINETICS: Absorption: Rapid; T_{max}=1 hr. **Distribution:** V_d=2L/kg; plasma protein binding (40%). **Metabolism:** Metabolized to hydroxymetabolites, which are excreted as glucoronides and ethereal sulfates. **Elimination:** Urine (35-40%), feces (6-9%); $T_{1/2}$=approximately 3-4 hrs, $T_{1/2}$=8 hrs (metabolites).

NURSING CONSIDERATIONS

Assessment: Assess for history of anaphylactic reaction, bronchial asthma, overt cardiac failure, cardiogenic shock, 2nd- or 3rd-degree heart block, severe bradycardia, bronchospastic disease, DM, thyrotoxicosis, LFTs, renal function, pregnancy/nursing status, and possible drug interactions. D/C drug well before any surgeries.

Monitoring: Monitor for anaphylactic reactions, LFTs, dizziness, fatigue, edema, dyspnea, muscle pain, heart block, hypotension, claudication, visual disturbances, impotence, CBC with differential and platelet count, Peyronie's disease, CHF, bronchospasm.

Patient Counseling: Instruct not to interrupt or d/c therapy without consulting physician. Counsel about signs/symptoms of CHF, bronchospasm, and other adverse effects; seek prompt medical assistance if any develop.

Administration: Oral route. **Storage:** Below 30°C (86°F); tight, light-resistant container.

PLAQUENIL

RX

hydroxychloroquine sulfate (Sanofi-Aventis)

Be familiar with complete prescribing information before prescribing hydroxychloroquine.

THERAPEUTIC CLASS: Quinine derivative

INDICATIONS: Suppression and treatment of acute attacks of malaria in adults and children. Treatment of discoid and systemic lupus erythematosus and rheumatoid arthritis (RA) in adults.

DOSAGE: *Adults:* Malaria Suppression: 400mg weekly. Begin 2 weeks before exposure and continue for 8 weeks after leaving endemic area. Give 400mg q6h for 2 doses if therapy is not begun before exposure. Acute Attack: 800mg, then 400mg 6-8 hrs later, then 400mg for 2 more days. RA: Initial:

P

400-600mg qd with food or milk; increase until optimum response. Maint: After 4-12 weeks, 200-400mg qd with food or milk. Lupus Erythematosus: Initial: 400mg qd-bid for several weeks depending on response. Maint: 200-400mg/day.

Pediatrics: Malaria Suppression: 5mg/kg (base) weekly, max 400mg/dose. Begin 2 weeks before exposure and continue for 8 weeks after leaving endemic area. Acute Attack: 10mg base/kg, max 800mg/dose; then 5mg base/kg, max 400mg/dose at 6, 24 and 48 hrs after 1st dose.

HOW SUPPLIED: Tab: 200mg (200mg tab=155mg base)

CONTRAINDICATIONS: Long term therapy in children or if retinal/visual field changes due to 4-aminoquinoline compounds.

WARNINGS/PRECAUTIONS: Caution with hepatic disease, G6PD deficiency, alcoholism, psoriasis, and porphyria. Perform baseline and periodic (3 months) ophthalmologic exams and blood cell counts with prolonged therapy. Test periodically for muscle weakness. D/C if blood disorders occur. Avoid if possible in pregnancy. D/C after 6 months if no improvement in RA.

ADVERSE REACTIONS: Headache, dizziness, diarrhea, loss of appetite, muscle weakness, nausea, abdominal cramps, bleaching of hair, dermatitis, ocular toxicity, visual field defects.

INTERACTIONS: Caution with hepatotoxic drugs.

PREGNANCY: Safety in pregnancy and nursing not known.

MECHANISM OF ACTION: Quinine derivative; has antimalarial action. Precise mechanism not established.

NURSING CONSIDERATIONS

Assessment: Assess for retinal or visual field defects, psoriasis, hepatic disease, alcoholism, G-6-PD deficiency, chloroquine-resistant strains of *P. falciparum*, auditory damage, pregnancy/nursing status. Note other diseases/conditions and drug therapies.

Monitoring: Monitor CBC with differential and platelet count, dermatologic reactions, chloroquine retinopathy, psychosis, irritability, myopathy, abnormal nerve conduction, depression of deep tendon reflexes, and allergic reactions.

Patient Counseling: Counsel about adverse effects and to d/c drug and seek medical attention if any signs/symptoms develop. Advise about need for periodic follow-up.

Administration: Oral route. **Storage:** Room temperature up to 30°C (86°F).

PLAVIX   RX
clopidogrel bisulfate (Bristol-Myers Squibb/Sanofi-Aventis)

> **Effectiveness is dependent on activation to an active metabolite via CYP2C19. Poor metabolizers of CYP2C19 treated with clopidogrel at recommended doses exhibit higher cardiovascular (CV) event rates following acute coronary syndrome (ACS) or undergoing percutaneous coronary intervention than patients with normal CYP2C19 function. Tests are available to identify a patient's CYP2C19 genotype and to determine therapeutic strategy. Consider alternative treatment in poor metabolizers.**

THERAPEUTIC CLASS: Platelet aggregation inhibitor

INDICATIONS: Reduction of rate of CV death, MI, stroke, or refractory ischemia in patients with non-ST-segment elevation ACS (unstable angina [UA]/non-ST-elevation MI [NSTEMI]), including those who are managed medically and those with coronary revascularization. Reduction of rate of death from any cause, re-infarction, or stroke in patients with ST-elevation MI (STEMI). Reduction in rate of new ischemic stroke or MI, and other vascular deaths in patients with history of recent MI or stroke, or established peripheral arterial disease (PAD).

DOSAGE: *Adults:* Recent MI/Stroke or PAD: 75mg qd. UA/NSTEMI: Initial: LD: 300mg. Maint: 75mg qd with aspirin (ASA) (75-325mg qd). STEMI: 75mg qd with ASA (75-325mg qd), with or without thrombolytics. May initiate with or without a LD.

HOW SUPPLIED: Tab: 75mg, 300mg

CONTRAINDICATIONS: Active pathological bleeding (eg, peptic ulcer, intracranial hemorrhage).

WARNINGS/PRECAUTIONS: Increased risk of bleeding; d/c 5 days before surgery if antiplatelet effect is not desired. Avoid therapy lapses; if need to temporarily d/c, restart as soon as possible; premature d/c increases risk of CV events. Thrombotic thrombocytopenic purpura (TTP) reported.

ADVERSE REACTIONS: TTP, bleeding, epistaxis, hematuria, bruising, hematoma, pruritus.

INTERACTIONS: Increased risk of bleeding with warfarin, NSAIDs, and ASA. Reduced platelet inhibition with CYP2C19 inhibitors (eg, omeprazole, pantoprazole); avoid with moderate to strong CYP2C19 inhibitors.

PREGNANCY: Category B, not for use in nursing.

MECHANISM OF ACTION: Platelet activation and aggregation inhibitor; irreversibly and selectively inhibits the binding of adenosine diphosphate (ADP) to its platelet $P2Y_{12}$ receptor and subsequent ADP-mediated activation of the glycoprotein GPIIb/IIIa complex.

PHARMACOKINETICS: Absorption: Rapid. Bioavailability (≥50%); T_{max}=30-60 min. **Metabolism:** Liver (extensive) via CYP450 (active thiol metabolite) and hydrolysis. **Elimination:** Urine (50%), feces (46%); $T_{1/2}$=6 hrs.

NURSING CONSIDERATIONS

Assessment: Assess for presence of active bleeding (eg, peptic ulcer, intracranial hemorrhage), previous hypersensitivity to the drug, reduced CYP2C19 function, pregnancy/nursing status, and possible drug interactions. Assess use in patients at risk for increased bleeding (eg, undergoing surgery).

Monitoring: Monitor for signs/symptoms of TTP (eg, thrombocytopenia, microangiopathic hemolytic anemia, neurological findings, renal dysfunction, fever) and bleeding.

Patient Counseling: Inform about the benefits and risks of treatment. Instruct to take exactly as prescribed and not to d/c without consulting the prescribing physician. Inform patients that they may bruise and/or bleed more easily and that bleeding will take longer than usual to stop. Report to physician any unanticipated, prolonged, or excessive bleeding, or blood in stool or urine. Inform that TTP, a rare but serious condition, has been reported; seek prompt medical attention if unexplained fever, weakness, extreme skin paleness, purple skin patches, yellowing of the skin or eyes, or neurological changes occur. Notify physician or dentist about therapy before scheduling any invasive procedure.

Administration: Oral route. **Storage:** 25°C (77°F); excursions permitted to 15-30°C (59-86°F).

PLETAL   RX
cilostazol (Otsuka America)

> Contraindicated with congestive heart failure (CHF) of any severity due to possible decrease in survival.

THERAPEUTIC CLASS: Phosphodiesterase III inhibitor

INDICATIONS: Reduction of symptoms with intermittent claudication.

DOSAGE: *Adults:* 100mg bid, 1/2 hr before or 2 hrs after breakfast and dinner. Concomitant CYP3A4 and CYP2C19 Inhibitors: Consider 50mg bid.

HOW SUPPLIED: Tab: 50mg, 100mg

CONTRAINDICATIONS: CHF of any severity. Haemostatic disorders or active pathologic bleeding (eg, peptic ulcer, intracranial bleeding).

WARNINGS/PRECAUTIONS: Risks not known in patients with severe underlying heart disease, moderate or severe hepatic impairment, or with long-term use. Rare cases of thrombocytopenia or leukopenia reported.

ADVERSE REACTIONS: Headache, palpitation, tachycardia, abnormal stool, diarrhea, peripheral edema, dizziness, infection, rhinitis, BP increase, aplastic anemia.

INTERACTIONS: Caution with CYP3A4 inhibitors (eg, ketoconazole, diltiazem, erythromycin) or CYP2C19 inhibitors (eg, omeprazole); may increase cilostazol levels. Avoid grapefruit juice.

PREGNANCY: Category C, not for use in nursing.

MECHANISM OF ACTION: Phosphodiesterase III inhibitor; not established. Inhibits phosphodiesterase activity and suppresses cyclic AMP (cAMP) degradation. Results in an increase of cAMP in platelets and blood vessels. Leads to reversible inhibition of platelet aggregation and produces vasodilation.

PHARMACOKINETICS: Distribution: Plasma protein binding (95-98%). **Metabolism:** Liver via CYP450 3A4 (primary), 2C19; 3,4-dehydro-cilostazol, 4'-trans-hydroxy-cilostazol (major active metabolites). **Elimination:** Urine (74%), feces (20%); $T_{1/2}$=11-13 hrs.

NURSING CONSIDERATIONS

Assessment: Assess for CHF, hemostatic disorders, presence of major bleeding (eg, peptic ulcer, intracranial bleeding), renal/hepatic function, pregnancy/nursing status, and drug interactions.

Monitoring: Monitor for signs/symptoms of thrombocytopenia, leukopenia, agranulocytosis, cardiovascular toxicity (eg, cardiovascular lesions), and headaches.

Patient Counseling: Advise to take at least 30 min before or 2 hrs after food. Inform that benefits of medication may not be immediate; treatment required for up to 12 weeks before beneficial effect.

Administration: Oral route. **Storage:** 25°C (77°F); excursions permitted to 15-30°C (59-86°F).

PNEUMOVAX 23   RX
pneumococcal vaccine polyvalent (Merck)

THERAPEUTIC CLASS: Vaccine

INDICATIONS: Immunization against pneumococcal disease caused by pneumococcal types included in the vaccine.

DOSAGE: *Adults:* Usual/Revaccination: Single 0.5mL dose SQ/IM in deltoid muscle or lateral mid-thigh.
Pediatrics: ≥2 yrs: Usual/Revaccination: Single 0.5mL dose SQ/IM in deltoid muscle or lateral mid-thigh.

HOW SUPPLIED: Inj: 0.5mL

WARNINGS/PRECAUTIONS: Will not prevent disease caused by capsular types of pneumococcus other than those contained in the vaccine. Should be given at least 2 weeks before elective splenectomy and immunosuppressive therapy. Avoid vaccination during chemotherapy or radiation. Suboptimal response may occur in immunocompromised patients. Intradermal administration may cause severe local reactions. Caution with severely compromised cardiovascular (CV) or pulmonary function in whom systemic reaction would be a significant risk. Delay vaccination with any febrile respiratory illness or other active infection. Prophylaxis with pneumococcal antibiotics should be continued. May not prevent pneumococcal meningitis in patients with chronic CSF leakage. Avoid routine revaccination of immunocompetent patients previously vaccinated with a 23-valent vaccine. Patients ≥2 yrs who are at highest risk for serious pneumococcal infections and likely to have a rapid decline in pneumococcal antibody levels may be revaccinated once.

ADVERSE REACTIONS: Local injection-site reactions (eg, soreness, warmth, erythema, swelling, induration), fever (≤102°F), asthenia, fatigue, myalgia, headache.

INTERACTIONS: Immunosuppressive therapies may reduce immune response; administer vaccine at least 2 weeks prior to the initiation of chemotherapy or other immunosuppresive therapies.

PREGNANCY: Category C, caution in nursing.

MECHANISM OF ACTION: Vaccine; bacterial capsular polysaccharides induce antibodies primarily by T-cell-independent mechanisms that protect against pneumococcal infection.

NURSING CONSIDERATIONS

Assessment: Assess hypersensitivity to any component of vaccine, health/immunity status, vaccination history, reaction to previous pneumococcal vaccine, compromised CV and pulmonary function, chronic CSF leakage, febrile respiratory illness or any active infection, pregnancy/nursing status, and possible drug interactions. Assess timing in chemotherapy and immunosuppressive therapy patients.

Monitoring: Monitor patients with compromised CV and pulmonary function. Monitor hypersensitivity reactions.

Patient Counseling: Inform about risks and benefits of vaccination. Inform that the vaccine may be administered at the same time as influenza vaccine (by separate injection in the other arm). Inform that vaccination may not offer 100% protection from pneumococcal infection. Inform that injection-site reactions may occur; advise to report any serious adverse reactions to physician/healthcare provider and if any serious adverse reactions develop. Advise routine vaccination for immunocompetent patients ≥65 yrs of age.

Administration: IM (preferably in deltoid muscle or lateral mid-thigh) and SQ route. Refer to PI for proper administration. **Storage:** 2-8°C (36-46°F).

PONSTEL   RX
mefenamic acid (Sciele)

> NSAIDs may cause an increased risk of serious cardiovascular thrombotic events, MI, stroke, and serious GI adverse events including bleeding, ulceration, and perforation of the stomach or intestines. Contraindicated for the treatment of perioperative pain in the setting of coronary artery bypass graft (CABG) surgery.

THERAPEUTIC CLASS: NSAID

INDICATIONS: Relief of mild to moderate pain in patients ≥14 yrs, when therapy will not exceed 7 days. Treatment of primary dysmenorrhea.

DOSAGE: *Adults:* Acute Pain: Usual: 500mg, then 250mg q6h prn up to 1 week. Primary Dysmenorrhea: Usual: 500mg, then 250mg q6h up to 3 days. Take with food.
Pediatrics: ≥14 yrs: Acute Pain: Usual: 500mg, then 250mg q6h prn up to 1 week. Primary Dysmenorrhea: Usual: 500mg, then 250mg q6h up to 3 days. Take with food.

HOW SUPPLIED: Cap: 250mg

CONTRAINDICATIONS: Pre-existing renal disease, active ulceration or chronic inflammation of the GI tract. Allergic-type reactions, including asthma and urticaria, after taking aspirin (ASA) or other NSAIDs. Treatment of perioperative pain in the setting of CABG surgery.

WARNINGS/PRECAUTIONS: May lead to onset of new HTN or worsening of pre-existing HTN; monitor BP closely. Fluid retention and edema reported; caution with fluid retention or heart failure. Renal papillary necrosis and other renal injury reported after long-term use. Not recommended for use with advanced renal disease. Anaphylactoid reactions may occur. May cause serious skin adverse events (eg, exfoliative dermatitis, Stevens-Johnson syndrome, and toxic epidermal necrolysis). Avoid in late pregnancy; may cause premature closure of ductus arteriosus. May cause elevations of LFTs; d/c if liver disease develops or systemic manifestations occur. Caution in elderly. Anemia may occur; with long-term use, monitor Hgb/Hct if signs or symptoms of anemia develop. May inhibit platelet aggregation and prolong bleeding

P

time; monitor with coagulation disorders. Caution with asthma and avoid with ASA-sensitive asthma.

ADVERSE REACTIONS: Abdominal pain, constipation, diarrhea, dyspepsia, flatulence, gross bleeding/perforation, heartburn, GI ulcers, N/V, anemia, dizziness, edema, headache, rash, tinnitus.

INTERACTIONS: Caution with CYP2C9 inhibitors. ASA may increase adverse effects; avoid use. Warfarin may increase GI bleeding. May prolong PT with oral anticoagulants. Decreases effects of ACE inhibitors, furosemide, and thiazides; monitor for renal toxicity. Increases lithium levels. Magnesium hydroxide may increase mefenamic acid levels. Enhances methotrexate toxicity; caution with concomitant use.

PREGNANCY: Category C, not for use in nursing.

MECHANISM OF ACTION: NSAID (fenamate derivative); suspected to inhibit prostaglandin synthetase, exerts anti-inflammatory, analgesic, and antipyretic actions.

PHARMACOKINETICS: Absorption: Rapid; C_{max}=10-20mcg/mL, T_{max}=2-4 hrs. **Distribution:** V_d=1.06L/kg; plasma protein binding (90%). **Metabolism**: Via CYP2C9. **Elimination:** Urine (52%), feces (20%); $T_{1/2}$=2 hrs.

NURSING CONSIDERATIONS

Assessment: Assess LFTs, renal function, CBC and coagulation profile. Assess for history of CABG surgery, asthma and allergic reactions to ASA or other NSAIDs, active ulceration or chronic inflammation of GI tract, CVD, pregnancy/nursing status. Note other diseases/conditions and drug therapies.

Monitoring: Monitor for hypersensitivity reactions, cardiac complications, stroke, GI bleeding, asthma, skin side effects. Monitor BP, LFT, renal functions, CBC with differential and platelet count and coagulation profile, hyperglycemia.

Patient Counseling: Counsel about side effects; seek medical attention if any develop. Avoid alcohol and smoking during treatment. Take drug as prescribed. Caution women against using medication late in pregnancy.

Administration: Oral route. **Storage:** 20-25°C (68-77°F); excursions permitted to 15-30°C (59-86°F).

PRADAXA   RX
dabigatran etexilate mesylate (Boehringer Ingelheim)

THERAPEUTIC CLASS: Thrombin inhibitor

INDICATIONS: To reduce risk of stroke and systemic embolism in patients with non-valvular atrial fibrillation.

DOSAGE: *Adults:* CrCl >30mL/min: 150mg bid. CrCl 15-30mL/min: 75mg bid. Conversion from Warfarin: D/C warfarin and start when INR is <2.0. Conversion from Parenteral Anticoagulants: Start 0-2 hrs before the time the next dose of parenteral drug was to have been administered or at the time of d/c of continuously administered parenteral drug (eg, IV unfractionated heparin). Surgery and Interventions: D/C 1-2 days for CrCl ≥50mL/min or 3-5 days for CrCl <50mL/min before invasive or surgical procedures. Refer to PI for conversion to warfarin and parenteral anticoagulants.

HOW SUPPLIED: Cap: 75mg, 150mg

CONTRAINDICATIONS: Active pathological bleeding.

WARNINGS/PRECAUTIONS: Increases risk of bleeding and can cause significant and sometimes, fatal bleeding; promptly evaluate for any signs/symptoms of blood loss (eg, drop in Hgb and/or Hct or hypotension). D/C use with active bleeding, elective surgery, or invasive procedures that may increase the risk of stroke. Avoid lapses in therapy; if therapy is temporarily d/c, restart as soon as possible. Caution with severe renal impairment (CrCl 15-30mL/min).

ADVERSE REACTIONS: Bleeding, GI reactions.

INTERACTIONS: Increased risk of bleeding with use of drugs that increase the risk of bleeding in general (eg, anti-platelet agents, heparin, fibrinolytics, chronic use of NSAIDs). Reduced exposure with P-gp inducers (eg, rifampin); avoid concomitant use. May increase concentrations when used concomitantly with ketoconazole, oral verapamil, amiodarone, quinidine, and clopidogrel.

PREGNANCY: Category C, caution in nursing.

MECHANISM OF ACTION: Direct thrombin inhibitor; prevents the development of a thrombus. Both free and clot-bound thrombin, and thrombin-induced platelet aggregation are inhibited by the active moieties.

PHARMACOKINETICS: Absorption: Absolute bioavailability (3-7%); T_{max}=1 hr (fasted). **Distribution:** Plasma protein binding (35%); V_d=50-70L. **Metabolism:** Hydrolysis, conjugation; acyl glucuronide (active metabolite). **Elimination:** Urine (7%), feces (86%); $T_{1/2}$=12-17 hrs. Refer to PI for estimated pharmacokinetic parameters by renal function.

NURSING CONSIDERATIONS

Assessment: Assess for active pathological bleeding, renal impairment, pregnancy/nursing status, and for possible drug interactions. Assess for ecarin clotting time (ECT), or activated partial thromboplastin time (aPTT) prior to invasive or surgical procedures. Assess risk factors for bleeding.

Monitoring: Monitor for bleeding, GI adverse reactions, and hypersensitivity reactions. Monitor for increased risk of stroke on temporary d/c.

Patient Counseling: Instruct to take exactly as prescribed and not to d/c without talking to physician. Advise not to chew, break or open caps and take the pellets alone. Inform patients that they may bleed longer and more easily; instruct to call healthcare provider for any signs/symptoms of bleeding. Call healthcare provider if signs/symptoms of dyspepsia or gastritis. Instruct patients to notify physician that they are taking dabigatran before any invasive procedure is scheduled.

Administration: Oral route. Swallow caps whole; do not break, chew or empty contents. **Storage:** 25°C (77°F); excursions permitted to 15-30°C (59-86°F). Store in the original package to protect from moisture. (Bottles) Once opened, must use within 30 days. Keep tightly closed.

PRANDIMET   RX
metformin HCl - repaglinide (Novo Nordisk)

> Lactic acidosis can occur due to metformin accumulation; increased risk with sepsis, dehydration, excess alcohol intake, hepatic impairment, renal impairment, and acute congestive heart failure (CHF). If acidosis suspected, d/c and hospitalize patient immediately.

THERAPEUTIC CLASS: Biguanide/Meglitinide

INDICATIONS: Adjunct to diet and exercise to improve glycemic control in adults with type 2 diabetes mellitus (DM) who are already treated with a meglitinide and metformin HCl, or who have inadequate glycemic control on a meglitinide alone or metformin HCl alone.

DOSAGE: *Adults:* Individualize dose. Administer 2-3 times a day up to 4mg-1000mg/meal. Take 15-30 min before meals. Max: 10mg-2500mg/day. Patient Inadequately Controlled on Metformin Monotherapy: Initial: 1mg-500mg bid with meals. Titrate: Gradually escalate dose to reduce risk of hypoglycemia. Patient Inadequately Controlled w/ Meglitinide Monotherapy: Initial: 500mg metformin bid. Titrate: Gradually escalate dose to reduce GI side effects. Concomitant use of Repaglinide/Metformin: Initiate at dose of repaglinide and metformin similar to (but not exceeding) current doses. Titrate to maximum daily dose as necessary to achieve targeted glycemic control.

HOW SUPPLIED: Tab: (Repaglinide-Metformin) 1mg-500mg, 2mg-500mg

CONTRAINDICATIONS: Renal impairment (eg, SrCr ≥1.5mg/dL [males], ≥1.4mg/dL [females], or abnormal CrCl). Acute or chronic metabolic acidosis, including diabetic ketoacidosis. Concomitant gemfibrozil.

WARNINGS/PRECAUTIONS: D/C temporarily prior to surgical procedures (except minor procedures not associated with restricted food and fluid intake); restart when oral intake resumed and if renal function is normal. D/C at the time of or prior to intravascular contrast studies with iodinated materials; withhold for 48 hrs subsequent to procedure and restart only if renal function is normal. Caution in elderly, debilitated, or malnourished patients and those with adrenal or pituitary insufficiency. May cause hypoglycemia, start on lowest repaglinide component. Loss of glycemic control may occur in patients with fever, infection, trauma or surgery; d/c and change to insulin temporarily. Promptly evaluate for lactic acidosis or ketoacidosis if a change in clinical status occurs in patients with previously controlled type 2 DM. May cause vitamin B_{12} deficiency; measure hematologic parameters annually. Avoid with hepatic impairment.

ADVERSE REACTIONS: Lactic acidosis, hypoglycemia, headache, diarrhea, N/V, upper respiratory tract infection.

INTERACTIONS: See Contraindications. (Metformin) Cationic drugs (eg, amiloride, digoxin, morphine, procainamide, quinidine, quinine, ranitidine, triamterene, trimethoprim, vancomycin) may increase levels. Increased levels with cimetidine, furosemide, nifedipine, ibuprofen. Decreased levels with propranolol. Alcohol potentiates effect of metformin. May decrease furosemide levels. Caution with drugs that may affect renal function or result in significant hemodynamic change or may interfere with the disposition of metformin. (Repaglinide) CYP2C8 inhibitors (eg, gemfibrozil, trimethoprim), CYP3A4 inhibitors (eg, itraconazole, ketaconazole), or CYP2C8/3A4 inducers (eg, rifampin) may alter the pharmacokinetics and pharmacodynamics of repaglinide. Not for use in combination with NPH insulin. May alter levels when used concomitantly with levonorgestrel/ethinyl estradiol. Increased levels with clarithromycin, ketoconazole, simvastatin, trimethoprim. Decreased levels with nifedipine, rifampin. May increase ethinyl estradiol levels. OATPIBI inhibitors (eg, cyclosporine) may increase plasma concentrations.

PREGNANCY: Category C, not for use in nursing.

MECHANISM OF ACTION: Metformin: Biguanide; improves glucose tolerance by lowering both basal and post prandial plasma glucose. Decreases hepatic glucose production, decreases intestinal absorption of glucose, and improves insulin sensitivity by increasing peripheral glucose uptake and utilization. Repaglinide: Meglitinide; lowers blood glucose levels by stimulating the release of insulin from the pancreas.

PHARMACOKINETICS: Absorption: Metformin: Absolute bioavailabilty (50%-60%); C_{max}=174.6-210.2ng/mL; AUC=1442-1494.6ng•h/mL. Repaglinide: Absolute bioavailability (56%); C_{max}=6.9-13.7ng/mL; AUC=6.6-13.3ng•h/mL. T_{max}=1 hr. **Distribution:** Metformin: V_d=654L. Repaglinide: V_d=31L; Plasma protein binding (>98%). **Metabolism:** Repaglinide: CYP2C8, CYP3A4; oxidation and direct conjugation; oxidized dicarboxylic acid (M2), aromatic amine (M1), acyl glucuronide (M7) (major metabolites). **Elimination:** Metformin: Urine (90%); $T_{1/2}$=6.2 hrs (plasma), 17.6 hrs (blood). Repaglinide: Feces (90%), urine (8%).

NURSING CONSIDERATIONS

Assessment: Assess for acute or chronic metabolic acidosis, renal/hepatic impairment, pregnancy/nursing status, possible drug interactions, or any other conditions where treatment is contraindicated or cautioned. Assess if scheduled to undergo any radiologic studies with iodinated materials, surgical procedure, or under any form of stress (eg, fever, infection, trauma). Obtain baseline vital signs and weight, FPG, HbA1c, renal function, LFTs, and hematological parameters (CBC).

Monitoring: Monitor for signs/symptoms of hypoglycemia, lactic acidosis, decreased Vitamin B_{12} levels, cardiovascular collapse (shock), acute CHF, acute MI, adrenal or pituitary insufficiency, and for renal/hepatic impairment. Perform periodic monitoring of vital signs and weight, physical activity, FPG, HbA1c, and LFTs, and hematologic parameters (CBC). Monitor renal function at least annually. Monitor serum electrolytes and ketones, blood pH, lactate, pyruvate, and metformin levels if clinical illness develops.

Patient Counseling: Inform about risks and benefits of therapy. Inform that drug is an adjunct to diet and should be taken 15-30 min before meals. If meal is skipped, instruct to skip dose for that meal. Counsel against excessive alcohol intake during therapy. Inform patient of importance of regular testing of blood glucose, HbA1c, renal function, and hematologic parameters. Advise that during periods of stress (eg, fever, trauma, infection, or surgery), medication requirements may change. Inform about the risks of hypoglycemia, its symptoms and treatment, and predisposing conditions. Inform of risk of lactic acidosis, and predisposing conditions; advise to d/c immediately and contact physician if unexplained hyperventilation, myalgia, malaise, unusual somnolence, or other nonspecific symptoms occur. Advise to notify physician of all concomitant medications and if pregnant or nursing.

Administration: Oral route. **Storage:** Do not store above 25°C (77°F). Protect from moisture. Keep bottles tightly closed.

PRANDIN RX
repaglinide (Novo Nordisk)

THERAPEUTIC CLASS: Meglitinide

INDICATIONS: Adjunct to diet and exercise to improve glycemic control in type 2 diabetes mellitus (DM).

DOSAGE: *Adults:* Initial: Treatment-Naive or HbA1c <8%: 0.5mg with each meal. Previous Therapy with Blood Glucose-Lowering Drugs and HbA1c ≥8%: 1-2mg with each meal. Titrate: May double preprandial dose up to 4mg at no less than 1-week intervals until response is achieved. Maint: 0.5-4mg with meals. May be dosed preprandially bid-qid in response to changes in meal pattern. Max: 16mg/day. Occurrence of Hypoglycemia with Metformin or Thiazolidinedione (TZD) Combination: Reduce repaglinide dose. Replacement Therapy of Other Oral Hypoglycemic Agents: Start repaglinide on the day after final dose is given. Severe Renal Impairment: CrCl 20-40mL/min: Initial: 0.5mg with each meal; titrate carefully. Hepatic Dysfunction: Longer intervals between dose adjustments. Take within 15-30 min before meals (bid-qid). Skip dose if skip meal and add dose if add meal.

HOW SUPPLIED: Tab: 0.5mg, 1mg, 2mg

CONTRAINDICATIONS: Diabetic ketoacidosis with or without coma, type 1 diabetes, coadministration of gemfibrozil.

WARNINGS/PRECAUTIONS: Risk of hypoglycemia, especially with renal/hepatic insufficiency, elderly, debilitated, malnourished, and adrenal/pituitary insufficiency. Loss of blood glucose control may occur when exposed to stress (eg, fever, trauma, infection, or surgery); may need to d/c therapy and administer insulin. Secondary failure can occur over a period of time. Caution with hepatic impairment.

ADVERSE REACTIONS: Hypoglycemia, upper respiratory infection, headache, rhinitis, sinusitis, bronchitis, arthralgia, back pain, N/V, diarrhea, dyspepsia, cardiovascular (CV) events, constipation, paresthesia, chest pain.

INTERACTIONS: See Contraindications. Avoid coadministering with NPH-insulin. Increased metabolism with CYP3A4 and/or 2C8 inducers (eg, rifampin, barbiturates, carbamazepine). CYP3A4 inhibitors (eg, ketoconazole, itraconazole, clarithromycin, erythromycin) and CYP2C8 inhibitors (eg, trimethoprim, gemfibrozil, and montelukast) may inhibit metabolism. Increased levels with Organic Anion Transporting Protein (OATP1B1) inhibitors (eg, cyclosporine). Potentiated hypoglycemia with alcohol, β-blockers, NSAIDs, other highly protein-bound drugs, salicylates, sulfonamides, cyclosporine, chloramphenicol, coumarins, probenecid, MAOIs, and other glucose-lowering agents. Risk of hyperglycemia with thiazides and other diuretics, corticosteroids, phenothiazines, thyroid products, estrogens, phenytoin, nicotinic acid, oral contraceptives, sympathomimetics, CCBs, and isoniazid (INH). β-blockers may mask hypoglycemia. Increased repaglinide, levonorgestrel, and ethinyl estradiol C_{max} and ethinyl estradiol AUC with levonorgestrel/ethinyl estradiol combination coadministration. Increased repaglinide C_{max} with simvastatin.

PREGNANCY: Category C, not for use in nursing.

MECHANISM OF ACTION: Meglitinide; lowers blood glucose levels by stimulating the release of insulin from the pancreas.

PHARMACOKINETICS: Absorption: Rapid and complete; absolute bioavailability (56%); (0.5mg) $C_{max0-5 hr}$=9.8ng/mL; (0.5mg) $AUC_{0-24 hr}$=68.9ng/mL•hr; T_{max}=1 hr. See PI for parameters for different doses. **Distribution:** (IV) V_d=31L; plasma protein binding (>98%). **Metabolism:** CYP2C8, 3A4; oxidation, glucuronidation; oxidized dicarboxylic acid (M2), aromatic amine (M1), acyl glucuronide (M7) (major metabolites). **Elimination:** Feces (90%), urine (8%); $T_{1/2}$=1 hr.

NURSING CONSIDERATIONS

Assessment: Assess for diabetic ketoacidosis, type 1 DM, concomitant use of gemfibrozil, CV risk factors, adrenal insufficiency, pituitary insufficiency, renal/hepatic insufficiency, pregnancy/nursing status, and possible drug interactions. Obtain baseline FPG, HbA1c, renal function, and LFTs.

Monitoring: Monitor for hypo/hyperglycemia, upper respiratory infection, headache, renal/hepatic insufficiency, and other adverse events that may occur. Monitor FPG, HbA1c every 3 months, renal function, and LFTs.

Patient Counseling: Inform about importance of adherence to dietary instructions, regular exercise program, regular blood glucose monitoring, and periodic HbA1c testing. Inform about risks/benefits of therapy, alternative modes of therapy, and primary/secondary failure. Inform about risks of hypoglycemia, its symptoms and treatment, and predisposing conditions. Instruct to inform physician if rhinitis, sinusitis, headache, and other adverse events occur. Instruct to take before meals. Instruct to skip dose if skipping a meal and add dose if adding a meal.

Administration: Oral route. **Storage:** Do not store above 25°C (77°F).

PRAVACHOL   RX
pravastatin sodium (Bristol-Myers Squibb)

THERAPEUTIC CLASS: HMG-CoA reductase inhibitor

INDICATIONS: Adjunct to diet in primary hypercholesterolemia and mixed dyslipidemia (Fredrickson Type IIa and IIb) to reduce elevated total-C, LDL-C, Apo B, TG levels, and to increase HDL-C. Treatment of primary dysbetalipoproteinemia (Fredrickson Type III) with inadequate response to diet. Adjunct to diet in the treatment of elevated TG levels (Fredrickson Type IV). Adjunct to diet and lifestyle modifications in heterozygous familial hypercholesterolemia in patients ≥8 years-old if LDL-C remains ≥190mg/dL, or LDL-C remains ≥160mg/dL (with positive family history of premature cardiovascular diseasae (CVD), or 2 or more other CVD risk factors present). Reduction of risk of MI, of undergoing myocardial revascularization procedures, and of cardiovascular mortality with no increase in death from non-cardiovascular causes in hypercholesterolemia without coronary heart disease (CHD). Reduction of risk of mortality by reducing coronary death, of undergoing myocardial revascularization procedures, and of MI, stroke, and transient ischemic attack (TIA) in clinically evident CHD and to slow progression of coronary atherosclerosis.

DOSAGE: *Adults:* ≥18 yrs: Initial: 40mg qd. Perform lipid tests within 4 weeks and adjust according to response and guidelines. Titrate: May increase to 80mg qd if needed. Significant Renal/Hepatic Dysfunction: Initial: 10mg qd. Concomitant Immunosuppressives (eg, cyclosporine): Initial:10mg qhs. Max: 20mg/day.
Pediatrics: Heterozygous Familial Hypercholesterolemia: 14-18 yrs: Initial: 40mg qd. Max: 40mg/day. 8-13 yrs: 20mg qd. Max: 20mg/day. Concomitant Immunosuppressives (eg, cyclosporine): Initial: 10mg qhs. Max: 20mg/day.

HOW SUPPLIED: Tab: 10mg, 20mg, 40mg, 80mg

CONTRAINDICATIONS: Active liver disease, unexplained persistent elevations of LFTs, pregnancy, nursing mothers.

WARNINGS/PRECAUTIONS: May cause biochemical abnormalities of liver function; perform LFTs before therapy, before dose increases, and if clinically indicated. Risk of myopathy, myalgia, and rhabdomyolysis. D/C if AST or ALT ≥3x ULN persists, if elevated CPK levels occur, or if myopathy diagnosed or suspected. Less effective with homozygous familial hypercholesterolemia. Monitor for endocrine dysfunction. Closely monitor with heavy alcohol use, recent history or signs of hepatic disease, or renal dysfunction.

ADVERSE REACTIONS: Rash, N/V, diarrhea, headache, chest pain, abdominal pain, dizziness, constipation, flatulence, fatigue, localized pain, common cold, rhinitis, dyspepsia/heartburn, musculoskeletal pain.

INTERACTIONS: Risk of myopathy with fibrates, niacin, cyclosporine, erythromycin. Increased levels with gemfibrozil, itraconazole. Avoid fibrates unless benefit outweighs drug combination risk. Decreased levels with concomitant cholestyramine/colestipol; take 1 hr before or 4 hrs after resins. Caution with drugs that diminish levels or activity of steroid hormones (eg, ketoconazole, spironolactone, cimetidine).

PREGNANCY: Category X, not for use in nursing.

MECHANISM OF ACTION: HMG-CoA reductase inhibitor; causes increased number of LDL-receptors on cell surfaces and enhanced receptor mediated catabolism and clearance of circulating LDL. Inhibits LDL production by inhibiting hepatic synthesis of VLDL, LDL precursor.

PHARMACOKINETICS: Absorption: Rapid. Absolute bioavailability (17%); T_{max}=1-1.5 hrs. **Distribution:** Plasma protein binding (50%). **Metabolism:** Liver. **Elimination:** Feces (70%), urine (20%); $T_{1/2}$=77 hrs.

NURSING CONSIDERATIONS

Assessment: Prior to initiation, assess secondary causes of hypercholesterolemia (eg, poorly controlled DM, hypothyroidism, nephrotic syndrome, dysproteinemias, obstructive liver disease, other drug therapy, alcoholism), active liver disease, elevations in serum transaminases, pregnancy/nursing status, and possible drug interactions. Obtain baseline lipid profile and LFTs.

Monitoring: Monitor for signs/symptoms of active liver disease, rhabdomyolysis with acute renal failure, myoglobinuria, myopathies. Monitor CPK and LFTs periodically, and lipid levels every 4 weeks to evaluate response.

Patient Counseling: Advise to report signs/symptoms of unexplained muscle pain, tenderness, or weakness, particularly with malaise or fever. Recommend standard cholesterol-lowering diet prior to and during treatment. Educate about pregnancy/nursing risks. Counsel to take with/without food.

Administration: Oral route. **Storage:** 25°C (77°F); excursions permitted to 15-30°C (59-86°F). Keep tightly closed, protect from light and moisture.

P

PRECEDEX   RX
dexmedetomidine HCl (Hospira)

THERAPEUTIC CLASS: Alpha$_2$-agonist

INDICATIONS: For sedation of initially intubated and mechanically ventilated patients during treatment in an intensive care setting. For sedation of non-intubated patients prior to and/or during surgical and other procedures.

DOSAGE: *Adults:* Individualize dose. Not indicated for infusions >24 hrs. ICU Sedation: Initial: Up to 1mcg/kg IV infusion over 10 min. Conversion from Alternate Sedative Therapy: Initial: A loading dose may be required. Maint: 0.2-0.7mcg/kg/hr. Adjust to achieve desired level of sedation. Procedural Sedation: Initial: 1mcg/kg IV infusion over 10 min. Maint: 0.6mcg/kg/hr. Titrate: 0.2-1mcg/kg/hr. Adjust to achieve desired level of sedation. Elderly (>65 yrs): Initial: 0.5mcg/kg IV infusion over 10 min. Less Invasive Procedures (eg, ophthalmic surgery): Initial: 0.5mcg/kg IV infusion over 10 min. Awake Fiberoptic Intubation: Initial: 1mcg/kg IV infusion over 10 min. Maint: 0.7mcg/kg/hr until endotracheal tube is secured. Elderly (>65 yrs)/Hepatic Impairment: Dose reduction should be considered.

HOW SUPPLIED: Inj: 100mcg/mL

WARNINGS/PRECAUTIONS: Should only be administered by persons skilled in the management of patients in an intensive care setting. Monitor patients continuously. Hypotension, bradycardia and sinus arrest reported; treat appropriately. Hypotension and/or bradycardia may be more pronounced in patients with hypovolemia, diabetes mellitus (DM), or chronic HTN and in elderly patients. Caution with advanced heart block and/or severe ventricular dysfunction. Transient HTN observed primarily during the loading dose. Arousability and alertness reported in some patients upon stimulation. Withdrawal events (eg, N/V, agitation) reported within 24-48 hrs after d/c therapy. If tachycardia and/or HTN occurs after d/c, supportive therapy is indicated. Use for >24 hrs associated with tolerance, tachyphylaxis, and a dose related increase in adverse events.

ADVERSE REACTIONS: Hypotension, HTN, bradycardia, dry mouth, respiratory depression, tachycardia, N/V, atrial fibrillation, fever, hyperglycemia, anemia, hypovolemia, hypoxia, atelectasis.

INTERACTIONS: Concurrent use with anesthetics, sedatives, hypnotics, and opioids (eg, sevoflurane, isoflurane, propofol, alfentanil, midazolam) may potentiate effects; consider dose reduction. Caution with concomitant use of other vasodilators or negative chronotropic agents; may have additive effects.

PREGNANCY: Category C, caution in nursing.

MECHANISM OF ACTION: Selective α_2-adrenergic agonist; possesses sedative properties.

PHARMACOKINETICS: Distribution: V_d=118L, plasma protein binding (94%). **Metabolism:** Liver via direct glucuronidation and CYP2A6 (aliphatic hydroxylation). **Elimination:** Feces (4%), urine (95%); $T_{1/2}$= 2 hrs.

NURSING CONSIDERATIONS

Assessment: Assess for advanced heart block, severe ventricular dysfunction, hepatic impairment, hypovolemia, DM, chronic HTN, pregnancy/nursing status, and for possible drug interactions. Obtain baseline vital signs, ECG, and LFTs.

Monitoring: Monitor for hypotension, bradycardia, sinus arrest, transient HTN. Monitor for tolerance and tachyphylaxis if use of therapy >24 hrs.

Patient Counseling: If infused for >6 hrs, instruct to report nervousness, agitation and headaches that may occur for up to 48 hrs. Instruct to report symptoms that may occur within 48 hrs after administration (eg, weakness, confusion, excessive sweating, weight loss, abdominal pain, salt cravings, diarrhea, constipation, dizziness or lightheadedness).

Administration: IV route. Refer to PI for preparation and administration instructions. **Storage:** 25°C (77°F); excursions allowed 15-30°C (59-86°F).

PRECOSE   RX
acarbose (Bayer Healthcare)

THERAPEUTIC CLASS: Alpha-glucosidase inhibitor

INDICATIONS: Adjunct to diet and exercise, to improve glycemic control in type 2 diabetes mellitus.

DOSAGE: *Adults:* Initial: 25mg tid with first bite of each main meal. To minimize GI effects: 25mg qd, increase gradually to 25mg tid. Titrate: After reaching 25mg tid, may increase at 4-8 week intervals. Maint: 50-100mg tid. Max: ≤60kg: 50mg tid. >60kg: 100mg tid. If no further reduction in postprandial glucose or HbA$_{1c}$ with 100mg tid, consider reducing dose.

HOW SUPPLIED: Tab: 25mg, 50mg, 100mg

CONTRAINDICATIONS: Diabetic ketoacidosis, cirrhosis, inflammatory bowel disease, colonic ulceration, partial or predisposition to intestinal obstruction, chronic intestinal disease with marked disorders of digestion or absorption, and conditions that may deteriorate from increased intestinal gas formation.

WARNINGS/PRECAUTIONS: Avoid with significant renal dysfunction (SrCr >2mg/dL). May need to d/c and give insulin with stress (eg, fever, trauma). Dose-related elevated serum transaminase levels reported. Monitor serum transaminases every 3 months for first year, then periodically. Reduce dose or d/c if elevated serum transaminases persist. Use glucose (dextrose) instead of sucrose (sugar cane) to treat mild to moderate hypoglycemia.

ADVERSE REACTIONS: Flatulence, diarrhea, abdominal pain.

INTERACTIONS: Risk of hyperglycemia with diuretics, corticosteroids, phenothiazines, thyroid products, estrogens, oral contraceptives, phenytoin, nicotinic acid, sympathomimetics, CCBs, and isoniazid. Reduced effect with intestinal adsorbents (eg, charcoal) and digestive enzymes containing carbo-hydrate-splitting enzymes (eg, amylase, pancreatin); avoid concomitant use. May affect digoxin bioavailability; may require dose adjustment of digoxin. Monitor for hypoglycemia with insulin or sulfonylureas.

PREGNANCY: Category B, not for use in nursing.

MECHANISM OF ACTION: α-glucosidase inhibitor; reversibly inhibits pan-creatic α-amylase and membrane-bound intestinal α-glucoside hydrolase enzymes.

PHARMACOKINETICS: Absorption: Poor; T_{max}=1 hr. **Metabolism:** GI tract by in-testinal bacteria or digestive enzymes; 4-methylpyrogallol derivatives (major metabolites). **Elimination:** Urine (unchanged); $T_{1/2}$=2 hrs.

NURSING CONSIDERATIONS

Assessment: Assess for renal dysfunction, cirrhosis, diabetic ketoacidosis, in-flammatory bowel disease, colonic ulceration or partial intestinal obstruction, chronic intestinal disease, pregnancy status, and possible drug interactions.

Monitoring: Monitor for hypoglycemia, FPG, HbA_{1c}, LFTs, renal function, diabetic ketoacidosis, GI symptoms (eg, abdominal pain, diarrhea, flatulence), hypersensitivity reactions. Monitor serum transaminases every 3 months for first year, then periodically.

Patient Counseling: Instruct to take three times daily at the start of each meal. Counsel about signs/symptoms of hypoglycemia. Inform about impor-tance of adhering to dietary instructions, a regular exercise program, and regular testing of urine and blood glucose.

Administration: Oral route. **Storage:** 25°C (77°F); protect from moisture; keep container tightly closed.

PRED FORTE   RX
prednisolone acetate (Allergan)

THERAPEUTIC CLASS: Corticosteroid

INDICATIONS: Treatment of inflammation of the palpebral and bulbar con-junctiva, cornea and anterior segment of the globe.

DOSAGE: *Adults:* 1-2 drops bid-qid. May dose more frequently during initial 24-48 hrs. Re-evaluate after 2 days if no improvement.

HOW SUPPLIED: Sus: 1% [1mL, 5mL, 10mL, 15mL]

CONTRAINDICATIONS: Viral diseases of the cornea and conjunctiva including epithelial herpes simplex keratitis, vaccinia, and varicella. Mycobacterial infec-tion and fungal diseases of the eye.

WARNINGS/PRECAUTIONS: Caution with glaucoma, herpes simplex, diseases causing thinning of cornea/sclera and other ocular viral infections. Prolonged use can cause glaucoma or secondary ocular infections (eg, fungal). Monitor IOP after 10 days of therapy. Re-evaluate if no response after 2 days. May delay healing and increase incidence of bleb formation after cataract surgery. Avoid abrupt withdrawal with chronic use. Contains sodium bisulfite.

ADVERSE REACTIONS: Elevation of IOP, glaucoma, infrequent optic nerve damage, posterior subcapsular cataract formation, delayed wound healing, burning/stinging upon instillation, ocular irritation, secondary infection, visual disturbance.

PREGNANCY: Category C, not for use in nursing.

MECHANISM OF ACTION: Glucocorticoid; anti-inflammatory agent; inhibits edema, fibrin deposition, capillary dilation, deposition of collagen, and scar formation.

NURSING CONSIDERATIONS

Assessment: Assess for viral disease of cornea and conjunctiva, dendritic keratitis, vaccinia and varicella, mycobacterial infection and/or fungal disease of ocular structures, glaucoma, mustard gas keratitis, Sjogren's keratocon-juctivitis, thinning of corneal/scleral epithelium, hypersensitivity to sulfite, asthma, cataract surgery, and pregnancy/nursing status.

Monitoring: Monitor for anaphylactic symptoms and asthma attacks. Frequent measuring of IOP and slit lamp microscopy exam where appropriate, fluorescein staining for monitoring of glaucoma with damage to the optic nerve with defects in visual acuity and fields of vision, posterior subcapsular cataract, delayed corneal healing, thinning of cornea and sclera, ulceration, perforation, and secondary ocular infections (or masking of existing infections).

Patient Counseling: Advise to d/c drug and consult physician if symptoms persist or worsen. Instruct to wait 15 min after instillation to wear soft contact lenses. Counsel to avoid touching bottle tip to eyelids or any other surface.

Administration: Ocular route. **Storage:** 25°C (77°F). Protect from freezing. Keep tightly closed.

PREDNISONE   RX
prednisone (Roxane)

THERAPEUTIC CLASS: Glucocorticoid

INDICATIONS: Steroid-responsive disorders.

DOSAGE: *Adults:* Initial: 5-60mg/day depending on disease and response. Maint: Decrease dose by small amounts to lowest effective dose. *Pediatrics:* Initial: 5-60mg/day depending on disease and response. Maint: Decrease dose by small amounts to lowest effective dose.

HOW SUPPLIED: Sol: 5mg/mL, 5mg/5mL; Tab: 1mg, 2.5mg, 5mg, 10mg, 20mg, 50mg

CONTRAINDICATIONS: Systemic fungal infections.

WARNINGS/PRECAUTIONS: May need to increase dose before, during, and after stressful situations. May mask signs of infection or cause new infections. Prolonged use may produce glaucoma, optic nerve damage, secondary ocular infections. Increases BP, salt/water retention, K$^+$ excretion. More severe/fatal course of infections reported with chickenpox, measles. Caution with latent TB, hypothyroidism, cirrhosis, ocular herpes simplex, HTN, diverticulitis, fresh intestinal anastomosis, ulcerative colitis, osteoporosis, myasthenia gravis, renal insufficiency, peptic ulcer disease. Growth and development of children on prolonged therapy should be monitored. Monitor for psychic disturbances. Avoid abrupt withdrawal.

ADVERSE REACTIONS: Fluid and electrolyte disturbances, HTN, osteoporosis, muscle weakness, cushingoid state, menstrual irregularities, nervousness, insomnia, impaired wound healing, DM, ulcerative esophagitis, excessive sweating, increased ICP, carbohydrate intolerance, glaucoma, cataracts, weight gain, nausea, malaise.

INTERACTIONS: Increases clearance of high dose aspirin (ASA); caution in hypoprothrombinemia. Increased insulin and oral hypoglycemic requirements in DM. Avoid smallpox vaccine, and live vaccines with immunosuppressive doses. Possible decreased vaccine response with killed or inactivated vaccines with immunosuppressive doses. Increased clearance with hepatic enzyme inducers. Decreased metabolism with troleandomycin, ketoconazole. Variable effect on oral anticoagulants.

PREGNANCY: Safety in pregnancy and nursing not known.

MECHANISM OF ACTION: Anti-inflammatory glucocorticoid; causes profound and varied metabolic effects and modifies the body's immune responses to diverse stimuli.

PHARMACOKINETICS: Absorption: Readily absorbed (GI tract).

NURSING CONSIDERATIONS

Assessment: Assess unusual stress, fungal/other current infections, active TB, thyroid status, vaccination status, hepatic/liver impairment, hypoprothrombinemia, psychiatric tendencies, ulcerative colitis, diverticulitis, peptic ulcer with/without impending perforation, intestinal anastamoses, HTN, osteoporosis, myasthenia gravis, pregnancy/nursing status, and possible drug interactions.

Monitoring: In pediatrics, monitor for hypoadrenalism, growth and development. Monitor for psychiatric derangements, infection, cataracts, fluid retention, adrenocortical insufficiency, intestinal perforation/peritoneal irritation, serum electrolytes, TSH, glucose, LFTs, BP, IOP.

Patient Counseling: Avoid exposure to chickenpox or measles; report immediately if exposed. Advise regarding dietary salt restriction and K⁺ supplementaion.

Administration: Oral route. **Storage:** 25°C (77°F); excursions permitted to 15-30°C.

PREMARIN TABLETS RX
conjugated estrogens (Wyeth)

> Estrogens increase the risk of endometrial cancer; perform adequate diagnostic measures to rule out malignancy. Estrogens, with or without progestins, should not be used for the prevention of cardiovascular (CV) disease or dementia. Increased risks of myocardial infarction (MI), stroke, invasive breast cancer, pulmonary embolism (PE), and deep vein thrombosis (DVT) in postmenopausal women (50-79 yrs of age). Increased risk of developing probable dementia in postmenopausal women ≥65. Prescribe at the lowest effective dose for the shortest duration consistent with treatment goals and risks for the individual woman.

THERAPEUTIC CLASS: Estrogen

INDICATIONS: Treatment of moderate to severe vasomotor symptoms and/or vulvar/vaginal atrophy due to menopause. Treatment of hypoestrogenism due to hypogonadism, castration, or primary ovarian failure. Palliative treatment of breast cancer in patients with metastatic disease. Palliative treatment of advanced androgen-dependent carcinoma of the prostate. Prevention of postmenopausal osteoporosis.

DOSAGE: *Adults:* Vasomotor Symptoms/Vulvar/Vaginal Atrophy: Initial: 0.3mg qd continuously or cyclically (eg, 25 days on, 5 days off). Subsequent dosage adjustment may be made based upon individual patient response. Osteoporosis Prevention: Initial: 0.3mg qd continuously or cyclically. Subsequent dosage adjustment may be made based upon the individual clinical and bone mineral density (BMD) response. Female Hypogonadism: 0.3 or 0.625mg qd cyclically (eg, 3 weeks on and 1 week off). Doses are adjusted depending on the severity of symptoms and responsiveness of the endometrium. Female Castration/Ovarian Failure: 1.25mg qd cyclically. Adjust dosage according to severity of symptoms and response. Breast Cancer (palliation): 10mg tid for minimum 3 months. Prostate Cancer (palliation): 1.25-2.5mg tid. Use lowest effective dose and for the shortest duration consistent with treatment goals and risk. Re-evaluate periodically as clinically appropriate (eg, 3 month to 6 month intervals) to determine if treatment is still necessary.

HOW SUPPLIED: Tab: 0.3mg, 0.45mg, 0.625mg, 0.9mg, 1.25mg.

CONTRAINDICATIONS: Pregnancy, undiagnosed abnormal genital bleeding, known, suspected or history of breast cancer unless being treated for metastatic disease, known or suspected estrogen-dependent neoplasia, active or history of DVT/PE, active or recent (eg, within past year) arterial thromboembolic disease (eg, stroke, MI), liver dysfunction or disease, thrombophilic disorders (eg, protein C, protein S, or antithrombin deficiency).

WARNINGS/PRECAUTIONS: May increase risk of MI, stroke, DVT, and PE; d/c immediately if any of these events occur or are suspected. May increase risk of breast/endometrial cancer, and gallbladder diseases. May lead to severe hypercalcemia with breast cancer and bone metastases; monitor and d/c if hypercalcemia occurs. Retinal vascular thrombosis reported; d/c pending an exam if sudden partial or complete loss of vision, or sudden onset of proptosis, diplopia, or migraine occur. D/C permanently if papilledema or retinal vascular lesions are found. Consider addition of a progestin if no hysterectomy. May elevate BP; monitor at regular intervals. May cause elevations of plasma triglycerides which may lead to pancreatitis in patients with pre-existing hypertriglyceridemia. Caution with history of cholestatic jaundice associated with past estrogen use or with pregnancy; d/c with recurrence. May lead to increased thyroid-binding globulin levels; monitor thyroid function. May cause fluid retention; caution with cardiac/renal dysfunction. Caution with severe hypocalcemia. May increase risk of ovarian cancer. May induce or exacerbate symptoms of angioedema, particularly in women with hereditary angioedema. May exacerbate endometriosis, asthma, DM, epilepsy, migraine, porphyria, systemic lupus erythematosus (SLE), and hepatic hemangiomas; use with caution.

ADVERSE REACTIONS: Abdominal pain, back pain, headache, infection, pain, arthralgia, leg cramps, breast pain, vaginal hemorrhage, vaginitis, flatulence, asthenia, flu syndrome, diarrhea, nausea.

INTERACTIONS: CYP3A4 inducers (eg, St. John's wort, phenobarbital, carbamazepine, rifampin) may decrease levels which may decrease therapeutic effects and/or change uterine bleeding profile. CYP3A4 inhibitors (eg, erythromycin, clarithromycin, ketoconazole, itraconazole, ritonavir, grapefruit juice) may increase levels which may result in side effects. Patients dependent on thyroid replacement therapy may require increased doses of their thyroid replacement therapy; estrogen leads to increased thyroid-binding globulin (TBG) levels.

PREGNANCY: Contraindicated in pregnancy, not for use in nursing.

MECHANISM OF ACTION: Estrogen; binds to nuclear receptors in estrogen-responsive tissues. Circulating estrogens modulate pituitary secretion of the gonadotropins, luteinizing hormone and follicle stimulating hormone, through negative feedback mechanism. Reduces elevated levels of these hormones in postmenopausal women.

PHARMACOKINETICS: Absorption: Well absorbed; oral administration of variable doses resulted in different parameters. **Distribution:** Largely bound to sex hormone binding globulin and albumin; found in breast milk. **Metabolism:** Liver, to estrone (metabolite) and estriol (major urinary metabolite); sulfate and glucuronide conjugation (liver); gut hydrolysis; CYP3A4 (partial metabolism). **Elimination:** Urine (parent drug and metabolites).

NURSING CONSIDERATIONS

Assessment: Assess for undiagnosed abnormal genital bleeding, presence or history of breast cancer, estrogen-dependent neoplasia, DVT or PE, or any other conditions where treatment is contraindicated or cautioned. Assess for pregnancy/nursing status and possible drug interactions. Assess need for progestin therapy in women who have not had a hysterectomy. Assess for cardiac or renal dysfunction.

Monitoring: Monitor for signs/symptoms of CV disorders, malignant neoplasms, dementia, gallbladder disease, hypercalcemia, visual abnormalities, BP elevations, elevations in plasma triglycerides, pancreatitis, hypothyroidism, fluid retention, exacerbation of endometriosis and other conditions (eg, asthma, DM, epilepsy, migraines, SLE). Perform annual breast exam. Monitor BP levels regularly and thyroid function in patients on thyroid replacement therapy. Perform periodic evaluation (every 3-6 months) including BMD to determine treatment need. If undiagnosed persistent or recurring genital bleeding occurs, perform adequate diagnostic measures (eg, endometrial sampling) to rule out malignancy.

Patient Counseling: Inform that drug increases risk for uterine cancer, heart attack, stroke, breast cancer, blood clots, and dementia. Report any breast lumps, unusual vaginal bleeding, dizziness and faintness, changes in speech, severe headaches, chest pain, SOB, leg pains, changes in vision, or vomiting. Advise to notify physician if planning surgery or bedrest. Instruct to take medication at same time daily and to perform monthly self breast exams. Counsel that if dose is missed, take as soon as possible; if almost time for next dose, skip dose, and go back to normal dosing schedule.

Administration: Oral route. **Storage:** 20-25°C (68-77°F); excursions permitted to 15-30°C (59-86°F); dispense in tightly closed container.

PREMARIN VAGINAL   RX
conjugated estrogens (Wyeth)

> Estrogens increase the risk of endometrial cancer. Should not be used, with or without progestins, for the prevention of cardiovascular (CV) disease or dementia. Increased risks of myocardial infarction (MI), stroke, invasive breast cancer, pulmonary embolism (PE), and deep vein thrombosis (DVT) in postmenopausal women (50-79 yrs of age) reported. Increased risk of developing probable dementia in postmenopausal women ≥65 yrs of age reported. Estrogens with or without progestins should be prescribed at the lowest effective dose and for the shortest duration consistent with treatment goals and risks for the individual woman.

THERAPEUTIC CLASS: Estrogen

INDICATIONS: Treatment of atrophic vaginitis, kraurosis vulvae, and moderate-to-severe dyspareunia due to menopause.

DOSAGE: *Adults:* Atrophic Vaginitis/Kraurosis Vulvae: Usual: 0.5g intravaginally qd cyclically (3 weeks on, 1 week off). Titrate: 0.5-2g based on individual response. Moderate To Severe Dyspareunia: 0.5g intravaginally twice weekly (eg, Monday and Thursday) continuous regimen or cyclically (3 weeks on, 1 week off).

HOW SUPPLIED: Cre: 0.625mg/g [42.5g]

CONTRAINDICATIONS: Pregnancy, undiagnosed abnormal genital bleeding, known or suspected or history of breast cancer, known or suspected estrogen-dependent neoplasia, active or history of DVT/PE, history of or active arterial thromboembolic disease (eg, stroke, MI), liver dysfunction or disease, thrombophilic disorders (eg, protein C, protein S, or antithrombin deficiency).

WARNINGS/PRECAUTIONS: May increase risk of breast/endometrial/ovarian cancer, dementia and gallbladder disease. May lead to severe hypercalcemia in women with breast cancer and bone metastases; monitor and d/c if hypercalcemia occurs. Retinal vascular thrombosis reported; d/c pending examination if sudden partial or complete loss of vision, sudden onset of proptosis, diplopia, migraine, or if examination reveals papilledema or retinal vascular lesions. Consider addition of a progestin if no hysterectomy. May elevate BP; monitor at regular intervals. May cause elevations of plasma triglycerides with pre-existing hypertriglyceridemia. Caution with history of cholestatic jaundice associated with past estrogen use or with pregnancy; d/c with recurrence. May lead to increased thyroid-binding globulin levels; monitor thyroid function. May cause fluid retention; caution with cardiac/renal dysfunction. Caution with severe hypocalcemia. May induce or exacerbate symptoms of angioedema, particularly in women with hereditary angioedema. May exacerbate endometriosis, asthma, diabetes mellitus (DM), epilepsy, migraine, porphyria, systemic lupus erythematosus (SLE), and hepatic hemangiomas; use with caution. May weaken and contribute to the failure of condoms, diaphragms, or cervical caps made of latex or rubber.

ADVERSE REACTIONS: Arthralgia, asthenia, pain, breast pain, abdominal pain, back pain, vaginitis, headache, nausea, insomnia, vasodilation, pharyngitis, infection, cough increased, diarrhea.

INTERACTIONS: CYP3A4 inducers (eg, St. John's wort, phenobarbital) may decrease levels and decrease therapeutic effects and/or change uterine bleeding profile. CYP3A4 inhibitors (eg, erythromycin, clarithromycin) may increase levels and result in side effects. Women dependent on thyroid replacement therapy may require higher doses of thyroid hormone; estrogen leads to increased thyroid-binding globulin (TBG) levels.

PREGNANCY: Contraindicated in pregnancy, caution in nursing.

MECHANISM OF ACTION: Estrogen; binds to nuclear receptors in estrogen-responsive tissues. Circulating estrogens modulate pituitary secretion of gonadotropins, luteinizing hormone and follicle stimulating hormone, through negative feedback mechanism. Reduces elevated levels of these hormones in postmenopausal women.

PHARMACOKINETICS: Absorption: Well-absorbed. **Distribution:** Largely bound to sex hormone binding globulin and albumin; found in breast milk. **Metabolism:** Liver to estrone (metabolite), estriol (major urinary metabolite); sulfate and glucuronide conjugation (liver); gut hydrolysis; CYP3A4 (partial metabolism). **Elimination:** Urine (parent compound and metabolites).

NURSING CONSIDERATIONS

Assessment: Assess for undiagnosed abnormal genital bleeding, presence or history of breast cancer, DVT or PE, or any other conditions where treatment is contraindicated or cautioned. Assess for pregnancy/nursing status and possible drug interactions. Assess need for progestin therapy in women who have not had a hysterectomy.

Monitoring: Monitor for signs/symptoms of CV disorders, malignant neoplasms, dementia, gallbladder disease, hypercalcemia, visual abnormalities, BP elevations, elevations in plasma TG, pancreatitis, hypothyroidism, fluid retention, angioedema, exacerbation of endometriosis and other conditions (eg, asthma, DM, epilepsy, migraines, SLE). Perform annual breast exam. Monitor BP levels at regular intervals and thyroid function in patients on thyroid replacement therapy. Perform periodic evaluation (every 3-6 months) to determine treatment need. If undiagnosed persistent or recurring genital bleeding occurs, perform adequate diagnostic measures (eg, endometrial sampling) to rule out malignancy.

Patient Counseling: Inform that drug increases risk for uterine cancer, heart attack, stroke, breast cancer, blood clots, and dementia. Report any breast lumps, unusual vaginal bleeding, dizziness and faintness, changes in speech, severe headaches, chest pain, SOB, leg pain, changes in vision, and vomiting. Advise on proper administration of medication; applicator should be cleansed with mild soap and warm water following application; do not boil or use hot water. Instruct to perform monthly self breast exams. Inform that medication may weaken barrier contraceptives (eg, latex condoms, diaphragms, cervical caps).

Administration: Intravaginal route. **Storage:** 20-25°C (68-77°F); excursions permitted to 15-30°C (59-86°F).

PREMPHASE   RX
medroxyprogesterone acetate - conjugated estrogens (Wyeth)

> Estrogens and progestins should not be used for prevention of cardiovascular (CV) disease or dementia. Increased risks of myocardial infarction (MI), stroke, invasive breast cancer, pulmonary embolism (PE), and deep vein thrombosis (DVT) in postmenopausal women (50-79 yrs of age) reported. Increased risk of developing probable dementia in postmenopausal women ≥65 yrs of age reported. Estrogens, with or without progestins, should be prescribed at the lowest effective doses and for the shortest duration consistent with treatment goals and risks. Increased risk of endometrial cancer in woman with a uterus who use unopposed estrogens.

THERAPEUTIC CLASS: Estrogen/progestogen combination

INDICATIONS: Treatment of moderate to severe vasomotor symptoms and/or vulvar/vaginal atrophy associated with menopause and prevention of postmenopausal osteoporosis in women with an intact uterus.

DOSAGE: *Adults:* Vasomotor Symptoms/Vulvar/Vaginal Atrophy/Osteoporosis Prevention: 0.625mg tab qd on Days 1-14 and 0.625mg-5mg tab qd on Days 15-28. Re-evaluate periodically.

HOW SUPPLIED: Tab: 0.625mg (Estrogens, Conjugated) and 0.625mg-5mg (Estrogens, Conjugated-Medroxyprogesterone)

CONTRAINDICATIONS: Pregnancy, undiagnosed abnormal genital bleeding, known/suspected or history of breast cancer, known or suspected estrogen-dependent neoplasia, active or history of DVT/PE, active or history of arterial thromboembolic disease (eg, stroke, MI), liver dysfunction or disease.

WARNINGS/PRECAUTIONS: May increase risk of gallbladder disease requiring surgery. May lead to severe hypercalemia in patients with breast cancer and bone metastases; monitor and d/c if hypercalemia occurs. Retinal vascular thrombosis reported; monitor and d/c if papilledema or retinal vascular lesions occur. Consider addition of a progestin if no hysterectomy. May elevate BP; monitor at regular intervals. May elevate plasma TG with pre-existing hypertriglyceridemia; d/c if pancreatitis occurs. Caution with history of cholestatic jaundice associated with past estrogen use or with pregnancy; d/c with recurrence. May lead to increased thyroid-binding globulin levels; monitor thyroid function. May cause fluid retention; caution with cardiac/renal dysfunction. Caution with hypoparathyroidism; hypocalcemia may result. May increase risk of ovarian cancer. May induce or exacerbate symptoms of angioedema, particularly in women with hereditary angioedema. May exacerbate endometriosis, asthma, DM, epilepsy, migraine, porphyria, systemic lupus erythematosus (SLE), and hepatic hemangiomas; use with caution.

ADVERSE REACTIONS: Abdominal pain, asthenia, flu syndrome, leukorrhea, pharyngitis, dysmenorrhea, breast pain, nausea, arthralgia, headache, depression, back pain, infection, pain, rhinitis.

INTERACTIONS: CYP3A4 inducers (eg, St. John's wort, phenobarbital) may decrease levels and decrease therapeutic effects and/or change uterine bleeding profile. CYP3A4 inhibitors (eg, erythromycin, clarithromycin) may increase levels and result in side effects. Concomitant aminoglutethimide may significantly depress bioavailability of medroxyprogesterone. Patients concomitantly receiving thyroid hormone replacement therapy and estrogens may require increased doses of their thyroid replacement therapy.

PREGNANCY: Contraindicated in pregnancy, not for use in nursing.

MECHANISM OF ACTION: Conjugated Estrogens: Estrogen; binds to nuclear receptors in estrogen-responsive tissues. Circulating estrogens modulate pituitary secretion of the gonadotropins, luteinizing hormone and follicle stimulating hormone, through negative feedback. Medroxyprogesterone (MPA): Progesterone derivative; inhibits gonadotropin production, which prevents follicular maturation and ovulation. Decreases nuclear estrogen receptors and suppresses epithelial DNA synthesis in endometrial tissue.

PHARMACOKINETICS: Absorption: Well-absorbed. Oral administration of various doses resulted in different parameters. **Distribution:** Found in breast milk. Estrogen: Largely bound to sex hormone binding globulin and albumin. Medroxyprogesterone (MPA): Plasma protein binding (90%). **Metabolism:** Estrogen: Liver, to estrone (metabolite) and estriol (major urinary metabolite); sulfate and glucuronide conjugation (liver); gut hydrolysis; CYP3A4 (partial metabolism). MPA: Liver, via hydroxylation, conjugation. **Elimination:** Estrogen: Urine (parent compound and metabolites); MPA: Urine (metabolites).

NURSING CONSIDERATIONS

Assessment: Assess for undiagnosed abnormal genital bleeding, presence or history of breast cancer, estrogen-dependent neoplasia, active or history of DVT/PE, or any conditions where treatment is contraindicated or cautioned. Asses for pregnancy/nursing status and possible drug interactions.

Monitoring: Monitor for signs/symptoms of CV disorders, malignant neoplasms, dementia, gallbladder disease, hypercalcemia, visual abnormalities, BP elevations, elevations in plasma triglycerides, pancreatitis, hypothyroidism, fluid retention, exacerbation of endometriosis and other conditions (eg, asthma, DM, epilepsy, migraines, SLE, hepatic hemangiomas, angioedema). Perform annual breast exam. Monitor BP levels at regular intervals and thyroid function if on thyroid replacement therapy. Perform periodic evaluation to determine treatment need. If undiagnosed persistent or recurring genital bleeding occurs, perform adequate diagnostic measures (eg, endometrial sampling) to rule out malignancy.

Patient Counseling: Inform of pregnancy risks. Seek medical attention if symptoms of hepatic dysfunction (jaundice), hypercalcemia, visual abnormalities (partial/complete loss of vision, diplopia), migraines, abnormal vaginal bleeding, hypersensitivity reactions, HTN, thromboembolic disorders, fluid retention, exacerbation of diseases, CV events, or dementia occur. Report breast lumps, dizziness and faintness, changes in vision/speech, chest pain and SOB, leg pains, or vomiting.

Administration: Oral route. **Storage:** 20-25°C (68-77°F); excursions permitted to 15-30°C (59-86°F).

PREMPRO   RX
medroxyprogesterone acetate - conjugated estrogens (Wyeth)

> Estrogens and progestins should not be used for prevention of cardiovascular (CV) disease or dementia. Increased risks of myocardial infarction (MI), stroke, invasive breast cancer, pulmonary embolism (PE), and deep vein thrombosis (DVT) in postmenopausal women (50-79 yrs of age) reported. Increased risk of developing probable dementia in postmenopausal women ≥65 yrs of age reported. Estrogens, with or without progestins, should be prescribed at the lowest effective doses and for the shortest duration consistent with treatment goals and risks. Increased risk of endometrial cancer in woman with a uterus who use unopposed estrogens.

THERAPEUTIC CLASS: Estrogen/progestogen combination

INDICATIONS: Treatment of moderate to severe vasomotor symptoms and/or vulvar/vaginal atrophy due to menopause. Prevention of postmenopausal osteoporosis in women with an intact uterus.

DOSAGE: *Adults:* Vasomotor Symptoms/Vulvar and Vaginal Atrophy/Osteoporosis Prevention: Initial: 0.3mg-1.5mg qd. Adjust dose based on individual response. Re-evaluate periodically.

HOW SUPPLIED: Tab: (Estrogens, Conjugated-Medroxyprogesterone) 0.3mg-1.5mg, 0.45mg-1.5mg, 0.625mg-2.5mg, 0.625mg-5mg

CONTRAINDICATIONS: Pregnancy, undiagnosed abnormal genital bleeding, known/suspected or history of breast cancer, known or suspected estrogen-dependent neoplasia, active or history of DVT/PE, active or history of arterial thromboembolic disease (eg, stroke, MI), liver dysfunction or disease.

WARNINGS/PRECAUTIONS: May increase risk of gallbladder disease requiring surgery. May lead to severe hypercalcemia in patients with breast cancer and bone metastases; monitor and d/c if hypercalcemia occurs. Retinal vascular thrombosis reported; monitor and d/c if papilledema or retinal vascular lesions occur. Consider addition of a progestin if no hysterectomy. May elevate BP; monitor at regular intervals. May elevate plasma TG with pre-existing hypertriglyceridemia; d/c if pancreatitis occurs. Caution with history of cholestatic jaundice associated with past estrogen use or with pregnancy; d/c with recurrence. May lead to increased thyroid-binding globulin levels; monitor thyroid function. May cause fluid retention; caution with cardiac/renal dysfunction. Caution with hypoparathyroidism; hypocalcemia may result. May increase risk of ovarian cancer. May induce or exacerbate symptoms of angioedema, particularly in women with hereditary angioedema. May exacerbate endometriosis, asthma, DM, epilepsy, migraine, porphyria, systemic lupus erythematosus (SLE), and hepatic hemangiomas; use with caution.

ADVERSE REACTIONS: Abdominal pain, asthenia, flu syndrome, leukorrhea, pharyngitis, dysmenorrhea, breast pain, nausea, arthralgia, headache, depression, back pain, infection, pain, rhinitis.

INTERACTIONS: CYP3A4 inducers (eg, St. John's wort, phenobarbital) may decrease levels, which may decrease effects and/or change uterine bleeding profile. CYP3A4 inhibitors (eg, erythromycin, clarithromycin) may increase levels and result in side effects. Concomitant aminoglutethimide may significantly depress bioavailability of medroxyprogesterone. Patients concomitantly receiving thyroid hormone replacement therapy and estrogens may require increased doses of their thyroid replacement therapy.

PREGNANCY: Contraindicated in pregnancy, not for use in nursing.

MECHANISM OF ACTION: Conjugated Estrogens: Estrogen; binds to nuclear receptors in estrogen-responsive tissues. Circulating estrogens modulate pituitary secretion of the gonadotropins, luteinizing hormone and follicle stimulating hormone, through negative feedback. Medroxyprogesterone (MPA): Progesterone derivative; inhibits gonadotropin production, which prevents follicular maturation and ovulation. Decreases nuclear estrogen receptors and suppresses epithelial DNA synthesis in endometrial tissue.

PHARMACOKINETICS: Absorption: Well absorbed. Oral administration of various doses resulted in different parameters. **Distribution**: Found in breast milk. Estrogen: Largely bound to sex hormone binding globulin and albumin. Medroxyprogesterone (MPA): Plasma protein binding (90%). **Metabolism**: Estrogen: Liver, to estrone (metabolite) and estriol (major urinary metabolite); sulfate and glucuronide conjugation (liver); gut hydrolysis; CYP3A4 (partial metabolism). MPA: Liver, via hydroxylation, conjugation. **Elimination**: Estrogen: Urine (parent compound and metabolites). MPA: Urine (metabolites).

NURSING CONSIDERATIONS

Assessment: Assess for undiagnosed abnormal genital bleeding, presence or history of breast cancer, estrogen-dependent neoplasia, active or history of DVT/PE, or any other conditions where treatment is contraindicated or cautioned. Assess for pregnancy/nursing status and possible drug interactions.

Monitoring: Monitor for signs/symptoms of CV disorders, malignant neoplasms, dementia, gallbladder disease, hypercalcemia, visual abnormalities, BP elevations, elevations in plasma TG, pancreatitis, hypothyroidism, fluid retention, exacerbation of endometriosis and other conditions (eg, asthma, DM, epilepsy, migraines, SLE, hepatic hemangiomas, angioedema). Perform annual breast exam. Monitor BP levels at regular intervals and thyroid function if on thyroid replacement therapy. Perform periodic evaluation to determine treatment need. If undiagnosed persistent or recurring genital bleeding occurs, perform adequate diagnostic measures (eg, endometrial sampling) to rule out malignancy.

Patient Counseling: Inform of pregnancy risks. Seek medical attention if symptoms of hepatic dysfunction (jaundice), hypercalcemia, visual abnormalities (partial/complete loss of vision, diplopia), migraines, abnormal vaginal bleeding, hypersensitivity reactions, HTN, thromboembolic disorders, fluid retention, exacerbation of diseases, CV events, or dementia occur. Report breast lumps, dizziness and faintness, changes in vision/speech, chest pain or SOB, leg pains or vomiting.

Administration: Oral route. **Storage**: 20-25°C (68-77°F); excursions permitted to 15-30°C (59-86°F).

PREVACID   RX
lansoprazole (Takeda)

OTHER BRAND NAMES: Prevacid Solutab (Takeda)

THERAPEUTIC CLASS: Proton pump inhibitor

INDICATIONS: Short-term treatment (for 4 weeks) for healing and symptom relief of active duodenal ulcer (DU). Maintenance of healed DU. Short term treatment (up to 8 weeks) for healing and symptom relief of active benign gastric ulcer (GU). Treatment of NSAID-associated GU in patients who continue NSAID use. Reduce risk of NSAID-associated GU in patients with history of documented GU who require the use of an NSAID. Treatment of heartburn and other symptoms associated with gastroesophageal reflux disease (GERD). Short term treatment (up to 8 weeks) for healing and symptom relief of all grades of erosive esophagitis (EE). Maintenance of healing of EE. Long-term treatment of pathological hypersecretory conditions (eg, Zollinger-Ellison syndrome). Combination therapy with amoxicillin +/- clarithromycin for *H. pylori* eradication in DU disease, to reduce risk of ulcer recurrence.

DOSAGE: *Adults:* DU: Short-Term Treatment: 15mg qd for 4 weeks. Maintenance of Healed: 15mg qd. Short-term Treatment Benign GU: 30mg

qd up to 8 weeks. NSAID-associated GU: Healing: 30mg qd for 8 weeks. Risk Reduction: 15mg qd for up to 12 weeks. GERD: Short-term Treatment of Symptomatic GERD: 15mg qd up to 8 weeks. Short-Treatment of EE: 30mg qd up to 8 weeks. May give for 8 more weeks if healing does not occur. If there is recurrence of EE, an additional 8 week course may be considered. Maintenance of Healing of EE: 15mg qd. Pathological Hypersecretory Conditions (including Zollinger-Ellison Syndrome): Initial: 60mg qd, then adjust to individual patient's needs. Max: 90mg bid. Divide dose if >120mg/day. *H. pylori* Eradication to Reduce Risk of DU Recurrence : Triple Therapy: 30mg + amoxicillin 1000mg + clarithromycin 500mg, all bid (q12h) for 10-14 days. Dual Therapy: 30mg + amoxicillin 1000mg both tid (q8h) for 14 days. Severe Hepatic Impairment: Consider dose reduction. Take before eating.
Pediatrics: 12-17 yrs: Short-Term Symptomatic GERD: Nonerosive GERD:15mg qd for up to 8 weeks. EE: 30mg qd for up to 8 weeks. 1-11 yrs: Short-Term Symptomatic GERD/EE: ≤30kg: 15mg qd for up to 12 weeks. Titrate: May increase after two or more weeks of treatment if remain symptomatic. Max: 30mg bid. >30kg: 30mg qd for up to 12 weeks. Titrate: May increase after two or more weeks of treatment if remain symptomatic. Max: 30mg bid. Severe Hepatic Impairment: Consider dose reduction. Take before eating.

HOW SUPPLIED: Cap, Delayed-Release: 15mg, 30mg; Tab, Disintegrating (SoluTab): 15mg, 30mg.

WARNINGS/PRECAUTIONS: Symptomatic response does not preclude the presence of gastric malignancy. May increase risk for osteoporosis-related fractures of the hip, wrist, or spine; risk of fracture may increase if receive high-dose and on long term therapy; consider using lowest dose and shortest duration appropriate to the condition being treated. Consider dose reduction with severe hepatic impairment. Contains phenylalanine.

ADVERSE REACTIONS: Abdominal pain, constipation, diarrhea, nausea, dizziness.

INTERACTIONS: May substantially decrease atazanavir concentrations which may lead to a loss of therapeutic effect; avoid concomitant use. May alter absorption of other drugs where gastric pH is an important determinant of oral bioavailability (eg, ketoconazole, ampicillin esters, digoxin, iron salts). May increase theophylline clearance; may require dosage adjustment. Monitor for increases in INR and prothrombin time (PT) with warfarin. May increase tacrolimus levels. Delayed absorption and reduced bioavailability with sucralfate; give at least 30 mins prior to sucralfate.

PREGNANCY: Category B, not for use in nursing.

MECHANISM OF ACTION: Proton pump inhibitor; suppresses gastric acid secretion by specific inhibition of the (H^+, K^+)-ATPase enzyme system at the secretory surface of the gastric parietal cell.

PHARMACOKINETICS: Absorption: Rapid; absolute bioavailability (>80%); T_{max}=1.7 hrs. **Distribution:** Plasma protein binding (97%). **Metabolism:** Liver (extensive). **Elimination:** Urine, feces, bile; $T_{1/2}$=<2 hrs. Refer to PI for pediatric parameters.

NURSING CONSIDERATIONS

Assessment: Assess for gastric malignancy, severe hepatic insufficiency, osteoporosis, phenylketonuria, pregnancy/nursing status, and for possible drug interactions.

Monitoring: Monitor for signs/symptoms of gastric malignancy and bone fractures.

Patient Counseling: Advise to contact physician if any adverse events develop while on therapy. Instruct to take before eating. Inform that caps should not be crushed or chewed. Inform of alternate methods of administration if unable to swallow caps whole.

Administration: Oral route, nasogastric route (delayed release cap). Swallow caps whole; do not crush or chew. Do not break or cut tabs. Refer to PI for further instruction on administration methods. **Storage:** 25°C (77°F); excursions permitted to 15-30°C (59-86°F).

PREVNAR RX
pneumococcal vaccine, diphtheria conjugate (Wyeth)

OTHER BRAND NAMES: Prevnar 13 (Wyeth)

THERAPEUTIC CLASS: Vaccine

INDICATIONS: Active immunization against invasive disease caused by *S. pneumoniae*. Active immunization of infants and toddlers against otitis media caused by serotypes included in the vaccine.

DOSAGE: *Pediatrics:* 6 weeks-2 months: 4 doses of 0.5mL IM. Give 3 doses at 2-month intervals and 4th dose at 12-15 months old. Unvaccinated Children: 7-11 months: 3 doses of 0.5mL IM. Give first 2 doses at least 4 weeks apart and 3rd dose after first birthday; separate from 2nd dose by at least 2 months. 12-23 months: 2 doses of 0.5mL IM at least 2 months apart. (Prevnar) ≥24 months-9 yrs, (Prevnar 13) 24 months-5 yrs: 0.5mL IM single dose. Prevnar 13 Vaccine Schedule for Previously Vaccinated With Prevnar: 15 months-5 yrs: Give 0.5mL IM single dose at least 8 weeks after the 4th dose of Prevnar.

HOW SUPPLIED: Inj: 0.5mL [1 dose prefilled syringe]

WARNINGS/PRECAUTIONS: Will not protect against *S. pneumoniae* disease caused by serotypes unrelated to those in the vaccine. Not a substitute for 23-valent pneumococcal vaccination. Impaired immune responses due to immunosuppressive therapy may cause reduced response. Have epinephrine (1:1000) or other agents available for control of immediate allergic reaction. (Prevnar) Fever and febrile seizures (rare) reported. Avoid with thrombocytopenia or coagulation disorder. Postpone if patient has acute, severe, febrile illness. Not a substitute for diphtheria or 23-valent pneumococcal vaccinations. (Prevnar 13) Apnea observed in some premature infants; administration should be based on medical status, potential benefits, and possible risks. Will not protect against other microorganisms and does not treat active infection.

ADVERSE REACTIONS: Injection-site reactions, irritability, decreased appetite, vomiting, diarrhea, fever. (Prevnar) Restless sleep, drowsiness. (Prevnar 13) Decreased/increased sleep, anaphylactic reactions, apnea.

INTERACTIONS: Suboptimal response with immunosuppressants (eg, large amounts of corticosteroids, antimetabolites, alkylating agents, cytotoxic agents). (Prevnar) Caution with anticoagulants.

PREGNANCY: Category C, not for use in nursing.

MECHANISM OF ACTION: Vaccine; elicits formation of antibodies that may protect against invasive pneumococcal disease and otitis media.

NURSING CONSIDERATIONS

Assessment: Assess age, health/immunity status, active infection, history of febrile convulsions, bleeding disorders, previous sensitivity/vaccination history, family history, and for possibile drug interactions.

Monitoring: Monitor for hypersensitivity reactions (eg, face edema, dyspnea, bronchospasm), injection site reactions (eg, redness, swelling, tenderness, and induration) fever, irritability, drowsiness, restless sleep, anorexia, vomiting, and diarrhea.

Patient Counseling: Inform parent/guardian of benefits/risks of therapy and the importance of completing the immunization series. Inform that vaccine will not protect against *S. pneumoniae* disease caused by serotypes unrelated to those in the vaccine, will not protect against other microorganisms, and does not treat active infection. Advise to report any adverse reactions to physician.

Administration: IM route. Inject into the anterolateral aspect of thigh (infants) or deltoid region (toddlers and young children). Do not inject IV, ID or SQ. Refer to PI for preparation for administration. **Storage**: Refrigerate at 2-8°C (36-46°F). Do not freeze; discard if has been frozen. Shake well.

PREVPAC   RX
amoxicillin - clarithromycin - lansoprazole (TAP)

THERAPEUTIC CLASS: *H.pylori* treatment combination

INDICATIONS: Treatment of *H.pylori* infection associated with active duodenal ulcer and to reduce the risk of duodenal ulcer recurrence.

DOSAGE: *Adults:* 1g amoxicillin, 500mg clarithromycin and 30mg lansoprazole, all bid (am and pm) before meals for 10 or 14 days. Swallow each pill whole. Renal Impairment (with or without hepatic impairment): Decrease clarithromycin dose or prolong intervals.

HOW SUPPLIED: Cap: (Amoxicillin) 500mg, Tab: (Clarithromycin) 500mg, Cap, Delayed-Release: (Lansoprazole) 30mg

CONTRAINDICATIONS: Concomitant use with cisapride, pimozide, astemizole, terfenadine, ergotamine or dihydroergotamine.

WARNINGS/PRECAUTIONS: Serious and occasional fatal hypersensitivity reactions reported in patients on penicillin therapy. Avoid if CrCl <30mL/min. Caution with cephalosporin/PCN allergy; anaphylactic reactions have been reported. Pseudomembranous colitis reported. D/C if superinfections occur. Caution in elderly. Do not use clarithromycin during pregnancy. Symptomatic response to lansoprazole does not preclude the presence of gastric malignancy. *Clostridium difficile*-associated diarrhea (CDAD) reported. D/C if confirmed. Exacerbation of symptoms with myasthenia gravis and new onset of myasthenic syndrome reported with clarithromycin.

ADVERSE REACTIONS: Diarrhea, taste perversion, headache, abdominal pain, dark stools, myalgia, confusion, respiratory disorders, skin reactions, vaginitis.

INTERACTIONS: See Contraindications. Lansoprazole: May interfere with absorption of drugs dependent on gastric pH for bioavailability (eg, atazanavir, ketoconazole, ampicillin esters, iron salts, digoxin). Monitor increase in INR and prothrombin time with concomitant use of warfarin. Amoxicillin: May decrease renal tubular secretion when coadministered with probenecid. May interfere with bactericidal effects of penicillin with chloramphenicol, macrolides, sulfonamides and tetracycline. Clarithromycin: May increase theophylline and carbamazepine levels. Simultaneous administration with zidovudine resulted in decreased steady-state zidovudine levels in HIV-infected patients. Elevated digoxin levels in patients receiving concomitant digoxin. May lead to increased exposure to colchicine when coadministered; monitor for toxicity. May increase or prolong both therapeutic and adverse effects with erythromycin. Torsades de pointes may occur with quinidine or disopyramide. May increase systemic exposure of sildenafil; consider dose reduction.

PREGNANCY: Category C, not for use in nursing.

MECHANISM OF ACTION: Lansoprazole: Substituted benzimidazole; inhibits gastric acid secretion. Amoxicillin: Semi-synthetic antibiotic; has broad spectrum of bactericidal activity against many gram-positive and gram-negative microorganisms. Clarithromycin: Semi-synthetic macrolide antibiotic.

PHARMACOKINETICS: Absorption: Lansoprazole: Rapidly absorbed; absolute bioavailability (80%); T_{max}=1.7 hrs. Amoxicillin: Rapidly absorbed. Clarithromycin: Rapidly absorbed; absolute bioavailability (50%); T_{max}=2-2.5 hrs. **Distribution:** Lansoprazole: Plasma protein binding (97%); found in breast milk. Amoxicillin: Plasma protein binding (approximately 20%). Clarithromycin: Found in breast milk. **Metabolism:** Lansoprazole: Liver (extensive). Clarithromycin: 14-OH clarithromycin (active metabolite). **Elimination:** Lansoprazole: Urine, feces; $T_{1/2}$=<2 hrs. Amoxicillin: Urine (60%); $T_{1/2}$=61.3 mins. Clarithromycin: Urine (30%); $T_{1/2}$=5-7 hrs; (metabolite) $T_{1/2}$=7-9 hrs.

NURSING CONSIDERATIONS

Assessment: Assess for hypersensitivity to other macrolides, PCNs, or cephalosporins. Assess for proper diagnosis of susceptible bacteria (eg, cultures), pregnancy/nursing status, renal impairment, gastric malignancy, presence of bacterial infection, and possible drug interactions.

Monitoring: Monitor for signs/symptoms of drug interactions (eg, cardiac arrhythmias), hypersensitivity reactions (eg, anaphylaxis), pseudomembranous colitis and CDAD, and development of superinfections.

Patient Counseling: Instruct to take each dose twice per day before eating; swallow pill whole. Notify physician of all medications currently being taken. Inform that drug treats bacterial, not viral, infections. Take exactly as directed; skipping doses may decrease effectiveness and increase antibiotic resistance. Instruct to avoid pregnancy/nursing during therapy and contact physician if diarrhea occurs.

Administration: Oral route. **Storage:** 20-25°C (68-77°F). Protect from light and moisture.

PREZISTA   RX
darunavir (Tibotec)

THERAPEUTIC CLASS: Protease inhibitor

INDICATIONS: Treatment of HIV-1 infection in adult and pediatric (≥6 yrs) patients in combination with ritonavir and other antiretroviral agents.

DOSAGE: *Adults:* Treatment-Naive/Treatment-Experienced With No Darunavir Resistance Associated Substitution: 800mg with ritonavir 100mg qd. Treatment Experienced With ≥1 Darunavir Resistance Associated Substitution: 600mg with ritonavir 100mg bid. Take with food.
Pediatrics: 6-<18 yrs: ≥20-<30kg (≥44-<66 lbs): 375mg with ritonavir 50mg bid. ≥30-<40kg (≥66-<88 lbs): 450mg with ritonavir 60mg bid. ≥40kg (≥88 lbs): 600mg with ritonavir 100mg bid. Take with food. Do not use qd dosing.

HOW SUPPLIED: Tab: 75mg, 150mg, 400mg, 600mg

CONTRAINDICATIONS: Concomitant use with dihydroergotamine, ergonovine, ergotamine, methylergonovine, cisapride, pimozide, oral midazolam, triazolam, St. John's wort, lovastatin, simvastatin, rifampin, alfuzosin, and sildenafil for treatment of pulmonary arterial HTN (PAH).

WARNINGS/PRECAUTIONS: Must be coadministered with ritonavir and food to achieve desired effect. Drug-induced hepatitis (eg, acute hepatitis, cytolytic hepatitis) and liver injury reported; consider interrupting or d/c therapy if evidence of new or worsening liver dysfunction occurs. Avoid in patients with severe hepatic impairment. Severe skin reactions, Stevens-Johnson syndrome (SJS), toxic epidermal necrolysis (TEN) reported; d/c if signs/symptoms of severe skin reactions develop. Caution with sulfonamide allergy. New onset diabetes mellitus (DM), exacerbation of pre-existing DM, and hyperglycemia reported. Redistribution/accumulation of body fat reported. Immune reconstitution syndrome may occur. Increased bleeding reported in patients with hemophilia type A and B. Do not give to patients <3 yrs old. Caution in elderly.

ADVERSE REACTIONS: Diarrhea, N/V, headache, abdominal pain, rash.

INTERACTIONS: See Contraindications. Increases plasma concentrations of CYP3A and CYP2D6 substrates. Increased clearance with CYP3A inducers. Decreased clearance with CYP3A inhibitors. Administer didanosine 1 hr before or 2 hrs after darunavir/ritonavir. Not recommended with lopinavir/ritonavir, and saquinavir. Increases concentrations of indinavir, colchicine, bosentan, salmeterol, maraviroc, antiarrhythmics (eg, bepridil, lidocaine (systemic), quinidine, amiodarone, flecainide, propafenone), digoxin, carbamazepine, trazodone, desipramine, clarithromycin, ketoconazole, itraconazole, rifabutin, 25-O-desacetylrifabutin, β-blockers (eg, metoprolol, timolol), midazolam, calcium channel blockers (eg, felodipine, nifedipine, nicardipine), fluticasone, pravastatin, atorvastatin, rosuvastatin, immunosuppressants (eg, cyclosporine, tacrolimus, sirolimus), norbuprenorphine, neuroleptics (eg, risperidone, thioridazine), and PDE-5 inhibitors (eg, sildenafil, vardenafil, tadalafil). Decreases concentrations of warfarin, phenytoin, phenobarbital, voriconazole, methadone, ethinyl estradiol, norethindrone, sertraline, and paroxetine. Decreased plasma concentrations with dexamethasone. Increased concentrations with indinavir, rifabutin, ketoconazole and itraconazole. May require dose adjustment of insulin/oral hypoglycemics. Refer to PI for a complete list of drug interactions.

PREGNANCY: Category C, not for use in nursing.

MECHANISM OF ACTION: Protease inhibitor; selectively inhibits the cleavage of HIV-1 encoded Gag-Pol polyproteins in infected cells, preventing the formation of mature virus particles.

PHARMACOKINETICS: Absorption: Darunavir: Absolute bioavailability (37%). Darunavir/Ritonavir: Absolute bioavailability (82%); T_{max} =2.5-4 hrs. **Distribution:** Darunavir: Plasma protein binding (95%). **Metabolism:** Darunavir: Hepatic (oxidation) via CYP3A. **Elimination:** Darunavir: Feces (41.2%), urine (7.7%). Darunavir/Ritonavir: Feces (79.5%), urine (13.9%). Darunavir/Ritonavir: $T_{1/2}$=15 hrs.

NURSING CONSIDERATIONS

Assessment: Assess for sulfonamide allergy, liver dysfunction (including chronic active hepatitis), hemophilia, pre-existing DM, pregnancy/nursing status, and for possible drug interactions. Assess ability to swallow tablets in pediatrics.

Monitoring: Monitor for signs/symptoms of severe skin reactions (eg, SJS, TEN), new onset DM, exacerbation of DM and hyperglycemia, LFT abnormalities, hemophilia, fat redistribution, immune reconstitution syndrome, laboratory abnormalities (eg, biochemistry, hematology), and for hepatic impairment. Perform therapeutic drug monitoring for drug interactions as recommended.

Patient Counseling: Inform that drug does not cure HIV and that opportunistic infections may continue to develop as well as other complications associated with HIV. Inform that sustained decrease in plasma HIV RNA is associated with reduced risk of progression to AIDS and death. Advise to take with food, swallow tab whole, and not to alter dose or d/c without consulting physician. Advise to take the next dose at regularly scheduled time if a dose is missed by 6 hrs; do not double next dose. Counsel to report use of any other Rx, OTC or herbal medication (eg, St. John's wort). Instruct to use alternative contraceptive measures if on estrogen-based contraceptive during therapy. Instruct to seek medical attention if symptoms of severe skin reactions (eg, erythema multiforme, SJS), exacerbation of DM and hyperglycemia, liver dysfunction, unexplained bleeding, fat redistribution, or if immune reconstitution syndrome occur.

Administration: Oral route. **Storage:** 25°C (77°F); excursions permitted to 15-30°C (59-86°F).

PRILOSEC   RX
omeprazole magnesium - omeprazole (AstraZeneca)

THERAPEUTIC CLASS: Proton pump inhibitor

INDICATIONS: Short-term treatment of active duodenal ulcer and active benign gastric ulcer in adults. Treatment of heartburn and other symptoms associated with gastroesophageal reflux disease (GERD) in adults and pediatrics. Short-term treatment and maintenance of healing of erosive esophagitis in adults and pediatrics. Long-term treatment of pathological hypersecretory conditions (eg, Zollinger-Ellison syndrome, multiple endocrine adenomas, systemic mastocytosis) in adults. Combination therapy with clarithromycin +/- amoxicillin for *H. pylori* eradication in *H. pylori* infection and duodenal ulcer disease and to reduce risk of recurrence in adults.

DOSAGE: *Adults:* Active Duodenal Ulcer: 20mg PO qd for 4 weeks; May require additional 4 weeks. GERD: Without Esophageal Lesions: 20mg PO qd for up to 4 weeks; With Erosive Esophagitis and Accompanying Symptoms: 4-8 weeks. Gastric Ulcer: 40mg PO qd for 4-8 weeks. Maint of Healing of Erosive Esophagitis: 20mg PO qd. Hypersecretory Conditions: Initial: 60mg PO qd for as long as clinically indicated, then adjust if needed. Divide dose if >80mg/day. Doses up to 120mg tid have been given. Some patients with Zollinger-Ellison syndrome have been treated for >5 yrs. *H. pylori* Eradication for Risk Reduction of Duodenal Ulcer Recurrence: Triple Therapy: omeprazole 20mg + clarithromycin 500mg + amoxicillin 1000mg, all bid for 10 days. Give additional 18 days of omeprazole 20mg qd if ulcer present at time of initial therapy. Dual Therapy: omeprazole 40mg qd + clarithromycin 500mg tid for 14 days. Give additional 14 days of omeprazole 20mg qd if ulcer present at time of initial therapy.

Pediatrics: 1-16 yrs: GERD/Maint of Healing of Erosive Esophagitis: ≥20kg: 20mg PO qd. 10 to <20kg: 10mg PO qd. 5 to <10kg: 5mg PO qd.

HOW SUPPLIED: Cap, Delayed-Release (omeprazole): 10mg, 20mg, 40mg; Sus, Delayed-Release (omeprazole magnesium): 2.5mg, 10mg granules/pkt

WARNINGS/PRECAUTIONS: Symptomatic response does not preclude the presence of gastric malignancy. Atrophic gastritis reported with long-term use. May increase risk for osteoporosis-related fractures of the hip, wrist, or spine. The risk of fracture was increased in patients who received high-dose and long term therapy; consider using lowest dose and shortest duration appropriate to the condition being treated.

ADVERSE REACTIONS: Headache, diarrhea, abdominal pain, N/V, flatulence; (pediatrics) fever, respiratory disorders.

INTERACTIONS: Avoid concomitant use with clopidogrel; co-administration with 80mg omeprazole reduces the pharmacological activity of clopidogrel. May prolong elimination of diazepam, warfarin, and phenytoin (drugs metabolized by oxidation in the liver). May increase INR and PT with concomitant warfarin. May alter with absorption of pH-dependent drugs (eg, ketoconazole, ampicillin esters, iron salts). Monitor patients taking drugs metabolized by CYP450 (eg, cyclosporine, disulfiram, benzodiazepines). When used with clarithromycin, the levels of both drugs may be increased. May increase levels with voriconazole. May change the absorption of antiretroviral drugs and/or interact via CYP2C19. May reduce plasma levels of atazanavir and nelfinavir; concomitant use is not recommended. May increase levels of tacrolimus, cilostazol, and saquinavir.

PREGNANCY: Category C, not for use in nursing.

MECHANISM OF ACTION: Proton pump inhibitor; suppresses gastric acid secretion by specific inhibition of the H^+/K^+ ATPase enzyme system at the secretory surface of the gastric parietal cell.

PHARMACOKINETICS: Absorption: (Cap) Rapid; absolute bioavailability (30-40%); T_{max}=0.5-3.5 hrs. **Distribution:** Plasma protein binding (95%); found in breast milk. **Metabolism:** Extensive via CYP450. **Elimination:** Urine (77%), feces; (cap) $T_{1/2}$=0.5-1 hr.

NURSING CONSIDERATIONS

Assessment: Assess for gastric malignancy, hepatic impairment, hypersensitivity, risk for osteoporosis-related fractures, history of atrophic gastritis with long term use of omeprazole, pregnancy/nursing status, and possible drug interactions. Obtain baseline LFTs.

Monitoring: Monitor for signs/symptoms of atrophic gastritis, hypersensitivity reactions, and other GI effects. Monitor LFTs. Monitor INR and PT when given with warfarin.

Patient Counseling: Inform about risks and benefits of therapy. Inform to take before eating, to swallow caps whole, and not to chew or crush. Instruct to empty contents of cap into 1 tbsp of applesauce if cannot swallow whole. Mix with applesauce and swallow immediately with cool glass of water; applesauce should not be hot and should be soft enough to be swallowed without chewing. Advise not chew or crush pellets; pellets/applesauce mixture should not be stored for future use. Sus may be given by NG or gastric tube.

Administration: Oral route. Taken before eating. (Cap) Swallow whole or empty contents into 1 tbsp of applesauce if cannot swallow whole. (Sus) Empty contents of 2.5mg pkt into 5mL of water or 10mg pkt into 15mL of water. Stir and leave 2-3 min to thicken. Stir and drink within 30 min. If any material remains, add more water, stir, and drink immediately. Sus may also be given with a NG or gastric tube (using a catheter tipped syringe) using a similar procedure; refer to PI. **Storage:** (Cap) 15-30°C (59-86°F); protect from light and moisture. (Sus) 25°C (77°F); excursions permitted to 15-30°C (59-86°F).

PRIMAXIN I.M. RX
cilastatin sodium - imipenem (Merck)

THERAPEUTIC CLASS: Thienamycin/dehydropeptidase I inhibitor

INDICATIONS: Treatment of lower respiratory tract (LRTI), skin and skin structure (SSSI), intra-abdominal, and gynecologic infections caused by susceptible strains of microorganisms.

DOSAGE: *Adults:* Mild to Moderate LRTI/SSSI/Gynecologic Infection: 500mg or 750mg IM q12h depending on severity. Mild to Moderate Intra-Abdominal Infection: 750mg IM q12h. Continue for at least 2 days after symptoms resolve; do not treat >14 days. Max: 1500mg/day. Elderly: Start at low end of dosing range.
Pediatrics: ≥12 yrs: Mild to Moderate LRTI/SSSI/Gynecologic Infections: 500mg or 750mg IM q12h depending on severity. Mild to Moderate Intra-Abdominal Infection: 750mg IM q12h. Continue for at least 2 days after symptoms resolve; do not treat >14 days. Max: 1500mg/day.

HOW SUPPLIED: Inj: (Imipenem-Cilastatin) 500mg-500mg, 750mg-750mg

CONTRAINDICATIONS: Severe shock, heart block, hypersensitivity to local anesthetics of amide type (due to lidocaine diluent).

WARNINGS/PRECAUTIONS: Serious, sometimes fatal, hypersensitivity (anaphylactic) reactions reported; d/c and institute appropriate therapy. Caution with history of hypersensitivity to PCN, cephalosporin or other allergens. *Clostridium difficile*-associated diarrhea (CDAD) reported; may need to d/c if suspected or confirmed. CNS adverse events (eg, myoclonic activity or seizures) reported with CNS disorders (eg, brain lesions or history of seizures) and renal dysfunction. Prolonged use may result in overgrowth of nonsusceptible organisms; if a superinfection occurs, institute appropriate therapy. Resistance may develop with use of therapy in the absence of a proven or strongly suspected infection. Avoid injection into blood vessel. Caution in elderly.

ADVERSE REACTIONS: Injection-site pain, N/V, diarrhea, rash.

INTERACTIONS: Minimal increases in plasma levels with probenecid; concomitant use not recommended. May decrease levels of valproic acid or divalproex sodium.

PREGNANCY: Category C, caution in nursing.

MECHANISM OF ACTION: (Imipenem) Thienamycin; inhibits cell-wall synthesis. (Cilastatin) Dehydropeptidase I inhibitor; prevents renal metabolism of imipenem.

PHARMACOKINETICS: Absorption: Imipenem: Bioavailability (75%), C_{max}=10mcg/mL (500mg), 12mcg/mL (750mg); T_{max}=2 hrs. Cilastatin: Bioavailability (95%), C_{max}=24mcg/mL (500mg), 33mcg/mL (750mg); T_{max}=1 hr. **Distribution:** Imipenem: Plasma protein binding (20%). Cilastatin: Plasma protein binding (40%). **Metabolism:** Imipenem: Kidneys. **Elimination:** Imipinem: Urine (50%); $T_{1/2}$=2-3 hrs. Cilastatin: Urine (75%).

NURSING CONSIDERATIONS

Assessment: Assess for severity and type of infection. Assess for hypersensitivity to local anesthetics (amide), PCN, cephalosporins, β-lactams, and other allergens. Assess for severe shock, heart block, CNS disorders (brain lesions, history of seizures), renal function, pregnancy/nursing status, and possible drug interactions.

Monitoring: Monitor for CNS adverse events (eg, seizures or myoclonic activity), hypersensitivity reactions, CDAD, and superinfections, and other possible adverse events.

Patient Counseling: Inform physician if taking valproic acid or divalproex sodium. Therapy only treats bacterial, not viral, infections. Take as directed; skipping doses or not completing full course may decrease effectiveness and increase resistance. May experience diarrhea; notify physician if watery/bloody stools (with or without stomach cramps and fever).

Administration: IM route. Administer by deep IM injection into large muscle mass (eg, gluteal muscles or lateral part of the thigh). Do not mix or physically add with other antibiotics; may be administered concomitantly but at separate sites with antibiotics such as aminoglycosides. Use within 1 hr after reconstitution. **Storage:** Below 25°C (77°F).

PRIMAXIN I.V. RX
cilastatin sodium - imipenem (Merck)

THERAPEUTIC CLASS: Thienamycin/dehydropeptidase I inhibitor

INDICATIONS: Treatment of lower respiratory tract, complicated and uncomplicated urinary tract (UTI), intra-abdominal, gynecologic, skin and skin structure, bone and joint, and polymicrobic infections, septicemia, and endocarditis caused by susceptible strains of microorganisms.

DOSAGE: *Adults:* Dose based on severity or type of infection. ≥70kg and CrCl ≥71mL/min: Uncomplicated UTI: 250mg q6h. Complicated UTI: 500mg q6h. Fully susceptible organisms (eg, gram-positive and gram-negative aerobes and anaerobes): Mild: 250mg q6h. Moderate: 500mg q8h or 500mg q6h. Severe: 500mg q6h. Moderately susceptible organisms (eg, P. aeruginosa): Mild: 500mg q6h. Moderate: 500mg q6h or 1g q8h. Severe: 1g q8h or 1g q6h. Max: 50mg/kg/day or 4g/day, whichever is lower. May use up to 90mg/kg/day, not exceeding 4g/day with cystic fibrosis. Renal Impairment (CrCl ≤70ml/min) and/or <70kg: Refer to PI. CrCl 6-20mL/min or CrCl ≤5mL/min with Hemodialysis: 125-250mg q12h.
Pediatrics: ≥3 months: Dose based on severity or type of infection. Non-CNS Infections: 15-25mg/kg q6h. Max: 2g/day if fully susceptible or 4g/day if moderately susceptible. May use up to 90mg/kg/day in older children (>12 yrs) with cystic fibrosis. 4 weeks-3 months and ≥1500g: 25mg/kg q6h. 1-4 weeks and ≥1500g: 25mg/kg q8h. <1 week and ≥1500g: 25mg/kg q12h.

HOW SUPPLIED: Inj: (Imipenem-Cilastatin) 250mg-250mg, 500mg-500mg

WARNINGS/PRECAUTIONS: Serious, sometimes fatal, hypersensitivity (anaphylactic) reactions reported; d/c and institute appropriate therapy. Caution with history of hypersensitivity to PCN, cephalosporin, β-lactam or other allergen. *Clostridium difficile*-associated diarrhea (CDAD) reported; may need to d/c if suspected or confirmed. CNS adverse events (eg, myoclonic activity, confusion, seizures) reported with CNS disorders (eg, brain lesions or history of seizures) and renal dysfunction. If focal tremors, myoclonus, or seizures occur, perform neurological evaluation, institute anticonvulsant therapy, and re-examine whether to decrease or d/c use. Caution with CrCl ≤20mL/min; may be at higher risk for seizure activity. Avoid with CrCl ≤5mL/min unless hemodialysis is instituted within 48 hrs. Prolonged use may result in overgrowth of nonsusceptible organisms; if superinfection occurs, institute appropriate measures. Not recommended in pediatric patients with CNS infections and <30kg with impaired renal function.

ADVERSE REACTIONS: Phlebitis/thrombophlebitis, convulsions, diarrhea, rash, fever, hypotension, seizures, dizziness, pruritus, urticaria, somnolence, N/V

INTERACTIONS: Seizures reported with ganciclovir; avoid concomitant use. Minimal increases in plasma levels with probenecid; concomitant use not recommended. May decrease levels of valproic acid or divalproex sodium.

PREGNANCY: Category C, caution in nursing.

MECHANISM OF ACTION: Imipenem: Thienamycin; inhibits cell-wall synthesis. Cilastatin: Dehydropeptidase I inhibitor; prevents renal metabolism of imipenem to achieve fully adequate antibacterial levels.

PHARMACOKINETICS: Absorption: Imipenem: 14-24mcg/mL (250mg), 21-58mcg/mL (500mg), 41-83mcg/mL (1000mg). Cilastatin: 15-25mcg/mL (250mg), 31-49mcg/mL (500mg), 56-88mcg/mL (1000mg). **Distribution:** Imipenem: Plasma protein binding (20%). Cilastatin: Plasma protein binding (40%). **Metabolism:** Imipenem: Kidneys. **Elimination:** Imipenem: Urine (70%). Cilastatin: Urine (70%).

NURSING CONSIDERATIONS

Assessment: Assess for severity and type of infection. Assess for organ system functions (eg, renal, hepatic, hematopoietic), weight, history of hypersensitivity to PCN, cephalosporins, β-lactams, and other allergens, use of hemodialysis, CNS disorders (eg, brain lesions, history of seizures), pregnancy/nursing status, and possible drug interactions. Obtain CrCl.

Monitoring: Monitor periodically organ system functions (eg, renal, hepatic, and hematopoietic). Monitor for CNS adverse events (eg, seizures, myoclonic activity and confusional states), hypersensitivity reactions, CDAD, and superinfections. Monitor electrolytes and CrCl.

Patient Counseling: Inform physician if taking valproic acid or divalproex sodium. Therapy only treats bacterial, not viral, infections. Take as directed; skipping doses or not completing full course may decrease effectiveness and increase resistance. May experience diarrhea; notify physician if watery/bloody stools (with or without stomach cramps and fever), hypersensitivity reactions, superinfections, CNS adverse events (myoclonic activity, confusion, seizures) occur.

Administration: IV route. Each 125mg, 250mg, 500mg dose infused over 20-30 min. Each 750mg, 1000mg dose infused over 40-60 min. Do not mix or physically add to other antibiotics; may be administered concomitantly with other antibiotics, such as aminoglycosides. **Storage:** Dry powder: Below 25°C (77°F). Reconstituted: Stable for 4 hrs at room temperature or for 24 hrs under refrigeration (5°C).

PRINIVIL   RX
lisinopril (Merck)

> ACE inhibitors can cause death/injury to the fetus during 2nd and 3rd trimesters. D/C therapy if pregnancy is detected.

THERAPEUTIC CLASS: ACE inhibitor

INDICATIONS: Treatment of HTN used alone as initial therapy or concomitantly with other antihypertensive agents. Adjunct therapy in heart failure inadequately responding to diuretics and digitalis. Adjunct therapy in stable patients within 24 hrs of acute myocardial infarction (AMI) to improve survival.

DOSAGE: *Adults:* HTN: Initial: 10mg qd. Usual: 20-40mg qd. Max: 80mg qd. CrCl 10-30mL/min: Initial: 5mg qd. CrCl <10mL/min: Initial: 2.5mg qd. Max: 40mg qd. Diuretic-Treated: Initial: 5mg qd. If possible, d/c diuretic 2-3 days prior to therapy. Resume diuretic if BP not controlled. Heart Failure: Initial: 5mg qd. Usual: 5-20mg qd. Hyponatremia or CrCl ≤30mL/min: Initial: 2.5mg qd. AMI: Initial: 5mg within 24 hrs, then 5mg after 24 hrs, then 10mg after 48 hrs, then daily. Use 2.5mg during first 3 days with low systolic BP. Maint: 10mg qd for 6 weeks. 2.5-5mg with hypotension. D/C with prolonged hypotension. Elderly/Renal Impairment: Caution with dose adjustment.
Pediatrics: ≥6 yrs: HTN: Initial: 0.07mg/kg qd (up to 5mg total). Adjust dose based on BP response. Max: 0.61mg/kg qd (up to 40mg qd).

HOW SUPPLIED: Tab: 5mg*, 10mg*, 20mg* *scored

CONTRAINDICATIONS: History of ACE inhibitor-associated angioedema and hereditary or idiopathic angioedema.

WARNINGS/PRECAUTIONS: Anaphylactoid reactions observed. Angioedema involving the face, extremities, lips, tongue, glottis, and/or larynx reported; d/c and monitor until symptoms resolve. Angioedema of tongue, glottis, or larynx may be fatal due to airway obstruction. Intestinal angioedema reported. More reports of angioedema in blacks than nonblacks. Rarely, a syndrome of cholestatic jaundice, fulminant necrosis and sometimes death occurs; d/c if angioedema, jaundice or marked LFT elevation occur. Excessive hypotension rarely seen with uncomplicated HTN but common with heart failure; caution when initiating therapy. Dose reduction or d/c if symptomatic hypotension develops. Rare cases of leukopenia/neutropenia and bone marrow depression revealed. Fetal/neonatal morbidity and death reported; d/c if pregnancy detected. Risk of hyperkalemia with diabetes mellitus (DM) and renal dysfunction. Persistent non-productive cough reported. Caution with renal artery stenosis/artery stenosis/hypertrophic cardiomyopathy, congestive heart failure (CHF), renal dysfunction, or if obstruction to left ventricle outflow tract.

ADVERSE REACTIONS: Hypotension, dizziness, headache, diarrhea, cough, chest pain, elevated BUN, elevated creatinine and hyperkalemia.

INTERACTIONS: Hypotension risk with diuretics. Increase hypoglycemic risk with antidiabetics (insulin, oral hypoglycemics). May further decrease renal function with NSAIDs including COX-2 inhibitors. Hyperkalemia with K⁺ sparing diuretics (eg, spironolactone, eplerenone, triamterene, or amiloride), K⁺ containing salt substitutes, or K⁺supplements. May increase lithium levels. Nitritoid reactions rarely reported with injectable gold. NSAIDs may diminish antihypertensive effects. May attenuate K⁺ loss with thiazide diuretics. Additive effect with HCTZ.

PREGNANCY: Category C (1st trimester) and D (2nd and 3rd trimesters), not for use in nursing.

MECHANISM OF ACTION: Angiotensin converting enzyme inhibitor; inhibition results in decreased plasma angiotensin II, which leads to decreased vasopressor activity and aldosterone secretion.

PHARMACOKINETICS: Absorption: Adults: 25%; T_{max}=7 hrs. **Pediatrics:** T_{max}=6 hrs. **Elimination: Adults:** Urine (unchanged); $T_{1/2}$=12 hrs. **Pediatrics:** Urine (28%).

NURSING CONSIDERATIONS

Assessment: Assess for aortic stenosis, hypertrophic cardiomyopathy, myocardial infarction, CHF, LFTs, renal artery stenosis, HTN, history of angioedema, hypotension in high-risk patients (eg, heart failure with systolic BP <100mmHg, surgery/anesthesia, hyponatremia, high-dose diuretic therapy, severe volume and/or salt depletion), ischemic heart/cerebrovascular disease, DM, renal function, hypersensitivity, pregnancy/nursing status, and possible drug interactions.

Monitoring: Monitor for head/neck and intestinal angioedema, anaphylactoid reactions and MI. Monitor vital signs and weight, CBC with platelet count and differential, FPG, urinalysis, ECG, cardiac markers (CPK-MB), serum K⁺, hepatic/renal function and serial ultrasound examinations.

Patient Counseling: Counsel about fetal risks during pregnancy, signs/symptoms of angioedema (eg, laryngeal/tongue edema, abdominal pain), adverse effects (eg, anaphylaxis, cough, hypotension, hyperkalemia). Inform that periodic monitoring of electrolytes and blood counts is required.

Administration: Oral route. **Storage:** 15-30°C (59-86°F); protect from moisture. Dispense in a tight container.

PRINZIDE   RX
lisinopril - hydrochlorothiazide (Merck)

> ACE inhibitors can cause death/injury to developing fetus during 2nd and 3rd trimesters. D/C if pregnancy is detected.

THERAPEUTIC CLASS: ACE inhibitor/thiazide diuretic

INDICATIONS: Treatment of HTN.

DOSAGE: *Adults:* Not Controlled with Lisinopril/HCTZ Monotherapy: Initial: 10mg-12.5mg or 20mg-12.5mg qd. Titrate: May increase after 2-3 weeks. Controlled on 25mg HCTZ qd with Hypokalemia: 10mg-12.5mg qd. Max: 80mg-50mg. Replacement Therapy: Substitute combination for titrated individual components. Elderly: Start at lower end of dosing range.

HOW SUPPLIED: Tab: (Lisinopril-HCTZ) 10mg-12.5mg, 20mg-12.5mg* *scored

CONTRAINDICATIONS: History of ACE inhibitor-associated angioedema, hereditary or idiopathic angioedema, anuria, hypersensitivity to other sulfonamide-derived drugs.

WARNINGS/PRECAUTIONS: Not for initial therapy of HTN. Angioedema of the face, extremities, lips, tongue, glottis, and larynx reported; d/c and administer appropriate therapy if this occurs. Intestinal angioedema reported; monitor for abdominal pain (with or without N/V). Anaphylactoid reactions reported during desensitization with hymenoptera venom and with dialysis with high-flux membranes and LDL apheresis with dextran sulfate absorption. Excessive hypotension observed. Neutropenia and bone marrow depression reported; monitor WBCs in patients with renal disease and collagen vascular disease. D/C if jaundice or marked elevations of hepatic enzymes occur. Caution with severe renal disease, hepatic dysfunction, left ventricular outflow obstruction, renal artery stenosis, and in elderly. May exacerbate or activate systemic lupus erythematosus (SLE). Risk of hyperkalemia with diabetes mellitus (DM) and renal insufficiency. Persistent nonproductive cough reported. Sensitivity reactions may occur in patients with/without history of allergy or bronchial asthma. Not recommended in patients with severe renal impairment (CrCl <30mL/min). May increase cholesterol and TG levels. Fluid/electrolyte imbalance, hypercalcemia, hyperglycemia, hypomagnesemia, and hyperuricemia may occur. Enhanced effects with postsympathectomy patients.

ADVERSE REACTIONS: Dizziness, headache, cough, fatigue, orthostatic effects, muscle cramps, angioedema, hypotension.

INTERACTIONS: Increased risk of lithium toxicity; avoid with lithium. Lisinopril: Hypotension risk with diuretics. NSAIDs, including selective COX-2 inhibitors, may diminish antihypertensive effect. May cause further deterioration of renal function in patients with compromised renal function taking NSAIDs, including selective COX-2 inhibitors. Increased risk of hyperkalemia with K^+-sparing diuretics, K^+ supplements, or K^+-containing salt substitutes. Nitritoid reactions with injectable gold. Hypotension may occur during anesthesia. HCTZ: Potentiation of orthostatic hypotension with alcohol, barbiturates, and narcotics. Dose adjustment of insulin or oral hypoglycemic agents may be required. Potentiation or additive effects with other antihypertensives. Reduced absorption with cholestyramine or colestipol. Increased risk of electrolyte depletion (eg, hypokalemia) with corticosteroids and ACTH. May decrease response to pressor amines (eg, norepinephrine). May increase responsiveness to nondepolarizing skeletal muscle relaxants (eg, tubocurarine). NSAIDs may reduce diuretic, natriuretic, and antihypertensive effects. May cause hypokalemia, which may lead to cardiac arrhythmia and sensitize or exaggerate the response of the heart to the toxic effects of digitalis.

PREGNANCY: Category C (1st trimester) and D (2nd and 3rd trimesters), not for use in nursing.

MECHANISM OF ACTION: Lisinopril: ACE inhibitor; decreases plasma angiotensin II, which leads to decreased vasopressor activity and decreased aldosterone secretion. HCTZ: Thiazide diuretic; not established. Affects distal renal tubular mechanism of electrolyte reabsorption. Increases excretion of Na^+ and Cl^-.

PHARMACOKINETICS: Absorption: Lisinopril: T_{max}=7 hrs. **Distribution:** Crosses placenta. HCTZ: Found in breast milk. **Elimination:** Lisinopril: Urine (unchanged); $T_{1/2}$=12 hrs. HCTZ: Renal (≥61% unchanged); $T_{1/2}$=5.6-14.8 hrs.

NURSING CONSIDERATIONS

Assessment: Assess for CHF, SLE, collagen vascular disease, renal artery stenosis, risk factors for hyperkalemia, histories of angioedema, allergy or bronchial asthma, and any other conditions where treatment is contraindicated or cautioned. Assess for hypersensitivity to drug, renal/hepatic function, pregnancy/nursing status, and possible drug interactions.

Monitoring: Monitor for angioedema, anaphylactoid reactions, hypotension, jaundice, sensitivity reactions, SLE, hyperglycemia, and hyperuricemia. Periodically monitor serum electrolytes and WBCs in patients with collagen vascular and renal diseases. Monitor BP, LFTs, renal function (BUN, SrCr), and cholesterol/TG levels.

Patient Counseling: Inform about fetal risks if taken during pregnancy; report pregnancies to physicians as soon as possible. Advise to use caution with excessive perspiration, dehydration, and other causes of volume depletion (eg, diarrhea, vomiting); may lead to fall in BP. Instruct to report lightheadedness, to d/c therapy if actual syncope occurs, not to use salt substitutes containing K⁺ without consulting physician, and to report immediately any signs/symptoms of neutropenia (eg, infections, fever, sore throat) and angioedema (swelling of face, extremities, eyes, lips, tongue, difficulty swallowing or breathing).

Administration: Oral route. **Storage:** 15-30°C (59-86°F). Protect from excessive light and humidity.

PRISTIQ   RX
desvenlafaxine (Wyeth)

> Antidepressants increased the risk of suicidal thinking and behavior (suicidality) in children, adolescents, and young adults in short-term studies of major depressive disorder (MDD) and other psychiatric disorders. Monitor and observe closely for clinical worsening, suicidality, or unusual changes in behavior. Not approved for use in pediatric patients.

THERAPEUTIC CLASS: Serotonin and norepinephrine reuptake inhibitor

INDICATIONS: Treatment of major depressive disorder (MDD).

DOSAGE: *Adults:* 50mg qd. 50-400mg/day shown to be effective, although no additional benefit at doses >50mg/day seen. Moderate Renal Impairment (CrCl 30-50mL/min): 50mg/day. Severe Renal Impairment (CrCl <30mL/min) or ESRD: 50mg qod. Do not give supplemental doses after dialysis. Do not escalate doses with moderate or severe renal impairment or ESRD. Hepatic Impairment: 50mg/day. Max: 100mg/day.

HOW SUPPLIED: Tab, Extended-Release: 50mg, 100mg

CONTRAINDICATIONS: Concomitant use of MAOIs or use within 14 days of taking an MAOI. Allow ≥7 days after stopping drug before starting an MAOI.

WARNINGS/PRECAUTIONS: Serotonin syndrome or neuroleptic malignant syndrome (NMS)-like reactions reported; d/c immediately and initiate supportive symptomatic treatment. May cause sustained increases in BP; consider dose reduction or d/c. Control pre-existing HTN prior to treatment. May increase risk of bleeding events. Mydriasis reported; monitor patients with increased intraocular pressure (IOP) or those at risk of acute narrow-angle glaucoma. Activation of mania/hypomania may occur; caution with history of mania/hypomania. Caution with cardiovascular (CV), cerebrovascular, lipid metabolism disorders; increased HR and lipid levels seen. Avoid abrupt withdrawal. D/C symptoms may occur; gradually taper dose. Assess risk of bipolar disorder before initiating therapy; not approved for use in bipolar depression treatment. Caution in moderate/severe renal impairment and with seizure disorder. May cause hyponatremia; d/c if symptomatic and institute appropriate intervention. Consider d/c if interstitial lung disease and eosinophilic pneumonia occur. Caution in elderly.

ADVERSE REACTIONS: Headache, N/V, dry mouth, diarrhea, dizziness, insomnia, somnolence, hyperhidrosis, constipation, anxiety, decreased appetite, male sexual function disorders, fatigue.

INTERACTIONS: See Contraindications. Caution with serotonergic drugs, triptans, antipsychotic agents and other dopamine antagonists; may increase risk of serotonin syndrome and NMS-like reactions; d/c immediately should these occur. Concomitant use with serotonin precursors (eg, tryptophan) is not recommended. Avoid use with alcohol and products containing venlafaxine. Increased risk of bleeding may occur with aspirin (ASA), NSAIDs, warfarin, and other anticoagulants. May increase levels with potent CYP3A4 inhibitors (eg, ketoconazole). May increase levels of CYP2D6 substrates (eg, desipramine). May decrease levels of CYP3A4 substrates (eg, midazolam). Caution with CNS-active drugs. Diuretics may increase risk of hyponatremia.

PREGNANCY: Category C, not for use in nursing.

MECHANISM OF ACTION: Selective serotonin and norepinephrine reuptake inhibitor; potentiates neurotransmitter activity in CNS by inhibiting neuronal serotonin and norepinephrine reuptake.

PHARMACOKINETICS: Absorption: Absolute bioavailability (80%); T_{max}=7.5 hrs. **Distribution:** Plasma protein binding (30%); V_d=3.4L/kg (IV); found in breast milk. **Metabolism:** Conjugation and via CYP3A4 mediated oxidation (minor). **Elimination:** Urine (45%, unchanged; 19% glucuronide metabolite, <5% oxidative metabolite); $T_{1/2}$=11 hrs.

NURSING CONSIDERATIONS

Assessment: Assess for bipolar disorder risk, pre-existing HTN, increased IOP, risk factors for acute-narrow angle glaucoma, history or family history of mania/hypomania; CV, cerebrovascular, or lipid metabolism disorders; hepatic/renal impairment, seizures, volume depletion, hypersensitivity to drug, pregnancy/nursing status, and possible drug interactions.

Monitoring: Monitor HR, BP, LFTs, renal function, serum lipid levels, signs/symptoms of clinical worsening, serotonin syndrome or NMS-like reactions, HTN, abnormal bleeding, mydriasis, activation of mania/hypomania, seizures, hyponatremia, interstitial lung disease, and eosinophilic pneumonia. If d/c therapy (particularly if abrupt), monitor for d/c symptoms. Periodically re-evaluate need for continued treatment.

Patient Counseling: Advise patients, families and caregivers about benefits and risks of therapy, its appropriate use, and to look for emergence of suicidality especially during dose adjustments. Inform physician of drug interactions and if allergic phenomena occur. Avoid taking with MAOIs or within 14 days of stopping MAOIs. Caution about risk of serotonin syndrome or NMS-like reactions and increased risk of bleeding. Advise to have BP monitored regularly, that mydriasis may occur in patients with increased IOP or those at risk of acute narrow-angle glaucoma, to observe for signs and symptoms of activation of mania/hypomania, to avoid alcohol, and that drug may be taken with or without food. Caution is advised with CV, cerebrovascular or lipid metabolism disorders. Do not d/c without notifying physician; d/c symptoms may occur. May impair physical/mental ability. May notice remains of tab passing in the stool. Notify physician if pregnant/nursing, become pregnant or intend to become pregnant.

Administration: Oral route. Do not divide, crush, chew, or dissolve tab. Swallow whole with fluid. Take at same time each day. **Storage:** 20-25°C (68-77°F); excursions permitted to 15-30°C (59-86°F).

ProAir HFA   RX
albuterol sulfate (Teva)

THERAPEUTIC CLASS: Beta₂-agonist

INDICATIONS: Treatment or prevention of bronchospasm in patients ≥4 yrs with reversible obstructive airway disease. Prevention of exercise-induced bronchospasm (EIB) in patients ≥4 yrs.

DOSAGE: *Adults*: Treatment/Prevention of Bronchospasm: 2 inh q4-6h or 1 inh q4h. EIB Prevention: 2 inh 15-30 min before exercise.
Pediatrics: ≥4 yrs: Treatment/Prevention of Bronchospasm: 2 inh q4-6h or 1 inh q4h. EIB Prevention: 2 inh 15-30 min before exercise.

HOW SUPPLIED: MDI: 90mcg/inh [8.5g]

WARNINGS/PRECAUTIONS: May produce paradoxical bronchospasm; d/c therapy immediately and institute alternative therapy. Asthma may deteriorate acutely over a period of hours or longer; re-evaluate patient and treatment regimen. Consider adding anti-inflammatory agents (eg, corticosteroids) to therapeutic regimen. May produce clinically significant cardiovascular effects; caution with cardiovascular (CV) disorders, especially coronary insufficiency, cardiac arrhythmias, and HTN. ECG changes reported. Fatalities reported with excessive use. Immediate hypersensitivity reactions may occur. Caution with convulsive disorders, hyperthyroidism, and diabetes mellitus (DM). May produce significant hypokalemia. Caution when administering higher doses with renal impairment.

ADVERSE REACTIONS: Pharyngitis, headache, rhinitis, dizziness, pain, tachycardia.

INTERACTIONS: Avoid use with other short-acting sympathomimetic aerosol bronchodilators. Caution with additional adrenergic drugs to avoid deleterious CV effects. Avoid β-blockers; if not possible, use cardioselective β-blockers with caution. Extreme caution with, or within 2 weeks of discontinuation of MAOIs and TCAs. Monitor digoxin levels. May worsen ECG changes and/or hypokalemia with non-K⁺-sparing diuretics (eg, loop diuretics, thiazide diuretics); consider monitoring K⁺ levels.

PREGNANCY: Category C, not for use in nursing.

MECHANISM OF ACTION: β_2-agonist; activates β_2-adrenergic receptors on airway smooth muscle. Activation of receptors leads to activation of adenylcyclase and increase in intracellular cyclic-3',5'-adenosine monophosphate (cAMP). Increased cAMP leads to activation of protein kinase A, which then leads to relaxation of smooth muscle of all airways, from the trachea to terminal bronchioles. Increased cAMP concentrations are also associated with inhibition of the release of mediators from mast cells in the airway.

PHARMACOKINETICS: **Absorption:** C_{max}=4,100pg/mL; AUC=28,426pg•hr/mL. (Pediatrics) C_{max}=1100pg/mL; AUC=5120pg•hr/mL. **Metabolism:** GI tract by SULTIA3 (sulfotransferase). **Elimination:** Urine (80-100%), feces (<20%); $T_{1/2}$=6 hrs.(Pediatrics) $T_{1/2}$=166 min.

NURSING CONSIDERATIONS

Assessment: Assess for convulsive disorders, hyperthyroidism, DM, CV disorders (eg, coronary insufficiency, cardiac arrhythmias, HTN), renal impairment, hypersensitivity, pregnancy/nursing status and possible drug interactions. Assess use in patients unusually responsive to sympathomimetic amines.

Monitoring: Monitor HR, BP, ECG changes, blood glucose, paradoxical bronchospasm, hypokalemia, hypersensitivity reactions, and deterioration of asthma.

Patient Counseling: Instruct to use as prescribed and not to increase dose or frequency of doses without consulting physician. Instruct on how to properly prime, clean, and use inhaler. Inform to take other concomitant drugs/asthma medications as directed. Counsel to report lack of response or the occurrence of any adverse side effect. Instruct to inform physician if pregnant or nursing. Counsel to keep out of reach of children.

Administration: Oral inhalation route. Shake well before use. 1) Prime inhaler before using for 1st time or if inhaler has not been used for 2 weeks by releasing 3 test sprays into air, away from face. 2) Clean mouthpiece at least once a week. Use actuator with supplied product only. 3) Discard inhaler after 200 sprays. Avoid spraying in eyes. **Storage:** 15-25°C (59-77°F). Protect from freezing and prolonged exposure to direct sunlight.

PROAMATINE RX
midodrine HCl (Shire)

> Can cause marked elevation of supine BP. Clinical benefits of improving ability to carry out activities of daily living have not been verified.

THERAPEUTIC CLASS: Alpha₁-agonist

INDICATIONS: Treatment of symptomatic orthostatic hypotension.

DOSAGE: *Adults:* Initial: 10mg tid; at 3-4 hr intervals, while awake. Max: 30mg/day. To avoid supine HTN during sleep, do not give <4 hrs before bedtime or after evening meal. Renal Dysfunction: Initial: 2.5mg tid.

HOW SUPPLIED: Tab: 2.5mg*, 5mg*, 10mg* *scored

CONTRAINDICATIONS: Severe organic heart disease, acute renal disease, urinary retention, pheochromocytoma, thyrotoxicosis, persistent and excessive supine HTN.

WARNINGS/PRECAUTIONS: Risk of supine HTN; monitor for symptoms of supine HTN (eg, pounding in ears, headache, blurred vision) and supine and standing BP; d/c if supine HTN persists. Caution with urinary retention, diabetes, renal or hepatic dysfunction. May decrease HR due to vagal reflex.

ADVERSE REACTIONS: Supine and sitting HTN, paresthesia, scalp pruritus, goosebumps, chills, urinary urge/retention/frequency.

INTERACTIONS: Caution with concomitant use of drugs that cause vasoconstriction (eg, phenylephrine, ephedrine, phenylpropanolamine, dihydroergotamine, pseudoephedrine); monitor BP. Fludrocortisone may potentiate supine HTN due to salt-retaining properties. OTC cold and diet products may potentiate pressor effects. Antagonized by alpha-blockers (eg, prazosin, terazosin, doxazosin). Metformin, cimetidine, ranitidine, procainamide, triamterene, flecainide, and quinidine may increase clearance. Caution with cardiac glycosides (eg, digitalis), psychopharmacologics, β-blockers, or other drugs that directly or indirectly reduce HR.

PREGNANCY: Category C, caution in nursing.

MECHANISM OF ACTION: Desglymidodrine (major metabolite); α_1-agonist; exerts its actions via activation of the α-adrenergic receptors of the arteriolar and venous vasculature, producing an increase in vascular tone and elevation of BP.

PHARMACOKINETICS: Absorption: Midodrine (prodrug): Rapid; absolute bioavailability (93%); T_{max}=1/2 hr. Desglymidodrine: T_{max}=1-2 hrs. **Distribution:** Poor; across blood-brain barrier. **Metabolism:** Liver via deglycination to desglymidodrine (major metabolite). **Elimination:** Urine (80%, metabolite); $T_{1/2}$=3-4 hrs (metabolite).

NURSING CONSIDERATIONS

Assessment: Assess for severe organic heart disease, acute renal impairment, urinary retention, hepatic impairment, pheochromocytoma or thyrotoxicosis, orthostatic hypotension with DM, history of visual problems, pregnancy/nursing status, and for possible drug interactions. Evaluate baseline renal and LFTs.

Monitoring: Monitor for signs/symptoms of supine HTN (eg, cardiac awareness, pounding in the ears, headache, blurred vision) and for bradycardia (eg, pulse slowing, increased dizziness, syncope, cardiac awareness). Monitor supine and sitting BP, HR, and renal/hepatic function.

Patient Counseling: Inform that certain OTC products (eg, cold remedies, diet aids) can elevate BP and may potentiate the pressor effect of the drug. Inform about the signs/symptoms of supine HTN; instruct to not take dose if supine for any length of time.

Administration: Oral route. Take during daytime, not to be taken after evening meals or <4 hrs before bedtime. **Storage:** 25°C (77°F); excursions permitted to 15-30°C (59-86°F).

PROCARDIA XL   RX
nifedipine (Pfizer)

THERAPEUTIC CLASS: Calcium channel blocker (dihydropyridine)

INDICATIONS: Management of vasospastic angina and chronic stable angina without evidence of vasospasm in patients who remain symptomatic despite adequate doses of β-blockers and/or organic nitrates or who cannot tolerate those agents. Treatment of HTN.

DOSAGE: *Adults:* Angina/HTN: Adjust dosage according to each patient's needs. Initial: 30-60mg qd. Titrate over 7-14 days. Max: 120mg qd. Caution if dose >90mg with angina.

HOW SUPPLIED: Tab, Extended-Release: 30mg, 60mg, 90mg

WARNINGS/PRECAUTIONS: May cause hypotension; monitor BP initially or with titration. May increase frequency, duration and/or severity of angina or acute myocardial infarction (MI), particularly those who have severe obstructive coronary artery disease (CAD), on starting or at time of dosage increase. Congestive heart failure (CHF) risk, especially with aortic stenosis or β-blockers. GI obstruction and bezoars reported; caution with altered GI anatomy and hypomotility disorders. Peripheral edema associated with vasodilation of dependent arterioles and small blood vessels may occur; in patients with angina or HTN complicated by CHF, rule out peripheral edema cause by left ventricular dysfunction. Transient elevations of enzymes (such as alkaline phosphatase, CPK, LDH, SGOT and SGPT), cholestasis with or without jaundice and allergic hepatitis reported (rare). Positive direct Coombs test with or without hemolytic anemia reported; casual relationship not determined. Rare, reversible elevation in BUN and SrCr reported with chronic renal insufficiency.

ADVERSE REACTIONS: Dizziness, headache, nausea, fatigue, constipation, edema.

INTERACTIONS: β-Blockers may increase risk of CHF, severe hypotension, or angina exacerbation; avoid abrupt β-blocker withdrawal. Possible hypotension with fentanyl and other narcotic analgesics. May increase digoxin levels; monitor digoxin levels when initiating, adjusting, and d/c nifedipine. May increase PT with coumarin anticoagulants. May increase levels with cimetidine. Decreased serum K^+ levels with diuretics. Monitor with antihypertensives. Increased risk of GI obstruction with H_2-histamine blockers, NSAIDs, laxatives, anticholinergic agents, and levothyroxine.

PREGNANCY: Category C, safety not known in nursing.

MECHANISM OF ACTION: Calcium channel blocker; inhibits calcium ion influx into cardiac muscle and smooth muscle. Angina: Has not been established; believed to act by relaxation and prevention of coronary artery spasm and reduction of oxygen utilization. HTN: Peripheral vasodilation and resulting reduction in peripheral resistance.

PHARMACOKINETICS: Absorption: Complete. Bioavailabilty (steady-state)= 86% relative to Procardia capsules. **Distribution:** Plasma protein binding (92-98%). **Metabolism:** Extensive; Hepatic biotransformation. **Elimination:** Urine (<0.1%, unchanged), feces; $T_{1/2}$=2 hrs.

NURSING CONSIDERATIONS

Assessment: Assess for hypersensitivity reactions, hepatic/renal impairment, severe obstructive CAD, severity of angina and/or MI, aortic stenosis, altered GI anatomy (severe GI narrowing, colon cancer, small bowel obstruction, bowel resection, gastric bypass, vertical banded gastroplasty, colostomy), hypomotility disorders (constipation, GERD, ileus, obesity, hypothyroidism, DM), CHF with left ventricular dysfunction, pregnancy/nursing status and possible drug interactions.

Monitoring: Monitor for hypersensitivity reactions, excessive hypotension, increased frequency, duration and/or severity of angina and/or acute MI (especially during initiation and dose titration), CHF, signs/symptoms of GI obstruction, peripheral edema (determine cause), cholestasis with or without jaundice and allergic hepatitis.

Patient Counseling: Advise to take exactly as prescribed. Instruct to swallow tablet whole; do not crush, divide, or chew. Inform that it is normal to occasionally observe a tablet like material in the stool. Counsel about adverse effects; advise to report any.

Administration: Oral route. Swallow whole. Do not chew, divide or crush tablet. **Storage:** Below 30°C (86°F). Protect from moisture and humidity.

PROCHLORPERAZINE   RX
prochlorperazine (Various)

Elderly patients with dementia-related psychosis treated with antipsychotic drugs are at an increased risk of death; most deaths appeared to be cardiovascular (CV) (eg, heart failure, sudden death) or infectious (eg, pneumonia) in nature. Treatment with conventional antipsychotic drugs may similarly increase mortality. Prochlorperazine is not approved for the treatment of patients with dementia-related psychosis.

THERAPEUTIC CLASS: Phenothiazine derivative

INDICATIONS: Severe N/V. Treatment of schizophrenia. (Maleate) Short-term treatment of generalized non-psychotic anxiety.

DOSAGE: *Adults:* Adjust dose according to individual response. N/V: Begin with the lowest recommended dosage. (Tab) Usual: 5-10mg PO tid-qid. Daily dose >40mg should only be used in resistant cases. (IM) Initial: 5-10mg IM q3-4h prn. Max: 40mg/day. (IV) 2.5-10mg slow IV or infusion at rate ≤5mg/min. Max: 10mg single dose and 40mg/day. N/V with Surgery: 5-10mg IM 1-2 hrs before induction of anesthesia (repeat once in 30 min if needed) or 5-10mg as slow IV injection or infusion 15-30 min before induction of anesthesia. To control acute symptoms during or after surgery, repeat once if needed. Max: 40mg/day. Non-Psychotic Anxiety: (Tab) Usual: 5mg tid-qid. Max: 20mg/day or ≤12 weeks. Psychotic Disorders (Schizophrenia): Mild/Outpatient: 5-10mg PO tid-qid. Moderate-Severe/Hospitalized: Initial: 10mg PO tid-qid. May increase dose gradually in small increments every 2-3 days. Severe: (PO) 100-150mg/day. (IM) Initial: 10-20mg, may repeat q2-4h prn (or, in resistant cases, every hr). Switch to oral after obtaining control at the same dosage level or higher. Prolonged Parenteral Therapy: 10-20mg IM q4-6h. Debilitated or Emaciated **Adults:** Titrate more gradually. Elderly: Use lower dosing range and titrate more gradually.

Pediatrics: ≥2 yrs and ≥20 lbs: N/V: Adjust dosage and frequency according to the severity of symptoms and response. (PO) 20-29 lbs: Usual: 2.5mg qd-bid. Max: 7.5mg/day. 30-39 lbs: 2.5mg bid-tid. Max: 10mg/day. 40-85 lbs: 2.5mg tid or 5mg bid. Max: 15mg/day. Severe N/V: (IM) 0.06mg/lb of body weight. Control is usually obtained with 1 dose. Psychotic Disorders (Schizophrenia): (PO) 2-12 yrs: Initial: 2.5mg bid-tid. Do not give >10mg on the first day. Increase dose based on patient's response. 2-5 yrs: Max: 20mg/day. 6-12 yrs: Max: 25mg/day. (IM) <12 yrs: 0.06mg/lb of body weight. Control is usually obtained with 1 dose. Switch to oral after obtaining control at the same dosage level or higher.

HOW SUPPLIED: Inj: (Edisylate) 5mg/mL [2mL, 10mL]; Tab: (Maleate) 5mg, 10mg

CONTRAINDICATIONS: Comatose states, concomitant large doses of CNS depressants (eg, alcohol, barbiturates, narcotics), pediatric surgery, pediatrics <2 yrs or <20 lbs.

WARNINGS/PRECAUTIONS: Secondary extrapyramidal symptoms can occur. Tardive dyskinesia (TD), may develop especially in elderly and during long term use. Neuroleptic malignant syndrome (NMS) reported; d/c if it occurs and institute appropriate treatment; caution during re-introduction of therapy. NMS recurrence reported. Avoid in patients with bone marrow depression, who have previously demonstrated a hypersensitivity reaction with a phenothiazine and in pregnant women, unless potential benefits outweigh the possible hazards. May impair mental and/or physical abilities, especially during the first few days of therapy. May mask symptoms of overdose of other drugs. May obscure diagnosis of intestinal obstruction, brain tumor, and Reye's syndrome; avoid in children and adolescents whose signs and symptoms suggest Reye's syndrome. May cause hypotension; caution with large doses and parenteral administration in patients with impaired CV systems. May interfere with thermoregulation; caution in patients exposed to extreme heat. May elevate prolactin levels; caution with prolactin-dependent tumors. Evaluate therapy periodically with prolonged use. Leukopenia/neutropenia/agranulocytosis reported. Caution with glaucoma. Caution in children with dehydration or acute illness and in the elderly. May lower seizure threshold. D/C 48 hrs before myelography; may resume after 24 hrs postprocedure. May produce α-adrenergic blockade.

ADVERSE REACTIONS: NMS, cholestatic jaundice, leukopenia, agranulocytosis, drowsiness, dizziness, amenorrhea, blurred vision, skin reactions, hypotension, motor restlessness, extrapyramidal symptoms, TD, dystonia, pseudoparkinsonism.

INTERACTIONS: See Contraindications. May intensify and prolong action of CNS depressants (opiates, alcohol, anesthetics, barbiturates, narcotics, analgesics, antihistamines), atropine and organophosphorus insecticides. May decrease oral anticoagulant effects. May produce α-adrenergic blockade. Thiazide diuretics accentuate orthostatic hypotension. Increased levels of both drugs with propranolol. Anticonvulsants may need dosage adjustment. May lower convulsive threshold. May interfere with metabolism of phenytoin and precipitate toxicity. Risk of encephalopathic syndrome occurs with lithium. May antagonize antihypertensive effects of guanethidine and related compounds. Avoid use prior to myelography with metrizamide; vomiting as a sign of toxicity of cancer chemotherapeutic drugs may be obscured by the anti-emetic effect. May reverse effect of epinephrine. May cause paradoxical further lowering of BP with other pressor agents (excluding norepinephrine bitartrate and phenylephrine HCl), including epinephrine. Avoid with stimulants that may cause convulsions (eg, picrotoxin or pentylenetetrazol) when treating overdose.

PREGNANCY: Safety is not known in pregnancy; caution in nursing.

MECHANISM OF ACTION: Phenothiazine derivative; anti-emetic and antipsychotic.

NURSING CONSIDERATIONS

Assessment: Assess for Reye's syndrome, TD, pregnancy/nursing status, possible drug interactions, impaired CV system, breast cancer, glaucoma, bone marrow depression, pre-existing low WBC count, history of drug induced leukopenia/neutropenia, history of psychosis, and seizure disorder. Assess use in children with acute illness or dehydration, elderly, debilitated or emaciated patients.

Monitoring: Monitor for extrapyramidal symptoms, signs/symptoms of TD, NMS, hypotension, fever, sore throat, infection, jaundice, motor restlessness, dystonia, pseudoparkinsonism, and hypersensitivity reactions. Monitor CBC, WBC, and prolactin levels. Conduct liver studies if fever with grippe-like symptoms occur.

Patient Counseling: Inform about the risks and benefits of therapy. Avoid engaging in hazardous activities (eg, operating vehicles or machinery) and exposure to extreme heat. Seek medical attention if symptoms of TD, NMS (hyperpyrexia, muscle rigidity, altered mental status), hypotension, mydriasis, encephalopathic syndrome (weakness, lethargy, fever), sore throat, infection, deep sleep, or hypersensitivity reactions occur.

Administration: IV, IM, Oral route. (Inj) Inspect visually for particulate matter and discoloration. Do not use if with marked discoloration. Inject deeply into upper, outer quadrant of the buttock. SQ is not advisable because of local irritation. May be administered either undiluted or diluted in isotonic solution. When given IV, do not use bolus injection. Do not mixed with other agents in the syringe. Avoid getting injection solution on hands or clothing because of potential contact dermatitis. **Storage:** Tab, Inj: 20-25°C (68-77°F). Protect from light. (Inj) Do not freeze.

PROCRIT   RX
epoetin alfa (Centocor)

> Increased mortality, serious cardiovascular (CV) events and stroke in CRF patients when administered to target Hgb levels of ≥13g/dL. Individualize dosing to achieve and maintain Hgb levels within range of 10-12g/dL. Shortened overall survival and/or increased risk of tumor progression or recurrence in patients with breast, non-small cell lung, head and neck, lymphoid, and cervical cancers. To decrease these risks, as well as risk of serious cardio- and thrombovascular events, use lowest dose needed to avoid RBC transfusions. Because of these risks, prescribers and hospitals must enroll in and comply with the ESA APPRISE Oncology Program to prescribe and/or dispense to patients with cancer. Use only for treatment of anemia due to concomitant myelosuppressive chemotherapy. Not indicated for patients receiving myelosuppressive therapy when anticipated outcome is cure. D/C following completion of chemotherapy course. Increased the rate of deep venous thromboses (DVT) in patients not receiving prophylactic anticoagulation during surgery. Consider DVT prophylaxis.

THERAPEUTIC CLASS: Erythropoiesis stimulator

INDICATIONS: Treatment of anemia of chronic renal failure (CRF); anemia related to therapy with zidovudine in HIV-infected patients; anemic patients (Hgb >10-≤13g/dL) who are at high risk for perioperative blood loss to reduce the need for allogeneic blood transfusions; anemia due to the effect of con-comitantly administered chemotherapy based on studies that have shown a reduction in the need for RBC transfusions in patients with metastatic, non-myeloid malignancies receiving chemotherapy for minimum of 2 months.

DOSAGE: *Adults:* CRF: (IV/SQ) Individualize dose. Initial: 50-100 U/kg TIW. See PI for dose adjustments based on Hgb levels. Maint: Individually titrate for each patient on dialysis; Hgb levels between 10-12g/dL. Median Maint: (Hemodialysis) 75 U/kg TIW with the range of 12.5-525 U/kg TIW. Zidovudine-Treated HIV Patients: If serum erythropoietin ≤500 mU/mL and zidovudine ≤4200mg/week give 100 U/kg IV/SQ TIW for 8 weeks. Titrate: Increase by 50-100 U/kg TIW after 8 weeks if necessary. Max: 300 U/kg TIW. Maint: If Hgb >12g/dL, d/c until Hgb <11g/dL, then reduce dose by 25% when therapy is resumed. Surgery Patients: Initial: (Hgb >10-≤13g/dL) 300 U/kg/day SQ for 10 days before, on day of, and for 4 days after surgery; or 600 U/kg SQ once weekly on 21, 14, and 7 days before surgery plus a fourth dose on the day of surgery. Cancer Patients on Chemotherapy: 150 U/kg SQ TIW or 40,000 U SQ weekly. Titrate: (TIW dosing) Increase to 300 U/kg TIW if response not satis-factory after 4 weeks to avoid need for RBC transfusion or (Weekly dosing) 60,000 U SQ weekly if Hgb is not increased by ≥1g/dL after 4 weeks. See PI for dose adjustments based on Hgb levels.
Pediatrics: CRF: (IV/SQ) Individualize dose. Initial: 50 U/kg TIW. See PI for dose adjustments based on Hgb levels. Median Maint (Hemodialysis and Peritoneal dialysis): 167 U/kg/week (49-447 U/kg/week) and 76 U/kg/week (24-323 U/kg/week) in divided doses (TIW or BIW). If transferrin saturation is >20%, dose may be increased. Maintain Hgb levels between 10-12g/dL; 75-150 U/kg/week maintains the Hct of 36%-38% for 6 months. Cancer Patients on Chemotherapy: 600 U/kg IV weekly. Titrate: If Hgb is not increased by ≥1g/dL after 4 weeks increase to 900 U/kg IV weekly. See PI for dose adjustments based on Hgb levels. Max: 60,000 U.

HOW SUPPLIED: Inj: 2000 U/mL, 3000 U/mL, 4000 U/mL, 10,000 U/mL, 40,000 U/mL [single dose]; 10,000 U/mL, 20,000 U/mL [multidose].

CONTRAINDICATIONS: Uncontrolled HTN. Hypersensitivity to mammalian cell-derived products and albumin (human).

WARNINGS/PRECAUTIONS: Contains benzyl alcohol; increased incidence of neurological and other complications in premature infants have been re-ported. Pure red cell aplasia (PRCA) and severe anemia (with or without other cytopenias) may occur. Evaluate etiology if lack/loss of response occurs; test for presence of antibodies to erythropoietin; if present d/c permanently. Should not be switched to other erythropoiesis-stimulating agents (ESAs) as antibodies may cross-react. Formulation with albumin may carry risk for trans-mission of viral diseases. Closely monitor and aggressively control BP in those treated and adjust dose in CRF patients on dialysis with clinically evident isch-emic heart disease or CHF. Seizures reported; BP and presence of premoni-tory neurologic symptoms should be monitored. Avoid potentially hazardous activities such as driving or operating heavy machinery. Exacerbation of por-phyria observed; caution in patients with known porphyria. Transient rashes occasionally observed. Decreased locoregional control/progression-free sur-vival and/or overall survival in patients with advanced head and neck cancer receiving radiation therapy, in patients receiving chemotherapy for metastatic breast cancer or lymphoid malignancy, and in patients with non-small cell lung cancer or various malignancies who were not receiving chemotherapy or radiotherapy. Functional iron deficiency may develop. Menses may resume during therapy. IV route recommended in hemodialysis patients.

ADVERSE REACTIONS: HTN, headache, fatigue, dizziness, insomnia, skin pain, pruritus, N/V, diarrhea, edema, pyrexia, constipation, cough, skin reac-tion at administration site, CV events.

INTERACTIONS: Adjust heparin and antihypertensive doses in dialysis patients.

PREGNANCY: Category C, caution in nursing.

MECHANISM OF ACTION: Erythropoiesis stimulator.

PHARMACOKINETICS: Absorption: (SQ) T_{max}=5-24 hrs. **Elimination:** (IV) $T_{1/2}$=4-13 hrs.

NURSING CONSIDERATIONS

Assessment: Assess for uncontrolled HTN, porphyria, history of HTN, CV disease (ischemic heart disease, CHF), renal failure, cancer, PRCA, seizure, pregnancy/nursing status, possible drug interactions, hypersensitivity to mammalian cell-derived products and albumin. Obtain baseline BP measurements and iron status (transferrin saturation, serum ferritin).

Monitoring: Monitor BP, Hct, CBC with differential and platelet count, iron status (transferrin saturation, serum ferritin) regularly. CRF: Serum chemistries (BUN, uric acid, creatinine, phosphorus, K+) regularly, Hgb twice weekly; HIV and cancer: Hgb once weekly. Monitor for signs/symptoms of CV events (MI, stroke, CHF), PRCA, severe anemia, viral diseases, seizures, lack/loss of response to therapy, and hypersensitivity reactions.

Patient Counseling: Instruct patients or their caregiver on how to safely and effectively administer the drug at home, and on proper dosage. Seek medical attention if symptoms of CV events, anemia, infections, seizures, or hypersensitivity reactions occur. Can increase the risk of having serious CV events, thromboembolic events and tumor progression or recurrence. Instruct on the importance of proper disposal and caution against the reuse of needles, syringes, or drug product. May impair physical/mental abilities. A puncture-resistant container should be available for disposal of used syringes and needles.

Administration: IV, SC route. **Storage:** 2-8°C (36-46°F). Do not freeze or shake. Protect from light.

PROGRAF   RX
tacrolimus (Astellas)

> Increased susceptibility to infection and development of lymphoma. Should only be prescribed by physicians experienced in immunosuppressive therapy and management of organ transplant patients. Should be managed in facilities equipped and staffed with adequate laboratory and supportive medical resources.

THERAPEUTIC CLASS: Macrolide immunosuppressant

INDICATIONS: Prophylaxis of organ rejection in allogeneic liver, kidney, or heart transplants with concomitant adrenal corticosteroids. In heart and kidney transplant patients, azathioprine or mycophenolate mofetil (MMF) coadministration is recommended. Because of the risk of anaphylaxis, injection should be reserved for patients unable to take capsules orally.

DOSAGE: *Adults:* (IV) Initial (no sooner than 6 hrs after transplantation): 0.03-0.05mg/kg/day (liver, kidney) or 0.01mg/kg/day (heart) as a continuous IV infusion if cannot tolerate PO. (PO) Liver Transplant: Initial: 0.10-0.15mg/kg/day q12h in two divided daily doses no sooner than 6 hrs after transplantation. In patient receiving an IV infusion, the first dose of oral therapy should be given 8-12 hrs after discontinuing IV infusion. Titrate based on clinical assessments of rejection and tolerability. Lower dosage may be sufficient as maintenance therapy. Adjunct therapy with adrenal corticosteroids is recommended early post-transplant. Kidney Transplant: Initial: 0.2mg/kg/day in combination with azathioprine or 0.1mg/kg/day in combination with MMF and IL-2 receptor antagonist q12h in two divided doses. May administer initial dose within 24 hrs of transplantation, but should be delayed until renal function has recovered. Black patients may require higher doses. Heart Transplant: Initial: 0.075mg/kg/day q12h in two divided daily doses no sooner than 6 hrs after transplantation. In patients receiving an IV infusion, the first dose of oral therapy should be given 8-12 hrs after discontinuing IV infusion. Titrate based on clinical assessments of rejection and tolerability. Lower dosage may be sufficient as maintenance therapy. Adjunct therapy with adrenal corticosteroids is recommended early post-transplant. Renal/Hepatic Impairment: Give lowest recommended dose. Severe Hepatic Impairment (Pugh ≥10): May require lower doses. Should be delayed up to 48 hrs or longer with post-operative oliguria.
Pediatrics: Liver Transplant: Initial: 0.03-0.05mg/kg/day IV or 0.15-0.2mg/kg/day PO. Dose adjustments may be required. Renal/Hepatic

Impairment: Give lowest recommended dose. Severe Hepatic Impairment (Pugh ≥10): May require lower doses. Should be delayed up to 48 hrs or longer with post-operative oliguria.

HOW SUPPLIED: Cap: 0.5mg, 1mg, 5mg; Inj: 5mg/mL

WARNINGS/PRECAUTIONS: Insulin-dependent post-transplant diabetes mellitus (DM), hyperglycemia, HTN, and hyperkalemia reported. Myocardial hypertrophy reported; if diagnosed, dosage reduction or discontinuation should be considered. Neurotoxicity reported, including development of posterior reversible encephalopathy syndrome (PRES); if PRES suspected or diagnosed, BP should be maintained & reduction of immunosuppression is advised. Nephrotoxicity reported; avoid co-administration with cyclosporine. Monitor drug levels frequently to prevent organ rejection and/or reduce potential toxicity. Monitor for anaphylaxis with infusion. Monitor closely and dosage adjustments should be considered with hepatic/renal impairment. Increased risk of latent viral infections with immunosupressed patients.

ADVERSE REACTIONS: HTN, headache, insomnia, infection, hyperglycemia, hyperkalemia, hypomagnesemia, diarrhea, N/V, tremor, paresthesia, anemia, abdominal pain, abnormal renal function.

INTERACTIONS: CYP450 3A inducers, carbamazepine, phenobarbital, phenytoin, rifabutin, caspofungin, rifampin, St. John's wort, sirolimus, may decrease blood concentrations. Caution with other nephrotoxic drugs (eg, aminoglycosides, amphotericin B, cisplatin, ganciclovir) and drugs metabolized by CYP450 3A (eg, nelfinavir, ritonavir). Avoid grapefruit juice. CYP450 3A inhibitors, diltiazem, nicardipine, nifedipine, verapamil, clotrimazole, fluconazole, itraconazole, ketoconazole, voriconazole, clarithromycin, erythromycin, troleandomycin, bromocriptine, chloramphenicol, cimetidine, cyclosporine, danazol, ethinyl estradiol, methylprednisolone, lansoprazole, omeprazole, protease inhibitors, nefazodone, magnesium-aluminum-hydroxide, cisapride, metoclopramide, nelfinavir may increase blood concentrations. Vaccination may be less effective. Avoid live vaccines, cyclosporine (when switching to tacrolimus, wait at least 24 hrs after last cyclosporine dose), K⁺-sparing diuretics, and sirolimus. Caution with calcium-channel blocking agents and immunosuppressant therapy. Additive/synergistic impairment of renal function with drugs that may be associated with renal dysfunction. Caution with drugs with castor oil derivatives with injection administration.

PREGNANCY: Category C, not for use in nursing.

MECHANISM OF ACTION: Macrolide immunosuppressant; not established. Suspected to inhibit T-lymphocyte activation. Binds to intracellular protein (FKBP-12). Complex of tacrolimus-FKBP-12, calcium, calmodulin, and calcineurin is then formed and phosphatase activity of calcineurin inhibited. Effect may prevent dephosphorylation and translocation of nuclear factor of activated T cells (NF-AT), a nuclear component responsible for initiating gene transcription for the formation of lymphokines. Results in inhibition of T-lymphocyte activation.

PHARMACOKINETICS: Absorption: (PO) Incomplete and variable; (Healthy Volunteers) absolute bioavailability (18%), C_{max}=29.7ng/mL, T_{max}=1.6 hrs, AUC=243ng•hr/mL; (IV) AUC=598ng•hr/mL. Refer to PI for detailed parameters. **Distribution:** Plasma protein binding (99%), found in breast milk. **Metabolism:** Hepatic, via CYP3A (demethylation and hydroxylation); 13-methyl tacrolimus (major metabolite); 31-demethyl (active metabolite). **Elimination:** (PO) Feces (92.6%), urine (2.3%); $T_{1/2}$=34.8 hrs. (IV) Feces (92.4%); $T_{1/2}$=34.2 hrs. Refer to PI for parameters in patients with renal, hepatic, and cardiac transplants.

NURSING CONSIDERATIONS

Assessment: Assess for hypersensitivity to HCO-60 (polyoxyl 60 hydrogenated castor oil), impaired hepatic/renal function, and possible drug interactions. Assess use in pregnant/nursing females.

Monitoring: Monitor for signs/symptoms of insulin dependent post-transplant DM, neurotoxicity, nephrotoxicity, hyperkalemia, lymphomas and other malignancies (eg, skin), lymphoproliferative disorder, anaphylactic reactions, HTN, myocardial hypertrophy, and latent viral infections. Monitor with renal impairment for dose adjustments. Perform regular evaluation of SrCr, K⁺, and fasting glucose. Monitor metabolic and hematologic systems as clinically warranted.

Patient Counseling: Inform that repeated lab testing required. Advise females about risks of use during pregnancy. Advise to avoid adjusting dose without consulting a physician. Inform about increased risk of neoplasia and DM. Instruct to contact physician if frequent urination, increased hunger, or thirst occur. Counsel to wear protective clothing, use sunscreen, and avoid exposure to sunlight/UV light to reduce risk of malignant skin changes.

Administration: Oral/IV routes. IV: Must be diluted with 0.9% NS or D5W to concentration between 0.004mg/mL and 0.02 mg/mL. Patients receiving IV formulation should be under continuous observation for at least first 30 min following start of infusion and at frequent intervals thereafter. **Storage:** Cap: 25°C (77°F); excursions permitted to 15-30°C (59-86°F). Inj: 5-25°C (41-77°F). Store diluted infusion in glass or polyethylene containers and discarded after 24 hrs.

PROLIA   RX
denosumab (Amgen)

THERAPEUTIC CLASS: IgG₂ Monoclonal antibody

INDICATIONS: Treatment of postmenopausal women with osteoporosis at high risk of fracture (eg, history of osteoporotic fracture, multiple risk factors for fracture) or patients who have failed or cannot tolerate other available osteoporosis therapy. Reduces the incidence of vertebral, nonvertebral, and hip fractures.

DOSAGE: *Adults:* 60mg as single SQ injection once q6 months. Administer in the upper arm, upper thigh, or abdomen. If a dose is missed, administer as soon as patient is available and schedule inj q6 months from date of last inj. All patients should receive calcium 1000mg daily and at least 400 IU vitamin D daily.

HOW SUPPLIED: Inj: 60mg/mL

CONTRAINDICATIONS: Hypocalcemia.

WARNINGS/PRECAUTIONS: Should be administered by a healthcare professional. Hypocalcemia may be exacerbated; correct pre-existing hypocalcemia prior to initiating therapy. Monitor calcium and mineral levels (phosphorus and magnesium) in patients predisposed to hypocalcemia and with disturbances of mineral metabolism (eg, history of hypoparathyroidism, thyroid/parathyroid surgery, malabsorption syndromes, excision of small intestines, severe renal impairment or receiving dialysis). Serious skin, abdomen, urinary tract, and ear infections leading to hospitalization reported; consider the benefit-risk profile prior to therapy. Caution in patients with impaired immune system; may be at increased risk for serious infections. Epidermal and dermal adverse events such as dermatitis, eczema, and rashes may occur; d/c if severe symptoms develop. Osteonecrosis of the jaw (ONJ) may occur; routine oral exam should be performed prior to initiation of treatment. Significant suppression of bone remodeling as evidenced by markers of bone turnover and bone histomorphometry reported.

ADVERSE REACTIONS: Back pain, anemia, vertigo, upper abdominal pain, peripheral edema, cystitis, upper respiratory tract infection, pneumonia, hypercholesterolemia, pain in extremity, musculoskeletal pain, bone pain, sciatica, insomnia.

INTERACTIONS: Immunosuppressant agents may increase the risk of serious infections. Concomitant use with chemotherapy and corticosteroids may increase risk of ONJ.

PREGNANCY: Category C, not for use in nursing.

MECHANISM OF ACTION: Receptor activator of nuclear factor kappa-B ligand (RANKL) inhibitor; prevents RANKL from activating its receptor, RANK, on the surface of osteoclasts and their precursors thereby decreasing

P

bone resorption and increasing bone mass and strength in both cortical and trabecular bone.

PHARMACOKINETICS: Absorption: (60mg SQ, after fasting) C_{max}=6.75mcg/mL; T_{max}=10 days; $AUC_{0-16\ weeks}$=316mcg•day/mL. **Elimination:** $T_{1/2}$=25.4 days.

NURSING CONSIDERATIONS

Assessment: Assess for pre-existing hypocalcemia, history of hypoparathyroidism, thyroid/parathyroid surgery, malabsorption syndromes, excision of small intestines, renal impairment or if receiving dialysis, risk factors for ONJ such as invasive dental procedures (eg, tooth extraction, dental implants, oral surgery) and oral hygiene, pregnancy/nursing status, and possible drug interactions.

Monitoring: Monitor for calcium and mineral levels (phosphorus and magnesium). Monitor for signs and symptoms of hypocalcemia, infections including cellulitis, and dermatological reactions (dermatitis, rashes, and eczema). Monitor for long-term consequences of the degree of suppression of bone remodeling (eg, ONJ, atypical fractures, delayed fracture healing).

Patient Counseling: Inform about the symptoms of hypocalcemia and the importance of maintaining calcium levels with adequate calcium and vitamin D supplementation. Advise patients to seek prompt medical attention if they develop signs and symptoms of hypocalcemia, infections including cellulitis, and dermatological reactions (dermatitis, rashes, and eczema). Advise to maintain good oral hygiene during treatment and to inform dentist prior to dental procedures that they are on treament; instruct to inform physician or dentist if experiencing persistent pain and/or slow healing of the mouth or jaw after dental surgery. If a dose is missed, administer injection as soon as convenient; thereafter, schedule injections every 6 months from the date of the last injection.

Administration: SQ route. Refer to PI for Preparation and Administration. **Storage:** 2-8°C (36-46°F). Do not freeze. Prior to administration, may be allowed to reach up to 25°C (77°F). Must be used within 14 days. Protect from direct light and heat. Avoid vigorous shaking.

PROMACTA   RX
eltrombopag (GlaxoSmithKline)

> May cause hepatotoxicity. Measure serum ALT, AST, and bilirubin prior to initiation, q2 weeks when adjusting dose and monthly after stabilizing dose. If bilirubin is elevated, perform fractionation. Evaluate abnormal serum liver tests with repeat testing within 3-5 days. If the abnormalities are confirmed, monitor weekly until the abnormality(ies) resolves, stabilizes, or returns to baseline levels. D/C if ALT levels increase to ≥3X ULN and are progressive, persistent for ≥4 weeks, accompanied by increased direct bilirubin, or accompanied by clinical symptoms of liver injury or evidence for hepatic decompensation. Available only through a restricted distribution program called **PROMACTA** *CARES*.

THERAPEUTIC CLASS: Thrombopoietin receptor agonist

INDICATIONS: Treatment of thrombocytopenia in patients with chronic immune (idiopathic) thrombocytopenia purpura (ITP) who have had an insufficient response to corticosteroids, immunoglobulins, or splenectomy.

DOSAGE: *Adults:* Initial: 50mg qd. East Asian Ancestry/Mild-to-Severe Hepatic Impairment (Child-Pugh Class A, B, C): Initial: 25mg qd. East Asian Ancestry with Hepatic Impairment (Child-Pugh Class A, B, C): Initial: 25mg qod. Titrate: Adjust to achieve and maintain platelet count ≥50 x 10⁹/L. Max: 75mg/day. Platelet Count <50 x 10⁹/L following ≥2 Weeks of Therapy: Increase daily dose by 25mg to max of 75mg/day. For patients taking 25mg qod, increase to 25mg/day before increasing dose by 25mg. Platelet Count ≥200 x 10⁹/L to ≤400 x 10⁹/L at Any Time: Decrease daily dose by 25mg. Wait 2 weeks to assess effects of this and any subsequent dose adjustments. Platelet count >400 x 10⁹/L: D/C therapy; increase monitoring of platelet count to twice weekly. Once platelet count falls to <150 x 10⁹/L, reinitiate therapy at a daily dose reduced by 25mg. Platelet Count >400 x 10⁹/L After 2

Weeks of Therapy at Lowest Dose: D/C therapy. Hepatic Impairment (Child-Pugh A, B, C): Increase dose after 3 weeks of initial therapy or after any subsequent dosing increase. D/C if no increase in platelet count to a sufficient level after 4 weeks at max dose or excessive platelet count responses, or important liver test abnormalities occur. Elderly: Start at lower end of dosing range.

HOW SUPPLIED: Tab: 25mg, 50mg, 75mg

WARNINGS/PRECAUTIONS: Use only in patients with ITP whose degree of thrombocytopenia and clinical condition increase the risk for bleeding; not to be used to normalize platelet counts. If discontinued due to ≥3X ULN ALT, reinitiation is not recommended; may cautiously reintroduce if potential benefit outweighs risk for hepatotoxicity. May increase risk for development or progression of reticulin fiber deposition within the bone marrow; d/c and consider bone marrow biopsy if morphological abnormalities or cytopenias occur. D/C may result in recurrence of thrombocytopenia which may increase risk of bleeding while the patient is on anticoagulants or antiplatelet agents. Excessive doses may increase platelet counts, producing thrombotic/thromboembolic complications; caution with risk factors for thromboembolism (eg, Factor V Leiden, ATIII deficiency, antiphospholipid syndrome, chronic liver disease). May increase the risk for hematological malignancies. Development or worsening of cataracts reported. Caution with hepatic impairment (Child-Pugh Class A, B, C) and in elderly.

ADVERSE REACTIONS: Headache, hyperbilirubinemia, fatigue, N/V, diarrhea, myalgia, cataracts, upper respiratory tract infection, urinary tract infection, pharyngitis, oropharyngeal pain, increased ALT/AST, hepatotoxicity.

INTERACTIONS: Monitor for signs/symptoms of excessive exposure with moderate/strong inhibitors of CYP1A2 (eg, ciprofloxacin, fluvoxamine) or CYP2C8 (eg, gemfibrozil, trimethoprim), moderate/strong inhibitors of breast cancer resistance protein (BCRP), and moderate/strong inhibitors of UGT1A1 or UGT1A3. Polyvalent cations (eg, iron, calcium, aluminum, magnesium, selenium, zinc) may reduce absorption due to chelation; do not take within 4 hrs of any medications or products containing polyvalent cations (eg, antacids, dairy products, and mineral supplements). Monitor closely for signs/symptoms of excessive exposure to substrates of UGTs where enzymes involved in the metabolism of multiple drugs (eg, acetaminophen, narcotics, NSAIDs). Caution with substrates of organic anion transporting polypeptide OATP1B1 and BCRP (eg, benzylpenicillin, atorvastatin, fluvastatin, pravastatin, rosuvastatin, methotrexate, nateglinide, repaglinide, rifampin, doxorubicin); consider dose reduction of these drugs.

PREGNANCY: Category C, not for use in nursing.

MECHANISM OF ACTION: Thrombopoietin (TPO)-receptor agonist; interacts with the transmembrane domain of the human TPO-receptor and initiates signaling cascades that induce proliferation and differentiation of megakaryocytes from bone marrow progenitor cells.

PHARMACOKINETICS: Absorption: T_{max}=2-6 hrs, AUC=108mcg•hr/mL (50mg), 168mcg•hr/mL (75mg). **Distribution:** Plasma protein binding (>99%). **Metabolism:** Cleavage, oxidation (via CYP1A2, CYP2C8), and conjugation with glucuronic acid (via UGT1A1, UGT1A3), glutathione, or cysteine. **Elimination:** Urine (31%), feces (59%, 20% unchanged); $T_{1/2}$=26-35 hrs (ITP).

NURSING CONSIDERATIONS

Assessment: Assess for degree of thrombocytopenia, risk factors for thromboembolism, hepatic function, pregnancy/nursing status, and possible drug interactions. Obtain baseline CBC (eg, platelet counts, peripheral blood smears, peripheral blood differential count), LFTs and eye exam.

Monitoring: Monitor for bone marrow reticulin deposition, worsening thrombocytopenia, thrombotic/thromboembolic complications, cataracts, hematologic malignancies, and other adverse reactions. Monitor LFTs, CBC (weekly during dose adjustment phase and then monthly after establishment of a stable dose), and after d/c for ≥4 weeks.

Patient Counseling: Inform about risks/benefits of therapy and to enroll in Promacta *CARES* program. Counsel that platelet counts and CBCs must be performed weekly until stable dose is achieved, then monthly while on therapy, and for ≥4 weeks after d/c. Inform that thrombocytopenia and risk of bleeding may recur following d/c, particularly when d/c while on anticoagulants/antiplatelet agents. Inform that therapy may be associated with hepatobiliary lab abnormalities; monitor LFTs prior to, during, and after therapy. Advise to avoid situations or medications that may increase risk for bleeding and to report any signs/symptoms of liver problem (eg, yellowing of the skin or the whites of the eyes, unusual darkening of the urine, unusual tiredness, right upper stomach area pain) to healthcare provider. Inform about the risk of reticulin fiber formation within bone marrow and risk for thrombotic/thromboembolic complications with excessive dose. Counsel to take on an empty stomach and to space ≥4 hrs between therapy and foods, mineral supplements, and antacids containing polyvalent cations. Advise pregnant women to enroll in pregnancy registry.

Administration: Oral route. Take on empty stomach (1 hr before or 2 hrs after meal). Do not take >1 dose within 24 hrs. **Storage:** 25°C (77°F); excursions permitted to 15-30°C (59-86°F).

PROMETHAZINE RX
promethazine HCl (Various)

Promethazine HCl should not be used in patients <2 yrs; potential for fatal respiratory depression. Caution when administering to patients ≥2 yrs; use lowest effective dose and avoid concomitant administration of respiratory depressants.

OTHER BRAND NAMES: Phenadoz (Paddock) - Promethegan (G & W Labs)

THERAPEUTIC CLASS: Phenothiazine derivative

INDICATIONS: Allergic and vasomotor rhinitis, allergic conjunctivitis, allergic reactions to blood or plasma, dermographism, mild allergic skin manifestation of urticaria and angioedema. Preoperative, postoperative, or obstetric sedation. Adjunct in anaphylactic reactions. Prevention and control of N/V with certain types of anesthesia and surgery. Active and prophylactic treatment of motion sickness. Sedation, relief of apprehension, production of light sleep. Adjunct with meperidine or other analgesics for postoperative pain. Antiemetic in postoperative patients.

DOSAGE: *Adults:* Allergy: Usual: 25mg qhs or 12.5mg ac and hs; may give 6.25-12.5mg tid. Adjust to lowest effective dose after initiation. Motion Sickness: Initial: 25mg 30-60 min before travel, repeat after 8-12 hrs prn. Maint: 25mg bid, on arising and before pm meal. Prevention/Control of N/V: Prevention: Usual: 25mg, may repeat q4-6h prn. Control: Usual: 25mg, then 12.5-25mg q4-6h prn. Sedation: 25-50mg qhs. Preoperative: 50mg night before surgery, then 50mg preoperatively. Postoperative/Adjunctive with analgesics: 25-50mg.
Pediatrics: ≥2 yrs: Allergy: Usual: 25mg qhs or 12.5mg ac and hs; may give 6.25-12.5mg tid. Adjust to lowest effective dose after initiation. Motion Sickness: 12.5-25mg bid. Prevention/Control of N/V: Prevention: Usual: 25mg, may repeat q4-6h prn. Control: Usual: 25mg or 0.5mg/lb, then 12.5-25mg q4-6h prn. Adjust dose based on patient age/weight and severity of condition. Sedation: 12.5-25mg hs. Preoperative: 12.5-25mg night before surgery, then 0.5mg/lb preoperatively. Postoperative/Adjunctive with analgesics: 12.5-25mg.

HOW SUPPLIED: Sup: (Phenadoz, Promethazine) 12.5mg, 25mg, (Promethegan) 50mg; Syrup: (Promethazine): 6.25mg/5mL [118mL, 237mL, 473mL] Tab: (Promethazine) 12.5mg*, 25mg*, 50mg *scored

CONTRAINDICATIONS: Treatment of lower respiratory tract symptoms including asthma. Comatose states, pediatric patients <2 yrs.

WARNINGS/PRECAUTIONS: Avoid in pediatrics whose signs and symptoms may suggest Reye's syndrome or other hepatic diseases. May impair mental/physical abilities. May lower seizure threshold; caution with seizure disorders. May lead to potentially fatal respiratory depression; avoid with compromised respiratory function (eg, COPD, sleep apnea). Caution with bone marrow depression; leukopenia and agranulocytosis reported. Neuroleptic malignant syndrome (NMS) reported; d/c immediately. Hallucinations and convulsions may occur in pediatrics. Acutely ill pediatrics who are dehydrated may have increased susceptibility to dystonias. Not recommended for uncomplicated vomiting in pediatrics; should be limited to prolonged vomiting of known etiology. Caution with narrow-angle glaucoma, prostatic hypertrophy, stenosing peptic ulcer, bladder-neck or pyloroduodenal obstruction, cardiovascular (CV) disease, hepatic impairment. Cholestatic jaundice reported. Caution in elderly.

ADVERSE REACTIONS: Drowsiness, sedation, blurred vision, dizziness, increased or decreased BP, urticaria, dry mouth, N/V, respiratory depression, hallucination, leukopenia, apnea, NMS.

INTERACTIONS: See Boxed Warning. May increase rates of extrapyramidal effects with concomitant MAOI use. May increase, prolong, or intensify the sedative action of other CNS depressants, such as alcohol, sedatives/hypnotics (including barbiturates), narcotics, narcotic analgesics, general anesthetics, TCAs, tranquilizers; avoid such agents or reduce dosages. Reduce barbiturate dose by at least one-half and narcotic analgesics by one-quarter to one-half. May reverse vasopressor effect of epinephrine. Caution with medications that may affect seizure threshold (eg, narcotics, local anesthetics). Caution with anticholinergics. Leukopenia and agranulocytosis reported, usually with marrow-toxic agents. NMS reported in combination with antipsychotics.

PREGNANCY: Category C, not for use in nursing.

MECHANISM OF ACTION: Phenothiazine derivative; H, receptor-blocking agent (antihistaminic action) and provides sedative and antiemetic effects.

PHARMACOKINETICS: Absorption: Well absorbed from GI tract. **Metabolism:** Liver; sulfoxides, N-demethylpromethazine (metabolites). **Elimination:** Urine.

NURSING CONSIDERATIONS

Assessment: Assess for drug hypersensitive or idiosyncratic reaction, or any other conditions where treatment is contraindicated or cautioned. Assess for pregnancy/nursing status and for possible drug interaction. Assess for signs/symptoms of Reye's syndrome, hepatic diseases, or encephalopathy in pediatrics.

Monitoring: Monitor for signs/symptoms of CNS/respiratory depression, NMS, seizures, cholestatic jaundice, leukopenia, agranulocytosis. Monitor for hallucinations, convulsions, extrapyramidal symptoms, respiratory depression, dystonias in pediatrics. Monitor for false positive and false negative pregnancy tests, blood glucose levels, and BP. Monitor platelet count in newborns when used in pregnant women within 2 weeks of delivery.

Patient Counseling: Inform that drowsiness or impairment of mental and/or physical abilities may occur. Counsel to report involuntary muscle movements. Instruct to avoid alcohol use, prolonged sun exposure, and concomitant use of other CNS depressants.

Administration: Oral and rectal route. **Storage:** (Tab) 20-25°C (68-77°F). Protect from light. (Sup) 2-8°C (36-46°F).

PROMETHAZINE DM   RX
dextromethorphan hbr - promethazine HCl (Various)

> Promethazine HCl should not be used in patients <2 yrs; potential for fatal respiratory depression. Caution when administering to patients ≥2 yrs; use lowest effective dose and avoid concomitant administration of respiratory depressants.

THERAPEUTIC CLASS: Phenothiazine derivative/antitussive

INDICATIONS: Temporary relief of coughs and upper respiratory symptoms associated with allergy or the common cold.

DOSAGE: *Adults:* 5mL q4-6h. Max: 30mL/24 hr. Elderly: Start at lower end of dosing range.
Pediatrics: ≥12 yrs: 5mL q4-6h. Max: 30mL/24hr. 6-<12 yrs: 2.5-5mL q4-6h. Max: 20mL/24hr. 2-<6 yrs: 1.25-2.5mL q4-6h. Max: 10mL/24hr.

HOW SUPPLIED: Syrup: (Dextromethorphan-Promethazine) 15mg-6.25mg/5mL

CONTRAINDICATIONS: Concomitant MAOIs, comatose states, treatment of lower respiratory tract symptoms (eg, asthma).

WARNINGS/PRECAUTIONS: Should be given to a pregnant woman only if clearly needed. Avoid prolonged exposure to sunlight. Promethazine: Caution in pediatrics ≥2 yrs. Respiratory depression and apnea, sometimes associated with death, are strongly associated with promethazine products and are not directly related to individualized weight-based dosing. Avoid in pediatric patients whose signs and symptoms may suggest Reye's syndrome or hepatic diseases. May impair mental/physical abilities. May lower seizure threshold; caution with seizure disorders. May lead to potentially fatal respiratory depression; avoid with compromised respiratory function (eg, chronic obstructive pulmonary disease [COPD], sleep apnea). Caution with bone marrow depression; leukopenia and agranulocytosis reported. Neuroleptic malignant syndrome (NMS) reported; d/c immediately. Hallucinations and convulsions may occur in pediatrics with therapeutic doses or overdoses. Acutely ill dehydrated pediatric patients may have increased susceptibility to dystonias. Caution with narrow-angle glaucoma, prostatic hypertrophy, stenosing peptic ulcer, bladder neck or pyloroduodenal obstruction, cardiovascular (CV) disease, hepatic impairment. Cholestatic jaundice reported. May increase blood glucose. Dextromethorphan: Caution in atopic children, sedated, or debilitated patients, and patients confined to supine position.

ADVERSE REACTIONS: Drowsiness, dizziness, sedation, blurred vision, dry mouth, increased or decreased BP, rash, N/V, respiratory depression, apnea, leukopenia, agranulocytosis, NMS.

INTERACTIONS: See Boxed Warning and Contraindications. Promethazine: May increase, prolong, or intensify the sedative action of other CNS depressants, such as alcohol, sedatives/hypnotics (including barbiturates), narcotics, narcotic analgesics, general anesthetics, TCAs, and tranquilizers; avoid such agents or administer in reduced dosages. Reduce barbiturate dose by at least one-half and narcotic analgesics by one-quarter to one-half. May reverse vasopressor effect of epinephrine. Caution with concomitant medications that may also affect seizure threshold (eg, narcotics, local anesthetics). Caution with concomitant use of other agents with anticholinergic properties. Leukopenia and agranulocytosis reported, usually when used in association with other marrow-toxic agents. NMS reported alone or in combination with antipsychotic drugs. Dextromethorphan: Hyperpyrexia, hypotension, and death have been reported coincident with the coadministration of MAOIs and products containing dextromethorphan.

PREGNANCY: Category C, caution in nursing.

MECHANISM OF ACTION: Dextromethorphan: Antitussive agent; acts centrally and elevates the threshold for coughing. Promethazine: Phenothiazine derivative; blocks H_1 receptor (antihistaminic action) and provides clinically useful sedative and antiemetic effects.

PHARMACOKINETICS: Absorption: Dextromethorphan: Rapid. Promethazine: Well-absorbed. **Metabolism:** Dextromethorphan: Liver via O-demethylation, N-demethylation, and partial conjugation with glucuronic acid and sulfate. Promethazine: Liver, sulfoxides and N-demethylpromethazine (metabolites). **Elimination:** Dextromethorphan: Urine [(+)-3-hydroxy-N-methylmorphinan, (+)-3-hydroxymorphinan, traces of unmetabolized drug]. Promethazine: Urine (sulfoxides and N-demethylpromethazine).

NURSING CONSIDERATIONS

Assessment: Assess for drug hypersensitivity or idiosyncrasy, or any other conditions where treatment is contraindicated or cautioned. Assess for pregnancy/nursing status and possible drug interactions. Assess use in atopic children, elderly, debilitated, and for signs/symptoms of Reye's syndrome, hepatic diseases, or encephalopathy in pediatrics.

Monitoring: Monitor for signs/symptoms of CNS/respiratory depression, NMS, seizures, cholestatic jaundice, leukopenia, agranulocytosis. Monitor children for hallucinations, convulsions, extrapyramidal symptoms, and dystonias.

Monitor for false positive and false negative pregnancy tests, blood glucose levels, and BP.

Patient Counseling: Inform that therapy may cause marked drowsiness or may impair mental and/or physical abilities required for performing hazardous tasks (eg, operating machinery, driving). Instruct to report involuntary muscle movements. Counsel to avoid the use of alcohol and other CNS depressants while on therapy. Instruct to avoid prolonged exposure to the sun.

Administration: Oral route. **Storage:** 20-25°C (68-77°F). Protect from light. Keep bottle tightly closed. Dispense in a tight, light-resistant container with a child-resistant closure.

PROMETHAZINE VC RX
phenylephrine HCl - promethazine HCl (Various)

> Promethazine HCl should not be used in patients <2 yrs; potential for fatal respiratory depression. Caution when administering to patients ≥2 yrs; use lowest effective dose and avoid concomitant administration of respiratory depressants.

THERAPEUTIC CLASS: Phenothiazine derivative/sympathomimetic

INDICATIONS: Temporary relief of upper respiratory symptoms including nasal congestion associated with allergy or the common cold.

DOSAGE: *Adults:* 5mL q4-6h. Max: 30mL/24 hr. Elderly: Start at low end of dosing range.
Pediatrics: ≥12 yrs: 5mL q4-6h. Max: 30mL/24 hr. 6-<12 yrs: 2.5-5mL q4-6h. Max: 30mL/24 hr. 2-<6 yrs: 1.25-2.5mL q4-6h.

HOW SUPPLIED: Syrup: (Promethazine-Phenylephrine) 6.25mg-5mg/5mL

CONTRAINDICATIONS: Concomitant use with MAOIs, comatose states, treatment of lower respiratory tract symptoms (eg, asthma), HTN, peripheral vascular insufficiency, pediatric patients <2 yrs.

WARNINGS/PRECAUTIONS: Should only be given to a pregnant woman if clearly needed. Caution with narrow-angle glaucoma, prostatic hypertrophy, stenosing peptic ulcer, and bladder neck or pyloroduodenal obstruction. Avoid prolonged exposure to sunlight. Promethazine: Caution with cardiovascular disease (CVD) or impaired liver function. Caution in pediatrics ≥2 yrs. Avoid in pediatric patients whose signs and symptoms may suggest Reye's syndrome or other hepatic diseases. May lead to potentially fatal respiratory depression; avoid with compromised respiratory function (eg, chronic obstructive pulmonary disease [COPD], sleep apnea). May impair mental/physical abilities. May lower seizure threshold; caution with seizure disorders. Hallucinations and convulsions may occur in pediatrics with therapeutic doses or overdoses. Acutely ill pediatric patients who are dehydrated may have increased susceptibility to dystonias. Caution with bone marrow depression; leukopenia and agranulocytosis reported. Neuroleptic malignant syndrome (NMS) reported; d/c immediately. Cholestatic jaundice reported. May increase blood glucose. Phenylephrine: Caution with HTN, DM, thyroid and heart diseases. Urinary retention may occur with symptomatic benign prostatic hypertrophy (BPH). May decrease cardiac output; use extreme caution with arteriosclerosis, elderly, and patients with poor cerebral or coronary circulation.

ADVERSE REACTIONS: Drowsiness, dizziness, anxiety, sedation, tremor, blurred vision, dry mouth, increased or decreased BP, N/V, respiratory depression, urinary retention, NMS, weakness, arrhythmia, convulsions.

INTERACTIONS: See Boxed Warning and Contraindications. Phenylephrine: Cardiac pressor response potentiated and possible acute hypertensive crisis with prior administration of MAOIs. Pressor response increased with TCAs and decreased with prior administration of phentolamine or other α-adrenergic blockers. Excessive rise in BP with ergot alkaloids. Tachycardia or other arrhythmias may occur with epinephrine or other sympathomimetics. Reflex bradycardia blocked and pressor response enhanced with atropine sulfate. Cardiostimulating effects blocked with prior administration of propranolol or other β-adrenergic blockers. Synergistic adrenergic response with diet preparations (eg, amphetamines, phenylpropanolamine). Promethazine: Caution with concomitant medications which may affect seizure threshold (eg, narcotics, local anesthetics). May increase, prolong, or intensify the sedative action of other CNS depressants such as alcohol, sedatives/hypnotics (including barbiturates), narcotics, narcotic analgesics, general anesthetics, TCAs, and tranquilizers; avoid such agents or administer in reduced dosages. Reduce barbiturate dose by at least one-half and narcotic analgesics by one-quarter to one-half. Leukopenia and agranulocytosis reported, usually when used in association with other marrow-toxic agents. Caution with concomitant use of other agents with anticholinergic properties. May reverse vasopressor effect of epinephrine. NMS reported alone or in combination with antipsychotic drugs.

PREGNANCY: Category C, caution in nursing.

MECHANISM OF ACTION: Promethazine: Phenothiazine derivative; blocks H_1-receptor (antihistaminic action) and provides sedative and antiemetic effects. Phenylephrine: Sympathomimetic amine; potent postsynaptic α-receptor agonist with little effect on β-receptors of heart; increases resistance and decreases capacitance of blood vessels; has mild central stimulant effect.

PHARMACOKINETICS: Absorption: Promethazine: Well absorbed (GI tract). Phenylephrine: Irregularly absorbed. **Metabolism:** Promethazine: Liver, sulfoxides and N-demethylpromethazine (metabolites). Phenylephrine: Liver and intestine via monoamine oxidase. **Elimination:** Promethazine: Urine (sulfoxides and N-demethylpromethazine).

NURSING CONSIDERATIONS

Assessment: Assess for drug hypersensitivity or idiosyncrasy, or any other conditions where treatment is contraindicated or cautioned. Assess BP, pregnancy/nursing status, and for possible drug interactions. Assess for Reye's syndrome, hepatic diseases, or encephalopathy in pediatric patients. Assess age of patient.

Monitoring: Monitor for signs/symptoms of CNS and respiratory depression, seizures, leukopenia, agranulocytosis, NMS, and for cholestatic jaundice. Monitor for urinary retention in men with BPH. Monitor pediatric patients for hallucinations, convulsions, and dystonias. Monitor for false positive and false negative pregnancy tests. Monitor blood glucose levels.

Patient Counseling: Inform that therapy may cause marked drowsiness or may impair mental and/or physical abilities required for performing hazardous tasks (eg, driving, operating machinery). Counsel to avoid alcohol and other CNS depressants while on therapy. Advise to report any involuntary muscle movements. Instruct to avoid prolonged exposure to the sun.

Administration: Oral route. **Storage:** 20-25°C (68-77°F). Keep tighly closed. Protect from light. Dispense in a tight, light-resistant container with a child-resistant closure.

PROMETHAZINE VC/CODEINE `CV`
phenylephrine HCl - promethazine HCl - codeine phosphate (Various)

> Combination of promethazine HCl, phenylephrine HCl and codeine phosphate is contraindicated in patients <6 yrs. Concomitant administration of promethazine products with other respiratory depressants is associated with respiratory depression, and sometimes death, in pediatrics. Respiratory depression, including fatalities, have been reported with use of promethazine HCl in patients <2 yrs; wide range of weight-based doses have resulted in respiratory depression.

THERAPEUTIC CLASS: Phenothiazine derivative/antitussive/sympathomimetic

INDICATIONS: Temporary relief of cough and upper respiratory symptoms (eg, nasal congestion) associated with allergy or the common cold.

DOSAGE: *Adults:* 5mL q4-6h. Max: 30mL/24hr. Elderly: Start at lower end of dosing range.
Pediatrics: ≥12 yrs: 5mL q4-6h. Max: 30mL/24hr. 6-<12 yrs: 2.5-5mL q4-6h. Max: 30mL/24hr.

HOW SUPPLIED: Syrup/Sol: (Promethazine-Codeine-Phenylephrine) 6.25mg-10mg-5mg/5mL

CONTRAINDICATIONS: Concomitant MAOIs, comatose states, treatment of lower respiratory tract symptoms (eg, asthma), HTN, peripheral vascular insufficiency, pediatric patients <6 yrs.

WARNINGS/PRECAUTIONS: Should only be given to a pregnant woman if clearly needed. Codeine: Do not increase dose if cough is unresponsive to treatment. Caution in atopic children. Capacity to elevate CSF pressure and respiratory depressant effects may be markedly exaggerated in head injury, intracranial lesions, or with pre-existing increased intracranial pressure (ICP). May obscure clinical course in patients with head injuries. Avoid with asthma, acute febrile illness with productive cough, or with chronic respiratory disease where interference with ability to clear tracheobronchial tree of secretions is critical. May produce orthostatic hypotension in ambulatory patients. May cause/aggravate constipation. Administer cautiously and with reduced initial dose in acute abdominal conditions, convulsive disorders, significant hepatic/renal impairment, fever, hypothyroidism, Addison's disease, ulcerative colitis, prostatic hypertrophy, recent GI or urinary tract surgery, and in the very young, elderly, and debilitated. Caution with narrow-angle glaucoma, stenosing peptic ulcer, pyloroduodenal or bladder-neck obstruction, cardiovascular disease (CVD), thyroid disease, diabetes mellitus (DM), heart disease and ultra-rapid metabolizers. Use lowest effective dose for the shortest period of time. Promethazine: May lead to potentially fatal respiratory depression; avoid with compromised respiratory function (eg, COPD, sleep apnea). May impair mental/physical abilities. May lower seizure threshold; caution with seizure disorders. Caution with bone marrow depression; leukopenia and agranulocytosis reported. Neuroleptic malignant syndrome (NMS) reported; d/c immediately. Excessively large doses in pediatric patients may cause sudden death. Hallucinations and convulsions have occurred in pediatrics. Cholestatic jaundice reported. May increase blood glucose. Caution with CVD or with impaired liver function. Phenylephrine: Urinary retention may occur with BPH. May decrease cardiac output; use extreme caution with arteriosclerosis, elderly, and patients with initially poor cerebral or coronary circulation.

ADVERSE REACTIONS: Drowsiness, dizziness, sedation, tremor, anxiety, blurred vision, dry mouth, increased or decreased BP, N/V, constipation, urinary retention, respiratory depression, NMS.

INTERACTIONS: See Boxed Warning and Contraindications. Promethazine: Caution with concomitant medications that may also affect seizure threshold (eg, narcotics, local anesthetics). May increase, prolong, or intensify the sedative action of other CNS depressants such as alcohol, sedatives/hypnotics (including barbiturates), narcotics, narcotic analgesics, general anesthetics, TCAs, and tranquilizers; avoid such agents or administer in reduced doses. Reduce barbiturate dose by at least one-half and narcotic analgesics by one-quarter to one-half. Leukopenia and agranulocytosis reported, usually when used in association with other marrow-toxic agents. Caution with concomitant use of other agents with anticholinergic properties. May reverse vasopressor effect of epinephrine. NMS reported alone or in combination with antipsychotic drugs. Phenylephrine: Pressor response increased with TCAs and decreased with phentolamine or other α-adrenergic blockers. Excessive rise in BP with ergot alkaloids. Tachycardia or other arrhythmias may occur with epinephrine or other sympathomimetics. Cardiostimulating effects blocked with propranolol or other β-adrenergic blockers. Reflex bradycardia blocked and pressor response enhanced with atropine. Synergistic adrenergic response with diet preparations (eg, amphetamines, phenylpropanolamine).

PREGNANCY: Category C, caution in nursing.

MECHANISM OF ACTION: Codeine: Narcotic analgesic/antitussive; primary effects are on CNS and GI tract. Promethazine: Phenothiazine derivative; blocks H_1 receptor (antihistaminic action) and provides sedative and antiemetic effects. Phenylephrine: Sympathomimetic amine; potent postsynaptic-α-receptor agonist with little effect on β-receptors of heart; increases resistance and decreases capacitance of blood vessels.

PHARMACOKINETICS: Absorption: Codeine: Well-absorbed. Promethazine: Well-absorbed (GI tract). Phenylephrine: Irregularly absorbed. **Distribution:**

Codeine: Crosses placental barrier, found in breast milk. **Metabolism:** Promethazine: Liver, sulfoxides and N-demethylpromethazine (metabolites). Phenylephrine: Liver and intestine via monoamine oxidase. Codeine: Liver via O-demethylation, N-demethylation, and partial conjugation with glucuronic acid. **Elimination:** Promethazine: Urine (sulfoxides and N-demethylpromethazine). Codeine: Urine (inactive metabolites and free/conjugated morphine), feces (parent compound and metabolites).

NURSING CONSIDERATIONS

Assessment: Assess for drug hypersensitivity or idiosyncracy, history of drug abuse/dependence, or any other conditions where treatment is contraindicated or cautioned. Assess BP, pregnancy/nursing status, and for possible drug interactions. Assess use in very young, elderly, debilitated, and in men with BPH.

Monitoring: Monitor for signs/symptoms of CNS/respiratory depression, constipation, leukopenia, agranulocytosis, cholestatic jaundice, seizures, NMS, and for orthostatic hypotension. Monitor for convulsions, hallucinations and dystonias in children. Monitor CBC and glucose levels. Monitor for overuse and vital signs including respiration, pulse, BP, temperature, and ECG in the case of overdosage. Re-evaluate 5 days or sooner if cough is unresponsive to treatment.

Patient Counseling: Advise not to increase dosage if cough fails to respond. Measure medication with an accurate measuring device; a household teaspoon is not an accurate measuring device. Inform that therapy may cause drowsiness and may impair mental and/or physical abilities required for performing potentially hazardous tasks (eg, driving, operating machinery). Inform about risks and the signs of morphine overdose (extreme sleepiness, confusion, shallow breathing). Advise to report any involuntary muscle movements. Avoid prolonged exposure to the sun. Counsel to avoid the use of alcohol and other CNS depressants while on therapy. Inform that therapy may produce orthostatic hypotension. Advise to notify physician if pregnant. Instruct nursing mothers to watch for signs of morphine toxicity in their infants (eg, increased sleepiness more than usual, difficulty breastfeeding, breathing difficulties, or limpness; notify pediatrician immediately if these signs are noticed or get emergency medical attention.

Administration: Oral route. **Storage:** 20-25°C (68-77°F). Dispense in a tight, light-resistant container with child-resistant closure.

PROMETHAZINE W/CODEINE `CV`
promethazine HCl - codeine phosphate (Various)

> **Combination of promethazine HCl and codeine phosphate is contraindicated in patients <6 yrs. Concomitant administration of promethazine products with other respiratory depressants is associated with respiratory depression, and sometimes death, in pediatrics. Respiratory depression, including fatalities, have been reported with use of promethazine HCl in patients <2 yrs; wide range of weight-based doses have resulted in respiratory depression.**

OTHER BRAND NAMES: Prometh w/ Codeine (Actavis)

THERAPEUTIC CLASS: Phenothiazine derivative/antitussive

INDICATIONS: Temporary relief of cough and upper respiratory symptoms associated with allergy or the common cold.

DOSAGE: *Adults:* 5mL q4-6h. Max: 30mL/24hr. Elderly: Start at lower end of dosing range.
Pediatrics: ≥12 yrs: 5mL q4-6h. Max: 30mL/24hr. 6-<12 yrs: 2.5-5mL q4-6h. Max: 30mL/24hr.

HOW SUPPLIED: Syrup: (Codeine-Promethazine) 10mg-6.25mg/5mL

CONTRAINDICATIONS: Comatose states, treatment of lower respiratory tract symptoms (eg, asthma), pediatric patients <6 yrs.

WARNINGS/PRECAUTIONS: Should only be given to a pregnant woman if clearly needed. Codeine: Do not increase dose if cough is unresponsive to treatment. Caution in atopic children. Capacity to elevate CSF pressure and respiratory depressant effects may be markedly exaggerated in head injury, intracranial lesions, or with pre-existing increased intracranial pressure (ICP). May obscure clinical course in patients with head injuries. May produce orthostatic hypotension in ambulatory patients. May cause/aggravate constipation. Administer cautiously and with reduced initial dose in acute abdominal conditions, convulsive disorders, significant hepatic/renal impairment, fever, hypothyroidism, Addison's disease, ulcerative colitis, prostatic hypertrophy, recent GI or urinary tract surgery, and in the very young, elderly, or debilitated. Caution with narrow-angle glaucoma, stenosing peptic ulcer, pyloroduodenal or bladder-neck obstruction, cardiovascular disease (CVD), and ultra-rapid metabolizers. Avoid in asthmatic patients, acute febrile illness associated with productive cough or in chronic respiratory disease where interference with ability to clear the tracheobronchial tree of secretions is critical. May increase biliary tract pressure with resultant increase in plasma lipase/amylase levels. Use lowest effective dose for the shortest period of time. Promethazine: May lead to potentially fatal respiratory depression; avoid with compromised respiratory function (eg, COPD, sleep apnea). May impair mental/physical abilities. May lower seizure threshold; caution with seizure disorders. Caution with bone marrow depression; leukopenia and agranulocytosis reported. Neuroleptic malignant syndrome (NMS) reported; d/c immediately. Excessively large doses in pediatric patients may cause sudden death. Hallucinations and convulsions have occurred in pediatrics with therapeutic doses and overdoses. Increased susceptibility to dystonias in pediatric patients who are acutely ill and who are dehydrated. Cholestatic jaundice reported. May increase blood glucose. Caution with CVD or with impaired liver function.

ADVERSE REACTIONS: Drowsiness, dizziness, sedation, blurred vision, dry mouth, increased or decreased BP, N/V, constipation, urinary retention, photosensitivity, leukopenia, agranulocytosis, respiratory depression, NMS.

INTERACTIONS: See Boxed Warning. Possible interaction with MAOIs (eg, increased incidence of extrapyramidal effects); consider initial small test dose. Promethazine: Caution with concomitant medications that affect seizure threshold (eg, narcotics, local anesthetics). May increase, prolong, or intensify the sedative action of other CNS depressants such as alcohol, sedative/hypnotics (including barbiturates), general anesthetics, TCAs, and tranquilizers; avoid such agents or administer in reduced doses. Leukopenia and agranulocytosis reported, usually when used in association with other marrow-toxic agents. Reduce barbiturate dose by at least one-half and narcotic analgesics by one-quarter to one-half. May reverse vasopressor effect of epinephrine. Caution with concomitant use of other agents with anticholinergic properties. NMS reported alone or in combination with antipsychotic drugs.

PREGNANCY: Category C, caution in nursing.

MECHANISM OF ACTION: Codeine: Narcotic analgesic and antitussive; primary effects are on CNS and GI tract. Promethazine: Phenothiazine derivative; blocks H_1 receptor (antihistaminic action) and provides sedative and antiemetic effects.

PHARMACOKINETICS: Absorption: Well-absorbed. **Distribution:** Codeine: Crosses placental barrier, found in breast milk. **Metabolism:** Promethazine: Liver, sulfoxides and N-demethylpromethazine (metabolites). Codeine: Liver via O-demethylation, N-demethylation, and partial conjugation with glucuronic acid. **Elimination:** Promethazine: Urine (sulfoxides and N-demethylpromethazine). Codeine: Urine (inactive metabolites and free/conjugated morphine), feces (parent compound and metabolites).

NURSING CONSIDERATIONS

Assessment: Assess for history of drug abuse/dependence or any other conditions where treatment is contraindicated or cautioned. Assess for hypersensitivity, pregnancy/nursing status, and for possible drug interactions. Assess use in very young, elderly, atopic children and debilitated patients.

Monitoring: Monitor for signs/symptoms of CNS/respiratory depression, constipation, cholestatic jaundice, seizures, leukopenia, agranulocytosis, NMS, and orthostatic hypotension. Monitor glucose levels. Re-evaluate 5 days or sooner if cough is unresponsive to treatment. Monitor for overuse and vital signs including respiration, pulse, BP, temperature, and EKG in the case of overdosage.

Patient Counseling: Advise not to increase dosage if cough fails to respond. Measure medication with an accurate measuring device; a household teaspoon is not an accurate measuring device. Inform that therapy may cause drowsiness and may impair mental and/or physical abilities required for performing potentially hazardous tasks (eg, driving, operating machinery). Inform about risks and the signs of morphine overdose (extreme sleepiness, confusion, shallow breathing). Advise to report any involuntary muscle movements. Avoid prolonged exposure to the sun. Counsel to avoid the use of alcohol and other CNS depressants while on therapy. Inform that therapy may produce orthostatic hypotension. Advise to notify physician if pregnant. Instruct nursing mothers to watch for signs of morphine toxicity in their infants (eg, increased sleepiness more than usual, difficulty breastfeeding, breathing difficulties, or limpness); notify pediatrician immediately if these signs are noticed or get emergency medical attention.

Administration: Oral route. **Storage:** 20-25°C (68-77°F). Dispense in a tight, light-resistant container.

PROPECIA   RX
finasteride (Merck)

THERAPEUTIC CLASS: Type II 5 alpha-reductase inhibitor

INDICATIONS: Treatment of male pattern hair loss (androgenetic alopecia) in men only.

DOSAGE: *Adults:* Usual: 1mg qd for ≥3 months. Continued use is recommended to sustain benefit; re-evaluate periodically. Withdrawal of treatment may lead to reversal of effect within 12 months.

HOW SUPPLIED: Tab: 1mg

CONTRAINDICATIONS: Pregnancy.

WARNINGS/PRECAUTIONS: Not for use in pediatrics or women. Efficacy not established in bitemporal recession. Caution with liver function abnormalities. Pregnant women or women who may potentially be pregnant should not handle crushed or broken tabs because of potential risk to a male fetus.

ADVERSE REACTIONS: Decreased libido, erectile dysfunction, decreased volume of ejaculate, ejaculation disorder.

PREGNANCY: Category X, not for use in nursing.

MECHANISM OF ACTION: Type II 5α-reductase inhibitor; blocks peripheral conversion of testosterone to 5α-dihydrotestosterone (DHT), resulting in significant decreases in serum and tissue DHT concentrations.

PHARMACOKINETICS: Absorption: Mean bioavailability (65%); C_{max}=9.2ng/mL; T_{max}=1-2 hrs; $AUC_{(0-24\ hr)}$=53ng•hr/mL. **Distribution:** V_d=76L; plasma protein binding (90%); crosses blood brain barrier. **Metabolism:** Liver (extensive); via CYP3A4. **Elimination:** (Oral) Urine (39% metabolites), feces (57%); $T_{1/2}$=4.5 hrs (IV), 5-6 hrs (18-60 yrs), 8 hrs (>70 yrs).

NURSING CONSIDERATIONS

Assessment: Assess for liver dysfunction and hypersensitivity to drug and its components.

Monitoring: Monitor for signs/symptoms of breast changes (eg, lumps, pain, nipple discharge, breast enlargement, tenderness, neoplasm). Monitor prostate-specific antigen levels.

Patient Counseling: Instruct pregnant or potentially pregnant females not to handle broken or crushed tabs due to potential risk to male fetus. Advise to notify physician if changes in breast (eg, lumps, pain, nipple discharge) occur. Inform of possible adverse reactions (eg, decreased volume of ejaculate, impotence, decreased libido).

Administration: Oral route. **Storage:** 15-30°C (59-86°F).

PROPRANOLOL   RX
propranolol HCl (Various)

THERAPEUTIC CLASS: Nonselective beta-blocker

INDICATIONS: (Tab) Management of HTN, angina pectoris, hypertrophic sub-aortic stenosis, atrial fibrillation (A-fib), reduction of cardiovascular mortality post-myocardial infarction (MI), and familial or hereditary essential tremor. Adjunct to control BP and reduce symptoms of pheochromocytoma. Common migraine headache prophylaxis. (Inj) For cardiac arrhythmias (supraventricular/ventricular tachycardia, tachyarrhythmia of digitalis intoxication, resistant tachyarrhythmia due to excessive catecholamine action during anesthesia).

DOSAGE: *Adults:* (Tab) Individualize dose. HTN: Initial: 40mg bid. Titrate: Increase gradually until adequate BP control. Maint: 120-240mg/day. Angina: 80-320mg/day bid-qid. To d/c, reduce gradually over several weeks. A-Fib: 10-30mg tid-qid before meals and hs. MI: Initial: 40mg tid. Titrate: 60-80mg tid after 1 month as tolerated. Usual: 180-240mg/day in divided doses. Max: 240mg/day. Migraine: Initial: 80mg/day in divided doses. Usual: 160-240mg/day. May increase gradually for optimum prophylaxis. D/C if unsatisfactory within 4-6 weeks after max dose; withdraw gradually over several weeks. Tremor: Initial: 40mg bid. Usual/Maint: 120mg/day. Hypertrophic Subaortic Stenosis: Usual: 20-40mg tid-qid, before meals and hs. Pheochromocytoma: Usual: 60mg/day in divided doses for 3 days before surgery with α-adrenergic blocker. Inoperable Tumor: Usual: 30mg/day in divided doses with α-adrenergic blocker. (Inj) Arrhythmia: Usual: 1-3mg IV at ≤1mg/min. May give 2nd dose if necessary after 2 min then avoid additional drugs <4 hrs. Hepatic Impairment: Consider lower dose. (Inj/Tab) Elderly: Start at lower end of dosing range.

HOW SUPPLIED: Inj: 1mg/mL; Tab: 10mg*, 20mg*, 40mg*, 60mg*, 80mg* *scored

CONTRAINDICATIONS: Cardiogenic shock, sinus bradycardia and >1st-degree block, bronchial asthma.

WARNINGS/PRECAUTIONS: Exacerbation of angina and MI following abrupt d/c reported. Caution with well-compensated cardiac failure, bronchospastic lung disease, Wolff-Parkinson-White (WPW) syndrome, tachycardia, and hepatic/renal impairment. Withdrawal before surgery is controversial. May mask acute hypoglycemia or hyperthyroidism signs/symptoms. Avoid abrupt d/c. May reduce intraocular pressure (IOP). May be more reactive to repeated challenge with history of severe anaphylactic reaction to variety of allergens; may be unresponsive to usual doses of epinephrine. Elevated serum K⁺, transaminases and alkaline phosphatase observed. Elevated BUN reported in severe heart failure. Not for treatment of hypertensive emergencies. Caution in elderly. (Inj) Risk of anaphylactic reaction. (Tab) Hypersensitivity reactions and cutaneous reactions (eg, Stevens-Johnson syndrome [SJS]) reported. Continued use in patients without history of heart failure may cause cardiac failure.

ADVERSE REACTIONS: Bradycardia, CHF, hypotension, lightheadedness, mental depression, N/V, agranulocytosis.

INTERACTIONS: Administration with CYP450 (2D6, 1A2, 2C19) substrates, inducers, and inhibitors may lead to clinically relevant drug interactions. Increased levels with CYP2D6 substrates/inhibitors (eg, amiodarone, cimetidine, delavirdine, fluoxetine, paroxetine, quinidine, ritonavir), CYP1A2 substrates/inhibitors (eg, imipramine, cimetidine, ciprofloxacin, fluvoxamine, isoniazid, ritonavir, theophylline, zileuton, zolmitriptan, rizatriptan), and CYP2C19 substrates/inhibitors (eg, fluconazole, cimetidine, fluoxetine, fluvoxamine, teniposide, tolbutamide). Decreased blood levels with hepatic enzyme inducers (eg, rifampin, ethanol, phenytoin, phenobarbital, cigarette smoking). Increased levels of propafenone, lidocaine, zolmitriptan, rizatriptan, diazepam and its metabolites. Increased levels with nisoldipine, nicardipine, chlorpromazine. Decreased theophylline clearance. Increased thioridazine plasma and metabolite concentrations with doses ≥160mg/day. Decreased levels with aluminum hydroxide gel, cholestyramine, colestipol, lovastatin, pravastatin.

P

Decreased levels of lovastatin, pravastatin. Increased warfarin levels and PT. Caution with drugs that slow AV nodal conduction (eg, digitalis, lidocaine, calcium channel blocker). Bradycardia, hypotension, high degree heart block, and heart failure reported with diltiazem. May cause hypotension with ACE inhibitors. May antagonize effects of clonidine. May prolong 1st dose hypotension with prazosin. Postural hypotension reported with terazosin or doxazosin. May reduce resting sympathetic nervous activity with catecholamine-depleting drugs (eg, reserpine). May experience uncontrolled HTN with epinephrine. Effects can be reversed by β-agonists (eg, dobutamine or isoproterenol). May reduce efficacy with indomethacin and NSAIDs. May depress myocardial contractility with methoxyflurane and trichloroethylene. Hypotension and cardiac arrest reported with haloperidol. May lower T_3 concentration with thyroxine. May exacerbate hypotensive effects of MAOIs or TCAs. May augment the risks of general anesthesia. May need to adjust dose of insulin. (Inj) Severe bradycardia, asystole, and heart failure reported with disopyramide. (Tab) Increased levels with alcohol.

PREGNANCY: Category C, caution in nursing.

MECHANISM OF ACTION: Nonselective β-adrenergic receptor blocker; not established. (Tab) Proposed to decrease cardiac output, inhibit renin release and lessen tonic sympathetic nerve outflow from vasomotor centers in the brain. (Inj) Decreases normal and ectopic pacemaker cells and AV nodal conduction velocity.

PHARMACOKINETICS: Absorption: (Tab) Almost complete; T_{max}=1-4 hrs. **Distribution:** V_d=4-5L/kg; plasma protein binding (90%). (Tab) Crosses placenta; (Inj/Tab) found in breast milk. **Metabolism:** CYP2D6 (hydroxylation), CYP1A2, 2D6 (oxidation), N-dealkylation, glucuronidation. Propranolol glucuronide, naphthyloxylactic acid, glucuronic acid, sulfate conjugates (major metabolites). **Elimination:** $T_{1/2}$=3-6 hrs (PO), 2-5.5 hrs (Inj).

NURSING CONSIDERATIONS

Assessment: Assess for bronchial asthma, sinus bradycardia, AV heart block, cardiogenic shock, CHF, bronchospastic disease, hyperthyroidism, diabetes mellitus, WPW syndrome, history of heart failure, hepatic/renal function, hypersensitivity to drug, pregnancy/nursing status, and possible drug interactions.

Monitoring: Monitor for signs/symptoms of cardiac failure, hypoglycemia, decreased IOP, thyrotoxicosis, withdrawal symptoms, hypersensitivity reactions, and other adverse reactions. (Inj) Monitor ECG and central venous pressure during anesthesia. (Tab) For HTN, measure BP near end of dosing interval to determine satisfactory BP control.

Patient Counseling: Instruct not to interrupt or d/c therapy without consulting physician. Advise to contact physician if symptoms of heart failure, withdrawal, or hypersensitivity reactions occur. May interfere with glaucoma screening test.

Administration: Oral and IV route. (Inj) Inspect visually for particulate matter/discoloration. **Storage:** 20-25°C (68-77°F). (Inj) Protect from freezing/excessive heat. (Tab) Dispense in tight, light-resistant container.

PROPYLTHIOURACIL   RX
propylthiouracil (Various)

> Severe liver injury and acute liver failure, in some cases fatal, reported; hepatic reactions include cases requiring liver transplantation in adults and pediatrics. Should be reserved for those who can not tolerate methimazole and in whom radioactive iodine therapy or surgery are not appropriate for the management of hyperthyroidism. May be treament of choice during or just prior to the first trimester of pregnancy due to risk of fetal abnormalities associated with methimazole.

THERAPEUTIC CLASS: Thiourea-derivative antithyroid agent

INDICATIONS: Patients with Grave's disease with hyperthydroidism or toxic multinodular goiter who are intolerant of methimazole and for whom surgery or radioactive iodine therapy is not an appropriate treatment option. To ameliorate symptoms of hyperthyroidism in preparation for thyroidectomy or radioactive iodine therapy in patients who are intolerant of methimazole.

DOSAGE: *Adults:* Initial: 300mg/day in 3 divided doses, q8h. Severe Hyperthyroidism/Very Large Goiters: Initial: 400mg/day in 3 divided doses, q8h; may give up to 600-900mg/day if needed. Usual Maint: 100-150mg/day in 3 divided doses, q8h.
Pediatrics: ≥6 yrs: Initial: 50mg/day. Titrate: Based on clinical response and evaluation of TSH and free T$_4$ levels.

HOW SUPPLIED: Tab: 50mg

WARNINGS/PRECAUTIONS: Not recommended for pediatric patients except when methimazole is not well-tolerated and surgery or radioactive iodine therapy are not appropriate therapies. D/C if symptoms of hepatic dysfunction (eg, anorexia, pruritus, RUQ pain) develop. Agranulocytosis, leukopenia, thrombocytopenia, and aplastic anemia (pancytopenia) may occur; d/c if agranulocytosis, aplastic anemia (pancytopenia), ANCA-positive vasculitis, hepatitis, interstitial pneumonitis, fever or exfoliative dermatitis develops; obtain bone marrow indices. May cause hypothyroidism; adjust dose to maintain euthyroidism. Fetal goiter and cretinism may occur when administered to a pregnant woman. May cause hypoprothrombinemia and bleeding.

ADVERSE REACTIONS: Agranulocytosis, liver injury, liver failure, thrombocytopenia, aplastic anemia, hepatitis, periarteritis, hypoprothrombinemia, skin rash, urticaria, N/V, epigastric distress, arthralgia, paresthesias.

INTERACTIONS: May increase activity of oral anticoagulants (eg, warfarin); consider additional monitoring of PT/INR. Hyperthyroidism may increase clearance of β-blockers; reduce β-blocker dose when patient becomes euthyroid. Increased digitalis glycoside levels when patient becomes euthyroid; reduce digitalis dose. May decrease theophylline clearance when patient becomes euthyroid; reduce theophylline dose. Caution with other drugs that cause agranulocytosis.

PREGNANCY: Category D, safety not known in nursing.

MECHANISM OF ACTION: Antithyroid agent; inhibits the synthesis of thyroid hormones; inhibits the conversion of thyroxine to triiodothyronine in peripheral tissues and may be an effective for treatment for thyroid storm.

PHARMACOKINETICS: Absorption: Readily absorbed. **Distribution:** Found in breast milk, crosses placental membranes. **Metabolism:** extensively metabolized. **Elimination:** Urine (35%).

NURSING CONSIDERATIONS

Assessment: Assess for hepatic impairment, pregnancy/nursing status, and for possible drug interactions.

Monitoring: Monitor for signs/symptoms of hepatic dysfunction (eg, anorexia, pruritus, RUQ pain), agranulocytosis (eg, fever, sore throat), leukopenia, thrombocytopenia, aplastic anemia, ANCA-positive vasculitis, interstitial pneumonitis, exfoliative dermatitis, and for hypothyroidism. Monitor CBC, PT, TSH, free T$_4$ levels, AST, ALT, bilirubin, and alkaline phosphatase.

Patient Counseling: Instruct to inform physician if pregnant/nursing or planning to become pregnant. Advise to report signs/symptoms of illness (eg, fever, sore throat, skin eruptions, headache, general malaise), and also hepatic dysfunction (anorexia, pruritus, upper quadrant pain). Inform about the risk of liver failure.

Administration: Oral route. **Storage:** 15-30°C (59-86°F).

P

PROQUAD   RX
varicella virus vaccine live - rubella vaccine live - measles vaccine live - mumps vaccine live (Merck)

THERAPEUTIC CLASS: Vaccine

INDICATIONS: Active immunization for the prevention of measles, mumps, rubella, and varicella in children 12 months through 12 yrs of age.

DOSAGE: *Pediatrics:* 12 months-12 yrs: 0.5mL SQ (1st dose usually at 12-15 months). If a 2nd dose is needed, administer at 4-6 yrs of age.

HOW SUPPLIED: Inj: 0.5mL

CONTRAINDICATIONS: Concomitant administration with immunosuppressive therapy (including high-dose corticosteroids) or immunosuppressant drugs. History of hypersensitivity to gelatin, history of anaphylactoid reaction to neomycin, blood dyscrasias, leukemia, lymphomas of any type, or other malignant neoplasms affecting the bone marrow or lymphatic systems, primary and acquired immunodeficiency states, including AIDS or other clinical manifestations of infection with human immunodeficiency virus (HIV); cellular immune deficiencies; hypogammaglobulinemic and dysgammaglobulinemic states, family history of congenital or hereditary immunodeficiency, active untreated tuberculosis (TB) or active febrile illness with fever >101.3°F; pregnancy.

WARNINGS/PRECAUTIONS: Higher rates of fever and febrile seizures at 5-12 days after vaccination in children 12-23 months old who have not been previously vaccinated against measles, mumps, rubella, or varicella. Caution with history of cerebral injury, individual or family history of convulsions or any other condition in which stress due to fever should be avoided. Caution with history of anaphylactic/anaphylactoid reactions to egg ingestion; may increase risk of immediate-type hypersensitivity reactions. Neomycin allergy manifested as a contact dermatitis is not a contraindication. Caution in children with thrombocytopenia or in those who experienced thrombocytopenia after vaccination with previous dose of measles, mumps, rubella, and/or varicella vaccine. Contains albumin; remote risk for transmission of viral diseases. Vaccine recipients should attempt to avoid close association with high-risk individuals susceptible to varicella for ≤6 weeks following vaccination; refer to PI for information on high-risk individuals. Defer vaccination for ≥3 months following blood or plasma transfusions, or administration of immune globulins (IG). Avoid pregnancy for 3 months following vaccination. May result in temporary depression of tuberculin skin sensitivity if given individually; administer test either any time before, simultaneously with, or ≥4-6 weeks after administration.

ADVERSE REACTIONS: Injection-site reactions (pain/tenderness/soreness, erythema, swelling), fever, irritability, measles-like rash, rubella-like rash, arthralgia, arthritis.

INTERACTIONS: See Contraindications. Avoid use of salicylates for 6 weeks after vaccination; Reye's syndrome reported. ≥1 month should elapse between a dose of measles-containing vaccine (eg, M-M-R II), and ≥3 months between a dose of varicella-containing vaccine.

PREGNANCY: Category C, not for use in nursing.

MECHANISM OF ACTION: Vaccine; stimulates immune system to elicit immune response to produce antibodies that may protect against measles, mumps, rubella, and varicella.

NURSING CONSIDERATIONS

Assessment: Assess for health status, immunization history, conditions where treatment is contraindicated or cautioned, and possible drug interactions. Assess for high-risk individuals susceptible to varicella.

Monitoring: Monitor for signs/symptoms of allergic reactions, fever, thrombocytopenia, Reye's syndrome, and injection-site reactions (eg, pain, tenderness, soreness, erythema, swelling, ecchymosis, rash).

Patient Counseling: Inform of potential benefits/risk associated with vaccination. Advise to avoid use of salicylates for 6 weeks after vaccination. Instruct post-pubertal females to postpone pregnancy for 3 months after vaccination. Inform that vaccination may not offer 100% protection. Instruct to report any adverse reactions to health care provider.

Administration: SQ route. Inspect for particulate matter and discoloration before administration. Inject SQ into the outer aspect of the deltoid region of the upper arm or into the higher anterolateral area of the thigh. Refer to PI for preparation/administration. **Storage:** Frozen between -50 to -15°C (-58 to +5°F) or refrigerate at 2-8°C (36-46°F) for up to 72 hrs prior to reconstitution. Discard if stored at 2-8°C and not used within 72 hrs of removal from 5°F (-15°C). Protect from light. Discard if reconstituted vaccine not used within 30 min and was stored at room temperature. Do not freeze reconstituted vaccine. Store diluent separately at room temperature 20-25°C (68-77°F), or refrigerate at 2-8°C (36-46°F). Refer to PI for more storage information.

PROQUIN XR   RX
ciprofloxacin (Depomed)

> Fluoroquinolones are associated with an increased risk of tendinitis and tendon rupture in all ages. Risk is further increased in patients >60 yrs, patients taking corticosteroids, and patients with kidney, heart or lung transplants. May exacerbate muscle weakness with myasthenia gravis; avoid in patients with known history of myasthenia gravis.

THERAPEUTIC CLASS: Fluoroquinolone

INDICATIONS: Treatment of uncomplicated urinary tract infections (UTI) (acute cystitis) caused by *E. coli* and *K. pneumoniae*.

DOSAGE: *Adults:* 500mg qd, preferably with pm meal, for 3 days.

HOW SUPPLIED: Tab, Extended-Release: 500mg

WARNINGS/PRECAUTIONS: D/C if experience pain, swelling, inflammation, or rupture of tendon. Convulsions, increased intracranial pressure (ICP), and toxic psychosis reported; d/c if CNS events (eg, dizziness, confusion, tremors, hallucinations, depression, or suicidal thoughts/acts) occur. Caution with CNS disorders or other risk factors that may predispose them to seizures or lower the seizure threshold. Severe and occasionally fatal hypersensitivity reactions reported; d/c immediately if signs of hypersensitivity appear. *Clostridium difficile*-associated diarrhea (CDAD) reported. Rare cases of sensory or sensorimotor axonal polyneuropathy reported; d/c if symptoms of neuropathy occur. Crystalluria and cylindruria reported; maintain adequate hydration. Photosensitivity/phototoxicity reactions may occur; d/c if phototoxicity occurs. Not interchangeable with other ciprofloxacin extended-release or immediate-release formulations. Caution with risk factors for torsades de pointes (eg, known QT prolongation, uncorrected hypokalemia). Caution in elderly and with renal impairment.

ADVERSE REACTIONS: Fungal infection, nasopharyngitis, headache, micturition urgency.

INTERACTIONS: See Boxed Warning. Increased levels of and serious and fatal reactions reported with theophylline; monitor levels and adjust dose. Magnesium- or aluminum-containing antacids, sucralfate, didanosine chewable/buffered tablets or pediatric powder, and products containing calcium, iron, or zinc decrease absorption; administer ≥4 hrs before or 2 hrs after these drugs. May alter serum levels of phenytoin. Severe hypoglycemia with glyburide (rare). Increased levels with probenecid. Reduced clearance of caffeine. Transient SrCr elevations with cyclosporine. Enhances oral anticoagulant effects of warfarin or its derivatives; monitor PT or other coagulation tests. May increase risk of methotrexate toxic reactions due to inhibition of renal tubular transport. High-dose quinolones shown to provoke convulsions with NSAIDs (not aspirin [ASA]). Caution with drugs that can result in prolongation of the QT interval (eg, class IA or III antiarrhythmics). Caution with concomitant use of drugs that may lower the seizure threshold. Avoid taking with milk products or calcium-fortified juices alone.

PREGNANCY: Category C, not for use in nursing.

MECHANISM OF ACTION: Fluoroquinolone; inhibits topoisomerase II (DNA gyrase) and topoisomerase IV (both type II topoisomerases), which are required for bacterial DNA replication, transcription, repair, and recombination.

PHARMACOKINETICS: Absorption: C_{max}=0.82mcg/mL; T_{max}=6.1 hrs; AUC=7.67mcg•hr/mL. **Distribution:** Plasma protein binding (9.9-36.6%). Found in breast milk. **Metabolism:** Desethyleneciprofloxacin, sulfociprofloxacin, oxociprofloxacin and formylciprofloxacin (metabolites). **Elimination:** Urine

(26.9%, unchanged) (over 24 hrs), (41%) (over 96 hrs), feces (43%); $T_{1/2}$=4.5 hrs.

NURSING CONSIDERATIONS

Assessment: Assess for risk factors for developing tendinitis and tendon rupture, myasthenia gravis, drug hypersensitivity, renal function, risk factors for torsades de pointes, CNS disorders or factors that may predispose to seizures or lower seizure threshold, pregnancy/nursing status, and possible drug interactions.

Monitoring: Monitor for tendinitis or tendon rupture, convulsions, increased ICP, toxic psychosis, CNS events, CDAD, peripheral neuropathy, photosensitivity reactions, and hypersensitivity reactions. Assess renal function.

Patient Counseling: Instruct to take exactly as directed; skipping doses or not completing full course may decrease effectiveness and increase bacterial resistance. Inform to notify healthcare provider if experience pain, swelling, or inflammation of a tendon, or weakness or inability to move joints; rest and refrain from exercise and d/c therapy. Instruct to d/c and notify physician if an allergic reaction, skin rash, watery and bloody stools, or symptoms of peripheral neuropathy. Notify prescriber if worsening muscle weakness or breathing problems, or sunburn-like reaction occurs, if pregnant/nursing, and all medications and supplements currently taking. Inform to take with main meal of day, preferably with evening meal. Instruct to avoid concomitant use with dairy products or calcium-fortified juices alone and to avoid breastfeeding. Avoid exposure to natural or artificial sunlight. Instruct to see how they react to therapy before engaging in activities that require mental alertness or coordination.

Administration: Oral route. Swallow whole; do not split, crush, or chew. Administer ≥4 hrs before or 2 hrs after magnesium- or aluminum-containing antacids, sucralfate, didanosine chewable/buffered tab or pediatric powder, metal cations (eg, iron), multivitamins with zinc. **Storage:** 25°C (77°F); excursions permitted to 15-30°C (59-86°F).

PROSCAR   RX
finasteride (Merck)

THERAPEUTIC CLASS: Type II 5 alpha-reductase inhibitor

INDICATIONS: Treatment of symptomatic benign prostatic hyperplasia (BPH) in men with an enlarged prostate to improve symptoms, reduce risk of acute urinary retention, and reduce risk of the need for surgery including transurethral resection of the prostate (TURP) and prostatectomy. To reduce risk of symptomatic progression of BPH (a confirmed ≥4 point increase in AUA symptom score) in combination with doxazosin.

DOSAGE: *Adults:* 5mg qd.

HOW SUPPLIED: Tab: 5mg

CONTRAINDICATIONS: Pregnancy.

WARNINGS/PRECAUTIONS: Not for use in pediatrics or women. Pregnant women or women who may potentially be pregnant should not handle crushed or broken tabs because of potential risk to a male fetus. Perform appropriate evaluation to identify other conditions that might mimic BPH (eg, infection, prostate cancer, stricture disease, hypotonic bladder or other neurogenic disorders). Patients with large residual urinary volume and/or severely diminished urinary flow may not be candidates for therapy; monitor for obstructive uropathy. Caution with liver dysfunction. May decrease serum prostate specific antigen (PSA) levels in patients with BPH or prostate cancer; any confirmed increase should be carefully evaluated.

ADVERSE REACTIONS: Impotence, decreased libido, decreased ejaculate volume, asthenia, postural hypotension, dizziness, abnormal ejaculation.

PREGNANCY: Category X, not for use in nursing.

MECHANISM OF ACTION: Type II 5α-reductase inhibitor; competitively inhibits type II 5α-reductase with which it forms a stable enzyme complex inhibiting metabolism of testosterone to 5α-dihydrotestosterone (DHT).

PHARMACOKINETICS: Absorption: Mean bioavailability (63%); C_{max}=37ng/mL; T_{max}=1-2 hrs. Refer to PI for different pharmacokinetic parameters of different age groups. **Distribution:** V_d=76L; plasma protein binding (90%). **Metabolism:** Liver (extensive) via CYP3A4. **Elimination:** (Oral) Urine (39% metabolites), feces (57%); $T_{1/2}$=6 hrs (45-60 yrs), 8 hrs (≥70 yrs).

NURSING CONSIDERATIONS

Assessment: Assess for pregnancy status, hypersensitivity to drug and its components, conditions which may mimic BPH and for liver function abnormalities. Assess for patients with large residual urinary volume and/or severely diminished urinary flow. Obtain baseline PSA levels.

Monitoring: Monitor for obstructive uropathy in patients with large residual urinary volume and/or severely diminished urinary flow. Monitor for hypersensitivity reactions and other adverse reactions. Monitor PSA levels.

Patient Counseling: Instruct pregnant or potentially pregnant females not to handle crushed or broken tabs due to potential risk to male fetus. Inform males that the volume of ejaculate may decrease and impotence/decrease libido may occur. Advise to notify physician if changes in breast (eg, lumps, pain, nipple discharge) occurs.

Administration: Oral route. **Storage:** <30°C (86°F).

PROTAMINE SULFATE
protamine sulfate (Various)

RX

> May cause severe hypotension, cardiovascular (CV) collapse, noncardiogenic pulmonary edema, catastrophic pulmonary vasoconstriction, and pulmonary HTN; risk factors include high dose/overdose, rapid/previous administration, repeated doses, and current/previous use of protamine-containing drugs. Risk to benefit of administration should be carefully considered with presence of any risk factors. Should not be given when bleeding occurs without prior heparin use.

THERAPEUTIC CLASS: Heparin antagonist

INDICATIONS: Management of heparin overdose.

DOSAGE: *Adults:* Administer as very slow IV infusion over 10 min in doses not to exceed 50mg. Determine dose by blood coagulation studies. Each mg neutralizes not less than 100 USP heparin units.

HOW SUPPLIED: Inj: 10mg/mL [5mL, 25mL]

WARNINGS/PRECAUTIONS: May cause allergic reactions with fish hypersensitivity. Rapid administration may cause severe hypotensive and anaphylactoid-like reactions. Caution in cardiac surgeries; hyperheparinemia or bleeding reported. Previous exposure to protamine/protamine-containing insulin may induce humoral immune response; severe hypersensitivity reaction, including life-threatening anaphylaxis reported. Increased risk of antiprotamine antibodies in infertile or vasectomized men.

ADVERSE REACTIONS: Hypotension, bradycardia, transitory flushing/feeling of warmth, lassitude, dyspnea, N/V, back pain, anaphylaxis that causes severe respiratory distress, circulatory collapse, noncardiogenic pulmonary edema, acute pulmonary HTN.

INTERACTIONS: Incompatible with certain antibiotics, such as cephalosporins and penicillins. Concomitant or previous use of protamine-containing drugs (eg, NPH insulin, protamine zinc insulin, certain beta-blockers) is risk factor for severe adverse events; see Boxed Warning.

PREGNANCY: Category C, caution in nursing.

MECHANISM OF ACTION: Heparin antagonist; has anticoagulant effects when administered alone, however, when given in presence of heparin, a stable salt is formed and anticoagulant activity of both drugs is lost.

P

NURSING CONSIDERATIONS

Assessment: Assess for fish allergy, previous vasectomy, previous exposure, severe left ventricular dysfunction, abnormal preoperative pulmonary hemodynamics, and possible drug interactions. Assess blood coagulation studies for appropriate dosage.

Monitoring: Monitor for hypersensitivity/allergic reactions, hypotension, CV collapse, pulmonary edema, and pulmonary HTN. Monitor blood coagulation studies.

Administration: Slow IV infusion. Large-size 25mL vials are designed for antiheparin treatment only when large doses of heparin have been given during surgery. **Storage:** 20-25°C (68-77°F). Do not freeze.

PROTONIX   RX
pantoprazole sodium (Wyeth)

OTHER BRAND NAMES: Protonix IV (Wyeth)

THERAPEUTIC CLASS: Proton pump inhibitor

INDICATIONS: (Tab/Sus) Short-term treatment (up to 8 weeks) in the healing and symptomatic relief of erosive esophagitis (EE) associated with gastroesophageal reflux disease (GERD) in adults and pediatric patients ≥5 yrs. Maintenance of healing of EE and reduction in relapse rates of daytime and nighttime heartburn symptoms in adult patients with GERD. Long-term treatment of pathological hypersecretory conditions including Zollinger-Ellison syndrome. (Inj) Short-term treatment (7-10 days) of GERD and a history of EE. Treatment of pathological hypersecretory conditions associated with Zollinger-Ellison syndrome or other neoplastic conditions.

DOSAGE: *Adults:* (Tab/Sus) Short-Term Treatment of EE associated with GERD: 40mg qd PO for up to 8 weeks. May repeat for 8 weeks if needed. Maintenance of Healing of EE: 40mg qd PO. Pathological Hypersecretory Conditions Including Zollinger-Ellison Syndrome: Initial: 40mg bid PO. Adjust to patient's needs and continue for as long as clinically indicated. Max: 240mg/day. If unable to swallow 40mg tab, take two 20mg tabs. Do not split, crush, or chew. (Sus) Administer 30 min prior to meal via PO administration in 1 tsp of apple juice or applesauce or NG tube in apple juice only. (Inj) GERD: 40mg qd IV infusion for 7-10 days. Pathological Hypersecretion Associated with Zollinger-Ellison Syndrome: 80mg q12h IV infusion. May adjust based on acid output. Max: 240mg/day. Duration >6 days not studied.
Pediatrics: ≥5 yrs: Short-Term Treatment of EE Associated with GERD: ≥15kg-<40kg: 20mg qd for up to 8 weeks. ≥40kg: 40mg qd for up to 8 weeks. If unable to swallow 40mg tab, take two 20mg tabs. Do not split, crush, or chew. (Sus) Administer 30 min prior to meal via PO administration in 1 tsp of apple juice or applesauce or NG tube in apple juice only. Do not divide 40mg pkt to create 20mg dosage for pediatrics unable to take tab.

HOW SUPPLIED: Inj: 40mg; Sus, Delayed-Release: 40mg (granules/pkt); Tab, Delayed-Release: 20mg, 40mg

WARNINGS/PRECAUTIONS: Associated with increased risk for osteoporosis-related fractures of hip, wrist, or spine. Increased risk in high-dose; use lowest dose and shortest duration appropriate to the condition being treated. Symptomatic response does not preclude the presence of gastric malignancy. (Tab/Sus) Atrophic gastritis has been noted with long-term therapy particularly in patients who were *H. pylori* positive. Vitamin B_{12} deficiency caused by hypo- or achlorhydria reported with long-term use (>3 yrs). (Inj) Anaphylaxis and thrombophlebitis reported. Mild, transient transaminase elevations observed in clinical studies. Consider zinc supplementation in patients who are prone to zinc deficiency. D/C as soon as the patient is able to resume treatment with delayed-release tabs.

ADVERSE REACTIONS: Abdominal pain, headache, nausea, dizziness, constipation, (Inj) dyspepsia, injection-site reactions, rhinitis, insomnia, (Tab/Sus) diarrhea, vomiting, flatulence, fever, upper respiratory infection (URI), rash.

INTERACTIONS: May alter absorption of pH-dependent drugs (eg, ketoconazole, ampicillin esters, and iron salts). May increase INR and PT with concomitant warfarin therapy. May substantially decrease atazanavir level; avoid concomitant use. (PO) Concomitant use with nelfinavir is not recommended. (Inj) Caution with other edetate disodium (EDTA)-containing products.

PREGNANCY: Category B, not for use in nursing.

MECHANISM OF ACTION: Proton pump inhibitor; suppresses final step in gastric acid production by covalently binding to the (H^+,K^+)-ATPase enzyme system of the gastric parietal cell.

PHARMACOKINETICS: Absorption: (Tab) Absolute bioavailability (77%); C_{max}=2.5µg/mL; T_{max}=2.5 hr; AUC=4.8µg•h/mL. (IV) C_{max}=5.52µg/mL; AUC=5.4µg•hr/mL. Refer to PI for PK parameters of delayed-release oral suspension and in children and adolescents (6-16 yrs). **Distribution:** V_d=11.0-23.6L; plasma protein binding (98%); found in breast milk. **Metabolism:** Liver (extensive) via CYP2C19 (demethylation), sulfation; CYP3A4 (oxidation). **Elimination:** Urine (71%), feces (18%); $T_{1/2}$=1 hr.

NURSING CONSIDERATIONS

Assessment: Assess for gastric malignancy, hepatic impairment, hypersensitivity, pregnancy/nursing status, and possible drug interactions.

Monitoring: Monitor for osteoporosis-related fractures of hip, wrist, or spine. (Tab/Sus) Monitor for signs/symptoms of GI tumors, vitamin B_{12} deficiency, and atrophic gastritis. (Inj) Monitor for hypersensitivity reaction (eg, anaphylaxis), injection-site reactions (eg, thrombophlebitis), zinc deficiency, acid output measurements, and hepatic effects (eg, elevations in transaminases).

Patient Counseling: (Inj) Switch treatment to PO formulation as soon as patient is able. Contact physician immediately if hypersensitivity or other adverse events occur; may require emergency medical treatment. (Tab) Swallow whole, with or without food in stomach; do not split, crush, or chew. Concomitant administration of antacids does not affect absorption. (Sus) Administer in applesauce or apple juice approximately 30 min before meal; do not place in water, other liquids, or food. Advise not to divide PO sus pkt to make smaller dose.

Administration: Oral, NG and IV route. (Tab) Swallow whole, with or without food. (Sus) Do not administer in liquids other than apple juice or foods other than applesauce. Refer to PI for proper administration. (Inj) Flush IV lines prior to and after administration with either 5% Dextrose Inj, USP, 0.9% NaCl Inj, USP, or Lactated Ringer's Inj, USP. Inspect visually for particulate matter and discoloration. May be administered over a period of 2-min or 15-min infusion. Refer to PI for reconstitution and dilution. **Storage:** 20-25°C (68-77°F); excursions permitted to 15-30°C (59-86°F). (Inj) Protect from light. Refer to PI for storage information regarding reconstituted solution.

PROTOPIC RX
tacrolimus (Astellas)

THERAPEUTIC CLASS: Macrolide immunosuppressant

INDICATIONS: Second-line therapy for short-term and noncontinuous chronic treatment of moderate to severe atopic dermatitis in nonimmunocompromised adults and children who are intolerant or unresponsive to conventional therapy.

DOSAGE: *Adults:* (0.03% or 0.1%) Apply thin layer to the affected skin bid. Rub in gently. Stop use when signs and symptoms resolve.
Pediatrics: ≥16 yrs: (0.03% or 0.1%) Apply thin layer to the affected skin bid. Rub in gently. 2-15 yrs: (0.03%) Apply thin layer to the affected skin bid. Rub in gently. Stop use when signs and symptoms resolve.

HOW SUPPLIED: Oint: 0.03%, 0.1% [30g, 60g, 100g]

WARNINGS/PRECAUTIONS: Do not use with occlusive dressings. Rare cases of malignancy (eg, skin and lymphoma) reported; avoid continuous long-term use and limit application to areas of involvement. Should not be used in immunocompromised adults and children. Avoid in premalignant and malignant skin conditions, Netherton's syndrome or other skin diseases where there is potential for increased systemic absorption. Increased risk of varicella zoster (chickenpox or shingles) and herpes simplex infection, or eczema herpeticum; resolve cutaneous bacterial or viral infections at treatment sites before commencing treatment. Lymphadenopathy reported; d/c if etiology of lymphadenopathy is unknown, or in presence of acute infectious mononucleosis. May cause local symptoms such as skin burning (eg, burning sensation, stinging, soreness) or pruritus. Minimize or avoid exposure to natural or artificial sunlight. Long-term safety not established. Rare cases of acute renal failure reported; caution in patients predisposed to renal impairment. Only 0.03% oint is indicated for use in children 2-15 yrs.

ADVERSE REACTIONS: Skin burning, pruritus, flu-like symptoms, allergic reaction, skin erythema, headache, skin infection, fever, herpes simplex, rhinitis, increased cough, asthma, pharyngitis, pustular rash.

INTERACTIONS: Caution with CYP3A4 inhibitors (eg, erythromycin, itraconazole, ketoconazole, fluconazole, CCBs, cimetidine) in widespread and/or erythrodermic disease.

PREGNANCY: Category C, not for use in nursing.

MECHANISM OF ACTION: Macrolide immunosuppressant; mechanism not known in atopic dermatitis. Inhibits T-lymphocyte activation by first binding to an intracellular protein, FKBP-12. A complex of tacrolimus-FKBP-12, calcium, calmodulin, and calcineurin is then formed and the phosphate activity of calcineurin is inhibited. This has been shown to prevent the dephosphorylation and translocation of nuclear factor of activated T-cells (NF-AT), a nuclear component thought to initiate gene transcription for the formation of lymphokines.

PHARMACOKINETICS: Absorption: Absolute bioavailability (0.5%), C_{max}=<2ng/mL (85% of population). **Distribution:** V_d=99%. **Metabolism:** CYP3A (extensive); demethylation and hydroxylation; 13-demethyl tacrolimus (major metabolite). **Elimination:** Feces (92.4% IV, 92.6% PO), urine (<1% unchanged IV, 2.3% PO). $T_{1/2}$=43.5% (IV), 48.4% (PO).

NURSING CONSIDERATIONS

Assessment: Assess for history of hypersensitivity to tacrolimus or any other component of the ointment, premalignant and malignant skin conditions, and renal impairment. Prior to initiation, resolve cutaneous bacterial or viral infections at treatment sites.

Monitoring: Monitor for varicella zoster virus infection (chickenpox or shingles), herpes simplex virus infection, eczema herpeticum, acute mononucleosis, lymphomas, skin malignancies (eg, cutaneous T-cell lymphoma), lymphadenopathy, and acute renal failure. Monitor improvement of signs/ symptoms of atopic dermatitis within 6 weeks.

Patient Counseling: Advise to consult physician if symptoms get worse, contracted an infection, or if symptoms do not improve within 6 weeks. Use as prescribed, apply a thin layer only on skin areas that have eczema and avoid getting in the eyes or mouth, use only for short periods, and if needed, treatment may be repeated with breaks in between. D/C when signs/symptoms of eczema (eg, itching, rash and redness) go away, and avoid exposure to ultraviolet therapy, sun lamps and tanning beds during treatment. Limit sun exposure, wear loose-fitting clothing that protects treated area from the sun, and do not cover treated skin with bandages, dressings, or wraps. Advise caregivers applying the ointment or patients not treating their hands to wash hands with soap and water after application. Advise patients not to bathe, shower or swim right after application. Counsel that ointment is not indicated for children <2 yrs old.

Administration: Topical route. **Storage:** 25°C (77°F); excursions permitted to 15-30°C (59-86°F).

PROVENGE
sipuleucel-T (Dendreon)

RX

THERAPEUTIC CLASS: Immunomodulatory agent

INDICATIONS: Treatment of asymptomatic or minimally symptomatic metastatic castrate resistant (hormone refractory) prostate cancer.

DOSAGE: *Adults:* Infuse 250mL over 60 min q2 weeks for 3 doses. If unable to administer a scheduled infusion, the patient will need to undergo an additional leukapheresis. Premedication: Oral acetaminophen and antihistamine (eg, diphenhydramine) 30 min prior to administration.

HOW SUPPLIED: Sus: 250mL

WARNINGS/PRECAUTIONS: For autologous use only. Acute infusion reactions (eg, fever, chills, respiratory events, N/V, fatigue, HTN, tachycardia) reported; infusion rate may be decreased or stopped depending on severity of reaction. Monitor closely with cardiac or pulmonary conditions. May transmit diseases to health care professionals handling the product; employ universal precautions.

ADVERSE REACTIONS: Chills, fatigue, fever, back pain, N/V, joint ache, headache, paresthesia, anemia, constipation, infusion reactions.

INTERACTIONS: Concurrent use of immunosuppressive agents may alter efficacy and/or safety of sipuleucel-T.

PREGNANCY: Safety in pregnancy and nursing not known.

MECHANISM OF ACTION: Immunomodulatory agent (autologous cellular immunotherapy). Precise mechanism is not established; induces an immune response targeted against prostatic acid phosphatase (PAP), an antigen expressed in prostatic cancer tissue.

NURSING CONSIDERATIONS

Assessment: Assess for history of cardiac or pulmonary conditions.

Monitoring: Monitor for signs and symptoms of infusion reactions especially with cardiac or pulmonary conditions. Monitor for infectious sequelae in patients with central venous catheters.

Patient Counseling: Counsel on adhering to preparation instructions for leukapheresis procedure, possible side effects, and post-procedure care. If a scheduled dose must be missed, the patient will have to undergo an additional leukapheresis. Report signs and symptoms of acute infusion reactions (eg, fever, chills, fatigue, breathing problems, dizziness, high blood pressure, N/V, headache or muscle aches) and symptoms suggestive of cardiac arrhythmia. Notify physician if taking immunosuppressive agents. Inform of the need for a central venous catheter placement if peripheral venous access is not adequate. Inform physician if fever or any swelling or redness around the catheter site occurs.

Administration: IV infusion. For autologous use only. Begin infusion prior to expiration date and time indicated on the product label. Do not infuse expired product. Infuse IV over 60 min. Observe patient for at least 30 min after each infusion. Refer to PI for preparation instructions. **Storage:** Infusion bag must remain within the insulated polyurethane container until the time of administration. Do not remove from the outer cardboard shipping box. Refer to PI for complete handling instructions.

PROVERA
medroxyprogesterone acetate (Pharmacia & Upjohn)

RX

> Estrogen and progestins should not be used for prevention of cardiovascular disease or dementia. Increased risk of myocardial infarction (MI), stroke, invasive breast cancer, pulmonary embolism (PE), and deep vein thrombosis (DVT) in postmenopausal women (50-79 yrs). Increased risk of developing probable dementia in postmenopausal women (≥65 yrs).

THERAPEUTIC CLASS: Progestogen

INDICATIONS: Treatment of secondary amenorrhea and abnormal uterine bleeding due to hormonal imbalance in the absence of organic pathology, such as fibroids or uterine cancer. Reduce incidence of endometrial hyperplasia in non-hysterectomized postmenopausal women receiving 0.625mg conjugated estrogen.

DOSAGE: *Adults:* Secondary Amenorrhea: 5-10mg qd for 5-10 days. Abnormal Uterine Bleeding: 5-10mg qd for 5-10 days beginning on Day 16 or 21 of cycle. Endometrial Hyperplasia: 5-10mg qd for 12-14 consecutive days per month beginning on Day 1 or 16 of cycle.

HOW SUPPLIED: Tab: 2.5mg*, 5mg*, 10mg* *scored

CONTRAINDICATIONS: Undiagnosed abnormal genital bleeding, breast cancer, estrogen- or progesterone-dependent neoplasia, active or history of DVT/PE, arterial thromboembolic disease (eg, stroke, MI), liver dysfunction or disease, missed abortion, pregnancy, as a diagnostic test for pregnancy.

WARNINGS/PRECAUTIONS: D/C if thrombotic events, malignancy, papilledema, or retinal vascular lesions develop. D/C pending exam with sudden onset of proptosis, partial or complete loss of vision, diplopia, or migraine. May elevate BP; monitor at regular intervals. May lower HDL and raise LDL levels as well as impair glucose tolerance. May increase plasma TG with pre-existing hypertriglyceridemia. Caution in patients with history of cholestatic jaundice associated with past estrogen use or pregnancy and with severe hypocalcemia. May cause fluid retention; caution with cardiac/renal dysfunction. May exacerbate asthma, DM, epilepsy, migraine, porphyria, systemic lupus erythematosus (SLE), and hepatic hemangiomas; use with caution.

ADVERSE REACTIONS: Abnormal uterine bleeding, breast tenderness, galactorrhea, urticaria, pruritus, edema, rash, thromboembolic phenomena, menstrual changes, change in weight, cervical changes, cholestatic jaundice, depression, insomnia, nausea.

INTERACTIONS: Patients on thyroid replacement therapy may require higher doses of thyroid hormone.

PREGNANCY: Category X, not for use in nursing.

MECHANISM OF ACTION: Progesterone derivative; transforms proliferative into secretory endometrium.

PHARMACOKINETICS: Absorption: (10mg) Rapid; C_{max}=0.71ng/mL; T_{max}=2.83 hrs; AUC=6.01ng•h/mL. **Distribution:** V_d=40564L; plasma protein binding (90%); Found in breast milk. **Metabolism:** hydroxylation, conjugation. **Elimination:** $T_{1/2}$= 16.6 hrs; Urine.

NURSING CONSIDERATIONS

Assessment: Assess for undiagnosed abnormal genital bleeding; known/suspected or history of breast cancer, estrogen- or progesterone-dependent neoplasia, pregnancy status, missed abortion, thromboembolic disease, CAD, asthma, DM, epilepsy, SLE, migraine, porphyria, hypocalcemia, cardiac or renal/hepatic impairment.

Monitoring: Monitor BP regularly; breast exam by physician yearly and self monthly; mammogram as required. Monitor for signs/symptoms of thromboembolic disease (eg, stroke, DVT, PE, MI), HTN, hypocalcemia, abnormal vaginal bleeding, dementia, visual abnormalities, hypersensitivity reactions, hepatic dysfunction, fluid retention, exacerbation of asthma, DM, epilepsy, SLE, migraine, and porphyria. Monitor thyroid function if on thyroid replacement therapy.

Patient Counseling: Inform of risks, including birth defects if exposed during 1st trimester, thromboembolic events, dementia and malignancy in postmenopausal use. Advise to seek medical attention if experience symptoms of hepatic dysfunction (jaundice), hypocalcemia, visual abnormalities (partial/complete loss of vision, diplopia, migraines), abnormal vaginal bleeding, hypersensitivity reactions, HTN, thromboembolic disease, fluid retention, exacerbation of diseases, or dementia.

Administration: Oral route. **Storage:** 20-25°C (68-77°F).

PROVIGIL
modafinil (Cephalon)

THERAPEUTIC CLASS: Wakefulness-promoting agent

INDICATIONS: To improve wakefulness in patients with excessive sleepiness associated with narcolepsy, obstructive sleep apnea (OSA), shift work disorder (SWD). As adjunct to standard treatment for underlying obstruction in OSA.

DOSAGE: *Adults:* ≥17 yrs: 200mg qd. Max: 400mg/day as single dose. Narcolepsy/OSA: Take as single dose in AM. SWD: Take 1 hr prior to start of work shift. Severe Hepatic Impairment: 100mg qd. Elderly: Consider dose reduction.

HOW SUPPLIED: Tab: 100mg, 200mg* *scored

WARNINGS/PRECAUTIONS: Rare cases of severe or life-threatening rash, including Stevens-Johnson syndrome (SJS), toxic epidermal necrolysis (TEN), and drug rash with eosinophilia and systemic symptoms (DRESS) reported; d/c treatment at first sign of rash. Angioedema, anaphylactoid reactions, multi-organ hypersensitivity and psychiatric adverse experiences reported; d/c treatment if symptoms develop. Caution with a history of psychosis, depression or mania. Caution if recent myocardial infarction (MI) or unstable angina. Avoid in patients with history of left ventricular hypertrophy or with mitral valve prolapse who have experienced mitral valve prolapse syndrome (eg, ischemic ECG changes, chest pain, arrhythmia) with CNS stimulants. May impair mental/physical abilities. Reduce dose with severe hepatic impairment. Use low dose in elderly. Doses up to 400mg/day have been well tolerated but there is no evidence that this dose confers additional benefit.

ADVERSE REACTIONS: Headache, nausea, nervousness, anxiety, insomnia, rhinitis, diarrhea, back pain, dizziness, dyspepsia, flu syndrome, dry mouth, anorexia, pharyngitis.

INTERACTIONS: Methylphenidate and dextroamphetamine may delay absorption. May reduce efficacy of steroidal contraceptives up to 1 month after d/c. Caution with MAOIs. CYP3A4 inducers (eg, carbamazepine, phenobarbital, rifampin) may decrease levels. CYP3A4 inhibitors (eg, ketoconazole, itraconazole) may increase levels. May increase levels of drugs metabolized by CYP2C19 (eg, diazepam, propranolol, phenytoin) or CYP2C9 (eg, warfarin). Monitor for toxicity with CYP2C19 substrates and PT/INR with warfarin. May increase levels of certain TCAs (eg, clomipramine, desipramine) and SSRIs in CYP2D6 deficient patients. May decrease levels of drugs metabolized by CYP3A4 (eg, cyclosporine, ethinyl estradiol, triazolam). May induce CYP1A2 and CYP2B6; caution with CYP1A2 and CYP2B6 substrates.

PREGNANCY: Category C, caution in nursing.

MECHANISM OF ACTION: Wakefulness promoting agent; not established. Binds to dopamine transporter, inhibits dopamine reuptake, and results in increased extracellular dopamine levels in some brain regions.

PHARMACOKINETICS: Absorption: Rapid. T_{max}=2-4 hrs, delayed by 1 hr (fed). **Distribution:** V_d=0.9L/kg; plasma protein binding (60%). **Metabolism:** Liver via hydrolytic deamination, S-oxidation, aromatic ring hydroxylation, and glucuronide conjugation; CYP3A4. **Elimination:** Feces (1%), urine (80%, <10% parent compound); $T_{1/2}$=15 hrs.

NURSING CONSIDERATIONS

Assessment: Assess for hypersensitivity, hepatic impairment, pregnancy/nursing status, possible drug interactions, and a history of psychosis, depression, mania, left ventricular hypertrophy, or mitral valve prolapse. Assess for a recent history of MI or unstable angina. Use only in patients who have had complete evaluation of their excessive sleepiness, and in whom a diagnosis of either narcolepsy, OSA, and/or SWD has been made.

Monitoring: Monitor for serious rash, SJS, TEN, DRESS, angioedema, hypersensitivity, multi-organ hypersensitivity reactions, psychiatric adverse symptoms, and other adverse reactions. Monitor BP. If used adjunctively with continuous positive airway pressure (CPAP), monitor for CPAP compliance. Periodically re-evaluate long-term usefulness if prescribed for an extended time.

Patient Counseling: Advise that this is not a replacement for sleep. Inform that drug may improve but does not eliminate sleepiness. Avoid taking alcohol during therapy. Caution against hazardous tasks (eg, driving, operating machinery) or performing other activities that require mental alertness. Notify physician if pregnant or intend to become pregnant or if nursing during therapy. Caution about increased risk of pregnancy when using steroidal contraceptives and for 1 month after d/c therapy. Inform physician if taking or planning to take any prescribed or OTC drugs. Contact physician if chest pain, rash, depression, anxiety, or signs of psychosis or mania develop. Inform of importance of continuing previously prescribed treatments. D/C and notify physician if rash, hives, mouth sores, blisters, peeling skin, trouble swallowing or breathing or other allergic reactions develop.

Administration: Oral route. **Storage:** 20-25°C (68-77°F).

PROZAC   RX
fluoxetine HCl (Lilly)

> Antidepressants increased the risk of suicidal thinking and behavior (suicidality) in short-term studies in children, adolescents, and young adults with major depressive disorder (MDD) and other psychiatric disorders. Monitor and observe closely for clinical worsening, suicidality, or unusual changes in behavior in patients who are started on antidepressant therapy. Fluoxetine is approved for use in pediatric patients with MDD and obsessive compulsive disorder (OCD).

THERAPEUTIC CLASS: Selective serotonin reuptake inhibitor

INDICATIONS: Treatment of major depressive disorder (MDD), obsessive compulsive disorder (OCD), bulimia nervosa, and panic disorder with or without agoraphobia. In combination with olanzapine, acute treatment of depressive episodes associated with bipolar I disorder, and treatment-resistant depression (MDD patients who failed to respond to 2 separate trials of different antidepressants) in adults.

DOSAGE: *Adults:* ≥18 yrs: MDD: Initial: 20mg qam; increase dose if no improvement after several weeks. Doses >20mg/day, give qam or bid (am and noon). Max: 80mg/day. OCD: Initial: 20mg qam; may increase dose if no significant improvement after several weeks. Maint: 20-60mg/day given qd-bid, am and noon. Max: 80mg/day. Bulimia Nervosa: 60mg qam. Max: 60mg/day. Panic Disorder: Initial: 10mg/day. May increase to 20mg/day after 1 week. May increase further after several weeks if no clinical improvement. Max: 60mg/day. Hepatic Impairment/Elderly: Use lower or less frequent dosage. Consider dose tapering for pregnant women during the third trimester. Combination with Olanzapine: Depressive Episodes Associated with Bipolar I Disorder/Treatment Resistant Depression: Initial: 20mg plus olanzapine 5mg qd in evening. Titrate: Adjust dose based on efficacy and tolerability. Usual: 25mg-50mg plus olanzapine 6mg-12mg (depressive episodes associated with Bipolar I disorder) or 6mg-18mg (treatment-resistant depression). Predisposed to Hypotensive Reactions/Hepatic Impairment/Factors to Slow Metabolism of Olanzapine or Fluoxetine in Combination: 20mg plus olanzapine 2.5mg-5mg.
Pediatrics: MDD: ≥8 yrs: Higher Wt Peds: Initial: 10 or 20mg/day. After 1 week at 10mg/day, may increase to 20mg/day. Lower Wt Peds: Initial: 10mg/day. Titrate: May increase to 20mg/day after several weeks if clinical improvement is not observed. OCD: ≥7 yrs: Adolescents and Higher Wt Peds: Initial: 10mg/day. Titrate: Increase to 20mg/day after 2 weeks. Consider additional dose increases after several more weeks if clinical improvement is not observed. Usual: 20-60mg/day. Lower Wt Peds: Initial: 10mg/day. Titrate: Consider additional dose increases after several weeks if clinical improvement is not observed. Usual: 20-30mg/day. Max: 60mg/day.

HOW SUPPLIED: Cap: 10mg, 20mg, 40mg; Sol (Generic): 20mg/5mL

CONTRAINDICATIONS: During or within 14 days of MAOI therapy. Thioridazine during or within 5 weeks of d/c. Concomitant use of pimozide.

WARNINGS/PRECAUTIONS: Avoid abrupt withdrawal. Serotonin syndrome and neuroleptic malignant syndrome (NMS)-like reactions reported. May increase risk of bleeding events. Activation of mania/hypomania, SIADH, hyponatremia, anxiety, insomnia, nervousness reported. D/C if unexplained allergic reaction occurs. Caution with diseases or conditions that could affect hemodynamic responses or metabolism, altered glucose levels, history of seizures or mania, suicidal tendencies. Monitor height and weight periodically in children. Altered appetite and weight loss reported. Caution in third trimester of pregnancy due to risk of serious neonatal complications. Caution with hepatic impairment. May impair mental/physical abilities. May precipitate mixed/manic episode in patients at risk for bipolar disorder. Fluoxetine monotherapy is not approved for use in treating bipolar depression.

ADVERSE REACTIONS: Abnormal dreams, abnormal ejaculation, anorexia, anxiety, asthenia, diarrhea, dry mouth, dyspepsia, flu syndrome, impotence, insomnia, decreased libido, nausea, nervousness, pharyngitis.

INTERACTIONS: See Contraindications. Caution with CYP2D6 substrates including antidepressants (eg, TCA), antipsychotics (eg, phenothiazines and most atypicals), and antiarrhythmics (eg, propafenone, flecainide). May increase levels of phenytoin, carbamazepine, haloperidol, clozapine, diazepam, imipramine, desipramine. Caution with CNS active drugs. May increase/decrease lithium levels; lithium toxicity and increased serotogenic effects reported. Caution with drugs that may affect serotogenic neurotransmitter systems (eg, triptans, linezolid, tramadol, lithium, St. John's wort). Avoid with other selective serotonin reuptake inhibitors (SSRIs), serotonin-norepinephrine reuptake inhibitors (SNRIs), or tryptophan. May cause a shift in plasma concentration with drugs that are tightly bound to protein (eg, warfarin, digoxin) resulting in an adverse effect. Increased risk of bleeding events with aspirin (ASA), NSAIDs, warfarin, and other anticoagulants. Greater risk of hyponatremia with diuretics. Increased risk of NMS-like reactions with serotogenic drugs (eg, triptans), MAOIs, antipsychotics, other dopamine antagonists. Antidiabetic drugs may need adjustment. Rare reports of prolonged seizures with combined electroconvulsive therapy.

PREGNANCY: Category C, not for use in nursing.

MECHANISM OF ACTION: SSRI; not established. Presumed to be linked to inhibition of CNS neuronal reuptake of serotonin.

PHARMACOKINETICS: Absorption: C_{max}=15-55ng/mL, T_{max}=6-8 hrs. **Distribution:** Plasma protein binding (94.5%); excreted in breast milk. **Metabolism:** Liver (extensive) via demethylation, norfluoxetine (active metabolite). **Elimination:** Urine; $T_{1/2}$=1-3 days (fluoxetine), 4-16 days (norfluoxetine).

NURSING CONSIDERATIONS

Assessment: Assess for risk of bipolar disorder, history of mania, history of seizures, disease/condition that alters metabolism or hemodynamic response, hepatic/renal impairment, MAOI, thioridazine, or pimozide therapy, pregnancy/nursing status, and possible drug interactions.

Monitoring: Monitor for signs/symptoms of clinical worsening, suicidality and unusual changes in behavior (especially during initial few months, and dosage changes), hypersensitivity reactions, serotonin syndrome, abnormal bleeding, altered appetite and weight, hyponatremia, seizures, hypo/hyperglycemia, and abrupt withdrawal symptoms.

Patient Counseling: Advise to avoid alcohol. Seek medical attention for symptoms of serotonin syndrome, abnormal bleeding (particularly if using NSAIDs or ASA), akathisia, hyponatremia, mydriasis, activation of mania, seizures, clinical worsening and discontinuation symptoms (eg, irritability, agitation, dizziness, anxiety, headache, insomnia). Caution against hazardous tasks (eg, operating machinery and driving). May notice improvement in 1-4 weeks; continue therapy as directed. Notify physician if pregnant/intend to become pregnant, or breastfeeding. Counsel about benefits and risks of therapy. Inform physician if taking, or plan to take any OTC prescriptions.

Administration: Oral route. **Storage:** 15-30°C (59-86°F). Protect from light.

PROZAC WEEKLY
fluoxetine HCl (Lilly)

RX

> Antidepressants increased the risk of suicidal thinking and behavior (suicidality) in short-term studies in children, adolescents, and young adults with major depressive disorder (MDD) and other psychiatric disorders. Monitor and observe closely for clinical worsening, suicidality, or unusual changes in behavior in patients who are started on antidepressant therapy. Fluoxetine is approved for use in pediatric patients with MDD and obsessive compulsive disorder (OCD).

THERAPEUTIC CLASS: Selective serotonin reuptake inhibitor

INDICATIONS: Treatment of major depressive disorder (MDD).

DOSAGE: *Adults:* One 90mg cap every week starting 7 days after last daily dose of fluoxetine 20mg.

HOW SUPPLIED: Cap, Delayed-Release: 90mg

CONTRAINDICATIONS: During or within 14 days of MAOI therapy. Thioridazine during or within 5 weeks of d/c. Concomitant use of pimozide.

WARNINGS/PRECAUTIONS: Avoid abrupt withdrawal. Serotonin syndrome and neuroleptic malignant syndrome (NMS)-like reactions reported. May increase risk of bleeding events. Activation of mania/hypomania, SIADH, hyponatremia, anxiety, insomnia, nervousness reported. D/C if unexplained allergic reaction occurs. Caution with diseases or conditions that could affect hemodynamic responses or metabolism, altered glucose levels, history of seizures or mania, suicidal tendencies. Monitor height and weight periodically in children. Altered appetite and weight loss reported. Caution in third trimester of pregnancy due to risk of serious neonatal complications. Caution with hepatic impairment. May impair mental/physical abilities. May precipitate mixed/manic episode in patients at risk for bipolar disorder. Fluoxetine monotherapy is not approved for use in treating bipolar depression.

ADVERSE REACTIONS: Abnormal dreams, abnormal ejaculation, anorexia, anxiety, asthenia, diarrhea, dry mouth, dyspepsia, flu syndrome, impotence, insomnia, decreased libido, nausea, nervousness, pharyngitis.

INTERACTIONS: See Contraindications. Caution with CYP2D6 substrates including antidepressants (eg, TCA), antipsychotics (eg, phenothiazines and most atypicals), and antiarrhythmics (eg, propafenone, flecainide). May increase levels of phenytoin, carbamazepine, haloperidol, clozapine, diazepam, imipramine, desipramine. Caution with CNS active drugs. May increase/decrease lithium levels; lithium toxicity and increased serotogenic effects reported. Caution with drugs that may affect serotogenic neurotransmitter systems (eg, triptans, linezolid, tramadol, lithium, St. John's wort). Avoid with other selective serotonin reuptake inhibitors (SSRIs), serotonin-norepinephrine reuptake inhibitors (SNRIs), or tryptophan. May cause a shift in plasma concentration with drugs that are tightly bound to protein (eg, warfarin, digoxin) resulting in an adverse effect. Increased risk of bleeding events with aspirin (ASA), nonsteroidal anti-inflammatory drugs (NSAID), warfarin, and other anti-coagulants. Greater risk of hyponatremia with diuretics. Increased risk of NMS-like reactions with serotogenic drugs (eg, triptans), MAOIs, antipsychotics, other dopamine antagonists. Antidiabetic drugs may need adjustment. Rare reports of prolonged seizures with combined electroconvulsive therapy.

PREGNANCY: Category C, not for use in nursing.

MECHANISM OF ACTION: SSRI; exact mechanism is not established. Believed to inhibit CNS neuronal reuptake of serotonin.

PHARMACOKINETICS: Absorption: Delayed onset by 1-2 hrs. **Distribution:** Plasma protein binding (94.5%). Excreted in breast milk. **Metabolism:** Liver (extensive) via demethylation, norfluoxetine (active metabolite). **Elimination:** Kidney. $T_{1/2}$=1-3 days (fluoxetine), 4-16 days (norfluoxetine).

NURSING CONSIDERATIONS

Assessment: Assess for risk of bipolar disorder, history of mania, history of seizures, disease/condition that alters metabolism or hemodynamic response, hepatic/renal impairment, MAOI, thioridazine, or pimozide therapy, pregnancy/nursing status, and possible drug interactions.

Monitoring: Monitor for signs/symptoms of clinical worsening, suicidality and unusual changes in behavior (especially during initial few months, and dosage changes), hypersensitivity reactions, serotonin syndrome, abnormal bleeding, altered appetite and weight, hyponatremia, seizures, hypo/hyperglycemia, and abrupt withdrawal symptoms.

Patient Counseling: Advise to avoid alcohol. Seek medical attention for symptoms of serotonin syndrome, abnormal bleeding (particularly if using NSAIDs or ASA), akathisia, hyponatremia, mydriasis, activation of mania, seizures, clinical worsening and d/c symptoms (irritability, agitation, dizziness, anxiety, headache, insomnia). Caution against hazardous tasks (eg, operating machinery and driving). May notice improvement in 1-4 weeks; continue therapy as directed. Notify physician if pregnant/intend to become pregnant, or breastfeeding. Counsel about benefits and risks of therapy. Inform physician if taking, or plan to take any over-the-counter prescriptions.

Administration: Oral route. **Storage:** 15-30°C (59-86°F). Protect from light.

PULMICORT RX
budesonide (AstraZeneca)

OTHER BRAND NAMES: Pulmicort Turbuhaler (AstraZeneca) - Pulmicort Respules (AstraZeneca) - Pulmicort Flexhaler (AstraZeneca)

THERAPEUTIC CLASS: Corticosteroid

INDICATIONS: (Flexhaler, Turbuhaler) Maintenance treatment of asthma as prophylactic therapy in patients ≥6 yrs. (Turbuhaler) For patients requiring oral corticosteroid therapy for asthma. (Respules) Maintenance treatment of asthma and as prophylactic therapy in children 12 months to 8 yrs.

DOSAGE: *Adults:* (Flexhaler) ≥18 yrs: Initial: 180-360mcg bid. Max: 720mcg bid. Individualize dose. Elderly: Start at low end of dosing range. (Turbuhaler) Bronchodilators Alone: Initial: 200-400mcg bid. Max: 400mcg bid. Inhaled Corticosteroids: Initial: 200-400mcg bid. Max: 800mcg bid. Oral Corticosteroids: 400-800mcg bid. Max: 800mcg bid.
Pediatrics: (Flexhaler) ≥6 yrs: Individualize dose. Initial: 180-360mcg bid. Max: 360mcg bid. (Turbuler) Bronchodilators Alone/Inhaled/Oral Corticosteroids: 400mcg bid. Max: 400mcg bid. (Respules) Administer via compressed air driven jet nebulizer only; 1-8 yrs: Previous Bronchodilator Only: Initial: 0.5mg qd or 0.25mg bid. Max: 0.5mg/day. Previous Inhaled Corticosteroid: 0.5mg qd or 0.25mg bid. Max: 1mg/day. Taper to lowest effective dose once desired clinical effect achieved. Previous Oral Corticosteroid: 1mg qd or 0.5mg bid. Max: 1mg/day. Gradually reduce PO corticosteroid dose after 1 week of budesonide. Not Responding to Non-Steroidal Therapy: Initial: 0.25mg qd.

HOW SUPPLIED: Powder, Inhalation: (Flexhaler) 90mcg/dose, 180mcg/dose; (Turbuhaler) 200mcg; Sus, Inhalation: (Respules) 0.25mg/2mL, 0.5mg/2mL, 1mg/2mL [2mL, 30ˢ]

CONTRAINDICATIONS: Primary treatment of status asthmaticus or other acute episodes of asthma where intensive measures are required. (Flexhaler) Hypersensitivity to milk proteins.

WARNINGS/PRECAUTIONS: Deaths due to adrenal insufficiency reported with transfer from systemic corticosteroids to inhaled corticosteroids. Not indicated for the rapid relief of bronchospasm or other acute episodes of asthma; resume oral corticosteroids during stress or severe asthma attack. Transfer from systemic to inhalation therapy may unmask allergic conditions (eg, rhinitis, conjunctivitis, arthritis, eosinophilic conditions, eczema). Observe for adrenal insufficiency, systemic corticosteroid withdrawal effects, and growth suppression (children). Increased susceptibility to infections (eg, chickenpox, measles), which may lead to serious/fatal course; if exposed, prophylaxis/treatment considered. Appearance of hypercorticism and adrenal suppression (including adrenal crisis); reduce dose slowly. Paradoxical bronchospasm may occur; d/c immediately. Caution with tuberculosis (TB), untreated systemic fungal, bacterial, viral or parasitic infections, ocular herpes simplex, patients with major risk factors for decreased bone mineral content. In rare cases may present with systemic eosinophilic conditions and vasculitis consistent with Churg-Strauss syndrome. Physicians should be alert to eo-sinophilia, vasculitic rash, worsening pulmonary symptoms, cardiac complications, and/or neuropathy. *Candida* infections of mouth and pharynx reported; treat and/or d/c if needed. Patients requiring oral corticosteroids should be weaned slowly from systemic corticosteroid use. Glaucoma, increased intraocular pressure (IOP) and cataracts reported. Caution in elderly. (Respules, Flexhaler) Hypersensitivity reactions including anaphylaxis, rash, contact dermatitis, urticaria, angioedema, and bronchospasm reported; d/c treatment if reactions occurs.

ADVERSE REACTIONS: (Flexhaler) Nasopharyngitis, headache, fever, sinusitis, back pain, respiratory infection, N/V, oral candidiasis, dyspepsia, rhinitis, insomnia, dry mouth, weight gain.(Turbuhaler) Respiratory infection, pharyngitis, sinusitis, headache, flu syndrome. (Respules) Respiratory infection, rhinitis, coughing, otitis media, viral infection.

INTERACTIONS: Oral ketoconazole increases plasma levels. Coadministration with CYP3A4 may inhibit the metabolism and increase the systemic exposure. Exercise caution when coadministered with ketoconazole and other known strong CYP3A4 inhibitors (eg, itraconazole, clarithromycin).

PREGNANCY: Category B, caution in nursing.

MECHANISM OF ACTION: Corticosteroid; not established. Shown to have inhibitory effects on multiple cell types (mast cells, eosinophils, neutrophils, macrophages and lymphocytes) and mediators (histamine, eicosanoids, leukotrienes and cytokines) involved in inflammatory and asthmatic response.

PHARMACOKINETICS: Absorption: Respules: (4-6 yrs) Absolute bioavailability (6%); C_{max}=2.6nmol/L, T_{max}=20 min. Flexhaler: (Adults) T_{max}=10 min, (180mcg qd) C_{max}=0.6nmol/L. (360mcg bid) C_{max}=1.6nmol/L. (Peds) T_{max}=15-30 min, (180mcg qd) C_{max}=0.4nmol/L. (360mcg bid) C_{max}=1.5nmol/L. **Distribution:** V_d=3L/kg; plasma protein binding (85-90%); found in breast milk (0.3-1%). **Metabolism:** Liver (extensive), via CYP450 and CYP3A4. **Elimination:** Urine and feces (metabolites); (Respules) $T_{1/2}$=2.3 hrs. (Flexhaler) (IV) Urine (60%); $T_{1/2}$=2-3 hrs.

NURSING CONSIDERATIONS

Assessment: Assess for concomitant diseases such as status asthmaticus, acute bronchospasm, other acute episodes of asthma, pulmonary TB, ocular herpes simplex, untreated systemic fungal, bacterial, parasitic or viral infections, hepatic dysfunction, milk protein hypersensitivity, pregnancy/nursing status, and possible drug interactions. Obtain baseline lung function, cortisol production, and LFTs prior to therapy.

Monitoring: Monitor lung function periodically. Perform periodic eye exams; monitor for development of glaucoma, increased IOP and cataracts. Monitor for localized oral infections with *Candida albicans*, decreased bone mass, worsening or acutely deteriorating asthma, height in children, development of adrenal insufficiency (eg, fatigue, weakness, N/V, hypotension), paradoxical bronchospasm, hepatic disease, and hypersensitivity reactions.

Patient Counseling: Effectiveness depends on regular use. Do not increase dosage or d/c inhaler abruptly unless directed by physician. Instruct patients whose chronic systemic corticosteroids have been reduced or withdrawn to carry a warning card indicating the need for supplemental systemic corticosteroid during periods of stress or severe asthma attack. Inform not to use for acute asthma symptoms. Inform that medication may cause reduction in growth rate (pediatrics) and may unmask allergies. Advise to seek medical attention if exposed to chickenpox or measles, worsening of existing TB, infections or ocular herpes simplex. Avoid exposure to chickenpox or measles. Instruct to notify healthcare provider if symptoms worsen or do not improve or if adrenal insufficiency, paradoxical bronchospasm, or hypersensitivity reactions occur. May decrease bone mineral density. (Flexhaler) Instruct not to repeat inhalation even if they did not feel medication when inhaling and to rinse the mouth after inhalation. May need to wait (Flexhaler) ≥1-2 weeks or (Respules) ≥4-6 weeks for maximum benefit.

Administration: Oral inhalation route. After use, rinse mouth with water without swallowing. (Flexhaler) Prime prior to initial use and inhale deeply and

forcefully each time the device is used. Refer to PI for proper administration.
Storage: (Flexhaler): 20-25°C (68-77°F). Cover tightly. Store in a dry place.
(Respules): 20-25°C (68-77°F). Protect from light. Do not freeze. After aluminum foil opened, stable for 2 weeks. Before use, gently shake using circular
motion. Once opened, use promptly.

PURINETHOL   RX
mercaptopurine (Gate)

THERAPEUTIC CLASS: Purine analog

INDICATIONS: Maintenance therapy of acute lymphatic (lymphocytic, lymphoblastic) leukemia as part of a combination therapy.

DOSAGE: *Adults:* Maint: Usual: 1.5-2.5mg/kg/day as single dose. Renal/
Hepatic Impairment: Reduce dose. Concomitant Allopurinol: Reduce mer-
captopurine dose by 1/3-1/4 of usual dose. Thiopurine-S-methyltransferase
(TPMT) Deficiency: Consider dose reduction. Elderly: Start at the low end of
the dosing range.
Pediatrics: Maint: Usual: 1.5-2.5mg/kg/day as single dose. Renal/Hepatic
Impairment: Reduce dose. Concomitant Allopurinol: Reduce mercaptopurine
dose by 1/3-1/4 of usual dose. TPMT Deficiency: Consider dose reduction.

HOW SUPPLIED: Tab: 50mg* *scored

CONTRAINDICATIONS: Prior resistance to mercaptopurine.

WARNINGS/PRECAUTIONS: Not effective for prophylaxis or treatment
of CNS leukemia. Not effective in acute myelogenous leukemia, chronic
lymphatic leukemia, the lymphomas (including Hodgkins disease), or solid tumors. Risk of dose-related bone marrow suppression. Monitor weekly platelet
counts, Hgb, Hct, total WBC with differential; increase monitoring frequency
during induction phase. Life-threatening infections and bleeding reported;
d/c at first sign on unexpectedly abnormal large fall in any formed elements
of the blood not attributable to other drugs or disease process. Increased
sensitivity to myelosuppressive effects with TPMT gene deficiency; consider
TPMT testing with evidence of severe toxicity. Risk of hepatotoxicity, anorexia,
diarrhea, jaundice, and ascites (especially with >2.5mg/kg dose). Hepatic
encephalopathy reported. Monitor LFTs weekly initially, then monthly; monitor
more frequently with pre-existing liver disease. D/C with deterioration of liver
function, toxic hepatitis and biliary stasis. Risk of immunosuppression; may
manifest decreased cellular hypersensitivities and decreased allograft rejection. May cause fetal harm. Monitor patient clinical status and modify therapy
depending on response and manifestations of toxicity. Caution in elderly,
renal, and hepatic impairment.

ADVERSE REACTIONS: Bone marrow toxicity, hepatotoxicity, hyperuricemia, hyperuricosuria, intestinal ulceration, rash, hyperpigmentation, alopecia,
oligospermia.

INTERACTIONS: Severe toxicity with allopurinol; reduce mercaptopurine dose
to 1/3 to 1/4 of the usual dose. Reduce dose with other myelosuppressants.
Enhanced bone marrow suppression reported with trimethoprim-sulfamethoxazole. Cross-resistance with thioguanine. Increased risk of bone marrow
toxicity with coadministration of drugs that inhibit TPMT (eg, olsalazine,
mesalazine, sulphasalazine). Inhibition of the anticoagulant effect of warfarin
reported when used concomitantly with mercaptopurine. Perform careful
clinical and biochemical monitoring of hepatic function when concomitantly
using other hepatoxic agents. Hepatotoxicity reported with concomitant use
of doxorubicin. Subnormal induction of immunity to vaccines may occur with
concomitant use.

PREGNANCY: Category D, not for use in nursing.

MECHANISM OF ACTION: Purine analog; competes with hypoxanthine and
guanine for hypoxanthine-guanine phosphoribosyltransferase and is converted to thioinosinic acid, which then inhibits glutamine-5-phosphoribosylpyro-
phosphate amidotransferase of the de novo pathway for purine ribonucleotide
synthesis.

P

PHARMACOKINETICS: Absorption: Incomplete. **Distribution:** Plasma protein binding (19%). **Elimination:** (PO) Urine (46%). (IV) $T_{1/2}$=21 min (pediatric); 47 min (adult).

NURSING CONSIDERATIONS

Assessment: Assess for CNS leukemia, acute myelogenous leukemia, chronic lymphatic leukemia, the lymphomas (including Hodgkins disease), solid tumors, prior drug resistance, pre-existing liver/renal disease, TPMT gene defect, pregnancy/nursing status, and for possible drug interactions. Obtain baseline WBC with differential, Hgb/Hct, platelet count, serum transaminase levels, alkaline phosphatase levels, bilirubin levels, and renal function.

Monitoring: Monitor for signs/symptoms of bone marrow toxicity, hepatoxicity, and immunosuppression. Monitor WBC with differential, Hgb/Hct, and platelet count weekly; increase monitoring frequency during induction phase. Monitor serum transaminase levels, alkaline phosphatase, and bilirubin levels weekly at beginning of therapy and then at monthly intervals thereafter; monitor more frequently with pre-existing liver disease. Perform bone marrow exam for evaluation of marrow status. Consider performing TPMT testing if evidence of severe bone marrow toxicity develops. Monitor patient clinical status and need to modify therapy based on response and manifestations of toxicity.

Patient Counseling: Inform of major toxicities related to therapy (eg, myelosuppression, hepatotoxicity, GI toxicity). Advise women of childbearing potential to avoid becoming pregnant while on therapy. Take under medical supervision. Seek medical attention if symptoms of fever, sore throat, jaundice, N/V, signs of local infection, bleeding from any site, or if symptoms suggestive of anemia develop.

Administration: Oral route. **Storage:** 15-25°C (59-77°F) in a dry place.

PYLERA
tetracycline HCl - bismuth subcitrate potassium - metronidazole (Axcan Scandipharm)

RX

> Unnecessary use of the drug should be avoided. Reserved only for the treatment of *Helicobacter pylori* infection and duodenal ulcer disease.

THERAPEUTIC CLASS: *H.pylori* treatment combination

INDICATIONS: Treatment *Helicobacter pylori* (*H. pylori*) infection and duodenal ulcer disease (in combination with omeprazole).

DOSAGE: *Adults:* Usual: 3 caps qid, after meals and at bedtime. Take with omeprazole 20mg bid after morning and evening meals for 10 days.

HOW SUPPLIED: Cap: (Bismuth Subcitrate Potassium-Metronidazole-Tetracycline HCl) 140mg-125mg-125mg [120].

CONTRAINDICATIONS: Pregnancy, nursing women, pediatric patients, and patients with renal or hepatic impairment.

WARNINGS/PRECAUTIONS: (Bismuth) Neurotoxicity (rare) associated with excessive doses reported. May interfere with x-ray diagnostics of the GI tract. (Metronidazole) Convulsive seizures and peripheral neuropathy reported. D/C if abnormal neurologic signs appear. Caution with CNS diseases, evidence or history of blood dyscrasia. Known or previously unrecognized candidiasis may present more prominent symptoms and requires treatment with an antifungal agent. (Tetracycline) May cause permanent discoloration (yellow-gray-brown) of the teeth during tooth development (last half of pregnancy, infancy, and childhood to the age of 8 yrs). Enamel hypoplasia reported; avoid in patients with enamel hypoplasia. Photosensitivity manifested by an exaggerated sunburn reaction, reported; d/c if skin erythema occurs. May increase blood urea nitrogen (BUN). Higher serum tetracycline levels may lead to azotemia, hyperphosphatemia, and acidosis in patients with renal impairment. May cause overgrowth of non-susceptible organisms, including fungi; d/c and appropriate therapy should be instituted. Pseudotumor cerebri (benign intracranial hypertension) reported.

ADVERSE REACTIONS: Darkening of the tongue and/or black stools, diarrhea, dyspepsia, abdominal pain, nausea, headache, flu syndrome, taste perversion, asthenia, vaginitis, dizziness, pain, infection, pharyngitis.

INTERACTIONS: (Metronidazole) Increase lithium levels and signs of lithium toxicity with high doses of lithium and short term therapy. Avoid alcoholic beverages for at least 1 day during therapy. Psychotic reactions reported in alcoholic patients when coadministered with disulfiram. May potentiate anticoagulant effect of warfarin and other oral coumarin anticoagulant. Inhibitors of liver enzymes (eg, cimetidine) may decrease microsomal liver enzyme activity, and may prolong half-life and decrease plasma clearance. Inducers of liver enzymes (eg, phenytoin or phenobarbital) may accelerate elimination and reduce plasma concentration. (Tetracycline) Fatal renal toxicity reported when coadministered with methoxyflurane. Concomitant use of oral contraceptives may become less effective and breakthrough bleeding reported. Anticoagulants may depress plasma prothrombin activity; monitor clotting times periodically and make appropriate dosage adjustment to anticoagulants. May interfere with bactericidal effects of penicillin; avoid coadministration. Antacids containing aluminum, calcium, or magnesium; preparations containing iron, zinc, or sodium bicarbonate; or milk or dairy products may impair absorption. Bismuth may reduce systemic absorption.

PREGNANCY: Category D, not for use in nursing.

MECHANISM OF ACTION: Antimicrobial agent. (Bismuth) Antibacterial action not well understood. (Metronidazole) Metabolized through reductive pathways into reactive intermediates that have cytotoxic action. (Tetracycline HCl) Interacts with 30S subunit of the bacterial ribosome and inhibits protein synthesis.

PHARMACOKINETICS: Absorption: Bismuth: AUC=56.5ng(hr)/mL, C_{max}=16.7ng/mL. Metronidazole: AUC= 84413ng(hr)/mL, C_{max}=8666.3ng/mL. Tetracycline: AUC=9987ng(hr)/mL, C_{max}=773.8ng/mL. **Distribution:** Bismuth: Orally absorbed bismuth is distributed throughout the entire body; plasma protein binding (90%). Metronidazole: Plasma protein binding (<20%); appears in CSF, saliva and breast milk in concentrations similar to the plasma. Tetracycline: Distributed into most body tissues and fluids. **Metabolism:** Metronidazole: Side chain oxidation and glucuronide conjugation. **Elimination:** Bismuth: $T_{1/2}$=5 days in blood and urine, elimination of bismuth is primarily through urinary biliary routes. Metronidazole: $T_{1/2}$=8 hrs, urine (60-80%), fecal (6-15%, 20% unchanged). Tetracycline: $T_{1/2}$=6-11 hrs, concentrated by the liver in the bile and excreted in the urine and feces in a biologically active form.

NURSING CONSIDERATIONS

Assessment: Assess for history of blood dyscrasia, known or previously unrecognized candidiasis, renal function, LFTs, BUN levels, pregnancy/nursing status, and possible drug interactions.

Monitoring: Monitor for BUN levels, renal/hepatic impairment, lithium levels in patients taking lithium, leucopenia, black stool, abnormal neurologic signs, skin erythema, candidiasis, photosensitivity, neuropathy, convulsive seizures, neurotoxicity, enamel hypoplasia, azotemia, hyperphosphatemia, and acidosis. Monitor for occult blood in stool if indicated.

Patient Counseling: Swallow capsules whole with full glass of water espically at bedtime to reduce the risk of esophagel irritation and ulceration. Co-administration with oral contraceptives may render birth control less effective; advise to use a different or additional form of contraception. Notify a physician immediately if pregnant/intend to become pregnant, or breast-feeding. Avoid exposure to sun or sun lamps. Avoid alcoholic beverages. Counsel about temporary and harmless darkening of the tongue and/or black stool. Stool darkening should not be confused with melena. Advise not to take double doses; missed doses may be made up by continuing normal dosing schedule until medication is gone.

Administration: Oral route. Swallow whole with a full glass of water (8 oz.). **Storage:** 20-25°C (68-77°F).

QUESTRAN
RX

cholestyramine (Par)

OTHER BRAND NAMES: Questran Light (Par)

THERAPEUTIC CLASS: Bile acid sequestrant

INDICATIONS: Adjunct to reduce elevated cholesterol in primary hypercholesterolemia not responding to diet or to reduce LDL in hypertriglyceridemia. Relief of pruritus associated with partial biliary obstruction.

DOSAGE: *Adults:* Initial: 1 pkt or scoopful qd or bid. Maint: 2-4 pkts or scoopfuls/day, given bid. Titrate: Adjust at no less than 4 week intervals. Max: 6 pkts/day or 6 scoopfuls/day. May also give as 1-6 doses/day. Mix with fluid or highly fluid food.
Pediatrics: Usual: 240mg/kg/day of anhydrous cholestyramine resin in 2-3 divided doses. Max: 8g/day.

HOW SUPPLIED: Powder: 4g/pkt [60ˢ, 378g], (Light) 4g/scoopful [60ˢ, 268g]

CONTRAINDICATIONS: Complete biliary obstruction.

WARNINGS/PRECAUTIONS: May produce hyperchloremic acidosis with prolonged use. Caution in renal insufficiency and volume depletion. Chronic use may produce or worsen constipation. Avoid constipation with symptomatic CAD. May increase bleeding tendency due to vitamin K deficiency. Serum or red cell folate reduced with chronic use. Constipation may aggravate hemorrhoids. Light formulation contains phenylalanine.

ADVERSE REACTIONS: Constipation, heartburn, N/V, abdominal pain, flatulence, diarrhea, anorexia, osteoporosis, rash, hyperchloremic acidosis (children), vitamin A and D deficiency, steatorrhea, hypoprothrombinemia (vitamin K deficiency).

INTERACTIONS: May interfere with absorption of fat-soluble vitamins (A, D, E, K), drugs that undergo enterohepatic circulation, and oral phosphate supplements. Take concomitant drugs 1hr before or 4-6 hrs after. Additive effects with HMG-CoA reductase inhibitors and nicotinic acid. Caution with spironolactone. May reduce or delay absorption of phenylbutazone, warfarin, thiazide diuretics, propranolol, tetracycline, penicillin G, phenobarbital, thyroid and thyroxine agents, estrogens, progestins, digitalis.

PREGNANCY: Category C, caution in nursing.

MECHANISM OF ACTION: Bile acid sequestrant; absorbs and combines with bile acids in intestine to form insoluble complex excreted in the feces, resulting in partial removal of bile acids from enterohepatic circulation by preventing their absorption. This leads to increased oxidation of cholesterol to bile acids and decreased plasma LDL and serum cholesterol levels.

PHARMACOKINETICS: Elimination: Feces.

NURSING CONSIDERATIONS

Assessment: Prior to initiation, assess secondary causes of hypercholesterolemia (eg, poorly controlled diabetes mellitus, hypothyroidism, nephrotic syndrome, dysproteinemias, obstructive liver disease, other drug therapy, alcoholism), presence of biliary obstruction, pregnancy/nursing status, and possible drug interactions. Obtain baseline serum, cholesterol, and TG levels.

Monitoring: Monitor for signs/symptoms of increased bleeding tendencies (vitamin K deficiency), hyperchloremic acidosis, and worsening of pre-existing constipation. Monitor serum cholesterol and TGs periodically.

Patient Counseling: Advise to drink plenty of fluids and to mix each 9g dose of Questran in at least 2-6 oz. of fluid or each 6.4g dose of Questran Light in at least 4-6 oz. of fluid. Instruct not to sip or hold suspension in mouth for prolonged periods; may lead to changes on surface of teeth (eg, discoloration, erosion of enamel, or decay). Advise to maintain good oral hygiene.

Administration: Oral route. **Storage:** Room temperature.

QUINIDINE GLUCONATE INJECTION   RX
quinidine gluconate (Various)

THERAPEUTIC CLASS: Class IA antiarrhythmic/schizonticide antimalarial

INDICATIONS: Treatment of life-threatening *Plasmodium falciparum* malaria. Conversion of atrial fibrillation/flutter (A-Fib/Flutter) to normal sinus rhythm. Treatment of ventricular arrhythmias.

DOSAGE: *Adults:* Malaria: LD: 15mg/kg base (24mg/kg gluconate) over 4 hrs. Maint: After 8 hrs, 7.5mg/kg (12mg/kg gluconate) IV q8h for 7 days. Alternate: Initial: 6.25mg/kg base (10mg/kg gluconate) IV over 1-2 hrs. Maint: 12.5mcg/kg/min base (20mcg/kg/min gluconate) for 72hr. A-Fib/Flutter: 0.25mg/kg/min. Max: 5-10mg/kg. Consider alternate therapy if conversion to sinus rhythm not achieved. Ventricular Arrhythmia: Dosing regimens not adequately studied. Generally similar to A-Fib/Flutter. Renal/Hepatic Impairment or CHF: Reduce dose. Elderly: Start at low end of dosing range.
Pediatrics: Malaria: LD: 15mg/kg base (24mg/kg gluconate) over 4 hrs. Maint: After 8 hrs, 7.5mg/kg (12mg/kg gluconate) IV q8h for 7 days. Alternate: Initial: 6.25mg/kg base (10mg/kg gluconate) IV over 1-2 hrs. Maint: 12.5mcg/kg/min base (20mcg/kg/min gluconate) for 72hr.

HOW SUPPLIED: Inj: 80mg/mL [10mL]

CONTRAINDICATIONS: In the absence of a functional artificial pacemaker any cardiac rhythm dependent upon a junctional or idioventricular pacemaker (including with complete atrioventricular [AV] block), thrombocytopenic purpura with previous treatment, patients adversely affected by anticholinergics (eg, myasthenia gravis).

WARNINGS/PRECAUTIONS: Rapid infusion can cause peripheral vascular collapse and severe hypotension. May prolong QTc interval and may lead to torsades de pointes. Paradoxical increase in ventricular rate in A-Fib/Flutter. Caution in those at risk of complete AV block without implanted pacemakers, renal/hepatic dysfunction, elderly, and congestive heart failure (CHF). Physical/pharmacologic maneuvers to terminate paroxysmal supraventricular tachycardia may be ineffective. Exacerbated bradycardia in sick sinus syndrome.

ADVERSE REACTIONS: Upper GI distress, lightheadedness, fatigue, palpitations, weakness, visual problems, N/V, diarrhea, changes in sleeping habits, rash, headache, diarrhea, angina-like pain.

INTERACTIONS: Urine alkalinizers (eg, carbonic anhydrase inhibitors, sodium bicarbonate, thiazide diuretics) reduce renal elimination. CYP3A4 inducers (eg, phenobarbital, phenytoin, rifampin) may accelerate elimination. Verapamil, diltiazem decrease clearance. Caution with drugs metabolized by CYP2D6 (eg, mexiletine, phenothiazines, polycyclic antidepressants, codeine, hydrocodone) or by CYP3A4 (eg, nifedipine, felodipine, nicardipine, nimodipine). β-blockers may decrease clearance. May slow metabolism of nifedipine. Increases levels of digoxin, digitoxin, procainamide and haloperidol. Increased levels with ketoconazole, amiodarone, cimetidine. Potentiates warfarin, depolarizing and nondepolarizing neuromuscular blockers. Additive effects with anticholinergics, vasodilators, and negative inotropes. Antagonistic effects with cholinergics, vasoconstrictors, and positive inotropes.

PREGNANCY: Category C, not for use in nursing.

MECHANISM OF ACTION: Antimalarial schizonticide and antiarrhythmic agent with class Ia activity. Slows phase-0 depolarization by depressing the inward depolarizing Na^+ current, which slows conduction, prolongs effective refractory period, and reduces automaticity in the heart. Also has anticholinergic activity, negative ionotropic activity, and acts peripherally as an α-adrenergic antagonist.

PHARMACOKINETICS: Absorption: T_{max} =<2 hrs. **Distribution:** V_d=2-3L/kg; plasma protein binding (80-88%) in adults and older children, (50-70%) in pregnant women, infants and neonates; found in breast milk. **Metabolism:** Liver, via CYP3A4 pathway. 3-hydroxy-quinidine (3HQ); major metabolite.

Elimination: Urine (20% unchanged); $T_{1/2}$=6-8 hrs (adults), 3-4 hrs (pediatrics), and 12 hrs (3HQ).

NURSING CONSIDERATIONS

Assessment: Assess for structural heart disease, pre-existing long-QT syndrome, implanted pacemaker, history of torsades de pointes, other conduction defects, thrombocytopenic purpura, CHF, renal/hepatic dysfunction, myasthenia gravis, pregnancy/nursing status, and possible drug/diet interactions.

Monitoring: Monitor for exacerbated bradycardia, paradoxical increase in ventricular rate in atrial flutter/fibrillation, torsades de pointes, life-threatening ventricular arrhythmia, hypotension, ventricular extrasystoles/tachycardia/ flutter and ventricular fibrillation. Continuously/carefully monitor ECG and BP.

Patient Counseling: Inform about risks/benefits of drug and report any adverse reactions. Notify physician if pregnant/nursing. Avoid grapefruit juice.

Administration: IV route. **Storage:** 25°C (77°F); excursions permitted to 15-30°C (59-86°F).

QUIXIN RX
levofloxacin (Vistakon)

THERAPEUTIC CLASS: Fluoroquinolone

INDICATIONS: Treatment of bacterial conjunctivitis.

DOSAGE: *Adults:* Days 1-2: 1-2 drops q2h while awake, up to 8x/day. Days 3-7: 1-2 drops q4h while awake, up to qid.
Pediatrics: ≥1 yr: Days 1-2: 1-2 drops q2h while awake, up to 8x/day. Days 3-7: 1-2 drops q4h while awake, up to qid.

HOW SUPPLIED: Sol: 0.5% [5mL]

WARNINGS/PRECAUTIONS: D/C if hypersensitivity or superinfection occurs. Avoid contact lenses with conjunctivitis.

ADVERSE REACTIONS: Transient ocular burning, decreased vision, fever, foreign body sensation, headache, ocular pain, pharyngitis, photophobia.

INTERACTIONS: Systemic quinolone therapy may increase theophylline levels, interfere with caffeine metabolism, enhance warfarin effects, and elevate SrCr with cyclosporine.

PREGNANCY: Category C, caution in nursing.

MECHANISM OF ACTION: Fluoroquinolone; antibacterial active against broad spectrum of gram-positive and gram-negative organisms. Responsible for inhibition of bacterial topoisomerase IV and DNA gyrase, enzymes required for DNA replication, transcription, repair, and recombination.

PHARMACOKINETICS: **Absorption:** C_{max}=0.94ng/mL (single dose), 2.15ng/mL (multiple doses).

NURSING CONSIDERATIONS

Assessment: Assess for proper diagnosis (eg, slit-lamp biomicroscopy, fluorescein staining), hypersensitivity to other quinolones, possible drug interactions, and use in pregnant/nursing females.

Monitoring: Monitor for signs/symptoms of hypersensitivity or anaphylactic reaction (eg, cardiovascular collapse, loss of consciousness, angioedema, airway obstruction, dyspnea, uticaria, and itching). With prolonged therapy, monitor for overgrowth of nonsusceptible organisms (eg, fungi) and for development of superinfection. Perform periodic exam of patient using magnification (eg, slit-lamp biomicroscopy, fluorescein staining).

Patient Counseling: Instruct to avoid touching applicator tip to material from eye, fingers, or other sources to prevent contamination. Advise not to wear contact lenses if there are signs/symptoms of bacterial conjunctivitis. Instruct to d/c medication and contact physician if signs of hypersensitivity reaction (eg, rash) develop.

Administration: Ocular route. Do not inject subconjunctivally or introduce directly into anterior chamber of eye. **Storage:** 15-25°C (59-77°F). Keep out of reach of children.

QUTENZA RX
capsaicin (NeurogesX)

THERAPEUTIC CLASS: Analgesic

INDICATIONS: Management of neuropathic pain associated with postherpetic neuralgia.

DOSAGE: *Adults:* Apply single patch for 60 min; up to 4 patches may be applied. May repeat q3 months or as warranted by the return of pain (not more frequently than q3 months). Apply to dry, intact skin.

HOW SUPPLIED: Patch: 179mg [8%]

WARNINGS/PRECAUTIONS: Do not apply to the face, scalp, or broken skin. Do not use near eyes or mucous membranes. Aerosolization may occur upon rapid removal; remove gently and slowly by rolling the adhesive side inward. If irritation of eyes or airways occur, flush with cool water. Inhalation can result in coughing or sneezing; provide supportive medical care if SOB develops. If skin not intended to be treated comes into contact with patch, apply cleansing gel for 1 min, then wipe off with dry gauze and wash with soap and water. May experience substantial procedural pain; treat with local cooling (eg, ice pack) and/or analgesic medication, such as opioids; use of opioids may impair mental/physical abilities. HTN reported; monitor periodically. Increased risk of cardiovascular (CV) effects with unstable/poorly controlled HTN and history of CV/cerebrovascular events.

ADVERSE REACTIONS: Application-site erythema, pain, pruritus, papules, edema, nasopharyngitis, N/V.

PREGNANCY: Category B, safety not known in nursing.

MECHANISM OF ACTION: TRPV1 channel agonist; causes an initial enhanced stimulation of the TRPV1-expressing cutaneous nociceptors that may be associated with painful sensations followed by pain relief thought to be mediated by a reduction in TRPV1-expressing nociceptive nerve endings.

PHARMACOKINETICS: Absorption: C_{max}=4.6ng/mL.

NURSING CONSIDERATIONS

Assessment: Assess application site, unstable/poorly controlled HTN, history of CV/cerebrovascular events, and pregnancy/nursing status.

Monitoring: Monitor for any hypersensitivity reactions and monitor BP periodically during treatment. Monitor for occurrence of possible side effects.

Patient Counseling: Inform that exposure of the skin to the patch may result in transient erythema and burning sensation. Instruct not to touch patch; may produce burning and/or stinging sensation. Inform physician if pregnant/breastfeeding, side effects becomes severe or if eye/airway irritation occurs. Inform that treated area may be heat sensitive (eg, hot showers/bath, direct sunlight, vigorous exercise) for a few days after treatment. Inform patients that they may be given medications such as opioids that may impair mental/physical abilities. Inform that a small transient increase in BP may occur during and shortly after treatment. Instruct to inform physician if have experienced any recent CV event.

Administration: Topical route. May cut patch to match size/shape of treatment. Refer to PI for instructions for use. **Storage:** 20-25°C (68-77°F); excursions permitted between 15-30°C (59-86°F). Keep in sealed pouch immediately before use.

QVAR   RX
beclomethasone dipropionate (Teva)

THERAPEUTIC CLASS: Corticosteroid

INDICATIONS: Maintenance treatment of asthma as prophylactic therapy in patients ≥5 yrs. To reduce or eliminate the need for systemic corticosteroids in asthma patients requiring systemic corticosteroids.

DOSAGE: *Adults:* Previous Bronchodilator Only: 40-80mcg bid. Max: 320mcg bid. Previous Inhaled Corticosteroid (CS) Therapy: 40-160mcg bid. Max: 320mcg bid. Maintained on Systemic CS: May attempt gradual reduction of systemic CS dose after 1 week on inhaled therapy. Elderly: Start at lower end of dosing range.
Pediatrics: ≥12 yrs: Previous Bronchodilator Only: 40-80mcg bid. Max: 320mcg bid. Previous Inhaled Corticosteroid (CS) Therapy: 40-160mcg bid. Max: 320mcg bid. 5-11 yrs: Previous Bronchodilator Only or Inhaled CS Therapy: 40mcg bid. Max: 80mcg bid. Maintained on Systemic CS: May attempt gradual reduction of systemic CS dose after 1 week on inhaled therapy.

HOW SUPPLIED: MDI: 40 mcg/inh, 80 mcg/inh [7.3g]

CONTRAINDICATIONS: Primary treatment of status asthmaticus or other acute episodes of asthma where intensive measures are required.

WARNINGS/PRECAUTIONS: Deaths due to adrenal insufficiency have occurred with transfer from systemic corticosteroids to inhaled corticosteroids. Resume oral corticosteroids during stress or severe asthma attack. Risk of adrenal insufficiency and withdrawal symptoms when replacing systemic corticosteroids. May unmask allergic conditions previously suppressed by systemic steroid therapy. Caution with tuberculosis (TB), ocular herpes simplex, or untreated systemic bacterial, fungal, parasitic, or viral infections. May suppress growth in children. Exposure to chickenpox or measles requires prophylactic treatment. Not for rapid relief of bronchospasm. Rare cases of glaucoma, increased intraocular pressure (IOP), and cataracts reported.

ADVERSE REACTIONS: Headache, pharyngitis, upper respiratory tract infection, rhinitis, increased asthma symptoms, sinusitis, dysphonia, dysmenorrhea, coughing.

PREGNANCY: Category C, not for use in nursing.

MECHANISM OF ACTION: Corticosteroid; shown to have inhibitory effects on multiple cell types (mast cells, eosinophils, neutrophils, macrophages and lymphocytes) and mediators (histamine, eicosanoids, leukotrienes and cytokines) involved in inflammatory and asthmatic response.

PHARMACOKINETICS: Absorption: C_{max} = 88pg/mL, T_{max} = 0.5 hr. **Metabolism:** Liver (biotransformation), via CYP3A4. **Elimination:** Feces, urine (<10%); $T_{1/2}$= 2.8 hrs.

NURSING CONSIDERATIONS

Assessment: Assess for history of IOP, glaucoma, cataracts, concomitant diseases such as status asthmaticus, active or quiescent pulmonary TB, ocular herpes simplex, untreated systemic fungal, bacterial, parasitic or viral infections, pregnancy/nursing status, and possible drug interactions.

Monitoring: Monitor for localized oral infections, asthma instability (serial objective measures of airflow), body height in children, development of glaucoma, increased IOP, cataracts, adrenal insufficiency (eg, fatigue, weakness, N/V, hypotension), paradoxical bronchospasm, and hypersensitivity reactions.

Patient Counseling: Advise that drug is not intended for treatment of acute asthma (sudden symptoms of SOB or acute bronchospasm). Advise to rinse mouth after using inhaler. Inform that medication may cause reduction in growth rate (pediatrics) and may also unmask allergies (eg, rhinitis, conjunctivitis, eczema). Avoid exposure to chickenpox or measles. Advise to seek medical attention if exposed to chickenpox or measles, worsening of existing TB, infections, ocular herpes simplex, symptoms do not improve or worsen, during periods of stress or severe asthmatic attack, adrenal insufficiency (eg, fatigue, weakness, N/V, hypotension), paradoxical bronchospasm or hypersensitivity reactions occur. Inform that the drug should be used at regular intervals as directed and should not be stopped abruptly.

Administration: Oral inhalation. Refer to PI for directions for use. **Storage:** 25°C (77°F); excursions permitted to 15-30° (59-86°F). For optimal results, canister should be at room temperature when used. Keep out of reach of children.

RANEXA   RX
ranolazine (Gilead Sciences)

THERAPEUTIC CLASS: Miscellaneous antianginal

INDICATIONS: Treatment of chronic angina; may be used with β-blockers, nitrates, calcium channel blockers, antiplatelet therapy, lipid-lowering therapy, ACE inhibitors, and angiotensin receptor blockers.

DOSAGE: *Adults:* Initial: 500mg bid. Titrate: May increase to 1000mg bid, prn, based on clinical symptoms. Max: 1000mg bid. Concurrent Use With Diltiazem/Verapamil/Other Moderate CYP3A Inhibitors: Max: 500mg bid. Concurrent Use With P-gp Inhibitors: Down titrate dose based on clinical response. If a dose is missed, take the dose at the next scheduled time; do not double the dose. Elderly: Start at the low end of dosing range.

HOW SUPPLIED: Tab, Extended-Release: 500mg, 1000mg

CONTRAINDICATIONS: Strong CYP3A inhibitors (eg, ketoconazole, itraconazole, clarithromycin, nefazodone, nelfinavir, ritonavir, indinavir, saquinavir), CYP3A inducers (eg, rifampin, rifabutin, rifapentin, phenobarbital, phenytoin, carbamazepine, St. John's wort), and clinically significant hepatic impairment.

WARNINGS/PRECAUTIONS: May prolong QTc interval in a dose-related manner. Increased plasma concentrations in mild and moderate hepatic impairment. Caution with renal impairment, and in the elderly. Produces small reductions in HbA1c; should not be considered a treatment for diabetes.

ADVERSE REACTIONS: Dizziness, headache, constipation, nausea.

INTERACTIONS: See Contraindications. Limit dose with moderate CYP3A inhibitors (eg, fluconazole, diltiazem, verapamil, aprepitant, erythromycin, grapefruit juice or grapefruit-containing products). Lower dose based on clinical response with P-gp inhibitors (eg, cyclosporine). Reduce dose of drugs metabolized by CYP2D6 (eg, tricyclic depressants, antipsychotics). Avoid with drugs that may prolong the QTc interval. Increases plasma levels of simvastatin & digoxin. Increased plasma concentrations with immediate-release metoprolol, ketoconazole and paroxetine (a potent CYP2D6 inhibitor). Decreased plasma concentrations with rifampin.

PREGNANCY: Category C, not for use in nursing.

MECHANISM OF ACTION: Antianginal; mechanism not established. Can inhibit the cardiac late sodium current (I_{NA}). Relationship of this inhibition to angina symptoms is uncertain.

PHARMACOKINETICS: Absorption: Highly variable; C_{max}=2600ng/mL; T_{max}=2-5 hrs. **Distribution:** Plasma protein binding (62%). **Metabolism:** Intestine and liver (extensive), via CYP3A and CYP2D6. **Elimination:** Urine (75%), feces (25%), (<5% unchanged in urine and feces); $T_{1/2}$=7 hrs.

NURSING CONSIDERATIONS

Assessment: Assess for renal/hepatic impairment, QT prolongation, pregnancy/nursing status, and for possible drug interactions.

Monitoring: Monitor for ECG changes (eg, prolongation of the QTc interval). Monitor for HbA1c and SrCr levels.

Patient Counseling: Inform that medication will not abate an acute angina episode and is not for use with liver dysfunction. Inform about risks/benefits of drug and not to exceed recommended dose. Instruct to swallow tab whole; do not crush, break, or chew. Medication may be taken with or without meals. If a dose is missed, take the prescribed dose at the next scheduled time; do not double the next dose. Counsel that grapefruit juice and grapefruit products should be limited while on therapy. Therapy may cause dizziness and lightheadedness and therefore caution should be use while performing hazardous tasks (eg, operating machinery, driving). Notify physician if concurrently taking any other medications including OTCs or if experience fainting spells while on therapy. Inform about possible drug interactions. Inform physician of any personal or family history of QTc prolongation, congenital long QT syndrome. Therapy may produce ECG changes.

Administration: Oral route. Swallow whole; do not crush, break, or chew.
Storage: 25°C (77°F); excursions permitted to 15-30°C (59-86°F).

Rapaflo   RX
silodosin (Watson)

THERAPEUTIC CLASS: Alpha$_1$-antagonist

INDICATIONS: Treatment of the signs and symptoms of benign prostatic hyperplasia (BPH).

DOSAGE: *Adults:* 8mg qd with a meal. Moderate Renal Impairment (CrCl 30-50mL/min): 4mg qd with a meal.

HOW SUPPLIED: Cap: 4mg, 8mg

CONTRAINDICATIONS: Severe renal impairment (CrCl<30mL/min), severe hepatic impairment (Child-Pugh score ≥10), and concomitant administration with strong CYP3A4 inhibitors (eg, ketoconazole, clarithromycin, itraconazole, ritonavir).

WARNINGS/PRECAUTIONS: Postural hypotension and syncope may occur. May impair mental/physical abilities. Caution in patients with moderate renal impairment. Patients thought to have BPH should be examined prior to therapy to rule out prostate cancer. Intraoperative floppy iris syndrome observed during cataract surgery in some patients on α$_1$-blockers or previously treated with α$_1$-blockers.

ADVERSE REACTIONS: Retrograde ejaculation, dizziness, diarrhea, orthostatic hypotension, headache, nasopharyngitis, nasal congestion.

INTERACTIONS: See Contraindications. Concomitant administration with moderate CYP3A4 inhibitors (eg, diltiazem, erythromycin, verapamil) may increase plasma concentrations. Caution with antihypertensives; monitor for possible adverse events. Avoid with strong P-gp inhibitors (eg, cyclosporine) and other α-blockers. Concomitant use with PDE5 inhibitors can potentially cause symptomatic hypotension.

PREGNANCY: Category B, safety not known in nursing.

MECHANISM OF ACTION: α$_1$-antagonist; blocks α$_1$-adrenoreceptors, causing relaxation of smooth muscles in the bladder neck and prostate, resulting in improved urine flow and reduction in BPH symptoms.

PHARMACOKINETICS: Absorption: Absolute bioavailability (32%), C_{max}=61.6ng/mL, T_{max}=2.6 hrs, AUC_{ss}=373.4ng•hr/mL. **Distribution:** V_d=49.5L; plasma protein binding (97%). **Metabolism:** Via glucuronidation, alcohol and aldehyde dehydrogenase, CYP3A4; KMD-3213G (main metabolite), KMD-3293 (second major metabolite). **Elimination:** Urine (33.5%), feces (54.9%); $T_{1/2}$=13.3 hrs.

NURSING CONSIDERATIONS

Assessment: Assess for severe renal/hepatic impairment, prostate cancer, and possible drug interactions.

Monitoring: Monitor for signs/symptoms of postural hypotension and adverse reactions. Monitor for degree of renal impairment.

Patient Counseling: Instruct to take medication with a meal. Counsel about possible symptoms of postural hypotension (eg, dizziness); caution about driving, operating machinery, or performing hazardous tasks. Inform that orgasm with reduced or no semen does not pose a safety concern and is reversible when drug is d/c. Notify ophthalmologist about the use of silodosin before cataract surgery or other eye procedures, even if no longer taking silodosin.

Administration: Oral route. **Storage:** Store at 25°C (77°F); excursions permitted to 15°-30°C (59°-86°F). Protect from light and moisture. Keep out of reach of children.

RAPAMUNE   RX
sirolimus (Wyeth)

> Increased susceptibility to infection and possible development of lymphoma and other malignancies may result. Only physicians experienced in immunosuppressive therapy and management of renal transplant patients should use sirolimus. Avoid use in liver or lung transplant patients. Excess mortality and graft loss in combination with tacrolimus reported in liver transplant patients. Increased hepatic artery thrombosis (HAT) with cyclosporine or tacrolimus in liver transplant patients. Cases of bronchial anastomotic dehiscence, most fatal, reported in lung transplant patients.

THERAPEUTIC CLASS: Macrocyclic lactone immunosuppressant

INDICATIONS: Prophylaxis of organ rejection in patients ≥13 yrs receiving renal transplants.

DOSAGE: *Adults:* Take initial dose as soon as possible after transplantation. Take 4 hours after cyclosporine. Maintain on a dose for at least 7-14 days before further dose adjustment. Refer to full PI for maintenance dose adjustments. Max: 40mg/day. If estimated dose is >40mg/day due to LD, LD should be administered over 2 days. Monitor trough concentration at least 3-4 days after LD. Low-Moderate Immunologic Risk: Initial: Take with cyclosporine and corticosteroids. Give LD equivalent to 3x the maintenance dose. D/C cyclosporine 2-4 months after transplantation over 4-8 weeks. Adjust dose to maintain blood trough concentration within target range. High-Immunologic Risk: Take with cyclosporine and corticosteroids for the first 12 months. LD: Up to 15mg on Day 1 post-transplantation. Maint: 5mg/day beginning on Day 2. Obtain trough level between Days 5 and 7 and adjust daily dose thereafter. Mild-Moderate Hepatic Impairment: Reduce maintenance dose by one-third. Severe Hepatic Impairment: Reduce maintenance by one-half. Elderly: Start at low end of dosing range. Low Body Weight (<40kg): Adjust initial dose based on BSA to 1mg/m²/day with a LD of 3mg/m².

Pediatrics: ≥13 yrs: Take initial dose as soon as possible after transplantation. Take 4 hours after cyclosporine. Maintain on a dose for at least 7-14 days before further dose adjustment. Refer to full PI for maintenance dose adjustments. Max: 40mg/day. If estimated dose is >40mg/day due to LD, Administer LD over 2 days. Monitor trough concentration at least 3-4 days after LD. Low-Moderate Immunologic Risk: Initial: Take with cyclosporine and corticosteroids. Give LD equivalent to 3x the maintenance dose. D/C cyclosporine 2-4 months after transplantation over 4-8 weeks. Adjust dose to maintain blood trough concentration within target range. High-Immunologic Risk: Take with cyclosporine and corticosteroids for the first 12 months. LD: Up to 15mg on Day 1 post-transplantation. Maint: 5mg/day beginning on Day 2. Obtain trough level between Days 5 and 7 and adjust daily dose thereafter. Mild-Moderate Hepatic Impairment: Reduce maintenance dose by one-third. Severe Hepatic Impairment: Reduce maintenance by one-half. Low Body Weight (<40kg): Adjust initial dose based on BSA to 1mg/m²/day with a LD of 3mg/m².

HOW SUPPLIED: Sol: 1mg/mL [60mL]; Tab: 0.5mg, 1mg, 2mg

WARNINGS/PRECAUTIONS: Hypersensitivity reactions reported. Associated with the development of angioedema. Impaired wound healing, lymphocele, wound dehiscence and fluid accumulation (eg, peripheral edema, lymphedema, pleural effusion, ascites, pericardial effusions) reported. May increase cholesterol and TG that may require treatment. May delay recovery of renal function in patients with delayed graft function. Proteinuria commonly observed. Increased risk for opportunistic infections, including activation of latent viral infections (eg, BK virus-associated nephropathy). Progressive multifocal leukoencephalopathy (PML) reported. Reduce immunosuppression

R

if BK virus nephropathy is suspected or PML develops. Interstitial lung disease (pneumonitis, bronchiolitis obliterans organizing pneumonia [BOOP], pulmonary fibrosis) reported. Safety and efficacy of *de novo* use without cyclosporine is not established in renal transplant patients. Provide 1 year prophylaxis for *Pneumocystis carinii* pneumonia (PCP) and 3 months for cytomegalovirus (CMV) after transplant. Patient sample concentration values from different assays may not be interchangeable. Increased risk of skin cancer; limit exposure to sunlight and UV light. Caution in elderly.

ADVERSE REACTIONS: Peripheral edema, hypertriglyceridemia, HTN, constipation, hypercholesterolemia, increased creatinine, abdominal pain, diarrhea, headache, fever, UTI, anemia, nausea, arthralgia, pain.

INTERACTIONS: See Boxed Warning. CYP3A4 and P-gp inducers may decrease sirolimus concentrations. CYP3A4 and P-gp inhibitors may increase sirolimus concentrations. Avoid with strong inhibitors (eg, ketoconazole, voriconazole, itraconazole, erythromycin, telithromycin, clarithromycin) and strong inducers (eg, rifampin, rifabutin) of CYP3A4 and P-gp. May increase levels with cyclosporine, bromocriptine, cimetidine, cisapride, clotrimazole, danazol, diltiazem, fluconazole, HIV-protease inhibitors (eg, ritonavir, indinavir), metoclopramide, nicardipine, troleandomycin, and verapamil. May decrease levels with carbamazepine, phenobarbital, phenytoin, rifapentine, St. John's wort. May increase verapamil concentration. Vaccines may be less effective; avoid live vaccines. Increased risk of angioedema with ACE inhibitors. Increase risk of calcineurin inhibitor-induced hemolytic uremic syndrome/thrombotic thrombocytopenic purpura/thrombotic microangiography. Do not dilute or take with grapefruit juice. Caution with other nephrotoxic drugs (eg, aminoglycosides, amphotericin B). Monitor for possible development of rhabdomyolysis with HMG-CoA inhibitor and/or fibrate.

PREGNANCY: Category C, not for use in nursing.

MECHANISM OF ACTION: Immunosuppressant; inhibits T-lymphocyte activation and proliferation that occurs in response to antigenic and cytokine (interleukin [IL]-2, IL-4, and IL-15) stimulation by a mechanism distinct from that of other immunosuppressants. Also inhibits antibody production. Prolongs allograft survival and suppresses immune-mediated events (animal study).

PHARMACOKINETICS: Absorption: (Sol) AUC=194ng•hr/mL, C_{max}=14.4ng/mL, T_{max}=2.1hrs. (Tab) AUC=230ng•hr/mL, C_{max}=15ng/mL, T_{max}=3.5hrs. **Distribution:** V_d=12L/kg; plasma protein binding (92%). **Metabolism:** CYP3A4 and P-gp, intestinal wall, liver (extensive) via O-demethylation and hydroxylation; hydroxy, demethyl and hydroxymethyl (major metabolites). **Elimination:** Feces (91%), urine (2.2%); $T_{1/2}$=62 hrs. Different pharmacokinetic data resulted from concentration-controlled trials of pediatric renal transplants.

NURSING CONSIDERATIONS

Assessment: Assess for drug hypersensitivity, immunologic risk, hepatic impairment, body weight/body mass index, hyperlipidemia, infections, pregnancy/nursing status and possible drug interactions.

Monitoring: Monitor trough concentrations especially in patients with altered drug metabolism, who weigh <40kg, and with hepatic impairment, and when a change is made during concurrent administration of strong CYP3A4 inducers or inhibitors. Monitor for infections including opportunistic infections and activation of latent infections, development of PML, lymphoma/lymphoproliferative disease, other malignancies particularly of the skin, signs and symptoms of graft loss, hypersensitivity reactions, interstitial lung disease, and hyperlipidemia. Monitor urinary protein excretion, renal/hepatic functions, cholesterol, TG, and BP.

Patient Counseling: Instruct to avoid prolonged exposure to sunlight and UV light. Instruct not to take during pregnancy/nursing. Instruct to use effective contraception prior to, during therapy and 12 weeks after therapy has been stopped. Inform to take with/without food, but do not crush, chew, or split.

Administration: Oral route. (Tab) Do not crush, chew or split. (Sol) Refer to PI for proper dilution and administration. **Storage:** (Sol) 2-8°C (36-46°F), should be used within 1 month once opened. May store at temperatures up to

25°C (77°F) for a short period of time (eg, ≤15 days). (Tab) 20-25°C (68-77°F). Protect from light.

RAZADYNE ER   RX
galantamine hbr (Ortho-McNeil)

OTHER BRAND NAMES: Razadyne (Ortho-McNeil)

THERAPEUTIC CLASS: Acetylcholinesterase inhibitor

INDICATIONS: Treatment of mild to moderate dementia of the Alzheimer's type.

DOSAGE: *Adults:* (Sol, Tab) Initial: 4mg bid with am and pm meals. Titrate: Increase to 8mg bid after 4 weeks if tolerated, then increase to 12mg bid after 4 weeks if tolerated. Usual: 16-24mg/day. Max: 24mg/day. (Cap, ER) Initial: 8mg qd with am meal. Titrate: Increase to 16mg qd after 4 weeks, then increase to 24mg qd after 4 weeks if tolerated. Usual: 16-24mg/day. Max: 24mg/day. If therapy is interrupted, restart at lowest dose and increase to current dose. Moderate Renal/Hepatic Impairment (Child-Pugh: 7-9): Caution during dose titration. Max: 16mg/day. Avoid use with severe renal (CrCl <9mL/min) and severe hepatic impairment (Child-Pugh: 10-15).

HOW SUPPLIED: Sol: (Razadyne) 4mg/mL [100mL]; Tab: (Razadyne) 4mg, 8mg, 12mg. Cap, Extended-Release: (Razadyne ER) 8mg, 16mg, 24mg.

WARNINGS/PRECAUTIONS: Vagotonic effects; caution with supraventricular conduction disorder. May cause bradycardia and/or heart block. Caution with asthma or obstructive pulmonary disease. Monitor for active or occult GI bleeding and ulcers due to increased gastric acid secretion. Risk of generalized convulsions or bladder outflow obstruction. Ensure adequate fluid intake during treatment. Deaths reported with mild cognitive impairment.

ADVERSE REACTIONS: N/V, diarrhea, anorexia, weight loss, fatigue, dizziness, headache, depression, insomnia, abdominal pain, dyspepsia, UTI.

INTERACTIONS: Potential to interfere with anticholinergics. Synergistic effect with succinylcholine, other cholinesterase inhibitors, similar neuromuscular blockers, or cholinergic agonists (eg, bethanechol). Increased levels with cimetidine, ketoconazole, and paroxetine. Caution with drugs that slow HR due to vagotonic effects. Monitor for GI bleeding with NSAIDs.

PREGNANCY: Category B, not for use in nursing.

MECHANISM OF ACTION: Unknown; suspected to inhibit acetylcholinesterase-enhancing cholinergic function by increasing concentration of acetylcholine through reversible inhibition of its hydrolysis.

PHARMACOKINETICS: Absorption: Rapid and complete, bioavailability: (90%), T_{max}=1 hr. **Distribution:** V_d=175L; plasma protein binding (18%). **Metabolism:** Liver (glucuronidation). CYP450 enzymes: 2D6, 3A4. **Elimination:** Urine (unchanged); $T_{1/2}$=7 hrs.

NURSING CONSIDERATIONS

Assessment: Assess for drug hypersensitivity, cardiovascular conduction defects, GI bleeding, ulcer disease, severe asthma or COPD, renal/hepatic function, and possible drug interactions.

Monitoring: Monitor closely for symptoms of active or occult GI bleeding, and cardiac conduction defects. Monitor for common adverse events (eg, N/V, anorexia, dizziness, syncope).

Patient Counseling: Take drug preferably with morning and evening meals. Ensure adequate fluid intake during treatment. If therapy has been interrupted for several days or longer, physician must restart patient at lowest dose and gradually increase to current dose. Report any adverse effects.

Administration: Oral route. **Storage:** 25°C (77°F); excursions permitted to 15-30°C (59-86°F). Do not freeze.

REBETOL

RX

ribavirin (Schering)

> Not for monotherapy treatment of chronic hepatitis C virus infection. Primary toxicity is hemolytic anemia. Anemia associated with therapy may result in worsening of cardiac disease that may lead to fatal and nonfatal myocardial infarction (MI). Avoid with significant or unstable cardiac disease. Contraindicated in pregnancy and male partners of pregnant women. Extreme care must be taken to avoid pregnancy during therapy and for 6 months after completion of treatment. Use ≥2 reliable forms of contraception during therapy and for 6 months after d/c.

THERAPEUTIC CLASS: Nucleoside analogue

INDICATIONS: In combination with interferon alfa-2b (pegylated and nonpegylated) for treatment of chronic hepatitis C in patients ≥3 yrs with compensated liver disease.

DOSAGE: *Adults:* ≥18 yrs: Combination Therapy with Peg-Intron: 800-1400mg/day PO based on body weight. Interferon Alpha-naive: Genotype 1: Treat for 48 weeks. Genotype 2 and 3: Treat for 24 weeks. Prior Retreatment: Treat for 48 weeks, regardless of HCV genotype. Combination Therapy with Intron A: ≤75kg: 400mg qam and 600mg qpm. >75kg: 600mg qam and 600mg qpm. Interferon Alpha-naive: Treat for 24-48 weeks. Retreatment: Treat for 24 weeks. Individualize duration of treatment depending on baseline disease characteristics, response to therapy and tolerability of regimen. Elderly: Start at lower end of dosing range. Refer to PI for dose modifications and discontinuation with Peg-Intron and Intron A.
Pediatrics: ≥3 yrs: Combination Therapy with Peg-Intron/Intron A: <47kg: 15mg/kg/day divided into two doses. 47-59kg: 400mg qam and 400mg qpm. 60-73kg: 400mg qam and 600mg qpm. >73kg: 600mg qam and 600mg qpm. May use sol regardless of body weight. Interferon Alpha-naive: Genotype 1: Treat for 48 weeks. Genotype 2 or 3: Treat for 24 weeks. Remain on pediatric dosing if reached 18th birthday while receiving therapy. Refer to PI for dose modifications and discontinuation.

HOW SUPPLIED: Cap: 200mg; Sol: 40mg/mL [100mL]

CONTRAINDICATIONS: Women who are or may become pregnant, male partners of pregnant women, autoimmune hepatitis, hemoglobinopathies (eg, thalassemia major, sickle cell anemia), CrCl <50mL/min, concomitant use with didanosine.

WARNINGS/PRECAUTIONS: Patients with the following characteristics are less likely to benefit from retreatment after failing a course of therapy: previous nonresponse, previous pegylated interferon treatment, significant bridging fibrosis or cirrhosis, and genotype 1 infection. Suspend therapy in patients with signs and symptoms of pancreatitis and d/c therapy in patients with confirmed pancreatitis. Pulmonary symptoms, including dyspnea, pulmonary infiltrates, pneumonitis, pulmonary HTN and pneumonia reported; closely monitor or d/c therapy if appropriate. May induce or aggravate ophthalmologic disorders (eg, decrease or loss of vision or retinopathy). Perform eye examination in all patients prior to therapy, periodically in patients with pre-existing ophthalmologic disorders (eg, diabetic or hypertensive retinopathy), and if symptoms develop during therapy. D/C if new or worsening ophthalmologic disorders develop. Severe decreases in neutrophil and platelet counts, and hematologic, endocrine (eg, TSH), and hepatic abnormalities may occur; perform hematology and blood chemistry testing prior to therapy and periodically thereafter. Dental/periodontal disorders reported with combination therapy. Weight loss and growth inhibition reported with combination therapy in pediatric patients. Significant adverse reactions may be caused by ribavirin/intron A, or pegintron therapy, including severe depression and suicidal ideation, suppression of bone marrow function, autoimmune and infectious disorders and diabetes. Caution with pre-existing cardiac disease and in elderly. (Cap) Not used for treatment of HIV infection, adenovirus, RSV, parainfluenza, or influenza infections.

ADVERSE REACTIONS: Hemolytic anemia, headache, fatigue/asthenia, rigors, fever, N/V, anorexia, myalgia, arthralgia, insomnia, irritability, depression, neutropenia.

INTERACTIONS: See Contraindications. Closely monitor for toxicities (hepatic decompensation, anemia) with nucleoside reverse transcriptase inhibitors (NRTIs); d/c NRTI, reduce dose or d/c interferon, ribavirin or both with worsening toxicities. Caution with lamivudine, stavudine and zidovudine. Induce severe pancytopenia and increase risk of myelotoxicity with azathioprine.

PREGNANCY: Category X, not for use in nursing.

MECHANISM OF ACTION: Nucleoside analogue; not established. Has direct antiviral activity in tissue culture against many RNA viruses; increases mutation frequency in the genomes of several viruses and ribavirin triphosphate inhibits HCV polymerase in a biochemical reaction.

PHARMACOKINETICS: Absorption: Rapid and extensive; (Cap) C_{max}=782ng/mL, T_{max}=1.7 hrs, AUC=13400ng•h/mL; absolute bioavailability (64%). (Sol) C_{max}=872ng/mL, T_{max}=1 hr, AUC=14098ng•h/mL. **Distribution:** (Cap) V_d=2825L. **Metabolism:** Nucleated cells (phosphorylation); deribosylation and amide hydrolysis. **Elimination:** Urine (61%), feces (12%). (Cap) $T_{1/2}$=43.6 hrs.

NURSING CONSIDERATIONS

Assessment: Assess for history of hemoglobinopathy (eg, thalassemia major, sickle-cell anemia), depression, hepatic/renal dysfunction, autoimmune hepatitis, autoimmune disorders, infections, pregnancy status (including female partners of male patients), nursing status, pre-existing ophthalmologic disorders, cardiac disease, and possible drug interactions. Prior to initiation, conduct pregnancy test, hematologic tests (CBC with differential, Hct, Hgb, neutrophil and platelet count), blood chemistries (LFTs, TSH), ECG, eye examination and renal function tests. Confirm use of ≥2 reliable forms of effective contraception.

Monitoring: Monitor CBC, LFTs, TSH, platelet and neutrophil count, ECG and HCV-RNA periodically. Monitor height and weight in pediatrics. Obtain Hct and Hgb (Week 2 and 4, more if needed). Perform pregnancy test monthly and 6 months after d/c of therapy (including female partners of male patients). Monitor the use of effective contraception during therapy and for 6 months after therapy. Schedule regular dental exams. Perform periodic ophthalmologic exams in patients with pre-existing ophthalmologic disorders. Monitor for anemia, worsening of cardiac disease, MI, pancreatitis, renal/hepatic dysfunction, cardiovascular deterioration, pulmonary impairment, new/worsening ophthalmologic disorders, dental/periodontal disorders, suicidal ideation, depression, bone marrow suppression, autoimmune and infectious disorders, diabetes and other adverse reactions. Monitor patients >50 yrs and those with impaired renal function with respect to development of anemia.

Patient Counseling: Counsel risk/benefits associated with treatment. Instruct to take with food and keep well hydrated; do not open, break or crush capsules before swallowing. Counsel that if dose is missed, take as soon as possible during same day; do not double dose. Inform of pregnancy risks. Use ≥2 forms of contraception during therapy and 6 months after d/c of therapy (including female partners of male patients). Advise to have a regular examination to reduce damage to teeth and oral membranes. Advise that laboratory evaluation are required prior to starting therapy and periodically thereafter. Seek medical attention if signs/symptoms of pancreatitis, hepatic dysfunction, depression (suicidal ideation), anemia, cardiac deterioration or pulmonary impairment occur.

Administration: Oral route. (Cap) Do not open, crush or break. **Storage:** Cap: 25°C (77°F); excursions permitted to 15-30°C (59-86°F). Sol: 2-8°C (36-46°F) or 25°C (77°F); excursions permitted to 15-30°C (59-86°F).

Rebif   RX
interferon beta-1a (EMD Serono)

THERAPEUTIC CLASS: Biological response modifier

INDICATIONS: Treatment of patients with relapsing forms of multiple sclerosis (MS).

DOSAGE: *Adults:* Initial: 20% of prescribed dose SQ 3x/week. Titrate: Increase over a 4-week period to either 22mcg or 44mcg SQ 3x/week. Refer to PI for full schedule for patient titration. Leukopenia/Elevated LFTs: Reduce dose until toxicity resolves. Administer dose at the same time every day (late afternoon, or evening) on the same 3 days/week at least 48 hrs apart.

HOW SUPPLIED: Inj: 22mcg, 44mcg; Titration Pack: 8.8mcg and 22mcg

WARNINGS/PRECAUTIONS: Caution with depression; increased frequency of depression and suicide reported; d/c if develops. Severe hepatic injury including hepatic failure and asymptomatic elevation of hepatic transaminases reported; reduce dose if serum SGPT >5X ULN. D/C if jaundice or other symptoms of liver dysfunction appear. Caution with active liver disease, alcohol abuse, increased serum SGPT (>2.5X ULN) or history of significant hepatic disease. Contains albumin; theoretical risk of viral disease transmission. Anaphylaxis reported; allergic reactions, some severe, have occurred after prolonged use. Seizures, leukopenia and new or worsening thyroid abnormalities reported; monitor regularly for these conditions.

ADVERSE REACTIONS: Injection-site disorders, influenza-like symptoms (eg, headache, fatigue, fever, rigors, chest pain, back pain, myalgia), abdominal pain, depression, elevation of liver enzymes, hematologic abnormalities.

INTERACTIONS: May cause neutropenia and lymphopenia with myelosuppressive agents. Potential for hepatic injury with hepatotoxic agents or new agents added to the regimen.

PREGNANCY: Category C, caution in nursing.

MECHANISM OF ACTION: Biological response modifier; mechanism in MS not established. Binding of interferon β to its receptors initiates a complex cascade of intracellular events that leads to the expression of numerous interferon-induced gene products and markers, including 2, 5-oligoadenylate synthetase, β 2-microglobulin and neopterin, which may mediate some of the biological activities.

PHARMACOKINETICS: Absorption: C_{max}=5.1 IU/mL, T_{max}=16 hrs, AUC_{0-96}=294 IU·h/mL. **Elimination:** $T_{1/2}$=69 hrs.

NURSING CONSIDERATIONS

Assessment: Assess for history of drug hypersensitivity, depression, liver disease, alcohol abuse, thyroid dysfunction, preexisting seizure disorder, myelosuppression, pregnancy/nursing status, and possible drug interactions.

Monitoring: Monitor blood cell counts and LFTs at 1, 3, and 6 months after initiation, then periodically. Monitor thyroid function tests every 6 months or as clinically indicated. Monitor depression, suicidal ideation, suicide attempts, hepatic dysfunction, allergic reaction, and seizures.

Patient Counseling: Instruct not to change dosage or schedule without consulting physician. Inform about risks/benefits of drug; report any adverse reactions. Notify if pregnant/nursing or planning to become pregnant; inform about the abortifacient potential of the drug. Instruct on aseptic technique when administering drug and on importance of proper syringe disposal. Inform of the importance of rotating injection sites.

Administration: SQ route. Rotate site of injection. **Storage:** 2-8°C (36-46°F). Do not freeze. If refrigerator is not available, store at or below 25°C (77°F) up to 30 days, away from heat and light.

Reclast   RX
zoledronic acid (Novartis)

THERAPEUTIC CLASS: Bisphosphonate

INDICATIONS: Treatment and prevention of osteoporosis in postmenopausal women. Treatment to increase bone mass in men with osteoporosis. Treatment and prevention of glucocorticoid-induced osteoporosis in men and women who are either initiating or continuing systemic glucocorticoids in a daily dosage equivalent to ≥7.5mg of prednisone and who are expected to remain on glucocorticoids for ≥12 months. Treatment of Paget's disease of bone in men and women.

DOSAGE: *Adults:* IV infusion over ≥15 min at a constant rate. Treatment of Osteoporosis (Men/Postmenopausal Women) and Treatment/Prevention of Glucocorticoid-Induced Osteoporosis: 5mg once a year. Paget's disease: 5mg. Prevention of Osteoporosis (Postmenopausal Women): 5mg once q2 yrs. CrCl ≥35mL/min: 5mg. Recommended Intake of Calcium in Osteoporosis: ≥1200mg/day. Recommended Intake of Vitamin D in Osteoporosis: 800-1000 IU/day. Recommended Intake of Calcium in Paget's Disease: 1500mg/day in 2-3 divided doses, particularly in 2 weeks following zoledronic acid administration. Recommended Intake of Vitamin D in Paget's Disease: 800 IU/day, particularly in 2 weeks following zoledronic acid administration.

HOW SUPPLIED: Sol: 5mg/100mL

CONTRAINDICATIONS: Hypocalcemia.

WARNINGS/PRECAUTIONS: Contains same active ingredient as Zometa; do not treat concomitantly. Treat pre-existing hypocalcemia and disturbances of mineral metabolism (eg, hypoparathyroidism, thyroid/parathyroid surgery, malabsorption syndromes, excision of small intestine) prior to treatment. Risk of hypocalcemia in Paget's disease. Avoid with severe renal impairment (CrCl <35mL/min). Renal impairment may occur, especially with pre-existing renal compromise or other risk factors (eg, severe dehydration); use with caution with other nephrotoxic drugs. Osteonecrosis of the jaw (ONJ) reported; perform routine oral exam prior to treatment and avoid invasive dental procedures if possible. Atypical, low-energy, or low trauma fractures of the femoral shaft reported; evaluate patients with thigh/groin pain to rule out incomplete femur fracture and consider interruption of therapy. Avoid pregnancy; may cause fetal harm. Musculoskeletal (bone, joint, muscle) pain reported; d/c if severe symptoms develop. Caution with aspirin (ASA)-sensitivity; may cause bronchoconstriction. Caution in elderly.

ADVERSE REACTIONS: Pain, chills, dizziness, osteoarthritis, fatigue, hypocalcemia, headache, HTN, influenza-like illness, myalgia, arthralgia, pyrexia, N/V, acute phase reaction, pain in extremity, eye inflammation.

INTERACTIONS: Caution with aminoglycosides; may have an additive effect to lower serum calcium levels for prolonged periods. Caution with loop diuretics; may increase risk of hypocalcemia. Caution with other nephrotoxic drugs (eg, NSAIDs) and diuretics. May increase risk of atypical femur fractures with glucocorticoids (eg, prednisone). Exposure to concomitant medications that are primarily renally excreted (eg, digoxin) may increase in patients with renal impairment.

PREGNANCY: Category D, not for use in nursing.

MECHANISM OF ACTION: Bisphosphonate; acts primarily on bone. Inhibits osteoclast-mediated bone resorption.

PHARMACOKINETICS: Distribution: Plasma protein binding (28% at 200ng/mL), (53% at 50ng/mL). **Elimination:** Urine (39% within 24 hrs); $T_{1/2}$=146 hrs.

NURSING CONSIDERATIONS

Assessment: Assess for hypocalcemia and disturbances of mineral metabolism, renal function, risk factors for developing renal impairment and ONJ, hypersensitivity, ASA sensitivity, pregnancy/nursing status, and possible drug interactions. Measure SrCr before each dose. Perform oral exam and consider appropriate preventive dentistry prior to treatment in patients with history of concomitant risk factors.

Monitoring: Monitor for signs and symptoms of hypocalcemia, acute phase reactions, ONJ, atypical femur fracture, musculoskeletal pain, bronchoconstriction, and other adverse events that may develop. Monitor renal function, serum calcium/mineral levels, and alkaline phosphatase.

Patient Counseling: Inform that Zometa contains same active ingredient and that concomitant use should be avoided. Inform about benefits and risks of therapy, and the importance of calcium and vitamin D supplementation. Notify physician if existing kidney problems, taking any other medications, unable to take calcium supplements, had surgery to remove some or all of parathyroid glands, had sections of intestine removed, and sensitive to ASA. Inform that drug may cause fetal harm; avoid becoming pregnant and breast-feeding. Advise on day of treatment to eat and drink normally (≥2 glasses of fluid, eg, water) within a few hours prior to infusion. Instruct to contact physician or dentist if persistent pain and/or non-healing sore of the mouth or jaw, fever, flu-like symptoms, myalgia, arthralgia, headache, bone/joint/muscle pain, and other adverse events develop.

Administration: IV route. Rehydrate prior to administration. Administration of acetaminophen following zoledronic acid may reduce incidence of acute phase reaction symptoms. Do not allow to come in contact with any calcium or other divalent cation-containing solutions. Administer as a single IV solution through a separate vented infusion line. Inspect visually for particulate matter and discoloration prior to administration. **Storage:** 25°C (77°F); excursions permitted to 15-30°C (59-86°F). Stable for 24 hrs at 2-8°C (36-46°F) after opening. If refrigerated, allow to reach room temperature before administration.

RECOMBIVAX HB   RX
hepatitis B (recombinant) (Merck)

OTHER BRAND NAMES: Recombivax HB Adult (Merck) - Recombivax HB Dialysis (Merck) - Recombivax HB Pediatric/Adolescent (Merck)

THERAPEUTIC CLASS: Vaccine

INDICATIONS: Vaccination against infection caused by all known subtypes of hepatitis B virus.

DOSAGE: *Adults:* ≥20 yrs: 3-Dose Regimen: 10mcg IM into deltoid muscle at 0, 1, 6 months. May be given SQ if at risk of hemorrhage. Predialysis/Dialysis (Dialysis Formulation): 40mcg at 0, 1, 6 months; consider booster/revaccination if anti-HBs level <10 mIU/mL 1-2 months after 3rd dose. Known/Presumed Exposure to HBsAg: Follow 3-Dose Regimen giving 1st dose within 7 days of exposure. Give 0.06mL/kg HBIG immediately after exposure or within 24 hrs IM at a separate site.
Pediatrics: Give IM into anterolateral thigh in infants/young children. May be given SQ if at risk of hemorrhage. 0-19 yrs: 3-Dose Regimen (Pediatric/Adolescent Formulation) 5mcg at 0, 1, 6 months. 11-15 yrs: 2-Dose Regimen (Adult Formulation): 10mcg at 0 and 4-6 months. Infants Born to HBsAg Positive/Unknown Status Mothers: Follow 3-Dose Regimen above. Give 0.5mL HBIG immediately in the opposite anterolateral thigh if the mother is determined to be HBsAg positive within 7 days of delivery.

HOW SUPPLIED: Inj: (Pediatric/Adolescent) 5mcg/0.5mL, (Adult) 10mcg/mL, (Dialysis) 40mcg/mL

CONTRAINDICATIONS: Yeast hypersensitivity.

WARNINGS/PRECAUTIONS: Do not continue therapy if hypersensitivity occurs after inj. May not prevent hepatitis B with unrecognized infection at time of vaccination. Epinephrine injection (1:1000) should be immediately available should an anaphylactoid reaction occur. May cause allergic reactions in latex-sensitive individuals; use with caution. Caution with severely compromised cardiopulmonary status and those where febrile or systemic reaction is a significant risk. Delay use with serious active infection (eg, febrile illness). Do not give intradermally or IV. Avoid injection of a blood vessel.

ADVERSE REACTIONS: Irritability, fever, diarrhea, fatigue/weakness, diminished appetite, rhinitis, inj-site reactions.

PREGNANCY: Category C, caution in nursing.

MECHANISM OF ACTION: Vaccine; may produce immune response for protection against infection caused by all known subtypes of hepatitis B virus.

NURSING CONSIDERATIONS

Assessment: Assess current health status, medical history, previous vaccination history, previous vaccine-related adverse reactions, hypersensitivity to yeast or any component of the vaccine, pregnancy/nursing status, and possible drug interactions.

Monitoring: Monitor for signs/symptoms of hypersensitivity reactions, inj-site reactions, and systemic reactions. Perform annual antibody testing in hemodialysis patients to assess the need for booster doses.

Patient Counseling: Inform about benefits and risks of therapy and the importance of completing the immunization series. Inform physician if inj-site reactions and any severe adverse reactions occur.

Administration: IM route. Shake well before use. Inspect for particulate matter and discoloration prior to administration. **Storage:** 2-8°C (36-46°F). Do not freeze.

REFLUDAN RX
lepirudin (Bayer Healthcare)

THERAPEUTIC CLASS: Thrombin inhibitor

INDICATIONS: Anticoagulant for heparin-induced thrombocytopenia (HIT) and associated thromboembolic disease.

DOSAGE: *Adults:* LD: 0.4mg/kg (max 44mg) IV over 15-20 seconds. Initial: 0.15mg/kg/hr (max 16.5mg/hr) continuous infusion for 2-10 days. Adjust dose based on aPTT. If aPTT is above target range, stop infusion for 2 hrs and restart at 50% of previous rate. Check aPTT 4 hrs later. If aPTT is below target range, increase rate in steps of 20% and check aPTT 4 hrs later. Do not exceed 0.21mg/kg/hr. Renal Impairment: LD: 0.2mg/kg. Initial: CrCl 45-60 mL/min: 0.075mg/kg/hr. CrCl 30-44mL/min: 0.045mg/kg/hr. CrCl 15-29 mL/min: 0.0225mg/kg/hr. CrCl <15mL/min/Hemodialysis: Avoid or stop infusion. Concomitant Thrombolytic Therapy: LD: 0.2mg/kg. Initial: 0.1mg/kg/hr.

HOW SUPPLIED: Inj: 50mg

WARNINGS/PRECAUTIONS: Risk of bleeding. Weigh risks/benefits with recent puncture of large vessels or organ biopsy, anomaly of vessels or organs, recent cerebrovascular accident (CVA), stroke, intracerebral surgery or other neuraxial procedures, severe uncontrolled HTN, bacterial endocarditis, advanced renal impairment, hemorrhagic diathesis, recent major surgery or bleeding. Avoid with baseline aPTT ≥2.5. Monitor aPTT 4 hrs after initiating infusion and at least once daily. Liver injury may enhance anticoagulant effects. Antihirudin antibodies reported; may increase anticoagulant effects.

ADVERSE REACTIONS: Hemorrhagic events (eg, bleeding, anemia, hematoma, hematuria, epistaxis, hemothorax), fever, liver dysfunction, pneumonia, sepsis, allergic skin reactions, multiorgan failure.

INTERACTIONS: Thrombolytics increase risk of life-threatening intracranial bleeding or other bleeding complications and may enhance the effect on aPTT prolongation. Increased risk of bleeding with coumarin derivatives and other drugs that affect platelet function.

PREGNANCY: Category B, not for use in nursing.

MECHANISM OF ACTION: Thrombin inhibitor; binds to thrombin and thereby blocks its thrombogenic activity.

PHARMACOKINETICS: Absorption: C_{max}=1500ng/mL. **Distribution:** V_d=12.2L. **Metabolism:** Catabolic hydrolysis. **Elimination:** Urine(48%); $T_{1/2}$=1.3 hrs.

NURSING CONSIDERATIONS

Assessment: Assess for bleeding risk (eg, recent puncture of large vessels, recent cerebrovascular accident, severe uncontrolled HTN, bacterial endocarditis, hemorrhagic diathesis), presence of hepatic/renal dysfunction, nursing status, and drug interactions. Obtain baseline aPTT ratio.

Monitoring: Monitor for signs/symptoms of bleeding complications (eg, intracranial bleeding) and allergic reactions (eg, anaphylactic reactions). Monitor aPTT ratio 4 hrs after start of infusion and perform once daily thereafter during treatment.

Patient Counseling: Instruct to notify physician immediately if develop any type of allergic reaction (eg, anaphylaxis). Advise about increased risk of bleeding during therapy. Laboratory monitoring is needed during therapy.

Administration: IV route. Do not mix with other drugs. Reconstitute: 1) Use Sterile Water for Inj, USP; or 0.9% for NaCl Inj, USP. 2) For rapid, complete reconstitution, inject 1mL of diluent into the vial and shake it gently. 3) Further dilute to final concentration of 5mg/mL. Dilute using 0.9% NaCl Inj USP, or 5% Dextrose Inj USP. 4) Warm to room temperature prior to administration.
Storage: Unopened vials: 2-25°C (35.6-77°F). Reconstituted: Use immediately; will remain stable for 24 hrs at room temperature.

REGLAN
metoclopramide HCl (Alaven)

RX

> May cause tardive dyskinesia (TD); d/c if signs/symptoms of TD develop; avoid use for >12 weeks of therapy unless benefit outweighs risk.

OTHER BRAND NAMES: Reglan Injection (Baxter)

THERAPEUTIC CLASS: Dopamine antagonist/prokinetic

INDICATIONS: (PO) Short-term therapy (4-12 weeks) for adults with symptomatic, documented gastroesophageal reflux disease (GERD) in patients who fail to respond to conventional therapy. (Inj, PO) Relief of symptoms associated with acute and recurrent diabetic gastric stasis in adults. (Inj) Prevention of postoperative or chemotherapy induced N/V. Facilitates intubation of small bowel in adults and pediatric patients in whom the tube does not pass the pylorus with conventional maneuvers. Stimulates gastric emptying and intestinal transit of barium in cases where delayed emptying interferes with radiological examination of the stomach and/or small intestines.

DOSAGE: *Adults:* GERD: 10-15mg PO up to qid ≥30 min ac and hs. (Sol, Tab) Sensitive to Metoclopramide/Elderly: 5 mg/dose. Max: 12 weeks of therapy. Intermittent Symptoms: Up to 20mg as single dose prior to provoking situation. If esophageal lesions are present, 15mg qid. Diabetic Gastroparesis: 10mg PO up to qid 30 min ac and hs for 2-8 weeks. If severe, begin with IM or IV. May give 10mg IV slowly over 1-2 min. May need inj up to 10 days before symptoms subside, at which time PO administration may be instituted. Antiemetic: (Post-op) 10-20mg IM near end of surgery. (Chemotherapy-Induced) 1-2mg/kg IV infusion over a period of not <15 min, 30 min before chemotherapy then q2h for 2 doses, then q3h for 3 doses. Give 2mg/kg for highly emetogenic drugs for initial 2 doses. Small Bowel Intubation/Radiological Exam: 10mg by slow IV as single dose (undiluted) over 1-2 min. CrCl <40mL/min: 50% of normal dose. Elderly: Start at the low end of dosing range. *Pediatrics:* Small Bowel Intubation: Administer single dose (undiluted) by slow IV over 1-2 min. >14 yrs: 10 mg. 6-14 yrs: 2.5-5mg. <6 yrs: 0.1mg/kg. CrCl <40mL/min: 50% of normal dose.

HOW SUPPLIED: Inj: 5mg/mL; Sol (Generic): 5mg/5mL; Tab: 5mg, 10mg*
*scored

CONTRAINDICATIONS: When GI motility stimulation is dangerous (eg, perforation, mechanical obstruction, GI hemorrhage), pheochromocytoma, epilepsy, and concomitant drugs that cause extrapyramidal symptoms (EPS).

WARNINGS/PRECAUTIONS: Neuroleptic malignant syndrome (NMS) reported; d/c and institute intensive symptomatic treatment and medical monitoring if NMS occurs. May cause acute dystonic reactions. May cause Parkinsonian-like symptoms; more common within first 6 months after beginning treatment; generally subside within 2-3 months of d/c; caution in patients with pre-existing Parkinson's disease. Mental depression may occur; caution in patients with prior history of depression. Caution with HTN, renal impairment, and/or in elderly. Risk of developing fluid retention and volume overload, especially with cirrhosis or congestive heart failure (CHF); d/c if these occur. May increase risk of developing methemoglobinemia and/or sulfhemoglobinemia with NADH-cytochrome b_5 reductase deficiency. May experience withdrawal symptoms after d/c. (Inj) IV injections of undiluted metoclopramide should be made slowly, allowing 1-2 min for 10mg to prevent transient intense feeling of anxiety and restlessness. Diluted administration should be slow, over a period of ≥15 min.

ADVERSE REACTIONS: Tardive dyskinesia (TD), fatigue, restlessness, lassitude, drowsiness.

INTERACTIONS: See Contraindications. May decrease gastric absorption of some drugs (eg, digoxin) and increase intestinal absorption of others (eg, acetaminophen, tetracycline, levodopa, ethanol, and cyclosporine). Additive sedation with alcohol, sedatives, hypnotics, narcotics, or tranquilizers. Caution with MAOIs; catecholamines released in patients with HTN. GI motility effect antagonized by anticholinergics and narcotic analgesics. Insulin dose or timing of dose may need adjustment to prevent hypoglycemia. Rare cases of hepatotoxicity with drugs with hepatotoxic potential. Avoid treating methemoglobinemia with methylene blue in patients with G6PD deficiency. Inhibits the central and peripheral effects of apomorphine.

PREGNANCY: Category B, caution in nursing (Inj, Sol, Tab).

MECHANISM OF ACTION: Dopamine antagonist/promotility agent; mechanism not established, appears to sensitize tissues to the action of acetylcholine; stimulates motility of upper GI tract and accelerates gastric emptying and intestinal transit without stimulating gastric, biliary or pancreatic secretions; increases resting tone of lower esophageal sphincter. Antiemetic; antagonizes central and peripheral dopamine receptors, thereby blocking stimulation of chemoreceptor trigger zone.

PHARMACOKINETICS: Absorption: Rapid and well absorbed; (IV) absolute bioavailability (80%), (PO) T_{max}=1-2 hrs. IV administration in pediatrics resulted in different parameters. **Distribution:** Plasma protein binding (30%); V_d=3.5L/kg; found in breast milk. **Elimination:** (PO) Urine (85%); $T_{1/2}$=5-6 hrs.

NURSING CONSIDERATIONS

Assessment: Assess for conditions when GI motility stimulation is dangerous (eg, GI hemorrhage, mechanical obstruction or perforation), CHF, cirrhosis, pheochromocytoma, sensitivity or tolerance to the drug, history of depression, Parkinson's disease, HTN, NADH-cytochrome b_5 reductase and G6PD deficiency, renal impairment, diabetes mellitus (DM), epilepsy, pregnancy/nursing status, and possible drug interactions.

Monitoring: Monitor for signs/symptoms of depression, extrapyramidal symptoms (EPS), Parkinsonian-like symptoms, TD, NMS, HTN, fluid retention/volume overload, and hypersensitivity reactions. (PO) Monitor for withdrawal symptoms (eg, dizziness, nervousness, and/or headaches).

Patient Counseling: Inform that drug may impair mental and physical abilities; use caution while operating machinery/driving. Inform that sedation may be more pronounced in elderly. Advise to seek medical attention if experience symptoms of depression, EPS (eg, involuntary movements of limbs, facial grimacing, torticollis), TD (eg, involuntary movements of tongue, face, mouth), NMS (eg, hyperthermia, muscle rigidity, altered consciousness), HTN, fluid retention, volume overload, or hypersensitivity reactions. Counsel about possible adverse reactions and drug interactions.

Administration: Oral, IV/IM route. Inj: Inspect for particulates and discoloration prior to administration. For doses >10mg, dilute in 50mL of parenteral solution. Refer to PI for IV admixture compatibilities. **Storage:** Tab, Inj, Sol: 20-25°C (68-77°F). Inj: If diluted with NaCl, may be stored frozen for up to 4 weeks. Diluted solutions may be stored up to 48 hrs (without freezing) if protected from light. In normal light conditions, may be stored up to 24 hrs.

RELENZA   RX
zanamivir (GlaxoSmithKline)

THERAPEUTIC CLASS: Neuraminidase inhibitor

INDICATIONS: Treatment of uncomplicated acute illness due to influenza A and B virus in adults and pediatric patients (≥7 yrs) symptomatic for ≤2 days. Prophylaxis of influenza in adults and pediatric patients ≥5 yrs.

DOSAGE: *Adults:* Treatment: 2 inh (10mg) q12h for 5 days. Take 2 doses on 1st day ≥2 hrs apart, then 12 hrs apart on subsequent days. Prophylaxis: Administer at same time every day. Community Outbreaks: 2 inh (10mg) qd for 28 days. Household Setting: 2 inh (10mg) qd for 10 days.
Pediatrics: Treatment: ≥7 yrs: 2 inh (10mg) q12h for 5 days. Take 2 doses on 1st day ≥2 hrs apart, then 12 hrs apart on subsequent days. Prophylaxis: Administer at same time every day. Community Outbreaks: ≥12 yrs: 2 inh (10mg) qd for 28 days. Household Setting: ≥5 yrs: 2 inh (10mg) qd for 10 days.

HOW SUPPLIED: Powder, Inhalation: 5mg/inh [4 blisters]

CONTRAINDICATIONS: History of allergic reaction to lactose (contains milk proteins).

WARNINGS/PRECAUTIONS: Not a substitute for annual influenza vaccination. Not recommended for use with underlying airways disease (eg, asthma, chronic obstructive pulmonary disease [COPD]). Serious cases of bronchospasm reported; d/c if bronchospasm or decline in respiratory function develops. D/C and institute appropriate treatment if allergic reaction occurs. Postmarketing neuropsychiatric events (eg, delirium, abnormal behavior) reported; if neuropsychiatric symptoms occur, evaluate risks and benefits of continuing treatment. Not shown to prevent complications secondary to influenza-like symptoms or concurrent bacterial infections. Must not be made into an extemporaneous solution for administration by nebulization or mechanical ventilation. Administer only using the Diskhaler device provided; evaluate the ability of young children to use the delivery system. Not studied in high-risk underlying medical conditions.

ADVERSE REACTIONS: Bronchospasm, headache, diarrhea, nausea, sinusitis, cough, ear/nose/throat infections, nasal symptoms, throat/tonsil discomfort and pain, muscle pain, malaise, fatigue, viral respiratory infection.

INTERACTIONS: Avoid administration of live attenuated influenza vaccine within 2 weeks before or 48 hrs after; may interfere with replication of live vaccine virus.

PREGNANCY: Category C, caution in nursing.

MECHANISM OF ACTION: Neuraminidase inhibitor; inhibits influenza virus neuraminidase, affecting release of viral particles.

PHARMACOKINETICS: Absorption: Absolute bioavailability (4-17%); C_{max}=17-142ng/mL; T_{max}=1-2 hrs; AUC_{inf}=111-1364ng•hr/mL. **Distribution:** Plasma protein binding (<10%). **Elimination:** Urine (unchanged), feces (unabsorbed); $T_{1/2}$=2.5-5.1 hrs.

NURSING CONSIDERATIONS

Assessment: Assess for history of allergic reaction to lactose, airway disease, pregnancy/nursing status, and possible drug interactions.

Monitoring: Monitor for signs/symptoms of bronchospasm, allergic-like reactions, and neuropsychiatric events. Monitor respiratory function in patients with underlying airways disease.

Patient Counseling: Advise to seek medical attention if symptoms of bronchospasm, allergic-like reactions, or neuropsychiatric events (unusual behavior) occur. If taking inhaled bronchodilators, counsel to use bronchodilators before drug. Inform that the use of the drug does not reduce the risk of transmission of influenza to others. Instruct on proper use of Diskhaler. Use only under adult supervision for children.

Administration: Oral inhalational route. Refer to PI on instructions for use.
Storage: 25°C (77°F); excursions permitted to 15-30°C (59-86°F).

RELISTOR   RX
methylnaltrexone bromide (Wyeth)

THERAPEUTIC CLASS: Opioid antagonist

INDICATIONS: Treatment of opioid-induced constipation in patients with advanced illness who are receiving palliative care, when response to laxative therapy has not been sufficient.

DOSAGE: *Adults:* Inject SQ in upper arm, abdomen, or thigh. Usual: One dose qod, prn. Max: 1 dose/24 hrs. Patient's Weight: 38-<62kg (84-<136 lbs): 8mg. 62-114kg (136-251 lbs): 12mg. Patients Outside These Ranges: 0.15mg/kg. To calculate inj volume for these patients, multiply weight in lbs by 0.0034 or weight in kg by 0.0075 and round up volume to nearest 0.1mL. Do not prescribe pre-filled syringes to patients requiring doses calculated on a mg/kg basis. CrCl <30mL/min: Reduce dose by one-half. Pre-filled Syringes: Only if body weight calculated dose is 8mg or 12mg.

HOW SUPPLIED: Inj: 12mg/0.6mL; Pre-filled Syringe: 8mg/0.4mL, 12mg/0.6mL

CONTRAINDICATIONS: Known or suspected mechanical GI obstruction.

WARNINGS/PRECAUTIONS: D/C therapy if severe/persistent diarrhea occurs and/or worsening abdominal symptoms develop during treatment. GI perforations (eg, stomach, duodenum, colon) reported in advanced illness associated with reduction of structural integrity in the wall of GI tract (eg, cancer, peptic ulcer, Ogilvie's syndrome). Caution with known or suspected lesions of the GI tract. Use has not been studied in patients with peritoneal catheters. Use beyond 4 months has not been studied.

ADVERSE REACTIONS: Abdominal pain, flatulence, nausea, dizziness, hyperhidrosis, diarrhea.

PREGNANCY: Category B, caution in nursing.

MECHANISM OF ACTION: Opioid antagonist; peripherally acting mu-opioid receptor antagonist in tissues such as GI tract, thereby decreasing constipating effects of opioids without impacting opioid-mediated analgesic effects on the CNS.

PHARMACOKINETICS: **Absorption:** Rapid; (0.15mg/kg) C_{max}=117ng/mL, AUC=175ng•hr/mL. (0.30mg/kg) C_{max}=239ng/mL, AUC=362ng•hr/mL. (0.50mg/kg) C_{max}=392ng/mL, AUC=582ng•hr/mL; T_{max}=0.5 hrs. **Distribution:** V_d=1.1L/kg; plasma protein binding (11-15.3%). **Metabolism:** Methyl-6-naltrexol isomers (5%), methylnaltrexone sulfate (1.3%) (metabolites). **Elimination:** 85% unchanged; urine (approximately 50%), feces (<50%); $T_{1/2}$=8 hrs.

NURSING CONSIDERATIONS

Assessment: Assess for mechanical GI obstruction, presence of peritoneal catheters, severe renal impairment (CrCl <30mL/min), presence of advanced illness associated with localized/diffused reduction of structural integrity of the GI tract wall (eg, cancer, peptic ulcer, Ogilvie's syndrome), patients with GI tract lesions, and pregnancy/nursing status.

Monitoring: Monitor for signs/symptoms of severe/persistent diarrhea and abdominal symptoms, and GI perforations (eg, stomach, duodenum, colon). Monitor CrCl.

Patient Counseling: Instruct that usual schedule is 1 dose qod, prn but no more frequently than 1 dose in a 24-hr period. Advise to be within close proximity to toilet facilities once drug is administered. Inform to d/c therapy if experiencing severe/persistent diarrhea and/or worsening abdominal symptoms; contact physician. Counsel that common side effects include transient abdominal pain, N/V. Inform to d/c if opioid pain medication is stopped. Advise to rotate sites for injection (thigh, abdomen, upper arm).

Administration: SQ route only. Rotate sites for injection (thigh, abdomen, upper arm). **Storage:** 20-25°C (68-77°F); excursions permitted to 15-30°C (59-86°F). Do not freeze. Protect from light. Once drawn into syringe, if immediate administration is not possible, store at ambient room temperature and administer within 24 hrs.

RELPAX

RX

eletriptan hydrobromide (Pfizer)

THERAPEUTIC CLASS: 5-HT$_{1B/1D}$ agonist

INDICATIONS: Acute treatment of migraine with or without aura.

DOSAGE: *Adults:* Initial: 20 or 40mg at onset of headache. If recurs after initial relief, may repeat after 2 hrs. Max: 40mg/dose or 80mg/day. Safety of treating >3 headaches/30 days not known. Severe Hepatic Impairment: Avoid use. Avoid within 72 hrs of potent CYP3A4 inhibitors.

HOW SUPPLIED: Tab: 20mg, 40mg

CONTRAINDICATIONS: Ischemic heart disease, cerebrovascular or periph-eral vascular syndromes, other significant cardiovascular disease (CVD), uncontrolled HTN, hemiplegic or basilar migraine, within 24 hrs of other 5-HT$_1$ agonist or ergot-type agent (eg, dihydroergotamine, methysergide), severe hepatic impairment.

WARNINGS/PRECAUTIONS: Potential to cause coronary artery vasospasm; do not give with documented ischemic/vasospastic coronary artery disease (CAD). Not for patients in whom unrecognized CAD is predicted by presence of risk factors (eg, HTN, hypercholesterolemia, smoker, obesity, diabetes, CAD family history, menopause, males >40 yrs) unless with a satisfactory cardio-vascular evaluation; administer 1st dose under medical supervision; obtain ECG to assess presence of cardiac ischemia. Monitor cardiovascular function with long-term intermittent use. May cause vasospastic reactions or cerebro-vascular events. Serotonin syndrome may occur; symptoms may include men-tal status changes, autonomic instability, neuromuscular aberrations, and GI symptoms. HTN and hypertensive crisis reported rarely. Caution with hepatic dysfunction. Avoid in elderly. Possible long-term ophthalmologic effects.

ADVERSE REACTIONS: Paresthesias, dizziness, drowsiness, malaise, throat and neck symptoms, pain/pressure sensation, N/V.

INTERACTIONS: See Contraindications. Avoid use within 72 hrs of potent CYP3A4 inhibitors (eg, ketoconazole, itraconazole, nefazodone, trolean-domycin, clarithromycin, ritonavir, nelfinavir). Serotonin syndrome reported with combined use of an SSRI or SNRI. Propranolol, erythromycin, verapamil, fluconazole may increase levels.

PREGNANCY: Category C, caution in nursing.

MECHANISM OF ACTION: Selective 5HT$_{1D/1B}$ agonist; binds with high affinity to 5HT$_{1D/1B/1F}$ receptors. Suspected to perform its action by (1) activation of 5-HT$_{1D/1B}$ receptors located on intracranial blood vessels, including those on arterio-venous anastomoses, which leads to vasoconstriction and is correlated with relief of migraine headache, or (2) activation of 5-HT$_{1D/1B}$ receptors in trigemi-nal system results in inhibition of pro-inflammatory neuropeptide release.

PHARMACOKINETICS: Absorption: Well-absorbed; absolute bioavailabil-ity (50%); T$_{max}$=1.5 hrs. **Distribution:** V$_d$=138L; plasma protein binding (85%). **Metabolism:** via CYP3A4; N-demethylated (active metabolite). **Elimination:** Urine. T$_{1/2}$= 4 hrs (parent drug), 13 hrs (metabolite).

NURSING CONSIDERATIONS

Assessment: Confirm diagnosis of migraine before therapy. Assess for ischemic heart disease (eg, angina pectoris, Prinzmetal's variant angina, MI or documented silent MI), ECG changes, or any other conditions where treat-ment is contraindicated or cautioned. Assess for hepatic/renal impairment, pregnancy/nursing status, and possible drug interactions.

Monitoring: Administration of 1st dose should be in physician's office or medi-cally staffed and equipped facility as cardiac ischemia may occur in absence of clinical symptoms; ECG should be obtained immediately during interval in those with risk factors. Monitor for signs/symptoms of cardiac events (eg, coronary vasospasm, acute MI, arrhythmia, ECG changes, follow-up coronary angiography), cerebrovascular events (eg, hemorrhage, stroke, TIAs), periph-eral vascular ischemia, colonic ischemia with bloody diarrhea and abdominal pain, serotonin syndrome (eg, mental status changes, autonomic instability, neuromuscular aberrations and/or GI symptoms), ophthalmic effects, increased BP, and anaphylaxis/anaphylactoid reactions.

Patient Counseling: Inform about potential risks of therapy (eg, symptoms of serotonin syndrome such as confusion, hallucinations, fast heartbeat, fever, sweating, muscle spasms, and diarrhea), especially if taken with SSRIs or SNRIs. Advise to take exactly as prescribed. Instruct to notify physician if pregnant/nursing or planning to become pregnant. Instruct to report adverse reactions to physician.

Administration: Oral route. **Storage:** 25°C (77°F); excursions permitted to 15-30°C (59-86°F).

REMERON RX
mirtazapine (Schering)

> Antidepressants increased the risk of suicidal thinking and behavior (suicidality) in short-term studies in children, adolescents, and young adults with major depressive disorder (MDD) and other psychiatric disorders. Monitor and observe closely for clinical worsening, suicidality, or unusual changes in behavior in patients who are started on antidepressant therapy. Mirtazapine is not approved for use in pediatric patients.

OTHER BRAND NAMES: Remeron SolTab (Schering)

THERAPEUTIC CLASS: Piperazino-azepine

INDICATIONS: Treatment of major depressive disorder.

DOSAGE: *Adults:* Initial: 15mg qhs. Titrate: May increase every 1-2 weeks. Max: 45mg/day. Swallow disintegrating tab with saliva; no water is needed. Do not split the disintegrating tab. Reassess periodically to determine the need for maintenance treatment.

HOW SUPPLIED: Tab: 15mg*, 30mg*, 45mg; Tab, Disintegrating: 15mg, 30mg, 45mg *scored

CONTRAINDICATIONS: Concomitant use within 14 days of initiating or discontinuing therapy with a monoamine oxidase inhibitor (MAOI).

WARNINGS/PRECAUTIONS: Risk of agranulocytosis and severe neutropenia; d/c if develop sore throat, fever, stomatitis, or other signs of infection, along with low WBC count. May rarely cause serotonin syndrome; d/c if combination of symptoms (eg, hyperthermia, rigidity, myoclonus, autonomic instability with possible rapid fluctuations of vital signs, mental status changes including confusion, irritability, extreme agitation progressing to delirium and coma) develop. Caution in patients with history of seizures, mania/hypomania, hepatic or renal impairment, altered metabolic or hemodynamic conditions. Caution in elderly, history of cerebrovascular or cardiovascular (CV) disease, or conditions that predispose to hypotension (eg, dehydration, hypovolemia). Somnolence, dizziness, akathisia, hyponatremia reported. Screen patients for bipolar disorder. Increased appetite and weight gain, elevation in cholesterol, triglycerides (TG), and ALT reported. Discontinuation symptoms reported; do not d/c abruptly.

ADVERSE REACTIONS: Somnolence, increased appetite, weight gain, dizziness, dry mouth, constipation, asthenia, flu syndrome, abnormal dreams, thinking abnormal, increased cholesterol and TG levels.

INTERACTIONS: See Contraindications. Caution with drugs that may affect serotonergic neurotransmitter systems (eg, tryptophan, triptans, linezolid, serotonin reuptake inhibitors, venlafaxine, lithium, tramadol, St. John's wort). Alcohol and diazepam increase cognitive and motor skill impairment. Caution with antihypertensive medications; orthostatic hypotension observed infrequently. Decreased levels with phenytoin, carbamazepine and other hepatic metabolism inducers (eg, rifampicin). Increased levels with cimetidine, ketoconazole. Caution with potent CYP3A4 inhibitors, HIV protease inhibitors, azole antifungals, erythromycin, or nefazodone. Increased INR with warfarin.

PREGNANCY: Category C, caution in nursing.

MECHANISM OF ACTION: Piperazino-azepine group; the mechanism of action is unknown. Acts as an antagonist at central presynaptic α_2 adrenergic

R

inhibitory autoreceptors and heteroreceptors, an action that is postulated to result in an increase in central noradrenergic and serotonergic activity.

PHARMACOKINETICS: Absorption: Rapidly and completely absorbed; Absolute bioavailability (50%); T_{max}=2 hrs. **Distribution:** Plasma protein binding (85%). **Metabolism:** Demethylation and hydroxylation via CYP2D6, CYP1A2, and CYP3A followed by glucuronide conjugation. **Elimination:** Urine (75%), feces (15%); $T_{1/2}$=20-40 hrs.

NURSING CONSIDERATIONS

Assessment: Assess for psychiatric history (including history of suicide, bipolar disorder, depression), CV or cerebrovascular diseases, renal/hepatic impairment, pregnancy/nursing status and for possible drug interactions.

Monitoring: Monitor for signs/symptoms of worsening of depression, emergence of suicidal ideation, unusual changes in behavior, signs of infection (eg, sore throat, fever, stomatitis), and serotonin syndrome. Monitor LFTs, renal function tests, absolute neutrophil count (ANC), and cholesterol and TG levels.

Patient Counseling: Inform about risks and benefits associated with the therapy. Advise families and caregivers of the need for close observation of clinical worsening and suicidal risks. Warn about risk of developing agranulocytosis. Caution against operating machinery/driving. Advise to continue therapy as directed, to inform physician on concomitant medications, and to avoid alcohol. Inform physician if pregnant/nursing or planning to become pregnant.

Administration: Oral route. **Storage:** 25°C (77°F); excursions permitted to 15-30°C (59-86°F). Protect from light and moisture.

REMICADE   RX
infliximab (Centocor)

> Increased risk for developing serious infections (eg, tuberculosis [TB], TB reactivation, invasive fungal infection, bacterial/viral infection, and other infections due to opportunistic pathogens) that may lead to hospitalization or death. Most patients were taking concomitant immunosuppressants (eg, methotrexate, [MTX] or corticosteroids). Evaluate for latent TB and treat prior to initiation of therapy. Monitor for development of signs and symptoms of infection during and after treatment. D/C if serious infection or sepsis develops. Lymphoma and other malignancies reported in children and adolescents. Hepatosplenic T-cell lymphoma (HSTCL) reported with concomitant azathioprine or 6-mercaptopurine at or prior to diagnosis.

THERAPEUTIC CLASS: Monoclonal antibody/TNF-alpha receptor blocker

INDICATIONS: Reduce signs/symptoms, induce and maintain clinical remission in adults and pediatric patients with moderately to severely active Crohn's disease when response to conventional therapy is inadequate. Reduce the number of draining enterocutaneous and rectovaginal fistulas and maintain fistula closure in adults with fistulizing Crohn's disease. Reduce signs/symptoms, induce and maintain clinical remission and mucosal healing, and eliminate corticosteroid use in patients with moderately to severely active ulcerative colitis who have had inadequate response to conventional therapy. Reduce signs/symptoms, inhibit progression of structural damage, and improve physical function in patients with moderately to severely active rheumatoid arthritis (RA) (in combination with MTX) and psoriatic arthritis. Reduce signs/symptoms of active ankylosing spondylitis. Treatment of adult patients with chronic, severe plaque psoriasis who are candidates for systemic therapy and when other systemic therapies are medically less appropriate.

DOSAGE: *Adults:* Crohn's Disease/Fistulizing Crohn's Disease: Induction Regimen: 5mg/kg IV at 0, 2 and 6 weeks. Maint: 5mg/kg q8 weeks. Patients Who Respond and Lose Their Response: May increase to 10mg/kg. Consider d/c if no response by Week 14. Ulcerative Colitis: Induction Regimen: 5mg/kg IV at 0, 2 and 6 weeks. Maint: 5mg/kg q8 weeks. RA (with MTX): Induction Regimen: 3mg/kg IV at 0, 2 and 6 weeks. Maint: 3mg/kg q8 weeks. Incomplete Response: May increase to 10mg/kg or give q4 weeks. Ankylosing Spondylitis: Induction Regimen: 5mg/kg IV at 0, 2 and 6 weeks. Maint:

5mg/kg q6 weeks. Psoriatic Arthritis: Induction Regimen: 5mg/kg IV at 0, 2 and 6 weeks. Maint: 5mg/kg q8 weeks. May be used with or without MTX. Plaque Psoriasis: Induction Regimen: 5mg/kg IV at 0, 2 and 6 weeks. Maint: 5mg/kg q8 weeks.
Pediatrics: ≥6 yrs: Crohn's Disease: Induction Regimen: 5mg/kg IV at 0, 2 and 6 weeks. Maint: 5mg/kg q8 weeks.

HOW SUPPLIED: Inj: 100mg [20mL]

CONTRAINDICATIONS: Hypersensitivity to murine proteins. Moderate to severe heart failure (NYHA Class III/IV) with doses >5mg/kg.

WARNINGS/PRECAUTIONS: Do not initiate with an active infection. Monitor for non-melanoma skin cancers in psoriasis patients. Caution in patients with chronic obstructive pulmonary disease (COPD). Hepatitis B virus (HBV) reactivation reported; if reactivation occurs, d/c and institute appropriate therapy. Severe hepatic reactions (eg, acute liver failure, jaundice, hepatitis, cholestasis) reported; d/c if jaundice or marked elevations of liver enzymes (eg, ≥5x ULN) develop. Caution in patients with heart failure; monitor and d/c if new or worsening symptoms develop. Leukopenia, neutropenia, thrombocytopenia, and pancytopenia reported. Hypersensitivity reactions reported; d/c if severe hypersensitivity reactions occur. Systemic vasculitis, seizures, and new onset or exacerbation of CNS demyelinating disorders reported; d/c if these disorders develop. Caution when switching from one biologic to another; overlapping biological activity may further increase the risk of infection. May cause autoantibody formation and lupus-like syndrome; d/c if lupus-like syndrome develops. All pediatric patients with Crohn's disease should be up to date with vaccinations prior to therapy. Caution in elderly.

ADVERSE REACTIONS: Infections, infusion reactions, nausea, rash, headache, sinusitis, pharyngitis, coughing, abdominal pain, diarrhea, bronchitis, dyspepsia, fatigue, HTN, arthralgia.

INTERACTIONS: See Boxed Warning. Do not give concurrently with live vaccines. Concomitant use with anakinra or abatacept is not recommended; may increase risk of serious infection. Avoid use with tocilizumab because of the possibility of increased immunosuppression and increased risk of infection. Concomitant MTX use may decrease the incidence of anti-infliximab antibody production and increase infliximab concentrations.

PREGNANCY: Category B, not for use in nursing.

MECHANISM OF ACTION: Monoclonal antibody/TNF-α receptor blocker; neutralizes biological activity of TNF-α by binding with high affinity to the soluble and transmembrane forms of TNF-α and inhibits binding of TNF-α with its receptors.

PHARMACOKINETICS: Elimination: $T_{1/2}$=7.7-9.5 days.

NURSING CONSIDERATIONS

Assessment: Assess for active/chronic/recurrent infection (eg, TB, HBV), TB exposure, recent travel in areas of endemic TB or endemic mycoses, underlying conditions that may predispose to infection, heart failure, history of heavy smoking, history of malignancy, moderate to severe COPD, inflammatory bowel disease, presence or history of significant hematologic abnormalities, neurologic disorders, pregnancy/nursing status, known hypersensitivity to murine proteins, and for possible drug interactions. Assess for vaccination history in pediatric patients. Perform test for latent infection (eg, TB).

Monitoring: Monitor for sepsis, TB (active, reactivation, or latent), invasive fungal infection, bacterial, viral and other infections caused by opportunistic pathogens during and after therapy. Monitor for development of lymphoma, hepatosplenic T-cell lymphoma, or other malignancies. Monitor for new or worsening symptoms of heart failure, active HBV infection, hepatotoxicity, hematological events, hypersensitivity reactions, and CNS demyelinating disorders, and lupus-like syndrome. Monitor LFTs.

Patient Counseling: Advise of potential risks and benefits of therapy. Inform that therapy may lower ability of the immune system to fight infections. Instruct to immediately contact physician if experience signs/symptoms of infection, including TB and HBV reactivation. Counsel about the risk of lymphoma and other malignancies. Advise to report signs of new or worsening medical conditions such as heart disease, neurological diseases, or autoimmune disorders. Advise to report any symptoms of cytopenia (eg, bruising, bleeding, persistent fever).

Administration: IV infusion route. Refer to PI for administration and preparation instructions. **Storage:** 2-8°C (36-46°F).

RENAGEL   RX
sevelamer HCl (Genzyme)

THERAPEUTIC CLASS: Phosphate binder

INDICATIONS: Control of serum phosphorus in patients with chronic kidney disease (CKD) on dialysis.

DOSAGE: *Adults:* Not Taking Phosphate Binder: Usual: 800-1600mg with each meal. Initial: Based on Serum Phosphorus: >5.5 to <7.5mg/dL: 800mg tid. ≥7.5 to <9mg/dL: 1200-1600mg tid. ≥9mg/dL: 1600mg tid. Titrate: Serum Phosphorus >5.5mg/dL: Increase by 1 tab per meal at 2-week intervals. 3.5-5.5mg/dL: Maintain dose. <3.5mg/dL: Decrease 1 tab per meal at 2-week intervals. Switching from Calcium Acetate (667mg tab): Adjust according to calcium dose. Calcium acetate 1 tab per meal: 800mg per meal. Calcium acetate 2 tabs per meal: 1200-1600mg per meal. Calcium acetate 3 tabs per meal: 2000mg-2400mg per meal. Elderly: Start at lower end of dosing range.

HOW SUPPLIED: Tab: 400mg, 800mg

CONTRAINDICATIONS: Hypophosphatemia or bowel obstruction.

WARNINGS/PRECAUTIONS: Caution with dysphagia, swallowing disorders, severe GI motility, constipation or GI surgery. Monitor bicarbonate and chloride levels. May reduce vitamin D, E and K levels. Caution in elderly.

ADVERSE REACTIONS: N/V, abdominal pain, constipation, diarrhea, flatulence, dyspepsia, peritonitis, intestinal obstruction, ileus, fecal impaction, intestinal perforation.

INTERACTIONS: May decrease ciprofloxacin bioavailability by 50%. Very rare cases of increased thyroid stimulating hormone (TSH) levels reported when coadministered with levothyroxine; monitor TSH levels. May bind other drugs; give drugs with narrow therapeutic index 1 hr before or 3 hrs after sevelamer. Caution with antiarrhythmic or anti-seizure medications.

PREGNANCY: Category C, safety in nursing not known.

MECHANISM OF ACTION: Phosphate binder; binds to phosphate in the dietary tract, decreasing absorption and lowering its serum concentration.

NURSING CONSIDERATIONS

Assessment: Assess for hypophosphatemia, bowel obstruction, dysphagia, swallowing disorders, severe GI motility disorders including severe constipation, major GI tract surgery, pregnancy/nursing status, peritoneal/hemodialysis patients and possible drug interactions.

Monitoring: Monitor serum chemistries (eg, bicarbonate and chloride levels), levels of vitamin D, E, and K (clotting factors) and folic acid, and for constipation.

Patient Counseling: Counsel to take with meals and adhere to prescribed diets. Dose separately from therapy if taken with concomitant medication. Report if new onset or worsening of existing constipation occurs.

Administration: Oral route. **Storage:** 25°C (77°F); excursions permitted to 15-30°C (59-86°F). Protect from moisture.

RENVELA   RX
sevelamer carbonate (Genzyme)

THERAPEUTIC CLASS: Phosphate binder

INDICATIONS: Control of serum phosphorus in patients with chronic kidney disease (CKD) on dialysis.

DOSAGE: *Adults:* Take with meals. Initial: Not Taking Phosphate Binder: Serum Phosphorus >5.5 and <7.5mg/dL: 0.8g tid. Serum Phosphorus ≥7.5mg/dL: 1.6g tid. Switching from Sevelamer HCl or Switching Between Sevelamer Carbonate Tab and Powder: Use same dose in grams. Further titration may be necessary to achieve desired phosphorus levels. Switching from Calcium Acetate (667mg tab) to Sevelamer Carbonate: Initial: If Previously Taking 1 Tab Calcium Acetate Per Meal: 0.8g per meal. If Previously Taking 2 Tabs Calcium Acetate Per Meal: 1.6g per meal. If Previously Taking 3 Tabs Calcium Acetate Per Meal: 2.4g per meal. Titrate: All Patients: May increase dose by 0.8g tid with meals at 2-week intervals as needed. Elderly: Start at low end of dosing range.

HOW SUPPLIED: Tab: 800mg; Powder: 0.8g, 2.4g

CONTRAINDICATIONS: Bowel obstruction.

WARNINGS/PRECAUTIONS: Caution in patients with GI disorders; safety not established in patients with dysphagia, swallowing disorders, severe GI motility disorders, or major GI tract surgery. Bowel obstruction and perforation reported. Monitor bicarbonate levels, chloride levels, and for reduced vitamins D, E, and K (clotting factors), and folic acid levels. Caution in elderly.

ADVERSE REACTIONS: N/V, diarrhea, dyspepsia, abdominal pain, flatulence, constipation.

INTERACTIONS: May decrease ciprofloxacin bioavailability by 50%. Rare cases of increased thyroid stimulating hormone (TSH) levels reported when when coadministered with levothyroxine; monitor TSH levels and for signs of hypothyroidism when used concomitantly. When giving oral medication where reduction in bioavailability would have a clinically significant effect on its safety or efficacy, administer the drug at least 1 hr before or 3 hrs after sevelamer carbonate and monitor blood levels of the drug when appropriate.

PREGNANCY: Category C, safety in nursing is not known.

MECHANISM OF ACTION: Phosphate binder; contains multiple amines separated by one carbon from the polymer backbone. Amines exist in a protonated form in the intestine and interact with phosphate molecules through ionic and hydrogen bonding. By binding phosphate in the GI tract and decreasing absorption, a lowering of the phosphate concentration in the serum (serum phosphorus) occurs.

NURSING CONSIDERATIONS

Assessment: Assess for presence of bowel obstruction and for other GI disorders (eg, dysphagia, swallowing disorders, GI motility disorders, GI tract surgery), pregnancy/nursing status, and for possible drug interactions.

Monitoring: Monitor bicarbonate and chloride levels and for reduced vitamins D, E, and K (clotting factors), and folic acid levels.

Patient Counseling: Inform to take with meals and adhere to prescribed diets. If taking an oral medication where reduced bioavailability would produce a clinically significant effect on safety or efficacy, advise to take medication at least 1 hr before or 3 hrs after sevelamer carbonate. Advise to report new onset or worsening of existing constipation to physician.

Administration: Oral route. Powder Preparation: Empty contents of packet in cup and mix throughly with appropriate amount of water. Minimum Amount of Water: 0.8g: 1 oz, 30mL, 6 tsp, or 2 tbsp. 2.4g: 2 oz, 60mL, or 4 tbsp. **Storage:** 25°C (77°C); excursions permitted to 15-30°C (59-86°F). Protect from moisture.

ReoPro

abciximab (Lilly)

RX

THERAPEUTIC CLASS: Glycoprotein IIb/IIIa inhibitor

INDICATIONS: Adjunct to percutaneous coronary intervention (PCI) for prevention of cardiac ischemic complications in patients undergoing PCI or with unstable angina unresponsive to conventional therapy when PCI is planned within 24 hrs. Intended for use with aspirin and heparin.

DOSAGE: *Adults:* PCI: 0.25mg/kg IV bolus given 10-60 min before start PCI, followed by 0.125mcg/kg/min IV infusion (Max: 10mcg/min) for 12 hrs. Unstable Angina: 0.25mg/kg IV bolus followed by 10mcg/min infusion for 18-24 hrs, concluding 1 hr after PCI.

HOW SUPPLIED: Inj: 2mg/mL

CONTRAINDICATIONS: Active internal bleeding, recent (within 6 weeks) significant GI or genitourinary (GU) bleeding, cerebrovascular accident (CVA) within 2 yrs, CVA with significant residual neurological deficit, bleeding diathesis, oral anticoagulants within 7 days (unless PT ≤1.2x control), thrombocytopenia, recent (within 6 weeks) major surgery or trauma, intracranial neoplasm, arteriovenous malformation, aneurysm, severe uncontrolled HTN, history of vasculitis, IV dextran use before PCI or during an intervention. Hypersensitivity to murine proteins.

WARNINGS/PRECAUTIONS: Increased risk of bleeding. Monitor all potential bleeding sites (eg, catheter insertion sites, arterial and venous puncture sites, cutdown sites). Arterial/venous punctures, intramuscular injections, and use of urinary catheters, nasotracheal intubation, nasogastric tubes, and automatic blood pressure cuffs should be minimized. When obtaining intravenous access, non-compressible sites (eg, subclavian or jugular veins) should be avoided. Minimize vascular and other trauma. D/C if serious, uncontrollable bleeding, thrombocytopenia, or emergency surgery occurs. Anaphylaxis may occur. Antibody (HACA) formation may occur; risk of hypersensitivity, thrombocytopenia, decreased benefit with readministration. Monitor platelets, PT, APTT, ACT before infusion.

ADVERSE REACTIONS: Bleeding, thrombocytopenia, hypotension, bradycardia, N/V, back/chest pain, headache.

INTERACTIONS: Caution with other drugs that affect hemostasis (eg, thrombolytics, heparin, oral anticoagulants, NSAIDs, dipyridamole, ticlopidine). Increased risk of bleeding with anticoagulants, thrombolytics, and antiplatelets. If have HACA titers, possible allergic reactions with monoclonal antibody agents.

PREGNANCY: Category C, caution in nursing.

MECHANISM OF ACTION: Glycoprotein IIb/IIIa inhibitor; binds to the GPIIb/IIIa receptor and inhibits platelet aggregation by preventing the binding of fibrinogen, von Willebrand factor, and other adhesive molecules to GPIIb/IIIa receptor sites on activated platelets. Also binds to vitronectin receptor, which mediates the procoagulant properties of platelets and the proliferative properties of vascular endothelial and smooth muscle cells.

PHARMACOKINETICS: Elimination: $T_{1/2}$=30 min.

NURSING CONSIDERATIONS

Assessment: Assess for active internal bleeding, recent GI or GU bleeding, history of CVA, bleeding diathesis, thrombocytopenia, recent major surgery or trauma, intracranial neoplasm, arteriovenous malformation, aneurysm, severe uncontrolled HTN, presence or history of vasculitis, pregnancy/nursing status, and drug interactions. Obtain baseline prothrombin time, ACT, aPTT, and platelet counts.

Monitoring: Monitor for signs/symptoms of bleeding; document and monitor vascular puncture sites. If hematoma develops, monitor for enlargement. Monitor for allergic reactions (eg, anaphylaxis) and thrombocytopenia. Check aPTT or ACT prior to arterial sheath removal; should not be removed unless aPTT ≤50 seconds or ACT ≤175 seconds. Monitor platelet counts 2-4 hrs following bolus dose and 24 hrs prior to discharge.

Patient Counseling: Counsel to contact physician if develop hypersensitivity reactions (eg, anaphylaxis). Inform patients that they will bleed and bruise more easily and take longer to stop bleeding. Instruct to report any unusual bleeding to physician.

Administration: IV infusion. In case of hypersensitivity reaction, epinephrine, dopamine, theophylline, antihistamines, and corticosteroids should be available for immediate use. **Storage:** Store at 2-8°C (36-46°F). Do not freeze. Do not shake. Discard any unused portion left in vial.

REQUIP

RX

ropinirole HCl (GlaxoSmithKline)

OTHER BRAND NAMES: Requip XL (GlaxoSmithKline)

THERAPEUTIC CLASS: Non-ergoline dopamine agonist

INDICATIONS: (Tab/Tab, Extended-Release) Treatment of signs and symptoms of idiopathic Parkinson's disease. (Tab) Treatment of moderate-to-severe primary Restless Legs Syndrome (RLS).

DOSAGE: *Adults:* Parkinson's: Tab: Initial: 0.25mg tid. Titrate: May increase weekly by 0.25mg tid (0.75mg/day) for 4 weeks. After week 4, may increase weekly by 1.5mg/day up to 9mg/day, then by 3mg/day weekly to 24mg/day. Max: 24mg/day. Withdrawal: Decrease dose to bid for 4 days, then qd for 3 days. Tab, XL: Initial: 2mg qd for 1-2 weeks. Titrate: May increase by 2mg/day at ≥1 week intervals, depending on therapeutic response and tolerability. Max: 24mg/day. Swallow whole; do not chew, crush, or divide. Switching from Immediate-Release (IR) to XL: Initial dose should match total daily dose of IR formulation. Refer to PI for conversion from IR to XL. RLS: Tab: Initial: 0.25mg qd, 1-3 hrs before bedtime. Titrate: 0.5mg qd days 3-7, 1mg qd week 2, then increase by 0.5mg weekly. Max: 4mg.

HOW SUPPLIED: Tab: 0.25mg, 0.5mg, 1mg, 2mg, 3mg, 4mg, 5mg; Tab, Extended-Release: (XL) 2mg, 4mg, 6mg, 8mg, 12mg

WARNINGS/PRECAUTIONS: (Tab/Tab, XL) Falling asleep during activities of daily living reported; if significant, d/c or warn patient to refrain from dangerous activities. Syncope, bradycardia, postural hypotension, and hallucinations reported. Caution with hepatic dysfunction. Symptom complex similar to neuroleptic malignant syndrome (NMS), fibrotic complications, and melanoma reported. (Tab, XL) May cause elevation of BP and changes in HR. May exacerbate psychosis.

ADVERSE REACTIONS: (Tab) Neuralgia, hallucinations, somnolence, vomiting, headache, edema, fatigue, syncope, orthostatic symptoms. (Tab, XL) Dyskinesia, nausea, dizziness, constipation, abdominal pain/discomfort, back pain.

INTERACTIONS: Adjust dose if CYP1A2 inhibitor or estrogen is stopped or started during treatment. Potentiated by ciprofloxacin. Decreased effects with dopamine antagonists (eg, phenothiazines, butyrophenones, thioxanthenes, metoclopramide). Caution with alcohol, CNS depressants, and sedatives which may increase drowsiness. May increase clearance with smoking. May potentiate dopaminergic side effects of L-dopa and cause or exacerbate pre-existing dyskinesia.

PREGNANCY: Category C, not for use in nursing.

MECHANISM OF ACTION: Non-ergoline dopamine agonist; believed to stimulate postsynaptic D_2-type receptors within the caudate-putamen in the brain.

PHARMACOKINETICS: Absorption: Rapid; absolute bioavailability (45-55%), T_{max}=1-2 hrs (IR), 6-10 hrs (XL). **Distribution:** V_d=7.5L/kg, plasma protein binding (40%). **Metabolism:** Liver via CYP1A2 (extensive); N-despropylation and hydroxylation. **Elimination:** Urine (<10%, unchanged), $T_{1/2}$=6 hrs.

NURSING CONSIDERATIONS

Assessment: Assess for presence of sleep disorder, history of cardiovascular disease, dyskinesia, major psychotic disorder, pregnancy/nursing status and possible drug interactions. Assess LFTs, renal function tests, and CBC.

Monitoring: Perform dermatological screening periodically. Monitor eye exams and for symptoms of NMS, impulse control symptoms (eg, compulsive behaviors such as pathological gambling and hypersexuality), fibrotic complications, melanomas, signs/symptoms of postural hypotension, hallucinations.

Patient Counseling: Caution while operating machinery/driving. Counsel on potential for drowsiness, daytime sleepiness, falling asleep during activity; d/c if these events occurs. Risk of symptomatic hypotension. Take as prescribed; avoid alcohol or concurrent CNS depressants. Report lack of response or severe adverse effects. Notify physician if new or increased gambling urges, increased sexual urges, or other intense urges occur.

Administration: Oral route. **Storage:** (Tab) 20-25°C (68-77°F). Protect from light and moisture. (Tab, Extended-Release) 25°C (77°F); excursions permitted to 15-30°C (59-86°F).

RESCRIPTOR   RX
delavirdine mesylate (Pfizer)

THERAPEUTIC CLASS: Non-nucleoside reverse transcriptase inhibitor

INDICATIONS: Treatment of HIV-1 infection in combination with at least two other active antiretrovirals.

DOSAGE: *Adults:* Usual: 400mg (four 100-mg or two 200-mg tab) tid. Take with acidic beverage (eg, orange juice) if achlorhydric.
Pediatrics: ≥16 yrs: Usual: 400mg (four 100-mg or two 200-mg tab) tid. Take with acidic beverage (eg, orange juice) if achlorhydric.

HOW SUPPLIED: Tab: 100mg, 200mg

CONTRAINDICATIONS: Concomitant use of astemizole, terfenadine, dihydro-ergotamine, ergonovine, ergotamine, methylergonovine, cisapride, pimozide, alprazolam, midazolam, triazolam.

WARNINGS/PRECAUTIONS: Severe rash (eg, erythema multiforme, Stevens-Johnson syndrome) reported; d/c use if this occurs. Immune reconstitution syndrome and redistribution/accumulation of body fat reported. May confer cross-resistance to the other NNRTIs. Caution with hepatic impairment and elderly.

ADVERSE REACTIONS: Headache, fatigue, N/V, diarrhea, increased ALT and AST, rash, maculopapular rash, pruritus, erythema, insomnia, upper respiratory infection.

INTERACTIONS: See Contraindications. Antacids decrease absorption; separate doses by ≥1 hr. H_2-antagonists may reduce absorption; avoid chronic use. CYP3A inducers (eg, rifampin) may decrease plasma levels; avoid concomitant use. Increased plasma levels of amprenavir and drugs metabolized by CYP3A. Certain antihistamines, sedative hypnotics, antiarrhythmics, CCBs, ergot agents, amphetamines, cisapride, and sildenafil (max: 25mg/48 hrs) may result in potentially serious and/or life-threatening adverse events. Avoid use with lovastatin, simvastatin and St. John's wort. Caution with other HMG-CoA reductase inhibitors (statins); increased risk of myopathy and rhabdomyolysis. Reduced effects of both delavirdine and didanosine when used together; separate doses by ≥1 hr. Increases saquinavir levels; consider dose reduction. Increases indinavir levels; consider reducing indinavir dose to 600mg tid. May increase levels of clarithromycin, warfarin, trazodone, amphetamines, immunosuppressants and methadone; adjust doses and perform therapeutic drug monitoring as appropriate. Refer to PI for complete information.

PREGNANCY: Category C, not for use in nursing.

MECHANISM OF ACTION: Non-nucleoside reverse transcriptase inhibitor (NNRTI); binds directly to reverse transcriptase (RT) and blocks RNA-dependent and DNA-dependent DNA polymerase activities.

PHARMACOKINETICS: Absorption: Rapid; (400mg tid) C_{max}=35µM, AUC=180µM•hr; T_{max}=1 hr. Bioavailability (relative to oral sol) (85%). **Distribution:** Plasma protein binding (98%). **Metabolism:** Hepatic (N-desalkylation, pyridine hydroxylation) via CYP3A (major), 2D6. **Elimination:** (300mg tid multiple dose) Urine (51%, <5% unchanged), Feces (44%); $T_{1/2}$=5.8 hrs (400mg tid).

NURSING CONSIDERATIONS

Assessment: Assess for hepatic dysfunction, hypersensitivity, achlorhydria, pregnancy/nursing status and possible drug interactions.

Monitoring: Monitor for severe rash or rash accompanied by symptoms such as fever, blistering, oral lesions, conjunctivitis, swelling, muscle and joint aches. Monitor for immune reconstitution syndrome, cross-resistance to other NNRTIs, and fat redistribution.

Patient Counseling: Instruct to read patient package insert before therapy. Inform that drug is not a cure for HIV-1 infection and that they may continue to acquire illnesses associated with HIV-1 infection (eg, opportunistic infections). Also it has not been shown to reduce the risk of HIV-1 transmission. Inform to take as prescribed, not to alter dose without consulting doctor. If a dose is missed, do not double next dose. Patients with achlorhydria should take with acidic beverage (orange/cranberry juice). Take ≥1 hr apart if taking antacids, and to take with/without food. D/C and seek medical attention if severe rash or rash with symptoms of fever, blistering, oral lesions, conjunctivitis, swelling, and muscle and joint aches occur. Fat redistribution may occur. Advise to report use of any prescription or nonprescription medication or herbal products, particularly St. John's wort. May be at an increased risk of sildenafil-associated adverse events. Notify physician if pregnant or breastfeeding. Encourage exposed pregnant women to enroll in an Antiretroviral Pregnancy Registry.

Administration: Oral route. May disperse 100-mg tab in ≥3 oz. of water (200-mg tab is not dispersible). Refer to PI on how to prepare dispersion. **Storage:** 20-25°C (68-77°F). Keep container tightly closed. Protect from high humidity.

RESERPINE   RX
reserpine (Various)

THERAPEUTIC CLASS: Rauwolfia alkaloid

INDICATIONS: Treatment of mild essential HTN and adjunct treatment of severe HTN. Relief of symptoms in agitated psychotic states.

DOSAGE: *Adults:* HTN: Initial: 0.5mg/day for 1-2 weeks. Maint: reduce to 0.1-0.25mg/day. Psychotic Disorders: Initial: 0.5mg/day. Range: 0.1-1mg/day.

HOW SUPPLIED: Tab: 0.1mg, 0.25mg

CONTRAINDICATIONS: Active or history of mental depression, active peptic ulcer, ulcerative colitis, current electroconvulsive therapy.

WARNINGS/PRECAUTIONS: Caution with renal insufficiency. May cause depression; d/c at 1st sign. Caution with history of peptic ulcer, ulcerative colitis, or gallstones.

ADVERSE REACTIONS: GI effects, dry mouth, hypersecretion, arrhythmia, syncope, edema, dyspnea, muscle aches, dizziness, depression, nervousness, impotence, gynecomastia, rash.

INTERACTIONS: Avoid MAOIs or use extreme caution. Prolonged effect of direct-acting sympathomimetics (eg, epinephrine, isoproterenol). May inhibit effects of indirect-acting sympathomimetics (eg, ephedrine, tyramine). Risk of arrhythmia with quinidine or digoxin. Titrate carefully with other antihypertensives. Decreased effect with TCAs.

PREGNANCY: Category C, not for use in nursing.

MECHANISM OF ACTION: Rauwolfia alkaloid; antihypertensive, depletes stores of catecholamine and 5-hydroxytryptamine in many organs including brain and adrenal medulla, resulting in decreased HR and lowering of arterial BP.

PHARMACOKINETICS: Absorption: (0.5mg) Absolute bioavailability (50%); C_{max}=1.1ng/mL; T_{max}=2.5 hrs. **Distribution:** Plasma protein binding (95%); found in breast milk. **Metabolism:** Complete. **Elimination:** Urine (1% unchanged); $T_{1/2}$=200 hrs.

R

NURSING CONSIDERATIONS

Assessment: Assess for hypersensivity, mental depression (suicidal tendencies), active peptic ulcer, ulcerative colitis, renal insufficiency, possible drug interactions, and pregnancy/nursing status.

Monitoring: Monitor for signs of mental depression (eg, despondency, early morning insomnia, loss of appetite, impotence, self-depreciation); d/c if any occur. Monitor BP, GI motility/secretion, and signs/symptoms of overdose (eg, flushing, pupillary constriction, hypotension, respiratory depression, impairment of consciousness, bradycardia).

Patient Counseling: Inform of possible adverse effects; immediately notify physician if any occur. Advise to take medication regularly and continuously as directed.

Administration: Oral route. **Storage:** 20-25°C (68-77°F). Protect from moisture. Preserve in tight, light-resistant container.

RESTASIS   RX
cyclosporine (Allergan)

THERAPEUTIC CLASS: Topical immunomodulator

INDICATIONS: To increase tear production in patients with suppressed tear production due to ocular inflammation associated with keratoconjunctivitis sicca.

DOSAGE: *Adults:* 1 drop bid, q12h. Concomitant Artificial Tears: Space by 15 min.
Pediatrics: ≥16 yrs: 1 drop bid, q12h. Concomitant Artificial Tears: Space by 15 min.

HOW SUPPLIED: Emul: 0.05% [0.4mL, 30ˢ]

CONTRAINDICATIONS: Active ocular infections.

WARNINGS/PRECAUTIONS: For ophthalmic use only. Not studied in patients with a history of herpes keratitis. Not to be given while wearing contact lenses; lenses may be reinserted 15 min following administration.

ADVERSE REACTIONS: Ocular burning, conjunctival hyperemia, discharge, epiphora, eye pain, foreign body sensation, pruritus, stinging, visual disturbance (eg, blurring).

PREGNANCY: Category C, caution in nursing.

MECHANISM OF ACTION: Topical immunomodulator; not established. Thought to act as a partial immunomodulator.

PHARMACOKINETICS: Distribution: Following systemic administration, found in breast milk.

NURSING CONSIDERATIONS

Assessment: Assess for presence of active ocular infection. Assess use in pregnancy/nursing and in patients with a history of herpes keratitis.

Monitoring: Monitor for signs/symptoms of ocular burning and other adverse reactions.

Patient Counseling: Inform to use single-use vial immediately after opening and discard remaining contents following use. Instruct not to allow tip of vial to touch eye or any surface to avoid contamination. Advise to remove contact lenses prior to use; inform that lenses may be reinserted 15 min following administration.

Administration: Ocular route. 1) Invert unit dose vial a few times to obtain uniform, white, opaque emulsion before using. 2) Instill 1 drop bid in each eye, approximately 12 hrs apart. May be used concomitantly with artificial tears, allowing 15 min interval between products. 3) Discard vial immediately after administration. **Storage:** 15-25°C (59-77°F).

RESTORIL

temazepam (Mallinckrodt)

THERAPEUTIC CLASS: Benzodiazepine

INDICATIONS: Short-term treatment of insomnia (7-10 days).

DOSAGE: *Adults:* Administer before retiring. Usual: 15mg. Range: 7.5-30mg. Transient Insomnia: 7.5mg. Elderly/Debilitated: Initial: 7.5mg.

HOW SUPPLIED: Cap: 7.5mg, 15mg, 22.5mg, 30mg

CONTRAINDICATIONS: Pregnancy and women who may become pregnant.

WARNINGS/PRECAUTIONS: Initiate only after careful evaluation; failure of insomnia to remit after 7-10 days of treatment may indicate primary psychiatric and/or medical illness. Worsening of insomnia and emergence of thinking or behavior abnormalities may occur especially in elderly; use lowest possible effective dose. Behavioral changes (eg, decreased inhibition, bizarre behavior, agitation, hallucinations, depersonalization) and complex behavior (eg, sleep-driving) reported; strongly consider d/c if sleep-driving episode occurs. Amnesia and other neuropsychiatric symptoms may occur unpredictably. Worsening of depression including suicidal thinking reported. Withdrawal symptoms may occur after abrupt d/c. Angioedema (eg, tongue, glottis, larynx) and anaphylaxis reported; do not rechallenge if angioedema develops. Caution with hepatic/renal impairment, chronic pulmonary insufficiency, debilitated, severe or latent depression, and elderly.

ADVERSE REACTIONS: Headache, dizziness, drowsiness, fatigue, nervousness, nausea, lethargy.

INTERACTIONS: Increased risk of complex behaviors with alcohol and CNS depressants. Potential additive effects with hypnotics and CNS depressants. Possible synergistic effect with diphenhydramine.

PREGNANCY: Category X, caution in nursing.

MECHANISM OF ACTION: Benzodiazepine hypnotic agent.

PHARMACOKINETICS: Absorption: Well absorbed; C_{max}=666-982ng/mL; T_{max}=1.2-1.6 hrs. **Distribution:** Plasma protein binding (96% unchanged); crosses placenta. **Elimination:** Urine (80-90%); $T_{1/2}$=3.5-18.4 hrs.

NURSING CONSIDERATIONS

Assessment: Assess for pregnancy, physical and/or psychiatric disorder, medical illness, severe or latent depression, impaired renal/hepatic function, chronic pulmonary insufficiency, nursing status, possible drug interactions, alcohol use, and if elderly or debilitated.

Monitoring: Monitor for worsening of insomnia, severe or latent depression with suicidal ideation, emergence of new abnormalities of thinking or behavior, physical/psychological dependence, withdrawal symptoms, and hypersensitivity reactions. Monitor LFTs.

Patient Counseling: Inform about the risks and possibility of physical/psychological dependence, memory problems, and complex behaviors (eg, sleep-driving). Caution against hazardous tasks (eg, operating machinery/driving). Advise not to drink alcohol. Instruct to notify physician if pregnant/planning to become pregnant. Counsel to take as directed by physician.

Administration: Oral route. **Storage:** 20-25°C (68-77°F). Dispense in a well-closed, light-resistant container with a child-resistant closure.

R

RETAVASE

RX

reteplase (EKR)

THERAPEUTIC CLASS: Thrombolytic agent

INDICATIONS: Management of acute myocardial infarction (AMI) in adults for the improvement of ventricular function following AMI, reduction of the incidence of congestive heart failure (CHF), and the reduction of mortality associated with AMI.

DOSAGE: *Adults:* Administer two 10 U bolus injections. Administer each bolus as IV inj over 2 mins. Give 2nd bolus 30 mins after 1st bolus inj. Do not administer other medications simultaneously via the same IV line.

HOW SUPPLIED: Inj: 10.4 U (18.1mg)

CONTRAINDICATIONS: Active internal bleeding; history of cerebrovascular accident (CVA); recent intracranial or intraspinal surgery or trauma; intracranial neoplasm; arteriovenous malformation, or aneurysm; known bleeding diathesis; severe uncontrolled HTN.

WARNINGS/PRECAUTIONS: Bleeding is the most common complication during therapy; careful attention to all potential bleeding sites is required. If arterial puncture is necessary during administration, use an upper extremity vessel that is accessible to manual compression. Avoid IM inj and nonessential handling of patients. Perform venipuncture carefully and only if required. Weigh benefits/risks of therapy with recent major surgery, previous puncture of noncompressible vessels, cerebrovascular disease, recent GI or genitourinary (GU) bleeding, recent trauma, HTN, high likelihood of left heart thrombus, acute pericarditis, subacute bacterial endocarditis, hemostatic defects, severe hepatic or renal dysfunction, pregnancy, diabetic hemorrhagic retinopathy or other hemorrhagic ophthalmic conditions, septic thrombophlebitis or occluded AV cannula at a seriously infected site, advanced age, any other condition in which bleeding would constitute a significant hazard or be difficult to manage. Cholesterol embolism reported. Coronary thrombolysis may result in arrhythmias associated with reperfusion. Do not administer second bolus if an anaphylactoid reaction occurs. May affect results of coagulation tests and/or measurements of fibrinolytic activity.

ADVERSE REACTIONS: Bleeding, allergic reactions.

INTERACTIONS: Increased risk of bleeding with heparin, vitamin K antagonists, and drugs that alter platelet function (eg, ASA, dipyridamole, abciximab) if administered before, during, or after therapy. Concomitant use of anticoagulant therapy should be terminated if serious bleeding occurs.

PREGNANCY: Category C, caution in nursing.

MECHANISM OF ACTION: Thrombolytic agent; recombinant plasminogen activator which catalyzes the cleavage of endogenous plasminogen to generate plasmin. Plasmin in turn degrades the fibrin matrix of the thrombus, thereby exerting its thrombolytic action.

PHARMACOKINETICS: Metabolism: Hepatic. **Elimination:** Renal; $T_{1/2}$=13-16 min.

NURSING CONSIDERATIONS

Assessment: Assess for active internal bleeding, history of CVA, or any other conditions where treatment is contraindicated or cautioned. Assess for age, renal/hepatic function, pregnancy/nursing status, and possible drug interactions.

Monitoring: Monitor for signs/symptoms of bleeding, internal and superficial bleeding sites, bleeding at recent puncture sites, cholesterol embolism (eg, livedo reticularis, "purple toe" syndrome, MI, cerebral infarction, HTN, gangrenous digits), and arrhythmias. Monitor renal/hepatic function.

Patient Counseling: Inform the patient about the risks and benefits of the therapy. Instruct to contact physician if any unusual bleeding occurs or if any other adverse reaction develops. Advise to avoid IM injections while on therapy.

Administration: IV route. Refer to the PI for administration and reconstitution instructions. **Storage:** Unused vial: 2-25°C (36-77°F). Box should remain sealed until use to protect the lyophilisate from exposure to light. Reconstituted: 2-30°C (36-86°F); use within 4 hrs.

RETIN-A

RX

tretinoin (Ortho Neutrogena)

OTHER BRAND NAMES: Retin-A Micro (Ortho Neutrogena)

THERAPEUTIC CLASS: Retinoid

INDICATIONS: Topical treatment of acne vulgaris.

DOSAGE: *Adults:* Cleanse area thoroughly, then apply qhs. May temporarily d/c or reduce dosing frequency if irritation occurs.
Pediatrics: ≥12 yrs: (Gel: 0.04%, 0.1%) Cleanse area thoroughly, then apply qhs. May temporarily d/c or reduce dosing frequency if irritation occurs.

HOW SUPPLIED: (Retin-A) Cre: 0.025%, 0.05%, 0.1% [20g, 45g]; Gel: 0.01%, 0.025% [15g, 45g]; Sol: 0.05% [28mL]; (Retin-A Micro) Gel: 0.04%, 0.1% [20g, 45g]

WARNINGS/PRECAUTIONS: Avoid eyes, lips, paranasal creases, mucous membranes, and sunburned skin. Acne exacerbation during 1st weeks of therapy may occur. D/C if sensitivity or irritation occurs. Severe irritation with eczematous skin. Causes photosensitivity. Extreme weather (eg, cold, wind) may irritate skin.

ADVERSE REACTIONS: Local skin reactions (red, edematous, blistered, crusted), photosensitivity, temporary skin pigmentation changes.

INTERACTIONS: Caution with topical agents with strong drying effects, high concentration of alcohol, astringents, spices, or lime. Caution with sulfur, resorcinol, or salicylic acid; allow effects of these agents to subside before application of tretinoin.

PREGNANCY: Category C, caution in nursing.

MECHANISM OF ACTION: Retinoic acid derivative; not established. Responsible for decreasing cohesiveness of follicular epithelial cells with decreased microcomedo formation. Also stimulates mitotic activity and increases turnover of follicular epithelial cells, causing extrusion of comedones.

NURSING CONSIDERATIONS

Assessment: Assess for presence of sunburn and eczematous skin, pregnancy/nursing status, and possible drug interactions.

Monitoring: Monitor for signs/symptoms of a skin sensitivity reaction (eg, red, edematous, blistered, or crusted skin) or chemical irritation.

Patient Counseling: Avoid exposure to sunlight/sunlamps during therapy. Advise using effective sunscreen when outdoors and protective clothing during extended sun exposure. If sunburn occurs, instruct to d/c until skin is recovered. Avoid excessive exposure to wind or cold. Medication is flammable; avoid fire, flame, or smoking during use. Keep away from eyes, mouth, angles of the nose, and mucous membranes. Notify physician if severe skin irritation occurs.

Administration: Topical administration. **Storage:** Retin A Liquid, Gel: Below 86°F; Retin A Cream: Below 80°F.

RETROVIR

RX

zidovudine (ViiV Healthcare)

> Associated with hematologic toxicity (eg, neutropenia, severe anemia), particularly with advanced HIV-1 disease. Symptomatic myopathy associated with prolonged use. Lactic acidosis and severe hepatomegaly with steatosis, including fatal cases, reported; suspend treatment if lactic acidosis or pronounced hepatotoxicity occur.

THERAPEUTIC CLASS: Nucleoside analogue

INDICATIONS: Treatment of HIV-1 infection in combination with other antiretrovirals. Prevention of maternal-fetal HIV-1 transmission.

DOSAGE: *Adults:* HIV-1 Infection: (Cap/Tab/Syrup) 600mg/day in divided doses in combination with other antiretroviral agents. (Inj) 1mg/kg IV over 1

R

hr 5-6 times/day. Use only until oral therapy can be administered. Maternal-Fetal HIV Transmission: >14 weeks pregnancy: Maternal Dosing: 100mg PO 5 times/day until start of labor. During Labor and Delivery: 2mg/kg IV over 1 hr followed by 1mg/kg/hr IV infusion until clamping of umbilical cord. End-Stage Renal Disease On Dialysis: 100mg PO q6-8h or 1mg/kg IV q6-8h. Significant Anemia/Neutropenia: May require dose interruption and adjunctive epoetin α therapy. Elderly: Start at low end of dosing range.

Pediatrics: HIV-1 Infection: 4 weeks - <18 yrs: (Cap/Tab/Syrup) BSA Based: 480mg/m² /day PO in divided doses (240mg/m² bid or 160mg/m² tid). Weight Based: 4 to <9kg: 12mg/kg bid or 8mg/kg tid. ≥9 to <30kg: 9mg/kg bid or 6mg/kg tid. ≥30kg: 300mg bid or 200mg tid. Maternal-Fetal HIV Transmission: Neonates: 2mg/kg PO q6h or 1.5mg/kg IV over 30 min q6h, starting within 12 hrs after birth and continuing through 6 weeks of age. End-Stage Renal Disease On Dialysis: 100mg PO q6-8h or 1mg/kg IV q6-8h. Significant Anemia/Neutropenia: May require dose interruption and adjunctive epoetin α therapy.

HOW SUPPLIED: Cap: 100mg; Inj: 10mg/mL [20mL]; Syrup: 50mg/5mL [240mL]; Tab: 300mg

WARNINGS/PRECAUTIONS: Adverse reactions increase with disease progression. Caution with compromised bone marrow (granulocyte count<1,000cells/mm³ or Hgb<9.5g/dL). Frequent blood counts are strongly recommended in patients with poor bone marrow reserve. D/C if neutropenia or anemia develops. Pancytopenia reported. Caution with known risk factors for liver disease, obesity, and prolonged exposure to antiretroviral nucleoside analogues; increased risk of lactic acidosis and hepatomegaly with steatosis; d/c if develops. Redistribution/accumulation of body fat observed. Immune reconstitution syndrome reported. Dose reduction in severe renal impairment (CrCl<15mL/min). Caution in elderly.

ADVERSE REACTIONS: Hematologic toxicity (eg, anemia, neutropenia), lactic acidosis, hepatomegaly with steatosis, hepatotoxicity, headache, N/V, malaise, anorexia, asthenia, constipation, abdominal pain/cramps, arthralgia, chills.

INTERACTIONS: Hepatic decompensation has occurred in HIV/HCV coinfected patients receiving combination antiretroviral therapy for HIV and interferon-α w/ or w/o ribavirin. Increased risk of hematologic toxicities with ganciclovir, interferon-α, ribavirin, bone marrow suppressives, and cytotoxic drugs. Possible increased levels with lamivudine, atovaquone, fluconazole, methadone, probenecid, and valproic acid. Possible decreased levels with nelfinavir, ritonavir, rifampin and clarithromycin. Avoid with stavudine, nucleoside analogues affecting DNA replication such as ribavirin, doxorubicin, and other combination products containing zidovudine. May decrease phenytoin levels.

PREGNANCY: Category C, not for use in nursing.

MECHANISM OF ACTION: Nucleoside analogue; inhibits reverse transcriptase via DNA chain termination.

PHARMACOKINETICS: Absorption: (PO): Rapid. Bioavailability (64%). T_{max}=0.5-1.5 hrs. (IV) C_{max}=1.06mcg/mL. **Distribution:** V_d=1.6L/kg; plasma protein binding (<38%); found in breast milk. **Metabolism:** Hepatic. 3'-azido-3'-deoxy-5'-*O*-β-*D*-glucopyranuronosylthymidine (major metabolite). **Elimination:** (PO): Urine (14% unchanged, 74% metabolite). $T_{1/2}$=0.5-3 hrs. (IV): Urine (18% unchanged, 60% metabolite). $T_{1/2}$=1.1 hrs. Refer to PI for pediatric and renal impairment pharmacokinetic parameters.

NURSING CONSIDERATIONS

Assessment: Assess for advanced symptomatic HIV disease, risk of liver disease, lactic acidosis, obesity, prolonged use of antiretrovial nucleoside analogues, signs/symptoms of bone marrow compromise, renal/hepatic function, drug hypersensitivity, ability to swallow cap or tab in children, pregnancy/nursing status, and possible drug interactions.

Monitoring: Monitor for signs/symptoms of lactic acidosis, severe hepatomegaly with steatosis, hypersensitivity reaction, myopathy, anemia, liver/renal dysfunction, bone marrow suppression, immune reconstitution syndrome, and other treatment-associated toxicities. Monitor for blood counts/hematologic indices periodically and need for dosage adjustment.

Patient Counseling: Inform that therapy is not cure for HIV, does not reduce risk of transmission of HIV and that opportunistic infections may develop. Inform that major toxicities are neutropenia and/or anemia; may require transfusions or drug d/c if toxicity develops. Inform of importance of frequent blood counts while on therapy. Inform that may cause myopathy, myositis, lactic acidosis with liver enlargement, redistribution/accumulation of body fat, headache, malaise, N/V, anorexia in adults, fever, cough, and digestive disorder in pediatrics. Consult physician if experience muscle weakness, SOB, symptoms of hepatitis or pancreatitis, or any other adverse events. Inform pregnant women that transmission may still occur despite therapy and not to breastfeed to prevent postnatal transmission. May enroll patients in the Antiretroviral Pregnancy Registry (1-800-258-4263) if they become pregnant while on treatment. Counsel about the use of other medications which may exacerbate toxicity. Instruct not to share medication and exceed recommended dose; take as prescribed. Inform that long-term effects are unknown at this time.

Administration: IV or oral route. (IV) Avoid rapid infusion and bolus injection. Should not be given IM. **Storage:** (IV): 15-25°C (59-77°F); protect from light. (Diluted): Stable for 24 hrs at room temperature. Stable for 48 hrs when refrigerated at 2-8°C (36-46°F). Administer within 8 hrs if stored at 25°C (77°F) or 24 hrs if refrigerated at 2-8°C to minimize contamination. (Cap, Tab, Syrup): 15-25°C (59-77°F); protect caps from moisture.

REVATIO   RX
sildenafil (Pfizer)

THERAPEUTIC CLASS: Phosphodiesterase type 5 inhibitor

INDICATIONS: Treatment of pulmonary arterial HTN (PAH) (WHO Group I) to improve exercise ability and delay clinical worsening.

DOSAGE: *Adults:* IV: 10mg IV bolus tid. PO: 20mg tid, 4-6 hrs apart. Max: 20mg tid.

HOW SUPPLIED: Inj: 10mg [12.5mL]; Tab: 20mg

CONTRAINDICATIONS: Coadministration with organic nitrates in any form, either regularly or intermittently.

WARNINGS/PRECAUTIONS: Caution with myocardial infarction (MI), stroke or life-threatening arrhythmia within last 6 months; coronary artery disease (CAD) causing unstable angina; and HTN (BP >170/110). Vasodilatory effects may adversely affect patients with resting hypotension (BP <90/50), fluid depletion, severe left ventricular outflow obstruction, or autonomic dysfunction. Not recommended with pulmonary veno-occlusive disease (PVOD); consider possibility of associated PVOD if signs of pulmonary edema occur. Caution in patients with bleeding disorders or active peptic ulceration. Non-arteritic anterior ischemic optic neuropathy (NAION) reported; seek immediate medical attention if sudden loss of vision in one or both eyes occurs. Caution with previous NAION in one eye and with retinitis pigmentosa. Sudden decrease or loss of hearing reported. Caution in patients with anatomical penile deformation or with predisposition to priapism. Penile tissue damage and permanent loss of potency may result if priapism is not immediately treated. Vaso-occlusive crises requiring hospitalization reported in patients with pulmonary HTN secondary to sickle cell disease. Caution in elderly.

ADVERSE REACTIONS: Epistaxis, headache, flushing, dyspepsia, insomnia, erythema, dyspnea exacerbated, rhinitis, diarrhea, myalgia, pyrexia, gastritis, sinusitis, paresthesia.

INTERACTIONS: See Contraindications. Reports of epistaxis with oral vitamin K antagonists. Retinal and eye hemorrhage reported with anticoagulants. May potentiate anti-aggregatory effect of sodium nitroprusside. Increased levels with ritonavir (a highly potent CYP3A inhibitor); avoid with ritonavir or other potent CYP3A inhibitors. CYP3A and CYP2C9 inhibitors may decrease sildenafil clearance. CYP3A and CYP2C9 inducers may increase sildenafil

R

clearance. Greater decrease in plasma levels with potent CYP3A inducers. Concomitant use with other protease inhibitors may increase sildenafil levels. Increased plasma concentrations with cimetidine. Increased AUC with erythromycin. Increased C_{max} and AUC with saquinavir. Slight decrease of sildenafil exposure with epoprostenol. Administration with CYP3A substrates and the combination of CYP3A substrates and β-blockers may reduce clearance or increase oral bioavailability of sildenafil. Caution with α-blockers (eg, doxazosin) due to its additive BP-lowering effects. Additional reduction of supine BP with oral amlodipine reported. Avoid concomitant use with other PDE5 inhibitors (eg, Viagra®). Caution with bosentan; concomitant administration decreased sildenafil AUC and C_{max} and increased bosentan AUC.

PREGNANCY: Category B, caution in nursing.

MECHANISM OF ACTION: Phosphodiesterase type-5 (PDE5) inhibitor; increases cGMP within pulmonary vascular smooth muscle cells resulting in relaxation. This can lead to vasodilation of pulmonary vascular bed and, to a lesser degree, vasodilation in the systemic circulation.

PHARMACOKINETICS: Absorption: (PO) Rapid; absolute bioavailability (41%); T_{max}=30-120 min. **Distribution:** V_d=105L; plasma protein binding (96%). **Metabolism:** CYP3A (major route) and CYP2C9 (minor route); N-desmethyl metabolite (active metabolite). **Elimination:** (PO) Feces (80%), urine (13%); $T_{1/2}$=4 hrs.

NURSING CONSIDERATIONS

Assessment: Assess for hypotension, fluid depletion, left ventricular outflow obstruction, autonomic dysfunction, PVOD, CAD causing unstable angina, HTN, active peptic ulceration or bleeding problems, previous NAION in one eye, retinitis pigmentosa, anatomical deformities of the penis, conditions predisposing to priapism, pulmonary HTN secondary to sickle cell disease, drug hypersensitivity, nursing/pregnancy status and possible drug interactions (eg, nitrates). Assess for MI, stroke or life-threatening arrhythmia within last 6 months. Obtain baseline BP.

Monitoring: Monitor for signs of pulmonary edema, decreased/sudden loss of vision or hearing, tinnitus, dizziness, epistaxis, priapism and hypersensitivity reactions. Monitor BP.

Patient Counseling: Inform about risks of drug and to consult physician if any adverse events occur. Inform that drug is also marketed as Viagra for male erectile dysfunction. Advise not to take Viagra or other PDE5 inhibitors during therapy. Inform of contraindication of regular and/or intermittent use of organic nitrates during therapy. Counsel about the increased risk of NAION with patients who already experienced NAION in one eye. Instruct to notify physician if sudden decrease/loss of vision or hearing occur. Instruct to seek immediate medical attention if an erection persists >4 hrs.

Administration: Oral, IV route. **Storage:** 25°C (77°F); excursions permitted to 15-30°C (59-86°F).

ReVia
naltrexone HCl (Duramed)

RX

THERAPEUTIC CLASS: Opioid antagonist

INDICATIONS: Treatment of alcohol dependence and to block effects of exogenously administered opioids.

DOSAGE: *Adults:* Alcoholism: 50mg qd up to 12 weeks. Opioid Dependence: Begin 7-10 days after opioid-free period and no signs of withdrawal. Initial: 25mg qd. Maint: 50mg qd. Naloxone Challenge Test: 0.2mg IV, observe for 30 sec, then 0.6mg IV, observe for 20 min; or 0.8mg SQ, observe for 20 min.

HOW SUPPLIED: Tab: 50mg* *scored

CONTRAINDICATIONS: Acute hepatitis or liver failure, failed naloxone challenge test or positive urine screen for opioids, opioid-dependent, concomitant opioid analgesics, acute opioid withdrawal.

WARNINGS/PRECAUTIONS: Hepatotoxicity with excessive doses; does not appear to be a hepatotoxin at recommended doses. Only treat patients opioid-free for 7-10 days. Attempting to overcome opiate blockade is very dangerous. More sensitive to lower doses of opioids after naltrexone is d/c. Safety in ultra-rapid opiate detoxification is not known. Increased risk of suicide in substance abuse patients. Severe opioid withdrawal syndromes reported with accidental ingestion in opioid-dependent patients. Monitor closely during blockade reversal. Caution in renal or hepatic impairment. Perform naloxone challenge test if question of opioid dependence.

ADVERSE REACTIONS: N/V, headache, dizziness, nervousness, fatigue, restlessness, insomnia, anxiety, somnolence.

INTERACTIONS: See Contraindications. Do not use with disulfiram unless benefits outweigh risk of hepatotoxicity. Lethargy and somnolence reported with thioridazine. Antagonizes opioid-containing cough and cold, antidiarrheal, and analgesic agents.

PREGNANCY: Category C, caution in nursing.

MECHANISM OF ACTION: Opioid antagonist; markedly attenuates or completely blocks (reversibly) the subjective effects of IV-administered opioids.

PHARMACOKINETICS: Absorption: Rapid and complete. Bioavailability (5-40%); T_{max}=1 hr. **Distribution:** V_d=1350L; plasma protein binding (21%). **Metabolism:** Liver , 6β-naltrexol (major metabolite). **Elimination:** Urine (2% unchanged), (43% conjugated); (naltrexone, β-naltrexol) $T_{1/2}$=4 hrs, 13 hrs.

NURSING CONSIDERATIONS

Assessment: Start treatment only under medical judgment of prescribing physician, assess potential of opioid use within past 7-10 days. If question of occult opioid dependence, perform naloxone challenge test. Assess for acute hepatitis or liver failure and possible drug interactions.

Monitoring: Monitor LFTs, symptoms/signs of respiratory depression, hepatotoxicity, idiopathic thrombocytopenic purpura, suicide attempts, withdrawal symptoms in opioid-dependent patients.

Patient Counseling: Instruct to take as prescribed. Drug treats alcoholism or drug dependence. Carry identification card to alert medical personnel of naltrexone use and to ensure adequate treatment in a medical emergency. Caution against taking heroin or any other opioid drug with therapy; may lead to serious injury, including coma. Notify physician if pregnant/nursing.

Administration: Oral route. **Storage:** 20-25°C (68-77°F).

REVLIMID
lenalidomide (Celgene)

RX

A known human teratogen that causes severe life-threatening human birth defects. Avoid during pregnancy; may cause birth defects or death to a developing baby. Women of childbearing potential should have 2 negative pregnancy tests prior to treatment and must use 2 forms of contraception or continuously abstain from heterosexual sex during and for 4 weeks after treatment. Available only under a restricted distribution program called "RevAssist". May cause neutropenia and thrombocytopenia. Patients on therapy for del 5q myelodysplastic syndromes (MDS) should have their CBC monitored weekly for the 1st 8 weeks of therapy and monthly thereafter; patients may require dose interruption and/or reduction and use of blood product support and/or growth factors. Increased risk of deep vein thrombosis (DVT) and pulmonary embolism (PE) in patients with multiple myeloma. Observe for signs and symptoms of thromboembolism.

THERAPEUTIC CLASS: Thalidomide Analog

INDICATIONS: Treatment for transfusion-dependent anemia due to low- or intermediate-1-risk myelodysplastic syndromes (MDS) associated with a deletion 5q cytogenetic abnormality with or without additional cytogenetic abnormalities. In combination with dexamethasone for the treatment of multiple myeloma (MM) in patients who have received at least 1 prior therapy.

DOSAGE: *Adults:* MDS: Initial: 10mg qd with water. Renal Impairment: Moderate (CrCl 30-60mL/min): 5mg q24h. Severe without Dialysis (CrCl <30mL/min): 5mg q48h. End Stage Renal Disease (ESRD) with Dialysis

(CrCl <30mL/min): 5mg 3x a week following each dialysis. MM: Initial: 25mg qd with water on Days 1-21 of repeated 28-day cycles. Give with dexamethasone 40mg qd on Days 1-4, 9-12, and 17-20 of each 28-day cycle for the 1st 4 cycles then on Days 1-4 every 28 days. Renal Impairment: Moderate (CrCl 30-60mL/min): 10mg q24h. Severe without Dialysis (CrCl <30mL/min): 15mg q48h. ESRD with Dialysis (CrCl <30mL/min): 5mg qd; on dialysis days, administer dose following dialysis. For Grade 3/4 toxicities, hold treatment and restart at next lower dose when toxicity resolved to ≤Grade 2. Refer to PI for dose adjustments for hematologic toxicities based on platelet and/or absolute neutrophil counts. Do not break, chew or open caps.

HOW SUPPLIED: Cap: 5mg, 10mg, 15mg, 25mg

CONTRAINDICATIONS: Pregnancy and childbearing potential.

WARNINGS/PRECAUTIONS: Angioedema and serious dermatologic reactions including Stevens-Johnson syndrome (SJS) and toxic epidermal necrolysis (TEN) reported. D/C if angioedema, SJS, TEN, Grade 4 rash, exfoliative or bullous rash develops. Consider treatment interruption or d/c for Grade 2-3 skin rash. Avoid with a prior history of Grade 4 rash associated with thalidomide treatment. Tumor lysis syndrome reported; caution in patients with high tumor burden prior to treatment and monitor closely. Tumor flare reaction (characterized by tender lymph node swelling, low grade fever, pain, rash) occurred during investigational use for chronic lymphocytic leukemia (CLL) and lymphoma; treatment of CLL or lymphoma outside a well-monitored clinical trial is discouraged. Caution with renal impairment.

ADVERSE REACTIONS: Thrombocytopenia, neutropenia, pruritus, rash, diarrhea, constipation, nausea, nasopharyngitis, fatigue, arthralgia, cough, pyrexia, peripheral edema, anemia, asthenia.

INTERACTIONS: May increase digoxin levels; monitor periodically. Caution in multiple myeloma with erythropoietic agents or other agents that may increase risk of thrombosis such as estrogen containing therapies.

PREGNANCY: Category X, not for use in nursing.

MECHANISM OF ACTION: Thalidomide analogue; not established, possesses antineoplastic, immunomodulatory and antiangiogenic properties. Inhibits secretion of pro-inflammatory cytokines such as tumor necrosis factor (TNF-α) from peripheral blood mononuclear cells and also inhibits expression of cyclooxygenase-2 (COX-2) in vitro.

PHARMACOKINETICS: Absorption: Rapid, T_{max}=0.625-1.5 hrs (healthy); T_{max}=0.5-4.0 hrs (multiple myeloma). **Distribution:** Plasma protein binding (30%). **Elimination:** Urine (2/3, unchanged); $T_{1/2}$=3 hrs.

NURSING CONSIDERATIONS

Assessment: Assess for pregnancy/nursing status, renal impairment, history of Grade 4 rash, patients with high tumor burden, hypersensitivity to the drug and possible drug interactions. Obtain pregnancy test (sensitivity of ≥50 mIU/mL) 10-14 days before and 24 hrs before initiating therapy. Confirm use of 2 forms of effective contraception beginning 4 weeks prior to therapy.

Monitoring: Monitor the use of effective contraception during therapy, during therapy interruptions and for 4 weeks after therapy. Perform pregnancy test weekly during the 1st month, then monthly thereafter in women with regular menstrual cycles and every 2 weeks with irregular menstrual cycles. Monitor CBC weekly for 1st 8 weeks of therapy and monthly thereafter (MDS); every 2 weeks for 1st 12 weeks and monthly thereafter (multiple myeloma). Monitor for signs/symptoms of hypersensitivity reactions, DVT, PE, thromboembolism, neutropenia, thrombocytopenia, angioedema, Grade 2-3 rash, exfoliative/bullous rash, SJS, TEN, tumor lysis syndrome, and tumor flare reaction. Monitor renal function, especially in elderly.

Patient Counseling: Instruct not to break, chew, or open caps. Counsel on potential risk of teratogenicity. Inform that treatment should only be initiated following a negative pregnancy and the importance of performing monthly pregnancy tests. Instruct to use 2 effective contraceptive methods during therapy, during therapy interruptions, and for at least 4 weeks after completing therapy. Instruct males receiving therapy to always use a latex condom during any sexual contact, even if with successful vasectomy; inform physician if he has had unprotected sexual contact with a woman who can become pregnant. Instruct to immediately d/c therapy if the patient becomes pregnant, misses her menstrual period, experiences unusual bleeding, stops taking birth control, or thinks that she may be pregnant. Inform that therapy is associated with significant neutropenia and thrombocytopenia. Instruct to seek medical attention if symptoms of thromboembolism, hypersensitivity reactions, or infection occur. Inform that the therapy in combination with dexamethasone has demonstrated significant increased risk of DVT and PE in multiple myeloma.

Administration: Oral route. Do not break, chew, or open the caps; wash thoroughly if powder gets in contact with the skin or mucous membranes.
Storage: 25°C (77°F); excursions permitted to 15-30°C (59-86°F). Dispense no more than a 28-day supply.

REYATAZ
atazanavir sulfate (Bristol-Myers Squibb)

RX

THERAPEUTIC CLASS: Protease inhibitor

INDICATIONS: Treatment of HIV-1 infection in combination with other antiretrovirals.

DOSAGE: *Adults:* Therapy-Naive: 300mg with ritonavir (RTV) 100mg qd. If intolerant to RTV, give atazanavir (ATV) 400mg qd. Therapy-Experienced: 300mg with RTV 100mg qd. Concomitant Therapy: Refer to PI for proper administration and dose adjustments. Therapy-Experienced 2nd/3rd Trimester Pregnancy with H_2-Receptor Antagonist or Tenofovir: 400mg with RTV 100mg qd. Therapy-Naive End Stage Renal Disease (ESRD) with Hemodialysis: 300mg with RTV 100mg. Moderate Hepatic Impairment (Child-Pugh Class B) Without Prior Virologic Failure: 300mg qd. Take with food. *Pediatrics:* ≥ 6 yrs: Therapy-Naive: 15 to <25kg: 150mg with RTV 80mg qd. 25 to <32kg: 200mg with RTV 100mg qd. 32 to <39kg: 250mg with RTV 100mg qd. ≥39kg: 300mg with RTV 100mg qd. ≥13 yrs and ≥39kg: If intolerant to RTV, give ATV 400mg qd. Therapy-Experienced: 25 to <32kg: 200mg with RTV 100mg qd. 32 to <39kg: 250mg with RTV 100mg qd. ≥39kg: 300mg with RTV 100mg qd. Max: 300mg with RTV 100mg. Do not exceed recommended adult dose. Take with food.

HOW SUPPLIED: Cap: 100mg, 150mg, 200mg, 300mg

CONTRAINDICATIONS: Concomitant use with drugs highly dependent on CYP3A or UGT1A1 for clearance: alfuzosin, rifampin, irinotecan, triazolam, orally administered midazolam, dihydroergotamine, ergotamine, ergonovine, methylergonovine, cisapride, St. John's wort (*Hypericum perforatum*), lovastatin, simvastatin, pimozide, indinavir, sildenafil (when dosed as Revatio for pulmonary arterial HTN).

WARNINGS/PRECAUTIONS: Not recommended without RTV for treatment-experienced patients with prior virologic failure and, during pregnancy and the postpartum period. Caution with mild to moderate hepatic impairment. Avoid with severe hepatic impairment. Should not be administered to HIV treatment-experienced patients with ESRD managed with hemodialysis. ATV/RTV is not recommended with hepatic impairment. May prolong PR-interval; caution with pre-existing conduction system diseases. May cause rash, including Stevens-Johnson syndrome (SJS), erythema multiforme and toxic skin eruptions; d/c if severe rash develops. May cause hyperbilirubinemia. Increased risk for further transaminase elevations or hepatic decompensation in patients with underlying hepatitis B or C infections or marked transaminase elevations; monitor prior to and during treatment. Nephrolithiasis reported; may temporarily interrupt or d/c therapy if symptoms occur. New onset or exacerbation of diabetes mellitus (DM), hyperglycemia, and diabetic ketoacidosis reported. Immune reconstitution syndrome reported. May cause redistribution/accumulation of body fat. Increased risk of bleeding may occur with hemophilia A and B. Various degrees of cross-resistance observed. Caution in elderly.

ADVERSE REACTIONS: Nausea, jaundice/scleral icterus, rash, myalgia.

R

INTERACTIONS: See Contraindications. Coadministration with drugs primarily metabolized by CYP3A or UGT1A1 may result in increased plasma concentrations of the other drug that could increase or prolong its therapeutic and adverse effects. Caution with drugs highly dependent on CYP2C8 with narrow therapeutic indices when administered without RTV. Decreased levels with CYP3A4 inducers, PPIs, antacids, buffered medications (give ATV 2 hrs before or 1 hr after), or H$_2$-receptor antagonists (space dosing by 10 hrs). Caution with other drugs that prolong the PR interval, including β-blockers, verapamil, and digoxin, especially those metabolized by CYP3A. May require dose adjustments of insulin or oral hypoglycemic agents. Increased diltiazem plasma concentration with an additive effect on PR interval. Decreased exposure with didanosine, efavirenz and nevirapine. Decreased plasma concentration with tenofovir. May increase concentration with RTV and voriconazole. Increased plasma concentration of saquinavir, protease inhibitors, TCAs, rifabutin, parenteral midazolam, immunosuppressants, clarithromycin, buprenorphine, norbuprenorphine, sildenafil, tadalafil and vardenafil. Increased plasma concentration of amiodarone, bepridil, lidocaine (systemic), quinidine, trazodone, CCBs and fluticasone proprionate; use with caution. Concomitant use with ATV/RTV increases plasma concentration of ketoconazole and itraconazole. Coadministration of ATV/RTV with other protease inhibitors is not recommended. Monitor INR with warfarin. Avoid with colchicine in patients with renal/hepatic impairment. Avoid with bosentan when administered without RTV. Increased risk of myopathy and rhabdomyolysis with atorvastatin and rosuvastatin. Caution with oral contraceptives. Coadministration with salmeterol is not recommended. Refer to PI for pharmacokinetic parameters with other coadministered drugs.

PREGNANCY: Category B, not for use in nursing.

MECHANISM OF ACTION: HIV-1 protease inhibitor; selectively inhibits virus-specific processing of viral Gag and Gag-Pol polyproteins in HIV-1 infected cells, preventing formation of mature virions.

PHARMACOKINETICS: Absorption: Rapid. C$_{max}$=5233ng/mL, T$_{max}$=2.5 hrs, AUC=53761ng•h/mL. **Distribution:** Plasma protein binding (86%). **Metabolism:** Liver; mono- and dioxygenation via CYP3A. **Elimination:** Urine (13%, 7% unchanged), feces (79%, 20% unchanged); T$_{1/2}$=7 hrs.

NURSING CONSIDERATIONS

Assessment: Assess renal/liver function. Assess for treatment history, hepatitis B or C infection, transaminase elevations, known hypersensitivity, DM, hemophilia, conduction system disease, pregnancy/nursing status, and possible drug interactions. Obtain baseline ECG.

Monitoring: Monitor for cardiac conduction abnormalities, PR interval prolongation, rash, hyperbilirubinemia, nephrolithiasis, new onset or exacerbation of DM, hyperglycemia, diabetic ketoacidosis, immune reconstitution syndrome, fat redistribution/accumulation, and cross-resistance among protease inhibitors. Monitor LFTs in patients with underlying hepatitis B or C infection and serum transaminase elevations. Monitor for bleeding in patients with hemophilia. Monitor closely for adverse events during the 1st 2 months after delivery.

Patient Counseling: Inform that therapy is not cure for HIV, does not reduce risk of transmission of HIV, that opportunistic infections may develop, and to take with food as prescribed. If dose is missed, take as soon as possible and return to normal schedule. Report use of any other medications or herbal products. Inform that mild rashes, asymptomatic elevations in indirect bilirubin, or redistribution and accumulation of body fat may occur. Seek medical attention if symptoms of PR interval prolongation (eg, dizziness or lightheadedness) occur.

Administration: Oral route. **Storage:** 25°C (77°F); excursions permitted to 15-30°C (59-86°F).

RHINOCORT AQUA

RX

budesonide (AstraZeneca)

THERAPEUTIC CLASS: Corticosteroid

INDICATIONS: Treatment of nasal symptoms of seasonal or perennial allergic rhinitis in adults and children ≥6 yrs.

DOSAGE: *Adults:* Initial: 1 spray/nostril qd. Max: 4 sprays/nostril qd.
Pediatrics: ≥12 yrs: Initial: 1 spray/nostril qd. Max: 4 sprays/nostril qd. 6-<12 yrs: Initial: 1 spray/nostril qd. Max: 2 sprays/nostril qd.

HOW SUPPLIED: Spray: 32mcg/spray [8.6g]

WARNINGS/PRECAUTIONS: Local nasal effects (eg, epistaxis, *Candida* infections of the nose and pharynx, nasal septal perforation, impaired wound healing) may occur. May need to d/c treatment when *Candida* infection develops. Avoid in patients with recent nasal surgery, trauma, or septal ulcers until healing has occurred. Hypersensitivity reactions may occur. May cause immunosuppresion; caution with active or quiescent tuberculosis (TB), untreated fungal, bacterial, systemic viral or parasitic infections; or ocular herpes simplex. Hypercorticism and adrenal suppression may appear with higher than recommended dose or in susceptible individuals at recommended dose; d/c slowly. Adrenal insufficiency and withdrawal symptoms may occur when replacing a systemic with a topical corticosteroid. May reduce growth velocity in pediatrics. Glaucoma, increased intraocular pressure (IOP) and cataracts reported; monitor closely in patients with change in vision, history of IOP, glaucoma, and/or cataracts. Caution with hepatic dysfunction.

ADVERSE REACTIONS: Pharyngitis, epistaxis, cough, bronchospasm, nasal irritation.

INTERACTIONS: Oral ketoconazole and other known strong CYP3A4 inhibitors (eg, ritonavir, atazanavir, clarithromycin, indinavir, itraconazole, nefazodone, nelfinavir, saquinavir, telithromycin) may increase plasma levels; use with caution.

PREGNANCY: Category B, caution in nursing.

MECHANISM OF ACTION: Corticosteroid; not established. Possesses a wide range of inhibitory activities against multiple cell types (eg, mast cells, eosinophils, neutrophils, macrophages, lymphocytes) and mediators (eg, histamine, leukotrienes, eicosanoids, cytokines) involved in allergic-mediated inflammation.

PHARMACOKINETICS: Absorption: Absolute bioavailability (34%); C_{max}=0.3nmol/L; T_{max}=0.5 hr. **Distribution:** V_d=2-3L/kg, plasma protein binding (85-90%), found in breast milk. **Metabolism:** Liver (rapid, extensive) via CYP3A4; 16α-hydroxyprednisolone and 6β-hydroxybudesonide (major metabolites). **Elimination:** Urine (2/3 metabolites), feces; $T_{1/2}$=2-3 hrs.

NURSING CONSIDERATIONS

Assessment: Assess for history of hypersensitivity, increased IOP, glaucoma and/or cataracts. Assess for recent nasal ulcers, surgery/trauma, active or quiescent TB, untreated local or systemic fungal or bacterial infections, systemic viral or parasitic infections, ocular herpes simplex, suppressed immune system, asthma or other conditions requiring chronic systemic corticosteroid therapy, pregnancy/nursing status, and possible drug interactions.

Monitoring: Monitor for acute adrenal insufficiency and withdrawal symptoms when replacing systemic corticosteroid with topical corticosteroid. Monitor for hypercorticism and/or HPA-axis suppression, disseminated infections (eg, chickenpox and measles), nasal or pharyngeal *Candida* infections, suppression of growth velocity in children, nasal septal perforation, epistaxis, glaucoma, increased IOP, and cataracts.

Patient Counseling: Inform about the benefits and risks of the treatment. Counsel to take as directed at regular intervals. Advise to avoid exposure to chickenpox or measles. Instruct to consult physician immediately if exposed to chickenpox or measles, if existing infection worsens, or if episodes of

R

epistaxis or nasal discomfort occur. Instruct to inform physician if a change in vision occurs.

Administration: Intranasal route. Shake gently before use. Refer to PI for further administration instructions. **Storage:** 20-25°C (68-77°F) with the valve up. Do not freeze. Protect from light.

RIASTAP RX
fibrinogen concentrate (human) (CSL Behring)

THERAPEUTIC CLASS: Plasma glycoprotein

INDICATIONS: Treatment of acute bleeding episodes in patients with congenital fibrinogen deficiency, including afibrinogenemia and hypofibrinogenemia.

DOSAGE: *Adults:* Individualize dose. Known Baseline Fibrinogen Level: Dose calculated based on the target plasma fibrinogen level based on bleeding type, actual measured plasma fibrinogen level, and body weight. Refer to PI for dose calculation based on target plasma fibrinogen level. Unknown Baseline Fibrinogen Level: Usual: 70mg/kg IV. Monitor fibrinogen level during treatment. A target fibrinogen level of 100mg/dL should be maintained until hemostasis is obtained.

HOW SUPPLIED: Inj: 900mg-1300mg [50mL]

WARNINGS/PRECAUTIONS: For IV use only. Reconstitute prior to use. Administer under supervision of a physician. Not indicated for dysfibrinogenemia. Allergic reactions may occur; d/c if symptoms of this or early signs of hypersensitivity (eg, hives, generalized urticaria, chest tightness, wheezing, hypotension, and anaphylaxis) occur. Thromboembolic events reported. May contain infectious agents (eg, viruses and Creutzfeldt-Jakob (CJD) agents) that may cause disease. Healthcare provider should report all infections thought to have been transmitted by this product to CSL Behring at 1-866-915-6958.

ADVERSE REACTIONS: Allergic-anaphylactic reactions, chills, fever, headache, N/V, thromboembolic episodes.

PREGNANCY: Category C, safety not known in nursing.

MECHANISM OF ACTION: Plasma glycoprotein; physiological substrate of thrombin, factor XIIIa, and plasmin. Replaces the missing or low coagulation factor.

PHARMACOKINETICS: Absorption: C_{max}=140mg/dL, AUC=124.3mg•hr/mL (70mg/kg dose). **Distribution:** V_d=52.7mL/kg. **Elimination:** $T_{1/2}$=78.7 hrs.

NURSING CONSIDERATIONS

Assessment: Assess for hypersensitivity reactions, dysfibrinogenemia, and pregnancy/nursing status. Assess fibrinogen levels.

Monitoring: Monitor for signs/symptoms of an allergic/hypersensitivity reaction, thrombosis, and for the transmission of infectious agents (eg, viruses, CJD agent). Monitor fibrinogen levels.

Patient Counseling: Notify physician immediately if experience allergic/hypersensitivity reactions (eg, hives, chest tightness, hypotension, wheezing, and anaphylaxis) or thrombotic events (eg, unexplained pleuritic, chest/leg pain or edema, hemoptysis, dyspnea, tachypnea or unexplained neurologic symptoms). Counsel about the risk of thrombosis with or without embolization. Inform that may contain infectious agents that can cause disease (eg, viruses and CJD agent). Symptoms of a possible viral infection include headache, fever, N/V, weakness, malaise, diarrhea, or, in the case of hepatitis, jaundice.

Administration: IV route. Use aseptic technique in preparing and reconstitution. Do not mix with other medicinal products or IV solutions, and should be administered through separate injection site. Administer at room temperature by slow IV injection at a rate not exceeding 5mL/min. Refer to PI for reconstitution instructions. **Storage:** Prior to Reconstitution: 2-25°C (36-77°F) up to 30 months. Protect from light. Do not freeze. Following Reconstitution: 20-25°C; stable for 24 hrs. Do not freeze.

RIFADIN   RX
rifampin (Sanofi-Aventis)

THERAPEUTIC CLASS: Rifamycin derivative

INDICATIONS: Treatment of all forms of tuberculosis (TB). Treatment of asymptomatic carriers of *Neisseria meningitidis* to eliminate meningococci from nasopharynx. (IV) For initial treatment and retreatment of TB when drug cannot be taken by mouth.

DOSAGE: *Adults:* TB: 10mg/kg PO/IV qd. Max: 600mg/day. Meningococcal Carriers: 600mg bid for 2 days. Take cap 1 hr before or 2 hrs after a meal with a full glass of water.
Pediatrics: TB: 10-20mg/kg PO/IV qd. Max: 600mg/day. Meningococcal Carriers: ≥1 month: 10mg/kg q12h for 2 days. Max: 600mg/dose. <1 month: 5mg/kg q12h for 2 days. Take cap 1 hr before or 2 hrs after a meal with a full glass of water.

HOW SUPPLIED: Cap: 150mg, 300mg; Inj: 600mg

CONTRAINDICATIONS: Patients who are receiving atazanavir, darunavir, fosamprenavir, saquinavir or tipranavir; may result in loss of antiviral efficacy and/or development of viral resistance. Patients who are taking ritonavir-boosted saquinavir due to an increased risk of severe hepatocellular toxicity.

WARNINGS/PRECAUTIONS: May produce liver dysfunction. Jaundice reported in patients with liver disease. Caution with impaired liver function. D/C if signs of hepatocellular damage occur. Hyperbilirubinemia and porphyria exacerbation reported. Not for treatment of meningococcal disease. Caution with history of diabetes mellitus (DM); diabetes management may be more difficult. Higher doses may result in higher incidence of adverse reactions including flu syndrome (fever, chills and malaise), hematopoietic reactions (leukopenia, thrombocytopenia, or acute hemolytic anemia), cutaneous, GI, and hepatic reactions, SOB, shock, anaphylaxis, renal failure. Not recommended for intermittent therapy; rare renal hypersensitivity reactions reported when therapy was resumed. Caution in elderly. (IV) For IV infusion only; do not administer IM or SQ. Avoid extravasation; d/c infusion if local irritation and inflammation occur and restart at another site.

ADVERSE REACTIONS: Heartburn, N/V, headache, fever, drowsiness, dizziness, muscle weakness, visual disturbances, menstrual disturbances, BUN elevation, serum uric acid elevation, flushing, rash, edema.

INTERACTIONS: See Contraindications. May accelerate the metabolism of the following drugs: anticonvulsants (eg, phenytoin), digitoxin, antiarrhythmics (eg, disopyramide, mexiletine, quinidine, tocainide), oral anticoagulants, antifungals (eg, fluconazole, itraconazole, ketoconazole), barbiturates, β-blockers, calcium channel blockers (eg, diltiazem, nifedipine, verapamil), chloramphenicol, clarithromycin, corticosteroids, cyclosporine, cardiac glycoside preparations, clofibrate, oral or other systemic hormonal contraceptives, dapsone, diazepam, doxycycline, fluoroquinolones (eg, ciprofloxacin), haloperidol, oral hypoglycemic agents (sulfonylureas), levothyroxine, methadone, narcotic analgesics, progestins, quinine, tacrolimus, theophylline, tricyclic antidepressants (eg, amitriptyline, nortriptyline) and zidovudine; dose adjustments of these drugs may be necessary. May need to change use of oral or other systemic hormonal contraceptives to nonhormonal methods of birth control. May increase requirements for anticoagulant drugs of the coumarin type; perform PT daily or as frequently as necessary to establish and maintain anticoagulant dose. Antacids may reduce absorption; give rifampin at least 1 hr before antacids. Increased risk of hepatotoxicity with halothane or isoniazid. Avoid concomitant use with halothane and monitor closely when given with isoniazid. Increased serum levels with probenecid and cotrimoxazole. Caution with other hepatotoxic agents. Concomitant use of ketoconazole decreases both drug serum levels. Decreased levels of enalapril, atovaquone. Increased levels with atovaquone. Plasma concentrations of sulfapyridine may be reduced following

R

the concomitant administration of sulfasalazine and rifampin. May accelerate elimination of cytochrome P-450 substrates; may require dose adjustments of drugs metabolized by these enzymes.

PREGNANCY: Category C, not for use in nursing.

MECHANISM OF ACTION: Rifamycin derivative; inhibits DNA-dependent RNA polymerase activity in susceptible *Mycobacterium tuberculosis* organisms. Interacts with bacterial RNA polymerase; does not inhibit the mammalian enzyme.

PHARMACOKINETICS: Absorption: Oral and IV administration resulted in different parameters; refer to PI for further information. **Distribution:** Distributed in body fluids and CSF; crosses the placenta; plasma protein binding (80%); (IV, 300mg, 600mg): V_d=0.66L/kg, 0.64L/kg;. **Metabolism:** Via deacetylation; 25-desacetyl-rifampin (major metabolite). **Elimination:** Urine (30%), bile; Elimination half-life varied based on age and dosing; refer to PI for further details.

NURSING CONSIDERATIONS

Assessment: Assess for liver and renal function, history of DM, meningococcal disease, drug hypersensitivity, nursing/pregnancy status and possible drug interactions. Document indications for therapy, culture and sensitivity. Obtain baseline measurement of LFTs (SGPT, SGOT), bilirubin, transaminase level, SrCr, CBC, and platelet count. Obtain bacteriologic cultures to confirm susceptibility of organism prior to therapy

Monitoring: Monitor SGPT and SGOT every 2-4 weeks with impaired liver function, bilirubin and/or transaminase levels, renal function, SrCr, serum uric acid, CBCs, and platelet count. Monitor treatment response by performing susceptibility tests. Monitor for adverse reactions. (IV) Monitor for local irritation and inflammation at infusion site.

Patient Counseling: Counsel that drug treats bacterial, and not viral infections. Instruct to comply with full course of therapy and not to miss doses; skipping doses or not completing full course of therapy may decrease effectiveness and increase likelihood of developing drug-resistance to the bacteria. Drug may produce reddish urine, sweat, sputum, and tears; soft contact lenses may be permanently stained. Take cap 1 hr before or 2 hrs after meal with full glass of water. Notify physician if fever, loss of appetite, malaise, N/V, darkened urine, yellowish discoloration of skin/eyes, and joint pain/swelling occur. Reliability of oral or systemic hormonal contraceptives may be affected; use alternate contraceptive measures.

Administration: Oral and IV route. Refer to PI for the proper preparation of IV infusion and extemporaneous oral suspension. **Storage:** Cap: Store in dry place. Avoid excessive heat. IV: Reconstituted Sol: Room temperature for 24 hrs. Dilutions in Dextrose 5% for Inj (D5W): Room temperature for up to 4 hrs. Dilutions in Normal Saline: Room temperature for up to 24 hrs. Prepare and use within this time. Avoid excessive heat (40-104°C). Protect from light.

RIFAMATE   RX
rifampin - isoniazid (Sanofi-Aventis)

> Isoniazid associated with severe and sometimes fatal hepatitis. Monitor LFTs on a monthly basis.

THERAPEUTIC CLASS: Isonicotinic acid hydrazide/rifamycin derivative

INDICATIONS: For pulmonary tuberculosis (TB). Not for initial therapy or prevention.

DOSAGE: *Adults:* 2 caps qd. Take 1 hr before or 2 hrs after meals. Give with pyridoxine in the malnourished, those predisposed to neuropathy (eg, alcoholics, diabetics), and adolescents.

HOW SUPPLIED: Cap: (Isoniazid-Rifampin) 150mg-300mg

CONTRAINDICATIONS: Previous isoniazid-associated hepatic injury, severe adverse reactions to isoniazid (eg, drug fever, chills, and arthritis), acute liver disease.

WARNINGS/PRECAUTIONS: Monitor LFTs before therapy, periodically thereafter. Not for intermittent therapy. Urine, feces, saliva, sputum, sweat, and tears may be colored red-orange; may stain soft contact lenses permanently. Caution with chronic liver disease or severe renal dysfunction. Perform periodic ophthalmoscopic exams.

ADVERSE REACTIONS: Headache, drowsiness, fatigue, ataxia, dizziness, confusion, visual disturbances, weakness, GI effects, peripheral neuropathy, pyridoxine deficiency, anorexia, nausea, renal or hepatic insufficiency, blood dyscrasias.

INTERACTIONS: Anticoagulants may need dose increase. May decrease activity of methadone, oral hypoglycemics, digitoxin, quinidine, disopyramide, dapsone, and corticosteroids. Higher incidence of isoniazid hepatitis with daily alcohol ingestion. Risk of phenytoin toxicity. Caution with other hepatotoxic agents and phenytoin. May decrease effects of oral contraceptives; use alternative measures.

PREGNANCY: Safety in pregnancy not known, caution in nursing.

MECHANISM OF ACTION: Isonicotinic acid hydrazide/rifamycin derivative. Isoniazid/Rifampin: Exhibits bacterial activity against intracellular and extracellular *Mycobacterium tuberculosis*. Inhibits DNA-dependent RNA polymerase activity in susceptible cells; interacts with bacterial RNA polymerase but does not inhibit the mammalian enzyme. Inhibits mycoloic acid synthesis and acts against actively growing tubercle bacilli.

PHARMACOKINETICS: Absorption: Rifampin: C_{max}=10mcg/mL, T_{max}=1.5-3 hrs. Isoniazid: T_{max}=1-2 hrs. **Distribution:** Isoniazid: Diffuses into body fluids; crosses placental barrier and into milk. **Metabolism:** Isoniazid: Acetylation and dehydrazination. **Elimination:** Rifampin: Bile, urine; $T_{1/2}$=3 hrs.

NURSING CONSIDERATIONS

Assessment: Assess for previous isoniazid-associated hepatic injury, acute liver disease, HIV status, pregnancy/nursing status, and drug interactions. Document reasons for therapy, culture and susceptibility.

Monitoring: Prior to therapy and periodically thereafter, measure hepatic enzymes (AST, ALT). D/C at first sign of hypersensitivity reactions (fever, skin eruptions, Stevens-Johnson syndrome, vasculitis, anaphylaxis). Monitor for peripheral neuropathy, convulsions, N/V, agranulocytosis, hemolytic anemia, systemic lupus erythematosus like syndrome, metabolic and endocrine reactions (hyperglycemia, pyridoxine deficiency, pellagra), visual disturbances, serum uric acid levels. Perform periodic ophthalmoscopic exams.

Patient Counseling: Advise to immediately report signs/symptoms consistent with liver damage or other adverse events (eg, unexplained anorexia, N/V, dark urine, icterus, rash, persistent paresthesias of the hands and feet, persistent fatigue, weakness or fever of >3 days duration and/or abdominal tenderness). Counsel not to administer with food, take as prescribed, take pyridoxine tablets if peripheral neuropathy develops. Inform that drug may produce reddish urine, sweat, sputum, and tears. Periodic eye exams are recommended when visual symptoms occur.

Administration: Oral route. **Storage:** Keep tightly closed. Store in a dry place. Avoid excessive heat.

RIFATER   RX
pyrazinamide - rifampin - isoniazid (Sanofi-Aventis)

> Isoniazid associated with severe and sometimes fatal hepatitis. Monitor LFTs on a monthly basis. D/C promptly if symptoms of hepatitis occur. Defer treatment in persons with acute hepatic diseases.

THERAPEUTIC CLASS: Isonicotinic acid hydrazide/rifamycin derivative/nicotinamide analogue

INDICATIONS: For initial phase of pulmonary tuberculosis (TB) treatment.

DOSAGE: *Adults:* ≤44kg: 4 tabs single dose qd. 45-54kg: 5 tabs single dose qd. ≥55kg: 6 tabs single dose qd. Give pyridoxine in malnourished, if predisposed to neuropathy (eg, alcoholics, diabetics), and adolescents. Take 1 hr before or 2 hrs after meals with full glass of water. Treatment usually lasts 2 months.

Pediatrics: ≥15 yrs: ≤44kg: 4 tabs single dose qd. 45-54kg: 5 tabs single dose qd. ≥55kg: 6 tabs single dose qd. Give pyridoxine in malnourished, if predisposed to neuropathy (eg, alcoholics, diabetics), and adolescents. Take 1 hr before or 2 hrs after meals with full glass of water. Treatment usually lasts 2 months.

HOW SUPPLIED: Tab: (Isoniazid-Pyrazinamide-Rifampin) 50mg-300mg-120mg

CONTRAINDICATIONS: Severe hepatic damage, adverse reactions to isoniazid (eg, drug fever, chills, arthritis), acute liver disease, acute gout. Concomitant administration of atazanavir, darunavir, fosamprenavir, saquinavir, tipranavir, and ritonavir-boosted saquinavir.

WARNINGS/PRECAUTIONS: Liver dysfunction, hyperbilirubinemia, and hyperuricemia with acute gouty arthritis reported. Caution in patients with impaired liver function; monitor LFTs (every 2-4 weeks) and serum uric acid. Perform regular ophthalmologic exams. Caution with diabetes mellitus (DM), severe renal dysfunction. Doses of rifampin >600mg given once daily or twice weekly resulted in higher incidence of adverse reactions ("flu syndrome", hematopoietic, cutaneous, GI, and hepatic reactions, SOB, shock, anaphylaxis, and renal failure). Rifampin is not recommended for intermittent therapy. May produce reddish coloration of urine, sweat, sputum, and tears. May permanently stain soft contact lenses. Caution in elderly.

ADVERSE REACTIONS: Cutaneous reactions, N/V, digestive pain, diarrhea, arthralgia, sweating, headache, insomnia, anxiety, tightness in chest, coughing, angina, palpitation, anxiety, phlebitis.

INTERACTIONS: See Contraindications. Rifampin may accelerate metabolism of anticonvulsants (eg, phenytoin), digitoxin, antiarrhythmics (eg, disopyramide, mexiletine, quinidine, tocainide), oral anticoagulants, antifungals (eg, fluconazole, itraconazole, ketoconazole), barbiturates, β-blockers, calcium channel blockers (eg, diltiazem, nifedipine, verapamil), chloramphenicol, clarithromycin, fluoroquinolones (eg, ciprofloxacin), corticosteroids, cyclosporine, cardiac glycosides, clofibrate, oral or other systemic hormonal contraceptives, dapsone, diazepam, doxycycline, haloperidol, oral hypoglycemics (eg, sulfonylureas), levothyroxine, methadone, narcotic analgesics, TCAs (eg, amitriptyline, nortriptyline), progestins, quinine, tacrolimus, theophylline and zidovudine. Decreased concentration of atovaquone, ketoconazole, enalaprilat and sulfapyridine. Increased rifampin concentrations with probenecid and cotrimoxazole. Antacids may reduce rifampin absorption. Avoid foods containing tyramine and histamine (eg, cheese, red wine, tuna). Anticoagulants may need dose increase. Higher incidence of isoniazid (INH) hepatitis with daily alcohol ingestion. Avoid halothane. Monitor renal function with enflurane. INH inhibits certain CYP450 enzymes; monitor with anticonvulsants, benzodiazepines, haloperidol, ketoconazole, theophylline and warfarin. Decreased levels with corticosteroids. Increased levels with para-aminosalicylic acid. Exaggerates CNS effects of meperidine, cycloserine, disulfiram. Excess catecholamine stimulation with L-dopa.

PREGNANCY: Category C, not for use in nursing.

MECHANISM OF ACTION: Rifampin: Rifamycin derivative; inhibits DNA-dependent RNA polymerase activity in susceptible *Mycobacterium tuberculosis* organism. Interacts with bacterial RNA polymerase, but does not inhibit the mammalian enzyme. Isoniazid: Isonicotinic acid hydrazide; inhibits the biosynthesis of mycolic acids, which are major component of the cell wall of *Mycobacterium tuberculosis*. Pyrazinamide: Nicotinamide analog; has not been established.

PHARMACOKINETICS: Absorption: Isoniazid: Bioavailability (100.6%), C_{max}=3.09mcg/mL, T_{max}=1-2 hrs. Rifampin: Bioavailability (88.8%), C_{max}=11.04mcg/mL. Pyrazinamide: Bioavailability (96.8%), C_{max}=28.02mcg/mL.

Distribution: Isoniazid: Passes through placental barrier and into milk. Pyrazinamide: Plasma protein binding (10%), distributed in liver, lungs, and CSF; found in breast milk. Rifampin: Protein binding (80%). **Metabolism:** Isoniazid: Acetylation and dehydrazination. Pyrazinamide: Liver, via hydroxylation; pyrazinoic acid (major active metabolite). Rifampin: Via deacetylation. **Elimination:** Rifampin: Urine (30%), bile; $T_{1/2}$=3.35 hrs. Pyrazinamide: Urine (70%), (4-14% unchanged); $T_{1/2}$=9-10 hrs. Isoniazid: Urine (50-70%); $T_{1/2}$=1-4 hrs.

NURSING CONSIDERATIONS

Assessment: Assess for previous isoniazid-associated hepatic injury, acute gout, HIV status, pregnancy/nursing status, DM, and drug interactions. Document reasons for therapy, culture and susceptibility.

Monitoring: Prior to therapy and periodically thereafter, measure hepatic enzymes (AST, ALT) every 2-4 weeks with impaired liver function. D/C at first sign of hypersensitivity reactions (fever, skin eruptions, Stevens-Johnson syndrome, vasculitis, anaphylaxis). Monitor for peripheral neuropathy, convulsions, N/V, agranulocytosis, hemolytic anemia, systemic lupus erythematosus-like syndrome, metabolic and endocrine reactions (hyperglycemia, pyridoxine deficiency, pellagra), visual disturbances, serum uric acid levels. Perform regular ophthalmologic exams.

Patient Counseling: Immediately report signs/symptoms consistent with liver damage or other adverse events (unexplained anorexia, N/V, dark urine, icterus, rash, persistent paresthesias of hands and feet, persistent fatigue, weakness or fever of >3 days' duration and/or abdominal tenderness). Do not administer with food; take as prescribed. Take pyridoxine tablets if peripheral neuropathy develops. Drug may produce reddish urine, sweat, sputum, and tears. Periodic ophthalmologic examination is recommended. Avoid tyramine- and histamine-containing foods. Effectiveness of oral contraceptives may be decreased; consider alternative contraceptive methods.

Administration: Oral route. **Storage:** 15-30°C (59-86°F). Protect from excessive humidity.

RILUTEK   RX
riluzole (Sanofi-Aventis)

THERAPEUTIC CLASS: Benzothiazole

INDICATIONS: Treatment of amyotrophic lateral sclerosis (ALS). Extends survival and/or time to tracheostomy.

DOSAGE: *Adults:* 50mg q12h. Take 1 hr before or 2 hrs after meals.

HOW SUPPLIED: Tab: 50mg

WARNINGS/PRECAUTIONS: Caution with hepatic impairment; monitor LFTs. D/C if ALT levels ≥5 x ULN or clinical jaundice develops. Clinical hepatitis reported. Neutropenia may occur; monitor WBC count with febrile illness. Interstitial lung disease reported; perform chest radiography if respiratory symptoms develop such as dry cough and/or dyspnea. May impair mental/physical abilities. Caution in elderly.

ADVERSE REACTIONS: Asthenia, N/V, dizziness, decreased lung function, diarrhea, abdominal pain, vertigo, circumoral paresthesia, anorexia, somnolence, headache, anorexia, rhinitis, HTN.

INTERACTIONS: Caution with concomitant use with potentially hepatotoxic drugs (eg, allopurinol, methyldopa, sulfasalazine). CYP1A2 inhibitors (eg, caffeine, phenacetin, theophylline, amitriptyline, quinolones) may decrease elimination. CYP1A2 inducers (eg, cigarette smoke, charcoal-broiled food, rifampicin, omeprazole) may increase elimination. Potential interaction may occur if riluzole is given concurrently with drugs metabolized by CYP1A2 (eg, theophylline, caffeine, tacrine).

PREGNANCY: Category C, not for use in nursing.

MECHANISM OF ACTION: Benzothiazole; mechanism not established. May inhibit the effect on glutamate release, inactivates voltage-dependent sodium channels, and interferes with intracellular events that follow transmitter binding at excitatory amino acid receptors.

PHARMACOKINETICS: Absorption: Well absorbed; absolute bioavailability (60%). **Distribution:** Plasma protein binding (96%). **Metabolism:** Extensive; liver via CYP450 by hydroxylation and glucuronidation; N-hydroxyriluzole (major metabolite). **Elimination:** Urine (90% metabolites, 2% unchanged), feces (5%); $T_{1/2}$=12 hrs.

NURSING CONSIDERATIONS

Assessment: Assess for hepatic impairment, pregnancy/nursing status, alcohol intake, hypersensitivity and possible drug interactions. Perform baseline LFTs.

Monitoring: Perform baseline LFTs before therapy, every month during first 3 months, every 3 months for the remainder of the first year, then periodically thereafter. Take WBC count and chest radiography if necessary. Monitor for signs/symptoms of febrile illness, liver toxicity, and hypersensitivity reactions.

Patient Counseling: Notify healthcare professional of any signs of febrile illness. Caution about hazardous tasks (eg, operating machinery/driving). Notify healthcare professional if cough or SOB occur. Avoid use with excessive intake of alcohol. Instruct patient if a dose is missed, take next tablet as originally planned.

Administration: Oral route. **Storage:** 20-25°C (68-77°F); protect from bright light.

Riomet   RX
metformin HCl (Ranbaxy)

> Lactic acidosis reported (rare); increased risk with increased age, DM, renal dysfunction, congestive heart failure (CHF), and conditions with risk of hypoperfusion and hypoxemia. Avoid use in patients ≥80 yrs unless renal function is normal. Withhold therapy in the presence of any condition associated with hypoxemia, dehydration, or sepsis. Avoid in patients with clinical or laboratory evidence of hepatic disease. Caution against excessive alcohol intake;may potentiate the effects of metformin on lactate metabolism. Temporarily D/C prior to any IV radiocontrast study or surgical procedures. D/C use and institute appropriate therapy if lactic acidosis occur.

THERAPEUTIC CLASS: Biguanide

INDICATIONS: Adjunct to diet and exercise, to improve glycemic control in type 2 diabetes mellitus (DM).

DOSAGE: *Adults:* Individualize dose. Initial: 500mg bid or 850mg qd with meals. Titrate: Increase by 500mg/week or 850mg every 2 weeks, or may increase from 500mg bid to 850mg bid after 2 weeks. Max: 2550mg/day. Give in 3 divided doses with meals if dose is >2g/day. With Insulin: Initial: 500mg qd. Titrate: Increase by 500mg/week. Max: 2500mg/day. Decrease insulin dose by 10-25% when FPG <120mg/dL. Elderly/Debilitated/Malnourished: Conservative dosing; do not titrate to max.
Pediatrics: 10-16 yrs: Individualize dose. Initial: 500mg bid with meals. Titrate: Increase by 500mg/week. Max: 2000mg/day, given in divided doses.

HOW SUPPLIED: Sol: 500mg/5mL

CONTRAINDICATIONS: Renal disease/dysfunction (eg, SrCr ≥1.5mg/dL [males], ≥1.4mg/dL [females], or abnormal CrCl), metabolic acidosis, diabetic ketoacidosis with or without coma. D/C temporarily (48 hrs) for radiologic studies with intravascular iodinated contrast materials.

WARNINGS/PRECAUTIONS: Avoid in renal/hepatic impairment. D/C therapy in the presence of hypoxemia (eg, acute CHF, acute MI, cardiovascular collapse), dehydration, sepsis, or if loss of blood glucose occurs due to stress (give insulin). Temporarily d/c therapy prior to any surgical procedure (except minor procedures not associated with restricted intake of food and fluids). May decrease serum vitamin B_{12} levels. Increased risk of hypoglycemia in elderly, debilitated/malnourished, adrenal or pituitary insufficiency, or alcohol intoxication.

ADVERSE REACTIONS: Lactic acidosis, diarrhea, N/V, flatulence, asthenia, abdominal discomfort, hypoglycemia, dizziness, dyspnea, taste disorder, chest discomfort, flu syndrome, palpitations, indigestion, headache.

INTERACTIONS: See Boxed Warning and Contraindications. Furosemide, nifedipine, cimetidine, cationic drugs (eg, digoxin, amiloride, procainamide, quinidine, quinine, ranitidine, trimethoprim, vancomycin, triamterene, morphine) may increase metformin levels. Thiazides, other diuretics, corticosteroids, phenothiazines, thyroid products, estrogens, oral contraceptives, phenytoin, nicotinic acid, sympathomimetics, CCBs, and isoniazid may cause hyperglycemia. May interact with highly protein-bound drugs (eg, salicylates, sulfonamides, chloramphenicol, probenecid). May decrease furosemide levels. Caution with drugs that may affect renal function or result in significant hemodynamic change or may interfere with the disposition of metformin. Hypoglycemia may occur with concomitant use of other glucose-lowering agents (eg, sulfonylureas, insulin).

PREGNANCY: Category B, not for use in nursing.

MECHANISM OF ACTION: Biguanide; decreases hepatic glucose production, decreases intestinal absorption of glucose, and improves insulin selectivity by increasing peripheral glucose uptake and utilization.

PHARMACOKINETICS: Absorption: Absolute bioavailability (50-60%); T_{max}=2.5 hrs. **Distribution:** V_d=654L. **Elimination:** Urine (90%); $T_{1/2}$=6.2 hrs (plasma), 17.6 hrs (blood).

NURSING CONSIDERATIONS

Assessment: Assess for renal/hepatic impairment, acute or chronic metabolic acidosis, presence of a hypoxic state (eg, CHF, acute MI, cardiovascular collapse), dehydration, sepsis, alcoholism, nutritional status, adrenal or pituitary insufficiency, pregnancy/nursing status, and for possible drug interactions. Assess baseline renal function, FPG, HbA1c, and hematological parameters (Hct, Hgb, red blood cell indices).

Monitoring: Monitor for lactic acidosis, ketoacidosis, hypoglycemia, hypoxemia (eg, cardiovascular collapse, acute CHF, acute MI), prerenal azotemia, and for decreases in Vitamin B_{12} levels. Monitor FPG, HbA1c, renal function (eg, SrCr), and hematological parameters (eg, Hgb, Hct, red blood cell indices).

Patient Counseling: Inform about the importance of adherence to dietary instructions and a regular exercise program. Inform of the risk of developing lactic acidosis during therapy; advise to d/c therapy immediately and contact physician if unexplained hyperventilation, myalgia, malaise, unusual somnolence, or other nonspecific symptoms occur. Instruct to avoid excessive alcohol intake. Inform that regular follow-up is needed. Counsel to take with meals.

Administration: Oral route. **Storage:** 15-30°C (59-86°F).

R

RISPERDAL   RX
risperidone (Ortho-Mcneil/Janssen)

> Elderly patients with dementia-related psychosis treated with antipsychotic drugs are at an increased risk of death; most deaths appeared to be cardiovascular (eg, heart failure, sudden death) or infectious (eg, pneumonia) in nature. Risperidone is not approved for treatment of patients with dementia-related psychosis.

OTHER BRAND NAMES: Risperdal M-Tab (Ortho-Mcneil/Janssen)

THERAPEUTIC CLASS: Benzisoxazole derivative

INDICATIONS: Acute and maintenance treatment of schizophrenia in adults. Treatment of schizophrenia in adolescents 13-17 yrs. Short-term treatment of acute manic or mixed episodes associated with bipolar I disorder as monotherapy (adults and in children and adolescents 10-17 yrs) or in combination with lithium or valproate (adults). Treatment of irritability associated with autistic disorder in children and adolescents 5-16 yrs, including symptoms of aggression toward others, deliberate self-injuriousness, temper tantrums, and quickly changing moods.

DOSAGE: *Adults:* Schizophrenia: Initial: 2mg/day qd or bid. Titrate: Adjust dose at intervals not <24 hrs, in increments of 1-2mg/day, as tolerated, to recommended dose of 4-8mg/day. Dosing Range: 4-16mg/day. Max: 16mg/day. Maint: 2-8mg/day. Periodically reassess need for maintenance treatment. Refer to PI for information on reinitiating treatment and switching from other antipsychotics. Bipolar Mania: Initial: 2-3mg qd. Titrate: Adjust dose at intervals not <24 hrs and in increments/decrements of 1mg/day. Dosing Range: 1-6mg/day. Max: 6mg/day. Elderly/Debilitated/Hypotension/Severe Renal or Hepatic Impairment: Initial: 0.5mg bid. Titrate: Adjust dose in increments not >0.5mg bid. Increases to doses >1.5mg bid should occur at intervals of ≥1 week. If qd dosing regimen in elderly or debilitated is being considered, titrate on bid regimen for 2-3 days at the target dose. Subsequent switches to a qd dosing regimen can be done thereafter. Coadministration w/ Enzyme Inducers/Fluoxetine/Paroxetine: May affect plasma concentrations; titrate accordingly.
Pediatrics: Schizophrenia: 13-17 yrs: Initial: 0.5mg qd in am or pm. Titrate: Adjust dose at intervals not <24 hrs in increments of 0.5 or 1mg/day, as tolerated, to recommended dose of 3mg/day. Dosing Range: 1-6mg/day. Max: 6mg/day. If with persistent somnolence, may administer half the daily dose bid. Refer to PI for information on reinitiating treatment and switching from other antipsychotics. Bipolar Mania: 10-17 yrs: Initial: 0.5mg qd in am or pm. Titrate: Adjust dose at intervals not <24 hrs in increments of 0.5 or 1mg/day, as tolerated, to recommended dose of 2.5mg/day. Dosing Range: 0.5-6mg/day. Max: 6mg/day. If with persistent somnolence, give half the daily dose bid. Irritability Associated With Autistic Disorder: 5-16 yrs: Individualize dose. Initial: <20kg: 0.25mg/day qd or bid; ≥20kg: 0.5mg/day qd or bid. Titrate: After at least 4 days, may increase dose to 0.5mg/day (<20kg) or 1mg/day (≥20kg). Maint: Minimum of 14 days. Inadequate Response: Increase at ≥2 weeks intervals: <20kg: Increase by 0.25mg/day; ≥20kg: Increase by 0.5mg/day. Caution in patients <15kg. Max: <20kg: 1mg/day; ≥20kg: 2.5mg/day; >45kg: 3mg/day. If with persistent somnolence, give qd dose hs or half the daily dose bid, or reduce dose. Coadministration w/ Enzyme Inducers/Fluoxetine/Paroxetine: May affect plasma concentrations; titrate accordingly.

HOW SUPPLIED: Sol: 1mg/mL [30mL]; Tab: 0.25mg, 0.5mg, 1mg, 2mg, 3mg, 4mg; Tab, Disintegrating: (M-Tab) 0.5mg, 1mg, 2mg, 3mg, 4mg.

WARNINGS/PRECAUTIONS: Neuroleptic malignant syndrome (NMS) reported. Tardive dyskinesia (TD) may occur. Hyperglycemia and diabetes mellitus (DM) reported. May elevate prolactin levels. May induce orthostatic hypotension; caution with cardiovascular disease (CVD), cerebrovascular disease, and conditions that predispose to hypotension. Leukopenia, neutropenia and agranulocytosis reported; d/c in cases of severe neutropenia (ANC<1000/mm³). May impair mental/physical abilities. Seizures reported; caution with history of seizures. Esophageal dysmotility and aspiration reported; caution in patients at risk for aspiration pneumonia. Priapism and thrombotic thrombocytopenic purpura (TTP) reported. May disrupt body temperature regulation; caution when exposed to extreme temperatures. May produce antiemetic effect that may mask signs/symptoms of overdosage with certain drugs or certain conditions (eg, intestinal obstruction, Reye's syndrome, brain tumor). Increased sensitivity to antipsychotic medications reported in patients with Parkinson's disease or dementia with Lewy bodies. Caution with diseases/conditions affecting metabolism or hemodynamic responses, renal/hepatic impairment, and in elderly.

ADVERSE REACTIONS: Somnolence, increased appetite, fatigue, N/V, cough, constipation, parkinsonism, upper abdominal pain, anxiety, dizziness, tremor, insomnia, sedation, akathisia.

INTERACTIONS: Caution with other centrally acting drugs and alcohol. May potentiate hypotensive effects of other drugs with this potential (eg, antihypertensives). May antagonize effects of levodopa and dopamine agonists. Increased bioavailability with cimetidine and ranitidine. Increased exposure with ranitidine. Decreased clearance with chronic use of clozapine. Increased valproate peak plasma concentrations. Increased concentrations with fluoxetine, paroxetine and other CYP2D6 inhibitors. Carbamazepine and other

CYP3A4 enzyme inducers (eg, phenytoin, rifampin, phenobarbital) may decrease concentrations. Increased mortality with furosemide in elderly patients with dementia-related psychosis.

PREGNANCY: Category C, not for use in nursing.

MECHANISM OF ACTION: Benzisoxazole derivative; not established. In schizophrenia, proposed to be mediated through a combination of dopamine Type 2 (D_2) and serotonin Type 2 ($5HT_2$) receptor antagonism.

PHARMACOKINETICS: Absorption: Well absorbed; Absolute Oral Bioavailability (70%). Risperidone T_{max}=1 hr; 9-hydroxyrisperidone T_{max}=3 hrs (extensive metabolizers), 17 hrs (poor metabolizers) **Distribution:** V_d=1-2L/kg; plasma protein binding (risperidone, 90%) (9-hydroxyrisperidone, 77%); found in breast milk. **Metabolism:** Liver; hydroxylation via CYP2D6 to 9-hydroxyrisperidone (major metabolite); N-dealkylation (minor pathway). **Elimination:** Urine (70%), feces (14%). Risperidone $T_{1/2}$=3 hrs (extensive metabolizers); 20 hrs (poor metabolizers). 9-hydroxyrisperidone $T_{1/2}$=21 hrs (extensive metabolizers); 30 hrs (poor metabolizers).

NURSING CONSIDERATIONS

Assessment: Assess for dementia-related psychosis, DM, or any other conditions where treatment is contraindicated or cautioned. Assess for hepatic/renal impairment, pregnancy/nursing status, and for possible drug interactions. Obtain baseline FPG in patients at risk for DM.

Monitoring: Monitor for NMS, TD, hyperprolactinemia, orthostatic hypotension, cognitive and motor impairment, seizures, esophageal dysmotility, aspiration, priapism, TTP, and for disruption of body temperature. Monitor for signs of hyperglycemia; perform periodic monitoring of FPG levels in patients with DM or at risk for DM. Monitor for signs/symptoms of leukopenia, neutropenia (eg, fever, infection), and agranulocytosis; perform frequent monitoring of CBC in patients with history of clinically significant low WBC or drug-induced leukopenia/neutropenia. Monitor liver/renal function.

Patient Counseling: Advise of risk of orthostatic hypotension and of non-pharmacologic interventions that will help reduce its occurrence. Inform that therapy has the potential to impair judgement, thinking, or motor skills; advise to use caution when operating hazardous machinery (eg, automobiles). Notify physician if pregnant or planning to become pregnant. Do not breastfeed while on therapy. Notify physician of all medications currently being taken. Avoid alcohol during treatment. Inform that disintegrating tab contains phenylalanine.

Administration: Oral route. Take with or without meals. Sol can be administered directly from the calibrated pipette or mixed with a compatible beverage. Do not push orally disintegrating tab through the foil. Place disintegrating tab on the tongue; do not split or chew tab. Disintegrating tab may be swallowed with or without liquid. **Storage**: 15-25°C (59-77°F). (Sol) Protect from light and freezing. (Tab) Protect from light and moisture.

R

RISPERDAL CONSTA   RX
risperidone (Ortho-Mcneil/Janssen)

> Elderly patients with dementia-related psychosis treated with antipsychotic drugs are at an increased risk of death; most deaths appeared to be cardiovascular (eg, heart failure [HF], sudden death) or infectious (eg, pneumonia) in nature. Risperidone is not approved for the treatment of patients with dementia-related psychosis.

THERAPEUTIC CLASS: Benzisoxazole derivative

INDICATIONS: Treatment of schizophrenia. As monotherapy or adjunctive therapy to lithium or valproate for maintenance treatment of bipolar I disorder.

DOSAGE: *Adults:* In risperidone naive patients, establish tolerability with oral risperidone prior to treatment with risperidone inj. Give 1st inj with oral risperidone or other antipsychotic, continue for 3 weeks, then d/c oral therapy. Upward dose adjustment should not be made more frequently than every 4 weeks. Schizophrenia/Bipolar I Disorder: 25mg IM every 2 weeks. Titrate: May increase to 37.5mg or 50mg based on response. Max: 50mg every 2 weeks. Hepatic or Renal Impairment: Prior to initiating IM therapy, administer oral dosage, 0.5mg po bid during the 1st week. Titrate: May increase oral dosage to 1mg po bid or 2mg po qd during the 2nd week of therapy. If total daily dose of 2mg po is tolerated, start at 12.5mg or 25mg IM every 2 weeks. Elderly: 25mg IM every 2 weeks. Reinitiation: Supplement with oral risperidone or other antipsychotic. Switching from Other Antipsychotics: Continue previous antpsychotic for 3 weeks after 1st risperidone inj. Poor Tolerability: Initial: 12.5mg IM. Coadministration w/ Enzyme Inducers/Fluoxetine/Paroxetine: May affect plasma concentrations; titrate accordingly.

HOW SUPPLIED: Inj: 12.5mg, 25mg, 37.5mg, 50mg

WARNINGS/PRECAUTIONS: Neuroleptic malignant syndrome (NMS) reported. Tardive dyskinesia (TD) may occur. Hyperglycemia and diabetes mellitus (DM) reported. May elevate prolactin levels. May induce orthostatic hypotension; caution with history of cardiovascular disease (CVD), cerebrovascular disease and conditions that predispose to hypotension. Leukopenia, neutropenia, and agranulocytosis reported; d/c in cases of severe neutropenia (ANC<1000/mm³). May impair mental/physical abilities. Seizures reported; caution with history of seizures. Esophageal dysmotility and aspiration reported; caution in patients with an increased risk of aspiration pneumonia. Priapism and thrombotic thrombocytopenic purpura (TTP) reported. May disrupt body temperature regulation; caution when exposed to extreme temperatures. Avoid inadvertent injection into a blood vessel. May have antiemetic effects that may mask the signs and symptoms of overdosage with certain drugs or conditions (eg, intestinal obstruction, Reye's syndrome, brain tumor). Increased risk of suicide attempt with bipolar disorder or schizophrenia. Increased sensitivity to antipsychotic medications reported in patients with Parkinson's disease or dementia with Lewy bodies. Caution with diseases/conditions affecting metabolism or hemodynamic responses, renal/hepatic impairment and in elderly.

ADVERSE REACTIONS: Headache, dizziness, constipation, dyspepsia, akathisia, parkinsonism, weight increase, dry mouth, fatigue, pain in extremity, tremor, nausea, sedation, cough, pain.

INTERACTIONS: Caution with other centrally acting drugs and alcohol. May potentiate hypotensive effects of other drugs with this potential (eg, antihypertensives). May antagonize effects of levodopa and dopamine agonists. Increases bioavailability of oral risperidone with concomitant use of cimetidine or ranitidine. Increased exposure with ranitidine. May decrease clearance with oral risperidone. Increased valproate peak plasma concentrations with concomitant use of oral risperidone. Increased concentrations with fluoxetine, paroxetine and other CYP2D6 inhibitors. Carbamazepine and other CYP3A4 enzyme inducers (eg, phenytoin, rifampin, phenobarbital) may decrease concentrations. Increase mortality with oral risperidone and furosemide in elderly patients with dementia-related psychosis.

PREGNANCY: Category C, not for use in nursing.

MECHANISM OF ACTION: Benzisoxazole derivative; not established. In schizophrenia, proposed to be mediated through a combination of dopamine Type 2 (D_2) and serotonin Type 2 ($5HT_2$) receptor antagonism.

PHARMACOKINETICS: Distribution: Rapid; V_d=1-2L/kg; plasma protein binding (risperidone, 90%), (9-hydroxyrisperidone, 77%); found in breast milk. **Metabolism**: Liver (extensive) via CYP2D6; hydroxylation, N-dealkylation; 9-hydroxyrisperidone (major metabolite). **Elimination**: Urine (70%), feces (14%); $T_{1/2}$=3-6 days.

NURSING CONSIDERATIONS

Assessment: Assess for dementia-related psychosis, DM, or any other conditions where treatment is contraindicated or cautioned. Assess for hepatic/renal impairment, pregnancy/nursing status, and for possible drug interactions. Obtain baseline FPG in patients at risk for DM.

Monitoring: Monitor for NMS, TD, hyperprolactinemia, orthostatic hypotension, cognitive and motor impairment, seizures, esophageal dysmotility, aspiration, priapism, TTP, and for disruption of body temperature. Monitor for signs of hyperglycemia; perform periodic monitoring of FPG levels in patients with DM or at risk for DM. Monitor for signs/symptoms of leukopenia, neutropenia (eg, fever, infection), and agranulocytosis; perform frequent monitoring of CBC in patients with history of clinically significant low WBC or drug-induced leukopenia/neutropenia. Monitor liver/renal function.

Patient Counseling: Advise of risk of orthostatic hypotension and of non-pharmacologic interventions that will help reduce its occurrence. Inform that therapy has the potential to impair judgement, thinking, or motor skills; advise to use caution when operating hazardous machinery (eg, automobiles). Notify physician if pregnant or planning to become pregnant. Do not breastfeed while on therapy and for at least 12 weeks after last inj. Notify physician of all medications currently being taken. Avoid alcohol during treatment.

Administration: IM route. Deep IM into the gluteal or deltoid muscle every 2 weeks. Not for IV use. Refer to PI for complete instructions for use. **Storage:** 2-8°C (36-46°F). Protect from light. If refrigeration is unavailable, store at ≤25°C (77°F) for ≤7 days prior to administration.

RITALIN CII
methylphenidate HCl (Novartis)

> Caution with a history of drug dependence or alcoholism. Marked tolerance and psychological dependence may result from chronic abusive use. Frank psychotic episodes may occur, especially with parenteral abuse. Supervision required for withdrawal from abusive use, since severe depression may occur. Withdrawal following chronic therapeutic use may unmask symptoms of underlying disorder that may require follow-up.

OTHER BRAND NAMES: Ritalin LA (Novartis) - Ritalin SR (Novartis)

THERAPEUTIC CLASS: Sympathomimetic amine

INDICATIONS: (Cap, Extended-Release) Treatment of Attention Deficit Hyperactivity Disorder (ADHD). (Tab; Tab, Sustained-Release) Treatment of Attention Deficit Disorders; treatment of narcolepsy.

DOSAGE: *Adults:* Individualize dose. Reduce dose or d/c if paradoxical aggravation of symptoms occurs. D/C if no improvement after appropriate dose adjustment over a 1-month period. (Tab) 10-60mg/day divided bid-tid 30-45 min ac. Take last dose before 6 pm if insomnia occurs. (Tab, SR) May use in place of immediate-release (IR) tab when the 8-hr dose corresponds to the titrated 8-hr IR dose. (Cap, ER) Initial: 10-20mg qam. Titrate: May adjust weekly by 10mg. Max: 60mg/day. Current Methylphenidate Therapy: May use in place of IR or SR tabs with a qd equivalent dose; refer to PI for recommended dosing. *Pediatrics:* ≥6 yrs: Individualize dose. Reduce dose or d/c if paradoxical aggravation of symptoms occurs. D/C if no improvement after appropriate dose adjustment over a 1-month period. (Tab) Initial: 5mg bid before breakfast and lunch. Titrate: Increase gradually by 5-10mg weekly. Max: 60mg/day. (Tab, SR) May use in place of IR tab when the 8-hr dose corresponds to the titrated 8-hr IR dose. (Cap, ER) Initial: 10-20mg qam. Titrate: May adjust weekly by 10mg. Max: 60mg/day. Current Methylphenidate Therapy: May use in place of IR or SR tabs with a qd equivalent dose; refer to PI for recommended dosing.

HOW SUPPLIED: Cap, Extended-Release (Ritalin LA): 10mg, 20mg, 30mg, 40mg; Tab (Ritalin): 5mg, 10mg*, 20mg*; Tab, Sustained-Release (Ritalin SR): 20mg *scored

CONTRAINDICATIONS: Marked anxiety, tension, and agitation; glaucoma; motor tics or family history or diagnosis of Tourette's syndrome; during or within 14 days of MAOI use.

WARNINGS/PRECAUTIONS: Sudden death, stroke, and myocardial infarction (MI) reported; avoid with known structural cardiac abnormalities, cardiomyopathy, serious heart abnormalities, coronary artery disease or other serious cardiac problems. May increase BP and HR; caution with pre-existing HTN, heart failure, MI, or ventricular arrhythmias. When symptoms suggestive of cardiac disease develop, prompt evaluation required. May exacerbate symptoms of behavior disturbance and thought disorder in patients with a pre-existing psychotic disorder. Caution with comorbid bipolar disorder; risk for induction of mixed/manic episode in such patients. May cause treatment-emergent psychotic or manic symptoms in children and adolescents without prior history of psychotic illness. Monitor for appearance and worsening of aggressive behavior or hostility during initial treatment. May cause growth suppression; monitor growth during therapy. May lower convulsive seizure threshold, especially with prior history of seizures or with prior EEG abnormalities; d/c if seizures occur. Accommodation difficulties and blurring of vision reported. Monitor CBC, differential, and platelet counts periodically during prolonged therapy. Not for use in children <6 yrs. (Tab/ Tab, SR) Patients with an element of agitation may react adversely; d/c therapy if necessary. Not indicated in all cases of behavioral syndrome. Not for use in symptoms associated with acute stress reactions.

ADVERSE REACTIONS: Nervousness, insomnia, anorexia, headache, abdominal pain, decreased appetite.

INTERACTIONS: See Contraindications. Caution with pressor agents. May decrease effectiveness of antihypertensives. May inhibit metabolism of coumarin anticoagulants, anticonvulsants (eg, phenobarbital, phenytoin, primidone), TCAs (eg, imipramine, clomipramine, desipramine); may adjust dose downward and monitor plasma drug levels when starting/stopping therapy. Possible occurrence of neuroleptic malignant syndrome (NMS) with concurrent therapies associated with NMS; single report of NMS-like event possibly related with concurrent use of venlafaxine. (Cap, ER) Antacids or acid suppressants may alter release of methylphenidate. May be associated with pharmacodynamic interaction when coadministered with direct and indirect dopamine agonists (including DOPA and tricyclic antidepressants) as well as dopamine antagonists (antipsychotics, eg, haloperidol).

PREGNANCY: Category C, caution in nursing.

MECHANISM OF ACTION: Sympathomimetic amine; CNS stimulant, mechanism has not been established. Suspected to block the reuptake of norepinephrine and dopamine into the presynaptic neuron and increase the release of monoamines into the extraneuronal space. Presumably activates the brain stem arousal system and cortex to produce stimulant effect.

PHARMACOKINETICS: Absorption: Extensive. **Adults:** (Cap, ER 20mg) T_{max1}=2 hrs, C_{max1}=5.3ng/mL, T_{max2}=5.5 hrs, C_{max2}=6.2ng/mL, AUC=45.8ng•h/mL. See PI for parameters in pediatric patients. **Distribution:** Plasma protein binding (10%-33%). (Cap, ER) d-methylphenidate: V_d=2.65L/kg, l-methylphenidate: V_d=1.8L/kg. **Metabolism:** α-phenyl-2-piperidine acetic acid (major metabolite). **Elimination:** (Cap, ER 20mg) **Adults:** $T_{1/2}$=3.5 hrs; Peds: $T_{1/2}$=2.5 hrs. (Tab) Urine (78-97% metabolites, <1% unchanged), feces (1-3% metabolites).

NURSING CONSIDERATIONS

Assessment: Assess for appropriate diagnosis. Assess for marked anxiety, tension, agitation, glaucoma, tics, family history of Tourette's syndrome, cardiovascular conditions, comorbid depression symptoms, bipolar disorder, psychosis, seizures, history of drug dependence or alcoholism, acute stress reactions, pregnancy/nursing status, and for possible drug interactions.

Monitoring: Monitor for signs and symptoms of cardiac disease, exacerbations of behavior disturbances and thought disorders, bipolar disorder, psychotic or manic symptoms, aggression, seizures, visual disturbances, CBC with differential and platelet counts. Monitor growth (height and weight) in children. D/C drug periodically to assess child's condition. Monitor cardiovascular status (BP and HR).

Patient Counseling: Inform about risks and benefits of treatment, appropriate use, and potential for drug abuse/dependence. Instruct to read medication guide and assist in understanding its contents.

Administration: Oral route. (Tab, SR) Swallow whole; do not crush or chew. (Cap, ER) Swallow whole or sprinkle contents over spoonful of applesauce; do not crush, chew, or divide. **Storage:** 25°C (77°F), excursions permitted to 15-30°C (59-86°F). (Tab) Protect from light. Dispense in tight, light-resistant container. (Tab, SR) Protect from moisture. Dispense in tight, light-resistant container. (Cap, ER) Dispense in a tight container.

RITUXAN

RX

rituximab (Genentech/Biogen Idec)

> Serious, including fatal, infusion reactions reported; deaths within 24 hrs of infusion have occurred. Acute renal failure, sometimes fatal, reported in the setting of tumor lysis syndrome (TLS) following treatment of non-Hodgkin's lymphoma (NHL). Severe, including fatal, mucocutaneous reactions may occur. JC virus infection resulting in progressive multifocal leukoencephalopathy (PML) and death may occur.

THERAPEUTIC CLASS: Monoclonal antibody/CD20-blocker

INDICATIONS: Treatment of NHL in patients with: 1) relapsed or refractory, low-grade or follicular, CD20-positive, B-cell NHL as a single agent; 2) previously untreated follicular, CD20-positive, B-cell NHL in combination with 1st-line chemotherapy and, in patients achieving a complete or partial response in combination with chemotherapy, as single agent maintenance therapy; 3) non-progressing (including stable disease), low-grade, CD20-positive, B-cell NHL, as a single agent, after 1st-line CVP chemotherapy; 4) previously untreated diffuse large B-cell, CD20-positive NHL in combination with CHOP or other anthracycline-based chemotherapy regimens. Treatment of previously untreated and previously treated CD20-positive chronic lymphocytic leukemia (CLL) in combination with fludarabine and cyclophosphamide (FC). Treatment of moderately to severely active rheumatoid arthritis (RA) (who had inadequate response to ≥1 TNF-antagonist therapies) in combination with methotrexate.

DOSAGE: *Adults:* Premedicate before each infusion with acetaminophen and antihistamine. Administer as IV infusion only. Relapsed/Refractory, Low-Grade/Follicular, CD20-Positive, B-Cell NHL: 375mg/m² once weekly for 4 or 8 doses. Retreatment: 375mg/m² once weekly for 4 doses. Previously Untreated, Follicular, CD20-Positive, B-Cell NHL: 375mg/m² on Day 1 of each chemotherapy cycle for ≤8 doses. Maint: Initiate therapy q8 weeks for 12 doses after completing 8 weeks of rituximab with chemotherapy. Non-progressing, Low-Grade, CD20-Positive, B-Cell NHL: After completion of 6-8 CVP chemotherapy cycles, give 375mg/m² once weekly for 4 doses at 6-month intervals to max of 16 doses. Diffuse Large B-Cell NHL: 375mg/m² on Day 1 of each chemotherapy cycle for ≤8 infusions. CLL: 375mg/m² the day prior to initiation of FC chemotherapy, then 500mg/m² on Day 1 of cycles 2-6 (q28 days). Refer to PI for dosing as a component of Zevalin. RA (with methotrexate): Two-1000mg separated by 2 weeks. Give methylprednisolone 100mg IV (or equivalent) 30 min prior to each infusion. Give subsequent courses q24 weeks or based on evaluation, but not sooner than q16 weeks.

HOW SUPPLIED: Inj: 100mg/10mL, 500mg/50mL

WARNINGS/PRECAUTIONS: Do not administer as IV push or bolus. Not recommended for use with severe, active infections. Hepatitis B virus (HBV) reactivation with fulminant hepatitis, hepatic failure, and death reported; d/c if viral hepatitis develops. Serious, including fatal, bacterial, fungal, and new/reactivated viral infections may occur during and ≤ 1 yr after complete therapy; d/c for serious infections and institute anti-infective therapy. D/C if serious/life-threatening cardiac arrhythmias occur. Perform cardiac monitoring during and after all infusions if arrhythmias develop with history of arrhythmias/angina. Severe renal toxicity reported in NHL; d/c if SrCr rises or oliguria occurs. *Pneumocystis jiroveci pneumonia* (PCP) and anti-herpetic viral prophylaxis is recommended for patients with CLL during treatment and for ≤12 months following treatment as appropriate. Potential for immunogenicity. Follow current immunization guidelines and administer non-live vaccines ≥4weeks prior to therapy for RA patients. Not recommended in patients with RA who have not had prior inadequate response to one or more TNF-antagonists and with severe active infections. Obtain CBC and platelet count prior to therapy, at weekly to monthly intervals (more frequently if cytopenia develops), and at 2-4 month intervals during therapy in RA patients. Abdominal pain, bowel obstruction and perforation may occur.

R

ADVERSE REACTIONS: Infusion reactions, mucocutaneous reactions, renal failure, JC virus infection, PML, fever, chills, rash, asthenia, lymphopenia, infection, leukopenia, neutropenia, headache, night sweats.

INTERACTIONS: Renal toxicity reported with cisplatin. Vaccination with live viral vaccines not recommended. Observe closely for signs of infection if biologic agents and/or DMARDs are used concomitantly.

PREGNANCY: Category C, caution in nursing.

MECHANISM OF ACTION: Chimeric murine/human monoclonal IgG$_1$ kappa antibody/CD20 antigen blocker; binds to CD20 antigen on B-lymphocytes and recruits immune effector functions to mediate B-cell lysis, possibly by complement-dependent cytotoxicity and antibody-dependent cell-mediated cytotoxicity.

PHARMACOKINETICS: Absorption: RA: C_{max}=157mcg/mL (1st infusion), 183mcg/mL (2nd infusion), 318mcg/mL (2x500mg dose), 381mcg/mL (2x1000mg dose). **Distribution:** RA: V_d=3.1L. **Elimination:** NHL: $T_{1/2}$=22 days, RA: $T_{1/2}$=18 days, CLL: $T_{1/2}$=32 days.

NURSING CONSIDERATIONS

Assessment: Assess for severe active infections, pre-existing cardiac/pulmonary conditions, high number of circulating malignant cells (>25,000/mm³), history of arrhythmias or angina, high tumor burden, electrolyte abnormalities, hematologic malignancies or autoimmune diseases, risk/pre-existing HBV infection, possible drug interactions, pregnancy/nursing status. Assess history of immunization, renal function, fluid and electrolyte balance, CBC, and platelet count.

Monitoring: Monitor fluid and electrolyte balance, cardiac/renal function, CBC and platelet count periodically. Monitor for signs/symptoms of HBV reactivation, viral hepatitis, infusion reactions, TLS, arrhythmias, bacterial, fungal, and new/reactivated viral infections, mucocutaneous reactions, PML, cytopenias, bowel obstruction/perforation, new-onset neurologic manifestations, and hypersensitivity reactions. Monitor closely for infusion reactions in patients with pre-existing cardiac/pulmonary conditions, and those with high numbers of circulating malignant cells. Monitor HBV infection in hepatitis B carriers.

Patient Counseling: Inform of risks of therapy and importance to assess overall health status at each visit. Drug is detectable in serum for up to 6 months following complete therapy. Use effective contraception during and for 12 months after therapy.

Administration: IV route. Do not administer as IV push/bolus; for IV infusion only. Refer to PI for infusion instructions and preparation for administration. **Storage:** 2-8°C (36-46°F). Protect from direct sunlight. Do not freeze or shake. Sol for infusion: 2-8°C (36-46°F) for 24 hrs. Stable for additional 24 hrs at room temperature.

ROBAXIN

RX

methocarbamol (Schwarz)

OTHER BRAND NAMES: Robaxin Injection (Baxter) - Robaxin-750 (Schwarz)

THERAPEUTIC CLASS: Muscular analgesic (central-acting)

INDICATIONS: Adjunct for relief of acute, painful musculoskeletal conditions.

DOSAGE: *Adults:* (PO) Initial: (500mg tab) 1500mg qid for 2-3 days. Maint: 1000mg qid. Initial: (750mg tab) 1500mg qid for 2-3 days. Maint: 750mg q4h or 1500mg tid. Max: 6g/d for 2-3 days; 8g/d if severe. (Inj) Moderate Symptoms: 10mL IV/IM. IV Max Rate: 3mL undiluted drug/min. IM Max: 5mL into each gluteal region. Severe/Post-Op Condition: Max: 20-30mL/day up to 3 consecutive days. If feasible, continue with PO. Tetanus: 10-20mL up to 30mL. May repeat q6h until NG tube can be inserted. Continue with crushed tabs. Max: 24g/day PO.
Pediatrics: Tetanus: Initial: 15mg/kg or 500mg/m². Repeat q6h prn. Max: 1.8g/m² for 3 consecutive days. Administer by injection into tubing or IV infusion.

HOW SUPPLIED: Inj: 100mg/mL [10mL]; Tab: 500mg, 750mg

CONTRAINDICATIONS: (Inj) Renal pathology with injection due to propylene glycol content.

WARNINGS/PRECAUTIONS: May impair mental/physical abilities. May cause color interference in certain screening tests for 5-hydroxy-indoleacetic acid (5-HIAA) and vanillylmandelic acid (VMA). Caution in epilepsy with the injection. Injection rate should not exceed 3mL/min. Avoid extravasation with injection. Avoid use of injection particularly during early pregnancy.

ADVERSE REACTIONS: Lightheadedness, dizziness, drowsiness, nausea, urticaria, pruritus, rash, conjunctivitis, nasal congestion, blurred vision, headache, fever, seizures, syncope, flushing.

INTERACTIONS: Additive adverse effects with alcohol and other CNS depressants. May inhibit effect of pyridostigmine; caution in patients with myasthenia gravis receiving anticholinergics.

PREGNANCY: Category C, caution in nursing.

MECHANISM OF ACTION: Carbamate derivative of guaifenesin; not established, suspected to have CNS depressant with sedative and musculoskeletal relaxant properties.

PHARMACOKINETICS: Distribution: Plasma protein binding (46-50%). **Distribution:** Found in breast milk. **Metabolism:** Via dealkylation, hydroxylation, and conjugation pathways. **Elimination:** Urine; $T_{1/2}$=1-2 hrs.

NURSING CONSIDERATIONS

Assessment: Assess for renal/hepatic impairment, myasthenia gravis, seizures, pregnancy/nursing status, alcohol intake, and drug interactions.

Monitoring: Monitor for congenital and fetal abnormalities if taken during pregnancy, for color interference in certain screening tests for 5-HIAA using nitrosonaphthol reagent and in screening tests for urinary VMA using Gitlow method.

Patient Counseling: Caution while performing hazardous tasks (operating machinery/driving). Avoid alcohol or other CNS depressants. Notify if pregnant/nursing or if planning to become pregnant.

Administration: Oral route, IV infusion, and IM; careful supervision of dose and rate of injection. **Storage:** 20-25°C (68-77°F), in tight container; excursions permitted to 15-30°C (59-86°F).

ROCALTROL   RX
calcitriol (Validus)

OTHER BRAND NAMES: Calcitriol (Various)

THERAPEUTIC CLASS: Vitamin D analog

INDICATIONS: Management of secondary hyperparathyroidism and resultant metabolic bone disease with moderate to severe chronic renal failure (CrCl 15-55mL/min) in patients not yet on dialysis. Management of hypocalcemia and resultant metabolic bone disease in patients undergoing chronic renal dialysis. Management of hypocalcemia and its clinical manifestations in patients with postsurgical hypoparathyroidism, idiopathic hypoparathyroidism, and pseudohypoparathyroidism.

DOSAGE: *Adults:* Predialysis: Initial: 0.25mcg/day. Max: 0.5mcg/day. Hypoparathyroidism: Initial: 0.25mcg/day every am. Titrate: May increase at 2- to 4-week intervals. Usual: 0.5-2mcg/day. Dialysis: Initial: 0.25mcg/day. Titrate: May increase by 0.25mcg/day at 4- to 8-week intervals. Patients with normal or slightly reduced calcium levels may respond to 0.25mcg qod. Usual: 0.5-1mcg/day. Monitor serum calcium levels at least twice weekly during titration. D/C with hypercalcemia; when calcium levels return to normal, continue therapy and decrease daily dose by 0.25mcg. Elderly: Start at lower end of dosing range.
Pediatrics: Predialysis: ≥3 yrs: Initial: 0.25mcg/day. Max: 0.5mcg/day. <3yrs: Initial: 10-15ng/kg/day. Hypoparathyroidism: ≥6 yrs: Usual: 0.5-2mcg/day

every am. 1-5yrs: Usual: 0.25-0.75mcg/day every am. Monitor serum calcium levels twice weekly during titration. D/C with hypercalcemia; when calcium levels return to normal, continue therapy and decrease daily dose by 0.25mcg.

HOW SUPPLIED: Cap: 0.25mcg, 0.5mcg; Sol: 1mcg/mL [15mL]

CONTRAINDICATIONS: Hypercalcemia or vitamin D toxicity.

WARNINGS/PRECAUTIONS: Administration in excess of daily requirements may cause hypercalcemia, hypercalciuria, and hyperphosphatemia. Chronic hypercalcemia can lead to generalized vascular calcification, nephrocalcinosis, and other soft tissue calcification. May increase inorganic phosphate levels in serum leading to ectopic calcification in renal failure; use non-aluminum phosphate binders and low phosphate diet to control serum phosphate in dialysis patients. Caution in elderly and immobilized patients. If treatment switched from ergocalciferol, may take several months for ergocalciferol level in blood to return to baseline. Avoid dehydration in patients with normal renal function. In patients with normal renal function, chronic hypercalcemia may be associated with an increase in SrCr. Maintain adequate calcium intake, at least 600mg/day.

ADVERSE REACTIONS: Weakness, N/V, dry mouth, constipation, muscle and bone pain, metallic taste, polyuria, polydipsia, weight loss, pancreatitis, photophobia, pruritus, decreased libido, hyperthermia, hypersensivity reactions.

INTERACTIONS: Avoid pharmacological doses of vitamin D products and derivatives during therapy. Avoid uncontrolled intake of additional calcium-containing preparations. Avoid concomitant administration with magnesium-containing preparations (eg, antacids) in patients on chronic renal dialysis because use may lead to hypermagnesemia. May reduce intestinal absorption with cholestyramine. May reduce endogenous plasma levels with phenytoin or phenobarbital. Concomitant use with thiazides may cause hypercalcemia. May reduce endogenous serum concentrations when used comcomitantly with ke-toconazole. Hypercalcemia may precipitate cardiac arrhythmias in patients on digitalis. Functional antagonism with corticosteroids. Dose of the phosphate binding agent may be need to be adjusted when used concomitantly with calcitriol.

PREGNANCY: Category C, not for use in nursing.

MECHANISM OF ACTION: Synthetic vitamin D analog; regulates absorption of calcium from the GI tract and its utilization in the body.

PHARMACOKINETICS: Absorption: Rapidly absorbed (intestine). T_{max}=3-6 hrs (adult); C_{max}=116pmol/L (pediatrics). **Distribution:** Plasma protein binding (99.9%); found in breast milk. **Metabolism:** Liver via hydroxylation. 1,25R(OH)$_2$-26, 23S-lactone D$_3$ (major metabolite). **Elimination:** Urine (16%), feces (49%); $T_{1/2}$=5-8 hrs (adult), 27.4 hrs (pediatrics).

NURSING CONSIDERATIONS

Assessment: Assess for hypercalcemia, evidence of vitamin D toxicity, renal dysfunction, presence of immobilization, pregnancy/nursing status, and for possible drug interactions. In predialysis patients, obtain baseline levels of serum calcium, phosphorus, alkaline phosphatase, creatinine, and iPTH.

Monitoring: Monitor for signs/symptoms of hypercalcemia, hypercalciuria, hyperphosphatemia, and for hypersensitivity reactions. If hypercalcemia develops d/c use and perform daily monitoring of serum calcium and phosphate levels. For dialysis patients, perform periodic monitoring of serum calcium, phosphorus, magnesium, and alkaline phosphatase. In hypoparathyroid patients, perform periodic monitoring of serum calcium, phosphorus, and 24-hr urinary calcium. In predialysis patients serum calcium, phosphorus, alkaline phosphatase and creatinine should be monitored monthly during the first 6 months of therapy and then periodically. Intact PTH (iPTH) should be evaluated every 3 to 4 months. During titration periods, serum calcium levels should be checked twice weekly.

Patient Counseling: Inform about compliance with dosage instructions, adherence to instructions about diet and calcium supplementation, and avoidance of the use of unapproved nonprescription drugs. Carefully inform about symptoms of hypercalcemia. Inform patients with normal renal function to avoid dehydration and maintain proper fluid intake during therapy. Advise to maintain adequate calcium intake, at least 600mg/day.

Administration: Oral route. **Storage:** 59-86°F (15-30°C) . Protect from light.

ROMAZICON RX
flumazenil (Roche Labs)

THERAPEUTIC CLASS: Benzodiazepine antagonist

INDICATIONS: Complete or partial reversal of sedative effects of benzodiazepines (BZDs) given with general anesthesia, or diagnostic and therapeutic procedures, and for the management of BZD overdose in adults. For reversal of BZD-induced conscious sedation in pediatrics (1-17 yrs old).

DOSAGE: *Adults:* Reversal of Conscious Sedation/General Anesthesia: Give IV over 15 seconds. Initial: 0.2mg. May repeat dose after 45 sec and again at 60 sec intervals up to a max of 4 additional times until reach desired level of consciousness. Max Total Dose: 1mg. In event of resedation, repeated doses may be given at 20-min intervals. Max: 1mg/dose (0.2mg/min) and 3mg/hr. BZD Overdose: Give IV over 30 sec. Initial: 0.2mg. May repeat with 0.3mg after 30 sec and then 0.5mg at 1-min intervals until reach desired level of consciousness. Max Total Dose: 3mg. In event of resedation, repeated doses may be given at 20-min intervals. Max: 1mg/dose (0.5mg/min); 3mg/hr.
Pediatrics: >1yr: Give IV over 15 sec. Initial: 0.01mg/kg (up to 0.2mg). May repeat dose after 45 sec and again at 60-sec intervals up to a max of 4 additional times until reach desired level of consciousness. Max Total Dose: 0.05mg/kg or 1mg, whichever is lower.

HOW SUPPLIED: Inj: 0.1mg/mL

CONTRAINDICATIONS: Patients given BZDs for life-threatening conditions (eg, control of ICP or status epilepticus), signs of serious cyclic antidepressant overdose.

WARNINGS/PRECAUTIONS: Caution in overdoses involving multiple drug combinations. Risk of seizures, especially with long-term BZD-induced sedation, cyclic antidepressant overdose, concurrent major sedative-hypnotic drug withdrawal, recent therapy with repeated doses of parenteral BZDs, myoclonic jerking or seizure prior to flumazenil administration. Monitor for resedation, respiratory depression, or other residual BZD effects (up to 2 hrs). Avoid use in the ICU; increased risk of unrecognized BZD dependence. Caution with head injury, alcoholism, and other drug dependencies. Does not reverse respiratory depression/hypoventilation or cardiac depression. May provoke panic attacks with history of panic disorder. Adjust subsequent doses in hepatic dysfunction. Not for use as treatment for BZD dependence or for management of protracted abstinence syndromes. May trigger dose-dependent withdrawal syndromes. Extravasation may occur; administer IV into a large vein.

ADVERSE REACTIONS: N/V, dizziness, injection-site pain, increased sweating, headache, abnormal or blurred vision, agitation.

INTERACTIONS: Avoid use until neuromuscular blockade effects are reversed. Toxic effects (eg, convulsions, cardiac dysrhythmias) may occur with mixed drug overdose (eg, cyclic antidepressants).

PREGNANCY: Category C, caution in nursing.

MECHANISM OF ACTION: Benzodiazepine receptor antagonist; inhibits activity at the benzodiazepine recognition site on the GABA/benzodiazepine receptor complex.

PHARMACOKINETICS: Absorption: C_{max}=24ng/mL; AUC=15ng•hr/mL. **Distribution:** V_d=1L/kg (steady state); plasma protein binding (50%). **Metabolism:** Complete (99%). **Elimination:** Urine (90-95%), feces (5-10%); $T_{1/2}$=54 min.

NURSING CONSIDERATIONS

Assessment: Assess patients using BZD for control of potentially life-threatening condition, those showing signs of serious cyclic antidepressant overdose. Assess for head injury, history of convulsions, panic disorders, lung disease, hepatic impairment, and possible drug interactions.

Monitoring: Monitor for occurrence of seizure, re-sedation, respiratory depression, or other residual BZD effects, dizziness, injection-site pain, increased sweating, headache, and abnormal or blurred vision.

Patient Counseling: Advise not to engage in activities requiring complete alertness (eg, operating machinery/driving) during first 24 hrs after discharge. Advise not to take alcohol or non-prescription drugs during first 24 hrs after flumazenil administration, or if effects of the benzodiazepine persist.

Administration: IV route. **Storage:** 25°C (77°F); excursions permitted to 15-30°C (59-86°F).

ROTATEQ

RX

rotavirus vaccine, live (Merck)

THERAPEUTIC CLASS: Vaccine

INDICATIONS: Prevention of rotavirus gastroenteritis in infants and children caused by the serotypes G1, G2, G3, and G4 when administered as a 3-dose series to infants between the ages of 6-32 weeks.

DOSAGE: *Pediatrics:* 6-32 weeks: Administer series of 3 doses. Initial: 2mL PO starting at 6-12 weeks of age, with subsequent doses at 4- to 10-weeks intervals. Third dose should not be given after 32 weeks of age.

HOW SUPPLIED: Sol: 2mL

CONTRAINDICATIONS: Severe Combined Immunodeficiency Disease (SCID).

WARNINGS/PRECAUTIONS: Caution with administration to potentially immunocompromised infants or to infants with a history of GI disorders. May increase risk of intussusception. Shedding and transmission of vaccine virus observed; caution when administering to individuals with immunodeficient close contacts (eg, with malignancies or primary immunodeficiency, immunocompromised, receiving immunosuppressants). Consider delaying use with febrile illness. May not protect all vaccine recipients against rotavirus. No clinical data available for postexposure prophylaxis and administration with incomplete regimen.

ADVERSE REACTIONS: Irritability, fever, diarrhea, vomiting, elevated temperature, bronchospasm, nasopharyngitis, otitis media, bronchiolitis, gastroenteritis, pneumonia, urinary tract infection (UTI), shedding, transmission.

INTERACTIONS: Immunosuppressive therapies including irradiation, antimetabolites, alkylating agents, cytotoxic drugs, and corticosteroids (used in greater than physiologic doses) may reduce the immune response to vaccines.

PREGNANCY: Category C, safety not known in nursing.

MECHANISM OF ACTION: Vaccine; exact immunologic mechanism is unknown. Replicates in small intestine and induces immunity.

NURSING CONSIDERATIONS

Assessment: Assess for previous hypersensitivity to the vaccine, SCID, immunization history, immunocompromised conditions (eg, blood dyscrasias, leukemia, lymphomas, malignant neoplasms, use of immunosuppressive therapy, primary/acquired immunodeficiency, cellular immune deficiencies, hypogammaglobulinemic and dysgammaglobulinemic states, received blood transfusion/blood products within 42 days), history of GI disorders (eg, active acute GI illness, chronic diarrhea, failure to thrive, and history of congenital abdominal disorders, abdominal surgery, and intussusception), febrile illness, and possible drug interactions.

Monitoring: Monitor for hypersensitivity reactions and possible adverse events.

Patient Counseling: Inform parent/guardian of potential benefits and risks. Instruct parent/guardian to inform physician of the current health status of patient and to report if patient has close contact with a family/household member who has weak immune system (eg, cancer or someone taking immunosuppressants). Advise to contact physician immediately if patient develops vomiting, diarrhea, severe stomach pain, blood in stool, or change in bowel movements. Instruct parents/guardians to report other adverse reaction to their health care provider.

Administration: Oral route. Administer as soon as possible after being removed from refrigeration. Do not mix with any other vaccines or solutions. Do not reconstitute or dilute. Refer to PI for instructions for use. **Storage:** 2-8°C (36-46°F). Protect from light.

Roxicet `CII`
oxycodone HCl - acetaminophen (Roxane)

THERAPEUTIC CLASS: Analgesic combination

INDICATIONS: Relief of moderate to moderately severe pain.

DOSAGE: *Adults:* Usual: (5mg-325mg): 1 tab or 5mL sol q6h prn. (5mg-500mg): 1 tab q6h prn. Titrate: May need to exceed usual dose based on individual response, pain severity and tolerance. Max: 12 tabs/day or 60mL/day. Do not exceed acetaminophen (APAP) 4g/day.

HOW SUPPLIED: (Oxycodone-Acetaminophen) Sol: 5mg-325mg/5mL [5mL, 500mL]; Tab: 5mg-325mg*, 5mg-500mg* *scored

CONTRAINDICATIONS: Oxycodone: Significant respiratory depression (in unmonitored settings or absence of resuscitative equipment), acute or severe bronchial asthma or hypercarbia, known/suspected paralytic ileus.

WARNINGS/PRECAUTIONS: May cause physical dependence and tolerance; d/c gradually to avoid withdrawal symptoms. Potential for misuse, abuse or diversion. May cause respiratory depression, induce or aggravate convulsions/seizures, produce severe hypotension in compromised patients and orthostatic hypotension in ambulatory patients. May decrease bowel motility. May obscure the diagnosis or clinical course with head injuries or acute abdominal conditions. Caution with circulatory shock, head injury, other intracranial lesions, pre-existing increase in intracranial pressure (ICP), elderly, debilitated, CNS depression, nontolerant patients, hepatic, pulmonary or renal impairment, liver disease, hypothyroidism, Addison's disease, prostatic hypertrophy, urethral stricture, acute alcoholism, delirium tremens, kyphoscoliosis with respiratory depression, myxedema, toxic psychosis, biliary tract disease (eg, acute pancreatitis). Caution with acute asthma, COPD, cor pulmonale, pre-existing respiratory impairment; may decrease respiratory drive leading to apnea even at therapeutic doses. May increase serum amylase levels. Anaphylactic reactions reported.

ADVERSE REACTIONS: Respiratory depression, apnea, respiratory arrest, circulatory depression, hypotension, shock, lightheadedness, dizziness, sedation, N/V, euphoria, dysphoria, constipation, pruritus.

INTERACTIONS: Oxycodone: May enhance neuromuscular-blocking action of skeletal muscle relaxants and increase respiratory depression. Additive CNS depression with other opioid analgesics, general anesthetics, centrally acting anti-emetics, phenothiazines, tranquilizers, sedative-hypnotics, alcohol and other CNS depressants; reduce dose of one or both agents. Agonist/antagonist analgesics (eg, pentazocine, nalbuphine and butorphanol) may reduce analgesic effect of oxycodone and/or may precipitate withdrawal symptoms; administer with caution. May produce paralytic ileus with anticholinergics. APAP: Hepatotoxicity occured in chronic alcoholics. Increase in glucuronidation, plasma clearance and decreased half-life with oral contraceptives. Increased effect with propranolol. Decreases loop diuretic effects. Reduces serum lamotrigine concentrations producing decreased therapeutic effects. Increases therapeutic effectiveness with probenecid. Decreased zidovudine pharmacologic effects.

PREGNANCY: Category C, not for use in nursing.

MECHANISM OF ACTION: Oxycodone: Pure opioid agonist; principal therapeutic effect is analgesia. Effects mediated by CNS receptors (eg, μ and kappa) for endogenous opioid-like compounds (eg, endorphins, enkephalins).

APAP: Non-opiate, non-salicylate; site and mechanism for analgesic effect not established. Antipyretic effect occurs through inhibition of endogenous pyrogen action on the hypothalamic heat-regulating centers.

PHARMACOKINETICS: Absorption: Oxycodone: Absolute bioavailability (87%). APAP: Rapid and almost complete. **Distribution:** Oxycodone: Plasma protein binding (45%); (IV) V_d=211.9L; found in breast milk. APAP: Plasma protein binding (20-50%) (variable); found in most body fluids, breast milk. **Metabolism:** Oxycodone: N-dealkylation to noroxycodone (metabolite); CYP2D6, O-demethylation to oxymorphone (metabolite). APAP: Liver via CYP450 (conjugation), N acetyl-p-benzoquinoneimine, N-acetylimidoquinone (NAPQI, toxic metabolite). **Excretion:** Oxycodone: Urine (parent compound and metabolites); $T_{1/2}$=3.51 hrs. APAP: Urine (90-100%).

NURSING CONSIDERATIONS

Assessment: Assess for level of pain intensity, type of pain, patient's general condition and medical status, or any other conditions where treatment is contraindicated or cautioned. Assess for history of hypersensitivity, pregnancy/nursing status, renal/hepatic function, and possible drug interactions.

Monitoring: Monitor for signs/symptoms of respiratory depression, anaphylactic reactions, elevations of CSF pressure, ileus, decreased bowel motility in postoperative patients, hypotension, hepatotoxicity, convulsions, anaphylactic reactions, sphincter of Oddi spasms, abuse, tolerance and physical dependence. Monitor serum amylase.

Patient Counseling: Instruct to keep out of reach of children. Dispose of unused drug down toilet. Do not adjust dosing without consulting physician. Drug may impair mental/physical abilities required to perform hazardous tasks (eg, operating machinery/driving). Avoid alcohol and other CNS depressants. If on medication for more than a few weeks, consult physician for gradual d/c dose schedule. Medication has potential for abuse; protect from theft. May interfere with home blood glucose measurement system and cross react with assays for detection of cocaine or cannabinoids (eg, marijuana) in human urine.

Administration: Oral route. **Storage:** (Sol/Tab) 20-25°C (68-77°F). Protect from moisture.

ROXICODONE
oxycodone HCl (Xanodyne)

`CII`

THERAPEUTIC CLASS: Opioid analgesic

INDICATIONS: Management of moderate to severe pain.

DOSAGE: *Adults:* Individualize dose. Initial: Opioid-Naive: 5-15mg q4-6h prn. Titrate: Based on individual response. For chronic pain, give around-the-clock. For severe chronic pain, give q4-6h at lowest effective dose. Conversion from Fixed Ratio Opioid/Non-Opioid Analgesic: D/C non-opioid analgesic; titrate dose in response to level of analgesia and adverse effects. Continuing Concomitant Non-Opioid Analgesic: Initial dose based upon most recent dose of opioid as a baseline for further titration. Conversion from Different Opioid: Consider potency of prior opioid in selection of total daily dose and adjust dosage based on patient's response. May administer supplemental analgesia for breakthrough or incident pain and titrate as needed. Re-assess the need for continued use. D/C gradually by decrements of 25-50% daily. If withdrawal symptoms occur, raise dose to previous level and titrate down more slowly.

HOW SUPPLIED: Sol: 5mg/5mL [500mL], 20mg/mL [30mL]; Tab: 5mg*, 15mg*, 30mg* *scored

CONTRAINDICATIONS: Significant respiratory depression (in unmonitored settings or the absence of resuscitative equipment), acute or severe bronchial asthma, hypercarbia, paralytic ileus.

WARNINGS/PRECAUTIONS: Potential for tolerance and physical dependence. May cause respiratory depression; caution in elderly/debilitated patients, significant COPD, cor pulmonale, decreased respiratory drive, hypoxia, hypercapnia or pre-existing respiratory depression. May markedly exaggerate respiratory depressant effects in head injuries, other intracranial lesions or increased ICP. May obscure the clinical course of patients with head injuries and acute abdominal conditions. May cause severe hypotension if with compromised ability to maintain BP due to depleted volume and orthostatic hypotension. May aggravate convulsions and seizures. Caution with acute alcoholism, adrenocortical insufficiency (eg, Addison's disease), convulsive disorders, CNS depression or coma, delirium tremens, kyphoscoliosis associated with respiratory depression, myxedema or hypothyroidism, prostatic hypertrophy or urethral stricture, severe hepatic or renal impairment, toxic psychosis and biliary tract disease (eg, acute pancreatitis). May increase serum amylase. Avoid giving to women during and prior to labor. Withdrawal symptoms reported. May impair mental/physical abilities.

ADVERSE REACTIONS: Respiratory depression/arrest, circulatory depression, cardiac arrest, hypotension, shock, N/V, constipation, headache, pruritus, insomnia, dizziness, asthenia, somnolence.

INTERACTIONS: Additive CNS depression with narcotic analgesics, general anesthetics, phenothiazines, tranquilizers, sedative-hypnotics, alcohol, and other CNS depressants; reduce dose. Mixed agonist/antagonist analgesics may reduce analgesic effect and/or cause withdrawal symptoms. May enhance effect of neuromuscular blockers. May intensify effects with MAOIs; avoid within 14 days of stopping MAOIs. Severe hypotension may occur with phenothiazines or other agents that compromise vasomotor tone. Possible interaction with CYP2D6 inhibitors (eg, certain cardiovascular drugs, antidepressants).

PREGNANCY: Category B, not for use in nursing.

MECHANISM OF ACTION: Opioid analgesic; pure opioid agonist whose principal therapeutic effect is analgesia. Precise mechanism of analgesic effect has not been established. Specific CNS opioid receptors for endogenous compounds with opioid-like activity are found in the brain and spinal cord and play a role in analgesic effects.

PHARMACOKINETICS: Absorption: Various doses resulted in different parameters; refer to PI. **Distribution:** Plasma protein binding (45%), (IV) V_d=2.6L/kg; found in breast milk. **Metabolism:** Hepatic (extensively); noroxycodone (major metabolite); CYP2D6 to oxymorphone (metabolite) and glucuronides. **Elimination:** Urine; $T_{1/2}$=3.5-4 hrs.

NURSING CONSIDERATIONS

Assessment: Assess for level of pain intensity, type of pain, patient's general condition and medical status or any other conditions where treatment is contraindicated or cautioned. Assess for history of hypersensitivity, pregnancy/nursing status, renal/hepatic function, and possible drug interactions.

Monitoring: Monitor for signs/symptoms of respiratory depression, hypotension, elevations in CSF pressure, convulsions/seizures, tolerance and physical dependence. Monitor serum amylase.

Patient Counseling: Report episodes of breakthrough pain and adverse events. Avoid adjusting dose without consulting physician. May impair mental/physical abilities required to perform hazardous tasks (eg, operating machinery/driving). Avoid alcohol consumption and other CNS depressants. Advise drug has potential for abuse. Counsel that if on medication for more than a few weeks and need to d/c therapy, taper dosing to avoid abrupt withdrawal. Women of childbearing potential should consult physician regarding analgesic effects and other drug use during pregnancy.

Administration: Oral route. **Storage:** 25°C (77°F); excursions permitted to 15-30°C (59-86°F). (Tab) Protect from moisture.

ROZEREM RX
ramelteon (Takeda)

THERAPEUTIC CLASS: Melatonin receptor agonist

INDICATIONS: Treatment of insomnia characterized by difficulty with sleep onset.

DOSAGE: *Adults:* 8mg within 30 min of hs. Max: 8mg/day.

HOW SUPPLIED: Tab: 8mg

CONTRAINDICATIONS: Avoid with fluvoxamine.

WARNINGS/PRECAUTIONS: Angioedema (eg, of the tongue, glottis, larynx) reported; do not rechallenge. Sleep disturbances may manifest as a physical and/or psychiatric disorder; symptomatic treatment of insomnia should be initiated after evaluation. Failure of insomnia to remit after 7-10 days of therapy may indicate presence of psychiatric and/or medical illness; evaluate. Abnormal thinking, behavioral changes, hallucinations, complex behaviors (eg, sleep-driving), worsening depression, suicidal ideation reported. D/C therapy if complex sleep behavior occurs. May impair mental/physical abilities. May affect reproductive hormones. Avoid with severe hepatic impairment and sleep apnea. Caution in moderate hepatic impairment.

ADVERSE REACTIONS: Somnolence, fatigue, dizziness, nausea, exacerbated insomnia.

INTERACTIONS: See Contraindications. Decreased efficacy with strong CYP inducers (eg, rifampin). Increased levels with donepezil and doxepin. Caution with less strong CYP1A2 inhibitors, strong CYP3A4 inhibitors (eg, ketoconazole), strong CYP2C9 inhibitors (eg, fluconazole). Additive effect with alcohol and CNS depressants; avoid alcohol use. Avoid taking with or directly after a high-fat meal.

PREGNANCY: Category C, caution in nursing.

MECHANISM OF ACTION: Melatonin receptor agonist; activity at receptors believed to contribute to sleep-promoting properties, as these receptors, acted upon by endogenous melatonin, are thought to be involved in the maintenance of the circadian rhythm underlying the normal sleep-wake cycle.

PHARMACOKINETICS: Absorption: Rapid; absolute bioavailabilty (1.8%); T_{max}=0.75 hr. **Distribution**: Plasma protein binding (82%); (IV) V_d=73.6L. **Metabolism**: Oxidation via CYP1A2 (major), CYP2C, CYP3A4 (minor). M-II (metabolite). **Elimination:** Urine and feces (<0.1% parent compound); $T_{1/2}$=1-2.6 hrs, (M-II) 2-5 hrs.

NURSING CONSIDERATIONS

Assessment: Assess for manifestations of physical or psychiatric disorders, hepatic impairment, sleep apnea, depression, other comorbid diagnoses, pregnancy/nursing status, and possible drug interactions.

Monitoring: Monitor for signs/symptoms of worsening of depression, suicidal ideation, exacerbations of insomnia, emergence of cognitive or behavioral abnormalities, complex sleep behaviors, and anaphylactic/anaphylactoid reactions.

Patient Counseling: Inform patients, families and caregivers about benefits and risks associated with treatment. Instruct to take within 30 min prior to bedtime on empty stomach. Caution against hazardous tasks (eg, operating machinery, driving). Seek medical attention if worsening of insomnia, symptoms of cognitive or behavioral abnormalities (eg, complex behavior), hypersensitivity reactions, cessation of menses, galactorrhea in females, decreased libido, or infertility occurs. Swallow tablet whole.

Administration: Oral route. Do not take with or after high-fat meal. **Storage**: 25°C (77°F); excursions permitted to 15-30°C (59-86°F). Protect from moisture and humidity.

RYTHMOL
propafenone HCl (GlaxoSmithKline)

> Increased rate of death or reversed cardiac arrest rate was seen in patients treated with encainide or flecainide (Class 1C antiarrhythmics) in a long-term, multi-center, randomized, double-blind study of patients with asymptomatic non-life-threatening ventricular arrhythmias who had a myocardial infarction >6 days but <2 yrs previously. Consider any 1C antiarrhythmics to have significant proarrhythmic risk in patients with structural heart disease. Avoid in patients with non-life-threatening ventricular arrhythmias, even if the patients are experiencing unpleasant, but not life-threatening signs or symptoms.

THERAPEUTIC CLASS: Class 1C antiarrhythmic

INDICATIONS: To prolong the time to recurrence of paroxysmal atrial fibrillation/flutter (PAF) and paroxysmal supraventricular tachycardia (PSVT) associated with disabling symptoms in patients without structural heart disease. Treatment of life-threatening documented ventricular arrhythmias (eg, sustained ventricular tachycardia).

DOSAGE: *Adults:* Initial: 150mg q8h. Titrate: Individualize based on response and tolerance. May increase at a minimum of 3-4 day intervals to 225mg q8h, then to 300mg q8h PRN. Max: 900mg/day. Elderly/Ventricular Arrhythmia with Marked Previous Myocardial Damage: Increase more gradually during initial phase. QRS Widening/2nd- or 3rd-degree AV Block: Reduce dose. Hepatic Dysfunction: Give 20%-30% of normal dose. Elderly: Start at the low end of dosing range.

HOW SUPPLIED: Tab: 150mg*, 225mg* *scored

CONTRAINDICATIONS: Uncontrolled congestive heart failure (CHF), cardiogenic shock, bradycardia, marked hypotension, bronchospastic disorders, electrolyte imbalance, and sinoatrial, atrioventricular (AV) and intraventricular disorders of impulse generation and/or conduction (eg, sick sinus node syndrome, AV block) in the absence of an artificial pacemaker.

WARNINGS/PRECAUTIONS: Do not use to control ventricular rate during AF or in bronchospastic disease. May cause new or worsened arrhythmias and CHF. Patients with CHF should be fully compensated before receiving therapy; d/c if CHF worsens (unless CHF is due to cardiac arrhythmia) and, if indicated, restart at lower dose. Caution with hepatic or renal dysfunction. Conduction disturbances (eg, 1st-degree heart block), agranulocytosis, positive ANA titers, and exacerbation of myasthenia gravis reported. D/C if persistent or worsening elevation of ANA titers detected. May alter pacing and sensing thresholds of artificial pacemakers. Reversible short-term drop (within normal range) in sperm count may occur. Caution in elderly.

ADVERSE REACTIONS: Unusual taste, N/V, dizziness, constipation, headache, fatigue, blurred vision, 1st-degree AV block, intraventricular conduction delay, weakness, dry mouth, dyspnea, diarrhea, proarrhythmia, angina.

INTERACTIONS: Increased levels with inhibitors of CYP2D6 (eg, desipramine, paroxetine, ritonavir, sertraline), CYP1A2 (eg, amiodarone), CYP3A4 (eg, ketoconazole, ritonavir, saquinavir, erythromycin, grapefruit juice); monitor closely. May increase levels of drugs metabolized by CYP2D6 (eg, desipramine, imipramine, haloperidol, venlafaxine). May increase CNS side effects of lidocaine. May increase levels of digoxin, propranolol, metoprolol, warfarin. Increased levels with cimetidine. May increase levels with fluoxetine in extensive metabolizers. Rifampin may decrease levels and may increase norpropafenone (an active metabolite) levels. Avoid with quinidine. Amiodarone can affect conduction and repolarization and is not recommended. May result in severe adverse events (eg, convulsion, AV block, and acute circulatory failure) with abrupt cessation of orlistat.

PREGNANCY: Category C, not for use in nursing.

MECHANISM OF ACTION: Class 1C antiarrhythmic; has local anesthetic effects and direct stabilizing action on myocardial membranes. Reduces upstroke velocity (phase 0) of the monophasic action potential. In Purkinje fibers, and to a lesser extent myocardial fibers, reduces the fast inward current carried by Na$^+$ ions. Diastolic excitability threshold is increased and effective refractory

R

period prolonged. Reduces spontaneous automaticity and depresses triggered activity.

PHARMACOKINETICS: Absorption: Complete; absolute bioavailability (3.4%, 150mg dose), (10.6%, 300mg dose); T_{max}=3.5 hrs. **Metabolism:** Liver (rapid, extensive) via CYP3A4, CYP1A2 and CYP2D6. 5-hydroxypropafenone, N-depropylpropafenone (active metabolites). **Elimination:** $T_{1/2}$=2-10 hrs.

NURSING CONSIDERATIONS

Assessment: Assess for HF; cardiogenic shock; sinoatrial, AV and intraventricular disorders of impulse generation or conduction (eg, sick sinus node syndrome, AV block); implanted functioning pacemaker; bradycardia; marked hypotension; bronchospastic disorders; marked electrolyte imbalance; myocardial infarction (MI); renal/hepatic dysfunction; pregnancy/nursing status; and possible drug interactions. Evaluate ECG prior to therapy.

Monitoring: Monitor for proarrhythmic effects, signs/symptoms of conduction disturbances, agranulocytosis (eg, fever, chills, sore throat, decrease in white cell count), HF, and exacerbation of myasthenia gravis. Monitor implanted pacemakers and defibrillators during and after therapy and re-program accordingly. Evaluate ECG during therapy. Monitor ANA titers, LFTs, and renal function.

Patient Counseling: Inform about risks/benefits of therapy. Advise to report signs of electrolyte imbalance or any adverse reactions to physician. Instruct to report the development of signs of infection such as fever, sore throat, or chills.

Administration: Oral route. **Storage:** 25°C (77°F); excursions permitted to 15-30°C (59-86°F).

RYTHMOL SR

RX

propafenone HCl (GlaxoSmithKline)

> Increased rate of death or reversed cardiac arrest rate was seen in patients treated with encainide or flecainide (Class 1C antiarrhythmics) in a long-term, multi-center, randomized, double-blind study of patients with asymptomatic non-life-threatening ventricular arrhythmias who had a myocardial infarction (MI) >6 days but <2 yrs previously. Consider any 1C antiarrhythmics to have significant proarrhythmic risk in patients with structural heart disease. Avoid in patients with non-life-threatening ventricular arrhythmias, even if the patients are experiencing unpleasant, but not life-threatening signs or symptoms.

THERAPEUTIC CLASS: Class IC antiarrhythmic

INDICATIONS: To prolong the time to recurrence of symptomatic atrial fibrillation (A-fib) in patients with episodic (most likely paroxysmal or persistent) A-fib who do not have structural heart disease.

DOSAGE: *Adults:* Initial: 225mg q12h. Titrate: Individualize based on response and tolerance. May increase at a minimum of 5-day interval to 325mg q12h, then to 425mg q12h if needed. Hepatic Impairment/QRS Widening/2nd- or 3rd-degree AV Block: Reduce dose.

HOW SUPPLIED: Cap, Extended-Release: 225mg, 325mg, 425mg

CONTRAINDICATIONS: Heart failure (HF), cardiogenic shock, bradycardia, marked hypotension, bronchospastic disorders or severe obstructive pulmonary disease, marked electrolyte imbalance, or sinoatrial, atrioventricular (AV) and intraventricular disorders of impulse generation or conduction (eg, sick sinus node syndrome, AV block) in the absence of an artificial pacemaker.

WARNINGS/PRECAUTIONS: Do not use to control ventricular rate during A-fib. Concomitant drugs that increase the functional AV nodal refractory period is recommended. May cause new or worsened arrhythmias (eg, ventricular fibrillation, ventricular tachycardia, asystole, torsade de pointes). May provoke overt HF. Caution with hepatic or renal dysfunction. Conduction disturbances (eg, 1st-degree AV block), agranulocytosis, positive antinuclear antibody (ANA) titers, and exacerbation of myasthenia gravis reported. D/C if persistent or worsening elevation of ANA titers detected. Reversible, short-term drop (within normal range) in sperm count may occur. May alter pacing and sensing thresholds of implanted pacemakers and defibrillators.

ADVERSE REACTIONS: Dizziness, chest pain, palpitations, taste disturbance, dyspnea, nausea, constipation, anxiety, fatigue, upper respiratory tract infection, influenza, edema.

INTERACTIONS: Withhold Class Ia and III antiarrhythmics for ≥5 half-lives prior to dosing with propafenone. Avoid with Class Ia and III antiarrhythmics (eg, quinidine, amiodarone). Inhibitors of CYP2D6 (eg, desipramine, paroxetine, ritonavir, sertraline) and CYP3A4 (eg, ketoconazole, ritonavir, saquinavir, erythromycin, grapefruit juice) may increase levels; avoid concomitant use with both a CYP2D6 inhibitor and a CYP3A4 inhibitor. Amiodarone can affect conduction and repolarization and is not recommended. May increase CNS side effects of lidocaine. May increase levels of digoxin, propranolol, metoprolol, and warfarin; monitor closely. Fluoxetine may increase levels in extensive metabolizers. Rifampin may decrease levels and may increase norpropafenone (an active metabolite) levels. May result in severe adverse events (eg, convulsion, AV block, and acute circulatory failure) with abrupt cessation of orlistat. Increased plasma levels with CYP1A2 inhibitors (eg, amiodarone, tobacco smoke) and cimetidine.

PREGNANCY: Category C, not for use in nursing.

MECHANISM OF ACTION: Class 1C antiarrhythmic; has local anesthetic effects and direct stabilizing action on myocardial membranes. Reduces upstroke velocity (Phase 0) of the monophasic action potential. In Purkinje fibers, and to a lesser extent myocardial fibers, propafenone reduces the fast inward current carried by Na^+ ions. Diastolic excitability is increased and effective refractory period is prolonged. Reduces spontaneous automaticity and depresses triggered activity.

PHARMACOKINETICS: Absorption: T_{max}=3-8 hrs. **Distribution:** V_d=252L (IV); plasma protein binding (>95%); found in breast milk. **Metabolism:** Rapid and extensive (>90% of patients), via CYP2D6, 3A4 and 1A2. 5-hydroxy-propafenone and N-depropylpropafenone (active metabolites). **Elimination:** $T_{1/2}$=2-10 hrs (>90% of patients), $T_{1/2}$=10-32 hrs (<10% of patients).

NURSING CONSIDERATIONS

Assessment: Assess for HF; cardiogenic shock; sinoatrial, AV and intraventricular disorders of impulse generation or conduction (eg, sick sinus node syndrome, AV block); implanted functioning pacemaker; bradycardia; marked hypotension; bronchospastic disorders or severe obstructive pulmonary disease; marked electrolyte imbalance; MI; renal/hepatic dysfunction; pregnancy/nursing status; and possible drug interactions. Evaluate ECG prior to therapy.

Monitoring: Monitor for proarrhythmic effects, signs/symptoms of conduction disturbances, agranulocytosis (eg, fever, chills, sore throat, decrease in white cell count), HF, impaired spermatogenesis, and exacerbation of myasthenia gravis. Monitor implanted pacemakers and defibrillators during and after therapy and re-program accordingly. Evaluate ECG during therapy. Monitor ANA titers, LFTs, and renal function.

Patient Counseling: Inform about risks/benefits of therapy. Instruct to report any signs of electrolyte imbalance (eg, excessive/prolonged diarrhea, sweating, vomiting, loss of appetite, thirst). Advise to notify physician of all prescription, herbal/natural preparations, and over-the-counter medications currently being taken or of any changes with these products. Instruct not to double the next dose if a dose is missed; take next dose at the usual time.

Administration: Oral route. Do not crush or further divide capsule contents. May take with or without food. **Storage:** 25°C (77°F); excursions permitted to 15-30°C (59-86°F).

RYZOLT

RX

tramadol HCl (Purdue Pharma)

THERAPEUTIC CLASS: Central acting analgesic

INDICATIONS: Management of moderate to moderately severe chronic pain.

DOSAGE: *Adults:* Individualize dose: Initial: 100mg/day. Titrate: 100mg every 2-3 days to achieve adequate pain control and tolerability. For patients requiring 300mg/day, titration should take at least 4 days. Usual: 200-300mg/day. Max: 300mg/day. Patients Currently on Tramadol IR Products: Calculate 24 hr IR dose and initiate on a total daily dose rounded down to next lowest 100mg increment. Max: 300mg/day. Elderly: Start at low end of dosing range. Swallow whole with liquid; do not split, chew, dissolve or crush.

HOW SUPPLIED: Tab, Extended-Release: 100mg, 200mg, 300mg

CONTRAINDICATIONS: Significant respiratory depression in unmonitored settings, acute or severe bronchial asthma, and hypercapnia.

WARNINGS/PRECAUTIONS: Seizures and anaphylactoid reactions reported. Avoid in suicidal or addiction-prone patients. May increase risk of serotonin syndrome (eg, mental changes, autonomic instability, neuromuscular aberrations, and GIT symptoms). Caution if at risk for respiratory depression, or with increased ICP or head trauma. May impair mental or physical abilities. Do not d/c abruptly; withdrawal symptoms may occur. May complicate acute abdominal conditions. Avoid in severe renal or hepatic impairment.

ADVERSE REACTIONS: Dizziness, N/V, constipation, headache, somnolence, pruritus, sweating, dry mouth, fatigue, anorexia, vertigo, insomnia, arthralgia, anxiety, hot flushes.

INTERACTIONS: CYP2D6 inhibitors (eg, quinidine, fluoxetine, paroxetine, amitriptyline) and CYP3A4 inhibitors (eg, ketoconazole, erythromycin) may reduce clearance of tramadol and increase risk for serious adverse events (eg, seizures, serotonin syndrome). Serotonergic drugs (eg, SSRIs, SNRIs, MAOIs, triptans, α_2-adrenergic blockers, linezolid, lithium, St. John's wort) may increase risk of seizures and/or serotonin syndrome; monitor closely, especially during treatment initiation and dose increases. Avoid with carbamazepine. Rare reports of digoxin toxicity and altered warfarin effects. Caution and reduce dose with CNS depressants (eg, alcohol, opioids, anesthetics, phenothiazines, tranquilizers, sedative hypnotics). Additive effects with alcohol and CNS depressants may occur.

PREGNANCY: Category C, safety in nursing not known.

MECHANISM OF ACTION: Centrally acting synthetic opioid analgesic; not fully understood. Shown to inhibit reuptake of norepinephrine and serotonin.

PHARMACOKINETICS: Absorption: Bioavailability (95%); T_{max}=4 hrs (drug) , 5 hrs (M1 metabolite); C_{max}=345ng/mL (drug), 71ng/mL (M1 metabolite); AUC_{0-24}=5991ng•h/mL (drug), 1361ng•h/mL (M1 metabolite). **Distribution:** V_d=2.6L/kg (male), 2.9L/kg (female); plasma protein binding (20%). **Metabolism:** Liver (extensive); through N-and O-demethylation and glucuronidation or sulfation pathways via CYP3A4, 2D6. M1 (active metabolite). **Elimination:** Urine (30% unchanged), (60% as metabolite); $T_{1/2}$=6.3 hrs (drug), 7.4 hrs (M1).

NURSING CONSIDERATIONS

Assessment: Assess for significant respiratory depression, acute or severe bronchial asthma, hypercapnia, seizure risk, epilepsy, risk for respiratory depression, increased ICP, acute abdominal conditions, renal/hepatic impairment, pregnancy/nursing status, and possible drug interactions.

Monitoring: Monitor for anaphylactoid reactions (eg, pruritus, hives, bronchospasm, angioedema, toxic epidermal necrolysis, and Stevens-Johnson syndrome), respiratory/CNS symptoms, physical dependence/abuse, seizures, serotonin syndrome, withdrawal symptoms with abrupt d/c (eg, anxiety, sweating, insomnia, rigors, upper respiratory symptoms, diarrhea, piloerection, and, rarely, hallucinations).

Patient Counseling: Advise to use caution while performing hazardous tasks (eg, operating machinery, driving). Do not take with alcohol, tranquilizers, or

R

hypnotics. Notify physician if pregnant/nursing or planning to become pregnant. Take as prescribed.

Administration: Oral route. **Storage:** Store at 25°C (77°F); excursions permitted between 15-30°C (59-86°F).

SABRIL   RX
vigabatrin (Lundbeck)

> Causes permanent vision loss in a high percentage of infants, children, and adults; timing of onset unpredictable. Causes progressive and permanent bilateral concentric visual field constriction in a high percentage of adult patients; in some cases may damage central retina and may reduce visual acuity. Risk increases with dose and cumulative exposure; use lowest effective dose and shortest exposure. Risk may persist after d/c therapy. D/C in patients who fail to show clinical benefit within 2-4 weeks (peds) or 3 months (adults) of initiation, or as soon as treatment failure is obvious. Vision testing is required at baseline, while on therapy, and after d/c. Unless benefit clearly outweighs the risk, avoid use with other drugs associated with serious adverse ophthalmic effects (eg, retinopathy, glaucoma) and in patients with, or at high risk of, other types of irreversible vision loss. Available only through restricted distribution program (SHARE).

THERAPEUTIC CLASS: GABA analog

INDICATIONS: (Powder) Monotherapy for pediatrics (1 month-2 yrs) with infantile spasms (IS) for whom the potential benefits outweigh the potential risk of vision loss. (Tab) Adjunctive therapy for adults with refractory complex partial seizures (CPS) who have inadequately responded to several alternative treatments and for whom the potential benefits outweigh the risk of vision loss.

DOSAGE: *Adults:* Refractory CPS: (Tab) Initial: 500mg bid (1g/day). Titrate: May increase in 500mg increments at weekly intervals depending on response. Maint: 1.5g bid (3g/day). Renal Impairment: CrCl >50-80mL/min: Decrease dose by 25%. CrCl >30-50mL/min: Decrease dose by 50%. CrCl >10-<30mL/min: Decrease dose by 75%. Withdraw gradually to d/c therapy. *Pediatrics:* 1 month-2 yrs: IS: (Powder) Initial: 50mg/kg/day in 2 divided doses. Titrate: May increase by 25-50mg/kg/day increments every 3 days. Max: 150mg/kg/day. Refer to PI for volume of individual doses. Renal Impairment: CrCl >50-80mL/min: Decrease dose by 25%. CrCl >30-50mL/min: Decrease dose by 50%. CrCl >10-<30mL/min: Decrease dose by 75%. Withdraw gradually to d/c therapy.

HOW SUPPLIED: Powder: 500mg/pkt [50^s]; Tab: 500mg* *scored

WARNINGS/PRECAUTIONS: Vision testing required no later than 4 weeks after starting, at least every 3 months during, and 3-6 months after d/c. Abnormal MRI changes involving thalamus, basal ganglia, brain stem, and cerebellum observed in some infants. May increase risk of suicidal thoughts/behavior. Monitor for worsening/emergence of depression and unusual changes in mood/behavior; risk observed as early as 1 week after initiation. May cause anemia, somnolence, fatigue, peripheral neuropathy, weight gain, and edema. Should be withdrawn gradually when necessary. Enroll all patients in SHARE; may be dispensed only to patients enrolled in, and who meet all conditions of, SHARE (1-888-45-SHARE).

ADVERSE REACTIONS: Vision loss/visual field defects, decreased AST/ALT activity, headache, fatigue, drowsiness, dizziness, irritability, nystagmus, upper respiratory tract infection, weight gain, diarrhea, abnormal coordination, fever, otitis media.

INTERACTIONS: See Boxed Warning. Decreases phenytoin plasma levels, probably due to induction of CYP450 2C enzymes. Increases C_{max} and decreases T_{max} of clonazepam. Decreased levels of sodium valproate and phenobarbital (from phenobarbital or primidone).

PREGNANCY: Category C, not for use in nursing.

MECHANISM OF ACTION: GABA analog; not established; may be due to irreversible inhibition of gamma-aminobutyric acid transaminase (GABA-T), which results in increased levels of GABA in the CNS.

S

PHARMACOKINETICS: Absorption: Complete; T_{max}=1 hr (Adults/Children), 2.5 hrs (Infants). **Distribution:** V_d=1.1L/kg. Found in breast milk. **Elimination:** Urine (95%); $T_{1/2}$=7.5 hrs (Adults), 5.7 hrs (Infants).

NURSING CONSIDERATIONS

Assessment: Perform baseline vision test. Assess renal function, pregnancy/nursing status, underlying suicidal behavior/ideation. Assess patient response to and continued need for treatment periodically.

Monitoring: Monitor worsening vision/visual field changes. Perform vision testing no later than 4 weeks after stopping therapy, q3 months during therapy and 3-6 months after d/c. Monitor for signs of hypersensitivity, signal changes on MRI, and any untoward effects (eg, suicidal thoughts/behavior, worsening/emergence of depression, thoughts of self-harm, change in mood/behavior). Monitor CBC, Hgb, Hct, LFTs, renal function, weight, and edema.

Patient Counseling: Inform patients of the risk of permanent vision loss and the need for vision monitoring. If changes in vision occur, instruct to notify healthcare provider. Drug may increase the risk of suicidal thoughts and behavior; behaviors of concern should be reported immediately to healthcare provider. Do not drive or operate complex machinery until familiar with effects of drug. Inform of the possibility of developing abnormal MRI signal changes. If pregnant or about to become pregnant, instruct to enroll in the North American Antiepileptic Drug (NAAED) Pregnancy Registry by calling 1-888-233-2334 go to aedpregnancyregistry.com. Instruct caregivers to withdraw gradually during d/c of therapy.

Administration: Oral route. (Powder) Empty contents of pkt into empty cup and dissolve with 10mL of cold/room temperature water using oral syringe. Final solution concentration should be 50mg/mL. Prepare each dose immediately prior to administration. Refer to PI for dilution table. **Storage:** 20-25°C (68-77°F).

SAMSCA   RX
tolvaptan (Otsuka America)

> Initiate and re-initiate therapy in hospitalized patients only; monitor serum sodium levels closely. Osmotic demyelination resulting in dysarthria, mutism, dysphagia, lethargy, affective changes, spastic quadriparesis, seizures, coma or death may occur due to rapid correction of hyponatremia (eg, >12mEq/L/24 hrs). Slower rates of correction may be advisable in susceptible patients with severe malnutrition, alcoholism, or advanced liver disease.

THERAPEUTIC CLASS: Arginine vasopressin antagonist

INDICATIONS: Treatment of clinically significant hypervolemic and euvolemic hyponatremia (eg, serum sodium <125mEq/L or less marked hyponatremia that is symptomatic and has resisted correction with fluid restriction), including patients with heart failure, cirrhosis, and Syndrome of Inappropraiate Antidiuretic Hormone (SIADH).

DOSAGE: *Adults:* Initial: 15mg qd. Titrate: May increase to 30mg qd after at least 24 hrs to maximum of 60mg qd until desired level of serum sodium is achieved. Max: 60mg qd.

HOW SUPPLIED: Tab: 15mg, 30mg

CONTRAINDICATIONS: Urgent need to raise serum sodium acutely, inability to auto-regulate fluid balance, hypovolemic hyponatremia, concomitant use of strong CYP3A inhibitors (eg, ketoconazole, clarithromycin, itraconazole, ritonavir, indinavir, nelfinavir, saquinavir, nefazodone, telithromycin), and anuria.

WARNINGS/PRECAUTIONS: D/C or interrupt therapy if patient develops rapid elevation of sodium acutely; consider hypotonic fluid administration. Avoid fluid restriction during the first 24 hrs of therapy. Monitor for changes in serum electrolytes and volume during initiation and titration of therapy. GI bleeding reported in patients with cirrhosis. Dehydration and hypovolemia may occur; interrupt or d/c therapy and provide supportive care with careful management of vital signs, fluid balance and electrolytes. Increased serum K+ levels reported; monitor serum K+ levels after initiation of therapy in patients with a serum K+ of >5mEq/L and with those receiving drugs known to increase potassium levels.

ADVERSE REACTIONS: Thirst, dry mouth, asthenia, constipation, pollakiuria, polyuria, hyperglycemia, pyrexia, anorexia.

INTERACTIONS: See Contraindications. Increased levels with ketoconazole and grapefruit juice. Avoid with moderate CYP3A inhibitors (eg, erythromycin, fluconazole, aprepitant, dilitiazem, and verapamil). Dose reduction with P-gp inhibitors (eg, cyclosporine). Avoid with CYP3A inducers (eg, rifampin, rifabutin, barbiturates, phenytoin, carbamazepine, and St. John's wort). Avoid with concomitant use of hypertonic saline. Higher adverse reactions of hyperkalemia with angiotensin receptor blockers, angiotensin converting enzyme inhibitors and K+ sparing diuretics.Increase levels of digoxin and lovastatin.

PREGNANCY: Category C, not for use in nursing.

MECHANISM OF ACTION: Selective vasopressin V2-receptor antagonist; antagonize the effect of vasopressin and cause increase in urine water excretion resulting in increase free water clearance (aquaresis), decrease urine osmolality and increase serum sodium levels.

PHARMACOKINETICS: Absorption: T_{max}=2-4 hrs. **Distribution:** V_d=3L/kg; plasma protein binding (99%). **Metabolism:** Via CYP3A. **Elimination:** $T_{1/2}$=12 hrs.

NURSING CONSIDERATIONS

Assessment: Assess for serum sodium levels, neurologic status, anuria, hypovolemia, cirrhosis, pregnancy/nursing status, and possible drug interactions.

Monitoring: Monitor for serum K+ levels, neurologic status, signs and symptoms of hypovolemia, GI bleeding in patients with cirrhosis, changes in serum sodium/volume status, vital signs, fluid balance and electrolytes.

Patient Counseling: Advise to continue ingestion of fluid in response to thirst. Instruct to avoid fluid restriction within 24 hrs of therapy. Inform physician if you are taking or planning to take any prescription or over-the-counter drugs, using strong or moderate CYP3A inhibitors, or P-gp inhibitors. Advise nursing mothers not to breastfeed. Keep out of reach of children.

Administration: Oral route. **Storage:** 25°C (77°F), excursions permitted between 15-30°C (59-86°F).

SANCTURA **XR**   **RX**
trospium chloride (Allergan)

OTHER BRAND NAMES: Sanctura (Allergan)

THERAPEUTIC CLASS: Muscarinic antagonist

INDICATIONS: Treatment of overactive bladder with symptoms of urge urinary incontinence, urgency, and urinary frequency.

DOSAGE: Adults: (Tab) 20mg bid ≥1 hr before meals or on empty stomach. CrCl<30mL/min: 20mg qhs. Elderly (≥75 yrs): May be reduced to 20mg qd based upon tolerability. (Cap, ER) 60mg qam with water on an empty stomach, ≥1 hr before meals.

HOW SUPPLIED: Cap, Extended-Release: 60mg; Tab: 20mg

CONTRAINDICATIONS: Active or risk of urinary/gastric retention and uncontrolled narrow-angle glaucoma.

WARNINGS/PRECAUTIONS: Angioedema of face, lips, tongue, and/or larynx reported; d/c if tongue, hypopharynx, or larynx involvement occurs and provide appropriate therapy/measures. Caution with significant bladder outflow obstruction, GI obstructive disorders, and moderate or severe hepatic dysfunction. May decrease GI motility; caution with ulcerative colitis, intestinal atony, and myasthenia gravis. Used only if benefits outweigh the risks in patients being treated for controlled narrow-angle glaucoma; monitor carefully. (Cap, ER) Not recommended for use with severe renal impairment (CrCl<30mL/min). Alcohol should not be consumed within 2 hours of administration.

S

ADVERSE REACTIONS: Dry mouth, constipation. (Cap, ER) Urinary tract infection. (Tab) Headache.

INTERACTIONS: May increase the frequency and/or severity of anticholinergic effects with other anticholinergic agents. May alter GI absorption of other drugs. May interact with some drugs that are actively secreted by the kidney by competing for renal tubular secretion (eg, procainamide, pancuronium, morphine, vancomycin, metformin, tenofovir). May enhance drowsiness with alcohol. (Cap, ER) May increase or decrease exposure with antacids containing aluminum hydroxide and magnesium carbonate.

PREGNANCY: Category C, caution in nursing.

MECHANISM OF ACTION: Antispasmodic, antimuscarinic agent; reduces tonus of smooth muscle in bladder by antagonizing effect of acetylcholine on muscarinic receptors.

PHARMACOKINETICS: Absorption: (Tab) Absolute bioavailability (9.6%); C_{max}=3.5ng/mL; T_{max}=5.3 hrs; AUC=36.4ng/mL•hr. (Cap, ER) C_{max}=2ng/mL; T_{max}=5 hrs; AUC=18ng•hr/mL. **Distribution:** (Tab) Plasma protein binding (50-85%); V_d=395L. (Cap, ER) Plasma protein binding (48-78%); V_d=>600L. **Metabolism:** Ester hydrolysis with subsequent conjugation. **Elimination:** (Tab) Feces (85.2%), urine (5.8%); $T_{1/2}$=18.3 hrs. (Cap, ER) $T_{1/2}$=36 hrs.

NURSING CONSIDERATIONS

Assessment: Assess for bladder outflow obstruction, urinary/gastric retention, narrow-angle glaucoma, GI obstructive disorder, ulcerative colitis, intestinal atony, myasthenia gravis, hepatic/renal impairment, pregnancy/nursing status, and possible drug interactions.

Monitoring: Monitor for signs/symptoms of angioedema, gastric retention, urinary retention, decreased gastric motility, and for hepatic/renal dysfunction. Carefully monitor use in patients being treated for narrow-angle glaucoma.

Patient Counseling: Inform that therapy may produce angioedema which could result in life-threatening airway obstruction. D/C therapy and seek immediate medical attention if edema of tongue or laryngopharynx, or difficulty breathing occurs. Heat prostration may occur when used in hot environment, and dry mouth, constipation, trouble emptying the bladder, dizziness and blurred vision may also be experienced. Do not take if urinary/gastric retention or uncontrolled narrow-angle glaucoma are present. Alcohol may enhance drowsiness effect. (Cap, ER) Avoid alcohol within 2 hrs of dosing of cap. Take cap in the am with water on an empty stomach or ≥1 hr before meals. (Tab) Instruct to take tab 1 hr prior to meals or on empty stomach. Take next dose 1 hr prior to next meal if a dose is skipped.

Administration: Oral route. **Storage:** 20-25°C (68-77°F); (Cap, ER) excursions permitted at 15-30°C.

SANCUSO   RX
granisetron (Prostrakan)

THERAPEUTIC CLASS: 5-HT$_3$ receptor antagonist

INDICATIONS: Prevention of N/V in patients receiving moderately and/or highly emetogenic chemotherapy for up to 5 consecutive days.

DOSAGE: *Adults:* Apply single patch to upper outer arm a minimum of 24 hrs before chemo. May be applied up to a maximum of 48 hrs before chemo. Remove patch a minimum of 24 hrs after completion of chemo. Patch can be worn for up to 7 days depending on duration of chemo regimen.

HOW SUPPLIED: Patch: 3.1mg/24 hrs

WARNINGS/PRECAUTIONS: May mask progressive ileus and/or gastric distention. Avoid placing on red, irritated, or damaged skin. Generalized skin reaction (eg, allergic rash, including erythematous, macular, papular rash, pruritus) may occur; d/c and remove patch immediately. Avoid direct natural or artificial sunlight. Cover application site in case of risk of exposure to sunlight throughout the period of wear and for 10 days following removal.

ADVERSE REACTIONS: Constipation, abdominal pain, diarrhea, HTN, hypotension, dizziness, insomnia, fever.

PREGNANCY: Category B, caution in nursing.

MECHANISM OF ACTION: 5-HT$_3$ receptor antagonist; blocks serotonin stimulation and subsequent vomiting after emetogenic stimuli such as cisplatin in animal studies.

PHARMACOKINETICS: Absorption: T$_{max}$=48 hrs. C$_{max}$=5.0ng/mL. AUC=527ng•hr/mL. **Distribution:** Plasma protein binding (65%). **Metabolism:** N-demethylation and aromatic ring oxidation mediated by hepatic CYP1A1 and CYP3A4. **Elimination:** Urine (12%, unchanged; 49%, metabolites), feces (34%).

NURSING CONSIDERATIONS

Assessment: Assess skin condition and GI history.

Monitoring: Monitor for abdominal pain and/or swelling, generalized skin reactions, and adverse events.

Patient Counseling: Apply to clean, dry, intact healthy skin on upper outer arm. Do not place on skin that is red, irritated, or damaged. Inform physician if abdominal pain and swelling occurs. Remove patch if severe skin or generalized skin reactions (eg, allergic rash, including erythematous macular, papular rash, or pruritus) occur. Cover patch application site when there is a risk of exposure to sunlight or sunlamps during the period of wear and for 10 days after removal. Patch should not be cut into pieces.

Administration: Topical route. Patch should be applied to clean, dry, intact healthy skin on the upper outer arm. **Storage:** Store at 20-25°C (68-77°F); excursions permitted between 15-30°C (59-86°F).

SANDIMMUNE
cyclosporine (Novartis)

RX

> Should only be prescribed by physicians experienced in immunosuppressive therapy and management of organ transplant. Patients should be managed at equipped facilities and staffed with adequate laboratory and supportive medical resources. Give with adrenal corticosteroids but not with other immunosuppressive agents. Increased susceptibility to infection and development of lymphoma may result from immunosuppression. Not bioequivalent to Neoral; not interchangeable without physician supervision. Monitor blood levels to avoid toxicity with chronic administration of soft gelatin caps and oral solution.

THERAPEUTIC CLASS: Cyclic polypeptide immunosuppressant

INDICATIONS: Prophylaxis of organ rejection in kidney, liver, and heart allogeneic transplants with concomitant adrenal corticosteroids. Treatment of chronic rejection in patients previously treated with other immunosuppressive agents.

DOSAGE: *Adults:* Adjunct therapy with adrenal corticosteroids; dosage adjustment must be made according to the clinical situation. Initial: PO: 15mg/kg single dose 4-12 hrs before transplant; continue same dose qd for 1-2 weeks. Titrate: Taper by 5% per week to 5-10mg/kg/day. IV: 1/3 PO dose. Initial: 5-6mg/kg/day single dose 4 to 12 hrs prior to transplantation. Continue single daily dose until PO forms are tolerated; switch to PO as soon as possible after surgery. Elderly: Start at lower end of dosing range.
Pediatrics: Adjunct therapy with adrenal corticosteroids; dosage adjustment must be made according to the clinical situation. Higher doses may be required. Initial: PO: 15mg/kg single dose 4-12 hrs before transplant; continue same dose qd for 1-2 weeks. Titrate: Taper by 5% per week to 5-10mg/kg/day. IV: 1/3 PO dose. Initial: 5-6mg/kg/day single dose 4 to 12 hrs prior to transplantation. Continue single daily dose until PO forms are tolerated; switch to PO as soon as possible after surgery.

HOW SUPPLIED: Cap: 25mg, 100mg; Inj: 50mg/mL; Sol: 100mg/mL [50mL]

CONTRAINDICATIONS: (Inj) Hypersensitivity to Cremophor EL (polyoxyethylated castor oil).

WARNINGS/PRECAUTIONS: Due to risk of anaphylaxis, only use injection if unable to take oral agents. May cause hepatotoxicity and nephrotoxicity. Convulsions, elevated SrCr, and BUN levels reported. Thrombocytopenia and microangiopathic hemolytic anemia, hyperuricemia, hyperkalemia, encephalopathy may develop. Increased risk for development of lymphomas and other malignancies. Anaphylactic reactions reported rarely with IV administration; observe for 30 min after start of infusion and frequently thereafter. Caution with malabsorption. HTN may occur and persist which may require antihypertensive therapy. Increased risk of opportunistic infections including activation of latent viral infection such as BK virus-associated nephropathy in patients receiving immunosuppressants. Caution in elderly.

ADVERSE REACTIONS: Renal dysfunction, tremor, hirsutism, HTN, gum hyperplasia, cramps, acne, convulsions, headache, diarrhea, hepatotoxity, abdominal discomfort, paresthesia, flushing, BK virus-associated nephropathy.

INTERACTIONS: Ciprofloxacin, gentamicin, tobramycin, vancomycin, trimethoprim with sulfamethoxazole, amphotericin B, ketoconazole, melphalan, diclofenac, azapropazon, sulindac, naproxen, colchicine, cimetidine, ranitidine, tacrolimus, bezafirate, fenofibrate may potentiate renal dysfunction. Diltiazem, nicardipine, colchicine, fluconazole, itraconazole, ketoconazole, voriconazole, verapamil, azithromycin, clarithromycin, erythromycin, quinupristin/dalfopristin, allopurinol, amiodarone, bromocriptine, danazol, imatinib, nefazodone, metoclopramide, oral contraceptives, methylprednisolone, grapefruit, grapefruit juice, HIV protease inhibitors (eg, indinavir, nelfinavir, ritonavir, and saquinavir) may increase levels. St. John's wort, carbamazepine, oxcarbazepine, bosentan, phenobarbital, phenytoin, rifampin, sulfinpyrazone, octreotide, orlistat, terbinafine, ticlopidine, and naficillin may decrease levels. Avoid with K^+-sparing diuretics. Digitalis toxicity reported with digoxin. Myotoxicity cases seen with statins (lovastatin, simvastatin, atorvastatin, pravastatin, fluvastatin). Frequent gingival hyperplasia with nifedipine, and convulsions with high dose methylprednisolone reported. Increased levels of sirolimus; give 4 hrs after cyclosporine. Avoid live vaccines during therapy. Caution with rifabutin, NSAIDs, angiotensin-converting enzyme inhibitors, angiotensin II receptor antagonists, K^+-containing drugs, and K^+-rich diet. Increase concentration of methotrexate, repaglinide. Increase/decrease levels with CYP3A4 or P-glycoprotein inhibitors/inducers. Dose adjustment with calcium antagonists. Increases concentration of CYP3A4 or P-glycoprotein substrates.

PREGNANCY: Category C, not for use in nursing.

MECHANISM OF ACTION: Cyclic polypeptide immunosuppressant; not fully established. May cause specific and reversible inhibition of immunocompetent lymphocytes in the G_0- or G_1-phase of the cell cycle. T lymphocytes are preferentially inhibited with T-helper cell as main target while also possibly suppressing T-suppressor cells. Also inhibits lymphokine production and release (eg, interleukin-2, T-cell growth factor).

PHARMACOKINETICS: Absorption: Incomplete and variable. Absolute bioavailability (30%)(PO); C_{max}=1ng/mL/mg; T_{max}=3.5 hrs. **Distribution:** Plasma protein binding (90%); found in breast milk. **Metabolism:** Extensively metabolized via hydroxylation, cyclic ether formation, and N-demethylation. **Elimination:** Urine (6%); $T_{1/2}$=19 hrs.

NURSING CONSIDERATIONS

Assessment: Prior to IV administration, assess that patient cannot take oral formulations and is on concomitant therapy with adrenal corticosteroids. Assess for hypersensitivity to Cremophor EL (polyoxyethylated castor oil), pregnancy/nursing status, possible drug interactions. Assess use of oral formulations in patients with malabsorption problems.

Monitoring: Patients receiving IV formulation should be under continuous observation for anaphylactic reactions for at least first 30 min following start of infusion and at frequent intervals thereafter. Monitor for signs/symptoms of hepatotoxicity, nephrotoxicity, thrombocytopenia, microangiopathic hemolytic anemia, HTN, hyperkalemia, glomerular capillary thrombosis, lymphomas, and other malignancies, convulsions, encephalopathy, and development of anaphylactic reactions (eg, facial flushing, non-cardiogenic pulmonary edema with acute respiratory distress, dyspnea, changes in BP, and tachycardia). Frequently monitor cyclosporine blood levels, especially when converting from Neoral to Sandimmune, as well as renal/hepatic function (eg, BUN, SrCr, serum bilirubin, liver enzymes).

Patient Counseling: Instruct to contact a physician before changing formulations of cyclosporine, which may require dose changes. Repeated tests are required while on medication. Drug may cause increased risk of neoplasias. Advise females about risks of use during pregnancy. Instruct patients using the oral syringe, that syringe should not be washed before or after use as that will cause variation in dosage.

Administration: Oral/IV routes. Oral solution may be mixed with milk, chocolate milk, or orange juice. IV concentrate should be administered by slow IV infusion over 2-6 hrs. **Storage:** Cap: 25°C (77°F); excursions permitted to 15-30°C (59-86°F). Oral Sol: Store in original container, below 30°C (86°F). Do not refrigerate. Protect from freezing. Once opened, use contents within 2 months. Inj: Below 30°C (86°F), protect from light. Discard diluted infusion after 24 hrs.

SANDOSTATIN LAR   RX
octreotide acetate (Novartis)

THERAPEUTIC CLASS: Somatostatin analog

INDICATIONS: Long-term maintenance therapy in acromegalic patients with inadequate response to surgery and/or radiotherapy or for whom surgery and/or radiotherapy is not an option. Long-term treatment of severe diarrhea and flushing associated with metastatic carcinoid tumors. Long-term treatment of profuse watery diarrhea associated with vasoactive intestinal peptide tumors (VIPomas).

DOSAGE: *Adults:* Administer intragluteally. Patients not currently receiving octreotide should begin therapy with Sandostatin injection; please see PI for dosing. Acromegaly: Initial: 20mg IM every 4 weeks for 3 months. Titrate: See PI for dose adjustment based on growth hormone (GH), IGF-1, and/or clinical symptoms. Max: 40mg every 4 weeks. Withdraw yearly for 8 weeks to assess disease activity after pituitary irradiation. Carcinoid Tumors/VIPomas: Initial: 20mg IM every 4 weeks for 2 months. Continue with Sandostatin injection SQ for at least 2 weeks. Titrate: If symptoms not controlled, increase to 30mg every 4 weeks. If symptoms controlled at 20mg, reduce to 10mg. If symptoms recur increase dose to 20mg every 4 weeks. Max: 30mg every 4 weeks. For exacerbation of symptoms, give Sandostatin Injection SQ for at least 2 weeks. Patients must be considered responders and tolerate the injection before switching to the depot. Renal Failure Requiring Dialysis/Cirrhotic patients: Initial: 10mg every 4 weeks.

HOW SUPPLIED: Inj, Depot: 10mg, 20mg, 30mg

WARNINGS/PRECAUTIONS: May inhibit gallbladder contractility and decrease bile secretions; increased risk of gallbladder abnormalities. May alter balance between insulin, glucagon, and GH and lead to hypoglycemia or hyperglycemia; monitor glucose tolerance and antidiabetic treatment periodically. May cause hypothyroidism; monitor thyroid levels periodically. Cardiac conduction and other cardiovascular (CV) abnormalities may occur; caution in patients at-risk. Depressed vitamin B_{12} levels, alteration in fat absorption and abnormal Schilling's test reported. Caution in the elderly and in patient on total parenteral nutrition (TPN).

ADVERSE REACTIONS: Diarrhea, N/V, abdominal discomfort, flatulence, constipation, hyperglycemia, injection-site pain, upper respiratory infection, flu-like symptoms, fatigue, dizziness, headache, malaise, fever.

INTERACTIONS: May alter absorption of orally administered drugs. May decrease cyclosporine effects. May need dose adjustments of insulin, oral hypoglycemics, and bradycardia-inducing drugs (eg, beta-blocker). Increased availability of bromocriptine. Caution in other drugs metabolized by CYP3A4 with a low therapeutic index (eg, quinidine, terfenadine).

PREGNANCY: Category B, caution in nursing.

S

MECHANISM OF ACTION: Somatostatin analog; long acting. Exerts similiar actions to natural hormone somatostatin, but is more potent in inhibiting GH, glucagon, and insulin. Like somatostatin, it also suppresses LH response to GnRH, decreases splanchnic blood flow and inhibits release of serotonin, gastrin, vasoactive intestinal peptide, secretin, motilin and pancreatic polypeptide.

PHARMACOKINETICS: Absorption: (SQ) Rapid, Complete. C_{max}=5.2ng/mL; T_{max}=0.4 hrs; Acromegaly: C_{max}=2.8ng/mL, T_{max}=0.7 hr. **Distribution:** V_d=13.6L; plasma protein binding (65%); Acromegaly: V_d=21.6L, plasma protein binding (41.2%). **Elimination:** Urine (32%, unchanged); $T_{1/2}$=1.7-1.9 hrs.

NURSING CONSIDERATIONS

Assessment: Assess GH and IGF-I levels, baseline renal function. Obtain baseline thyroid function tests (TSH, total and/or free T4). Assess use with cardiac dysfunction, for glycemic control with diabetes mellitus (DM), and for possible drug interactions.

Monitoring: Monitor for signs/symptoms of biliary tract abnormalities (eg, gallstones, biliary duct dilatation), hypo/hyperglycemia, hypothyroidism, cardiac conduction abnormalities, and pancreatitis. With acromegaly: Monitor GH and IGF-1 levels. With carcinoids: Monitor 5-HIAA (urinary 5-hydroxyin-doleacetic acid), plasma serotonin levels, and plasma Substance P levels. With VIPoma: Monitor VIP levels. Monitor zinc levels if receiving TPN.

Patient Counseling: Advise patients with carcinoid tumors and VIPomas to adhere closely to scheduled return visits for reinjection to minimize exacerbation of symptoms. Advise patients with acromegaly to adhere to return visit schedule to help ensure steady control of GH and IGF-1 levels.

Administration: IM route. Do not directly inject diluent without preparing sus. Never administer via IV/SQ routes. Sandostatin LAR depot drug product kit should remain at room temperature for 30-60 min prior to preparation of drug sus. Administer sus immediately after preparation. **Storage:** Refrigerate between 2-8°C (36-46°F) and protect from light until time of use.

SAPHRIS

RX

asenapine (Merck)

> Elderly patients with dementia-related psychosis treated with antipsychotic drugs are at an increased risk of death; most deaths appeared to be cardiovascular (eg, heart failure, sudden death) or infectious (eg, pneumonia) in nature. Not approved for treatment of dementia-related psychosis.

THERAPEUTIC CLASS: Dibenzapine derivative

INDICATIONS: Treatment of schizophrenia. As monotherapy or adjunctive therapy with either lithium or valproate for the acute treatment of manic or mixed episodes associated with bipolar I disorder.

DOSAGE: *Adults:* Schizophrenia: Initial/Usual: 5mg bid. Titrate: May increase to 10mg bid after 1 week based on tolerability. Max: 10mg bid. Bipolar Disorder: Monotherapy: Initial/Usual/Max: 10mg bid. Titrate: May decrease to 5mg bid if needed. Adjunctive Therapy (with lithium/valproate): Initial/Usual: 5mg bid. Titrate: May increase to 10mg bid based on response and tolerability. Max: 10mg bid. Continue treatment beyond acute response.

HOW SUPPLIED: Tab, SL: 5mg, 10mg

WARNINGS/PRECAUTIONS: Neuroleptic malignant syndrome (NMS) reported; d/c therapy, institute intensive treatment and medical monitoring, and treat any concomitant illness if it occurs. Tardive dyskinesia (TD) may occur; consider d/c therapy. Hyperglycemia reported; caution with diabetes mellitus (DM) or if at risk for DM. May cause weight gain. May induce orthostatic hypotension and syncope; monitor orthostatic vital signs and consider dose reduction if hypotension occurs. Caution with cardiovascular disease (CVD), cerebrovascular disease, or conditions that predispose to hypotension. Leukopenia, neutropenia, agranulocytosis reported; d/c with severe neutropenia (<1000/mm³) or at 1st sign of decline in WBC. May prolong QTc interval; avoid use with history of cardiac arrhythmias or in circumstances that may increase risk of torsades de pointes. May elevate prolactin levels. Seizures reported; caution with history of seizures or conditions that lower seizure threshold. Caution with elderly. May impair physical/mental abilities. May disrupt body's ability to reduce core body temperature; caution with strenuous exercise, exposure to extreme heat, or being subject to dehydration. Caution with those at risk for suicide. May cause dysphagia and esophageal dysmotility. Avoid with risk of aspiration pneumonia. Not recommended with severe hepatic impairment (Child-Pugh C). Minimize period of overlapping antipsychotic administration.

ADVERSE REACTIONS: Somnolence, insomnia, headache, dizziness, extrapyramidal symptoms, akathisia, vomiting, oral hypoesthesia, constipation, weight increase, fatigue, increased appetite, anxiety.

INTERACTIONS: Avoid use with other drugs known to prolong QTc. Caution with fluvoxamine; may increase concentrations. Increased concentrations with imipramine. Decreased concentrations with paroxetine, cimetidine, and carbamazepine. Caution with other centrally acting drugs, alcohol, drugs that are both substrates and inhibitors of CYP2D6, and drugs that can induce hypotension, bradycardia, respiratory or central nervous system depression. May enhance effects of antihypertensive agents. May elevate core body temperature if used concomitantly with anticholinergic medications.

PREGNANCY: Category C, not for use in nursing.

MECHANISM OF ACTION: Dibenzapine derivative; not established. Suggested that efficacy may be mediated through a combination of antagonist activity at D_2 and 5-HT$_{2A}$ receptors.

PHARMACOKINETICS: Absorption: Rapid; (5mg) absolute bioavailability (35%); C_{max}=4ng/mL; T_{max}=1 hr. **Distribution:** V_d=20-25L/kg; plasma protein binding (95%). **Metabolism:** Glucuronidation via UGT1A4 and oxidation via CYP1A2. **Elimination:** Urine (50%), feces (40%); $T_{1/2}$=24 hrs.

NURSING CONSIDERATIONS

Assessment: Assess for conditions where treatment is cautioned. Assess for hepatic function, pregnancy/nursing status, and possible drug interactions. Obtain baseline FBG in patients with DM or at risk for DM. Perform baseline CBC if at risk for leukopenia/neutropenia.

Monitoring: Monitor for QT prolongation, NMS, TD, orthostatic hypotension, seizures, esophageal dysmotility, aspiration, suicidal ideation. Monitor renal function, prolactin levels, serum transaminases, creatine kinase, total-C, TG, and CBC, especially for decline of WBC with signs/symptoms of infection. Monitor for symptoms of hyperglycemia. Monitor regularly for FBG and worsening of glucose control in DM patients. Monitor orthostatic vital signs and weight regularly. Periodically reassess to determine the need for maintenance treatment.

Patient Counseling: Inform that tab should not be chewed, crushed, or swallowed; place under tongue and allow to dissolve. Instruct to avoid eating or drinking for 10 min after administration. Inform that therapy is not approved for elderly with dementia-related psychosis. Inform about risk of developing NMS and counsel about its signs and symptoms (eg, hyperpyrexia, muscle rigidity, altered mental status, autonomic instability). Inform the need to monitor blood glucose in patients with DM or risk factors of diabetes. Advise that weight gain may be experienced. Inform about risk of developing orthostatic hypotension. Instruct that CBC should be monitored in patients with preexisting WBC or history of drug-induced leukopenia/neutropenia. Caution about performing activities requiring mental alertness (eg, driving/operating machinery). Instruct to avoid overheating or dehydration. Advise to notify physician if taking or plan to take any prescription or OTC medications, or if pregnant or intend to become pregnant. Advise not to breastfeed and avoid alcohol use while on therapy.

Administration: SL route. Place under tongue and allow to dissolve completely. Do not crush, chew, or swallow. Do not eat or drink for 10 min after administration. **Storage:** 15-30°C (59-86°F).

SAVELLA
RX

milnacipran HCl (Forest)

> Antidepressants increased the risk of suicidal thinking and behavior (suicidality) in children, adolescents, and young adults in short-term studies of major depressive disorder (MDD) and other psychiatric disorders. Depression and other psychiatric disorders are associated with increases in the risk of suicide. Monitor appropriately and observe closely for clinical worsening, suicidality, or unusual behavioral changes. Families and caregivers should be advised to observe closely and communicate with the prescriber. Not approved for use in treatment of MDD and in pediatric patients.

THERAPEUTIC CLASS: Serotonin and norepinephrine reuptake inhibitor

INDICATIONS: Management of fibromyalgia.

DOSAGE: *Adults:* 100mg qd (50mg bid). Titrate: Day 1: 12.5mg qd. Days 2-3: 25mg qd (12.5mg bid). Days 4-7: 50mg qd (25mg bid). After Day 7: 100mg qd (50mg bid). May increase dose to 200mg qd (100mg bid) based on individual patient response. Max: 200mg/day. Severe Renal Impairment (CrCl 5-29mL/min): Reduce maintenance dose by 50% to 50mg/day (25mg bid). Titrate: May increase dose to 100mg/day (50mg bid) based on individual patient response.

HOW SUPPLIED: Tab: 12.5mg, 25mg, 50mg, 100mg

CONTRAINDICATIONS: Uncontrolled narrow-angle glaucoma and concomitant use with monoamine oxidase inhibitors (MAOIs) or within 14 days of stopping an MAOI.

WARNINGS/PRECAUTIONS: Serotonin syndrome symptoms, neuroleptic malignant syndrome (NMS)-like reactions, increased BP, HR, liver enzymes, and severe liver injury reported. Caution with hypertension (HTN) or cardiac disease. If sustained increase in BP or HR occurs; reduce dose or d/c therapy. Caution with history of seizure disorder. D/C if jaundice or liver dysfunction occurs. Avoid with substantial alcohol use or chronic liver disease. Withdrawal and physical dependence reported; avoid abrupt d/c. Taper after long-term use. Hyponatremia may occur; d/c in symptomatic patients. Increased risk of bleeding events. Caution with history of mania, dysuria, prostatic hypertrophy, prostatitis, and other lower urinary tract obstructive disorders. Males may experience testicular pain or ejaculation disorders. Mydriasis reported; caution with controlled narrow-angle glaucoma. Caution with moderate renal and severe hepatic impairment. Contains FD and C Yellow No. 5 (tartrazine) which may cause allergic reactions (including bronchial asthma) in susceptible persons.

ADVERSE REACTIONS: N/V, headache, constipation, hot flushes, insomnia, hyperhidrosis, palpitations, upper respiratory infection, increased HR, dry mouth, HTN, anxiety, dizziness.

INTERACTIONS: See Contraindications. Risk of serotonin syndrome with lithium, serotonergic drugs (eg, triptans and tramadol), antipsychotics, and dopamine antagonists. Concurrent use with epinephrine and norepinephrine may increase risks of paroxysmal HTN and possible arrhythmia. Concomitant use with other serotonin reuptake inhibitors may result in HTN and coronary artery vasoconstriction. Digoxin may potentiate adverse hemodynamic effects. Risks of postural hypotension and tachycardia with IV digoxin. May inhibit antihypertensive effect of clonidine. Switch from clomipramine may increase risk of euphoria and postural hypotension. Caution with other centrally acting drugs. Avoid with serotonin precursors (eg, tryptophan). Concurrent use of aspirin, NSAIDs, warfarin, and other anticoagulants may increase risk of bleeding events.

PREGNANCY: Category C, not for use in nursing.

MECHANISM OF ACTION: Selective serotonin and norepinephrine reuptake inhibitor; exact mechanism is not established. Hypothesized to be associated with the various anticholinergic, sedative, and cardiovascular effects seen with other psychotropic drugs.

PHARMACOKINETICS: Absorption: Well absorbed; absolute bioavailability (85%-90%); T_{max}=2-4 hrs. **Distribution:** V_d=400L; plasma protein binding

(13%). **Metabolism:** Liver; *l*-milnacipran carbamoyl-O-glucuronide (major metabolite). **Elimination:** Urine (55%, unchanged). T$_{1/2}$=6-8 hrs.

NURSING CONSIDERATIONS

Assessment: Assess for suicidality, worsening of depression, uncontrolled narrow-angle glaucoma, concomitant MAOIs, pre-existing tachyarrhythmias, other cardiac diseases, history of seizure disorder, pre-existing liver disease, renal impairment, dysuria, prostatic hypertrophy, prostatitis, other lower urinary tract obstructive disorders, pregnancy/nursing status, and possible drug interactions. Assess BP, HR, and LFTs (eg, AST, ALT).

Monitoring: Monitor BP, HR, LFTs, sodium levels. Monitor for emergence of agitation, irritability, unusual changes in behavior, serotonin syndrome (eg, mental status changes, autonomic instability, neuromuscular aberrations, GIT symptoms), NMS-like signs and symptoms (eg, hyperthermia, muscle rigidity, autonomic instability with possible rapid fluctuation of vital signs), withdrawal symptoms, physical dependence, hyponatremia, and abnormal bleeding.

Patient Counseling: Counsel patients, families, and caregivers about the risks and benefits of therapy. Instruct families and caregivers of patients to notify a healthcare provider if experience agitation, irritability, suicidality, or unusual changes in behavior. Inform patients about the risk of serotonin syndrome with concomitant use of triptans, tramadol, or other serotonergic agents. Advise to monitor BP and PR periodically. Caution about the increased risk of abnormal bleeding with concomitant use of NSAIDs, aspirin, and other anticoagulation drugs. Caution against operating machinery or driving motor vehicles until effects of drug known. Avoid consumption of alcohol. Advise that withdrawal symptoms may occur with abrupt d/c. Notify physician if pregnant or intend to become pregnant, or if breastfeeding.

Administration: Oral route. **Storage:** 25°C (77°F); excursions permitted to 15-30°C (59-86°F).

SEASONALE   RX
ethinyl estradiol - levonorgestrel (Duramed)

> Cigarette smoking increases the risk of serious cardiovascular (CV) side effects. Risk increases with age (>35yrs) and with heavy smoking (≥15 cigarettes/day). Women who use oral contraceptives should be strongly advised not to smoke.

OTHER BRAND NAMES: Quasense (Watson)

THERAPEUTIC CLASS: Estrogen/progestogen combination

INDICATIONS: Prevention of pregnancy.

DOSAGE: *Adults:* 1 tab qd for 91 days, then repeat. Start 1st Sunday after menses begin or on 1st day of menses if menses begins on a Sunday.
Pediatrics: Postpubertal adolescents: 1 tab qd for 91 days, then repeat. Start 1st Sunday after menses begin or on 1st day of menses if menses begins on a Sunday.

HOW SUPPLIED: Tab: (Ethinyl Estradiol-Levonorgestrel) 0.03mg/0.15mg

CONTRAINDICATIONS: Thrombophlebitis or past history of deep vein thrombophlebitis, thromboembolic disorders or past history of thromboembolic disorders, current or history of cerebrovascular or coronary artery disease (CAD), valvular heart disease with thrombogenic complications, uncontrolled HTN, diabetes with vascular involvement, headaches with focal neurological symptoms, major surgery with prolonged immobilization, breast carcinoma (current or past history), carcinoma of the endometrium or other known or suspected estrogen-dependent neoplasia, undiagnosed abnormal genital bleeding, cholestatic jaundice of pregnancy or jaundice with prior pill use, hepatic adenomas or carcinomas or active liver disease, known or suspected pregnancy.

WARNINGS/PRECAUTIONS: Increased risk of myocardial infarction (MI), vascular disease, thromboembolism, stroke, HTN, and gallbladder disease, and hepatic neoplasia. May increase risk of breast cancer and cancer of the reproductive organs. Retinal thrombosis reported; d/c if unexplained partial or complete loss of vision, onset of proptosis or diplopia, papilledema, or retinal vascular lesions develop. May cause glucose intolerance, fluid retention, breakthrough bleeding, and spotting. May increase BP, elevate LDL cholesterol levels or cause other lipid changes. May cause or exacerbate migraine headaches. Refer to an ophthalmologist if develop visual changes with contact lenses or changes in lens tolerance. Increased risk of morbidity and mortality with certain inherited thrombophilias, HTN, hyperlipidemia, obesity, and diabetes. D/C if jaundice, significant depression, or recurrent/persistent new headache patterns develop. Not indicated for use before menarche. May affect certain endocrine, LFTs, and blood components. Does not protect against HIV infection (AIDS) or other STDs. Weigh benefit of fewer planned menses against inconvenience of increased intermenstrual bleeding or spotting.

ADVERSE REACTIONS: N/V, breakthrough bleeding, GI symptoms (eg, abdominal cramps, bloating), spotting, amenorrhea, migraine, depression, vaginal candidiasis, edema, weight changes, changes in cervical erosion and secretion.

INTERACTIONS: Reduced effects resulting in breakthrough bleeding or unintended pregnancy may occur when coadministered with antibiotics (eg, ampicillin, tetracycline), anticonvulsants and other drugs that increase the metabolism of contraceptive steroids (eg, rifampin, barbiturates, phenylbutazone, phenytoin, carbamazepine, felbamate, oxcarbazepine, griseofulvin, topiramate, St. John's wort). Atorvastatin, ascorbic acid, acetaminophen (APAP), CYP3A4 inhibitors (eg, itraconazole, ketoconazole) may increase hormone levels. HIV protease inhibitors may increase or decrease levels. May increase levels of cyclosporine, prednisolone, theophylline. May decrease levels of APAP. Increases clearance of temazepam, ASA, morphine, clofibric acid. May significantly decrease plasma levels of lamotrigine; dosage adjustment of lamotrigine may be necessary.

PREGNANCY: Category X, not for use in nursing.

MECHANISM OF ACTION: Estrogen/progestogen combination oral contraceptive; acts by suppression of gonadotropins. Primarily inhibits ovulation. Also produces other alterations including changes in the cervical mucus (increases difficulty of sperm entry into uterus) and endometrium (reduces likelihood of implantation).

PHARMACOKINETICS: Absorption: Levonorgestrel: Rapid and complete. Absolute bioavailability (100%), C_{max}=5.6ng/mL, T_{max}=1.4 hrs, AUC=60.8ng•hr/mL. Ethinyl estradiol: Rapid. Absolute bioavailability (43%), C_{max}=145pg/mL, T_{max}=1.6 hrs, AUC=1307pg•hr/mL. **Distribution:** Found in breast milk. Levonorgestrel: V_d=1.8L/kg, plasma protein binding (97.5-99%). Ethinyl estradiol: V_d=4.3L/kg, plasma protein binding (95-97%). **Metabolism:** Levonorgestrel: Sulfate and glucuronide conjugates. Ethinyl estradiol: First-pass metabolism, hepatic via CYP3A4 (hydroxylation), methylation, conjugation. **Elimination:** Levonorgestrel: Urine (45%), feces (32%); $T_{1/2}$=30 hrs. Ethinyl estradiol: Urine, feces; $T_{1/2}$=15 hrs.

NURSING CONSIDERATIONS

Assessment: Assess for current or history of thrombophlebitis or thromboembolic disorders, or any other conditions where treatment is contraindicated or cautioned. Assess for pregnancy/nursing status and for possible drug interactions. Assess use in patients ≥35 yrs who smoke ≥15 cigarettes/day.

Monitoring: Monitor for venous or arterial thrombotic or thromboembolic events (eg, MI, thromboembolism, stroke), hepatic neoplasia, ocular lesions, bleeding irregularities, fluid retention, onset or exacerbation of migraine headaches, gallbladder disease, HTN, and hypertriglyceridemia. Monitor glucose levels in DM and prediabetic patients, lipid levels with history of hyperlipidemia, signs of liver dysfunction (eg, jaundice), and signs of worsening depression with a history. Refer patients with contact lenses to ophthalmologist if visual changes occur. Perform periodic history and physical exam.

Patient Counseling: Inform that drug does not protect against HIV infection (AIDS) and other STDs. Counsel about potential adverse effects. Inform about possible serious CV and pulmonary effects. Advise to avoid smoking while on medication. Counsel to take medication at same time daily. Instruct that if miss 1 pill, take as soon as possible; take next dose at regular time. Advise that stomach upset, spotting, or light bleeding may develop when initiating therapy; continue taking medication. Advise to notify physician if bleeding lasts longer than 7 days. If vomiting or diarrhea occurs or if taking other medications, may need backup form of contraception. Inform patient will have 4 menstrual periods per yr while on medication.

Administration: Oral route. 1) Take 1 pill at same time every day until last pill in dispenser taken. 2) After taking last white pill, start first pink pill from new extended-cycle tab dispenser the next day regardless of when period started. This should be on a Sunday. **Storage:** 20-25°C (68-77°F).

SEASONIQUE   RX
ethinyl estradiol - levonorgestrel (Duramed)

> Cigarette smoking increases the risk of serious cardiovascular (CV) events from combination oral contraceptive (COC) use. Risk increases with age (>35 yrs) and with heavy smoking (≥15 cigarettes/day). Women who are >35 yrs and smoke should not use COCs.

THERAPEUTIC CLASS: Estrogen/progestogen combination

INDICATIONS: Prevention of pregnancy.

DOSAGE: *Adults:* Take 1 blue-green tab qd for 84 consecutive days, followed by 1 yellow tab qd for 7 days. Begin taking on first Sunday after the onset of menstruation. If menses begin on Sunday, start on that day. Postpartum women who choose not to breastfeed should start COC no earlier than 4-6 weeks postpartum.
Pediatrics: Postpubertal adolescents: Take 1 blue-green tab qd for 84 consecutive days, followed by 1 yellow tab qd for 7 days. Begin taking on first Sunday after the onset of menstruation. If menses begin on Sunday, start on that day.

HOW SUPPLIED: Tab: (Ethinyl Estradiol-Levonorgestrel) 0.03mg-0.15mg (blue-green); Tab: (Ethinyl Estradiol) 0.01mg (yellow)

CONTRAINDICATIONS: Patients with high risk of arterial or venous thrombotic diseases (eg, women who smoke, if over age 35; presence or history of deep vein thrombosis or pulmonary embolism; cerebrovascular or coronary artery disease; thrombogenic valvular or thrombogenic rhythm diseases of the heart such as subacute bacterial endocarditis with valvular disease, or atrial fibrillation; inherited or acquired hypercoagulopathies; uncontrolled HTN; diabetes with vascular disease; headaches with focal neurological symptoms or migraines with or without aura if over age 35), undiagnosed abnormal genital bleeding, presence or history of breast cancer or other estrogen- or progestin-sensitive cancer, liver tumors or liver disease, and pregnancy.

WARNINGS/PRECAUTIONS: Increased risk of venous and arterial thromboembolism (eg, myocardial infarction (MI)), and cerebrovascular events (thrombotic or hemorrhagic stroke). D/C if arterial or deep venous thrombotic events, unexplained loss of vision, proptosis, diplopia, papilledema, or retinal vascular lesions occur. D/C at least 4 weeks before and through 2 weeks after major surgery or other surgeries with an elevated risk of thromboembolism. May increase risk of cervical cancer or intraepithelial neoplasia and gallbladder disease. Hepatic adenoma and increased risk of hepatocellular carcinoma reported; d/c if jaundice develops. Cholestasis may occur with history of pregnancy-related cholestasis. Increased BP reported; for well-controlled HTN, monitor BP and d/c if BP rises significantly. May decrease glucose tolerance (dose-related). Consider alternative contraception with uncontrolled dyslipidemias. Increased risk of pancreatitis with hypertriglyceridemia or history thereof. May increase frequency or severity of migraine; d/c if new headaches are recurrent, persistent or severe. Unscheduled (breakthrough) bleeding and spotting may occur; if bleeding persists, check for causes (eg, pregnancy or malignancy). Should not be used to test for pregnancy. Caution in history of depression; d/c if depression recurs or worsens. May change results of laboratory tests (eg, coagulation factors, lipids, glucose tolerance and binding proteins). Caution with hereditary angioedema; exogenous estrogens may induce or exacerbate symptoms of angioedema. Chloasma may occur es-

S

pecially with history of chloasma; avoid sun exposure or ultraviolet radiation. Not indicated for use before menarche.

ADVERSE REACTIONS: Irregular and/or heavy uterine bleeding, weight gain, acne, migraine, cholecystitis, cholelithiasis, pancreatitis, abdominal pain, major depressive disorder.

INTERACTIONS: Reduced effectiveness, decreased plasma concentrations of contraceptive hormones or increased incidence of breakthrough bleeding with drugs or herbal products that induce enzymes (eg, CYP3A4) that metabolize contraceptive hormones (eg, barbiturates, bosentan, carbamazepine, felbamate, griseofulvin, oxcarbazepine, phenytoin, rifampin, St. John's wort, topiramate). Significant changes (increase or decrease) in plasma levels with protease inhibitors or non-nucleoside reverse transcriptase inhibitors. Pregnancy reported with use of hormonal contraceptives and antibiotics. Increased levels with atorvastatin, ascorbic acid, acetaminophen, and CYP3A4 inhibitors (eg, itraconazole, ketoconazole). Decreases levels of lamotrigine and may reduce seizure control; may require dosage adjustment of lamotrigine. May need to increase dose of thyroid hormone in patients on thyroid hormone replacement therapy due to increased thyroid binding globulin.

PREGNANCY: Contraindicated in pregnancy; not for use in nursing.

MECHANISM OF ACTION: Estrogen/progestogen combination oral contraceptive; primarily suppresses ovulation. May change cervical mucus (inhibiting sperm penetration) and endometrium (reducing likelihood of implantation).

PHARMACOKINETICS: Absorption: T_{max}=2 hrs; Levonorgestrel: Complete; absolute bioavailability (100%). Ethinyl estradiol: Absolute bioavailability (43%). Oral administration of variable doses resulted in different parameters. **Distribution:** Levonorgestrel: V_d=1.8L/kg; plasma protein binding (97.5-99%). Ethinyl estradiol: V_d=4.3L/kg; plasma protein binding (95-97%). **Metabolism:** Levonorgestrel: Sulfate and glucuronide conjugates. Ethinyl estradiol: 1st pass metabolism in gut wall, Hepatic, via CYP3A4 (hydroxylation), methylation, conjugation. **Elimination:** Levonorgestrel: Urine (45%), feces (32%); $T_{1/2}$=34 hrs. Ethinyl estradiol: Urine, feces; $T_{1/2}$=18 hrs.

NURSING CONSIDERATIONS

Assessment: Assess for risk of arterial or venous thrombotic diseases (eg, smokers >35 yrs of age, presence or history of deep vein thrombosis or pulmonary embolism), uncontrolled dyslipidemias, hypertriglyceridemia, or any other conditions where treatment is contraindicated or cautioned. Assess for pregnancy/nursing status and for possible drug interactions.

Monitoring: Monitor for venous or arterial thrombotic and thromboembolic events (eg, MI, stroke), cervical cancer or intraepithelial neoplasia, retinal vein thrombosis (eg, loss of vision, proptosis, diplopia, papilledema, retinal vascular lesions), increasing BP, jaundice, acute or chronic disturbances in liver function, worsening headaches or migraines, and unscheduled bleeding or spotting. Monitor for cholestasis with history of pregnancy related cholestasis, glucose levels in DM or prediabetes, and recurrence of depression with previous history.

Patient Counseling: Inform that drug does not protect against HIV infection and other STDs. Cigarette smoking increases the risk of serious cardiovascular events from COC use, and women who are >35 yrs and smoke should not use COCs. Counsel on Warnings and Precautions associated with COCs. Instruct to take at the same time everyday, what to do in the event pills are missed, and to use a backup or alternative method of contraception when enzyme inducers are used with COCs. COCs may reduce breast milk production if breastfeeding. Counsel any patient who starts COCs postpartum, and who has not yet had a period, to use an additional method of contraception until she has taken a light blue-green tablet for 7 consecutive days. Pregnancy should be considered if amenorrhea occurs and should be ruled out if amenorrhea is associated with symptoms of pregnancy (eg, morning sickness or unusual breast tenderness).

Administration: Oral route. **Storage:** 20-25°C (68-77°F).

SECTRAL

RX

acebutolol HCl (Promius Pharma)

THERAPEUTIC CLASS: Selective beta₁-blocker

INDICATIONS: Management of HTN alone or in combination with other antihypertensive agents (eg, thiazide diuretics). Management of ventricular premature beats.

DOSAGE: *Adults:* HTN: Mild-Moderate: Initial: 400mg/day, given qd-bid. Usual: 200-800mg/day. Severe: 1200mg/day, given bid. Ventricular Arrhythmia: Initial: 200mg bid. Maint: Increase gradually to 600-1200mg/day. CrCl <50mL/min: Decrease daily dose by 50%. CrCl <25mL/min: Decrease daily dose by 75%. Elderly: Start at low end of dosing range. Max: 800mg/day.

HOW SUPPLIED: Cap: 200mg, 400mg

CONTRAINDICATIONS: Persistently severe bradycardia, 2nd- and 3rd-degree heart block, overt cardiac failure, cardiogenic shock.

WARNINGS/PRECAUTIONS: Withdrawal before surgery is controversial. Caution with bronchospastic disease, peripheral vascular disease (PVD), hepatic or renal dysfunction. May mask hypoglycemia or hyperthyroidism symptoms. Avoid in overt cardiac failure. Exacerbation of ischemic heart disease (eg, angina pectoris, myocardial infarction [MI]) reported; avoid abrupt withdrawal. Risk of anaphylactic reaction may occur in patients with previous history of severe anaphylaxis to a variety of allergens. May develop antinuclear antibodies (ANA).

ADVERSE REACTIONS: Fatigue, dizziness, headache, constipation, diarrhea, dyspepsia, flatulence, nausea, dyspnea, micturition, insomnia.

INTERACTIONS: Possible additive effects with catecholamine-depleting drugs (eg, reserpine); monitor closely for hypotension and bradycardia. NSAIDs may reduce antihypertensive effects. Exaggerated hypertensive responses with alpha adrenergic stimulants. May antagonize epinephrine. May potentiate insulin-induced hypoglycemia. Digitalis glycosides increase risk of bradycardia. Use lowest possible dose with anesthetic agents that depress the myocardium (eg, ether, cyclopropane, trichlorethylene).

PREGNANCY: Category B, not for use in nursing.

MECHANISM OF ACTION: Cardioselective β-adrenoreceptor blocking agent; reduction in resting heart rate and decrease in exercise-induced tachycardia, reduction in cardiac output at rest and after exercise, reduction of systolic and diastolic BP at rest and post exercise, and inhibition of isoproterenol-induced tachycardia.

PHARMACOKINETICS: Absorption: Well-absorbed; absolute bioavailability (40%); T_{max}=2.5 hrs. **Distribution:** Plasma protein binding (26%); crosses placental barrier; secreted in breast milk. **Metabolism:** Diacetolol (major metabolite). **Elimination:** Renal (30-40%), nonrenal (50-60%). $T_{1/2}$=3-4 hrs (acebutolol), 8-13 hrs (diacetolol).

NURSING CONSIDERATIONS

Assessment: Assess for bradycardia, cardiogenic shock, 2nd- and 3rd-degree heart block, overt cardiac failure, impaired hepatic/renal function, bronchospastic disease, PVD, diabetes mellitus, thyrotoxicosis, valvular heart disease, nursing status, and possible drug interactions.

Monitoring: Monitor for cardiac failure, HTN, renal dysfunction, exacerbation of ischemia following abrupt withdrawal, bronchospastic disease, PVD, ANA, anaphylactoid reactions, hypersensitivity reactions.

Patient Counseling: Instruct not to interrupt or d/c therapy without consulting physician. Advise to consult physician if signs/symptoms of impending CHF or unexplained respiratory symptoms develop. Inform about hypertensive reactions from concomitant use of α-adrenergic stimulants, such as nasal decongestants used in OTC cold preparations.

Administration: Oral route. **Storage:** 20-25°C (68-77°F). Protect from light.

SELZENTRY

maraviroc (Pfizer)

RX

> Hepatotoxicity reported; may be preceded by evidence of systemic allergic reaction (eg, pruritic rash, eosinophilia, elevated IgE). Evaluate patients immediately if exhibiting signs or symptoms of hepatitis or allergic reaction.

THERAPEUTIC CLASS: CCR5 co-receptor antagonist

INDICATIONS: Combination with other antiretroviral agents for adults infected with only CCR5-tropic HIV-1.

DOSAGE: *Adults:* ≥16 yrs: Concomitant Potent CYP3A Inhibitors (with/without Potent CYP3A Inducer): 150mg bid. Other Concomitant Medications (Tipranavir/Ritonavir, Nevirapine, Raltegravir, NRTIs, and Enfuvirtide): 300mg bid. Concomitant Potent CYP3A Inducers (without a Potent CYP3A Inhibitor): 600mg bid. Refer to PI for concomitant medications and Dosing Regimen Based on Renal Funtion.

HOW SUPPLIED: Tab: 150mg, 300mg

CONTRAINDICATIONS: Severe renal impairment or end-stage renal disease (ESRD) (CrCl <30mL/min) who are taking potent CYP3A inhibitors or inducers.

WARNINGS/PRECAUTIONS: Caution with pre-existing liver dysfunction. D/C if signs or symptoms of hepatitis or increased liver transaminases occur along with rash or other systemic symptoms. Myocardial ischemia and/or infarction, and postural hypotension reported; caution in patients with increased risk for cardiovascular (CV) events and history of postural hypotension. Increased risk of postural hypotension in patients with severe renal insufficiency or ESRD. Immune reconstitution syndrome reported. May increase risk of developing infections; monitor closely for evidence of infections. May affect immune surveillance and may lead to increased risk of malignancy. Caution in elderly .

ADVERSE REACTIONS: Upper respiratory tract infections, cough, pyrexia, rash, dizziness/postural dizziness, sleep disturbance, appetite disorders, herpes infection, sinusitis, bronchitis, constipation, pain/discomfort, paresthesias/dysesthesias, hepatotoxicity.

INTERACTIONS: See Contraindications. Decreased concentration with St. John's wort; concomitant use not recommended. Caution with medication known to lower BP. Increased C_{max} and AUC with CYP3A/Pgp inhibitors (eg, ketoconazole, lopinavir, ritonavir, darunavir, saquinavir, and atazanavir). Decreased C_{max} and AUC with CYP3A inducers (eg, rifampin, etravirine, efavirenz). Dose adjustment may be required when coadministered with CYP3A inhibitors/inducers and Pgp inhibitors/inducers. Increased metabolic ratio of debrisoquine at 600mg maraviroc; potential CYP2D6 inhibition at high dose.

PREGNANCY: Category B, not for use in nursing.

MECHANISM OF ACTION: CCR5 co-receptor antagonist; selectively binds to human chemokine receptor CCR5 present on cell membrane, preventing interaction of HIV-1 gp120 and CCR5 necessary for CCR5-tropic HIV-1 to enter cells.

PHARMACOKINETICS: Absorption: T_{max}=0.5-4 hrs (1-1200mg in uninfected volunteers); Absolute bioavailability 100mg (23%), 300mg (33%). Refer to PI for other pharmacokinetic parameters. **Distribution:** V_d=194L; plasma protein binding (76%). **Metabolism:** CYP3A (major); secondary amine (metabolite) via N-dealkynation. **Elimination:** Urine (20%, 8% unchanged), feces (76%, 25% unchanged); $T_{1/2}$=14-18 hrs.

NURSING CONSIDERATIONS

Assessment: Assess renal and liver dysfunction or co-infection with HBV or HCV, history of postural hypotension or concomitant medication known to lower BP, risk of CV events, pregnancy/nursing status, and possible drug interactions. May conduct tropism testing to identify appropriate patients.

Monitoring: Monitor for signs/symptoms of hepatotoxicity, allergic reactions, immune reconstitution syndrome, CV events, symptoms of postural hypotension, infections, and development of malignancy.

Patient Counseling: Inform that therapy is not a cure for HIV, does not reduce risk of transmission of HIV, and that opportunistic infections may develop. Instruct patient to use caution with history of postural hypotension or concomitant medication that lowers BP; avoid driving/operating machinery if dizziness occurs. Seek medical attention if signs/symptoms of hepatitis or allergic reactions (yellow eyes/skin, dark urine, vomiting, abdominal pain). Instruct to take as prescribed and in combination with other antiretroviral drugs; do not change dose or dosing schedule without consulting a physician. Take at the same time(s) each day. Notify physician if taking prescription, non-prescription, or herbal medications, pregnant, planning to become pregnant or become pregnant while taking therapy. Advise patients to ask their doctor or pharmacist to refill their medicine when supply starts to run low. When dose is missed, instruct to take the next dose as soon as possible and take next scheduled dose at regular time. If <6 hrs before next scheduled dose, do not take missed dose; wait and take the next dose at regular time.

Administration: Oral route. **Storage:** 25°C (77°F); excursions permitted 15-30°C (59-86°F). Shelf life: 24 months.

SENSIPAR

RX

cinacalcet (Amgen)

THERAPEUTIC CLASS: Calcimimetic agent

INDICATIONS: Treatment of secondary hyperparathyroidism (HPT) in patients with chronic kidney disease (CKD) on dialysis, of hypercalcemia in patients with parathyroid carcinoma, and of severe hypercalcemia in patients with primary HPT who are unable to undergo parathyroidectomy.

DOSAGE: *Adults:* Individualize dose. Secondary HPT with CKD on Dialysis: Initial: 30mg qd. Titrate: Increase no more frequently than q2-4 weeks through sequential doses of 30, 60, 90, 120, and 180mg qd to target intact parathyroid hormone (iPTH) of 150-300pg/mL. Measure serum calcium (Ca) and phosphorus within 1 week and iPTH between 1-4 weeks after initiation or dose adjustment. May be used alone or in combination with vitamin D sterols and/or phosphate binders. Hypercalcemia with Parathyroid Carcinoma/Primary HPT: Initial: 30mg bid. Titrate: Increase q2-4 weeks through sequential doses of 30mg bid, 60mg bid, 90mg bid, and 90mg tid-qid prn to normalize serum Ca levels.

HOW SUPPLIED: Tab: 30mg, 60mg, 90mg

CONTRAINDICATIONS: Hypocalcemia.

WARNINGS/PRECAUTIONS: Lowers serum Ca; monitor for hypocalcemia. If serum Ca <8.4mg/dL but remains >7.5mg/dL, or if symptoms of hypocalcemia occur, Ca-containing phosphate binders and/or vitamin D sterols can be used to raise serum Ca. If serum Ca <7.5 mg/dL, or if symptoms of hypocalcemia persist and dose of vitamin D cannot be increased, d/c therapy until Ca levels reach 8mg/dL or symptoms of hypocalcemia are resolved. Avoid use in patients with CKD not on dialysis. Seizures reported; monitor serum Ca particularly in patients with history of seizure disorder. Hypotension, worsening heart failure (HF), and/or arrhythmia reported in patients with impaired cardiac function. Adynamic bone disease may develop with iPTH levels <100pg/mL; reduce dose or d/c therapy if iPTH levels <150pg/mL. Monitor patients with moderate and severe hepatic impairment throughout treatment.

ADVERSE REACTIONS: N/V, diarrhea, myalgia, dizziness, asthenia, anorexia, paresthesia, fatigue, fracture, hypercalcemia, dehydration, anemia, arthralgia, depression.

INTERACTIONS: May require dose adjustment with drugs metabolized by CYP2D6 (eg, desipramine, metoprolol, carvedilol) and particularly those with narrow therapeutic index (eg, flecainide and most TCAs). May require dose adjustment if a patient initiates or d/c therapy with strong CYP3A4 inhibitors (eg, ketoconazole, itraconazole); closely monitor iPTH and serum Ca levels. Increased AUC and C_{max} with ketoconazole. Decreased AUC with calcium carbonate and sevelamer HCl. Increased AUC and decreased C_{max} with pantoprazole. Increased AUC and C_{max} of desipramine, amitriptyline, and nortriptyline. Decreased C_{max} of warfarin. Increased AUC and decreased C_{max} of midazolam.

PREGNANCY: Category C, not for use in nursing.

MECHANISM OF ACTION: Calcimimetic agent; lowers PTH levels by increasing the sensitivity of the Ca-sensing receptor to extracellular Ca.

PHARMACOKINETICS: Absorption: T_{max}=2-6 hrs. **Distribution:** V_d=1000L; plasma protein binding (93-97%). **Metabolism:** (Liver) Rapid and extensive via CYP3A4, 2D6, and 1A2; hydrocinnamic acid and glucuronidated dihydrodiols (major metabolites). **Elimination:** Urine (80%), feces (15%); $T_{1/2}$=30-40 hrs.

NURSING CONSIDERATIONS

Assessment: Assess for hypocalcemia, a history of seizure disorder, hepatic impairment, cardiac function, pregnancy/nursing status, and possible drug interactions. Assess serum Ca levels prior to administration.

Monitoring: Monitor for seizures, signs/symptoms of hypocalcemia, and adynamic bone disease. In patients with impaired cardiac function, monitor for hypotension, worsening HF, and/or arrhythmias. For patients with CKD on dialysis, monitor serum Ca and phosphorus levels within 1 week after initiation of therapy or dose adjustment and iPTH levels 1-4 weeks after initiation of therapy or dose adjustment. After maintenance dose is reached, measure serum Ca and phosphorus levels monthly and iPTH levels q1-3 months. For patients with parathyroid carcinoma/primary HPT, measure serum Ca levels within 1 week after drug initiation or dose adjustment; measure serum Ca levels q2 months after maintenance dose levels have been established. Monitor iPTH/Ca/phosphorus levels with moderate and severe hepatic impairment.

Patient Counseling: Advise to take with food or shortly after a meal; instruct to take whole and not to divide. Inform of the importance of regular blood tests. Advise to report N/V and potential symptoms of hypocalcemia (eg, tingling/numbness of the skin, muscle pain/cramping). Advise to report to their physician if taking medication to prevent seizures, have had seizures in the past, and experience any seizure episodes while on therapy.

Administration: Oral route. Swallow whole; do not divide. Take with food or shortly after a meal. **Storage:** 25°C (77°F); excursions permitted to 15-30°C (59-86°F).

Septra   RX
sulfamethoxazole - trimethoprim (King)

OTHER BRAND NAMES: Septra DS (King) - Sulfatrim Pediatric (Alpharma)

THERAPEUTIC CLASS: Sulfonamide/tetrahydrofolic acid inhibitor

INDICATIONS: Treatment of urinary tract infections (UTI), acute otitis media, acute exacerbations of chronic bronchitis (AECB), *Pneumocystis carinii* pneumonia (PCP), traveler's diarrhea, and shigellosis caused by susceptible strains of microorganisms.

DOSAGE: *Adults:* UTI/Shigellosis: 800mg-160mg PO q12h for 10-14 days (UTI) or 5 days (shigellosis). AECB: 800mg-160mg PO q12h for 14 days. Traveler's Diarrhea: 800mg-160mg PO q12h for 5 days. PCP Treatment: 15-20mg/kg TMP and 75-100mg/kg SMX per 24 hrs given PO q6h for 14-21 days. PCP Prophylaxis: 800mg-160mg PO qd. Renal Impairment: CrCl 15-30mL/min: 50% usual dose. CrCl <15mL/min: Not recommended.
Pediatrics: ≥2 months: UTI/Otitis Media/Shigellosis: 4mg/kg TMP and 20mg/kg SMX q12h for 10 days (UTI/otitis media) or 5 days (shigellosis). PCP Treatment: 15-20mg/kg TMP and 75-100mg/kg SMX per 24 hrs given q6h for 14-21 days. PCP Prophylaxis: 150mg/m²/day TMP and 750mg/m²/day SMX PO given bid, on 3 consecutive days per week. Max: 320mg TMP and 1600mg SMX per day. Renal Impairment: CrCl 15-30mL/min: 50% usual dose. CrCl <15mL/min: Not recommended.

HOW SUPPLIED: (Sulfamethoxazole [SMX]-Trimethoprim [TMP]) Sus: (Sulfatrim Pediatric, Septra) 200mg-40mg/5mL [100mL, 473mL]; Tab: (Septra) 400mg-80mg*; Tab, DS: (Septra DS) 800mg-160mg* *scored

CONTRAINDICATIONS: Megaloblastic anemia due to folate deficiency, pregnancy at term, nursing, infants <2 months old.

WARNINGS/PRECAUTIONS: Fatal hypersensitivity reactions (eg, Stevens-Johnson syndrome [SJS], toxic epidermal necrolysis [TEN], fulminant hepatic necrosis, agranulocytosis, aplastic anemia) may occur. Cough, SOB, and pulmonary infiltrates reported. Avoid with group A β-hemolytic streptococcal infections. *Clostridium difficile*-associated diarrhea (CDAD) reported. Caution with hepatic/renal impairment, elderly, folate deficiency (eg, chronic alcoholics, anticonvulsants, malabsorption, malnutrition), bronchial asthma, and other allergies. In G6PD deficiency, hemolysis may occur. Increased incidence of adverse events in AIDS patients. Maintain adequate fluid intake.

ADVERSE REACTIONS: Anorexia, N/V, rash, urticaria, cough, SOB, cholestatic jaundice, agranulocytosis, anemia, hyperkalemia, renal failure, interstitial nephritis, hyponatremia, convulsions.

INTERACTIONS: Increased risk of thrombocytopenia with purpura with diuretics (especially thiazides) in the elderly. Caution with warfarin; may prolong PT. Increased effects of phenytoin, methotrexate. Concomitant ACE inhibitor therapy may cause hyperkalemia.

PREGNANCY: Category C, not for use in nursing.

MECHANISM OF ACTION: Sulfamethoxazole: Inhibits bacterial synthesis of dihydrofolic acid by competing with para-aminobenzoic acid (PABA). Trimethoprim: Blocks production of tetrahydrofolic acid from dihydrofolic acid by binding to and reversibly inhibiting required enzyme, dihydrofolate reductase; thus drug blocks 2 consecutive steps in biosynthesis of nucleic acids and proteins essential to many bacteria.

PHARMACOKINETICS: Absorption: Rapid; T_{max}=1-4 hrs. **Distribution:** Trimethoprim: Plasma protein binding (44%); Sulfamethoxazole: Plasma protein binding (70%). Crosses placenta, found in breast milk. **Metabolism:** Sulfamethoxazole: N_4 acetylation. Trimethoprim: 1-and 3-oxide, 3'-and 4'-hydroxy derivative (principal metabolites). **Elimination:** Urine, trimethoprim (66.8%), sulfamethoxazole (84.5%; 30% as free and remaining as N_4 acetylated metabolite); $T_{1/2}$=10 hrs (sulfamethoxazole), 8-10 hrs (trimethoprim).

NURSING CONSIDERATIONS

Assessment: Assess for previous drug hypersensitivity, megaloblastic anemia, renal/hepatic impairment, folate deficiency (eg, elderly, chronic alcoholics, patients on anticonvulsants, malabsorption syndrome, malnutrition states), G6PD deficiency, severe allergy or bronchial asthma, pregnancy/nursing status, and possible drug interactions.

Monitoring: Monitor for severe reactions (eg, SJS, TEN, fulminant hepatic necrosis, agranulocytosis), CDAD (may range from mild diarrhea to fatal colitis), development of drug resistance, superinfection, signs of bone marrow depression or specific decrease in platelets with or without pupura, hyperkalemia, hyponatremia, kernicterus, and clinical signs (eg, skin rash, sore throat, fever, arthralgia, pallor, jaundice) that may be early indications of serious reactions. Monitor CBC; d/c if significant reduction is noted. Perform urinalysis with careful microscopic exam and renal function tests (particularly for renal impairment).

Patient Counseling: Inform that drug only treats bacterial, not viral, infections. Take exactly as directed; skipping doses or not completing full course may decrease effectiveness and increase resistance. Maintain adequate fluid intake to prevent crystalluria and stone formation. Inform about potential benefits/risks of therapy. D/C and notify physician if skin rash, watery/bloody diarrhea (with/without muscle cramps), or fever occurs (may occur up to 2 months after therapy). Notify if pregnant/nursing.

Administration: Oral route. **Storage:** 15-25°C (59-77°F); protect from light.

SEREVENT

RX

salmeterol xinafoate (GlaxoSmithKline)

> Long-acting β₂-adrenergic agonists (LABA), such as salmeterol, may increase the risk of asthma-related deaths. Use for asthma without concomitant use of a long-term asthma control medication, such as an inhaled corticosteroid, is contraindicated. Do not use for patients whose asthma is adequately controlled on low- or medium-dose inhaled corticosteroids. LABA may increase the risk of asthma-related hospitalization in pediatric and adolescent patients. For pediatric and adolescent patients with asthma who require addition of a LABA to an inhaled corticosteroid, a fixed-dose combination product containing both an inhaled corticosteroid and a LABA should be used to ensure adherence with both drugs.

THERAPEUTIC CLASS: Beta₂-agonist

INDICATIONS: Treatment of asthma and prevention of bronchospasm only as concomitant therapy with a long-term asthma control medication, such as an inhaled corticosteroid, in patients ≥4 yrs with reversible obstructive airway disease, including patients with symptoms of nocturnal asthma. Prevention of exercise-induced bronchospasm (EIB) in patients ≥4 yrs. For the long-term, bid (am and pm) administration in the maintenance treatment of bronchospasm associated with chronic obstructive pulmonary disease (COPD) (including emphysema and chronic bronchitis).

DOSAGE: *Adults:* Asthma/COPD: 1 inh bid, am and pm (12 hrs apart). EIB Prevention: 1 inh ≥30 min before exercise (additional doses should not be used for 12 hrs after administration of this drug; do not give preventive doses if already on bid dose).
Pediatrics: ≥4 yrs: Asthma: 1 inh bid, am and pm (12 hrs apart). EIB Prevention: 1 inh ≥30 min before exercise (additional doses should not be used for 12 hrs after administration of this drug; do not give preventive doses if already on bid dose).

HOW SUPPLIED: Disk (Inhalation): 50mcg/inh [28, 60 blisters]

CONTRAINDICATIONS: Treatment of asthma without concomitant use of long-term asthma control medication, such as an inhaled corticosteroid. Primary treatment of status asthmaticus or other acute episodes of asthma or COPD where intensive measures are required. Severe hypersensitivity to milk proteins.

WARNINGS/PRECAUTIONS: Should not be initiated during rapidly deteriorating or potentially life-threatening episodes of asthma or COPD. Increased use of inhaled, short-acting β₂-agonists (SABA) is a marker of deteriorating asthma; re-evaluate and reassess treatment regimen. Should not be used for relief of acute symptoms; use SABA to relieve acute symptoms. At treatment initiation, regular use of an inhaled SABA should be d/c. Not a substitute for oral/inhaled corticosteroids. Should not be used more often or at higher doses than recommended or in conjunction with other medications containing LABA; cardiovascular (CV) effects and fatalities reported with excessive use. May produce paradoxical bronchospasm; d/c immediately, treat, and institute alternative therapy. Caution with cardiovascular disorders (CVDs) (eg, coronary insufficiency, cardiac arrhythmias, and HTN), convulsive disorders, thyrotoxicosis, hepatic disease, diabetes mellitus (DM), those who are unusually responsive to sympathomimetic amines, and in elderly. ECG changes (eg, flattening of T wave, QTc interval prolongation, and ST segment depression) reported. Immediate hypersensitivity reactions, hypokalemia, and dose-related changes in blood glucose and/or serum K⁺ may occur.

ADVERSE REACTIONS: Nasal/sinus congestion, pharyngitis, cough, viral respiratory infection, musculoskeletal pain, HTN, rhinitis, headache, tracheitis/bronchitis, influenza, throat irritation, skin rashes, N/V.

INTERACTIONS: Concomitant use with strong CYP3A4 inhibitors (eg, ketoconazole, ritonavir, atazanavir, clarithromycin, indinavir, itraconazole, nefazodone, nelfinavir, saquinavir, telithromycin) is not recommended. Increased exposure with ketoconazole. Caution with non-K⁺-sparing diuretics (eg, loop or thiazide diuretics). Caution with β-blockers; may produce severe bronchospasm. Extreme caution with MAOIs or TCAs or within 2 weeks of d/c with these agents. Increased C_max with erythromycin.

PREGNANCY: Category C, caution in nursing.

MECHANISM OF ACTION: Selective long-acting β_2-adrenergic agonist; increases cAMP levels causing relaxation of bronchial smooth muscles and inhibits the release of mediators of immediate hypersensitivity from mast cells.

PHARMACOKINETICS: Absorption: C_{max}=167pg/mL; T_{max}=20 min. **Distribution:** Plasma protein binding (96%). **Metabolism:** Liver (aliphatic oxidation) via CYP3A4. (Metabolite) α-hydroxysalmeterol. **Elimination:** Urine (25%), feces (60%); $T_{1/2}$=5.5 hrs.

NURSING CONSIDERATIONS

Assessment: Assess for asthma control. Assess for hypersensitivity to milk proteins, acute bronchospasm, rapidly deteriorating asthma or COPD, CVD (eg, coronary insufficiency, cardiac arrhythmia, HTN), convulsive disorder, thyrotoxicosis, hepatic disease, pregnancy/nursing status, and possible drug interactions. Obtain baseline lung function before therapy.

Monitoring: Monitor lung function periodically. Monitor patients with hepatic disease. Monitor for upper airway symptoms (eg, laryngeal spasm, irritation, swelling), worsening or acutely deteriorating asthma (increased use of inhaled β_2-agonist, decreased lung function), paradoxical bronchospasm, CV effects, and hypersensitivity reactions. Monitor serum K^+ and glucose levels.

Patient Counseling: Inform that drug may increase risk of asthma-related death. Should only be used as additional therapy when long-term asthma control medications do not adequately control asthma symptoms. Diskus is not meant to relieve acute asthma or exacerbations of COPD symptoms and extra doses should not be used for that purpose; and is not a substitute for oral or inhaled corticosteroids. Instruct to notify physician immediately if signs of seriously worsening asthma or COPD occur. Instruct not to change dosage or stop therapy unless directed by physician/healthcare provider. Additional LABA should not be used while on therapy. Inform of adverse effects (eg, palpitations, chest pain, rapid HR, tremor, or nervousness). Inform patients treated for EIB that additional doses should not be used for 12 hrs and not to use additional doses.

Administration: Oral inhalation. Refer to PI for proper administration and use. **Storage:** 20-25°C (68-77°F). Keep in dry place, away from direct heat or sunlight. Discard 6 weeks after removal from pouch or after all blisters have been used (when the dose indicator reads "0"), whichever comes first. Do not attempt to take the Diskus apart.

SEROQUEL   RX
quetiapine fumarate (AstraZeneca)

> Elderly patients with dementia-related psychosis treated with antipsychotic drugs are at an increased risk of death; most deaths appeared to be cardiovascular (eg, heart failure, sudden death) or infectious (eg, pneumonia) in nature. Quetiapine is not approved for the treatment of patients with dementia-related psychosis. Antidepressants increased the risk of suicidal thinking and behavior (suicidality) in short-term studies in children, adolescents, and young adults with major depressive disorder (MDD) and other psychiatric disorders. Monitor and observe closely for clinical worsening, suicidality, or unusual changes in behavior in patients who are started on antidepressant therapy. Quetiapine is not approved for use in pediatric patients <10 yrs.

THERAPEUTIC CLASS: Dibenzapine derivative

INDICATIONS: Treatment of schizophrenia in adults and adolescents (13-17 yrs). Acute treatment of manic episodes associated with bipolar I disorder, both as monotherapy and as an adjunct therapy to lithium or divalproex in adults and pediatrics (10-17 yrs). Monotherapy for acute treatment of depressive episodes associated with bipolar disorder in adults. Maintenance treatment of bipolar I disorder as adjunct therapy to lithium or divalproex in adults.

DOSAGE: *Adults:* Schizophrenia: Initial: 25mg bid. Titrate: Increase in total daily dose of 25-50mg divided bid-tid on the 2nd and 3rd day, as tolerated, to 300-400mg/day by the 4th day. Adjust doses by 25-50mg bid at intervals of ≥2 days if indicated. Max: 800mg/day. Maint: Responding patients should continue beyond acute response at lowest dose to maintain remission. Reassess periodically to determine the need for maintenance treatment. Bipolar I Disorder: Manic Episodes: Monotherapy/Adjunct: 100mg/day bid on Day 1, increase to 400mg/day bid on Day 4 in increments of up to 100mg/day and further adjust to 800mg/day bid by Day 6 in increments of ≤200mg/day. Max: 800mg/day. Maint: 400-800mg/day given bid as adjunct therapy to lithium or divalproex. Depressive Episodes: Day 1: 50mg qhs. Day 2: 100mg qhs. Day 3: 200mg qhs. Day 4: 300mg qhs. Patients receiving 600 mg: Day 5: 400mg qhs. Day 8: 600mg qhs. Elderly/Debilitated/Predisposition to Hypotension: Consider slower rate of dose titration and lower target dose. Hepatic Impairment: Initial: 25mg/day. Titrate: May increase by 25-50mg/day to an effective dose, depending on response and tolerability. Reinitiation of Treatment: If d/c >1 week: Follow initial titration schedule. If off <1 week: No titration required, may reinitiate maintenance dose. Switching from Depot Antipsychotics: Initiate therapy in place of the next scheduled injection. *Pediatrics:* Schizophrenia: 13-17 yrs: Administer bid or tid. Day 1: 50mg/day. Day 2: 100mg/day. Day 3: 200mg/day. Day 4: 300mg/day. Day 5: 400mg/day. Adjust dose based on response and tolerability within recommended range of 400-800mg/day with increments of ≤100mg/day. Max: 800mg/day. Bipolar I Disorder: Manic Episodes: 10-17 yrs: Administer bid or tid. Day 1: 50mg/day. Day 2: 100mg/day. Day 3: 200mg/day. Day 4: 300mg/day. Day 5: 400mg/day. After Day 5, adjust dose based on response and tolerability within recommended range of 400-600mg/day with increments of ≤100mg/day. Max: 600mg/day. Maint: Responding patients should continue beyond acute response at lowest dose to maintain remission. Periodically reassess to determine the need for maintenance treatment. Debilitated/Predisposition to Hypotension: Consider slower rate of dose titration and lower target dose. Hepatic Impairment: Initial: 25mg/day. Titrate: May increase by 25-50mg/day to an effective dose, depending on response and tolerability. Reinitiation of Treatment: If d/c >1 week: Follow initial titration schedule. If d/c <1 week: No titration required, may reinitiate the maintenance dose. Switching from Depot Antipsychotics: Initiate therapy in place of the next scheduled injection.

HOW SUPPLIED: Tab: 25mg, 50mg, 100mg, 200mg, 300mg, 400mg

WARNINGS/PRECAUTIONS: Neuroleptic malignant syndrome (NMS) reported; d/c and treat immediately. Hyperglycemia reported; monitor FPG regularly in diabetes mellitus (DM) patients. Undesirable alterations in lipids reported; monitor lipid levels periodically. Weight gain observed; monitor weight regularly. Tardive dyskinesia (TD) may develop; if signs and symptoms appear d/c therapy or treat with the smallest dose in the shortest duration if chronic therapy required. May induce orthostatic hypotension; caution with cardiovascular (CV) disease, cerebrovascular disease, or conditions that predispose to hypotension (eg, dehydration, hypovolemia). HTN and hypertensive crisis in children and adolescents reported; monitor BP. Leukopenia, neutropenia, and agranulocytosis reported; caution with pre-existing low WBC count or history of drug-induced leukopenia/neutropenia and d/c if absolute neutrophil count (ANC) <1000/mm³. Lenticular changes (eg, cataracts) reported; monitor with slit lamp exam or other methods at initiation and every 6-months. Seizures reported; caution with history of seizures or with conditions that potentially lower the seizure threshold (eg, Alzheimer's dementia). Decrease in total and free thyroxine (T4); elevations in prolactin and serum transaminase may occur. May impair mental/physical abilities. May disrupt body's ability to reduce core body temperature. Priapism, esophageal dysmotility, aspiration pneumonia in elderly may develop. Acute withdrawal symptoms (eg, N/V, insomnia) may occur after abrupt cessation; gradual withdrawal is advised.

ADVERSE REACTIONS: Headache, somnolence, dizziness, dry mouth, constipation, dyspepsia, tachycardia, asthenia, agitation, pain, weight gain, ALT increased, abdominal pain, back pain, N/V.

INTERACTIONS: Caution with other centrally acting drugs. Avoid with alcohol; may increase cognitive and motor effects. May antagonize effects of levodopa and dopamine agonists. May enhance hypotensive effects of antihypertensives. Caution with drugs known to cause electrolyte imbalance or to increase QT interval. Increased clearance with thioridazine, phenytoin, and other hepatic enzyme inducers (eg, carbamazepine, barbiturates, rifampin, glucocorticoids). Increased concentration with divalproex. Reduced clearance of ketoconazole; caution with CYP3A inhibitors (eg, itraconazole, fluconazole, protease inhibitors, erythromycin). Decreased clearance with cimetidine. Decreases clearance of lorazepam. Increase clearance of divalproex. Caution with neuroleptics and drugs with anticholinergic activity.

PREGNANCY: Category C, not for use in nursing.

MECHANISM OF ACTION: Dibenzothiazepine derivative; not established. Suspected to mediate through a combination of dopamine type 2 (D_2) and serotonin type 2 ($5HT_2$) antagonism.

PHARMACOKINETICS: Absorption: Rapid, T_{max}=1.5 hrs. **Distribution:** V_d=10L/kg; plasma protein binding (83%). **Metabolism:** Liver (extensive) via sulfoxidation and oxidation; CYP3A4; N-desalkyl quetiapine (active metabolite). **Elimination:** Urine (73%), feces (20%); $T_{1/2}$=6 hrs.

NURSING CONSIDERATIONS

Assessment: Assess for history of dementia-related psychosis, MDD, bipolar mania, DM, or any other conditions where treatment is contraindicated or cautioned. Assess for pregnancy/nursing status and possible drug interactions. Perform baseline vital signs and weight, CBC, FBG, lipid profile, LFTs, ECG, thyroid function tests, prolactin levels, and ophthalmologic examination.

Monitoring: Monitor for signs/symptoms of TD, clinical manifestations of NMS, extrapyramidal symptoms, hyperglycemia, suicide attempts, orthostatic hypotension, worsening depression, behavioral changes, agitation, irritability, priapism, esophageal dysmotility, and aspiration. Monitor for acute withdrawal symptoms (eg, N/V, insomnia) with abrupt withdrawal. Monitor vital signs and weight, CBC, FPG in DM patients, lipid profile, LFTs, ECG, thyroid function tests, prolactin levels, and ophthalmologic examination (eg, lenticular changes at 6-month intervals during chronic treatment).

Patient Counseling: Inform about risks and benefits of therapy. Advise patient, family, and caregivers to be alert of signs of behavior changes, suicidal ideation, worsening of depression, muscle stiffness, high fever, overheating, dehydration, weight gain, dizziness, lightheadedness upon standing, orthostatic hypotension, and hyperglycemia; notify physician if these and other adverse reaction occur. Counsel to avoid activities requiring mental alertness (eg, operating machinery/driving). Instruct to notify physician if taking other drugs, pregnant or intend to become pregnant. Instruct to avoid breastfeeding and alcohol intake.

Administration: Oral route. **Storage:** 25°C (77°F); excursions permitted to 15-30°C (59-86°F).

SEROQUEL XR   RX
quetiapine fumarate (AstraZeneca)

Elderly patients with dementia-related psychosis treated with antipsychotic drugs are at an increased risk of death; most deaths appeared to be cardiovascular (eg, heart failure, sudden death) or infectious (eg, pneumonia) in nature. Quetiapine is not approved for the treatment of patients with dementia-related psychosis. Antidepressants increased the risk of suicidal thinking and behavior (suicidality) in short-term studies in children, adolescents, and young adults with major depressive disorder (MDD) and other psychiatric disorders. Monitor and observe closely for clinical worsening, suicidality, or unusual changes in behavior in patients who are started on antidepressant therapy. Quetiapine is not approved for use in pediatric patients.

THERAPEUTIC CLASS: Dibenzapine derivative

INDICATIONS: Treatment of schizophrenia. Acute treatment of manic or mixed episodes associated with bipolar I disorder, both as monotherapy and as an adjunct to lithium or divalproex. Acute treatment of depressive episodes associated with bipolar disorder. Maintenance treatment of bipolar I disorder as adjunct therapy to lithium or divalproex. Adjunctive therapy to antidepressants for treatment of MDD.

DOSAGE: *Adults:* Schizophrenia: Give qd in pm. Initial: 300mg/day. Titrate: Within range of 400-800mg/day depending on response and tolerance.

Dose increases may be made at intervals as short as 1 day and in increments up to 300mg/day. Maint: 400-800mg/day for 16 weeks. Max: 800mg/day. Reassess periodically the need for maintenance treatment and the appropriate dose. Bipolar Disorder: Bipolar Mania: Monotherapy/Adjunct: Give qd in pm. Day 1: 300mg/day. Day 2: 600mg/day. Titrate: May adjust dose between 400-800mg beginning on Day 3 depending on response and tolerance. Maint: 400-800mg/day as adjunct therapy to lithium or divalproex. Periodically reassess the need for maintenance treatment and the appropriate dose. Depressive Episodes: Give qd in pm. Day 1: 50mg/day. Day 2: 100mg/day. Day 3: 200mg/day. Day 4: 300mg/day. MDD, Adjunctive Therapy with Antidepressants: Initial: 50mg qd in pm. Day 3: Increase dose to 150mg qd. Range: 150-300mg/day. Max: 300mg/day. Elderly/Hepatic Impairment: Initial: 50mg/day. Titrate: May increase in increments of 50mg/day depending on response and tolerance. Elderly/Debilitated/Predisposition to Hypotension: Consider slower rate of dose titration and lower target dose. Reinitiation of Treatment: If off >1 week: Follow initial dosing schedule. If off <1 week: No dose escalation required, may reinitiate maintenance dose. Switching from Seroquel: May switch at equivalent total daily dose taken qd. Switching from Depot Antipsychotics: Initiate in place of next scheduled injection. Swallow tab whole; do not split, crush, or chew. Take without food or with a light meal (approximately 300cal).

HOW SUPPLIED: Tab, Extended-Release: 50mg, 150mg, 200mg, 300mg, 400mg

WARNINGS/PRECAUTIONS: Neuroleptic malignant syndrome (NMS) reported; d/c and treat immediately. Hyperglycemia reported; monitor FPG regularly on diabetes mellitus (DM) patients. Undesirable alterations in lipids reported; monitor lipid levels periodically. Weight gain observed; monitor weight regularly. Tardive dyskinesia (TD) may develop; if signs and symptoms appear d/c therapy or treat with the smallest dose in the shortest duration if chronic therapy required. May induce orthostatic hypotension; caution with cardiovascular (CV) disease, cerebrovascular disease, or conditions that predispose to hypotension (eg, dehydration, hypovolemia). HTN and hypertensive crisis in children and adolescents reported; monitor BP. Leukopenia, neutropenia, and agranulocytosis reported; caution with pre-existing low WBC count or history of drug-induced leukopenia/neutropenia and d/c if absolute neutrophil count (ANC) <1000/mm^3. Lenticular changes (eg, cataracts) reported; slit lamp exam or other appropriate sensitive methods at initiation and every 6-months recommended. Seizures reported; caution with history of seizures or with conditions that potentially lower the seizure threshold (eg, Alzheimer's dementia). Decrease in total and free thyroxine (T_4); elevations in prolactin and serum transaminase may occur. May impair mental/physical abilities. May disrupt body's ability to reduce core body temperature. Priapism, esophageal dysmotility, aspiration pneumonia in elderly may develop. Acute withdrawal symptoms (eg, N/V, insomnia) may occur after abrupt cessation; gradual withdrawal is advised.

ADVERSE REACTIONS: Dry mouth, constipation, dyspepsia, somnolence, dizziness, orthostatic hypotension, weight gain, fatigue, dysarthria, nasal congestion, extrapyramidal symptoms, increased appetite, back pain, abnormal dreams, irritability.

INTERACTIONS: Caution with other centrally acting drugs. Avoid with alcohol; may increase cognitive and motor effects. May antagonize effects of levodopa and dopamine agonists. May enhance hypotensive effects of antihypertensives. Caution with drugs known to cause electrolyte imbalance or to increase QT interval. Increased clearance with thioridazine, phenytoin, and other hepatic enzyme inducers (eg, carbamazepine, barbiturates, rifampin, glucocorticoids). Increased concentration with divalproex. Reduced clearance of ketoconazole; caution with CYP3A inhibitors (eg, itraconazole, fluconazole, protease inhibitors, erythromycin). Decreased clearance with cimetidine. Decreases clearance of lorazepam. Increase clearance of divalproex. Caution with neuroleptics and drugs with anticholinergic activity.

PREGNANCY: Category C, caution in nursing.

MECHANISM OF ACTION: Dibenzothiazepine derivative; not established. Suspected to mediate through a combination of dopamine type 2 (D_2) and serotonin type 2A ($5HT_2A$) antagonism.

PHARMACOKINETICS: Absorption: T_{max}=6 hrs. **Distribution:** V_d=10L/kg; plasma protein bound (83%); found in breast milk. **Metabolism:** Liver (extensive) via sulfoxidation and oxidation; CYP3A4; norquetiapine (active metabolite). **Elimination:** Urine (73%), feces (20%); $T_{1/2}$=7 hrs.

NURSING CONSIDERATIONS

Assessment: Assess for history of dementia-related psychosis, MDD, bipolar mania, DM, or any other conditions where treatment is contraindicated or cautioned. Assess for pregnancy/nursing status and possible drug interactions. Perform baseline vital signs and weight, CBC, FPG, lipid profile, LFTs, ECG, thyroid function tests, prolactin levels, and ophthalmologic examination.

Monitoring: Monitor for signs/symptoms of TD, clinical manifestations of NMS, EPS, hyperglycemia, suicide attempts, orthostatic hypotension, worsening depression, behavioral changes, agitation, irritability, priapism, esophageal dysmotility, and aspiration. Monitor for acute withdrawal symptoms (eg, N/V, insomnia) with abrupt withdrawal, Monitor vital signs and weight, CBC, FPG in DM patients, lipid profile, LFTs, ECG, thyroid function tests, prolactin levels, and ophthalmologic examination (eg, lenticular changes at 6-month intervals during chronic treatment).

Patient Counseling: Inform about risks and benefits of therapy. Advise patient, family and caregivers to be alert for the emergence of behavior changes, suicidal ideation, worsening of depression, signs of NMS (eg, muscle stiffness, high fever), overheating, signs of dehydration, weight gain, risk of orthostatic hypotension, and hyperglycemia; notify physician if these and other adverse reaction occur. Counsel to avoid activities requiring mental alertness (eg, operating machinery/driving). Instruct to notify physician if taking other drugs, pregnant or intend to become pregnant. Instruct to avoid breastfeeding and alcohol intake.

Administration: Oral route. Swallow tab whole; do not split, crush, or chew. Take without food or with a light meal (approximately 300cal). **Storage:** Store at 25°C (77°F); excursions permitted to 15-30°C (59-86°F).

SEROSTIM   RX
somatropin (EMD Serono)

THERAPEUTIC CLASS: Human growth hormone

INDICATIONS: Treatment of HIV patients with wasting or cachexia to increase lean body mass and weight, and improve physical endurance with concomitant use of antiretroviral therapy.

DOSAGE: *Adults:* Usual: 0.1mg/kg (up to 6mg) SQ qhs. Dosing Recommendations: >55kg: 6mg SQ qhs. 45-55kg: 5mg SQ qhs. 35-45kg: 4mg SQ qhs. <35kg: 0.1mg/kg SQ qhs. Increased Risk for Adverse Effects Related to Therapy: Initial: 0.1mg/kg qod. Dose Reductions Due to Side Effects: Reduce total daily dose or number of doses/week. Rotate injection sites.

HOW SUPPLIED: Inj: 4mg, 5mg, 6mg, 8.8mg

CONTRAINDICATIONS: Acute critical illness due to complications following open heart or abdominal surgery, multiple accidental trauma or acute respiratory failure; active neoplasia; benzyl alcohol sensitivity.

WARNINGS/PRECAUTIONS: Benzyl alcohol associated with toxicity in newborns; if sensitivity occurs, may reconstitute with sterile water for injection (SWFI). Inadequate nutritional intake, malabsorption, and hypogonadism may contribute to catabolism and weight loss and should be diagnosed and treated. Potential for acceleration of HIV virus replication; patients should be maintained on antiretroviral therapy for duration of treatment. Carpal tunnel syndrome reported; d/c if symptoms do not resolve after decreasing weekly number of doses. Increased tissue turgor (eg, swelling of hands and feet) and musculoskeletal discomfort (eg, pain, swelling, stiffness) may occur during treatment. Seek prompt medical attention if allergic reaction occurs. Hyperglycemia may occur; monitor for glucose intolerance during therapy. Cases of new-onset impaired glucose tolerance, new onset type 2 DM, exacerbation of pre-existing DM, diabetic ketoacidosis, and diabetic coma reported. Intracranial hypertension syndrome with papilledema, visual changes, headache, and N/V reported with growth hormone products; perform funduscopic evaluation at the initiation and during therapy. May be associated with acute pancreatitis. Therapy should be carried out under the regular guidance of a physician who is experienced in HIV infection diagnosis and management.

ADVERSE REACTIONS: Peripheral edema, fatigue, rhinitis, arthralgia, extremity pain, myalgia, hyperglycemia, arthrosis, diarrhea, headache, paresthesia, insomnia, upper respiratory tract infection, joint swelling, gynecomastia.

INTERACTIONS: May unmask previously undiagnosed hypoadrenalism requiring glucocorticoid therapy; increase glucocorticoid dose with concomitant use. Monitor effectiveness of drugs known to be metabolized by CYP3A4 hepatic enzymes (eg, antiretroviral drugs) when coadministered. May increase dose if taking oral estrogen replacement concomitantly. Adjust dose of antidiabetics while on therapy.

PREGNANCY: Category B, caution in nursing.

MECHANISM OF ACTION: Human growth hormone; anabolic and anticatabolic agent exerting influence by interacting with specific receptors on variety of cell types. Some effects are mediated by insulin-like growth factor-1 (IGF-1).

PHARMACOKINETICS: Absorption: (SQ) Absolute bioavailability (70-90%). **Distribution:** (IV) V_d=12.0L. **Metabolism:** Liver, kidneys. **Elimination:** Urine; (SQ) $T_{1/2}$=3.94 hrs, (IV) $T_{1/2}$=0.58 hrs.

NURSING CONSIDERATIONS

Assessment: Assess for known benzyl alcohol sensitivity, acute critical illness due to complications of surgery, multiple accidental trauma, acute respiratory failure, active malignancy, inadequate nutritional intake-malabsorption, hypogonadism, risk factors for glucose intolerance, preexisting DM, nursing status, and possible drug interactions. Obtain baseline vital signs and weight, FPG, LFTs, renal function, and fundoscopic exam.

Monitoring: Monitor for signs/symptoms of carpal tunnel syndrome, increased tissue turgor, musculoskeletal discomfort, hypersensitivity/allergic reactions, diabetic ketoacidosis/coma, and acute pancreatitis. Monitor periodically vital signs and weight, FPG, LFTs, renal function, and fundoscopic exam.

Patient Counseling: Inform about benefits and risks of therapy. Inform that allergic reactions, swelling of hands and feet, muscle pain/swelling/stiffness, visual changes, headache, N/V may develop; instruct to contact physician if these or any side effects or discomfort occur. Instruct to use sterile, disposable syringes/needles and caution against reuse. Inform on the importance of proper disposal. Instruct to rotate injection sites.

Administration: SQ route. Rotate injection sites. Refer to PI for proper reconstitution. **Storage:** Before reconstitution: 15-30°C (59-86°F). After Reconstitution with SWFI: Use immediately and discard any unused portion. After Reconstitution with Bacteriostatic Water for Injection: 2-8°C (36-46°F); stable for 14 days. Avoid freezing reconstituted solution.

SF ROWASA   RX
mesalamine (Alaven)

OTHER BRAND NAMES: Rowasa (Alaven)

THERAPEUTIC CLASS: 5-Aminosalicylic acid derivative

INDICATIONS: Treatment of active mild to moderate distal ulcerative colitis, proctosigmoiditis or proctitis.

DOSAGE: *Adults:* Usual: 60mL units in one rectal instillation qhs for 3-6 weeks. Retain for 8 hrs.

HOW SUPPLIED: Sus: 4g/60mL

WARNINGS/PRECAUTIONS: Acute intolerance syndrome (eg, cramping, bloody diarrhea, abdominal pain, headache) may develop; d/c if signs and symptoms occur. Re-evaluate history of sulfasalazine intolerance; if rechallenge is considered, perform under close supervision. Caution with sulfasalazine hypersensitivity; d/c if rash or fever occurs. Carefully monitor with pre-existing renal disease; obtain baseline/periodic urinalysis, BUN, and creatinine. Worsening of colitis or symptoms of inflammatory bowel disease, including melena and hematochezia, may occur. Pancolitis, pericarditis (rare) reported. (Rowasa) Contains potassium metabisulfite; caution with sulfite sensitivity especially in asthmatics.

ADVERSE REACTIONS: Abdominal pain/cramps/discomfort, headache, flatulence, flu, fever, nausea, malaise/fatigue.

PREGNANCY: Category B, not for use in nursing.

MECHANISM OF ACTION: 5-aminosalicylic acid; has not been established. Suspected to diminish inflammation by blocking cyclo-oxygenase and inhibiting prostaglandin production in the colon.

PHARMACOKINETICS: Absorption: Colon: Poor. Extent dependent on retention time. **Metabolism:** Acetylation, N-acetyl-5-ASA (Metabolite). **Elimination:** Urine (10-30%), feces, $T_{1/2}$=0.5-1.5 hrs.

NURSING CONSIDERATIONS

Assessment: Assess for history of sulfasalazine intolerance, pre-existing renal disease, hypersensitivity, pregnancy/nursing status, and possible drug interactions. Obtain baseline urinalysis, BUN, and creatinine. (Rowasa) Assess for history of asthma or atopic allergies.

Monitoring: Monitor urinalysis, BUN, and creatinine periodically. Monitor for signs/symptoms of acute intolerance syndrome (cramping, acute abdominal pain, bloody diarrhea), hypersensitivity or allergic reaction (rash, fever).

Patient Counseling: Instruct on how to use: 1) Shake bottle well and remove sheath from tip. 2) Lie either on left side with left leg extended and right leg flexed or "knee-chest" position. 3) Gently insert lubricated tip into rectum, slightly toward navel; grasp firmly, tilt so nozzle aimed at back and squeeze slowly to instill drug. 4) Remain in position for 30 min to allow distribution. Retain all night if possible. Advise that best results achieved if bowel emptied immediately before administration. Advise to seek medical attention if symptoms of acute intolerance syndrome (cramping, acute abdominal pain, bloody diarrhea), hypersensitivity or allergic reactions occur. If signs of rash or fever develop, d/c therapy. Advise to choose a suitable location for administration.

Administration: Rectal route. **Storage:** 20-25°C (68-77°F). Excursions permitted. Discard unwrapped bottles after 14 days and products with dark brown contents.

SILENOR   RX   S
doxepin (Somaxon)

THERAPEUTIC CLASS: H₁-antagonist

H_1-antagonist

INDICATIONS: Treatment of insomnia characterized by difficulties with sleep maintenance.

DOSAGE: *Adults:* Individualized. Do not take within 3 hrs of a meal. Initial: 6mg qd within 30 min of bedtime. May decrease to 3mg. Max: 6mg/day. Elderly: ≥65 yrs: Initial: 3mg qd. May increase to 6mg. Hepatic Impairment: Initial 3mg. Concomitant use with Cimetidine: Max: 3mg.

HOW SUPPLIED: Tab: 3mg, 6mg

CONTRAINDICATIONS: Avoid with or within 2 weeks of MAOIs. Untreated narrow angle glaucoma, severe urinary retention.

WARNINGS/PRECAUTIONS: Evaluate comorbid diagnoses prior to initiation of treatment. Failure of remission after 7 to 10 days may indicate the presence of primary psychiatric and/or medical illness that should be evaluated. Complex behaviors (eg, sleep-driving), amnesia, anxiety and other neuropsychiatric symptoms reported; consider d/c if sleep-driving episode occurs. Worsening of depression, including suicidal thoughts and actions reported. May impair physical/mental abilities. Caution in patients with compromised respiratory function. Avoid in patient with severe sleep apnea.

ADVERSE REACTIONS: Somnolence, sedation, upper respiratory tract infection, nasopharyngitis, HTN, gastroenteritis, dizziness, N/V.

INTERACTIONS: See Contraindications. Alcohol, CNS depressants, sedating antihistamines may potentiate sedative effects. Increased exposure with inhibitors of CYP2C19, CYP2D6, CYP1A2, and CYP2C9. Doubled exposure with cimetidine. Hypoglycemia reported when oral doxepin was added to tolazamide therapy. Increased blood concentration and decreased psychomotor function with sertraline.

PREGNANCY: Category C, caution in nursing.

MECHANISM OF ACTION: H_1-antagonist; mechanism unknown but is believed to exert its sleep maintenance effect by antagonizing the H_1 receptor.

PHARMACOKINETICS: Absorption: T_{max} = 3.5 hrs; **Distribution:** V_d = 11,930L; plasma protein binding (80%); found in breast milk. **Metabolism:** Extensive by oxidation and demethylation via CYP2C19, CYP2D6, CYP1A2, CYP2C9; N-desmethyldoxepin (nordoxepin)(primary metabolite). **Elimination:** Urine (<3%); $T_{1/2}$ = 15.3 hrs (doxepin), 31 hrs (nordoxepin).

NURSING CONSIDERATIONS

Assessment: Assess for untreated narrow angle glaucoma, urinary retention, presence of a primary psychiatric and/or medical illness that may cause insomnia, depression, hepatic impairment, sleep apnea, pregnancy/nursing status, and possible drug interactions.

Monitoring: Monitor treatment response, sleep-driving, and worsening of depression such as suicidal thinking and actions.

Patient Counseling: Inform of benefits and risks associated with therapy. Counsel on appropriate use of medication. Instruct to contact physician if "sleep driving" occurs or if patient performs other complex behaviors while not fully awake. Seek medical attention if worsening of insomnia, symptoms of cognitive or behavioral abnormalities. Medication may cause sedation; caution against operating machinery (eg, automobiles) during therapy. Inform that use of alcohol, sedating antihistamines, or other CNS depressants may potentiate sedative effects of drug.

Administration: Oral route. Storage: 20°-25°C (68°-77°F). Protect from light.

SILVADENE RX
silver sulfadiazine (Monarch Pharmaceuticals Inc.)

OTHER BRAND NAMES: SSD (Par)

THERAPEUTIC CLASS: Sulfonamide

INDICATIONS: Adjunct for prevention and treatment of wound sepsis in patients with 2nd- and 3rd-degree burns.

DOSAGE: *Adults:* Apply under sterile conditions qd-bid to thickness of approximately 1/16 inch. Re-apply if removed by patient activity. Continue until wound is healed.

HOW SUPPLIED: Cre: 1% [20g, 50g, 85g, 400g, 1000g]

CONTRAINDICATIONS: Late pregnancy, premature infants, newborns during first 2 months of life.

WARNINGS/PRECAUTIONS: Potential cross-sensitivity with other sulfonamides. Hemolysis may occur in G6PD deficient patients. Drug accumulation with hepatic and renal dysfunction. Monitor renal function and serum sulfa levels with extensive burns. Fungal proliferation, including superinfection, has been reported.

ADVERSE REACTIONS: Transient leukopenia, skin necrosis, erythema multiforme, skin discoloration, burning sensation, rash, interstitial nephritis, systemic sulfonamide reactions.

INTERACTIONS: May inactivate topical proteolytic enzymes. Leukopenia increased with cimetidine.

PREGNANCY: Category B, not for use in nursing.

MECHANISM OF ACTION: Topical antimicrobial of sulfonamide class; acts on cell membrane and cell wall of many gram-negative and gram-positive bacteria and yeast to produce bactericidal effect.

NURSING CONSIDERATIONS

Assessment: Assess pregnancy/nursing status, renal/hepatic dysfunction, glucose-6-phosphate dehydrogenase deficiency, and for possible drug interactions.

Monitoring: Monitor fungal proliferation, renal/hepatic function, urine to identify sulfa crystals, serum sulfa concentrations with wounds involving extensive body surface areas, and signs/symptoms of sulfonamide reaction (eg, agranulocytosis, aplastic anemia, thrombocytopenia, leukopenia, Stevens-Johnson syndrome, exfoliative dermatitis, hepatitis and hepatocellular necrosis, CNS reactions, and toxic nephrosis).

Patient Counseling: Instruct to clean wound with soap and water and dry thoroughly prior to application. Instruct patient to reapply to any areas from which the cream has been removed by patient's activity. Inform patients that dressings can be used if needed. Instruct patient to continue therapy until satisfactory healing has occurred, burn site is ready for graft, or serious adverse events occur.

Administration: Topical. **Storage:** At room temperature.

SIMCOR   RX
simvastatin - niacin (Abbott)

THERAPEUTIC CLASS: HMG-CoA reductase inhibitor/Nicotinic acid

INDICATIONS: Adjunct to diet to reduce total-C, LDL-C, Apo B, non-HDL-C, TG, or to increase HDL-C with primary hypercholesterolemia and mixed dyslipidemia and to reduce TG with hypertriglyceridemia when treatment with simvastatin monotherapy or niacin extended-release monotherapy is considered inadequate.

DOSAGE: *Adults:* Not Currently on Niacin Extended-Release or Switching from Non-Extended-Release Niacin: Initial: 500mg-20mg qhs. With Simvastatin 20-40mg Who Need Additional Lipid Level Management: Initial: 500mg-40mg qhs. Titrate: Increase by ≤500mg q4 weeks. After Week 8, titrate to patient response and tolerance. Do not increase daily dose by >500mg in any 4-week period. Maint: 1000mg-20mg to 2000mg-40mg qd depending on tolerability and lipid levels. Max: 2000mg-40mg qd. Severe Renal Dysfunction: Do not start unless already tolerating ≥10mg simvastatin. Take with a low-fat snack. Do not break, crush, or chew.

HOW SUPPLIED: Tab: (Niacin Extended-Release-Simvastatin) 500mg-20mg, 500mg-40mg, 750mg-20mg, 1000mg-20mg, 1000mg-40mg

CONTRAINDICATIONS: Active liver disease (unexplained persistent elevations in hepatic transaminase levels), active peptic ulcer disease, arterial bleeding, women who are pregnant or may become pregnant, and nursing mothers.

WARNINGS/PRECAUTIONS: Severe hepatic toxicity, including fulminant hepatic necrosis, occurred when substituting sustained-release niacin for immediate-release niacin at equivalent doses. Do not substitute for equivalent dose of immediate-release (crystalline) niacin. Myopathy and rhabdomyolysis reported; monitor serum creatine kinase (CK) periodically. D/C therapy if myopathy is suspected or diagnosed, if transaminase levels >3X ULN persist or if transaminase elevations are associated with nausea, fever, and/or malaise, or prior to elective major surgery and when any major acute medical or surgical condition supervenes. Caution with heavy alcohol users, past history of liver disease, renal impairment, and those predisposed to gout. Perform LFTs prior to therapy, q12 weeks for the 1st 6 months and periodically thereafter. May cause reductions in platelet counts and increase in blood glucose. Caution with diabetic or potentially diabetic patients; monitor closely during therapy.

ADVERSE REACTIONS: Flushing, headache, back pain, diarrhea, nausea, pruritus.

INTERACTIONS: Adjust hypoglycemic therapy in diabetics. Avoid ingestion of alcohol, hot drinks, or spicy foods around time of administration; may increase flushing and pruritus. (Simvastatin) Avoid use with concomitant potent CYP3A4 inhibitors (eg, itraconazole, ketoconazole, and other antifungal azoles, macrolide antibiotics [eg, erythromycin, clarithromycin], telithromycin, HIV protease inhibitors, nefazodone, grapefruit juice [>1 quart/day]), cyclosporine, danazol, gemfibrozil, and fibrates); increased risk of myopathy/rhabdomyolysis. Concurrent use of simvastatin >20mg daily with amiodarone or verapamil should be avoided unless clinical benefit is likely to outweigh the increased risk of myopathy. Decreased simvastatin levels with concomitant use of propranolol. Potentiated the effect of coumarin anticoagulants; monitor PT. May increase digoxin levels; monitor appropriately. (Niacin) Aspirin (ASA) may decrease metabolic clearance. Binding to bile acid sequestrants (eg, cholestyramine and colestipol) reported; separate administration by 4-6 hrs. May potentiate the effects of ganglionic blocking agents and vasoactive drugs, resulting in hypotension. Nutritional supplements containing large doses of niacin or related compounds may potentiate adverse effects.

PREGNANCY: Category X, not for use in nursing.

MECHANISM OF ACTION: HMG-CoA reductase inhibitor/nicotinic acid. Niacin: Nicotinic acid; not well established. May partially inhibit release of free fatty acids from adipose tissue and increase lipoprotein lipase activity, which increases rate of chylomicron TG removal from plasma. Decreases rate of hepatic synthesis of VLDL-C and LDL-C. Simvastatin: HMG-CoA reductase inhibitor; lipid-lowering agent. Inhibits conversion of HMG-CoA to mevalonate. Also reduces VLDL, TG and increases HDL-C.

PHARMACOKINETICS: Absorption: C_{max}=3.29ng/mL, T_{max}=6.56 hrs, $AUC_{(0-t)}$=30.81ng•hs/mL'simvastatin acid). Niacin: T_{max}=4.6-4.9 hrs. Simvastatin: T_{max}=1.9-2 hrs. **Metabolism:** Niacin: Nicotinamide adenine dinucleotide (NAD) and other metabolites; conjugation to nicotinuric acid (NUA) (metabolite). Simvastatin: CYP3A4. Liver (1st pass); β-hydroxyacid, 6'-hydroxy, 6'-hydroxymethyl, and 6'-exomethylene derivatives (major active metabolites). **Elimination:** Urine (54% niacin and metabolites); $T_{1/2}$=4.2-4.9 hrs (simvastatin), 4.6-5 hrs (simvastatin acid). Niacin: Urine (53-77%, 7.7% unchanged after multiple dosing). Simvastatin: Feces (60%), urine (13%).

NURSING CONSIDERATIONS

Assessment: Assess for hypersensitivity reaction, conditions where treatment is contraindicated or cautioned, and possible drug interactions. Obtain baseline lipid profile and LFTs.

Monitoring: Monitor for signs/symptoms of myopathy, rhabdomyolysis, hepatotoxicity. Monitor platelet counts, PT, uric acid, and phosphorus levels. Periodically monitor lipid profile, CK, and blood glucose levels. Monitor LFTs q12 weeks for the 1st 6 months and q6 months thereafter. With increased transaminase levels, perform a 2nd liver function evaluation to confirm finding, and follow-up with frequent LFTs until abnormality returns to normal.

Patient Counseling: Instruct to take at bedtime after a low-fat snack. Advise to swallow tab whole; do not break, crush, or chew. Inform that flushing may occur but should subside after several weeks of therapy; taking ASA 30 min prior may minimize flushing. if awakened at night, rise slowly, especially if dizzy. Instruct to avoid alcohol, hot drinks, and spicy foods during administration time to minimize flushing. Instruct to contact physician prior to restarting therapy if dosing is interrupted. Notify physician if taking vitamins or other nutritional supplements containing niacin or nicotinamide. Contact physician promptly if any unexplained muscle pain, tenderness, or weakness and if dizziness occurs. If diabetic, notify physician of changes in blood glucose. Instruct to use an effective method of birth control to prevent pregnancy while on therapy; if pregnant or nursing, d/c therapy.

Administration: Oral route. Avoid taking on an empty stomach. **Storage:** 20-25°C (68-77°F).

SIMPONI   RX
golimumab (Centocor)

> Increased risk for developing serious infections (eg, tuberculosis [TB], TB reactivation, invasive fungal infection, bacterial/viral infection, and other infections due to opportunistic pathogens) that may lead to hospitalization or death. Most patients were taking concomitant immunosuppressants (eg, methotrexate [MTX] or corticosteroids). Evaluate for latent TB and treat prior to initiation of therapy. Monitor for development of signs and symptoms of infection during and after treatment. D/C if serious infection develops. Lymphoma and other malignancies reported in children and adolescents.

THERAPEUTIC CLASS: Monoclonal antibody/TNF-alpha receptor blocker

INDICATIONS: Treatment of adults with moderate to severe active rheumatoid arthritis (RA) in combination with MTX, active psoriatic arthritis (PsA), alone or in combination with MTX, and active ankylosing spondylitis (AS).

DOSAGE: *Adults:* RA: 50mg SQ once a month in combination with MTX. PsA/AS: 50mg SQ once a month with or without MTX or other nonbiologic Disease Modifying Antirheumatic Drugs (DMARDs). May continue corticosteroids, nonbiologic DMARDs, and/or NSAIDs during treatment.

HOW SUPPLIED: Inj: 50mg/0.5mL

WARNINGS/PRECAUTIONS: Avoid with active infection. Monitor chronic hepatitis B virus (HBV) carriers; if reactivation occurs, d/c and start antiviral therapy. Worsening congestive heart failure (CHF) and new onset CHF reported; monitor closely and d/c if new/worsening symptoms appear. Cases of new onset or exacerbation of CNS demyelinating disorders (eg, multiple sclerosis [MS]) and peripheral demyelinating disorders (eg, Guillain-Barre syndrome) reported; caution with central or peripheral nervous system demyelinating disorders and consider d/c if these develop. Pancytopenia, leukopenia, neutropenia, aplastic anemia, and thrombocytopenia reported; caution with significant cytopenias. Prefilled syringe/autoinjector contains dry natural rubber, a derivative of latex; caution with latex sensitivity. Caution when switching from one biologic to another. Caution in elderly.

ADVERSE REACTIONS: Serious infection, lymphoma, upper respiratory tract infection, nasopharyngitis, injection site reactions.

INTERACTIONS: See Boxed Warning. Avoid with live vaccines. Increased risk of serious infections with abatacept, anakinra, and rituximab; concomitant use with abatacept or anakinra is not recommended. Caution with CYP450 substrates with a narrow therapeutic index; monitor effect (eg, warfarin) or drug concentration (eg, cyclosporine, theophylline) upon initiation or d/c of therapy; may need dose adjustments.

PREGNANCY: Category B, not for use in nursing.

MECHANISM OF ACTION: Monoclonal antibody/TNF-α receptor blocker; binds to both the soluble and transmembrane bioactive forms of human TNFα preventing binding of TNFα to its receptors, thereby inhibiting the biological activity of TNFα.

PHARMACOKINETICS: Absorption: C_{max}=2.5µg/mL; T_{max}=2-6 days; absolute bioavailability (53%). **Distribution:** (IV) V_d=58-126mL/kg. **Elimination:** $T_{1/2}$=2 weeks.

NURSING CONSIDERATIONS

Assessment: Assess for active/chronic/recurrent infection, TB exposure, recent travel in areas of endemic TB or mycoses, history of opportunistic infection, underlying conditions that may predispose to infection, chronic HBV carriers, known malignancies, CHF, demyelinating disorder, significant cytopenia, latex sensitivity, pregnancy/nursing status, and possible drug interactions. Perform test for active TB/latent infection and treat if necessary.

Monitoring: Monitor for signs/symptoms of infection, HBV reactivation, malignancies, new or worsening CHF, new onset/exacerbation of CNS

S

demyelinating disorders, hematological events (eg, aplastic anemia, pancy-topenia, leukopenia, neutropenia, thrombocytopenia), lupus-like syndrome, and other adverse reactions. Periodically evaluate for active TB and test for latent infection during therapy.

Patient Counseling: Advise of potential risks and benefits of the drug. Instruct to read Medication Guide before initiation of therapy and each time the prescription is renewed. Inform that therapy may lower ability of the immune system to fight infections. Instruct to contact physician if any symptoms of infection develop. Counsel about the risk of lymphoma and other malignancies. Advise latex-sensitive patients that the needle cover contains dry natural rubber, a derivative of latex. Advise to report signs of new/worsening medical conditions (eg, CHF, demyelinating disorders, autoimmune disease, liver disease, cytopenias, or psoriasis).

Administration: SQ route. Refer to PI for administration instructions. Rotate injection sites; avoid areas where skin is tender, bruised, red, or hard. Do not use if discolored, cloudy, or if foreign particles are present. **Storage:** 2-8°C (36-46°F). Do not freeze or shake. Protect from light.

SINEMET CR   RX
levodopa - carbidopa (Mylan)

OTHER BRAND NAMES: Sinemet (Mylan)

THERAPEUTIC CLASS: Dopa-decarboxylase inhibitor/dopamine precursor

INDICATIONS: Treatment of symptoms of idiopathic Parkinson's disease (paralysis agitans), post-encephalitic parkinsonism, and symptomatic parkinsonism.

DOSAGE: *Adults:* Individualize dose. (Tab): Initial: (25mg-100mg) 1 tab tid. Titrate: Increase by 1 tab qd or qod until 8 tabs/day. 10mg-100mg: Initial: 1 tab tid-qid. Titrate: Increase 1 tab qd or qod until 2 tabs qid. 70-100mg/day carbidopa required. Max: 200mg/day carbidopa. Conversion from levodopa (d/c ≥12 hr before starting): <1500mg: (25mg-100mg) 1 tab tid or qid. >1500mg: (25mg-250mg) 1 tab tid or qid. (Tab, Extended-Release) No Prior Levodopa Use: Initial: 1 tab 50mg-200mg bid at intervals ≥6 hrs. Titrate: Increase or decrease dose or interval accordingly. Adjust dose at interval ≥3 days. Usual: 400-1600mg/day levodopa, given in 4-8 hr intervals while awake. Refer to PI for conversion to Extended-Release Tabs, addition of other antiparkinsonian medication and interruption of therapy.

HOW SUPPLIED: Tab: (Carbidopa-Levodopa) 10mg-100mg, 25mg-100mg, 25mg-250mg; Tab, Sustained-Release: (Carbidopa-Levodopa) 25mg-100mg, 50mg-200mg

CONTRAINDICATIONS: Nonselective MAOIs during or within 14 days of use; narrow-angle glaucoma; suspicious, undiagnosed skin lesions; history of melanoma.

WARNINGS/PRECAUTIONS: Dyskinesias may occur; consider dose reduction. May cause mental disturbances; carefully observe for development of depression with suicidal tendencies. Caution with past or current psychoses, severe cardiovascular (CV) or pulmonary disease, bronchial asthma, renal, hepatic or endocrine disease. Caution with history of myocardial infarction (MI) with residual arrhythmias; monitor cardiac function carefully during initial dose adjustment. May increase possibility of upper GI hemorrhage in patients with history of peptic ulcer. Neuroleptic malignant syndrome (NMS)-like symptoms reported during dose reduction or d/c. Caution with chronic wide-angle glaucoma; monitor intraocular pressure (IOP) changes during therapy. May cause somnolence and sudden onset of sleep; caution while driving or operating machines. Monitor for development of melanoma. May cause false (+) ketonuria or false (-) glucosuria (glucose-oxidase method).

ADVERSE REACTIONS: Dyskinesia, nausea, hallucination, confusion.

INTERACTIONS: See Contraindications. Caution with neuroleptics. Risk of postural hypotension with antihypertensives and selegiline. HTN and dyskinesia reported with TCAs. Reduced effects with dopamine D_2 antagonists (eg, phenothiazines, butyrophenones, risperidone) and isoniazid (INH). Antagonized by phenytoin, papaverine and metoclopramide. Reduced bio-availability with iron salts and high-protein diets. Pyridoxine (vitamin B_6) may reverse the effects of levodopa; carbidopa inhibits this action of pyridoxine.

PREGNANCY: Category C, caution in nursing.

MECHANISM OF ACTION: Dopa-decarboxylase inhibitor/dopamine precursor. Carbidopa: Inhibits decarboxylation of peripheral levodopa. Levodopa: Crosses blood-brain barrier and presumably converted to dopamine in brain.

PHARMACOKINETICS: Absorption: Administration of variable doses resulted in different parameters. **Distribution:** Levodopa: Crosses the placenta; found in breast milk. **Elimination:** Levodopa: $T_{1/2}$=50 min, 1.5 hrs (in the presence of carbidopa).

NURSING CONSIDERATIONS

Assessment: Assess for glaucoma, suspicious or undiagnosed skin lesions, history of melanoma, MI and peptic ulcer, arrhythmia, CV, pulmonary and endocrine diseases, bronchial asthma, hepatic/renal function, psychosis, previous hypersensitivity to drug, pregnancy/nursing status, and possible drug interaction.

Monitoring: Monitor for cardiac function during initial dosage adjustment period, depression and suicidal ideations, dyskinesia, upper GI hemorrhage, NMS, IOP changes, and hypersensitivity. Periodically monitor LFTs, CBC, CV and renal function during extended therapy. Monitor for melanomas frequently and on a regular basis; periodic skin examinations should be performed by a dermatologist.

Patient Counseling: Instruct to take as prescribed. Caution while operating machinery/driving. Instruct to notify physician if wearing-off effect poses a problem to lifestyle, appearance or worsening of involuntary movements occur, and gambling, sexual or other urges intensify. Advise that discoloration of body fluids may occur. Inform that high-protein diet, excessive acidity, and iron salts reduce clinical effectiveness. Instruct to swallow extended-release tab without chewing or crushing.

Administration: Oral route. **Storage:** 25°C (77°F); excursions permitted to 15-30°C (59-86°F). Store in tightly closed container. Protect from light and moisture.

SINGULAIR   RX
montelukast sodium (Merck)

THERAPEUTIC CLASS: Leukotriene receptor antagonist

INDICATIONS: Prophylaxis and chronic treatment of asthma in adults and pediatric patients ≥12 months. Relief of symptoms of seasonal allergic rhinitis in patients ≥2 yrs and perennial allergic rhinitis in patients ≥6 months. Prevention of exercise-induced bronchoconstriction (EIB) in patients ≥15 yrs.

DOSAGE: *Adults:* Asthma: 10mg qpm. Rhinitis: 10mg qd. EIB: 10mg at least 2 hrs before exercise. Do not take additional dose within 24 hrs of previous dose.
Pediatrics: Asthma: ≥15 yrs: 10mg qpm. 6-14 yrs: 5mg qpm. 2-5 yrs: 4mg tab or 4mg oral granules pkt qpm. 12-23 months: 4mg oral granules pkt qpm. Seasonal/Perennial Allergic Rhinitis: ≥15 yrs: 10mg qd. 6-14yrs: 5mg qd. 2-5 yrs: 4mg tab or 4mg oral granules pkt qd. Perennial Allergic Rhinitis: 6-23 months: 4mg oral granules pkt qd. EIB: ≥15 yrs: 10mg at least 2 hrs before exercise. Do not take additional dose within 24 hrs of previous dose. Granules may be mixed with applesauce, carrots, rice, or ice cream; give within 15 min of opening pkt.

HOW SUPPLIED: Granules: 4mg/pkt; Tab, Chewable: 4mg, 5mg; Tab: 10mg

WARNINGS/PRECAUTIONS: Not for use in the reversal of bronchospasm in acute asthma attacks, including status asthmaticus. Avoid abrupt substitution for inhaled or oral corticosteroids. Continue therapy during acute exacerbations of asthma; have a short-acting inhaled β-agonists available. Systemic

S

eosinophilic conditions reported. Neuropsychiatric events (eg, agitation, aggressive behavior or hostility, anxiousness, depression, dream abnormalities, hallucinations, insomnia, irritability, restlessness, somnambulism, suicidal thinking and behavior, and tremor) reported. Chewable tabs contains phenylalanine; caution with phenylketonuria. Avoid aspirin (ASA) and nonsteroidal anti-inflammatory agents (NSAIDs) with known ASA sensitivity.

ADVERSE REACTIONS: Headache, pharyngitis, influenza, fever, sinusitis, diarrhea, upper respiratory tract infection, cough, abdominal pain, otitis media, rhinorrhea.

INTERACTIONS: Monitor with potent CYP450 inducers (eg, phenobarbital, rifampin). Cases of cholestatic hepatitis, hepatocellular liver injury, and mixed-pattern liver injury reported with alcohol.

PREGNANCY: Category B, caution in nursing.

MECHANISM OF ACTION: Leukotriene receptor antagonist; binds to cysteinyl leukotriene receptors found on airway smooth muscle cells and macrophages and other pro-inflammatory cells (eg, eosinophils and certain myeloid stem cells). Inhibits physiologic actions of leukotrienes.

PHARMACOKINETICS: Absorption: Rapid. (10mg) Bioavailability (64%) T_{max}=3-4 hrs. (5mg) T_{max}=2-2.5 hrs. Bioavailability (73%, fasted), (63%, fed). Fasted 2-5 yrs: (4mg Chewable) T_{max}=2 hrs. (4mg Granules) T_{max}=2.3 hrs (fasted), 6.4 hrs (fed). **Distribution:** V_d=8-11L; plasma protein binding (99%). **Metabolism:** Liver (extensive); CYP3A4, 2C9. **Elimination:** Biliary (major); $T_{1/2}$=2.7-5.5 hrs.

NURSING CONSIDERATIONS

Assessment: Assess for hepatic dysfunction, history of phenylketonuria, history of ASA sensitivity, bronchospasm (status asthmaticus), pregnancy/nursing status, and possible drug interactions. Obtain baseline LFTs.

Monitoring: Monitor for signs/symptoms of eosinophilia, vasculitic rash, worsening pulmonary symptoms, cardiac complications, neuropathy, neuropsychiatric events, and hypersensitivity reactions.

Patient Counseling: Inform not to use for treatment of acute asthma attacks and EIB; appropriate rescue drug (eg, short acting $β_2$-agonist) should be available to prevent worsening. Seek medical attention if short acting bronchodilators are needed more than usual while on therapy. Take daily as prescribed, even if asymptomatic, as well as during periods of worsening asthma. Take directly or mix granules with applesauce, carrots, rice, or ice cream. Advise phenylketonuric patients that chewable tablets contain phenylalanine. Instruct not to decrease dose or d/c other anti-asthma medications unless instructed by physician. Seek medical attention if symptoms of eosinophilia, vasculitic rash, worsening pulmonary symptoms, cardiac complications, neuropathy, neuropsychiatric events, and hypersensitivity reactions occur. Advise patients with ASA sensitivity to continue avoiding ASA and NSAIDs.

Administration: Oral route. **Storage:** 25°C (77°F); excursions permitted to 15-30°C (59-86°F). Protect from light and moisture.

SKELAXIN   RX
metaxalone (King)

THERAPEUTIC CLASS: Muscular analgesic (central-acting)

INDICATIONS: Adjunct to rest, physical therapy, and other measures for the relief of discomforts associated with acute, painful musculoskeletal conditions.

DOSAGE: *Adults:* 800mg tid-qid.
Pediatrics: >12 yrs: 800mg tid-qid.

HOW SUPPLIED: Tab: 800mg* *scored

CONTRAINDICATIONS: Known tendency for drug-induced, hemolytic, and other anemias. Significantly impaired renal/hepatic function.

WARNINGS/PRECAUTIONS: Caution with pre-existing liver damage; perform serial liver function studies. False-positive Benedict's tests reported. May impair mental/physical abilities. Caution in elderly.

ADVERSE REACTIONS: N/V, GI upset, drowsiness, dizziness, headache, irritability, nervousness.

INTERACTIONS: Additive sedative effects with other CNS depressants (eg, alcohol, benzodiazepines, opioids, tricyclic antidepressants); use caution. Administration with high-fat meals may increase C_{max} & AUC, and delay T_{max} and $T_{1/2}$.

PREGNANCY: Not for use in pregnancy or nursing.

MECHANISM OF ACTION: Centrally acting muscular analgesic; mechanism not established; activity may be due to general depression of CNS.

PHARMACOKINETICS: **Absorption:** (400mg) C_{max}=983ng/mL, T_{max} = 3.3 hrs, AUC=7479ng•hr/mL. (800mg) C_{max}=1816ng/mL, T_{max}=3 hrs, AUC=15044ng•hr/mL. **Distribution:** V_d=800L. **Metabolism:** Liver; via CYP1A2, CYP2D6, CYP2E1, CYP3A4 and to a lesser extent, CYP2C8, CYP2C9, CYP2C19. **Elimination:** Urine (metabolites); (400mg) $T_{1/2}$=9 hrs. (800mg) $T_{1/2}$=8 hrs.

NURSING CONSIDERATIONS

Assessment: Assess for drug-induced, hemolytic or other anemias, renal/hepatic impairment, pregnancy/nursing status, alcohol intake, hypersensitivity and possible drug interactions.

Monitoring: Perform serial monitoring of LFTs. Monitor for signs/symptoms of CNS depression.

Patient Counseling: Caution against performing hazardous tasks (operating machinery/driving). Advise to avoid alcohol or other CNS depressants. Instruct to notify if pregnant/nursing or planning to become pregnant.

Administration: Oral route. May enhance CNS depression with food intake.
Storage: 15-30°C (59-86°F).

SKELID   RX
tiludronate disodium (Sanofi-Aventis)

THERAPEUTIC CLASS: Bisphosphonate

INDICATIONS: Treatment of Paget's disease of bone when serum alkaline phosphatase is ≥2x ULN, or if symptomatic, or if at risk for future complications.

DOSAGE: *Adults:* 400mg qd for 3 months. After therapy, wait 3 months to assess response. Take with 6-8 oz of plain water. Do not take within 2 hrs of food. Do not lie down for at least 30 min after medication.

HOW SUPPLIED: Tab: 200mg

CONTRAINDICATIONS: Inability to stand or sit upright for at least 30 min.

WARNINGS/PRECAUTIONS: May cause local irritation of the upper GI mucosa. Caution with active upper GI problems (eg, Barrett's esophagus, dysphagia, other esophageal diseases, gastritis, duodenitis, or ulcers). Esophageal adverse experiences (eg, esophagitis, esophageal ulcers, esophageal erosions) reported; d/c if dysphagia, odynophagia, retrosternal pain, or new or worsening heartburn develop. Post-marketing reports of gastric and duodenal ulcers observed. Avoid in severe renal failure. May cause osteonecrosis, primarily in jaw; caution with cancer, concomitant therapies (eg, chemotherapy, radiotherapy, corticosteroids) and co-morbid disorders (eg, anemia, coagulopathy, infection, pre-existing dental disease). If osteonecrosis of the jaw develops, dental surgery may exacerbate the condition. Bone, joint, and/or muscle pain may occur.

ADVERSE REACTIONS: Pain, headache, dizziness, paresthesia, diarrhea, N/V, dyspepsia, rhinitis, upper respiratory infection, sinusitis, influenza-like symptoms.

S

INTERACTIONS: Increased bioavailability with indomethacin; space dosing by 2 hrs. Decreased bioavailability with calcium supplements, aspirin (ASA), and aluminum- or magnesium-containing antacids; space dosing by 2 hrs.

PREGNANCY: Category C, caution in nursing.

MECHANISM OF ACTION: Bisphosphonate; acts primarily on bone to inhibit osteoclastic activity, with a probable reduction in the enzymatic and transport processes that lead to resorption of mineralized matrix. Inhibits osteoclasts through inhibiting protein-tyrosine-phosphatase and through inhibition of the osteoclastic proton pump.

PHARMACOKINETICS: Absorption: Rapid; C_{max}=3mg/L; T_{max}=2 hrs. **Distribution:** Plasma protein binding (90%). **Elimination:** Urine (60%); $T_{1/2}$=150 hrs.

NURSING CONSIDERATIONS

Assessment: Assess for severe renal impairment (eg, CrCl <30mL/min), risk of osteonecrosis (eg, cancer, anemia, pre-existing dental disease), pregnancy/nursing status, and for. possible drug interactions.

Monitoring: Monitor for signs/symptoms of an upper GI disorder (eg, gastritis, duodenitis, dysphagia), esophageal complications (eg, esophagitis, esophageal ulcers, esophageal erosions), osteonecrosis (eg, jaw), and musculoskeletal pain.

Patient Counseling: Instruct to take with 6-8 oz. of plain water. Counsel to not lie down for at least 30 min after medication. Advise not to take within 2 hrs of food. Instruct to maintain vitamin D and calcium intake. Inform not to take calcium supplements, ASA, and indomethacin 2 hrs before or 2 hrs after medication. If aluminum- or magnesium-containing antacids are needed, take at least 2 hrs after medication. Therapy should be taken for a period of 3 months, followed by another 3 months to assess response.

Administration: Oral route. **Storage:** 25°C (77°F); excursions permitted to 15-30°C (59-86°F). Do not remove tablets from foil strips until ready to be used.

SOLIRIS   RX
eculizumab (Alexion)

> Increases risk of meningococcal infections; may become fatal if not recognized and treated early. Vaccinate 2 weeks prior to receiving first dose; revaccinate according to current guidelines. Monitor for early signs of meningococcal infections, evaluate, and treat if necessary.

THERAPEUTIC CLASS: Monoclonal antibody/Protein C5 blocker

INDICATIONS: Treatment of paroxysmal nocturnal hemoglobinuria (PNH) to reduce hemolysis.

DOSAGE: *Adults:* Initial: 600mg every 7 days for first 4 weeks, then 900mg as 5th dose 7 days later, then 900mg every 14 days thereafter. Do not administer as an IV push or bolus injection; administer by IV infusion over 35 min.

HOW SUPPLIED: Inj: 10mg/mL [30mL]

CONTRAINDICATIONS: Patients with unresolved serious *Neisseria meningitidis* infection and patients not vaccinated against it.

WARNINGS/PRECAUTIONS: Monitor for early signs and symptoms of meningococcal infections; d/c during treatment of serious meningococcal infections. Increased susceptibility to infection reported; caution in patients with systemic infection. Monitor for signs and symptoms of hemolysis (eg, LDH increase) for at least 8 weeks after discontinuation. Infusion reactions, including anaphylaxis and hypersensitivity, reported. Administration should be interrupted in patients experiencing severe infusion reaction and appropriate therapy administered.

ADVERSE REACTIONS: Meningococcal infections, headache, nasopharyngitis, back pain, nausea, fatigue, cough, herpes simplex infections, sinusitis, respiratory tract infection, constipation, myalgia, pain in extremities, influenza-like illness.

PREGNANCY: Category C, caution in nursing.

MECHANISM OF ACTION: Monoclonal antibody/protein C5 blocker; binds to the complement C5 with high affinity, thereby inhibiting its cleavage to C5a and C5b and preventing the generation of the terminal complement C5b-9. Inhibits terminal complement-mediated intravascular hemolysis in PNH patient.

PHARMACOKINETICS: Absorption: C_{max} (week 26)=194mcg/mL. **Distribution:** V_d=7.7L. **Elimination:** $T_{1/2}$=272 hrs.

NURSING CONSIDERATIONS

Assessment: Assess for signs and symptoms of *Neisseria meningitidis* infection and other serious infection; meningococcal vaccination status; pregnancy and nursing status. Obtain baseline serum LDH, Hgb, and SrCr.

Monitoring: Monitor for signs and symptoms of meningococcal infections; other serious infections; signs and symptoms of hemolysis (eg, LDH increased with any of the following: >25% absolute decrease in PNH clone size in ≤1 week, Hgb <5 gm/dL or decrease of >4 mg/dL in ≤1 week, angina, change in mental status, 50% increase in SrCr level); infusion reactions including anaphylaxis and hypersensitivity reaction.

Patient Counseling: Counsel about possible risks and benefits in particular the risk of meningococcocal infection. Inform patients they are required to receive meningococcal vaccination at least 2 weeks prior to receiving the first dose of eculizumab if not previously vaccinated and revaccinated according to current medical guidelines. Inform that vaccination may not prevent meningococcal infection. Educate about the signs and symptoms of meningococcal infection and advise to seek immediate medical attention if these signs or symptoms occur. Inform that there is a potential for serious hemolysis when d/c'd and that they will be monitored for at least 8 weeks following d/c.

Administration: IV route. **Storage:** Refrigerate at 2-8°C (36-46°F) and protect from light. Do not freeze or shake.

SOLODYN
minocycline HCl (Medicis)

RX

THERAPEUTIC CLASS: Tetracycline derivative

INDICATIONS: Treatment of inflammatory lesions of non-nodular moderate to severe acne vulgaris in patients ≥12 yrs.

DOSAGE: *Adults:* 1mg/kg qd for 12 weeks. Refer to PI for dose equivalents based on body weight. Renal Impairment: Reduce dose or extend time intervals between doses. Elderly: Start at the low end of the dosing range. Swallow tab whole; do not crush, chew, or split tab.
Pediatrics: ≥12 yrs: 1mg/kg qd for 12 weeks. Refer to PI for dose equivalents based on body weight. Renal Impairment: Reduce dose or extend time intervals between doses. Swallow tab whole; do not crush, chew, or split tab.

HOW SUPPLIED: Tab, Extended-Release: 45mg, 55mg, 65mg, 80mg, 90mg, 105mg, 115mg, 135mg

WARNINGS/PRECAUTIONS: May cause fetal harm during pregnancy. May cause permanent discoloration of the teeth or enamel hypoplasia; avoid use during tooth development (last half of pregnancy, infancy, <8yrs). Reversible decrease in bone growth in premature infants reported. May cause pseudomembranous colitis; d/c therapy and treat appropriately. May cause an increase in BUN, resulting in azotemia, hyperphosphatemia and acidosis; caution in patients with renal impairment. CNS effects (eg, light-headedness, dizziness, vertigo) reported. Pseudotumor cerebri reported; question for visual disturbances prior to treatment and routinely check for papilledema during treatment. Use may result in overgrowth of drug-resistant bacteria; d/c if superinfection develops. Long-term use has been associated with development of autoimmune syndromes, including drug-induced lupus-like syndrome, autoimmune hepatitis and vasculitis; d/c if any of these occur. May induce tissue hyperpigmentation. Serious liver injury (eg, irreversible drug-induced hepatitis, fulminant hepatic failure), anaphylaxis, serious skin reactions (eg,

Stevens-Johnson syndrome [SJS], erythema multiforme), photosensitivity reported. Caution in elderly. No effect on non-inflammatory acne lesions. Safety beyond 12 weeks of use has not been established.

ADVERSE REACTIONS: Headache, fatigue, dizziness, pruritus, malaise, mood alteration.

INTERACTIONS: May require downward adjustments of anticoagulant dosage. May interfere with bactericidal action of penicillin; avoid concurrent use when possible. Concomitant use with methoxyflurane may result in fatal renal toxicity. Antacids containing aluminum, calcium or magnesium, and iron-containing preparations may impair absorption. May interfere with the effectiveness of oral contraceptives; female patients should use second form of contraception during treatment. Avoid concurrent use with isotretinoin.

PREGNANCY: Category D, not for use in nursing.

MECHANISM OF ACTION: Tetracycline derivative; not established.

PHARMACOKINETICS: Absorption: C_{max}=2.63mcg/mL; T_{max}=3.5-4 hrs; AUC_{0-24}=33.32mcg•hr/mL. **Distribution:** Crosses the placenta and found in breast milk.

NURSING CONSIDERATIONS

Assessment: Assess pregnancy/nursing status, hepatic/renal impairment, hypersensitivity, and for possible drug interactions. Assess for visual disturbances. Obtain baseline BUN, LFTs, ANA and CBC.

Monitoring: Monitor for signs/symptoms of pseudomembranous colitis (eg, diarrhea), hepatoxicity, superinfection, pseudotumor cerebri, papilledema, anaphylaxis, serious skin reactions (eg, SJS), CNS effects, and autoimmune syndromes (eg, drug-induced lupus-like syndrome, autoimmune hepatitis, vasculitis). Perform periodic laboratory monitoring of organ systems including hematopoietic, renal, and hepatic studies. In patients showing symptoms of an autoimmune syndrome, perform appropriate tests (eg, LFTs, ANA, CBC).

Patient Counseling: Inform that photosensitivity reactions (eg, exaggerated sunburn reaction) may occur; advise to minimize/avoid exposure to sunlight and to wear loose-fitting clothes when outdoors. Counsel about CNS symptoms (eg, dizziness, lightheadedness); may impair mental/physical abilities. Advise to seek medical help if persistent headache/blurred vision is experienced. Inform females that drug may render oral contraceptives less effective, and avoid if pregnant or nursing; use a second form of contraception during treatment. Avoid use if planning to conceive (male and female). Autoimmune syndromes may occur; d/c therapy if symptoms (eg, arthralgia, fever, rash, and malaise) are experienced. Counsel that discoloration of skin, scars, teeth, or gums may arise during therapy. Pseudomembranous colitis may occur; seek medical attention if watery/bloody stools develop. Counsel about possibility of hepatoxicity (eg, loss of appetite, fatigue, jaundice). Take exactly as directed; skipping doses or not taking as directed may decrease effectiveness of therapy and create bacterial resistance. Swallow tab whole; do not crush, chew, or split. Keep out of reach of children.

Administration: Oral route. **Storage:** 25°C (77°F); excursions permitted to 15-30°C (59-86°F). Dispense in tight, light, child-resistant container. Protect from light, moisture, excessive heat.

SOLU-CORTEF   RX
hydrocortisone sodium succinate (Pharmacia & Upjohn)

THERAPEUTIC CLASS: Glucocorticoid

INDICATIONS: Steroid-responsive disorders.

DOSAGE: *Adults:* Individualize dose. Initial: 100-500mg IV/IM, depending on disease. May repeat dose at 2, 4, or 6 hrs based on clinical response. High-dose therapy should continue only until patient is stabilized, usually not beyond 48-72 hrs. Maint: Decrease initial dosage in small decrements at appropriate time intervals until the lowest dosage to maintain an adequate clinical response is reached. Withdraw gradually after long-term therapy. Acute

Exacerbations of Mutliple Sclerosis: 800mg qd for 1 week followed by 320mg qod for 1 month.

Pediatrics: Dosage requirements are variable and must be individualized on basis of disease under treatment and response. Initial: 0.56-8mg/kg/day IV/IM in 3-4 divided doses (20-240mg/m²bsa/day).

HOW SUPPLIED: Inj: 100mg, 250mg, 500mg, 1000mg

CONTRAINDICATIONS: Systemic fungal infections, IM preparations are contraindicated with idiopathic thrombocytopenic purpura, intrathecal administration.

WARNINGS/PRECAUTIONS: May result in dermal and/or subdermal changes, forming depressions in the skin at the injection site. Exercise caution not to exceed recommended doses. May need to increase dose before, during, and after stressful situations. High doses should not be used for the treatment of traumatic brain injury. Anaphylactoid reactions (rare) may occur. Increases BP, salt/water retention, K⁺ and Ca excretion. Caution in patients with recent myocardial infarction (MI). Monitor for hypothalamic-pituitary adrenal (HPA) axis suppression, Cushing's syndrome, and hyperglycemia with chronic use. May produce reversible HPA axis suppression with the potential for gluco-corticosteroid insufficiency after withdrawal of treatment. May mask signs of infection or cause new infections; avoid use intra-articularly, intrabursally or for intratendinous administration for local effect in the presence of acute local infection. May exacerbate systemic fungal infections; avoid use unless needed to control drug reactions. Rule out latent or active amebiasis before initiating therapy. Caution with strongyloides, active or latent tuberculosis (TB), HTN, congestive heart failure (CHF), renal insufficiency, osteoporosis, ocular herpes simplex, myasthenia gravis. Caution with active or latent peptic ulcers, diverticulitis, fresh intestinal anastomoses and nonspecific ulcerative colitis; may increased risk of perforation. Enhanced effect with cirrhosis. More severe/fatal course of infections reported with chickenpox, measles. Not for use in cerebral malaria, active ocular herpes simplex, and optic neuritis. Reports of severe medical events have been associated with intrathecal administration. May produce posterior subcapsular cataracts, glaucoma with possible damage to the optic nerves, and may enhance the establishment of secondary ocular infections due to bacteria, fungi, or viruses. Kaposi's sarcoma reported. Change in thyroid status may necessitate dose adjustment. May decrease bone formation and increase bone resorption. Acute myopathy with high doses. Elevation of creatinine kinase may occur. Psychic derangements may appear and existing emotional instability or psychotic tendencies may be aggravated. May elevate IOP; monitor IOP if steroid therapy >6 weeks. Avoid abrupt withdrawal.

ADVERSE REACTIONS: Fluid and electrolyte disturbances, HTN, osteoporosis, muscle weakness, cushingoid state, menstrual irregularities, insomnia, impaired wound healing, diabetes mellitus (DM), ulcerative esophagitis, excessive sweating, increased intracranial pressure, carbohydrate intolerance, glaucoma, cataracts.

INTERACTIONS: Administration of live or live, attenuated vaccines is contraindicated in patients receiving immunosuppressive doses. Killed or inactivated vaccines may be administered, although response is unpredictable. Use with aminoglutethimide may lead to a loss of corticosteroid-induced adrenal suppression. May develop hypokalemia with K⁺-depleting agents (eg, amphotericin-B, diuretics). Case reports of cardiac enlargement and CHF when hydrocortisone is used with amphotericin-B. Anticholinesterase agents may produce severe weakness in patients with myasthenia gravis. Use with digitalis glycosides may increase risk of arrhythmias. Aspirin or NSAIDs may increase risk of GI side effects. Convulsions reported with cyclosporine use. Macrolide antibiotics may cause a significant decrease in clearance. Coadministration with hepatic enzyme inhibitors (eg, ketoconazole, erythromycin, and troleandomycin) may increase plasma concentrations. Cholestyramine may increase clearance. Hepatic enzyme inducers (eg, barbiturates, phenytoin, carbamazepine, rifampin) may enhance metabolism and require dosage increase. May inhibit response to warfarin; frequently monitor coagulation indices. Estrogens, including oral contraceptives, may decrease hepatic metabolism and enhance effect. Serum concentration of isoniazid may be decreased.

S

Steroids may increase blood glucose concentrations, dosage adjustments of antidiabetic agents may be required.

PREGNANCY: Category C, not for use in nursing.

MECHANISM OF ACTION: Anti-inflammatory glucocorticoid; causes profound and varied metabolic effects and modifies the body's immune responses to diverse stimuli.

NURSING CONSIDERATIONS

Assessment: Assess for systemic fungal infections, other current infections, active TB, vaccination status, hypersensitivity to drug, unusual stress, ulcerative colitis, diverticulitis, HTN, recent MI, intestinal anastomoses, active or latent peptic ulcer, osteoporosis, myasthenia gravis, psychotic tendencies, pregnancy/nursing status and possible drug interactions.

Monitoring: Monitor for HPA axis suppression, Cushing's syndrome, and hyperglycemia with chronic use. Monitor for anaphylactoid reactions, growth/development (in pediatrics), intestinal perforation and hemorrhage, infections, cataracts, osteoporosis, psychic derangement, Kaposi's sarcoma, acute myopathy. Monitor BP, HR, ECG, glucose, TSH, LFTs, creatinine kinase, serum electrolytes, IOP.

Patient Counseling: Warn not to d/c use abruptly or without medical supervision. Instruct to avoid exposure to chickenpox and measles; report immediately if exposed, or for fever/signs of infection. Advise regarding dietary salt restriction and K+ supplementation.

Administration: IM/IV routes. Avoid injection into deltoid muscle. Refer to PI for preparation and administration. **Storage:** 20-25°C (68-77°F). Protect from light. Unused solution should be discarded after 3 days.

SOLU-MEDROL   RX
methylprednisolone sodium succinate (Pharmacia & Upjohn)

THERAPEUTIC CLASS: Glucocorticoid

INDICATIONS: Steroid-responsive disorders.

DOSAGE: *Adults:* Dosage requirements are variable and must be individualized on basis of disease under treatment and the response. Initial: 10-40mg IV/IM, depending on disease. Maint: Decrease initial dosage in small decrements at appropriate time intervals until the lowest dosage that will maintain an adequate clinical response is reached. Withdraw gradually after long-term therapy. High-Dose Therapy: 30mg/kg IV over at least 30 min, may repeat q4-6h for 48 hrs, usually not beyond 48-72 hrs. Acute Exacerbations of Multiple Sclerosis: 160mg qd for 1 week followed by 64mg qod for 1 month.
Pediatrics: Initial: 0.11-1.6mg/kg/day in 3-4 divided doses (3.2-48mg/m²bsa/day); Asthma: 1-2mg/kg/day in single or divided doses. Continue short-course ("burst" therapy) until patient achieves a peak expiratory flow rate of 80% of his/her personal best or symptoms resolve (usually 3-10 d).

HOW SUPPLIED: Inj: 40mg, 125mg, 500mg, 1g, 2g

CONTRAINDICATIONS: Premature infants (due to benzyl alcohol diluent), idiopathic thrombocytopenic purpura (IM preparations) and intrathecal administration.

WARNINGS/PRECAUTIONS: Product contains benzyl alcohol, which is potentially toxic when administered locally to neural tissue. Excessive amounts of benzyl alcohol have been associated with toxicity, particularly in neonates, and an increased incidence of kernicterus, particularly in small preterm infants. May cause dermal and/or subdermal changes, forming depression in the skin at the injection site. Avoid injection into deltoid muscle. May need to increase dose before, during and after stressful situations. High doses should not be used for the treatment of traumatic brain injury. Anaphylactoid reactions (rare) may occur. Increases BP, salt/water retention; K+ and Ca excretion may occur. Caution with recent myocardial infarction (MI); left ventricular free wall rupture associated with corticosteroid therapy. Monitor for hypothalamic-pituitary adrenal (HPA) axis suppression, Cushing's syndrome, and hyperglycemia with chronic use. May produce reversible HPA axis suppression with the potential for glucocorticosteroid insufficiency following withdrawal. May mask signs of infection or cause new infections; avoid use intra-articularly, intrabursally or for intratendinous administration for local effect in the presence of acute local infection. May exacerbate systemic fungal infections; avoid use unless needed to control drug reactions. Rule out latent amebiasis or active amebiasis before initiating therapy. Caution with *Strongyloides*, active or latent tuberculosis (TB), HTN, congestive heart failure (CHF), renal insufficiency, osteoporosis, ocular herpes simplex, myasthenia gravis. Caution with active or latent peptic ulcers, diverticulitis, fresh intestinal anastomoses and nonspecific ulcerative colitis; may increase risk of perforation. Enhanced effect with cirrhosis. More severe/fatal course of infections reported with chickenpox, measles. Not for use in cerebral malaria, active ocular herpes simplex and optic neuritis. Reports of severe medical events with intrathecal administration. May produce posterior subcapsular cataracts, glaucoma with possible damage to the optic nerves, and enhance the establishment of secondary ocular infections due to bacteria, fungi or viruses. Kaposi's sarcoma reported. Changes in thyroid status may necessitate dose adjustment. May decrease bone formation and increase bone resorption. Acute myopathy with high doses. Elevation of creatinine kinase may occur. Psychic derangements may appear and existing emotional instability or psychotic tendencies may be aggravated. May elevate IOP; monitor IOP if steroid therapy >6 weeks. Avoid abrupt withdrawal.

ADVERSE REACTIONS: Fluid and electrolyte disturbances, HTN, osteoporosis, muscle weakness, cushingoid state, menstrual irregularities, insomnia, impaired wound healing, diabetes mellitus (DM), ulcerative esophagitis, excessive sweating, increased intracranial pressure, carbohydrate intolerance, glaucoma, cataracts.

INTERACTIONS: Administration of live or live, attenuated vaccines is contraindicated in patients receiving immunosuppressive doses. Killed or inactivated vaccines may be administered, though response unpredictable. Use with aminoglutethimide may lead to a loss of corticosteroid-induced adrenal suppression. May develop hypokalemia with K⁺-depleting agents (eg, amphotericin-B, diuretics). Case reports of cardiac enlargement and CHF when hydrocortisone is used with amphotericin-B. Anticholinesterase agents may produce severe weakness in patients with myasthenia gravis. Use with digitalis glycosides may increase risk of arrhythmias. Aspirin or NSAIDs may increase risk of GI side effects. Convulsions reported with cyclosporine use. Macrolide antibiotics may cause a significant decrease in clearance. Coadministration with hepatic enzyme inhibitors (eg, ketoconazole, erythromycin and troleandomycin) may increase plasma concentrations. Cholestyramine may increase clearance. Hepatic enzyme inducers (eg, barbiturates, phenytoin, carbamazepine, rifampin) may enhance metabolism and require dosage increase. May inhibit response to warfarin; frequently monitor coagulation indices. Estrogens, including oral contraceptives, may decrease hepatic metabolism and enhance effect. Serum concentration of isoniazid may be decreased. Steroids may increase blood glucose concentrations, dosage adjustments of antidiabetic agents may be required.

PREGNANCY: Category C, not for use in nursing.

MECHANISM OF ACTION: Anti-inflammatory glucocorticoid; causes profound and varied metabolic effects and modifies the body's immune responses to diverse stimuli.

NURSING CONSIDERATIONS

Assessment: Assess for hypersensitivity to drug, unusual stress, infection, active TB, vaccination status, thyroid status, hepatic/renal impairment, HTN, ulcerative colitis, diverticulitis, intestinal anastomoses, active or latent peptic ulcer, osteoporosis, myasthenia gravis, psychotic tendencies, glaucoma, pregnancy/nursing status and possible drug interactions.

Monitoring: Monitor for anaphylactic reactions. In pediatrics, monitor for gasping syndrome, hypoadrenalism, growth and development. Monitor for Cushing's syndrome, hyperglycemia, adrenocortical insufficiency, infection, intestinal perforation and hemorrhage, cataracts, acute myopathy, psychiatric derangement, Kaposi's sarcoma, creatinine kinase, BP, HR, serum electrolytes, IOP, TSH, LFTs, glucose, and ECG for cardiac arrhythmias and bradycardia.

Patient Counseling: Warn not to discontinue use abruptly or without medical supervision. Instruct to avoid exposure to chickenpox and measles; report immediately if exposed, or for fever/signs of infection. Advise regarding dietary salt restriction and K⁺ supplementation.

Administration: IM/IV routes. **Storage:** 20-25°C (68-77°F) for unreconstituted product and solution. Use within 48 hrs after mixing.

Soma RX
carisoprodol (Meda)

THERAPEUTIC CLASS: Skeletal muscle relaxant (central-acting)

INDICATIONS: Relief of discomfort associated with acute, painful musculoskeletal conditions.

DOSAGE: *Adults:* ≥16 yrs: 250-350mg tid and hs for up to 2-3 weeks.

HOW SUPPLIED: Tab: 250mg, 350mg

CONTRAINDICATIONS: History of acute intermittent porphyria.

WARNINGS/PRECAUTIONS: May impair mental/physical abilities. Drug abuse, dependence, and withdrawal reported with prolonged use. Withdrawal symptoms reported following abrupt cessation after prolonged use. Seizures reported in postmarketing surveillance. Caution with hepatic or renal dysfunction and in addiction-prone patients. Not studied in patients >65 yrs.

ADVERSE REACTIONS: Drowsiness, dizziness, headache.

INTERACTIONS: Additive sedative effects with other CNS depressants (eg, alcohol, benzodiazepines, opioids, TCAs); caution when coadministering. Concomitant use with meprobamate is not recommended. Increased exposure of carisoprodol and decreased exposure of meprobamate with CYP2C19 inhibitors (eg, omeprazole, fluvoxamine). Decreased exposure of carisoprodol and increased exposure of meprobamate with CYP2C19 inducers (eg, rifampin, St. John's wort). Induction effect on CYP2C19 seen with low dose aspirin.

PREGNANCY: Category C, caution in nursing.

MECHANISM OF ACTION: Centrally acting muscle relaxant; not established. Suspected to be associated with altered interneuronal activity in the spinal cord and the descending reticular formation of the brain. Meprobamate, a metabolite, has anxiolytic and sedative properties.

PHARMACOKINETICS: Absorption: Carisoprodol: (250mg) C_{max}=1.2mcg/mL, T_{max}=1.5 hrs, AUC=4.5mcg•hr/mL; (350mg) C_{max}=1.8mcg/mL, T_{max}=1.7 hrs, AUC=7.0mcg•hr/mL. Meprobamate: (250mg) C_{max}=1.8mcg/mL, T_{max}= 3.6 hrs, AUC=32mcg•hr/mL; (350mg) C_{max}=2.5mcg/mL, T_{max}=4.5 hrs, AUC=46mcg•hr/mL. **Distribution:** Found in breast milk. **Metabolism:** Liver via CYP2C19. Meprobamate (metabolite). **Elimination:** Renal/Nonrenal route, Carisoprodol: $T_{1/2}$=1.7 hrs (250mg), 2.0 hrs (350mg). Meprobamate: $T_{1/2}$=9.7 hrs (250mg), 9.6 hrs (350mg).

NURSING CONSIDERATIONS

Assessment: Assess for acute intermittent porphyria, renal/hepatic impairment, seizures, addiction-prone patients, use of alcohol/illegal drugs/drugs of abuse, pregnancy/nursing status, and possible drug interactions.

Monitoring: Monitor for signs/symptoms of CNS depression, drug abuse/dependence, and seizures.

Patient Counseling: Advise that drug may cause drowsiness and/or dizziness; avoid taking carisoprodol before engaging in hazardous tasks (operating machinery/driving). Avoid alcohol, illegal drugs, drugs of abuse, or other CNS depressants. Drug is limited to acute use. Notify physician if musculoskeletal symptoms persist. Inform of drug dependence/abuse potential.

Administration: Oral route. **Storage:** 20-25°C (68-77°F).

SOMATULINE DEPOT
lanreotide (Ipsen/Tercica)

RX

THERAPEUTIC CLASS: Somatostatin analog

INDICATIONS: Long-term treatment of acromegalic patients who have had inadequate response to surgery and/or radiotherapy, or for whom surgery and/or radiotherapy is not an option.

DOSAGE: *Adults:* Initial: 90mg deep SQ at 4 week intervals for 3 months. Titrate: Adjust dose based on IGF-1 and GH levels. GH >1 to ≤2.5ng/mL, IGF-1 Normal and Controlled Clinical Symptoms: 90mg every 4 weeks. GH >2.5ng/mL, IGF-1 Elevated and/or Clinical Symptoms Uncontrolled: 120mg every 4 weeks. GH ≤1ng/mL, IGF-1 Normal and Clinical Symptoms Controlled: 60mg every 4 weeks. Moderate to Severe Renal Impairment/Moderate to Severe Hepatic Impairment: Initial: 60mg deep SQ at 4 week intervals for 3 months.

HOW SUPPLIED: Inj: 60mg, 90mg, 120mg

WARNINGS/PRECAUTIONS: May reduce gallbladder motility and lead to gallstone formation; monitor periodically. Hypo- and/or hyperglycemia may occur; monitor glucose levels. Decreased thyroid function reported. Caution in patients with bradycardia. Sinus bradycardia, bradycardia, and HTN reported.

ADVERSE REACTIONS: Diarrhea, N/V, constipation, flatulence, abdominal pain, injection-site reactions, bradycardia, cholelithiasis, arthralgia.

INTERACTIONS: May decrease cyclosporine levels. May reduce intestinal absorption of concomitant drugs. Dose adjustments for concomitant antidiabetic treatment and drugs that induce bradycardia (eg, beta-blockers) may be needed. Caution with drugs metabolized by CYP3A4 and have a low therapeutic index (eg, quinidine, terfenadine). Drugs metabolized by liver may need dose reduction.

PREGNANCY: Category C, not for use in nursing.

MECHANISM OF ACTION: Somatostatin analog; acts mainly at the human somatostatin receptors (SSTR) 2 and 5 to inhibit growth hormone. Like somatostatin, lanreotide is an inhibitor of various endocrine, neuroendocrine, exocrine, and paracrine functions.

PHARMACOKINETICS: Absorption: SQ administration of variable doses resulted in different parameters. **Elimination:** Urine (<5%), feces (<0.5% unchanged). Biliary excretion.

NURSING CONSIDERATIONS

Assessment: Assess for cardiac disease, diabetes mellitus, impaired hepatic/renal function, pregnancy/nursing status and possible drug interactions.

Monitoring: Monitor for cholethiasis, gallbladder sludge, hyper/hypoglycemia, hypothyroidism, and cardiovascular abnormalities. Monitor blood glucose levels when dosages are adjusted. Monitor serum GH, and IGF-1 levels to assess effectiveness of treatment. Monitor thyroid function.

Patient Counseling: Instruct to report any adverse reactions or if condition persists or worsens. Provide a copy of FDA-Approved Patient Labeling and review the contents with the patient.

Administration: SQ. In the superior external quadrant of the buttock. Rotate injection-site between right and left side. **Storage:** Refrigerate at 2-8°C (36-46°F). Protect from light in its original package. Remove sealed pouch from refrigerator 30 min prior to injection. Keep pouch sealed until injection.

SOMAVERT
pegvisomant (Pharmacia & Upjohn)

RX

THERAPEUTIC CLASS: Growth hormone receptor antagonist

INDICATIONS: Treatment of acromegaly in those who have had an inadequate response to surgery and/or radiation therapy, and/or other medical therapies, or for whom these therapies are not appropriate.

DOSAGE: *Adults:* LD: 40mg SQ. Maint: 10mg SQ qd. Titrate: Adjust dose by 5mg increments/decrements, based on IGF-I levels, every 4-6 weeks. Max: 30mg/day. LFTs ≥3x/<5x ULN (without symptoms of liver dysfunction): Monitor LFTs weekly. LFTs ≥5x ULN or Transaminase Elevations ≥3x ULN: D/C immediately and evaluate. Do not initiate if baseline LFTs >3x ULN until cause is determined.

HOW SUPPLIED: Inj: 10mg, 15mg, 20mg

WARNINGS/PRECAUTIONS: Tumors that secrete growth hormone (GH) may expand and cause complications; monitor with periodic imaging scans of the sella turcica. May increase glucose tolerance and risk of hypoglycemia in diabetics. May result in functional GH deficiency. AST/ALT elevations reported; obtain baseline ALT, AST, total bilirubin (TBIL), and alkaline phosphatase (ALP) levels prior to initiation. Monitor LFTs monthly for first 6 months, quarterly for next 6 months, then biannually; monitor more frequently if elevations occur. D/C if liver injury confirmed. Monitor IGF-I levels 4-6 weeks after initiation or dose adjustments; every 6 months after levels are normalized. Interferes with the measurement of serum GH levels by commercially available GH assays; do not adjust dosage based on serum GH levels.

ADVERSE REACTIONS: Infection, abnormal LFTs, pain, injection-site reactions, back pain, diarrhea, nausea, flu syndrome, chest pain, dizziness, paresthesia, HTN, sinusitis, peripheral edema.

INTERACTIONS: May need to reduce dosage of insulin and/or hypoglycemic agents. Concomitant opioids may increase dosage requirements of pegvisomant.

PREGNANCY: Category B; caution in nursing.

MECHANISM OF ACTION: Growth hormone receptor antagonist; selectively binds to GH receptors on cell surfaces, where it blocks binding of endogenous GH and interferes with GH signal transduction. This decreases serum concentrations of insulin-like growth factor-I (IGF-I), as well as other GH-responsive proteins, including IGF binding protein-3 (IGFBP-3), and acid labile subunit (ALS).

PHARMACOKINETICS: Absorption: Absolute bioavailability (57%). **Distribution:** V_d=7L. **Elimination:** Urine (<1%); $T_{1/2}$=6 days.

NURSING CONSIDERATIONS

Assessment: Assess for latex allergy before therapy (stopper on vial contains latex). Assess use with tumors that secrete GH. Assess proper glucose control with diabetic patients prior to therapy. Obtain baseline serum liver tests (ALT, AST, TBIL, ALP). Assess for possible drug interactions.

Monitoring: Monitor for tumor growth in patients who have GH-secreting tumors. Perform periodic image scans of the sella turcica. Monitor for increased glucose tolerance while on anti-diabetic medication (hypoglycemia). Monitor for signs/symptoms of a GH-deficient state. Serum IGF-I concentrations should be evaluated 4-6 weeks after initiation of treatment, or when dose adjustments are made, and at least every 6 months after IGF-I levels have normalized. Monitor for signs/symptoms of liver dysfunction. Evaluate periodic serum levels of ALT, AST, TBIL, and ALP.

Patient Counseling: Counsel on signs/symptoms of liver dysfunction. If jaundice develops, immediately contact physician and d/c therapy. Serial monitoring of LFTs will be required. Instruct on how to properly administer drug. Periodic monitoring of serial IGF-1 levels is required in order to adjust dosing.

Administration: SQ route. Administer within 6 hrs after reconstitution. **Storage:** 2-8°C (36-46°F). Protect from freezing.

S

SONATA
zaleplon (King) `CIV`

THERAPEUTIC CLASS: Pyrazolopyrimidine (non-benzodiazepine)

INDICATIONS: Short-term treatment of insomnia.

DOSAGE: *Adults:* Individualize dose. Insomnia: 10mg qhs. Low Weight Patients: 5mg qhs. Max: 20mg/day. Elderly/Debilitated: 5mg qhs. Max: 10mg/day. Mild to Moderate Hepatic Dysfunction/Concomitant Cimetidine: 5mg qhs. Take immediately prior to bedtime.

HOW SUPPLIED: Cap: 5mg, 10mg

WARNINGS/PRECAUTIONS: Failure to remit after 7-10 days of treatment may indicate the presence of a primary psychiatric and/or medical illness that should be evaluated. Use the lowest effective dose. Abnormal thinking and behavior changes including bizarre behavior, agitation, hallucinations and de-personalization reported. Complex behaviors such as sleep-driving reported; d/c if sleep-driving occurs. Amnesia and other neuropsychiatric symptoms may occur unpredictably. Caution with depressed patients; worsening of depression, suicidal thoughts and actions reported. Anaphylaxis (eg, dyspnea, throat closing, N/V) and angioedema of the tongue, glottis and larynx leading to airway obstruction may occur. Patients who develop angioedema after treatment should not be rechallenged with the drug. May result in short-term memory impairment, hallucinations, impaired coordination, dizziness and lightheadedness when taken while still up. Caution in elderly. Abuse potential exists; avoid abrupt withdrawal. Caution with diseases or conditions affecting metabolism or hemodynamic responses, compromised respiratory function, and mild-to-moderate hepatic insufficiency. Not for use in severe hepatic impairment. May impair mental/physical abilities. Contains tartrazine, which may cause allergic reactions including bronchial asthma.

ADVERSE REACTIONS: Headache, dizziness, nausea, asthenia, abdominal pain, somnolence, amnesia, eye pain, dysmenorrhea, paresthesia.

INTERACTIONS: Coadministration with other psychotropic medications, anticonvulsants, antihistamines, narcotic analgesics, anesthetics, ethanol, and other CNS depressants may produce additive CNS-depressant effects. Avoid with alcohol. CYP3A4 inducers (eg, rifampin, phenytoin, carbamazepine and phenobarbital) increase clearance. CYP3A4 inhibitors (eg, erythromycin and ketoconazole) decrease clearance. Caution when coadministered with pro-methazine, imipramine, or thioridazine. Cimetidine reduces clearance.

PREGNANCY: Category C, not for use in nursing.

MECHANISM OF ACTION: Pyrazolopyrimidine class. Hypnotic agent; interacts with GABA-benzodiazepine receptor complex.

PHARMACOKINETICS: Absorption: Rapid and complete. Absolute bioavailability (30%); T_{max}=1 hr. **Distribution:** (IV) V_d=1.4L/kg; plasma protein binding (60%); found in breastmilk. **Metabolism:** Liver (extensive) via aldehyde oxidation. **Elimination:** Urine (<1% unchanged, 70% within 48 hrs, 71% within 6 days), feces (17% within 6 days); (IV, oral) $T_{1/2}$=1 hr.

NURSING CONSIDERATIONS

Assessment: Assess for primary psychiatric and/or medical illness, diseases/conditions affection metabolism or hemodynamic responses, compromised respiratory function (COPD, sleep apnea), depression, suicidal tendencies, hepatic/renal impairment, drug abuse/addiction, alcohol intake, pregnancy/nursing status, hypersensitivity and possible drug interactions.

Monitoring: Monitor for anaphylaxis (eg, dyspnea, throat closing, N/V), angioedema of the tongue, glottis and larynx, worsening of insomnia, abnormal thinking and behavior changes (eg, bizarre behavior, agitation, hallucina-tions, depersonalization), complex behaviors (eg, sleep-driving), amnesia, neuropsychiatric symptoms, worsening of depression, suicidal thoughts/actions, memory impairment, impaired coordination, dizziness, lightheaded-ness, physical/psychological dependence, withdrawal symptoms, hepatic and pulmonary functions and possible drug interactions. Monitor elderly and debilitated patients closely.

Patient Counseling: Take drug immediately prior to bedtime. Caution against hazardous tasks (eg, operating machinery/driving). Instruct to notify physician if sleep-driving or other complex behaviors occur. Inform about the benefits/risks, possibility of physical/psychological dependence and memory disturbances. Notify if pregnant/nursing or planning to become pregnant. Do not increase dose or d/c drug before consulting physician. Avoid alcohol.

Administration: Oral route. Take immediately prior to bedtime. **Storage:** 20-25°C (68-77°F). Dispense in a light-resistant container.

SORIATANE   RX
acitretin (Stiefel)

> Avoid in pregnancy or becoming pregnant ≤3 yrs after d/c of therapy; use two reliable forms of contraception simultaneously. Only use in females of reproductive potential with severe psoriasis unresponsive to or contraindicated with other therapies. Patient must have two negative urine/serum pregnancy tests with a sensitivity of at least 25 mIU/mL before receiving initial prescription. Contraception counseling should be done on a regular basis. It is not known whether residual acitretin in seminal fluid poses risk to fetus with male patients during or after therapy. Females should avoid ethanol during and 2 months after therapy because it may increase the duration of teratogenic potential; severe birth defects reported. Interferes with contraceptive effect of microdosed progestin "minipill" oral contraceptives. Caution not to self-medicate with herbal St. John's wort because a possible interaction has been suggested with hormonal contraceptives based on reports of breakthrough bleeding. Potential to induce hepatotoxicity; elevations of AST (SGOT), ALT (SGPT), GGT (GGTP) or LDH reported. D/C if hepatotoxicity is suspected.

THERAPEUTIC CLASS: Retinoid

INDICATIONS: Treatment of severe psoriasis in adults.

DOSAGE: *Adults:* Intersubject variation in pharmacokinetics, clinical efficacy, and incidence of side effects exists. Individualize dose. Initial: 25-50mg single dose qd with main meal. Maint: 25-50mg qd may be given dependent upon response to initial treatment. May treat relapses as outlined for initial therapy. Decrease concomitant phototherapy dose dependent on patient's individual response.

HOW SUPPLIED: Cap: 10mg, 17.5mg, 25mg

CONTRAINDICATIONS: See Boxed Warning. Pregnancy, severely impaired liver or kidney function and in patients with chronic abnormally elevated blood lipid values. Combined use with methotrexate; increased risk of hepatitis. Combined use with tetracyclines; can cause increased intracranial pressure.

WARNINGS/PRECAUTIONS: Risk of hyperostosis, pancreatitis, and pseudotumor cerebri. D/C if visual difficulties occur; decreased night vision and reduced tolerance to contact lenses reported. Bone abnormalities of the vertebral column, knees, and ankles reported. Increases TG and cholesterol and decreases HDL; perform lipid tests before therapy every 1-2 weeks until lipid response established. Caution with severe hepatic/renal impairment. Transient worsening of psoriasis may occur initially. Do not donate blood during and for 3 yrs after therapy. Avoid sun lamps and excessive sun exposure. Depression and/or psychiatric symptoms (eg, aggressive feelings, thoughts of self-harm) reported. Thinning of the skin observed. Lower dose of phototherapy is required. Caution in elderly.

ADVERSE REACTIONS: Cheilitis, rhinitis, dry mouth, epistaxis, alopecia, dry skin, skin peeling, nail disorder, pruritus, paresthesia, paronychia, skin atrophy, sticky skin, xerophthalmia, arthralgia.

INTERACTIONS: See Boxed Warning and Contraindications. Potentiates the blood glucose lowering effect of glibenclamide; careful supervision of diabetic patients is recommended. Reduced protein binding effect of phenytoin. Avoid use with vitamin A or other oral retinoids; may increase risk of hypervitaminosis A.

PREGNANCY: Category X, not for use in nursing.

MECHANISM OF ACTION: Retinoid; antipsoriatic action not established.

PHARMACOKINETICS: Absorption: C_{max}=416ng/mL; T_{max}=2-5 hrs.
Distribution: Plasma protein binding (99.9%); found in breast milk.
Metabolism: Extensive; via isomerization to cis-acitretin; metabolized with the parent drug into chain-shortened breakdown products and conjugates.
Elimination: Metabolites and conjugates: feces (34-54%), urine (16-53%).
Acitretin: $T_{1/2}$=49 hrs. Cis-acitretin: $T_{1/2}$=63 hrs.

NURSING CONSIDERATIONS

Assessment: Assess for pregnancy/reproductive status, renal/liver impairment, elevated blood lipid values, diabetes, obesity, alcohol intake, or a familial history of these conditions. Assess cardiovascular status, pre-existing abnormalities of the spine or extremities, and possible drug interactions (eg, tetracyclines). Blood lipids and LFT levels should be evaluated prior to therapy and again at intervals of 1-2 weeks.

Monitoring: Monitor for hepatotoxicity, hyperostosis, hypertriglyceridemia, radiological changes of pre-existing abnormalities of the spine (eg, degenerative spurs, anterior bridging of spinal vertebrae, diffuse idiopathic skeletal hyperostosis, ligament calcification, and narrowing/destruction of the cervical disc space), MI or other thromboembolic events, pancreatitis, psychiatric problems, and signs/symptoms of pseudotumor cerebri (eg, headache, N/V, visual disturbances, papilledema). Monitor eyes for dryness, lash loss, irritation, Bell's palsy, blepharitis, blurred vision and cataracts. Perform LFTs, lipids and blood sugar determination. Pregnancy test must be repeated every month during therapy and for at least 3 yrs after d/c.

Patient Counseling: Inform about the Pregnancy Prevention Actively Required During and After Treatment (*Do Your P.A.R.T*) program and about the risks of therapy. Advise to use two effective forms of contraception simultaneously at least 1 month prior to initiation of therapy. Advise against donating blood during or at least 3 yrs following completion of therapy. Inform that it is required by law that medication guide must be given to patient each time therapy is dispensed. Instruct not to ingest beverages or products containing ethanol while taking therapy and for 2 months after d/c of therapy. Notify physician if nursing. Caution when driving or operating a vehicle at night. Caution against taking vitamin A supplements to avoid additive toxic effects. Avoid excessive exposure to sunlight. Keep medication away from children.

Administration: Oral route. Take with food. **Storage:** 15-25°C (59-77°F). Protect from light. Avoid exposure to high temperatures and humidity after the bottle is opened.

SORILUX   RX
calcipotriene (Stiefel)

THERAPEUTIC CLASS: Vitamin D_3 derivative

INDICATIONS: Treatment of plaque psoriasis in adults.

DOSAGE: *Adults:* Apply thin layer bid to the affected areas and rub in gently and completely.

HOW SUPPLIED: Foam: 0.005% [60g]

CONTRAINDICATIONS: Hypercalcemia.

WARNINGS/PRECAUTIONS: Propellant in drug is flammable; avoid fire, flame, and/or smoking during and immediately following application. Hypercalcemia may occur; d/c treatment until normal calcium levels are restored. Avoid exposure of treated areas to natural or artificial sunlight (eg, tanning booths, sun lamps). Limit or avoid use of phototherapy. Use not evaluated with erythrodermic, exfoliative, or pustular psoriasis. Avoid contact with eyes.

ADVERSE REACTIONS: Erythema, hypercalcemia.

PREGNANCY: Category C; caution in nursing.

MECHANISM OF ACTION: Vitamin D_3 analog; mechanism not established.

NURSING CONSIDERATIONS

Assessment: Assess for hypercalcemia and pregnancy/nursing status. Confirm that psoriasis is a plaque type and not erythrodermic, exfoliative or pustular type.

Monitoring: Monitor serum calcium levels.

Patient Counseling: Do not place the product in the refrigerator or freezer. Avoid excessive exposure of the treated areas to natural or artificial sunlight (eg, tanning booths, sun lamps). If the foam gets in or near the eyes, advise to rinse thoroughly with water. Consult physician if there are no improvements after 8 weeks of treatment. Advise to wash hands after application. Avoid fire, flame, or smoking during and immediately following application. Advise to keep out of reach of children.

Administration: Topical route. Not for oral, ophthalmic, or intravaginal use.
Storage: 25°C (77°F); excursions permitted to 15-30°C (59-86°F). Do not puncture or incinerate. Do not expose to >49°C (120°F).

SPIRIVA RX
tiotropium bromide (Boehringer Ingelheim/Pfizer)

THERAPEUTIC CLASS: Anticholinergic bronchodilator

INDICATIONS: Long-term, once-daily, maintenance treatment of bronchospasm associated with chronic obstructive pulmonary disease (COPD), including chronic bronchitis and emphysema. Reduction of exacerbations in COPD patients.

DOSAGE: *Adults:* 2 inhalations of the contents of 1 cap (18mcg) qd, with HandiHaler device. Do not swallow caps.

HOW SUPPLIED: Cap, Inhalation: 18mcg

WARNINGS/PRECAUTIONS: Not for initial treatment of acute episodes of bronchospasm. D/C if hypersensitivity (eg, angioedema, itching, rash) or paradoxical bronchospasm occurs. Caution with hypersensitivity to milk proteins. Caution with narrow-angle glaucoma; alert patients for eye pain/discomfort, blurred vision, visual halos or colored images in association with red eyes from conjunctival congestion. Caution with urinary retention; alert patients for prostatic hyperplasia, bladder-neck obstruction (eg, difficulty passing urine, painful urination). Monitor for anticholinergic effects with moderate to severe renal impairment (CrCl ≤50mL/min).

ADVERSE REACTIONS: Dry mouth, sinusitis, constipation, abdominal pain, urinary tract infection, upper respiratory tract infection, chest pain, edema, vomiting, myalgia, moniliasis, rash, dyspepsia, pharyngitis, rhinitis.

INTERACTIONS: Avoid with other anticholinergic-containing drugs (eg, ipratropium).

PREGNANCY: Category C, caution in nursing.

MECHANISM OF ACTION: Anticholinergic bronchodilator; inhibits M_3-receptors on smooth muscle leading to bronchodilation.

PHARMACOKINETICS: **Absorption:** Absolute bioavailability (19.5%); T_{max}=5 min. **Distribution:** V_d=32L/kg; plasma protein binding (72%). **Metabolism:** Liver (oxidation, conjugation) via CYP2D6, 3A4. **Elimination:** Urine (14%, inhalation) (74%, IV). $T_{1/2}$=5-6 days.

NURSING CONSIDERATIONS

Assessment: Assess for hypersensitivity to atropine or its derivatives, narrow-angle glaucoma, prostatic hyperplasia, bladder-neck obstruction, renal impairment, pregnancy/nursing status and possible drug interactions.

Monitoring: Monitor for urinary retention, acute narrow-angle glaucoma, paradoxical bronchospasm and hypersensitivity reactions (angioedema of tongue, lips or throat; itching; rash).

Patient Counseling: Inform that contents of capsule are for oral inhalation only and must not be swallowed. Administer only via the HandiHaler device and the device should not be used for other medications. Do not increase dose or frequency, or use as a rescue medication for immediate relief of breathing problems. Seek medical attention if with symptoms of precipitation or worsening of narrow-angle glaucoma (increased IOP, acute eye pain/discomfort, blurring of vision, visual halos or colored images with red eyes from conjunctival, corneal congestion), or of prostatic hyperplasia or bladder neck obstruction (difficulty in passing urine, dysuria), with paradoxical bronchospasm, or allergic/hypersensitivity reactions. Inform not to allow the powder to enter into the eyes.

Administration: Oral inhalation. 1) Open HandiHaler device and blister. 2) Insert the capsule. 3) Press green piercing button. 4) Inhale through the mouthpiece. Refer to PI for illustrative and detailed administration procedures. **Storage:** 25°C (77°F); excursions permitted to 15°-30°C (59°-86°F). Do not expose cap to extreme temperatures or moisture. Do not store cap in Handihaler device.

SPORANOX   RX

itraconazole (Janssen/Ortho Biotech)

> Contraindicated with cisapride, pimozide, quinidine, dofetilide, levacetylmethadol. Serious cardiovascular events (eg, QT prolongation, torsades de pointes, ventricular tachycardia, cardiac arrest, and/or sudden death) reported with cisapride, pimozide, quinidine, levacetylmethadol. Do not use cap for onychomycosis with ventricular dysfunction such as congestive heart failure (CHF) or history of CHF. D/C use if signs/symptoms of CHF occur.

THERAPEUTIC CLASS: Azole antifungal

INDICATIONS: (Cap) Onychomycosis of the toenail and fingernail in immunocompetent patients. (Cap/Inj) Treatment of blastomycosis (pulmonary/extrapulmonary) and histoplasmosis (eg, chronic cavitary pulmonary disease, disseminated non-meningeal), and aspergillosis (pulmonary/extrapulmonary) if refractory to or intolerant of amphotericin B therapy. (Sol) Treatment of oropharyngeal and esophageal candidiasis. (Sol/Inj) Empiric therapy of febrile neutropenic patients (ETFN) with suspected fungal infections.

DOSAGE: *Adults:* Cap: Take with full meal. If patient has achlorhydria or taking gastric acid suppressors, give with cola beverage. Aspergillosis: 200-400mg/day. Blastomycosis/Histoplasmosis: 200mg qd. May increase in 100-mg increments if no improvement. Max: 400mg/day. Give bid if dose >200mg/day. Life-Threatening Situations: LD: 200mg tid for 1st 3 days. Continue for at least 3 months and until infection subsides. Onychomycosis: Toenail: 200mg qd for 12 consecutive weeks. Fingernail: 200mg bid for 1 week, skip 3 weeks, then repeat. Sol: Take on empty stomach. Swish 10mL at a time for several seconds, then swallow. Candidiasis: Oropharyngeal: 200mg/day for 1-2 weeks. If unresponsive/refractory to fluconazole, give 100mg bid. Esophageal: 100-200mg/day for at least 3 weeks. Continue for 2 weeks following resolution of symptoms. IV: ETFN: 200mg bid over 1 hr infusion for 4 doses, followed by 200mg qd for 14 days. Continue with oral solution 200mg bid until resolution of clinically significant neutropenia. Blastomycosis/Histoplasmosis/Aspergillosis: 200mg bid over 1 hr infusion for four doses, followed by 200mg qd. Continue for at least 3 months until active fungal infection subsides.

HOW SUPPLIED: Cap: 100mg [Pulsepak, 7 x 4 caps]; Inj: 10mg/mL [25mL]; Sol: 10mg/mL [150mL]

CONTRAINDICATIONS: Cisapride, oral midazolam, nisoldipine, pimozide, quinidine, dofetilide, triazolam and levacetylmethadol (levomethadyl), HMG CoA-reductase inhibitors (eg, lovastatin, simvastatin), ergot alkaloids (eg, dihydroergotamine, ergometrine, ergotamine and methylergometrine). (Cap) Treatment of pregnant patients or those contemplating pregnancy. (Cap/Sol) Evidence of ventricular dysfunction (eg, CHF/history of CHF). (Inj) Severe renal impairment (CrCl <30mL/min). Contraindicated when use of sodium chloride injection is contraindicated.

WARNINGS/PRECAUTIONS: Rare cases of hepatotoxicity reported. Monitor LFTs; d/c if hepatic dysfunction develops. Avoid with liver disease. D/C if neuropathy or CHF occurs. Sol and caps not interchangeable. Avoid with ventricular dysfunction. Caution with ischemic/valvular disease, pulmonary disease, renal failure, hepatic impairment, and other edematous disorders. Transient or permanent hearing loss reported, d/c if hearing loss symptoms occur. Caution in elderly. CHF, peripheral edema and pulmonary edema reported in patients treated for onychomycosis and/or systemic fungal infections. (Sol) Consider alternative therapy if unresponsive in patients with cystic fibrosis. Not recommended for initiation of treatment in patients at immediate risk of systemic candidiasis.

ADVERSE REACTIONS: N/V, diarrhea, abdominal pain, fever, cough, rash, increased sweating, headache, hypokalemia, myalgia, pruritus, rhinitis, sinusitis, dyspepsia.

INTERACTIONS: See Contraindications. Increased levels of antiarrhythmics (eg, digoxin, quinidine, dofetilide, disopyramide), warfarin, carbamazepine, rifabutin, antineoplastics (eg, busulfan, docetaxel, vinca alkaloids), benzodiazepines (eg, alprazolam, diazepam, midazolam), calcium channel blockers (eg, dihydropyridines, verapamil), cisapride, immunosuppressants (eg, cyclosporine, tacrolimus, sirolimus), oral hypoglycemics, protease inhibitors (eg, indinavir, ritonavir, saquinavir), HMG CoA-reductase inhibitors (eg, atorvastatin, cerivastatin, lovastatin, simvastatin), halofantrine, alfentanil, buspirone, methylprednisolone, budesonide, dexamethasone, fluticasone, trimetrexate, cilostazol, eletriptan and fentanyl. Anticonvulsants (eg, carbamazepine, phenobarbital, phenytoin), antimycobacterials (eg, isoniazid, rifabutin, rifampin), gastric acid suppressors/neutralizers (eg, antacids, H$_2$-receptor antagonists, proton pump inhibitors) and nevirapine decrease levels of itraconazole. Macrolide antibiotics (eg, clarithromycin, erythromycin) and protease inhibitors (eg, indinavir, ritonavir) increase levels of itraconazole. Severe hypoglycemia with oral hypoglycemics. Additive negative inotropic effects with CCBs. Edema reported with dihydropyridine CCBs; adjust dose. Decreased absorption of caps with antacids or gastric secretion suppressors. Prolonged QT interval may occur with halofantrine, pimozide, levacetylmethadol (levomethadyl). Fatal respiratory depression reported with fentanyl. May inhibit metabolism of glucocorticoids (eg, budesonide, dexamethasone, fluticasone), CCBs (eg, nifedipine, felodipine), trimetrexate. May increase concentration of ergot alkaloids, causing ergotism. Enhanced anticoagulant effect of coumarin-like drugs (eg, warfarin). Prior treatment with itraconazole may reduce activity of polyenes (eg, amphotericin B).

PREGNANCY: Category C, not for use in nursing.

MECHANISM OF ACTION: Azole antifungal agent; inhibits the CYP450-dependent synthesis of ergosterol, which is a vital component of fungal cell membranes.

PHARMACOKINETICS: Absorption: (Cap/Sol) Absolute bioavailabilty (55%). Oral administration of variable doses resulted in different parameters; refer to respective PIs for further details. (IV) C_{max}=2856ng/mL; T_{max}=1.08 hr; AUC=30605ng•hr/mL. **Metabolism:** Liver via CYP3A4; hydroxyitraconazole (major metabolite). **Distribution:** Plasma protein binding (99.8%) itraconazole, (99.5%) hydroxyitraconazole; found in breast milk. (IV) V_d=796L. **Elimination:** (Cap/Sol) Urine (40%, inactive metabolites), feces (3-18%). (Inj) Urine (35%), feces (54%, inactive metabolites).

NURSING CONSIDERATIONS

Assessment: Assess for proper diagnosis of fungal infection (eg, cultures, microscopic studies), hepatic/renal impairment, cardiac function (eg, ventricular dysfunction, CHF) prior to administration. Assess pregnancy/nursing status prior to use. Assess for possible drug interactions.

Monitoring: Monitor for signs/symptoms of CHF, QT prolongation, torsades de pointes, ventricular tachycardia, cardiac arrest, liver dysfunction, and LFTs. Blood glucose concentrations should also be monitored when coadminstered with hypoglycemic agents. Monitor for SrCr levels and prolongation of sedative effect of midazolam.

Patient Counseling: Instruct to take cap with a full meal and oral solution in fasted state and not to interchange caps and oral solution. Counsel on signs/symptoms of CHF and liver dysfunction (eg, unusual fatigue, anorexia, N/V, jaundice, dark urine or pale stools). Avoid pregnancy while on medication and remain on contraceptives for 2 months following completion of therapy. Contact physician before taking concomitant meds with drug. D/C therapy if hearing loss occurs.

Administration: Oral/IV route. Not for IV bolus injection. **Storage:** (Cap): 15-25°C (59-77°F). Protect from light and moisture. (Sol): 25°C (77°F). Do not freeze. (Inj): 25°C (77°F). Protect from light and freezing.

SPRYCEL   RX
dasatinib (Bristol-Myers Squibb)

THERAPEUTIC CLASS: Kinase inhibitor

INDICATIONS: Treatment of adults with newly diagnosed Philadelphia chromosome-positive (Ph+) chronic myeloid leukemia (CML) in chronic phase. Treatment of adults with chronic, accelerated, or myeloid or lymphoid blast phase Ph+ CML with resistance or intolerance to prior therapy including imatinib. Treatment of adults with Ph+ acute lymphoblastic leukemia (ALL) with resistance or intolerance to prior therapy.

DOSAGE: *Adults:* Chronic Phase CML: Initial: 100mg qd. Titrate: If no response, increase to 140mg qd. Accelerated Phase CML/Myeloid or Lymphoid Blast Phase CML/Ph+ ALL: Initial: 140mg qd. Titrate: If no response, increase to 180mg qd. Concomitant Strong CYP3A4 Inducers: Avoid use. If use is necessary, consider dose increase. Concomitant Strong CYP3A4 Inhibitors: Consider dose decrease to 20mg if taking 100mg qd; 40mg if taking 140mg qd. Refer to PI for dose adjustments for neutropenia and thrombocytopenia.

HOW SUPPLIED: Tab: 20mg, 50mg, 70mg, 80mg, 100mg, 140mg

WARNINGS/PRECAUTIONS: Severe thrombocytopenia, neutropenia, and anemia reported; monitor CBC weekly for 1st 2 months, then monthly thereafter. Severe CNS and GI hemorrhage, including fatalities, have occurred; other cases of severe hemorrhage reported. Severe fluid retention including severe ascites, generalized edema, and severe pulmonary edema reported. Perform chest x-ray if symptoms of pleural effusion develop (eg, dyspnea, dry cough). May prolong QT interval; caution in patients at risk (eg, hypokalemia or hypomagnesemia, congenital long QT syndrome). Correct hypokalemia or hypomagnesemia prior to administration. Cardiac adverse reactions reported; monitor for signs and symptoms consistent with cardiac dysfunction and treat appropriately. Elderly are more likely to experience toxicity. May cause fetal harm if used during pregnancy. Caution with hepatic impairment.

ADVERSE REACTIONS: Myelosuppression, fluid retention, diarrhea, N/V, headache, abdominal pain, hemorrhage, pyrexia, pleural effusion, dyspnea, skin rash, fatigue.

INTERACTIONS: Increased levels with CYP3A4 inhibitors (eg, ketoconazole, itraconazole, voriconazole, clarithromycin, ritonavir, atazanavir, indinavir, nefazodone, nelfinavir, saquinavir, telithromycin). Avoid strong CYP3A4 inhibitors or consider dose decrease if use is necessary. Grapefruit juice may also increase levels and should be avoided. Decreased levels with CYP3A4 inducers (eg, dexamethasone, phenytoin, carbamazepine, rifampin, rifabutin, phenobarbital). Avoid strong CYP3A4 inducers or consider dose increase if use is necessary. St. John's wort may decrease dasatinib levels unpredictably and should be avoided. Avoid antacids (eg, aluminum hydroxide/magnesium hydroxide); if necessary, separate dose by 2 hrs. Reduced exposure with H_2 blockers (eg, famotidine) or proton pump inhibitors (PPIs) (eg, omeprazole); concomitant use is not recommended. May increase simvastatin mean C_{max} and AUC. Caution with CYP3A4 substrates with narrow therapeutic index (eg, alfentanil, astemizole, terfenadine, cisapride, cyclosporine, fentanyl, pimozide, quinidine, sirolimus, tacrolimus, ergot alkaloids [eg, ergotamine, dihydroergotamine]). Caution with anticoagulants or medications that inhibit platelet function. May increase risk of QT prolongation with concomitant antiarrhythmics, other QT-prolonging agents, and cumulative high-dose anthracycline therapy.

PREGNANCY: Category D, not for use in nursing.

S

MECHANISM OF ACTION: Kinase inhibitor; inhibits BCR-ABL, SRC family, c-KIT, EPHA2, and PDGFRβ kinases.

PHARMACOKINETICS: Absorption: T_{max}=0.5-6 hrs. **Distribution:** V_d=2505L; plasma protein binding (96% [parent], 93% [active metabolite]). **Metabolism:** Extensive, primarily via CYP3A4. **Elimination:** Urine (4%), feces (85%); $T_{1/2}$=3-5 hrs.

NURSING CONSIDERATIONS

Assessment: Assess for hepatic impairment, prolonged QTc, lactose intolerance, hypokalemia, hypomagnesemia, pregnancy/nursing status, and possible drug interactions. Obtain baseline CBC, LFTs, and electrolytes.

Monitoring: Monitor for signs/symptoms of hemorrhage, myelosuppression, pleural/pericardial effusion, fluid retention, and QT prolongation. If symptoms of pleural effusion (eg, dyspnea, dry cough) are present, perform chest x-ray. Monitor CBC weekly for 1st 2 months and monthly afterward and LFTs periodically.

Patient Counseling: Instruct to swallow whole; do not break, cut, or crush. May take with or without food in am or pm. Inform of pregnancy risks and advise to avoid becoming pregnant during therapy. Seek medical attention if experiencing symptoms of hemorrhage (eg, unusual bleeding, easy bruising), myelosuppression (eg, fever, infection), pleural effusion (eg, dyspnea, dry cough), fluid retention (eg, swelling, weight gain, SOB), significant N/V, diarrhea, headache, musculoskeletal pain, fatigue, or rash. Inform that product contains lactose. In case of missed dose, advise not to take two doses at the same time; take next scheduled dose at its regular time.

Administration: Oral route. Swallow whole; do not crush or cut. **Storage:** 25°C (77°F); excursions permitted between 15-30°C (59-86°F).

STALEVO   RX
entacapone - levodopa - carbidopa (Novartis)

THERAPEUTIC CLASS: Dopa-decarboxylase inhibitor/dopamine precursor/COMT inhibitor

INDICATIONS: Treatment of idiopathic Parkinson's disease; to substitute for equivalent doses of carbidopa/levodopa and entacapone previously administered as individual products or to replace carbidopa/levodopa (without entacapone) for those experiencing signs and symptoms of end-of-dose "wearing off" (only for those taking ≤600mg/day levodopa without dyskinesias).

DOSAGE: *Adults:* ≤75 yrs: Individualize dose. Titrate: Adjust according to desired therapeutic response. Currently Taking Carbidopa/Levodopa and Entacapone: May switch directly to corresponding strength of Stalevo with same amounts of carbidopa/levodopa. Currently Taking Carbidopa/Levodopa without Entacapone: Titrate individually with carbidopa/levodopa and an entacapone, then transfer to corresponding dose once stabilized. Maint: Less Levodopa Required: Decrease strength of Stalevo at each administration or decrease frequency by extending time between doses. More Levodopa Required: Take next higher strength of Stalevo and/or increase frequency of doses. Max: 8 tabs/day (Stalevo 50, 75, 100, 125, 150); 6 tabs/day (Stalevo 200). Refer to PI for further dosing information when used concomitantly with other antiparkinsonian medications or general anesthesia.

HOW SUPPLIED: Tab: (Carbidopa-Levodopa-Entacapone): Stalevo 50: 12.5mg-50mg-200mg; Stalevo 75: 18.75mg-75mg-200mg; Stalevo 100: 25mg-100mg-200mg; Stalevo 125: 31.25mg-125mg-200mg; Stalevo 150: 37.5mg-150mg-200mg; Stalevo 200: 50mg-200mg-200mg

CONTRAINDICATIONS: Narrow-angle glaucoma, suspicious, undiagnosed skin lesions, history of melanoma. Nonselective MAOIs (eg, phenelzine, tranylcypromine); d/c nonselective MAOIs ≥2 weeks prior to therapy.

WARNINGS/PRECAUTIONS: CNS adverse effects may occur; may require dose reduction if dyskinesia or exacerbation of preexisting dyskinesia develop; monitor for depression and suicidal tendencies. May cause mental disturbances. Caution with biliary obstruction, severe cardiovascular (CV)/ pulmonary disease, bronchial asthma, renal/hepatic/endocrine disease, past or current psychoses, history of myocardial infarction with residual arrhythmias, chronic wide-angle glaucoma. Caution with history of peptic ulcer; may increase the risk of upper GI hemorrhage. Symptom complex resembling neuroleptic malignant syndrome (NMS) reported; observe carefully if dose is reduced abruptly or d/c. Syncope, hypotension, hallucinations, rhabdomyolysis, hyperpyrexia, confusion, and fibrotic complications reported. Diarrhea and colitis may develop; d/c with prolonged diarrhea and institute appropriate therapy. Melanomas may develop; perform periodic skin examination. Caution when d/c combination therapy; slowly withdraw therapy if necessary. Abnormalities in laboratory tests, including elevated LFTs, decreased BUN, creatinine and uric acid levels, positive Coomb's test, false-positive reaction for urinary ketone bodies, false-negative glucose oxidase test, may occur. Caution when interpreting plasma and urine levels of catecholamines and metabolites; falsely diagnosed pheochromocytoma reported. May decrease serum iron concentrations. May depress prolactin secretion and increase growth hormone levels.

ADVERSE REACTIONS: Dyskinesia, N/V, hyperkinesia, diarrhea, urine discoloration, hypokinesia, dizziness, abdominal pain, constipation, fatigue, back pain, dry mouth, dyspnea.

INTERACTIONS: See Contraindications. May result in increased HR, arrhythmias, and BP changes with drugs metabolized by catechol-O-methyltransferase (COMT) (eg, isoproterenol, epinephrine, norepinephrine, dopamine, dobutamine, α-methyldopa, apomorphine, isoetherine, bitolterol); use with caution. Caution with drugs known to interfere with biliary excretion, glucuronidation, and intestinal β-glucuronidase which includes probenecid, cholestyramine, and some antibiotics (eg, erythromycin, rifampicin, ampicillin, chloramphenicol). Symptomatic postural hypotension reported when added with antihypertensives. Concomitant therapy with selegiline may be associated with severe orthostatic hypotension. HTN and dyskinesia may occur with TCAs. Reduced effect with phenytoin, papaverine, metoclopramide, isoniazid, dopamine D2 antagonists (eg, phenothiazines, butyrophenones, risperidone). Reduced bioavailability with iron salts. Observe carefully when dose is reduced abruptly or d/c, especially with neuroleptics.

PREGNANCY: Category C, caution in nursing.

MECHANISM OF ACTION: Dopa-decarboxylase inhibitor/dopamine precursor/COMT inhibitor. Carbidopa: Inhibits the decarboxylation of peripheral levodopa, making more levodopa available for transport to the brain. Levodopa: Crosses blood-brain barrier and presumably converted to dopamine in brain. Entacapone: Sustains plasma levels of levodopa, resulting in more constant dopaminergic stimulation in brain.

PHARMACOKINETICS: Absorption: Levodopa: Rapid. (PO) Administration of variable doses resulted in different parameters. Entacapone: Rapid. C_{max}=1200-1500ng/mL; T_{max}=0.8-1.2 hrs; AUC=1250-1750ng•hr/mL. Carbidopa: Slower; C_{max}=40-225ng/mL; T_{max}=2.5-3.4 hrs; AUC=170-1200ng•hr/mL. **Distribution:** Plasma protein binding: Levodopa: (10-30%); Entacapone: (98%); Carbidopa: (36%). Crosses the placenta (levodopa). **Metabolism:** Levodopa: Extensive decarboxylation by dopa decarboxylase and O-methylation by COMT. Entacapone: Almost complete. Isomerization; cis-isomer (active metabolite). Carbidopa: α-methyl-3-methoxy-4-hydroxyphenylpropionic acid, α-methyl-3,4-dihydroxyphenylpropionic acid (metabolites). **Elimination:** Levodopa: $T_{1/2}$=1.7 hrs. Entacapone: Feces (90%), urine (10%, 0.2% unchanged); $T_{1/2}$=0.8-1 hr. Carbidopa: Urine (30%, unchanged); $T_{1/2}$=1.6-3 hrs.

NURSING CONSIDERATIONS

Assessment: Assess for narrow-angle or chronic wide-angle glaucoma, pre-existing dyskinesia, or any other conditions where treatment is contraindicated or cautioned. Assess for pregnancy/nursing status and possible drug interactions. Obtain intraocular pressure (IOP) in patients with chronic wide-angle glaucoma. Assess renal/hepatic function.

Monitoring: Monitor hematopoietic, CV/renal/hepatic function, and uric acid levels. Perform skin examination periodically. Monitor for signs/symptoms of mental disturbances, depression, suicidal tendencies, new/exacerbation of dyskinesia, NMS, rhabdomyolysis, diarrhea, colitis, upper GI hemorrhage, syncope, hypotension, melanomas, hallucinations, fibrotic complications, confusion and hyperpyrexia. Monitor IOP in chronic wide-angle glaucoma. Monitor closely and adjust other dopaminergic treatments PRN if d/c therapy.

Patient Counseling: Advise to take as prescribed. Inform that drug begins release of ingredients within 30 min after ingestion. Instruct to take at regular intervals, not to change dose regimen, and not to add any additional antiparkinsonian medications, including other carbidopa-levodopa preparations. Advise that "wearing-off" effect may occur at end of dosing interval; notify physician for possible treatment adjustments. Discoloration of saliva, urine or sweat may occur after ingestion. High-protein diet, excessive acidity, and iron salts may reduce clinical effectiveness. Hallucinations, postural (orthostatic) hypotension, dizziness, nausea, syncope, sweating, diarrhea and increase in dyskinesia may occur. Caution against rising rapidly after sitting or lying down, especially if for prolonged periods. Avoid operating machinery/driving until sufficient experience is gained on therapy. Caution when taking other CNS depressants due to its additive sedative effects. Notify physician if pregnant, intend to be pregnant or breastfeeding. Inform physician if new or increased gambling, sexual, or other intense urges develop.

Administration: Oral route. Do not fractionate tab. Administer only 1 tab at each dosing interval. **Storage:** 25°C (77°F); excursions permitted to 15-30°C (59-86°F). Dispense in tight container.

STARLIX

RX

nateglinide (Novartis)

THERAPEUTIC CLASS: Meglitinide

INDICATIONS: Adjunct to diet and exercise, to improve glycemic control in adults with type 2 diabetes.

DOSAGE: *Adults:* Initial/Maint: 120mg tid before meals (with or without metformin or TZD). Take 1-30 min before meals. May use 60mg tid (with or without metformin or TZD) in patients near goal HbA1c.

HOW SUPPLIED: Tab: 60mg, 120mg

CONTRAINDICATIONS: Type 1 diabetes, diabetic ketoacidosis.

WARNINGS/PRECAUTIONS: Caution in moderate to severe hepatic impairment. Transient loss of glucose control with trauma, surgery, fever, and infection; may need insulin therapy. Secondary failure may occur in prolonged therapy. Hypoglycemia risk in elderly, debilitated, malnourished, strenuous exercise, and with adrenal or pituitary insufficiency. Autonomic neuropathy may mask hypoglycemia.

ADVERSE REACTIONS: Upper respiratory infection, flu symptoms, dizziness, arthropathy, diarrhea, hypoglycemia, back pain, jaundice, cholestatic hepatitis, elevated liver enzymes.

INTERACTIONS: Potentiated hypoglycemia with alcohol, NSAIDs, salicylates, MAOIs, and non-selective β-blockers. Risk of hyperglycemia with thiazides, corticosteroids, thyroid products, and sympathomimetics. May potentiate tolbutamide. Peak plasma levels reduced with liquid meals. β-blockers may mask hypoglycemic effects. Caution with highly protein-bound drugs.

PREGNANCY: Category C, not for use in nursing.

MECHANISM OF ACTION: Meglitinide; lowers blood glucose levels by stimulating insulin secretion from the pancreas.

PHARMACOKINETICS: Absorption: Absolute bioavailability (73%); T_{max} =1 hr. **Distribution:** V_d =10L; plasma protein binding (98%). **Metabolism:** CYP2C9, 3A4; hydroxylation, glucuronide conjugation. **Elimination:** Urine (75%), feces; $T_{1/2}$ =1.5 hrs.

NURSING CONSIDERATIONS

Assessment: Assess FPG, HbA1c, renal function, LFTs, diabetic ketoacidosis, pregnancy/nursing status, and for possible drug interactions.

Monitoring: Monitor FPG, HbA1c, renal function, LFTs, and uric acid levels. Monitor for diabetic ketoacidosis, upper respiratory infection, back pain, flu symptoms, dizziness, arthropathy, diarrhea, bronchitis, or coughing.

Patient Counseling: Inform about importance of adherence to meal planning, regular physical activity, regular blood glucose monitoring, periodic HbA1c testing, recognition and management of hypo/hyperglycemia, and periodic assessment for diabetes complications. During periods of stress (eg, trauma, infection, surgery) medication requirements may change; seek prompt medical advice. Instruct to take 30 min before meals.

Administration: Oral route. **Storage:** 25°C (77°F); excursions permitted to 15-30°C (59-86°F).

STAVZOR   RX
valproic acid (Noven)

> Hepatotoxicity, including fatalities, usually during first 6 months of treatment. Children under the age of 2 yrs are at considerably higher risk of fatal hepatotoxicity. Monitor patients closely and perform liver function tests (LFTs) prior to therapy and at frequent intervals thereafter. Teratogenicity reported, including neural tube defects. Pancreatitis reported, including fatal hemorrhagic cases.

THERAPEUTIC CLASS: Carboxylic acid derivative

INDICATIONS: Monotherapy and adjunctive therapy of complex partial seizures that occur in isolation or in association with other types of seizures in patients ≥10 yrs. Treatment of simple and complex absence seizures as sole and adjunctive therapy and adjunctively in patients with multiple seizure types that include absence seizures. Treatment of manic episodes associated with bipolar disorder. Prophylaxis of migraine headaches.

DOSAGE: *Adults:* Mania: Initial: 750mg/day in divided doses. Titrate: Increase dose rapidly to achieve clinical effect. Max: 60mg/kg/day. Complex Partial Seizures: Monotherapy/Conversion to Monotherapy/Adjunctive Therapy: Initial: 10-15mg/kg/day. Titrate: Increase weekly by 5-10mg/kg/day until optimal response. Max: 60mg/kg/day. When converting to monotherapy, reduce concomitant antiepilepsy drug by 25% every 2 weeks at the start of therapy or 1-2 weeks after. Simple and Complex Absence Seizures: Initial: 15mg/kg/day. Titrate: Increase weekly by 5-10mg/kg/day until optimal response. Max: 60mg/kg/day. If dose >250mg/day, give in 2-3 doses. Migraine: Initial: 250mg bid. Max: 1000mg/day. Elderly: Reduce initial dose and titrate slowly. Consider dose reduction or d/c in patients with decreased food or fluid intake or if excessive somnolence occurs.
Pediatrics: ≥10 yrs: Complex Partial Seizures: Monotherapy/Conversion to Monotherapy/Adjunctive Therapy: Initial: 10-15mg/kg/day until optimal response. Max: 60mg/kg/day. When converting to monotherapy, reduce concomitant antiepilepsy drug by 25% every 2 weeks at the start of therapy or 1-2 weeks after.

HOW SUPPLIED: Cap, Delayed-Release: 125mg, 250mg, 500mg

CONTRAINDICATIONS: Hepatic disease, significant hepatic dysfunction, and known urea cycle disorders (UCD).

WARNINGS/PRECAUTIONS: Increased risk of suicidal thoughts or behavior; monitor for the emergence of worsening and/or any unusual changes in mood or behavior. Hyperammonemic encephalopathy in UCD patients; d/c if this occurs. If unexplained lethargy, hypothermia, vomiting, or mental status changes occur, measure ammonia levels. Caution with hepatic disease; d/c if hepatic failure suspected or apparent. Caution in the elderly; monitor fluid/nutritional intake and for dehydration/somnolence. Dose-related thrombocytopenia and elevated liver enzymes reported. Monitor platelet and coagulation tests prior to therapy, then periodically. Altered thyroid function tests and urine ketone

S

tests. May stimulate replication of HIV and CMV. Avoid abrupt d/c. Multi-organ hypersensitivity reactions and hypothermia reported.

ADVERSE REACTIONS: Headache, asthenia, rash, N/V, dyspepsia, diarrhea, anorexia, somnolence, tremor, dizziness, diplopia, flu syndrome.

INTERACTIONS: Drugs that affect level of expression of hepatic enzymes (eg, phenytoin, carbamazepine, phenobarbital, primidone) may increase valproate clearance. Concomitant use with aspirin (ASA) decreases protein binding and metabolism. Carbapenem antibiotics (eg, ertapenem, imipenem, meropenem) may reduce serum concentration to subtherapeutic levels, resulting in loss of seizure control. Rifampin increases oral clearance and may require valproate dosage adjustment. Concomitant use with felbamate leads to an increase in valproate C_{max}. Reduces the clearance of amitriptylline, nortriptyline, and lorazepam. Induces metabolism of carbamazepine. Inhibits metabolism of diazepam, ethosuximide, phenobarbital and phenytoin; monitor drug serum concentrations and adjust dose appropriately. Breakthrough seizures reported with concomitant valproate and phenytoin use. Administration with clonazepam may induce absence status in patients with absence seizures. Increases $T_{1/2}$ of lamotrigine; serious skin reactions reported. Concomitant use with topiramate associated with hyperammonemia, with or without encephalopathy, and hypothermia. May displace protein-bound warfarin; monitor coagulation tests. Additive CNS depression with other CNS depressants (eg, alcohol). May decrease clearance of zidovudine in HIV-seropositive patients.

PREGNANCY: Category D, not for use in nursing.

MECHANISM OF ACTION: Carboxylic acid derivative; proposed to increase brain concentrations of GABA.

PHARMACOKINETICS: Absorption: T_{max}=2 hrs (fasting), 4.8 hrs (fed). **Distribution:** V_d=11L/1.73m^2, plasma protein binding (10% at 40mcg/mL and 18.5% at 130mcg/mL), CSF distribution (10%). Found in breast milk. **Metabolism:** Liver via glucuronidation, mitochondrial β-oxidation. **Elimination:** Urine (30-50% glucuronide conjugate, <3% unchanged); $T_{1/2}$=9-16 hrs.

NURSING CONSIDERATIONS

Assessment: Assess LFTs prior to therapy, CBC with platelets, pancreatitis, plasma ammonia levels, hepatic dysfunction/disease, and pregnancy/nursing status. Note other diseases/conditions and drug therapies. Prior to therapy, evaluate for UCD in high-risk patients (eg, history of unexplained encephalopathy, coma, etc.).

Monitoring: Monitor LFTs (at frequent intervals during first 6 months), CBC with platelets, coagulation parameters, pancreatitis, ketone and thyroid function tests, plasma drug levels, hyperammonemia, and hypersensitivity reactions. Monitor for emergence/worsening of depression, suicidality, unusual changes in behavior.

Patient Counseling: Inform to take exactly as prescribed to get the most benefit and to reduce side effects. Instruct to swallow whole; do not chew. Counsel about signs/symptoms of hepatotoxicity, pancreatitis, and hyperammonemic encephalopathy. Avoid CNS depressants (eg, alcohol). Instruct that a fever associated with other organ system involvement (rash, lymphadenopathy, etc.) may be drug-related and should be reported to physician immediately. Advise not to engage in hazardous activities (driving or operating machinery). Notify physician if suicidal thoughts, behavior, or thoughts about self harm emerge. Advise to enroll in North American Antiepileptic Drug (NAAED) Pregnancy Registry.

Administration: Oral route. **Storage:** 25°C (77°F); excursions permitted to 15-30°C (59-86°F).

STAXYN
vardenafil HCl (GlaxoSmithKline)

THERAPEUTIC CLASS: Phosphodiesterase type 5 inhibitor

INDICATIONS: Treatment of erectile dysfunction (ED).

DOSAGE: *Adults:* 10mg PO prn 60 min before sexual activity. Max: 1 tab/day. Place on tongue to disintegrate. Take without liquid.

HOW SUPPLIED: Tab, Disintegrating: 10mg

CONTRAINDICATIONS: Concomitant nitrates or nitric oxide donors.

WARNINGS/PRECAUTIONS: Avoid when sexual activity is inadvisable due to underlying cardiovascular (CV) status. Increased sensitivity to vasodilatation effects with left ventricular outflow obstruction. Decrease in supine BP reported. Avoid with unstable angina, hypotension (SBP<90 mmHg), uncontrolled HTN (>170/100 mmHg), recent history of stroke, life-threatening arrhythmia, myocardial infarction (MI) within last 6 months, severe cardiac failure, moderate or severe hepatic impairment (Child-Pugh B or C), renal dialysis, hereditary degenerative retinal disorders including retinitis pigmentosa, congenital QT prolongation, phenylketonuria, fructose intolerance. Caution with bleeding disorders, active peptic ulcers, anatomical deformation of the penis (eg, angulation, cavernosal fibrosis, Peyronie's disease) or predisposition to priapism (eg, sickle cell anemia, multiple myeloma, leukemia). Rarely, non-arteritic anterior ischemic optic neuropathy (NAION) has been reported. Sudden decrease or loss of hearing accompanied by tinnitus and dizziness reported. Contains aspartame and sorbitol.

ADVERSE REACTIONS: Headache, flushing, nasal congestion, dyspepsia, dizziness.

INTERACTIONS: See Contraindications. Avoid use with Class IA (eg, quinidine, procainamide) or Class III (eg, amiodarone, sotalol) antiarrhythmics and other treatments for ED. Increased levels with moderate or potent CYP3A4 inhibitors (eg, ritonavir, indinavir, saquinavir, atazanavir, ketoconazole, itraconazole, clarithromycin, erythromycin). Additive hypotensive effect, which may lead to symptomatic hypotension when used with α-blockers or other antihypertensive agents. Reduced clearance with CYP3A4 and CYP2C9 inhibitors. Caution with medications known to prolong QT interval.

PREGNANCY: Category B, not for use in nursing.

MECHANISM OF ACTION: Phosphodiesterase Type 5 inhibitor; enhances erectile function by increasing the amount of cyclic guanosine monophosphate (cGMP), which triggers smooth muscle relaxations, allowing increased blood flow into the penis, resulting in erection.

PHARMACOKINETICS: Absorption: T_{max}=1.5 hrs. **Distribution:** V_{ss}=208L; plasma protein binding (95%). **Metabolism:** Via CYP3A4, CYP3A5, CYP2C. M1 (major metabolite). **Excretion:** Feces (91%-95%), urine (2%-6%); $T_{1/2}$=4-6 hrs (vardenafil), 3-5 hrs (M1).

NURSING CONSIDERATIONS

Assessment: Assess for CV disease, long QT syndrome, retinitis pigmentosa, bleeding disorders, active peptic ulceration, anatomical deformation of the penis, renal/hepatic impairment. Assess potential underlying causes of erectile dysfunction, and for possible drug interactions.

Monitoring: Monitor for potential cardiac risk due to sexual activity, postural hypotension, vision changes or other eye adverse events (eg, NAION), hypersensitivity reactions and hearing impairment. Monitor therapeutic effect when used in combination with other drugs.

Patient Counseling: Discuss the risk and benefits of the therapy. Counsel patient that use of nitrates and α-blockers could cause hypotension resulting in dizziness, syncope, or even heart attack or stroke. Contact the physician or healthcare provider if not satisfied with the quality of sexual performance or in case of unwanted effect. Priapism may occur; if not treated immediately penile tissue damage and permanent loss of potency may result. Stop the medication if experiencing sudden hearing loss, NAION, loss of vision in one or both eye. Therapy does not protect against sexually transmitted diseases.

Administration: Oral route. Place on tongue to distinegrate. Take without liquid. **Storage:** 25°C (77°F); excursions permitted to 15-30°C (59-86°F).

STELARA
ustekinumab (Centocor)

RX

THERAPEUTIC CLASS: Monoclonal antibody

INDICATIONS: Treatment of adult patients (≥18 yrs) with moderate to severe plaque psoriasis who are candidates for phototherapy or systemic therapy.

DOSAGE: *Adults:* ≤100kg: Initial: 45mg SQ and 4 weeks later, followed by 45mg q12 weeks. >100kg: Initial: 90mg SQ and 4 weeks later, followed by 90mg q12 weeks.

HOW SUPPLIED: Inj: 45mg/0.5mL, 90mg/1mL

WARNINGS/PRECAUTIONS: May increase risk of infections, and reactivate latent infections. Serious bacterial, fungal, and viral infections reported. Do not give with active infection or until infection resolves or adequately treated. Caution in patients with chronic infection or history of recurrent infection. Caution with interleukin (IL)-12/IL-23-deficiency; disseminated infections from mycobacteria (including nontuberculous, environmental mycobacteria), salmonella (including nontyphi strains), and Bacillus Calmette-Guerin (BCG) vaccinations may occur. Evaluate for tuberculosis (TB) infection prior to, during and after treatment; avoid with active TB. Consider anti-TB therapy prior to initiation in patients with history of latent or active TB when adequate treatment cannot be confirmed. May increase risk of malignancy. Serious allergic reactions (eg, angioedema, anaphylaxis) reported; d/c if occur. Reversible posterior leukoencephalopathy syndrome (RPLS) reported; d/c if suspected. Needle cover on prefilled syringe contains dry natural rubber; caution in latex sensitive individuals.

ADVERSE REACTIONS: Infection, nasopharyngitis, upper respiratory infection, headache, fatigue, malignancies, RPLS.

INTERACTIONS: Avoid with live vaccines; BCG vaccines should not be given during treatment or for 1 yr prior to initiating treatment or 1 yr following d/c of treatment. Non-live vaccinations received during course of therapy may not elicit an immune response sufficient to prevent disease. Caution in patients receiving or who have received allergy immunotherapy, may decrease protective effect of allergy immunotherapy and may increase risk of allergic reaction to allergen immunotherapy dose. Monitor therapeutic effect (eg, warfarin) or drug concentration (eg, cyclosporine) of coadministered CYP450 substrates.

PREGNANCY: Category B, caution in nursing.

MECHANISM OF ACTION: Monoclonal antibody; binds with high affinity and specificity to the p40 protein subunit used by both the IL-12 and IL-23 cytokines. In vitro models show ustekinumab may disrupt IL-12 and IL-23 mediated signaling and cytokine cascades by disrupting the interaction of these cytokines with a shared cell-surface receptor chain, IL-12 β1.

PHARMACOKINETICS: Absorption: (SQ) T_{max}=13.5 days (45mg), 7 days (90mg). **Distribution:** (SQ) V_d=161mL/kg (45mg), 179mL/kg (90mg). (IV) V_d=56.1-82.1mL/kg. Found in breast milk. **Elimination:** $T_{1/2}$=14.9-45.6 days.

NURSING CONSIDERATIONS

Assessment: Assess for active/chronic infections, TB, history of recurrent infections, IL-12/IL-23 deficiency, immunization history including BCG immunization, pregnancy/nursing status, and for possible drug interactions.

Monitoring: Monitor for infections (eg, cellulitis, diverticulitis, osteomyelitis, viral infections, gastroenteritis, pneumonia, and urinary tract infections), reactivation of latent infections, TB during and after treatment, malignancies, serious allergic reactions (eg, angioedema, anaphylaxis), and for RLPS (eg, headache, seizures, confusion, visual disturbances) Perform appropriate diagnostic test (eg, tissue culture and stool culture). Monitor all patients closely after administration.

Patient Counseling: Instruct patient to seek medical advice if signs or symptoms suggestive of an infection or serious allergic reaction occur. Inform of the risks and benefits of therapy. Therapy may lower the ability of the immune system to fight infections. Counsel about the risk of malignancies while on therapy. Instruct patients of the importance of communicating any history of infections and contacting their physician if they develop any symptoms of infection. Advise latex-sensitive individuals not to handle the needle cover of prefilled syringe since it contains a derivative of latex. Instruct to read the Medication Guide before starting the therapy and to reread it each time the prescription is renewed.

Administration: SQ route. Refer to PI for general considerations and instructions for administration. **Storage:** Store upright at 2-8°C (36-46°F). Protect from light. Do not freeze or shake. Discard any unused portion.

STRATTERA   RX
atomoxetine HCl (Lilly)

> Increased risk of suicidal ideation in short-term studies in children or adolescents with ADHD; balance this risk with the clinical need. Closely monitor for suicidality (suicidal thinking and behavior), clinical worsening, or unusual changes in behavior. Close observation and communication with the prescriber by families and caregivers is advised. Not approved for major depressive disorder.

THERAPEUTIC CLASS: Selective norepinephrine reuptake inhibitor

INDICATIONS: Treatment of Attention-Deficit/Hyperactivity Disorder (ADHD).

DOSAGE: *Adults:* Initial: 40mg/day. Titrate: Increase after a minimum of 3 days to target dose of about 80mg/day given qam or as evenly divided doses in the am and late afternoon/early pm. May increase to 100mg/day after 2-4 weeks if optimum response is not achieved. Max: 100mg/day. Refer to PI for dose modifications for hepatic impairment and concomitant use of CYP2D6 inhibitors.
Pediatrics: ≥6 yrs: ≤70kg: Initial: 0.5mg/kg/day. Titrate: Increase after a minimum of 3 days to target dose of about 1.2mg/kg/day given qam or as evenly divided doses in the am and late afternoon/early pm. Max: 1.4mg/kg/day or 100mg, whichever is less. >70kg: Initial: 40mg/day. Titrate: Increase after a minimum of 3 days to target dose of about 80mg/day given qam or as evenly divided doses in the am and late afternoon/early pm. Max: 100mg/day. May increase to 100mg/day after 2-4 weeks if optimal response is not achieved. Refer to PI for dose modifications for hepatic impairment and concomitant use of CYP2D6 inhibitors.

HOW SUPPLIED: Cap: 10mg, 18mg, 25mg, 40mg, 60mg, 80mg, 100mg

CONTRAINDICATIONS: Concomitant use with MAOI during or within 2 weeks after d/c of therapy, narrow-angle glaucoma, and with known/history of pheochromocytoma.

WARNINGS/PRECAUTIONS: Not intended for use with symptoms secondary to environmental factors and/or other primary psychiatric disorders, including psychoses. May cause severe liver injury in rare cases; monitor liver enzymes and d/c with jaundice or laboratory evidence of liver injury, and should not be restarted. Reports of myocardial infarction (MI), stroke, and sudden death in adults. Avoid use with known structural cardiac abnormalities, cardiomyopathy, serious heart rhythm abnormalities, coronary artery disease (CAD), or other serious cardiac problems; physical exam and evaluation of patient history is necessary. May increase BP and HR; caution with HTN, tachycardia, cardiovascular (CV) or cerebrovascular disease. Orthostatic hypotension and syncope reported; caution in any condition that may predispose to hypotension or with abrupt HR or BP changes. Raynaud's phenomenon reported. May cause treatment-emergent psychotic or manic symptoms (eg, hallucinations, delusional thinking, mania) in children and adolescents without prior history of psychotic illness at usual doses. Screen for risk for bipolar disorder

S

(including psychiatric history, family history of suicide, bipolar disorder, and depression). Monitor for appearance/worsening of aggressive behavior or hostility. Allergic reactions (eg, anaphylactic reactions, angioneurotic edema, urticaria, and rash) reported (uncommon). May increase risk of urinary retention and hesitation. Rare cases of priapism reported. Monitor growth in children. Caution with hepatic impairment.

ADVERSE REACTIONS: Abdominal pain, N/V, fatigue, decreased appetite, somnolence, dizziness, headache, dry mouth, insomnia, constipation, hot flushes, urinary hesitation/retention, dysmenorrhea, dyspepsia, erectile dysfunction.

INTERACTIONS: See Contraindications. May potentiate the CV effects of systemically administered albuterol or other β_2 agonists. Caution with pressor agents (eg, dopamine, dobutamine). Increased levels with CYP2D6 inhibitors (eg, paroxetine, fluoxetine, quinidine); may need dose adjustment.

PREGNANCY: Category C, caution in nursing.

MECHANISM OF ACTION: Selective norepinephrine reuptake inhibitor; mechanism not established. May selectively inhibit the presynaptic norepinephrine transporter.

PHARMACOKINETICS: Absorption: Rapid; well absorbed; absolute bioavailability (extensive metabolizers [63%], poor metabolizers [94%]); T_{max}=1-2 hrs. **Distribution:** V_d=0.85L/kg; plasma protein binding (98%). **Metabolism:** Via CYP2D6; 4-hydroxyatomoxetine (major metabolite). **Elimination:** Urine (>80% [4-hydroxyatomoxetine-O-glucuronide] and <3% [unchanged]), feces (<17%); $T_{1/2}$=5 hrs.

NURSING CONSIDERATIONS

Assessment: Assess for MDD, psychosis, other primary psychiatric disorders, and other conditions where treatment is contraindicated or cautioned. Assess for pregnancy/nursing status and possible drug interactions. Assess BP, HR, hepatic/renal function.

Monitoring: Monitor for cardiac abnormalities or symptoms of cardiac disease, mixed/manic episode in patients at risk for bipolar disorder, suicidality, clinical worsening or unusual changes in behavior, and other adverse effects. Monitor growth in children. Monitor HR and BP at dose increases, and periodically during therapy. Perform LFTs at the 1st sign of liver dysfunction. Periodically reevaluate long-term usefulness of therapy.

Patient Counseling: Inform about risks of treatment and appropriate use. Encourage patients, their families and caregivers to be alert for the emergence of depression, suicidal ideation and other unusual changes in behavior. Advise to contact physician if symptoms of liver injury or priapism occur. Drug is an ocular irritant; avoid contact with eyes. Caution while operating machinery/driving. Avoid late evening doses to prevent insomnia. Instruct to contact physician if increase in aggression or hostility, and priapism occurs. Instruct to consult physician if taking or planning to take any prescription or OTC medicines, dietary supplements, and herbal medicines or if nursing, pregnant or planning to be pregnant. If patients miss a dose, advise to take it as soon as possible, but should not take more than the total daily dose in any 24-hr period.

Administration: Oral route. Take whole with or without food; do not open cap. **Storage:** 25°C (77°F); excursions permitted to 15-30°C (59-86°F).

STRIANT   CIII
testosterone (Columbia Labs)

THERAPEUTIC CLASS: Androgen

INDICATIONS: Testosterone replacement therapy in males with primary or hypogonadotropic hypogonadism, congenital or acquired.

DOSAGE: *Adults:* 30mg q12h to gum region, just above the incisor tooth on either side of mouth. Rotate sites with each application. Hold system in place for 30 seconds. If buccal system falls off within the 12-hr dosing interval or falls out of position within 4 hrs prior to next dose, remove and apply new system. Do not chew or swallow.

HOW SUPPLIED: Tab, Buccal: 30mg [6 blister packs, 10 buccal systems/blister]

CONTRAINDICATIONS: Women. Carcinoma of the breast or known or suspected carcinoma of the prostate. Hypersensitivity to soy products.

WARNINGS/PRECAUTIONS: Caution in elderly; increased risk of prostatic hyperplasia/carcinoma. Risk of edema with pre-existing cardiac, renal, or hepatic disease; d/c if edema occurs. May potentiate sleep apnea, especially with obesity or chronic lung diseases. Monitor Hgb, Hct, LFTs, prostate specific antigen (PSA), cholesterol, lipids, serum testosterone. Gynecomastia frequently develops and occasionally persists.

ADVERSE REACTIONS: Gum/mouth irritation, bitter taste, gum pain/tenderness, headache, gynecomastia.

INTERACTIONS: May elevate oxyphenbutazone levels. May decrease blood glucose and, therefore, insulin requirements. ACTH/corticosteroids may enhance edema formation; caution with cardiac or hepatic disease.

PREGNANCY: Category X, not for use in nursing.

MECHANISM OF ACTION: Androgen; responsible for normal growth and development of male sex organs and maintenance of secondary sex characteristics.

PHARMACOKINETICS: Absorption: T_{max}=10-12 hrs. **Distribution:** Sex hormone-binding globulin (40%), plasma protein binding. **Metabolism:** Estradiol, dihydrotestosterone (metabolites). **Elimination:** Urine, feces; $T_{1/2}$=10-100 min.

NURSING CONSIDERATIONS

Assessment: Assess for hypersensitivity to soy products, breast or prostate carcinoma, cardiac or renal/hepatic disease, obesity, chronic lung disease, diabetes mellitus, and possible drug interactions.

Monitoring: Periodically monitor Hgb, Hct, LFTs, PSA, cholesterol and HDL. Obtain serum testosterone levels 4-12 weeks after initiation of therapy. Monitor for signs/symptoms of hypersensitivity reactions, edema with/without CHF, gynecomastia, prostatic hyperplasia/carcinoma in geriatrics, and potentiation of sleep apnea.

Patient Counseling: Instruct to apply against gums above incisors; if it fails to adhere, replace with new system. If system falls out 4 hrs prior to next dose, replace with a new one until next scheduled dose. Advise to regularly inspect gums where applying system. Contact physician if abnormal findings on gums, too frequent or persistent erections, N/V, changes in skin color, ankle swelling, breathing disturbances, or hypersensitivity reactions occur.

Administration: Buccal route. Place rounded side surface of system against gum above incisor tooth and hold firmly in place with finger over lip and against product for 30 seconds. To remove, slide gently downwards towards tooth to avoid scratching gums. **Storage:** 20-25°C (68-77°F). Protect from heat and moisture.

SUBLIMAZE
fentanyl citrate (Taylor)

CII

THERAPEUTIC CLASS: Opioid analgesic

INDICATIONS: For analgesic action of short duration during the anesthetic periods, premedication, induction and maintenance, and in the immediate postoperative period (recovery room) as the need arises. For use as a narcotic analgesic supplement in general or regional anesthesia. For administration with a neuroleptic as an anesthetic premedication, for the induction of anesthesia and as an adjunct in the maintenance of general and regional anesthesia. For use as an anesthetic agent with oxygen in selected high-risk patients, such as those undergoing open heart surgery or certain complicated neurological or orthopedic procedures.

DOSAGE: *Adults:* Individualized: Premedication: 50-100mcg IM 30-60 min prior to surgery. Adjunct to General Anesthesia: Low-Dose: Total Dose: 2mcg/kg for minor surgery. Maint: 2mcg/kg. Moderate Dose: Total Dose: 2-20mcg/kg for major surgery. Maint: 2-20mcg/kg or 25-100mcg IM or IV if surgical stress or lightening of analgesia. High-Dose: Total Dose: 20-50mcg/kg for open heart surgery, complicated neurosurgery, or orthopedic surgery. Maint: 20-50mcg/kg. Additional dosage selected must be individualized, especially if the anticipated remaining operative time is short. Adjunct to Regional Anesthesia: 50-100mcg IM or slow IV over 1-2 min. Post-op: 50-100mcg IM, repeat q1-2 hrs PRN. General Anesthetic: 50-100mcg/kg with oxygen and a muscle relaxant, up to 150mcg/kg may be used. Elderly/Debilitated patient: Start at low end of dosing range.
Pediatrics: 2-12 yrs: Individualized: Induction/Maint: 2-3mcg/kg.

HOW SUPPLIED: Inj: 50mcg/mL

WARNINGS/PRECAUTIONS: Administer only by persons specifically trained in the use of IV anesthetics and management of the respiratory effects of potent opioids. An opioid antagonist, resuscitative and intubation equipment and oxygen should be readily available. Fluids and other countermeasures to manage hypotension should be available when used with tranquilizers. Initial dose reduction recommended with narcotic analgesia for recovery. May cause muscle rigidity particularly with muscles used for respiration. Adequate facilities should be available for postoperative monitoring and ventilation. Caution in respiratory depression-susceptible patients (eg, comatose patients with head injury or brain tumor). May cause euphoria, miosis, bradycardia and bronchoconstriction and obscure the clinical course of patients with head injury. Reduce dose for elderly and debilitated patients. Caution with obstructive pulmonary disease, decreased respiratory reserve, liver and kidney dysfunction, cardiac bradyarrhythmias. Monitor vital signs routinely.

ADVERSE REACTIONS: Respiratory depression, apnea, rigidity, bradycardia.

INTERACTIONS: Severe and unpredictable potentiation by MAOIs has been reported; appropriate monitoring and availability of vasodilators and β-blockers for HTN treatment is indicated. Additive or potentiating effects with other CNS depressants (eg, barbiturates, tranquilizers, narcotics, general anesthetics); reduce dose of other CNS depressants. Reports of cardiovascular (CV) depression with nitrous oxide. Alteration of respiration with certain forms of conduction anesthesia (eg, spinal anesthesia, some peridural anesthesia). Decreased pulmonary arterial pressure and hypotension with tranquilizers. May cause CV depression with diazepam. Elevated BP, with and without HTN, reported in combination with a neuroleptic; neuroleptic agents should be administered with extreme caution in the presence of risk factors for development of prolonged QT syndrome and torsades de pointes.

PREGNANCY: Category C, caution with nursing.

MECHANISM OF ACTION: Narcotic analgesic; produces analgesic and sedative effects. Alters respiratory rate and alveolar ventilation, which may last longer than analgesic effects.

PHARMACOKINETICS: Distribution: V_d=4L/kg. **Metabolism:** Liver. **Elimination:** Urine (75%, <10% unchanged), feces (9%); $T_{1/2}$=219 min.

NURSING CONSIDERATIONS

Assessment: Assess level of pain intensity, patient's general condition and medical status, or any other conditions where treatment is contraindicated or cautioned. Assess for history of hypersensitivity, pregnancy/nursing status, renal/hepatic function, and possible drug interactions. Assess use in the elderly and debilitated patient.

Monitoring: Monitor for signs/symptoms of respiratory depression, muscle rigidity, medication abuse, and drug dependence. If given with nitrous oxide, monitor for CV depression. If administered with a tranquilizer, monitor for hypotension and hypovolemia. If combined with a neuroleptic, monitor for increases in BP; perform ECG monitoring. Perform routine monitoring of vital signs.

Patient Counseling: Inform drug should be administered by persons specifically trained in use of IV anesthetics and management of respiratory effects of potent opioids. Notify physician prior to surgery if with impaired respiration (eg, COPD), liver/kidney dysfunction, and CV problems (eg, bradyarrhythmias).

Administration: IM/IV route. **Storage:** 20-25°C (68-77°F). Protect from light. (Generic) Excursions permitted 15-30°C (59-86°F).

SUBOXONE CIII
buprenorphine HCl - naloxone HCl dihydrate (Reckitt Benckiser)

OTHER BRAND NAMES: Subutex (Reckitt Benckiser)

THERAPEUTIC CLASS: Partial opioid agonist/opioid antagonist

INDICATIONS: Opioid dependence.

DOSAGE: *Adults:* Give either agent SL as a single daily dose in the range of 12-16mg/day. Hold tabs under tongue until dissolved; swallowing tabs reduces bioavailability. Induction: Subutex: Give at least 4 hrs after last short-acting opioid (eg, heroin) use or preferably when early signs of opioid withdrawal appear. Maint: Suboxone: Range: 4mg-24mg/day. Target dose: 16mg/day. Titrate: Adjust by 2mg or 4mg to a level that maintains treatment and suppresses opioid withdrawal effects. Hepatic Impairment: Adjust dose and observe for precipitated opioid withdrawal. Concomitant CNS Depressants: Consider dose reduction.
Pediatrics: ≥16 yrs: Give either agent SL as a single daily dose in the range of 12-16mg/day. Hold tabs under tongue until dissolved; swallowing tabs reduces bioavailability. Induction: Subutex: Give at least 4 hrs after last short-acting opioid (eg, heroin) use or preferably when early signs of opioid withdrawal appear. Maint: Suboxone: Range: 4mg-24mg/day. Target dose: 16mg/day. Titrate: Adjust by 2mg or 4mg to a level that maintains treatment and suppresses opioid withdrawal effects. Hepatic Impairment: Adjust dose and observe for precipitated opioid withdrawal. Concomitant CNS Depressants: Consider dose reduction.

HOW SUPPLIED: Suboxone (Buprenorphine-Naloxone) Tab, SL: 2mg-0.5mg, 8mg-2mg. Subutex (Buprenorphine) Tab, SL: 2mg, 8mg

WARNINGS/PRECAUTIONS: Significant respiratory depression reported with buprenorphine; caution with compromised respiratory function. Naloxone may not be effective in reversing any respiratory depression produced by buprenorphine. Cytolytic hepatitis and hepatitis with jaundice reported. Obtain LFTs prior to initiation and periodically thereafter. Acute and chronic hypersensitivity reactions reported. May increase CSF pressure; caution with head injury, intracranial lesions. May cause miosis, changes in level of consciousness, and orthostatic hypotension. Caution with elderly, debilitated, myxedema, hypothyroidism, acute alcoholism, Addison's disease, CNS depression or coma, toxic psychoses, prostatic hypertrophy, urethral stricture, delirium tremens, kyphoscoliosis, biliary tract dysfunction or severe hepatic/renal/pulmonary impairment. Suboxone may cause opioid withdrawal symptoms. May obscure diagnosis of acute abdominal conditions. May produce dependence.

ADVERSE REACTIONS: Headache, infection, pain (general, abdomen, back), withdrawal syndrome, constipation, nausea, insomnia, sweating, asthenia, anxiety, depression, rhinitis.

INTERACTIONS: May need dose reduction with CYP3A4 inhibitors (eg, azole antifungals, macrolides and HIV protease inhibitors). General anesthetics, other narcotic analgesics, benzodiazepines, phenothiazines, other tranquilizers, sedative/hypnotics or other CNS depressants (including alcohol) may increase risk of CNS depression; consider dose reduction of one or both agents. Monitor closely with CYP3A4 inducers (eg, phenobarbital, carbamazepine, phenytoin, rifampicin).

PREGNANCY: Category C, not for use in nursing.

MECHANISM OF ACTION: Buprenorphine: Partial agonist at the μ-opioid receptor, antagonist at the kappa-opioid receptor. Naloxone: Inhibits μ-opioid receptor activity.

PHARMACOKINETICS: Absorption: (Suboxone 16mg) C_{max}=5.95ng/mL, AUC=34.89 hr•ng/mL. (Subutex 16mg) C_{max}=5.47ng/mL, AUC=32.63 hr•ng/mL. Refer to PI for more detailed information. **Distribution:** Plasma protein binding 96% (buprenorphine), 45% (naloxone). **Metabolism:** Buprenorphine: Through N-dealkylation and glucuronidation pathways; norbuprenorphine (active metabolite). Naloxone: Through glucuronidation, N-dealkylation, and reduction. **Elimination:** Urine (30%), feces (69%); $T_{1/2}$=37 hrs (Buprenorphine), 1.1 hrs (Naloxone).

NURSING CONSIDERATIONS

Assessment: Assess for hepatic/renal and pulmonary impairment, myxedema or hypothyroidism, Addison's disease, toxic psychosis, CNS depression or coma, prostatic hypertrophy or urethral stricture, biliary tract dysfunction, acute abdominal conditions, pregnancy/nursing status, head injury or intracranial lesions, increased CSF, alcohol intake, possible drug interactions. Perform LFTs prior to therapy and periodically thereafter.

Monitoring: Monitor LFTs. Monitor for signs/symptoms of respiratory/CNS depression, drug dependence, hepatitis, allergic reactions or anaphylactic shock, orthostatic hypotension, elevation of CSF.

Patient Counseling: Caution against hazardous tasks (eg, operating machinery/driving). Notify if pregnant/nursing. Concurrent administration of sedatives or alcohol may lead to serious overdose or death. Notify if taking or planning to take other medication.

Administration: Oral route. **Storage:** 25°C (77°F); excursions permitted to 15-30°C (59-86°F).

SUBOXONE SUBLINGUAL FILM `CIII`

buprenorphine - naloxone (Reckitt Benckiser)

THERAPEUTIC CLASS: Partial opioid agonist/opioid antagonist

INDICATIONS: Maintenance treatment of opioid dependence.

DOSAGE: *Adults:* Target Maint Dose: 16mg-4mg, as a single daily dose SL in patients initially inducted using Subutex (buprenorphine) SL tab. Titrate: Adjust in increments/decrements of 2mg-0.5mg or 4mg-1mg to maintain treatment and suppress opioid withdrawal effects. Range: 4mg-1mg to 24mg-6mg/day. Switching Between SL Tab and SL Film: Start on the same dosage as the previously administered product, then adjust dose PRN. Hepatic Impairment: Adjust dose. Elderly: Start at low end of dosing range.

HOW SUPPLIED: Film, SL: (Buprenorphine-Naloxone) 2mg-0.5mg, 8mg-2mg

WARNINGS/PRECAUTIONS: Potential for abuse. Re-establish adequate ventilation in case of overdose. May use higher doses and repeated administration of naloxone PRN to manage buprenorphine overdose. Caution with compromised respiratory function. Accidental pediatric exposure can cause fatal respiratory depression. Chronic use produces physical dependence. Cytolytic hepatitis and hepatitis with jaundice reported; obtain LFTs prior to therapy and monitor during treatment. Hypersensitivity reactions reported. May cause opioid withdrawal symptoms. Neonatal withdrawal reported when used during pregnancy. Not appropriate as an analgesic. May impair mental/physical abilities. May cause orthostatic hypotension in ambulatory patients. May elevate CSF pressure; caution with head injuries, intracranial lesions, and other circumstances when CSF pressure may be increased. May produce miosis and changes in the level of consciousness. May increase intracholedochal pressure; caution with biliary tract dysfunction. May obscure the diagnosis or clinical course of acute abdominal conditions. Caution in elderly, debilitated, myxedema/hypothyroidism, adrenal cortical insufficiency (eg, Addison's disease), CNS depression/coma, toxic psychoses, prostatic hypertrophy/urethral stricture, acute alcoholism, delirium tremens, or kyphoscoliosis.

ADVERSE REACTIONS: Oral hypoesthesia, constipation, glossodynia, oral mucosal erythema, vomiting, intoxication, disturbance in attention, palpitations, insomnia, withdrawal syndrome, hyperhidrosis, blurred vision.

INTERACTIONS: May need dose reduction with CYP3A4 inhibitors (eg, azoles such as ketoconazole, macrolides such as erythromycin, HIV protease inhibitors). Concomitant use with other potentially hepatotoxic drugs may increase risk of hepatitis or other hepatic events. Opioid analgesics, general anesthetics, benzodiazepines, phenothiazines, other tranquilizers, sedative/hypnotics or other CNS depressants (including alcohol) may increase CNS depression; consider dose reduction of one or both agents. Monitor closely for signs and symptoms of opioid withdrawal with CYP3A4 inducers (eg, efavirenz, phenobarbital, carbamazepine, phenytoin, rifampicin). Monitor dose with non-nucleoside reverse transcriptase inhibitors (NNRTIs). Some antiretroviral protease inhibitors with CYP3A4 inhibitory activity (nelfinavir, lopinavir/ritonavir, ritonavir) have little effect on pharmacokinetics. Increased levels and sedation with atazanavir, atazanavir/ritonavir. Caution with drugs that act on the CNS.

PREGNANCY: Category C, not for use in nursing.

MECHANISM OF ACTION: Buprenorphine: Partial agonist at the μ-opioid receptor and antagonist at the kappa-opioid receptor. Naloxone: Potent antagonist at the μ-opioid receptor.

PHARMACOKINETICS: Absorption: Administration of variable doses resulted in different pharmacokinetic parameters. **Distribution:** Plasma protein binding (96% buprenorphine; 45% naloxone); found in breast milk (buprenorphine). **Metabolism:** Buprenorphine: N-dealkylation via CYP3A4 and glucuronidation; norbuprenorphine (major metabolite). Naloxone: Glucuronidation, N-dealkylation, and reduction; naloxone-3-glucoronide (metabolite). **Elimination:** Buprenorphine: Urine (30%), feces (69%); $T_{1/2}$=24-42 hrs. Naloxone: $T_{1/2}$=2-12 hrs.

NURSING CONSIDERATIONS

Assessment: Assess for previous hypersensitivity, pregnancy/nursing status, possible drug interactions, and conditions where treatment is cautioned. Obtain baseline LFTs.

Monitoring: Monitor for signs/symptoms of respiratory/CNS depression, drug dependence, illicit drug use, hepatitis, hypersensitivity reactions, orthostatic hypotension, and elevation of CSF and intracholedochal pressure. Periodically monitor LFTs. Observe for signs and symptoms of precipitated opioid withdrawal in patients with hepatic impairment. Monitor for over-medication when switching from SL tab to SL film and withdrawal and under-dosing when switching from SL film to SL tab.

Patient Counseling: Warn patient on danger of self-administration of benzodiazepines and other CNS depressants including alcohol while taking Suboxone. Advise that the drug contains opioid that can be a target for abuse; keep films in safe place protected from theft and children. Seek medical attention immediately upon pediatric exposure to the drug. Never give the film to anyone else; selling or giving away of Suboxone is against the law. Drug may impair mental/physical abilities; use caution when performing hazardous tasks (eg, operating machinery/driving). Take film qd and do not change dose without consulting physician. Treatment can cause dependence and withdrawal syndrome may occur upon d/c. Caution about possibility of orthostatic hypotension in ambulatory individuals. Report to physician all medications prescribed or currently being used. Advise women regarding possible effects during pregnancy and not to breastfeed. Instruct family members that, in event of emergency, the treating physician or staff should be informed that patient is physically dependent on an opioid. Advise to dispose unopened drugs as soon as they are no longer needed by removing the film from its foil pouch and flushing them in the toilet.

Administration: Sublingual route. If additional SL film is necessary, place it on the opposite side from the first film in a manner to minimize overlapping. Keep under tongue until completely dissolved. Do not chew, swallow, or move film after placement. **Storage:** 25°C (77°F); excursions permitted to 15-30°C (59-86°F).

S

SUFENTA

sufentanil citrate (Akorn)

CII

THERAPEUTIC CLASS: Opioid analgesic

INDICATIONS: Analgesic adjunct in the maintenance of balanced general anesthesia in patients who are intubated and ventilated. Primary anesthetic agent of the induction and maintenance of anesthesia with 100% oxygen in patients undergoing major surgical procedures who are intubated or ventilated, such as cardiovascular surgery or neurosurgical procedures in the sitting position, to provide favorable myocardial and cerebral oxygen balance or when extended postoperative ventilation is anticipated. For epidural administrations an analgesic combined with low dose bupivacaine, usually 12.5mg per administration during labor and vaginal delivery.

DOSAGE: *Adults:* Individualize dose. Premedication: Based on patients needs. Analgesic: Total Dose: 1-8mcg/kg. Maint: Incremental: 10-50mcg. Infusion: Based on induction dose not to exceed 1mcg/kg/hr. Anesthetic: Total Dose: 8-30mcg/kg. Maint: Incremental 0.5-10mcg/kg. Infusion: Based on induction dose not to exceed 30mcg/kg. Epidural: 10-15mcg with 10mL bupivacaine 0.125% with or without epinephrine. May repeat for a total of 3 doses in not less than 1 hour intervals.
Pediatrics: Individualize dose. ≥12 yrs: Use same dose as adults. <12 yrs: 10-25mcg/kg with 100% oxygen. Maint: 25-50mcg supplemental doses.

HOW SUPPLIED: Inj: 50mcg/mL

WARNINGS/PRECAUTIONS: Should only be administered by persons specifically trained in the use of IV and epidural anesthetics and management of the respiratory effects of potent opioids. An opioid antagonist, resuscitative and intubation equipment and oxygen should be readily available. Prior to catheter insertion, the physician should be familiar with patient conditions (such as infection at the injection site, bleeding diathesis, anticoagulation therapy) which call for special evaluation of the benefit versus risk potential. May cause muscle rigidity of the neck and extremities. Adequate facilities should be available for postoperative monitoring and ventilation. Monitor vital signs routinely. Reduce dose for elderly and debilitated patients. Caution with pulmonary disease, decreased respiratory reserve, liver and kidney dysfunction, cardiac bradyarrhythmias. Reports of bradycardia responsive to atropine. May obscure clinical course of patients with head injuries.

ADVERSE REACTIONS: Respiratory depression, skeletal muscle rigidity, bradycardia, HTN, hypotension, chest wall rigidity, somnolence, pruritus, N/V.

INTERACTIONS: Reports of cardiovascular depression with nitrous oxide. High doses of pancuronium may produce increase in HR. Reports of bradycardia and hypotension with other muscle relaxants. Greater incidence and degree of bradycardia and hypotension with chronic CCB and β-blocker therapy. Additive or potentiating effects with other CNS depressants (eg, barbiturates, tranquilizers, narcotics, general anesthetics). Reduce dose of either agent. Decrease in mean arterial pressure and systemic vascular resistance with benzodiazepines.

PREGNANCY: Category C, caution in nursing.

MECHANISM OF ACTION: An opioid analgesic.

PHARMACOKINETICS: Distribution: Plasma protein binding (healthy males: 93%, mothers: 91%, neonates: 79%). **Elimination:** $T_{1/2}$=164 min (adults), 97 min (neonates).

NURSING CONSIDERATIONS

Assessment: Assess for pulmonary disease, decreased respiratory reserve, hepatic/renal dysfunction, cardiac bradyarrhythmias, head injury, pregnancy/nursing status, and possible drug interactions.

Monitoring: Monitor for cardiovascular depression (eg, bradycardia and hypotension), respiratory depression, muscle rigidity of the neck and extremities, N/V, chills, arrhythmias, chest wall rigidity. Monitor vital signs routinely. Appropriate postoperative monitoring should ensure that adequate spontaneous breathing is established and maintained prior to discharging patient.

Patient Counseling: Counsel about side effects of drug and abuse potential.

Absorption: IV and epidural route. **Storage:** 20-25°C (68-77°F). Protect from light.

SULAR
nisoldipine (Sciele)

RX

THERAPEUTIC CLASS: Calcium channel blocker (dihydropyridine)

INDICATIONS: Treatment of HTN alone or in combination with other antihypertensive agents.

DOSAGE: *Adults:* Initial: 17mg qd. Titrate: Increase by 8.5mg weekly or longer. Maint: 17-34mg qd. Max: 34mg/day. Elderly (>65 yrs)/Hepatic Dysfunction: Initial: Do not exceed 8.5mg/day. Take on an empty stomach (1 hr ac or 2 hrs pc). Swallow whole.

HOW SUPPLIED: Tab, Extended-Release: 8.5mg, 17mg, 25.5mg, 34mg

WARNINGS/PRECAUTIONS: May increase angina or myocardial infarction (MI) in patients with severe obstructive coronary artery disease (CAD). May cause hypotension; monitor BP initially or with titration. Caution with heart failure or compromised ventricular function, especially with concomitant β-blockers. Caution with severe hepatic dysfunction or in elderly.

ADVERSE REACTIONS: Peripheral edema, headache, dizziness, pharyngitis, vasodilation, sinusitis, palpitations.

INTERACTIONS: Increased AUC and C_{max} with cimetidine. Avoid phenytoin or CYP3A4 inducers and inhibitors. Decreased bioavailability with quinidine. Avoid high-fat meals as they increase peak drug levels. Avoid grapefruit juice.

PREGNANCY: Category C, not for use in nursing.

MECHANISM OF ACTION: Calcium channel antagonist (dihydropyridine); inhibits transmembrane influx of calcium into vascular smooth muscle and cardiac muscle resulting in dilation of arterioles and decreased peripheral vascular resistance.

PHARMACOKINETICS: Absorption: Well absorbed; absolute bioavailability (5%); T_{max}=9.2 hrs. **Metabolism:** CYP3A4 via hydroxylation. **Elimination:** Urine: (60-80%); $T_{1/2}$=13.7 hrs.

NURSING CONSIDERATIONS

Assessment: Assess for CAD, CHF, LFTs, BP, pregnancy/nursing status, and possible drug interactions.

Monitoring: Monitor BP, LFTs. Monitor for peripheral edema, headache, dizziness, vasodilation, chest pain, rash, CBC with differential and platelet count, diabetes mellitus, thyroiditis, atrial fibrillation, hypokalemia, hematuria, sinusitis.

Patient Counseling: Instruct to swallow whole; do not chew, divide, or crush. Counsel about adverse effects; seek medical attention if any develop. Avoid concomitant intake of high-fat meal. Do not take with grapefruit juice.

Administration: Oral route. **Storage:** 20-25°C (68-77°F); excursions permitted to 15-30°C (59-86°F). Protect from moisture. Dispense in tight, light-resistant container.

SULINDAC
sulindac (Various)

RX

NSAIDs may cause an increased risk of serious cardiovascular (CV) thrombotic events, myocardial infarction (MI), stroke, and serious GI adverse events including bleeding, ulceration, and perforation of the stomach or intestines. Contraindicated for the treatment of perioperative pain in the setting of coronary artery bypass graft (CABG) surgery.

S

OTHER BRAND NAMES: Clinoril (Merck)

THERAPEUTIC CLASS: NSAID

INDICATIONS: Acute or long-term use in the relief of signs and symptoms of: osteoarthritis (OA), rheumatoid arthritis (RA), ankylosing spondylitis (AS), acute painful shoulder (acute subacromial bursitis/supraspinatus tendinitis) and acute gouty arthritis.

DOSAGE: *Adults:* Take with food bid. Max: 400mg/day. OA/RA/AS: Initial: 150mg bid. Titrate: May increase or reduce dose depending on clinical response. Acute Painful Shoulder: 200mg bid for 7-14 days. Acute Gouty Arthritis: 200mg bid for 7 days.

HOW SUPPLIED: Tab: 200mg* (Generic) 150mg, 200mg* *scored

CONTRAINDICATIONS: Asthma, urticaria, or allergic-type reaction after taking aspirin (ASA) or other NSAIDs. Treatment of perioperative pain in the setting of CABG surgery.

WARNINGS/PRECAUTIONS: May lead to onset of new HTN or worsening of pre-existing HTN. Caution in patients with HTN; monitor BP closely. Fluid retention and edema reported; caution in patients with fluid retention or heart failure (HF). Renal papillary necrosis and other renal injury reported after long-term use. Renal toxicity also reported in patients in whom renal prostaglandins have a compensatory role in the maintenance of renal perfusion; caution with impaired renal function, HF, liver dysfunction, volume-depleted patients, and the elderly. Not recommended for use with advanced renal disease; if therapy must be initiated, monitor renal function. Extreme caution with prior history of ulcer disease or GI bleeding. May cause anaphylactic/anaphylactoid reactions and serious skin adverse events (eg, exfoliative dermatitis, Stevens-Johnson syndrome [SJS], toxic epidermal necrolysis [TEN]); d/c if fever, skin rash or other evidence of hypersensitivity occurs. Avoid in patients with the ASA triad. Avoid in late pregnancy; may cause premature closure of ductus arteriosus. May cause elevation of LFTs; d/c if abnormal LFTs persist/worsen, liver disease develops, or systemic manifestations (eg, eosinophilia, rash) occur. Not a substitute for corticosteroids or for treatment of corticosteroid insufficiency. Anemia may occur; monitor Hgb/Hct with long-term use. May inhibit platelet aggregation and prolong bleeding time; monitor with coagulation disorders. Caution with asthma and avoid with ASA-sensitive asthma. Caution with history of renal lithiasis; keep patients well hydrated. Pancreatitis reported; d/c and institute appropriate medical therapy. Adverse eye findings reported; perform ophthalmologic tests if eye complaints develop. Monitor closely with poor liver function and consider dose reduction. May increase risk of aseptic meningitis in patients with systemic lupus erythematosus (SLE) and mixed connective tissue disease.

ADVERSE REACTIONS: GI pain, dyspepsia, N/V, diarrhea, constipation, rash, dizziness, headache, tinnitus, flatulence, anorexia, GI cramps, pruritus, nervousness.

INTERACTIONS: Avoid use with DMSO, ASA, and other NSAIDs. May increase methotrexate (MTX) and cyclosporine toxicities. Probenecid may increase plasma levels. Diflunisal may decrease plasma levels. Concomitant use of ACE inhibitors or angiotensin II antagonists may diminish antihypertensive effect and may cause further deterioration of renal function in patients with compromised renal function. May impair response to thiazides or loop diuretics; may reduce natriuretic effect of furosemide and thiazide diuretics; monitor for renal failure. Monitor patients on oral hypoglycemic agents. May elevate plasma lithium levels; monitor for toxicity. Increased risk of GI bleeding with anticoagulants (eg, warfarin), alcohol and oral corticosteroids. May increase PT with oral anticoagulants.

PREGNANCY: Category C, not for use in nursing.

MECHANISM OF ACTION: NSAID; mechanism not established; suspected to inhibit prostaglandin synthetase; exerts anti-inflammatory, analgesic, and antipyretic actions.

PHARMACOKINETICS: Absorption: Refer to PI; administration of variable doses resulted in different parameters. **Distribution:** Penetrates placental and blood brain barrier. Plasma protein binding: Sulindac (93.1%), sulindac sulfone (95.4%), sulindac sulfide (97.9%). **Metabolism:** Via oxidation and reduction.

Elimination: Urine (50%), feces (25%, metabolites); $T_{1/2}$(sulindac, sulindac sulfide)=7.8, 16.4 hrs.

NURSING CONSIDERATIONS

Assessment: Assess for history of a hypersensitivity reaction to ASA or other NSAIDs, CV disease (eg, pre-existing HTN, CHF) or risk factors for CVD, or any other conditions where treatment is contraindicated or cautioned. Assess for pregnancy/nursing status and for possible drug interactions. Assess use in elderly, volume depleted and debilitated. Obtain baseline LFTs, renal function, BP, and CBC.

Monitoring: Monitor for signs/symptoms of CV thrombotic events, new onset or worsening pre-existing HTN, GI events, fluid retention and edema, renal effects, hepatic reactions, anaphylactic/anaphylactoid reactions, skin reactions, fever, rash, hypersensitivity, hematological effects, bronchospasm, renal calculi, pancreatitis, and for ocular effects. Monitor for aseptic meningitis in patients with SLE. Monitor BP. Perform periodic monitoring of CBC, chemistry profile (eg, serum and urine amylase, amylase/CrCl ratio, electrolytes, serum calcium, glucose, lipase), renal function, and LFTs.

Patient Counseling: Instruct to seek medical attention for symptoms of GI ulceration or bleeding (eg, epigastric pain, dyspepsia, melena, hematemesis), hepatotoxicity (eg, nausea, fatigue, jaundice, pruritus, lethargy, right upper quadrant tenderness and "flu-like" symptoms), anaphylactic/anaphylactoid reactions (eg, difficulty breathing, swelling of the face/throat), skin reactions (eg, rash, blisters, fever) or other hypersensitivity (eg, itching), CV events (eg, chest pain, SOB, weakness, slurring of speech), or if unexplained weight gain or edema occurs. Counsel on the importance of medical follow up. Inform of risks if used during pregnancy.

Administration: Oral route. **Storage:** 15-30°C (59-86°F). Store in a well-closed container.

SUMAVEL DOSEPRO   RX
sumatriptan (Zogenix, Inc)

THERAPEUTIC CLASS: 5-HT$_{1B/1D}$ agonist

INDICATIONS: Acute treatment of migraine attacks, with or without aura, and acute treatment of cluster headache episodes.

DOSAGE: *Adults:* Initial: 6mg SQ. May repeat after 1 hr. Max: 12mg/24 hrs. Administer to the abdomen or thigh.

HOW SUPPLIED: Inj: 6mg/0.5mL

CONTRAINDICATIONS: IV route, ischemic heart disease (eg, angina pectoris, history of myocardial infarction (MI), or documented silent ischemia) or symptoms/findings consistent with ischemic heart disease, coronary artery vasospasm (eg, Prinzmetal's variant angina), or other significant underlying cardiovascular (CV) disease, cerebrovascular syndromes (eg, stroke, TIA), peripheral vascular disease (eg, ischemic bowel disease), uncontrolled HTN, or hemiplegic or basilar migraine, administration of any ergot-type agents (eg, dihydroergotamine or methysergide) or other 5-HT$_1$ agonists (eg, triptan) within 24 hrs.

WARNINGS/PRECAUTIONS: Not for IM/IV use. Serious adverse cardiac events (eg, acute MI, life-threatening arrhythmias), cerebrovascular events, and vasospastic reactions (eg, coronary artery vasospasm, peripheral vascular ischemia, colonic ischemia) reported. Evaluate coronary artery disease (CAD) before use and administer first dose with supervision; consider ECG monitoring. Sensations of tightness, pain, pressure, and heaviness in the precordium, throat, neck, and jaw are common after therapy. Seizures reported; caution with history of epilepsy or lowered seizure threshold. Caution with controlled HTN. Elevation in BP including hypertensive crisis reported. Corneal opacities may occur. Avoid in elderly.

ADVERSE REACTIONS: Injection-site reactions, tingling, warm/hot sensation, burning sensation, feeling of heaviness, pressure sensation, feeling of tightness, numbness, flushing, chest tightness, weakness, dizziness/vertigo, drowsiness/sedation, paresthesia, N/V.

INTERACTIONS: See Contraindications. Avoid use with MAOIs; reduced sumatriptan clearance. May cause additive prolonged vasospastic reactions with ergot-containing drugs. Serotonin syndrome (eg, mental status changes, autonomic instability, neuromuscular aberrations, GI symptoms) reported with combined use of SSRIs, SNRIs, or triptans.

PREGNANCY: Category C, caution in nursing.

MECHANISM OF ACTION: Selective 5-HT$_{1B/1D}$ agonist; binds to vascular 5-HT$_1$-type receptors in cranial arteries, basilar artery, and vasculature of isolated dura mater, which causes vasoconstriction.

PHARMACOKINETICS: Absorption: Absolute Bioavailability (97%); C_{max}=71.9ng/mL (thigh), 78.6ng/mL (abdomen); T_{max}=12 min. **Distribution:** Plasma protein binding (14-21%). **Elimination:** $T_{1/2}$=103 min (thigh), 102 min (abdomen).

NURSING CONSIDERATIONS

Assessment: Assess for presence/history of ischemic heart disease, CAD, cerebrovascular or peripheral vascular disease, uncontrolled HTN, hemiplegic or basilar migraines, history of epilepsy, pregnancy/nursing status, and possible drug interactions. Establish proper diagnosis of migraine; exclude other potentially serious neurological condition.

Monitoring: Monitor for signs/symptoms of cardiac events, colonic ischemia, bloody diarrhea, serotonin syndrome (eg, mental status changes), hypersensitivity reactions, jaw/neck tightness, seizures, exacerbation of headache, and ophthalmic changes (eg, corneal opacities). For patients on long-term therapy or with CAD risk factors, perform periodic monitoring of CV function. If patients with no risk factors develop signs/symptoms of angina after administration, stop and reevaluate for CAD or other cardiac disease. If clinical response does not occur following administration of first dose, reassess diagnosis.

Patient Counseling: Inform about possible adverse events; consult physician if symptoms such as chest pain, abdominal pain, SOB, mental status changes, trouble walking, tight muscles, fast heartbeat, changes in BP, flushing, vision changes, N/V, diarrhea and/or hypersensitivity reactions occur. Caution about the risk of serotonin syndrome. Advise to notify physician if pregnant or breastfeeding. Counsel regarding proper use; for SQ administration to the abdomen or thigh only and not to be administered within 2 inches of the navel or to the arm. Advise not to use device if the tip is tilted or broken off upon removal from packaging.

Administration: SQ route. Refer to PI for administration. **Storage:** 20-25°C (68-77°F), with excursions permitted between 15-30°C (59-86°F). Do not freeze.

SUPARTZ   RX
sodium hyaluronate (Smith & Nephew)

THERAPEUTIC CLASS: Hyaluronan

INDICATIONS: Treatment of pain in osteoarthritis of the knee in patients who have failed to respond adequately to conservative non-pharmacologic therapy and simple analgesics (eg, APAP).

DOSAGE: *Adults:* Administer 2.5mL by intra-articular injection once a week for a total of 5 injections. Some patients may experience benefit with 3 injections given at weekly intervals. Use strict aseptic technique.

HOW SUPPLIED: Inj: 2.5mL

CONTRAINDICATIONS: Avoid with knee infections or skin diseases in the area of the injection site.

WARNINGS/PRECAUTIONS: Avoid disinfectants containing quaternary ammonium salts for skin preparation; hyaluronic acid can precipitate in their presence. Transient pain and/or swelling of the injected joint may occur.

Safety and effectiveness in joints other than the knee or concomitantly with other intra-articular injectables have not been established. Caution in patients who are allergic to avian proteins, feathers, and egg products. Avoid any strenuous activities or prolonged (eg, more than 1 hr) weight-bearing activities within 48 hours following the intra-articular injection. Remove any joint effusion before injecting.

ADVERSE REACTIONS: Arthralgia, arthropathy, arthrosis, arthritis, back pain, pain (non-specific), injection-site reaction, headache, injection-site pain.

PREGNANCY: Safety in pregnancy and nursing not known.

MECHANISM OF ACTION: Hyaluronan.

NURSING CONSIDERATIONS

Assessment: Assess for skin infections or disease in area of injection site, use of disinfectants containing quaternary ammonium salts, knee joint infections, and pregnancy/nursing status.

Monitoring: Monitor for knee joint swelling/effusion and local skin reaction.

Patient Counseling: Inform that drug may cause transient pain/swelling at injection site. Avoid strenuous activities or prolonged weight-bearing activities (jogging, tennis) within 48 hrs following injection.

Administration: Intra-articular. **Storage:** Below 25°C (77°F). Do not freeze. Shelf life is 42 months.

SUPRAX   RX
cefixime (Lupin)

THERAPEUTIC CLASS: Cephalosporin (3rd generation)

INDICATIONS: Otitis media, pharyngitis, tonsillitis, acute bronchitis, acute exacerbation of chronic bronchitis, uncomplicated urinary tract infections (UTIs), and cervical/urethral gonorrhea caused by susceptible strains.

DOSAGE: *Adults:* Usual: 400mg qd. Gonorrhea: 400mg single dose. CrCl 21-60mL/min/Hemodialysis: Give 75% of standard dose. CrCl <20mL/min/CAPD: Give 50% of standard dose.
Pediatrics: >12 yrs or >50kg: (Tab/Sus) Usual: 400mg qd. ≥6 months: (Sus) 8mg/kg qd or 4mg/kg bid. Treat for at least 10 days for *S.pyogenes*. CrCl 21-60mL/min/Hemodialysis: Give 75% of standard dose. CrCl <20mL/min/CAPD: Give 50% of standard dose.

HOW SUPPLIED: Tab: 400mg; Sus: 100mg/5mL [50mL, 75mL, 100mL]

WARNINGS/PRECAUTIONS: Caution with PCN or other allergy, GI disease (eg, colitis). Anaphylactic/anaphylactoid reactions, pseudomembranous colitis reported. May cause false (+) direct Coombs' test or false (+) reaction for urinary glucose using Benedict's/Fehling's solution or Clinitest.

ADVERSE REACTIONS: Diarrhea, abdominal pain, nausea, dyspepsia, flatulence, superinfection.

INTERACTIONS: May increase carbamazepine levels. Increased PT with anticoagulants (eg, warfarin).

PREGNANCY: Category B, not for use in nursing.

MECHANISM OF ACTION: 3rd generation cephalosporin; inhibits cell-wall synthesis.

PHARMACOKINETICS: Absorption: 40-50%. C_{max}=2mcg/mL (200mg tab), 3.7mcg/mL (400mg tab), 3mcg/mL (200mg sus), 4.6mcg/mL (400mg sus); T_{max}=2-6 hrs (200mg tab, 400mg tab/sus), 2-5 hrs (200mg sus). **Distribution:** Serum protein binding (65%). **Elimination:** Urine (50% unchanged); $T_{1/2}$=3-4 up to 9 hrs.

NURSING CONSIDERATIONS

Assessment: Assess for previous hypersensitivity to cephalosporins/PCNs or other drugs, renal/hepatic impairment, GI tract disease (eg, colitis), nutritional status, those receiving protracted course of antibiotics or anticoagulants, pregnancy/nursing status, possible drug interactions.

Monitoring: Monitor for PT with vitamin K administration as indicated. Monitor for signs/symptoms of anaphylatic/anaphylactoid reactions, pseudomembranous colitis or *Clostridium difficile* associated diarrhea (CDAD), development of drug resistance, superinfection, pancytopenia, agranulocytosis and lab test interference (eg, false (+) reaction of urinary ketones if using nitroprusside, false (+) reaction for urinary glucose if using Clinitest, Benedict's or Fehling's solution, false (+) Coombs' test). Monitor renal function tests, LFTs, LDH, and CBC.

Patient Counseling: Inform that therapy only treats bacterial, not viral, infections. Take exactly as directed; skipping doses or not completing full course may decrease effectiveness and increase resistance. Inform about benefits/risks. D/C and notify physician if diarrhea or allergic reactions occur. Notify if pregnant/nursing.

Administration: Oral route. **Storage:** Sus/Tab, 20-25°C (68-77°F). After mixing, store sus at room temperature or under refrigeration for 14 days; keep tightly closed and shake well before use.

Suprep   RX
sodium sulfate - potassium sulfate - magnesium sulfate (Braintree)

THERAPEUTIC CLASS: Bowel cleanser

INDICATIONS: Cleansing of colon as a preparation of colonoscopy in adults.

DOSAGE: *Adults:* Day Prior to Colonoscopy: May consume light breakfast or have only clear liquids. Early in evening prior to colonoscopy, dilute one bottle with 16 oz. of water and drink entire amount. Drink additional 32 oz. of water over the next hour. Day of Colonoscopy: Have only clear liquids until after colonoscopy. Morning of Colonoscopy (10-12 hrs after pm dose): Repeat steps taken on day prior with second bottle. Complete all Suprep Bowel Prep Kit and required water at least 1 hr prior to colonoscopy.

HOW SUPPLIED: Sol: (Sodium Sulfate-Potassium Sulfate-Magnesium Sulfate) 17.5g-3.13g-1.6g

CONTRAINDICATIONS: GI obstruction, bowel perforation, gastric retention, ileus, toxic colitis or toxic megaocolon.

WARNINGS/PRECAUTIONS: Hydrate adequately before, during, and after use. If significant vomiting or signs of dehydration occur, consider performing post-colonoscopy tests (electrolytes, creatinine, BUN). Correct electrolyte abnormalities prior to use. Caution with conditions that may increase the risk of fluid/electrolyte disturbances and renal impairment. May increase uric acid levels; caution in patients with gout or uric acid metabolism disorders. Serious arrhythmias reported rarely; caution in patients at increased risk of arrhythmias (eg, history of prolonged QT, uncontrolled arrhythmias, recent MI, unstable angina, CHF, cardiomyopathy). Generalized tonic-clonic seizures and/or loss of consciousness reported; caution in patients with a history of seizures and in patients at increased risk of seizures (eg, hyponatremia, alcohol or benzodiazepine withdrawal). May produce colonic mucosal aphthous ulcerations and ischemic colitis. If suspected, rule out GI obstruction or perforation prior to administration. Caution in patients with impaired gag reflex and patients prone to regurgitation or aspiration; observe during administration. Not for direct ingestion.

ADVERSE REACTIONS: Overall discomfort, abdominal distention, abdominal pain, N/V.

INTERACTIONS: Caution with concomitant use of medications that increase the risk for fluid and electrolyte disturbances or increase the risk of seizures (eg, tricyclic antidepressants), arrhythmias and prolonged QT. Caution with medications that may affect renal function (eg, diuretics, angiotensin converting enzyme inhibitors, angiotensin receptor blockers, NSAIDs). Concurrent use with stimulant laxatives may increase risk of colonic mucosal ulcerations and ischemic colitis. Absorption of oral medications may not occur if administered within an hour of the start of a Suprep dose.

PREGNANCY: Category C, caution in nursing.

MECHANISM OF ACTION: Bowel cleanser: sulfate salts provide sulfate anions that are poorly absorbed. The osmotic effect of the unabsorbed sulfate anions and the associated cations causes water to be retained within the GI tract.

PHARMACOKINETICS: Absorption: T_{max} = 17 hrs (1st dose), 5 hrs (2nd dose). **Elimination:** Feces (primary), $T_{1/2}$ = 8.5 hrs.

NURSING CONSIDERATIONS

Assessment: Assess for GI obstruction, bowel perforation, or any other conditions where treatment is contraindicated or cautioned. Assess for pregnancy/nursing status, and for possible drug interactions. Obtain baseline electrolytes, creatinine, and BUN in patients with renal impairment. Perform baseline ECGs in patients at risk for arrhythmias.

Monitoring: Monitor for electrolyte abnormalities, cardiac arrhythmias, seizures, loss of consciousness, colonic mucosal ulcerations, ischemic colitis and for aspiration. Perform ECG in patients at increased risk of serious cardiac arrhythmias. Monitor electrolytes, creatinine, and BUN in patients with renal impairment.

Patient Counseling: Instruct to notify physician if have difficulty swallowing or are prone to regurgitation or aspiration. Inform to dilute each bottle with water prior to ingestion and drink additional water as directed by instructions. Advise that ingestion of undiluted solution may increase risk of N/V and dehydration. Inform that oral medications may not be absorbed properly if they are taken within 1 hr of starting each dose of Suprep Bowel Kit. Instruct not to take additional laxatives.

Administration: Oral Route. **Storage:** 20-25°C (68-77°F); excursions permitted between 15-30°C (59-86°F).

SUSTIVA   RX
efavirenz (Bristol-Myers Squibb)

THERAPEUTIC CLASS: Non-nucleoside reverse transcriptase inhibitor

INDICATIONS: Treatment of HIV-1 infection in combination with other antiretrovirals.

DOSAGE: *Adults:* Initial: 600mg qd with a protease inhibitor and/or nucleoside analogue reverse transcriptase inhibitors (NRTIs). Concomitant Voriconazole: 300 mg qd; increase voriconazole maintenance dose to 400 mg q12h. Take on an empty stomach hs.
Pediatrics: ≥3 yrs: 10-<15kg: 200mg qd. 15-<20kg: 250mg qd. 20-<25kg: 300mg qd. 25-<32.5kg: 350mg qd. 32.5-<40kg: 400mg qd. ≥40kg: 600mg qd. Take on an empty stomach hs.

HOW SUPPLIED: Cap: 50mg, 200mg; Tab: 600mg

CONTRAINDICATIONS: Concomitant use with bepridil, cisapride, midazolam, triazolam, pimozide, ergot derivatives (dihydroergotamine, ergonovine, ergotamine, methylergonovine), St. John's wort.

WARNINGS/PRECAUTIONS: Not for use as monotherapy or added on as a sole agent to a failing regimen to avoid virus resistance or cross-resistance with other agents. Do not give with other efavirenz-containing products. Serious psychiatric events reported; immediate medical evaluation is recommended if symptoms occur. CNS symptoms reported; may dose at bedtime to improve tolerability. Skin rash reported; give appropriate treatment or prophylaxis if rash occurs. D/C therapy if severe rash develops. Avoid with moderate or severe hepatic impairment. Caution in patients with mild hepatic impairment or in elderly. Monitor liver enzymes before and during treatment with underlying hepatic disease or periodically without pre-existing conditions. Caution with history of seizures; convulsions reported. Increased total cholesterol (TC) and triglycerides (TG) levels reported. Immune reconstitution

S

syndrome and body fat redistribution/accumulation observed. Fetal harm can occur during first trimester of pregnancy; avoid use during pregnancy.

ADVERSE REACTIONS: Dizziness, headache, insomnia, anxiety, desquamation, depression, rash, N/V, increased ALT/AST levels, abnormal dream, fatigue, erythema, CNS symptoms.

INTERACTIONS: See Contraindications. Inhibits CYP2C9, 2C19, and 3A4 isozymes; may alter plasma concentrations of drugs primarily metabolized by these isozymes. CYP3A inducers (eg, phenobarbital, rifampin, rifabutin) may increase the clearance. May decrease levels of amprenavir, atazanavir, indinavir, lopinavir, saquinavir, efavirenz, sertraline, calcium channel blockers (diltiazem, felodipine, nicardipine, nifedipine, verapamil), atorvastatin, pravastatin, simvastatin, itraconazole, ketoconazole, voriconazole, maraviroc, clarithromycin, rifabutin, active metabolites of norgestimate, progestin (norelgestromin, levonorgestrel), etonogestrel, CYP3A substrates. May decrease posaconazole levels; avoid concomitant use unless benefit outweighs risks. May decrease levels of immunosuppressants (cyclosporine, tacrolimus, sirolimus); close monitoring of immunosuppressant concentrations for ≥2 weeks and/or dose adjustment is recommended. May decrease methadone levels; monitor for signs of withdrawal. May increase ritonavir and nelfinavir levels. May alter warfarin levels. May decrease anticonvulsants levels (carbamazepine, phenytoin, phenobarbital). May increase levels with ritonavir, clarithromycin, voriconazole, fluconazole, diltiazem, sertraline. May decrease levels with anticonvulsants, nelfinavir, saquinavir, rifampin, simvastatin, carbamazepine. Additive CNS effects with alcohol or psychoactive drugs. For appropriate dose adjustments with concomitant agents, refer to PI.

PREGNANCY: Category D, not for use in nursing.

MECHANISM OF ACTION: Non-nucleoside reverse transcriptase inhibitor (NNRTI); mediated predominantly by noncompetitive inhibition of HIV-1 reverse transcriptase (RT).

PHARMACOKINETICS: Absorption: (600 mg qd) C_{max}=12.9 μM. **Distribution:** Plasma protein binding (99.5-99.75%). **Metabolism:** CYP3A, 2B6 (hydroxylation, glucuronidation). **Elimination:** Urine (14-34%, <1% unchanged), feces (16-61%); $T_{1/2}$=40-55 hrs (multiple dose), 52-76 hrs (single dose).

NURSING CONSIDERATIONS

Assessment: Assess for underlying hepatic disease, HBV/HCV infection, marked transaminase elevations or those treated with other medications associated with liver toxicity, history of injection drug use, history of seizures, psychiatric history, previous hypersensitivity to the drug, pregnancy/nursing status, and possible drug interactions. Perform pregnancy test prior to therapy. Obtain baseline serum transaminase levels (eg, ALT, AST), gamma-glutamyltransferase (GGT), amylase, glucose levels, TC and TG levels, and neutrophil count.

Monitoring: Monitor for psychiatric events, CNS symptoms, skin rash, pregnancy, convulsions, immune reconstitution syndrome, infection, hypersensitivity reactions, and other adverse reactions. Monitor LFTs before and during treatment with hepatic impairment or periodically without pre-existing conditions. Monitor TC and TG levels before and periodically after therapy. Check drug levels of concomitant anticonvulsants metabolized by the liver.

Patient Counseling: Advise to report to physician use of any other prescription/nonprescription medication or herbal products, particularly St. John's wort. Inform that therapy is not cure for HIV, does not reduce risk of transmission of HIV and that opportunistic infections may develop. Take every day as prescribed. CNS symptoms (eg, dizziness, insomnia, impaired concentration, abnormal dreams) may occur during 1st weeks of therapy. Avoid potentially hazardous tasks such as driving or operating machinery. Seek medical attention if symptoms of seizures, rash, serious psychiatric events (severe depression, suicidal ideation, aggressive behavior), severe infection or hypersensitivity reactions occur. Notify physician of any history of mental illness or substance abuse. Inform of pregnancy risks; use of reliable barrier and oral contraception during therapy and 12 weeks after d/c of therapy is recommended. Apprise of the potential harm to fetus if used during 1st trimester of pregnancy. Register pregnant patients in the Antiretroviral Pregnancy Registry while on treatment by calling 1-800-258-4263. Advise that redistribution or accumulation of body fat may occur.

Administration: Oral route. Do not break tab. **Storage:** 25°C (77°F); excursions permitted to 15-30°C (59-86°F).

SUTENT   RX
sunitinib malate (Pfizer)

> Hepatotoxicity has been observed; may be severe, and deaths reported.

THERAPEUTIC CLASS: Multikinase inhibitor

INDICATIONS: Treatment of gastrointestinal stromal tumor (GIST) after disease progression on or intolerance to imatinib mesylate. Treatment of advanced renal cell carcinoma (RCC).

DOSAGE: *Adults:* 50mg qd; 4 weeks on, 2 weeks off. Dose increase/reduction in 12.5mg increments is recommended. Concomitant Strong CYP3A4 Inhibitors: Consider dose reduction to minimum of 37.5mg daily. Concomitant CYP3A4 Inducer: Consider dose increase to maximum of 87.5mg daily.

HOW SUPPLIED: Cap: 12.5mg, 25mg, 50mg

WARNINGS/PRECAUTIONS: Decreased left ventricular ejection fraction (LVEF) reported. Patients with cardiac risk factors should be carefully monitored for signs and symptoms of CHF; baseline and periodic evaluation of LVEF should be considered. D/C if clinical manifestations of CHF occur. Interrupt and/or reduce in patients without clinical evidence of CHF but ejection fraction <50% and >20% below baseline. Cardiovascular (CV) events (eg, heart failure, myocardial disorders, cardiomyopathy) reported. Prolongation of QT interval and torsades de pointes observed; consider monitoring ECG and electrolytes (Mg^{2+}, K^+). Hemorrhagic events (eg, GI, respiratory, tumor, urinary tract, brain) reported. Serious, sometimes fatal GI complications including GI perforation have occurred with intra-abdominal malignancies. HTN reported; monitor and treat as needed with standard antihypertensive therapy. Temporary suspension recommended if severe HTN occurs. Adrenal toxicity reported; monitor for adrenal insufficiency with stress, trauma, or severe infection. Hypothyroidism reported; monitor thyroid function and treat if signs/symptoms suggest thyroid dysfunction. May cause fetal harm; avoid pregnancy.

ADVERSE REACTIONS: Fatigue, asthenia, diarrhea, N/V, mucositis/stomatitis, dyspepsia, abdominal pain, HTN, rash, hand-foot syndrome, skin discoloration, altered taste, anorexia, bleeding.

INTERACTIONS: Concomitant CYP3A4 inhibitors (eg, ketoconazole, itraconazole, clarithromycin, atazanavir, indinavir, nefazodone, nelfinavir, ritonavir, saquinavir, telithromycin, voriconazole) and grapefruit may increase plasma concentrations; consider dose reduction. CYP3A4 inducers (eg, dexamethasone, phenytoin, carbamazepine, rifampin, rifabutin, rifapentin, phenobarbital, St. John's wort) may decrease plasma concentrations; consider dose increase while monitoring for toxicity.

PREGNANCY: Category D, not for use in nursing.

MECHANISM OF ACTION: Multikinase inhibitor; inhibits multiple receptor tyrosine kinases, implicated in tumor growth, pathologic angiogenesis, and metastatic cancer progression.

PHARMACOKINETICS: **Absorption:** T_{max}=6-12 hrs. **Distribution:** V_d=2230L; plasma protein binding (95%). **Metabolism:** CYP3A4. **Elimination:** Feces (61%), renal (16%); $T_{1/2}$=40-60 hrs, 80-110 hrs (metabolite).

NURSING CONSIDERATIONS

Assessment: Assess for risk factors or history of CV events (eg, LVEF, QT prolongation, bradycardia, HTN, myocardial infarction, coronary artery bypass graft), seizures, renal/hepatic dysfunction, hypothyroidism, pregnancy/nursing status, and possible drug interactions. Obtain baseline vital signs,

S

ECG, thyroid function, CBC with platelet count, serum electrolytes, phosphate levels, LFTs, and renal function.

Monitoring: Monitor for signs/symptoms of CVD, electrolyte imbalance, hemorrhagic events, hypothyroidism, adrenal insufficiency, reversible posterior leukoencephalopathy syndrome (RPLS), pancreatitis, muscle toxicity, hepatotoxicity, hypersensitivity reactions, renal/hepatic dysfunction, venous thromboembolic events. Monitor LVEF, chemistries (Mg^{2+}, K^+, phosphate) vital signs, ECG, thyroid function, LFTs (eg, ALT, AST, bilirubin), and renal function. CBCs with platelet count and serum chemistries including phosphate should be performed at the beginning of each treatment cycle.

Patient Counseling: Inform of pregnancy risks. May be taken with or without food. Do not to take with grapefruit juice or grapefruit. Seek medical attention if GI disorders (eg, diarrhea, N/V, stomatitis, dyspepsia), skin discoloration, fatigue, HTN, bleeding, swelling, mouth pain/irritation, taste disturbance, dermatological effects (eg, dryness, thickness or cracking of skin, blister, rash on palms of hands and soles of the feet) occur. Inform healthcare provider of all concomitant medications, including OTC medications and dietary supplements.

Administration: Oral route. **Storage:** 25°C (77°F); excursions permitted to 15-30°C (59-86°F).

SYMBICORT   RX
formoterol fumarate dihydrate - budesonide (AstraZeneca)

> Long-acting β₂-adrenergic agonists (LABA), such as formoterol, may increase the risk of asthma-related death. LABA may increase the risk of asthma-related hospitalization in pediatric and adolescent patients. Symbicort should only be used for patients not adequately controlled on a long-term asthma-control medications or whose disease severity clearly warrants initiation of treatment with both inhaled coticosteroids and LABA. Do not use Symbicort in patients whose asthma is adequately controlled on low or medium dose inhaled corticosteroids.

THERAPEUTIC CLASS: Corticosteroid/beta₂ agonist

INDICATIONS: Treatment of asthma in patients ≥12 yrs. Symbicort 160/4.5: Maintenance treatment of airflow obstruction in patients with chronic obstructive pulmonary disease (COPD) including chronic bronchitis and emphysema.

DOSAGE: *Adults:* Asthma: Initial: 2 inh bid (am/pm q12h). Individualize dose based on asthma severity. Max: 160/4.5mcg bid. Patients not responding to the starting dose after 1-2 weeks of therapy with 80/4.5, replace with 160/4.5 for better asthma control. COPD (160/4.5 only): 2 inh bid. If asthma symptoms or SOB occur in the period between doses, use short-acting β₂-agonist for immediate relief. Rinse mouth with water after use.
Pediatrics: ≥12 yrs: Asthma: Initial: 2 inh bid (am/pm q12h). Individualize dose based on asthma severity. Max: 160/4.5mcg bid. Patients not responding to the starting dose after 1-2 weeks of therapy with 80/4.5, replace with 160/4.5 for better asthma control. If asthma symptoms occur in the period between doses, use short-acting β₂-agonist for immediate relief. Rinse mouth with water after use.

HOW SUPPLIED: MDI: (Budesonide-Formoterol Fumarate Dihydrate)(80/4.5) 80mcg-4.5mcg/inh, (160/4.5) 160mcg-4.5mcg/inh [60 inhalations, 120 inhalations]

CONTRAINDICATIONS: Primary treatment of status asthmaticus or other acute asthma attacks or COPD requiring intensive measures.

WARNINGS/PRECAUTIONS: Should not be initiated during acutely/rapidly deteriorating or potentially life-threatening episodes of asthma or COPD. Increase use of inhaled, short-acting β₂-agonists is a marker of deteriorating asthma; re-evaluate and reassess treatment regimen. Should not be used for relief of acute symptoms; inhaled short-acting β₂-agonists should be used. At treatment initiation, regular use of oral/inhaled short-acting β₂-agonists should be d/c. Should not be use more than recommended or at higher doses than recommended; cardiovascular (CV) effects & fatalities reported.

Localized infection of the mouth and pharynx with *Candida albicans* reported; if develops, treat accordingly. Lower respiratory tract infections (eg, pneumonia) reported in patients with COPD. Increased susceptibility to infections; avoid exposure to chicken pox and measles. Caution in patients with active/quiescent tuberculosis, untreated systemic fungal, bacterial, viral, or parasitic infections, or ocular herpes simplex. Deaths due to adrenal insufficiency have occurred with transfer from systemic to inhaled corticosteroids. If withdrawn from systemic corticosteroids, resume oral corticosteroids during stress or severe asthma attack. Wean slowly from systemic corticosteroid use after transferring. Transferring from oral to inhalation therapy may unmask conditions (eg, rhinitis, conjunctivitis, eczema) previously suppressed by corticosteroids. Monitor for systemic corticosteroid effects such as hypercorticism and adrenal suppression (including adrenal crisis); if effects occur reduce dose slowly. May cause paradoxical bronchospasm; d/c immediately and institute alternative therapy. Immediate hypersensitivity reactions (eg, urticaria, angioedema, rash, bronchospasm) reported. CV effects may occur; caution with CV disorder (eg, coronary insufficiency, arrhythmia, HTN). Prolonged use may result in decrease bone mineral density, glaucoma, increased IOP and cataracts. May cause reduction in growth velocity in pediatric patients. Rare cases of eosinophilic conditions (eg, Churg-Strauss syndrome) reported. Caution with convulsive disorders, thyrotoxicosis, and hepatic impairment. May aggravate pre-existing diabetes mellitus and ketoacidosis. Hypokalemia and hyperglycemia may occur.

ADVERSE REACTIONS: Asthma: Nasopharyngitis, headache, upper respiratory tract infections, sinusitis, influenza, back pain, nasal congestion, stomach discomfort. COPD: nasopharyngitis, oral candidiasis, bronchitis, sinusitis, upper respiratory tract infection.

INTERACTIONS: Caution with concomitant use of strong CYP3A4 inhibitors (eg, ketoconazole, ritonavir, atazanavir, indinavir, nefazodone, nelfinavir, saquinavir, telithromycion, itraconazole, clarithromycin); may inhibit the metabolism and increase systemic exposure of budesonide. Caution with monoamine oxidase inhibitors or tricyclic antidepressants, or within 2 weeks of discontinuation of such agents. Concomitant use with β-blockers may block the pulmonary effect of formoterol and may produce severe bronchospasm in patients with asthma. Caution with non-K$^+$-sparing diuretics (eg, loop or thiazide); ECG changes and/or hypokalemia may develop. Do not use any additional inhaled LABAs for any reason, including prevention of exercise-induced bronchospasm or treatment of asthma or COPD. Caution with chronic use of drugs that can reduce bone mass (eg, anticonvulsants, oral corticosteroids).

PREGNANCY: Category C, not for use in nursing.

MECHANISM OF ACTION: Budesonide: Corticosteroid with anti-inflammatory activity; shown to have inhibitory effects on multiple cell types (eg, mast cells, eosinophils, neutrophils, macrophages, lymphocytes) and mediators (eg, histamine, eicosanoids, leukotrienes, cytokines) involved in allergic and non-allergic mediated inflammation. Formoterol: Long-acting selective $β_2$-adrenergic agonist; stimulates intracellular adenyl cyclase which catalyzes conversion of ATP to cAMP to produce relaxation of bronchial smooth muscle and inhibition of release of mediators of immediate hypersensitivity from cells, especially mast cells.

PHARMACOKINETICS: Absorption: (Asthma) Budesonide: Rapidly absorbed. C_{max}=4.5nmol/L; T_{max}=20 min. Formoterol: Rapidly absorbed. C_{max}=136pmol; T_{max}=10 min. (COPD) Budesonide: Rapid (lungs). C_{max}=3.3nmol/L; T_{max}=30 min. Formoterol: Rapid (GI). C_{max}=167pmol/L; T_{max}=15 min. **Distribution:** Budesonide: V_d=3L/kg; plasma protein binding (85-90%). Formoterol: Plasma protein binding (RR enantiomer, 46%), (SS enantiomer, 58%). **Metabolism:** Budesonide: Liver (rapid; extensive) via CYP3A4. Formoterol: Liver (direct glucuronidation and O-demethylation) via CYP2D6, CYP2C. **Elimination:** Budesonide: Urine (60%); feces. $T_{1/2}$=2-3 hrs. Formoterol: Urine (62%); feces (24%).

NURSING CONSIDERATIONS

Assessment: Assess if asthma controlled by inhaled corticosteroids and occasional use of short-acting $β_2$-agonists. Assess for risk factors for decreased bone mineral content (eg, tobacco use, advanced age, sedentary lifestyle, family history of osteoporosis, drugs that decrease bone mass), or any other conditions where treatment is contraindicated or cautioned. Assess for pregnancy/nursing status and for possible drug interactions. Obtain baseline bone mineral density and lung function prior to therapy.

Monitoring: Monitor bone mineral density and lung function periodically. Perform periodic eye exams. Monitor for localized oral infections with *Candida albicans*, decreased bone mass, upper airway symptoms, worsening or acutely deteriorating asthma, asthma instability (serial objective measures of airflow), body height in children, development of glaucoma, increased IOP, posterior subcapsular cataracts, adrenal insufficiency, paradoxical bronchospasm, eosinophilic conditions, pneumonia, and hypersensitivity reactions.

Patient Counseling: Inform about increased risk of asthma-related death and asthma-related hospitalization in pediatric and adolescent patients. Symbicort is not meant to relieve acute asthma symptoms or exacerbations of COPD and extra doses should not be used for that purpose. Notify physician immediately if experience decrease effectiveness of therapy, need more inhalations than usual, or significant decrease in lung function. Do not d/c without physician's guidance. Do not use with other long-acting β₂-agonists for asthma and COPD. Rinse the mouth after inhalation. Contact physician if develop symptoms of pneumonia. Avoid exposure to chicken pox or measles and, if exposed, consult physician without delay. Inform of potential worsening of existing tuberculosis, fungal, bacterial, viral, or parasitic infections, or ocular herpes simplex. Inform about risks of hypercorticism and adrenal suppression, decreased bone mineral density, cataracts or glaucoma and reduced growth velocity. Taper slowly from systemic corticosteroids if transferring to Symbicort. Inform of adverse effects associated with β₂-agonists, such as palpitations, chest pain, rapid HR, tremor, or nervousness. Keep out of reach of children.

Administration: Oral inhalation. Prime before use for the first time by releasing 2 test sprays into the air away from face; shake well for 5 sec before each spray. Prime again if inhaler has not been used for >7 days or when it has been dropped. Shake well for 5 sec before using. **Storage:** 20-25°C (68-77°F). Canister should be at room temperature before use. Store with mouthpiece down.

SYMBYAX   RX
fluoxetine HCl - olanzapine (Lilly)

> Antidepressants increased the risk of suicidal thinking and behavior (suicidality) in short-term studies in children, adolescents, and young adults with Major Depressive Disorder (MDD) and other psychiatric disorders. Monitor and observe closely for clinical worsening, suicidality or unusual changes in behavior in patients who are started on antidepressant therapy. Elderly patients with dementia-related psychosis treated with antipsychotic drugs are at an increased risk of death; most deaths appeared to be cardiovascular (eg, heart failure, sudden death) or infectious (eg, pneumonia) in nature. Symbyax is not approved for pediatric use or for the treatment of patients with dementia-related psychosis.

THERAPEUTIC CLASS: Thienobenzodiazepine/selective serotonin reuptake inhibitor

INDICATIONS: Acute treatment of depressive episodes associated with bipolar I disorder and treatment-resistant depression MDD patients who do not respond to 2 separate trials of different antidepressants of adequate dose and duration in the current episode) in adults.

DOSAGE: *Adults:* Depressive Episodes Associated with Bipolar I Disorder/Treatment Resistant Depression: Initial: 6mg-25mg qd in the evening. Adjust dose based on efficacy and tolerability. Dosing Range: Depressive Episodes Associated with Bipolar I Disorder: 6mg-12mg (olanzapine) to 25mg-50mg (fluoxetine). Treatment Resistant Depression: 6mg-18mg to 25mg-50mg. Max: 18mg-75mg/day. Periodically re-examine the need for continued pharmacotherapy. Hypotension Risk/Hepatic Impairment/Slow Metabolizers/Olanzapine-Sensitive: Initial: 3mg-25mg to 6mg-25mg qd in evening. Titrate:

Increase cautiously. Pregnant: Use lower dose during 3rd trimester. Elderly: Start at the low end of dosing range.

HOW SUPPLIED: Cap: (Olanzapine-Fluoxetine HCl): 3mg-25mg, 6mg-25mg, 6mg-50mg, 12mg-25mg, 12mg-50mg

CONTRAINDICATIONS: During or within 14 days of d/c therapy with a mono-amine oxidase inhibitor (MAOI), during or within 5 weeks of d/c of thioridazine use, and concomitant pimozide use.

WARNINGS/PRECAUTIONS: Neuroleptic malignant syndrome (NMS) reported; d/c and instill intensive symptomatic treatment and monitoring. May cause hyperglycemia; caution in patients with diabetes mellitus (DM) or having borderline increased blood glucose levels. Obtain FPG at the beginning of treatment and periodically during treatment. Hyperlipidemia reported; obtain lipid levels at baseline and periodically thereafter. May cause weight gain; regularly monitor weight. Serotonin syndrome or NMS-like reactions reported; d/c treatment and initiate supportive therapy. Anaphylactoid and pulmonary reactions reported; d/c if unexplained allergic reaction occurs. Tardive dyskinesia (TD) may develop; consider d/c if signs and symptoms of TD appear. Activation of mania/hypomania, hyponatremia, hyperprolactine-mia reported. May cause orthostatic hypotension; caution with cardiovascular disease, cerebrovascular disease, or conditions that predispose to hypotension. Leukopenia, neutropenia, and agranulocytosis reported; d/c at first sign of clinically significant decline in WBC without causative factor or if severe neutropenia (absolute neutrophil count <1000/mm³) develops. May cause esophageal dysmotility and aspiration. Not approved for treatment in patients with Alzheimer's disease. Caution in patients with history of seizures or with conditions that potentially lower the seizure threshold. May increase risk of bleeding events. May impair physical/mental abilities. May disrupt body's ability to reduce core body temperature. Caution with clinically significant prostatic hypertrophy, narrow-angle glaucoma, history of paralytic ileus or related conditions, diseases or conditions affecting hemodynamic responses, hepatic impairment, and elderly. Avoid abrupt withdrawal.

ADVERSE REACTIONS: Asthenia, somnolence, weight gain, increased appetite, disturbance in attention, peripheral edema, tremor, dry mouth, arthralgia, blurred vision, sedation, fatigue, flatulence, restlessness, hypersomnia.

INTERACTIONS: See Contraindications. Caution with CYP2D6 substrates including antidepressants (eg, tricyclic antidepressants (TCA)), antipsychotics (eg, phenothiazines and most atypicals), vinblastine and antiarrhythmics (eg, propafenone, flecainide). Monitor TCA (eg, imipramine, desipramine) and lithium levels. Caution with CNS-active drugs, hepatotoxic drugs, and anticholinergic drugs. May potentiate effects of certain antihypertensive agents. May antagonize levodopa, dopamine agonists. May potentiate orthostatic hypotension with diazepam and alcohol. May increase levels of phenytoin, carbamazepine, haloperidol, clozapine, alprazolam. Caution with other drugs that may affect the serotonergic neurotransmitter systems (eg, triptans, linezolid, lithium, tramadol, St. John's wort), and antipsychotics and other dopamine antagonists; risk for serotonin syndrome. Avoid with SSRIs, SNRIs, and tryptophan. Inducers of CYP1A2 or glucuronyl transferase (eg, carbamazepine, omeprazole, rifampin) may increase olanzapine clearance. CYP1A2 inhibitors (eg, fluvoxamine, some fluoroquinolone antibiotics) may decrease olanzapine clearance. Increased risk of bleeding events with aspirin, NSAIDs, warfarin, and other anti-coagulants. May cause a shift in plasma concentration with drugs that are tightly bound to protein (eg, warfarin, digitoxin) resulting in an adverse effect. May prolong half-life of diazepam. Concomitant use with diuretics, may increase the risk of hyponatremia. Rare reports of prolonged seizures with combined use of electroconvulsive therapy.

PREGNANCY: Category C, not for use in nursing.

MECHANISM OF ACTION: SSRI/Thienobenzodiazepine; unknown. Proposed that activation of 3 monoaminergic neural systems (serotonin, norepinephrine, and dopamine) is responsible for its enhanced antidepressant effect. Fluoxetine: SSRI; inhibits serotonin transport; weak inhibitor of norepinephrine and dopamine transporters. Olanzapine: Thienobenzodiazepine; psychotropic agent with high affinity binding to $5HT_{2a/2c}$, $5HT_6$, D_{1-4}, H_1, and adrenergic $(\alpha)_1$-receptors.

PHARMACOKINETICS: Absorption: Fluoxetine: C_{max}=15-55ng/mL, T_{max}=6-8 hrs. Olanzapine: Well absorbed; T_{max}=6 hrs. **Distribution:** Found in breast milk. Fluoxetine: Crosses placenta; plasma protein binding (94.5%). Olanzapine: V_d=1000L; plasma protein binding (93%). **Metabolism:** Fluoxetine: Liver (extensive) via CYP2D6 pathway; norfluoxetine (active metabolite). Olanzapine: Via direct glucuronidation and CYP450 mediated oxidation; 10-N-glucuronide and 4'-N-desmethyl olanzapine (major metabolites). **Elimination:** Fluoxetine: Kidneys; (acute administration) $T_{1/2}$=1-3 days; (chronic administration) $T_{1/2}$=4-6 days. Olanzapine: Urine (57%), feces (30%); $T_{1/2}$=21-54 hrs.

NURSING CONSIDERATIONS

Assessment: Assess for MDD, bipolar mania, DM, renal/hepatic impairment, or any other conditions where treatment is contraindicated or cautioned. Assess for pregnancy/nursing status, and for possible drug interactions. Assess for dementia-related psychosis and Alzheimer's disease in the elderly. Obtain baseline lipid panel, CBC and FBG levels.

Monitoring: Monitor for signs/symptoms of NMS, serotonin syndrome, hyperglycemia, hyperlipidemia, weight gain, TD, orthostatic hypotension, and other adverse effects. Perform periodic monitoring of FPG, lipid levels, and weight of patient. Perform frequent monitoring of CBC in patients with a history of clinically significant low WBC or drug-induced leukopenia/neutropenia. In patient with clinically significant neutropenia, monitor for fever or other symptoms or signs of infection. In high-risk patients, monitor closely for a suicide attempt.

Patient Counseling: Inform about the benefits and risk of therapy. Treatment may induce clinical worsening and suicide risks. Treatment is not approved for elderly patients with dementia-related psychosis. Advise of risk of orthostatic hypotension. Avoid hazardous tasks (eg, operating machinery/driving), alcohol use, overheating, and dehydration. Notify physician if taking, planning to take, or have stopped taking any prescription or over the counter drugs including herbal supplements. Notify physician if pregnant or intend to become pregnant. Instruct not to breastfeed while on therapy. Instruct to notify physician if rash or hives develop. Hyponatremia may occur. Counsel to take exactly as prescribed; instruct to continue even if symptoms improve. Advise to regularly have FPG, lipid profile, and weight monitored. Seek medical care if experienced serotonin syndrome or NMS-like reactions, increased or unusual bruising or bleeding.

Administration: Oral route. **Storage:** 25°C (77°F); excursions permitted to 15-30°C (59-86°F). Keep tightly closed; protect from moisture.

SYMLIN   RX
pramlintide acetate (Amylin)

> Use with insulin. Risk of insulin-induced severe hypoglycemia, particularly with type 1 DM. Severe hypoglycemia usually occurs within 3 hrs of injection. Serious injuries may occur if severe hypoglycemia occurs while operating a motor vehicle, heavy machinery, or other high-risk activities. Appropriate patient selection, careful patient instruction, and insulin dose adjustments are necessary to reduce this risk.

OTHER BRAND NAMES: SymlinPen (Amylin)

THERAPEUTIC CLASS: Synthetic amylin analog

INDICATIONS: Adjunct treatment in patients with type 1 or type 2 diabetes mellitus (DM) who use mealtime insulin therapy and who have failed to achieve desired glucose control despite optimal insulin therapy. May be used with or without sulfonylurea and/or metformin in type 2 DM.

DOSAGE: *Adults:* Before initiating therapy, reduce insulin dose by 50%. Monitor blood glucose frequently. Adjust insulin dose once target dose of pramlintide is maintained. Type 2 DM: Initial: 60mcg SQ immediately prior to meals. Titrate: 120mcg as tolerated. Type 1 DM: Initial: 15mcg SQ immediately prior to meals. Titrate: Increase by 15mcg increments to 30mcg or 60mcg as tolerated.

HOW SUPPLIED: Inj: 600mcg/mL [5mL]; Pen injector: 1000mcg/mL [1.5mL, 2.7mL]

CONTRAINDICATIONS: Confirmed diagnosis of gastroparesis; hypoglycemia unawareness.

WARNINGS/PRECAUTIONS: Do not mix with insulin; administer as separate injections.

ADVERSE REACTIONS: N/V, headache, anorexia, abdominal pain, fatigue, dizziness, coughing, pharyngitis.

INTERACTIONS: Do not administer with agents that alter GI motility (eg, anticholinergic agents such as atropine), and agents that slow intestinal absorption of nutrients (eg, α-glucosidase inhibitors). Administer analgesics and other oral agents that require rapid onset 1 hr before or 2 hrs after injection.

PREGNANCY: Category C, caution in nursing.

MECHANISM OF ACTION: Amylinomimetic agent that modulates gastric emptying, prevents postprandial rise in plasma glucagon, and produces satiety, which leads to a decreased caloric intake.

PHARMACOKINETICS: Absorption: Absolute bioavailability (30-40%); SQ administration of variable doses resulted in different parameters. **Distribution:** Not extensively bound to blood cells or albumin (40% unbound). **Metabolism:** Kidneys (primarily). Des-lys pramlintide (primary active metabolite). **Elimination:** $T_{1/2}$=48 min.

NURSING CONSIDERATIONS

Assessment: Assess patient does not have confirmed diagnosis of gastroparesis or hypoglycemia unawareness. Evaluate patient's HbA1c, recent blood glucose monitoring data, history of insulin-induced hypoglycemia, current insulin regimen, and body weight. Assess if patient has failed to achieve proper glycemic control despite individualized insulin management. Assess use in patients with visual or dexterity impairment. Assess for possible drug interactions and pregnancy/nursing status.

Monitoring: Monitor for signs/symptoms of hypoglycemia (eg, hunger, headache, sweating, tremor) when using in combination with insulin. Monitor proper glucose control through serum blood glucose levels and HbA1c test.

Patient Counseling: Instruct to never mix with insulin and not to transfer from pen-injector to syringe. If dose missed, wait until next scheduled dose and administer usual amount. Administer immediately prior to each major meal (≥250 calories or ≥30g of carbohydrates). Insulin dose adjustments should be made only by healthcare professional. Patients should have fast-acting sugar (eg, hard candy, glucose tablet, juice) at all times. Self-glucose monitoring should be done on a daily basis. Counsel about signs/symptoms of hypoglycemia (eg, hunger, headache, sweating, tremor, irritability). Instruct regarding the critical importance of maintaining proper glucose control, especially when operating heavy machinery (eg, motor vehicles).

Administration: SQ injection to abdomen or thigh; administration to the arm is not recommended because of variable absorption. Rotate injection sites and injection site should be distinct from site for any concomitant insulin injection. Allow to come to room temperature before injecting. **Storage:** Pen injectors and vials not in use: 2-8°C (36-40°F). Do not freeze. Do not use if frozen. Pen-injectors and vials in use: After 1st use, refrigerate or keep at a temperature <30°C (86°F). Use within 30 days.

SYNAGIS   RX
palivizumab (MedImmune)

THERAPEUTIC CLASS: Monoclonal antibody/RSV F-protein blocker

INDICATIONS: Prevention of serious lower respiratory tract disease caused by respiratory syncytial virus (RSV) in pediatrics at high risk of RSV disease.

DOSAGE: *Pediatrics:* 15mg/kg IM; give 1st dose before start of RSV season, then monthly throughout season. Give monthly also if develop RSV infection.

Patients Undergoing Cardiopulmonary Bypass: Give a dose as soon as possible after procedure then monthly thereafter. Inj volumes >1mL: Give as divided dose.

HOW SUPPLIED: Inj: 50mg/0.5mL, 100mg/1mL

WARNINGS/PRECAUTIONS: Cases of anaphylaxis and anaphylactic shock reported; d/c if severe hypersensitivity reactions occur. Administer appropriate medications (eg, epinephrine) and provide supportive care if anaphylaxis or severe allergic reactions occur. Caution with thrombocytopenia or any coagulation disorder. Safety and efficacy not demonstrated for treatment of established RSV disease.

ADVERSE REACTIONS: Upper respiratory infection, otitis media, rash, increased SGOT, cyanosis, arrhythmia, anaphylaxis, fever, rhinitis, hernia, gastroenteritis, wheezing, cough, vomiting, diarrhea.

PREGNANCY: Category C, safety not known in nursing.

MECHANISM OF ACTION: Monoclonal antibody; exhibits neutralizing and fusion-inhibitory activity against RSV.

PHARMACOKINETICS: Elimination: $T_{1/2}$=20 days.

NURSING CONSIDERATIONS

Assessment: Assess for previous hypersensitivity to the drug, thrombocytopenia or any coagulation disorder.

Monitoring: Monitor for anaphylaxis or acute hypersensitivity reactions. Monitor platelet count.

Patient Counseling: Counsel parents/caregivers about risks and benefits of therapy. Advise to seek medical attention if hypersensitivity reaction occurs. Advise to keep all appointments and if missed, to schedule another as soon as possible.

Administration: IM route. Administer preferably in the anterolateral aspect of the thigh. The gluteal muscle should not be used routinely as an inj site because of the risk of damage to the sciatic nerve. Administer immediately after withdrawal from vial; do not re-enter vial. Do not dilute, shake, or vigorously agitate the vial. **Storage:** 2-8°C (35.6-46.4°F). Do not freeze.

SYNERA   RX
tetracaine - lidocaine (Endo)

THERAPEUTIC CLASS: Acetamide local anesthetic

INDICATIONS: For use on intact skin to provide local dermal analgesia for superficial venous access and superficial dermatological procedures such as excision, electrodessication, and shave biopsy of skin lesions.

DOSAGE: *Adults:* Venipuncture or IV Cannulation: Apply to intact skin for 20-30 min prior to procedure. Superficial Dermatological Procedures: Apply to intact skin for 30 min prior to procedure.
Pediatrics: ≥3 yrs: Venipuncture or IV Cannulation: Apply to intact skin for 20-30 min prior to procedure. Superficial Dermatological Procedure: Apply to intact skin for 30 min prior to procedure.

HOW SUPPLIED: Patch: (Lidocaine-Tetracaine) 70mg-70mg

CONTRAINDICATIONS: PABA hypersensitivity.

WARNINGS/PRECAUTIONS: Serious adverse events may occur in children or pets if ingested. Caution in acutely ill or debilitated. Risk of allergic/anaphylactoid reactions (eg, urticaria, angioedema, bronchospasm, shock). Increased risk of toxicity in severe hepatic disease. Avoid broken or inflamed skin, eye contact, larger area or longer duration than recommended.

ADVERSE REACTIONS: Erythema, blanching, edema, urticaria, angioedema, bronchospasm, shock.

INTERACTIONS: Additive toxic effect with concomitant Class I antiarrhythmics (eg, tocainide, mexiletine). Consider total amount absorbed from all formulations with other local anesthetics.

PREGNANCY: Category B, caution in nursing.

MECHANISM OF ACTION: Lidocaine: Amide-type local anesthetic; blocks Na^+ channels required for initiation and conduction of neuronal impulses. Tetracaine: Ester-type local anesthetic; blocks Na^+ channels required for initiation and conduction of neuronal impulses.

PHARMACOKINETICS: Absorption: C_{max}=1.7ng/mL (lidocaine), <0.9ng/mL (tetracaine); T_{max}=1.7 hrs. (lidocaine). **Distribution:** Lidocaine: V_d=0.8-1.3 L/kg; plasma protein binding (75%); crosses placenta. **Metabolism:** Lidocaine: CYP1A2, CYP3A4 (N-deethylation). Monoethylglycinexylidide, glycinexylidide (active metabolites). Tetracaine: Plasma esterases (hydrolysis). **Elimination:** Lidocaine: Urine; $T_{1/2}$=1.8 hrs.

NURSING CONSIDERATIONS

Assessment: Assess for pseudocholinesterase deficiency, possible drug interactions, cardiac and hepatic impairment.

Monitoring: Monitor for allergic or anaphylactoid reactions (eg, erythema, blanching, edema), cardiac and hepatic dysfunction.

Patient Counseling: Inform that use may lead to diminished or blocked sensation in treated skin. Instruct to wash hands after application; avoid contact with eyes; remove patch before MRI.

Administration: Transdermal route. **Storage:** 25°C (77°F) excursions permitted to 15-30°C (59-86°F).

SYNERCID   RX
dalfopristin - quinupristin (Monarch Pharmaceuticals Inc.)

THERAPEUTIC CLASS: Streptogramin

INDICATIONS: Treatment of complicated skin and skin structure infections (cSSSI) caused by *Staphylococcus aureus* (methicillin-susceptible) or *Streptococcus pyogenes*.

DOSAGE: *Adults:* Usual: 7.5mg/kg IV q12h for at least 7 days. Hepatic Cirrhosis (Child Pugh A or B): May need dose reduction. Infuse over 60 min. *Pediatrics:* ≥12 yrs: Usual: 7.5mg/kg IV q12h for at least 7 days. Hepatic Cirrhosis (Child Pugh A or B): May need dose reduction. Infuse over 60 min.

HOW SUPPLIED: Inj: (Dalfopristin-Quinupristin) 350mg-150mg

WARNINGS/PRECAUTIONS: *C. difficile*-associated diarrhea (CDAD) reported and may range in severity from mild diarrhea to fatal colitis. Flush vein with 5% dextrose following infusion to minimize venous irritation; do not flush with saline or heparin. Arthralgia, myalgia, and total bilirubin elevation reported. Superinfections may occur.

ADVERSE REACTIONS: Infusion-site reactions (eg, inflammation, pain, edema), N/V, pain, rash, hyperbilirubinemia, arthralgia, myalgia.

INTERACTIONS: Caution with drugs metabolized by CYP3A4; may increase plasma levels (eg, cyclosporine A, tacrolimus, midazolam, dihydropyridine calcium channel blockers [eg, nifedipine], verapamil, diltiazem, astemizole, terfenadine, delaviridine, nevirapine, indinavir, ritonavir, vinca alkaloids [eg, vinblastine], docetaxel, paclitaxel, diazepam, cisapride, HMG-CoA reductase inhibitors [eg, lovastatin], methylprednisolone, carbamazepine, quinidine, lidocaine, disopyramide). Monitor cyclosporine levels. Avoid drugs metabolized by CYP3A4 that prolong QTc interval. May inhibit gut metabolism of digoxin.

PREGNANCY: Category B, caution in nursing.

MECHANISM OF ACTION: Streptogramin antibiotic; components act synergistically on bacterial ribosome. Dalfopristin: Inhibits the early phase of protein synthesis. Quinupristin: Inhibits the late phase of protein synthesis.

PHARMACOKINETICS: Absorption: Quinupristin: C_{max}=3.2μg/mL, AUC=7.2μg•hr/mL; Dalfopristin: C_{max}=7.96μg/mL, AUC=10.57μg•hr/mL. **Distribution:** Quinupristin: V_d=0.45L/kg; Dalfopristin: V_d=0.24L/kg. **Metabolism:** Quinupristin: 2 conjugated active metabolites (1 with glutathione; 1 with cysteine); Dalfopristin: 1 nonconjugated active metabolite, via hydrolysis. **Elimination:** Urine: 15% (quinupristin), 19% (dalfopristin), feces (75-77%); T$_{1/2}$=0.85 hrs (quinupristin), 0.70 hrs (dalfopristin).

NURSING CONSIDERATIONS

Assessment: Assess for hepatic impairment, pregnancy/nursing status, and for possible drug interactions (eg, concurrent administration with cyclosporine).

Monitoring: Monitor for CDAD, venous irritation, arthralgia, myalgia, superinfection, and for hyperbilirubinemia. Monitor liver and renal function.

Patient Counseling: Inform about risks/benefits of therapy. Instruct to notify physician if any adverse reactions occur such as watery and bloody stools (with or without stomach cramps and fever) develop, if pregnant/nursing, and of all prescription/ non-prescription drugs being taken.

Administration: IV route. Infuse over 60 min; flush only with D5W to minimize venous irritation. Inspect for particulate matter prior to administration. Do not dilute with saline solution. Refer to PI for detailed preparation and information on compatibility. **Storage:** Before reconstitution, store in refrigerator at 2-8°C (36-46°F); diluted solution stable for 5 hrs at room temperature or for 54 hrs if refrigerated at 2-8°C (36-46°F). Do not freeze.

SYNTHROID   RX
levothyroxine sodium (Abbott)

THERAPEUTIC CLASS: Thyroid replacement hormone

INDICATIONS: Replacement or supplemental therapy in congenital or acquired hypothyroidism except transient hypothyroidism during the recovery phase of subacute thyroiditis. As a pituitary TSH suppressant in the treatment and prevention of euthyroid goiters, including thyroid nodules, lymphocytic thyroiditis, and multinodular goiter. Adjunct to surgery and radioiodine therapy for thyrotropin-dependent well-differentiated thyroid cancer.

DOSAGE: *Adults:* Individualize. Given as a single dose, preferably 30 min to 1 hr before breakfast. Should be taken at least 4 hrs apart from drugs that are known to interfere with its absorption. Hypothyroidism: Usual: 1.7mcg/kg/day PO. >200mcg/day (seldom). Patients ≥50 yrs/<50 yrs With Cardiac Disease: Initial: 25-50mcg/day. Gradually increase every 6-8 weeks until euthyroid. Elderly With Cardiac Disease: Initial: 12.5-25mcg qd PO. Titrate: Increase by 12.5-25mcg every 4-6 weeks until euthyroid. Severe Hypothyroidism: Initial: 12.5-25mcg/day. Titrate: Increase by 25mcg/day every 2-4 weeks until TSH level normalized. Secondary (Pituitary) or Tertiary (Hypothalamic) Hypothyroidism: Titrate: Increase until clinically euthyroid and the serum free-T$_4$ level is restored to the upper half of the normal range. Pregnancy: May require increased doses. Subclinical Hypothyroidism: Lower doses required. Well-Differentiated (papillary or follicular) Thyroid Cancer: >2mcg/kg/day (target level for TSH suppression may be <0.1 mU/L). In high risk patients, target level for TSH suppression may be <0.01 mU/L.
Pediatrics: Individualize. Given as a single dose, preferably 30 min to 1 hr before breakfast. May crush tab and sprinkle over food (applesauce) or mix with 5-10mL water, formula (non-soy), or breast milk. Should be taken at least 4 hrs apart from drugs that are known to interfere with its absorption. Hypothyroidism: Growth/Puberty Complete: 1.7mcg/kg/day. >12 yrs (growth/ puberty incomplete): 2-3mcg/kg/day. 6-12 yrs: 4-5mcg/kg/day. 1-5 yrs: 5-6mcg/kg/day. 6-12 months: 6-8mcg/kg/day. 3-6 months: 8-10mcg/kg/day. 0-3 months: 10-15mcg/kg/day. Cardiac Risk: Lower starting dose and increased based on clinical and laboratory response to treatment. Minimize Hyperactivity in Older Children: Initial: 1/4 recommended dose. Titrate: Increased weekly by 1/4 recommended dose until full recommended dose is reached. Chronic/Severe Hypothyroidism: Children: 25mcg/day. Titrate: Increase by 25mcg for 2 weeks then every 2-4 weeks until euthyroid. Infants with Serum T$_4$ <5mcg/dL: Initial: 50mcg/day.

HOW SUPPLIED: Tab: 25mcg*, 50mcg*, 75mcg*, 88mcg*, 100mcg*, 112mcg*, 125mcg*, 137mcg*, 150mcg*, 175mcg*, 200mcg*, 300mcg* *scored

CONTRAINDICATIONS: Untreated subclinical or overt thyrotoxicosis of any etiology, acute myocardial infarction (MI), uncorrected adrenal insufficiency.

WARNINGS/PRECAUTIONS: Do not use in the treatment of obesity or for weight loss; larger doses in euthyroid patients can cause serious or even life-threatening toxicity. Not for the treatment of infertility unless associated with hypothyroidism. Monitor closely to avoid undertreatment or overtreatment. Long-term therapy has been associated with increased bone resorption, thereby decreasing bone mineral density, especially in post-menopausal women on greater than replacement doses or in women who are receiving suppressive doses. Caution in patients with cardiovascular (CV) disorders and elderly; reduce or withhold dose for a week if cardiac symptoms develops. Caution in patients with nontoxic diffuse goiter or nodular thyroid disease; avoid use if TSH is already suppressed. Patients with concomitant adrenal insufficiency should be treated with replacement glucocorticoids prior to initiation of treatment.

ADVERSE REACTIONS: Fatigue, weight loss, headache, hyperactivity, anxiety, tremors, muscle weakness, palpitations, arrhythmias, diarrhea, hair loss, flushing, decreased bone mineral density, pseudotumor cerebri in pediatrics, hypersensitivity reactions.

INTERACTIONS: Increased risk of coronary insufficiency with sympathomimetics and coronary artery disease (CAD). May potentiate oral anticoagulant effects; adjust dose and monitor PT/INR. Increased antidiabetic or insulin requirements. Dopamine/dopamine agonists (≥1mcg/kg/min), glucocorticoids (hydrocortisone ≥100mg/day or equivalent) and octreotide (>100mcg/day) may reduce TSH secretion. Decreased absorption with aluminum and magnesium antacids, simethicone, cholestyramine, colestipol, calcium carbonate, kayexalate, ferrous sulfate, orlistat, and sucralfate; administer at least 4 hours apart. Aminoglutethimide, lithium, methimazole, propylthiouracil (PTU), sulfonamides and tolbutamide decrease thyroid hormone secretion. Amiodarone and iodide (including iodine-containing radiographic contrast agents) may increase or decrease thyroid hormone secretion. Clofibrate, estrogens, estrogen-containing oral contraceptives, heroin/methadone, 5-FU, mitotane and tamoxifen increase TBG concentrations. Androgens/anabolic steroids, asparaginase, glucocorticoids and slow-release nicotinic acid decrease serum TBG concentrations. Furosemide, heparin, hydantoins, fenamates, phenylbutazone and salicylates may cause protein-binding site displacement. Carbamazepine, hydantoins, phenobarbital and rifampin increase hepatic metabolism, resulting in hypothyroidism. Amiodarone, β-adrenergic antagonists, glucocorticoids, and PTU decrease T$_4$ 5'-deiodinase activity. Increase therapeutic and toxic effects of both drugs with tri/tetracyclic antidepressants. Reduced therapeutic effect of digitalis glycosides. Development of antithyroid microsomal antibodies, hypothyroidism and hyperthyroidism with interferon-α. Transient painless thyroiditis reported with interleukin-2. Increase thyroid hormone requirement with sertraline. HTN and tachycardia reported with ketamine. Decreased clearance of theophylline in hypothyroid state. Decreased uptake of iodine-containing radiolabeled ions. Excessive use with somatrem/somatropin may accelerate epiphyseal closure. Chloral hydrate, diazepam, ethionamide, lovastatin, metoclopromide, 6-mercaptopurine, nitroprusside, para-aminosalicylate sodium, perphenazine, resorcinol (excessive topical use) and thiazide diuretics have been associated with thyroid hormone and/or TSH level alterations. Avoid mixing crushed tabs with foods/formula with large amounts of iron, soybean or fiber.

PREGNANCY: Category A, caution in nursing.

MECHANISM OF ACTION: Thyroid hormone; not understood, suspected to control DNA transcription and protein synthesis.

PHARMACOKINETICS: Absorption: Absolute bioavailability (40%-80%). **Distribution:** Plasma protein binding (99%); crosses placenta; found in breast milk. **Metabolism:** Sequential deiodination in the liver (mainly), kidneys, and other tissues. T$_3$ (active metabolite) **Elimination:** Urine; feces (approximately 20% unchanged). (T$_4$) T$_{1/2}$=6-7 days; (T$_3$) T$_{1/2}$≤2 days.

NURSING CONSIDERATIONS

Assessment: Assess for suppressed TSH level with normal T_3 and T_4 or overt thyrotoxicosis, hypersensitivity history, CV disease (angina or acute MI), uncorrected adrenal insufficiency, thyroid diseases (nontoxic diffuse or nodular goiter), endocrine disorders (hypothalamic/pituitary hormone deficiencies and/or autoimmune polyglandular disorders), DM, clotting status, upcoming surgery and possible drug and test interactions. Assess infants for associated congenital anomalies, pregnancy/nursing status.

Monitoring: Perform frequent lab tests and clinical evaluation of thyroid functions (TSH and free T_4 levels), glucose/lipid metabolism, blood and/or urinary glucose in diabetics, and clotting parameters in patients on anticoagulants. Monitor for effects on CV system (eg, arrhythmia, coronary insufficiency), growth development, bone metabolism, cognitive function, emotional status, GI functions, reproductive functions, and signs/symptoms of thyrotoxicosis.

Patient Counseling: Counsel to notify prescriber of any allergies or concomitant medications including OTCs. Notify physician of any comorbidities. Counsel diabetic patients to monitor blood/urinary glucose closely and to report any changes. Advise patients on anticoagulants to monitor clotting parameters frequently. Except in cases of transient hypothyroidism, levothyroxine is to be taken for life and not to be taken for the treatment of obesity or weight reduction. Take 30 min to 1 hr prior to breakfast on an empty stomach with a full glass of water. Inform that it may take several weeks before a noticeable improvement. Notify the prescriber if toxicity occurs (eg, rapid/irregular heartbeat, irritability, sleeplessness, heat intolerance, etc.). Notify prescriber if pregnant/nursing or planning to become pregnant. Notify surgeon or dentist of levothyroxine use prior to procedure. Partial, temporary hair loss rarely occurs during first few months of therapy.

Administration: Oral route. **Storage:** Store at 25°C (77°F); excursions permitted to 15-30°C (59-86°F). Protect from light and moisture.

SYNVISC   RX
hylan G-F 20 (Wyeth)

THERAPEUTIC CLASS: Hylan polymer

INDICATIONS: Treatment of osteoarthritis (OA) knee pain inadequately responsive to conservative nonpharmacologic therapy and simple analgesics.

DOSAGE: *Adults:* Usual: Intra-articular injection once weekly (one week apart) for total of three injections.

HOW SUPPLIED: Inj: 8mg/mL

CONTRAINDICATIONS: Knee joint infections, hyaluronan hypersensitivity, skin diseases or infections in injection site area.

WARNINGS/PRECAUTIONS: Avoid with skin disinfectants containing quaternary ammonium salts; hyaluronan can precipitate in their presence. Do not inject extra-articularly or into synovial tissue and capsule. Intravascular injections may cause systemic adverse events. Caution with allergies to avian proteins, feathers, and egg products. Avoid with severely inflamed knee joints. Remove synovial fluid or effusion, if present, before injecting. Follow strict aseptic administration. Caution with lymphatic or venous stasis. Avoid strenuous activity or prolonged weight-bearing activities after injection. Packaging contains dry natural rubber latex.

ADVERSE REACTIONS: Injection-site pain, knee swelling/effusion, rash, calf cramps, ankle edema, muscle pain.

INTERACTIONS: Do not inject anesthetics or other drugs into knee joint during therapy.

PREGNANCY: Safety in pregnancy and nursing not known.

MECHANISM OF ACTION: Hylan polymer.

NURSING CONSIDERATIONS

Assessment: Assess for knee joint infection, skin disease, or infection in area of injection site, pregnancy/nursing status, lymphatic or venous stasis.

Monitoring: Monitor for signs/symptoms of allergic reaction (eg, rash, hives, itching, fever), knee joint effusion/swelling, and local skin reactions.

Patient Counseling: Inform that use may cause transient pain/swelling of injected joint. Instruct to avoid any strenuous or prolonged weight-bearing activity (eg, jogging, tennis) within 48 hrs of injection. Seek medical attention if symptoms of allergic reaction occur.

Administration: Intra-articular. **Storage:** 30°C (86°F). Do not freeze. Protect from light.

TACHOSIL
absorbable fibrin sealant (Baxter)

RX

THERAPEUTIC CLASS: Topical thrombin/fibrinogen

INDICATIONS: Adjunct to hemostasis for use in cardiovascular surgery when control of bleeding by standard surgical techniques (such as suture, ligature or cautery) is ineffective or impractical.

DOSAGE: Apply the yellow, active side of the patch to the bleeding area and hold in place with gentle pressure for ≥3 min. Number of patches to be applied should be determined by the size of the bleeding area. Max: 7 patches sized 9.5 x 4.8cm, 14 patches sized 4.8 x 4.8cm, or 42 patches sized 3.0 x 2.5cm.

HOW SUPPLIED: Patch: (Human fibrinogen-Human thrombin) 5.5mg-2.0 U/cm² [9.5cm x 4.8cm, 1ˢ; 4.8cm x 4.8cm, 2ˢ; 3.0cm x 2.5cm, 1ˢ 5ˢ]

CONTRAINDICATIONS: Intravascular application.

WARNINGS/PRECAUTIONS: Do not use in renal pelvis or ureter procedures, the closure of skin incisions, or neurological procedures. Not to be used for the treatment of severe or brisk arterial bleeding and not intended as a substitute for meticulous surgical technique and proper application of suture, ligature, or conventional procedures for hemostasis. Hypersensitivity or allergic/anaphylactoid reactions may occur with first-time or repetitive application. Do not leave patch in an infected or contaminated space; may potentiate existing infection. When placing into cavities or closed spaces, exercise care to avoid overpacking. Use only minimum amount of patches necessary to achieve hemostasis. Unattached pieces should be carefully removed. May carry risk of transmitting infectious agents, including viruses and Creutzfeldt-Jakob disease (CJD) agents.

ADVERSE REACTIONS: Atrial fibrillation, pyrexia, pleural effusion, hemorrhagic anemia, tachyarrhythmia, pericardial effusion, post-procedural hemorrhage.

PREGNANCY: Category C, caution in nursing.

MECHANISM OF ACTION: Topical thrombin/fibrinogen; soluble fibrinogen transformed into fibrin, by enzymatic action of thrombin, which polymerizes into a fibrin clot that adheres the collagen patch to the wound surface and achieves hemostasis.

NURSING CONSIDERATIONS

Assessment: Assess for previous hypersensitivity reactions, site of bleeding, and pregnancy/nursing status.

Monitoring: Monitor for signs/symptoms of an allergic/hypersensitivity reactions, and for the transmission of infectious agents (eg, viruses, CJD).

Patient Counseling: Advise patients that patch is made from human blood, and it may carry a risk of transmitting infectious agents, (eg, viruses, CJD agents). Instruct to consult physician if symptoms of B19 virus infection appear (fever, drowsiness, chills, and runny nose followed about 2 weeks later by a rash and joint pain).

Administration: Topical route. Refer to PI for preparation and application of patch. **Storage:** 2-25°C. Do not freeze.

TAMBOCOR

RX

flecainide acetate (Graceway)

An excessive mortality or non-fatal cardiac arrest was reported in patients with asymptomatic non-life-threatening ventricular arrhythmias with MI >6 days but <2 yrs prior. Class 1C antiarrhythmic unacceptable without life-threatening ventricular arrhythmias. Not recommended for chronic atrial fibrillation. Case reports of ventricular proarrhythmic effects with atrial fibrillation/flutter.

THERAPEUTIC CLASS: Class IC antiarrhythmic

INDICATIONS: Prevention of paroxysmal supraventricular tachycardias (PSVT), paroxysmal atrial fibrillation/flutter (PAF) associated with disabling symptoms in patients without structural heart disease. Prevention of documented ventricular arrhythmias such as sustained ventricular tachycardia (VT).

DOSAGE: *Adults:* PSVT/PAF: Initial: 50mg q12h. Titrate: May increase by 50mg bid every 4 days. Max: 300mg/day. Sustained VT: Initial: 100mg q12h. Titrate: May increase by 50mg bid every 4 days. Max: 400mg/day. CrCl ≤35mL/min: Initial: 100mg qd or 50mg bid. Reduce dose by 50% with amiodarone. *Pediatrics:* <6 months: Initial: 50mg/m²/day given bid-tid. ≥6 months: Initial: 100mg/m²/day given bid-tid. Max: 200mg/m²/day. Reduce dose by 50% with amiodarone.

HOW SUPPLIED: Tab: 50mg, 100mg*, 150mg* *scored

CONTRAINDICATIONS: Right bundle branch block associated with left hemiblock (without a pacemaker), pre-existing 2nd- or 3rd-degree atrioventricular (AV) block, cardiogenic shock.

WARNINGS/PRECAUTIONS: Ventricular proarrhythmic effects may occur with atrial fibrillation/flutter. May cause or worsen congestive heart failure (CHF) and arrhythmias. Slows cardiac conduction; dose related increases in PR, QRS, and QT intervals reported. Conduction changes may cause sinus pause, sinus arrest, bradycardia, 2nd- or 3rd-degree AV block. Extreme caution with sick sinus syndrome. May increase endocardial pacing thresholds and suppress ventricular escape with pacemakers. Correct hypokalemia or hyperkalemia before therapy. Monitor with significant hepatic impairment. Initiate treatment of sustained VT in the hospital.

ADVERSE REACTIONS: Arrhythmias, hepatic dysfunction, cardiac arrest, CHF, dizziness, visual disturbances, headache, fatigue, N/V, dyspnea.

INTERACTIONS: Additive negative inotropic effects with β-blockers (eg, propranolol). Potentiated by cimetidine, amiodarone, CYP2D6 inhibitors (eg, quinidine). Increases digoxin levels. Increased elimination with phenytoin, phenobarbital, carbamazepine. Diltiazem, nifedipine, verapamil, disopyramide not recommended.

PREGNANCY: Category C, safety not known in nursing.

MECHANISM OF ACTION: Class 1C antiarrhythmic agent with local anesthetic activity; decreases intracardiac conduction in all parts of the heart with greatest effect on His-Purkinje system (H-V conduction).

PHARMACOKINETICS: Absorption: Complete. T_{max}=3 hrs. **Distribution:** Plasma protein binding (40%). Found in human milk. **Metabolism:** Extensive, via CYP2D6. Meta-O-dealkylated flecainide (active metabolite). **Elimination:** Urine (30% unchanged), feces (5%); $T_{1/2}$=20 hrs, 29 hrs (at birth), 11-12 hrs (3 months), 6 hrs (1 yr), 8 hrs (1-12 yrs), and 11-12 hrs (12-15 yrs).

NURSING CONSIDERATIONS

Assessment: Assess for pre-existing 2nd- or 3rd-degree AV block, right bundle branch block associated with a left hemiblock, implanted pacemaker, cardiogenic shock, myocardial infarction (MI), asymptomatic non-life threatening ventricular arrhythmia, atrial fibrillation/flutter, cardiomyopathy, pre-existing severe HF or low ejection fraction, sick sinus syndrome, supraventricular tachycardia, hypersensitivity, pregnancy/nursing status, and possible drug interactions. Correct hypokalemia or hyperkalemia prior to therapy.

Monitoring: Determine pacing threshold in patients with pacemaker prior to therapy, after 1 week, and at regular intervals thereafter. Periodically monitor plasma levels with renal/hepatic impairment, CHF, and/or those on concurrent amiodarone therapy. Monitor for HR, ECG changes, paradoxical increase in ventricular rate, proarrhythmic effects (new or worsened supraventricular or ventricular arrhythmia), worsening of CHF, effects on cardiac conduction, bradycardia, and hypersensitivity reactions.

Patient Counseling: Advise about importance of initiating therapy in hospital with continuous rhythmic monitoring. Inform about risks/benefits and report any adverse reactions to physician.

Administration: Oral route. **Storage:** 15-30°C (59-86°F). Store in tight, light-resistant containers.

TAMIFLU RX
oseltamivir phosphate (Genentech)

THERAPEUTIC CLASS: Neuraminidase inhibitor

INDICATIONS: Treatment of uncomplicated acute illness due to influenza in patients ≥1 yr who have been symptomatic for no more than 2 days. Prophylaxis of influenza in patients ≥1 yr.

DOSAGE: *Adults:* Prophylaxis: Begin within 2 days of exposure. 75mg qd for ≥10 days. Community Outbreak: May use up to 6 weeks. CrCl 10-30mL/min: 75mg qod or 30mg qd. Treatment: Begin within 2 days of symptom onset. 75mg bid for 5 days. CrCl 10-30mL/min: 75mg qd for 5 days.
Pediatrics: Prophylaxis: ≥13 yrs: Begin within 2 days of exposure. 75mg qd for ≥10 days. ≥1 yr: 10-Day Regimen: ≤15kg: 30mg qd. >15-23kg: 45mg qd. >23-40kg: 60mg qd. >40kg: 75mg qd. Community Outbreak: May use up to 6 weeks. Treatment: ≥13 yrs: Begin within 2 days of symptom onset. 75mg bid for 5 days. ≥1 yr: 5-Day Regimen: ≤15kg: 30mg bid. >15-23kg: 45mg bid. >23-40kg: 60mg bid. >40kg: 75mg bid.

HOW SUPPLIED: Cap: 30mg, 45mg, 75mg; Sus: 12mg/mL [25 mL]

WARNINGS/PRECAUTIONS: Anaphylaxis and serious skin reactions (eg, toxic epidermal necrolysis, Stevens-Johnson syndrome, erythema multiforme) reported; d/c and initiate appropriate treatment. Postmarketing neuropsychiatric events (eg, delirium, abnormal behavior) reported. Does not prevent complications of influenza (eg, serious bacterial infection). Efficacy in patients with chronic cardiac disease, respiratory disease or immunocompromised patients has not been established. No evidence for efficacy in any illness caused by agents other than influenza viruses Type A and B.

ADVERSE REACTIONS: N/V, diarrhea, cough, headache, fatigue, abdominal pain, otitis media, asthma, epistaxis.

INTERACTIONS: Avoid administration of live attenuated influenza vaccine within 2 weeks before or 48 hrs after; may inhibit replication of live vaccine virus. May increase exposure to oseltamivir carboxylate when coadministered with probenecid.

PREGNANCY: Category C, caution in nursing.

MECHANISM OF ACTION: Neuraminidase inhibitor; inhibits influenza virus neuraminidase, affecting release of viral particles.

PHARMACOKINETICS: Absorption: Readily absorbed. Oseltamivir: C_{max}=65ng/mL; AUC_{0-12h}=112ng•h/mL. Oseltamivir carboxylate (metabolite): C_{max}=348ng/mL; AUC_{0-12h}=2719ng•h/mL. **Distribution:** Oseltamivir carboxylate: (IV) V_d=23-26L; plasma protein binding (3%). Oseltamivir: Plasma protein binding (42%). **Metabolism:** Hepatic (esterases). Oseltamivir carboxylate (metabolite). **Elimination:** Oseltamivir carboxylate: Renal (>99%); feces (<20%); $T_{1/2}$=6-10 hrs. Oseltamivir: $T_{1/2}$=1-3 hrs.

NURSING CONSIDERATIONS

Assessment: Assess for drug hypersensitivity, renal impairment, hereditary fructose intolerance, pregnancy/nursing status, and possible drug interactions.

Monitoring: Monitor for signs/symptoms of neuropsychiatric events (eg, delirium, abnormal behavior) and anaphylaxis/serious skin reactions.

Patient Counseling: Instruct to begin treatment as soon as 1st appearance of flu symptoms or as soon as possible after exposure for prevention. Take missed doses as soon as possible, unless next scheduled dose is within 2 hrs. Medication is not a substitute for flu vaccination and that it may be taken with or without food. Seek medical attention if symptoms of neuropsychiatric events (eg, abnormal behavior) or severe allergic reactions occur. Counsel that medication contains more than max limit of sorbitol and may cause dyspepsia or diarrhea in hereditary fructose intolerance.

Administration: Oral route. If oral sus is not available, may open caps and mix with sweetened liquids (eg, chocolate syrup). Refer to PI for Emergency Compounding of a PO sus from caps. **Storage:** Powder/Cap: 25°C (77°F); excursions permitted to 15-30°C (59-86°F). Sus: Constituted: 2-8°C (36-46°F) up to 17 days, or 25°C (77°F) for up to 10 days; excursions permitted to 15-30°C (59-86°F). Do not freeze.

TAMOXIFEN RX
tamoxifen citrate (Various)

> For women with ductal carcinoma in situ (DCIS) and women at high risk for breast cancer; serious and life-threatening events including uterine malignancies (eg, endometrial adenocarcinoma, uterine sarcoma), stroke, and pulmonary embolism (PE) reported. Some of these events were fatal. Discuss the potential benefits vs. the potential risks of these serious events with women at high risk of breast cancer and women with DCIS. The benefits of tamoxifen outweigh risks in women already diagnosed with breast cancer.

THERAPEUTIC CLASS: Antiestrogen

INDICATIONS: Treatment of metastatic breast cancer in women and men. Use as an alternative to oophorectomy or ovarian irradiation in premenopausal women with metastatic breast cancer. Treatment of node-positive and axillary node-negative breast cancer in women following mastectomy, axillary dissection, and breast irradiation. To reduce risk of invasive breast cancer in women with DCIS following breast surgery and radiation. Reduction of breast cancer incidence in high risk women. ("High risk," defined as ≥35 yrs of age with 5 yrs predicted risk of breast cancer ≥1.67%, as calculated by the Gail Model). Use for up to 5 yrs.

DOSAGE: *Adults:* Breast Cancer Treatment: 20-40mg qd. Divide daily dosages >20mg into AM and PM doses. Breast Cancer Risk Reduction/DCIS: 20mg qd for 5 yrs.

HOW SUPPLIED: Tab: 10mg, 20mg

CONTRAINDICATIONS: Women who require coumarin-type anticoagulant therapy or who have a history of deep vein thrombosis (DVT), PE.

WARNINGS/PRECAUTIONS: Hypercalcemia reported in patients with bone metastases. Increased incidence of uterine malignancies (eg, endometrial carcinoma, uterine sarcoma) and endometrial changes including hyperplasia and polyps with use. Endometriosis, fibroids, ovarian cysts, and menstrual irregularities also reported. Increased incidence of thromboembolic events (eg, DVT, PE). Malignant and nonmalignant (eg, changes in liver enzyme levels) effects on the liver reported. Ocular disturbances reported. Leukopenia, anemia, thrombocytopenia, neutropenia, pancytopenia reported. Promptly evaluate abnormal vaginal bleeding if receiving or previously received tamoxifen. Patients receiving or who have previously received tamoxifen should have annual gynecological examinations and should promptly notify physician if experience any abnormal gynecological symptoms (eg, menstrual irregularities, abnormal vaginal bleeding, changes in vaginal discharge, pelvic pain or pressure). May cause fetal harm during pregnancy; avoid pregnancy within 2 months of d/c therapy. May cause hyperlipidemia; periodic monitoring of plasma TG and cholesterol may be indicated in patients with pre-existing hyperlipidemia. Does not cause infertility even with menstrual irregularity. Perform periodic CBC, including platelet counts and periodic LFTs. Second primary tumors reported.

ADVERSE REACTIONS: Hot flashes, vaginal discharge, fatigue/asthenia, mood disturbances, insomnia, pharyngitis, N/V, irregular menses, fluid retention, pain, infection, flu syndrome, HTN, (men) loss of libido, impotence.

INTERACTIONS: Increases effects of coumarin-type anticoagulants. Increased risk of thromboembolic events with cytotoxic agents. Decreases letrozole and anastrozole levels; avoid coadministration with anastrozole. Increased levels with bromocriptine. Decreased levels with rifampin, aminoglutethimide, medroxyprogesterone, and phenobarbital. Erythromycin, cyclosporine, nifedipine and diltiazem may inhibit metabolism.

PREGNANCY: Category D, not for use in nursing.

MECHANISM OF ACTION: Non-steroidal antiestrogen; competes with estrogen for binding sites in target tissues.

PHARMACOKINETICS: Absorption: C_{max}=40ng/mL; T_{max}=5 hrs. N-desmethyl tamoxifen: C_{max}=15ng/mL. **Metabolism:** N-desmethyl tamoxifen (major metabolite). **Elimination:** Feces (primary); $T_{1/2}$=5-7 days.

NURSING CONSIDERATIONS

Assessment: Assess for history of DVT and PE, hepatic impairment, hyperlipidemia, pregnancy/nursing status, risk factors (eg, age, family history of breast cancer, breast biopsy results), and possible drug interactions. Perform baseline breast exam, mammogram, and gynecologic exam.

Monitoring: Monitor for signs/symptoms of hypercalcemia, uterine malignancies, endometrial changes, thromboembolic events (eg, PE, DVT), ocular disturbances, and for hypersensitivity reactions. Monitor CBC with platelets and LFTs periodically. Monitor PT when used with coumarin-type anticoagulants. Perform breast exam, mammogram, and gynecologic exam routinely. Perform periodic monitoring of plasma TG and cholesterol levels in patients with pre-existing hyperlipidemia.

Patient Counseling: Inform of pregnancy risks; advise to use nonhormonal contraception during therapy and for 2 months after d/c. Instruct women to seek medical attention if they experience symptoms of new breast lumps, abnormal vaginal bleeding, gynecological symptoms (eg, menstrual irregularities, changes in vaginal discharge, pelvic pain or pressure), leg swelling/tenderness, unexplained SOB, or changes in vision.

Administration: Oral route. **Storage:** 20-25°C (68-77°F). Dispense in a well-closed, light-resistant container with a child-resistant closure.

TAPAZOLE   RX
methimazole (King)

THERAPEUTIC CLASS: Thyroid hormone synthesis inhibitor

INDICATIONS: Treatment of hyperthyroidism. To ameliorate hyperthyroidism prior to subtotal thyroidectomy or radioactive iodine therapy. Also indicated when thyroidectomy is contraindicated or not advisable.

DOSAGE: *Adults:* PO: Given in 3 equal doses at 8-hr intervals. Initial: Mild: 15mg/day. Moderately Severe: 30-40mg/day. Severe: 60mg/day. Maint: 5-15mg/day.
Pediatrics: PO: Given in 3 equal doses at 8-hr intervals. Initial: 0.4mg/kg/day. Maint: 1/2 of initial dose.

HOW SUPPLIED: Tab: 5mg*, 10mg* *scored

CONTRAINDICATIONS: Nursing mothers.

WARNINGS/PRECAUTIONS: Can cause fetal harm. Agranulocytosis, leukopenia, thrombocytopenia, aplastic anemia (pancytopenia) may occur; monitor bone marrow function. D/C with agranulocytosis, aplastic anemia (pancytopenia), hepatitis or exfoliative dermatitis. Fulminant hepatitis, hepatic necrosis, and encephalopathy reported; d/c with liver abnormality, including transaminases >3x ULN. Monitor thyroid function periodically. May cause hypoprothrombinemia and bleeding; monitor PT.

ADVERSE REACTIONS: Agranulocytosis, granulocytopenia, thrombocytopenia, aplastic anemia, drug fever, lupus-like syndrome, insulin autoimmune syndrome, hepatitis, periarteritis, hypoprothrombinemia, skin rash, urticaria, N/V, epigastric distress.

INTERACTIONS: May potentiate oral anticoagulants. β-blockers, digitalis, theophylline may need dose reduction when patient becomes euthyroid. Caution with other drugs that cause agranulocytosis.

PREGNANCY: Category D, contraindicated in nursing.

MECHANISM OF ACTION: Inhibits synthesis of thyroid hormones.

PHARMACOKINETICS: Absorption: Readily absorbed (GI tract). **Distribution:** Crosses placenta and found in breast milk. **Elimination:** Urine.

NURSING CONSIDERATIONS

Assessment: Assess for drug hypersensitivity, pregnancy/nursing status, and possible drug interactions.

Monitoring: Monitor for signs of illness (eg, fever, sore throat, malaise, skin eruptions, headache), and hepatic dysfunction (eg, anorexia, upper quadrant pain). Monitor CBC, LFTs, PT and bone marrow function. Monitor thyroid function periodically.

Patient Counseling: Instruct to inform physician if pregnant/nursing or planning to become pregnant. Instruct to report signs/symptoms of illness (eg, fever, general malaise, sore throat) to physician.

Administration: Oral route. **Storage:** 15-30°C (59-86°F).

TARCEVA   RX
erlotinib (Genentech/OSI)

THERAPEUTIC CLASS: Epidermal growth factor receptor tyrosine kinase inhibitor

INDICATIONS: Treatment of locally advanced or metastatic non-small cell lung cancer (NSCLC) after failure of at least one prior chemotherapy regimen. Maintenance treatment of locally advanced or metastatic NSCLC whose disease has not progressed after four cycles of platinum-based first-line chemotherapy. First-line treatment of locally advanced, unresectable, or metastatic pancreatic cancer in combination with gemcitabine.

DOSAGE: *Adults:* NSCLC: 150mg qd. Pancreatic Cancer: 100mg qd in combination with gemcitabine. Continue until disease progression or unacceptable toxicity. Take at least 1 hr before or 2 hrs after ingestion of food. Severe Diarrhea/Severe Skin Reactions: May require dose reduction or temporary interruption of therapy. When dose reduction is necessary, reduce dose in 50-mg decrements. Concomitant Use With Strong CYP3A4 Inhibitors or Inhibitors of Both CYP3A4 and CYP1A2: Reduce dose if severe adverse events occur. Concomitant Use With CYP3A4 Inducers (Rifampicin): Consider alternative treatment or increase the dose at 2-week intervals. Max: 450mg. Cigarette Smoker: Increase the dose. Max: 300mg.

HOW SUPPLIED: Tab: 25mg, 100mg, 150mg

WARNINGS/PRECAUTIONS: Serious interstitial lung disease (ILD)-like events, including fatalities, reported; d/c if ILD diagnosed. Hepatotoxicity, hepatorenal syndrome, renal failure/insufficiency reported. Perform periodic LFTs; interrupt or d/c if total bilirubin >3X ULN and/or transaminases >5X ULN if pretreatment values normal and if with severe LFT changes. If dehydration occurs, interrupt therapy and intensively rehydrate; periodically monitor renal function and serum electrolytes. Caution with history of peptic ulceration or diverticular disease; d/c if GI perforation develops. Bullous, blistering, and exfoliative skin conditions, corneal perforation/ulceration reported; interrupt or d/c if symptoms develop or worsen. May cause myocardial infarction (MI)/ischemia, cerebrovascular accident (CVA), microangiopathic hemolytic anemia with thrombocytopenia, and fetal harm. INR elevations and infrequent bleeding events reported.

ADVERSE REACTIONS: Rash, diarrhea, anorexia, fatigue, dyspnea, cough, N/V, infection, stomatitis, pruritus, dry skin, conjunctivitis, keratoconjunctivitis sicca, abdominal pain, decreased weight.

INTERACTIONS: Increased concentrations with ketoconazole and other strong CYP3A4 inhibitors including ciprofloxacin, atazanavir, clarithromycin, indinavir, itraconazole, nefazodone, nelfinavir, ritonavir, saquinavir, telithromycin, troleandomycin, voriconazole, and grapefruit or grapefruit juice. CYP3A4 inducers may decrease plasma concentrations; use of CYP3A4 inducers (eg, rifampin, rifabutin, rifapentine, phenytoin, carbamazepine, phenobarbital, St. John's wort) is not recommended unless alternative therapy is unavailable. Cigarette smoking may reduce AUC. May decrease the AUC of CYP3A4 substrate midazolam. Drugs that alter pH of upper GI tract may alter solubility and bioavailability; concomitant use of proton pump inhibitors should be avoided. PT or INR changes with warfarin or other coumarin-derivative anticoagulants. Use with anti-angiogenic agents, corticosteroids, NSAIDs, and/or taxane-based chemotherapy may increase risk of GI perforation.

PREGNANCY: Category D, not for use in nursing.

MECHANISM OF ACTION: Kinase inhibitor; inhibits the intracellular phosphorylation of tyrosine kinase associated with epidermal growth factor receptor (EGFR).

PHARMACOKINETICS: Absorption: T_{max}=4 hrs. **Distribution:** V_d=232L; plasma protein binding (93%). **Metabolism:** CYP3A4 (major); CYP1A2, 1A1 (minor). **Elimination:** Feces (83%), urine (8%); $T_{1/2}$=36.2hrs.

NURSING CONSIDERATIONS

Assessment: Assess for lung disease/infection, hepatic/renal impairment, dehydration, history of peptic ulceration or diverticular disease, pregnancy/nursing status, and possible drug interactions. Obtain baseline LFTs and renal function. If taking warfarin or other coumarin anticoagulants, obtain baseline PT/INR.

Monitoring: Monitor for signs and symptoms of ILD (eg, dyspnea, cough, fever), hepatotoxicity, hepatorenal syndrome, renal failure/insufficiency, and dehydration. Monitor LFTs (transaminases, bilirubin, alkaline phosphatase), renal function and serum electrolytes if there is risk of dehydration. Monitor for signs/symptoms of GI perforation, bullous and exfoliative skin disorders, MI/ischemia, CVA, microangiopathic hemolytic anemia with thrombocytopenia, and ocular disorders (eg, corneal perforation/ulceration). If taking concomitant warfarin or coumarin anticoagulants, monitor PT/INR.

Patient Counseling: Inform of risks of therapy. Instruct to notify physician if notice onset or worsening of skin rash, severe or persistent diarrhea, N/V, anorexia, SOB, cough, or if eye irritation occurs. Avoid sun exposure; recommend use of sunscreen. Advise to stop smoking and to avoid becoming pregnant while on therapy.

Administration: Oral route. **Storage:** 25°C (77°F); excursions permitted to 15-30° (59-86°F).

TARKA

verapamil HCl - trandolapril (Abbott)   **RX**

> ACE inhibitors can cause death/injury to developing fetus during 2nd and 3rd trimesters. D/C if pregnancy is detected.

THERAPEUTIC CLASS: ACE inhibitor/calcium channel blocker (nondihydropyridine)

INDICATIONS: Treatment of HTN.

DOSAGE: *Adults:* Replacement Therapy: 1 tab qd with food.

HOW SUPPLIED: Tab: (Trandolapril-Verapamil) 2mg-180mg, 1mg-240mg, 2mg-240mg, 4mg-240mg

CONTRAINDICATIONS: Severe left ventricular dysfunction, hypotension, cardiogenic shock, sick sinus syndrome or 2nd- or 3rd-degree atrioventricular

(AV) block (except with functioning ventricular pacemaker), Atrial fibrillation (A-Fib)/atrial flutter (A-flutter) with an accessory bypass tract, history of ACE inhibitor-associated angioedema.

WARNINGS/PRECAUTIONS: Monitor for hypotension with surgery or anesthesia. Risk of hyperkalemia with renal insufficiency, diabetes mellitus (DM). D/C if jaundice develops. Avoid with moderate to severe cardiac failure and ventricular dysfunction if taking a β-blocker. May cause angioedema, cough, fetal/neonatal morbidity and death, hypotension, AV block, anaphylactoid reactions, transient bradycardia, PR-interval prolongation. Monitor LFTs periodically. Reduce dose with severe hepatic dysfunction. Caution with congestive heart failure (CHF), hypertrophic cardiomyopathy, renal or hepatic dysfunction. Decrease dose in those with decreased neuromuscular transmission. Monitor WBCs with collagen-vascular disease and/or renal disease. Not for initial treatment.

ADVERSE REACTIONS: AV block, constipation, cough, dizziness, fatigue, headache, increased hepatic enzymes, chest pain, upper respiratory tract infection (URI)/congestion.

INTERACTIONS: Additive effects on HR, AV conduction, and contractility with β-blockers. Potentiates other antihypertensives. May increase digoxin, carbamazepine, theophylline, and cyclosporine levels. Avoid disopyramide within 48 hrs before or 24 hrs after verapamil. Additive negative inotropic effects and AV conduction prolongation with flecainide. Avoid quinidine with hypertrophic cardiomyopathy. Monitor lithium. Increased clearance with phenobarbital. Rifampin may reduce oral bioavailability. May potentiate neuromuscular blockers; both agents may need dose reduction. Risk of hyperkalemia with K⁺-sparing diuretics, K⁺ supplements. Caution with inhalation anesthetics. Risks of hypotension, bradyarrhythmias, and lactic acidosis with clarithromycin and erythromycin ethylsuccinate. Nitritoid reactions (eg, facial flushing, N/V, hypotension) reported rarely with injectable gold.

PREGNANCY: Category C (1st trimester) and D (2nd and 3rd trimesters), not for use in nursing.

MECHANISM OF ACTION: Trandolapril: ACE inhibitor; inhibition results in decreased plasma angiotensin II, which leads to decreased vasopressor activity and decreased aldosterone secretion. Verapamil: Calcium channel blocker; modulates influx of ionic calcium across the cell membrane of the arterial smooth muscle as well as in conductile and contractile myocardial cells. Decreases systemic vascular resistance, usually without orthostatic decreases in BP or reflex tachycardia.

PHARMACOKINETICS: Absorption: Verapamil: Absolute bioavailability (20-35%), T_{max}=4-15 hrs. Trandolopril: Absolute bioavailability (approximate 10%), T_{max}=0.5-2 hrs. **Distribution:** Verapamil: Plasma protein binding (90%). Trandolapril: Plasma protein binding (80%). **Metabolism:** Verapamil: Liver. **Elimination:** Verapamil: Urine (70% metabolite, 3-4% unchanged), feces (16% metabolite). Trandolapril: Urine (33% metabolite, <1% unchanged), feces (66% metabolite).

NURSING CONSIDERATIONS

Assessment: Assess for severe left ventricular dysfunction, hypotension, cardiogenic shock, sick sinus syndrome, 2nd- or 3rd-degree AV block, A-fib/A-flutter with an accessory bypass tract, history of angioedema, heart failure, hypotension, LFTs, renal function, CHF, accessory bypass tract, hypertrophic cardiomyopathy, CBC with platelets and differential, pregnancy/nursing status, neuromuscular disorders (Duchenne's), and possible drug interactions.

Monitoring: Monitor for angioedema, cough, anaphylactoid reactions, LFTs, renal function, headaches, URI, heart block, chest pains, CBC with platelets and differential count, serum electrolytes.

Patient Counseling: Counsel regarding adverse effects (eg, angioedema, neutropenia, jaundice) and instruct to report any signs/symptoms. Inform of risks when taken during pregnancy. Educate about need for periodic follow-ups and blood tests to rule out adverse effects and to monitor therapeutic effects.

Administration: Oral route. **Storage:** 15-25°C (59-77°F). Dispense in tightly closed container with safety closure.

TASIGNA RX
nilotinib (Novartis)

> Prolongs QT interval. Sudden deaths reported. Avoid with hypokalemia, hypomagnesemia, or long QT syndrome. Correct hypokalemia or hypomagnesemia prior to administration and monitor periodically. Avoid drugs known to prolong the QT interval and strong CYP3A4 inhibitors. Avoid food 2 hrs before and 1 hr after taking dose. Caution with hepatic impairment; dose reduction recommended. Monitor QTc at baseline, 7 days after initiation, and periodically thereafter, as well as following any dose adjustments.

THERAPEUTIC CLASS: Kinase inhibitor

INDICATIONS: Treatment of adult patients with newly diagnosed Philadelphia chromosome positive chronic myeloid leukemia (Ph+CML) in chronic phase. Treatment of chronic phase and accelerated phase Philadelphia chromosome positive chronic myelogenous leukemia (CML) in adult patients resistant or intolerant to prior therapy that included imatinib.

DOSAGE: *Adults:* Newly Diagnosed Ph+ CML-CP: 300mg PO bid. Resistant or Intolerant Ph+ CML-CP/CML-AP: 400mg PO bid at approximately 12 hr intervals. Avoid food 2 hrs before and 1 hr after taking dose. Refer to PI for dosage adjustments based on hematologic and non hematologic toxicities, QT prolongation, hepatic impairment, and drug interactions.

HOW SUPPLIED: Cap: 150mg, 200mg

CONTRAINDICATIONS: Hypokalemia, hypomagnesemia, or long QT syndrome.

WARNINGS/PRECAUTIONS: Myelosuppression associated with neutropenia, thrombocytopenia, and anemia may occur; perform CBC every 2 weeks for the first 2 months, then monthly. Myelosuppression may be reversed by reducing or withholding dose. May increase serum lipase; monitor periodically and use caution with history of pancreatitis. May elevate bilirubin, AST/ALT, and alkaline phosphatase; monitor LFTs periodically. May cause hypophosphatemia, hypokalemia, hyperkalemia, hypocalcemia, hyponatremia; correct electrolyte abnormalities prior to initiation and monitor periodically. Cap contains lactose; avoid with hereditary problems of galactose intolerance, severe lactase deficiency, or glucose-galactose malabsorption. Caution in patients with relevant cardiac disorders (eg, recent myocardial infarction (MI), congestive heart failure (CHF), unstable angina, clinically significant bradycardia). Exposure increased in patients with impaired hepatic function; dose reduction is recommended and QT interval should be monitored. Caution in patients with total gastrectomy; consider frequent follow-up and dose increase or alternative therapy. Laboratory monitoring (eg, CBC, lipid profile, ECG) should be performed periodically. May cause fetal harm when administered to a pregnant woman.

ADVERSE REACTIONS: QT prolongation, rash, pruritus, N/V, fatigue, myalgia, headache, constipation, diarrhea, thrombocytopenia, neutropenia, anemia.

INTERACTIONS: See Boxed Warning. May increase levels of drugs eliminated by CYP3A4 (eg, midazolam), CYP2C8, CYP2C9, CYP2D6, and UGT1A1 enzymes. Caution when coadministering with substrates of CYP3A4 or CYP2C9 enzymes that have a narrow therapeutic index. May induce CYP2B6, CYP2C8, and CYP2C9 enzymes and thereby decrease levels of drugs eliminated by these enzymes. May increase levels of drugs that are substrates of P-glycoprotein (Pgp); caution when coadministering. Concomitant administration of strong inhibitors (eg, ketoconazole) or inducers (eg, rifampicin) of CYP3A4 may increase or decrease levels significantly; avoid concomitant use. Drugs that inhibit Pgp may increase levels; caution when coadministering. Avoid concomitant use with antiarrhythmic drugs and other drugs that may prolong the QT interval. Concomitant use with imatinib may increase the AUC of both drugs. Avoid St. John's wort and grapefruit products. Caution when coadministered with proton pump inhibitors, H2 blockers, and antacids.

PREGNANCY: Category D, not for use in nursing.

MECHANISM OF ACTION: Kinase inhibitor; binds to and stabilizes the inactive conformation of the kinase domain of Abl protein.

PHARMACOKINETICS: Absorption: T_{max} =3 hrs. **Distribution:** plasma protein binding (98%). **Metabolism:** Via oxidation and hydroxylation. **Elimination:** Feces (93%, 69% unchanged), $T_{1/2}$ = 17 hours.

NURSING CONSIDERATIONS

Assessment: Assess for long QT syndrome, history of pancreatitis and total gastrectomy, hepatic impairment, galactose intolerance, severe lactase deficiency, glucose-galactose malabsorption, relevant cardiac disorders, pregnancy/nursing status, possible drug interactions. Assess for electrolyte abnormalities and correct prior to therapy. Perform baseline ECG.

Monitoring: Monitor for myelosuppression; perform CBC every 2 weeks for the first 2 months of therapy and then monthly thereafter. Check chemistry panels, including lipid profile periodically. Monitor for signs/symptoms of QT prolongation; obtain ECG 7 days after initiating treatment and then periodically thereafter, including after dose adjustments. Monitor for electrolyte abnormalities; measure serum electrolytes periodically. Monitor for elevations in serum lipase; test serum lipase levels monthly or as clinically indicated. Monitor for signs/symptoms of hepatotoxicity, AST/ALT, and alkaline phosphatase; perform periodic measurements of LFTs.

Patient Counseling: Take dose on empty stomach (no food should be consumed 2 hrs before or 1 hr after dose is taken). Take twice daily approximately 12 hrs apart and swallow capsules whole with water. Advise not to consume grapefruit products and other foods known to inhibit CYP3A4 at all times during treatment. Counsel about possible drug interactions. Advise women of childbearing potential to use effective contraceptive methods while on therapy. Take as prescribed and not to d/c therapy or change dose without consulting physician. In cases of missed doses, advise patients to take the next dose as scheduled and not to make up for a missed dose.

Administration: Oral route. Swallow whole with water. **Storage:** 25°C (77°F); excursions permitted between 15-30°C (59-86°F).

TASMAR   RX
tolcapone (Valeant)

> Risk of fatal, acute fulminant liver failure. Withdraw if patients fail to show benefit within 3 weeks of initiation. D/C if hepatotoxicity develops, and do not consider retreatment. Perform LFTs before therapy, then every 2 weeks for 1st year, every 4 weeks for next 6 months, then every 8 weeks thereafter. Perform LFTs before increase dose to 200mg tid. Avoid with liver disease or if LFTs ≥2X ULN. Caution with severe dyskinesia or dystonia.

THERAPEUTIC CLASS: COMT inhibitor

INDICATIONS: Adjunct to levodopa/carbidopa for the treatment of symptoms of idiopathic Parkinson's disease.

DOSAGE: *Adults:* Initial: 100mg tid. Use 200mg tid only if clinical benefit is justified. May need to decrease levodopa dose.

HOW SUPPLIED: Tab: 100mg, 200mg

CONTRAINDICATIONS: Liver disease, patients withdrawn from therapy due to drug-induced hepatocellular injury. History of non-traumatic rhabdomyolysis, hyperpyrexia or confusion related to medication.

WARNINGS/PRECAUTIONS: Dyskinesia, hypotension/syncope, rhabdomyolysis, hallucinations, hyperpyrexia, confusion, diarrhea, hematuria, fibrotic complications reported. Avoid with liver dysfunction. Caution with severe renal dysfunction. Closely monitor when d/c therapy. Increased risk of melanoma with Parkinson's disease; monitor periodically.

ADVERSE REACTIONS: Dyskinesia, dystonia, anorexia, muscle cramps, orthostatic complaints, diarrhea, confusion, hallucination, N/V, constipation, fatigue, increased sweating, xerostomia, urine discoloration, hepatotoxicity.

INTERACTIONS: α-methyldopa, dobutamine, apomorphine and isoproterenol may need a dose reduction. Avoid non-selective MAOIs (eg, phenelzine, tranylcypromine). May increase risk of orthostatic hypotension and dyskinesia with levodopa. Caution with tolbutamide, desipramine, warfarin.

PREGNANCY: Category C, caution in nursing.

MECHANISM OF ACTION: Catecol-*O*-methyltransferase inhibitor; suspected to alter the plasma pharmacokinetics of levodopa, leading to more sustained plasma levels of drug.

PHARMACOKINETICS: Absorption: (PO) Rapidly absorbed; absolute bioavailability (65%); T_{max}=2 hrs; C_{max}=3mcg/mL (100mg); C_{max}=6mcg/mL (200mg). **Distribution:** V_d=9L; plasma protein binding (>99.9%). **Metabolism:** Liver (glucuronidation) via CYP450 enzymes 3A4, 2A6. **Elimination:** Urine (60%, 0.5% unchanged), feces (40%); $T_{1/2}$=2-3 hrs.

NURSING CONSIDERATIONS

Assessment: Assess LFTs, renal function test, dyskinesia, psychosis, depression, cardiovascular complications, pregnancy/nursing status, and for possible drug interactions.

Monitoring: LFTs (SGPT/ALT, SGOT/AST), renal function test, hypotension/syncope, diarrhea, dyskinesia, rhabdomyolysis, hematuria, hyperpyrexia, confusion, melanoma, fibrotic complications, hallucinations, and depression.

Patient Counseling: Instruct to take as prescribed. Caution while operating machinery/driving. Regular follow-up needed. Avoid alcohol, OTC agents, and CNS depressants. Report adverse effects. Inform about signs/symptoms of onset of hepatic injury. Advise that hallucinations and nausea may occur. Inform the possibility of increased dyskinesia and dystonia. Notify physician if new or increased gambling urges, sexual urges or other intense urges occur.

Administration: Oral route. **Storage:** 20-25°C (68-77°F). Keep in tight container.

TAXOTERE RX
docetaxel (Sanofi-Aventis)

> Increased treatment-related mortality reported with hepatic dysfunction, high-dose therapy, in non-small cell lung carcinoma (NSCLC) and prior platinum-based chemotherapy with docetaxel at 100mg/m². Avoid if neutrophils <1500 cells/mm³, bilirubin >ULN, or AST/ALT >1.5X ULN with alkaline phosphatase >2.5X ULN; may increase risk for the development of grade 4 neutropenia, febrile neutropenia, infections, severe thrombocytopenia, severe stomatitis, severe skin toxicity, and toxic death. Obtain LFTs before each treatment cycle and frequent blood counts to monitor for neutropenia. Severe hypersensitivity reactions reported with dexamethasone premedication; d/c immediately if rash/erythema, hypotension, bronchospasm or anaphylaxis occur. Contraindicated with history of severe hypersensitivity reactions to docetaxel or to drugs formulated with polysorbate 80. Severe fluid retention may occur despite dexamethasone.

THERAPEUTIC CLASS: Antimicrotubule agent

INDICATIONS: Treatment of locally advanced or metastatic breast cancer (BC) and NSCLC after failure of prior chemotherapy. In combination with doxorubicin and cyclophosphamide for the adjuvant treatment of operable node-positive breast cancer. In combination with cisplatin for treatment of unresectable, locally advanced or metastatic NSCLC who have not previously received chemotherapy for this condition. In combination with prednisone for treatment of androgen-independent (hormone refractory) metastatic prostate cancer (HRPC). In combination with cisplatin and fluorouracil for the treatment of advanced gastric adenocarcinoma (GC), including adenocarcinoma of the gastroesophageal junction, in patients who have not received prior chemotherapy for advanced disease. In combination with cisplatin and fluorouracil for the induction treatment of patients with locally advanced squamous cell carcinoma of the head and neck (SCCHN).

DOSAGE: *Adults:* Premedicate with corticosteroids (eg, dexamethasone 8mg bid for 3 days); start 1 day prior to docetaxel (premedication regimen different with HRPC). BC: 60-100mg/m² IV over 1 hr every 3 weeks. Adjuvant to Operable Node-Positive BC: 75mg/m² 1 hr after doxorubicin 50mg/m² and cyclophosphamide 500mg/m² every 3 weeks for 6 courses. G-CSF may be given as prophylaxis. NSCLC: After Platinum Therapy Failure: 75mg/m² IV over 1 hr every 3 weeks. Chemotherapy-naive: 75mg/m² IV over 1 hr followed by cisplatin 75mg/m² over 30-60 min every 3 weeks. HRPC: 75mg/m² IV over 1 hr every 3 weeks with prednisone 5mg bid. Premedicate with oral dexamethasone 8mg at 12 hrs, 3 hrs and 1 hr before docetaxel. GC: 75mg/m² IV over 1 hr, followed by cisplatin 75mg/m² IV over 1-3 hrs (both on Day 1 only), followed by fluorouracil 750mg/m²/day IV over 24 hrs for 5 days, starting at end of cisplatin infusion. Repeat treatment every 3 weeks. SCCHN: Induction Followed by Radiotherapy: 75mg/m² IV over 1 hr, followed by cisplatin 75mg/m² IV over 1 hr, on Day 1, followed by fluorouracil as a continuous IV infusion at 750mg/m²/day for 5 days. Administer every 3 weeks for 4 cycles. Induction Followed by Chemoradiotherapy: 75mg/m² IV over 1 hr on Day 1, followed by cisplatin 100mg/m² IV over 30 min to 3 hrs, followed by fluorouracil 1000mg/m²/day as a continuous IV infusion from Day 1 to Day 4. Administer every 3 weeks for 3 cycles. Premedicate patients receiving cisplatin with antiemetics and provide appropriate hydration. Refer to PI for dosage adjustments during treatment.

HOW SUPPLIED: Inj: 20mg/0.5mL, 80mg/2mL

CONTRAINDICATIONS: Neutrophils <1500 cells/mm³.

WARNINGS/PRECAUTIONS: Monitor CBC and avoid subsequent cycles until neutrophils recover to level >1500 cells/mm³ and platelets to >100000 cells/mm³. Localized erythema of extremities with edema and desquamation, severe asthenia, severe peripheral motor neuropathy reported. Adjust dose or consider d/c if severe neurosensory symptoms (eg, paresthesia, dysesthesia, pain) develop. Acute myeloid leukemia or myelodysplasia may occur in adjuvant therapy. Monitor from the first dose for possible exacerbation of pre-existing effusions. Can cause fetal harm. Caution in elderly.

ADVERSE REACTIONS: Arthralgia, myalgia, alopecia, stomatitis, N/V, diarrhea, nail changes, cutaneous and neurosensory reactions, fluid retention, thrombocytopenia, anemia, neutropenia, fever.

INTERACTIONS: Avoid with strong CYP3A4 inhibitors (eg, ketoconazole, itraconazole, clarithromycin, atazanavir, indinavir, nefazodone, nelfinavir, ritonavir, saquinavir, telithromycin and voriconazole). Caution with CYP3A4 inducers, inhibitors and substrates. Increased exposure with protease inhibitors (eg, ritonavir).

PREGNANCY: Category D, not for use in nursing.

MECHANISM OF ACTION: Antimicrotubule agent; acts by disrupting the microtubular network in cells that is essential for mitotic and interphase cellular functions. Binds to free tubulin and promotes assembly of tubulin into stable microtubules while simultaneously inhibiting their disassembly which results in the inhibition of mitosis in cells.

PHARMACOKINETICS: Distribution: V_d=113L; plasma protein binding (94%). **Metabolism:** CYP3A4. **Elimination:** Urine (6%), feces (75%, within 7 days) (80%, 1st 48 hrs); $T_{1/2}$=11.1 hrs.

NURSING CONSIDERATIONS

Assessment: Assess for NSCLC, pre-existing effusion, weight gain, hepatic impairment, hypersensitivity/allergy, pregnancy/nursing status, and possible drug interactions. Obtain baseline vital signs and weight, CBC with platelets and differential count, LFTs.

Monitoring: Monitor for fluid retention, diarrhea, stomatitis, mucositis, cutaneous reactions, exacerbation of effusions, neurosensory symptoms, hepatic impairment and hypersensitivity reactions. Check vital signs and weight, CBC with platelets and differential count, and LFTs.

Patient Counseling: Inform about risks and benefits of therapy. May cause fetal harm; avoid becoming pregnant and use effective contraceptives. Explain the significance of oral corticosteroids such as dexamethasone administration to help facilitate compliance; instruct to report if not compliant. Report signs of hypersensitivity reaction, fluid retention (eg, peripheral edema in the lower extremities), weight gain, dyspnea, myalgia, cutaneous, neurologic reactions, and other adverse events (eg, N/V, diarrhea, constipation, fatigue, excessive tearing, infusion site reactions, hair loss) that may occur. Explain the significance of routine blood cell counts. Monitor temperature frequently and immediately report any occurrence of fever.

Administration: IV route. Refer to PI for preparation and administration procedures/precautions. **Storage:** 2-25°C (36-77°F). Protect from bright light.

TAZICEF RX
ceftazidime (Hospira)

THERAPEUTIC CLASS: Cephalosporin (3rd generation)

INDICATIONS: Treatment of lower respiratory tract (eg, pneumonia), skin and skin structure (SSSI), bone and joint, gynecologic, intra-abdominal, CNS (eg, meningitis), and urinary tract infections (UTI), bacterial septicemia, and sepsis caused by susceptible strains of microorganisms.

DOSAGE: *Adults:* Usual: 1g IV q8-12h. Uncomplicated UTI: 250mg IM/IV q12h. Complicated UTI: 500mg IM/IV q8-12h. Bone and Joint Infections: 2g IV q12h. Uncomplicated Pneumonia/SSSI: 500mg-1g IM/IV q8h. Gynecological/Intra-Abdominal/Meningitis/Severe Life-Threatening Infection: 2g IV q8h. Lung Infection caused by *Pseudomonas* in Cystic Fibrosis (normal renal function): 30-50mg/kg IV q8h. Max: 6g/day. Renal Impairment: CrCl 31-50mL/min: 1g q12h. CrCl 16-30mL/min: 1g q24h. CrCl 6-15mL/min: 500mg q24h. CrCl <5mL/min: 500mg q48h. For severe infections (6g/day), increase renal impairment dose by 50% or increase dosing interval. Apply reduced dosage recommendations after initial 1g LD is given. Hemodialysis: Give 1g LD before and 1g after each hemodialysis period. Intra-Peritoneal Dialysis/Continuous Ambulatory Peritoneal Dialysis: Give 1g LD followed by 500mg q24h, or add to fluid at 250mg/2L.
Pediatrics: Neonates (0-4 weeks): 30mg/kg IV q12h. 1 month-12 yrs: 30-50mg/kg IV q8h. Max: 6g/day. Higher doses for patients with cystic fibrosis or when treating meningitis.

HOW SUPPLIED: Inj: 1g, 2g. Also available as a Pharmacy Bulk Package. Refer to individual package insert for more information

WARNINGS/PRECAUTIONS: Monitor renal function; potential for nephrotoxicity. May result in overgrowth of nonsusceptible organisms. Possible cross-sensitivity between PCNs, cephalosporins, and β-lactams. Pseudomembranous colitis reported. Elevated levels with renal insufficiency can lead to seizures, encephalopathy, asterixis, and neuromuscular excitability. Possible decrease in PT; caution with renal or hepatic impairment, poor nutritional state; monitor PT and give vitamin K if needed. Caution with colitis and other GI diseases. Distal necrosis may occur after inadvertent intra-arterial administration. Continue for 2 days after signs/symptoms of infection resolve; may require longer therapy with complicated infections. Caution in elderly.

ADVERSE REACTIONS: Phlebitis and inflammation at injection site, pruritus, rash, fever, diarrhea, N/V.

INTERACTIONS: Nephrotoxicity reported with aminoglycosides or potent diuretics (eg, furosemide). Avoid with chloramphenicol; may decrease effect of β-lactam antibiotics.

PREGNANCY: Category B, caution in nursing.

MECHANISM OF ACTION: 3rd-generation cephalosporin; inhibits enzymes responsible for cell-wall synthesis.

PHARMACOKINETICS: Absorption: C_{max}=90mcg/mL (1g IV), 39mcg/mL (1g IM); see PI for detailed info. **Distribution:** Plasma protein binding (<10%); found in breast milk. **Elimination:** Urine (80-90% unchanged); $T_{1/2}$=1.9 hrs (IV).

NURSING CONSIDERATIONS

Assessment: Assess for previous hypersensitivity reaction to cephalosporins/PCNs or other drugs, renal/hepatic impairment, poor nutritional status, patients receiving protracted course of antibiotics, GI disease (particularly colitis), pregnancy/nursing status, and possible drug interactions.

Monitoring: Monitor PT; vitamin K administration as indicated. Monitor for signs/symptoms of allergic reactions (eg, Stevens-Johnson syndrome, toxic epidermal necrolysis), pseudomembranous colitis or *C.difficile*-associated diarrhea (may range in severity from mild diarrhea to fatal colitis), development of drug resistance, overgrowth of nonsusceptible organisms, seizures, encephalopathy, asterixis, neuromuscular excitability, distal necrosis in inadvertent intra-atrial injection, lab test interactions (eg, false (+) urinary glucose test), (+) Coombs' test without hemolysis, LFTs, renal function tests, and CBCs.

Patient Counseling: Only treats bacterial, not viral, infections. Take exactly as directed; skipping doses or not completing full course may decrease effectiveness and increase resistance. Inform about risks/benefits. D/C and notify physician if experience allergic reaction or diarrhea. Notify if pregnant/nursing.

Administration: IV and IM route. Do not use flexible container in series connections. **Storage:** Dry state 20-25°C (68-77°F), reconstituted solution for 24 hrs at room temperature, or for 7 days at 5°C; stable for 3 months if frozen at -20°C; thawed solution, store for up to 8 hrs at room temperature or for 4 days at 5°C; do not refreeze thawed solution.

TAZORAC

RX

tazarotene (Allergan)

THERAPEUTIC CLASS: Retinoid

INDICATIONS: (Gel 0.05%, 0.1%) Treatment of stable plaque psoriasis of up to 20% BSA involvement. (Gel 0.1%) Treatment of mild to moderate facial acne vulgaris. (Cre 0.05%, 0.1%) Treatment of plaque psoriasis. (Cre 0.1%) Treatment of acne vulgaris.

DOSAGE: *Adults:* ≥18 yrs: (Gel/Cre) Psoriasis: Start with 0.05% gel/cre, increase to 0.1% if tolerated and medically indicated. Apply thin film (enough to cover lesion) to psoriatic lesions qpm. Use gel only to ≤20% BSA. Acne: Cleanse and dry skin. Apply thin film (enough to cover affected area) of 0.1% gel/cre to acne lesions qpm.
Pediatrics: ≥12 yrs: (Gel) Psoriasis: Start with 0.05% gel, increase to 0.1% if tolerated and medically indicated. Apply thin film (enough to cover lesion and ≤20% BSA) to psoriatic lesions qpm. (Gel/Cre) Acne: Cleanse and dry skin. Apply thin film (enough to cover affected area) of 0.1% gel/cre to acne lesions qpm.

HOW SUPPLIED: Gel: 0.05%, 0.1% [30g, 100g]; Cre: 0.05%, 0.1% [30g, 60g]

CONTRAINDICATIONS: Women who are or may become pregnant.

WARNINGS/PRECAUTIONS: Not for ophthalmic, oral, or intravaginal use. Use adequate birth-control measures in women of child-bearing potential. Obtain negative pregnancy test result (sensitivity down to ≥50 mIU/mL for human chorionic gonadotropin [hCG]) within 2 weeks prior to therapy; initiate therapy during normal menstrual period. Apply only to affected area; for external use only. May cause severe irritation; do not use on eczematous skin. Avoid exposure to sunlight (including sunlamps); if exposure is necessary, use sunscreens (SPF ≥15) and protective clothing. Avoid with sunburn. May cause excessive pruritus, burning, skin redness, or peeling; d/c or reduce dosing interval if these occur, and patients with psoriasis being treated with 0.1% concentration can be switched to lower concentration. Weather extremes (eg, wind, cold) may cause irritation. (Gel) Not for use in >20% of BSA.

ADVERSE REACTIONS: Pruritus, burning/stinging, erythema, worsening of psoriasis, irritation, skin pain, desquamation, dry skin, rash, contact dermatitis, skin inflammation; (Cre) eczema, pertriglyceridemia; (Gel) fissuring, bleeding.

INTERACTIONS: Avoid dermatologic medications and cosmetics that have a strong drying effect. Caution with photosensitizers (eg, thiazides, tetracyclines, fluoroquinolones, phenothiazines, sulfonamides). Apply emollients ≥1 hr before gel/cream application.

PREGNANCY: Category X, caution in nursing.

MECHANISM OF ACTION: Retinoid. Psoriasis: not established; suppresses expression of MRP8, a marker of inflammation; inhibits cornified envelope formation; induces expression of a gene which may be a growth suppressor in keratinocytes and may inhibit epidermal hyperproliferation in treated plaques. Acne: not established; may be due to anti-hyperproliferative, normalizing-of-differentiation and anti-inflammatory actions.

PHARMACOKINETICS: Absorption: (Gel): After 7 days: Cmax=0.72ng/mL; Tmax=9 hrs after last dose; AUC=10.1ng•hr/mL. (Cre): After 14 Days: Cmax=2.31ng/mL; Tmax=8 hrs after last dose; AUC=31.2ng•hr/mL. **Distribution:** Tazarotenic Acid: Plasma protein binding (>99%). **Metabolism:** Esterase hydrolysis to form tazarotenic acid (active metabolite). **Excretion:** Urine, feces; Tazarotenic Acid: $T_{1/2}$=18 hrs.

NURSING CONSIDERATIONS

Assessment: Assess for eczematous skin, sunburn, considerable sun exposure due to occupation, sunlight sensitivity, hypersensitivity, pregnancy/nursing status, and possible drug interactions. Obtain negative pregnancy test result (sensitivity down to ≥50 mIU/mL for hCG) within 2 weeks prior to therapy.

Monitoring: Monitor for excessive pruritus, burning, skin redness, or peeling. Monitor application frequency, clinical therapeutic response, and skin tolerance.

Patient Counseling: Instruct to avoid contact with eyes, eyelids, and mouth; if contact occurs, rinse with water. Do not cover treated areas with dressings or bandages. Instruct to wash hands following administration. Advise not to take if pregnant, planning to become or suspected to be pregnant. Instruct females to use effective form of contraception while on medication; advise to begin therapy during menstrual period. Instruct to avoid exposure to sunlight/sunlamps while on therapy; wear protective clothing and use sunscreen (SPF ≥15) when exposed to sunlight. Instruct not to use with sunburn. Inform that exposure to weather extremes (eg, wind, cold) may cause skin irritation. Contact physician if excessive skin irritation develops. Counsel that if dose is missed, do not make it up; return to normal dosing schedule.

Administration: Topical route. Refer to PI for proper administration. **Storage:** 25°C (77°F); excursions permitted to (Gel) 15-30°C (59-86°F), (Cre) -5 to 30°C (23-86°F).

TEFLARO   RX
ceftaroline fosamil (Forest)

THERAPEUTIC CLASS: Cephalosporin

INDICATIONS: Treatment of acute bacterial skin and skin structure infections (ABSSSI) and community-acquired bacterial pneumonia (CABP) caused by susceptible isolates of microorganisms.

DOSAGE: *Adults:* ≥18 yrs: ABSSSI: 600mg q12h IV infusion over 1 hr for 5-14 days. CABP: 600mg q12h IV infusion over 1 hr for 5-7 days. Renal Impairment: CrCl>30-≤50mL/min: 400mg IV (over 1 hr) q12h. CrCl ≥15-≤30mL/min: 300mg IV (over 1 hr) q12h. End-stage Renal Disease (CrCl<15mL/min)/Hemodialysis: 200mg IV (over 1 hr) q12h. Elderly: Adjust dosage based on renal function.

HOW SUPPLIED: Inj: 400mg, 600mg

WARNINGS/PRECAUTIONS: Serious fatal hypersensitivity and skin reactions reported. Caution with penicillin (PCN) or other β-lactam-allergy; cross sensitivity may occur. D/C and institute appropriate therapy if allergic reaction occurs. *Clostridium difficile*-associated diarrhea (CDAD) reported. Seroconversion from negative to positive direct Coombs' test reported. If anemia develops, consider drug induced hemolytic anemia; perform diagnostic studies including a direct Coombs' test. Use in the absence of a proven or strongly suspected bacterial infection is unlikely to provide benefit and may increase risk of drug-resistant bacteria. Caution in elderly and renally impaired.

ADVERSE REACTIONS: Diarrhea, nausea, rash.

PREGNANCY: Category B, caution in nursing.

MECHANISM OF ACTION: Cephalosporin; bactericidal action is mediated through binding to essential penicillin-binding proteins (PBPs)

PHARMACOKINETICS: Absorption: C_{max}=19mcg/mL (single 600mg dose), 21.3mcg/mL (multiple 600mg doses); T_{max}=1.00 hrs (single 600mg dose); 0.92 hrs (multiple 600mg doses); AUC=56.8mcg•hr/mL (single 600mg dose); 56.3mcg•hr/mL (multiple 600mg doses). **Distribution:** V_d=20.3 L (single 600mg dose); plasma protein binding (20%). **Metabolism:** via phosphatase enzyme; via hydrolysis to ceftaroline M-1 (inactive metabolite). **Elimination:** Urine (88%); feces (6%). $T_{1/2}$=1.6 hrs (single 600mg dose), 2.66 hrs (multiple 600mg doses).

NURSING CONSIDERATIONS

Assessment: Assess for PCN or other β-lactam-allergy, renal impairment, pregnancy/nursing status, and for possible drug interactions. Obtain appropriate specimens for microbiological examination to identify pathogen and determine susceptibility.

Monitoring: Monitor for signs and symptoms of hypersensitivity reactions, skin reactions, CDAD, and anemia. Perform diagnostic studies including direct Coombs' test. Monitor renal function especially in elderly.

Patient Counseling: Advise that allergic reactions could occur and that serious reactions require immediate treatment; report any previous hypersensitivity reactions to other β-lactams (including cephalosporins) or other allergens. Antibacterial drugs should be used to treat only bacterial infections; they do not treat viral infections (eg, common cold). Although it is common to feel better early in the course of therapy, the medication should be taken as directed; skipping doses or not completing the full course of therapy may decrease the effectiveness and increase the likelihood that bacteria will develop resistance. Diarrhea is common and is usually resolved when drug is d/c. Frequent watery or bloody diarrhea may occur and may be a sign of a more serious intestinal infection; notify physician if this develops.

Administration: IV route. Refer to PI for further information on preparation and administration. **Storage:** 2-8°C (36-46°F). Use constituted sol within 6 hrs when stored at room temperature or within 24 hrs when stored under 2-8°C (36-46°F). Unrefrigerated/Unreconstituted: Store at temperatures not exceeding 25°C (77°F) for ≤7 days.

TEGRETOL   RX
carbamazepine (Novartis)

> Serious and fatal dermatologic reactions, including toxic epidermal necrolysis (TEN), Stevens-Johnson syndrome (SJS) reported; increased risk with presence of HLA-B*1502 allele; screen prior to initiation of therapy. Aplastic anemia and agranulocytosis reported. Obtain complete pretreatment hematological testing as a baseline. D/C if evidence of bone marrow depression develops.

OTHER BRAND NAMES: Epitol (Teva) - Tegretol-XR (Novartis)

THERAPEUTIC CLASS: Carboxamide

INDICATIONS: Treatment of partial seizures with complex symptomatology (psychomotor, temporal lobe), generalized tonic-clonic seizures (grand mal), and mixed seizure patterns of these, or other partial or generalized seizures. Treatment of pain associated with true trigeminal or glossopharyngeal neuralgia.

DOSAGE: *Adults:* Epilepsy: Initial: (Tab/Tab, ER) 200mg bid or (Sus) 100mg qid. Titrate: Increase weekly by adding up to 200mg/day given bid (Tab, ER) or tid-qid (Tab/Sus/Tab, Chewable) until optimal response. Maint: 800-1200mg/day. Max: 1200mg/day but doses up to 1600mg/day have been used in rare instances. With Other Anticonvulsants: Add gradually while other anticonvulsants are maintained or gradually decreased (except phenytoin, which may have to be increased). Trigeminal Neuralgia: Initial (Day 1): (Tab/Tab, ER) 100mg bid or (Sus) 50mg qid. Titrate: May increase by up to 200mg/day using

increments of 100mg q12h (Tab/Tab, ER) or 50mg qid (Sus) PRN. Maint: 400-800mg/day. Max: 1200mg/day. Re-evaluate every 3 months. Conversion from Tab to Sus: Give same mg/day in smaller, more frequent doses.
Pediatrics: Epilepsy: >12 yrs: Initial: (Tab/Tab, ER) 200mg bid or (Sus) 100mg qid. Titrate: Increase weekly by adding up to 200mg/day given bid (Tab, ER) or tid-qid (Tab/Sus/Tab, Chewable) until optimal response. Maint: 800-1200mg/day. Max: >15 yrs: 1200mg/day; 12-15 yrs: 1000mg/day. 6-12 yrs: Initial: (Tab/Tab, ER) 100mg bid or (Sus) 50mg qid. Titrate: Increase weekly by adding up to 100mg/day given bid (Tab, ER) or tid-qid (Tab/Sus/Tab, Chewable) until optimal response. Maint: 400-800mg/day. Max: 1000mg/day. <6 yrs: Initial: 10-20mg/kg/day given bid-tid (Tab) or qid (Sus). Titrate: (Tab/Sus) Increase weekly tid-qid. Max: 35mg/kg/day. With Other Anticonvulsants: Add gradually while other anticonvulsants are maintained or gradually decreased (except phenytoin, which may have to be increased). Conversion from Tab to Sus: Give same mg/day in smaller, more frequent doses.

HOW SUPPLIED: Sus: (Tegretol) 100mg/5mL [450mL]; Tab, Extended-Release: (Tegretol-XR) 100mg, 200mg, 400mg; (Tegretol) Tab, Chewable: 100mg*; (Tegretol, Epitol) Tab: 200mg* *scored

CONTRAINDICATIONS: History of bone marrow depression, MAOI use within 14 days, hypersensitivity to tricyclic compounds (eg, amitriptyline, desipramine, imipramine, protriptyline, nortriptyline, etc). Coadministration with nefazodone.

WARNINGS/PRECAUTIONS: Increased risk of suicidal thoughts or behavior. Caution in patients with history of cardiac conduction disturbance; cardiac, hepatic, or renal damage; adverse hematologic or hypersensitivity reactions to other drugs; increased intraocular pressure (IOP); mixed seizure disorder; previously interrupted course of carbamazepine. Atrioventricular heart block, slight elevations in LFTs, rare cases of liver failure. Multiorgan hypersensitivity reactions reported; consider d/c if hypersensitivity develops. May cause activation of latent psychosis and, in the elderly, confusion or agitation. Avoid with history of hepatic porphyria (eg, acute intermittent porphyria, variegate porphyria, porphyria cutanea tarda); acute attacks reported. Withdraw gradually to minimize potential increase in seizure frequency. May cause fetal harm with pregnancy. May impair physical/mental abilities. Avoid suspension in patients with fructose intolerance; start on lower doses and increase slowly. Not for relief of trivial aches or pains.

ADVERSE REACTIONS: Dizziness, drowsiness, unsteadiness, N/V, bone marrow depression, multiorgan hypersensitivity, aplastic anemia, agranulocytosis, leukopenia, eosinophilia, Stevens-Johnson syndrome (SJS), toxic epidermal necrolysis (TEN), liver dysfunction, cardiovascular complications.

INTERACTIONS: See Contraindications. Do not give suspension with other medicinal liquids or diluents. CYP3A4 inhibitors (eg, cimetidine, macrolides, azoles) may increase plasma concentration. CYP3A4 inducers (eg, cisplatin, rifampin, theophylline) may decrease plasma concentration. Increases plasma levels of clomipramine, phenytoin, and primidone. Decreases levels of CYP3A4 substrates (eg, APAP, alprazolam, warfarin). May render hormonal contraceptives (eg, oral, levonorgestrel subdermal implant) less effective. Increased risk of neurotoxic side effects with lithium. Alteration of thyroid function with other anticonvulsants. Increased isoniazid-induced hepatotoxicity with isoniazid. Symptomatic hyponatremia with some diuretics (eg, HCTZ, furosemide). Antagonizes effects of nondepolarizing muscle relaxants (eg, pancuronium).

PREGNANCY: Category D, not for use in nursing.

MECHANISM OF ACTION: Carboxamide; anticonvulsant: reduce polysynaptic response and block post-tetanic potentiation. Neuralgia: Depresses thalamic potential and bulbar and polysynaptic reflexes.

PHARMACOKINETICS: Absorption: T_{max}=1.5 hrs (Sus), 4-5 hrs (Tab), 3-12 hrs (Tab, ER). **Distribution:** Plasma protein binding (76%). Crosses placenta; found in breast milk. **Metabolism:** Liver via CYP3A4 to carbamazepine-10,11-epoxide (active metabolite). **Elimination:** Urine (72%; 3% unchanged), feces (28%); $T_{1/2}$=25-65 hrs (single dose); $T_{1/2}$=12-17 hrs (multiple doses).

NURSING CONSIDERATIONS

Assessment: Assess for history of bone marrow depression, hepatic porphyria, hypersensitivity to any tricyclic compound, increased IOP, previous
adverse hematological and dermatological reactions with other medications,
history of mixed seizure disorders, cardiac damage or cardiac conduction
disturbances, depression, suicidal behavior and ideation, pregnancy/nursing
status, and possible drug interactions. Assess renal function (eg, complete
urinalysis, BUN), CBC (eg, platelets, reticulocytes), serum iron, presence of
HLA-B*1502, LFTs; perform eye exam (eg, slit-lamp, funduscopy, tonometry)
prior to therapy. (Cre) eczema, pertriglyceridemia; (Gel) fissuring, bleeding.

Monitoring: Monitor for hepatic failure, multiorgan hypersensitivity reactions,
bone marrow depression, aplastic anemia, agranulocytosis, dermatological reactions (eg, SJS, TEN), latent psychosis, and confusion or agitation in elderly
patients. Monitor for emergence of suicidal behavior and ideation, signs and
symptoms of depression. Monitor LFTs, SrCr, BUN, IOP.

Patient Counseling: Counsel about signs/symptoms of hematological, dermatological, and hepatic complications (eg, fever, sore throat, easy bruising,
jaundice); instruct to report any occurrence to physician. May cause drowsiness or dizziness; caution against using heavy machinery/driving. Avoid with
alcohol or abrupt d/c. Notify physician if worsening of depression, unusual
changes in mood or behavior, or suicidal thoughts/behavior occurs. Notify
physician if pregnant or intend to become pregnant. Encourage pregnant
patients to enroll in North American Antiepileptic Drug (NAAED) Pregnancy
Registry by calling 1-888-233-2334 or go to http://www.aedpregnancyregis-
try.org/.

Administration: Oral route. (Sus) Shake well before using. (Tab, ER) Swallow
whole; do not chew or crush. **Storage:** (Sus): ≤30°C (86°F); dispense in tight,
light-resistant container. (Tab & Tab, Chewable): ≤30°C (86°F); Protect from
light and moisture; dispense in tight, light-resistant container. (Tab, ER): 15-
30°C (59-86°F). Protect from moisture. Dispense in tight container.

TEKTURNA   RX
aliskiren (Novartis)

> Drugs that act directly on the renin-angiotensin system can cause injury and death to the devel-
> oping fetus. D/C therapy when pregnancy is detected.

THERAPEUTIC CLASS: Renin inhibitor

INDICATIONS: Treatment of HTN as monotherapy or with other
antihypertensives.

DOSAGE: *Adults:* Usual: 150mg qd. May increase daily dose to 300mg if BP is
not adequately controlled. Max: 300mg/day.

HOW SUPPLIED: Tab: 150mg, 300mg

WARNINGS/PRECAUTIONS: Angioedema of the face, extremities, lips,
tongue, glottis, and/or larynx reported; d/c therapy and do not readminister
if angioedema occurs. In patients with an activated renin-angiotensin system
(eg, volume- and/or salt-depleted patients), symptomatic hypotension may
occur. Monitor for electrolyte imbalances particularly with severe renal impairment. May increase serum K+. Caution with severe renal impairment.

ADVERSE REACTIONS: Angioedema, diarrhea, cough, headache, nasopharyngitis, dizziness, fatigue, upper respiratory tract infection, back pain.

INTERACTIONS: Increased levels with cyclosporine and itraconazole; avoid
concomitant use. Caution with K+-sparing diuretics, K+ supplements, salt
substitutes containing K+, or other drugs that increase K+ levels; may lead to
increases in serum K+. May cause excessive fall in BP with other antihypertensives and symptomatic hypotension with high doses of diuretics. May cause
hyperkalemia with angiotensin-converting enzyme inhibitors in diabetic
population. Additive hyperuricemia with HCTZ. Potential interaction with Pgp
inhibitors.

PREGNANCY: Category C (1st trimester) and D (2nd and 3rd trimesters); not for use in nursing.

MECHANISM OF ACTION: Renin inhibitor; decreases plasma renin activity and inhibits conversion of angiotensinogen to angiotensin I.

PHARMACOKINETICS: Absorption: Poorly absorbed; T_{max}=1-3 hrs; bioavailability (2.5%). **Metabolism:** Via CYP3A4 enzyme. **Elimination:** Urine (25% of absorbed dose as parent drug).

NURSING CONSIDERATIONS

Assessment: Assess for diabetes, severe renal impairment, renal artery stenosis, history of angioedema, activated renin-angiotensin system (volume-/salt-depletion), pregnancy/nursing status, and possible drug interactions. Obtain baseline BP.

Monitoring: Monitor BP, serum electrolytes, renal functions, and serum K^+, BUN, and SrCr levels. Monitor for angioedema, airway obstruction, hypotension, hypokalemia, and electrolyte imbalances in diabetic patients.

Patient Counseling: Counsel about fetal risks during pregnancy and advise to report pregnancies as soon as possible. Inform that angioedema (eg, laryngeal edema) may occur anytime during therapy; advise to report any signs/symptoms of angioedema immediately (eg, swelling of face, extremities, eyes, lips, tongue, difficulty swallowing/breathing). Inform that lightheadedness can occur. Advise to consult physician and to d/c treatment if syncope occurs. Inform that inadequate fluid intake, excessive perspiration, diarrhea, or vomiting can lead to an excessive fall in BP. Instruct patients not to use K^+ supplements or salt substitutes containing K^+ without consulting their physician. Advise patients to establish a routine pattern for taking medication with regard to meals and inform that high-fat meals decrease absorption substantially.

Administration: Oral route. **Storage:** 25°C (77°F); excursions permitted to 15-30°C (59-86°F).

TEKTURNA HCT   RX
aliskiren - hydrochlorothiazide (Novartis)

> Drugs that act directly on the renin-angiotensin system can cause injury and even death to the developing fetus. D/C therapy when pregnancy is detected.

THERAPEUTIC CLASS: Renin inhibitor/thiazide diuretic

INDICATIONS: Treatment of HTN in patients whose BP is not controlled with monotherapy, is controlled with HCTZ alone but who experience hypokalemia, and in patients who experience dose-limiting adverse reactions on either component alone. As a replacement therapy for the titrated components and as initial therapy in patients likely to need multiple drugs to achieve BP goals.

DOSAGE: *Adults*: Initial Therapy/Not Controlled On Monotherapy: Initial: 150mg-12.5mg qd. Titrate: May increase up to 300mg-25mg qd if uncontrolled after 2-4 weeks. Replacement Therapy: May substitute for individually titrated components. May administer with other antihypertensive agents. CrCl >30mL/min: Follow usual regimen. CrCl <30mL/min: Avoid use. Elderly: May not require adjustment of initial dose.

HOW SUPPLIED: Tab: (Aliskiren-HCTZ) 150mg-12.5mg, 150mg-25mg, 300mg-12.5mg, 300mg-25mg

CONTRAINDICATIONS: Anuria, hypersensitivity to sulfonamide-derived drugs.

WARNINGS/PRECAUTIONS: Angioedema of the face, extremities, lips, tongue, glottis and/or larynx reported; d/c therapy and do not readminister if angioedema occurs. In patients with an activated renin-angiotensin system (eg, volume- and/or salt-depleted patients), symptomatic hypotension may occur. Avoid with severe renal impairment (GFR <30mL/min). May develop hypokalemia or hyperkalemia; monitor serum electrolytes periodically to detect possible electrolyte imbalance. Do not use as initial therapy with intravascular volume depletion. (HCTZ) May precipitate azotemia and hepatic coma; up-titrate slowly with renal/hepatic impairment. May cause hypersensitivity reactions, exacerbation or activation of systemic lupus erythematosus (SLE).

ADVERSE REACTIONS: Fetal injury, head and neck angioedema, dizziness, influenza, diarrhea, cough, vertigo, asthenia, arthralgia

INTERACTIONS: K^+-sparing diuretics, K^+ supplements, salt substitutes containing K^+, or other drugs that increase K^+ levels may increase serum K^+. (Aliskiren) Ketoconazole, atorvastatin, cyclosporine, verapamil and itraconazole may increase plasma levels. Avoid concomitant use with cyclosporine or itraconazole. Irbesartan may reduce levels. May diminish the effects of furosemide. (HCTZ) Potentiation of orthostatic hypotension may occur with alcohol, barbiturates, and narcotics. Dosage adjustment of insulin or oral hypoglycemic agents may be required. Potentiate effects of other antihypertensives. Cholestyramine and colestipol resins may reduce absorption. Corticosteroids and ACTH deplete electrolytes especially K^+. May decrease response to pressor amines (eg, norepinephrine). May increase responsiveness to skeletal muscle relaxants (eg, tubucurarine). Increased risk of lithium toxicity; avoid concurrent use. NSAIDs may reduce diuretic, natriuretic, and antihypertensive effects.

PREGNANCY: Category D, not for use in nursing.

MECHANISM OF ACTION: Aliskiren: Direct renin inhibitor; lowers BP by decreasing plasma renin activity, and inhibiting conversion of angiotensinogen to angiotensin I. HCTZ: Thiazide diuretic; affects renal tubular mechanisms of electrolyte reabsorption, directly increasing excretion of Na^+ and Cl^- in approximately equivalent amounts. Mechanism of antihypertensive effect is unknown.

PHARMACOKINETICS: Absorption: Aliskiren: T_{max}=1 hr. HCTZ: T_{max}=2.5 hrs. **Distribution:** HCTZ: Crosses the placenta; found in breast milk. **Metabolism:** Aliskiren: CYP3A4 enzyme. HCTZ: Not metabolized. **Elimination:** Aliskiren: Urine (25%, unchanged). HCTZ: Urine (≥61%, unchanged), $T_{1/2}$=5.8-18.9 hrs.

NURSING CONSIDERATIONS

Assessment: Assess for hepatic/renal function, serum electrolytes, anuria, sulfonamide hypersensitivity, volume- and/or salt depletion, allergy or bronchial asthma, SLE, pregnancy/nursing status, and possible drug interactions.

Monitoring: Monitor for hypersensitivity and anaphylactic reactions, anuria, urticaria, rapid weight gain, head/neck angioedema. Monitor BP, renal function, LFTs, serum uric acid, BUN, SrCr, CBC and electrolytes. Perform serial ultrasound examinations and routine fetal testing in pregnant patients under therapy.

Patient Counseling: Instruct to read the patient package insert before starting therapy. Notify physician or pharmacist if any unusual symptoms develop or if any known symptoms persist or worsen. Inform females of childbearing age on hazards to the developing fetus; ask to report pregnancies immediately; discuss other treatment options if planning to become pregnant. Lightheadedness may occur, especially during first days of therapy. If syncope occurs, d/c until physician consulted. Inadequate fluid intake, excessive perspiration, diarrhea, or vomiting can lead to an excessive fall in BP leading to lightheadedness and possible syncope. Do not use K^+ supplements or salt substitutes containing K^+ without consulting a physician. Establish routine pattern for taking medication with regard to meals. High-fat meals decrease absorption substantially.

Administration: Oral route. Establish routine pattern when taking with regard to meals. **Storage:** 25°C (77°F); excursions permitted to 15-30°C (59-86°F). Protect from moisture.

Temodar

temozolomide (Merck)

RX

THERAPEUTIC CLASS: Alkylating agent (imidazotetrazine derivative)

INDICATIONS: Treatment of newly diagnosed glioblastoma multiforme (GBM) concomitantly with radiotherapy and as maintenance treatment. Treatment of refractory anaplastic astrocytoma (eg, patients experiencing disease progression on a drug regimen containing nitrosourea and procarbazine).

DOSAGE: *Adults:* (IV/PO) Adjust according to nadir neutrophil and platelet counts of previous cycle and at time of initiating next cycle. Newly Diagnosed High Grade GBM: 75mg/m² qd for 42 days with focal radiotherapy. Maint: Cycle 1 (28 days): 150mg/m² qd for 1st 5 days of each 28-day cycle. Cycle 2-6 (28 days): Refer to PI for specific dosing. Refractory Anaplastic Astrocytoma: Initial: 150mg/m² qd for 5 consecutive days per 28-day cycle. May continue therapy until disease progression. Refer to PI for dose modifications for hematologic and nonhematologic toxicities.

HOW SUPPLIED: Cap: 5mg, 20mg, 100mg, 140mg, 180mg, 250mg; Inj: 100mg [vial]

CONTRAINDICATIONS: Hypersensitivity to DTIC (dacarbazine).

WARNINGS/PRECAUTIONS: Myelosuppression may occur, including prolonged pancytopenia, which may result in aplastic anemia. Greater risk of myelosuppression in women and elderly. Cases of myelodysplastic syndrome and secondary malignancies, including myeloid leukemia, reported. *Pneumocystis carinii* pneumonia (PCP) prophylaxis required in all patients with newly diagnosed GBM receiving concomitant radiotherapy for 42-day regimen; higher occurrence of PCP when administered during a longer dosing regimen. Perform weekly blood counts until recovery if ANC <1.5 x 10⁹/L and platelet count <100 x 10⁹/L. May cause fetal harm in pregnancy. Caution in elderly and severe renal/hepatic impairment. (IV) Increased risk of infusion-related adverse reactions and suboptimal dosing with shorter or longer infusion time.

ADVERSE REACTIONS: Fatigue, alopecia, myelosuppression (eg, thrombocytopenia, neutropenia), N/V, anorexia, headache, constipation, fever, rash, convulsions, hemiparesis.

INTERACTIONS: May decrease clearance with valproic acid. Monitor all patients for the development of PCP, especially those receiving steroids. Concomitant use of medications associated with aplastic anemia, including carbamazepine, phenytoin, sulfamethoxazole/trimethoprim, complicate assessment.

PREGNANCY: Category D, not for use in nursing.

MECHANISM OF ACTION: Alkylating agent (imidazotetrazine derivative); exerts action by alkylation of DNA. Alkylation (methylation) occurs mainly at the O^6 and N^7 positions of guanine.

PHARMACOKINETICS: Absorption: (PO) Rapid and complete, T_{max}=1 hr; C_{max}= 7.5mcg/mL, 282ng/mL (MTIC); AUC=23.4mcg•hr/mL, 864ng•hr/mL (MTIC). (IV) C_{max}=7.3mcg/mL, 276ng/mL (MTIC); AUC=24.6mcg•hr/mL, 891ng•hr/mL (MTIC). **Distribution:** V_d=0.4L/kg; plasma protein binding (15%). **Metabolism:** Via spontaneous hydroxylation; 5-(3-methyltriazen-1-yl)-imidazole-4-carboxamide (MTIC) (major metabolite) to 5-amino-imidazole-4-carboxamide (AIC). **Elimination:** Urine (37.7%, 5.6% unchanged), feces (0.8%); $T_{1/2}$=1.8 hrs.

NURSING CONSIDERATIONS

Assessment: Assess for previous hypersensitivity, hypersensitivity to DTIC, myelosuppression, hepatic/renal functions, pregnancy/nursing status, and possible drug interactions. Obtain baseline CBC, platelet count, and ANC.

Monitoring: Monitor for CBC on Day 22 (21 days after 1st dose) or within 48 hrs of that day; repeat weekly until ANC >1.5 x 10⁹/L and platelet count >100 x 10⁹/L. Monitor for myelosuppression, pancytopenia, aplastic anemia, PCP, myelodysplastic syndrome, secondary malignancies, myeloid leukemia, infusion-related reactions, and other adverse reactions.

Patient Counseling: Take as prescribed; swallow cap whole and do not open or chew. Instruct not to open capsule; if accidentally opened or damaged, take rigorous precautions to avoid inhalation or contact with skin or mucous membranes. Counsel about adverse effects (eg, N/V); seek medical attention if any develop.

Administration: Oral and IV route. See PI for preparation and administration techniques. Swallow cap whole with water. **Storage:** (Cap) 25°C (77°F); excursions permitted to 15-30°C (59-96°F). (IV) 2-8°C (36-46°F). After reconstitution, store at 25°C (77°F); use reconstituted product within 14 hrs including infusion time.

TEMOVATE   RX
clobetasol propionate (GlaxoSmithKline)

OTHER BRAND NAMES: Temovate Scalp (GlaxoSmithKline) - Temovate-E (GlaxoSmithKline)

THERAPEUTIC CLASS: Corticosteroid

INDICATIONS: Corticosteroid-responsive dermatoses. Temovate-E is also used to treat moderate to severe plaque-type psoriasis.

DOSAGE: *Adults:* Apply bid. Max: 50g/week or 50mL/week. Moderate-Severe Psoriasis: (Temovate-E) Apply bid for up to 4 weeks. May use on 5-10% of BSA. Max: 50g/week. Limit treatment to 2 consecutive weeks. Avoid with occlusive dressings.
Pediatrics: ≥12 yrs: Apply bid. Max: 50g/week or 50mL/week. Moderate-Severe Psoriasis: ≥16 yrs: (Temovate-E) Apply bid for up to 4 weeks. May use on 5-10% of BSA. Max: 50g/week. Limit treatment to 2 consecutive weeks. Avoid with occlusive dressings.

HOW SUPPLIED: (Temovate) Cre, Oint: 0.05% [15g, 30g, 45g, 60g]; Gel: 0.05% [15g, 30g, 60g]; Sol: 0.05% [25mL]; (Temovate-E) Cre: 0.05% [15g, 30g, 60g]; (Temovate Scalp) Sol: 0.05% [25mL, 50mL]

CONTRAINDICATIONS: (Scalp Sol) Primary scalp infections.

WARNINGS/PRECAUTIONS: Not for use on face, groin, or axillae, or for treatment of rosacea or perioral dermatitis. May produce reversible HPA axis suppression, manifestations of Cushing's syndrome, hyperglycemia, and glucosuria. Use appropriate antifungal or antibacterial agent with dermatological infections; d/c if infection does not clear. Pediatric patients may be more susceptible to systemic toxicity. Avoid eyes. D/C if irritation occurs.

ADVERSE REACTIONS: Burning, stinging, pruritus, skin atrophy, cracking/fissuring of the skin, erythema, folliculitis, numbness of fingers, telangiectasia, tingling (Sol), folliculitis (Sol).

PREGNANCY: Category C, caution in nursing.

MECHANISM OF ACTION: Corticosteroid; possesses anti-inflammatory, antipruritic, and vasoconstrictive properties. Anti-inflammatory effects not established. Suspected to act by induction of phospholipase A_2 inhibitory proteins, lipocortins. Lipocortins control biosynthesis of potent inflammation mediators (eg, prostaglandins, leukotrienes) by inhibiting release of their common precursor, arachidonic acid.

PHARMACOKINETICS: Absorption: Occlusion, inflammation, other disease states may increase absorption. Use of occlusive dressings ≤24 hrs does not increase penetration, use for 96 hrs markedly enhances penetration.

NURSING CONSIDERATIONS

Assessment: Assess medication not for treatment of perioral dermatitis or rosacea. Assess pregnancy/nursing status.

Monitoring: Monitor for signs/symptoms of reversible HPA-axis suppression, Cushing's syndrome, hyperglycemia, glucosuria, skin irritation, allergic contact dermatitis (eg, failure to heal), and concomitant skin infections (eg, fungal, bacterial). With large doses or use of occlusive dressings, perform periodic monitoring for HPA-axis suppression using ACTH stimulation, A.M. plasma cortisol, and urinary free cortisol tests. Following d/c, monitor for glucocorticosteroid insufficiencies. In pediatric patients, monitor for systemic toxicity, HPA-axis suppression (linear growth retardation, delayed weight gain), Cushing's syndrome, and intracranial HTN.

Patient Counseling: Counsel to use externally and exactly as directed; avoid contact with eyes, face, groin, or axillae. Advise not to bandage, cover, or wrap treated skin area. Contact physician if adverse reactions occur or improvement not seen after 2 weeks of therapy.

Administration: Topical route. **Storage:** 15-30°C (59-86°F). Do not refrigerate.

TENORETIC RX
chlorthalidone - atenolol (AstraZeneca)

THERAPEUTIC CLASS: Selective beta₁-blocker/monosulfamyl diuretic

INDICATIONS: Treatment of HTN.

DOSAGE: *Adults:* Initial: 50mg-25mg tab qd. May increase to 100mg-25mg tab qd. CrCl 15-35mL/min: Max: 50mg atenolol/day. CrCl <15mL/min: Max: 50mg atenolol qod.

HOW SUPPLIED: Tab: (Atenolol-Chlorthalidone) 50mg-25mg, 100mg-25mg

CONTRAINDICATIONS: Sinus bradycardia, >1st-degree heart block, cardiogenic shock, overt cardiac failure, anuria, sulfonamide hypersensitivity.

WARNINGS/PRECAUTIONS: Withdrawal before surgery is not recommended. Caution with bronchospastic disease, conduction abnormalities, left ventricular dysfunction. Caution in patients with impaired renal and hepatic function. Can cause heart failure with prolonged use; d/c if cardiac failure continues despite adequate treatment. Caution with diabetes mellitus (DM); may mask tachycardia occuring with hypoglycemia. May mask hypoglycemia or hyperthyroidism symptoms. Latent DM may become manifest. Avoid abrupt d/c; exacerbation of angina and myocardial infarction (MI) reported. Avoid with untreated pheochromocytoma. Possible fetal harm in pregnancy. May aggravate peripheral arterial circulatory disorders. Enhanced effects in postsympathectomy patient. Electrolyte imbalance (eg, hyponatremia, hypochloremic alkalosis, and hypokalemia) and hyperuricemia may develop. Hypercalcemia and hypophosphatemia observed. Acute gout, hepatic coma, and azotemia may be precipitated. Caution in congestive heart failure (CHF) controlled by digitalis and/or diuretics.

ADVERSE REACTIONS: Bradycardia, dizziness, fatigue, nausea.

INTERACTIONS: Additive effects with catecholamine-depleting drugs (eg, reserpine), CCBs, amiodarone, and digitalis. Bradycardia and heart block can occur with verapamil or diltiazem. Exacerbates rebound HTN with clonidine withdrawal. Prostaglandin synthase inhibitors (eg, indomethacin) may decrease hypotensive effects. Caution with anesthetic agents. May block epinephrine effects. May decrease arterial response to norepinephrine. May increase risk of lithium toxicity. Possible hypokalemia with corticosteroids or ACTH. May alter insulin requirements. May increase responsiveness to tubocurarine. Class I antiarrhythmic drugs (eg, disopyramide) may have a potentiating effect on atrial conduction time and induce negative inotropic effect.

PREGNANCY: Category D, caution in nursing.

MECHANISM OF ACTION: Atenolol: Cardioselective β-adrenoreceptor blocking agent; has not been established. Suspected to competitively antagonize catecholamines at peripheral adrenergic neuron sites, leading to decreased cardiac output; a central effect leading to reduced sympathetic outflow to the periphery and suppression of renin activity. Chlorthalidone: Monosulfamyl diuretic; acts on distal convoluted tubule and produces diuresis with increased excretion of Na⁺ and Cl⁻.

PHARMACOKINETICS: Absorption: (Atenolol): Rapid, incomplete, T_{max}=2-4 hrs. **Distribution:** (Atenolol): Plasma protein binding (6-16%). **Elimination:** (Atenolol): Renal excretion; feces (unchanged); $T_{1/2}$=6-7 hrs.

NURSING CONSIDERATIONS

Assessment: Assess for bradycardia, cardiogenic shock, 2nd- and 3rd-degree heart block, overt cardiac failure, impaired renal/hepatic function, bronchospastic disease, PVD, DM, thyrotoxicosis, pheochromocytoma, anuria, hypersensitivity to sulfonamide-derived drugs, serum electrolytes, parathyroid disease, pregnancy/nursing status, SLE, and possible drug interactions.

Monitoring: Monitor for cardiac failure, HTN, renal function, exacerbation of ischemia following abrupt withdrawal, bronchospastic disease, arrhythmias, CBC with platelets and differential count, hypersensitivity reactions, mesenteric arterial thrombosis, reversible mental depression, hyperuricemia or acute gout, signs/symptoms of electrolyte imbalance, serum glucose, lipid profile, toxic epidermal necrolysis (TEN), impotence, HR, orthostatic hypotension, pancreatitis, LFTs.

Patient Counseling: Instruct not to interrupt or d/c therapy without consulting physician. Notify physician if signs/symptoms of impending CHF or unexplained respiratory symptoms develop. Counsel about signs/symptoms of electrolyte imbalance (eg, dry mouth, thirst, weakness, lethargy, drowsiness, restlessness, muscle pains/cramps, muscular fatigue, hypotension, oliguria, tachycardia, N/V), and advise to seek prompt medical attention.

Administration: Oral route. **Storage:** 20-25°C (68-77°F).

TENORMIN   RX
atenolol (AstraZeneca)

THERAPEUTIC CLASS: Selective beta$_1$-blocker

INDICATIONS: Management of HTN. Long-term management of angina pectoris. Management of hemodynamically stable patients with definite or suspected acute myocardial infarction (AMI) to reduce cardiovascular mortality.

DOSAGE: *Adults:* HTN: Initial: 50mg qd. Titrate: May increase after 1-2 weeks. Max: 100mg qd. Angina: Initial: 50mg qd. Titrate: May increase to 100mg after 1 week. Max: 200mg qd. AMI: Initial: 5mg IV over 5 min, repeat 10 min later. If tolerated, give 50mg PO 10 min after the last IV dose, followed by another 50mg PO 12 hrs later. Maint: 100mg qd or 50mg bid for 6-9 days. Renal Impairment/Elderly: HTN: Initial: 25mg qd. HTN/Angina/AMI: Max: CrCl 15-35mL/min: 50mg/day. CrCl <15mL/min: 25mg/day. Hemodialysis: 25-50mg after each dialysis.

HOW SUPPLIED: Tab: 25mg, 50mg*, 100mg *scored

CONTRAINDICATIONS: Sinus bradycardia, >1st-degree heart block, cardiogenic shock, overt cardiac failure.

WARNINGS/PRECAUTIONS: Avoid abrupt d/c of therapy in coronary artery disease. Severe exacerbation of angina and occurrence of MI and ventricular arrhythmias reported in angina patients following abrupt d/c of therapy with β-blockers. When d/c is planned, patients should be monitored and advised to limit activity. Withdrawal before surgery is not recommended. Caution with bronchospastic disease, conduction abnormalities, left ventricular dysfunction, heart failure controlled by digitalis and/or diuretics, renal or hepatic dysfunction. Can cause heart failure with prolonged use. Caution with diabetes mellitus (DM). May mask tachycardia occuring with hypoglycemia or hyperthyroidism symptoms. Avoid abrupt d/c. Avoid with untreated pheochromocytoma. Possible fetal harm in pregnancy. May aggravate peripheral arterial circulatory disorders. Caution in elderly.

ADVERSE REACTIONS: Bradycardia, hypotension, dizziness, fatigue, nausea, depression, dyspnea, wheezing, tiredness.

INTERACTIONS: Additive effects with catecholamine-depleting drugs (eg, reserpine), CCBs, amiodarone, and digitalis. Use with disopyramide may be associated with severe bradycardia, asystole, and heart failure. Bradycardia and heart block can occur with verapamil or diltiazem. Exacerbates rebound HTN with clonidine withdrawal. Prostaglandin synthase inhibitors (eg, indomethacin) may decrease hypotensive effects. Caution with drugs that depress myocardium (eg, anesthesia). May block epinephrine effects. Concomitant use with digitalis glycosides may increase risk of bradycardia. Coadministration of isoproterenol or dobutamine can reverse effects of beta-blockers.

PREGNANCY: Category D, caution in nursing.

MECHANISM OF ACTION: Cardioselective β-adrenoreceptor blocking agent; has not been established. Suspected to competitively antagonize catecholamines at peripheral adrenergic neuron sites, leading to decreased cardiac output; a central effect leading to reduced sympathetic outflow to the periphery and suppression of renin activity.

PHARMACOKINETICS: Absorption: Rapid, incomplete; T_{max}= 2-4 hrs. **Distribution:** Plasma protein binding (6-16%). **Elimination:** Kidneys; urine (50%); $T_{1/2}$=6-7 hrs.

NURSING CONSIDERATIONS

Assessment: Assess for bradycardia, cardiogenic shock, 2nd- and 3rd-degree heart block, overt cardiac failure, impaired renal/hepatic function, bronchospastic disease, PVD, DM, thyrotoxicosis, pregnancy/nursing status, pheochromocytoma, and possible drug interactions.

Monitoring: Monitor for cardiac failure, HTN, renal function, exacerbation of ischemia following abrupt withdrawal, bronchospastic disease, arrhythmias, CBC with platelets and differential count, hypersensitivity reactions, mesenteric arterial thrombosis, reversible mental depression.

Patient Counseling: Instruct not to interrupt or d/c therapy without consulting physician. Notify physician if signs/symptoms of impending CHF or unexplained respiratory symptoms develop. Educate about signs/symptoms of adverse effects.

Administration: Oral route. **Storage:** 20-25°C (68-77°F). Dispense in tightly closed, light-resistant containers.

TERAZOL 3 RX
terconazole (Ortho-McNeil)

THERAPEUTIC CLASS: Azole antifungal

INDICATIONS: Local treatment of vulvovaginal candidiasis (moniliasis).

DOSAGE: *Adults:* Administer 1 full applicator or sup intravaginally qhs for 3 nights.

HOW SUPPLIED: Cre: 0.8% [20g]; Sup: 80mg [2.5g] [3°]

WARNINGS/PRECAUTIONS: D/C and do not retreat if sensitization, irritation, fever, chills, or flu-like symptoms occur. Confirm diagnosis by KOH smears and/or cultures; reconfirm if no response. Base in suppository may interact with certain rubber or latex products (eg, vaginal contraceptive diaphragms); avoid concurrent use.

ADVERSE REACTIONS: Sup: Localized burning, pruritus, genital pain, headache. Cre: Dysmenorrhea, headache, pruritus, burning, abdominal pain.

PREGNANCY: Category C, not for use in nursing.

MECHANISM OF ACTION: Azole antifungal; uncertain. Suspected to exert antifungal activity by disruption of normal fungal cell membrane permeability.

PHARMACOKINETICS: Absorption: C_{max}=5.9ng/mL, T_{max}=6.6 hrs. **Distribution:** Plasma protein binding (94.9%).

NURSING CONSIDERATIONS

Assessment: Assess for proper diagnosis with appropriate microbiologic studies (KOH smears and/or culture). Assess for hypersensitivity and pregnancy/nursing status.

Monitoring: Monitor for signs/symtoms of sensitization, irritation, fever, chills, and flu-like symptoms. Monitor for response to treatment; if lack of response, standard KOH smear and cultures should be repeated to confirm diagnosis.

Patient Counseling: Counsel to use as prescribed, even if symptoms improve. Do not use suppository concurrently with rubber or latex products (eg, condoms, diaphragms), or with tampons. Consult physician if partner has penile itching, redness or discomfort. Do not douche unless otherwise directed by physician. Notify physician of all medications currently being taken.

T

Administration: Intravaginal route. 1) Lie on back, knees drawn up toward chest. 2) Cre: Insert filled applicator into vagina and press plunger to release cre into vagina. Sup: Insert sup into vagina with finger at hs as directed by physician. **Storage:** 15-30°C (59-86°F).

TERAZOL 7   RX
terconazole (Ortho-McNeil)

THERAPEUTIC CLASS: Azole antifungal

INDICATIONS: Local treatment of vulvovaginal candidiasis (moniliasis).

DOSAGE: *Adults:* Administer 1 full applicator intravaginally qhs for 7 nights.

HOW SUPPLIED: Cre: 0.4% [45g]

WARNINGS/PRECAUTIONS: D/C and do not retreat if sensitization, irritation, fever, chills, or flu-like symptoms occur. Confirm diagnosis by KOH smears and/or cultures; reconfirm if no response.

ADVERSE REACTIONS: Headache, body pain, burning, itching, irritation.

PREGNANCY: Category C, not for use in nursing.

MECHANISM OF ACTION: Azole antifungal; uncertain. Suspected to exert antifungal activity by disruption of normal fungal cell membrane permeability

PHARMACOKINETICS: Absorption: 5-8% (hysterectomized), 12-16% (non-hysterectomized); C_{max}=5.9ng/mL, T_{max}=6.6 hrs. **Distribution:** Plasma protein binding (94.9%).

NURSING CONSIDERATIONS

Assessment: Assess for proper diagnosis with appropriate microbiologic studies (KOH smears and/or culture). Assess for hypersensitivity and pregnancy/nursing status.

Monitoring: Monitor for signs/symptoms of sensitization, irritation, fever, chills, flu-like symptoms. Monitor for response to treatment; if lack of response, standard KOH smear and cultures should be repeated to confirm diagnosis.

Patient Counseling: Counsel to use as prescribed, even if symptoms improve. Consult physician if partner has penile itching, redness, or discomfort. Do not use tampons while on medication or douche unless otherwise directed by physician. Notify physician of all medications currently being taken.

Administration: Intravaginal route. 1) Lie on back with knees drawn up towards chest. 2) Insert filled applicator into vagina as far as it will comfortably go. 3) Press plunger to release cre into vagina. 4) Apply at bedtime as directed by doctor. **Storage:** 15-30°C (59-86°F).

TERAZOSIN HCL   RX
terazosin HCl (Various)

THERAPEUTIC CLASS: Alpha$_1$-blocker (quinazoline)

INDICATIONS: Treatment of HTN and symptomatic benign prostatic hyperplasia (BPH).

DOSAGE: *Adults:* HTN: Initial: 1mg hs, then slowly increase dose. Usual: 1-5mg/day. Max: 20mg/day. If response is substantially diminished at 24 hrs, may increase dose or use bid regimen. BPH: Initial: 1mg qhs. Titrate: Increase stepwise to 2mg, 5mg, or 10mg qd prn. Usual: 10mg/day. May increase to 20mg/day after 4-6 weeks. Max: 20mg/day. If d/c for several days, restart at initial dose.

HOW SUPPLIED: Cap: 1mg, 2mg, 5mg, 10mg

WARNINGS/PRECAUTIONS: Monitor for orthostatic hypotension and syncope initially, with dose increase, or introduction of additional antihypertensive agent. May impair physical/mental abilities. Rule out prostate cancer. Priapism (rare) reported. Intraoperative floppy iris syndrome observed during cataract surgery. Significant decreases in Hct, Hgb, WBC, total protein and albumin were observed, possibly due to hemodilution. Examine patients with BPH prior to initiation of therapy.

ADVERSE REACTIONS: Asthenia, postural hypotension, headache, dizziness, dyspnea, nasal congestion/rhinitis, somnolence, blurred vision, palpitations, nausea, peripheral edema, priapism, thrombocytopenia.

INTERACTIONS: Caution with other antihypertensive agents (eg, verapamil). Hypotension reported when coadministering with PDE-5 inhibitors. May need dose reduction or retitration of either agent with other antihypertensive agents.

PREGNANCY: Category C, caution with nursing.

MECHANISM OF ACTION: Alpha$_1$-blocker; (BPH) antagonizes α_1-receptors in bladder neck and prostate, relaxing smooth muscle; (HTN) antagonizes α_1-receptors decreasing total peripheral vascular resistance, causing decreased BP.

PHARMACOKINETICS: Absorption: Complete; T_{max}=1 hr. **Distribution:** Plasma protein binding (90-94%). **Elimination:** Feces (20%), urine (10%); $T_{1/2}$=12 hrs.

NURSING CONSIDERATIONS

Assessment: Assess for HTN, BPH, pregnancy/nursing status and possible drug interactions. Rule out prostate cancer.

Monitoring: Monitor for Hct, Hgb, WBC, total protein/albumin, and BP periodically. Monitor for signs/symptoms of hypotension, priapism.

Patient Counseling: Inform of possibility of syncope and orthostatic symptoms, especially at initiation of therapy. Caution against driving or hazardous tasks for 24 hrs after first dose, dosage increase, or when resuming therapy after interruption. Avoid situations where injury could result should syncope occur. Advise to sit or lie down when symptoms of low BP occur. Inform of possibility of priapism; advise to seek medical attention if it occurs.

Administration: Oral route. **Storage:** 20°-25°C (68°-77°F). Protect from light and moisture.

TESSALON   RX
benzonatate (Pfizer)

THERAPEUTIC CLASS: Non-narcotic antitussive

INDICATIONS: Symptomatic relief of cough.

DOSAGE: *Adults:* Usual: 100mg or 200mg tid PRN. Max: 600mg/day in 3 divided doses.
Pediatrics: >10 yrs: Usual: 100mg or 200mg tid PRN. Max: 600mg/day in 3 divided doses.

HOW SUPPLIED: Cap: 200mg, (Perle) 100mg

WARNINGS/PRECAUTIONS: Severe hypersensitivity reactions (eg, bronchospasm, laryngospasm, cardiovascular collapse) reported. Swallow capsules without sucking/chewing to avoid local anesthesia adverse effects. Accidental ingestion resulting in death reported in children <10 yrs; keep out of reach of children. May cause adverse CNS effects; caution with prior sensitivity to related agents such as para-amino-benzoic acid based anesthetics (eg, procaine, tetracaine).

ADVERSE REACTIONS: Hypersensitivity reactions, sedation, headache, constipation, nausea, GI upset, pruritus, skin eruptions, nasal congestion, numbness of the chest.

INTERACTIONS: Bizarre behavior (eg, mental confusion and visual hallucinations) reported when used concomitantly with other prescribed drugs. May cause adverse CNS effects when used concomitantly with other medications.

PREGNANCY: Category C, caution in nursing.

MECHANISM OF ACTION: Non-narcotic antitussive agent; acts peripherally by anesthetizing the stretch receptors located in the respiratory passages, lungs, and pleura by dampening their activity, thereby reducing cough reflex at its source.

NURSING CONSIDERATIONS

Assessment: Assess for previous sensitivity to related compounds such as para-amino-benzoic acid based anesthetics (eg, procaine, tetracaine), pregnancy/nursing status, and for possible drug interactions.

Monitoring: Monitor for hypersensitivity reactions (eg, bronchospasm, laryngospasm, cardiovascular collapse), mental confusion, visual hallucinations, overdose signs/symptoms (eg, restlessness, tremors, clonic convulsions followed by profound CNS depression).

Patient Counseling: Advise not to break, chew, dissolve, cut, or crush the drug and to swallow it whole. Instruct to avoid food or liquid ingestion if numbness or tingling of the tongue, mouth, throat, or face occurs; if symptoms worsen, advise to seek medical attention. Instruct to keep out of reach of children. Inform that overdosage may occur in adults; advise not to exceed single dose and total daily dose and not to take two doses at a time.

Administration: Oral route. Swallow whole; do not break, chew, dissolve, cut, or crush. **Storage:** 25°C (77°F); excursions permitted to 15-30°C (59-86°F).

TESTIM
CIII
testosterone (Auxilium)

> Virilization reported in children secondarily exposed to testosterone gel. Children should avoid contact with unwashed or unclothed application sites in men using testosterone gel. Healthcare providers should advise patients to strictly adhere to recommended use instructions.

THERAPEUTIC CLASS: Androgen

INDICATIONS: Testosterone replacement in males with primary or hypogonadotropic hypogonadism.

DOSAGE: *Adults:* ≥18 yrs: Initial: Apply 5g qd, preferably in the am, to clean, dry, intact skin of shoulders and/or upper arms. Allow to dry prior to dressing. Titrate: May increase to 10g qd if response not achieved or serum concentration is below normal range. Do not apply to genitals or abdomen; wash hands after application. To maintain serum testosterone levels, do not wash application site for at least 2 hrs.

HOW SUPPLIED: Gel: 1% [5g/tube, 30s]

CONTRAINDICATIONS: Breast or prostate carcinoma in men. Not for use by women. Pregnant and nursing women should avoid skin contact with application sites on men. Hypersensitivity to soy products.

WARNINGS/PRECAUTIONS: Increases risk for worsening of BPH. Increases risk for prostate cancer in men treated with androgens; evaluate for prostate cancer prior to therapy especially in elderly patients. Risk of virilization in women (eg, changes in body hair distribution, significant increase in acne) due to secondary skin exposure from contact with men using testosterone-containing gel products; d/c until cause of virilization has been identified. Risk of edema with pre-existing cardiac, renal, or hepatic disease; d/c if edema occurs, diuretic therapy may be required. Gynecomastia may develop. May potentiate sleep apnea especially with obesity or chronic lung diseases. Advise patients to report persistent penis erections, changes in skin color, ankle swelling, unexplained N/V, or breathing disturbances.

ADVERSE REACTIONS: Application-site reactions, virilization from secondary exposure.

INTERACTIONS: May elevate oxyphenbutazone levels. May decrease blood glucose and insulin requirements. ACTH or corticosteroids may enhance edema; caution with cardiac or hepatic disease.

PREGNANCY: Category X, not for use in nursing.

MECHANISM OF ACTION: Endogenous androgen; responsible for normal growth and development of male sex organs and for maintenance of secondary sex characteristics.

PHARMACOKINETICS: Absorption: 10% absorbed systemically. **Distribution:** Sex hormone-binding globulin (SHBG) binding (40%), albumin- and plasma protein-binding (58%), unbound (2%). **Metabolism:** Skin, liver, male urogenital tract via 5α-reductase; estradiol and dihydrotestosterone (metabolites). **Elimination:** Urine (90%), feces (6%); $T_{1/2}$=10-100 min.

NURSING CONSIDERATIONS

Assessment: Assess for hypersensitivity to soy, breast or prostate carcinoma, BPH, cardiac or renal/hepatic disease, obesity, chronic lung disease, polycythemia, pregnancy/nursing status of female partner, and possible drug interactions.

Monitoring: Perform periodic monitoring of Hgb, Hct, LFTs, PSA, HDL, and serum testosterone levels. Obtain serum testosterone levels 14 days after initiation of therapy. Monitor for signs/symptoms of hypersensitivity reactions, edema with/without CHF, gynecomastia, BPH, prostate carcinoma in geriatrics, and potentiation of sleep apnea.

Patient Counseling: Inform of pregnancy risks; avoid contact with application sites in children and women or if pregnant/nursing. If contact occurs, wash area immediately with soap and water. Instruct not to apply to the scrotum, penis, or abdomen. Cover application site with clothing after gel dries; wash application site with soap and water prior to direct skin-to-skin contact. Advise not to wash or swim until ≥2 hrs after application. Contact physician if experience changes in body hair distribution, increase in acne, virilization of female partner or child, too frequent or persistent erections, changes in skin color, ankle swelling, unexplained N/V, breathing disturbances, or hypersensitivity reactions. Advise to carefully read Medication Guide. Apply qd at approximately the same time each day. Avoid if have known/suspected prostate or breast cancer. Keep out of reach of children. Inform that drug is flammable.

Administration: Topical route. Apply every day at same time to clean, dry skin of shoulder or upper arms. Wash hands thoroughly after application. **Storage:** 25°C (77°F); excursions permitted to 15-30°C (59-86°F). Discard used tubes.

TESTRED | CIII
methyltestosterone (Valeant)

THERAPEUTIC CLASS: Androgen

INDICATIONS: Testosterone replacement therapy in males with primary hypogonadism or hypogonadotropic hypogonadism. To stimulate puberty in males with delayed puberty. Secondary treatment of advancing inoperable metastatic (skeletal) breast cancer in females 1-5 yrs postmenopausal.

DOSAGE: *Adults:* Dose based on age, sex and diagnosis. Adjust dose according to clinical response and adverse events. Male Replacement Therapy: 10-50mg/day. Breast Carcinoma: 50-200mg/day.
Pediatrics: Dose based on age, sex and diagnosis. Adjust dose according to clinical response and adverse events. Delayed Puberty: Use lower range of 10-50mg/day for 4-6 months. Caution in children.

HOW SUPPLIED: Cap: 10mg

CONTRAINDICATIONS: Pregnancy. Males with breast or prostate carcinoma.

WARNINGS/PRECAUTIONS: D/C if hypercalcemia occurs in breast cancer; monitor calcium levels. Monitor for virilization in females. Risk of compromised stature in children; monitor bone growth every 6 months. Risk of hepatic damage with long-term use. D/C if jaundice, cholestatic hepatitis occur. Risk of edema; caution with pre-existing cardiac, renal or hepatic disease. Caution in the elderly; increased risk of prostatic hypertrophy and prostatic carcinoma. Should not be used for enhancement of athletic performance. Monitor LFTs, Hct, and Hgb periodically.

ADVERSE REACTIONS: Amenorrhea, virilization, menstrual irregularities, gynecomastia, excessive frequency/duration of penile erections, male-pattern baldness, increased/decreased libido, oligospermia, hirsutism, acne, fluid and electrolyte disturbances, nausea, hypercholesterolemia, clotting factor suppression, polycythemia, altered LFTs, priapism, anxiety, depression.

INTERACTIONS: Potentiates oral anticoagulants and oxyphenbutazone. May decrease blood glucose and insulin requirements in diabetics.

PREGNANCY: Category X, not for use in nursing.

MECHANISM OF ACTION: Endogenous androgen (derivative of testosterone); responsible for normal growth and development of male sex organs and maintenance of secondary sex characteristics.

PHARMACOKINETICS: Metabolism: Gut, liver. **Elimination:** Urine, feces; $T_{1/2}$=10-100 min.

NURSING CONSIDERATIONS

Assessment: Assess for known or suspected carcinoma of prostate or male breast, pregnancy status, pre-existing cardiac or renal/hepatic disease, and possible drug interactions.

Monitoring: Periodically monitor urine and serum calcium levels (female breast cancer), LFTs, Hgb and Hct, and bone age of left wrist and hand every 6 months (bone maturation in pediatrics). Monitor for signs/symptoms of hypersensitivity reactions, peliosis hepatis, hepatic dysfunction, prostatic hyperplasia/carcinoma in geriatrics, edema (with or without CHF), hypercalcemia, and virilization of females.

Patient Counseling: Inform of pregnancy risks. Instruct to contact physician if any hypersensitivity reactions, N/V, ankle swelling, changes in skin color, symptoms of hepatotoxicity, frequent or persistent erections (males), hoarseness (females), acne, changes in menstrual periods (females), or more facial hair occur.

Administration: Oral route. **Storage:** 25°C (77°F); excursions permitted to 15-30°C (59-86°F).

TETANUS & DIPHTHERIA TOXOIDS ADSORBED   RX
diphtheria toxoid - tetanus toxoid (Various)

THERAPEUTIC CLASS: Toxoid combination

INDICATIONS: Active immunization for the prevention of tetanus and diphtheria (Td) in persons ≥ 7 yrs.

DOSAGE: *Adults:* Primary immunization: 0.5mL IM (deltoid) in a series of three doses. The first 2 doses are administered 4-8 weeks apart. Administer 3rd dose 6-12 months after 2nd dose. Routine booster immunization in persons who have completed primary immunization every 10 yrs thereafter. Tetanus prophylaxis in wound management: Preparation containing Td toxoids is preferred. Refer to PI for proper guide to tetanus prophylaxis in routine wound management. May be used for post-exposure diphtheria prophylaxis in persons who have not completed primary vaccination, whose vaccination status is unknown, or have not been vaccinated with diphtheria toxoid within the previous 5 yrs.

Pediatrics: ≥7 yrs: Primary immunization: 0.5mL IM (deltoid) in a series of three doses. The first 2 doses are administered 4-8 weeks apart. Administer 3rd dose 6-12 months after 2nd dose. Routine booster immunization in children 7 yrs and older who have completed primary immunization. Routine booster is recommended in children 11-12 yrs and every 10 yrs thereafter. Tetanus prophylaxis in wound management: Preparation containing Td toxoids is preferred. Refer to PI for proper guide to tetanus prophylaxis in routine wound management. May be used for post-exposure diphtheria prophylaxis in children 7 yrs and older who have not completed primary vaccination, whose vaccination status is unknown, or have not been vaccinated with diphtheria toxoid within the previous 5 yrs.

HOW SUPPLIED: Inj: (Diptheria toxoid - Tetanus toxoid) 2Lf-2Lf/0.5mL

WARNINGS/PRECAUTIONS: Immune response may not be obtained in immunocompromised patients. Increased incidence and severity of adverse reactions with more frequent administration. Do not give more frequently than every 10 yrs in persons who experienced an Arthus-type hypersensitivity reaction following a prior dose of a tetanus toxoid-containing vaccine. Have epinephrine (1:1000) and other appropriate agents and equipment available for anaphylactic reactions. Caution with tetanus toxoid-related Guillain-Barre syndrome. Not for pediatrics <7 yrs.

ADVERSE REACTIONS: Injection-site reactions, malaise, nausea, arthralgia, pyrexia, peripheral edema, dizziness, headache, convulsion, myalgia, musculo-skeletal stiffness or pain, rash, cellulitis.

INTERACTIONS: May have reduced immune response with immunosuppressive therapy, including alkylating agents, antimetabolite, cytotoxic drugs, irradiation, or corticosteroids (used in greater than physiologic doses).

PREGNANCY: Category C, caution in nursing.

MECHANISM OF ACTION: Toxoid combination; activates neutralizing antibodies to diphtheria and tetanus toxins for protection against diphtheria and tetanus.

NURSING CONSIDERATIONS

Assessment: Assess history of vaccination to determine necessity of boosters. In cases of wound care, determine the necessity of tetanus prophylaxis. Assess for history of hypersensitivity reactions following previous dose of vaccine, current health status and health history, pregnancy/nursing status, and possible drug interaction. Assess for history of Arthus-type hypersensitivity reaction and Guillain-Barre syndrome following prior dose of a tetanus toxoid-containing vaccine.

Monitoring: Monitor for increased incidence and severity of adverse reactions and hypersensitivity reactions.

Patient Counseling: Inform of the benefits and risks of immunization and of importance of completing the primary immunization series or receiving recommended booster doses. Instruct to report any adverse reactions to healthcare provider.

Administration: IM route (deltoid). Inspect for particulate matter and/or discoloration prior to administration. Shake well before withdrawing each dose. Avoid into gluteal areas. Do not administer IV, SQ, or ID. **Storage:** 2-8°C (36-46°F). Do not freeze. Do not use after expiration date.

TEVETEN   RX
eprosartan mesylate (Abbott)

Can cause death/injury to developing fetus during 2nd and 3rd trimesters. D/C therapy if pregnancy detected.

THERAPEUTIC CLASS: Angiotensin II receptor antagonist

INDICATIONS: Treatment of HTN, alone or with other antihypertensives (eg, diuretics, calcium channel blockers).

DOSAGE: *Adults:* Initial (as monotherapy in non-volume depleted patients): 600mg qd. Usual: 400-800mg/day, given qd-bid. Max: 800mg/day. Moderate to Severe Renal Impairment: Max: 600mg qd. Max BP reduction in most patients may take 2-3 weeks.

HOW SUPPLIED: Tab: 400mg, 600mg

WARNINGS/PRECAUTIONS: May cause symptomatic hypotension in patients with activated renin-angiotensin system (eg, volume- and/or salt-depleted patients); correct volume- or salt- depletion prior to therapy or monitor closely. Renal function changes reported which may be reversible upon d/c. Oliguria, progressive azotemia, and acute renal failure (rare) may occur in renin-angiotensin-aldosterone system (RAAS) dependent patients (eg, severe congestive heart failure (CHF)). Increase in SrCr or BUN reported with renal artery stenosis.

ADVERSE REACTIONS: Upper respiratory tract infection, rhinitis, pharyngitis, cough.

INTERACTIONS: Risk of hypotension with diuretics.

PREGNANCY: Category C (1st trimester) and D (2nd and 3rd trimesters), not for use in nursing.

MECHANISM OF ACTION: Angiotensin II receptor antagonist; blocks vasoconstrictor and aldosterone-secreting effects of angiotensin II by selectively blocking binding of angiotensin II to AT_1 receptor found in many tissues.

PHARMACOKINETICS: Absorption: (single 300mg oral dose) Absolute bioavailability: approximately 13% ; T_{max}=1-2 hrs. **Distribution:** V_d=308L; plasma protein binding (approximately 98%). **Elimination:** Feces (90%), urine (7%; 80%, unchanged); (multiple 600mg oral dose) $T_{1/2}$=20 hrs.

NURSING CONSIDERATIONS

Assessment: Assess for volume/salt depletion, renal function, BP, CHF, unilateral or bilateral renal stenosis, previous hypersensitivity, pregnancy/nursing status and possible drug interaction.

Monitoring: Monitor BP, LFTs and other laboratory abnormalities (eg, K⁺, WBC, Hgb), changes in renal function and volume/salt depletion.

Patient Counseling: Counsel about signs/symptoms of adverse effects; advise to seek prompt medical attention. Inform about fetal risks if taken during pregnancy. Ask to report pregnancy to physician immediately so that treatment may be d/c under medical supervision. Instruct to take with or without food.

Administration: Oral route. **Storage:** 20-25°C (68-77°F).

TEVETEN HCT   RX
eprosartan mesylate - hydrochlorothiazide (Abbott)

> Can cause death/injury to developing fetus during 2nd and 3rd trimesters. D/C therapy if pregnancy detected.

THERAPEUTIC CLASS: Angiotensin II receptor antagonist/thiazide diuretic

INDICATIONS: Treatment of HTN alone or with other antihypertensives (eg, calcium channel blocker).

DOSAGE: *Adults:* May substitute for individual components; begin combination therapy only after failure with monotherapy. Refer to PI for monotherapy dosing. Replacement Therapy: Usual: 600mg-12.5mg qd. Titrate: May increase to 600mg-25mg qd. Max: 600mg-25mg qd. If additional BP control required, or to maintain bid dosing of monotherapy, 300mg qpm eprosartan may be added. Moderate to Severe Renal Impairment: Max: 600mg qd. Max BP reduction in most patients may take 2-3 weeks.

HOW SUPPLIED: Tab: (Eprosartan-HCTZ) 600mg-12.5mg, 600mg-25mg

CONTRAINDICATIONS: Anuria, hypersensitivity to sulfonamide-derived drugs.

WARNINGS/PRECAUTIONS: May cause symptomatic hypotension in patients with activated renin-angiotensin system (eg, volume- and/or salt-depleted patients); correct volume- or salt- depletion prior to therapy or monitor closely. HCTZ: May precipitate hepatic coma; caution with impaired hepatic function or progressive liver disease. Hypersensitivity reactions may occur and are more likely with history of allergy or bronchial asthma. Exacerbation or activation of systemic lupus erythematosus (SLE) reported. Hypercalcemia, hypomagnesemia, hypokalemia, hyponatremia, and hypochloremic alkalosis may occur; monitor electrolytes periodically. Hyperuricemia or precipitation of frank gout may occur. May cause hyperglycemia, thus latent diabetes mellitus (DM) may become manifest. Enhanced antihypertensive effects in post-sympathectomy patients. Renal function changes reported, which may be reversible upon d/c. Oliguria, progressive azotemia, and acute renal failure (rare) may occur in renin-angiotensin-aldosterone system (RAAS) dependent patients (eg, severe congestive heart failure (CHF)). Increase in SrCr and BUN may occur with renal artery stenosis. Withhold or d/c with evident progressive renal impairment. Not for initial therapy.

ADVERSE REACTIONS: Dizziness, headache, back pain, fatigue, myalgia, upper respiratory tract infection, sinusitis, viral infection.

INTERACTIONS: (Eprosartan) Increased risk of hyperkalemia with K^+-sparing diuretics, K^+ supplements, or K^+-containing salt substitutes. Risk of hypotension with diuretics. (HCTZ) Potentiates orthostatic hypotension with alcohol, barbiturates, and narcotics. May need to adjust dosages of insulin and oral antidiabetic drugs. Impaired absorption with cholestyramine and colestipol resins. Corticosteroids and ACTH intensify electrolyte depletion. May decrease response to pressor amines (eg, norepinephrine). Potentiated effect with other antihypertensives. May increase responsiveness to nondepolarizing skeletal muscle relaxants (eg, tubocurarine). Risk of lithium toxicity; avoid use. NSAIDs may decrease diuretic, natriuretic, and antihypertensive effects. May sensitize or exaggerate response of the heart to toxic effects of digitalis.

PREGNANCY: Category C (1st trimester) and D (2nd and 3rd trimesters), not for use in nursing.

MECHANISM OF ACTION: Eprosartan: Angiotensin II receptor antagonist; blocks vasoconstrictor and aldosterone-secreting effects of angiotensin II by selectively blocking binding of angiotensin II to AT_1 receptor found in many tissues (eg, vascular smooth muscle, adrenal gland). HCTZ: Thiazide diuretic; mechanism not established. Affects renal tubular mechanisms of electrolyte reabsorption, directly increasing excretion of Na^+ and Cl^- and indirectly reducing plasma volume.

PHARMACOKINETICS: Absorption: Eprosartan: Absolute bioavailability (approximately 13%); T_{max}=1-2 hrs. **Distribution:** Eprosartan: V_d=308L; plasma protein binding (approximately 98%). HCTZ: Crosses placenta; excreted in breast milk. **Elimination:** Eprosartan: Feces (90%), urine (7%; 80%, unchanged); $T_{1/2}$=20 hrs. HCTZ: Urine (61%, unchanged); $T_{1/2}$=5.6-14.8 hrs.

NURSING CONSIDERATIONS

Assessment: Assess for anuria, hypersensitivity to other sulfonamide-derived drugs, renal/hepatic insufficiency, allergy or bronchial asthma, volume/salt depletion, renal function, SLE, CHF, unilateral or bilateral renal stenosis, DM, electrolyte imbalance, post-sympathectomy, pregnancy/nursing status, and possible drug interactions.

Monitoring: Perform periodic measurements of serum electrolytes. Monitor response and renal function. Monitor for signs and symptoms of fluid or electrolyte imbalance, hypotension, hyperuricemia or precipitation of gout, exacerbation or activation of SLE, hypersensitivity reactions, hyperglycemia, BP, CBC, renal/hepatic dysfunction, and other adverse effects.

Patient Counseling: Inform of risks if taken during pregnancy. Report pregnancy to physician immediately so that treatment may be d/c under medical supervision. Lightheadedness can occur especially during first days of therapy and should be reported to physician. D/C treatment and consult physician if syncope occurs. Inadequate fluid intake, excessive perspiration, diarrhea, or vomiting can lead to an excessive fall in BP, leading to lightheadedness or possible syncope. Do not use K^+ supplements or salt substitutes containing K^+ without consulting physician. Inform about signs/symptoms of adverse effects and advise to seek prompt medical attention.

Administration: Oral route. **Storage:** 20-25°C (68-77°F).

T

THALOMID

RX

thalidomide (Celgene)

> May cause severe, life-threatening birth defects or death to an unborn baby, if taken during pregnancy. Women of childbearing potential should have a pregnancy test within 24 hrs before starting therapy. Once treatment started, pregnancy testing should occur weekly for the first 4 weeks, then pregnancy testing should be repeated at 4 weeks in women with regular menstrual cycles. Pregnancy testing should occur every 2 weeks in women with irregular menstrual cycles; d/c immediately if pregnancy occurs. Two reliable forms of contraception must be used simultaneously unless continuous abstinence from heterosexual sexual contact is the chosen method. Males must use latex condoms during sexual contact with females of childbearing potential. Effective contraception must be used 4 weeks before, during, and 4 weeks after therapy. Only prescribers and pharmacists registered with the *S.T.E.P.S.*® distribution program can prescribe and dispense. Use in multiple myeloma results in an increased risk of venous thromboembolic events (eg, DVT, PE). Seek immediate medical care if symptoms of thromboembolism (eg, SOB, chest pain, arm or leg swelling) develop. Immediately report any suspected fetal exposure to the FDA and the manufacturer.

THERAPEUTIC CLASS: Immunomodulatory agent

INDICATIONS: Acute treatment of the cutaneous manifestations of moderate to severe erythema nodosum leprosum (ENL). Maintenance therapy for prevention and suppression of the cutaneous manifestations of ENL recurrence. In combination with dexamethasone for the treatment of newly diagnosed multiple myeloma.

DOSAGE: *Adults:* Acute ENL: Initial: 100-300mg qd. <50kg: Start at lower end of dosing range. If severe cutaneous ENL reaction or if previously required higher doses, may initiate at higher doses up to 400mg/day. In moderate to severe neuritis associated with a severe ENL reaction, may use with concomitant corticosteroid therapy. Taper steroid when neuritis is ameliorated. Usual duration: 2 weeks, or until signs/symptoms have subsided. Taper Dose: Decrease by 50mg every 2-4 weeks. Maintenance Therapy for Prevention/Suppression of ENL Recurrence: Use minimum dose to control reaction. Taper Dose: Every 3-6 months, attempt to decrease dose by 50mg every 2-4 weeks. Multiple Myeloma: 200mg qd. Give with dexamethasone in 28-day treatment cycles (40mg po on days 1-4, 9-12, and 17-20). Take with water, preferably at hs, and at least 1hr after the evening meal.
Pediatrics: ≥12 yrs: Initial: 100-300mg qd. <50kg: Start at lower end of dosing range. If severe cutaneous ENL reaction or if previously required higher doses, may initiate at higher doses up to 400mg/day. In moderate to severe neuritis associated with a severe ENL reaction, may use with concomitant corticosteroid therapy. Taper steroid when neuritis is ameliorated. Usual duration: 2 weeks, or until signs/symptoms have subsided. Taper Dose: Decrease by 50mg every 2-4 weeks. Maintenance Therapy for Prevention/Suppression of ENL Recurrence: Use minimum dose to control reaction. Taper Dose: Every 3-6 months, attempt to decrease dose by 50mg every 2-4 weeks. Multiple Myeloma: 200mg qd. Give with dexamethasone in 28-day treatment cycles (40mg po on days 1-4, 9-12, and 17-20). Take with water, preferably at hs, and at least 1hr after the evening meal.

HOW SUPPLIED: Cap: 50mg, 100mg, 150mg, 200mg

CONTRAINDICATIONS: Pregnancy and women of childbearing potential unless alternative therapies are considered inappropriate and if precautions are taken to avoid pregnancy. Sexually mature males unless they comply with the *S.T.E.P.S.*® program and mandatory contraceptive measures.

WARNINGS/PRECAUTIONS: May impair mental/physical abilities. May cause irreversible peripheral neuropathy; monitor for neuropathy during the first 3 months of therapy and periodically thereafter; d/c immediately if drug-induced neuropathy develops. May cause dizziness and orthostatic hypotension; sit upright for a few minutes prior to standing. If hypersensitivity reaction occurs (eg, erythematous macular rash); d/c drug. Serious dermatological reactions including Stevens-Johnson syndrome (SJS) and toxic epidermal necrolysis (TEN) reported. Decreased WBC, including neutropenia reported; do not initiate if absolute neutrophil count <750/mm³. Measure viral load of HIV patients after 1st and 3rd month of therapy and every 3 months thereafter.

T

Bradycardia and seizures, including grand mal convulsions, reported. Not indicated as monotherapy for cutaneous manifestations of moderate/severe ENL in the presence of moderate/severe neuritis.

ADVERSE REACTIONS: Drowsiness/somnolence, peripheral neuropathy, dizziness, orthostatic hypotension, neutropenia, increased HIV viral load, rash, constipation, hypocalcemia, thrombosis/embolism, dyspnea.

INTERACTIONS: Enhanced sedation with barbiturates, alcohol, chlorpromazine, and reserpine. Caution with drugs associated with peripheral neuropathy. Concomitant use with chemotherapeutic agents such as dexamethasone may increase risk for thromboembolic events (DVT, PE).

PREGNANCY: Category X, not for use in nursing.

MECHANISM OF ACTION: Immunomodulatory agent; not fully established. Possesses immunomodulatory, anti-inflammatory, and anti-angiogenic properties. Immunologic effects may be caused by suppression of excessive TNF-α production and down-modulation of selected cell surface adhesion molecules involved in leukocyte migration. Also causes suppression of macrophage involvement in prostaglandin synthesis and modulation of interleukin-10 and 12 production by peripheral blood mononuclear cells. In multiple myeloma, increased circulating natural killer cells and plasma levels of interleukin-2 and INF-gamma are also seen.

PHARMACOKINETICS: Absorption: Slow; T_{max}=2.9-5.7 hrs, variable doses resulted in different parameters. **Distribution:** Plasma protein binding (55-66%); found in semen. **Metabolism:** Non-enzymatic hydrolysis. **Elimination:** Urine (<0.7% unchanged); $T_{1/2}$=5-7 hrs.

NURSING CONSIDERATIONS

Assessment: Assess use in those capable of reproduction. Assess that females of child-bearing potential are committed to either abstaining from heterosexual contact or willing to use 2 forms of reliable contraception including 1 highly effective method (eg, IUD, hormonal contraception, tubal ligation, partner's vasectomy) and 1 additional effective method (eg, latex condom, diaphragm, cervical cap) beginning 4 weeks prior to treatment, during treatment, and continuing 4 weeks after treatment. Prior to therapy, assess that males will wear latex condom during any sexual contact with women of childbearing potential, even if they have undergone a vasectomy. Assess pregnancy status 24 hrs prior to therapy. Assess nursing status, absolute neutrophil count (ANC), and for drug interactions.

Monitoring: Monitor for signs/symptoms of venous thromboembolic events, drowsiness, somnolence, peripheral neuropathy, dizziness, orthostatic hypotension, neutropenia, hypersensitivity reactions (eg, erythematous macular rash), bradycardia, seizures, serious dermatological reactions (eg, SJS, TEN). Perform periodic monitoring of WBC count with differential. Perform pregnancy test weekly during first 4 weeks of therapy, then at 4-week intervals (regular menstrual cycle) or every 2 weeks (irregular menstrual cycle). Monitor for missed periods or abnormal menstrual bleeding. In HIV patients, monitor viral load after first and third months of therapy and every 3 months thereafter.

Patient Counseling: Instruct females they must use 2 forms of contraception beginning 4 weeks prior to treatment, during treatment, and 4 weeks following end of therapy. Instruct males to use latex condom during any heterosexual contact. Counsel to not extensively handle caps and maintain medication in blister packs until ingestion. Therapy may cause drowsiness and somnolence and impair mental/physical abilities. Avoid hazardous tasks (eg, operating machinery/driving) and alcohol or medications which may cause drowsiness. Advise that therapy may cause dizziness; sit upright for a few minutes prior to standing up from recumbent position. Instruct about signs/symptoms of peripheral neuropathies (eg, numbness, tingling) and thromboembolism (eg, SOB, chest pain, leg or arm swelling). Inform that blood donation is not allowed and males are not allowed to donate sperm while on medication.

Administration: Oral route. **Storage:** 25°C (77°F); excursions permitted to 15-30°C (59-86°F). Protect from light.

T

TIAZAC   RX

diltiazem HCl (Forest)

OTHER BRAND NAMES: Taztia XT (Andrx)

THERAPEUTIC CLASS: Calcium channel blocker (nondihydropyridine)

INDICATIONS: Treatment of HTN alone or in combination with other antihypertensives. Treatment of chronic stable angina.

DOSAGE: *Adults:* HTN: Usual: 120-240mg qd. Titrate: Adjust at 2-week intervals. Max: 540mg qd. Angina: Initial: 120-180mg qd. Titrate: Increase over 7-14 days. Max: 540mg qd. Elderly: Start at low end of dosing range.

HOW SUPPLIED: Cap, Extended-Release: 120mg, 180mg, 240mg, 300mg, 360mg; (Tiazac) 420mg

CONTRAINDICATIONS: Sick sinus syndrome and 2nd- or 3rd-degree atrioventricular (AV) block (except with a functioning pacemaker), severe hypotension (<90mmHg systolic), acute myocardial infarction (AMI), pulmonary congestion documented by x-ray.

WARNINGS/PRECAUTIONS: Prolongs AV node refractory periods. May develop asystole with Prinzmetal's angina. Caution in patients with pre-existing ventricular dysfunction; worsening of congestive heart failure (CHF) reported. Symptomatic hypotension may occur. Mild elevations of transaminases (eg, alkaline phosphatase, bilirubin, LDH, SGOT, SGPT) reported. Acute hepatic injury reported. Caution in patients with impaired renal or hepatic function. Monitor LFTs and renal function with prolonged use. D/C if persistent dermatologic reactions (eg, skin eruptions progressing to erythema multiforme and/or exfoliative dermatitis) occur. Caution in elderly.

ADVERSE REACTIONS: Peripheral edema, dizziness, headache, infection, pain, pharyngitis, dyspepsia, dyspnea, bronchitis, AV block, asthenia, vasodilation.

INTERACTIONS: Potential additive effects with agents known to affect cardiac contractility and/or conduction. Increased levels of carbamazepine, midazolam, triazolam, lovastatin, and propranolol; monitor closely. Increased levels of diltiazem with cimetidine. Monitor digoxin and cyclosporine levels if used concomitantly. Potentiates cardiac contractility, conductivity, and automaticity, and vascular dilation with anesthetics. Additive cardiac conduction effects with digitalis or β-blockers. Avoid rifampin and other CYP3A4 inducers. Additive antihypertensive effect when used concomitantly with other antihypertensive agents. Other drugs that are specific substrates, inhibitors, or inducers of CYP3A4 may have a significant impact on the efficacy and side effect profile of diltiazem. (Tiazac) Increased levels of buspirone and quinidine. Increased risk of myopathy and rhabdomyolysis with statins (eg, lovastatin, simvastatin). Sinus bradycardia reported with the use of clonidine concurrently; monitor HR.

PREGNANCY: Category C, not for use in nursing.

MECHANISM OF ACTION: Calcium channel blocker; inhibits cellular influx of calcium ions during membrane depolarization of cardiac and vascular smooth muscle. HTN: Primarily by relaxation of vascular smooth muscle and the resultant decrease in peripheral vascular resistance. Angina: Reduces myocardial oxygen demand and inhibits coronary artery spasms.

PHARMACOKINETICS: Absorption: Well-absorbed; Absolute bioavailability (40%). **Distribution:** Plasma protein binding (70-80%); found in breast milk. **Metabolism:** Hepatic; desacetyldiltiazem, desmethyldiltiazem (major metabolites). **Elimination:** Urine (2%-4%, unchanged); bile; $T_{1/2}$=4-9.5 hrs.

NURSING CONSIDERATIONS

Assessment: Assess for sick sinus syndrome and 2nd- or 3rd-degree AV block without a functional ventricular pacemaker, severe hypotension, acute MI, pulmonary congestion (documented by x-ray), CHF, ventricular dysfunction, renal/hepatic function, drug hypersensitivity, pregnancy/nursing status and possible drug interactions.

Monitoring: Monitor LFTs (eg, alkaline phosphatase, bilirubin, LDH, SGOT, SGPT), BP, HR, renal/hepatic/cardiac function, ECG abnormalities. Monitor for signs/symptoms of angina and dermatological reactions (eg, skin eruptions progressing to erythema multiforme and/or exfoliative dermatitis).

Patient Counseling: Counsel about signs/symptoms of adverse effects. Instruct to take as prescribed. Educate about need for routine checkup and lab exams. When administering with applesauce, it should not be hot and should be soft enough to swallow without chewing.

Administration: Oral route. May be administered by opening the capsule and sprinkling contents on a spoonful of applesauce. The applesauce should be swallowed immediately without chewing and followed with a glass of water. Do not divide contents. **Storage:** (Taztia XT) 20-25°C (68-77°F). (Tiazac) 25°C (77°F); excursions permitted to 15-30°C (59-86°F). Avoid excessive humidity.

TICLOPIDINE RX
ticlopidine HCl (Various)

> Can cause life-threatening hematological adverse reactions, including neutropenia/agranulocytosis, thrombotic thrombocytopenic purpura (TTP), and aplastic anemia. Monitor for evidence of neutropenia or TTP during first 3 months; d/c if any seen.

THERAPEUTIC CLASS: Platelet aggregation inhibitor

INDICATIONS: To reduce risk of thrombotic stroke in stroke patients or those with stroke precursors who are aspirin (ASA) intolerant, allergic, or failed ASA therapy. Adjunct to ASA to reduce incidence of subacute stent thrombosis in patients undergoing successful coronary artery stent implantation.

DOSAGE: *Adults:* Stroke: 250mg bid. Coronary Artery Stenting: 250mg bid with ASA up to 30 days after stent implant.

HOW SUPPLIED: Tab: 250mg

CONTRAINDICATIONS: Hematopoietic disorders (eg, neutropenia, thrombocytopenia), history of TTP or aplastic anemia, hemostatic disorders, active pathological bleeding, severe liver impairment.

WARNINGS/PRECAUTIONS: Monitor for hematologic toxicity before treatment, then every 2 weeks for 1st 3 months, and 2 weeks after discontinuation. Monitor more frequently if signs of hematological adverse reactions; d/c if neutrophils <1200/mm³, aplastic anemia or TTP occurs. D/C 10-14 days before surgery. Caution in trauma, surgery, bleeding disorders. May need dose adjustment with renal or hepatic impairment. May elevate LFTs, TG, and cholesterol.

ADVERSE REACTIONS: Diarrhea, rash, nausea, GI pain, dyspepsia, neutropenia.

INTERACTIONS: Adjust dose with drugs metabolized by CYP450 with low therapeutic ratios or with hepatic impairment. Potentiates ASA and NSAIDs effect on platelet aggregation. Antacids reduce plasma levels. Cimetidine reduces clearance. Decreases digoxin plasma levels. Significant decrease of theophylline plasma clearance. Caution with phenytoin, propranolol. D/C anticoagulants or fibrinolytics. Increased bioavailability with food.

PREGNANCY: Category B, not for use in nursing.

MECHANISM OF ACTION: Platelet aggregation inhibitor; interferes with platelet membrane function by inhibiting ADP-induced platelet fibrinogen binding and subsequent platelet-platelet interactions. Effect on platelet function is irreversible. Responsible for prolonging bleeding time.

PHARMACOKINETICS: Absorption: Rapid; T_{max}=2 hrs. **Distribution:** Plasma protein binding (98%). **Metabolism:** Liver (extensive). **Elimination:** Urine (60%), feces (23%); $T_{1/2}$=12.6 hrs (single dose), 4-5 days (multiple dose).

NURSING CONSIDERATIONS

Assessment: Assess for presence of hematopoietic disorders (eg, neutropenia, thrombocytopenia), history of TTP, aplastic anemia, presence of hemostatic disorder or active bleeding (eg, bleeding peptic ulcer, intracranial bleeding), severe liver impairment, renal impairment, nursing status, and drug interactions. Obtain baseline CBC including ANC, platelet count, and peripheral smear.

Monitoring: Monitor for signs/symptoms of thrombocytopenia, TTP (eg, weakness, petechiae, purpura, dark urine, neurological changes), aplastic anemia, agranulocytosis, pancytopenia, leukemia, liver dysfunction, and serum cholesterol elevations. During first 3 months of therapy, monitor CBC including ANC, platelet count, and peripheral smear every 2 weeks. If therapy d/c before 3 months, monitor for 2 weeks following d/c. If liver dysfunction suspected, perform liver function testing (eg, ALT, AST, GGT).

Patient Counseling: Counsel about possible adverse effects (eg, thrombocytopenia, neutropenia). Contact physician immediately if any signs/symptoms of infection or TTP syndrome (eg, fever, weakness, difficulty speaking, seizures, yellowing of skin or eyes, bloody urine, petechiae) develop. Lab testing is required during therapy. It may take longer than usual to stop bleeding while on medication; contact physician if any unusual bleeding occurs. Notify all other physicians of medication. Take with food.

Administration: Oral route. Take with food. **Storage:** 15-30°C (59-86°F).

TIGAN   RX
trimethobenzamide HCl (Various)

THERAPEUTIC CLASS: Emetic response modifier

INDICATIONS: Treatment of postoperative nausea and vomiting (PONV) and for nausea associated with gastroenteritis.

DOSAGE: *Adults:* (Cap) 300mg tid-qid. (Inj) 200mg IM tid-qid. Renal Impairment (GFR ≤ 70mL/min/1.73m²): Reduce dose or increase dosing interval. Elderly: Start at low end of dosing range.

HOW SUPPLIED: Cap: 300mg; Inj: 100mg/mL

CONTRAINDICATIONS: (Inj) Pediatric patients.

WARNINGS/PRECAUTIONS: May impair physical/mental abilties. Caution with acute febrile illness, encephalitides, gastroenteritis, dehydration, electrolyte imbalance and in elderly; CNS reactions reported. Caution with renal impairment. May produce drowsiness. May obscure diagnosis of appendicitus and signs of toxicity due to overdosage of other drugs. (Cap) Caution in children; may cause extrapyramidal syndrome, which may be confused with CNS signs of undiagnosed primary disease (eg, Reye's syndrome) and may unfavorably alter the course of Reye's syndrome due to hepatotoxic potential.

ADVERSE REACTIONS: Parkinson's-like symptoms, blood dyscrasias, blurred vision, coma, convulsions, mood depression, diarrhea, disorientation, dizziness, drowsiness, headache, jaundice, muscle cramps, opisthotonos.

INTERACTIONS: Caution with CNS agents (eg, phenothiazines, barbiturates, belladonna derivatives) in acute febrile illness, encephalitides, gastroenteritis, dehydration, and electrolyte imbalance. Adverse drug interactions reported with alcohol.

PREGNANCY: Safety in pregnancy and nursing not known.

MECHANISM OF ACTION: Not established; thought to involve chemoreceptor trigger zone, an area in medulla oblongata through which emetic impulses are conveyed to vomiting center (direct impulses to vomiting center apparently not similarly inhibited).

PHARMACOKINETICS: Absorption: T_{max}=30 min (IM 200mg), 45 min (cap 300mg). **Metabolism:** Oxidation, trimethobenzamide N-oxide (major metabolite). **Elimination:** Urine (30-50%, unchanged); $T_{1/2}$=7-9 hrs.

NURSING CONSIDERATIONS

Assessment: Assess for renal/hepatic impairment, Reye's syndrome in children, pregnancy/nursing status, alcohol intake, acute febrile illness, encephalitides, gastroenteritis, dehydration, electrolyte imbalance, appendicitis, toxicity, possible drug interactions.

Monitoring: Monitor renal function, for signs of hepatotoxicity, CNS reactions (eg, opisthotonos, convulsions, coma), EPS, and cerebral edema. Reduce dose in elderly and in patients with renal impairment (CrCl: ≤70ml/min/1.73m²).

Patient Counseling: Caution against performing hazardous tasks (operating machinery/driving). Notify if pregnant/nursing.

Administration: Oral and IM route. **Storage:** 25°C (77°F); excursions permitted to 15-30°C (59-86°F).

TIKOSYN   RX
dofetilide (Pfizer)

To minimize risk of arrhythmia, place patients initiated or reinitiated on therapy for minimum of 3 days in a facility that can provide CrCl, ECG monitoring, and cardiac resuscitation. Dofetilide is available only to hospitals and prescribers who have received appropriate dofetilide dosing and treatment initiation education.

THERAPEUTIC CLASS: Class III antiarrhythmic

INDICATIONS: Conversion to and maintenance of normal sinus rhythm in patients with atrial fibrillation/flutter.

DOSAGE: *Adults:* Individualize dose base on CrCl or QT interval (if HR <60bpm). Start: CrCl >60mL/min: 500mcg bid. CrCl 40-60mL/min: 250mcg bid. CrCl 20 to <40mL/min: 125mcg bid. Determine QTc interval 2-3 hrs after 1st dose and adjust dose if QTc >500msec or if >15% increase from baseline. QTc/Renal Dose Adjustment: Reduce 500mcg bid to 250mcg bid. Reduce 250mcg bid to 125mcg bid. Reduce 125mcg bid to 125mcg qd. Max: CrCl >60mL/min: 500mcg bid. D/C any time after 2nd dose if QTc >500msec (550msec with ventricular conduction abnormalities). Refer to PI for step by step instruction for dose initiation.

HOW SUPPLIED: Cap: 125mcg, 250mcg, 500mcg

CONTRAINDICATIONS: Long QT syndromes, baseline QT interval or QTc >440msec (500msec with ventricular conduction abnormalities). Severe renal impairment (CrCl <20mL/min). Concomitant verapamil, HCTZ, and inhibitors of renal cation transport system (eg, cimetidine, trimethoprim, ketoconazole, megesterol, prochlorperazine).

WARNINGS/PRECAUTIONS: Can cause serious ventricular arrhythmias, primarily torsade de pointes (TdP). Calculate CrCl before 1st dose; adjust dose based on CrCl. Caution in severe hepatic impairment. Maintain normal K⁺ levels. Patients with atrial fibrillation should be anticoagulated prior to cardioversion. Rehospitalize patient for 3 days anytime lower dose is increased. Allow 2 days washout period before start of other drugs. Caution with elderly.

ADVERSE REACTIONS: Headache, chest pain, dizziness, ventricular arrhythmia, dyspnea, nausea, insomnia, ventricular tachycardia, TdP, respiratory tract infection, flu syndrome, back pain, diarrhea, rash, abdominal pain.

INTERACTIONS: See Contraindications. Hypokalemia or hypomagnesemia may occur with K⁺-depleting diuretics. CYP3A4 inhibitors (eg, macrolides, protease inhibitors, azole antifungals, etc) may potentiate dofetilide. Caution with drugs actively secreted by cationic secretion (eg, amiloride, triamterene, metformin). Not recommended with drugs that prolong the QT interval. Hold Class I and III antiarrhythmics for at least 3 half-lives before initiating dofetilide. Reduce amiodarone to <0.3mcg/mL or withdraw at least 3 months before initiating dofetilide. Higher occurrence of TdP with digoxin.

PREGNANCY: Category C, not for use in nursing.

MECHANISM OF ACTION: Class III antiarrhythmic; blocks cardiac ion channel carrying rapid component of delayed rectifier K⁺ current, I_{Kr}.

PHARMACOKINETICS: Absorption: Bioavailability (>90%); T_{max}=2-3 hrs. **Distribution:** V_d=3L/kg; plasma protein binding (60-70%). **Metabolism:** Liver via CYP3A4 through N-dealkylation and N-oxidation pathways. **Elimination:** Urine (80% unchanged), (20% metabolites); $T_{1/2}$=10 hrs.

NURSING CONSIDERATIONS

Assessment: Assess for congenital or acquired long QT syndrome, ventricular arrhythmia, CHF, recent MI, structural heart disease, atrial flutter/fibrillation, baseline QT interval or QTc ≥440 msec (500 msec with ventricular conduction abnormalities), sick sinus syndrome, heart block, renal/hepatic impairment, pregnancy/nursing status, and possible drug interactions. Correct K⁺ levels prior to therapy.

Monitoring: Patient should be in a facility for minimum of 3 days where CrCl, continuous ECG monitoring, and cardiac resuscitation are available. Monitor for ventricular arrhythmias (eg, torsade de pointes and polymorphic ventricular tachycardia associated with QT interval prolongation).

Patient Counseling: Inform about risks/benefits and need for compliance with prescribed dosing. Periodic monitoring of QTc and renal function required. Notify physician if pregnant/nursing or if taking any OTC medications. Counsel to report immediately any symptoms associated with electrolyte imbalance (eg, excessive/prolonged diarrhea, sweating, vomiting, loss of appetite, thirst). Instruct not to double the next dose if a dose is missed.

Administration: Oral route. **Storage:** 15-30°C (59-86°F). Protect from humidity and moisture.

TIMENTIN   RX
ticarcillin disodium - clavulanate potassium (GlaxoSmithKline)

THERAPEUTIC CLASS: Broad-spectrum penicillin/beta-lactamase inhibitor

INDICATIONS: Treatment of septicemia (including bacteremia), lower respiratory tract, bone and joint, skin and skin structure, urinary tract (UTI), gynecologic, and intra-abdominal infections, caused by susceptible strains of microorganisms.

DOSAGE: *Adults:* ≥60kg: UTI/Systemic Infection: 3.1g q4-6h. Gynecologic Infections: (Based on ticarcillin content) Moderate: 200mg/kg/day in divided doses q6h. Severe: 300mg/kg/day in divided doses q4h. <60kg: (Based on ticarcillin content) 200-300mg/kg/day in divided doses q4-6h. Administer by IV over 30 min for 10-14 days but may prolong duration for difficult/complicated infections; continue for ≥2 days after signs/symptoms of infection disappear. Persistent Infections: May require treatment for several weeks; do not use smaller doses than indicated above. Renal Impairment: Refer to PI. *Pediatrics:* ≥3 months: ≥60kg: Mild to Moderate Infections: 3.1g (3g ticarcillin, 100mg clavulanate) q6h. Severe Infections: 3.1g (3g ticarcillin, 100mg clavulanate) q4h. <60kg: (Based on ticarcillin content): Usual: 50mg/kg/dose. Mild to Moderate Infections: 200mg/kg/day in divided doses q6h. Severe: 300mg/kg/day in divided doses q4h. Administer by IV over 30 min for 10-14 days but may prolong duration for difficult/complicated infections; continue for ≥2 days after signs/symptoms of infection disappear. Persistent Infections: May require treatment for several weeks; do not use smaller doses than indicated above. Renal Impairment: Refer to PI.

HOW SUPPLIED: Inj: (Ticarcillin-Clavulanate) 3g-100mg (3.1g) [Vial, Add-Vantage]; 3g-100mg/100mL [Galaxy]. Also available as a Pharmacy Bulk Package. Refer to individual package insert for more information.

WARNINGS/PRECAUTIONS: Serious, fatal hypersensitivity reactions reported; d/c and institute appropriate therapy if allergic reaction occurs. *Clostridium difficile*-associated diarrhea (CDAD) reported. Risk of convulsions with high doses, especially with renal impairment. Bleeding manifestations associated with coagulation tests abnormalities (eg, clotting time, platelet aggregation, PT) may occur, especially with renal impairment; d/c therapy if occur. Hypokalemia reported; caution with fluid and electrolyte imbalance. Periodically monitor serum K⁺ with prolonged therapy. Consider the salt content of the drug (4.51mEq/g) in patients requiring restricted salt intake. Prolonged use may result in superinfections with mycotic or bacterial pathogens. Caution in elderly.

ADVERSE REACTIONS: Hypersensitivity reactions, headache, giddiness, taste/smell disturbances, stomatitis, N/V, diarrhea, thrombocytopenia, leukopenia, elevated AST/ALT, elevated SrCr/BUN, hemorrhagic cystitis.

INTERACTIONS: Increased serum levels and prolonged $T_{1/2}$ with probenecid. May reduce efficacy of combined oral estrogen/progesterone contraceptives. Inactivates aminoglycoside when mixed together in solutions for parenteral administration.

PREGNANCY: Category B, caution in nursing.

MECHANISM OF ACTION: Ticarcillin: Broad-spectrum penicillin (PCN) with bactericidal activity against many gram-positive and -negative aerobic and anaerobic bacteria. Clavulanic acid: β-lactamase inhibitor; possesses ability to inactivate wide range of β-lactamase enzymes.

PHARMACOKINETICS: Absorption: Ticarcillin: C_{max}=330mcg/mL, 324mcg/mL (Galaxy), AUC=485mcg•hr/mL (adults), 339mcg•hr/mL (infants/children). Clavulanic acid: C_{max}=8mcg/mL, AUC=8.2mcg•hr/mL (adults), 7mcg•hr/mL (infants/children). **Distribution:** Plasma protein binding (45%, ticarcillin), (25%, clavulanic acid). **Elimination:** Ticarcillin: Urine (60-70%, unchanged); $T_{1/2}$=1.1 hrs (adults), 4.4 hrs (neonates), 1 hr (infants/children). Clavulanic acid: Urine (35-45%, unchanged); $T_{1/2}$=1.1 hrs (adults), 1.9 hrs (neonates), 0.9 hr (infants/children).

NURSING CONSIDERATIONS

Assessment: Assess for organisms causing the infection and their susceptibility to drug, previous hypersensitivity reactions to cephalosporins, PCNs, or other allergens, renal/hepatic impairment, presence of fluid/electrolyte imbalance, restricted salt intake, pregnancy/nursing status, and possible drug interactions.

Monitoring: Periodically monitor renal, hepatic, hematopoietic function, and serum K^+ levels with prolonged use. Monitor for signs/symptoms of anaphylactic/allergic reactions, CDAD, drug resistance or superinfection, bleeding manifestations, and electrolyte abnormalities.

Patient Counseling: Counsel that drug only treats bacterial, not viral (eg, common cold), infections. Instruct to take as directed; skipping doses or not completing full course may decrease effectiveness and increase resistance. Inform that diarrhea is a common problem and usually ends when antibiotic is d/c. Advise that watery and bloody stools (with or without stomach cramps and fever) may develop even as late as ≥2 months after last dose; notify physician immediately if occurs.

Administration: IV route; infuse over 30 min. Refer to individual PI for compatibility, stability, and directions for use. **Storage:** Vial: ≤24°C (75°F). Galaxy: -20°C (-4°F). Thawed Sol: 22°C (72°F) for 24 hrs or 4°C (39°F) for 7 days.

TIMOLOL   RX
timolol maleate (Various)

THERAPEUTIC CLASS: Nonselective beta-blocker

INDICATIONS: Treatment of HTN. To reduce cardiovascular mortality and risk of reinfarction with previous myocardial infarction (MI). Migraine prophylaxis.

DOSAGE: *Adults:* HTN: Initial: 10mg bid. Maint: 20-40mg/day. Wait at least 7 days between dose increases. Max: 60mg/day given bid. MI: 10mg bid. Migraine: Initial: 10mg bid. Maint: 20mg qd. Max: 30mg/day in divided doses. May decrease to 10mg qd. D/C if inadequate response after 6-8 weeks with max dose.

HOW SUPPLIED: Tab: 5mg, 10mg*, 20mg* *scored

CONTRAINDICATIONS: Active or history of bronchial asthma, severe chronic obstructive pulmonary disease (COPD), sinus bradycardia, 2nd- and 3rd-degree atrioventricular (AV) block, overt cardiac failure, cardiogenic shock.

WARNINGS/PRECAUTIONS: Caution with well-compensated cardiac failure, diabetes mellitus (DM), mild to moderate COPD, bronchospastic disease, dialysis, hepatic/renal impairment, or cerebrovascular insufficiency. Exacerbation of ischemic heart disease with abrupt cessation. May mask hyperthyroidism or hypoglycemia symptoms. Withdrawal before surgery is controversial. May potentiate weakness with myasthenia gravis. Can cause cardiac failure. Caution and consider monitoring renal function in elderly.

ADVERSE REACTIONS: Fatigue, headache, nausea, arrhythmia, pruritus, dizziness, dyspnea, asthenia, bradycardia.

INTERACTIONS: Possible additive effects and hypotension and/or marked bradycardia with catecholamine-depleting drugs. NSAIDs may reduce antihypertensive effects. Quinidine may potentiate β-blockade. AV conduction time prolonged with digitalis and either diltiazem or verapamil. Hypotension, AV conduction disturbances, left ventricular failure reported with oral calcium antagonists. Caution with IV calcium antagonists, insulin, oral hypoglycemics. Avoid calcium antagonists with cardiac dysfunction. May exacerbate rebound HTN following clonidine withdrawal. May block effects of epinephrine.

PREGNANCY: Category C, not for use in nursing.

MECHANISM OF ACTION: β_1 and β_2 adrenergic receptor blocking agent; reduces cardiac output and plasma renin activity.

PHARMACOKINETICS: Absorption: (PO) Completely absorbed (90%); T_{max}=2 hrs. **Metabolism:** Partially, by liver. **Excretion:** Kidneys; $T_{1/2}$= 4 hrs.

NURSING CONSIDERATIONS

Assessment: Assess for bradycardia, cardiogenic shock, 2nd- and 3rd-degree heart block, overt cardiac failure, impaired hepatic/renal function, bronchospastic disease, PVD, DM, thyrotoxicosis, valvular heart disease, pregnancy/nursing status and possible drug interactions.

Monitoring: Monitor for cardiac failure, HTN, renal function, exacerbation of ischemia following abrupt withdrawal, bronchospastic disease, anaphylactoid reactions, hypersensitivity reactions.

Patient Counseling: Counsel if signs suggest reduced cerebral blood flow; may need to d/c therapy. Instruct not to interrupt or d/c therapy without consulting physician. Counsel about signs/symptoms of congestive heart failure (CHF); notify physician if signs/symptoms of impending CHF or unexplained respiratory symptoms occur.

Administration: Oral route. **Storage:** 20-25°C (68-77°F); tight, light-resistant container.

TIMOPTIC   RX
timolol maleate (Aton)

OTHER BRAND NAMES: Timoptic-XE (Aton) - Timoptic in Ocudose (Aton)

THERAPEUTIC CLASS: Nonselective beta-blocker

INDICATIONS: Treatment of elevated intraocular pressure (IOP) in patients with ocular HTN or open-angle glaucoma. (Ocudose) May be used when a patient is sensitive to the preservative in timolol maleate ophthalmic sol, benzalkonium chloride, or when use with a preservative free topical medication is advisable.

DOSAGE: *Adults:* (Sol/Ocudose) Initial: 1 drop (0.25%) in affected eye(s) bid. If clinical response is not adequate, may change to 1 drop (0.5%) in affected eye(s) bid. Maint: 1 drop (0.25-0.5%) in affected eye(s) qd. Max: 1 drop (0.5%) bid. (XE) Initial: 1 drop (0.25 or 0.5%) in the affected eye(s) qd. Max: 1 drop (0.5%) qd. Dose of other topically applied ophthalmic drugs should be administered at least 10 mins prior to gel forming drops. (Sol/Ocudose/XE) Concomitant therapy can be instituted if IOP is still not at a satisfactory level. Evaluate IOP after 4 weeks.

HOW SUPPLIED: Sol: (Timoptic) 0.25% [5mL], 0.5% [5mL, 10mL]; Sol: (Timoptic Ocudose) 0.25%, 0.5% [0.2mL, 60's]; Sol, Gel Forming: (Timoptic-XE) 0.25%, 0.5% [5mL]

CONTRAINDICATIONS: Bronchial asthma, history of bronchial asthma, severe chronic obstructive pulmonary disease (COPD), sinus bradycardia, 2nd- or 3rd-degree atrioventricular (AV) block, overt cardiac failure, cardiogenic shock.

WARNINGS/PRECAUTIONS: Severe cardiac and respiratory reactions, including death, due to bronchospasm in patients with asthma and, rarely, death associated with cardiac failure reported. Caution with cardiac failure; d/c at 1st sign/symptom of cardiac failure. May mask the signs and symptoms of acute hypoglycemia; caution in patients subject to spontaneous hypoglycemia or diabetes mellitus (DM). May mask certain clinical signs (eg, tachycardia) of hyperthyroidism; carefully manage patients suspected of developing thyrotoxicosis. Avoid with COPD (eg, chronic bronchitis, emphysema), history/known bronchospastic disease. Not for use alone in angle-closure glaucoma. May potentiate muscle weakness consistent with myasthenic symptoms (eg, diplopia, ptosis, generalized weakness); caution with myasthenia gravis or patients with myasthenic symptoms. Caution with cerebrovascular insufficiency; consider alternative therapy if signs/symptoms of reduced cerebral blood flow develop. Choroidal detachment after filtration reported. Caution in patients with history of atopy or history of severe anaphylactic reactions to a variety of allergens. (Sol/XE) Bacterial keratitis with the use of multiple dose containers reported.

ADVERSE REACTIONS: Burning/stinging upon instillation. (XE) Ocular: blurred vision, pain, conjunctivitis, discharge, foreign-body sensation, itching, tearing. Systemic: headache, dizziness, upper respiratory infections.

INTERACTIONS: May potentiatially produce additive effects if used concomitantly with systemic β-blockers. Concomitant use of two topical β-adrenergic blocking agents is not recommended. Caution with oral/IV calcium antagonists because of possible AV conduction disturbances, left ventricular failure, or hypotension. Avoid oral/IV calcium antagonists with impaired cardiac function. Possible additive effects, production of hypotension and/or marked bradycardia may occur when used concomitantly with catecholamine depleting drugs (eg, reserpine). Concomitant use with calcium antagonists and digitalis may cause additive effects in prolonging AV conduction time. Potentiated systemic β-blockade reported with concomitant use of CYP2D6 inhibitors (eg, quinidine, SSRIs). Mydriasis reported occasionally with epinephrine. May augment risks of general anesthesia in surgical procedures; protracted severe hypotension and difficulty in restarting and maintaining heartbeat reported; gradual withdrawal recommended. Caution with insulin or oral hypoglycemic agents.

PREGNANCY: Category C, not for use in nursing.

MECHANISM OF ACTION: Nonselective β-blocker; reduces elevated and normal IOP, whether or not accompanied by glaucoma. Ocular hypotensive action not clearly established; may be related to reduced aqueous formation and a slight increase in outflow capacity.

PHARMACOKINETICS: Absorption: (Sol/Ocudose) C_{max}=0.46ng/mL (morning dose), 0.35ng/mL (afternoon dose); (XE) C_{max}=0.28ng/mL (morning dose). **Distribution:** Found in breast milk.

NURSING CONSIDERATIONS

Assessment: Assess for presence or history of bronchial asthma, COPD (eg, bronchitis, emphysema), or any other conditions where treatment is contraindicated or cautioned. Assess for pregnancy/nursing status and possible drug interactions. Assess if planning to undergo major surgery. (Sol/XE) Assess for corneal disease or disruption of the ocular epithelial surface.

Monitoring: Monitor for signs/symptoms of cardiac failure, masking of signs/symptoms of hypoglycemia, masking of hyperthyroidism, thyrotoxicosis, reduced cerebral blood flow, choroidal detachment, and for anaphylaxis. Monitor BP, HR, IOP. Evaluate IOP after 4 weeks of treatment. (Sol/XE) Monitor for bacterial keratitis.

Patient Counseling: Advise not to use product if have presence or history of bronchial asthma, severe chronic obstructive pulmonary disease, sinus bradycardia, second or third degree AV block, or if have cardiac failure. (Sol/XE)

Instruct to avoid touching tip of container to eye or surrounding structures. Counsel to seek physician's advice on continued use of product if underwent ocular surgery or develop intercurrent ocular condition (eg, trauma or infection). Handle ocular solutions properly to avoid contamination; using contaminated solution may result in serious eye damage. (Sol) Contains benzalkonium chloride which may be absorbed by soft contact lenses. Remove contact lenses prior to administration and reinsert 15 min following administration. (Ocudose) Instruct about proper administration. Advise to use immediately after opening, and discard the individual unit and any remaining contents immediately after use. (XE) Invert the closed container and shake once before each use. Administer at least 10 mins apart with other topical ophthalmic medications. May impair ability to perform hazardous task (eg, operating machinery, driving motor vehicle).

Administration: Ocular route. **Storage:** 15-30°C (59-86°F). Avoid freezing. Protect from light. (Ocudose) Keep unit dose container in protective foil overwrap and use within 1 month after opening.

TINDAMAX   RX
tinidazole (Mission)

> Carcinogenicity has been seen in mice and rats treated chronically with metronidazole. Although not reported for tinidazole, the two drugs are structurally related and have similar biologic effects. Use only for approved indications.

THERAPEUTIC CLASS: Antiprotozoal agent

INDICATIONS: Treatment of trichomoniasis caused by *Trichomonas vaginalis*, giardiasis caused by *Giardia duodenalis*, intestinal amebiasis and amebic liver abscess caused by *Entamoeba histolytica*, and bacterial vaginosis in non-pregnant women.

DOSAGE: *Adults:* Take with food. Trichomoniasis/Giardiasis: 2g single dose. For trichomoniasis, treat sexual partner with same dose and at same time. Amebiasis: Intestinal: 2g qd for 3 days. Amebic Liver Abscess: 2g qd for 3-5 days. Bacterial Vaginosis: 2g qd for 2 days or 1g qd for 5 days. Hemodialysis: If given on same day and prior to hemodialysis, give additional dose equivalent to one-half of recommended dose at the end of dialysis.
Pediatrics: >3 yrs: Take with food. Giardiasis: 50mg/kg single dose. Amebiasis: Intestinal: 50mg/kg qd for 3 days. Amebic Liver Abscess: 50mg/kg qd for 3-5 days. Max (for all): 2g/day. May crush tabs in cherry syrup.

HOW SUPPLIED: Tab: 250mg*, 500mg* *scored

CONTRAINDICATIONS: Treatment during 1st trimester of pregnancy, nursing mothers during therapy and 3 days following last dose.

WARNINGS/PRECAUTIONS: Seizures, peripheral neuropathy reported. D/C if abnormal neurologic signs occur. Caution with hepatic impairment or blood dyscrasias. May develop vaginal candidiasis. May develop drug resistance if prescribed in absence of proven or strongly suspected bacterial infection. Caution in elderly.

ADVERSE REACTIONS: Metallic/bitter taste, N/V, vaginal fungal infection, anorexia, headache, dizziness, constipation, dyspepsia, cramps/epigastric discomfort, weakness, fatigue, malaise, convulsions, peripheral neuropathy.

INTERACTIONS: Avoid alcohol during therapy and for 3 days after use. Do not give if taken disulfiram within the last 2 weeks. May potentiate oral anticoagulants. May prolong $T_{1/2}$ and reduce clearance of phenytoin (IV). May decrease clearance of fluorouracil causing increased side effects; if concomitant use needed, monitor for toxicities. May increase levels of lithium, cyclosporine, tacrolimus. Separate dosing with cholestyramine. Phenobarbital, rifampin, phenytoin, fosphenytoin and other CYP3A4 inducers may decrease levels. Cimetidine, ketoconazole, other CYP3A4 inhibitors may increase levels. Therapeutic effect antagonized by oxytetracycline.

PREGNANCY: Category C, not for use in nursing.

MECHANISM OF ACTION: Antiprotozoal, antibacterial agent; nitro group of tinidazole is reduced by cell extracts of *Trichomonas*. Free nitro radical

ASE

generated as a result of this reduction may be responsible for antiprotozoal activity.

PHARMACOKINETICS: Absorption: Rapid, complete. (Fasted) C_{max}=47.7mcg/mL, T_{max}=1.6 hrs, AUC=901.6mcg.hr/mL at 72 hours. **Distribution:** V_d=50L; plasma protein binding (12%); crosses blood-brain and placental barrier; found in breast milk. **Metabolism:** Mainly via oxidation, hydroxylation, conjugation; CYP3A4 mainly involved. **Elimination:** Urine (20-25% unchanged), feces (12%); $T_{1/2}$=12-14 hrs.

NURSING CONSIDERATIONS

Assessment: Assess for blood dyscrasias, seizures, pregnancy/nursing status, hypersensitivity and possible drug interactions. Assess for proven or strongly suspected bacterial infection to avoid drug resistance.

Monitoring: Monitor for convulsive seizures, peripheral neuropathy, vaginal candidiasis, drug resistance, hypersensitivity reactions (urticaria, pruritis, angioedema, erythema multiforme, Stevens-Johnson syndrome).

Patient Counseling: Advise to take with food to minimize epigastric discomfort and other GI side effects. Avoid alcohol and preparations containing ethanol and propylene glycol during therapy and for 3 days afterward to prevent abdominal cramps, N/V, headache, and flushing. Therapy only treats bacterial, not viral, infections (eg, common cold). Instruct to take as directed; skipping doses or not completing full course may decrease effectiveness and increase resistance.

Administration: Oral route. **Storage:** 20-25°C (68-77°F); excursions permitted to 15-30°C (59-86°F). Protect contents from light.

TNKASE   RX
tenecteplase (Genentech)

THERAPEUTIC CLASS: Thrombolytic agent

INDICATIONS: To reduce mortality with acute myocardial infarction (AMI).

DOSAGE: *Adults:* Administer as single IV bolus over 5 sec. <60kg: 30mg. ≥60 to <70kg: 35mg. ≥70 to <80kg: 40mg. ≥80 to <90kg: 45mg. ≥90kg: 50mg. Max: 50mg/dose.

HOW SUPPLIED: Inj: 50mg

CONTRAINDICATIONS: Active internal bleeding, history of cerebrovascular accident (CVA), intracranial or intraspinal surgery or trauma within 2 months, intracranial neoplasm, arteriovenous malformation, aneurysm, bleeding diathesis, severe uncontrolled HTN .

WARNINGS/PRECAUTIONS: Weigh benefits/risks with recent major surgery, cerebrovascular disease, recent GI or genitourinary (GU) bleeding, recent trauma, HTN (systolic BP ≥180mmHg and/or diastolic BP ≥110mmHg), left heart thrombus, acute pericarditis, subacute bacterial endocarditis, hemostatic defects, severe hepatic dysfunction, pregnancy, diabetic hemorrhagic retinopathy or other hemorrhagic ophthalmic conditions, septic thrombophlebitis or occluded atriventricular (AV) cannula at a seriously infected site, elderly, any other bleeding condition that is difficult to manage. Cholesterol embolism and internal/superficial bleeding reported. Arrhythmias may occur with reperfusion. Avoid IM injection, noncompressible arterial puncture, and internal jugular or subclavian venous puncture. Caution with readministration.

ADVERSE REACTIONS: Bleeding.

INTERACTIONS: Increased risk of bleeding with heparin, vitamin K antagonists, and drugs that alter platelet function (eg, ASA, dipyridamole, GP IIb/IIIa inhibitors) before or after therapy. Weigh benefits/risks with oral anticoagulants, GP IIb/IIIa inhibitors.

PREGNANCY: Category C, caution in nursing.

MECHANISM OF ACTION: Thrombolytic agent; modified form of human tissue plasminogen activator (tPA) that binds to fibrin and converts plasminogen to plasmin.

PHARMACOKINETICS: Metabolism: Liver. **Elimination:** T$_{1/2}$=90-130 min.

NURSING CONSIDERATIONS

Assessment: Assess for active internal bleeding, history of CVA, or any other condition where treatment is contraindicated or cautioned. Assess for hepatic function, pregnancy/nursing status, advanced age, and drug interactions.

Monitoring: Check for signs/symptoms of bleeding; if serious bleeding occurs, concomitant heparin or antiplatelet agents should be discontinued immediately. Monitor for cholesterol embolization (eg, livedo reticularis, "purple toe" syndrome, acute renal failure), arrhythmia, and hypersensitivity reactions (eg, anaphylaxis).

Patient Counseling: Counsel about increased risk of bleeding while on therapy. Contact physician if any type of unusual bleeding or hypersensitivity reactions develop.

Administration: IV route. Reconstitute just prior to use. 1) Inject 10mL of SWFI into vial. 2) Do not shake; gently swirl until contents completely dissolved. 3) May be administered as reconstituted solution (5mg/mL). **Storage:** Lyophilized vial: Store at controlled room temperature not exceeding 30°C (86°F), or under refrigeration 2-8°C (36-46°F). Reconstituted: 2-8°C (36-46°F); use within 8 hrs.

TOBRADEX   RX
tobramycin - dexamethasone (Alcon)

OTHER BRAND NAMES: TobraDex ST (Alcon)

THERAPEUTIC CLASS: Aminoglycoside/corticosteroid

INDICATIONS: Steroid-responsive inflammatory ocular condition and superficial bacterial ocular infection caused by susceptible strains of microorganisms.

DOSAGE: *Adults:* (Sus) 1-2 drops into the conjunctival sac(s) q4-6h. (ST) 1 drop into conjunctival sac(s) q4-6h. Titrate: May increase to 1-2 drops q2h for first 24-48 hrs. Not more than 20mL should be initially prescribed. (Oint) Apply 1/2 inch ribbon in conjunctival sac(s) up to tid-qid. Not more than 8g should be initially prescribed.
Pediatrics: ≥2 yrs: (Sus) 1-2 drops into the conjunctival sac(s) q4-6h. (ST) 1 drop into conjunctival sac(s) q4-6h. Titrate: May increase to 1-2 drops q2h for first 24-48 hrs. Not more than 20mL should be initially prescribed. (Oint) Apply 1/2 inch ribbon in conjunctival sac(s) up to tid-qid. Not more than 8g should be initially prescribed.

HOW SUPPLIED: Oint: (Tobramycin-Dexamethasone) 0.3-0.1% [3.5g]; Sus: 0.3-0.1% [2.5mL, 5mL, 10mL]; Sus (ST): 0.3%-0.05% [2.5mL, 5mL, 10mL]

CONTRAINDICATIONS: Viral diseases of the cornea and conjunctiva, epithelial herpes simplex keratitis (dendritic keratitis), vaccinia, and varicella. Mycobacterial infection and fungal diseases of the eye.

WARNINGS/PRECAUTIONS: Not for injection into the eye. Prolonged use may result in glaucoma, optic nerve damage, visual acuity and field of vision defects, posterior subcapsular cataract formation. Monitor for intraocular pressure (IOP) if to be used for ≥10 days (Sus, ST). Routinely monitor IOP (Oint/Sus). May delay healing and increase incidence of bleb formation after cataract surgery. Caution with diseases causing thinning of the cornea or sclera; perforations may occur. Prolonged use may suppress host response and increase risk of secondary ocular infections. May mask/enhance existing infection in acute purulent conditions. Re-evaluate after 2 days if patient fails to improve. Caution with history of herpes simplex. May prolong the course and exacerbate severity of many viral infections of the eye (including herpes simplex). Fungal infections of the cornea may occur; consider fungus invasion in any persistent corneal ulceration. Cross-sensitivity to other aminoglycoside antibiotics may occur; d/c if hypersensitivity develops.

ADVERSE REACTIONS: Hypersensitivity, localized ocular toxicity (including lid itching and swelling, conjunctival erythema), secondary infection.

PREGNANCY: Category C, caution in nursing.

MECHANISM OF ACTION: Tobramycin: Aminoglycoside antibiotic; provides action against susceptible organisms. Dexamethasone: Corticoid; suppresses inflammatory response and probably delays or slows healing.

NURSING CONSIDERATIONS

Assessment: Assess for epithelial herpes simplex keratitis (dendritic keratitis), vaccinia, varicella, other viral diseases of cornea or conjunctiva, mycobacterial infection and fungal diseases of eye, diseases that may cause thinning of cornea or sclera, other existing infections, glaucoma, history of herpes simplex, pregnancy/nursing status, and hypersensitivity reactions.

Monitoring: Routinely monitor IOP (>10 days). Monitor for signs/symptoms of hypersensitivity reactions, glaucoma, defects in visual acuity and fields of vision, posterior subcapsular cataracts, perforations, exacerbation of many viral infections of the eye, secondary infection, delayed wound healing, incidence of bleb formation and superinfections.

Patient Counseling: Instruct not to touch dropper or tube tip to any surface to avoid contaminating contents and not to wear contact lenses during therapy. Advise to seek medical attention if symptoms of glaucoma, defects in vision, perforations, or superinfections occur. Inform to consult physician if signs and symptoms fail to improve after 2 days. Advise that care should be taken not to d/c therapy prematurely.

Administration: Ocular route. Shake well before use. **Storage:** 8-27°C (46-80°F). Store upright. (Sus, ST): 2-25°C (36-77°F). Protect from light.

TOBREX
RX
tobramycin (Alcon)

THERAPEUTIC CLASS: Aminoglycoside

INDICATIONS: External infections of the eye and its adnexa.

DOSAGE: *Adults:* Mild to Moderate Infection: Apply half-inch oint bid-tid or 1-2 drops q4h. Severe Infection: Apply half-inch oint q3-4h or 2 drops hourly until improvement, reduce frequency prior to discontinuation.

HOW SUPPLIED: Oint: 0.3% [3.5g]; Sol: 0.3% [5mL]

WARNINGS/PRECAUTIONS: Oint may retard corneal wound healing. Cross-sensitivity to other aminoglycoside antibiotics may occur.

ADVERSE REACTIONS: Hypersensitivity, lid itching, swelling, conjunctival erythema, superinfection.

PREGNANCY: Category B, not for use in nursing.

MECHANISM OF ACTION: Aminoglycoside antibiotic; inhibits synthesis of proteins in bacterial cells.

NURSING CONSIDERATIONS

Assessment: Assess for proper diagnosis of causative organisms. Assess use in pregnancy/nursing.

Monitoring: Monitor for sensitivity reactions while on therapy. With prolonged therapy, monitor for overgrowth of nonsusceptible organisms (eg, fungi) and for development of superinfection. Monitor total serum drug concentrations with concomitant systemic aminoglycoside antibiotics.

Patient Counseling: Advise not to wear contact lenses if signs/symptoms of ocular infections develop. Instruct to notify physician if any sensitivity reactions occur. To avoid contamination, avoid touching tube or dropper tip to any surface.

Administration: Ocular route. Do not inject into eye. **Storage:** 8-27°C (46-80°F).

T

TOFRANIL

RX

imipramine HCl (Mallinckrodt)

> Antidepressants increased the risk of suicidal thinking and behavior (suicidality) in short-term studies in children, adolescents, and young adults with major depressive disorder (MDD) and other psychiatric disorders. Monitor and observe closely for clinical worsening, suicidality, or unusual changes in behavior in patients who are started on antidepressant therapy. Imipramine HCl is not approved for use in pediatric patients except for patients with nocturnal enuresis.

THERAPEUTIC CLASS: Tricyclic antidepressant

INDICATIONS: Treatment of depression. Temporary adjunct in childhood enuresis in ≥6 yrs.

DOSAGE: *Adults:* Depression: Initial: (Inpatient) 100mg/day in divided doses. Titrate: Increase to 200mg/day; up to 250-300mg/day after 2 weeks if needed. (Outpatient) 75mg/day. Titrate: Increase to 150mg/day. Maint: 50-150mg/day. Max: 200mg/day. Elderly/Adolescents: Initial: 30-40mg/day. Max: 100mg/day.
Pediatrics: Depression: Adolescents: Initial: 30-40mg/day. Max: 100mg/day. Enuresis: ≥6 yrs: Initial: 25mg/day 1 hour before bedtime. Titrate: 6-12 yrs: If inadequate response in 1 week, increase to 50mg before bedtime. ≥12 yrs: Increase to 75mg before bedtime after 1 week if needed. Max: 2.5mg/kg/day.

HOW SUPPLIED: Tab: 10mg, 25mg, 50mg

CONTRAINDICATIONS: Within 14 days of MAOI therapy, or during acute recovery period following MI.

WARNINGS/PRECAUTIONS: Caution with elderly, serious depression, CV disease, hyperthyroidism, urinary retention, narrow-angle glaucoma, increased IOP, seizure disorders, renal and hepatic impairment. May activate psychosis in schizophrenia; reduce dose. Limit electroshock therapy. May alter blood glucose levels. Photosensitivity reported. D/C prior to elective surgery, or with hypomanic or manic episodes. D/C with pathological neutrophil depression.

ADVERSE REACTIONS: Orthostatic hypotension, HTN, confusion, hallucinations, numbness, tremors, dry mouth, urticaria, N/V, diarrhea, gynecomastia (male), breast enlargement (female), galactorrhea.

INTERACTIONS: See Contraindications. Increased levels with methylphenidate, CYP2D6 inhibitors (eg, quinidine, cimetidine, SSRIs) and enzyme substrates (eg, phenothiazines, other antidepressants, propafenone, flecainide). Wait 5 weeks after d/c SSRIs before initiating TCAs. Decreased levels with enzyme inducers (eg, barbiturates, phenytoin). May block effects of clonidine, guanethidine. Additive effects with anticholinergics, CNS depressants, alcohol. Caution with drugs that lower BP and thyroid drugs. Paralytic ileus with anticholinergics. Avoid preparations that contain a sympathomimetic amine (eg, epinephrine, norepinephrine); may potentiate catecholamine effect.

PREGNANCY: Safety in pregnancy not known; not for use in nursing.

MECHANISM OF ACTION: Tricyclic antidepressant; mechanism unknown. Suspected to potentiate adrenergic synapses by blocking uptake of norepinephrine at nerve endings.

NURSING CONSIDERATIONS

Assessment: Assess renal/hepatic function, LFTs, ECG, IOP, major depressive disorder, and for seizures. Note other diseases/conditions and drug therapies.

Monitoring: Monitor for clinical worsening, suicidality, or unusual changes in behavior, seizures, increased restlessness, agitation, anxiety, insomnia, neuropsychiatric signs/symptoms (eg, delusions, hallucinations, psychosis, concentration disturbances, paranoia, confusion), ECG, CBC with differential and platelets, blood sugar levels.

Patient Counseling: Advise families and caregivers of need for close observation of clinical worsening and suicidal risks. Avoid alcohol, sedatives, OTC agents. Caution against operating machinery/driving. Report adverse reactions. Consult physician before taking any other medications. Avoid excessive exposure to sunlight.

Administration: Oral route. **Storage:** 20-25°C (68-77°F).

TOPAMAX   RX
topiramate (Ortho-McNeil)

OTHER BRAND NAMES: Topamax Sprinkle Capsules (Ortho-McNeil)

THERAPEUTIC CLASS: Sulfamate-substituted monosaccharide antiepileptic

INDICATIONS: Initial monotherapy in patients ≥10 yrs with partial onset or primary generalized tonic-clonic seizures. Adjunct therapy in adults and pediatric patients ages 2-16 yrs with partial onset seizures or primary generalized tonic-clonic seizures and in patients ≥2 yrs with seizures associated with Lennox-Gastaut syndrome. Migraine headache prophylaxis in adults.

DOSAGE: *Adults:* Monotherapy: Partial Onset/Primary Generalized Tonic-Clonic Seizures: Initial: Week 1: 25mg bid. Titrate: Week 2: 50mg bid. Week 3: 75mg bid. Week 4: 100mg bid. Week 5: 150mg bid. Week 6: 200mg bid. Adjunct Therapy: Partial Onset/Primary Generalized Tonic-Clonic Seizures/Lennox-Gastaut Syndrome: ≥17 yrs: Initial: 25-50mg/day. Titrate: Increments of 25-50mg/day qweek. Partial Onset: Usual: 200-400mg/day in 2 divided doses. Tonic-Clonic: Usual: 400mg/day in 2 divided doses. Max: 1600mg/day. Migraine Prophylaxis: Initial: Week 1: 25mg qpm. Titrate: Week 2: 25mg bid. Week 3: 25mg qam and 50mg qpm. Week 4: 50mg bid. Usual: 100mg in 2 divided doses. Renal Dysfunction (CrCl <70mL/min/1.73m²): 50% of usual dose. Hemodialysis: May need supplemental dose. Elderly: May need dose adjustment. Swallow caps whole or sprinkle over food.
Pediatrics: Monotherapy: Partial Onset/Primary Generalized Tonic-Clonic Seizures: ≥10 yrs: Initial: Week 1: 25mg bid. Titrate: Week 2: 50mg bid. Week 3: 75mg bid. Week 4: 100mg bid. Week 5: 150mg bid. Week 6: 200mg bid. Adjunct Therapy: Partial Onset/Primary Generalized Tonic-Clonic Seizures/Lennox-Gastaut Syndrome: 2-16 yrs: Initial: 1-3mg/kg qpm (≤25mg/day) for 1st week. Titrate: Increase q1-2 weeks by 1-3mg/kg/day (in 2 divided doses) increments. Usual: 5-9mg/kg/day in 2 divided doses. Swallow caps whole or sprinkle over food.

HOW SUPPLIED: Cap, Sprinkle: 15mg, 25mg; Tab: 25mg, 50mg, 100mg, 200mg

WARNINGS/PRECAUTIONS: A syndrome consisting of acute myopia associated with secondary angle-closure glaucoma reported; d/c immediately if occurs. Oligohidrosis infrequently resulting in hospitalization reported mostly in pediatrics. May increase the risk of suicidal thoughts or behavior; monitor for the emergence or worsening of depression, suicidal thoughts or behavior, and/or any unusual changes in mood or behavior. Hyperchloremic, non-anion gap, metabolic acidosis reported. Cognitive-related dysfunction, psychiatric/behavioral disturbances, somnolence, or fatigue reported. May cause fetal harm in pregnancy. Avoid abrupt d/c. Sudden unexplained death in epilepsy (SUDEP) and hyperammonemia with or without encephalopathy reported. Kidney stones reported; hydration is recommended to reduce new stone formation. Paresthesia reported. Caution with renal/hepatic impairment.

ADVERSE REACTIONS: Anorexia, anxiety, dizziness, diarrhea, fatigue, weight decrease, concentration/memory difficulty, paresthesia, psychomotor slowing, somnolence, taste perversion, nausea, nervousness, confusion.

INTERACTIONS: Decreased levels with phenytoin, carbamazepine, lamotrigine, and valproic acid. May cause hyperammonemia with or without encephalopathy with valproic acid. Increased levels with HCTZ, diltiazem, and risperidone. Increased levels of amitriptyline, lithium, phenytoin, carbamazepine, lamotrigine, primidone, phenobarbital. Decreases levels of pioglitazone, risperidone, digoxin, diltiazem, glyburide. May cause CNS depression and cognitive/neuropsychiatric adverse events with alcohol and other CNS depressants; use with extreme caution. May decrease contraceptive efficacy with combination oral contraceptives. Caution with drugs that predispose patient to heat-related disorder (eg, carbonic anhydrase inhibitors, drugs with anticholinergic effect). Increased risk of renal stones and worsening of metabolic acidosis with other carbonic anhydrase inhibitors (eg, zonisamide, acetazolamide or dichlorphenamide). May cause metabolic acidosis, a condition which the use of metformin is contraindicated. Avoid with other drugs that produce metabolic acidosis.

PREGNANCY: Category D, caution in nursing.

MECHANISM OF ACTION: Sulfamate-substituted monosaccharide; unknown mechanism. Suspected to block voltage-dependent sodium channels, augment activity of the neurotransmitter gamma-aminobutyrate at some subtypes of the GABA-A receptor, antagonizes the AMPA/kainate subtype of the glutamate receptor, and inhibits the carbonic anhydrase enzyme, particularly isoenzymes II and IV.

PHARMACOKINETICS: Absorption: Rapid; T_{max}=2 hrs (400mg). **Distribution:** Plasma protein binding (15-41%). **Metabolism:** Hydroxylation, hydrolysis, glucuronidation. **Elimination:** Urine: (70% unchanged); $T_{1/2}$=21 hrs.

NURSING CONSIDERATIONS

Assessment: Assess for renal/hepatic function, predisposing factors for metabolic acidosis, inborn errors of metabolism, reduced hepatic mitochondrial activity, pregnancy/nursing status, and possible drug interactions. Obtain baseline serum bicarbonate.

Monitoring: Monitor for signs/symptoms of acute myopia, secondary angle glaucoma, oligohidrosis, hyperthermia, cognitive or neuropsychiatric impairment, kidney stones, renal dysfunction, metabolic acidosis, paresthesias, emergence or worsening of suicidal behavior/ideation or depression, unusual changes in mood/behavior, and hyperammonemia. Monitor serum bicarbonate level.

Patient Counseling: Advise to seek immediate medical attention if blurred vision, visual disturbances, periorbital pain, or suicidal thoughts or behavior occurs and to closely monitor for decreased sweating and increased body temperature. Warn about risk for metabolic acidosis. Use caution when engaging in activities (eg, driving or operating machinery). Inform about risk for hyperammonemia with or without encephalopathy; contact physician if unexplained lethargy, vomiting, or mental status changes develops. Maintain adequate fluid intake to minimize risk of kidney stones. Medication may decrease efficacy of oral contraceptives. Inform of pregnancy risks/benefits. Encourage to enroll in the North American Antiepileptic Drug (NAAED) Pregnancy Registry if patient becomes pregnant by calling 1-888-233-2334. Can be taken with or without food. May swallow sprinkle caps whole or open cap and sprinkle contents on small amount (tsp) of soft food; do not chew.

Administration: Oral route. **Storage:** Protect from moisture. Tab: 15-30°C (59-86°F). Cap, Sprinkle: ≤25°C (77°F).

TOPICORT   RX
desoximetasone (Taro)

OTHER BRAND NAMES: Topicort LP (Taro)

THERAPEUTIC CLASS: Corticosteroid

INDICATIONS: Relief of the inflammatory and pruritic manifestations of corticosteroid-responsive dermatoses.

DOSAGE: *Adults:* Apply bid to affected area.
Pediatrics: (Cre, Gel) Apply bid to affected area. ≥10 yrs: (Oint) Apply bid to affected area.

HOW SUPPLIED: Cre: (LP) 0.05% [15g, 60g, 100g], 0.25% [15g, 60g, 100g]; Gel: 0.05% [15g, 60g]; Oint: 0.25% [15g, 60g, 100g]

WARNINGS/PRECAUTIONS: May produce reversible hypothalamic-pituitary-adrenal (HPA) axis suppression, manifestations of Cushing's syndrome, hyperglycemia, and glucosuria. If HPA axis suppression noted, d/c or reduce frequency of application or substitute a less potent steroid. Steroid withdrawal may occur upon d/c. Caution when applied to large surface areas or under occlusive dressings. Use appropriate antifungal or antibacterial agent with dermatological infections; d/c if infection does not clear or if irritation occurs.

Avoid contact with eyes. Pediatric patients may be more susceptible to systemic toxicity; chronic therapy may interfere with growth and development.

ADVERSE REACTIONS: Burning, itching, irritation, dryness, folliculitis, hypertrichosis, acneiform eruptions, hypopigmentation, perioral dermatitis, allergic contact dermatitis, skin maceration, secondary infection, skin atrophy, striae, miliaria.

PREGNANCY: Category C, caution in nursing.

MECHANISM OF ACTION: Corticosteroid; possesses anti-inflammatory, anti-pruritic, and vasoconstrictive properties. Anti-inflammatory activity not established.

PHARMACOKINETICS: Absorption: Percutaneous; occlusion, inflammation, and other disease states may increase absorption. **Metabolism:** Liver. **Excretion:** Urine (major), bile. Cre 0.25% (men): Urine (4.1%), Feces (1.1%); $T_{1/2}$=15-17 hrs.

NURSING CONSIDERATIONS

Assessment: Assess for hypersensitivity, dermatological infection, and pregnancy/nursing status.

Monitoring: Monitor for signs/symptoms of reversible HPA-axis suppression, Cushing's syndrome, hyperglycemia, glucosuria, skin irritation, and for dermatological infections. In patients on large doses or using occlusive dressings, monitor for HPA-axis suppression by using urinary free cortisol and ACTH stimulation tests. Following d/c, monitor for signs of steroid withdrawal. In pediatrics, monitor for signs/symptoms of systemic toxicity, HPA-axis suppression (eg, linear growth retardation, delayed weight gain), Cushing's syndrome, and intracranial HTN.

Patient Counseling: Instruct to use externally and exactly as directed; avoid contact with eyes. Report local adverse reactions, especially under occlusive dressings. Do not bandage, cover, or wrap treated skin unless directed by physician. Advise caregivers of pediatric patients not to use tight-fitting diapers or plastic pants on treatment area.

Administration: Topical route. **Storage:** Cre, Gel: 20-25°C (68-77°F). Oint: 15-30°C (59-86°F).

TOPROL-XL   RX
metoprolol succinate (AstraZeneca)

> Following abrupt cessation of therapy, exacerbation of angina pectoris and, in some cases, MI have occurred. When d/c chronically administered metoprolol, particularly in patients with ischemic heart disease, dosage should be gradually reduced over a period of 1-2 weeks and patients should be monitored carefully. If angina markedly worsens or acute coronary insufficiency develops, reinstate therapy promptly, at least temporarily, and take other appropriate measures. Avoid interruption or d/c of therapy without physician's advice.

THERAPEUTIC CLASS: Selective beta₁-blocker

INDICATIONS: Treatment of HTN; may be used alone or in combination with other antihypertensive agents. Long-term treatment of angina pectoris. Treatment of stable symptomatic (NYHA Class II or III) heart failure (HF) of ischemic, hypertensive, or cardiomyopathic origin.

DOSAGE: *Adults:* Individualize dose. HTN: Initial: 25-100mg qd. Titrate: May increase at weekly (or longer) intervals until optimum BP reduction is achieved. Max: 400mg/day. Angina: Initial: 100mg qd. Titrate: May increase weekly until optimum clinical response has been obtained or there is pronounced slowing of heart rate. Max: 400mg/day. HF: Initial: (NYHA Class II) 25mg qd for 2 weeks. Severe HF: 12.5mg qd for 2 weeks. Titrate: Double dose every 2 weeks as tolerated. Max: 200mg/day. Reduce dose if experiencing symptomatic bradycardia. Dose should not be increased until symptoms of worsening HF have been stabilized. Hepatic Impairment: May require lower initial dose; gradually increase dose to optimize therapy. Elderly: Start at low initial dose. Do not crush or chew; tablet may be divided. *Pediatrics:* ≥6 yrs: HTN: Initial: 1mg/kg qd up to 50mg/day. Adjust dose

T

according to BP response. Max: 2.0mg/kg (or up to 200mg) qd. Do not crush or chew; tablet may be divided.

HOW SUPPLIED: Tab, Extended-Release: 25mg*, 50mg*, 100mg*, 200mg* *scored

CONTRAINDICATIONS: Severe bradycardia, 2nd or 3rd degree heart block, cardiogenic shock, sick sinus syndrome (unless a pacemaker is present), decompensated cardiac failure.

WARNINGS/PRECAUTIONS: May precipitate or aggravate symptoms of arterial insufficiency in patients with peripheral vascular disease (PVD). May mask symptoms of hyperthyroidism and hypoglycemia. Abrupt withdrawal may precipitate thyroid storm. Avoid initiation of high-dose regimen in patients undergoing non-cardiac surgery. Worsening cardiac failure may occur during up-titration; lower dose or temporarily d/c. Caution with hepatic impairment. If used in the setting of pheochromocytoma, give in combination with and after initiation of an alpha blocker; may cause paradoxical increase in BP when given alone. Should generally be avoided with bronchospastic disease; may be used only with those who do not respond to or cannot tolerate other antihypertensive treatment. Caution in elderly.

ADVERSE REACTIONS: Bradycardia, SOB, tiredness, dizziness, depression, diarrhea, rash.

INTERACTIONS: Additive effects with catecholamine-depleting drugs (eg, reserpine, MAOIs). May block epinephrine effects when used to treat an allergic reaction. CYP2D6 inhibitors (eg, quinidine, fluoxetine, paroxetine, propafenone) may increase levels. May exacerbate rebound HTN following clonidine withdrawal. Caution when used with calcium channel blockers of the verapamil and diltiazem type. Concomitant use with digitalis glycosides, clonidine, diltiazem, and verapamil may increase the risk of bradycardia.

PREGNANCY: Category C, caution in nursing.

MECHANISM OF ACTION: β_1-selective adrenergic receptor blocker; not established. Proposed to competitively antagonize catecholamines at peripheral adrenergic-neuronal sites leading to decreased cardiac output, has central effect leading to reduced symptomatic outflow to periphery, and suppression of renin activity.

PHARMACOKINETICS: Absorption: Rapid and complete. **Distribution:** Plasma protein binding (12%); found in breast milk; crosses blood-brain barrier. **Metabolism:** Metabolized via CYP2D6. **Elimination:** Liver; Urine (<5% unchanged); $T_{1/2}$=3-7 hrs.

NURSING CONSIDERATIONS

Assessment: Assess for bradycardia, heart block, cardiogenic shock, cardiac failure, sick sinus syndrome, presence of pacemaker, ischemic heart disease, bronchospastic disease, DM, hyperthyroidism, PVD, arterial insufficiency, impaired hepatic function, pheochromocytoma, upcoming surgery, anaphylactic reactions, pregnancy/nursing status, and possible drug interactions. Obtain baseline vital signs and LFTs.

Monitoring: Monitor vital signs and LFTs. Monitor difficulty of breathing in patients with bronchospastic disease, signs/symptoms of worsening of cardiac failure during up-titration in patients with DM, thyroid function in patients with hyperthyroidism, arterial insufficiency in patients with PVD, and anaphylactic reactions.

Patient Counseling: Inform about risks/benefits of therapy. Instruct not to interrupt or d/c therapy without consulting physician. Advise to take drug regularly and continuously, as directed, preferably with or immediately following meals. If dose is missed, take only next scheduled dose (without doubling). Avoid engaging in tasks requiring mental alertness (eg, operating machinery/driving). Contact physician if any difficulty in breathing occurs. Inform physician or dentist of medication use before any type of surgery. Advise HF patients to consult physician if experience signs/symptoms of worsening HF (eg, weight gain, increasing SOB).

Administration: Oral route. Do not crush or chew; tablet may be divided. **Storage:** 25°C (77°F); excursions permitted to 15-30°C (59-86°F).

TORISEL
temsirolimus (Wyeth)

THERAPEUTIC CLASS: mTOR inhibitor

INDICATIONS: Treatment of advanced renal cell carcinoma.

DOSAGE: *Adults:* 25mg IV over 30-60 min once a week. Premedication: Diphenhydramine IV (or similar antihistamine) 25-50mg 30 min before the start of each dose. Hold if ANC <1,000/mm³, platelet count <75,000/mm³, or NCI CTCAE ≥Grade 3 adverse reactions. Once toxicities resolve to ≤Grade 2, restart with dose reduced by 5mg/week to a dose ≥15mg/week. Mild Hepatic Impairment: Reduce dose to 15mg/week. Concomitant Strong CYP3A4 Inhibitors: Consider dose reduction to 12.5mg/week. If strong inhibitor is d/c, allow wash-out period of about 1 week before dose re-adjustment. Concomitant Strong CYP3A4 Inducers: Consider dose increase to 50mg/week.

HOW SUPPLIED: Inj: 25mg/mL

CONTRAINDICATIONS: Patients with bilirubin >1.5X ULN.

WARNINGS/PRECAUTIONS: Hypersensitivity reactions observed; if develop, d/c infusion and observe for 30-60 min. Give H1 antihistamine before starting infusion. Hyperglycemia may occur; monitor blood glucose. Infections may result from immunosuppression. Monitor for interstitial lung disease (ILD); d/c if suspected. Increases in serum TG and cholesterol reported; test before and during therapy. Bowel perforation may occur. Renal failure reported; monitor renal function. May cause abnormal wound healing; caution during perioperative period. Caution with CNS tumors due to increased risk of intracerebral hemorrhage. Monitor CBC weekly and chemistry panel every 2 weeks. May cause fetal harm. Caution with hepatic impairment; may need dose reduction.

ADVERSE REACTIONS: Rash, asthenia, mucositis, nausea, edema, anorexia.

INTERACTIONS: Strong inducers of CYP3A4/5 may decrease levels. Strong CYP3A4 inhibitors may increase levels. Concomitant use with sunitinib may result in dose-limiting toxicity. Angioneurotic edema-type reactions may occur with concomitant ACE inhibitors. Avoid concurrent use of live vaccines.

PREGNANCY: Category D, not for use in nursing.

MECHANISM OF ACTION: mTOR inhibitor; inhibits activity of mTOR that controls cell division, resulting in G1 growth arrest in treated tumor cells, inability to phosphorylate p70S6k and S6 ribosomal protein, and reduced levels of hypoxia-inducible factors HIF-1 and HIF-2 α, and the vascular endothelial growth factor.

PHARMACOKINETICS: Absorption: C_{max} =585ng/mL, AUC=1627ng•h/mL. **Distribution:** V_d=172L. **Metabolism:** Liver, via CYP3A4; sirolimus (active metabolite). **Elimination:** Urine (4.6%), feces (78%); $T_{1/2}$=17.3 hrs (temsirolimus), 54.6 hrs (sirolimus).

NURSING CONSIDERATIONS

Assessment: Assess for renal/hepatic impairment, CNS tumors, surgery within a few weeks prior to therapy, pregnancy/nursing status, and for possible drug interactions. Obtain baseline vital signs and weight, CBC, renal/hepatic function, serum glucose and cholesterol, TG.

Monitoring: Monitor for hypersensitivity reactions, infections, ILD, bowel perforation, renal/hepatic impairment, intracerebral bleeding, wound healing complications, and other adverse events that may occur. Monitor vital signs and weight, CBC, serum glucose, cholesterol, TG levels.

Patient Counseling: Inform of possible serious allergic reactions despite premedication with antihistamines; report if facial swelling or difficulty of breathing occurs. Women of childbearing potential should use reliable contraception throughout treatment and continue for 3 months after last dose. Blood glucose, TG and/or cholesterol levels may increase. Counsel on the risk of developing ILD, renal failure, abnormal wound healing, intracerebral bleeding, bowel perforation, and infections. Inform physician if any adverse events occur.

Administration: IV route. Refer to PI for proper preparation and administration. **Storage:** 2-8°C (36-46°F). Protect from light.

TORSEMIDE RX
torsemide (Various)

OTHER BRAND NAMES: Demadex (Meda)

THERAPEUTIC CLASS: Loop diuretic

INDICATIONS: Treatment of edema associated with congestive heart failure (CHF), renal disease, chronic renal failure (CRF) or hepatic disease. Treatment of HTN, alone or with other antihypertensive agents. (Inj) Indicated when a rapid onset of diuresis is desired or when oral administration is impractical.

DOSAGE: *Adults:* PO/IV (bolus over 2 min or continuous infusion): CHF: Initial: 10-20mg qd. Titrate: Double dose until desired response. Max: 200mg single dose. Chronic Renal Failure: Initial: 20mg qd. Titrate: Double dose until desired response. Max: 200mg single dose. Hepatic Cirrhosis: Initial: 5-10mg qd with aldosterone antagonist or K⁺-sparing diuretic. Titrate: Double dose until desired response. Max: 40mg single dose. HTN: Initial: 5mg qd. Titrate: May increase to 10mg qd in 4-6 weeks, then may add additional antihypertensive agent if needed.

HOW SUPPLIED: Inj: 10mg/mL [2mL, 5mL]; Tab: (Demadex) 5mg*, 10mg*, 20mg*, 100mg* *scored

CONTRAINDICATIONS: Anuria.

WARNINGS/PRECAUTIONS: Caution with cirrhosis and ascites in hepatic disease. Tinnitus and hearing loss (usually reversible) reported. Excessive diuresis may cause dehydration, blood-volume reduction, and possible thrombosis and embolism especially in elderly. Monitor for electrolyte imbalance, hypovolemia, or prerenal azotemia; if symptoms occur, d/c until corrected and restart at lower dose. Increased risk of hypokalemia with liver cirrhosis, brisk diuresis, and inadequate oral intake of electrolytes. May develop arrhythmias in patients with cardiovascular disease (CVD). Hyperglycemia, hypokalemia, hypomagnesemia, hypercalcemia and symptomatic gout reported. May increase BUN, SrCr, serum uric acid, cholesterol and TG.

ADVERSE REACTIONS: Headache, excessive urination, dizziness, hypomagnesemia.

INTERACTIONS: Caution with high-dose salicylates, aminoglycosides, ethacrynic acid, lithium and digitalis glycoside. Indomethacin partially inhibits natriuretic effect. Avoid simultaneous cholestyramine administration; may decrease oral drug absorption. Probenecid decreases effects. Reduces spironolactone clearance. Risk of hypokalemia with ACTH and corticosteroids. Possible renal dysfunction with NSAIDs (including aspirin). Increased levels with digoxin.

PREGNANCY: Category B, caution in nursing.

MECHANISM OF ACTION: Loop diuretic; acts within lumen of thick ascending part of loop of Henle, inhibiting Na⁺/K⁺/Cl⁻-carrier system.

PHARMACOKINETICS: Absorption: (Tab) Absolute bioavailability (80%); (Tab) T_{max}=1 hr. **Distribution:** V_d=12-15L; plasma protein binding (>99%). **Metabolism:** Liver; Carboxylic acid (major metabolite). **Elimination:** Urine (20%); $T_{1/2}$=3.5 hrs.

NURSING CONSIDERATIONS

Assessment: Assess for history of hypersensitivity to the drug or to sulfonylureas, anuria, CVD, renal/hepatic impairment, pregnancy/nursing status and possible drug interactions.

Monitoring: Monitor serum electrolytes (serum K⁺, magnesium, calcium), BUN, creatinine, uric acid, blood glucose, TG, cholesterol, alkaline phosphatase, CBC. Monitor for signs/symptoms of hypokalemia, electrolyte imbalance, hypovolemia, prerenal azotemia, arrhythmias, tinnitus, hearing loss, hypersensitivity reactions and renal/hepatic dysfunction.

Patient Counseling: Discuss risks and benefits of therapy. Advise to seek medical attention if symptoms of hypokalemia, electrolyte imbalance, hypersensitivity reactions, hearing loss or tinnitus occur.

Administration: IV and Oral route. (Inj) Visually inspect for particulate matter and discoloration prior to administration. Flush IV line with normal saline before and after administration. **Storage:** (Inj) 20-25°C (68-77°F); do not freeze. (Tab) 15-30°C (59-86°F).

TOVIAZ   RX
fesoterodine fumarate (Pfizer)

THERAPEUTIC CLASS: Muscarinic antagonist

INDICATIONS: Treatment of overactive bladder with symptoms of urge urinary incontinence, urgency, and frequency.

DOSAGE: *Adults:* Initial: 4mg qd. Titrate: May increase to 8mg qd based on individual response and tolerability. Severe Renal Impairment (CrCl <30mL/min)/With Potent CYP3A4 Inhibitors: Max: 4mg/day.

HOW SUPPLIED: Tab, Extended Release: 4mg, 8mg

CONTRAINDICATIONS: Urinary retention, gastric retention, or uncontrolled narrow-angle glaucoma.

WARNINGS/PRECAUTIONS: Angioedema of the face, lips, tongue and/or larynx reported; d/c and provide appropriate therapy and/or measures if airway patency compromised.Caution with significant bladder outlet obstruction, decreased GI motility such as those with severe constipation, myasthenia gravis, and patients treated for narrow-angle glaucoma. Avoid with severe renal/hepatic impairment (Child-Pugh C).

ADVERSE REACTIONS: Dry mouth, constipation, urinary tract infection, dry eyes.

INTERACTIONS: Other antimuscarinic agents may increase the frequency and/or severity of anticholinergic pharmacologic effects (eg, dry mouth, constipation, urinary retention). May alter the absorption of some concomitantly administered drugs due to effects on GI motility. Doses >4mg are not recommended with concomitant administration of potent CYP3A4 inhibitors (eg, ketoconazole, itraconazole, clarithromycin). Careful assessment of dose tolerability with weak or moderate CYP3A4 inhibitors (eg, erythromycin).

PREGNANCY: Category C, caution in nursing.

MECHANISM OF ACTION: Competitive muscarinic receptor antagonist; inhibits muscarinic receptors in the bladder which affects contractions of urinary bladder smooth muscle and stimulation of salivary secretion.

PHARMACOKINETICS: Absorption: Well absorbed; T_{max}=5 hrs. **Distribution:** Plasma protein binding (50%), (IV) V_d=169L. **Metabolism:** Rapid and extensive hydrolysis. Metabolite in liver via CYP2D6 and CYP3A4 (carboxylation). **Excretion:** (PO) Urine (70%), feces (7%); (PO) $T_{1/2}$=7 hrs, (IV) $T_{1/2}$=4 hrs. Refer to PI for pharmacokinetic parameters for extensive and poor CYP2D6 metabolizers.

NURSING CONSIDERATIONS

Assessment: Assess for previous hypersensitivity, other conditions where treatment is contraindicated or cautioned, hepatic/renal function, pregnancy/nursing status, and for possible drug interactions.

Monitoring: Monitor for angioedema (eg, face, lips, tongue, larynx, hypopharynx), and other adverse reactions.

Patient Counseling: Instruct to take with liquids and swallow whole; do not chew, divide, or crush. Inform patients that therapy may produce angioedema which could result to life-threatening airway obstruction; d/c and seek medical attention if edema of tongue or laryngopharynx, or difficulty of breathing occur. Counsel about clinically significant adverse effects (eg, constipation and urinary retention). Inform that blurred vision may occur; advise to exercise caution until effects have been determined. Inform that heat prostration may occur when used in a hot environment. Advise that alcohol may enhance drowsiness.

Administration: Oral route. Take with liquid and swallow whole; do not crush, chew or divide. **Storage:** 20-25°C (68-77°F); excursions permitted between 15-30°C (59-86°F). Protect from moisture.

TRACLEER
bosentan (Actelion)

RX

Potential liver injury; monitor LFTs before therapy, then monthly. Avoid use with elevated aminotransferases (>3X ULN); d/c use when elevated aminotransferases are accompanied by clinical symptoms of liver injury (eg, N/V, fever, abdominal pain, jaundice, unusual lethargy, fatigue) or increases in bilirubin ≥2X ULN. Hepatic cirrhosis reported with prolonged use and liver failure. Contraindicated in pregnancy; likely to cause major birth defects if used during pregnancy. Exclude pregnancy before treatment, throughout treatment, and for one month after d/c. Obtain monthly pregnancy tests. Females of childbearing potential must use two reliable methods of contraception unless have had tubal sterilization or Copper T 380A IUD or LNg 20 IUS inserted, in which case, no other contraception is needed. Available only through Tracleer Access Program (T.A.P.).

THERAPEUTIC CLASS: Endothelin receptor antagonist

INDICATIONS: Treatment of pulmonary arterial hypertension (PAH) (WHO Group 1) to improve exercise ability and decrease clinical worsening in patients with (NYHA) Functional Class II-IV symptoms and etiologies of idiopathic or heritable PAH, PAH associated with connective tissue diseases, and PAH associated with congenital systemic-to-pulmonary shunts.

DOSAGE: *Adults:* Initial: 62.5mg bid for 4 weeks. Titrate/Maint/Max: Increase to 125mg bid. Low Weight (<40kg): Initial/Maint: 62.5mg bid. Adjust if develop LFT Abnormality: >3 and ≤5X ULN: Reconfirm LFTs. Reduce daily dose to 62.5mg bid or interrupt therapy. Monitor LFTs ≥ every 2 weeks. If LFTs return to pre-treatment levels, reintroduce at starting dose or continue therapy. >5 and ≤8X ULN: Reconfirm LFTs. Stop treatment and monitor LFTs ≥ every 2 weeks. If LFTs return to pre-treatment values, may reintroduce therapy at starting dose. >8X ULN: D/C; do not reintroduce. With Ritonavir for ≥10 Days: Initial: 62.5mg qd or qod based on individual tolerability. Adding Ritonavir: d/c use ≥36 hrs prior to initiation of ritonavir, after ≥10 days resume therapy at 62.5mg qd or qod. D/C: gradual dose reduction (62.5mg bid for 3-7 days). *Pediatrics:* >12 yrs: <40kg: Initial/Maint: 62.5mg bid.

HOW SUPPLIED: Tab: 62.5mg, 125mg

CONTRAINDICATIONS: Pregnancy, use with cyclosporine A, use with glyburide.

WARNINGS/PRECAUTIONS: May decrease Hgb and Hct. Avoid with moderate to severe hepatic impairment. Fluid retention and peripheral edema reported; d/c if necessary. Consider intervention with diuretic, fluid management, or hospitalization for decompensating heart failure. If signs of pulmonary edema occur, consider possibility of associated pulmonary veno-occlusive disease (PVOD) and d/c therapy. Decreased sperm count reported after 3 or 6 months of therapy. Caution with mildly impaired liver function and elderly.

ADVERSE REACTIONS: Liver injury, birth defects, decreased Hgb, oligospermia, respiratory tract infection, headache, ALT/AST elevations, edema, chest pain, syncope, flushing, hypotension, sinusitis, arthralgia.

INTERACTIONS: See Contraindications. May decrease plasma levels of oral hypoglycemic agents metabolized by CYP2C9 or CYP3A, sildenafil, both S-warfarin (a CYP2C9 substrate) and R-warfarin (a CYP3A substrate), CYP3A or CYP2C9 substrates, simvastatin or other statins metabolized by CYP3A (eg, lovastatin, atorvastatin). Hormonal contraceptives (eg, oral, injectable, transdermal, implantable forms) may not be reliable when coadministered with bosentan. May decrease levels of estrogens and progestins in hormonal contraceptives; use additional forms of contraception. Increased levels with ritonavir/lopinavir; adjust dose of bosentan. Caution with tacrolimus. Rifampin may increase trough levels of bosentan after first dose, but decrease levels at steady-state; measure LFTs weekly for first 4 weeks before reverting to normal monitoring. Increased levels with CYP2C9 inhibitors (eg, fluconazole, amiodarone), strong CYP3A inhibitors (eg, ketoconazole, itraconazole), and CYP3A inhibitors (eg, amprenavir, erythromycin, fluconazole, diltiazem) and sildenafil.

PREGNANCY: Category X, not for use in nursing.

MECHANISM OF ACTION: Endothelin receptor antagonist; specific and competitive antagonist at endothelin receptor types ET_A and ET_B with slightly higher affinity for ET_A receptors than ET_B receptors.

PHARMACOKINETICS: Absorption: Absolute bioavailability (50%); T_{max}=3-5 hrs. **Distribution:** V_d=18L; plasma protein binding (>98%). **Metabolism:** Liver. **Elimination:** Biliary, urine (<3%); $T_{1/2}$=5 hrs.

NURSING CONSIDERATIONS

Assessment: Assess serum aminotransferase levels, pregnancy test, that female patients of child bearing potential are on two forms of reliable contraception, have had tubal sterilization, or a Copper T 380A IUD or LNg 20 IUS is inserted. Assess for pulmonary HTN, chronic heart failure, hepatic impairment, nursing status, and for possible drug interactions.

Monitoring: Monitor for liver injury; perform monthly measurements. Perform monthly pregnancy tests in women of childbearing potential. In male patients, monitor for decreased sperm counts. Monitor for fluid retention, decompensating heart failure, pulmonary edema, and PVOD. Monitor for decreased Hgb, and Hct; measure Hgb concentrations after 1 and 3 months of therapy and then every 3 months thereafter.

Patient Counseling: Advise to consult Medication Guide for safe use. Discuss the importance of monthly monitoring of serum aminotransferases. Medication is likely to cause birth defects and is not to be used during pregnancy. Notify physician if pregnancy is suspected. Advise women of childbearing potential to have monthly pregnancy tests and to use 2 forms of contraception during therapy and for one month after d/c therapy. Inform females that had tubal ligation or Copper T 380A IUD or LNg 20 IUS that they can use these forms of contraception alone. Inform about possible drug interactions and discuss importance of disclosing all concomitant or new medications.

Administration: Oral route. **Storage:** 20-25°C (68-77°F); excursions permitted to 15-30°C (59-86°F).

TRANDATE   RX
labetalol HCl (Prometheus)

THERAPEUTIC CLASS: Nonselective beta-blocker/alpha₁ blocker

INDICATIONS: Management of HTN alone or in combination with other antihypertensives especially thiazide and loop diuretics.

DOSAGE: *Adults:* Individualize dose. Initial: 100mg bid. Titrate: May increase by 100mg bid every 2-3 days. Maint: 200-400mg bid. Severe HTN: 1200-2400mg/day given bid-tid. Titrate: Do not increase by >200mg bid. Elderly: Initial: 100mg bid. Titrate: May increase by 100mg bid. Maint: 100-200mg bid.

HOW SUPPLIED: Tab: 100mg*, 200mg*, 300mg* *scored

CONTRAINDICATIONS: Bronchial asthma, overt cardiac failure, greater than first degree heart block, cardiogenic shock, severe bradycardia, other conditions associated with severe and prolonged hypotension.

WARNINGS/PRECAUTIONS: Hepatic injury, hepatic necrosis and death reported. Caution with hepatic dysfunction. Avoid abrupt withdrawal; may exacerbate ischemic heart disease. Intraoperative floppy iris syndrome (IFIS) reported during cataract surgery. Caution with latent cardiac insufficiency. Avoid in overt CHF. Avoid with bronchospastic disease; use caution if patient does not respond to or cannot tolerate other antihypertensives. Paradoxical HTN in pheochromocytoma reported. May prevent the appearance of premonitory signs and symptoms of acute hypoglycemia. Do not withdraw routinely prior to surgery.

ADVERSE REACTIONS: Dizziness, fatigue, N/V, dyspepsia, paresthesia, nasal stuffiness, ejaculation failure, impotence, edema, dyspnea, headache, vertigo, postural hypotension, increased sweating.

INTERACTIONS: Increased tremor with TCAs. Antagonizes effects of β-agonists (bronchodilators). Potentiated by cimetidine; may need to reduce dose. Synergistic effects with halothane anesthesia. Synergistic antihypertensive effects blunts the reflex tachycardia with nitroglycerin. Caution with calcium antagonists. May need to adjust dose of antidiabetic drugs (eg, insulin). Increase risk of bradycardia with digitalis glycosides.

PREGNANCY: Category C, caution in nursing.

MECHANISM OF ACTION: Selective α_1-adrenergic and nonselective β-adrenergic receptor blocking agent.

PHARMACOKINETICS: Absorption: Complete; T_{max}=1-2 hrs; absolute bioavailability (25%). **Distribution:** Plasma protein binding (50%); crosses placenta. **Metabolism:** Liver (conjugation, glucuronidation). **Elimination:** Feces, urine (55-60%); $T_{1/2}$=6-8 hrs.

NURSING CONSIDERATIONS

Assessment: Assess for bradycardia, heart block, cardiogenic shock, cardiac failure, ischemic heart disease, severe hypotension, bronchospastic disease, DM, pheochromocytoma, anaphylactic reactions, pregnancy/nursing status and possible drug interactions.

Monitoring: Monitor for cardiac failure, HTN, renal function, exacerbation of ischemia following abrupt withdrawal, bronchospastic disease, arrhythmias, hypersensitivity reactions, CBC with platelets and differential, anaphylactic reactions.

Patient Counseling: Instruct not to interrupt or d/c without consulting physician. Report signs/symptoms of cardiac failure or hepatic dysfunction (eg, pruritus, dark urine, persistent anorexia, jaundice, right upper quadrant (RUQ) tenderness, or unexplained flu-like symptoms). Transient scalp itching may occur, usually when treatment initiated.

Administration: Oral route. **Storage:** 2-30°C (36-86°F); protect from excessive moisture.

TRANSDERM SCOP   RX
scopolamine (Novartis Consumer)

THERAPEUTIC CLASS: Anticholinergic

INDICATIONS: Prevention of nausea and vomiting associated with motion sickness or recovery from anesthesia and surgery.

DOSAGE: *Adults:* Motion Sickness: Apply 1 patch 4 hrs before travel. Replace after 3 days. Post-OP N/V: Apply 1 patch the evening before surgery or 1 hr prior to cesarean section. Keep in place for 24 hrs. Apply patch to a hairless area behind the ear. Do not cut patch in half.

HOW SUPPLIED: Patch: 0.33mg/24 hrs [4s]

CONTRAINDICATIONS: Angle-closure (narrow angle) glaucoma, hypersensitivity to belladonna alkaloids.

WARNINGS/PRECAUTIONS: Monitor IOP with open-angle glaucoma. Not for use in children. Caution with pyloric obstruction, urinary bladder neck or intestinal obstruction, and in elderly. Increased CNS effects with liver or kidney dysfunction. May aggravate seizures or psychosis. Idiosyncratic reactions reported (rare). Remove patch before MRI.

ADVERSE REACTIONS: Dry mouth, drowsiness, blurred vision, dilation of pupils, dizziness, disorientation, confusion.

INTERACTIONS: Caution with anticholinergic drugs (eg, other belladonna alkaloids, antihistamines, TCAs, and muscle relaxants). Increased CNS effects with sedatives, tranquilizers, and alcohol. May decrease absorption of oral medications due to delayed gastric emptying or decreased gastric motility.

PREGNANCY: Category C, caution in nursing.

MECHANISM OF ACTION: Anticholinergic agent; acts as competitive inhibitor at postganglionic muscarinic receptor sites of parasympathetic nervous system and on smooth muscle that responds to acetylcholine but lacks cholinergic innervation. Acts in the CNS by blocking cholinergic transmission from vestibular nuclei to higher centers in the CNS and from reticular formation to the vomiting center.

PHARMACOKINETICS: Absorption: Well-absorbed; C_{max}=87pg/mL (free), 354pg/mL (total); T_{max}=24 hrs. **Distribution:** Crosses placenta and blood brain barrier; plasma protein binding (reversibly bound); found in breast milk. **Metabolism:** Extensively metabolized. **Elimination:** Urine (10%) parent and metabolite, (5%, unchanged); $T_{1/2}$=9.5 hrs.

NURSING CONSIDERATIONS

Assessment: Assess for angle-closure/chronic open-angle glaucoma, pyloric obstruction or urinary bladder neck obstruction, intestinal obstruction, hepatic/renal impairment, pregnancy/nursing status, seizures, psychosis, alcohol intake, and possible drug interactions.

Monitoring: Monitor for interference with gastric secretion test, IOP and glaucoma therapy in chronic open-angle glaucoma during patch use, acute toxic psychosis (eg, confusion, agitation, rambling speech, hallucinations, paranoid behaviors, delusions), drowsiness, and disorientation.

Patient Counseling: Caution against performing hazardous tasks (eg, operating machinery/driving). Wash hands thoroughly with soap and water immediately after handling patch; remove patch and consult physician if symptoms of acute-angle glaucoma or difficulty in urinating occur. Dispose properly and keep away from children or pets.

Administration: Transdermal route; apply on hairless area behind ear. Do not cut patch. **Storage:** 20-25°C (68-77°F).

TRANXENE T-TAB
clorazepate dipotassium (Lundbeck)

CIV

THERAPEUTIC CLASS: Benzodiazepine

INDICATIONS: Management of anxiety disorders or for the short-term relief of the symptoms of anxiety. Adjunctive therapy in the management of partial seizures. Symptomatic relief of acute alcohol withdrawal.

DOSAGE: *Adults:* Anxiety: Initial: 15mg qhs. Usual: 30mg/day in divided doses. Max: 60mg/day. Elderly/Debilitated: Initial: 7.5-15mg/day. Alcohol Withdrawal: Day 1: 30mg, then 30-60mg/day. Day 2: 45-90mg/day. Day 3: 22.5-45mg/day. Day 4: 15-30mg. Give in divided doses. Reduce dose and continue with 7.5-15mg/day; d/c when stable. Max: 90mg/day. Antiepileptic Adjunct: Max Initial: 7.5mg tid. Titrate: Increase by no more than 7.5mg/week. Max: 90mg/day. *Pediatrics:* ≥9 yrs: Anxiety: Initial: 15mg qhs. Usual: 30mg/day in divided doses. Max: 60mg/day. Antiepileptic Adjunct: >12 yrs: Max Initial: 7.5mg tid. Titrate: Increase by no more than 7.5mg/week. Max: 90mg/day. 9-12 yrs: Max Initial: 7.5mg bid. Titrate: Increase by no more than 7.5mg/week. Max: 60mg/day.

HOW SUPPLIED: Tab: 3.75mg*, 7.5mg*, 15mg* *scored

CONTRAINDICATIONS: Acute narrow-angle glaucoma.

WARNINGS/PRECAUTIONS: Avoid with depressive neuroses or psychotic reactions. May impair mental/physical abilities. Withdrawal symptoms (eg, delirium, tremors, abdominal and muscle cramps, insomnia, irritability, memory impairment) may occur following abrupt withdrawal; taper gradually following extended therapy. Caution with known drug dependency, renal/hepatic impairment. May increase the risk of suicidal thoughts and behavior; monitor for emergence or worsening of depression, suicidal thoughts or behavior and/or any unusual changes in mood or behavior. Suicidal tendencies may be present in patients who have depression along with anxiety; least amount of drug that is feasible should be available to such patients. Monitor LFTs and blood counts periodically with long-term therapy. Caution in elderly/debilitated; use lowest effective dose and dose adjustments should be made slowly to preclude ataxia or excessive sedation.

ADVERSE REACTIONS: Drowsiness, dizziness, GI complaints, nervousness, blurred vision, dry mouth, headache, mental confusion.

INTERACTIONS: Additive CNS depression with CNS depressants, alcohol. Potentiated by barbiturates, narcotics, phenothiazines, monoamine oxidase inhibitors (MAOIs), other antidepressants. Increased sedation with hypnotics.

PREGNANCY: Safety in pregnancy not known, not for use in nursing.

MECHANISM OF ACTION: Benzodiazepine; antianxiety/hypnotic agent which has CNS depressant effect.

PHARMACOKINETICS: Distribution: (Nordiazepam) Found in breast milk; Plasma protein binding (97-98%). **Metabolism:** Liver; rapidly decarboxylated to nordiazepam (primary metabolite); hydroxylation. **Elimination:** Urine (62-67%), feces (15-19%); (Nordiazepam)$T_{1/2}$=40-50 hrs.

NURSING CONSIDERATIONS

Assessment: Assess for acute narrow-angle glaucoma, renal/hepatic impairment, depressive neurosis, psychotic reactions, pregnancy/nursing status, and for possible drug interactions. Assess psychological potential for drug dependence.

Monitoring: Monitor for signs/symptoms of depression, suicidal thoughts or behavior, unusual changes in mood or behavior, and for drug dependence. Monitor for withdrawl symptoms (eg, delirium, tremors, abdominal and muscle cramps, insomnia, irritability, memory impairment) following abrupt withdrawl. In patients on prolonged therapy, monitor blood counts and LFTs periodically.

Patient Counseling: Inform about benefits/risks and appropriate use of therapy. Advise to read Medication Guide. Counsel patients, caregivers, and family members that therapy may increase the risk of suicidal thoughts and behavior and advise of the need to be alert for the emergence or worsening of the signs and symptoms of depression, any unusual changes in mood/behavior, suicidal thoughts/behavior, or thoughts about self-harm; instruct to immediately report behaviors of concern to healthcare provider. Caution against engaging in hazardous tasks requiring mental alertness (eg, operating machinery/driving). Inform that therapy may produce psychological and physical dependence; instruct to contact physician before either increasing the dose or discontinuing therapy. Advise patients to enroll in North American Antiepileptic Drug (NAAED) Pregnancy Registry if they become pregnant.

Administration: Oral route. **Storage:** 20-25°C (68-77°F). Protect from moisture; keep bottle tightly closed.

TRAVATAN   RX
travoprost (Alcon)

OTHER BRAND NAMES: Travatan Z (Alcon)

THERAPEUTIC CLASS: Prostaglandin analog

INDICATIONS: Reduction of elevated intraocular pressure (IOP) in patients with open-angle glaucoma or ocular HTN.

DOSAGE: *Adults:* 1 drop in affected eye(s) qd in pm. Space dosing with other ophthalmic drugs by at least 5 min.

HOW SUPPLIED: Sol: 0.004% [2.5mL, 5mL]

WARNINGS/PRECAUTIONS: Changes to pigmented tissues, including increased pigmentation of iris (may be permanent), eyelids and eyelashes (may be reversible). Regularly examine patients with noticeably increased iris pigmentation. May cause changes to eyelashes and vellus hair in the treated eye. Macular edema, including cystoid macular edema, reported. Caution with active intraocular inflammation (eg, uveitis), aphakic patients, pseudopha-kic patients with torn posterior lens capsule, and patients at risk of macular edema. Treatment of angle-closure, inflammatory, or neovascular glaucoma has not been evaluated. Bacterial keratitis reported with multi-dose container. Remove contact lenses prior to use and reinsert 15 min after administration.

ADVERSE REACTIONS: Ocular hyperemia, foreign body sensation, decreased visual acuity, eye discomfort/pruritus/pain.

PREGNANCY: Category C, caution in nursing.

MECHANISM OF ACTION: Prostaglandin analog; has not been established. Believed to reduce IOP by increasing uveoscleral outflow.

PHARMACOKINETICS: Absorption: C_{max}=0.018ng/mL; T_{max}=30 min. **Metabolism:** Cornea, via esterases to active free acid and systemically to inactive metabolites via β-oxidation and reduction. **Elimination:** Urine (2%); $T_{1/2}$=45 min.

NURSING CONSIDERATIONS

Assessment: Assess for active intraocular inflammation (uveitis); active macu-lar edema; aphakic/pseudophakic patient with torn posterior lens capsule; angle-closure, inflammatory, or neovascular glaucoma; pregnancy/nursing status.

Monitoring: Monitor for increased pigmentation of the iris, periorbital tissue (eyelid); changes in eyelashes (eg, increased length, thickness, and number of lashes); macular edema (including cystoid macular edema); and bacterial keratitis.

Patient Counseling: Inform about risk of brown pigmentation of iris, which may be permanent, and darkening of eyelid skin which may be reversible after d/c. Avoid touching tip of applicator to eye or surrounding areas. Remove contact lenses prior to administration; reinsert 15 min after administration. Administer at least 5 min apart if using >1 topical ophthalmic drugs. Consult physician if having ocular surgery or developed intercurrent ocular condi-tions (eg, trauma or infection) or ocular reactions. Inform of the possibility of eyelash and vellus hair changes.

Administration: Ocular route. **Storage:** 2-25°C (36-77°F).

TRAZODONE   RX
trazodone HCl (Various)

> Antidepressants increased the risk of suicidal thinking and behavior (suicidality) in short-term studies in children and adolescents with major depressive disorder (MDD) and other psychiatric disorders. Monitor and observe closely for clinical worsening, suicidality and unusual changes in behavior in patients who are started on antidepressant therapy. Trazodone is not approved for use in pediatric patients.

THERAPEUTIC CLASS: Triazolopyridine derivative

INDICATIONS: Treatment of depression.

DOSAGE: *Adults:* Initial: 150mg/day in divided doses pc. Titrate: May increase by 50mg/day every 3-4 days. Max: (Outpatient) 400mg/day in divided doses, (Inpatient) 600mg/day in divided doses. Maint: Lowest effective level, and may gradually reduce if adequate response is achieved.

HOW SUPPLIED: Tab: 50mg*, 100mg*, 150mg*, 300mg*, *scored

WARNINGS/PRECAUTIONS: Monitor for clinical worsening and/or suicidal ideation and behavior (suicidality), especially at initiation of therapy or dose changes. Consideration should be given to changing the therapeutic regimen, including possibly d/c medication if depression is persistently worse or if experience emergent suicidality or symptoms that may be precursors to wors-ening depression or suicidality. Prior to treatment, adequately screen for bipo-lar disorder; not approved for use in treating bipolar depression. May cause priapism; d/c use if prolonged or inappropriate erections occur. Not recom-mended for use during the initial recovery phase of myocardial infarction (MI). Cardiac arrhythmias may occur; caution in patients with pre-existing cardiac disease, and monitor closely. Hypotension, including orthostatic hypotension, and syncope reported. D/C therapy prior to elective surgery. Occasional low WBC and low neutrophil count reported. May impair physical/mental abilities.

ADVERSE REACTIONS: Dry mouth, edema, constipation, blurred vision, fatigue, nervousness, drowsiness, dizziness, headache, insomnia, N/V, musculoskeletal pain, hypotension, confusion, priapism.

INTERACTIONS: CYP3A4 inhibitors (eg, ritonavir, ketoconazole, indinavir, itraconazole, nefazodone) may increase levels; a lower dose of trazodone may be required when used with potent CYP3A4 inhibitors. Carbamazepine decreases levels; monitor to determine if dosage increase of trazodone is required. Increases digoxin and phenytoin serum levels. Caution with MAOIs. May enhance response to alcohol, barbiturates and other CNS depressants. May affect PT in patients on warfarin. Concomitant use with antihypertensive therapy, may require a dose reduction of the antihypertensive drug. Avoid electroshock therapy. May interact with general anesthetics.

PREGNANCY: Category C, caution in nursing.

MECHANISM OF ACTION: Triazolopyridine derivative; suspected to selectively inhibit serotonin uptake by brain synaptosomes and potentiate behavioral changes induced by the serotonin precursor, 5-hydroxytryptophan.

PHARMACOKINETICS: Absorption: Well absorbed; T_{max}=1 hr (taken on an empty stomach), 2 hrs (taken with food). **Metabolism:** Liver via CYP3A4 to m-chlorophenylpiperazine (active metabolite).

NURSING CONSIDERATIONS

Assessment: Assess for bipolar disorder, cardiac disease or recent MI, pregnancy/nursing status, and for possible drug interactions. Prior to initiating treatment, assess if patient is planning to undergo surgery.

Monitoring: Monitor for signs/symptoms of clinical worsening, suicidality, unusual changes in behavior, priapism, cardiac arrhythmias, and for hypotension.

Patient Counseling: Inform about the benefits and risks of therapy. Advise patients, families, and caregivers of need to observe for signs/symptoms of clinical worsening and suicidal risks (eg, anxiety, agitation, panic attacks, mania, changes in behavior, suicidal ideation); contact physician if such symptoms occur. Avoid alcohol, sedatives, and other CNS depressants. Instruct males to d/c use and contact physician if develop a prolonged or inappropriate penile erection. Inform that may impair the mental and/or physical ability required for performing potentially hazardous tasks (eg, driving). Take shortly after a meal or light snack.

Administration: Oral route. **Storage:** 20-25°C (68-77°F). Protect from temperatures above 40°C (104°F). Dispense in tight, light-resistant container.

TREANDA   RX
bendamustine HCl (Cephalon)

THERAPEUTIC CLASS: Alkylating agent

INDICATIONS: Treatment of chronic lymphocytic leukemia (CLL) and indolent B-cell non-Hodgkin's lymphoma (NHL) that has progressed during or within six months of treatment with rituximab or a rituximab-containing regimen.

DOSAGE: *Adults:* CLL: 100mg/m² IV over 30 min on Days 1 and 2, of a 28-day cycle. Max: 6 cycles. Delay treatment for Grade 4 hematologic toxicity or clinically significant ≥Grade 2 non-hematologic toxicity. ≥Grade 3 Hematologic Toxicity: Reduce dose to 50mg/m² on Days 1 and 2 of each cycle; if ≥Grade 3 toxicity recurs, reduce dose to 25mg/m² on Days 1 and 2 of each cycle. ≥Grade 3 Non-hematologic Toxicity: Reduce dose to 50mg/m² on Days 1 and 2 of each cycle. Consider dose re-escalation in subsequent cycles. NHL: 120mg/m² IV over 60 min on Days 1 and 2 of a 21-day cycle. Max: 8 cycles. Delay treatment for Grade 4 hematologic toxicity or clinically significant ≥Grade 2 non-hematologic toxicity. Grade 4 Hematologic Toxicity: Reduce dose to 90mg/m² on Days 1 and 2 of each cycle; if Grade 4 toxicity recurs, reduce dose to 60mg/m² on Days 1 and 2 of each cycle. ≥Grade 3 Non-hematologic Toxicity: Reduce dose to 90mg/m² on Days 1 and 2 of each cycle; if ≥Grade 3 toxicity recurs, reduce dose to 60mg/m² on Days 1 and 2 of each cycle.

HOW SUPPLIED: Inj: 25mg, 100mg

CONTRAINDICATIONS: Hypersensitivity to mannitol.

WARNINGS/PRECAUTIONS: Myelosuppression may occur; monitor blood counts including leukocytes, platelets, Hgb and neutrophils closely. Infection, including pneumonia and sepsis, reported. Increased susceptibility to infection with myelosuppression. May cause infusion reactions; monitor clinically and consider d/c with Grade 3 or 4 infusion reactions. May cause tumor lysis syndrome; maintain adequate volume status and monitor blood chemistry, particularly K⁺ and uric acid levels. Skin reactions, including rash, toxic skin reactions, and bullous exanthema, reported; if severe or progressive, withhold or d/c treatment. Pre-malignant and malignant diseases (eg, myelodysplastic syndrome, myeloproliferative disorders, acute myeloid leukemia, bronchial carcinoma) reported. Do not use with moderate or severe hepatic impairment; caution with mild hepatic impairment. Do not use if CrCl <40mL/min; caution with lesser degrees of renal impairment. Extravasation reported resulting in hospitalizations from erythema, marked swelling, and pain; take precautions to avoid extravasation and monitor infusion site for redness, swelling, pain, infection and necrosis. Can cause fetal harm.

ADVERSE REACTIONS: Lymphopenia, leukopenia, neutropenia, anemia, thrombocytopenia, N/V, fatigue, diarrhea, fever, constipation, anorexia, cough, headache, weight loss, rash.

INTERACTIONS: CYP1A2 inducers (eg, omeprazole, smoking) may decrease plasma concentrations and increase plasma concentrations of active metabolites. CYP1A2 inhibitors (eg, fluvoxamine, ciprofloxacin) may increase plasma concentrations and decrease plasma concentrations of active metabolites. Cases of Stevens-Johnson syndrome (SJS) and toxic epidermal necrolysis (TEN) reported with allopurinol and other medications known to cause these syndromes. Skin reactions including rash, toxic skin reactions and bullous exanthema may occur when used concomitantly with other anticancer agents.

PREGNANCY: Category D, not for use in nursing.

MECHANISM OF ACTION: Bifunctional mechlorethamine derivative. Mechanism not established; forms electrophilic alkyl groups which form co-valent bonds with electron-rich nucleophilic moieties, resulting in interstrand DNA crosslinks. Bifunctional covalent linkage can lead to cell death via several pathways. Active against both quiescent and dividing cells.

PHARMACOKINETICS: Distribution: Plasma protein binding (94-96%); V_d=25L. **Metabolism:** Hydrolysis; M3, M4 (minor metabolites) via CYP1A2. **Elimination:** Feces (90%); $T_{1/2}$=40 min (bendamustine 120mg/m²); $T_{1/2}$=3 hrs, 30 min (M3, M4).

NURSING CONSIDERATIONS

Assessment: Assess for hypersensitivity to mannitol, myelosuppression, premalignant or malignant disease, renal and hepatic impairment, pregnancy/nursing status and possible drug interactions. Obtain baseline blood counts including WBC, neutrophil, platelet count, Hgb/Hct, LFTs, CrCl.

Monitoring: Monitor CBCs, blood chemistry particularly K⁺ and uric acid levels, LFTs, SrCr levels, and renal/hepatic function periodically. Monitor for development of premalignant or malignant disease. Monitor for signs/symptoms of severe anaphylactic and anaphylactoid reactions, skin reactions, infusion reactions (eg, fever, chills, pruritus and rash) and IV infusion-site reactions (eg, redness, swelling, pain, infection, necrosis), severe myelosuppression (eg, neutropenic sepsis, alveolar hemorrhage with Grade 3 thrombocytopenia, and cytomegalovirus [CMV]), tumor lysis syndrome, infections, impaired hepatic/renal function, pregnancy/nursing status and possible drug interactions.

Patient Counseling: Contact physician if an allergic reaction (eg, rash, facial swelling, difficulty breathing during or soon after infusion) develops. Therapy may cause decrease in WBCs, platelets, and RBCs; advise to contact physician if SOB, significant fatigue, bleeding, fever, or other signs of infection develop. Advise women to avoid becoming pregnant throughout the treatment and for 3 months after the therapy; immediately report pregnancy. Avoid nursing while on therapy. Men should use reliable contraception while on therapy. May cause tiredness; avoid driving any vehicle or operating any dangerous tools or machinery. May cause N/V, diarrhea, and rash. Report any adverse reactions immediately to physician. Mild rash or itching may occur; report immediately for severity or worsening.

Administration: IV route. Administer as IV infusion only. Refer to PI for further instructions on preparation of reconstituted solution, dilution, and administration. **Storage:** 25°C (77°F); excursions permitted up to 30°C (86°F). Retain in original carton until time of use to protect from light. Sol for infusion: Stable for 24 hrs when refrigerated (2-8°C or 36°-47°F) or for 3 hrs when stored at room temperature (15-30°C or 59-86°F) and room light. Refer to PI for procedures for safe handling and disposal.

TRECATOR   RX
ethionamide (Wyeth)

THERAPEUTIC CLASS: Peptide synthesis inhibitor

INDICATIONS: Treatment of active tuberculosis (TB) in patients with *M.tuberculosis* resistant to isoniazid or rifampin, or where there is intolerance to other drugs.

DOSAGE: *Adults:* 15-20mg/kg qd with food. May give in divided doses with poor GI tolerance. Max: 1g/day. Alternate Regimen: Initial: 250mg qd then titrate gradually to optimal doses as tolerated, or 250mg qd for 1-2 days, then 250mg bid for 1-2 days, then 1g/day in 3-4 divided doses. Continue therapy until bacteriological conversion has become permanent and maximal clinical improvement occurs.
Pediatrics: ≥12 yrs: 10-20 mg/kg/day in divided doses given bid or tid with food, or 15mg/kg/day as single dose. Continue therapy until bacteriological conversion has become permanent and maximal clinical improvement occurs.

HOW SUPPLIED: Tab: 250mg

CONTRAINDICATIONS: Severe hepatic impairment.

WARNINGS/PRECAUTIONS: Give with pyridoxine. Rapid development of resistance if used alone; should be used with at least 1 or 2 other drugs. Perform ophthalmologic exams before and periodically during therapy. Measure serum transaminases prior to initiation and monthly thereafter. Risk of hypoglycemia in diabetics; monitor blood glucose prior to initiation then periodically. Hypothyroidism reported; monitor TFTs.

ADVERSE REACTIONS: N/V, diarrhea, abdominal pain, excessive salivation, metallic taste, stomatitis, anorexia, psychotic disturbances, drowsiness, dizziness, hypersensitivity reactions, increase in serum bilirubin, SGOT or SGPT.

INTERACTIONS: D/C all antituberculous medication with elevated serum transaminases until resolved; reintroduce sequentially to determine which drug is responsible. May raise isoniazid levels. May potentiate adverse effects of other antituberculous drugs. Convulsions reported with cycloserine. Risk of psychotic reactions with excessive ethanol ingestion.

PREGNANCY: Category C, not for use in nursing.

MECHANISM OF ACTION: Peptide synthesis inhibitor; may be bacteriostatic or bactericidal in action.

PHARMACOKINETICS: Absorption: Completely absorbed; C_{max}=2.16mcg/mL, T_{max}=1.02 hrs, AUC=7.67mcg•hr/mL. **Distribution:** V_d=93.5L; plasma protein binding (30%); widely distributed into body tissues. **Metabolism:** Liver (extensive). **Elimination:** Urine ≤1%; $T_{1/2}$=1.92 hrs.

NURSING CONSIDERATIONS

Assessment: Assess for severe hepatic impairment, diabetes mellitus, susceptibility test, pregnancy/nursing status and possible drug interactions.

Monitoring: Monitor for hypersensitivity reactions (eg, rash, photosensitivity), GI (eg, N/V, diarrhea) and psychotic disturbances (eg, mental depression).

Determination of serum transaminases (SGOT, SGPT), blood glucose, thyroid function, and eye exams should be done periodically.

Patient Counseling: Advise to report vision loss or blurriness, with/without eye pain. Instruct to avoid excessive ethanol ingestion to avoid psychotic reaction. Take as directed; skipping doses or not completing full course may decrease effectiveness and increase resistance.

Administration: Oral route. **Storage:** 20-25°C (68-77°F). Dispense in tight container.

TRELSTAR   RX
triptorelin pamoate (Watson)

THERAPEUTIC CLASS: Synthetic gonadotropin releasing hormone analog

INDICATIONS: Palliative treatment of advanced prostate cancer.

DOSAGE: *Adults:* 3.75mg IM q4 weeks, 11.25mg IM q12 weeks, or 22.5mg IM q24 weeks as single dose in either buttock. Alternate injection site periodically.

HOW SUPPLIED: Inj: 3.75mg, 11.25mg, 22.5mg

CONTRAINDICATIONS: Women who are or may become pregnant.

WARNINGS/PRECAUTIONS: Anaphylactic shock, hypersensitivity, angioedema reported; d/c immediately and administer appropriate supportive and symptomatic care if these occur. May cause transient increase in serum testosterone levels. Worsening/onset of new signs/symptoms (eg, bone pain, neuropathy, hematuria, urethral/bladder outlet obstruction) may occur during 1st weeks of treatment. Spinal cord compression reported. Institute standard treatment or immediate orchiectomy in extreme cases if spinal cord compression or renal impairment develops. Closely monitor patients with metastatic vertebral lesions and/or urinary tract obstruction during 1st few weeks of therapy. Hyperglycemia, increased risk of developing diabetes/myocardial infarction (MI), sudden cardiac death, and stroke reported in men receiving gonadotropin-releasing hormone (GnRH) agonists. Monitor response by measuring serum levels of testosterone periodically and as indicated. May suppress pituitary-gonadal system in therapeutic dose and mislead diagnostic tests of pituitary-gonadotropic and gonadal functions during treatment.

ADVERSE REACTIONS: Hot flushes, HTN, headache, skeletal pain, dysuria, leg edema, back pain, impotence, erectile dysfunction, testicular atrophy.

INTERACTIONS: Avoid hyperprolactinemic drugs.

PREGNANCY: Category X, not for use in nursing.

MECHANISM OF ACTION: Synthetic decapeptide agonist analog of GnRH; initially increases circulating levels of luteinizing hormone (LH), follicle-stimulating hormone (FSH), testosterone, and estradiol; chronic and continuous administration causes a sustained decrease in LH and FSH secretion and marked reduction of testicular steroidogenesis.

PHARMACOKINETICS: Absorption: (IM) C_{max} (3.75mg, 11.25mg, 22.5mg)=28.4ng/mL, 38.5ng/mL, 44.1ng/mL; T_{max}=1-3 hrs. **Distribution**: V_d (0.5mg IV)=30-33L. **Elimination**: Liver and kidneys; Urine (41.7%, unchanged); $T_{1/2}$=3 hrs.

NURSING CONSIDERATIONS

Assessment: Assess pregnancy/nursing status, metastatic vertebral lesions, urinary tract obstruction, hypersensitivity to drug, cardiovascular disease (CVD), diabetes mellitus (DM), renal/hepatic impairment, and for possible drug interactions. Obtain baseline serum testosterone, prostate specific antigen (PSA) levels, blood glucose levels, LFTs.

Monitoring: Monitor response to drug and for signs/symptoms of worsening prostate cancer, spinal cord compression, renal impairment, hypersensitivity reactions (eg, anaphylactic shock, angioedema), signs/symptoms suggestive of development of CVD, and other adverse reactions. Periodically monitor serum testosterone, PSA levels, blood glucose and/or glycosylated Hgb (HbA1c), LFTs.

Patient Counseling: Inform that patients may experience worsening of symptoms of prostate cancer during the 1st weeks of treatment. Advise that the symptoms should decline 3-4 weeks following administration of therapy. Inform of the increased risk of developing DM, MI, sudden cardiac death, and stroke. Allergic reactions could occur and serious reactions require immediate treatment. Report any previous hypersensitivity to drug and its components and contact physician if any side effects develop.

Administration: IM route. Inspect visually for particulate matter/discoloration prior to administration. Refer to PI for reconstitution instructions. **Storage:** 20-25°C (68-77°F). Do not freeze with Mixject.

TRENTAL RX
pentoxifylline (Sanofi-Aventis)

THERAPEUTIC CLASS: Blood viscosity reducer

INDICATIONS: Treatment of intermittent claudication due to chronic occlusive arterial disease of the limbs.

DOSAGE: *Adults:* 400mg tid with meals for at least 8 weeks. Reduce to 400mg bid if digestive and CNS side effects occur; d/c if side effects persist.

HOW SUPPLIED: Tab, Extended-Release: 400mg

CONTRAINDICATIONS: Recent cerebral and/or retinal hemorrhage, intolerance to methylxanthines (eg, caffeine, theophylline, theobromine).

WARNINGS/PRECAUTIONS: Monitor Hgb and Hct with risk factors complicated by hemorrhage (eg, recent surgery, peptic ulceration, cerebral/retinal bleeding). Occasional reports of angina, hypotension, and arrhythmia in patients with concurrent coronary artery and cerebrovascular diseases.

ADVERSE REACTIONS: Bloating, dyspepsia, N/V, dizziness, headache.

INTERACTIONS: Increase risk of bleeding with warfarin; monitor PT/INR more frequently. May increase theophylline levels; risk of theophylline toxicity. May increase effect of antihypertensives.

PREGNANCY: Category C, not for use in nursing.

MECHANISM OF ACTION: Blood viscosity reducer; not established. Increases blood flow to affected microcirculation and enhances tissue oxygenation. Improves erythrocyte flexibility, increases leukocyte deformability, and inhibits neutrophil adhesion and activation.

PHARMACOKINETICS: Absorption: T_{max}=1 hr. **Distribution:** Found in breast milk. **Metabolism:** 1st pass; metabolites (major): Metabolite 1(1-[5-hydroxyhexyl]-3,7-dimethylxanthine); metabolite V (1-[3-carboxypropyl]-3,7-dimethylxanthine). **Elimination:** Urine (major), feces (<4%); $T_{1/2}$=0.4-0.8 hrs; $T_{1/2}$=0.4-0.8 hrs (metabolites).

NURSING CONSIDERATIONS

Assessment: Assess for recent cerebral and/or retinal hemorrhage, hypersensitivity to methylxanthines (eg, caffeine, theophylline, theobromine), nursing/pregnancy status, renal function, and drug interactions.

Monitoring: In presence of concurrent coronary artery disease and cerebrovascular disease, monitor for signs/symptoms of angina, arrhythmia, and hypotension. If on concomitant warfarin therapy, perform more frequent monitoring of PT time. If risk for bleeding (eg, recent surgery, peptic ulceration, recent cerebral and/or retinal bleeding), periodically monitor Hgb and/or Hct. Perform periodic monitoring of renal function in the elderly (≥65 yrs).

Patient Counseling: Inform to take with meals. Instruct to report if any digestive (eg, dyspepsia, nausea) or CNS (eg, headaches) side effects develop; dose adjustment may be needed. Report any signs/symptoms of angina or hypotension.

Administration: Oral administration. **Storage**: 15-30°C (59-86°F). Dispense in well-closed, light-resistant container. Protect blisters from light.

TREXIMET
RX

naproxen sodium - sumatriptan succinate (GlaxoSmithKline)

> May cause increased risk of serious cardiovascular (CV) thrombotic events, myocardial infarction (MI), and stroke, which can be fatal. Risk may increase with duration of use. Patients with or have risk factors for CV disease may be at greater risk. May increase the risk of serious GI adverse events including bleeding, ulceration, and perforation of stomach or intestines, which can be fatal. Can occur at any time during use and without warning. Elderly patients at greater risk.

THERAPEUTIC CLASS: 5-HT$_1$-agonist/NSAID

INDICATIONS: Acute treatment of migraine attacks with or without aura.

DOSAGE: *Adults:* Initial: 1 tab. Max: 2 tabs/24 hrs. Dosing should be at least 2 hrs apart.

HOW SUPPLIED: Tab: (Naproxen-Sumatriptan): 500mg-85mg [9^s]

CONTRAINDICATIONS: History, symptoms, or signs of ischemic cardiac (eg, angina pectoris, MI, silent myocardial ischemia), cerebrovascular (eg, stroke, transient ischemic attacks), or peripheral vascular syndromes (eg, ischemic bowel disease). Other significant cardiovascular (CV) disease, coronary artery bypass graft (CABG) surgery, hepatic impairment, uncontrolled HTN, hemiplegic or basilar migraine. MAOIs during or within 2 weeks of administration. Use within 24 hrs of ergotamine-containing agents, ergot-type drugs, or other 5-HT$_1$ agonists. Presence or history of NSAID/ASA-related asthma, nasal polyps, urticaria, or hypotension.

WARNINGS/PRECAUTIONS: Establish clear diagnosis of migraine. Caution in patients with controlled HTN; monitor closely during initiation and throughout course of therapy. Caution in patients with fluid retention and heart failure. Serotonin syndrome may occur. Caution in patients with prior history of ulcer disease or GI bleed, impaired renal function, asthma, elderly, taking ACE inhibitors or diuretics, diseases that may alter absorption/metabolism/excretion, history of epilepsy or condition that lowers seizure threshold. Not recommended in patients with advanced renal disease or hepatic impairment. Anaphylactic/anaphylactoid reactions, serious skin reaction such as exfoliative dermatitis, Stevens-Johnson syndrome (SJS) and toxic epidermal necrolysis (TEN) may occur. Chest, jaw, or neck pain/discomfort reported. May cause vision disturbances. Caution in those with coagulation disorders or receiving anticoagulants and in those with pre-existing asthma. May decrease platelet aggregation and prolong bleeding time.

ADVERSE REACTIONS: Dizziness, somnolence, nausea, chest/neck/throat/jaw pain, tightness, pressure.

INTERACTIONS: See Contraindications. Avoid use with ASA. (Naproxen) Caution when administered concomitantly with methotrexate (MTX) due to elevated and prolonged serum MTX levels. NSAIDs can reduce the effect of furosemides and thiazides. Use with ACE inhibitors may potentiate renal disease states. May cause lithium toxicity when administered concurrently with lithium. Probenecid may extend naproxen plasma half-life. May reduce the antihypertensive effect of propranolol and other β-blockers. Increases GI bleeding with warfarin, alcohol, oral corticosteroids and anticoagulants. (Sumatriptan) Combined use with SSRIs, SNRIs, and triptans may cause serotonin syndrome.

PREGNANCY: Category C, not for use in nursing.

MECHANISM OF ACTION: Naproxen: NSAID; inhibits the synthesis of inflammatory mediators and prostaglandin synthetase. Sumatriptan: 5-HT$_1$ receptor agonist; mediates vasoconstriction of human basilar artery and vasculature of human dura mater, which correlates with the relief of migraine headache.

PHARMACOKINETICS: Absorption: Naproxen: Absolute bioavailability (95%), T_{max} =5 hrs; Sumatriptan: Absolute bioavailability (15%), T_{max} =1 hr. **Distribution:** Naproxen: V_d = 0.16L/kg. Plasma protein binding (>99%); Sumatriptan: V_d =2.4L/kg. Plasma protein binding (14-21%). **Metabolism:** Naproxen: Extensively metabolized to 6-0-desmethyl naproxen; Sumatriptan: via monoamine oxidase. **Elimination:** Naproxen: Urine (95%), $T_{1/2}$ =19 hrs; Sumatriptan: Renal (60%), feces (40%); $T_{1/2}$ =2 hrs.

NURSING CONSIDERATIONS

Assessment: Assess for presence/history of cardiac ischemic syndrome, cerebrovascular syndrome, or peripheral vascular syndrome, uncontrolled HTN, presence of hemiplegic or basilar migraines, hepatic/renal impairment, history of epilepsy, pregnancy/nursing status, and possible drug interactions. Establish diagnosis of migraine headaches and history of asthma. Evaluate for fluid retention, edema, and risk factors for GI events.

Monitoring: Monitor for signs/symptoms of cardiac events (eg, MI, cardiac rhythm disturbances, peripheral vascular ischemia, hypertensive crisis, chest tightness), colonic ischemia, bloody diarrhea, serotonin syndrome (eg, mental status changes), hypersensitivity reactions, jaw/neck tightness, seizures, exacerbation of headache, ophthalmic changes (eg, corneal opacities), and clinical response. In patients on long-term therapy and in patients with CAD risk factors, perform periodic monitoring of CV function. If clinical response does not occur following administration of first dose, reassess diagnosis. Monitor BP, CBC, LFTs, renal function, and chemistries periodically. Monitor for signs and symptoms of GI events (eg, bleeding, ulceration, perforation), renal/liver dysfunction.

Patient Counseling: Inform about possible adverse events and to consult physician if such symptoms of CV events (eg, chest or abdominal pain, SOB, weakness, slurring of speech), ulcerations and bleeding (eg, epigastric pain, dyspepsia, melena, hematemesis), serious skin side effects (eg, exfoliative dermatitis, SJS, TEN, skin rash, blister, fever), other signs of hypersensitivity reactions (eg, itching), hepatotoxicity (eg, nausea, fatigue, lethargy, pruritus, jaundice, etc), anaphylactic/anaphylactoid reactions (eg, difficulty breathing, swelling of the face or throat), unexplained weight gain, or edema occur. Inform that risk of developing an ulcer or bleeding increases with use of corticosteroids and anticoagulants, extended or more frequent use, smoking, drinking alcohol, older age, and poor health. Caution with activities that requires alertness if they experience drowsiness, dizziness, vertigo or depression. May enroll patients in the Treximet pregnancy registry if they become pregnant while on treatment.

Administration: Oral route. Do not split, crush, or chew. **Storage:** 25°C (77°F); excusions permitted to 15-30°C (59-86°F).

TRIBENZOR   RX

olmesartan medoxomil - hydrochlorothiazide - amlodipine (Daiichi Sankyo)

> Drugs that act directly on the renin-angiotensin system can cause injury and even death to the developing fetus. D/C if pregnancy is detected.

THERAPEUTIC CLASS: ARB/Calcium channel blocker (dihydropyridine)/Thiazide diuretic

INDICATIONS: Treatment of HTN.

DOSAGE: *Adults:* 1 tab qd. Titrate: May increase after 2 weeks. Max: 40mg-10mg-25mg qd. Replacement Therapy: May be substituted for its individually titrated components. May be used as add-on/switch therapy to provide additional BP lowering if not adequately controlled on agents from two of the following antihypertensive classes: angiotensin receptor blockers, CCBs, and diuretics.

HOW SUPPLIED: Tab: (Olmesartan-Amlodipine-HCTZ) 20mg-5mg-12.5mg, 40mg-5mg-12.5mg, 40mg-5mg-25mg, 40mg-10mg-12.5mg, 40mg-10mg-25mg

CONTRAINDICATIONS: Anuria, sulfonamide hypersensitivity.

WARNINGS/PRECAUTIONS: Not for initial therapy of HTN. Renal impairment reported. Avoid use with severe renal impairment (CrCl ≤30mL/min). Olmesartan: May cause symptomatic hypotension; caution in patients with activated renin-angiotensin system (eg, volume-and/or salt depletion). Increased SrCr and BUN levels reported with unilateral/bilateral renal artery stenosis. Oliguria, azotemia and rarely acute renal failure and/or death reported in patients whose renal function may depend upon the activity of the renin-angiotensin-aldosterone system. Increased blood creatinine levels and hyperkalemia reported. Amlodipine: May increase frequency, duration, or severity of angina or acute MI, particularly those with severe obstructive coronary artery disease (CAD). Rare reports of acute hypotension; caution with severe aortic stenosis. Hepatic enzyme elevations reported. HCTZ: May precipitate azotemia in patients with renal disease. Monitor for signs of fluid or electrolyte imbalance; minor alterations of fluid or electrolyte may precipitate hepatic coma. Hypokalemia may develop when severe cirrhosis is present or after prolonged therapy. Metabolic acidosis, dilutional hyponatremia, hyperuricemia, hyperglycemia, hypomagnesemia and hypersensitivity reactions may occur. May decrease urinary calcium excretion. D/C before carrying out test for parathyroid function. May exacerbate or activate systemic lupus erythematosus (SLE). May increase cholesterol and triglyceride levels.

ADVERSE REACTIONS: Dizziness, peripheral edema, headache, fatigue, nasopharyngitis, muscle spasms, nausea, upper respiratory tract infection, diarrhea, UTI, joint swelling.

INTERACTIONS: HCTZ: Alcohol, barbiturates, narcotics may potentiate orthostatic hypotension. Antidiabetic drugs (eg, oral agents, insulin) dosage adjustments may be required. Cholestyramine and colestipol resins decrease absorption from the GI tract. Corticosteroids and ACTH may intensify electrolyte depletion, particularly hypokalemia. Possible decreased response to pressor amines (eg, norepinephrine) but not sufficient to preclude their use. Lithium clearance may be decreased; monitor for toxicity. NSAIDS can reduce antidiuretic, natriuretic, and antihypertensive effects; observe for desired diuretic effect. Possible increased responsiveness to non-depolarizing muscle relaxants (eg, tubocurarine). Additive effect or potentiation with other antihypertensives.

PREGNANCY: Category C (1st trimester), D (2nd and 3rd trimesters), not for use in nursing.

MECHANISM OF ACTION: ARB/Calcium channel blocker (dihydropyridine)/Thiazide diuretic. Amlodipine: Dihydropyridine Calcium antagonist (calcium ion antagonist or slow-channel block); inhibits transmembrane influx of calcium ions into vascular smooth muscle and cardiac muscle. Olmesartan: Angiotensin II receptor antagonist; blocks vasoconstrictor effects of angiotensin II by selectively blocking binding of angiotensin II to AT_1 receptor in vascular smooth muscle. HCTZ: Thiazide diuretic; affects renal tubular mechanism of electrolyte reabsorption, directly increasing excretion of Na^+ and Cl^- and indirectly reducing plasma volume.

PHARMACOKINETICS: Absorption: Olmesartan: Rapid and complete; absolute bioavailability (26%); T_{max}=1-2 hrs. Amlodipine: Absolute bioavailability (64%-90%); T_{max}=6-12 hrs. HCTZ: T_{max}=1.5-2 hrs. **Distribution:** Olmesartan: Plasma protein binding (99%); V_d=17L. Amlodipine: Plasma protein binding (93%). HCTZ: Crosses placental barrier; found in breast milk. **Metabolism:** Olmesartan: Ester hydrolysis. Amlodipine: Hepatic (extensive). **Excretion:** Olmesartan: Urine (35-50%), feces; $T_{1/2}$=13 hrs. Amlodipine: Urine (60% metabolites), $T_{1/2}$=30-50 hrs. HCTZ: Urine (≥61% unchanged).

NURSING CONSIDERATIONS

Assessment: Assess for anuria, volume and/or salt depletion, renal/hepatic impairment, renal/aortic stenosis, CAD, congestive heart failure (CHF), cirrhosis, post-sympathectomy, history of allergy or bronchial asthma, recent MI, SLE, pregnancy/nursing status and possible drug interactions.

Monitoring: Monitor for hyperuricemia, hyperglycemia, hypomagnesemia, hypercalcemia, hypotension, angina, MI, renal/hepatic impairment, oliguria, azotemia, renal artery stenosis, and frank gout. Monitor cholesterol levels, triglyceride levels, SrCr, BUN, and LFTs. Observe for signs and symptoms of fluid or electrolyte imbalance.

Patient Counseling: Instruct to notify physician if pregnant/planning to become pregnant or breastfeeding. Inform that lightheadedness can occur, especially during first days of therapy; D/c and consult physician if syncope occurs. Inadequate fluid intake, excessive perspiration, diarrhea, and vomiting may lead to an excessive fall in BP.

Administration: Oral route. **Storage:** 25°C (77°F); excursions permitted to 15-30°C (59-86°F).

TRICOR
fenofibrate (Abbott)

RX

THERAPEUTIC CLASS: Fibric acid derivative

INDICATIONS: Adjunct to diet in primary hypercholesterolemia, mixed dyslipidemia (Fredrickson Types IIa and IIb), and hypertriglyceridemia (Fredrickson Types IV and V hyperlipidemia).

DOSAGE: *Adults:* Primary Hypercholesterolemia/Mixed Hyperlipidemia: Initial: 145mg/day. Hypertriglyceridemia: Initial: 48-145mg/day. Titrate: Adjust if needed after repeat lipid determinations at 4-8 week intervals. Max: 145mg/day. Mild to Moderate Renal Dysfunction: Initial: 48mg/day. Titrate: Increase only after evaluation of effects on renal function and lipid levels at this dose. Elderly: Base on renal function. Take without regard to meals. Withdraw therapy if an adequate response is not achieved after 2 months of treatment with max dose.

HOW SUPPLIED: Tab: 48mg, 145mg

CONTRAINDICATIONS: Preexisting gallbladder disease, unexplained persistent liver function abnormality, hepatic or severe renal dysfunction (including primary biliary cirrhosis).

WARNINGS/PRECAUTIONS: Increased serum transaminases (AST/ALT) reported; d/c if >3x ULN. Hepatocellular, chronic active and cholestatic hepatitis and cirrhosis reported. Perform periodic determinations of lipid levels during initial therapy to establish lowest effective dose. May cause cholelithiasis; d/c if gallstones found. Ascertain that lipid levels are consistently abnormal prior to initiating therapy. May cause myositis, myopathy, or rhabdomyolysis; d/c if myopathy/myositis or marked CPK elevation occurs. Decreased Hgb, Hct, WBCs, thrombocytopenia, and agranulocytosis reported; monitor CBC during first 12 months of therapy. Acute hypersensitivity reactions (eg, Stevens-Johnson syndrome [SJS], toxic epidermal necrolysis [TEN]), elevated SrCr, and pancreatitis reported. Avoid use with severe renal impairment; reduce dose in mild to moderate renal impairment. Higher rates of pulmonary embolus (PE) and deep vein thrombosis (DVT) reported. Caution in the elderly.

ADVERSE REACTIONS: Abnormal LFTs, respiratory disorder, abdominal pain, back pain, headache, increased creatinine phosphokinase.

INTERACTIONS: Potentiates coumarin anticoagulants; reduce anticoagulant dose and monitor PT/INR. Avoid HMG-CoA reductase inhibitors unless benefits outweigh risks. Bile acid sequestrants may impede absorption; take at least 1 hr before or 4-6 hrs after the resin. Evaluate benefits/risks with immunosuppressants (eg, cyclosporine) and other nephrotoxic agents. May decrease atorvastatin exposure. May increase exposure to fluvastatin. May increase glimepiride exposure and pravastatin levels. Decreased levels with pravastatin.

PREGNANCY: Category C, not for use in nursing.

MECHANISM OF ACTION: Fibric acid derivative; activates peroxisome proliferator activated receptor α (PPARα), increasing lipolysis and elimination of triglyceride-rich particles from plasma by activating lipoprotein lipase and reducing production of apoprotein C-III (lipoprotein lipase activity inhibitor). Activation of PPARα also induces an increase in synthesis of apoproteins A-I, A-II, and HDL-cholesterol.

PHARMACOKINETICS: Absorption: Well absorbed; T_{max}=6-8 hrs. **Distribution:** Plasma protein binding (99%). **Metabolism:** Hydrolysis, conjugation; fenofibric acid (active metabolite). **Elimination:** Urine (60%), feces (25%); $T_{1/2}$=20 hrs.

NURSING CONSIDERATIONS

Assessment: Assess for hepatic/renal dysfunction (eg, primary biliary cirrhosis), preexisting gallbladder disease, contributory diseases of lipid abnormalities (eg, diabetes mellitus [DM], hypothyroidism), pregnancy/nursing status, and for possible drug interactions. Obtain baseline lipid levels.

Monitoring: Monitor for signs/symptoms of liver dysfunction, cholelithiasis, gallstones, pancreatitis, hypersensitivity reactions (eg, SJS, TEN), hematological changes (eg, thrombocytopenia, agranulocytosis), myopathy, myositis, rhabdomyolysis, PE, DVT, and elevations in SrCr. Periodically monitor LFTs, cholesterol levels, and blood counts. Evaluate CPK levels in patients suspected of having myopathy. Monitor for clinical response; if adequate response not seen after 2 months with maximum dose, d/c therapy.

Patient Counseling: Advise to immediately contact physician if unexplained muscle pain, tenderness, or weakness develops, particularly when accompanied by malaise or fever. Follow appropriate lipid-lowering diet. Instruct to take with/without meals. Notify physician if pregnant/nursing and of all prescription and non-prescription medications currently being taken.

Administration: Oral route. **Storage:** 25°C (77°F); excursions permitted to 15-30°C (59-86°F). Protect from moisture.

TRIGLIDE RX
fenofibrate (Sciele)

THERAPEUTIC CLASS: Fibric acid derivative

INDICATIONS: Adjunct to diet for treatment of hypertriglyceridemia (Types IV and V). Reduction of LDL-C, Total-C, TG, and Apo B in primary hypercholesterolemia or mixed dyslipidemia (Types IIa and IIb).

DOSAGE: *Adults:* Hypercholesterolemia/Mixed Hyperlipidemia: 160mg qd. Hypertriglyceridemia: Initial: 50-160mg/day. Titrate: Adjust if needed after repeat lipid levels at 4-8 week intervals. Max: 160mg/day. Renal Dysfunction/Elderly: Initial: 50mg/day. Take without regard to meals.

HOW SUPPLIED: Tab: 50mg, 160mg

CONTRAINDICATIONS: Severe renal dysfunction, hepatic dysfunction (including primary biliary cirrhosis and unexplained persistent liver function abnormality), pre-existing gallbladder disease.

WARNINGS/PRECAUTIONS: Increased serum transaminases (AST/ALT) reported; d/c if >3x ULN. Hepatocellular, chronic active and cholestatic hepatitis and cirrhosis reported. Monitor LFTs regularly; d/c if >3x ULN. May cause cholelithiasis; d/c if gallstones found. May cause myositis, myopathy, or rhabdomyolysis; d/c if myopathy/myositis or marked CPK elevation occurs. Decreased Hgb, Hct, WBCs, thrombocytopenia, and agranulocytosis reported; monitor CBC during first 12 months of therapy. Acute hypersensitivity reactions (eg, Stevens-Johnson syndrome [SJS], toxic epidermal necrolysis [TEN]), elevated SrCr, and pancreatitis reported. Higher rates of pulmonary embolus (PE) and deep vein thrombosis (DVT) reported. Caution in the elderly. Monitor lipids periodically initially; d/c if inadequate response after 2 months on 160mg/day. Caution in elderly.

ADVERSE REACTIONS: Abdominal pain, back pain, headache, abnormal LFTs, respiratory disorder, increased creatinine phosphokinase/SGPT/SGOT.

INTERACTIONS: May potentiate coumarin anticoagulants; reduce anticoagulant dose and monitor PT/INR. Avoid HMG-CoA reductase inhibitors unless benefits outweigh risks. Bile acid sequestrants may impede absorption; take at least 1 hr before or 4-6 hrs after the resin. Evaluate benefits/risks with immunosuppressants (eg, cyclosporine) and other nephrotoxic agents; use lowest effective dose.

PREGNANCY: Category C, not for use in nursing.

MECHANISM OF ACTION: Fibric acid derivative; activates peroxisome proliferator-activated receptor alpha (PPARα). Causes an increase in lipolysis and elimination of triglyceride-rich particles from plasma by activating lipoprotein lipase and reducing production of apoprotein C-III. Induces an increase in apoprotein A-I, A-II and HDL cholesterol synthesis. Reduces serum uric acid levels by increasing urinary excretion of uric acid.

PHARMACOKINETICS: Absorption: Well absorbed; T_{max}=3 hrs. **Distribution:** Plasma protein binding (99%). **Metabolism:** Hydrolysis, conjugation; fenofibric acid (active metabolite). **Elimination:** Urine (60%), feces (25%); $T_{1/2}$=16 hrs.

NURSING CONSIDERATIONS

Assessment: Assess for hepatic/renal dysfunction, primary biliary cirrhosis, unexplained persistent liver function abnormality, persistent elevation of lipid levels, hypothyroidism, pre-existing gallbladder disease, and DM. Assess pregnancy/nursing status and possible drug interactions. Check baseline liver function and lipid levels.

Monitoring: Periodically monitor lipid levels, LFTs, CPK, PT, INR, CBC. Monitor for signs of myopathy (eg, unexplained muscle pain, tenderness, or weakness, with fever or malaise), cholelithiasis/cholecystitis, pancreatitis, hepatocellular, chronic active and cholestatic hepatitis, liver cirrhosis, malignancy, and hypersensitivity reaction or severe skin rash.

Patient Counseling: Advise to immediately contact physician if unexplained muscle pain, tenderness, or weakness with malaise or fever. Recommend appropriate lipid-lowering diet. May be taken with/without food.

Administration: Oral route. **Storage:** 20-25°C (68-77°F); excursions permitted between 15-30°C (59-86°F). Protect from light and moisture.

TRILEPTAL   RX
oxcarbazepine (Novartis)

THERAPEUTIC CLASS: Dibenzazepine

INDICATIONS: Monotherapy or adjunctive therapy in the treatment of partial seizures in adults, and as monotherapy in children aged ≥4 yrs with epilepsy and adjunctive therapy in children aged ≥2 yrs with epilepsy.

DOSAGE: *Adults:* Monotherapy: Initial: 300mg bid. Titrate: Increase by 300mg/day every 3rd day. Maint: 1200mg/day. Adjunct Therapy: Initial: 300mg bid. Titrate: Increase weekly by a max of 600mg/day. Maint: 1200mg/day. Conversion to Monotherapy: Initial: 300mg bid while reducing other AEDs. Titrate: Increase weekly by a max of 600mg/day. Withdraw other AEDs over 3-6 weeks. Maint: 2400mg/day. Renal Impairment: CrCl <30mL/min: Initial: 300mg qd. Titrate: Increase gradually.
Pediatrics: 4-16yrs: Monotherapy: Initial: 4-5mg/kg bid. Titrate: Increase by 5mg/kg/day every 3rd day. Maint (mg/day): Refer to PI for Dosing Chart. Adjunct Therapy: Initial: 4-5mg/kg bid. Max: 600mg/day. Titrate: Increase over 2 weeks. Maint: 20-29kg: 900mg/day. 29.1-39kg: 1200mg/day. >39kg: 1800mg/day. Conversion to Monotherapy: Initial: 4-5mg/kg bid while reducing other AEDs. Titrate: Increase weekly by max of 10mg/kg/day to target dose. Withdraw other AEDs over 3-6 weeks. Renal Impairment: CrCl <30mL/min: Initial: 300mg qd. Titrate: Increase gradually. Pediatrics 2-<4yrs: Adjunct Therapy: Initial: 4-5mg/kg bid. Max: 600mg/day. <20kg: Initial: 8-10mg/kg bid. Max: 60mg/kg/day. Titrate: 2-4 weeks until maximum dose achieved.

HOW SUPPLIED: Sus: 300mg/5mL [250mL]. Tab: 150mg*, 300mg*, 600mg* *scored.

WARNINGS/PRECAUTIONS: May develop hyponatremia. Cross-sensitivity with carbamazepine. D/C if anaphylaxis and angioedema involving the larynx, glottis, lips and eyelids develop. Serious dermatologic reactions (eg, Stevens-Johnson syndrome [SJS], toxic epidermal necrolysis [TEN]) and multi-organ hypersensitivity reported. Increased risk of suicidal thoughts or behavior; monitor unusual changes in mood and behavior. Withdraw gradually to minimize the potential of increased seizure frequency. Associated with CNS adverse effects (cognitive symptoms, somnolence or fatigue, coordination disturbances). Rare reports of agranulocytosis, aplastic anemia and pancytopenia; d/c if any evidence of hematologic events. Caution in patients with hepatic and/or renal impairment.

ADVERSE REACTIONS: Dizziness, somnolence, diplopia, fatigue, N/V, ataxia, abnormal vision, tremor, abnormal gait, dyspepsia, abdominal pain.

INTERACTIONS: Additive sedative effect with alcohol. Verapamil, carbamazepine, phenytoin, phenobarbital and valproic acid may decrease levels. Decreased plasma levels of felodipine, oral contraceptives and dihydropyridine calcium antagonists. May induce metabolism of CYP3A4/5 substrates. Increased plasma levels of phenytoin and phenobarbital. Decreased plasma levels of oxcarbazepine with AEDs that are CYP450 inducers.

PREGNANCY: Category C, not for use in nursing.

MECHANISM OF ACTION: Dibenzazepine; mechanism unknown. Oxcarbazepine and 10-monohydroxy metabolite (MHD) suspected to exert antiseizure effects through blockade of voltage-sensitive Na^+ channels, resulting in stabilization of hyperexcited neural membranes, inhibition of repetitive neuronal firing, and diminution of propagation of synaptic impulses. Also, increased K^+ conductance and modulation of high-voltage activated calcium channels may contribute to anticonvulsant activity.

PHARMACOKINETICS: Absorption: Completely absorbed. T_{max}=4.5 hrs (Tab), 6 hrs (Sus). **Distribution:** V_d=49L (MHD); plasma protein binding (40%) (MHD); found in breast milk. **Metabolism:** Liver; reduced to MHD (active metabolite), then conjugated. **Elimination:** Urine (>95%), feces (<4%); $T_{1/2}$=2 hrs (parent drug), 9 hrs (MHD). Refer to PI for pediatric parameters.

NURSING CONSIDERATIONS

Assessment: Assess hepatic and renal function. Assess history of hypersensitivity reaction to carbamazepine, depression, pregnancy/nursing status and possible drug interactions.

Monitoring: Monitor serum Na^+ levels with maintenance treatment, particularly with other medications also known to reduce levels. Monitor T_4 levels. Monitor for signs/symptoms of hyponatremia, anaphylaxis and angioedema, severe dermatological reactions, cognitive or neuropsychiatric events, multi-organ hypersensitivity, and hematological effects (eg, agranulocytosis, aplastic anemia). Monitor for the emergence or worsening of depression, suicidal thoughts or behavior, and/or any unusual changes in mood or behavior. Monitor for adverse reactions and hypersensitivity reactions.

Patient Counseling: Advise to patients, their caregivers and families to be alert for the emergence or worsening of signs/symptoms of depression, any unusual changes in mood or behavior, or the emergence of suicidal thoughts, behavior, or thoughts about self-harm. Immediately report signs/symptoms suggesting angioedema. Notify physician if fever with other organ system involvement or serious skin reaction develops. Counsel females that efficacy of oral contraceptives may decrease; use another form of contraception. Avoid operating heavy machinery until gauging effects of drug and avoid alcohol. Medication can be taken with/without food. If pregnant, encourage to enroll in the North American Antiepileptic Drug (NAAED) Pregnancy Registry at 888-233-2334 or aedpregnancyregistry.org.

Administration: Oral route. **Storage:** 25°C (77°F); excursions permitted to 15-30°C (59-86°F). Tab: Dispense in tight container. Sus: Use within 7 weeks after opening. Shake well before use.

TRILIPIX   RX
fenofibric acid (Abbott)

THERAPEUTIC CLASS: Fibric acid derivative

INDICATIONS: Adjunctive therapy to diet to reduce TG in patients with severe hypertriglyceridemia. Adjunctive therapy to diet to reduce elevated LDL-C, Total-C, TG, and Apo B, and to increase HDL-C in patients with primary hyperlipidemia or mixed dyslipidemia. Adjunct to diet in combination with a statin to reduce TG and increase HDL-C in patients with mixed dyslipidemia and coronary heart disease (CHD) or a CHD risk equivalent who are on optimal statin therapy to achieve LDL-C goal.

DOSAGE: *Adults:* Max: 135mg qd. Severe Hypertriglyceridemia: Individualize dose. Initial: 45-135mg qd. Titrate: May adjust dose if necessary following repeat lipid determinations at 4-8 week intervals. Primary Hyperlipidemia/ Mixed Dyslipidemia: 135mg qd. Mixed Dyslipidemia With Statins: 135mg qd. Mild-to-Moderate Renal Impairment: Initial: 45mg qd. Titrate: May increase after evaluation of effects on renal function and lipid levels.

HOW SUPPLIED: Cap, Delayed-Release: 45mg, 135mg

CONTRAINDICATIONS: Severe renal impairment (including dialysis), active liver disease (including primary biliary cirrhosis and unexplained persistent liver function abnormalities), nursing mothers, and pre-existing gallbladder disease.

WARNINGS/PRECAUTIONS: Increases risk of myositis/myopathy and rhabdomyolysis; d/c therapy if myopathy or marked creatine phosphokinase (CPK) elevation occurs. Reversible elevations in SrCr reported; monitor renal function in patients at risk for renal insufficiency. Increase in serum transaminases reported; monitor liver function, and d/c therapy if enzyme levels persist >3X ULN. Hepatocellular, chronic active, and cholestatic hepatitis and cirrhosis (rare) reported. May cause cholelithiasis; d/c if gallstones are found. Acute hypersensitivity reactions and pancreatitis reported. Decreased Hgb, Hct, WBCs, rare thrombocytopenia and agranulocytosis reported. May cause venothromboembolic disease (eg, pulmonary embolism [PE], deep vein thrombosis [DVT]). Avoid in severe renal impairment. Not indicated for patients with elevated chylomicrons and plasma TG but with normal VLDL levels.

ADVERSE REACTIONS: Headache, back pain, nasopharyngitis, nausea, myalgia, diarrhea, upper respiratory tract infection, abnormal liver function test, abdominal pain, arthralgia, dizziness, dyspepsia, sinusitis.

INTERACTIONS: May potentiate anticoagulant effects of oral coumarin anticoagulants; caution with use and monitor PT/INR frequently. Bile acid resins may impede absorption; take ≥1 hr before or 4-6 hrs after the bile acid resin. Evaluate benefits/risks with immunosuppressants (eg, cyclosporine) and other potentially nephrotoxic agents; use lowest effective dose. Changes in exposure with atorvastatin, ezetimibe, fluvastatin, glimepiride, metformin, omeprazole, pravastatin, rosiglitazone, rosuvastatin, and simvastatin. Weak inhibitor of CYP2C8, 2C19, 2A6 and mild-to-moderate inhibitor of CYP2C9. Increased risk of rhabdomyolysis with statins.

PREGNANCY: Category C, not for use in nursing.

MECHANISM OF ACTION: Fibric acid derivative; activates peroxisome proliferator-activated receptor α (PPARα). Increases lipolysis and elimination of TG-rich particles from plasma by activating lipoprotein lipase and reducing production of APO C-III. Also induces an increase in the synthesis of HDL-C and Apo AI and AII.

PHARMACOKINETICS: Absorption: Well-absorbed; absolute bioavailability (81%); T_{max}=4-5 hrs. **Distribution:** Plasma protein binding (99%). **Metabolism:** Conjugation with glucuronic acid. **Elimination:** Urine; $T_{1/2}$=20 hrs.

NURSING CONSIDERATIONS

Assessment: Assess for renal impairment, active liver disease, pre-existing gallbladder disease, pregnancy/nursing status, and for possible drug interactions. Obtain baseline LFTs and lipid levels.

Monitoring: Monitor for signs/symptoms of myositis, myopathy, and rhabdomyolysis; measure CPK levels if myopathy is suspected. Monitor for elevations in SrCr, increase in serum transaminase levels, hepatitis, pancreatitis, hypersensitivity reactions, hematological changes (eg, agranulocytosis, thrombocytopenia), DVT, and PE. Monitor PT/INR if on concomitant oral anticoagulants. Monitor for signs and symptoms of cholelithiasis. Monitor renal function in patients with or at risk for renal impairment. Perform periodic monitoring of LFTs, CBC, and lipid levels.

Patient Counseling: Inform of benefits and risks of therapy and medications that should be avoided during treatment. Instruct to take qd, without regard to food. Inform that if on statin therapy, both drugs may be taken at the same time. Advise to follow appropriate lipid-modifying diet during therapy. Notify physician of all medications, supplements, and herbal preparations taken and any changes in medical conditions, any muscle pain, tenderness, or weakness, onset of abdominal pain or if any other new symptoms develop. Read Medication Guide.

Administration: Oral route. **Storage:** 25°C (77°F); excursions permitted to 15-30°C (59-86°F). Protect from moisture.

TRI-NORINYL   RX
ethinyl estradiol - norethindrone (Watson)

> Cigarette smoking increases the risk of serious cardiovascular (CV) side effects. Risk increases with age (>35 yrs) and with heavy smoking (≥15 cigarettes/day). Women who use oral contraceptives should be strongly advised not to smoke.

THERAPEUTIC CLASS: Estrogen/progestogen combination

INDICATIONS: Prevention of pregnancy.

DOSAGE: *Adults:* 1 tab qd for 28 days, then repeat. Start 1st Sunday after menses begin or 1st day of menses.
Pediatrics: Postpubertal: 1 tab qd for 28 days, then repeat. Start 1st Sunday after menses begin or 1st day of menses.

HOW SUPPLIED: Tab: (Ethinyl Estradiol-Norethindrone) 0.035mg-0.5mg, 0.035mg-1mg

CONTRAINDICATIONS: Thrombophlebitis, DVT or thromboembolic disorders, pregnancy, cerebrovascular or coronary artery disease, undiagnosed abnormal genital bleeding, cholestatic jaundice of pregnancy or jaundice with prior pill use, hepatic adenomas or carcinomas, breast cancer or other estrogen-dependent neoplasia.

WARNINGS/PRECAUTIONS: Increased risk of MI, vascular disease, thromboembolism, stroke and gallbladder disease. Retinal thrombosis, hepatic neoplasia, carcinoma of breast and reproductive organs reported. May cause glucose intolerance. May increase BP, elevate LDL levels or cause other lipid changes, fluid retention, breakthrough bleeding, and spotting. May cause or exacerbate migraine. May develop visual changes with contact lens. Increased risk of MI with HTN, hyperlipidemia, obesity, and diabetes. D/C if jaundice, significant depression or ophthalmic irregularities develop. Perform annual physical exam. Not indicated for use before menarche. May affect certain endocrine, LFTs and blood components.

ADVERSE REACTIONS: N/V, breakthrough bleeding, spotting, amenorrhea, migraine, depression, vaginal candidiasis, edema, weight changes.

INTERACTIONS: Reduced effects, increased breakthrough bleeding, and menstrual irregularities with rifampin, barbiturates, phenylbutazone, phenytoin, and possibly with griseofulvin, ampicillin, and tetracyclines.

PREGNANCY: Category X, not for use in nursing.

MECHANISM OF ACTION: Combination oral contraceptive; acts by suppressing gonadotropins. Primarily inhibits ovulation. Also causes changes in cervical mucus (increases difficulty of sperm entry into uterus) and endometrium (reduces likelihood of implantation).

NURSING CONSIDERATIONS

Assessment: Assess family history of breast cancer, presence of certain inherited or acquired thrombophilias, HTN, hyperlipidemia, obesity, DM, renal disease, depression, heavy smoking, and potential drug interactions. Conduct personal and family history and complete physical exam.

Monitoring: Monitor for MI, thromboembolism, cerebrovascular disease, benign hepatic adenomas, retinal thrombosis, HTN, headache, bleeding irregularities, jaundice, fluid retention, and emotional disorders. Conduct periodic complete physical exam with emphasis on BP, breasts, abdomen, and pelvic organs including cervical cytology and relevant lab tests (eg, TG, prothrombin clotting factors such as VII, VIII, IX, and X, renal/hepatic functions, TBG, sex steroid binding globulins).

Patient Counseling: Inform drug does not protect against HIV infection (AIDS) and other STDs. Inform of potential risks/benefits of oral contraceptives. Do not smoke while on treatment. Take 1 pill at same time daily.

Administration: Oral route. **Storage:** 15-25°C (59-77°F).

TRIPEDIA RX

pertussis vaccine, acellular - diphtheria toxoid - tetanus toxoid (Sanofi Pasteur)

THERAPEUTIC CLASS: Vaccine/toxoid combination

INDICATIONS: Active immunization against diphtheria, tetanus, and pertussis in pediatrics 6 weeks to 7 yrs of age (prior to 7th birthday). Combined with ActHIB for active immunization in pediatrics 15-18 months previously immunized against diphtheria, tetanus, and pertussis with 3 doses of whole-cell pertussis DTP or acellular pertussis vaccine and 3 or fewer doses of ActHIB® within 1st year of life for prevention of *H. influenzae* type b, diphtheria, tetanus, and pertussis.

DOSAGE: *Pediatrics:* ≥6 weeks up to 7 yrs: Primary Series: 3 doses of 0.5mL IM at 4-8 week intervals. 1st dose usually at 2 months, but can give at 6 weeks up to 7th birthday. Booster: 4th dose (0.5mL IM) at 15-20 months, at least 6 months after 3rd dose, 5th dose at 4-6 yrs; prior to school entry. May give to complete 4th or 5th dose of primary series of 3 doses of whole-cell pertussis DTP (4th dose at 15-20 months and 5th dose before school if 4th dose not given on or before 4th birthday). May combine with ActHIB® for 4th dose at 15-18 months.

HOW SUPPLIED: Inj: 0.5mL

CONTRAINDICATIONS: Hypersensitivity to thimerosal and gelatin, immediate anaphylactic reaction associated with previous dose, encephalopathy not due to an identifiable cause within 7 days of prior pertussis immunization. Defer during poliomyelitis outbreak or acute febrile illness.

WARNINGS/PRECAUTIONS: Caution if within 48 hrs of previous whole-cell DTP or acellular DTP vaccine, fever ≥105°F not due to another identifiable cause, collapse or shock-like state, or inconsolable crying lasting ≥3 hrs occurs, or if convulsions occur within 3 days. For high seizure risk, give APAP at time of vaccination and q4-6h for 24 hrs. Caution with neurologic or CNS disorders. Avoid with coagulation disorders. Have epinephrine available. Suboptimal response may occur in immunocompromised patients.

ADVERSE REACTIONS: Local erythema and swelling, irritability, drowsiness, anorexia, fever.

INTERACTIONS: Avoid with anticoagulants. Immunosuppressive therapy (eg, irradiation, antimetabolites, alkylating agents, cytotoxic drugs, corticosteroids) may decrease response. Do not combine through reconstitution with any vaccine for infants <15 months.

PREGNANCY: Category C, safety in nursing not known.

MECHANISM OF ACTION: Active immunization against diphtheria, tetanus, and pertussis (whooping cough).

NURSING CONSIDERATIONS

Assessment: Review current health status, previous sensitivity/immunization events (eg, fever, shock, persistent crying, convulsions, Guillain-Barre syndrome), and possible drug interactions.

Monitoring: Monitor for Arthus-type hypersensitivity reactions, injection-site for erythema, swelling, and tenderness, fever, irritability, drowsiness, anorexia, N/V, high-pitched/persistent crying, and neurological complications.

Patient Counseling: Inform of potential benefits/risks; report any adverse reactions to physician. May not offer 100% protection.

Administration: IM route. Inject into anterolateral aspect of thigh or deltoid region. **Storage:** 2-8°C (36-46°F). Do not freeze.

TRIVORA   RX
ethinyl estradiol - levonorgestrel (Watson)

> Cigarette smoking increases risk of serious cardiovascular (CV) effects. This risk increases with age (>35 yrs) and with heavy smoking (≥15 cigarettes/day). Women who use oral contraceptives should be strongly advised not to smoke.

OTHER BRAND NAMES: Enpresse (Barr)

THERAPEUTIC CLASS: Estrogen/progestogen combination

INDICATIONS: Prevention of pregnancy.

DOSAGE: *Adults:* 1 tab qd for 28 days, then repeat. Start 1st Sunday after menses begin or 1st day of menses.
Pediatrics: Postpubertal: 1 tab qd for 28 days, then repeat. Start 1st Sunday after menses begin or 1st day of menses.

HOW SUPPLIED: Tab: (Ethinyl Estradiol-Levonorgestrel) 0.03mg-0.05mg, 0.04mg-0.075mg, 0.03mg-0.125mg

CONTRAINDICATIONS: Thrombophlebitis, deep vein thrombophlebitis, thromboembolic disorders, pregnancy, cerebrovascular or coronary artery disease, undiagnosed abnormal genital bleeding, cholestatic jaundice of pregnancy or jaundice with prior pill use, hepatic carcinoma, benign liver tumor, breast cancer, endometrial cancer, or other estrogen-dependent neoplasia.

WARNINGS/PRECAUTIONS: Increased risk of MI, vascular disease, thromboembolism, stroke, and gallbladder disease. Retinal thrombosis, hepatic neoplasia reported. May cause glucose intolerance. May increase BP, elevate LDL levels or cause other lipid changes, fluid retention, breakthrough bleeding, and spotting. May cause or exacerbate migraine. May develop visual changes with contact lens. Morbidity and mortality risk increased with HTN, hyperlipidemia, obesity, and diabetes. D/C if jaundice, significant depression or ophthalmic irregularities develop. Perform annual physical exam. Not indicated for use before menarche. May affect certain endocrine, LFTs, and blood components.

ADVERSE REACTIONS: N/V, breakthrough bleeding, spotting, amenorrhea, migraine, depression, vaginal candidiasis, edema, weight changes.

INTERACTIONS: Reduced effects, increased breakthrough bleeding, and menstrual irregularities with rifampin, barbiturates, phenylbutazone, phenytoin, and possibly with griseofulvin, ampicillin, and tetracyclines.

PREGNANCY: Category X, not for use in nursing.

MECHANISM OF ACTION: Combination oral contraceptive; acts by suppressing gonadotropins, primarily inhibits ovulation. Also causes changes in cervical mucus (increasing difficulty of sperm entry into uterus) and endometrium (reducing likelihood of implantation).

PHARMACOKINETICS: Absorption: Triphasic pharmacokinetic parameters varied according to variable dosing. Levonorgestrel: Rapidly and completely absorbed. Absolute bioavailability (100%). Ethinyl Estradiol: Rapid and almost completely absorbed. Absolute bioavailabilty (38-48%). **Distribution:** Found in breast milk. Levonorgestrel: SHBG binding (60%). Ethinyl Estradiol: Albumin binding (97%). **Metabolism:** Levonorgestrel: Via hydroxylation and conjugation. Ethinyl Estradiol: Liver via CYP3A4 enzyme through hydroxylation, methylation and glucuronidation. **Elimination:** Levonorgestrel: Urine (40-68%), feces (16-48%); $T_{1/2}$=36 hrs. Ethinyl Estradiol: Urine, feces; $T_{1/2}$=18 hrs.

NURSING CONSIDERATIONS

Assessment: Assess family history of breast cancer, presence of inherited or acquired thrombophilias, HTN, hyperlipidemia, obesity, DM, renal disease, depression, heavy smoking, and potential drug interactions. Conduct personal/family history and complete physical exam.

Monitoring: Monitor for MI, thromboembolism, cerebrovascular disease, benign hepatic adenomas, retinal thrombosis, HTN, headache, bleeding irregularites, jaundice, fluid retention, and emotional disorders. Conduct periodic complete physical exam with emphasis on BP, breasts, abdomen, and pelvic organs, including cervical cytology and relevant lab tests.

Patient Counseling: Inform that drug does not protect against HIV infection and other STDs. Counsel on benefits/risks of drug. Advise to avoid smoking while taking medication. Instruct to take 1 pill at same time daily.

Administration: Oral route. **Storage:** 20-25°C (68-77°F).

TRIZIVIR   RX
abacavir sulfate - zidovudine - lamivudine (ViiV Healthcare)

(Abacavir) Serious and sometimes fatal hypersensitivity reactions (multi-organ clinical syndrome) reported; d/c as soon as suspected and never restart therapy with any abacavir containing product. Patients with HLA-B*5701 allele at high risk. (Zidovudine) Associated with hematologic toxicity (eg, neutropenia, severe anemia), particularly with advanced HIV-1 disease. Symptomatic myopathy associated with prolonged use. Lactic acidosis and severe hepatomegaly with steatosis, including fatal cases reported with use of nucleoside analogues alone or in combination with , including abacavir, lamivudine, zidovudine, and other antiretrovirals. (lamivudine) Severe acute exacerbations of hepatitis B (HBV) reported in coinfected with HBV-1 and who d/c therapy; monitor hepatic function closely for at least several months after d/c and initiate anti-hepatic therapy if needed.

THERAPEUTIC CLASS: Nucleoside analog combination

INDICATIONS: Treatment of HIV-1 infection alone or in combination with other antiretrovirals.

DOSAGE: *Adults:* >40kg and CrCl >50mL/min: 1 tab bid.
Pediatrics: Adolescents: >40kg and CrCl >50mL/min: 1 tab bid.

HOW SUPPLIED: Tab: (Abacavir Sulfate-Lamivudine-Zidovudine) 300mg-150mg-300mg

CONTRAINDICATIONS: Hepatic impairment.

WARNINGS/PRECAUTIONS: Treatment is not recommended for HLA-B*5701-positive patients. Caution with bone marrow compromise; monitor blood counts. If anemia or neutropenia develops, dose interruption may be needed. Obesity and prolonged nucleoside exposure may be risk factors to lactic acidosis and severe hepatomegaly with steatosis; suspend therapy if clinical findings develop. Immune reconstitution syndrome reported. Redistribution/accumulation of body fat may occur. Increased risk of myocardial infarction (MI); caution in patients with underlying risk of coronary heart disease. Hepatic decompensation has occurred in HIV-1/HCV coinfected patients receiving combination antiretroviral therapy for HIV and interferon α, with or without ribavirin. Consider d/c or dose reduction of concurrent therapy if worsening of clinical toxicity occurs. Exacerbation of anemia reported in HIV-1/HCV coinfected patients with ribavirin and zidovudine. Cross-resistance potential with nucleoside reverse transcriptase inhibitors (NRTIs) reported. Use with other products with same ingredients should be avoided. Caution in elderly. Avoid use in adolescents weighing <40 kg, in patients requiring dose adjustments (eg, CrCl <50mL/min) and with renal impairment.

ADVERSE REACTIONS: N/V, headache, malaise, fatigue, hypersensitivity reaction, diarrhea, fever, chills, depressive disorders, musculoskeletal pain, skin rashes, ear/nose/throat infections, viral respiratory infections.

INTERACTIONS: Abacavir (ABC): Ethanol decreases elimination. Additive activity with didanosine. Zidovudine (AZT): Ganciclovir, interferon α, and other bone marrow suppressants or cytotoxic agents may increase hematologic toxicity. Antagonistic effects with stavudine. Avoid use with some nucleoside analogues affecting DNA replications (eg, ribavirin). Avoid use of doxorubicin. Synergistic activity with indinavir, delavirdine and nevirapine. Lamivudine (3TC): Increased 3TC exposure with trimethoprim 160mg/sulfamethoxazole 800mg. Avoid zalcitabine. Hepatic decompensation reported in patients on combination antiretroviral therapy for HIV and interferon α w/ or w/o ribavirin; monitor closely for treatment-associated toxicities. Avoid concomitant use with other ABC-, 3TC- or AZT-containing products including emtricitabine, tenofovir and efavirenz. Suspected Stevens-Johnson syndrome (SJS) and toxic epidermal necrolysis (TEN) reported when given in combination with medications known to be associated SJS and TEN.

PREGNANCY: Category C, not for use in nursing.

MECHANISM OF ACTION: Abacavir: Carbocyclic nucleoside analogue; inhibits HIV-1 reverse transcriptase (RT) by competing with natural substrate dGTP and incorporating into viral DNA. Lamivudine/Zidovudine: Nucleoside analogue; inhibits RT via DNA chain termination.

PHARMACOKINETICS: Absorption: Abacavir/Lamivudine: Rapid; bioavailability (86%). Zidovudine: Rapid; bioavailability (64%). **Distribution:** Abacavir: V_d=0.86L/kg; plasma protein binding (50%). Lamivudine: V_d=1.3L/kg; plasma protein binding (low). Zidovudine: V_d=1.6L/kg; plasma protein binding (low). **Metabolism:** Abacavir: Hepatic, via alcohol dehydrogenase and glucuronyl transferase. Lamivudine: Trans-sulfoxide (metabolite); found in breast milk. Zidovudine: Hepatic, via glucuronyl transferase; 3'-azido-3'-deoxy-5'-O-β-D-glucopyranuronosylthymidine (GZDV) (major metabolite); found in breast milk. **Elimination:** Abacavir: $T_{1/2}$=1.45 hrs. Lamivudine: (IV): Urine (70%); $T_{1/2}$=5-7 hrs. Zidovudine: Urine (14%); (GZDV): Urine (74%); $T_{1/2}$=0.5-3 hrs.

NURSING CONSIDERATIONS

Assessment: Assess for history of hypersensitivity, hepatic/renal impairment, risk factors for lactic acidosis, risk factors for liver and coronary heart disease, bone marrow compromise, pregnancy/nursing status, and possible drug interactions. Assess for HLA-B*5701 allele type. Assess for prior exposure to any abacavir-containing product.

Monitoring: Monitor for signs and symptoms of hypersensitivity reactions, hematologic toxicity, lactic acidosis, hepatomegaly with steatosis, exacerbation of HBV, myopathy, immune reconstitution syndrome, fat redistribution, and MI. Monitor hepatic/renal function, blood counts, LFTs, CPK, SrCr. Follow-up LFTs for several months after d/c therapy.

Patient Counseling: Inform patients regarding hypersensitivity reactions with abacavir (ABC). Inform patient that lactic acidosis (with hepatomegaly), hepatic dysfunction (eg, decompensation, failure), fat redistribution may occur. Instruct not to take with other ABC- or lamivudine-containing agents. Inform that the important toxicities associated with zidovudine are neutropenia and anemia; have blood counts closely monitored. May enroll patients in the Antiretroviral Pregnancy Registry if they become pregnant while on treatment. Advise that therapy has not been shown to reduce the risk of transmission of HIV to others through sexual contact or blood contamination. Inform patients to take all HIV medications exactly as prescribed.

Administration: Oral route. **Storage:** 25°C (77°F); excursions permitted to 15-30°C (59-86°F).

TRUSOPT   RX
dorzolamide HCl (Merck)

THERAPEUTIC CLASS: Carbonic anhydrase inhibitor

INDICATIONS: Treatment of elevated intraocular pressure (IOP) in open-angle glaucoma and ocular HTN.

DOSAGE: *Adults:* 1 drop in the affected eye(s) tid. Space dosing of other ophthalmic drugs by 10 min.
Pediatrics: 1 drop in the affected eye(s) tid. Space dosing of other ophthalmic drugs by 10 min.

HOW SUPPLIED: Sol: 2% [10mL]

WARNINGS/PRECAUTIONS: Systemically absorbed. Rare fatalities have occured due to severe sulfonamide reactions. Avoid with sulfonamide allergy or severe renal impairment (CrCl <30mL/ min). Caution with hepatic impairment. Not studied in acute angle-closure glaucoma. Local ocular adverse effects (eg, conjunctivitis, lid reactions) reported with chronic use; d/c use and evaluate patient before considering restarting therapy. Bacterial keratitis reported with contaminated containers. Choroidal detachment reported following filtration procedures. Increased potential for corneal edema in patients with low endothelial cell counts.

ADVERSE REACTIONS: Ocular burning, stinging, discomfort, bitter taste, superficial punctate keratitis, ocular allergic reactions, conjunctivitis, lid reactions, blurred vision, eye redness, tearing, dryness, photophobia.

INTERACTIONS: Acid-base disturbances reported with oral carbonic anhydrase inhibitors; caution with high-dose salicylates. Avoid with oral carbonic anhydrase inhibitors due to additive effects.

PREGNANCY: Category C, not for use in nursing.

MECHANISM OF ACTION: Carbonic anhydrase inhibitor; inhibition of carbonic anhydrase in the ciliary processes of the eye decreases aqueous humor secretion, presumably by slowing the formation of bicarbonate ions with subsequent reduction in sodium and fluid transport. The result is a reduction in IOP.

PHARMACOKINETICS: Distribution: Plasma protein binding (33%). **Metabolism:** Metabolites: N-desethyl. **Elimination:** Urine (unchanged, metabolite).

NURSING CONSIDERATIONS

Assessment: Assess for sulfonamide hypersensitivity reaction or history of sulfonamide hypersensitivity, acute angle-closure glaucoma, renal/hepatic dysfunction, pregnancy/nursing status, and possible drug interactions.

Monitoring: Monitor for sulfonamide hypersensitivity reactions (eg, Stevens-Johnson syndrome, toxic epidermal necrolysis, fulminant hepatic necrosis, agranulocytosis, aplastic anemia, blood dyscrasias). If using chronically, monitor for ocular reactions (eg, conjunctivitis and lid reactions); d/c therapy and evaluate patient if such reactions occur. Monitor for bacterial keratitis if using multiple dose container. Monitor for choroidal detachment following filtration procedures.

Patient Counseling: Advise to d/c and notify physician if signs of hypersensitivity or ocular reactions (eg, conjunctivitis, lid reactions) occur. Contact physician if patient has ocular surgery or develops an intercurrent ocular condition (eg, trauma, infection). Avoid allowing tip of dispensing container to contact eye or surrounding structures. If container becomes contaminated, serious damage to the eye and loss of vision may result. Remove contact lenses and reinsert 15 min after administration. Space dosing of other ophthalmic drugs by 10 min.

Administration: Ocular route. **Storage:** 15-30°C (59-86°F). Protect from light.

TRUVADA   RX
tenofovir disoproxil fumarate - emtricitabine (Gilead)

> Lactic acidosis and severe hepatomegaly with steatosis, including fatal cases, reported with nucleoside analogs alone or with concomitant antiretrovirals. Severe acute exacerbations of hepatitis B (HBV) reported in patients coinfected with HBV and HIV-1 upon d/c of therapy. Monitor hepatic function closely for at least several months in patients who are coinfected with HIV-1 and HBV. If appropriate, initiation of anti-HBV therapy may be warranted.

THERAPEUTIC CLASS: Nucleoside analog combination

INDICATIONS: Treatment of HIV-1 infection in combination with other antiretrovirals.

DOSAGE: *Adults:* CrCl ≥50mL/min: 1 tab qd. CrCl 30-49mL/min: 1 tab q48h.

HOW SUPPLIED: Tab: (Emtricitabine-Tenofovir Disoproxil Fumarate) 200mg-300mg

WARNINGS/PRECAUTIONS: Obesity and prolonged nucleoside exposure may be risk factors for lactic acidosis and severe hepatomegaly with steatosis. Caution in patients with risk factors for liver disease. Suspend therapy in any patients who develop clinical or laboratory findings suggestive of lactic acidosis or pronounced hepatotoxicity. Test for HBV infection before initiating therapy; safety and efficacy has not been established with coinfection. Avoid in patients with CrCl <30mL/min or patients requiring hemodialysis. Renal impairment, including cases of acute renal failure and Fanconi syndrome, reported. All patients should have CrCl calculated prior to and during therapy as clinically appropriate. Monitor serum phosphorus in patients at risk for renal impairment. May decrease bone mineral density; monitor patients with history of pathologic bone fracture or who are at risk for osteopenia. Possible redistribution/accumulation of body fat. Immune reconstitution syndrome reported. Carefully monitor patients utilizing a triple nucleoside-only regimen and consider treatment modification. Caution in elderly.

ADVERSE REACTIONS: Diarrhea, nausea, fatigue, sinusitis, upper respiratory tract infections, nasopharyngitis, headache, dizziness, depression, insomnia, rash.

INTERACTIONS: May increase levels of didanosine (ddI); caution when coadministering, monitor for ddI-associated adverse effects and d/c if these develop. Atazanavir (ATV) and lopinavir/ritonavir (LPV/r) may increase tenofovir concentrations; monitor for associated adverse effects. ATV without ritonavir should not be coadministered. Coadministration with drugs eliminated by active tubular secretion may increase levels of emtricitabine, tenofovir or the coadministered drug (eg, acyclovir, adefovir dipivoxil, cidofovir, ganciclovir, valacyclovir, valganciclovir). Drugs that decrease renal function may increase concentrations of emtricitabine and/or tenofovir; avoid with concurrent or recent use of a nephrotoxic agent. Do not coadminister with Atripla, Emtriva or Viread and other drugs containing lamivudine. Do not give with adefovir dipivoxil. See PI for complete information.

PREGNANCY: Category B, not for use in nursing.

MECHANISM OF ACTION: Emtricitabine: Synthetic nucleoside analog of cytidine. Inhibits activity of HIV-1 reverse transcriptase (RT) by competing with natural substrate deoxycytidine 5'-triphosphate and by being incorporated into nascent viral DNA, which results in chain termination. Tenofovir disoproxil: Acyclic nucleoside phosphonate diester analog of adenosine monophosphate. Inhibits activity of HIV-1 RT by competing with the natural substrate deoxyadenosine 5'-triphosphate and after incorporation into DNA, by DNA chain termination.

PHARMACOKINETICS: Absorption: Emtricitabine: Rapid. Bioavailability (92%), C_{max}=1.8mcg/mL, T_{max}=1-2 hrs, AUC=10mcg•h/mL. Tenofovir disoproxil: Bioavailability (25%), C_{max}=0.3mcg/mL, T_{max}=1 hr, AUC=2.29mcg•h/mL. **Distribution:** Emtricitabine: Plasma protein binding (<4%). Tenofovir disoproxil: Plasma protein binding (<0.7%). **Elimination:** Emtricitabine: Urine (86%); $T_{1/2}$=10 hrs. Tenofovir disoproxil: (IV) Urine (70-80%); $T_{1/2}$=17 hrs.

NURSING CONSIDERATIONS

Assessment: Assess for risk factors for lactic acidosis, liver disease, HBV status, renal impairment, history of pathologic bone fracture or risk of osteopenia, pregnancy/nursing status and for possible drug interactions. Obtain baseline CrCl.

Monitoring: Monitor for signs/symptoms of lactic acidosis, hepatomegaly with steatosis, new onset or worsening renal impairment, decreases in bone mineral density, redistribution/accumulation of body fat, and for immune reconstitution syndrome. In patients coinfected with HBV, upon d/c of therapy, monitor hepatic function closely and monitor for signs/symptoms of acute exacerbation of hepatitis B. Monitor CrCl and monitor serum phosphorus in patients at risk for renal impairment.

Patient Counseling: Inform that therapy is not cure for HIV, does not reduce risk of transmission of HIV and that opportunistic infections may develop. Advise of risks and benefits of therapy and counsel to continue to practice safe sex and to use latex or polyurethane condoms. Never reuse or share needles. It is important to follow regular dosing schedule and to avoid missing doses. Seek medical attention if symptoms of lactic acidosis, hepatotoxicity, exacerbation of HBV, renal impairment, fat redistribution/accumulation or immune reconstitution syndrome occur.

Administration: Oral route. **Storage:** 25°C (77°F), excursions permitted to 15-30°C (59-86°F).

T

TUSSIONEX PENNKINETIC
hydrocodone polistirex - chlorpheniramine polistirex (UCB)

THERAPEUTIC CLASS: Opioid antitussive/antihistamine

INDICATIONS: Relief of cough and upper respiratory symptoms associated with allergy and cold.

DOSAGE: *Adults:* 5mL q12h. Max: 10mL/24 hrs.
Pediatrics: ≥12 yrs: 5mL q12h. Max: 10mL/24 hrs. 6-11 yrs: 2.5mL q12h. Max: 5mL/24 hrs.

HOW SUPPLIED: Sus, Extended-Release: (Chlorpheniramine-Hydrocodone) 8mg-10mg/5mL [473mL]

CONTRAINDICATIONS: Children <6 yrs of age due to risk of fatal respiratory depression.

WARNINGS/PRECAUTIONS: May produce dose-related respiratory depression. May suppress cough reflex. Caution with pulmonary disease, post-surgery, depressed ventilatory function, narrow-angle glaucoma, asthma, prostatic hypertrophy, elderly, debilitated, severely impaired hepatic/renal function, hypothyroidism, Addison's disease or urethral stricture. May exaggerate respiratory depressant effects and elevations of CSF pressure in patients with head injury, intracranial lesions or pre-existing increase in intracranial pressure. May obscure clinical course of head injuries and acute abdominal conditions. May cause obstructive bowel disease especially with underlying intestinal motility disorder. Consider risk/benefit ratio in pediatrics, especially with respiratory embarrassment (eg, croup). Consider use of narcotic antagonist (eg, naloxone) and other supportive measures when indicated.

ADVERSE REACTIONS: Sedation, drowsiness, lethargy, anxiety, dysphoria, euphoria, dizziness, rash, pruritus, N/V, ureteral spasm, urinary retention, dryness of the pharynx, tightness of the chest.

INTERACTIONS: Additive CNS depression with narcotics, antihistaminics, antipsychotics, antianxiety agents, and other CNS depressants (including alcohol); reduce dose of one or both agents when combined therapy is contemplated. Increased effect of antidepressant or hydrocodone with MAOIs or TCAs. Concurrent anticholinergics may cause paralytic ileus. Increased risk of respiratory depression in pediatrics with other respiratory depressants.

PREGNANCY: Category C, not for use in nursing.

MECHANISM OF ACTION: Hydrocodone: Opioid antitussive/analgesic; not established. Believed to act directly on cough center. Chlorpheniramine: H_1-receptor antagonist; possesses anticholinergic and sedative activity. Prevents released histamine from dilating capillaries and causing edema of the respiratory mucosa.

PHARMACOKINETICS: Absorption: Hydrocodone: C_{max}=22.8ng/mL, T_{max}=3.4 hrs. Chlorpheniramine: C_{max}=58.4ng/mL, T_{max}=6.3 hrs. **Elimination:** Hydrocodone: $T_{1/2}$=4 hrs. Chlorpheniramine: $T_{1/2}$=16 hrs.

NURSING CONSIDERATIONS

Assessment: Assess that patient is ≥6 yrs. Assess use in postoperative patients, elderly/debilitated, severe hepatic/renal impairment, hypothyroidism, Addison's disease, prostatic hypertrophy, urethral stricture. Assess for presence of pulmonary disease, depressed ventilatory function, head injury, intracranial lesions, increased intracranial pressure, acute abdominal conditions, intestinal motility disorder, respiratory embarrassment, narrow-angle glaucoma, asthma, pregnancy/nursing status, and possible drug interactions.

Monitoring: Monitor for signs/symptoms of respiratory depression and development of obstructive bowel disease.

Patient Counseling: Inform medication may produce drowsiness and impair mental/physical abilities; use caution when performing hazardous tasks (eg, operating machinery/driving). Instruct not to dilute with fluids or mix with other drugs. Advise to measure suspension with accurate measuring device; a household teaspoon is not accurate and could lead to overdosage.

A pharmacist can recommend an appropriate measuring device and provide instructions. Advise to keep out of reach of children.

Administration: Oral route. Shake well before use. **Storage:** 20-25°C (68-77°F); excursions permitted to 15-30°C (59-86°F). Dispense in a well-closed container.

TWINJECT   RX
epinephrine (Verus)

THERAPEUTIC CLASS: Sympathomimetic catecholamine

INDICATIONS: Emergency treatment of severe allergic reactions (type 1) including anaphylaxis to insect stings or bites, allergens, foods, drugs, diagnostic testing substances, as well as idiopathic or exercise-induced anaphylaxis.

DOSAGE: *Adults:* Administer SQ or IM into thigh. 15-30kg: (Twinject 0.15mg) 0.15mg. May repeat if needed. ≥30kg: (Twinject 0.3mg) 0.3mg. May repeat if needed.
Pediatrics: Administer SQ or IM into thigh. 15-30kg: (Twinject 0.15mg) 0.15mg. May repeat if needed. ≥30kg: (Twinject 0.3mg) 0.3mg. May repeat if needed.

HOW SUPPLIED: Inj: (Twinject 0.15mg, Twinject 0.3mg) 1mg/mL

WARNINGS/PRECAUTIONS: Inject into anterolateral aspect of thigh; avoid injecting into hands, feet, or buttock. Avoid IV use. Contains sodium bisulfite. Caution with cardiac arrhythmias, coronary artery or organic heart disease, or HTN. May precipitate/aggravate angina pectoris or produce ventricular arrhythmias with coronary insufficiency or ischemic heart disease. Light-sensitive; store in tube provided.

ADVERSE REACTIONS: Anxiety, apprehensiveness, restlessness, tremor, weakness, dizziness, sweating, palpitations, pallor, N/V, headache, respiratory difficulties, HTN.

INTERACTIONS: Monitor for cardiac arrhythmias with cardiac glycosides or diuretics. Effects may be potentiated by TCAs, MAOIs, levothyroxine, and certain antihistamines (notably chlorpheniramine, tripelennamine, diphenhydramine). Cardiostimulating and bronchodilating effects antagonized by β-adrenergic blockers (eg, propranolol). Vasoconstricting and hypertensive effects antagonized by α-adrenergic blockers (eg, phentolamine). Ergot alkaloids and phenothiazines may reverse pressor effects.

PREGNANCY: Category C, safety in nursing not known.

MECHANISM OF ACTION: Acts on α- and β-adrenergic receptors.

NURSING CONSIDERATIONS

Assessment: Assess for arrhythmias, ischemic/organic heart disease, HTN, DM, hyperthyroidism, pregnancy/nursing status, Parkinson's disease, and drug interactions (eg, medications that may sensitize heart to arrhythmia such as digitalis).

Monitoring: Monitor BP, HR, blood glucose, signs of cerebral hemorrhage, ventricular arrhythmia, HTN, and anginal pain.

Patient Counseling: Inform about side effects of therapy (eg, increased pulse rate, sense of forceful heartbeat, palpitations, throbbing headache, pallor, anxiety, shakiness). Side effects may subside rapidly, especially with rest, quiet, and recumbency but may be severe or persistent with HTN or hyperthyroidism. Never inject into buttocks or by IV route.

Administration: IM or SQ route. Inject into anterolateral administration. **Storage:** 20-25°C (68-77°F); excursions permitted to 15-30°C (59-86°F). Protect from light. Avoid freezing or refrigeration. Discard if discolored.

TWINRIX   RX
hepatitis A vaccine (inactivated) - hepatitis B (recombinant) (GlaxoSmithKline)

THERAPEUTIC CLASS: Vaccine

INDICATIONS: Active immunization against disease caused by hepatitis A virus and infection by all known subtypes of hepatitis B virus in patients ≥18 yrs of age.

DOSAGE: *Adults:* 3-Dose Schedule: 1mL IM in deltoid region at 0, 1, and 6 months. Alternative 4-Dose Schedule: 1mL IM in deltoid region on Days 0, 7, and 21-30, followed by booster dose at 12 months.

HOW SUPPLIED: Inj: 1mL [vial, prefilled syringes]

CONTRAINDICATIONS: Hypersensitivity to yeast or neomycin.

WARNINGS/PRECAUTIONS: Rare reports of anaphylaxis/anaphylactoid reactions. Tip cap and rubber plunger of prefilled syringes contain natural latex rubber; allergic reactions may occur in latex-sensitive individuals. Epinephrine and other appropriate medical treatment should be immediately available for the control of immediate allergic reactions. May not prevent hepatitis A or B in individuals who have unrecognized hepatitis A or B at time of vaccination. Hepatitis A and B infection may not be prevented in individuals who do not achieve protective antibody titers. Delay administration with moderate or severe acute illness. Caution with bleeding disorders (eg, hemophilia, thrombocytopenia); take steps to avoid hematoma. Suboptimal response may occur in immunocompromised patients.

ADVERSE REACTIONS: Injection-site reactions (eg, soreness, redness, swelling, induration), upper respiratory infection, headache, fatigue, diarrhea, N/V, fever.

INTERACTIONS: Caution with anticoagulants. Immunosuppressive therapy may reduce response.

PREGNANCY: Category C, caution in nursing.

MECHANISM OF ACTION: Bivalent vaccine; produces immune response against hepatitis A and all known subtypes of hepatitis B virus.

NURSING CONSIDERATIONS

Assessment: Assess for hypersensitivity to yeast, neomycin, and to latex rubber. Assess for moderate or severe acute illness, bleeding disorders, pregnancy/nursing status, and for possible drug interactions. Review current health status (immunosuppression, unrecognized hepatitis A or B infection), medical history, immunization history, and previous vaccination-related adverse reactions.

Monitoring: Monitor for anaphylaxis/anaphylactoid reactions, injection site reactions, immune response, or possible adverse events. Monitor antibody titers.

Patient Counseling: Advise of potential benefits/risks of therapy. Inform that immunization will not cause hepatitis A or B infection. Instruct to contact physician if severe or unusual adverse reactions occur. Encourage and inform pregnant women who received vaccination to register with the pregnancy registry. Counsel on importance of completing vaccination series.

Administration: IM route. Do not inject via IV, intradermally, or in gluteal region. Shake well before withdrawal and use. Inspect visually for particulate matter and discoloration prior to administration; if any of these conditions exist, do not administer. Do not mix with any other vaccine in the same syringe or administer on the same site. **Storage:** 2-8°C (36-46°F). Do not freeze; discard if has been frozen.

TWYNSTA   RX
telmisartan - amlodipine (Boehringer Ingelheim)

> **D/C therapy when pregnancy is detected. Drugs that act directly on the renin-angiotensin system can cause injury and even death to the developing fetus.**

THERAPEUTIC CLASS: ARB/Calcium channel blocker (dihydropyridine)

INDICATIONS: Treatment of HTN alone or with other antihypertensive agents. Initial therapy for HTN in patients likely to need multiple agents to achieve BP goal.

DOSAGE: *Adults:* Individualize dosing. Initial: 5mg-40mg qd. Patients Requiring Large BP Reduction: Initial: 5mg-80mg qd. Titrate: Adjust dose if needed after 2 weeks. Max: 10mg-80mg qd. Hepatic Impairment/Patients ≥75 yrs: Not recommended for initial therapy. Severe Renal Impairment: Titrate slowly. Add-On Therapy: May be used to provide additional BP lowering when not adequately controlled on amlodipine or telmisartan alone. Patients treated with amlodipine 10mg who experience dose-limiting adverse reactions may switch to 5mg-40mg qd. Replacement Therapy: May be substituted for individual components. When substituting for individual components, the dose may be increased if needed.

HOW SUPPLIED: Tab: (Amlodipine-Telmisartan) 5mg-40mg, 10mg-40mg, 5mg-80mg, 10mg-80mg

WARNINGS/PRECAUTIONS: May increase frequency, duration or severity of angina or acute myocardial infarction (MI) in patients with severe obstructive coronary artery disease (CAD). Hypotension reported; correct volume/salt depletion prior to initiation or start therapy under medical supervision with a reduced dose. Risk of hyperkalemia with renal dysfunction/heart failure; periodically monitor serum electrolytes. Caution with renal/hepatic dysfunction, severe aortic/renal artery stenosis, biliary obstructive disorders and in elderly. Closely monitor patients with heart failure.

ADVERSE REACTIONS: Peripheral edema, dizziness, back pain.

INTERACTIONS: May increase digoxin levels; monitor digoxin levels during concurrent use. May increase lithium levels/toxicity; monitor lithium levels during concurrent use. Increased levels of ramipril/ramiprilat noted during concomitant use, whereas telmisartan levels are decreased; concomitant use not recommended. Dual blockade of the renin-angiotensin-aldosterone system with ACE inhibitors. Increased risk of hyperkalemia with K^+-sparing diuretics, K^+ supplements or K^+-containing salt substitutes or drugs that increase K^+ levels. Symptomatic hypotension may occur with high doses of diuretics. Possible inhibition of the metabolism of drugs metabolized by CYP2C19.

PREGNANCY: Category C (1st trimester) and D (2nd and 3rd trimester), not for use in nursing.

MECHANISM OF ACTION: Amlodipine: Dihydropyridine calcium channel blocker; inhibits transmembrane influx of calcium ions into vascular smooth muscle and cardiac muscle. Telmisartan: Angiotensin II receptor antagonist; blocks vasoconstrictor and aldosterone-secreting effects of angiotensin II by selectively blocking the binding of angiotensin II to the AT_1 receptor in many tissues, such as vascular smooth muscle and adrenal gland.

PHARMACOKINETICS: Absorption: Amlodipine: Absolute bioavailability (64-90%); T_{max}=6-12 hrs. Telmisartan: Absolute bioavailability (42%, 40mg), (58%, 160mg); T_{max}=0.5-1 hr. **Distribution:** Amlodipine: V_d=21L/kg; plasma protein binding (93%). Telmisartan: V_d=500L; plasma protein binding (>99.5%). **Metabolism:** Amlodipine: Liver. Telmisartan: Conjugation. **Elimination:** Amlodipine: Urine (10%, parent compound), (60%, metabolites); $T_{1/2}$=30-50 hrs. Telmisartan: Feces (>97%, unchanged), urine (0.91%); $T_{1/2}$=24 hrs.

NURSING CONSIDERATIONS

Assessment: Assess for angina, MI, severe obstructive CAD, severe aortic/renal artery stenosis, congestive heart failure (CHF), volume/salt depletion, hepatic/renal function, pregnancy/nursing status, and possible drug interactions. Assess for baseline BP levels.

Monitoring: Monitor hepatic/renal function, and other adverse reactions. Monitor BP, ECG, serum electrolytes especially K^+ levels.

Patient Counseling: Inform of pregnancy risk. Advise to notify physician as soon as possible if pregnant. Inform patients of side effects and to seek medical attention if any occur.

Administration: Oral route. **Storage:** 25°C (77°F); excursions permitted to 15-30°C (59-86°F). Do not remove from blisters until immediately before administration. Protect from light and moisture.

TYGACIL RX
tigecycline (Wyeth)

THERAPEUTIC CLASS: Glycylcycline

INDICATIONS: Treatment of complicated skin and skin structure infections (cSSSI), complicated intra-abdominal infections (cIAI), and community-acquired bacterial pneumonia (CABP) caused by susceptible strains of indicated pathogens in patients ≥18 yrs.

DOSAGE: *Adults:* Initial: 100mg IV over 30-60 min. Maint: 50mg q12h over 30-60 min for 5-14 days (cSSSI/cIAI) or for 7-14 days (CABP). Severe Hepatic Impairment (Child-Pugh C): Initial: 100mg IV over 30-60 min. Maint: 25mg q12h over 30-60 min.

HOW SUPPLIED: Inj: 50mg/5mL, 50mg/10mL [vial]

WARNINGS/PRECAUTIONS: Anaphylaxis/anaphylactoid reactions reported. Structurally similar to tetracyclines and may have similar adverse effects: photosensitivity, pseudotumor cerebri, pancreatitis, and anti-anabolic action (may lead to increased BUN, azotemia, acidosis, and hyperphosphatemia). Caution with known hypersensitivity to tetracyclines. Isolated cases of significant hepatic dysfunction and failure reported; evaluate risk/benefit of continued therapy if hepatic function worsens. Efficacy in hospital-acquired pneumonia not demonstrated; greater mortality seen in ventilator-associated pneumonia. Acute pancreatitis reported. Consider stopping therapy if suspected. May cause fetal harm in pregnant women and permanent tooth discoloration (yellow-gray-brown) when administered during tooth development (last half of pregnancy to 8 yrs). *Clostridium difficile*-associated diarrhea (CDAD) reported. Caution when used for cIAI secondary to clinically apparent intestinal perforations. May result in overgrowth of nonsusceptible organisms, including fungi; monitor during therapy.

ADVERSE REACTIONS: N/V, diarrhea, abdominal pain, infection, headache, anemia, hypoproteinemia, increased liver enzymes, anaphylaxis/anaphylactoid reactions, acute pancreatitis, asthenia, elevated BUN, dizziness, phlebitis.

INTERACTIONS: Decreased effectiveness of oral contraceptives. Monitor PT with warfarin.

PREGNANCY: Category D, caution in nursing.

MECHANISM OF ACTION: Glycylcycline; inhibits protein translation in bacteria by binding to the 30S ribosomal subunit and blocking entry of amino-acyl tRNA molecules into the A site of the ribosome.

PHARMACOKINETICS: Absorption: IV infusion of variable doses resulted in different parameters. **Distribution:** V_d=7-9L/kg; plasma protein binding (71-89%). **Metabolism:** Liver. **Elimination:** Bile (primary), urine (22%, unchanged); $T_{1/2}$=27.1 hrs (single dose), 42.4 hrs (multiple dose).

NURSING CONSIDERATIONS

Assessment: Assess for known hypersensitivity to tetracycline antibiotics, hepatic impairment, cIAI secondary to clinically apparent intestinal perforation, culture and susceptibility testing, pregnancy/nursing status, and possible drug interactions.

Monitoring: Monitor for signs/symptoms of hypersensitivity reactions, hepatic impairment, pancreatitis, photosensitivity, superinfection, and CDAD. Monitor PT with warfarin.

Patient Counseling: Inform of fetal harm during pregnancy and that therapy treats bacterial, not viral, infections. Take as directed; skipping doses or not completing full course of therapy may decrease effectiveness and increase resistance. May experience diarrhea; notify physician if with watery/bloody stools even as late as >2 months after last dose.

Administration: IV route. Refer to PI for reconstitution. Reconstituted solution should be yellow to orange in color; if not, discard solution. **Storage:** Powder: 20-25°C (68-77°F); excursions permitted to 15-30°C (59-86°F). Solution: Room temperature up to 24 hrs (up to 6 hrs in vial and remaining time in IV bag); refrigerated 2-8°C (36-46°F) up to 48 hrs following immediate transfer of reconstituted solution into IV bag.

TYKERB   RX
lapatinib (GlaxoSmithKline)

> Hepatotoxicity may occur; may be severe and deaths have been reported.

THERAPEUTIC CLASS: Kinase inhibitor

INDICATIONS: In combination with capecitabine for the treatment of patients with advanced or metastatic breast cancer whose tumors overexpress HER2 and who have received prior therapy including an anthracycline, a taxane, and trastuzumab. In combination with, letrozole for the treatment of postmenopausal women with hormone receptor positive metastatic breast cancer that overexpresses the HER2 receptor for whom hormonal therapy is indicated.

DOSAGE: *Adults:* HER2 Positive Metastatic Breast Cancer: Usual: 1250mg qd on Days 1-21 continuously with capecitabine 2000mg/m²/day (2 doses 12 hrs apart) on Days 1-14 in a repeating 21-day cycle. Do not double the dose the next day, if a day's dose is missed. Continue treatment until disease progresses or unacceptable toxicity occurs. Hormone Receptor Positive, HER2 Positive Metastatic Breast Cancer: Usual: 1500mg qd continuously with letrozole 2.5mg qd. ≥Grade 2 Left Ventricular Ejection Fraction (LVEF): D/C dose. If LVEF recovers to normal and asymptomatic after 2 weeks, restart at 1000mg/day with capecitabine and 1250mg/day with letrozole. Hepatic Impairment (Child-Pugh Class C): Reduce dose from 1250mg/day to 750mg/day (HER2 positive metastatic breast cancer) or from 1500mg/day to 1000mg/day (hormone receptor positive, HER2 positive breast cancer). Concomitant Strong CYP3A4 Inhibitors: Reduce dose to 500mg/day. Concomitant Strong CYP3A4 Inducers: Titrate gradually from 1250mg/day up to 4500mg/day (HER2 positive metastatic breast cancer) and 1500mg/day up to 5500mg/day (hormone receptor positive, HER2 positive breast cancer) based on tolerability. ≥Grade 2 NCI CTCAE Toxicity: D/C or interrupt dose and restart with 1250mg/day when toxicity <Grade 1. Restart at 1000mg/day (with capecitabine) or 1250mg/day (with letrozole) if toxicity recurs. Dividing daily dosing not recommended. Take at least 1 hr before or after meal.

HOW SUPPLIED: Tab: 250mg

WARNINGS/PRECAUTIONS: Decreased LVEF reported; confirm normal LVEF prior to therapy and evaluate during treatment. Caution in patients with conditions that may impair left ventricular function. Monitor LFTs prior to initiation of treatment, every 4-6 weeks during therapy, and as clinically indicated; d/c therapy if severe LFT changes. Reduce dose with severe pre-existing hepatic impairment. Diarrhea reported; manage with antidiarrheals, replace electrolytes/fluids, and interrupt or d/c therapy if severe diarrhea occurs. QT prolongation observed. Caution with hypokalemia/hypomagnesemia, and congenital long QT syndrome; correct hypokalemia/hypomagnesemia prior to administration. Associated with interstitial lung disease and pneumonitis in monotherapy or in combination with other chemotherapies; d/c if pulmonary symptoms indicative of interstitial lung disease/pneumonitis ≥Grade 3. May cause fetal harm.

ADVERSE REACTIONS: Diarrhea, N/V, stomatitis, dyspepsia, palmar-plantar erythrodysesthesia, rash, dry skin, mucosal inflammation, pain in extremity, back pain, dyspnea, insomnia, fatigue, anorexia, asthenia.

INTERACTIONS: Caution with CYP3A4 or CYP2C8 substrates; consider dose reduction. Avoid with strong CYP3A4 inhibitors (eg, ketoconazole, itraconazole, clarithromycin, atazanavir, indinavir, nefazodone, nelfinavir, ritonavir, saquinavir, telithromycin, voriconazole) and inducers (eg, dexamethasone, phenytoin, carbamazepine, rifampin, rifabutin, rifapentin, phenobarbital, St. John's wort); if unavoidable, consider dose reduction with concomitant CYP3A4 inhibitors, and gradual dose increase with concomitant CYP3A4 inducers. May increase plasma concentrations with grapefruit; avoid coadministration. Caution with concomitant use of anti-arrhythmic medications or

T

medications which lead to QT prolongation and with cumulative high-dose anthracycline therapy. May increase concentrations with P-glycoprotein inhibitors. May increase concentrations of P-glycoprotein substrates and paclitaxel.

PREGNANCY: Category D, not for use in nursing.

MECHANISM OF ACTION: Kinase inhibitor; inhibits intracellular tyrosine kinase domains of both Epidermal Growth Factor Receptor (EGFR) and Human Epidermal Receptor Type 2 (HER2) receptors.

PHARMACOKINETICS: Absorption: Incomplete and variable. C_{max}=2.43mcg/mL, T_{max}=4 hrs, AUC=36.2mcg•hr/mL. **Distribution**: Plasma protein binding (>99%). **Metabolism**: (Major) CYP3A4, CYP3A5; (Minor) CYP2C19, CYP2C8. **Elimination**: Feces (27%), urine (<2%); $T_{1/2}$=14.2 hrs (single dose), 24 hrs (multiple dose).

NURSING CONSIDERATIONS

Assessment: Assess for severe hepatic impairment, decreased LVEF or conditions which may impair left ventricular function, QT prolongation, hypokalemia, hypomagnesemia, pregnancy/nursing status, and for possible drug interactions. Obtain baseline ECG, LFTs, serum K+, and magnesium levels.

Monitoring: Monitor for signs/symptoms of hepatotoxicity, diarrhea, interstitial lung disease, hypokalemia, hypomagnesemia, and for QT prolongation. Monitor ECG and electrolytes. Monitor LFTs every 4-6 weeks during therapy and as clinically indicated.

Patient Counseling: Notify physician if SOB, palpitations, fatigue or diarrhea occurs. Advise that diarrhea is a common side effect and explain how it should be managed. Report use of any Rx/OTC drugs or herbal products. Avoid grapefruit products and take at least 1 hr before or 1 hr after a meal; take capecitabine with food or within 30 min after food. Take once daily and inform that dividing daily dose is not recommended.

Administration: Oral route. **Storage**: 25°C (77°F); excursions permitted to 15-30°C (59-86°F).

TYLENOL WITH CODEINE   CIII
codeine phosphate - acetaminophen (Ortho-McNeil)

THERAPEUTIC CLASS: Opioid analgesic

INDICATIONS: Relief of mild to moderately severe pain.

DOSAGE: *Adults:* (Sol) Usual: 15mL PO q4h prn. (Tab) Usual: 15-60mg codeine/dose, 300-1000mg APAP/dose up to q4h prn. Adjust according to severity of pain and response of the patient. Max: 360mg codeine/day, 4g APAP/day.
Pediatrics: (Sol) Usual: 0.5mg/kg/dose. 7-12 yrs: 10mL PO tid-qid. 3-6 yrs: 5mL PO tid-qid. Adjust according to severity of pain and response of the patient.

HOW SUPPLIED: (APAP-Codeine) Elix/Sol (generic): (CV) 120mg-12mg/5mL; Tab: (#3, CIII) 300mg-30mg, (#4, CIII) 300mg-60mg

WARNINGS/PRECAUTIONS: Respiratory depressant effects may be exacerbated with head injury or increased ICP. May obscure head injuries, acute abdominal conditions. Potential for physical dependence and tolerance. Caution in the elderly, debilitated, severe hepatic or renal dysfunction, hypothyroidism, Addison's disease, prostatic hypertrophy, or urethral stricture. Tab contains sodium metabisulfite; may cause allergic-type reactions including anaphylactic symptoms and life-threatening or less severe asthmatic episodes in certain susceptible patients. Extreme sleepiness, confusion or shallow breathing may occur with ultra-rapid metabolizers of codeine; choose the lowest effective dose for the shortest period of time.

ADVERSE REACTIONS: Drowsiness, lightheadedness, dizziness, sedation, SOB, N/V.

INTERACTIONS: May enhance the effects of other narcotic analgesics, alcohol, general anesthetics, tranquilizers (eg, chlordiazepoxide), sedative-hypnotics, or other CNS depressants causing increased CNS depression.

PREGNANCY: Category C, not for use in nursing.

MECHANISM OF ACTION: Codeine: Opiate analgesic and antitussive; produces centrally acting analgesic effects. APAP: Non-opiate, non-salicylate analgesic and antipyretic; produces peripherally acting analgesic effects.

PHARMACOKINETICS: Absorption: Rapid; T_{max}=2 hrs. **Distribution:** Codeine: Rapid; to liver, spleen and kidneys. Crosses blood-brain barrier; found in fetal tissue and breast milk. APAP: Found in breast milk. **Metabolism:** APAP: Liver (conjugation). **Elimination:** Codeine: Urine (90%, parent and metabolites); $T_{1/2}$=2.9 hrs. APAP: Urine (85%); $T_{1/2}$=1.25-3 hrs.

NURSING CONSIDERATIONS

Assessment: Assess for head injury or other intracranial lesions, presence of increased ICP, acute abdominal conditions, asthma, hypersensitivity to sulfite and other ingredients of the formulation, presence of renal/hepatic impairment, hypothyroidism, urethral stricture, Addison's disease, prostatic hypertrophy, pregnancy/nursing status, and possible drug interactions.

Monitoring: Monitor for signs/symptoms of respiratory depression, elevations in CSF pressure, drowsiness, allergic type reactions (eg, anaphylaxis), elevations in serum amylase levels, medication abuse, and medication dependence. Monitor hepatic/renal function with severe hepatic/renal disease.

Patient Counseling: Inform that drug may be habit-forming; take only for as long as prescribed, in amounts prescribed, and no more frequently than prescribed. Caution to avoid performing hazardous tasks (eg, operating machinery/driving) while on therapy. Counsel to avoid alcohol and other CNS depressants during therapy. Counsel about possible adverse events if used during pregnancy/nursing.

Administration: Oral route. **Storage:** (Sol) 15-30°C (59-86°F); (Tab) 20-25°C (68-77°F). Do not refrigerate. Dispense in tight, light-resistant container.

TYSABRI RX
natalizumab (Elan)

> Increases risk of progressive multifocal leukoencephalopathy (PML). Because of risk of PML, natalizumab is available only through a special restricted distribution program called the TOUCH® Prescribing Program. Administer only to patients who are enrolled in and meet all conditions of the TOUCH® Prescribing Program. Monitor patients for any new signs or symptoms that may be suggestive of PML. Dosing should be withheld immediately at the first sign or symptom suggestive of PML.

THERAPEUTIC CLASS: Monoclonal antibody/VCAM-1 blocker

INDICATIONS: Treatment of patients with relapsing forms of multiple sclerosis (MS) to delay the accumulation of physical disability and reduce the frequency of clinical exacerbations. Treatment for inducing and maintaining clinical response and remission in adult patients with moderately to severely active Crohn's disease (CD) with evidence of inflammation who have had an inadequate response to, or are unable to tolerate, conventional CD therapies and TNF-α inhibitors.

DOSAGE: *Adults:* MS/CD: 300mg IV infusion over 1 hr every 4 weeks. (CD) D/C therapy if no therapeutic benefit by 12 weeks, if patient cannot be tapered off corticosteroids within 6 months, or in patients who require additional steroid use that exceeds 3 months within a calendar year to control their CD.

HOW SUPPLIED: Inj: 300mg/15mL

CONTRAINDICATIONS: Progressive multifocal leukoencephalopathy (PML).

WARNINGS/PRECAUTIONS: Hypersensitivity reactions, including anaphylaxis reported; d/c and do not retreat. Liver injury reported; d/c with jaundice or evidence of liver injury. Induces increases in circulating lymphocytes, monocytes, eosinophils, basophils, and nucleated RBCs. Additional cases of PML reported in patients with MS who were not receiving concomitant immunomodulatory therapy. Avoid in patients with serious medical conditions resulting in significantly compromised immune system function. Immune reconstitution inflammatory syndrome (IRIS) reported with PML and subsequent d/c of natalizumab; monitor for development of IRIS and treat appropriately. May increase risk for infections.

ADVERSE REACTIONS: Headache, fatigue, urinary tract infection (UTI), depression, lower/upper respiratory tract infection, arthralgia, abdominal discomfort, rash, gastroenteritis, vaginitis, urinary urgency/frequency, irregular menstruation/dysmenorrhea, dermatitis, abnormal LFTs.

INTERACTIONS: Avoid with concomitant immunomodulatory therapy, immunosuppressants (eg, 6-mercaptopurine, azathioprine, cyclosporine, or methotrexate) or inhibitors of TNF-α. Taper corticosteroids in CD patients when starting natalizumab therapy. Concurrent use with antineoplastic, immunosuppressive, or immunomodulating agents may further increase risk of infections, including PML and other opportunistic infections.

PREGNANCY: Category C, safety not known in nursing.

MECHANISM OF ACTION: Monoclonal antibody/VCAM-1 blocker; recombinant humanized IgG4k monoclonal antibody that binds to α4-subunit of α4β1 and α4β7 integrins expressed on surface of all leukocytes except neutrophils. Inhibits α4-mediated adhesion of leukocytes to their counter-receptor(s).

PHARMACOKINETICS: Absorption: (MS) C_{max}=110mcg/mL; (CD) C_{max}=101mcg/mL **Distribution:** Found in breast milk; (MS) V_d=5.7L; (CD) V_d=5.2L. **Elimination:** (MS) $T_{1/2}$=11 days; (CD) $T_{1/2}$=10 days.

NURSING CONSIDERATIONS

Assessment: Assess for risk of PML, history of chronic immunosuppressant or immunomodulatory therapy and immunocompromised status, drug hypersensitivity, pregnancy/nursing status, and drug interactions. Perform MRI prior to initiating therapy in MS. Obtain baseline MRI in patients with CD.

Monitoring: Monitor for PML, anaphylactic reactions, hypersensitivity reactions, infections, hepatotoxicity, and development of IRIS. Antibody testing recommended if presence of persistent antibodies suspected. Monitor CBC, LFTs, and bilirubin.

Patient Counseling: Inform about TOUCH® Prescribing Program. Educate on risks/benefits. Instruct to report signs of infections, hypersensitivity reactions, liver toxicity. Counsel on importance of follow-up schedule (3 and 6 months after 1st infusion, then every 6 months). Instruct to contact their physician if symptoms suggestive of PML develop; includes progressive weakness on one side of the body or clumsiness of the limbs, disturbance of vision, and changes in thinking, memory, and orientation leading to confusion and personality changes.

Administration: IV route. Refer to PI for dilution/administration instructions.
Storage: 2-8°C (36-46°F). Administer within 8 hrs of preparation. Do not shake or freeze. Protect from light.

TYVASO   RX
treprostinil (United Therapeutics)

THERAPEUTIC CLASS: Pulmonary and systemic vasodilator

INDICATIONS: Treatment of pulmonary arterial hypertension (PAH) (WHO Group 1) in patients with NYHA Class III symptoms and etiologies of idiopathic or heritable PAH or PAH associated with connective tissue diseases to improve exercise ability.

DOSAGE: *Adults:* Initial: 3 breaths (18mcg) per treatment session qid. Reduce to 1-2 breaths if not tolerated and subsequently increase to 3 breaths, as tolerated. Maint: Increase by an additional 3 breaths at approx 1-2 week intervals, if tolerated, to a target dose of 9 breaths (54mcg) per treatment session qid. Max: 9 breaths per treatment session qid. Hepatic/Renal Insufficiency: Titrate slowly.

HOW SUPPLIED: Sol: 0.6mg/mL [2.9mL]

WARNINGS/PRECAUTIONS: Safety and efficacy not established with significant underlying lung disease (eg, asthma or chronic obstructive pulmonary disease [COPD]). Caution with acute pulmonary infections; monitor carefully to detect worsening of lung disease and loss of drug effect. May produce symptomatic hypotension in patients with low systemic arterial pressure. Caution with hepatic or renal impairment. May increase risk of bleeding. Caution in elderly.

ADVERSE REACTIONS: Headache, cough, throat irritation/pharyngolaryngeal pain, nausea, flushing, syncope.

INTERACTIONS: Increased risk of bleeding with anticoagulants. Increased risk of symptomatic hypotension with diuretics, antihypertensive agents, or other vasodilators. Increased exposure with CYP2C8 inhibitors (eg, gemfibrozil); decreased exposure with CYP2C8 inducers (eg, rifampin).

PREGNANCY: Category B, caution in nursing.

MECHANISM OF ACTION: Pulmonary and systemic vasodilator; causes direct vasodilation of pulmonary and systemic arterial vascular beds. Inhibits platelet aggregation.

PHARMACOKINETICS: Absorption: Absolute bioavailability (64%) (18mcg), (72%) (36mcg); (54mcg)C_{max}=0.91-1.32ng/mL, T_{max}=0.12-0.25 hr, AUC=0.81-0.97ng•hr/mL. **Distribution:** (parenteral infusion) V_d=14L/70kg; plasma protein binding (91%). **Metabolism:** Liver via CYP2C8. **Elimination:** (SQ) Urine (79%, 4% unchanged), feces (13%); $T_{1/2}$=4 hrs.

NURSING CONSIDERATIONS

Assessment: Assess for lung disease (eg, asthma, COPD), acute pulmonary infections, low systemic arterial pressure, hepatic/renal insufficiency, pregnancy/nursing status, and possible drug interactions. Obtain baseline LFTs, renal and lung functions.

Monitoring: Monitor for worsening of lung disease, loss of drug effect, hepatic/renal insufficiency, and symptomatic hypotension. Monitor LFTs, renal and lung functions.

Patient Counseling: Counsel for proper administration process including dosing, set-up, operation, cleaning, and maintenance, according to the instruction for use. Advise to have back-up Optineb-ir device to avoid potential interruptions in drug delivery. Inform that therapy should be resumed as soon as possible if treatment session is missed or interrupted. Advise to immediately rinse with water if in contact with skin or eyes.

Administration: Oral inhalation route. Refer to PI for proper administration. **Storage:** 25°C (77°F); excursions permitted to 15-30°C (59-86°F). If opened or transferred in a device, solution should remain for no >1 day. Use within 7 days if foil pack is opened. Protect from light; store unopened ampules in foil pouch.

TYZEKA   RX
telbivudine (Novartis)

> Lactic acidosis and severe hepatomegaly with steatosis, including fatal cases, reported. Severe acute exacerbations of hepatitis B reported in patients who discontinued therapy; monitor hepatic function closely.

THERAPEUTIC CLASS: Nucleoside analogue

INDICATIONS: Treatment of chronic hepatitis B in adults with evidence of viral replication and either evidence of persistent elevations in serum aminotransferases (ALT or AST) or histologically active disease.

DOSAGE: *Adults:* Usual: 600mg or 30mL qd. Dose Adjustment: CrCl 30-49mL/min: 600mg q48h or 20mL qd. CrCl <30mL/min (not requiring dialysis): 600mg q72h or 10mL qd. ESRD: 600mg q96h.
Pediatrics: ≥16 yrs: Usual: 600mg or 30mL qd. Dose Adjustment: CrCl 30-49mL/min: 600mg q48h or 20mL qd. CrCl <30mL/min (not requiring dialysis): 600mg q72h or 10mL qd. ESRD: 600mg q96h.

HOW SUPPLIED: Tab: 600mg; Sol: 100mg/5mL [300mL]

WARNINGS/PRECAUTIONS: Myopathy/myositis and peripheral neuropathy reported; interrupt therapy if suspected and d/c if diagnosed. Rhabdomyolysis and uncomplicated myalgia reported. Caution with known factors for liver disease. Oral solution contains sodium and should be used cautiously in patients with sodium-restricted diet. Caution in elderly.

ADVERSE REACTIONS: Abdominal pain, arthralgia, cough, diarrhea, dizziness, elevated blood creatinine kinase levels, fatigue, headache, myalgia, nausea, fever, lactic acidosis, hepatomegaly, steatosis, exacerbation of hepatitis.

INTERACTIONS: Drugs that alter renal function may alter plasma concentrations of telbivudine. Combination with pegylated interferon alfa-2a and other interferons may be associated with risk of peripheral neuropathy.

PREGNANCY: Category B, not for use in nursing.

MECHANISM OF ACTION: Thymidine nucleoside analogue; inhibits HBV DNA polymerase by competing with thymidine 5'-triphosphate and causes DNA chain termination.

PHARMACOKINETICS: Absorption: C_{max}=3.69mcg/mL, T_{max}=1-4 hrs, 2 hrs (median), AUC=26.1mcg•h/mL; administration with varying degrees of renal function resulted in different pharmacokinetic parameters. **Distribution:** Plasma protein binding (3.3%). **Elimination:** Urine; $T_{1/2}$=40-49 hrs.

NURSING CONSIDERATIONS

Assessment: Assess for renal/hepatic impairment, pregnancy/nursing status, and possible drug interactions. Check if patient on low-sodium diet.

Monitoring: Monitor LFTs periodically and for several months after d/c. Monitor for signs/symptoms of exacerbation of HBV after d/c, unexplained muscle pain, tenderness, weakness, hepatotoxicity, hypersensitivity reactions, and myopathy.

Patient Counseling: Advise to report promptly unexplained muscle weakness, tenderness or pain, numbness, tingling, and/or burning sensations in the arms and/or legs with or without difficulty walking. The medication is not a cure for hepatitis B and long-term treatment benefits are unknown. Deterioration of liver disease may occur in some cases if treatment is discontinued. Therapy has not shown to reduce risk of transmission of HBV to other through sexual contact or blood contamination. Encourage pregnant women to enroll in the Antiretroviral Pregnancy Registry by calling 1-800-258-4263.

Administration: Oral route. **Storage:** 25°C (77°F); excursions permitted to 15-30°C (59-86°F). (Sol) Use within two months after opening. Do not freeze.

ULORIC   RX
febuxostat (Takeda)

THERAPEUTIC CLASS: Xanthine oxidase inhibitor

INDICATIONS: Chronic management of hyperuricemia in patients with gout.

DOSAGE: *Adults:* Initial: 40mg qd. Titrate: If serum uric acid (sUA) is not <6mg/dL after 2 weeks, increase dose to 80mg qd. Range: 40-80mg qd.

HOW SUPPLIED: Tab: 40mg, 80mg

CONTRAINDICATIONS: Patients being treated with azathioprine or mercaptopurine.

WARNINGS/PRECAUTIONS: Not for treatment of asymptomatic hyperuricemia. Increase in gout flares observed; concurrent prophylactic treatment (NSAIDs or colchicine) recommended. Increased rate of cardiovascular (CV) thromboembolic events (eg, CV deaths, myocardial infarction (MI), stroke) reported; monitor for signs and symptoms of MI and stroke. Elevated serum transaminase levels (ALT, AST) reported; monitor LFTs periodically. Caution with severe hepatic impairment (Child-Pugh Class C) and severe renal impairment (CrCl<30mL/min). Avoid in patients or use in whom the rate of urate formation is greatly increased (eg, malignant disease and its treatment, Lesch-Nyhan syndrome).

ADVERSE REACTIONS: Liver function abnormalities, nausea, arthralgia, rash.

INTERACTIONS: See Contraindications. Caution with theophylline. Delay absorption and decreased levels with antacid containing magnesium hydroxide and aluminum hydroxide. Increased levels with colchicine and naproxen. Increase levels of desipramine. Change the concentration of colchicine, naproxen, HCTZ, and indomethacin.

PREGNANCY: Category C, caution in nursing.

MECHANISM OF ACTION: Xanthine oxidase inhibitor; achieves therapeutic effect by decreasing sUA.

PHARMACOKINETICS: Absorption: (40mg) C_{max}=1.6mcg/mL; (80mg) C_{max}=2.6mcg/mL; T_{max}=1-1.5 hrs. **Distribution:** V_d=50L; plasma protein binding (99.2%). **Metabolism:** Conjugation via uridine diphosphate glucuronosyltransferase (UGT), and oxidation via CYP450 enzymes. **Elimination:** Urine (49%), feces (45%); $T_{1/2}$=5-8 hrs.

NURSING CONSIDERATIONS

Assessment: Assess for secondary/asymptomatic hyperuricemia, hepatic/renal impairment, malignant disease, Lesch-Nyhan syndrome, pregnancy/nursing status and possible drug interactions. Obtain baseline sUA and LFTs.

Monitoring: Monitor sUA levels (as early as 2 weeks after initiation), LFTs 2, 4 months following initiation and periodically thereafter, and for signs/symptoms of MI and stroke.

Patient Counseling: Inform that medication may be taken without regard to food or antacid use. Counsel about potential benefits and risks. Gout flares, elevated liver enzymes, and adverse CV events may occur. Notify physician if rash, chest pain, SOB, or neurologic symptoms suggesting stroke occur. Inform physician of any other medications, including over-the-counter drugs currently being taken.

Administration: Oral route. **Storage:** 25°C (77°F); excursions permitted to 15-30°C (59-86°F). Protect from light.

ULTIVA `CII`
remifentanil HCl (Abbott)

THERAPEUTIC CLASS: Opioid analgesic

INDICATIONS: As an analgesic agent for use during the induction and maintenance of general anesthesia. For continuation as an analgesic into the immediate postoperative period in adults under the direct supervision of an anesthesia practitioner in a postoperative anesthesia care unit or intensive care setting. As an analgesic component of monitored anesthesia care in adults.

DOSAGE: *Adults:* Continuous IV Infusion: Induction: 0.5-1mcg/kg/min. Maint: 0.4mcg/kg/min with nitrous oxide 66%; 0.25mcg/kg/min with isoflurane (0.4-1.25 MAC); 0.25mcg/kg/min with propofol (100-200mcg/kg/min). Post-Op Continuation: 0.1mcg/kg/min. CABG: Induction/Maint/Continuation: 1mcg/kg/min. Elderly (>65 yrs): Use 50% of adult dose. Titrate carefully. *Pediatrics:* Anesthesia Maint: Continuous IV Infusion: 1-12 yrs: 0.25mcg/kg/min with halothane (0.3-1.5 MAC), sevoflurane (0.3-1.5 MAC), or isoflurane (0.4-1.5 MAC). Range: 0.05-1.3mcg/kg/min. Birth-2 months: 0.4mcg/kg/min. Range: 0.4-1mcg/kg/min.

HOW SUPPLIED: Inj: 1mg, 2mg, 5mg

CONTRAINDICATIONS: Epidural or intrathecal administration, hypersensitivity to fentanyl analogs.

WARNINGS/PRECAUTIONS: Administer only with infusion device. IV bolus administration should be used only during the maintenance of general anesthesia. Interruption of infusion will result in rapid offset of effect. Use associated with apnea and respiratory depression. Not for use in diagnostic or therapeutic procedures outside the monitored anesthesia care setting. Resuscitative and intubation equipment, oxygen, and opioid antagonist must be readily available. May cause skeletal muscle rigidity and is related to the dose and speed of administration. Do not administer into the same IV tubing with blood due to potential inactivation by nonspecific esterases in blood

U

products. Continuously monitor vital signs and oxygenation. Bradycardia, hypotension, intraoperative awareness reported. Not recommended as sole agent for induction of anesthesia.

ADVERSE REACTIONS: N/V, hypotension, muscle rigidity, bradycardia, shivering, fever, dizziness, visual disturbances, respiratory depression, apnea.

INTERACTIONS: Synergism with thiopental, propofol, isoflurane, midazolam; reduce doses of these drugs by up to 75%.

PREGNANCY: Category C, caution in nursing.

MECHANISM OF ACTION: Opioid analgesic.

PHARMACOKINETICS: Distribution: V_d=100mL/kg, 350mL/kg (initial, steady-state), plasma protein binding (70%). **Metabolism**: Hydrolysis via nonspecific blood and tissue esterases to carboxylic acid metabolite. **Elimination**: $T_{1/2}$=10-20 min.

NURSING CONSIDERATIONS

Assessment: Assess for pulmonary disease, decreased respiratory reserve, pregnancy/nursing status, and possible drug interactions.

Monitoring: Monitor for cardiovascular depression (eg, bradycardia, hypotension), respiratory depression, muscle rigidity of neck and extremities, N/V, chills, arrhythmias, chest wall rigidity. Monitor vital signs routinely. Appropriate post-op monitoring should ensure adequate spontaneous breathing is established and maintained prior to discharge.

Patient Counseling: Advise to use caution while performing potentially hazardous tasks (eg, operating machinery/driving). Counsel about side effects of drug and abuse potential.

Administration: IV infusion. Continuous infusions should only be administered using an infusion device. **Storage**: 2-25°C (36-77°F).

ULTRACET   RX
tramadol HCl - acetaminophen (Ortho-McNeil)

THERAPEUTIC CLASS: Analgesic combination

INDICATIONS: Short-term (≤5 days) management of acute pain.

DOSAGE: *Adults:* 2 tabs q4-6h prn for 5 days or less. Max: 8 tabs/24 hrs. CrCl <30mL/min: Max: 2 tabs q12h. Elderly: Start at lower end of dosing range.

HOW SUPPLIED: Tab: (Tramadol-APAP) 37.5mg-325mg

CONTRAINDICATIONS: Acute intoxication with any of the following: alcohol, hypnotics, narcotics, centrally acting analgesics, opioids, or psychotropic drugs.

WARNINGS/PRECAUTIONS: Increased risk of convulsion in patients with history of seizures and epilepsy. Avoid use with suicidal, depressed or addiction-prone patients. Seizures and anaphylactic reactions reported. May complicate clinical assessment with acute abdominal conditions. Caution with risk of respiratory depression, increased intracranial pressure (ICP), or head injury. May impair mental or physical abilities. Avoid abrupt withdrawal and overdosage. Caution in elderly. Avoid use in opioid-dependent patients and with hepatic impairment.

ADVERSE REACTIONS: Constipation, diarrhea, nausea, somnolence, anorexia, increased sweating, dizziness.

INTERACTIONS: See Contraindications. Caution and reduce dose with CNS depressants (eg, alcohol, opioids, anesthetics, phenothiazines, tranquilizers, narcotics, sedative hypnotics, muscle relaxants); may increase risk of CNS and respiratory depression. May reduce analgesic effects with carbamazepine; not recommended. Possible digoxin toxicity and altered warfarin effects; monitor PT periodically. CYP2D6 inhibitors (eg, fluoxetine, paroxetine, amitriptyline) may inhibit metabolism of tramadol. CYP3A4 inhibitors (eg, ketoconazole, erythromycin) and CYP3A4 inducers (eg, rifampin, St, John's wort) may alter tramadol exposure. May potentiate seizure risk with MAOIs, SSRIs, naloxone (with overdose), TCAs, tricyclics (eg, cyclobenzaprine, promethazine), neuroleptics, other opioids, and drugs that lower seizure threshold. May cause serotonin syndrome with serotonergic agents (eg, SSRIs, SNRIs, TCAs, MAOIs, triptans) and drugs that impair metabolism of tramadol (CYP2D6, 3A4 inhibitors). Avoid alcohol and other tramadol- or APAP-containing products.

PREGNANCY: Category C, not for use in nursing.

MECHANISM OF ACTION: Tramadol: Centrally acting synthetic opioid analgesic; mechanism not fully understood. Binds to μ-opioid receptors and inhibits reuptake of norepinephrine and serotonin. APAP: Nonopiate, nonsalicylate analgesic.

PHARMACOKINETICS: Absorption: Tramadol: Bioavailability (75%), T_{max}=2 hrs, 3 hrs (M1). APAP: Small intestines; T_{max}=1 hr. **Distribution:** (IV) Tramadol: V_d=2.6L/kg (male), 2.9L/kg (female); found in breast milk (0.1%); plasma protein binding (20%). APAP: V_d=0.9L/kg; plasma protein binding (20%). **Metabolism:** Tramadol: CYP2D6, 3A4 (N- and O-demethylation, glucuronidation, or sulfation); M1 (active metabolite). APAP: CYP2E1, 1A2, 3A4 (glucuronidation, sulfation, oxidation). **Elimination:** Tramadol: $T_{1/2}$=5-6 hrs, 7 hrs (M1); urine (30%, unchanged), (60%, metabolites). APAP: $T_{1/2}$=2-3 hrs; urine (<9%, unchanged).

NURSING CONSIDERATIONS

Assessment: Assess for acute intoxication, CNS/respiratory depression, seizures, serotonin syndrome, head trauma, metabolic disorders, CNS infection, acute abdominal conditions, increased ICP, drug abuse, opioid dependence, renal/hepatic impairment, pregnancy/nursing status, and possible drug interactions.

Monitoring: Monitor for signs/symptoms of seizures, serotonin syndrome, respiratory depression, withdrawal symptoms, hepatotoxicity, and hypersensitivity reactions.

Patient Counseling: Inform that drug may cause seizures and/or serotonin syndrome with concomitant use of serotonergic agents. Caution when taking tranquilizers, hypnotics, or other opiate-containing analgesics. Caution when driving and operating machinery. Instruct to avoid alcohol. Advise to seek medical attention if experience symptoms of seizures, respiratory depression, hypersensitivity reactions, hepatotoxicity, or withdrawal symptoms (eg, anxiety, sweating, insomnia, rigors). Warn not to exceed the recommended dose. Instruct to inform physician if pregnant or are trying to become pregnant.

Administration: Oral route. **Storage:** 25°C (77°F); excursions permitted to 15-30°C (59-86°F).

ULTRAM   RX
tramadol HCl (Ortho-McNeil)

OTHER BRAND NAMES: Ultram ER (PRICARA)

THERAPEUTIC CLASS: Central acting analgesic

INDICATIONS: Management of moderate to moderately severe pain.

DOSAGE: *Adults:* ≥17 yrs: (Tab) Initial: 25mg qam. Titrate: Increase by 25mg every 3 days to 25mg qid, then increase by 50mg every 3 days to 50mg qid. Usual: 50-100mg q4-6h as needed. Max: 400mg/day. Individualize dose. CrCl <30mL/min: Dose q12h. Max: 200mg/day. Cirrhosis: 50mg q12h. Elderly: Start at low end of dosing range. >75 yrs: Max: 300mg/day. ≥18 yrs: (Tab, ER) Initial: 100mg qd. Titrate: Increase by 100mg every 5 days. Max: 300mg/day. Elderly: Start at low end of dosing range.

HOW SUPPLIED: Tab: 50mg*; Tab, Extended-Release: 100mg, 200mg, 300mg *scored

CONTRAINDICATIONS: Any situation where opioids are contraindicated including acute intoxication with any of the following: alcohol, hypnotics, narcotics, centrally acting analgesics, opioids or psychotropic drugs.

WARNINGS/PRECAUTIONS: Seizures and anaphylactoid reactions reported. Do not prescribe for suicidal or addiction-prone patients. Caution with patients at risk for respiratory depression, with increased intracranial pressure (ICP), or head trauma. May complicate clinical assessment of acute abdominal conditions. Do not d/c abruptly. Adjust dose with renal/hepatic impairment and patients older than 75 yrs of age. Development of serotonin syndrome including mental status changes, autonomic instability, neuromuscular aberrations, and GI symptoms reported. May impair physical or mental abilities.

ADVERSE REACTIONS: Dizziness, N/V, constipation, headache, somnolence, sweating, asthenia, dyspepsia, dry mouth, diarrhea, CNS stimulation, pruritus.

INTERACTIONS: See Contraindications. Caution and reduce dose with CNS depressants (eg, alcohol, opioids, anesthetics, phenothiazines, tranquilizers, sedatives, hypnotics). Avoid with carbamazepine. Possible digoxin toxicity and altered warfarin effects. Increased risk of adverse events with CYP2D6 inhibitors (eg, quinidine, fluoxetine, paroxetine, amtriptyline), CYP3A4 inhibitors (eg, ketoconazole, erythromycin), TCAs and other tricyclic compounds (eg, cyclobenzaprine, promethazine, etc), other opioids, neuroleptics, and drugs that reduce seizure threshold. Caution with SSRIs, MAOIs, triptans, linezolid, lithium, or St. John's wort; increased risk of serotonin syndrome. Increased levels with quinidine.

PREGNANCY: Category C, not for use in nursing.

MECHANISM OF ACTION: Centrally acting synthetic opioid analgesic; not established. Binding of parent and M1 metabolite to μ-opioid receptors and weak inhibition of norepinephrine and serotonin reuptake.

PHARMACOKINETICS: Absorption: (100mg) Bioavailability (75%); T_{max}=2 hrs (drug), 3 hrs (M1). **Distribution:** V_d=2.6L/kg (male), 2.9L/kg (female); plasma protein binding (20%). **Metabolism:** Liver (extensive); through N-and O-demethylation and glucuronidation or sulfation pathways via CYP3A4, 2D6. M1 (active metabolite). **Elimination:** Urine: (30% unchanged), (60% as metabolite); $T_{1/2}$=6.3 hrs (drug), 7.4 hrs (M1).

NURSING CONSIDERATIONS

Assessment: Assess for acute intoxication with alcohol, hypnotics, centrally acting analgesics, opioids, or psychotropic drugs. Assess for epilepsy, risk for seizure (eg, head trauma, metabolic disorders, alcohol and drug withdrawal, CNS infections), risk for respiratory depression, increased ICP, renal/hepatic impairment, pregnancy/nursing status, and possible drug interactions.

Monitoring: Monitor for anaphylactoid reactions (eg, pruritus, hives, bronchospasm, angioedema, toxic epidermal necrolysis and Stevens-Johnson syndrome), respiratory/CNS depression, physical dependence/abuse, seizures, serotonin syndrome, withdrawal symptoms with abrupt d/c (eg, anxiety, sweating, insomnia, rigors, upper respiratory symptoms, diarrhea, piloerection and rarely, hallucinations).

Patient Counseling: Advise to use caution while performing hazardous tasks (operating machinery/driving). Do not take with alcohol, tranquilizers, or hypnotics. Notify physician if pregnant/nursing or planning to become pregnant.

Administration: Oral route. **Storage:** 25°C (77°F); excursions permitted to 15-30°C (59-86°F).

ULTRAVATE   RX
halobetasol propionate (Ranbaxy)

THERAPEUTIC CLASS: Corticosteroid

INDICATIONS: Relief of the inflammatory and pruritic manifestations of corticosteroid-responsive dermatoses.

DOSAGE: *Adults:* Apply a thin layer to affected skin qd-bid ud. Rub in gently and completely. Do not use >2 weeks. Max: 50g/week. Reassess if no improvement within 2 weeks.

Pediatrics: ≥12 yrs: Apply a thin layer to affected skin qd-bid ud. Rub in gently and completely. Do not use >2 weeks. Max: 50g/week. Reassess if no improvement within 2 weeks.

HOW SUPPLIED: Cre, Oint: 0.05% [15g, 50g]

WARNINGS/PRECAUTIONS: Systemic absorption may produce reversible hypothalamic-pituitary-adrenal (HPA) axis suppression, manifestations of Cushing's syndrome, hyperglycemia, and glucosuria. Pediatric patients may be more susceptible to systemic toxicity and drug may interfere with their growth and development. Caution when applied to large surface areas or under occlusive dressings; evaluate periodically for HPA suppression. Do not use for >2 weeks at a time and treat only small areas at any one time. If HPA axis suppression occurs, reduce application frequency, substitute less potent corticosteroid, or attempt to withdraw drug. Use appropriate antifungal or antibacterial agent with concomitant dermatological infections; d/c if no prompt favorable response until infection is controlled. HPA axis suppression (eg, low plasma cortisol, no response to ACTH stimulation), linear growth retardation, delayed weight gain, Cushing's syndrome and intracranial HTN (eg, bulging fontanelles, headache, bilateral papilledema) reported in pediatrics. Not recommended for treatment of rosacea or perioral dermatitis. Do not use on face, groin, or axillae. D/C if irritation occurs and institute appropriate therapy. Failure to heal may indicate allergic contact dermatitis; corroborate with appropriate patch testing. Signs and symptoms of glucocorticosteroid insufficiency may occur after treatment withdrawal; may require supplemental systemic corticosteroids. Reassess if no improvement after 2 weeks. D/C when control is achieved. Not for ophthalmic use.

ADVERSE REACTIONS: Stinging, burning, itching, acneiform eruptions, secondary infection, miliaria, striae, folliculitis, allergic contract dermatitis, perioral dermatitis, hypertrichosis, hypopigmentation.

PREGNANCY: Category C, caution in nursing.

MECHANISM OF ACTION: Corticosteroid; possesses anti-inflammatory, antipruritic, and vasoconstrictive properties. Anti-inflammatory activity not established; suspected to act by induction of phospholipase A_2 inhibitory proteins called lipocortins. Lipocortins control biosynthesis of potent inflammation mediators (eg, prostaglandins, leukotrienes) by inhibiting release of their common precursor, arachidonic acid.

PHARMACOKINETICS: Absorption: Percutaneous; extent of absorption determined by vehicle, integrity of skin, occlusion, inflammation, and other disease states. **Distribution:** Systemically administered corticosteroids are found in breast milk.

NURSING CONSIDERATIONS

Assessment: Assess for age in pediatric patients, rosacea or perioral dermatitis, presence of concomitant skin infections, hypersensitivity and pregnancy/nursing status. Assess skin integrity at application site.

Monitoring: Monitor for signs/symptoms of HPA axis suppression, Cushing's syndrome, hyperglycemia, glucosuria, treatment-site irritation, allergic contact dermatitis (eg, failure to heal), dermatological infections, and for hypersensitivity reactions. Following withdrawal of therapy, monitor for glucocorticosteroid insufficiency. If applying to large area or to areas under occlusion, perform periodic monitoring for HPA axis suppression using ACTH stimulation, A.M. plasma cortisol and urinary free cortisol tests. In pediatric patients, monitor for signs/symptoms of systemic toxicity, HPA axis suppression, linear growth retardation, delayed weight gain, Cushing's syndrome and intracranial HTN. Monitor for signs of clinical improvement; if no improvement within 2 weeks, reassess diagnosis.

Patient Counseling: Instruct to use externally and as directed; avoid contact with eyes and avoid use on face, groin or axillae. Do not bandage or wrap treatment area so as to be occlusive unless directed by physician. Report signs of local adverse reactions (eg, irritation). Do not use for any disorder other than for which it was used/prescribed.

Administration: Topical route. **Storage**: 15-30°C (59-86°F).

U

UNASYN
ampicillin sodium - sulbactam sodium (Pfizer)

RX

THERAPEUTIC CLASS: Semisynthetic penicillin/beta-lactamase inhibitor

INDICATIONS: Treatment of skin and skin structure (SSSI), intra-abdominal, and gynecological infections caused by susceptible microorganisms.

DOSAGE: *Adults:* 1.5-3g (ampicillin+sulbactam) IM/IV q6h. Max: 4g sulbactam/day. Renal Impairment: CrCl ≥30mL/min: 1.5-3g q6-8h. CrCl 15-29mL/min: 1.5-3g q12h. CrCl 5-14mL/min: 1.5-3g q24h.
Pediatrics: ≥1 yr: 300mg/kg/day (ampicillin+sulbactam) IV in equally divided doses q6h. Max: 4g sulbactam/day. ≥40kg: Dose according to adult recommendations.

HOW SUPPLIED: Inj: (Ampicillin-Sulbactam) 1g-0.5g, 2g-1g. Also available as a Pharmacy Bulk Package. Refer to individual package insert for more information

WARNINGS/PRECAUTIONS: Serious, sometimes fatal, hypersensitivity reactions reported with PCN therapy; d/c use and initiate appropriate therapy. *Clostridium difficile*-associated diarrhea (CDAD) reported; if suspected or confirmed d/c ongoing antibiotics not for *C.difficile*. Increased risk of skin rash with mononucleosis; use alternate agent. Possible superinfections with mycotic or bacterial pathogens; d/c therapy if superinfection occurs. Use in the absence of a proven or strongly suspected bacterial infection or a prophylactic indication is unlikely to provide benefit and increases the risk of drug resistant bacteria. False positive reactions may occur when using Benedict's or Fehling solution for urinary glucose test. Decreases in total conjugated estriol, estriol-glucoronide, conjugated estrone, and estradiol reported in pregnant women.

ADVERSE REACTIONS: Injection-site pain, thrombophlebitis, diarrhea.

INTERACTIONS: Probenecid may increase and prolong blood levels and decreases renal tubular secretion. Increased incidence of rash with allopurinol. Do not reconstitute with aminoglycosides; ampicillin component may inactivate aminoglycosides.

PREGNANCY: Category B, caution in nursing.

MECHANISM OF ACTION: Ampicillin: Semi-synthetic penicillin; acts through inhibition of cell wall mucopeptide biosynthesis. Has a broad spectrum of bactericidal activity against many gram-positive and gram-negative aerobic and anaerobic bacteria. Sulbactam: beta-lactamase inhibitor: provides good inhibitory activity against clinically important plasmid mediated β-lactamases most frequently responsible for transferred drug resistance.

PHARMACOKINETICS: **Absorption:** IV/IM administration of variable doses resulted in different parameters. **Distribution:** Plasma protein binding (28% ampicillin), (38% sulbactam); found in breast milk. **Elimination:** Urine (75-85% unchanged); $T_{1/2}$=1 hr.

NURSING CONSIDERATIONS

Assessment: Assess for history of hypersensitivity to cephalosporins/PCNs or other allergens, nursing status, mononucleosis, renal impairment, and for possible drug interactions. Document indications for therapy, culture, and susceptibility testing.

Monitoring: Monitor for signs/symptoms of hypersensitivity reactions (eg, anaphylaxis), CDAD, superinfection, GI changes, hematological changes (eg, agranulocytosis), and for changes in hepatic/renal function. Monitor for changes in estrogen levels in pregnant women and for false positive reactions when testing for glucose in urine if using Clinitest, Benedict's Solution, or Fehling's Solution.

Patient Counseling: Inform that drug only treats bacterial, not viral infections. Take as directed; skipping doses or not completing full course may decrease effectiveness and increase resistance. May experience diarrhea. Contact physician if GIsymptoms including watery/bloody stools develop or if allergic reaction develops.

Administration: IV/IM route. IV: Refer to PI for reconstitution instructions. IM: Reconstitute with sterile water for injection (SWFI) or lidocaine 0.5% or 2%. For 1.5g vial, add 3.2mL diluent; withdrawal volume is 4mL. For 3g vial, add 6.4mL diluent; withdrawal volume is 8mL. **Storage:** Prior to reconstitution: 30°C (86°F). IV Reconstituted Solution: Refer to PI for storage requirements. IM Reconstituted Solution: Use only freshly prepared solutions and administer within 1 hr after preparation.

UNIPHYL   RX
theophylline (Purdue Pharmaceutical)

THERAPEUTIC CLASS: Xanthine bronchodilator

INDICATIONS: Treatment of the symptoms and reversible airflow obstruction associated with chronic asthma and other chronic lung disease (eg, emphysema, chronic bronchitis).

DOSAGE: *Adults:* ≥16 yrs: Initial: 300-400mg qd for 3 days with meals. Titrate: Increase to 400-600mg qd. After 3 days and if needed/tolerated, increase dose according to blood levels. Tab may be split in half; do not chew or crush. Renal Dysfunction/Elderly (>60 yrs): Max: 400mg/day. Conversion from Immediate-Release Theophylline: Give same daily dose as once daily. *Pediatrics:* 12-15 yrs: (<45kg): Initial: 12-14mg/kg/day up to 300mg qd for 3 days with meals. Titrate: Increase to 16mg/kg/day up to 400mg qd. After 3 days if needed/tolerated increase to 20mg/kg/day up to 600mg qd. (>45kg): Follow adult dose schedule. Tab may be split in half; do not chew or crush. Conversion from Immediate-Release Theophylline: ≥12 yrs: Give same daily dose as once daily. Renal Dysfunction: Max: 400mg qd.

HOW SUPPLIED: Tab, Extended-Release: 400mg, 600mg

WARNINGS/PRECAUTIONS: Extreme caution in peptic ulcer disease, seizure disorders, and/or cardiac arrhythmias (except bradycardia). Caution in neonates, children <1 yr, and the elderly. Caution in pulmonary edema, CHF, fever ≥102°F for 24 hrs, cor pulmonale, hypothyroidism, liver disease, reduced renal function, sepsis, shock, and HTN. If toxicity develops (eg, repetitive vomiting), monitor serum levels and adjust dosage.

ADVERSE REACTIONS: Vomiting, headache, insomnia, diarrhea, restlessness, tremors, hematemesis, hypokalemia, hyperglycemia, tachycardia, hypotension/shock, nervousness, disorientation, arrhythmias, seizures.

INTERACTIONS: Diminished effects with charcoal-broiled food, phenytoin, carbamazepine, phenobarbital, hydantoins, rifampin, ritonavir, aminoglutethimide, barbiturates, ketoconazole, sulfinpyrazone, INH, loop diuretics, sympathomimetics, high protein/low carbohydrate diet, alcohol, St. John's wort. Potentiated by propranolol, allopurinol, erythromycin, troleandomycin, ciprofloxacin, quinolone antibiotics, oral contraceptives, CCBs, corticosteroids, disulfiram, ephedrine, influenza virus vaccine, interferon, macrolides, mexiletine, thiabendazole, thyroid hormones, carbamazepine, loop diuretics, high carbohydrate/low protein diet and parenteral nutrition.

PREGNANCY: Category C, caution in nursing.

MECHANISM OF ACTION: Methylxanthine; acts via smooth muscle relaxation and suppression of airway response to stimuli. Bronchodilatation suggested to be mediated by inhibiting isozymes of phosphodiesterase. Also increases the force of contraction of diaphragmatic muscles due to enhancement of calcium uptake through adenosine-mediated channel.

PHARMACOKINETICS: Absorption: Rapid, complete; (800 qam, fed) C_{max}=12.1mcg/mL, T_{max}=8.8 hrs, AUC=203mcg•hr/mL. (600 qd, fed) C_{max}=12.91mcg/mL, T_{max}=8.62 hrs, AUC=209mcg•hr/mL. Bioavailability Ratio 600/400: 98.8%. **Distribution:** V_d = 0.45L/kg; plasma protein binding (40%). **Metabolism:** Extensive; CYP1A2, 2E1, 3A3; Caffeine and 3-methylxanthine (active metabolites). **Elimination:** Urine (10% unchanged), $T_{1/2}$=8 hrs.

U

NURSING CONSIDERATIONS

Assessment: Assess risk of exacerbation of concurrent conditions (eg, active PUD, seizure disorder, cardiac arrhythmias). Assess use with any conditions where treatment is contraindicated or cautioned. Assess known hypersensitivity, renal/hepatic functions, pregnancy/nursing status, and possible drug interactions.

Monitoring: Carefully monitor serum drug levels (target unbound concentration: 6-12mcg/mL) for dose adjustments, drug toxicity, worsening of chronic illness, hepatic dysfunction. Monitor plasma glucose, uric acid, free fatty acids, cholesterol, HDL, LDL, LFTs, and urine free cortisol excretion. If toxicity develops (eg, repetitive vomiting), adjust dosage based on serum levels.

Patient Counseling: Instruct to seek medical attention if N/V, persistent headache, insomnia, or rapid heartbeat occur. Counsel not to take St. John's wort concurrently; may result in decreased drug levels. Take once daily in morning or evening. Consistently take with/without food, do not chew or crush, and inform physician if new illness (especially if accompanied with persistent fever) or worsening of chronic illness occurs. Inform all physicians of theophylline use especially if medication is being added or removed from treatment.

Administration: Oral route. **Storage:** 25°C (77°F); excursions permitted to 15-30°C (59-86°F).

UNIRETIC   RX
moexipril HCl - hydrochlorothiazide (Schwarz)

> ACE inhibitors can cause death/injury to developing fetus during 2nd and 3rd trimesters. D/C if pregnancy detected.

THERAPEUTIC CLASS: ACE inhibitor/thiazide diuretic

INDICATIONS: Treatment of HTN. Not for initial therapy.

DOSAGE: *Adults:* Initial (if not controlled on moexipril/HCTZ monotherapy): Switch to 7.5mg-12.5mg tab, 15mg-12.5mg tab, or 15mg-25mg tab qd. Titrate: Based on clinical response. May increase after 2-3 weeks. Initial (if controlled on 25mg HCTZ/day with hypokalemia): 3.75mg-6.25mg (1/2 of 7.5mg-12.5mg tab). If excessive reduction with 7.5mg-12.5mg tab, may switch to 3.75mg-6.25mg. Replacement Therapy: Substitute combination for titrated components. Take 1 hr before meals.

HOW SUPPLIED: Tab: (Moexipril-HCTZ) 7.5mg-12.5mg*, 15mg-12.5mg*, 15mg-25mg* *scored

CONTRAINDICATIONS: History of ACE inhibitor-associated angioedema, anuria, sulfonamide hypersensitivity.

WARNINGS/PRECAUTIONS: Angioedema involving the face, extremities, lips, tongue, glottis, and/or larynx reported; d/c if it occurs as it may be fatal due to airway obstruction. Intestinal angioedema reported. Can cause symptomatic hypotension; caution in patients with ischemic heart disease, aortic stenosis, cerebrovascular disease. Caution in patients with severe renal disease; may precipitate azotemia. Monitor WBCs in renal and collagen vascular disease. Fetal/neonatal morbidity and death reported. Risk of hyperkalemia with DM, renal dysfunction. Persistent nonproductive cough reported. Anaphylactoid reactions reported. Rarely, associated with syndrome that starts with cholestatic jaundice and progresses to fulminant necrosis and sometimes death; d/c if experience jaundice or marked elevations of hepatic enzymes. Caution in patients with hepatic impairment or progressive liver disease. May exacerbate or activate SLE. May cause electrolyte imbalance (hyperkalemia, hypokalemia, hyponatremia, hypochloremic alkalosis, hypomagnesemia, hypercalcemia); monitor electrolytes. May reduce glucose tolerance and increase cholesterol, TG.

ADVERSE REACTIONS: Cough.

INTERACTIONS: Increase risk of hyperkalemia with K+-sparing diuretics, K+ supplements, or K+-containing salt substitutes. Potentiates orthostatic hypotension with alcohol, barbiturates, and narcotics. Adjust antidiabetic drugs.

Reduced absorption with cholestyramine, colestipol. Corticosteroids, ACTH deplete antihypertensives. May decrease response to pressor amines. Potentiates other antihypertensives. May increase responsiveness to skeletal muscle relaxants. Risk of lithium toxicity. NSAIDs reduce effects. Increased absorption of HCTZ with guanabenz and propantheline. Nitritoid reactions have been reported rarely with injectable gold (sodium aurothiomalate).

PREGNANCY: Category C (1st trimester) and D (2nd and 3rd trimesters), not for use in nursing.

MECHANISM OF ACTION: Moexipril: ACE inhibitor; inhibition results in decreased plasma angiotensin II, leading to decreased vasopressor activity and decreased aldosterone secretion. HCTZ: Thiazide diuretic; affects renal tubular mechanism of electrolyte reabsorption, directly increasing excretion of Na^+ and Cl^-.

PHARMACOKINETICS: Absorption: Moexipril-HCTZ: T_{max}=0.8 hrs. Moexipril: Incomplete; bioavailability (13%), T_{max}= 1.5 hrs. **Distribution:** Moexiprilat: V_d=2.8L/kg; plasma protein binding (50%). HCTZ: V_d=1.5-4.2L/kg; crosses the placenta; found in breast milk; plasma protein binding (21-24%). **Metabolism:** Moexiprilat (active metabolite). **Elimination:** Urine (7% moexiprilat, 1% moexipril, 5% other metabolites), feces (52% moexiprilat, 1% moexipril); $T_{1/2}$=2-9 hrs (Moexiprilat). HCTZ: Renal excretion; $T_{1/2}$=5.6-14.8 hrs.

NURSING CONSIDERATIONS

Assessment: Assess BP, history of angioedema, collagen-vascular disease, hepatic/renal function, CHF, renal artery stenosis, SLE, serum electrolytes, pregnancy/nursing status, history of allergy to sulfonamides, bronchial asthma, parathyroid disorders, and possible drug interactions. Obtain baseline electrolytes (K+, Na, Cl, Mg), blood glucose, cholesterol, TG and uric acid.

Monitoring: Monitor for signs of angioedema (face, extremities, lips, glottis, and/or larynx), hypotension, infections, electrolyte imbalance (hyperkalemia, hypokalemia, hyponatremia, hypochloremic alkalosis, hypomagnesemia, hypercalcemia). Monitor BP, WBC counts, electrolytes (K+, Na, Cl, Mg), blood glucose, cholesterol, TG and uric acid.

Patient Counseling: Inform about fetal risks if taken during pregnancy. Inadequate fluid intake, excessive perspiration, diarrhea, or vomiting can lead to excessive fall in BP. Lightheadedness and possible syncope may occur, especially during first few days of therapy. Do not use K+ supplements or salt substitutes containing K+ without consulting physician. Counsel about signs/symptoms of neutropenia (eg, infections, sore throat, fever), angioedema, electrolyte imbalance (eg, thirst, weakness, lethargy), and other adverse effects; advise to seek prompt medical attention if any occur. Take medication 1 hr before meals.

Administration: Oral route. **Storage:** 20-25°C (68-77°F). Protect from excessive moisture.

UNITHROID   RX
levothyroxine sodium (Lannett)

THERAPEUTIC CLASS: Thyroid replacement hormone

INDICATIONS: Hypothyroidism. As a pituitary TSH suppressant in the treatment and prevention of euthyroid goiters, including thyroid nodules, lymphocytic thyroiditis, and multinodular goiter. Adjunct to surgery and radioiodine therapy for thyrotropin-dependent well-differentiated thyroid cancer.

DOSAGE: *Adults:* Take in AM at least 1/2-1 hr before food. Hypothyroid: Usual: 1.7mcg/kg/day. >200mcg/day (seldom). >50 yrs/<50 yrs with Cardiac Disease: Initial: 25-50mcg/day. Titrate: Increase by 12.5-25mcg/day every 6-8 weeks until euthyroid. Elderly with Cardiac Disease: Initial: 12.5-25mcg/day. Titrate: Increase by 12.5-25mcg/day every 4-6 weeks until euthyroid. Severe Hypothyroidism: Initial: 12.5-25mcg/day. Titrate: Increase by 25mcg/day every 2-4 weeks until euthyroid. Pregnancy: May increase dose requirements. Subclinical Hypothyroidism: Lower doses required.

Pediatrics: Take in AM at least 1/2-1 hr before food. Hypothyroidism: 0-3 months: 10-15mcg/kg/day. 3-6 months: 8-10mcg/kg/day. 6-12 months: 6-8mcg/kg/day. 1-5 yrs: 5-6mcg/kg/day. 6-12 yrs: 4-5mcg/kg/day. >12 yrs: 2-3mcg/kg/day. Growth/Puberty Complete: 1.7mcg/kg/day. Cardiac Risk: Initial: Use lower dose. Titrate: Increase dose every 4-6 weeks until euthyroid. Infants with Serum T_4 <5mcg/dL: Initial: 50mcg/day. Chronic/Severe Hypothyroidism: Children: Initial: 25mcg/day. Titrate: Increase by 25mcg/day every 2-4 weeks until desired effect. Minimize Hyperactivity in Older Children: Initial: Give 1/4 of full replacement dose. Titrate: Increase by same amount weekly until full dose achieved. May crush tab and mix with 5-10mL water.

HOW SUPPLIED: Tab: 25mcg*, 50mcg*, 75mcg*, 88mcg*, 100mcg*, 112mcg*, 125mcg*, 150mcg*, 175mcg*, 200mcg*, 300mcg* *scored

CONTRAINDICATIONS: Untreated thyrotoxicosis, acute MI, uncorrected adrenal insufficiency.

WARNINGS/PRECAUTIONS: Do not use in the treatment of obesity; larger doses in euthyroid patients can cause serious or even life threatening toxicity. Caution with cardiovascular disease, CAD, adrenal insufficiency, autonomous thyroid tissue, hypothalamic/pituitary hormone deficiencies, and the elderly with risk of occult cardiac disease. Carefully titrate dose to avoid over or under treatment. Decreased bone mineral density with long term use. With adrenal insufficiency supplement with glucocorticoids before therapy.

INTERACTIONS: Sympathomimetics may increase risk of coronary insufficiency with CAD. Upward dose adjustments needed for insulin and oral hypoglycemic agents. Decreased absorption with soybean flour (infant formula), cotton seed meal, walnuts, and fiber. May potentiate oral anticoagulant effects; adjust dose and monitor PT/INR. May decrease levels and effects of digitalis glycosides. Cholestyramine, colestipol, ferrous sulfate, aluminum hydroxide, sodium polystyrene, sucralfate may decrease absorption. Reduced TSH secretion with dopamine/dopamine agonists, glucocorticoids, octreotide. Decreased thyroid hormone secretion with aminoglutethimide, amiodarone, iodine (including iodine-containing radiographic contrast agents), lithium, methimazole, PTU, sulfonamides, tolbutamide. Increased thyroid hormone secretion with amiodarone, iodide (including iodine-containing radiographic contrast agents). Decreased T_4 absorption with antacids (aluminum & magnesium hydroxides), simethicone, bile acid sequestrants (cholestyramine, colestipol), calcium carbonate, cation exchange resins (eg, Kayexalate), ferrous sulfate, sucralfate. Increased serum TBG concentration with clofibrate, estrogens, heroin/methadone, 5-FU, mitotane, tamoxifen. Decreased serum TBG concentration with androgens/anabolic steroids, asparaginase, glucocorticoids, nicotinic acid (slow-release). Protein-binding site displacement with furosemide, heparin, hydantoins, NSAIDs, salicylates. Increased hepatic metabolism with carbamazepine, hydantoins, phenobarbital, rifampin. Decreased conversion of T_4 to T_3 levels with amiodarone, β-adrenergic antagonists (propranolol >160mg/day), glucocorticoids (dexamethasone >4mg/day), PTU. Additive effects of both agents with antidepressants. Interferon-(alpha) may cause development of antithyroid microsomal antibodies causing transient hypothyroidism, hyperthyroidism, or both. Interleukin-2 has been associated with transient painless thyroiditis. Excessive use with growth hormones may accelerate epiphyseal closure. Ketamine use may produce marked HTN and tachycardia. May reduce uptake of iodine-containing radiographic contrast agents. Altered levels of thyroid hormone and/or TSH level with choral hydrate, diazepam, ethionamide, lovastatin, metoclopramide, 6-mercaptopurine, nitroprusside, para-aminosalicylate sodium, perphenazine, resorcinol (excessive topical use), thiazide diuretics.

PREGNANCY: Category A, caution in nursing.

MECHANISM OF ACTION: Thyroid hormone; not understood, suspected to control DNA transcription and protein synthesis.

PHARMACOKINETICS: Distribution: Plasma protein binding (99%), found in breast milk. **Metabolism:** Liver via sequential deiodination (major pathway), conjugation in liver (mainly), kidneys, other tissues. **Elimination:** Urine, feces (20% unchanged); (T_4) $T_{1/2}$=6-7 days, (T_3) $T_{1/2}$≤2days.

NURSING CONSIDERATIONS

Assessment: Assess for suppressed serum TSH with normal T_3 and T_4 levels, overt thyrotoxicosis, thyroid diseases (eg, nontoxic diffuse or nodular goiter), endocrine disorders (eg, hypothalmic/pituitary hormone deficiencies, autoimmune polyglandular disorders), infants for congenital anomalies, cardiovascular diseases (eg, angina pectoris, acute MI), DM, hypersensitivity history, clotting status, upcoming surgery, and for possible drug and test interactions.

Monitoring: Perform frequent lab tests and clinical evaluations of thyroid functions (TSH and free T_4 levels, lipid metabolism, blood/urinary glucose in DM, clotting parameters). Monitor cardiovascular signs (eg, arrhythmias, coronary insufficiency), growth/development, bone metabolism, cognitive function, emotional status, GI functions, reproductive functions, partial hair loss in infants, and signs/symptoms of thyroid toxicity.

Patient Counseling: Inform that drug is to be taken for life and not for treatment of obesity or weight loss. Take on empty stomach, 1 hr before breakfast with full glass of water. Notify physician if pregnant/nursing or planning to become pregnant. Notify if taking any other drugs. Do not d/c or change dosage unless directed by physician. Report any signs/symptoms of thyroid toxicity to physician.

Administration: Oral route. **Storage:** 20-25°C (68-77°F); excursions permitted to 15-30°C (59-86°F).

UNIVASC RX
moexipril HCl (Schwarz)

> ACE inhibitors can cause death/injury to developing fetus during 2nd and 3rd trimesters. D/C if pregnancy detected.

THERAPEUTIC CLASS: ACE inhibitor

INDICATIONS: Treatment of HTN alone or in combination with thiazide diuretics.

DOSAGE: *Adults:* D/C diuretic 2-3 days prior to therapy if possible. Take 1 hr before meals. Initial: 7.5mg qd, 3.75mg with concomitant diuretic therapy. Maint: 7.5-30mg/day given qd-bid. Resume diuretic if BP not controlled. Max: 60mg/day. CrCl ≤40mL/min: Initial: 3.75mg qd. Max: 15mg/day. Elderly: Start at lower end of dosing range.

HOW SUPPLIED: Tab: 7.5mg*, 15mg* *scored

CONTRAINDICATIONS: History of ACE inhibitor-associated angioedema.

WARNINGS/PRECAUTIONS: Angioedema involving the face, extremities, lips, tongue, glottis, and/or larynx reported; d/c if it occurs. Angioedema associated with involvement of tongue, glottis, or larynx, may be fatal due to airway obstruction. Can cause symptomatic hypotension; caution in patients with ischemic heart disease, aortic stenosis, cerebrovascular disease. Monitor WBCs in renal and collagen vascular disease. Fetal and neonatal injury and death reported. Rarely, associated with syndrome that starts with cholestatic jaundice and progresses to fulminant necrosis and sometimes death; d/c if experience jaundice or marked elevations of hepatic enzymes. Caution in patients with impaired renal function, CHF, and renal artery stenosis. Risk of hyperkalemia with DM, renal dysfunction. Persistent nonproductive cough reported. Minor increases in BUN or SrCr reported.

ADVERSE REACTIONS: Cough, dizziness, diarrhea, flu syndrome.

INTERACTIONS: May increase lithium levels. Hypotension risk with diuretics. Increased risk of hyperkalemia with K^+-sparing diuretics, K^+-containing salt substitutes, or K^+ supplements. Nitritoid reactions reported rarely with injectable gold (sodium aurothiomalate).

PREGNANCY: Category C (1st trimester) and D (2nd and 3rd trimesters), caution in nursing.

MECHANISM OF ACTION: ACE inhibitor; inhibition results in decreased plasma angiotensin II, which leads to decreased vasopressor activity, increased plasma renin activity, and decreased aldosterone secretion.

U

PHARMACOKINETICS: Absorption: Incomplete; bioavailability (13%). **Distribution:** V_d=183L; plasma protein binding (50%). **Metabolism:** Moexiprilat (active metabolite). **Elimination:** Urine (7% moexiprilat, 1% moexipril, 5% other metabolites), feces (52% moexiprilat, 1% moexipril); $T_{1/2}$=2-9 hrs.

NURSING CONSIDERATIONS

Assessment: Assess for history of angioedema, BP, LFTs, renal function, CHF, renal artery stenosis, pregnancy/nursing status, and possible drug interactions. Obtain baseline serum K^+, Na^+, WBC count, LFTs, SrCr, BUN, uric acid.

Monitoring: Monitor BP, LFTs, renal function, WBC, BUN, SrCr, serum electrolytes, and serum K^+ levels. Monitor for MI, CHF, head/neck and intestinal angioedema, anaphylactoid reactions, hepatic failure, hypersensitivity reactions, cough, N/V, dizziness, oliguria and azotemia.

Patient Counseling: Counsel about fetal risks during pregnancy and signs/symptoms of angioedema (eg, laryngeal/tongue edema, abdominal pain); advise to seek prompt medical attention if symptoms develop. Inform about adverse effects (eg, anaphylaxis, cough, hypotension, hyperkalemia, neutropenia). Inform about need for periodic monitoring of electrolytes and blood counts. Caution that inadequate fluid intake, excessive perspiration, diarrhea, vomiting may lead to excessive fall in BP, resulting in lightheadedness and possible syncope. Advise not to use K^+ supplements or salt substitutes. Instruct to take 1 hr before meals.

Administration: Oral route. **Storage:** Room temperature; protect from excessive moisture.

UROXATRAL   RX
alfuzosin HCl (Sanofi-Aventis)

THERAPEUTIC CLASS: Alpha$_1$-antagonist

INDICATIONS: Treatment of signs and symptoms of benign prostatic hyperplasia (BPH).

DOSAGE: *Adults:* 10mg qd, with same meal each day. Swallow tab whole; do not chew or crush.

HOW SUPPLIED: Tab, Extended-Release: 10mg

CONTRAINDICATIONS: Moderate or severe hepatic impairment (Child-Pugh categories B and C), concomitant use of potent CYP3A4 inhibitors (eg, ketoconazole, itraconazole, ritonavir).

WARNINGS/PRECAUTIONS: Postural hypotension with or without symptoms may develop within few hours after administration; caution with symptomatic hypotension. Syncope may occur. Rule out the presence of prostatic cancer prior to therapy. D/C with new or worsening of angina pectoris symptoms. Caution with severe renal impairment, mild hepatic impairment, and congenital or acquired QT prolongation. Intraoperative floppy iris syndrome (IFIS) observed in some patients during cataract surgery. Priapism (rare) associated with use; may lead to permanent impotence if not properly treated. May impair mental/physical abilities. Not for treatment of HTN.

ADVERSE REACTIONS: Dizziness, upper respiratory tract infection, headache, fatigue.

INTERACTIONS: See Contraindications. Avoid use with other α-blockers. Increased levels with cimetidine, atenolol, and moderate CYP3A4 inhibitors (eg, diltiazem). Increased risk of hypotension/postural hypotension and syncope with nitrates and other antihypertensives. Caution with medications that prolong the QT interval. Caution with PDE5 inhibitors; may potentially cause symptomatic hypotension.

PREGNANCY: Category B, safety not known in nursing.

MECHANISM OF ACTION: α$_1$-antagonist; inhibits α$_1$-adrenergic receptors in lower urinary tract causing smooth muscle in bladder neck and prostate to relax, which results in improved urine flow and decreased symptoms of BPH.

PHARMACOKINETICS: Absorption: Absolute bioavailability (49%), C_{max}=13.6ng/mL, T_{max}=8 hrs, AUC_{0-24}=194ng•hr/mL. **Distribution:** V_d=3.2L/kg (IV); plasma protein binding (82-90%). **Metabolism:** Liver (extensive) via CYP3A4 (oxidation, O-demethylation, N-dealkylation). **Elimination:** Feces (69%), urine (24%, 11% unchanged); $T_{1/2}$=10 hrs.

NURSING CONSIDERATIONS

Assessment: Assess for BPH, prostatic cancer, symptomatic hypotension, history of QT prolongation, hepatic/renal impairment, cataract surgery, hypersensitivity, and possible drug interactions.

Monitoring: Monitor for postural hypotension, syncope, hypersensitivity reactions, IFIS, QT prolongation, hepatic/renal dysfunction, adverse reactions, and urine flow.

Patient Counseling: Inform about possible occurrence of symptoms related to postural hypotension such as dizziness. Caution about driving, operating machinery, or performing hazardous tasks during initial treatment. Tell ophthalmologist about using the product before cataract surgery or other procedures involving the eyes. Advise about the possibility of priapism resulting from treatment; seek immediate medical attention. Take the drug with food and with the same meal each day. Do not crush or chew tablets. Keep out or reach of children.

Administration: Oral route. Swallow tab whole; do not chew or crush.
Storage: 25°C (77°F); excursions permitted to 15-30°C (59-86°F). Protect from light and moisture.

VAGIFEM   RX
estradiol (Novo Nordisk)

> Estrogens increase the risk of endometrial cancer. Perform adequate diagnostic measures, including directed or random endometrial sampling when indicated, to rule out malignancy in postmenopausal women with undiagnosed persistent or recurring abnormal genital bleeding. Do not use as monotherapy or concomitant with progestin for the prevention of cardiovascular (CV) disease or probable dementia. Increased risk of stroke, deep vein thrombosis (DVT), pulmonary embolism (PE), myocardial infarction (MI), and invasive breast cancer in postmenopausal women. Should be prescribed at lowest effective doses and for shortest duration consistent with treatment goals and risks for individual women.

THERAPEUTIC CLASS: Estrogen

INDICATIONS: Treatment of atrophic vaginitis due to menopause.

DOSAGE: *Adults:* Initial: Insert 1 tab vaginally qd for 2 weeks. Maint: Insert 1 tab twice weekly. Generally, women should be started at the 10mcg dosage strength.

HOW SUPPLIED: Tab, Vaginal: 10mcg

CONTRAINDICATIONS: Breast carcinoma or other estrogen-dependent neoplasia, abnormal genital bleeding, pregnancy, active DVT, PE, arterial thromboembolic disease (eg, stroke, MI) or history of these conditions, and liver dysfunction or disease.

WARNINGS/PRECAUTIONS: Risk of gallbladder disease, thromboembolism, thrombotic disease, retinal vascular disease. May elevate BP, thyroid binding globulin levels, and plasma TG leading to pancreatitis. Monitor for hypercalcemia in breast cancer and bone metastases. Caution in asthma, epilepsy, migraine, porphyria, systemic lupus erythematosus, diabetes mellitus (DM), hepatic hemangiomas, cardiac or renal dysfunction due to fluid retention, liver dysfunction and metabolic bone disease associated with hypercalcemia. Few cases of local abrasion and malignant transformation of residual endometrial implants reported. Caution in young patients. For vaginal administration only.

ADVERSE REACTIONS: Headache, abdominal pain, respiratory infection, genital moniliasis, back pain, diarrhea, vulvovaginal mycotic infection, vulvovaginal pruritis.

INTERACTIONS: Reduced plasma concentration resulting in decrease in therapeutic effects and/or changes in uterine bleeding profile with CYP3A4 inducers (eg, St. Johns wort, phenobarbital, carbamazepine, rifampin). Increases plasma concentrations, which may result in side effects with CYP3A4 inhibitors (eg, erythromycin, clarithromycin, ketoconazole, itraconazole, ritonavir, and grapefruit juice).

PREGNANCY: Contraindicated in pregnancy. Caution in nursing.

MECHANISM OF ACTION: Estrogen (estradiol); acts through binding to nuclear receptors in estrogen-responsive tissues. Reduce elevated levels of gonodotropins, luteinizing hormone (LH), and follicle-stimulating hormone (FSH) seen in postmenopausal women through a negative feedback mechanism.

PHARMACOKINETICS: Absorption: Well absorbed. **Metabolism:** Liver; estrone, estriol (metabolites). **Elimination:** Urine.

NURSING CONSIDERATIONS

Assessment: Assess for abnormal genital bleeding, strong family history of breast cancer, abnormal mammograms, or any other conditions where treatment is contraindicated or cautioned. Assess for hepatic/renal impairment, pregnancy status, and possible drug interactions. Perform exam of breast, and pelvic organs; obtain BP, serum TG, and calcium levels.

Monitoring: Monitor BP, serum TG, and calcium levels periodically; perform exams routinely. Monitor for abnormal vaginal bleeding, gallbladder disease, HTN, hyperglycemia, fluid retention, trauma from applicator, hypercalcemia, hepatic dysfunction, and hypersensitivity reactions.

Patient Counseling: Advise to seek medical attention for symptoms of abnormal vaginal bleeding, gallbladder disease, abdominal pain/tenderness, HTN, hyperglycemia, fluid retention, trauma from applicator, hypercalcemia, hepatic dysfunction (eg, jaundice), or hypersensitivity reactions. Instruct to insert applicator carefully if atrophic vaginal mucosa present.

Administration: Intravaginal route. **Storage:** 25°C (77°F); excursions permitted to 15-30°C (59-86°F). Do not refrigerate.

VALCYTE   RX
valganciclovir HCl (Genentech)

> Granulocytopenia, anemia, and thrombocytopenia reported. Carcinogenic, teratogenic, and may cause aspermatogenesis based on animal studies.

THERAPEUTIC CLASS: Synthetic guanine derivative nucleoside analogue

INDICATIONS: (Tab) Treatment of cytomegalovirus (CMV) retinitis in adult patients with AIDS and prevention of CMV disease in adult kidney, heart, or kidney-pancreas transplant patients at high risk (donor CMV seropositive/recipient CMV seronegative). (Tab/Sol) Prevention of CMV disease in kidney or heart transplant patients (4 months-16 yrs of age) at high risk.

DOSAGE: *Adults:* Treatment of CMV Retinitis: Initial: 900mg bid for 21 days. Maint: 900mg qd. Prevention of CMV Disease: Heart/Kidney-Pancreas Transplant: 900mg qd starting within 10 days of transplantation until 100 days post-transplantation. Kidney Transplant: 900mg qd starting within 10 days of transplantation until 200 days post-transplantation. Renal Impairment: CrCl ≥60mL/min: Initial: 900mg bid. Maint: 900mg qd. CrCl 40-59mL/min: Initial: 450mg bid. Maint: 450mg qd. CrCl 25-39mL/min: Initial: 450mg qd. Maint: 450mg every 2 days. CrCl 10-24mL/min: Initial: 450mg every 2 days. Maint: 450mg 2X weekly. Elderly: Start at low end of dosing range. Take with food.

Pediatrics: 4 months-16 yrs: Prevention of CMV Disease: Recommended once-daily dose starting within 10 days of transplantation until 100 days post-transplantation is based on body surface area (BSA) and creatinine clearance (CrCl) derived from modified Schwartz formula. Refer to PI for dose calculations.

HOW SUPPLIED: Tab: 450mg; Sol: 50mg/mL

WARNINGS/PRECAUTIONS: Severe leukopenia, neutropenia, anemia, thrombocytopenia, pancytopenia, bone marrow aplasia, and aplastic anemia reported. Avoid if absolute neutrophil count <500cells/μL, platelet count <25,000/μL, or Hgb <8g/dL. Cytopenia may occur; caution with pre-existing cytopenias. Acute renal failure may occur in elderly and in patients without adequate hydration; maintain adequate hydration; caution in elderly and reduce dose in renal impairment. Do not substitute Valcyte tab for ganciclovir caps on a 1-to-1 basis.

ADVERSE REACTIONS: Diarrhea, N/V, pyrexia, neutropenia, anemia, cough, HTN, constipation, upper respiratory tract infection, tremor, graft rejection, thrombocytopenia.

INTERACTIONS: Greater risk for neutropenia and anemia with zidovudine. Monitor for toxicity with probenecid. Increased levels of mycophenolate mofetil metabolites and ganciclovir in patients with renal impairment. Caution with myelosuppressive drugs or irradiation. Increased risk of didanosine toxicity. Acute renal failure may occur in patients receiving nephrotoxic drugs; caution with use.

PREGNANCY: Category C, not for use in nursing.

MECHANISM OF ACTION: Guanine derivative antiviral; L-valyl ester (prodrug) of ganciclovir. Inhibits viral DNA polymerase synthesis, resulting in inhibition of human CMV replication.

PHARMACOKINETICS: Absorption: Absolute bioavailability (59.4%, Adult) (60%, Pediatrics); C_{max}=5.61μg/mL; T_{max}=1-3 hrs; AUC=29.1μg•h/mL (Tab). **Distribution:** (Ganciclovir) V_d=0.703L/kg; plasma protein binding (1-2%). **Metabolism:** Intestinal wall, liver (hydrolysis). **Elimination:** Renal; $T_{1/2}$=4.08 hrs. Refer to PI for different parameters.

NURSING CONSIDERATIONS

Assessment: Assess for renal impairment, pre-existing cytopenia, pregnancy/nursing status, prior/current irradiation, and possible drug interactions. Obtain baseline ANC, platelet count and Hgb.

Monitoring: Monitor CBC with differential and platelet counts frequently. Perform ophthalmologic exams every 4-6 weeks during therapy. Monitor for signs/symptoms of drug toxicity (eg, granulocytopenia, anemia, thrombocytopenia), cytopenia, infertility, renal dysfunction, and hypersensitivity reactions.

Patient Counseling: Counsel to avoid direct contact of broken or crushed tab and oral solution with skin or mucous membranes; if contact occurs, wash thoroughly with soap and water. Advise not to substitute Valcyte tablet for ganciclovir capsules on a 1-to-1 basis. Instruct adults to use tablets, not the oral solution. Inform patients of major toxicities (eg, granulocytopenia, anemia, thrombocytopenia) and possible elevations in SrCr; may need to adjust dose or d/c. Instruct to take with food. Advise patients of possible decreased fertility. Advise women not to use during pregnancy/breast-feeding. Advise women of childbearing potential to use effective contraception during and for at least 30 days following treatment. Consider the drug a potential carcinogen. Therapy may impair physical/mental ability. May continue to experience progression of CMV retinitis during or following treatment. Have ophthalmologic exams every 4-6 weeks while being treated. Keep out of reach of children.

Administration: Oral route. Take with food; do not break or crush tabs. **Storage:** Tab/Dry Powder: 25°C (77°F); excursions permitted to 15-30°C (59-86°F). Reconstituted Sol: 2-8°C (36-46°F) for no longer than 49 days. Do not freeze.

V

VALIUM

CIV

diazepam (Roche Labs)

THERAPEUTIC CLASS: Benzodiazepine

INDICATIONS: Management of anxiety disorders and short-term relief of anxiety symptoms. Symptomatic relief of acute alcohol withdrawal. Adjunct therapy for convulsive disorders and relief of skeletal muscle spasms.

DOSAGE: *Adults:* Individualize dose. Anxiety Disorders/Anxiety Symptoms: 2-10mg bid-qid. Acute Alcohol Withdrawal: 10mg tid-qid for 24 hrs. Reduce to 5mg tid-qid prn. Skeletal Muscle Spasm: 2-10mg tid-qid. Convulsive Disorders: 2-10mg bid-qid. Elderly/Debilitated: 2-2.5mg qd-bid initially. May increase gradually prn if tolerated.
Pediatrics: ≥6 months: 1-2.5mg tid-qid initially. May increase gradually prn if tolerated.

HOW SUPPLIED: Tab: 2mg*, 5mg*, 10mg* *scored

CONTRAINDICATIONS: Acute narrow-angle glaucoma, patients <6 months, myasthenia gravis, severe respiratory insufficiency, severe hepatic insufficiency, sleep apnea syndrome.

WARNINGS/PRECAUTIONS: Not recommended for the treatment of psychotic patients. Increase in frequency and/or severity of grand mal seizures may occur during adjunctive therapy and may require an increase in the dose of the standard anticonvulsant medication. May temporarily increase frequency and/or severity of seizures during abrupt withdrawal. Psychiatric and paradoxical reactions may occur; d/c if these occur. Lower dose with chronic respiratory insufficiency. Caution with history of alcohol and drug abuse. Prolonged use may result in loss of response to the effects of benzodiazepines.

ADVERSE REACTIONS: Drowsiness, fatigue, muscle weakness, ataxia, confusion, vertigo, constipation, blurred vision, dizziness, hypotension, stimulation, agitation, incontinence, skin reactions, hypersalivation.

INTERACTIONS: Mutually potentiates effects with phenothiazines, antipsychotics, anxiolytics/sedatives, hypnotics, anticonvulsants, narcotic analgesics, anesthetics, sedative antihistamines, narcotics, barbiturates, MAOIs, and other antidepressants. Alcohol enhances sedative effects; avoid concomitant use. Increased and prolonged sedation with cimetidine, ketoconazole, fluvoxamine, fluoxetine, and omeprazole. Diazepam decreases metabolic elimination of phenytoin.

PREGNANCY: Category D, not for use in nursing.

MECHANISM OF ACTION: Benzodiazepine; exerts anxiolytic, sedative, muscle-relaxant, anticonvulsant, and amnestic effects. Facilitates GABA, an inhibitory neurotransmitter in the CNS.

PHARMACOKINETICS: Absorption: T_{max}=1-1.5 hrs. **Distribution:** V_d=0.8-1.0L/kg; plasma protein binding (98%); crosses blood-brain/placental barrier, and appears in breast milk. **Metabolism:** Via N-demethylation and hydroxylation by CYP3A4 and CYP2C19 enzymes, glucuronidation; N-desmethyldiazepam, temazepam, oxazepam (active metabolites). **Elimination:** Urine; $T_{1/2}$=48 hrs, 100 hrs (N-desmethyldiazepam).

NURSING CONSIDERATIONS

Assessment: Assess for anxiety disorders/symptoms, acute alcohol withdrawal, skeletal muscle spasm, convulsive disorders, depression, and other conditions where treatment is contraindicated or cautioned. Assess for pregnancy/nursing status and possible drug interactions.

Monitoring: Monitor for hypersensitivity reactions, rebound or withdrawal symptoms, seizures, psychiatric and paradoxical reactions, and respiratory depression.

Patient Counseling: Advise to consult physician before increasing dose or abruptly d/c the drug. Advise against simultaneous ingestion of alcohol and other CNS depressants during therapy. Caution against engaging in hazardous occupations requiring complete mental alertness, such as operating machinery or driving a motor vehicle.

Administration: Oral route. **Storage:** 15-30°C (59-86°F).

VALSTAR

RX

valrubicin (Endo)

THERAPEUTIC CLASS: Anthracycline

INDICATIONS: Intravesical therapy of BCG-refractory carcinoma *in situ* (CIS) of the urinary bladder in patients for whom immediate cystectomy would be associated with unacceptable morbidity or mortality.

DOSAGE: *Adults:* 800mg intravesically once weekly for 6 weeks. Delay administration for at least 2 weeks after transurethral resection and/or fulguration. The patient should retain the drug for 2 hrs before voiding.

HOW SUPPLIED: Inj: 40mg/mL

CONTRAINDICATIONS: Concurrent UTI, small bladder capacity (unable to tolerate a 75mL instillation).

WARNINGS/PRECAUTIONS: Avoid in patients with a perforated bladder or to those in whom the integrity of the bladder mucosa has been compromised. Caution with severe irritable bladder symptoms. Bladder spasm and spontaneous discharge of the intravesical instillate may occur; clamping of urinary catheter is not advised and, if performed, should be executed under medical supervision and with caution. Skin reactions and eye irritation may occur with accidental exposure; caution in handling and preparing the solution. If there is not a complete response of CIS to treatment after 3 months or if CIS recurs, cystectomy must be reconsidered.

ADVERSE REACTIONS: Asthenia, headache, malaise, urinary frequency, urinary retention, urinary incontinence, dysuria, urinary urgency, bladder spasm, hematuria, bladder pain, cystitis, local burning symptoms, UTI, nausea.

PREGNANCY: Category C, not for use in nursing.

MECHANISM OF ACTION: Anthracycline; inhibits the incorporation of nucleosides into nucleic acids, causing extensive chromosomal damage, and arresting cell cycle in G_2.

PHARMACOKINETICS: Absorption: $AUC_{0-6\,hrs}$=78nmol/L•hr (900mg), 788nmol/L•hr (800mg)

NURSING CONSIDERATIONS

Assessment: Assess status of bladder, urinary tract infection, pregnancy and nursing status.

Monitoring: Monitor for local bladder symptoms, disease recurrence or progression, hypersensitivity reactions and pregnancy during treatment. Cystoscopy, biopsy, and urine cytology are recommended every 3 months.

Patient Counseling: Counsel on the risk/benefits associated with treatment. Instruct to maintain adequate hydration. Advise to report immediately prolonged irritable bladder symptoms or prolonged passage of red-colored urine. Inform men to refrain from procreative activities. Advise women of childbearing potential not to become pregnant and to use effective contraception method during treatment period.

Administration: Intravesical route. Use gloves during preparation and administration. **Storage:** (Vials) 2-8°C (36-46°F). Vials should not be heated. Diluted Solution: Stable for 12 hrs up to 25°C (77°F). Valrubicin should not be mixed with other drugs. Do not freeze.

V

VALTREX

RX

valacyclovir HCl (GlaxoSmithKline)

THERAPEUTIC CLASS: Nucleoside analogue

INDICATIONS: Treatment of herpes labialis (cold sores) in patients ≥12 yrs. Treatment of herpes zoster (shingles) in immunocompetent adults. Treatment of initial and recurrent episodes of genital herpes in immunocompetent adults, chronic suppressive therapy of recurrent episodes of genital herpes in immunocompetent and in HIV-infected adults, and reduction of transmission of genital herpes in immunocompetent adults. Treatment of chickenpox in immunocompetent patients 2 to <18 yrs.

DOSAGE: *Adults:* Herpes Zoster: 1g tid for 7 days. Start within 48 hrs after onset of rash. CrCl 30-49mL/min: 1g q12h. CrCl 10-29mL/min: 1g q24h. CrCl <10mL/min: 500mg q24h. Genital Herpes: Initial Episode: 1g bid for 10 days. Start within 48 hrs after onset of symptoms. CrCl 10-29mL/min: 1g q24h. CrCl <10mL/min: 500mg q24h. Recurrent Episodes: Treatment: 500mg bid for 3 days. Start at 1st sign/symptom of episode. CrCl ≤10-29mL/min: 500mg q24h. Suppressive Therapy w/ Normal Immune Function: 1g qd. CrCl ≤10-29mL/min: 500mg q24h. Alternative: (≤9 episodes/yr) 500mg qd. CrCl ≤10-29mL/min: 500mg q48h. Suppressive Therapy with HIV and CD4 ≥100 cells/mm³: 500mg q12h. CrCl ≤10-29mL/min: 500mg q24h. Reduction of Transmission of Genital Herpes (≤9 episodes/yr): 500mg qd for the source partner. Herpes Labialis: 2g q12h for 1 day. Start at earliest symptom of cold sore. CrCl 30-49mL/min: 1g q12h. CrCl 10-29mL/min: 500mg q12h. CrCl <10mL/min: 500mg single dose. Do not exceed 1 day of treatment. *Pediatrics:* Herpes Labialis: ≥12 yrs: 2g q12h for 1 day. Start at earliest symptom of cold sore. Chickenpox: 2 to <18 yrs: 20mg/kg tid for 5 days. Max: 1g tid. Initiate at the earliest sign/symptom of chickenpox.

HOW SUPPLIED: Tab: 500mg, 1g* *partially scored

WARNINGS/PRECAUTIONS: Thrombotic thrombocytopenic purpura/ hemolytic uremic syndrome (TTP/HUS) reported with advanced HIV disease, allogeneic bone marrow transplants, and in renal transplant patients. Cases of acute renal failure reported in elderly patients with or without reduced renal function, in patients with underlying renal disease who receive higher than recommended doses of valacyclovir for their level of renal function, and in patients without adequate hydration; reduce dose with renal dysfunction and maintain adequate hydration. Caution in elderly. CNS adverse reactions (eg, agitation, hallucinations, confusion, delirium, seizures, encephalopathy) are more likely in elderly but are also reported in adult and pediatric patients with or without reduced renal function and in patients with underlying renal disease; d/c if these occur.

ADVERSE REACTIONS: Headache, N/V, abdominal pain, dysmenorrhea, arthralgia, nasopharyngitis, fatigue, rash, upper respiratory tract infections, pyrexia, decreased neutrophil counts, diarrhea, elevated ALT/AST.

INTERACTIONS: Caution with other potentially nephrotoxic drugs.

PREGNANCY: Category B, caution in nursing.

MECHANISM OF ACTION: Nucleoside analogue; converted to acyclovir which inhibits replication of herpes viral DNA by competitively inhibiting viral DNA polymerase, incorporating and terminating growing viral DNA chain, and inactivating viral DNA polymerase.

PHARMACOKINETICS: Absorption: Rapid (GI tract); Acyclovir absolute bioavailability (54.5%). Oral administration of variable doses resulted in different parameters. **Distribution:** Valacyclovir: Plasma protein binding (13.5-17.9%). Acyclovir: Plasma protein binding (9-33%). Found in breast milk. **Metabolism:** Hepatic/Intestinal (1st pass) to acyclovir and L-valine. **Elimination:** Urine (46%), feces (47%); $T_{1/2}$=2.5-3.3 hrs.

NURSING CONSIDERATIONS

Assessment: Assess for renal impairment, age of patient, pregnancy/nursing status, hydration status, and for possible drug interactions. Assess for presence of advanced HIV disease, an allogeneic bone transplant, and for the presence of a renal transplant.

Monitoring: Monitor for signs/symptoms of renal toxicity. Monitor for signs/ symptoms of TTP/HUS in patients with advanced HIV disease, allogeneic bone marrow transplant patients, and in patients who are renal transplant recipients. Monitor for CNS effects such as agitation, hallucinations, confusion, delirium, seizures and encephalopathy.

Patient Counseling: Advise to maintain adequate hydration. Inform that product is not a cure for cold sores or genital herpes. In patients with genital herpes, instruct to avoid contact with lesions or sexual intercourse when lesions and/or symptoms are present to avoid infecting partner(s); use safe sex practice in combination with suppressive therapy. In patients with cold sores, instruct to initiate treatment at earliest symptom of a cold sore (eg, tingling, itching, burning); treatment should not exceed 1 day (2 doses) and that doses should be taken 12 hrs apart. In patients with herpes zoster, advise to initiate treatment as soon as possible after diagnosis. In patients with chickenpox, advise to initiate treatment at the earliest sign or symptom of chickenpox.

Administration: Oral route. **Storage:** 15-25°C (59-77°F). Dispense in well-closed container.

VALTROPIN   RX
somatropin (LG Life)

THERAPEUTIC CLASS: Human growth hormone

INDICATIONS: Treatment of pediatric patients who have growth failure due to inadequate secretion of endogenous growth hormone. Treatment of growth failure associated with Turner syndrome in pediatric patients who have open epiphyses. Long-term replacement therapy in adults with growth hormone deficiency (GHD) of either adult or childhood onset etiology.

DOSAGE: *Adults:* Individualize dose. Initial: 0.33mg/day SQ 6 days a week. Dosage may be increased to individual patient requirement to maximum of 0.66mg/day after 4 weeks. Alternative Dosing: 0.2mg/day (Range: 0.15-0.3mg/day). May increase gradually every 1-2 months by 0.1-0.2mg/day based on individual patient requirements.
Pediatrics: Individualize dose. Divide weekly dose into equal amounts given either daily or 6 days a week by SQ injection. GHD: 0.17-0.3mg/kg of body weight/week. Turner Syndrome: Up to 0.375mg/kg of body weight/week.

HOW SUPPLIED: Inj: 5mg

CONTRAINDICATIONS: Pediatrics with closed epiphyses. Active proliferative and severe non-proliferative diabetic retinopathy. Presence of active malignancy. Acute critical illness due to complications following open heart surgery, abdominal surgery, or multiple accidental trauma, or those with acute respiratory failure. Patients with Prader-Willi syndrome who are severely obese or have severe respiratory impairment.

WARNINGS/PRECAUTIONS: Known sensitivity to supplied diluent (meta-cresol). Caution in pediatric pateints with Prader-Willi syndrome with 1 or more risk factors (severe obesity, history of upper airway destruction or sleep apnea, or unidentified respiratory infection). May decrease insulin sensitivity. Patients with GHD secondary to intracranial lesion should be monitored closely for progression or recurrence of underlying disease process. Intracranial HTN reported. Monitor closely with DM, glucose intolerance, hypopituitarism. Funduscopic exam recommended at initiation and periodically during course of therapy. Monitor carefully for any malignant transformation of skin lesions.

ADVERSE REACTIONS: Headache, pyrexia, cough, respiratory tract infection, diarrhea, vomiting, pharyngitis.

INTERACTIONS: Growth-promoting effects may be inhibited by glucocorticoids. May alter clearance of compounds metabolized by CYP450 liver enzymes (eg, corticosteroids, sex steroids, anticonvulsants, cyclosporine); monitor closely. May need insulin adjustment.

PREGNANCY: Category B, caution in nursing.

MECHANISM OF ACTION: Human growth hormone; stimulates linear growth synthesis, metabolizes lipids, reduces body fat stores by increasing cellular protein, and increases plasma fatty acids.

PHARMACOKINETICS: Absorption: C_{max}=43.97ng/mL, T_{max}=4 hrs, AUC=369.9ng•hr/mL. **Metabolism:** Liver, kidneys (protein catabolism). **Elimination:** $T_{1/2}$=3.03 hrs.

NURSING CONSIDERATIONS

Assessment: Assess for hypersensitivity to benzyl alcohol, history of scoliosis, pre-existing papilledema, hypothyroidism, diagnostic imaging (pituitary or intracranial tumor), hypopituitarism, possible drug interactions, and any other

V

condition where treatment is contraindicated or cautioned. Obtain baseline funduscopic exam. Prader-Willi syndrome: Evaluate for signs of upper airway obstruction or sleep apnea before initiation. Turner syndrome: Evaluate for otitis media or other ear disorders, and CV disorders before initiation.

Monitoring: Monitor fasting blood glucose and thyroid function tests periodically, periodic fundoscopic exam, weight control (Prader-Willi syndrome), signs/symptoms of malignant transformation of skin lesions, intracranial HTN, slipped capital femoral epiphysis (eg, onset of limp, hip or knee pain), hypersensitivity/allergic reactions, respiratory infections (Prader-Willi syndrome), otitis media or ear disorders, CV disorders and progression of scoliosis.

Patient Counseling: Instruct thoroughly as to proper usage and disposal. Caution against any reuse of needles and syringes. Seek medical attention if signs/symptoms of slipped capital femoral epiphysis (eg, onset of limp, hip or knee pain), hypersensitivity/allergic reactions, respiratory infections (Prader-Willi syndrome), otitis media or CV disorders or progression of scoliosis occur.

Administration: SQ route (thighs). **Storage:** Before reconstitution: 2-8°C (36-46°F). Do not freeze. After reconstitution: 2-8°C (36-46°F) for up to 21 days. Do not freeze.

VALTURNA
RX

aliskiren - valsartan (Novartis)

> When used in pregnancy during the 2nd and 3rd trimesters, drugs that act directly on the renin-angiotensin-aldosterone system (RAAS) can cause injury and death to the developing fetus; d/c immediately if pregnancy is detected.

THERAPEUTIC CLASS: Renin inhibitor/angiotensin II receptor antagonist

INDICATIONS: Treatment of HTN. May be used as an add-on therapy in patients whose BP is not adequately controlled with aliskiren alone or valsartan (or another angiotensin receptor blocker) alone. May be substituted for titrated components. May be used as initial therapy in patients who are likely to need multiple drugs to achieve BP goals.

DOSAGE: *Adults:* Add-on/Initial Therapy: 150mg-160mg qd. Titrate: May increase up to 300mg-320mg if BP remains uncontrolled after 2-4 weeks. Max: 300mg-320mg qd. Replacement Therapy: May substitute for individually titrated components.

HOW SUPPLIED: Tab: (Aliskiren-Valsartan) 150mg-160mg, 300mg-320mg

WARNINGS/PRECAUTIONS: Angioedema of the face, extremities, lips, tongue, glottis and/or larynx reported; d/c immediately and do not readminister if angioedema develops. May cause symptomatic hypotension with activated RAAS (eg, volume-/salt-depleted patients); correct condition prior to therapy. Caution with heart failure (HF) or recent myocardial infarction (MI) and in those undergoing surgery/dialysis. Not recommended for use as initial therapy in patients with intravascular volume depletion. Increases in BUN and SrCr reported in patients with unilateral/bilateral renal artery stenosis. Changes in renal function may occur in volume-depleted patients. Clearance of valsartan lowered in patients with mild-to-moderate hepatic impairment, including biliary obstructive disorders. Minor and transient increases in BUN, SrCr, and K+ may occur in patients with HF and pre-existing renal impairment; dose reduction and/or d/c may be required. Hyperkalemia reported; periodic determinations of serum electrolytes is recommended.

ADVERSE REACTIONS: Hyperkalemia, fatigue, nasopharyngitis, diarrhea, upper respiratory tract infection, urinary tract infection, influenza, vertigo.

INTERACTIONS: Symptomatic hypotension may occur in volume- and/or salt-depleted patients receiving high doses of diuretics. (Aliskiren) Avoid with cyclosporine or itraconazole. Potential drug interaction with p-glycoprotein inhibitors. (Valsartan) May increase systemic exposure with inhibitors of the hepatic uptake transporter OATP1B1 (rifampin, cyclosporine) or the hepatic efflux transporter MRP2 (ritonavir). Increased serum K+ levels and increased SrCr in HF patients with K+ sparing diuretics, K+ supplements, salt substitutes containing K⁺ or other drugs that increase K⁺ levels; caution when coadministering.

PREGNANCY: Category D, not for use in nursing.

MECHANISM OF ACTION: Aliskiren: Renin inhibitor; lowers BP by directly inhibiting renin, decreasing plasma renin activity, and inhibiting conversion of angiotensinogen to angiotensin I. Valsartan: Angiotensin II receptor antagonist; blocks vasoconstrictor and aldosterone-secreting effects of angiotensin II by selectively blocking the binding of angiotensin II to the AT_1 receptor.

PHARMACOKINETICS: Administration: T_{max}=1 hr (aliskiren), 3 hrs (valsartan). **Distribution:** (Valsartan) (IV) V_d=17L; plasma protein binding (95%). **Metabolism:** (Aliskiren) Via CYP3A4. (Valsartan) Via CYP2C9; Valeryl-4-hydroxy valsartan (primary metabolite). **Elimination:** (Aliskiren) Urine (25%, unchanged). (Valsartan) (PO) Feces (83%), urine (13%); (IV) $T_{1/2}$=6 hrs.

NURSING CONSIDERATIONS

Assessment: Assess for history of angioedema, activated RAAS, renal artery stenosis, renal/hepatic impairment, surgery/dialysis, HF, recent/post-MI, biliary obstructive disorders, pregnancy/nursing status, and possible drug interactions. Obtain baseline BP and renal function.

Monitoring: Monitor for angioedema of throat, tongue, glottis and/or larynx, airway obstruction, hypotension, and hyperkalemia. Monitor BP, serum electrolytes, and renal function, including BUN, SrCr, and K⁺ levels.

Patient Counseling: Instruct to inform doctor or pharmacist if any unusual symptoms develop, or if any known symptoms persist or worsen. Drug may cause fetal harm; report pregnancies to physicians immediately. Lightheadedness may occur, especially during the 1st days of therapy; report immediately to physician and d/c if syncope occurs. Inadequate fluid intake, excessive perspiration, diarrhea, or vomiting can lead to an excessive fall in BP, with the same consequences of lightheadedness and possible syncope. Avoid taking K⁺ supplements or salt substitutes containing K⁺ without consulting a physician. Establish a routine pattern for taking medication with regard to meals; high-fat meals decrease absorption substantially.

Administration: Oral route. **Storage:** 25°C (77°F); excursions permitted to 15-30°C (59-86°F).

VANCOCIN ORAL   RX
vancomycin HCl (Viro Pharma)

THERAPEUTIC CLASS: Tricyclic glycopeptide antibiotic

INDICATIONS: Treatment of enterocolitis caused by *Staphylococcus aureus* and antibiotic-associated pseudomembranous colitis caused by *Clostridium difficile*.

DOSAGE: *Adults:* 500mg-2g/day given tid-qid for 7-10 days. Elderly: Start at lower end of dosing range.
Pediatrics: 40mg/kg/day given tid-qid for 7-10 days. Max: 2g/day.

HOW SUPPLIED: Cap: 125mg, 250mg

WARNINGS/PRECAUTIONS: Use in the absence of a proven or strongly suspected bacterial infection or a prophylactic indication is unlikely to provide benefit and increases the risk of drug-resistant bacteria. Monitoring serum concentrations may be appropriate in some instances (eg, renal insufficiency and/or colitis). Not effective for other types of infection. Caution with inflammatory disorders of intestinal mucosa, renal impairment; may have increased systemic absorption and may be at risk for development of adverse reactions associated with parenteral administration of vancomycin. Ototoxicity reported; caution in patients with underlying hearing loss; consider performing serial tests of auditory function during use to minimize ototoxicity risk. Monitor renal function in patients with underlying renal dysfunction. May cause overgrowth of nonsusceptible organisms; take appropriate measures if superinfection develops. Caution in elderly.

V

ADVERSE REACTIONS: Nephrotoxicity, ototoxicity, reversible neutropenia, anaphylactoid reactions (hypotension, wheezing, "Red Man syndrome," pruritus).

INTERACTIONS: Monitor renal function with aminoglycosides. Increased risk of ototoxicity when used concurrently with other ototoxic agents (eg, aminoglycosides).

PREGNANCY: Category B, caution in nursing.

MECHANISM OF ACTION: Tricyclic glycopeptide antibiotic; inhibits cell-wall biosynthesis. Also alters bacterial cell membrane permeabilty and RNA synthesis.

PHARMACOKINETICS: Absorption: Poor. **Elimination:** Urine, feces.

NURSING CONSIDERATIONS

Assessment: Assess for inflammatory intestinal disorders, renal dysfunction, hearing disturbances, pregnancy/nursing status, and for possible drug interactions. Document indications for therapy, culture, and susceptibility testing.

Monitoring: Monitor signs/symptoms of ototoxicity, superinfection, and for anaphylactoid reactions. Monitor drug levels when appropriate (eg, renal insufficiency and/or colitis). Monitor renal function in patients with underlying renal dysfunction.

Patient Counseling: Inform that therapy treats bacterial, not viral infections. Instruct to take as directed; inform that skipping doses or not completing full course may decrease effectiveness and increase resistance.

Administration: Oral route. **Storage:** 59-86°F (15-30°C).

VANCOMYCIN HCL   RX
vancomycin HCl (Various)

THERAPEUTIC CLASS: Tricyclic glycopeptide antibiotic

INDICATIONS: Treatment of serious or severe infections caused by susceptible strains of methicillin-resistant (β-lactam resistant) staphylococci. Indicated for penicillin-allergic patients who cannot receive or have failed to respond to other drugs, and for infections caused by vancomycin-susceptible organisms that are resistant to other antimicrobials. Initial therapy when methicillin-resistant staphylococci are suspected. Effective in the treatment of staphylococcal endocarditis, other infections due to staphylococci, including septicemia, bone infections, lower respiratory tract infections, and skin and skin-structure infections. Effective alone or in combination with an aminoglycoside for endocarditis caused by *S.viridans* or *S.bovis*. Effective only in combination with an aminoglycoside for endocarditis caused by enterococci (eg, *E.faecalis*). Effective for treatment of diphtheroid endocarditis. Successfully used in combination with either rifampin, an aminoglycoside, or both in early-onset prosthetic valve endocarditis caused by *S.epidermidis* or diphtheroids. Parenteral form may be administered orally for treatment of antibiotic-associated pseudomembranous colitis produced by *C.difficile* and for staphylococcal enterocolitis.

DOSAGE: *Adults*: Usual: 500mg IV q6h or 1g IV q12h. Administer at no more than 10mg/min or over at least 60 min, whichever is longer. Renal Impairment: Initial: Not <15mg/kg. Dosage per day in mg is about 15X the GFR in mL/min (refer to dosage table in PI). Elderly: Require greater dose reductions than expected. Functionally Anephric Patients: Initial: 15mg/kg, then 1.9mg/kg/24 hrs. Marked Renal Impairment: 250-1000mg once every several days. Anuria: 1000mg every 7-10 days. For PO Administration: 500-2000mg/day in 3-4 divided doses for 7-10 days. Max: 2000mg/day. May dilute in 1 oz. of water. May also be administered via NG tube.
Pediatrics: Usual: 10mg/kg IV q6h. Infants/Neonates: Initial: 15mg/kg, then 10mg/kg q12h for neonates in 1st week of life and q8h thereafter until 1 month of age. Administer over at least 60 min. Renal Impairment: Initial: Not <15mg/kg. Dosage per day in mg is about 15X the GFR in mL/min (refer to table in PI). Premature Infants: Requires longer dosing intervals. ADD-Vantage

vials should not be used in neonates, infants, and pediatrics who require doses <500mg. For PO Administration: 40mg/kg/day in 3-4 divided doses for 7-10 days. Max: 2000mg/day. May dilute in 1 oz. of water. May also be administered via NG tube.

HOW SUPPLIED: Inj: 500mg, 1g

WARNINGS/PRECAUTIONS: Not effective by the oral route for other types of infections. Rapid bolus administration may cause hypotension and cardiac arrest (rare); administer in diluted solution over a period not <60 min. Ototoxicity reported; caution with underlying hearing loss. Caution with renal insufficiency and adjust dose with renal dysfunction. Pseudomembranous colitis reported. Prolonged use may result in overgrowth of nonsusceptible organisms. Reversible neutropenia reported; monitor leukocyte count periodically. Administer via IV route. Thrombophlebitis may occur; infuse slowly and rotate injection sites. Safety and efficacy of administration via the intraperitoneal and intrathecal (intralumbar and intraventricular) routes have not been established. Administration via intraperitoneal route during continuous ambulatory peritoneal dialysis (CAPD) has resulted in a syndrome of chemical peritonitis. Caution in elderly.

ADVERSE REACTIONS: Infusion-related events, hypotension, wheezing, pruritus, chest and back muscle spasm or pain, dyspnea, urticaria, nephrotoxicity, pseudomembranous colitis, ototoxicity, neutropenia, phlebitis.

INTERACTIONS: Concomitant use of anesthetic agents associated with erythema, histamine-like flushing, and anaphylactoid reactions. Concurrent and/or sequential systemic or topical use of other potentially neurotoxic and/or nephrotoxic drugs (eg, amphotericin B, aminoglycosides, bacitracin, polymyxin B, colistin, viomycin, cisplatin) requires careful monitoring. Increased risk of ototoxicity with concomitant ototoxic agents (eg, aminoglycoside). Periodic leukocyte count monitoring with drugs that may cause neutropenia. Serial monitoring of renal function and particular care following appropriate dosing to minimize risk of nephrotoxicity with concomitant aminoglycoside.

PREGNANCY: Category C, not for use in nursing.

MECHANISM OF ACTION: Tricyclic glycopeptide antibiotic; inhibits cell-wall biosynthesis, alters bacterial cell membrane permeability and RNA synthesis.

PHARMACOKINETICS: **Absorption:** (1g at 2 hrs) C_{max} =23mcg/mL; (500mg at 2 hrs) C_{max} =19mcg/mL. **Distribution:** Serum protein binding (55%). **Elimination:** Urine (75%); $T_{1/2}$=4-6 hrs.

NURSING CONSIDERATIONS

Assessment: Assess for renal function, underlying hearing loss, pregnancy/nursing status and possible drug interactions. Perform culture and susceptibility testing.

Monitoring: Monitor for hypersensitivity reactions (eg, Stevens-Johnson syndrome, vasculitis), infusion reactions (eg, hypotension, arrhythmias, "Red Neck"), thrombophlebitis, ototoxicity, renal function, diarrhea, pseudomembranous colitis, neutropenia, superinfection, and chemical peritonitis (intraperitoneal route). Monitor leukocyte count periodically.

Patient Counseling: Inform that drug treats bacterial, not viral, infections. Take as directed; skipping doses or not completing full course may decrease effectiveness and increase bacterial resistance. May experience diarrhea; notify physician if watery/bloody stools, hypersensitivity reactions, or superinfection develops.

Administration: IV, Oral route. Refer to PI for preparation for IV use. Intermittent infusion recommended. Physically incompatible with β-lactam antibiotics. Diluted sol may be given via NGT. (PO) Common flavoring syrup may be added to improve taste. **Storage:** 20-25°C (68-77°F). After reconstitution: may refrigerate for 14 days. After further dilution: may refrigerate for 14 days or 96 hrs depending on diluent used (refer to PI).

V

VANOS

RX

fluocinonide (Medicis)

THERAPEUTIC CLASS: Corticosteroid

INDICATIONS: To relieve inflammatory and pruritic manifestations of corticosteroid-responsive dermatoses in patients ≥12 yrs.

DOSAGE: *Adults:* Psoriasis/Corticosteroid Responsive Dermatoses: Apply thin layer to affected areas qd-bid ud. Atopic Dermatitis: Apply thin layer to affected areas qd ud. Max: 60g/week. Do not use >2 weeks. D/C when control is achieved. Reassess if no improvement seen within 2 weeks.
Pediatrics: ≥12 yrs: Psoriasis/Corticosteroid Responsive Dermatoses: Apply thin layer to affected areas qd-bid ud. Atopic Dermatitis: Apply thin layer to affected areas qd ud. Max: 60g/week. Do not use >2 weeks. D/C when control is achieved. Reassess if no improvement seen within 2 weeks.

HOW SUPPLIED: Cre: 0.1% [30g, 60g, 120g]

WARNINGS/PRECAUTIONS: Systemic absorption may produce reversible hypothalamic-pituitary-adrenal (HPA) axis suppression, Cushing's syndrome, hyperglycemia, and unmask latent diabetes mellitus (DM). May suppress immune system if used >2 weeks. Caution when used over large surface areas, over prolonged periods, under occlusion, on an altered skin barrier, and with liver failure; evaluate periodically for HPA axis suppression. If HPA-axis suppression occurs, withdraw drug, reduce application frequency, or substitute less potent corticosteroid. Pediatric patients may be more susceptible to systemic toxicity. Local adverse reactions may occur. Use appropriate antifungal or antibacterial agent for skin infections; d/c if favorable response does not occur. D/C if irritation occurs. HPA axis suppression, linear growth retardation, delayed weight gain, Cushing's syndrome and intracranial HTN reported in children. Not for rosacea, perioral dermatitis or application on face, groin, or axillae. Not for ophthalmic, oral or intravaginal use.

ADVERSE REACTIONS: Headache, application site burning, nasopharyngitis, nasal congestion.

INTERACTIONS: Use of >1 corticosteroid-containing product at the same time may increase total systemic absorption of topical corticosteroids.

PREGNANCY: Category C, not for use in nursing.

MECHANISM OF ACTION: Corticosteroid; possesses anti-inflammatory and antipruritic actions. Plays a role in cellular signaling, immune function inflammation, and protein regulation; precise mechanism has not been established.

PHARMACOKINETICS: Absorption: Percutaneous; extent of absorption determined by vehicle, integrity of skin and use of occlusive dressings. **Distribution:** Systemically administered corticosteroids are found in breast milk.

NURSING CONSIDERATIONS

Assessment: Assess for age of the patient, rosacea or perioral dermatitis, skin infections, inflammation or other skin diseases, liver function, previous hypersensitivity, concomitant corticosteroid use, and pregnancy/nursing status.

Monitoring: Monitor for signs/symptoms of HPA-axis suppression, Cushing's syndrome, hyperglycemia, unmasking of latent DM, skin irritation, allergic contact dermatitis (eg, failure to heal), and for development of skin infections. In pediatric patients, also monitor for linear growth retardation, delayed weight gain, and intracranial HTN. Monitor for HPA-axis suppression using an ACTH stimulation test especially with use over large surface areas, over prolonged periods, under occlusion, with altered skin barrier or with liver failure. Following withdrawal of therapy, monitor for glucocorticoid insufficiency. Monitor for signs of clinical improvement; if no improvement within 2 weeks, reassess diagnosis.

Patient Counseling: Advise to use ud by physician and not to use for any other disorder other than for which it was prescribed. Avoid contact with eyes and do not use on face, groin, and underarms. Do not use >60g/week or cover, wrap, or bandage treatment areas unless directed by physician.

Wash hands following application. Contact physician if adverse reactions (eg, burning, itching, irritation) occur or no clinical improvement seen in 2 weeks. Contact physician before using other corticosteroid-containing products. Notify physician if planning surgery during therapy. D/C therapy when control is achieved.

Administration: Topical route. **Storage:** 15-30°C (59-86°F).

VANTAS

RX

histrelin acetate (Endo)

THERAPEUTIC CLASS: Synthetic gonadotropin releasing hormone analog

INDICATIONS: Palliative treatment of advanced prostate cancer.

DOSAGE: *Adults:* Usual: 1 implant SQ (into the inner aspect of the upper arm) for 12 months. Remove after 12 months and replace with new implant.

HOW SUPPLIED: Implant: 50mg

CONTRAINDICATIONS: Women who are or may become pregnant.

WARNINGS/PRECAUTIONS: May cause transient increase in serum testosterone during 1st week of treatment; patient may experience worsening or new onset of symptoms (eg, bone pain, neuropathy, hematuria, or ureteral or bladder outlet obstruction). Spinal cord compression and ureteral obstruction reported; observe closely during 1st few weeks in patients with metastatic vertebral lesions and/or urinary tract obstruction. Difficulty in locating or removing implant may be experienced. Hyperglycemia and increased risk of developing diabetes reported; monitor blood glucose periodically. Increased risk of developing MI, sudden cardiac death, and stroke reported.

ADVERSE REACTIONS: Hot flashes, fatigue, implant-site reaction (bruising/pain/soreness/tenderness), testicular atrophy, renal impairment, gynecomastia, constipation, erectile dysfunction.

PREGNANCY: Category X, not for use in nursing.

MECHANISM OF ACTION: Synthetic gonadotropin-releasing hormone analog; acts as potent inhibitor of gonadotropin secretion when given continuously in therapeutic doses. Desensitizes responsiveness of pituitary gonadotropin, causing reduction in testicular steroidogenesis.

PHARMACOKINETICS: Absorption: C_{max}=1.1ng/mL; T_{max}=12 hrs. **Distribution:** V_d=58.4L. **Metabolism:** C-terminal dealkylation and hydrolysis. **Elimination:** $T_{1/2}$=3.92 hrs.

NURSING CONSIDERATIONS

Assessment: Assess for previous hypersensitivity, pregnancy/nursing status, metastatic vertebral lesions, urinary tract obstruction, diabetes mellitus (DM), and cardiovascular (CV) risk factors. Obtain baseline serum testosterone and prostate-specific antigen (PSA) levels.

Monitoring: Monitor for anaphylactic reactions, transient worsening or onset of new symptoms, implant-site reactions, signs/symptoms suggestive of development of CV disease, and other adverse reactions. Periodically monitor serum testosterone and PSA levels, and blood glucose and HbA1c in patients with DM.

Patient Counseling: Instruct to refrain from wetting arm for 24 hrs and from heavy lifting or strenuous exertion of arm for 7 days after implant insertion. Inform that anaphylactic reactions, transient worsening of symptoms and implant-site reactions may occur. Instruct to report to physician if the implant was expelled from the body and if the patient is experiencing unusual bleeding, redness, or pain at insertion site.

Administration: SQ implant. Refer to PI for full instructions on implant insertion/removal. **Storage:** Implant: 2-8°C (36-46°F); excursions permitted to 25°C (77°F) for 7 days. Keep in the original packaging until day of insertion. Protect from light. Do not freeze. Implantation Kit: Room temperature.

V

VAQTA RX
hepatitis A vaccine (inactivated) (Merck)

THERAPEUTIC CLASS: Vaccine

INDICATIONS: Prevention of disease caused by hepatitis A virus (HAV) in persons ≥12 months. For postexposure prophylaxis when given with immune globulin (IG).

DOSAGE: *Adults:* ≥19 yrs: 1mL IM followed by a booster of 1mL 6-18 months later. May be given as a booster dose at 6-12 months following the primary dose of another inactivated hepatitis A vaccine.
Pediatrics: 1-18 yrs: 0.5mL IM followed by a booster of 0.5mL 6-18 months later.

HOW SUPPLIED: Inj: 25 U/0.5mL, 50 U/mL

CONTRAINDICATIONS: Previous allergic reaction to neomycin.

WARNINGS/PRECAUTIONS: May not prevent hepatitis A in patients who have unrecognized hepatitis A infection at time of vaccination. Medical treatment and supervision must be available to manage possible hypersensitivity reactions. Caution when vaccinating latex-sensitive individuals; may cause allergic reactions. Immunocompromised persons may have diminished response and may not be protected against HAV infection after vaccination.

ADVERSE REACTIONS: Injection-site pain, tenderness, soreness, warmth, or redness; asthenia, myalgia, fever, headache, cough, diarrhea, upper respiratory tract infection, irritability, nausea, fatigue.

INTERACTIONS: Immunosuppressive therapy may reduce immune response.

PREGNANCY: Category C, caution in nursing.

MECHANISM OF ACTION: Vaccine; presence of antibodies confers protection against HAV infection.

NURSING CONSIDERATIONS

Assessment: Assess for hypersensitivity reactions after previous dose of hepatitis A vaccine, hypersensitivity to neomycin, immunization status/vaccination history, latex sensitivity, presence of immunosuppression, pregnancy/nursing status, and possible drug interaction.

Monitoring: Monitor for signs/symptoms of hypersensitivity reactions (eg, anaphylaxis), injection-site reactions, immune response, fever, or other possible adverse effects.

Patient Counseling: Inform of potential risks and benefits of immunization. Inform about the potential for adverse events that have been temporally associated with the vaccination. Report severe or unusual adverse events to physician or clinic where the vaccine was administered.

Administration: IM route. Shake well before use. Refer to PI for proper administration procedures. For adults, adolescents, and children >2 yrs, inject preferably into deltoid muscle. For children 12-23 months, inject at the anterolateral area of the thigh. Do not mix with any other vaccine in the same syringe or vial. **Storage:** 2-8°C (36-46°F). Do not freeze.

VARIVAX RX
varicella virus vaccine live (Merck)

THERAPEUTIC CLASS: Vaccine

INDICATIONS: Vaccination against varicella in individuals ≥12 months of age.

DOSAGE: *Adults:* 0.5mL SQ at elected date; repeat 4-8 weeks later.
Pediatrics: ≥13 yrs: 0.5mL SQ at elected date; repeat 4-8 weeks later.
12 months-12 yrs: 0.5mL SQ. If a second dose is given, administer a minimum of 3 months later.

HOW SUPPLIED: Inj: 0.5mL

CONTRAINDICATIONS: Individuals receiving immunosuppressive therapy or immunosuppressant doses of corticosteroids, history of hypersensitivity to gelatin, anaphylactoid reaction to neomycin, blood dyscrasias, leukemia, lymphomas of any type, or other malignant neoplasms affecting the bone marrow or lymphatic systems, primary and acquired immunodeficiency states, including association with AIDS or other clinical manifestations of infection with HIV, cellular immune deficiencies, and hypogammaglobulinemic and dysgammaglobulinemic states, family history of congenital or hereditary immunodeficiency, active untreated tuberculosis (TB), febrile respiratory illness or other active febrile infection, and pregnancy.

WARNINGS/PRECAUTIONS: Anaphylactoid reaction may occur; have epinephrine (1:1000) available. Defer vaccine for ≥5 months after blood or plasma transfusions, or administration of immune globulin or varicella zoster immune globulin. Defer vaccine with family history of congenital, hereditary immunodeficiency until immune system evaluated. Vaccine virus transmission may occur; avoid close association with susceptible high-risk individuals for ≤6 weeks (eg, immunocompromised patients, pregnant women without history of chickenpox). Do not inject into a blood vessel. Use separate needle and syringe for administration of each dose to prevent transfer of infectious disease. May not result in protection of all vaccinees. Pregnancy should be avoided for 3 months following vaccination.

ADVERSE REACTIONS: Fever, injection-site complaints (eg, pain/soreness, swelling and/or erythema, rash, pruritus, hematoma, induration, stiffness), varicella-like rashes.

INTERACTIONS: See Contraindications. Avoid immune globulins including varicella zoster immune globulin (VZIG) for 2 months after vaccination; defer vaccination for ≥5 months following administration of immune globulin including VZIG. Avoid salicylates for 6 weeks after vaccination.

PREGNANCY: Category C, caution in nursing.

MECHANISM OF ACTION: Vaccine; induces cell-mediated immune response against varicella zoster virus (VZV) infection.

NURSING CONSIDERATIONS

Assessment: Assess for any other conditions where treatment is contraindicated or cautioned, pregnancy/nursing status and possible drug interactions. Obtain previous immunization history and previous reaction to vaccine or similar products.

Monitoring: Monitor for signs/symptoms of allergic reactions, inj-site reactions (eg, pain, swelling, rash, hematoma, pruritus), fever, and thrombocytopenia.

Patient Counseling: Inform of potential benefits and risks of vaccination. Advise to report any adverse reactions to physician. Inform that the vaccine may not result in protection of all vaccinees. Avoid use of salicylates for 6 weeks after vaccination and avoid pregnancy 3 months after vaccination.

Administration: SQ route. Inject preferably into outer aspect of deltoid or anterolateral thigh. Refer to PI for reconstitution. Administer immediately after reconstitution; discard if not used within 30 min. **Storage:** -15°C (5°F) or colder. Prior to Reconstitution: 2-8°C (36-46°F) for ≤72 continuous hrs; discard if not used. Before reconstitution, protect from light. Diluent: 20-25°C (68-77°F), or in the refrigerator.

VASOTEC   RX
enalapril maleate (Merck)

> ACE inhibitors can cause death/injury to developing fetus during 2nd and 3rd trimesters. D/C therapy if pregnancy detected.

THERAPEUTIC CLASS: ACE inhibitor

INDICATIONS: Treatment of HTN, alone or with other antihypertensive agents (thiazide diuretics). Treatment of symptomatic chronic heart failure (CHF) usually in combination with diuretics and digitalis. To decrease overt heart failure development and hospitalization in stable asymptomatic left ventricular dysfunction.

DOSAGE: *Adults:* HTN: If possible, d/c diuretic 2-3 days prior to therapy. Initial: 5mg qd, 2.5mg qd with concomitant diuretic. Usual: 10-40mg/day given qd or bid. Resume diuretic if BP not controlled. CrCl >80mL/min: Initial: 5mg qd. CrCl >30mL-≤80/min: Initial: 5mg qd. CrCl ≤30mL/min: Initial: 2.5mg qd. Dialysis: Initial: 2.5mg qd on dialysis days. Max: 40mg qd. Heart Failure: Initial: 2.5mg qd. Usual: 2.5-20mg given bid. Max: 40mg qd. Asymptomatic Left Ventricular Dysfunction: Initial: 2.5mg bid. Titrate: Increase to 20mg qd. Hyponatremia or SrCr 1.6mg/dL with Heart Failure: Initial: 2.5mg qd. Titrate: Increase to 2.5mg bid, then 5mg bid. Max: 40mg qd.
Pediatrics: HTN: Initial: 0.08mg/kg (up to 5mg) qd. Titrate: Adjust according to response. Max: 0.58mg/kg/dose (or 40mg/dose). Avoid if GFR <30mL/min/1.73m².

HOW SUPPLIED: Tab: 2.5mg*, 5mg*, 10mg,* 20mg* *scored

CONTRAINDICATIONS: History of ACE inhibitor-associated angioedema and hereditary or idiopathic angioedema.

WARNINGS/PRECAUTIONS: D/C if angioedema, jaundice, or if marked LFT elevation occurs. Risk of hyperkalemia with DM, renal dysfunction. Persistent nonproductive cough reported. Monitor WBCs in renal or collagen vascular disease. Anaphylactoid reactions reported. Fetal/neonatal morbidity and death reported. Monitor for hypotension in high-risk patients (heart failure, surgery/anesthesia, hyponatremia, high-dose diuretic therapy, severe volume and/or salt depletion, etc). Caution with CHF, obstruction to left ventricle outflow tract, renal dysfunction, and renal artery stenosis. Less effective on BP in blacks and more reports of angioedema than nonblacks. Intestinal angioedema reported. Oliguria, progressive azotemia, acute renal failure, and death (rare) may occur in patients at high risk for hypotension.

ADVERSE REACTIONS: Fatigue, headache, dizziness, hypotension.

INTERACTIONS: May increase lithium levels. Hypotension risk with diuretics. May further decrease renal dysfunction with NSAIDs. Increased risk of hyperkalemia with K⁺-sparing diuretics, K⁺-containing salt substitutes, or K⁺ supplements. Augmented effect by antihypertensives that cause renin release (eg, thiazides). NSAIDs may diminish antihypertensive effect. Nitritoid reactions (eg, facial flushing, N/V, hypotension) reported rarely with injectable gold. Concomitant use of diuretic may increase blood urea and SrCr with HTN or CHF.

PREGNANCY: Category C (1st trimester) and D (2nd and 3rd trimesters), not for use in nursing.

MECHANISM OF ACTION: ACE inhibitor; inhibition results in decreased plasma angiotensin II, which leads to decreased vasopressor activity and decreased aldosterone secretion.

PHARMACOKINETICS: Absorption: T_{max}=1, 3-4 hrs (enalapril, enalaprilat). **Metabolism:** Via hydrolysis, enalaprilat (metabolite). **Elimination:** Urine,/feces (94%); $T_{1/2}$=11 hrs (enalaprilat).

NURSING CONSIDERATIONS

Assessment: Assess BP, LFTs, renal function, CHF, renal artery stenosis, pregnancy/nursing status, history of angioedema, and possible drug interactions.

Monitoring: Monitor BP, LFTs, renal function, CBC with platelet count and differential, serum K⁺ levels. Monitor for MI, CHF, angioedema (head, neck, intestinal), anaphylactoid reactions, hepatic failure, hypersensitivity reactions, cough, N/V, dizziness.

Patient Counseling: Counsel about fetal risks during pregnancy and signs/symptoms of angioedema (eg, laryngeal/tongue edema, abdominal pain); advise to seek prompt medical attention if symptoms develop. Inform about adverse effects (eg, anaphylaxis, cough, hypotension, hyperkalemia). Infants with histories of *in utero* exposure should be closely observed for hypotension, oliguria, hyperkalemia. Inform about need for periodic monitoring of electrolytes and blood counts. Caution that inadequate fluid intake, excessive perspiration, diarrhea, vomiting may lead to excessive fall in BP, which can result in lightheadedness or possible syncope. Advise not to use K⁺ supplements or salt substitutes containing K⁺ without consulting physician. Advise patient to report any signs of infection.

Administration: Oral route. **Storage:** (Cap) 25°C (77°F); excursions permitted to 15-30°C (59-86°F). Protect from moisture. Dispense in tight container.

VASOTEC I.V.   RX
enalaprilat (Merck)

> ACE inhibitors can cause death/injury to developing fetus during 2nd and 3rd trimesters. Stop therapy if pregnancy detected.

THERAPEUTIC CLASS: ACE inhibitor

INDICATIONS: Treatment of HTN when oral therapy is not practical.

DOSAGE: *Adults:* Administer IV over 5 min. Usual: 1.25mg q6h for no longer than 48 hrs. Max: 20mg/day. Concomitant Diuretic/CrCl ≤30mL/min: Initial: 0.625mg, may repeat after 1 hr. Maint: 1.25mg q6h. Risk of Excessive Hypotension: Initial: 0.625mg over 5 min to 1 hr. PO/IV Conversion: Give 5mg/day PO for 1.25mg IV q6h and 2.5mg/day PO for 0.625mg q6h IV.

HOW SUPPLIED: Inj: 1.25mg/mL

CONTRAINDICATIONS: History of ACE inhibitor associated angioedema and hereditary or idiopathic angioedema.

WARNINGS/PRECAUTIONS: D/C if angioedema, jaundice, or if marked LFT elevation occurs. Risk of hyperkalemia with DM, renal dysfunction. Persistent nonproductive cough reported. Monitor WBCs in renal or collagen vascular disease. Anaphylactoid reactions reported. Fetal/neonatal morbidity and death reported. Monitor for hypotension in high risk patients (heart failure, surgery/anesthesia, hyponatremia, high dose diuretic therapy, severe volume and/or salt depletion, etc). Caution with CHF, obstruction to left ventricle outflow tract, renal dysfunction, and renal artery stenosis. Less effective on BP in blacks and more reports of angioedema than nonblacks. Oliguria, progressive azotemia, acute renal failure, and death (rare) may occur in patients at high risk for hypotension.

ADVERSE REACTIONS: Hypotension, headache, angioedema, myocardial infarction, fatigue, dizziness, fever, rash, constipation, cough.

INTERACTIONS: May increase lithium levels. Hypotension risk with diuretics. May further decrease renal dysfunction with NSAIDs. Increase risk of hyperkalemia with K⁺-sparing diuretics, K⁺-containing salt substitutes or K⁺ supplements. Augmented effect by antihypertensives that cause renin release (eg, thiazides). NSAIDs may diminish antihypertensive effect.

PREGNANCY: Category C (1st trimester) and D (2nd and 3rd trimesters), not for use in nursing.

MECHANISM OF ACTION: ACE inhibitor; inhibition results in decreased plasma angiotensin II, which leads to decreased vasopressor activity and decreased aldosterone secretion.

PHARMACOKINETICS: Absorption: (PO) Poorly absorbed. **Elimination:** Urine (90% unchanged); $T_{1/2}$=11 hrs.

NURSING CONSIDERATIONS

Assessment: Assess BP, LFTs, renal function, CVD (eg, aortic stenosis, cardiomyopathy), renal artery stenosis, pregnancy/nursing status, and possible drug interactions.

Monitoring: Monitor BP, LFTs, renal function, CBC with platelet count and differential, serum K⁺ levels. Monitor for MI, CHF, angioedema (head, neck, intestinal), anaphylactoid reactions, hepatic failure, hypersensitivity reactions, cough, N/V, dizziness.

Patient Counseling: Counsel about fetal risks during pregnancy and signs/symptoms of angioedema (eg, laryngeal/tongue edema, abdominal pain);

seek prompt medical attention if any develop. Inform about adverse effects (eg, anaphylaxis, cough, hypotension, hyperkalemia, neutropenia). Infants with histories of *in utero* exposure should be closely observed for hypotension, oliguria, hyperkalemia. Inform about need for periodic monitoring of electrolytes and blood counts. Advise not to use K⁺ supplements or salt substitutes containing K⁺ without consulting physician.

Administration: IV route; inject over 5 min. **Storage:** Store below 30°C (86°F).

VECTIBIX   RX
panitumumab (Amgen)

> Dermatologic toxicities and severe infusion reactions reported. Fatal infusion reactions occurred in postmarketing experience.

THERAPEUTIC CLASS: Monoclonal antibody/EGFR-blocker

INDICATIONS: Treatment as a single agent of epidermal growth factor receptor (EGFR)-expressing, metastatic colorectal carcinoma (mCRC) with disease progression on or following fluoropyrimidine-, oxaliplatin-, and irinotecan-containing chemotherapy regimens.

DOSAGE: *Adults:* 6mg/kg IV infusion over 60 min q14 days. Infuse doses >1000mg over 90 min. Reduce infusion rate by 50% with mild or moderate (Grade 1 or 2) infusion reaction for duration of that infusion. Terminate infusion if experiencing severe infusion reactions. Depending on the severity and/or persistence of the reaction, permanently d/c treatment. Withhold for dermatologic toxicities that are ≥Grade 3 or considered intolerable. If toxicity does not improve to ≤Grade 2 within 1 month, permanently d/c. If dermatologic toxicity improves to ≤Grade 2 and symptoms improve after withholding no more than 2 doses, treatment may be resumed at 50% of original dose. If toxicities recur, permanently d/c. If toxicities do not recur, subsequent doses may be increased by increments of 25% of original dose until recommended dose of 6mg/kg is reached.

HOW SUPPLIED: Inj: 20mg/mL [5mL, 10mL, 20mL]

WARNINGS/PRECAUTIONS: D/C if severe dermatologic toxicities and infusion reactions occur. Pulmonary fibrosis reported; d/c therapy in patients developing interstitial lung disease, pneumonitis, or lung infiltrates. Hypomagnesemia and hypocalcemia may occur; monitor periodically during and for 8 weeks after completion of therapy and institute appropriate treatment such as oral or IV electrolyte repletion. Exacerbation of dermatologic toxicity upon sun exposure; wear sunscreen, hats and limit exposure while on therapy. EGFR protein expression is necessary for appropriate selection of patients. Refer to PI for FDA-approved test kits.

ADVERSE REACTIONS: Skin toxicities (eg, erythema, dermatitis acneiform, pruritus, exfoliation, rash, fissures), hypomagnesemia, paronychia, fatigue, abdominal pain, N/V, diarrhea, constipation.

INTERACTIONS: Avoid use in combination with chemotherapy.

PREGNANCY: Category C, not for use in nursing.

MECHANISM OF ACTION: IgG2 kappa monoclonal antibody; binds specifically to EGFR on both normal and tumor cells, and competitively inhibits binding of ligands for EGFR.

PHARMACOKINETICS: Absorption: C_{max}=213mcg/mL, AUC=1306mcg•day/mL. **Elimination:** $T_{1/2}$=7.5 days.

NURSING CONSIDERATIONS

Assessment: Assess electrolyte baseline levels, EGFR protein expression, pulmonary disease, and pregnancy/nursing status.

Monitoring: Monitor electrolytes periodically during and for 8 weeks after therapy. Monitor for signs/symptoms of dermatologic toxicities (eg, dermatitis acneiform, pruritus, erythema, rash, skin exfoliation, paronychia, dry skin, skin fissures), severe infusion reactions (eg, anaphylactic reactions, bronchospasm, fever, chills, hypotension), angioedema, and pulmonary fibrosis.

Patient Counseling: Advise to report skin/ocular changes, signs and symptoms of infusion reactions (eg, fever, chills, or breathing problems), persistent/recurrent coughing, wheezing, dyspnea, or new onset facial swelling and if pregnant or nursing. Advise of need for adequate contraception in both males and females during and for 6 months after therapy. Limit sun exposure (use sunscreen, wear hats) during and for 2 months after the last dose of therapy to prevent exacerbation of skin reactions. D/C nursing during and 2 months after therapy. Report severe cases of diarrhea and dehydration.

Administration: IV infusion; do not administer as bolus or push. Refer to PI for preparation and administration of solution. **Storage:** 2-8°C (36-46°F). Protect from sunlight. (Diluted): Room temperature; use within 6 hrs, or at 2-8°C (36-46°F); stable for 24 hrs. Do not freeze.

VECTICAL   RX
calcitriol (Galderma)

THERAPEUTIC CLASS: Vitamin D analog

INDICATIONS: Topical treatment of mild to moderate plaque psoriasis in adults >18 yrs.

DOSAGE: *Adults:* Apply to affected area(s) bid, am and pm. Max: 200g week. Do not apply to the eyes, lips, or facial skin.

HOW SUPPLIED: Oint: 3mcg/g [5g, 100g]

WARNINGS/PRECAUTIONS: Not for oral, ophthalmic, or intravaginal use. D/C therapy if aberrations in parameters of calcium metabolism occur. Avoid excessive exposure of treated areas to either natural or artificial sunlight (eg, tanning booths, sun lamps). May enhance the ability of ultraviolet radiation to induce skin tumors (animal studies).

ADVERSE REACTIONS: Laboratory test abnormality, urine abnormality, psoriasis, hypercalciuria, and pruritus.

INTERACTIONS: Caution with thiazide diuretics and calcium supplements or high doses of vitamin D; may increase serum calcium levels.

PREGNANCY: Category C, caution in nursing.

MECHANISM OF ACTION: Vitamin D analog; mechanism of action in the treatment of psoriasis is not established.

NURSING CONSIDERATIONS

Assessment: Assess for hypercalcemia/hypercalciuria, pregnancy/nursing status, and possible drug interactions. Assess for serum and urinary calcium levels.

Monitoring: Monitor for hypercalcemia/hypercalciuria, psoriasis, pruritus, and possible skin tumors.

Patient Counseling: For external use only; not for oral, ophthalmic, or intravaginal use. Apply only to areas of the skin affected by psoriasis. Instruct to rub the skin gently. Notify physician if adverse reactions occur.

Administration: Topical route. **Storage:** Store at 25°C (77°F); excursions permitted to 15°-30°C(59°-86°F). Do not freeze or refrigerate.

VELTIN GEL   RX
clindamycin phosphate - tretinoin (Stiefel)

THERAPEUTIC CLASS: Lincosamide derivative/retinoid

INDICATIONS: Topical treatment of acne vulgaris in patients ≥12 yrs.

DOSAGE: *Adults:* Apply pea-sized amount qd in pm. Gently rub the medication to lightly cover the entire affected area. Avoid the eyes, lips and mucous membranes.
Pediatrics: ≥12 yrs: Apply pea-sized amount qd in pm. Gently rub the medica-

tion to lightly cover the entire affected area. Avoid the eyes, lips and mucous membranes.

HOW SUPPLIED: Gel: (Clindamycin phosphate-Tretinoin) 1.2%-0.025% [30g, 60g]

CONTRAINDICATIONS: Regional enteritis, ulcerative colitis, or history of antibiotic-associated colitis.

WARNINGS/PRECAUTIONS: Systemic absorption of clindamycin has been demonstrated following topical use. Diarrhea, bloody diarrhea, and colitis reported with clindamycin; d/c if significant diarrhea occurs. Severe colitis reported up to several weeks following cessation of therapy. Avoid exposure to sunlight, including sunlamps. Avoid use if sunburn present. Daily use of sunscreen products and protective apparel are recommended. Weather extremes (eg, wind, cold) may be irritating while under treatment.

ADVERSE REACTIONS: Local site reactions (eg, dryness, irritation, exfoliation, erythema).

INTERACTIONS: Avoid with erythromycin-containing products due to possible antagonism to clindamycin. Caution with neuromuscular blocking agents. Antiperistaltic agents (eg, opiates, diphenoxylate with atropine) may prolong and/or worsen severe colitis. Skin irritation may increase when used concomitantly with other topical products with strong drying effects (eg, soaps, cleansers).

PREGNANCY: Category C, caution in nursing.

MECHANISM OF ACTION: Clindamycin: Lincosamide antibiotic; binds to the 50S ribosomal subunit of susceptible bacteria and prevents elongation of peptide chains by interfering with peptidyl transfer, thereby suppressing protein synthesis. Found to have activity against *P. acnes*. Tretinoin: Retinoid; not established; suspected to decrease the cohesiveness of follicular epithelial cells with decreased microcomedone formation. Also, stimulates mitotic activity and increased turnover of follicular epithelial cells causing extrusion of the comedones.

PHARMACOKINETICS: Absorption: Clindamycin: C_{max} = 8.73ng/mL; T_{max} = 4 hrs.

NURSING CONSIDERATIONS

Assessment: Assess for regional enteritis, ulcerative colitis or history of antibiotic-associated colitis, pre-existing sunburns, pregnancy/nursing status, and for possible drug interactions. Assess use in patients whose occupations required considerable sun exposure.

Monitoring: Monitor for signs/symptoms of diarrhea, bloody diarrhea and colitis (including pseudomembranous colitis). If diarrhea, abdominal cramps, or passage of blood or mucus, perform stool culture for *Clostridium difficile* and stool assay for *C. difficile* toxin. Monitor for local skin reactions (eg, erythema, scaling, burning, dryness, itching).

Patient Counseling: Instruct to gently wash face with a mild soap and water prior to application. Do not use more than a pea-sized amount to lightly cover the face and not to apply more than once daily only at bedtime. Avoid exposure to sunlight, sunlamps, and ultraviolet light; daily use of sunscreen products and protective apparel are recommended. Avoid other topical medications that may increase sensitivity to sunlight. Do not use other topical products that may cause an increase in skin irritation. Therapy may cause irritation such as erythema, scaling, itching, burning, or stinging. Contact physician if experience diarrhea or GI discomfort. Advise to keep out of the reach of children.

Administration: Topical route. Not for oral, ophthalmic or intravaginal use.
Storage: 25°C (77°F); excursions permitted to 15-30°C (59-86°F). Protect from light, heat and freezing. Keep tube tightly closed.

VENTAVIS   RX
iloprost (Actelion)

THERAPEUTIC CLASS: Prostaglandin analog

INDICATIONS: Treatment of pulmonary arterial hypertension (PAH) (WHO Group I) to improve a composite endpoint consisting of exercise tolerance, symptoms (NYHA Class), and lack of deterioration in patients with NYHA Functional Class III-IV symptoms and etiologies of idiopathic or heritable PAH or PAH associated with connective tissue diseases.

DOSAGE: *Adults:* Administer via I-neb™ or Prodose™ AAD* Systems. Initial: 2.5mcg. Titrate: May increase to 5mcg and maintain if well tolerated; otherwise maintain at 2.5mcg. Should be taken 6-9 times/day (no more than once q2h). Max: 45mcg/day. Child Pugh Class B or C Hepatic Impairment: Increase dosing interval (eg, 3-4 hrs between doses). Elderly: Start at lower end of dosing range.

HOW SUPPLIED: Sol, Inhalation: 10mcg/mL [1mL], 20mcg/mL [1mL]

WARNINGS/PRECAUTIONS: Avoid contact with skin or eyes. Avoid oral ingestion. Do not initiate in patients with systolic BP <85mmHg; monitor for vital signs. Exertional syncope may reflect therapeutic gap or insufficient efficacy; consider adjusting dose or changing therapy if it occurs. D/C if signs of pulmonary edema occur. May induce bronchospasm. Bronchospasm may be more severe or frequent in patients with history of hyperreactive airways. Caution in patients with COPD, severe asthma, or pulmonary infections, hepatic/renal impairment, and in the elderly.

ADVERSE REACTIONS: Increased cough, headache, vasodilation/flushing, flu syndrome, N/V, trismus, hypotension, syncope, insomnia, palpitations, increased alkaline phosphatase/GGT, back pain.

INTERACTIONS: May increase hypotensive effect of vasodilators and antihypertensive agents. Increased risk of bleeding with anticoagulants or platelet inhibitors.

PREGNANCY: Category C, not for use in nursing.

MECHANISM OF ACTION: Synthetic analogue of prostacyclin PGI_2; dilates systemic and pulmonary arterial vascular beds. Affects platelet aggregation; relevance of this effect is unknown.

PHARMACOKINETICS: Absorption: C_{max}=150pg/mL. **Distribution:** (IV) V_d=0.7-0.8L/kg; plasma protein binding (60%). **Metabolism:** Via β-oxidation. Tetranor-iloprost (main metabolite). **Elimination:** Urine (68%), feces (12%); $T_{1/2}$=20-30 min.

NURSING CONSIDERATIONS

Assessment: Assess for history of hyperreactive airways, COPD, severe asthma, acute pulmonary infection, renal/hepatic impairment, pregnancy/nursing status, and possible drug interactions. Obtain baseline BP and vitals prior to initiation of therapy.

Monitoring: Monitor for vital signs, signs and symptoms pulmonary edema, exertional syncope, bleeding, and bronchospasm.

Patient Counseling: Counsel to use as prescribed with either I-neb™ or Prodose™ AAD* Systems. Instruct on proper administration techniques. Advise that a drop in BP during therapy is possible and may cause dizziness or fainting; advise to stand up slowly when getting out of a chair or bed. Consult a physician if fainting gets worse. Inform that medication should be inhaled at intervals of not <2 hrs and that acute benefits of therapy may not last 2 hours. Inform that patients may adjust times of administration to cover planned activities. Counsel to avoid mixing with other medications.

Administration: Inhalation route. Refer to PI for preparation instructions. **Storage:** 20-25°C (68-77°F); excursions permitted to 15-30°C (59-86°F).

VENTOLIN HFA

RX

albuterol sulfate (GlaxoSmithKline)

THERAPEUTIC CLASS: Beta$_2$-agonist

INDICATIONS: Treatment or prevention of bronchospasm in patients with reversible obstructive airway disease. Prevention of exercise-induced bronchospasm (EIB).

DOSAGE: *Adults:* Bronchospasm: 2 inh q4-6h or 1 inh q4h. EIB: 2 inh 15-30 min before exercise. Elderly: Start at lower end of dosing range. *Pediatrics:* ≥4 yrs: Bronchospasm: 2 inh q4-6h or 1 inh q4h. EIB: 2 inh 15-30 min before exercise.

HOW SUPPLIED: MDI: 90mcg/inh [8g, 18g]

WARNINGS/PRECAUTIONS: D/C if paradoxical bronchospasm or CV events occur. Avoid excessive use; may be marker of destabilization of asthma and require reevaluation of the patient. Caution with convulsive disorders, coronary insufficiency, arrhythmias, HTN, diabetes mellitus (DM), hyperthyroidism, sensitivity to sympathomimetics. Hypersensitivity reactions may occur. Fatalities reported with excessive use. May need concomitant corticosteroids. May produce significant hypokalemia. Caution in elderly.

ADVERSE REACTIONS: Throat irritation, viral respiratory infections, upper respiratory inflammation, cough, musculoskeletal pain, parodoxical bronchospasm, hoarseness, arrhythmias, hypersensitivity reactions, hypokalemia, HTN, peripheral vasodilation, angina, tremor.

INTERACTIONS: Avoid other short-acting sympathomimetic bronchodilators; caution with oral sympathomimetics. Extreme caution with MAOIs, TCAs during or within 2 weeks of d/c. β-blockers may block pulmonary effects and cause severe bronchospasm. Decreases digoxin levels. ECG changes and/or hypokalemia caused by non-K$^+$-sparing diuretics (eg, loop or thiazide diuretics) may be worsened.

PREGNANCY: Category C, caution in nursing.

MECHANISM OF ACTION: β$_2$-adrenergic agonist; activates β$_2$-adrenergic receptors on airway smooth muscle leading to the activation of adenylcyclase and to an increase in the intracellular concentration of cAMP. This increase of cAMP leads to the activation of protein kinase A, which inhibits the phosphorylation of myosin and lowers intracellular ionic calcium concentrations, resulting in relaxation of the smooth muscles of all airways, from the trachea to the terminal bronchioles.

PHARMACOKINETICS: Absorption: C$_{max}$=3ng/mL; T$_{max}$=0.42 hrs. **Elimination:** T$_{1/2}$=4.6 hrs.

NURSING CONSIDERATIONS

Assessment: Assess renal/hepatic function, history of hypersensitivity to drug, CVD (eg, coronary insufficiency, HTN, cardiac arrhythmias), convulsive disorders, hyperthyroidism, DM and ketoacidosis, pregnancy/nursing status, and possible drug interactions. Assess use in patients unusually responsive to sympathomimetic amines.

Monitoring: Monitor for possible paradoxical bronchospasm, deterioration of asthma, CV effects, hypokalemia, immediate hypersensitivity reactions and common adverse effects (eg, palpitation, rapid HR, tremor and nervousness. Monitor BP, HR, ECG changes and blood glucose.

Patient Counseling: Advise to seek medical attention if treatment becomes less effective for symptomatic relief, symptoms become worse, or usage becomes more frequent than usual. Take as directed and report lack of response or adverse side effects. Instruct how to properly prime, clean and use inhaler. Prime inhaler before using for first time or if inhaler has not been used for 2 weeks, or if it has been dropped by releasing 4 test sprays into air, away from face. Clean inhaler at least once a week, wash the actuator with warm water and let it air-dry completely. Use only with actuator supplied with product. Refill prescription when the counter reads 020 or discard when the counter reads 000 or if it is 12 months after removal from the moisture-protective foil pouch, whichever comes first. Advise to never immerse the canister in water to determine the amount of drug remaining in the canister. Avoid spraying in eyes and shake well before each spray.

Administration: Oral inhalation route. **Storage:** 15-25°C (59-77°F). Keep out of the reach of children. Do not puncture. Do not use or store near heat or open flame. Exposure to temperatures above 120°F may cause bursting. Store inhaler with mouthpiece down.

VERAMYST   RX
fluticasone furoate (GlaxoSmithKline)

THERAPEUTIC CLASS: Corticosteroid

INDICATIONS: Treatment of the symptoms of seasonal and perennial allergic rhinitis in patients ≥2 yrs.

DOSAGE: *Adults:* Initial: 2 sprays per nostril qd. Titrate to minimum effective dose. Maint: 1 spray per nostril qd. Elderly: Start at low end of dosing range. *Pediatrics:* ≥12 yrs: Initial: 2 sprays per nostril qd. Titrate to minimum effective dose. Maint: 1 spray per nostril qd. 2-11 yrs: Initial: 1 spray per nostril qd. Titrate: May increase to 2 sprays per nostril qd if inadequate, then return to initial dose when symptoms are controlled.

HOW SUPPLIED: Spray: 27.5mcg/spray [10g]

WARNINGS/PRECAUTIONS: May cause local nasal effects (eg, epistaxis, nasal ulceration, *Candida* infection, nasal septum perforation, and impaired wound healing). Avoid with recent nasal ulcers, surgery, or trauma. May result in glaucoma and/or cataracts. Hypersensitivity reactions may occur. May increase susceptibility to infections; caution with active or quiescent tuberculosis (TB), untreated fungal or bacterial infections, systemic viral or parasitic infections or ocular herpes simplex. Avoid exposure to chickenpox and measles. May cause hypercorticism and adrenal suppression. Risk of adrenal insufficiency and withdrawal symptoms when replacing systemic corticosteroids with topical corticosteroids. Potential for reduced growth velocity in pediatrics. Caution with severe hepatic impairment and elderly.

ADVERSE REACTIONS: Headache, epistaxis, pharyngolaryngeal pain, nasal ulceration, back pain, pyrexia, cough.

INTERACTIONS: Increased exposure with ritonavir; avoid coadministration. Reduced cortisol levels with ketoconazole. Caution with ketoconazole or other potent CYP3A4 inhibitors.

PREGNANCY: Category C, caution in nursing.

MECHANISM OF ACTION: Corticosteroid; not established. Shown to have a wide range of actions on multiple cell types (eg, mast cells, eosinophils, neutrophils, macrophages, lymphocytes) and mediators (eg, histamine, eicosanoids, leukotrienes, cytokines) involved in inflammation.

PHARMACOKINETICS: Absorption: Incomplete; absolute bioavailability (0.5%). **Distribution:** V_d=608L. Plasma protein binding (>99%). **Metabolism:** Hepatic via CYP3A4; hydrolysis. **Elimination:** Feces; (IV) $T_{1/2}$=15.1 hrs.

NURSING CONSIDERATIONS

Assessment: Assess for previous hypersensitivity to the drug, active or quiescent TB, untreated fungal/bacterial infection, systemic viral infection, ocular herpes simplex, history of increased IOP, glaucoma or cataracts, recent nasal ulcers/surgery/trauma, hepatic impairment, pregnancy/nursing status, and possible drug interactions.

Monitoring: Monitor for hypercorticism, chickenpox, measles, nasal *Candida* infections, epistaxis, nasal ulceration, nasal septal perforation, hypoadrenalism (in infants born to mother who received corticosteroids during pregnancy), suppression of growth velocity in children, vision changes, glaucoma, cataracts, and hypersensitivity reactions.

Patient Counseling: Counsel to take as directed. Inform the patient for possible local nasal effects, cataracts, glaucoma, immunosuppression, and

V

hypersensitivity reactions. Advise not to use with recent nasal ulcers, surgery, or trauma until healing has occurred. Instruct to d/c if hypersensitivity reaction occurs. Instruct to avoid exposure to chickenpox and measles. Instruct to consult physician if symptoms do not improve, the condition worsens, or change in vision occurs. Advise to avoid spraying into eyes. Inform of potential drug interactions.

Administration: Intranasal route. Prime pump before 1st time use, if not used >30 days, or cap left off >5 days. Shake well before each use. **Storage:** 15-30°C (59-86°F). Store device in upright position with cap in place. Do not freeze or refrigerate.

VERDESO   RX
desonide (Stiefel)

THERAPEUTIC CLASS: Corticosteroid

INDICATIONS: Treatment of mild to moderate atopic dermatitis in patients ≥3 months.

DOSAGE: *Adults:* Apply thin layer to affected area(s) bid. D/C when control is achieved. Max Duration: 4 consecutive weeks. Dispense smallest amount necessary to adequately cover affected area with thin layer.
Pediatrics: ≥3 months: Apply thin layer to affected area(s) bid. D/C when control is achieved. Max Duration: 4 consecutive weeks. Dispense smallest amount necessary to adequately cover affected area with thin layer.

HOW SUPPLIED: Foam: 0.05% [50g, 100g]

WARNINGS/PRECAUTIONS: May produce reversible hypothalamic-pituitary-adrenal (HPA) axis suppression, manifestations of Cushing's syndrome, hyperglycemia, facial swelling, glucosuria, withdrawal syndrome, and growth retardation in children. Caution when applied to large surface areas, upon prolonged use, or addition of occlusive dressing. Periodic evaluation of HPA suppression required due to potential for systemic absorption; withdraw, reduce frequency, or substitute with a less potent steroid if adrenal suppression is noted. Pediatric patients may be more susceptible to systemic toxicity. If concomitant skin infections are present or develop, institute an appropriate antifungal, antibacterial or antiviral agent. D/C if local skin adverse reactions (eg, irritation and allergic contact dermatitis) occur. Flammable; avoid fire, flame and smoking during and immediately following application. Caution in elderly.

ADVERSE REACTIONS: Application-site reactions (eg, burning), adrenal suppression, upper respiratory tract infection, cough.

INTERACTIONS: Concomitant therapy with topical corticosteroids may produce cumulative effect; use with caution.

PREGNANCY: Category C, caution in nursing.

MECHANISM OF ACTION: Corticosteroid; possesses anti-inflammatory, antipruritic, and vasoconstrictive properties. Anti-inflammatory activity not established. Suspected to act by induction of phospholipase A_2 inhibitory proteins, lipocortins. Lipocortins control biosynthesis of potent mediators of inflammation (eg, prostaglandins, leukotrienes) by inhibiting release of their common precursor, arachidonic acid.

PHARMACOKINETICS: Absorption: Extent of percutaneous absorption is determined by product formulation, integrity of the epidermal barrier, and age. **Distribution:** Systemically administered corticosteroids found in breast milk. **Metabolism:** Liver. **Elimination:** Kidneys, bile.

NURSING CONSIDERATIONS

Assessment: Assess use in pregnant/nursing females and for possible drug interaction with concomitant topical corticosteroids.

Monitoring: Monitor for signs/symptoms of reversible HPA-axis suppression, Cushing's syndrome, hyperglycemia, facial swelling, glucosuria, withdrawal syndrome, growth retardation, delayed weight gain, and intracranial HTN in children. If using medication on large body surface area, prolonged use or using occlusive dressing, perform periodic monitoring of HPA-axis suppression using cosyntropin (ACTH$_{1-24}$) stimulation test. Monitor for irritation, concomitant skin infections.

Patient Counseling: Instruct to use as directed; avoid contact with eyes or other mucous membranes. Foam is not for oral, ophthalmic, or intravaginal use. Instruct not to dispense directly on the face; dispense in hands and gently massage. For other treatment areas, medication may be directly dispensed onto affected area. Wash hands after administration and do not bandage, wrap, or cover treatment areas unless directed by physician. Contact physician if signs of local or systemic adverse reactions develop or if no improvement seen within 4 weeks of starting therapy. Contact physician if contemplating surgery. D/C when control is achieved. Medication is flammable; avoid contact with fire, flames, or smoking during and immediately following application. Do not use other corticosteroid-containing products while on therapy without consulting physician. Do not use for any disorder other than for which it was prescribed.

Administration: Topical route. Not for oral, ophthalmic, or intravaginal use. Shake can before use and dispense by inverting the can. Do not dispense directly on face; dispense in hands and gently massage. Do not use occlusive dressing unless directed by physician. **Storage:** 20-25°C (68-77°F). Do not expose containers to heat, and/or store at temperatures above 49°C (120°F).

VERELAN
verapamil HCl (Schwarz Pharma)
RX

THERAPEUTIC CLASS: Calcium channel blocker (nondihydropyridine)

INDICATIONS: Management of essential HTN.

DOSAGE: *Adults:* Individualize dose. Usual: 240mg qam. Elderly/Small People: Initial: 120mg qam. Titrate: If inadequate response with 120mg, increase to 180mg qam, then 240mg qam, then 360mg qam, then 480mg qam. Upward titration should be based on the therapeutic efficacy and safety evaluated approximately 24 hrs after the previous dose. Swallow whole; do not crush or chew. May be opened and sprinkled on applesauce.

HOW SUPPLIED: Cap, Extended-Release: 120mg, 180mg, 240mg, 360mg

CONTRAINDICATIONS: Severe left ventricular dysfunction, hypotension (SBP <90mmHg), cardiogenic shock, sick sinus syndrome, 2nd- or 3rd-degree AV block (except with functioning ventricular pacemaker), A-fib/flutter with an accessory bypass tract (Wolff-Parkinson-White, Lown-Ganong-Levine syndromes).

WARNINGS/PRECAUTIONS: Congestive heart failure (CHF) or pulmonary edema reported. Avoid use with severe left ventricular dysfunction (eg, ejection fraction <30% or moderate to severe symptoms of cardiac failure) and any degree of ventricular dysfunction if taking β-blockers. May cause hypotension, AV block, transient bradycardia, PR interval prolongation. Elevated transaminases (eg, elevations in alkaline phosphatase, SGOT, SGPT and bilirubin) reported; monitor LFTs periodically. Hepatocellular injury reported. Ventricular fibrillation has occurred in patients with A-fib/flutter and an accessory bypass tract. Sinus bradycardia, 2nd-degree AV block, pulmonary edema, hypotension, and sinus arrest reported in patients with hypertrophic cardiomyopathy. Caution with impaired hepatic function; give 30% of normal dose with severe hepatic dysfunction. Caution with renal impairment; monitor for abnormal PR interval prolongation. Decrease dose in those with decreased neuromuscular transmission. May cause worsening of myasthenia gravis.

ADVERSE REACTIONS: Constipation, dizziness, headache, lethargy.

INTERACTIONS: CYP3A4 inhibitors (eg, erythromycin, ritonavir) or grapefruit juice may increase levels. CYP3A4 inducers (eg, rifampin) may lower levels. Hypotension and bradyarrhythmias reported with telithromycin. Additive negative effects on HR, AV conduction, and contractility with β-blockers. Asymptomatic bradycardia with atrial pacemaker has been observed with concomitant use of timolol eye drops. Decreased clearance of metoprolol if given concomitantly with administration. Sinus bradycardia resulting in

V

hospitalization and pacemaker insertion has been reported with concomitant use of clonidine; monitor HR. May increase digoxin, carbamazepine, cyclosporine and alcohol levels. Potentiates effects of other antihypertensives (eg, vasodilators, ACE inhibitors, diuretics). Excessive reduction in BP with concurrent use of prazosin. Avoid disopyramide within 48 hrs before or 24 hrs after verapamil. Additive negative inotropic effects and AV conduction prolongation with flecainide. Avoid quinidine with hypertrophic cardiomyopathy. Increased bleeding time with ASA. Coadministration with cimetidine may either reduce or not change the clearance of verapamil. Increased sensitivity to effects of lithium; monitor lithium levels. Increased clearance with phenobarbital. Rifampin may reduce oral bioavailability. Caution with inhalation anesthetics. May potentiate neuromuscular blockers; both agents may need dose reduction.

PREGNANCY: Category C, not for use in nursing.

MECHANISM OF ACTION: Calcium ion influx inhibitor (calcium ion antagonist or slow-channel blocker); decreases systemic vascular resistance without orthostatic decreases in BP or reflex tachycardia.

PHARMACOKINETICS: Absorption: T_{max}=7-9 hrs; administration of variable doses resulted in different parameters. **Distribution:** Plasma protein binding (90%); crosses placenta; found in breast milk. **Metabolism:** Liver (extensive), norverapamil (metabolite). **Elimination:** Urine (70%; 3-4% unchanged), feces (≥16%); $T_{1/2}$=12 hrs.

NURSING CONSIDERATIONS

Assessment: Assess for left ventricular dysfunction, hypotension, cardiogenic shock, sick sinus syndrome, 2nd- or 3rd-degree AV block, atrial flutter/fibrillation, presence of functional artificial ventricular pacemaker, accessory bypass tract (eg, Wolff-Parkinson-White, Lown-Ganong-Levine syndromes), LFTs, hypertrophic cardiomyopathy, Duchenne's muscular dystrophy, myasthenia gravis, hepatic/renal impairment, hypersensitivity, pregnancy/nursing status and possible drug interactions.

Monitoring: Monitor signs/symptoms of hypotension, CHF, heart block, ventricular fibrillation, renal/hepatic dysfunction, abnormal prolongation of PR interval and hypersensitivity reactions. Periodically monitor LFTs (SGOT, SGPT, alkaline phosphatase, bilirubin) BP, ECG changes and HR.

Patient Counseling: Advise to swallow cap whole; do not crush or chew. May administer by opening and sprinkling pellets on spoonful of applesauce (should not be hot), and swallowed immediately without chewing, with a glass of cool water. Subdividing contents of capsule not recommended.

Administration: Oral route. **Storage:** 20-25°C (68-77°F). Avoid excessive heat. Brief digressions above 25°C, while not detrimental, should be avoided. Protect from moisture.

Verelan PM   RX
verapamil HCl (Schwarz Pharma)

THERAPEUTIC CLASS: Calcium channel blocker (nondihydropyridine)

INDICATIONS: Management of essential HTN.

DOSAGE: *Adults:* Individualize dose. Usual: 200mg qhs. Renal or Hepatic Dysfunction/Elderly/Low-Weight Patients: Initial: 100mg qhs. If Inadequate Response with 200mg: May increase to 300mg qhs, then 400mg qhs. Upward titration should be based on the therapeutic efficacy and safety evaluated approximately 24 hrs after the previous dose. May sprinkle on applesauce. Swallow whole; do not crush or chew.

HOW SUPPLIED: Cap, Extended-Release: 100mg, 200mg, 300mg

CONTRAINDICATIONS: Severe left ventricular dysfunction, hypotension (SBP <90mmHg), cardiogenic shock, sick sinus syndrome or 2nd- or 3rd-degree AV block (except in patients with a functioning ventricular pacemaker), A-fib/A-flutter and an accessory bypass tract (eg, Wolff-Parkinson-White, Lown-Ganong-Levine syndromes).

WARNINGS/PRECAUTIONS: Congestive heart failure (CHF) or pulmonary edema may develop. Avoid use with severe left ventricular dysfunction (eg, ejection fraction <30% or moderate to severe symptoms of cardiac failure) and any degree of ventricular dysfunction if taking β-blockers. May cause hypotension, AV block, transient bradycardia, PR interval prolongation. Elevated transaminases (eg, elevations in alkaline phosphate, SGOT, SGPT and bilirubin) have occurred; monitor LFTs periodically. Hepatocellular injury reported. Ventricular fibrillation has occurred in patients with A-flutter or A-fib and a coexisting accessory AV pathway. Reduce dose or d/c therapy if marked first-degree AV block or progression to 2nd- or 3rd-degree AV block occurs. Sinus bradycardia, pulmonary edema, severe hypotension, 2nd-degree AV block, sinus arrest occurred in patients with hypertrophic cardiomyopathy. Caution with impaired hepatic function; give 30% of normal dose with severe hepatic dysfunction. Caution with renal impairment; monitor for abnormal PR interval prolongation. Decrease dose in those with decreased neuromuscular transmission. May cause worsening of myasthenia gravis.

ADVERSE REACTIONS: Headache, infection, constipation, flu syndrome, peripheral edema, dizziness, pharyngitis, sinusitis.

INTERACTIONS: Additive negative effects on HR, AV conduction, and cardiac contractility with β-blockers. Additive effects with other antihypertensives (eg, vasodilators, ACE inhibitors, diuretics). May increase digoxin, metoprolol, propranolol, quinidine, carbamazepine, theophylline, cyclosporine, alcohol and doxorubicin levels. May alter levels of atenolol. Sinus bradycardia resulting in hospitalization and pacemaker insertion has been reported in association with the use of clonidine; monitor HR. Hypotension and bradyarrhythmias have been observed in patients receiving concurrent telithromycin. Avoid disopyramide within 48 hrs before or 24 hrs after administration. Additive negative inotropic effects and AV conduction prolongation with flecainide. Avoid quinidine with hypertrophic cardiomyopathy. May increase sensitivity to neurotoxic effects of lithium with or without an increase in serum lithium levels. Increased clearance with phenobarbital. CYP3A4 inducers (eg, rifampin) may reduce the levels of verapamil. Rifampin may reduce oral bioavailability. May potentiate neuromuscular blockers (eg, curare-like and depolarizing); both agents may need dose reduction. Caution with inhalation anesthetics. May increase bleeding time with ASA. Reduced absorption with COPP and VAC cytotoxic drug regimens. May decrease clearance of paclitaxel and digitoxin. CYP3A4 inhibitors (eg, erythromycin, ritonavir) or grapefruit juice may increase levels. Asymptomatic bradycardia with a wandering atrial pacemaker has been observed with concomitant use of timolol eye drops. Excessive reduction in BP with concurrent use of prazosin. Reduced or unchanged clearance with cimetidine.

PREGNANCY: Category C, not for use in nursing.

MECHANISM OF ACTION: Calcium channel blocker (nondihydropyridine); inhibits transmembrane influx of ionic calcium into arterial smooth muscle as well as in conductile and contractile myocardial cells without altering serum calcium concentrations.

PHARMACOKINETICS: Absorption: T_{max}=11 hrs. Bioavailability (33-65%, R-enantiomer), (13-34%, S-enantiomer). C_{max}=(77.8ng/mL, R-enantiomer), (16.8ng/mL, S-enantiomer). AUC_{0-24}=(1037ng•h/mL, R-enantiomer), (195ng•h/mL, S-enantiomer). **Distribution:** Plasma protein binding (94%, R-enantiomer), (88%, S-enantiomer); found in breast milk, crosses placenta. **Metabolism:** Liver (extensive); via CYP450; norverapamil (active metabolite). **Elimination:** Urine (70%, metabolites), (3-4%, unchanged), feces (16%, metabolites).

NURSING CONSIDERATIONS

Assessment: Assess for left ventricular dysfunction, hypotension, cardiogenic shock, sick sinus syndrome, 2nd- or 3rd-degree AV block, A-fib/A-flutter (eg, Wolff-Parkinson-White, Lown-Ganong-Levine syndromes), accessory bypass tract, CHF, LFTs, hypertrophic cardiomyopathy, Duchenne's muscular dystrophy, myasthenia gravis, impaired hepatic/renal function, pregnancy/nursing status, and possible drug interactions.

Monitoring: Monitor signs/symptoms of hypotension, CHF, heart block, ventricular fibrillation, renal/hepatic dysfunction, abnormal prolongation of

PR interval and hypersensitivity reactions. Periodically monitor LFTs (SGOT, SGPT, alkaline phosphatase, bilirubin), BP, ECG changes, and HR.

Patient Counseling: Advise to immediately seek medical help if a drop in BP, chest pain, headache, dizziness, N/V, or edema occurs. Swallow capsule whole; do not crush or chew. May administer by opening and sprinkling pellets onto a spoonful of applesauce (should not be hot), and swallow immediately, without chewing, with a glass of cool water. Subdividing contents of capsule not recommended.

Administration: Oral route. **Storage:** 25°C (77°F); excursions permitted to 15-30°C (59-86°F). Protect from moisture. Dispense in tight, light-resistant container.

VESIcare
solifenacin succinate (Astellas/GlaxoSmithKline)

RX

THERAPEUTIC CLASS: Muscarinic antagonist

INDICATIONS: Treatment of overactive bladder with symptoms of urge urinary incontinence, urgency, and urinary frequency.

DOSAGE: *Adults:* Usual: 5mg qd. Titrate: May increase to 10mg qd if 5mg dose is well tolerated. Max: 10mg qd. Severe Renal Impairment (CrCl <30mL/min)/ Moderate Hepatic Impairment (Child-Pugh B)/Ketoconazole or other Potent CYP3A4 Inhibitors: Max: 5mg qd. Take with water and swallow tab whole.

HOW SUPPLIED: Tab: 5mg, 10mg

CONTRAINDICATIONS: Urinary retention, gastric retention, uncontrolled narrow-angle glaucoma.

WARNINGS/PRECAUTIONS: Angioedema of the face, lips, tongue, and/or larynx reported. Angioedema associated with upper airway swelling may be life threatening; d/c immediately and provide appropriate therapy if involvement of tongue, hypopharynx, or larynx occurs. Caution with bladder outflow obstruction, decreased GI motility and narrow-angle glaucoma. Caution with renal/hepatic impairment. Avoid with severe hepatic impairment (Child-Pugh C). Caution with history of QT interval prolongation.

ADVERSE REACTIONS: Dry mouth, constipation, nausea, dyspepsia, urinary tract infection, blurred vision.

INTERACTIONS: Do not exceed 5mg daily dose when administered with therapeutic doses of ketoconazole or other potent CYP3A4 inhibitors. Decreased concentration with inducers of CYP3A4. Caution with medications known to prolong the QT interval.

PREGNANCY: Category C, not for use in nursing.

MECHANISM OF ACTION: Muscarinic receptor antagonist; play an important role in several major cholinergically mediated functions, including contractions of urinary bladder smooth muscle and stimulation of salivary secretion.

PHARMACOKINETICS: Absorption: Absolute bioavailabilty (90%); T_{max}=3-8 hrs. **Distribution:** V_d=600L; plasma protein binding (98%). **Metabolism:** Liver (extensive) via CYP3A4 (N-oxidation, 4R-hydroxylation; 4R-hydroxy solifenacin (active metabolite). **Elimination:** Urine (<15%), feces; $T_{1/2}$=45-68 hrs.

NURSING CONSIDERATIONS

Assessment: Assess for bladder outflow obstruction, urinary retention, gastric retention, narrow-angle glaucoma, decreased GI motility, known history of QT prolongation, drug hypersensitivity, pregnancy/nursing status, and possible drug interactions. Assess renal/hepatic function.

Monitoring: Monitor for signs/symptoms of angioedema, urinary retention, QT prolongation, and renal/hepatic impairment.

Patient Counseling: Inform that therapy has been associated with constipation and blurred vision. Caution against potentially dangerous activities. Advise to seek medical attention if symptoms of severe abdominal pain or constipation (≥3 days) occurs. Inform that heat prostration (due to decreased sweating) may occur when used in a hot environment. Inform that it may produce angioedema resulting in fatal airway obstruction; d/c therapy and seek medical help if tongue/laryngopharyngeal edema, or difficulty breathing occurs. Advise to take with water and swallow whole; may be administered with or without food.

Administration: Oral route. **Storage:** 25°C (77°F); excursions permitted to 15-30°C (59-86°F).

VFEND RX
voriconazole (Pfizer)

THERAPEUTIC CLASS: Azole antifungal

INDICATIONS: Treatment of invasive aspergillosis, esophageal candidiasis. Treatment of candidemia in nonneutropenic patients and the following *Candida* infections: disseminated infections in skin and infections in abdomen, kidney, bladder wall, and wounds. Treatment of serious fungal infections caused by *Scedosporium apiospermum* and *Fusarium* spp. including *Fusarium solani* in patients intolerant of, or refractory to, other therapy.

DOSAGE: *Adults:* Invasive Aspergillosis/Scedosporiosis/Fusariosis: LD: 6mg/kg IV q12h for the first 24 hrs. Maint: IV: 4mg/kg q12h. PO: ≥40kg: 200mg q12h; 300mg q12h if inadequate response. <40kg: 100mg q12h; 150 mg q12h if inadequate response. Candidemia in Nonneutropenic Patients and other Deep Tissue *Candida* Infections: LD: 6mg/kg IV q12h for the first 24 hrs. Maint: IV: 3-4mg/kg q12h. PO: ≥40kg: 200mg q12h; 300mg q12h if inadequate response. <40kg: 100mg q12h; 150mg q12h if inadequate response. Treat for ≥14 days after resolution of symptoms or last positive culture, whichever is longer. Esophageal Candidiasis: Maint: PO: ≥40kg: 200mg q12h; 300mg q12h if inadequate response. <40kg: 100mg q12h; 150mg q12h if inadequate response. Treat for ≥14 days and for ≥7 days after resolution of symptoms. Intolerant to Maint dose: IV: Reduce to 3mg/kg q12h. PO: Reduce by 50mg steps to minimum of 200mg q12h for >40kg or 100mg q12h for <40kg. Concomitant Phenytoin: Maint: IV: 5mg/kg q12h. PO: ≥40kg: 400mg q12h. <40kg: 200mg q12h. Concomitant Efavirenz: Maint: 400mg q12h and efavirenz should be decreased to 300mg q24h. Mild to Moderate Hepatic Cirrhosis: Maint: 1/2 of usual maint dose. CrCl <50mL/min: Use PO. Hemodialysis: 4-hr session does not remove sufficient amount of voriconazole to warrant dosage adjustment. Give PO 1 hr before or 1 hr after a meal. Base duration of therapy on severity of underlying disease, recovery from immunosuppression, and clinical response. *Pediatrics:* ≥12 yrs: Invasive Aspergillosis/Scedosporiosis/Fusariosis: LD: 6mg/kg IV q12h for the first 24 hrs. Maint: IV: 4mg/kg q12h. PO: ≥40kg: 200mg q12h; 300mg q12h if inadequate response. <40kg: 100mg q12h; 150 mg q12h if inadequate response. Candidemia in Nonneutropenic Patients and other Deep Tissue *Candida* Infections: LD: 6mg/kg IV q12h for the first 24 hrs. Maint: IV: 3-4mg/kg q12h. PO: ≥40kg: 200mg q12h; 300mg q12h if inadequate response. <40kg: 100mg q12h; 150mg q12h if inadequate response. Treat for ≥14 days after resolution of symptoms or last positive culture, whichever is longer. Esophageal Candidiasis: Maint: PO: ≥40kg: 200mg q12h; 300mg q12h if inadequate response. <40kg: 100mg q12h; 150mg q12h if inadequate response. Treat for ≥14 days and for ≥7 days after resolution of symptoms. Intolerant to Maint dose: IV: Reduce to 3mg/kg q12h. PO: Reduce by 50mg steps to minimum of 200mg q12h for >40kg or 100mg q12h for <40kg. Concomitant Phenytoin: Maint: IV: 5mg/kg q12h. PO: ≥40kg: 400mg q12h. <40kg: 200mg q12h. Concomitant Efavirenz: Maint: 400mg q12h and efavirenz should be decreased to 300mg q24h. Mild to Moderate Hepatic Cirrhosis: Maint: 1/2 of usual maint dose. CrCl <50mL/min: Use PO. Hemodialysis: 4-hr session does not remove sufficient amount of voriconazole to warrant dosage adjustment. Give PO 1 hr before or 1 hr after a meal. Base duration of therapy on severity of underlying disease, recovery from immunosuppression, and clinical response.

HOW SUPPLIED: Inj: 200mg; Sus: 40mg/mL; Tab: 50mg, 200mg

CONTRAINDICATIONS: Concomitant CYP3A4 substrates, terfenadine, astemizole, cisapride, pimozide, quinidine, sirolimus, rifampin, carbamazepine, long-acting barbiturates, high-dose ritonavir (400mg q12h), rifabutin, ergot alkaloids (ergotamine and dihydroergotamine), St. John's wort. Low-dose ritonavir (100mg q12h) should be avoided unless an assessment of benefit/risk justifies the use.

WARNINGS/PRECAUTIONS: Optic neuritis and papilledema reported; monitor visual function with treatment >28 days. Hepatic reactions (clinical hepatitis, cholestasis, fulminant hepatic failure) reported; monitor LFTs at initiation and during therapy. D/C if liver disease develops. May cause fetal harm. Tabs contain lactose; avoid with galactose intolerance, Lapp lactase deficiency, or glucose-galactose malabsorption. May prolong QT interval; caution with proarrhythmic conditions. Correct electrolyte imbalance before starting therapy. Anaphylactoid-type reactions reported with infusion; consider d/c of therapy if reactions occur. Acute renal failure observed in severely ill patients; monitor renal function. Monitor pancreatic function in patients with risk factors for pancreatitis. May cause serious exfoliative cutaneous reactions (eg, Stevens-Johnson syndrome) and photosensitivity skin reaction; d/c if exfoliative cutaneous reaction or skin lesion develops.

ADVERSE REACTIONS: Visual disturbances, fever, chills, rash, headache, N/V, sepsis, peripheral edema, abdominal pain, respiratory disorder, diarrhea, increased alkaline phosphatase.

INTERACTIONS: See Contraindications. Reduced levels with efavirenz, phenytoin. Increased levels with cimetidine, omeprazole, oral contraceptives (containing ethinyl estradiol and norethindrone), HIV protease inhibitors (eg, saquinavir, amprenavir, nelfinavir), non-nucleoside reverse transcriptase inhibitors (NNRTIs) (eg, delavirdine), fluconazole. Increased levels of efavirenz, oral contraceptives, cyclosporine, fentanyl, alfentanil, oxycodone, NSAIDs (including ibuprofen and diclofenac), tacrolimus, phenytoin, statins (eg, lovastatin), benzodiazepines (eg, midazolam, triazolam, alprazolam), calcium channel blockers (eg, felodipine), sulfonylureas (eg, tolbutamide, glipizide, glyburide), vinca alkaloids (eg, vincristine, vinblastine), prednisolone, omeprazole, HIV protease inhibitors, NNRTIs, proton pump inhibitors, methadone. Reduce dose of opiates metabolized by CYP3A4 (eg, sufentanil). Increased PT with warfarin, oral coumarin anticoagulants. Inhibitors or inducers of CYP2C19, CYP2C9, and CYP3A4 may increase or decrease voriconazole systemic exposure. May increase systemic exposure of other drugs metabolized by CYP2C9 and CYP2C19. Must not be infused concomitantly with any blood products or short-term infusion of concentrated electrolytes. Carefully monitor for NSAID-related adverse events and toxicity with other NSAIDs (eg, celecoxib, naproxen, lornoxicam, meloxicam).

PREGNANCY: Category D, not for use in nursing.

MECHANISM OF ACTION: Triazole antifungal agent; inhibits fungal CYP450 mediated 14 α-lanosterol demethylation, an essential step in fungal ergosterol biosynthesis. Accumulation of 14 α-methyl-sterols correlates with subsequent loss of ergosterol in fungal cell wall and may be responsible for antifungal activity of voriconazole.

PHARMACOKINETICS: Absorption: Administration of different doses led to varying parameters. T_{max}=1-2 hrs, oral bioavailability (96%). **Distribution:** V_d=4.6L/kg; plasma protein binding (58%). **Metabolism:** Hepatic, via CYP2C19/2C9/3A4; N-oxide (major metabolite). **Elimination:** Urine (80-83%, <2% unchanged).

NURSING CONSIDERATIONS

Assessment: Obtain fungal cultures prior to therapy to properly identify causative organisms. Assess for proarrhythmic conditions, hematological malignancy, known hypersensitivity to drug or excipient, hereditary problems of galactose intolerance, Lapp lactase deficiency or glucose-galactose malabsorption, history of cardiotoxic chemotherapy, cardiomyopathy, hypokalemia, arrhythmias, hepatic/renal insufficiency, and electrolyte disturbances. Assess for pregnancy/nursing status and possible drug interactions. Obtain baseline LFTs.

Monitoring: Monitor visual acuity, visual field, and color perception with therapy for >28 days. Monitor for infusion-related reactions, hepatotoxicity, arrhythmias, QT prolongation, acute renal failure, pancreatitis and dermatological reactions (eg, Stevens-Johnson syndrome, exfoliative cutaneous reactions, skin lesions). Monitor for drug toxicity with hepatic insufficiencies. Monitor renal function (SrCr) and hepatic function (LFTs, bilirubin) during therapy.

Patient Counseling: Counsel to take tabs or oral suspension at least 1 hr before or after a meal. Avoid driving at night; drug may affect vision. Counsel to avoid hazardous tasks such as driving or operating machinery if with visual changes. Advise to avoid exposure to strong, direct sunlight. Inform that oral suspension contains sucrose and is not recommended with rare problems of fructose intolerance, sucrase-isomaltase deficiency, or glucose-galactose malabsorption. Counsel females to use proper contraception during therapy.

Administration: Oral and IV route. Tab/Sus: Take at least 1 hr before, or 1 hr after a meal. IV: Do not infuse concomitantly into same line or cannula with other drug infusions, including parenteral nutrition. Visually inspect for particulate matter and discoloration prior to administration. Refer to PI for IV reconstitution and dilution instructions. Reconstitute suspension by adding 46mL of water to bottle and shaking. **Storage:** Vial: Unreconstituted: 15-30°C (59-86°F). Reconstituted: 2-8°C (36-46°F) for 24 hrs. Tab: 15-30°C (59-86°F). Oral Sus: Unreconstituted: 2-8°C (36-46°F). Reconstituted: 15-30°C (59-86°F) for 14 days. Do not refrigerate or freeze. Keep container tightly closed.

VIAGRA   RX
sildenafil citrate (Pfizer)

THERAPEUTIC CLASS: Phosphodiesterase type 5 inhibitor

INDICATIONS: Treatment of erectile dysfunction (ED).

DOSAGE: *Adults:* Usual: 50mg PRN 1 hr (recommended) or 0.5-4 hrs prior to sexual activity up to qd. Titrate: May decrease to 25mg or increase to 100mg qd based on effectiveness and tolerance. Max: 100mg qd. Elderly/Hepatic Impairment/CrCl <30mL/min/Concomitant Potent CYP3A4 Inhibitors (eg, ketoconazole, itraconazole, erythromycin, saquinavir): Initial: 25mg qd. Concomitant Ritonavir: Max: 25mg q48h. Concomitant α-blocker: Patient should be on stable α-blocker therapy. Initiate sildenafil at lowest dose.

HOW SUPPLIED: Tab: 25mg, 50mg, 100mg

CONTRAINDICATIONS: Organic nitrates, either taken regularly and/or intermittently, in any form.

WARNINGS/PRECAUTIONS: Potential for cardiac risk of sexual activity in patients with cardiovascular disease (CVD); avoid in men where sexual activity is inadvisable due to underlying cardiovascular status. Decrease in supine BP reported; caution in patients with left ventricular outflow obstruction (eg, aortic stenosis, idiopathic hypertrophic subaortic stenosis) and severely impaired autonomic control of BP. Prolonged erection (>4 hrs) and priapism reported. Caution with myocardial infarction (MI), stroke, or life-threatening arrhythmia within last 6 months; resting hypotension (BP<90/50) or HTN (BP>170/110), unstable angina due to cardiac failure or coronary artery disease (CAD), retinitis pigmentosa, sickle cell or related anemias, anatomical penile deformation (eg, angulation, cavernosal fibrosis, Peyronie's disease), and predisposition to priapism (eg, multiple myeloma, leukemia). Not indicated for use in newborns, children, and women. Safety not known in patients with bleeding disorders and active peptic ulceration. Rare reports of non-arteritic anterior ischemic optic neuropathy (NAION) with PDE5 inhibitors. Cases of sudden decrease or loss of hearing reported.

ADVERSE REACTIONS: Headache, flushing, dyspepsia, nasal congestion, urinary tract infection, abnormal vision (eg, color tinge, increased light sensitivity, blurred vision), diarrhea.

INTERACTIONS: See Contraindications. Contraindicated with nitric oxide donors. Increased levels with CYP3A4 inhibitors (eg, ketoconazole, itraconazole, erythromycin), protease inhibitors (eg, ritonavir, saquinavir) and cimetidine. Reduced clearance with CYP2C9 inhibitors. Increased clearance with CYP3A4 inducers (eg, rifampin, bosentan) and CYP2C9 inducers. Increased levels of bosentan. Additional supine BP reduction with amlodipine reported. Additive hypotensive effect with α-blockers (eg, doxazosin) and vasodilators (eg, minoxidil). May augment BP lowering effect of other antihypertensives. Avoid with other treatments for ED. Loop and K⁺-sparing diuretics and nonselective β-blockers increase AUC of N-desmethyl sildenafil. May potentiate antiaggregatory effect of sodium nitroprusside.

PREGNANCY: Category B, not for use in nursing.

MECHANISM OF ACTION: Phosphodiesterase type 5 (PDE5) inhibitor; enhances effect of nitric oxide by inhibiting PDE5, which then increase the levels of cGMP in corpus cavernosum, resulting in smooth muscle relaxation and inflow of blood to corpus cavernosum.

PHARMACOKINETICS: Absorption: Rapid; absolute bioavailability (41%). Fasted state: T_{max}=30-120 min. High fat meal: T_{max}=delayed 60 min; C_{max}=reduction of 29%. **Distribution:** V_d=105L; plasma protein binding (96%). **Metabolism:** Liver, via CYP450 3A4 (major), 2C9 (minor); N-desmethyl sildenafil (major metabolite). **Elimination:** Feces (80% metabolites), urine (13%); $T_{1/2}$=4 hrs.

NURSING CONSIDERATIONS

Assessment: Assess for previous hypersensitivity to drug, CVD, left ventricular outflow obstruction, impaired autonomic control of BP; history of MI, stroke, or arrhythmia; resting hypotension or HTN, cardiac failure, CAD, sickle cell anemia, predisposing conditions to priapism, retinitis pigmentosa, bleeding disorders, active peptic ulceration, anatomical deformation of penis, renal/hepatic impairment, potential underlying causes of ED, and possible drug interactions.

Monitoring: Monitor potential for hypersensitivity reactions, abnormalities in vision, decrease/loss of hearing, prolonged erection, priapism and other adverse reactions.

Patient Counseling: Instruct to seek medical assistance if erection persists >4 hrs. Inform of potential BP-lowering effect with α-blockers and antihypertensive drugs, and potential cardiac risk of sexual activity in patients with preexisting CV risk factors. Instruct not to take with other PDE5 inhibitors and organic nitrates. Counsel about protective measures necessary to guard against STDs, including HIV. Instruct to d/c and seek medical attention if sudden decrease/loss of vision or hearing occur. Counsel to take a tab 1 hr before sexual activity.

Administration: Oral route. **Storage:** 25°C (77°F); excursions permitted to 15-30°C (59-86°F).

VIBATIV   RX
telavancin (Astellas)

Women of childbearing potential should have a serum pregnancy test prior to administration. Avoid use during pregnancy unless potential benefit to the patient outweighs the potential risk to the fetus. Potential adverse developmental outcomes in humans may occur.

THERAPEUTIC CLASS: Antibacterial agent

INDICATIONS: Treatment of adult patients with complicated skin and skin structure infections (cSSSI) caused by susceptible Gram-positive microorganisms.

DOSAGE: *Adults:* cSSSI: Initial: 10mg/kg IV q24h for 7-14 days. Administer over a 60-minute period by IV infusion. Duration of therapy depend on the severity, site of infection, and patient's clinical and bacteriologial process. Renal Impairment: CrCl 30-50mL/min: 7.5 mg/kg q24h. CrCl 10-<30mL/min: 10mg/kg q48h.

HOW SUPPLIED: Inj: 250mg, 750mg

WARNINGS/PRECAUTIONS: New onset or worsening of renal impairment may occur; monitor renal function. Decreased efficacy with moderate/severe baseline renal impairment (CrCl ≤50mL/min). Infusion-related reactions (eg, "Red-man Syndrome"-like reactions) may occur with rapid infusion. *Clostridium difficile*-associated diarrhea (CDAD) reported; may range from mild diarrhea to fatal colitis. May increase the risk of the development of drug-resistant bacteria if used in the absence of a proven or strongly suspected bacterial infection. May cause overgrowth of nonsusceptible organisms (eg, fungi); monitor for superinfection. QTc interval prolongation reported; avoid in patients with congenital long QT syndrome, known prolongation of the QTc interval, uncompensated heart failure, or severe left ventricular hypertrophy. May interfere with coagulation tests such as PT, INR, activated partial thromboplastin time (aPTT), activated clotting time, and coagulation based factor Xa; collect sample as close as possible prior to next dose.

ADVERSE REACTIONS: Taste disturbance, N/V, foamy urine, rigors, pruritus (generalized), diarrhea, dizziness, decreased appetite, rash, infusion site pain, infusion site erythema.

INTERACTIONS: Caution with drugs known to prolong QT interval. Higher renal adverse events rate with concomitant medications known to affect kidney function (eg, NSAIDs, ACE inhibitors, loop diuretics).

PREGNANCY: Category C, caution in nursing.

MECHANISM OF ACTION: Antibacterial agent: Lipoglycopeptide; inhibits bacterial cell wall synthesis by interfering with the polymerization and cross-linking of peptidoglycan. Binds to the bacterial membrane and disrupts membrane barrier function.

PHARMACOKINETICS: Absorption: (Single dose) C_{max}=93.6mcg/mL; AUC=747mcg•hr/mL, (Multiple Dose) C_{max}=108mcg/mL. **Distribution:** Plasma protein binding (90%). (Single dose) V_d=145mL/kg. (Multiple dose) V_d=133mL/kg. **Excretion:** Urine (76%), feces (<1%); (Single dose) $T_{1/2}$=8 hr. (Multiple dose) $T_{1/2}$=8.1 hr.

NURSING CONSIDERATIONS

Assessment: Assess for renal impairment, renal impairment risk (eg, pre-existing renal disease, DM, CHF, HTN), congenital long QT syndrome, known prolongation of the QTc interval, uncompensated heart failure, severe left ventricular hypertrophy, concomitant drugs that prolong QTc interval, nursing status, and possible drug interactions. Perform pregnancy test prior to initiation. Obtain baseline SrCr, CrCl and ECG.

Monitoring: Monitor renal function (eg, SrCr). Monitor for CDAD, superinfection, and infusion-related reactions (eg, "Red-man Syndrome"-like reactions).

Patient Counseling: Inform patients of risk of fetal harm when used during pregnancy; perform pregnancy test prior to administration. Encourage women capable of child-bearing to use contraceptives while on therapy. Advise to notify health care provider if pregnancy occurs and encourage patients to enroll themselves in pregnancy registry. Inform physicians if watery and bloody stools (with or without stomach cramps or fever) occur as late as 2 months after the last dose of antibiotics. Antibacterial drugs should only be used to treat bacterial infections and not to treat viral infection. Take as directed. Skipping doses or failure to complete the full course of therapy may decrease effectiveness of immediate treatment and may increase the development of drug-resistant bacteria. Counsel about the common adverse effects; notify physician if any unusual or known symptoms persist or worsens.

Administration: IV route. Infuse over 60 min. Refer to PI for preparation and reconstitution. Additives or other medications should not be added to single-use vials or infused simultaneously through the same IV line. If same IV line is used for sequential infusion of additional medications, the line should be flushed before and after infusion. **Storage:** 2-8°C (36-46°F); excursions permitted to ambient temperature (up to 25°C [77°F]). Avoid excessive heat. (Diluted/Reconstituted) Use within 4 hrs when stored at room temperature or within 72 hrs when stored under refrigeration at 2-8°C (36-46°F).

V

VIBRAMYCIN   RX
doxycycline calcium - doxycycline hyclate - doxycycline monohydrate (Pfizer)

OTHER BRAND NAMES: Vibra-Tabs (Pfizer)
THERAPEUTIC CLASS: Tetracycline derivative

VIBRAMYCIN

INDICATIONS: Treatment of the following infections caused by susceptible microorganisms: Rocky Mountain spotted fever, typhus fever and the typhus group, Q fever, rickettsialpox, tick fevers, respiratory tract infections, lymphogranuloma venereum, psittacosis (ornithosis), trachoma, inclusion conjunctivitis, uncomplicated urethral, endocervical, or rectal infections, nongonococcal urethritis, relapsing fever, chancroid, plague, tularemia, cholera, *Campylobacter fetus* infections, brucellosis, bartonellosis, granuloma inguinale, respiratory/urinary tract infections, anthrax. Treatment of infections caused by *Escherichia coli, Enterobacter aerogenes, Shigella* species, *Acinetobacter* species. When penicillin is contraindicated, treatment of the following infections caused by susceptible microorganisms: uncomplicated gonorrhea, syphilis, yaws, listeriosis, Vincent's infection, actinomycosis, infections caused by *Clostridium* species. Adjunct in acute intestinal amebiasis and severe acne. Prophylaxis of malaria.

DOSAGE: *Adults:* Usual: 100mg q12h on Day 1. Maint: 100mg qd. Severe Infections (Chronic UTI): 100mg q12h. Treat for 10 days with strep infection. Uncomplicated Gonococcal Infection (Except Anorectal in Men): 100mg bid for 7 days or 300mg once followed by 300mg stat in 1 hr. May be taken with food, including milk or carbonated beverage, as required. Uncomplicated Urethral/Endocervical/Rectal Infection and Nongonococcal Urethritis: 100mg bid for 7 days. Early Syphilis: 100mg bid for 2 weeks. Syphilis for >1 yr: 100mg bid for 4 weeks. Acute Epididymo-orchitis: 100mg bid for at least 10 days. Malaria Prophylaxis: 100mg qd. Begin 1-2 days before travel and continue for 4 weeks after leaving malarious area. Inhalational Anthrax (Post-Exposure): 100mg bid for 60 days.
Pediatrics: >8 yrs: ≤100 lbs: 1mg/lb bid on Day 1 then 1mg/lb qd or divided into 2 doses, on subsequent days. Severe Infections: Maint: 2mg/lb. >100 lbs: Usual: 100mg q12h on Day 1 then 100mg qd. Severe Infections (Chronic UTI): 100mg q12h. Malaria Prophylaxis: >8 yrs: 2mg/kg qd. Max: 100mg/day. Begin 1-2 days before travel and continue for 4 weeks after leaving malarious area. Treat for 10 days with strep infection. Inhalation Anthrax (Post-Exposure): <100 lbs (45kg): 1mg/lb (2.2mg/kg) bid for 60 days. ≥100 lbs: 100mg bid for 60 days.

HOW SUPPLIED: Cap: (Doxycycline Hyclate) 100mg; Syrup: (Doxycycline Calcium) 50mg/5mL [473mL]; Sus: (Doxycycline Monohydrate) 25mg/5mL [60mL]; Tab: (Vibra-Tabs) 100mg

WARNINGS/PRECAUTIONS: May cause permanent tooth discoloration during tooth development (last half of pregnancy, infancy, and children <8 yrs). *Clostridium difficile*-associated diarrhea (CDAD) reported; if suspected/confirmed, appropriate fluid and electrolyte management, protein supplementation, antibiotic treatment of CDAD, and surgical evaluation should be instituted as clinically indicated. Enamel hypoplasia reported. May increase BUN. Photosensitivity manifested by sunburn reaction reported; d/c at first evidence of skin erythema. Superinfection may occur; d/c antibiotic and institute proper therapy. Syrup contains sodium metabisulfite that may cause allergic-type reactions, including anaphylactic symptoms and life-threatening or less severe asthmatic episodes. Bulging fontanels in infants and benign intracranial HTN in adults reported.

ADVERSE REACTIONS: Anorexia, N/V, diarrhea, maculopapular/erythematous rash, Stevens Johnson syndrome, toxic epidermal necrolysis, photosensitivity, increased BUN, hypersensitivity reactions, hemolytic anemia, thrombocytopenia, neutropenia, eosinophilia.

INTERACTIONS: May decrease PT, adjust anticoagulants. May interfere with bactericidal agents (eg, penicillin). May decrease effects of oral contraceptives. Aluminum-, calcium-, iron-, and magnesium-containing products and bismuth subsalicylate impair absorption. Decreased half-life with barbiturates, carbamazepine, and phenytoin. Fatal renal toxicity with methoxyflurane.

PREGNANCY: Category D, not for use in nursing.

MECHANISM OF ACTION: Tetracycline derivative; thought to inhibit protein synthesis.

PHARMACOKINETICS: Absorption: (PO) completely absorbed, C_{max}=2.6 mcg/mL, T_{max}=2 hrs. **Distribution:** Crosses placenta. Found in breast milk. **Elimination:** Urine, feces; $T_{1/2}$=18-22 hrs.

NURSING CONSIDERATIONS

Assessment: Assess for age, history of exposure to direct sunlight or UV light, diarrhea, pregnancy/nursing status, possible drug interactions, and renal impairment. Perform incision and drainage in conjunction with antibiotic therapy when indicated. Document indications for therapy, culture, and susceptibility testing. Obtain baseline CBC, serum electrolytes if with diarrhea, LFTs, and renal function.

Monitoring: Monitor for signs/symptoms of hypersensitivity reactions, photosensitivity, superinfection, CDAD, vaginal candidiasis, benign intracranial HTN. In venereal disease with coexistent syphilis, conduct dark field exam before treatment and monthly for 4 months. Perform periodic laboratory evaluation of organ systems including hematopoietic (eg, CBC), renal, and hepatic studies in long-term therapy.

Patient Counseling: Inform of pregnancy risks and photosensitivity reactions (d/c at 1st sign of skin erythema). Avoid excessive sunlight and UV light and use sunscreen/sunblock. Drink fluids liberally to reduce risk of esophageal irritation or ulceration. Therapy only treats bacterial, not viral, infections. Take as directed; skipping doses or not completing full course may decrease effectiveness and increase resistance. Inform that diarrhea may be experienced and to notify physician if watery/bloody stools (with or without stomach cramps and fever) even as late as ≥2 months after last dose), hypersensitivity reactions, superinfections, photosensitivity, or benign intracranial HTN occur. Avoid foods with calcium. Advise patients on malaria prophylaxis to avoid being bitten by mosquitoes by using personal protective measures that help avoid contact with mosquitoes. Counsel to begin therapy 1-2 days before travel to the malarious area, continue while in malarious area, and 4 weeks after returning from area. Therapy should not exceed 4 months. Take adequate fluids with caps or tabs to reduce esophageal irritation or take with food or milk if GI irritation occurs.

Administration: Oral route. Take adequate fluids with caps or tabs to reduce esophageal irritation. Take with food or milk if GI irritation occurs. **Storage:** Below 30°C (86°F).

VICODIN

CIII

hydrocodone bitartrate - acetaminophen (Abbott)

OTHER BRAND NAMES: Vicodin HP (Abbott) - Vicodin ES (Abbott)

THERAPEUTIC CLASS: Opioid analgesic

INDICATIONS: Relief of moderate to moderately severe pain.

DOSAGE: *Adults:* Usual: Vicodin: 1-2 tabs q4-6h prn. Max: 8 tabs/day. Vicodin HP: 1 tab q4-6h prn. Max: 6 tabs/day. Vicodin ES: 1 tab q4-6h prn. Max: 5 tabs/day.

HOW SUPPLIED: (Hydrocodone-APAP) Tab: Vicodin: 5mg-500mg*; Vicodin HP: 10mg-660mg*; Vicodin ES: 7.5mg-750mg* *scored

WARNINGS/PRECAUTIONS: Caution in elderly, debilitated, severe hepatic or renal dysfunction, hypothyroidism, Addison's disease, prostatic hypertrophy, urethral stricture, pulmonary disease and postoperative use. May obscure acute abdominal conditions or head injuries. May produce dose-related respiratory depression. Monitor for tolerance. Suppresses cough reflex.

ADVERSE REACTIONS: Lightheadedness, dizziness, sedation, N/V, constipation, rash, respiratory depression.

INTERACTIONS: Additive CNS depression with other narcotic analgesics, antihistamines, antipsychotics, antianxiety agents, alcohol and other CNS depressants. Increased effect of antidepressant or hydrocodone with MAOIs or TCAs.

PREGNANCY: Category C, not for use in nursing.

V

MECHANISM OF ACTION: Hydrocodone: Opioid analgesic; precise mechanism not known. Suspected to relate to existence of opiate receptors in CNS. APAP: Nonopiate, nonsalicylate analgesic and antipyretic. Analgesic action involves peripheral influences; specific mechanism not established. Antipyretic activity mediated through hypothalmic heat-regulating centers. Inhibits prostaglandin synthetase.

PHARMACOKINETICS: Absorption: Hydrocodone: C_{max}=23.6ng/mL; T_{max}=1.3 hrs. APAP: Rapidly absorbed. **Distribution:** APAP: Found in breast milk. **Metabolism:** Hydrocodone: O-demethylation, N-demethylation and 6-keto reduction. APAP: Liver (conjugation). **Elimination:** Hydrocodone: $T_{1/2}$=3.8 hrs. APAP: Urine (85%) (parent compound and metabolites); $T_{1/2}$=1.25-3 hrs.

NURSING CONSIDERATIONS

Assessment: Assess for hypersensitivity to other opioids, head injury or other intracranial lesions, elevated ICP, acute abdominal conditions, pulmonary disease, presence of debilitation (eg, elderly), hepatic/renal impairment, hypothyroidism, Addison's disease, prostatic hypertrophy or urethral stricture, nursing/pregnancy status, potential for misuse or abuse, and possible drug interactions.

Monitoring: Monitor for signs/symptoms of respiratory depression, elevations in CSF pressure, drug abuse, and drug dependence. In presence of severe hepatic/renal disease, monitor serial liver and/or renal function tests.

Patient Counseling: Caution that may impair mental/physical abilities required for performance of potentially hazardous tasks (eg, operating machinery). Avoid alcohol and other CNS depressants. Advise that drug may be habit forming; should only take for as long as prescribed, in amounts prescribed, and no more frequently than prescribed.

Administration: Oral route. **Storage:** 25°C (77°F); excursions permitted to 15-30°C (59-86°F). Dispense in tight, light-resistant container.

VICOPROFEN   `CIII`
hydrocodone bitartrate - ibuprofen (Abbott)

OTHER BRAND NAMES: Reprexain (Centrix)

THERAPEUTIC CLASS: Opioid analgesic

INDICATIONS: Short-term (generally <10 days) management of acute pain.

DOSAGE: *Adults:* Usual: 1 tab q4-6h prn. Max: 5 tabs/day. Elderly: Use lowest effective dose or longest dosing interval.
Pediatrics: ≥16 yrs: Usual: 1 tab q4-6h prn. Max: 5 tabs/day.

HOW SUPPLIED: (Hydrocodone-Ibuprofen) Tab: (Vicoprofen) 7.5mg-200mg; (Reprexain) 2.5mg-200mg, 5mg-200mg, 10m-200mg

CONTRAINDICATIONS: ASA or other NSAID allergy that precipitates asthma, urticaria, or other allergic reactions. Peri-operative pain in the setting of coronary artery bypass graft (CABG) surgery.

WARNINGS/PRECAUTIONS: May produce dose-related respiratory depression. May obscure acute abdominal conditions or the clinical course of patients with head injuries. May elevate cerebrospinal fluid pressure in the presence of head injury, intracranial lesions or a pre-existing increase in intracranial pressure. Avoid with ASA triad, late pregnancy, advanced renal disease, ASA-sensitive asthma. Caution in elderly, debilitated, renal disease, coagulation disorders, severe hepatic dysfunction, asthma, hypothyroidism, Addison's disease, prostatic hypertrophy, urethral stricture, heart failure, HTN, ulcer disease. May be habit-forming. Suppresses cough reflex; use caution postoperatively and in pulmonary disease. Risk of GI ulceration, bleeding, perforation. Anemia, fluid retention, edema, severe hepatic reactions reported. Possible risk of aseptic meningitis, especially in SLE patients. Increased risk of serious cardiovascular thrombotic events, myocardial infarction (MI), and stroke. Skin reactions (eg, exfoliative dermatitis, TEN, SJS) can occur.

ADVERSE REACTIONS: Headache, somnolence, dizziness, constipation, dyspepsia, N/V, infection, edema, nervousness, anxiety, pruritus, diarrhea, asthenia, abdominal pain, insomnia.

INTERACTIONS: Additive CNS depression with other narcotics, antihistamines, antipsychotics, antianxiety agents, alcohol, CNS depressants. Increased effect of antidepressant or hydrocodone with MAOIs or TCAs. May produce paralytic ileus with anticholinergics. May decrease effects of furosemide and thiazide diuretics, ACE-inhibitors. Avoid ASA. Risk of serious GI bleeding with warfarin. May enhance methotrexate toxicity. Monitor for lithium toxicity. May enhance neuromuscular blocking action of skeletal muscle relaxants.

PREGNANCY: Category C, not for use in nursing.

MECHANISM OF ACTION: (Hydrocodone): Opioid analgesic; not established. Suspected to relate to existence of opiate receptors in CNS. (Ibuprofen): Non-steroidal anti-inflammatory agent; not established. Suspected to inhibit cyclooxygenase activity and prostaglandin synthesis. Possesses analgesic and antipyretic activity.

PHARMACOKINETICS: Absorption: Hydrocodone: C_{max}=27ng/mL; T_{max}=1.7 hrs. Ibuprofen: C_{max}=30mcg/mL; T_{max}=1.8 hrs. **Distribution:** Ibuprofen: Plasma protein binding (99%). **Metabolism:** Hydrocodone: CYP2D6, via O-demethylation to hydromorphone (active metabolite); CYP3A4 via N-demethylation; 6-keto reduction. Ibuprofen: Interconversion from R-isomer to S-isomer; (+)-2-4'-(2-hydroxy-2-methyl-propyl) phenyl propionic acid and (+)-2-4-(2-carboxypropyl) phenyl propionic acid (primary metabolites). **Elimination:** Hydrocodone: Urine (primary); $T_{1/2}$=4.5 hrs. Ibuprofen: Urine (50-60% metabolites, 15% unchanged, conjugate), $T_{1/2}$=2.2 hrs.

NURSING CONSIDERATIONS

Assessment: Assess for hypersensitivity to other opioids, previous reaction to ASA or NSAIDs (eg, asthma, urticaria), type of pain (eg, CABG surgery), or any other conditions where treatment is contraindicated or cautioned. Assess for renal/hepatic function, pregnancy/nursing status, and possible drug interactions. Obtain baseline BP.

Monitoring: Monitor for signs/symptoms of CV thrombotic events, MI, stroke, HTN, fluid retention and edema, drug abuse and dependence, respiratory depression, elevations in cerebrospinal fluid pressure, GI effects, renal effects (eg, renal papillary necrosis), anaphylactoid reactions, skin reactions, hepatic effects (eg, elevations in hepatic enzymes, jaundice, liver necrosis), hematological effects (eg, anemia), bronchospasm, and aseptic meningitis. If signs/symptoms of anemia develop, evaluate Hgb/Hct. Monitor BP while on therapy. If on long-term therapy, perform periodic monitoring of CBC and chemistry profile.

Patient Counseling: Inform drug cannot be substitute for corticosteroids or treat corticosteroid insufficiency. Caution that may impair mental and/or physical abilities required to perform potentially hazardous tasks (eg, operating machinery/driving). Avoid alcohol and other CNS depressants while on therapy. Drug may be habit-forming; only take for as long as prescribed, and not more frequently than prescribed. Contact physician if CV events (eg, chest pain, SOB, slurring of speech), GI effects (eg, ulcers, bleeding), edema, or weight gain occur. Immediately stop therapy and contact physician if signs/symptoms of skin reactions or hepatotoxicity (eg, nausea, fatigue, jaundice) develop. Seek immediate medical attention if any anaphylactoid reactions (eg, difficulty breathing, facial swelling) develop. Report any signs of blurred vision or other eye symptoms.

Administration: Oral route. **Storage:** 25°C (77°F); excursions permitted to 15-30°C (59-86°F). Dispense in a tight, light-resistant container.

Victoza RX

liraglutide (rdna origin) (Novo Nordisk)

> Causes dose-dependent and treatment-duration-dependent thyroid C-cell tumors at clinically relevant exposure in animal studies. It is unknown whether drug causes thyroid C-cell tumors, (eg, medullary thyroid carcinoma [MTC]) in humans. Contraindicated in patients with a personal or family history of MTC and with multiple endocrine neoplasia syndrome type 2 (MEN 2). It is unknown whether monitoring with serum calcitonin or thyroid ultrasound will mitigate human risk of thyroid C-cell tumors. Counsel patients on risks and symptoms of thyroid tumors.

THERAPEUTIC CLASS: Incretin mimetic

INDICATIONS: Adjunct to diet and exercise to improve glycemic control in adults with type 2 diabetes mellitus (DM).

DOSAGE: *Adults:* Initial: 0.6mg qd SQ for 1 week. Titrate: Increase to 1.2mg after 1 week, then to 1.8mg if acceptable glycemic control is not achieved.

HOW SUPPLIED: Inj: 0.6mg, 1.2mg, 1.8mg (6mg/mL)

CONTRAINDICATIONS: MEN 2; personal or family history of MTC.

WARNINGS/PRECAUTIONS: Not recommended as 1st-line therapy with inadequate glycemic control on diet and exercise. Not a substitute for insulin; do not use in type 1 DM or for treatment of diabetic ketoacidosis. Refer patient to an endocrinologist if thyroid nodule and/or elevated calcitonin level are detected. Pancreatitis reported; observe for signs and symptoms (eg, persistent severe abdominal pain, sometimes radiating to the back with or without vomiting) after initiation and dose increases; d/c if suspected and do not restart if confirmed. Caution with history of pancreatitis and with renal/hepatic impairment. Concurrent use with insulin has not been studied. No clinical studies reported establishing conclusive evidence of macrovascular risk reduction. Slows gastric emptying; caution with pre-existing gastroparesis.

ADVERSE REACTIONS: N/V, diarrhea, constipation, upper respiratory tract infection, headache, antibody formation, influenza, urinary tract infection, dizziness, sinusitis, nasopharyngitis, back pain, HTN.

INTERACTIONS: Sulfonylureas or other insulin secretagogues may increase the risk of hypoglycemia. May delay gastric emptying; use caution with concomitant oral medications. Interferes with exposure of digoxin, lisinopril, atorvastatin, acetaminophen, griseofulvin, ethinyl estradiol and levonorgestrel.

PREGNANCY: Category C, not for use in nursing.

MECHANISM OF ACTION: Human glucagon-like peptide-1 (GLP-1) receptor agonist; increases intracellular cyclic AMP (cAMP) leading to insulin release in presence of elevated glucose concentrations. Also decreases glucagon secretion in a glucose-dependent manner and delays gastric emptying.

PHARMACOKINETICS: Absorption: Absolute bioavailability (55%); T_{max}=8-12 hrs; (0.6mg) C_{max}=35ng/mL, AUC= 960ng•hr/mL. **Distribution:** Plasma protein binding (>98%); V_d=13L. **Elimination:** Urine (6%); feces (5%); $T_{1/2}$=13 hrs.

NURSING CONSIDERATIONS

Assessment: Assess for thyroid nodules, MEN 2, personal or family history of MTC, history of pancreatitis, type I DM, diabetic ketoacidosis, pre-existing gastroparesis, renal/hepatic impairment, pregnancy/nursing status, and possible drug interactions. Obtain baseline serum calcitonin, blood glucose, and HbA1c levels.

Monitoring: Monitor for signs and symptoms of thyroid tumor, pancreatitis, and hypoglycemia. Monitor blood glucose and HbA1c levels.

Patient Counseling: Counsel regarding the risks for MTC and to report symptoms of thyroid tumors (eg, a lump in the neck, dysphagia, dyspnea, hoarseness). Inform that persistent severe abdominal pain, sometimes radiating to the back with or without vomiting is the hallmark symptom of acute pancreatitis and advise to d/c therapy promptly and contact physician if persistent severe abdominal pain occurs. Advise not to share pen to prevent transmission of infection. Counsel on potential risks and benefits of treatment, alternative modes of therapy, importance of adhering to dietary instructions, regular physical activity, periodic blood glucose monitoring and HbA1c testing, recognition/management of hypoglycemia/hyperglycemia, and assessment for diabetes complications. Inform that the most common side effects are headache, nausea and diarrhea and that nausea mostly decreases over time. Inform doctor or pharmacist if any unusual symptom develops or if any known symptom persists or worsens. Instruct to read the Medication Guide before starting. Advise to seek medical advice during periods of stress (eg, fever, trauma, infection, or surgery) as medication requirements may change.

Administration: SQ route (abdomen, thigh, or upper arm). Inj site and timing can be changed without dose adjustment. Inspect sol before administration; should be clear, colorless, and contain no particles. **Storage:** Prior to 1st use: 2-8°C (36-46°F). Do not freeze. After 1st use: 15-30°C (59-86°F) or 2-8°C (36-46°F) for 30 days. Keep the pen cap on when not in use. Protect from excessive heat and sunlight.

VIDAZA　　　　　　　　　　　　　　　RX
azacitidine (Celgene)

THERAPEUTIC CLASS: Pyrimidine nucleoside analog

INDICATIONS: Treatment of myelodysplastic syndrome subtypes: refractory anemia (RA) or refractory anemia with ringed sideroblasts (if accompanied by neutropenia or thrombocytopenia or requiring transfusions), refractory anemia with excess blasts (RAEB), refractory anemia with excess blasts in transformation (RAEB-T), and chronic myelomonocytic leukemia (CMMoL).

DOSAGE: *Adults:* Initial: 75mg/m² SQ or IV daily for 7 days. Repeat cycle every 4 weeks. May increase to 100mg/m² after 2 cycles if no beneficial effect and no toxicity other than N/V. Treat for a minimum of 4-6 cycles. Premedicate for N/V. If administer IV, administer over 10-40 min. Adjust dose based on hematology lab values, renal function, and serum electrolytes; refer to PI for further detail.

HOW SUPPLIED: Inj: 100mg

CONTRAINDICATIONS: Advanced malignant hepatic tumors and hypersensitivity to mannitol.

WARNINGS/PRECAUTIONS: Anemia, neutropenia and thrombocytopenia may occur; monitor CBC periodically (at minimum, before each cycle). Potentially hepatotoxic in patients with severe pre-existing hepatic impairment; caution with liver disease. Renal abnormalities reported; reduce dose or hold for unexplained reductions in serum bicarbonate <20mEq/L or elevations of BUN or SrCr occur. Monitor for toxicity with renal impairment. Obtain liver chemistries and SrCr prior to initiation of therapy. May cause fetal harm; avoid pregnancy in women of childbearing potential. Men should not father a child while receiving treatment.

ADVERSE REACTIONS: (SQ) N/V, anemia, thrombocytopenia, pyrexia, leukopenia, diarrhea, fatigue, injection-site erythema, constipation, neutropenia, ecchymosis. (IV) Petechiae, rigors, weakness, hypokalemia.

PREGNANCY: Category D, not for use in nursing.

MECHANISM OF ACTION: Pyrimidine nucleoside analogue; believed to exert its antineoplastic effects by causing hypomethylation of DNA and direct cytotoxicity on abnormal hematopoietic cells in the bone marrow.

PHARMACOKINETICS: Absorption: (SQ) Rapid; Bioavailability (89%). C_{max}=750ng/mL; T_{max}=0.5 hr. **Distribution:** (IV) V_d=76L. **Elimination:** (SQ) $T_{1/2}$=41 min.

NURSING CONSIDERATIONS

Assessment: Assess for hypersensitivity to mannitol, advanced malignant hepatic tumors, renal/hepatic impairment, pregnancy/nursing status, and for possible drug interactions. Obtain baseline CBC, LFTs, and SrCr.

Monitoring: Monitor for signs/symptoms of renal/hepatic dysfunction, anemia, neutropenia, and for thrombocytopenia. Perform periodic monitoring of CBC, liver chemistries, and SrCr.

Patient Counseling: Instruct to notify physician of any underlying liver or renal disease. Inform of pregnancy risks; advise women to avoid pregnancy and men not to father children while on therapy.

Administration: IV/SQ route. **Storage:** 25°C (77°F); excursions permitted to 15-30°C (59-86°F). Reconstituted: Vials: Stable for 1 hr at 25°C (77°F); stable for 8 hrs at 2-8°C (36-46°F).

VIDEX   RX
didanosine (Bristol-Myers Squibb)

> Fatal and nonfatal pancreatitis reported when used alone or part of a combination regimen. Suspend therapy in patients with suspected pancreatitis and d/c with confirmed pancreatitis. Lactic acidosis and severe hepatomegaly with steatosis, including fatal cases, reported with nucleoside analogs alone or in combination. Fatal lactic acidosis reported in pregnant women who received the combination of stavudine and didanosine with other antiretroviral agents.

OTHER BRAND NAMES: Videx EC (Bristol-Myers Squibb)

THERAPEUTIC CLASS: Nucleoside analogue

INDICATIONS: Treatment of HIV-1 infection in combination with other antiretrovirals.

DOSAGE: *Adults:* >18yrs: ≥60kg: (Cap) 400mg qd; (Sol) 200mg bid or 400mg qd. 25-<60kg: (Cap) 250mg qd. <60kg: (Sol) 125mg bid or 250mg qd. 20-<25kg: (Cap) 200mg qd. Renal Impairment: CrCl ≥60mL/min: ≥60kg: (Cap) 400mg qd; (Sol) 400mg qd or 200mg bid. <60kg: (Cap) 250mg qd; (Sol) 250mg qd or 125mg bid. CrCl 30-59mL/min: ≥60kg: (Cap) 200mg qd; (Sol) 200mg qd or 100mg bid. <60kg: (Cap) 125mg qd; (Sol) 150mg qd or 75mg bid. CrCl 10-29mL/min: ≥60kg: (Cap) 125mg qd; (Sol) 150mg qd. <60kg: (Cap) 125mg qd; (Sol) 100mg qd. CrCl <10mL/min: ≥60kg: (Cap) 125mg qd; (Sol) 100mg qd. <60kg: (Sol) 75mg qd. Continous Ambulatory Peritoneal Dialysis/Hemodialysis: CrCl <10mL/min: ≥60kg: (Cap) 125mg qd; (Sol) 100mg qd. <60kg: (Sol) 75mg qd. Concomitant Therapy with Tenofovir Disoproxil Fumarate: CrCl ≥60mL/min: ≥60kg: 250mg qd; <60kg: 200mg qd.
Pediatrics: (Cap) ≥60kg: 400mg qd. 25-<60kg: 250mg qd. 20-<25kg: 200mg qd. (Sol) 2 weeks-8 months: 100mg/m² bid. >8 months: 120mg/m² bid. Do not exceed adult dosing recommendations. Renal Impairment: (cap) dose reduction recommended. Refer to PI for more information.

HOW SUPPLIED: Sol: (powder) 2g, 4g; Cap, Delayed-Release: (Videx EC) 125mg, 200mg, 250mg, 400mg

CONTRAINDICATIONS: Concomitant use with allopurinol and ribavirin.

WARNINGS/PRECAUTIONS: Retinal changes and optic neuritis reported; perform periodic retinal exams. Peripheral neuropathy and non-cirrhotic portal hypertension reported; d/c if occur. May cause fat redistribution. Immune reconstitution syndrome reported in patients treated with combination antiretroviral therapy. Caution with pre-existing liver dysfunction.

ADVERSE REACTIONS: Pancreatitis, lactic acidosis, hepatomegaly with steatosis, diarrhea, neuropathy, headache, N/V, rash.

INTERACTIONS: See Contraindications. Extreme caution with drugs that may cause pancreatitis. Increased risk of peripheral neuropathy with neurotoxic agents (eg, stavudine); use with caution. Ganciclovir, metoclopramide, ranitidine, rifabutin, trimethoprim may increase didanosine (ddI) levels. Methadone, ciprofloxacin, indinavir, ketoconazole, loperamide, ritonavir may decrease ddI levels. DDI may decrease levels of ganciclovir, ranitidine, sulfamethoxazole, zidovudine and increase the AUC, decrease the C_{max} of trimethoprim. Avoid with stavudine. Administer nelfinavir 1 hr after ddI. (Sol) Aluminum- and magnesium-containing antacids may potentiate adverse events. May decrease ketoconazole or itraconazole concentration; administer azole antifungals (eg, ketoconazole or itraconazole) at least 2 hrs before ddI. May decrease quinolone antibiotic concentrations; administer ddI at least 2 hrs after or 6 hrs before ciprofloxacin. May decrease delavirdine concentrations; administer ddI 1 hr after delavirdine. Administer ddI at least 1 hr after indinavir. May decrease tetracycline antibiotic concentrations.

PREGNANCY: Category B, not for use in nursing.

MECHANISM OF ACTION: Synthetic purine nucleoside analogue; inhibits activity of HIV-1 reverse transcriptase both by competing with natural substrate deoxyadenosine 5'-triphosphate and by incorporation into viral DNA, causing termination of viral DNA chain elongation.

PHARMACOKINETICS: Absorption: Rapid. T_{max}=0.25-1.5 hrs. **Distribution:** Plasma protein binding (<5%). (Sol) V_d= (Adults) 43.70L/m²; (Pediatrics, 8 months-19 yrs) 28L/m². Different parameters based on body weight, refer to PI. **Elimination:** (Sol) $T_{1/2}$= (Adults) 1.5 hrs; (**Pediatrics:** 8 months-19 yrs) 0.8 hrs; (**Pediatrics:** 2 weeks-4 months) 1.2 hrs.

NURSING CONSIDERATIONS

Assessment: Assess for pre-existing liver dysfunction, known risk factors for liver disease/pancreatitis, renal impairment, obesity, prolonged nucleoside exposure, advanced HIV disease, history of neuropathy, pregnancy/nursing status, and possible drug interactions.

Monitoring: Monitor for signs/symptoms of pancreatitis, lactic acidosis, hepatomegaly with steatosis, peripheral neuropathy, portal hypertension, retinal changes, optic neuritis, immune reconstitution syndrome, and for fat redistribution. Closely monitor renal/hepatic function. Perform periodic retinal exams. Perform laboratory testing including liver enzymes, serum bilirubin, albumin, CBC, INR, and ultrasonography. May enroll patients in the antiretroviral pregnancy registry if they become pregnant while on treatment.

Patient Counseling: Inform about possible serious toxicity of pancreatitis and about signs/symptoms of lactic acidosis, hepatotoxicity including fatal hepatic events, and peripheral neuropathy. Inform about retinal changes/optic neuritis and non-cirrhotic portal hypertension, including cases leading to liver transplant or death. Caution about use of medications or other substances, including alcohol. Inform about fat redistribution effect. Medication does not cure HIV and may continue to develop opportunistic infections and other complications of HIV. Advise HIV-infected females to avoid nursing to reduce the risk of transmission. Instruct not to miss a dose but if they do, take medication immediately. Continue to practice safe sex and take precautions to prevent from coming in contact with infected blood and other body fluids. Contact poison control center or emergency room right away in case of overdose. (Sol) Take on empty stomach, at least 30 min ac or 2 hrs pc. (Cap) Swallow capsule whole and do not open.

Administration: Oral route. Cap: Take on empty stomach; swallow caps whole. Pediatric Powder for Oral Sol: 1) Reconstitute dry powder with purified water, USP, to initial concentration of 20mg/mL. 2) Immediately mix resulting sol with antacids to final concentration of 10mg/mL. Take on empty stomach, at least 30 min ac or 2 hrs pc. **Storage:** Cap: 25°C (77°F); excursions permitted 15-30°C (59-86°F). Store in tightly closed container. Powder: 15-30°C (59-86°F). Admixture: May be stored up to 30 days in refrigerator at 2-8°C (36-46°F). Discard unused medication after 30 days.

VIGAMOX   RX
moxifloxacin HCl (Alcon)

THERAPEUTIC CLASS: Fluoroquinolone

INDICATIONS: Treatment of bacterial conjunctivitis.

DOSAGE: *Adults:* 1 drop tid for 7 days.
Pediatrics: ≥1 yr: 1 drop tid for 7 days.

HOW SUPPLIED: Sol: 0.5% [3mL]

WARNINGS/PRECAUTIONS: Not for injection. Do not inject subconjunctivally or into the anterior chamber of the eye. Superinfection may result with prolonged use. Fatal hypersensitivity reactions reported after first dose of systemic quinolone therapy. Avoid contact lenses when symptoms are present.

V

ADVERSE REACTIONS: Conjunctivitis, decreased visual acuity, dry eye, keratitis, ocular discomfort/hyperemia, ocular pain/pruritus, subconjunctival hemorrhage, tearing.

PREGNANCY: Category C, caution in nursing.

MECHANISM OF ACTION: Fluoroquinolone antibiotic; inhibits topoisomerase II (DNA gyrase) and topoisomerase IV. DNA gyrase is essential enzyme involved in replication, transcription, and repair of bacterial DNA. Topoisomerase IV is enzyme known to play key role in partitioning of chromosomal DNA during bacterial cell division.

PHARMACOKINETICS: Absorption: C_{max}=2.7ng/mL; AUC=45ng•hr/mL. **Distribution:** Presumed to be excreted in breast milk.

NURSING CONSIDERATIONS

Assessment: Assess for proper diagnosis of causative organisms (eg, slit lamp biomicroscopy, fluorescein staining). Assess for allergies to other quinolones. Assess use in pregnant/nursing females.

Monitoring: Monitor for signs/symptoms of hypersensitivity or anaphylactic reactions (eg, cardiovascular collapse, angioedema, airway obstruction, dyspnea, urticaria). With prolonged therapy, monitor for overgrowth of nonsusceptible organisms (eg, fungi) and for development of superinfection.

Patient Counseling: Instruct to avoid contaminating applicator tip with material from eye, fingers, or other sources. Instruct to d/c medication and contact physician if rash or allergic reaction occurs. Advise not to wear contact lenses with bacterial conjunctivitis.

Administration: Ocular route. Do not inject into eye. **Storage:** Store at 2-25°C (36-77°F).

VIIBRYD   RX
vilazodone HCl (Trovis)

> Antidepressants increased the risk of suicidal thinking and behavior (suicidality) in children, adolescents, and young adults in short-term studies of major depressive disorder (MDD) and other psychiatric disorders. Monitor and observe closely for clinical worsening, suicidality, or unusual changes in behavior. Not approved for use in pediatric patients.

THERAPEUTIC CLASS: Selective serotonin reuptake inhibitor/5-HT$_{1A}$-receptor partial agonist

INDICATIONS: Treatment of major depressive disorder.

DOSAGE: *Adults:* Initial: 10mg qd for 7 days. Titrate: Increase to 20mg qd for an additional 7 days, and then an increase to 40mg qd. Usual: 40mg qd. Reassess periodically to determine the need for maintenance treatment and the appropriate dose for treatment. D/C of Therapy: Gradual dose reduction is recommended. If intolerable symptoms occur following a dose decrease or upon d/c, consider resuming previously prescribed dose and decreasing the dose at a more gradual rate. Take with food.

HOW SUPPLIED: Tab: 10mg, 20mg, 40mg

CONTRAINDICATIONS: During or within 14 days of MAOI therapy.

WARNINGS/PRECAUTIONS: Serotonin syndrome or Neuroleptic Malignant Syndrome (NMS)-like reactions may occur; d/c and initiate supportive treatment. Caution with seizure disorder. May increase the risk of bleeding events. Mania/hypomania reported; caution with a history or family history of bipolar disorder, mania, or hypomania. May increase the likelihood of mixed/manic episode in patients at risk for bipolar disorder; screen for bipolar disorder prior to initiating treatment. Reports of adverse events with abrupt d/c; reduce dose gradually whenever possible. Hyponatremia may occur in association with the syndrome of inappropriate antidiuretic hormone secretion (SIADH); greater risk in elderly.

ADVERSE REACTIONS: Diarrhea, N/V, dizziness, dry mouth, insomnia, abnormal dreams, libido decreased, fatigue, arthralgia, dyspepsia, flatulence, gastroenteritis, somnolence, paresthesia, restlessness.

INTERACTIONS: See Contraindications. May increase risk of serotonin syndrome and NMS-like reactions with serotonergic drugs (eg, triptans, SSRIs, SNRIs, buspirone, tramadol), drugs that impair metabolism of serotonin (including MAOIs), antipsychotics or other dopamine antagonists. Caution with CNS-active drugs. Not recommended with serotonin precursors (eg, tryptophan). Increased risk of bleeding may occur with psychotropic drugs, aspirin (ASA), NSAIDs, warfarin, and other anticoagulants. Increased levels with strong CYP3A4 inhibitors (eg, ketoconazole). Reduce dose for patients with intolerable adverse events if coadministered with moderate inhibitors of CYP3A4 (eg, erythromycin). Decreased levels with CYP3A4 inducers. May increase the biotransformation of mephenytoin. May inhibit the biotransformation of substrates of CYP2C8. Diuretics may increase risk of hyponatremia. Increased free concentrations with other highly protein bound drugs.

PREGNANCY: Category C, not for use in nursing.

MECHANISM OF ACTION: SSRI and 5-HT$_{1A}$ receptor partial agonist; mechanism not established; thought to enhance serotonergic activity in the CNS through selective inhibition of serotonin reuptake.

PHARMACOKINETICS: Absorption: Absolute bioavailability (72%, with food); C_{max}=156ng/mL (fed), AUC=1645ng•h/mL (fed), T_{max}=4-5 hrs. **Distribution:** Plasma protein binding (96-99%). **Metabolism:** CYP and non-CYP pathways (possibly by carboxylesterase). **Elimination:** Urine (1%, unchanged), feces (2%, unchanged); $T_{1/2}$=25 hrs.

NURSING CONSIDERATIONS

Assessment: Assess for history or family history of mania/hypomania, seizures, volume depletion, pregnancy/nursing status, and possible drug interactions. Screen for bipolar disorder. Evaluate for history of drug abuse.

Monitoring: Monitor for clinical worsening, suicidality, unusual changes in behavior, serotonin syndrome or NMS-like reactions, abnormal bleeding, activation of mania/hypomania, hyponatremia. If d/c therapy (particularly if abrupt), monitor for d/c symptoms. Monitor for signs of drug misuse or abuse (eg, development of tolerance, drug-seeking behavior, increases in dose).

Patient Counseling: Counsel about benefits and risks of therapy. Look for the emergence of suicidality, especially early during treatment and when the dose is adjusted up or down. Take with food. Do not take with an MAOI or within 14 days of stopping an MAOI and allow 14 days after stopping vilazodone HCl before starting an MAOI. Caution about risk of serotonin syndrome or NMS-like reactions, and increased risk of bleeding. Caution about use if with history of seizures. Observe for signs and symptoms of activation of mania/hypomania. Patients treated with diuretics, are volume depleted, or elderly may be at greater risk of developing hyponatremia. Avoid alcohol. Notify physician if allergic reactions (eg, rash, hives, swelling, or difficulty breathing) occur. Do not d/c without notifying physician. Therapy may impair physical/mental ability. Notify physician if pregnant/nursing, become pregnant or intend to become pregnant during therapy.

Administration: Oral route. **Storage:** 25°C (77°F); excursions permitted to 15-30°C (59-86°F).

VIMOVO

RX

esomeprazole magnesium - naproxen (AstraZeneca)

THERAPEUTIC CLASS: NSAID/Proton Pump Inhibitor

INDICATIONS: Relief of signs and symptoms of osteoarthritis, rheumatoid arthritis, and ankylosing spondylitis and to decrease the risk of developing gastric ulcers in patients at risk of developing NSAID-associated gastric ulcers.

DOSAGE: *Adults:* 375mg/20mg bid or 500mg/20mg bid. Take ≥30 min before meals. Use lowest dose at the shortest possible duration. Do not split, chew, crush, or dissolve tab. Elderly: Start at lowest effective dose.

HOW SUPPLIED: Tab, Delayed-Release: (Naproxen-Esomeprazole): 375mg-20mg, 500mg-20mg

CONTRAINDICATIONS: Patients who have experienced asthma, urticaria, or allergic-type reactions after taking aspirin (ASA) or other NSAIDs. Patients in the late stages of pregnancy. Treatment of peri-operative pain in the setting of coronary artery bypass graft (CABG) surgery.

WARNINGS/PRECAUTIONS: Can lead to onset/worsening of HTN; monitor BP. Fluid retention, edema, and peripheral edema has been observed; caution in patients with fluid retention or congestive heart failure (CHF). Caution with history of ulcer, GI bleeding; increased risk for GI bleeding with longer duration of therapy, smoking, old age, debilitated condition, and poor health status. Caution with history of inflammatory bowel disease (ulcerative colitis, Crohn's disease) as their condition may be exacerbated. D/C with active bleeding. Long-term use resulted in renal papillary necrosis and other renal injury. Risk of renal toxicity with impaired renal function, hypovolemia, heart failure, liver dysfunction, and salt depletion. Severe hepatic reactions (eg, jaundice, hepatitis, necrosis and hepatic failure) reported rarely; d/c if liver disease develops. May cause anaphylactoid reactions; not recommended for use in patients with the ASA triad. May cause serious skin adverse events (eg, exfoliative dermatitis, Stevens-Johnson syndrome [SJS], toxic epidermal necrolysis [TEN]); d/c at first appearance of skin rash or any other sign of hypersensitivity. May cause premature closure of the ductus arteriosus in late pregnancy. May cause anemia and prolonged bleeding time; monitor Hgb/Hct if signs of anemia present. Caution with asthma and ASA-sensitive asthma. Increased risk for osteoporosis-related fractures; adequate vitamin D and calcium intake is recommended. May mask signs of inflammation and fever. Not recommended for initial treatment of acute pain.

ADVERSE REACTIONS: Flatulence, hiatus hernia, gastritis, diarrhea, nausea, abdominal distension, constipation, esophagitis, GI bleeding/perforation, dyspepsia, upper respiratory tract infection, gastric ulcer, upper abdominal pain, erosive gastritis.

INTERACTIONS: Increased risk for GI bleeding with oral corticosteroids, anticoagulants (eg, warfarin), antiplatelets (including low dose ASA), SSRIs, alcohol and smoking. Upper GI bleeding may occur with psychotropic drugs that interfere with serotonin reuptake. Increased risk of adverse reactions with ASA and non-ASA NSAIDs. Diminished antihypertensive effect of ACE inhibitors, propranolol, and other β-blockers. Cholestyramine can delay absorption of naproxen. Reduced natriuretic effect of furosemide, thiazides, and loop diuretics. Elevates lithium plasma levels; observe for signs of lithium toxicity. Caution with methotrexate. Potential interaction with albumin-bound drugs (eg, sulphonylureas/sulphonamides, hydantoins). Increased plasma levels with probenecid. Interferes with absorption of pH-dependent drugs (eg, ketoconazole, iron salts, digoxin). Decreased plasma levels of atazanavir, nelfinavir. Increased plasma levels of saquinavir, diazepam, cilostazol. Voriconazole may double esomeprazole exposure.

PREGNANCY: Category C (<30 weeks gestation) and D (≥30 weeks gestation), not for use in nursing.

MECHANISM OF ACTION: Naproxen: NSAID; prostaglandin synthetase inhibition. Esomeprazole: Proton pump inhibitor; suppresses gastric acid secretion by specific inhibition of the H^+/K^+ ATPase in the gastric parietal cell.

PHARMACOKINETICS: Absorption: Naproxen: Bioavailability (95%); T_{max}=3 hrs. Esomeprazole: Rapid; T_{max}=0.43-1.2 hrs. **Distribution:** Naproxen: V_d=0.16L/kg; plasma protein binding (>99%); found in breast milk. Esomeprazole: V_d=16L; plasma protein binding (97%); . **Metabolism:** Naproxen: Liver (extensive) via CYP2C9 and CYP1A2 into 6-O-desmethyl naproxen (metabolite). Esomeprazole: Liver (extensive) via CYP2C19 into hydroxyl- and desmethyl metabolites, and via CYP3A4 into sulphone (major metabolite). **Elimination:** Naproxen: Urine (95%), feces (≤3%); $T_{1/2}$=15 hrs. Esomeprazole: Urine (80%, <1% unchanged), feces; $T_{1/2}$=1.2-1.5 hrs.

NURSING CONSIDERATIONS

Assessment: Assess for hypersensitivity, aspirin (ASA) triad, history of asthma, inflammatory bowel syndrome (ulcerative colitis, Crohn's disease), CV thrombotic events (eg, MI, stroke), HTN, CHF, fluid retention, pregnancy/ nursing status, risk factors for GI events (eg, bleeding, ulceration, perforation), possible drug interactions, renal/hepatic dysfunction, and risk of osteoporosis-related fractures. Obtain baseline vital signs, CBC with platelet count, chemistry profile, LFTs, renal function.

Monitoring: Monitor for signs/symptoms of GI events (eg, bleeding, ulceration, perforation), CHF, edema, HTN. Monitor for serious skin adverse events and anaphylactic reactions. Monitor vital signs, PT/INR, CBC with platelet count, chemistry profile, LFTs and renal function periodically.

Patient Counseling: Inform about benefits and risks of therapy. Therapy may cause CV side effects (eg, MI, stroke), GI side effects (eg, discomfort, ulcers, bleeding) and skin side effects (eg, exfoliative dermatitis, SJS, TEN). Ask for medical advice if with chest pain, SOB, weakness, slurring of speech, epigastric pain, dyspepsia, melena, hematemesis, skin rash/blisters, fever, and itching. Promptly report signs of unexplained weight gain or edema, anaphylactoid reaction (eg, difficulty breathing, swelling of face or throat). D/C therapy if signs/symptoms of hepatotoxicity (eg, nausea, fatigue, jaundice, right upper quadrant tenderness, flu-like symptoms). Avoid in late stages of pregnancy. Caution against activities requiring alertness if patient experiences drowsiness, dizziness, vertigo, or depression. Inform physician of history of asthma or ASA-sensitive asthma. Instruct to swallow tab whole with liquid, to take 30 min before meals, and not to split, chew, crush or dissolve tab.

Administration: Oral route. Swallow whole with liquid. Do not split, chew, crush, or dissolve tab. **Storage:** 25°C (77°F); excursions permitted to 15-30°C (59-86°F). Store in original container; keep tightly closed. Protect from moisture.

VIMPAT `CV`
lacosamide (Schwarz Pharma)

THERAPEUTIC CLASS: Sodium channel inactivator

INDICATIONS: (Tab/Sol) Adjunctive therapy for the treatment of partial-onset seizures in patients ≥17 yrs with epilepsy. (Inj) Adjunctive therapy for the treatment of partial-onset seizures in patients ≥17 yrs with epilepsy when oral administration is temporarily not feasible.

DOSAGE: *Adults:* Partial-Onset Seizures: Initial: 50mg bid (100mg/day). Titrate: May increase at weekly intervals by 100mg/day given as two divided doses. Maint: 200-400mg/day based on response and tolerability. Mild/ Moderate Hepatic Impairment/Severe Renal Impairment (CrCl ≤30mL/min)/ End-Stage Renal Disease (ESRD): Max: 300mg/day. Switching from Oral to IV Dosing: Initial total daily IV dosage should be equivalent to total daily dosage and frequency of PO dosing and infused over 30-60 min. Switching from IV to Oral Dosing: Give at equivalent daily dosage and frequency of IV treatment. *Pediatrics:* ≥17 yrs: Partial-Onset Seizures: Initial: 50mg bid (100mg/day). Titrate: May increase, at weekly intervals by 100mg/day given as two divided doses. Maint: 200-400mg/day based on response and tolerability. Mild/ Moderate Hepatic Impairment/Severe Renal Impairment (CrCl ≤30mL/min)/ End-Stage Renal Disease (ESRD): Max: 300mg/day. Switching from Oral to IV Dosing: Initial total daily IV dosage should be equivalent to total daily dosage and frequency of PO dosing and infused over 30-60 min. Switching from IV to Oral Dosing: Give at equivalent daily dosage and frequency of IV treatment.

HOW SUPPLIED: Inj: 200mg/20mL; Sol: 10mg/mL; Tab: 50mg, 100mg, 150mg, 200mg

V

WARNINGS/PRECAUTIONS: May increase risk of suicidal thoughts or behavior; monitor emergence or worsening of depression, suicidal thoughts/behavior and/or unusual changes in mood/behavior. May cause dizziness and ataxia; may impair physical/mental abilities. Prolongations in PR interval reported. Caution with known conduction abnormalities (eg, AV block, sick sinus syndrome without pacemaker) or severe cardiac disease (eg, myocardial ischemia, heart failure). May predispose to atrial arrhythmias especially in patients with diabetic neuropathy and/or cardiovascular disease (CVD). Syncope or loss of consciousness reported in patients with diabetic neuropathy. Withdraw gradually over minimum of 1 week to minimize potential of increased seizure frequency in patients with seizure disorders. Multi-organ hypersensitivity reactions (Drug Reaction with Eosinophilia and Systemic Symptoms [DRESS]) may occur; d/c if suspected. Avoid use with severe hepatic impairment. Monitor closely during dose titration with co-existing hepatic or renal impairment; abnormalities in LFTs reported. Caution in elderly. Oral solution Contains aspartame, a source of phenylalanine.

ADVERSE REACTIONS: Dizziness, headache, N/V, fatigue, diplopia, vertigo, somnolence, ataxia, tremor, skin laceration, nystagmus, balance disorder, diarrhea, contusion.

INTERACTIONS: Caution with drugs known to induce PR interval prolongation. Small decreases in concentrations with carbamazepine, phenobarbital or phenytoin. Possibility of pharmacodynamic interactions with drugs that affect the heart conduction system. Abnormality in LFTs with concomitant anti-epileptic drugs.

PREGNANCY: Category C, not for use in nursing.

MECHANISM OF ACTION: Sodium channel inactivator, not established. Selectively enhances slow inactivation of voltage-gated sodium channels, resulting in stabilization of hyperexcitable neuronal membranes and inhibition of repetitive neuronal firing. Binds to collapsin response mediator protein-2 (CRMP-2), which is mainly expressed in the nervous system and is involved in neuronal differentiation and control of axonal outgrowth.

PHARMACOKINETICS: Absorption: Complete; Absolute Bioavailability (100%); T_{max}=1-4 hrs. **Distribution:** V_d=0.6L/kg; plasma protein binding (<15%). **Metabolism:** CYP2C19; O-desmethyl-lacosamide (major metabolite). **Elimination:** Urine (95%), feces (<0.5%); $T_{1/2}$=13 hrs.

NURSING CONSIDERATIONS

Assessment: Assess hepatic/renal function. Assess history of depression, conduction problems and/or cardiovascular disease, diabetic neuropathy, phenylketonuria (PKU), pregnancy/nursing status, and possible drug interactions. Obtain baseline LFTs, and ECG.

Monitoring: Monitor renal/hepatic function, ECG abnormalities, emergence or worsening of depression, suicidal thoughts or behavior and/or any unusual changes in mood or behavior, dizziness, ataxia, prolongation in PR interval, syncope or loss of consciousness and DRESS. Monitor if pregnant or intend to get pregnant.

Patient Counseling: Instruct to take only as prescribed with or without food. Oral solution contains aspartame, a source of phenylalanine. Counsel about high risk of suicidal thoughts and behavior. Carefully monitor emergence or worsening symptoms of depression, any unusual changes in behavior or mood, suicidal thoughts, behavior or self-harm. Counsel about dizziness, double vision, abnormal coordination and balance, and somnolence. Do not engage in hazardous activities (eg, driving/operating complex machinery) until effects of drug are known. ECG changes may predispose to irregular HR and syncope. Medication may cause hypersensitivity reactions affecting multiple organs such as liver and kidney and d/c therapy if suspected. Seek consultation if symptoms of liver toxicity (eg, fatigue, jaundice, dark urine) occur. Notify physician if pregnant or intend to get pregnant; encourage to enroll in the North American Antiepileptic Drug Pregnancy Registry.

Administration: Oral/IV route. Inj: May be administered without further dilution or may be mixed with diluents. Refer to PI for compatability. **Storage:** 20-25°C (68-77°F); excursions permitted between 15-30°C (59-86°F). Inj mixed with diluents: Stable for at least 24 hrs and stored in glass or PVC bags at ambient room temperature 15-30°C (59-86°F). Inj/Sol: Do not freeze. Sol: Discard any unused contents remaining after 7 weeks of first opening the bottle.

VIRACEPT   RX
nelfinavir mesylate (Agouron)

THERAPEUTIC CLASS: Protease inhibitor

INDICATIONS: Treatment of HIV infection in combination with other antiretroviral agents.

DOSAGE: *Adults:* 1250mg bid (five 250mg or two 625mg tabs) or 750mg tid (three 250mg tabs). Max: 2500 mg/day. Take with meal. May dissolve whole tab in small amount of water. Once dissolved, mix cloudy liquid well and consume immediately. Rinse glass with water and swallow rinse to ensure that entire dose is consumed.
Pediatrics: 2-13 yrs: 45-55mg/kg bid or 25-35mg/kg tid. Take with meal. May mix powder with small amount of water, milk, formula, soy formula/milk, or dietary supplements; once mixed, entire contents must be consumed in order to obtain the full dose. If mixture is not consumed immediately, refrigerate ≤6 hrs. Acidic food or juice are not recommended to be used in combination (eg, orange juice, apple juice, applesauce). Do not reconstitute powder with water in its original container. Refer to PI for further dosing guidelines.

HOW SUPPLIED: Sus: (powder) 50mg/g [144g]; Tab: 250mg, 625mg

CONTRAINDICATIONS: Concomitant use with alfuzosin, amiodarone, quinidine, dihydroergotamine, ergonovine, ergotamine, methylergonovine, pimozide, sildenafil (for the treatment of pulmonary arterial hypertension), midazolam, triazolam.

WARNINGS/PRECAUTIONS: Powder contains phenylalanine; caution in patients with phenylketonuria. New-onset diabetes mellitus (DM), exacerbation of DM, and hyperglycemia reported. Do not use in patients with moderate or severe hepatic impairment. HIV cross-resistance between protease inhibitors reported. Increased bleeding reported in patients with hemophilia A and B (eg, hematomas, hemarthrosis). Fat redistribution/accumulation and immune reconstitution syndrome reported.

ADVERSE REACTIONS: Diarrhea, N/V, flatulence, rash, redistribution of body fat, jaundice, allergic reactions, bilirubinemia, hyperglycemia, metabolic acidosis, anemia, anxiety, rhinitis, pruritus.

INTERACTIONS: See Contraindications. CYP3A or CYP2C19 inducers (eg, rifampin) may decrease plasma levels and reduce therapeutic effect. Use with rifampin may lead to loss of virologic response and possible resistance to nelfinavir or other coadministered antiretroviral agents. CYP3A or CYP2C19 inhibitors may increase plasma levels. Avoid lovastatin or simvastatin; caution with other HMG-CoA reductase inhibitors that are metabolized by CYP3A. Reduce dose of rifabutin to 50% of the usual dose when coadministering. May increase sildenafil or other PDE5 inhibitor levels and adverse effects. Avoid St. John's wort; may decrease levels of nelfinavir. May increase levels of drugs metabolized by CYP3A (eg, dihydropyridine CCBs, immunosuppressants, etc). Caution with drugs metabolized by CYP3A and that prolong the QT interval. Use alternative or additional contraception with oral contraceptives. May increase levels of cyclosporine, tacrolimus, sirolimus, atorvastatin, rosuvastatin, fluticasone, azithromycin, trazodone. Carbamazepine, phenobarbital may decrease levels of nelfinavir. May decrease levels of phenytoin, methadone. Give didanosine 1 hr before or 2 hrs after nelfinavir. Concomitant use with indinavir may increase nelfinavir and indinavir concentrations. Concomitant use with ritonavir may increase nelfinavir concentrations. Concomitant use with saquinavir may increase saquinavir levels. Concomitant use with delavirdine may increase nelfinavir levels, decrease delavirdine levels and decrease nelfinavir C_{min}. Coadministration with amprenavir may decrease C_{max} of amprenavir and increase the C_{min} of amprenavir. Omeprazole decreases levels of nelfinavir; concomitant use with proton pump inhibitors may lead to loss

V

of virologic response and development of resistance. May increase colchicine levels; should not be given in combination in patients with renal or hepatic impairment. May increase bosentan levels; consider dose adjustment. See PI for complete information.

PREGNANCY: Category B, not for use in nursing.

MECHANISM OF ACTION: HIV-1 protease inhibitor; prevents cleavage of *gag* and *gag*-Pol polyprotein resulting in production of immature, noninfectious virus.

PHARMACOKINETICS: Absorption: 28 days: (1250mg bid) C_{max}=4mg/L; AUC=52.8mg•h/L. (750mg tid) C_{max}=3mg/L; AUC=43.6mg•h/L. 14 days: (1250mg bid) C_{max}=4.7mg/L; AUC=35.3mg•h/L. **Distribution:** V_d=2-7L/kg; plasma protein binding (>98%). **Metabolism:** Liver via CYP3A, 2C19 (oxidation). **Elimination:** Feces (78%, metabolites), (22%, unchanged), urine (1-2%); $T_{1/2}$=3.5-5 hrs.

NURSING CONSIDERATIONS

Assessment: Assess for previous hypersensitivity, hepatic impairment, DM, hemophilia, pregnancy/nursing status, and for possible drug interactions. Assess for phenylketonuria if planning to use oral powder formulation. Obtain baseline ECG, ALT, AST, GGT, CPK, uric acid levels.

Monitoring: Monitor for signs/symptoms of hypersensitivity reactions, new onset or exacerbation of DM and hyperglycemia, immune reconstitution syndrome, fat redistribution/accumulation, and hepatic dysfunction. In patients with hemophilia, monitor for signs/symptoms of increased bleeding (eg, hematomas, hemarthrosis). Monitor ECG, ALT, AST, GGT, CPK, uric acid levels. May enroll patients in the Antiretroviral Pregnancy Registry if they become pregnant while on treatment.

Patient Counseling: Inform that therapy does not cure HIV; may continue to acquire illnesses including opportunistic infections. Inform that therapy does not reduce risk of transmitting HIV. Inform that fat redistribution/accumulation may occur. Instruct to take with food; do not alter dose or d/c without consulting physician. Instruct to notify physician if using other prescription, non-prescription or herbal products particularly St. John's wort. Advise to use alternative or additional contraceptive measures if taking oral contraceptives. Inform that most frequent adverse effect is diarrhea; may use non-prescription drugs (eg, loperamide) if occurs.

Administration: Oral route. **Storage:** Tab/Oral Powder: 15-30°C (59-86°F). Keep container tightly closed.

VIRAMUNE   RX
nevirapine (Boehringer Ingelheim)

> Severe, life-threatening, in some cases fatal, hepatotoxicity and skin reactions (eg, Stevens-Johnson syndrome, toxic epidermal necrolysis, hypersensitivity) reported. Hepatic failure reported in patients without HIV taking nevirapine for post-exposure prophylaxis (PEP). Use for occupational and non-occupational PEP is contraindicated. Women, including pregnant women, and/or patients with higher CD4 counts are at higher risk of hepatotoxicity. Seek medical evaluation and d/c if signs or symptoms of hepatitis, increased transaminases combined with rash or other systemic symptoms, severe skin or hypersensitivity reactions and any rash with systemic symptoms develop. The 14-day lead-in period with 200mg qd dosing must be followed; decrease incidence of rash. Monitoring during the first 18 weeks of therapy is essential; extra vigilance is warranted during the first 6 weeks of therapy. Do not restart following severe hepatic, skin or hypersensitivity reactions.

OTHER BRAND NAMES: Viramune XR (Boehringer Ingelheim)

THERAPEUTIC CLASS: Non-nucleoside reverse transcriptase inhibitor

INDICATIONS: Treatment of HIV-1 infection in combination with other antiretrovirals.

DOSAGE: *Adults:* 200mg qd for 14 days (lead-in period), then 200mg bid. If dosing interrupted for >7 days, restart using 200mg qd for 14 days (lead-in period), then 200mg bid. Total duration of the once daily lead-in dosing period should not exceed 28 days. Additional 200mg dose following each dialysis treatment for patients requiring dialysis.

Pediatrics: ≥15 days: 150mg/m² qd for 14 days, followed by 150mg/m² bid. Max: 400mg/day. If dosing interrupted for >7 days, restart using 150mg/m² qd for 14 days, followed by 150mg/m² bid. Total duration of the once daily lead-in dosing period should not exceed 28 days. Additional 200mg dose following each dialysis treatment for patients requiring dialysis. Refer to PI for dose calculation based on BSA.

HOW SUPPLIED: Sus: 50mg/5mL [240mL]; Tab: 200mg

CONTRAINDICATIONS: Moderate or severe (Child-Pugh Class B or C) hepatic impairment. Use as part of occupational and non-occupational PEP regimens.

WARNINGS/PRECAUTIONS: Caution in adult females with CD4⁺ cell counts >250cells/mm³ or in adults males with CD4⁺ cell counts >400cells/mm³. Hepatic injury progresses despite discontinuation. Co-infection with Hepatitis B or C and/or increased transaminase elevations at the start of therapy are associated with a greater risk of later symptomatic events and asymptomatic increases in AST or ALT. Serious hepatotoxicity reported in HIV uninfected individual receiving multiple doses for post-exposure prophylaxis. Caution in hepatic fibrosis or cirrhosis. Rhabdomyolysis reported in some patients experiencing skin and/or liver reactions. If mild-to-moderate rash occurs during 14-day lead-in period, do not increase dose until rash resolves. Delay in stopping nevirapine treatment after the onset of rash may result in a more serious reaction. Women appear to be at higher risk than men of developing rash. Do not use as single agent to treat HIV or add on as a sole agent to a failing regimen. Resistant virus emerges rapidly when administered as monotherapy. Immune reconstitution syndrome reported. Possible fat redistribution/accumulation.

ADVERSE REACTIONS: Nausea, headache, fatigue, neutropenia, anemia, hepatotoxicity, rash, asymptomatic transaminase elevations, liver enzyme abnormalities.

INTERACTIONS: Avoid use of prednisone for prevention of therapy-associated rash. Decreased levels of CYP3A and 2B6 substrates. Decreased levels of clarithromycin; reduce activity against MAC; consider alternatives. Decreased levels of indinavir, nelfinavir and amprenavir. May decrease effectiveness of oral contraceptives and other hormonal contraceptives; use alternate or additional method of contraception. Increased levels with fluconazole; monitor for adverse effects. Avoid use with ketoconazole, St. John's wort or St. John's wort-containing products, efavirenz and atazanavir. Decreased levels of lopinavir; adjust lopinavir/ritonavir doses. May decrease levels of methadone; monitor for signs of withdrawal. Increased levels of rifabutin; use caution. Decreased plasma concentration with rifampin; avoid concomitant use. May decrease plasma concentrations of antiarrhythmics (eg, amiodarone, disopyramide, lidocaine), anticonvulsants (eg, carbamazepine, clonazepam, ethosuximide), azole antifungals (eg, itraconazole), CCBs (eg, diltiazem, nifedipine, verapamil), cancer chemotherapy (eg, cyclophosphamide), ergot alkaloids (eg, ergotamine), immunosuppressants (eg, cyclosporine, tacrolimus, sirolimus), motility agents (eg, cisapride), opiate agonist (eg, fentanyl). Monitor anticoagulation levels with warfarin.

PREGNANCY: Category B, not for use in nursing.

MECHANISM OF ACTION: Non-nucleoside reverse transcriptase inhibitor; binds directly to reverse transcriptase and blocks RNA-dependent DNA polymerase activities by causing disruption of the enzyme's catalytic site.

PHARMACOKINETICS: Absorption: Absolute bioavailability: 93% (tab), 91% (sol); C_{max}=2mcg/mL; T_{max}=4 hrs. **Distribution:** V_d=1.21L/Kg; plasma protein binding (60%); readily crosses placenta; found in breast milk. **Metabolism:** Liver (extensive); oxidative metabolism, via CYP3A and CYP2B6. **Elimination:** Urine (<3% excreted as parent drug); $T_{1/2}$=45 hrs.

NURSING CONSIDERATIONS

Assessment: Assess for CD4, LFTs, hepatic disease/impairment, Hepatitis B or C co-infection, pregnancy/nursing status and possible drug interactions.

Monitoring: Monitor for signs/symptoms of hepatitis and severe skin reactions or hypersensitivity reactions especially during the first 6-18 weeks of

V

treatment; check transaminase immediately if suggestive signs or symptoms appear. Perform LFTs prior to dose escalation and 2 weeks following dose escalation. Monitor patients on methadone for evidence of narcotic withdrawal. Monitor therapeutic effects of the hormonal therapy. May enroll patients in the Antiretroviral Pregnancy Registry if they become pregnant while on medication.

Patient Counseling: Counsel about signs/symptoms of hepatoxicity. Notify physician immediately if any rash or skin reactions develop. May experience redistribution or accumulation of fat tissue. Take as prescribed. Drug does not cure HIV and may continue to develop opportunistic infections and other complications of HIV. Instruct females to avoid nursing to reduce transmission risk. Inform females that oral contraceptives and other hormonal methods of birth control should not be used as sole method of birth control since drug may lower plasma levels of those medications. Report to doctor if using any Rx, OTC or herbal products.

Administration: Oral route. (Sus) Shake prior to administration. Use of oral dosing syringe is recommended. If dosing cup is used, rinsed thoroughly with water and the rinse should also be administered to patient. **Storage:** 25°C (77°F); excursions permitted to 15-30°C (59-86°F).

VIRAZOLE   RX
ribavirin (Valeant)

> Sudden deterioration of respiratory function associated with initiation in infants. Monitor respiratory function carefully. Not for use in adults. Use with mechanical ventilator assistance with staff familiar with mode of administration and specific type of ventilator.

THERAPEUTIC CLASS: Nucleoside analogue

INDICATIONS: Treatment of hospitalized infants and young children with severe lower respiratory tract infections due to respiratory syncytial virus.

DOSAGE: *Pediatrics:* Continuous aerosol administration of 20mg/mL in the drug reservoir of the SPAG-2 unit for 12-18 hrs/day for 3-7 days.

HOW SUPPLIED: Sol, Inhalation: 6g

CONTRAINDICATIONS: Women who are or may become pregnant during exposure to drug.

WARNINGS/PRECAUTIONS: Monitor respiratory function and fluid status according to SPAG-2 manual. Accumulation of drug precipitate can result in mechanical ventilator dysfunction and associated increased pulmonary pressures.

ADVERSE REACTIONS: Worsening of respiratory status, bronchospasm, pulmonary edema, hypoventilation, cyanosis, dyspnea, bacterial pneumonia, pneumothorax, apnea, atelectasis, ventilator dependence, cardiac arrest, hypotension, bradycardia.

INTERACTIONS: Digoxin toxicity reported.

PREGNANCY: Category X, safety in nursing not known.

MECHANISM OF ACTION: Nucleoside analogue; mechanism unknown. Suspected to be analogue of guanosine or xanthosine.

PHARMACOKINETICS: Elimination: $T_{1/2}$=9.5 hrs.

NURSING CONSIDERATIONS

Assessment: Assess for pregnancy status and possible drug interactions.

Monitoring: Monitor respiratory function and fluid status periodically.

Administration: Inhalation route. **Storage:** 25°C (77°F); excursions permitted to 15-30°C (68-86°F). Reconstituted: 20-30°C (68-86°F); stable for 24 hrs.

VIREAD   RX
tenofovir disoproxil fumarate (Gilead)

> Lactic acidosis and severe hepatomegaly with steatosis, including fatal cases, reported with nucleoside analogs, including tenofovir disoproxil fumarate, in combination with other antiretrovirals. Severe acute exacerbations of hepatitis reported in hepatitis B virus (HBV)-infected patients who have d/c anti-HBV therapy including tenofovir disoproxil fumarate. Monitor hepatic function closely for at least several months in patients who d/c anti-HBV therapy. If appropriate, resumption of anti-HBV therapy may be warranted.

THERAPEUTIC CLASS: Nucleotide analog reverse transcriptase inhibitor

INDICATIONS: Treatment of HIV-1 infections in combination with other antiretroviral agents in adults and pediatrics ≥12 yrs. Treatment of chronic hepatitis B in adults.

DOSAGE: *Adults:* 300mg qd without regard to food. Renal Impairment: CrCl 30-49mL/min: 300mg q48h. CrCl 10-29mL/min: 300mg q72-96h. Hemodialysis: 300mg every 7 days or after a total of approximately 12 hrs of dialysis.
Pediatrics: ≥12 yrs: ≥35kg (≥77 lbs): 300mg qd without regard to food.

HOW SUPPLIED: Tab: 300mg

WARNINGS/PRECAUTIONS: Obesity and prolonged nucleoside exposure may be risk factors for lactic acidosis and severe hepatomegaly with steatosis. Caution with known risk factors for hepatic disease. Renal impairment, including cases of acute renal failure and Fanconi syndrome reported; calculate CrCl prior to and during therapy. Monitor CrCl and serum phosphorus levels with renal impairment. Adjust dose and monitor renal function with CrCl <50mL/min. Use only in HIV-1 and HBV coinfected patients as part of an appropriate antiretroviral combination regimen. HIV-1 antibody testing should be offered to all HBV-infected patients before initiating therapy. Prior to treatment, all patients with HIV-1 should be tested for the presence of chronic HBV. Consider bone mineral density (BMD) assessment with history of pathologic bone fracture or other risk factors for osteoporosis or bone loss. Cases of osteomalacia reported. Fat redistribution/accumulation including central obesity, dorsocervical fat enlargement, peripheral wasting, facial wasting, breast enlargement, and "cushingoid appearance" may develop. Immune reconstitution syndrome reported. Early virological failure and high rates of resistance substitutions reported with certain regimens that only contain three nucleoside reverse transcriptase inhibitors (NRTIs); triple nucleoside regimens should be used with caution and treatment modifications should be considered. Caution in elderly.

ADVERSE REACTIONS: Lactic acidosis, hepatomegaly with steatosis, acute exacerbations of hepatitis, N/V, diarrhea, depression, asthenia, headache, pain, rash, elevated cholesterol levels, elevated creatine kinase, elevated serum amylase, increased AST/ALT.

INTERACTIONS: Increases levels of didanosine, use caution when coadministered and monitor for didanosine-associated adverse events. Concomitant use with atazanavir may increase tenofovir (TDF) levels and decrease atazanavir levels; monitor for TDF-associated adverse reactions and d/c if any develop. Levels of renally eliminated drugs (eg, cidofovir, acyclovir, valacyclovir, ganciclovir, valganciclovir) may increase, along with TDF. Lopinavir/ritonavir, and drugs that decrease renal function may increase TDF levels. Concomitant use with indinavir may decrease indinavir levels and increase TDF levels. Concomitant use with saquinavir/ritonavir may increase saquinavir levels and increase the C_{min} of ritonavir and TDF. Concomitant use with tacrolimus may increase levels. Concomitant use with emtricitabine may increase the C_{min} of emtricitabine. Concomitant use with entecavir may increase the AUC of entecavir. May decrease lamivudine plasma levels. May increase C_{max} of abacavir. Avoid with concurrent or recent use of nephrotoxic agents. Do not use concomitantly with fixed-dose combination products containing TDF or with adefovir.

PREGNANCY: Category B, not for use in nursing.

MECHANISM OF ACTION: Nucleotide analog reverse transcriptase inhibitor (NRTI); inhibits activity of HIV-1 reverse transcriptase and HBV polymerase by competing with natural substrate deoxyadenosine 5'-triphosphate and, after incorporation into DNA, by DNA termination.

PHARMACOKINETICS: Absorption: (Fasted) C_{max}=0.30mcg/mL; T_{max}=1 hr; AUC=2.29mcg•hr/mL. **Distribution:** Serum protein bound (7.2%), human plasma bound (<0.7%); V_d=1.3L/kg (1mg/kg IV dose); V_d=1.2L/kg (3mg/kg IV dose). **Elimination:** Urine (70-80% unchanged) (IV), (32%) (multiple oral doses); (PO) $T_{1/2}$=17 hrs.

NURSING CONSIDERATIONS

Assessment: Assess for renal impairment, risk factors for liver disease, pregnancy/nursing status, and for possible drug interactions. Assess BMD in patient with a history of pathologic bone fracture or other risk factors for osteoporosis or bone loss. Calculate CrCl in all patients prior to initiating therapy. In HBV-infected patients, perform HIV-1 antibody testing. In HIV-1 patients, perform testing for presence of chronic HBV.

Monitoring: Monitor for signs/symptoms of lactic acidosis, severe hepatomegaly with steatosis and immune reconstitution syndrome. Upon d/c of therapy in HBV patients, monitor clinical and laboratory follow-up for acute exacerbations of hepatitis. Monitor BMD with history of pathologic bone fracture. Monitor renal function in all patients with CrCl <50mL/min. Monitor calculated CrCl and serum phosphorus levels especially in patients at risk for renal impairment.

Patient Counseling: Inform that medication is not a cure for HIV-1 infection and may continue to experience illness associated with HIV-1 infection, including opportunistic infections. Medication has not been shown to reduce the risk of transmission of HIV-1 or HBV to others through sexual contact or blood contamination; advise to continue to practice safe sex and to use latex or polyurethane condoms. Never reuse or share needles. Tablets are for oral ingestion only. Do not d/c without informing physician. Counsel about the importance of adherence to regimen and avoid missing doses. Patients with HIV should be tested for HBV prior to therapy and patients with HBV should be tested for HIV antibodies prior to therapy. Decreases in bone mineral density may occur. Lactic acidosis, severe hepatomegaly, and severe acute exacerbations of hepatitis may occur. Avoid use of nephrotoxic agents. Do not combine drug with adefovir or fixed-dose combination products containing tenofovir.

Administration: Oral route. **Storage:** 25°C (77°F); excursions permitted to 15-30°C (59-86°F).

VIROPTIC RX

trifluridine (Monarch Pharmaceuticals Inc.)

THERAPEUTIC CLASS: Fluorinated pyrimidine nucleoside antiviral

INDICATIONS: Treatment of primary keratoconjunctivitis and recurrent epithelial keratitis due to herpes simplex virus, types 1 and 2.

DOSAGE: *Adults:* 1 drop into cornea of the affected eye q2h while awake until corneal ulcer has completely re-epithelialized. Max: 9 drops/day. Following Re-epithelialization: 1 drop q4h while awake for 7 days; minimum of 5 drops/day. If no improvement after 7 days or if complete re-epithelialization has not occurred after 14 days, consider other forms of therapy. Avoid using >21 days. *Pediatrics:* ≥6 yrs: 1 drop into cornea of the affected eye q2h while awake until corneal ulcer has completely re-epithelialized. Max: 9 drops/day. Following Re-epithelialization: 1 drop q4h while awake for 7 days; minimum of 5 drops/day. If no improvement after 7 days or if complete re-epithelialization has not occurred after 14 days, consider other forms of therapy. Avoid using >21 days.

HOW SUPPLIED: Sol: 1% [7.5mL]

WARNINGS/PRECAUTIONS: Only use with a clinical diagnosis of herpetic keratitis. May cause transient, mild local irritation of the conjunctiva and cornea when instilled. Possibility of development of viral resistance.

ADVERSE REACTIONS: Burning, stinging, palpebral edema, superficial punctate keratopathy, epithelial keratopathy, hypersensitivity reaction, stromal edema, irritation, keratitis sicca, hyperemia, increased IOP.

PREGNANCY: Category C, not for use in nursing.

MECHANISM OF ACTION: Fluorinated pyrimidine nucleoside antiviral; unknown, suspected to interfere with DNA synthesis.

PHARMACOKINETICS: Absorption: Intraocular penetration; decreased corneal integrity or stromal/uveal inflammation may enhance penetration into the aqueous humor.

NURSING CONSIDERATIONS

Assessment: Assess for clinical diagnosis of herpetic keratitis and for pregnancy/nursing status.

Monitoring: Monitor for clinical signs of improvement after 7 days of therapy and complete re-epithelialization after 14 days of therapy. Monitor for signs/symptoms of mild local irritation of conjunctiva and cornea. Monitor for possible viral resistance and hypersensitivity reactions.

Patient Counseling: Advise that recommended dosage and frequency of administration should not be exceeded. Inform that continuous administration for periods exceeding 21 days should be avoided because of potential for ocular toxicity. Instruct to report any adverse reactions that develop.

Administration: Ocular route. **Storage:** Store under refrigeration 2-8°C (36-46°F).

Visicol   RX
sodium phosphate (Salix)

> Serious acute phosphate nephropathy (rare) reported. Some cases resulted in permanent renal impairment requiring long-term dialysis. Increased risk of acute phosphate nephropathy may occur with increased age, hypovolemia, increased bowel transit time (eg, bowel obstruction), active colitis or baseline kidney disease and using medicines that affect renal perfusion or function (eg, diuretics, ACE inhibitors, ARBs, and possibly NSAIDs). Use the recommended dose and dosing regimen (pm/am split dose).

THERAPEUTIC CLASS: Bowel cleanser

INDICATIONS: For cleansing the colon in preparation for colonoscopy in adults ≥18 yrs.

DOSAGE: *Adults:* ≥18 yrs: Adequately hydrate before, during, and after use. Evening Before Colonoscopy Procedure: 3 tabs with 8 oz. clear liquids every 15 min for total of 20 tabs (last dose is 2 tabs). Day of Colonoscopy Procedure: Repeat dosing on day of exam 3-5 hrs before procedure. May re-treat after 7 days.

HOW SUPPLIED: Tab: (Sodium Phosphate Monobasic Monohydrate-Sodium Phosphate Dibasic Anhydrous) 1.102g-0.398g

CONTRAINDICATIONS: Patients with biopsy-proven acute phosphate nephropathy.

WARNINGS/PRECAUTIONS: Fatalities reported due to significant fluid shift, severe electrolyte imbalances and arrhythmias with administration of sodium phosphate products. Caution with severe renal insufficiency (CrCl <30 mL/min), CHF, ascites, unstable angina, acute bowel obstruction, bowel perforation, toxic megacolon, gastric retention, ileus, pseudo-obstruction of the bowel, severe chronic constipation, acute colitis, gastric bypass, stapling surgery or hypomotility syndrome. Caution with impaired renal function, history of acute phosphate nephropathy, known or suspected electrolyte disturbances (eg, dehydration). Correct electrolyte disturbance before use. Reports of generalized tonic-clonic seizures and/or loss of consciousness in patients with no prior history of seizures. Caution in patients with history of seizures and in patients at high risk of seizure (eg, withdrawing from alcohol or benzodiazepines, known or suspected hyponatremia). Caution in patients with higher risk of arrhythmias (eg, history of cardiomyopathy, prolonged QT interval,

V

uncontrolled arrhythmias, recent MI). Pre-dose and post-colonoscopy ECGs should be done in patients with high risk of serious, cardiac arrhythmias. May induce colonic mucosal aphthous ulcerations and exacerbate IBD. Difficulty of swallowing may occur in patients with a history of difficulties or anatomic narrowing of the esophagus (eg, stricture). Caution with recent cardiac surgery (eg, coronary artery bypass graft surgery). Caution in elderly.

ADVERSE REACTIONS: N/V, abdominal bloating, abdominal pain, hyperphosphatemia, hypocalcemia, hypokalemia, acute phosphate nephropathy (rare).

INTERACTIONS: See Box Warning. May reduce absorption of other drugs. Caution with agents that prolong QT interval or affect electrolyte levels. Avoid use of additional purgative or laxative (eg, other sodium phosphate-containing products) agents. Caution with concomitant use of medications lowering seizure threshold (eg, TCAs).

PREGNANCY: Category C, safety not known in nursing.

MECHANISM OF ACTION: Osmotic laxative; causes large amounts of water to be drawn into colon, promoting colon evacuation.

NURSING CONSIDERATIONS

Assessment: Assess for acute phosphate nephropathy, known hypersensitivity to sodium phosphates, cardiac arrhythmias, severe electrolyte abnormalities, severe renal insufficiency, CHF, unstable angina, bowel obstruction, bowel perforation, gastric retention, severe chronic constipation, acute colitis, history of seizures, pregnancy/nursing status and possible drug interactions. Perform baseline ECG, phosphate, calcium, K⁺, Na⁺, creatinine and BUN levels.

Monitoring: Monitor CrCl, ECG, phosphate, calcium, K⁺, Na⁺, creatinine and BUN levels post-colonoscopy. Watch out for vomiting, arrhythmias and seizures.

Patient Counseling: Discuss the benefits and risks of therapy. Inform healthcare provider of any concomitant medical condition or medication being taken. Instruct to follow the dose and dosing regimen. Drink 8 oz. clear liquid with each 3-tab dose. Ingest total of 3.6 quarts clear liquid. Do not use within 7 days of previous administration. Do not take additional laxatives or purgatives.

Administration: Oral route. **Storage:** 25°C (77°F); excursions permitted to 15-30°C (59-86°F). Discard any unused portion.

VISTIDE

RX

cidofovir (Gilead)

> Renal impairment is a major toxicity; prehydrate with IV normal saline (NS) and administer probenecid with each dose. Monitor serum creatinine (SrCr) and urine protein within 48 hrs prior to each dose. Modify dose with renal function changes. Contraindicated with nephrotoxic agents. Neutropenia reported; monitor neutrophils. Carcinogenic, teratogenic, and hypospermatic in animal studies.

THERAPEUTIC CLASS: Viral DNA synthesis inhibitor

INDICATIONS: Treatment of cytomegalovirus (CMV) retinitis in AIDS patients.

DOSAGE: *Adults:* IV: Induction: 5mg/kg once weekly for 2 weeks. Maint: 5mg/kg once every 2 weeks. Reduce maint from 5mg/kg to 3mg/kg for an increase in SrCr of 0.3-0.4mg/dL above baseline. D/C with increase in SrCr ≥0.5mg/dL above baseline or ≥3+ proteinuria. Administer probenecid 2g PO 3 hrs before cidofovir, then 1g at 2 hrs and 8 hrs after completion of cidofovir infusion. Administer at least 1L normal saline (NS) immediately before infusion. If tolerated, give 2nd liter at start of or immediately after infusion.

HOW SUPPLIED: Inj: 75mg/mL

CONTRAINDICATIONS: SrCr >1.5mg/dL, CrCl ≤55mL/min, or urine protein ≥100mg/dL (≥2+ proteinuria) with therapy initiation. Nephrotoxic agents (d/c at least 7 days before therapy), severe hypersensitivity to probenecid or other sulfa-containing agents, direct intraocular use.

WARNINGS/PRECAUTIONS: Dose-dependent nephrotoxicity. Monitor IOP, visual acuity, ocular symptoms, uveitis/iritis, and renal function periodically. Monitor WBC with differential before each dose. Avoid during pregnancy. Adequate contraception for both sexes during and following treatment is advised. May cause male infertility. Potentially carcinogenic.

ADVERSE REACTIONS: N/V, neutropenia, proteinuria, decreased IOP/ocular hypotony, anterior uveitis/iritis, metabolic acidosis, nephrotoxicity, pneumonia, dyspnea, infection, fever, creatinine ≥2mg/dL, decreased sodium bicarbonate.

INTERACTIONS: Avoid nephrotoxic agents (aminoglyosides, amphotericin B, foscarnet, IV pentamidine, vancomycin, and NSAIDs); d/c nephrotoxic agents at least 7 days before therapy. Temporarily d/c zidovudine or decrease zidovudine by 50% with probenecid.

PREGNANCY: Category C, not for use in nursing.

MECHANISM OF ACTION: Viral DNA synthesis inhibitor; suppresses CMV replication by selective inhibition of viral DNA synthesis.

PHARMACOKINETICS: Administration: Variable doses resulted in altered parameters. **Absorption:** 5mg/kg: AUC=28.3mcg•mL/hr (without probenecid), AUC=40.8mcg•mL/hr (with probenecid), C_{max}=11.5mcg/mL (without probenecid), C_{max}=19.6mcg/mL (with probenecid); 3mg/kg: AUC=20.0mcg•mL/hr (without probenecid), AUC=25.7mcg•mL/hr (with probenecid); C_{max}=7.3mcg/mL (without probenecid), C_{max}=9.8mcg/mL (with probenecid). **Distribution:** V_d=537mL/kg (without probenecid), V_d= 410mL/kg (with probenecid); Plasma protein binding (≤6%). **Elimination:** Urine (80-100% unchanged).

NURSING CONSIDERATIONS

Assessment: Assess renal function, pregnancy/nursing status, and possible drug interactions prior to therapy.

Monitoring: Monitor renal function, SrCr, urine protein, WBC, neutrophils, serum bicarbonate, IOP, and visual acuity. Monitor for signs/symptoms of nephrotoxicity, metabolic acidosis, uveitis, or iritis. Monitor for allergic reactions when using in combination with probenecid.

Patient Counseling: Counsel to take full course of probenecid with drug. If nausea develops, take with food. Inform drug does not cure CMV retinitis; may continue to experience progression of retinitis during, and following, treatment. Advise for regular follow-up ophthalmologic exams. Advise females to use proper contraception while on medication and to continue using contraception for at least 1 month following therapy. Counsel males to use proper contraception while on medication and for 3 months following therapy. Advise drug is not for direct intraocular injection.

Administration: IV route. 1) Inspect for particulate matter and discoloration. 2) Add appropriate volume to 100mL NS. 3) Infuse over 1 hr at constant rate. 4) Probenecid and IV saline prehydration must be administered with each infusion. **Storage:** Vial: 20-25°C (68-77°F). Admixture: Under refrigeration, 2-8°C, for no more than 24 hrs. If refrigerated, allow admixture to reach room temperature prior to use.

VISUDYNE   RX
verteporfin (QLT)

THERAPEUTIC CLASS: Photosensitizing agent

INDICATIONS: Treatment of predominantly classic subfoveal choroidal neovascularization due to age-related macular degeneration, pathologic myopia, or presumed ocular histoplasmosis.

DOSAGE: *Adults:* 6mg/m² diluted in 5% Dextrose for Inj to a total of 30mL IV over 10 min at 3mL/min. Initiate 689nm wavelength laser light therapy with nonthermal diode laser 15 min after start of 10-min IV infusion. In choroidal neovascularization, recommended light dose is 50J/cm² of neovascular lesion at an intensity of 600mW/cm² over 83 sec. Re-evaluate every 3 months and repeat if choroidal neovascular leakage detected on fluorescein angiography. Concurrent Bilateral Treatment: More aggressive lesion should be treated 1st at 15 min after start of infusion. 1 week after the 1st course, if no significant safety issues are identified, treat the 2nd eye using the same treatment regimen. Evaluate after 3 months and start concurrent therapy following a new infusion if both lesions show evidence of leakage.

HOW SUPPLIED: Inj: 15mg

CONTRAINDICATIONS: Porphyria.

WARNINGS/PRECAUTIONS: Avoid exposure of skin or eyes to direct sunlight or bright indoor light for 5 days following injection. If extravasation occurs, d/c infusion immediately; protect area from direct light until swelling and discoloration fade. Protect from intense light if surgery within 48 hrs after therapy is necessary. Do not retreat if severe vision decrease of ≥4 lines within 1 week after therapy occurs. Only use compatible lasers. Caution with moderate to severe hepatic dysfunction or biliary obstruction. Reduced effects with increasing age. Complement activation reported; supervise during infusion.

ADVERSE REACTIONS: Injection-site reactions (eg, pain, edema, inflammation, extravasation, rashes, hemorrhage, discoloration), visual disturbances (eg, blurred vision, flashes of light, decreased visual acuity, visual field defects, including scotoma).

INTERACTIONS: Calcium channel blockers, polymyxin B, and radiation therapy may enhance rate of uptake by vascular endothelium. Increased photosensitivity reactions with other photosensitizing agents (eg, tetracyclines, sulfonamides, phenothiazines, sulfonylurea hypoglycemic agents, thiazide diuretics, and griseofulvin). Decreased effects with compounds that quench active oxygen species or scavenge radicals (eg, dimethyl sulfoxide, β-carotene, ethanol, formate, mannitol) and drugs that decrease clotting, vasoconstriction, or platelet aggregation (eg, thromboxane A_2 inhibitors).

PREGNANCY: Pregnancy C, not for use in nursing.

MECHANISM OF ACTION: Photosensitizing agent; activated by light in presence of oxygen; light activation causes local damage to neovascular endothelium, subsequently leading to vessel occlusion. Damaged endothelium releases procoagulant and vasoactive factors through lipo-oxygenase and cyclo-oxygenase pathways, resulting in platelet aggregation, fibrin clot formation, and vasoconstriction.

PHARMACOKINETICS: Distribution: Found in breast milk. **Metabolism:** Liver and plasma esterases; diacid metabolite. **Elimination:** Feces (major), urine (<0.01%); $T_{1/2}$=5-6 hrs.

NURSING CONSIDERATIONS

Assessment: Assess for drug hypersensitivity, porphyria, hepatic dysfunction, biliary obstruction, pregnancy/nursing status, and possible drug interactions.

Monitoring: Monitor for signs/symptoms of extravasation or injection site reactions, severe decreases in vision, and hypersensitivity reactions. Monitor that IV line is free-flowing.

Patient Counseling: Instruct to avoid exposure of unprotected skin, eyes, or other body organs to direct sunlight, bright indoor light (eg, tanning salon, bright halogen lighting, high powered lighting), or light-emitting medical devices (eg, pulse oximeters) for 5 days following therapy; instruct to wear wristband to remind them to avoid direct sunlight. Instruct to protect eyes and skin if going outdoors during 1st 5 days following treatment. UV sunscreens are ineffective in protecting against photosensitive reactions. Advise to avoid staying in dark when indoors; skin should be exposed to ambient indoor lighting. Inform that visual disturbances may occur; instruct to avoid using machinery/driving.

Administration: IV route. Inspect for particulate matter and discoloration prior to administration. Do not use normal saline or other parenteral solutions, except 5% Dextrose for Inj for dilution. Do not mix with other drugs in the same solution. **Storage:** 20-25°C (68-77°F). Following dilution, protect from light and use within maximum of 4 hrs.

VITRASERT   RX
ganciclovir (Bausch & Lomb)

THERAPEUTIC CLASS: Nucleoside analogue

INDICATIONS: Treatment of cytomegalovirus (CMV) retinitis in AIDS patients.

DOSAGE: *Adults:* Each implant releases 4.5mg over 5-8 months. Remove and replace when evidence of retinitis progression.
Pediatrics: ≥9 yrs: Each implant releases 4.5mg over 5-8 months. Remove and replace when evidence of retinitis progression.

HOW SUPPLIED: Implant: 4.5mg

CONTRAINDICATIONS: Hypersensitivity to acyclovir, patients with contraindication for intraocular surgery (eg, external infection, severe thrombocytopenia).

WARNINGS/PRECAUTIONS: For intravitreal implantation only. Monitor for extraocular CMV disease. Implant does not treat systemic CMV. Complications from surgery include vitreous loss or hemorrhage, cataract formation, retinal detachment, uveitis, endophthalmitis, decrease in visual acuity. Immediate decrease in visual acuity will last 2-4 weeks postop. Maintain sterility of the surgical field, implant. Handle implant by suture tab to avoid damage to polymer coating. Handling and disposal of the implant should follow guidelines for antineoplastics.

ADVERSE REACTIONS: Visual acuity loss, vitreous hemorrhage, retinal detachments, cataract formation/lens opacities, macular abnormalities, IOP spikes, optic disk/nerve changes, uveitis, hyphemas.

PREGNANCY: Category C, not for use in nursing.

MECHANISM OF ACTION: Nucleoside analogue antiviral; inhibits replication of herpes viruses.

NURSING CONSIDERATIONS

Assessment: Assess for proper diagnosis of CMV retinitis (eg, indirect opthalmoscopy). Assess patient does not have contraindications for intraocular surgery (eg, external infection, severe thrombocytopenia) and does not have allergy to acyclovir. Assess use in pregnancy/nursing.

Monitoring: Monitor for extraocular CMV disease and infections (eg, pneumonitis, colitis), vitreous loss or hemorrhage, cataract formation, retinal detachment, uvelitis, intraocular infection, and decrease in visual acuity.

Patient Counseling: Advise that implant is not a cure for CMV retinitis; some patients may continue to experience progression of retinitis. Counsel about potential complications following intraocular surgery (eg, intraocular infection, retina detachment, formation of cataracts). Inform patient will experience immediate and temporary decrease in visual acuity for 2-4 weeks after surgery and will require follow-up ophthalmological exams at regular intervals following surgery. Inform medication may cause infertility and may be carcinogenic.

Administration: Ocular implant. **Storage:** 15-30°C (59-86°F). Protect from freezing, excessive heat, and light.

VIVELLE   RX
estradiol (Novartis)

Estrogens increase risk of endometrial cancer in postmenopausal women. Estrogens, with or without progestins, should not be used for the prevention of cardiovascular disease. Increased risks of MI, stroke, invasive breast cancer, PE, and DVT in postmenopausal women (50-79 yrs of age) reported. Increased risk of developing probable dementia in postmenopausal women ≥65 yrs of age reported.

OTHER BRAND NAMES: Vivelle-Dot (Novartis)
THERAPEUTIC CLASS: Estrogen

INDICATIONS: Treatment of moderate to severe vasomotor symptoms and/or vulvar/vaginal atrophy associated with menopause. Treatment of hypoestrogenism due to hypogonadism, castration, or primary ovarian failure. Prevention of postmenopausal osteoporosis.

DOSAGE: *Adults:* Vasomotor Symptoms/Vulvar/Vaginal Atrophy: Initial: 0.0375mg/day twice weekly. Titrate: Adjust after at least 1 month. D/C or taper at 3-6 month intervals. Wait 1 week after withdrawal of oral therapy before initiating therapy. Osteoporosis Prevention: Minimum Effective Dose: 0.025mg/day twice weekly. Apply to clean, dry area of the trunk; avoid breasts and waistline. Rotate sites; allow 1 week between same site. Without intact uterus, may give continuously; with intact uterus, may give cyclically (3 weeks on, 1 week off) with a progestin.

HOW SUPPLIED: Patch: (Vivelle) 0.05mg/day, 0.1mg/day [8ˢ, 48ˢ]; (Vivelle-Dot) 0.025mg/day, 0.0375mg/day, 0.05mg/day, 0.075mg/day, 0.1mg/day [8ˢ, 24ˢ]

CONTRAINDICATIONS: Pregnancy, undiagnosed abnormal genital bleeding, breast cancer, estrogen dependent neoplasia, DVT/PE, active or recent (eg, within past year) arterial thromboembolic disease (eg, stroke, MI), liver dysfunction or disease.

WARNINGS/PRECAUTIONS: May increase risk of cardiovascular events (eg, MI, stroke), venous thrombosis, and PE; d/c immediately if any of these events occur or are suspected. May increase risk of breast/endometrial cancer and gallbladder disease. May lead to severe hypercalcemia with breast cancer and bone metastases; monitor and d/c if hypercalcemia occurs. Retinal vascular thrombosis reported; monitor and d/c if papilledema or retinal vascular lesions occur. Consider addition of a progestin if no hysterectomy. May elevate BP; monitor at regular intervals. May cause elevations of plasma triglycerides with pre-existing hypertriglyceridemia. Caution with history of cholestatic jaundice associated with past estrogen use or with pregnancy; d/c with recurrence. May lead to increased thyroid-binding globulin levels; monitor thyroid function. May cause fluid retention; caution with cardiac/renal dysfunction. Caution with severe hypocalcemia. May increase risk of ovarian cancer. May exacerbate endometriosis, asthma, DM, epilepsy, migraine, porphyria, SLE, and hepatic hemangiomas; use with caution.

ADVERSE REACTIONS: Altered vaginal bleeding, vaginal candidiasis, breast tenderness/enlargement, N/V, melasma, headache, weight changes, edema, altered libido.

INTERACTIONS: CYP3A4 inducers (eg, St. John's wort, phenobarbital, carbamazepine, rifampin) may decrease levels which may decrease therapeutic effects and/or change uterine bleeding profile. CYP3A4 inhibitors (eg, erythromycin, clarithromycin, ketoconazole, itraconazole, ritonavir, grapefruit juice) may increase levels which may result in side effects.

PREGNANCY: Contraindicated in pregnancy, caution in nursing.

MECHANISM OF ACTION: Estrogen; responsible for development and maintenance of female reproductive system, and secondary sexual characteristics by modulating pituitary secretion of gonadotropins, LH and FSH.

PHARMACOKINETICS: Absorption: Transdermal administration of variable doses resulted in different parameters. **Metabolism**: Liver, estrone (metabolite), estriol (major urinary metabolite). **Elimination**: Urine; $T_{1/2}$=4.4 hrs, 5.9-7.7 hrs (Dot).

NURSING CONSIDERATIONS

Assessment: Assess for abnormal bleeding, breast or estrogen-dependent neoplasia, CAD, asthma, endometriosis, DM, epilepsy, migraine, porphyrias, SLE, hypothyroidism, pregnancy/nursing status, thromboembolic disease, hypocalcemia, and hepatic impairment.

Monitoring: Monitor BP regularly; TFTs periodically. Breast exam by physician yearly and self-exam monthly; mammogram as required. Monitor for signs/symptoms of dementia, gallbladder disease, hypercalcemia, CV events (eg, MI, stroke), abnormal vaginal bleeding, thromboembolic disorders, fluid retention, visual abnormalities, hypersensitivity reactions, hepatic dysfunction, exacerbation of asthma, DM, epilepsy, SLE, migraines, and porphyria.

Patient Counseling: Inform of pregnancy risks. Advise to seek medical attention if symptoms of hepatic dysfunction (eg, jaundice), hypercalcemia, visual abnormalities (eg, partial/complete loss of vision, diplopia), migraines, abnormal vaginal bleeding, hypersensitivity reactions, HTN, thromboembolic disorders, fluid retention, exacerbation of diseases, CV events, or dementia occur.

Administration: Transdermal route. Apply immediately after removed from pouch. **Storage:** Below 30°C (86°F). Dot: 25°C (77°F).

VIVITROL
naltrexone (Alkermes)

RX

> May cause hepatocellular injury with excessive doses. Contraindicated in acute hepatitis or liver failure; caution with active liver disease. Does not appear to be a heptatotoxin at recommended doses. Warn patient of the risk of hepatic injury and advise to seek medical attention if symptoms of acute hepatitis occur. D/C in the event of symptoms and/or signs of acute hepatitis.

THERAPEUTIC CLASS: Opioid antagonist

INDICATIONS: Treatment of alcohol dependence in patients who are able to abstain from alcohol in an outpatient setting prior to initiation of therapy. Prevention of relapse to opioid dependence, following opioid detoxification.

DOSAGE: *Adults:* 380mg IM gluteal inj q4 weeks or once a month, alternating buttocks.

HOW SUPPLIED: Inj, Extended-Release: 380mg

CONTRAINDICATIONS: Acute hepatitis or liver failure, concomitant opioid analgesics, physiologic opioid dependence, acute opioid withdrawal, positive urine screen for opioids or failed naloxone challenge test.

WARNINGS/PRECAUTIONS: Cases of eosinophilic pneumonia and hypersensitivity reactions including anaphylaxis reported. May precipitate opioid withdrawal in alcohol-dependent patients using or dependent on opioids. Must be opioid-free for ≥7-10 days prior to initiation of therapy. Perform naloxone challenge test if there is a risk of precipitating withdrawal. May respond to lower doses of opioids than previously used. Opioid overdose with fatal outcomes reported in patients who use opioids at the end of a dosing interval or when missing a dose. Attempts to overcome opioid blockade could lead to fatal overdose. Monitor for development of depression or suicidal thinking. In emergency situation, suggested plan for pain management is regional analgesia or use of non-opioid analgesics. If opioid therapy is required, monitor continuously in an anesthesia care setting. Caution in renal/hepatic impairment. Does not eliminate or diminish alcohol withdrawal symptoms. Injection-site reactions reported; inadvertent SQ injection may increase likelihood of severe injection-site reactions. As with any IM inj, caution with thrombocytopenia or any coagulation disorder (eg, hemophilia, severe hepatic failure). May cross-react with certain immunoassay methods for the detection of drugs of abuse in urine.

ADVERSE REACTIONS: N/V, diarrhea, insomnia, depression, injection-site reactions, somnolence, anorexia, muscle cramps, dizziness, syncope, appetite disorder, hepatic enzyme abnormalities, nasopharyngitis, toothache.

INTERACTIONS: See Contraindications. Antagonizes effects of opioid-containing medicines (eg, cough and cold remedies, antidiarrheals, opioid analgesics).

PREGNANCY: Category C, not for use in nursing.

MECHANISM OF ACTION: Opioid antagonist; blocks the effects of opioids by competitive binding at opioid receptors.

PHARMACOKINETICS: Absorption: T_{max}=2-3 days. **Distribution:** Plasma protein binding (21%); (PO) found in breast milk. **Metabolism:** Extensive, via dihydrodiol dehydrogenase, 6β-naltrexol (primary metabolite). **Elimination:** Urine; $T_{1/2}$=5-10 days.

V

NURSING CONSIDERATIONS

Assessment: Assess for hepatic failure, hepatitis or active liver disease, opioid use or dependence thrombocytopenia, coagulation disorder (eg, hemophilia, severe hepatic failure), renal impairment, pre-existing subclinical abstinence syndrome, hypersensitivity, pregnancy/nursing status, alcohol intake, and for possible drug interactions. Assess patient's body habitus to assure the needle length is adequate.

Monitoring: Monitor for severe injection-site reactions, signs/symptoms of acute hepatitis, unintended opioid withdrawal, opioid intoxication (respiratory compromise/arrest, circulatory collapse), eosinophilic pneumonia, depression, suicidal thinking, and hypersensitivity reactions. Monitor LFTs and CPK.

Patient Counseling: Alert families and caregivers to monitor for emergence of symptoms of depression and call a doctor immediately. Carry documentation to alert medical personnel to therapy. Concomitant large doses of opioids may lead to serious injury, coma, or death. If previously used opioids, may be more sensitive to lower doses of opioids after naltrexone is d/c. Notify if pregnant/nursing or planning to become pregnant, experience respiratory symptoms (eg, dyspnea, coughing, or wheezing), allergic reactions. Inform that injection-site reactions may occur and to seek medical attention for worsening skin reactions. Avoid opioids for ≥7-10 days before therapy and inform doctor of any prior opioid use. May cause liver injury if liver disease develops from other cause. Notify physician if signs/symptoms of liver disease and pneumonia develop. Therapy treats alcohol dependence only when used as part of treatment program. May impair mental/physical abilities. May cause nausea, which tends to subside. Instruct to receive the next dose as soon as possible if a dose is missed.

Administration: IM route; gluteal region. Must be administered by healthcare professional. Not for IV/SQ use. Inspect for particulate matter and discoloration prior to use. Refer to PI for preparation and administration instructions.
Storage: 2-8°C (36-46°F). Do not freeze. Can be stored at <25°C (77°F) for <7 days prior administration.

VOLTAREN GEL   RX
diclofenac sodium (Novartis Consumer)

> NSAIDs may cause an increased risk of serious cardiovascular (CV) thrombotic events, MI, stroke and serious GI adverse events including bleeding, ulceration, and perforation of the stomach or intestines. Contraindicated for the treatment of perioperative pain in the setting of coronary artery bypass graft (CABG) surgery.

THERAPEUTIC CLASS: NSAID

INDICATIONS: Relief of the pain of osteoarthritis of joints amenable to topical treatment, such as knees and hands.

DOSAGE: *Adults:* Measure onto enclosed dosing card to appropriate 2g or 4g line. Lower Extremities: Apply 4g to affected foot, knee, or ankle qid. Max: 16g/day to any single joint. Upper Extremities: Apply 2g to affected hand, elbow, or wrist qid. Max: 8g/day to any single joint. Total dose should not exceed 32g/day over all affected joints. Avoid showering or bathing for at least 1 hour after application. Avoid open wounds, eyes, mucous membranes, external heat, and/or occlusive dressings. Avoid wearing clothing or gloves for at least 10 min after application.

HOW SUPPLIED: Gel: 1%

CONTRAINDICATIONS: ASA or other NSAID allergy that precipitates asthma, urticaria, or allergic-type reactions. Treatment of perioperative pain in the setting of CABG surgery.

WARNINGS/PRECAUTIONS: Not evaluated for use on spine, hip, or shoulder. May lead to onset of new HTN or worsening of pre-existing HTN; monitor BP closely. Fluid retention and edema reported; caution with fluid retention or heart failure. Renal papillary necrosis and other renal injury reported after long-term use. Not recommended for use with advanced renal disease; if therapy must be initiated, monitor renal function. Anaphylactoid reactions may occur. May cause serious skin adverse events (eg, exfoliative dermatitis, Stevens-Johnson syndrome [SJS], and toxic epidermal necrolysis [TEN]). Avoid in late pregnancy; may cause premature closure of ductus arteriosus. May cause elevations of LFTs; d/c if liver disease develops or systemic manifestations occur. To minimize the potential for adverse liver-related events, use the lowest effective dose for the shortest duration possible. Caution in elderly. Anemia may occur; with long-term use, monitor Hgb/Hct if signs or symptoms of anemia develop. May inhibit platelet aggregation and prolong bleeding time; monitor with coagulation disorders. Caution with asthma and avoid with ASA-sensitive asthma. Patients should minimize or avoid exposure to natural or artificial sunlight on treated areas. Caution in patients with prior history of ulcer or GI bleeding; monitor for signs or symptoms of GI bleeding. May diminish utility of diagnostic signs (eg, inflammation, fever) in detecting infectious complications of presumed noninfectious, painful conditions.

ADVERSE REACTIONS: Application-site reactions, dermatitis.

INTERACTIONS: May enhance methotrexate toxicity and cyclosporine nephrotoxicity; caution when coadministering. May diminish antihypertensive effect of ACE-inhibitors. May reduce natriuretic effect of furosemide and thiazides; monitor for renal failure. May increase lithium levels; monitor for toxicity. Synergistic effects on GI bleeding with anticoagulants (eg, warfarin). Avoid concomitant use with other topical products, including topical medications, sunscreens, lotions, moisturizers, and cosmetics, on the same skin site; may alter tolerability and absorption. Coadministration with oral NSAIDs or ASA may result in increased adverse NSAID effects. Caution with concomitant hepatotoxic drugs (eg, antibiotics, anti-epileptics).

PREGNANCY: Category C, not for use in nursing.

MECHANISM OF ACTION: NSAID; inhibits cyclooxygenase, resulting in reduced formation of prostaglandins, thromboxanes, and prostacylin.

PHARMACOKINETICS: Absorption: (4g) C_{max}=15ng/mL; T_{max}=14 hrs; AUC=233ng•h/mL. (12g) C_{max}=53.8ng/mL; T_{max}=10 hrs; AUC=807ng•h/mL.

NURSING CONSIDERATIONS

Assessment: Assess for hypersensitivity to ASA or NSAIDs, history of ulcer or GI bleeding, HTN, fluid retention, CHF, asthma, CV disease (or risk factors), renal/hepatic impairment, pregnancy/nursing status and possible drug interactions. Obtain baseline BP.

Monitoring: Monitor BP, LFTs, and renal function periodically. Monitor for signs/symptoms of CV events, GI events (eg, ulcerations, bleeding), hepatotoxicity, renal dysfunction, HTN, skin reactions, anemia, blood loss and hypersensitivity reactions.

Patient Counseling: Instruct to avoid contact with eyes and mucous membranes; if contact occurs, wash with water or saline and if irritation persists for >1 hr call physician. Advise to minimize sun exposure. Inform to avoid late in pregnancy. Seek medical attention for symptoms of CV events (eg, chest pain, SOB, weakness, slurring of speech), GI events (eg, epigastric pain, dyspepsia, melena, hematemesis), hepatotoxicity (eg, RUQ pain, pruritus, fatigue), unexplained weight gain or edema, skin reactions (eg, rash, blisters, fever, SJS, TEN, exfoliative dermatitis) or hypersensitivity reactions (eg, difficulty breathing, swelling of face/throat); d/c at first appearance of rash/hypersensitivity reactions.

Administration: Topical route. **Storage:** 25°C (77°F), excursions permitted to 15-30°C (59-86°F). Avoid freezing.

VOLTAREN OPHTHALMIC   RX
diclofenac sodium (Novartis Ophthalmics)

THERAPEUTIC CLASS: NSAID

INDICATIONS: Treatment of postoperative inflammation following cataract surgery. Temporary relief of pain and photophobia in corneal refractive surgery.

DOSAGE: *Adults:* Cataract Surgery: 1 drop qid, start 24 hrs after surgery and continue for 2 weeks. Corneal Refractive Surgery: 1-2 drops within 1 hr prior to, and within 15 min after surgery. Continue qid for up to 3 days.

HOW SUPPLIED: Sol: 0.1% [2.5mL, 5mL]

WARNINGS/PRECAUTIONS: May delay wound healing. Caution with bleeding tendencies. Monitor for 1 yr after use in corneal refractive procedures. May increase bleeding of ocular tissues. No significant increase in tumor incidence.

ADVERSE REACTIONS: Transient burning/stinging, keratitis, elevated IOP, lacrimation, abnormal vision, conjunctivitis, eyelid swelling, discharge, iritis, itching.

INTERACTIONS: Caution with agents that prolong bleeding time (eg, NSAIDs). Potential for cross-sensitivity to acetylsalicylic acid, phenylacetic acid derivatives, and other NSAIDs.

PREGNANCY: Category C, safety in nursing not known.

MECHANISM OF ACTION: NSAID; anti-inflammatory and analgesic that inhibits the enzyme cyclo-oxygenase, which is essential for biosynthesis of prostaglandins.

PHARMACOKINETICS: Absorption: C_{max} <10ng/mL; T_{max}=4 hrs.

NURSING CONSIDERATIONS

Assessment: Assess for hypersensitivity or cross-sensitivity with some drugs (eg, ASA), history of complicated or repeated ocular surgeries, corneal denervation, corneal epithelial defects, DM, ocular surface diseases (eg, dry eye syndrome), RA, bleeding tendencies, pregnancy/nursing status, and history of concomitant use of medications that may prolong bleeding time or delay wound healing.

Monitoring: Monitor for corneal thinning, erosion, ulceration, or perforation and for hypersensitivity reactions, wound healing problems, keratitis, increased bleeding time, bleeding of ocular tissues (hyphemas) in conjunction with ocular surgery, and increased IOP after cataract surgery.

Patient Counseling: Instruct not to administer while wearing contact lenses.

Administration: Ocular route. **Storage:** 15-25°C (59-77°F).

VOLTAREN-XR   RX
diclofenac sodium (Novartis)

NSAIDs may cause an increased risk of serious cardiovascular thrombotic events, MI, stroke and serious GI adverse events including inflammation, bleeding, ulceration, and perforation of the stomach or intestines, which may be fatal. Contraindicated for the treatment of perioperative pain in the setting of coronary artery bypass graft (CABG) surgery.

THERAPEUTIC CLASS: NSAID

INDICATIONS: Relief of signs and symptoms of osteoarthritis (OA), and rheumatoid arthritis (RA).

DOSAGE: *Adults:* OA: 100mg qd. RA: 100mg qd-bid.

HOW SUPPLIED: Tab, Extended-Release: 100mg

CONTRAINDICATIONS: ASA or other NSAID allergy that precipitates asthma, urticaria, or allergic-type reactions. Treatment of perioperative pain in the setting of CABG surgery.

WARNINGS/PRECAUTIONS: Not a substitute for corticosteroids or to treat corticosteroid insufficiency. May lead to onset of new HTN or worsening of pre-existing HTN; monitor BP closely. Fluid retention and edema reported; caution with fluid retention or heart failure. Caution with considerable dehydration. Renal papillary necrosis and other renal injury reported after long-term use. Not recommended for use with advanced renal disease; if therapy must be initiated, monitor renal function. Anaphylactoid reactions may occur. May cause serious skin adverse events (eg, exfoliative dermatitis, Stevens-Johnson syndrome [SJS], toxic epidermal necrolysis). Avoid in late pregnancy. May cause elevations of LFTs; d/c if liver disease develops or systemic manifestations occur. Caution in elderly. Anemia may occur; with long-term use, monitor Hgb/Hct if signs or symptoms of anemia develop. May inhibit platelet aggregation and prolong bleeding time; monitor with coagulation disorders. Caution with asthma and avoid with ASA-sensitive asthma.

ADVERSE REACTIONS: Abdominal pain, constipation, diarrhea, dyspepsia, flatulence, gross bleeding/perforation, heartburn, N/V, GI ulcers (gastric/duodenal), renal function abnormalities, anemia, dizziness, edema, elevated liver enzymes, headaches.

INTERACTIONS: Increased adverse effects with ASA; avoid use. May enhance methotrexate toxicity and increase nephrotoxicity of cyclosporine; caution with coadministration. May diminish antihypertensive effect of ACE-inhibitors and impair response of loop diuretics (eg, furosemide) and thiazides. ACE inhibitors and diuretics may precipitate overt renal decompensation. May increase lithium levels; monitor for toxicity. Synergistic effects with warfarin on GI bleeding. May increase risk of GI bleeding with oral corticosteroids, anticoagulants, tobacco or alcohol use. Caution with hepatotoxic drugs (eg, antibiotics, anti-epileptics). Caution with CYP2C9 inhibitors or inducers (eg, voriconazole, rifampin); dosage adjustment may be warranted.

PREGNANCY: Category C, not for use in nursing.

MECHANISM OF ACTION: NSAID; not known, suspected to inhibit prostaglandin synthetase.

PHARMACOKINETICS: Absorption: Absolute bioavailability (55%); T_{max}=5.3 hrs. **Distribution:** V_d=1.4L/kg; plasma protein binding (99%). **Metabolism:** Liver (glucuronidation and sulfation). **Elimination:** Urine (65%), bile (35%); $T_{1/2}$=2.3 hrs.

NURSING CONSIDERATIONS

Assessment: Assess for history of hypersensitivity to ASA or other NSAIDs, history of asthma, cardiovascular thrombotic events, CABG surgery, stroke, MI, CVD (eg, pre-existing HTN, CHF) or risk factors, fluid retention, edema, conditions affected by platelet function alterations (eg, coagulation disorders), pregnancy/nursing status, GI events (eg, bleeding, ulceration, perforation) or risk factors, possible drug interactions, renal/hepatic impairment. Assess baseline LFTs, renal function, and CBC.

Monitoring: Monitor BP, CBC, LFTs, renal/hepatic function, and chemistry profile periodically. Monitor for signs/symptoms of GI events (eg, bleeding, ulceration, perforation), cardiovascular thrombotic events, CHF, HTN, allergic or skin reactions (eg, rash, eosinophilia, SJS), hematological effects (eg, anemia, prolongation of bleeding time), renal papillary necrosis or other renal injury/toxicity, hepatotoxicity.

Patient Counseling: Advise to seek medical attention if symptoms of hepatotoxicity (eg, nausea, fatigue, pruritus), anaphylactic/anaphylactoid reactions (eg, difficulty breathing, swelling of face/throat), hypersensitivity reactions (eg, rash), cardiovascular events (eg, chest pain, SOB, weakness, slurring of speech), GI ulceration or bleeding (eg, epigastric pain, dyspepsia, melena, hematemesis), weight gain, or edema occur. Inform of pregnancy risks.

Administration: Oral route. **Storage:** Below 30°C (86°F).

VoSpire ER
albuterol sulfate (Dava)

RX

THERAPEUTIC CLASS: Beta$_2$-agonist

INDICATIONS: Treatment of bronchospasm in reversible obstructive airway disease.

DOSAGE: *Adults:* Usual: 4-8mg q12h. Low Body Weight: Initial: 4mg q12h. Titrate: May increase to 8mg q12h. Max: 32mg/day in divided doses. Swallow whole with liquids; do not chew or crush.
Pediatrics: >12 yrs: Usual: 4-8mg q12h. Low Body Weight: Initial: 4mg q12h. Titrate: May increase to 8mg q12h. Max: 32mg/day in divided doses. 6-12 yrs:

Usual: 4mg q12h. Max: 24mg/day in divided doses. Swallow whole with liquids; do not chew or crush.

HOW SUPPLIED: Tab, Extended-Release: 4mg, 8mg

WARNINGS/PRECAUTIONS: Hypersensitivity reactions reported. Caution with cardiovascular disorders, especially coronary insufficiency, arrhythmias and HTN. Increased doses may signify need for concomitant corticosteroids. Can produce paradoxical bronchospasm. Caution with DM, hyperthyroidism, seizures. May produce transient hypokalemia. Erythema multiforme and Stevens-Johnson syndrome (rare) reported in children.

ADVERSE REACTIONS: Tremor, headache, nervousness, tachycardia, palpitations, N/V, muscle cramps.

INTERACTIONS: Avoid oral sympathomimetic agents. Extreme caution within 14 days of MAOI or TCA therapy. Monitor digoxin. May worsen ECG changes and/or hypokalemia with non-K$^+$-sparing diuretics. Antagonized by β-blockers.

PREGNANCY: Category C, not for use in nursing.

MECHANISM OF ACTION: β$_2$-adrenergic bronchodilator; stimulates adenyl cylase, enzyme that catalyzes formation of cAMP from ATP. Increased cAMP levels associated with relaxation of bronchial smooth muscle and inhibition of release of mediators of immediate hypersensitivity.

PHARMACOKINETICS: Absorption: C$_{max}$=13.7ng/mL; T$_{max}$=6 hrs; AUC=134ng•hr/mL. **Elimination:** T$_{1/2}$=9.3 hrs.

NURSING CONSIDERATIONS

Assessment: Assess for renal/hepatic functions, history of hypersensitivity to drug, cardiovascular disorder (coronary insufficiency, HTN, cardiac arrhythmias), convulsive disorders, hyperthyroidism, DM and ketoacidosis, pregnancy/nursing status, and possible drug interactions.

Monitoring: Monitor for possible paradoxical bronchospasm, asthma deterioration, cardiovascular effects, immediate hypersensitivity reactions, CBC with differential count, ketoacidosis, hypokalemia, serum glucose concentrations, tremors.

Patient Counseling: Instruct to swallow tablet; do not chew or crush. Report lack of response or adverse effects.

Administration: Oral route. **Storage:** Store at 20-25°C (68-77°F). Dispense in well-closed, light-resistant container.

VOTRIENT   RX

pazopanib (GlaxoSmithKline)

> Severe and fatal hepatotoxicity reported; monitor hepatic function and interrupt, reduce, or d/c dosing as recommended.

THERAPEUTIC CLASS: Tyrosine kinase inhibitor

INDICATIONS: Treatment of advanced renal cell carcinoma (RCC).

DOSAGE: *Adults:* Usual: 800mg PO qd without food (at least 1 hr before or 2 hrs after a meal). Max: 800mg. Dose Modification: Initial: Reduce to 400mg. Additional adjustment should be in 200-mg steps based on tolerability. Max: 800mg. Moderate Hepatic Impairment: Reduce to 200mg/day. Concomitant Strong CYP3A4 Inhibitors (eg, ketoconazole, ritonavir, clarithromycin): Reduce to 400mg. Further dose reductions may be needed if adverse effects occur during therapy. If a dose is missed, do not take it if it is <12 hrs until the next dose. Do not crush tablets.

HOW SUPPLIED: Tab: 200mg

WARNINGS/PRECAUTIONS: Increased serum ALT, AST, and bilirubin reported; monitor baseline LFTs, once every 4 weeks for 4 months and then periodically. D/C if ALT elevations >3X ULN occur concurrently with bilirubin elevations >2X ULN. Avoid with severe hepatic impairment. Caution with history of QT prolongation, and those with relevant pre-existing cardiac disease; monitor baseline and periodic ECG and maintain electrolytes. Hemorrhagic events reported; avoid with history of hemoptysis, or cerebral or GI hemorrhage in the past 6 months. MI, angina, ischemic stroke, and TIA reported; caution in patients at risk or who have history of these events and avoid use if occurred within the past 6 months. GI perforation/fistula reported. Hypothyroidism reported; monitor thyroid function tests proactively. Proteinuria reported; monitor basline and periodic urinalysis during therapy. D/C if Grade 4 proteinuria develops. HTN reported; control BP prior to therapy. D/C if severe and persistent HTN occurs despite antihypertensive therapy and dose reduction. May impair wound healing; d/c at least 7 days prior to surgery and with wound dehiscence. May cause fetal harm.

ADVERSE REACTIONS: Diarrhea, HTN, hair color changes, N/V, anorexia, fatigue, asthenia, abdominal pain, headache, alopecia, chest pain, dysgeusia, dyspepsia, proteinuria, severe/fatal hepatotoxicity.

INTERACTIONS: May increase concentrations when coadministered with strong inhibitors of CYP3A4 (eg, ketoconazole, ritonavir, clarithromycin); consider dose reduction of pazopanib. Avoid grapefruit juice. May decrease plasma concentrations with CYP3A4 inducers (eg, rifampin). Coadministration of agents with narrow therapeutic windows that are metabolized by CYP3A4, CYP2D6, or CYP2C8 is not recommended. Caution with anti-arrhythmics or other medications that may prolong QT interval. May increase concentrations of drugs eliminated by UGT1A1 and OATP1B1.

PREGNANCY: Category D, not for use in nursing.

MECHANISM OF ACTION: Tyrosine kinase inhibitor; inhibits vascular endothelial growth factor receptor (VEGFR)-1, VEGFR-2, VEGFR-3, platelet-derived growth factor receptor (PDGFR) -α and -β, fibroblast growth factor receptor (FGFR) -1 and -3, cytokine receptor (Kit), interleukin 2 receptor inducible T-cell kinase (Itk), leukocyte-specific protein tyrosine kinase (Lck), and transmembrane glycoprotein receptor tyrosine kinase (c-Fms).

PHARMACOKINETICS: Absorption: T_{max}=2-4 hrs; (800mg dose) AUC=1037 hr•mcg/mL; C_{max}=58.1mcg/mL. **Distribution:** Plasma protein binding (>99%). **Metabolism:** CYP3A4 (major), CYP1A2/CYP2C8 (minor). **Elimination:** Feces, urine (<4% of the administered dose); (800 mg dose) $T_{1/2}$=30.9 hrs.

NURSING CONSIDERATIONS

Assessment: Assess for RCC, history of QT interval prolongation, pre-existing cardiac disease, history of hemoptysis, history of cerebral or GI hemorrhage, MI, angina, ischemic stroke, TIA, HTN, impaired wound healing, pregnancy/nursing status, and for possible drug interactions. Obtain baseline BP, LFTs, ECG, electrolytes, urinalysis.

Monitoring: Monitor for signs/symptoms of hepatotoxicity, QT prolongation, hemorrhagic events, arterial thrombotic events (MI, angina, ischemic stroke, TIA), GI perforation or fistula, HTN, impaired wound healing, and hypothyroidism. Monitor for LFTs once every 4 weeks for at least the 1st 4 months and then periodically. Monitor ECG, electrolytes, urinalysis, and thyroid function tests.

Patient Counseling: Advise that laboratory monitoring will be required prior to and while on therapy. Contact physician if develop any signs/symptoms suggestive of liver problems (eg, yellowing of the skin or whites of the eyes, unusual darkening of the urine, unusual tiredness, right upper stomach pain). Advise on how to manage diarrhea and to notify healthcare provider if moderate to severe diarrhea occurs. Counsel women of childbearing potential that therapy may be a potential hazard to the fetus and pregnancy should be avoided while on therapy. Inform healthcare providers of all concomitant medications, vitamins, or dietary and herbal supplements. Depigmentation of the hair or skin may occur during treatment. Take medication without food (at least 1 hr or 2 hrs after a meal) and do not crush the tablet.

Administration: Oral route. **Storage:** 25°C (77°F); excursions permitted to 15-30°C (59-86°F).

V

VPRIV
velaglucerase alfa (Shire)

RX

THERAPEUTIC CLASS: Enzyme

INDICATIONS: Long-term enzyme replacement therapy (ERT) in pediatric and adult patients with type 1 Gaucher's disease.

DOSAGE: *Adults:* 60 U/kg administered every other week as a 60-min IV infusion. Switching from Imiglucerase Therapy: Begin at the same dose when switching from imiglucerase to velaglucerase alfa. Adjust dose based on therapeutic goals.
Pediatrics: 4-17 yrs: 60 U/kg administered every other week as a 60-min IV infusion. Switching from Imiglucerase Therapy: Begin at the same dose when switching from imiglucerase to velaglucerase alfa. Adjust dose based on therapeutic goals.

HOW SUPPLIED: Inj: 200 U, 400 U

WARNINGS/PRECAUTIONS: Hypersensitivity reactions reported; appropriate medical support should be readily available during administration. Infusion-related reactions reported; management should be based on the severity of the reaction (eg, slowing the infusion rate, treatment with antihistamines, antipyretics, and/or corticosteroids, and/or increasing the infusion time). Caution in elderly.

ADVERSE REACTIONS: Headache, dizziness, abdominal pain, nausea, back pain, joint pain, upper respiratory tract infection, prolonged PT, infusion-related reaction, pyrexia, asthenia/fatigue.

PREGNANCY: Category B, caution in nursing.

MECHANISM OF ACTION: β-glucocerebrosidase; catalyzes hydrolysis of the sphingolipid glucocerebroside to glucose and ceramide.

PHARMACOKINETICS: Distribution: V_d=82-108mL/kg. **Elimination:** $T_{1/2}$=11-12 min.

NURSING CONSIDERATIONS

Assessment: Assess for hypersensitivity and pregnancy/nursing status.

Monitoring: Monitor for headache, dizziness, infusion-related reactions, and hypersensitivity reactions.

Patient Counseling: Inform that it should be administered under the supervision of healthcare professional. Advise that may cause hypersensitivity or infusion-related reactions.

Administration: IV route (IV infusion). Refer to PI for preparation and administration instructions. **Storage:** 2-8°C (36-46°F). Do not freeze. Protect from light.

VYTORIN
simvastatin - ezetimibe (Merck/Schering-Plough)

RX

THERAPEUTIC CLASS: Cholesterol absorption inhibitor/HMG-CoA reductase inhibitor

INDICATIONS: When treatment with both components is appropriate, used as an adjunct to diet for the reduction of elevated total-C, LDL-C, Apo B, TG, non-HDL-C, and to increase HDL-C in primary hyperlipidemia (heterozygous familial and non-familial) or mixed hyperlipidemia. For the reduction of elevated total-C, LDL-C in homozygous familial hypercholesterolemia, as an adjunct to other lipid-lowering treatments or if such treatments are unavailable.

DOSAGE: *Adults:* Initial: 10mg-20mg qd. Take qpm, with or without food. Less Aggressive LDL-C Reductions: Initial: 10mg-10mg qd. LDL-C Reduction >55%: Initial: 10mg-40mg qd. Titrate: Adjust at ≥2 weeks. Homozygous Familial Hypercholesterolemia: 10mg-40mg or 10mg-80mg qpm. Severe Renal Insufficiency: Avoid unless tolerant of ≥5mg of simvastatin; monitor closely. Chinese Patients taking Lipid-Modifying Doses (≥1g/day Niacin) of Niacin-containing Products: Avoid 10mg-80mg. Concomitant Bile Acid Sequestrant: Take either ≥2 hrs before or ≥4 hrs after bile acid sequestrant. Concomitant Cyclosporine/Danazol: Avoid unless tolerant of ≥5mg of simvastatin. Max: 10mg-10mg/day. Concomitant Amiodarone/Verapamil: Max: 10mg-20mg/day. Concomitant Diltiazem: Max: 10mg-40mg/day.

HOW SUPPLIED: Tab: (Ezetimibe-Simvastatin) 10mg-10mg, 10mg-20mg, 10mg-40mg, 10mg-80mg

CONTRAINDICATIONS: Active liver disease, unexplained persistent elevations in hepatic transaminase, pregnancy, lactation.

WARNINGS/PRECAUTIONS: Rhabdomyolysis (rare), myopathy reported. Predisposing risk factors for myopathy include advanced age (≥65 yrs), uncontrolled hypothyroidism, and renal impairment. D/C therapy if myopathy is suspected or diagnosed, if AST or ALT ≥3X ULN persists, a few days prior to major surgery, or when any major medical or surgical condition supervenes. Monitor LFTs prior to therapy and thereafter when clinically indicated. With 10mg-80mg dose, monitor LFTs prior to titration, 3 months after titration, and periodically thereafter for 1st yr. Caution with heavy alcohol use, severe renal insufficiency, or history of hepatic disease. Avoid use in moderate or severe hepatic insufficiency. Caution in elderly and in severe renal impairment. Females of childbearing potential should use effective contraception. D/C if pregnancy occurs.

ADVERSE REACTIONS: Myopathy/rhabdomyolysis, liver enzyme abnormalities (eg, transaminase elevations), headache, upper respiratory tract infection, myalgia.

INTERACTIONS: Use with CYP3A4 inhibitors may increase simvastatin levels and increase risk for myopathy and rhabdomyolysis. Avoid use with the following CYP3A4 inhibitors: antifungal azoles (eg, itraconazole, ketoconazole), erythromycin, clarithromycin, telithromycin, HIV protease inhibitors, nefazodone, grapefruit juice [>1 quart/day], and other strong CYP3A4 inhibitors. Increased risk for myopathy/rhabdomyolysis with fibrates (eg, gemfibrozil), niacin, amiodarone, verapamil, cyclosporine, danazol, diazepam. Avoid use with fibrates. If used with gemfibrozil, dose should not exceed 10mg-10mg daily. Monitor cyclosporine levels. Caution with ≥1g/day of niacin. Reduced ezetimibe levels with cholestyramine; incremental LDL-C reduction with concomitant use may be reduced. May increase plasma digoxin concentrations. Simvastatin may potentiate effect of coumarin anticoagulants; monitor PT levels. Use with cimetidine may increase ezetimibe levels. Use with aluminum and magnesium hydroxide antacids may decrease ezetimibe levels. Lovastatin and ezetimibe levels may be increased when used concomitantly. Use with pravastatin may increase ezetimibe levels and decrease pravastatin levels. Use with atorvastatin may affect ezetimibe and atorvastatin levels. Use with rosuvastatin may increase ezetimibe and rosuvastatin levels. Concomitant use with fluvastatin may affect ezetimibe levels and fluvastatin levels. Use with glipizide may affect ezetimibe and glipizide levels. May decrease ethinyl estradiol & levonorgestrel levels. Use with warfarin may affect warfarin levels. Fenofibrate and ezetimibe levels may be increased when used concomitantly.

PREGNANCY: Category X, not for use in nursing.

MECHANISM OF ACTION: Ezetimibe: Cholesterol absorption inhibitor. Reduces blood cholesterol by inhibiting absorption of cholesterol by small intestine. Molecular target is sterol transporter, Niemann-Pick C1-Like 1 (NPC1L1), which is involved in intestinal uptake of cholesterol and phytosterols. Simvastatin: HMG-CoA reductase inhibitor. Inhibits conversion of HMG-CoA to mevalonate. Also reduces VLDL, TG, and increases HDL-C.

PHARMACOKINETICS: Absorption: Simvastatin: T_{max}=4 hrs. **Distribution:** Ezetimibe: Plasma protein binding (>90%). Simvastatin: Plasma protein binding (95%). **Metabolism:** Ezetimibe: Small intestine, liver via glucuronide conjugation; ezetimibe-glucuronide (active metabolite). Simvastatin: Liver (1st pass); β-hydroxyacid, 6'-hydroxy, 6'-hydroxymethyl, and 6'-exomethylene (major active metabolites). **Elimination:** Ezetimibe: Feces (78%), urine (11%); $T_{1/2}$=22 hrs. Simvastatin: Feces (60%), urine (13%).

NURSING CONSIDERATIONS

Assessment: Assess for active liver disease or unexplained persistent eleva-tions in hepatic transaminases, pregnancy/nursing status, risk factors for developing myopathy (eg, advanced age, uncontrolled hypothyroidism, renal impairment), severe renal impairment, and for possible drug interactions. Assess use in patients who consume substantial quantities of alcohol and/ or have a past history of liver disease. Obtain baseline lipid profile (total-C, LDL-C, HDL-C, TG) and liver function (eg, AST, ALT) parameters.

Monitoring: Monitor for signs/symptoms of myopathy (unexplained muscle pain, tenderness, weakness), rhabdomyolysis, and for liver dysfunction. Perform periodic monitoring of CK levels, LFTs, and lipid profile. Patients titrated to 80mg dose should have LFTs evaluated prior to titration, 3 months after titration, and periodically thereafter.

Patient Counseling: Recommend cholesterol-lowering diet while taking drug. Advise to adhere to the National Cholesterol Education Program (NCEP) recommended diet, regular exercise program, and periodic testing of a fasting lipid panel. Take in evening, with/without food. Contact physician immediately if unexplained muscle pain, tenderness, or weakness develops. Advise about possible drug interactions and interaction with grapefruit juice. D/C therapy if pregnant or planning to become pregnant. Females of childbearing potential should use effective contraception. Do not use if breastfeeding. Inform physi-cian if taking other medications.

Administration: Oral route. **Storage:** 20-25°C (68-77°F). Store in original package. If package is subdivided, repackage into tightly closed, light-resis-tant container.

VYVANSE `CII`
lisdexamfetamine dimesylate (Shire)

> High abuse potential; prolonged use may lead to dependence. Misuse of amphetamines may cause sudden death and serious cardiovascular (CV) events.

THERAPEUTIC CLASS: Sympathomimetic amine

INDICATIONS: Treatment of attention deficit hyperactivity disorder (ADHD).

DOSAGE: *Adults:* Individualize dose. Initial: 30mg qam. Titrate: May increase by 10- or 20mg/day at weekly intervals. Max: 70mg/day.
Pediatrics: 6-17 yrs: Individualize dose. Initial: 30mg qam. Titrate: May increase by 10- or 20mg/day at weekly intervals. Max: 70mg/day.

HOW SUPPLIED: Cap: 20mg, 30mg, 40mg, 50mg, 60mg, 70mg

CONTRAINDICATIONS: Advanced arteriosclerosis, symptomatic CV disease, moderate to severe HTN, hyperthyroidism, glaucoma, agitated states, history of drug abuse, use during or within 14 days following MAOI use.

WARNINGS/PRECAUTIONS: Sudden death, stroke, myocardial infarction (MI) reported; avoid use with known cardiac and heart rhythm abnormali-ties, cardiomyopathy, coronary artery disease (CAD) or other serious cardiac problems. May increase BP and HR; caution with conditions that could be compromised by BP or HR elevation. Promptly evaluate when symptoms suggestive of cardiac disease develop. May exacerbate symptoms of behavior disturbance and thought disorder in psychotic patients. May induce mixed/manic episode in patients with bipolar disorder. May need to d/c if psychotic or manic symptoms emerge. Aggressive behavior or hostility reported. May lower convulsive threshold; d/c if seizure develops. Visual disturbances re-ported. May exacerbate motor and phonic tics and Tourette's syndrome. May slow growth rate in children; may need to d/c if patients are not growing or gaining weight as expected.

ADVERSE REACTIONS: N/V, insomnia, rash, upper abdominal pain, de-creased appetite, dizziness, dry mouth, irritability, weight loss, affect lability, anxiety, anorexia, diarrhea, jittery feeling.

INTERACTIONS: See Contraindications. Urinary acidifying agents (eg, ammo-nium chloride, sodium acid phosphate) and methenamine lower blood levels.

May reduce effects of adrenergic blockers, antihistamines, antihypertensives, and veratrum alkaloids. Urinary alkalinizing agents (eg, acetazolamide and some thiazides) may increase levels. A furazolidone metabolite may cause headaches and other signs of hypertensive crisis. Antagonized by chlorpromazine, haloperidol, and lithium carbonate. May delay absorption of ethosuximide, phenobarbital, phenytoin. May potentiate effects of meperidine, norepinephrine, phenobarbital, phenytoin, TCAs, sympathomimetics. Potentiated by propoxyphene overdose; fatal convulsions may occur. May increase levels of extended release guanfacine and corticosteroids. One report of congenital anomalies in a baby born to woman who took dextroamphetamine sulfate with lovastatin during 1st trimester of pregnancy. Caution with other sympathomimetic drugs.

PREGNANCY: Category C, not for use in nursing.

MECHANISM OF ACTION: Sympathomimetic amine; prodrug of dextroamphetamine. Therapeutic action in ADHD not known; suspected to block reuptake of norepinephrine and dopamine into presynaptic neuron and increase the monoamine release into extraneuronal space.

PHARMACOKINETICS: Absorption: Rapid; T_{max}=1 hr. **Distribution:** Found in breast milk. **Metabolism:** 1st-pass intestinal and/or hepatic metabolism. Dextroamphetamine, L-lysine (metabolites). **Elimination:** Urine (96%), feces (0.3%); $T_{1/2}$<1 hr.

NURSING CONSIDERATIONS

Assessment: Assess for psychiatric history (eg, family history of suicide, bipolar disorder, depression, drug abuse or alcoholism), agitation, glaucoma, tics or Tourette's syndrome, seizure, CV conditions (eg, advanced arteriosclerosis, moderate to severe HTN, cardiac structural abnormalities, cardiomyopathy, arrhythmias, HF, recent MI), hyperthyroidism, hypersensitivity or idiosyncratic reactions to other sympathomimetic amines, pregnancy/nursing status, and possible drug interactions. Assess for family history of sudden death and ventricular arrhythmia. Obtain baseline vital signs, weight and height in children, ECG, EEG.

Monitoring: Monitor for CV abnormalities, exacerbation of behavioral disturbances and thought disorders, aggression, hostility, seizures, visual disturbances and other adverse events. In patients with bipolar disorder, monitor for mixed/manic episode. Monitor vital signs, weight and height in children, ECG, EEG.

Patient Counseling: Inform about benefits and risks of treatment, appropriate use, and drug abuse/dependence. Advise about serious CV risks (eg, sudden death, MI, stroke and HTN). Instruct to notify physician if exertional chest pain, unexplained syncope, other symptoms suggestive of cardiac disease, or psychotic or manic symptoms occur. Notify physician if pregnant/planning to become pregnant and to avoid breastfeeding. Use caution while operating machinery/vehicles. Instruct to read Medication Guide and assist in understanding of its contents.

Administration: Oral route. May be taken with or without food. Swallow caps whole or dissolve contents in glass of water; do not store once dissolved. Do not divide dose of single cap. Avoid afternoon doses. **Storage:** 25°C (77°F); excursions permitted to 15-30°C (59-86°F). Keep in tight, light-resistant container.

WELCHOL   RX
colesevelam HCl (Daiichi Sankyo)

THERAPEUTIC CLASS: Bile acid sequestrant

INDICATIONS: Adjunct to diet and exercise to reduce elevated LDL-C in adults with primary hyperlipidemia (Fredrickson Type IIa) as monotherapy or with an HMG-CoA reductase inhibitor. As monotherapy or in combination with a statin to reduce LDL-C levels in boys and postmenarchal girls 10-17 yrs old with heterozygous familial hypercholesterolemia if after an adequate trial of diet therapy, LDL-C remains ≥190mg/dL or ≥160mg/dL and there is a positive family history of premature cardiovascular disease (CVD), or ≥2 other CVD risk factors are present. Adjunct to diet and exercise to improve glycemic control in adults with type 2 diabetes mellitus (DM).

DOSAGE: *Adults:* Hyperlipidemia/Type 2 DM: 3 tabs bid or 6 tabs qd. Take with meal and liquid. Sus: 3.75g qd or 1.875g bid in 4-8 oz. of water. Stir well and drink. Take with meals. May be dosed at the same time as a statin or the 2 drugs can be dosed apart.
Pediatrics: 10-17 yrs: Hyperlipidemia: Sus: 3.75g qd or 1.875g bid in 4-8 oz. of water. Stir well and drink. Take with meals. May be dosed at the same time as a statin or the 2 drugs can be dosed apart.

HOW SUPPLIED: Sus: 1.875g, 3.75g [pkt]; Tab: 625mg

CONTRAINDICATIONS: History of bowel obstruction, history of hypertriglyceridemia-induced pancreatitis, serum TG concentrations >500mg/dL.

WARNINGS/PRECAUTIONS: May cause increases in serum TG concentrations; d/c if TG levels >500mg/dL or if patient develops hypertriglyceridemia-induced pancreatitis. May cause constipation; avoid use in patients with gastroparesis, GI motility disorders, major GI tract surgery, and those at risk for bowel obstruction. Caution in patients with TG levels >300mg/dL; susceptibility to deficiencies of vitamin K (eg, malabsorption syndromes) or other fat-soluble vitamins. Caution with use of tabs in patients with dysphagia or swallowing disorders. Has not been studied in type 2 DM as monotherapy or in combination with dipeptidyl peptidase 4 inhibitor and thiazolidinediones, and in Fredrickson Type I, III, IV or V dyslipidemias. Not for use in treatment of type 1 DM or for diabetic ketoacidosis. (Sus) Contains phenylalanine, caution with phenylketonurics.

ADVERSE REACTIONS: Asthenia, constipation, dyspepsia, nausea, rhinitis, fatigue, flu syndrome, nasopharyngitis, headache, influenza, pharyngitis, upper respiratory tract infection.

INTERACTIONS: May increase TG levels when used with insulin or sulfonylureas. May decrease levels of glyburide, levothyroxine, and oral contraceptives containing ethinyl estradiol and norethindrone, cyclosporine, repaglinide and verapamil sustained-release. Concomitant use with warfarin decreases INR; monitor INR. May elevate TSH in patients receiving thyroid hormone replacement therapy. May increase seizure activity or decrease phenytoin levels. May decrease absorption of vitamins A, D, E, and K.

PREGNANCY: Category B, safety not known in nursing.

MECHANISM OF ACTION: Bile acid sequestrant; non-absorbed, lipid-lowering polymer that binds bile acids in intestine, impeding their reabsorption. Consequently, compensatory effects lead to increased LDL-C clearance from blood, resulting in decreased serum LDL-C levels.

PHARMACOKINETICS: Absorption: Not hydrolyzed by digestive enzymes and not absorbed. **Distribution:** Limited to GI tract. **Excretion:** Urine (0.05%).

NURSING CONSIDERATIONS

Assessment: Assess for history/risk of bowel obstruction, gastroparesis or other GI motility disorders, history of major GI tract surgery or hypertriglyceridemia-induced pancreatitis; susceptibility to deficiencies of vitamin K or other fat soluble vitamins; dysphagia or swallowing disorders; pregnancy/nursing status; possible drug interactions. Obtain baseline lipid parameters (eg, TG, non-HDL-C).

Monitoring: Monitor for hypertriglyceridemia-induced pancreatitis, hypoglycemia, dysphagia, and for esophageal obstruction. Periodically monitor lipid profile (eg, TG, non-HDL-C), blood glucose and coadministered drug levels.

Patient Counseling: Instruct to take with meal/liquid and consume diet that promotes bowel regularity; inform to take drugs that may interact (eg, cyclosporine, glyburide, levothyroxine, oral contraceptives) ≥4 hrs prior. Promptly d/c and seek medical attention if severe abdominal pain/constipation, or symptoms of acute pancreatitis (eg, severe abdominal pain with or without N/V) occur. Adhere to the recommended diet of National Cholesterol Education Program (NCEP), to dietary instructions, regular exercise program, and regular testing of blood glucose. Therapy may increase serum TG concentrations. Dysphagia or esophageal obstruction may occur because of tab size; caution with swallowing disorders. (Sus) Mix with water before ingesting and avoid taking in its dry form.

Administration: Oral route. Do not take suspension in its dry form to avoid esophageal distress. **Storage:** (Tab/Sus) 25°C (77°F); excursions permitted to 15-30°C (59-86°F). Protect from moisture. (Tab) Brief exposure to 40°C does not affect the product.

WELLBUTRIN SR   RX
bupropion HCl (GlaxoSmithKline)

> Antidepressants increased the risk of suicidal thinking and behavior (suicidality) in short-term studies in children, adolescents, and young adults with major depressive disorder (MDD) and other psychiatric disorders. Bupropion is not approved for use in pediatric patients. Wellbutrin, Wellbutrin SR, and Wellbutrin XL are not approved for smoking cessation treatment but bupropion under the name Zyban is approved for this use. Serious neuropsychiatric events including depression, suicidal ideation, suicide attempt, and completed suicide reported in patients taking bupropion for smoking cessation. Monitor and observe closely for clinical worsening, suicidality, or unusual changes in behavior and for neuropsychiatric symptoms (eg, behavioral changes, hostility, agitation, depressed mood, and suicide-related events) or worsening of pre-existing psychiatric illness. D/C if psychiatric symptoms observed.

OTHER BRAND NAMES: Wellbutrin (GlaxoSmithKline)

THERAPEUTIC CLASS: Aminoketone

INDICATIONS: Treatment of MDD.

DOSAGE: *Adults:* (Tab, Sustained-Release) Initial: 150mg qam. May increase to 150mg bid on Day 4. There should be an interval of at least 8 hrs between successive doses. Usual: 150mg bid. Max: 200mg bid. Maint: Reassess periodically to determine the need for maintenance treatment and the appropriate dose. Severe Hepatic Cirrhosis: Max: 100mg/day or 150mg qod. Mild-Moderate Hepatic Cirrhosis/Renal Impairment: Consider reduced frequency and/or dose. Swallow whole; do not crush, divide or chew. (Tab) Initial: 100mg bid. May increase to 100mg tid, no sooner than 3 days after beginning therapy. Increases should not exceed 100mg/day in a 3-day period. Usual: 100mg tid, preferably with at least 6 hrs between successive doses. Max: 450mg/day, given in divided doses of not more than 150mg each (eg, 100mg qid with at least 4 hrs between successive doses). Severe Hepatic Cirrhosis: Max: 75mg qd. Mild-Moderate Hepatic Cirrhosis/Renal Impairment: Consider reduced frequency and/or dose.

HOW SUPPLIED: Tab: 75mg, 100mg; Tab, Sustained-Release: 100mg, 150mg, 200mg

CONTRAINDICATIONS: Seizure disorders, bulimia or anorexia nervosa, patients treated with other medications that contain bupropion, use of MAOIs or within 14 days of use, and patients undergoing abrupt d/c of alcohol or sedatives (including benzodiazepines).

WARNINGS/PRECAUTIONS: Dose-related risk of seizures. D/C and do not restart if seizure occurs. Extreme caution with history of seizure, cranial trauma, CNS tumor, or other predisposition(s) toward seizure, and severe hepatic cirrhosis. Screen for bipolar disorder; not approved for use in treating bipolar depression. May precipitate mixed/manic episodes in bipolar disorder patients. Restlessness, agitation, anxiety, and insomnia reported after initiation of treatment. Neuropsychiatric signs and symptoms (eg, delusions, hallucinations, psychosis, concentration disturbance, paranoia, confusion) reported. Caution with recent MI, unstable heart disease, renal impairment, and hepatic impairment. D/C if anaphylactoid/anaphylactic reactions occur. Altered appetite/weight and HTN reported. Potential for hepatotoxicity.

ADVERSE REACTIONS: Dry mouth, excessive sweating, headache/migraine, insomnia, tremor, agitation, weight loss, N/V, constipation, dizziness, sedation, blurred vision, decreased libido, anorexia, neuropsychiatric events.

INTERACTIONS: See Contraindications. Extreme caution with drugs that lower seizure threshold (eg, antidepressants, antipsychotics, theophylline,

W

systemic steroids). Increased seizure risk with opioids, cocaine, or stimulant addiction, use of OTC stimulants or anorectics, oral hypoglycemics, insulin. Caution with levodopa and amantadine. Inhibits CYP2D6; caution with drugs that are metabolized by CYP2D6 (eg, SSRIs, TCAs, antipsychotics, β-blockers, type 1C antiarrhythmics); use low initial dose and gradually titrate. Monitor for HTN with nicotine replacement therapy. Caution with CYP2B6 substrates or inhibitors/inducers (eg, orphenadrine, cyclophosphamide, thiotepa, ticlopidine, and clopidogrel). Carbamazepine, phenytoin, and phenobarbital may induce metabolism of bupropion. Hemorrhagic or thrombotic complications reported with warfarin. Minimize or avoid alcohol. Increase dose with ritonavir. Caution with concomitant use of cimetidine.

PREGNANCY: Category C, not for use in nursing.

MECHANISM OF ACTION: Aminoketone antidepressant; unknown. Suspected to inhibit neuronal uptake of norepinephrine and dopamine.

PHARMACOKINETICS: Absorption: T_{max}=3 hrs. **Distribution:** Plasma protein binding (84%); found in breast milk. **Metabolism:** Extensive. Hydroxylation, hydroxybupropion (active metabolite)(CYP2B6); Reduction of carbonyl group, threohydrobupropion (active metabolite), eythrohydrobupropion (active metabolite). **Elimination:** Urine (87%), feces (10%), (0.5% unchanged); $T_{1/2}$=21 hrs, 20 hrs, 33 hrs, 37 hrs (bupropion, hydroxybupropion, erythrohydrobupropion, threohydrobupropion, respectively).

NURSING CONSIDERATIONS

Assessment: Assess for seizure disorder, presence of increased seizure risk (eg, head trauma, excessive use of alcohol or sedatives, addiction to opiates, cocaine, or stimulants, use of OTC stimulants and anorectics, use of insulin or oral hypoglycemics), pre-existing psychiatric illness, bulimia/anorexia nervosa, history of MI or unstable heart disease, renal/hepatic impairment, pregnancy/nursing status, and possible drug interactions. Note other diseases/conditions.

Monitoring: Monitor for clinical worsening, suicidality, or unusual changes in behavior, seizures, increased restlessness, agitation, anxiety, insomnia, neuropsychiatric signs/symptoms (eg, delusions, hallucinations, psychosis, concentration disturbance, paranoia, confusion), changes in weight or appetite, anaphylactoid/anaphylactic reactions (eg, pruritus, urticaria, angioedema, dyspnea), delayed hypersensitivity reactions (eg, arthralgia, myalgia, fever with rash), and HTN.

Patient Counseling: Advise patients and caregivers of need for close observation for clinical worsening and/or suicidal risks. D/C and do not restart if experience a seizure while on therapy. Excessive use or abrupt d/c of alcohol or sedatives may alter seizure threshold; advise to minimize or avoid alcohol use. May impair the ability to perform tasks requiring judgment or motor or cognitive skills; use caution while operating hazardous machinery/driving. Report to physician all prescription or OTC medications being taken. Contact physician if become pregnant or planning to become pregnant during therapy.

Administration: Oral route. Avoid bedtime dosing to minimize insomnia. (SR Tab) Swallow whole; do not crush, divide or chew. **Storage:** Tab: 15-25°C (59-77°F); protect from light and moisture. SR Tab: 20-25°C (68-77°F); dispense in a tight, light-resistant container.

WELLBUTRIN XL   RX
bupropion HCl (GlaxoSmithKline)

Antidepressants increased the risk of suicidal thinking and behavior (suicidality) in short-term studies in children, adolescents, and young adults with major depressive disorder (MDD) and other psychiatric disorders. Bupropion is not approved for use in pediatric patients. Wellbutrin, Wellbutrin SR, and Wellbutrin XL are not approved for smoking cessation treatment but bupropion under the name Zyban is approved for this use. Serious neuropsychiatric events including depression, suicidal ideation, suicide attempt, and completed suicide reported in patients taking bupropion for smoking cessation. Monitor and observe closely for clinical worsening, suicidality, or unusual changes in behavior and for neuropsychiatric symptoms (eg, behavioral changes, hostility, agitation, depressed mood, and suicide-related events) or worsening of pre-existing psychiatric illness. D/C if psychiatric symptoms observed.

THERAPEUTIC CLASS: Aminoketone

INDICATIONS: Treatment of MDD and prevention of seasonal major depressive episodes in patients diagnosed with seasonal affective disorder (SAD).

DOSAGE: *Adults:* Give in AM. MDD: Initial: 150mg qd. May increase to 300mg qd on Day 4. There should be an interval of at least 24 hrs between successive doses. Usual: 300mg qd. Max: 450mg qd. Maint: Reassess periodically to determine the need for maintenance treatment and the appropriate dose for such. SAD: The timing of initiation and duration of treatment should be individualized based on the patient's historical pattern of SAD episodes. Start in autumn; stop in early spring. Initial: 150mg qd. May increase to 300mg after 1 week. If the 300mg dose is not adequately tolerated, the dose can be reduced to 150mg/day. Usual/Max: 300mg qd. Taper dose to 150mg for 2 weeks prior to d/c. Mild-Moderate Hepatic Cirrhosis/Renal Impairment: Reduce frequency and/or dose. Severe Hepatic Cirrhosis: Max: 150mg qod. Switching from Wellbutrin Tablet/Wellbutrin SR: Give the same total daily dose when possible. Swallow whole; do not chew, divide, or crush tablets.

HOW SUPPLIED: Tab, Extended-Release: 150mg, 300mg

CONTRAINDICATIONS: Seizure disorder, bulimia or anorexia nervosa, within 14 days of MAOIs, patients treated with other medications that contain bupropion, and abrupt d/c of alcohol or sedatives.

WARNINGS/PRECAUTIONS: Dose-related risk of seizures. D/C and do not restart if seizure occurs. Risk of seizure may be minimized if daily dose does not exceed 450mg and if the rate of incrementation of dose is gradual. Extreme caution with history of seizures, cranial trauma, CNS tumor, severe hepatic cirrhosis. Screen for bipolar disorder; not approved for use in treating bipolar depression. May precipitate manic episodes in bipolar disorder patients. Restlessness, agitation, anxiety, and insomnia reported after initiation of treatment. Neuropsychiatric signs and symptoms (eg, delusions, hallucinations, psychosis, concentration disturbance, paranoia, confusion) reported. Caution with recent MI, unstable heart disease, and renal and hepatic impairment. D/C if anaphylactoid/anaphylactic reactions occur. Altered appetite/weight and HTN reported. Potential for hepatotoxicity.

ADVERSE REACTIONS: Headache, dry mouth, nausea, insomnia, dizziness, nasopharyngitis, flatulence, tremor, upper respiratory infection, sinusitis, cough, myalgia, anxiety, constipation, neuropsychiatric events.

INTERACTIONS: See Contraindications. Extreme caution with drugs that lower seizure threshold (eg, antidepressants, antipsychotics, theophylline, systemic steroids). Increased seizure risk with opioid, cocaine, or stimulant addiction, OTC stimulants or anorectics; oral hypoglycemics; insulin. Caution with levodopa, and amantadine. Inhibits CYP2D6; caution with drugs that are metabolized by CYP2D6 (eg, SSRIs, TCAs, antipsychotics, β-blockers, type 1C antiarrhythmics); use low initial dose and gradually titrate. Monitor for HTN with transdermal nicotine replacement therapy. Caution with CYP2B6 substrates or inhibitors/inducers (eg, orphenadrine, cyclophosphamide, thiotepa, ticlopidine, and clopidogrel). Carbamazepine, phenytoin, cimetidine, and phenobarbital may induce metabolism of bupropion. Hemorrhagic or thrombotic complications reported with warfarin. Increase dose with ritonavir.

PREGNANCY: Category C, not for use in nursing.

W

1319

MECHANISM OF ACTION: Aminoketone antidepressant; suspected to inhibit neuronal uptake of norepinephrine and dopamine.

PHARMACOKINETICS: Absorption: T_{max} =5 hrs. **Distribution**: Plasma protein binding (84%); found in breast milk. **Metabolism**: Extensive to hydroxybupropion (CYP2B6) via hydroxylation; threohydrobupropion, eythrohydrobupropion via reduction of carbonyl group. **Elimination**: Urine (87%), feces (10%), (0.5% unchanged); $T_{1/2}$=21 hrs, 20 hrs, 33 hrs, 37 hrs (bupropion, hydroxybupropion, erythrohydrobupropion, threohydrobupropion respectively).

NURSING CONSIDERATIONS

Assessment: Assess for seizure disorder, presence of increased seizure risk (eg, head trauma, excessive use of alcohol or sedatives, addiction to opiates, cocaine, or stimulants, use of OTC stimulants and anorectics, use of insulin or oral hypoglycemics), pre-existing psychiatric illness, bulimia/anorexia nervosa, history of MI or unstable heart disease, renal/hepatic impairment, pregnancy/nursing status, and possible drug interactions. Note other diseases/conditions.

Monitoring: Monitor for clinical worsening, suicidality, or unusual changes in behavior, seizures, increased restlessness, agitation, anxiety, insomnia, neuropsychiatric signs/symptoms (eg, delusions, hallucinations, psychosis, concentration disturbance, paranoia, confusion), changes in weight or appetite, anaphylactoid/anaphylactic reactions (eg, pruritus, urticaria, angioedema, dyspnea), delayed hypersensitivity reactions (eg, arthralgia, myalgia, fever with rash), and HTN.

Patient Counseling: Advise patients and caregivers of need for close observation for clinical worsening and/or suicidal risks. D/C and do not restart if experience seizures while on therapy. Excessive use or abrupt d/c of alcohol or sedatives may alter seizure threshold; advise to minimize or avoid alcohol use. May impair the ability to perform tasks requiring judgment or motor or cognitive skills; use caution while operating hazardous machinery/driving. Report to physician all prescription or OTC medications being taken. Contact physician if become pregnant or planning to become pregnant during therapy. Swallow tablets whole; do not chew, divide, or crush.

Administration: Oral route. Avoid bedtime dosing to minimize insomnia. Swallow whole; do not chew, divide or crush tablets. **Storage**: 25°C (77°F); excursions permitted to 15-30°C (59-86°F).

XALATAN   RX
latanoprost (Pharmacia & Upjohn)

THERAPEUTIC CLASS: Prostaglandin analog

INDICATIONS: Reduction of elevated intraocular pressure (IOP) in patients with open-angle glaucoma or ocular HTN.

DOSAGE: *Adults:* Usual: 1 drop in affected eye(s) qd in pm. Max: Once-daily dosing. Space dosing with other ophthalmic drugs by at least 5 min.

HOW SUPPLIED: Sol: 0.005% [2.5mL]

WARNINGS/PRECAUTIONS: Changes to pigmented tissues, increased pigmentation of iris (may be permanent), eyelids and eyelashes (may be reversible), growth of eyelashes reported. Regularly exam patients with noticeably increased iris pigmentation. Macular edema, including cystoid macular edema, reported; mainly occurred in aphakic patients, pseudophakic patients with a torn posterior lens capsule, and patients at risk for macular edema. Caution with history of intraocular inflammation (iritis/uveitis), patients without an intact posterior capsule, and at risk of macular edema. Avoid with active intraocular inflammation. Limited experience in treating angle-closure, inflammatory, or neovascular glaucoma. Bacterial keratitis reported with multi-dose container. Contains benzalkonium chloride; remove contact lenses prior to use and reinsert 15 min after administration.

ADVERSE REACTIONS: Eyelash changes, eyelid skin darkening, intraocular inflammation, iris pigmentation changes, macular edema, blurred vision, ocular burning/stinging, conjunctival hyperemia, foreign body sensation, ocular itching, punctuate epithelial keratopathy.

INTERACTIONS: Avoid with other prostaglandins or prostaglandin analogs; may decrease the IOP lowering effect or cause paradoxical IOP elevations.

PREGNANCY: Category C, caution in nursing.

MECHANISM OF ACTION: Selective FP prostanoid receptor agonist; believed to reduce IOP by increasing outflow of aqueous humor.

PHARMACOKINETICS: Absorption: T_{max}=2 hrs. **Distribution:** V_d=0.16L/kg. **Metabolism:** Cornea, via esterases to active acid; liver, via fatty acid β-oxidation to 1,2-dinor and 1,2,3,4-tetranor (metabolites). **Elimination:** Urine (88-98%); $T_{1/2}$=17 min.

NURSING CONSIDERATIONS

Assessment: Assess for hypersensitivity, intraocular inflammation (iritis/uveitis), active or high risk for macular edema, aphakic or pseudophakic patients with torn posterior lens capsule, patients without an intact posterior capsule, active intraocular inflammation, angle-closure, inflammatory or neovascular glaucoma, pregnancy/nursing status, and possible drug interactions.

Monitoring: Monitor for increased brown pigmentation of iris, periorbital tissue (eyelid); changes in eyelashes (eg, increased length, thickness, or growth; brown pigmentation; change in number of lashes; misdirected growth of lashes); macular edema (eg. cystoid macular edema); active intraocular inflammation, bacterial keratitis, and hypersensitivity reactions.

Patient Counseling: Inform about risk of brown pigmentation of iris, (may be permanent); darkening of eyelid skin; eyelashes and vellus hair changes. Avoid touching tip of applicator to eye or surrounding areas. Contains benzalkonium chloride; remove contact lenses prior to administration; reinsert 15 min after administration. Administer at least 5 min apart if using >1 topical ophthalmic drug. Consult physician if having ocular surgery, if intercurrent ocular condition (eg, trauma or infection) develops, or if ocular reaction (conjunctivitis, lid reactions) occurs.

Administration: Ocular route. Continue with the next dose as normal if one dose is missed. **Storage:** 2-8°C (36-46°F); may store opened bottle for 6 weeks at room temperature up to 25°C (77°F). During shipment to the patient, may maintain up to 40°C (104°F) for a period not exceeding 8 days. Protect from light.

XANAX
alprazolam (Pharmacia & Upjohn)

THERAPEUTIC CLASS: Benzodiazepine

INDICATIONS: Anxiety disorders and short-term relief of anxiety symptoms. Panic disorder with or without agoraphobia.

DOSAGE: *Adults:* Anxiety: Initial: 0.25-0.5mg tid. Titrate: May increase every 3-4 days. Max: 4mg/day. Elderly/Advanced Liver Disease/Debilitated: Initial: 0.25mg bid-tid. Titrate: Increase gradually as tolerated. Panic Disorder: Initial: 0.5mg tid. Titrate: Increase by no more than 1mg/day every 3-4 days; slower titration if ≥4mg/day. Usual: 1-10mg/day. Decrease dose slowly (no more than 0.5mg every 3 days).

HOW SUPPLIED: Tab: 0.25mg*, 0.5mg*, 1mg*, 2mg* *scored

CONTRAINDICATIONS: Acute narrow-angle glaucoma, untreated open angle-glaucoma, concomitant ketoconazole or itraconazole.

WARNINGS/PRECAUTIONS: Risk of dependence. Withdrawal symptoms, including seizures, reported with dose reduction or abrupt d/c; avoid abrupt withdrawal. Caution with impaired renal, hepatic, or pulmonary function, severe depression, obesity, elderly, and debilitated. May cause fetal harm. Hypomania/mania reported with depression. Weak uricosuric effect. Periodically reassess usefulness.

X

ADVERSE REACTIONS: Drowsiness, lightheadedness, depression, headache, confusion, insomnia, dry mouth, constipation, diarrhea, N/V, tachycardia/palpitations, blurred vision, nasal congestion.

INTERACTIONS: See Contraindications. Increases plasma levels of imipramine, desipramine. Additive CNS depressant effects with psychotropics, anticonvulsants, antihistamines, ethanol. Potentiated by fluoxetine, fluvoxamine, nefazodone, cimetidine, oral contraceptives. Decreased levels with CYP3A inducers (eg, carbamazepine) and propoxyphene. Caution with diltiazem, isoniazid, macrolides, grapefruit juice, sertraline, paroxetine, ergotamine, cyclosporine, amiodarone, nicardipine, nifedipine and other CYP3A inhibitors. Avoid azole antifungals.

PREGNANCY: Category D, not for use in nursing.

MECHANISM OF ACTION: Benzodiazepine; mechanism unknown, suspected to bind at stereo specific receptors at several sites within the CNS.

PHARMACOKINETICS: Absorption: (PO) Readily absorbed; T_{max}=1-2 hrs; C_{max}(0.5-3mg)=8-37ng/mL. **Distribution:** Plasma protein binding (80%). **Metabolism:** Liver via CYP3A4; 4-hydroxyalprazolam and α-hydroxyalprazolam (metabolites). **Elimination:** Urine; $T_{1/2}$=11.2 hrs.

NURSING CONSIDERATIONS

Assessment: Assess for acute narrow-angle glaucoma, renal/hepatic/pulmonary function, pregnancy/nursing status. Note other diseases/conditions and drug therapies.

Monitoring: Monitor hypersensitivity reactions, rebound/withdrawal symptoms (eg, seizures), renal function, LFTs, pulmonary function tests, HR, insomnia.

Patient Counseling: Avoid alcohol, sedatives, smoking. Caution while operating machinery/driving. Take as directed. Counsel about drug abuse/dependence and potential side effects, and advise to report if any signs/symptoms occur.

Administration: Oral route. **Storage:** 20-25°C (68-77°F).

XANAX XR   CIV
alprazolam (Pharmacia & Upjohn)

THERAPEUTIC CLASS: Benzodiazepine

INDICATIONS: Panic disorder with or without agoraphobia.

DOSAGE: *Adults:* Initial: 0.5-1mg qd, preferably in the am. Titrate: Increase by no more than 1mg/day every 3-4 days. Maint: 1-10mg/day. Usual: 3-6mg/day. Decrease dose slowly (no more than 0.5mg every 3 days). Elderly/Advanced Liver Disease/Debilitated: Initial: 0.5mg qd.

HOW SUPPLIED: Tab, Extended-Release: 0.5mg, 1mg, 2mg, 3mg

CONTRAINDICATIONS: Acute narrow-angle glaucoma, untreated open-angle glaucoma, concomitant ketoconazole or itraconazole.

WARNINGS/PRECAUTIONS: Risk of dependence. Withdrawal symptoms, including seizures, reported with dose reduction or abrupt d/c; avoid abrupt withdrawal. Caution with impaired renal, hepatic, or pulmonary function, severe depression, obesity, elderly, and debilitated. May cause fetal harm. Hypomania/mania reported with depression. Weak uricosuric effect. Periodically reassess usefulness.

ADVERSE REACTIONS: Sedation, somnolence, memory impairment, dysarthria, abnormal coordination, fatigue, depression, constipation, mental impairment, ataxia, dry mouth, decreased libido, increased/decreased appetite.

INTERACTIONS: See Contraindications. Increases plasma levels of imipramine, desipramine. Additive CNS depressant effects with psychotropics, anticonvulsants, antihistamines, ethanol. Potentiated by fluoxetine, fluvoxamine, nefazodone, cimetidine, oral contraceptives. Decreased levels with CYP3A inducers (eg, carbamazepine) or propoxyphene. Caution with diltiazem, isoniazid, macrolides, grapefruit juice, sertraline, paroxetine, ergotamine, cyclosporine, amiodarone, nicardipine, nifedipine and other CYP3A inhibitors. Avoid azole antifungals.

PREGNANCY: Category D, not for use in nursing.

MECHANISM OF ACTION: Benzodiazepine; mechanism unknown, suspected to bind at stereo specific receptors at several sites within the CNS.

PHARMACOKINETICS: Absorption: Readily absorbed; absolute bioavailability (90%); C_{max}(0.5-3mg)=8-37ng/mL; T_{max}=1-2 hrs. **Distribution:** Plasma protein binding (80%). **Metabolism:** Liver, via CYP3A4; 4-hydroxyalprazolam and α-hydroxyalprazolam (metabolites). **Elimination:** Urine (unchanged and metabolites); $T_{1/2}$=10.7-15.58 hrs.

NURSING CONSIDERATIONS

Assessment: Assess for acute narrow-angle glaucoma, seizures, renal/hepatic/pulmonary function, and pregnancy/nursing status. Note other diseases/conditions and drug therapies.

Monitoring: Monitor for hypersensitivity reactions, rebound or withdrawal symptoms, seizures, LFTs, renal/pulmonary function tests, HR, insomnia.

Patient Counseling: Instruct to avoid alcohol, sedatives, smoking. Caution while operating machinery/driving. Take as directed. Counsel about drug abuse/dependence and side effects, and advise to report if any signs/symptoms occur. Advise to take in the AM; do not crush or chew tabs.

Administration: Oral route. **Storage:** 25°C (77°F); excursions permitted to 15-30°C (59-86°F).

XELODA   RX
capecitabine (Genentech)

Altered coagulation parameters and/or bleeding, including death, reported with concomitant coumarin-derivative anticoagulants (eg, warfarin, phenprocoumon). Monitor PT and INR frequently to adjust anticoagulant dose. Postmarketing reports showed clinically significant increases in PT and INR in patients who were stabilized on anticoagulants at start of therapy. Age >60 and diagnosis of cancer independently predispose to increased risk of coagulopathy.

THERAPEUTIC CLASS: Fluoropyrimidine carbamate

INDICATIONS: First-line treatment of metastatic colorectal carcinoma and adjuvant treatment in patients with Dukes' C colon cancer who have undergone complete resection of the primary tumor when treatment with fluoropyrimidine therapy alone is preferred. Treatment of metastatic breast cancer in combination with docetaxel after failure of prior anthracycline-containing chemotherapy. Treatment of metastatic breast cancer in patients resistant to paclitaxel and anthracycline-containing chemotherapy or resistant to paclitaxel and for whom further anthracycline therapy is not indicated.

DOSAGE: *Adults:* Individualize dose. Monotherapy: Metastatic Colorectal Cancer/Metastatic Breast Cancer: Usual: 1250mg/m² bid for 2 weeks followed by 1-week rest period given as 3-week cycles. Combination with Docetaxel: Usual: 1250mg/m² bid for 2 weeks followed by 1-week rest period, combined with docetaxel 75mg/m² as 1 hr IV q3 weeks. Adjuvant Dukes' C Colon Cancer Treatment: 1250mg/m² bid for 2 weeks followed by 1-week rest period, given as 3-week cycles for total of 8 cycles (24 weeks). CrCl 30-50mL/min: Reduce to 75% of starting dose. Interrupt and/or reduce dose if toxicity occurs. Readjust according to adverse effects. Refer to PI for dose calculation according to body surface area, dose modification recommendations, and docetaxel dose reduction schedule. Swallow whole. Take with water within 30 min after am and pm meals.

HOW SUPPLIED: Tab: 150mg, 500mg

CONTRAINDICATIONS: Hypersensitivity to 5-fluorouracil (5-FU), dihydropyrimidine dehydrogenase (DPD) deficiency, severe renal impairment (CrCl <30mL/min).

WARNINGS/PRECAUTIONS: May induce diarrhea; give fluid and electrolyte replacement with severe diarrhea. Interrupt therapy if grade 2/3/4 diarrhea occurs until diarrhea resolves or decreases intensity to grade 1. Necrotizing enterocolitis reported. Caution with elderly; ≥80 yrs may experience greater incidence of grade 3/4 adverse events. Hand-and-foot syndrome may occur; interrupt therapy if grade 2/3 symptoms occur until event resolves or decreases intensity to grade 1. Cardiotoxicity (eg, myocardial infarction [MI]/ischemia, angina, dysrhythmias, cardiac arrest/failure, cardiomyopathy) observed. Hyperbilirubinemia reported; interrupt therapy if grade 3/4 elevations in bilirubin occur until hyperbilirubinemia decreases to ≤3X ULN. Neutropenia, thrombocytopenia, and decrease in hemoglobin reported. Avoid with baseline neutrophil counts of <1.5X10⁹/L and/or thrombocyte counts of <100X10⁹/L; interrupt therapy with grade 3/4 hematologic toxicity. Rarely, severe toxicity (eg, stomatitis, diarrhea, neutropenia, neurotoxicity) associated with 5-FU has been attributed to DPD deficiency. May cause fetal harm. Caution with mild to moderate hepatic dysfunction due to liver metastases. Caution with renal insufficiency.

ADVERSE REACTIONS: Diarrhea, hand-and-foot syndrome, pyrexia, anemia, N/V, fatigue/weakness, dermatitis, thrombocytopenia, constipation, taste disturbance, stomatitis, alopecia, abdominal pain, decreased appetite.

INTERACTIONS: See Boxed Warning. May increase phenytoin levels; reduce phenytoin dose and monitor carefully. Leucovorin may increase levels and toxicity of 5-FU. May increase the mean AUC of S-warfarin. Use in combination with irinotecan has not been adequately studied. Caution with CYP2C9 substrates. May increase levels with aluminum/magnesium hydroxide antacids.

PREGNANCY: Category D, not for use in nursing.

MECHANISM OF ACTION: Fluoropyrimidine carbamate; binds to thymidylate synthetase forming covalently bound ternary complex that inhibits formation of thymidylate from 2'-deoxyuridylate, inhibits DNA synthesis/cell division and interferes with RNA processing and protein synthesis.

PHARMACOKINETICS: Absorption: T_{max} =1.5 hrs. **Distribution:** Plasma protein binding (<60%); primarily bound to human albumin (approximately 35%). **Metabolism:** Extensive enzymatic conversion to 5-FU; hydrogenated to less toxic metabolite (FUH_2) by dihydropyrimidine dehydrogenase; cleavage of pyrimidine ring to 5-fluoro-ureido-propionic acid (FUPA); cleavage to α-fluoro-β-alanine (major metabolite). **Elimination:** Urine (95.5%) (3% unchanged) (57% major metabolite), feces (2.6%); $T_{1/2}$=0.75 hr.

NURSING CONSIDERATIONS

Assessment: Assess for hypersensitivity to 5-FU, DPD deficiency, severe renal impairment (CrCl <30mL/min), hepatic function, history of CAD, pregnancy/nursing status, and possible drug interactions. Obtain baseline neutrophil/thrombocyte counts.

Monitoring: Monitor for cardiotoxicity, severe diarrhea, hand-and-foot syndrome, hypersensitivity reactions, renal/hepatic impairment, necrotizing enterocolitis, neutropenia, thrombocytopenia, and decreases in Hgb. Perform periodic monitoring of LFTs, CBC, and renal function.

Patient Counseling: Instruct to d/c therapy if moderate/severe toxicity occurs. Inform that toxicities may include diarrhea, N/V, hand-and-foot syndrome, and stomatitis. Instruct to seek medical attention if fever (≥100.5°F) or infection occurs. Counsel about pregnancy risks; instruct to avoid pregnancy during therapy. Advise of possible drug and food interactions. Instruct to take with water within 30 min after a meal.

Administration: Oral route. Swallow whole. Do not cut or crush. **Storage:** 25°C (77°F); excursions permitted to 15-30°C (59-86°F). Keep tightly closed.

XENICAL   RX
orlistat (Genentech)

THERAPEUTIC CLASS: Lipase inhibitor

INDICATIONS: For obesity management including weight loss and weight maintenance when used in conjunction with a reduced-calorie diet. To reduce risk for weight regain after prior weight loss. Indicated for obese patients with initial BMI ≥30kg/m² or ≥27kg/m² in the presence of other risk factors (eg, HTN, diabetes, dyslipidemia).

DOSAGE: *Adults:* 120mg tid with each main meal containing fat. Max: 120mg tid. Take during or ≤1 hr after meals. Omit dose if meal is missed or contains no fat.
Pediatrics: ≥12 yrs: 120mg tid with each main meal containing fat. Max: 120mg tid. Take during or ≤1 hr after meals. Omit dose if meal is missed or contains no fat.

HOW SUPPLIED: Cap: 120mg

CONTRAINDICATIONS: Chronic malabsorption syndrome or cholestasis.

WARNINGS/PRECAUTIONS: Exclude organic causes of obesity (eg, hypothyroidism). GI effects may increase with a high-fat diet (>30% total daily calories from fat). May increase levels of urinary oxalate; caution with history of hyperoxaluria or calcium oxalate nephrolithiasis. Weight loss may improve metabolic control in diabetics. May increase risk of cholelithiasis due to substantial weight loss. Severe liver injury with hepatocellular necrosis or acute hepatic failure reported with some resulting in liver transplant and death. Potential for misuse in inappropriate patients (eg, patients with anorexia nervosa or bulimia). Safety and effectiveness beyond 4 yrs have not been determined.

ADVERSE REACTIONS: Oily spotting, flatus with discharge, fecal urgency, fatty/oily stool, oily evacuation, increased defecation, fecal incontinence.

INTERACTIONS: Monitor changes in coagulation parameters with warfarin. Decreased prothrombin, increased INR and unbalanced anticoagulant treatment with anticoagulants. Reduced levels of cyclosporine; take cyclosporine dose ≥2 hrs before or after administration and consider more frequent monitoring of cyclosporine levels if levels are being measured. Reduced absorption of fat-soluble vitamins and β-carotene. Hypothyroidism reported with levothyroxine; administer at least 4 hrs apart. May require reduction in dosage of oral hypoglycemic agents or insulin in diabetics.

PREGNANCY: Category B, not for use in nursing.

MECHANISM OF ACTION: Lipase inhibitor; inhibits absorption of dietary fats. Acts in lumen of stomach and small intestine by forming a covalent bond with the active serine residue site of gastric and pancreatic lipases, inactivating enzymes making them unavailable to hydrolyze dietary fats.

PHARMACOKINETICS: Absorption: Minimal. T_{max}=8 hrs. **Distribution:** Plasma protein binding (>99%). **Metabolism:** GI wall; M1 and M3 (metabolites). **Elimination:** Feces (97%, 83% unchanged), urine (<2%); $T_{1/2}$=1-2 hrs.

NURSING CONSIDERATIONS

Assessment: Assess for chronic malabsorption or cholestasis, history of hyperoxaluria or calcium oxalate nephrolithiasis, anorexia nervosa, bulimia, HTN, diabetes, dyslipidemia, organic causes of obesity (eg, hypothyroidism), pregnancy/nursing status and possible drug interactions. Obtain baseline vital signs, weight, blood glucose, lipid profile, urinary oxalate levels, LFTs and thyroid function tests.

Monitoring: Monitor for symptoms of hepatic dysfunction, hepatic failure, cholelithiasis, coagulation parameters with warfarin, changes in thyroid function with levothyroxine, signs/symptoms of hypersensitivity reactions and other adverse events. Monitor periodic vital signs, weight, blood glucose, lipid profile, urinary oxalate levels, and LFTs.

Patient Counseling: Inform about risks and benefits of therapy. Inform that GI events may increase when taken with high-fat diet. Advise that daily intake of fat, carbohydrates, and protein should be distributed over 3 main meals. Instruct to take during or up to 1 hr after meals and omit dose if meal is missed or contains no fat. Instruct patients to report symptoms of hepatic dysfunction (eg, anorexia, pruritus, jaundice, dark urine, light colored stools, or right upper quadrant pain); d/c therapy and other suspect medications immediately. Encourage patients to take multivitamin supplement containing fat-soluble vitamins at least 2 hrs before or after administration, such as at bedtime.

X

Administration: Oral route. **Storage:** 25°C (77°F); excursions permitted to 15-30°C (59-86°F). Keep bottle tightly closed.

XGEVA   RX
denosumab (Amgen)

THERAPEUTIC CLASS: IgG$_2$ Monoclonal antibody

INDICATIONS: Prevention of skeletal-related events in patients with bone metastases from solid tumors.

DOSAGE: *Adults:* 120mg SQ q4 weeks in the upper arm, upper thigh or abdomen. Administer calcium and vitamin D prn to treat or prevent hypocalcemia.

HOW SUPPLIED: Inj: 70mg/mL

WARNINGS/PRECAUTIONS: Not indicated for the prevention of skeletal-related events with multiple myeloma. May cause severe hypocalcemia; correct pre-existing hypocalcemia, monitor calcium levels and administer calcium, magnesium, and vitamin D prn. Patients with CrCl <30mL/min or receiving dialysis are at greater risk of severe hypocalcemia. Osteonecrosis of the jaw (ONJ) reported; avoid invasive dental procedures during therapy. Perform oral exam with appropriate preventive dentistry prior to and during treatment.

ADVERSE REACTIONS: Fatigue/asthenia, hypophosphatemia, nausea, dyspnea, diarrhea, hypocalcemia, cough, headache.

INTERACTIONS: Caution with drugs that can lower calcium levels.

PREGNANCY: Category C, not for use in nursing.

MECHANISM OF ACTION: IgG2 monoclonal antibody; binds to RANKL and prevents it from activating its receptor, RANK, on the surface of osteoclasts and their precursors. Increased osteoclast activity, stimulated by RANKL, is a mediator of bone pathology in solid tumors with osseous metastases.

PHARMACOKINETICS: **Absorption:** Bioavailability (62%). **Elimination:** $T_{1/2}$=28 days.

NURSING CONSIDERATIONS

Assessment: Assess for hypocalcemia, renal function, pregnancy/nursing status, and possible drug interactions. Perform oral exam and appropriate preventive dentistry prior to initiation of therapy.

Monitoring: Monitor calcium levels, CrCl, serum phosphorus, and possible adverse events (eg, ONJ). Perform oral exam and appropriate preventive dentistry.

Patient Counseling: Advise to contact a healthcare professional for any of the following: symptoms of hypocalcemia (eg, paresthesias or muscle stiffness, twitching, spasms, cramps), symptoms of ONJ (eg, pain, numbness, swelling of or drainage from the jaw, mouth, or teeth), persistent pain or slow healing of the mouth or jaw after dental surgery, or pregnancy/nursing. Advise patients of the need for: proper oral hygiene and routine dental care, informing their dentist that they are receiving denosumab, and avoiding invasive dental procedures during treatment. Advise that denosumab is also marketed as Prolia™; inform healthcare provider if used.

Administration: SQ route. Inspect for particulate matter/discoloration prior to administration. Do not use if discolored, cloudy or contains many particles or foreign particulate matter. Refer to PI for more details. **Storage:** Refrigerate at 2-8°C (36-46°F); do not freeze. Once removed from the refrigerator, do not expose to >25°C (77°F) or direct light. Discard if not used within 14 days. Protect from heat. Avoid vigorous shaking.

XIAFLEX   RX
collagenase clostridium histolyticum (Auxilium)

THERAPEUTIC CLASS: Debriding/Healing Agent

INDICATIONS: Treatment of adult patients with Dupuytren's contracture with a palpable cord.

DOSAGE: *Adults:* Initial: Inject 0.58mg (0.25mL) into a palpable cord with a contracture of a metacarpophalangeal (MP) joint or 0.58mg (0.20mL) for proximal interphalangeal (PIP) joint. After 24 hrs, perform finger extension procedure if contracture persists. After 4 weeks, if MP or PIP contracture remains, re-inject 0.58mg (0.25mL or 0.20mL) single dose; may repeat finger extension procedure after 24 hrs. Injection and finger extension procedures may be administered up to 3x/cord at approx. 4-week intervals. Please refer to PI for reconstition/preparation, injection, and finger extension procedures.

HOW SUPPLIED: Inj: 0.9mg/vial

WARNINGS/PRECAUTIONS: Tendon rupture, ligament damage, and serious local reactions (eg, pulley rupture, complex regional pain syndrome, sensory abnormality of the hand) reported. Avoid injecting into tendons, nerves, blood vessels, or other collagen-containing structures of the hand. Severe allergic reactions may occur.

ADVERSE REACTIONS: Tendon rupture, ligament damage, peripheral edema, contusion, injection-site hemorrhage, extremity pain, lymphadenopathy, tenderness, pruritus, skin laceration, injection-site reaction, skin laceration, lymph node pain, tenderness, axillary pain.

INTERACTIONS: Caution in patients receiving concomitant anticoagulants (except low-dose aspirin).

PREGNANCY: Category B, caution in nursing.

MECHANISM OF ACTION: Debriding/healing agent; enzymatically disrupts collagen.

NURSING CONSIDERATIONS

Assessment: Assess for coagulation disorders, anticoagulant medication, pregnancy/nursing status, hypersensitivity, possible drug interactions.

Monitoring: Monitor for signs/symptoms of hypersensitivity reactions, tendon/ligament injury and bleeding.

Patient Counseling: Advise that serious complications may occur. After injection, instruct to limit motion of treated finger and keep injected hand elevated until bedtime. Instruct not to disrupt injected cord by self-manipulation and to return for follow-up the next day. After finger extension and split fitting procedure, instruct to avoid strenuous activity with injected hand, wear splint at bedtime up to 4 months, and perform finger flexion and extension exercises each day. Notify of pregnancy/nursing status.

Administration: IV, or intralesional route. Must be reconstituted with the provided diluent prior to use. Refer to PI for preparation of reconstituted solution, dilution and administration. Inject only one cord at a time; inject other cords with contractures in sequential order. **Storage:** Lyophilized Powder: Refrigerate at 2-8°C (36-46°F) Do not freeze. Reconstituted solution: May keep at room temperature 20-25°C (68-77°F) up to 1 hr or refrigerate at 2-8°C (36-46°F) up to 4 hrs prior to administration.

XIBROM   RX
bromfenac (Ista)

THERAPEUTIC CLASS: NSAID

INDICATIONS: Treatment of postoperative inflammation and reduction of ocular pain who have undergone cataract extraction.

DOSAGE: *Adults:* 1 drop bid in affected eye(s), start 24 hrs post-op and continue for 2 weeks.

HOW SUPPLIED: Sol: 0.09% [2.5mL, 5mL]

WARNINGS/PRECAUTIONS: Contains Na sulfite; may cause allergic-type reactions including anaphylactic symptoms and life-threatening or less severe asthmatic episodes. Potential cross-sensitivity to acetylsalicylic acid, phenylacetic acid derivatives, and other NSAIDs. May cause increased bleeding of ocular tissues and may slow or delay healing. May result in keratitis. Continued use may lead to sight-threatening epithelial breakdown, corneal thinning, corneal erosion, corneal ulceration, corneal perforation; d/c if this occurs and monitor for corneal health. Caution in complicated ocular surgeries, corneal denervation, corneal epithelial defects, diabetes mellitus (DM), ocular surface diseases (eg, dry eye syndrome), rheumatoid arthritis (RA), repeat ocular surgeries within a short period of time, or with known bleeding tendencies. Increased risk for occurrence and severity of corneal adverse events if used >24 hrs prior to surgery or use beyond 14 days post-surgery. Avoid use during late pregnancy because of the known effects on fetal CV system (closure of ductus arteriosus).

ADVERSE REACTIONS: Abnormal sensation in eye, conjunctival hyperemia, eye irritation (burning/stinging), eye pain, eye pruritus, eye redness, headache, iritis.

INTERACTIONS: Concomitant use of topical NSAIDs and topical steroids may increase potential for healing problems. Caution with other medications which may prolong bleeding time.

PREGNANCY: Category C, caution in nursing.

MECHANISM OF ACTION: NSAID; thought to block prostaglandin synthesis by inhibiting cyclooxygenase 1 and 2.

NURSING CONSIDERATIONS

Assessment: Assess for hypersensitivity reactions (eg, Na sulfite) or cross-sensitivity, history of complicated or repeated ocular surgeries, corneal denervation, corneal epithelial defects, DM, ocular surface diseases (eg, dry eye syndrome), RA, bleeding tendencies, and concomitant medications that may prolong bleeding time or delay wound-healing, pregnancy/nursing status and possible drug interactions.

Monitoring: Monitor for anaphylactic symptoms, severe asthma attacks, wound-healing problems, keratitis, corneal thinning, corneal erosion/ulceration/perforation, increased bleeding time, and bleeding of ocular tissues (hyphemas) in conjunction with ocular surgery.

Patient Counseling: Advise not to wear contact lenses during therapy.

Administration: Ocular route. **Storage:**15-25°C (59-77°F).

XIFAXAN   RX
rifaximin (Salix)

THERAPEUTIC CLASS: Semisynthetic rifampin analog

INDICATIONS: Treatment of travelers' diarrhea caused by noninvasive strains of *E.coli* in patients ≥12 yrs. For reduction in risk of overt hepatic encephalopathy (HE) recurrence in patients ≥18 yrs.

DOSAGE: *Adults:* Travelers' Diarrhea: 200mg tid for 3 days. Hepatic Encephalopathy: 550mg bid.
Pediatrics: Travelers' Diarrhea: ≥12 yrs: 200mg tid for 3 days.

HOW SUPPLIED: Tab: 200mg, 550mg

WARNINGS/PRECAUTIONS: Do not use for diarrhea complicated by fever or blood in the stool or diarrhea due to pathogens other than *E.coli*; d/c if diarrhea symptoms worsen or persist >24-48 hrs and consider alternative antibiotic therapy. *Clostridium difficile*-associated diarrhea (CDAD) reported and may range in severity from mild diarrhea to fatal colitis; d/c if suspected or confirmed and institute appropriate management/therapy. Use in the absence of a proven or strongly suspected bacterial infection or a prophylactic indication is unlikely to provide benefit and may increase the risk of the development of drug-resistant bacteria. Caution with severe hepatic impairment (Child-Pugh C); may increase systemic exposure.

ADVERSE REACTIONS: Flatulence, headache, abdominal pain, rectal tenesmus, nausea, peripheral edema, dizziness, fatigue, ascites, muscle spasms, pruritus, abdominal distention, anemia, cough, depression.

PREGNANCY: Category C, not for use in nursing.

MECHANISM OF ACTION: Semisynthetic rifampin analog; binds to β-subunit of bacterial DNA-dependent RNA polymerase, resulting in inhibition of bacterial RNA synthesis.

PHARMACOKINETICS: Absorption: Administration with consecutive dosing, fasting/fed conditions, and Child-Pugh Class (A, B, C) resulted in different pharmacokinetic parameters. **Distribution:** Plasma protein binding; 550mg: (67.5%, healthy), (62%, hepatic impairment). **Elimination:** Feces (96.62%, unchanged), urine (0.32%), (0.03%, unchanged).

NURSING CONSIDERATIONS

Assessment: Assess for presence of diarrhea complicated by fever or blood in stool, diarrhea caused by pathogens other than *E. coli* (eg, *Campylobacter jejuni*, *Shigella* spp. *Salmonella* spp.), hepatic impairment (Child-Pugh C), and pregnancy/nursing status.

Monitoring: Monitor for signs/symptoms of a hypersensitivity reaction (eg, exfoliative dermatitis, angioneurotic edema, anaphylaxis), CDAD, development of drug resistant bacteria, and for worsening of symptoms.

Patient Counseling: Instruct to d/c if diarrhea persists for more than 24-48 hrs or worsens if being treated for traveler's diarrhea; advise to seek medical care for fever or blood in the stool. CDAD may develop; contact physician if diarrhea occurs after therapy or does not improve or worsens during therapy. The drug may be taken with or without food. The drug only treats bacterial infections, not viral infections. Take as directed and avoid skipping doses or not completing the full course of therapy. There is an increase in systemic exposure in patients with severe hepatic impairment.

Administration: Oral route. **Storage:** 20-25°C (68-77°F); excursions permitted to 15-30°C (59-86°F).

XIGRIS   RX
drotrecogin alfa (Lilly)

THERAPEUTIC CLASS: Activated protein C

INDICATIONS: For reduction of mortality in adult patients with severe sepsis (sepsis associated with acute organ dysfunction) at a high risk of death (eg, as determined by APACHE II score ≥25).

DOSAGE: *Adults:* Infuse at 24mcg/kg/hr IV for 96 hrs (based on actual body weight). Dose adjustment, dose escalation or bolus doses are not recommended. If infusion interrupted, restart at same rate.

HOW SUPPLIED: Inj: 5mg, 20mg

CONTRAINDICATIONS: Clinical conditions where bleeding could lead to significant morbidity or death, namely active internal bleeding, hemorrhagic stroke within 3 months, intracranial or intraspinal surgery or severe head trauma within 2 months, trauma with an increased risk of life-threatening bleeding, presence of an epidural catheter, or intracranial neoplasm, mass lesion or evidence of cerebral herniation.

WARNINGS/PRECAUTIONS: Not indicated for adult patients with severe sepsis and lower risk of death or for pediatric patients. May not be indicated in patients with single organ dysfunction and recent surgery. Carefully evaluate and anticipate the benefits against potential risks of therapy. Increased risk of bleeding with therapy in patients with platelets <30,000 x 10^6/L (even if count is increased by transfusions), PT/INR >3.0, GI bleed within 6 weeks, ischemic stroke within 3 months, intracranial arteriovenous malformation or aneurysm, known bleeding diathesis, chronic severe hepatic disease, and conditions where bleeding is a significant hazard or difficult to manage due to location. If bleeding occurs, stop infusion. D/C 2 hrs before invasive surgical procedures or procedures with risk of bleeding. Restart 12 hrs after surgery and major invasive procedures. Minimize arterial and central venous puncture. Avoid noncompressible puncture sites. Prolongs activated partial thromboplastin time (APTT). Monitor coagulopathy with prothrombin time (PT).

ADVERSE REACTIONS: Bleeding, GI bleeding, intrathoracic bleeding, retroperitoneal bleeding, immunogenicity.

INTERACTIONS: Caution with drugs that affect hemostasis; increased risk of bleed with therapeutic heparin, thrombolytic therapy within 3 days, and oral anticoagulants, ASA >650mg per day, platelet inhibitors or glycoprotein IIb/IIIa inhibitors within 7 days.

PREGNANCY: Category C, not for use in nursing.

MECHANISM OF ACTION: Activated protein C; exerts antithrombotic effect by inhibiting Factors Va and VIIIa.

NURSING CONSIDERATIONS

Assessment: Assess for any conditions where treatment is contraindicated, platelet count, bleeding diathesis, LFTs, GI bleeding, recent administration of heparin, ASA, thrombolytic therapy, oral anticoagulants. Assess for possible drug interactions.

Monitoring: Monitor for hypersensitivity reactions and active bleeding. Monitor PT and platelet count.

Patient Counseling: Advise to report any side effects. Counsel about the potential risk and benefits associated with therapy.

Administration: IV route. Administer via dedicated IV line or lumen of a multilumen venous catheter; compatible with 0.9% sodium chloride injection, lactated Ringer's injection, dextrose injection, and dextrose sodium chloride injection. Refer to PI for preparation of concentrated solution, dilution and administration instructions for IV infusion pump and syringe pump. **Storage:** Do not freeze. Protect from light. Lyophilized Powder: Refrigerate at 2-8°C (36-46°F). Reconstituted Solution: Avoid exposure to heat and/or direct sunlight. Prepare IV solution immediately after reconstitution; may keep at room temperature 20-25°C (68-77°F) but use within 3 hrs. Infusion solution with an infusion bag or syringe pump: IV solution should be used at controlled room temperature 20-25°C (68-77°F) within 12 hrs. May refrigerate at 2-8°C (36-46°F) up to 12 hrs. If prepared solution is refrigerated prior to administration, may use within 24 hrs (maximum time limit).

XOLAIR   RX
omalizumab (Genentech/Novartis)

> Anaphylaxis, presenting as bronchospasm, hypotension, syncope, urticaria, and/or angioedema of the throat or tongue has been reported as early as after the first dose or beyond 1 yr. Monitor closely for an appropriate time period after administration.

THERAPEUTIC CLASS: Monoclonal antibody/IgE-blocker

INDICATIONS: For adults and adolescents (≥12 yrs) with moderate-severe persistent asthma with a positive skin test or in vitro reactivity to a perennial aeroallergen and whose symptoms are inadequately controlled with inhaled corticosteroids.

DOSAGE: *Adults:* 150-375mg SQ q2 or 4 weeks based on body weight (kg) and pretreatment serum total IgE level (IU/mL). Max: 150mg/site. 30-90kg & IgE ≥30-100 IU/mL: 150mg q4 weeks. >90-150kg and IgE ≥30-100 IU/mL or 30-90kg and IgE >100-200 IU/mL or 30-60kg and IgE >200-300 IU/mL: 300mg q4 weeks. >90-150kg and IgE >100-200 IU/mL or >60-90kg and IgE >200-300 IU/mL or 30-70kg and IgE >300-400 IU/mL: 225mg q2 weeks. >90-150kg and IgE >200-300 IU/mL or >70-90kg and IgE >300-400 IU/mL or 30-70kg and IgE >400-500 IU/mL or 30-60kg and IgE >500-600 IU/mL: 300mg q2 weeks. >70-90kg and IgE >400-500 IU/mL or >60-70kg and IgE >500-600 IU/mL or 30-60kg and IgE >600-700 IU/mL: 375mg q2 weeks. Refer to PI for dosing adjustments.
Pediatrics: ≥12 yrs: 150-375mg SQ q2 or 4 weeks based on body weight (kg) and pretreatment serum total IgE level (IU/mL). Max: 150mg/site. 30-90kg & IgE ≥30-100 IU/mL: 150mg q4 weeks. >90-150kg and IgE ≥30-100 IU/mL or 30-90kg and IgE >100-200 IU/mL or 30-60kg and IgE >200-300 IU/mL: 300mg q4 weeks. >90-150kg and IgE >100-200 IU/mL or >60-90kg and IgE

>200-300 IU/mL or 30-70kg and IgE >300-400 IU/mL: 225mg q2 weeks. >90-150kg and IgE >200-300 IU/mL or >70-90kg and IgE >300-400 IU/mL or 30-70kg and IgE >400-500 IU/mL or 30-60kg and IgE >500-600 IU/mL: 300mg q2 weeks. >70-90kg and IgE >400-500 IU/mL or >60-70kg and IgE >500-600 IU/mL or 30-60kg and IgE >600-700 IU/mL: 375mg q2 weeks. Refer to PI for dosing adjustments.

HOW SUPPLIED: Inj: 150mg [5mL]

WARNINGS/PRECAUTIONS: Malignant neoplasms reported. Not for use in treatment of acute bronchospasm or status asthmaticus. Do not abruptly d/c systemic or inhaled corticosteroids when initiating therapy. Rarely, serious systemic eosinophilia reported with clinical features of vasculitis consistent with Churg-Strauss syndrome; caution with worsening pulmonary symptoms, cardiac complications, and/or neuropathy, especially upon reduction of oral corticosteroids. Geohelminth (eg, roundworm, hookworm, whipworm, threadworm) infections reported in patients at high risk. D/C if constellation of signs/symptoms (arthritis/arthralgia, rash, fever, lymphadenopathy) with an onset 1-5 days after the first or subsequent injections develop.

ADVERSE REACTIONS: Anaphylaxis, malignancies, injection-site reactions, viral infections, upper respiratory infection, sinusitis, headache, pharyngitis, pain, fatigue, arthralgia, leg pain, dizziness.

PREGNANCY: Category B, caution in nursing.

MECHANISM OF ACTION: Monoclonal antibody/IgE blocker; inhibits binding of IgE to the high-affinity IgE receptor on the surface of mast cells and basophils; limits degree of mediator release of allergic response.

PHARMACOKINETICS: Absorption: Absolute bioavailability (62%); T_{max}=7-8 days. **Distribution:** V_d=78mL/kg. **Elimination:** $T_{1/2}$=26 days.

NURSING CONSIDERATIONS

Assessment: Assess for acute bronchospasm or status asthmaticus, malignancies, hypersensitivity, risk of geohelminth infections, and pregnancy/nursing status. Obtain baseline vital signs and weight, CBC (eg, eosinophils), stool exam, IgE levels.

Monitoring: Monitor for anaphylaxis, hypersensitivity reactions, injection-site reactions, viral infections, headaches, malignancies, upper respiratory tract infections, geohelminth infections (eg, roundworm, hookworm, whipworm, threadworm), arthritis/arthralgia, rash (eg, urticaria or other forms), fever, worsening pulmonary symptoms, cardiac complications, and/or neuropathy, especially upon reduction of oral corticosteroids. Periodically reassess need for continued therapy based upon disease severity and level of asthma control. Monitor vital signs and weight, CBC (eg, eosinophils), stool exam, IgE levels.

Patient Counseling: Only to be administered by healthcare providers. Advise about risk of life-threatening anaphylaxis. Injection-site reactions (eg, bruising, redness, warmth, burning, stinging) may occur; notify physician immediately if these adverse reactions develop. Do not decrease dose, or stop taking any other asthma medications unless otherwise instructed by the physician. Immediate improvement may not be seen after beginning of therapy. Encourage pregnant women to enroll in the Pregnancy Exposure Registry.

Administration: SQ route. Refer to PI for proper preparation and administration procedures. **Storage:** 2-8°C (36-46°F). Reconstituted vial may be stored at 2-8°C (36-46°F) for up to 8 hrs or 4 hrs at room temperature. Protect reconstituted vial from direct sunlight.

XOLEGEL RX
ketoconazole (Stiefel)

THERAPEUTIC CLASS: Azole antifungal

INDICATIONS: Topical treatment of seborrheic dermatitis in immunocompetent adults and pediatrics ≥12 yrs.

DOSAGE: *Adults:* Apply qd to affected area for 2 weeks.
Pediatrics: ≥12 yrs: Apply qd to affected area for 2 weeks.

HOW SUPPLIED: Gel: 2% [45g]

WARNINGS/PRECAUTIONS: Not for oral, ophthalmic or intravaginal use. Avoid fire, flame or smoking during and immediately following application. D/C therapy if irritation occurs or disease worsens. Use caution when applying to the chest during lactation to avoid accidental ingestion by the infant.

ADVERSE REACTIONS: Application-site burning.

PREGNANCY: Category C, caution in nursing.

MECHANISM OF ACTION: Azole antifungal; not established.

PHARMACOKINETICS: Absorption: Day 7: C_{max}=1.35ng/mL; T_{max}=8 hrs; AUC_{0-24}=20.8ng•h/mL. Day 14: C_{max}=0.80ng/mL; T_{max}=7 hrs; AUC_{0-24}=15.6ng•h/mL.

NURSING CONSIDERATIONS

Assessment: Assess for immunocompetence and pregnancy/nursing status.

Monitoring: Monitor for irritation, worsening of seborrheic dermatitis and application-site burning/reactions.

Patient Counseling: Instruct to use only as directed; for external use only. Avoid contact with eyes, nostrils and mouth. Advise to wash hands after application. Notify healthcare provider of any signs of adverse reactions.

Administration: Topical route. **Storage:** 25°C (77°F); excursions permitted to 15-30°C (59-86°F). Contents are flammable.

XOPENEX   RX
levalbuterol HCl (Sunovion)

THERAPEUTIC CLASS: Beta$_2$-agonist

INDICATIONS: Treatment or prevention of bronchospasm in patients ≥6 yrs with reversible obstructive airway disease.

DOSAGE: *Adults:* Initial: 0.63mg tid q6-8h. Inadequate Response/Severe Asthma: 1.25mg tid. Administer by nebulizer.
Pediatrics: ≥12 yrs: Initial: 0.63mg tid q6-8h. Inadequate Response/Severe Asthma: 1.25mg tid. 6-11 yrs: 0.31mg tid. Max: 0.63mg tid. Administer by nebulizer.

HOW SUPPLIED: Sol, Inhalation: 0.31mg/3mL, 0.63mg/3mL, 1.25mg/3mL [24^s]

WARNINGS/PRECAUTIONS: May produce paradoxical bronchospasm; d/c immediately and institute alternative therapy. May produce cardiovascular effects and BP changes; caution with cardiovascular diseases (CVD), especially coronary insufficiency, arrhythmias, and HTN. ECG changes reported. Fatalities reported with excessive use. Immediate hypersensitivity reactions may occur. Caution with convulsive disorders, hyperthyroidism, and diabetes mellitus (DM), and in patients unusually responsive to sympathomimetic amines. May produce significant hypokalemia. Caution when administering higher doses with renal impairment.

ADVERSE REACTIONS: Nervousness, tremor, rhinitis, increased cough, diarrhea, flu syndrome, viral infection, sinusitis, fever, headache, lymphadenopathy, pharyngitis, rash, asthenia, pain.

INTERACTIONS: Caution with other short-acting sympathomimetic aerosol bronchodilators or epinephrine. Caution with additional adrenergic drugs to avoid deleterious cardiovascular effects. Antagonized by β-blockers. Extreme caution with or within 2 weeks of d/c of MAOIs and TCAs due to potentiation. Decreased digoxin levels reported. May worsen ECG changes and/or hypokalemia with non-K$^+$-sparing diuretics (eg, loop and thiazide diuretics).

PREGNANCY: Category C, not for use in nursing.

MECHANISM OF ACTION: β_2-adrenergic agonist; stimulates adenylcyclase, the enzyme that catalyzes formation of cAMP from ATP. Increased cAMP levels are associated with relaxation of smooth muscles of the airway and inhibition of release of mediators from mast cells.

PHARMACOKINETICS: Absorption: Administration of variable doses in different age groups resulted in different pharmacokinetic parameters. **Metabolism:** GI tract via SULT1A3 (sulfotransferase). **Elimination:** Urine (25-46%), feces (<20%); ≥12 yrs: $T_{1/2}$=3.3 hrs (1.25mg), 4 hrs (5mg).

NURSING CONSIDERATIONS

Assessment: Assess for history of hypersensitivity to drug, CVD, convulsive disorders, hyperthyroidism, DM, renal impairment, pregnancy/nursing status and possible drug interactions. Assess use in patients unusually responsive to sympathomimetic amines.

Monitoring: Monitor for paradoxical bronchospasm, deterioration of asthma, CV effects, hypokalemia, and immediate hypersensitivity reactions. Monitor BP, HR, and ECG changes.

Patient Counseling: Instruct not to increase dose/frequency of doses without consulting physician. Seek immediate medical attention if treatment becomes less effective for symptomatic relief, symptoms worsen, or need to use the product more frequently than usual. Counsel on common side effects (eg, chest pain, palpitations, rapid HR, tremor, nervousness). Notify physician if pregnant/nursing. Take concurrent inhaled/asthma medications only as directed. Vials should be used within 2 weeks once foil pouch is opened and within 1 week if not used immediately after removal from pouch. Discard vial if solution is not colorless.

Administration: Inhalation route. Refer to PI for proper administration. **Storage:** 20-25°C (68-77°F). Protect from light and excessive heat.

XOPENEX HFA   RX
levalbuterol tartrate (Sunovion)

THERAPEUTIC CLASS: Beta$_2$-agonist

INDICATIONS: Treatment or prevention of bronchospasm in patients ≥4 yrs with reversible obstructive airway disease.

DOSAGE: *Adults:* 2 inh (90mcg) q4-6h or 1 inh (45mcg) q4h. Elderly: Start at low end of dosing range.
Pediatrics: ≥4 yrs: 2 inh (90mcg) q4-6h or 1 inh (45mcg) q4h.

HOW SUPPLIED: MDI: 45mcg/inh [8.4g, 15g]

WARNINGS/PRECAUTIONS: May produce paradoxical bronchospasm; d/c immediately and institute alternative therapy. May produce clinically significant cardiovascular effects and BP changes; caution with cardiovascular diseases (CVD), especially coronary insufficiency, arrhythmias, and HTN. ECG changes reported. Fatalities reported with excessive use. Immediate hypersensitivity reactions may occur. Caution with convulsive disorders, hyperthyroidism, and diabetes mellitus (DM), and in patients unusually responsive to sympathomimetic amines. May produce significant hypokalemia. Caution when administering higher doses with renal impairment. Caution in elderly.

ADVERSE REACTIONS: Pharyngitis, rhinitis, pain, vomiting.

INTERACTIONS: Caution with other short-acting sympathomimetic aerosol bronchodilators or epinephrine. Caution with additional adrenergic drugs to avoid deleterious cardiovascular effects. Antagonized by β-blockers. Extreme caution with or within 2 weeks of d/c of MAOIs and TCAs due to potentiation. Decreased digoxin levels reported. May worsen ECG changes and/or hypokalemia with non-K$^+$-sparing diuretics (eg, loop and thiazide diuretics).

PREGNANCY: Category C, not for use in nursing.

MECHANISM OF ACTION: β$_2$-adrenergic agonist; stimulates adenylate cyclase, the enzyme that catalyzes formation of cAMP from ATP. Increased cAMP levels are associated with relaxation of smooth muscles of the airway and inhibition of release of mediators from mast cells.

X

PHARMACOKINETICS: Absorption: C_{max}=0.199ng/mL (≥12 yrs), 0.163ng/mL (4-11 yrs); T_{max}=0.54 hrs (≥12 yrs), 0.76 hrs (4-11 yrs); AUC=0.695ng•hr/mL (≥12 yrs), 0.579ng•hr/mL (4-11 yrs). **Metabolism:** GI tract via SULT1A3 (sulfo-transferase). **Elimination:** Urine (25-46%), feces (<20%).

NURSING CONSIDERATIONS

Assessment: Assess for history of hypersensitivity to drug, CVD, convulsive disorders, hyperthyroidism, DM, renal impairment, pregnancy/nursing status and possible drug interactions. Assess use in patients unusually responsive to sympathomimetic amines.

Monitoring: Monitor for paradoxical bronchospasm, deterioration of asthma, CV effects, hypokalemia, and immediate hypersensitivity reactions. Monitor BP, HR, and ECG changes.

Patient Counseling: Instruct not to increase dose/frequency of doses without consulting physician. Seek immediate medical attention if treatment becomes less effective for symptomatic relief, symptoms worsen, or need to use the product more frequently than usual. Keep plastic mouthpiece clean to prevent medication build-up and blockage; wash, shake to remove excess water, and air dry thoroughly at least once a week. Counsel on common side effects (eg, chest pain, palpitations, rapid HR, tremor, nervousness). Notify physician if pregnant/nursing. Keep out of reach of children. Avoid spraying in eyes and shake well before each spray. Prime inhaler before using if using for the 1st time or inhaler has not been used for >3 days.

Administration: Oral inhalation. Refer to PI for proper administration. Shake well before use. Prime inhaler by releasing 4 test sprays into the air, away from face. **Storage:** 20-25°C (68-77°F). Store with mouthpiece down. Protect from freezing and direct sunlight. Contents under pressure. Do not puncture or incinerate. Exposure to >49°C (120°F) may cause bursting.

XYLOCAINE INJECTION   RX
lidocaine HCl (APP Pharmaceuticals)

OTHER BRAND NAMES: Xylocaine-MPF (Abraxis)

THERAPEUTIC CLASS: Local anesthetic

INDICATIONS: For production of local or regional anesthesia by infiltration techniques such as percutaneous injection and IV regional anesthesia by peripheral nerve block techniques such as brachial plexus and intercostal and by central neural techniques such as lumbar and caudal epidural blocks.

DOSAGE: *Adults:* Individualize dose. Dosage varies depending on procedure, depth of anesthesia, degree of muscular relaxation, duration of anesthesia required, and the physical condition of the patient. Max: 4.5mg/kg or total daily dose of 300mg (without epinephrine), 7mg/kg or total daily dose of 500mg (with epinephrine). Continuous Epidural/Caudal Anesthesia: Max: Intervals not less than 90 min. Paracervical Block: Max: 200mg/90 min. Administer 1/2 of the dose slowly to each side, 5 minutes between sides. Regional Anesthesia: IV: Max: 4mg/kg. Elderly/Debilitated/Cardiac or Liver Disease: Reduce dose. Refer to PI for recommended dosing for various types of anesthetic procedures.
Pediatrics: Dosage varies with age and weight. Regional Anesthesia: IV: Max: 3mg/kg. Use lowest effective concentration and lowest effective dose at all times.

HOW SUPPLIED: Inj: 0.5%, 1%, 2%; (MPF) 0.5%, 1%, 1.5%, 2%

WARNINGS/PRECAUTIONS: Should only be employed by clinicians well versed in diagnosis and management of dose related toxicity and other acute emergencies which might arise; oxygen, other resuscitative drugs, and cardiopulmonary equipment should be available for immediate use. Acidosis, cardiac arrest, and death may occur if there is a delay in toxicity management. Intra-articular infusion following arthroscopic and other surgical procedures is an unapproved use and chondrolysis reported in patients who received such infusions. Local anesthetic solutions containing antimicrobial preservatives (eg, methylparaben) should not be used for epidural or spinal anesthesia. Syringe aspiration should be performed to avoid intravascular injection. Use lowest effective dose. During epidural anesthesia, administer initial test dose and monitor for CNS and cardiovascular toxicity as well as for signs of unintended intrathecal administration. Repeated doses may cause significant increases in blood levels with each repeated dose. Reduce dose with debilitated, elderly, acutely ill, and children. Extreme caution when using lumbar and caudal epidural anesthesia with existing neurological disease, spinal deformities, septicemia, and severe HTN. May trigger malignant hyperthermia. Monitor cardiovascular and respiratory vital signs and state of consciousness after each injection. Caution with hepatic disease, cardiovascular disorders, and in patients with known drug sensitivities. Small doses injected into the head and neck area including retrobulbar, dental and stellate ganglion blocks, may produce adverse reactions similiar to systemic toxicity seen with unintentional intravascular injection of larger doses; circulation and respiration should be constantly monitored and observed.

ADVERSE REACTIONS: Lightheadedness, nervousness, euphoria, confusion, dizziness, drowsiness, blurred vision, vomiting, heat/cold/numbness sensations, tremors, convulsions, respiratory depression, bradycardia, hypotension, urticaria

INTERACTIONS: Use of CNS stimulants and depressants affects the CNS levels of lidocaine required to produce overt systemic effects. Concurrent administration of vasopressor drugs (for the treatment of hypotension related to obstetric blocks) and ergot-type oxytocic drugs may cause severe, persistent HTN or CVA.

PREGNANCY: Category B, caution in nursing.

MECHANISM OF ACTION: Anesthetic; stabilizes neuronal membrane by inhibiting ionic fluxes required for initiation and conduction of impulses, thereby effecting local anesthetic action.

PHARMACOKINETICS: Absorption: Complete. **Distribution:** Crosses blood-brain and placental barriers. **Metabolism:** Liver (rapid), oxidative N-alkylation (major pathway), yields monoethylglycinexylidide and glycinexylidide (metabolites). **Elimination:** Urine, (90% metabolites), (<10% unchanged); $T_{1/2}$=1.5-2.0 hrs.

NURSING CONSIDERATIONS

Assessment: Assess for drug sensitivities, presence of debilitation, hepatic/renal disease, pregnancy/nursing status, and for possible drug interactions. If planning to use for lumbar or caudal epidural anesthesia, assess for neurological disease, spinal deformities, septicemia, and severe HTN.

Monitoring: Monitor for allergic-type reactions, CNS toxicity, and cardiotoxiciy. Monitor for increased creatine phosphokinase levels following IM injection. Perform careful and constant monitoring of cardiovascular and respiratory vital signs and the patient's state of consciousness following each injection.

Patient Counseling: Inform about possible adverse reactions. Counsel about possibilty of temporary loss of sensation and motor activity, usually in the lower half of the body, following proper administration of epidural anesthesia.

Administration: Infiltration, peripheral nerve block, central neural block.
Storage: 25°C (77°F). Protect from light.

XYLOCAINE VISCOUS RX
lidocaine HCl (AstraZeneca)

THERAPEUTIC CLASS: Acetamide local anesthetic

INDICATIONS: Production of topical anesthesia of irritated or inflamed mucous membranes of the mouth and pharynx. Also useful for reducing gagging during the taking of x-ray pictures and dental impressions.

DOSAGE: *Adults:* Irritated/Inflamed Mucous Membranes: Usual: 15mL undiluted. (Mouth) Swish and spit out. (Pharynx) Gargle and may swallow. Do not administer in <3-hr intervals. Max: 8 doses/24 hr; (Single Dose) 4.5mg/kg and

should not in any case exceed a total of 300mg.
Pediatrics: >3 yrs: Max: Determine by age and weight. Infants - <3 yrs: Apply 1/4 tsp with cotton-tipped applicator to immediate area. Do not administer in <3-hr intervals. Max: 4 doses/24 hr.

HOW SUPPLIED: Sol: 2% [100mL, 450mL]

WARNINGS/PRECAUTIONS: Excessive dosage or too frequent administration may result in high plasma levels and serious adverse effects requiring resuscitative measures. Use lowest effective dose. Tolerance varies with the status of the patient. Extreme caution if mucosa in the treatment area has been severely traumatized; risk of rapid systemic absorption. Elderly, debilitated, acutely ill, and children should be given reduced doses commensurate with their age, weight, and physical condition. Caution with severe shock or heart block, and in patients with known drug sensitivities. Overdose reported in pediatrics due to inappropriate dosing. Acidosis affects the CNS levels of lidocaine required to produce overt systemic effects.

ADVERSE REACTIONS: Lightheadedness, nervousness, confusion, euphoria, dizziness, drowsiness, blurred vision, tremors, convulsions, respiratory depression, bradycardia, hypotension, urticaria, edema, anaphylactoid reactions.

INTERACTIONS: Use of CNS stimulants and depressants affects the CNS levels of lidocaine required to produce overt systemic effects.

PREGNANCY: Category B, caution in nursing.

MECHANISM OF ACTION: Local anesthetic; stabilizes the neuronal membrane by inhibiting the ionic fluxes required for the initiation and conduction of impulses, thereby effecting local anesthetic action.

PHARMACOKINETICS: Absorption: Rate and extent of absorption is dependent on the concentration and total dose administered, the specific site of application, and duration of exposure. Well-absorbed from the GI tract. **Distribution:** Crosses blood-brain and placental barriers; plasma protein binding (60-80%). **Metabolism:** Liver (rapid), oxidative N-dealkylation, ring hydroxylation, cleavage of amide linkage, conjugation; monoethylglycinexylidide and glycinexylidide (metabolites). **Elimination:** Urine; $T_{1/2}$=1.5-2 hrs.

NURSING CONSIDERATIONS

Assessment: Assess for traumatized mucosa in the area of application, acidosis, renal/hepatic dysfunction, debilitation or acute illness, severe shock or heart block, known drug sensitivities, pregnancy/nursing status, and for possible drug interactions.

Monitoring: Monitor for signs/symptoms of CNS manifestations (eg, lightheadedness, nervousness, euphoria, confusion, dizziness, tremors, convulsions, unconsciousness, respiratory depression), cardiovascular manifestations (eg, bradycardia, hypotension, cardiovascular collapse), and for allergic reactions (eg, urticaria, edema, anaphylactoid reactions).

Patient Counseling: Inform that when topical anesthetics are used in the mouth or throat, that swallowing may be impaired and consequently the danger of aspiration may be enhanced; instruct not to ingest food or drink within 60 min of using local anesthetics in mouth or throat area. Advise that numbness of tongue or buccal mucosa may enhance danger of unintentional biting trauma. Counsel to strictly adhere to dosing instructions and keep out of reach of children.

Administration: Topical route. **Storage**: 15-30°C (59-86°F).

XYREM CIII

sodium oxybate (Jazz Pharmaceuticals, Inc.)

THERAPEUTIC CLASS: CNS Depressant

INDICATIONS: Treatment of excessive daytime sleepiness and cataplexy in patients with narcolepsy.

DOSAGE: *Adults:* Initial: 2.25g qhs at least 2 hrs pc, then take 2.25g 2.5-4 hrs later. Titrate: Increase by 1.5g/night (0.75g/dose) every 1-2 weeks. Range: 6-9g/night. Max: 9g/night. Hepatic Insufficiency: Initial: Decrease by 50%. Titrate dose increments to effect.
Pediatrics: ≥16 yrs: Initial: 2.25g qhs at least 2 hrs pc, then take 2.25g 2.5-4 hrs later. Titrate: Increase by 1.5g/night (0.75g/dose) every 1-2 weeks. Range: 6-9g/night. Max: 9g/night. Hepatic Insufficiency: Initial: Decrease by 50%. Titrate dose increments to effect.

HOW SUPPLIED: Sol: 500mg/mL [180mL]

CONTRAINDICATIONS: Concomitant use with sedative hypnotic agents and patients with succinic semialdehyde dehydrogenase deficiency.

WARNINGS/PRECAUTIONS: Rapid onset of CNS depressant effects; ingest only at bedtime and while in bed. May impair physical/mental abilities. May impair respiratory drive and cause sleep apnea; caution with compromised respiratory function. Confusion, sleepwalking, and other neuropsychiatric events (eg, psychosis, paranoia, hallucinations, agitation, thought disorders and/or behavior abnormalities) may occur; evaluate patients and consider appropriate intervention. Depressive symptoms reported; monitor patients with previous history of depressive illness and/or suicide attempt. Rule out underlying etiologies, including worsening sleep apnea or nocturnal seizures if urinary/fecal incontinence develops. Daily Na^+ intake ranges from 0.5g (with 3g dose) to 1.6g (with 9g dose); caution with heart failure (HF), HTN, or renal impairment. Caution with hepatic insufficiency and in elderly.

ADVERSE REACTIONS: Headache, N/V, dizziness, pain, somnolence, nasopharyngitis, diarrhea, urinary incontinence, sleepwalking, depression.

INTERACTIONS: See Contraindications. Avoid with alcohol and other CNS depressants.

PREGNANCY: Category B, caution in nursing.

MECHANISM OF ACTION: CNS depressant; effect on cataplexy not established.

PHARMACOKINETICS: Absorption: Rapid, incomplete; absolute bioavailabiltiy (25%). C_{max}=78mcg/mL (1st peak), 142mcg/mL (2nd peak); T_{max}=0.5-1.25 hr. **Distribution:** V_d=190-384mL/kg; plasma protein binding (<1%). **Metabolism:** Kreb's cycle, β-oxidation. **Elimination:** By transformation to CO_2 eliminated by expiration. Urine (<5%), feces; $T_{1/2}$=0.5-1 hr.

NURSING CONSIDERATIONS

Assessment: Assess for compromised respiratory function, history of depressive illness or suicide attempt, sleep apnea, seizures, HF, HTN, hepatic/renal impairment, pregnancy/nursing status, alcohol intake, and possible drug interactions.

Monitoring: Monitor for signs/symptoms of CNS depression, confusion, sleep apnea, psychosis, suicide attempt, urinary/fecal incontinence, sleepwalking, dosage monitoring in hepatic/renal dysfunction. Perform antinuclear antibody (ANA) test.

Patient Counseling: Inform about the Xyrem Patient Success Program, which includes detailed information about safe/proper use of therapy as well as information to help prevent accidental use or abuse of therapy by others. See a prescriber frequently during treatment to review dose titration, symptom response, and adverse reaction. Food significantly decreases the bioavailability of the drug and may affect both the efficacy and safety of therapy; first dose should be taken several hrs after meal. Urinary/fecal incontinence may occur. Lie down and sleep after each dose and do not take the drug at any time other than at night, immediately before bedtime and then 2.5-4 hrs later. Do not take with alcohol or other sedative hypnotics while on therapy. Notify if pregnant/nursing or planning to become pregnant. Keep out of reach of children.

Administration: Oral route. Prepare both doses prior to bedtime, and place 2nd dose in close proximity to the patient's bed. Dilute each dose with 2 oz. of water prior to ingestion. Take 1st dose at least 2 hrs pc. Take both doses while

seated in bed. After ingestion, patient should lie down and remain in bed.
Storage: 25°C (77°F); excursions permitted 15°-30°C (59-86°F); consume diluted solution within 24 hrs; provided with a child-resistant cap.

XYZAL   RX
levocetirizine dihydrochloride (Sanofi-Aventis/UCB)

THERAPEUTIC CLASS: H_1-antagonist

INDICATIONS: Relief of symptoms associated with allergic rhinitis: seasonal (for adults and children ≥2 yrs) and perennial (for adults and children ≥6 months of age). Treatment of uncomplicated skin manifestations of chronic idiopathic urticaria in adults and children ≥6 months of age.

DOSAGE: *Adults:* 5mg (1 tab or 2 tsp [10mL] oral sol) qd in evening. Mild Renal Impairment (CrCl 50-80mL/min): 2.5mg qd. Moderate Renal Impairment (CrCl 30-50mL/min): 2.5mg qod. Severe Renal Impairment (CrCl 10-30mL/min): 2.5mg twice weekly (administered q3-4 days). Elderly: Start at lower end of dosing range.
Pediatrics: ≥12 yrs: 5mg (1 tab or 2 tsp [10mL] oral sol) qd in evening. Mild Renal Impairment (CrCl 50-80mL/min): 2.5mg qd. Moderate Renal Impairment (CrCl 30-50mL/min): 2.5mg qod. Severe Renal Impairment (CrCl 10-30mL/min): 2.5mg twice weekly (administered q3-4 days). 6-11 yrs: Usual/Max: 2.5mg (1/2 tab or 1 tsp [5mL] oral sol) qd in evening. 6 months-5 yrs: Usual/Max: 1.25mg (1/2 tsp [2.5mL] oral sol) qd in evening.

HOW SUPPLIED: Sol: 0.5mg/mL; Tab: 5mg* *scored

CONTRAINDICATIONS: End-stage renal disease (ESRD) (CrCl <10mL/min) and patients undergoing hemodialysis, pediatrics 6-11 yrs with renal impairment.

WARNINGS/PRECAUTIONS: Somnolence, fatigue, and asthenia reported. May impair mental/physical abilities. Adjust dose in patients with both renal/hepatic impairment. Adjust dose and dosing intervals based on CrCl in patients with renal impairment. Caution in the elderly; start at low end of dosing range.

ADVERSE REACTIONS: Somnolence, fatigue, nasopharyngitis, dry mouth, constipation, diarrhea, cough, drowsiness, pyrexia, vomiting, pharyngitis, otitis media.

INTERACTIONS: Avoid alcohol and CNS depressants. Decreased clearance with theophylline and ritonavir. Increased plasma concentration with ritonavir.

PREGNANCY: Category B, not for use in nursing.

MECHANISM OF ACTION: H_1-Antagonist; antihistamine that selectively inhibits H_1-receptors.

PHARMACOKINETICS: Absorption: Rapid, extensive; C_{max}=270ng/mL (single dose), 308ng/mL (multiple doses); T_{max}=0.9 hr (tab), 0.5 hr (oral sol). **Distribution:** V_d=0.4L/kg; plasma protein binding (91-92%); found in breast milk. **Metabolism:** < 14% metabolized through aromatic oxidation (via CYP 450 system), N- and O- dealkylation (via CYP3A4) and taurine conjugation pathways. **Elimination:** Urine (85.4%), feces (12.9%); $T_{1/2}$=8-9 hrs. Refer to PI for pharmacokinetic parameters of different populations.

NURSING CONSIDERATIONS

Assessment: Assess for ESRD or patients on hemodialysis, hypersensitivity to the drug, renal function, pregnancy/nursing status, and possible drug interactions.

Monitoring: Monitor for adverse reactions. Monitor renal function in elderly.

Patient Counseling: Instruct to use caution against performing hazardous tasks requiring mental alertness and motor coordination (eg, operating machinery, driving). Instruct to avoid use of alcohol or other CNS depressants since additional reduction in mental alertness may occur. Advise not to ingest more than the recommended dose.

Administration: Oral route. **Storage:** 20-25°C (68-77°F), excursions permitted to 15-30°C (59-86°F).

YASMIN RX

drospirenone - ethinyl estradiol (Bayer Healthcare)

> Cigarette smoking increases the risk of serious cardiovascular (CV) side effects from oral contraceptive use. Risk increases with age (>35 yrs) and with heavy smoking (≥15 cigarettes/day). Women who use oral contraceptives should be strongly advised not to smoke.

OTHER BRAND NAMES: Ocella (Various)

THERAPEUTIC CLASS: Estrogen/progestogen combination

INDICATIONS: Prevention of pregnancy.

DOSAGE: *Adults:* 1 yellow tab (active) qd for 21 consecutive days, followed by 1 white tab (inert) on Days 22-28. Start 1st Sunday after menses begins or 1st day of menses. To be taken at the same time each day, preferably after evening meal or at bedtime. Begin next and all subsequent regimens on the same day of the week that the first regimen began.
Pediatrics: Postpubertal: 1 yellow tab (active) qd for 21 consecutive days, followed by 1 white tab (inert) on Days 22-28. Start 1st Sunday after menses begin or 1st day of menses. To be taken at the same time each day, preferably after evening meal or at bedtime. Begin next and all subsequent regimens on the same day of the week that the first regimen began.

HOW SUPPLIED: Tab: (Ethinyl Estradiol-Drospirenone) 0.03mg-3mg

CONTRAINDICATIONS: Renal or adrenal insufficiency, hepatic dysfunction, thrombophlebitis, thromboembolic disorders, history of deep vein thrombophlebitis or thromboembolic disorders, cerebral-vascular or coronary artery disease (CAD), valvular heart disease with thrombogenic complications, severe HTN, diabetes with vascular involvement, headaches with focal neurological symptoms, known or suspected breast carcinoma, endometrial carcinoma, estrogen-dependent neoplasia, undiagnosed abnormal genital bleeding, cholestatic jaundice of pregnancy or jaundice with prior pill use, liver tumor (benign or malignant) or active liver disease, pregnancy, heavy smoking (≥15 cigarettes daily) and >35 yrs.

WARNINGS/PRECAUTIONS: May cause hyperkalemia in high-risk patients; avoid use in patients predisposed to hyperkalemia (eg, renal insufficiency, hepatic dysfunction, adrenal insufficiency). Monitor K⁺ levels during first cycle with conditions predisposed to hyperkalemia. Increased risk of myocardial infarction (MI), thromboembolic and thrombotic disease, cerebrovascular diseases, vascular disease, breast cancer, cancer of the reproductive organs, gallbladder disease, and hepatic neoplasia. Increased risk of morbidity and mortality in patients with HTN, hyperlipidemia, obesity, and diabetes mellitus (DM). Benign hepatic adenomas and hepatocellular carcinoma reported (rare). Retinal thrombosis reported; d/c use if unexplained partial or complete loss of vision occurs, or onset of proptosis or diplopia, papilledema, or retinal vascular lesions develop. May cause glucose intolerance; monitor prediabetic and diabetic patients. May cause fluid retention and increase BP; monitor closely with HTN and d/c if significant elevation of BP occurs. D/C with onset or exacerbation of migraine or development of headache with new pattern which is persistent, recurrent and severe. Breakthrough bleeding and spotting reported; rule out malignancy or pregnancy. Monitor closely with hyperlipidemias. Caution in patient with impaired liver function; d/c if jaundice develops. Monitor closely with depression and d/c if depression recurs to serious degree. Contact lens wearers may develop visual changes. Perform annual physical exam. Should not be used to induce withdrawal bleeding as a test for pregnancy or to treat threatened or habitual abortion during pregnancy. Not indicated for use before menarche. May affect certain endocrine, LFTs, and blood components in laboratory tests. Does not protect against HIV infection (AIDS) and other STDs.

ADVERSE REACTIONS: N/V, breakthrough bleeding, spotting, amenorrhea, migraine, depression, vaginal candidiasis, edema, weight changes, breast changes, GI symptoms (abdominal cramps and bloating), menstrual flow changes.

INTERACTIONS: Concomitant use with rifampin, anticonvulsants (eg, phenobarbital, phenytoin, carbamazepine), or phenylbutazone may reduce contraceptive effectiveness and increase menstrual irregularities. Pregnancy reported with antimicrobials (eg, ampicillin, tetracycline, griseofulvin). St. John's wort may reduce contraceptive effectiveness and cause breakthrough bleeding. Increased levels with atorvastatin, ascorbic acid and APAP. Risk of hyperkalemia with ACE inhibitors, angiotensin-II receptor antagonists, K⁺-sparing diuretics, heparin, aldosterone antagonists, and NSAIDs; monitor K⁺ levels during 1st cycle. May increase levels of cyclosporine, prednisolone, and theophylline. May decrease APAP levels and increase clearance of temazepam, salicylic acid, morphine, and clofibric acid.

PREGNANCY: Category X, not for use in nursing.

MECHANISM OF ACTION: Estrogen/progestogen oral contraceptive; suppresses gonadotropins. Inhibits ovulation and produces changes in cervical mucus (increasing difficulty of sperm entry into uterus) and endometrium (reducing likelihood of implantation).

PHARMACOKINETICS: Absorption: Drospirenone (DRSP): Absolute bioavailability (76%); (Cycle 13/Day 21) C_{max}=78.7ng/mL; T_{max}=1.6 hrs; AUC=968ng•h/mL. Ethinyl estradiol (EE): Absolute bioavailability (40%); (Cycle 13/Day 21) C_{max}=90.5pg/mL; T_{max}=1.6 hrs; AUC=469.5pg•h/mL. **Distribution:** Found in breast milk; DRSP: V_d=4L/kg; serum protein binding (97%). EE: V_d=4-5L/kg; serum albumin binding (98.5%). **Metabolism:** DRSP: Liver, via CYP3A4 (minor). EE: Hydroxylation (via CYP3A4), conjugation (glucuronidation and sulfation). **Elimination:** DRSP: Urine, feces; $T_{1/2}$=30 hrs. EE: Urine, feces; $T_{1/2}$=24 hrs.

NURSING CONSIDERATIONS

Assessment: Assess for presence or history of breast cancer, estrogen dependent neoplasia, abnormal genital bleeding, active liver disease, and known/suspected pregnancy or any other conditions where treatment is cautioned or contraindicated. Assess use in patients who are >35 yrs and heavy smokers (≥15 cigarettes/day). Assess use with HTN, hyperlipidemias, obesity, DM, or in patients at increased risk for thrombosis. Assess for possible drug interactions.

Monitoring: Monitor bleeding irregularities, thromboembolic events, onset or exacerbation of headaches or migraines, and ectopic pregnancy. Monitor fasting blood glucose levels in DM and prediabetic patients, BP with history of HTN, lipid levels with a history of hyperlipidemia. Monitor for signs of liver dysfunction (eg, jaundice) and signs of depression with previous history. Refer patients with contact lenses to an ophthalmologist if visual changes occur. Perform annual history and physical exam

Patient Counseling: Inform that drug does not protect against HIV infection (AIDS) and other STDs. Inform of potential risks/benefits of oral contraceptives. Counsel not to smoke while on treatment. Instruct to take medication at the same time daily. Inform that there may be spotting, light bleeding, or nausea during first 1-3 packs; advise not to d/c medication and if symptoms persist, notify physician.

Administration: Oral route. **Storage:** 25°C (77°F); excursions permitted to 15-30° (59-86°F).

YAZ   RX
drospirenone - ethinyl estradiol (Bayer Healthcare)

> Cigarette smoking increases risk of serious cardiovascular side effects; risk increases with age (especially >35 yrs) and heavy smoking (≥15 cigarettes/day). Advise women who use oral contraceptives not to smoke.

THERAPEUTIC CLASS: Estrogen/progestogen combination

INDICATIONS: Prevention of pregnancy. Treatment of symptoms of premenstrual dysphoric disorder (PMDD). Treatment of moderate acne vulgaris in women ≥14 yrs.

DOSAGE: *Adults:* Start 1st Sunday after menses begin or 1st day of menses. Contraception/Premenstrual Dysphoric Disorder: 1 light pink tab (active) qd for 24 consecutive days, followed by 1 white tab (inert) on days 25-28. Take at the same time each day, preferably pm pc or qhs. Begin next and all subsequent regimens on the same day of the week that the first regimen began. Acne: 1 light pink tab (active) qd for 24 consecutive days, followed by 1 white tab (inert) days 25-28. After 28 tablets are taken, start new course the next day.
Pediatrics: Postpubertal: Start 1st Sunday after menses begin or 1st day of menses. Contraception/Premenstrual Dysphoric Disorder: 1 light pink tab (active) qd for 24 consecutive days, followed by 1 white tab (inert) days 25-28. Take at the same time each day, preferably pm pc or qhs. Begin next and all subsequent regimens on the same day of the week that the first regimen began. ≥14 yrs: Acne: 1 light pink tab (active) qd for 24 consecutive days, followed by 1 white tab (inert) days 25-28. After 28 tablets are taken, start new course the next day.

HOW SUPPLIED: Tab: (Ethinyl Estradiol-Drospirenone) 0.02mg-3mg

CONTRAINDICATIONS: Renal or adrenal insufficiency, hepatic dysfunction, thrombophlebitis, thromboembolic disorders, history of deep vein thrombophlebitis or thromboembolic disorders, cerebral-vascular or coronary artery disease (current or history), valvular heart disease with thrombogenic complications, severe HTN, DM with vascular involvement, headaches with focal neurological symptoms, major surgery with prolonged immobilization, known or suspected carcinoma of the breast, carcinoma of the endometrium or other known or suspected estrogen-dependent neoplasia, undiagnosed abnormal genital bleeding, cholestatic jaundice of pregnancy or jaundice with prior pill use, liver tumor (benign or malignant), active liver disease, pregnancy, heavy smoking (≥15 cigarettes daily) and age >35 yrs.

WARNINGS/PRECAUTIONS: May cause hyperkalemia in high-risk patients; avoid use in patients predisposed to hyperkalemia (eg, renal insufficiency, hepatic dysfunction, adrenal insufficiency). Monitor K+ levels during 1st cycle with conditions predisposing to hyperkalemia. Increased risk of myocardial infarction (MI), thromboembolic and thrombotic disease, cerebrovascular diseases, vascular disease, breast cancer, cancer of the reproductive organs, gallbladder disease and hepatic neoplasia. Increased risk of morbidity and mortality in patients with HTN, hyperlipidemia, obesity, and diabetes mellitus (DM). Retinal thrombosis reported; d/c use if unexplained partial or complete loss of vision occurs, onset of proptosis or diplopia, papilledema, or retinal vascular lesions develop. Contact-lens wearers may develop visual changes or changes in lens tolerance; recommend assessment by ophthalmologist. May cause glucose intolerance; monitor prediabetic and diabetic patients. May cause fluid retention and increase BP; monitor closely with HTN and d/c if significant elevation of BP occurs. May cause onset or exacerbation of migraine or development of headaches. Breakthrough bleeding and spotting reported; rule out malignancy or pregnancy. Monitor closely with hyperlipidemias. D/C if jaundice develops. Monitor closely with depression and d/c if depression recurs to serious degree. May develop visual changes with contact lens. Perform annual physical exam. Use before menarche is not indicated. Does not protect against HIV infection (AIDS) and other sexually transmitted diseases. Caution with history of depression; d/c if depression recurs to serious degree. May affect certain endocrine, LFTs, and blood components in laboratory tests. Should not be used to induce withdrawal bleeding as a test for pregnancy, or to treat threatened or habitual abortion during pregnancy.

ADVERSE REACTIONS: N/V, breakthrough bleeding, spotting, amenorrhea, migraine, vaginitis, edema, depression, decrease in serum folate levels, aggravation of varicose veins, breast changes, mood changes, cholestatic jaundice, rash.

INTERACTIONS: Concomitant use with rifampin, anticonvulsants (eg, phenobarbital, phenytoin, carbamazepine), phenylbutazone, and antimicrobials (eg, ampicillin, tetracycline, griseofulvin) may reduce contraceptive effectiveness

Y

and increase breakthrough bleeding. Increased levels with atorvastatin, ascorbic acid and APAP. Risk of hyperkalemia with ACE inhibitors, angiotensin-II receptor antagonists, K⁺-sparing diuretics, heparin, aldosterone antagonists, and NSAIDs; monitor K⁺ levels during 1st cycle. May increase levels with cyclosporine, prednisolone, and theophylline. May decrease APAP levels and increase clearance of temazepam, salicylic acid, morphine, and clofibric acid. Caution with minocycline. St. John's Wort may reduce contraceptive effectiveness and cause breakthrough bleeding.

PREGNANCY: Category X, not for use in nursing.

MECHANISM OF ACTION: Estrogen/progestogen oral contraceptive; suppresses gonadotropins, inhibiting ovulation. Also causes changes in cervical mucus (increases difficulty of sperm entry into uterus) and endometrium (reduces likelihood of implantation).

PHARMACOKINETICS: Absorption: Drospirenone (DRSP): Absolute bioavailability (76%); (Cycle 1/Day 21) C_{max}=70.3ng/mL; T_{max}=1.5 hrs; AUC=763ng•h/mL. Ethinyl estradiol (EE): Absolute bioavailability (40%); (Cycle 1/Day 21) C_{max}=45.1pg/mL; T_{max}=1.5 hrs; AUC=220pg•h/mL. **Distribution:** DRSP: V_d=4L/kg; serum protein binding (97%). EE: V_d=4-5L/kg; serum albumin binding (98.5%). **Metabolism:** DRSP: Liver, via CYP3A4 (minor). EE: Hydroxylation (via CYP3A4), conjugation with glucuronide and sulfate. **Elimination:** DRSP: Urine, feces; $T_{1/2}$=30 hrs. EE: Urine, feces; $T_{1/2}$=24 hrs.

NURSING CONSIDERATIONS

Assessment: Assess for renal or adrenal insufficiency, hepatic dysfunction, thrombophlebitis, thromboembolic disorders, history of deep vein thrombophlebitis or thromboembolic disorders, cerebral-vascular or CAD (current or history), valvular heart disease with thrombogenic complications, severe HTN, DM with vascular involvement, headaches with focal neurological symptoms, major surgery with prolonged immobilization, known or suspected carcinoma of the breast, carcinoma of the endometrium or other known or suspected estrogen-dependent neoplasia, abnormal genital bleeding, cholestatic jaundice of pregnancy or jaundice with prior pill use, liver tumor (benign or malignant), active liver disease, mental depression, migraines, pregnancy/nursing status, and for possible drug interactions. Assess use in patients with HTN, contact lenses wearer, DM, hyperlipidemias, and obesity.

Monitoring: Monitor for signs/symptoms of MI, thromboembolism, cerebrovascular disease, carcinoma of the breast, cervical intraepithelial neoplasia, hepatic neoplasia, onset or exacerbation of a migraine headache, gallbladder disease, ocular lesions, hyperlipidemia, bleeding irregularities, jaundice, and fluid retention. Monitor for signs of worsening depression in patients with a history of depression. Monitor lipid levels in patients with a history of hyperlipidemia. Monitor blood glucose levels in patients with DM. Monitor BP in patients with HTN. Perform annual history and physical exam. Monitor K+ levels in patients at risk for hyperkalemia. Refer patients with contact lenses to an ophthalmologist if visual changes or changes in contact lens tolerance occur.

Patient Counseling: Inform that drug does not protect against HIV infection (AIDS) and other STDs. Inform of potential risks/benefits of oral contraceptives. Counsel not to smoke while on treatment. Instruct to take 1 pill at same time daily. Inform that if dose is missed, take as soon as possible; take next dose regularly scheduled time. Inform there may be spotting, light bleeding, or nausea during 1-3 packs of pills; advise not to d/c medication and if symptoms persist, notify physician.

Administration: Oral route. **Storage:** 25°C (77°F); excursions permitted to 15-30°C (59-86°F).

ZANAFLEX

RX

tizanidine HCl (Acorda)

THERAPEUTIC CLASS: Alpha$_2$-agonist

INDICATIONS: Short-term treatment of spasticity.

DOSAGE: *Adults:* Initial: 4mg single dose q6-8h. Titrate: Increase by 2-4mg. Usual: 8mg single dose q6-8h. Max: 3 doses/24h or 36mg/day.

HOW SUPPLIED: Cap: 2mg, 4mg, 6mg; Tab: 2mg*, 4mg* *scored

CONTRAINDICATIONS: Concomitant use with fluvoxamine, ciprofloxacin or potent inhibitors of CYP1A2.

WARNINGS/PRECAUTIONS: May prolong QT interval. May cause liver damage; monitor baseline LFTs at and at 1, 3, and 6 months. Retinal degeneration and corneal opacities reported. Caution with renal impairment or elderly. May cause hypotension; caution with antihypertensives. Use with extreme caution in patients with hepatic impairment. May cause sedation and hallucinations. When discontinuing, taper dose to avoid withdrawal and rebound HTN, tachycardia, and hypertonia.

ADVERSE REACTIONS: Dry mouth, somnolence, asthenia, dizziness, UTI, urinary frequency, flu-like syndrome, rhinitis.

INTERACTIONS: See Contraindications. Potentiated depressant effect with alcohol. Potentiated by oral contraceptives; avoid concomitant use. Avoid α-adrenergic agonists. Avoid with CYP1A2 inhibitors.

PREGNANCY: Category C, caution in nursing.

MECHANISM OF ACTION: Centrally acting α_2-adrenergic agonist: reduces spasticity by increasing presynaptic inhibition of motor neurons.

PHARMACOKINETICS: Absorption: Complete; (Fasting) T_{max}=1 hr. (Fed) Absolute bioavailability (40%); C_{max} increased by 30%; T_{max}=1.25 hrs. **Distribution:** V_d=2.4L/kg; plasma protein binding (30%); excreted in breast milk. **Metabolism:** CYP1A2. **Elimination:** Urine (60%), feces (20%); $T_{1/2}$=2.5 hrs.

NURSING CONSIDERATIONS

Assessment: Assess for hypersensitivity, hypotension, hepatic/renal dysfunction, corneal opacities, retinal degeneration, CVD, QT prolongation, pregnancy/nursing status, and possible drug interactions. Obtain baseline LFTs.

Monitoring: Monitor for hypotension, bradycardia, lightheadedness/dizziness, syncope, hepatic impairment, sedation, hallucinosis/psychotic-like symptoms, corneal opacities, retinal degeneration, dry mouth, somnolence, asthenia, and withdrawal symptoms (eg, rebound HTN, tachycardia, hypertonia). Evaluate LFTs at 1, 3, and 6 months, BP, HR, ECG.

Patient Counseling: Counsel to take exactly as directed, not to increase dose unless directed by physician, and about possibility of orthostatic hypotension. Caution against performing hazardous tasks (eg, operating machinery/driving). To avoid withdrawal symptoms, do not suddenly d/c therapy. Avoid alcohol and CNS depressants. Advise that food changes absorption; may lead to potentiation in efficacy and adverse effects. Instruct to inform physician if taking oral contraceptives, fluvoxamine, ciprofloxacin, or if pregnant/nursing.

Administration: Oral route. **Storage:** 25°C (77°F); excursions permitted to 15-30°C (59-86°F). Dispense in tight, child-resistant container.

ZANTAC   RX
ranitidine HCl (GlaxoSmithKline)

THERAPEUTIC CLASS: H_2-blocker

INDICATIONS: (PO) Short-term treatment of active duodenal ulcer (DU) and benign gastric ulcer (GU). Maintenance therapy for DU and GU. Treatment of pathological hypersecretory conditions (eg, Zollinger-Ellison syndrome and systemic mastocytosis) and gastroesophageal reflux disease (GERD). Treatment and maintenance of erosive esophagitis. (Inj) Hospitalized patients with pathological hypersecretory conditions or intractable DU. Short-term alternative to oral therapy in patients who are unable to take oral medication.

DOSAGE: *Adults:* (PO) DU/GU/GERD: 150mg bid or (DU) 300mg after pm meal or qhs. Maint: 150mg qhs. Erosive Esophagitis: 150mg qid. Maint: 150mg bid. Intractable DU/Hypersecretory Conditions: 150mg bid. May give ≤6g/day with severe disease. (Inj) Usual: 50mg IV/IM q6-8h or 6.25mg/hr continuous

IV. IV Bolus: Inject at a rate ≤4mL/min. Intermittent Infusion: Infuse at a rate ≤5-7mL/min (15-20 min). Max: 400mg/day. Zollinger Ellison: Initial: 1mg/kg/hr. Titrate: May increase after 4 hrs by 0.5mg/kg/hr increments if >10 mEq/hr gastric output or patient becomes symptomatic. Max: 2.5mg/kg/hr and 220mg/hr infusion rate. CrCl <50mL/min: 50mg IV q18-24h or 150mg PO q24h. May increase dosing frequency to q12h if necessary. Hemodialysis: Give dose at the end of treatment.

Pediatrics: 1 month-16 yrs: (PO) DU/GU: 2-4mg/kg bid. Max: 300mg/day. Maint: 2-4mg/kg qd. Max: 150mg/day. GERD/Erosive Esophagitis: 5-10mg/kg/day given as 2 divided doses. (Inj) DU: 2-4mg/kg/day IV given q6-8h. Max: 50mg q6-8h. CrCl <50mL/min: 50mg IV q18-24h or 150mg PO q24h. May increase dosing frequency to q12h if necessary. <1 month: Patients on Extracorporeal Membrane Oxygenation (ECMO): 2mg/kg IV q12-24h or as continuous infusion.

HOW SUPPLIED: Inj: 25mg/mL, 50mg/50mL; Syrup: 15mg/mL; Tab: 150mg, 300mg; Tab, Effervescent: 25mg. Also available as a Pharmacy Bulk Package. Refer to individual package insert for more information

WARNINGS/PRECAUTIONS: Symptomatic response does not preclude the presence of gastric malignancy. Caution with hepatic/renal dysfunction. Avoid with history of acute porphyria. Caution in elderly. (IV) Do not exceed recommended infusion rates; bradycardia reported with rapid infusion. SGPT elevations reported; monitor SGPT if on IV therapy for ≥5 days at dose >100mg qid.

ADVERSE REACTIONS: Headache, constipation, diarrhea, N/V, abdominal discomfort, hepatitis, blood dyscrasias, rash, injection-site reactions (IV/IM).

INTERACTIONS: Increased absorption of triazolam, midazolam, and glipizide. Decreased absorption of ketoconazole, atazanavir, delaviridine, and gefitinib. Procainamide plasma levels increased with high doses. Altered anticoagulant effects with warfarin; monitor PT closely. Avoid chronic use with delavirdine. Monitor for prolonged sedation with midazolam and triazolam. Caution with gefitinib and atazanavir. (PO) Delayed and increased peak blood levels with propantheline. Decreased absorption in fasting subjects with high potency antacids.

PREGNANCY: Category B, caution with nursing.

MECHANISM OF ACTION: H_2-blocker; competitive, reversible inhibitor of histamine at histamine H_2-receptors, including those found on gastric cells.

PHARMACOKINETICS: Absorption: (PO, 150mg) C_{max}=440-545ng/mL, T_{max}=2-3 hrs; bioavailability (50%). (IM) Rapid; C_{max}=576ng/mL, T_{max}=15 min; bioavailability (90-100%). **Distribution:** V_d=1.4L/kg; plasma protein binding (15%); found in breast milk. **Metabolism:** Liver, N-oxide (principal metabolite). **Elimination:** Feces, Urine: (PO) (30% unchanged), (IV) (70% unchanged); (PO) $T_{1/2}$=2.5-3 hrs, (IV) $T_{1/2}$=2-2.5 hrs. Refer to PI for pediatric parameters.

NURSING CONSIDERATIONS

Assessment: Assess for hypersensitivity to drug, renal/hepatic function, gastric malignancy, history of acute porphyria, pregnancy/nursing status, and possible drug interactions.

Monitoring: Monitor for signs/symptoms of hepatic effects (eg, elevations in SGPT values), cardiovascular (CV) effects, headache, GI effects (eg, constipation, diarrhea), hypersensitivity reactions, and other adverse reactions. In patients receiving IV formulation at dosages ≥100mg qid for ≥5 days, monitor SGPT daily from Day 5 to the conclusion of IV therapy.

Patient Counseling: Inform that antacids may be given as pain relief for GI symptoms. Inform that efferdose tab contains phenylalanine. If taking efferdose tab formulation, instruct not chew tab, swallow whole, or dissolve on tongue; should be completely dissolved in ≥5mL of water before administration; may be given by medicine dropper or oral syringe. Notify physician if any adverse events develop.

Administration: Oral/IM/IV routes. Do not chew, swallow whole, or dissolve efferdose tab in tongue. Dissolve 1 tablet in ≥5 mL of water in an appropriate measuring cup. Wait until the tablet is completely dissolved before administering the solution to the infant/child. (IV) Inspect visually for particulate matter and discoloration prior to administration. Refer to PI for stability instructions and premixed inj preparation. **Storage:** Tab: 15-30°C (59-86°F). Efferdose Tab: 2-30°C (36-86°F). Syrup: 4-25°C (39-77°F). Inj: 4-25°C (39-77°F); excursions permitted to 30°C (86°F). Protect from light. Premixed Inj: 2-25°C (36-77°F). Protect from light. Protect from freezing.

ZARAH   RX
drospirenone - ethinyl estradiol (Watson)

> Cigarette smoking increases the risk of serious cardiovascular (CV) side effects from oral con-
> traceptive use. Risk increases with age (>35 yrs) and with heavy smoking (≥15 cigarettes/day).
> Women who use oral contraceptives should be strongly advised not to smoke.

THERAPEUTIC CLASS: Estrogen/progestogen combination

INDICATIONS: Prevention of pregnancy.

DOSAGE: *Adults:* 1 blue tab (active) qd for 21 consecutive days, followed by 1 peach tab (inert) on Days 22-28. Start 1st Sunday after menses begins or 1st day of menses. Should be taken at the same time each day, preferably pm pc or qhs. Begin next and all subsequent regimens on the same day of the week on which the first regimen began.
Pediatrics: Postpubertal: 1 blue tab (active) qd for 21 consecutive days, fol-lowed by 1 peach tab (inert) on Days 22-28. Start 1st Sunday after menses begins or 1st day of menses. Should be taken at the same time each day, preferably pm pc or qhs. Begin next and all subsequent regimens on the same day of the week on which first regimen began.

HOW SUPPLIED: Tab: (Ethinyl Estradiol-Drospirenone) 0.03mg-3mg

CONTRAINDICATIONS: Renal or adrenal insufficiency, hepatic dysfunction, thrombophlebitis, thromboembolic disorders, history of deep vein throm-bophlebitis or thromboembolic disorders, cerebral-vascular or coronary artery disease (CAD), valvular heart disease with thrombogenic complica-tions, severe HTN, diabetes with vascular involvement, headaches with focal neurological symptoms, known or suspected breast carcinoma, endometrial carcinoma or other known or suspected estrogen-dependent neoplasia, undiagnosed abnormal genital bleeding, cholestatic jaundice of pregnancy or jaundice with prior pill use, liver tumor (benign or malignant) or active liver disease, pregnancy, heavy smoking (>15 cigarettes daily) and >35 yrs.

WARNINGS/PRECAUTIONS: May cause hyperkalemia in high-risk patients; avoid use in patients predisposed to hyperkalemia (eg, renal insufficiency, hepatic dysfunction, adrenal insufficiency). Monitor K⁺ levels during first treatment cycle with conditions predisposed to hyperkalemia. Increased risk of myocardial infarction (MI), thromboembolism, stroke, gallbladder disease, vascular disease, and hepatic neoplasia. Increased risk of morbidity and mortality in patients with HTN, hyperlipidemia, obesity, and diabetes mellitus (DM). May increase risk of breast cancer and cervical intraepithelial neoplasia. Retinal thrombosis reported; d/c use if unexplained partial or complete loss of vision, onset of proptosis or diplopia, papilledema, or retinal vascular lesions develop. May cause glucose intolerance; monitor prediabetic and diabetic patients. May cause fluid retention. May increase BP; monitor closely with HTN and d/c if significant elevation of BP occurs. D/C with onset or exacerbation of migraine or development of headache with new pattern which is persistent, recurrent and severe. Breakthrough bleeding and spotting reported; rule out malignancy or pregnancy. Monitor closely with hyperlipidemias. D/C if jaun-dice develops. Monitor closely with depression and d/c if depression recurs to serious degree. Contact lens wearers may develop visual changes. Perform annual physical exam. Should not be used to induce withdrawal bleeding as a test for pregnancy or to treat threatened or habitual abortion during preg-nancy. Not indicated for use before menarche. May affect certain endocrine, LFTs, and blood components in laboratory tests. Does not protect against HIV infection (AIDS) and other STDs.

ADVERSE REACTIONS: N/V, breakthrough bleeding, spotting, amenorrhea, migraine, depression, vaginal candidiasis, edema, weight changes, breast changes, GI symptoms (abdominal cramps and bloating), menstrual flow changes.

Z

INTERACTIONS: Concomitant use with rifampin, anticonvulsants (eg, phenobarbital, phenytoin, carbamazepine), or phenylbutazone may reduce contraceptive effectiveness and increase menstrual irregularities. Pregnancy reported with antimicrobials (eg, ampicillin, tetracycline, griseofulvin). St. John's wort may reduce contraceptive effectiveness and cause breakthrough bleeding. Increased levels with atorvastatin, ascorbic acid and acetaminophen (APAP). Risk of hyperkalemia with ACE inhibitors, angiotensin-II receptor antagonists, K⁺-sparing diuretics, heparin, aldosterone antagonists, and NSAIDs; monitor K⁺ levels during 1st cycle. May increase levels of cyclosporine, prednisolone, and theophylline. May decrease APAP levels and increase clearance of temazepam, salicylic acid, morphine, and clofibric acid.

PREGNANCY: Category X, not for use in nursing.

MECHANISM OF ACTION: Estrogen/progestogen oral contraceptive; suppresses gonadotropins. Inhibits ovulation and produces changes in cervical mucus (increasing difficulty of sperm entry into uterus) and endometrium (reducing likelihood of implantation).

PHARMACOKINETICS: Absorption: Drospirenone (DRSP): Absolute bioavailability (76%); (Cycle 13/Day 21) C_{max}=78.7ng/mL; T_{max}=1.6 hrs; AUC=968ng•h/mL. Ethinyl estradiol (EE): Absolute bioavailability (40%); (Cycle 13/Day 21) C_{max}=90.5pg/mL; T_{max}=1.6 hrs; AUC=469.5pg•h/mL. **Distribution:** Found in breast milk; DRSP: V_d=4L/kg; serum protein binding (97%). EE: V_d=4-5L/kg; serum albumin binding (98.5%). **Metabolism:** DRSP: Liver, via CYP3A4 (minor). EE: Hydroxylation (via CYP3A4), conjugation (glucuronidation and sulfation). **Elimination:** DRSP: Urine, feces; $T_{1/2}$=30 hrs. EE: Urine, feces; $T_{1/2}$=24 hrs.

NURSING CONSIDERATIONS

Assessment: Assess for current or history of thrombophlebitis or thromboembolic disorders, cerebrovascular disorders, or any other conditions where treatment is contraindicated or cautioned. Assess for pregnancy/nursing status and for possible drug interactions. Assess use in patients with contact lenses, HTN, DM, hyperlipidemia, and obesity.

Monitoring: Monitor for signs/symptoms of MI, thromboembolism, cerebrovascular disease, carcinoma of the breast, cervical intraepithelial neoplasia, hepatic neoplasia, onset or exacerbation of a migraine headache, gallbladder disease, ocular lesions, hypertriglyceridemia, HTN, bleeding irregularities, jaundice, and for fluid retention. Monitor for signs of worsening depression in patients with a history of depression. Monitor lipid levels in patients with a history of hyperlipidemia. Monitor blood glucose levels in patients with DM. Monitor BP in patients with HTN. Perform annual history and physical exam. Monitor K⁺ levels in patients at risk for hyperkalemia. Refer patients with contact lenses to an ophthalmologist if visual changes or changes in contact lens tolerance occur.

Patient Counseling: Inform that drug does not protect against HIV infection (AIDS) and other STDs. Inform of potential risks/benefits of oral contraceptives. Counsel not to smoke while on treatment. Instruct to take medication at the same time daily. Inform that there may be spotting, light bleeding, or nausea during first 1-3 packs; advise not to d/c medication and if symptoms persist, notify physician. If started later than the first day of the menstrual cycle, it should not be considered effective as a contraceptive until after first 7 consecutive days of administration. Instruct what to do in the event pills are missed.

Administration: Oral route. **Storage:** 20-25°C (68-77°F).

ZARONTIN CAPSULES   RX
ethosuximide (Parke-Davis)

OTHER BRAND NAMES: Zarontin Oral Solution (Parke-Davis)

THERAPEUTIC CLASS: Succinimide

INDICATIONS: Control of absence (petit mal) epilepsy.

DOSAGE: *Adults:* Initial: 500mg qd. Individualize dose according to response. Titrate: May increase daily dose by 250mg q4-7 days until control is achieved with minimal effects. Other Forms of Epilepsy with Absence (Petit Mal): Administer in combination with other anticonvulsants. Max: 1.5g/day. *Pediatrics:* ≥6 yrs: Initial: 500mg qd. 3-6 yrs: Initial: 250mg qd. Individualize dose according to response. Titrate: May increase daily dose by 250mg q4-7 days until control is achieved with minimal side effects. Other Forms of Epilepsy With Absence (Petit Mal): Administer in combination with other anticonvulsants. Usual Optimal Dose: 20mg/kg/day. Max: 1.5g/day.

HOW SUPPLIED: Cap: 250mg; Syrup: 250mg/5mL

WARNINGS/PRECAUTIONS: Abnormal renal and liver function studies reported; extreme caution with known liver or renal disease; perform periodic urinalysis and LFTs. Systemic lupus erythematosus (SLE) reported. Blood dyscrasias reported; monitor blood counts periodically. Increased risk of suicidal thoughts or behavior reported; monitor for worsening of depression and any unusual changes in mood or behavior. May increase grand mal seizures in mixed types of epilepsy when used alone. May precipitate absence (petit mal) status; adjust dose slowly and avoid abrupt withdrawal. Cases of birth defects reported. Caution in nursing women. Dosage exceeding 1.5g/day in divided doses should be administered only under physician's supervision. May impair physical/mental abilities.

ADVERSE REACTIONS: Anorexia, N/V, abdominal pain, leukopenia, drowsiness, headache, urticaria, SLE, myopia, vaginal bleeding, diarrhea, euphoria, hirsutism, hematuria.

INTERACTIONS: May interact with concurrently administered antiepileptic drugs, periodic serum level determinations of these drugs may be necessary (eg, may elevate phenytoin serum levels and valproic acid reported to both increase and decrease ethosuximide levels).

PREGNANCY: Safety not known in pregnancy/caution in nursing.

MECHANISM OF ACTION: Succinimide; suppresses the paroxysmal three-cycle-per-second spike and wave activity associated with lapses of consciousness, which is common in absence (petit mal) seizures. Frequency of attacks is reduced through depression of motor cortex and elevation of the CNS threshold to convulsive stimuli.

PHARMACOKINETICS: Distribution: Crosses placenta, found in breast milk.

NURSING CONSIDERATIONS

Assessment: Assess for presence of mental depression, renal/hepatic impairment, pregnancy/nursing status, and for possible drug interactions. Obtain baseline CBC, urinalysis, renal/hepatic function prior to therapy.

Monitoring: Monitor for blood dyscrasias, signs/symptoms of SLE, and infection (eg, sore throat, fever). Monitor for occurrence of grand mal seizures in patients with mixed types of epilepsy who are on monotherapy. Monitor CBC, urinalysis, renal/hepatic function. Monitor for worsening of depression, suicidal thoughts or behavior and/or any unusual changes in mood or behavior.

Patient Counseling: Inform of the importance of strictly adhering to prescribed dosage regimen. Read the Medication Guide. Contact physician if any signs/symptoms of infection (eg, sore throat, fever) and if other adverse events develop. Contact physician if worsening of depression or any unusual changes in mood or behavior develop. May impair mental/physical abilities. If pregnant, encourage to enroll in North American Antiepileptic Drug (NAAED) Pregnancy Registry.

Administration: Oral route. **Storage:** (Oral Sol) 20-25°C (68-77°F). Preserve in tight containers. Protect from freezing and light. (Caps) 25°C (77°F); excursions permitted to 15-30°C (59-86°F).

Z

ZAROXOLYN RX
metolazone (Celltech)

> Do not interchange rapid and complete bioavailability metolazone formulations for other slow and incomplete bioavailability metolazone formulations; they are not therapeutically equivalent.

THERAPEUTIC CLASS: Quinazoline diuretic

INDICATIONS: Treatment of HTN and of salt and water retention in edema accompanying CHF or renal disease.

DOSAGE: *Adults:* Edema: 5-20mg qd. HTN: 2.5-5mg qd. Elderly: Start at low end of dosing range.

HOW SUPPLIED: Tab: 2.5mg, 5mg, 10mg

CONTRAINDICATIONS: Anuria, hepatic coma or precoma.

WARNINGS/PRECAUTIONS: Risk of hypokalemia, orthostatic hypotension, hypercalcemia, hyperuricemia, azotemia, and rapid-onset hyponatremia. Cross-allergy with sulfonamide-derived drugs, thiazides, or quinethazone. Sensitivity reactions may occur with 1st dose. Monitor electrolytes. May cause hyperglycemia and glycosuria in diabetics. Caution in elderly or severe renal impairment. May exacerbate or activate SLE.

ADVERSE REACTIONS: Chest pain/discomfort, orthostatic hypotension, syncope, neuropathy, necrotizing angiitis, hepatitis, jaundice, pancreatitis, blood dyscrasias, joint pain.

INTERACTIONS: Furosemide and other loop diuretics prolong fluid and electrolyte loss. Adjust dose of other antihypertensives. Potentiates hypotensive effects of alcohol, barbiturates, and narcotics. Lithium, digitalis toxicity. Corticosteroids and ACTH increase hypokalemia and salt and water retention. Enhanced neuromuscular blocking effects of curariform drugs. Salicylates and NSAIDs decrease effects. Decreased arterial response to norepinephrine. Decrease in methenamine efficacy. Adjust anticoagulants, antidiabetics.

PREGNANCY: Category B, not for use in nursing.

MECHANISM OF ACTION: Quinazoline diuretic; acts primarily to inhibit Na^+ reabsorption at cortical diluting site and, to a lesser extent, in proximal convoluted tubule.

PHARMACOKINETICS: Absorption: T_{max}=8 hrs. **Elimination:** Urine (unchanged).

NURSING CONSIDERATIONS

Assessment: Assess for anuria, SLE, DM, sulfonamide hypersensitivity, history of allergy or bronchial asthma, hepatic/renal impairment, possible drug interactions.

Monitoring: Monitor serum electrolytes periodically. Monitor for signs/symptoms of electrolyte imbalance, exacerbation or activation of SLE, hyperglycemia, hyperuricemia or precipitation of gout, hypersensitivity reactions (eg, angioedema, bronchospasm, toxic epidermal necrolysis, Stevens-Johnson syndrome), orthostatic hypotension, renal/hepatic dysfunction.

Patient Counseling: Counsel to take medication as directed and promptly report adverse reactions. Advise not to interchange formulations. Instruct to seek medical attention if symptoms of electrolyte imbalance (eg, dry mouth, thirst, weakness) or hypersensitivity reactions occur.

Administration: Oral route. **Storage:** 25°C (77°F); excursions permitted to 15-30°C (59-86°F). Protect from light.

ZEBETA RX
bisoprolol fumarate (Duramed)

THERAPEUTIC CLASS: Selective beta₁-blocker

INDICATIONS: Management of HTN alone or in combination with other antihypertensive agents.

DOSAGE: *Adults:* Individualize dose. Initial: 5mg qd. Titrate: May increase to 10mg and then, if necessary, to 20mg qd. Bronchospastic Disease: Initial: 2.5mg qd. Hepatic/Renal Dysfunction (CrCl <40mL/min): Initial: 2.5mg qd; caution with dose titration.

HOW SUPPLIED: Tab: 5mg*, 10mg *scored

CONTRAINDICATIONS: Cardiogenic shock, overt cardiac failure, 2nd- or 3rd-degree atrioventricular (AV) block, marked sinus bradycardia.

WARNINGS/PRECAUTIONS: Avoid abrupt withdrawal; exacerbation of angina pectoris, myocardial infarction (MI) and ventricular arrhythmia in patients with coronary artery disease (CAD), and exacerbation of symptoms of hyperthyroidism or precipitation of thyroid storm reported. Reinstitute temporary therapy if withdrawal symptoms occur. May mask manifestations of hypoglycemia or clinical signs of hyperthyroidism (eg, tachycardia). Caution with compensated cardiac failure, diabetes mellitus (DM), bronchospastic disease, and hepatic/renal impairment. May precipitate cardiac failure; d/c at the 1st signs/symptoms of heart failure (HF) or continue therapy while HF is treated with other drugs. Caution with peripheral vascular disease (PVD); may precipitate or aggravate symptoms of arterial insufficiency. Caution with history of severe anaphylactic reaction to a variety of allergens; reactivity may increase with repeated challenge.

ADVERSE REACTIONS: Headache, upper respiratory infection (URI), peripheral edema, fatigue, ALT/AST elevation.

INTERACTIONS: Patients with a history of severe anaphylactic reaction to a variety of allergens taking β-blockers may be unresponsive to usual doses of epinephrine. D/C several days before withdrawal of clonidine. Excessive reduction of sympathetic activity with catecholamine-depleting drugs (eg, reserpine, guanethidine); monitor closely. Avoid with other β-blockers. Caution with myocardial depressants or inhibitors of AV conduction such as calcium antagonists (eg, verapamil, diltiazem) or antiarrhythmics (eg, disopyramide). Increased risk of bradycardia with digitalis glycosides. Increased clearance with rifampin. Caution with insulin or oral hypoglycemic agents. Reversed effects with bronchodilator therapy. Additive BP lowering effects in mild to moderate HTN with HCTZ.

PREGNANCY: Category C, caution in nursing.

MECHANISM OF ACTION: β_1-selective adrenoreceptor blocking agent; not established. May decrease cardiac output, inhibit renin release by the kidneys, and diminution of tonic sympathetic outflow from the vasomotor centers in the brain.

PHARMACOKINETICS: Absorption: (10mg) Absolute bioavailability (80%); C_{max}= (5mg) 16ng/mL, (20mg) 70ng/mL; (5-20mg) T_{max}=2-4 hrs. **Distribution:** Plasma protein binding (30%). **Elimination:** Urine (50%, unchanged), feces (<2%); $T_{1/2}$=9-12 hrs.

NURSING CONSIDERATIONS

Assessment: Assess for conditions where treatment is contraindicated or cautioned, pregnancy/nursing status, and possible drug interactions.

Monitoring: Monitor for hypoglycemia, hyperthyroidism, hepatic/renal function, signs/symptoms of HF, withdrawal and arterial insufficiency. Monitor HR, ECG, CBC with platelet and differential count.

Patient Counseling: Instruct not to interrupt or d/c therapy without consulting physician. Notify physician if difficulty in breathing, signs/symptoms of CHF or excessive bradycardia develop. Educate about signs/symptoms of drug's potential adverse effects. Advise to exercise caution while driving, operating machinery or other tasks requiring alertness.

Administration: Oral route. **Storage:** 20-25°C (68-77°F). Protect from moisture. Dispense in tight container.

Z

ZEGERID RX
sodium bicarbonate - omeprazole (Santarus)

THERAPEUTIC CLASS: Proton pump inhibitor/Antacid

INDICATIONS: Short-term treatment of erosive esophagitis diagnosed by endoscopy, active duodenal ulcer, and active benign gastric ulcer. Treatment of heartburn and other symptoms associated with gastroesophageal reflux disease (GERD). Maintain healing of erosive esophagitis. (Sus 40mg-1680mg) Reduction of risk of upper GI bleeding in critically ill patients.

DOSAGE: *Adults:* Cap/Sus: Duodenal Ulcer: 20mg qd for 4-8 weeks. Gastric Ulcer: 40mg qd for 4-8 weeks. GERD with no esophogeal lesions: 20mg qd for up to 4 weeks and for 4-8 weeks with erosive esophagitis. May give up to an additional 4 weeks if with no response to 8 weeks of therapy or may consider additional 4-8 week courses if there is recurrence of erosive esophagitis or GERD symptoms. Maintenance of Healing Erosive Esophagitis: 20mg qd. (Sus 40mg-1680mg): Risk Reduction of Upper GI Bleeding in Critically Ill Patients: Initial: 40mg, followed by 40mg after 6-8 hrs. Maint: 40mg qd for 14 days.

HOW SUPPLIED: (Omeprazole-Sodium Bicarbonate) Cap: 20mg-1100mg, 40mg-1100mg; Sus: (powder) 20mg-1680mg/pkt, 40mg-1680mg/pkt

WARNINGS/PRECAUTIONS: Atrophic gastritis reported with long-term use. Symptomatic response to therapy does not preclude the presence of gastric malignancy. Consider Na^+ content when administering to patients on a Na^+-restricted diet. Caution with Bartter's syndrome, hypokalemia, hypocalcemia, and acid-base balance problems due to Na^+ bicarbonate content. Chronic use of Na^+ bicarbonate may lead to systemic alkalosis, and increased Na^+ intake producing edema and weight increase. May increase risk of osteoporosis-related fractures of the hips, wrist or spine with high doses and long-term PPI therapy; use lowest dose and shortest duration of PPI therapy.

ADVERSE REACTIONS: Abdominal pain, diarrhea, headache, N/V, upper respiratory infection, dizziness, fever, thrombocytopenia, hypokalemia, hypomagnesemia, hyperglycemia, nosocomial pneumonia, HTN, hypotension.

INTERACTIONS: May reduce plasma levels of atazanavir; concurrent use not recommended. May interfere with the absorption of drugs where gastric pH is an important determinant of bioavailability (eg, ketoconazole, ampicillin esters, iron salts). May prolong elimination of diazepam, warfarin, phenytoin, and drugs metabolized by hepatic oxidation. May increase PT and INR if given concomitantly with warfarin. Monitor when given with drugs metabolized by CYP450 (eg, cyclosporine, disulfiram, benzodiazepines). May increase levels of tacrolimus, clarithromycin, saquinavir. May decrease levels of nelfinavir. Reported interaction with some antiretroviral drugs. Concomitant administration with voriconazole resulted in more than doubling of the omeprazole exposure. Long-term use of bicarbonate with calcium or milk can cause milk-alkali syndrome.

PREGNANCY: Category C, not for use in nursing.

MECHANISM OF ACTION: Omeprazole: Proton-pump inhibitor; suppresses gastric acid secretion by specific inhibition of the (H^+/K^+)-ATPase enzyme system at secretory surface of gastric parietal cell. Sodium Bicarbonate: Antacid; raises gastric pH and thus protects omeprazole from acid degradation.

PHARMACOKINETICS: Absorption: Omeprazole: Rapid; T_{max}=30 min; (Sus) Absolute bioavailability (30-40%), C_{max}=1954ng/mL, $AUC_{(0-inf)}$=1665ng•hr/mL (after dose 1), 3356ng•hr/mL (after dose 2). (Cap) C_{max}=1526ng/mL; (Tab) C_{max}=1763 ng/mL. **Distribution:** Omeprazole: Plasma protein binding (95%); found in breast milk. **Metabolism:** Omeprazole: Hydroxyomeprazole and corresponding carboxylic acid (metabolites). **Elimination:** Omeprazole: Urine (77% as metabolites), feces; $T_{1/2}$=1 hr.

NURSING CONSIDERATIONS

Assessment: Assess for hepatic impairment, gastric malignancy, Na^+-restricted diet, acid-base balance problems, hypocalcemia, Bartter's syndrome, hypokalemia, risk for osteoporosis-related fractures of the hip, wrist, and spine, hypersensitivity to the drug or its components, pregnancy/nursing status, and possible drug interactions. Assess dosing in Asian patients, particularly in maintenance of healing of erosive esophagitis.

Monitoring: Monitor for hypersensitivity reactions, signs/symptoms of atrophic gastritis, osteoporosis-related fractures of the hip, wrist, and spine. Monitor for milk-alkali syndrome with long-term use of bicarbonate with calcium or milk. Monitor for systemic alkalosis, edema or weight increase due to increased Na$^+$ intake with chronic use.

Patient Counseling: Instruct to take on empty stomach at least 1 hr before meals. Instruct about proper dosing and directions for use. Different formulations are not bioequivalent and can not be used as substitute of one for the other. Advise patients on a Na$^+$-restricted diet or patients at risk of developing CHF that drug contains Na$^+$. Chronic use may increase Na$^+$ intake causing swelling and weight gain. Counsel pregnant women of the harmful effects of therapy on the fetus. Notify physician if regularly taking calcium supplements. Counsel about the most frequent adverse events. Medication is not approved for patients <18 yrs.

Administration: Oral route. Take at least 1 hr prior to meals. (Caps) Swallow intact with water; do not open caps and sprinkle contents into food; do not use other liquids. (Powder) Empty pkt contents to 1-2 tbsp of water, stir well and drink immediately; refill cup with water and drink; do not use other liquids or foods. Refer to PI for administration in patients receiving continuous naso-gastric/orogastric tube feeding. **Storage:** 25°C (77°F); excursions permitted to 15-30°C (59-86°F). Protect from light and moisture.

ZEGERID OTC   OTC
sodium bicarbonate - omeprazole (Schering-Plough)

THERAPEUTIC CLASS: Proton pump inhibitor/Antacid

INDICATIONS: Treatment of frequent heartburn (≥2 days per week).

DOSAGE: *Adults:* ≥18 yrs: 1 cap qd (q24h) for 14 days. Take with glass of water in am 1 hr before food. May repeat q4 months. Do not crush, chew, open cap and sprinkle on food. Do not take >1 cap a day.

HOW SUPPLIED: Cap: (Omeprazole-Sodium Bicarbonate) 20mg-1100mg

WARNINGS/PRECAUTIONS: Each capsule contains sodium 303mg. Do not use if patient has hypersensitivity to omeprazole. Not for immediate relief of heartburn. D/C if heartburn continues or worsens, if need to take for >14 days or if need to take >1 course of treatment every 4 months. Avoid use if having trouble/pain in swallowing food, vomiting with blood or have bloody/black stools; these may be signs of a serious condition.

INTERACTIONS: Caution with warfarin, diazepam, digoxin, antifungals/anti-yeast, tacrolimus and antiretroviral agents. Sodium bicarbonate may interact with certain prescription drugs.

PREGNANCY: Safety in pregnancy and nursing not known.

MECHANISM OF ACTION: Omeprazole: Proton pump inhibitor; stops stomach acid production at the acid pump. Sodium Bicarbonate: Antacid; allows absorption of omeprazole.

NURSING CONSIDERATIONS

Assessment: Assess for proper diagnosis, hypersensitivity to omeprazole, difficulty/pain in swallowing, vomiting with blood, bloody/black stools, pregnancy/nursing status and possible drug interactions. Assess for heartburn that lasts >3 months, lightheadedness, sweating, dizziness, chest/shoulder pain with SOB, pain radiating to the arms, neck or shoulders, frequent chest pain/wheezing, unexplained weight loss, N/V, stomach pain and if on sodium-restricted diet.

Monitoring: Monitor for continuing/worsening of heartburn, treatment that lasts >14 days, >1 treatment course every 4 months, allergic/hypersensitivity reactions and relief of symptoms.

Z

Patient Counseling: Instruct to take 1 hr before breakfast; do not chew, crush, or open and sprinkle on food. Notify that drug may take 1 to 4 days for full effect. Advise not to take >14 days or more often than every 4 months unless directed by a doctor. Consult a physician if heartburn continues/worsens. Inform of any other medications being taken. Seek medical help or contact a poison control center if overdosage occurs. Notify physician if pregnant/breastfeeding. Keep out of reach of children.

Administration: Oral route. Swallow cap with a glass of water in am 1 hr before food. Do not chew, crush or open cap and sprinkle on food. Do not use if blue band around cap is missing/broken or if foil inner seal is missing/open/broken. **Storage:** 20-25°C (68-77°F). Keep out of high heat and humidity. Protect from moisture.

ZELAPAR RX
selegiline HCl (Valeant)

THERAPEUTIC CLASS: Monoamine oxidase inhibitor (Type B)

INDICATIONS: Adjunct in the management of Parkinson's disease in patients exhibiting a deteriorated response to levodopa/carbidopa therapy.

DOSAGE: *Adults:* 1.25mg qd for 6 weeks. Titrate: After 6 weeks, may increase to 2.5mg if desired benefit not achieved. Max: 2.5mg/day.

HOW SUPPLIED: Tab, Orally Disintegrating: 1.25mg

CONTRAINDICATIONS: Concomitant meperidine, tramadol, methadone, propoxyphene, dextromethorphan, and other MAOIs.

WARNINGS/PRECAUTIONS: Do not exceed 2.5mg/day; risk of non-selective MAO inhibition. Greater risk of orthostatic hypotension and dizziness in geriatric patients. Decrease levodopa/carbidopa to prevent exacerbation of levodopa side effects (eg, pre-existing dyskinesias). Melanoma reported; perform periodic dermatologic screening. May increase frequency of mild oropharyngeal abnormality. Caution with renal or hepatic impairment. Neuroleptic malignant syndrome reported in association with rapid dose reduction, withdrawal of, or changes in antiparkinsonian therapy. Compulsive behaviors (eg, intense urges to gamble, increased sexual urges) reported.

ADVERSE REACTIONS: Nausea, dizziness, pain, headache, insomnia, rhinitis, skin disorders, dyskinesia, backache, dyspepsia, stomatitis, constipation, hallucinations, pharyngitis, rash.

INTERACTIONS: See Contraindications. Serious, sometimes fatal, reactions have been precipitated with meperidine, tramadol, methadone, and propoxyphene; avoid concomitant use. Episodes of psychosis or bizarre behavior reported with dextromethorphan; avoid concomitant use. Severe toxicity reported with SSRIs or TCAs; avoid concurrent use and allow 2 weeks between d/c of selegiline and initiation of TCAs or SSRIs. Allow 5 weeks for fluoxetine due to a longer half-life. Caution with sympathomimetics and CYP3A4 inducers (eg, phenytoin, carbamazepine, nafcillin, phenobarbital, and rifampin).

PREGNANCY: Category C, not for use in nursing.

MECHANISM OF ACTION: Irreversible MAO inhibitor; blocks catabolism of dopamine and increases net amount of dopamine available.

PHARMACOKINETICS: Absorption: C_{max}(1.25mg, 2.5mg, 5mg)=3.34, 4.47, 1.12ng/mL. T_{max}(1.25mg, 2.5mg, 5mg)=10-15 min, 10-15 min, 40-90 min. **Distribution:** Plasma protein binding (85%). **Metabolism:** Liver (1st-pass metabolism). **Elimination:** Urine; $T_{1/2}$=10 hrs (steady state).

NURSING CONSIDERATIONS

Assessment: Assess renal function, LFTs, dyskinesia, phenylalanine levels, BP, melanomas, pregnancy/nursing status, and possible drug interactions.

Monitoring: Monitor LFTs, renal function, BP, exacerbation of pre-existing dyskinesia, melanomas, hyperpyrexia, hallucinations, compulsive behaviors (eg, pathological gambling, hypersexuality).

Patient Counseling: Should be taken every morning before breakfast without liquid. Do not remove blister from outer pouch until just prior to dosing. Report any side effects. Notify physician if new or increased gambling urges, sexual urges, or other urges occur.

Administration: Oral route; dissolve on tongue. **Storage:** 25°C (77°F); excursions permitted to 15-30°C (59-86°F). Use within 3 months after opening.

ZEMPLAR ORAL RX
paricalcitol (Abbott)

THERAPEUTIC CLASS: Vitamin D analog

INDICATIONS: Prevention and treatment of secondary hyperparathyroidism associated with Stage 3 and 4 chronic kidney disease (CKD), and CKD Stage 5 on hemodialysis or peritoneal dialysis.

DOSAGE: *Adults:* CKD Stages 3 and 4: Initial: Baseline iPTH Level ≤500pg/mL: 1mcg qd or 2mcg 3X/week. Baseline iPTH Level >500pg/mL: 2mcg qd or 4mcg 3X/week. Administer the 3X/week dose not more often than qod. Dose Titration: Individualize dose and base dose on serum or plasma iPTH levels. Refer to PI for further dose titration recommendations. CKD Stage 5: Initial: Based on baseline iPTH level (pg/mL)/80. Should only be treated after baseline SrCa adjusted to ≤9.5mg/dL. Titration: Individualize dose. May need to decrease dose by 2-4mcg lower than the calculated baseline iPTH level/80 if SrCa levels or CaxP are elevated. If further dose reduction is required, reduce dose or withhold until parameters are normalized. Refer to PI for further recommendations on dose titration.

HOW SUPPLIED: Cap: 1mcg, 2mcg, 4mcg

CONTRAINDICATIONS: Vitamin D toxicity, hypercalcemia.

WARNINGS/PRECAUTIONS: Excessive administration may cause over suppression of PTH, hypercalcemia, hypercalciuria, hyperphosphatemia, and adynamic bone disease. Overdose may cause progressive hypercalcemia. Exacerbation of cardiac arrhythmias and seizures may occur in acute hypercalcemia. Chronic hypercalcemia may cause generalized vascular calcification and other soft-tissue calcification. During initial dosing as well as during dose adjustments, monitor SrCa, serum phosphorus, and serum or plasma iPTH every 2 weeks for 3 months, then monthly for 3 months, then every 3 months thereafter.

ADVERSE REACTIONS: Pain, allergic reactions, headache, hypotension, infection, HTN, diarrhea, N/V, constipation, edema, arthritis, dizziness, rhinitis, rash.

INTERACTIONS: Digitalis toxicity potentiated by hypercalcemia; caution with concomitant use of digitalis products. Caution with strong CYP3A inhibitors (eg, ketoconazole, atazanavir, clarithromycin, indinavir, itraconazole, nefazodone, nelfinavir, ritonavir, saquinavir, telithromycin, voriconazole). Drugs that may impair intestinal absorption of fat-soluble vitamins (eg, cholestyramine) may interfere with absorption. Avoid regular administration of aluminum. Withhold pharmacologic doses of vitamin D and its derivatives to avoid hypercalcemia. High intake of calcium and phosphate may cause serum abnormalities. Mineral oil or other substances that may affect absorption of fat may impair absorption.

PREGNANCY: Category C, not for use in nursing.

MECHANISM OF ACTION: Synthetic vitamin D_2 analog; binds to vitamin D receptor (VDR), which results in selective activation of vitamin D responsive pathways. Shown to reduce parathyroid hormone levels by inhibiting PTH synthesis and secretion.

PHARMACOKINETICS: Absorption: Absolute bioavailability (72%-86%). Refer to PI for different pharmacokinetic parameters of CKD Stages. **Distribution:** V_d=34L (healthy); 44-46L (CKD Stages 3 and 4); plasma protein binding (≥99.8%). **Metabolism:** Hepatic (extensive), via hydroxylation and glucuronidation; metabolized by CYP24, as well as CYP3A4, UGT1A4. 24(R)-hydroxy paricalcitol (minor metabolite). **Elimination:** Hepatobiliary excretion (primary);

Z

urine (18%), feces: (70%), (2%, unchanged). $T_{1/2}$=4-6 hrs (healthy), 14-20 hrs (CKD Stages 3, 4, 5).

NURSING CONSIDERATIONS

Assessment: Assess for vitamin D toxicity or hypercalcemia, pregnancy/nursing status, and for possible drug interactions. Obtain baseline values of serum calcium, serum phosphorus and serum/plasma iPTH.

Monitoring: Monitor for signs/symptoms of hypercalcemia (eg, cardiac arrhythmias, seizures, vascular calcification, soft tissue calcification). Monitor for over suppression of PTH, hypercalciuria, hyperphosphatemia and adynamic bone disease. Monitor serum calcium, serum phosphorus, and serum/plasma iPTH every 2 weeks for 3 months, then monthly for 3 months, then every 3 months thereafter during initiation or following dosage adjustment.

Patient Counseling: Counsel about possible side effects such as diarrhea, infection, HTN and dizziness. Comply with dosage instructions, proper diet, phosphorus restrictions, and avoid unapproved OTC drugs. Contact healthcare provider if symptoms of elevated calcium (eg, feeling tired, difficulty thinking clearly, loss of appetite, N/V, constipation, increased thirst, increased urination, weight loss) develop. Frequent monitoring is necessary during initiation of therapy, following dose changes or when potentially interacting medications are started or d/c. Notify physician of all medications, Rx/OTC drugs, supplements, and herbal preparations currently taken. Medication may be taken without regard to food.

Administration: Oral route. **Storage:** 25°C (77°F); excursions permitted to 15-30°C (59-86°F).

ZENAPAX   RX
daclizumab (Roche Labs)

> Should only be prescribed by physicians experienced in immunosuppressive therapy and management of organ transplant patients. Physician should have complete information requisite for the follow-up of the patient. Only healthcare personnel trained in the administration of the drug who have adequate laboratory and supportive medical resources available should administer.

THERAPEUTIC CLASS: Interleukin-2 receptor antagonist

INDICATIONS: For prophylaxis of acute organ rejection in renal transplants, in combination with cyclosporine and corticosteroids.

DOSAGE: *Adults:* 1mg/kg IV over 15 min for 5 doses. Administer 1st dose no more than 24 hrs prior to transplant and remaining four doses at 14-day intervals.
Pediatrics: ≥11 months: 1mg/kg IV over 15 min for 5 doses. Administer 1st dose no more than 24 hrs prior to transplant and remaining 4 doses at 14-day intervals.

HOW SUPPLIED: Inj: 25mg/5mL

WARNINGS/PRECAUTIONS: May be associated with increased risk in mortality, lymphoproliferative disorder, and opportunistic infections; monitor accordingly. Hypersensitivity reactions including anaphylaxis reported on initial and re-exposure. Postmarketing reports of cytokine release syndrome. D/C if severe hypersensitivity reaction occurs. Caution in elderly. Re-administration after initial course of therapy has not been studied in humans.

ADVERSE REACTIONS: GI disorders, constipation, N/V, diarrhea, abdominal pain, pyrosis, dyspepsia, abdominal distention, epigastric pain, edema extremities, edema, tremor, headache, dizziness, oliguria.

INTERACTIONS: Immunosuppressive regimens including cyclosporine, mycophenolate mofetil, and corticosteroids are associated with an increase in mortality, particularly in patients receiving anti-lymphocyte antibody therapy and who develop severe infections. Very limited experience exists with tacrolimus, muromonab-CD3, antithymocyte globulin, and anti-lymphocyte globulin.

PREGNANCY: Category C, not for use in nursing.

MECHANISM OF ACTION: IL-2 receptor antagonist; binds with high affinity to the Tac subunit of the high affinity IL-2 receptor complex and inhibits IL-2 binding.

PHARMACOKINETICS: Absorption: C_{max}=21mcg/mL (adult); 16mcg/mL (pediatric). **Elimination:** $T_{1/2}$=20 days (adult), 13 days (pediatric).

NURSING CONSIDERATIONS

Assessment: Assess for drug hypersensitivity, DM, pregnancy/nursing status, and possible drug interactions.

Monitoring: Monitor for hypersensitivity reactions (eg, hypotension, bronchospasm, wheezing, laryngeal edema, pulmonary edema, cyanosis, hypoxia, respiratory arrest, cardiac arrhythmia, cardiac arrest, peripheral edema, loss of consciousness, fever, rash, urticaria, diaphoresis, pruritus, injection-site reactions), lymphoproliferative disorders, infectious episodes (eg, viral and fungal infections, bacteremia, and septicemia), pneumonia, and opportunistic infections (eg, CMV, cellulitis, and wound infection). Monitor FPG.

Patient Counseling: Inform about potential risks/benefits. Instruct not to take while pregnant/nursing.

Administration: IV route. Not for direct injection; dilute with 50mL of 0.9% NaCl solution and administer via central or peripheral vein for 15 min. When mixing, invert the bag without shaking. **Storage:** 2-8°C (36-46°F). Do not shake or freeze. Protect diluted solution against direct light. Diluted medication is stable for 24 hrs at 4°C or for 4 hrs at room temp.

ZENPEP   RX
pancrelipase (Eurand Pharmaceuticals, Inc.)

THERAPEUTIC CLASS: Pancreatic enzyme supplement

INDICATIONS: Treatment of exocrine pancreatic insufficiency due to cystic fibrosis (CF) or other conditions.

DOSAGE: *Adults:* Individualize dose. Titrate: May increase dose based on clinical symptoms, degree of steatorrhea present, and fat content of diet. Initial: 500 lipase U/kg/meal. Max: 2,500 lipase U/kg/meal (≤10,000 lipase U/kg/day) or <4,000 lipase U/g fat ingested/day. Usual: Half the dose used for meals should be given with each snack. Approximately 3 meals plus 2 or 3 snacks/day should reflect as the total daily dose.
Pediatrics: Individualize dose. Titrate: May increase dose based on clinical symptoms, degree of steatorrhea present, and fat content of diet. ≥4 yrs: Initial: 500 lipase U/kg/meal. Max: 2,500 lipase U/kg/meal (≤10,000 lipase U/kg/day) or <4,000 lipase U/g fat ingested/day. Usual: Half the dose used for meals should be given with each snack. >12 mth-<4 yrs: Initial: 1,000 lipase U/kg/meal. Max: 2,500 lipase U/kg/meal (≤10,000 lipase U/kg/day) or <4,000 lipase U/g fat ingested/day. Infants ≤12 mth: 2,000-4,000 lipase U/120 mL of formula or per breastfeeding.

HOW SUPPLIED: Cap, Delayed-Release: (Amylase-Lipase-Protease) (Zenpep 5) 27,000 U-5,000 U-17,000 U, (Zenpep 10) 55,000 U-10,000 U-34,000 U, (Zenpep 15) 82,000 U-15,000 U-51,000 U, (Zenpep 20) 109,000 U-20,000 U-68,000 U

WARNINGS/PRECAUTIONS: Fibrosing colonopathy reported; Monitor closely for progression to stricture formation. Caution in doses >2500 lipase U/kg/meal (>10,000 lipase U/kg/day). When receiving doses >6,000 lipase U/kg/meal, patients should be examined and dosage either immediately decreased or titrated downward to a lower range. May irritate oral mucosa; ensure that no drug is retained in the mouth. Do not crush, chew, or mix in foods with a pH >4.5. Caution with gout, renal impairment, or hyperuricemia; may increase serum uric acid levels. Risk for transmission of viral disease, including diseases caused by novel or unidentified viruses. Caution with a known allergy to porcine protein. Allergic reactions (eg, anaphylaxis, asthma, hives, pruritus) may occur. Do not interchange with any other pancrelipase products. Not rec-

Z

ommended to mix directly with milk formula or breast milk. Decrease dosing in older patients.

ADVERSE REACTIONS: Abdominal pain, flatulence, headache, cough, weight loss, early satiety, contusion, steatorrhea, GI disorders, skin disorders.

PREGNANCY: Category C, caution in nursing.

MECHANISM OF ACTION: Pancreatic enzyme supplement; catalyzes the hydrolysis of fats to monoglycerol, glycerol and fatty acids, protein into peptides and amino acids, and starch into dextrins and short chain sugars in the duodenum and proximal small intestine, thereby acting like digestive enzymes physiologically secreted by the pancreas.

NURSING CONSIDERATIONS

Assessment: Assess for gout, renal impairment, hyperuricemia, known allergy to porcine proteins, and pregnancy/nursing status. Obtain baseline serum uric acid levels and renal function.

Monitoring: Monitor for fibrosing colonopathy, colonic strictures, renal impairment, oral mucosa irritation, hyperuricemia, viral diseases, gout, steatorrhea, and allergic reactions. Monitor serum uric acid levels and renal function.

Patient Counseling: Instruct to take as prescribed and follow dosing instructions. If dose is missed, take the next dose with the next meal/snack as directed; do not double the dose. Maximum total daily dose is 10,000 lipase U/kg/day unless clinically indicated. Take with food and swallow cap whole with adequate amount of liquid; do not crush, chew, or mix directly with formula or breast milk. If cannot swallow intact cap, may be opened carefully and the contents may be added or sprinkled onto a small amount of acidic soft food (pH ≤4.5) (eg, applesauce). Care should be taken to ensure that no drug is retained in the mouth to avoid oral mucosa irritation. Notify physician if pregnant or intend to become pregnant during treatment. Immediately contact physician if allergic reactions occur.

Administration: Oral route. Administer to infants immediately prior to each feeding. Swallow whole; do not crush or chew. Refer to PI for proper administration. **Storage:** 20-25°C (68-77°F); excursions permitted to 15-40°C (59-104°F). Keep tightly closed. Protect from moisture.

ZENTRIP   OTC
meclizine HCl (Sato)

THERAPEUTIC CLASS: Antihistamine

INDICATIONS: Prevention and treatment of N/V, or dizziness associated with motion sickness.

DOSAGE: *Adults:* Dissolve 1-2 strips on tongue qd or ud. Prevention: ≥1 hr prior to travel.
Pediatrics: ≥12 yrs: Dissolve 1-2 strips on tongue qd or ud. Prevention: ≥1 hr prior to travel.

HOW SUPPLIED: Strip, Oral: 25mg

WARNINGS/PRECAUTIONS: Avoid use in children <12 yrs of age. Caution with glaucoma, breathing problems (eg, emphysema, chronic bronchitis), and difficulty in urination due to an enlarged prostate gland. D/C use and consult physician if rash, redness, itching, or difficulty in urination occurs, or if symptoms of dry mouth continue or increase. Drowsiness may occur and may impair mental/physical abilities.

ADVERSE REACTIONS: Drowsiness

INTERACTIONS: Alcohol, sedatives, and tranquilizers may increase drowsiness. Avoid alcohol use.

PREGNANCY: Safety not known in pregnancy and nursing.

MECHANISM OF ACTION: Antihistamine.

Z

NURSING CONSIDERATIONS

Assessment: Assess for breathing problems (eg, emphysema, chronic bronchitis), glaucoma, difficulty in urination due to an enlarged prostate gland, pregnancy/nursing status, and possible drug interactions.

Monitoring: Monitor for drowsiness, rash, redness, itching, difficulty in urination and increased/continued symptoms of dry mouth.

Patient Counseling: Inform that drowsiness may occur; caution when driving a vehicle or operating machinery. Avoid alcohol use. D/C and consult physician if rash, redness, itching, or difficulty in urination occurs, or if symptoms of dry mouth continue or increase. Consult physician before use if taking sedatives or tranquilizers and if pregnant/nursing. Keep out of reach of children; in case of overdose, get medical help or contact a Poison Control Center right away.

Administration: Oral route. **Storage:** 20-30°C (68-86°F). Protect from light. Use only if safety seal intact.

ZERIT   RX
stavudine (Bristol-Myers Squibb)

> Lactic acidosis and severe hepatomegaly with steatosis, including fatal cases, reported with nucleoside analogues alone or in combination with other antiretrovirals. Fatal lactic acidosis reported in pregnant women who received the combination of stavudine and didanosine with other antiretroviral agents. Use with caution in pregnancy when coadministered with didanosine. Fatal and nonfatal pancreatitis reported when part of a combination regimen that included didanosine.

THERAPEUTIC CLASS: Synthetic thymidine nucleoside analogue

INDICATIONS: Treatment of HIV-1 infection in combination with other antiretrovirals.

DOSAGE: *Adults:* ≥60kg: 40mg q12h. <60kg: 30mg q12h. Renal Impairment: CrCl >50mL/min: ≥60kg: 40mg q12h. <60kg: 30mg q12h. CrCl 26-50mL/min: ≥60kg: 20mg q12h. <60kg: 15mg q12h. CrCl 10-25mL/min/Hemodialysis: ≥60kg: 20mg q24h. <60kg: 15mg q24h.
Pediatrics: ≥60kg: 40mg q12h. ≥30-<60kg: 30mg q12h. ≥14 Days & <30kg: 1mg/kg q12h. Birth-13 Days: 0.5mg/kg q12h.

HOW SUPPLIED: Cap: 15mg, 20mg, 30mg, 40mg; Sol: 1mg/mL [200mL]

WARNINGS/PRECAUTIONS: Suspend therapy in patients who develop clinical or laboratory findings suggestive of symptomatic hyperlactatemia, lactic acidosis or pronounced hepatotoxicity. Caution in patients with risk factors for liver disease. Patients with pre-existing liver dysfunction have an increased frequency of liver function abnormalities (eg, severe and fatal hepatic adverse events); monitor accordingly and interrupt or d/c if worsening of liver disease is evident. Motor weakness reported rarely; d/c if this develops. Peripheral sensory neuropathy reported; consider permanent d/c if this develops. Redistribution/accumulation of body fat reported; monitor for signs/symptoms of lipoatrophy or lipodystrophy. Immune reconstitution syndrome reported. Caution in elderly and renal impairment.

ADVERSE REACTIONS: Peripheral neuropathy, rash, headache, diarrhea, N/V, pancreatitis, lactic acidosis, increased AST/ALT, increased GGT/amylase/lipase/bilirubin, hepatomegaly.

INTERACTIONS: See Boxed Warning. Avoid with zidovudine, which inhibits intracellular phosphorylation of drug. Increased risk of peripheral neuropathy and hepatotoxicity may occur when concomitantly used in combination with didanosine with or without hydroxyurea; avoid concomitant use. Fatal hepatic decompensation may occur in HIV/HCV co-infected patients with concomitant use of interferon/ribavirin; monitor for clinical toxicities. Caution with concomitant use of doxorubicin or ribavirin. Incidence of peripheral neuropathy may occur more frequently if receiving other drugs that have been associated with neuropathy. D/C use with agents that are toxic to the pancreas in patients with suspected pancreatitis. Increased concentration with lamivudine.

Z

PREGNANCY: Category C, not for use in nursing.

MECHANISM OF ACTION: Synthetic thymidine nucleoside analogue; inhibits activity of HIV-1 reverse transcriptase (RT) by competing with natural substrate thymidine triphosphate and by causing DNA chain termination following incorporation into viral DNA. Inhibits cellular DNA polymerases β and gamma and markedly reduces synthesis of mitochondrial DNA.

PHARMACOKINETICS: Absorption: Rapid; C_{max}=536ng/mL; T_{max}=1 hr; AUC_{0-24}=2,568ng•hr/mL. **Distribution:** V_d=46L (adults), 0.73L/kg (5 weeks-15 yrs). **Metabolism:** Oxidized stavudine, glucuronide conjugates and N-acetylcysteine conjugate (minor metabolites). **Elimination:** Feces (62%), urine (73.7%). $T_{1/2}$=2.3 hrs.

NURSING CONSIDERATIONS

Assessment: Assess for drug hypersensitivity, liver dysfunction, renal impairment, pancreatitis, pregnancy/nursing status and for possible drug interactions.

Monitoring: Monitor for signs/symptoms of lactic acidosis, severe hepatomegaly with steatosis, pancreatitis, immune reconstitution syndrome, motor weakness, peripheral neuropathy, redistribution/accumulation of body fat and for evidence of worsening liver disease. Monitor LFTs and renal function.

Patient Counseling: Inform that therapy is not cure for HIV, does not reduce risk of HIV transmission and that illnesses associated with HIV-1 may develop. Increased risk of hepatotoxicity with didanosine and hydroxyurea; instruct to avoid this combination. Increased risk of pancreatitis with didanosine. Avoid alcohol while on therapy. Seek medical attention if symptoms of hyperlactatemia or lactic acidosis syndrome (eg, unexplained weight loss, abdominal discomfort, N/V, fatigue, dyspnea, motor weakness) occurs. Peripheral neuropathy may develop; contact physician if symptoms of numbness, tingling or pain in the hands or feet occur. Redistribution/accumulation of fat tissue may occur. Enroll patients in the Antiretroviral Pregnancy Registry if they become pregnant while on therapy. If dose is missed, take as soon as possible; continue the regular dosing schedule if it is almost time for the next dose.

Administration: Oral route. Refer to PI for preparation of oral solution. **Storage:** Cap, Sol: 25°C (77°F); excursions permitted between 15-30°C (59-86°F) in a tightly closed container. Sol: Protect from excessive moisture. After reconstitution, refrigerate at 2-8°C (36-46°F). Discard any unused portion after 30 days.

ZESTORETIC   RX
lisinopril - hydrochlorothiazide (AstraZeneca)

> ACE inhibitors can cause death/injury to developing fetus during 2nd and 3rd trimesters. D/C if pregnancy is detected.

THERAPEUTIC CLASS: ACE inhibitor/thiazide diuretic

INDICATIONS: Treatment of HTN.

DOSAGE: *Adults:* Not Controlled with Lisinopril/HCTZ Monotherapy: Initial: 10mg-12.5mg or 20mg-12.5mg qd depending on current monotherapy dose. Titrate: May increase HCTZ dose after 2-3 weeks. May reduce dose of lisinopril after addition of diuretic. Controlled on 25mg HCTZ qd with Hypokalemia: Switch to 10mg-12.5mg qd. Replacement Therapy: Substitute combination for titrated individual components. Elderly: Start at lower end of dosing range.

HOW SUPPLIED: Tab: (Lisinopril-HCTZ) 10mg-12.5mg, 20mg-12.5mg, 20mg-25mg

CONTRAINDICATIONS: History of ACE inhibitor-associated angioedema, hereditary or idiopathic angioedema, anuria, hypersensitivity to other sulfonamide-derived drugs.

WARNINGS/PRECAUTIONS: Not for initial therapy of HTN. Angioedema of the face, extremities, lips, tongue, glottis, and/or larynx reported; d/c and administer appropriate therapy if this occurs. Intestinal angioedema reported;

monitor for abdominal pain (with or without N/V). Anaphylactoid reactions reported during desensitization with hymenoptera venom, with dialysis with high-flux membranes, and LDL apheresis with dextran sulfate absorption. Excessive hypotension may occur. Leukopenia/neutropenia and bone marrow depression reported; monitor WBCs in patients with renal and collagen vascular disease. D/C if jaundice or marked elevations of hepatic enzymes occur. Caution with severe renal disease, hepatic dysfunction, left ventricular outflow obstruction, renal artery stenosis, and in elderly. May exacerbate or activate systemic lupus erythematosus (SLE). Risk of hyperkalemia with diabetes mellitus (DM) and renal insufficiency. Persistent nonproductive cough reported. Sensitivity reactions may occur in patients with/without history of allergy or bronchial asthma. May increase cholesterol and TG levels. Fluid/electrolyte imbalance, hyperglycemia, and hyperuricemia may occur. Enhanced effects with postsympathectomy patients. (Zestoretic) May cause idiosyncratic reaction, resulting in acute transient myopia and acute angle-closure glaucoma.

ADVERSE REACTIONS: Dizziness, headache, cough, fatigue, orthostatic effects, angioedema, hypotension.

INTERACTIONS: Increased risk of lithium toxicity; avoid with lithium. Lisinopril: Hypotension risk with diuretics. Indomethacin may reduce effects. May cause further deterioration of renal function in patients with compromised renal function taking NSAIDs. Increased risk of hyperkalemia with K^+-sparing diuretics, K^+ supplements, or K^+-containing salt substitutes. Nitritoid reactions with injectable gold reported. Hypotension may occur during anesthesia. HCTZ: Potentiation of orthostatic hypotension with alcohol, barbiturates, and narcotics. Dose adjustment of insulin or oral hypoglycemic agents may be required. Potentiation or additive effects with other antihypertensives. Reduced absorption with cholestyramine or colestipol. Increased risk of electrolyte depletion (eg, hypokalemia) with corticosteroids and ACTH. May decrease response to pressor amines (eg, norepinephrine). May increase responsiveness to nondepolarizing skeletal muscle relaxants (eg, tubocurarine). NSAIDs may reduce diuretic, natriuretic, and antihypertensive effects. May cause hypokalemia, which may lead to cardiac arrhythmia and sensitize or exaggerate the response of the heart to the toxic effects of digitalis.

PREGNANCY: Category C (1st trimester) and D (2nd and 3rd trimesters), not for use in nursing.

MECHANISM OF ACTION: Lisinopril: ACE inhibitor; decreases plasma angiotensin II, which leads to decreased vasopressor activity and decreased aldosterone secretion. HCTZ: Thiazide diuretic; not established. Affects distal renal tubular mechanism of electrolyte reabsorption. Increases excretion of Na^+ and Cl^-.

PHARMACOKINETICS: Absorption: Lisinopril: T_{max}=7 hrs. **Distribution:** HCTZ: Crosses placenta, found in breast milk. **Elimination:** Lisinopril: Urine (unchanged); $T_{1/2}$=12 hrs. HCTZ: Kidneys (≥61% unchanged); $T_{1/2}$=5.6-14.8 hrs.

NURSING CONSIDERATIONS

Assessment: Assess for congestive heart failure, SLE, collagen vascular disease, renal artery stenosis, risk factors for hyperkalemia, histories of angioedema, allergy or bronchial asthma, and any other conditions where treatment is contraindicated or cautioned. Assess for hypersensitivity to drug, renal/hepatic function, pregnancy/nursing status, and possible drug interactions.

Monitoring: Monitor for angioedema, anaphylactoid reactions, hypotension, jaundice, sensitivity reactions, SLE, hyperglycemia, and hyperuricemia. Periodically monitor serum electrolytes and WBCs in patients with collagen vascular and renal diseases. Monitor BP, LFTs, renal function (BUN, SrCr), and cholesterol/TG levels.

Patient Counseling: Inform about fetal risks if taken during pregnancy; report pregnancies to physicians as soon as possible. Advise to be cautioned with excessive perspiration, dehydration, and other causes of volume depletion (eg, diarrhea, vomiting); may lead to fall in BP. Instruct to report lightheadedness, to d/c therapy if actual syncope occurs, not to use salt substitutes containing K^+ without consulting physician, and to report immediately any signs/symptoms of leukopenia/neutropenia (eg, infections, fever, sore throat)

Z

1359

and angioedema (eg, swelling of face, extremities, eyes, lips, tongue, difficulty swallowing or breathing).

Administration: Oral route. **Storage:** 20-25°C (68-77°F). Protect from excessive light and humidity.

ZESTRIL RX
lisinopril (AstraZeneca)

> ACE inhibitors can cause injury/death to developing fetus during 2nd and 3rd trimesters. D/C if pregnancy is detected.

THERAPEUTIC CLASS: ACE inhibitor

INDICATIONS: Treatment of HTN alone as initial therapy or concomitantly with other classes of antihypertensive. Adjunct therapy in heart failure if inadequately controlled by diuretics and digitalis. Treatment of stable patients within 24 hrs of AMI to improve survival.

DOSAGE: *Adults:* HTN: Initial: 10mg qd. Adjust dose according to BP response. Usual: 20-40mg qd. Max: 80mg/day. May add a low-dose diuretic if BP not controlled. Diuretic-Treated Patients: D/C diuretic 2-3 days prior to therapy to reduce likelihood of hypotension. Adjust dose according to BP response. If diuretic cannot be d/c; give initial dose of 5mg under medical supervision for at least 2 hrs and BP stabilized for 1 hr. Renal Impairment: CrCl 10-30mL/min: Initial: 5mg/day. CrCl <10mL/min: Initial: 2.5mg/day. Titrate up until BP is controlled. Max: 40mg/day. Heart Failure: Initial: 5mg qd. Usual: 5-40mg qd. May increase by 10mg every 2 weeks. Max: 40mg/day. Heart failure/Hyponatremia or CrCl ≤30mL/min or SrCr >3mg/dL: Initial: 2.5mg qd under close medical supervision. AMI: Initial: 5mg within 24 hrs, then 5mg after 24 hrs, then 10mg after 48 hrs, then 10mg qd for 6 weeks. Patients with low SBP (≤120mmHg) when treatment is started or during the 1st 3 days after the infarct: Give 2.5mg PO. Maint: 5mg qd may be given with temporary reductions to 2.5mg prn if prolonged hypotension (SBP≤100mmHg) occurs. D/C with prolonged hypotension (SBP<90mmHg for more than 1 hr). Dose Adjustment with MI with Renal Impairment: Initiate treatment with caution. Elderly: Start at low end of the dosing range.
Pediatrics: ≥6 yrs: HTN: Initial: 0.07mg/kg qd up to 5mg total. Adjust dose according to response. Max: 0.61mg/kg or 40mg.

HOW SUPPLIED: Tab: 2.5mg, 5mg, 10mg, 20mg, 30mg, 40mg

CONTRAINDICATIONS: History of ACE inhibitor-associated angioedema, hereditary or idiopathic angioedema.

WARNINGS/PRECAUTIONS: Anaphylactoid reactions during membrane exposure, and angioedema of the head and neck (rarely with fatalities) and of the intestines reported. Rarely, syndrome of cholestatic jaundice progressing to fulminant necrotic hepatitis and death reported. D/C if angioedema, jaundice, or marked LFT elevation occur. Risk of hyperkalemia, hypoglycemia with DM, renal dysfunction. Persistent nonproductive cough reported; resolves upon d/c. Monitor WBCs in renal and collagen vascular disease; agranulocytosis and bone marrow depression may occur. Monitor for hypotension in high-risk patients (heart failure with SBP <100mmHg, surgery/anesthesia, hyponatremia, high-dose diuretic therapy, severe volume, and/or salt depletion, etc.). Fetal/neonatal morbidity and death reported. Caution with CHF, aortic stenosis/hypertrophic cardiomyopathy, renal dysfunction, and renal artery stenosis. Less effective on BP and higher rates of angioedema reported in blacks than non-blacks. Not recommended in pediatric patients with GFR <30mL/min/1.73min².

ADVERSE REACTIONS: Chest pain, cough, diarrhea, dizziness, headache, hyperkalemia, hypotension, syncope, angioedema, increased creatinine and non-protein nitrogen.

INTERACTIONS: May increase lithium levels. Hypotension risk with diuretics. Concomitant use with antidiabetic agents or insulin may increase risk of hypoglycemia. Coadministration with NSAIDs in patients with compromised renal function may cause further deterioration. Increased risk of hyperkalemia with K⁺-sparing diuretics, K⁺-containing salt substitutes, or K⁺ supplements. Indomethacin may reduce effects. Nitritoid reactions (eg, facial flushing, N/V, hypotension) rarely reported when used concomitantly with injectable gold.

PREGNANCY: Category C (1st trimester) and D (2nd and 3rd trimesters), not for use in nursing.

MECHANISM OF ACTION: ACE inhibitor; inhibition results in decreased plasma angiotensin II, which leads to decreased vasopressor activity and aldosterone secretion.

PHARMACOKINETICS: Absorption: T_{max}=7 hrs. **Distribution:** Crosses placenta. **Elimination:** Urine (unchanged); $T_{1/2}$=12 hrs.

NURSING CONSIDERATIONS

Assessment: Assess BP, LFTs, renal function, CVD (eg, aortic stenosis, cardio-myopathy), renal artery stenosis, pregnancy/nursing status, and for possible drug interactions.

Monitoring: Monitor BP, LFTs, renal function, CBC with platelet count and differential, serum K⁺ levels. Monitor for MI, CHF, angioedema (head, neck, intestinal), anaphylactoid reactions, hepatic failure, hypoglycemia, hypersen-sitivity reactions, cough, N/V, dizziness, mood alterations.

Patient Counseling: Inform about fetal risks during pregnancy. Advise to report if pregnant. Watch for signs/symptoms of angioedema (laryngeal/ tongue edema, abdominal pain); seek prompt medical attention if symptoms develop. Inform about potential adverse effects (eg, anaphylaxis, cough, hypotension, hyperkalemia, diarrhea, dizziness, headaches, mood alterations). Report any indication of infection (eg, sore throat, fever) which may be a sign of leukopenia/neutropenia. Inform about need for periodic monitoring of electrolytes and blood counts. Caution that inadequate fluid intake, excessive perspiration, diarrhea, vomiting may lead to excessive fall in BP, which can re-sult in lightheadedness or possible syncope. Do not use K⁺ supplements or salt substitutes containing K⁺ without consulting physician. Monitor for hypoglyce-mia in diabetics during the first month of combined use with oral antidiabetic agents or insulin.

Administration: Oral route. Refer to PI for preparation of suspension. **Storage:** 20-25°C (68-77°F). Protect from moisture, freezing, and excessive heat.

ZETIA   RX
ezetimibe (Merck/Schering-Plough)

THERAPEUTIC CLASS: Cholesterol absorption inhibitor

INDICATIONS: Adjunct to diet, as monotherapy or with concomitant HMG-CoA reductase inhibitors (statins), to reduce total cholesterol (total-C), low-density lipoprotein cholesterol (LDL-C), and apolipoprotein B (Apo B) levels in primary (heterozygous familial and non-familial) hyperlipidemia. Adjunct to diet, with concomitant fenofibrate, to reduce elevated total-C, LDL-C, Apo B, and non-high-density lipoprotein cholesterol (non-HDL-C) in adults with mixed hyperlipidemia. Adjunct to other lipid-lowering treatments (eg, LDL apheresis) or if such treatments are unavailable, with concomitant atorvasta-tin or simvastatin, to reduce total-C and LDL-C in homozygous familial hyper-cholesterolemia (HoFH). Adjunct to diet, to reduce sitosterol and campesterol levels in homozygous familial sitosterolemia.

DOSAGE: *Adults:* 10mg qd. May give with a statin (with primary hyperlipi-demia) or fenofibrate (with mixed hyperlipidemia); daily dose may be taken at the same time as statin or fenofibrate. Concomitant Bile Acid Sequestrant: Give either ≥2 hrs before or ≥4 hrs after bile acid sequestrant.

HOW SUPPLIED: Tab: 10mg

CONTRAINDICATIONS: When used with a statin, contraindicated in pregnan-cy, nursing, and with active liver disease or unexplained persistent elevations in hepatic transaminase levels.

WARNINGS/PRECAUTIONS: Concurrent statin therapy may lead to transami-nase elevations; monitor LFTs. May increase risk of rhabdomyolysis/myopathy

Z

especially during concomitant use with fibrate or statin therapy; d/c use of ezetimibe, fibrate, or statin if myopathy is suspected. Not recommended with moderate or severe hepatic impairment.

ADVERSE REACTIONS: Upper respiratory tract infection, diarrhea, arthralgia.

INTERACTIONS: Concomitant use with cyclosporine, may increase exposure to both ezetimibe and cyclosporine; monitor cyclporine levels. Use with fenofibrate may increase fenofibrate and ezetimibe levels; use with fenofibrate may cause cholelithiasis requiring gallbladder studies and alternate lipid-lowering therapy. Use with gemfibrozil may increase ezetimibe levels and may decrease gemfibrozil levels; avoid concomitant use with fibrates other than fenofibrate. Use with cholestyramine may decrease ezetimibe levels; incremental LDL-C reduction may be reduced by this interaction. Monitor INR levels when administered with warfarin. Use with aluminum and magnesium hydroxide may decrease ezetimibe levels. Use with cimetidine may increase ezetimibe levels. Use with glipizide may cause a decrease in ezetimibe and glipizide levels. May decrease digoxin levels. May decrease ethinyl estradiol and levonorgestrel levels. Use with lovastatin may increase ezetimibe and lovastatin levels. Concomitant use with pravastatin may increase ezetimibe levels and decrease pravastatin levels. Use with atorvastatin may increase atorvastatin and ezetimibe levels. Use with rosuvastatin may increase ezetimibe and rosuvastatin levels. Use with fluvastatin may increase ezetimibe levels and decrease fluvastatin levels.

PREGNANCY: Category C, caution in nursing.

MECHANISM OF ACTION: Cholesterol absorption inhibitor; inhibits absorption of cholesterol by the small intestine. Targets the sterol transporter, Neimann-Pick C1-like 1 (NPC1L1), which is involved in intestinal uptake of cholesterol and phytosterols; inhibited cholesterol absorption leads to a decrease in delivery of intestinal cholesterol to the liver, causing reduction of hepatic cholesterol stores and increase in clearance of cholesterol from the blood.

PHARMACOKINETICS: Absorption: (Fasted) Ezetimibe: C_{max}=3.4-5.5ng/mL; T_{max}=4-12 hrs. Ezetimibe-glucuronide (active metabolite) C_{max}=45-71ng/mL; T_{max}=1-2 hrs. **Distribution:** Plasma protein binding (>90%). **Metabolism:** Small intestine, liver via glucuronide conjugation; Ezetimibe-glucuronide (major active metabolite). **Elimination:** Feces (78%), urine (11%); $T_{1/2}$=22 hrs.

NURSING CONSIDERATIONS

Assessment: Assess for hepatic impairment, pregnancy/nursing status, and for possible drug interactions. If using in combination with statin therapy, assess for risk factors for skeletal muscle toxicity (eg, use with higher doses of statins, advanced age, hypothyroidism, renal impairment, concomitant drug use). Obtain baseline lipid profile (total-C, LDL-C, HDL-C, TG). If using in combination with statin therapy, obtain baseline LFTs.

Monitoring: Monitor for signs/symptoms of elevated liver enzymes, myopathy, and rhabdomyolysis. Periodically monitor LFTs during concomitant therapy with statin therapy. Perform periodic monitoring of lipid profile.

Patient Counseling: Instruct to adhere to proper diet and exercise regimen. Counsel about risk of myopathy; contact physician promptly if any unexplained muscle pain, tenderness, or weakness occurs. Periodic liver tests will be required if taking concomitant statin therapy. If used in combination with statin therapy, an effective method of birth control should be used to prevent pregnancy. Do not breastfeed if using with statin therapy. May take with/without food.

Administration: Oral route. **Storage:** 25°C (77°F); excursions permitted to 15-30°C (59-86°F). Protect from moisture.

Z

ZEVALIN

RX

ibritumomab tiuxetan (Spectrum)

> Serious infusion reactions, some fatal, may occur within 24 hrs of rituximab infusion; d/c if reaction occurs. May cause severe and prolonged cytopenias; avoid if ≥25% lymphoma marrow involvement and/or impaired bone marrow reserve. Severe cutaneous and mucocutaneous reactions, some fatal, may occur; d/c rituximab, In-111 ibritumomab, and Y-90 ibritumomab if this occurs. Do not exceed the 32mCi (1184MBq). Do not administer to patients with altered biodistribution.

THERAPEUTIC CLASS: Monoclonal antibody/CD20-blocker

INDICATIONS: Treatment of relapsed or refractory, low-grade or follicular B-cell non-Hodgkin's lymphoma (NHL) and for previously untreated follicular NHL in patients who achieve partial or complete response to first-line chemotherapy.

DOSAGE: *Adults:* Day 1: Administer rituximab 250mg/m^2 IV initially at 50mg/hr. Escalate in 50mg/hr-increments q30 mins to max of 400mg/hr in absence of infusion reactions. Give 5mCi In-111 ibritumomab IV over 10 min within 4 hrs following completion of rituximab infusion. Days 7-9: Verify that expected biodistribution is present at 48-72 hrs after In-111. Refer to PI for instructions for image acquisition and biodistribution determination. If acceptable, administer rituximab 250mg/m^2 IV initially at 100mg/hr and increase rate by 100mg/hr-increments at 30 min to max of 400mg/hr. If infusion reactions occurred on Day 1, administer only at 50mg/hr and escalate in 50mg/hr increments q30 mins to max of 400mg/hr. Give Y-90 ibritumomab 0.4mCi/kg if platelets ≥150,000/mm^3 (or 0.3mCi/kg if platelets 100,000-149,000 cells/mm^3) over 10 min IV within 4 hours. Do not administer >32mCi (1184 MBq). Premedicate with acetaminophen 650mg PO and diphenhydramine 50mg PO prior to rituximab infusion.

HOW SUPPLIED: Inj: 3.2mg/2mL

WARNINGS/PRECAUTIONS: Myelodysplastic syndrome (MDS) and/or acute myelogenous leukemia (AML) reported. May cause fetal harm. Monitor closely for extravasation; d/c infusion if experience signs or symptoms occur and restart in another limb. Minimize radiation exposure to patients during and after treatment. Contains albumin; carries remote risk for transmission of viral disease and Creutzfeldt-Jakob disease (CJD). Potential for immunogenicity.

ADVERSE REACTIONS: Infusion reactions, cytopenias (neutropenia, leukopenia, thrombocytopenia, anemia, lymphopenia), severe cutaneous and mucocutaneous reactions, fatigue, abdominal pain, nausea, nasopharyngitis, asthenia, diarrhea, cough, pyrexia, myalgia, anorexia, night sweats, influenza-like illness.

INTERACTIONS: Avoid with live vaccines. Caution with medications that interfere with platelet function or coagulation; monitor for thrombocytopenia more frequently.

PREGNANCY: Category D, not for use in nursing.

MECHANISM OF ACTION: Human monoclonal IgG1 kappa antibody/CD20 antigen blocker; binds specifically to CD20 antigen, which is expressed on pre-B and mature B lymphocytes, and on B-cell non-Hodgkin's lymphomas. The β emission from Y-90 induces cellular damage by the formation of free cell radicals in the target and neighboring cells.

PHARMACOKINETICS: Distribution: Expected to be present in breast milk. **Elimination:** Urine (7.2%); T$_{1/2}$=30 hrs.

NURSING CONSIDERATIONS

Assessment: Assess for lymphoma marrow involvement, impaired bone marrow reserve, cytopenia, hemorrhage, severe infections, biodistribution, pregnancy/nursing status and for possible drug interactions.

Monitoring: Monitor for infusion reactions within 24 hrs of rituximab infusion. Monitor for severe cutaneous and mucocutaneous reactions and extravasation during infusion. Monitor for cytopenias and complications (eg, febrile neutropenia, hemorrhage) and CBC and platelet counts following weekly regimen until levels recover or as clinically indicated.

Z

Patient Counseling: Advise to contact physician if experience signs/symptoms of infusion reactions, cytopenias (eg, bleeding, easy bruising, petechiae or purpura, pallor, weakness or fatigue), infection (eg, pyrexia), diffuse rash, bullae, or desquamation of skin or oral mucosa. Advise to take premedications as prescribed and avoid medications that interfere with platelet function. Counsel female patients of childbearing potential to avoid pregnancy/nursing and to use effective contraceptive methods during treatment and for a minimum of 12 months following therapy. Caution against immunization with live vaccines.

Administration: IV route. Refer to PI for directions for medication preparation, radiochemical purity determination and radiation dosimetry. **Storage:** 2-8°C (36-46°F). Do not freeze.

ZIAC RX
bisoprolol fumarate - hydrochlorothiazide (Duramed)

THERAPEUTIC CLASS: Selective beta$_1$-blocker/thiazide diuretic

INDICATIONS: Management of HTN.

DOSAGE: *Adults:* Initial: 2.5mg-6.25mg qd. Maint: May increase every 14 days. Max: 20mg-12.5mg/day. Replacement therapy: Substitute for titrated individual components. Renal/Hepatic Dysfunction: Caution in dosing/titrating. Cessation of therapy: Withdraw gradually over 2 weeks.

HOW SUPPLIED: Tab: (Bisoprolol-HCTZ) 2.5mg-6.25mg, 5mg-6.25mg, 10mg-6.25mg

CONTRAINDICATIONS: Cardiogenic shock, overt cardiac failure, 2nd- or 3rd-degree AV block, marked sinus bradycardia, anuria, sulfonamide hypersensitivity.

WARNINGS/PRECAUTIONS: Caution with compensated cardiac failure, diabetes mellitus (DM), bronchospastic disease, impaired hepatic function or progressive liver disease, or peripheral vascular disease (PVD). Caution with impaired renal function; d/c if progressive renal impairment becomes apparent. Avoid abrupt withdrawal; exacerbation of angina pectoris, myocardial infarction (MI), and ventricular arrhythmias observed. Abrupt withdrawl may exacerbate the symptoms of hyperthyroidism or may precipitate thyroid storm. Monitor for fluid/electrolyte imbalance; hypokalemia, hypercalcemia, hypophosphatemia reported. May activate/exacerbate systemic lupus erythematosus (SLE). Enhanced effects in post-sympathectomy patients. May mask hyperthyroidism or hypoglycemia symptoms. Sensitivity reactions may occur with or without a history of allergy or bronchial asthma. Photosensitivity reactions reported. May precipitate hyperuricemia, acute gout, cardiac failure. May impair physical/mental abilities.

ADVERSE REACTIONS: Diarrhea, headache, dizziness, fatigue.

INTERACTIONS: Alcohol, barbiturates, or narcotics may potentiate orthostatic hypotension. Antidiabetic drugs (eg, oral agents, insulin) may require dosage adjustments. Potentiates other antihypertensives. Avoid other β-blockers. Impaired absorption with cholestyramine and colestipol resins. Corticosteroids, ACTH intensify electrolyte depletion. May decrease response to pressor amines (eg, norepinephrine). May increase response to nondepolarizing skeletal muscle relaxants (eg, tubocurarine). Risk of lithium toxicity. NSAIDs may reduce effects. May block epinephrine effects. Excessive reduction of sympathetic activity with catecholamine-depleting drugs (eg, reserpine, guanethidine). Caution with clonidine withdrawal. Increased clearance with rifampin. Caution with myocardial depressants or inhibitors of AV conduction (eg, CCBs, antiarrhythmics, anesthetic agents). Digitalis glycosides and β-blockers slow atrioventricular conduction and decrease HR; concomitant use can increase the risk of bradycardia.

PREGNANCY: Category C, not for use in nursing.

MECHANISM OF ACTION: Bisoprolol: β$_1$-selective, cardioselective, adrenoreceptor-blocking agent; not established. Proposed to decrease cardiac output, inhibit renin release, and lessen tonic sympathetic nerve outflow. HCTZ:

Thiazide diuretic; not established. Affects renal tubular mechanisms of electrolyte reabsorption and increases excretion of Na⁺ and Cl⁻.

PHARMACOKINETICS: Absorption: Bisoprolol: Absolute bioavailability (80%); (2.5mg) C_{max}=9ng/mL, T_{max}=3 hrs. HCTZ: Well-absorbed; C_{max}=30ng/mL, T_{max}=2.5 hrs. **Distribution**: Bisoprolol: Plasma protein binding (30%). HCTZ: Plasma protein binding (40-68%); found in breast milk. **Elimination:** Bisoprolol: $T_{1/2}$=7-15 hrs; urine (55% unchanged). HCTZ: $T_{1/2}$=4-10 hrs; urine (60% unchanged).

NURSING CONSIDERATIONS

Assessment: Assess for bradycardia, cardiogenic shock, 2nd- or 3rd-degree heart block, overt cardiac failure, impaired renal/hepatic function, bronchospastic disease, PVD, DM, thyrotoxicosis, anuria, sulfonamide hypersensitivity, history of allergy or bronchial asthma, SLE, parathyroid disease, pregnancy/nursing status, and for possible drug interactions.

Monitoring: Monitor for cardiac failure, symptoms of arterial insuffiency, hypoglycemia, azotemia, hepatic coma, fluid or electrolyte disturbances (eg, hyponatremia, hypochloremic alkalosis, hypokalemia, hypomagnesemia), hyperuricemia or precipitation of gout, hypersensitivity reactions, photosensitivity reactions, and for exacerbation or activation of SLE. Following abrupt withdrawl, monitor for exacerbations of angina pectoris, MI, ventricular arrhythmias, exacerbation of symptoms of hyperthyroidism or precipitation of thyroid storm. Perform periodic monitoring of serum electrolytes.

Patient Counseling: Instruct not to interrupt or d/c therapy without consulting a physician. Counsel to notify physician if signs/symptoms of impending CHF or unexplained respiratory symptoms develop. Advise to exercise caution while operating machinery/driving. Advise to seek medical attention if symptoms of electrolyte imbalance (eg, dry mouth, thirst, weakness) or hypersensitivity/photosensitivity reactions occur. Inform diabetics that drug may mask symptoms of hypoglycemia.

Administration: Oral route. **Storage:** 20-25°C (68-77°F).

ZIAGEN   RX
abacavir sulfate (GlaxoSmithKline)

> Serious and sometimes fatal hypersensitivity reactions reported (multi-organ clinical syndrome); d/c as soon as suspected and never restart therapy with any abacavir containing product. Patients with HLA-B*5701 allele at high risk. Lactic acidosis and severe hepatomegaly with steatosis, including fatal cases reported.

THERAPEUTIC CLASS: Synthetic carbocyclic nucleoside analogue

INDICATIONS: Treatment of human immunodeficiency virus (HIV-1) infection in combination with other antiretroviral agents.

DOSAGE: *Adults:* 300mg bid or 600mg qd. Mild Hepatic Impairment (Child-Pugh: 5-6): Tab: 200mg bid. Oral Sol: 10mL bid.
Pediatrics: Oral Sol: ≥3 months: 8mg/kg bid. Max: 300mg bid. Tab: 14-21 kg: 150mg (1/2 tab) bid (am and pm). >21-<30 kg: 150mg (1/2 tab) in am, 300mg (1 tab) in pm. ≥30 kg: 300mg (1 tab) bid (am and pm). Mild Hepatic Impairment (Child-Pugh: 5-6): Tab: 200mg bid. Oral Sol: 10mL bid.

HOW SUPPLIED: Sol: 20mg/mL [240mL]; Tab: 300mg* *scored

CONTRAINDICATIONS: Moderate or severe hepatic impairment.

WARNINGS/PRECAUTIONS: Symptoms of hypersensitivity that may occur include lethargy, myolysis, edema, abnormal chest x-ray findings, paresthesia, lymphadenopathy, mucous membrane lesions, and rash. Screen for HLA-B*5701 allele prior to therapy. Caution in patients with known risk factors for liver disease. Suspend therapy in any patient who develops clinical or laboratory findings suggestive of lactic acidosis or pronounced hepatotoxicity. Immune reconstitution syndrome reported. Redistribution/accumulation of body fat including central obesity, dorsocervical fat enlargement, peripheral wasting, facial wasting, breast enlargement, and "cushingoid appearance" reported. Increased risk of myocardial infarction (MI) reported; caution in

Z

patients with underlying risk factors for coronary heart disease (eg, hyperlipidemia, HTN, DM, smoking). Caution in elderly.

ADVERSE REACTIONS: Hypersensitivity reaction, lactic acidosis, severe hepatomegaly, N/V, headache, malaise, fatigue, diarrhea, dream/sleep disorders, fever, chills, skin rashes, ear/nose/throat infection.

INTERACTIONS: Concomitant use with ethanol may decrease the elimination of abacavir and increase the overall exposure. Concomitant use with methadone may increase the clearance of methadone and may require an increased dose of methadone.

PREGNANCY: Category C, not for use in nursing.

MECHANISM OF ACTION: Carbocyclic nucleoside analogue; inhibits HIV-1 reverse transcriptase (RT) by competing with natural substrate dGTP and its incorporation into viral DNA.

PHARMACOKINETICS: Absorption: Rapid and extensive; Absolute bioavailability (83%). (300 mg bid) C_{max}= 3mcg/mL, AUC_{0-12h}=6.02mcg•hr/mL. (600 mg qd) C_{max} = 4.26mcg/mL, AUC=11.95mcg•hr/mL. **Distribution:** (IV) V_d=0.86L/kg; plasma protein binding (50%). **Metabolism:** Via alcohol dehydrogenase and glucuronyl transferase. **Elimination:** Urine (1.2%, abacavir), (30%, 5'-carboxylic acid metabolite), (36%, 5'glucuronide metabolite), (15% unidentified minor metabolites); feces (16%); $T_{1/2}$=1.54 hrs (single dose).

NURSING CONSIDERATIONS

Assessment: Assess for hepatic impairment, risk factors for coronary heart disease (eg, HTN, hyperlipidemia, DM, smoking), risk factors for lactic acidosis (eg, obesity), pregnancy/nursing status, and for possible drug interactions. Screen for HLA-B*5701 allele prior to initiation of therapy and prior to reinitiation of therapy.

Monitoring: Monitor for signs/symptoms of hypersensitivity (eg, fever, rash, N/V, diarrhea, generalized malaise, fatigue, dyspnea, cough), immune reconstitution syndrome, fat redistribution/accumulation, lactic acidosis, MI, and for hepatomegaly with steatosis. Monitor creatine phosphokinase (CPK), creatinine, LFTs, and triglycerides. Monitor for lymphopenia.

Patient Counseling: Inform that therapy is not cure for HIV, does not reduce risk of transmission of HIV and that opportunistic infections may develop. Inform if treatment is interrupted, do not restart or replace with any drug containing abacavir without medical consultation. Instruct to seek medical attention if experience symptoms of hypersensitivity (eg, fever, rash, N/V, diarrhea, generalized malaise, fatigue, dyspnea, cough), lactic acidosis, hepatomegaly, immune reconstitution syndrome, or fat redistribution/accumulation.

Administration: Oral route. **Storage**: 20-25°C (68-77°F). Sol: Do not freeze. May be refrigerated.

ZIANA   RX
clindamycin phosphate - tretinoin (Medicis)

THERAPEUTIC CLASS: Lincosamide derivative/retinoid

INDICATIONS: Topical treatment of acne vulgaris in patients ≥12 yrs.

DOSAGE: *Adults:* Apply at hs, a pea-sized amount onto 1 fingertip, dot onto the chin, cheeks, nose, and forehead, then gently rub over entire face. Avoid the eyes, lips and mucous membranes.
Pediatrics: ≥12 yrs: Apply at hs, a pea-sized amount onto 1 fingertip, dot onto the chin, cheeks, nose, and forehead, then gently rub over entire face. Avoid the eyes, lips and mucous membranes.

HOW SUPPLIED: Gel: (Clindamycin-Tretinoin) 1.2%-0.025% [2g, 30g, 60g]

CONTRAINDICATIONS: Regional enteritis, ulcerative colitis, or history of antibiotic-associated colitis.

WARNINGS/PRECAUTIONS: Systemic absorption of clindamycin has been demonstrated following topical use. Diarrhea, bloody diarrhea, and colitis (including pseudomembranous colitis) reported with clindamycin; d/c if

significant diarrhea occurs. Severe colitis reported following oral and parenteral administration up to several weeks following cessation of therapy. Avoid
exposure to sunlight, including sunlamps. Avoid use if sunburn is present.
Daily use of sunscreen products and protective apparel are recommended.
Weather extremes (eg, wind, cold) may be irritating while under treatment.

ADVERSE REACTIONS: Nasopharyngitis, erythema, scaling, itching, burning,
GI symptoms.

INTERACTIONS: Caution with concomitant topical medications, medicated/
abrasive soaps and cleansers, soaps/cosmetics with strong drying effect,
products with high concentrations of alcohol, astringents, spices, or lime.
Avoid with erythromycin-containing products. Caution with neuromuscular
blocking agents. Antiperistaltic agents (eg, opiates, diphenoxylate with atropine) may prolong and/or worsen severe colitis.

PREGNANCY: Category C, not for use in nursing.

MECHANISM OF ACTION: Clindamycin: Lincosamide antibiotic; binds to 50S
ribosomal subunits of susceptible bacteria and prevents elongation of peptide
chains by interfering with peptidyl transfer, thereby suppressing bacterial
protein synthesis. Found to have activity against *P. acnes*. Tretinoin: Retinoid;
has not been established. Suspected to decrease cohesiveness of follicular
epithelial cells with decreased microcomedo formation. Also, stimulates
mitotic activity and increased turnover of follicular epithelial cells, causing
extrusion of comedones.

PHARMACOKINETICS: Absorption: Tretinoin: Percutaneous (minimal).
Metabolism: Tretinoin: 13-cis-retinoic acid and 4-oxo-13-cis-retinoic acid
(metabolites).

NURSING CONSIDERATIONS

Assessment: Assess for regional enteritis, ulcerative colitis, or history of
antibiotic-associated colitis, pregnancy/nursing status, and for possible drug
interactions. Assess use in patients whose occupations require considerable
sun exposure.

Monitoring: Monitor for signs/symptoms of diarrhea, bloody diarrhea, and
colitis. Monitor for signs/symptoms of skin irritation (eg, erythema, scaling,
burning, stinging).

Patient Counseling: Instruct to wash face gently with mild soap and warm
water at hs before applying. Advise not to use more than recommended
amount and not to apply more than once daily. Instruct to apply sunscreen
every morning and reapply over the course of the day PRN. Advise to avoid
exposure to sunlight, sunlamp, UV light, and other medicines that may
increase sensitivity to sunlight. Inform that medication may cause irritation
(eg, erythema, scaling, itching, burning, stinging). Instruct to d/c therapy
and contact physician if severe diarrhea or GI discomfort occurs. Keep out ot
reach of children.

Administration: Topical route. **Storage:** 25°C (77°F); excursions permitted to
15-30°C (59-86°F). Protect from light and freezing. Keep away from heat.

ZINACEF   RX
cefuroxime (GlaxoSmithKline)

THERAPEUTIC CLASS: Cephalosporin (2nd generation)

INDICATIONS: Treatment of septicemia; meningitis; gonorrhea; lower respiratory tract, urinary tract, skin and skin structure (SSSI), and bone and joint
infections caused by susceptible strains of microorganisms. For preoperative
and perioperative surgical prophylaxis.

DOSAGE: *Adults:* Usual: 750mg-1.5g q8h for 5-10 days. Uncomplicated
Pneumonia and UTI/SSSI/Disseminated Gonococcal Infections: 750mg q8h.
Severe/Complicated Infections: 1.5g q8h. Bone and Joint Infections: 1.5g q8h.
Life-Threatening Infections/Infections With Susceptible Organisms: 1.5g q6h.
Meningitis: Max: 3g q8h. Uncomplicated Gonococcal Infection: 1.5g IM single
dose at 2 different sites with 1g PO probenecid. Surgical Prophylaxis: 1.5g IV

Z

0.5-1 hr before incision, then 750mg IM/IV q8h with prolonged procedure. Open Heart Surgery (Perioperative): 1.5g IV at induction of anesthesia and q12h thereafter, for total of 6g. Renal Impairment: CrCl 10-20mL/min: 750mg q12h. CrCl <10mL/min: 750mg q24h. Hemodialysis: Give further dose at end of dialysis.

Pediatrics: >3 months: Usual: 50-100mg/kg/day in divided doses q6-8h. Severe Infections: 100mg/kg/day (not to exceed max adult dose). Bone and Joint Infections: 150mg/kg/day in divided doses q8h (not to exceed max adult dose). Meningitis: 200-240mg/kg/day IV in divided doses q6-8h. Renal Insufficiency: Modify dosing frequency consistent with adult recommendations.

HOW SUPPLIED: Inj: 750mg, 1.5g, 7.5g, 750mg/50mL, 1.5g/50mL

WARNINGS/PRECAUTIONS: Caution with use in penicillin-sensitive patients or patients who have demonstrated some form of allergy, particularly to drugs. D/C use if an allergic reaction occurs. *Clostridium difficile*-associated diarrhea (CDAD) reported, ranging in severity from mild diarrhea to fatal colitis. Monitor renal function. Prolonged use may result in overgrowth of non-susceptible organisms; take appropriate measures if superinfection develops. Caution with history of GI disease, particularly colitis. Hearing loss reported in peds being treated for meningitis. Risk of decreased prothrombin activity with renal or hepatic impairment, poor nutritional state, or protracted course of therapy. Use in the absence of a proven or strongly suspected bacterial infection or a prophylactic indication is unlikely to provide benefit and increases the risk of the development of drug-resistant bacteria. False (+) urine glucose with copper reduction tests and false (-) with ferricyanide test.

ADVERSE REACTIONS: Thrombophlebitis, GI symptoms, decreased Hgb and Hct, eosinophilia. Transient rise in SGOT, SGPT, alkaline phosphatase, bilirubin, and LDH.

INTERACTIONS: Possible nephrotoxicity with concomitant administration of aminoglycosides. Caution with potent diuretics; may adversely affect renal function. May decrease prothrombin activity; caution with anticoagulants. May affect the gut flora, leading to lower estrogen reabsorption and reduced efficacy of combined estrogen/progesterone oral contraceptives. Concomitant oral administration of probenecid with cefuroxime may increase peak serum levels and the serum-half life.

PREGNANCY: Category B, caution in nursing.

MECHANISM OF ACTION: 2nd-generation cephalosporin; inhibits cell-wall synthesis.

PHARMACOKINETICS: Absorption: C_{max}(750mg IM, IV)=27mcg/mL, 50mcg/mL; T_{max}(750mg IM, IV)=45 min, 15 min. **Distribution:** Plasma protein binding (50%); found in breast milk. **Elimination**: Urine; $T_{1/2}$=80 min.

NURSING CONSIDERATIONS

Assessment: Assess for presence of allergies including allergy to penicillin, renal/hepatic impairment, nutritional status, history of GI disease (eg, colitis), pregnancy/nursing status, and for possible drug interactions. Document indications for therapy, culture, and susceptibility testing.

Monitoring: Monitor for signs/symptoms of an allergic reaction, CDAD, and for overgrowth of nonsusceptible organisms. In pediatric patients with meningitis, monitor for hearing loss. Monitor renal function and PT.

Patient Counseling: Inform therapy only treats bacterial, not viral, infections. Instruct to take as directed. Advise that skipping doses or not completing full course may decrease effectiveness and increase resistance. Inform that may experience diarrhea. Instruct to notify physician if watery/bloody stools, superinfections, or an allergic reaction develops.

Administration: IV/IM routes. Refer to PI for administration procedures.
Storage: (Dry State) 15-30°C (59-86°F). Protect from light. (Frozen Premixed Solution) Should not be stored above -20°C.

Z

ZINECARD RX

dexrazoxane (Pharmacia & Upjohn)

THERAPEUTIC CLASS: EDTA derivative

INDICATIONS: To reduce the incidence and severity of cardiomyopathy associated with doxorubicin in women with metastatic breast cancer who received a cumulative doxorubicin dose of 300mg/m² and who will continue doxorubicin therapy to maintain tumor control.

DOSAGE: *Adults:* IV: 10:1 ratio of dexrazoxane:doxorubicin (eg, 500mg/m² dexrazoxane:50mg/m² doxorubicin). Moderate to Severe Renal Dysfunction (CrCl <40mL/min): 5:1 ratio of dexrazoxane:doxorubicin (eg, 250mg/m² dexrazoxane:50mg/m² doxorubicin). Hepatic Impairment: Reduce dose proportionally (maintaining the 10:1 ratio). Administer via rapid IV drip infusion. Give doxorubicin within 30 min after start of infusion.

HOW SUPPLIED: Inj: 250mg, 500mg

CONTRAINDICATIONS: Chemotherapy regimens not containing an anthracycline.

WARNINGS/PRECAUTIONS: Not for use with initiation of fluorouracil, doxorubicin, and cyclophosphamide (FAC) therapy. Monitor cardiac function. Secondary malignancies (primarily acute myeloid leukemia) reported. Obtain frequent CBCs. Caution with moderate or severe renal insufficiency; reduce dose by 50% if CrCl <40mL/min. Caution in elderly.

ADVERSE REACTIONS: Alopecia, N/V, fatigue, malaise, anorexia, stomatitis, fever, infection, diarrhea, pain on injection, sepsis, neurotoxicity, streaking/erythema.

INTERACTIONS: Avoid during initiation of FAC (fluorouracil, doxorubicin, cyclophosphamide) therapy; may reduce antitumor efficacy. Additive myelosuppression with other chemotherapies.

PREGNANCY: Category C, not for use in nursing.

MECHANISM OF ACTION: EDTA derivative; not established. Suspected to interfere with iron-mediated free radical generation thought to be responsible, in part, for anthracycline induced cardiomyopathy.

PHARMACOKINETICS: Absorption: (500mg) C_{max} = 36.5µg/mL. **Distribution:** (500mg) V_d=22.4L/m². (600mg) V_d=22L/m². **Elimination:** Urine (42%). (500mg) $T_{1/2}$=2.5 hrs. (600mg) $T_{1/2}$=2.1 hrs.

NURSING CONSIDERATIONS

Assessment: Assess cardiac function (eg, left ventricular ejection fraction), renal function, hepatic function, pregnancy/nursing status, and for possible drug interactions. Obtain baseline CBC, LFTs, and renal function test (eg, creatinine, BUN). Should not be used with chemotherapy regimens that do not contain an anthracycline.

Monitoring: Monitor cardiac function, myelosuppression, secondary malignancies (eg, acute myeloid leukemia), CBC with differential and platelet count and renal/hepatic function.

Patient Counseling: Instruct to avoid nursing during therapy. Discuss signs/symptoms of adverse side effects and advise to report any if they develop.

Administration: IV route. Do not administer via IV push. Reconstitute with sterile water for injection. Further dilute with lactated ringers injection. Refer to PI for details. Discard unused solutions. Do not mix with other drugs. **Storage:** 25°C (77°F); excursions permitted to 15-30°C (59-86°F). Reconstituted solution: stable for 30 min at room temperature or 3 hrs under 2°-8°C (36° to 46°F). Infusion solution: stable for 1 hr at room temperature or 4 hrs under 2°-8°C (36° to 46°F).

Z

ZIPSOR

RX

diclofenac potassium (Xanodyne)

> NSAIDs may cause an increased risk of serious cardiovascular thrombotic events, MI, stroke, and serious GI adverse events including bleeding, ulceration, and perforation of the stomach or intestines. Contraindicated for the treatment of perioperative pain in the setting of coronary artery bypass graft (CABG) surgery.

THERAPEUTIC CLASS: NSAID

INDICATIONS: Relief of mild to moderate acute pain in adults ≥18 yrs.

DOSAGE: *Adults:* ≥18 yrs: 25mg qid. Elderly: Start at low end of dosing range.

HOW SUPPLIED: Cap: 25mg

CONTRAINDICATIONS: Asthma, urticaria, or allergic reactions after taking aspirin (ASA) or other NSAIDs. Hypersensitivity to bovine protein. Treatment of perioperative pain in the setting of CABG surgery.

WARNINGS/PRECAUTIONS: May lead to onset of new HTN or worsening of pre-existing HTN; monitor BP closely. Fluid retention and edema reported; caution with fluid retention or heart failure. Caution in patients with considerable dehydration. Renal papillary necrosis and other renal injury reported after long-term use. Not recommended for use with advanced renal disease. If therapy must be initiated, monitor renal function. Anaphylactoid reactions may occur. Contraindicated in ASA-triad patients. May cause serious skin adverse events (eg, exfoliative dermatitis, Stevens-Johnson syndrome, and toxic epidermal necrolysis). Avoid in late pregnancy; may cause premature closure of ductus arteriosus. May cause elevations of LFTs; d/c if liver disease develops or systemic manifestations occur. Caution in elderly and debilitated. Anemia may occur; with long-term use, monitor Hgb/Hct if signs or symptoms of anemia develop. May inhibit platelet aggregation and prolong bleeding time; monitor with coagulation disorders. Caution with asthma and avoid with ASA-sensitive asthma. May mask symptoms of infection (eg, fever, inflammation). Caution in patients with history of ulcer disease or GI bleeding, or with risk factors (eg, concomitant oral corticosteroids or anticoagulants, smoking, alcohol). Not a substitute for corticosteroids or to treat corticosteroid insufficiency.

ADVERSE REACTIONS: Abdominal pain, constipation, diarrhea, dyspepsia, N/V, dizziness, headache, somnolence, pruritus, increased sweating.

INTERACTIONS: Avoid use with other diclofenac products. Increased adverse effects with ASA. May impair therapeutic response to ACE inhibitors, thiazides or loop diuretics; monitor for renal failure. Avoid acetaminophen unless prescribed. Synergistic effects on GI bleeding with warfarin. May increase lithium levels; monitor for toxicity. May enhance methotrexate toxicity; caution when coadministering. May increase nephrotoxicity of cyclosporine; caution when coadministering. Caution with coadministration of other drugs that are substrates or inhibitors of CYP2C9.

PREGNANCY: Category C <30 weeks gestation, Category D after 30 weeks. Not for use in nursing.

MECHANISM OF ACTION: NSAID (benzeneacetic acid derivative); suspected to inhibit prostaglandin synthetase, exerts anti-inflammatory, analgesic, and antipyretic actions.

PHARMACOKINETICS: Absorption: Mean absolute bioavailability (50%), C_{max}=1087ng/mL, AUC=597ng•h/mL, T_{max}=0.5 hr. **Distribution:** V_d=1.3L/kg; serum protein binding (>99%). **Metabolism:** Metabolites: 4'-hydroxy-, 5-hydroxy-, 3'-hydroxy-, 4',5-dihydroxy- and 3'-hydroxy-4'-methoxy diclofenac. **Elimination:** Urine (65%), bile (35%); $T_{1/2}$= approximately 1 hr.

NURSING CONSIDERATIONS

Assessment: Assess LFTs, renal function, CBC and coagulation profile. Assess for history of CABG surgery, asthma and allergic reactions to ASA or other NSAIDS, active ulceration, bleeding or chronic inflammation of GI tract, cardiovascular disease (CVD), pregnancy/nursing status, and possible drug interactions. Note other diseases/conditions and drug therapies.

Monitoring: Monitor for hypersensitivity reactions, cardiac complications, stroke, GI bleeding, asthma, skin side effects. Monitor BP, LFTs, renal function, CBC with differential and platelet count, coagulation profile (especially if on anticoagulation therapy), hyperglycemia.

Patient Counseling: Counsel about potential CV, GI, hepatotoxic and dermatological events, as well as possible weight gain/edema. Take as prescribed. Caution women against using late in pregnancy.

Administration: Oral route. **Storage:** 25°C (77°F); excursions permitted to 15-30°C (59-86°F). Protect from moisture. Dispense in tight container.

ZIRGAN   RX
ganciclovir (Bausch & Lomb)

THERAPEUTIC CLASS: Synthetic guanine derivative

INDICATIONS: Treatment of acute herpetic keratitis (dendritic ulcers).

DOSAGE: *Adults:* 1 drop in affected eye 5X per day (q3h while awake) until corneal ulcer heals, then 1 drop tid for 7 days.
Pediatrics: ≥2 yrs: 1 drop in affected eye 5X per day (q3h while awake) until corneal ulcer heals, then 1 drop tid for 7 days.

HOW SUPPLIED: Gel: 0.15% [5g]

WARNINGS/PRECAUTIONS: For topical ophthalmic use only. Avoid wearing contact lenses during the course of treatment or if signs and symptoms of herpetic keratitis are present.

ADVERSE REACTIONS: Blurred vision, eye irritation, punctate keratitis, conjunctival hyperemia.

PREGNANCY: Category C, caution in nursing.

MECHANISM OF ACTION: Guanosine derivative; competitive inhibition of viral DNA-polymerase and direct incorporation into viral primer strand DNA, resulting in DNA chain termination and prevention of replication.

NURSING CONSIDERATIONS

Assessment: Assess for signs and symptoms of herpetic keratitis, and pregnancy/nursing status.

Monitoring: Monitor for eye pain, redness, itching or inflammation, and possible adverse reactions.

Patient Counseling: Counsel regarding proper use; for topical use only. Advise that dropper tip should not touch any surface, as this may contaminate gel. Advise to consult physician if pain develops, or if redness, itching, or inflammation becomes aggravated. Instruct not to wear contact lenses during treatment.

Administration: Ocular route. **Storage:** 15-25°C (59-77°F). Do not freeze.

ZITHROMAX   RX
azithromycin (Pfizer)

THERAPEUTIC CLASS: Macrolide

INDICATIONS: Treatment of the following infections caused by susceptible microorganisms: (PO) Acute bacterial exacerbations of chronic obstructive pulmonary disease (COPD), acute bacterial sinusitis (ABS), community-acquired pneumonia (CAP), pharyngitis/tonsillitis, uncomplicated skin and skin structure infections (SSSIs), urethritis/cervicitis, genital ulcer disease (men), acute otitis media. Prevention of disseminated *Mycobacterium avium* complex (MAC) disease, alone or in combination with rifabutin, in persons with advanced HIV infection. Treatment of disseminated MAC disease in combination

Z

with ethambutol in persons with advanced HIV infection. (IV) CAP and pelvic inflammatory disease (PID).

DOSAGE: *Adults:* IV: CAP: 500mg IV qd for ≥2 days, then 500mg PO (two 250mg tab) qd to complete 7-10-day course. PID: 500mg IV qd for 1-2 days, then 250mg PO qd to complete 7-day course. PO: CAP (mild severity)/ Pharyngitis/Tonsillitis (2nd-line therapy)/SSSI (uncomplicated): 500mg single dose on Day 1, then 250mg qd on Days 2-5. Acute Bacterial Exacerbation of COPD (mild-moderate): 500mg qd for 3 days or 500mg single dose on Day 1, then 250mg qd on Days 2-5. ABS: 500mg qd for 3 days. Genital Ulcer Disease (Chancroid)/Nongonococcal Urethritis/Cervicitis: 1g single dose. Gonococcal Urethritis/Cervicitis: 2g single dose. Prevention of Disseminated MAC Infections: 1200mg once weekly. May be combined with rifabutin. Treatment of Disseminated MAC Infections: 600mg qd in combination with ethambutol at 15mg/kg/day.

Pediatrics: IV: ≥16 yrs: CAP: 500mg IV qd for ≥2 days, then 500mg PO (two 250mg tab) qd to complete 7-10-day course. PID: 500mg IV qd for 1-2 days, then 250mg PO qd to complete 7-day course. Sus: ≥2 yrs: Pharyngitis/ Tonsillitis: 12mg/kg qd for 5 days. ≥6 months: Acute Otitis Media: 30mg/kg single dose, or 10mg/kg qd for 3 days, or 10mg/kg single dose on Day 1, then 5mg/kg/day on Days 2-5. CAP: 10 mg/kg single dose on Day 1, then 5mg/kg on Days 2-5. ABS: 10mg/kg qd for 3 days.

HOW SUPPLIED: Inj: 500mg; Sus: 100mg/5mL [15mL], 200mg/5mL [15mL, 22.5mL, 30mL], 1g; Tab: 250mg, 500mg, 600mg

CONTRAINDICATIONS: History of cholestatic jaundice/hepatic dysfunction with prior use of azithromycin.

WARNINGS/PRECAUTIONS: Serious allergic reactions (eg, angioedema, anaphylaxis) and dermatologic reactions (eg, Stevens-Johnson syndrome [SJS] and toxic epidermal necrolysis [TEN]) rarely reported. D/C if allergic reaction occurs and institute appropriate therapy; reappearance of allergic symptoms may occur with d/c of symptomatic therapy. Abnormal liver function, hepatitis, cholestatic jaundice, hepatic necrosis, and hepatic failure reported; d/c immediately if signs/symptoms of hepatitis occur. *Clostridium difficile*-associated diarrhea (CDAD) reported. D/C if CDAD is suspected or confirmed; institute appropriate therapy as clinically indicated. Caution with hepatic impairment and in GFR <10mL/min. May increase risk of developing cardiac arrhythmia and torsades de pointes; caution in patients at increased risk for prolonged cardiac repolarization. Myasthenia gravis exacerbation and new onset of myasthenic syndrome reported. Increased risk of development of drug-resistant bacteria in absence of proven or strongly suspected bacterial infection or prophylactic indication. (PO) Should not be relied on to treat syphilis. Avoid in patients with pneumonia who are inappropriate for PO therapy because of moderate to severe illness or risk factors such as cystic fibrosis, nosocomially acquired infections, known/suspected bacteremia, patients requiring hospitalization, elderly or debilitated patients, or significant underlying health problems that may compromise ability to respond to illness (eg, immunodeficiency or functional asplenia). Do not use single-dose packet to administer doses other than 1000mg; not for pediatrics. (IV) Local inj-site reactions reported.

ADVERSE REACTIONS: Diarrhea/loose stools, N/V, abdominal pain. (IV) Pain at site, local inflammation.

INTERACTIONS: Monitor terfenadine, cyclosporine, hexobarbital, phenytoin levels. May increase digoxin levels. May potentiate effects of oral anticoagulants; monitor for prothrombin time. Increased serum concentrations with nelfinavir. May produce modest effect on pharmacokinetics of atorvastatin, carbamazepine, cetirizine, didanosine, efavirenz, fluconazole, indinavir, midazolam, rifabutin, sildenafil, theophylline (PO and IV), triazolam, trimethoprim/ sulfamethoxazole, and zidovudine. Efavirenz or fluconazole may have a modest effect on pharmacokinetics of azithromycin. Aluminum- and magnesium-containing antacids may reduce PO levels. Acute ergot toxicity may occur with ergotamine or dihydroergotamine. (IV) Increased side effects reported (N/V, abdominal pain, etc) with metronidazole.

PREGNANCY: Category B, caution in nursing.

MECHANISM OF ACTION: Macrolide; inhibits protein synthesis by binding to the 50S ribosomal subunits of susceptible organisms, thus interfering with microbial protein synthesis.

PHARMACOKINETICS: Absorption: Administration of variable doses resulted in different parameters. **Distribution:** (PO) V_d=31.1L/kg. **Elimination:** Biliary (major), urine; $T_{1/2}$=68 hrs.

NURSING CONSIDERATIONS

Assessment: Assess for history of cholestatic jaundice, liver/renal dysfunction, myasthenia gravis, pregnancy/nursing status, and possible drug interactions. Assess use in patients at risk for prolonged cardiac repolarization. In patients with sexually transmitted urethritis or cervicitis, perform serologic test for syphilis and perform appropriate cultures for gonorrhea at the time of diagnosis. In all patients, perform appropriate culture and susceptibility tests prior to treatment. (PO) Assess for pneumonia, cystic fibrosis, nosocomial infections, known or suspected bacteremia, patients requiring hospitalization, age, debilitated condition, and underlying health problems.

Monitoring: Monitor for signs/symptoms of allergic reactions, CDAD, arrhythmias, torsades de pointes, hepatic dysfunction, hepatitis, cholestatic jaundice, hepatic necrosis, hepatic failure, and for new onset of myasthenic syndrome or exacerbation of myasthenia gravis. Monitor PT with oral anticoagulants. (IV) Monitor for inj-site reactions.

Patient Counseling: Inform patient to d/c immediately and contact physician if allergic reaction occurs. Inform that therapy treats bacterial, not viral, infections. Instruct to take as directed; skipping doses or not completing full course may decrease effectiveness and increase resistance. May experience diarrhea; notify physician if watery and bloody stools occur. (PO) Advise patient to not take aluminum- or magnesium-containing antacids simultaneously.

Administration: Oral/IV routes. (IV) Refer to PI for reconstitution and dilution instructions. Infusate concentration and rate of infusion should either be 1mg/mL over 3 hrs or 2mg/mL over 1 hr. Do not give as a bolus or as an IM injection. Do not give with other IV substances, additives, or medications or infuse simultaneously through the same IV line. (Sus) Shake well before use. (Single-dose packet) Mix entire content of packet with 2 oz. of water. Drink completely. **Storage:** (Tab) 15-30°C (59-86°F); (600mg tab) ≤30°C (86°F). (Sus) Dry Powder: <30°C (86°F); Constituted: 5-30°C (41-86°F); use within 10 days. (Single-dose packet) 5-30°C (41-86°F). Reconstituted Inj: ≤30°C (86°F) for 24 hrs or <5°C (41°F) for 7 days.

ZMAX   RX
azithromycin (Pfizer)

THERAPEUTIC CLASS: Macrolide

INDICATIONS: Treatment of mild to moderate community-acquired pneumonia (CAP) in adults and children ≥6 months and acute bacterial sinusitis in adults caused by susceptible bacteria.

DOSAGE: *Adults:* 2g single dose. Take on empty stomach (at least 1 hr before or 2 hrs after a meal).
Pediatrics: ≥6 months: 60mg/kg single dose. Take on empty stomach (at least 1 hr before or 2 hrs after a meal). Patients weighing >34kg should receive adult dose (2g). See PI for specific pediatric dosage guidelines.

HOW SUPPLIED: Sus, Extended-Release: 2g (27mg/mL)

CONTRAINDICATIONS: Hypersensitivity to macrolide or ketolide antibiotics.

WARNINGS/PRECAUTIONS: Rare reports of serious allergic reactions including angioedema, anaphylaxis, Stevens-Johnson syndrome (SJS), and toxic epidermal necrolysis. Institute appropriate therapy if allergic reaction occurs. Allergic symptoms may recur after initial successful symptomatic treatment. *Clostridium difficile*-associated diarrhea (CDAD) reported; d/c if CDAD is suspected or confirmed. Caution with severe renal dysfunction. Exacerbation

Z

of symptoms of myasthenia gravis and new onset of myasthenia syndrome reported. GI disturbances, prolonged cardiac repolarization and QT interval reported. Increased risk of developing drug-resistant bacteria when taken in the absence of a proven or strongly suspected bacterial infection.

ADVERSE REACTIONS: Diarrhea/loose stools, N/V, abdominal pain, headache, rash.

INTERACTIONS: May potentiate the effect of oral anticoagulants such as warfarin; monitor PT. Increased AUC and C_{max} with nelfinavir. Monitor carefully when used with drugs such as digoxin, ergotamine or dihydroergotamine, cyclosporine, hexobarbital and phenytoin.

PREGNANCY: Category B, caution in nursing.

MECHANISM OF ACTION: Macrolide antibiotic; inhibits microbial protein synthesis by binding to the 50S ribosomal subunits of susceptible organisms.

PHARMACOKINETICS: Absorption: Oral administration of variable doses resulted in different parameters. **Distribution:** V_d=31.1L/kg; plasma protein binding (7-51%). **Elimination:** Bile (major route), urine (6%, unchanged); $T_{1/2}$=59 hrs.

NURSING CONSIDERATIONS

Assessment: Assess for hypersensitivity to erythromycin, any macrolide or ketolide antibiotic. Assess for pregnancy/nursing status, renal/hepatic function, LFTs, prolonged QT interval, and possible drug interactions. Document indications for therapy, culture and susceptibility testing.

Monitoring: Monitor for signs/symptoms of hypersensitivity reactions (eg, angioedema, SJS), CDAD, diarrhea/loose stools, QT prolongation, cardiac repolarization, neutropenia, arrhythmia, jaundice, LFTs, hearing loss, seizures, and myasthenia gravis.

Patient Counseling: Inform to take on empty stomach. Immediately report any signs of allergic reaction. Contact physician if vomiting occurs within 1st hr. Keep bottle tightly closed, use within 12 hrs of reconstitution, shake well before use, and consume entire contents of bottle. Therapy treats bacterial, not viral, infections. Take as directed; skipping doses or not completing full course may decrease effectiveness and increase resistance. May experience diarrhea; notify physician if watery/bloody stools, superinfection, or hypersensitivity reactions occur.

Administration: Oral route. Reconstitute with 60mL water. Shake well. **Storage:** Store dry powder at or below 30°C (86°F). Reconstituted sus should be consumed within 12 hrs and stored at 25°C (77°F); excursions permitted to 15-30°C (59-86°F). Do not refrigerate or freeze.

ZOCOR   RX
simvastatin (Merck)

THERAPEUTIC CLASS: HMG-CoA reductase inhibitor

INDICATIONS: Adjunct to diet in patients with, or at high-risk for coronary heart disease (CHD), in patients with existing diabetes, peripheral vessel disease, history of stroke or other cerebrovascular disease, to reduce risk of total mortality by reducing CHD deaths, risk of non-fatal MI and stroke, need for revascularization procedures. To reduce elevated total cholesterol (total-C), LDL-C, apolipoprotein B (Apo B), triglycerides (TG), and increase HDL-C in primary hyperlipidemia (Fredrickson Type IIa, heterozygous familial and nonfamilial) or mixed dyslipidemia (Fredrickson Type IIb): To reduce elevated TG in hypertriglyceridemia (Fredrickson Type IV hyperlipidemia). To reduce elevated TG and VLDL-C in primary dysbetalipoproteinemia (Fredrickson Type III hyperlipidemia). To reduce total-C, LDL-C in homozygous familial hypercholesterolemia as an adjunct to other lipid-lowering agents or if such treatments are unavailable. Adjunct to diet to reduce total-C, LDL-C, Apo B levels in adolescents who are at least 1 yr postmenarche, 10-17 yrs of age, with heterozygous familial hypercholesterolemia (HeFH) if after an adequate trial of diet therapy the following findings are present: LDL remains ≥190mg/dL;

or LDL remains ≥160mg/dL and there is positive family history of premature cardiovascular disease (CVD) or 2 or more other CVD risk factors are present.

DOSAGE: *Adults:* Initial: 20-40mg qpm. Usual: 5-80mg qd. High Risk for CHD Events: Initial: 40mg qd. Perform lipid determinations after 4 weeks and periodically thereafter. Homozygous Familial Hypercholesterolemia: 40mg qpm or 80mg qd given as 20mg bid plus 40mg qpm. Chinese Patients taking Lipid-Modifying Doses (≥1g/day niacin) of Niacin-containing Products: Avoid 80mg. Concomitant Cyclosporine/Danazol: Initial: 5mg qd. Max: 10mg qd. Concomitant Gemfibrozil: Max: 10mg qd. Concomitant Amiodarone/Verapamil: Max: 20mg qd. Concomitant Diltiazem: Max: 40mg qd. Severe Renal Impairment: Initial: 5mg qd; monitor closely.
Pediatrics: HeFH: 10-17 yrs (at least 1 yr postmenarchal): Initial: 10mg qpm. Usual: 10-40mg qd. Doses should be individualize according to goal of therapy. Adjust at ≥4-week intervals. Max: 40mg qd. Severe Renal Impairment: Initial: 5mg qd; monitor closely. Chinese Patients taking Lipid-Modifying Doses (≥1g/day niacin) of Niacin-containing Products: Avoid 80mg. Concomitant Gemfibrozil: Max: 10mg qd. Concomitant Cyclosporine/Danazol: Initial: 5mg qd. Max: 10mg qd. Concomitant Amiodarone/Verapamil: Max: 20mg qd. Concomitant Diltiazem: Max: 40mg qd.

HOW SUPPLIED: Tab: 5mg, 10mg, 20mg, 40mg, 80mg

CONTRAINDICATIONS: Active liver disease, which may include unexplained persistent elevations of hepatic transaminases, pregnancy, and nursing mothers.

WARNINGS/PRECAUTIONS: May cause myopathy/rhabdomyolysis (dose-related). Predisposing risk factors for myopathy include advanced age (≥65 yrs), uncontrolled hypothyroidism and renal impairment. D/C therapy if myopathy is suspected or diagnosed. D/C a few days before elective major surgery and when any major acute medical or surgical condition supervenes. Persistent increases in serum transaminases reported; monitor LFTs before and during treatment when clinically indicated. With 80mg dose, monitor LFTs prior to titration, 3 months after titration, and periodically thereafter for the 1st yr. D/C if increases in ALT/AST persist. Caution with heavy alcohol use, severe renal insufficiency or history of hepatic disease. Caution in elderly.

ADVERSE REACTIONS: Abdominal pain, headache, myalgia, constipation, nausea, atrial fibrillation, gastritis, DM, insomnia, vertigo, bronchitis, eczema, upper respiratory tract and urinary tract infections.

INTERACTIONS: Avoid concomitant use with itraconazole, ketoconazole, other azole antifungals, erythromycin, clarithromycin, telithromycin, HIV protease inhibitors, nefazodone, grapefruit juice (>1 quart/day); increased risk of myopathy/rhabdomyolysis. Coadministration with gemfibrozil, cyclosporine, danazol, amiodarone, verapamil, or diltiazem may increase the risk of myopathy/rhabdomyolysis. Caution with other fibrates, ≥1g/day of niacin. May elevate digoxin levels; monitor patients taking digoxin. Concomitant use with coumarin anticoagulants prolongs INR; monitor INR prior to and during therapy.

PREGNANCY: Category X, not for use in nursing.

MECHANISM OF ACTION: HMG-CoA reductase inhibitor; specific inhibitor of 3-hydroxy-3-methylglutaryl-coenzyme A (HMG-CoA) reductase, the enzyme that catalyzes the conversion of HMG-CoA to mevalonate, an early and rate limiting step in the biosynthetic pathway for cholesterol. Reduces VLDL and TG and increases HDL-C.

PHARMACOKINETICS: Absorption: T_{max}=1.3-2.4 hrs. **Distribution:** Plasma protein binding (95%). **Metabolism:** Liver (1st pass); β-hydroxyacid, 6'-hydroxy. 6'-hydroxymethyl, 6'-exomethylene (active metabolites). **Elimination:** Feces (60%), urine (13%).

NURSING CONSIDERATIONS

Assessment: Assess for active liver disease or unexplained elevations in serum transaminases, risk factors for developing myopathy (eg, advanced age, uncontrolled hypothyroidism, renal impairment) severe renal impairment, pregnancy/nursing status and possible drug interactions. Assess use in patients who consume substantial quantities of alcohol and/or have a past

Z

history of liver disease. Obtain baseline lipid profile (total-C, HDL-C, TG) and LFTs.

Monitoring: Monitor for signs/symptoms of myopathy (eg, muscle pain, tenderness, weakness), rhabdomyolysis, liver dysfunction. Periodically monitor lipid levels (LDL-C), creatine kinase levels (CK). Monitor liver enzymes before and during treatment. Patients titrated to 80mg dose should have LFTs evaluated prior to titration, 3 months after titration, and periodically thereafter for the first year.

Patient Counseling: Recommend standard cholesterol-lowering diet while taking drug. Advise to adhere to their National Cholesterol Education Program (NCEP) recommended diet, regular exercise program, and periodic testing of a fasting lipid panel. Contact physician immediately if unexplained muscle pain, tenderness, or weakness occurs. Advise about possible drug interactions and interaction with grapefruit juice. Notify all physicians of all concurrently taken medications. Use effective contraceptives in women of childbearing potential. Stop taking medication if pregnant or planning to become pregnant. Counsel about risks during pregnancy/nursing.

Administration: Oral route. **Storage:** 5-30°C (41-86°F). Dispense in a tightly closed container.

ZOFRAN   RX
ondansetron HCl - ondansetron (GlaxoSmithKline)

OTHER BRAND NAMES: Zofran ODT (GlaxoSmithKline)

THERAPEUTIC CLASS: 5-HT$_3$ receptor antagonist

INDICATIONS: (Inj) Prevention of nausea and vomiting (N/V) associated with initial and repeat courses of emetogenic cancer chemotherapy, including high-dose cisplatin. Prevention of postoperative nausea and/or vomiting (PONV). (Sol/Tab) Prevention of N/V associated with: highly emetogenic cancer chemotherapy, including cisplatin ≥50mg/m²; initial and repeat courses of moderately emetogenic cancer chemotherapy; and radiotherapy in patients receiving either total body irradiation, single high-dose fraction to the abdomen, or daily fractions to the abdomen.

DOSAGE: *Adults:* Prevention of Chemotherapy-Induced N/V: (Inj) 32mg single IV dose or three 0.15mg/kg IV doses; give 1st dose (over 15 min) 30 min before chemotherapy. For the three-dose regimen, give subsequent two doses 4 and 8 hrs after 1st dose. Prevention of N/V Associated with Highly Emetogenic Chemotherapy: (Tab) 24mg (given as three 8mg tabs) 30 min before chemotherapy. Prevention of N/V Associated with Moderately Emetogenic Chemotherapy: (Sol/Tab) 8mg bid; give 1st dose 30 min before chemotherapy, then 8 hrs later, then q12h for 1-2 days after completion of chemotherapy. Prevention of PONV: (Inj) 4mg IM/IV undiluted immediately before induction of anesthesia or post-op if N/V occurs. As IV, infuse over 2-5 min. (Sol/Tab) 16mg 1 hr before induction of anesthesia. Prevention of N/V Associated with Radiation Therapy: (Sol/Tab) Usual: 8mg tid. Total Body Irradiation: 8mg 1-2 hrs before each fraction of radiotherapy administered each day. Single High-Dose Therapy Fraction Radiotherapy to Abdomen: 8mg 1-2 hrs before therapy then q8h after 1st dose for 1-2 days after completion of therapy. Daily Fractionated Radiotherapy Therapy to Abdomen: 8mg 1-2 hrs before therapy then q8h after 1st dose for each day radiotherapy is given. Severe Hepatic Dysfunction (Child-Pugh ≥10): Max: 8mg/day. (Inj) IV single dose over 15 min; give 30 min before chemotherapy.
Pediatrics: Prevention of Chemotherapy-Induced N/V: (Inj) 6 months-18 yrs: Three 0.15mg/kg doses; infuse over 15 min. Give 1st dose 30 min before chemotherapy, then 4 and 8 hrs after the 1st dose. (Sol/Tab) Prevention of N/V Associated with Moderately Emetogenic Cancer Chemotherapy: ≥12 yrs: 8mg bid; give 1st dose 30 min before chemotherapy, then 8 hrs later, then bid for 1-2 days after completion of chemotherapy. 4-11 yrs: 4mg tid; give 1st dose 30 min before chemotherapy, then 4 and 8 hrs after 1st dose, then q8h for 1-2 days after completion of chemotherapy. Prevention of PONV: (Inj) 1 month-12 yrs: ≤40kg: 0.1mg/kg IV single dose. >40kg: 4mg IV single dose.

Infuse over 2-5 min immediately before or after induction of anesthesia or post-op if N/V occurs. Severe Hepatic Dysfunction (Child Pugh ≥10): Max: 8mg/day. (Inj) IV single dose over 15 min; give 30 min before chemotherapy.

HOW SUPPLIED: Inj: 2mg/mL [2, 20mL]; Sol: 4mg/5mL [50mL]; Tab: 4mg, 8mg; Tab, Disintegrating: (ODT) 4mg, 8mg

CONTRAINDICATIONS: Concomitant use of apomorphine; profound hypotension and loss of consciousness reported.

WARNINGS/PRECAUTIONS: Hypersensitivity reactions reported in those hypersensitive to other 5-HT$_3$ receptor antagonists. Does not stimulate gastric or intestinal peristalsis; do not use instead of nasogastric suction. May mask progressive ileus or gastric distension. Rarely and predominantly with IV administration, transient ECG changes including QT interval prolongation reported. Orally disintegrating tabs contain phenylalanine; caution in phenylketonurics.

ADVERSE REACTIONS: Headache, diarrhea, dizziness, constipation, wound problem, drowsiness/sedation, pyrexia, shivering, anxiety/agitation, LFT abnormalities, urinary retention.

INTERACTIONS: See Contraindications. Inducers or inhibitors of CYP3A4, CYP2D6, CYP1A2 may change the clearance and half-life of ondansetron. Concomitant use with tramadol may be associated with an increase in patient-controlled administration of tramadol. Potent inducers of CYP3A4 (ie, phenytoin, carbamazepine and rifampicin) significantly increased the clearance of ondansetron.

PREGNANCY: Category B, caution in nursing.

MECHANISM OF ACTION: Selective 5-HT$_3$ receptor blocker; not established. Blocks 5-HT$_3$ receptors from serotonin, which may stimulate vagal afferents through the 5-HT$_3$ receptors and initiate the vomiting reflex.

PHARMACOKINETICS: Absorption: Various age groups resulted in different parameters. PO: Well-absorbed from GI tract; bioavailability (56%) **Distribution:** Plasma protein binding (70-76%). **Metabolism:** Hydroxylation (primary), glucuronide/sulfate conjugation. **Elimination:** Urine (5%).

NURSING CONSIDERATIONS

Assessment: Assess for hepatic impairment, pregnancy/nursing status, hypersensitivity, and for possible drug interactions. If planning to use ODT, assess for phenylketonuria.

Monitoring: Monitor signs/symptoms of ECG changes, hypersensitivity reactions, and LFT abnormalities. In patients who recently underwent abdominal surgery or in patients with chemotherapy-induced N/V, monitor for masking of signs of a progressive ileus and/or gastric distension.

Patient Counseling: Do not remove disintegrating tab from blister until just prior to dosing; do not push through foil. Use dry hands to peel blister backing completely off blister. Remove gently and immediately place on tongue to dissolve and swallow; taking with liquid not necessary. Inform that disintegrating tab contains phenylalanine. Advise to seek medical attention if symptoms of hypersensitivity reactions, progressive ileus, or gastric distention occur.

Administration: IM/IV/Oral routes. Inj: Refer to PI for reconstitution procedures. **Storage:** Inj/Tab: 2-30°C (36-86°F). Protect from light. Sol: 15-30°C (59-86°F). Protect from light; store upright.

ZOLADEX 1-MONTH

RX

goserelin acetate (AstraZeneca)

THERAPEUTIC CLASS: Synthetic gonadotropin releasing hormone analog

INDICATIONS: Palliative treatment of advanced prostatic carcinoma and advanced breast cancer in pre- and perimenopausal women. In combination with flutamide for management of locally confined Stage T2b-T4 (Stage B2-C) prostatic carcinoma. Management of endometriosis, including pain relief and reduction of endometriotic lesions. Use as an endometrial-thinning agent prior to endometrial ablation for dysfunctional uterine bleeding.

Z

DOSAGE: *Adults:* Inject SQ every 28 days into anterior abdominal wall below navel line. Advanced Prostatic Carcinoma/Breast Cancer: 3.6mg every 28 days. Stage B2-C Prostatic Carcinoma: 3.6mg starting 8 weeks before radio-therapy, then 10.8mg formulation 28 days after 1st injection, or 3.6mg at 28-day intervals for 4 doses (2 before and 2 during radiotherapy). Endometriosis: 3.6mg every 28 days for 6 months. Endometrial Thinning: 3.6mg then surgery 4 weeks later, or 2 doses of 3.6mg (given 4 weeks apart) followed by surgery 2-4 weeks after 2nd dose.

HOW SUPPLIED: Implant: 3.6mg

CONTRAINDICATIONS: Pregnancy (unless used for palliative treatment of advanced breast cancer).

WARNINGS/PRECAUTIONS: Premenopausal women should use nonhormonal contraception during therapy and for 12 weeks post-therapy. Transient wors-ening of symptoms or occurrence of additional signs/symptoms of prostate/breast cancer may occur during initial therapy. Temporary increase in bone pain may occur. Ureteral obstruction and spinal cord compression reported with prostate cancer. Hyperglycemia, increased risk of developing diabetes/myocardial infarction (MI), sudden cardiac death, and stroke reported in men. Hypercalcemia reported in prostate/breast cancer patients with bone metas-tases; initiate appropriate treatment measures if it occurs. Hypersensitivity, antibody formation, and acute anaphylactic reactions may occur. Caution when dilating the cervix for endometrial ablation; may increase cervical resis-tance. Retreatment cannot be recommended for management of endometrio-sis; consider monitoring bone mineral density (BMD) if further treatment is contemplated. May suppress pituitary-gonadal system in therapeutic doses; normal function is usually restored 12 weeks after d/c treatment.

ADVERSE REACTIONS: Hot flushes, sexual dysfunction, decreased erections, seborrhea, peripheral edema, breast enlargement/atrophy, pain, vaginitis, emotional lability, decreased libido, sweating, depression, headache, acne.

INTERACTIONS: Ovarian hyperstimulation syndrome reported with other gonadotropins.

PREGNANCY: Category X (endometriosis and endometrial thinning), Category D (advanced breast cancer), not for use in nursing.

MECHANISM OF ACTION: Synthetic decapeptide analog of GnRH; acts as an inhibitor of pituitary gonadotropin secretion. In males, causes initial increase in serum LH and FSH levels, causing subsequent increases in serum testos-terone levels; chronic administration suppresses pituitary gonadotropins, causing fall in testosterone levels to post-castration levels. In females, chronic exposure causes decrease in serum estradiol to levels consistent with post-menopausal state, leading to reduction of ovarian size and function, reduction in size of uterus and mammary gland, and regression of sex hormone-respon-sive tumors.

PHARMACOKINETICS: Absorption: (Males) C_{max}=2.84ng/mL, T_{max}=12-15 days, AUC=27.8ng•day/mL; (Females) C_{max}=1.46ng/mL, T_{max}=8-22 days, AUC=18.5ng•day/mL. **Distribution:** V_d=44.1L (Males), 20.3L (Females); plasma protein binding (27.3%). **Metabolism:** Hydrolysis of C-terminal amino acids. **Elimination:** Urine (>90%, 20% unchanged); $T_{1/2}$=4.2 hrs (Sol).

NURSING CONSIDERATIONS

Assessment: Assess for hypersensitivity, cardiovascular disease (CVD), dia-betes mellitus (DM), bone metastases, ureteral obstruction, spinal cord com-pression, pregnancy/nursing status, and possible drug interactions. Obtain baseline vital signs and weight, serum testosterone/cholesterol/blood glucose levels, PSA, LFTs.

Monitoring: Monitor for tumor flare, ureteral obstruction, spinal cord com-pression, renal impairment, hypersensitivity reactions, pituitary apoplexy, sexual dysfunction, occurrence/worsening of signs/symptoms of prostate/breast cancer, bone pain, signs/symptoms suggestive of development of CVD, and hypercalcemia. Monitor BMD, serum testosterone/cholesterol/blood glucose levels, glycosylated Hgb (HbA$_{1c}$), PSA, LFTs.

Patient Counseling: Inform men that risk of developing ureteral obstruction, spinal cord compression, reduction in BMD, DM or loss of glycemic control with DM, MI, sudden cardiac death, and stroke may occur. Inform women that menstruation should stop with effective doses. Counsel women about potential side effects (regular menstrual bleeding, allergic reactions, hypoestrogenism, reduction in BMD, and amenorrhea); seek medical attention if any occur. Advise against pregnancy and/or breastfeeding except for palliative treatment of advanced breast cancer. Instruct to d/c use if pregnancy occurs during treatment for endometriosis/endometrial thinning. Advise premenopausal women to use nonhormonal contraception during and 12 weeks after treatment ends. Counsel to avoid initiating treatment with abnormal vaginal bleeding or known allergy. Advise to avoid use for periods >6 months in treatment of benign gynecological conditions.

Administration: SQ route. Inject into anterior abdominal wall below navel line. See PI for extensive details of administration. **Storage:** <25°C (77°F).

ZOLADEX 3-MONTH RX
goserelin acetate (AstraZeneca)

THERAPEUTIC CLASS: Synthetic gonadotropin releasing hormone analog

INDICATIONS: Palliative treatment of advanced prostatic carcinoma. In combination with flutamide for management of locally confined Stage T2b-T4 (Stage B2-C) prostatic carcinoma.

DOSAGE: *Adults:* Inject SQ q12 weeks into anterior abdominal wall below navel line. Stage B2-C Prostatic Carcinoma: Use 3.6mg formulation starting 8 weeks before radiotherapy, then 10.8mg formulation 28 days after 1st injection. Advanced Prostatic Carcinoma: 10.8mg q12 weeks.

HOW SUPPLIED: Implant: 10.8mg

CONTRAINDICATIONS: Pregnancy.

WARNINGS/PRECAUTIONS: Goserelin 10.8mg is not indicated in women. Tumor flare phenomenon observed; transient worsening of symptoms (or occurrence of additional signs/symptoms) of prostate cancer with initial therapy. Ureteral obstruction and spinal cord compression reported. Temporary increase in bone pain may occur. Hypersensitivity, antibody formation, and acute anaphylactic reactions may occur. Hyperglycemia, increased risk of developing diabetes/myocardial infarction (MI), sudden cardiac death, and stroke reported. May suppress pituitary-gonadal system in therapeutic doses and mislead diagnostic tests of pituitary-gonadotropic and gonadal functions during treatment.

ADVERSE REACTIONS: Hot flashes, diarrhea, pain, asthenia, gynecomastia, pelvic/bone pain, erectile/sexual dysfunction and lower urinary tract symptoms.

PREGNANCY: Category X, not for use in nursing.

MECHANISM OF ACTION: Synthetic decapeptide analog of GnRH; acts as an inhibitor of pituitary gonadotropin secretion. In males, causes initial increase in serum LH and FSH levels, causing subsequent increases in serum testosterone levels; chronic administration suppresses pituitary gonadotropins, causing fall in testosterone levels to postcastration levels.

PHARMACOKINETICS: Absorption: C_{max}=8.85ng/mL; T_{max}=1.8 hrs. **Distribution:** V_d=44.1L; plasma protein binding (27%). **Metabolism:** Hydrolysis of C-terminal amino acids. **Elimination:** Urine (>90%, 20% unchanged); $T_{1/2}$=4.2 hrs.

NURSING CONSIDERATIONS

Assessment: Assess for hypersensitivity, history of cardiovascular disease (CVD), diabetes mellitus (DM), bone metastases, ureteral obstruction, spinal cord compression, and possible drug interactions. Obtain baseline serum testosterone/cholesterol/blood glucose levels, prostate-specific antigen (PSA), LFTs.

Monitoring: Monitor for signs/symptoms of worsening prostate cancer, tumor flare, ureteral obstruction, spinal cord compression, renal impairment, hypersensitivity reactions, pituitary apoplexy, signs/symptoms of CVD, and

Z

hypercalcemia, bone mineral density, serum testosterone/cholesterol/blood glucose levels, glycosylated Hgb (HbA$_{1c}$), PSA, and LFTs.

Patient Counseling: Inform men of the risk of developing ureteral obstruction, spinal cord compression, reduction in BMD, DM or loss of glycemic control with DM, MI, sudden cardiac death, and stroke. Advise to inform physician if other adverse events occur.

Administration: SQ route. Inject into anterior abdominal wall below navel line. Refer to PI for proper administration. **Storage:** <25°C (77°F).

ZOLINZA   RX
vorinostat (Merck)

THERAPEUTIC CLASS: Histone deacetylase inhibitor

INDICATIONS: Treatment of cutaneous manifestations in patients with cutaneous T-cell lymphoma who have progressive, persistent, or recurrent disease on or following 2 systemic therapies.

DOSAGE: *Adults:* 400mg PO qd. Intolerant to Therapy: May reduce to 300mg PO qd. May further reduce to 300mg PO qd for 5 consecutive days each week. Take with food.

HOW SUPPLIED: Cap: 100mg

WARNINGS/PRECAUTIONS: Pulmonary embolism and deep vein thrombosis (DVT) reported. Dose-related thrombocytopenia and anemia may occur; modify dose or d/c therapy if platelet counts and/or Hgb are reduced. GI disturbances (eg, N/V, diarrhea) reported; replace fluid and electrolytes to prevent dehydration. Adequately control pre-existing N/V and diarrhea before beginning therapy. Hyperglycemia observed; monitor serum glucose, especially in diabetics or potentially diabetics. Monitor blood cell counts and chemistry tests, including electrolytes (eg, K+, magnesium, calcium), glucose, and SrCr every 2 weeks during 1st 2 months of therapy and monthly thereafter. May cause fetal harm. Caution with renal/hepatic impairment.

ADVERSE REACTIONS: Diarrhea, fatigue, N/V, thrombocytopenia, anorexia, dysgeusia, decreased weight, muscle spasms, alopecia, dry mouth, increased SrCr, chills, constipation, hyperglycemia, proteinuria.

INTERACTIONS: Prolongation of PT and INR observed with coumarin-derivative anticoagulants. Severe thrombocytopenia and GI bleeding reported with other histone deacetylase inhibitors (eg, valproic acid).

PREGNANCY: Category D, not for use in nursing.

MECHANISM OF ACTION: Histone deacetylase inhibitor; inhibits activity of histone deacetylases (HDACs) allowing for accumulation of acetyl groups on the histone lysine residues, resulting in open chromatin structure and transcriptional activation.

PHARMACOKINETICS: Absorption: (Fasted) C_{max}=1.2µM, T_{max}=1.5 hrs, AUC=4.2µM•hr. (Fed) C_{max}=1.2µM, T_{max}=4 hrs, AUC=6.0µM•hr. **Distribution:** Plasma protein binding (71%). **Metabolism:** Liver, via glucuronidation, hydrolysis, and β-oxidation. **Elimination:** Urine (<1% unchanged); $T_{1/2}$=2 hrs.

NURSING CONSIDERATIONS

Assessment: Assess for renal/hepatic impairment, history of thromboembolism, GI disturbances, diabetes, fluid imbalance, cardiac symptoms, pregnancy/nursing status, and possible drug interactions. Assess for hypokalemia and hypomagnesemia; correct prior to therapy.

Monitoring: Monitor for signs/symptoms of pulmonary embolism; monitor for signs and symptoms particularly in patients with prior history of thromboembolic events. Monitor for DVT, thrombocytopenia, anemia, GI disturbances, dehydration, and hyperglycemia. Monitor blood cell counts, chemistry tests, electrolytes, serum glucose, and SrCr every 2 weeks for 1st 2 months and monthly thereafter.

Patient Counseling: Inform about risks and benefits of therapy. Counsel to take with food, not to open or crush, and to drink ≥2L/day of fluid to prevent dehydration. Instruct to contact physician if excessive vomiting, diarrhea, unusual bleeding, signs of DVT, and if other adverse events develop. Instruct to read patient insert carefully.

Administration: Oral route. Do not open or crush. Avoid direct contact of powder in caps with skin or mucous membranes. Avoid exposure to crushed and/or broken caps. **Storage:** 20-25°C (68-77°F); excursions permitted between 15-30°C (59-86°F).

ZOLOFT   RX
sertraline HCl (Pfizer)

Antidepressants increased the risk of suicidal thinking and behavior (suicidality) in short-term studies in children, adolescents, and young adults with major depressive disorder (MDD) and other psychiatric disorders. Monitor and observe closely for clinical worsening, suicidality, or unusual changes in behavior in patients who are started on antidepressant therapy. Sertraline HCl is not approved for use in pediatric patients except for patients with obsessive compulsive disorder (OCD).

THERAPEUTIC CLASS: Selective serotonin reuptake inhibitor

INDICATIONS: Treatment of major depressive disorder (MDD), social anxiety disorder (SAD), obsessive compulsive disorder (OCD), panic disorder with or without agoraphobia, premenstrual dysphoric disorder (PMDD) and post-traumatic stress disorder (PTSD).

DOSAGE: *Adults:* MDD/OCD: 50mg qd. Reassess to determine need for maintenance treatment. Max: 200mg/day. Panic Disorder/PTSD/SAD: Initial: 25mg qd. Titrate: Increase to 50mg qd after 1 week. Adjust dose at intervals no less than 1 week. Max: 200mg/day. PMDD: Initial: 50mg qd continuous or limited to luteal phase of cycle. Titrate: Increase 50mg/cycle if needed up to 150mg/day for continuous or 100mg/day for luteal phase dosing. If 100mg/day is established for luteal phase dosing, a 50mg/day titration step for 3 days should take place at the beginning of each luteal phase dosing period. Hepatic Impairment: Use lower or less frequent doses.
Pediatrics: OCD: Initial: 6-12 yrs: 25mg qd. 13-17 yrs: 50mg qd. Titrate: Adjust dose at intervals no less than 1 week. Max: 200mg/day. Hepatic Impairment: Use lower or less frequent doses.

HOW SUPPLIED: Sol: 20mg/mL [60mL]; Tab: 25mg*, 50mg*, 100mg* *scored

CONTRAINDICATIONS: Concomitant use of MAOIs or pimozide. Concomitant disulfiram with concentrate solution.

WARNINGS/PRECAUTIONS: May increase risk of bleeding events. Screen for bipolar disorder prior to initiation (eg, psychiatric history, family history of suicide, bipolar disorder, depression). Activation of mania/hypomania, SIADH, altered platelet function reported. Hyponatremia reported; caution in elderly and volume-depleted patients. Caution with diseases or conditions that could affect hemodynamic responses or metabolism, seizure disorder, suicidal tendencies. Monitor for emergence of agitation, irritability, unusual changes in behavior, or clinical worsening and/or suicidality, especially at initiation of therapy or dose changes. Decreased appetite and weight loss reported. Caution in third trimester of pregnancy due to risk of serious neonatal complications. Serotonin syndrome (eg, mental status changes, autonomic instability, neuromuscular aberrations, GI symptoms) and neuroleptic malignant syndrome (NMS)-like reactions reported. Dysphoric mood, irritability, agitation, dizziness, sensory disturbances, anxiety, confusion, headache, lethargy, emotional lability, insomnia, hypomania reported upon d/c; avoid abrupt withdrawal. May impair mental/physical abilities.

ADVERSE REACTIONS: Ejaculation failure, dry mouth, increased sweating, somnolence, tremor, anorexia, dizziness, headache, diarrhea, dyspepsia, N/V, agitation, insomnia, nervousness, abnormal vision.

INTERACTIONS: See Contraindications. Avoid alcohol, tryptophans, other SNRIs, and SSRIs. Caution with other centrally acting drugs, TCAs. May shift concentrations with plasma-bound drugs (eg, warfarin, digitoxin). May alter warfarin effects. Increased levels with cimetidine. Decreases clearance of tolbutamide. Rare reports of weakness, hyperreflexia, incoordination with an SSRI and sumatriptan. May potentiate drugs metabolized by CYP2D6 (eg, TCAs, Type 1C antiarrhythmics). Monitor lithium. Caution with OTC products. May induce metabolism of cisapride. Increased risk of bleeding with NSAIDs, ASA, warfarin. Concomitant use of serotonergic drugs and drugs that impair metabolism of serotonin may cause serotonin syndrome. Caution with other agents that may affect serotonergic neurotransmitter systems (eg, triptans, linezolid, tramadol, or St. John's wort).

PREGNANCY: Category C, caution in nursing.

MECHANISM OF ACTION: SSRI; inhibits CNS neuronal uptake of serotonin.

PHARMACOKINETICS: Absorption: T_{max}=4.5-8.4 hrs. **Distribution:** Plasma protein binding (98%). **Metabolism:** Liver (extensive). **Elimination:** Feces (12-14% unchanged), urine (minor); $T_{1/2}$=26 hrs.

NURSING CONSIDERATIONS

Assessment: Assess for risk of bipolar disorder, history of seizures, disease/condition that alters metabolism or hemodynamic response, volume depletion, hepatic/renal impairment, MAOI or pimozide therapy, pregnancy/nursing status, and possible drug interactions. Obtain baseline vital signs and weight.

Monitoring: Monitor for worsening of depression, emergence of suicidal ideation, or unusual changes in behavior. Monitor for possible serotonin syndrome (eg, mental status changes, tachycardia, hyperthermia, N/V, diarrhea, incoordination), NMS-like reactions, hyponatremia (eg, headache, difficulty concentrating, memory impairment, confusion, weakness, and unsteadiness, which may lead to falls), and other adverse events that may occur. Monitor vital signs and weight, platelets, serum Na^+.

Patient Counseling: Counsel about benefits and risks of therapy. Advise to avoid alcohol. Caution about risk of serotonin syndrome with concomitant use of SNRIs and SSRIs including sertraline, triptans, tramadol, or other serotonergic agents. Seek medical attention for symptoms of serotonin syndrome, abnormal bleeding, hyponatremia, activation of mania, seizures, clinical worsening, d/c symptoms (eg, irritability, agitation, dizziness, anxiety, headache, insomnia), and if other adverse events occur. Caution with concomitant use with NSAIDs, aspirin, warfarin, and other drugs that affect coagulation. Caution with hazardous tasks (eg, operating machinery, driving). May notice improvement in 1-4 weeks; advise to continue therapy as directed. Notify physician if pregnant, intend to become pregnant, or breastfeeding. Inform physician if taking, or plan to take any over-the-counter prescriptions.

Administration: Oral route. Mix sol with 4 oz. water, ginger ale, lemon/lime soda, lemonade, or orange juice; do not mix with any other liquids. Dose should be taken immediately after mixing. **Storage:** 25°C (77°F); excursions permitted to 15-30°C (59-86°F).

ZOLPIMIST

zolpidem tartrate (NovaDel Pharma)

THERAPEUTIC CLASS: Imidazopyridine hypnotic

INDICATIONS: Short-term treatment of insomnia characterized by difficulties with sleep initiation.

DOSAGE: *Adults:* Individualize dose. 10mg qhs. Max: 10mg/day. Elderly/Debilitated/Hepatic Insufficiency: 5mg qhs.

HOW SUPPLIED: Spray: 5mg/spray [8.2g]

WARNINGS/PRECAUTIONS: Evaluate for primary psychiatric and/or medical illness if insomnia fails to remit after 7-10 days of treatment. Severe anaphylactic and anaphylactoid reactions reported. Visual/auditory hallucinations, complex behavior (eg, sleep-driving), abnormal thinking and behavior changes reported. Worsening of depression, including suicidal thoughts and actions have been reported in depressed patients. Caution with conditions that could affect metabolism or hemodynamic responses, sleep apnea syndrome, myasthenia gravis, and worsening depression. Signs and symptoms of withdrawal reported with abrupt d/c of sedative/hypnotics. Monitor elderly and debilitated patients for impaired motor and/or cognitive performance.

ADVERSE REACTIONS: Drowsiness, dizziness, headache, N/V, diarrhea.

INTERACTIONS: CNS-active drugs may potentially enhance effects; downward dose adjustment may be necessary. Additive effects seen with alcohol use. Decreased alertness observed with combination use of imipramine/chlorpromazine. Ketoconazole may enhance sedative effects; consider lowering dose when given with ketoconazole.

PREGNANCY: Category C, safety not known in nursing.

MECHANISM OF ACTION: Imidazopyridine, non-benzodiazepine hypnotic; interacts with a GABA-BZ receptor complex and preferentially binds to the BZ_1 receptor subtype at the α_1/α_5 subunits.

PHARMACOKINETICS: Absorption: Rapid; (5mg) C_{max}=114ng/mL, (10mg) C_{max}=210ng/mL; T_{max}=0.9 hrs. **Distribution:** Plasma protein binding (92.5%). **Elimination:** Renal; (5mg) $T_{1/2}$=2.7 hrs, (10mg) $T_{1/2}$= 3.

NURSING CONSIDERATIONS

Assessment: Assess for primary psychiatric and/or medical illness, pre-existing respiratory impairment (eg, sleep apnea syndrome), myasthenia gravis, hypersensitivity reactions, hepatic impairment, possible drug interactions, history of alcohol abuse, and pregnancy/nursing status.

Monitoring: Monitor for anaphylactic/anaphylactoid reactions, abnormal thinking, behavioral changes, complex behavior (eg, sleep-driving, hallucinations). Monitor patients with hepatic impairment, and those on long-term treatment for drug abuse/dependence.

Patient Counseling: Instruct not to take with or immediately after meals. Counsel to take just before bedtime (prior to a full 7-8 hrs of sleep) without food and do not take with alcohol. Caution against hazardous tasks (eg, driving/operating machines). Inform about risks/benefits of use.

Administration: Oral route. **Storage:** Store upright at 25°C (77°F); with excursions permitted to 15-30°C (59-86°F). Do not freeze. Avoid prolonged exposure to heat.

ZOMETA   RX
zoledronic acid (Novartis)

THERAPEUTIC CLASS: Bisphosphonate

INDICATIONS: Treatment of hypercalcemia of malignancy. Treatment of multiple myeloma and bone metastases of solid tumors, in conjunction with antineoplastic therapy.

DOSAGE: *Adults:* Hypercalcemia of Malignancy: Max: 4mg IV infused over no less than 15 min. Retreatment (if necessary): Wait ≥7 days from initial dose. Multiple Myeloma/Bone Metastases: 4mg IV infused over no less than 15 min q3-4 weeks. CrCl 50-60mL/min: 3.5mg; CrCl 40-49mL/min: 3.3mg; CrCl 30-39mL/min: 3mg. Measure SrCr prior to each dose. Withhold treatment with renal deterioration; resume when SrCr returns to within 10% of baseline. Take with oral calcium 500mg qd and vitamin D 400 IU qd.

HOW SUPPLIED: Inj: 4mg/5mL

WARNINGS/PRECAUTIONS: Contains same active ingredient as Reclast; do not treat concomitantly. Rehydrate before use with hypercalcemia of malignancy. Monitor hypercalcemia-related metabolic parameters (eg, serum calcium, phosphate and magnesium). Use with caution for treatment of hypercalcemia of malignancy in patients with severe renal impairment. Avoid with bone metastases with severe renal impairment. Osteonecrosis of the jaw (ONJ) reported; perform dental exam prior to therapy and maintain good oral hygiene. Avoid invasive dental procedures during therapy. Avoid during pregnancy; may cause fetal harm. Severe and incapacitating bone, joint, and/or muscle pain reported; d/c if severe symptoms develop. Bronchoconstriction

Z

in aspirin-sensitive patients reported. Caution with hepatic/renal insufficiency and in the elderly.

ADVERSE REACTIONS: Fever, bone pain, hypophosphatemia, N/V, abnormal SrCr, fatigue, anemia, constipation, dyspnea, arthralgia, diarrhea, weakness, myalgia, hypocalcemia.

INTERACTIONS: Caution with aminoglycosides; may have an additive effect to lower serum calcium level for prolonged periods. Loop diuretics may increase risk of hypocalcemia; do not use until patient is rehydrated. Caution with other nephrotoxic drugs.

PREGNANCY: Category D, not for use in nursing.

MECHANISM OF ACTION: Bisphosphonate; inhibits bone resorption by inhibiting osteoclastic activity and induces osteoclast apoptosis. Also blocks osteoclastic resorption of mineralized bone and cartilage through binding to bone.

PHARMACOKINETICS: Distribution: Plasma protein binding (28-53%). **Elimination:** Urine (39%), feces (<3%); $T_{1/2}$=146 hrs.

NURSING CONSIDERATIONS

Assessment: Assess for hypersensitivity, aspirin hypersensitivity, asthma, pregnancy/nursing status, possible drug interactions, and risk factors for osteonecrosis of the jaw. Assess renal function (eg, SrCr), hydration status and perform dental exam prior to treatment.

Monitoring: Monitor renal function, standard hypercalcemia-related parameters, hydration status, dental status. Monitor for ONJ, local infection, osteomyelitis, musculoskeletal pain, bronchoconstriction and hypersensitivity reactions. Assess SrCr prior to each treatment.

Patient Counseling: Instruct to notify physician of kidney problems. Inform about importance of blood tests, to avoid if pregnant/breastfeeding, and to take oral calcium supplement of 500mg and vitamin D 400 IU daily if with multiple myeloma or bone metastasis of solid tumor. Patients should maintain good oral hygiene, have dental exam prior to therapy, and avoid invasive dental procedures. Inform about the most common adverse events that may develop.

Administration: IV route. Rehydrate prior to administration. Inspect for particulate matter and discoloration before use. Refer to PI for proper preparation of sol. Do not mix with calcium or other divalent cation-containing infusion sol. **Storage:** 25°C (77°F); excursions permitted to 15-30°C (59-86°F). Reconstituted Sol: 2-8°C (36-46°F) for ≤24 hrs. Equilibrate to room temperature before administration if refrigerated.

ZOMIG   RX
zolmitriptan (AstraZeneca)

OTHER BRAND NAMES: Zomig Nasal Spray (AstraZeneca) - Zomig-ZMT (AstraZeneca)

THERAPEUTIC CLASS: 5-HT$_{1B/1D}$ agonist

INDICATIONS: Acute treatment of migraine attacks with or without aura.

DOSAGE: *Adults:* (Spray) 5mg single dose; may repeat once after 2 hrs. Max: 10mg/24 hrs. Safety of treating >4 headaches/30 days unknown. (Tab) Initial: 2.5mg or lower (2.5mg tab may be broken in 1/2); may repeat after 2 hrs. Max: 10mg/24 hrs. Safety of treating >3 headaches/30 days unknown. (ZMT) 2.5mg single dose; may repeat after 2 hrs. Max: 10mg/24 hrs. Dissolve on tongue without water. Safety of treating >3 headaches/30 days unknown. Hepatic Impairment: Use low dose and monitor blood pressure.

HOW SUPPLIED: Nasal Spray: 5mg [0.1mL, 6^s]; Tab: 2.5mg*, 5mg; Tab, Disintegrating: (ZMT) 2.5mg, 5mg *scored

CONTRAINDICATIONS: Ischemic heart disease, coronary artery vasospasm (eg, Prinzmetal's angina), uncontrolled HTN, cerebrovascular syndromes, other significant cardiovascular disease, hemiplegic or basilar migraine, MAOI use during or within 14 days, other 5-HT$_1$ agonist or ergot containing medications/ergot-type agent (eg, dihydroergotamine, methysergide) use within 24 hrs.

WARNINGS/PRECAUTIONS: Confirm migraine diagnosis. Supervise 1st dose and monitor cardiac function in those at risk of CAD (eg, HTN, hypercholesterolemia, smoker, obesity, diabetes, CAD family history, postmenopausal women, males >40 yrs). Serious adverse cardiac events, cerebrovascular events, vasospastic reactions reported with 5-HT$_1$ agonists. Disintegrating tabs contain phenylalanine. Caution with hepatic dysfunction. Reconsider diagnosis before 2nd dose, if no response seen after 1st dose. Serotonin syndrome symptoms (eg, mental status changes, autonomic instability, neuromuscular aberrations, and GI symptoms) reported. Avoid in patients with symptomatic Wolff-Parkinson-White syndrome or arrhythmias associated with other cardiac accessory conduction pathway disorders.

ADVERSE REACTIONS: Paresthesia, hyperesthesia, asthenia, warm/cold sensation, neck/throat/jaw pain, dry mouth, nausea, dizziness, somnolence, unusual taste (nasal spray).

INTERACTIONS: See Contraindications. Ergot-containing agents may prolong vasospastic reactions. Serotonin syndrome reported with combined use of an SSRI or SNRI. Half-life and AUC doubled with cimetidine.

PREGNANCY: Category C, caution in nursing.

MECHANISM OF ACTION: 5-HT$_{1D/1B}$ agonist; binds with high affinity to 5-HT$_{1D/1B}$ receptors on intracranial vessels (including arteriovenous anastomoses) and sensory nerves of trigeminal system, which results in cranial vessel constriction and inhibition of pro-inflammatory neuropeptide release.

PHARMACOKINETICS: Absorption: Well-absorbed; absolute bioavailability (40%); T$_{max}$=3 hrs (ODT/Nasal Spray), 1.5 hrs (Tab). **Distribution:** (Oral) V$_d$=7L/kg, (Nasal Spray) V$_d$=8.4L/kg. Plasma protein binding (25%). **Metabolism:** N-desmethyl (active metabolite). **Elimination:** Urine (65%, 8% unchanged), feces (30% Oral); T$_{1/2}$=3 hrs (Nasal Spray).

NURSING CONSIDERATIONS

Assessment: Confirm diagnosis of migraine before therapy. Assess for ischemic heart disease (eg, angina pectoris, Prinzmetal's variant angina, MI or documented silent MI), HTN, hemiplegic or basilar migraine, presence of risk factors for CAD (eg, hypercholesterolemia, smoking, obesity, DM, strong family history of CAD, female with surgical or physiological menopause, or male >40 yrs), ECG changes, hepatic/renal impairment, pregnancy/nursing status, and possible drug interactions.

Monitoring: Administration of 1st dose should be in physician's office or medically staffed and equipped facility as cardiac ischemia may occur in absence of clinical symptoms. ECG should be obtained immediately after administration in those with risk factors. Monitor for signs/symptoms of cardiac events (eg, coronary vasospasm, acute MI, arrhythmia, ECG changes, follow-up coronary angiography), cerebrovascular events (eg, hemorrhage, stroke, TIAs), peripheral vascular ischemia, colonic ischemia with bloody diarrhea and abdominal pain, serotonin syndrome (eg, mental status changes, autonomic instability, neuromuscular aberrations and/or GI symptoms), ophthalmic effects, and increased BP.

Patient Counseling: Inform about risk of serotonin syndrome, especially if taken with SSRIs or SNRIs. Advise to notify physician if pregnant/nursing or planning to become pregnant. Counsel on proper administration technique for nasal spray.

Administration: Oral/Nasal routes. ODT: Immediately prior to dosing, remove blister from outer pouch with dry hands. Dissolve on tongue and swallow. **Storage:** 20-25°C (68-77°F).

ZONEGRAN RX

zonisamide (Eisai)

THERAPEUTIC CLASS: Sulfonamide anticonvulsant

INDICATIONS: Adjunctive therapy in the treatment of partial seizures in adults with epilepsy.

DOSAGE: *Adults:* Initial: 100mg qd for 2 weeks. Titrate: May increase to 200mg/day in ≥2 weeks. May then increase to 300mg/day, then to 400mg/day in ≥2-week intervals. Elderly: Start at low end of dosing range. Swallow caps whole.
Pediatrics: ≥16 yrs: Initial: 100mg qd for 2 weeks. Titrate: May increase to 200mg/day in ≥2 weeks. May then increase to 300mg/day, then to 400mg/day in ≥2-week intervals. Swallow caps whole.

HOW SUPPLIED: Cap: 25mg, 100mg

CONTRAINDICATIONS: Hypersensitivity to sulfonamides.

WARNINGS/PRECAUTIONS: Fatal sulfonamide reactions (eg, Stevens-Johnson syndrome [SJS], toxic epidermal necrolysis [TEN], fulminant hepatic necrosis, blood dyscrasias) rarely reported; d/c if signs of hypersensitivity (eg, unexplained rash) and other serious reactions occur. Increased risk of suicidal thoughts or behavior reported; monitor for emergence/worsening of depression and any unusual changes in mood or behavior. Increased risk of oligohidrosis and hyperthermia in pediatrics; monitor for decreased sweating and increased body temperature. May cause dose-dependent metabolic acidosis; d/c or reduce dose if metabolic acidosis develops/persists. Avoid abrupt withdrawal; may precipitate increased seizure frequency or status epilepticus. Advise females to use effective contraception during therapy. May cause cognitive/neuropsychiatric adverse events. May impair physical/mental abilities. Caution with renal/hepatic impairment. Kidney stones formation, increased SrCr and BUN reported; d/c if acute renal failure or if a sustained increase in BUN/SrCr develops. Do not use with renal failure (GFR <50mL/min). Status epilepticus observed. Creatinine phosphokinase elevation and pancreatitis reported rarely; taper dose or d/c if occurs. Caution in elderly.

ADVERSE REACTIONS: Headache, abdominal pain, anorexia, nausea, dizziness, ataxia, confusion, concentration/memory difficulties, agitation/irritability, insomnia, somnolence, fatigue, depression, diplopia.

INTERACTIONS: Liver enzyme inducers increase metabolism and clearance and decrease half-life of zonisamide. Concomitant administration of phenytoin and carbamazepine increases zonisamide plasma clearance and decreases the half-life of zonisamide. Concomitant use with phenobarbital or valproate decreases the half-life of zonisamide. Caution with drugs that predispose patients to heat-related disorders (eg, carbonic anhydrase inhibitors, anticholinergic drugs). Drugs that induce or inhibit CYP3A4 may alter zonisamide serum concentrations. Caution with alcohol or other CNS depressants due to the potential of zonisamide to cause CNS depression and other cognitive/neuropsychiatric adverse events.

PREGNANCY: Category C, not for use in nursing.

MECHANISM OF ACTION: Sulfonamide anticonvulsant; mechanism not established. Found to block Na^+ channels and reduce voltage-dependent, transient inward currents (T-type Ca^{2+} currents), consequently stabilizing neuronal membranes and suppressing neuronal hypersynchronization. Facilitates both dopaminergic and serotonergic neurotransmission.

PHARMACOKINETICS: **Absorption:** C_{max}=2-5mcg/mL; T_{max}=2-6 hrs (fasting), 4-6 hrs (fed). **Distribution:** V_d=1.45L/kg; plasma protein binding (40%); found in breast milk. **Metabolism:** Liver, via reduction by CYP3A4 and acetylation; N-acetyl zonisamide, 2-sulfamoylacetyl phenol (metabolites). **Elimination**: Urine (62%), feces (3%); $T_{1/2}$=63 hrs.

NURSING CONSIDERATIONS

Assessment: Assess hepatic function, hypersensitivity to sulfonamides, history of depression, suicidal thoughts or behavior, pregnancy/nursing status, and possible drug interactions. Obtain baseline CBC, renal function (SrCr, BUN), serum bicarbonate.

Monitoring: Monitor for signs/symptoms of sulfonamide reactions (eg, SJS, TEN, fulminant hepatic necrosis, agranulocytosis, aplastic anemia, other blood dyscrasias), oligohidrosis, hyperthermia, emergence or worsening of depression, suicidal thoughts or behavior, cognitive or other neuropsychiatric disorders (eg, psychosis, psychomotor slowing, somnolence), kidney stones, and status epilepticus. If abruptly withdrawn from therapy, monitor for increased seizure frequency. Monitor renal function (SrCr, BUN), serum bicarbonate periodically. Monitor for severe muscle pain and/or weakness.

Patient Counseling: Advise that caps should be swallowed whole. May produce drowsiness; do not drive or operate complex machinery until accustomed to effects of medication. Contact physician if skin rash develops or seizures worsen. Contact physician if develop signs or symptoms that could indicate a kidney stone (eg, sudden back pain, abdominal pain, blood in urine). Increasing fluid intake and urine output may decrease risk of kidney stones. Contact physician if a child has been taking zonisamide and is not sweating as usual with or without a fever. Notify physician if develop any signs or symptoms of hematological complications (eg, fever, sore throat, oral ulcers, easy bruising). Counsel patients, caregivers and families that zonisamide may increase the risk of suicidal thoughts and behavior; contact physician if develop emergence or worsening symptoms of depression, changes in mood or behavior, or the emergence of suicidal thoughts or behavior. Contact physician if fast breathing, fatigue/tiredness, loss of appetite, irregular heart beat or palpitations develop. Inform females to use proper contraception while on therapy. Contact physician if they became pregnant, intend to become pregnant, are breastfeeding or plan to breastfeed during therapy. Advise to enroll in NAAED Pregnancy Registry at aedpregnancyregistry.org or by calling 888-233-2334. Contact physician if severe muscle pain and/or weakness occurs.

Administration: Oral route. **Storage:** 25°C (77°F); excursions permitted to 15-30°C (59-86°F). Store in a dry place and protected from light.

ZORBTIVE RX
somatropin (EMD Serono)

THERAPEUTIC CLASS: Human growth hormone

INDICATIONS: Treatment of short bowel syndrome in patients receiving specialized nutritional support.

DOSAGE: *Adults:* 0.1mg/kg qd SC for 4 weeks. Max: 8mg qd. Rotate injection site.

HOW SUPPLIED: Inj: 8.8mg

CONTRAINDICATIONS: Acute critical illness due to complications following open heart or abdominal surgery, multiple accidental trauma, or acute respiratory failure; active neoplasia (either newly diagnosed or recurrent); benzyl alcohol sensitivity.

WARNINGS/PRECAUTIONS: Associated with acute pancreatitis. New onset impaired glucose intolerance, new onset type 2 DM, exacerbation of pre-existing DM, ketoacidosis, diabetic coma reported; closely monitor with risk factors for glucose intolerance. Perform funduscopic evaluations periodically. Increased tissue turgor, musculoskeletal discomfort, and carpal tunnel syndrome may occur.

ADVERSE REACTIONS: Peripheral/facial edema, chest/back pain, fever, flu-like disorder, malaise, flatulence, abdominal pain, N/V, viral infection, dizziness, headache, rash.

PREGNANCY: Category B, caution in nursing.

MECHANISM OF ACTION: Human growth hormone; anabolic and anticatabolic agent, exerts influence by interacting with specific receptors. On gut, actions may be direct or mediated via local or systemic production of IGF-1; also enhances transmucosal transport of water, electrolytes, and nutrients.

PHARMACOKINETICS: Absorption: (SQ) Absolute bioavailability (70-90%). **Distribution:** V_d=12.0L. **Metabolism:** Liver, kidneys. **Elimination:** Urine; (SQ) $T_{1/2}$=3.94 hrs. (IV) $T_{1/2}$=0.58 hrs.

NURSING CONSIDERATIONS

Assessment: Assess for acute critical illness (eg, complications after open heart or abdominal surgery, multiple accidental trauma, acute respiratory failure), active malignancy, hypersensitivity to benzyl alcohol, and possible drug interactions. Perform baseline fundoscopic exam.

Monitoring: Perform fundoscopic exam periodically. Monitor for signs/symptoms of impaired glucose intolerance, new onset type 2 DM, exacerbation of pre-existing DM, diabetic ketoacidosis, diabetic coma, carpal tunnel syndrome, acute pancreatitis, tissue atrophy at injection site, increased tissue turgor (swelling), musculoskeletal discomfort (eg, pain, swelling, stiffness), and hypersensitivity/allergic reactions.

Patient Counseling: Instruct thoroughly as to proper usage and disposal; caution against any reuse of needles or syringes. Advise to seek medical attention if symptoms of impaired glucose intolerance, new onset type 2 DM, exacerbation of pre-existing DM, diabetic ketoacidosis, diabetic coma, carpal tunnel syndrome, acute pancreatitis, tissue atrophy at injection site, increased tissue turgor (swelling), musculoskeletal discomfort (pain, swelling, stiffness), or hypersensitivity/allergic reactions occur.

Administration: SQ route. **Storage:** (Before reconstitution): 15-30°C (59-86°F). (After reconstitution): Refrigerate; 2-8°C (36-46°F) for up to 14 days. Avoid freezing.

ZORTRESS   RX
everolimus (Novartis)

> Increased susceptibility to infection and possible development of malignancies such as lymphoma and skin cancer. Only physicians experienced in immunosuppressive therapy and management of transplant patients may prescribe everolimus. Increased nephrotoxicity may occur with use of standard doses of cyclosporine; reduce dose of cyclosporine and monitor levels in order to reduce renal dysfunction. Increased risk of kidney arterial and venous thrombosis leading to graft loss, mostly within the first 30 days post-transplantation.

THERAPEUTIC CLASS: Macrolide immunosuppressant

INDICATIONS: Prophylaxis for organ rejection in adult patients at low-moderate immunologic risk receiving a kidney transplant in combination with basiliximab induction and concurrently with reduced doses of cyclosporine and corticosteroids.

DOSAGE: *Adults:* Initial: 0.75mg bid (1.5mg/day). Administer immediately after transplantation in combination with reduced dose of cyclosporine. Titrate: May adjust dose at 4-5 day intervals based on blood concentrations achieved, tolerability, individual response, change in concomitant medications and clinical situation. Moderate Hepatic Impairment (Child-Pugh Class B): Reduce daily dose by one-half the recommended initial daily dose. Do not crush; swallow whole with a glass of water.

HOW SUPPLIED: Tab: 0.25mg, 0.5mg, 0.75mg

WARNINGS/PRECAUTIONS: Increased risk of developing bacterial, viral, fungal, and protozoal infections, including opportunistic infections (eg, polyoma virus infections); caution with combination immunosuppressant therapy. Angioedema and fluid accumulation reported. Delayed wound healing and increased wound-related complications reported; may require surgical intervention. Increased serum cholesterol and TG levels following initiation; may require anti-lipid therapy. BK virus associated nephropathy (BKVAN) may lead to renal dysfunction and graft loss. Non-infectious pneumonitis and male infertility reported. May increase risk of new-onset diabetes mellitus (DM) after transplant; monitor blood glucose concentrations. Avoid with rare hereditary problems of galactose intolerance (Lapp lactase deficiency, glucose-galactose malabsorption); diarrhea and malabsorption may occur. Increased risk for proteinuria, nephrotoxicity, thrombotic microangiopathy/thrombotic thrombocytopenic purpura/hemolytic uremic syndrome with standard use of cyclosporine; reduce dose.

ADVERSE REACTIONS: Peripheral edema, constipation, HTN, nausea, anemia, UTI, hyperlipidemia, diarrhea, increased blood creatinine, pyrexia, hyperkalemia, headache, hypercholesterolemia, insomnia, upper respiratory tract infections.

INTERACTIONS: See Boxed Warning. Caution with concomitant use of other drugs known to impair renal function. Avoid concurrent treatment with strong inhibitors (eg, ketoconazole, itraconazole, voriconazole, clarithromycin, telithromycin, ritonavir) and inducers (eg, rifampin, rifabutin) of CYP3A4. Inhibitors of P-glycoprotein may increase concentrations. Caution with CYP3A4 and CYP2D6 substrates with a narrow therapeutic index. Dose adjustment may be needed if cyclosporine dose is altered. Moderate inhibitors of CYP3A4 and P-gp (eg, fluconazole, macrolide antibiotics, nicardipine, diltiazem, nelfinavir, indinavir, amprenavir) may increase levels. CYP3A4 inducers (eg, St. John's wort, carbamazepine, phenobarbital, phenytoin, efavirenz, nevirapine) may decrease levels. Monitor blood concentrations and adjust dose with erythromycin and verapamil. Monitor for the development of rhabdomyolysis with atorvastatin and pravastatin. Avoid with HMG-CoA reductase inhibitors such as simvastatin and lovastatin. Avoid with grapefruit and grapefruit juice. Avoid with live vaccines. Increased clearance with rifampin; avoid concurrent use. Increased risk of developing angioedema with ACE inhibitors.

PREGNANCY: Category C, not for use in nursing.

MECHANISM OF ACTION: Macrolide immunosuppressant; inhibits antigenic and interleukin (IL-2 and IL-15) stimulated activation and proliferation of T and B lymphocytes. Binds to a cytoplasmic protein, the FK506 Binding Protein-12 (FKBP-12), to form an immunosuppressive complex (everolimus: FKBP-12) in cells.

PHARMACOKINETICS: Absorption: (0.75mg bid dose) AUC=75ng•h/mL, C_{max} =11.1ng/mL, T_{max} =1-2 hrs. **Distribution:** Plasma protein binding (74%). **Metabolism:** via CYP3A4 and P-gp (monohydroxylations and O-dealkylations). **Elimination:** Feces (80%), urine (5%). $T_{1/2}$ =30 hrs.

NURSING CONSIDERATIONS

Assessment: Assess for hereditary problems of galactose intolerance, hepatic impairment, pregnancy/nursing status, and for possible drug interactions. Obtain lipid profile, fasting serum glucose, CBC.

Monitoring: Monitor for serious infections, angioedema, thrombosis, wound-related complications, lymphomas, hyperlipidemia, hepatic impairment, nephrotoxicity, DM, proteinuria, BKVAN, hematologic parameters, and blood glucose concentrations.

Patient Counseling: Inform to take orally bid approximately 12 hrs apart consistently. Swallow whole with a glass of water; do not crush. Avoid grapefruit and grapefruit juice. Counsel of risk of developing lymphomas/other malignancies and infections. Limit exposure to sunlight and UV light by wearing protective clothing and using sunscreen with high protective factor. Notify physician if have hereditary disorders of galactose intolerance (Lapp lactase deficiency or glucose-galactose malabsorption). Inform of risks of impaired kidney function with cyclosporine and the importance of serum creatinine monitoring. Avoid pregnancy throughout treatment and for 8 weeks after d/c. Notify physician of all medications and herbal/dietary supplements being taken. The drug has been associated with increased serum cholesterol and TG; treatment and monitoring of blood lipid concentrations may be required. Avoid live vaccines. Inform physician if symptoms of infection, pneumonia, DM, angioedema develop.

Administration: Oral route. Do not crush; swallow whole with a glass of water. **Storage:** 25°C (77°F); excursions permitted to 15-30°C (59-86°F). Protect from light and moisture.

ZOSTAVAX   RX
zoster vaccine live (Merck)

THERAPEUTIC CLASS: Vaccine

INDICATIONS: Prevention of herpes zoster (shingles) in individuals ≥50 yrs.

DOSAGE: *Adults:* ≥50 yrs: Single 0.65mL SQ in the deltoid region of upper arm.

Z

HOW SUPPLIED: Inj: 0.65mL

CONTRAINDICATIONS: Anaphylactic/anaphylactoid reactions to gelatin or neomycin. Immunosuppression or immunodeficiency, including history of primary or acquired immunodeficiency states, leukemia, lymphoma or other malignant neoplasms affecting the bone marrow or lymphatic system, AIDS or other clinical manifestations of infection with HIV, and those on immunosuppressive therapy. Pregnant women.

WARNINGS/PRECAUTIONS: Avoid pregnancy for 3 months following administration.Not indicated for treatment of zoster or postherpetic neuralgia or prevention of primary varicella infection (chickenpox). Serious adverse reactions, including anaphylaxis, reported; adequate treatment provisions, including epinephrine inj (1:1000), should be available for immediate use should an anaphylactic/anaphylactoid reaction occur. Transmission of vaccine virus may occur between vaccinees and susceptible contacts. Consider deferral in acute illness (eg, fever) or with active untreated tuberculosis (TB). Duration of protection >4 yrs after vaccination is unknown. May not result in protection of all vaccine recipients. Do not use in children and adolescents.

ADVERSE REACTIONS: Injection-site reactions (erythema, pain, tenderness, swelling, pruritus, warmth), headache.

INTERACTIONS: See Contraindications. Reduced immune response with pneumococcal vaccine polyvalent; consider administration of 2 vaccines separated by ≥4 weeks.

PREGNANCY: Contraindicated in pregnancy, caution in nursing.

MECHANISM OF ACTION: Live attenuated vaccine; boosts varicella-zoster virus (VZV) specific immunity; hence protects against zoster and its complications.

NURSING CONSIDERATIONS

Assessment: Assess age, acute illness (eg, fever), active untreated TB, previous hypersensitivity to the vaccine, anaphylactic/anaphylactoid reactions to gelatin or neomycin, immunosuppression/immunodeficiency, pregnancy/nursing status, and possible drug interactions.

Monitoring: Monitor for anaphylactic/anaphylactoid reactions, injection-site reactions, headache, and other adverse events that may occur.

Patient Counseling: Ask about reactions to previous vaccines. Inform about benefits/risks of vaccine, including potential risk of transmitting vaccine virus to susceptible individuals (eg, immunosuppressed/immunodeficient individuals, pregnant women who have not had chickenpox). Instruct to report any adverse reactions or any symptoms of concern to their healthcare professional.

Administration: SQ route. Administer immediately after reconstitution. Refer to PI for proper preparation, reconstitution, and administration. **Storage:** Frozen between -50°C and -15°C (-58°F and +5°F) until reconstituted. Store diluent at 20-25°C (68-77°F) or 2-8°C (36-46°F). Store and/or transport at 2-8°C (36-46°F) up to 72 hrs; discard if not used within 72 hrs of removal from -15°C (+5°F). Do not freeze reconstituted vaccine. Protect from light.

ZOSYN   RX
tazobactam sodium - piperacillin sodium (Wyeth)

THERAPEUTIC CLASS: Broad-spectrum penicillin/beta-lactamase inhibitor

INDICATIONS: Treatment of appendicitis, peritonitis, uncomplicated/complicated skin and skin structure infections, postpartum endometritis, pelvic inflammatory disease (PID), moderate community-acquired pneumonia (CAP), and moderate to severe nosocomial pneumonia caused by susceptible strains of microorganisms.

DOSAGE: *Adults:* Usual: 3.375g q6h. CrCl 20-40mL: 2.25g q6h. CrCl <20mL/min: 2.25g q8h. Hemodialysis/CAPD: 2.25g q12h. Give 1 additional 0.75 g dose after each dialysis period. Nosocomial Pneumonia: 4.5g q6h for 7-14 days plus aminoglycoside. CrCl 20-40mL/min: 3.375g q6h. CrCl <20mL/min: 2.25g

q6h. Hemodialysis/CAPD: 2.25g q8h. Give 1 additional 0.75 g dose after each dialysis period. Elderly: Start at low end of dosing range.
Pediatrics: Appendicitis/Peritonitis: ≤40kg: ≥9 months: 100mg piperacillin-12.5mg tazobactam/kg q8h. 2-9 months: 80mg piperacillin-10mg tazobactam/kg q8h. >40kg: Use adult dose.

HOW SUPPLIED: Inj: (Piperacillin-Tazobactam) 2g-0.25g, 3g-0.375g, 4g-0.5g, 2g-0.25g/50mL, 3g-0.375g/50mL, 4g-0.5g/100mL. Also available as a Pharmacy Bulk Package. Refer to individual package insert for more information

CONTRAINDICATIONS: History of allergic reactions to penicillins, cephalosporins or β-lactamase inhibitors.

WARNINGS/PRECAUTIONS: Serious, fatal hypersensitivity (anaphylactic/anaphylactoid) reactions including shock reported; if these occur d/c and institute appropriate therapy. Hypersensitivity reactions more likely to occur with history of penicillin allergy or history of sensitivity to multiple allergens. *Clostridium difficile*-associated diarrhea (CDAD) reported. D/C if bleeding manifestations occur. Superinfection may develop; take appropriate measures if this occurs. May experience neuromuscular excitability or convulsions with higher than recommended dose. Caution with restricted salt intake. Increased incidence of rash and fever in cystic fibrosis reported. Monitor electrolytes periodically with low K⁺ reserves. Caution with renal impairment (CrCl ≤40mL/min). Caution in elderly.

ADVERSE REACTIONS: Diarrhea, headache, constipation, N/V, insomnia, rash, dyspepsia, pruritus, allergic reactions, stool changes, fever, agitation, pain.

INTERACTIONS: May inactivate aminoglycosides. Probenecid prolongs half-life. Monitor coagulation parameters with high doses of heparin, oral anticoagulants, or other drugs which may affect blood coagulation system or thrombocyte function. (Piperacillin) May prolong neuromuscular blockade of vecuronium or any non-depolarizing muscle relaxant. Increase risk of hypokalemia with cytotoxic therapy or diuretics. May reduce methotrexate clearance.

PREGNANCY: Category B, caution in nursing.

MECHANISM OF ACTION: Piperacillin: Broad-spectrum penicillin; exerts bactericidal activity by inhibiting septum formation and cell wall synthesis of susceptible bacteria. Tazobactam: β-lactamase enzyme inhibitor.

PHARMACOKINETICS: Absorption: Piperacillin (2.25g, 3.375g, 4.5g): C_{max} = 134μg/mL, 242μg/mL, 298μg/mL. Tazobactam (2.25g, 3.375g, 4.5g): C_{max}= 15μg/mL, 24μg/mL, 34μg/mL. T_{max} = 30 min. **Distribution:** Plasma protein binding (30%); wide distribution into tissues and bodily fluids; crosses placental barrier. Piperacillin: V_d=0.243L/kg, found in breast milk. **Elimination:** Kidneys; $T_{1/2}$=0.7-1.2 hrs. Piperacillin: Urine (68% unchanged). Tazobactam: Urine (80% unchanged, 20% as single metabolite).

NURSING CONSIDERATIONS

Assessment: Assess for previous hypersensitivity reaction to cephalosporins, penicillins, β-lactamase inhibitors or other allergens, history of bleeding disorder, conditions with restricted salt intake, cystic fibrosis, renal impairment, hypokalemia, pregnancy/nursing status, and for possible drug interactions.

Monitoring: Monitor hematopoietic and renal function, and serum electrolytes periodically. Monitor for signs/symptoms of electrolyte imbalance (eg, hypokalemia), hypersensitivity reactions, CDAD, superinfections, leukopenia/neutropenia, bleeding manifestations, neuromuscular excitability or convulsions, rash and fever in cystic fibrosis patients.

Patient Counseling: Inform about risks/benefits of therapy. Counsel that drug only treats bacterial, not viral, infections. Take as directed; skipping doses or not completing full course may decrease effectiveness and increase resistance. D/C and notify physician if allergic reaction or watery/bloody diarrhea (with or without stomach cramps and fever) occur. Notify physician if pregnant/nursing.

Administration: IV route. Administer as infusion over 30 min. **Storage:** 20-25°C (68-77°F); discard any unused portion of reconstituted solution after 24 hrs. 2-8°C (36-46°F); discard after 48 hrs. Do not freeze after reconstitution.

ZOVIRAX CREAM

acyclovir (Biovail)

RX

THERAPEUTIC CLASS: Nucleoside analogue

INDICATIONS: Treatment of recurrent herpes labialis (cold sores).

DOSAGE: *Adults:* Apply 5X/day for 4 days. Initiate with 1st sign/symptom. *Pediatrics:* ≥12 yrs: Apply 5X/day for 4 days. Initiate with 1st sign/symptom.

HOW SUPPLIED: Cre: 5% [2g, 5g]

WARNINGS/PRECAUTIONS: Cutaneous use only; not for use in the eye, mouth or nose.

ADVERSE REACTIONS: Dry lips, desquamation, dryness of skin, cracked lips, burning skin, pruritus, flakiness of skin, stinging on skin.

PREGNANCY: Category B, caution in nursing.

MECHANISM OF ACTION: Synthetic purine nucleoside analogue; possesses inhibitory activity against herpes simplex virus types 1 and 2, and varicella-zoster virus. Stops replication of herpes viral DNA by competitive inhibition of viral DNA polymerase, incorporation into and termination of growing viral DNA chain, and inactivation of viral DNA polymerase.

PHARMACOKINETICS: Absorption: Minimal systemic absorption.

NURSING CONSIDERATIONS

Assessment: Assess nursing status and for immunocompromised state.

Monitoring: Monitor for signs/symptoms of irritation and contact sensitization.

Patient Counseling: Inform that medication is for treatment of cold sores. Medication is for external use only; avoid application to eyes, inside mouth or nose, or unaffected skin areas. Drug is not for treatment of genital herpes and not a cure for cold sores. Use at first sign of cold sore (eg, tingling, redness, bump, or itch). Wash hands prior to and following administration, apply to clean/dry skin, and do not cover cold sores with bandages or dressings unless directed by physician. Avoid applying another type of skin product (eg, cosmetics, sunscreen, lip balms) or medication to cold sore area during therapy, unless directed by physician. Do not bathe, shower, or swim immediately after application.

Administration: Topical route. **Storage:** 25°C (77°F); excursions permitted to 15-30°C (59-86°F).

ZOVIRAX INJECTION

acyclovir sodium (GlaxoSmithKline)

RX

THERAPEUTIC CLASS: Nucleoside analogue

INDICATIONS: Treatment of neonatal herpes simplex infections and herpes simplex encephalitis. Treatment of varicella-zoster (shingles), initial and recurrent mucosal and cutaneous herpes simplex in immunocompromised patients. Treatment of severe initial clinical episodes of herpes genitalis in immunocompetent patients.

DOSAGE: *Adults:* Initiate with 1st sign/symptom. Max: 20mg/kg q8h for any patient. Mucosal/Cutaneous Herpes Simplex Infections: 5mg/kg q8h for 7 days. Herpes Genitalis: 5mg/kg q8h for 5 days. Herpes Simplex Encephalitis: 10mg/kg q8h for 10 days. Varicella Zoster: 10mg/kg q8h for 7 days. Obese Patients: Dose according to IBW. CrCl 25-50mL/min: Give 100% of recommended dose q12h. CrCl 10-25: Give 100% of recommended dose q24h. CrCl 0-10mL/min: Give 50% of recommended dose q24h. Elderly: Reduce dose and monitor renal function.

Pediatrics: Initiate with 1st sign/symptom. Max: 20mg/kg q8h for any patient. Mucosal/Cutaneous Herpes Simplex: ≥12 yrs: 5mg/kg q8h for 7 days. <12 yrs: 10mg/kg q8h for 7 days. Herpes Genitalis: ≥12 yrs: 5mg/kg q8h for 5 days. Herpes Simplex Encephalitis: ≥12 yrs: 10mg/kg q8h for 10 days. 3 months-12 yrs: 20mg/kg q8h for 10 days. Neonatal Herpes Simplex: Birth-3 months: 10mg/kg q8h for 10 days. Varicella Zoster: ≥12 yrs: 10mg/kg q8h for 7 days. <12 yrs: 20mg/kg q8h for 7 days. Obese Patients: Dose according to IBW. CrCl 25-50mL/min: Give 100% of recommended dose q12h. CrCl 10-25: Give 100% of recommended dose q24h. CrCl 0-10mL/min: Give 50% of recommended dose q24h.

HOW SUPPLIED: Inj: 500mg, 1000mg

CONTRAINDICATIONS: Hypersensitivity to valacyclovir.

WARNINGS/PRECAUTIONS: Do not administer topically, IM, PO, SQ, or in the eye. Adjust dose in renal impairment and the elderly. Renal failure and death reported. Thrombotic thrombocytopenic purpura/hemolytic uremic syndrome in immunocompromised patients reported. Patient must be adequately hydrated. Caution with underlying neurologic abnormalities, electrolyte abnormalities, significant hypoxia, and serious renal or hepatic abnormalities. Infusion must not be given over <1 hr.

ADVERSE REACTIONS: Injection-site inflammation, phlebitis, transient serum creatinine and BUN elevations, N/V.

INTERACTIONS: Increased serum levels with probenecid. Avoid with nephrotoxic drugs.

PREGNANCY: Category B, caution in nursing.

MECHANISM OF ACTION: Synthetic purine nucleoside analogue; possesses inhibitory activity against herpes simplex virus types 1 and 2, and varicella-zoster virus. Stops replication of herpes viral DNA by competitive inhibition of viral DNA polymerase, incorporation into and termination of growing viral DNA chain, and inactivation of viral DNA polymerase.

PHARMACOKINETICS: Absorption: C_{max}=9.8mcg/mL (5mg/kg), 22.9mcg/mL (10mg/kg). **Distribution:** Plasma protein binding (9-33%); found in breast milk. **Metabolism:** 9-carboxymethoxymethylguanine (major metabolite). **Elimination:** Urine (62-91% unchanged) (14.1% metabolite). Refer to PI for detailed info regarding renal function and pediatrics.

NURSING CONSIDERATIONS

Assessment: Assess for immunosuppression, renal/hepatic disease, electrolyte abnormalities, significant hypoxia, pregnancy/nursing status, hydration status, possible drug interactions.

Monitoring: Monitor for signs/symptoms of renal failure, thrombocytopenic purpura/hemolytic uremic syndrome, encephalopathic changes (eg, lethargy, obtundation, tremors, confusion, hallucinations, agitation, seizures, or coma). Monitor renal function (CrCl), LFTs, and CBC.

Patient Counseling: Notify physician if pregnant/nursing. Inform about potential risks of therapy and advise to report any adverse reactions.

Administration: IV route. Infuse over period of ≥1 hr to reduce risk of renal tubular damage, with adequate hydration. Not for topical, IM, oral, ocular, or SQ use. **Storage:** 15-25°C (59-77°F).

ZOVIRAX OINTMENT   RX
acyclovir (Biovail)

THERAPEUTIC CLASS: Nucleoside analogue

INDICATIONS: Management of initial genital herpes and in limited non-life-threatening mucocutaneous herpes simplex infections in immunocompromised patients.

DOSAGE: *Adults:* Apply to all lesions q3h, 6X/day for 7 days. Apply with finger cot or rubber glove to prevent autoinoculation and transmission. Initiate with 1st sign/symptom.

Z

HOW SUPPLIED: Oint: 5% [15g]

WARNINGS/PRECAUTIONS: Not for use for the prevention of recurrent HSV infections. Cutaneous use only; avoid eyes.

ADVERSE REACTIONS: Pain with application, transient burning and stinging, pruritus.

PREGNANCY: Category B, not for use in nursing.

MECHANISM OF ACTION: Synthetic purine nucleoside analogue; possesses inhibitory activity against herpes simplex virus types 1 and 2, and varicella-zoster virus. Stops replication of herpes viral DNA by competitive inhibition of viral DNA polymerase, incorporation into and termination of growing viral DNA chain, and inactivation of viral DNA polymerase.

PHARMACOKINETICS: Absorption: Minimal systemic absorption.

NURSING CONSIDERATIONS

Assessment: Assess for active signs/symptoms of herpes simplex virus. Assess nursing status.

Monitoring: Monitor for signs/symptoms of mild pain (eg, transient burning, stinging) and for pruritus at treatment site.

Patient Counseling: Counsel that ointment is for cutaneous administration only; should not be used in eyes. Advise to initiate as soon as possible following onset of signs/symptoms; not to use in absence of signs/symptoms. Counsel to use finger cot or rubber glove when applying to prevent autoinoculation of other body sites and transmission of infection to others.

Administration: Topical route. **Storage:** 15-25°C (59-77°F); store in dry place.

ZOVIRAX ORAL   RX
acyclovir (GlaxoSmithKline)

THERAPEUTIC CLASS: Nucleoside analogue

INDICATIONS: Acute treatment of herpes zoster (shingles). Treatment of initial and recurrent episodes of genital herpes. Treatment of chickenpox (varicella).

DOSAGE: *Adults:* Herpes Zoster: 800mg q4h, 5x/day for 7-10 days. Start within 72 hrs after onset of rash. Genital Herpes: Initial: 200mg q4h, 5x/day for 10 days. Chronic Therapy: 400mg bid or 200mg 3-5x/day up to 12 months, then re-evaluate. Intermittent Therapy: 200mg q4h, 5x/day for 5 days. Start with 1st sign/symptom of recurrence. Chickenpox: 800mg qid for 5 days. CrCl 10-25mL/min: For a dose of 800mg q4h, give 800mg q8h. CrCl 0-10mL/min: For a dose of 200mg q4h, give 200mg q12h. For a dose of 400mg q12h, give 200mg q12h. For a dose of 800mg q4h, give 800mg q12h. Elderly: Reduce dose.
Pediatrics: ≥2 yrs: Chickenpox: ≤40kg: 20mg/kg qid for 5 days. >40kg: 800mg qid for 5 days.

HOW SUPPLIED: Cap: 200mg; Sus: 200mg/5mL; Tab: 400mg, 800mg

CONTRAINDICATIONS: Hypersensitivity to valacyclovir.

WARNINGS/PRECAUTIONS: Adjust dose in renal impairment, elderly. Renal failure and death reported. Thrombotic thrombocytopenic purpura/hemolytic uremic syndrome in immunocompromised patients reported.

ADVERSE REACTIONS: Nausea, diarrhea, headache, malaise, renal dysfunction, seizures, tremors, anemia, leukopenia, elevated LFTs.

INTERACTIONS: Probenecid increased levels of IV formulation. Caution with potentially nephrotoxic agents.

PREGNANCY: Category B, caution in nursing.

MECHANISM OF ACTION: Synthetic purine nucleoside analogue; possesses inhibitory activity against herpes simplex virus types 1 and 2, and varicella-zoster virus. Stops replication of herpes viral DNA by competitive inhibition of viral DNA polymerase, incorporation into and termination of growing viral DNA chain, and inactivation of viral DNA polymerase.

PHARMACOKINETICS: Absorption: Absolute bioavailability (10-20%). Oral administration of variable doses resulted in different parameters. **Distribution:** Plasma protein binding (9-33%). **Elimination:** $T_{1/2}$=2.5-3.3 hrs.

NURSING CONSIDERATIONS

Assessment: Assess for immunocompromised state (eg, transplant, advanced HIV, AIDS), renal impairment, nursing status, and possible drug interactions.

Monitoring: Monitor for signs/symptoms of thrombotic thrombocytopenic purpura/hemolytic syndrome. Check renal function, LFTs, BUN, and SrCr.

Patient Counseling: Inform medication may be taken with/without food and to maintain adequate hydration. Advise to avoid contact when lesions or symptoms are present to avoid infecting partners. Advise to use safe sex practice in combination with suppressive therapy. Instruct to initiate treatment at earliest symptom of cold sores (eg, tingling, itching, burning).

Administration: Oral route. **Storage:** 15-25°C (59-77°F); protect from moisture.

ZUPLENZ   RX
ondansetron (Par)

THERAPEUTIC CLASS: 5-HT$_3$ receptor antagonist

INDICATIONS: Prevention of N/V associated with highly emetogenic cancer chemotherapy, including cisplatin ≥50mg/m^2; moderately emetogenic cancer chemotherapy with initial and repeat courses; radiotherapy in patients receiving either total body irradiation, single high-dose fraction to abdomen, or daily fractions to the abdomen. Prevention of postoperative N/V (PONV).

DOSAGE: *Adults:* Prevention of N/V Associated with Highly Emetogenic Chemotherapy: 24mg 30 min before chemotherapy. Prevention of N/V Associated with Moderately Emetogenic Chemotherapy: 8mg bid; give 1st dose 30 min before chemotherapy, then 8 hrs later, then bid (q12h) for 1-2 days after completion of chemotherapy. Prevention of N/V Associated with Radiotherapy: 8mg tid. Total Body Irradiation: 8mg 1-2 hrs before each fraction of radiotherapy administered each day. Single High-Dose Fraction Radiotherapy to Abdomen: 8mg 1-2 hrs before therapy then q8h after 1st dose for 1-2 days after completion of therapy. Daily Fractionated Radiotherapy to Abdomen: 8mg 1-2 hrs before therapy then q8h after 1st dose for each day radiotherapy is given. Prevention of PONV: 16mg 1 hr before induction of anesthesia. Severe Hepatic Dysfunction (Child-Pugh ≥10): Max: 8mg/day. *Pediatrics:* ≥12 yrs: Prevention of N/V Associated with Moderately Emetogenic Chemotherapy: 8mg bid; give 1st dose 30 min before chemotherapy, then 8 hrs later, then bid (q12h) for 1-2 days after completion of chemotherapy. 4-11 yrs: 4mg tid; give 1st dose 30 min before chemotherapy, then 4 and 8 hrs later, then tid (q8h) for 1-2 days after completion of chemotherapy. Severe Hepatic Dysfunction (Child-Pugh ≥10): Max: 8mg/day.

HOW SUPPLIED: Film, Oral: 4mg, 8mg

CONTRAINDICATIONS: Concomitant use of apomorphine.

WARNINGS/PRECAUTIONS: Hypersensitivity reactions, including anaphylaxis and bronchospasm reported. QT interval prolongation reported with IV administration. May mask progressive ileus and/or gastric distension. Does not stimulate gastric or intestinal peristalsis; do not use instead of nasogastric suction.

ADVERSE REACTIONS: Headache, diarrhea, malaise/fatigue, constipation, hypoxia, pyrexia, dizziness, gynecological disorder, anxiety/agitation, urinary retention, pruritus.

INTERACTIONS: See Contraindications. Apomorphine may cause profound hypotension and loss of consciousness. Inducers and inhibitors of CYP3A4, CYP2D6, and CYP1A2 may change the clearance and half-life of ondansetron. Potent inducers of CYP3A4 (eg, phenytoin, carbamazepine, rifampicin) significantly increased the clearance of ondansetron. Concomitant use with tramadol may result in reduced analgesic activity of tramadol.

Z

PREGNANCY: Category B, caution in nursing.

MECHANISM OF ACTION: Serotonin 5-HT$_3$ receptor antagonist; mechanism has not been established. Blocks 5-HT$_3$ receptors from serotonin, which may stimulate vagal afferents through 5-HT$_3$ receptors, which initiate vomiting reflex.

PHARMACOKINETICS: Absorption: Well-absorbed from GI tract. T$_{max}$=1.3 hrs; AUC=225ng•hr/mL, C$_{max}$=37.28ng/mL. **Distribution:** Plasma protein binding (70-76%). **Metabolism:** CYP1A2, CYP2D6, CYP3A4; hydroxylation, conjugation. **Elimination:** Urine (5% unchanged); T$_{1/2}$=4.6 hrs.

NURSING CONSIDERATIONS

Assessment: Assess for hepatic impairment, pregnancy/nursing status, previous hypersensitivity, and for possible drug interactions.

Monitoring: Monitor signs/symptoms of ECG changes, hypersensitivity reactions, and LFT abnormalities. In patients who recently underwent abdominal surgery or in patients with chemotherapy-induced N/V, monitor for masking of signs of a progressive ileus and/or gastric distension.

Patient Counseling: Inform patients they may experience headache, malaise/fatigue, constipation, and diarrhea. Inform to report any hypersensitivity reactions, some as severe as anaphylaxis and bronchospasm and the use of all concurrent medications, especially apomorphine. Instruct on proper administration techniques and not to chew or swallow the film whole.

Administration: Oral route. Allow each film to dissolve completely before giving the next film. Refer to PI for proper administration. **Storage:** 20-25°C (68-77°F). Store pouches in carton. Keep product in pouch until ready to use.

Zyban   RX
bupropion HCl (GlaxoSmithKline)

> Serious neuropsychiatric events including depression, suicidal ideation, suicide attempt, and completed suicide have been reported. Some cases may be complicated by nicotine withdrawal symptoms. Advise patients and caregivers that the patient should stop taking bupropion and contact a healthcare provider immediately if agitation, hostility, depressed mood, changes in behavior, suicidal ideation, or suicidal behavior occur. Although Zyban is not indicated for the treatment of depression, it contains the same active ingredient found in antidepressant medications. Antidepressants increase the risk of suicidal thinking and behavior in children, adolescents, and young adults with major depressive disorder (MDD) and other psychiatric disorders.

THERAPEUTIC CLASS: Aminoketone

INDICATIONS: Aid to smoking cessation treatment.

DOSAGE: *Adults:* Initial: 150mg qd for 3 days. Usual: 150mg bid. Max: 300mg/day. Separate doses by at least 8 hrs. Initiate treatment while patient is still smoking. Patients should set a "target quit date" within the first 2 weeks of treatment. Treat for 7 to 12 weeks; d/c at 7 weeks if no progress seen. Renal Dysfunction: Reduce frequency of dosing. Severe Hepatic Cirrhosis: Max: 150mg qod. Swallow whole, do not crush, chew, or divide.

HOW SUPPLIED: Tab, Sustained-Release: 150mg

CONTRAINDICATIONS: Seizure disorder, current or prior history of bulimia or anorexia nervosa, use of MAOIs or within 14 days of use, other forms of bupropion, abrupt d/c of alcohol or sedatives (including benzodiazepines).

WARNINGS/PRECAUTIONS: Patients with major depressive disorder (MDD) may experience worsening of depression and/or emergence of suicidal ideation and behavior (suicidality) or unusual changes in behavior; monitor appropriately especially during the initial few months of a course of drug therapy, or during dosing changes. Screen for bipolar disorder; may precipitate onset of mixed/manic episode in patients at risk. Dose-dependent risk of seizures; do not prescribe doses over 300mg/day for smoking cessation. D/C use and do not restart if seizure occurs. Extreme caution with history of seizure, cranial trauma, or other predisposition toward seizures, and with severe hepatic cirrhosis. Potential for hepatotoxicity. Allergic reactions (eg, anaphylactoid/anaphylactic), insomnia, and HTN reported. Caution with use in hepatic impairment, recent history of myocardial infarction (MI), unstable heart disease, and renal impairment.

ADVERSE REACTIONS: Insomnia, dry mouth, dizziness, disturbed concentration, dream abnormality, rhinitis, rash, nervousness, nausea, diarrhea, anorexia, constipation, arthralgia, anxiety, myalgia.

INTERACTIONS: See Contraindications. Caution with drugs that lower seizure threshold. Increased seizure risk with opioid, cocaine, or stimulant addiction, use of OTC stimulants and anorectics, oral hypoglycemics or insulin, and excessive use of alcohol or sedatives. Caution with levodopa and amantadine. Caution with drugs that are metabolized by CYP2D6. Monitor HTN with nicotine replacement. Caution with CYP2B6 substrates or inhibitors. Carbamazepine, phenytoin, and phenobarbital may induce metabolism. Cimetidine may inhibit metabolism. May alter PT and/or INR with warfarin. May increase citalopram level. Ritonavir/lopinavir may decrease levels. Paroxetine, sertraline, norfluoxetine, fluvoxamine, nelfinavir, and efavirenz may inhibit metabolism.

PREGNANCY: Pregnancy C, not for use in nursing.

MECHANISM OF ACTION: Aminoketone: unknown; suspected to inhibit neuronal uptake of norepinephrine and dopamine.

PHARMACOKINETICS: Absorption: C_{max}=136ng/mL; T_{max}=3 hrs. **Distribution:** V_d=1,950L; plasma protein binding (84%); found in breast milk. **Metabolism:** Extensive to hydroxybupropion (CYP2B6) via hydroxylation; threohydrobupropion, erythrohydrobupropion via reduction of carbonyl group. **Elimination:** Urine (87%), feces (10%); $T_{1/2}$=21 hrs.

NURSING CONSIDERATIONS

Assessment: Assess for hepatic/renal impairment, seizure disorder, risk of seizure development, presence or history of bulimia or anorexia nervosa, MDD, bipolar disorder, recent MI, presence of unstable heart disease, pregnancy/nursing status, and possible drug interactions. Detailed psychiatric history should be taken.

Monitoring: Monitor signs and symptoms of neuropsychiatric events, hepatotoxicity, allergic reactions, insomnia, activation of psychosis and/or mania, HTN, and seizures.

Patient Counseling: Inform about the benefits and risks of therapy. Advise patients and caregivers to d/c therapy and notify physician if agitation, hostility, depressed mood, changes in thinking or behavior, or if suicidal ideation or suicidal behavior occur. Inform patient to notify physician if pregnant/nursing. Instruct to swallow whole and not to crush, divide, or chew tablet.

Administration: Oral route. **Storage:** 20-25°C (68-77°F); dispense in a tight, light-resistant container.

ZYCLARA   RX
imiquimod (Graceway)

THERAPEUTIC CLASS: Immune response modifier

INDICATIONS: Topical treatment of clinically typical visible or palpable actinic keratoses (AK) of the full face or balding scalp in immunocompetent adults. Treatment of external genital and perianal warts (EGW)/condyloma acuminata in patients ≥12 yrs.

DOSAGE: *Adults:* Apply as a thin film qd before hs. Wash off after 8 hrs with mild soap and water. May suspend use for several days to manage local reactions. AK: Apply to affected area (face or balding scalp) for two 2-week treatment cycles separated by a 2-week no treatment period. Rub until no longer visible. Max: 2 pkts/application; 56 pkts/treatment course. EGW/Perianal Warts: Apply to warts until total clearance or up to 8 weeks. Max: 1 pkt/application; 56 pkts/treatment course.
Pediatrics: ≥12 yrs: EGW/Perianal Warts: Apply as a thin film to warts qd before hs until total clearance or up to 8 weeks. Max: 1 pkt/application; 56 pkts/

treatment course. Wash off after 8 hrs with mild soap and water. May suspend use for several days to manage local reactions.

HOW SUPPLIED: Cre: 3.75% [28 x 250mg pkts]

WARNINGS/PRECAUTIONS: Not for oral, ophthalmic, intra-anal, or intravaginal use. Interruption of dosing should be considered if systemic reactions (eg, flu-like signs/symptoms) or local skin reactions (eg, skin weeping/erosion) occur. May exacerbate inflammatory skin conditions, including chronic graft versus host disease. Use not recommended until the skin is healed from any previous drug or surgical treatment. Lymphadenopathy reported. Avoid or minimize natural or artificial sunlight exposure; not for use with sunburn until fully recovered. Caution with inherent sensitivity to sunlight and patients who may have considerable sun exposure. Caution with pre-existing autoimmune conditions. Avoid concomitant use of any other imiquimod creams.

ADVERSE REACTIONS: Local skin reactions (erythema, scabbing/crusting, flaking/scaling/dryness, edema, erosion/ulceration, weeping/exudate), headache, application site pruritus, pain and irritation.

PREGNANCY: Category C, caution in nursing.

MECHANISM OF ACTION: Toll-like receptor 7 agonist; mechanism unknown. Activates immune cells; associated with increases in markers for cytokines and immune cells.

PHARMACOKINETICS: Absorption: (AK) C_{max}=0.323ng/mL, T_{max}=9 hrs. (EGW) C_{max}=0.488ng/mL, T_{max}=12 hrs. **Elimination:** (AK) $T_{1/2}$=29.3 hrs. (EGW) $T_{1/2}$=24.1 hrs.

NURSING CONSIDERATIONS

Assessment: Assess for age, pre-existing autoimmune and inflammatory skin conditions, immunosuppression, human papilloma viral disease, superficial basal cell carcinoma, xeroderma pigmentosum, inherent sensitivity to sunlight, current sunburn, pregnancy/nursing status and if previously treated for AK.

Monitoring: Monitor for signs/symptoms of local skin and systemic reactions, and clinical signs of improvement.

Patient Counseling: Instruct to use as directed. Avoid contact with eyes, lips, nostrils, anus, and vagina. Wash hands before and after application. Treatment area should not be bandaged or otherwise occluded. Avoid exposure to natural or artificial sunlight (eg, sunlamps) and use protective clothing (eg, hat) or sunscreen when using medication. Local skin/systemic reactions may occur; contact your doctor if these occur. (AK treatment) Do not extend treatment cycle beyond 2 weeks due to missed doses or rest periods. Continue use for the full treatment course even if all AK appear to be gone. (EGW treatment) Do not extend treatment beyond 8 weeks due to missed doses or rest periods. Advise female patients to take special care during application at the vaginal opening. New warts may develop during therapy. Avoid sexual contact while cream is on the skin. Drug may weaken condoms and vaginal diaphragms; concurrent use not recommended. Instruct uncircumcised males treating warts under the foreskin to retract the foreskin and clean the area daily. The effect on transmission of genital/perianal warts is unknown.

Administration: Topical route. **Storage:** 25°C (77°F); excursions permitted to 15-30°C (59-86°F). Avoid freezing.

ZYDONE

CIII

hydrocodone bitartrate - acetaminophen (Endo)

THERAPEUTIC CLASS: Opioid analgesic

INDICATIONS: Relief of moderate to moderately severe pain.

DOSAGE: *Adults:* (5/400): 1-2 tabs q4-6h prn. Max: 8 tabs/day. (7.5/400, 10/400): 1 tab q4-6h prn. Max: 6 tabs/day.

HOW SUPPLIED: Tab: (Hydrocodone-APAP) 5mg-400mg, 7.5mg-400mg, 10mg-400mg

WARNINGS/PRECAUTIONS: May produce dose-related respiratory depression. May obscure diagnosis of acute abdominal conditions or head injuries. Caution in elderly, debilitated, severe hepatic or renal dysfunction, hypothyroidism, Addison's disease, prostatic hypertrophy, urethral stricture, pulmonary disease, and postoperative use. May be habit-forming. May impair mental/physical abilities. Suppresses cough reflex.

ADVERSE REACTIONS: Lightheadedness, dizziness, sedation, N/V.

INTERACTIONS: Additive CNS depression with opioids, antihistamines, antipsychotics, antianxiety agents, or other CNS depressants (including alcohol). Increased effect of antidepressant or hydrocodone with MAOIs or TCAs.

PREGNANCY: Category C, not for use in nursing.

MECHANISM OF ACTION: Hydrocodone: Opioid analgesic and antitussive; not established. Possibly related to existence of opiate receptors in CNS. Most actions involve CNS and smooth muscle. APAP: Nonopiate, nonsalicylate analgesic and antipyretic. Mechanism of analgesic effect not established; involves peripheral influences. Antipyretic activity mediated through hypothalamic heat-regulating centers. Inhibits prostaglandin synthetase.

PHARMACOKINETICS: Absorption: Hydrocodone: C_{max}=23.6ng/mL; T_{max}=1.3 hrs. APAP: Rapidly absorbed. **Distribution:** APAP: Found in breast milk. **Metabolism:** Hydrocodone: O-demethylation, N-demethylation and 6-keto reduction. APAP: Liver (conjugation). **Elimination:** Hydrocodone: $T_{1/2}$=3.8 hrs. APAP: Urine (85%); $T_{1/2}$=1.25-3 hrs.

NURSING CONSIDERATIONS

Assessment: Assess for hypersensitivity to other opioids, head injury or other intracranial lesions, presence of increased ICP, acute abdominal conditions, presence of debilitation (eg, elderly), hepatic/renal impairment, hypothyroidism, Addison's disease, prostatic hypertrophy or urethral stricture, pulmonary disease, pregnancy/nursing status, and possible drug interactions.

Monitoring: Monitor for signs/symptoms of respiratory depression, elevations in CSF pressure, hepatic/renal dysfunction, drug abuse and dependence.

Patient Counseling: Inform that drug may impair mental/physical abilities required for performing potentially hazardous tasks (eg, operating machinery/driving). Advise to avoid alcohol and other CNS depressants. Counsel drug may be habit forming; take only as long as prescribed, in amounts prescribed, and no more frequently than prescribed.

Administration: Oral route. **Storage:** 25°C (77°F); excursions permitted to 15-30°C (59-86°F). Dispense in a tight, light-resistant container with child-resistant closure.

ZYFLO CR RX
zileuton (Cornerstone)

OTHER BRAND NAMES: Zyflo (Cornerstone)

THERAPEUTIC CLASS: Leukotriene inhibitor

INDICATIONS: Prophylaxis and chronic treatment of asthma in adults and children ≥12 yrs.

DOSAGE: *Adults:* (Tab) 600mg qid. Max: 2400mg/day. May take with meals and at hs. (Tab, ER) 1200mg bid within 1 hr after am and pm meals. Max: 2400mg/day. Do not chew, cut, or crush.
Pediatrics: ≥12 yrs: (Tab) 600mg qid. Max: 2400mg/day. May take with meals and at hs. (Tab, ER) 1200mg bid within 1 hr after am and pm meals. Max: 2400mg/day. Do not chew, cut, or crush.

HOW SUPPLIED: Tab: 600mg; Tab, Extended-Release: 600mg

CONTRAINDICATIONS: Active liver disease or transaminase elevations (≥3x ULN).

WARNINGS/PRECAUTIONS: Not for use in reversal of bronchospasm in acute attacks and status asthmaticus. Elevations of one or more LFTs and bilirubin may occur; monitor serum ALT prior to therapy, once a month for

Z

first 3 months, every 2-3 months for remainder of 1st yr, and periodically thereafter. Symptomatic hepatitis with jaundice may develop. Increased risk for ALT elevation in females >65 yrs and those with pre-existing transaminase elevations. D/C and follow transaminase levels until normal if signs of liver dysfunction (eg, RUQ pain, nausea, fatigue, lethargy, pruritus, jaundice, or flulike symptoms) or serum transaminase ≥5x ULN occur. Caution in patients who consume substantial quantities of alcohol and/or have a past history of liver disease. Neuropsychiatric events including sleep disorders and behavior changes reported; evaluate risks and benefits of continuing treatment. Not appropriate for children <12 yrs.

ADVERSE REACTIONS: Headache, elevation of hepatic function enzyme (ALT) and bilirubin, nausea, myalgia, upper respiratory tract infection, sinusitis, pharyngolaryngeal pain, diarrhea.

INTERACTIONS: May increase theophylline and propranolol concentrations; monitor levels and reduce dose as necessary. May increase warfarin levels; monitor PT or other coagulation tests and adjust dose appropriately. (IR) Avoid concomitant use with terfenadine. Monitor use with B-blockers and drugs metabolized by CYP3A4 (eg, dihydropyridine, calcium channel blockers, cyclosporine, cisapride and astemizole). (Tab, ER) Monitor use with CYP3A4 inhibitors such as ketoconazole.

PREGNANCY: Category C, not for use in nursing.

MECHANISM OF ACTION: Leukotriene inhibitor; antiasthmatic agent, inhibits leukotriene (LTB_4, LTC_4, LTD_4, and LTE_4) formation by inhibiting the enzyme 5-lipoxygenase.

PHARMACOKINETICS: Absorption: (IR) Rapid; T_{max}=1.7 hrs, C_{max}=4.98μg/ml, AUC=19.2mcg•hr/ml; (Tab, ER) T_{max}=2.1 hrs (without food), T_{max}=4.3 hrs (with food). **Distribution:** (IR) V_d=1.2L/kg; plasma protein binding (93%). **Metabolism:** Liver, via oxidation by CYP1A2, CYP2C9, CYP3A4. **Elimination:** Urine, feces; (IR) $T_{1/2}$=2.5 hrs; (Tab,ER) $T_{1/2}$=3.2 hrs.

NURSING CONSIDERATIONS

Assessment: Assess LFTs and for active or history of liver disease prior to initiation and periodically thereafter. Assess for acute asthma attacks, status asthmaticus, age (female >65 yrs), pre-existing transaminase elevation, neuropsychiatric conditions, alcohol use, hypersensitivity, pregnancy/nursing status and possible drug interactions.

Monitoring: Monitor for LFTs and bilirubin levels. Monitor serum ALT prior to therapy, once a month for first 3 months, every 2-3 months for remainder of 1st yr, and periodically thereafter. Monitor for signs/symptoms of hepatitis, jaundice, liver dysfunction (eg, RUQ pain, nausea, fatigue, lethargy, pruritus or flu-like symptoms), neuropsychiatric events (eg, sleep disorders, behavior changes). Monitor alcohol consumption, pregnancy/nursing status and possible drug interactions. Monitor for signs of worsening asthma.

Patient Counseling: Inform that drug is indicated for chronic treatment, not for acute episodes, of asthma. Advise not to reduce dose or d/c other antiasthma medications unless instructed. If a dose is missed, take the next dose at the scheduled time and do not double the dose. Instruct to notify healthcare provider if signs/symptoms of liver dysfunction (eg, RUQ pain, nausea, fatigue, lethargy, pruritus, jaundice, "flu-like" symptoms) or neuropsychiatric events (eg, sleep disorders, behavior changes) occur. Consult physician before starting or stopping any prescription or OTC medications. Counsel about potential for liver damage and need for liver enzyme monitoring on regular basis. Avoid alcohol. (Tab, ER) Take regularly as prescribed; within 1 hr after morning and evening meals. Do not cut, crush or chew.

Administration: Oral route. **Storage:** 20-25°C (68-77°F); excursions permitted to 15-30°C (59-86°F). Protect from light.

ZYLET   RX
loteprednol etabonate - tobramycin (Bausch & Lomb)

THERAPEUTIC CLASS: Aminoglycoside/corticosteroid

INDICATIONS: Treatment of steroid-responsive inflammatory ocular conditions for which a corticosteroid is indicated and where superficial bacterial ocular infection or a risk of bacterial ocular infection exists.

DOSAGE: *Adults:* Initial: 1-2 drops q4-6h into conjunctival sac of affected eye(s). Titrate: May increase to 1-2 drops q1-2h for first 24-48 hrs. Max: 20mL for initial Rx.

HOW SUPPLIED: Sus: (Loteprednol etabonate-Tobramycin) 0.5%-0.3% [2.5mL, 5mL, 10mL]

CONTRAINDICATIONS: Viral diseases of the cornea and conjunctiva including epithelial herpes simplex keratitis (dendritic keratitis), vaccinia, and varicella, and also in mycobacterial infection of the eye and fungal diseases of ocular structures.

WARNINGS/PRECAUTIONS: Not for injection into the eye. Prolonged use may result in glaucoma with optic nerve damage, visual acuity and fields of vision defects, posterior subcapsular cataract formation, secondary ocular infections, superinfections (including fungi). Fungal cultures should be taken when appropriate. Thinning of the cornea or sclera may occur. May exacerbate the severity of many viral infections of the eye (including herpes simplex). May delay healing and increase incidence of bleb formation after cataract surgery. Caution with glaucoma and history of herpes simplex. May mask infection or enhance existing infection. D/C if sensitivity reactions occurred. Re-evaluate after 2 days if patient failed to improve. Monitor for intraocular pressure (IOP) if to be used for ≥10 days. Cross-sensitivity to other aminoglycosides may occur, d/c if hypersensitivity occurs.

ADVERSE REACTIONS: Injection and superficial punctate keratitis, increased IOP, burning, stinging, headache, secondary infection, vision disorders, discharge, itching, lacrimation disorder, photophobia, corneal deposits, ocular discomfort, eyelid disorder.

PREGNANCY: Category C, caution in nursing.

MECHANISM OF ACTION: Loteprednol etabonate: Corticosteroid; has not been established. Suspected to act by induction of phospholipase A_2 inhibitory proteins (lipocortins), which control the biosynthesis of potent inflammatory mediators. Tobramycin: Aminoglycoside antibiotic; provides action against susceptible organisms.

NURSING CONSIDERATIONS

Assessment: Assess for viral disease of cornea and conjunctiva (eg, dendritic keratitis, vaccinia, varicella), mycobacterial infection or fungal disease of eye, glaucoma, history of herpes simplex, pregnancy/nursing status, and possible drug interactions.

Monitoring: Routinely monitor IOP (use ≥10 days). Monitor for signs/symptoms of hypersensitivity reactions, glaucoma, defects in visual acuity and fields of vision, posterior subcapsular cataracts, perforations, exacerbation of many viral infections of the eye, secondary infection, delayed wound healing, incidence of bleb formation, and superinfections.

Patient Counseling: Instruct not to touch dropper tip to any surface to avoid contamination and not to wear contact lenses during therapy. Seek medical attention if pain develops, or if itching/inflammation become aggravated, or if hypersensitivity reactions, defects in vision, glaucoma, perforations, or superinfections occur. Consult the physician if signs and symptoms fail to improve after 2 days. Care should be taken not to d/c therapy prematurely. Keep out of reach of children.

Administration: Ocular route. Shake vigorously before using. **Storage:** 15-25°C (59-77°F). Protect from freezing; store upright.

Z

ZYLOPRIM

RX

allopurinol (Prometheus)

THERAPEUTIC CLASS: Xanthine oxidase inhibitor

INDICATIONS: Management of symptoms of primary and secondary gout (acute attacks, tophi, joint destruction, uric acid lithiasis, and/or nephropathy). Management of hyperuricosuria and hyperuricemia in patients with leukemia, lymphoma and malignancies due to chemotherapy. Management of recurrent calcium oxalate calculi in those with hyperuricosuria (uric acid excretion >800mg/day in males and >750mg/day in females).

DOSAGE: *Adults:* Individualize dose. Reduction of Flare-Up of Acute Gouty Attacks: Initial: 100mg/day. Titrate: Increase by 100mg/week until serum uric acid level is ≤6mg/dL. Mild Gout: Usual: 200-300mg/day. Moderately Severe Tophaceous Gout: Usual: 400-600mg/day. Max: 800mg/day. Concomitant Colchicine/Anti-Inflammtatory Agents: While adjusting dose of allopurinol, continue therapy until serum uric acid normal and no acute gouty attacks for months. Transfer from a Uricosuric Agent: Gradually reduce dose of uricosuric agent over several weeks while gradually increasing allopurinol to the required dose. Recurrent Calcium Oxalate Stones: Usual: 200-300mg/day in divided doses or as single equivalent. Prevention of Uric Acid Nephropathy with Chemotherapy: Usual: 600-800mg/day for 2-3 days with high fluid intake. CrCl 10-20mL/min: 200mg/day. CrCl <10mL/min: Max: 100mg/day. CrCl <3mL/min: Also increase dosing intervals. Take after meals. Divide dose if >300mg.
Pediatrics: Hyperuricemia with Malignancies: 6-10 yrs: 300mg/day. <6 yrs: 150mg/day. Evaluate response after 48 hrs. Take after meals.

HOW SUPPLIED: Tab: 100mg*, 300mg* *scored

WARNINGS/PRECAUTIONS: Not for treatment of asymptomatic hyperuricemia. D/C at first appearance of skin rash or other signs of allergic reaction. Severe hypersensitivity reactions, hepatotoxicity, and bone marrow depression reported. Monitor LFTs during early stages of therapy with liver disease. Caution with activities that require alertness. Caution with renal impairment. Renal failure reported with hyperuricemia secondary to neoplastic diseases; caution with multiple myeloma and congestive myocardial disease. Fluid intake should yield ≥2L of urinary output/day. Maintain neutral or slightly alkaline urine. Acute gouty attacks increase during early stages of therapy; give colchicine or anti-inflammatory agents.

ADVERSE REACTIONS: Acute gout attacks, rash, diarrhea, SGOT/SGPT increase, alkaline phosphatase increase, nausea.

INTERACTIONS: Increased toxicity with thiazide diuretics; monitor renal function. Reduce mercaptopurine or azathioprine to 1/3 or 1/4 of usual dose with concomitant use. Prolongs half-life of dicumarol and chlorpropamide. May increase cyclosporine levels. Decreased effects with uricosuric agents. Increased skin rash with ampicillin and amoxicillin. Enhanced bone marrow suppression by cyclophosphamide and other cytotoxic agents among patients with neoplastic disease, except leukemia. Caution with sulfinpyrazone.

PREGNANCY: Category C, caution in nursing.

MECHANISM OF ACTION: Xanthine oxidase inhibitor; acts on purine catabolism; reduces production of uric acid by inhibiting biochemical reactions immediately preceding its formation.

PHARMACOKINETICS: Absorption: C_{max}=3mcg/mL, T_{max}=1.5 hrs. Oxipurinol: C_{max}=6.5mcg/mL, T_{max}=4.5 hrs. **Metabolism:** Oxidation to oxipurinol (metabolite). **Elimination:** Kidneys, feces (20%); $T_{1/2}$=1-2 hrs. Oxipurinol: $T_{1/2}$=15 hrs.

NURSING CONSIDERATIONS

Assessment: Assess for HTN, DM, multiple myeloma, congestive myocardial diseases, pre-existing hepatic/renal disease, pregnancy/nursing status and possible drug interactions.

Monitoring: Monitor LFTs, serum uric acid, and renal function periodically. Monitor for signs/symptoms of hepatotoxicity, hypersensitivity/allergic reaction, bone marrow depression, and renal dysfunction.

Patient Counseling: Inform that full benefit will not be seen until after 2-6 weeks of therapy. Increase fluid intake during therapy to prevent renal stones. Instruct to take after meals to minimize gastric irritation. Caution that drowsiness may occur and physical/mental abilities may be impaired. Caution about possible drug interactions. Advise to seek medical attention immediately at 1st sign of allergic reaction (skin rash), painful urination, blood in urine, irritation of eyes, swelling of lips/mouth, or hepatotoxicity (anorexia, weight loss, pruritus).

Administration: Oral route. **Storage:** 15-25°C (59-77°F); store in dry place and protect from light.

ZYMAR   RX
gatifloxacin (Allergan)

THERAPEUTIC CLASS: Fluoroquinolone

INDICATIONS: Treatment of bacterial conjunctivitis.

DOSAGE: *Adults:* 1 drop q2h while awake, up to 8x/day for 2 days; then 1 drop up to qid while awake for 5 days.
Pediatrics: ≥1 yr: 1 drop q2h while awake, up to 8x/day for 2 days; then 1 drop up to qid while awake for 5 days.

HOW SUPPLIED: Sol: 0.3% [5mL]

WARNINGS/PRECAUTIONS: Not for injection. Do not inject subconjunctivally or into the anterior chamber of the eye. Superinfection may result with prolonged use. Fatal hypersensitivity reactions reported after 1st dose of systemic quinolone therapy. Avoid contact lenses when symptoms are present.

ADVERSE REACTIONS: Conjunctival irritation, increased lacrimation, keratitis, papillary conjunctivitis, chemosis, conjunctival hemorrhage, dry eye, eye discharge/irritation/pain, red eye, eyelid edema, headache, reduced visual acuity, taste disturbance.

INTERACTIONS: Systemic quinolone therapy may increase theophylline levels, interfere with caffeine metabolism, enhance warfarin effects, and elevate SrCr with cyclosporine.

PREGNANCY: Category C, caution in nursing.

MECHANISM OF ACTION: Fluoroquinolone antibiotic; inhibits topoisomerase II (DNA gyrase) and topoisomerase IV. DNA gyrase is an essential enzyme involved in replication, transcription, and repair of bacterial DNA. Topoisomerase IV is an enzyme known to play a key role in partitioning of chromosomal DNA during bacterial cell division.

NURSING CONSIDERATIONS

Assessment: Assess for proper diagnosis of causative organisms (eg, slit lamp biomicroscopy, fluorescein staining). Assess for hypersensitivity to other quinolones, possible drug interactions, and use in pregnancy/nursing.

Monitoring: Monitor for signs/symptoms of hypersensitivity or anaphylactic reactions (eg, cardiovascular collapse, loss of consciousness, angioedema). Monitor for overgrowth of nonsusceptible organisms (eg, fungi) with prolonged therapy.

Patient Counseling: Advise to avoid contaminating applicator tip with material from eye, fingers, or other sources. Instruct to d/c therapy and contact physician at first sign of rash or allergic reaction. Advise not to wear contact lenses if there are signs/symptoms of bacterial conjunctivitis.

Administration: Ocular route. Do not inject into eye. **Storage:** Store at 15-25°C (59-77°F). Protect from freezing.

ZYMAXID
gatifloxacin (Allergan)

RX

THERAPEUTIC CLASS: Fluoroquinolone

INDICATIONS: Treatment of bacterial conjunctivitis caused by susceptible strains of organisms.

DOSAGE: *Adults:* 1 drop q2h while awake, up to 8X on Day 1, then 1 drop bid-qid while awake on Days 2-7.
Pediatrics: ≥1 yr: 1 drop q2h while awake, up to 8X on Day 1, then 1 drop bid-qid while awake on Days 2-7.

HOW SUPPLIED: Sol: 0.5% [2.5mL]

WARNINGS/PRECAUTIONS: For ophthalmic use only; should not be introduced directly into the anterior chamber of the eye. Overgrowth of non-susceptible organisms, including fungi, may result with prolonged use. D/C use and institute alternative therapy if superinfection occurs. Avoid wearing contact lenses if there are signs and symptoms of bacterial conjunctivitis or during the course of therapy.

ADVERSE REACTIONS: Worsening of the conjunctivitis, eye irritation, dysgeusia, eye pain.

PREGNANCY: Category C, caution in nursing.

MECHANISM OF ACTION: Fluoroquinolone antibiotic; inhibition of DNA gyrase and topoisomerase IV. DNA gyrase is an essential enzyme involved in replication, transcription, and repair of bacterial DNA. Topoisomerase IV is an enzyme known to play a key role in partitioning of chromosomal DNA during bacterial cell division.

NURSING CONSIDERATIONS

Assessment: Assess for conjunctivitis, proper diagnosis of causative organisms (eg, slit lamp biomicroscopy, fluorescein staining), and pregnancy/nursing status.

Monitoring: Monitor for adverse events and overgrowth of nonsusceptible organisms (eg, fungi) with prolonged therapy.

Patient Counseling: Inform that solution is for ophthalmic use only and should not be introduced directly into the anterior chamber of the eye. Advise not to wear contact lenses if there are signs and symptoms of bacterial conjunctivitis and during course of therapy. Instruct to avoid contaminating the applicator tip with material from the eyes, fingers or other sources.

Administration: Ocular route. **Storage:** 15-25°C (59-77°F). Protect from freezing.

ZYPREXA
olanzapine (Lilly)

RX

> Elderly patients with dementia-related psychosis treated with antipsychotic drugs are at an increased risk of death. Most deaths reported appeared to be cardiovascular (eg, heart failure, sudden death) or infectious (eg, pneumonia) in nature. Olanzapine is not approved for the treatment of patients with dementia-related psychosis. When using olanzapine and fluoxetine in combination, refer to the Boxed Warning section of the PI for Symbyax.

OTHER BRAND NAMES: Zyprexa IntraMuscular (Lilly) - Zyprexa Zydis (Lilly)

THERAPEUTIC CLASS: Thienobenzodiazepine

INDICATIONS: (PO) Treatment of schizophrenia in adults and adolescent patients (ages 13-17 yrs). Acute treatment of manic or mixed episodes associated with bipolar I disorder and maintenance treatment of bipolar I disorder in adults and adolescent patients (ages 13-17 yrs). Adjunct to lithium or valproate for the treatment of manic or mixed episodes associated with bipolar I disorder in adults. In combination with fluoxetine for the treatment of depressive episodes associated with bipolar I disorder and for the treatment of treatment-resistant depression. (IM) Treatment of acute agitation associated with schizophrenia and bipolar I mania.

DOSAGE: *Adults:* (PO) Schizophrenia: Initial/Usual: 5-10mg qd. Target dose: 10mg/day. Titrate: Adjust by dose increments/decrements of 5mg qd at intervals of not <1 week. Max: 20mg/day. Debilitated/Hypotension Risk/Slow Metabolizers/Sensitive to Effects: Initial: 5mg qd. Titrate: Increase cautiously. Maint: 10-20mg/day. Periodically reevaluate. Bipolar I Disorder (Manic or Mixed Episodes): Initial: 10-15mg qd. Titrate: Adjust by dose increments/decrements of 5mg qd at intervals of not <24 hrs. Maint: 5-20mg/day. Periodically reevaluate. Max: 20mg/day. With Lithium or Valproate: Initial/Usual: 10mg qd. Max: 20mg/day. Concomitant Use with Fluoxetine: Depressive Episodes Associated with Bipolar I Disorder/Resistant Depression: Initial: 5mg with 20mg fluoxetine qpm. Titrate: Adjust dose based on efficacy and tolerability. Usual: 5-12.5mg with 20-50mg fluoxetine (depressive episodes associated with Bipolar I disorder) or 5-20mg with 20-50mg fluoxetine (resistant depression). Max: 18mg with 75mg fluoxetine. Hypotension Risk/Hepatic Impairment/Slow Metabolizers/Sensitive to Effects: Initial: 2.5-5mg with 20mg fluoxetine qd. Titrate: Increase cautiously. (IM) Agitation: Usual: 10mg IM. Dosing range: 2.5-10mg IM. Assess for orthostatic hypotension prior to subsequent dosing. Max: 3 doses of 10mg IM q2-4h. May initiate PO therapy in a range of 5-20mg/day when clinically appropriate. Elderly: 5mg IM. Debilitated/Hypotension Risk/Sensitive to Effects: 2.5mg IM.
Pediatrics: 13-17 yrs: (PO) Schizophrenia/Bipolar I Disorder (Manic or Mixed Episodes): Initial: 2.5-5mg qd. Target dose: 10mg/day. Titrate: Adjust by dose increments/decrements of 2.5-5mg. Max: 20mg/day. Periodically reassess to determine the need for maintenance treatment. Use lowest dose to maintain remission.

HOW SUPPLIED: Inj: 10mg; Tab: 2.5mg, 5mg, 7.5mg, 10mg, 15mg, 20mg; Tab, Disintegrating: (Zydis) 5mg, 10mg, 15mg, 20mg

WARNINGS/PRECAUTIONS: May cause hyperglycemia; caution in patients with diabetes mellitus (DM) or in patients with borderline increased blood glucose levels and monitor for worsening of glucose control. Obtain fasting blood glucose (FBG) levels at beginning of treatment and periodically during treatment. Supervision should accompany therapy if patients are at high risk of attempted suicide. Neuroleptic malignant syndrome (NMS) reported; d/c if symptoms occur and instill intensive symptomatic treatment and monitoring. Tardive dyskinesia reported; d/c if signs/symptoms develop unless treatment is required despite the presence of syndrome. Hyperlipidemia reported; obtain lipid levels at baseline and periodically thereafter. May cause weight gain; perform regular monitoring of weight. May cause orthostatic hypotension; caution with cardiovascular (CV) disease, cerebrovascular disease and conditions that would predispose to hypotension. May cause esophageal dysmotility and aspiration. Not approved for use in patients with Alzheimer's disease. Seizures reported; caution in patients with history of seizures or with conditions that lower the seizure threshold (eg, Alzheimer's dementia). Leukopenia, neutropenia, and agranulocytosis reported; d/c in first sign of clinically significant decline in WBC without causative factors or if severe neutropenia (ANC<1000/mm^3) develops. May cause cognitive and motor impairment. Hyperprolactinemia reported. May cause disruption of body temperature regulation. Caution in patients with clinically significant prostatic hypertrophy, narrow-angle glaucoma, a history of paralytic ileus or related conditions, hepatic impairment, and the elderly.

ADVERSE REACTIONS: Postural hypotension, constipation, dry mouth, weight gain, somnolence, dizziness, personality disorder, akathisia, asthenia, dyspepsia, tremor, increased appetite, abdominal pain, headache, insomnia.

INTERACTIONS: May potentiate orthostatic hypotension with diazepam and alcohol. May enhance effects of certain antihypertensive agents. Increased clearance with carbamazepine (CYP1A2 inducer). Caution with other CNS-acting drugs. May antagonize effects of levodopa and dopamine agonists. Inducers of CYP1A2 or glucuronyl transferase (eg, omeprazole, rifampin) may increase clearance. CYP1A2 inhibitors (eg, fluvoxamine) and CYP2D6 inhibitors (eg, fluoxetine) may decrease clearance. Caution with concomitant use of drugs whose effects can induce hypotension, bradycardia, or respiratory

Z

or CNS depression. Caution in patients receiving concomitant therapy with potentially hepatotoxic drugs. Caution when prescribing with anticholinergic drugs; may contribute to elevation in core body temperature. (IM) Concomitant administration with parenteral benzodiazepines is not recommended. Coadministration with IM lorazepam may increase the incidence of somnolence. (PO) Activated charcoal may decrease oral olanzapine levels.

PREGNANCY: Category C, not for use in nursing.

MECHANISM OF ACTION: Thienobenzodiazepine; not established. Proposed that the mechanism of action for the treatment of schizophrenia is mediated through a combination of dopamine and serotonin type 2 ($5HT_2$) antagonism.

PHARMACOKINETICS: Absorption: (PO) Well-absorbed, T_{max}=6 hrs; (IM) Rapid, T_{max}=15-45 min. **Distribution:** Found in breast milk. (PO) V_d=1000L; plasma protein binding (93%). **Metabolism:** Via CYP450 mediated oxidation and direct glucuronidation; 10-N-glucuronide, 4'-N-desmethyl olanzapine (major metabolites). **Elimination:** (PO) Urine (57%, 7% unchanged), feces (30%); $T_{1/2}$=21-54 hrs.

NURSING CONSIDERATIONS

Assessment: Assess for DM, CV disease, cerebrovascular disease, risk of hypotension, history of seizures or conditions that could lower the seizure threshold, prostatic hypertrophy, narrow-angle glaucoma, history of paralytic ileus, hepatic impairment, history of drug abuse, pregnancy/nursing status, and possible drug interactions. Assess for dementia-related psychosis and Alzheimer's disease in the elderly. Assess for debilitated, slow metabolizers and those pharmacodynamically sensitive to olanzapine. Obtain baseline lipid panel, CBC, and FBG levels.

Monitoring: Monitor for signs/symptoms of NMS, hyperglycemia, hyperlipidemia, weight gain, tardive dyskinesia, and other adverse effects. Perform periodic monitoring of FBG, lipid levels, and weight of patient. Perform frequent monitoring of CBC in patients with a history of clinically significant low WBC or drug-induced leukopenia/neutropenia. In patients with clinically significant neutropenia, monitor for fever or other symptoms or signs of infection. In high-risk patients, monitor closely for suicide attempt.

Patient Counseling: Advise of benefits/risks of therapy. Counsel about signs and symptoms of NMS. Inform of potential risk of hyperglycemia-related adverse events. Medication may cause hyperlipidemia and weight gain. Medication may cause orthostatic hypotension; instruct to contact physician if dizziness, fast or slow heart beat, or fainting occurs. Medication may impair judgment, thinking, or motor skills; instruct to use caution when operating hazardous machinery. Avoid overheating and dehydration. Avoid alcohol. Olanzapine orally disintegrating tab contains phenylalanine. Notify physician if taking, planning to take, or have stopped taking any prescription or over-the-counter (OTC) products, including herbal supplements. Notify physician if pregnant or planning to become pregnant during treatment. Avoid breastfeeding during therapy.

Administration: Oral/IM routes. (Inj) Do not administer IV or SQ. See PI for proper reconstitution procedures. (Tab, Disintegrating) After opening sachet, peel back foil on blister. Do not push tab through foil. Upon opening the blister, remove tab and place entire tab in the mouth using dry hands. **Storage:** Tab/Tab, Disintegrating/Inj (Before reconstitution): 20-25°C (68-77°F); excursions permitted between 15-30°C (59-86°F). Reconstituted Inj: May be stored at 20-25°C (68-77°F) for up to 1 hr; excursions permitted between 15-30°C (59-86°F). Tab/Tab, Disintegrating: Protect from light and moisture. Inj: Protect from light. Do not freeze.

ZYPREXA RELPREVV   RX
olanzapine (Lilly)

> Elderly patients with dementia-related psychosis treated with antipsychotic drugs are at an increased risk of death. Most deaths reported appeared to be cardiovascular (eg, heart failure, sudden death) or infectious (eg, pneumonia) in nature. Not approved for the treatment of patients with dementia-related psychosis. Post-inj delirium and sedation (including coma) reported. Must be administered in a registered healthcare facility with ready access to emergency response services. Observe patient for ≥3 hrs after each inj. Available only through a restricted distribution program called Zyprexa Relprevv Patient Care Program and requires prescriber, healthcare facility, patient, and pharmacy enrollment.

THERAPEUTIC CLASS: Thienobenzodiazepine

INDICATIONS: Treatment of schizophrenia.

DOSAGE: *Adults:* Usual: 150-300mg IM q2 weeks or 405mg IM q4 weeks. Max: 405mg IM q4 weeks or 300mg IM q2 weeks. Debilitated/Hypotension Risk/ Slow Metabolizers/Sensitive to Effects: Initial: 150mg IM q4 weeks. Titrate: Increase cautiously. Establish tolerability with oral olanzapine prior to initiating treatment. Refer to PI for recommended dosing based on corresponding oral olanzapine doses.

HOW SUPPLIED: Inj, Extended-Release: 210mg, 300mg, 405mg

WARNINGS/PRECAUTIONS: May cause hyperglycemia; caution in patients with diabetes mellitus (DM) or borderline increased blood glucose levels; monitor for worsening of glucose control. Obtain fasting blood glucose (FBG) levels at beginning of treatment and periodically during treatment. Supervision should accompany therapy if patients are at high risk of attempted suicide. Neuroleptic malignant syndrome (NMS) reported; d/c if symptoms occur and instill intensive symptomatic treatment and monitoring. Tardive dyskinesia reported; d/c if signs/symptoms develop. Hyperlipidemia reported; obtain lipid levels at baseline and periodically thereafter. May cause weight gain; perform regular monitoring of weight. May induce orthostatic hypotension; caution with known cardiovascular (CV) disease, cerebrovascular disease, and conditions that would predispose to hypotension. May cause esophageal dysmotility and aspiration. Not approved for use in patients with Alzheimer's disease. Seizures reported; caution with history of seizures or with conditions that potentially lower the seizure threshold. Leukopenia, neutropenia, and agranulocytosis reported; d/c in first sign of clinically significant decline in WBC without causative factor or if severe neutropenia (ANC <1000/mm³) develops. May cause cognitive and motor impairment. Hyperprolactinemia reported. May cause disruption of body temperature regulation. Caution in patients with clinically significant prostatic hypertrophy, narrow-angle glaucoma, history of paralytic ileus or related conditions, hepatic impairment, and elderly. Not for IV or SQ use.

ADVERSE REACTIONS: Headache, sedation, dizziness, diarrhea, back pain, N/V, nasal congestion, dry mouth, nasopharyngitis, weight increased, abdominal pain, fatigue, somnolence, increased appetite.

INTERACTIONS: May potentiate orthostatic hypotension with diazepam and alcohol. May enhance effects of certain antihypertensive agents. Increased clearance with carbamazepine, a CYP1A2 inducer. Caution with other CNS-acting drugs. May antagonize effects of levodopa and dopamine agonists. Omeprazole and rifampin, inducers of CYP1A2 or glucuronyl transferase may increase clearance. Fluvoxamine, a CYP1A2 inhibitor and fluoxetine, a CYP2D6 inhibitor may decrease clearance. Caution with concomitant use of drugs whose effects can induce hypotension, bradycardia, respiratory or CNS depression. Caution with parenteral benzodiazepines. Coadministration with IM lorazepam may potentiate somnolence. Caution in patients receiving concomitant therapy with potentially hepatotoxic drugs. Caution when prescribing with anticholinergic drugs; may contribute to elevation in core body temperature.

PREGNANCY: Category C, not for use in nursing.

Z

MECHANISM OF ACTION: Thienobenzodiazepine; not established. Proposed that efficacy in schizophrenia is mediated through a combination of dopamine and serotonin type 2 ($5HT_2$) antagonism.

PHARMACOKINETICS: Absorption: (IM) Rapid, T_{max}=15-45 min. **Distribution:** (PO) Found in breast milk; V_d=1000L; plasma protein binding (93%). **Metabolism:** (PO) Via CYP450 mediated oxidation and direct glucuronidation; 10-N-glucuronide, 4'-N-desmethyl olanzapine (major metabolites). **Elimination:** (PO) Urine (57%, 7% unchanged), feces (30%); $T_{1/2}$=30 days (IM).

NURSING CONSIDERATIONS

Assessment: Assess for tolerability with oral olanzapine, DM, hyperlipidemia, CV or cerebrovascular disease, risk of hypotension, history of seizures or conditions that could lower the seizure threshold, prostatic hypertrophy, narrow-angle glaucoma, history of paralytic ileus, hepatic impairment, pregnancy/nursing status, and possible drug interactions. Assess for dementia-related psychosis and Alzheimer's disease in elderly. Assess for debilitated, slow metabolizers and those pharmacodynamically sensitive to olanzapine. Obtain baseline lipid panel, CBC and FBG levels.

Monitoring: Monitor for sedation and/or delirium for ≥3 hrs post-inj. Monitor for signs/symptoms of NMS, hyperglycemia, hyperlipidemia, weight gain, tardive dyskinesia, and other adverse effects. Perform periodic monitoring of FBG, lipid levels, and weight of patient. Perform frequent monitoring of CBC in patients with a history of clinically significant low WBC or drug-induced leukopenia/neutropenia. In patients with clinically significant neutropenia, monitor for fever or other symptoms or signs of infection. In high-risk patients, monitor closely for a suicide attempt.

Patient Counseling: Advise of benefits/risks of therapy. Advise of the risk of post-inj delirium/sedation syndrome following administration. Inform that drug is not approved for elderly with dementia-related psychosis. Counsel about the signs/symptoms of NMS. Inform of potential risk of hyperglycemia-related adverse events. Medication may cause hyperlipidemia and weight gain. Medication may cause orthostatic hypotension; instruct to contact physician if dizziness, fast or slow heart beat, or fainting occurs. Medication may impair judgment, thinking, or motor skills; instruct to use caution when operating hazardous machinery. Avoid alcohol. Notify physician if taking, planning to take, or have stopped taking any prescription or over-the-counter (OTC) drugs, including herbal supplements. Notify physician if pregnant or planning to become pregnant during treatment. Avoid breastfeeding during therapy. Advise regarding appropriate care in avoiding overheating and dehydration. Reassess periodically to determine the need for continued treatment.

Administration: IM route. See PI for proper reconstitution and administration technique. **Storage:** Room temperature ≤30°C (86°F). Reconstituted Sol: May store at room temperature for 24 hrs.

ZYRTEC-D OTC

pseudoephedrine HCl - cetirizine HCl (McNeil Consumer)

THERAPEUTIC CLASS: Antihistamine/decongestant

INDICATIONS: Relief of nasal and non-nasal symptoms associated with seasonal or perennial allergic rhinitis in patients ≥12 yrs.

DOSAGE: *Adults:* 1 tab bid. Hepatic Impairment/Renal Dysfunction (CrCl <31mL/min): 1 tab qd. Swallow whole.
Pediatrics: ≥12 yrs: 1 tab bid. Hepatic Impairment/Renal Dysfunction (CrCl <31mL/min): 1 tab qd. Swallow whole.

HOW SUPPLIED: Tab, Extended-Release: (Cetirizine-Pseudoephedrine) 5mg-120mg

CONTRAINDICATIONS: Narrow-angle glaucoma, urinary retention, MAOIs during or within 14 days of use, severe HTN, severe CAD, hypersensitivity to adrenergics.

WARNINGS/PRECAUTIONS: Caution with HTN, DM, ischemic heart disease, increased IOP, hyperthyroidism, renal impairment, or prostatic hypertrophy. May produce CNS stimulation with convulsions or cardiovascular collapse. May impair mental/physical abilities. The elderly are more likely to have adverse reactions.

ADVERSE REACTIONS: Insomnia, dry mouth, fatigue, somnolence.

INTERACTIONS: See Contraindications. Avoid alcohol or other CNS depressants due to additional reduction in alertness and CNS impairment. May reduce antihypertensive effects of antihypertensive drugs that interfere with sympathetic activity (eg, methyldopa, mecamylamine, reserpine). Caution with sympathomimetic amines; combined effects on the cardiovascular system may be harmful. Theophylline may decrease clearance of cetirizine; larger doses may have greater effect. Increased ectopic pacemaker may occur when pseudoephedrine is used concomitantly with digitalis.

PREGNANCY: Category C, not for use in nursing.

MECHANISM OF ACTION: Cetirizine: Antihistamine; selectively inhibits H_1-receptors. Pseudoephedrine: decongestant; Orally active sympathomimetic amine; exerts a decongestant effect on the nasal mucosa.

PHARMACOKINETICS: Absorption: Cetirizine: C_{max}=114ng/mL (single dose), 178ng/mL (multiple doses); T_{max}=2.2 hrs. Pseudoephedrine: C_{max}=309ng/mL, 526ng/mL (multiple doses); T_{max}=4.4 hrs. **Distribution:** Cetirizine: Plasma protein binding (93%). Pseudoephedrine: V_d=2.6-3.3L/kg. **Metabolism:** Cetirizine: Oxidative-O-dealkylation. Pseudoephedrine: N-demethylation; (1%-7%) metabolized to norpseudoephedrine. **Elimination:** Cetirizine: Urine (70%), feces (10%); $T_{1/2}$=7.9 hrs. Pseudoephedrine: $T_{1/2}$=6 hrs.

NURSING CONSIDERATIONS

Assessment: Assess for narrow-angle glaucoma, urinary retention, current or recent use (within 14 days) of MAO inhibitors, severe HTN, and CAD. Assess use in pregnant/nursing females, patients with idiosyncratic reactions to adrenergic agents or other drugs with similiar structures, patients with HTN, DM, ischemic heart disease, increased IOP, hyperthyroidism, renal impairment, prostatic hypertrophy, and in elderly patients. Assess for possible drug interactions.

Monitoring: Monitor for manifestations of idiosyncrastic reactions to adrenergic agents (eg, insomnia, dizziness, weakness, tremor, or arrhythmia).

Patient Counseling: Inform drug may cause somnolence and decreased alertness; caution when operating machinery/driving. Advise to avoid concurrent use with alcohol or other CNS depressants. Instruct to swallow whole, do not chew or break. May be given with/without food.

Administration: Oral route. **Storage:** 20-25°C (68-77°F); excursions permitted to 15-30°C (59-86°F).

ZYVOX   RX
linezolid (Pharmacia & Upjohn)

THERAPEUTIC CLASS: Oxazolidinone class antibacterial

INDICATIONS: Treatment of vancomycin-resistant *Enterococcus faecium* (VRE) infections including cases with concurrent bacteremia, nosocomial pneumonia, complicated skin and skin structure infections (SSSI) including diabetic foot infections without concomitant osteomyelitis, uncomplicated SSSI, community-acquired pneumonia (CAP) including concurrent bacteremia caused by susceptible strains of designated microorganisms.

DOSAGE: *Adults:* Complicated SSSI/CAP (including concurrent bacteremia)/Nosocomial Pneumonia: 600mg IV/PO q12h for 10-14 days. VRE (including concurrent bacteremia): 600mg IV/PO q12h for 14-28 days. Uncomplicated SSSI: 400mg PO q12h for 10-14 days. Methicillin-Resistant *Staphylococcus Aureus* (MRSA) infection: 600mg q12h.
Pediatrics: Complicated SSSI/CAP (including concurrent bacteremia)/Nosocomial Pneumonia: Treat for 10-14 days. ≥12 yrs: 600mg IV/PO q12h.

Birth-11 yrs: 10mg/kg IV/PO q8h. VRE (including concurrent bacteremia): Treat for 14-28 days: ≥12 yrs: 600mg IV/PO q12h; Birth-11 yrs: 10mg/kg IV/PO q8h. Uncomplicated SSSI: Treat for 10-14 days: ≥12 yrs: 600mg PO q12h; 5-11 yrs: 10mg/kg PO q12h; <5 yrs: 10mg/kg PO q8h. Neonates <7 days: Initiate with dosing regimen of 10mg/kg q12h; may increase to 10mg/kg q8h if suboptimal response. All neonatal patients should receive 10mg/kg q8h by 7 days of life.

HOW SUPPLIED: Inj: 2mg/mL [100mL, 200mL, 300mL]; Sus: 100mg/5mL [240mL]; Tab: 600mg

CONTRAINDICATIONS: MAOIs A or B (eg, phenelzine, isocarboxazid) or within two weeks after taking such drugs; uncontrolled HTN, pheochromocytoma, thyrotoxicosis, and/or taking directly and indirectly acting sympathomimetic agents (eg, pseudoephedrine), vasopressive agents (eg, epinephrine, norepinephrine), dopaminergic agents (eg, dopamine, dobutamine); carcinoid syndrome and/or taking SSRIs, TCAs, serotonin 5-HT$_1$ receptor agonists (triptans), meperidine or buspirone.

WARNINGS/PRECAUTIONS: Myelosuppression (eg, anemia, thrombocytopenia, pancytopenia, leukopenia) reported; monitor CBC weekly and d/c if myelosuppression develops or worsens. *Clostridium difficile*-associated diarrhea (CDAD) reported; if suspected or confirmed, d/c treatment and institute appropriate treatment. Peripheral/optic neuropathy and visual impairment (eg, visual acuity and color vision changes, blurred vision, visual field defect) may occur; prompt ophthalmic evaluation recommended and monitor visual function if for extended treatment periods (≥3 months). Lactic acidosis and convulsions reported. May promote overgrowth of nonsusceptible organisms. Not approved for treatment of catheter-related bloodstream infections, catheter-site infections, or gram-negative infections. Oral suspension contains phenylalanine.

ADVERSE REACTIONS: Diarrhea, headache, N/V, fever, sepsis, anemia, thrombocytopenia, upper respiratory infection, trauma.

INTERACTIONS: See Contraindications. Avoid large quantities of tyramine-containing foods or beverages. Reduced plasma concentration with rifampin. Caution with drugs that produce bone marrow suppression or antibiotic therapy.

PREGNANCY: Category C, caution in nursing.

MECHANISM OF ACTION: Oxazolidinone antibacterial; inhibits bacterial protein synthesis; binds to a site on the bacterial 23S ribosomal RNA of the 50S subunit and prevents formation of functional 70S initiation complex, which is an essential component of the bacterial translation process.

PHARMACOKINETICS: Absorption: Rapid/extensive; absolute bioavailability (100%); IV and PO administration of variable doses resulted in different parameters. T_{max}=1-2 hrs. **Distribution:** V_d=40-50L; plasma protein binding (31%); distributes to well-perfused tissues. **Metabolism:** Via oxidation; aminoethoxy-acetic acid (A), hydroxyethyl glycine (B) (inactive metabolites). **Elimination:** Urine (30% as parent drug, 40% as B, 10% as A), feces (6% as B, 3% as A).

NURSING CONSIDERATIONS

Assessment: Assess for pre-existing myelosuppression (including anemia, leukopenia, pancytopenia, thrombocytopenia), concomitant drugs that produce myelosuppression, presence of chronic infections, previous or concomitant antibiotic therapy, catheter-related bloodstream infections or catheter-site infections, pregnancy/nursing status, uncontrolled HTN, carcinoid syndrome, pheochromocytoma, untreated hyperthyroidism, phenylketonuria, renal/hepatic impairment, and possible drug interactions (eg, SSRIs).

Monitoring: Perform weekly monitoring of CBC. Monitor for signs/symptoms of myelosuppression (eg, anemia, leukopenia, pancytopenia, thrombocytopenia), pseudomembranous colitis or CDAD (may range from mild diarrhea to fatal colitis), lactic acidosis with repeated N/V, convulsions, development of drug resistance or superinfection, serotonin syndrome (eg, cognitive dysfunction, hyperpyrexia, hyperreflexia, incoordination), blurred vision, optic/peripheral neuropathy. Monitor visual function with long-term therapy or if new visual symptoms occur.

Patient Counseling: Inform about risks/benefits of therapy. May be taken with or without food. Notify if pregnant/nursing, have history of seizures or HTN, or if taking cold remedies, decongestants or SSRIs. Watery and bloody stools (with or without stomach cramps and fever) may occur as late as ≥2 months after last dose; inform physician if these develop. Notify physician if visual changes or other side effects occur. Drug treats bacterial, not viral, infections. Take drug exactly as directed and do not skip doses to prevent drug resistance and maintain effectiveness. Avoid large quantities of food or beverages with high tyramine content.

Administration: IV/Oral routes. (IV) Administer over a period of 30-120 min. Do not use in series connections. Flush line before and after infusion if same IV line is used for sequential infusion of several drugs. Refer to PI for compatible IV solutions. (Sus) Refer to PI for proper constitution. (IV) Administer over a period of 30-120 min. Do not use in series connections. **Storage:** 25°C (77°F); excursions permitted to 15-30°C (59-86°F). (IV) Keep infusion bags in the overwrap until ready to use. Protect from freezing. (Tab/Sus) Store in tightly closed bottles to protect from moisture. Protect from light.

Appendix: Reference Tables

ABBREVIATIONS, ACRONYMS, AND SYMBOLS

ABBREVIATIONS	DESCRIPTIONS
- (eg, 6-8)	to (eg, 6 to 8)
/	per
<	less than
>	greater than
≤	less than or equal to
≥	greater than or equal to
α	alpha
β	beta
5-FU	5-fluorouracil
5-HT	5-hydroxytryptamine (serotonin)
ABECB	acute bacterial exacerbation of chronic bronchitis
aa	of each
ACTH	adrenocorticotrophic hormone
ad	right ear
ADHD	attention-deficit/hyperactivity disorder
A-fib	atrial fibrillation
A-flutter	atrial flutter
AIDS	acquired immunodeficiency syndrome
ALT	alanine transaminase (SGPT)
am or AM	morning
AMI	acute myocardial infarction
ANA	antinuclear antibodies
ANC	absolute neutrophil count
APAP	acetaminophen
as	left ear
ASA	aspirin
AST	aspartate transaminase (SGOT)
au	each ear
AUC	area under the curve
AV	atrioventricular
bid	twice daily
BMI	body mass index
BP	blood pressure
BPH	benign prostatic hypertrophy
BSA	body surface area
BUN	blood urea nitrogen
CABG	coronary artery bypass graft
CAD	coronary artery disease
Cap	capsule or gelcap
CAP	community-acquired pneumonia
CBC	complete blood count
CF	cystic fibrosis
CHF	congestive heart failure
cm	centimeter
CMV	cytomegalovirus
C_{max}	peak plasma concentration
CNS	central nervous system
COPD	chronic obstructive pulmonary disease
CrCl	creatinine clearance
Cre	cream
CRF	chronic renal failure

(Continued)

ABBREVIATIONS	DESCRIPTIONS
CSF	cerebrospinal fluid
CVA	cerebrovascular accident
CVD	cardiovascular disease
CYP450	cytochrome P450
d/c or D/C	discontinue
DHEA	dehydroepiandrosterone
DM	diabetes mellitus
DVT	deep vein thrombosis
ECG	electrocardiogram
EEG	electroencephalogram
eg	for example
EPS	extrapyramidal symptom
ESRD	end-stage renal disease
FPG	fasting plasma glucose
FSH	follicle-stimulating hormone
g	gram
GABA	gamma-aminobutyric acid
GAD	general anxiety disorder
GERD	gastroesophageal reflux disease
GFR	glomerular filtration rate
GI	gastrointestinal
GnRH	gonadotropin-releasing hormone
GVHD	graft versus host disease
HCG	human chorionic gonadotropin
Hct	hematocrit
HCTZ	hydrochlorothiazide
HDL	high-density lipoprotein
Hgb	hemoglobin
HIV	human immunodeficiency virus
HMG-CoA	3-hydroxy-3-methylglutaryl-coenzyme A
HR	heart rate
hr or hrs	hour or hours
hs	bedtime
HSV	herpes simplex virus
HTN	hypertension
IBD	inflammatory bowel disease
IBS	irritable bowel syndrome
ICH	intracranial hemorrhage
ICP	intracranial pressure
IM	intramuscular
INH	isoniazid
Inj	injection
INR	international normalized ratio
IOP	intraocular pressure
IU*	international units
IV	intravenous/intravenously
K+	potassium
kg	kilogram
KIU	kallikrein inhibitor unit
L	liter
lbs	pounds
LD	loading dose
LDL	low-density lipoprotein
LFT	liver function test

(Continued)

ABBREVIATIONS	DESCRIPTIONS
LH	luteinizing hormone
LHRH	luteinizing-hormone releasing hormone
Lot	lotion
Loz	lozenge
LVH	left ventricular hypertrophy
M	molar
MAC	mycobacterium avium complex
Maint	maintenance
MAOI	monoamine oxidase inhibitor
Max	maximum
mcg	microgram
mEq	milli-equivalent
mg	milligram
MI	myocardial infarction
min	minute (usually as mL/min)
mL	milliliter
mm	millimeter
mM	millimolar
MRI	magnetic resonance imaging
MS	multiple sclerosis
msec	millisecond
MTX	methotrexate
Na	sodium
NaCl	sodium chloride
NG	nasogastric
NKA	no known allergies
NMS	neuroleptic malignant syndrome
NPO	nothing by mouth
NSAID	nonsteroidal anti-inflammatory drug
NV or N/V	nausea and vomiting
OA	osteoarthritis
OCD	obsessive-compulsive disorder
od	right eye
Oint	ointment
os	left eye
ou	each eye
PAT	paroxysmal atrial tachycardia
pc	after meals
PCN	penicillin
PCP	*Pneumocystis carinii* pneumonia
PD	Parkinson's disease
PID	pelvic inflammatory disease
pkt, pkts	packet, packets
pm	evening
po or PO	orally
PONV	postoperative nausea and vomiting
pr	rectally
prn	as needed
PSA	prostate-specific antigen
PSVT	paroxysmal supraventricular tachycardia
PT	prothrombin time
PTSD	post-traumatic stress disorder
PTT	partial thromboplastin time
PTU	propylthiouracil

ABBREVIATIONS	DESCRIPTIONS
PUD	peptic ulcer disease
PVD	peripheral vascular disease
q4h, q6h, q8h, etc.	every four hours, every six hours, every eight hours, etc.
qd*	once daily
qh	every hour
qid	four times daily
qod*	every other day
qs	a sufficient quantity
qs ad	a sufficient quantity up to
RA	rheumatoid arthritis
RBC	red blood cells
RDS	respiratory distress syndrome
REM	rapid eye movement
SAH	subarachnoid hemorrhage
SBP	systolic blood pressure
sec	second(s)
SGOT	serum glutamic-oxaloacetic transaminase (AST)
SGPT	serum glutamic-pyruvic transaminase (ALT)
SIADH	syndrome of inappropriate antidiuretic hormone secretion
SLE	systemic lupus erythematosus
SOB	shortness of breath
Sol	solution
SQ, SC	subcutaneous
SrCr	serum creatinine
SSRI	selective serotonin reuptake inhibitor
SSSI	skin and skin structure infection
STD	sexually transmitted disease
Sup or supp	suppository
Sus	suspension
SVT	supraventricular tachycardia
$T_{1/2}$	half-life
Tab	tablet or caplet
Tab, SL	sublingual tablet
TB	tuberculosis
TBG	thyroxine binding globulin
tbl or tbsp	tablespoonful
TCA	tricyclic antidepressant
TD	tardive dyskinesia
TFT	thyroid function test
TG	triglyceride
tid	three times daily
T_{max}	time to maximum concentration
TNF	tumor necrosis factor
TPN	total parenteral nutrition
TSH	thyroid stimulating hormone
tsp	teaspoonful
TTP	thrombotic thrombocytopenic purpura

(Continued)

ABBREVIATIONS	DESCRIPTIONS
U*	unit
ud	as directed
ULN	upper limit of normal
URTI/URI	upper respiratory tract infection
UTI	urinary tract infection
UV	ultraviolet
WBC	white blood cell count
V_d	volume of distribution
VTE	venous thromboembolism
X	times (eg, >2X ULN)
yr or yrs	year or years

* According to JCAHO these abbreviations are not recommended for use and should be written out to reduce errors.

CALCULATIONS AND FORMULAS

WEIGHTS AND MEASURES

METRIC MEASURES

1 kilogram (kg)	1000 g
1 gram (g)	1000 mg
1 milligram (mg)	0.001 g
1 microgram (mcg or µg)	0.001 mg; 1 x 10⁻⁶ g
1 liter (L)	1000 mL
1 milliliter (mL)	0.001 L; 1 cc (cubic centimeter)

APOTHECARY MEASURES (AP)

1 scruple	20 grains (gr)
1 drachm	3 scruples; 60 gr
1 ounce (oz)	8 drachms; 24 scruples; 480 gr
1 pound (lb)	12 oz; 96 drachms; 288 scruples; 5760 gr

U.S. FLUID MEASURES

1 fluidrachm	60 minim
1 fluid ounce	8 fluidrachm; 480 minim
1 pint (pt)	16 fl oz; 7680 minim
1 quart (qt)	2 pt; 32 fl oz
1 gallon (gal)	4 qt; 128 fl oz

AVOIRDUPOIS WEIGHT (AV)

1 ounce	437.5 gr
1 pound	16 oz

CONVERSION FACTORS

1 gram	15.4 gr
1 grain	64.8 mg
1 ounce (Av)	28.35 g; 437.5 gr
1 ounce (Ap)	31.1 g; 480 gr
1 pound (Av)	453.6 g; 2.68 lb (Ap); 2.20 lb (Av)
1 fluid ounce	29.57 mL
1 fluidrachm	3.697 mL
1 minim	0.06 mL

COMMON MEASURES

1 teaspoonful	5 mL; ⅛ fl oz
1 tablespoonful	15 mL; ½ fl oz
1 wineglassful	60 mL; 2 fl oz
1 teacupful	120 mL; 4 fl oz
1 gallon	3800 mL; 128 fl oz
1 quart	960 mL; 32 fl oz
1 pint	480 mL; 16 fl oz (exactly 473.2 mL)
8 fluid ounces	240 mL
4 fluid ounces	120 mL
2.2 lb	1 kg

DOSE EQUIVALENTS

WEIGHT (METRIC)	WEIGHT (APOTHECARY)
30 g	1 ounce
15 g	4 drams
10 g	2 ½ drams
7.5 g	2 drams
6 g	90 grains
5 g	75 grains
4 g	60 grains; 1 dram
3 g	45 grains
2 g	30 grains; ½ dram
1.5 g	22 grains
1 g	15 grains
750 mg	12 grains
600 mg	10 grains
500 mg	7 ½ grains
400 mg	6 grains
300 mg	5 grains
250 mg	4 grains

(Continued)

DOSE EQUIVALENTS *(Continued)*	
WEIGHT (METRIC)	**WEIGHT (APOTHECARY)**
200 mg	3 grains
150 mg	2 ½ grains
125 mg	2 grains
100 mg	1 ½ grains
75 mg	1 ¼ grains
60 mg	1 grain
50 mg	¾ grain
40 mg	⅔ grain
30 mg	½ grain
25 mg	⅜ grain
20 mg	⅓ grain
15 mg	¼ grain
12 mg	⅕ grain
10 mg	⅙ grain
8 mg	⅛ grain
6 mg	¹/₁₀ grain
5 mg	¹/₁₂ grain
4 mg	¹/₁₅ grain
3 mg	¹/₂₀ grain
2 mg	¹/₃₀ grain
1.5 mg	¹/₄₀ grain
1.2 mg	¹/₅₀ grain
1 mg	¹/₆₀ grain
LIQUID MEASURES (METRIC)	**LIQUID MEASURES (APOTHECARY)**
1000 mL	1 quart
750 mL	1 ½ pints
500 mL	1 pint
230 mL	8 fluid ounces
200 mL	7 fluid ounces
100 mL	3 ½ fluid ounces
50 mL	1 ¾ fluid ounces
30 mL	1 fluid ounce
15 mL	4 fluid drams
10 mL	2 ½ fluid drams
8 mL	2 fluid drams
5 mL	1 ¼ fluid drams
4 mL	1 fluid dram
3 mL	45 minims
2 mL	30 minims
1 mL	15 minims
0.75 mL	12 minims
0.6 mL	10 minims
0.5 mL	8 minims
0.3 mL	5 minims
0.25 mL	4 minims
0.2 mL	3 minims
0.1 mL	1 ½ minims
0.06 mL	1 minim
0.05 mL	¾ minim
0.03 mL	½ minim

MILLIEQUIVALENT (mEq) AND MILLIMOLE (mmol)

CALCULATIONS

moles = $\dfrac{\text{weight of a substance (grams)}}{\text{molecular weight of that substance (grams)}}$	**OR**	$= \dfrac{\text{equivalent}}{\text{valence of ion}}$	
millimoles = $\dfrac{\text{weight of a substance (milligrams)}}{\text{molecular weight of that substance (milligrams)}}$	**OR**	$= \dfrac{\text{milliequivalents}}{\text{valence of ion}}$	**OR** $= \text{moles x 1000}$
equivalents = moles x valence of ion			
milliequivalents = millimoles x valence of ion	**OR**	= equivalents x 1000	

(Continued)

CONVERSIONS

mg/100mL to mEq/L	$mEq/L = \dfrac{(mg/100mL) \times 10 \times valence}{atomic\ weight}$
mEq/L to mg/100mL	$mg/100mL = \dfrac{(mEq/L) \times atomic\ weight}{10 \times valence}$
mEq/L to volume percent of a gas	$volume\ \% = \dfrac{(mEq/L) \times 22.4}{10}$

ACID-BASE ASSESSMENT

DEFINITIONS

PIO_2	Oxygen partial pressure of inspired gas (mmHg); 150 mmHg in room air at sea level
FiO_2	Fractional pressure of oxygen in inspired gas (0.21 in room air)
PAO_2	Alveolar oxygen partial pressure
$PACO_2$	Alveolar carbon dioxide partial pressure
PaO_2	Arterial oxygen partial pressure
$PaCO_2$	Arterial carbon dioxide partial pressure
R	Respiratory exchange quotient (typically 0.8, increases with high carbohydrate diet, decreases with high fat diet)

HENDERSON-HASSELBALCH EQUATION

$pH = 6.1 + \log [HCO_3^- / (0.03) (pCO_2)]$

ALVEOLAR GAS EQUATION

$PIO_2 = FiO_2 \times$ (total atmospheric pressure - vapor pressure of H_2O at 37°C)
$\quad\quad = FiO_2 \times$ (760 mmHg - 47 mmHg)
$PaO_2 = PIO_2 - PaCO_2/R$

ALVEOLAR/ARTERIAL OXYGEN GRADIENT

$PAO_2 - PaO_2$

ACID-BASE DISORDERS

Disorder	pH	HCO_3^-	PCO_2	Compensation
Metabolic acidosis	< 7.35	Primary decrease	Compensatory decrease	1.2-mmHg decrease in PCO_2 for every 1-mmol/L decrease in HCO_3^- **or** $PCO_2 = (1.5 \times HCO_3^-) + 8\ (\pm 2)$ **or** $PCO_2 = HCO_3^- + 15$ **or** $PCO_2 =$ last 2 digits of pH x 100
Metabolic alkalosis	> 7.45	Primary increase	Compensatory increase	0.6-0.75 mmHg increase in PCO_2 for every 1-mmol/L increase in HCO_3^-. PCO_2 should not rise above 60 mm Hg in compensation.
Respiratory acidosis	< 7.35	Compensatory increase	Primary increase	*Acute:* 1-2 mmol decrease in HCO_3^-. for every 10-mmHg decrease in PCO_2. *Chronic:* 3-4 mmol increase in HCO_3^-. for every 10-mmHg increase in PCO_2.
Respiratory alkalosis	> 7.45	Compensatory decrease	Primary decrease	*Acute:* 1-2 mmol increase in HCO_3^-. for every 10-mmHg increase in PCO_2. *Chronic:* 4-5 mmol decrease in HCO_3^-. for every 10-mmHg decrease in PCO_2.

ACID-BASE EQUATION

H^+ (in mEq/L) = (24 x $PaCO_2$) divided by HCO_3^-

(Continued)

OTHER CALCULATIONS

ANION GAP

Anion gap = Na^+ - (Cl^- + HCO_3^- measured)

ALVEOLAR-ARTERIAL GRADIENT

Aa gradient [(713) (FiO_2 - ($PaCO_2$ divided by 0.8))] - PaO_2

OSMOLALITY

Definition:
Osmolality is a measure of the total number of particles in a solution.

U.S. units (sodium as mEq/L, BUN (blood urea nitrogen) and glucose as (mg/dL)
Plasma osmolality (mOsm/kg) = 2([Na^+] + [K^+]) + ([BUN]/2.8) + ([glucose]/18)

SI units (all variables in mmol/L):
Plasma osmolality (mOsm/kg) = 2[Na^+] + [urea] + [glucose]
Normal range plasma osmolality: 280 - 303 mOsm/kg

Corrected Sodium
Corrected Na+ = measured Na^+ + [1.5 x (glucose - 150 divided by 100)]*
*Do not correct for glucose <150.

Total Serum Calcium Corrected for Albumin Level
[(Normal albumin - patient's albumin) x 0.8] + patient's measured total calcium

Water Deficit
Water deficit = 0.6 x body weight [1 - (140 divided by Na^+)]*
*Body weight is estimated weight in kg; Na^+ is serum or plasma sodium.

Bicarbonate Deficit
HCO_3^- deficit = [0.4 x weight (kg)] x (HCO_3^- desired - HCO_3^- measured)

CHILD-PUGH SCORE

The Child-Pugh classification is used to assess the prognosis of chronic liver disease, mainly cirrhosis. Child-Pugh is also used to determine the required strength of treatment and the necessity of liver transplantation.
Score:
The score employs five clinical measures of liver disease. Each measure is scored 1-3, with 3 indicating the most severe derangement.

Measure	1 point	2 points	3 points	Units
Bilirubin (total)*	<34 (<2)	34-50 (2-3)	>50 (>3)	mol/L (mg/dL)
Serum albumin	>35	28-35	<28	mg/L
INR**	<1.7	1.71-2.20	>2.20	no unit
Ascites	None	Suppressed with medication	Refractory	no unit
Hepatic encephalopathy	None	Grade I-II (or suppressed with medication)	Grade III-IV (or refractory)	no unit

* In primary sclerosing cholangitis and primary biliary cirrhosis, the bilirubin references are changed to reflect the fact that these diseases feature high conjugated bilirubin levels. The upper limit for 1 point is 68 mol/L (4 mg/dL) and the upper limit for 2 points is 170 mol/L (10 mg/dL).

** Some older reference works substitute PT prolongation for INR.

Interpretation:
Chronic liver disease is classified into Child-Pugh class A to C, employing the added score from above.

Points	Class	One-year survival	Two-year survival
5-6	A	100%	85%
7-9	B	81%	57%
10-15	C	45%	35%

CREATININE CLEARANCE

Clinically, creatinine clearance is a useful measure for estimating the glomerular filtration rate (GFR) of the kidneys.

Factors	Abbreviations
Creatinine clearance	Cl_{Cr}
Plasma creatinine concentration	P_{Cr}
Serum creatinine concentration	S_{Cr}
Urine creatinine concentration	U_{Cr}
Urine flow rate	V

(Continued)

CREATININE CLEARANCE (Continued)

Calculations:

$$Cl_{Cr} = \frac{U_{Cr} \times V}{P_{Cr}}$$

Example:
Patient with P_{Cr} 1 mg/dL, U_{Cr} 60 mg/dL, and V of 0.5 dL/hr.

$$Cl_{Cr} = \frac{60 \text{ mg/dL} \times 0.5 \text{ dL/hr}}{1 \text{ mg/dL}} = 30 \text{ dL/hr}$$

Cockcroft-Gault formula: Estimates creatinine clearance (mL/min).

Male:

$$Cl_{Cr} = \frac{(140 - \text{age}) \times \text{mass (kg)}}{72 \times S_{Cr} \text{ (mg/dL)}}$$

Example:
Male patient, 67 years of age, weight 75 kg, and S_{Cr} 1 mg/dL.

$$Cl_{Cr} = \frac{(140 - 67) \times 75}{72 \times 1} = 76 \text{ mL/min}$$

Female:

$$Cl_{Cr} = \frac{(140 - \text{age}) \times \text{mass (kg)} \times 0.85}{72 \times S_{Cr} \text{ (mg/dL)}}$$

Example:
Female patient, 67 years of age, weight 75 kg, and S_{Cr} 1 mg/dL.

$$Cl_{Cr} = \frac{(140 - 67) \times 75}{72 \times 1} \times 0.85 = 64.6 \text{ mL/min}$$

Note: Using actual body weight (ABW) in obese patients can significantly overestimate creatinine clearance. Adjusted ideal body weight (IBW) can provide a more approximate estimate. Adjusted IBW = IBW + 0.4 (ABW - IBW).

BASAL ENERGY EXPENDITURE (BEE)

Basal energy expenditure: the amount of energy required to maintain the body's normal metabolic activity (eg, respiration, maintenance of body temperature, etc).

H = height (cm), W = weight (kg), A = age (years)

Male:
BEE = 66.67 + 13.75W + 5H - 6.76A

Female:
BEE = 665.1 + 9.56W + 1.85H - 4.68A

BODY MASS INDEX (BMI)

$$BMI = \frac{\text{weight (kg)}}{[\text{height (m)}]^2}$$

BODY SURFACE AREA (BSA)

$$BSA \text{ (m}^2) = \sqrt{\frac{\text{height (in)} \times \text{weight (lb)}}{3131}} \quad \textbf{OR} \quad BSA \text{ (m}^2) = \sqrt{\frac{\text{height (cm)} \times \text{weight (kg)}}{3600}}$$

IDEAL BODY WEIGHT (IBW)

Adults (18 years and older; IBW is in kg):
IBW (male) = 50 + (2.3 x height [inches] over 5 feet)
IBW (female) = 45.5 + (2.3 x height [inches] over 5 feet)

Children (IBW is in kg; height is in cm):
1-18 years of age:

$$IBW = \frac{(\text{height}^2 \times 1.65)}{100}$$

5 feet and taller:
IBW (male) = 39 + (2.27 x height [inches] over 5 feet)
IBW (female) = 42.2 + (2.27 x height [inches] over 5 feet)

(Continued)

POUNDS/KILOGRAM CONVERSION

1 pound = 0.45359 kilogram				1 kilogram = 2.2 pounds			
lb	kg	lb	kg	lb	kg	lb	kg
1	0.45	105	47.63	210	95.25	315	142.88
5	2.27	110	49.89	215	97.52	320	145.15
10	4.54	115	52.16	220	99.79	325	147.42
15	6.80	120	54.43	225	102.06	330	149.68
20	9.07	125	56.70	230	104.33	335	151.95
25	11.34	130	58.97	235	106.59	340	154.22
30	13.61	135	61.23	240	108.86	345	156.49
35	15.88	140	63.50	245	111.13	350	158.76
40	18.14	145	65.77	250	113.40	355	161.02
45	20.41	150	68.04	255	115.67	360	163.29
50	22.68	155	70.31	260	117.93	365	165.56
55	24.95	160	72.57	265	120.20	370	167.83
60	27.22	165	74.84	270	122.47	375	170.10
65	29.48	170	77.11	275	124.74	380	172.36
70	31.75	175	79.38	280	127.01	385	174.63
75	34.02	180	81.65	285	129.27	390	176.90
80	36.29	185	83.91	290	131.54	395	179.17
85	38.56	190	86.18	295	133.81	400	181.44
90	40.82	195	88.45	300	136.08	405	183.70
95	43.09	200	90.72	305	138.34	410	185.97
100	45.36	205	92.99	310	140.61	415	188.24

TEMPERATURE CONVERSION

Fahrenheit to Celsius = (°F - 32) x 5/9 = °C				Celsius to Fahrenheit = (°C x 9/5) + 32 = °F			
°F	°C	°F	°C	°C	°F	°C	°F
0.0	-17.8	92.0	33.3	0.0	32.0	49.0	120.2
5.0	-15.0	93.0	33.9	5.0	41.0	50.0	122.0
10.0	-12.2	94.0	34.4	10.0	50.0	51.0	123.8
15.0	-9.4	95.0	35.0	15.0	59.0	52.0	125.6
20.0	-6.7	96.0	35.6	20.0	68.0	53.0	127.4
25.0	-3.9	97.0	36.1	25.0	77.0	54.0	129.2
30.0	-1.1	98.0	36.7	30.0	86.0	55.0	131.0
35.0	1.7	98.6	37.0	35.0	95.0	56.0	132.8
40.0	4.4	99.0	37.2	36.0	96.8	57.0	134.6
45.0	7.2	100.0	37.8	37.0	98.6	58.0	136.4
50.0	10.0	101.0	38.3	38.0	100.4	59.0	138.2
55.0	12.8	102.0	38.9	39.0	102.2	60.0	140.0
60.0	15.6	103.0	39.4	40.0	104.0	65.0	149.0
65.0	18.3	104.0	40.0	41.0	105.8	70.0	158.0
70.0	21.1	105.0	40.6	42.0	107.6	75.0	167.0
75.0	23.9	106.0	41.1	43.0	109.4	80.0	176.0
80.0	26.7	107.0	41.7	44.0	111.2	85.0	185.0
85.0	29.4	108.0	42.2	45.0	113.0	90.0	194.0
90.0	32.2	109.0	42.8	46.0	114.8	95.0	203.0
91.0	32.8	110.0	43.3	47.0	116.6	100.0	212.0
				48.0	118.4	105.0	221.0

(Continued)

PEDIATRIC DOSAGE ESTIMATION FORMULAS

The following formulas can be used to estimate the approximate pediatric dosage of a medication. These formulas are based on the adult dose and either the child's age or weight. These formulas should be used with caution as the response to any drug is not always directly proportional to the age or weight of the child relative to the usual adult dose. Dosage will also vary based on the formula used. Care should be taken when using any of these methods to calculate the child's dosage. Some products have FDA-approved pediatric indications and dosages; always refer to the full prescribing information first before calculating a pediatric dosage.

BASED ON WEIGHT

Augsberger's Rule:

$$\frac{[(1.5 \times \text{weight [kg]}) + 10]}{100} \times \text{adult dose} = \text{approximate child's dose}$$

Example: If the child's weight is 15 kg (33 lb) and the adult dose is 50 mg then the child's dose is 16.25 mg.

$$\frac{[(1.5 \times 15 \text{ kg}) + 10]}{100} \times 50 \text{ mg} = 0.325 \times 50 \text{ mg} = 16.25 \text{ mg}$$

Clark's Rule:

(weight [lb]/150) × adult dose = approximate child's dose

Example: If the child's weight is 15 kg (33 lb) and the adult dose is 50 mg then the child's dose is 11 mg.

(33/150) × 50 mg = 0.22 × 50 mg = 11 mg

BASED ON AGE

Augsberger's Rule:

$$\frac{[(4 \times \text{age [years]}) + 20]}{100} \times \text{adult dose} = \text{approximate child's dose}$$

Example: If the child's age is 8 years and the adult dose is 50 mg then the child's dose is 26 mg.

[(4 × 8) + 20)/100] × 50 mg = 0.52 × 50 mg = 26 mg

Dilling's Rule:

(age [years]/20) × adult dose = approximate child's dose

Example: If the child's age is 8 years and the adult dose is 50 mg then the child's dose is 20 mg.

(8/20) × 50 mg = 0.40 × 50 mg = 20 mg

Cowling's Rule:

$$\frac{[\text{age at next birthday (years)}]}{24} \times \text{adult dose} = \text{approximate child's dose}$$

Example: If the child is going to turn 8 years old in a few months and the adult dose is 50 mg then the child's dose is 16.7 mg. (8/24) × 50 mg = 0.33 × 50 mg = 16.7 mg

Young's Rule:

$$\frac{[\text{age (years)}]}{\text{age} + 12} \times \text{adult dose} = \text{approximate child's dose}$$

Example: If the child's age is 8 years and the adult dose is 50 mg then the child's dose is 20 mg.

[8/(8+12)] × 50 mg = 0.4 × 50 mg = 20 mg

Fried's Rule (younger than 1 year):

$$\frac{[\text{age (months)}]}{150} \times \text{adult dose} = \text{approximate infant's dose}$$

Example: If the child's age is 10 months and the adult dose is 50 mg then the child's dose is 3.33 mg.

(10/150) × 50 mg = 0.067 × 50 mg = 3.33 mg

TABLES FOR PHARMACY CALCULATIONS

WEIGHTS AND MEASURES

Metric Measure
Weight

1 kilogram (kg)	=	1,000 g
1 gram (g)	=	1,000 mg
1 milligram (mg)	=	0.001 g
1 microgram (mcg)	=	0.001 mg
1 gamma	=	1 mcg

Liquid

1 liter (L)	=	1,000 mL
1 milliliter (mL)	=	1 cc (cubic centimeter)

Apothecary (Ap)
Weight

1 scruple	=	20 grains (gr)
1 drachm	=	3 scruples
	=	60 gr
1 ounce (oz)	=	8 drachms
	=	24 scruples
	=	480 gr
1 pound (lb)	=	16 oz
	=	96 drachms
	=	288 scruples
	=	5,760 gr

U.S. Fluid Measure

1 fluidrachm	=	60 minim (min)
1 fluid ounce	=	8 fld drachm
	=	480 min
1 pint (pt)	=	16 fl oz
	=	7,680 min
1 quart (qt)	=	2 pt
	=	32 fl oz
1 gallon (gal)	=	4 qts
	=	128 fl oz

Avoirdupois (Av)
Weight

1 ounce	=	437.5 gr
1 pound	=	16 oz

Conversion Factors

1 gram	=	15.4 gr
1 grain	=	64.8 mg
1 ounce (Av)	=	28.35 g
	=	437.5 gr
1 ounce (Ap)	=	31.1 g
	=	480 gr
1 pound (Av)	=	453.6 g
1 kilogram	=	2.68 pounds Ap
	=	2.20 lbs Av
1 fluid ounce	=	29.57 mL
1 fluidrachm	=	3.697 mL
1 minim	=	0.06 mL

Converting °F to °C
For °F to °C, the formula is:
$$°C = \tfrac{5}{9}(°F - 32)$$
For °C to °F, the formula is:
$$°F = (\tfrac{9}{5} \times °C) + 32$$

Common Measures

1 teaspoonful	=	5 mL
	=	⅙ fl oz
1 tablespoonful	=	15 mL
	=	½ fl oz
1 wineglassful	=	60 mL
	=	2 fl oz
1 teacupful	=	120 mL
	=	4 fl oz

TABLE OF SATURATED SOLUTIONS

This table shows the quantity of the substance and milliliters (mL) of water for 100 mL of a saturated solution at about 25° C.

Substance	Gram	mL Water
Alum	13.00	92.0
Ammonium Carbonate	22.00	88.0
Ammonium Chloride	28.30	79.3
Ammonium Nitrate	90.20	41.8
Ammonium Sulfate	53.10	71.7
Borax	5.90	98.0
Boric Acid	5.10	97.0
Calcium Lactate	5.00	96.0
Chloral Hydrate	120.00	31.0
Citric Acid	88.60	42.7
Copper Sulfate	22.30	98.7
Dextrose	59.00	60.0
Ferric Chloride	125.00	29.0
Ferrous Sulfate	52.80	72.7
Lactose	17.00	90.0
Lead Acetate	55.00	79.0
Lithium Chloride	59.50	70.2
Lithium Sulfate	33.00	88.5
Magnesium Sulfate	72.00	58.5
Manganese Chloride	90.00	54.0
Mercuric Chloride	6.96	98.5
Methylene Blue	4.30	97.0
Oxalic Acid	10.30	94.2
Potassium Bromide	56.00	82.0
Potassium Carbonate	82.20	73.5
Potassium Chloride	8.41	96.6
Potassium Citrate	92.00	56.5
Potassium Iodide	103.20	69.1
Potassium Nitrate	33.40	86.0
Potassium Permanganate	7.43	97.3
Resorcinol	67.20	47.2
Rochelle Salt	51.90	78.8
Silver Nitrate	164.00	65.5
Sodium Acetate	65.00	53.0
Sodium Benzoate	41.50	73.9
Sodium Bicarbonate	8.80	97.6
Sodium Bromide	73.00	78.0
Sodium Carbonate	27.50	96.0
Sodium Chloride	31.50	88.1
Sodium Citrate	55.50	72.5
Sodium Iodide	124.30	67.7
Sodium Nitrate	62.30	73.8
Sodium Salicylate	67.00	58.0
Sodium Sulfate	33.30	87.0
Sodium Thiocyanate	87.00	51.0
Sodium Thiosulfate	93.00	46.0
Tartaric Acid	76.90	54.7
Urea	62.00	53.5
Zinc Sulfate	93.00	56.0

DOSE EQUIVALENTS

These approximate dose equivalents have been adopted by U.S.P. XXII, N.F. XVII. They are approved by the Food and Drug Administration.

When converting specific quantities of a prescription that requires compounding, or when converting a pharmaceutical formula from one system of weights or measures to the other, the following must be used.

Weight

Metric	Apothecary
030 g	1 ounce
015 g	4 drachms
010 g	2½ drachms
07.5 g	2 drachms
006 g	90 grains
005 g	75 grains
004 g	60 grains (1 drachm)
003 g	45 grains
002 g	30 grains (½ drachm)
01.5 g	22 grains
001 g	15 grains
750 mg	12 grains
600 mg	10 grains
500 mg	7½ grains
400 mg	6 grains
300 mg	5 grains
250 mg	4 grains
200 mg	3 grains
150 mg	2½ grains
125 mg	2 grains
100 mg	1½ grains
75 mg	1¼ grains
60 mg	1 grain
50 mg	¾ grain
40 mg	⅔ grain
30 mg	½ grain
25 mg	⅜ grain
20 mg	⅓ grain
15 mg	¼ grain
12 mg	⅕ grain
10 mg	⅙ grain
08 mg	⅛ grain
06 mg	¹/₁₀ grain
05 mg	¹/₁₂ grain
04 mg	¹/₁₅ grain
03 mg	¹/₂₀ grain
02 mg	¹/₃₀ grain
1.5 mg	¹/₄₀ grain
1.2 mg	¹/₅₀ grain
01 mg	¹/₆₀ grain

(Continued)

TABLES FOR PHARMACY CALCULATIONS

Liquid Measure					
Metric	**Apothecary**	0030 mL	1 fluid ounce	00.6 mL	10 minims
		0015 mL	4 fluidrachms	00.5 mL	8 minims
1000 mL	1 quart	0010 mL	2½ fluidrachms	00.3 mL	5 minims
0750 mL	1½ pints	0008 mL	2 fluidrachms	0.25 mL	4 minims
0500 mL	1 pint	0005 mL	1¼ fluidrachms	00.2 mL	3 minims
0250 mL	8 fluid ounces	0004 mL	1 fluidrachm	00.1 mL	1½ minims
0200 mL	7 fluid ounces	0003 mL	45 minims	0.06 mL	1 minim
0100 mL	3½ fluid ounces	0002 mL	30 minims	0.05 mL	¾ minim
0050 mL	1¾ fluid ounces	0001 mL	15 minims	0.03 mL	½ minim
		0.75 mL	12 minims		

POISON CONTROL CENTERS

The American Association of Poison Control Centers (AAPCC) uses a single, nationwide emergency number to automatically link callers with their regional poison center. This toll-free number, **800-222-1222**, also works for **teletype lines (TTY)** for the hearing-impaired and **telecommunication devices (TDD)** for individuals who are deaf. However, a few local poison centers and the ASPCA/Animal Poison Control Center are not part of this nationwide system and continue to use separate numbers.

Most of the centers listed below are accredited by the AAPCC. **Certified centers are marked by an asterisk after the name.** Each has to meet certain criteria. It must, for example, serve a large geographic area; it must be open 24 hours a day and provide direct-dial or toll-free access; it must be supervised by a medical director; and it must have registered pharmacists or nurses available to answer questions from the public.

Within each state, centers are listed alphabetically by city. Some state poison centers also list their original emergency numbers (including TTY/TDD) that only work within that state. For these listings, callers may use either the state number or the nationwide 800 number.

ALABAMA

BIRMINGHAM

Regional Poison Control Center (*)
Children's Hospital of Alabama

1600 7th Ave South
Birmingham AL 35233-1711
Business: 205-939-6334
Emergency: 800-222-1222
               800-462-0800 (AL)

www.chsys.org

TUSCALOOSA

Alabama Poison Center (*)

2503 Phoenix Dr
Tuscaloosa AL 35405-8546
Business: 205-345-0600
Emergency: 800-222-1222
               800-462-1222 (AL)

www.alapoisoncenter.org

ALASKA

JUNEAU

Alaska Poison Control System
Section of Injury Prevention and
EMS

410 Willoughby Ave – Room 113
Box 110616
Juneau AK 99811-0616
Business: 907-465-3027
Emergency: 800-222-1222

www.chems.alaska.gov

(PORTLAND, OR)

Oregon Poison Center (*)
Oregon Health and Science
University

3181 SW Sam Jackson Park Rd –
Suite CB550
Portland OR 97239-3011
Business: 503-494-8600
Emergency: 800-222-1222

www.oregonpoison.com

ARIZONA

PHOENIX

Banner Poison Control Center (*)

901 E Willetta St-Suite 200
Phoenix AZ 85006-2767
Business: 602-253-3334
Emergency: 800-222-1222

www.bannerpoisoncontrol.com

TUCSON

Arizona Poison and Drug
Information Center (*)
Arizona Department of Health
Services
University of Arizona College of
Pharmacy

1295 N Martin Ave – Room B308
Tucson AZ 85721-0202
Business: 520.626.6016
Emergency: 800-222-1222
               800-362-0101
               (Tucson)

www.pharmacy.arizona.edu/
outreach/poison

ARKANSAS

LITTLE ROCK

Arkansas Poison and Drug
Information Center (*)
College of Pharmacy – UAMS

4301 W Markham St – MS 522-2
Little Rock AR 72205-7101
Business: 501-686-6161
Emergency: 800-222-1222
               800-376-4766 (AR)
TDD/TTY: 800-641-3805

www.uamshealth.com

ASPCA/Animal Poison Control Center

1717 S Philio Rd – Suite 36
Urbana IL 61802-6044
Business: 217-337-5030
Emergency: 888-426-4435

http://www.aspca.org

CALIFORNIA

FRESNO/MADERA

California Poison Control System
UCSF School of Pharmacy
Fresno/Madera Division (*)
Children's Hospital Central
California

9300 Valley Children's Place – MB 15
Madera CA 93636-8761
Business: 559-622-2300
Emergency: 800-222-1222
               800-876-4766 (CA)
TDD/TTY: 800-972-3323

www.calpoison.org

SACRAMENTO

California Poison Control System
UCSF School of Pharmacy
Sacramento Division (*)
UC Davis Medical Center

2315 Stockton Blvd – Suite 1024
Sacramento CA 95817-2201
Business: 916-227-1400
Emergency: 800-222-1222
               800-876-4766 (CA)
TDD/TTY: 800-972-3323

www.calpoison.org

SAN DIEGO

California Poison Control System
UCSF School of Pharmacy
San Diego Division (*)
UC San Diego Medical Center

200 W Arbor Dr
San Diego CA 92103-8925
Business: 858-715-6300
Emergency: 800-222-1222
               800-876-4766 (CA)
TDD/TTY: 800-972-3323

www.calpoison.org

SAN FRANCISCO

California Poison Control System
UCSF School of Pharmacy
San Francisco Division (*)

UC San Francisco
UCSF Box 1369
San Francisco CA 94143-0001
Business: 415-502-6000
Emergency: 800-222-1222
              800-876-4766 (CA)
TDD/TTY: 800-972-3323
www.calpoison.org

COLORADO

DENVER

Rocky Mountain Poison and Drug Center (*)

Physical Address: 999 Bannock St
Denver CO 80204-4028
Mailing Address: 777 Bannock St –
MC 0180
Denver CO 80204-4507
Business: 303-739-1100
Emergency: 800-222-1222
TDD/TTY: 303-739-1127 (CO)
www.rmpdc.org

CONNECTICUT

FARMINGTON

Connecticut Poison Control Center (*)
University of Connecticut Health Center

263 Farmington Ave
Farmington CT 06030-5365
Business: 860-679-4540
Emergency: 800-222-1222
TDD/TTY: 866-218-5372
http://poisoncontrol.uchc.edu

DELAWARE

(PHILADELPHIA, PA)

The Poison Control Center (*)
Children's Hospital of Philadelphia

34th St & Civic Center Blvd
Philadelphia PA 19104-4399
Business: 215-590-2003
Emergency: 800-222-1222
TDD/TTY: 215-590-8789
www.poisoncontrol.chop.edu

DISTRICT OF COLUMBIA

WASHINGTON, DC

National Capital Poison Center (*)

3201 New Mexico Ave NW –
Suite 310
Washington DC 20016-2739
Business: 202-362-3867
Emergency: 800-222-1222
www.poison.org

FLORIDA

JACKSONVILLE

Florida/USVI Poison Information Center (*)
Jacksonville Division

655 W 8th St – Box C23
Jacksonville FL 32209-6511
Business: 904-244-4465
Emergency: 800-222-1222
http://fpicjax.org

MIAMI

Florida/USVI Poison Information Center (*)
Miami Division

1611 NW 12th Ave – Institute Annex
– 3rd Floor
Miami FL 33136-1005
Business: 305-585-5250
Emergency: 800-222-1222
www.med.miami.edu/poisoncontrol

TAMPA

Florida/USVI Poison Information Center (*)
Tampa Division

Physical Address: 1 Davis Blvd –
Suite 203
Tampa FL 33606-3422
Mailing Address: PO Box 1289
Tampa FL 33601-1289
Business: 813-844-4444
Emergency: 800-222-1222
www.poisoncentertampa.org

GEORGIA

ATLANTA

Georgia Poison Control Center: Metro Atlanta (*)
Hughes Spalding Children's Hospital Emory University at Grady Health System

80 Jesse Hill Jr. Dr SE
PO Box 26066
Atlanta GA 30303-3050
Business: 404-616-1000
Emergency: 800-222-1222
              404-616-9000
              (Atlanta)
TDD: 404-616-9287
www.georgiapoisoncenter.org

HAWAII

(DENVER, CO)

Rocky Mountain Poison and Drug Center (*)

Physical Address: 999 Bannock St
Denver CO 80204-4028
Mailing Address: 777 Bannock St –
MC 0180
Denver CO 80204-4507
Business: 303-739-1100
Emergency: 800-222-1222
TDD/TTY: 303-739-1127 (CO)
www.rmpdc.org

IDAHO

(DENVER, CO)

Rocky Mountain Poison and Drug Center (*)

Physical Address: 999 Bannock St
Denver CO 80204-4028
Mailing Address: 777 Bannock St –
MC 0180
Denver CO 80204-4507
Business: 303-739-1100
Emergency: 800-222-1222
TDD/TTY: 303-739-1127 (CO)
www.rmpdc.org

ILLINOIS

CHICAGO

Illinois Poison Center (*)

222 S Riverside Plaza – Suite 1900
Chicago IL 60606-6010
Business: 312-906-6136
Emergency: 800-222-1222
TDD/TTY: 312-906-6185
www.mchc.org/ipc

INDIANA

INDIANAPOLIS

Indiana Poison Center (*)
Emergency Medicine and Trauma Center
Indiana University Health Methodist Hospital

I-65 at 21st Street
Indianapolis, IN 46206-1367
Business: 317-962-2335
Emergency: 800-222-1222
              800-382-9097 (IN)
              317-962-2323
              (Indianapolis)
TTY   317-929-2336
http://iuhealth.org/metholidst/
poisoning

IOWA

SIOUX CITY

Iowa Statewide Poison Control Center (*)
Iowa Health System and the University of Iowa Hospitals and Clinics

401 Douglas St – Suite 402
Sioux City IA 51101-1471
Business: 712-279-3710
Emergency: 800-222-1222
    712-277-2222 (IA)
www.iowapoison.org

KANSAS

KANSAS CITY

Mid-America Kansas Poison Control Center
University of Kansas Medical Center

3901 Rainbow Blvd – DELP – Room 40403
Kansas City KS 66160-7231
Business: 913-588-6638
Emergency: 800-222-1222
    800-332-6633 (KS)
www.kumed.com/poison

KENTUCKY

LOUISVILLE

Kentucky Regional Poison Center (*)
Kosair Children's Hospital

234 E Gray St – Suite 847
Louisville KY 40202-1909
Business: 502-629-7264
Emergency: 800-222-1222
    502-589-8222 (KY)
www.krpc.com

LOUISIANA

SHREVEPORT

Louisiana Poison Center (*)
LSUHC Shreveport
Emergency Medicine – Clinical Toxicology

1455 Wilkinson St
Shreveport LA 71130-3733
Business: 318-813-3314
Emergency: 800-222-1222
www.ems.lsuhscshreveport.edu/poison-control

MAINE

PORTLAND

Northern New England Poison Center (*)

22 Bramhall St
Portland ME 04102-3134
Business: 207-662-7042
Emergency: 800-222-1222
    800-442-6035 (ME)
    207-871-2879 (ME)
TDD/TTY   207-662-2879 (ME)
www.nnepc.org

MARYLAND

BALTIMORE

Maryland Poison Center (*)
University of Maryland at Baltimore School of Pharmacy

220 Arch St – Office Level 01
Baltimore MD 21201-1531
Business: 410-706-7701
Emergency: 800-222-1222
TDD: 410-528-7530
www.mdpoison.com

(WASHINGTON, DC)

National Capital Poison Center (*)

3201 New Mexico Ave NW – Suite 310
Washington DC 20016-2739
Business: 202-362-3867
Emergency: 800-222-1222
www.poison.org

MASSACHUSETTS

BOSTON

Regional Center for Poison Control and Prevention (*)

300 Longwood Ave
Boston MA 02115-5724
Business: 617-355-6609
Emergency: 800-222-1222
TDD/TTY   888-244-5313
www.maripoisoncenter.com

MICHIGAN

DETROIT

Regional Poison Control Center (*)
Children's Hospital of Michigan

4160 John R Harper Professional Office Bldng – Ste 616
Detroit MI 48201-2022
Business: 313-745-5335
Emergency: 800-222-1222
    313-745-5711
    [Detroit]
www.mitoxic.org/pcc

MINNESOTA

MINNEAPOLIS

Minnesota Poison Control System (*)
Hennepin County Medical Center

701 Park Avenue, Mail Code RL
Minneapolis, MN 55415-1623
Business: 612-873-3144
Emergency: 800-222-1222
www.mnpoison.org

MISSISSIPPI

JACKSON

Mississippi Regional Poison Control Center
University of Mississippi Medical Center

2500 N State St
Jackson MS 39216-4500
Business: 601-984-1680
Emergency: 800-222-1222
http://poisoncontrol.umc.edu

MISSOURI

ST LOUIS

Missouri Regional Poison Center (*)

7980 Clayton Rd – Suite 200
St Louis MO 63117-1354
Business: 314-772-8300
Emergency: 800-222-1222
www.cardinalglennon.com

MONTANA

(DENVER, CO)

Rocky Mountain Poison and Drug Center (*)

Physical Address: 999 Bannock St
Denver CO 80204-4028
Mailing Address: 777 Bannock St – MC 0180
Denver CO 80204-4507
Business: 303-739-1100
Emergency: 800-222-1222
TDD/TTY: 303-739-1127 (CO)
www.rmpdc.org

NEBRASKA

OMAHA

Nebraska Regional Poison Center (*)

8401 W Dodge Rd – Suite 115
Omaha NE 68114-3494
Business: 402-390-5555
Emergency: 800-222-1222
www.nebraskapoison.com

NEVADA

(DENVER, CO)

Rocky Mountain Poison and Drug Center (*)

Physical Address: 999 Bannock St
Denver CO 80204-4028
Mailing Address: 777 Bannock St –
MC 0180
Denver CO 80204-4507
Business: 303-739-1100
Emergency: 800-222-1222
TDD/TTY: 303-739-1127 (CO)
www.rmpdc.org

NEW HAMPSHIRE

(PORTLAND, ME)

Northern New England Poison Center (*)

22 Bramhall St
Portland ME 04102-3134
Business: 207-662-7042
Emergency: 800-222-1222
www.nnepc.org

NEW JERSEY

NEWARK

New Jersey Poison Information and Education System (*)
UMDNJ

140 Bergen St
PO Box 1709
Newark NJ 07101-2425
Business: 973-972-9280
Emergency: 800-222-1222
TDD/TTY: 973-926-8008
www.njpies.org

NEW MEXICO

ALBUQUERQUE

New Mexico Poison and Drug Information Center (*)

1 University of New Mexico
Albuquerque NM 87131-0001
Business: 505-272-4261
Emergency: 800-222-1222
http://hsc.unm.edu/pharmacy/poison

NEW YORK

NEW YORK CITY

New York City Poison Control Center (*)
NYC Bureau of Public Health

455 1st Ave – Room 123 – Box 81
New York NY 10016-9102
Business: 212-447-8152
English
Emergency: 800-222-1222
               212-340-4494
               212-POISONS
               (212-764-7667)
TDD: 212-689-9014
Spanish
Emergency: 212-venemos
               (212-836-3667)
www.nyc.gov/html/doh/html/poison/
poisons.html

SYRACUSE

Upstate New York Poison Center (*)
SUNY Upstate Medical University

750 E Adams St
Syracuse NY 13210-1834
Business: 315-464-7078
Emergency: 800-222-1222
TTY: 315-464-5424
www.upstatepoison.org

NORTH CAROLINA

CHARLOTTE

Carolinas Poison Center (*)
Carolinas Medical Center

Physical Address: 4400 Golf Acres Dr
– Suite B2
Charlotte NC 28208-5990
Mailing Address: PO Box 32861
Charlotte NC 28232-2861
Business: 704-512-3795
Emergency: 800-222-1222
www.ncpoisoncenter.org

NORTH DAKOTA

(MINNEAPOLIS, MN)

Minnesota Poison Control System (*)
Hennepin County Medical Center

701 Park Avenue, Mail Code RL
Minneapolis, MN 55415-1623
Business: 612-873-3144
Emergency: 800-222-1222
www.mnpoison.org

OHIO

CINCINNATI

Cincinnati Drug and Poison Information Center (*)

3333 Burnett Ave – MLC 9004
Cincinnati OH 45229-3026
Business: 513-636-5063
Emergency: 800-222-1222
               513-558-5111
               (Cincinnati)
www.cincinnatichildrens.org/dpic

CLEVELAND

Greater Cleveland/Northern Ohio Poison Control Center
Rainbow Babies and Children's Hospital

11100 Euclid Ave – B261 MP6007
Cleveland OH 44106-6010
Business: 216-844-1573
Emergency: 800-222-1222
www.uhhospitals.org/rainbow
children/tabid/195/default.aspx

COLUMBUS

Central Ohio Poison Center (*)

700 Children's Dr
Columbus OH 43205-2664
www.bepoisonsmart.com

OKLAHOMA

OKLAHOMA CITY

Oklahoma Poison Control Center (*)
OU Health Science Center

940 NE 13th St – Room 3N3510
Oklahoma City OK 73104-5008
Business: 405-271-5062
Emergency: 800-222-1222
www.oklahomapoison.org

OREGON

PORTLAND

Oregon Poison Center (*)
Oregon Health and Science University

3181 SW Sam Jackson Park Rd –
Suite CB550
Portland OR 97239-3011
Business: 503-494-8600
Emergency: 800-222-1222
www.oregonpoison.com

PENNSYLVANIA

PHILADELPHIA

The Poison Control Center (*)
Children's Hospital of Philadelphia

34th St & Civic Center Blvd
Philadelphia PA 19104-4399
Business: 215-590-2003
Emergency: 800-222-1222
TDD/TTY: 215-590-8789
www.poisoncontrol.chop.edu

PITTSBURGH

Pittsburgh Poison Center (*)
UPMC

200 Lothrop Street - BIR 010701
Pittsburgh, PA 15213-2536
Business: 412-390-3300
Emergency: 800-222-1222
               412-681-6669
               [Pittsburgh]
www.upmc.com/services/
poisoncenter

RHODE ISLAND

(BOSTON, MA)

Regional Center for Poison Control and Prevention (*)

300 Longwood Ave
Boston MA 02115-5724
Business: 617-355-6609
Emergency: 800-222-1222
TDD/TTY   888-244-5313
www.maripoisoncenter.com

SOUTH CAROLINA

COLUMBIA

Palmetto Poison Center (*)
South Carolina College of Pharmacy
University of South Carolina

1215 Blossom St
Columbia SC 29208-2900
Business: 803-777-7909
Emergency: 800-222-1222
http://poisonsc.edu

SOUTH DAKOTA

(MINNEAPOLIS, MN)

Minnesota Poison Control System (*)
Hennepin County Medical Center

701 Park Ave
Minneapolis MN 55415-1623
Business: 612-873-3144
Emergency: 800-222-1222
www.mnpoison.org

TENNESSEE

NASHVILLE

Tennessee Poison Center (*)

501 Oxford House – 1161 21st Ave
Nashville TN 37232-4632
Business: 615-936-0760
Emergency: 800-222-1222
www.tnpoisoncenter.org

TEXAS

AMARILLO

Texas Panhandle Poison Center (*)
Texas Poison Center Network

1501 S Coulter Dr
Amarillo TX 79106-1770
Business: 806-354-1630
Emergency: 800-222-1222
www.poisoncontrol.org

DALLAS

North Texas Poison Center (*)
Texas Poison Center Network
Parkland Memorial Hospital

5201 Harry Hines Blvd
Dallas TX 75235-7708
Business: 214-589-0911
Emergency: 800-222-1222
www.poisoncontrol.org

EL PASO

West Texas Regional Poison Center (*)
Texas Poison Center Network
University Medical Center of El Paso

4815 Alameda Ave
El Paso TX 79905-2705
Business: 915-534-3802
Emergency: 800-222-1222
www.poisoncontrol.org

GALVESTON

Southeast Texas Poison Center (*)
Texas Poison Center Network
The University of Texas Medical Branch

3.112 Trauma Center
Galveston TX 77555-1175
Business: 409-772-3307
Emergency: 800-222-1222
www.utmb.edu/setpc

SAN ANTONIO

South Texas Poison Center (*)
Texas Poison Center Network
The University of Texas Health Science
Center at San Antonio
Department of Surgery

7703 Floyd Curl Dr-MSC 7849
San Antonio TX 78229-3900
Business: 210-567-5762
Emergency: 800-222-1222
www.texaspoison.com

TEMPLE

Central Texas Poison Center (*)
Texas Poison Center Network
Scott & White Memorial Hospital

2401 S 31st St
Temple TX 76808-0001
Business: 254-724-7405
Emergency: 800-222-1222
www.swmail.sw.org

UTAH

SALT LAKE CITY

Utah Poison Control Center (*)
University of Utah

585 Komas Dr – Suite 200
Salt Lake City UT 84108-1234
Business: 801-587-0600
Emergency: 800-222-1222
http://uuhsc.utah.edu/poison

VERMONT

(PORTLAND, ME)

Northern New England Poison Center (*)

22 Bramhall St
Portland ME 04102-3134
Business: 207-662-7042
Emergency: 800-222-1222
www.nnepc.org

VIRGINIA

CHARLOTTESVILLE

Blue Ridge Poison Center (*)
Jefferson Park Place

Physical Address: 1222 Jefferson Pl
Charlottesville VA 22908-0774
Mailing Address: PO Box 800774
Charlottesville VA 22908-0774
Business: 434-924-0347
Emergency: 800-222-1222
www.healthsystem.virginia.edu/brpc

RICHMOND

Virginia Poison Center (*)
Medical College of Virginia Hospitals
Virginia Commonwealth University Health System

Physical Address: 600 E Broad St
Richmond VA 23219-1832
Mailing Address: PO Box 980522
Richmond VA 23298-0522
Bus Emergency: 800-222-1222
www.poison.vcu.edu

WASHINGTON

SEATTLE

Washington Poison Control Center (*)

155 NE 100th St
Seattle WA 98125-8007
Business: 206-517-2350
Emergency: 800-222-1222
www.wapc.org

WEST VIRGINIA

CHARLESTON

West Virginia Poison Center (*)
WVU Charleston Division

3110 MacCorkle Ave SE
Charleston WV 25304-1210
Business: 304-347-1212
Emergency: 800-222-1222
www.wvpoisoncenter.org

WISCONSIN

MILWAUKEE

Wisconsin Poison Center

PO Box 1997 – Mail Station 660
Milwaukee WI 53201-1997
Business: 414-266-6973
Emergency: 800-222-1222
www.wisconsinpoison.org

WYOMING

(OMAHA, NE)

Nebraska Regional Poison Center (*)

8401 W Dodge Rd – Suite 115
Omaha NE 68114-3494
Business: 402-390-5555
Emergency: 800-222-1222
www.nebraskapoison.com

CERTIFICATION PROGRAMS FOR NURSES

Organization	Website
American Nurses Credentialing Center (ANCC)	www.nursecredentialing.org

- Acute Care Nurse Practitioner
- Adult Health Clinical Nurse Specialist (formerly Med-Surg)
- Adult Nurse Practitioner
- Adult Psychiatric & Mental Health Clinical Nurse Specialist
- Adult Psychiatric & Mental Health Nurse Practitioner
- Ambulatory Care Nurse
- Cardiac Rehabilitation Nurse
- Cardiac Vascular Nurse
- Case Management Nurse
- Child/Adolescent Psychiatric & Mental Health Clinical Nurse Specialist
- Clinical Nurse Specialist (CNS) Core Exam
- College Health Nurse
- Community Health Nurse
- Diabetes Management, Advanced
- Family Nurse Practitioner
- Family Psychiatric & Mental Health Nurse Practitioner
- General Nursing Practice
- Gerontological Clinical Nurse Specialist
- Gerontological Nurse
- Gerontological Nurse Practitioner
- High-Risk Perinatal Nurse
- Home Health Clinical Nurse Specialist
- Home Health Nurse
- Informatics Nurse
- Medical-Surgical Nurse
- Nurse Executive (formerly Nursing Administration)
- Nurse Executive, Advanced (formally Nursing Administration, Advanced)
- Nursing Professional Development
- Pain Management
- Pediatric Clinical Nurse Specialist
- Pediatric Nurse
- Pediatric Nurse Practitioner
- Perinatal Nurse
- Psychiatric and Mental Health Nurse
- Public/Community Health Clinical Nurse Specialist
- Public Health Nurse, Advanced
- School Nurse

Organization	Website
American Academy of Medical Esthetic Professionals (AAMEP)	www.amen-usa.org

- Medical Esthetics-Certified (ME-C)

Organization	Website
Association for the Advancement of Medical Instrumentation (AAMI)	www.aami.org

- Biomedical Equipment Technicians (CBET)
- Clinical Laboratory Equipment Specialists (CLES)
- Radiology Equipment Specialists (CRES)

Organization	Website
American Society of Ophthalmic Registered Nurses (ASORN)	http://webeye.ophth.uiowa.edu/asorn

- Ophthalmic Registered Nurses (CORN)

Organization	Website
American Board of Certification for Gastroenterology Nurses (ABCGN)	www.abcgn.org

- Certified Gastroenterology Registered Nurses (CGRN)

Organization	Website
National Council of State Boards of Nursing (NCSBN)	www.ncsbn.org

- Nurse Practitioner Certification
- Nurse Licensure Compact (NLC)

Organization	Website
National Certification Board for Diabetes Educators (NCBDE)	www.ncbde.org

- Certified Diabetes Educator

Organization	Website
Board of Certification for Emergency Nursing (BCEN)	www.ena.org/bcen

- Certified Emergency Nursing (CEN)
- Certified Flight Registered Nurse (CFRN)

Organization	Website
HIV/AIDS Nursing Certification Board (HANCB)	www.hancb.org

- HIV/AIDS Nursing

Organization	Website
Certification Board of Infection Control & Epidemiology (CBIC)	www.cbic.org

- Infectious Disease Nursing

Organization	Website
Infusion Nurses Society (INS) • Infusion Nursing	**www.ins1.org**
National Certification Corporation (NCC) • Inpatient Obstetric (INPT) • Maternal Newborn (MN) • Low-Risk Neonatal (LRN) • Neonatal Intensive Care (NIC) • Neonatal Nurse Practitioner • Women's Health Care Nurse Practitioner • Electronic Fetal Monitoring • Neonatal Pediatric Transport	**www.nccwebsite.org**
Oncology Nursing Certification Corporation • Oncology Certified Nurse (OCN®) • Certified Pediatric Hematology Oncology Nurse (CPHON®) • Advanced Oncology Certified Nurse Practitioner (AOCNP®) • Advanced Oncology Certified Clinical Nurse Specialist (AOCNS®) • Certified Breast Care Nurse (CBCN®) • Certified Pediatric Oncology Nurse (CPON®) • Advanced Oncology Certified Nurse (AOCN®)	**www.oncc.org**
American Academy of Pain Management (AAPM) • Credentialed Pain Practitioner (CPP)	**www.aapainmanage.org**
Competency & Credentialing Institute (CCI) • Perioperative Nursing (CNOR & CRNFA)	**www.cc-institute.org**
American Society of Plastic Surgical Nurses (ASPSN) • Certified Plastic Surgical Nurse (CPSN)	**www.aspsn.org**
American Board of Perianesthesia Nursing Certification (ABPANC) • Certified Post Anesthesia Nurse (CPAN®) • Certified Ambulatory Perianesthesia Nurse (CAPA®)	**www.cpancapa.org**
National Board for Certification of School Nurses (NBCSN) • School Nursing (NBCSN)	**www.nbcsn.com**
Genetic Nursing Credentialing Commission (GNCC) • Advanced Practice Nurse in Genetics (APNG) • Genetics Clinical Nurse (GCN)	**www.geneticnurse.org**
Center for Nursing Education and Testing (C-NET®) • Dermatology Nurses Certification Board (DNCB) • Certified Dermatology Nurse (DNC) • Certified Dermatology Nurse Practitioner (DCNP) • Certified Medical-Surgical Nurse (CMSRN) • Certified Hemodialysis Technician (CCHT) • Certified Dialysis Nurse (CDN) • Certified Nephrology Nurse (CNN) • Certified Nephrology Nurse Practitioner (CNN-NP) • Plastic Surgical Nursing Certification Board (PSNCB) • Radiological Nurse (RNC) • Certified Board for Urology Nurses & Associates (CBUNA) • Certified Board Urology Associate (CUA) • Certified Urology Registered Nurse (CURN) • Certified Urology Nurse Practitioner (CUNP)	**www.cnetnurse.com**
Prepared Childbirth Educators, Inc. • Certified Breastfeeding Counselor (CBC) • Certified Childbirth Educator (CCE) • Certified Labor Support Specialist (CLSS) • Certified Prenatal/Postnatal Fitness Instructor • Certified Infant Massage Instructor/Educator	**www.childbirtheducation.org**
American Association of Nurse Anesthetists • Certified Registered Nurse Anesthetist (CRNA)	**www.aana.com**

PROFESSIONAL ASSOCIATIONS FOR NURSES

COMMUNITY HEALTH

American Academy of Ambulatory Care Nursing
East Holly Ave – Box 56
Pitman NJ 08071-0056
800-262-6877
www.aaacn.org

American Public Health Association
800 I St NW
Washington DC 20001-3710
202-777-APHA (2742)
www.apha.org

CRITICAL CARE

American Association of Critical-Care Nurses
101 Columbia
Aliso Viejo CA 92656-4109
800-899-2226
www.aacn.org

Northeast Pediatric Cardiology Nurses Association
PO Box 261
Brookline MA 02446-0261
www.npcna.org

Society of Critical Care Medicine
500 Midway Dr
Mount Prospect IL 60056-5811
847-827-6869
www.sccm.org

EMERGENCY NURSING

Air & Surface Transport Nurses
7995 E Prentice Ave – Suite 100
Greenwood Village CO 80111-2710
800-897-6362
www.astna.org

Emergency Nurses Association
915 Lee St
Des Plaines IL 60016-6569
800-900-9659
www.ena.org

GERIATRICS

The American Geriatrics Society
The Empire State Building
350 5th Ave – Suite 801
New York NY 10118-0801
212-308-1414
www.americangeriatrics.org

Gerontological Advanced Practice Nurses Association
East Holly Ave – Box 56
Pitman NJ 08071-0056
800-262-6877
www.gapna.org

The Gerontological Society of America
1220 L St NW – Suite 901
Washington DC 20005-4001
202-842-1275
www.geron.org

MIDWIFERY

American College of Nurse-Midwives
8403 Colesville Rd – Suite 1550
Silver Spring MD 20910-6374
240-485-1800
www.acnm.org

NEONATAL

Association of Women's Health, Obstetric & Neonatal Nurses
2000 L St NW – Suite 740
Washington DC 20036-4912
800-673-8499
www.awhonn.org

National Association of Neonatal Nurses
4700 W Lake Ave
Glenview IL 60025-1468
800-451-3795
www.nann.org

NEPHROLOGY

American Nephrology Nurses' Association
East Holly Ave – Box 56
Pitman NJ 08071-0056
800-262-6877
www.annanurse.org

National Kidney Foundation
30 E 33rd St
New York NY 10016-5337
800-622-9010
www.kidney.org

NEUROSCIENCE

American Association of Neuroscience Nurses
4700 W Lake Ave
Glenview IL 60025-1468
800-557-2266
www.aann.org

American Association of Spinal Cord Injury Professionals (Paralyzed Veterans of America)
801 18th St NW
Washington DC 20006-3585
202-416-7704
www.nurses-ascipro.org

ONCOLOGY

Association of Pediatric Hematology/Oncology Nurses
4700 W Lake Ave
Glenview IL 60025-1485
800-375-4724
www.aphon.org

Oncology Nursing Society
125 Enterprise Dr
Pittsburgh PA 15275-1214
866-257-4ONS (4667)
www.ons.org

PALLIATIVE CARE

Hospice and Palliative Nurses Association
One Penn Center West – Suite 229
Pittsburgh PA 15276-0100
412-787-9301
www.hpna.org

PEDIATRICS

Pediatric Nursing Certification Board
800 S Frederick Ave – Suite 204
Gaithersburg MD 20877-4152
888-641-2767
www.pncb.org

PREOPERATIVE & PERIOPERATIVE

American Association of Nurse Anesthetists
222 S Prospect Ave
Park Ridge IL 60068-4037
847-692-7050
www.aana.com

American Society of PeriAnesthesia Nurses
90 Frontage Rd
Cherry Hill NJ 08034-1424
877-737-9696
www.aspan.org

American Society of Plastic Surgical Nurses
7794 Grow Dr
Pensacola FL 32514-7072
800-272-0136
www.aspsn.org

Association of Perioperative Registered Nurses (AORN)
2170 S Parker Rd – Suite 400
Denver CO 80231-5734
800-755-2676
www.aorn.org

PSYCHIATRIC

**American Psychiatric Nurses
Association**
1555 Wilson Blvd – Suite 530
Arlington VA 22209-2405
866-243-2443
www.apna.org

REHABILITATION

Association of Rehabilitation Nurses
4700 W Lake Ave
Glenview IL 60025-1468
800-229-7530
www.rehabnurse.org

SCHOOL NURSING

American School Health Association
4340 East West Hwy – Suite 403
Bethesda MD 20814-4494
301-652-8072
www.ashaweb.org

**National Association of School
Nurses**
8484 Georgia Ave – Suite 420
Silver Spring MD 20910-5623
240-821-1130
www.nasn.org

STATE ASSOCIATIONS/ANESTHETISTS

**California Association of Nurse
Anesthetists**
PO Box 1426
Boyes Hot Springs CA 95416-1426
707-480-0096
www.canainc.org

**Connecticut Association of Nurse
Anesthetists**
377 Research Pkwy – Suite 2D
Meriden CT 06450-7155
203-238-1207
www.ctnurses.org

**New York State Association of Nurse
Anesthetists**
1450 Western Ave – Suite 101
Albany NY 12203-3539
518-861-8876
www.nysana.com

**Pennsylvania Association of Nurse
Anesthetists**
234 N 3rd St
Harrisburg PA 17101-1516
800-495-7262
www.pana.org

**Texas Association of Nurse
Anesthetists**
PO Box 40775
Austin TX 78704-0775
512-495-9004
www.txana.org

STUDENT NURSING

**National Student Nurses'
Association**
45 Main St – Ste 606
Brooklyn NY 11201-1099
718-210-0705
www.nsna.org

WOUND CARE
Wound, Ostomy and Continence
Nurses Society
15000 Commerce Pkwy – Suite C
Mt Laurel NJ 08054-2212
888-224-WOCN (9626)
www.wocn.org

NURSE PRACTITIONER PROGRAMS BY STATE

ALABAMA

University of Alabama-Huntsville
College of Nursing
Nursing Building – Room 207
301 Sparkman Dr NW
Huntsville AL 35899-1911
256-824-6345
http://onlinenurse.nb.uah.edu

ARIZONA

Arizona State University
College of Nursing & Health Innovation
500 N 3rd St
Phoenix AZ 85004-2135
602-496-2264
http://nursingandhealth.asu.edu

University of Arizona
College of Nursing
1305 N Martin St
PO Box 210203
Tucson AZ 85721
520-626-6154
www.nursing.arizona.edu

CALIFORNIA

Azusa Pacific University
School of Nursing
PO Box 7000
Azusa CA 91702-7000
626-815-5386
www.apu.edu/nursing

California State University-Bakersfield
Department of Nursing
9001 Stockdale Hwy – 29RNC
Bakersfield CA 93311-1022
661-654-3110
www.csub.edu/nursing

California State University-Fresno
Department of Nursing
College of Health & Human Services
2345 E San Ramon – M/S MH26
Fresno CA 93740-8031
559-278-4004
www.csufresno.edu/chhs

California State University-Long Beach
Department of Nursing
College of Health & Human Services
1250 Bellflower Blvd
Long Beach CA 90840-0301
562-985-4194
www.csulb.edu/colleges/chhs

Loma Linda University
School of Nursing West Hall
11001 Hill Dr
Loma Linda CA 92354-2725
800-422-4558
909-558-4923
www.llu.edu/llu/nursing

UCLA School of Nursing
Factor Building
700 Tiverton Ave
Los Angeles CA 90095-8361
310-825-7181
www.nursing.ucla.edu

University of California – San Francisco
School of Nursing
2 Koret Way – N319X
UCSF Box 0602
San Francisco CA 94113-0602
415-476-9710
www.nurseweb.ucsf.edu

University of San Diego
Hahn School of Nursing & Health Science
5998 Alcala Park
San Diego CA 92110-8001
619-260-4600
www.sandiego.edu/academics/nursing

University of San Francisco
School of Nursing
2130 Fulton St
San Francisco CA 94117-1080
415-422-6681
www.usfca.edu/nursing

COLORADO

Regis University Loretto Heights
School of Nursing
Rueckert-Hartman College for Health Professions
3333 Regis Blvd – Mail Code G9
Denver CO 80221-1099
303-458-4126
www.regis.edu

University of Colorado Denver
College of Nursing
Campus Box C288 – Education 2 North
13120 E 19th Ave
Aurora CO 80045-2568
303-724-1812
www.nursing.ucdenver.edu

CONNECTICUT

Quinnipiac University
Department of Nursing
275 Mount Carmel Ave
Hamden CT 06518-1908
203-582-5397
www.quinnipiac.edu

Saint Joseph College
Division of Nursing
1678 Asylum Ave
West Hartford CT 06117-2791
860-231-5211
http://www.sjc.edu/academics/schools/school-of-health-and-natural-sciences/nursing/

Yale University
School of Nursing
100 Church St S
PO Box 9740
New Haven CT 06536-0740
203-785-2389
www.nursing.yale.edu

DELAWARE

University of Delaware
College of Health Sciences
School of Nursing
McDowell Hall
25 N College
Newark DE 19716-3799
302-831-1253
www.udel.edu/nursing

DISTRICT OF COLUMBIA

Catholic University of America
School of Nursing
125 Gowan Hall
620 Michigan Ave NE
Washington DC 20064
202-319-5400
http://nursing.cua.edu

Georgetown University
School of Nursing & Health Studies
St Mary's Hall
3700 Reservoir Rd NW at 38th St
PO Box 571107
Washington DC 20057-1107
202-687-4647
http://snhs.georgetown.edu

FLORIDA

Barry University
School of Nursing
11300 NE 2nd Ave
Miami Shores FL 33161-6695
305-899-3800
http://www.barry.edu/nursing

Florida State University
College of Nursing
Vivian M Duxbury Hall
98 Varsity Way
PO Box 3064310
Tallahassee FL 3206-4310
850-644-3296
www.nursing.fsu.edu

University of Miami
School of Nursing & Health Studies
PO Box 248153
Coral Gables FL 33124-8153
305-284-3666
www.miami.edu/sonhs

GEORGIA

Emory University
Nell Hodgson Woodruff School of
Nursing
1520 Clifton Rd NE
Atlanta GA 30322-4207
404-727-7980
www.nursing.emory.edu

Georgia State University
Byrdine F Lewis School of Nursing
PO Box 4019
Atlanta GA 30303-4019
404-413-1200
http://chhs.gsu.edu/nursing

HAWAII

Hawaii Pacific University
School of Nursing
45-045 Kamehameha Hwy
Kaneohe HI 96744-5297
808-236-3552
www.hpu.edu/nursing

IDAHO

Boise State University
Department of Nursing
1910 University Drive
Boise ID 83725-1840
208-426-4143
http://nursing.boisestate.edu

Idaho State University
School of Nursing
921 S 8th Ave – MS 8101
Pocatello ID 83209-8101
208-282-2132
www.isu.edu/nursing

ILLINOIS

De Paul University
Lincoln Park Campus
Department of Nursing
990 W Fullerton Pkwy
Chicago IL 60614
773-325-7280
http://las.depaul.edu/nursing/
Programs/MastersEntryProgram/
index.asp

North Park University
School of Nursing
3225 W Foster Ave
Chicago IL 60625-4895
773-244-5680
http://www.northpark.edu/Academics/
School-of-Nursing

Southern Illinois University –
Edwardsville
School of Nursing
Alumni Hall
PO Box 1066 – Room 2117
Edwardsville IL 62026-2117
800-234-4844
www.siue.edu/nursing

University of Illinois – Chicago
College of Nursing
845 S Damen Ave – MC 802
Chicago IL 60612-3727
312-996-7800
www.uic.edu/nursing

INDIANA

Indiana Wesleyan University – Marion
School of Nursing
4201 S Washington St
Marion IN 46953-4974
888-876-6498
www.indwes.edu/nursing

Purdue University
College of Health and Human
Sciences
School of Nursing
502 N University St
West Lafayette IN 47907-2069
765-494-4004
www.nursing.purdue.edu

KENTUCKY

University of Kentucky
College of Nursing
315 College of Nursing Building
Lexington KY 40536-0232
859-323-5108
www.mc.uky.edu/nursing

LOUISIANA

Louisiana State University
School of Nursing
1900 Gravier St – 4th Floor
New Orleans LA 70112-2262
504-568-4106
http://nursing.lsuhsc.edu

MARYLAND

Johns Hopkins University
School of Nursing
525 N Wolfe St
Baltimore MD 21205-2110
410-955-7548
www.son.jhmi.edu

MASSACHUSETTS

Northeastern University
College of Health Sciences
School of Nursing
102 Robinson Hall
Boston MA 02115-5005
617-373-3649
http://www.northeastern.edu/bouve/
nursing/index.html

University of Massachusetts –
Dartmouth
College of Nursing
285 Old Westport Rd
North Dartmouth MA 02747-2300
508-999-8586
http://umassd.edu/nursing

University of Massachusetts –
Worcester
Graduate School of Nursing
55 Lake Ave N
Worcester MA 01655-0002
508-856-5801
http://www.umassmed.edu/gsn/
index.aspx

MICHIGAN

Michigan State University
College of Nursing
Life Sciences Building A117
East Lansing MI 48824-1317
800-605-6424
www.nursing.msu.edu

University of Michigan
School of Nursing Building
400 N Ingalls
Ann Arbor MI 48109-5482
734-763-5985
www.nursing.umich.edu

University of Michigan – Flint
School of Health Professions &
Studies
2180 William S White Building
303 East Kearsley St
Flint MI 48502-1950
810-237-6503
www.umflint.edu/nursing

MINNESOTA

University of Minnesota
School of Nursing
5-140 Weaver-Densford Hall
308 Harvard St SE
Minneapolis MN 55455-7602
612-624-9600
www.nursing.umn.edu

MISSOURI

Missouri State University
Department of Nursing
Professional Building – Suite 300
901 S National Ave
Springfield MO 65897-0027
417-836-5310
www.missouristate.edu/nursing

Saint Louis University
School of Nursing
3525 Caroline St
St Louis MO 63104-
314-977-8995
www.slu.edu/nursing

University of Missouri – Kansas City
School of Nursing
Health Sciences Building
2464 Charlotte
Kansas City MO 64108-2718
816-235-1700
http://nursing.umkc.edu

NEBRASKA

Creighton University
School of Nursing
2500 California Plaza
Omaha NE 68178-0002
800-544-5071
www.creighton.edu/nursing

NEW JERSEY

The College of New Jersey
Department of Nursing
Paul Loser Hall 206
PO Box 7718
Ewing NJ 08628-0718
609-771-2591
http://www.tcnj.edu/~nursing/
nursing.html

Felician College
Division of Health Sciences
Nursing & Health Management
262 S Main St
Lodi NJ 07644-2117
201-559-6000
www.felician.edu

Monmouth University
School of Nursing & Health Studies
400 Cedar Ave
West Long Branch NJ 07764-1898
732-571-3443
http://www.monmouth.edu/acade-
mics/departments/nursing.asp

Ramapo College of New Jersey
Nursing Programs at Ramapo
School of Theoretical & Applied
Science
505 Ramapo Valley Rd
Mahwah NJ 07430-1623
201-684-7737
www.ramapo.edu/nursing

Rutgers College of Nursing
Ackerson Hall – Room 102
180 University Ave
Newark NJ 07102-
973-353-1157
http://nursing.rutgers.edu

NEW MEXICO

New Mexico State University
School of Nursing
MSC 3185
PO Box 30001
Las Cruces NM 88003-8001
575-646-3812
http://www.nmsu.edu/~nursing/

University of New Mexico
College of Nursing
1 University of New Mexico
MSCO9 5350
Albuquerque NM 87131-0001
505-272-4223
http://hsc.unm.edu/consg

NEW YORK

Adelphia University
School of Nursing
One South Ave
PO Box 0701
Garden City NY 11530-0701
516-877-4540
http://nursing.adelphi.edu

SUNY Binghamton University
Decker School of Nursing
PO Box 6000
Binghamton NY 13902-6000
607-777-4954
http://www.binghamton.edu/dson

College of Mount Saint Vincent
Department of Nursing
6301 Riverdale Ave
Riverdale NY 10471-1046
718-405-3365
http://www.mountsaintvincent.edu/
nursing

Columbia University
School of Nursing
630 W 168th St
PO Box 6
New York NY 10032-0006
212-305-5756
http://cumc.columbia.edu/dept/
nursing

D'Youville College
Nursing Department
320 Porter Ave
Buffalo NY 14201-9985
716-829-7613
http://www.dyc.edu/academics/
nursing/index.asp

Long Island University – Brooklyn
School of Nursing
1 University Plaza
Brooklyn NY 11201-8423
718-488-1508
http://www.liu.edu/Brooklyn/
Academics/Schools/SON.aspx

Long Island University – Brookville
C W Post Campus Department of
Nursing
720 Northern Blvd
Brookville NY 11548-1319
516-299-11548
http://www.liu.edu/CWPost/
Academics.aspx

New York University
College of Nursing
726 Broadway – 10th Floor
New York NY 10003-9502
212-998-5300
http://www.nyu.edu/nursing

Pace University
Lienhard School of Nursing
41 Park Row – Room 300
New York NY 10038-1508
914-773-3552
http://www.pace.edu/lienhard

SUNY Institute of Technology at
Utica/Rome
School of Nursing & Health Systems
PO Box 3050
Utica NY 13504-3050
315-792-7295
http://www.sunyit.edu/nursing

University of Buffalo
School of Nursing
Wende Hall
3435 Main St
Buffalo NY 14214-3010
716-829-2533
www.nursing.buffalo.edu

University of Rochester
School of Nursing
601 Elmwood Ave
Rochester NY 14642-0001
585-273-2375
www.son.rochester.edu

NORTH CAROLINA

University of North Carolina – Chapel
Hill
School of Nursing
301 Carrington Hall – CB7460
Chapel Hill NC 27599-7460
919-966-3638
http://nursing.ce.unc.edu

University of North Carolina –
Charlotte
School of Nursing
9201 University City Blvd
Charlotte NC 28223-0001
704-687-7952
www.nursing.uncc.edu

OHIO

Case Western Reserve University
Frances Payne Bolton School of
Nursing
10900 Euclid Ave
Cleveland OH 44106-1712
216-368-2529
http://fpb.case.edu

Kent State University
College of Nursing
113 H Henderson Hall
Petrarca Dr
Kent OH 44242-0001
330-672-7930
www.kent.edu/nursing

Ohio State University
College of Nursing
Newton Hall
1585 Neil Ave
Columbus OH 43210-1216
614-292-8900
www.con.ohio-state.edu

University of Akron
College of Nursing
Mary Gladwin Hall
209 Carroll St
Akron OH 44325-3701
330-972-7551
www.uakron.edu/nursing

University of Toledo
College of Nursing
2801 W Bancroft
Toledo OH 43606-3390
800-586-5336
www.utoledo.edu/nursing

OKLAHOMA

University of Oklahoma
College of Nursing
PO Box 26901
1100 N Stonewall Ave
Oklahoma City OK 73117-6901
877-367-6876
http://nursing.ouhsc.edu

OREGON

Oregon Health & Sciences University
School of Nursing
3455 SW US Veterans Hospital Rd
Portland OR 97239-3076
866-223-1811
http://www.ohsu.edu/xd/education/
schools/school-of-nursing/about

University of Portland
School of Nursing
5000 N Willamette Blvd
Portland OR 97203-5798
503-943-7211
www.nursing.up.edu

PENNSYLVANIA

Bloomsburg University
Department of Nursing
3121 McCormick Center for Human
Services
400 E 2nd St
Bloomsburg PA 17815-1301
570-389-4615
http://bloomu.edu/nursing

Drexel University
College of Nursing & Health
Professions
245 N 15th St
Philadelphia PA 19102-1192
215-895-2000
http://www.drexel.edu/cnhp

Millersville University
Department of Nursing
127 Caputo Hall
PO Box 1002
1 S George St
Millersville PA 17551-1002
717-872-3410
www.millersville.edu/nursing

Pennsylvania State University
School of Nursing Graduate Programs
201 Health & Human Development
East
201 Old Main
University Park PA 16802-1589
814-863-0245
www.psu.edu/nursing

Temple University
College of Health Professions
Nursing Department
3307 N Broad St
Philadelphia PA 19140-5101
215-707-4686
www.temple.edu/nursing

University of Pennsylvania
School of Nursing
Claire M Fagin Hall
418 Curie Blvd
Philadelphia PA 19104-4217
215-898-8281
www.nursing.upenn.edu

University of Pittsburgh
School of Nursing
3500 Victoria St
Victoria Building
Pittsburgh PA 152261-2543
412-624-4586
www.nursing.pitt.edu

Villanova University
College of Nursing
800 Lancaster Ave
Villanova PA 19085-1690
610-519-4933
www.villanova.edu/nursing

TENNESSEE

Belmont University
Gordon E Inman College of Health
Sciences and Nursing
School of Nursing
1900 Belmont Blvd
Nashville TN 37212-3757
615-460-6781
www.belmont.edu/nursing

East Tennessee State University
College of Nursing
310 Roy S Nicks Hall
PO Box 70617
Johnson City TN 37614-0617
423-439-4578
www.etsu.edu/nursing

Union University
School of Nursing
Nursing Admissions Coordinator
1050 Union University Dr
Jackson TN 38305-3656
731-661-5538
www.uu.edu/nursing

University of Tennessee – Memphis
College of Nursing
877 Madison Ave
Memphis TN 38163-3408
800-733-2498
www.uthsc.edu/nursing

Vanderbilt University
School of Nursing
Godchaux Hall 207
461 21st Ave S
Nashville TN 37240-1104
888-333-9192
www.nursing.vanderbilt.edu

TEXAS

Texas A&M University – Corpus
Christi
College of Nursing & Health Sciences
6300 Ocean Dr
Corpus Christi TX 78412-5804
361-825-2648
www.tamucc.edu

University of Texas – Austin
School of Nursing
1700 Red River St – D0100
Austin TX 78701-1412
512-471-7311
www.utexas.edu/nursing

VIRGINIA

Marymount University
School of Health Professions
Department of Nursing
2807 N Glebe Rd
Arlington VA 22207-4224
703-284-1580
http://www.marymount.edu/acade-
mics/programs/nursingBSN

Shenandoah University
Division of Nursing
1775 N Sector Ct
Winchester VA 22601-2859
540-678-4374
http://www.su.edu/academics/0B875
B3A348444769D87E900A02AF363.asp

University of Virginia
School of Nursing
McLeod Hall
PO Box 800782
Charlottesville VA 22908-0782
434-924-0063
www.nursing.virginia.edu

Virginia Commonwealth University
School of Nursing
PO Box 980567
1100 E Leigh St
Richmond VA 23298-0567
800-828-9421
www.nursing.vcu.edu

WASHINGTON

Gonzaga University
Department of Nursing
502 E Boone Ave
Spokane WA 99528-0102
509-313-3569
www.gonzaga.edu/nursing

Pacific Lutheran University
School of Nursing
Ramstad Building 214
Tacoma WA 98447-0001
253-535-7672
http://www.plu.edu/nursing

Seattle University
College of Nursing
901 12th Ave
PO Box 222000
Seattle WA 98122-
206-296-5660
www.seattleu.edu/nursing

University of Washington
School of Nursing
PO Box 357260
Seattle WA 98195-7260
206-543-8736
http://nursing.uw.edu

Washington State University
Intercollegiate College of Nursing
PO Box 1495
Spokane WA 99210-1495
509-324-7360
www.nursing.wsu.edu

WISCONSIN

University of Wisconsin – Milwaukee
College of Nursing
1921 E Hartford Ave
PO Box 413
Milwaukee WI 53201
414-229-4801
www.uwm.edu/nursing

WYOMING

University of Wyoming
College of Health Sciences
Fay W Whitney School of Nursing
Department 3065
1000 E University Ave
Laramie WY 82071-2000
307-766-4312
www.uwyo.edu/nursing

PROFESSIONAL ASSOCIATIONS FOR NPs

NATIONAL ASSOCIATIONS

American Academy of Nurse Practitioners
PO Box 12846
Austin TX 78711-2846
512-442-4262
www.aanp.org

Gerontological Advanced Practice Nurses Association
East Holly Ave – Box 56
Pitman NJ 08071-0056
800-262-6877
www.gapna.org

National Association of Pediatric Nurse Practitioners
20 Brace Rd – Suite 200
Cherry Hill NJ 08034-2634
856-857-9700
www.napnap.org

Nurse Practitioners in Women's Health
505 C St NE
Washington DC 20002-5809
202-543-9693
www.npwh.org

STATE ASSOCIATIONS

ALABAMA
North Alabama Nurse Practitioner Association
PO Box 14055
Huntsville AL 35815-4055
www.northalabamanpa.com

ALASKA
Alaska Nurse Practitioner Association
3701 E Tudor Rd – Suite 208
Anchorage AK 99507-1259
907-222-6847
www.alaskanp.org

ARIZONA
Arizona Nurse Practitioner Council
1850 E Southern Ave – Suite 1
Tempe AZ 85282-5882
480-831-0404
www.arizonanp.com

ARKANSAS
Arkansas Nurses Association
1123 S University – Suite 1015
Little Rock AR 72204-1617
501-244-2363
www.arna.org

CALIFORNIA
California Association for Nurse Practitioners
1415 L Street – Suite 200
Sacramento CA 95814-3962
916-441-1361
www.canpweb.org

COLORADO
Colorado Society of Advanced Practice Nurses
PO Box 100158
Denver CO 80250-0158
303-757-7483
www.csapn.org

CONNECTICUT
Connecticut Advanced Practice Registered Nurse Society
2842 Main St - PO Box 323
Glastonbury CT 06033-1077
www.ctaprns.org

DELAWARE
Delaware Nurses Association
5586 Kirkwood Hwy
Wilmington DE 19808-5002
302-998-3141
www.denurses.org

DISTRICT OF COLUMBIA
Nurse Practitioner Association of DC
PO Box 77424
Washington DC 20013-7424
www.npadc.org

FLORIDA
Florida Nurses Association
PO Box 536985
Orlando FL 32803-6985
407-896-3261
www.floridanurses.org

Florida Nurse Practitioner Network
PO Box 25422
Tampa FL 33622-5422
866-535-3676
www.fnpn.org

GEORGIA
Nurse Practitioner Council of Coastal Georgia
PO Box 14046
Savannah GA 31416-4046
912-351-7800
www.npcouncilofcoastalga.org

IDAHO
Nurse Practitioners of Idaho
5120-5129 W Overland – PMB 218
Boise ID 83705-2680
208-914-0138
www.npidaho.org

ILLINOIS
Illinois Nurses Association
105 W Adams St – Ste 1420
Chicago IL 60603-6253
312-419-2900
www.illinoisnurses.com

INDIANA
Coalition of Advanced Practice Nurses of Indiana
PO Box 502858
Indianapolis IN 46250-2858
www.capni.org

IOWA
Iowa Nurse Practitioner Society
Hoskins Geriatrics
www.iowanpsociety.org

KENTUCKY
Kentucky Coalition of Nurse Practitioners and Nurse Midwives
1017 Ash St
Louisville KY 40217-1229
502.333-0076
www.kcnpnm.org

LOUISIANA
Louisiana Association of Nurse Practitioners
5713 Superior Dr – Suite A5
Baton Route LA 70816-8015
www.lanp.org

MAINE
Maine Nurse Practitioner Association
11 Columbia St
Augusta ME 04330-6809
207-621-0313
www.mnpa.us

MARYLAND
Nurse Practitioner Association of Maryland
PO Box 540
Ellicott City MD 21041-0540
888-405-NPAM (6726)
www.npamonline.org

MASSACHUSETTS
Massachusetts Coalition of Nurse Practitioners
PO Box 1153
Littleton MA 01460-1153
781-575-1565
www.mcnpweb.org

MICHIGAN
Michigan Council of Nurse Practitioners
PO Box 87934
Canton MI 48187-7934
734-432-9881
www.micnp.org

MINNESOTA
Association of Southeast Minnesota Nurse Practitioners
www.asmnp.org

MISSISSIPPI
Mississippi Nurses Association
31 Woodgreen Pl
Madison MS 39110-9531
601-898-0670

MISSOURI
Missouri Nurses Association
1904 Bubba Ln
PO Box 105228
1904 Bubba Ln
Jefferson City MO 65110-5634
573-636-4623
www.missourinurses.org

MONTANA
Montana Nurses Association
20 Old Mountain State Hwy
Clancy MT 59634
406-442-6710
www.mtnurses.org

NEVADA
Nevada Nurses Association
PO Box 34660
Reno NV 89533-4660
757-747-2333
www.nvnurses.org

NEW HAMPSHIRE
New Hampshire Nurse Practitioner
Association
603-648-2233

NEW JERSEY
New Jersey State Nurses Association
1479 Pennington Rd
Trenton NJ 08618-2661
888-UR-NJSNA (876-5752)
www.njsna.org

NEW MEXICO
New Mexico Nurse Practitioner Council
PO Box 40682
Albuquerque NM 87196-0682
505-697-1680
www.nmnpc.org

NEW YORK
The Nurse Practitioner Association
New York State
12 Corporate Dr
Clifton Park NY 12065-8645
518-348-0719
www.thenpa.org

NORTH CAROLINA
North Carolina Nurses Association
PO Box 12025
Raleigh NC 27605-2025
800-626-2153
www.ncnurses.org

OHIO
Ohio Association of Advanced Practice
Nurses
5818 Wilmington Pike – Suite 300
Dayton OH 45459
866-668-3839
www.oaapn.org

OKLAHOMA
Oklahoma Nurse Practitioners
Association
337 NE 4th
Oklahoma City OK 73104-4027
405-445-4874
www.npofoklahoma.com

OREGON
Nurse Practitioners of Oregon
18765 SW Boones Ferry Rd –
Suite 200
Tualatin OR 97062-8498
800-634-3552
503-293-0011
www.nursepractitionersoforegon.org

PENNSYLVANIA
Pennsylvania Coalition of Nurse
Practitioners
PO Box 1071
Jenkintown PA 19046-1071
866-800-6206
www.pacnp.org

SOUTH DAKOTA
Nurse Practitioner Association of
South Dakota
PO Box 2822
Rapid City SD 57709-2822
www.npasd.org

TENNESSEE
Tennessee Nurses Association
545 Mainstream Dr – Suite 405
Nashville TN 37228-1296
615-254-0350
www.tnaonline.org

TEXAS
Texas Nurse Practitioners
4425 S Mopac Expswy – Bldg III –
Suite 405
Austin TX 78735-6701
512-291-6224
www.texasnp.org

UTAH
Utah Nurse Practitioners
PO Box 581084
Salt Lake City UT 84108-1084
www.utahnp.org

VERMONT
Vermont Nurse Practitioners
PO Box 64773
Burlington VT 05406-4773
www.vtnpa.org

VIRGINIA
Virginia Council of Nurse Practitioners
600 Peter Jefferson Pkwy – Suite 300
Charlottesville VA 22911-8837
434-977-3716
www.vcnp.net

WASHINGTON
ARNPs United of Washington State
10024 SE 240th St – Suite 230
Kent WA 98031-5124
253-480-1035
www.auws.org

WEST VIRGINIA
West Virginia Nurses Association
1007 Bigley Ave – Suite 308
Charleston WV 25302-3536
800-400-1226
304-342-1169
www.wvnurses.org

WISCONSIN
Wisconsin Nurses Association
6117 Monona Dr – Suite 1
Monona WI 53716-4304
608-221-0383
www.wisconsinnurses.org

ANTIPYRETIC PRODUCTS

BRAND	INGREDIENT/STRENGTH	DOSE
ACETAMINOPHEN		
Anacin Extra Strength Aspirin Free Tablets	Acetaminophen 500mg	**Adults & Peds ≥12 yrs:** 2 tabs q6h. **Max:** 8 tabs q24h.
FeverAll Childrens' Suppositories	Acetaminophen 120mg	**Peds 3-6 yrs:** 1 supp q4-6h. **Max:** 6 supp q24h.
FeverAll Infants' Suppositories	Acetaminophen 80mg	**Peds 6-11 months:** 1 supp q6h. **12-36 months:** 1 supp q4h. **Max:** 6 supp q24h.
FeverAll Jr. Strength Suppositories	Acetaminophen 325mg	**Peds 6-12 yrs:** 1 supp q4-6h. **Max:** 6 supp q24h.
Tylenol 8 Hour Caplets	Acetaminophen 650mg	**Adults & Peds ≥12 yrs:** 2 tabs q8h prn. **Max:** 6 tabs q24h.
Tylenol Arthritis Caplets	Acetaminophen 650mg	**Adults:** 2 tabs q8h prn. **Max:** 6 tabs q24h.
Tylenol Arthritis Gelcaps	Acetaminophen 650mg	**Adults:** 2 caps q8h prn. **Max:** 6 caps q24h.
Tylenol Arthritis Geltabs	Acetaminophen 650mg	**Adults:** 2 tabs q8h prn. **Max:** 6 tabs q24h.
Tylenol Children's Meltaways Tablets*	Acetaminophen 80mg	**Peds 2-3 yrs (24-35 lbs):** 2 tabs. **4-5 yrs (36-47 lbs):** 3 tabs. **6-8 yrs (48-59 lbs):** 4 tabs. **9-10 yrs (60-71 lbs):** 5 tabs. **11 yrs (72-95 lbs):** 6 tabs. May repeat q4h. **Max:** 5 doses q24h.
Tylenol Children's Suspension*	Acetaminophen 160mg/5mL	**Peds 2-3 yrs (24-35 lbs):** 1 tsp (5mL). **4-5 yrs (36-47 lbs):** 1.5 tsp (7.5mL). **6-8 yrs (48-59 lbs):** 2 tsp (10mL). **9-10 yrs (60-71 lbs):** 2.5 tsp (12.5mL). **11 yrs (72-95 lbs):** 3 tsp (15mL). May repeat q4h. **Max:** 5 doses q24h.
Tylenol Extra Strength Caplets	Acetaminophen 500mg	**Adults & Peds ≥12 yrs:** 2 tabs q4-6h prn. **Max:** 8 tabs q24h.
Tylenol Extra Strength Cool Caplets	Acetaminophen 500mg	**Adults & Peds ≥12 yrs:** 2 tabs q4-6h prn. **Max:** 8 tabs q24h.
Tylenol Extra Strength EZ Tablets	Acetaminophen 500mg	**Adults & Peds ≥12 yrs:** 2 tabs q4-6h prn. **Max:** 8 tabs q24h.
Tylenol Extra Strength Rapid Blast Liquid	Acetaminophen 500mg/15mL	**Adults & Peds ≥12 yrs:** 2 tbl (30mL) q4-6h prn. **Max:** 8 tbl (120mL) q24h.
Tylenol Extra Strength Rapid Release Gelcaps	Acetaminophen 500mg	**Adults & Peds ≥12 yrs:** 2 caps q4-6h prn. **Max:** 8 caps q24h.
Tylenol Infants' Drops*	Acetaminophen 160mg/1.6mL	**Peds 2-3 yrs (24-35 lbs):** 1.6 mL q4h prn. **Max:** 5 doses (8mL) q24h.
Tylenol Junior Meltaways Tablets*	Acetaminophen 160mg	**Peds 6-8 yrs (48-59 lbs):** 2 tabs. **9-10 yrs (60-71 lbs):** 2.5 tabs. **11 yrs (72-95 lbs):** 3 tabs. **12 yrs (≥96 lbs):** 4 tabs. May repeat q4h. **Max:** 5 doses q24h.
Tylenol Regular Strength Tablets	Acetaminophen 325mg	**Adults & Peds ≥12 yrs:** 2 tabs q4-6h prn. **Max:** 12 tabs q24h. **Peds 6-11 yrs:** 1 tab q4-6h. **Max:** 5 tabs q24h.

(Continued)

BRAND	INGREDIENT/STRENGTH	DOSE
NONSTEROIDAL ANTI-INFLAMMATORY DRUGS (NSAIDs)		
Advil Caplets	Ibuprofen 200mg	**Adults & Peds ≥12 yrs:** 1-2 tabs q4-6h. **Max:** 6 tabs q24h.
Advil Children's Suspension	Ibuprofen 100mg/5mL	**Peds 2-3 yrs (24-35 lbs):** 1 tsp (5mL). **4-5 yrs (36-47 lbs):** 1.5 tsp (7.5mL). **6-8 yrs (48-59 lbs):** 2 tsp (10mL). **9-10 yrs (60-71 lbs):** 2.5 tsp (12.5mL). **11 yrs (72-95 lbs):** 3 tsp (15mL). May repeat q6-8h. **Max:** 4 doses q24h.
Advil Gel Caplets	Ibuprofen 200mg	**Adults & Peds ≥12 yrs:** 1-2 tabs q4-6h. **Max:** 6 tabs q24h.
Advil Infants' Concentrated Drops*	Ibuprofen 50mg/1.25mL	**Peds 6-11 months (12-17 lbs):** 1.25mL. **12-23 months (18-23 lbs):** 1.875mL. May repeat q6-8h. **Max:** 4 doses q24h.
Advil Liqui-Gels	Ibuprofen 200mg	**Adults & Peds ≥12 yrs:** 1-2 caps q4-6h. **Max:** 6 caps q24h.
Advil Tablets	Ibuprofen 200mg	**Adults & Peds ≥12 yrs:** 1-2 tabs q4-6h. **Max:** 6 tabs q24h.
Aleve Caplets	Naproxen Sodium 220mg	**Adults & Peds ≥12 yrs:** 1 tab q8-12h. May take 1 additional tab within 1 hour of first dose. **Max:** 2 tabs q8-12h or 3 tabs q24h.
Aleve Liquid Gels	Naproxen Sodium 220mg	**Adults & Peds ≥12 yrs:** 1 cap q8-12h. May take 1 additional cap within 1 hour of first dose. **Max:** 2 caps q8-12h or 3 caps q24h.
Aleve Tablets	Naproxen Sodium 220mg	**Adults & Peds ≥12 yrs:** 1 tab q8-12h. May take 1 additional tab within 1 hour of first dose. **Max:** 2 tabs q8-12h or 3 tabs q24h.
Motrin Children's Suspension*†	Ibuprofen 100mg/5mL	**Peds 2-3 yrs (24-35 lbs):** 1 tsp (5mL). **4-5 yrs (36-47 lbs):** 1.5 tsp (7.5mL). **6-8 yrs (48-59 lbs):** 2 tsp (10mL). **9-10 yrs (60-71 lbs):** 2.5 tsp (12.5mL). **11 yrs (72-95 lbs):** 3 tsp (15mL). May repeat q6-8h. **Max:** 4 doses q24h.
Motrin IB Caplets	Ibuprofen 200mg	**Adults & Peds ≥12 yrs:** 1-2 tabs q4-6h. **Max:** 6 tabs q24h.
Motrin IB Tablets	Ibuprofen 200mg	**Adults & Peds ≥12 yrs:** 1-2 tabs q4-6h. **Max:** 6 tabs q24h.
Motrin Infants' Drops*†	Ibuprofen 50mg/1.25mL	**Peds 6-11 months (12-17 lbs):** 1.25mL. **12-23 months (18-23 lbs):** 1.875mL. May repeat q6-8h. **Max:** 4 doses q24h.
Motrin Junior Strength Caplets*†	Ibuprofen 100mg	**Peds 6-8 yrs (48-59 lbs):** 2 tabs. **9-10 yrs (60-71 lbs):** 2.5 tabs. **11 yrs (72-95 lbs):** 3 tabs. May repeat q6-8h. **Max:** 4 doses q24h.
Motrin Junior Strength Chewable Tablets*†	Ibuprofen 100mg	**Peds 2-3 yrs (24-35 lbs):** 1 tab. **4-5 yrs (36-47 lbs):** 1.5 tabs. **6-8 yrs (48-59 lbs):** 2 tabs. **9-10 yrs (60-71 lbs):** 2.5 tabs. **11 yrs (72-95 lbs):** 3 tabs. May repeat q6-8h. **Max:** 4 doses q24h.

(Continued)

BRAND	INGREDIENT/STRENGTH	DOSE
SALICYLATES		
Bayer Aspirin Extra Strength Caplets	Aspirin 500mg	**Adults & Peds ≥12 yrs:** 1-2 tabs q4-6h. **Max:** 8 tabs q24h.
Bayer Aspirin Safety Coated Caplets	Aspirin 325mg	**Adults & Peds ≥12 yrs:** 1-2 tabs q4h. **Max:** 12 tabs q24h.
Bayer Genuine Aspirin Tablets	Aspirin 325mg	**Adults & Peds ≥12 yrs:** 1-2 tabs q4h or 3 tabs q6h. **Max:** 12 tabs q24h.
Bayer Low-Dose Aspirin Chewable Tablets*	Aspirin 81mg	**Adults & Peds ≥12 yrs:** 4-8 tabs q4h. **Max:** 48 tabs q24h.
Bayer Low-Dose Aspirin Safety Coated Tablets	Aspirin 81mg	**Adults & Peds ≥12 yrs:** 4-8 tabs q4h. **Max:** 48 tabs q24h.
Ecotrin Low Strength Tablets	Aspirin 81mg	**Adults:** 4-8 tabs q4h. **Max:** 48 tabs q24h.
Ecotrin Regular Strength Tablets	Aspirin 325mg	**Adults & Peds ≥12 yrs:** 1-2 tabs q4h. **Max:** 12 tabs q24h.
Halfprin 162mg Tablets	Aspirin 162mg	**Adults & Peds ≥12 yrs:** 2-4 tabs q4h. **Max:** 24 tabs q24h.
Halfprin 81mg Tablets	Aspirin 81mg	**Adults & Peds ≥12 yrs:** 4-8 tabs q4h. **Max:** 48 tabs q24h.
St. Joseph Aspirin Chewable Tablets	Aspirin 81mg	**Adults & Peds ≥12 yrs:** 4-8 tabs q4h. **Max:** 48 tabs q24h.
St. Joseph Enteric Safety-Coated Tablets	Aspirin 81mg	**Adults & Peds ≥12 yrs:** 4-8 tabs q4h. **Max:** 48 tabs q24h.
SALICYLATES, BUFFERED		
Bayer Extra Strength Plus Caplets	Aspirin 500mg Buffered with Calcium Carbonate	**Adults & Peds ≥12 yrs:** 1-2 tabs q4-6h. **Max:** 8 tabs q24h.
Bayer Women's Low Dose Aspirin Caplets	Aspirin 81mg Buffered with Calcium Carbonate 777mg	**Adults & Peds ≥12 yrs:** 4-8 tabs q4h. **Max:** 10 tabs q24h.
Bufferin Extra Strength Tablets	Aspirin 500mg Buffered with Calcium Carbonate/Magnesium Oxide/Magnesium Carbonate	**Adults & Peds ≥12 yrs:** 2 tabs q6h. **Max:** 8 tabs q24h.
Bufferin Tablets	Aspirin 325mg Buffered with Benzoic Acid/Citric Acid	**Adults & Peds ≥12 yrs:** 2 tabs q4h. **Max:** 12 tabs q24h.
Bufferin Low Dose Tablets	Aspirin 81mg Buffered with Calcium Carbonate/Magnesium Oxide/Magnesium Carbonate	**Adults & Peds ≥12 yrs:** 4-8 tabs q4h. **Max:** 48 tabs q24h.

*Multiple flavors available.
†Product currently on recall, available in generic form.

INSOMNIA PRODUCTS

BRAND	INGREDIENT/STRENGTH	DOSE
DIPHENHYDRAMINE		
Nytol Quick Caps Caplets	Diphenhydramine 25mg	**Adults & Peds ≥12 yrs:** 2 tabs qhs.
Simply Sleep Nighttime Sleep Aid Caplets	Diphenhydramine 25mg	**Adults & Peds ≥12 yrs:** 2 tabs qhs.
Sominex Original Formula	Diphenhydramine 25mg	**Adults & Peds ≥12 yrs:** 2 tabs qhs.
Sominex Maximum Strength Formula	Diphenhydramine 50mg	**Adults & Peds ≥12 yrs:** 1 tab qhs.
Unisom Nighttime Sleep-Aid Sleep Gels	Diphenhydramine 50mg	**Adults & Peds ≥12 yrs:** 1 cap qhs.
Unisom Sleep Melts	Diphenhydramine 25mg	**Adults & Peds ≥12 yrs:** 2 tabs qhs.
DIPHENHYDRAMINE COMBINATION		
Advil PM Caplets	Ibuprofen/Diphenhydramine Citrate 200mg-38mg	**Adults & Peds ≥12 yrs:** 2 tabs qhs.
Advil PM Liqui-Gels	Ibuprofen/Diphenhydramine HCl 200mg-25mg	**Adults & Peds ≥12 yrs:** 2 caps qhs.
Bayer PM Relief Caplets	Aspirin/Diphenhydramine Citrate 500mg-38.3mg	**Adults & Peds ≥12 yrs:** 2 tabs qhs.
Doan's Extra Strength PM Caplets	Magnesium Salicylate Tetrahydrate/ Diphenhydramine 580mg-25mg	**Adults & Peds ≥12 yrs:** 2 tabs qhs.
Excedrin PM Caplets	Acetaminophen/Diphenhydramine Citrate 500mg-38mg	**Adults & Peds ≥12 yrs:** 2 tabs qhs.
Excedrin PM Express Gels	Acetaminophen/Diphenhydramine Citrate 500mg-38mg	**Adults & Peds ≥12 yrs:** 2 caps qhs.
Goody's PM Powder	Acetaminophen/Diphenhydramine Citrate 1000mg-76mg/dose	**Adults & Peds ≥12 yrs:** 1 packet (2 powders) qhs.
Motrin PM Caplets	Ibuprofen/Diphenhydramine Citrate 200-38mg	**Adults & Peds ≥12 yrs:** 2 tabs qhs.
Tylenol PM Caplets	Acetaminophen/Diphenhydramine HCl 500mg-25mg	**Adults & Peds ≥12 yrs:** 2 tabs qhs.
Tylenol PM Rapid Release Gelcaps	Acetaminophen/Diphenhydramine HCl 500mg-25mg	**Adults & Peds ≥12 yrs:** 2 caps qhs.
Tylenol PM Geltabs	Acetaminophen/Diphenhydramine HCl 500mg-25mg	**Adults & Peds ≥12 yrs:** 2 tabs qhs.
Tylenol PM Liquid	Acetaminophen/Diphenhydramine HCl 1000mg-50mg/30mL	**Adults & Peds ≥12 yrs:** 2 tbl (30mL) qhs.
Unisom PM Pain SleepCaps	Acetaminophen/Diphenhydramine HCl 325mg-50mg	**Adults & Peds ≥12 yrs:** 1 cap qhs.
DOXYLAMINE		
Unisom Nighttime Sleep-Aid Sleep Tabs	Doxylamine Succinate 25mg	**Adults & Peds ≥12 yrs:** 1 tab 30 min before hs.

SMOKING CESSATION PRODUCTS

BRAND	INGREDIENT/STRENGTH	DOSE
NicoDerm CQ Step 1 Clear Patch	Nicotine 21mg	**Adults:** If smoking >10 cigarettes/day. **Weeks 1 to 6:** Apply one 21mg patch/day. **Weeks 7 to 8:** Apply one 14mg patch/day. **Weeks 9 to 10:** Apply one 7mg patch/day.
NicoDerm CQ Step 2 Clear Patch	Nicotine 14mg	**Adults:** If smoking >10 cigarettes/day. **Weeks 1 to 6:** Apply one 21mg patch/day. **Weeks 7 to 8:** Apply one 14mg patch/day. **Weeks 9 to 10:** Apply one 7mg patch/day. If smoking ≤10 cigarettes/day. **Weeks 1 to 6:** Apply one 14mg patch/day. **Weeks 7 to 8:** Apply one 7mg patch/day.
NicoDerm CQ Step 3 Clear Patch	Nicotine 7mg	**Adults:** Apply 1 patch qd Weeks 9 to 10 if smoking >10 cigarettes/day or Weeks 7 to 8 if smoking ≤10 cigarettes/day.
Nicorette 2mg	Nicotine Polacrilex 2mg	**Adults:** If smoking <25 cigarettes/day use 2mg gum. **Weeks 1 to 6:** 1 piece q1-2h. **Weeks 7 to 9:** 1 piece q2-4h. **Weeks 10 to 12:** 1 piece q4-8h. **Max:** 24 pieces/day.
Nicorette 4mg	Nicotine Polacrilex 4mg	**Adults:** If smoking ≥25 cigarettes/day use 4mg gum. **Weeks 1 to 6:** 1 piece q1-2h. **Weeks 7 to 9:** 1 piece q2-4h. **Weeks 10 to 12:** 1 piece q4-8h. **Max:** 24 pieces/day.
Nicorette Stop Smoking 2mg Lozenges	Nicotine Polacrilex 2mg	**Adults:** If smoking first cigarette >30 minutes after waking up use 2mg lozenge. **Weeks 1 to 6:** 1 lozenge q1-2h. **Weeks 7 to 9:** 1 lozenge q2-4h. **Weeks 10 to 12:** 1 lozenge q4-8h. **Max:** 5 lozenges/6 hours; 20 lozenges/day. Stop using at the end of 12 weeks.
Nicorette Stop Smoking 4mg Lozenges	Nicotine Polacrilex 4mg	**Adults:** If smoking first cigarette within 30 minutes after waking up use 4mg lozenge. **Weeks 1 to 6:** 1 lozenge q1-2h. **Weeks 7 to 9:** 1 lozenge q2-4h. **Weeks 10 to 12:** 1 lozenge q4-8h. **Max:** 5 lozenges/6 hours; 20 lozenges/day. Stop using at the end of 12 weeks.
Habitrol Nicotine Transdermal System Patch Step 1	Nicotine 21mg/24hr	**Adults:** If smoking >10 cigarettes/day. **Weeks 1 to 4:** Apply one 21mg patch/day. **Weeks 5 to 6:** Apply one 14mg patch/day. **Weeks 7 to 8:** Apply one 7mg patch/day.
Habitrol Nicotine Transdermal System Patch Step 2	Nicotine 14mg/24hr	**Adults:** If smoking >10 cigarettes/day. **Weeks 1 to 4:** Apply one 21mg patch/day. **Weeks 5 to 6:** Apply one 14mg patch/day. **Weeks 7 to 8:** Apply one 7mg patch/day. If smoking ≤10 cigarettes/day. **Weeks 1 to 6:** Apply one 14 mg patch/day. **Weeks 7 to 8:** Apply one 7mg patch/day.
Habitrol Nicotine Transdermal System Patch Step 3	Nicotine 7mg/24hr	**Adults:** If smoking >10 cigarettes/day. **Weeks 1 to 4:** Apply one 21mg patch/day. **Weeks 5 to 6:** Apply one 14mg patch/day. **Weeks 7 to 8:** Apply one 7mg patch/day. If smoking ≤10 cigarettes/day. **Weeks 1 to 6:** Apply one 14mg patch/day. **Weeks 7 to 8:** Apply one 7mg patch/day.

WEIGHT MANAGEMENT PRODUCTS

BRAND	DOSE
Alli Weight-Loss Aid	**Adults:** 1 cap with each fat-containing meal. **Max:** 3 caps per day.
Applied Nutrition Carb Blocker	**Adults:** Take 2 caps with meals bid.
Applied Nutrition Green Tea Fat Burner	**Adults:** Take 2 caps with meals bid.
Applied Nutrition Green Tea Triple Fat Burner	**Adults:** Take 2 caps with meals bid.
Applied Nutrition Natural Fat Burner Capsules	**Adults:** Take 2 caps with meals bid.
Applied Nutrition Resveratol Rapid Calorie Burn	**Adults:** Take 2 tabs qam and 2 tabs qpm.
Aqua-Ban Maximum Strength Diuretic Tablets	**Adults:** Take 1 tab qid. **Max:** 4 tabs q24h.
BioMD Nutraceuticals Metabolism T3 Capsules	**Adults:** Take 2 caps with meals bid-tid. **Max:** 6 caps q24h.
Biotest Hot-Rox Capsules	**Adults:** Take 1-2 caps bid. **Max:** 6 caps q24h.
Carb Cutter Original Formula Tablets	**Adults:** Take 1-2 tabs with a glass of water 15 mins prior to carbohydrate foods.
Carb Cutter Phase 2 Starch Neutralizer Tablets	**Adults:** Take 1-2 tabs with meals bid.
Dexatrim Max	**Adults:** Take 1-2 caps with water, one in AM and one in afternoon. **Max:** 2 caps q24h.
Dexatrim Max Daytime Appetite Control	**Adults:** Take 1-2 caps daily. **Max:** 2 caps q24h.
Dexatrim Max Slim Packs	**Adults:** Dissolve 1 packet in 16.9 ounces of water. **Max:** 6 packs q24h.
Dexatrim Natural Extra Energy Formula Caplets	**Adults:** Take 1 tab with meals tid. **Max:** 3 tabs q24h.
Dexatrim Natural Green Tea Formula Caplets	**Adults:** Take 1 tab with meals tid. **Max:** 3 tabs q24h.
Dexatrim Max Complex 7	**Adults:** Take 2 caps qam. Second serving mid-afternoon. **Max:** 4 caps q24h.
EAS CLA Capsules	**Adults:** Take 2 caps with meals tid.
Estrin-D Capsules	**Adults:** Take 2 caps 30 min before meals. **Max:** 6 caps q24h.
Isatori MX-LS7 Maximum Strength Lean System 7	**Adults: Men/Women <200 lbs:** Day 1 to 6: 2 caps bid. Day 7 & on: 3 caps bid. **Men >200 lbs:** Day 1 to 6: 2 caps bid. Day 7 to 14: 3 caps bid. Day 14 & on: 4 caps bid. **Max:** 4 caps q4h.
Metabolife Break Through	**Adults:** Take 2 tabs 1 hr before meals tid, at least 3-4 hrs apart. **Max:** 6 tabs q24h.
Metabolife Extreme Energy	**Adults:** Take 1-2 tabs tid at least 3-4 hrs apart. **Max:** 4 tabs q8h.
Metabolife Ultra Caplets	**Adults:** Take 2 tabs tid 30-60 min before meals, at least 3-4 hrs apart. **Max:** 6 tabs q24h.
Metabolife Caffeine Free Caplets	**Adults:** Take 2 tabs tid 30-60 min before meals, at least 3-4 hrs apart. **Max:** 6 tabs q24h.
Metabolife Green Tea	**Adults:** Take 2 tabs tid 30-60 min before meals, at least 3-4 hrs apart. **Max:** 6 tabs q24h.
MHP TakeOff, Hi-Energy Fat Burner Capsules	**Adults:** Take 2 caps qd or bid.
Natrol Carb Intercept with Phase 2 Starch Neutralizer Capsules	**Adults:** Take 2 caps before carbohydrate-containing meals.
Natrol Green Tea 500mg Capsules	**Adults:** Take 1 cap with meals qd.
Natural Balance Fat Magnet Capsules	**Adults:** Take 2 caps with meals bid.
Nature Made Chromium Picolinate, Extra Strength	**Adults:** Take 1 tab qd.
Nunaturals LevelRight for Blood Sugar Management Capsules	**Adults:** Take 1 cap with meals tid.
Prolab Enhanced CLA	**Adults:** Take 3 caps with meals qd.
Stacker 2 Ephedra Free Capsules	**Adults:** Take 1 cap after meals. **Max:** 3 caps q24h.
Stacker 3 Ephedra Free Formula with Chitosan Capsules	**Adults:** Take 1 cap after meals. **Max:** 3 caps q24h.
Stacker 3 XPLC Extreme Performance Formula Ephedra Free	**Adults:** Take 1 cap after meals. **Max:** 3 caps q24h.

(Continued)

BRAND	DOSE
Tetrazene ES-50 Ultra High-Energy Weight Loss Catalyst Capsules	**Adults:** Take 2 caps with meals tid. **Max:** 6 caps q24h.
Tetrazene KGM-90 Rapid Weight Loss Catalyst Capsules	**Adults:** Take 2 caps with meals tid. **Max:** 6 caps q24h.
Twinlab CLA Fuel	**Adults:** Take 1 cap tid.
Twinlab GTF Chromium	**Adults:** Take 1 tab qd.
Twinlab Mega L-Carnitine	**Adults:** Take 1 tab daily on an empty stomach.
Twinlab Metabolift, Ephedra Free Formula Capsules	**Adults:** Take 2 caps before each meal. **Max:** 6 caps q24h.
Twinlab Ripped Fuel 5X	**Adults:** Take 1 tab before meals bid.
Twinlab Ripped Fuel Ephedra Free	**Adults:** Take 2 caps before each meal. **Max:** 6 caps q24h.
Twinlab Ripped Fuel Extreme	**Adults:** Take 2 caps bid.
Twinlab Ripped Fuel Xtendr	**Adults:** Take 2 tabs 30 min before meals. **Max:** 6 tabs q24h.
Twinlab 7-Keto Fuel	**Adults:** Take 2-4 caps daily.
Ultra Diet Pep Tablets	**Adults:** Take 1 tab with meals bid.
XtremeLean Advanced Formula, Ephedra Free Capsules	**Adults:** Take 2 caps before meals bid.
Zantrex 3, Ephedrine Free	**Adults:** Take 2 caps with meals qd. **Max:** 6 caps q24h.
Zantrex 3 High Energy Fat Burner	**Adults:** Take 2 caps qam and 2 caps with main meal. **Max:** 4 caps q24h.
Zantrex 3 Power Crystals	**Adults:** Add 1 packet to 16 oz of water. **Max:** 3 packets q24h.

ANTIFUNGAL PRODUCTS

BRAND	INGREDIENT/STRENGTH	DOSE
BUTENAFINE		
Lotrimin Ultra Athlete's Foot Cream	Butenafine HCl 1%	**Adults & Peds ≥12 yrs:** Athlete's Foot: Apply bid for 1 week or qd for 4 weeks. Jock Itch/Ringworm: Apply qd for 2 weeks.
Lotrimin Ultra Jock Itch Cream	Butenafine HCl 1%	**Adults & Peds ≥12 yrs:** Apply qd for 2 weeks.
CLOTRIMAZOLE		
Desenex Antifungal Cream	Clotrimazole 1%	**Adults & Peds ≥2 yrs:** Athlete's Foot/Ringworm: Apply bid for 4 weeks. Jock Itch: Apply bid for 2 weeks.
FungiCure Anti-Fungal Liquid Pump Spray	Clotrimazole 1%	**Adults & Peds ≥2 yrs:** Athlete's Foot/Ringworm: Apply bid for 4 weeks. Jock Itch: Apply bid for 2 weeks.
FungiCure Intensive Anti-Fungal Treatment	Clotrimazole 1%	**Adults & Peds ≥2 yrs:** Athlete's Foot/Ringworm: Apply bid for 4 weeks. Jock Itch: Apply bid for 2 weeks.
Lotrimin AF Athlete's Foot Cream	Clotrimazole 1%	**Adults & Peds ≥2 yrs:** Athlete's Foot/Ringworm: Apply bid for 4 weeks. Jock Itch: Apply bid for 2 weeks.
Lotrimin AF For Her Athlete's Foot Cream	Clotrimazole 1%	**Adults & Peds ≥2 yrs:** Apply bid for 4 weeks.
Lotrimin AF Jock Itch Cream	Clotrimazole 1%	**Adults & Peds ≥2 yrs:** Apply bid for 2 weeks.
Lotrimin AF Ringworm Cream	Clotrimazole 1%	**Adults & Peds ≥2 yrs:** Apply bid for 4 weeks.
MICONAZOLE		
Clearly Confident Antifungal Cream	Miconazole Nitrate 2%	**Adults & Peds ≥2 yrs:** Apply bid for 4 weeks.
Desenex Antifungal Liquid Spray	Miconazole Nitrate 2%	**Adults & Peds ≥2 yrs:** Apply bid for 4 weeks.
Desenex Antifungal Powder	Miconazole Nitrate 2%	**Adults & Peds ≥2 yrs:** Athlete's Foot/Ringworm: Apply bid for 4 weeks. Jock Itch: Apply bid for 2 weeks.
Desenex Antifungal Spray Powder	Miconazole Nitrate 2%	**Adults & Peds ≥2 yrs:** Apply bid for 4 weeks.
Lotrimin AF Athlete's Foot Deodorant Powder Spray	Miconazole Nitrate 2%	**Adults & Peds ≥2 yrs:** Athlete's Foot/Ringworm: Apply bid for 4 weeks. Jock Itch: Apply bid for 2 weeks.
Lotrimin AF Athlete's Foot Liquid Spray	Miconazole Nitrate 2%	**Adults & Peds ≥2 yrs:** Athlete's Foot/Ringworm: Apply bid for 4 weeks. Jock Itch: Apply bid for 2 weeks.
Lotrimin AF Athlete's Foot Powder	Miconazole Nitrate 2%	**Adults & Peds ≥2 yrs:** Athlete's Foot/Ringworm: Apply bid for 4 weeks. Jock Itch: Apply bid for 2 weeks.
Lotrimin AF Athlete's Foot Powder Spray	Miconazole Nitrate 2%	**Adults & Peds ≥2 yrs:** Athlete's Foot/Ringworm: Apply bid for 4 weeks. Jock Itch: Apply bid for 2 weeks.

(Continued)

BRAND	INGREDIENT/STRENGTH	DOSE
MICONAZOLE *(Continued)*		
Lotrimin AF Jock Itch Powder Spray	Miconazole Nitrate 2%	**Adults & Peds ≥2 yrs:** Apply bid for 2 weeks.
Micatin Cream	Miconazole Nitrate 2%	**Adults & Peds ≥2 yrs:** Athlete's Foot/Ringworm: Apply bid for 4 weeks. Jock Itch: Apply bid for 2 weeks.
Miranel AF Antifungal Treatment	Miconazole Nitrate 2%	**Adults & Peds ≥12 yrs:** Athlete's Foot: Apply bid for 4 weeks.
Ting Spray Powder	Miconazole Nitrate 2%	**Adults & Peds ≥2 yrs:** Athlete's Foot/Ringworm: Apply bid for 4 weeks. Jock Itch: Apply bid for 2 weeks.
Zeasorb-AF Antifungal Drying Gel	Miconazole Nitrate 2%	**Adults & Peds ≥2 yrs:** Athlete's Foot/Ringworm: Apply bid for 4 weeks. Jock Itch: Apply bid for 2 weeks.
Zeasorb-AF Super Absorbent Antifungal Powder	Miconazole Nitrate 2%	**Adults & Peds ≥2 yrs:** Athlete's Foot/Ringworm: Apply bid for 4 weeks. Jock Itch: Apply bid for 2 weeks.
TERBINAFINE		
Lamisil AT Antifungal Continuous Spray, Athlete's Foot	Terbinafine HCl 1%	**Adults & Peds ≥12 yrs:** Athlete's Foot (between toes): Apply bid for 1 week. Jock Itch/Ringworm: Apply qd for 1 week.
Lamisil AT Antifungal Continuous Spray, Jock Itch	Terbinafine HCl 1%	**Adults & Peds ≥12 yrs:** Apply qd for 1 week.
Lamisil AT Athlete's Foot Treatment Cream	Terbinafine HCl 1%	**Adults & Peds ≥12 yrs:** Athlete's Foot (between toes): Apply bid for 1 week. Athlete's Foot (on side or bottom of foot): Apply bid for 2 weeks. Jock Itch/Ringworm: Apply qd for 1 week.
Lamisil AT Athlete's Foot Treatment Gel	Terbinafine HCl 1%	**Adults & Peds ≥12 yrs:** Athlete's Foot (between toes): Apply qhs for 1 week. Jock Itch/Ringworm: Apply qd for 1 week.
TOLNAFTATE		
Flexitol Medicated Foot Cream	Tolnaftate 1%	**Adults & Peds ≥2 yrs:** Apply bid for 4 weeks.
Tinactin Athlete's Foot Cream	Tolnaftate 1%	**Adults & Peds ≥2 yrs:** Apply bid for 4 weeks.
Tinactin Deodorant Powder Spray	Tolnaftate 1%	**Adults & Peds ≥2 yrs:** Athlete's Foot: Apply bid for 4 weeks. Prevention: Apply qd-bid.
Tinactin Jock Itch Cream	Tolnaftate 1%	**Adults & Peds ≥2 yrs:** Apply bid for 2 weeks.
Tinactin Jock Itch Powder Spray	Tolnaftate 1%	**Adults & Peds ≥2 yrs:** Apply bid for 2 weeks.
Tinactin Liquid Spray	Tolnaftate 1%	**Adults & Peds ≥2 yrs:** Athlete's Foot: Apply bid for 4 weeks. Prevention: Apply qd-bid.
Tinactin Powder Spray	Tolnaftate 1%	**Adults & Peds ≥2 yrs:** Athlete's Foot: Apply bid for 4 weeks. Prevention: Apply qd-bid.
Tinactin Pump Spray	Tolnaftate 1%	**Adults & Peds ≥2 yrs:** Athlete's Foot: Apply bid for 4 weeks. Prevention: Apply qd-bid.

(Continued)

BRAND	INGREDIENT/STRENGTH	DOSE
TOLNAFTATE (Continued)		
Tinactin Super Absorbent Powder	Tolnaftate 1%	**Adults & Peds ≥2 yrs:** Athlete's Foot: Apply bid for 4 weeks. Prevention: Apply qd-bid.
Ting Antifungal Cream	Tolnaftate 1%	**Adults & Peds ≥2 yrs:** Athlete's Foot/Ringworm: Apply bid for 4 weeks. Jock Itch: Apply bid for 2 weeks.
Ting Spray Liquid	Tolnaftate 1%	**Adults & Peds ≥2 yrs:** Apply bid for 4 weeks.
UNDECYLENIC ACID		
DiabetiDerm Toenail & Foot Fungus Antifungal Cream	Undecylenic Acid 10%	**Adults & Peds ≥2 yrs:** Athlete's Foot/Ringworm: Apply bid for 4 weeks. Jock Itch: Apply bid for 2 weeks.
Flexitol Anti-Fungal Liquid	Undecylenic Acid 25%	**Adults & Peds ≥2 yrs:** Athlete's Foot/Ringworm: Apply bid.
Fungi Nail Anti-Fungal Solution	Undecylenic Acid 25%	**Adults & Peds ≥2 yrs:** Athlete's Foot/Ringworm: Apply bid.
Fungi Nail Anti-Fungal Pen	Undecylenic Acid 25%	**Adults & Peds ≥2 yrs:** Athlete's Foot/Ringworm: Apply bid.
FungiCure Extra Strength Anti-Fungal Liquid	Undecylenic Acid 10%	**Adults & Peds ≥2 yrs:** Athlete's Foot/Ringworm: Apply bid for 4 weeks.
FungiCure Professional Formula Anti-Fungal Liquid	Undecylenic Acid 15%	**Adults & Peds ≥2 yrs:** Athlete's Foot/Ringworm: Apply bid for 4 weeks.
Tineacide Antifungal Cream	Undecylenic Acid 13%	**Adults & Peds ≥12 yrs:** Athlete's Foot (between toes): Apply bid for 4 weeks. Jock Itch/Ringworm: Apply bid for 2 weeks.

CONTACT DERMATITIS PRODUCTS

BRAND	INGREDIENT/STRENGTH	DOSE
ANTIHISTAMINE		
Benadryl Itch Stopping Extra Strength Gel	Diphenhydramine HCl 2%	**Adults & Peds ≥2 yrs:** Apply to affected area tid-qid.
ANTIHISTAMINE COMBINATION		
Benadryl Extra Strength Itch Stopping Cream	Diphenhydramine HCl/Zinc Acetate 2%-0.1%	**Adults & Peds ≥2 yrs:** Apply to affected area tid-qid.
Benadryl Extra Strength Spray	Diphenhydramine HCl/Zinc Acetate 2%-0.1%	**Adults & Peds ≥2 yrs:** Apply to affected area tid-qid.
Benadryl Extra Strength Itch Relief Stick	Diphenhydramine HCl/Zinc Acetate 2%-0.1%	**Adults & Peds ≥2 yrs:** Apply to affected area tid-qid.
Benadryl Original Strength Itch Stopping Cream	Diphenhydramine HCl/Zinc Acetate 1%-0.1%	**Adults & Peds ≥2 yrs:** Apply to affected area tid-qid.
Benadryl Readymist Itch Stopping Spray	Diphenhydramine/Zinc Acetate 2%-0.1%	**Adults & Peds ≥2 yrs:** Apply to affected area tid-qid.
CalaGel Anti-Itch Gel	Diphenhydramine HCl/Zinc Acetate/ Benzenthonium Chloride 2%-0.215%-0.15%	**Adults & Peds ≥2 yrs:** Apply to affected area no more than tid.
Ivarest Double Relief Formula	Diphenhydramine HCl/Benzyl Alcohol/ Calamine 2%-10.5%-14%	**Adults & Peds ≥2 yrs:** Apply to affected area tid-qid.
ASTRINGENT		
Domeboro Astringent Solution Powder Packets	Aluminum Acetate (combination of Calcium Acetate 952mg and Aluminum Sulfate 1347mg)	**Adults & Peds:** Dissolve 1-3 pkts and apply to affected area for 15-30 min tid.
Ivy-Dry Cream	Zinc Acetate/Benzyl Alcohol 2%-10%	**Adults & Peds ≥6 yrs:** Apply to affected area tid.
ASTRINGENT COMBINATION		
Aveeno Calamine and Pramoxine HCl Anti-Itch Cream	Calamine/Camphor/Pramoxine HCl 3%-0.5%-1%	**Adults & Peds ≥2 yrs:** Apply to affected area tid-qid.
Aveeno Anti-Itch Concentrated Lotion	Calamine/Camphor/Pramoxine HCl 3%-0.47%-1%	**Adults & Peds ≥2 yrs:** Apply to affected area qid.
Caladryl Clear Anti-Itch Lotion	Zinc Acetate/Pramoxine HCl 0.1%-1%	**Adults & Peds ≥2 yrs:** Apply to affected area tid-qid.
Caladryl Anti-Itch Lotion	Calamine/Pramoxine HCl 8%-1%	**Adults & Peds ≥2 yrs:** Apply to affected area tid-qid.
Calamine Lotion (generic)	Calamine/Zinc Oxide 8%-8%	**Adults & Peds:** Apply to affected area prn.
Cortaid Poison Ivy Care Treatment Kit	(Scrub) Water, polyethylene, laureth-4, sodium lauryl sarcosinate, glycol distearate, acrylates/ C10-30, alkyl acrylate crosspolymer, coco-glucoside, sodium hydroxide, microcrystalline wax, tetrasodium EDTA, glyceryl oleate, glyceryl stearate, quaternium-15, chromium hydroxide green, tocopherol (Spray) Zinc Acetate/Pramoxine 0.12%-1%	**Adults & Peds:** (Scrub) Apply quarter-sized amount into hand and rub onto affected area for 30 seconds. Rinse area thoroughly and pat dry. (Spray) Apply to affected area tid-qid.
CLEANSER		
Cortaid Poison Ivy Care Toxin Removal Cloths	Water, laureth-4, sodium lauryl sarcosinate, glycerin, DMDM, hydantoin, methylparaben, tetrasodium EDTA, *Aloe barbadensis* leaf extract, citric acid	**Adults & Peds:** Wipe affected area at least 15 seconds. Rinse or wipe dry.
Ivarest Poison Ivy Cleansing Foam	Menthol 1%	**Adults & Peds ≥2 yrs:** Gently rub into affected area and rinse under running water.

(Continued)

BRAND	INGREDIENT/STRENGTH	DOSE
CORTICOSTEROID		
Aveeno 1% Hydrocortisone Anti-Itch Cream	Hydrocortisone 1%	**Adults & Peds ≥2 yrs:** Apply to affected area tid-qid.
Cortaid Advanced 12-Hour Anti-Itch Cream	Hydrocortisone 1%	**Adults & Peds ≥2 yrs:** Apply to affected area tid-qid.
Cortaid Intensive Therapy Cooling Spray	Hydrocortisone 1%	**Adults & Peds ≥2 yrs:** Apply to affected area tid-qid.
Cortaid Intensive Therapy Moisturizing Cream	Hydrocortisone 1%	**Adults & Peds ≥2 yrs:** Apply to affected area tid-qid.
Cortaid Maximum Strength Cream	Hydrocortisone 1%	**Adults & Peds ≥2 yrs:** Apply to affected area tid-qid.
Cortaid Maximum Strength Ointment	Hydrocortisone 1%	**Adults & Peds ≥2 yrs:** Apply to affected area tid-qid.
Cortizone-10 Easy Relief Applicator	Hydrocortisone 1%	**Adults & Peds ≥2 yrs:** Apply to affected area tid-qid.
Cortizone-10 Cooling Relief Gel	Hydrocortisone 1%	**Adults & Peds ≥2 yrs:** Apply to affected area tid-qid.
Cortizone-10 Creme	Hydrocortisone 1%	**Adults & Peds ≥2 yrs:** Apply to affected area tid-qid.
Cortizone-10 Ointment	Hydrocortisone 1%	**Adults & Peds ≥2 yrs:** Apply to affected area tid-qid.
Cortizone-10 Creme Plus	Hydrocortisone 1%	**Adults & Peds ≥2 yrs:** Apply to affected area tid-qid.
Cortizone-10 Intensive Healing Formula	Hydrocortisone 1%	**Adults & Peds ≥2 yrs:** Apply to affected area tid-qid.
Cortizone-10 Intensive Healing Eczema Lotion	Hydrocortisone 1%	**Adults & Peds ≥2 yrs:** Apply to affected area tid-qid.
Cortizone-10 Hydraintensive Anti-Itch Soothing Lotion	Hydrocortisone 1%	**Adults & Peds ≥2 yrs:** Apply to affected area tid-qid.
Cortizone-10 Hydraintensive Anti-Itch Healing Lotion	Hydrocortisone 1%	**Adults & Peds ≥2 yrs:** Apply to affected area tid-qid.
Corticool 1% Hydrocortisone Anti-Itch Gel	Hydrocortisone 1%	**Adults & Peds ≥2 yrs:** Apply to affected area tid-qid.
COUNTERIRRITANT		
Gold Bond Medicated Maximum Strength Anti-Itch Cream	Menthol/Pramoxine HCl 1%-1%	**Adults & Peds ≥2 yrs:** Apply to affected area tid-qid.
Ivy Block Lotion	Bentoquatam 5%	**Adults & Peds ≥6 yrs:** Apply 15 minutes before exposure risk and q4h for continued protection.
LOCAL ANESTHETIC		
Solarcaine Aloe Extra Burn Relief Gel	Lidocaine HCl 0.5%	**Adults & Peds ≥2 yrs:** Apply to affected area tid-qid.
Solarcaine Aloe Extra Burn Relief Spray	Lidocaine HCl 0.5%	**Adults & Peds ≥2 yrs:** Apply to affected area tid-qid.
Solarcaine First Aid Medicated Spray	Benzocaine/Triclosan 20%-0.13%	**Adults & Peds ≥2 yrs:** Apply to affected area qd-tid.
LOCAL ANESTHETIC COMBINATION		
Bactine Pain Relieving Cleansing Spray	Lidocaine HCl/Benzalkonium Chloride 2.5%-0.13%	**Adults & Peds ≥2 yrs:** Apply to affected area qd-tid.
Bactine Original First Aid Liquid	Lidocaine HCl/Benzalkonium Chloride 2.5%-0.13%	**Adults & Peds ≥2 yrs:** Apply to affected area qd-tid.
Lanacane Maximum Strength Cream	Benzocaine/Benzethonium Chloride 20%-0.2%	**Adults & Peds ≥2 yrs:** Apply to affected area qd-tid.
Lanacane Antibacterial First Aid Spray	Benzocaine/Benzethonium Chloride 20%-0.2%	**Adults & Peds ≥2 yrs:** Apply to affected area qd-tid.

(Continued)

BRAND	INGREDIENT/STRENGTH	DOSE
SKIN PROTECTANT		
Aveeno Skin Relief Moisturizing Cream	Dimethicone 2.5%	**Adults & Peds ≥2 yrs:** Apply to affected area prn.
Aveeno Skin Relief Moisturizing Lotion	Dimethicone 1.3%	**Adults & Peds:** Apply to affected area prn.
Vaseline Intensive Rescue Clinical Therapy Lotion	Dimethicone 1%	**Adults & Peds:** Apply to affected area prn.
SKIN PROTECTANT COMBINATION		
Gold Bond Extra Strength Medicated Body Lotion	Dimethicone/Menthol 5%-0.5%	**Adults & Peds:** Apply to affected area tid-qid.
Gold Bond Medicated Body Lotion	Dimethicone/Menthol 5%-0.15%	**Adults & Peds:** Apply to affected area prn.
Gold Bond Medicated Powder	Zinc Oxide/Menthol 1%-0.15%	**Adults & Peds ≥2 yrs:** Apply to affected area tid-qid.
Gold Bond Extra Strength Medicated Powder	Zinc Oxide/Menthol 5%-0.8%	**Adults & Peds ≥2 yrs:** Apply to affected area tid-qid.
Gold Bond Medicated Baby Powder	Cornstarch/Kaolin/Zinc Oxide 79%-4%-15%	**Adults & Peds ≥2 yrs:** Apply to affected area tid-qid.

DIAPER RASH PRODUCTS

BRAND	INGREDIENT/STRENGTH	DOSE
WHITE PETROLATUM		
Balmex Multi-Purpose Healing Ointment	White Petrolatum 51.1%	**Peds:** Apply prn.
Desitin Multi-Purpose Skin Protectant and Diaper Rash Ointment	White Petrolatum 60.4%	**Peds:** Apply prn.
Vaseline Petroleum Jelly	White Petrolatum 100%	**Peds:** Apply prn.
ZINC OXIDE		
Aveeno Baby Soothing Relief Diaper Rash Cream	Zinc Oxide 13%	**Peds:** Apply prn.
Balmex Prevention Baby Powder with ActivGuard	Zinc Oxide 11.3%	**Adults & Peds ≥2 yrs:** Apply tid-qid. **Peds <2 yrs:** Apply prn.
Boudreaux's Butt Paste, Diaper Rash Ointment	Zinc Oxide 16%	**Peds:** Apply prn.
California Baby Calming Diaper Rash Cream	Zinc Oxide 12%	**Peds:** Apply prn.
Canus Li'l Goat's Milk Ointment	Zinc Oxide 40%	**Peds:** Apply prn.
Desitin Rapid Relief Cream	Zinc Oxide 13%	**Peds:** Apply prn.
Desitin Maximum Strength Original Paste	Zinc Oxide 40%	**Peds:** Apply prn.
Johnson's Baby Powder Medicated with Aloe & Vitamin E Medicated	Zinc Oxide 10%	**Peds:** Apply prn.
Mustela Bebe Vitamin Barrier Cream	Zinc Oxide 10%	**Peds:** Apply prn.
Triple Paste Medicated Ointment	Zinc Oxide 12.8%	**Peds:** Apply prn.
COMBINATION PRODUCTS		
A+D Original Ointment	Petrolatum/Lanolin 53.4%-15.5%	**Peds:** Apply prn.
A+D Zinc Oxide Cream	Dimethicone/Zinc Oxide 1%-10%	**Peds:** Apply prn.
Balmex Diaper Rash Cream with ActivGuard	Cornstarch/Zinc Oxide 83.6%-11.3%	**Peds:** Apply prn.
Lansinoh Diaper Rash Ointment	Dimethicone/USP Modified Lanolin/ Zinc Oxide 5.0%-15.5%-5.5%	**Peds:** Apply prn.

PSORIASIS PRODUCTS

BRAND	INGREDIENT/STRENGTH	DOSE
COAL TAR		
DHS Tar Gel Shampoo	Coal Tar 0.5%	Use at least biw.
DHS Tar Shampoo	Coal Tar 0.5%	Use at least biw.
Ionil Plus Shampoo	Coal Tar 2%	Use at least biw.
Ionil-T Plus Shampoo	Coal Tar 2%	Use at least biw.
Ionil-T Shampoo	Coal Tar 2%	Use at least biw.
MG217 Medicated Tar Lotion	Coal Tar 1%	Apply to affected area qd-qid.
MG217 Medicated Tar Ointment	Coal Tar 2%	Apply to affected area qd-qid.
MG217 Medicated Tar Shampoo	Coal Tar 3%	Use at least biw.
Neutrogena T/Gel Shampoo Extra Strength	Coal Tar 1%	Use at least biw.
Neutrogena T/Gel Shampoo Original Formula	Coal Tar 0.5%	Use at least biw.
Neutrogena T/Gel Shampoo Stubborn Itch Control	Coal Tar 0.5%	Use at least biw.
Psoriasin Gel	Coal Tar 1.25%	**Adults:** Apply to affected area qd-qid.
Psoriasin Liquid For Skin & Scalp	Coal Tar 0.66%	**Adults:** Apply to affected area qd-qid.
Psoriasin Ointment	Coal Tar 2%	**Adults:** Apply to affected area qd-qid.
CORTICOSTEROID		
Aveeno 1% Hydrocortisone Anti-Itch Cream	Hydrocortisone 1%	**Adults & Peds ≥2 yrs:** Apply to affected area tid-qid.
Cortaid Advanced 12-Hour Anti-Itch Cream	Hydrocortisone 1%	**Adults & Peds ≥2 yrs:** Apply to affected area tid-qid.
Cortaid Intensive Therapy Cooling Spray	Hydrocortisone 1%	**Adults & Peds ≥2 yrs:** Apply to affected area tid-qid.
Cortaid Intensive Therapy Moisturizing Cream	Hydrocortisone 1%	**Adults & Peds ≥2 yrs:** Apply to affected area tid-qid.
Cortaid Maximum Strength Cream	Hydrocortisone 1%	**Adults & Peds ≥2 yrs:** Apply to affected area tid-qid.
Cortaid Maximum Strength Ointment	Hydrocortisone 1%	**Adults & Peds ≥2 yrs:** Apply to affected area tid-qid.
Corticool 1% Hydrocortisone Anti-Itch Gel	Hydrocortisone 1%	**Adults & Peds ≥2 yrs:** Apply to affected area tid-qid.
Cortizone-10 Cooling Relief Gel	Hydrocortisone 1%	**Adults & Peds ≥2 yrs:** Apply to affected area tid-qid.
Cortizone-10 Creme	Hydrocortisone 1%	**Adults & Peds ≥2 yrs:** Apply to affected area tid-qid.
Cortizone-10 Creme Plus	Hydrocortisone 1%	**Adults & Peds ≥2 yrs:** Apply to affected area tid-qid.
Cortizone-10 Ointment	Hydrocortisone 1%	**Adults & Peds ≥2 yrs:** Apply to affected area tid-qid.
Cortizone-10 Easy Relief Applicator	Hydrocortisone 1%	**Adults & Peds ≥2 yrs:** Apply to affected area tid-qid.
Cortizone-10 Intensive Healing Formula	Hydrocortisone 1%	**Adults & Peds ≥2 yrs:** Apply to affected area tid-qid.
SALICYLIC ACID		
Dermarest Psoriasis Medicated Moisturizer	Salicylic Acid 2%	**Adults & Peds:** Apply to affected area qd-qid.
Dermarest Psoriasis Medicated Scalp Treatment	Salicylic Acid 3%	**Adults & Peds:** Apply to affected area qd-qid.
Dermarest Psoriasis Medicated Shampoo Plus Conditioner	Salicylic Acid 3%	**Adults & Peds:** Use at least biw.
Dermarest Psoriasis Medicated Skin Treatment	Salicylic Acid 3%	**Adults & Peds:** Apply to affected area qd-qid.

(Continued)

BRAND	INGREDIENT/STRENGTH	DOSE
SALICYLIC ACID (Continued)		
DHS Sal Shampoo	Salicylic Acid 3%	**Adults & Peds:** Use at least biw.
MG217 Sal-Acid Ointment	Salicylic Acid 3%	**Adults & Peds:** Apply to affected area qd-qid.
Neutrogena T/Gel Therapeutic Conditioner	Salicylic Acid 2%	**Adults & Peds:** Use at least biw.
Neutrogena T/Sal Therapeutic Shampoo	Salicylic Acid 3%	**Adults & Peds:** Use at least tiw.
Psoriasin Therapeutic Shampoo and Body Wash	Salicylic Acid 3%	**Adults & Peds:** Use at least biw.

WOUND CARE PRODUCTS

BRAND	INGREDIENT/STRENGTH	DOSE
NEOMYCIN/POLYMYXIN B/BACITRACIN COMBINATIONS		
Bacitracin Ointment	Bacitracin 500 U	**Adults & Peds:** Apply to affected area qd-tid.
Neosporin First Aid Antibiotic Ointment	Neomycin/polymyxin B/bacitracin 3.5mg-5,000 U-400 U	**Adults & Peds:** Apply to affected area qd-tid.
Neosporin Neo To Go! Single Use Packets	Neomycin/polymyxin B/bacitracin 3.5mg-5,000 U-400 U	**Adults & Peds:** Apply to affected area qd-tid.
Neosporin Plus Pain Relief Cream	Neomycin/polymyxin B/pramoxine HCl 3.5mg-10,000 U-10mg	**Adults & Peds** ≥2 yrs: Apply to affected area qd-tid.
Neosporin Plus Pain Relief Ointment	Neomycin/polymyxin B/bacitracin/pramoxine HCl 3.5mg-10,000 U-400 U-10mg	**Adults & Peds** ≥2 yrs: Apply to affected area qd-tid.
Polysporin First Aid Antibiotic Ointment	Polymyxin B/bacitracin 10,000 U-500 U	**Adults & Peds:** Apply to affected area qd-tid.
Polysporin First Aid Antibiotic Powder	Polymyxin B/bacitracin 10,000 U-500 U	**Adults & Peds:** Apply to affected area qd-tid.
BENZALKONIUM CHLORIDE COMBINATIONS		
Bactine Original First Aid Liquid	Benzalkonium chloride/lidocaine HCl 0.13%-2.5%	**Adults & Peds** ≥2 yrs: Use to clean affected area qd-tid.
Bactine Pain Relieving Cleansing Spray	Benzalkonium chloride/lidocaine HCl 0.13%-2.5%	**Adults & Peds** ≥2 yrs: Use to clean affected area qd-tid.
Band-Aid Hurt Free Antiseptic Wash	Benzalkonium chloride/lidocaine HCl 0.13%-2%	**Adults & Peds** ≥2 yrs: Use to clean affected area qd-tid.
Neosporin Neo To Go! First Aid Antiseptic/Pain Relieving Spray	Benzalkonium chloride/pramoxine HCl 0.13%-1%	**Adults & Peds** ≥2 yrs: Use to clean affected area qd-tid.
BENZETHONIUM CHLORIDE COMBINATIONS		
Gold Bond Quick Spray	Benzethonium chloride/menthol 0.13%-1%	**Adults & Peds** ≥2 yrs: Apply to affected area qd-tid.
Lanacane Anti-Bacterial First Aid Spray	Benzethonium chloride/benzocaine 0.2%-20%	**Adults & Peds** ≥2 yrs: Apply to affected area qd-tid.
Lanacane Maximum Strength Pain & Intense Itch Anti-Itch Cream	Benzethonium chloride/benzocaine 0.2%-20%	**Adults & Peds** ≥2 yrs: Apply to affected area qd-tid.
Lanacane Original Strength Itch & Irritation Anti-Itch Cream	Benzethonium chloride/benzocaine 0.2%-6%	**Adults & Peds** ≥2 yrs: Apply to affected area qd-tid.
CHLORHEXIDINE GLUCONATE		
Hibiclens	Chlorhexidine gluconate 4%	**Adults:** Apply sparingly to affected area and wash.
Hibistat	Chlorhexidine gluconate/isopropyl alcohol 0.5%-70%	**Adults:** Rub vigorously with the towelette for about 15 seconds.
IODINE		
Betadine Skin Cleanser	Povidone-iodine 7.5%	**Adults & Peds:** Apply to affected area, wash vigorously for 15 seconds, rinse and dry.
Betadine Solution	Povidone-iodine 10%	**Adults & Peds:** Apply to affected area qd-tid.
MISCELLANEOUS		
Aquaphor Healing Ointment	Petrolatum (41%), mineral oil, ceresin, lanolin alcohol, panthenol, glycerin, bisabolol	**Adults & Peds:** Apply to affected area prn.
Wound Wash Saline	Sterile 0.9% sodium chloride solution	**Adults & Peds:** Use to clean affected area prn.

ANTACID AND HEARTBURN PRODUCTS

BRAND	INGREDIENT/STRENGTH	DOSE
ANTACID		
Alka-Seltzer Gold Tablets	Citric Acid/Potassium Bicarbonate/Sodium Bicarbonate 1000mg-344mg-1050mg	**Adults ≥60 yrs:** 2 tabs q4h prn. **Max:** 6 tabs q24h. **Adults & Peds ≥12 yrs:** 2 tabs q4h prn. **Max:** 8 tabs q24h. **Peds ≤12 yrs:** 1 tab q4h prn. **Max:** 4 tabs q24h.
Alka-Seltzer Heartburn Relief Tablets	Citric Acid/Sodium Bicarbonate 1000mg-1940mg	**Adults ≥60 yrs:** 2 tabs q4h prn. **Max:** 4 tabs q24h. **Adults & Peds ≥12 yrs:** 2 tabs q4h prn. **Max:** 8 tabs q24h.
Alka-Seltzer Lemon Lime Tablets	Aspirin/Citric Acid/Sodium Bicarbonate 325mg-1000mg-1700mg	**Adults ≥60 yrs:** 2 tabs q4h prn. **Max:** 4 tabs q24h. **Adults & Peds ≥12 yrs:** 2 tabs q4h prn. **Max:** 8 tabs q24h.
Alka-Seltzer Tablets, Extra-Strength	Aspirin/Citric Acid/Sodium Bicarbonate 500mg-1000mg-1985mg	**Adults ≥60 yrs:** 2 tabs q6h prn. **Max:** 3 tabs q24h. **Adults & Peds ≥12 yrs:** 2 tabs q6h prn. **Max:** 7 tabs q24h.
Alka-Seltzer Tablets, Original	Aspirin/Citric Acid/Sodium Bicarbonate 325mg-1000mg-1916mg	**Adults ≥60 yrs:** 2 tabs q4h prn. **Max:** 4 tabs q24h. **Adults & Peds ≥12 yrs:** 2 tabs q4h prn. **Max:** 8 tabs q24h.
Brioschi Powder	Sodium Bicarbonate/Tartaric Acid 2.69g-2.43g/dose	**Adults & Peds ≥12 yrs:** 1 capful (6g) dissolved in 4-6 oz water q1h. **Max:** 6 doses q24h. **Adults ≥60 yrs:** 1 capful (6g) dissolved in 4-6 oz water q1h. **Max:** 3 doses q24h.
Gaviscon Extra Strength Liquid	Aluminum Hydroxide/Magnesium Carbonate 254mg-237.5mg/5mL	**Adults:** 2-4 tsp (10-20mL) qid.
Gaviscon Extra Strength Tablets	Aluminum Hydroxide/Magnesium Carbonate 160mg-105mg	**Adults:** 2-4 tabs qid. **Max:** 16 doses q24h.
Gaviscon Regular Strength Liquid	Aluminum Hydroxide/Magnesium Carbonate 95mg-358mg/15mL	**Adults:** 1-2 tbl (15-30mL) qid. **Max:** 8 tbl q24h.
Gaviscon Regular Strength Tablets	Aluminum Hydroxide/Magnesium Trisilicate 80mg-14.2mg	**Adults:** 2-4 tabs qid. **Max:** 16 tabs q24h.
Maalox Children's Relief Chewables	Calcium Carbonate 400mg	**Peds 6-11 yrs (48-95 lbs):** 2 tabs prn. **Max:** 6 tabs q24h. **Peds 2-5 yrs (24-47 lbs):** 1 tab prn. **Max:** 3 tabs q24h.
Maalox Regular Strength Chewable Tablets	Calcium Carbonate 600mg	**Adults:** 1-2 tabs prn. **Max:** 12 tabs q24h.
Mylanta, Children's	Calcium Carbonate 400mg	**Peds 6-11 yrs (48-95 lbs):** Take 2 tabs prn. **Max:** 6 tabs q24h. **Peds 2-5 yrs (24-47 lbs):** Take 1 tab prn. **Max:** 3 tabs q24h.
Mylanta Supreme Antacid Liquid	Calcium Carbonate/Magnesium Hydroxide 400mg-135mg/5mL	**Adults:** 2-4 tsp (10-20mL) qid (between meals & hs). **Max:** 18 tsp (90mL) q24h.
Mylanta Ultimate Strength Chewable Tablets	Calcium Carbonate/Magnesium Hydroxide 700mg-300mg	**Adults:** 2-4 tabs qid (between meals & hs). **Max:** 10 tabs q24h for ≤2 weeks.
Mylanta Ultimate Strength Liquid	Aluminum Hydroxide/Magnesium Hydroxide 500mg-500mg/5mL	**Adults & Peds ≥12 yrs:** 2-4 tsp (10-20mL) qid (between meals & hs). **Max:** 9 tsp (45mL) q24h for ≤2 weeks.
Pepto Bismol Children's Pepto Chewable Tablets	Calcium Carbonate 400mg	**Peds 6-11 yrs (48-95 lbs):** Take 2 tabs prn. **Max:** 6 tabs q24h. **Peds 2-5 yrs (24-47 lbs):** Take 1 tab prn. **Max:** 3 tabs q24h.
Rolaids Extra Strength Softchews	Calcium Carbonate 1177mg	**Adults:** 2-3 chews q1h prn. **Max:** 6 chews q24h.
Rolaids Extra Strength Tablets	Calcium Carbonate/Magnesium Hydroxide 675mg-135mg	**Adults:** 2-4 tabs q1h prn. **Max:** 10 tabs q24h.

(Continued)

BRAND	INGREDIENT/STRENGTH	DOSE
ANTACID *(Continued)*		
Rolaids Regular Strength Tablets	Calcium Carbonate/Magnesium Hydroxide 550mg-110mg	**Adults:** 2-4 tabs q1h prn. **Max:** 12 tabs q24h.
Titralac Instant Relief Tablets	Calcium Carbonate 420mg	**Adults:** 2 tabs q2-3h prn. **Max:** 19 tabs q24h.
Tums Regular Strength Tablets	Calcium Carbonate 500mg	**Adults:** 2-4 tabs prn. **Max:** 15 tabs q24h.
Tums E-X 750 Chewable Tablets	Calcium Carbonate 750mg	**Adults:** 2-4 tabs prn. **Max:** 10 tabs q24h.
Tums E-X 750 Sugar Free Chewable Tablets	Calcium Carbonate 750mg	**Adults:** 2-4 tabs prn. **Max:** 9 tabs q24h.
Tums Kids Chewable Tablets	Calcium Carbonate 750mg	**Peds 5-11 yrs:** 1 tab prn. **Max:** 4 tabs q24h. **Peds 2-4 yrs:** 1/2 tab prn. **Max:** 2 tabs q24h.
Tums Smoothies Tablets	Calcium Carbonate 750mg	**Adults:** 2-4 tabs prn. **Max:** 10 tabs q24h.
Tums Ultra 1000 Chewable Tablets	Calcium Carbonate 1000mg	**Adults:** 2-3 tabs prn. **Max:** 7 tabs q24h for ≤2 weeks.
ANTACID/ANTIFLATULANT		
Gelusil Chewable Tablets	Aluminum Hydroxide/Magnesium Hydroxide/Simethicone 200mg-200mg-25mg	**Adults:** 2-4 tabs q1h prn. **Max:** 12 tabs q24h.
Maalox Advanced Maximum Strength Chewable Tablets	Calcium Carbonate/Simethicone 1000mg-60mg	**Adults & Peds ≥12 yrs:** 1-2 tabs prn. **Max:** 8 tabs q24h.
Maalox Advanced Maximum Strength Liquid	Aluminum Hydroxide/Magnesium Hydroxide/Simethicone 400mg-400mg-40mg/5mL	**Adults & Peds ≥12 yrs:** 2-4 tsp (10-20mL) bid. **Max:** 8 tsp (40mL) q24h.
Maalox Advanced Regular Strength Liquid	Aluminum Hydroxide/Magnesium Hydroxide/Simethicone 200mg-200mg-20mg/5mL	**Adults & Peds ≥12 yrs:** 2-4 tsp (10-20mL) qid. **Max:** 16 tsp (80mL) q24h.
Maalox Junior Relief Chewables	Calcium Carbonate/Simethicone 400mg-24mg	**Peds 6-11 yrs:** 2 tabs prn. **Max:** 6 tabs q24h.
Mylanta Maximum Strength Liquid	Aluminum Hydroxide/Magnesium Hydroxide/Simethicone 400mg-400mg-40mg/5mL	**Adults & Peds ≥12 yrs:** 2-4 tsp (between meals and hs) (10-20mL) qid. **Max:** 12 tsp (60mL) q24h.
Mylanta Regular Strength Liquid	Aluminum Hydroxide/Magnesium Hydroxide/Simethicone 200mg-200mg-20mg/5mL	**Adults & Peds ≥12 yrs:** 2-4 tsp (between meals and hs) (10-20mL) qid. **Max:** 24 tsp (120mL) q24h.
Rolaids Extra Strength Plus Gas Soft Chews	Calcium Carbonate/Simethicone 1177mg-80mg	**Adults:** 2-3 chews q1h prn. **Max:** 6 chews q24h.
Rolaids Multi-Symptom Chewable Tablets	Calcium Carbonate/Magnesium Hydroxide/Simethicone 675mg-135mg-60mg	**Adults:** 2-4 tabs q1h prn. **Max:** 8 tabs q24h.
Titralac Plus Chewable Tablets	Calcium Carbonate/Simethicone 420mg-21mg	**Adults:** 2 tabs q2-3h prn. **Max:** 19 tabs q24h.
BISMUTH SUBSALICYLATE		
Maalox Total Relief Maximum Strength Liquid	Bismuth Subsalicylate 525mg/15mL	**Adults & Peds ≥12 yrs:** 2 tbl (30mL) q1h prn. **Max:** 8 tbl (120mL) q24h.
Pepto Bismol Caplets	Bismuth Subsalicylate 262mg	**Adults & Peds ≥12 yrs:** 2 tabs q1/2-1h prn. **Max:** 8 doses q24h.
Pepto Bismol Chewable Tablets	Bismuth Subsalicylate 262mg	**Adults & Peds ≥12 yrs:** 2 tabs q1/2-1h prn. **Max:** 8 doses q24h.

(Continued)

BRAND	INGREDIENT/STRENGTH	DOSE
BISMUTH SUBSALICYLATE *(Continued)*		
Pepto Bismol Liquid	Bismuth Subsalicylate 262mg/15mL	**Adults & Peds ≥12 yrs:** 2 tbl (30mL) q1/2-1h prn. **Max:** 8 doses (240mL) q24h.
Pepto Bismol Liquid Max	Bismuth Subsalicylate 525mg/15mL	**Adults & Peds ≥12 yrs:** 2 tbl (30mL) q1h prn. **Max:** 4 doses (120mL) q24h.
H₂-RECEPTOR ANTAGONIST		
Axid AR	Nizatidine 75mg	**Adults & Peds ≥12 yrs:** 1 tab qd. **Max:** 2 tabs q24h.
Pepcid AC Maximum Strength EZ Chews	Famotidine 20mg	**Adults & Peds ≥12 yrs:** 1 tab qd. **Max:** 2 tabs q24h.
Pepcid AC Maximum Strength Tablets	Famotidine 20mg	**Adults & Peds ≥12 yrs:** 1 tab qd. **Max:** 2 tabs q24h.
Pepcid AC Tablets	Famotidine 10mg	**Adults & Peds ≥12 yrs:** 1 tab qd. **Max:** 2 tabs q24h.
Tagamet HB Tablets	Cimetidine 200mg	**Adults & Peds ≥12 yrs:** 1 tab qd. **Max:** 2 tabs q24h.
Zantac 75 Tablets	Ranitidine 75mg	**Adults & Peds ≥12 yrs:** 1 tab qd. **Max:** 2 tabs q24h.
Zantac 150 Tablets	Ranitidine 150mg	**Adults & Peds ≥12 yrs:** 1 tab qd. **Max:** 2 tabs q24h.
H₂-RECEPTOR ANTAGONIST/ANTACID		
Pepcid Complete Chewable Tablets	Famotidine/Calcium Carbonate/ Magnesium Hydroxide 10mg-800mg-165mg	**Adults & Peds ≥12 yrs:** 1 tab qd. **Max:** 2 tabs q24h.
Tums Dual Action	Famotidine/Calcium Carbonate/ Magnesium Hydroxide 10mg-800mg-165mg	**Adults & Peds ≥12 yrs:** 1 tab qd. **Max:** 2 tabs q24h.
PROTON PUMP INHIBITOR		
Prevacid 24HR	Lansoprazole 15mg	**Adults:** 1 cap qd x 14 days. May repeat 14-day course q4 months.
Prilosec OTC Tablets	Omeprazole 20mg	**Adults:** 1 tab qd x 14 days. May repeat 14-day course q4 months.
Zegerid OTC	Omeprazole/Sodium bicarbonate 20mg-1100mg	**Adults:** 1 cap qd x 14 days. May repeat 14-day course q4 months.

ANTIDIARRHEAL PRODUCTS

BRAND	INGREDIENT/STRENGTH	DOSE
ABSORBENT AGENTS		
Equalactin Chewable Tablets	Calcium Polycarbophil 625mg	**Adults & Peds ≥12 yrs:** 2 tabs/dose. **Max:** 8 tabs q24h. **Peds 6-12 yrs:** 1 tab/dose. **Max:** 4 tabs q24h. **Peds 2 to ≤6 yrs:** 1 tab/dose. **Max:** 2 tabs q24h.
Fibercon Caplets	Calcium Polycarbophil 625mg	**Adults & Peds ≥12 yrs:** 2 tabs qd. **Max:** 8 tabs q24h.
Konsyl Fiber Caplets	Calcium Polycarbophil 625mg	**Adults & Peds ≥12 yrs:** 2 tabs qd-qid. **Peds 6-12 yrs:** 1 tab qd-tid. **Max:** 8 tabs q24h.
ANTIPERISTALTIC AGENTS		
Imodium A-D Caplets	Loperamide HCl 2mg	**Adults & Peds ≥12 yrs:** 2 tabs after first loose stool; 1 tab after each subsequent loose stool. **Max:** 4 tabs q24h. **Peds 9-11 yrs (60-95 lbs):** 1 tab after first loose stool; ½ tab after each subsequent loose stool. **Max:** 3 tabs q24h. **Peds 6-8 yrs (48-59 lbs):** 1 tab after first loose stool; ½ tab after each subsequent loose stool. **Max:** 2 tabs q24h.
Imodium A-D E-Z Chews	Loperamide HCl 2mg	**Adults & Peds ≥12 yrs:** 2 tabs after first loose stool; 1 tab after each subsequent loose stool. **Max:** 4 tabs q24h. **Peds 9-11 yrs (60-95 lbs):** 1 tab after first loose stool; ½ tab after each subsequent loose stool. **Max:** 3 tabs q24h. **Peds 6-8 yrs (48-59 lbs):** 1 tab after first loose stool; ½ tab after each subsequent loose stool. **Max:** 2 tabs q24h.
Imodium A-D Liquid	Loperamide HCl 1mg/7.5mL	**Adults & Peds ≥12 yrs:** 4 tsp (20mL) after first loose stool; 2 tsp (10mL) after each subsequent loose stool. **Max:** 8 tsp (40mL) q24h. **Peds 9-11 yrs (60-95 lbs):** 2 tsp (10mL) after the first loose stool; 1 tsp (5mL) after each subsequent loose stool. **Max:** 6 tsp (30mL) q24h. **Peds 6-8 yrs (48-59 lbs):** 2 tsp (10mL) after the first loose stool; 1 tsp (5mL) after each subsequent loose stool. **Max:** 4 tsp (20mL) q24h.
Imodium A-D Liquid For Use In Children (Mint Flavor)	Loperamide HCl 1mg/7.5mL	**Adults & Peds ≥12 yrs:** 6 tsp (30mL) after first loose stool; 3 tsp (15mL) after each subsequent loose stool. **Max:** 12 tsp (60mL) q24h. **Peds 9-11 yrs (60-95 lbs):** 3 tsp (15mL) after the first loose stool; 1½ tsp (7.5mL) after each subsequent loose stool. **Max:** 9 tsp (45mL) q24h. **Peds 6-8 yrs (48-59 lbs):** 3 tsp (15mL) after first loose stool; 1½ tsp (7.5mL) after each subsequent loose stool. **Max:** 6 tsp (30mL) q24h.

(Continued)

BRAND	INGREDIENT/STRENGTH	DOSE
ANTIPERISTALTIC/ANTIFLATULENT AGENTS		
Imodium Multi-Symptom Relief Caplets	Loperamide HCl/Simethicone 2mg-125mg	**Adults & Peds ≥12 yrs:** 2 tabs after first loose stool; 1 tab after each subsequent loose stool. **Max:** 4 tabs q24h. **Peds 9-11 yrs (60-95 lbs):** 1 tab after first loose stool; ½ tab after each subsequent loose stool. **Max:** 3 tabs q24h. **6-8 yrs (48-59 lbs):** 1 tab after first loose stool; ½ tab after each subsequent loose stool. **Max:** 2 tabs q24h.
Imodium Multi-Symptom Relief Chewable Tablets	Loperamide HCl/Simethicone 2mg-125mg	**Adults & Peds ≥12 yrs:** 2 tabs with 4-8 oz water after first loose stool; 1 tab with 4-8 oz water after each subsequent loose stool. **Max:** 4 tabs q24h. **Peds 9-11 yrs (60-95 lbs):** 1 tab with 4-8 oz water after first loose stool; ½ tab after each subsequent loose stool. **Max:** 3 tabs q24h. **Peds 6-8 yrs (48-59 lbs):** 1 tab with 4-8 oz water after first loose stool; ½ tab with 4-8 oz water after each subsequent loose stool. **Max:** 2 tabs q24h.
BISMUTH SUBSALICYLATE		
Kaopectate Extra Strength Liquid	Bismuth Subsalicylate 525mg/15mL	**Adults & Peds ≥12 yrs:** 2 tbl (30mL) q1h prn. **Max:** 4 doses (8 tbl) q24h.
Kaopectate Liquid	Bismuth Subsalicylate 262mg/15mL	**Adults & Peds ≥12 yrs:** 2 tbl (30mL) q½-1h prn. **Max:** 8 doses (16 tbl) q24h.
Maalox Total Relief Liquid	Bismuth Subsalicylate 525mg/15mL	**Adults & Peds ≥12 yrs:** 2 tbl (30mL) q1h prn. **Max:** 4 doses (8 tbl) q24h.
Pepto Bismol Caplets	Bismuth Subsalicylate 262mg	**Adults & Peds ≥12 yrs:** 2 tabs q½-1h. **Max:** 8 doses (16 tabs) q24h.
Pepto Bismol Chewable Tablets	Bismuth Subsalicylate 262mg	**Adults & Peds ≥12 yrs:** 2 tabs q½-1h. **Max:** 8 doses (16 tabs) q24h.
Pepto Bismol Liquid	Bismuth Subsalicylate 262mg/15mL	**Adults & Peds ≥12 yrs:** 2 tbl (30mL) q½-1h prn. **Max:** 8 doses (16 tbl) q24h.
Pepto Bismol Liquid Max	Bismuth Subsalicylate 525mg/15mL	**Adults & Peds ≥12 yrs:** 2 tbl (30mL) q1h prn. **Max:** 4 doses (8 tbl) q24h.

LAXATIVE PRODUCTS

BRAND	INGREDIENT/STRENGTH	DOSE
BULK-FORMING		
Citrucel Caplets	Methylcellulose 500mg	**Adults & Peds ≥12 yrs:** 2 tabs qd prn. **Max:** 12 tabs q24h. **Peds 6-11 yrs:** 1 tab qd prn. **Max:** 6 tabs q24h.
Citrucel Sugar Free Powder	Methylcellulose 2g/tbl	**Adults & Peds ≥12 yrs:** 1 tbl (11.5g) qd-tid. **Peds 6-11 yrs:** ½ tbl (5.75g) qd.
Equalactin Chewable Tablets	Calcium Polycarbophil 625mg	**Adults & Peds ≥12 yrs:** 2 tabs qd. **Max:** 8 tabs q24h. **Peds 6-11 yrs:** 1 tab qd. **Max:** 4 tabs q24h. **Peds 2-5 yrs:** 1 tab qd. **Max:** 2 tabs q24h.
Fibercon Caplets	Calcium Polycarbophil 625mg	**Adults & Peds ≥12 yrs:** 2 tabs qd. **Max:** 8 tabs qd.
Konsyl Easy Mix Powder	Psyllium 4.3g/tsp	**Adults & Peds ≥12 yrs:** 1 tsp qd-tid. **Peds 6-11 yrs:** ½ tsp qd-tid.
Konsyl Fiber Caplets	Calcium Polycarbophil 625mg	**Adults:** 2 tabs qd-qid. **Max:** 8 tabs q24h. **Peds 6-12 yrs:** 1 tab qd-tid. **Max:** 3 tabs q24h.
Konsyl Orange Powder	Psyllium 3.4g/tbl	**Adults & Peds ≥12 yrs:** 1 tbl qd-tid. **Peds 6-11 yrs:** ½ tbl qd-tid.
Konsyl Original Powder	Psyllium 6g/tsp	**Adults & Peds ≥12 yrs:** 1 tsp qd-tid. **Peds 6-11 yrs:** ½ tsp qd-tid.
Konsyl-D Powder	Psyllium 3.4g/tsp	**Adults & Peds ≥12 yrs:** 1 tsp qd-tid. **Peds 6-11 yrs:** ½ tsp qd-tid.
Metamucil Capsules	Psyllium 0.52g	**Adults & Peds ≥12 yrs:** 5 caps qd-tid.
Metamucil Original Texture Powder (multi-flavor)	Psyllium 3.4g/tbl	**Adults & Peds ≥12 yrs:** 1 tbl up to tid. **Peds 6-11 yrs:** ½ tbl up to tid.
Metamucil Smooth Texture Powder (multi-flavor)	Psyllium 3.4g/tbl	**Adults & Peds ≥12 yrs:** 1 tbl up to tid. **Peds 6-11 yrs:** ½ tbl up to tid.
Metamucil Wafers	Psyllium 3.4g/dose	**Adults & Peds ≥12 yrs:** 2 wafers qd-tid. **Peds 6-11 yrs:** 1 wafer qd-tid.
HYPEROSMOTICS		
Colace Glycerin Suppositories for Adults and Children	Glycerin 2.1g	**Adults & Peds ≥6 yrs:** 1 supp **Max:** 1 supp q24h.
Colace Glycerin Suppositories for Infants and Children	Glycerin 1.2g	**Peds 2-5 yrs:** 1 supp **Max:** 1 supp q24h.
Dulcolax Balance	Polyethylene Glycol 3350, 17g	**Adults & Peds ≥17 yrs:** 1 capful (17g) qd. **Max:** 7 days.
Fleet Glycerin Suppositories	Glycerin 2g	**Adults & Peds ≥6 yrs:** 1 supp ud.
Fleet Liquid Glycerin Suppositories	Glycerin 5.6g	**Adults & Peds ≥6 yrs:** 1 supp ud.
Fleet Mineral Oil Enema	Mineral Oil 118mL	**Adults & Peds ≥12 yrs:** 1 bottle (118mL). **Peds 2-11 yrs:** ½ bottle (59mL).
Fleet Pedia-Lax Glycerin Suppositories	Glycerin 1g	**Peds 2-6 yrs:** 1 supp ud.
Fleet Pedia-Lax Liquid Glycerin Suppositories	Glycerin 2.8g	**Peds 2-6 yrs:** 1 supp ud.

(Continued)

BRAND	INGREDIENT/STRENGTH	DOSE
SALINES		
Fleet Enema	Monobasic Sodium Phosphate/Dibasic Sodium Phosphate 19g-7g/118mL	**Adults & Peds ≥12 yrs:** 1 bottle (118mL).
Fleet Enema Extra	Monobasic Sodium Phosphate/Dibasic Sodium Phosphate 19g-7g/197mL	**Adults & Peds ≥12 yrs:** 1 bottle (197mL).
Fleet Pedia-Lax Chewable Tablets	Magnesium Hydroxide 400mg	**Peds 6-<12 yrs:** 3-6 tabs qd. **Max:** 6 tabs q24h. **Peds 2-<6 yrs:** 1-3 tabs qd. **Max:** 3 tabs q24h.
Fleet Pedia-Lax Enema	Monobasic Sodium Phosphate/Dibasic Sodium Phosphate 9.5g-3.5g/59mL	**Peds 5-11 yrs:** 1 bottle (59mL). **Peds 2-<5 yrs:** ½ bottle (29.5mL).
Magnesium Citrate Solution	Magnesium Citrate 1.75g/30mL	**Adults & Peds ≥12 yrs:** 300mL. **Peds 6-<12 yrs:** 90-210mL. **Peds 2-<6 yrs:** 60mL.
Little Phillips' Milk of Magnesia Safe and Gentle	Magnesium Hydroxide 800mg/5mL	**Adults & Peds ≥12 yrs:** 3-6 tsp qd. **Peds 6-11 yrs:** 1.5-3 tsp qd. **Peds 2-5 yrs:** 1/2-1.5 tsp qd.
Phillips' Antacid/Laxative Chewable Tablets	Magnesium Hydroxide 311mg	**Adults & Peds ≥12 yrs:** 8 tabs qd. **Peds 6-11 yrs:** 4 tabs qd. **Peds 3-5 yrs:** 2 tabs qd.
Phillips' Laxative Caplets	Magnesium 500mg	**Adults & Peds ≥12 yrs:** Take 2-4 tabs qd. **Max:** 4 tabs q24h.
Phillips' M-O	Magnesium Hydroxide 300mg/5mL	**Adults & Peds ≥12 yrs:** 3-4 tbl qd. **Peds 6-11 yrs:** 4-6 tsp qd.
Phillips' Concentrated Milk of Magnesia Liquid	Magnesium Hydroxide 800mg/5mL	**Adults & Peds ≥12 yrs:** 1-2 tbl qd. **Peds 6-11 yrs:** ½-1 tbl qd.
Phillips' Milk of Magnesia Liquid	Magnesium Hydroxide 400mg/5mL	**Adults & Peds ≥12 yrs:** 2-4 tbl qd. **Peds 6-11 yrs:** 1-2 tbl qd.
SALINE COMBINATION		
Phillips' M-O Liquid	Magnesium Hydroxide/Mineral Oil 300mg-1.25mL/5mL	**Adults & Peds ≥12 yrs:** 3-4 tbl qd. **Peds 6-11 yrs:** 4-6 tsp qd.
STIMULANTS		
Alophen Enteric Coated Stimulant Laxative Pills	Bisacodyl 5mg	**Adults & Peds ≥12 yrs:** Take 1-3 tabs qd. **Peds 6-11 yrs:** Take 1 tab qd.
Carter's Laxative, Sodium Free Pills	Bisacodyl 5mg	**Adults & Peds ≥12 yrs:** Take 1-3 tabs (usually 2 tabs) qd. **Peds 6-<12 yrs:** Take 1 tab qd.
Castor Oil	Castor Oil	**Adults & Peds ≥12 yrs:** 15-60mL. **Peds 2-<12 yrs:** 5-15mL. **Peds <2 yrs:** 1-5 mL.
Dulcolax Suppository	Bisacodyl 10mg	**Adults & Peds ≥12 yrs:** 1 supp qd. **Peds 6-<12 yrs:** ½ supp qd.
Dulcolax Tablets	Bisacodyl 5mg	**Adults & Peds ≥12 yrs:** 1-3 tabs qd. **Peds 6-<12 yrs:** 1 tab qd.
Ex-Lax Maximum Strength Tablets	Sennosides 25mg	**Adults & Peds ≥12 yrs:** 2 tabs qd-bid. **Peds 6-<12 yrs:** 1 tab qd-bid.
Ex-Lax Tablets	Sennosides 15mg	**Adults & Peds ≥12 yrs:** 2 tabs qd-bid. **Peds 6-<12 yrs:** 1 tab qd-bid.
Ex-Lax Ultra Stimulant Laxative Tablets	Bisacodyl 5mg	**Adults & Peds ≥12 yrs:** 1-3 tabs qd. **Peds 6-<12 yrs:** 1 tab qd-bid.
Fleet Bisacodyl Enema	Bisacodyl 10mg/30mL	**Adults & Peds ≥12 yrs:** 1 bottle (30mL).
Fleet Bisacodyl Suppositories	Bisacodyl 10mg	**Adults & Peds ≥12 yrs:** 1 supp qd. **Peds 6-<12 yrs:** ½ supp qd.

(Continued)

BRAND	INGREDIENT/STRENGTH	DOSE
STIMULANTS (Continued)		
Fleet Pedia-Lax Quick Dissolve Strips	Sennosides 8.6mg	**Peds 6-<12 yrs:** 2 strips. **Max:** 4 strips q24h. **Peds 2-<6 yrs:** 1 strip. **Max:** 2 strips q24h.
Fleet Stimulant Laxative Tablets	Bisacodyl 5mg	**Adults & Peds ≥12 yrs:** 1-3 tabs qd. **Peds 6-<12 yrs:** 1 tab qd.
Perdiem Overnight Relief Tablets	Sennosides 15mg	**Adults & Peds ≥12 yrs:** 2 tabs qd-bid. **Peds 6-<12 yrs:** 1 tab qd-bid.
Senokot Tablets	Sennosides 8.6mg	**Adults & Peds ≥12 yrs:** 2 tabs qd. **Max:** 4 tabs bid. **Peds 6-<12 yrs:** 1 tab qd. **Max:** 2 tabs bid. **Peds 2-<6 yrs:** ½ tab bid. **Max:** 1 tab bid.
SenokotXTRA Tablets	Sennosides 17.2mg	**Adults & Peds ≥6 yrs:** Starting dose 1 tab qd. **Max:** 2 tabs bid. **Peds 2-<6 yrs:** ½ tab qd. **Max:** 1 tab bid.
STIMULANT COMBINATIONS		
Peri-Colace Tablets	Sennosides/Docusate 8.6mg-50mg	**Adults & Peds ≥12 yrs:** 2-4 tabs qd. **Peds 6-<12 yrs:** 1-2 tabs qd. **Peds 2-5 yrs:** 1 tab qd.
Senna Prompt	Psyllium/Sennosides 500mg-9mg	**Adults & Peds ≥12 yrs:** 1-5 caps qd-bid.
Senokot S Tablets	Sennosides/Docusate 8.6mg-50mg	**Adults ≥12 yrs:** 2 tabs qd. **Max:** 4 tabs bid. **Peds 6-<12 yrs:** 1 tab qd. **Max:** 2 tabs bid. **Peds 2-<6 yrs:** ½ tab qd. **Max:** 1 tab bid.
SURFACTANTS (STOOL SOFTENERS)		
Colace Capsules	Docusate Sodium 100mg	**Adults & Peds ≥12 yrs:** 1-3 caps qd. **Peds 2-<12 yrs:** 1 cap qd.
Colace Capsules	Docusate Sodium 50mg	**Adults & Peds ≥12 yrs:** 1-6 caps qd. **Peds 2-<12 yrs:** 1-3 caps qd.
Colace Liquid	Docusate Sodium 10mg/mL	**Adults & Peds ≥12 yrs:** 5-15mL qd-bid. **Peds 2-<12 yrs:** 5-15mL qd.
Colace Syrup	Docusate Sodium 60mg/15mL	**Adults & Peds ≥12 yrs:** 1-6 tbl qd. **Peds 2-<12 yrs:** 1-2½ tbl qd.
Docusol Constipation Relief, Mini Enemas	Docusate Sodium 283mg	**Adults & Peds ≥12 yrs:** Take 1-3 units qd. **Peds 6-12:** Take 1 unit qd.
Dulcolax Stool Softener Capsules	Docusate Sodium 100mg	**Adults & Peds ≥12 yrs:** 1-3 caps qd. **Peds 2-<12 yrs:** 1 cap qd.
Fleet Pedia-Lax Liquid Stool Softener	Docusate 50mg/15mL	**Peds 2-12 yrs:** 1-3 tbl qd. **Max:** 3 tbl q24h.
Fleet Sof-Lax	Docusate 100mg	**Adults & Peds ≥12 yrs:** 1-3 caps qd. **Peds 2-<12 yrs:** 1 cap qd.
Kaopectate Liqui-Gels	Docusate Calcium 240mg	**Adults & Peds ≥12 yrs:** 1 cap qd until normal bowel movement.
Phillips' Stool Softener Capsules	Docusate Sodium 100mg	**Adults & Peds ≥12 yrs:** 1-3 caps qd. **Peds 6-<12 yrs:** 1 cap qd.

ALLERGIC RHINITIS PRODUCTS

BRAND	INGREDIENT/STRENGTH	DOSE
ANTIHISTAMINE		
Alavert Quick Dissolving Tablets	Loratadine 10mg	**Adults & Peds ≥6 yrs:** 1 tab qd. **Max:** 1 tab q24h.
Alavert For Kids 6+	Loratadine 10mg	**Adults & Peds ≥6 yrs:** 1 tab qd. **Max:** 1 tab q24h.
Benadryl Allergy Quick Dissolve Strips	Diphenhydramine HCl 25mg	**Adults & Peds ≥12 yrs:** Dissolve 1-2 strips on tongue q4-6h. **Peds 6-<12 yrs:** Dissolve 1 strip on tongue q4-6h. **Max:** 6 doses q24h.
Benadryl Allergy Kapgels	Diphenhydramine HCl 25mg	**Adults & Peds ≥12 yrs:** 1-2 caps q4-6h. **Peds 6-<12 yrs:** 1 cap q4-6h. **Max:** 6 doses q24h.
Benadryl Allergy Ultratab Tablets	Diphenhydramine HCl 25mg	**Adults & Peds ≥12 yrs:** 1-2 tabs q4-6h. **Peds 6-<12 yrs:** 1 tab q4-6h. **Max:** 6 doses q24h.
Benadryl Dye-Free Allergy Liqui-Gels	Diphenhydramine HCl 25mg	**Adults & Peds ≥12 yrs:** 1-2 caps q4-6h. **Peds 6-<12 yrs:** 1 cap q4-6h. **Max:** 6 doses q24h.
Children's Benadryl Allergy Fastmelt Tablets	Diphenhydramine HCl 12.5mg	**Adults & Peds ≥12 yrs:** 2-4 tabs q4-6h. **Peds 6-<12 yrs:** 1-2 tabs q4-6h. **Max:** 6 doses q24h.
Children's Benadryl Perfect Measure Pre-Filled Single Use Spoons	Diphenhydramine HCl 12.5mg/5mL	**Adults & Peds ≥12 yrs:** 2-4 pre-filled spoons (10-20mL) q4-6h. **Peds 6-<12 yrs:** 1-2 pre-filled spoons (5-10mL) q4-6h. **Max:** 6 doses q24h.
Children's Benadryl Allergy Liquid	Diphenhydramine HCl 12.5mg/5mL	**Peds 6-<12 yrs:** 1-2 tsp (5-10mL) q4-6h. **Max:** 6 doses q24h.
Children's Benadryl Dye-Free Allergy Liquid	Diphenhydramine HCl 12.5mg/5mL	**Peds 6-<12 yrs:** 1-2 tsp (5-10mL) q4-6h. **Max:** 6 doses q24h.
Claritin Tablets	Loratadine 10mg	**Adults & Peds ≥6 yrs:** 1 tab qd. **Max:** 1 tab q24h.
Claritin Liqui-Gels	Loratadine 10mg	**Adults & Peds ≥6 yrs:** 1 cap qd. **Max:** 1 cap q24h.
Claritin RediTabs 24-Hour	Loratadine 10mg	**Adults & Peds ≥6 yrs:** 1 tab qd. **Max:** 1 tab q24h.
Claritin 12-Hour RediTabs	Loratadine 5mg	**Adults & Peds ≥6 yrs:** 1 tab q12h. **Max:** 2 tabs q24h.
Claritin 24-Hour RediTabs For Kids	Loratadine 10mg	**Adults & Peds ≥6 yrs:** 1 tab qd. **Max:** 1 tab q24h.
Claritin 12-Hour RediTabs For Kids	Loratadine 5mg	**Adults & Peds ≥6 yrs:** 1 tab q12h. **Max:** 2 tabs q24h.
Children's Claritin Chewables	Loratadine 5mg	**Adults & Peds ≥6 yrs:** 2 tabs qd. **Max:** 2 tabs q24h. **Peds 2-<6 yrs:** 1 tab qd. **Max:** 1 tab q24h.
Children's Claritin Syrup	Loratadine 5mg/5mL	**Adults & Peds ≥6 yrs:** 2 tsp (10mL) qd. **Max:** 2 tsp q24h. **Peds 2-<6 yrs:** 1 tsp (5mL) qd. **Max:** 1 tsp q24h.
Zyrtec Tablets	Cetirizine HCl 10mg	**Adults & Peds 6-<65 yrs:** 1 tab qd. **Max:** 1 tab q24h.
Children's Zyrtec Chewable 10mg	Cetirizine HCl 10mg	**Adults & Peds 6-<65 yrs:** 1 tab qd. **Max:** 1 tab q24h.
Children's Zyrtec Perfect Measure	Cetirizine HCl 5mg/5mL	**Adults & Peds 6-<65 yrs:** 1-2 prefilled spoons (5-10mL) qd. **Max:** 2 prefilled spoons q24h. **Adults ≥65 yrs:** 1 prefilled spoon (5mL) qd. **Max:** 1 prefilled spoon q24h.

(Continued)

BRAND	INGREDIENT/STRENGTH	DOSE
ANTIHISTAMINE *(Continued)*		
Children's Zyrtec Allergy Syrup	Cetirizine HCl 5mg/5mL	**Adults & Peds 6-<65 yrs:** 1-2 tsp (5-10mL) qd. **Max:** 2 tsp q24h. **Adults ≥65 yrs:** 1 tsp qd. **Max:** 1 tsp q24h. **Peds 2-<6 yrs:** ½-1 tsp (2.5-5mL) qd or ½ tsp q12h. **Max:** 1 tsp q24h.
ANTIHISTAMINE COMBINATIONS		
Advil Allergy Sinus Caplets	Chlorpheniramine Maleate/ Ibuprofen/Pseudoephedrine HCl 2mg-200mg-30mg	**Adults & Peds ≥12 yrs:** 1 tab q4-6h. **Max:** 6 tabs q24h.
Alavert Allergy & Sinus D-12	Loratadine/Pseudoephedrine Sulfate 5mg-120mg	**Adults & Peds ≥12 yrs:** 1 tab q12h. **Max:** 2 tabs q24h.
Allerest PE	Chlorpheniramine Maleate/ Phenylephrine HCl 4mg-10mg	**Adults & Peds ≥12 yrs:** 1 tab q4h. **Peds 6-<12 yrs:** ½ tab q4h **Max:** 6 doses q24h.
Benadryl-D Allergy Plus Sinus	Diphenhydramine HCl/ Phenylephrine HCl 25mg-10mg	**Adults & Peds ≥12 yrs:** 1 tab q4h. **Max:** 6 tabs q24h.
Benadryl Severe Allergy Plus Sinus Headache Caplets	Diphenhydramine HCl/ Acetaminophen/Phenylephrine HCl 25mg-325mg-5mg	**Adults & Peds ≥12 yrs:** 2 tabs q4h. **Max:** 12 tabs q24h.
Benadryl Severe Allergy Plus Sinus Headache Kapgels	Diphenhydramine HCl/ Acetaminophen/Phenylephrine HCl 12.5mg-325mg-5mg	**Adults & Peds ≥12 yrs:** 2 caps q4h. **Max:** 12 caps q24h.
Benadryl Severe Allergy Plus Cold Kapgels	Diphenhydramine HCl/ Acetaminophen/Phenylephrine HCl 12.5mg-325mg-5mg	**Adults & Peds ≥12 yrs:** 2 caps q4h. **Max:** 12 caps q24h.
Children's Benadryl-D Allergy & Sinus Liquid	Diphenhydramine HCl/ Phenylephrine HCl 12.5mg-5mg/5mL	**Adults & Peds ≥12 yrs:** 2 tsp (10mL) q4h. **Peds 6-<12 yrs:** 1 tsp (5mL) q4h. **Max:** 6 doses q24h.
Claritin-D 12 Hour	Loratadine/Pseudoephedrine Sulfate 5mg-120mg	**Adults & Peds ≥12 yrs:** 1 tab q12h. **Max:** 2 tabs q24h.
Claritin-D 24 Hour	Loratadine/Pseudoephedrine Sulfate 10mg-240mg	**Adults & Peds ≥12 yrs:** 1 tab qd. **Max:** 1 tab q24h.
Children's Dimetapp Cold & Allergy Chewable Tablets	Brompheniramine Maleate/ Phenylephrine HCl 1mg-2.5mg	**Peds 6-<12 yrs:** 2 tabs q4h. **Max:** 6 doses q24h.
Children's Dimetapp Cold & Allergy Syrup	Brompheniramine Maleate/ Phenylephrine HCl 1mg-2.5mg/5mL	**Adults & Peds ≥12 yrs:** 4 tsp (20mL) q4h. **Peds 6-<12 yrs:** 2 tsp (10mL) q4h. **Max:** 6 doses q24h.
Zyrtec-D Tablets	Cetirizine HCl/ Pseudoephedrine HCl 5mg-120mg	**Adults & Peds 12-<65 yrs:** 1 tab q12h. **Max:** 2 tabs q24h.
TOPICAL NASAL DECONGESTANTS		
4-Way Fast Acting Nasal Decongestant Spray	Phenylephrine HCl 1%	**Adults & Peds ≥12 yrs:** Instill 2-3 sprays per nostril q4h.
4-Way Mentholated Nasal Decongestant Spray	Phenylephrine HCl 1%	**Adults & Peds ≥12 yrs:** Instill 2-3 sprays per nostril q4h.
Afrin Original 12 Hour Pump Mist	Oxymetazoline HCl 0.05%	**Adults & Peds ≥6 yrs:** Instill 2-3 sprays per nostril q10-12h. **Max:** 2 doses q24h.
Afrin Extra Moisturizing 12 Hour Pump Mist	Oxymetazoline HCl 0.05%	**Adults & Peds ≥6 yrs:** Instill 2-3 sprays per nostril q10-12h. **Max:** 2 doses q24h.
Afrin All Night 12 Hour Pump Mist	Oxymetazoline HCl 0.05%	**Adults & Peds ≥6 yrs:** Instill 2-3 sprays per nostril q10-12h. **Max:** 2 doses q24h.
Afrin Sinus 12 Hour Pump Mist	Oxymetazoline HCl 0.05%	**Adults & Peds ≥6 yrs:** Instill 2-3 sprays per nostril q10-12h. **Max:** 2 doses q24h.

(Continued)

BRAND	INGREDIENT/STRENGTH	DOSE
TOPICAL NASAL DECONGESTANTS *(Continued)*		
Afrin Severe Congestion 12 Hour Pump Mist	Oxymetazoline HCl 0.05%	**Adults & Peds ≥6 yrs:** Instill 2-3 sprays per nostril q10-12h. **Max:** 2 doses q24h.
Benzedrex Inhaler	Propylhexedrine 250mg	**Adults & Peds ≥6 yrs:** Inhale 2 sprays per nostril q2h. **Max:** Do not use >3 days.
Dristan 12-hr Nasal Spray	Oxymetazoline HCl 0.05%	**Adults & Peds ≥12 yrs:** Instill 2-3 sprays per nostril q10-12h. **Max:** 2 doses q24h.
Little Noses Decongestant Nose Drops	Phenylephrine HCl 0.125%	**Peds 2-<6 yrs:** Instill 2-3 sprays per nostril q4h. **Max:** 2 doses q24h.
Mucinex Moisture Smart Nasal Spray	Oxymetazoline HCl 0.05%	**Adults & Peds ≥6 yrs:** Instill 2-3 sprays per nostril q10-12h. **Max:** 2 doses q24h.
Mucinex Full Force Nasal Spray	Oxymetazoline HCl 0.05%	**Adults & Peds ≥6 yrs:** Instill 2-3 sprays per nostril q10-12h. **Max:** 2 doses q24h.
Neo-Synephrine Regular Strength Nasal Spray	Phenylephrine HCl 0.5%	**Adults & Peds ≥12 yrs:** Instill 2-3 sprays per nostril q4h.
Neo-Synephrine Extra Strength Nasal Spray	Phenylephrine HCl 1%	**Adults & Peds ≥12 yrs:** Instill 2-3 sprays per nostril q4h.
Neo-Synephrine Nighttime Nasal Spray	Oxymetazoline HCl 0.05%	**Adults & Peds ≥6 yrs:** Instill 2-3 sprays per nostril q10-12h. **Max:** 2 doses q24h.
Nostrilla Fast Relief	Oxymetazoline HCl 0.05%	**Adults & Peds ≥6 yrs:** Instill 2-3 sprays per nostril q10-12h. **Max:** 2 doses q24h.
Nostrilla Complete Congestion Relief	Oxymetazoline HCl 0.05%	**Adults & Peds ≥6 yrs:** Instill 2-3 sprays per nostril q10-12h. **Max:** 2 doses q24h.
Privine Nasal Drops	Naphazoline HCl 0.05%	**Adults & Peds ≥12 yrs:** Instill 1-2 sprays per nostril q6h.
Privine Nasal Spray	Naphazoline HCl 0.05%	**Adults & Peds ≥12 yrs:** Instill 1-2 sprays per nostril q6h.
Sudafed OM Sinus Congestion Spray	Oxymetazoline HCl 0.05%	**Adults & Peds ≥6 yrs:** Instill 2-3 sprays per nostril q10-12h. **Max:** 2 doses q24h.
Vicks Sinex 12-Hour Decongestant UltraFine Mist	Oxymetazoline HCl 0.05%	**Adults & Peds ≥6 yrs:** Instill 2-3 sprays per nostril q10-12h. **Max:** 2 doses q24h.
Vicks Sinex VapoSpray 12-Hour Decongestant Nasal Spray	Oxymetazoline HCl 0.05%	**Adults & Peds ≥6 yrs:** Instill 2-3 sprays per nostril q10-12h. **Max:** 2 doses q24h.
Vicks VapoInhaler	Levmetamfetamine 50mg	**Adults & Peds ≥12 yrs:** Inhale 2 sprays per nostril q2h. **Peds 6-<12 yrs:** Inhale 1 spray per nostril q2h.
Zicam Extreme Congestion Relief Nasal Gel	Oxymetazoline HCl 0.05%	**Adults & Peds ≥6 yrs:** Instill 2-3 sprays per nostril q10-12h. **Max:** 2 doses q24h.
Zicam Intense Sinus Relief Nasal Gel	Oxymetazoline HCl 0.05%	**Adults & Peds ≥6 yrs:** Instill 2-3 sprays per nostril q10-12h. **Max:** 2 doses q24h.
TOPICAL NASAL MOISTURIZERS		
4-Way Saline Moisturizing Mist	Water, Boric Acid, Glycerin, Sodium Chloride, Sodium Borate, Eucalyptol, Menthol, Polysorbate 80, Benzalkonium Chloride	**Adults & Peds ≥2 yrs:** Instill 2-3 sprays per nostril prn.

(Continued)

BRAND	INGREDIENT/STRENGTH	DOSE
TOPICAL NASAL MOISTURIZERS (Continued)		
Afrin PureSea Medium Stream	Sea Water	**Adults & Peds ≥2 yrs:** Use to rinse nostrils qid.
Afrin PureSea Gentle Mist	Sea Water	**Adults & Peds ≥2 yrs:** Use to rinse nostrils qid.
Afrin PureSea Ultra-Gentle Mist	Sea Water	**Peds ≥6 mos:** Use to rinse nostrils qid.
Ayr Saline Nasal Mist	Sodium Chloride 0.65%	**Adults & Peds:** Instill 1 spray per nostril prn.
Ayr Saline Nasal Drops	Sodium Chloride 0.65%	**Adults & Peds:** Instill 2-6 drops per nostril prn
Ayr Allergy & Sinus Hypertonic Saline Nasal Mist	Sodium Chloride 2.65%	**Adults & Peds:** Instill 2 sprays per nostril bid-tid
Baby Ayr Saline Nose Spray/Drops	Sodium Chloride 0.65%	**Peds:** Instill 2-6 drops per nostril.
Ayr Saline Nasal Gel No-Drip Sinus Spray	Water, Sodium Carbomethyl Starch, Propylene Glycol, Glycerin, *Aloe Barbadensis* Leaf Juice (Aloe Vera), Sodium Chloride, Cetylpyridinium Chloride, Citric Acid, Disodium EDTA, *Glycine Soja* (Soybean) Oil, Tocopheryl Acetate, Benzyl Alcohol, Benzalkonium Chloride, *Geranium Maculatum* Oil	**Adults & Peds:** Instill 1 spray per nostril.
Ayr Saline Nasal Gel	Water, Methyl Gluceth-10, Propylene Glycol, Glycerin, Glyceryl Polymethacrylate, Triethanolamine, *Aloe Barbadensis* Leaf Juice (Aloe Vera Gel), PEG/PPG-18/18 Dimethicone, Carbomer, Poloxamer 184, Sodium Chloride, Xanthan Gum, Diazolidinyl Urea, Methylparaben, Propylparaben, *Glycine Soja* (Soybean) Oil, *Geranium Maculatum* Oil, Tocopheryl Acetate, Blue 1	**Adults & Peds:** Apply around nostrils and under nose prn.
Ayr Saline Nasal Gel Swabs	Water, Methyl Gluceth-10, Propylene Glycol, Glycerin, Glyceryl Polymethacrylate, Triethanolamine, *Aloe Barbadensis* Leaf Juice (Aloe Vera Gel), PEG/PPG-18/18 Dimethicone, Carbomer, Poloxamer 184, Sodium Chloride, Xanthan Gum, Diazolidinyl Urea, Methylparaben, Propylparaben, *Glycine Soja* (Soybean) Oil, *Geranium Maculatum* Oil, Tocopheryl Acetate, Blue 1	**Adults & Peds:** Apply around nostrils and under nose prn.
Little Noses Saline Spray/Drops	Sodium Chloride 0.65%	**Adults & Peds:** Instill 2-6 drops/sprays per nostril prn.
Little Noses Sterile Saline Nasal Mist	Sodium Chloride 0.9%	**Adults & Peds:** Instill 1-3 short sprays per nostril prn.
Nostrilla Conditioning Double-Moisture	Benzalkonium Chloride Solution, Carboxymethylcellulose Sodium, Eucalyptol, Glycine, Hyaluronic Acid Sodium, Polyethylene Glycol, Povidone, Propylene Glycol, Sodium Chloride (as 1.9% saline solution), Spearmint Oil, Wintergreen Oil, Water	**Adults & Peds:** Instill 1-2 sprays per nostril bid.
Ocean Gel Ultra Moisturizing Gel	Purified water, Glycerin, Carbomer 940, Trolamine, Hyaluronan, Methylparaben, Propylparaben	**Adults & Peds:** Apply around nostrils and under nose prn.

(Continued)

BRAND	INGREDIENT/STRENGTH	DOSE
TOPICAL NASAL MOISTURIZERS *(Continued)*		
Ocean Complete Sinus Irrigation	Purified Water, Glycerin, Sodium Chloride, Monobasic Sodium Phosphate, Dibasic Sodium Phosphate, Potassium Chloride, Calcium Chloride, Magnesium Chloride	**Adults & Peds:** Attach white actuator and spray into each nostril prn.
Ocean Ultra Sterile Saline Mist	Purified Water, Glycerin, Sodium Chloride, Monobasic Sodium Phosphate, Sodium Hyaluronan, Dibasic Sodium Phosphate, Potassium Chloride, Calcium Chloride, Magnesium Chloride	**Adults & Peds:** Spray into each nostril prn.
Ocean for Kids Premium Saline Nasal Spray	Sodium Chloride 0.65%, Purified Water, Glycerin, Sodium Phosphate Monobasic, Sodium Hydroxide, Benzalkonium Chloride	**Peds:** Instill 2 sprays per nostril prn.
Ocean Premium Saline Nasal Spray	Sodium Chloride 0.65%	**Adults & Peds:** Instill 2 sprays per nostril prn.
Simply Saline Nasal Mist	Sodium Chloride 0.9%	**Adults & Peds:** Spray into each nostril prn.
Baby Simply Saline Sterile Saline Mist	Sodium Chloride 0.9%	**Peds:** Spray into each nostril prn.
Simply Saline Nasal Moist Gel	Propylene Glycol, Hydroxyethyl-cellulose, Aloe Vera, Sodium Chloride, Allantoin, Methylparaben, Propylparaben, Purified Water	**Adults & Peds:** Apply around nostrils and under nose prn.
MISCELLANEOUS		
NasalCrom Nasal Spray	Cromolyn Sodium 5.2 mg	**Adults & Peds ≥2 yrs:** Instill 1 spray per nostril q4-6h. **Max:** 6 doses q24h.
Similasan Relief Nasal Spray	*Cardiospermum* 6X, *Galphimia glauca* 6X, *Luffa operculata* 6X, *Sabadilla* 6X	**Adults & Peds:** Instill 1-3 sprays per nostril prn.
SinoFresh Nasal & Sinus Care	*Eucalyptus Globulus* 20x, *Kalium Bichromicum* 30x	**Adults:** Instill 1-2 sprays per nostril every morning and evening. Gently sniff to distribute solution. Blow nose to clear it of loosened debris and mucus. Re-apply 1 spray to each nostril.
Zicam Allergy Relief Nasal Gel	*Luffa Operculata* (4x, 12x, 30x), *Galphimia Glauca* (12x, 30x), *Histaminum Hydrochloricum* (12x, 30x, 200x), *Sulphur* (12x, 30x, 200x)	**Adults & Peds ≥12 yrs:** Instill 1 spray per nostril q4h.
Zicam Allergy Relief Gel Swabs	*Galphimia Glauca* (12x, 30x), *Histaminum Hydrochloricum* (12x, 30x, 200x), *Luffa Operculata* (4x, 12x, 30x), *Sulphur* (12x, 30x, 200x)	**Adults & Peds ≥6 yrs:** Apply medication just inside first nostril. Remove swab and press lightly on the outside of first nostril for 5 sec. Re-dip swab in tube and repeat with 2nd nostril.

IS IT A COLD, THE FLU, OR AN ALLERGY?

	COLD	FLU	AIRBORNE ALLERGY
SYMPTOMS			
Chest discomfort	Mild to moderate	Common; can become severe	Sometimes
Cough	Common (hacking cough)	Sometimes	Sometimes
Diarrhea	Never	Sometimes (more common in children)	Never
Duration	3-14 days	Days to weeks	Weeks (eg, 6 weeks for ragweed or grass pollen seasons)
Extreme exhaustion	Never	Early and prominent	Never
Fatigue, weakness	Sometimes	Can last up to 2-3 weeks	Sometimes
Fever	Rare	Characteristic, high (100-102°F); lasts 3-4 days	Never
General aches, pains	Slight	Usual; often severe	Never
Headache	Rare	Common	Sometimes
Itchy eyes	Rare or never	Rare or never	Common
Runny nose	Common	Common	Common
Sneezing	Usual	Sometimes	Usual
Sore throat	Common	Sometimes	Sometimes
Stuffy nose	Common	Sometimes	Common
Vomiting	Never	Sometimes (more common in children)	Never
TREATMENT			
	Antihistamines*	Amantadine	Antihistamines*
	Decongestants*	Rimantadine	Nasal steroids*
	Nonsteroidal anti-inflammatories*	Oseltamivir	Decongestants*
		Zanamivir	
PREVENTION			
	Wash your hands often; avoid close contact with anyone with a cold	Annual vaccination Amantadine Rimantadine Oseltamivir	Avoid allergens such as pollen, house flies, dust mites, mold, pet dander, cockroaches
COMPLICATIONS			
	Sinus infection	Bronchitis	Sinus infections
	Middle ear infection	Pneumonia	Asthma
	Asthma	Can be life-threatening	

Adapted from the National Institute of Allergy and Infectious Diseases, November 2008 and CDC.gov.

*Used only for temporary relief of cold symptoms.

COUGH-COLD-FLU PRODUCTS

BRAND NAME	ANALGESIC	ANTIHISTAMINE	DECONGESTANT	COUGH SUPPRESSANT	EXPECTORANT	DOSE
ANTIHISTAMINE + DECONGESTANT						
Actifed Cold & Allergy Tablets		Chlorpheniramine Maleate 4mg	Phenylephrine HCl 10mg			**Adults & Peds ≥12 yrs:** 1 tab q4h. **Max:** 6 tabs q24h.
Benadryl-D Allergy Plus Sinus		Diphenhydramine HCl 25mg	Phenylephrine HCl 10mg			**Adults & Peds ≥12 yrs:** 1 tab q4h. **Max:** 6 tabs q24h.
Children's Benadryl-D Allergy & Sinus Liquid		Diphenhydramine HCl 12.5mg/5mL	Phenylephrine HCl 5mg/5mL			**Adults ≥12 yrs:** 2 tsp (10mL) q4h. **Peds 6–<12 yrs:** 1 tsp (5mL) q4h. **Max:** 6 doses q24h.
Children's Dimetapp Cold & Allergy Chewable Tablets		Brompheniramine Maleate 1mg	Phenylephrine HCl 2.5mg			**Peds ≥12 yrs:** 4 tabs q4h. **6–<12 yrs:** 2 tabs q4h. **Max:** 6 doses q24h.
Children's Dimetapp Cold & Allergy Syrup		Brompheniramine Maleate 1mg/5mL	Phenylephrine HCl 2.5mg/5mL			**Adults & Peds ≥12 yrs:** 4 tsp (20mL) q4h. **Peds 6–<12 yrs:** 2 tsp (10mL) q4h. **Max:** 6 doses q24h.
Children's Dimetapp Nighttime Cold & Congestion Liquid		Diphenhydramine HCl 6.25mg/5mL	Phenylephrine HCl 2.5mg/5mL			**Adults & Peds ≥12 yrs:** 4 tsp (20mL) q4h. **Peds 6–<12 yrs:** 2 tsp (10mL) q4h. **Max:** 6 doses q24h.
Pediacare Children's Allergy & Cold		Diphenhydramine HCl 12.5mg/5mL	Phenylephrine HCl 5mg/5mL			**Peds 6-11 yrs:** 1 tsp (5mL) q4h. **Max:** 6 doses q24h.
Robitussin Night Time Cough & Cold		Diphenhydramine HCl 6.25mg/5mL	Phenylephrine HCl 2.5mg/5mL			**Adults & Peds ≥12 yrs:** 4 tsp (20mL) q4h. **Max:** 6 doses q24h.
Sudafed PE Maximum Strength Sinus & Allergy Tablets		Chlorpheniramine Maleate 4mg	Phenylephrine HCl 10mg			**Adults & Peds ≥12 yrs:** 1 tab q4h. **Max:** 6 tabs q24h.
Night Time Triaminic Thin Strips Cold & Cough		Diphenhydramine HCl 12.5mg/strip	Phenylephrine HCl 5mg/strip			**Peds 6-12 yrs:** 1 strip q4h. **Max:** 6 strips q24h.
Triaminic Night Time Cold & Cough		Diphenhydramine HCl 6.25mg/5mL	Phenylephrine HCl 2.5mg/5mL			**Peds 6–<12 yrs:** 2 tsp (10mL) q4h. **Max:** 6 doses q24h.
Triaminic Syrup Cold & Allergy		Chlorpheniramine Maleate 1mg/5mL	Phenylephrine HCl 2.5mg/5mL			**Peds 6–<12 yrs:** 2 tsp (10mL) q4h. **Max:** 6 doses q24h.

BRAND NAME	ANALGESIC	ANTIHISTAMINE	DECONGESTANT	COUGH SUPPRESSANT	EXPECTORANT	DOSE
ANTIHISTAMINE + DECONGESTANT + ANALGESIC						
Advil Allergy Sinus Caplets	Ibuprofen 200mg	Chlorpheniramine Maleate 2mg	Pseudoephedrine HCl 30mg			**Adults & Peds ≥12 yrs:** 1 tab q4-6h. **Max:** 6 tabs q24h.
Alka-Seltzer Plus Cold Formula Effervescent Tablets	Aspirin 325mg	Chlorpheniramine Maleate 2mg	Phenylephrine Bitartrate 7.8mg			**Adults & Peds ≥12 yrs:** 2 tabs q4h. **Max:** 8 tabs q24h.
Alka-Seltzer Plus Fast Crystal Packs	Acetaminophen 650mg/packet	Chlorpheniramine HCl 4mg/packet	Phenylephrine HCl 10mg/packet			**Adults & Peds ≥12 yrs:** 1 pkt q4h. **Max:** 6 pkts q24h.
Benadryl Severe Allergy Plus Cold Kapgels	Acetaminophen 325mg	Diphenhydramine HCl 12.5mg	Phenylephrine HCl 5mg			**Adults & Peds ≥12 yrs:** 2 caps q4h. **Max:** 12 caps q24h.
Benadryl Severe Allergy Plus Sinus Headache Caplets	Acetaminophen 325mg	Diphenhydramine HCl 25mg	Phenylephrine HCl 5mg			**Adults & Peds ≥12 yrs:** 2 tabs q4h. **Max:** 12 tabs q24h.
Benadryl Severe Allergy Plus Sinus Headache Kapgels	Acetaminophen 325mg	Diphenhydramine HCl 12.5mg	Phenylephrine HCl 5mg			**Adults & Peds ≥12 yrs:** 2 caps q4h. **Max:** 12 caps q24h.
Comtrex Severe Cold & Sinus Caplets	Acetaminophen 325mg	Chlorpheniramine Maleate 2mg	Phenylephrine HCl 5mg			**Adults & Peds ≥12 yrs:** 2 tabs q4h. **Max:** 12 tabs q24h.
Contac Cold Plus Flu	Acetaminophen 500mg	Chlorpheniramine Maleate 2mg	Phenylephrine HCl 5mg			**Adults & Peds ≥12 yrs:** 2 tabs q4-6h. **Max:** 8 tabs q24h.
Dristan Cold Multi-Symptom Formula Tablets	Acetaminophen 325mg	Chlorpheniramine Maleate 2mg	Phenylephrine HCl 5mg			**Adults & Peds ≥12 yrs:** 2 tabs q4h. **Max:** 12 tabs q24h.
Sudafed PE Severe Cold Formula Caplets	Acetaminophen 325mg	Diphenhydramine HCl 12.5mg	Phenylephrine HCl 5mg			**Adults & Peds ≥12 yrs:** 2 tabs q4h. **Max:** 12 tabs q24h. **Peds 6–<12 yrs:** 1 tab q4h. **Max:** 5 tabs q24h.
Theraflu Cold & Sore Throat Hot Liquid	Acetaminophen 325mg/packet	Pheniramine Maleate 20mg/packet	Phenylephrine HCl 10mg/packet			**Adults & Peds ≥12 yrs:** 1 pkt q4h. **Max:** 6 pkts q24h.
Theraflu Nighttime Severe Cold & Cough Hot Liquid	Acetaminophen 650mg/packet	Diphenhydramine HCl 25mg/packet	Phenylephrine HCl 10mg/packet			**Adults & Peds ≥12 yrs:** 1 pkt q4h. **Max:** 6 pkts q24h.
Theraflu Sugar Free Nighttime Severe Cold & Cough Hot Liquid	Acetaminophen 650mg/packet	Diphenhydramine HCl 25mg/packet	Phenylephrine HCl 10mg/packet			**Adults & Peds ≥12 yrs:** 1 pkt q4h. **Max:** 6 pkts q24h.
Theraflu Flu & Sore Throat Hot Liquid	Acetaminophen 650mg/packet	Pheniramine Maleate 20mg/packet	Phenylephrine HCl 10mg/packet			**Adults & Peds ≥12 yrs:** 1 pkt q4h. **Max:** 6 pkts q24h.

(Continued)

BRAND NAME	ANALGESIC	ANTIHISTAMINE	DECONGESTANT	COUGH SUPPRESSANT	EXPECTORANT	DOSE
ANTIHISTAMINE + DECONGESTANT + ANALGESIC *(Continued)*						
Theraflu Warming Relief Nighttime Severe Cough & Cold	Acetaminophen 325mg/15mL	Diphenhydramine HCl 12.5mg/15mL	Phenylephrine HCl 5mg/15mL			**Adults & Peds ≥12 yrs:** 2 tbl (30mL) q4h. **Max:** 6 doses (12 tbl or 180mL) q24h.
Theraflu Warming Relief Flu & Sore Throat	Acetaminophen 325mg/15mL	Diphenhydramine HCl 12.5mg/15mL	Phenylephrine HCl 5mg/15mL			**Adults & Peds ≥12 yrs:** 2 tbl (30mL) q4h. **Max:** 6 doses (12 tbl or 180mL) q24h.
Children's Tylenol Plus Cold	Acetaminophen 160mg/5mL	Chlorpheniramine Maleate 1mg/5mL	Phenylephrine HCl 2.5mg/5mL			**Peds 6-11 yrs (48-95 lbs):** 2 tsp (10mL) q4h. **Max:** 5 doses q24h.
Children's Tylenol Plus Cold and Allergy	Acetaminophen 160mg/5mL	Diphenhydramine HCl 12.5mg/5mL	Phenylephrine HCl 2.5mg/5mL			**Peds 6-11 yrs (48-95 lbs):** 2 tsp (10mL) q4h. **Max:** 5 doses q24h.
Tylenol Allergy Multi-Symptom*	Acetaminophen 325mg	Chlorpheniramine Maleate 2mg	Phenylephrine HCl 5mg			**Adults & Peds ≥12 yrs:** 2 tabs q4h. **Max:** 12 tabs q24h.
Tylenol Allergy Multi-Symptom Nighttime*	Acetaminophen 325mg	Diphenhydramine HCl 25mg	Phenylephrine HCl 5mg			**Adults & Peds ≥12 yrs:** 2 tabs q4h. **Max:** 12 tabs q24h.
Tylenol Sinus Congestion & Pain Nighttime*	Acetaminophen 325mg	Chlorpheniramine Maleate 2mg	Phenylephrine HCl 5mg			**Adults & Peds ≥12 yrs:** 2 tabs q4h. **Max:** 12 tabs q24h.
Vicks NyQuil Sinex LiquiCaps	Acetaminophen 325mg	Doxylamine Succinate 6.25mg	Phenylephrine HCl 5mg			**Adults & Peds ≥12 yrs:** 2 caps q4h. **Max:** 4 doses q24h.
COUGH SUPPRESSANT						
Children's Delsym Cough Medicine				Dextromethorphan HBr 30mg/5mL		**Adults & Peds ≥12 yrs:** 2 tsp (10mL) q12h. **Max:** 4 tsp (20mL) q24h. **Peds 6-<12 yrs:** 1 tsp (5mL) q12h. **Max:** 2 tsp (10mL) q24h. **Peds 4-<6 yrs:** 1/2 tsp (2.5mL) q12h. **Max:** 1 tsp (5mL) q24h.
Delsym Cough Medicine				Dextromethorphan HBr 30mg/5mL		**Adults & Peds ≥12 yrs:** 2 tsp (10mL) q12h. **Max:** 4 tsp (20mL) q24h. **Peds 6-<12 yrs:** 1 tsp (5mL) q12h. **Max:** 2 tsp (10mL) q24h. **Peds 4-<6 yrs:** 1/2 tsp (2.5mL) q12h. **Max:** 1 tsp (5mL) q24h.

BRAND NAME	ANALGESIC	ANTIHISTAMINE	DECONGESTANT	COUGH SUPPRESSANT	EXPECTORANT	DOSE
COUGH SUPPRESSANT *(Continued)*						
Children's Robitussin Cough Long-Acting				Dextromethorphan HBr 7.5mg/5mL		**Adults & Peds ≥12 yrs:** 4 tsp (20mL) q6-8h. **Peds 6-<12 yrs:** 2 tsp (10mL) q6-8h. **Peds 4-<6 yrs:** 1 tsp (5mL) q6-8h. **Max:** 4 doses q24h.
Robitussin Cough Long-Acting				Dextromethorphan HBr 15mg/5mL		**Adults & Peds ≥12 yrs:** 2 tsp (10mL) q6-8h. **Max:** 4 doses q24h.
Robitussin CoughGels				Dextromethorphan HBr 15mg		**Adults & Peds ≥12 yrs:** 2 caps q6-8h. **Max:** 8 caps q24h.
Triaminic Long-Acting Cough				Dextromethorphan HBr 7.5mg/5mL		**Peds 6-<12 yrs:** 2 tsp (10mL) q6-8h. **Peds 4-<6 yrs:** 1 tsp (5mL) q6-8h. **Max:** 4 doses q24h.
Triaminic Thin Strips Long-Acting Cough				Dextromethorphan HBr 7.5mg/strip		**Peds 6-<12 yrs:** 2 strips q6-8h. **Peds 4-<6 yrs:** 1 strip q6-8h. **Max:** 4 doses q24h.
Vicks DayQuil Cough				Dextromethorphan HBr 15mg/15mL		**Adults & Peds ≥12 yrs:** 2 tbl (30mL) q6-8h. **Peds 6-12 yrs:** 1 tbl (15mL) q6-8h. **Max:** 4 doses q24h.
Vicks Formula 44 Custom Care Dry Cough Suppressant				Dextromethorphan HBr 30mg/15mL		**Adults & Peds ≥12 yrs:** 1 tbl (15mL) q6-8h. **Peds 6-<12 yrs:** 1½ tsp (7.5mL) q6-8h. **Max:** 4 doses q24h.
Vicks BabyRub				Petrolatum, fragrance, aloe extract, eucalyptus oil, lavender oil, rosemary oil		**Peds:** Gently massage on the chest, neck, and back to help soothe and comfort.
Vicks VapoRub Topical Cream				Camphor 5.2%, Menthol 2.8%, Eucalyptus 1.2%		**Adults & Peds ≥2 yrs:** Apply to chest and throat. **Max:** tid per 24h.
Vicks VapoRub Topical Ointment				Camphor 4.8%, Menthol 2.6%, Eucalyptus 1.2%		**Adults & Peds ≥2 yrs:** Apply to chest and throat. **Max:** tid per 24h.
Vicks VapoSteam				Camphor 6.2%		**Adults & Peds ≥2 yrs:** 1 tbl/quart q8h or 1½ tsp/pint q8h (for use in a hot steam vaporizer). **Max:** tid per 24h.

(Continued)

BRAND NAME	ANALGESIC	ANTIHISTAMINE	DECONGESTANT	COUGH SUPPRESSANT	EXPECTORANT	DOSE
COUGH SUPPRESSANT (Continued)						
Vicks Vapodrops				Menthol 1.7mg (cherry), Menthol 3.3mg (menthol)		**Peds ≥5 years:** 3 drops (cherry), **Peds >5 years:** 2 drops (menthol).
COUGH SUPPRESSANT + ANTIHISTAMINE						
Coricidin HBP Cough & Cold		Chlorpheniramine Maleate 4mg		Dextromethorphan HBr 30mg		**Adults & Peds ≥12 yrs:** 1 tab q6h. **Max:** 4 tabs q24h.
Children's Dimetapp Long-Acting Cough Plus Cold		Chlorpheniramine Maleate 1mg/5mL		Dextromethorphan HBr 7.5mg/5mL		**Adults & Peds ≥12 yrs:** 4 tsp (20mL) q6h. **6–<12 yrs:** 2 tsp (10mL) q6h. **Max:** 4 doses q24h.
Children's Robitussin Cough & Cold Long-Acting		Chlorpheniramine Maleate 1mg/5mL		Dextromethorphan HBr 7.5mg/5mL		**Adults & Peds ≥12 yrs:** 4 tsp (20mL) q6h. **Peds 6–<12 yrs:** 2 tsp (10mL) q6h. **Max:** 4 doses q24h.
Robitussin Cough & Cold Long-Acting		Chlorpheniramine Maleate 2mg/5mL		Dextromethorphan HBr 15mg/5mL		**Adults & Peds ≥12 yrs:** 2 tsp (10mL) q6h. **Max:** 4 doses q24h.
Triaminic Softchews Cough and Runny Nose		Chlorpheniramine Maleate 1mg		Dextromethorphan HBr 5mg		**Peds 6–<12 yrs:** 2 tabs q4-6h. **Max:** 5 doses q24h.
Vicks Children's NyQuil		Chlorpheniramine Maleate 2mg/15mL		Dextromethorphan HBr 15mg/15mL		**Adults & Peds ≥12 yrs:** 2 tbl (30mL) q6h. **Peds 6-11 yrs:** 1 tbl (15mL) q6h. **Max:** 4 doses q24h.
Vicks NyQuil Cough		Doxylamine Succinate 6.25mg/15mL		Dextromethorphan HBr 15mg/15mL		**Adults & Peds ≥12 yrs:** 2 tbl (30mL) q6h. **Max:** 4 doses q24h.
COUGH SUPPRESSANT + ANALGESIC						
Pediacare Children's Fever Reducer Plus Cough and Sore Throat with APAP	Acetaminophen 160mg/5mL			Dextromethorphan 5mg/5mL		**6-11 yrs (48-95 lbs):** 2 tsp (10ml) q4h. **Max:** 5 times in 24 hrs.
Triaminic Cough & Sore Throat	Acetaminophen 160mg/5mL			Dextromethorphan HBr 5mg/5mL		**Peds 6–<12 yrs:** 2 tsp (10mL) q4h. **Peds 4–<6 yrs:** 1 tsp (5mL) q4h. **Max:** 5 doses q24h.

BRAND NAME	ANALGESIC	ANTIHISTAMINE	DECONGESTANT	COUGH SUPPRESSANT	EXPECTORANT	DOSE
COUGH SUPPRESSANT + ANALGESIC *(Continued)*						
Children's Tylenol Plus Cough and Sore Throat	Acetaminophen 160mg/5mL			Dextromethorphan HBr 5mg/5mL		**Peds 6-11 yrs (48-95 lbs):** 2 tsp (10mL) q4h. **Peds 4-5 yrs (36-47 lbs):** 1 tsp (5mL) q4h. **Max:** 5 doses q24h.
Tylenol Cough & Sore Throat Daytime*	Acetaminophen 1000mg/30mL			Dextromethorphan HBr 30mg/30mL		**Adults & Peds ≥12 yrs:** 2 tbl (30mL) q6h. **Max:** 8 tbl q24h.
COUGH SUPPRESSANT + ANTIHISTAMINE + ANALGESIC						
Alka-Seltzer Plus Flu Formula Effervescent Tablets	Aspirin 500mg	Chlorpheniramine Maleate 2mg		Dextromethorphan HBr 15mg		**Adults & Peds ≥12 yrs:** 2 tabs q6h. **Max:** 8 tabs q24h.
Coricidin HBP Day & Night Multi-Symptom Cold	Acetaminophen 500mg (nighttime dose only)	Chlorpheniramine Maleate 2mg (nighttime dose only)		Dextromethorphan HBr 10mg (daytime dose), 15mg (nighttime dose)	Guaifenesin 200mg (daytime dose only)	**Adults & Peds ≥12 yrs:** 2 tabs hs and q6h prn. **Max:** 4 tabs q12h.
Coricidin HBP Maximum Strength Flu	Acetaminophen 500mg	Chlorpheniramine Maleate 2mg		Dextromethorphan HBr 15mg		**Adults & Peds ≥12 yrs:** 2 tabs q6h. **Max:** 8 tabs q24h.
Coricidin HBP Nighttime Multi-Symptom Cold Relief Liquid	Acetaminophen 500mg/15mL	Doxylamine 6.25mg/15mL		Dextromethorphan HBr 15mg/15mL		**Adults & Peds ≥12 yrs:** 2 tbl (30mL) q6h. **Max:** 4 doses q24h.
Pediacare Children's Fever Reducer Plus Cough and Runny Nose with Acetaminophen	Acetaminophen 160mg/5mL	Chlorpheniramine Maleate 1mg/5mL		Dextromethorphan HBr 5mg/5mL		**6-11 yrs (48-95 lbs):** 2 tsp (10mL) q4h. **Max:** 5 times in 24 hrs.
Triaminic Multisymptom Fever	Acetaminophen 160mg/5mL	Chlorpheniramine Maleate 1mg/5mL		Dextromethorphan HBr 7.5mg/5mL		**Peds 6-<12 yrs:** 2 tsp (10mL), q6h. **Max:** 4 doses q24h.
Children's Tylenol Plus Cough & Runny Nose	Acetaminophen 160mg/5mL	Chlorpheniramine Maleate 1mg/5mL		Dextromethorphan HBr 5mg/5mL		**Peds 6-11 yrs (48-95 lbs):** 2 tsp (10mL) q4h. **Max:** 5 doses q24h.
Tylenol Cold and Cough Nighttime Liquid Burst	Acetaminophen 500mg/15mL	Doxylamine 6.25mg/15mL		Dextromethorphan HBr 15mg/15mL		**Adults & Peds ≥12 yrs:** 2 tbl (30mL) q6h. **Max:** 8 tbl q24h.
Vicks Formula 44 Custom Care Cough & Cold PM	Acetaminophen 650mg/15mL	Chlorpheniramine Maleate 4mg/15mL		Dextromethorphan HBr 30mg/15mL		**Adults & Peds ≥12 yrs:** 1 tbl q6h. **Max:** 4 doses q24h.
Vicks NyQuil Cold & Flu Relief Liquid	Acetaminophen 500mg/15mL	Doxylamine Succinate 6.25mg/15mL		Dextromethorphan HBr 15mg/15mL		**Adults & Peds ≥12 yrs:** 2 tbl (30mL) q6h. **Max:** 4 doses q24h.
Vicks NyQuil Cold & Flu Relief LiquiCaps	Acetaminophen 325mg	Doxylamine Succinate 6.25mg		Dextromethorphan HBr 15mg		**Adults & Peds ≥12 yrs:** 2 caps q6h. **Max:** 4 doses q24h.
Vicks NyQuil Cold & Flu Symptom Relief Plus Vitamin C	Acetaminophen 325mg	Doxylamine Succinate 6.25mg		Dextromethorphan HBr 15mg		**Adults & Peds ≥12 yrs:** 2 caps q6h. **Max:** 4 doses q24h.

(Continued)

COUGH-COLD-FLU PRODUCTS

BRAND NAME	ANALGESIC	ANTIHISTAMINE	DECONGESTANT	COUGH SUPPRESSANT	EXPECTORANT	DOSE
COUGH SUPPRESSANT + ANTIHISTAMINE + ANALGESIC *(Continued)*						
Alcohol Free NyQuil, Cold and Flu Relief Liquid	Acetaminophen 325mg/15mL	Chlorpheniramine Maleate 2mg/15mL		Dextromethorphan 15mg/15mL		**Adults & Peds ≥12 yrs:** 2 tbl (30mL) q6h. **Max:** 4 doses q24h.
COUGH SUPPRESSANT + ANTIHISTAMINE + ANALGESIC + DECONGESTANT						
Alka-Seltzer Plus Cold & Cough Formula Effervescent Tablets	Aspirin 325mg	Chlorpheniramine Maleate 2mg	Phenylephrine Bitartrate 7.8mg	Dextromethorphan HBr 10mg		**Adults & Peds ≥12 yrs:** 2 tabs q4h. **Max:** 8 tabs q24h.
Alka-Seltzer Plus Cold & Cough Formula Liquid Gels	Acetaminophen 325mg	Chlorpheniramine Maleate 2mg	Phenylephrine HCl 5mg	Dextromethorphan HBr 10mg		**Adults & Peds ≥12 yrs:** 2 caps q4h. **Max:** 12 caps q24h.
Alka-Seltzer Plus Night Cold Formula Effervescent Tablets	Aspirin 500mg	Doxylamine Succinate 6.25mg	Phenylephrine Bitartrate 7.8mg	Dextromethorphan HBr 10mg		**Adults & Peds ≥12 yrs:** 2 tabs q4-6h. **Max:** 8 tabs q24h.
Alka-Seltzer Plus Night Cold Formula Liquid Gels	Acetaminophen 325mg	Doxylamine Succinate 6.25mg	Phenylephrine HCl 5mg	Dextromethorphan HBr 10mg		**Adults & Peds ≥12 yrs:** 2 caps q4h. **Max:** 12 caps q24h.
Comtrex Nighttime Cough & Cold Caplets	Acetaminophen 325mg	Chlorpheniramine Maleate 2mg	Phenylephrine HCl 5mg	Dextromethorphan HBr 10mg		**Adults & Peds ≥12 yrs:** 2 tabs q4h. **Max:** 12 tabs q24h.
Robitussin Night Time Cough, Cold & Flu	Acetaminophen 160mg/5mL	Chlorpheniramine Maleate 1mg/5mL	Phenylephrine HCl 2.5mg/5mL	Dextromethorphan HBr 5mg/5mL		**Adults & Peds ≥12 yrs:** 4 tsp (20mL) q4h. **Max:** 6 doses q24h.
Theraflu Nighttime Severe Cold & Cough Caplets	Acetaminophen 325mg	Chlorpheniramine Maleate 2mg	Phenylephrine HCl 5mg	Dextromethorphan HBr 10mg		**Adults & Peds ≥12 yrs:** 2 tabs q4h. **Max:** 12 tabs q24h.
Children's Tylenol Plus Multi-Symptom Cold	Acetaminophen 160mg/5mL	Chlorpheniramine Maleate 1mg/5mL	Phenylephrine HCl 2.5mg/5mL	Dextromethorphan HBr 5mg/5mL		**Peds 6-11 yrs (48-95 lbs):** 2 tsp (10mL) q4h. **Max:** 5 doses q24h.
Tylenol Cold Head Congestion Nighttime	Acetaminophen 325mg	Chlorpheniramine Maleate 2mg	Phenylephrine HCl 5mg	Dextromethorphan HBr 10mg		**Adults & Peds ≥12 yrs:** 2 tabs q4h. **Max:** 12 tabs q24h.
Tylenol Cold Multi-Symptom Nighttime Gelcaps	Acetaminophen 325mg	Chlorpheniramine Maleate 2mg	Phenylephrine HCl 5mg	Dextromethorphan HBr 10mg		**Adults & Peds ≥12 yrs:** 2 tabs q4h. **Max:** 12 tabs q24h.
Tylenol Cold Multi-Symptom Nighttime Liquid	Acetaminophen 325mg/15mL	Doxylamine Succinate 6.25mg/30mL	Phenylephrine HCl 5mg/15mL	Dextromethorphan HBr 10mg/15mL		**Adults & Peds ≥12 yrs:** 2 tbl (30mL) q4h. **Max:** 12 tbl (180mL) q24h.
Vicks NyQuil D	Acetaminophen 500mg/15mL	Doxylamine Succinate 6.25mg/15mL	Pseudoephedrine HCl 30mg/15mL	Dextromethorphan HBr 15mg/15mL		**Adults & Peds ≥12 yrs:** 2 tbl (30mL) q6h. **Max:** 4 doses q24h.

BRAND NAME	ANALGESIC	ANTIHISTAMINE	DECONGESTANT	COUGH SUPPRESSANT	EXPECTORANT	DOSE
COUGH SUPPRESSANT + ANTIHISTAMINE + DECONGESTANT						
Children's Dimetapp Cold & Cough		Brompheniramine Maleate 1mg/5mL	Phenylephrine HCl 2.5mg/5mL	Dextromethorphan HBr 5mg/5mL		**Adults & Peds ≥12 yrs:** 4 tsp (20mL) q4h. **Peds 6–<12 yrs:** 2 tsp (10mL) q4h. **Max:** 6 doses q24h.
Theraflu Cold & Cough Hot Liquid		Pheniramine Maleate 20mg/packet	Phenylephrine HCl 10mg/packet	Dextromethorphan HBr 20mg/packet		**Adults & Peds ≥12 yrs:** 1 pkt q4h. **Max:** 6 pkts q24h.
Triaminic-D Multi-Symptom Cold		Chlorpheniramine Maleate 1mg/5mL	Pseudoephedrine HCl 15mg/5mL	Dextromethorphan HBr 7.5mg/5mL		**Peds 6–<12 yrs:** 2 tsp q6h. **Max:** 4 doses q24h.
COUGH SUPPRESSANT + DECONGESTANT						
PediaCare Children's Multi-Symptom Cold			Phenylephrine HCl 2.5mg/5mL	Dextromethorphan HBr 5mg/5mL		**Peds 6-11 yrs:** 2 tsp (10mL) q4h. **Peds 4-5 yrs:** 1 tsp (5mL) q4h. **Max:** 6 doses q24h.
Children's Sudafed PE Cold & Cough Liquid			Phenylephrine HCl 2.5mg/5mL	Dextromethorphan HBr 5mg/5mL		**Peds 6-11 yrs:** 2 tsp (10mL) q4h. **Peds 4-5 yrs:** 1 tsp (5mL) q4h. **Max:** 6 doses q24h.
Day Time Triaminic Thin Strips Cold & Cough			Phenylephrine HCl 2.5mg/strip	Dextromethorphan HBr 5mg/strip		**Peds 6–<12 yrs:** 2 strips q4h. **Peds 4–<6 yrs:** 1 strip q4h. **Max:** 6 doses q24h.
Triaminic Day Time Cold & Cough			Phenylephrine HCl 2.5mg/5mL	Dextromethorphan HBr 5mg/5mL		**Peds 6–<12 yrs:** 2 tsp (10mL) q4h. **Peds 4–<6 yrs:** 1 tsp (5mL) q4h. **Max:** 6 doses q24h.
Vicks Formula 44 Custom Care Congestion			Phenylephrine HCl 10mg/15mL	Dextromethorphan HBr 20mg/15mL		**Adults & Peds ≥12 yrs:** 1 tbl (15mL) q4h. **Peds 6–<12 yrs:** 1½ tsp (7.5mL) q4h. **Max:** 6 doses q24h.
COUGH SUPPRESSANT + DECONGESTANT + ANALGESIC						
Alka-Seltzer Plus Day Non-Drowsy Cold Formula Liquid Gels	Acetaminophen 325mg		Phenylephrine HCl 5mg	Dextromethorphan HBr 10mg		**Adults & Peds ≥12 yrs:** 2 caps q4h. **Max:** 12 caps q24h.
Alka-Seltzer Plus Day & Night Cold Formula Liquid Gels	Acetaminophen 325mg	Doxylamine 6.25mg (nighttime dose only)	Phenylephrine HCl 5mg	Dextromethorphan HBr 10mg		**Adults & Peds ≥12 yrs:** 2 caps q4h. **Max:** 12 caps q24h.
Alka-Seltzer Plus Day & Night Cold Formula Effervescent Tablets	Aspirin 325mg	Doxylamine 6.25mg (nighttime dose only)	Phenylephrine Bitartrate 7.8mg	Dextromethorphan HBr 10mg		**Adults & Peds ≥12 yrs:** 2 tabs q4h. **Max:** 8 tabs q24h.

(Continued)

A83

BRAND NAME	ANALGESIC	ANTIHISTAMINE	DECONGESTANT	COUGH SUPPRESSANT	EXPECTORANT	DOSE
COUGH SUPPRESSANT + DECONGESTANT + ANALGESIC (Continued)						
Theraflu Daytime Severe Cold & Cough Caplets	Acetaminophen 325mg		Phenylephrine HCl 5mg	Dextromethorphan HBr 10mg		**Adults & Peds ≥12 yrs:** 2 tabs q4h. **Max:** 12 tabs q24h.
Theraflu Daytime Severe Cold & Cough Hot Liquid	Acetaminophen 650mg/packet		Phenylephrine HCl 10mg/packet	Dextromethorphan HBr 20mg/packet		**Adults & Peds ≥12 yrs:** 1 pkt q4h. **Max:** 6 pkts q24h.
Theraflu Warming Relief Daytime Severe Cough & Cold	Acetaminophen 325mg/15mL		Phenylephrine HCl 5mg/15mL	Dextromethorphan HBr 10mg/15mL		**Adults & Peds ≥12 yrs:** 2 tbl (30mL) q4h. **Max:** 6 doses q24h.
Children's Tylenol Plus Cold & Cough	Acetaminophen 160mg/5mL		Phenylephrine HCl 2.5mg/5mL	Dextromethorphan HBr 5mg/5mL		**Peds 6-11 yrs (48-95 lbs):** 2 tsp (10mL) q4h. **Peds 4-5 yrs (36-47 lbs):** 1 tsp (5mL) q4h. **Max:** 5 doses q24h.
Tylenol Cold Head Congestion Daytime	Acetaminophen 325mg		Phenylephrine HCl 5mg	Dextromethorphan HBr 10mg		**Adults & Peds ≥12 yrs:** 2 caps q4h. **Max:** 12 caps q24h.
Tylenol Cold Multi-Symptom Daytime Gelcaps/Caplets	Acetaminophen 325mg		Phenylephrine HCl 5mg	Dextromethorphan HBr 10mg		**Adults & Peds ≥12 yrs:** 2 caps q4h. **Max:** 12 caps q24h.
Tylenol Cold Multi-Symptom Daytime Liquid	Acetaminophen 325mg/15mL		Phenylephrine HCl 5mg/15mL	Dextromethorphan HBr 10mg/15mL		**Adults & Peds ≥12 yrs:** 2 tbl (30mL) q4h. **Max:** 12 tbl (180mL) q24h.
Vicks DayQuil Cold & Flu Relief LiquiCaps	Acetaminophen 325mg		Phenylephrine HCl 5mg	Dextromethorphan HBr 10mg		**Adults & Peds ≥12 yrs:** 2 doses q4h. **Max:** 6 doses q24h.
Vicks DayQuil Cold & Flu Relief Liquid	Acetaminophen 325mg/15mL		Phenylephrine HCl 5mg/15mL	Dextromethorphan HBr 10mg/15mL		**Adults & Peds ≥12 yrs:** 2 tbl (30 mL) q4h. **Max:** 6 doses q24h. **Peds 6-<12 yrs:** 1 tbl (15mL) q4h. **Max:** 5 doses q24h.
Vicks DayQuil Cold & Flu Symptom Relief Plus Vitamin C	Acetaminophen 325mg		Phenylephrine HCl 5mg	Dextromethorphan HBr 15mg		**Adults & Peds ≥12 yrs:** 2 caps q4h. **Max:** 6 doses q24h.
COUGH SUPPRESSANT + DECONGESTANT + EXPECTORANT						
Children's Robitussin Cough & Cold CF			Phenylephrine HCl 2.5mg/5mL	Dextromethorphan HBr 5mg/5mL	Guaifenesin 50mg/5mL	**Adults & Peds ≥12 yrs:** 4 tsp (20mL) q4h. **Peds 6-<12 yrs:** 2 tsp (10mL) q4h. **Peds 4-<6 yrs:** 1 tsp (5mL) q4h. **Max:** 6 doses q24h.
Robitussin Cough & Cold CF			Phenylephrine HCl 5mg/5mL	Dextromethorphan HBr 10mg/5mL	Guaifenesin 100mg/5mL	**Adults & Peds ≥12 yrs:** 2 tsp (10mL) q4h. **Max:** 6 doses q24h.
Children's Mucinex, Multi-Symptom Cold Liquid (Very Berry Flavor)			Phenylephrine 2.5mg	Dextromethorphan 5mg	Guaifenesin 100mg	**Peds 6-<12 yrs:** 10mL q4h. **Peds 4-6 yrs:** 5mL q4h.

BRAND NAME	ANALGESIC	ANTIHISTAMINE	DECONGESTANT	COUGH SUPPRESSANT	EXPECTORANT	DOSE
COUGH SUPPRESSANT + DECONGESTANT + EXPECTORANT (Continued)						
Robitussin To Go Cough & Cold CF			Phenylephrine HCl 10mg/10mL	Dextromethorphan HBr 20mg/10mL	Guaifenesin 200mg/10mL	**Adults & Peds ≥12 yrs:** 1 pre-filled spoon (10 mL) q4h. **Max:** 6 doses q24h.
COUGH SUPPRESSANT + DECONGESTANT + EXPECTORANT + ANALGESIC						
Sudafed PE Cold & Cough Caplets	Acetaminophen 325mg		Phenylephrine HCl 5mg	Dextromethorphan HBr 10mg	Guaifenesin 100mg	**Adults & Peds ≥12 yrs:** 2 tabs q4h. **Max:** 12 tabs q24h.
Tylenol Cold Multi-Symptom Severe Liquid	Acetaminophen 325mg/15mL		Phenylephrine HCl 5mg/15mL	Dextromethorphan HBr 10mg/15mL	Guaifenesin 200mg/15mL	**Adults & Peds ≥12 yrs:** 2 tbl (30mL) q4h. **Max:** 12 tbl (180mL) q24h.
Tylenol Cold Severe Head Congestion	Acetaminophen 325mg		Phenylephrine HCl 5mg	Dextromethorphan HBr 10mg	Guaifenesin 200mg	**Adults & Peds ≥12 yrs:** 2 tabs q4h. **Max:** 12 tabs q24h.
COUGH SUPPRESSANT + EXPECTORANT						
Alka-Seltzer Plus Mucus & Congestion Liquid Gels				Dextromethorphan HBr 10mg	Guaifenesin 200mg	**Adults & Peds ≥12 yrs:** 2 caps q4h. **Max:** 12 caps q24h.
Coricidin HBP Chest Congestion & Cough				Dextromethorphan HBr 10mg	Guaifenesin 200mg	**Adults & Peds ≥12 yrs:** 1-2 caps q4h. **Max:** 12 caps q24h.
Maximum Strength Mucinex DM				Dextromethorphan HBr 60mg	Guaifenesin 1200mg	**Adults & Peds ≥12 yrs:** 1 tab q12h. **Max:** 2 tabs q24h.
Mucinex Cough Liquid (Cherry Flavor)				Dextromethorphan HBr 5mg/5mL	Guaifenesin 100mg/5mL	**Peds 6-<12 yrs:** 1-2 tsp (5-10mL) q4h. **Peds 4-<6yrs:** ½-1 tsp (2.5-5mL) q4h. **Max:** 6 doses q24h.
Mucinex Cough Mini-Melts (Orange Crème Flavor)				Dextromethorphan HBr 5mg	Guaifenesin 100mg	**Adults & Peds ≥12 yrs:** 2-4 pkts q4h. **Peds 6-<12 yrs:** 1-2 pkts q4h. **Peds 4-<6yrs:** 1 pkt q4h. **Max:** 6 doses q24h.
Mucinex DM				Dextromethorphan HBr 30mg	Guaifenesin 600mg	**Adults & Peds ≥12 yrs:** 1-2 tabs q12h. **Max:** 4 tabs q24h.
Robitussin Cough & Chest Congestion DM Max				Dextromethorphan HBr 10mg/5mL	Guaifenesin 200mg/5mL	**Adults & Peds ≥12 yrs:** 2 tsp (10mL) q4h. **Max:** 6 doses q24h.
Robitussin Cough & Chest Congestion DM				Dextromethorphan HBr 10mg/5mL	Guaifenesin 100mg/5mL	**Adults & Peds ≥12 yrs:** 2 tsp (10mL) q4h. **Max:** 6 doses q24h.
Robitussin Cough & Chest Congestion Sugar-Free DM				Dextromethorphan HBr 10mg/5mL	Guaifenesin 100mg/5mL	**Adults & Peds ≥12 yrs:** 2 tsp (10mL) q4h. **Max:** 6 doses q24h.

(Continued)

A85

BRAND NAME	ANALGESIC	ANTIHISTAMINE	DECONGESTANT	COUGH SUPPRESSANT	EXPECTORANT	DOSE
COUGH SUPPRESSANT + EXPECTORANT *(Continued)*						
Robitussin To Go Cough & Chest Congestion DM				Dextromethorphan HBr 20mg/10mL	Guaifenesin 200mg/10mL	**Adults & Peds ≥12 yrs:** 1 pre-filled spoon (10mL) q4h. **Max:** 6 doses q24h.
Vicks DayQuil Mucus Control DM				Dextromethorphan HBr 10mg/15mL	Guaifenesin 200mg/15mL	**Adults & Peds ≥12 yrs:** 2 tbl (30mL) q4h. **Peds 6-12 yrs:** 1 tbl (15mL) q4h. **Max:** 6 doses q24h.
Vicks Formula 44 Custom Care Chesty Cough				Dextromethorphan HBr 20mg/15mL	Guaifenesin 200mg/15mL	**Adults & Peds ≥12 yrs:** 1 tbl (15mL) q4h. **Peds 6-<12 yrs:** 1½ tsp (7.5mL) q4h. **Max:** 6 doses q24h.
DECONGESTANT						
Contac-D Cold Decongestant Tablets			Phenylephrine HCl 10mg			**Adults & Peds ≥12 yrs:** 1 tab q4h. **Max:** 6 tabs q24h.
Mucinex Moisture Smart Nasal Spray			Oxymetazoline HCl 0.05%			**Adults & Peds ≥12 yrs:** 2-3 sprays in each nostril q10-12h. **Max:** 2 doses q24h.
Mucinex Full Force Nasal Spray			Oxymetazoline HCl 0.05%			**Adults & Peds ≥12 yrs:** 2-3 sprays in each nostril q10-12h. **Max:** 2 doses q24h.
PediaCare Children's Decongestant			Phenylephrine HCl 2.5mg/5mL			**Peds 6-11 yrs:** 2 tsp (10mL) q4h. **Peds 4-5 yrs:** 1 tsp (5mL) q4h. **Max:** 6 doses q24h.
Children's Sudafed Nasal Decongestant Liquid			Pseudoephedrine HCl 15mg/5mL			**Peds 6-11 yrs:** 2 tsp (10mL) q4-6h. **Peds 4-5 yrs:** 1 tsp (5mL) q4-6h. **Max:** 4 doses q24h.
Children's Sudafed PE Nasal Decongestant Liquid			Phenylephrine HCl 2.5mg/5mL			**Peds 6-11 yrs:** 2 tsp (10mL) q4h. **Peds 4-5 yrs:** 1 tsp (5mL) q4h. **Max:** 6 doses q24h.
Sudafed 12-Hour Tablets			Pseudoephedrine HCl 120mg			**Adults & Peds ≥12 yrs:** 1 tab q12h. **Max:** 2 tabs q24h.
Sudafed 24-Hour Tablets			Pseudoephedrine HCl 240mg			**Adults & Peds ≥12 yrs:** 1 tab q24h. **Max:** 1 tab q24h.

BRAND NAME	ANALGESIC	ANTIHISTAMINE	DECONGESTANT	COUGH SUPPRESSANT	EXPECTORANT	DOSE
DECONGESTANT (Continued)						
Sudafed Nasal Decongestant Tablets			Pseudoephedrine HCl 30mg			**Adults ≥12 yrs:** 2 tabs q4-6h. **Max:** 8 tabs q24h. **Peds 6-12 yrs:** 1 tab q4-6h. **Max:** 4 tabs q24h.
Sudafed OM Sinus Congestion Spray			Oxymetazoline HCl 0.05%			**Adults & Peds ≥6 yrs:** 2-3 sprays in each nostril q10-12h. **Max:** 2 doses q24h.
Sudafed PE Nasal Decongestant Tablets			Phenylephrine HCl 10mg			**Adults & Peds ≥12 yrs:** 1 tab q4h. **Max:** 6 tabs q24h.
Triaminic Thin Strips Cold with Stuffy Nose			Phenylephrine HCl 2.5mg/strip			**Peds 6-<12 yrs:** 2 strips q4h. **Peds 4-<6 yrs:** 1 strip q4h. **Max:** 6 doses q24h.
Vicks Sinex VapoSpray 4-Hour*			Phenylephrine HCl 0.5%			**Adults & Peds ≥12 yrs:** Instill 2-3 sprays per nostril q4h.
Vicks Sinex VapoSpray 12-Hour Decongestant Nasal Spray			Oxymetazoline HCl 0.05%			**Adults & Peds ≥6 yrs:** Instill 2-3 sprays per nostril q10-12h. **Max:** 2 doses q24h.
Vicks Sinex VapoSpray 12-Hour Decongestant UltraFine Mist			Oxymetazoline HCl 0.05%			**Adults & Peds ≥6 yrs:** Instill 2-3 sprays per nostril q10-12h. **Max:** 2 doses q24h.
Vicks VapoInhaler			Levmetamfetamine 50mg			**Adults & Peds ≥12 yrs:** 2 inhalations q2h. **Max:** 24 inhalations q24h. **Peds 6-<12 yrs:** 1 inhalation q2h.
DECONGESTANT + ANALGESIC						
Children's Advil Cold Suspension	Ibuprofen 100mg/5mL		Pseudoephedrine HCl 15mg/5mL			**Peds 6-11 yrs (48-95 lbs):** 2 tsp (10mL) q6h. **2-5 yrs (24-47 lbs):** 1 tsp (5mL) q6h. **Max:** 4 doses q24h.
Advil Cold & Sinus Caplets/Liqui-Gels	Ibuprofen 200mg		Pseudoephedrine HCl 30mg			**Adults & Peds ≥12 yrs:** 1-2 caps q4-6h. **Max:** 6 caps q24h.
Alka-Seltzer Plus Sinus Formula Effervescent Tablets	Aspirin 325mg		Phenylephrine Bitartrate 7.8mg			**Adults & Peds ≥12 yrs:** 2 tabs q4h. **Max:** 8 tabs q24h.

(Continued)

BRAND NAME	ANALGESIC	ANTIHISTAMINE	DECONGESTANT	COUGH SUPPRESSANT	EXPECTORANT	DOSE
DECONGESTANT + ANALGESIC *(Continued)*						
Contac Cold Plus Flu	Acetaminophen 500mg		Phenylephrine HCl 5mg			**Adults & Peds ≥12 yrs:** 2 tabs q4-6h. **Max:** 8 tabs q24h.
Children's Motrin Cold*	Ibuprofen 100mg/5mL		Pseudoephedrine HCl 15mg/5mL			**Peds 6-11 yrs (48-95 lbs):** 2 tsp (10mL) q6h. **2-5 yrs (24-47 lbs):** 1 tsp (5mL) q6h. **Max:** 4 doses q24h.
Sinutab Sinus Caplets	Acetaminophen 325mg		Phenylephrine HCl 5mg			**Adults & Peds ≥12 yrs:** 2 tabs q4h. **Max:** 12 tabs q24h.
Sudafed PE Sinus Headache Caplets	Acetaminophen 325mg		Phenylephrine HCl 5mg			**Adults & Peds ≥12 yrs:** 2 tabs q4h. **Max:** 12 tabs q24h.
Sudafed Sinus Pain 12 Hour Caplets	Naproxen Sodium 220mg		Pseudoephedrine HCl 120mg			**Adults & Peds ≥12 yrs:** 1 tab q12h. **Max:** 2 tabs q24h.
Children's Tylenol Plus Cold & Stuffy Nose	Acetaminophen 160mg/5mL		Phenylephrine HCl 2.5mg/5mL			**Peds 6-11 yrs (48-95 lbs):** 2 tsp (10mL) q4h. **Peds 4-5 yrs (36-47 lbs):** 1 tsp (5mL) q4h. **Max:** 5 doses q24h.
Tylenol Sinus Congestion & Pain Daytime	Acetaminophen 325mg		Phenylephrine HCl 5mg			**Adults & Peds ≥12 yrs:** 2 caps q4h. **Max:** 12 caps q24h.
DECONGESTANT + EXPECTORANT						
Maximum Strength Mucinex D			Pseudoephedrine HCl 120mg		Guaifenesin 1200mg	**Adults & Peds ≥12 yrs:** 1 tab q12h. **Max:** 2 tabs q24h.
Mucinex Cold Liquid (Mixed Berry Flavor)			Phenylephrine HCl 2.5mg/5mL		Guaifenesin 100mg/5mL	**Peds 6-<12 yrs:** 2 tsp (10mL) q4h. **Peds 4-<6 yrs:** 1 tsp (5mL) q4h. **Max:** 6 doses q24h.
Mucinex D			Pseudoephedrine HCl 60mg		Guaifenesin 600mg	**Adults & Peds ≥12 yrs:** 2 tabs q12h. **Max:** 4 tabs q24h.
Sudafed PE Non-Drying Sinus Caplets			Phenylephrine HCl 5mg		Guaifenesin 200mg	**Adults & Peds ≥12 yrs:** 2 tabs q4h. **Max:** 12 tabs q24h.
Triaminic Chest & Nasal Congestion			Phenylephrine HCl 2.5mg/5mL		Guaifenesin 50mg/5mL	**Peds 6-<12 yrs:** 2 tsp (10mL) q4h. **Peds 4-<6 yrs:** 1 tsp (5mL) q4h. **Max:** 6 doses q24h.

BRAND NAME	ANALGESIC	ANTIHISTAMINE	DECONGESTANT	COUGH SUPPRESSANT	EXPECTORANT	DOSE
DECONGESTANT + EXPECTORANT + ANALGESIC						
Sudafed PE Triple Action Caplets	Acetaminophen 325mg		Phenylephrine HCl 5mg		Guaifenesin 200mg	**Adults & Peds ≥12 yrs:** 2 tabs q4h. **Max:** 12 tabs q24h.
Sudafed Triple Action Caplets	Acetaminophen 325mg		Pseudoephedrine HCl 30mg		Guaifenesin 200mg	**Adults & Peds ≥12 yrs:** 2 tabs q4-6h. **Max:** 8 tabs q24h.
Theraflu Warming Relief Cold & Chest Congestion	Acetaminophen 325mg/15mL		Phenylephrine HCl 5mg/15mL		Guaifenesin 200mg/15mL	**Adults & Peds ≥12 yrs:** 2 tbl (30mL) q4h. **Max:** 6 doses q24h.
Tylenol Sinus Severe Congestion & Pain*	Acetaminophen 325mg		Phenylephrine HCl 5mg		Guaifenesin 200mg	**Adults & Peds ≥12 yrs:** 2 tabs q4h. **Max:** 12 tabs q24h.
Tylenol Sinus Severe Congestion Daytime*	Acetaminophen 325mg		Pseudoephedrine HCl 30mg		Guaifenesin 200mg	**Adults & Peds ≥12 yrs:** 2 tabs q4-6h. **Max:** 8 tabs q24h.
EXPECTORANT						
Maximum Strength Mucinex					Guaifenesin 1200mg	**Adults & Peds ≥12 yrs:** 1 tab q12h. **Max:** 2 tabs q24h.
Mucinex					Guaifenesin 600mg	**Adults & Peds ≥12 yrs:** 1-2 tabs q12h. **Max:** 4 tabs q24h.
Mucinex Liquid (Grape Flavor)					Guaifenesin 100mg/5mL	**Peds 6-<12 yrs:** 1-2 tsp (5-10mL) q4h. **Peds 4-<6 yrs:** ½-1 tsp (2.5-5mL) q4h. **Max:** 6 doses q24h.
Mucinex Mini-Melts (Bubble Gum Flavor)					Guaifenesin 100mg/pkt	**Adults & Peds ≥12 yrs:** 2-4 pkts q4h. **Peds 6-<12 yrs:** 1-2 pkts q4h. **Peds 4-<6 yrs:** 1 pkt q4h. **Max:** 6 doses q24h.
Mucinex Mini-Melts (Grape Flavor)					Guaifenesin 50mg/pkt	**Peds 6-<12 yrs:** 2-4 pkts q4h. **Peds 4-<6 yrs:** 1-2 pkts q4h. **Max:** 6 doses q24h.
Robitussin Chest Congestion					Guaifenesin 100mg/5mL	**Adults & Peds ≥12 yrs:** 2-4 tsp (10-20mL) q4h. **Max:** 6 doses q24h.
Vicks DayQuil Mucus Control Liquid					Guaifenesin 200mg/15mL	**Adults & Peds ≥12 yrs:** 2 tbl (30mL) q4h. **Peds 6-<12 yrs:** 1 tbl (15mL) q4h. **Max:** 6 doses q24h.

(Continued)

A89

BRAND NAME	ANALGESIC	ANTIHISTAMINE	DECONGESTANT	COUGH SUPPRESSANT	EXPECTORANT	DOSE
EXPECTORANT + ANALGESIC						
Comtrex Deep Chest Cold Caplets	Acetaminophen 325mg				Guaifenesin 200mg	**Adults & Peds ≥12 yrs:** 2 tabs q4h. **Max:** 12 tabs q24h.
Theraflu Flu & Chest Congestion Hot Liquid	Acetaminophen 1000mg/packet				Guaifenesin 400mg/packet	**Adults & Peds ≥12 yrs:** 1 pkt q6h. **Max:** 4 pkts q24h.
ANTIHISTAMINE + ANALGESIC						
Advil PM Caplets/Liqui-Gels	Ibuprofen 200mg	Diphenhydramine Citrate 38mg				**Adults & Peds ≥12 yrs:** 2 caps hs. **Max:** 2 caps q24h.
Coricidin HBP Cold & Flu	Acetaminophen 325mg	Chlorpheniramine Maleate 2mg				**Adults & Peds ≥12 yrs:** 2 tabs q4-6h. **Max:** 12 tabs q24h. **Peds 6-<12 yrs:** 1 tab q4-6h. **Max:** 5 tabs q24h.
Motrin PM	Ibuprofen 200mg	Diphenhydramine Citrate 38mg				**Adults & Peds ≥12 yrs:** 2 tabs hs. **Max:** 2 tabs q24h.
Tylenol Severe Allergy*	Acetaminophen 500mg	Diphenhydramine HCl 12.5mg				**Adults & Peds ≥12 yrs:** 2 tabs q4-6h. **Max:** 8 tabs q24h.

*Product currently on recall but generic forms may be available.

ANALGESIC PRODUCTS

BRAND	INGREDIENT/STRENGTH	DOSE
ACETAMINOPHEN		
Anacin Extra Strength Aspirin Free Tablets	Acetaminophen 500mg	**Adults & Peds ≥12 yrs:** 2 tabs q6h. **Max:** 8 tabs q24h.
FeverAll Children's Suppositories	Acetaminophen 120mg	**Peds 3-6 yrs:** 1 supp q4-6h. **Max:** 6 supp q24h.
FeverAll Infants' Suppositories	Acetaminophen 80mg	**Peds 6-11 months:** 1 supp q6h. **12-36 months:** 1 supp q4h. **Max:** 6 supp q24h.
FeverAll Jr. Strength Suppositories	Acetaminophen 325mg	**Peds 6-12 yrs:** 1 supp q4-6h. **Max:** 6 supp q24h.
Tylenol 8 Hour Caplets	Acetaminophen 650mg	**Adults & Peds ≥12 yrs:** 2 tabs q8h prn. **Max:** 6 tabs q24h.
Tylenol Arthritis Caplets	Acetaminophen 650mg	**Adults:** 2 tabs q8h prn. **Max:** 6 tabs q24h.
Tylenol Arthritis Gelcaps	Acetaminophen 650mg	**Adults:** 2 caps q8h prn. **Max:** 6 caps q24h.
Tylenol Arthritis Geltabs	Acetaminophen 650mg	**Adults:** 2 tabs q8h prn. **Max:** 6 tabs q24h.
Tylenol Children's Meltaways Tablets*	Acetaminophen 80mg	**Peds 2-3 yrs (24-35 lbs):** 2 tabs. **4-5 yrs (36-47 lbs):** 3 tabs. **6-8 yrs (48-59 lbs):** 4 tabs. **9-10 yrs (60-71 lbs):** 5 tabs. **11 yrs (72-95 lbs):** 6 tabs. May repeat q4h. **Max:** 5 doses q24h.
Tylenol Children's Suspension*	Acetaminophen 160mg/5mL	**Peds 2-3 yrs (24-35 lbs):** 1 tsp (5mL). **4-5 yrs (36-47 lbs):** 1.5 tsp (7.5mL). **6-8 yrs (48-59 lbs):** 2 tsp (10mL). **9-10 yrs (60-71 lbs):** 2.5 tsp (12.5mL). **11 yrs (72-95 lbs):** 3 tsp (15mL). May repeat q4h. **Max:** 5 doses q24h.
Tylenol Extra Strength Caplets	Acetaminophen 500mg	**Adults & Peds ≥12 yrs:** 2 tabs q4-6h prn. **Max:** 8 tabs q24h.
Tylenol Extra Strength Cool Caplets	Acetaminophen 500mg	**Adults & Peds ≥12 yrs:** 2 tabs q4-6h prn. **Max:** 8 tabs q24h.
Tylenol Extra Strength Rapid Release Gelcaps	Acetaminophen 500mg	**Adults & Peds ≥12 yrs:** 2 caps q4-6h prn. **Max:** 8 caps q24h.
Tylenol Extra Strength Rapid Blast Liquid	Acetaminophen 500mg/15mL	**Adults & Peds ≥12 yrs:** 2 tbl (30mL) q4-6h prn. **Max:** 8 tbl (120mL) q24h.
Tylenol Extra Strength EZ Tablets	Acetaminophen 500mg	**Adults & Peds ≥12 yrs:** 2 tabs q4-6h prn. **Max:** 8 tabs q24h.
Tylenol Infants' Drops*	Acetaminophen 160mg/1.6mL	**Peds 2-3 yrs (24-35 lbs):** 1.6 mL q4h prn. **Max:** 5 doses (8mL) q24h.
Tylenol Junior Meltaways Tablets*	Acetaminophen 160mg	**Peds 6-8 yrs (48-59 lbs):** 2 tabs. **9-10 yrs (60-71 lbs):** 2.5 tabs. **11 yrs (72-95 lbs):** 3 tabs. **12 yrs (≥96 lbs):** 4 tabs. May repeat q4h. **Max:** 5 doses q24h.
Tylenol Regular Strength Tablets	Acetaminophen 325mg	**Adults & Peds ≥12 yrs:** 2 tabs q4-6h prn. **Max:** 12 tabs q24h. **Peds 6-11 yrs:** 1 tab q4-6h. **Max:** 5 tabs q24h.
ACETAMINOPHEN COMBINATIONS		
Excedrin Back & Body Caplets	Acetaminophen/Aspirin Buffered 250mg-250mg	**Adults & Peds ≥12 yrs:** 2 tabs q6h. **Max:** 8 tabs q24h.
Excedrin Extra Strength Caplets	Acetaminophen/Aspirin/Caffeine 250mg-250mg-65mg	**Adults & Peds ≥12 yrs:** 2 tabs q6h. **Max:** 8 tabs q24h.

(Continued)

BRAND	INGREDIENT/STRENGTH	DOSE
ACETAMINOPHEN COMBINATIONS *(Continued)*		
Excedrin Extra Strength Geltabs	Acetaminophen/Aspirin/Caffeine 250mg-250mg-65mg	**Adults & Peds ≥12 yrs:** 2 tabs q6h. **Max:** 8 tabs q24h.
Excedrin Extra Strength Express Gels	Acetaminophen/Aspirin/Caffeine 250mg-250mg-65mg	**Adults & Peds ≥12 yrs:** 2 tabs q6h. **Max:** 8 tabs q24h.
Excedrin Extra Strength Tablets	Acetaminophen/Aspirin/Caffeine 250mg-250mg-65mg	**Adults & Peds ≥12 yrs:** 2 tabs q6h. **Max:** 8 tabs q24h.
Excedrin Menstrual Complete Express Gels	Acetaminophen/Aspirin/Caffeine 250mg-250mg-65mg	**Adults & Peds ≥12 yrs:** 2 tabs q4-6h. **Max:** 8 tabs q24h.
Excedrin Migraine Caplets	Acetaminophen/Aspirin/Caffeine 250mg-250mg-65mg	**Adults:** 2 tabs prn. **Max:** 2 tabs q24h.
Excedrin Migraine Geltabs	Acetaminophen/Aspirin/Caffeine 250mg-250mg-65mg	**Adults:** 2 tabs prn. **Max:** 2 tabs q24h.
Excedrin Migraine Tablets	Acetaminophen/Aspirin/Caffeine 250mg-250mg-65mg	**Adults:** 2 tabs prn. **Max:** 2 tabs q24h.
Excedrin Sinus Headache Caplets	Acetaminophen/Phenylephrine HCl 325mg-5mg	**Adults & Peds ≥12 yrs:** 2 tabs q4h. **Max:** 12 tabs q24h.
Excedrin Tension Headache Caplets	Acetaminophen/Caffeine 500mg-65mg	**Adults & Peds ≥12 yrs:** 2 tabs q6h. **Max:** 8 tabs q24h.
Excedrin Tension Headache Express Gels	Acetaminophen/Caffeine 500mg-65mg	**Adults & Peds ≥12 yrs:** 2 caps q6h. **Max:** 8 caps q24h.
Excedrin Tension Headache Geltabs	Acetaminophen/Caffeine 500mg-65mg	**Adults & Peds ≥12 yrs:** 2 tabs q6h. **Max:** 8 tabs q24h.
Goody's Body Pain Powder	Acetaminophen/Aspirin 325mg-500mg	**Adults & Peds ≥12 yrs:** 1 powder q4-6h. **Max:** 4 powders q24h.
Goody's Cool Orange	Acetaminophen/Aspirin/Caffeine 325mg-500mg-65mg	**Adults & Peds ≥12 yrs:** 1 powder q6h. **Max:** 4 powders q24h.
Goody's Extra Strength Headache Powder	Acetaminophen/Aspirin/Caffeine 260mg-520mg-32.5mg	**Adults & Peds ≥12 yrs:** 1 powder q4-6h. **Max:** 4 powders q24h.
Midol Menstrual Complete Caplets	Acetaminophen/Caffeine/Pyrilamine Maleate 500mg-60mg-15mg	**Adults & Peds ≥12 yrs:** 2 tabs q6h. **Max:** 8 tabs q24h.
Midol Menstrual Complete Gelcaps	Acetaminophen/Caffeine/Pyrilamine Maleate 500mg-60mg-15mg	**Adults & Peds ≥12 yrs:** 2 caps q6h. **Max:** 8 caps q24h.
Midol Teen Formula Caplets	Acetaminophen/Pamabrom 500mg-25mg	**Adults & Peds ≥12 yrs:** 2 tabs q6h. **Max:** 8 tabs q24h.
Pamprin Cramp Caplets	Acetaminophen/Magnesium Salicylate/ Pamabrom 250mg-250mg-25mg	**Adults & Peds ≥12 yrs:** 2 tabs q4-6h. **Max:** 8 tabs q24h.
Pamprin Max Caplets	Acetaminophen/Aspirin/Caffeine 250mg-250mg-65mg	**Adults & Peds ≥12 yrs:** 2 tabs q4-6h. **Max:** 8 tabs q24h.
Pamprin Multi-Symptom Caplets	Acetaminophen/Pamabrom/Pyrilamine 500mg-25mg-15mg	**Adults & Peds ≥12 yrs:** 2 tabs q4-6h. **Max:** 8 tabs q24h.
Premsyn PMS Caplets	Acetaminophen/Pamabrom/Pyrilamine 500mg-25mg-15mg	**Adults & Peds ≥12 yrs:** 2 tabs q4-6h. **Max:** 8 tabs q24h.
Vanquish Caplets	Acetaminophen/Aspirin/Caffeine 194mg-227mg-33mg	**Adults & Peds ≥12 yrs:** 2 tabs q6h. **Max:** 8 tabs q24h.
ACETAMINOPHEN/SLEEP AIDS		
Excedrin PM Caplets	Acetaminophen/Diphenhydramine Citrate 500mg-38mg	**Adults & Peds ≥12 yrs:** 2 tabs qhs. **Max:** 2 tabs q24h.
Excedrin PM Express Gels	Acetaminophen/Diphenhydramine Citrate 500mg-38mg	**Adults & Peds ≥12 yrs:** 2 tabs qhs. **Max:** 2 tabs q24h.
Goody's PM Powder	Acetaminophen/Diphenhydramine 1000mg-76mg/dose	**Adults & Peds ≥12 yrs:** 1 packet (2 powders) qhs.
Tylenol PM Caplets	Acetaminophen/Diphenhydramine 500mg-25mg	**Adults & Peds ≥12 yrs:** 2 tabs qhs. **Max:** 2 tabs q24h.
Tylenol PM Rapid Release Gels	Acetaminophen/Diphenhydramine 500mg-25mg	**Adults & Peds ≥12 yrs:** 2 caps qhs. **Max:** 2 caps q24h.
Tylenol PM Geltabs	Acetaminophen/Diphenhydramine 500mg-25mg	**Adults & Peds ≥12 yrs:** 2 tabs qhs. **Max:** 2 tabs q24h.

(Continued)

BRAND	INGREDIENT/STRENGTH	DOSE
NSAIDs		
Advil Caplets	Ibuprofen 200mg	**Adults & Peds ≥12 yrs:** 1-2 tabs q4-6h. **Max:** 6 tabs q24h.
Advil Children's Suspension	Ibuprofen 100mg/5mL	**Peds 2-3 yrs (24-35 lbs):** 1 tsp (5mL). **4-5 yrs (36-47 lbs):** 1.5 tsp (7.5mL). **6-8 yrs (48-59 lbs):** 2 tsp (10mL). **9-10 yrs (60-71 lbs):** 2.5 tsp (12.5mL). **11 yrs (72-95 lbs):** 3 tsp (15mL). May repeat q6-8h. **Max:** 4 doses q24h.
Advil Gel Caplets	Ibuprofen 200mg	**Adults & Peds ≥12 yrs:** 1-2 tabs q4-6h. **Max:** 6 tabs q24h.
Advil Infants' Concentrated Drops	Ibuprofen 50mg/1.25mL	**Peds 6-11 months (12-17 lbs):** 1.25mL. **12-23 months (18-23 lbs):** 1.875mL. May repeat q6-8h. **Max:** 4 doses q24h.
Advil Liqui-Gels	Ibuprofen 200mg	**Adults & Peds ≥12 yrs:** 1-2 caps q4-6h. **Max:** 6 caps q24h.
Advil Migraine Capsules	Ibuprofen 200mg	**Adults:** 2 caps prn. **Max:** 2 caps q24h.
Advil Tablets	Ibuprofen 200mg	**Adults & Peds ≥12 yrs:** 1-2 tabs q4-6h. **Max:** 6 tabs q24h.
Aleve Caplets	Naproxen Sodium 220mg	**Adults & Peds ≥12 yrs:** 1 tab q8-12h. May take 1 additional tab within 1h of first dose. **Max:** 2 tabs q8-12h or 3 tabs q24h.
Aleve Liquid Gels	Naproxen Sodium 220mg	**Adults & Peds ≥12 yrs:** 1 cap q8-12h. May take 1 additional cap within 1h of first dose. **Max:** 2 caps q8-12h or 3 caps q24h.
Aleve Tablets	Naproxen Sodium 220mg	**Adults & Peds ≥12 yrs:** 1 tab q8-12h. May take 1 additional tab within 1h of first dose. **Max:** 2 tabs q8-12h or 3 tabs q24h.
Midol Liquid Gels	Ibuprofen 200mg	**Adults & Peds ≥12 yrs:** 1-2 caps q4-6h. **Max:** 6 caps q24h.
Midol Extended Relief Caplets	Naproxen Sodium 220mg	**Adults & Peds ≥12 yrs:** 1-2 tabs q8-12h. **Max:** 2 tabs q8-12h or 3 tabs q24h.
Motrin Children's Suspension**	Ibuprofen 100mg/5mL	**Peds 2-3 yrs (24-35 lbs):** 1 tsp (5mL). **4-5 yrs (36-47 lbs):** 1.5 tsp (7.5mL). **6-8 yrs (48-59 lbs):** 2 tsp (10mL). **9-10 yrs (60-71 lbs):** 2.5 tsp (12.5mL). **11 yrs (72-95 lbs):** 3 tsp (15mL). May repeat q6-8h. **Max:** 4 doses q24h.
Motrin IB Caplets	Ibuprofen 200mg	**Adults & Peds ≥12 yrs:** 1-2 tabs q4-6h. **Max:** 6 tabs q24h.
Motrin IB Tablets	Ibuprofen 200mg	**Adults & Peds ≥12 yrs:** 1-2 tabs q4-6h. **Max:** 6 tabs q24h.
Motrin Infants' Drops**	Ibuprofen 50mg/1.25mL	**Peds 6-11 months (12-17 lbs):** 1.25mL. **12-23 months (18-23 lbs):** 1.875mL. May repeat q6-8h. **Max:** 4 doses q24h.
Motrin Junior Strength Caplets**	Ibuprofen 100mg	**Peds 6-8 yrs (48-59 lbs):** 2 tabs. **9-10 yrs (60-71 lbs):** 2.5 tabs. **11 yrs (72-95 lbs):** 3 tabs. May repeat q6-8h. **Max:** 4 doses q24h.

(Continued)

BRAND	INGREDIENT/STRENGTH	DOSE
NSAIDs *(Continued)*		
Motrin Junior Strength Chewable Tablets**	Ibuprofen 100mg	**Peds 2-3 yrs (24-35 lbs):** 1 tab. **4-5 yrs (36-47 lbs):** 1.5 tabs. **6-8 yrs (48-59 lbs):** 2 tabs. **9-10 yrs (60-71 lbs):** 2.5 tabs. **11 yrs (72-95 lbs):** 3 tabs. May repeat q6-8h. **Max:** 4 doses q24h.
Pamprin All Day Caplets	Naproxen Sodium 220mg	**Adults & Peds ≥12 yrs:** 1-2 tabs q8-12h. **Max:** 2 tabs q8-12h or 3 tabs q24h.
NSAID SLEEP AIDS		
Advil PM Caplets	Ibuprofen/Diphenhydramine Citrate 200mg-38mg	**Adults & Peds ≥12 yrs:** 2 tabs qhs. **Max:** 2 tabs q24h.
Advil PM Liqui-Gels	Ibuprofen/Diphenhydramine 200mg-25mg	**Adults & Peds ≥12 yrs:** 2 caps qhs. **Max:** 2 caps q24h.
Motrin PM Caplets	Ibuprofen/Diphenhydramine Citrate 200mg-38mg	**Adults & Peds ≥12 yrs:** 2 tabs qhs. **Max:** 2 tabs q24h.
SALICYLATES		
Bayer Aspirin Extra Strength Caplets	Aspirin 500mg	**Adults & Peds ≥12 yrs:** 1-2 tabs q4-6h. **Max:** 8 tabs q24h.
Bayer Aspirin Safety Coated Caplets	Aspirin 325mg	**Adults & Peds ≥12 yrs:** 1-2 tabs q4h. **Max:** 12 tabs q24h.
Bayer Low Dose Aspirin Chewable Tablets*	Aspirin 81mg	**Adults & Peds ≥12 yrs:** 4-8 tabs q4h. **Max:** 48 tabs q24h.
Bayer Low Dose Aspirin Safety Coated Tablets	Aspirin 81mg	**Adults & Peds ≥12 yrs:** 4-8 tabs q4h. **Max:** 48 tabs q24h.
Bayer Genuine Aspirin Tablets	Aspirin 325mg	**Adults & Peds ≥12 yrs:** 1-2 tabs q4h or 3 tabs q6h. **Max:** 12 tabs q24h.
Doan's Extra Strength Caplets	Magnesium Salicylate Tetrahydrate 580mg	**Adults & Peds ≥12 yrs:** 2 tabs q6h. **Max:** 8 tabs q24h.
Ecotrin Low Strength Tablets	Aspirin 81mg	**Adults:** 4-8 tabs q4h. **Max:** 48 tabs q24h.
Ecotrin Regular Strength Tablets	Aspirin 325mg	**Adults & Peds ≥12 yrs:** 1-2 tabs q4h. **Max:** 12 tabs q24h.
Halfprin 162mg Tablets	Aspirin 162mg	**Adults & Peds ≥12 yrs:** 2-4 tabs q4h. **Max:** 24 tabs q24h.
Halfprin 81mg Tablets	Aspirin 81mg	**Adults & Peds ≥12 yrs:** 4-8 tabs q4h. **Max:** 48 tabs q24h.
St. Joseph Chewable Aspirin Tablets	Aspirin 81mg	**Adults & Peds ≥12 yrs:** 4-8 tabs q4h. **Max:** 48 tabs q24h.
St. Joseph Enteric Safety-Coated Tablets	Aspirin 81mg	**Adults & Peds ≥12 yrs:** 4-8 tabs q4h. **Max:** 48 tabs q24h.
SALICYLATES, BUFFERED		
Alka-Seltzer Lemon-Lime Tablets	Aspirin/Citric Acid/Sodium Bicarbonate 325mg-1000mg-1700mg	**Adults & Peds ≥12 yrs:** 2 tabs q4h. **Max:** 8 tabs q24h. **≥60 yrs:** **Max:** 4 tabs q24h.
Alka-Seltzer Original Effervescent Tablets	Aspirin/Citric Acid/Sodium Bicarbonate 325mg-1000mg-1916mg	**Adults & Peds ≥12 yrs:** 2 tabs q4h. **Max:** 8 tabs q24h. **≥60 yrs:** **Max:** 4 tabs q24h.
Alka-Seltzer Extra Strength Effervescent Tablets	Aspirin/Citric Acid/Sodium Bicarbonate 500mg-1000mg-1985mg	**Adults & Peds ≥12 yrs:** 2 tabs q6h. **Max:** 7 tabs q24h. **≥60 yrs:** **Max:** 3 tabs q24h.
Ascriptin Maximum Strength Tablets	Aspirin 500mg Buffered with Aluminum Hydroxide/Calcium Carbonate/Magnesium Hydroxide	**Adults:** 2 tabs q6h. **Max:** 8 tabs q24h.
Ascriptin Regular Strength Tablets	Aspirin 325mg Buffered with Aluminum Hydroxide/Calcium Carbonate/Magnesium Hydroxide	**Adults:** 2 tabs q4h. **Max:** 12 tabs q24h.

(Continued)

BRAND	INGREDIENT/STRENGTH	DOSE
SALICYLATES, BUFFERED *(Continued)*		
Bayer Extra Strength Plus Caplets	Aspirin 500mg Buffered with Calcium Carbonate	**Adults & Peds ≥12 yrs:** 1-2 tabs q4-6h. **Max:** 8 tabs q24h.
Bayer Women's Low Dose Aspirin Caplets	Aspirin 81mg Buffered with Calcium Carbonate 777mg	**Adults & Peds ≥12 yrs:** 4-8 tabs q4h. **Max:** 10 tabs q24h.
Bufferin Extra Strength Tablets	Aspirin 500mg Buffered with Calcium Carbonate/Magnesium Oxide/Magnesium Carbonate	**Adults & Peds ≥12 yrs:** 2 tabs q6h. **Max:** 8 tabs q24h.
Bufferin Tablets	Aspirin 325mg Buffered with Benzoic Acid/Citric Acid	**Adults & Peds ≥12 yrs:** 2 tabs q4h. **Max:** 12 tabs q24h.
SALICYLATE COMBINATIONS		
Anacin Max Strength Tablets	Aspirin/Caffeine 500mg-32mg	**Adults & Peds ≥12 yrs:** 2 tabs q6h. **Max:** 8 tabs q24h.
Anacin Regular Strength Caplets	Aspirin/Caffeine 400mg-32mg	**Adults & Peds ≥12 yrs:** 2 tabs q6h. **Max:** 8 tabs q24h.
Anacin Tablets	Aspirin/Caffeine 400mg-32mg	**Adults & Peds ≥12 yrs:** 2 tabs q6h. **Max:** 8 tabs q24h.
Bayer Back & Body Pain Caplets	Aspirin/Caffeine 500mg-32.5mg	**Adults & Peds ≥12 yrs:** 2 tabs q6h. **Max:** 8 tabs q24h.
Bayer AM Extra Strength Tablets	Aspirin/Caffeine 500mg-65mg	**Adults & Peds ≥12 yrs:** 2 tabs q6h. **Max:** 8 tabs q24h.
BC Arthritis Strength Powders	Aspirin/Caffeine 1000mg-65mg	**Adults & Peds ≥12 yrs:** 1 powder q6h. **Max:** 4 powders q24h.
BC Original Formula Powders	Aspirin/Caffeine 845mg-65mg	**Adults & Peds ≥12 yrs:** 1 powder q6h. **Max:** 4 powders q24h.
SALICYLATE/SLEEP AID		
Bayer PM Caplets	Aspirin/Diphenhydramine Citrate 500mg-38.3mg	**Adults & Peds ≥12 yrs:** 2 tabs qhs.
Doan's Extra Strength PM Caplets	Magnesium Salicylate Tetrahydrate/Diphenhydramine 580mg-25mg	**Adults & Peds ≥12 yrs:** 2 tabs qhs.

*Multiple flavors available
**Currently on recall, generics available

ACE INHIBITORS

DRUG (BRAND)	PEAK PLASMA LEVEL	FOOD EFFECT ON AMOUNT ABSORBED	HYPERTENSION DOSING*	HEART FAILURE DOSING	RENAL DOSE ADJUSTMENT
Benazepril (Lotensin)	1-2 hrs (fasting**); 2-4 hrs (non-fasting**)	None	**Initial:** 10mg qd. **Usual:** 20-40mg/day given qd-bid. **Max:** 80mg/day.†	Not FDA approved.	CrCl<30mL/min/1.73m²: **Initial:** 5mg qd. **Max:** 40mg/day.
Captopril (Capoten)****	1 hr	Reduced***	**Initial:** 25mg bid-tid. **Usual:** 25-150mg bid-tid. **Max:** 450mg/day.	**Initial:** 25mg tid. **Usual:** 50-100mg tid. **Max:** 450mg/day.	**Significant Renal Dysfunction:** Lower initial dose and titrate slowly.
Enalapril (Vasotec)****	3-4 hrs**	None	**Initial:** 5mg qd. **Usual:** 10-40mg/day given qd-bid. **Max:** 40mg/day.†	**Initial:** 2.5mg qd. **Usual:** 2.5-20mg given bid. **Max:** 40mg/day.	HTN: CrCl ≤30mL/min: **Initial:** 2.5mg qd. **Max:** 40mg/day. **Dialysis:** 2.5mg/day on dialysis day. HF: SCr >1.6mg/dL: **Initial:** 2.5mg qd. **Max:** 40mg/day.
Fosinopril (Monopril)	3 hrs**	None	**Initial:** 10mg qd. **Usual:** 20-40mg/day. **Max:** 80mg/day.†	**Initial:** 10mg qd. **Usual:** 20-40mg qd. **Max:** 40mg/day.	HTN: No dosage adjustment needed. HF: Moderate to severe renal failure/vigorous diuresis: initial: 5mg qd.
Lisinopril (Prinivil, Zestril)****	7 hrs	None	**Initial:** 10mg qd. **Usual:** 20-40mg/day. **Max:** 80mg/day.†	(Prinivil) **Initial:** 5mg qd. **Usual:** 5-20mg qd. (Zestril) **Initial:** 5mg qd. **Usual:** 5-40mg qd. **Max:** 40mg/day.	HTN: CrCl 10-30mL/min: **Initial:** 5mg qd. **Max:** 40mg/day. CrCl <10mL/min: **Initial:** 2.5mg qd. **Max:** 40mg/day. HF: CrCl ≤30mL/min: **Initial:** 2.5mg qd.
Moexipril (Univasc)	1.5 hrs**	Reduced***	**Initial:** 7.5mg qd. **Usual:** 7.5-30mg/day given qd-bid. **Max:** 60mg/day.	Not FDA approved.	CrCl ≤40mL/min/1.73m²: **Initial:** 3.75mg qd. **Max:** 15mg/day.
Perindopril (Aceon)****	3-7 hrs**	None	**Initial:** 4mg qd. **Usual:** 4-8mg/day given qd-bid. **Max:** 16mg/day.	Not FDA approved.	CrCl >30mL/min: **Initial:** 2mg qd. **Max:** 8mg/day.
Quinapril (Accupril)	2 hrs**	Reduced (after high-fat meals)	**Initial:** 10-20mg qd. **Usual:** 20-80mg/day given qd-bid.	**Initial:** 5mg bid. **Usual:** 10-20mg bid.	CrCl 30-60mL/min: **Initial:** 5mg qd. CrCl 10-30mL/min: **Initial:** 2.5mg/day.
Ramipril (Altace)****	2-4 hrs**	None	**Initial:** 2.5mg qd. **Usual:** 2.5-20mg/day given qd-bid.	**Post MI:** **Initial:** 2.5mg bid; 1.25mg bid if hypotensive. Titrate to 5mg bid.	HTN: **Initial:** 1.25mg qd. **Max:** 5mg/day. **Post MI:** **Initial:** 1.25mg qd. **Max:** 2.5mg bid.
Trandolapril (Mavik)****	4-10 hrs**	None	**Initial:** 1mg qd in non-black patients. 2mg qd in black patients. **Usual:** 2-4mg/day. **Max:** 8mg/day.	**Post MI:** **Initial:** 1mg qd. Titrate to 4mg qd if tolerated.	CrCl <30mL/min: **Initial:** 0.5mg qd. Titrate slowly.

* Note: Dosages may need to be adjusted when used in combination with other antihypertensives (ie, diuretics). Monitor patient closely. For more information, refer to monograph listings or drug's FDA-approved labeling.
** Peak effect of active metabolite.
*** Administer 1 hour before meals.
**** There are additional indications found in the FDA-approved labeling.
† Refer to monograph for pediatric dosing.

ANTIARRHYTHMIC AGENTS

DRUG (BRAND)	HOW SUPPLIED	INDICATION	DOSAGE	HEPATIC/RENAL DOSE ADJUSTMENT*
Class IA Antiarrhythmics				
Disopyramide (Norpace, Norpace CR)	Cap: (Norpace) 100mg, 150mg; Cap, ER: (Norpace CR) 100mg, 150mg	Treatment of documented life-threatening ventricular arrhythmias.	**Adults:** Usual: 400-800mg/day in divided dose. Recommended: 150mg q6h immediate-release (IR) or 300mg q12h extended-release (CR). Adjust dose with anticholinergic effects. Rapid Control of Ventricular Arrhythmia: 300mg IR (200mg if <110 lbs). Follow with maint dose. Cardiomyopathy/Cardiac Decompensation: Initial: 100mg q6-8h IR. Adjust gradually. See labeling if no response or toxicity occurs. **Elderly:** Start at low end of dosing range. **Pediatrics:** <1 yr: 10-30mg/kg/day. 1-4 yrs: 10-20mg/kg/day. 4-12 yrs: 10-15mg/kg/day. 12-18 yrs: 6-15mg/kg/day. Give in equally divided doses q6h. Hospitalize patient during initial therapy. Start dose titration at lower end of range.	Weight <110 lbs/Moderate Hepatic or Renal Insufficiency (CrCl >40mL/min): 100mg q6h IR or 200mg q12h CR. Severe Renal Insufficiency (with or without initial 150mg LD): CrCl 30-40mL/min: 100mg q8h IR. CrCl 30-15mL/min: 100mg q12h IR. CrCl <15mL/min: 100mg q24h IR.
Procainamide	Inj: 100mg/mL, 500mg/mL	Treatment of documented life-threatening ventricular arrhythmias.	**Adults:** IM: Initial: 50mg/kg/day. Divide into fractional doses of 1/8-1/4 to be injected q3-6h. If >3 doses given, assess patient factors and adjust dose for individual. Arrhythmias Associated with Anesthesia/Surgical Operation: 100-500mg. IV: 100mg q5min until arrhythmia suppressed or 500mg administered. Wait ≥10 min before resuming. Max: 50mg/min. Alternate Regimen: LD: 20mg/mL at 1mL/min for 25-30min to deliver 500-600mg. Max: 1g. Maint: 2mg/mL at 1-3mL/min. Limited Daily Total Fluid Intake: 4mg/mL at 0.5-1.5mL/min to deliver 2-6mg/min.	May need dose adjustment for hepatic/renal impairment.
Quinidine Gluconate	Tab, ER: 324mg; Inj: 80mg/mL	Conversion of symptomatic atrial fibrillation/flutter (A-Fib/Flutter) to normal sinus rhythm, and suppression of ventricular arrhythmias. Tab: reduction of relapse frequency into A-Fib/Flutter.	**Adults:** A-Fib/Flutter Conversion: Initial: 2 tabs q8h. Titrate: Increase cautiously if no effect after 3-4 doses. Alternate Regimen: 1 tab q8h for 2 days, then 2 tabs q12h for 2 days, then 2 tabs q8h up to 4 days. A-Fib/Flutter Relapse Reduction: 1 tab q8-12h. Titrate: Increase cautiously if needed.* May break tab in half. Do not chew or crush. IV: A-Fib/Flutter: 0.25mg/kg/min. Max: 5-10mg/kg.* Consider alternate therapy if conversion to sinus rhythm not achieved. Elderly: Start at low end of dosing range.	Renal/Hepatic Impairment or CHF: Reduce dose.

DRUG (BRAND)	HOW SUPPLIED	INDICATION	DOSAGE	HEPATIC/RENAL DOSE ADJUSTMENT*
Class IA Antiarrhythmics *(Continued)*				
Quinidine Sulfate	Tab: 200mg, 300mg; (ER) 300mg	Conversion of symptomatic A-fib/flutter to normal sinus rhythm, reduction of relapse frequency into A-fib/flutter, and suppression of ventricular arrhythmias.	**Adults:** A-Fib/Flutter Conversion: Initial: 400mg q6h. Titrate: Increase cautiously if no effect after 4-5 doses. (ER): 300mg q8-12h. Titrate: Increase dose cautiously if needed. A-Fib/Flutter Relapse Reduction: 200mg q6h. (ER): 300mg q8-12h. Titrate: Increase cautiously if needed.*	Renal/Hepatic impairment or CHF: Reduce dose.
Class IB Antiarrhythmics				
Lidocaine and Dextrose	Inj: 0.4%-5%, 0.8%-5%	Acute management of ventricular arrhythmias occurring during cardiac manipulations and life-threatening arrhythmias which are ventricular in origin.	**Adults:** Initial: 50-100mg IV bolus of lidocaine injection. If arrhythmias recur or incapable of receiving oral antiarrhythmics, continue with 1-4mg/min IV infusion of lidocaine and dextrose (0.4% sol given at 15-60mL/hr; 0.8% sol given at 7.5-30mL/hr). Determine dose by patient response. Should rarely be necessary to continue IV infusions >24 hrs. **Pediatrics:** Initial: 1mg/kg as IV bolus followed by 30mg/kg/min IV infusion. Should rarely be necessary to continue IV infusions >24 hrs.	
Mexiletine	Cap: 150mg, 200mg, 250mg	Treatment of life-threatening ventricular arrhythmias.	**Adults:** Initial: 200mg q8h when rapid control is not essential. Titrate: Adjust by 50-100mg, not less than every 2-3 days. Usual: 200-300mg q8h. Max: 1200mg/day. If control with ≤300mg q8h, then may divide daily dose and give q12h. Max: 450mg q12h. For Rapid Control: LD: 400mg, then 200mg in 8 hrs. Transfer from Class I Oral Agents: Initial: 200mg and titrate as above, 6-12 hrs after last quinidine sulfate or disopyramide dose, 3-6 hrs after last procainamide dose, or 8-12 hrs after last tocainide dose. Take with food or antacid.	Severe Hepatic Disease: May need lower dose.
Class IC Antiarrhythmics				
Flecainide (Tambocor)	Tab: 50mg, 100mg*, 150mg* *scored	Prevention of paroxysmal supraventricular tachycardias (PSVT), paroxysmal atrial fibrillation/flutter (PAF) associated with disabling symptoms in patients without structural heart disease. Prevention of life-threatening ventricular arrhythmias (VT).	**Adults:** PSVT/PAF: Initial: 50mg q12h. Titrate: May increase by 50mg bid every 4 days. Max: 300mg/day. Sustained VT: Initial: 100mg q12h. Titrate: May increase by 50mg bid every 4 days. Max: 400mg/day. Reduce dose by 50% with amiodarone. **Pediatrics:** <6 months: Initial: 50mg/m²/day given bid-tid. >6 months: Initial: 100mg/m²/day given bid-tid. Max: 200mg/m²/day. Reduce dose by 50% with amiodarone.	CrCl ≤35mL/min: Initial: 100mg qd or 50mg bid. Less Severe Renal Disease: Initial: 100mg q12h.

(Continued)

DRUG (BRAND)	HOW SUPPLIED	INDICATION	DOSAGE	HEPATIC/RENAL DOSE ADJUSTMENT*
Class IC Antiarrhythmics *(Continued)*				
Propafenone (Rythmol, Rythmol SR)	Tab: 150mg*, 225mg*; (generic) 300mg*; *scored (SR) Cap, ER: 225mg, 325mg, 425mg	To prolong the time to recurrence of paroxysmal atrial fibrillation/flutter (PAF) and paroxysmal supraventricular tachycardia (PSVT) associated with disabling symptoms in patients without structural heart disease. Treatment of life-threatening documented ventricular arrhythmias. (SR) To prolong time to recurrence of symptomatic atrial fibrillation (AF) in patients with episodic AF without structural heart disease.	**Adults:** Initial: 150mg q8h. Titrate: May increase at minimum 3-4 day intervals to 225mg q8h, then to 300mg q8h if needed. Max: 900mg/day. Elderly/Marked Myocardial Damage: Increase more gradually during initial phase. **SR: Adults:** Initial: 225mg q12h. Titrate: May increase at minimum 5-day intervals to 325mg q12h, then to 425mg q12h if needed. QRS Widening/2nd- or 3rd-degree AV Block: Reduce dose.	Hepatic Dysfunction: Give 20-30% of normal dosage. (SR) Hepatic Impairment: Reduce dose.
Class II Antiarrhythmics (Beta-Blockers)				
Acebutolol (Sectral)	Cap: 200mg, 400mg	Management of hypertension and ventricular premature beats.	**Adults:** Ventricular Arrhythmia: Initial: 200mg bid. Maint: In-crease gradually to 600-1200mg/day. Elderly: Lower daily doses. Max: 800mg/day.	CrCl <50mL/min: Decrease daily dose by 50%. CrCl <25mL/min: Decrease daily dose by 75%.
Esmolol (Brevibloc)	Inj: 10mg/mL, 20mg/mL	For rapid control of ventricular rate in atrial fibrillation or atrial flutter in perioperative, postoperative, or other emergent circumstances. For non-compensatory sinus tachycardia.	**Adults:** Supraventricular Tachycardia: Titrate dose based on ventricular rate. LD: 0.5mg/kg over 1 min. Maint: 0.05mg/kg/min for next 4 min. May continue at 0.05mg/kg/min or increase stepwise with each step maintained for ≥4 min to max 0.2mg/kg/min. Rapid slowing of ventricular response: Repeat 0.5mg/kg LD over 1 min, then 0.1mg/kg/min for 4 min. If needed, another (final) LD of 0.5mg/kg over 1 min, then 0.15mg/kg/min for 4 min then up to 0.2mg/kg/min if needed. May continue infusions for 24 hrs. Intraoperative/Postoperative Tachycardia: Immediate Control: Initial: 80mg bolus over 30 sec. Maint: 0.15mg/kg/min. May titrate up to 0.3mg/kg/min. Gradual Control: Initial: 0.5mg/kg/min over 1 min. Maint: 0.05mg/kg/min for 4 min. Then, if needed, may repeat LD and increase maintenance infusion to 0.1mg/kg/min.	
Propranolol	Inj: 1mg/mL; Tab: 10mg*, 20mg*, 40mg*, 60mg*, 80mg* *scored	(Inj) For cardiac arrhythmias (supraventricular, ventricular tachy-cardia, tachyarrhythmia of digitalis intoxication, resistant tachyarrhythmia). (Tab) To control ventricular rate in patients with atrial fibrillation and a rapid ventricular response.	**Adults:** (Inj) 1-3mg IV at 1mg/min. May give 2nd dose after 2 min, subsequent doses ≥4 hrs later. A Fib: (Tab) 10-30mg PO tid-qid ac and hs.	Hepatic insufficiency: May need to lower dose.

DRUG (BRAND)	HOW SUPPLIED	INDICATION	DOSAGE	HEPATIC/RENAL DOSE ADJUSTMENT*
Class II Antiarrhythmics (Beta-Blockers) *(Continued)*				
Sotalol (Betapace)†	Tab: 80mg*, 120mg*, 160mg* *scored	Treatment of documented life threatening ventricular arrhythmias.	**Adults:** Initial: 80mg bid. Titrate: Increase to 120-160mg bid if needed. Allow 3 days between dose increments. Usual: 160-320mg/day given bid-tid. Refractory Patients: 480-640mg/day. **Pediatrics:** ≥2 yrs: Initial: 30mg/m² tid. Titrate: Wait at least 36 hrs between dose increases. Guide dose by response, HR, and QTc. Max: 60mg/m². <2 yrs: See dosing chart in PI. Reduce dose or d/c if QTc >550msec.	**Adults:** CrCl 30-59mL/min: Dose q24h. CrCl 10-29mL/min: Dose q36-48h. CrCl <10mL/min: Individualize dose. May increase dose with renal impairment after at least 5-6 doses at appropriate intervals. **Pediatrics:** Renal Impairment: Reduce dose or increase interval.
Sotalol (Betapace AF)†	Tab: 80mg*, 120mg*, 160mg* *scored	Maintenance of normal sinus rhythm with symptomatic atrial fibrillation/atrial flutter (AFIB/AFL) in patients who are currently in sinus rhythm.	**Adults:** Initiate with continuous ECG monitoring. Give dose qd for CrCl 40-60mL/min and bid for CrCl >60mL/min. Initial: 80mg. Monitor QT 2-4 hrs after each dose. Reduce dose or d/c if QT ≥500msec. If QT <500msec after 3 days (after 5th or 6th dose if receiving qd dosing), discharge on current treatment. Alternately, may increase dose to 120mg during hospitalization, and follow for 3 days with bid dose and for 5 or 6 doses if receiving qd dose. Max: 160mg qd or bid depending on CrCl. **Pediatrics:** ≥2 yrs: Initial: 30mg/m² tid. Titrate: Wait at least 36 hrs between dose increases. Guide dose by response, heart rate and QTc. Max: 60mg/m². <2 yrs: See dosing chart in PI. Reduce dose or d/c if QTc >550msec.	Renal Impairment: Reduce dose or increase interval.
Class III Antiarrhythmics				
Amiodarone (Cordarone, Nexterone, Pacerone)	Tab: 100mg, 200mg*, (generic) 400mg* *scored; Inj: 1.5mg/mL, 1.8mg/mL, 50mg/mL	Treatment and prophylaxis (inj) of documented, life-threatening recurrent ventricular fibrillation and recurrent hemodynamically unstable ventricular tachycardia.	**Adults:** Give LD in hospital. LD: 800-1600mg/day for 1-3 weeks. Give in divided doses with meals for total daily dose ≥1000mg or if GI intolerance occurs. After control is achieved, then 600-800mg/day for 1 month. Maint: 400mg/day; up to 600mg/day if needed. Use lowest effective dose. Take consistently with regards to meals. Elderly: Start at low end of dosing range. **IV: Adults:** LD: 150mg over 1st 10 min (15mg/min), then 360mg over next 6 hrs (1mg/min), then 540mg over remaining 18 hrs (0.5mg/min). Maint: 0.5mg/min for 2-3 weeks. Breakthrough Ventricular Tachycardia/Ventricular Fibrillation: 150mg supplement IV over 10 min. Increase rate to achieve suppression. Max Infusion Rate: 30mg/min (initial); 2mg/mL (>1 hr, unless central venous catheter used). See PI for transition to oral amiodarone. Elderly: Start at low end of dosing range.	

(Continued)

DRUG (BRAND)	HOW SUPPLIED	INDICATION	DOSAGE	HEPATIC/RENAL DOSE ADJUSTMENT*
Class III Antiarrhythmics *(Continued)*				
Dofetilide (Tikosyn)	Cap: 125mcg, 250mcg, 500mcg	Conversion to and maintenance of normal sinus rhythm in atrial fibrillation/flutter.	**Adults:** Individualize dose based on CrCl and QTc. Use QT interval if HR <60 beats/min. Initiate with continuous ECG monitoring. CrCl >60mL/min: 500mcg bid. Determine QTc interval 2-3 hrs after 1st dose and adjust dose if QTc >500msec (550msec with ventricular conduction abnormalities) or if >15% increase from baseline. QTc Adjustment: Reduce 500mcg bid to 250mcg bid. Reduce 250mcg bid to 125mcg bid. Reduce 125mcg bid to 125mcg qd. Max: CrCl >60mL/min: 500mcg bid. D/C anytime after 2nd dose if QTc >500msec (550msec with ventricular conduction abnormalities).	CrCl 40-60mL/min: 250mcg bid. CrCl 20 to <40mL/min: 125mcg bid. CrCl <20mL/min: do not use. Monitor ECG.
Dronedarone (Multaq)**	Tab: 400mg	Reduces risk of cardiovascular hospitalization with paroxysmal or persistent atrial fibrillation (AF) or atrial flutter (AFL), with a recent episode of AF/AFL and associated cardiovascular risk factors, who are in sinus rhythm or who will be cardioverted.	**Adults:** 400mg bid (with morning and evening meals).	
Ibutilide (Corvert)	Inj: 0.1mg/mL	For rapid conversion of atrial fibrillation or flutter (A-Fib/Flutter) of recent onset to sinus rhythm.	**Adults:** ≥60kg: 1mg over 10 min. <60kg: 0.01mg/kg over 10 min. If arrhythmia still present within 10 min after the end of the initial infusion, repeat infusion 10 min after completion of 1st infusion. Continuous ECG monitoring for 4 hrs after infusion or until QTc returns to baseline.	
Class IV Antiarrhythmics (Calcium Channel Blockers)				
Diltiazem Injection	Inj: 5mg/mL	Temporary control of rapid ventricular rate in atrial fibrillation/flutter (A-Fib/Flutter). Rapid conversion of paroxysmal supraventricular tachycardia (PSVT) to sinus rhythm.	**Adults:** Bolus: 0.25mg/kg IV over 2 min. If no response after 15 minutes, may give 2nd dose of 0.35mg/kg over 2 min. Continuous Infusion: 0.25-0.35mg/kg IV bolus, then 10mg/hr. Titrate: Increase by 5mg/hr. Max: 15mg/hr and duration up to 24 hrs.	

DRUG (BRAND)	HOW SUPPLIED	INDICATION	DOSAGE	HEPATIC/RENAL DOSE ADJUSTMENT*
Class IV Antiarrhythmics (Calcium Channel Blockers) *(Continued)*				
Verapamil (Calan)	Tab: 40mg*, 80mg*, 120mg* *scored Inj: 2.5mg/mL (generic)	(Tab): With digitalis, for control of ventricular rate at rest and during stress in patients with chronic atrial flutter and/or atrial fibrillation and prophylaxis of repetitive PSVT. (Inj): Rapid conversion of PSVT to sinus rhythm, including those associated with accessory bypass tracts and temporary control of rapid ventricular rate in A-fib/flutter except when associated with accessory bypass tracts.	**Adults:** A-Fib (Digitalized): Usual: 240-320mg/day PO given tid-qid. PSVT Prophylaxis (Non-Digitalized): 240-480mg/day PO given tid-qid. Max: 480mg/day. (Inj): **Adults:** Initial: 5-10mg IV bolus over 2 min. If 1st dose not adequate, repeat 10mg over 2 min 30 min after first dose. Elderly: Administer dose over at least 3 min. **Pediatrics:** Continuously monitor ECG. ≤1 yr: 0.1-0.2mg/kg IV bolus over 2 min. If 1st dose not adequate, repeat 0.1-0.2mg/kg over 2 min 30 min after 1st dose. **1-15 yrs:** 0.1-0.3 mg/kg IV bolus over 2 min. Max: 5mg. If 1st dose not adequate, repeat 0.1-0.3mg/kg over 2 min 30 min after 1st dose. Max: 10mg single dose.	Severe hepatic dysfunction: (Tab) Give 30% of normal dose.
Class V Antiarrhythmics				
Adenosine (Adenocard)	Inj: 3mg/mL	Conversion of paroxysmal supraventricular tachycardia (including that associated with accessory bypass tracts) to sinus rhythm (SR).	**Adults:** 6mg rapid IV bolus over 1-2 sec. If not converted to SR within 1-2 min, give 12mg rapid IV bolus; may give 2nd 12mg rapid IV bolus if needed. Max: 12mg/dose. **Pediatrics:** <50kg: 0.05-0.1mg/kg rapid IV bolus. If not converted to SR within 1-2 min, give incrementally increasing amount by 0.05-0.1mg/kg. Follow each bolus with a saline flush. Continue process until SR or a maximum single dose of 0.3mg/kg is used. ≥50kg: 6mg rapid IV bolus over 1-2 sec. If not converted to SR within 1-2 min, give 12mg rapid IV bolus; may give 2nd 12mg dose if needed. Max: 12mg/dose.	
Digoxin (Lanoxin)	Inj: (Pediatric Inj) 0.1mg/mL, 0.25mg/mL; Sol: (generic) 0.05mg/mL; Tab: 0.125mg*, 0.25mg* *scored	Treatment of mild to moderate heart failure and to control ventricular response rate with chronic atrial fibrillation.	**Adults:** Rapid Digitalization: LD: (Inj) 0.4-0.6mg IV single dose or (Tab) 0.5-0.75mg PO, may give additional (Inj) 0.1-0.3mg or (Tab) 0.125-0.375mg at 6-8 hr intervals until clinical effect. Maint: (Tab) 0.125-0.5mg qd. A-Fib: Titrate to minimum effective dose for desired response. (Sol) Initial: 3mcg/kg/day. Refer to PI for details. **Pediatrics:** See PI for full pediatric dosing information.	Elderly (>70 yrs)/Renal Dysfunction: Initial: 0.125mg qd. Marked Renal Dysfunction: Initial: 0.0625mg qd. Titrate every 2 weeks based on response.

* Ventricular Arrhythmia: Dosing regimens not adequately studied. Generally similar to A-Fib/Flutter.
** Has antiarrhythmic properties of all four classes.
† Also has Class III properties.
ER: Extended-Release

ARBs* AND COMBINATIONS

DRUG	BRAND	USUAL HTN† DOSAGE RANGE	HOW SUPPLIED
ANGIOTENSIN II RECEPTOR BLOCKERS			
Candesartan	Atacand	8–32mg/day.‡	**Tab:** 4mg, 8mg, 16mg, 32mg
Eprosartan	Teveten	400–800mg/day.	**Tab:** 400mg, 600mg
Irbesartan	Avapro	150–300mg/day.	**Tab:** 75mg, 150mg, 300mg
Losartan	Cozaar	25–100mg/day.‡	**Tab:** 25mg, 50mg, 100mg
Olmesartan	Benicar	20–40mg/day.‡	**Tab:** 5mg, 20mg, 40mg
Telmisartan	Micardis	20–80mg/day.	**Tab:** 20mg, 40mg, 80mg
Valsartan	Diovan	80–320mg/day.‡	**Tab:** 40mg, 80mg, 160mg, 320mg
COMBINATIONS			
Candesartan-Hydrochlorothiazide	Atacand HCT	16/12.5–32/25mg/day.	**Tab:** 16mg-12.5mg, 32mg-12.5mg, 32mg-25mg
Eprosartan-Hydrochlorothiazide	Teveten HCT	600/12.5–600/25mg/day.	**Tab:** 600mg-12.5mg, 600mg-25mg
Irbesartan-Hydrochlorothiazide	Avalide	150/12.5–300/25mg/day.	**Tab:** 150mg-12.5mg, 300mg-12.5mg, 300mg-25mg
Losartan-Hydrochlorothiazide	Hyzaar	50/12.5–100/25mg/day.	**Tab:** 50mg-12.5mg, 100mg-12.5mg, 100mg-25mg
Olmesartan-Amlodipine	Azor	20/5-40/10mg/day.	**Tab:** 20mg-5mg, 20mg-10mg, 40mg-5mg, 40mg-10mg
Olmesartan-Amlodipine-Hydrochlorothiazide	Tribenzor	Individualize dose up to 40/10/25mg/day.§	**Tab:** 20mg-5mg-12.5mg, 40mg-5mg-12.5mg, 40mg-5mg-25mg, 40mg-10mg-12.5mg, 40mg-10mg-25mg
Olmesartan-Hydrochlorothiazide	Benicar HCT	20/12.5–40/25mg/day.	**Tab:** 20mg-12.5mg, 40mg-12.5mg, 40mg-25mg
Telmisartan-Amlodipine	Twynsta	40/5-80/10mg/day.	**Tab:** 40mg-5mg, 40mg-10mg, 80mg-5mg, 80mg-10mg
Telmisartan-Hydrochlorothiazide	Micardis HCT	40/12.5–160/25mg/day.	**Tab:** 40mg-12.5mg, 80mg-12.5mg, 80mg-25mg
Valsartan-Amlodipine	Exforge	160/5-320/10mg/day.	**Tab:** 160mg-5mg, 160mg-10mg, 320mg-5mg, 320mg-10mg
Valsartan-Amlodipine-Hydrochlorothiazide	Exforge HCT	Individualize dose up to 320/10/25mg/day.§	**Tab:** 160mg-5mg-12.5mg, 160mg-5mg-25mg, 160mg-10mg-12.5mg, 160mg-10mg-25mg, 320mg-10mg-25mg
Valsartan-Hydrochlorothiazide	Diovan HCT	160/12.5–320/25mg/day.	**Tab:** 80mg-12.5mg, 160mg-12.5mg, 160mg-25mg, 320mg-12.5mg, 320mg-25mg

*ARBs: Angiotensin II receptor blockers.

†HTN: Hypertension.

‡Refer to monograph for pediatric dosing.

§Exforge HCT and Tribenzor are not indicated for initial therapy of hypertension. May be used for patients not adequately controlled on any two of the following antihypertensive classes: calcium channel blockers, angiotensin receptor blockers, and diuretics.

Adapted from the Seventh Report of the Joint National Committee on Prevention, Detection, Evaluation, and Treatment of High Blood Pressure (JNC 7); http://www.nhlbi.nih.gov/guidelines/hypertension/jnc7full.htm.

BETA-BLOCKERS

DRUG	BRAND	HOW SUPPLIED	HYPERTENSION DOSING	ANGINA DOSING	POST-MI DOSING
NONSELECTIVE BETA-BLOCKERS					
Nadolol	Corgard	**Tab:** 20mg, 40mg, 80mg	**Initial:** 40mg qd. **Usual:** 40mg–80mg qd. **Max:** 320mg/day.	**Initial:** 40mg qd. **Usual:** 40mg–80mg qd. **Max:** 240mg/day.	Not FDA approved
Penbutolol sulfate	Levatol	**Tab:** 20mg	**Initial** and **Usual:** 20mg qd.	Not FDA approved	Not FDA approved
Pindolol	Various generics	**Tab:** 5mg, 10mg	**Initial:** 5mg bid. **Max:** 60mg/day.	Not FDA approved	Not FDA approved
Propranolol HCl***	Various generics†	**Tab:** 10mg, 20mg, 40mg, 60mg, 80mg	**Initial:** 40mg bid. **Usual:** 120mg–240mg/day. **Max:** 640mg/day.	**Usual:** 80mg–320mg/day.	**Initial:** 40mg tid. **Usual:** 180mg–240mg/day. **Max:** 240mg/day.
	Inderal LA†	**Cap, LA:** 60mg, 80mg, 120mg, 160mg	**Initial:** 80mg qd. **Usual:** 120mg–160mg qd. **Max:** 640mg/day.	**Initial:** 80mg qd. **Usual:** 160mg qd. **Max:** 320mg.	Not FDA approved
	Innopran XL	**Cap, ER:** 80mg, 120mg	**Initial:** 80mg qhs. **Max:** 120mg qhs.	Not FDA approved	Not FDA approved
Timolol maleate	Various generics	**Tab:** 5mg, 10mg 20mg	**Initial:** 10mg bid. **Usual:** 20mg–40mg/day. **Max:** 60mg/day.	Not FDA approved	**Usual:** 10mg bid (post acute MI).
SELECTIVE BETA₁-BLOCKERS					
Acebutolol	Sectral†	**Cap:** 200mg, 400mg	**Initial:** 400mg qd or bid. **Usual:** 400mg–800mg/day. **Max:** 1200mg/day.	Not FDA approved	Not FDA approved
Atenolol	Tenormin	**Tab:** 25mg, 50mg, 100mg	**Initial:** 50mg qd. **Max:** 100mg qd.	**Initial:** 50mg qd. **Usual:** 100mg qd. **Max:** 200mg qd.	**Usual:** 50mg bid or 100mg qd for 6–9 days post MI.
Betaxolol HCl	Various generics	**Tab:** 10mg, 20mg	**Initial:** 10mg qd. **Max:** 20–40mg qd.	Not FDA approved	Not FDA approved
Bisoprolol fumarate	Zebeta	**Tab:** 5mg, 10mg	**Initial:** 2.5mg–5mg qd. **Usual:** 2.5mg–20mg qd. **Max:** 20mg qd.	Not FDA approved	Not FDA approved
Esmolol	Brevibloc†	**Inj:** 10mg/mL, 20mg/mL	**Immediate Control:** **Initial:** 80mg bolus over 30 sec. **Maint:** 0.15mg/kg/min. May titrate up to 0.3mg/kg/min. **Gradual Control:** **Initial:** 0.5mg/kg/min over 1 min. **Maint:** 0.05mg/kg/min for 4 min. If needed, may repeat loading dose. **Maint:** follow with increase to 0.1mg/kg/min.**	Not FDA approved	Not FDA approved
Metoprolol succinate	Toprol-XL†	**Tab, XL:** 25mg, 50mg, 100mg, 200mg	**Initial:** 25mg–100mg qd. **Max:** 400mg/day.	**Initial:** 100mg qd. **Max:** 400mg/day.	Not FDA approved

(Continued)

DRUG	BRAND	HOW SUPPLIED	HYPERTENSION DOSING	ANGINA DOSING	POST-MI DOSING
SELECTIVE BETA₁-BLOCKERS *(Continued)*					
Metoprolol tartrate***	Lopressor	**Tab:** 50mg, 100mg	**Initial:** 100mg qd or in divided doses. **Usual:** 100mg–450mg/day. **Max:** 450mg/day.	**Initial:** 50mg bid. **Usual:** 100mg–400mg/day. **Max:** 400mg/day.	**Usual Maint:** 100mg bid for at least 3 months.
	Various generics	**Tab:** 25mg, 50mg 100mg	**Initial:** 100mg qd or in divided doses. **Usual:** 100mg–450mg/day. **Max:** 450mg/day.	**Initial:** 50mg bid. **Usual:** 100mg–400mg/day. **Max:** 400mg/day.	**Usual Maint:** 100mg bid for at least 3 months.
Nebivolol	Bystolic	**Tab:** 2.5mg, 5mg 10mg, 20mg	**Initial:** 5mg qd. **Titrate:** May increase dose if needed at 2-week intervals. **Max:** 40mg.	Not FDA approved	Not FDA approved
MIXED ALPHA- AND BETA-BLOCKERS					
Carvedilol	Coreg†	**Tab:** 3.125mg, 6.25mg, 12.5mg, 25mg	**Initial:** 6.25mg bid. **Max:** 25mg bid.	Not FDA approved	Left Ventricular Dysfunction post MI: **Initial:** 6.25mg bid, then increase to 12.5mg bid after 3-10 days. **Usual Target:** 25mg bid.
	Coreg CR†	**Cap, ER:** 10mg, 20mg, 40mg, 80mg	**Initial:** 20mg qd. **Max:** 80mg/day.	Not FDA approved	Left Ventricular Dysfunction post MI: **Initial:** 10mg–20mg qd. **Usual:** 80mg qd.
Labetalol HCl***	Trandate	**Tab:** 100mg, 200mg, 300mg	**Initial:** 100mg bid. **Usual:** 200mg–400mg bid.	Not FDA approved	Not FDA approved
COMBINATIONS					
Atenolol/ Chlorthalidone	Tenoretic	**Tab:** 50mg/25mg, 100mg/25mg	**Initial:** 50mg/25mg qd. **Max:** 100mg/25mg/day.	Not FDA approved	Not FDA approved
Nadolol/ Bendroflumethiazide	Corzide	**Tab:** 40mg/5mg, 80mg/5mg	**Initial:** 40mg/5mg qd. **Max:** 80mg/5mg/day.	Not FDA approved	Not FDA approved
Bisoprolol/ fumarate/ HCTZ*	Ziac	**Tab:** 2.5mg/ 6.25mg, 5mg/ 6.25mg, 10mg/ 6.25mg	**Initial:** 2.5mg/ 6.25mg qd. **Max:** 20mg/12.5mg/day.	Not FDA approved	Not FDA approved

(Continued)

DRUG	BRAND	HOW SUPPLIED	HYPERTENSION DOSING	ANGINA DOSING	POST-MI DOSING
COMBINATIONS *(Continued)*					
Metoprolol tartrate/ HCTZ*	Lopressor HCT	**Tab:** 50mg/25mg, 100mg/25mg, (generic) 100mg/50mg	Individualize dose. **Lopressor Usual Initial:** 100mg/day qd or in divided doses. **Lopressor Max:** 450mg/day. **HCTZ Usual:** 12.5mg-50mg/day. HCTZ dose >50mg/day not recommended.	Not FDA approved	Not FDA approved
Propranolol/ HCTZ*	Various generics	**Tab:** 40mg/25mg, 80mg/25mg	Individualize dose. **Propranolol Alone Initial:** 80mg/day. **Usual:** 160mg-480mg/day. **HCTZ Alone Usual:** 12.5-50mg/day. **Inderide Max Dose:** 160mg/50mg.	Not FDA approved	Not FDA approved

*Hydrochlorothiazide.

**Brevibloc is used for the treatment of tachycardia and hypertension that occur during induction and tracheal intubation, during surgery, on emergence from anesthesia, and in the postoperative period.

***For additional dosage forms, refer to FDA-approved labeling.

†For additional indications, refer to FDA-approved labeling.

Note: Sotalol (Betapace) is indicated for ventricular arrhythmias. Refer to FDA-approved labeling for dosing and additional information.

Source: FDA-approved labeling.

CALCIUM CHANNEL BLOCKERS

DRUG	BRAND	HOW SUPPLIED	HYPERTENSION DOSING*	ANGINA DOSING*
DIHYDROPYRIDINES				
Amlodipine besylate	Norvasc	**Tab:** 2.5mg, 5mg, 10mg	**Initial:** 5mg qd. **Max:** 10mg qd.	**Usual:** 5-10mg qd.
Clevidipine butyrate	Cleviprex	**Inj:** 0.5mg/mL	**Initial:** 1-2mg/hr. **Maint:** 4-6mg/hr. **Max:** 21mg/hr or 1000mL per 24 hrs.	Not FDA approved
Felodipine	Generic	**Tab, ER:** 2.5mg, 5mg, 10mg	**Initial:** 5mg qd. **Usual:** 2.5-10mg qd.	Not FDA approved
Isradipine	DynaCirc CR, Generic	**Tab, CR:** 5mg, 10mg **Cap:** 2.5mg, 5mg	**Initial:** Cap: 2.5mg bid or (CR): 5mg qd. **Max:** 20mg/day.	Not FDA approved
Nicardipine HCl**	Generic	**Cap:** 20mg, 30mg	**Initial:** 20mg tid. **Usual:** 20-40mg tid.	**Initial:** 20mg tid. **Usual:** 20-40mg tid.
	Cardene SR	**Cap, ER:** 30mg, 45mg, 60mg	**Initial:** 30mg bid. **Usual:** 30-60mg bid.	Not FDA approved
Nifedipine	Adalat CC	**Tab, ER:** 30mg, 60mg, 90mg	**Initial:** 30mg qd. **Usual:** 30-60mg qd. **Max:** 90mg/day.	Not FDA approved
	Afeditab CR, Nifediac CC	**Tab, ER:** 30mg, (Afeditab CR) 60mg	**Initial:** 30mg qd. **Usual:** 30-60mg qd. **Max:** 90mg/day.	Not FDA approved
	Procardia	**Cap:** 10mg, 20mg	Not FDA approved	**Initial:** 10mg tid. **Usual:** 10-20mg tid. **Max:** 180mg/day.
	Procardia XL	**Tab, ER:** 30mg, 60mg, 90mg	**Initial:** 30-60mg qd. **Max:** 120mg/day.	**Initial:** 30-60mg qd. **Max:** 90-120mg/day.
Nisoldipine	Generic	**Tab, ER:** 20mg, 30mg, 40mg	**Initial:** 20mg qd. **Usual:** 20-40mg qd. **Max:** 60mg/day.	Not FDA approved
	Sular	**Tab, ER:** 8.5mg, 17mg, 25.5mg, 34mg	**Initial:** 17mg qd. **Usual:** 17-34mg qd. **Max:** 34mg/day.	Not FDA approved
NON-DIHYDROPYRIDINES				
Diltiazem HCl**	Cardizem	**Tab:** 30mg, 60mg, 90mg, 120mg	Not FDA approved	**Initial:** 30mg qid. **Usual:** 180-360mg/day.
	Cardizem CD, Cartia XT, Dilt-CD	**Cap, ER:** 120mg, 180mg, 240mg, 300mg, (Cardizem CD) 360mg	**Initial:** 180-240mg qd. **Usual:** 240-360mg qd. **Max:** 480mg qd.	**Initial:** 120-180mg qd. **Max:** 480mg/day.
	Cardizem LA	**Tab, ER:** 120mg, 180mg, 240mg, 300mg, 360mg, 420mg	**Initial:** 180-240mg qd. **Max:** 540mg/day.	**Initial:** 180mg qd. **Max:** 360mg/day.
	Dilacor XR, Diltia XT	**Cap, ER:** 120mg, 180mg, 240mg	**Initial:** 180-240mg qd. **Usual:** 180-480mg qd. **Max:** 540mg/day.	**Initial:** 120mg qd. **Max:** 480mg/day.
	Diltzac, Tiazac, Taztia XT	**Cap, ER:** 120mg, 180mg, 240mg, 300mg, 360mg, (Tiazac) 420mg	**Initial:** 120-240mg qd. **Usual:** 120-540mg qd. **Max:** 540mg qd.	**Initial:** 120-180mg qd. **Max:** 540mg/day.

(Continued)

CALCIUM CHANNEL BLOCKERS

DRUG	BRAND	HOW SUPPLIED	HYPERTENSION DOSING*	ANGINA DOSING*
NON-DIHYDROPYRIDINES *(Continued)*				
Verapamil HCl**	Calan***	**Tab:** 40mg, 80mg, 120mg	**Initial:** 80mg tid. **Usual:** 360–480mg/day.	**Usual:** 80-120mg tid. **Max:** 480mg/day.
	Calan SR	**Cap, ER:** 120mg, 180mg, 240mg	**Initial:** 180mg qam. **Max:** 480mg/day.	Not FDA approved
	Covera HS	**Tab, ER:** 180mg, 240mg	**Initial:** 180mg qhs. **Max:** 480mg qhs.	**Initial:** 180mg qhs. **Max:** 480mg qhs.
	Isoptin SR	**Tab, ER:** 120mg, 180mg, 240mg	**Initial:** 180mg qam. **Max:** 480mg/day.	Not FDA approved
	Verelan	**Cap, ER:** 120mg, 180mg, 240mg, 360mg	**Usual:** 240mg qam. **Max:** 480mg qam.	Not FDA approved
	Verelan PM	**Cap, ER:** 100mg, 200mg, 300mg	**Usual:** 200mg qhs. **Max:** 400mg qhs.	Not FDA approved

* NOTE: Adult dosing shown is for monotherapy. Dosage needs to be adjusted by titration to individual patient needs. Dosages may need to be reduced in the elderly, or in patients with renal/hepatic impairment. When used in combination with other antihypertensives, the dosage of the calcium channel blocker or the concomitant antihypertensive agent may need to be adjusted due to possible additive effects. Monitor the patient closely. For more information, refer to the monograph listings or the drug's FDA-approved labeling.
** For additional dosage forms, refer to the monograph listings or the drug's FDA-approved labeling.
*** For additional indications, refer to the monograph listings or the drug's FDA-approved labeling.

CHOLESTEROL-LOWERING AGENTS

BRAND (GENERIC)	HOW SUPPLIED (MG)*	USUAL DOSAGE RANGE**	T-CHOL (% DECREASE)	LDL (% DECREASE)	HDL (% INCREASE)	TG (% DECREASE)
HMG-CoA REDUCTASE INHIBITORS (STATINS)						
Altoprev (Lovastatin)	**Tab, ER:** 20, 40, 60	20-60mg/day	20.9 to 29.2	29.6 to 40.8	11.6 to 13.1	9.9 to 25.1
Crestor (Rosuvastatin)	**Tab:** 5, 10, 20, 40	5-40mg/day	33 to 46	45 to 63	8 to 14	10 to 35
Lescol (Fluvastatin)	**Cap:** 20, 40	20-80mg/day	17 to 27	22 to 36	3 to 6	12 to 18
Lescol XL (Fluvastatin)	**Tab, ER:** 80	80mg/day	25	35	7	19
Lipitor (Atorvastatin)	**Tab:** 10, 20, 40, 80	10-80mg/day	29 to 45	39 to 60	5 to 9	19 to 37
Livalo (Pitavastatin)	**Tab:** 1, 2, 4	1-4mg/day	23 to 31	32 to 43	5 to 8	15 to 19
Mevacor (Lovastatin)	**Tab:** 10 (generic), 20, 40	10-80mg/day given qd or bid	17 to 29	24 to 40	6.6 to 9.5	10 to 19
Pravachol (Pravastatin)	**Tab:** 10, 20, 40, 80	40-80mg/day qd; renal/hepatic dysfunction: Initial: 10mg qd	16 to 27	22 to 37	2 to 12	11 to 24
Zocor (Simvastatin)	**Tab:** 5, 10, 20, 40, 80	5-80mg/day	19 to 36	26 to 47	8 to 16	12 to 33
FIBRATES* **						
Antara (Fenofibrate)	**Cap:** 43, 130	43-130mg/day	16.8 to 22.4	20.1 to 31.4	9.8 to 14.6	23.5 to 35.9
Fenoglide (Fenofibrate)	**Tab:** 40, 120	40-120mg/day	16.8 to 22.4	20.1 to 31.4	9.8 to 14.6	23.5 to 35.9
Fibricor (Fenofibric acid)	**Tab:** 35, 105	35-105mg/day	16.8 to 22.4	20.1 to 31.4	9.8 to 14.6	23.5 to 35.9
Lipofen (Fenofibrate)	**Cap:** 50, 150	50-150mg/day	16.8 to 22.4	20.1 to 31.4	9.8 to 14.6	23.5 to 35.9
Lofibra (Fenofibrate)	**Tab:** 54, 160; **Cap:** 67, 134, 200	54-160mg/day, 67-200mg/day	16.8 to 22.4	20.1 to 31.4	9.8 to 14.6	23.5 to 35.9
Lopid (Gemfibrozil)	**Tab:** 600	1200mg/day in divided doses	n/a	4.1	12.6	Not specified-but decrease
Tricor (Fenofibrate)	**Tab:** 48, 145	48-145mg/day	16.8 to 22.4	20.1 to 31.4	9.8 to 14.6	23.5 to 35.9
Triglide (Fenofibrate)	**Tab:** 50, 160	50-160mg/day	16.8 to 22.4	20.1 to 31.4	9.8 to 14.6	23.5 to 35.9
Trilipix (Fenofibric acid)	**Cap, Delayed-Release:** 45, 135	45-135mg/day	12.4	5.1	16.3	31
BILE-ACID SEQUESTRANTS						
Colestid (Colestipol)	**Granules:** 5g/pkt or scoop; **Tab:** 1000	**Granules:** 1-6 pkts or scoopfuls/day given qd or in divided doses; **Tab:** 2-16g/day given qd or in divided doses	Not specified-but decrease	Not specified-but decrease	Not specified	Not specified
Prevalite, Questran, Questran Light (Cholestyramine)	**Powder:** 4g/pkt or scoop	2-4 pkts or scoopfuls daily (8-16g) divided into two doses	7.2	10.4	n/a	n/a
Welchol (Colesevelam HCl)	**Tab:** 625 **Sus:** 3.75g, 1.875g [pkt]	3750mg/day given qd or bid	7	15	3	+10

(Continued)

BRAND (GENERIC)	HOW SUPPLIED (MG)*	USUAL DOSAGE RANGE**	T-CHOL (% DECREASE)	LDL (% DECREASE)	HDL (% INCREASE)	TG (% DECREASE)
CHOLESTEROL ABSORPTION INHIBITOR						
Zetia (Ezetimibe)	**Tab:** 10	10mg qd	13	18	1	8
NICOTINIC ACID DERIVATIVE						
Niaspan (Niacin, ER)	**Tab, ER:** 500, 750, 1000	1-2g qhs	3 to 10	5 to 14	18 to 22	13 to 28
LIPID-REGULATING AGENT						
Lovaza (Omega-3-Acid Ethyl Esters)	**Cap:** 1000	4g/day given qd or bid	9.7	+44.5	9.1	44.9
COMBINATIONS						
Advicor (Niacin ER/ Lovastatin)	**Tab:** 500/20, 750/20, 1000/20, 1000/40	500/20mg to 2000/40mg	Not specified	30 to 42	20 to 30	32 to 44
Caduet (Amlodipine/ Atorvastatin)	**Tab:** 2.5/10, 2.5/20, 2.5/40, 5/10, 5/20, 5/40, 5/80, 10/10, 10/ 20, 10/40, 10/80	5/10mg to 10/80mg	n/a	36.6 to 49.1	n/a	n/a
Simcor (Niacin ER/ Simvastatin)	**Tab:** 500/20, 500/40, 750/20, 1000/20, 1000/40	500/20mg to 2000/40mg	8.8 to 11.1	11.9 to 14.3	20.7 to 29	26.5 to 38.0
Vytorin (Ezetimibe/ Simvastatin)	**Tab:** 10/10, 10/20, 10/40, 10/80	10/10 to 10/80mg/day	31 to 43	45 to 60	6 to 10	23 to 31

* Unless otherwise indicated.

** NOTE: Dosage shown is for adults and may need to be adjusted to individual patient needs. For pediatric dosing and additional information, please refer to the individual monograph listing or the drug's FDA-approved labeling. According to NCEP-ATP III guidelines, lipid-altering agents should be used in addition to a diet restricted in saturated fat and cholesterol only when the response to diet and other nonpharmacological measures has been inadequate.

*** Refer to the drug's FDA-approved labeling for the lipid parameter changes observed for the treatment of hypertriglyceridemia; LDL increases reported.

Abbreviation: ER: Extended-Release.

Major Contraindications (refer to the FDA-approved labeling for a complete list of warnings and precautions)

Statins: Active liver disease or unexplained persistent elevations of hepatic transaminase levels; pregnancy; nursing mothers.

Fibrates: Hepatic or severe renal dysfunction, including primary biliary cirrhosis; pre-existing gallbladder disease; combination therapy with repaglinide; nursing mothers.

Bile-acid sequestrants: History of bowel obstruction; serum triglycerides >500 mg/dL; history of hypertriglyceridemia-induced pancreatitis.

Cholesterol absorption inhibitors: Statin contraindications apply when used with a statin; active liver disease or unexplained persistent elevations in hepatic transaminase levels; pregnancy; nursing mothers.

Nicotinic acid derivatives: Active liver disease or unexplained persistent elevations in hepatic transaminases; active peptic ulcer disease; arterial bleeding.

Combinations: Refer to individual therapeutic class contraindications.

COAGULATION MODIFIERS

DRUG (BRAND)	HOW SUPPLIED	INDICATIONS	DOSAGE	HEPATIC/RENAL IMPAIRMENT
THROMBOLYTICS				
Alteplase (Activase)	Inj: 50mg, 100mg	To improve ventricular function, reduce incidence of congestive heart failure, and reduce mortality with acute myocardial infarction (AMI). Management of acute ischemic stroke and acute massive pulmonary embolism (PE).	AMI: Accelerated Infusion: >67kg: 15mg IV bolus, then 50mg over next 30 min, and then 35mg over next 60 min. ≤67kg: 15mg IV bolus, then 0.75mg/kg (max 50mg) over next 30 min, then 0.5mg/kg (max 35mg) over next 60 min. Max: 100mg total dose. 3-Hr Infusion: ≥65kg: 60mg in 1st hr (give 6-10mg as IV bolus), then 20mg over 2nd hr, then 20mg over 3rd hr. <65kg: 1.25mg/kg over 3 hrs as described above. Stroke: 0.9mg/kg IV over 1 hr (max 90mg total dose). Administer 10% of total dose as IV bolus over 1 min. PE: 100mg IV over 2 hrs. Start heparin at end or immediately after infusion when PTT or thrombin time ≤2× normal.	
Reteplase (Retavase)	Inj: 10.4 U	To improve ventricular function following acute myocardial infarction (AMI), reduce the incidence of congestive heart failure (CHF) and reduce the mortality associated with AMI.	10 U IV over 2 min. Repeat in 30 min.	
Tenecteplase (TNKase)	Inj: 50mg	To reduce mortality with AMI.	Administer as single IV bolus over 5 seconds. <60kg: 30mg. 60 to <70kg: 35mg. 70 to <80kg: 40mg. 80 to <90kg: 45mg. ≥90kg: 50mg. Max: 50mg/dose.	
PLATELET AGGREGATION INHIBITORS				
Abciximab (Reopro)	Inj: 2mg/mL	Adjunct to percutaneous coronary intervention (PCI) for prevention of cardiac ischemic complications in patients undergoing PCI or with unstable angina unresponsive to conventional therapy when PCI is planned within 24 hrs. Intended for use with aspirin and heparin.	PCI: 0.25mcg/kg IV bolus given 10-60 min before start PCI, followed by 0.125mcg/kg/min IV infusion (Max: 10mcg/min) for 12 hrs. Unstable Angina: 0.25mcg/kg IV bolus followed by 10mcg/min infusion for 18-24 hrs, concluding 1 hr after PCI.	
Anagrelide (Agrylin)	Cap: 0.5mg, (generic) 1mg	Treatment of thrombocythemia secondary to myeloproliferative disorders, to reduce the elevated platelet count and the risk of thrombosis and to ameliorate associated symptoms including thrombo-hemorrhagic events.	Initial: 0.5mg qid or 1mg bid for at least 1 week. Titrate: Increase by no more than 0.5mg/day per week. Max: 10mg/day or 2.5mg/dose. Adjust to lowest effective dose to reduce and maintain platelets <600,000/mcL. Monitor platelets every 2 days during first week, then weekly thereafter until reach maintenance dose. **Pediatrics:** Initial: 0.5mg qd. Titrate: Increase by no more than 0.5mg/day per week. Max:10mg/day or 2.5mg/dose. Adjust to lowest effective dose to reduce and maintain platelets <600,000/mcL. Monitor platelets every 2 days during first week, then weekly thereafter until reach maintenance dose.	Moderate Hepatic Impairment: Initial: 0.5mg qd for at least 1 week. Titrate: Increase by no more than 0.5mg/day per week. Max: 10mg/day or 2.5mg/dose.

(Continued)

DRUG (BRAND)	HOW SUPPLIED	INDICATIONS	DOSAGE	HEPATIC/RENAL IMPAIRMENT
PLATELET AGGREGATION INHIBITORS *(Continued)*				
Aspirin (Halfprin)	Tab, Delayed-Release: 81mg, 162mg	To reduce the risk of vascular mortality and fatal and nonfatal cardiovascular and cerebrovascular events in patients with a suspected acute MI.	162mg as soon as MI suspected. May need to continue as prophylaxis for recurrent MI. Chew and swallow the 1st dose.	
Cilostazol (Pletal)	Tab: 50mg, 100mg	Reduction of symptoms with intermittent claudication.	100mg bid, ½ hr before or 2 hrs after breakfast and dinner. Concomitant CYP3A4 and CYP2C19 inhibitors: Consider 50mg bid.	
Clopidogrel (Plavix)	Tab: 75mg, 300mg	For reduction of thrombotic events in those with recent stroke or MI, established peripheral arterial disease (PAD); or with non-ST-segment elevation acute coronary syndrome (unstable angina (UA)/non-ST-elevation MI (STEMI)); and patients with ST-segment elevation myocardial infarction (STEMI).	MI/Stroke/PAD: 75mg qd. Acute Coronary Syndrome: UA/NSTEMI: Initial: LD: 300mg. Maint: 75mg qd with 75-325mg ASA qd. STEMI: 75mg, with 75-325mg ASA, qd with or without LD and thrombolytics.	
Dipyridamole (Persantine)	Tab: 25mg, 50mg, 75mg	Adjunct to coumarin anticoagulants for prevention of postoperative thromboembolic complications of cardiac valve replacement.	75-100mg qid.	
Dipyridamole and aspirin (Aggrenox)	Cap: (Dipyridamole Extended-Release/ASA) 200mg-25mg	Reduce risk of stroke in patients with transient brain ischemia or complete ischemic stroke due to thrombosis.	1 cap bid (am and pm).	
Eptifibatide (Integrilin)	Inj: 0.75mg/mL, 2mg/mL	Treatment of acute coronary syndrome (ACS) in patients being medically managed or undergoing percutaneous coronary intervention (PCI) or treatment of patients undergoing PCI, including intracoronary stenting.	ACS: 180mcg/kg IV bolus, then 2mcg/kg/min IV infusion until discharge, initiation of CABG, or up to 72 hrs. If undergoing PCI, continue until discharge or up to 18-24 hrs post-PCI allowing up to 96 hrs of therapy. PCI: 180mcg/kg IV bolus immediately before PCI, then 2mcg/kg/min IV infusion. Give 2nd bolus of 180mcg/kg 10 min after 1st bolus. Continue until discharge or up to 18-24 hrs post-PCI. Minimum of 12 hrs of infusion recommended. See PI for concomitant ASA and heparin doses.	ACS: CrCl <50mL/min: 180mcg/kg IV bolus, then 1mcg/kg/min IV infusion. PCI: CrCl <50mL/min: 180mcg/kg IV bolus immediately before PCI, then 1mcg/kg/min IV infusion. Give 2nd bolus of 180mcg/kg 10 min after 1st bolus.
Prasugrel (Effient)	Tab: 5mg, 10mg	Reduction of thrombotic CV events (eg, stent thrombosis) in patients with ACS (eg, unstable angina, non ST-elevation MI, ST-elevation MI) who are to be managed with percutaneous coronary intervention (PCI).	LD: 60mg PO single dose. Maint: 10mg qd. <60kg: Reduce to 5mg qd. Should be taken with ASA 75mg-325mg qd.	

DRUG (BRAND)	HOW SUPPLIED	INDICATIONS	DOSAGE	HEPATIC/RENAL IMPAIRMENT
PLATELET AGGREGATION INHIBITORS *(Continued)*				
Ticlopidine	Tab: 250mg	To reduce risk of thrombotic stroke in stroke patients or those with stroke precursors who are ASA intolerant, allergic, or failed ASA therapy. Adjunct to ASA to reduce incidence of subacute stent thrombosis in patients undergoing successful coronary artery stent implantation.	Take with food. Stroke: 250mg bid. Coronary Artery Stenting: 250mg bid with ASA for up to 30 days after stent implant.	May need dose adjustment with hepatic/renal impairment.
Tirofiban (Aggrastat)	Inj: 0.05mg/mL	In combination with heparin, for treatment of acute coronary syndrome, in patients being medically managed or undergoing PTCA or atherectomy.	Initial: 0.4mcg/kg/min IV for 30 min. Maint: 0.1mcg/kg/min IV. Continue through angiography and for 12-24 hrs after angioplasty or atherectomy.	CrCl <30mL/min: Administer half of the usual rate of infusion.
COAGULATION FACTOR INHIBITORS				
Dalteparin (Fragmin)	Inj: (Syringe) 2,500 IU/0.2mL, 5,000 IU/ 0.2mL, 7,500 IU/0.3mL, 10,000 IU/0.4mL, 10,000 IU/1mL, 12,500 IU/0.5mL, 15,000 IU/ 0.6mL, 18,000 IU/ 0.72mL; (MDV) 25,000 IU/mL [3.8mL], 10,000 IU/mL [9.5mL]	Prophylaxis of ischemic complications in unstable angina and non-Q-wave MI with concurrent ASA therapy. Prophylaxis of DVT in hip replacement surgery, abdominal surgery in patients who are at high risk for thromboembolic complications, and for those at risk for thromboembolic complications due to severely restricted mobility during acute illness. Extended treatment of symptomatic VTE (proximal DVT and/or PE) to reduce the recurrence of VTE in patients with cancer.	Administer SQ. Unstable Angina/Non-Q-Wave MI: 120 IU/kg up to 10,000 IU q12h with ASA (75-165mg/day) for 5-8 days. Hip Surgery: Pre-Op Start: Initial (if start 2 hrs pre-op): 2500 IU within 2 hrs pre-op, then 2500 IU 4-8 hrs post-op. Initial (if start 10-14 hrs pre-op): 5000 IU 10-14 hrs pre-op, then 5000 IU 4-8 hrs post-op. Maint (for either initial dose): 5000 IU SQ qd for 5-10 days post-op (up to 14 days). Post-Op Start: Initial: 2500 IU 4-8 hrs after last dose for 2 hrs pre-op start regimen). Allow 24 hrs between doses for 10-14 hrs pre-op start regimen. Post-Op Start: 2500 IU 4-8 hrs post-op. Maint: 5000 IU qd for 5-10 days post-op (up to 14 days). Abdominal Surgery: 2500 IU 1-2 hrs pre-op. Maint: 2500 IU qd for 5-10 days post-op. Abdominal Surgery with High Risk: 5000 IU evening before surgery. Maint: 5000 IU qd for 5-10 days post-op. Abdominal Surgery with Malignancy: Initial: 2500 IU 1-2 hrs pre-op, then 2500 IU 12 hrs later. Maint: 5000 IU qd for 5-10 days post-op. Severely Restricted Mobility During Acute Illness: 5000 IU qd for 12-14 days. Symptomatic VTE in Cancer Patients: 200 IU/kg qd for first 30 days, then 150 IU/kg qd for months 2-6. Max: 18,000 IU/day. Platelet Count 50,000-100,000/mm³: Reduce dose by 2500 IU until platelet count ≥100,000/mm³. Platelet Count <50,000/mm³: D/C therapy until platelet count >50,000/mm³.	Symptomatic VTE in Cancer Patients: Renal Impairment (CrCl <30mL/min): Monitor anti-Xa levels to determine appropriate dose.

(Continued)

DRUG (BRAND)	HOW SUPPLIED	INDICATIONS	DOSAGE	HEPATIC/RENAL IMPAIRMENT
COAGULATION FACTOR INHIBITORS *(Continued)*				
Enoxaparin (Lovenox)	Inj: (MDV) 300mg/3mL; (Syringe) 30mg/0.3mL, 40mg/0.4mL, 60mg/0.6mL, 80mg/0.8mL, 100mg/mL, 120mg/0.8mL, 150mg/mL	Prophylaxis of DVT in hip or knee replacement surgery, abdominal surgery, or with severely restricted mobility during acute illness. With concomitant warfarin, inpatient treatment of acute DVT with or without PE and outpatient treatment of DVT without PE. Prophylaxis of ischemic complications in unstable angina and non-Q-wave MI with concurrent ASA therapy. Treatment of acute ST-segment elevation MI (STEMI) in patients receiving thrombolysis and being managed medically or with percutaneous coronary intervention (PCI) with concurrent ASA therapy.	Hip/Knee Surgery: 30mg SQ q12h, starting 12-24 hrs post-op, for 7-10 days (up to 14 days) or 40mg SQ qd, starting 12 hrs pre-op for hip surgery for 3 weeks. Abdominal Surgery: 40mg SQ qd, starting 2 hrs pre-op, for 7-10 days (up to12 days). DVT with or without PE treatment: (inpatient/outpatient) 1mg/kg SQ q12h or (inpatient) 1.5mg/kg SQ qd with warfarin (start within 72 hrs) for 7 days (up to 17 days). Acute Illness: 40mg SQ qd for 6-11 days (up to 14 days). Unstable Angina/Non-Q-Wave MI: 1mg/kg SQ q12h with 100-325mg/day of ASA for 2-8 days (up to 12.5 days). Acute STEMI (<75 yrs): 30mg single IV bolus plus a 1mg/kg SQ dose followed by 1mg/kg SQ q12h with ASA. Max: 100mg for 1st 2 doses only. Acute STEMI (≥75 yrs): 0.75mg/kg SQ q12h (no initial bolus) with ASA. Max: 75mg for 1st 2 doses only. When given with thrombolytic, give enoxaparin dose between 15 min before and 30 min after start of fibrinolytic therapy. With PCI, if last enoxaparin SQ dose was given >8 hrs before balloon inflation, an IV bolus of 0.3mg/kg of enoxaparin should be given.	CrCl <30mL/min: Surgery/Acute Illness: 30mg SQ qd. DVT with or without PE treatment (inpatient/outpatient)/Unstable Angina/Non-Q-Wave MI: 1mg/kg SQ qd. Acute STEMI <75 yrs: 30mg single IV bolus plus a 1mg/kg SQ dose followed by 1mg/kg SQ qd. ≥75 yrs: 1mg/kg SQ qd (no initial bolus)
Fondaparinux (Arixtra)	Inj: (Syringe) 2.5mg/0.5mL, 5mg/0.4mL, 7.5mg/0.6mL, 10mg/0.8mL	Prophylaxis of DVT in patients undergoing hip fracture surgery, including extended prophylaxis; hip replacement surgery; knee replacement surgery; abdominal surgery who are at risk of thromboembolic complications. With concomitant warfarin, treatment of acute PE when initial therapy is administered in hospital and acute DVT.	DVT Prophylaxis: 2.5mg SQ qd, starting 6-8 hrs post-op for 5-9 days (up to 11 days). Hip Fracture Surgery: Extended prophylaxis up to 24 additional days is recommended. DVT/PE Treatment: <50kg: 5mg SQ qd. 50-100kg: 7.5mg SQ qd. >100kg: 10mg SQ qd. Add concomitant warfarin ASAP (usually within 72 hrs) and continue for 5-9 days (up to 26 days) until INR=2-3.	CrCl <30mL/min: Avoid use.
Heparin	Inj: 1,000 U/mL, 5000 U/mL, 10,000 U/mL, 20,000 U/mL	Prophylaxis and treatment of venous thrombosis and its extension, PE in atrial fibrillation. Prevention of postoperative DVT and PE. Diagnosis and treatment of acute and chronic consumptive coagulopathies, for prevention of clotting in arterial and cardiac surgery. Anticoagulant in blood transfusions, extracorporeal circulation, and dialysis procedures and in blood samples.	Based on 68kg: Initial: 5000 U IV, then 10,000-20,000 U SQ. Maint: 8000-10,000 U SQ q8h or 15,000-20,000 U SQ q12h. Intermittent IV Injection: Initial: 10,000 U. Maint: 5000-10,000 U q4-6h. Continuous IV Infusion: Initial: 5000U. Maint: 20,000-40,000 U/24 hrs. Adjust to coagulation test results. See PI for details in specific disease states. Pediatrics: Initial: 50 U/kg IV infusion. Maint: 100 U/kg IV infusion q4h or 20,000 U/m²/24 hrs continuously.	

DRUG (BRAND)	HOW SUPPLIED	INDICATIONS	DOSAGE	HEPATIC/RENAL IMPAIRMENT
COAGULATION FACTOR INHIBITORS *(Continued)*				
Protein C Concentrate (Human) (Ceprotin)	Inj: 500 IU, 1,000 IU	Prevention and treatment of venous thrombosis and purpura fulminans in patients with severe congenital Protein C deficiency. Also indicated as replacement therapy for pediatric and adult patients.	Individualize dose. Acute Episodes/Short-Term Prophylaxis: Initial: 100-120 IU/kg. Subsequent 3 Doses: 60-80 IU/kg q6h. Maint: 45-60 IU/kg q6h or q12h. Adjust dose to maintain target peak protein C activity of 100%. After resolution of acute episode, continue on same dose to maintain trough protein C activity level above 25% for duration of treatment. Long-Term Prophylaxis: Maint: 45-60 IU q12h. Higher peak protein C activity levels may be warranted in situations of increased risk of thrombosis. Maintenance of trough protein C activity levels above 25% is recommended.	
Tinzaparin (Innohep)	Inj: 20,000 anti-Xa IU/mL	Treatment of acute symptomatic DVT with or without PE with concomitant warfarin.	175 anti-Xa IU/kg SQ qd for at least 6 days and until anticoagulated with warfarin (INR is at least 2.0 for 2 consecutive days). Begin warfarin within 1-3 days of therapy.	
Warfarin (Coumadin, Jantoven)	Inj: (Coumadin) 5mg; Tab: (Coumadin, Jantoven) 1mg*, 2mg*, 2.5mg*, 3mg*, 4mg*, 5mg*, 6mg*, 7.5mg*, 10mg*. *scored	Prophylaxis and treatment of venous thrombosis and its extension PE, and thromboembolic complications associated with atrial fibrillation and/or cardiac valve replacement. To reduce risk of death, recurrent MI, and thromboembolic events after MI.	Adjust dose based on PT/INR. Give IV as alternate to PO. Initial: 2-5mg qd. Usual: 2-10mg qd. Venous Thromboembolism (including DVT and PE): Target INR: 2.5 (INR range 2-3). Atrial Fibrillation: INR 2-3. Post-MI: INR 2.5-3.5. See PI. Mechanical/Bioprosthetic Heart Valve: See PI for specific target INRs for each valve type. Valvular Disease Associated with Atrial Fibrillation/Mitral Stenosis/Recurrent Systemic Embolism of Unknown Etiology: INR 2-3.	
THROMBIN INHIBITORS				
Antithrombin (Recombinant) (ATryn)	Inj: 1750 IU	Prevention of peri-operative and peri-partum thromboembolic events in hereditary antithrombin deficient patients.	Individualize dose. Goal of treatment is to restore and maintain functional AT activity levels between 80%-120% of normal (0.8-1.2 IU/mL). Administer as IV infusion over 15 min, followed by continuous infusion of maint dose. Surgical Patients: LD: (100-baseline AT activity level) × body weight (BW) (kg)/2.3. Maint (IU/hr): (100-baseline AT activity level) × BW (kg)/10.2. Pregnant Women: LD: (100-baseline AT activity level) × BW (kg)/1.3. Maint (IU/hr): (100-baseline AT activity level) × BW (kg)/5.4. Refer to PI for monitoring and adjustments.	
Antithrombin III (Human) (Thrombate III)	Inj: 500 IU	Treatment of patients with hereditary antithrombin III deficiency in connection with surgical or obstetrical procedures or when they suffer from thromboembolism.	Individualize LD, maintenance doses, and dosing intervals based on the individual clinical conditions, response to therapy, and actual plasma AT-III levels achieved. Dose: units required (IU)=[(desired - baseline AT-III level) x weight (kg)]/1.4. Refer to PI for further dosing information.	

(Continued)

DRUG (BRAND)	HOW SUPPLIED	INDICATIONS	DOSAGE	HEPATIC/RENAL IMPAIRMENT
THROMBIN INHIBITORS *(Continued)*				
Argatroban	Inj: 100mg/mL	Prophylaxis or treatment of thrombosis in heparin-induced thrombocytopenia (HIT). As an anticoagulant in patients with or at risk for HIT undergoing percutaneous coronary intervention (PCI).	Thrombosis: D/C heparin and obtain baseline aPTT. Initial: 2mcg/kg/min IV. Check aPTT after 2 hrs. Titrate: Increase dose until aPTT is 1.5-3× the initial baseline. Max: 10mcg/kg/min. PCI: Initial: 350mcg/kg bolus with 25mcg/kg/min IV. Check activated clotting time (ACT) 5-10 min after bolus. Proceed with PCI if ACT >300 seconds. See PI for detailed information for dose adjustment.	Thrombosis: Moderate Hepatic Impairment: Initial: 0.5mcg/kg/min
Bivalirudin (Angiomax)	Inj: 250mg	Adjunct to aspirin for anticoagulation in patients with unstable angina undergoing percutaneous transluminal coronary angioplasty (PTCA) or percutaneous coronary intervention (PCI). Patients with, or at risk of, HIT/HITTS undergoing PCI.	Initial: 0.75mg/kg IV bolus, then 1.75mg/kg/hr for duration of PCI procedure. Additional bolus of 0.3mg/kg can be given if needed based on ACT (patients who do not have HIT/HITTS). Continuation of infusion for up to 4 hrs post-procedure is optional. After 4 hrs, if needed, an additional 0.2mg/kg/hr IV for up to 20 hrs may be initiated.	Renal Impairment: CrCl <30mL/min: 1mg/kg/hr infusion. Hemodialysis: 0.25mg/kg/hr infusion. Reduction in bolus dose not necessary; monitor anticoagulation.
Dabigatran (Pradaxa)	Cap: 75mg, 150mg	To reduce the risk of stroke and systemic embolism in patients with non-valvular atrial fibrillation.	CrCl >30mL/min: 150mg bid. Refer to PI for surgery and interventions and for conversion from or to warfarin and parenteral anticoagulants.	CrCl 15-30mL/min: 75mg bid.
Lepirudin (Refludan)	Inj: 50mg	Anticoagulant for heparin-induced thrombocytopenia (HIT) and associated thromboembolic disease.	LD: 0.4mg/kg (max 44mg) IV over 15-20 seconds. Initial: 0.15mg/kg/hr (max 16.5mg/hr) continuous infusion for 2-10 days. Adjust dose based on aPTT. Concomitant Thrombolytic Therapy: LD: 0.2mg/kg. Initial: 0.1mg/kg/hr. See PI for monitoring and adjusting therapy details.	Renal Impairment: LD: 0.2mg/kg. Initial: CrCl 45-60 mL/min: 0.075mg/kg/hr. CrCl 30-44mL/min: 0.045mcg/kg/hr. CrCl 15-29 mL/min: 0.0225mg/kg/hr. CrCl <15mL/min/Hemodialysis: Avoid or stop infusion.
MISCELLANEOUS				
Aminocaproic Acid (Amicar)	Inj: (generic) 250mg/mL; Syrup: 1.25g/5mL; Tab: 500mg*, 1,000mg* *scored	To enhance hemostasis when fibrinolysis contributes to bleeding.	IV: 16-20mL (4-5g) in 250mL diluent during 1st hr, then 4mL/hr (1g) in 50mL of diluent. PO: 5g during 1st hr, then 5mL (syr) or 1g (tabs) per hr. Continue IV/PO therapy for 8 hrs or until bleeding is controlled.	
Fibrinogen and Thrombin (Human) (TachoSil)	Patch: (Human fibrinogen-Human thrombin) 5.5mg-2.0 U/cm²	Adjunct to hemostasis for use in cardiovascular surgery when control of bleeding by standard surgical techniques (such as suture, ligature or cautery) is ineffective or impractical.	Apply the yellow, active side of the patch to the bleeding area and hold in place with gentle pressure for ≥3 min. Number of patches applied should be determined by the size of the bleeding area. Max: 7 patches sized 9.5 × 4.8cm, 14 patches sized 4.8 × 4.8cm, or 42 patches sized 3.0 × 2.5cm.	

DRUG (BRAND)	HOW SUPPLIED	INDICATIONS	DOSAGE	HEPATIC/RENAL IMPAIRMENT
MISCELLANEOUS (Continued)				
Pentoxifylline (Trental)	Tab, Extended-Release: 400mg	Treatment of intermittent claudication due to chronic occlusive arterial disease of the limbs.	400mg tid with meals for at least 8 weeks. Reduce to 400mg bid if digestive and CNS side effects occur; d/c if side effects persist.	
Phytonadione (Mephyton)	Tab: 5mg* *scored; Inj: (generic) 1mg/0.5 mL	For coagulation disorders caused by vitamin K deficiency or interference with vitamin K activity, including anticoagulant-induced prothrombin deficiency caused by coumarin or indanedione derivatives; and hypoprothrombinemia secondary to antibacterials, salicylates, obstructive jaundice, or biliary fistulas.	(Tab): Anticoagulant-Induced Prothrombin Deficiency: Initial: 2.5-10mg up to 25mg (rarely 50mg). May repeat if PT is still elevated 12-48 hrs after initial dose. Hypoprothrombinemia Due to Other Causes: 2.5-25mg or more (rarely up to 50mg). Give bile salts when endogenous bile supply to GIT is deficient. **Adults** (Inj): Administer SQ/IM when possible. Anticoagulant-Induced PT Deficiency: Initial: 2.5-10mg up to 25mg (rarely 50mg). May repeat if PT is still elevated 6-8 hrs after initial dose. Hypoprothrombinemia Due to Other Causes: 2.5-25mg or more (rarely up to 50mg); route depends on severity of condition and response. **Pediatrics** (Inj): Prophylaxis of Hemorrhagic Disease in Newborn: 0.5-1mg IM within 1 hr of birth. Treatment of Hemorrhagic Disease in Newborn: 1mg SQ/IM (may need higher dose if mother has received oral anticoagulants).	
Thrombin (Recombinant) (Recothrom)	Powder: 5,000 IU, 20,000 IU	Aid to hemostasis whenever oozing blood and minor bleeding from capillaries and small venules is accessible and control of bleeding by standard surgical techniques is ineffective or impractical. May be used in conjunction with an absorbable gelatin sponge, USP.	Apply directly on the surface of bleeding tissue or in conjunction with absorbable gelatin sponge. Required amount depends upon the tissue area to be treated. Reconstitute with sterile isotonic saline at a recommended concentration of 1000 IU/mL.	
Topical Thrombin (Thrombin-JMI)	Powder: 5,000 IU, 20,000 IU; Kit: 5,000 IU [Epistaxis Kit], 20,000 IU [Spray; Syringe Spray]	An aid to hemostasis whenever oozing blood and minor bleeding from capillaries and small venules is accessible. In various types of surgery, may be used in conjuction with an absorbable gelatin sponge, USP for hemostasis.	Spray topically on surface of bleeding tissue. Reconstitute with sterile isotonic saline at a recommended concentration of 1,000-2,000 IU/mL. Profuse Bleeding: Use 1,000 IU/mL. General use (eg, plastic surgery, dental extractions, skin grafting): 100 IU/mL. Intermediate strengths may be prepared by diluting in appropriate isotonic saline volume if needed. Oozing surfaces: Use dry form. May be used with FlowSeal™ NT.	
Topical Thrombin (Thrombi-Gel)	Gelatin Sponge/Pad: ≥1,000 U (Thrombi-Gel 10, Thrombi-Gel 40), ≥2,000 U (Thrombi-Gel 100)	Trauma dressing for temporary control of moderate to severely bleeding wounds and for the control of surface bleeding from vascular access sites and percutaneous catheters and tubes.	Wet the Thrombi-Gel with sterile normal saline or sterile water for injection. See PI for further preparation instructions. Knead the wetted Thrombi-Gel. Place directly over source of bleeding and apply adjunct manual compression until hemostasis is achieved. May be used up to 3 hrs after preparation.	
Topical Thrombin (Thrombi-Pad)	Pad: ≥200 U	Trauma dressing for temporary control of moderate to severely bleeding wounds and for the control of surface bleeding from vascular access sites and percutaneous catheters and tubes.	May be used dry or wet. If wetting, apply up to 10mL of sterile normal saline (may use up to 1 hr after preparation) to the pad. Apply directly over source of bleeding and apply adjunct manual pressure. May be left in place for up to 24 hrs.	

DIURETICS

DRUG	BRAND	USUAL HYPERTENSION DOSAGE RANGE	HOW SUPPLIED
ALDOSTERONE-RECEPTOR BLOCKERS			
Eplerenone	Inspra	50mg qd or bid.	**Tab:** 25mg, 50mg
Spironolactone	Aldactone	50mg–100mg/day.	**Tab:** 25mg, 50mg, 100mg
LOOP DIURETICS			
Bumetanide**	—	***	**Tab:** 0.5mg, 1mg, 2mg
Furosemide**	Lasix	40mg bid.†	**Tab:** 20mg, 40mg, 80mg
Torsemide**	Demadex	5mg–10mg qd.	**Tab:** 5mg, 10mg, 20mg, 100mg
POTASSIUM-SPARING DIURETICS			
Amiloride	Midamor	5mg–10mg qd.	**Tab:** 5mg
Triamterene	Dyrenium	***	**Cap:** 50mg, 100mg
THIAZIDE DIURETICS			
Chlorothiazide**	Diuril	**Sus:** 0.5–1g/day.†	**Sus:** 250mg/5mL
	Various generics	**Tab:** 0.5g–1g/day.†	**Tab:** 250mg, 500mg
Chlorthalidone	Thalitone	15mg–50mg qd.	**Tab:** 15mg
	Various generics	25mg–100mg qd.	**Tab:** 25mg, 50mg
Hydrochlorothiazide	Microzide	12.5mg–50mg qd.	**Cap:** 12.5mg
	Various generics	12.5mg–50mg qd.†	**Cap:** 12.5mg; **Tab:** 12.5mg, 25mg, 50mg
Indapamide	Various generics	1.25mg–5mg qd.	**Tab:** 1.25mg, 2.5mg
Methyclothiazide	—	2.5–5mg qd.	**Tab:** 5mg
QUINAZOLINE DIURETIC			
Metolazone	Zaroxolyn	2.5mg–5mg qd.	**Tab:** 2.5mg, 5mg, 10mg
COMBINATION DIURETICS*			
Amiloride-Hydrochlorothiazide	Various generics	1-2 tabs qd (5/50mg–10/100mg/day).	**Tab:** 5/50mg
Spironolactone-Hydrochlorothiazide	Aldactazide	50/50mg–100/100mg/day.	**Tab:** 25/25mg, 50/50mg
Triamterene-Hydrochlorothiazide	Dyazide, Maxzide	37.5mg/25mg–75/50mg/day.	**Cap:** 37.5/25mg **Tab:** 37.5/25mg, 75/50mg

* Fixed combination drugs are indicated for the treatment of hypertension in patients who develop hypokalemia on hydrochlorothiazide alone.

** For additional dosage forms refer to monograph listings or drug's FDA-approved labeling.

*** Not indicated for hypertension. For other indications refer to monograph listings or drug's FDA-approved labeling.

† Pediatric dosing available.

PSORIASIS MANAGEMENT: SYSTEMIC THERAPIES

DRUG (BRAND)	HOW SUPPLIED	DOSAGE	SIDE EFFECTS
ANTIMETABOLITE			
Methotrexate	**Inj:** 25mg/mL; **Tab:** 2.5mg	**Initial:** 10-25mg weekly until response or use divided oral dose schedule, 2.5mg at 12-hr intervals for 3 doses. **Titrate:** Increase gradually until optimal response. **Maint:** Reduce to lowest effective dose. **Max:** 30mg/wk.	Ulcerative stomatitis, leukopenia, nausea, abdominal distress, malaise, fatigue, chills, fever, dizziness, decreased resistance to infection.
IMMUNOSUPPRESSIVES			
Alefacept (Amevive)	**Inj:** (IM) 15mg	15mg IM once wkly for 12 wks. May repeat cycle 12 wks after first cycle complete. Adjust dose, D/C, based on CD4+ T-lymphocyte counts.	Lymphopenia, injection-site reactions, influenza-like symptoms, pruritus, hypersensitivity reactions.
Cyclosporine (Gengraf, Neoral)	(Gengraf, Neoral) **Cap:** 25mg, 100mg; **Sol:** 100mg/mL [50mL]	**Initial:** 1.25mg/kg bid for 4 wks. **Titrate:** May increase by 0.5mg/kg/day every 2 wks. **Max:** 4mg/kg/day.	Infection, renal dysfunction, HTN, malignancy risk w/certain psoriasis therapies, hirsutism, muscle cramps, acne, tremor, headache, gingival hyperplasia, diarrhea, nausea, vomiting.
MONOCLONAL ANTIBODY			
Ustekinumab (Stelara)	**Inj:** 45mg/0.5mL, 90mg/1mL	≤100kg: **Initial:** 45mg SQ and 4 wks later, followed by 45mg q12 wks. >100kg: **Initial:** 90mg SQ and 4 wks later, followed by 90mg q12 wks.	Infection, malignancies, RPLS, nasopharyngitis, upper respiratory infection, headache, fatigue.
MONOCLONAL ANTIBODIES/TNF BLOCKERS			
Adalimumab (Humira)	**Inj:** 20mg/0.4mL, 40mg/0.8mL	**Initial:** 80mg. **Maint:** 40mg every other week starting 1 wk after initial dose.	URI, injection-site pain/reactions, headache, rash, sinusitis, nausea, UTI, flu syndrome, abdominal pain, hyperlipidemia, hypercholesterolemia, back pain, hematuria, HTN, immunogenicity.
Infliximab (Remicade)	**Inj:** 100mg	5mg/kg IV infusion; repeat at 2 and 6 weeks. **Maint:** 5mg/kg every 8 wks.	Infusion reactions, nausea, infections, URI, pruritus, headache, sore throat, potential risk of reactivating TB, hepatotoxicity.
PSORALENS			
Methoxsalen* (8-Mop, Oxsoralen-Ultra)	**Cap:** 10mg	**Initial:** <30kg: 10mg. 30-50kg: 20mg. 51-65kg: 30mg. 66-80kg: 40mg. 81-90kg: 50mg. 91-115kg: 60mg. >115kg: 70mg. Take 2 hrs before UVA exposure. **Titrate:** May increase by 10mg after 15th treatment under certain conditions. **Max:** Do not treat more often than qod. Take with food or milk.	Nausea, nervousness, insomnia, depression, pruritus, erythema.
RETINOID			
Acitretin (Soriatane)	**Cap:** 10mg, 17.5mg, 25mg	**Initial:** 25-50mg qd w/food. Individualize dose. **Maint:** 25-50mg qd. May treat relapses as outlined for initial therapy.	Ophthalmologic effects, cheilitis, rhinitis, dry mouth, epistaxis, alopecia, dry skin, rash, skin peeling, nail disorder, pruritus, paresthesia, paronychia, skin atrophy, sticky skin, xerophthalmia, arthralgia.

DRUG (BRAND)	HOW SUPPLIED	DOSAGE	SIDE EFFECTS
TNF-BLOCKING AGENT			
Etanercept (Enbrel)	**Inj:** 25mg [vial], 25mg/0.5mL [syringe] 50mg/mL [autoinjector, syringe]	**Initial:** 50mg SQ twice weekly for 3 months. May begin with 25-50mg/wk. **Maint:** 50mg/wk.	Injection-site reactions, infections, diarrhea.

* Oxsoralen-Ultra and 8-MOP are not interchangeable due to significantly greater bioavailability and earlier photosensitization onset time of Oxsoralen-Ultra.

Sources: FDA-approved product labeling.

PSORIASIS MANAGEMENT: TOPICAL THERAPIES

DRUG (BRAND)	HOW SUPPLIED	DOSAGE	SIDE EFFECTS
TOPICAL IMMUNOSUPPRESSANT			
Pimecrolimus (Elidel)	Cre: 1% [30g, 60g, 100g]	Apply bid.	Stinging, soreness, burning, headache, nasopharyngitis, pyrexia, influenza, bacterial and viral skin infections
TOPICAL STEROIDS			
Betamethasone (Luxiq)	Foam: 0.12% [50g, 100g]	Apply bid.	Burning, itching, stinging, pruritus, paresthesia, acne, alopecia, conjunctivitis
Clobetasol (Temovate, Temovate-E, Clobex, Olux, Olux-E)	(Temovate) Cre, Oint: 0.05% [15g, 30g, 45g, 60g]; Gel: 0.05% [15g, 30g, 60g]; Sol: 0.05% [50mL]; (Temovate-E) Cre: 0.05% [60g]; (Clobex) Lot: 0.05% [59mL, 118mL]; Shampoo: 0.05% [118mL]; Spray: 0.05% [2oz, 4.25oz]; (Olux) Foam: 0.05% [50g, 100g] (Olux-E) Foam: 0.05% [50g, 100g]	Apply bid.	Hypopigmentation, tachyphylaxis, striae, skin atrophy. Other common side effects: burning, stinging, pruritus, erythema, folliculitis, cracking/ fissures of the skin, numbness in fingers, tenderness
Fluocinolone	Cre: 0.01%, 0.025% [15g, 60g]; Oint: 0.025% [15g, 60g]; Sol: 0.01% [60mL]	Apply tid-qid.	Dryness, folliculitis, acne, skin atrophy, burning, itching, irritation
Fluocinonide (Vanos)	(Generic) Cre: 0.05% [15g, 30g, 60g,120g] Cre (Emulsified base): 0.05% [15g, 30g, 60g, 120g] Gel, Oint: 0.05% [15g, 30g, 60g] Sol: 0.05% [20mL, 60mL] (Vanos) Cre: 0.1% [30mg, 60mg, 120mg]	(Generic) Apply bid-qid. (Vanos) Apply qd-bid.	Burning, itching, irritation, dryness, folliculitis, acne, hypopigmentation, skin atrophy
Halcinonide (Halog)	Cre: 0.1% [1.5g, 30g, 60g, 216g]; Oint: 0.1% [15g, 30g, 60g]	Apply bid-tid.	Burning, itching, irritation, dryness, folliculitis, hypopigmentation, contact dermatitis, skin maceration
Hydrocortisone (Anusol-HC, Locoid, Locoid Lipocream, Pandel, Proctocort, Westcort)	(Anusol-HC) Cre: 2.5% [30g]; (Locoid 0.1%) Cre, Oint: [15g, 45g], Sol: [20mL, 60mL]; (Locoid Lipocream) Cre: 0.1% [15g, 45g, 60g]; (Pandel) Cre: 0.1% [15g, 45g, 80g]; (Proctocort) Cre: 1% [1oz]; (Westcort) Cre, Oint: 0.2% [15g, 45g, 60g]	(Anusol-HC) Apply bid-qid. (Locoid, Locoid Lipocream) Cre, Oint, Sol: Apply bid-tid. (Pandel) qd-bid. (Proctocort) Apply bid-qid. (Westcort) Apply bid-tid.	Burning, stinging, moderate paresthesia, itching, dryness, folliculitis, hypopigmentation, skin atrophy
Hydrocortisone/ Pramoxine (Epifoam, Novacort, Pramosone)	(Epifoam) Foam: (Hydrocortisone-Pramoxine) 1%-1% [10g]; (Novacort) Gel: 2%-1% [29g]; (Pramosone) Cre: 1%-1%, 2.5%-1% [30g, 60g]; Lot: 1%-1% [60mL, 120mL, 240mL], 2.5%-1% [60mL, 120mL]; Oint: 1%-1%, 2.5%-1% [30g]	Apply tid-qid.	Burning, itching, irritation, dryness, folliculitis, hypopigmentation, maceration, skin atrophy
Mometasone (Elocon)	Cre, Oint: 0.1% [15g, 45g]; Lot: 0.1% [30mL, 60mL]	Apply qd.	Burning, pruritus, skin atrophy, rosacea, acneiform reaction, tingling, stinging, furunculosis, folliculitis

(Continued)

DRUG (BRAND)	HOW SUPPLIED	DOSAGE	SIDE EFFECTS
TOPICAL STEROIDS *(Continued)*			
Prednicarbate (Dermatop)	Cre, Oint: 0.1% [15g, 60g]	Apply bid.	Burning, itching, irritation, dryness, folliculitis, hypertrichosis, acneiform eruptions, hypopigmentation
Triamcinolone (Kenalog)	(Generic) Cre, Oint: 0.025%, 0.1% [15g, 80g, 454g], 0.5% [15g]; (Generic) Lot: 0.025%, 0.1% [60mL]; 0.1%: [15g, 60g]; Spray: 0.147mg/g [63g]	(Kenalog) Cre, Lot, Oint: Apply 0.025% bid-qid. Apply 0.1% or 0.5% bid-tid. Spray: Apply tid-qid.	Burning, itching, irritation, dryness, folliculitis, hypopigmentation, allergic contact dermatitis
Tazarotene (Avage, Tazorac)	(Avage) Cre: 0.1% [30g] (Tazorac) Cre: 0.05%, 0.1% [30g, 60g]; Gel: 0.05%, 0.1% [30g, 100g]	Apply hs.	Pruritus, erythema, irritation, dry skin, rash, skin discoloration
VITAMIN D DERIVATIVES & COMBINATIONS			
Calcitriol (Vectical)	Oint: 3mcg/g [5g, 100g]	Apply to affected area(s) bid, am and pm.	Laboratory test abnormality, urine abnormality, psoriasis, hypercalciuria, pruritus
Calcipotriene (Dovonex, Dovonex Scalp, Sorilux)	(Dovonex) Cre, 0.005% [60g, 120g]; (Dovonex Scalp) Sol: 0.005% [60mL]; (Sorilux) Foam: 0.005% [60g]	Apply bid.	Skin irritation, pruritus, burning, hypercalcemia, erythema
Calcipotriene/ betamethasone (Taclonex, Taclonex Scalp)	Oint: (Calcipotriene-Betamethasone) 0.005%-0.064% [60g, 100g] Scalp Sus: [30g, 60g]	(Oint) Apply qd up to 4 wks. (Scalp Sus) Apply qd for 2 wks or until cleared (up to 8 wks).	Pruritus, headache
MISCELLANEOUS AGENTS			
Anthralin (Anthra-Derm, Zithranol-RR)	Cre: 1% [50g] (Zithranol-RR) Cre: 1.2% [45g]	Apply qd-bid. (Zithranol-RR) Apply qd.	Skin irritation, erythema, staining (skin and clothing), odor
Coal Tar (Zetar)	Sol 10%: 2% [3.8oz]	Apply hs.	Skin irritation, folliculitis, odor, staining of clothing
Urea (Carmol 40)	Cre: 40% [28.35g, 85g, 198.6g]; Gel: 40% [15mL]; Lot: 40% [236.6mL]	Apply bid.	Transient stinging, burning, itching, irritation

Sources:
FDA-approved drug labeling.
Luba KM, Stulberg DL. Chronic plaque psoriasis. *Am Fam Physician*. 2006 Feb 15;73(4):636-44. Review.

TOPICAL CORTICOSTEROIDS

STEROID	DOSAGE FORM(S)	STRENGTH (%)	POTENCY	FREQUENCY
Alclometasone Dipropionate (Aclovate)	Cre, Oint	0.05	Low-Med	bid/tid
Amcinonide	Cre, Lot	0.1		bid/tid
	Oint	0.1	High*	bid/tid
Augmented Betamethasone Dipropionate (Diprolene, Diprolene AF)	Lot, Oint	0.05	Very High	qd/bid
	Cre	0.05	High	qd/bid
Betamethasone Dipropionate	Cre, Lot, Oint	0.05	High	qd/bid
Betamethasone Valerate (Luxiq)	Cre, Lot	0.1	Medium*	qd/tid, bid (Lot)
	Foam (Luxiq)	0.12	Medium	bid
	Oint	0.1	Medium	qd/tid
Clobetasol Propionate (Clobevate, Clobex, Cormax, Embeline E, Olux, Olux E, Temovate, Temovate-E)	Cre, Foam (Olux)	0.05	Very High	bid
	Cream (Embeline E), Foam, Gel (Clobevate), Lotion (Clobex), Oint, Shampoo (Clobex), Sol	0.05	Very High	qd (shampoo)
Clocortolone Pivalate (Cloderm)	Cre	0.1	Med	tid
Desonide (Desonate, DesOwen, Verdeso)	Cre, Foam, Gel (Desonate), Lot, Oint	0.05	Low-Med	bid/tid
Desoximetasone (Topicort, Topicort LP)	Cre	0.05	Medium	bid
	Cre, Oint	0.25	High	bid
	Gel	0.05	High	bid
Diflorasone Diacetate (Apexicon)	Cre, Oint	0.05	High-Very High*	qd/tid
Fluocinolone Acetonide (Capex, Derma-Smoothe/FS)	Cre, Oint	0.025	Medium	tid/qid
	Cre, Sol	0.01	Medium	tid/qid
	Oil (Derma-Smoothe/FS)	0.01	Low-Med	qd hs
	Shampoo (Capex)	0.01	Low-Med	qd
Fluocinonide (Vanos)	Cre, Gel, Oint, Sol	0.05	High	bid/qid
	Cre (Vanos)	0.1	Very High	qd/bid
Flurandrenolide (Cordran, Cordran SP)	Cre, Oint	0.025	Medium	bid/tid
	Cre, Lot, Oint	0.05	Medium	bid/tid
	Tape	4mcg/cm²	Medium	qd/bid
Fluticasone Propionate (Cutivate)	Cre, Lot	0.05	Medium	qd/bid
	Oint	0.005	Medium	bid
Halcinonide (Halog)	Cre, Oint	0.1	High	bid/tid
Halobetasol Propionate (Ultravate, Ultravate PAC)	Cre, Oint	0.05	Very High	qd/bid
Hydrocortisone (Anusol HC, Hytone, Proctocort)	Cre, Lot	1	Low	tid/qid
	Cre, Lot, Oint	2.5	Low	bid/qid
Hydrocortisone Acetate (Alacort, U-cort)	Cre	1		bid/qid
Hydrocortisone Butyrate (Locoid, Locoid Lipo Cream)	Cre, Lot, Oint, Sol	0.1	Medium	bid/tid
Hydrocortisone Probutate (Pandel)	Cre	0.1	Medium	qd/bid
Hydrocortisone Valerate (Westcort)	Cre, Oint	0.2	Medium	bid/tid
Mometasone Furoate (Elocon)	Cre, Lot, Oint	0.1	Medium	qd
Prednicarbate (Dermatop)	Cre, Oint	0.1	Medium	bid
Triamcinolone Acetonide (Kenalog, Triderm)	Cre, Lot, Oint	0.025	Medium	bid/qid
	Cre, Lot, Oint	0.1	Medium	bid/tid
	Cre, Oint	0.5	High	bid/tid
	Spray	0.147	Medium	bid/qid

*Source: Fougera & Co. website: Available at: www.fougera.com/knowledge_center/steroidpotency.asp.

INSULIN FORMULATIONS

TYPE OF INSULIN	BRAND	ONSET*	PEAK* (hrs)	DURATION* (hrs)
Rapid-acting Insulin glulisine Insulin lispro Insulin aspart	Apidra Humalog Novolog	5 to 15 minutes	0.5 to 1.5	<5
Short-acting Regular Insulin	Humulin R† Novolin R	0.5 to 1 hr	2 to 3	5 to 8
Intermediate-acting NPH (Isophane)	Humulin N Novolin N	2 to 4 hrs	4 to 10	10 to 16
Long-acting Insulin glargine Insulin detemir	Lantus Levemir	Not applicable	Relatively flat	up to 24
Combinations Isophane insulin suspension (70%)/ regular insulin (30%)	Humulin 70/30 Novolin 70/30	0.5 to 1 hr	Dual	10 to 16
Insulin aspart protamine (70%)/ insulin aspart (30%)	Novolog Mix 70/30	5 to 15 minutes	Dual	10 to 16
Insulin lispro protamine (50%)/ insulin lispro (50%)	Humalog Mix 50/50		0.75 to 2	
Insulin lispro protamine (75%)/ insulin lispro (25%)	Humalog Mix 75/25	5 to 15 minutes	Dual	10 to 16

*Assumes 0.1-0.2 units/kg/injection. Onset and duration may vary by injection site.

Niswender K. Early and Aggressive Initiation of Insulin Therapy for Type 2 Diabetes: What Is the Evidence? Clinical Diabetes Spring 2009 27:60-68; doi:10.2337/diaclin.27.2.60.

†Also available as 500 U/mL for insulin-resistant patients (rapid onset; up to 24-hr duration).

ORAL ANTIDIABETIC AGENTS

DRUG	HOW SUPPLIED	INITIAL* & (MAX) DOSE	USUAL DOSE RANGE*
BIGUANIDES			
Metformin HCl			
Fortamet	**Tab: ER:** 500mg, 1000mg	1000mg qd with evening meal (2500mg/day).	500-2500mg qd.
Glumetza	**Tab: ER:** 500mg, 1000mg	1000mg qd with evening meal (2000mg/day).	1000mg-2000mg/day.
Glucophage, Riomet	**Tab:** 500mg, 850mg, 1000mg **Sol:** 500mg/5mL	500mg bid or 850mg qd with meals (2550mg/day).	850mg-2000mg/day qd or divided doses.
Glucophage XR	**Tab: ER:** 500mg, 750mg	500mg qd with evening meal (2000mg/day).	500-2000mg/day qd or divided doses.
BILE-ACID SEQUESTRANT			
Colesevelam HCl			
Welchol	**Tab:** 625mg **Sus:** 3.75g, 1.875g [pkt]	1875mg bid or 3750mg qd (3750mg/day).	3750mg qd.
DIPEPTIDYL PEPTIDASE-4 INHIBITORS			
Saxagliptin			
Onglyza	**Tab:** 2.5mg, 5mg	2.5-5mg qd.	2.5-5mg qd.
Sitagliptin			
Januvia	**Tab:** 25mg, 50mg, 100mg	100mg qd.	100mg qd.
GLUCOSIDASE INHIBITORS			
Acarbose			
Precose	**Tab:** 25mg, 50mg, 100mg	25mg tid at start of each meal (≤60kg: 50mg tid, >60kg: 100mg tid).	50-100mg tid.
Miglitol			
Glyset	**Tab:** 25mg, 50mg, 100mg	25mg tid at start of each meal (300mg/day).	50-100mg tid.
MEGLITINIDES			
Nateglinide			
Starlix	**Tab:** 60mg, 120mg	120mg tid before meals (360mg/day).	120mg tid.
Repaglinide			
Prandin	**Tab:** 0.5mg, 1mg, 2mg	0.5-2mg with each meal (16mg/day).	0.5-4mg with each meal.
SULFONYLUREAS			
Chlorpropamide Diabinese	**Tab:** 100mg, 250mg	Initial: 250mg qd. Elderly: 100-125mg qd. (750mg/day).	<100-500mg qd. Most patients controlled with 250mg qd.
Glimepiride Amaryl	**Tab:** 1mg, 2mg, 4mg	1-2mg qd w/breakfast or first main meal (8mg/day).	1-4mg qd.
Glipizide			
Glucotrol	**Tab:** 5mg, 10mg	5mg qd before breakfast (40mg/day).	5-40mg qd or divided if >15mg/day.
Glucotrol XL	**Tab, ER:** 2.5mg, 5mg, 10mg	5mg qd w/breakfast (20mg/day).	5-10mg qd.
Glyburide Diabeta	**Tab:** 1.25mg, 2.5mg, 5mg	2.5-5mg qd w/breakfast or first main meal (20mg/day).	1.25-20mg qd or divided doses.
Glyburide Micronized Glynase PresTab	**Tab:** 1.5mg, 3mg, 6mg	1.5-3mg qd w/breakfast or first main meal (12mg/day).	0.75-12mg qd or divided doses.
Tolazamide	**Tab:** 250mg, 500mg	100-250mg qd with breakfast or first main meal (1000mg/day).	100-1000mg qd or divided if >500mg/day.

(Continued)

DRUG	HOW SUPPLIED	INITIAL* & (MAX) DOSE	USUAL DOSE RANGE*
SULFONYLUREAS (*Continued*)			
Tolbutamide	**Tab:** 250mg, 500mg	1000-2000mg qd or divided doses (3000mg/day).	250-3000mg/day qd or divided doses.
THIAZOLIDINEDIONES			
Pioglitazone HCl Actos	**Tab:** 15mg, 30mg, 45mg	15-30mg qd (45mg/day).	15-30mg qd.
Rosiglitazone maleate Avandia	**Tab:** 2mg, 4mg, 8mg	2mg bid or 4mg qd (8mg/day).	4-8mg qd.
COMBINATIONS			
Glipizide/ Metformin HCl Metaglip	**Tab:** 2.5mg/250mg, 2.5mg/500mg, 5mg/500mg	2.5mg/250mg qd w/meals or 2.5mg/500mg bid (20mg/ 2000mg/day).	2.5mg/250mg qd-5mg/500mg bid.
Glyburide/ Metformin HCl Glucovance	**Tab:** 1.25mg/250mg, 2.5mg/500mg, 5mg/500mg	1.25mg/250mg qd or bid with meals (20mg/2000mg/day).	1.25mg/250mg qd-5mg/500mg bid.
Pioglitazone/ Glimepiride Duetact	**Tab:** 30mg/2mg, 30mg/4mg	30mg/2mg qd or 30mg/4mg with first meal qd. Do not give more than once daily at any of the tablet strengths.	1 tab qd.
Pioglitazone/ Metformin HCl Actoplus Met	**Tab:** 15mg/500mg, 15mg/850mg	15mg/500mg or 15mg/850mg qd-bid with food (45mg/ 2550mg/day).	1 tab qd-bid.
Actoplus Met XR	**Tab: ER:** 15mg/1000mg, 30mg/1000mg	15mg/1000mg or 30mg/1000mg qd with evening meal (45mg/2000mg/day).	1 tab qd.
Repaglinide/ Metformin HCl PrandiMet	**Tab:** 1mg/500mg, 2mg/500mg	1mg/500mg bid before meals or 2mg/500mg bid before meals (10mg/2500/day).	1 tab bid-tid.
Rosiglitazone/ Glimepiride Avandaryl	**Tab:** 4mg/1mg, 4mg/2mg, 4mg/4mg, 8mg/2mg, 8mg/4mg	4mg/1mg qd or 4mg/2mg qd w/first meal (8mg/4mg/day).	1 tab qd.
Rosiglitazone/ Metformin HCl Avandamet	**Tab:** 2mg/500mg, 4mg/500mg, 2mg/1000mg, 4mg/1000mg	Individualize - 2mg/500mg bid w/meals (8mg/2000mg/day).	1 tab bid.
Saxagliptin/ Metformin HCl Kombiglyze XR	**Tab: ER:** 5mg/500mg, 5mg/1000mg, 2.5mg/1000mg	5mg/500mg or 2.5mg/1000mg qd with evening meal (5mg/2000mg).	1 tab qd.
Sitagliptin/ Metformin Janumet	**Tab:** 50mg/500mg, 50mg/1000mg	50mg/500mg or 50mg/1000mg bid w/meals (100mg/2g/day).	1 tab bid.

*NOTE: Usual dose ranges are derived from the drug's FDA-approved labeling. There is no fixed dosage regimen for the management of diabetes mellitus with any hypoglycemic agent. The initial and maintenance dosing should be conservative, depending on the patient's individual needs, especially in elderly, debilitated or malnourished patients, and with impaired renal or hepatic function. Management of type 2 diabetes should include blood glucose and HbA1c monitoring, nutritional counseling, exercise, and weight reduction as needed. For more detailed information, refer to the individual monograph listings or the drug's FDA-approved labeling.

ANTIEMETICS

DRUG (BRAND)	INDICATIONS	HOW SUPPLIED	ADULT DOSING	PEDIATRIC DOSING
Anticholinergic Agent				
Scopolamine (Transderm Scop)	Prevention of nausea and vomiting associated with motion sickness or recovery from anesthesia and surgery.	Patch: 1mg/72 hrs [4⁵]	PONV: Apply 1 patch the evening before surgery or 1 hr prior to cesarean section. Keep in place for 24 hrs following surgery. Motion Sickness: Apply patch to a hairless area behind the ear at least 4 hrs before needed. Do not cut patch in half.	
Antihistamines				
Dimenhydrinate	Prevention and treatment of nausea, vomiting, or vertigo caused by motion sickness.	Inj: 50mg/mL	(Inj) 50mg q4h, may increase to 100mg q4h if drowsiness is desirable. For IV administration, dilute each mL of solution in 10mL of 0.9% sodium chloride and inject over 2 minutes. IM injection is administered undiluted.	(IM) 1.25mg/kg or 37.5mg/m² body surface area qid. Max: 300mg/day.
Meclizine HCl (Antivert)	Management of nausea, vomiting and dizziness associated with motion sickness. Management of vertigo associated with diseases affecting the vestibular system.	Tab: 12.5mg, 25mg, 50mg* *scored	Motion Sickness: 25-50mg 1 hr prior to trip/departure, repeat q24h prn.	≥12 yrs: Motion Sickness: 25-50mg 1 hr prior to trip/departure, repeat q24h prn. Vertigo: 25-100mg/day in divided doses.
Promethazine HCl (Phenadoz, Phenergan, Promethegan)	Prevention and control of nausea and vomiting associated with certain types of anesthesia and surgery. Active and prophylactic treatment of motion sickness. Postoperative antiemetic therapy.	Liq: 6.25/5mL [473mL, 118mL]; Sup: 12.5mg, 25mg, 50mg; Tab: 12.5mg*, 25mg*, 50mg *scored Inj: 25mg/mL, 50mg/mL	Nausea/Vomiting: 12.5-25mg q4-6h. Do not give IV administration >25mg/mL and at a rate >25mg/min. Motion Sickness: 25mg 0.5-1h prior to trip/departure, repeat after 8-12 hrs if needed. Maint: 25mg bid.	≥2 yrs: Motion Sickness: 12.5-25mg bid. Nausea/vomiting: 12.5-25mg may be repeated at 4-6h intervals. Usual: 0.5mg/lb; adjust for patient's age and weight and condition severity. Dose should not exceed half of adult dose. Do not give IV administration >25mg/mL and at a rate >25mg/min.
Cannabinoids				
Dronabinol (Marinol)	Treatment of nausea and vomiting associated with chemotherapy when conventional treatment has failed.	Cap: 2.5mg, 5mg, 10mg	Initial: 5mg/m² given 1-3 hrs before chemotherapy, then q2-4h after chemotherapy, up to 4-6 doses/day. Titrate: May increase by 2.5mg/m² increments. Max: 15mg/m²/dose.	Initial: 5mg/m² given 1-3 hrs before chemotherapy, then q2-4h after chemotherapy, up to 4-6 doses/day. Titrate: May increase by 2.5mg/m² increments. Max: 15mg/m²/dose. Use caution because of psychoactive effects.

(Continued)

DRUG (BRAND)	INDICATIONS	HOW SUPPLIED	ADULT DOSING	PEDIATRIC DOSING
Cannabinoids *(Continued)*				
Nabilone (Cesamet)	Treatment of the nausea and vomiting associated with chemotherapy when conventional treatment has failed.	Cap: 1mg	Usual: 1 or 2mg bid. Give initial dose 1-3 hrs before chemotherapy. A dose of 1 or 2mg the night before may be useful. May be given bid-tid during chemotherapy cycle and, if needed, for 48 hrs after the last dose of each cycle. Max: 6mg/day given in divided doses tid.	
5-HT₃ Antagonists				
Dolasetron mesylate (Anzemet)	(Inj) Prevention and treatment of post-op nausea/vomiting (PONV). (Tab) Prevention of nausea/vomiting associated with moderately emetogenic cancer chemotherapy and prevention of PONV.	Inj: 20mg/mL; Tab: 50mg, 100mg	(Inj) Prevention/Treatment of PONV: 12.5mg IV single dose 15 min before cessation of anesthesia or as soon as nausea/vomiting presents. (Tab) Prevention of CINV: 100mg PO within 1 hr before chemotherapy. Prevention of PONV: 100mg PO within 2 hrs before surgery.	**2-16 yrs:** (Inj) Prevention/Treatment of PONV: 0.35mg/kg IV single dose 15 min before cessation of anesthesia or as soon as nausea/vomiting presents. Max: 12.5mg single dose. May mix 1.2mg/kg in apple or grape juice and take orally within 2 hrs before surgery. Max: 100mg/dose. (Tab) Prevention of CINV: 1.8mg/kg PO within 1 hr before chemotherapy. Max: 100mg. Prevention of PONV: 1.2mg/kg PO within 2 hrs before surgery. Max: 100mg.
Granisetron HCl (Kytril)	(Inj, Sol, Tab) Prevention of nausea and vomiting associated with chemotherapy including high-dose cisplatin. (Sol, Tab) Prevention of nausea and vomiting associated with radiation. (Inj) Prevention and treatment of post-op nausea and vomiting (PONV).	Inj: 0.1mg/mL, 1mg/mL; Sol: 2mg/10mL [30mL]; Tab: 1mg	(Sol/Tab) Prevention of Chemotherapy-Induced Nausea/Vomiting (CINV): 2mg qd up to 1 hr before chemotherapy or 1mg bid (up to 1 hr before chemotherapy and 12 hrs later). (Inj) 10mcg/kg within 30 min before chemotherapy. Prevention with Radiation: (Sol/Tab) 2mg within 1 hr of radiation. Prevention and treatment of PONV: (Inj) Administer 1mg over 30 sec before induction of anesthesia or immediately before anesthesia reversal.	**2-16 yrs:** Prevention of CINV: 10mcg/kg IV within 30 min before chemotherapy.
Granisetron transdermal system (Sancuso)	Prevention of nausea and vomiting in patients receiving moderately and/or highly emetogenic chemotherapy regimens of up to 5 consecutive days duration.	Patch: 3.1mg/24hrs [1ˢ]	Apply patch to upper outer arm 24 hrs prior to chemotherapy. The patch may be applied up to a maximum of 48 hrs before chemotherapy. Remove patch a minimum of 24 hrs after completion of chemotherapy. Patch can be worn for up to 7 days depending on duration of chemotherapy regimen.	

DRUG (BRAND)	INDICATIONS	HOW SUPPLIED	ADULT DOSING	PEDIATRIC DOSING

5-HT₃ Antagonists *(Continued)*

DRUG (BRAND)	INDICATIONS	HOW SUPPLIED	ADULT DOSING	PEDIATRIC DOSING
Ondansetron (Zuplenz)	Prevention of nausea and vomiting (N/V) associated with: Highly emetogenic cancer chemotherapy, including cisplatin ≥50mg/m²; moderately emetogenic cancer chemotherapy with initial and repeat courses; radiotherapy in patients receiving either total body irradiation, single high-dose fraction to the abdomen, or daily fractions to the abdomen. Prevention of postoperative nausea and/or vomiting (PONV).	Film, Oral: 4mg, 8mg	Prevention of N/V Associated with Highly Emetogenic Chemotherapy: 24mg 30 min before chemotherapy. Prevention of N/V Associated with Moderately Emetogenic Chemotherapy: 8mg bid; give 1st dose 30 min before chemotherapy, then 8 hrs later, then bid (q12h) for 1-2 days after completion of chemotherapy. Prevention of N/V Associated with Radiotherapy: 8mg tid. Total Body Irradiation: 8mg 1-2 hrs before each fraction of radiotherapy administered each day. Single High-Dose Fraction Radiotherapy to Abdomen: 8mg 1-2 hrs before therapy then q8h after 1st dose for 1-2 days after completion of therapy. Daily Fractionated Radiotherapy to Abdomen: 8mg 1-2 hrs before therapy then q8h after 1st dose for each day radiotherapy is given. Prevention of PONV: 16mg 1 hr before induction of anesthesia. Severe Hepatic Dysfunction (Child-Pugh ≥10): Max: 8mg/day.	**≥12 yrs:** Prevention of N/V Associated with Moderately Emetogenic Chemotherapy: 8mg bid; give 1st dose 30 min before chemotherapy, then 8 hrs later, then bid (q12h) for 1-2 days after completion of chemotherapy. **4-11 yrs:** 4mg tid: give 1st dose 30 min before chemotherapy, then 4 and 8 hrs later, then tid (q8h) for 1-2 days after chemotherapy. Severe Hepatic Dysfunction (Child-Pugh ≥10): Max: 8mg/day.
Ondansetron HCl (Zofran)	(Inj) Prevention of nausea and vomiting associated with initial and repeat courses of emetogenic cancer chemotherapy, including post-op nausea and/or vomiting (PONV). (Sol/Tab) Prevention of nausea and vomiting associated with: highly emetogenic cancer chemotherapy, including cisplatin ≥50mg/m²; initial and repeat courses of moderately emetogenic cancer chemotherapy; and radiotherapy in patients receiving either total body irradiation, single high-dose fraction to the abdomen, or daily fractions to the abdomen. Prevention of PONV.	Inj: 2mg/mL; Sol: 4mg/5mL [50mL]; Tab: 4mg, 8mg; Tab, Disintegrating: 4mg, 8mg	Prevention of Chemotherapy-Induced Nausea/Vomiting (CINV): (Inj) 32mg single dose or three 0.15mg/kg doses; give 1st dose (over 15 min) 30 min before chemotherapy. For three-dose regimen, give subsequent two doses 4 and 8 hrs after 1st dose. Prevention of CINV, Highly Emetogenic Therapy: (Tab) 24mg given as three 8mg tablets administered 30 min before chemotherapy. Prevention of CINV, Moderately Emetogenic Therapy: (Sol/Tab) 8mg bid, 1st dose 30 min before chemotherapy, then 8 hrs later, then bid for 1-2 days after chemotherapy. Prevention of PONV: (Inj) 4mg undiluted IM/IV immediately before anesthesia or post-op if nausea or vomiting occurs; as IV, infuse over 2-5 min. (Sol/Tab) 16mg 1 hr before anesthesia. Prevention of Nausea/Vomiting Associated with Radiation Therapy: (Sol/Tab) Usual: 8mg tid. Total Body Irradiation: 8mg 1-2 hrs before each fraction of therapy daily. Single High-Dose Therapy To Abdomen: 8mg 1-2 hrs before therapy then q8h after 1st dose for 1-2 days after completion of therapy. Daily Fractionated Therapy To Abdomen: 8mg 1-2 hrs before therapy then q8h after 1st dose for each day radiotherapy is given. Severe Hepatic Dysfunction (Child-Pugh ≥10): Max: 8mg/day IV single dose infused over 15 min, start 30 min before chemotherapy or 8mg/day PO.	Prevention of CINV: (Inj) **6 months-18 yrs:** Three 0.15mg/kg doses, 1st dose 30 min before chemotherapy, then 4 and 8 hrs after the 1st dose. Infuse over 15 min. (Sol/Tab) Prevention of CINV, Moderately Emetogenic Therapy: **≥12 yrs:** 8mg bid, 1st dose 30 min before chemotherapy, then 8mg 8 hrs later, then bid for 1-2 days after chemotherapy. **4-11 yrs:** 4mg tid, 1st dose 30 min before chemotherapy, then 4 and 8 hrs after 1st dose, then tid for 1-2 days after chemotherapy. Prevention of PONV: (Inj) **1 month-12 yrs:** ≤40kg: 0.1mg/kg single dose. >40kg: 4mg single dose. Infuse over 2-5 min immediately before or after anesthesia induction or post-op if N/V occurs. Severe Hepatic Dysfunction: Max: 8mg/day IV single dose infused over 15 min, start 30 min before chemotherapy or 8mg/day PO.

(Continued)

DRUG (BRAND)	INDICATIONS	HOW SUPPLIED	ADULT DOSING	PEDIATRIC DOSING
5-HT₃ Antagonists *(Continued)*				
Palonosetron HCl (Aloxi)	(Inj) Prevention of acute and delayed nausea and vomiting associated with initial and repeat courses of moderately emetogenic cancer chemotherapy and prevention of acute N/V associated with initial and repeat courses of highly emetogenic cancer chemotherapy. Prevention of post-op nausea and vomiting (PONV) for up to 24 hrs following surgery.	Inj: 0.25mg/5mL, 0.075mg/1.5mL	Chemo-Induced N/V: 0.25mg IV single dose over 30 sec 30 min before start of chemotherapy. PONV: 0.075mg IV single dose 10 sec before induction of anesthesia.	
Miscellaneous				
Droperidol	To reduce incidence of nausea and vomiting associated with surgical and diagnostic procedures.	Inj: 2.5mg/mL	Initial (Max): 2.5mg IM/IV. May give additional 1.25mg cautiously to achieve desired effect. Lower initial doses in elderly, debilitated, poor-risk patients.	2-12 yrs: Initial (Max): 0.1 mg/kg IM/IV. May give additional dose cautiously. Lower initial doses in debilitated, poor-risk patients.
Metoclopramide (Reglan)	Prevention of post-op or chemo-induced nausea/vomiting.	Inj: 5mg/mL	Postoperative: 10-20mg IM near end of surgery. Chemotherapy-Induced: 1-2mg/kg IV over not less than 15 min, 30 min before chemotherapy then q2h for two doses, then q3h for three doses. Give 2mg/kg for highly emetogenic drugs for initial 2 doses. For CrCl <40mL/min: Give approx. half the recommended dosage.	
Trimethobenzamide HCl (Tigan)	Treatment of postoperative nausea and vomiting and for nausea associated with gastroenteritis.	Cap: 300mg; Inj: 100mg/mL	(Cap) 300mg tid-qid. (Inj) 200mg IM tid-qid. Renal Impairment (CrCl ≤70mL/min/1.73m²): Reduce dose or increase dosing interval.	
Phenothiazine Derivative				
Prochlorperazine (Compro)	Control of severe nausea and vomiting.	Inj: (Edisylate) 5mg/mL; Supp: (Compro) 25mg; Tab: (Maleate) 5mg, 10mg	Nausea/Vomiting: (Tab) Usual: 5-10mg tid-qid. >40mg/day only in resistant cases. (Supp) 25mg bid. (IM) 5-10mg IM q3-4h prn. Max: 40mg/day. (IV) 2.5-10mg IV (not bolus) at rate ≤5mg/min. Max: 10mg single dose and 40mg/day. Nausea/Vomiting with Surgery: 5-10mg IM 1-2 hrs or 5-10mg IV (not bolus) at rate ≤5mg/min 15-30 min before anesthesia (repeat once in 30 min if needed for IM), or to control acute symptoms during or after surgery; repeat once if needed. Max: 10mg single dose and 40mg/day.	Nausea/Vomiting: ≥2 yrs and ≥20 lbs: (PO/PR) 20-29 lbs: Usual: 2.5mg qd-bid. Max: 7.5mg/day. 30-39 lbs: 2.5mg bid-tid. Max: 10mg/day. 40-85 lbs: 2.5mg tid or 5mg bid. Max: 15mg/day. (IM) 0.06mg/lb, usually single dose for control.

DRUG (BRAND)	INDICATIONS	HOW SUPPLIED	ADULT DOSING	PEDIATRIC DOSING
Substance P/Neurokinin 1 Receptor Antagonists				
Aprepitant (Emend)	In combination with other antiemetics for prevention of acute and delayed nausea and vomiting associated with initial and repeat courses of highly emetogenic cancer chemotherapy (eg, high-dose cisplatin) or moderately emetogenic cancer chemotherapy. For the prevention of post-op nausea and vomiting (PONV).	Cap: 40mg, 80mg, 125mg; Tri-Pak: (one 125mg & two 80mg caps)	Prevention of Chemotherapy-Induced Nausea/Vomiting: Day 1: 125mg 1 hr prior to chemotherapy. Days 2 and 3: 80mg qam. Regimen should include a corticosteroid and a 5-HT$_3$ antagonist. Prevention of PONV: 40mg within 3 hrs prior to induction of anesthesia.	
Fosaprepitant Dimeglumine (Emend for injection)	In combination with other antiemetics for prevention of acute and delayed nausea and vomiting associated with initial and repeat courses of highly emetogenic cancer chemotherapy (eg, high-dose cisplatin) or moderately emetogenic cancer chemotherapy.	Powder (Vial): 115mg, 150mg	Prevention of Highly Emetogenic Chemotherapy-Induced Nausea/Vomiting: 3-Day Dosing Regimen: 115mg IV over 15 min initiated 30 min prior to chemotherapy on day 1 only of a 3-day regimen, in addition to corticosteroid and 5-HT$_3$ antagonist. Single-Dose Regimen: 150mg IV over 20-30 min initiated 30 min prior to chemotherapy, in addition to a corticosteroid and 5-HT$_3$ antagonist. Prevention of Moderately Emetogenic Chemotherapy-Induced Nausea/Vomiting: 3-Day Dosing Regimen: 115mg IV over 15 min 30 min prior to chemotherapy on day 1 only of a 3-day regimen, in addition to corticosteroid and 5-HT$_3$ antagonist.	

H₂ ANTAGONISTS AND PPIS COMPARISON§

	DRUG	HOW SUPPLIED	Heart-burn	PUD	GERD	Esophagitis	Zollinger-Ellison	H.pylori	NSAID† Induced	Upper GI‡ Bleeding
H₂ ANTAGONISTS	**CIMETIDINE**									
	Generic	**Inj:** 150mg/mL, 300mg/50mL* **Sol:** 300mg/5mL* **Tab:** 200mg, 300mg, 400mg, 800mg*		X	X	X	X			X
	FAMOTIDINE									
	Pepcid	**Inj:** 0.4mg/mL, 10mg/mL* **Sus:** 40mg/5mL; **Tab:** 20mg, 40mg		X	X	X	X			
	NIZATIDINE									
	Axid	**Cap:** 150mg, 300mg **Sol:** 15mg/mL	X	X	X	X				
	RANITIDINE									
	Zantac	**Inj:** 1mg/mL, 25mg/mL **Syrup:** 15mg/mL **Tab:** 150mg, 300mg **Tab, Effervescent:** 25mg	X	X	X	X	X			
PROTON PUMP INHIBITORS	**DEXLANSOPRAZOLE**									
	Dexilant (formerly known as Kapidex)	**Cap, DR:** 30mg, 60mg	X		X	X				
	ESOMEPRAZOLE									
	Nexium	**Cap, DR:** 20mg, 40mg; **Inj:** 20mg, 40mg **Sus, DR:** 10mg, 20mg, 40mg (granules/packet)	X	X	X	X	X	X	X	
	Vimovo	**Tab, DR:** (Esomeprazole Magnesium-Naproxen) 20mg-375mg, 20mg-500mg							X	
	LANSOPRAZOLE									
	Prevacid	**Cap, DR:** 15mg, 30mg; **Tab, Disintegrating:** 15mg, 30mg	X	X	X	X	X	X	X	
	Prevpac	**Cap:** (Amoxicillin) 500mg **Tab:** (Clarithromycin) 500mg **Cap, DR:** (Lansoprazole) 30mg						X		
	OMEPRAZOLE									
	Prilosec	**Cap, DR:** 10mg, 20mg, 40mg; **Sus, DR:** 2.5mg, 10mg (granules/packet)	X	X	X	X	X	X		
	Zegerid	(Omeprazole-Sodium Bicarbonate); **Cap:** 20mg-1100mg, 40mg-1100mg; **Pow:** 20mg-1680mg/packet, 40mg-1680mg/packet **Tab:** (Omeprazole-Sodium Bicarbonate-Magnesium Hydroxide) 20mg-750mg-343mg, 40mg-750mg-343mg*	X	X	X	X				X
	PANTOPRAZOLE									
	Protonix	**Inj:** 40mg; **Tab, DR:** 20mg, 40mg **Sus, DR:** 40mg (granules/packet)	X		X	X	X			
	RABEPRAZOLE									
	Aciphex	**Tab, DR:** 20mg	X	X	X		X	X		

DR=Delayed-Release   *Product available generically only.   †Prevention of NSAID-induced gastric ulcers.
‡Prevention of upper GI bleeding in critically ill patients.
§Rx products only. For OTC products, refer to Antacid and Heartburn Products on page A59.

DRUG TREATMENTS FOR COMMON STDs*

DISEASE	DRUG	RECOMMENDED DOSAGE
Bacterial Vaginosis Nonpregnant Women	Metronidazole (Flagyl) or Clindamycin cream (Cleocin) or Metronidazole gel (MetroGel)	500mg PO bid x 7d. 2%, 1 full applicator intravaginally qhs x 7d. 0.75%, 1 full applicator intravaginally qd x 5d.
Alternative Regimens (Nonpregnant Women)	Clindamycin or Clindamycin ovules	300mg PO bid x 7d. 100mg intravaginally qhs x 3d.
	Tinidazole	2g PO QD x 2d or 1g PO QD x 5d.
Pregnant Women	Metronidazole or Clindamycin	250mg PO tid x 7d (metronidazole) or 500mg PO bid x 7d. 300mg PO bid x 7d (clindamycin).
Chancroid	Azithromycin (Zithromax) or Ceftriaxone (Rocephin) or Ciprofloxacin (Cipro) or Erythromycin base	1g PO single dose. 250mg IM single dose. 500mg PO bid x 3d. 500mg PO tid x 7d.
Chlamydial Infection Nonpregnant Women	Azithromycin (Zithromax) or Doxycycline (Vibramycin)	1g PO single dose. 100mg PO bid x 7d.
Alternative Regimens (Nonpregnant/pregnant)	Erythromycin base or Erythromycin Ethylsuccinate or Ofloxacin (Floxin) or Levofloxacin (Levaquin)	500mg PO qid x 7d or 250mg PO qid x 14d (pregnancy). 800mg PO qid x 7d or 400mg PO qid x 14d (pregnancy). 300mg PO bid x 7d (nonpregnant). 500mg PO qd x 7d (nonpregnant).
Pregnant Women	Azithromycin (Zithromax) or Amoxicillin	1g PO single dose. 500mg PO tid x 7d.
Epididymitis Gonococcal or Chlamydial Infection	Ceftriaxone (Rocephin) plus Doxycycline (Vibramycin)	250mg IM single dose. 100mg PO bid x 10d.
Enteric organisms, negative gonococcal culture, or nucleic acid amplification test	Ofloxacin (Floxin) or Levofloxacin (Levaquin)	300mg PO bid x 10d. 500mg PO qd x 10d.
Granuloma Inguinale	Doxycycline (Vibramycin)	100mg PO bid for at least 3 weeks.
Alternative Regimens	Ciprofloxacin (Cipro) or Erythromycin base (during pregnancy) or Azithromycin (Zithromax) Trimethoprim/Sulfamethoxazole (Bactrim, Septra) plus (if no improvement w/in first few days) Aminoglycoside (ie, gentamicin)	750mg PO bid for at least 3 weeks. 500mg PO qid for at least 3 weeks. 1g PO once weekly for at least 3 weeks. 1 tab (DS) PO bid for at least 3 weeks. 1mg/kg IV q8h for at least 3 weeks.
Herpes Simplex Virus (HSV) First Episode	Acyclovir (Zovirax) or Famciclovir (Famvir) or Valacyclovir (Valtrex)	400mg PO tid x 7-10d or 200mg PO 5x/d x 7-10d. 250mg PO tid x 7-10d. 1g PO bid x 7-10d.
Recurrent Episodes	Acyclovir or Famciclovir or Valacyclovir	400mg PO tid x 5d or 800mg PO bid x 5d or 800mg PO tid x 2d. 1g bid x 1d or 125mg PO bid x 5d or 500mg once followed by 250mg bid x 2d. 500mg PO bid x 3d or 1g PO qd x 5d.
Daily Suppressive Therapy	Acyclovir or Famciclovir or Valacyclovir	400mg PO bid. 250mg PO bid. 500mg PO qd (<10 episodes/yr) or 1g PO qd.

(Continued)

DISEASE	DRUG	RECOMMENDED DOSAGE
Human Papillomavirus (HPV) Infection		
External Genital Area	Podofilox (Condylox) *or*	0.5% sol or gel (patient-applied) bid x 3d, wait 4d, repeat as necessary x 4 cycles. Limit application to 0.5mL/day and to <10cm² wart area.
	Imiquimod (Aldara)	5% cre (patient-applied) hs, 3 times a wk for up to 16 wks.
	Sinecatechins (Veregen)	15% oint tid (0.5cm strand/wart) x ≤16 wks.
	Cryotherapy *or* Podophyllum resin	Physician-applied every 1-2 wks. 10-25% (physician-applied) qwk if necessary. Limit application to 0.5mL/day and to <10cm² wart area. Do not apply to area with open lesions or wounds.
	Trichloroacetic acid *or* Bichloroacetic acid *or* Surgical removal	80-90% (physician-applied) qwk if necessary. 80-90% (physician-applied) qwk if necessary.
Alternative Regimens	Intralesional interferon *or* photodynamic therapy *or* topical cidofovir	
Vaginal warts	Cryotherapy *or* Trichloroacetic acid *or* Bichloroacetic acid	With liquid nitrogen. 80-90% (physician-applied) qwk if necessary. 80-90% (physician-applied) qwk if necessary.
Urethral Meatus warts	Cryotherapy *or* Podophyllum	With liquid nitrogen. 10-25% (physician-applied) qwk if necessary.
Anal warts	Cryotherapy Trichloroacetic acid *or* Bichloroacetic acid *or* Surgical removal	With liquid nitrogen. 80-90% (physician-applied) qwk if necessary. 80-90% (physician-applied) qwk if necessary.
Lymphogranuloma Venereum	Doxycycline (Vibramycin)	100mg PO bid x 21d.
Alternative Regimen (including pregnancy)	Erythromycin base	500mg PO qid x 21d.
Nongonococcal Urethritis	Azithromycin (Zithromax) *or* Doxycycline (Vibramycin)	1g PO single dose. 100mg PO bid x 7d.
Alternative Regimens	Erythromycin base *or* Erythromycin ethylsuccinate *or* Ofloxacin (Floxin) *or* Levofloxacin (Levaquin)	500mg PO qid x 7d. 800mg PO qid x 7d. 300mg PO bid x 7d. 500mg PO qd x 7d.
Recurrent and Persistent Urethritis	Metronidazole *or* Tinidazole *plus* Azithromycin	2g PO single dose. 2g PO single dose. 1g PO single dose (if not used for initial episodes).
Pediculosis Pubis	Permethrin cream (NIX)	1% cre: Apply to affected area & wash off after 10 min.
	Pyrethrins with piperonyl butoxide (compounded by pharmacist)	Apply to affected area and wash off after 10 min.
Alternative Regimens	Malathion Ivermectin	0.5% lotion: Apply for 8-12 hours and wash off. 250µg/kg repeat in 2 weeks.
Pelvic Inflammatory Disease		
Parenteral Regimen A	Cefotetan (Cefotan) *or* Cefoxitin (Mefoxin) *plus* Doxycycline (Vibramycin)	2g IV q12h. 2g IV q6h. 100mg IV q12h.
Parenteral Regimen B	Clindamycin (Cleocin) *plus* Gentamicin	900mg IV q8h. LD: 2mg/kg IM/IV. MD: 1.5mg/kg IM/IV q8h (may substitute single daily dosing).
Alternative Regimen	Ampicillin/Sulbactam *plus* Doxycycline	3g IV q6h. 100mg PO/IV q12h.
Oral Regimen	Ceftriaxone (Rocephin) *plus* Doxycycline w/ or w/o Metronidazole *or* Cefoxitin *plus*	250mg IM single dose. 100mg PO bid x 14d. 500mg PO bid x 14d. 2g IM single dose with probenecid 1g PO single dose.
	Doxycycline w/ or w/o Metronidazole *or* 3rd Gen Cephalosporin *plus* Doxycycline w/ or w/o Metronidazole	100mg PO bid x 14d. 500mg PO bid x 14d. Given IV/IM 100mg PO bid x 14d. 500mg PO bid x 14d.
Alternative Oral Regimen (Use only if negative NAAT test or negative gonococcal culture)	Levofloxacin *or* Ofloxacin w/ or w/o Metronidazole	500mg PO qd x 14d. 400mg PO bid x 14d. 500mg PO bid x 14d.

(Continued)

DISEASE	DRUG	RECOMMENDED DOSAGE
Proctitis, Proctocolitis & Enteritis	Ceftriaxone (Rocephin) *plus* Doxycycline (Vibramycin)	250mg IM. 100mg PO bid x 7d.
Scabies	Permethrin cream (Elimite) or Ivermectin	5% cre: Apply to body from the neck down & wash off after 8-14h; re-evaluate in 1 week. 200mcg/kg PO; repeat in 2 weeks.
Alternative Regimens	Lindane (Kwell)	1% lot or cre: Apply 1oz lotion or 30g cream to body from the neck down & wash off after 8h; re-evaluate in 1 wk (not recommended in pregnancy, lactating women or children <2 yrs).
Syphilis Primary & Secondary Disease	Benzathine Penicillin G	**Adults:** 2.4 MU IM single dose. **Pediatrics:** 50,000 U/kg IM single dose. **Max:** 2.4 MU/dose.
Penicillin Allergy	Doxycycline (Vibramycin) *or* Tetracycline	100mg PO bid x 14d. 500mg PO tid x 14d.
Early Latent Disease	Benzathine Penicillin G	**Adults:** 2.4 MU IM single dose. **Pediatrics:** 50,000 U/kg IM single dose. **Max:** 2.4 MU/dose.
Late Latent, Unknown Duration	Benzathine Penicillin G	**Adults:** 2.4 MU IM qwk x 3 doses. **Pediatrics:** 50,000 U/kg IM qwk x 3 doses. **Max:** 2.4 MU/dose.
Tertiary Disease	Benzathine Penicillin G	2.4 MU IM qwk x 3 doses.
Neurosyphilis	Aqueous Crystalline Penicillin G	3-4 MU IV q4h or continuous infusion x 10-14d.
Alternative Regimen	Procaine Penicillin *plus* Probenecid	2.4 MU IM qd x 10-14d. 500mg PO qid x 10-14d.
Trichomoniasis	Metronidazole (Flagyl) Tinidazole (Tindamax)	2g PO single dose. 2g PO single dose.
Alternative Regimen	Metronidazole	500mg PO bid x 7d.
Pregnant Women	Metronidazole (CI in 1st trimester)	2g PO single dose.
Uncomplicated Gonococcal Infections Cervix, Urethra, and Rectum *Recommended Regimens*	Ceftriaxone or Cefixime or Single-dose injectible cephalosporin regimens Plus Azithromycin (Zithromax) or Doxycyline (Vibramycin)	250mg IM single dose. 400mg PO single dose. 1g PO single dose. 100mg PO bid x7d.
Alternative Regimens	*Cephalosporin regimens:* Ceftizoxime *or* Cefotaxime *or* Cefoxitin plus Probenecid	500mg IM single dose. 500mg IM single dose. 2g IM. 1g PO.
Pharynx *Recommended Regimens*	Ceftriaxone *plus* Azithromycin (Zithromax) or Doxycycline (Vibramycin)	250mg IM single dose. 1g PO single dose. 100mg PO bid x 7d.

(Continued)

DISEASE	DRUG	RECOMMENDED DOSAGE
Vulvovaginal Candidiasis		
Intravaginal Agents	Butoconazole *or*	2% cre, 5g intravaginally x 3d. (OTC)
	Butoconazole *or*	2% cre, 5g intravaginally single dose. (Rx)
	Clotrimazole *or*	1% cre, 5g intravaginally x 7-14d.
	Clotrimazole *or*	2% cre, 5g intravaginally x 3d.
	Miconazole *or*	2% cre, 5g intravaginally qd x 7d.
	Miconazole	4% cre, 5g intravaginally x 3d.
	Miconazole *or*	200mg vaginal supp qd x 3d.
	Miconazole *or*	100mg vaginal supp qd x 7d.
	Miconazole	1200mg vaginal supp single dose.
	Nystatin *or*	100,000-U vaginal tab qd x 14d.
	Tioconazole *or*	6.5% oint, 5g intravaginally single dose.
	Terconazole *or*	0.4% cre, 5g intravaginally x 7d.
	Terconazole *or*	0.8% cre, 5g intravaginally x 3d.
	Terconazole	80mg vaginal supp qd x 3d.
Oral Agent	Fluconazole	150mg tab PO single dose.

*Adapted from: Centers for Disease Control and Prevention. Sexually Transmitted Diseases Treatment Guidelines 2010.
MMWR 2010; 59 (No. RR-12): 1-109.

HIV/AIDS PHARMACOTHERAPY

DRUG	BRAND	HOW SUPPLIED	USUAL DOSE	FOOD EFFECT
CCR5 ANTAGONIST				
Maraviroc (MVC)	Selzentry	**Tab:** 150mg, 300mg	**Adults ≥16 yrs:** Give in combination with other anti-retroviral medications. With Strong CYP3A Inhibitors (with or without CYP3A inducers) Including PIs (except tipranavir/ritonavir), Delavirdine, Ketoconazole, Itraconazole, Clarithromycin, Others (eg, Nefazodone, Telithromycin): 150mg bid. With NRTIs, Tipranavir/Ritonavir, Nevirapine, Raltegravir, Enfuvirtide, Other Drugs That Are Not Strong CYP3A Inhibitors/Inducers: 300mg bid. With Strong CYP3A Inducers (without strong CYP3A inhibitor) Including Efavirenz, Rifampin, Etravirine, Carbamazepine, Phenobarbital, Phenytoin: 600mg bid.	Take without regard to meals.
HIV INTEGRASE STRAND TRANSFER INHIBITOR				
Raltegravir	Isentress	**Tab:** 400mg	**Adults:** 400mg bid. With Rifampin: 800mg bid.	Take without regard to meals.
NUCLEOSIDE REVERSE TRANSCRIPTASE INHIBITORS (NRTIs)				
Abacavir (ABC)	Ziagen	**Sol:** 20mg/mL [240mL]; **Tab:** 300mg	**Adults:** 300mg bid or 600 mg qd. **Pediatrics ≥3 months:** 8mg/kg bid. **Max:** 300mg bid.	Take without regard to meals.
Didanosine (ddI)	Videx Powder for Oral Sol; Videx EC	**Powder for Sol:** 10mg/mL [2g, 4g]; **Cap, Delayed Release:** (Videx EC) 125mg, 200mg, 250mg, 400mg	**Adults ≥60kg: (Cap)** 400mg qd; **(Sol)** 200mg bid or 400mg qd. With TDF: 250mg qd. **<60kg: (Sol)** 125mg bid. or 250mg qd. 25-60 kg; **(Cap)** 250mg qd. 20-25 kg: **(Cap)** 200mg qd. With TDF: 200mg qd. **Pediatrics 2 weeks-8 months: (Sol)** 100mg/m² bid. **>8 months:** 120mg/m² bid.	Take on empty stomach at least 30 minutes before or 2 hrs after meals. Swallow caps whole.
Emtricitabine (FTC)	Emtriva	**Cap:** 200mg; **Sol:** 10mg/mL [170mL]	**Adults ≥18 yrs: Cap:** 200 mg qd. **Sol:** 240mg (24mL) qd. **Pediatrics 0-3 mos:** 3mg/kg qd. **3 mos-17 yrs: Cap:** >33kg: 200mg qd. **Sol:** 6mg/kg qd. **Max:** 240mg (24mL) qd.	Take without regard to meals.
Lamivudine	Epivir	**Sol:** 10mg/mL [240mL]; **Tab:** 150mg, 300mg	**Adults >16 yrs:** 150mg bid or 300mg qd. **Pediatrics 3 months-16 yrs:** 4mg/kg bid. **Max:** 150mg bid.	Take without regard to meals.
Stavudine (d4T)	Zerit	**Cap:** 15mg, 20mg, 30mg, 40mg; **Sol:** 1mg/mL [200mL]	**Adults ≥60kg:** 40mg q12h. **<60kg:** 30mg q12h. **Pediatrics ≥60kg:** 40mg q12h. **30-59kg:** 30mg q12h. **≥14 days and <30kg:** 1mg/kg q12h. **Birth-13 days:** 0.5mg/kg q12h.	Take without regard to meals.

(Continued)

DRUG	BRAND	HOW SUPPLIED	USUAL DOSE	FOOD EFFECT
NUCLEOSIDE REVERSE TRANSCRIPTASE INHIBITORS (NRTIs) *(Continued)*				
Tenofovir Disoproxil Fumarate (TDF)	Viread	**Tab:** 300mg	**Adults/Pediatrics ≥12 yrs: ≥35kg:** 300mg once daily.	Take without regard to meals.
Zidovudine (AZT, ZDV)	Retrovir	**Cap:** 100mg; **Inj:** 10mg/mL; **Syrup:** 50mg/5mL [240mL]; **Tab:** 300mg	**Adults: (Cap, Tab, Syrup)** 600mg/day in divided doses (300mg bid or 200mg tid). (Inj) 1mg/kg IV over 1 hr 5-6 times/day. **Pediatrics ≥4 weeks: (Cap, Tab, Syrup) BSA Based:** 480mg/m²/day in divided doses. **Weight Based: 4 to <9kg:** 12mg/kg bid or 8mg/kg tid. **≥9 to <30kg:** 9mg/kg bid or 6mg/kg tid. **≥30kg:** 300mg bid or 200mg tid.	Take without regard to meals.
NON-NUCLEOSIDE REVERSE TRANSCRIPTASE INHIBITORS (NNRTIs)				
Delavirdine (DLV)	Rescriptor	**Tab:** 100mg, 200mg	**Adults: Usual:** 400mg tid. **Pediatrics ≥16 yrs: Usual:** 400mg tid.	Take without regard to meals. Separate doses from antacids by 1 hr.
Efavirenz (EFV)	Sustiva	**Cap:** 50mg, 200mg; **Tab:** 600mg	**Adults Initial:** 600mg qd at bedtime. **Pediatrics ≥3 yrs: 10 to <15kg:** 200mg qd. **15 to <20kg:** 250mg qd. **20 to <25kg:** 300mg qd. **25 to <32.5kg:** 350mg qd. **32.5 to <40kg:** 400mg qd. **≥40kg:** 600mg qd at bedtime.	Take on an empty stomach.
Etravirine (ETR)	Intelence	**Tab:** 100mg, 200mg	**Adults:** 200mg bid.	Take following a meal.
Nevirapine (NVP)	Viramune	**Sus:** 50mg/5mL [240mL]; **Tab:** 200mg* *scored	**Adults ≥16 yrs:** 200mg qd for 14 days (lead-in period), then 200mg bid. **Pediatrics >15 days:** 150mg/m² qd for 14 days, then 150mg/m² bid. **Max:** 400mg/day.	Take without regard to meals.
PROTEASE INHIBITORS (PIs)				
Atazanavir (ATV)	Reyataz	**Cap:** 100mg, 150mg, 200mg, 300mg	**Adults:** Therapy-naive: 400mg qd or (ATV 300mg + RTV 100mg) qd. With EFV: (ATV 400mg + RTV 100mg) qd. Therapy Experienced: (ATV 300mg + RTV 100mg) qd. **Pediatrics: ≥6 yrs:** Therapy-naive: ≥39kg: ATV 300mg + RTV 100mg qd (or ATV 400mg qd if ≥13 yrs and RTV intolerant). 32-<39kg: ATV 250mg + RTV 100mg qd. 25-<32kg: ATV 200mg + RTV 100mg qd. 15-<25kg: ATV 150mg + RTV 80mg qd. Therapy Experienced: ≥39kg: ATV 300mg + RTV 100mg qd. 32-<39kg: ATV 250mg + RTV 100mg qd. 25-<32kg: ATV 200mg + RTV 100mg qd.	Take with food; avoid taking with antacids.

(Continued)

PROTEASE INHIBITORS (PIs) *(Continued)*

DRUG	BRAND	HOW SUPPLIED	USUAL DOSE	FOOD EFFECT
Darunavir (DRV)	Prezista	**Tab:** 75mg, 150mg, 300mg, 400mg, 600mg	**Adults:** Therapy-naïve or ARV-experienced patients with no DRV mutations: (DRV 800mg + RTV 100mg) qd. Therapy-experienced patients with at least 1 DRV mutation: (DRV 600mg + RTV 100mg) bid. **Pediatrics: (6 to <18 yrs):** ≥**40kg:** (DRV 600mg + RTV 100mg) bid. ≥**30-<40kg:** (DRV 450mg + RTV 60mg) bid. ≥**20-<30kg:** (DRV 375mg + RTV 50mg) bid. **Max:** (DRV 600mg + RTV 100mg) bid.	Take with food.
Fosamprenavir (FPV)	Lexiva	**Tab:** 700mg **Sus:** 50mg/mL [225mL]	**Adults:** Therapy-naïve: FPV 1,400mg bid OR FPV 1400mg qd + RTV 200mg qd OR FPV 1400mg qd + RTV 100mg qd OR FPV 700mg bid + RTV 100mg bid. PI-experienced: FPV 700mg bid + RTV 100mg bid. **Pediatrics:** (Sus): Therapy-naïve: **(2-5 yrs)** FPV 30mg/kg bid **Max:** FPV 1,400mg bid. **(≥6 yrs):** FPV 30mg/kg bid **Max:** FPV 1,400mg bid. OR FPV 18mg/kg bid + RTV 3mg/kg bid **Max:** FPV 700mg bid + RTV 100mg bid. Therapy-experienced: **(≥6 yrs)** FPV 18mg/kg bid + RTV 3mg/kg bid **Max:** FPV 700mg bid + RTV 100mg bid.	**Tab:** Take w/o regard to meals (if not boosted with RTV tab). **Sus: Adults:** Take w/o food. **Pediatrics:** Take with food. FPV with RTV Tab: Take with meals.
Indinavir (IDV)	Crixivan	**Cap:** 100mg, 200mg, 400mg	**Adults:** 800mg q8h RTV Boost: (IDV 800mg + RTV 100 or 200mg) q12h.	Take 1 hr before or 2 hr after meals; may take with skim milk or low-fat meal. (RTV Boost) Take w/o regard to meals.
Nelfinavir (NFV)	Viracept	**Sus:** (powder) 50mg/g [144g] **Tab:** 250mg, 625mg	**Adults:** 1250mg bid or 750mg tid. **Pediatrics 2-13 yrs:** 45-55mg/kg bid; 25-35mg/kg tid. **Max:** 2500mg/day.	Take with meals.
Ritonavir (RTV)	Norvir	**Cap, Tab:** 100mg **Sol:** 80mg/mL [240mL]	**Adults: Initial:** 300mg bid. **Titrate:** Increase every 2-3 days by 100mg bid. **Maint:** 600mg bid. **Pediatrics >1 month: Initial:** 250mg/m² po bid. **Titrate:** Increase by 50mg/m² bid every 2-3 days. **Maint:** 350-400mg/m² po bid or highest tolerated dose. **Max:** 600mg bid.	**Cap, Sol:** Take with food, may improve tolerability. **Tab:** Take with food.
Saquinavir (SQV)	Invirase	**Cap:** 200mg **Tab:** 500mg	**Adults/Pediatrics >16 yrs:** 1000mg bid with RTV 100mg bid OR 1000mg bid with LPV/RTV 400/100mg bid (no additional RTV).	Take within 2 hrs after a meal when taken with RTV.

(Continued)

DRUG	BRAND	HOW SUPPLIED	USUAL DOSE	FOOD EFFECT
PROTEASE INHIBITORS (PIs) *(Continued)*				
Tipranavir (TPV)	Aptivus	**Cap:** 250mg **Sol:** 100mg/mL	**Adults:** (500mg + RTV 200mg) bid. **Pediatrics** ≥2 yrs: 14mg/kg + RTV 6mg/kg (or 375mg/m² + RTV 150 mg/m²) bid. **Max:** (500mg + RTV 200mg) bid.	(TPV taken with RTV tab) Take with meals. (TPV taken with RTV cap or sol) Take w/o regard to meals.
FUSION INHIBITOR				
Enfuvirtide (T20)	Fuzeon	**Inj:** 90mg/mL [60ˢ]	**Adults:** 90mg SQ bid. **Pediatrics 6-16 yrs:** 2mg/kg SQ bid. **Max:** 90mg bid. 11-15.5kg: 27mg bid. 15.6-20.0kg: 36mg bid. 20.1-24.5kg: 45mg bid. 24.6-29.0kg: 54mg bid. 29.1-33.5kg: 63mg bid. 33.6-38.0kg: 72mg bid. 38.1-42.5kg: 81mg bid. ≥42.6kg: 90mg bid.	
COMBINATIONS				
EFV/FTC/TDF	Atripla	**Tab:** (Efavirenz-Emtricitabine-Tenofovir DF) 600mg-200mg-300mg	**Adults ≥18 yrs:** 1 tab qd, preferably at bedtime. Do not give if CrCl <50mL/min.	Take on empty stomach.
3TC/ZDV	Combivir	**Tab:** (Lamivudine-Zidovudine) 150mg-300mg	**Adults/Pediatrics:** (≥30kg) 1 tab bid. Do not give if CrCl <50mL/min or if <30kg weight.	Take without regard to meals.
ABC/3TC	Epzicom	**Tab:** (Abacavir Sulfate-Lamivudine) 600mg-300mg	**Adults ≥18 yrs:** CrCl ≥50 mL/min: 1 tab qd. Do not give if CrCl <50mL/min.	Take without regard to meals.
LPV/RTV	Kaletra	**Tab:** (LPV-RTV) 200mg-50mg; 100mg-25mg; **Sol:** (LPV-RTV) 80mg-20mg/mL [160mL]	**Adults:** 400/100mg bid or 800/200mg qd. With EFV or NVP (PI-naïve or PI-experienced patients): 500mg/125mg tab bid or 533mg/133mg sol bid. **Pediatrics:** **Sol:** (14 days-6 months) LPV/RTV 16/4 mg/kg or 300/75 mg/m² bid. (6 months-18 yrs) LPV/RTV 230/57.5 mg/m² bid or weight-based (<15kg) 12/3 mg/kg bid (≥15-40kg) 10/2.5 mg/kg bid. **Max:** 400/100mg bid. See PI for additional pediatric dosing.	**Tab:** Take without regard to meals. **Sol:** Take with meals.
ABC/ZDV/3TC	Trizivir	**Tab:** (Abacavir-Lamivudine-Zidovudine) 300mg-150mg-300mg	**Adults/Adolescents:** ≥40kg and CrCl ≥50mL/min: 1 tab bid.	Take without regard to meals.
FTC/TDF	Truvada	**Tab:** (Emtricitabine-Tenofovir Disoproxil Fumarate) 200mg-300mg	**Adults ≥18 yrs:** CrCl ≥50mL/min: 1 tab qd. CrCl 30-49mL/min: 1 tab q48h.	Take without regard to meals.

Sources: FDA-approved Labeling; Guidelines for the Use of Antiretroviral Agents in HIV-1-Infected Adults and Adolescents - January 11, 2011.

HIV/AIDS COMPLICATIONS THERAPY

HIV/AIDS DISEASE-RELATED COMPLICATIONS	GENERIC (BRAND)	RECOMMENDED DOSAGE
ASPERGILLOSIS, INVASIVE		
Recommended Treatment Regimen	Voriconazole (Vfend)*	**Adults: LD:** 6mg/kg q12h for 1st 24 hrs. **MD:** (IV) 4mg/kg q12h or (PO) ≥40kg: 200mg q12h. <40kg: 100mg q12h. For a minimum of 14 days and for at least 7 days following resolution of symptoms.
Alternative Treatment Regimen	Amphotericin B Liposome (AmBisome)	**Adults/Pediatrics:** (1 month-16 yrs): 3-5mg/kg/day IV controlled infusion over 1-2 hrs.
	Amphotericin B (Amphotec)	**Adults/Pediatrics:** 3-4mg/kg qd at 1mg/kg/hr over 2 hrs.
	Amphotericin B Lipid Complex (Abelcet)	**Adults/Pediatrics ≥16 yrs:** 5mg/kg at 2.5mg/kg/hr.
	Caspofungin (Cancidas)	**Adults: LD:** 70mg slow IV infusion over 1 hr on Day 1. **MD:** 50mg IV qd. **Pediatrics:** (3 months-17 yrs): **LD:** 70mg/m² slow IV infusion over 1 hr on Day 1. **MD:** 50mg/m² qd. **Max:** LD and MD should not exceed 70mg.
	Itraconazole (Sporanox)	**Adults:** 200-400mg PO qd for a minimum of 3 months and until infection subsides.
	Posaconazole (Noxafil)	**Adults/Pediatrics ≥13 yrs:** 200mg PO tid. Duration of treatment based on neutropenia/immunosuppression.
CANDIDIASIS		
Prevention/Treatment	Amphotericin B Liposome (AmBisome)	**Adults/Pediatrics:** 3-5mg/kg/day IV controlled infusion over 1-2 hrs.
	Amphotericin B Lipid Complex (Abelcet)	**Adults/Pediatrics ≥16 yrs:** 5mg/kg at 2.5mg/kg/hr.
	Anidulafungin (Eraxis)	**Esophageal: Adults: LD:** 100mg IV at rate of no more than 1.1mg/min on Day 1. **MD:** 50mg IV qd for a minimum of 14 days and for at least 7 days following resolution of symptoms.
	Caspofungin (Cancidas)	**Adults: LD:** 70mg slow IV infusion over 1 hr on Day 1. **MD:** 50mg IV qd. **Esophageal:** 50mg/day slow IV infusion over 1 hr. For 7-14 days after symptoms resolution. **Pediatrics:** (3 months-17 yrs): **LD:** 70mg/m² slow IV infusion over 1 hr on Day 1. **MD:** 50mg/m² qd. **Max:** LD and MD should not exceed 70mg.
	Fluconazole (Diflucan)†	**Oropharyngeal: Adults:** 200mg PO Day 1, then 100mg qd for at least 2 weeks. **Pediatrics:** 6mg/kg Day 1, then 3mg/kg qd q2 weeks. **Esophageal: Adults:** 200mg Day 1, then 100mg qd for a minimum of 3 weeks and for at least 2 weeks after resolution of symptoms. **Max:** 400mg/day. **Pediatrics:** 6mg/kg Day 1, then 3mg/kg qd for a minimum of 3 weeks and for at least 2 weeks following resolution of symptoms. **Max:** 12mg/kg/day.
	Itraconazole (Sporanox)	**Oropharyngeal: Adults:** Swish and swallow 200mg (20mL) oral solution qd x 1-2 weeks. **Esophageal: Adults:** 200mg qd x 14-21 days.
	Micafungin (Mycamine)	**Esophageal: Adults:** 150mg IV qd over 1 hr x 10-30 days.
	Posaconazole (Noxafil)	**Oropharyngeal: ≥13 yrs:** 100mg bid Day 1, then 100mg qd x 13d. **Refractory to fluconazole:** 400mg bid. Duration of therapy individualized.
	Voriconazole (Vfend)*	**Esophageal: Adults: ≥40kg:** 200mg PO q12h. <40kg: 100mg PO q12h. For a minimum of 14 days and for at least 7 days following resolution of symptoms.

(Continued)

HIV/AIDS DISEASE-RELATED COMPLICATIONS	GENERIC (BRAND)	RECOMMENDED DOSAGE
CMV RETINITIS		
Treatment	Cidofovir (Vistide)†	**Adults:** Induction: 5mg/kg IV infusion over 1 hr q week x 2 weeks. **Maint:** 5mg/kg IV over 1 hr q2 weeks.
	Foscarnet†	**Adults:** Induction: 90mg/kg over 1.5-2 hrs IV infusion q12h or 60mg/kg 1 hr IV infusion q8h x 2-3 weeks. **Maint:** 90-120mg/kg/day IV over 2 hrs.
	Ganciclovir (Cytovene)†	**Adults:** Induction: 5mg/kg IV over 1hr q12h x 14-21days. **Maint:** 5mg/kg IV over 1 hr qd x 7 days/week or 6mg/kg IV qd x 5 days/week.
	Ganciclovir (Vitrasert)	**Adults/Pediatrics ≥9 yrs:** One implant q5-8 months.
	Valganciclovir (Valcyte)	**Adults:** Induction: 900mg PO bid x 21 days w/ food. **Maint:** 900mg PO qd w/ food.
CRYPTOCOCCAL MENINGITIS		
Treatment	Amphotericin B Liposome (AmBisome)	**Adults:** 6mg/kg/day IV over 1-2 hrs.
	Fluconazole (Diflucan)	**Adults:** 400mg on Day 1, then 200-400mg qd x 10-12 weeks after the cerebrospinal fluid becomes culture negative. For suppression of relapse: 200mg qd. **Pediatrics:** 12mg/kg on Day 1, then 6-12mg/kg qd x 10-12 weeks after the cerebrospinal fluid becomes culture negative. For suppression of relapse: 6mg/kg qd.
HSV		
Recommended Regimen for Daily Suppressive Therapy	Acyclovir or Famciclovir (Famvir) or Valacyclovir	400-800mg PO bid-tid. 500mg PO bid. 1000mg PO bid.
Recommended Regimen for Episodic Infection	Acyclovir or Famiciclovir† or Valacyclovir	400mg PO tid x 5-10 days. 500mg PO bid x 5-10 days. 1g PO bid x 5-10 days.
KAPOSI'S SARCOMA		
Treatment	Alitretinoin (Panretin)	**0.1% gel: Adults: Initial:** Apply bid to lesions. Can increase to tid-qid based on individual lesion tolerance.
	Daunorubicin (DaunoXome)±	**Adults:** 40mg/m² IV over 60 min q2 weeks.
	Doxorubicin (Doxil)	**Adults:** 20mg/m² IV q3 weeks. Initial rate: 1mg/min. May be increased to administer over 1 hr if tolerated.
	Interferon alfa-2b (Intron A)†	**Adults:** 30 MIU/m²/dose SQ/IM tiw until max response achieved after 16 weeks.
	Paclitaxel (Taxol)	**Adults:** 135mg/m² IV over 3 hrs q3 weeks or 100mg/m2 IV over 3 hrs q2 weeks. Dose Intensity: 45-50mg/m²/week.
MAC		
Prevention/Treatment	Azithromycin (Zithromax)	**Adults:** Prevention: 1200mg once weekly. Treatment: 600mg PO qd with ethambutol 15mg/kg PO qd.
Prevention/Treatment	Clarithromycin (Biaxin)	**Adults:** 500mg PO bid. **Pediatrics:** 7.5mg/kg bid up to 500mg bid.
Prevention	Rifabutin (Mycobutin)†	**Adults:** 300mg PO qd. N/V/GI upset: 150mg bid w/ food.
PCP		
Prevention/Treatment	Atovaquone (Mepron)	**Adults/Pediatrics ≥13 yrs:** Prevention: 1500mg PO qd w/ meals. **Adults/Pediatrics ≥13 yrs:** Treatment (mild-moderate): 750mg PO bid w/ meals x 21 days. TDD: 1500mg.
	TMP/SMX (Bactrim)	**Adults/Pediatrics:** Treatment: 15-20mg/kg/day TMP and 75-100mg/kg/day SMX in divided doses q6h x 14-21days.
	TMP/SMX DS (Bactrim DS)	**Adults:** Prevention: 1 DS tab (160/800mg) qd. **Pediatrics:** Prevention: 150mg/m²/day TMP with 750mg/m²/day SMX PO bid in equally divided doses on 3 consecutive days/week. TDD: 1600mg SMX/320mg TMP.

(Continued)

HIV/AIDS DISEASE-RELATED COMPLICATIONS	GENERIC (BRAND)	RECOMMENDED DOSAGE
VISCERAL LEISHMANIASIS		
Treatment	Amphotericin B Liposome (AmBisome)	**Adults:** Immunocompetent: 3mg/kg/day IV Days 1-5, then on Days 14 and 21. Immunocompromised: 4mg/kg/day IV Days 1-5, then on Days 10, 17, 24, 31, and 38.
WEIGHT LOSS		
Anorexia	Dronabinol (Marinol)	**Adults:** 2.5mg PO bid; before lunch and hs. **Max:** 20mg/day in divided doses.
Anorexia, cachexia, unexplained weight loss	Megesterol (Megace)	**Adults:** Initial: 800mg/d. **Usual:** 400-800mg/day.
Cachexia/Wasting	Somatropin (Serostim)	**Adults:** >55kg: 6mg SQ qhs. 45-55kg: 5mg SQ qhs. 35-45kg: 4mg SQ qhs. <35kg: 0.1mg/kg SQ qhs. **Max:** 6mg/day.

Abbreviations: CMV=cytomegalovirus; HSV=herpes simplex virus; MAC=*Mycobacterium avium* complex; PCP=*Pneumocystis carinii* pneumonia.
*Use cautiously in patients on protease inhibitors and efavirenz.
†For dosing in special populations, see the complete prescribing information.
±Withhold therapy if the absolute granulocyte count is less than 750 cells/mm^3
Sources: Prescribing information; Guidelines for prevention and treatment of opportunistic infections in HIV-infected adults and adolescents. MMWR; Vol 59, No. RR-12. April 10, 2009.

MANAGEMENT OF HEPATITIS B

BRAND NAME (GENERIC)	HOW SUPPLIED	DOSAGE	COMMENTS
Acyclic Nucleotide Analog			
Hepsera (Adefovir dipivoxil)	**Tab:** 10mg	**Adults/Pediatrics ≥12 yrs:** 10mg QD PO without regard to food.	Renal Impairment: CrCl 30-49mL/min: 10mg q48h. CrCl 10-29mL/min: 10mg q72h. Hemodialysis Patients: 10mg every 7 days following dialysis.
Biological Response Modifier			
Intron-A (Interferon alfa-2b, recombinant)	**Inj:** 10 MIU, 18 MIU, 50 MIU [Powder], 3 MIU/0.2mL, 5 MIU/0.2mL, 10 MIU/0.2mL [Pen], 3MIU/0.5mL, 5MIU/0.5mL [Vial]	**Adults ≥18 yrs:** IM/SQ: 30-35 MIU per week; 5 MIU 3x/week or 10 MIU IM/SQ 3x/week for 16 weeks. **Pediatrics 1-17yrs:** 3 MIU/m² SQ 3x/week for 1 week, then 6 MIU/m² 3x/week (max 10 MIU/m²) for total therapy of 16-24 weeks.	Adjust dose according to severe adverse reactions and laboratory abnormalities (See PI for more information). Reduce dose by 50% or stop therapy with severe reactions. Adjust based on WBC, granulocyte, and/or platelet counts.
Guanosine Nucleoside Analogue			
Baraclude (Entecavir)	**Sol:** 0.05mg/mL; **Tab:** 0.5mg, 1mg	**Adults/Pediatrics >16 yrs:** Compensated Liver Disease; Nucleoside-Treatment-Naive: 0.5mg qd. CrCl 30 to <50mL/min: 0.25mg qd or 0.5mg q48h. CrCl 10 to <30mL/min: 0.15mg qd or 0.5mg q72h. CrCl <10mL/min, hemodialysis or peritoneal dialysis: 0.05mg qd or 0.5mg q7 days. History of Hepatitis B Viremia while receiving Lamivudine or Known Lamivudine or Telbivudine Resistance Mutation: 1mg qd. CrCl 30 to <50mL/min: 0.5mg qd or 1mg q48h. CrCl 10 to <30mL/min: 0.3mg qd or 1mg q72h. CrCl <10mL/min, hemodialysis or peritoneal dialysis: 0.1mg qd or 1mg q7 days. Decompensated liver disease: 1mg qd.	Take on empty stomach (at least 2 hrs after a meal and 2 hrs before next meal).
Immune Globulin			
Nabi-HB (Hepatitis B immune globulin, human)	**Inj:** >312 IU/1mL, >1560 IU/5mL	**Adults:** 0.06mL/kg IM and should begin the hepatitis B vaccine series.	See PI for special populations.
Nucleoside Analogues			
Epivir-HBV (Lamivudine)	**Sol:** 5mg/mL [240mL]; **Tab:** 100mg	**Adults:** 100mg qd. CrCl 30-49mL/min: 100mg Day 1, then 50mg qd. CrCl: 15-29mL/min: 100mg Day 1, then 25mg qd. CrCl 5-14mL/min: 35mg Day 1, then 15mg qd. CrCl <5mL/min: 35mg Day 1, then 10mg qd. **Pediatrics 2-17 yrs:** 3mg/kg qd. Max: 100mg/day.	

(Continued)

BRAND NAME (GENERIC)	HOW SUPPLIED	DOSAGE	COMMENTS
Nucleoside Analogues *(Continued)*			
Tyzeka (Telbivudine)	**Tab:** 600mg; **Sol:** 100mg/5mL [300mL]	**Adults/Pediatrics ≥16 yrs: Tab:** CrCL ≥50mL/min: 600mg qd. CrCL 30-49mL/min: 600mg every 48 hrs. CrCL <30mL/min (not requiring dialysis): 600mg every 72 hrs. ESRD: 600mg every 96 hrs. **Sol:** CrCL ≥50mL/min: 30mL qd. CrCL 30-49mL/min: 20mL qd. CrCL <30mL/min (not requiring dialysis): 10mL qd. ESRD: 6mL qd.	Take with or without food. When administered on hemodialysis days, administer Tyzeka after hemodialysis.
Viread (Tenofovir disoproxil fumarate)	**Tab:** 300mg	**Adults/Pediatrics ≥12 yrs and ≥35 kgs:** 300mg qd without regard to food. Renal Impairment: CrCl 30-49mL/min: 300mg q48 hrs. CrCl 10-29mL/min: 300mg q72-96 hrs. Hemodialysis: 300mg every 7 days after approximately 12 hrs of dialysis.	
Pegylated Virus Proliferation Inhibitor			
Pegasys (Peginterferon alfa-2a)	**Inj:** Prefilled syringe: 180mcg/0.5mL; **Single Dose Vial:** 180mcg/mL	**Monotherapy:** 180mcg SQ in abdomen or thigh once weekly for 48 wks.	Adjust dose based on hematological parameters, depression severity, and renal/hepatic dysfunction (see PI for dose modifications).
Vaccines			
Engerix-B (Hepatitis B vaccine [recombinant])	**Inj:** Prefilled syringes: 10mcg/0.5mL, 20mcg/mL	**Adults ≥20 yrs:** 20mcg/1mL IM at 0, 1, 6 months. Hemodialysis: 40mcg/2mL IM at 0, 1, 2, 6 months. Booster: 20mcg IM. Hemodialysis Booster: 40mcg IM. May give SQ with risk of hemorrhage. **Pediatrics ≤19 yrs:** 10mcg/0.5mL IM at 0, 1, 6 months. Booster: ≤10 yrs: 10mcg IM. ≥11 yrs: 20mcg IM.	See PI for special populations. May give SQ with risk of hemorrhage. The preferred administration site is the anterolateral aspect of the thigh for infants <1 yr and the deltoid muscle in older children and adults.
Recombivax HB, Recombivax HB Adult, Recombivax HB Dialysis, Recombivax HB Pediatric/Adolescent (Hepatitis B vaccine [recombinant])	**Inj:** Pediatric/Adolescent Formulation Preservative-Free: 5mcg/0.5mL, Adult Formulation Preservative-Free: 10mcg/1mL, Dialysis Formulation Preservative-Free: 40mcg/1mL	**Adults:** IM into deltoid muscle. If at risk of hemorrhage with IM injection, give SQ. ≥20 years (Adult Formulation): 10mcg at 0, 1, 6 months. Predialysis/Dialysis (Dialysis Formulation): 40mcg at 0, 1, 6 months; consider booster dose or revaccination if anti-HBs level <10mlU/mL 1 to 2 months after the 3rd dose. **Pediatrics:** IM injection into anterolateral thigh in infants and young children. Give SQ if risk of hemorrhage following IM injection. 0-19 years (Pediatric/Adolescent Formulation): 5mcg at 0, 1, 6 months. 11-15 years (Adult Formulation): 10mcg as first dose, then 10mcg 4-6 months later.	

BRAND NAME (GENERIC)	HOW SUPPLIED	DOSAGE	COMMENTS
Combination Vaccines			
Comvax (*Haemophilus* B conjugate [Meningococcal protein conjugate] and Hepatitis B [recombinant] vaccine)	**Inj:** 7.5mcg PRP polysaccaride conjugated to about 125mcg OMPC and 5 mcg HBsAg [0.5mL]	**Pediatrics ≥6 weeks:** 0.5mL IM at 2, 4, and 12-15 months of age. If schedule cannot be followed, wait at least 6 wks between 1st 2 doses. The 2nd and 3rd dose should be close to 8-11 months apart.	See PI for special populations.
Pediarix (Diphtheria and tetanus toxoids and acellular pertussis adsorbed, Hepatitis B [recombinant] and Inactivated poliovirus vaccine combined)	**Inj:** 0.5mL	**Pediatrics ≥6 weeks to <7 yrs:** 3 doses of 0.5mL IM at 2, 4, and 6 months of age (at 6-8 wk intervals). Start at 2 months old or as early as 6 wks old.	Preferred site is anterolateral aspect of the thigh for children <1yr. In older children, deltoid muscle. May use to complete primary series in infants who have received 1 or 2 doses of Infanrix or IPV or to complete a hepatitis B vaccine (recombinant) series. Not recommended for completion of the first 3 doses of the DTaP vaccination series initiated with a DTaP vaccine from a different manufacturer.
Twinrix Hepatitis A inactivated & Hepatitis B [recombinant] vaccine)	**Inj:** (Hepatitis A-Hepatitis B) 720 ELISA U-20mcg/mL [1.0mL]	**Adults ≥18 yrs:** 3-Dose Schedule: 1mL IM in deltoid region at 0, 1, and 6 months. Alternative 4-Dose Schedule: 1 mL IM in deltoid region on Days 0, 7, and 21-30, followed by booster dose at 12 months.	

MANAGEMENT OF HEPATITIS C

BRAND NAME (GENERIC)	HOW SUPPLIED	DOSAGE	COMMENTS
Biological Response Modifiers			
Infergen (Interferon alfacon-1)	**Inj:** 9mcg/0.3mL, 15mcg/0.5mL	**Adults ≥18 yrs:** 9mcg 3x/week (TIW) SQ for 24 wks. If No Response or Relapse: 15mcg TIW SQ as a single injection for up to 48 wks.	Hold dose temporarily in presence of severe adverse effects and reduce to 7.5mcg.
Intron-A (Interferon alfa-2b, recombinant)	**Inj:** 10 MIU, 18 MIU, 50 MIU **[Powder]**, 3 MIU/0.2mL, 5 MIU/0.2mL, 10 MIU/0.2mL **[Pen]**, 3MIU/0.5mL, 5MIU/0.5mL **[Vial]**	**Adults ≥18 yrs:** 3 MIU IM/SQ TIW for 18-24 months.	If severe adverse reactions develop, reduce dose by 50% or temporarily stop therapy.
Nucleoside Analog			
Copegus (Ribavirin)	**Tab:** 200mg	**Adults ≥18 yrs:** Give bid in divided doses. Treat for 24-48 wks with Pegasys 180mcg. Genotypes 1 and 4: <75kg: 1000mg/day for 48 wks. ≥75kg: 1200mg/day for 48 wks. Genotypes 2 and 3: 800mg/day for 24 wks. HCV/HIV: 800mg PO QD. Treat for 48 wks with Pegasys 180mcg SQ once weekly.	**Dose Modifications:** Reduce to 600mg/day for Copegus if Hgb <10g/dL with no cardiac history, or if Hgb decreases by ≥2g/dL during a 4-week period with stable cardiac disease. D/C Copegus if Hgb <8.5g/dL with no cardiac history or if Hgb <12g/dL after 4 wks of dose reduction with stable cardiac disease. After dose modification, may restart Copegus at 600mg/day, then may increase to 800mg/day. CrCl <50mL/min: Avoid use.
Rebetol (Ribavirin)	**Cap:** 200mg; **Sol:** 40mg/mL [100mL]	**Adults ≥18 yrs:** With Intron A: ≤75kg: 400mg qam and 600mg qpm PO. >75kg: 600mg qam and 600mg qpm PO. Treat for 24-48 wks in interferon-naive patients. In relapsed patients, treat for 24 wks. With Peg-Intron: use in divided doses. ≤65kg: 800mg/day (400mg qam and 400mg qpm). 66-80kg: 1000mg/day (400mg qam and 600mg qpm). 81-105kg: 1200mg/day (600mg qam and 600mg qpm). >105kg: 1400mg/day (600mg qam and 800mg qpm). **Pediatrics ≥3 yrs:** Use in divided doses qam and qpm. <47kg: 15mg/kg/day (use oral solution). 47-59kg: 800mg/day (400mg qam and 400mg qpm). 60-73kg: 1g/day (400mg qam and 600mg qpm). >73kg: 1.2g/day (600mg qam and 600mg qpm). Genotype 1: Treat for 48 wks. Genotype 2/3: Treat for 24 wks. See PI for more detailed dosage information.	**Adults:** Reduce by 200mg/day (or 400mg/day if receiving 1400mg dose) and by 200mg/day again, if needed, if Hgb <10g/dL with no cardiac history. Reduce by 200mg/day if Hgb decreases by ≥2g/dL during a 4 week-period with a cardiac history. **Adults/Peds:** D/C if Hgb <8.5g/dL with no cardiac history or if Hgb <12g/dL after 4 wks of dose reduction with a cardiac history. CrCl <50mL/min: Avoid use.

(Continued)

BRAND NAME (GENERIC)	HOW SUPPLIED	DOSAGE	COMMENTS
Nucleoside Analog *(Continued)*			
Ribasphere (Ribavirin)	**Tab:** 200mg, 400mg, 600mg; **Cap:** 200mg	**Adults ≥18 yrs:** Give bid in divided doses. Treat for 24-48 wks with Pegasys 180mcg. Genotypes 1 and 4: <75kg: 1000mg/day for 48 wks. ≥75kg: 1200mg/day for 48 wks. Genotypes 2 and 3: 800mg/day for 24 wks. HCV/HIV: 800mg PO QD. Treat for 48 wks with Pegasys 180mcg SQ once weekly.	**Dose Modifications:** Reduce to 600mg/day for Ribasphere if Hgb <10g/dL with no cardiac history, or if Hgb decreases by ≥2g/dL during a 4-week period with stable cardiac disease. D/C Ribasphere if Hgb <8.5g/dL with no cardiac history or if Hgb <12g/dL after 4 wks of dose reduction with stable cardiac disease. After dose modification, may restart Ribasphere at 600mg/day, then may increase to 800mg/day. CrCl <50mL/min: Avoid use.
Pegylated Virus Proliferation Inhibitor			
Pegasys (Peginterferon alfa-2a)	**Inj:** Prefilled syringe: 180mcg/0.5mL; Single Dose Vial: 180mcg/mL	**Adults ≥18 yrs:** Monotherapy: 180mcg SQ (in abdomen or thigh) once weekly for 48 weeks. Combination Therapy With Copegus: 180mcg SQ once weekly for 24 weeks with Genotypes 2 and 3 or 48 wks with Genotypes 1 and 4. HCV/HIV: Monotherapy: 180mcg SQ in abdomen or thigh once weekly for 48 weeks. Combination Therapy with Copegus: 180mcg SQ once weekly for 48 wks, regardless of genotype.	Adjust dose based on hematological parameters and depression severity (see PI for dose modifications).
PegIntron (Peginterferon alpha-2b)	**Inj:** 50mcg/0.5mL, 80mcg/0.5mL, 120mcg/0.5mL, 150mcg/0.5mL	**Adults ≥18 yrs:** Monotherapy: 1mcg/kg/wk SQ for 1 yr administered on the same day of the week. Combination Therapy With Rebetol: 1.5mcg/kg/wk plus Rebetol 800-1400mg/day PO based on patient's body weight for 48 wks in Genotype 1, and 24 wks in Genotype 2 and 3 patients. CrCl <50mL/min: D/C therapy. Adjust dose based on hematological parameters and depression severity (see PI for dose modifications). **Pediatrics 3-17 yrs:** Combination Therapy With Rebetol: 60mcg/m²/wk SQ plus Rebetol 15mg/kg/day in 2 divided doses for 48 wks in Genotype 1, and 24 weeks in Genotype 2 and 3 patients.	**Adults:** Renal Impairment: CrCl 30-50mL/min: Reduce PegIntron dose by 25%. CrCl 10-29mL/min: Reduce PegIntron dose by 50%. D/C therapy if renal function decreases, if there is not at least a 2 $\log_{10}$ drop or loss of HCV-RNA at 12 wks, or whose HCV-RNA levels remain detectable after 24 wks of therapy. CrCl <50mL/min: D/C therapy. Adjust dose based on hematological parameters and depression severity (see PI for dose modifications). **Pediatrics:** Renal Impairment: CrCl 30-50mL/min: Reduce PegIntron dose by 25%. CrCl 10-29mL/min: Reduce PegIntron dose by 50%. D/C if renal function decreases, HCV-RNA dropped <2 $\log_{10}$ at 12 wks, or HCV-RNA levels remain detectable after 24 wks.

ORAL AND SYSTEMIC ANTIBIOTICS

DRUG	BRAND	HOW SUPPLIED	INDICATIONS
AMINOGLYCOSIDES			
Amikacin sulfate	Amikacin	**Inj:** 50mg/mL, 250mg/mL	Short-term treatment of serious infections caused by gram-negative bacteria such as septicemia, and respiratory tract, bone/joint, CNS (including meningitis), skin and soft tissue, and intra-abdominal infections; burns and postoperative infections; complicated and recurrent urinary tract infections (UTI); and staphylococcal disease. Concomitant therapy with a penicillin-type drug as treatment of certain severe infections such as neonatal sepsis.
Gentamicin sulfate		**Inj:** 10mg/mL, 40mg/mL	Treatment of bacterial neonatal sepsis, bacterial septicemia, and serious bacterial infections of the CNS (meningitis), urinary tract, respiratory tract, GI tract (including peritonitis), skin, bone and soft tissue (including burns) caused by susceptible strains of microorganisms.
Streptomycin sulfate		**Inj:** 1g	Treatment of moderate to severe infections such as mycobacterium tuberculosis (TB) and non-TB infections (eg, plague, tularemia, chancroid, brucella, donovanosis, granuloma inguinale, *H. influenzae* infections, *K. pneumoniae* pneumonia, UTI, gram-negative bacillary bacteremia, endocardial infections).
Tobramycin	TOBI	**Sol:** 60mg/mL (300mg/ampule)	Management of cystic fibrosis patients with *P. aeruginosa*.
Tobramycin sulfate		**Inj:** l0mg/mL, 40mg/mL, 1.2g	Treatment of infections including serious lower respiratory tract, CNS (eg, meningitis), intra-abdominal, bone, skin and skin structure, and complicated/recurrent UTIs; and septicemia caused by susceptible strains of microorganisms.
CARBAPENEMS			
Doripenem	Doribax	**Inj:** 250mg, 500mg	Treatment of infections such as complicated intra-abdominal infections and UTIs, including pyelonephritis, caused by susceptible microorganisms.
Ertapenem sodium	Invanz	**Inj:** 1g	Treatment of complicated intra-abdominal infections, SSSI (including diabetic foot infections without osteomyelititis), CAP, complicated UTI (including pyelonephritis), and acute pelvic infections (including postpartum endomyometritis, septic abortion, and post surgical gynecologic infections); also used in prophylaxis of surgical-site infection following elective colorectal surgery.
Meropenem	Merrem	**Inj:** 500mg, 1g	Treatment of intra-abdominal infections, bacterial meningitis (in pediatric patients ≥3 months), and complicated SSSI caused by susceptible strains of microorganisms.
CEPHALOSPORINS, FIRST GENERATION			
Cefadroxil monohydrate		**Cap:** 500mg; **Sus:** 250mg/5mL [50mL, 100mL], 500mg/5mL [50mL, 75mL, 100mL]; **Tab:** 1g	Treatment of SSSI and UTI, pharyngitis, and tonsillitis.
Cefazolin sodium		**Inj:** 500mg, 1g, 10g, 20g	Treatment of respiratory tract, UTI, SSSI, biliary tract, bone and joint, and genital infections, septicemia, and endocarditis caused by susceptible strains of microorganisms. Perioperative prophylaxis for surgical procedures classified as contaminated or potentially contaminated.
Cephalexin	Keflex	**Cap:** 250mg, 500mg, 750mg; (Generic) **Sus:** 125mg/5mL, 250mg/5mL [100mL, 200mL]; **Tab:** 250mg, 500mg	Treatment of otitis media and SSSI; bone, genitourinary tract, and respiratory tract infections.

(Continued)

DRUG	BRAND	HOW SUPPLIED	INDICATIONS
CEPHALOSPORINS, SECOND GENERATION			
Cefaclor		**Cap:** 250mg, 500mg; **Sus:** 125mg/5mL [75mL, 150mL], 187mg/5mL [50mL, 100mL], 250mg/5mL [75mL, 150mL], 375mg/5mL [50mL, 100mL]	Treatment of otitis media, pharyngitis, tonsillitis, lower respiratory tract infections, UTI, and SSSI caused by susceptible strains of microorganisms.
Cefaclor ER		**Tab, Extended-Release:** 500mg	Acute bacterial exacerbation of chronic bronchitis (ABECB), secondary bacterial infections of acute bronchitis, pharyngitis, tonsillitis, and uncomplicated SSSI caused by susceptible strains of microorganisms.
Cefotetan		**Inj:** 1g, 2g, 10g	Treatment of SSSI, UTI, lower respiratory tract, gynecologic, intra-abdominal, bone and joint infections, and surgical prophylaxis. May use with an aminoglycoside for sepsis or other serious infections in which causative organism has not been identified.
Cefoxitin sodium		**Inj:** 1g, 2g, 10g	Treatment of lower respiratory tract, UTI, intra-abdominal, gynecological, SSSI, and bone and joint infections, and septicemia. For surgical prophylaxis.
Cefprozil		**Sus:** 125mg/5mL, 250mg/5mL [50mL, 75mL, 100mL]; **Tab:** 250mg, 500mg	Mild to moderate pharyngitis/tonsillitis, otitis media, acute sinusitis, secondary bacterial infection of acute bronchitis, ABECB, and uncomplicated SSSI.
Cefuroxime	Zinacef	**Inj:** 750mg, 1.5g, 7.5g, 750mg/50mL, 1.5g/50mL	Treatment of septicemia; meningitis; gonorrhea; lower respiratory tract, UTI, SSSI, and bone and joint infections caused by susceptible strains of microorganisms. For preoperative and perioperative surgical prophylaxis.
Cefuroxime axetil	Ceftin	**Sus:** 125mg/5mL [100mL], 250mg/5mL [50mL, 100mL]; **Tab:** 250mg, 500mg	(Sus/Tab) Pharyngitis/tonsillitis, acute bacterial otitis media (Sus) Impetigo. (Tab) Uncomplicated SSSI and UTI, uncomplicated gonorrhea, early Lyme disease, acute bacterial maxillary sinusitis, ABECB, and secondary bacterial infections of acute bronchitis.
CEPHALOSPORINS, THIRD GENERATION			
Cefdinir		**Cap:** 300mg; **Sus:** 125mg/5mL, 250mg/5mL [60mL, 100mL]	In adults and adolescents, used to treat CAP, ABECB, acute maxillary sinusitis, pharyngitis/tonsillitis, uncomplicated SSSI; in pediatric patients, used to treat acute bacterial otitis media, pharyngitis/tonsillitis, uncomplicated SSSI.
Cefditoren pivoxil	Spectracef	**Tab:** 200mg, 400mg	Treatment of ABECB, pharyngitis/tonsillitis, CAP, and uncomplicated SSSI in adults and adolescents >12 yrs.
Cefixime	Suprax	**Sus:** 100mg/5mL [50mL, 75mL, 100mL], 200mg/5mL [25mL, 37.5mL, 50mL, 75mL, 100mL]; **Tab:** 400mg	(Sus/Tab) Pharyngitis, tonsillitis, acute bronchitis, ABECB, uncomplicated UTIs, and cervical/urethral gonorrhea caused by susceptible strains. Otitis media should be treated with suspension.
Cefotaxime sodium	Claforan	**Inj:** 500mg, 1g, 2g, 10g	Treatment of lower respiratory tract, genitourinary, gynecologic, intra-abdominal, SSSI, bone and joint, and CNS infections (eg, meningitis), as well as bacteremia and septicemia; administered preoperatively to reduce incidence of certain infection from surgical procedures (abdominal hysterectomy, GI and genitourinary tract surgery) that may be classified as contaminated/potentially contaminated; administered during cesarean section postoperatively and intraoperatively (after clamping the umbilical cord) to reduce certain postoperative infections.

(Continued)

DRUG	BRAND	HOW SUPPLIED	INDICATIONS
CEPHALOSPORINS, THIRD GENERATION *(Continued)*			
Cefpodoxime proxetil		**Sus:** 50mg/mL [50mL, 100mL], 100mg/5mL [50mL, 100mL]; **Tab:** 100mg, 200mg	Acute otitis media, pharyngitis/tonsillitis, CAP, ABECB, acute uncomplicated urethral and cervical gonorrhea, acute uncomplicated ano-rectal infections in women, uncomplicated SSSI, acute maxillary sinusitis, uncomplicated UTI.
Ceftazidime	Tazicef	**Inj:** 1g, 2g, 6g; (Generic) 500mg, 1g, 2g, 6g	Treatment of infections such as lower respiratory tract (eg, pneumonia), SSSI, bone and joint, gynecologic, CNS (eg, meningitis), intra-abdominal, and complicated and uncomplicated UTI, and bacterial septicemia. Treatment of sepsis.
Ceftazidime	Fortaz	**Inj:** 500mg, 1g, 1g/50mL, 2g, 2g/50mL, 6g	Treatment of infections such as lower respiratory tract (eg, pneumonia), SSSI, bone and joint, gynecologic, CNS (eg, meningitis), intra-abdominal, and complicated and uncomplicated UTI, and bacterial septicemia. Treatment of sepsis.
Ceftibuten	Cedax	**Cap:** 400mg; **Sus:** 90mg/5mL [60mL, 90mL, 120mL]	Treatment of individuals with mild-to-moderate infections caused by susceptible strains of the designated microorganisms in ABECB, acute bacterial otitis media, pharyngitis and tonsillitis.
Ceftriaxone sodium	Rocephin	**Inj:** 500mg, 1g; (Generic) 250mg, 500mg, 1g, 2g, 10g	Treatment of lower respiratory tract infections, SSSI, bone and joint infections, intra-abdominal infections, acute otitis media, uncomplicated gonorrhea, pelvic inflammatory disease, UTI, bacterial septicemia, and meningitis. For surgical prophylaxis.
CEPHALOSPORINS, FOURTH GENERATION			
Cefepime HCl	Maxipime	**Inj:** 500mg, 1g, 2g	Treatment of uncomplicated/complicated UTI, uncomplicated SSSI, and complicated intra-abdominal infections, and (moderate to severe) pneumonia. Empiric therapy for febrile neutropenia.
CEPHALOSPORINS, FIFTH GENERATION			
Ceftaroline fosamil	Teflaro	**Inj:** 400mg, 600mg	Treatment of acute bacterial SSSI and community-acquired bacterial pneumonia (CABP) caused by susceptible strains of microorganisms.
FLUOROQUINOLONES			
Ciprofloxacin HCl	Cipro	**Sus:** 250mg/5mL, 500mg/5mL [100mL]; **Tab:** 250mg, 500mg, 750mg	(Adults) Treatment of infections such as lower respiratory tract (LRTI), complicated intra-abdominal, SSSI, bone and joint, and UTI; acute exacerbations of chronic bronchitis, acute sinusitis, acute uncomplicated cystitis in females, chronic bacterial prostatitis, infectious diarrhea, typhoid fever, uncomplicated cervical and urethral gonorrhea; (Adults/Pediatrics): Post-exposure inhalation anthrax; (Pediatrics): Complicated UTIs and pyelonephritis.
Ciprofloxacin HCl	Proquin XR	**Tab, Extended-Release:** 500mg	Treatment of uncomplicated UTIs (acute cystitis) caused by *E. coli* and *K. pneumoniae*.
Ciprofloxacin	Cipro IV	**Inj:** 10mg/mL, 200mg/100mL, 400mg/200mL	(Adults) Treatment of SSSI, bone and joint, complicated intra-abdominal infections, LRTI, and UTI; nosocomial pneumonia, acute sinusitis, chronic bacterial prostatitis, and empirical therapy for febrile neutropenia; (Adults/Pediatrics) Post-exposure inhalation anthrax; (Pediatrics) Complicated urinary tract infections and pyelonephritis.
Ciprofloxacin	Cipro XR	**Tab, Extended-Release:** 500mg, 1000mg	Uncomplicated (acute cystitis) and complicated UTI, and acute uncomplicated pyelonephritis due to *E. coli*.
Gemifloxacin	Factive	**Tab:** 320mg	Treatment of mild to moderate CAP, including multi-drug resistant *Streptococcus pneumoniae* (MDRSP), and ABECB.

(Continued)

DRUG	BRAND	HOW SUPPLIED	INDICATIONS
FLUOROQUINOLONES *(Continued)*			
Levofloxacin	Levaquin	**Inj:** 5mg/mL, 25mg/mL; **Sol:** 25mg/mL; **Tab:** 250mg, 500mg, 750mg [Leva-pak, 5s]	Uncomplicated and complicated SSSI, uncomplicated and complicated UTI, acute bacterial sinusitis, ABECB, CAP, nosocomial pneumonia, chronic bacterial prostatitis (CBP), and acute pyelonephritis caused by susceptible strains of microorganisms. To reduce the incidence or progression of disease of inhalational anthrax following exposure to *Bacillus anthracis*.
Moxifloxacin HCl	Avelox	**Inj:** 400mg/250mL; **Tab:** 400mg	Acute bacterial sinusitis, ABECB, uncomplicated and complicated SSSI, complicated intra-abdominal infections (cIAI), and CAP (including multidrug resistant *S. pneumoniae*).
Norfloxacin	Noroxin	**Tab:** 400 mg	Treatment of adults with uncomplicated (including cystitis) and complicated UTI, prostatitis, and uncomplicated cervical and urethral gonorrhea, caused by susceptible strains of microorganisms.
Ofloxacin		**Tab:** 200mg, 300mg, 400mg	Treatment of complicated UTI and uncomplicated SSSI, ABECB, CAP, acute uncomplicated urethral and cervical gonorrhea, nongonococcal urethritis and cervicitis, mixed infections of the urethra and cervix, acute pelvic inflammatory disease (PID), uncomplicated cystitis, prostatitis.
MACROLIDES			
Azithromycin	Zithromax	**Inj:** 500mg; **Sus:** 100mg/5mL [15mL], 200mg/5mL [15mL, 22.5mL, 30mL], 1g/pkt [3s 10s]; **Tab:** 250mg [Z-Pak, 6 tabs], 500mg [Tri-Pak, 3 tabs], 600mg	(PO): 600mg tab: Treatment of nongonococcal urethritis and cervicitis due to *Chlamydia trachomatis*, as well as prophylaxis (with or without rifabutin) and treatment (in combination with ethambutol) of disseminated Mycobacterium Avium Complex disease in advanced HIV infection; 100mg/5mL, 200mg/5mL, and 250 & 500mg tabs: (Adults) Treatment of acute bacterial exacerbations of COPD, acute bacterial sinusitis (ABS), CAP, pharyngitis/tonsillitis, uncomplicated SSSI, urethritis/cervicitis, genital ulcer disease (men); (Pediatrics): Acute otitis media, pharyngitis/tonsillitis, CAP; (IV) Treatment of CAP and pelvic inflammatory disease.
Azithromycin	Zmax	**Sus, Extended-Release:** 2g	Treatment of mild to moderate acute bacterial sinusitis in adults and treatment of CAP in adults and pediatric patients (6 months and older) caused by susceptible strains of microorganisms.
Clarithromycin	Biaxin	**Sus:** 125mg/5mL, 250mg/5mL [50mL, 100mL]; **Tab:** 250mg, 500mg	(Adults) Pharyngitis/tonsillitis, acute maxillary sinusitis, ABECB, CAP, uncomplicated SSSI, disseminated mycobacterial infections, (Tab) combination therapy for *H. pylori* infection with duodenal ulcers; Mycobacterium Avium Complex (MAC) prophylaxis in advanced HIV. (Pediatrics): Pharyngitis/tonsillitis, CAP, acute maxillary sinusitis, acute otitis media, uncomplicated SSSI, disseminated mycobacterial infections, MAC prophylaxis in advanced HIV.
Clarithromycin	Biaxin XL	**Tab, Extended-Release:** 500mg [PAC 14s, 60s, 100s]	Treatment of acute maxillary sinusitis, CAP, and ABECB.
Erythromycin	ERYC	**Cap, Delayed-Release:** 250mg	Mild to moderate upper and lower RTI and SSSI, listeriosis, pertussis, diphtheria, erythrasma, intestinal amebiasis, acute pelvic inflammatory disease (PID) (*N. gonorrhoeae*), primary syphilis (caused by *Treponema pallidum*) in PCN allergy, Legionnaires' disease, chlamydial infections (eg, newborn conjunctivitis, pneumonia of infancy, urogenital infections during pregnancy, urethral, endocervical, or rectal, etc), and nongonococcal urethritis (caused by *Ureaplasma urealyticum*). Used for prevention of initial and recurrent attacks of rheumatic fever with PCN allergy.

(Continued)

DRUG	BRAND	HOW SUPPLIED	INDICATIONS
MACROLIDES *(Continued)*			
Erythromycin	Ery-Tab	**Tab, Delayed-Release:** 250mg, 333mg, 500mg	Mild to moderate upper and lower RTIs, SSSIs, listeriosis, pertussis, diphtheria, erythrasma, intestinal amebiasis, acute pelvic inflammatory disease (PID) (*N. gonorrhoeae*), primary syphilis in PCN allergy, Legionnaires' disease, chlamydial infections (eg, newborn conjunctivitis, pneumonia of infancy, urogenital infections during pregnancy, urethral, endocervical, rectal, etc), and nongonococcal urethritis (when tetracyclines are contraindicated or not tolerated). Prevention of initial and recurrent attacks of rheumatic fever with PCN allergy.
Erythromycin		**Cap, Delayed-Release:** 250mg	Mild to moderate upper and lower RTIs, SSSIs, listeriosis, pertussis, diphtheria, erythrasma, intestinal amebiasis, acute pelvic inflammatory disease (PID) (*N. gonorrhoeae*), primary syphilis in PCN allergy, Legionnaires' disease, chlamydial infections (eg, newborn conjunctivitis, pneumonia of infancy, urogenital infections during pregnancy, urethral, endocervical, rectal, etc), and nongonococcal urethritis (when tetracyclines are contraindicated or not tolerated). Prevention of initial and recurrent attacks of rheumatic fever with PCN allergy.
Erythromycin	PCE	**Tab:** 333mg, 500mg	Mild to moderate upper and lower RTIs, SSSIs, listeriosis, pertussis, diphtheria, erythrasma, intestinal amebiasis, acute pelvic inflammatory disease (PID) (*N. gonorrhoeae*), primary syphilis in PCN allergy, Legionnaires' disease, chlamydial infections (eg, newborn conjunctivitis, pneumonia of infancy, urogenital infections during pregnancy, urethral, endocervical, rectal, etc), and nongonococcal urethritis (when tetracyclines are contraindicated or not tolerated). Prevention of initial and recurrent attacks of rheumatic fever with PCN allergy.
Erythromycin Base		**Tab:** 250mg, 500mg	Mild to moderate upper and lower RTI, SSSI, listeriosis, pertussis, diphtheria, erythrasma, intestinal amebiasis, acute pelvic inflammatory disease (PID) (*N. gonorrhoeae*), primary syphilis in PCN allergy, Legionnaires' disease, chlamydial infections (eg, newborn conjunctivitis, pneumonia of infancy, urogenital infections during pregnancy, urethral, endocervical, rectal, etc), and nongonococcal urethritis (when tetracyclines are contraindicated or not tolerated). Prevention of initial and recurrent attacks of rheumatic fever with PCN allergy.
Erythromycin ethylsuccinate	E.E.S.	**Sus (in liquid and granule premix form):** 200mg/5mL, 400mg/5mL (100mL, 480mL); **Tab:** 400mg	Mild to moderate upper and lower RTIs, SSSI, listeriosis, pertussis, diphtheria, erythrasma, intestinal amebiasis, acute pelvic inflammatory disease (PID) (*N. gonorrhoeae*), primary syphilis in PCN allergy, Legionnaires' disease, chlamydial infections (eg, newborn conjunctivitis, pneumonia of infancy, urogenital infections during pregnancy, urethral, endocervical, rectal, etc), and nongonococcal urethritis (when tetracyclines are contraindicated or not tolerated). Prevention of initial and recurrent attacks of rheumatic fever with PCN allergy.
Erythromycin ethylsuccinate	EryPed	**Sus:** 200mg/5mL, 400mg/5mL [5mL, 100mL, 200mL]; **(Drops)** 200mg/5mL [50mL]	Mild to moderate upper and lower RTI, SSSI, listeriosis, pertussis, diphtheria, erythrasma, intestinal amebiasis, acute pelvic inflammatory disease (PID) (*N. gonorrhoeae*), primary syphilis in PCN allergy, Legionnaires' disease, chlamydial infections (eg, newborn conjunctivitis, pneumonia of infancy, urogenital infections during pregnancy, urethral, endocervical, rectal, etc), and nongonococcal urethritis (when tetracyclines are contraindicated or not tolerated). Prevention of initial and recurrent attacks of rheumatic fever with PCN allergy.

(Continued)

DRUG	BRAND	HOW SUPPLIED	INDICATIONS
MACROLIDES *(Continued)*			
Erythromycin ethylsuccinate/ Sulfisoxazole acetyl		**Sus:** 200mg-600mg/ 5mL [100mL, 150mL, 200mL]	For treatment of acute otitis media in children that is caused by susceptible strains of *Haemophilus influenzae.*
Erythromycin lactobionate	Erythrocin	**Inj:** 500mg, 1g	Mild to moderate upper and lower RTIs, SSSI, diphtheria, erythrasma, acute pelvic inflammatory disease (PID) (*N. gonorrhoeae*), and Legionnaires' disease. Prevention of initial attacks of rheumatic fever with PCN allergy.
Erythromycin stearate	Erythrocin	**Tab:** 250mg, 500mg	Mild to moderate upper and lower RTIs, SSSI, listeriosis, pertussis, diphtheria, erythrasma, intestinal amebiasis, acute pelvic inflammatory disease (PID) (*N. gonorrhoeae*), primary syphilis in PCN allergy, Legionnaires' disease, chlamydial infections (eg, newborn conjunctivitis, pneumonia of infancy, urogenital infections during pregnancy, urethral, endocervical, rectal, etc), and nongonococcal urethritis (when tetracyclines are contraindicated or not tolerated). Prevention of initial and recurrent attacks of rheumatic fever with PCN allergy.
MONOBACTAM			
Aztreonam	Azactam	**Inj:** 1g, 2g, 1g/50mL, 2g/50mL	Treatment of septicemia and lower RTIs (eg, pneumonia, bronchitis), SSSIs (eg, postoperative wounds, ulcers, burns), complicated/uncomplicated UTIs including pyelonephritis and initial/ recurrent cystitis, gynecologic infections (eg, endometritis, pelvic cellulitis), and intra-abdominal (eg, peritonitis) infections caused by susceptible microorganisms. Adjunct therapy to surgery for management of infections caused by susceptible microorganisms (eg, abscesses, hollow viscus perforation infections, cutaneous infections, infections of serous surfaces).
Aztreonam	Cayston	**Sol (for inhalation):** 75mg/vial (Lyophilized)	To improve respiratory symptoms in cystic fibrosis patients with *Pseudomonas aeruginosa.*
PENICILLINS			
Amoxicillin		**Cap:** 250mg, 500mg; **Sus:** 125mg/5mL [80mL, 100mL, 150mL], 200mg/5mL [50mL, 75mL, 100mL], 250mg/5mL [80mL, 100mL, 150mL], 400mg/5mL [50mL, 75mL, 100mL]; **Tab:** 500mg, 875mg; **Tab, Chewable:** 125mg, 200mg, 250mg, 400mg; **Tab, Dispersible:** 200mg, 400mg	Infections of the ear, nose, throat, genitourinary tract, SSSI, and lower RTI due to susceptible (beta-lactamase negative) organisms, as well as gonorrhea (acute, uncomplicated). Also used in combination therapy for *H. pylori* eradication to reduce the risk of duodenal ulcer recurrence.
Amoxicillin	Moxatag	**Tab, Extended Release:** 775mg	Treatment of tonsillitis and/or pharyngitis secondary to *Streptococcus pyogenes* in adults and pediatric patients ≥12 yrs.
Amoxicillin-Clavulanate potassium	Augmentin	**(Amoxicillin-Clavulanate) Sus:** 125-31.25mg/5mL [75mL, 100mL, 150mL] (Generic) 200-28.5mg/ 5mL [50mL, 75mL, 100mL], 250-62.5mg/ 5mL [75mL, 100mL, 150mL], (Generic) 400-57mg/ 5mL [50mL, 75mL, 100mL]; **Tab:** 250-125mg, 500-125mg, 875-125mg; (Generic) **Tab, Chewable:** 200-28.5mg, 400-57mg	Treatment of lower RTI, SSSI, and UTI, as well as otitis media and sinusitis.

(Continued)

DRUG	BRAND	HOW SUPPLIED	INDICATIONS
PENICILLINS (Continued)			
Amoxicillin-Clavulanate potassium		**Sus:** (Amoxicillin-Clavulanate) 600mg-42.9mg/5mL [75mL, 125mL, 200mL]	Treatment of pediatric patients with recurrent or persistent acute otitis media.
Amoxicillin-Clavulanate potassium	Augmentin XR	**Tab, Extended-Release:** (Amoxicillin-Clavulanate) 1000mg-62.5mg	Treatment of CAP or acute bacterial sinusitis due to confirmed or suspected β-lactamase producing pathogens and *S. pneumoniae* with reduced susceptibility to penicillin.
Ampicillin		**Cap:** 250mg, 500mg; **Sus:** 125mg/5mL, 250mg/5mL [100mL, 200mL]	Treatment of meningitis, and infections of genitourinary tract (GU) (including gonorrhea), respiratory tract, and GI tract caused by susceptible strains of microorganisms.
Ampicillin sodium	Ampicillin	**Inj:** 125mg, 250mg, 500mg, 1g, 2g, 10g	Treatment of respiratory tract, urinary tract, and GI infections, bacterial meningitis, septicemia, endocarditis.
Ampicillin sodium/Sulbactam sodium	Unasyn	**Inj:** (Ampicillin-Sulbactam) 1g-0.5g, 2g-1g, 10g-5g	Treatment of SSSI, intra-abdominal, and gynecological infections caused by susceptible microorganisms.
Dicloxacillin sodium		**Cap:** 250mg, 500mg	Infections caused by penicillinase-producing staphylococci.
Penicillin G benzathine-Penicillin G procaine	Bicillin C-R	**Inj:** (Penicillin G Benzathine-Penicillin G Procaine) 600,000-600,000 U/2mL	Treatment of moderately severe to severe URTI and skin and soft-tissue infections (SSTI), scarlet fever and erysipelas due to streptococci. Treatment of moderately severe pneumonia and otitis media due to pneumococci.
Penicillin G benzathine-Penicillin G procaine	Bicillin C-R 900/300	**Inj:** (Penicillin G Benzathine-Penicillin G Procaine) 900,000-300,000 U/2mL	Treatment of moderately severe to severe URTI and SSTI, scarlet fever and erysipelas due to streptococci. Treatment of moderately severe pneumonia and otitis media due to pneumococci.
Penicillin G benzathine	Bicillin L-A	**Inj:** 600,000 U/mL, 1,200,000 U/2mL, 2,400,000 U/4mL	Treatment of mild to moderate URTI due to streptococci, and venereal infections (eg, syphilis, yaws, bejel, pinta); prophylaxis to prevent recurrence of rheumatic fever or chorea. As follow-up prophylactic therapy for rheumatic heart disease and acute glomerulonephritis.
Penicillin G benzathine	Permapen	**Inj:** 600,000 U/mL	Treatment of microorganisms susceptible to low and very prolonged serum levels in upper respiratory tract infections (streptococci group A, without bacteremia), syphilis, yaws, bejel, and pinta; prophylaxis for rheumatic fever and/or chorea. Follow-up prophylactic therapy for rheumatic heart disease and acute glomerulonephritis.
Penicillin G potassium	Pfizerpen	**Inj:** 5 MU, 20 MU	For therapy of severe infections when rapid and and high blood levels of penicillin required. Management of streptococcal, pneumococcal, staphylococcal, clostridial, fusospirochetal, listeria, gram negative bacillary, and pasteurella infections. For anthrax, actinomycosis, diphtheria, erysipeloid endocarditis, meningitis (including meningococci), endocarditis, bacteremia, rat-bite fever, syphilis, and gonorrheal endocarditis and arthritis; with combined oral therapy, prophylaxis against endocarditis in patients with congenital heart disease, rheumatic disease, or other acquired valvular heart disease undergoing dental procedures or surgical procedures of upper respiratory tract.
Penicillin V potassium	Penicillin VK	**Sus:** 125mg/5mL, 250mg/5mL [100mL, 200mL]; **Tab:** 250mg, 500mg	Mild to moderately severe bacterial infections including scarlet fever, mild erysipelas, mild to moderate infections of the respiratory tract, mild to moderately severe oropharynx infections, and mild infections of skin and soft tissue. Prevention of recurrence following rheumatic fever and/or chorea. May be useful as prophylaxis against bacterial endocarditis in patients with congenital heart disease or rheumatic or other acquired valvular heart disease who are undergoing dental procedures and surgical procedures of the upper respiratory tract.

(Continued)

DRUG	BRAND	HOW SUPPLIED	INDICATIONS
PENICILLINS *(Continued)*			
Piperacillin		**Inj:** 2g, 3g, 4g, 40g	Treatment of serious intra-abdominal, urinary tract, gynecologic, lower respiratory tract, SSSI, bone and joint, and uncomplicated gonococcal infections; septicemia, and perioperative surgical prophylaxis.
Piperacillin sodium/ Tazobactam sodium	Zosyn	**Inj:** 2g-0.25g, 3g-0.375g, 4g-0.5g, 2g-0.25g/50mL, 3g-0.375g/50mL, 4g-0.5g/100mL, 36g-4.5g	Treatment of appendicitis, peritonitis, uncomplicated/complicated SSSIs, postpartum endometritis, pelvic inflammatory disease, moderate severity of CAP, and moderate to severe nosocomial pneumonia.
Ticarcillin-Clavulanate potassium	Timentin	**Inj:** (Ticarcillin-Clavulanate) 3g-100mg, 30g-1g	Treatment of lower respiratory tract, bone and joint, SSS, uncomplicated/complicated UTI, gynecologic, and intra-abdominal infections, as well as septicemia.
TETRACYCLINES			
Demeclocycline HCl		**Tab:** 150mg, 300mg	Treatment of susceptible infections including illness due to *Rickettsiae*, respiratory infections, lymphogranuloma venereum, trachoma, inclusion conjunctivitis, psittacosis, nongonococcal urethritis, relapsing fever, chancroid, plague, tularemia, cholera, *Campylobacter fetus* infections, brucellosis, bartonellosis, and granuloma inguinale. Treatment of gram-negative infections (eg, respiratory, urinary tract) and gram-positive infections (eg, upper respiratory tract, skin and soft tissue). When PCN is contraindicated, treatment of gonococcal infections, syphilis, yaws, listeriosis, anthrax, Vincent's infection, actinomycosis, and clostridial disease. Adjunct therapy in acute intestinal amebiasis and severe acne.
Doxycycline	Oracea	**Cap:** 40mg	Treatment of only inflammatory lesions (papules and pustules) of rosacea in adults.
Doxycycline	Vibramycin	**Cap:** (Doxycycline Hyclate) 50mg, 100mg; **Syrup:** (Doxycycline Calcium) 50mg/5mL; **Sus:** (Doxycycline Mono hydrate) 25mg/5mL [60mL]	Treatment of susceptible infections including respiratory, urinary, lymphogranuloma venereum, psittacosis, trachoma, inclusion conjunctivitis, uncomplicated urethral/endocervical/rectal infections, relapsing fever, nongonococcal urethritis, illnesses caused by *Rickettsiae*, chancroid, tularemia, plague, cholera, *Campylobacter fetus* infections, brucellosis, bartonellosis, and granuloma inguinale. Treatment of anthrax. When penicillin is contraindicated, treatment of uncomplicated gonorrhea, syphilis, listeriosis, *Clostridium* species infections, actinomycosis, yaws, and Vincent's infection. Adjunct therapy for amebiasis (adjunct to amebicides) and severe acne. Prophylaxis of malaria.
Doxycycline hyclate		**Inj:** 100mg	Treatment of *Rickettsiae*, *Mycoplasma pneumoniae*, psittacosis, ornithosis, lymphogranuloma venereum, granuloma inguinale, relapsing fever, chancroid, *Pasteurella pestis*, *Pasturella tularensis*, *Bartonella bacilliformis*, *Bacteroides* species, *Vibrio comma*, *Vibrio fetus*, *Brucella* species, *E.coli*, *Enterobacter aerogenes*, Shigella species, Mima species, Herellea species, *Haemophilus influenzae*, *Klebsiella* species, *Streptococcus* species, *Diplococcus* pneumoniae, *Staphylococcus aureus*, anthrax, and trachoma. When PCN is contraindicated; treatment of *Neisseria gonorrhoeae*, *N.meningitis*, syphilis, yaws, *Listeria monocytogenes*, *Clostridium* species, *Fusobacterium fusiforme*, and *Actinomyces* species. Adjunct therapy for amebiasis.

(Continued)

DRUG	BRAND	HOW SUPPLIED	INDICATIONS
TETRACYCLINES *(Continued)*			
Doxycycline hyclate	Doryx	**Tab, Delayed-Release:** 75mg, 100mg, 150mg	Treatment of susceptible infections including RTI, UTI, uncomplicated urethral/endocervical/rectal, lymphogranuloma venereum, psittacosis, trachoma, inclusion conjunctivitis, relapsing fever due to *Borrelia recurrentis*, nongonococcal urethritis, *Rickettsiae*, chancroid, plague, granuloma inguinale, cholera, brucellosis, bartonellosis, *Campylobacter fetus* infections, tularemia, inhalation anthrax (post exposure). When penicillin is contraindicated, treatment of syphilis, yaws, Vincent's infection, actinomycosis, and infections from *Clostridium* species. Adjunct therapy for amebiasis and severe acne. Prophylaxis of malaria.
Doxycycline hyclate	Periostat	**Tab:** 20mg	Adjunct to scaling and root planing to promote attachment level gain and reduces pocket depth in patients with adult periodontitis.
Doxycycline hyclate	Vibra-tabs	**Tab:** 100mg	Treatment of susceptible infections including respiratory, urinary, lymphogranuloma venereum, psittacosis, trachoma, inclusion conjunctivitis, uncomplicated urethral/endocervical/rectal infections, relapsing fever, nongonococcal urethritis, illnesses caused by *Rickettsiae*, chancroid, tularemia, plague, cholera, *Campylobacter fetus* infections, brucellosis, bartonellosis, and granuloma inguinale. Treatment of anthrax. When penicillin is contraindicated, treatment of uncomplicated gonorrhea, syphilis, listeriosis, *Clostridium* species infections, actinomycosis, yaws, and Vincent's infection. Adjunct therapy for amebiasis (adjunct to amebicides) and severe acne. Prophylaxis of malaria.
Doxycycline monohydrate	Monodox	**Cap:** 50mg, 75mg, 100mg	Treatment of RTI, UTI, and SSSIs, uncomplicated urethral/endocervical/rectal infection caused by *C. trachomatis*, illnesses due to *Rickettsiae*, relapsing fever, nongonococcal urethritis caused by *U. urealyticum*, lymphogranuloma venereum, psittacosis, trachoma & inclusion conjunctivitis caused by *C. trachomatis*, chancroid, plague, cholera, brucellosis, tularemia, *Campylobacter fetus* infections, bartonellosis, and granuloma inguinale. Treatment of anthrax. Treatment of uncomplicated gonorrhea, syphilis, listeriosis, *Clostridium* species infections, actinomycosis, Vincent's infection, and yaws, all when PCN is contraindicated. Adjunct therapy for amebicides (adjunct to amebicides) and severe acne.
Minocycline HCl	Dynacin	**Tab:** 50mg, 75mg, 100mg	Treatment of respiratory tract, urinary tract, and skin and skin structure infections, lymphogranuloma venereum, psittacosis, trachoma, endocervical/rectal infection, nongonococcal urethritis, chancroid, plague, tularemia, cholera, brucellosis, inclusion conjunctivitis, bartonellosis, *Campylobacter fetus* infections, granuloma inguinale, relapsing fever, and illnesses due to *Rickettsiae*. When PCN is contraindicated, treatment of urethritis in men, gonococcal infections, syphilis, listeriosis, anthrax, *Clostridium* species infections, yaws, Vincent's infection, actinomycosis. Adjunct therapy for amebicides (in acute intestinal amebiasis) and severe acne. Treatment of *Mycobacterium marinum* and asymptomatic carriers of *Neisseria meningitidis*.

(Continued)

DRUG	BRAND	HOW SUPPLIED	INDICATIONS
TETRACYCLINES *(Continued)*			
Minocycline HCl	Minocin	**Cap:** 50mg, 100mg; **Inj:** 100mg/vial	Treatment of inclusion conjunctivitis, trachoma, relapsing fever, lymphogranuloma vereneum, *Rickettsiae*, plague, tularemia, cholera, *Campylobacter fetus* infections, brucellosis, bartonellosis, granuloma inguinale, nongonococcal urethritis, and other infections (eg, respiratory tract, endocervical, rectal, urinary tract, skin and skin structure) caused by susceptible strains of microorganisms. When PCN is contraindicated, treatment of yaws, listeriosis, Vincent's infection, actinomycosis, syphilis, anthrax, and *Clostridium* species infections. Adjunctive therapy in acute intestinal amebiasis and severe acne. (PO) Treatment of Mycobacterium marinum and asymptomatic carriers of *Neisseria meningitidis*. Treatment of chancroid. When PCN is contraindicated, treatment of uncomplicated urethritis and other gonococcal infections. (Inj) When PCN is contraindicated, treatment of meningitis.
Minocycline HCl	Solodyn	**Tab, Extended-Release:** 45mg, 55mg, 65mg, 80mg, 90mg, 105mg, 115mg, 135mg	Treatment of inflammatory lesions of non-nodular moderate to severe acne vulgaris in patients ≥12 yrs.
Tetracycline HCl		**Cap:** 250mg, 500mg	Treatment of RTI, UTI, and SSSIs, lymphogranuloma, psittacosis, trachoma, uncomplicated urethral/ endocervical/rectal infection caused by Chlamydia, nongonococcal urethritis, chancroid, plague, tularemia, cholera, brucellosis, inclusion conjunctivitis, bartonellosis, *Campylobacter fetus* infections, granuloma inguinale, relapsing fever, and illnesses due to *Rickettsiae*. When PCN is contraindicated, treatment of *N. gonorrhoeae* infections, syphilis, listeriosis, anthrax, *Clostridium* species infections, yaws, Vincent's infection, actinomycosis. Adjunct therapy for amebicides (in acute intestinal amebiasis) and severe acne.
MISCELLANEOUS			
Clindamycin	Cleocin	**Cap:** (HCl) 75mg, 150mg, 300mg; **Inj:** (Phosphate) 150mg/mL, 300mg/50mL, 600mg/50mL, 900mg/50mL; **Pediatric Solution:** palmitate (HCl) 75mg/5mL [100mL]	Serious infections caused by anaerobes, streptococci, pneumococci, and staphylococci.
Colistimethate sodium	Coly-Mycin M	**Inj:** 150mg	Treatment of acute or chronic infections due to certain gram-negative bacilli (eg, *Pseudomonas aeruginosa, Enterobacter aerogenes*, E. coli, *Klebsiella pneumoniae*).
Dalfopristin-Quinupristin	Synercid	**Inj:** (Dalfopristin-Quinupristin) 350mg-150mg per 500mg vial	Treatment of complicated SSSI caused by *Staphylococcus aureus* (methicillin susceptible) or *Streptococcus pyogenes*.
Dapsone	Dapsone	**Tab:** 25mg, 100mg	Treatment of leprosy and dermatitis herpetiformis.
Daptomycin	Cubicin	**Inj:** 500mg/vial	Susceptible complicated SSSI. *Staphylococcus aureus* bloodstream infections (bacteremia).
Fosfomycin tromethamine	Monurol	**Pow:** 3g/sachet	Uncomplicated UTI (acute cystitis) in women due to susceptible strains of *Escherichia coli* and *Enterococcus faecalis*.
Isoniazid-Rifampin	Rifamate	**Cap:** (Isoniazid-Rifampin) 150mg-300mg	For pulmonary TB when patient has been titrated on the individual components and it has been established that fixed dosage is therapeutically effective. Not for initial therapy or prevention of TB.
Isoniazid-Rifampin-Pyrazinamide	Rifater	**Tab:** (Isoniazid-Pyrazinamide-Rifampin) 50mg-300mg-120mg	For initial phase of short-course treatment of pulmonary TB.

(Continued)

DRUG	BRAND	HOW SUPPLIED	INDICATIONS
MISCELLANEOUS (Continued)			
Lincomycin HCl	Lincocin	**Inj:** 300mg/mL	Treatment of serious infections due to streptococci, pneumococci, and staphylococci. Reserve for PCN allergy or if PCN is inappropriate.
Linezolid	Zyvox	**Inj:** 2mg/mL [100mL, 200mL, 300mL]; **Sus:** 100mg/5mL; **Tab:** 600mg	Vancomycin-resistant *Enterococcus faecium* (VRE) infections, nosocomial pneumonia caused by *S. aureus* (methicillin-susceptible and resistant strains) or *S. pneumoniae* (including multidrug-resistant strains [MDRSP]), complicated SSSI including diabetic foot infections without concomitant osteomyelitis (caused by *S. aureus* [methicillin-susceptible and resistant strains], *S. pyogenes*, or *S. agalactiae*), uncomplicated SSSIs caused by *S. aureus* (methicillin-susceptible only) or *S. pyogenes*, CAP caused by *S. pneumoniae* (MDRSP) or *S. aureus* (methicillin-susceptible strains only).
Methenamine hippurate	Hiprex	**Tab:** 1g	Prophylaxis or suppression of recurrent UTIs when long-term therapy is necessary. For use only after infection is eradicated by other appropriate antimicrobials.
Metronidazole	Flagyl	**Cap:** 375mg; **Tab:** 250mg, 500mg	Treatment of symptomatic and asymptomatic trichomoniasis, asymptomatic consorts, amebiasis, and anaerobic bacterial infections (following IV metronidazole therapy for serious infections). Treatment of intra-abdominal, SSSI, gynecologic, bone and joint, CNS (eg, meningitis), and lower RTIs, as well as endocarditis and bacterial septicemia.
Metronidazole HCl	Flagyl IV	**Inj:** 500mg/100mL	Treatment of anaerobic intra-abdominal, SSSI, gynecologic, bone and joint, CNS, and lower respiratory tract infections, as well as endocarditis and bacterial septicemia. Prophylaxis preoperatively, intraoperatively, and postoperatively to reduce incidence of postoperative infection in patients undergoing contaminated or potentially contaminated elective colorectal surgery. Effective against *B. fragilis* infections resistant to clindamycin, chloramphenicol, and PCN.
Nitrofurantoin	Furadantin	**Sus:** 25mg/5mL	Treatment of UTIs when due to susceptible strains of *Escherichia coli*, enterococci, *Staphylococcus aureus*, and certain susceptible strains of *Klebsiella* and *Enterobacter* species.
Nitrofurantoin macrocrystals	Macrodantin	**Cap:** 25mg, 50mg, 100mg	Treatment of UTIs when due to susceptible strains of *Escherichia coli*, enterococci, *Staphylococcus aureus*, and certain susceptible strains of *Klebsiella* and *Enterobacter* species.
Nitrofurantoin macrocrystals/ Nitrofurantoin monohydrate	Macrobid	**Cap:** 100mg	Treatment of acute uncomplicated UTIs (acute cystitis) caused by susceptible strains of *Escherichia coli* or *Staphylococcus saprophyticus*.
Rifampin	Rifadin	**Cap:** 150mg, 300mg; **Inj:** 600mg	Treatment of all forms of TB. Treatment of asymptomatic carriers of *Neisseria meningitidis* to eliminate *meningococci* from the nasopharynx. (Inj) For initial treatment and retreatment of TB when drug cannot be taken by mouth.

(Continued)

DRUG	BRAND	HOW SUPPLIED	INDICATIONS
MISCELLANEOUS *(Continued)*			
Sulfamethoxazole-Trimethoprim	Bactrim, Bactrim DS, Septra, Septra DS, Sulfatrim	Sulfamethoxazole ([SMX]-Trimethoprim [TMP]) **Inj:** 80mg-16mg/mL; **Sus:** 200mg-40mg/5mL [100mL, 473mL]; **Tab:** 400mg-80mg; **Tab, DS:** 800mg-160mg (Generic available in tablet and DS form, as well as Suspension. Inj available as generic.)	(PO and Inj) Treatment of UTI, PCP, and enteritis caused by *Shigella.* (PO) Treatment of AECB, travelers' diarrhea, and acute otitis media.
Telavancin	Vibativ	**Inj:** 250mg, 750mg	Treatment of adult patients with complicated SSSI caused by susceptible gram-positive microorganisms.
Telithromycin	Ketek	**Tab:** 300mg, 400mg	Treatment of mild to moderate community-acquired pneumonia (CAP) due to *S. pneumoniae* (including MDRSP), *H. influenzae, M. catarrhalis, C. pneumoniae,* or *M. pneumoniae* for patients ≥18 yrs.
Tigecycline	Tygacil	**Inj:** 50mg/5mL, 50mg/10mL [vial]	Treatment of complicated SSSI, complicated intra-abdominal infections (cIAI), and community-acquired bacterial pneumonia (CABP) caused by susceptible strains of indicated pathogens in patients ≥18 yrs.
Trimethoprim		**Tab:** 100mg, 200mg	Treatment of initial episodes of uncomplicated UTIs due to susceptible organisms.
Trimethoprim HCl	Primsol	**Sol:** 50mg/5mL	Treatment of acute otitis media in pediatrics and UTI in adults.
Vancomycin HCl		**Inj:** 500mg/vial, 750mg/vial, 1g/vial, 5g/vial, 10g/vial	Treatment of severe infections caused by susceptible strains of methicillin-resistant staphylococci. Indicated for penicillin-allergic patients, those who cannot receive or have failed to respond to other drugs, and for vancomycin-susceptible organisms that are resistant to other antimicrobials.
Vancomycin HCl	Vancocin Oral	**Cap:** 125mg, 250mg	Treatment of enterocolitis caused by *Staphylococcus aureus* (including methicillin-resistant strains) and antibiotic-associated pseudomembranous colitis caused by *C. difficile.*

SYSTEMIC ANTIFUNGALS

GENERIC	BRAND	INDICATION	DOSAGE FORM	DOSAGE*
Amphotericin B		Progressive, potentially life-threatening fungal infections: Aspergillosis, cryptococcosis, North American blastomycosis, systemic candidiasis, coccidioidomycosis, histoplasmosis, zygomycosis, sporotrichosis, and infections due to *Conidiobolus* and *Basidiobolus* species. May be useful for treatment of American mucocutaneous leishmaniasis.	**Inj:** 50mg	Initial: 0.25mg/kg. Titrate: Increase by 5-10mg/day, depending on cardio-renal status, up to 0.5-0.7mg/kg/day. Max: 1mg/kg/day or 1.5mg/kg/day when given on alternate days.
Amphotericin B cholesteryl sulfate	Amphotec	Treatment of invasive aspergillosis in patients with renal impairment, unacceptable toxicity, or previous failure to amphotericin deoxycholate.	**Inj:** 50mg, 100mg	3-4mg/kg/day IV at 1mg/kg/hr.
Amphotericin B lipid complex injection	Abelcet	Invasive fungal infections in patients who are refractory to or intolerant of conventional amphotericin B therapy.	**Inj:** 5mg/mL	Single infusion 5mg/kg at 2.5mg/kg/hr.
Amphotericin B liposome injection	AmBisome	Treatment of patients with *Aspergillus* species, *Candida* species, and/or *Cryptococcus* species infections refractory to amphotericin B deoxycholate or in patients where renal impairment or unacceptable toxicity precludes the use of amphotericin B deoxycholate. Treatment of visceral leishmaniasis. Empirical therapy for presumed fungal infections in febrile neutropenic patients. Treatment of cryptococcal meningitis in HIV-infected patients.	**Inj:** 50mg	3-6mg/kg/day. Empiric therapy = 3mg/kg/day IV. Systemic infections (*Aspergillus, Candida, Cryptococcus*): 3-5mg/kg/day IV. Cryptococcal Meningitis in HIV: 6mg/kg/day IV. Visceral Leishmaniasis for Immunocompetent patients: 3mg/kg/day on Days 1-5 and 3mg/kg/day on Days 14, 21. Visceral Leishmaniasis in Immunocompromised patients: 4mg/kg/day on Days 1-5 and 4mg/kg/day on Days 10, 17, 24, 31, 38.
Anidulafungin	Eraxis	Treatment of candidemia and other forms of *Candida* infections, esophageal candidiasis.	**Inj:** 50mg, 100mg	Candidemia: LD 200mg on Day 1, MD 100mg qd. Treat for at least 14 days after last positive culture. Esophageal Candidiasis: LD 100mg qd x 1 day then 50mg qd. Treat for minimum of 14 days and for at least 7 days after symptoms resolve.
Caspofungin Acetate	Cancidas	Treatment of candidemia and the following *Candida* infections: intra-abdominal abscesses, peritonitis and pleural space infections. Treatment of esophageal candidiasis. Treatment of invasive aspergillosis in patients who are refractory to or intolerant of other therapies. Empirical therapy for presumed fungal infections in febrile, neutropenic patients.	**Inj:** 50mg, 70mg	70mg LD on Day 1 and then 50mg qd. Esophageal candidasis: 50mg qd.

(Continued)

GENERIC	BRAND	INDICATION	DOSAGE FORM	DOSAGE*
Clotrimazole	Mycelex Troche	Oropharyngeal candidiasis. To prevent oropharyngeal candidiasis in immuno-compromised conditions.	**Loz/Troche:** 10mg	1 troche in mouth 5 times/day for 14 days. Prophylaxis: 1 troche tid for duration of chemo-therapy or until steroids reduced to maintenance levels.
Fluconazole	Diflucan	Treatment of vaginal candidiasis, oropharyngeal, and esophageal, candidiasis. The treatment of *Candida* urinary tract infections, peritonitis, and systemic *Candida* infections including candidemia, disseminated candidiasis, and pneumonia. Treatment of cryptococcal meningitis. Prophylaxis in patients undergoing BMT.	**Inj:** 200mg/100mL, 400mg/200mL; **Sus:** 350mg/35mL, 1400mg/35mL [35mL]; **Tab:** 50mg, 100mg, 150mg, 200mg	Vaginal Candidiasis: 150mg po single dose. Cryptococcal Meningitis: 400mg on Day 1, then 200mg qd. Prophylaxis in Patients Undergoing Bone Marrow Transplantation: 400mg qd. Oropharyngeal Candidiasis: 200mg on Day 1, then 100 mg qd. Esophageal Candidiasis: 200mg on Day 1, then 100mg qd. Max: 400mg/day. Systemic Candida Infections: Up to 400mg/day. UTI/Peritonitis: 50-200mg/day.
Flucytosine	Ancobon	Treatment of septicemia, endo-carditis, and urinary tract infections caused by *Candida*. Treatment of meningitis and pulmonary infection caused by *Cryptococcus*.	**Cap:** 250mg, 500mg	50-150mg/kg/day given q6h.
Griseofulvin	Grifulvin V	Treatment of ringworm.	**Sus:** 125mg/5mL [120mL]; **Tab:** 500mg	0.5-1g qd.
Griseofulvin	Gris-PEG	Treatment of ringworm.	**Tab (ultramicro-size):** 125mg, 250mg	375mg as a single dose or in divided doses.
Itraconazole	Sporanox	(Cap) Onychomycosis of the toenail and fingernail. (Cap/Inj) Treatment of blastomycosis and histoplasmosis. Treatment of aspergillosis if refractory to or intolerant of amphotericin B. (Sol) Treatment of oropharyn-geal and esophageal candidiasis. (Sol/Inj) Empiric therapy of febrile neutropenic patients with suspected fungal infections (ETFN).	**Cap:** 100mg; **Inj:** 10mg/mL; **Sol:** 10mg/mL [150mL]	**(Cap)** Blastomycosis/Histoplasmosis: 200mg qd. Titrate: 100mg increments. Max: 400mg/day given bid. Asper-gillosis: 200-400mg/day. Onychomycosis: Toenail: 200mg qd for 12 weeks. Fingernail: 200mg bid for 1 week, skip 3 weeks, then repeat. **(Sol)** Oropharyngeal Candidiasis: 200mg/day for 1-2 weeks. Swish 10mL at a time for several sec and swallow. Esophageal Candidiasis: 100-200mg/day for at least 3 weeks. **(Inj)** ETFN: 200mg bid for 4 doses, then 200mg qd for 14 days. Continue with po solution 200mg bid until resolution of clinically significant neutropenia. Blastomycosis/Histoplas-mosis/Aspergillosis: 200mg bid for 4 doses, then 200mg qd.

(Continued)

GENERIC	BRAND	INDICATION	DOSAGE FORM	DOSAGE*
Ketoconazole	Nizoral	Candidiasis, chronic mucocutaneous candidiasis, oral thrush, candiduria, blastomycosis, coccidioidomycosis, histoplasmosis, chromomycosis, and paracoccidioidomycosis. Treatment of patients with severe recalcitrant cutaneous dermatophyte infections not responsive to topical therapy or oral griseofulvin. Not for treatment of fungal meningitis.	**Tab:** 200mg	200mg qd. Max: 400mg qd.
Micafungin sodium	Mycamine	Esophageal candidiasis and prophylaxis of *Candida* infection in HSCT patients. Treatment of candidemia, acute disseminated candidiasis, *Candida* peritonitis, and abscesses.	**Inj:** 50mg, 100mg	Treatment of Candidemia, Acute Disseminated Candidiasis, *Candida* Peritonitis and Abscesses: 100mg IV qd (usual range 10-47 days). Treatment of Esophageal Candidiasis: 150mg/day (usual range 10-30 days); Prophylaxis (HSCT): 50mg IV qd (usual range 6-51 days).
Miconazole	Oravig	Local treatment of oropharyngeal candidiasis.	**Tab, Buccal:** 50mg	Apply 1 buccal tab to upper gum region qd for 14 days.
Nystatin		(Sus) Treatment of oral candidiasis. (Tab) Treatment of non-esophageal mucous membrane GI candidiasis.	**Sus:** 100,000 U/mL [60mL, 480mL]; **Tab:** 500,000 U	**(Sus)** Oral Candidiasis: 2-3mL in each side of mouth qid. Retain in mouth as long as possible before swallowing. **(Tab)** Non-Esophageal GI Candidiasis: 1-2 tab tid.
Posaconazole	Noxafil	Prophylaxis of invasive *Aspergillus* and *Candida* infections. Treatment of oropharyngeal candidiasis, including oropharyngeal candidiasis refractory to itraconazole and/or fluconazole.	**Sus:** 40mg/mL [105mL]	Prophylaxis: 200mg tid. Oropharyngeal Candidiasis: 100mg bid x 1 day, 100mg qd x 13 days. Oropharyngeal Candidiasis refractory to itraconazole and/or fluconazole = 400mg bid.
Terbinafine HCl	Lamisil	(Tab): Onychomycosis of the toenail or fingernail. (Granules): Tinea capitis in patients ≥4 years old.	**Tab:** 250mg; **Granules:** 125mg/packet and 187.5mg/packet	**(Tab)** 250mg po qd for 6 weeks for fingernail and 12 weeks for toenail. **(Gran)** <25kg: 125mg/day, 25-35kg: 187.5mg/day, >35kg: 250mg/day. Take for 6 weeks.
Voriconazole	Vfend	Invasive aspergillosis, esophageal candidiasis, serious fungal infections caused by *Scedosporium apiospermum* and *Fusarium* spp. including *Fusarium solani*, candidemia in nonneutropenic patients, and disseminated candidiasis	**Inj:** 200mg; **Sus:** 40mg/mL **Tab:** 50mg, 200mg	IV LD: 6mg/kg q12h for first 24h. IV MD: 3-4mg/kg q12h. PO MD: ≥40kg: 200mg q12h. May increase to 300mg q12h. <40kg: 100mg q12h. May increase to 150mg q12h.

*Refer to FDA-approved labeling for more specific dosing information, such as the duration of treatment.

ANKYLOSING SPONDYLITIS AGENTS

DRUG (BRAND)	HOW SUPPLIED	USUAL DOSE RANGE	MAX DOSE
COX-2 INHIBITOR			
Celecoxib (Celebrex)	**Cap:** 50mg, 100mg, 200mg, 400mg	200mg qd or 100mg bid.	400mg/day with food.
MONOCLONAL ANTIBODIES/TNF-RECEPTOR BLOCKERS			
Adalimumab (Humira)	**Inj:** 20mg/0.4mL, 40mg/0.8mL	40mg SQ every other wk.	n/a
Golimumab (Simponi)	**Inj:** 50mg/0.5mL	50mg SQ every month.	n/a
Infliximab (Remicade)	**Inj:** 100mg [20mL]	5mg/kg as IV infusion repeat at 2 and 6 wks then every 6 wks thereafter.	20mg/kg.
NSAIDs			
Diclofenac sodium	**Tab, Delayed-Release:** 25mg, 50mg, 75mg	25mg qid and 25mg qhs prn.	125mg/day.
Indomethacin (Indocin)	**Cap:** 25mg, 50mg; **Sus:** 25mg/5mL [237mL]; **Cap, Extended-Release:** (Generic) 75mg	Take with food. **Cap/Sus:** 25mg bid-tid; may increase by 25-50mg/day at wkly intervals. **ER:** 75mg qd; may increase by 75mg/day.	**Cap/Sus:** 150-200mg/ day. **ER:** 150mg/day.
Naproxen (EC-Naprosyn, Naprosyn)	**Sus:** 25mg/mL; **Tab:** 250mg, 375mg, 500mg; **Tab, Delayed-Release:** (EC) 375mg, 500mg	250mg, 375mg, or 500mg bid.	1500mg/day.
Naproxen sodium (Anaprox)	**Tab:** 275mg	275mg bid or 550mg bid.	1500mg/day.
(Anaprox DS)	**Tab:** 550mg*	275mg bid or 550mg bid.	1500mg/day.
(Naprelan)	**Tab, Extended-Release:** 375mg, 500mg, 750mg	750mg-1g qd.	1500mg/day.
Sulindac (Clinoril)	**Tab:** 150mg, 200mg*	150mg bid with food.	400mg/day with food.
TNF-RECEPTOR BLOCKER			
Etanercept (Enbrel)	**Inj:** 25mg [vial], 50mg/mL [syringe]	50mg SQ per wk	50mg/wk.
*Scored.			

BONE MINERAL DENSITY CLASSIFICATION/TESTS

World Health Organization (WHO) Definition of Osteoporosis	
Normal	Bone mineral density within 1 standard deviation (SD) of the young adult mean (T-score ≥ -1.0)
Osteopenia (low bone mass)	Bone mineral density between 1.0 and 2.5 SD below the young adult mean ($-2.5 <$ T-score < -1.0)
Osteoporosis	Bone mineral density 2.5 SD or more below the young adult mean (T-score ≤ -2.5)

Note: The definitions above should not be applied to premenopausal women, men <50 years of age, and children.

Bone mineral density (BMD) tests

- BMD tests provide a measurement of T-score for bone density at hip and spine to:
  —Establish and confirm a diagnosis of osteoporosis
  —Predict future fracture risk
  —Measure response to osteoporosis treatment
- BMD is measured in grams of mineral per square centimeter scanned (g/cm^2) and compared to the expected BMD for the patient's age and sex (Z-score) or compared with "normal adults" of the same sex (T-score).
- The difference between the patient's score and the optimal BMD is expressed in standard deviations (SD) above and below the mean. Usually 1 SD equals about 10-15% of the bone density value in g/cm^2.
- Negative values for T-score, such as -1.5, -2, or -2.5, indicate low bone mass.
- The greater the negative score, the greater the risk of fracture.

DIETARY CALCIUM INTAKE

Recommended Calcium Intakes*

Age	Daily Intake (mg)
Birth-6 months	210
6 months-1 year	270
1-3 years	500
4-8 years	800
9-18 years	1,300
19-50 years	1,000
Over 50 years	1,200
Pregnant or Lactating	
14-18 years	1,300
19-50 years	1,000

*Source: National Institute of Arthritis and Musculoskeletal and Skin Diseases (NIAMS); National Institutes of Health

Estimating Daily Dietary Calcium Intake

Step 1: Estimate calcium intake from calcium-rich foods.*

Product	Servings/Day	Calcium/Serving (mg)		Calcium (mg)
Milk (8 oz)	_____	× 300	=	_____
Yogurt (8 oz)	_____	× 300	=	_____
Cheese (1 oz, or 1 cubic inch)	_____	× 200	=	_____
Fortified foods or juices	_____	× 80-1,000**	=	_____

Step 2: Total from above + 250 mg for nondairy sources = total dietary calcium.

* About 75-80% of the calcium consumed in American diets is from dairy products.
** Calcium content of fortified foods varies.

Factors related to vitamin D that may affect calcium absorption:

- National Osteoporosis Foundation recommends an intake of 800 to 1,000 International Units (IU) of vitamin D_3 per day for adults over age 50 and 400 to 800 IU of Vitamin D_3 for <50 years of age
- Desired level for the average adult's serum 25(OH)D concentration is 30 ng/mL (75 nmol/L) or higher
- Safe upper limit for vitamin D intake for normal adult population was set at 4,000 IU per day
- Patients with malabsorption (eg, celiac disease) or chronic renal insufficiency, or those who are housebound, chronically ill, or have limited sun exposure, may need vitamin D supplements

Source: National Institute of Arthritis and Musculoskeletal and Skin Diseases (NIAMS), National Institutes of Health, National Osteoporosis Foundation.

GOUT AGENTS

DRUG (BRAND)	HOW SUPPLIED	USUAL DOSE RANGE	MAX DOSE
ALKALINIZING AGENTS			
Citric Acid/ Potassium Citrate (Cytra-K Crystals)	1002mg-3300mg/pack [100ˢ]	1 packet qid, pc and hs. Reconstitute with at least 6 oz of cool water or juice.	
Citric Acid Monohydrate/ Potassium Citrate Monohydrate/ Sodium Citrate Dihydrate (Cytra-3)	**Syr:** (Citric Acid Monohydrate-Potassium Citrate Monohydrate-Sodium Citrate Dihydrate) 334mg-550mg-500mg/5mL	15-30mL diluted with water, qid, pc and hs.	
Citric Acid Monohydrate/ Potassium Citrate Monohydrate (Cytra-K)	(Citric Acid Monohydrate-Potassium Citrate Monohydrate) 334mg-1100mg/5mL	10-15mL diluted with a glassful of water, qid, pc and hs.	
CORTICOSTEROIDS			
Hydrocortisone sodium succinate (A-Hydrocort)	**Inj:** 100mg/2mL	**Acute Gout:** Individualized dosing. May repeat dose at intervals of 2,4, or 6 hrs based on patient response.	
Hydrocortisone (Cortef)	**Tab:** 5mg, 10mg, 20mg	**Acute Gout:** Individualized dosing.	
Methylprednisolone (Medrol)	**Tab:** 4mg, 8mg, 16mg, 32mg	**Acute Gout:** Individualized dosing.	
Prednisone	**Tab:** 1mg, 2.5mg, 5mg, 10mg, 20mg, 50mg; **Sol:** 5mg/mL, 5mg/5mL	**Acute Gout:** Individualized dosing.	
NSAIDs			
Indomethacin (Indocin)	**Cap:** (Generic) 25mg, 50mg; **Sus:** 25mg/5mL [237mL]	**Acute Gout:** 50mg PO tid until pain is tolerable, then d/c.	
Naproxen (Naprosyn)	**Sus:** 25mg/mL; **Tab:** 250mg*, 375mg, 500mg*	**Acute Gout:** 750mg followed by 250mg q8h until attack subsides.	
Naproxen Sodium (Anaprox)	**Tab:** 275mg	**Acute Gout:** 825mg followed by 275mg q8h.	
(Anaprox DS)	**Tab:** 550mg*	**Acute Gout:** 825mg followed by 275mg q8h.	
(Naprelan)	**Tab, Controlled-Release:** 375mg, 500mg, 750mg	**Acute Gout:** 1-1.5g qd x 1 day, then 1g qd until attack subsides.	1.5g/day.
Sulindac (Clinoril)	**Tab:** (Generic) 150mg (Clinoril, Generic) 200mg*	**Acute Gout:** 200mg bid, usually for 7 days.	400mg/day.
PHENANTHRENE DERIVATIVE			
(Colcrys)	**Tab:** 0.6mg	**Acute Gout:** 1.2mg at first sign of flare, then 0.6mg one hr later. **Prophylaxis:** 0.6mg qd-bid.	1.8mg over 1 hr period. 1.2mg/day.
RECOMBINANT URICASE			
Pegloticase (Krystexxa)	**Inj:** 8mg/mL	**Chronic Gout:** 8mg IV infusion every 2 wks.	
URICOSURIC AGENT			
Probenecid	**Tab:** 500mg	**Initial:** 250mg bid x 1 wk. **Maint:** 500mg bid. **Titrate:** May increase by 500mg every 4 wks.	2g/day.

(Continued)

GOUT AGENTS

DRUG (BRAND)	HOW SUPPLIED	USUAL DOSE RANGE	MAX DOSE
XANTHINE OXIDASE INHIBITORS			
Allopurinol (Zyloprim)	**Tab:** 100mg*, 300mg*	**Mild Gout:** 200-300mg/day. **Moderately-Severe Gout:** 400-600mg/day.	800mg/day.
Febuxostat (Uloric)	**Tab:** 40mg, 80mg	**Initial:** 40mg qd. Increase to 80mg qd if serum uric acid >6mg/dL after 2 wks.	
COMBINATION			
Colchicine/ Probenecid	**Tab:** (Colchicine-Probenecid) 0.5mg-500mg	1 tab qd x 1 wk, then 1 tab bid. **Titrate:** May increase by 1 tab/day every 4 wks.	4 tabs/day.
*Scored.			

OSTEOARTHRITIS AGENTS

DRUG (BRAND)	HOW SUPPLIED	USUAL DOSE RANGE	MAX DOSE
COX-2 INHIBITOR			
Celecoxib (Celebrex)	**Cap:** 50mg, 100mg, 200mg, 400mg	200mg qd or 100mg bid.	
NSAIDs			
Diclofenac epolamine (Flector)	**Patch:** 180mg [5ˢ]	Apply 1 patch to most painful area bid.	1 patch bid.
Diclofenac potassium (Cataflam)	**Tab:** 50mg	50mg bid-tid.	150mg/day.
Diclofenac sodium (Generic)	**Tab, Delayed-Release:** 25mg, 50mg, 75mg	50mg bid-tid or 75mg bid.	150mg/day.
(Voltaren-XR)	**Tab, Extended-Release:** 100mg	100mg qd.	100mg/day.
(Voltaren Gel)	**Gel:** 1% [20g, 100g]	Measure onto enclosed dosing card to appropriate 2g or 4g line. Lower Extremities: Apply 4g to affected foot, knee, or ankle qid. Upper Extremities: Apply 2g to affected hand, elbow, or wrist qid.	Lower Extremities: 16g/day to any single joint. Upper Extremities: 8g/day to any single joint. 32g/day over all affected joints.
(Pennsaid)	1.5% [15mL, 150mL]	40 drops per knee qid.	
Diflunisal	**Tab:** 500mg	500mg-1g qd in two divided doses.	1500mg/day.
Etodolac	**Cap:** 200mg, 300mg; **Tab:** 400mg, 500mg	300mg bid-tid or 400-500mg bid.	1000mg/day.
(Etodolac XR)	**Tab, Delayed-Release:** 400mg, 500mg, 600mg	400-1000mg qd.	1000mg/day.
Fenoprofen calcium (Nalfon)	**Cap:** (Nalfon) 200mg, 400mg; **Tab:** (Generic) 600mg	400-600mg tid-qid.	3200mg/day.
Flurbiprofen (Ansaid)	**Tab:** 50mg, 100mg	200-300mg/day given bid, tid or qid.	300mg/day or 100mg/dose.
Ketoprofen	**Cap:** 50mg, 75mg; **Cap, Extended-Release:** 100mg, 150mg, 200mg	75mg tid or 50mg qid. **ER:** 200mg qd.	300mg/day. **ER:** 200mg/day.
Ibuprofen	**Sus:** 100mg/5mL [120mL, 473mL]	300mg qid or 400mg, 600mg, or 800mg tid-qid.	3200mg/day.
	Tab: 400mg, 600mg, 800mg	300mg qid or 400mg, 600mg, or 800mg tid-qid.	3200mg/day.
(Motrin IB)	**Tab:** 200mg	200mg q4-6h. 400mg if no response.	
Indomethacin (Indocin)	**Cap:** (Generic) 25mg, 50mg; **Cap, Extended-Release:** (Generic) 75mg; **Sus:** (Indocin) 25mg/5mL	**Initial:** 25mg bid. **Titrate:** Increase by 25 or 50mg at weekly intervals until reach satisfactory response. **ER: Initial:** 75mg qd. **Titrate:** May increase to 75mg bid.	200mg/day. **ER:** 150mg/day.
Meclofenamate sodium	**Cap:** 50mg, 100mg	200-400mg/day in 3-4 divided doses.	400mg/day.
Meloxicam (Mobic)	**Sus:** 7.5mg/5mL; **Tab:** 7.5mg, 15mg	7.5mg qd.	15mg/day.
Nabumetone	**Tab:** 500mg, 750mg	1000mg qd.	2000mg/day.
Naproxen (Naprosyn)	**Sus:** 25mg/mL; **Tab:** 250mg, 375mg, 500mg.	250, 375, or 500mg bid.	1500mg/day.
(EC-Naprosyn)	**Tab, Delayed-Release:** 375mg, 500mg	375 or 500mg bid.	1500mg/day.
Naproxen sodium (Anaprox)	**Tab:** 275mg	275mg bid.	1500mg/day.
(Anaprox DS)	**Tab:** 550mg*	550mg bid.	1500mg/day.
(Naprelan)	**Tab, Extended-Release:** 375mg, 500mg, 750mg	750mg-1g qd.	1.5g/day.

(Continued)

OSTEOARTHRITIS AGENTS

DRUG (BRAND)	HOW SUPPLIED	USUAL DOSE RANGE	MAX DOSE
NSAIDs *(Continued)*			
Oxaprozin (Daypro)	**Tab:** 600mg*	1200mg qd.	1800mg/day or 26mg/kg/day in divided doses (whichever is lower)
Piroxicam (Feldene)	**Cap:** 10mg, 20mg	20mg qd or 10mg bid.	20mg/day
Sulindac (Clinoril)	**Tab:** (Generic) 150mg, (Clinoril, generic) 200mg*	150mg bid with food.	400mg/day with food.
Tolmetin	**Cap:** 400mg; **Tab:** 200mg*, 600mg	200-600mg tid.	1800mg/day.
NSAID COMBINATION			
Diclofenac sodium/Misoprostol (Arthrotec)	**Tab:** 50mg-0.2mg, 75mg-0.2mg	50mg tid. Do not crush, chew or divide.	**Diclofenac:** 150mg/day; **Misoprostol:** 200mcg/dose, 800mcg/day.
NON-SALICYLATE ANALGESIC			
Acetaminophen (Tylenol Arthritis Pain)	**Tab, Extended-Release:** 650mg	1300mg q8h.	3900mg/day (6 caps/day)
SALICYLATES			
Aspirin (Genuine Bayer Aspirin)	**Tab:** 325mg	1-2 tabs every 4 hrs or 3 tabs every 6 hrs.	12 tabs/day.
(Extra Strength Bayer Aspirin)	**Tab:** 500mg	1-2 tabs every 4-6 hrs.	8 tabs/24 hrs.
Salsalate	**Tab:** 500mg, 750mg	3000mg daily, given as 1500mg bid or 1000mg tid.	
MISCELLANEOUS			
Botanical/Mineral substances (Traumeel Inj)	**Inj:** 2.2mL amps [10s]	1 amp qd for acute disorders, otherwise 1 amp 1-3 times per week. May administer IV, IM, SQ, intradermally, or periarticularly.	NA
Flavocoxid (Limbrel)	**Cap:** 250mg, 500mg	250-500mg q12h.	500-1000mg/day.
Hyaluronan (Euflexxa)	**Inj:** 1% [2mL]	Inject 2mL intra-articularly into the knee at weekly intervals for 3 wks. Total 3 injections.	3 injections.
(Hyalgan)	**Inj:** 2mL	2mL by intra-articular injection once a wk for 5 injections. Some patients may experience benefit with 3 injections given at weekly intervals.	5 injections.
(Orthovisc)	**Inj:** 30mg/2mL	30mg intra-articularly once a wk. Total 3-4 injections.	3-4 injections.
(Supartz)	**Inj:** 2.5mL	2.5mL by intra-articular injection once a wk. Total 5 injections. Some patients may experience benefit with 3 injections given at weekly intervals.	5 injections.
Hylan G-F 20 (Synvisc)	**Inj:** 8mg/mL	Intra-articular injection once weekly (one wk apart). Total 3 injections.	3 injections.
(Synvisc-One)	**Inj:** 8mg/mL	Single intra-articular injection.	1 injection.

*Scored

OSTEOPOROSIS AGENTS

DRUG (BRAND)	INDICATIONS	HOW SUPPLIED	DOSAGE
BISPHOSPHONATES & COMBINATIONS			
Alendronate Sodium (Fosamax)	Treatment and prevention of osteoporosis in postmenopausal women. Treatment to increase bone mass in men with osteoporosis. Treatment of glucocorticoid-induced osteoporosis.	Sol: 70mg [75mL]; Tab: 5mg, 10mg, 35mg, 40mg, 70mg	Osteoporosis: Treatment: 70mg once weekly or 10mg qd. Prevention: 35mg once weekly or 5mg qd. Increase bone mass in men with osteoporosis: 70mg once weekly or 10mg qd. Glucocorticoid-Induced: 5mg qd; 10mg qd for post-menopausal women not on estrogen. Take at least 30 min before the first food, beverage (other than plain water), or medication. Take tabs with 6-8 oz plain water or 2oz with oral sol. Do not lie down for at least 30 min and until after 1st food of day.
Alendronate Sodium/ Cholecalciferol (Fosamax Plus D)	Treatment of osteoporosis in postmenopausal women. Treatment to increase bone mass in men with osteoporosis.	Tab: (Alendronate Sodium-Cholecalciferol) 70mg-2800 IU, 70mg-5600 IU	Adults: 1 tab (70mg/5600 IU or 70mg/2800 IU) once weekly. Take at least 30 min before 1st food, beverage (other than plain water), or medication. Do not lie down for at least 30 min and until after 1st food of day.
Ibandronate Sodium (Boniva)	(Inj) Treatment of osteoporosis in postmenopausal women. (PO) Treatment and prevention of postmenopausal osteoporosis.	Inj: 3mg/3mL; Tab: 150mg	Inj: 3mg IV over 15-30 sec every 3 months. PO: 150mg once monthly. Swallow whole with 6-8 oz plain water. Do not lie down for 60 min after dose. Take at least 60 min before 1st food, drink (other than plain water), medication, or supplementation.
Risedronate Sodium (Actonel)	Prevention and treatment of osteoporosis in postmenopausal women, glucocorticoid-induced osteoporosis in men and women. Treatment to increase bone mass in men with osteoporosis.	Tab: 5mg, 30mg, 35mg, 150mg	Postmenopausal Osteoporosis Prevention/Treatment: 5mg qd or 35mg once weekly or 150mg once a month. Glucocorticoid-Induced Osteoporosis: 5mg qd. Increase Bone Mass in Men with Osteoporosis: 35mg once weekly. Take at least 30 min before the first food or drink of the day other than water. Swallow tab in upright position with 6-8 oz of plain water. Do not lie down for 30 min after dose.
Risedronate Sodium (Atelvia)	Treatment of osteoporosis in postmenopausal women.	Tab, Delayed-Release: 35mg	Postmenopausal Osteoporosis Treatment: 35mg once weekly; take in am immediately after breakfast. Swallow tab in upright position with 4 oz of plain water. Do not lie down for 30 min after dose.
Zoledronic Acid (Reclast)	Treatment and prevention of osteoporosis in post-menopausal women. Treatment to increase bone mass in men with osteoporosis. Treatment and prevention of glucocorticoid-induced osteoporosis in men and women.	Sol: 5mg/100mL [100mL]	Osteoporosis (Men and Post-menopausal Women): 5mg IV once a year over >15 min at a constant infusion rate. Prevention of Osteoporosis (Postmenopausal Women): 5mg IV given every 2 yrs over >15 min at a constant infusion rate. Treatment/Prevention of Glucocorticoid-Induced Osteoporosis: 5mg IV once a year over >15 min at a constant infusion rate.

(Continued)

DRUG (BRAND)	INDICATIONS	HOW SUPPLIED	DOSAGE
HORMONE THERAPY			
Conjugated Estrogens (Premarin Tabs)	Prevention of postmenopausal osteoporosis.	Tab: 0.3mg, 0.45mg, 0.625mg, 0.9mg, 1.25mg	0.3mg qd continuous or cyclically (eg, 25 days on, 5 days off).
Conjugated Estrogens/ Medroxyprogesterone Acetate (Premphase)	Prevention of postmenopausal osteoporosis in women with intact uterus.	Tab: 0.625mg (Estrogens, Conjugated) and 0.625mg-5mg (Estrogens, Conjugated-Medroxyprogesterone)	0.625mg tab qd on Days 1-14 and 0.625mg-5mg tab qd on Days 15-28. Re-evaluate periodically.
Conjugated Estrogens/ Medroxyprogesterone Acetate (Prempro)	Prevention of postmenopausal osteoporosis in women with intact uterus.	Tab: (Estrogens, Conjugated-Medroxyprogesterone) 0.3mg-1.5mg, 0.45mg-1.5mg, 0.625mg-2.5mg, 0.625mg-5mg	Take 1 tab qd. Re-evaluate periodically.
Estradiol (Alora)	Prevention of postmenopausal osteoporosis.	Patch: 0.025mg/ 24 hrs [8ˢ], 0.05mg/ 24 hrs [8ˢ, 24ˢ], 0.075mg/24 hrs, 0.1mg/24 hrs [8ˢ]	Apply to lower abdomen, upper quadrant of the buttocks or the hip; avoid breasts and waistline. Rotate application sites. Osteoporosis: Apply 0.025mg/day twice weekly. Titrate: May increase depending on bone mineral density and adverse events.
Estradiol (Climara)	Prevention of postmenopausal osteoporosis.	Patch: 0.025mg/day, 0.0375mg/day, 0.05mg/day, 0.06mg/day, 0.075mg/day, 0.1mg/day [4ˢ]	Apply 1 patch weekly to lower abdomen or upper area of buttocks (avoid breasts and waistline). Rotate application sites. Minimum Effective Dose: 0.025mg/day once weekly. Re-evaluate as clinically appropriate.
Estradiol (Estrace)	Prevention of osteoporosis.	Tab: 0.5mg*, 1mg*, 2mg* *scored	Lowest effective dose has not been determined. When prescribing solely for the prevention of postmenopausal osteoporosis, therapy should be considered only for women at significant risk of osteoporosis and for whom non-estrogen medications are not considered to be appropriate.
Estradiol (Estraderm)	Prevention of postmenopausal osteoporosis.	Patch: 0.05mg/24 hrs, 0.1mg/24 hrs [8ˢ, 24ˢ]	Initial: 0.05mg/day. May give continuously without intact uterus. May give cyclically (3 weeks on, 1 week off) with intact uterus. Apply to clean, dry area on trunk of body. Do not apply to breast or waistline. Replace twice weekly. Rotate application site.
Estradiol (Menostar)	Prevention of postmenopausal osteoporosis.	Patch: 14mcg/day [4ˢ]	Apply 1 patch weekly to lower abdomen (avoid breasts, waistline, and areas where sitting would dislodge the patch). Rotate application sites.
Estradiol (Vivelle, Vivelle-Dot)	Prevention of postmenopausal osteoporosis.	Patch: (Vivelle) 0.05mg/day, 0.1mg/day [8ᶜ]; (Vivelle-Dot) 0.025mg/day, 0.0375mg/day, 0.05mg/day, 0.075mg/day, 0.1mg/day [8ᶜ, 24ᶜ]	Minimum Effective Dose: 0.025mg/day twice weekly. Apply to clean, dry area of the trunk; avoid breasts and waistline. Rotate sites; allow 1 week between same site. Without intact uterus, may give continuously; with intact uterus, may give cyclically (3 weeks on, 1 week off) with a progestin.

DRUG (BRAND)	INDICATIONS	HOW SUPPLIED	DOSAGE
HORMONE THERAPY (Continued)			
Estradiol/Levonorgestrel (Climara Pro)	Prevention of postmenopausal osteoporosis.	Patch: (Estradiol-Levonorgestrel): 0.045mg-0.015mg/day [4^s]	Apply 1 patch weekly to lower abdomen (avoid breasts and waistline). Rotate application site; allow 1 week between same site. Re-evaluate periodically (3-6 month intervals).
Estradiol/Norethindrone (Activella)	Prevention of postmenopausal osteoporosis in women with intact uterus.	Tab: (Estradiol-Norethindrone) 1mg-0.5mg, 0.5mg-0.1mg	1 tab qd.
Estradiol/Norgestimate (Prefest)	Prevention of postmenopausal osteoporosis in women with intact uterus.	Tab: (Estradiol) 1mg and (Estradiol-Norgestimate) 1mg-0.09mg	1 estradiol (pink color) tab for three days followed by 1 estradiol-norgestimate (white color) tab for three days. Repeat regimen continuously.
Estropipate	Prevention of postmenopausal osteoporosis.	Tab: 0.75mg*, 1.5mg*, 3mg* *scored	0.75mg (as estropipate) qd for 25 days of 31-day cycle.
Ethinyl Estradiol/ Norethindrone (Femhrt)	Prevention of postmenopausal osteoporosis in women with intact uterus.	Tab: (Ethinyl Estradiol-Norethindrone) 2.5mcg-0.5mg, 5mcg-1mg	1 tab qd. Assess response by measuring bone mineral density.
MISCELLANEOUS			
Calcitonin-Salmon (Miacalcin)	Treatment of postmenopausal osteoporosis in females >5 yrs postmenopause.	Inj: 200 IU/mL; Nasal Spray: 200 IU/inh	(Inj) 100 IU IM/SQ every other day. If >2mL, use IM injection. (Spray) 200 IU qd intranasally. Alternate nostrils daily. Take with supplemental calcium and vitamin D for postmenopausal osteoporosis.
Calcitonin-Salmon (Fortical)	Treatment of postmenopausal osteoporosis in females >5 yrs postmenopause in conjunction with an adequate calcium and vitamin D intake.	Nasal Spray: 200 IU/inh	200 IU qd intranasally. Alternate nostrils daily.
Denosumab (Prolia)	Treatment of postmenopausal women with osteoporosis at high risk of fracture (eg, history of osteoporotic fracture, multiple risk factors for fracture) or patients who have failed or cannot tolerate other available osteoporosis therapy.	Inj: 60mg/mL	60mg as single SQ injection once q6 months. Administer in the upper arm, upper thigh, or abdomen. All patients should receive calcium 1000mg and 400 IU vitamin D qd.
Raloxifene (Evista)	Treatment and prevention of osteoporosis in postmenopausal women.	Tab: 60mg	60mg qd.
Teriparatide (Forteo)	Treatment of postmeno-pausal women with osteo-porosis at high risk for fracture. To increase bone mass in men with primary or hypogonadal osteoporosis at high risk for fracture. Treatment of men and women with glucocorticoid-induced osteoporosis at high risk for fracture.	Inj: 250mcg/mL [2.4mL pen]	20mcg qd SQ into thigh or abdominal wall. Administer initially under circumstances where patient can sit or lie down if symptoms of orthostatic hypotension occur. Discard pen after 28 days.

OSTEOPOROSIS RISK FACTORS

Nonmodifiable risk factors	
Gender	Women > men
Age	Older age > younger age
Body size	Low body weight (small and thin) > high or overweight
Ethnicity	Caucasian, Asian, or Hispanic/Latino descent > African heritage
Family history	History of fractures or osteoporosis
Sex hormones	Females: delayed puberty, amenorrhea, early menopause, removal of ovaries, low estrogen levels
	Males: low testosterone
Modifiable risk factors	
Lifestyle	Cigarette smoking, excessive alcohol (≥3 drinks/day), excessive caffeine intake, high salt intake
Exercise	Inactive or bedridden
Vitamins	Low intake of calcium, vitamin D, phosphorous, magnesium, vitamin K, vitamin B_6, vitamin B_{12}; excessive intake of vitamin A

Drugs associated with increased risk of osteoporosis*

- Anticoagulants (heparin)
- Anticonvulsants
- Aromatase inhibitors
- Barbiturates
- Cancer chemotherapeutic drugs
- Cyclosporine A and tacrolimus
- Depo-medroxyprogesterone
- Glucocorticoids (≥5 mg/d of prednisone or equivalent for ≥3 mo)
- Gonadotropin releasing hormone agonists
- Lithium

Diseases/conditions associated with increased risk of osteoporosis*

Genetic factors

Cystic fibrosis	Homocystinuria	Osteogenesis imperfecta
Ehlers-Danlos	Hypophosphatasia	Parental history of hip fratrure
Gaucher's disease	Idiopathic hypercalciuria	Porphyria
Glycogen storage diseases	Marfan syndrome	Riley-Day syndrome
Hemochromatosis	Menkes steely hair syndrome	

Hypogonadal states

Androgen insensitivity	Hyperprolactinemia	Turner's & Klinefelter's syndromes
Anorexia nervosa and bulimia	Panhypopituitarism	
Athletic amenorrhea	Premature ovarian failure	

Endocrine disorders

Adrenal insufficiency	Diabetes mellitus	Thyrotoxicosis
Cushing's syndrome	Hyperparathyroidism	

Gastrointestinal disorders

Celiac disease	Inflammatory bowel disease	Pancreatic disease
Gastric bypass	Malabsorption	Primary biliary cirrhosis

Hematologic disorders

Hemophilia	Multiple myeloma	Systemic mastocytosis
Leukemia and lymphomas	Sickle cell disease	Thalassemia

Rheumatic and autoimmune disorders

Ankylosing spondylitis	Lupus	Rheumatoid arthritis

Miscellaneous conditions and diseases

Alcoholism	Emphysema	Muscular dystrophy
Amyloidosis	End stage renal disease	Parenteral nutrition
Chronic metabolic acidosis	Epilepsy	Post-transplant bone disease
Congestive heart failure	Idiopathic scoliosis	Prior fracture as an adult
Depression	Multiple sclerosis	Sarcoidosis

*This list is not inclusive of all drugs, diseases/conditions that may increase the risk factors for osteoporosis.
Sources: National Osteoporosis Foundation and World Health Organization.

RHEUMATOID ARTHRITIS AGENTS

DRUG (Brand)	HOW SUPPLIED	USUAL DOSE RANGE	MAX DOSE
5-AMINOSALICYLIC ACID DERIVATIVE			
Sulfasalazine (Azulfidine EN)	**Tab, Delayed-Release:** 500mg	1g bid.	3g/day.
COPPER CHELATING AGENT			
Penicillamine (Cuprimine, Depen)	**Cap:** (Cuprimine) 250mg; **Tab:** (Depen) 250mg*	**Initial:** 125-250mg/day. **Maint:** 500-750mg/day.	1.5g/day.
COX-2 INHIBITOR			
Celecoxib (Celebrex)	**Cap:** 50, 100mg, 200mg, 400mg	100-200mg bid.	
DIHYDROFOLIC ACID REDUCTASE INHIBITOR			
Methotrexate sodium (Trexall)	**Inj:** (Generic) 25mg/mL; **Tab:** (Generic) 2.5mg, (Trexall) 5mg, 7.5mg, 10mg, 15mg	7.5mg once weekly.	20mg/wk.
GOLD AGENT			
Auranofin (Ridaura)	**Cap:** 3mg	6mg qd or 3mg bid.	9mg/day.
IMMUNOSUPPRESSANTS			
Azathioprine (Imuran)	**Tab:** 50mg*; **Inj:** (Generic) 100mg/20mL	**Initial:** 1mg/kg/day given qd-bid. **Titrate:** Increase by 0.5mg/kg/day after 6-8 wks, then at 4 wk intervals.	2.5mg/kg/day.
Cyclosporine (Neoral)	**Cap:** 25mg, 100mg; **Sol:** 100mg/mL [50mL]	**Initial:** 1.25mg/kg bid. **Titrate:** Increase by 0.5-0.75mg/kg/day after 8 wks, again after 12 wks. D/C if no benefit by wk 16.	4mg/kg/day.
INTERLEUKIN-1 RECEPTOR ANTAGONIST			
Anakinra (Kineret)	**Inj:** 100mg/0.67mL	100mg SQ qd.	
INTERLEUKIN-6 RECEPTOR ANTAGONIST			
Tocilizumab (Actemra)	**Inj:** 20mg/mL [80mg/4mL, 200mg/10mL, 400mg/20mL]	**Initial:** 4mg/kg every 4 wks. as 60 min infusion. **Titrate:** Increase to 8mg/kg based on response.	800mg/infusion.
MONOCLONAL ANTIBODIES/CD20-BLOCKER			
Rituximab (Rituxan)	**Inj:** 10mg/mL	Two-1000mg IV infusions separated by 2 wks, with MTX. Give subsequent courses every 24 wks or based on clinical evaluation, but not sooner than every 16 wks.	400mg/hr infusion rate. See PI for initial rates.
MONOCLONAL ANTIBODIES/TNF-BLOCKERS			
Adalimumab (Humira)	**Inj:** 20mg/0.4mL, 40mg/0.8mL [Prefilled Glass Syringe], 40mg/0.8mL [Prefilled Pen]	40mg SQ every other wk.	40mg every wk. w/o MTX.
Golimumab (Simponi)	**Inj:** 50mg/0.5mL	50mg SQ once a month. Give with MTX.	
Infliximab (Remicade)	**Inj:** 100mg/20mL	3mg/kg IV infusion then repeat at 2 and 6 wks. **Maint:** 3mg/kg every 8 wks.	10mg/kg or every 4 wks.

(Continued)

DRUG (Brand)	HOW SUPPLIED	USUAL DOSE RANGE	MAX DOSE
NONSTEROIDAL ANTI-INFLAMMATORY DRUGS (NSAIDs)			
Diclofenac Potassium (Cataflam)	**Tab:** 50mg	50mg tid-qid.	200mg/day.
Diclofenac Sodium	**Tab, Delayed-Release:** 25mg, 50mg, 75mg	50mg tid-qid or 75mg bid.	200mg/day.
(Voltaren XR)	**Tab, Extended-Release:** 100mg	100mg qd-bid.	200mg/day.
Diflunisal	**Tab:** 500mg	500mg-1g/day in two divided doses.	1500mg/day.
Etodolac	**Cap:** 200mg, 300mg **Tab:** 400mg, 500mg	300mg bid-tid or 400-500mg bid.	1000mg/day.
(Etodolac XR)	**Tab, Extended-Release:** 400mg, 500mg, 600mg	400-1000mg qd.	1000mg/day.
Fenoprofen Calcium (Nalfon)	**Cap:** (Nalfon) 200mg, 400mg **Tab:** (Generic) 600mg	400-600mg tid-qid. 300-600mg tid-qid.	3200mg/day. 3200mg/day.
Flurbiprofen (Ansaid)	**Tab:** 50mg, 100mg	200-300mg/day given bid, tid or qid.	300mg/day 100mg/dose.
Ibuprofen	**Sus:** 100mg/5mL [120mL, 473mL]	300mg qid or 400mg, 600mg, or 800mg tid-qid.	3200mg/day.
	Tab: 400mg, 600mg, 800mg	300mg qid or 400mg, 600mg, or 800mg tid-qid.	3200mg/day.
(Motrin IB)	**Tab:** 200mg	200mg q4-6h. 400mg if no response.	1200mg/day.
Indomethacin (Indocin)	**Cap:** (Generic) 25mg, 50mg **Cap, Extended-Release:** (Generic) 75mg **Sus:** (Indocin) 25mg/5mL	**Initial:** 25mg bid-tid **Titrate:** Increase by 25mg or 50mg at weekly intervals until reach satisfactory response. **ER: Initial:** 75mg qd. **Titrate:** May increase to 75mg bid.	200mg/day **ER:** 150mg/day.
Ketoprofen	**Cap:** 50mg, 75mg; **Cap, Extended-Release:** 100mg, 150mg, 200mg	75mg tid or 50mg qid. **ER:** 200mg qd	300mg/day. **ER:** 200mg/day.
Meclofenamate Sodium	**Cap:** 50mg, 100mg	200-400mg/day in 3-4 divided doses.	400mg/day.
Meloxicam (Mobic)	**Sus:** 7.5mg/5mL; **Tab:** 7.5mg, 15mg	7.5mg qd.	15mg/day.
Nabumetone	**Tab:** 500mg, 750mg	1000mg qd.	2000mg/day.
Naproxen (Naprosyn)	**Sus:** 25mg/mL; **Tab:** 250mg, 375mg, 500mg	250, 375, or 500mg bid.	1500mg/day.
(EC-Naprosyn)	**Tab, Delayed-Release:** 375mg, 500 mg	375 or 500mg bid.	1500mg/day.
Naproxen Sodium (Anaprox)	**Tab:** 275mg	275mg bid.	1500mg/day.
(Anaprox DS)	**Tab:** 550mg*	550mg bid.	1500mg/day.
(Naprelan)	**Tab, Extended-Release:** 375mg, 500mg, 750mg	750mg-1g qd.	1.5g/day.
Oxaprozin (Daypro)	**Tab:** 600mg*	1200mg qd.	1800mg/day or 26mg/kg/day (whichever is lower)
Piroxicam (Feldene)	**Cap:** 10mg, 20mg	20mg qd or 10mg bid.	20mg/day.
Sulindac (Clinoril)	**Tab:** (Generic) 150mg, (Clinoril, Generic) 200mg*	150mg bid with food.	400mg/day.
Tolmetin	**Cap:** 400mg; **Tab:** 200mg*, 600mg	200-600mg tid.	1800mg/day.

(Continued)

DRUG (Brand)	HOW SUPPLIED	USUAL DOSE RANGE	MAX DOSE
NSAID/PROSTAGLANDIN E$_1$ ANALOGUE			
Diclofenac/Misoprostol (Arthrotec)	**Tab:** (Diclofenac-Misoprostol) 50mg-0.2mg, 75mg-0.2mg	50mg tid-qid. Do not crush, chew, or divide.	**Diclofenac:** 225mg/day **Misoprostol:** 800mcg/day 200mcg/dose
PYRIMIDINE SYNTHESIS INHIBITOR			
Leflunomide (Arava)	**Tab:** 10mg, 20mg, 100mg	**Load:** 100mg qd for 3 days. **Maint:** 20mg/day.	20mg/day
SALICYLATE			
Aspirin (Genuine Bayer Aspirin)	**Tab:** 325mg	1-2 tabs every 4 hrs or 3 tabs every 6 hrs.	12 tabs/day.
(Extra Strength Bayer Aspirin)	**Tab:** 500mg	1-2 tabs every 4-6 hrs.	8 tabs/24 hrs.
(Ecotrin)	**Tab, Delayed-Release:** 81mg, 325mg	(81mg) 4-8 tabs every 4 hrs. (325mg) 1-2 tabs every 4 hrs.	(81mg) 48 tabs/ day. (325mg) 12 tabs/day.
Salsalate	**Tab:** 500mg, 750mg	3000mg daily, given as 1500mg bid or 1000mg tid.	3000mg/day.
SELECTIVE COSTIMULATION MODULATOR			
Abatacept (Orencia)	**Inj:** 250mg	**Initial:** <60kg: 500mg; 60-100kg: 750mg; >100kg: 1g. **Maint:** Give at 2 and 4 wks after initial infusion, then q 4 wks thereafter.	
TNF-RECEPTOR BLOCKERS			
Certolizumab pegol (Cimzia)	**Inj:** 200mg/mL	**Initial:** 400mg SQ and at wks. 2 and 4, followed by 200mg every other wk. **Maint:** 400mg SQ every 4 wks.	
Etanercept (Enbrel)	**Inj:** 25mg [vial], 50mg/mL [syringe]	50mg SQ per wk.	50mg/week.
MISCELLANEOUS			
Hydroxychloroquine (Plaquenil)	**Tab:** 200mg	**Initial:** 400-600mg qd. **Maint:** When good response is obtained (usually in 4-12 wks), 200-400mg qd with meal or milk.	

*scored

ADHD Agents

BRAND (GENERIC)	HOW SUPPLIED	ADULT DOSE	PEDIATRIC DOSE
Adderall (Amphetamine plus dextroamphetamine)	Tab: 5mg*, 7.5mg*, 10mg*, 12.5mg*, 15mg*, 20mg*, 30mg* *scored		**3-5 yrs:** Initial: 2.5mg qd. Titrate: May increase by 2.5mg weekly. **≥6 yrs:** Initial: 5mg qd-bid. May increase by 5mg weekly. Give 1st dose upon awakening and add'l doses q4-6h. Max (usual): 40mg/day.
Adderall XR* (Amphetamine salt combo)	Cap: 5mg, 10mg, 15mg, 20mg, 25mg, 30mg	Initial: 20mg qam. Currently Using Adderall: Switch to Adderall XR at the same total daily dose, taken once daily. Titrate at weekly intervals as needed.	**≥6 yrs:** Initial: 10mg qam. Titrate: May increase weekly by 5-10mg/day. Max: 30mg/day. **13-17 yrs:** Initial: 10mg/day. Titrate: May increase to 20mg/day after one week. Currently Using Adderall: Switch to Adderall XR at the same total daily dose, taken once daily. Titrate at weekly intervals as needed.
Concerta** (Methylphenidate HCl)	Tab, ER: 18mg, 27mg, 36mg, 54mg	Methylphenidate-Naive or Receiving Other Stimulant: Initial: 18 or 36mg qam. Titrate: Adjust dose at weekly intervals. Previous Methylphenidate Use: Initial: 18mg qam if previous dose 10-15mg/day; 36mg qam if previous dose 20-30mg/day; 54mg qam if previous dose 30-45mg/day; 72mg qam if previous dose 40-60mg/day. Initial conversion should not exceed 72mg/day. Titrate: Adjust dose at weekly intervals. Max: 72mg/day. Reduce dose or d/c if paradoxical aggravation of symptoms occur. D/C if no improvement after appropriate dosage adjustments over 1 month.	**≥6 yrs:** Methylphenidate-Naive or Receiving Other Stimulant: Initial: 18mg qam. Titrate: Adjust dose at weekly intervals. Max: **6-12 yrs:** 54mg/day. **13-17 yrs:** 18-72mg/day not to exceed 2mg/kg/day. Previous Methylphenidate Use: Initial: 18mg qam if previous dose 10-15mg/day; 36mg qam if previous dose 20-30mg/day; 54mg qam if previous dose 30-45mg/day; 72mg qam if previous dose 40-60mg/day. Initial conversion should not exceed 72mg/day. Titrate: Adjust dose at weekly intervals. Max: 72mg/day. Reduce dose or d/c if paradoxical aggravation of symptoms occur. D/C if no improvement after appropriate dosage adjustments over 1 month.
Daytrana (Methylphenidate transdermal system)	Patch: 10mg/9 hrs, 15mg/9 hrs, 20mg/9 hrs, 30mg/9 hrs [30S]	Individualize dose. Apply to hip area 2 hrs before effect is needed and remove 9 hrs after application. Recommended Titration Schedule: Week 1: 10mg/9 hrs. Week 2: 15mg/9 hrs. Week 3: 20mg/9 hrs. Week 4: 30mg/9 hrs.	**≥6 yrs:** Individualize dose. Apply to hip area 2 hrs before effect is needed and remove 9 hrs after application. Recommended Titration Schedule: Week 1: 10mg/9 hrs. Week 2: 15mg/9 hrs. Week 3: 20mg/9 hrs. Week 4: 30mg/9 hrs.
Desoxyn (Methamphetamine HCl)	Tab: 5mg		**≥6 yrs:** Initial: 5mg qd-bid. Titrate: Increase weekly by 5mg/day until optimum response. Usual: 20-25mg/day; may be given in 2 divided doses.
Dexedrine (Dextroamphetamine sulfate)	Cap, ER: (Spansules) 5mg, 10mg, 15mg		**≥6 yrs:** 5mg qd-bid. Titrate: Increase weekly by 5mg/day. Max: 40mg/day.

(Continued)

BRAND (GENERIC)	HOW SUPPLIED	ADULT DOSE	PEDIATRIC DOSE
(Dextroamphetamine sulfate)	Tab: 5mg*, 10mg* **scored		**3-5 yrs:** Initial: 2.5mg/day. Titrate: Increase weekly by 2.5mg/day until optimum response. **≥6 yrs:** Initial: 5mg qd-bid. Titrate: Increase weekly by 5mg/day until optimum response. Give 1st dose upon awakening, and additional doses q4-6h.
Focalin (Dexmethylphenidate HCl)	Tab: 2.5mg, 5mg, 10mg	Take bid at least 4 hrs apart. Methylphenidate-Naive: Initial: 2.5mg bid. Titrate: Increase weekly by 2.5-5mg/day. Max: 20mg/day. Currently on Methylphenidate: Initial: Take ½ of methylphenidate dose. Max: 20mg/day. Reduce or d/c if paradoxical aggravation of symptoms occur. D/C if no improvement after appropriate dosage adjustments over 1 month.	**≥6 yrs:** Take bid at least 4 hrs apart. Methylphenidate-Naive: Initial: 2.5mg bid. Titrate: Increase weekly by 2.5-5mg/day. Max: 20mg/day. Currently on Methylphenidate: Initial: Take ½ of methylphenidate dose. Max: 20mg/day. Reduce or d/c if paradoxical aggravation of symptoms occur. D/C if no improvement after appropriate dosage adjustments over 1 month.
Focalin XR* (Dexmethylphenidate HCl)	Cap, ER: 5mg, 10mg, 5mg, 20mg, 130mg, 40mg	Methylphenidate-Naive: Initial: 10mg/day. Titrate: May adjust weekly by 10mg/day Max: 40mg/day. Currently on Methylphenidate: Initial: Take ½ of methylphenidate dose. Max: 40mg/day. Currently on Focalin: May switch to same daily dose of Focalin XR. Reduce or d/c if paradoxical aggravation of symptoms occur. D/C if no improvement after appropriate dosage adjustments over 1 month.	**≥6 yrs:** Methylphenidate-Naive: Initial: 5mg/day. Titrate: May adjust weekly by 5mg/day Max: 30mg/day. Currently on Methylphenidate: Initial: Take ½ of methylphenidate dose. Max: 30mg/day. Currently on Focalin: May switch to same daily dose of Focalin XR. Reduce or d/c if paradoxical aggravation of symptoms occur. D/C if no improvement after appropriate dosage adjustments over 1 month.
Intuniv** (Guanfacine)	Tab, ER: 1mg, 2mg, 3mg, 4mg		**6-17 yrs:** Initial: 1mg/day. Titrate: Adjust dose by increments of ≤1mg/week. Maint: 1-4mg/day based on clinical response and tolerability. Range: 0.05-0.08mg/kg/day. If well tolerated, doses up to 0.12mg/kg/day may provide additional benefit. Max: 4mg/day. D/C in decrements of no more than 1mg every 3 to 7 days. Reinitiation: Consider titration based on tolerability. Renal/Hepatic Impairment: Consider dose adjustment.
Kapvay** (Clonidine HCl)	Tab, ER: 0.1mg, 0.2mg		**6-17 yrs:** Initial: 0.1mg hs. Titrate: Adjust in increments of 0.1mg/day at weekly intervals until desired response is achieved. Max: 0.4mg/day. D/C in decrements of no more than 0.1mg every 3 to 7 days. Doses should be taken bid with equal or higher split dose given hs.
Metadate CD* (Methylphenidate HCl)	Cap, ER: 10mg, 20mg, 30mg, 40mg, 50mg, 60mg	Usual: 20mg qam before breakfast. Titrate: Increase weekly by 10-20mg depending on tolerability/efficacy. Max: 60mg/day. Reduce dose or d/c if paradoxical aggravation of symptoms occur. D/C if no improvement after appropriate dose adjustments over 1 month.	**≥6 yrs:** Usual: 20mg qam before breakfast. Titrate: Increase weekly by 10-20mg depending on tolerability/efficacy. Max: 60mg/day. Reduce dose or d/c if paradoxical aggravation of symptoms occur. D/C if no improvement after appropriate dose adjustments over 1 month.

BRAND (GENERIC)	HOW SUPPLIED	ADULT DOSE	PEDIATRIC DOSE
Metadate ER*** (Methylphenidate HCl)	Tab, ER: 10mg, 20mg	(Immediate-Release Methylphenidate) 10-60mg/day given bid-tid 30-45 min ac. If insomnia occurs, take last dose before 6 pm.†	≥6 yrs: (Immediate-Release Methylphenidate) Initial: 5mg bid before breakfast and lunch. Titrate: Increase gradually by 5-10mg weekly. Max: 60mg/day. Reduce dose or d/c if paradoxical aggravation of symptoms occur. D/C if no improvement after appropriate dose adjustment over 1 month.†
Methylin*** (Methylphenidate HCl)	Sol: 5mg/5mL [500mL], 10mg/5mL [500mL]; Tab: 5mg, 10mg, 20mg; Tab, Chewable: 2.5mg, 5mg, 10mg; Tab, Extended-Release: 10mg, 20mg	(Sol/Tab/Tab, Chewable) 10-60mg/day given bid-tid 30-45 min ac. If insomnia occurs, take last dose before 6 pm.†	≥6 yrs: (Sol/Tab/Tab, Chewable) Initial: 5mg bid before breakfast and lunch. Titrate: Increase gradually by 5-10mg weekly. Max: 60mg/day. Reduce dose or d/c if paradoxical aggravation of symptoms occur. D/C if no improvement after appropriate dose adjustment over 1 month.†
Ritalin, Ritalin LA*, Ritalin SR***** (Methylphenidate HCl)	Cap, ER (Ritalin LA): 10mg, 20mg, 30mg, 40mg; Tab (Ritalin): 5mg, 10mg*, 20mg**; Tab, ER (Ritalin SR): 20mg *scored*	(Tab) 10-60mg/day given bid-tid 30-45 min ac. Take last dose before 6 pm if insomnia occurs. (Cap, ER) Initial: 20mg qam. Titrate: Adjust weekly by 10mg. Max: 60mg qam. Previous Methylphenidate Use: May use as qd in place of IR dosed bid or daily dose of methylphenidate-SR. Reduce dose or d/c if no improvement after appropriate dose adjustment over 1 month.†	≥6 yrs: (Tab) Initial: 5mg bid before breakfast and lunch. Titrate: Increase gradually by 5-10mg weekly. Max: 60mg/day. (Cap, ER) Initial: 20mg qam. Titrate: Adjust weekly by 10mg. Max: 60mg qam. Previous Methylphenidate Use: May use as qd in place of IR dosed bid or daily dose of methylphenidate-SR. Reduce dose or d/c if paradoxical aggravation of symptoms occur. D/C if no improvement after appropriate dose adjustment over 1 month.†
Strattera (Atomoxetine HCl)	Cap: 10mg, 18mg, 25mg, 40mg, 60mg, 80mg, 100mg	Initial: 40mg given qam or evenly divided doses in the am and late afternoon/early evening. Titrate: Increase after minimum of 3 days to target dose of about 80mg/day. After 2-4 weeks, may increase to max of 100mg/day. Max: 100mg/day. Dose adjust in hepatic insufficiency and when used with concomitant CYP450 2D6 inhibitors. See PI for detailed dosing information.	≥6 yrs: ≤70kg: Initial: 0.5mg/kg/day given qam or evenly divided doses in the am and late afternoon or early evening. Titrate: Increase after minimum of 3 days to target dose of about 1.2mg/kg/day. Max: 1.4mg/kg/day or 100mg, whichever is less. >70kg: Initial: 40mg/day given qam or evenly divided doses in the am and late afternoon/early evening. Titrate: Increase after minimum of 3 days to target dose of about 80mg/day. After 2-4 weeks, may increase to max of 100mg/day. Max: 100mg/day. Dose adjust in hepatic insufficiency and when used with concomitant CYP450 2D6 inhibitors. See PI for detailed dosing information.
Vyvanse (Lisdexamfetamine dimesylate)	Cap: 20mg, 30mg, 40mg, 50mg, 60mg, 70mg	Individualize dose. Usual: 30mg qam. Titrate: If needed, may increase in increments of 10mg or 20mg at weekly intervals. Max: 70mg/day. Swallow caps or dissolve contents in glass of water; do not store once dissolved. Re-evaluate periodically.	6-17 yrs: Individualize dose. Usual: 30mg qam. Titrate: If needed, may increase in increments of 10mg or 20mg at weekly intervals. Max: 70mg/day. Swallow caps or dissolve contents in glass of water; do not store once dissolved. Re-evaluate periodically.

ADHD = attention-deficit/hyperactivity disorder.
* Swallow cap whole or open cap and sprinkle contents on applesauce; do not chew beads.
** Swallow whole; do not chew, crush, or divide.
†Tab, Extended-Release (ER): May use in place of immediate-release tabs when the 8-hr dose corresponds to the titrated 8-hr immediate-release dose.

ALZHEIMER'S DISEASE AGENTS

DRUG (BRAND)	INDICATIONS	HOW SUPPLIED	DOSAGE	SIDE EFFECTS
Donepezil HCl (Aricept)	Treatment of dementia of the Alzheimer's type.	Tab: 5mg, 10mg, 23mg; Tab, Disintegrating: 5mg, 10mg	Mild to Moderate Alzheimer's Disease: Initial: 5mg qd. Usual: 5-10mg. Titrate: May increase to 10mg after 4-6 weeks. Moderate to severe Alzheimer's Disease: Initial: 5mg qd. Usual: 10-23mg qd. Titrate: May increase to 10mg after 4-6 weeks, then to 23mg after ≥3 months.	Nausea, diarrhea, insomnia, vomiting, muscle cramps, fatigue, anorexia, dizziness, depression, weight decrease, infection, HTN, back pain, abnormal dreams, ecchymosis
Ergoloid Mesylates (Ergoloid mesylates)	Treatment of symptomatic decline in mental capacity of unknown etiology (eg, Alzheimer's dementia, multi-infarct dementia).	Tab: 1mg	Usual: 1mg tid.	Transient nausea, gastric disturbances
Galantamine HBr (Razadyne, Razadyne ER)	Treatment of mild to moderate dementia of the Alzheimer's type.	Sol: (Razadyne) 4mg/mL [100mL]; Tab: (Razadyne) 4mg, 8mg, 12mg. Cap, Extended-Release: (Razadyne ER) 8mg, 16mg, 24mg	(Sol, Tab) Initial: 4mg bid with am and pm meals. Titrate: Increase to 8mg bid after 4 weeks if tolerated, then increase to 12mg bid after 4 weeks if tolerated. Usual: 16-24mg/day. Max: 24mg/day. (Cap, ER) Initial: 8mg qd with am meal. Titrate: Increase to 16mg qd after 4 weeks, then increase to 24mg qd after 4 weeks if tolerated. Usual: 16-24mg/day. Max: 24mg/day. If therapy is interrupted, restart at lowest dose and increase to current dose. See PI for dose modification in moderate renal/hepatic impairment.	Nausea, vomiting, diarrhea, anorexia, weight loss, fatigue, dizziness, headache, depression, insomnia, abdominal pain, dyspepsia
Memantine HCl (Namenda, Namenda XR)	Treatment of moderate to severe dementia of the Alzheimer's type.	Sol: 2mg/mL [360mL]; Tab: 5mg, 10mg; Titration-Pak: 5mg [28*], 10mg [21*]. Cap, Extended-Release: (Namenda XR) 7mg, 14mg, 21mg, 28mg	(Sol/Tab) Initial: 5mg qd. Titrate: Increase at intervals of at least one week to 5mg bid, then 5mg and 10mg as separate doses, then to 10mg bid. Severe Renal Impairment: Target dose: 5mg bid. (Cap, ER) Initial: 7mg qd. Titrate: Increase at intervals of at least 1 week in 7mg increments to 28mg qd. Max: 28mg qd. Severe Renal Impairment: Target dose: 14mg/day. See PI for switching from Namenda to Namenda XR.	Dizziness, confusion, headache, constipation, coughing, HTN, pain, vomiting, somnolence, hallucinations
Rivastigmine tartrate (Exelon)	Treatment of mild to moderate dementia of the Alzheimer's type.	Cap: 1.5mg, 3mg, 4.5mg, 6mg; Sol: 2mg/mL [120mL]; Patch: 4.6mg/24 hrs, 9.5 mg/24 hrs [30*]	Initial: 1.5mg bid. Titrate: May increase by 1.5mg bid every 2 weeks. Max: 12mg/day. If not tolerating, suspend therapy for several doses and restart at same or next lower dose. If interrupted longer than several days, reinitiate with lowest daily dose and titrate as above. (Patch) Initial: Apply 4.6mg/24 hrs patch qd to clean, dry, hairless intact skin. Maint: Increase dose after 4 weeks. Max: 9.5mg/24 hrs if well tolerated. Switching from Capsules/Oral Sol: Total Oral Daily Dose <6mg: Switch to 4.6mg/24 hrs patch. Total Oral Daily Dose 6-12mg: Switch to 9.5mg/ 24 hrs patch. Apply 1st patch on day following last oral dose.	Nausea, vomiting, abdominal pain, dyspepsia, constipation, somnolence, anorexia, asthenia, headache, dizziness, fatigue, diarrhea, tremor, depression

ANTIPARKINSON'S AGENTS

DRUG (BRAND)	INDICATIONS	HOW SUPPLIED	DOSAGE	SIDE EFFECTS
Amantadine HCl	Treatment of idiopathic Parkinson's disease (Paralysis Agitans), post-encephalitic parkinsonism, and symptomatic parkinsonism. Treatment of drug-induced extrapyramidal reactions.	Cap, Tab: 100mg; Syr: 50mg/5mL	Parkinsonism: Initial: 100mg bid. Serious Associated Illness/ Concomitant High-Dose Antiparkinson Agent: Initial: 100mg qd. Titrate: May increase to 100mg bid after 1 to several weeks. Max: 400mg/day.	Nausea, dizziness, insomnia, depression, anxiety and irritability, hallucinations, confusion, anorexia, dry mouth, constipation, ataxia, livedo reticularis, peripheral edema, orthostatic hypotension, headache, somnolence, nervousness, dream abnormality, agitation, dry nose, diarrhea, fatigue
Apomorphine HCl (Apokyn)	Indicated for the acute, intermittent treatment of hypomobility, "off" episodes ("end-of-dose wearing off" and unpredictable "on/off" episodes) associated with advanced Parkinson's disease. Apokyn has been studied as an adjunct to other medications.	Inj: 10mg/mL [3mL]	Test Dose: 0.2mL (2mg) SQ to patients in an 'off' state; closely monitor BP. See PI for details. Titrate: Increase by 0.1mL (1mg) every few days, if needed; assess efficacy/tolerability. Max: 0.6mL (6mg)/dose. Renal Impairment: Test Dose/Initial: 0.1mL SQ.	Yawning, dyskinesias, nausea, vomiting, somnolence, dizziness, rhinorrhea, hallucinations, edema, chest pain, increased sweating, flushing, pallor
Benztropine mesylate (Cogentin)	Adjunct in all forms of parkinsonism. Control of drug-induced extrapyramidal disorders.	Inj: 1mg/mL₁ (Generic) Tab: 0.5mg, 1mg, 2mg	Idiopathic Parkinsonism: Initial: 0.5-1mg PO or IV/IM qhs. Postencephalitic Parkinsonism: 2mg/day PO or IV/IM given in 1 or more doses. Titrate: May increase every 5-6 days by 0.5mg. Usual: 1-2mg PO or IV/IM qhs. Max: 6mg/day.	Tachycardia, paralytic ileus, constipation, vomiting, nausea, dry mouth, confusion, blurred vision, urinary retention, heat stroke, hyperthermia, fever
Bromocriptine mesylate (Parlodel)	Treatment of signs and symptoms of idiopathic or postencephalitic Parkinson's disease. May provide additional therapeutic benefits as adjunctive treatment to levodopa.	Tab, Snap: 2.5mg*; Cap: 5mg *scored	Initial: 1.25mg bid. Titrate: If needed, increase by 2.5mg/day every 2-4 weeks. Max: 100mg/day. Take with food. See PI for detailed dosing information with levodopa.	Headache, dizziness, GI effects, orthostatic hypotension, fatigue, insomnia, hallucinations, abnormal involuntary movements, depression, syncope, shortness of breath, visual disturbance, asthenia

DRUG (BRAND)	INDICATIONS	HOW SUPPLIED	DOSAGE	SIDE EFFECTS
Carbidopa (Lodosyn)	For use with Sinemet or levodopa in treatment of symptoms of idiopathic Parkinson's disease, post-encephalitic parkinsonism, and symptomatic parkinsonism. For use in patients for whom the dosage of Sinemet provides less than adequate daily dosage (usually 70mg daily) of carbidopa. For use with levodopa in the patient whose dosage requirement of carbidopa and levodopa necessitates separate titration of each entity. Use with Sinemet or levodopa to permit the administration of lower doses of levodopa with reduced nausea and vomiting, more rapid dosage titration, and with a somewhat smoother response.	Tab: 25mg* *scored	With Sinemet or levodopa: Determine dose by careful titration. Most patients respond to a 1:10 proportion of carbidopa: levodopa provided carbidopa dose is ≥70mg/day. Max: 200mg/day. Consider amount of carbidopa in Sinemet when calculating dose. See PI for detailed dosing information.	Dyskinesia, psychotic episodes, delusions, hallucinations, paranoid ideation, depression with or without suicidal tendencies, dementia
Carbidopa/levodopa (Parcopa)	Treatment of symptoms of idiopathic Parkinson's disease, post-encephalitic parkinsonism, and symptomatic parkinsonism.	Tab, Disintegrating: (Carbidopa-Levodopa) 10mg-100mg*, 25mg-100mg*, 25mg-250mg* *scored	25mg-100mg tab: Initial: 1 tab tid. Titrate: Increase by 1 tab qd or qod up to 8 tabs/day. 10mg-100mg tab: Initial: 1 tab tid-qid. Titrate: Increase by 1 tab qd or qod up to 2 tabs qid. 70-100mg/day carbidopa required. Max: 200mg/day carbidopa. Conversion from levodopa: See PI.	Dyskinesia, nausea, cardiac irregularities, hypotension, dark saliva, GI bleeding, psychotic episodes, NMS, confusion, agitation, dizziness, somnolence, dream abnormalities, hemolytic and nonhemolytic anemia
Carbidopa/levodopa (Sinemet, Sinemet CR)	Treatment of symptoms of idiopathic Parkinson's disease, post-encephalitic parkinsonism, and symptomatic parkinsonism.	Tab: (Carbidopa-Levodopa) 10mg-100mg*, 25mg-100mg*, 25mg-250mg*; Tab, Extended Release: (Carbidopa-Levodopa) 25mg-100mg, 50mg-200mg* *scored	(Tab) 25mg-100mg tab: Initial: 1 tab tid. Titrate: Increase by 1 tab qd or qod up to 8 tabs/day, 10mg-100mg tab: Initial: 1 tab tid-qid. Titrate: Increase by 1 tab qd or qod up to 2 tabs qid. 70-100mg/day carbidopa required. Max: 200mg/day carbidopa. Conversion from levodopa: See PI. (Tab, Extended-Release) No Prior Levodopa Use: Initial: 1 50mg-200mg tab bid at intervals ≥6 hrs. Titrate: Increase or decrease dose or interval accordingly. Adjust dose at interval of ≥3 days. Usual: 400-1600mg/day levodopa, given in 4-8 hr intervals while awake. Conversion to Extended-Release Tabs: See PI.	Dyskinesia, nausea, cardiac irregularities, hypotension, dark saliva, GI bleeding, psychotic episodes, NMS, confusion, agitation, dizziness, somnolence, dream abnormalities

(Continued)

DRUG (BRAND)	INDICATIONS	HOW SUPPLIED	DOSAGE	SIDE EFFECTS
Carbidopa/levodopa/ entacapone (Stalevo)	Treatment of idiopathic Parkinson's disease to substitute for equivalent doses of immediate-release carbidopa/levodopa and entacapone previously administered as individual products, or to replace immediate-release carbidopa/ levodopa (without entacapone) for those experiencing signs and symptoms of end-of-dose "wearing off" and taking up to 600mg/day levodopa without experiencing dyskinesias.	Tab: (Carbidopa/Levodopa/ Entacapone): Stalevo 50: 12.5mg/50mg/200mg; Stalevo 75: 18.75mg/75mg/ 200 mg; Stalevo 100: 25mg/ 100mg/200mg; Stalevo 125: 31.25mg/125mg/200mg; Stalevo 150: 37.5mg/150mg/ 200mg; Stalevo 200: 50mg/ 200mg/200mg	Currently Taking Carbidopa/Levodopa and Entacapone: May switch directly to corresponding strength of levodopa/carbidopa/ entacapone. Currently Taking Carbidopa/Levodopa, but not Entacapone: First, titrate individually with carbidopa/levodopa product and entacapone product, then transfer to corresponding dose. Max dose: 8 tabs/day except Stalevo 200. Stalevo 200 Max: 6 tabs/day.	Dyskinesia, hyperkinesia, hypokinesia, dizziness, nausea, diarrhea, abdominal pain, constipation, vomiting, urine discoloration, back pain, fatigue
Diphenhydramine HCl Injection	For parkinsonism when oral therapy is not possible or contraindicated, as follows: elderly who are unable to tolerate more potent agents, mild cases of parkinsonism in other age groups, and in combination with centrally acting anticholinergic agents.	Inj: 50mg/mL	Usual: 10-50mg IV at ≤25 mg/min or up to 100mg IM if needed. Max: 400mg/day.	Sedation, drowsiness, dizziness, disturbed coordination, epigastric distress, thickening of bronchial secretions
Entacapone (Comtan)	Adjunct to levodopa/carbidopa for treatment of idiopathic Parkinson's disease if experience signs and symptoms of end-of-dose "wearing-off."	Tab: 200mg	200mg with each levodopa/carbidopa dose: Max: 1600mg/day. Withdraw slowing for discontinuation.	Sweating, back pain, dyskinesia, hyperkinesia, hypokinesia, nausea, diarrhea, abdominal pain, urine discoloration
Hyoscyamine sulfate (Levsin, Levbid, NuLev)	To reduce rigidity and tremors of Parkinson's disease and to control associated sialorrhea and hyperhidrosis.	(Levbid) Tab, Extended-Release: 0.375mg. (Levsin) Tab: 0.125mg; Tab, Sublingual: 0.125mg. (NuLev) Tab, Chewable: 0.125mg. Drops: 0.125mg/mL; Elixir: 0.125mg/5mL	May also chew or swallow SL tab. May also place on tongue and disintegrate chewable tab. Levsin and NuLev: 0.125mg-0.25mg q4h or prn. Max: 1.5mg/24 hrs. Levbid: 0.375-0.75mg q12h. Max: 1.5mg/24 hrs. Do not crush or chew. Drops: 1-2mL q4h or prn. Max: 12mL/24 hrs. Elixir: 1-2tsp q4h or prn. Max: 12tsp/24 hrs.	Anticholinergic effects, drowsiness, headache, nervousness

DRUG (BRAND)	INDICATIONS	HOW SUPPLIED	DOSAGE	SIDE EFFECTS
Pramipexole dihydrochloride (Mirapex)	Treatment of signs and symptoms of idiopathic Parkinson's disease.	Tab: 0.125mg, 0.25mg*, 0.5mg*, 0.75mg, 1mg*, 1.5mg* *scored	Initial: 0.125mg tid. Titrate: May increase every 5-7 days (eg, Week 2: 0.25mg tid; Week 3: 0.5mg tid; Week 4: 0.75mg tid; Week 5: 1mg tid; Week 6: 1.25mg tid; Week 7: 1.5mg tid). Maint: 0.5-1.5mg tid. Max: 1.5mg tid.†	Nausea, dizziness, somnolence, insomnia, constipation, asthenia, hallucinations, vision abnormalities, peripheral edema, arthritis, dry mouth, postural hypotension, chest pain, malaise, fatigue, headache
(Mirapex ER)		(Tab, ER): 0.375mg, 0.75mg, 1.5mg, 3mg, 4.5mg	(Tab, ER) Initial: 0.375mg qd. Titrate: May increase gradually not more frequently than q 5-7 days, first to 0.75mg/day and then by 0.75mg increments based on efficacy and tolerability. Max: 4.5mg/day. Refer to PI for more detailed dosing information.†	(Tab, ER) Somnolence, N/V, constipation, dizziness, fatigue, hallucinations, dry mouth, muscle spasms, peripheral edema
Rasagiline mesylate (Azilect)	Treatment of signs and symptoms of idiopathic Parkinson's disease as initial monotherapy and adjunct therapy to levodopa.	Tab: 0.5mg, 1mg	Monotherapy: 1mg qd. Adjunctive Therapy: Initial: 0.5mg qd. Titrate: May increase to 1mg qd. Adjust dose of levodopa with concomitant use. Concomitant Ciprofloxacin or Other CYP1A2 Inhibitors/Mild Hepatic Impairment: 0.5mg qd.	Headache, arthralgia, depression, fall, flu syndrome, dyskinesia, nausea, weight loss, constipation, postural hypotension, vomiting, dry mouth, rash, somnolence
Rivastigmine (Exelon)	Treatment of mild to moderate dementia associated with Parkinson's disease.	Cap: 1.5mg, 3mg, 4.5mg, 6mg; Patch: 4.6mg/24h, 9.5mg/24h; Sol: 2mg/mL (120mL)	(Cap, Sol): Initial: 1.5mg bid with meals in am and pm. Titrate: May increase at 4-week intervals to 3mg bid, then 4.5mg bid, and 6mg bid if tolerable. Usual: 1.5-6mg bid. Patch: Initial: 4.6mg/24h. Titrate: After 4 weeks, may increase to 9.5mg/24h if tolerated. Max: 9.5mg/24h.	Nausea, vomiting, anorexia, tremor, chest pain, dyskinesia, dyspepsia, back pain
Ropinirole HCl (Requip) (Requip XL)	Treatment of signs and symptoms of idiopathic Parkinson's disease.	Tab: 0.25mg, 0.5mg, 1mg, 2mg, 3mg, 4mg, 5mg Tab, ER: 2mg, 4mg, 6mg, 8mg, 12mg	Initial: 0.25mg tid. Titrate: May increase weekly by 0.25mg tid (0.75mg/day) for 4 weeks. After Week 4, may increase weekly by 1.5mg/day up to 9mg/day, then by 3mg/day weekly to 24mg/day. Max: 24mg/day. Withdrawal: Decrease dose to bid for 4 days, then qd for 3 days. (Requip XL). Tab. Extended-Release: Initial: 2mg qd for 1-2 weeks. Swallow whole. Titrate: May increase at ≥1 week intervals by 2mg/day. Max: 24mg/day. Levodopa dose may be gradually decreased as tolerated. Switching from IR to ER: Closely match total daily IR dose with initial extended-release dose. See PI for detailed information.	Neuralgia, increased BUN, hallucinations, somnolence, vomiting, headache, sweating, asthenia, edema, fatigue, syncope, orthostatic symptoms, dizziness, nausea, viral infection, confusion, abnormal vision

(Continued)

DRUG (BRAND)	INDICATIONS	HOW SUPPLIED	DOSAGE	SIDE EFFECTS
Selegiline HCl (Eldepryl)	Adjunct in the management of Parkinsonian patients being treated with levodopa/carbidopa who exhibit deterioration in the quality of their response to this therapy.	Cap: 5mg; (Generic) Tab: 5mg	5mg bid, at breakfast and lunch. Max: 10mg/day. May attempt to reduce levodopa/carbidopa by 10–30% after 2–3 days of therapy. May reduce further with continued therapy.	Nausea, dizziness, lightheadedness, fainting, abdominal pain, confusion, hallucinations, dry mouth
Selegiline HCl (Zelapar)	Adjunct in the management of patients with Parkinson's disease being treated with levodopa/carbidopa who exhibit deterioration in the quality of their response to this therapy.	Tab, Orally Disintegrating: 1.25mg	1.25mg qd for 6 weeks. Titrate: After 6 weeks, may increase to 2.5mg if desired benefit not achieved. Max: 2.5mg/day.	Nausea, dizziness, pain, headache, insomnia, rhinitis, skin disorders, dyskinesia, backache, dyspepsia, stomatitis, constipation, hallucinations, pharyngitis, rash
Tolcapone (Tasmar)	Adjunct to levodopa/carbidopa for the treatment of symptoms of idiopathic Parkinson's disease.	Tab: 100mg, 200mg	Initial: 100mg tid. Use 200mg tid only if clinical benefit is justified. May need to decrease levodopa dose.	Dyskinesia, nausea, dystonia, excessive dreaming, anorexia, muscle cramps, orthostatic complaints, diarrhea, dizziness, headache, hepatotoxicity
Trihexyphenidyl HCl	Adjunct treatment for all forms of parkinsonism (postencephalitic, arteriosclerotic, and idiopathic). For control of extrapyramidal disorders caused by CNS drugs.	Sol: 2mg/5mL [473mL]; Tab: 2mg*, 5mg* *scored	Idiopathic Parkinsonism: 1mg on Day 1. Titrate: Increase by 2mg every 3–5 days. Usual: 6–10mg/day. Max: 15mg/day. Drug-Induced Parkinsonism: Initial: 1mg. If extrapyramidal manifestations not controlled in a few hrs, increase dose until achieve control. Usual: 5–15mg/day. Concomitant Levodopa or Other Parasympathetic Inhibitors: See PI.	Dry mouth, blurred vision, dizziness, nausea, nervousness, constipation, drowsiness, urinary hesitancy/retention, tachycardia, pupil dilation, increased intraocular tension, vomiting, weakness, headache

†For specific dosing information on different creatinine clearance values, see full Prescribing Information.

OPIOID PRODUCTS

GENERIC	BRAND	DOSAGE FORMS	ORAL EQUI-ANALGESIC DOSE	EQUI-ANALGESIC DOSE**	USUAL ADULT DOSE	MAX DOSE	INDICATION	DEA SCHEDULE
Codeine		**Tab:** 15mg, 30mg, 60mg	200mg.	130mg.	PO, IM, SQ 15-60mg up to q4h prn.	360mg/24 hrs.	Relief of mild to moderately severe pain.	Schedule II
Codeine phosphate/ Acetaminophen		**Elixir:** 12mg-120mg/5mL			15mL q4h prn. 15-60mg codeine/dose and 300-1000mg APAP. Doses may be repeated q4h.	Codeine: 360mg/day. APAP: 4g/day.	Relief of mild to moderately severe pain.	Schedule V
		Tab: 15mg-300mg						Schedule III
	Tylenol #3	**Tab:** 30mg-300mg						Schedule III
	Tylenol #4	**Tab:** 60mg-300mg						Schedule III
Dihydrocodeine bitartrate/Aspirin/ Caffeine	Synalgos-DC	**Cap:** 16mg-356.4mg-30mg			2 caps q4h prn.		Relief of moderate to moderately severe pain.	Schedule III
Fentanyl	Abstral	**Tab, SL:** 100mcg, 200mcg, 300mcg, 400mcg, 600mcg, 800mcg			Initial: 100mcg. Individually titrate.	2 doses/episode of breakthrough pain separated by 30 min. Wait 2 hrs between episodes.	Management of breakthrough pain in cancer patients ≥18 years who are already receiving, and who are tolerant to, opioid therapy for their underlying persistent cancer pain.	Schedule II
	Duragesic	**Patch:** 12mcg/hr, 25mcg/hr, 50mcg/hr, 75mcg/hr, 100mcg/hr			Initial: 25mcg/hr for 72 hrs. Individualize dose.		Management of persistent, moderate to severe chronic pain that requires continuous, around-the-clock opioid administration for an extended period of time, and cannot be managed by other means such as non-steroidal analgesics, opioid combination products, or immediate-release opioids.	Schedule II

(Continued)

GENERIC	BRAND	DOSAGE FORMS	ORAL EQUI-ANALGESIC DOSE	EQUI-ANALGESIC DOSE**	USUAL ADULT DOSE	MAX DOSE	INDICATION	DEA SCHEDULE
Fentanyl citrate	Actiq	**Loz:** 200mcg, 400mcg, 600mcg, 800mcg, 1200mcg, 1600mcg			200mcg. Dispense no more than 6 units. Individually titrate.	2 doses/episode of breakthrough pain separated by 15 min. Wait 4 hrs between episodes. 4 units/day.	Management of breakthrough cancer pain in patients with malignancies who are already receiving and are tolerant to around-the-clock opioid therapy for their underlying persistent cancer pain.	Schedule II
	Fentora	**Tab, Buccal:** 100mcg, 200mcg, 400mcg, 600mcg, 800mcg			Initial:100mcg. Converting from Actiq doses ≥600mcg: 200mcg; proceed using multiples of this strength. Titrate: If 100mcg Initial Dose: Give two 100-mcg tabs (one on each side of mouth); may increase to four 100-mcg tabs (two on each side of the mouth). Use multiples of 200-mcg tabs for doses >400mcg.	2 doses/episode of breakthrough pain separated by 30 min. Wait 4 hrs between episodes. Not more than 4 tabs simultaneously.	Management of breakthrough pain in patients with cancer who are already receiving and are tolerant to around-the-clock opioid therapy for their underlying persistent cancer pain.	
	Onsolis	**Film, Buccal:** 200mcg, 400mcg, 600mcg, 800mcg, 1200mcg			Initial: 200mcg. Titrate: Use multiples of 200-mcg films. Increase by 200mcg per subsequent episode until effect.	Not more than four 200-mcg films simultaneously. If no adequate pain relief and tolerant to 800mcg, give one 1200-mcg film. Single doses are given 2 hrs apart; use once per breakthrough pain episode.	Management of breakthrough pain in patients with cancer, ≥18 yrs who are already receiving and are tolerant to opioid therapy for their underlying persistent cancer pain.	

Hydrocodone bitartrate/ Acetaminophen	**Tab:** 5mg-325mg, 7.5mg-325mg, 5mg-500mg, 7.5mg-650mg		(5/325, 5/500) 1-2 tabs q4-6h. (7.5/325, 7.5/650) 1 tab q4-6h.	(5/325, 5/500): 8 tabs/day, (7.5/325, 7.5/650): 6 tabs/day.	Relief of moderate to moderately severe pain.	Schedule III
	Co-gesic	**Cap:** 5mg-500mg	1-2 caps q4-6h prn.	8 caps/day.		
		Tab: 5mg-500mg	1-2 tab q4-6h prn.	8 tab(s)/day.		
	Hycet	**Sol:** 7.5mg-325mg/15mL	1 tbsp q4-6h prn.	6 tbsp/day.		
	Lorcet Plus, Lorcet 10/650	**Tab:** (Plus) 7.5mg-650mg, (10/650) 10mg-650mg	1 tab q4-6h prn.	6 tabs/day.		
	Lortab Elixir Lortab	**Sol:** 7.5mg-500mg/15mL **Tab:** 2.5mg-500mg, 5mg-500mg, 7.5mg-500mg, 10mg-500mg	(Sol) 1 tbsp q4-6h prn. (2.5/500, 5/500): 1-2 tabs q4-6h prn. (7.5/500,10/500): 1 tab q4-6h prn.	(Sol) 6 tbsp/day. (2.5/500, 5/500): 8 tabs/day. (7.5/500, 10/500): 6 tabs/day.		
	Maxidone	**Tab:** 10mg-750mg	1 tab q4-6h prn.	5 tabs/day.		
	Norco	**Tab:** 5mg-325mg, 7.5mg-325mg, 10mg-325mg	(5/325): 1-2 tabs q4-6h prn. (7.5/325, 10/325): 1 tab q4-6h prn.	(5/325): 8 tabs/day. (7.5/325): 6 tabs/day. (10/325): 6 tabs/day.		
	Vicodin	**Tab:** 5mg-500mg	1-2 tabs q4-6h prn.	8 tabs/day.		
	Vicodin ES	**Tab:** 7.5mg-750mg	1 tab q4-6h prn.	5 tabs/day.		
	Vicodin HP	**Tab:** 10mg-660mg	1 tab q4-6h prn.	6 tabs/day.		
	Zydone	**Tab:** 5mg-400mg, 7.5mg-400mg, 10mg-400mg	(5/400): 1-2 tabs q4-6h prn. (7.5/400, 10/400): 1 tab q4-6h prn.	(5/400): 8 tabs/day. (7.5/400, 10/400): 6 tabs/day.		
Hydrocodone bitartrate/ibuprofen	Reprexain	**Tab:** 2.5mg-200mg, 5mg-200mg, 10mg-200mg	1 tab q4-6h prn.	5 tabs/day.	Short-term (generally <10 days) management of acute pain.	Schedule III
	Vicoprofen	**Tab:** 7.5-200mg	1 tab q4-6h prn.	5 tabs/day.		
Hydromorphone HCl	Dilaudid, Dilaudid-HP	**Tab:** 2mg, 4mg, 8mg; **Sol:** 1mg/mL; **Inj:** 1mg/mL, 2mg/mL, 4mg/mL; **HP:** 10mg/mL, **Pow:** 250mg	7.5mg.	1.5mg.	**Tab:** 2-4mg, PO q4-6h. **Sol:** 2.5-10mL q3-6h as directed. **Inj:** 1-2mg SQ or IM q4-6h. HP: Individualized for each patient.	Management of pain. (HP) Relief of moderate to severe pain in opioid-tolerant patients who require larger than usual doses of opioids to provide adequate pain relief.	Schedule II

(Continued)

GENERIC	BRAND	DOSAGE FORMS	ORAL EQUI-ANALGESIC DOSE	EQUI-ANALGESIC DOSE**	USUAL ADULT DOSE	MAX DOSE	INDICATION	DEA SCHEDULE
Hydromorphone HCl (continued)	Exalgo	Tab, ER: 8mg, 12mg, 16mg			Dose range: 8-64mg. Administer once q24h. Individualize dose.		Management of moderate to severe pain in opioid-tolerant patients requiring continuous, around-the-clock opioid analgesia for an extended period of time.	
Meperidine HCl		Syr: 50mg/5mL		75mg.	50-150mg q3-4h prn.		Moderate to severe pain. Inj: also for preoperative medication, anesthesia support, and obstetrical analgesia.	Schedule II
	Demerol	Tab: 50mg, 100mg; Inj: 25mg/mL, 50mg/mL, 75mg/mL, 100mg/mL			Tab: 50-150mg q3-4h prn. Inj: 50-150mg IM/SQ q3-4h prn; 50-100mg IM/SQ 30-90 min prior to anesthesia for pre-op use or at 1- to 3-hr intervals during obstetrical analgesia.		Relief of moderate to severe pain.	
Methadone HCl	Dolophine,* Methadose*	Inj: 10mg/mL Tab: 5mg, 10mg	20mg.	10mg.	2.5mg to 10mg q8-12h, slowly titrated to effect.		To treat moderate to severe pain not responsive to non-narcotic analgesics.	Schedule II
Morphine sulfate	Astramorph PF	Inj: 0.5mg/mL, 1mg/mL	30-60mg.	10mg.	IV: 2-10mg/70kg of body weight. Epidural: Initial: 5mg. Titrate: If inadequate pain relief in 1 hr, administer incremental doses of 1-2mg at intervals sufficient to assess effectiveness. Continuous Infusion: 2-4mg/24 hrs. IT: 0.2-1mg single dose.	Epidural: 10mg/24h.	Management of pain not responsive to non-narcotic analgesics.	Schedule II

GENERIC	BRAND	DOSAGE FORMS	ORAL EQUI-ANALGESIC DOSE	EQUI-ANALGESIC DOSE**	USUAL ADULT DOSE	MAX DOSE	INDICATION	DEA SCHEDULE
Morphine sulfate *(continued)*	Avinza	**Cap, ER:** 30mg, 45mg, 60mg, 75mg, 90mg, 120mg			30mg q24h. Individualize dose.	1600mg/day.	Relief of moderate to severe pain requiring continuous, around-the-clock opioid therapy for an extended period of time.	
	Depodur	**Inj:** 10mg/mL			Epidural: 10-15mg		Treatment of pain following major surgery.	
	Duramorph	**Inj:** 0.5mg/mL, 1mg/mL			IV: 2-10mg/70kg of body weight. Epidural: Initial: 5mg. Titrate: If inadequate pain relief in 1 hr, administer incremental doses of 1-2mg at intervals sufficient to assess effectiveness. IT: 0.2-1mg single dose.	Epidural: 10mg/24h.	Management of pain not responsive to non-narcotic analgesics.	
	Infumorph	**Inj:** 10mg/mL (200mg), 25mg/mL (500mg)			IT: 0.2-10mg/day. Epidural: 3.5-30mg/day. Individualize dose.		Treatment of intractable chronic pain in microinfusion devices.	
	Kadian	**Cap, ER:** 10mg, 20mg, 30mg, 50mg, 60mg, 80mg, 100mg, 200mg			Give 50% of daily oral morphine dose q12h or give 100% oral morphine dose q24h.	Do not give more frequently than q12h.	Management of moderate to severe pain when a continuous, around-the-clock opioid analgesic is needed for an extended period of time.	
	MS Contin	**Tab, ER:** 15mg, 30mg, 60mg, 100mg, 200mg			Give 50% of pts 24-hr immediate-release oral morphine requirement q12h or ¹/₃ of pts 24-hr requirement q8h.		Management of moderate to severe pain when a continuous, around-the-clock analgesic is needed for an extended period of time.	
	Oramorph SR	**Tab, ER:** 15mg, 30mg, 60mg, 100mg			Single dose is 1/2 of daily oral morphine requirement q12h.		Relief of pain in patients who require opioid analgesics for more than a few days.	

(Continued)

GENERIC	BRAND	DOSAGE FORMS	ORAL EQUI-ANALGESIC DOSE	EQUI-ANALGESIC DOSE**	USUAL ADULT DOSE	MAX DOSE	INDICATION	DEA SCHEDULE
Morphine sulfate/ Naltrexone HCl	Embeda	**Cap, ER:** 20mg–0.8mg, 30mg–1.2mg, 50mg–2mg, 60mg–2.4mg, 80mg–3.2mg, 100mg–4mg			May be administered qd or bid. The lowest dose should be used. Titrate no more frequently than qod.		Management of moderate to severe pain when a continuous, around-the-clock opioid analgesic is needed for an extended period of time.	Schedule II
Oxycodone/ Acetaminophen	Percocet	**Tab:** 2.5mg–325mg, 5mg–325mg, 7.5mg–325mg, 7.5mg–500mg,10mg–325mg, 10mg–650mg			(2.5/325): 1-2 tabs q6h. (5/325): 1 tab q6h prn. (7.5/500): 1 tab q6h prn. (10/650): 1 tab q6h prn. (7.5/325): 1 tab q6h prn. (10/325): 1 tab q6h prn.	(2.5/325): 12 tabs/day. (5/325):12 tabs/day. (7.5/500): 8 tabs/day. (10/650) 6 tabs/day. (7.5/325): 8 tabs/day. (10/325): 6 tabs/day.	Relief of moderate to moderately severe pain.	Schedule II
	Roxicet	**Tab:** 5mg–325mg, 5mg–500mg **Sol:** 5mg–325mg/5mL			Tab: 1 tab q6h prn. Sol: 5mL q6h prn.	Tab: 12 tabs/day. Sol: 60mL/day. APAP: 4g/day.		
	Tylox	**Cap:** 5mg–500mg			1 cap q6h prn.	APAP: 4g/day.		
Oxycodone/Ibuprofen	Combunox	**Tab:** 5mg–400mg			1 tab/dose.	4 tabs/day. Do not exceed 7 days.	Short term (<7 days) management of acute, moderate to severe pain.	Schedule II
Oxycodone HCl	OxyContin	**Tab, ER:** 10mg, 15mg, 20mg, 30mg, 40mg, 60mg, 80mg	20mg.		10mg q12h. Titrate. May increase the q12h dose (not the dosing frequency). May increase the total daily dose by 25-50% of the current dose every 1-2 days.		Management of moderate to severe pain when a continuous, around-the-clock opioid analgesic is needed for an extended period. Only for postoperative use in patients already receiving the drug before surgery or those expected to have moderate-severe postoperative pain for an extended period of time.	Schedule II
		Cap, IR: 5mg; **Sol:** 20mg/mL.			Cap, IR: 5mg q6h prn; Sol: Individualize based on previous analgesic treatment.			

GENERIC	BRAND	DOSAGE FORMS	ORAL EQUI-ANALGESIC DOSE	EQUI-ANALGESIC DOSE**	USUAL ADULT DOSE	MAX DOSE	INDICATION	DEA SCHEDULE
Oxycodone HCl *(continued)*	Roxicodone	**Tab:** 5mg, 15mg, 30mg			Tab: 5-15mg q4-6h prn.		Relief of moderate to moderately severe pain. (Sol) Management of moderate to severe chronic pain in opioid-tolerant patients.	
Oxycodone HCl/ Aspirin	Percodan	**Tab:** 4.8355mg-325mg			1 tab q6h prn.	12 tabs/day or ASA 4g/day.	Relief of moderate to moderately severe pain.	Schedule II
Oxymorphone HCl	Opana	**Inj:** 1mg/1mL **Tab:** 5mg, 10mg	10mg (PR).	1mg.	Inj: SQ/IM: 1-1.5mg q4-6h prn, IV: 0.5mg initial. Labor Analgesia: 0.5-1mg IM. Tab: 10-20mg q4-6h.		(Inj) Relief of moderate to severe acute pain. For pre-operative medication, for support of anesthesia, for obstetrical analgesia, and for relief of anxiety in patients with dyspnea associated with pulmonary edema secondary to acute left ventricular dys-function. (Tab) Relief of moderate to severe acute pain. (Tab, ER) Relief of moderate to severe acute pain in patients requiring continuous, around-the-clock opioid treatment for extended period of time.	Schedule II
	Opana ER	**Tab, ER:** 5mg, 10mg, 20mg, 30mg, 40mg			5mg q12h. Titrate individually at increments of 5-10mg q12h every 3-7 days.			
Tapentadol	Nucynta	**Tab:** 50mg, 75mg, 100mg			50mg, 75mg, or 100mg q4-6 hrs depending upon pain intensity. A second dose may be given 1hr after first dose.	700mg/day on first day of therapy; 600mg/day on sub-sequent days of therapy.	Relief of moderate to severe acute pain in patients ≥18 yrs.	Schedule II

*Other formulations are available.

**IM

Refer to individual product's prescribing information for more detailed dosing.

ORAL ANTICONVULSANTS

DRUG (BRAND)	INDICATIONS	USUAL ADULT DOSE*	THERAPEUTIC SERUM LEVELS
BARBITURATES			
Mephobarbital (Mebaral)	Grand mal and petit mal epilepsy	400-600mg/day	NA
Phenobarbital	Generalized and partial	60-200mg/day	10-40mcg/mL
Primidone (Mysoline)	Tonic-clonic, psychomotor, focal	750-2000mg/day	5-12mcg/mL
BENZODIAZEPINES			
Clonazepam (Klonopin)	Myoclonic, akinetic, Lennox-Gastaut syndrome, absence seizures (if failed succinimides)	1.5-20mg/day	NA
Clorazepate dipotassium (Tranxene T-Tab)	Adjunct therapy in partial seizures	22.5-90mg/day	NA
Diazepam (Valium)	Adjunct in convulsive disorders	4-40mg/day	NA
HYDANTOINS			
Ethotoin (Peganone)	Tonic-clonic, complex partial (psychomotor)	2000-3000mg/day	N/A
Phenytoin (Dilantin, Phenytek)	Tonic-clonic, complex partial (psychomotor, temporal lobe), prevent/treat seizures during/following neurosurgery. (Suspension) Tonic-clonic, psychomotor (temporal lobe) seizures	300-600mg/day (Suspension) 375-625mg/day	10-20mcg/mL
SUCCINIMIDES			
Ethosuximide (Zarontin)	Absence	500-1500mg/day	40-100mcg/mL
Methsuximide (Celontin)	Absence	300-1200mg/day	Toxic level: >40mcg/mL
MISCELLANEOUS			
Carbamazepine (Carbatrol, Tegretol)	Tonic-clonic, mixed, partial (psychomotor, temporal lobe)	800-1200mg/day	4-12mcg/mL
Divalproex sodium (Depakote, Depakote ER, Depakote Sprinkles) **Valproic acid** (Depakene, Stavzor)	Absence, complex partial, adjunct in multiple seizure types	10-60mg/kg/day	50-100mcg/mL
Felbamate** (Felbatol)	Partial with or w/o generalization (adults), partial/generalized with Lennox-Gastaut syndrome (pediatrics)	1200-3600mg/day	NA
Gabapentin (Neurontin)	Partial with and without secondary generalization (>12 yrs), partial (3-12 yrs)	900-1800mg/day	NA
Lacosamide (Vimpat)	Partial	200-400mg/day	NA
Lamotrigine (Lamictal, Lamictal CD, Lamictal ODT, Lamictal XR)	Partial, generalized seizures of Lennox-Gastaut syndrome, tonic-clonic (≥2 yrs). (Lamictal XR) Partial with and without secondary generalization, tonic-clonic (≥13 yrs)	100-500mg/day (Lamictal XR) 200-600mg/day	NA

(Continued)

DRUG (BRAND)	INDICATIONS	USUAL ADULT DOSE*	THERAPEUTIC SERUM LEVELS
MISCELLANEOUS (Continued)			
Levetiracetam (Keppra, Keppra XR)	Partial, myoclonic, primary generalized tonic-clonic (Keppra XR): Partial	1000-3000mg/day	NA
Oxcarbazepine (Trileptal)	Partial	600-2400mg/day	NA
Pregabalin (Lyrica)	Partial	150-600mg/day	NA
Rufinamide (Banzel)	Lennox-Gastaut syndrome	400-3200mg/day	NA
Tiagabine (Gabitril)	Partial	32-56mg/day	NA
Topiramate (Topamax, Topamax Sprinkle)	Partial, tonic-clonic, Lennox-Gastaut syndrome (≥2 yrs)	200-400mg/day	NA
Vigabatrin (Sabril)	Refractory complex partial seizures. (Powder) Infantile spasms (1 month-2 yrs)	3000mg	NA
Zonisamide (Zonegran)	Partial	100-400mg/day	NA

*Please refer to complete monograph for pediatric dosing.
**For severe epilepsy refractory to other treatment where the risk of aplastic anemia and/or liver failure is deemed acceptable. Fully advise patient and obtain written, informed consent before treatment. Closely monitor patient.
NA = Not Available.

TRIPTANS FOR ACUTE MIGRAINE

DRUG	BRAND	HOW SUPPLIED	INITIAL & (MAX) DOSE*	HEPATIC/RENAL DOSE ADJUSTMENT*
Almotriptan malate	Axert	Tab: 6.25mg, 12.5mg	6.25-12.5mg. May repeat after 2 hrs. (25mg/24 hrs.)	Initial: 6.25mg. Max: 12.5mg/24 hrs.
Eletriptan HBr	Relpax	Tab: 20mg, 40mg	20-40mg. May repeat after 2 hrs. (40mg/dose or 80mg/day)	Severe Hepatic Impairment: Avoid use.
Frovatriptan succinate	Frova	Tab: 2.5mg	2.5mg. May repeat after 2 hrs. (7.5mg/day)	No adjustment.
Naratriptan HCl	Amerge	Tab: 1mg, 2.5mg	1-2.5mg. May repeat after 4 hrs. (5mg/24 hrs.)	Severe Renal/Hepatic Impairment: Avoid use. Mild-Moderate Renal/Hepatic Impairment: Use lower dose. Max: 2.5mg/24 hrs.
Rizatriptan benzoate	Maxalt	Tab: 5mg, 10mg	5-10mg. May repeat after 2 hrs. (30mg/24 hrs.)	No adjustment.
	Maxalt-MLT	Tab, Disintegrating: 5mg, 10mg	5-10mg. May repeat after 2 hrs. (30mg/24 hrs.)	No adjustment.
Sumatriptan	Alsuma, Imitrex, Sumavel DosePro	(Alsuma, Imitrex, Sumavel DosePro) Inj**: 6mg/0.5mL, (Imitrex) Inj**,stat dose system: 4mg, 6mg	(Alsuma, Imitrex, Sumavel DosePro) 6mg SQ. May repeat after 1 hr. (6mg/dose or 12mg/24 hrs.)	(Imitrex) Severe Hepatic Impairment: Avoid use.
		Nasal Spray: 5mg, 20mg	5mg, 10mg, or 20mg single dose into 1 nostril. May repeat after 2 hrs. (40mg/24 hrs.)	Severe Hepatic Impairment: Avoid use.
		Tab: 25mg, 50mg, 100mg	25-100mg. May repeat after 2 hrs. (200mg/24 hrs.)	Severe Hepatic Impairment: Avoid use. Hepatic Disease: Max: 50mg/single dose.
Zolmitriptan	Zomig	Nasal Spray: 5mg	5mg. May repeat after 2 hrs. (10mg/24 hrs.)	Hepatic Impairment: Use doses <2.5mg of alternate formulation.
		Tab: 2.5mg, 5mg	2.5mg or lower. May repeat after 2 hrs. (10mg/24 hrs.)	Hepatic Impairment: Use lower dose.
	Zomig-ZMT	Tab, Disintegrating: 2.5mg, 5mg	2.5mg. May repeat after 2 hrs. (10mg/24 hrs.)	Hepatic Impairment: Use lower dose.
COMBINATION DRUG				
Naproxen-Sumatriptan	Treximet	Tab: (Naproxen-Sumatriptan): 500mg/85mg [9°]	1 tab; may repeat after 2 hrs. (2 tabs/24 hrs.) Do not split, crush, or chew.	Hepatic Impairment/Advanced Renal Disease (CrCl <30mL/min): Avoid use.

*NOTE: Dosages shown are for adults ≥18 yrs. For more detailed information, refer to the individual monograph or the drug's FDA-approved labeling.

**Also indicated for acute treatment of cluster headaches.

FERTILITY AGENTS

DRUG (BRAND)	INDICATIONS	HOW SUPPLIED	DOSAGE
Cetrorelix acetate (Cetrotide)	For inhibition of premature LH surges in women undergoing controlled ovarian stimulation.	Inj: 0.25mg, 3mg	Multiple-Dose Regimen: 0.25mg SQ qd; start on stimulation day 5 (AM or PM) or day 6 (AM). Continue until hCG administration. Single-Dose Regimen: 3mg SQ single dose when estradiol level indicates appropriate stimulation response, usually on stimulation Day 7. If hCG not given within 4 days, then give 0.25mg SQ qd until day of hCG administration.
Choriogonadotropin alfa (Ovidrel)	For induction of final follicular maturation and early luteinization in infertile women who have undergone pituitary desensitization and have been appropriately pretreated with follicle stimulating hormone in an Assisted Reproductive Technology program. To induce ovulation and pregnancy in anovulatory, infertile women in whom infertility is functional and is not due to primary ovarian failure.	Inj: 250mcg/0.5mL	250mcg SQ 1 day following the last dose of follicle stimulating agent. Withhold if excessive ovarian response.
Chorionic gonadotropin (Novarel)	To induce ovulation and pregnancy in anovulatory, infertile women in whom anovulation is not due to primary ovarian failure and who have been pretreated with human menotropins.	Inj: 10,000 U	5000-10,000 U IM 1 day after last dose of menotropins.
Chorionic gonadotropin (Pregnyl)	To induce ovulation and pregnancy in anovulatory, infertile women in whom anovulation is not due to primary ovarian failure and who have been pretreated with human menotropins.	Inj: 10,000 U	5000-10,000 U IM 1 day after last dose of menotropins.
Clomiphene citrate (Clomid)	Treatment of ovulatory dysfunction in women desiring pregnancy.	Tab: 50mg* *scored	Initial: 50mg/day for 5 days. Start any time if no recent uterine bleeding. If progestin-induced bleeding is intended, or if spontaneous uterine bleeding occurs, start on the 5th day of the cycle. If ovulation does not occur, increase to 100mg qd for 5 days, 30 days after the 1st course. Max: 100mg qd for 5 days. If ovulation does not occur after 3 courses, further treatment is not recommended. Long-term cyclic therapy is not recommended beyond total of about 6 cycles.
Clomiphene citrate (Serophene)	Treatment of ovulatory dysfunction in women desiring pregnancy.	Tab: 50mg* *scored	Initial: 50mg/day for 5 days. Start any time if no recent uterine bleeding. If progestin-induced bleeding is intended, or if spontaneous uterine bleeding occurs, start on the 5th day of the cycle. If ovulation does not occur, increase to 100mg qd for 5 days, 30 days after the 1st course. Max: 100mg qd for 5 days. If ovulation does not occur after 3 courses, further treatment is not recommended. Long-term cyclic therapy is not recommended beyond total of about 6 cycles.

DRUG (BRAND)	INDICATIONS	HOW SUPPLIED	DOSAGE
Follitropin alfa (Gonal-F)	For development of multiple follicles in ovulatory patients participating in Assisted Reproductive Technology (ART) program. For the induction of ovulation and pregnancy in anovulatory infertile patients in whom the cause of infertility is functional and not due to primary ovarian failure. (Men) For induction of spermatogenesis in primary and secondary hypogonadotropic hypogonadism in whom the cause of infertility is not due to primary testicular failure.	Inj: 450 IU, 1050 IU	Individualize dose. Oligo-Anovulation: Initial: 75 IU/day SQ. Titrate: May make incremental adjustment in dose of up to 37.5 IU after 14 days. Further increases of same magnitude every 7 days if needed. Give hCG 5000 U 1 day after last dose. Do not exceed 35 days of therapy unless an E2 rise indicates imminent follicular development. Max: 300 IU/day. ART: Initial: 150 IU/day SQ on cycle Day 2 or 3 (early follicular phase). In most cases, should not exceed 10 days. If gonadotropins suppressed, initiate at 225 IU/day. Titrate: Adjust after 5 days if needed, then at intervals no less than 3-5 days and not exceeding 75-150 IU/adjustment. Max: 450 IU/day. Once follicular development is evident, give hCG 5000-10,000 U. Hypogonadotropic Hypogonadism: Pretreat with hCG 1000-2250 U 2-3x/week to achieve normal serum testosterone levels. When normal, give 150 IU SQ and hCG 1000 IU 3x/week. Max: 300 IU 3x/week.
Follitropin alfa (Gonal-F RFF)	For development of multiple follicles in ovulatory patients participating in Assisted Reproductive Technology (ART) program. For induction of ovulation and pregnancy in oligo-anovulatory infertile patients in whom the cause of infertility is functional and not due to primary ovarian failure.	Inj: 75 IU; 300 IU/0.5mL, 450 IU/0.75mL, 900 IU/ 1.5mL [prefilled pen]	Individualize dose. Oligo-Anovulation: Initial: 75 IU/day SQ. Titrate: May make incremental adjustment in dose of up to 37.5 IU after 14 days. Further dose increases of the same magnitude every 7 days if needed. Do not exceed 35 days of therapy unless an E2 rise indicates imminent follicular development. Give hCG after last dose. Max: 300 IU/day. ART: Initial: 150 IU/day SQ on cycle Day 2 or 3 (early follicular phase). In most cases, therapy should not exceed 10 days. If gonadotropin levels are suppressed, initiate at 150 IU/day for patients <35 yrs and 225 IU/day for patients ≥35 yrs. Titrate: Adjust after 5 days if needed, then at intervals no less than 3-5 days and not >75-150 IU/adjustment. Max: 450 IU/day. Administer hCG if follicular development is evident and withhold if ovaries are abnormally enlarged on the last day.
Follitropin beta (Follistim AQ)	For the development of multiple follicles in ovulatory patients participating in Assisted Reproductive Technology (ART). For the induction of ovulation and pregnancy in anovulatory infertile patients in whom the cause of infertility is functional and not due to primary ovarian failure. (Men) Induction of spermatogenesis in primary and secondary hypogonadotropic hypogonadism in whom the cause infertility is not due to primary testicular failure.	Cartridge: 150 IU, 300 IU, 600 IU, 900 IU. Inj: 75 IU, 150 IU	Individualize dose. Ovulation Induction: Cartridge: Initial: 50 IU SQ qd for 7 days. Titrate: Increase by 25-50 IU/week. Max: 250 IU qd. Inj: 75 IU IM/SQ for 7 days. Titrate: Increase by 25-50 IU/week. Max 300 IU qd. Administer hCG 5000-10,000 IU when pre-ovulatory conditions are reached. ART: Cartridge: Initial: 125-175 IU SQ qd for 4 days. Titrate: Adjust based upon ovarian response. See PI. Max: 500 IU qd. Inj: Initial: 150 to 225 IU SQ/IM qd for 4 days. Titrate: Adjust based upon ovarian response. See PI. Max: 600 IU qd. Administer hCG 5000-10,000 IU when a sufficient number of follicles of adequate size are present. Induction of Spermatogenesis: Pretreat with hCG: Initial: 1500 IU of hCG 2x/week to achieve normal serum testosterone levels. Increase hCG to 3000 IU 2x/week if serum testosterone levels not normal after 8 Weeks. When normal, give Follistim AQ 450 IU/week SQ (225 IU 2x/week or 150 IU 3x/week). Consider lower dose with cartridge. Continue concomitant therapy for 3-4 months.

(Continued)

DRUG (BRAND)	INDICATIONS	HOW SUPPLIED	DOSAGE
Ganirelix acetate	For inhibition of premature LH surges in women undergoing controlled ovarian hyperstimulation.	Inj: 250mcg/0.5mL	After initiating FSH therapy on Day 2 or 3 of the cycle give 250mg SQ qd during the mid to late follicular phase. Continue until hCG administration.
Lutropin alfa (Luveris)	Used in combination with Gonal-F (follitropin alfa) for stimulation of follicular development in infertile hypogonadotropic hypogonadal women with profound luteinizing hormone deficiency (LH <1.2 IU/L).	Inj: 75 IU	Initial: 75 IU with 75-150 IU of Gonal-F qd SQ as two separate injections. Give hCG 1 day after last dose. Do not exceed 14 days of therapy unless signs of imminent follicular development. Do not exceed 225 IU/day of Gonal-F.
Menotropins (Repronex)	With hCG, for multiple follicular development and ovulation induction in women who received pituitary suppression.	Inj: (FSH-LH) 75 IU-75 IU	Oligo-Anovulation: Individualize dose. Initial: 150 IU SQ/IM qd for 5 days. Adjust subsequent dose to individual response at intervals no less than every 2 days and not exceeding 75-150 IU/adjustment. Max: 450 IU/day. Dosing >12 days is not recommended. May repeat course if inadequate response. ART: Initial: 225 IU SQ/IM. Adjust subsequent dose to individual response at intervals no less than every 2 days and not exceeding 75-150 IU/adjustment. Max: 450 IU/day. Dosing >12 days is not recommended. If adequate response, give 5000-10,000 U hCG.
Menotropins (Menopur)	Development of multiple follicles and pregnancy in the ovulatory patients participating in an ART program.	Inj: (FSH-LH) 75 IU-75 IU	Initial: 225 IU SQ. Titrate: Adjust subsequent dosing to individual response at intervals no less than every 2 days and not exceeding 150 IU/adjustment. Max: 450 IU/day. Dosing >20 days not recommended. If adequate response, administer hCG. Withhold hCG if ovaries abnormally enlarged last day of therapy.
Progesterone (Crinone, Prochieve)	(4%) Treatment of secondary amenorrhea. (8%) Progesterone replacement or supplementation in Assisted Reproductive Technology (ART), and treatment of secondary amenorrhea after failure to respond to 4%.	Gel: (Crinone, Prochieve) 4% [45mg, 6s], (Crinone, Prochieve) 8% [90mg, 6s 15s 18s]	ART: 90mg of 8% intravaginally qd if require progesterone supplementation. 90mg of 8% intravaginally bid with partial or complete ovarian failure requiring progesterone replacement. If pregnancy occurs, continue until placental autonomy is achieved, up to 10-12 weeks.
Progesterone (Endometrin)	To support embryo implantation and early pregnancy by supplementation of corpus luteal function as part of an Assisted Reproductive Technology (ART) treatment program for infertile women.	Vaginal Insert: 100mg [21s]	100mg vaginally bid or tid starting the day after oocyte retrieval and continuing for up to 10 weeks.
Urofollitropin (Bravelle)	With hCG, to induce ovulation in patients who previously received pituitary suppression. With hCG, for multiple follicular development (controlled ovarian stimulation) during assisted reproductive technologies (ART) cycles in patients who previously received pituitary suppression.	Inj: 75 IU	Ovulation Induction: Initial: 150 IU SQ/IM qd for 1st 5 days. Adjust subsequent dose to individual response at intervals no less than every 2 days and not exceeding 75-150 IU/adjustment. Max: 450 IU/day. Dosing >12 days is not recommended. If adequate response, give 5000-10,000 U hCG 1 day following last dose. May repeat course if inadequate follicle development or ovulation without pregnancy occurs. ART: 225 IU SQ qd for 1st 5 days. Adjust subsequent dose to individual response at intervals no less than every 2 days and not exceeding 75-150 IU/adjustment. Max: 450 IU/day. Dosing >12 days is not recommended. If adequate follicular development, give 5000-10,000 U hCG to induce final follicular maturation in preparation for oocyte retrieval.

GYNECOLOGICAL ANTI-INFECTIVES

DRUG	CLASS	FORMULATION	ROUTE	RECOMMENDED DOSAGE
ANTIBACTERIALS				
Clindamycin Cleocin Vaginal	RX	**Cream:** 2%	Vaginal	**Bacterial Vaginosis: Adults:** 1 applicatorful qhs x 3-7 days (non-pregnant) or x 7 days (2nd or 3rd trimester).
Cleocin Vaginal Ovules	RX	**Sup:** 100mg	Vaginal	**Bacterial Vaginosis: Adults:** 1 sup qhs x 3 days (non-pregnant).
Clindesse	RX	**Cream:** 2%	Vaginal	**Bacterial Vaginosis: Adults:** 1 applicatorful once (non-pregnant).
Metronidazole Flagyl	RX	**Cap:** 375mg **Tab:** 250mg, 500mg	Oral	**Trichomoniasis: Adults: (Cap)** 375mg bid or **(Tab)** 250mg tid x 7 days. **Alternate Regimen (Tab):** If non-pregnant, 2g as single or divided dose. Contraindicated in 1st trimester.
Flagyl ER	RX	**Tab, ER:** 750mg	Oral	**Bacterial Vaginosis: Adults:** 750mg qd x 7 days. Contraindicated in 1st trimester.
MetroGel Vaginal	RX	**Gel:** 0.75%	Vaginal	**Bacterial Vaginosis: Adults:** 1 applicatorful qd-bid x 5 days. For qd dosing, administer qhs.
Vandazole	RX	**Gel:** 0.75%	Vaginal	**Bacterial Vaginosis: Adults:** 1 applicatorful qhs x 5 days (non-pregnant).
MISCELLANEOUS				
Tindamax	RX	**Tab:** 250mg, 500mg	Oral	**Bacterial Vaginosis:** 2g qd for 2 days or 1g qd for 5 days. **Trichomoniasis:** 2g single dose. Treat sexual partner with same dose and at same time.
ANTIFUNGALS: CANDIDIASIS TREATMENT				
Butoconazole Gynazole-1	RX	**Cream:** 2%	Vaginal	**Adults:** 1 applicatorful single dose.
Clotrimazole Gyne-Lotrimin 3	OTC	**Cream:** 2%	Vaginal	**Adults/Pediatrics ≥12 yrs:** 1 applicatorful qhs x 3 days.
Gyne-Lotrimin 7	OTC	**Cream:** 1%	Vaginal	**Adults/Pediatrics ≥12 yrs:** 1 applicatorful qhs x 7 days.
Fluconazole Diflucan	RX	**Tab:** 150mg	Oral	**Adults:** 150mg single dose.
Miconazole Monistat 1 Combination Pack	OTC	**Cream:** 2% + **Ovule Insert:** 1200mg	Vaginal	**Adults/Pediatrics ≥12 yrs:** 1 sup single dose. Apply cream externally bid up to 7 days prn.
Monistat 3	OTC	**Cream:** 4% + **External Cream:** 2%	Vaginal	**Adults/Pediatrics ≥12 yrs:** 1 applicatorful qhs x 3 days. (External Cream) Apply cream bid externally up to 7 days prn.
Monistat 3 Combination Pack	OTC	**Cream:** 2% + **Ovule Insert:** 200mg	Vaginal	**Adults/Pediatrics ≥12 yrs:** 1 applicatorful qhs x 3 days. Apply cream bid externally up to 7 days prn.
Monistat 7	OTC	**Cream:** 2%	Vaginal	**Adults/Pediatrics ≥12 yrs:** 1 applicatorful qhs x 7 days. Apply cream bid externally up to 7 days prn.
Monistat 7 Combination Pack	OTC	**Cream:** 2% + **External Cream:** 2%	Vaginal	**Adults/Pediatrics ≥12 yrs:** 1 applicatorful qhs x 7 days. (External Cream) Apply cream bid externally up to 7 days prn.

(Continued)

DRUG	CLASS	FORMULATION	ROUTE	RECOMMENDED DOSAGE
ANTIFUNGALS: CANDIDIASIS TREATMENT *(Continued)*				
Sulfanilamide AVC	RX	**Cream:** 15%	Vaginal	**Adults:** 1 applicatorful qd-bid x 30 days.
Terconazole Terazol 3	RX	**Cream:** 0.8% **Sup:** 80mg	Vaginal	**Adults:** 1 applicatorful or 1 sup qhs x 3 days.
Terazol 7	RX	**Cream:** 0.4%	Vaginal	**Adults:** 1 applicatorful qhs x 7 days.
Tioconazole Monistat 1, Vagistat 1	OTC	**Oint:** 6.5%	Vaginal	**Adults/Pediatrics ≥12 yrs:** 1 applicatorful single dose hs.

HORMONE THERAPY

DRUG	BRAND	STRENGTH (mg)†
INTRAMUSCULAR ESTROGEN PRODUCTS		
Estradiol valerate	Delestrogen	10mg/mL, 20mg/mL, 40mg/mL
Estradiol cypionate	Depo-Estradiol	5mg/mL
ORAL ESTROGEN PRODUCTS		
Conjugated equine estrogens	Premarin	0.3, 0.45, 0.625, 0.9, 1.25
	Enjuvia	0.3, 0.45, 0.625, 0.9, 1.25
ORAL SYNTHETIC CONJUGATED ESTROGEN PRODUCTS		
Estradiol acetate	Femtrace	0.45, 0.9, 1.8
Synthetic conjugated estrogens	Cenestin	0.3, 0.45, 0.625, 0.9, 1.25
Esterified estrogens	Menest	0.3, 0.625, 1.25, 2.5
Micronized 17β-estradiol	Estrace	0.5, 1, 2
Estropipate	(Generic)	0.75 (0.625), 1.5 (1.25), 3 (2.5)
TRANSDERMAL ESTROGEN PRODUCTS		
17β-estradiol matrix patch	Alora	0.025, 0.05, 0.075, 0.1
	Climara	0.025, 0.0375, 0.05, 0.06, 0.075, 0.1
	Vivelle, Vivelle-Dot	0.025, 0.0375, 0.05, 0.075, 0.1
Estradiol	Divigel	0.1% gel
17β-estradiol reservoir patch	Estraderm	0.05, 0.1
17β-estradiol	Elestrin	0.06% gel
17β-estradiol	Estrogel	0.06% gel
Estradiol hemihydrate	Estrasorb	(emulsion): 4.35mg/1.74g
17β-estradiol	Evamist	(spray): 1.53mg/spray
VAGINAL ESTROGEN PRODUCTS		
Vaginal Creams 17β-estradiol	Estrace Vaginal Cream	0.01%
Conjugated equine estrogens	Premarin Vaginal Cream	0.625mg/g
Estropipate	Ogen Vaginal Cream	1.5mg/g
Vaginal Ring 17β-estradiol	Estring	0.0075mg/day
	Femring	0.05 or 0.1mg/day
Vaginal Tablet Estradiol hemihydrate	Vagifem	10mcg
ORAL PROGESTOGEN ONLY PRODUCTS		
Medroxyprogesterone acetate	Provera	2.5, 5, 10
Norethindrone acetate	Aygestin	5
Progesterone USP (in peanut oil)	Prometrium	100, 200
ESTROGEN + PROGESTOGEN COMBINATIONS		
Oral continuous-cyclic regimen Conjugated equine estrogens (E) + Medroxyprogesterone acetate (P)	Premphase	0.625mg (E), 5mg (P)
17β-estradiol (E) + Norgestimate (P)	Prefest	1mg (E), 0.09mg (P)

(Continued)

HORMONE THERAPY

DRUG	BRAND	STRENGTH (mg)[†]		
ORAL ESTROGEN + PROGESTOGEN COMBINATIONS (Continued)				
Oral continuous-combined regimen Conjugated equine estrogens (E) + Medroxyprogesterone (P)	Prempro	0.3mg (E) + 1.5mg (P)	0.45mg + 1.5mg	0.625mg + 2.5 or 5mg
Estradiol (E) + Drospirenone (P)	Angeliq	1mg (E) + 0.5mg (P)		
Ethinyl estradiol (E) + Norethindrone acetate (P)	Femhrt	2.5mcg (E) + 0.5mg (P); 5mcg (E) + 1mg (P)		
17ß-estradiol (E) + Norethindrone acetate (P)	Activella	1mg (E) + 0.5mg (P); 0.5mg (E) + 0.1mg (P)		
Transdermal continuous-cyclic or continuous-combined regimen 17ß-estradiol (E) + Norethindrone acetate (P)	CombiPatch	0.05mg/day (E) + 0.14 or 0.25mg/day (P)		
Estradiol (E) + Levonorgestrel (P)	Climara Pro	0.045mg/day (E) + 0.015mg/day (P)		

NOTE: This list is not inclusive of all estrogen and progestogen products available. Indications vary among the different products. For more detailed information please refer to the individual monograph listings or the drug's FDA-approved labeling. Unopposed estrogen replacement therapy (ERT) is for use in women without an intact uterus. For women with an intact uterus, progestin must be added to the estrogen (HRT) for protection against estrogen-induced endometrial cancer. As with any therapy, the lowest possible effective dosage should be used. Re-evaluate periodically.

[†] Units are in mg unless stated otherwise.

ORAL CONTRACEPTIVES

DRUG	ESTROGEN	PROGESTIN	STRENGTH (ESTROGEN/PROGESTIN)
MONOPHASIC			
Aviane 28, Lessina 28, Lutera, Sronyx 28**	Ethinyl Estradiol	Levonorgestrel	20mcg/0.1mg
Beyaz†, YAZ (Gianvi**)	Ethinyl Estradiol	Drospirenone	20mcg/3mg
Brevicon, Modicon (Necon 0.5/35, Nortrel 0.5/35**)	Ethinyl Estradiol	Norethindrone	35mcg/0.5mg
Desogen, Ortho-Cept (Apri, Reclipsen, Solia**)	Ethinyl Estradiol	Desogestrel	30mcg/0.15mg
Femcon Fe, Ovcon 35, Balziva (Zenchent**)	Ethinyl Estradiol	Norethindrone	35mcg/0.4mg
Loestrin 21 1/20, Loestrin Fe 1/20, Loestrin 24 Fe (Junel, Microgestin**)	Ethinyl Estradiol	Norethindrone Acetate	20mcg/1mg
Loestrin 21 1.5/30, Loestrin Fe 1.5/30 (Junel, Microgestin**)	Ethinyl Estradiol	Norethindrone Acetate	30mcg/1.5mg
Lo/Ovral (Cryselle, Low-Ogestrel-28**)	Ethinyl Estradiol	Norgestrel	30mcg/0.3mg
Lybrel*	Ethinyl Estradiol	Levonorgestrel	20mcg/0.09mg
Nordette-28 (Jolessa, Levlen, Levora, Portia 28**)	Ethinyl Estradiol	Levonorgestrel	30mcg/0.15mg
Norinyl 1/35, Ortho-Novum 1/35 (Necon 1/35, Nortrel 1/35**)	Ethinyl Estradiol	Norethindrone	35mcg/1mg
Norinyl 1/50, (Necon 1/50**)	Mestranol	Norethindrone	50mcg/1mg
Ortho-Cyclen (MonoNessa, Previfem, Sprintec**)	Ethinyl Estradiol	Norgestimate	35mcg/0.25mg
Ovcon 50*	Ethinyl Estradiol	Norethindrone	50mcg/1mg
Ogestrel 28**	Ethinyl Estradiol	Norgestrel	50mcg/0.5mg
Safyral†, Yasmin (Ocella, Zarah**)	Ethinyl Estradiol	Drospirenone	30mcg/3mg
Seasonale (Quasense**)	Ethinyl Estradiol	Levonorgestrel	30mcg/0.15mg
Zovia 1/35E**	Ethinyl Estradiol	Ethynodiol Diacetate	35mcg/1mg
Zovia 1/50E**	Ethinyl Estradiol	Ethynodiol Diacetate	50mcg/1mg

(Continued)

DRUG	ESTROGEN	PROGESTIN	STRENGTH (ESTROGEN/PROGESTIN)
BIPHASIC			
Mircette (Kariva**)	Ethinyl Estradiol	Desogestrel	**Phase 1:** 20mcg/0.15mg **Phase 2:** 10mcg/NONE
Lo Loestrin Fe*	Ethinyl Estradiol	Norethindrone Acetate	**Phase 1:** 10mcg/1mg **Phase 2:** 10mcg/NONE
Loseasonique*	Ethinyl Estradiol	Levonorgestrel	**Phase 1:** 20mcg/0.1mg **Phase 2:** 10mcg/NONE
Necon 10/11**	Ethinyl Estradiol	Norethindrone	**Phase 1:** 35mcg/0.5mg **Phase 2:** 35mcg/1mg
Seasonique*	Ethinyl Estradiol	Levonorgestrel	**Phase 1:** 30mcg/0.15mg **Phase 2:** 10mcg/NONE
TRIPHASIC			
Cyclessa (Cesia, Velivet**)	Ethinyl Estradiol	Desogestrel	**Phase 1:** 25mcg/0.1mg **Phase 2:** 25mcg/0.125mg **Phase 3:** 25mcg/0.15mg
Estrostep Fe (Tilia Fe, Tri-legest Fe**)	Ethinyl Estradiol	Norethindrone Acetate	**Phase 1:** 20mcg/1mg **Phase 2:** 30mcg/1mg **Phase 3:** 35mcg/1mg
Ortho-Novum 7/7/7 (Nortrel 7/7/7**)	Ethinyl Estradiol	Norethindrone	**Phase 1:** 35mcg/0.5mg **Phase 2:** 35mcg/0.75mg **Phase 3:** 35mcg/1mg
Ortho Tri-Cyclen (Tri-Previfem, Trinessa, Tri-Sprintec**)	Ethinyl Estradiol	Norgestimate	**Phase 1:** 35mcg/0.18mg **Phase 2:** 35mcg/0.215mg **Phase 3:** 35mcg/0.25mg
Ortho Tri-Cyclen Lo*	Ethinyl Estradiol	Norgestimate	**Phase 1:** 25mcg/0.18mg **Phase 2:** 25mcg/0.215mg **Phase 3:** 25mcg/0.25mg
Trivora 28, Enpresse 28**	Ethinyl Estradiol	Levonorgestrel	**Phase 1:** 30mcg/0.05mg **Phase 2:** 40mcg/0.075mg **Phase 3:** 30mcg/0.125mg
Tri-Norinyl (Leena**)	Ethinyl Estradiol	Norethindrone	**Phase 1:** 35mcg/0.5mg **Phase 2:** 35mcg/1mg **Phase 3:** 35mcg/0.5mg
FOUR-PHASE			
Natazia*	Estradiol Valerate	Dienogest	**Phase 1:** 3mg/NONE **Phase 2:** 2mg/2mg **Phase 3:** 2mg/3mg **Phase 4:** 1mg/NONE
PROGESTIN ONLY			
Nor-Q.D. (Camila, Errin, Jolivette, Nora-BE**) Ortho-Micronor		Norethindrone	0.35mg
Plan B (Next Choice**)		Levonorgestrel	0.75mg
Plan B One Step		Levonorgestrel	1.5mg
MISCELLANEOUS			
Ella***		Ulipristal Acetate (Progestin agonist/antagonist)	30mg

*Currently NO generics available.
**Other branded generics.
***selective progesterone receptor modulator
†Also contains levomefolate calcium.

BREAST CANCER RISK FACTORS

Unmodifiable risk factors	
Gender	Women > men
Age	1 out of 8 breast cancer diagnoses are among women <45 yrs, while about 2 out of 3 occur in women ≥55 yrs
Genetic	BRCA1 and BRCA2, ATM gene, CHEK2 gene, p53 tumor suppressor gene, PTEN gene mutations, CDH1
Race	Whites > African Americans
Family history	Having a first-degree relative with breast cancer doubles risk; having 2 first-degree relatives increases risk about 3-fold
Personal history of breast cancer	Women with cancer in one breast have 3- to 4-fold increased risk of developing a new cancer in another area of the same breast or in the opposite breast
Abnormal breast biopsy	Nonproliferative lesions, proliferative lesions with or without atypia
Early menarche	Women who started menstruating at an early age (<12 yrs)
Age at menopause	Women who went through menopause at a late age (>55 yrs)
Personal history of breast abnormalities	Women with lobular carcinoma in situ (LCIS) have a 7- to 11-fold increased risk of developing cancer in either breast
Earlier breast radiation exposure	Women who had radiation therapy to the chest area as treatment for another cancer
Breast density	Women with a higher proportion of dense breast tissue (eg, connective and milk duct tissue)

Lifestyle factors associated with increased risk of breast cancer

- Alcohol (2 drinks/day)
- High body mass index
- Not having children or having them when >30 yrs
- Lack of physical activity
- Not breastfeeding

Drugs associated with increased risk of breast cancer

- Birth control pills
- DES (diethylstilbestrol)
- Postmenopausal hormone therapy or hormone replacement therapy

Uncertain risk factors

- Antiperspirants
- Bras
- Breast implants
- High-fat diets
- Induced abortion
- Miscarriages
- Night work
- Pollution (chemicals)
- Smoking (active or passive)

Sources: American Cancer Society and National Cancer Institute.

BREAST CANCER TREATMENT OPTIONS

DRUG (BRAND)	INDICATIONS	HOW SUPPLIED	DOSAGE
ANDROGENS			
Fluoxymesterone (Androxy)	Secondarily used in women with advancing inoperable metastatic (skeletal) mammary cancer who are 1-5 yrs postmenopausal.	Tab: 10mg* *scored	10-40mg/day in divided doses. Continue therapy for at least 3 months for objective response. Advanced Mammary Carcinoma: Duration depends on response and appearance of adverse effects.
Methyltestosterone (Testred)	Secondary treatment of advancing inoperable metastatic (skeletal) breast cancer in females who are 1-5 yrs postmenopausal.	Cap: 10mg	50-200mg/day.
Testosterone (Delatestryl)	Secondary treatment of advancing inoperable metastatic (skeletal) mammary cancer who are 1-5 years postmenopausal.	Inj: 200mg/mL [5mL]	200-400mg every 2-4 weeks.
ANTIESTROGEN			
Fulvestrant[†] (Faslodex)	Treatment of hormone receptor positive metastatic breast cancer in postmenopausal women with disease progression following anti-estrogen therapy.	Inj: 50mg/mL [5mL]	500mg IM into the buttocks slowly as two 5mL injections, one in each buttock, on days 1, 15, 29 and once monthly thereafter.
ESTROGENS			
Conjugated estrogens (Premarin Tablets)	Palliative treatment of breast cancer in selected patients with metastatic disease.	Tab: 0.3mg, 0.45mg, 0.625mg, 0.9mg, 1.25mg	10mg tid for minimum 3 months.
Esterified estrogens (Menest)	Palliative therapy of breast cancer in selected patients with metastatic disease.	Tab: 0.3mg, 0.625mg, 1.25mg, 2.5mg	10mg tid for at least 3 months.
Estradiol (Estrace)	Palliative treatment of breast cancer in selected patients with metastatic disease.	Tab: 0.5mg*, 1mg*, 2mg* *scored	10mg tid for at least 3 months.
LHRH AGONIST			
Goserelin (Zoladex 1-Month)	Palliative treatment of advanced breast cancer in pre-and perimenopausal women.	Implant: 3.6mg	3.6mg SQ every 28 days into anterior abdominal wall below navel line.
PROGESTIN			
Megestrol acetate	Palliative treatment of advanced breast carcinoma (eg, recurrent, inoperable or metastatic disease).	Tab: 20mg*, 40mg* *scored	40mg qid for a minimum of 2 months.
SELECTIVE ESTROGEN RECEPTOR MODULATORS			
Raloxifene (Evista)	Reduction in risk of invasive breast cancer in post-menopausal women with osteoporosis or at high risk for invasive breast cancer.	Tab: 60mg	60mg qd.

(Continued)

BREAST CANCER TREATMENT OPTIONS

DRUG (BRAND)	INDICATIONS	HOW SUPPLIED	DOSAGE
SELECTIVE ESTROGEN RECEPTOR MODULATORS *(continued)*			
Tamoxifen citrate	Treatment of metastatic breast cancer in women and men. Treatment of node-positive and axillary node-negative breast cancer in women following mastectomy, axillary dissection and breast irradiation. To reduce risk of invasive breast cancer in women with DCIS (Ductal carcinoma in-situ) following breast surgery and radiation. Reduction of breast cancer incidence in high risk women. Use for up to 5 yrs.	Tab: 10mg, 20mg	20-40mg qd. Divide dosages >20mg into AM and PM doses. Risk Reduction/DCIS: 20mg qd for 5 yrs.
Toremifene (Fareston)	Treatment of metastatic breast cancer in post-menopausal women with estrogen-receptor positive or unknown tumors.	Tab: 60mg	60mg qd. Treat until disease progression is evident.
SELECTIVE NONSTEROIDAL AROMATASE INHIBITORS (POSTMENOPAUSAL WOMEN ONLY)			
Anastrozole (Arimidex)	Adjuvant treatment of post-menopausal women with hormone-receptor positive early breast cancer. First-line treatment of post-menopausal women with hormone-receptor positive or hormone-receptor unknown locally advanced or metastatic breast cancer. Second line treatment of advanced breast cancer in postmenopausal women with disease progression following tamoxifen therapy.	Tab: 1mg	1mg qd. Continue until tumor progression with advanced breast cancer.
Letrozole (Femara)	Adjuvant treatment of postmenopausal women with hormone-receptor positive early breast cancer. Extended adjuvant treatment of early breast cancer in postmenopausal women who have received 5 yrs of adjuvant tamoxifen therapy. First-line treatment of hormone-receptor positive or unknown locally advanced or metastatic breast cancer in post-menopausal women. Treatment of advanced breast cancer with disease progression following antiestrogen therapy in postmenopausal women.	Tab: 2.5mg	2.5mg qd. Continue until tumor progression is evident. Cirrhosis/Severe Liver Dysfunction: 2.5mg every other day.

(Continued)

DRUG (BRAND)	INDICATIONS	HOW SUPPLIED	DOSAGE
CHEMOTHERAPY AGENTS			
ANTHRACYCLINES			
Doxorubicin[†] (Adriamycin)	To produce regression in disseminated neoplastic conditions such as breast carcinoma. Adjuvant therapy in women with evidence of axillary lymph node involvement following resection of primary breast cancer.	Inj: (2mg/mL) 10mg, 20mg, 50mg, 200mg	Monotherapy: 60-75mg/m² IV every 21 days. Use the lower dose with inadequate bone marrow reserves due to old age, prior therapy, or neoplastic marrow infiltration. Concomitant Chemotherapy: 40-60mg/m² IV every 21-28 days.
Epirubicin[†] (Ellence)	Adjuvant treatment in patients with evidence of axillary node tumor involvement following resection of primary breast cancer.	Inj: 2mg/mL [25mL, 100mL]	Initial: 100-120mg/m² IV infusion, repeat at 3-4 week cycles. May give total dose on Day 1 of each cycle or divide equally on Days 1 and 8. Bone Marrow Dysfunction: Initial: 75-90mg/m².
ANTIMICROTUBULE AGENT			
Erbulin[†] (Halaven)	Treatment of metastatic breast cancer in patients who have previously received ≥2 chemothera-peutic regimens (should have included anthracycline and a taxane) for the treat-ment of metastatic disease.	Inj: 0.5mg/mL [2mL]	Administer IV over 2-5 min on Days 1 and 8 of a 21-day cycle. Usual: 1.4mg/m².
Ixabepilone[†] (Ixempra)	In combination with capecitabine for treatment of patients with metastatic or locally advanced breast cancer resistant to treatment with an anthracycline and a taxane, or whose cancer is taxane resistant and for whom further anthracycline therapy is contraindicated. As monotherapy for treat-ment of metastatic or locally advanced breast cancer in patients whose tumors are resistant or refractory to anthracyclines, taxanes, and capecitabine.	Inj: 15mg, 45mg	40mg/m² IV infusion over 3 hrs every 3 weeks. Premedicate with H_1-antagonist (eg, diphenhydramine 50mg PO) and H_2-antagonist (eg, ranitidine 150-300mg PO) approximately 1 hr before infusion. Also premedicate with corticosteroid (eg, dexamethasone 20mg, IV 30 min before infusion or PO 60 min before infusion) if prior hypersensitivity reaction to ixabepilone.
KINASE INHIBITOR			
Lapatinib[†] (Tykerb)	Treatment of patients with advanced or metastatic breast cancer, in combination with capecitabine, whose tumors overexpress HER2 and received prior therapy including an anthracycline, a taxane, and trastuzumab. In combination with letrozole for treatment of postmenopausal women with hormone receptor positive metastatic breast cancer overexpressing HER2 receptor, for whom hormone therapy is indicated.	Tab: 250mg	HER2 Positive Metastatic Breast Cancer: Usual: 1250mg qd on Days 1-21 continuously with capecitabine 2000mg/m²/day (2 doses 12 hrs apart) on Days 1-14 in a repeating 21-day cycle. Give at least 1 hr before or 1 hr after a meal (however, give capecitabine with food).

(Continued)

BREAST CANCER TREATMENT OPTIONS

DRUG (BRAND)	INDICATIONS	HOW SUPPLIED	DOSAGE
MISCELLANEOUS			
Capecitabine[†] (Xeloda)	Treatment of metastatic breast cancer in combination with docetaxel after failure of prior anthracycline-containing chemotherapy. Treatment of metastatic breast cancer in patients resistant to paclitaxel and anthracycline-containing chemotherapy or resistant to paclitaxel and for whom further anthracycline therapy is not indicated.	Tab: 150mg, 500mg	Usual: 1250mg/m² bid for 2 weeks, then 1 week off. Give as 3-week cycles. Combination with Docetaxel: Usual: 1250mg/m² bid for 2 weeks followed by 1-week rest period, combined with docetaxel 75mg/m² as 1 hr IV infusion q3 weeks. Take with water within 30 min after meals.
Cyclophosphamide (Cytoxan)	Treatment of breast carcinoma.	Inj (Lyophilized): 500mg, 1g, 2g; Tab: 25mg, 50mg	Malignant Diseases (Without Hematologic Deficiency): Monotherapy: Initial: 40-50mg/kg IV in divided doses over 2-5 days, or 10-15mg/kg IV given every 7-10 days, or 3-5mg/kg twice weekly. Oral Dosing: Initial/Maint: 1-5mg/kg/day PO. Adjust dose according to antitumor activity and/or leukopenia. May need to reduce dose when combined with other cytotoxic drugs.
Dexrazoxane (Zinecard)	To reduce the incidence and severity of cardiomyopathy associated with doxorubicin in women with metastatic breast cancer who received a cumulative doxorubicin dose of 300mg/m² and who will continue doxorubicin therapy to maintain tumor control.	Inj: 250mg, 500mg	IV: 10:1 ratio of dexrazoxane: doxorubicin (eg, 500mg/m² dexrazoxane: 50mg/m² doxorubicin). Hepatic Impairment: Reduce dose proportionally. Give by slow IV push or rapid IV infusion. Give doxorubicin within 30 min after start of infusion. If CrCl <40 mL/min, the recommended dosage ratio is 5:1 (dexrazoxane: doxorubicin).
Fluorouracil	Palliative management of breast carcinoma.	Inj: 50mg/mL, [10mL]	12mg/kg IV qd for 4 days. Max: 800mg/day. If no toxicity, give 6mg/kg IV on 6th, 8th, 10th, and 12th days. Skip Days 5, 7, 9, and 11. Discontinue therapy at the end of Day 12. Inadequate Nutritional State: 6mg/kg IV for 3 days. If no toxicity, give 3mg/kg IV on 5th, 7th, and 9th days. Max: 400mg/day. Skip Days 4, 6, and 8. Maint (Use Schedule 1 or Schedule 2): Schedule 1: If no toxicity, repeat 1st course every 30 days after last day of previous course. Schedule 2: When toxic signs from initial course subside, give 10-15mg/kg/week IV single dose; do not exceed 1g/week.
Methotrexate (Methotrexate)	Alone or in combination with other anticancer agents in treatment of breast cancer.	Inj: 25mg/mL, Tab: 2.5mg* *scored	40mg/m² IV on Days 1 and 8. (Refer to PI or NCCN guidelines for regimen details.)

(Continued)

DRUG (BRAND)	INDICATIONS	HOW SUPPLIED	DOSAGE
MONOCLONAL ANTIBODY/HER2 BLOCKER			
Trastuzumab (Herceptin)	Adjuvant treatment of HER2-overexpressing node-positive/negative breast cancer. 1st-line treatment of HER2-over-expressing metastatic breast cancer in combination with paclitaxel. Single agent for adjuvant treatment of HER2-overexpressing breast cancer in patients who received 1 or more chemotherapy regimens for metastatic disease.	Inj: 440mg	Adjuvant Treatment: During and following paclitaxel, docetaxel, or docetaxel/carboplatin for 52 weeks total: IV infusion: Initial: 4mg/kg over 90 min. Maint: 2mg/kg over 30 min weekly during chemotherapy for the first 12 weeks (paclitaxel or docetaxel) or 18 weeks (docetaxel/carboplatin). 1 week following the last weekly dose of Herceptin: 6mg/kg IV infusion over 30-90 min every 3 weeks. Following completion of multimodality, anthracycline-based regimens as a single agent: Initial: 8mg/kg IV infusion over 90 min. Maint: 6mg/kg over 30-90 min every 3 weeks. Metastatic breast cancer: Alone or with paclitaxel: Initial: 4mg/kg over 90 min, then 2mg/kg weekly over 30 min until disease progression.
NUCLEOSIDE ANALOGUE/ANTIMETABOLITE			
Gemcitabine (Gemzar)	Adjunct with paclitaxel for 1st-line treatment of metastatic breast cancer after failure of prior anthracycline-containing adjuvant chemotherapy, unless anthracyclines were clinically contraindicated.	Inj: 200mg, 1g	1250mg/m^2 IV on Days 1 and 8 of each 21-day cycle. Give paclitaxel 175mg/m^2 IV on Day 1 before gemcitabine. All IV infusions given over 30 min. Adjust dose based on hematologic toxicity.
TAXANES			
Docetaxel (Taxotere)	Treatment of locally advanced or metastatic breast cancer after failure of prior chemotherapy. In combination with doxorubicin and cyclophosphamide for the adjuvant treatment of operable, node-positive breast cancer.	Inj: 20mg/mL, 80mg/4mL; (Generic) 20mg/2mL, 80mg/8mL; 160mg/16mL	Premedicate with oral corticosteroids. Adjust dose based on febrile neutropenia, neutrophil count, cutaneous reactions, peripheral neuropathy, neurosensory signs/symptoms, or GI toxicities (see PI). Breast Cancer: 60-100mg/m^2 IV over 1 hr every 3 weeks. Adjuvant Treatment Operable Node-Positive Breast CA: 75mg/m^2 1 hr after doxorubicin 50mg/m^2 and cyclophosphamide 500mg/m^2 every 3 weeks for 6 courses. Administer every 3 weeks for 3 cycles.
Paclitaxel	Treatment of breast cancer after failure with combination chemotherapy for metastatic disease or relapse within 6 months of adjuvant chemotherapy; prior therapy should have included an anthracycline unless clinically contraindicated. Adjuvant treatment of node-positive breast cancer ad-ministered sequentially to doxorubicin-containing chemotherapy.	Inj: 6mg/mL	Adjuvant treatment of node-positive: 175mg/m^2 over 3 hrs every 3 weeks for 4 courses given sequentially to doxorubicin-containing chemo-therapy. Failure of initial chemo-therapy for metastatic disease or relapse: 175mg/m^2 over 3 hrs every 3 weeks. Reduce dose of subsequent courses by 20% if neutrophils <500 cells/mm^3 for ≥1 week or severe peripheral neuropathy occurs. Premedicate prior to administration with appropriate medications; see PI for additional information.

(Continued)

DRUG (BRAND)	INDICATIONS	HOW SUPPLIED	DOSAGE
TAXANES (continued)			
Paclitaxel protein-bound particle for injectable suspension (Abraxane)	Treatment of breast cancer after failure of combination chemotherapy for metastatic disease or relapse within 6 months of adjuvant chemotherapy. Prior therapy should have included an anthracycline unless clinically contraindicated.	Inj: 100mg	260mg/m^2 IV over 30 min every 3 weeks. Severe neutropenia (neutrophil <500 cells/mm^3 for week or longer) or severe sensory neuropathy (Grade 3 or 4): Hold dose until neutrophil >1500 cells/mm^3 or sensory neuropathy resolves to Grade 1 or 2. Reduce subsequent courses to 220mg/m^2, if recurrence occurs reduce subsequent courses to 180mg/m^2.
VASCULAR ENDOTHELIAL GROWTH INHIBITOR			
Bevacizumab (Avastin)	Treatment of patients who have not received chemotherapy for metastatic HER2 negative breast cancer, in combination with paclitaxel.	Inj: 25mg/mL [4mL, 16mL]	10mg/kg every 2 weeks. Give as IV infusion over 90 min, if 1st infusion is well tolerated, give 2nd infusion over 60 min and subsequent doses over 30 min.
VINCA ALKALOID			
Vinblastine	Palliative treatment of breast carcinoma unresponsive to appropriate endocrine surgery and hormonal therapy.	Inj: 1mg/mL [10mL]	Dose at intervals of ≥7 days. 1st Dose: 3.7mg/m^2. 2nd Dose: 5.5mg/m^2. 3rd Dose: 7.4mg/m^2. 4th Dose: 9.25mg/m^2. 5th Dose: 11.1mg/m^2. Max: 18.5mg/m^2. Do not increase dose after that dose which reduces WBC to 3000 cells/mm^3. Maint: Use dose of 1 increment smaller than this dose at weekly intervals. Reduce to 50% dose if direct serum bilirubin >3mg/100mL. Only dose if WBC ≥4000 cells/mm^3.

†Refer to complete prescribing information for dosage adjustment.

*National Comprehensive Cancer Network Clinical Practice (NCCN) Guidelines in Oncology, 2011.

CHEMOTHERAPY REGIMENS*†

CANCER TYPE	PREFERRED THERAPIES	ALTERNATIVE REGIMENS
Bladder	*Non-muscle invasive:* Bacillus Calmette-Guerin (BCG) *Neoadjuvant, adjuvant, and metastatic:* Gemcitabine/cisplatin (preferred); or Methotrexate/ vinblastine/doxorubicin/cisplatin (MVAC)	*Non-muscle invasive:* Mitomycin C (MMC) *Neoadjuvant, adjuvant, and metastatic:* Carboplatin and taxane-based therapy or single-agent therapy
Breast		
Adjuvant (trastuzumab containing)	Doxorubicin/cyclophosphamide followed by paclitaxel + trastuzumab (AC → T + trastuzumab) Docetaxel, carboplatin, trastuzumab (TCH)	Docetaxel + trastuzumab → fluorouracil/epirubicin/ cyclophosphamide (FEC) Chemotherapy followed by trastuzumab sequentially Doxorubicin/cyclophosphamide (AC) → docetaxel + trastuzumab
Adjuvant (non-trastuzumab containing)	Docetaxel/doxorubicin/cyclophosphamide (TAC) Dose-dense doxorubicin/cyclophosphamide (AC) → paclitaxel every 2 weeks Doxorubicin/cyclophosphamide (AC) → weekly paclitaxel Docetaxel and cyclophosphamide (TC) Doxorubicin/cyclophosphamide (AC)	Fluorouracil/doxorubicin/ cyclophosphamide (FAC/CAF) Cyclophosphamide/epirubicin/ fluorouracil (FEC/CEF) Cyclophosphamide/methotrexate/ fluorouracil (CMF) Doxorubicin/cyclophosphamide (AC) → docetaxel every 3 weeks Epirubicin/cyclophosphamide (EC) Doxorubicin followed by paclitaxel followed by cyclophosphamide (every 2-week regimen) with filgrastim support (A → T → C) Fluorouracil/epirubicin/ cyclophosphamide followed by docetaxel (FEC → T) Fluorouracil/epirubicin/ cyclophosphamide (FEC) followed by weekly paclitaxel
Neoadjuvant	Paclitaxel + trastuzumab followed by cyclo-phosphamide/epirubicin/fluorouracil + trastuzumab (T + trastuzumab → CEF + trastuzumab)	
Recurrent or metastatic	*Single agents:* Anthracyclines: Doxorubicin, epirubicin, pegylated liposomal doxorubicin. Taxanes: paclitaxel, docetaxel, albumin-bound paclitaxel. Antimetabolites: capecitabine, gemcitabine. Other microtubule inhibitors: vinorelbine, eribulin *Combinations:* Cyclophosphamide/doxorubicin/ fluorouracil (CAF/FAC); fluorouracil/epirubicin/ cyclophosphamide (FEC); doxorubicin/ cyclophosphamide (AC); epirubicin/cyclo-phosphamide (EC); doxorubicin/docetaxel, doxorubicin/paclitaxel (AT); cyclophosphamide/ methotrexate/fluorouracil (CMF); docetaxel/ capecitabine; gemcitabine/paclitaxel (GT); bevacizumab + paclitaxel	*Other single agents:* Cyclophosphamide, mitoxantrone, cisplatin, etoposide (po), vinblastine, fluorouracil CI, ixabepilone *Other combinations:* ixabepilone + capecitabine
HER2-positive metastatic disease	1) Trastuzumab + (paclitaxel ± carboplatin) or (docetaxel) or (vinorelbine) or (capecitabine) 2) *Trastuzumab-exposed:* Lapatinib + capecitabine or trastuzumab + (other first-line agents) or (capecitabine) or (lapatinib) (without cytotoxic therapy)	

(Continued)

CANCER TYPE	PREFERRED THERAPIES	ALTERNATIVE REGIMENS
Colorectal	*Adjuvant Stage III:* 5-FU + oxaliplatin + leucovorin (FOLFOX)	*Adjuvant Stage III:* 5-FU/LV or capecitabine
	Metastatic: Intensive-Therapy Appropriate: Initial Therapy: 5-FU + oxaliplatin + leucovorin (FOLFOX) ± bevacizumab or CapeOX ± bevacizumab or 2) FOLFOX ± cetuximab or panitumumab (KRAS wild-type [WT] gene only) or 3) FOLFIRI + bevacizumab or 4) FOLFIRI ± cetuximab or panitumumab (KARS WT gene only) or 5-FU/LV or capecitabine ± bevacizumab or 5) FOLFOXIRI. *Refer to NCCN guidelines for therapy after first and second progression and for non–intensive-therapy appropriate patients.* Bevacizumab + 1) 5-FU + oxaliplatin + leucovorin (FOLFOX) or 2) irinotecan + leucovorin + 5-FU (FOLFIRI) or 3) oxaliplatin + capecitabine (CapeOX) or 4) 5-FU/LV	
Esophageal		
Definitive chemoradiation	Cisplatin + 5-FU	Cisplatin + 1) irinotecan or 2) paclitaxel or carboplatin or 3) docetaxel Docetaxel or paclitaxel + fluoropyrimidine (5-FU or capecitabine) Oxaliplatin + fluoropyrimidine (5-FU or capecitabine)
Locally advanced or metastatic	Docetaxel/cisplatin/5-FU (DCF) Epirubicin/cisplatin/5-FU (ECF)	Irinotecan + cisplatin or fluoropyrimidine (5-FU or capecitabine) Oxaliplatin + fluoropyrimidine (5-FU or capecitabine) Paclitaxel-based regimen Trastuzumab
Leukemia		
Acute lymphocytic leukemia (ALL) - Adults	*Induction:* Vincristine/anthracycline prednisone with or without asparaginase**	*Induction:* Imatinib mesylate (Ph1 positive ALL) *Recurrent:* Dasatinib (imatinib-resistant BCR/ABL mutants)
Acute myeloid leukemia (AML)	*Induction:* (pt <60) Cytarabine + 1) daunorubicin or 2) idarubicin *Induction:* (pt ≥60) Cytarabine + idarubicin or daunorubicin or mitoxantrone *Post-induction:* (pt <60) High-dose cytarabine; or standard-dose cytarabine + idarubicin or daunorubicin *Post-induction:* (pt ≥60) Standard-dose cytarabine + idarubicin or daunorubicin or mitoxantrone	*Induction:* (pt <60) High-dose cytarabine (HiDAC) + idarubicin or daunorubicin *Induction:* (pt ≥60) Low-intensity subQ cytarabine or 5-azacitidine or decitabine; or intermediate-intensity clofarabine; or best supportive care (hydroxyurea)
Acute promyelocytic leukemia (APL)	*Induction:* Able to tolerate anthracyclines: All-trans retinoic acid (ATRA) + daunorubicin + cytarabine. Not able to tolerate anthracyclines: ATRA + arsenic trioxide *Relapse:* Arsenic trioxide ± ATRA	
Chronic lymphocytic leukemia (CLL)	*First-line therapy (without 17p del or del 11q):* (pt ≥70 or younger pts with co-morbidities) Chlorambucil ± prednisone; bendamustine, rituximab (BR); cyclophosphamide, prednisone ± rituximab; alemtuzumab; rituximab; fludarabine ± rituximab; cladribine. (pt <70 or older pts without co-morbidities) Fludarabine, cyclophosphamide, rituximab (FCR); fludarabine, rituximab (FR); pentostatin, cyclophosphamide, rituximab (PCR); bendamustine, rituximab (BR) *Refer to guidelines for relapsed/refractory therapy and therapy for CLL with del (17p) or del (11q).*	

(Continued)

CANCER TYPE	PREFERRED THERAPIES	ALTERNATIVE REGIMENS
Chronic myelogenous leukemia (CML)	*Primary Treatment:* Imatinib 400mg or Nilotinib 300mg bid or Dasatinib 100mg	*Follow-up Therapy:* Imatinib 400mg or Nilotinib 300mg bid or Dasatinib 100mg
Hairy cell leukemia	Cladribine or pentostatin	Interferon alfa
Liver (hepatocellular carcinoma)	Sorafenib (Child-Pugh Class A [category 1] or B)	
Lung		
Non-small cell	*First-line:* Chemotherapy; or bevacizumab + chemotherapy; or cisplatin/pemetrexed; or erlotinib for EGFR mutation positive. *Second-line:* Docetaxel; or pemetrexed; or erlotinib *Third-line:* Erlotinib	*First-line:* Cetuximab/vinorelbine/cisplatin *Second-line:* Docetaxel; or pemetrexed; or erlotinib; or platinum doublet ± bevacizumab
Small cell	*Limited stage:* Cisplatin or carboplatin + etoposide *Extensive stage:* Cisplatin or carboplatin + etoposide; cisplatin or carboplatin + irinotecan. *Refer to guidelines for subsequent chemotherapy for relapses.*	
Lymphoma		
Hodgkin's disease/ lymphoma	Doxorubicin/bleomycin/vinblastine/dacarbazine (ABVD) Doxorubicin/vinblastine/mechlorethamine/ etoposide/vincristine/bleomycin/prednisone (Stanford V)	Bleomycin/etoposide/doxorubicin/ cyclophosphamide/vincristine/ procarbazine/prednisone (BEACOPP)
Non-Hodgkin's lymphoma		
Follicular lymphoma	Bendamustine + rituximab; cyclophosphamide (monotherapy); cyclophosphamide, doxorubicin, vincristine, prednisone (CHOP) + rituximab; cyclophosphamide, vincristine, prednisone (CVP) + rituximab; fludarabine + rituximab; fludarabine, mitoxantrone, dexamethasone (FND)+ rituximab; rituximab (monotherapy); radioimmunotherapy	Bendamustine (monotherapy); fludarabine, cyclophosphamide, mitoxantrone, rituximab (FCMR); radioimmunotherapy
Mantle cell lymphoma	Aggressive therapy: HyperCVAD (Cyclophosphamide, vincristine, doxorubicin, dexamethasone alternating with high-dose methotrexate + cytarabine) + rituximab; rituximab + cyclophosphamide, vincristine, doxorubicin, prednisone [maxi-CHOP] alternating with rituximab + high-dose cytarabine; CALGB (rituximab+ methotrexate with augmented CHOP); sequential RCHOP/RICE (rituximab, cyclo-phosphamide, doxorubicin, vincristine, prednisone) (rituximab, ifosfamide, carboplatin, etoposide) Less aggressive therapy: bendamustine ± rituximab; CHOP ± rituximab; cladribine + rituximab; CVP (cyclophosphamide, vincristine, prednisone) ± rituximab; dose-adjusted EPOCH (etoposide, prednisone, vincristine, cyclophosphamide, doxorubicin) + rituximab; modified rituximab-HyperCVAD with rituximab maintenance in pts >65	*Second-Line Therapy:* Bendamustine ± rituximab; bortezomib ± rituximab; cladribine ± rituximab; FC (fludarabine, cyclophosphamide) ± rituximab; FCMR (fludarabine, cyclophosphamide, mitoxantrone, rituximab); FMR (fludarabine, mitoxantrone, rituximab); lenalidomide ± rituximab; PCR (pentostatin, cyclophosphamide, rituximab); PEPC (prednisone, etoposide, procarbazine, cyclophosphamide) ± rituximab
Diffuse large B-cell	Rituximab + Cyclophosphamide/doxorubicin/ vincristine/prednisone (CHOP) Dose dense CHOP 14 + rituximab Dose adjusted EPOCH + rituximab *Refer to guidelines for therapy with poor left ventricular function.*	Dexamethasone/cisplatin/cytarabine (DHAP) ± rituximab Etoposide/methylprednisone/ cytarabine/cisplatin (ESHAP) ± rituximab Gemcitabine/dexamethasone/ cisplatin (GDP) ± rituximab Gemcitabine/oxaliplatin (GemOx) ± rituximab Ifosfamide/carboplatin/etoposide (ICE) ± rituximab Mesna/ifosfamide/mitoxantrone/ etoposide (MINE) ± rituximab

(Continued)

CANCER TYPE	PREFERRED THERAPIES	ALTERNATIVE REGIMENS
Burkitt's	*Low risk-combination:* CALGB 9251 regimen: Cyclophosphamide + prednisone → ifosfamide or cyclophosphamide; high-dose methotrexate, LV, vincristine, dexamethasone, and doxorubicin or etoposide or cytarabine; or intrathecal triple therapy (methotrexate, cytarabine, hydrocortisone). Cyclophosphamide/vincristine/doxorubicin/ intrathecal methotrexate and cytarabine → high-dose systemic methotrexate ± rituximab (CODOX-M). Dose-adjusted EPOCH: (etoposide, prednisone, vincristine, cyclophosphamide, doxorubicin) + rituximab (min 3 cycles plus one additional beyond CR) + intrathecal methotrexate. (HyperCVAD) alternating with high-dose methotrexate + cytarabine + rituximab *High risk-combination:* CALGB 9521 regimen. Cyclophosphamide/vincristine/doxorubicin/ intrathecal methotrexate and cytarabine → high-dose systemic methotrexate (CODOX-M) alternating with ifosfamide/etoposide and/cytarabine/ intrathecal methotrexate (IVAC) ± rituximab. Dose-adjusted EPOCH + rituximab. (Hyper CVAD) alternating with high-dose methotrexate and cytarabine + rituximab	*Second-Line Therapy:* Dose-adjusted EPOCH + rituximab; rituximab, ifosfamide, cytarabine, etoposide, intrathecal methotrexate (RIVAC); rituximab, gemcitabine, dexamethasone, cisplatin (RGDP); high-dose cytarabine (HDAC)
Lymphoblastic	Standard BFM (Berlin-Frankfurt-Munster) regimen Augmented BFM regimen CALGB ALL regimen HyperCAVD regimen LMB-86 regimen Maintenance chemotherapy *Refer to guidelines for specific information on each regimen.*	
Peripheral T-cell	Cyclophosphamide/doxorubicin/vincristine/ prednisone (CHOP) Cyclophosphamide/doxorubicin/vincristine/ etoposide/prednisone (CHOEP) CHOP every 2 or 3 weeks CHOP followed by ifosfamide/carboplatin/ etoposide (ICE) CHOP followed by ifosfamide/etoposide/epirubicin (IVE) alternating with intermediate dose methotrexate Cyclophosphamide/vincristine/doxorubicin/ dexamethasone (HyperCVAD) alternating with high-dose methotrexate + cytarabine	Dexamethasone/cisplatin/cytarabine (DHAP) Etoposide/methylprednisolone/ cytarabine/cisplatin (ESHAP) Gemcitabine/dexamethasone/ cisplatin (GDP) Gemcitabine/oxaliplatin (GemOX) Ifosfamide/carboplatin/etoposide (ICE) Mesna/ifosfamide/mitoxantrone/ etoposide (MINE) Pralatrexate *Refer to guidelines for regimens in non-candidates for high-dose therapy with stem-cell rescue.*
Ovarian	*Primary Chemotherapy/Adjuvant:* Paclitaxel/ carboplatin	Docetaxel/carboplatin Paclitaxel/cisplatin
Germ cell tumor	Bleomycin/etoposide/cisplatin (BEP)	Paclitaxel/ifosfamide/cisplatin (TIP)
Pancreatic	Locally advanced or metastatic: 5-FU/LV/irinotecan/ oxaliplatin (FOLFIRINOX) Gemcitabine Gemcitabine based-combination therapy Capecitabine	Gemcitabine or fluoropyrimidine based therapy Capecitabine or 5-FU/LV or CapeOX
Prostate	Docetaxel/prednisone *Refer to guidelines for androgen deprivation therapy.*	Mitoxantrone/prednisone

Abbreviations: MTX: methotrexate; 5-FU: 5-fluorouracil; LV: leucovorin.

* Selected cancers. For more detailed information, refer to the individual monograph listings or the drug's FDA-approved labeling.

**Refer to www.cancer.gov for more information, such as therapies for CNS prophylaxis.

† Source: National Comprehensive Cancer Network Clinical Practice (NCCN) Guidelines in Oncology, 2011.

COLORECTAL CANCER TREATMENT OPTIONS

DRUG (BRAND)	INDICATIONS	HOW SUPPLIED	DOSAGE
Bevacizumab (Avastin)	First- or second-line treatment of metastatic carcinoma of the colon or rectum, in combination with 5-fluorouracil-based chemotherapy.	Inj: 25mg/mL [4mL, 16mL]	5mg/kg (in combination with bolus IFL) or 10 mg/kg (in combination with FOLFOX4) given once every 14 days. Give as IV infusion over 90 min; if 1st infusion is well tolerated, give 2nd infusion over 60 min and subsequent doses over 30 min.
Capecitabine (Xeloda)	First-line treatment of metastatic colorectal carcinoma when fluoropyrimidine therapy alone is preferred. Adjuvant treatment in patients with Dukes' C colon cancer who have undergone complete resection of the primary tumor when treatment with fluoropyrimidine therapy alone is preferred.	Tab: 150mg, 500mg	1250mg/m² bid for 2 weeks followed by 1-week rest period given as 3-week cycles. Take with water within 30 min after therapy alone is preferred. Dukes' C Colon Cancer: Give as 3-week cycles for a total of 8 cycles (24 weeks). CrCl 30-50mL/min: Reduce to 75% of starting dose. Interrupt and/or reduce dose if toxicity occurs; readjust based on toxicity grade (refer to PI for details).
Cetuximab (Erbitux)	In combination with irinotecan for the treatment of epidermal growth factor receptor (EGFR)-expressing, metastatic colorectal carcinoma in patients who are refractory to irinotecan-based chemotherapy. As monotherapy, for the treatment of EGFR-expressing, metastatic colorectal carcinoma after failure of both irinotecan- and oxaliplatin-based regimens or in patients intolerant to irinotecan-based therapy.	Inj: 2mg/mL [50mL, 100mL]	Premedication with H₁ antagonist (eg, diphenhydramine 50mg) IV 30-60 min prior to 1st dose is recommended. Initial: 400mg/m² IV infusion over 120 min. Maint: 250mg/m² IV infusion over 60 min once weekly. Max Infusion Rate: 10mg/min. Refer to PI for dose modifications with infusion reactions and severe acneiform rash.
Fluorouracil	Palliative management of colon, rectum, breast, stomach, and pancreatic carcinomas.	Inj: 50mg/mL [10mL, 20mL]	12mg/kg IV qd for 4 days. Max: 800mg/day. If no toxicity, give 6mg/kg IV on 6th, 8th, 10th, and 12th days. Skip Days 5, 7, 9, and 11. Inadequate Nutritional State: 6mg/kg IV for 3 days. If no toxicity, give 3mg/kg IV on 5th, 7th, and 9th days. Max: 400mg/day. Skip Days 4, 6, and 8. Maint (Use Schedule 1 or Schedule 2): Schedule 1: If no toxicity, repeat 1st course every 30 days after last day of previous course. Schedule 2: When toxic signs from initial course subside, give 10-15mg/kg/ week IV single dose; do not exceed 1g/week.
Irinotecan hydrochloride (Camptosar)	First-line therapy in combination with 5-fluorouracil (5-FU) and leucovorin (LV) for metastatic colon or rectal carcinomas, and for disease that has progressed or recurred following initial 5-FU-based therapy.	Inj: 20mg/mL [2mL, 5mL, 15mL]	Refer to PI for dosage regimens and dose modifications: Combination Therapy (6-week cycle with bolus 5-FU/LV): 125mg/m² IV over 90 min on days 1, 8, 15, 22; or (6-week cycle with infusional 5-FU/LV) 180mg/m² IV over 90 min on days 1, 15, and 29. Both regimens: Begin next cycle on Day 43. Single Therapy: 125mg/m² IV over 90 min on days 1, 8, 15, 22, followed by a 2-week rest; or 350mg/m² IV over 90 min once every 3 weeks. Premedicate with antiemetics at least 30 min prior to therapy. Dose modifications for reduced UGT1A1 activity, neutropenia, diarrhea, and other toxicities: Refer to PI. All dose modifications should be based on worst preceding toxicity.

(Continued)

DRUG (BRAND)	INDICATIONS	HOW SUPPLIED	DOSAGE
Leucovorin calcium	Adjunct to 5-fluorouracil (5-FU) for palliative treatment of advanced colorectal cancer.	Inj: 50mg, 100mg, 200mg, 350mg, 500mg	$200mg/m^2$ slow IV push over 3 min followed by 5-FU $370mg/m^2$ IV qd for 5 days, or $20mg/m^2$ IV qd followed by 5-FU $425mg/m^2$ IV qd for 5 days. Administer leucovorin and 5-FU separately to avoid precipitation. May repeat at 4-week intervals for 2 courses, then at 4-5 week intervals. May increase 5-FU dose by 10% if no toxicity. Reduce 5-FU dose by 20% with moderate GI/hematologic toxicity and by 30% with severe toxicity.
Oxaliplatin (Eloxatin)	In combination with infusional 5-fluorouracil (5-FU) and leucovorin (LV) for treatment of advanced colorectal cancer and adjuvant treatment of Stage III colon cancer patients who have undergone complete resection of the primary tumor.	Inj: 50mg, 100mg, 200mg	Advanced Disease: Day 1: $85mg/m^2$ IV with LV $200mg/m^2$ IV in separate bags using a Y-line; followed by 5-FU $400mg/m^2$ bolus over 2-4 min, then 5-FU $600mg/m^2$ as a 22 hr-infusion. Day 2: LV $200mg/m^2$ over 120 min; followed by 5-FU $400mg/m^2$ bolus over 2-4 min, then 5-FU $600mg/m^2$ as a 22 hr-infusion. Repeat cycle every 2 weeks until disease progression or unacceptable toxicity. See PI for dose modifications for persistent grade 2 neurosensory events, grade 3 or 4 GI or grade 4 hematologic toxicity. Adjuvant Therapy: Recommended cycle every 2 weeks for 6 months (12 cycles).
Panitumumab (Vectibix)	Treatment of EGFR-expressing, metastatic colorectal carcinoma with disease progression on or following fluoro-pyrimidine-, oxaliplatin-, and irinotecan-containing chemo-therapy regimens.	Inj: 20mg/mL [5mL, 10mL, 20mL]	6mg/kg IV infusion over 60 min every 14 days. Infuse doses >1000mg over 90 min. Refer to PI for dose modifications with mild or severe infusion reactions and dermatologic toxicities.

LUNG CANCER TREATMENT OPTIONS

DRUG (BRAND)	INDICATIONS	HOW SUPPLIED	DOSAGE
ANTIMICROTUBULE AGENTS			
Docetaxel (Taxotere)	Treatment of NSCLC after failure of prior chemotherapy. In combination with cisplatin for treatment of unresectable, locally advanced or metastatic NSCLC who have not previously received chemotherapy for this condition.	Inj: 20mg/0.5mL, 80mg/2mL	NSCLC: After Platinum Therapy Failure: 75mg/m² IV over 1 hr every 3 weeks.
Paclitaxel	First-line (with cisplatin) for subsequent treatment of NSCLC. First-line treatment of NSCLC in combination with cisplatin in patients who are not candidates for potentially curative surgery and/or radiation therapy.	Inj: 30mg/5mL, 100mg/16.7mL, 150mg/25mL, 300mg/50mL	NSCLC: 135mg/m² over 24 hrs every 3 weeks followed by cisplatin.
PODOPHYLLOTOXIN DERIVATIVES			
Etoposide Phosphate (Etopophos)	First-line combination therapy for management of SCLC.	Inj: 100mg	SCLC: (Range) 35mg/m²/day for 4 days to 50mg/m²/day for 5 days.
Etoposide	First-line combination therapy for management of SCLC.	Cap: 50mg	SCLC: 2x the IV dose rounded to nearest 50mg. Eg, Two times 35mg/m²/day IV for 4 days to 50mg/m²/day for 5 days.
VINCA ALKALOID			
Vinorelbine Tartrate (Navelbine)	Single agent or in combination with cisplatin for 1st-line treatment of unresectable, advanced NSCLC, including Stage IV NSCLC. For use in combination with cisplatin for Stage III NSCLC.	Inj: 10mg/mL	Single-Agent: 30mg/m² IV weekly over 6-10 min. With Cisplatin: 25mg/m² weekly with cisplatin 100mg/m² every 4 weeks, or 30mg/m² weekly with cisplatin 120mg/m² on Days 1 and 29, then every 6 weeks.
DIHYDROFOLIC ACID REDUCTASE INHIBITOR			
Methotrexate Sodium	Treatment of neoplastic diseases such as lung cancer.	Inj: 25mg/mL; Tab: 2.5mg* *scored	Oral administration in tablet form is often preferred when low doses are being administered since absorption is rapid and effective serum levels are obtained. Methotrexate injection may be given by the intramuscular, intravenous or intra-arterial route. Refer to PI for more information.
NUCLEOSIDE ANALOGUE METABOLITE			
Gemcitabine HCl (Gemzar)	Combination with cisplatin for 1st-line treatment of inoperable, locally advanced (Stage IIIA or IIIB), or metastatic (Stage IV) NSCLC.	Inj: 200mg, 1 g	4-Week Cycle: 1000mg/m² IV over 30 min on Days 1, 8, and 15 of each 28-day cycle. Give cisplatin 100mg/m² IV on Day 1 after gemcitabine HCl infusion. 3-Week Cycle: 1250mg/m² IV over 30 min on Days 1 and 8 of each 21-day cycle. Give cisplatin 100mg/m² IV on Day 1 after gemcitabine HCl infusion.
NITROGEN MUSTARD ALKYLATING AGENT			
Mechlorethamine HCl (Mustargen)	(IV) Palliative treatment of bronchogenic carcinoma.	Inj: 10mg	IV: 0.4mg/kg/course given as a single dose or in divided doses of 0.1-0.2mg/kg/day.

(Continued)

LUNG CANCER TREATMENT OPTIONS

DRUG (BRAND)	INDICATIONS	HOW SUPPLIED	DOSAGE
ANTHRACYCLINE			
Doxorubicin HCl	To produce regression in disseminated neoplastic conditions such as bronchogenic carcinoma.	**Inj:** 10mg, 20mg, 50mg; 2mg/mL [5mL, 10mL, 25mL], **MDV:** 2mg/mL [100mL]	Monotherapy: 60-75mg/m^2 IV q21 days. Concomitant Chemotherapy: 40-60mg/m^2 IV every 21-28 days. Refer to PI for studied doses.
PHOTOSENSITIZER			
Porfimer Sodium (Photofrin)	Reduction of obstruction and palliation of symptoms in patients with completely or partially obstructive endobronchial NSCLC. Treatment of microinvasive endobronchial NSCLC in patients for whom surgery and radiotherapy are not indicated.	**Inj:** (powder) 75mg	Photodynamic Therapy (PDT) for Esophageal/Endobronchial Cancer or HGD in BE: 2mg/kg IV over 3-5 min. Deliver laser light therapy (refer to PI for details) 40-50 hrs following injection. A second laser light treatment may be given 96-120 hrs following injection. Max: 3 courses of PDT separated by 30-day (esophageal/endobronchial cancer) or 90-day (HGD in BE) intervals.
TOPOISOMERASE I INHIBITORS			
Topotecan HCl (Hycamtin Injection)	Treatment of initial or subsequent chemotherapy and SCLC sensitive disease after 1st-line chemotherapy failure.	**Inj:** 4mg	SCLC: 1.5mg/m^2 IV qd over 30 min for 5 days, starting on Day 1 of 21-day course. Minimum of 4 courses recommended in absence of tumor progression.
Topotecan HCl (Hycamtin Capsules)	Treatment of relapsed SCLC patients with a prior complete or partial response and who are at least 45 days from the end of first-line chemotherapy.	**Cap:** 0.25mg, 1mg	SCLC: 2.3mg/m^2/day PO qd for 5 consecutive days, repeated every 21 days. Round calculated dose to nearest 0.25mg and give minimum number of 1mg and 0.25mg caps.
ANTIFOLATE			
Pemetrexed Disodium (Alimta)	In combination with cisplatin for the initial treatment of locally advanced or metastatic nonsquamous NSCLC. Maintenance treatment in patients with locally advanced or metastatic nonsquamous NSCLC whose disease has not progressed after 4 cycles of platinum-based first-line chemotherapy. Single agent for the treatment of patients with locally advanced or metastatic nonsquamous NSCLC after prior chemotherapy. In combination with cisplatin for the treatment of patients with malignant pleural mesothelioma whose disease is unresectable or who are otherwise not candidates for curative surgery.	**Inj:** 100mg, 500mg	Combination with Cisplatin: Nonsquamous NSCLC/Mesothelioma: 500mg/m^2 IV infused over 10 min on Day 1 of each 21-day cycle. Give cisplatin 75mg/m^2 infused over 2 hrs beginning 30 min after the end of administration. Patient should receive appropriate hydration prior to and/or after receiving cisplatin. Single Agent: Nonsquamous NSCLC: 500mg/m^2 IV infused over 10 min on Day 1 of each 21-day cycle. Refer to PI for dose adjustments for hematologic, nonhematologic, and neurotoxicities. Give pre-medications (eg, dexamethsone, folic acid) as necessary.
VASCULAR AND ENDOTHELIAL GROWTH FACTOR INHIBITOR			
Bevacizumab (Avastin)	1st-line treatment of unresectable, locally advanced, recurrent or metastatic non-squamous NSCLC, in combination with carboplatin and paclitaxel.	**Inj:** 100mg/4mL, 400mg/16mL	NSCLC: 15mg/kg q3 weeks (in combination with carboplatin/paclitaxel).

(Continued)

DRUG (BRAND)	INDICATIONS	HOW SUPPLIED	DOSAGE
EPIDERMAL GROWTH FACTOR TYROSINE KINASE INHIBITOR			
Erlotinib HCl (Tarceva)	Treatment of locally advanced or metastatic NSCLC after failure of at least one prior chemotherapy regimen. Maintenance treatment of locally advanced or metastatic NSCLC whose disease has not progressed after four cycles of platinum-based first-line chemotherapy.	**Tab:** 25mg, 100mg, 150mg	NSCLC: 150mg qd.

*NSCLC: Non Small Cell Lung Cancer
*SCLC: Small Cell Lung Cancer

PROSTATE CANCER TREATMENT OPTIONS

DRUG (BRAND)	INDICATIONS	HOW SUPPLIED	DOSAGE
BISPHOSPHONATE			
Zoledronic acid (Zometa)	Treatment of documented bone metastases from solid tumors (progressive prostate cancer after treatment with one hormonal therapy), in conjunction with standard antineoplastic therapy.	**Inj:** 4mg/5mL	4mg as a single-dose IV infusion over ≥15 min q3-4wks with CrCl >60mL/min. Reduce with renal impairment. Coadminister calcium 500mg orally and 400 IU vitamin D daily.
CHEMOTHERAPY AGENTS			
Cabazitaxel (Jevtana)	In combination with prednisone for the treatment of patients with hormone refractory metastatic prostate cancer previously treated with a docetaxel-containing treatment regimen.	60mg/1.5mL	25mg/m^2 administered as a 1 hr IV infusion q3 weeks in combination with prednisone 10mg po administered qd. Premedicate at least 30 min prior to each dose. See PI for dose modifications for adverse effects.
Docetaxel (Taxotere)	Treatment of androgen-independent (hormone refractory) metastatic prostate cancer in combination with prednisone.	**Inj:** 20mg/mL, 80mg/4mL	Premedicate with oral corticosteroids. Adjust dose based on febrile neutropenia, neutrophil count, cutaneous reactions, peripheral neuropathy, neurosensory signs/symptoms, or GI toxicities (see PI). Usual: 75mg/m^2 q3 weeks over 1 hr; administer with prednisone 5mg bid continuously.
Estramustine phosphate sodium (Emcyt)	Palliative treatment of metastatic and/or progressive prostate carcinoma.	**Cap:** 140mg	Usual: 14mg/kg/day given tid-qid. Take with water at least 1 hr before or 2 hrs after meals. Treat for 30-90 days before determining possible benefits of continued therapy.
Mitoxantrone (Novantrone)	Initial treatment of patients with pain related to advanced hormone-refractory prostate cancer in combination with corticosteroids.	**Inj:** 2mg/mL	12-14mg/m^2/day IV every 21 days.
Sipuleucel-T (Provenge)	Treatment of asymptomatic or minimally symptomatic metastatic castrate resistant (hormone refractory) prostate cancer.	**Sus:** 250mL	Infuse 250mL over 60 min every 2 weeks for 3 doses. Premedicate 30 min prior to administration.
ESTROGENS			
Conjugated estrogens tablets (Premarin)	Palliative treatment of advanced androgen-dependent carcinoma of the prostate.	**Tab:** 0.3mg, 0.45mg, 0.625mg, 0.9mg, 1.25mg	1.25-2.5mg tid. Effectiveness of therapy judged by phosphatase determinations and symptomatic improvement.
Esterified estrogens tablets (Menest)	Palliative therapy for advanced prostatic carcinoma.	**Tab:** 0.3mg, 0.625mg, 1.25mg, 2.5mg	1.25-2.5mg tid. Effectiveness of therapy judged by phosphatase determinations and symptomatic improvement.
Estradiol tablets (Estrace)	Palliative treatment of advanced androgen-dependent prostate carcinoma.	**Tab:** 0.5mg*, 1mg*, 2mg* *scored	1-2mg tid. Effectiveness of therapy judged by phosphatase determinations and symptomatic improvement.
Estradiol valerate injection (Delestrogen)	Palliative treatment of advanced androgen-dependent prostate carcinoma.	**Inj:** 10mg/mL, 20mg/mL, 40mg/mL	30mg or more every 1 or 2 weeks.

(Continued)

PROSTATE CANCER TREATMENT OPTIONS

DRUG (BRAND)	INDICATIONS	HOW SUPPLIED	DOSAGE
GnRH ANALOGUES			
Goserelin acetate implant (Zoladex 3.6mg)	Palliative treatment of advanced prostatic carcinoma. Adjunct to and during radiotherapy, and in combination with flutamide, for management of locally confined Stage B2-C prostate cancer.	**Implant:** 3.6mg	Inject SQ into anterior abdominal wall below navel line. Advanced Prostatic Carcinoma: 3.6mg every 28 days. Stage B2-C Prostatic Carcinoma: 3.6mg starting 8 weeks before radiotherapy, then 10.8mg depot formulation 28 days after 1st injection, or 4 doses of 3.6mg at 28-day intervals (2 before and 2 during radiotherapy).
Goserelin acetate implant (Zoladex 10.8mg)	Palliative treatment of advanced prostate cancer. Adjunct to radiotherapy and flutamide for management of locally confined Stage B2-C prostate cancer.	**Implant:** 10.8mg	Inject SQ into anterior abdominal wall below navel line. Advanced Prostate Cancer: 10.8mg every 12 weeks. Stage B2-C Prostate Cancer: 3.6mg depot formulation 8 weeks before radiotherapy, followed by 10.8mg 28 days after 1st injection.
GnRH ANTAGONIST			
Degarelix for injection (Firmagon)	Treatment of advanced prostate cancer.	**Inj:** 80mg, 120mg	Initial: 240mg (as two SQ injections of 120mg) at 40mg/mL concentration. Maint: 80mg SQ every 28 days at 20mg/mL concentration.
LHRH AGONISTS			
Histrelin implant (Vantas)	Palliative treatment of advanced prostate cancer.	**Implant:** 50mg	50mg every 12 months. Inject SQ into inner aspect of the upper arm. Refrain from wetting the inserted arm for 24 hrs. Refrain from heavy lifting or strenuous exercise of the inserted arm for 7 days after implant insertion. Must remove after 12 months of therapy and replace with new implant.
Leuprolide acetate (Eligard)	Palliative treatment of advanced prostate cancer.	**Inj:** 7.5mg, 22.5mg, 30mg, 45mg	7.5mg SQ monthly, 22.5mg SQ every 3 months, 30mg SQ every 4 months, or 45mg SQ every 6 months. Rotate injection sites.
Leuprolide acetate	Palliative treatment of advanced prostate cancer.	**Inj:** 5mg/mL	1mg SQ qd. Rotate injection sites.
Leuprolide acetate (Lupron Depot)	Palliative treatment of advanced prostate cancer.	**Inj:** (1-month) 7.5mg, (3-month) 22.5mg, (4-month) 30mg	7.5mg IM as single dose monthly, 22.5mg IM single dose every 3 months, or 30mg IM single dose every 4 months. Rotate injection site.
Triptorelin pamoate injection, suspension (Trelstar)	Palliative treatment of advanced prostate cancer.	**Inj:** (Depot) 3.75mg, (LA) 11.25mg, 22.5mg	(Depot) 3.75mg IM q4wks or (LA) 11.25mg IM q12wks 22.5mg IM q24wks.
NONSTEROIDAL ANTIANDROGENS			
Bicalutamide (Casodex)	Treatment of Stage D2 metastatic carcinoma of the prostate in combination with an LHRH analogue.	**Tab:** 50mg	50mg qd at same time (morning or evening). Initiate simultaneously with an LHRH analogue.
Flutamide	Treatment of locally confined Stage B2-C and Stage D2 metastatic carcinoma of the prostate in combination with an LHRH analogue.	**Cap:** 125mg	250mg q8h. Max: 750mg/day.
Nilutamide (Nilandron)	Treatment of Stage D2 metastatic prostatic cancer in combination with surgical castration.	**Tab:** 150mg	Initial: 300mg/day for 30 days beginning on the day of, or on the day after, surgical castration. Maint: 150mg qd.

Abbreviations: LHRH = luteinizing hormone-releasing hormone; GnRH = gonadotropin-releasing hormone.

Sources:
FDA-approved product labeling.
Initial hormonal management of androgen-sensitive metastatic, recurrent, or progressive prostate cancer: 2007 update of an American Society of Clinical Oncology Practice Guideline. *J Clin Oncol.* 2007;25:1596-1605.
National Comprehensive Cancer Network Clinical Practice Guidelines in Oncology; Prostate Cancer. Version 1.2010.

ANTIDEPRESSANTS

DRUG (BRAND)	HOW SUPPLIED	DAILY DOSE Initial (I), Usual (U), Max (M)	TITRATE
AMINOKETONES			
Bupropion HCl (Wellbutrin)	**Tab:** 75mg, 100mg	**(I)**200mg **(U)**300mg **(M)**450mg	Increase by 100mg/d q3d.
(Wellbutrin SR)	**Tab, SR:** 100mg, 150mg, 200mg	**(I)**150mg **(U)**300mg **(M)**400mg	Increase to 300mg/d as early as day 4 of dosing if tolerated. Increase to 400mg/d after several wks if no clinical improvement.
(Wellbutrin XL)	**Tab, ER:** 150mg, 300mg	**(I)**150mg **(U)**300mg **(M)**450mg	Increase to 300mg/d as early as day 4 of dosing if tolerated. Increase to 450mg/d after several wks if no clinical improvement.
Bupropion HBr (Aplenzin)	**Tab, ER:** 174mg, 348mg, 522mg	**(I)**174mg **(U)**348mg **(M)**522mg	Increase to 348mg/d as early as day 4 of dosing if tolerated. Increase to 522mg/d after several wks if no clinical improvement.
MONOAMINE OXIDASE INHIBITORS			
Isocarboxazid (Marplan)	**Tab:** 10mg*	**(I)**20mg **(M)**60mg	Increase by 10mg q2-4d to 40mg/d by end of first wk. then increase by increments of up to 20mg/wk if needed.
Phenelzine (Nardil)	**Tab:** 15mg	**(I)**45mg **(U)**15mg qd or qod	Increase rapidly to 60-90mg/d then decrease to maintenance dose.
Selegiline (Emsam)	**Patch:** 6mg/24 hrs, 9mg/24 hrs, 12mg/24 hrs	**(I,U)**6mg/24 hrs **(M)**12mg/24 hrs	Increase by 3mg/24 hrs q2wks.
Tranylcypromine (Parnate)	**Tab:** 10mg	**(I,U)**30mg **(M)**60mg	Increase by 10mg/d q1-3wks.
PHENYLPIPERAZINE			
Nefazodone	**Tab:** 50mg, 100mg*, 150mg*, 200mg, 250mg	**(I)**200mg **(U)**300-600mg **(M)**600mg	Increase by 100-200mg/d in no less than 1 wk.
SELECTIVE SEROTONIN NOREPINEPHRINE REUPTAKE INHIBITORS			
Desvenlafaxine (Pristiq)	**Tab, ER:** 50mg, 100mg	**(I,U)**50mg **(M)**400mg	N/A
Duloxetine (Cymbalta)	**Cap, DR:** 20mg, 30mg, 60mg	**(I,U)**40-60mg **(M)**120mg	N/A
Venlafaxine (Effexor)	**Tab:** 25mg*, 37.5mg*, 50mg*, 75mg*, 100mg*	**(I)**75mg **(M)**375mg	Increase by 75mg/d-q4d.
(Effexor XR)	**Cap, ER:** 37.5mg, 75mg, 150mg	**(I)**37.5-75mg **(M)**225mg	Increase by 75mg/d q4d.
SELECTIVE SEROTONIN REUPTAKE INHIBITOR/5-HT$_{1A}$ PARTIAL AGONIST			
Vilazodone HCl (Viibryd)	**Tab:** 10mg, 20mg, 40mg	**(I)**10mg **(U)**40mg	Increase to 20mg/d after 1 wk then to 40mg/d after 1 wk.
SELECTIVE SEROTONIN REUPTAKE INHIBITORS			
Citalopram (Celexa)	**Sol:** 10mg/5mL; **Tab:** 10mg, 20mg*, 40mg*	**(I)**20mg **(U)**40mg **(M)**40-60mg	Increase by 20mg/d qwk.
Escitalopram (Lexapro)	**Sol:** 5mg/5mL; **Tab:** 5mg, 10mg*, 20mg*	**(I)**10mg **(U)**10-20mg **(M)**20mg	Increase to 20mg/d after 1 wk.
Fluoxetine (Prozac) (Prozac Weekly)	**Cap:** 10mg, 20mg, 40mg; **Sol:** (generic) 20mg/5mL; **Tab:** (generic) 10mg*, 20mg* **Cap, DR:** 90mg	**(I)**20mg **(U)**20-80mg **(M)**80mg 90mg weekly capsule initiated 7 days after the last dose of 20mg	Consider after several wks of therapy.

(Continued)

DRUG (BRAND)	HOW SUPPLIED	DAILY DOSE Initial (I), Usual (U), Max (M)	TITRATE
SELECTIVE SEROTONIN REUPTAKE INHIBITORS *(Continued)*			
Paroxetine (Paxil)	**Sus:** 10mg/5mL; **Tab:** 10mg*, 20mg*, 30mg, 40mg	**(I)**20mg **(M)**50mg	Increase by 10mg/d qwk.
(Paxil CR)	**Tab, CR:** 12.5mg, 25mg, 37.5mg	**(I)**25mg **(M)**62.5mg	Increase by 12.5mg/d qwk.
(Pexeva)	**Tab:** 10mg, 20mg*, 30mg, 40mg	**(I)**20mg **(M)**50mg	Increase by 10mg/d qwk.
Sertraline (Zoloft)	**Sol:** 20mg/mL; **Tab:** 25mg*, 50mg*, 100mg*	**(I)**50mg **(M)**200mg	Increase at 1-wk intervals.
TETRACYCLICS			
Maprotiline	**Tab:** 25mg*, 50mg*, 75mg*	**(I)**OP: 25mg-75mg maintain for 2 wks IP:100mg-150mg **(U)**OP: 75mg-150mg IP:150mg-225mg **(M)**OP: 150mg-225mg IP: 225mg	Increase by 25mg gradually.
Mirtazapine (Remeron) (Remeron SolTab)	**Tab:** 15mg*, 30mg*, 45mg; **Tab, Disintegrating:** 15mg, 30mg, 45mg	**(I)**15mg **(M)**45mg	Increase q1-2wk.
TRIAZOLOPYRIDINE			
Trazodone (Generic)	**Tab:** 50mg*, 100mg*, 150mg*, 300mg*	**(I)**150mg **(M)**OP: 400mg IP: 600mg	Increase by 50mg/d q3-4d.
(Oleptro)	**Tab ER:** 150mg*, 300mg*	**(I)**150mg **(U)**150-375mg **(M)**375mg	Increase by 75mg/d q3d.
TRICYCLICS			
Amitriptyline	**Tab:** 10mg, 25mg, 50mg, 75mg, 100mg, 150mg	**(I)**OP: 50-100mg, IP: 100mg **(U)**50-100mg **(M)**OP: 150mg, IP: 300mg	OP: Increase by 25-50mg/d. IP: Increase to 200mg/d.
Amoxapine	**Tab:** 25mg*, 50mg*, 100mg*, 150mg*	**(I)**100-150mg **(U)**200-300mg **(M)**OP: 400mg IP: 600mg	Increase to 100mg bid-tid by end of first wk.
Clomipramine (Anafranil)	**Cap:** 25mg, 50mg, 75mg	**(I)**25mg **(U)**100-250mg **(M)**250mg	Increase to 100mg/d in 2 wks, then increase gradually.
Desipramine (Norpramin)	**Tab:** 10mg, 25mg, 50mg, 75mg, 100mg, 150mg	**(I,U)**100-200mg **(M)**300mg	N/A
Doxepin	**Cap:** 10mg, 25mg, 50mg, 75mg, 100mg, 150mg; **Sol:** 10mg/mL	**(I)**75mg **(U)**75-150mg **(M)**300mg	Increase gradually.
Imipramine (Tofranil PM)	**Cap:** 75mg, 100mg, 125mg, 150mg	**(I)**OP: 75mg, IP: 100-150mg **(U)**75-150mg **(M)**OP: 200mg, IP: 250-300mg	OP: Increase to 150mg/d. IP: Increase to 200mg/d.
(Tofranil)	**Tab:** 10mg, 25mg, 50mg	**(I)**OP: 75mg IP: 100mg **(U)**50-150mg **(M)**OP: 200mg, IP: 250-300mg	OP: Increase to 150mg/d. IP: Increase to 200mg/d.
Nortriptyline (Pamelor)	**Cap:** 10mg, 25mg, 50mg, 75mg; **Sol:**10mg/5mL	**(I,U)**75-100mg **(M)**150mg	N/A
Protriptyline (Vivactil)	**Tab:** 5mg, 10mg	**(I)**15mg **(I,U)**15-40mg **(M)**60mg	Titrate morning dose.
Trimipramine (Surmontil)	**Cap:** 25mg, 50mg, 100mg	**(I)**OP: 75mg, IP: 100mg **(U)**OP: 50-150mg, IP: 200mg **(M)**OP: 200mg, IP: 250-300mg	OP: Increase to 150mg/d. IP: Increase to 200mg/d.

Abbreviations: IP=Inpatient; OP=Outpatient   *Scored.

ANTIPSYCHOTIC AGENTS

DRUG (BRAND)	HOW SUPPLIED (mg)*	INITIAL & (MAX) DOSE**	USUAL DOSE RANGE**
ATYPICAL			
Aripiprazole (Abilify)	**Tab:** 2, 5, 10, 15, 20, 30 **Sol:** 1mg/mL; **Inj:** 7.5mg/mL	10-15mg qd (30mg/day)	10-15mg qd
(Abilify Discmelt)	**Tab, Orally Disintegrating:** (Discmelt) 10, 15	10-15mg qd (30mg/day)	10-15mg qd
Asenapine (Saphris)	**Tab, SL:** 5, 10	5mg bid (20mg/day)	5-10mg bid
Clozapine (Clozaril)	**Tab:** 12.5†, 25, 50†, 100, 200†	12.5mg qd-bid (900mg/day)	100-900mg/day given tid
(Fazaclo)	**Tab, Orally Disintegrating:** 12.5, 25, 100, 150, 200	12.5mg qd-bid (900mg/day)	100-900mg/day given tid
Iloperidone (Fanapt)	**Tab:** 1, 2, 4, 6, 8, 10, 12	Schizophrenia: Initial: 1mg bid. Titrate: Must titrate dose slowly to avoid orthostatic hypotension. Day 2: 2mg bid. Day 3: 4mg bid. Day 4: 6mg bid. Day 5: 8mg bid. Day 6: 10mg bid. Day 7: 12mg bid. Max: 12mg bid (24mg/day)	6-12mg bid
Lurasidone HCl (Latuda)	**Tab:** 40, 80	40mg qd (80mg/day)	40-80mg qd
Olanzapine (Zyprexa, Zyprexa Zydis)	**Tab:** 2.5, 5, 7.5, 10, 15, 20 **Tab, Orally Disintegrating:** 5, 10, 15, 20	Schizophrenia: 5-10mg qd Bipolar Mania: 10-15mg qd (20mg/day for both)	Schizophrenia: 10-20mg qd Bipolar Mania: 5-20mg qd
(Zyprexa IntraMuscular)	**Inj:** 10	Agitation: 10mg IM (3 doses)	Agitation: 2.5-10mg IM
(Zyprexa Relprevv)	**Inj, Extended-Release:** 210, 300, 405	Establish tolerability with oral olanzapine prior to initiating treatment. (405mg q4 wks or 300mg q2 wks)	150-300mg/2 wks or 405mg/4 wks
Paliperidone (Invega)	**Tab, Extended-Release:** 1.5, 3, 6, 9	6mg qd (12mg/day)	3-12mg/day
(Invega Sustenna)	**Inj, Extended-Release:** 39, 78, 117, 156, 234	234mg IM on treatment Day 1 and 156mg IM after 1 week. (234mg IM)	39mg to 234mg IM
Quetiapine fumarate (Seroquel)	**Tab:** 25, 50, 100, 200, 300, 400	Schizophrenia: 25mg bid Bipolar Mania: 50mg bid (800mg/day for both)	Schizophrenia: 150-750mg/day Bipolar Mania: 400-800mg/day
(Seroquel XR)	**Tab, Extended-Release:** 50, 150, 200, 300, 400	Initial: 300mg/day (800mg/day)	400-800mg/day
Risperidone (Risperdal)	**Sol:** 1mg/mL **Tab:** 0.25, 0.5, 1, 2, 3, 4	Schizophrenia: 2mg/day given qd-bid (16mg/day) Bipolar Mania: 2-3mg qd (6mg/day)	Schizophrenia: 4-8mg/day Bipolar Mania: 1-6mg/day
(Risperdal M-Tab)	**Tab, Orally Disintegrating:** 0.5, 1, 2, 3, 4	Schizophrenia: 2mg/day given qd-bid (16mg/day) Bipolar Mania: 2-3mg qd (6mg/day)	Schizophrenia: 4-8mg/day Bipolar Mania: 1-6mg/day
(Risperdal Consta)	**Inj:** 12.5, 25, 37.5, 50	Schizophrenia: 25mg IM q2wk (50mg IM q2wks)	Schizophrenia: 25-50mg IM q2wks

(Continued)

DRUG (BRAND)	HOW SUPPLIED (mg)*	INITIAL & (MAX) DOSE**	USUAL DOSE RANGE**
ATYPICAL *(Continued)*			
Ziprasidone HCI (Geodon)	**Cap:** 20, 40, 60, 80	Schizophrenia: 20mg bid (80mg bid) Bipolar Mania: 40mg bid	Schizophrenia: 20-80mg bid Bipolar Mania: 40-80mg bid
Ziprasidone mesylate (Geodon) for Injection)	**Inj:** 20mg/mL	10mg IM q2h or 20mg IM q4h (40mg/day)	Switch to oral for long-term therapy.
CONVENTIONAL			
Chlorpromazine	**Inj:** 25mg/mL; **Tab:** 10, 25, 50, 100, 200	10mg tid-qid or 25mg bid-tid or 25mg IM (1000mg/day PO)	PO: 30-800mg/day IM: Additional 25-50mg IM in 1 hr. Increase subsequent doses over several days until patient is controlled.‡ Switch to PO when controlled.
Fluphenazine HCI	**Elixir:** 2.5mg/5mL **Sol, Conc:** 5mg/mL **Tab:** 1, 2.5, 5, 10 **Inj:** 2.5mg/mL	2.5mg-10mg/day in divided doses (40mg/day) 1.25mg IM q6-8h (10mg/day)	1-5mg qd Individualize to patient. Switch to PO when controlled.
Fluphenazine decanoate	**Inj:** 25mg/mL	12.5-25mg IM/SQ (100mg/dose)	Individualize to patient.
Haloperidol	**Sol, Conc:** 2mg/mL **Tab:** 0.5, 1, 2, 5, 10, 20	Moderate: 0.5-2mg bid-tid Sev/Resist: 3-5mg bid-tid (100mg/day)	Reduce to minimum effective dose.
Haloperidol lactate (Haldol)	**Inj:** 5mg/mL	2-5mg IM q4-8h or hourly if needed	Individualize to patient.
Haloperidol decanoate (Haldol Decanoate)	**Inj:** 50mg/mL, 100mg/mL	10-20x daily oral dose up to 100mg/dose (450mg/month)	10-15x daily oral dose
Loxapine succinate	**Cap:** 5, 10, 25, 50	10mg bid, up to 50mg/day (250mg/day)	60-100mg/day
Perphenazine	**Tab:** 2, 4, 8, 16	Non-hospitalized: 4-8mg tid Hospitalized: 8-16mg bid-qid. (64mg/day)	Reduce dose as soon as possible to minimum effective dose.
Prochlorperazine edisylate	**Inj:** 5mg/mL	10-20mg IM q2-4h or hourly if needed	Switch to PO when controlled.
Prochlorperazine maleate	**Tab:** 5, 10	5-10mg tid-qid	Moderate/Severe: 50-75mg/day Severe: 100-150mg/day
Thioridazine HCI	**Tab:** 10, 25, 50, 100	50-100mg tid (800mg/day)	200-800mg/day given bid-qid
Thiothixene	**Cap:** 1, 2, 5, 10, 20	Mild: 2mg tid Severe: 5mg bid (60mg/day)	20-30mg/day
Trifluoperazine HCI	**Tab:** 1, 2, 5, 10	2-5mg bid (40mg/day or higher if needed)	15-20mg/day

Note: This list is not inclusive of all antipsychotic agents. Indications may vary among the different products.

 * Unless otherwise indicated.

 ** Doses shown are for adults. For pediatric dosing and additional information please refer to the individual monograph listings or the drug's FDA-approved labeling. Dosages need to be adjusted by titration to individual patient needs and may need to be reduced in the elderly, debilitated, or with renal/hepatic impairment. Periodically reassess to determine the need for maintenance treatment.

 † Available only in generic forms.

 ‡ Severe cases may require up to 2g/day or 400mg/dose IM.

BIPOLAR DISORDER PHARMACOTHERAPY

DRUG	BRAND	HOW SUPPLIED	USUAL DOSE	INDICATIONS
MOOD STABILIZER				
Lithium	Lithobid	(generic) **Cap:** 150mg, 300mg, 600mg; (generic) **Tab:** 300mg; **Tab, Extended-Release:** (Lithobid) 300mg, (generic) 450mg; (generic) **Sol:** 8mEq/5mL	**Adults/Pediatrics: ≥12 yrs:** Acute Mania: 600mg or 10mL tid or (300mg ER tab) 900mg bid (am & pm) or 600mg tid to achieve effective serum levels of 1-1.5mEq/L; monitor levels twice a week until stabilized. Maint: 300mg or 5mL tid-qid or (300mg ER tab) 600mg bid (am & pm) or administered on tid dosing interval up to 1200mg/d or (450mg ER tab) 450mg bid to maintain serum levels of 0.6-1.2 mEq/L; monitor levels every 2 months. Elderly: Start at lower end of dosing range. Do not crush or chew ER tab.	Treatment of manic episodes of bipolar disorder and mainte-nance treatment of bipolar disorder.
ANTICONVULSANTS				
Carbamazepine	Equetro	**Cap, Extended-Release:** 100mg, 200mg, 300mg	**Adults:** Initial: 400mg/day, given in divided doses, bid. Titrate: Adjust in increments of 200mg/day. **Max:** 1600mg/day. Do not crush or chew.	Treatment of acute manic and mixed episodes associated with bipolar I disorder.
Divalproex sodium	Depakote ER	**Tab, Extended-Release:** 250mg, 500mg	**Adults:** Mania: Initial: 25mg/kg/day given once daily. Titrate: Increase dose rapidly to clinical effect. **Max:** 60mg/kg/day. Conversion from Depakote: Administer Depakote ER qd using a dose 8-20% higher than the total daily dose of Depakote. If cannot directly convert to Depakote ER, consider increasing to next higher Depakote total daily dose be-fore converting to appropriate total daily Depakote ER dose. Elderly: Give lower initial dose and titrate slowly. Decrease dose or discontinue if decreased food or fluid intake or if excessive somnolence occurs. Swal-low whole; do not crush or chew.	Acute manic or mixed episodes associated with bipolar disorder.
	Depakote	**Tab, Delayed-Release:** 125mg, 250mg, 500mg	**Adults:** Mania: 750mg daily in divided doses. Titrate: Increase dose rapidly to clinical effect. **Max:** 60mg/kg/day. Elderly: Give lower initial dose and titrate slowly. Decrease dose or discontinue if decreased food or fluid intake or if excessive somnolence occurs.	Treatment of manic episodes associated with bipolar disorder.
Lamotrigine	Lamictal	**Tab:** 25mg*, 100mg*, 150mg*, 200mg* *scored **Tab, Chewable:** (Lamictal CD) 2mg, 5mg, 25mg **Tab, Disintegrating:** (Lamictal ODT) 25mg, 50mg, 100mg, 200mg	**Adults:** Bipolar Disorder: Patients not taking carbamazepine, other enzyme-inducing drugs (EIDs) or VPA: **Weeks 1 and 2:** 25mg qd. **Weeks 3 and 4:** 50mg qd. **Week 5:** 100mg qd. **Weeks 6 and 7:** 200mg qd. Patients taking VPA: **Weeks 1 and 2:** 25mg every other day. **Weeks 3 and 4:** 25mg qd. **Week 5:** 50mg qd. **Weeks 6 and 7:** 100mg qd. Patients taking carbama-zepine (or other EIDs) and not taking VPA: **Weeks 1 and 2:** 50mg qd. **Weeks 3 and 4:** 100mg qd (divided doses). **Week 5:** 200mg qd (divided doses). **Week 6:** 300mg qd (divided doses). **Week 7:** Up to 400mg qd (divided doses). After discontinuation	Maintenance treatment of bipolar I disorder to delay the time to occurrence of mood episodes (depression, mania, hypomania, mixed episodes) in patients treated for acute mood episodes with standard therapy.

(Continued)

DRUG	BRAND	HOW SUPPLIED	USUAL DOSE	INDICATIONS
ANTICONVULSANTS *(Continued)*				
Lamotrigine *(continued)*			of psychotropic drugs excluding VPA, carbamazepine, or other EIDs: Maintain current dose. After discontinuation of VPA and current lamotrigine dose of 100mg qd: **Week 1:** 150mg qd. **Week 2 and onward:** 200mg qd. After discontinuation of carbamazepine or other EIDs and current lamotrigine dose of 400mg qd: **Week 1:** 400mg qd. **Week 2:** 300mg qd. **Week 3 and onward:** 200mg. Refer to PI for additional dosing information.	
Valproic Acid	**Stavzor**	**Cap, Delayed Release:** 125mg, 250mg, 500mg	**Adults:** Mania: Initial: 750mg daily in divided doses. Titrate: Increase rapidly to produce the desired clinical effect. **Max:** 60mg/kg/day.	Treatment of manic episodes associated with bipolar disorder.
CONVENTIONAL ANTIPSYCHOTIC				
Chlorpromazine HCl	**Generic**	**Inj:** 25mg/mL; **Tab:** 10mg, 25mg, 50mg, 100mg, 200mg	**Adults:** Inpatient: Acute Schizophrenic/ Manic State: 25mg IM, then 25-50mg IM in 1 hr if needed. Titrate: Increase over several days up to 400mg q4-6h until controlled then switch to PO. Usual: 500mg/day PO. **Max:** 1000mg/day PO (gradual increases to 2000mg/day or more may be necessary). Less acutely disturbed: 25mg PO tid. Titrate: Increase gradually to 400mg/day. Outpatient: 10mg PO tid-qid or 25mg PO bid-tid. More Severe: 25mg PO tid. Titrate: After 1-2 days, increase by 20-50mg semi-weekly until calm. Prompt control of severe symptoms: 25mg IM, may repeat in 1 hr then 25-50mg PO tid.	Control manifestations of manic type of manic-depressive illness.
ATYPICAL ANTIPSYCHOTICS				
Aripiprazole	**Abilify**	**Tab:** 2mg, 5mg, 10mg, 15mg, 20mg, 30mg; **Tab, Disintegrating:** 10mg, 15mg, (Discmelt) **Sol:** 1mg/mL [150mL]. **Inj:** 7.5mg/mL	**Adults:** (PO) Bipolar Disorder Monotherapy: Initial: 15mg/day. Adjunct: 10-15mg qd. Target: 15mg/day. **Max:** 30mg/day. (Inj) Agitation: 9.75mg IM. Range: 5.25-15mg IM. **Max:** 30mg/day; initiate PO therapy as soon as possible. **Pediatrics:** Bipolar Disorder (Monotherapy or Adjunct) 10-17 yrs: Initial: 2mg/day. Titrate: 5mg/day after 2 days. Target: 10mg/day after 2 additional days. May adjust dose in 5mg/day increments. Periodically reassess need for maintenance therapy. Oral sol can be substituted for tabs on mg-per-mg basis up to 25mg. Patients receiving 30mg tabs should receive 25mg of oral sol. Concomitant Strong CYP3A4 Inhibitors (eg, ketoconazole, clarithromycin)/ Concomitant CYP2D6 Inhibitors (eg, quinidine, fluoxetine, paroxetine): Reduce usual aripiprazole dose by 50%. Concomitant CYP3A4 Inducers (eg, carbamazepine):	(PO) Acute and maintenance treatment of manic and mixed episodes associated with bipolar I disorder, both as monotherapy and as an adjunct to lithium or valproate, in adults and pediatrics aged 10-17 yrs. (Inj) Acute treatment of agitation associated with bipolar disorder, manic or mixed, in adults.

(Continued)

DRUG	BRAND	HOW SUPPLIED	USUAL DOSE	INDICATIONS
ATYPICAL ANTIPSYCHOTICS *(Continued)*				
Aripiprazole *(continued)*			Double aripiprazole dose. When d/c CYP3A4 inducer, reduce aripiprazole dose to 10-15mg of usual dose. Concomitant Strong, Moderate, or Weak CYP3A4 and CYP2D6 Inhibitors: Reduce aripiprazole dose to 25% of usual dose and then adjust to favorable clinical response. See PI for more details.	
Asenapine	**Saphris**	**Tab, SL:** 5mg, 10mg	**Adults:** Monotherapy: **Initial/Usual/ Max:** 10mg bid SL. May decrease to 5mg bid if needed. Adjunctive Therapy (with lithium/valproate): Initial: 5mg bid SL. Titrate: May increase to 10mg bid based on response and tolerability. **Max:** 10mg bid. Recommended to continue treatment beyond acute response.	As monotherapy or adjunctive therapy with either lithium or valproate for the acute treatment of manic or mixed episodes associated with bipolar I disorder.
Olanzapine	**Zyprexa, Zyprexa Zydis**	**Inj:** 10mg; **Tab:** 2.5mg, 5mg, 7.5mg, 10mg, 15mg, 20mg; **Tab, Disintegrating:** (Zydis) 5mg, 10mg, 15mg, 20mg	**Adults:** Bipolar I Disorder (Manic or Mixed Episodes): Initial: 10-15mg qd. Titrate: May increase/decrease dose by 5mg daily at intervals of not less than 24 hrs. Maint: 5-20mg/day. Periodically re-evaluate. **Max:** 20mg/day. With Lithium or Valproate: Initial/Usual: 10mg qd. **Max:** 20mg/day. Concomitant Use with Fluoxetine: Depressive Episodes Associated with Bipolar I Disorder: Initial: 5mg with 20mg fluoxetine qd in the evening. Titrate: Adjust dose based on efficacy and tolerability. Usual: 5-12.5mg with 20-50mg fluoxetine. **Max:** 18mg plus fluoxetine 75mg. Hypotension Risk/Hepatic Impairment/Slow Metabolizers/Sensitivity to Olanzapine Effects: Initial: 2.5-5mg plus fluoxetine 20mg qd. Titrate: Increase cautiously. (IM) Agitation: Initial: 10mg IM. Usual: 2.5-10mg IM. Assess for orthostatic hypotension prior to subsequent dosing. **Max:** 30mg/day or 3 doses of 10mg IM q 2-4h. Elderly: 5mg IM. Debilitated/Hypotension Risk/ Sensitivity to Olanzapine Effects: 2.5mg IM. May initiate PO therapy when clinically appropriate. **Pediatrics:** Bipolar I Disorder (Manic or Mixed Episodes): Initial: 2.5-5mg qd. Target dose: 10mg/day. Titrate: Adjust by dose increments/ decrements of 2.5-5mg. **Max:** 20mg/day. Periodically re-evaluate.	Acute treatment of manic or mixed episodes associated with bipolar I disorder and maintenance treatment of bipolar I disorder in adults and adolescent patients (ages 13-17 yrs). Adjunct to lithium or valproate for the treatment of manic episodes or mixed episodes associated with bipolar I disorder in adults. (Inj) Treatment of acute agitation associated with bipolar I mania.
Olanzapine-fluoxetine	**Symbyax**	**Cap:** (Olanzapine-Fluoxetine): 3-25mg, 6-25mg, 6-50mg, 12-25mg, 12-50mg	Initial: 6mg-25mg qd in evening. Range: 6-12mg (olanzapine)-25-50mg (fluoxetine). Adjust dose based on efficacy and tolerability. **Max:** 18mg-75mg/day. Re-examine the need for continued pharmaco-therapy periodically. Hypotension	Acute treatment of depressive episodes associated with bipolar I disorder in adults.

(Continued)

DRUG	BRAND	HOW SUPPLIED	USUAL DOSE	INDICATIONS
ATYPICAL ANTIPSYCHOTICS (Continued)				
Olanzapine-fluoxetine (continued)			Risk/Hepatic Impairment/Slow Metabolizers/Olanzapine-Sensitive: Initial: 3mg-25mg to 6mg-25mg qd in evening. Titrate: Increase cautiously. Pregnant: Use lower dose during 3rd trimester.	
Quetiapine	**Seroquel**	**Tab:** 25mg, 50mg, 100mg, 200mg, 300mg, 400mg	**Adults:** Bipolar I Disorder: Manic Episodes: Monotherapy/Adjunct: Give bid. Day 1: 100mg/day, increase to 400mg/day on Day 4 in increments of up to 100mg/day and further adjust to 800mg/day by Day 6 in increments ≤200mg/day. **Max:** 800mg/day. Depressive Episodes: Give qd at hs. Day 1: 50mg/day. Day 2: 100mg/day. Day 3: 200mg/day. Day 4: 300mg/day. Maint (Bipolar I Disorder): 400-800mg/day given bid as adjunct therapy to lithium or divalproex. Hepatic Impairment: Initial: 25mg/day. Titrate: May increase by 25-50mg/day to an effective dose, depending on response and tolerability. See PI for more details. **Pediatrics:** Bipolar I Disorder: Manic Episodes: 10-17 yrs: Administer bid or tid based on response and tolerability. Day 1: 50mg/day. Day 2: 100mg/day. Day 3: 200mg/day. Day 4: 300mg/day. Day 5: 400mg/day. After Day 5, adjust dose based on response and tolerability within recommended range of 400-600mg/day with increments of ≤100mg/day. **Max:** 600mg/day. See PI for more details.	Acute treatment of manic episodes associated with bipolar I disorder, both as monotherapy and as an adjunct therapy to lithium or divalproex in adults and pediatrics (10-17 yrs). Monotherapy for acute treatment of depressive episodes associated with bipolar disorder in adults. Maintenance treatment of bipolar I disorder as adjunct therapy to lithium or divalproex.
Quetiapine	**Seroquel XR**	**Tab, Extended Release:** 50mg, 150mg, 200mg, 300mg, 400mg	**Adults:** Bipolar Disorder: Bipolar Mania: Monotherapy/Adjunct: Give qd in pm. Day 1: 300mg/day. Day 2: 600mg/day. Titrate: May adjust dose between 400-800mg beginning on Day 3 depending on response and tolerance. Depressive Episodes: Give qd in pm. Day 1: 50mg/day. Day 2: 100mg/day. Day 3: 200mg/day. Day 4: 300mg/day. Maint (Bipolar I Disorder): 400-800mg/day as adjunct therapy to lithium or divalproex. Periodically reassess the need for maintenance treatment and the appropriate dose. Elderly/Hepatic Impairment: Initial: 50mg/day. Titrate: May increase in increments of 50mg/day depending on response and tolerance. See PI for more details.	Acute treatment of manic or mixed episodes associated with bipolar I disorder, both as monotherapy and as an adjunct to lithium or divalproex. Acute treatment of depressive episodes associated with bipolar disorder. Maintenance treatment of bipolar I disorder as adjunct therapy to lithium or divalproex.
Risperidone	**Risperdal**	**Sol:** 1mg/mL [30mL]; **Tab:** 0.25mg, 0.5mg, 1mg, 2mg, 3mg, 4mg; **Tab, Disintegrating:** (M-Tab) 0.5mg, 1mg, 2mg, 3mg, 4mg **Inj:** (Risperdal Consta) 12.5mg, 25mg, 37.5mg, 50mg	**Adults:** Bipolar Mania: Initial: 2-3mg qd. Titrate: Adjust dose at intervals not <24 hrs and in increments/decrements of 1mg/day. Range: 1-6mg/day. **Max:** 6mg/day. **Pediatrics:** 10-17 yrs: Bipolar Mania: Initial: 0.5mg qd in morning or evening. Titrate: Adjust dose, if needed, in increments of 0.5 or 1mg/day and at intervals not <24 hrs, as tolerated, to recommended dose of 2.5mg/day. **Max:** 6mg/day. Elderly/Debilitated/Hypotension/Severe Renal or Hepatic Impairment: Initial: 0.5mg bid. Titrate: Adjust dose	Short-term treatment of acute manic or mixed episodes associated with bipolar I disorder as monotherapy (adults and pediatrics 10-17 yrs) or in combination with lithium or valproate (adults). Inj: Maintenance treatment of bipolar I disorder as monotherapy or in combination with lithium or valproate.

(Continued)

DRUG	BRAND	HOW SUPPLIED	USUAL DOSE	INDICATIONS
ATYPICAL ANTIPSYCHOTICS *(Continued)*				
Risperidone *(continued)*			in increments not >0.5mg bid. Increases to doses >1.5mg bid should occur at intervals of ≥1 week. Periodically reassess to determine maintenance treatment. Inj: Establish PO tolerability prior to IM treatment. Give 1st inj with PO risperidone or other antipsychotic, continue for 3 weeks, then d/c PO therapy. Usual: 25mg IM q2 weeks. Titrate: Upward dose adjustment should not be more frequent than q4 weeks. **Max:** 50mg IM q2 weeks. See PI for additional dosing information.	
Ziprasidone	**Geodon**	**Cap:** (HCl) 20mg, 40mg, 60mg, 80mg	**Adults:** Initial: 40mg bid with food. Titrate: Increase to 60-80mg bid on 2nd day of treatment, then adjust dose based on tolerance and efficacy. Maint: 40-80mg bid.	Monotherapy for acute treatment of manic or mixed episodes associated with bipolar I disorder. Adjunct to lithium or valproate for the maintenance treatment of bipolar I disorder.
Source: FDA-approved labeling.				

ADMINISTRATION GUIDELINES FOR DIFFERENT FORMS OF DRY POWDER INHALERS

Guidelines for Specific Products

Foradil Aerolizer Administration

1. Remove Aerolizer inhaler cover. Hold the base of Aerolizer and twist the mouthpiece in direction of arrow to open.
2. Place the Foradil capsule in capsule chamber. **Note:** Do not place capsule directly in mouthpiece. Twist mouthpiece back to the closed position.
3. Hold the mouthpiece upright and press both buttons at the same time once, then release. You should hear a click as the capsule is pierced. **Note:** If the buttons stay depressed, grasp the wings on the buttons and pull them out. Do not push the buttons a second time.
4. Exhale fully. **Note:** Do not exhale into Aerolizer mouthpiece.
5. Tilt head back slightly and keep inhaler level with blue buttons to left and right (not up and down).
6. Raise the inhaler to your mouth and close your lips tightly around the mouthpiece. Inhale quickly and deeply. **Note:** You will hear a whirring noise and experience a sweet taste.
7. Remove inhaler from the mouth. Continue to hold your breath as long as you can then exhale.
8. Open the inhaler and check that the capsule is empty. If not, close inhaler and repeat steps 4-7.
9. Remove and discard the empty capsule. Close mouthpiece and replace cover for storage.

Counseling Tips:

- Never take the Aerolizer apart.
- Use Aerolizer in a level position.
- If you do not hear whirring noise, the capsule may be stuck. Open inhaler and loosen the capsule. **Note:** Do not press the buttons again. Repeat steps 4 to 7 to get your dose.
- Do not wash Aerolizer inhaler. Keep inhaler and Foradil capsules in a dry place.
- Do not store the capsules in the Aerolizer inhaler.
- Use new Aerolizer inhaler with each refill.

Source: Foradil Aerolizer Prescribing Information.

General Administration Guidelines of a Diskus® inhaler:

1. Hold the Diskus in one hand and place the thumb of the other hand on the thumb grip.
2. Push the thumb grip away from you as far as it will go until the mouthpiece appears and it snaps into position.
3. Hold the Diskus in a level, flat position with the mouthpiece facing you.
4. Slide the lever away from you as far as it will go until it clicks. Make sure you don't tip your Diskus. The medicine is now ready to be inhaled.
5. Before inhaling the medication, breathe out gently to empty your lungs. Be sure to hold the Diskus level and away from your mouth when doing this. **Note:** Never breathe out into the Diskus mouthpiece.
6. Place the mouthpiece in your mouth and close your lips around it.
7. Breathe in deeply and quickly through your mouth until you have taken a full breath. Your breath will pull in the medicine. **Note:** Do not breathe through your nose.
8. Remove the Diskus from your mouth, holding your breath for approximately 10 seconds.
9. Relax and breathe out slowly. **Note:** Do not breathe out into the Diskus.
10. If another inhalation is prescribed, repeat steps 3 through 8.
11. When you are finished, close the Diskus by placing your thumb on the thumb grip and sliding it back and toward you until it clicks shut. The lever will return to its original position and reset.
12. Rinse out your mouth with water and spit the water out. Do not swallow.

Counseling Tips:

- Never wash the mouthpiece or any part of the Diskus.
- The Diskus features a built-in counter. Always check the number in the dose counter window to see how many doses are left.
- If you drop your Diskus or breathe into it after its dose had been loaded, you may cause the dose to be lost. If either of these things happen, reload the device before using it. Reloading the device will not result in an extra or larger dose.
- Never take the diskus apart.
- Do not use with a spacer device

**The Diskus inhaler is used with medicines such as Advair®, Serevent® and Flovent®. These may come with slightly different instructions. Please refer to product-specific Medication Guide for more information.

(Continued)

Pulmicort Flexhaler Administration

Loading a dose:

1. Turn the cover and lift it off.
2. Hold the Flexhaler upright, with mouthpiece up in order to load the correct dose.
3. Do not hold the mouthpiece when you load the inhaler.
4. Twist the brown grip fully in one direction as far as it will go and twist back again in the opposite direction as far as it will go until it clicks. **Note:** It does not matter which way you turn it first.

Inhaling the dose:

1. Turn your head away from the Flexhaler and breathe out completely. **Note:** Do not shake the inhaler after loading it.
2. Place the mouthpiece in your mouth, close your lips around the mouthpiece, and inhale deeply and forcefully.
3. Remove the Flexhaler from the mouth and breathe out. **Note:** Do not blow or exhale into the mouthpiece.
4. Replace the cover and twist shut when finished.
5. Rinse mouth with water after each dose. Spit out the water after last puff and do not swallow the water.

Counseling Tips:

- A new Flexhaler needs to be primed once before its first use. No further priming is indicated, even if it has been put aside for a long time.
- Flexhaler will deliver only one dose at a time, regardless of number of times you click the brown grip. **Note:** The dose indicator will continue to advance.
- Do not repeat inhalations even if you do not feel the sensation of medication when inhaling.
- Do not use with a spacer device.
- Do not chew or bite on the mouthpiece.
- Do not use Flexhaler if it has been damaged or if the mouthpiece has become detached.
- Wipe the outside of the mouthpiece once a week with a dry tissue.
- Keep the Flexhaler in a dry place, away from heat.

Source: Pulmicort Prescribing Information.

Spiriva HandiHaler Administration

1. Open the dust cap of the HandiHaler by pressing the green piercing button. Pull the dust cap upward.
2. Open the mouthpiece by pulling it upward and away from the base.
3. Insert one Spiriva capsule in the center chamber of the HandiHaler device. Close the mouthpiece firmly until you hear a click. Leave the dust cap open.
4. Hold the HandiHaler device with the mouthpiece upward and press the green button until it is flush against the base, then release. Only press the green button once. **Note:** Do not block the air intake vents.
5. Exhale completely. **Note:** Do not exhale into the HandiHaler mouthpiece.
6. Raise the HandiHaler device to your mouth and close your lips tightly around the mouthpiece.
7. Keep your head upright and breathe in slowly and deeply until your lungs are full. You should hear or feel the Spiriva capsule vibrate.
8. Hold your breath as long as is comfortable and remove the HandiHaler from your mouth. Breathe normally again.
9. To get the full dose of Spiriva, exhale completely and inhale medication again as in steps 6-8.
10. Remove and discard empty capsule. Close mouthpiece and replace dust cap for storage.

Counseling Tips:

- Spiriva capsules should not be removed from the package until ready to use. Do not store the capsules in the HandiHaler device. Discard any unused capsules that are exposed to the air.
- Do not swallow Spiriva capsules.
- If you do not hear or feel the capsule vibrate, hold the HandiHaler upright and tap the device gently on a hard surface. Check to see that the mouthpiece is completely closed and continue steps.
- Clean the HandiHaler device at least once a month. Rinse with warm water and allow to air dry completely for 24 hours. **Note:** Do not use cleaning agents.
- Keep the HandiHaler device and Spiriva capsules in a dry place.

Source: Spiriva HandiHaler Prescribing Information.

(Continued)

Asmanex Twisthaler® Administration

1. Hold the Twisthaler straight up with the colored portion (the base) on the bottom. This is important to make sure you get the right amount of medicine with each dose.

2. Remove the cap from the Twisthaler by twisting off the cap.

3. As you lift off the cap the dose counter on the base will count down by one. This action gets the medicine ready for you to inhale.

4. Hold the Twisthaler away from your mouth and gently breathe out. Seal your lips around the mouthpiece. Inhale rapidly and deeply. Continue to take a full, deep breath. **Note:** Since the medicine is a very fine powder, you may not be able to taste, smell, or feel it after inhalation.

5. Remove the Twisthaler out of your mouth. Hold your breath for 10 seconds.

6. Resume normal breathing. Do not breathe out into the Twisthaler.

7. Close the Twisthaler by twisting on the cap. The indented arrow on the case should line up with the dose counter when the Twisthaler is closed. Keep the cap on the Twisthaler when not in use. This will keep the Twisthaler clean and dry.

8. Repeat steps 1-6 when more than one puff is prescribed.

9. Rinse your mouth and spit out the water after inhaling the medication.

Counseling Tips:

- The Twisthaler has a dose counter on the colored base.

- The dose counter will show the doses of medicine left. When the dose counter shows 01, there is one dose left.

- When the Twisthaler is empty, the dose counter will show 00 and the pink base will not turn. Start using a new Twisthaler.

Source: Asmanex Prescribing Information.

ADMINISTRATION GUIDELINES FOR METERED-DOSE INHALERS

General Guidelines

1. Remove dust cap and hold inhaler upright.

2. Shake canister well before each use.

3. Prime the inhaler before using the first time and in cases where the inhaler has not been used for extended periods of time.*

4. Tilt head back slightly and breathe out slowly and completely.

5. For **closed mouth** technique: Place mouthpiece in mouth and close lips tightly around (not recommended for steroid inhaler). For **open mouth** technique: Hold inhaler 1 to 2 inches from open mouth (about the width of 2 fingers).

6. Inhale slowly and deeply, and press down on the inhaler to release the medication. (The slower the breath, the greater the likelihood that the drug will reach the smaller airways.) **NOTE:** If needed, a spacer or holding chamber can be used in children or elderly patients having difficulty with coordination of technique. If using a spacer, put the mouthpiece of the spacer between teeth, and into mouth. Then, close mouth around the spacer. With the device in place, actuate the inhaler once and inhale the medication immediately after actuating the aerosol.

7. Breathe in slowly and hold breath for about 10 seconds to allow the medication to go into lungs.

8. Breathe out slowly and wait about 30 seconds to 1 minute before administering second inhalation. **NOTE:** Expect relief of symptoms within 5 to 15 minutes. Seek medical attention if symptomatic relief takes longer than 20 minutes (this should occur with short-acting medications like albuterol).

9. If using a steroid inhaler, rinse mouth with water after use. **NOTE:** Spit out the water after last puff; do not swallow.

Counseling Tips:

- Rinse only the inhaler mouthpiece and cap with warm running water and air dry. Do not wash the canister or immerse in water.
- Keep the dust cap over the mouthpiece of the inhaler when not in use.
- Do not puncture the canister. The contents are under pressure.
- Store the canister at room temperature (15°C to 30°C), away from heat (>48.9°F) or open flames.

*Refer to product-specific Prescribing Information for complete instructions.

Adapted from http://www.nhlbi.nih.gov/guidelines/asthma/asthgdln.htm.

ASTHMA & COPD MANAGEMENT

DRUG (BRAND)	DOSAGE FORM	ADULT DOSE	CHILD DOSE
ANTICHOLINERGICS			
Ipratropium (Atrovent HFA)†	**MDI:** 0.017mg/inh	2 inh qid. **Max:** 12 inh/24 hrs.	
Tiotropium (Spiriva)†	**Cap, Inhalation:** 18mcg	2 inh of contents of 1 cap qd.	
COMBINATION AGENTS			
Budesonide/Formoterol (Symbicort)*	**MDI:** (Budesonide-Formoterol) 80mcg-4.5mcg/inh, 160mcg-4.5mcg/inh	**Asthma: Initial:** 2 inh bid (am/pm q12h). **Max:** 160mcg-4.5mcg bid. **COPD:** 2 inh of 160mcg-4.5mcg bid.	≥**12 yrs:** 2 inh bid (am/pm q12h). **Max:** 160mcg-4.5mcg bid.
Fluticasone/Salmeterol (Advair Diskus)*	**DPI:** (Fluticasone-Salmeterol) 100mcg-50mcg/inh, 250mcg-50mcg/inh, 500mcg-50mcg/inh	**Asthma:** 1 inh bid (am/pm q12h). **Max:** 500mcg-50mcg bid. **COPD:** 1 inh of 250mcg-50mcg bid (am/pm q12h).	≥**12 yrs:** 1 inh bid (am/pm q12h). **Max:** 500mcg-50mcg bid. **4-11 yrs:** 1 inh of 100mcg-50mcg bid (am/pm q12h).
Fluticasone/Salmeterol (Advair HFA)	**MDI:** (Fluticasone-Salmeterol) 45mcg-21mcg/inh, 115mcg-21mcg/inh, (230mcg-21mcg/inh	**Initial:** 2 inh bid (am/pm q12h). **Max:** 2 inh of 230mcg-21mcg bid.	≥**12 yrs: Initial:** 2 inh bid (am/pm q12h). **Max:** 2 inh of 230mcg-21mcg bid.
Ipratropium/Albuterol (Combivent)†	**MDI:** (Albuterol-Ipratropium) 0.09mg-0.018mg/inh	2 inh qid. **Max:** 12 inh/24 hrs.	
Ipratropium/Albuterol (Duoneb)†	**Sol, Inhalation:** (Albuterol-Ipratropium) 3mg-0.5mg/3mL	3mL qid via nebulizer with up to 2 additional 3mL doses/day.	
Mometasone/Formoterol (Dulera)	**MDI:** (Mometasone-Formoterol) 100mcg-5mcg/inh, 200mcg-5mcg/inh	2 inh bid (am/pm). **Previous Corticosteroid Therapy: Inhaled Medium-Dose Corticosteroids: Initial:** 2 inh of 100mcg-5mcg bid. **Max:** 400mcg-20mcg/day. **Inhaled High-Dose Corticosteroids: Initial:** 2 inh of 200mcg-5mcg bid. **Max:** 800mcg-20mcg/day.	≥**12 yrs:** 2 inh bid (am/pm). **Previous Corticosteroid Therapy: Inhaled Medium-Dose Corticosteroids: Initial:** 2 inh of 100mcg-5mcg bid. **Max:** 400mcg-20mcg/day. **Inhaled High-Dose Corticosteroids: Initial:** 2 inh of 200mcg-5mcg bid. **Max:** 800mcg-20mcg/day.
COMBINATION AGENT—MISCELLANEOUS			
Dyphylline/Guaifenesin (Lufyllin-GG)	**Sol:** (Dyphylline-Guaifenesin) 100mg-100mg/15mL	30mL qid.	>**6 yrs:** 15-30mL tid-qid.
CORTICOSTEROIDS			
Beclomethasone dipropionate HFA (QVAR)	**MDI:** 40mcg/inh, 80mcg/inh	**Initial:** 40-160mcg bid. **Max:** 320mcg bid.	**Adolescents: Initial:** 40-160mcg bid. **Max:** 320mcg bid. **5-11 yrs: Initial:** 40mcg bid. **Max:** 80mcg bid.
Budesonide DPI (Pulmicort Flexhaler)	**DPI:** 90mcg/inh, 180mcg/inh	**Initial:** 180-360mcg bid. **Max:** 720mcg bid.	≥**6 yrs: Initial:** 180-360mcg bid. **Max:** 360mcg bid.
Budesonide Neb (Pulmicort Respules)	**Sus, Inhalation:** 0.25mg/2mL, 0.5mg/2mL, 1mg/2mL		**12 months to 8 yrs: Initial:** 0.25mg/day-1mg/day via nebulizer. **Max:** 0.5-1mg/day.
Ciclesonide (Alvesco)	**MDI:** 80 mcg/inh, 160mcg/inh	**Initial:** 80mcg bid-320mcg bid. **Max:** 160mcg bid-320mcg bid.	≥**12 yrs: Initial:** 80mcg bid-320mcg bid. **Max:** 160mcg bid-320mcg bid.
Flunisolide (Aerospan)	**MDI:** 78mcg/inh	**Initial:** 160mcg bid. **Max:** 320mcg bid.	≥**12 yrs: Initial:** 160mcg bid. **Max:** 320mcg bid. **6-11 yrs: Initial:** 80mcg bid. **Max:** 160mcg bid.

(Continued)

DRUG (BRAND)	DOSAGE FORM	ADULT DOSE	CHILD DOSE
CORTICOSTEROIDS *(Continued)*			
Fluticasone propionate (Flovent Diskus)	**DPI:** 50mcg/inh, 100mcg/inh, 250mcg/inh	**Initial:** 100mcg bid-1000mcg bid. **Max:** 500mcg bid-1000mcg bid.	**≥12 yrs: Initial:** 100mcg bid-1000mcg bid. **Max:** 500mcg bid-1000mcg bid. **4-11 yrs: Initial:** 50mcg bid. **Max:** 100 mcg bid.
Fluticasone propionate (Flovent HFA)	**MDI:** 44mcg/inh, 110mcg/inh, 220mcg/inh	**Initial:** 88mcg bid-440mcg bid. **Max:** 440mcg bid- 880mcg bid.	**≥12 yrs: Initial:** 88mcg bid-440mcg bid. **Max:** 440mcg-880mcg bid. **4-11 yrs: Initial/Max:** 88mcg bid.
Mometasone furoate (Asmanex Twisthaler)	**DPI:** 110mcg/inh, 220mcg/inh	**Initial:** 220mcg qd hs-440mcg bid. **Max:** 440mcg-880mcg/day.	**≥12 yrs: Initial:** 220mcg qd hs-440mcg bid. **Max:** 440mcg-880mcg/day. **4-11 yrs: Initial/Max:** 110mcg qd hs.
Triamcinolone acetonide (Azmacort)	**MDI:** 75mcg/inh	**Initial:** 150mcg tid-qid or 300mcg bid. **Max:** 1200mcg/day.	**6-12 yrs: Initial:** 75-150 mcg tid-qid or 150mcg-300mcg bid. **Max:** 900mcg/day.
MAST CELL STABILIZER			
Cromolyn	**Sol, Inhalation:** 10mg/mL	20mg nebulized qid.	**≥2 yrs:** 20mg nebulized qid.
LEUKOTRIENE MODIFIERS			
Montelukast (Singulair)	**Tab:** 10mg; **Tab, Chewable:** 4mg, 5mg; **Granules:** 4mg	10mg qpm.	**≥15 yrs:** 10mg qpm. **6-14 yrs:** 5mg chewable tab qpm. **2-5 yrs:** 4mg chewable tab or 4mg oral granules pkt qpm. **12-23 months:** 4mg oral granules pkt qpm.
Zafirlukast (Accolate)	**Tab:** 10mg, 20mg	20mg bid.	**≥12 yrs:** 20mg bid. **5-11 yrs:** 10mg bid.
Zileuton (Zyflo, Zyflo CR)	**Tab:** 600mg; **Tab, Extended-Release:** 600mg	(Tab): 600mg qid. **Max:** 2400mg/day. (Tab, Extended-Release) 1200mg bid. **Max:** 2400mg/day.	**≥12 yrs:** (Tab): 600mg qid. **Max:** 2400mg/day. (Tab, Extended-Release) 1200mg bid. **Max:** 2400mg/day.
LONG-ACTING β₂-AGONISTS			
Arformoterol (Brovana)†	**Sol, Inhalation:** 15mcg/2mL	15mcg bid via nebulizer. **Max:** 30mcg/day.	
Formoterol (Foradil) *	**Cap, Inhalation:** 12mcg	1 cap (inh) q12 hrs. **Max:** 24mcg/day.	**≥5 yrs:** 1 cap (inh) q12 hrs. **Max:** 24mcg/day.
Formoterol (Foradil Certihaler)	**DPI:** 10mcg/inh	1 inh q12 hrs. **Max:** 1 inh bid.	**≥5 yrs:** 1 inh q12 hrs. **Max:** 1 inh bid.
Formoterol (Perforomist)†	**Sol, Inhalation:** 20mcg/2mL	2mL q12 hrs via nebulizer. **Max:** 40mcg/day.	
Metaproterenol	**Syrup:** 10mg/5mL; **Tab:** 10mg, 20mg; **Sol, Inhalation:** 0.4%, 0.6%,	20mg tid-qid. (Sol) one vial per nebulization tid-qid.	**6-9 yrs or <60 lbs:** 10mg tid-qid. **>9 yrs or >60 lbs:** 20mg tid-qid. **Sol (≥12 yrs):** one vial per nebulization tid-qid.
Salmeterol (Serevent) *	**DPI:** 50mcg/inh	1 inh q12 hrs.	**≥4 yrs:** 1 inh q12 hrs.
Terbutaline	**Tab:** 2.5mg, 5mg; **Inj:** 1mg/mL	(PO) 2.5-5mg q6 hrs, tid **Max:** 15mg/day. (Inj) 0.25mg SQ. May repeat in 15-30 min if no improvement. **Max:** 0.5mg/4hrs.	(PO) **12-15 yrs:** 2.5mg tid. **Max:** 7.5mg/day. (Inj) **≥12 yrs:** 0.25mg SQ. May repeat in 15-30 min if no improvement. **Max:** 0.5mg/4hrs.

(Continued)

DRUG (BRAND)	DOSAGE FORM	ADULT DOSE	CHILD DOSE
METHYLXANTHINE			
Theophylline (Elixophyllin)	Elixir: 80mg/15mL	**Adults & Children >45 kg** **Initial:** 300mg/day divided q6-8 hrs. After 3 days if tolerated: 400mg/day divided q6-8 hrs. After 3 more days if tolerated: 600mg/day divided q6-8 hrs.	**1-15 yrs (<45 kg):** **Initial:** 12-14mg/kg/day. (**Max:** 300mg/day divided q4-6 hrs.) After 3 days if tolerated: 16mg/kg/day. (**Max:** 400mg/day divided q4-6 hrs.) After 3 more days if tolerated: 20mg/kg/day. (**Max:** 600mg/day divided q4-6 hrs.) See PI for infant dose.
Theophylline (Theo-24)	Cap, Extended Release: 100mg, 200mg, 300mg, 400mg	**Adults & Children >45 kg** **Initial:** 300-400mg/day q24 hrs. After 3 days if tolerated: 400-600mg/day q24 hrs. After 3 more days if tolerated and needed: Doses >600mg should be titrated according to blood levels (See PI).	**12-15 yrs (<45 kg):** **Initial:** 12-14mg/kg/day. (**Max:** 300mg/day q24 hrs.) After 3 days if tolerated: 16mg/kg/day. (**Max:** 400mg/day q24 hrs.) After 3 more days if tolerated and needed: 20mg/kg/day. (**Max:** 600mg/day q24 hrs.)
Theophylline	Tab, Extended Release: (generic) 100mg, 200mg, 300mg, 400mg, 450mg, 600mg	**Adults & Children >45 kg** **Initial:** 300mg/day divided q12 hrs. After 3 days if tolerated: increase to 400mg/day divided q12 hrs. After 3 more days if tolerated and needed: increase to 600mg/day divided q12 hrs. Doses >600mg should be titrated according to blood levels (See PI).	**6-15 yrs (<45 kg):** **Initial:** 12-14mg/kg/day. (**Max:** 300mg/day divided q12 hrs.) After 3 days if tolerated: 16mg/kg/day. (**Max:** 400mg/day divided q12 hrs.) After 3 more days if tolerated and needed: 20mg/kg/day. **Max:** (600mg/day divided q12 hrs.)
Theophylline (Uniphyl)	Tab, Extended Release: 400mg, 600mg	**Adults & Children >45 kg** **Initial:** 300-400mg/day. After 3 days if tolerated: 400-600mg/day. After 3 more days if tolerated and needed: Doses >600mg should be titrated according to blood levels (See PI).	**12-15 yrs (<45 kg):** **Initial:** 12-14mg/kg/day. (**Max:** 300mg/day). After 3 days if tolerated: 16mg/kg/day. (**Max:** 400mg/day). After 3 more days if tolerated and needed: 20mg/kg/day. (**Max:** 600mg/day).
MONOCLONAL ANTIBODY/IgE-BLOCKER			
Omalizumab (Xolair)	Inj: 150mg	150-375mg SQ q2 or 4 weeks. Determine dose and dosing frequency by serum total IgE level (IU/mL), measured before the start of treatment, and body weight (kg). See PI for dose determination charts.	**≥12 yrs:** 150-375mg SQ q2 or 4 weeks. Determine dose and dosing frequency by serum total IgE level (IU/mL), measured before the start of treatment, and body weight (kg). See PI for dose determination charts.

(Continued)

DRUG (BRAND)	DOSAGE FORM	ADULT DOSE	CHILD DOSE
PHOSPHODIESTERASE₄ INHIBITOR			
Roflumilast (Daliresp)†	**Tab:** 500mcg	500mcg qd.	
SHORT-ACTING β₂-AGONISTS			
Albuterol	**Sol, Inhalation:** 0.083%, 0.5%; **Syrup:** 2mg/5mL; **Tab:** 2mg*, 4mg*; **Tab, Extended-Release:** 4mg, 8mg *scored	**(Tab, Extended-Release) Initial:** 4-8mg q12h. **Max:** 32mg/day. **(Sol)** 2.5mg tid-qid via nebulizer. **(Syrup, Tab)** 2-4mg tid-qid. **Max:** 8mg qid.	**>14 yrs: (Syrup) Initial:** 2-4mg tid-qid. **Max:** 8mg qid. **>12 yrs: (Tab) Initial:** 2-4mg tid-qid. **Max:** 8mg qid. **(Tab, Extended-Release) Initial:** 4-8mg q12h. **Max:** 32mg/day. **6-14 yrs: (Syrup) Initial:** 2mg tid-qid. **Max:** 24mg/day. **6-12 yrs: (Tab, Extended-Release) Initial:** 4mg q12h. **Max:** 24mg/day. **(Tabs) Initial:** 2mg tid-qid. **Max:** 24mg/day. **2-12 yrs: (Sol) ≥15 kg:** 2.5mg tid-qid via nebulizer. **<15 kg:** Use 0.5% solution for <2.5mg/dose. **2-6 yrs: (Syrup) Initial:** 0.1mg/kg tid (not to exceed 2mg tid). **Titrate:** May increase to 0.2mg/kg tid. **Max:** 4mg tid.
Albuterol Sulfate (AccuNeb)	**Sol, Inhalation:** 0.63mg/3mL, 1.25mg/3mL		**2-12 yrs:** 0.63mg or 1.25mg tid-qid via nebulizer.
Albuterol Sulfate (ProAir HFA, Proventil HFA, Ventolin HFA)	**MDI:** 90mcg/inh	2 inh q4-6h or 1 inh q4h.	**≥4 yrs:** 2 inh q4-6h or 1 inh q4h.
Levalbuterol (Xopenex, Xopenex HFA)	**Sol, Inhalation:** 0.31mg/3mL, 0.63mg/3mL, 1.25mg/3mL (HFA) 45mcg/inh	0.63mg tid q6-8h via nebulizer. (HFA) 2 inh (90mcg) q4-6h or 1 inh (45mcg) q4h.	**≥12 yrs:** 0.63mg tid q6-8h via nebulizer. **6-11 yrs:** 0.31mg tid (max: 0.63mg tid) q6-8h. **≥4 yrs:** (HFA) 2 inh (90mcg) q4-6h or 1 inh (45mcg) q4h.
Pirbuterol (Maxair)	**MDI:** 0.2mg/inh	1-2 inh q4-6h. **Max:** 12 inh/day.	**≥12 yrs:** 1-2 inh q4-6h. **Max:** 12 inh/day.
SYSTEMIC CORTICOSTEROIDS			
Methylprednisolone	**Tab:** 2, 4, 8, 16, 32mg	7.5-60mg qd in a single dose or qod prn for control. Short course "burst": 40-60 mg/day as single dose or 2 divided doses for 3-10 days.	**≥12 yrs:** 7.5-60mg qd in a single dose or qod prn for control. Short course "burst": 40-60mg/day as single dose or 2 divided doses for 3-10 days. **≤11 yrs:** 0.25-2mg/kg qd in a single dose or qod prn for control. Short course "burst": 1-2mg/kg/day. **Max:** 60mg/day or 3-10 days.
Prednisolone	**Tab:** 5mg; **Liq:** 5mg/5mL, 15mg/5mL		
Prednisone	**Tab:** 1, 2.5, 5, 10, 20, 50mg **Liq:** 5mg/mL, 5mg/5mL		

MDI: metered-dose inhaler; DPI: dry powder inhaler.
†Indicated for COPD only
*Indicated for Asthma & COPD
Adopted from: The NAEPP Expert Panel Report: Guidelines for the Diagnosis and Management of Asthma–Update on Selected Topics 2007. http://www.nhlbi.nih.gov/guidelines/asthma/asthsumm.htm

ASTHMA TREATMENT PLAN

CLASSIFICATION	LUNG FUNCTION	STEPWISE APPROACH TO THERAPY IN PATIENTS ≥12 YEARS OF AGE
Intermittent • Symptoms ≤2 days a week • Short-acting ß₂-agonist use for symptom control ≤2 days a week • Nighttime awakenings ≤2 times/month • Interference with normal activity - none	• Normal FEV_1 b/w exacerbations • FEV_1 >80% predicted • FEV_1/FVC - normal	**Step 1** • **Short-acting inhaled ß₂-agonists as needed.** • Severe exacerbations may occur, separated by long periods of normal lung function and no symptoms; a course of systemic corticosteroids is recommended.
Mild persistent • Symptoms >2 days/week but not daily • Short-acting ß₂-agonist use for symptom control >2 days/wk but not daily, and not more than 1x on any day • Nighttime awakenings 3-4x/month • Interference with normal activity - minor limitation	• FEV_1 >80% predicted • FEV_1/FVC - normal	**Step 2** • **Low-dose ICS.** • **Short-acting inhaled ß₂-agonists as needed.** ALTERNATIVE TREATMENT: • Cromolyn, LTRA, nedocromil OR theophylline
Moderate persistent • Daily symptoms • Short-acting ß₂-agonist use for symptom control daily • Nighttime awakenings >1x/wk but not nightly • Interference with normal activity - some limitation	• FEV_1 >60% but <80% predicted • FEV_1/FVC reduced 5%	**Step 3** • **Low-dose ICS + LABA OR medium-dose ICS.** AND • **Short-acting inhaled ß₂-agonists as needed.** ALTERNATIVE TREATMENT: • Low-dose ICS + either LTRA, theophylline, OR Zileuton
Severe persistent • Symptoms throughout the day • Short-acting ß₂-agonist use for symptom several times per day • Nighttime awakenings often >7x/week • Interference with normal activity - extreme limitation	• FEV_1 <60% predicted • FEV_1/FVC reduced >5%	**Step 4, Step 5 or Step 6** • **Medium-dose ICS + LABA OR** • **High-dose ICS + LABA OR** • **High-dose ICS + LABA + oral corticosteroid** AND • Consider Omalizumab for patients who have allergies • **Short-acting inhaled ß₂-agonists as needed.** ALTERNATIVE TREATMENT: • Medium-dose ICS + either LTRA, Theophylline, OR Zileuton

Note: Preferred treatments are in bold.
Key Points:
- Stepwise approach presents general guidelines. Review treatment every 1 to 6 months; a gradual stepwise reduction in treatment may be possible. If control is not maintained, consider step up.
- The presence of one of the features of severity is sufficient to place a patient in that category. An individual should be assigned to the most severe grade in which any feature occurs (PEF is % of personal best; FEV is % predicted).
- Short-acting ß₂-agonists as needed for symptoms. Intensity of treatment will depend on severity of exacerbation; up to 3 treatments at 20-minute intervals as needed. Course of systemic corticosteroids may be needed.
- Use of short-acting beta₂-agonists >2 days/week for symptom relief generally indicates inadequate control and the need to step up treatment
- Airflow obstruction is indicated by reduced FEV_1 and FEV_1/FVC values relative to reference or predicted values.
- Abnormalities of lung function are categorized as restrictive and obstructive defects. A reduced ratio of FEV_1/FVC (eg, <65%) indicates obstruction to the flow of air from the lungs, whereas a reduced FVC with a normal or increased FEV_1/FVC ratio suggests a restrictive pattern.

Abbreviations: FEV_1: Forced expiratory volume in one second. FVC: Forced vital capacity. ICS: Inhaled corticosteroid. LABA: Long-acting inhaled beta₂-agonist; LTRA: Leukotriene receptor antagonist.

*Adapted from the Full Report 2007 *Guidelines for the Diagnosis and Management of Asthma.* NAEPP Expert Panel Report III.

ERECTILE DYSFUNCTION TREATMENT

DRUG (BRAND)	HOW SUPPLIED	DOSING
PROSTAGLANDINS		
Alprostadil (Caverject, Caverject Impulse)	**Inj:** 5, 10, 20, 40mcg (sterile powder); **Inj:** 10, 20mcg (Impulse)	Vasculogenic, Psychogenic, or Mixed Etiology: Initiate: 2.5mcg. Increase to 5mcg within 1 hr if partial response. Max 2 doses during initial titration within 24 hrs. Increase by 5-10mcg if additional titration required ≥24 hrs apart until erection of 1 hr max duration. No Response to 2.5mcg: Initiate: 7.5mcg within 1 hr. Max 2 doses during initial titration within 24 hrs. Increase by 5-10mcg if additional titration required ≥24 hrs apart until erection. Pure Neurogenic Etiology (Spinal Cord Injury): Initiate: 1.25mcg. Increase to 2.5mcg within 1 hr. Max 2 doses during initial titration within 24 hrs. If additional titration required, give 5mcg within next 24 hrs. Thereafter, give 5mcg doses ≥24 hrs apart until erection of 1 hr max duration. Patient must stay in physician's office until complete detumescence. Max: 60mcg/dose. Maint: Give no more than 3 times weekly; allow 24 hrs between doses.
Alprostadil (Edex)	**Inj:** 10, 20, 40mcg (sterile powder)	Vasculogenic, Psychogenic, or Mixed Etiology: Initiate: 2.5mcg. Increase to 5mcg, then by 5-10mcg based on response until erection of 1 hr max duration. No Response to 2.5mcg: Initiate: 7.5mcg, followed by 5-10mcg increments. Pure Neurogenic Etiology (Spinal Cord Injury): Initiate: 1.25mcg. Increase to 2.5mcg, followed by a 5mcg dose, then increase by 5mcg increments until erection of 1 hr max duration. Patient must stay in physician's office until complete detumescence. If no response, give next higher dose within 1 hr. If response, min 24 hrs before next dose. Dose range: 1-40mcg. Give injection over 5-10 second interval. Maint: Give no more than 3 times weekly; allow 24 hrs between doses.
Alprostadil (Muse)	**Suppositories, Urethral:** 125, 250, 500, 1000mcg	Initial: 125-250mcg. Titration: Increase or decrease dose based on individual response. Max: 2 administrations within 24 hrs.
PHOSPHODIESTERASE INHIBITORS		
Sildenafil (Viagra)	**Tablets:** 25, 50, 100mg	Usual: 50mg prn 1 hr prior to sexual activity. Titration: Increase to 100mg qd or decrease to 25mg qd based on efficacy/tolerability.
Tadalafil (Cialis)	**Tablets:** 2.5, 5, 10, 20mg	PRN use: Initial: 10mg prior to sexual activity qd. Titration: Increase to 20mg qd or decrease to 5mg qd based on efficacy/tolerability. QD use: 2.5mg qd. Titration: Increase to 5mg qd based on efficacy/tolerability.
Vardenafil (Levitra)	**Tablets:** 2.5, 5, 10, 20mg	Usual: 10mg 1 hr prior to sexual activity qd. Titration: Increase to 20mg qd or decrease to 5mg qd based on efficacy/tolerability.
Vardenafil (Staxyn)	**Tab, Disintegrating:** 10mg	10mg 1 hr prior to sexual activity PRN. Max: 1 tab qd. Place on tongue to disintegrate. Take without liquid.

UROLOGICAL THERAPIES

OVERACTIVE BLADDER AGENTS

DRUG	BRAND	HOW SUPPLIED	DOSING	COMMENTS
Darifenacin	Enablex	**Tab, ER:** 7.5mg, 15mg	**Initial:** 7.5mg qd. **Max:** 15mg qd.	Swallow whole. Moderate Hepatic Impairment/ Concomitant Potent CYP3A4 Inhibitors: Do not exceed 7.5mg/day. Severe Hepatic Impairment: Avoid use.
Fesoterodine	Toviaz	**Tab, ER:** 4mg, 8mg	**Initial:** 4mg qd. **Max:** 8mg/day	Swallow whole. CrCl <30mL/min/ Concomitant Potent CYP3A4 Inhibitors: Do not exceed 4mg/day. Severe Hepatic Impaiment: Avoid use.
Oxybutynin	Ditropan	**(Generic) Syrup:** 5mg/5mL **Tab:** 5mg	**Usual:** 5mg bid-tid. **Max:** 5mg qid.	A lower starting dose of 2.5mg bid-tid is recommended for elderly patients. Pediatrics >5 yrs: 5mg bid. Max: 5mg tid.
	Ditropan XL	**Tab, ER:** 5mg, 10mg, 15mg	**Initial:** 5mg or 10mg qd. **Max:** 30mg/day.	Swallow whole. Increase dose by 5mg weekly if needed. Pediatrics ≥6 yrs: 5mg qd. Max: 20mg/day.
	Gelnique	**Gel:** 10% (1g/pkt)	Apply contents of 1 pkt qd to skin on abdomen, upper arms/shoulders, or thighs.	Rotate application sites.
	Oxytrol	**Patch:** 3.9mg/day	**Usual:** Apply 1 patch twice weekly (every 3-4 days).	Rotate application sites.
Solifenacin	VESIcare	**Tab:** 5mg, 10mg	**Usual:** 5mg qd. **Max:** 10mg qd.	Swallow whole. Renal (CrCl <30mL/min)/Hepatic (Child Pugh B)/Concomitant Potent CYP3A4 Inhibitors: Do not exceed 5mg/day. Hepatic (Child Pugh C): Avoid use.
Tolterodine	Detrol	**Tab:** 1mg, 2mg	**Initial:** 2mg bid.	Decrease dose to 1mg bid if needed. Significant Hepatic/Renal Dysfunction/Concomitant CYP3A4 Inhibitors: 1mg bid.
	Detrol LA	**Cap, ER:** 2mg, 4mg	**Initial:** 4mg qd.	Swallow whole. Decrease dose to 2mg qd if needed. Mild-Moderate Hepatic/Significant Renal Dysfunction/Concomitant CYP3A4 Inhibitors: 2mg qd. Severe Hepatic Impairment/CrCl <10mL/min: Avoid use.
Trospium	Sanctura	**Tab:** 20mg	**Usual:** 20mg bid.	Take 1 hr before meals or on empty stomach. CrCl <30mL/min: 20mg qhs. Elderly ≥75 yrs: May titrate to 20mg qd based upon tolerability.
	Sanctura XR	**Cap, ER:** 60mg	**Usual:** 60mg qam	Take on empty stomach, 1 hr before meal. CrCl <30mL/min: Avoid use.

(Continued)

BENIGN PROSTATIC HYPERTROPHY AGENTS

DRUG	BRAND	HOW SUPPLIED	DOSING	COMMENTS
ALPHA-BLOCKERS				
Alfuzosin	Uroxatral	**Tab, ER:** 10mg	**Usual:** 10mg qd.	Take dose immediately with the same meal each day. Swallow whole.
Doxazosin	Cardura	**Tab:** 1mg, 2mg, 4mg, 8mg	**Initial:** 1mg qd. **Max:** 8mg/day.	Stepwise titration every 1-2 weeks if needed.
	Cardura XL	**Tab, ER:** 4mg, 8mg	**Initial:** 4mg qd. **Max:** 8mg qd.	Take with breakfast. Swallow whole. Titrate after 3-4 weeks if needed.
Silodosin	Rapaflo	**Cap:** 4mg, 8mg	**Usual:** 8mg qd.	Take with food. CrCl 30-50mL/min: 4mg qd.
Tamsulosin	Flomax	**Cap:** 0.4mg	**Initial:** 0.4mg qd. **Max:** 0.8mg qd.	Take dose ½ hour after the same meal each day. Titrate after 2-4 weeks if needed. Restart at initial dose if therapy is interrupted. Do not use in combination with strong CYP3A4 inhibitors.
Terazosin	Generic	**Cap:** 1mg, 2mg, 5mg, 10mg	**Initial:** 1mg qhs. **Usual:** 10mg/day. **Max:** 20mg/day.	Increase stepwise as needed. Restart at initial dose if therapy is interrupted.
5-ALPHA-REDUCTASE INHIBITORS				
Dutasteride	Avodart	**Cap:** 0.5mg	**Usual:** 0.5mg qd.	Swallow whole. May be administered with tamsulosin.
Finasteride	Proscar	**Tab:** 5mg	**Usual:** 5mg qd.	May be administered with doxazosin with or without meals.
COMBINATION				
Dutasteride/ Tamsulosin	Jalyn	**Cap:** 0.5mg/0.4mg	**Usual:** 1 cap qd.	Swallow whole. Take dose 30 min after the same meal each day. Do not use in combination with strong CYP3A4 Inhibitors.

RECOMMENDED IMMUNIZATION SCHEDULE FOR PERSONS AGED 0-6 YEARS

Vaccine ▼ Age ▶	Birth	1 month	2 months	4 months	6 months	12 months	15 months	18 months	19–23 months	2–3 years	4–6 years
Hepatitis B[1]	HepB	HepB				HepB					
Rotavirus[2]			RV	RV	RV[2]						
Diphtheria, Tetanus, Pertussis[3]			DTaP	DTaP	DTaP	see footnote[3]	DTaP				DTaP
Haemophilus influenzae type b[4]			Hib	Hib	Hib[4]	Hib					
Pneumococcal[5]			PCV	PCV	PCV	PCV				PPSV	
Inactivated Poliovirus[6]			IPV	IPV		IPV					IPV
Influenza[7]						Influenza (Yearly)					
Measles, Mumps, Rubella[8]						MMR		see footnote[8]			MMR
Varicella[9]						Varicella		see footnote[9]			Varicella
Hepatitis A[10]						HepA (2 doses)				HepA Series	
Meningococcal[11]											MCV4

■ Range of recommended ages for all children ■ Range of recommended ages for certain high-risk groups

This schedule includes recommendations in effect as of December 21, 2010. Any dose not administered at the recommended age should be administered at a subsequent visit, when indicated and feasible. The use of a combination vaccine generally is preferred over separate injections of its equivalent component vaccines. Considerations should include provider assessment, patient preference, and the potential for adverse events. Providers should consult the relevant Advisory Committee on Immunization Practices statement for detailed recommendations: **http://www.cdc.gov/vaccines/pubs/acip-list.htm**. Clinically significant adverse events that follow immunization should be reported to the Vaccine Adverse Event Reporting System (VAERS) at **http://www.vaers.hhs.gov** or by telephone, **800-822-7967**.

1. **Hepatitis B vaccine (HepB).** (Minimum age: birth)
   At birth:
   - Administer monovalent HepB to all newborns before hospital discharge.
   - If mother is hepatitis B surface antigen (HBsAg)-positive, administer HepB and 0.5 mL of hepatitis B immune globulin (HBIG) within 12 hours of birth.
   - If mother's HBsAg status is unknown, administer HepB within 12 hours of birth. Determine mother's HBsAg status as soon as possible and, if HBsAg positive, administer HBIG (no later than age 1 week).
   Doses following the birth dose:
   - The second dose should be administered at age 1 or 2 months. Monovalent HepB should be used for doses administered before age 6 weeks.
   - Infants born to HBsAg-positive mothers should be tested for HBsAg and antibody to HBsAg 1 to 2 months after completion of at least 3 doses of the HepB series, at age 9 through 18 months (generally at the next well-child visit).
   - Administration of 4 doses of HepB to infants is permissable when a combination vaccine containing HepB is administered after the birth dose.
   - Infants who did not receive a birth dose should receive 3 doses of HepB on a schedule of 0, 1, and 6 months.
   - The final (3rd or 4th) dose in the HepB series should be administered no earlier than age 24 weeks.

2. **Rotavirus vaccine (RV).** (Minimum age: 6 weeks)
   - Administer the first dose at age 6 through 14 weeks (maximum age: 14 weeks 6 days). Vaccination should not be initiated for infants 15 weeks 0 days or older.
   - The maximum age for the final dose in the series is 8 months 0 days.
   - If Rotarix is administered at ages 2 and 4 months, a dose at 6 months is not indicated.

3. **Diphtheria and tetanus toxoids and acellular pertussis vaccine (DTaP).** (Minimum age: 6 weeks)
   - The fourth dose may be administered as early as age 12 months, provided at least 6 months have elapsed since the third dose.

4. **Haemophilus influenzae type b conjugate vaccine (Hib).** (Minimum age: 6 weeks)
   - If PRP-OMP (PedvaxHIB or Comvax [HepB-Hib]) is administered at ages 2 and 4 months, a dose at age 6 months is not indicated.
   - Hiberix should not be used for doses at ages 2, 4, or 6 months for the primary series but can be used as the final dose in children aged 12 months through 4 years.

5. **Pneumococcal vaccine.** (Minimum age: 6 weeks for pneumococcal conjugate vaccine [PCV]; 2 years for pneumococcal polysaccharide vaccine [PPSV])
   - PCV is recommended for all children aged younger than 5 years. Administer 1 dose of PCV to all healthy children aged 24 through 59 months who are not completely vaccinated for their age.
   - A PCV series begun with 7-valent PCV (PCV7) should be completed with 13-valent PCV (PCV13).
   - A single supplemental dose of PCV13 is recommended for all children aged 14 through 59 months who have received an age-appropriate series of PCV7.

(Continued)

- A single supplemental dose of PCV13 is recommended for all children aged 60 through 71 months with underlying medical conditions who have received an age-appropriate series of PCV7.
- The supplemental dose of PCV13 should be administered at least 8 weeks after the previous dose of PCV7. See MMWR 2010:59(No. RR-11).
- Administer PPSV at least 8 weeks after last dose of PCV to children aged 2 years or older with certain underlying medical conditions, including a cochlear implant.

6. **Inactivated poliovirus vaccine (IPV)** (Minimum age: 6 weeks)

- If 4 or more doses are administered prior to age 4 years an additional dose should be administered at age 4 through 6 years.
- The final dose in the series should be administered on or after the fourth birthday and at least 6 months following the previous dose.

7. **Influenza vaccine (seasonal).** (Minimum age: 6 months for trivalent inactivated influenza vaccine [TIV]; 2 years for live, attenuated influenza vaccine [LAIV])

- For healthy children aged 2 years and older (i.e., those who do not have underlying medical conditions that predispose them to influenza complications), either LAIV or TIV may be used, except LAIV should not be given to children aged 2 through 4 years who have had wheezing in the past 12 months.
- Administer 2 doses (separated by at least 4 weeks) to children aged 6 months through 8 years who are receiving seasonal influenza vaccine for the first time or who were vaccinated for the first time during the previous influenza season but only received 1 dose.
- Children aged 6 months through 8 years who received no doses of monovalent 2009 H1N1 vaccine should receive 2 doses of 2010–2011 seasonal influenza vaccine. See MMWR 2010;59 (No. RR-8):33–34.

8. **Measles, mumps, and rubella vaccine (MMR).** (Minimum age: 12 months)

- The second dose may be administered before age 4 years, provided at least 4 weeks have elapsed since the first dose.

9. **Varicella vaccine.** (Minimum age: 12 months)

- The second dose may be administered before age 4 years, provided at least 3 months have elapsed since the first dose.
- For children aged 12 months through 12 years the recommended minimum interval between doses is 3 months. However, if the second dose was administered at least 4 weeks after the first dose, it can be accepted as valid.

10. **Hepatitis A vaccine (HepA).** (Minimum age: 12 months)

- Administer 2 doses at least 6 months apart.
- HepA is recommended for children aged older than 23 months who live in areas where vaccination programs target older children, who are at increased risk for infection, or for whom immunity against hepatitis A is desired.

11. **Meningococcal conjugate vaccine, quadrivalent (MCV4).** (Minimum age: 2 years)

- Administer 2 doses of MCV4 at least 8 weeks apart to children aged 2 through 10 years with persistent complement component deficiency and anatomic or functional asplenia, and 1 dose every 5 years thereafter.
- Persons with human immunodeficiency virus (HIV) infection who are vaccinated with MCV4 should receive 2 doses at least 8 weeks apart.
- Administer 1 dose of MCV4 to children aged 2 through 10 years who travel to countries with highly endemic or epidemic disease and during outbreaks caused by a vaccine serogroup.
- Administer MCV4 to children at continued risk for meningococcal disease who were previously vaccinated with MCV4 or meningococcal polysaccharide vaccine after 3 years if the first dose was administered at age 2 through 6 years.

The Recommended Immunization Schedules for Persons Aged 0 Through 18 Years are approved by the Advisory Committee on Immunization Practices (http://www.cdc.gov/vaccines/recs/acip), the American Academy of Pediatrics (http://www.aap.org), and the American Academy of Family Physicians (http://www.aafp.org). U.S. Department of Health and Human Services • Centers for Disease Control and Prevention

RECOMMENDED IMMUNIZATION SCHEDULE FOR PERSONS AGED 7-18 YEARS

Vaccine ▼ Age ▶	7–10 years	11–12 years	13–18 years
Tetanus, Diphtheria, Pertussis[1]		Tdap	Tdap
Human Papillomavirus[2]	see footnote[2]	HPV (3 doses)(females)	HPV series
Meningococcal[3]	MCV4	MCV4	MCV4
Influenza[4]	Influenza (Yearly)		
Pneumococcal[5]	Pneumococcal		
Hepatitis A[6]	HepA Series		
Hepatitis B[7]	Hep B Series		
Inactivated Poliovirus[8]	IPV Series		
Measles, Mumps, Rubella[9]	MMR Series		
Varicella[10]	Varicella Series		

▨ Range of recommended ages for all children   ▨ Range of recommended ages for catch-up immunization   ▨ Range of recommended ages for certain high-risk groups

This schedule includes recommendations in effect as of December 21, 2010. Any dose not administered at the recommended age should be administered at a subsequent visit, when indicated and feasible. The use of a combination vaccine generally is preferred over separate injections of its equivalent component vaccines. Considerations should include provider assessment, patient preference, and the potential for adverse events. Providers should consult the relevant Advisory Committee on Immunization Practices statement for detailed recommendations: **http://www.cdc.gov/vaccines/pubs/acip-list.htm**. Clinically significant adverse events that follow immunization should be reported to the Vaccine Adverse Event Reporting System (VAERS) at **http://www.vaers.hhs.gov** or by telephone, **800-822-7967**.

1. **Tetanus and diphtheria toxoids and acellular pertussis vaccine (Tdap).** (Minimum age: 10 years for Boostrix and 11 years for Adacel)

   - Persons aged 11 through 18 years who have not received Tdap should receive a dose followed by Td booster doses every 10 years thereafter.
   - Persons aged 7 through 10 years who are not fully immunized against pertussis (including those never vaccinated or with unknown pertussis vaccination status) should receive a single dose of Tdap. Refer to the catch-up schedule if additional doses of tetanus and diphtheria toxoid–containing vaccine are needed.
   - Tdap can be administered regardless of the interval since the last tetanus and diphtheria toxoid–containing vaccine.

2. **Human papillomavirus vaccine (HPV).** (Minimum age: 9 years)

   - Quadrivalent HPV vaccine (HPV4) or bivalent HPV vaccine (HPV2) is recommended for the prevention of cervical precancers and cancers in females.
   - HPV4 is recommended for prevention of cervical precancers, cancers, and genital warts in females.
   - HPV4 may be administered in a 3-dose series to males aged 9 through 18 years to reduce their likelihood of acquiring genital warts.
   - Administer the second dose 1 to 2 months after the first dose and the third dose 6 months after the first dose (at least 24 weeks after the first dose).

3. **Meningococcal conjugate vaccine, quadrivalent (MCV4).** (Minimum age: 2 years)

   - Administer MCV4 at age 11 through 12 years with a booster dose at age 16 years.
   - Administer 1 dose at age 13 through 18 years if not previously vaccinated.
   - Persons who received their first dose at age 13 through 15 years should receive a booster dose at age 16 years.
   - Administer 1 dose to previously unvaccinated college freshmen living in a dormitory.
   - Administer 2 doses at least 8 weeks apart to children aged 2 through 10 years with persistent complement component deficiency and anatomic or functional asplenia, and 1 dose every 5 years thereafter.
   - Persons with HIV infection who are vaccinated with MCV4 should receive 2 doses at least 8 weeks apart.
   - Administer 1 dose of MCV4 to children aged 2 through 10 years who travel to countries with highly endemic or epidemic disease and during outbreaks caused by a vaccine serogroup.
   - Administer MCV4 to children at continued risk for meningococcal disease who were previously vaccinated with MCV4 or meningococcal polysaccharide vaccine after 3 years (if first dose administered at age 2 through 6 years) or after 5 years (if first dose administered at age 7 years or older).

4. **Influenza vaccine (seasonal).**

   - For healthy nonpregnant persons aged 7 through 18 years (i.e., those who do not have underlying medical conditions that predispose them to influenza complications), either LAIV or TIV may be used.
   - Administer 2 doses (separated by at least 4 weeks) to children aged 6 months through 8 years who are receiving seasonal influenza vaccine for the

(Continued)

first time or who were vaccinated for the first time during the previous influenza season but only received 1 dose.

- Children 6 months through 8 years of age who received no doses of monovalent 2009 H1N1 vaccine should receive 2 doses of 2010-2011 seasonal influenza vaccine. See *MMWR* 2010;59(No. RR-8): 33–34.

5. Pneumococcal vaccines.

- A single dose of 13-valent pneumococcal conjugate vaccine (PCV13) may be administered to children aged 6 through 18 years who have functional or anatomic asplenia, HIV infection or other immunocompromising condition, cochlear implant or CSF leak. See *MMWR* 2010;59(No. RR-11).

- The dose of PCV13 should be administered at least 8 weeks after the previous dose of PCV7.

- Administer pneumococcal polysaccharide vaccine at least 8 weeks after the last dose of PCV to children aged 2 years or older with certain underlying medical conditions, including a cochlear implant. A single revaccination should be administered after 5 years to children with functional or anatomic asplenia or an immunocompromising condition.

6. Hepatitis A vaccine (HepA).

- Administer 2 doses at least 6 months apart.

- HepA is recommended for children aged older than 23 months who live in areas where vaccination programs target older children, who are at increased risk for infection, or for whom immunity against hepatitis A is desired.

7. Hepatitis B vaccine (HepB).

- Administer the 3-dose series to those not previously vaccinated. For those with incomplete vaccination, follow the catch-up recommendations (Table).

- A 2-dose series (separated by at least 4 months) of adult formulation Recombivax HB is licensed for children aged 11 through 15 years.

8. Inactivated poliovirus vaccine (IPV).

- The final dose in the series should be administered on or after the fourth birthday and at least 6 months following the previous dose.

- If both OPV and IPV were administered as part of a series, a total of 4 doses should be administered, regardless of the child's current age.

9. Measles, mumps, and rubella vaccine (MMR).

- The minimum interval between the 2 doses of MMR is 4 weeks.

10. Varicella vaccine.

- For persons aged 7 through 18 years without evidence of immunity (see *MMWR* 2007;56[No. RR-4]), administer 2 doses if not previously vaccinated or the second dose if only 1 dose has been administered.

- For persons aged 7 through 12 years, the recommended minimum interval between doses is 3 months. However, if the second dose was administered at least 4 weeks after the first dose, it can be accepted as valid.

- For persons aged 13 years and older, the minimum interval between doses is 4 weeks.

The Recommended Immunization Schedules for Persons Aged 0 Through 18 Years are approved by the Advisory Committee on Immunization Practices **(http://www.cdc.gov/vaccines/recs/acip)**, the American Academy of Pediatrics **(http://www.aap.org)**, and the American Academy of Family Physicians **(http://www.aafp.org)**. U.S. Department of Health and Human Services • Centers for Disease Control and Prevention

CATCH-UP IMMUNIZATION SCHEDULE FOR PERSONS AGED 4 MONTHS-18 YEARS WHO START LATE OR WHO ARE MORE THAN 1 MONTH BEHIND

Vaccine	Minimum Age for Dose 1	Minimum Interval Between Doses			
		Dose 1 to Dose 2	Dose 2 to Dose 3	Dose 3 to Dose 4	Dose 4 to Dose 5
PERSONS AGED 4 MONTHS THROUGH 6 YEARS					
Hepatitis B[1]	Birth	4 weeks	8 weeks (and at least 16 weeks after first dose)		
Rotavirus[2]	6 wks	4 weeks	4 weeks[2]		
Diphtheria, Tetanus, Pertussis[3]	6 wks	4 weeks	4 weeks	6 months	6 months[3]
Haemophilus influenzae type b[4]	6 wks	4 weeks if first dose administered at younger than age 12 months / 8 weeks (as final dose) if first dose administered at age 12-14 months / No further doses needed if first dose administered at age 15 months or older	4 weeks[4] if current age is younger than 12 months / 8 weeks (as final dose)[4] if current age is 12 months or older and first dose administered at younger than age 12 months and second dose administered at younger than 15 months / No further doses needed if previous dose administered at age 15 months or older	8 weeks (as final dose) This dose only necessary for children aged 12 months through 59 months who received 3 doses before age 12 months	
Pneumococcal[5]	6 wks	4 weeks if first dose administered at younger than age 12 months / 8 weeks (as final dose for healthy children) if first dose administered at age 12 months or older or current age 24 through 59 months / No further doses needed for healthy children if first dose administered at age 24 months or older	4 weeks if current age is younger than 12 months / 8 weeks (as final dose for healthy children) if current age is 12 months or older / No further doses needed for healthy children if previous dose administered at age 24 months or older	8 weeks (as final dose) This dose only necessary for children aged 12 months through 59 months who received 3 doses before age 12 months or for children at high risk who received 3 doses at any age	
Inactivated Poliovirus[6]	6 wks	4 weeks	4 weeks	6 months[6]	
Measles, Mumps, Rubella[7]	12 mos	4 weeks			
Varicella[8]	12 mos	3 months			
Hepatitis A[9]	12 mos	6 months			
PERSONS AGED 7 THROUGH 18 YEARS					
Tetanus, Diphtheria / Tetanus, Diphtheria, Pertussis[10]	7 yrs[10]	4 weeks	4 weeks if first dose administered at younger than age 12 months / 6 months if first dose administered at 12 months or older	6 months if first dose administered at younger than age 12 months	
Human Papillomavirus[11]	9 yrs		Routine dosing intervals are recommended (females)[11]		
Hepatitis A[9]	12 mos	6 months			
Hepatitis B[1]	Birth	4 weeks	8 weeks (and at least 16 weeks after first dose)		
Inactivated Poliovirus[6]	6 wks	4 weeks	4 weeks[6]	6 months[6]	
Measles, Mumps, Rubella[7]	12 mos	4 weeks			
Varicella[8]	12 mos	3 months if person is younger than age 13 years / 4 weeks if person is aged 13 years or older			

The table above provides catch-up schedules and minimum intervals between doses for children whose vaccinations have been delayed. A vaccine series does not need to be restarted, regardless of the time that has elapsed between doses. Use the section appropriate for the child's age.

1. **Hepatitis B vaccine (HepB).**
   - Administer the 3-dose series to those not previously vaccinated.
   - The minimum age for the third dose of HepB is 24 weeks.
   - A 2-dose series (separated by at least 4 months) of adult formulation Recombivax HB is licensed for children aged 11 through 15 years.

2. **Rotavirus vaccine (RV).**
   - The maximum age for the first dose is 14 weeks 6 days. Vaccination should not be initiated for infants aged 15 weeks 0 days or older.
   - The maximum age for the final dose in the series is 8 months 0 days.
   - If Rotarix was administered for the first and second doses, a third dose is not indicated.

3. **Diphtheria and tetanus toxoids and acellular pertussis vaccine (DTaP).**
   - The fifth dose is not necessary if the fourth dose was administered at age 4 years or older.

4. ***Haemophilus influenzae* type b conjugate vaccine (Hib).**
   - 1 dose of Hib vaccine should be considered for unvaccinated persons aged 5 years or older who have sickle cell disease, leukemia, or HIV infection, or who have had a splenectomy.
   - If the first 2 doses were PRP-OMP (PedvaxHIB or Comvax), and administered at age 11 months or younger, the third (and final) dose should be administered at age 12 through 15 months and at least 8 weeks after the second dose.
   - If the first dose was administered at age 7 through 11 months, administer the second dose at least 4 weeks later and a final dose at age 12 through 15 months.

5. **Pneumococcal vaccine.**
   - Administer 1 dose of 13-valent pneumococcal conjugate vaccine (PCV13) to all healthy children aged 24 through 59 months with any incomplete PCV schedule (PCV7 or PCV13).

(Continued)

A277

- For children aged 24 through 71 months with underlying medical conditions, administer 1 dose of PCV13 if 3 doses of PCV were received previously or administer 2 doses of PCV13 at least 8 weeks apart if fewer than 3 doses of PCV were received previously.

- A single dose of PCV13 is recommended for certain children with underlying medical conditions through 18 years of age. See age-specific schedules for details.

- Administer pneumococcal polysaccharide vaccine (PPSV) to children aged 2 years or older with certain underlying medical conditions, including a cochlear implant, at least 8 weeks after the last dose of PCV. A single revaccination should be administered after 5 years to children with functional or anatomic asplenia or an immunocompromising condition. See *MMWR* 2010;59(No. RR-11).

6. Inactivated poliovirus vaccine (IPV).

- The final dose in the series should be administered on or after the fourth birthday and at least 6 months following the previous dose.

- A fourth dose is not necessary if the third dose was administered at age 4 years or older and at least 6 months following the previous dose.

- In the first 6 months of life, minimum age and minimum intervals are only recommended if the person is at risk for imminent exposure to circulating poliovirus (i.e., travel to a polio-endemic region or during an outbreak).

7. Measles, mumps, and rubella vaccine (MMR).

- Administer the second dose routinely at age 4 through 6 years. The minimum interval between the 2 doses of MMR is 4 weeks.

8. Varicella vaccine.

- Administer the second dose routinely at age 4 through 6 years.

- If the second dose was administered at least 4 weeks after the first dose, it can be accepted as valid.

9. Hepatitis A vaccine (HepA).

- HepA is recommended for children aged older than 23 months who live in areas where vaccination programs target older children, who are at increased risk for infection, or for whom immunity against hepatitis A is desired.

10. Tetanus and diphtheria toxoids vaccine (Td) and tetanus and diphtheria toxoids and acellular pertussis vaccine (Tdap).

- Doses of DTaP are counted as part of the Td/Tdap series.

- Tdap should be substituted for a single dose of Td in the catch-up series for children aged 7 through 10 years or as a booster for children aged 11 through 18 years; use Td for other doses.

11. Human papillomavirus vaccine (HPV).

- Administer the series to females at age 13 through 18 years if not previously vaccinated.

- Quadrivalent HPV vaccine (HPV4) may be administered in a 3-dose series to males aged 9 through 18 years to reduce their likelihood of genital warts.

- Use recommended routine dosing intervals for series catch-up (i.e., the second and third doses should be administered at 1 to 2 and 6 months after the first dose). The minimum interval between the first and second doses is 4 weeks. The minimum interval between the second and third doses is 12 weeks, and the third dose should be administered at least 24 weeks after the first dose.

Information about reporting reactions after immunization is available online at **http://www.vaers.hhs.gov** or by telephone, 800-822-7967. Suspected cases of vaccine-preventable diseases should be reported to the state or local health department. Additional information, including precautions and contraindications for immunization, is available from the National Center for Immunization and Respiratory Diseases at **http://www.cdc.gov/vaccines** or telephone, **800-CDC-INFO (800-232-4636)**. U.S. Department of Health and Human Services • Centers for Disease Control and Prevention

RECOMMENDED ADULT IMMUNIZATION SCHEDULE

Recommended adult immunization schedule, by vaccine and age group

VACCINE ▼ AGE GROUP ►	19–26 years	27–49 years	50–59 years	60–64 years	≥65 years
Influenza[1]	1 dose annually				
Tetanus, diphtheria, pertussis (Td/Tdap)[2]	Substitute 1-time dose of Tdap for Td booster; then boost with Td every 10 yrs				Td booster every 10 yrs
Varicella[3]	2 doses				
Human papillomavirus (HPV)[4]	3 doses (females)				
Zoster[5]				1 dose	
Measles, mumps, rubella (MMR)[6]	1 or 2 doses				
Pneumococcal (polysaccharide)[7,8]	1 or 2 doses				1 dose
Meningococcal[9]	1 or more doses				
Hepatitis A[10]	2 doses				
Hepatitis B[11]	3 doses				

*Covered by the Vaccine Injury Compensation Program.

For all persons in this category who meet the age requirements and who lack evidence of immunity (e.g., lack documentation of vaccination or have no evidence of previous infection)

Recommended if some other risk factor is present (e.g., based on medical, occupational, lifestyle, or other indications)

No recommendation

Report all clinically significant postvaccination reactions to the Vaccine Adverse Event Reporting System (VAERS). Reporting forms and instructions on filing a VAERS report are available at **http://www.vaers.hhs.gov** or by telephone, 800-822-7967.

Information on how to file a Vaccine Injury Compensation Program claim is available at **http://www.hrsa.gov/vaccinecompensation** or by telephone, 800-338-2382. Information about filing a claim for vaccine injury is available through the U.S. Court of Federal Claims, 717 Madison Place, N.W., Washington, D.C. 20005; telephone, 202-357-6400.

Additional information about the vaccines in this schedule, extent of available data, and contraindications for vaccination also is available at **http://www.cdc.gov/vaccines** or from the CDC-INFO Contact Center at 800-CDC-INFO (800-232-4636) in English and Spanish, 24 hours a day, 7 days a week.

Use of trade names and commercial sources is for identification only and does not imply endorsement by the U.S. Department of Health and Human Services.

The recommendations in this schedule were approved by:
Centers for Disease Control and Prevention's (CDC)
Advisory Committee on Immunization Practices (ACIP)
American Academy of Family Physicians (AAFP)
American College of Obstetricians and Gynecologists (ACOG)
American College of Physicians (ACP).

Vaccines that might be indicated for adults based on medical and other indications

INDICATION ► / VACCINE ▼	Pregnancy	Immunocompromising conditions (excluding human immunodeficiency virus [HIV])[3,5,6,13]	HIV infection[3,6,12,13] CD4+ T lymphocyte count		Diabetes, heart disease, chronic lung disease, chronic alcoholism	Asplenia[12] (including elective splenectomy) and persistent complement component deficiencies	Chronic liver disease	Kidney failure, end-stage renal disease, receipt of hemodialysis	Healthcare personnel
			<200 cells/µL	>200 cells/µL					
Influenza[1]	1 dose TIV annually								1 dose TIV or LAIV annually
Tetanus, diphtheria, pertussis (Td/Tdap)[2]	Td	Substitute 1-time dose of Tdap for Td booster; then boost with Td every 10 yrs							
Varicella[3]	Contraindicated				2 doses				
Human papillomavirus (HPV)[4]	3 doses through age 26 yrs								
Zoster[5]	Contraindicated				1 dose				
Measles, mumps, rubella (MMR)[6]	Contraindicated				1 or 2 doses				
Pneumococcal (polysaccharide)[7,8]	1 or 2 doses								
Meningococcal[9]	1 or more doses								
Hepatitis A[10]	2 doses								
Hepatitis B[11]	3 doses								

*Covered by the Vaccine Injury Compensation Program.

For all persons in this category who meet the age requirements and who lack evidence of immunity (e.g., lack documentation of vaccination or have no evidence of previous infection)

Recommended if some other risk factor is present (e.g., based on medical, occupational, lifestyle, or other indications)

No recommendation

These schedules indicate the recommended age groups and medical indications for which administration of currently licensed vaccines is commonly indicated for adults ages 19 years and older, as of January 1, 2011. For all vaccines being recommended on the adult immunization schedule, a vaccine series does not need to be restarted, regardless of the time that has elapsed between doses. Licensed combination vaccines may be used whenever any components of the combination are indicated and when the vaccine's other components are not contraindicated. For detailed recommendations on all vaccines, including those used primarily for travelers or that are issued during the year, consult the manufacturers' package inserts and the complete statements from the Advisory Committee on Immunization Practices (**http://www.cdc.gov/vaccines/pubs/acip-list.htm**).

(Continued)

1. **Influenza vaccination.** Annual vaccination against influenza is recommended for all persons aged 6 months and older, including all adults. Healthy, non-pregnant adults aged less than 50 years without high-risk medical conditions can receive either intranasally administered live, attenuated influenza vaccine (FluMist), or inactivated vaccine. Other persons should receive the inactivated vaccine. Adults aged 65 years and older can receive the standard influenza vaccine or the high-dose (Fluzone) influenza vaccine. Additional information about influenza vaccination is available at **http://www.cdc.gov/vaccines/vpd-vac/flu/default.htm**.

2. **Tetanus, diphtheria, and acellular pertussis (Td/Tdap) vaccination.** Administer a one-time dose of Tdap to adults aged less than 65 years who have not received Tdap previously or for whom vaccine status is unknown to replace one of the 10-year Td boosters, and as soon as feasible to all 1) postpartum women, 2) close contacts of infants younger than age 12 months (e.g., grandparents and childcare providers), and 3) healthcare personnel with direct patient contact. Adults aged 65 years and older who have not previously received Tdap and who have close contact with an infant aged less than 12 months also should be vaccinated. Other adults aged 65 years and older may receive Tdap. Tdap can be administered regardless of interval since the most recent tetanus or diphtheria-containing vaccine.

   Adults with uncertain or incomplete history of completing a 3-dose primary vaccination series with Td-containing vaccines should begin or complete a primary vaccination series. For unvaccinated adults, administer the first 2 doses at least 4 weeks apart and the third dose 6–12 months after the second. If incompletely vaccinated (i.e., less than 3 doses), administer remaining doses. Substitute a one-time dose of Tdap for one of the doses of Td, either in the primary series or for the routine booster, whichever comes first.

   If a woman is pregnant and received the most recent Td vaccination 10 or more years previously, administer Td during the second or third trimester. If the woman received the most recent Td vaccination less than 10 years previously, administer Tdap during the immediate postpartum period. At the clinician's discretion, Td may be deferred during pregnancy and Tdap substituted in the immediate postpartum period, or Tdap may be administered instead of Td to a pregnant woman after an informed discussion with the woman.

   The ACIP statement for recommendations for administering Td as prophylaxis in wound management is available at **http://www.cdc.gov/vaccines/pubs/acip-list.htm**.

3. **Varicella vaccination.** All adults without evidence of immunity to varicella should receive 2 doses of single-antigen varicella vaccine if not previously vaccinated or a second dose if they have received only 1 dose, unless they have a medical contraindication. Special consideration should be given to those who 1) have close contact with persons at high risk for severe disease (e.g., healthcare personnel and family contacts of persons with immunocompromising conditions) or 2) are at high risk for exposure or transmission (e.g., teachers; child-care employees; residents and staff members of institutional settings, including correctional institutions; college students; military personnel; adolescents and adults living in households with children; nonpregnant women of childbearing age; and international travelers).

   Evidence of immunity to varicella in adults includes any of the following: 1) documentation of 2 doses of varicella vaccine at least 4 weeks apart; 2) U.S.-born before 1980 (although for healthcare personnel and pregnant women, birth before 1980 should not be considered evidence of immunity); 3) history of varicella based on diagnosis or verification of varicella by a healthcare provider (for a patient reporting a history of or having an atypical case, a mild case, or both, healthcare providers should seek either an epidemiologic link with a typical varicella case or to a laboratory-confirmed case or evidence of laboratory confirmation, if it was performed at the time of acute disease); 4) history of herpes zoster based on diagnosis or verification of herpes zoster by a healthcare provider; or 5) laboratory evidence of immunity or laboratory confirmation of disease.

   Pregnant women should be assessed for evidence of varicella immunity. Women who do not have evidence of immunity should receive the first dose of varicella vaccine upon completion or termination of pregnancy and before discharge from the health-care facility. The second dose should be administered 4–8 weeks after the first dose.

4. **Human papillomavirus (HPV) vaccination.** HPV vaccination with either quadrivalent (HPV4) vaccine or bivalent vaccine (HPV2) is recommended for females at age 11 or 12 years and catch-up vaccination for females aged 13 through 26 years. Ideally, vaccine should be administered before potential exposure to HPV through sexual activity; however, females who are sexually active should still be vaccinated consistent with age-based recommendations. Sexually active females who have not been infected with any of the four HPV vaccine types (types 6, 11, 16, and 18, all of which HPV4 prevents) or any of the two HPV vaccine types (types 16 and 18, both of which HPV2 prevents) receive the full benefit of the vaccination. Vaccination is less beneficial for females who have already been infected with one or more of the HPV vaccine types. HPV4 or HPV2 can be administered to persons with a history of genital warts, abnormal Papanicolaou test, or positive HPV DNA test, because these conditions are not evidence of previous infection with all vaccine HPV types.

   HPV4 may be administered to males aged 9 through 26 years to reduce their likelihood of genital warts. HPV4 would be most effective when administered before exposure to HPV through sexual contact.

   A complete series for either HPV4 or HPV2 consists of 3 doses. The second dose should be administered 1–2 months after the first dose; the third dose should be administered 6 months after the first dose.

   Although HPV vaccination is not specifically recommended for persons with the medical indications described in Figure 2, "Vaccines that might be indicated for adults based on medical and other indications," it may be administered to these persons because the HPV vaccine is not a live-virus vaccine. However, the immune response and vaccine efficacy might be less for persons with the medical indications described in Figure 2 than in persons who do not have the medical indications described or who are immunocompetent.

5. **Herpes zoster vaccination.** A single dose of zoster vaccine is recommended for adults aged 60 years and older regardless of whether they report a previous episode of herpes zoster. Persons with chronic medical conditions may be vaccinated unless their condition constitutes a contraindication.

(Continued)

6. **Measles, mumps, rubella (MMR) vaccination.**
Adults born before 1957 generally are considered immune to measles and mumps. All adults born in 1957 or later should have documentation of 1 or more doses of MMR vaccine unless they have a medical contraindication to the vaccine, laboratory evidence of immunity to each of the three diseases, or documentation of provider-diagnosed measles or mumps disease. For rubella, documentation of provider-diagnosed disease is not considered acceptable evidence of immunity.
Measles component: A second dose of MMR vaccine, administered a minimum of 28 days after the first dose, is recommended for adults who 1) have been recently exposed to measles or are in an outbreak setting; 2) are students in postsecondary educational institutions; 3) work in a healthcare facility; or 4) plan to travel internationally. Persons who received inactivated (killed) measles vaccine or measles vaccine of unknown type during 1963–1967 should be revaccinated with 2 doses of MMR vaccine.
Mumps component: A second dose of MMR vaccine, administered a minimum of 28 days after the first dose, is recommended for adults who 1) live in a community experiencing a mumps outbreak and are in an affected age group; 2) are students in postsecondary educational institutions; 3) work in a healthcare facility; or 4) plan to travel internationally. Persons vaccinated before 1979 with either killed mumps vaccine or mumps vaccine of unknown type who are at high risk for mumps infection (e.g. persons who are working in a healthcare facility) should be revaccinated with 2 doses of MMR vaccine.
Rubella component: For women of childbearing age, regardless of birth year, rubella immunity should be determined. If there is no evidence of immunity, women who are not pregnant should be vaccinated. Pregnant women who do not have evidence of immunity should receive MMR vaccine upon completion or termination of pregnancy and before discharge from the healthcare facility.
Healthcare personnel born before 1957: For unvaccinated healthcare personnel born before 1957 who lack laboratory evidence of measles, mumps, and/or rubella immunity or laboratory confirmation of disease, healthcare facilities should 1) consider routinely vaccinating personnel with 2 doses of MMR vaccine at the appropriate interval (for measles and mumps) and 1 dose of MMR vaccine (for rubella), and 2) recommend 2 doses of MMR vaccine at the appropriate interval during an outbreak of measles or mumps, and 1 dose during an outbreak of rubella. Complete information about evidence of immunity is available at **http://www. cdc.gov/vaccines/ recs/provisional/default.htm**.

7. **Pneumococcal polysaccharide (PPSV) vaccination.** Vaccinate all persons with the following indications:
Medical: Chronic lung disease (including asthma); chronic cardiovascular diseases; diabetes mellitus; chronic liver diseases; cirrhosis; chronic alcoholism; functional or anatomic asplenia (e.g., sickle cell disease or splenectomy [if elective splenectomy is planned, vaccinate at least 2 weeks before surgery]); immunocompromising conditions (including chronic renal failure or nephrotic syndrome); and cochlear implants and cerebrospinal fluid leaks. Vaccinate as close to HIV diagnosis as possible.
Other: Residents of nursing homes or long-term care facilities and persons who smoke cigarettes. Routine use of PPSV is not recommended for American Indians/Alaska Natives or persons aged less than 65 years unless they have underlying medical conditions that are PPSV indications. However, public health authorities may consider recommending PPSV for American Indians/Alaska Natives and persons aged 50 through 64 years who are living in areas where the risk for invasive pneumococcal disease is increased.

8. **Revaccination with PPSV.** One-time revaccination after 5 years is recommended for persons aged 19 through 64 years with chronic renal failure or nephrotic syndrome; functional or anatomic asplenia (e.g., sickle cell disease or splenectomy); and for persons with immunocompromising conditions. For persons aged 65 years and older, one-time revaccination is recommended if they were vaccinated 5 or more years previously and were aged less than 65 years at the time of primary vaccination.

9. **Meningococcal vaccination.** Meningococcal vaccine should be administered to persons with the following indications:
Medical: A 2-dose series of meningococcal conjugate vaccine is recommended for adults with anatomic or functional asplenia, or persistent complement component deficiencies. Adults with HIV infection who are vaccinated should also receive a routine 2-dose series. The 2 doses should be administered at 0 and 2 months.
Other: A single dose of meningococcal vaccine is recommended for unvaccinated first-year college students living in dormitories; microbiologists routinely exposed to isolates of *Neisseria meningitidis*; military recruits; and persons who travel to or live in countries in which meningococcal disease is hyperendemic or epidemic (e.g., the "meningitis belt" of sub-Saharan Africa during the dry season [December through June]), particularly if their contact with local populations will be prolonged. Vaccination is required by the government of Saudi Arabia for all travelers to Mecca during the annual Hajj.
Meningococcal conjugate vaccine, quadrivalent (MCV4) is preferred for adults with any of the preceding indications who are aged 55 years and younger; meningococcal polysaccharide vaccine (MPSV4) is preferred for adults aged 56 years and older. Revaccination with MCV4 every 5 years is recommended for adults previously vaccinated with MCV4 or MPSV4 who remain at increased risk for infection (e.g., adults with anatomic or functional asplenia, or persistent complement component deficiencies).

10. **Hepatitis A vaccination.** Vaccinate persons with any of the following indications and any person seeking protection from hepatitis A virus (HAV) infection:
Behavioral: Men who have sex with men and persons who use injection drugs.
Occupational: Persons working with HAV-infected primates or with HAV in a research laboratory setting.
Medical: Persons with chronic liver disease and persons who receive clotting factor concentrates.
Other: Persons traveling to or working in countries that have high or intermediate endemicity of hepatitis A (a list of countries is available at **http:// wwww.cdc.gov/travel/ contentdiseases.aspx**). Unvaccinated persons who anticipate close personal contact (e.g., household or regular babysitting) with an international adoptee during the first 60 days after arrival in the United States from a

(Continued)

country with high or intermediate endemicity should be vaccinated. The first dose of the 2-dose hepatitis A vaccine series should be administered as soon as adoption is planned, ideally 2 or more weeks before the arrival of the adoptee.

Single-antigen vaccine formulations should be administered in a 2-dose schedule at either 0 and 6–12 months (Havrix), or 0 and 6–18 months (Vaqta). If the combined hepatitis A and hepatitis B vaccine (Twinrix) is used, administer 3 doses at 0, 1, and 6 months; alternatively, a 4-dose schedule may be used, administered on days 0, 7, and 21–30, followed by a booster dose at month 12.

11. **Hepatitis B vaccination.** Vaccinate persons with any of the following indications and any person seeking protection from hepatitis B virus (HBV) infection:

Behavioral: Sexually active persons who are not in a long-term, mutually monogamous relationship (e.g., persons with more than one sex partner during the previous 6 months); persons seeking evaluation or treatment for a sexually transmitted disease (STD); current or recent injection-drug users; and men who have sex with men.

Occupational: Healthcare personnel and public-safety workers who are exposed to blood or other potentially infectious body fluids.

Medical: Persons with end-stage renal disease, including patients receiving hemodialysis; persons with HIV infection; and persons with chronic liver disease.

Other: Household contacts and sex partners of persons with chronic HBV infection; clients and staff members of institutions for persons with developmental disabilities; and international travelers to countries with high or intermediate prevalence of chronic HBV infection (a list of countries is available at **http://wwwn.cdc.gov/travel/contentdiseases. aspx**).

Hepatitis B vaccination is recommended for all adults in the following settings: STD treatment facilities; HIV testing and treatment facilities; facilities providing drug-abuse treatment and prevention services; healthcare settings targeting services to injection-drug users or men who have sex with men; correctional facilities; end-stage renal disease programs and facilities for chronic hemodialysis patients; and institutions and nonresidential day-care facilities for persons with developmental disabilities.

Administer missing doses to complete a 3-dose series of hepatitis B vaccine to those persons not vaccinated or not completely vaccinated. The second dose should be administered 1 month after the first dose; the third dose should be given at least 2 months after the second dose (and at least 4 months after the first dose). If the combined hepatitis A and hepatitis B vaccine (Twinrix) is used, administer 3 doses at 0, 1, and 6 months; alternatively, a 4-dose Twinrix schedule, administered on days 0, 7, and 21 to 30, followed by a booster dose at month 12 may be used.

Adult patients receiving hemodialysis or with other immunocompromising conditions should receive 1 dose of 40 µg/mL (Recombivax HB) administered on a 3-dose schedule or 2 doses of 20 µg/mL (Engerix-B) administered simultaneously on a 4-dose schedule at 0, 1, 2, and 6 months.

12. **Selected conditions for which Haemophilus influenzae type b (Hib) vaccine may be used.** 1 dose of Hib vaccine should be considered for persons who have sickle cell disease, leukemia, or HIV infection, or who have had a splenectomy, if they have not previously received Hib vaccine.

13. **Immunocompromising conditions.** Inactivated vaccines generally are acceptable (e.g., pneumococcal, meningococcal, influenza [inactivated influenza vaccine]) and live vaccines generally are avoided in persons with immune deficiencies or immunocompromising conditions. Information on specific conditions is available at **http://www. cdc.gov/vaccines/pubs/acip-list.htm**.

ADMINISTRATION GUIDELINES FOR EYE DROPS & OINTMENT

Administration guidelines for eye drops:

1. Wash hands thoroughly.
2. Tilt head back.
3. Gently pull the lower eyelid away from the eye to create a pocket.
4. Hold the bottle upside down and look up just before applying a single drop. **NOTE:** To prevent contamination, do not let the tip of the eye drop applicator touch any surface (including the eye or eyelid). When not in use, keep the container tightly closed.
5. After applying the drop, look down for several seconds (still holding the eyelid away from the eye).
6. Slowly release the eyelid and close the eyes for 1 to 2 minutes. Do not blink.
7. Gently press on the inside corner of the eye (where the eyelid meets the nose) with a finger.
8. Blot excessive solution from around the eye with a tissue.

Administration guidelines for eye ointment:

1. Wash hands thoroughly.
2. Tilt head back.
3. Gently grasp lower outer eyelid below lashes, and pull eyelid away from the eye.
4. Place ointment tube over eye by directly looking at it. With a sweeping motion, place ¼ to ½-inch of ointment inside the lower eyelid by gently squeezing the tube. **NOTE:** To prevent contamination, do not let the tip of the tube touch any surface (including the eye or eyelid). When not in use, keep the tube tightly closed.
5. Slowly release eyelid and close eyes for 1 to 2 minutes.
6. Blot excessive ointment from around the eye with a tissue.
7. Vision may be temporarily blurred. Until vision clears, avoid activities requiring good visual ability.

Counseling tips:

- If having difficulty determining whether an eye dropper has touched the eye surface, keep the dropper in a refrigerator (not in a freezer).
- If more than one drop is needed, wait at least 5 minutes before instilling the next drop to prevent flushing away or diluting the first drop.
- If both eye drop and ointment therapy are needed, instill the eye drop at least 10 minutes before the ointment.
- Contact lenses should be removed unless the product is designed specifically for use with contact lenses.

ADMINISTRATION GUIDELINES FOR EAR DROPS

1. Wash hands thoroughly with soap and water.

2. Carefully wash and dry outside of the ear, taking care not to get water into the ear canal.

3. Warm ear drops to body temperature by holding the container in the palm of your hand for a few minutes.

4. Tilt head to the side, or lie down with the affected ear up. Use gentle restraint for an infant or a young child.

5. Position the dropper tip near, but not inside, the ear canal opening. **NOTE:** To prevent contamination and avoid injuring the ear, do not allow the dropper to touch the ear.

6. Pull ear backward and upward to open the ear canal and place the proper number of drops into the ear canal. Replace the cap on the container.

7. Gently press the small, flat skin flap over the ear canal opening to force out air bubbles and to push the drops down the ear canal.

8. Stay in the same position for the length of time indicated on the product instructions, or gently place a clean piece of cotton into the ear to prevent draining of medication. Do not leave it in the ear longer than one hour.

9. Repeat the procedure in the other ear, if needed.

10. Gently wipe the medication off the outside of the ear, using caution to avoid getting moisture in the ear canal.

11. Do not rinse the dropper after use. Wipe the tip of the dropper with a clean tissue and keep the container tightly closed.

12. Wash hands.

Counseling tips:

- If the drops are a suspension or if the label indicates, shake well before using.
- Do not warm the eardrop container in warm water. Hot ear drops can cause ear pain, nausea, and dizziness.
- Avoid contaminating applicator tip to preserve the sterility of the dropper.

ALCOHOL-FREE PRODUCTS

The following is a selection of alcohol-free products grouped by therapeutic category. This list is not comprehensive. Generic and alternate brands may exist. Always check product labeling for definitive information on specific ingredients.

Analgesics

Advil Children's Suspension	Pfizer Consumer
Advil Infant's Suspension	Pfizer Consumer
APAP Elixir	Bio-Pharm
Motrin Children's Cold Suspension	McNeil Consumer
Motrin Children's Suspension	McNeil Consumer
Motrin Infants' Suspension	McNeil Consumer
Silapap Children's Liquid	Silarx
Silapap Infant's Drops	Silarx
Tylenol Children's Suspension	McNeil Consumer
Tylenol Extra Strength Solution	McNeil Consumer
Tylenol Infant's Suspension	McNeil Consumer

Antiasthmatic Agent

Dy-G Liquid	Cypress

Anticonvulsant

Zarontin Syrup	Pfizer

Antiviral Agent

Epivir Oral Solution	ViiV

Cough/Cold/Allergy Preparations

Alacol Solution	Ballay
Alacol DM Syrup	Ballay
Allanhist PDX Syrup	Allan
Baltussin Solution	Ballay
Banophen Elixir	Major
Benadryl Allergy Solution	McNeil Consumer
Benadryl-D Allergy & Sinus Children's Liquid	McNeil Consumer
Bromaline Syrup	Rugby
Bromaline DM Elixir	Rugby
Bromphenex DM Solution	Breckenridge
Bromphenex HD Solution	Breckenridge
Bromplex DM Solution	Prasco
Bromtuss DM Solution	Breckenridge
Broncotron Liquid	Seyer Pharmatec
Broncotron-D Suspension	Seyer Pharmatec
B-Tuss Liquid	Blansett
Carbaphen 12 Ped Suspension	Gil
Carbaphen 12 Suspension	Gil
Carbatuss Liquid	GM
Carbatuss-12 Suspension	GM
Carbetaplex Solution	Breckenridge
Carbetaplex TS Suspension	Breckenridge
Children's Dimetapp Cold & Allergy Solution	Pfizer Consumer
Children's Dimetapp Long Acting Cough Plus Cold Solution	Pfizer Consumer
Children's Dimetapp Multi-Symptom Cold & Flu Solution	Pfizer Consumer
Children's Dimetapp Nighttime Cold & Congestion Solution	Pfizer Consumer
Children's Dimetapp Nighttime Flu Syrup	Pfizer Consumer
Children's Dimetapp DM Cold & Cough Solution	Pfizer Consumer
Children's Mucinex Cold Solution	Reckitt Benckiser
Children's Mucinex Cough Syrup	Reckitt Benckiser
Children's Mucinex Syrup	Reckitt Benckiser
Coughtuss Solution	Breckenridge
Crantex HC Syrup	Breckenridge
Crantex Syrup	Breckenridge
Creomulsion Cough Syrup	Summit Industries
Creomulsion for Children Syrup	Summit Industries
Dacex-DM Solution	Cypress
Dallergy Solution	Laser
De-Chlor DR Solution	Cypress
Dehistine Syrup	Cypress
Despec Liquid	International Ethical
Diabetic Tussin Cough Lozenges	Health Care Products
Diabetic Tussin Night Time Formula Solution	Health Care Products
Diabetic Tussin Solution	Health Care Products
Diabetic Tussin DM Solution	Health Care Products
Diabetic Tussin DM Maximum Strength Liquid	Health Care Products
Donatussin Solution	Laser
Donatussin DC Syrup	Laser
Donatussin DM Syrup	Laser
Double-Tussin DM Liquid	Reese
Dynatuss HC Solution	Breckenridge
Father John's Medicine Plus Drops	Oakhurst
Gani-Tuss NR Liquid	Cypress
Genebronco-D Liquid	PGD
Genecof-HC Liquid	PGD
Genecof-XP Liquid	PGD
Genecof-XP Syrup	PGD
Genedel Syrup	PGD
Genedotuss-DM Liquid	PGD
Genepatuss Liquid	PGD
Genetuss-2 Liquid	PGD
Genexpect-DM Liquid	PGD
Genexpect-PE Liquid	PGD
Genexpect-SF Liquid	PGD

Cough/Cold/Allergy Preparations (Continued)

Giltuss Liquid	Gil
Giltuss Ped-C Solution	Gil
H-C Tussive Syrup	Bryant Ranch
Histinex HC Syrup	Ethex
Histinex PV Syrup	Ethex
Hydramine Elixir	Quality Care Products
Hydro-Tussin HC Syrup	Ethex
Hydro-Tussin HD Liquid	Ethex
Hydro-Tussin XP Syrup	Ethex
Lohist D Syrup	Larken
Marcof Expectorant Syrup	Marnel
M-Clear Solution	McNeil, R.A.
Mintuss G Syrup	Breckenridge
Mintuss MR Syrup	Breckenridge
Mintuss MS Syrup	Breckenridge
Mintuss NX Solution	Breckenridge
Motrin Cold Children's Suspension	McNeil Consumer
Myhist-PD Solution	Larken
Nalex DH Liquid	Blansett Pharmacal
Nalex-A Liquid	Blansett Pharmacal
Neo AC Syrup	Laser
Neo DM Drops	Laser
Neo DM Suspension	Laser
Neo DM Syrup	Laser
Neotuss S/F Liquid	A.G. Marin
Neotuss-D Liquid	A.G. Marin
PediaCare Allergy Liquid	Prestige
PediaCare Allergy & Cold Liquid	Prestige
PediaCare Children's Fever Reducer & Pain Reliever Liquid	Prestige
PediaCare Cough & Congestion Liquid	Prestige
PediaCare Decongestant Liquid	Prestige
PediaCare Fever Reducer Plus Cough & Runny Nose Liquid	Prestige
PediaCare Fever Reducer Plus Cough & Sore Throat Liquid	Prestige
PediaCare Fever Reducer Plus Flu Liquid	Prestige
PediaCare Fever Reducer Plus Multi-Symptom Cold Liquid	Prestige
PediaCare Infant's Fever Reducer & Pain Reliever Liquid	Prestige
PediaCare Multi-Symptom Cold Liquid	Prestige
Pedia-Relief Liquid	Major
Phena-HC Solution	GM
Phena-S Liquid	GM
Poly Hist HC Solution	Poly
Poly Hist PD Solution	Poly
Poly-Tussin Solution	Poly
Poly-Tussin AC	Poly
Poly-Tussin DHC	Poly
Poly-Tussin HD Syrup	Poly
Poly-Tussin XP Solution	Poly
Q-Tussin Liquid	Qualitest
Rescon-DM Liquid	Capellon
Rescon-GG Liquid	Capellon
Rindal HD Liquid	Breckenridge
Rindal HD Plus Solution	Breckenridge
Robitussin Children's Cough & Cold CF Solution	Pfizer Consumer
Robitussin Children's Cough & Cold Long-Acting Solution	Pfizer Consumer
Robitussin Children's Cough Long-Acting Liquid	Pfizer Consumer
Robitussin Cold & Chest Congestion DM Max Liquid	Pfizer Consumer
Robitussin Cough & Chest Congestion Liquid	Pfizer Consumer
Robitussin Cough & Chest Congestion Sugar-Free Liquid	Pfizer Consumer
Robitussin Cough & Cold CF Syrup	Pfizer Consumer
Robitussin Cough & Cold Long-Acting Liquid	Pfizer Consumer
Robitussin Cough & Cold Nighttime Liquid	Pfizer Consumer
Robitussin To Go Cough & Cold CF Liquid	Pfizer Consumer
Robitussin To Go Cough & Congestion DM Liquid	Pfizer Consumer
Scot-Tussin Diabetes CF Liquid	Scot-Tussin
Scot-Tussin DM Solution	Scot-Tussin
Scot-Tussin Expectorant Solution	Scot-Tussin
Scot-Tussin Senior Solution	Scot-Tussin
Siladryl Allergy Solution	Silarx
Sildec Syrup	Silarx
Sildec-PE Solution	Silarx
Sildec PE-DM Solution	Silarx
Siltussin DAS Liquid	Silarx
Siltussin DM DAS Cough Formula Syrup	Silarx
Siltussin SA Syrup	Silarx
Sudafed Children's Solution	McNeil Consumer
Sudatuss DM Syrup	PGD
Sudatuss-2 Liquid	PGD
Sudatuss-SF Liquid	PGD
Theracof Plus	Reese
Tussi-Pres Liquid	Kramer-Novis
Tussi-Pres Pediatric Solution	Kramer-Novis
Tylenol Children's Liquid	McNeil Consumer
Tylenol Cold & Cough Daytime Liquid	McNeil Consumer

Cough/Cold/Allergy Preparations (Continued)

Tylenol Cold & Cough Nighttime Liquid	McNeil Consumer
Tylenol Cold & Flu Severe Liquid	McNeil Consumer
Tylenol Cold & Sore Throat Liquid	McNeil Consumer
Tylenol Flu Children's Suspension	McNeil Consumer
Tylenol Infants' Drops	McNeil Consumer
Tylenol Multi-Symptom Cold Children's Liquid	McNeil Consumer
Tylenol Plus Cold & Allergy Children's Liquid	McNeil Consumer
Tylenol Plus Cold & Cough Children's Suspension	McNeil Consumer
Tylenol Plus Cold & Cough Liquid	McNeil Consumer
Tylenol Plus Cold & Runny Nose Liquid	McNeil Consumer
Tylenol Plus Cough & Sore Throat Liquid	McNeil Consumer
Tylenol Plus Cold & Stuffy Nose Liquid	McNeil Consumer
Vazol Solution	Wraser Pharm
Vicks 44 Custom Care Chesty Cough Liquid	Procter & Gamble
Vicks 44 Custom Care Congestion Liquid	Procter & Gamble
Vicks 44 Custom Care Cough & Cold Liquid	Procter & Gamble
Vicks 44 Custom Care Dry Cough Suppressant Liquid	Procter & Gamble
Vicks Dayquil Cold & Flu Relief Liquid	Procter & Gamble
Vicks Dayquil Cough Liquid	Procter & Gamble
Vicks Dayquil Mucus Control Liquid	Procter & Gamble
Vicks Dayquil Mucus Control DM Liquid	Procter & Gamble
Vicks Dayquil Multi-Symptom Liquid	Procter & Gamble
Vicks Nyquil Children's Liquid	Procter & Gamble
Vicks Nyquil Cold & Flu Relief Liquid	Procter & Gamble
V-Tann Suspension	Breckenridge
Z-Cof 8 DM Suspension	Pernix
Z-Tuss DM Syrup	Magna

Ear/Nose/Throat Products

4-Way Saline Moisturizing Mist Spray	Bristol-Myers
Ayr Baby Saline Spray	Ascher
Bucalcide Spray	Seyer Pharmatec
Bucalsep Solution	Gil
Bucalsep Spray	Gil
Cheracol Sore Throat Spray	Lee
Fresh N Free Solution	Geritrex
Gly-Oxide Solution	GlaxoSmithKline
Listermint Solution	McNeil Consumer
Nasal Moist Gel	Blairex
Orajel Baby Day & Night Gel	Del
Orajel Baby Nighttime Teething Pain Medicine Gel	Del
OraMagic Plus Powder	MPM Medical
OraMagicRx Powder	MPM Medical
Tanac Liquid	Del
Throto-Ceptic Spray	S.S.S.
Triaminic Sore Throat Spray	Novartis Consumer
Vicks Sinex Spray	P&G Company
Vicks Sinex 12 Hour Spray	P&G Company
Zilactin Baby Extra Strength Gel	Zila

Gastrointestinal Agents

Axid Solution	Braintree
Colidrops Pediatric Drops	A.G. Marin
Colace Solution	Purdue
Gas Relief Solution	Amerisource Bergen
Imogen Liquid	PGD
Mylicon Infants' Drops	Johnson & Johnson/ Merck

Topical Products

Dermatone Lips N Face Protector Ointment	Dermatone
Dermatone Moisturizing Sunblock Cream	Dermatone
Dermatone Skin Protector Cream	Dermatone
Fresh & Pure Douche Solution	Unico
Handclens Solution	Woodward
Neutrogena Acne Wash Liquid	Neutrogena
Neutrogena Antiseptic Solution	Neutrogena
Neutrogena Clear Pore Gel	Neutrogena
Neutrogena T/Derm Liquid	Neutrogena
Neutrogena Toner Solution	Neutrogena
Podiclens Spray	Woodward
Sea Breeze Foaming Face Wash Gel	Clairol
Sportz Bloc Cream	Med-Derm
Tiger Balm Arthritis Rub Lotion	Prince of Peace

Vitamins/Minerals/Supplements

Adaptosode For Stress Liquid	HVS
Adaptosode R+R For Acute Stress Liquid	HVS
Apetigen Elixir	Kramer-Novis
Biosode Liquid	HVS
Detoxosode Products Liquid	HVS
Genesupp-500 Liquid	PGD
Genetect Plus Liquid	PGD
Multi-Delyn Liquid	Silarx
Multi-Delyn w/Iron Liquid	Silarx

ALCOHOL-FREE PRODUCTS

Vitamins/Minerals/Supplements (Continued)

Nutrivit Solution	Llorens
Poly-Vi-Sol Drops	Mead Johnson
Poly-Vi-Sol w/Iron Drops	Mead Johnson
Protect Plus Liquid	Gil
Strovite Forte Syrup	Everett
Supervite Liquid	Seyer Pharmatec
Suplevit Liquid	Gil
Tri-Vi-Sol w/Iron Drops	Mead Johnson
Vitafol Syrup	Everett

Miscellaneous

Cytra-2 Solution	Cypress
Cytra-K Solution	Cypress
Fluorinse Solution	Oral B
Namenda Solution	Forest
Primsol Solution	FSC

COMMON LABORATORY TEST VALUES

Listed below are generally accepted normal values for a selection of common laboratory assays conducted on serum, plasma, and blood. Remember that norms may vary from laboratory to laboratory in accordance with the methodology and quality control measures employed by the facility. When in doubt, check with the laboratory that performed the analysis.

"SI range" refers to Système International d'Unités, a uniform system of reporting numerical values that permits interchangeability of information among nations and disciplines.

TEST	US RANGE	SI RANGE
Acid phosphatase	≤2.5 ng/mL	≤2.5 µg/L
Prostatic Total	≤5.8 U/L	<97 nkat/L
Alanine aminotransferase [ALT] (SGPT)	≤48 U/L	≤0.8 µkat/L
Albumin, serum	3.5-5.5 g/dL	35-55 g/L
Alkaline phosphatase	20-125 U/L	0.33-2.08 µkat/L
Ammonia [NH_3^+]	10-80 µg/dL	6-47 µmol/L
Amylase, serum	60-180 U/L	0.8-3.2 µkat/L
Antinuclear antibodies (ANA)	Negative at 1:40 dilution	
Aspartate aminotransferase (AST) (SGOT)	≤42 U/L	<0.7 µkat/L
Bilirubin		
Total	0.3-1.0 mg/dL	5.1-17 µmol/L
Direct	0.1-0.3 mg/dL	1.7-5.1 µmol/L
Indirect	0.2-0.7 mg/dL	3.4-12 µmol/L
Blood urea nitrogen/creatinine ratio	10:1-20:1	Average 15:1
Calcium, plasma	9-10.5 mg/dL	2.2-2.6 mmol/L
Calcium, ionized	4.5-5.6 mg/dL	1.1-1.4 mmol/L
Chloride, serum	95-108 mEq/L	95-108 mmol/L
Cholesterol (total plasma)		
Desirable level	<200 mg/dL	<5.20 mmol/L
Moderate risk	200-240 mg/dL	5.2-6.3 mmol/L
High risk	>240 mg/dL	>6.3 mmol/L
Copper	70-140 µg/dL	11-22 µmol/L
Cortisol, serum		
0800 hours	5-25 µg/dL	140-690 nmol/L
1600 hours	3-12 µg/dL	80-330 nmol/L
Creatinine kinase (CK)		
Isoenzymes	CK-MM: 97-100% of total	CK-MM: 0.97-1.00 of total
	CK-MB: <3% of total	CK-MB: <0.03 of total
	CK-BB: 0% of total	CK-BB: 0 of total
Total	Male: ≤235 U/L	Male: ≤3.92 µkat/L
	Female: ≤190 U/L	Female: ≤3.17 µkat/L
Creatinine, serum	<1.5 mg/dL	<133 µmol/L
Creatinine clearance	75-125 mL/min	1.24-2.08 mL/sec
Digoxin		
Therapeutic	0.8-2.0 ng/mL	1.0-2.6 nmol/L
Toxic	>2.5 ng/mL	>3.2 nmol/L
Erythrocyte count (RBC)	$4.15\text{-}4.90 \times 10^6/mm^3$	$4.15\text{-}4.90 \times 10^{12}/L$
Erythrocyte sedimentation rate (ESR)		
Male	0-20 mm/hr	0-20 mm/hr
Female	0-30 mm/hr	0-30 mm/hr
Ferritin		
Male	15-400 ng/mL	15-400 µg/L
Female	10-200 ng/mL	10-200 µg/L
Folic acid	3-16 ng/mL	7-36 nmol/L

COMMON LABORATORY TEST VALUES

TEST	US RANGE	SI RANGE
Follicle-stimulating hormone (FSH)		
Female	1.4-9.6 mIU/mL	1.4-9.6 IU/L
Ovulation	2.3-21 mIU/mL	2.3-21 IU/L
Postmenopausal	34-96 mIU/mL	34-96 IU/L
Male	0.9-15 mIU/mL	0.9-15 IU/L
Gamma-glutamyl transferase (GGT)		
Male	≤65 U/L	≤1.08 µkat/L
Female	≤45 U/L	≤0.75 µkat/L
Gases, arterial blood		
pO_2	80-100 mmHg	11-13 kPa
pCO_2	35-45 mmHg	4.7-6 kPa
Glucose, plasma		
Fasting	75-115 mg/dL	4.2-6.4 mmol/L
Postprandial (2 h)	<120 mg/dL	<7.8 mmol/L
Immunoglobulins (Ig)		
IgG	800-1500 mg/dL	8.0-15.0 g/L
IgA	90-325 mg/dL	0.9-3.2 g/L
IgM	45-150 mg/dL	0.45-1.5 g/L
IgD	0-8 mg/dL	0-0.08 g/L
IgE	<0.025 mg/dL	<0.00025 g/L
Iron, serum	50-150 µg/dL	9-27 µmol/L
Iron binding capacity	250-370 µg/dL	45-66 µmol/L
Iron saturation	20-45%	
Lactic acid (plasma, venous)	9-16 mg/dL	1.0-1.8 mmol/L
Lactic dehydrogenase (LDH)	100-190 U/L	1.7-3.2 µkat/L
Lead	<20 µg/dL	1.0 µmol/L
Leukocyte count (WBC)	4.3-10.8 × 10³	4.3-10.8 × 10⁹/L
Lipase	0-160 U/L	0-2.66 µkat/L
Lipoproteins (desirable levels)		
Low density (LDL)	<130 mg/dL	<3.36 mmol/L
High density (HDL)	>60 mg/dL	>1.55 mmol/L
Lithium ion (therapeutic)	0.6-1.2 mEq/L	0.6-1.2 mmol/L
Luteinizing hormone		
Female	0.8-26 mIU/mL	0.8-26 IU/L
Ovulation	25-57 mIU/mL	25-57 IU/L
Postmenopausal	40-104 mIU/mL	40-104 IU/L
Male	1.3-13 mIU/mL	1.3-13 IU/L
Osmolality, plasma	285-295 mOsm/kg	285-295 mmol/kg
Phenytoin		
Therapeutic	10-20 mg/L	40-80 µmol/L
Toxic	>30 mg/L	>120 µmol/L
Phosphorus, serum	2.5-4.5 mg/dL	0.8-1.45 mmol/L
Potassium, serum	3.5-5 mEq/L	3.5-5 mmol/L
Prolactin	2-15 ng/mL	2-15 µg/L
Prostate-specific antigen (PSA)	≤4 ng/mL	≤4 µg/L
Protein		
Total	5.5-8.0 g/dL	55-80 g/L
Albumin	3.5-5.5 g/dL	35-55 g/L
Globulin	2.0-3.5 g/dL	20-35 g/L
Reticulocyte count	0.5-2.3% of RBCs	0.005-0.023 of RBCs
Rheumatoid factor	<40 IU/mL	<40 kIU/L
Sodium, serum	136-145 mEq/L	136-145 mmol/L
Theophylline (therapeutic)	10-20 mg/L	55-110 µmol/L
Thyroxine-binding globulin (TBG)	16-34 mg/L	16-34 mg/L

TEST	US RANGE	SI RANGE
Thyroid-stimulating hormone (TSH)	0.4-5 μU/mL	0.4-5 mU/L
Thyroxine (T_4)		
Free	0.8-1.8 ng/dL	10-23 pmol/L
Total	4.5-12.5 μg/dL	58-161 nmol/L
Transferrin	230-390 μg/dL	2.3-3.9 mg/L
Triglycerides	<160 μg/dL	<1.8 mmol/L
Triiodothyronine (T_3)	70-190 ng/dL	1.1-2.9 nmol/L
T_3 uptake	25-35%	0.25-0.35 (proportion of 1.0)
Urea nitrogen, blood (BUN)	7-30 mg/dL	2.5-10.7 mmol/L
Uric acid		
Male	4.0-8.5 mg/dL	238-506 μmol/L
Female	2.5-7.5 mg/dL	149-446 μmol/L
Vitamin B_{12}	200-600 pg/mL	148-443 pmol/L

SOURCES:

Beers MH, Porter RS, Jones TV, et al. *Merck Manual of Diagnosis and Therapy,* ed 18. Whitehouse Station, NJ: Merck Research Laboratories; 2006.

Fauci AS, Braunwald E, Kasper DL, et al. *Harrison's Principles of Internal Medicine,* ed 17. New York, NY: McGraw Hill; 2008.

CYTOCHROME P450 ENZYMES: SUBSTRATES, INDUCERS, AND INHIBITORS

SUBSTRATES	INDUCERS	INHIBITORS
CYP1A2		
Acetaminophen	Broccoli	Alatrofloxacin Mesylate
Alatrofloxacin Mesylate	Brussel Sprouts	Amiodarone HCl
Aminophylline	Carbamazepine	Anastrozole
Amitriptyline HCl	Charbroiled Food	Cimetidine HCl
Amoxapine	Citalopram Hydrobromide	Ciprofloxacin
Anagrelide HCl	Diltiazem HCl	Clarithromycin
Caffeine	Erythromycin	Desogestrel
Chlordiazepoxide	Escitalopram Oxalate	Enoxacin
Cimetidine HCl	Esomeprazole	Ethinyl Estradiol
Ciprofloxacin	Fluvoxamine Maleate	Fluvoxamine Maleate
Clomipramine HCl	Hypericum Perforatum	Gatifloxacin
Clopidogrel Bisulfate	Insulin	Gemifloxacin Mesylate
Clozapine	Lansoprazole	Grapefruit
Cyclobenzaprine	Nafcillin Sodium	Grepafloxacin HCl
Desipramine HCl	Nicotine	Isoniazid
Diazepam	Omeprazole	Ketoconazole
Diltiazem HCl	Phenobarbital	Levofloxacin
Doxepin HCl	Phenytoin	Levonorgestrel
Enoxacin	Primidone	Lomefloxacin HCl
Erythromycin	Rifampicin	Mestranol
Estradiol	Rifampin	Methoxsalen
Ethinyl Estradiol	Ritonavir	Mexiletine HCl
Flutamide	Tobacco	Mibefradil DiHCl
Fluticasone Propionate		Moxifloxacin HCl
Fluvoxamine Maleate		Nalidixic Acid
Grepafloxacin HCl		Norethindrone
Haloperidol		Norfloxacin
Imipramine		Norgestrel
Levobupivacaine HCl		Ofloxacin
Lomefloxacin HCl		Omeprazole
Maprotiline HCl		Paroxetine
Methadone HCl		Ranitidine HCl
Mexiletine HCl		Ritonavir
Mirtazapine		Sildenafil Citrate
Moxifloxacin HCl		Sparfloxacin
Nafcillin Sodium		Tacrine HCl
Naproxen		Ticlopidine HCl
Nicotine		Troleandomycin
Norethindrone		Trovafloxacin Mesylate
Norfloxacin		Vardenafil HCl
Nortriptyline HCl		Zileuton
Ofloxacin		
Olanzapine		
Ondansetron		
Phenobarbital		
Phenytoin		
Propafenone HCl		
Propranolol HCl		
Protriptyline HCl		
Riluzole		
Ritonavir		

(Continued)

SUBSTRATES	INDUCERS	INHIBITORS
CYP1A2 *(Continued)*		
Ropinirole HCl		
Ropivacaine HCl		
Tacrine HCl		
Tamoxifen Citrate		
Theobromine		
Theophylline		
Tizanidine		
Tizanidine HCl		
Trimethaphan Camsylate		
Trimipramine Maleate		
Trovafloxacin Mesylate		
Verapamil HCl		
Warfarin Sodium		
Zileuton		
Zolmitriptan		
CYP2C18		
Naproxen		Cimetidine HCl
Omeprazole		
Piroxicam		
Propranolol HCl		
Tretinoin		
Warfarin Sodium		
CYP2C19		
Amitriptyline HCl	Carbamazepine	Cimetidine HCl
Amoxapine	Norethindrone	Citalopram Hydrobromide
Carisoprodol	Phenobarbital	Delavirdine Mesylate
Cilostazol	Phenytoin	Desogestrel
Citalopram Hydrobromide	Prednisone	Efavirenz
Clomipramine HCl	Rifampin	Esomeprazole
Cyclophosphamide		Ethinyl Estradiol
Desipramine HCl		Ethynodiol Diacetate
Dextromethorphan		Felbamate
Diazepam		Fluoxetine
Divalproex Sodium		Fluvastatin Sodium
Doxepin HCl		Fluvoxamine Maleate
Esomeprazole		Indomethacin
Ethosuximide		Isoniazid
Ethotoin		Ketoconazole
Felbamate		Lansoprazole
Formoterol Fumarate		Letrozole
Fosphenytoin Sodium		Levonorgestrel
Gabapentin		Mestranol
Imipramine		Modafinil
Indomethacin		Norethindrone
Lamotrigine		Norethynodrel
Lansoprazole		Norgestimate
Levetiracetam		Norgestrel
Maprotiline HCl		Omeprazole
Mephenytoin		Oxcarbazepine
Mephobarbital		Paroxetine HCl
Meprobamate		Quinidine
Methsuximide		Ritonavir
Midazolam HCl		Sertraline HCl
Nelfinavir Mesylate		Sildenafil Citrate
Nilutamide		Sulfaphenazole

(Continued)

SUBSTRATES	INDUCERS	INHIBITORS
CYP2C19 *(Continued)*		
Nortriptyline HCl		Telmisartan
Omeprazole		Ticlopidine HCl
Oxcarbazepine		Tolbutamide
Pantoprazole Sodium		Topiramate
Paramethadione		Tranylcypromine Sulfate
Pentamidine Isethionate		Vardenafil HCl
Phenacemide		Voriconazole
Phenobarbital		
Phensuximide		
Phenytoin		
Primidone		
Progesterone		
Proguanil HCl		
Propranolol HCl		
Protriptyline HCl		
Rabeprazole Sodium		
Sertraline HCl		
Teniposide		
Thioridazine HCl		
Tiagabine HCl		
Tolbutamide		
Topiramate		
Trimethadione		
Trimipramine Maleate		
Valproate Sodium		
Valproic Acid		
Voriconazole		
Warfarin Sodium		
Zonisamide		
CYP2C8		
Amiodarone HCl	Carbamazepine	Anastrozole
Amitriptyline HCl	Phenobarbital	Cimetidine HCl
Amoxapine	Primidone	Gemfibrozil
Benzphetamine HCl	Rifabutin	Nicardipine HCl
Carbamazepine	Rifampin	Omeprazole
Clomipramine HCl		Quercetin
Desipramine HCl		Sulfaphenazole
Diazepam		Sulfinpyrazone
Diclofenac		Trimethoprim
Docetaxel		
Doxepin HCl		
Fluvastatin Sodium		
Imipramine		
Isotretinoin		
Maprotiline HCl		
Mephobarbital		
Nortriptyline HCl		
Omeprazole		
Paclitaxel		
Phenytoin		
Pioglitazone HCl		
Protriptyline HCl		
Repaglinide		
Rosiglitazone Maleate		
Rosiglitazone/Metformin		

(Continued)

CYTOCHROME P450 ENZYMES: SUBSTRATES, INDUCERS, AND INHIBITORS

SUBSTRATES	INDUCERS	INHIBITORS
CYP2C8 *(Continued)*		
Tolbutamide		
Tretinoin		
Trimipramine Maleate		
Verapamil HCI		
Vitamin A		
Warfarin Sodium		
Zopiclone		
CYP2C9		
Acarbose	Aprepitant	Amiodarone HCl
Amitriptyline HCl	Carbamazepine	Anastrozole
Candesartan Cilexetil	Dexamethasone	Bendroflumethiazide
Carbamazepine	Phenobarbital	Chloramphenicol
Carvedilol	Phenytoin	Chlorothiazide
Celecoxib	Primidone	Chlorpropamide
Chlorpropamide	Rifampin	Cimetidine HCl
Clomipramine HCl	Rifapentine	Clopidogrel Bisulfate
Desogestrel	Secobarbital Sodium	Clotrimazole
Dextromethorphan		Diclofenac
Diazepam		Disulfiram
Diclofenac		Efavirenz
Dronabinol		Fenofibrate
Eprosartan Mesylate		Fluconazole
Etodolac		Fluorouracil
Fenoprofen Calcium		Fluoxetine
Fluoxetine		Flurbiprofen
Flurbiprofen		Fluvastatin Sodium
Fluvastatin Sodium		Fluvoxamine Maleate
Glimepiride		Gemfibrozil
Glipizide		Glipizide
Ibuprofen		Glyburide
Imipramine HCl		Hydrochlorothiazide
Indomethacin		Hydroflumethiazide
Irbesartan		Imatinib Mesylate
Ketoprofen		Isoniazid
Ketorolac Tromethamine		Itraconazole
Lansoprazole		Ketoconazole
Losartan Potassium		Ketoprofen
Meclofenamate Sodium		Leflunomide
Mefenamic Acid		Lovastatin
Meloxicam		Methyclothiazide
Metformin HCl		Metronidazole
Miglitol		Miconazole
Mirtazapine		Modafinil
Montelukast Sodium		Nifedipine
Nabumetone		Omeprazole
Naproxen		Oxiconazole Nitrate
Nateglinide		Paroxetine HCl
Nifedipine		Phenylbutazone
Omeprazole		Polythiazide
Oxaprozin		Ritonavir
Phenylbutazone		Sertraline HCl
Phenytoin		Sildenafil Citrate
Pioglitazone HCl		Sulfacytine
Piroxicam		Sulfamethizole
Repaglinide		Sulfamethoxazole

(Continued)

SUBSTRATES	INDUCERS	INHIBITORS
CYP2C9 *(Continued)*		
Rofecoxib		Sulfasalazine
Rosiglitazone Maleate		Sulfinpyrazone
Sildenafil Citrate		Sulfisoxazole Acetyl
Sulfamethoxazole		Terconazole
Sulindac		Ticlopidine HCl
Suprofen		Tolazamide
Tamoxifen Citrate		Tolbutamide
Telmisartan		Troglitazone
Tolazamide		Vardenafil HCl
Tolbutamide		Voriconazole
Tolmetin Sodium		Zafirlukast
Torsemide		
Troglitazone		
Valdecoxib		
Valsartan		
Vardenafil HCl		
Verapamil HCl		
Voriconazole		
Warfarin Sodium		
Zafirlukast		
Zileuton		
CYP2D6		
Amitriptyline HCl	Carbamazepine	Amiodarone HCl
Amphetamine	Ethanol	Amitriptyline HCl
Atomoxetine HCl	Hypericum Perforatum	Amoxapine
Bisoprolol Fumarate	Phenobarbital	Bupropion HCl
Captopril	Phenytoin	Celecoxib
Carvedilol	Primidone	Chloroquine
Cevimeline HCl	Rifampin	Chlorpheniramine
Chlorpromazine HCl	Ritonavir	Cimetidine HCl
Chlorpropamide		Citalopram Hydrobromide
Clomipramine HCl		Clomipramine HCl
Clozapine		Cocaine HCl
Codeine Phosphate		Desipramine HCl
Cyclobenzaprine HCl		Diphenhydramine
Debrisoquine		Doxepin HCl
Desipramine HCl		Escitalopram Oxalate
Dexfenfluramine HCl		Fluoxetine
Dextroamphetamine		Fluphenazine
Dextromethorphan		Fluvoxamine Maleate
Dolasetron Mesylate		Halofantrine HCl
Donepezil HCl		Haloperidol
Doxepin HCl		Hydroxychloroquine Sulfate
Encainide HCl		Imatinib Mesylate
Esomeprazole		Imipramine HCl
Fentanyl		Maprotiline HCl
Flecainide Acetate		Methadone HCl
Fluoxetine		Mibefradil DiHCl
Fluphenazine		Moclobemide
Fluvoxamine Maleate		Nortriptyline HCl
Formoterol Fumarate		Paroxetine
Galantamine Hydrobromide		Perphenazine
Haloperidol		Propafenone HCl
Hydrocodone Bitartrate		Propoxyphene

(Continued)

CYTOCHROME P450 ENZYMES: SUBSTRATES, INDUCERS, AND INHIBITORS

SUBSTRATES	INDUCERS	INHIBITORS
CYP2D6 (Continued)		
Imipramine HCl		Protriptyline HCl
Indoramin HCl		Quinacrine HCl
Labetalol HCl		Quinidine
Lidocaine		Ranitidine HCl
Maprotiline HCl		Ritonavir
Meperidine HCl		Sertraline HCl
Methadone HCl		Sildenafil Citrate
Methamphetamine HCl		Terbinafine HCl
Methoxyphenamine		Thioridazine HCl
Metoprolol Succinate		Trimipramine Maleate
Mexiletine HCl		Vardenafil HCl
Mirtazapine		
Morphine Sulfate		
Nelfinavir Mesylate		
Nortriptyline HCl		
Olanzapine		
Omeprazole		
Ondansetron		
Oxycodone HCl		
Paroxetine HCl		
Pindolol		
Propafenone HCl		
Propoxyphene		
Propranolol HCl		
Quetiapine Fumarate		
Quinidine		
Risperidone		
Ritonavir		
Tamoxifen Citrate		
Teniposide		
Testosterone		
Thioridazine HCl		
Timolol Maleate		
Tolterodine Tartrate		
Tramadol HCl		
Trazodone HCl		
Triazolam		
Trimipramine Maleate		
Venlafaxine HCl		
Vinblastine Sulfate		
Zonisamide		
CYP3A4		
Alfentanil HCl	Allium sativum	**Potent inhibitors**
Alprazolam	Aminoglutethimide	Amprenavir
Amiodarone HCl	Aprepitant	Atazanavir Sulfate
Amitriptyline HCl	Betamethasone	Clarithromycin
Amlodipine Besylate	Bosentan	Delavirdine Mesylate
Aprepitant	Carbamazepine	Delavirine
Astemizole	Ciprofloxacin	Fosamprenavir Calcium
Atorvastatin Calcium	Cisplatin	Indinavir Sulfate
Belladonna Ergotamine	Cortisone Acetate	Itraconazole
Buspirone HCl	Dexamethasone	Ketoconazole
Busulfan	Doxorubicin HCl	Lopinavir
Carbamazepine	Efavirenz	Nefazodone HCl

(Continued)

SUBSTRATES	INDUCERS	INHIBITORS
CYP3A4 *(Continued)*		
		Potent inhibitors, cont.
Cerivastatin Sodium	Ethosuximide	Nelfinavir Mesylate
Chlorpheniramine	Felbamate	Posaconazole
Cisapride	Fludrocortisone Acetate	Ritonavir
Clarithromycin	Fosphenytoin Sodium	Saquinavir Mesylate
Cyclosporine	Garlic	Telithromycin
Dapsone	Hydrocortisone	Troleandomycin
Desogestrel	Hypericum Perforatum	Voriconazole
Diazepam	Mephenytoin	
Dihydroergotamine Mesylate	Methsuximide	**Inhibitors (potency not specified)**
Diltiazem HCl	Methylprednisolone	Acetazolamide
Disopyramide Phosphate	Modafinil	Amiodarone HCl
Disulfiram	Nafcillin Sodium	Amprenavir
Doxorubicin HCl	Nevirapine	Anastrozole
Dronabinol	Oxcarbazepine	Aprepitant
Ergonovine Maleate	Phenobarbital	Atazanavir Sulfate
Ergotamine Tartrate	Phenytoin	Cimetidine HCl
Erythromycin	Prednisolone	Ciprofloxacin
Esomeprazole	Prednisone	Clarithromycin
Estradiol	Primidone	Clotrimazole
Ethinyl Estradiol	Rifabutin	Conivaptan HCl
Ethosuximide	Rifampicin	Cyclosporine
Ethynodiol Diacetate	Rifampin	Dalfopristin
Etoposide	Rifapentine	Danazol
Felodipine	Sulfinpyrazone	Darunavir
Fentanyl	Theophyllinate	Dasatinib
Haloperidol	Theophylline	Delavirdine Mesylate
Indinavir Sulfate	Triamcinolone	Delavirine
Isradipine	Troglitazone	Desloratadine
Itraconazole		Diltiazem HCl
Ixabepilone		Efavirenz
Ketoconazole		Erythromycin
Levonorgestrel		Fluconazole
Lidocaine		Fluoxetine
Lovastatin		Fluvoxamine Maleate
Mestranol		Fosamprenavir Calcium
Methadone HCl		Grapefruit
Midazolam HCl		Imatinib Mesylate
Nefazodone HCl		Indinavir Sulfate
Nelfinavir Mesylate		Isoniazid
Nicardipine HCl		Itraconazole
Nifedipine		Ketoconazole
Nimodipine		Lapatinib
Nisoldipine		Lopinavir
Nitrendipine		Loratadine
Norethindrone		Metronidazole
Norgestrel		Miconazole
Omeprazole		Mifepristone
Ondansetron		Nefazodone HCl
Paclitaxel		Nelfinavir Mesylate
Pimozide		Nevirapine
Polyestradiol Phosphate		Niacin
Quinidine		Niacinamide
Quinine		Nicotinamide

(Continued)

CYTOCHROME P450 ENZYMES: SUBSTRATES, INDUCERS, AND INHIBITORS

SUBSTRATES	INDUCERS	INHIBITORS
CYP3A4 *(Continued)*		
Rifabutin		**Inhibitors**
Ritonavir		**(potency not specified, cont.)**
Saquinavir Mesylate		Nifedipine
Sertraline HCl		Norfloxacin
Sildenafil Citrate		Omeprazole
Simvastatin		Paroxetine
Sirolimus		Posaconazole
Tacrolimus		Propoxyphene
Tadalafil		Quinidine
Tamoxifen Citrate		Quinine
Terfenadine		Quinupristin
Theophylline		Ranitidine HCl
Tiagabine HCl		Ritonavir
Tolterodine Tartrate		Saquinavir Mesylate
Trazodone HCl		Sertraline HCl
Triazolam		Sildenafil Citrate
Vardenafil HCl		Telithromycin
Verapamil HCl		Troglitazone
Vinblastine Sulfate		Troleandomycin
Vincristine Sulfate		Valproate Sodium
Warfarin Sodium		Vardenafil HCl
		Verapamil HCl
		Voriconazole
		Zafirlukast
		Zileuton
CYP3A		
Alfentanil HCl	Allium sativum	Amiodarone HCl
Alprazolam	Aprepitant	Amprenavir
Aminophylline	Carbamazepine	Aprepitant
Amitriptyline HCl	Dexamethasone	Atazanavir Sulfate
Amlodipine Besylate	Efavirenz	Cimetidine HCl
Aprepitant	Ethosuximide	Ciprofloxacin
Astemizole	Hypericum Perforatum	Clarithromycin
Atorvastatin Calcium	Modafinil	Cyclosporine
Bromocriptine Mesylate	Nevirapine	Delavirdine Mesylate
Buspirone HCl	Phenobarbital	Delavirine
Busulfan	Phenytoin	Diltiazem HCl
Carbamazepine	Rifabutin	Efavirenz
Cerivastatin Sodium	Rifampicin	Erythromycin
Chlorpheniramine	Rifampin	Fluconazole
Cilostazol	Rifapentine	Fluoxetine
Cisapride		Fluvoxamine Maleate
Clarithromycin		Fosamprenavir Calcium
Cyclosporine		Grapefruit
Desogestrel		Indinavir Sulfate
Dexamethasone		Isoniazid
Diazepam		Itraconazole
Dihydroergotamine Mesylate		Ketoconazole
Diltiazem HCl		Lopinavir
Disopyramide Phosphate		Metronidazole
Doxorubicin HCl		Miconazole
Dronabinol		Nefazodone HCl
Dyphylline		Nelfinavir Mesylate
Ergotamine Tartrate		Nifedipine
Erythromycin		Norfloxacin
Estrogen		Paroxetine HCl

(Continued)

SUBSTRATES	INDUCERS	INHIBITORS
CYP3A *(Continued)*		
Ethinyl Estradiol		Quinine
Ethosuximide		Ritonavir
Ethynodiol Diacetate		Saquinavir Mesylate
Etoposide		Sertraline HCl
Felodipine		Troleandomycin
Fentanyl		Venlafaxine HCl
Glyburide		Verapamil HCl
Haloperidol		Voriconazole
Imipramine HCl		Zafirlukast
Indinavir Sulfate		Zileuton
Isradipine		
Itraconazole		
Ketoconazole		
Levonorgestrel		
Lidocaine		
Lovastatin		
Mestranol		
Methadone HCl		
Methylprednisolone		
Midazolam HCl		
Nefazodone HCl		
Nelfinavir Mesylate		
Nicardipine HCl		
Nifedipine		
Nimodipine		
Nisoldipine		
Norethindrone		
Norgestrel		
Ondansetron		
Paclitaxel		
Pimozide		
Quinidine		
Quinine		
Rifabutin		
Ritonavir		
Saquinavir Mesylate		
Sertraline HCl		
Sildenafil Citrate		
Simvastatin		
Sirolimus		
Tacrolimus		
Tamoxifen Citrate		
Terfenadine		
Testosterone		
Theophylline		
Tiagabine HCl		
Tolterodine Tartrate		
Trazodone HCl		
Triazolam		
Venlafaxine HCl		
Verapamil HCl		
Vinblastine Sulfate		
Vincristine Sulfate		
Warfarin Sodium		

Note: This list is not comprehensive. For more information, refer to the specific product's full Prescribing Information.

DRUGS EXCRETED IN BREAST MILK

The following list is not comprehensive; generic forms and alternate brands of some products may be available. When recommending drugs to pregnant or nursing patients, always check product labeling for specific precautions.

Abstral
Accolate
Accuretic
Aciphex
Actiq
Activella
Actonel
ActoPlus Met
Adalat
Adderall XR
Advicor
Aggrenox
Aldactazide
Aldactone
Alfenta
Allegra-D
Aloprim
Alsuma
Altace
Altavera
Ambien
Amerge
Amturnide
Anafranil
Anaprox
Androderm
Aplenzin
Aralen
Arthrotec
Asacol
Ativan
Augmentin
Avalide
Avandamet
Axid
Azactam
Azasan
Azathioprine
Azulfidine
Bactrim
Baraclude
Benadryl
Bentyl
Betapace
Bexxar
Beyaz
Boniva
Brevicon
Butrans
Byetta
Caduet
Cafergot
Calan
Campral
Capoten
Capozide
Captopril
Carbatrol
Cardizem
Cataflam
Catapres

Cayston
Ceftin
Celebrex
Celexa
Ceredase
Cipro
Ciprodex
Claforan
Clarinex
Claritin
Claritin-D
Cleocin
Climara
Clozaril
Codeine
Combigan
CombiPatch
Combivir
Combunox
Compro
Cordarone
Corgard
Cortisporin
Corzide
Cosopt
Coumadin
Covera-HS
Cozaar
Crestor
Crinone
Cyclessa
Cymbalta
Cytomel
Cytotec
Dapsone
Daraprim
Darvon
Demerol
Depacon
Depakene
Depakote
DepoDur
Depo-Provera
Desogen
Desoxyn
Dexedrine
D.H.E. 45
Diabinese
Diastat
Diflucan
Dilacor
Dilantin
Dilaudid
Diovan
Diprivan
Diuril
Dolophine
Doral
Doryx
Droxia
Duraclon

Duragesic
Duramorph
Dyazide
Dyrenium
E.E.S.
EC-Naprosyn
Ecotrin
Effexor
Elavil
EMLA
Enduron
Epzicom
Equetro
ERYC
Ery-Tab
Erythrocin
Erythromycin
Esgic-plus
Estrogel
Estrostep
Evista
Exalgo
Factive
FazaClo
Felbatol
Feldene
femhrt
Fiorinal
Flagyl
Foradil
Fortamet
Fortaz
Fosamax
Furosemide
Gabitril
Gablofen
Galzin
Glucophage
Glucovance
Glumetza
Glyset
Gralise
Halcion
Haldol
Helidac
Hycamtin
Ifex
Imitrex
Imuran
Inderal
Indocin
INFeD
InnoPran XL
Inspra
Invanz
Invega
Janumet
Jenloga
Kadian
Kaletra
Kapvay

Keflex
Keppra
Ketek
Klonopin
Lamictal
Lamisil
Lamprene
Lanoxin
Lescol
Letairis
Levitra
Levora
Levothroid
Levoxyl
Lexapro
Lexiva
Lialda
Lindane
Lioresal
Lithium
Lithobid
Lo Loestrin Fe
Lo/Ovral
Loestrin
Lomotil
Lopressor
Lortab
Lotensin
Lotrel
Luminal
Luvox
Lyrica
Macrobid
Macrodantin
Makena
Marinol
Maxipime
Maxzide
Menostar
Metaglip
Methergine
Methotrexate
MetroCream/Gel/Lotion
Micronor
Microzide
Migranal
Minocin
Mirapex
Mircette
M-M-R II
Mobic
Modicon
Monodox
Monopril
Morphine
MS Contin
Myambutol
Mycamine
Mysoline
Namenda
Naprelan

(Continued)

Naprosyn
Nascobal
Natazia
Neoral
Neurontin
Nexiclon XR
Niaspan
Nicotrol
Niravam
Nizoral
Norco
Nor-QD
Nordette
Noritate
Norpace
Norpramin
Novantrone
Oramorph
Ortho-Cept
Ortho-Cyclen
Ortho Tri-Cyclen
Ovcon
Oxistat
OxyContin
Pacerone
Pamelor
Paxil
PCE
Pediapred
Pediotic
Pentasa
Pepcid
Periostat
Persantine
Pfizerpen
Phenytek
Phrenilin
Plan B
Ponstel
Prandimet
Pravachol
Premphase
Prempro
Prevacid

PREVPAC
Prinzide
Pristiq
Prograf
Prometrium
Propofol
Prosed/DS
Protonix
Provera
Prozac
Pseudoephedrine
Pulmicort
Pyrazinamide
Quinine
Reglan
Relpax
Requip
Reserpine
Restoril
Retrovir
Rifadin
Rifamate
Rifater
Risperdal
Rocephin
Rozerem
Safyral
Sanctura
Sanctura XR
Sandimmune
Sarafem
Seconal
Sectral
Semprex-D
Septra
Seroquel
Seroquel XR
Silenor
Soma
Sonata
Soriatane
Spiriva
Sprycel
Stadol

Stavzor
Streptomycin
Stromectol
Suboxone
Symbyax
Synthroid
Tagamet
Tambocor
Tapazole
Tarka
Tasigna
Tazicef
Tegretol
Tenoretic
Tenormin
Thalitone
Theo-24
Tiazac
Timoptic
Tindamax
Tobi
Tofranil
Toprol-XL
Toradol
Trandate
Tranxene
Trental
Tribenzor
Tricor
Triglide
Trileptal
Tri-Norinyl
Triostat
Trisenox
Trivora
Trizivir
Truvada
Tygacil
Tylenol
Tylenol with Codeine
Ultane
Ultram
Unasyn
Uniretic

Unithroid
Valium
Valtrex
Vancocin
Vaseretic
Vasotec
Ventavis
Verelan
Vibramycin
Vibra-Tabs
Vicodin
Vigamox
Vimovo
Viramune
Voltaren
Vytorin
Vyvanse
Wellbutrin
Xanax
Xolair
Zantac
Zarontin
Zaroxolyn
Zegerid
Zemplar
Zestoretic
Zetia
Ziac
Zinacef
Zithromax
Zoloft
Zomig
Zonalon
Zonegran
Zosyn
Zovia
Zovirax
Zyban
Zydone
Zyloprim
Zyprexa
Zyrtec

DRUGS THAT MAY CAUSE PHOTOSENSITIVITY

The drugs in this table are known to cause photosensitivity in some individuals. Effects can range from itching, scaling, rash, and swelling to skin cancer, premature skin aging, skin and eye burns, cataracts, reduced immunity, blood vessel damage, and allergic reactions. The list is not all-inclusive, and shows only representative brands of each generic. When in doubt, always check specific product labeling. Individuals should be advised to wear protective clothing and to apply sunscreens while taking the medications listed below.

GENERIC	BRAND	GENERIC	BRAND
Acamprosate calcium	Campral	Carbamazepine	Carbatrol, Epitol, Equetro, Tegretol, Tegretol-XR
Acetazolamide	Diamox		
Acitretin	Soriatane		
Acyclovir	Zovirax	Carbinoxamine Maleate	Palgic
Alendronate Sodium	Fosamax	Carvedilol	Coreg
Alendronate Sodium/ Cholecalciferol	Fosamax Plus D	Carvedilol Phosphate	Coreg CR
		Celecoxib	Celebrex
Aliskiren/Amlodipine/HCTZ	Amturnide	Cetirizine HCl/ Pseudoephedrine HCl	Zyrtec-D 12 Hour
Aliskiren/HCTZ	Tekturna HCT		
Almotriptan Malate	Axert	Cevimeline HCl	Evoxac
Amiloride HCl/HCTZ		Chloroquine Phosphate	Aralen
Aminolevulinic Acid HCl	Levulan Kerastick	Chlorothiazide	Diuril
Amiodarone HCl	Cordarone, Pacerone	Chlorpheniramine Maleate/ Dextromethorphan HBr/ Pseudoephedrine HCl	Atuss DS Tannate Suspension
Amitriptyline HCl			
Amitriptyline HCl/ Chlordiazepoxide	Limbitrol, Limbitrol DS		
		Chlorpheniramine Maleate/ Pseudoephedrine HCl	Sudal-12
Amitriptyline HCl/Perphenazine			
Amlodipine/HCTZ/ Olmesartan Medoxomil	Tribenzor	Chlorpheniramine Tannate/ Dextromethorphan Tannate/ Pseudoephedrine Tannate	Dicel DM
Amlodipine Besylate/HCTZ/ Valsartan	Exforge HCT		
		Chlorpromazine HCl	
Amoxapine		Chlorpropamide	Diabinese
Amphetamine Aspartate/ Amphetamine Sulfate/ Dextroamphetamine Saccharate/ Dextroamphetamine Sulfate	Adderall XR	Chlorthalidone	Thalitone
		Chlorthalidone/Clonidine HCl	Clorpres
		Cidofovir	Vistide
		Ciprofloxacin	Cipro, Cipro XR, Proquin XR
Anagrelide HCl	Agrylin		
Aripiprazole	Abilify	Citalopram HBr	Celexa
Atenolol/Chlorthalidone	Tenoretic	Clemastine Fumarate	
Atovaquone/Proguanil HCl	Malarone	Clindamycin Phosphate	Clindagel
Azithromycin	Zithromax, Zmax	Clomipramine HCl	Anafranil
Benazepril HCl	Lotensin	Clozapine	Clozaril, FazaClo
Benazepril HCl/HCTZ	Lotensin HCT	Codeine Phosphate/ Phenylephrine HCl/ Promethazine HCl	Promethazine VC with Codeine
Bendroflumethiazide/Nadolol	Corzide		
Benzoyl Peroxide/Erythromycin	Benzamycin Pak		
Bexarotene	Targretin	Codeine Phosphate/ Promethazine HCl	Promethazine with Codeine
Bismuth Subcitrate Potassium/ Metronidazole/Tetracyline HCl	Pylera		
		Cromolyn Sodium	Gastrocrom
		Cyclobenzaprine HCl	Flexeril
Bismuth Subsalicylate/ Metronidazole/Tetracycline HCl	Helidac Therapy	Cyproheptadine HCl	
		Dacarbazine	DTIC-Dome
		Dasatinib	Sprycel
Bisoprolol Fumarate/HCTZ	Ziac	Demeclocycline HCl	Declomycin
Brompheniramine Maleate/ Carbetapentane Citrate/ Phenylephrine HCl	Vazotan Tannate	Desipramine HCl	Norpramin
		Desvenlafaxine	Pristiq
		Dextromethorphan HBr/ Promethazine HCl	Promethazine DM
Brompheniramine Maleate/ Phenylephrine HCl	Vazobid Tannate		
		Diclofenac Potassium	Cambia, Cataflam, Zipsor
Brompheniramine Maleate/ Dextromethorphan HBr/ Phenylephrine HCl	Alacol DM Syrup		
		Diclofenac Sodium/Misoprostol	Arthrotec
		Diclofenac Sodium	Solaraze, Voltaren-XR
Bupropion HBr	Aplenzin		
Bupropion	Budeprion SR, Budeprion XL, Buproban, Wellbutrin SR, Wellbutrin XL, Zyban	Diflunisal	Dolobid
		Diltiazem HCl	Cardizem, Cardizem LA, Tiazac
		Diphenhydramine HCl	Benadryl
		Dipivefrin HCl	Propine
Candesartan Cilexetil/HCTZ	Atacand HCT	Divalproex Sodium	Depakote, Depakote ER
Capecitabine	Xeloda		
Captopril	Capoten	Doxepin HCl	Silenor, Sinequan
Captopril/HCTZ	Capozide	Doxorubicin HCl	

(Continued)

DRUGS THAT MAY CAUSE PHOTOSENSITIVITY

GENERIC	BRAND	GENERIC	BRAND
Doxycycline Calcium	Vibramycin	HCTZ/Metoprolol Tartrate	Lopressor HCT
Doxycycline Hyclate	Doryx, PerioStat, Vibramycin, Vibra-Tabs	HCTZ/Moexipril HCl	Uniretic
		HCTZ/Propranolol HCl	
		HCTZ/Quinapril HCl	Accuretic
Doxycycline Monohydrate	Monodox, Oracea, Vibramycin	HCTZ/Spironolactone	Aldactazide
		HCTZ/Telmisartan	Micardis HCT
Duloxetine HCl	Cymbalta	HCTZ/Triamterene	Dyazide, Maxzide
Efavirenz/Emtricitabine/ Tenofovir Disoproxil Fumarate	Atripla	HCTZ/Valsartan	Diovan HCT
		Hydroxocobalamin	Cyanokit
Enalapril Maleate		Hydroxychloroquine Sulfate	Plaquenil
Enalapril Maleate/HCTZ		Ibuprofen	Motrin
Enalaprilat		Imatinib Mesylate	Gleevec
Epirubicin HCl	Ellence	Imipramine HCl	Tofranil
Eprosartan Mesylate/HCTZ	Teveten HCT	Imipramine Pamoate	Tofranil-PM
Erythromycin Ethylsuccinate/ Sulfisoxazole Acetyl		Indapamide	
		Interferon Alfa-2b	Intron A
Escitalopram Oxalate	Lexapro	Interferon Alfa-N3	Alferon N
Esomeprazole Magnesium	Nexium	Isocarboxazid	Marplan
Esomeprazole Magnesium/ Naproxen	Vimovo	Isoniazid/Pyrazinamide/Rifampin	Rifater
		Isotretinoin	Amnesteem, Claravis, Sotret
Esomeprazole Sodium	Nexium I.V.	Itraconazole	Sporanox
Estazolam	ProSom	Ketoprofen, Ketoprofen ER	
Estradiol Cypionate	Depo- Estradiol	Ketorolac Tromethamine	Toradol
Eszopiclone	Lunesta	Lamotrigine	Lamictal, Lamictal XR
Ethinyl Estradiol/Norelgestromin	Ortho Evra	Leuprolide Acetate	Lupron, Lupron Depot
Ethionamide	Trecator		
Etodolac, Etodolac ER		Levofloxacin	Levaquin
Ezetimibe/Simvastatin	Vytorin	Lisinopril	Prinivil, Zestril
Febuxostat	Uloric	Losartan Potassium	Cozaar
Felbamate	Felbatol	Lovastatin/Niacin	Advicor
Fenofibrate	Antara, Lipofen, Lofibra, Tricor, Triglide	Lovastatin	Altoprev, Mevacor
		Maprotiline HCl	
		Mefenamic Acid	Ponstel
Floxuridine	Sterile FUDR	Meloxicam	Mobic
Flucytosine	Ancobon	Mesalamine	Pentasa
Fluorouracil, Topical	Efudex	Methotrexate Sodium	
Fluoxetine HCl	Prozac, Sarafem	Methylclothiazide	
Fluoxetine HCl/Olanzapine	Symbyax	Methyl Aminolevulinate	Metvixia
Fluphenazine Decanoate		Metolazone	Zaroxolyn
Fluphenazine HCl		Metoprolol Succinate	Toprol-XL
Flurbiprofen	Ansaid	Metoprolol Tartrate	Lopressor
Flutamide	Eulexin	Minocycline HCl	Arestin, Dynacin, Minocin, Solodyn
Fluvastatin Sodium	Lescol, Lescol XL		
Fluvoxamine Maleate	Luvox CR	Mirtazapine	Remeron, RemeronSolTab
Fosinopril Sodium	Monopril		
Fosinopril Sodium/HCTZ	Monopril-HCT	Moexipril HCl	Univasc
Fosphenytoin Sodium	Cerebyx	Moxifloxacin HCl	Avelox
Furosemide	Lasix	Nabilone	Cesamet
Gabapentin	Neurontin	Nabumetone	
Gemfibrozil	Lopid	Naproxen	EC-Naprosyn, Naprosyn
Gemifloxacin Mesylate	Factive		
Gentamicin Sulfate		Naproxen Sodium	Anaprox, Anaprox DS, Naprelan
Glatiramer Acetate	Copaxone		
Glimepiride	Amaryl		
Glimepiride/Pioglitazone HCl	Duetact	Naratriptan HCl	Amerge
Glimepiride/Rosiglitazone Maleate	Avandaryl	Nefazodone HCl	
		Nifedipine	Adalat CC, Nifediac CC, Nifedical XL, Procardia, Procardia XL
Glipizide	Glucotrol		
Glyburide	DiaBeta, Glynase PresTab		
Griseofulvin	Grifulvin V, Gris-PEG		
Haloperidol Decanoate	Haldol Decanoate	Nilotinib	Tasigna
Haloperidol Lactate	Haldol	Nisoldipine	Sular
Hexachlorophene	pHisoHex Detergent	Norfloxacin	Noroxin
HCTZ	Microzide	Nortriptyline HCl	Pamelor
HCTZ/Irbesartan	Avalide	Ofloxacin	Floxin
HCTZ/Lisinopril	Prinzide, Zestoretic	Olanzapine	Zyprexa, Zyprexa ZYDIS
HCTZ/Losartan Potassium	Hyzaar		
HCTZ/Methyldopa		Olsalazine Sodium	Dipentum

GENERIC	BRAND	GENERIC	BRAND
Omeprazole	Prilosec	Sibutramine HCl Monohydrate	Meridia
Omeprazole/Sodium Bicarbonate	Zegerid	Sildenafil Citrate	Viagra
Oxaprozin	Daypro, Daypro Alta	Simvastatin	Zocor
Oxcarbazepine	Trileptal	Sotalol HCl	Betapace, Betapace AF
Oxycodone HCl	Roxicodone	Sulfamethoxazole/Trimethoprim	Bactrim, Bactrim DS,
Paclitaxel	Abraxane		Septra, Septra DS,
Panitumumab	Vectibix		Sulfatrim
Pantoprazole Sodium	Protonix	Sulfasalazine	Azulfidine, Azulfidine
Paroxetine HCl	Paxil, Paxil CR		EN-tabs
Paroxetine Mesylate	Pexeva	Sulindac	Clinoril
Pentosan Polysulfate Sodium	Elmiron	Sumatriptan	Alsuma,
Perphenazine			Imitrex Nasal Spray,
Phenylephrine HCl/	Promethazine VC		Sumavel DosePro
Promethazine HCl		Sumatriptan Succinate	Imitrex
Pilocarpine HCl	Salagen	Tacrolimus	Prograf
Pimozide	Orap	Tetracycline HCl	Sumycin
Piroxicam	Feldene	Thalidomide	Thalomid
Poly-L-Lactic Acid	Sculptra	Thioridazine HCl	
Polymyxin B Sulfate/	Polytrim	Thiothixene	Navane
Trimethoprim Sulfate		Tiagabine HCl	Gabitril
Porfimer Sodium	Photofrin	Tigecycline	Tygacil
Pramipexole DiHCl	Mirapex, Mirapex ER	Tipranavir	Aptivus
Pravastatin Sodium	Pravachol	Tolazamide	
Pregabalin	Lyrica	Tolbutamide	
Prochlorperazine	Compro	Topiramate	Topamax
Prochlorperazine Edisylate		Trazodone HCl	Oleptro
Prochlorperazine Maleate		Tretinoin	Avita
Promethazine HCl	Phenadoz, Phenergan,	Triamcinolone Acetonide	Azmacort
	Promethegan	Triamterene	Dyrenium
Protriptyline HCl	Vivactil	Trifluoperazine HCl	
Pyrazinamide		Trimipramine Maleate	Surmontil
Quetiapine Fumarate	Seroquel	Valacyclovir HCl	Valtrex
Quinapril HCl	Accupril	Valproate Sodium	Depacon
Quinidine Gluconate		Valproic Acid	Depakene, Stavzor
Quinidine Sulfate		Vardenafil HCl	Levitra
Quinine Sulfate	Qualaquin	Varenicline	Chantix
Ramipril	Altace	Venlafaxine HCl	Effexor, Effexor XR
Rasagiline Mesylate	Azilect	Verteporfin	Visudyne
Riluzole	Rilutek	Voriconazole	Vfend
Ritonavir	Norvir	Zaleplon	Sonata
Rizatriptan Benzoate	Maxalt, Maxalt-MLT	Ziprasidone HCl	Geodon
Ropinirole HCl	Requip	Zolmitriptan	Zomig, Zomig-ZMT
Selegiline	Emsam	Zolpidem Tartrate	Ambien, Ambien CR,
Selegiline HCl	Eldepryl		Edluar, Zolpimist
Sertraline HCl	Zoloft		

HCTZ: Hydrochlorothiazide
HCl: hydrochloride

DRUGS THAT SHOULD NOT BE CRUSHED

Listed below are various slow-release as well as enteric-coated products that should not be crushed or chewed. Slow-release (sr) represents products that are controlled-release, extended-release, long-acting, or timed-release. Enteric-coated (ec) represents products that are delayed-release.

In general, capsules containing slow-release or enteric-coated particles may be opened and their contents administered on a spoonful of soft food. Instruct patients not to chew the particles, though. (Patients should, in fact, be discouraged from chewing any medication unless it is specifically formulated for that purpose.)

This list should not be considered all-inclusive. Generic and alternate brands of some products may exist. Tablets intended for sublingual or buccal administration (not included in this list) should also be administered only as intended, in an intact form.

DRUG	MANUFACTURER	FORM	DRUG	MANUFACTURER	FORM
AcipHex	Eisai	ec	Cardura XL	Pfizer	sr
Actoplus met XR	Takeda	sr	Cartia XT	Watson	sr
Adalat CC	Bayer Healthcare	sr	Cemill 500	Miller	sr
Adderall XR	Shire U.S.	sr	Cemill 1000	Miller	sr
Advicor	Abbott	sr	Certuss-D	Capellon	sr
Afeditab CR	Watson	sr	Chlorex-A	Cypress	sr
Aggrenox	Boehringer Ingelheim	sr	Chlor-Phen	Truxton	sr
Aleve Cold & Sinus	Bayer Healthcare	sr	Chlor-Trimeton Allergy	Schering Plough	sr
Aleve Sinus & Headache	Bayer Healthcare	sr	Cipro XR	Schering Plough	sr
Allegra-D 12 Hour	sanofi-aventis	sr	Clarinex-D 24 Hour	Schering Plough	sr
Allegra-D 24 Hour	sanofi-aventis	sr	Claritin-D	Schering	sr
Allerx	Cornerstone	sr	Claritin-D 12 Hour	Schering	sr
Allfen	MCR American	sr	Claritin-D 24 Hour	Schering	sr
Allfen-DM	MCR American	sr	Concerta	Ortho-McNeil-Janssen	sr
Alophen	Numark	ec	Contac 12-Hour	GlaxoSmithKline	sr
Altoprev	Watson	sr	Correctol	Schering Plough	ec
Ambien CR	sanofi-aventis	sr	Coreg CR	GlaxoSmithKline	sr
Ampyra ER	Acorda Therapeutics	sr	Covera-HS	Pfizer	sr
Amrix	Cephalon	sr	CPM 8/PE 20/MSC 1.25	Cypress	sr
Aplenzin	sanofi-aventis	sr	Creon 5	Solvay	ec
Apriso	Salix	sr	Creon 10	Solvay	ec
Arthrotec	Pfizer	ec	Creon 20	Solvay	ec
Asacol	Procter & Gamble	ec	Cymbalta	Eli Lilly	ec
Asacol HD	Procter & Gamble	ec	Dairycare	Plainview	ec
Ascriptin Enteric	Novartis Consumer	ec	Deconsal II	Cornerstone	sr
Augmentin XR	GlaxoSmithKline	sr	Deconex DM	Poly	sr
Avinza	King	sr	Depakote	Abbott	ec
Azulfidine Entabs	Pfizer	ec	Depakote ER	Abbott	sr
Bayer Aspirin Regimen	Bayer Healthcare	ec	Depakote Sprinkles	Abbott	ec
Biaxin XL	Abbott	sr	Despec SR	International Ethical	sr
Bidex-A	SJ Pharmaceuticals	sr	Detrol LA	Pfizer	sr
Blanex-A	Blansett	sr	Dexedrine Spansules	GlaxoSmithKline	sr
Bontril Slow-Release	Valeant	sr	Dexilant	Takeda	sr
Bromfed-PD	Victory	sr	Diamox Sequels	Duramed	sr
Bromfenex PD	Quality Care	sr	Dilacor XR	Watson	sr
Budeprion SR	Teva	sr	Dilantin	Pfizer	sr
Budeprion XL	Teva	sr	Dilantin Kapseals	Pfizer	sr
Buproban	Teva	sr	Dilatrate-SR	UCB	sr
Calan SR	Pfizer	sr	Diltia XT	Watson	sr
Campral	Forest	ec	Dilt-CD	Apotex	sr
Carbatrol	Shire U.S.	sr	Ditropan XL	Ortho-McNeil-Janssen	sr
Cardene SR	EKR Therapeutics	sr	Donnatal Extentabs	PBM	sr
Cardizem CD	Biovail	sr	Doryx	Warner Chilcott	ec
Cardizem LA	Abbott	sr	D-Phen 1000	Midlothian	sr

Enteric-coated = ec   Slow-released = sr

DRUG	MANUFACTURER	FORM	DRUG	MANUFACTURER	FORM
Dulcolax	Boehringer Ingelheim	ec	Iberet-Folic-500	Abbott	sr
Duomax	Capellon	sr	Icar-C Plus SR	Hawthorn	sr
Duratuss	Physicians Total Care	sr	Inderal LA	Akrimax	sr
Duratuss DA	Victory	sr	Indocin SR	Forte Pharma	sr
Dynacirc CR	GlaxoSmithKline	sr	Innopran XL	GlaxoSmithKline	sr
Dynex LA	Athlon	sr	Intuniv	Shire	sr
Dynex VR	Athlon	sr	Invega	Ortho-McNeil-Janssen	sr
Dytan-CS	Hawthorn	sr	Isochron	Forest	sr
Easprin	Rosedale	ec	Isoptin SR	Ranbaxy	sr
EC Naprosyn	Genentech	ec	Kadian	Actavis	sr
Ecotrin	GlaxoSmithKline	ec	Kapvay ER	Shionogi	sr
Ecotrin Adult Low Strength	GlaxoSmithKline	ec	Kaon-Cl 10	Savage	sr
			Keppra XR	UCB	sr
Ecotrin Maximum Strength	GlaxoSmithKline	ec	Klor-Con 8	Upsher-Smith	sr
			Klor-Con 10	Upsher-Smith	sr
Ecpirin	Prime Marketing	ec	Klor-Con M10	Upsher-Smith	sr
Ed A-Hist	Edwards	sr	Klor-Con M15	Upsher-Smith	sr
Effexor-XR	Wyeth	sr	Klor-Con M20	Upsher-Smith	sr
Embeda	King	sr	Kombiglyze ER	BMS/AztraZeneca	se
Enablex	Novartis	sr	K-Tab	Abbott	sr
Entercote	Global Source	ec	K-Tan	Prasco	sr
Entocort EC	Prometheus	ec	Lamictal XR	GlaxoSmithKline	sr
Equetro	Validus	sr	Lescol XL	Novartis	sr
ERYC	Warner Chilcott	sr	Levall G	Auriga	sr
Ery-Tab	Abbott	ec	Levbid	Alaven	sr
Exalgo	Mallinckrodt	sr	Levsinex	Alaven	sr
Extress-30	Key	sr	Lialda	Shire	ec
Extress-60	Key	sr	Lipram 4500	Global	ec
Feen-A-Mint	Schering Plough	ec	Lipram-PN10	Global	ec
Femilax	G & W	ec	Lipram-PN16	Global	ec
Fero-Folic-500	Abbott	sr	Lipram-PN20	Global	ec
Fero-Grad-500	Abbott	sr	Liquibid-D	Capellon	sr
Ferro-Sequels	Inverness Medical	sr	Liquibid-D 1200	Capellon	sr
Ferrous Fumarate DS	Vita-Rx	sr	Lithobid	Noven Therapeutics	sr
Fetrin	Lunsco	sr	Lohist-12	Larken	sr
Flagyl ER	Pharmacia	sr	Luvox CR	Jazz Pharmaceuticals	sr
Fleet Bisacodyl	Fleet, C.B.	ec	Mag Delay	Major	ec
Focalin XR	Novartis	sr	Mag64	Rising	ec
Folitab 500	Rising	sr	Mag-Tab SR	Niche	sr
Fortamet	Shionogi Pharma	sr	Maxifed	MCR American	sr
Fumatinic	Laser	sr	Maxifed DM	MCR American	sr
Genacote	Teva	ec	Maxifed DMX	MCR American	sr
GFN 600/ Phenylephrine 20	Cypress	sr	Maxifed-G	MCR American	sr
			Medent PE	SJ Pharmaceuticals	sr
Gilphex TR	Gil	sr	Mega-C	Merit	sr
Glucophage XR	Bristol-Myers Squibb	sr	Menopause Trio	Mason Vitamins	sr
Glucotrol XL	Pfizer	sr	Mestinon Timespan	Valeant	sr
Glumetza	Depomed	sr	Metadate CD	UCB	sr
Guaifenex GP	Ethex	sr	Metadate ER	UCB	sr
Guaifenex PSE 60	Ethex	sr	Methylin ER	Mallinckrodt	sr
Guaifenex PSE 80	Ethex	sr	Micro-K	Ther-Rx	sr
Guaifenex PSE 85	Ethex	sr	Micro-K 10	Ther-Rx	sr
Guaifenex PSE 120	Ethex	sr	Mild-C	Carlson, J.R.	sr
Halfprin	Kramer	ec	Mirapex ER	Boehringer Ingelheim	sr
Hemax	Pronova	sr	Moxatag	Victory	sr
Histacol LA	Breckenridge	sr	MS Contin	Purdue	sr
Iberet-500	Abbott	sr			

DRUG	MANUFACTURER	FORM	DRUG	MANUFACTURER	FORM
Mucinex	Reckitt Benckiser	sr	Pristiq	Wyeth	sr
Mucinex D	Reckitt Benckiser	sr	Procardia XL	Pfizer	sr
Mucinex DM	Reckitt Benckiser	sr	Prolex PD	Blansett	sr
Mydocs	Centurion	sr	Prolex-D	Blansett	sr
Myfortic	Novartis	ec	Proquin XR	Depomed	sr
Nalex-A	Blansett	sr	Protid	Lunsco	sr
Namenda XR	Forest	sr	Protonix	Wyeth	ec
Naprelan	Victory	sr	Prozac Weekly	Eli Lilly	ec
New Ami-Tex LA	Actavis	sr	Pseudocot-C	Truxton	sr
Nexium	AstraZeneca	ec	Pseudocot-G	Truxton	sr
Nexiclon XR	Next Wave	sr	Pseudovent DM	Ethex	sr
Niaspan	Abbott	sr	Ralix	Cypress	sr
Nifediac CC	Teva	sr	Ranexa	Gilead	sr
Nifedical XL	Teva	sr	Razadyne ER	Ortho-McNeil-Janssen	sr
Nitro-Time	Time-Cap	sr	Requip XL	GlaxoSmithKline	sr
Norel SR	U.S. Pharmaceutical	sr	Rescon-Jr	Capellon	sr
Norpace CR	Pfizer	sr	Respa-AR	Respa	sr
Obstetrix EC	Seyer Pharmatec	ec	Respa-BR	Respa	sr
Oleptro	LaboPharm	sr	Respaire-120 SR	Laser	sr
Opana ER	Endo	sr	Rhinacon A	Breckenridge	sr
Oramorph SR	Xanodyne	sr	Ritalin LA	Novartis	sr
Oracea	Galderma	sr	Ritalin-SR	Novartis	sr
Oxycontin	Purdue	sr	Rodex Forte	Legere	sr
Palcaps 10	Breckenridge	ec	Ru-Tuss	Carwin	sr
Palcaps 20	Breckenridge	ec	Rythmol SR	GlaxoSmithKline	sr
Pancreaze	Ortho-McNeil-Janssen	ec	Ryzolt	Purdue	sr
Pancrecarb MS-4	Digestive Care	ec	SAM-e	Pharmavite	ec
Pancrecarb MS-8	Digestive Care	ec	Sanctura XR	Allergan	sr
Pancrecarb MS-16	Digestive Care	ec	Seroquel XR	AstraZeneca	sr
Pangestyme CN-10	Ethex	ec	Simcor	Abbott	sr
Pangestyme CN-20	Ethex	ec	Sinemet CR	Bristol-Myers Squibb	sr
Pangestyme EC	Ethex	ec	Slo-Niacin	Upsher-Smith	sr
Pangestyme MT16	Ethex	ec	Slow Fe	Novartis Consumer	sr
Pangestyme UL12	Ethex	ec	Slow Fe With Folic Acid	Novartis Consumer	sr
Pangestyme UL18	Ethex	ec	Slow-Mag	Purdue	ec
Pangestyme UL20	Ethex	ec	Solodyn	Medicis	sr
Panocaps	Breckenridge	ec	St. Joseph Pain Reliever	McNeil Consumer	ec
Panocaps MT 16	Breckenridge	ec	Stahist	Magna	sr
Panocaps MT 20	Breckenridge	ec	Stavzor	Noven	sr
Paser	Jacobus	sr	Sudafed 12 Hour	McNeil Consumer	sr
Pavacot	Truxton	sr	Sudafed 24 Hour	McNeil Consumer	sr
Paxil CR	GlaxoSmithKline	sr	Sular	Shionogi Pharma	sr
PCE Dispertab	Abbott	sr	Sulfazine EC	Qualitest	ec
PCM LA	Cypress	sr	Symax Duotab	Capellon	sr
Pendex	Cypress	sr	Symax-SR	Capellon	sr
Pentasa	Shire U.S.	sr	Tarka	Abbott	sr
Pentoxil	Upsher-Smith	sr	Taztia XT	Watson	sr
Phenavent D	Ethex	sr	Tegretol-XR	Novartis	sr
Phenytek	Mylan	sr	Theo-24	UCB	sr
Phlemex-PE	Cypress	sr	Theochron	Carac	sr
Poly Hist Forte	Poly	sr	Theo-Time	Major	sr
Poly-Vent	Poly	sr	Tiazac	Forest	sr
Prehist D	Marnel	sr	Toprol XL	AstraZeneca	sr
Prevacid	Takeda	ec	Totalday	National Vitamin	sr
Prilosec	AstraZeneca	ec	Toviaz	Pfizer	sr
Prilosec OTC	Procter & Gamble	sr	Trental	sanofi-aventis	sr

DRUGS THAT SHOULD NOT BE CRUSHED

DRUG	MANUFACTURER	FORM	DRUG	MANUFACTURER	FORM
Treximet	GlaxoSmithKline	ec	Vospire ER	Dava	sr
Trilipix	Abbott	ec	Votrient	GlaxoSmithKline	ec
Tussicaps	Mallinckrodt	sr	Wellbutrin SR	GlaxoSmithKline	sr
Tylenol Arthritis	McNeil Consumer	sr	Wellbutrin XL	GlaxoSmithKline	sr
Ultram ER	Valeant	sr	Wobenzym N	Marlyn	ec
Urocit-K 5	Mission	sr	Xanax XR	Pfizer	sr
Urocit-K 10	Mission	sr	Xedec II	Cypress	sr
Uroxatral	sanofi-aventis	sr	Xpect-AT	Hawthorn	sr
Utira	Hawthorn	sr	Xpect-HC	Hawthorn	sr
Veracolate	Numark	ec	Xpect PE	Hawthorn	sr
Verelan	UCB	sr	Zenpep	Eurand	ec
Verelan PM	UCB	sr	Zmax	Pfizer	sr
Videx EC	Bristol-Myers Squibb	ec	Zyban	GlaxoSmithKline	sr
Vimovo	AstraZeneca	ec	Zyflo CR	Cornerstone	sr
Vivitrol	Alkermes	sr	Zyrtec-D	McNeil Consumer	sr
Voltaren-XR	Novartis	sr			

LACTOSE- AND GALACTOSE-FREE DRUGS

The following is a selection of lactose- and galactose-free products. The list is not comprehensive. Generic and alternate brands may exist. Always check product labeling for definitive information on specific ingredients.

TRADE NAME (OTC)	FORM	TRADE NAME (OTC)	FORM	TRADE NAME (OTC)	FORM
Advil	Tablets, Caplets, Gel Caplets, Liquigels	Dramamine Chewable	Tablets	Mylicon Infants'	Drops
		Elecare	Powder	Nepro	Liquid
Advil PM	Liquigels	Enfamil ProSobee	Liquid, Powder	Ocuvite Vitamin and Mineral Supplement	Tablets
Advil Cold and Sinus	Caplets, Liquigels	Ensure	Liquid, Powder	One-A-Day Cholesterol Plus	Tablets
		Ensure Bone Health	Liquid	One-A-Day Energy	Tablets
Aleve	Tablets	Ensure Clinical Strength	Liquid	One-A-Day Essential	Tablets
Aleve Smooth Gels	Gel Tablets	Ensure Fiber	Liquid	One-A-Day Gummies	Gummies
Alka-Mints	Tablets	Ensure High Calcium	Liquid	One-A-Day Maximum	Tablets
Alka-Seltzer	Effervescent Tablets	Ensure High Protein	Liquid	One-A-Day Men's	Tablets
Alka-Seltzer Plus Cold	Effervescent Tablets, Softgels	Ensure Immune Health	Liquid	One-A-Day Men's Health Formula	Tablets
		Ensure Muscle Health	Liquid		
Alka-Seltzer Plus Cherry Burst Formula	Effervescent Tablets	Ensure Plus	Liquid	One-A-Day Men's 50+ Advantage	Tablets
Alka-Seltzer Plus Cold and Cough Formula	Effervescent Tablets, Liquigels	Excedrin Extra-Strength	Caplets, Capsules, Tablets	One-A-Day Men's Pro Edge	Tablets
		Excedrin Migraine	Capsules, Tablets, Gel Tablets	One-A-Day Menopause Formula	Tablets
Alka-Seltzer Plus Day and Night Cold Formula	Effervescent Tablets, Liquigels	Excedrin Menstrual Complete	Capsules	One-A-Day Teen Advantage	Tablets
				One-A-Day Women's	Tablets
Alka-Seltzer Plus Flu Formula	Effervescent Tablets	Excedrin Tension Headache	Caplets, Capsules, Tablets	One-A-Day Women's 50+ Advantage	Tablets
Alka-Seltzer Plus Mucus and Congestion	Liquigels	Excedrin Back and Body	Caplets	One-A-Day Women's Active Mind & Body	Tablets
		Excedrin PM	Caplets, Gel Tablets		
Alka-Seltzer Plus Night Cold Formula	Effervescent Tablets, Liquigels	Ex-Lax Maximum Strength	Tablets	One-A-Day Women's Active Metabolism	Tablets
		Ex-Lax Regular Strength	Tablets		
Alka-Seltzer Plus Orange Zest Formula	Effervescent Tablets	Ex-Lax Regular Strength Chocolate	Chewable	One-A-Day Women's Prenatal	Tablets
				Pepto-Bismol	Suspension, Tablets
Alka-Seltzer Plus Sinus Formula	Effervescent Tablets	Fergon	Tablets		
		Gaviscon Regular Strength	Tablets	Pepto-Bismol Instacool Chewable	Tablets
Ascriptin	Tablets	Imodium A-D	Liquid, Tablets		
Axid	Tablets	Imodium A-D EZ Chews	Tablets	Pepto-Bismol Max. Strength	Suspension
Axid AR	Tablets	Imodium Multi Symptom Relief Chewable	Tablets		
Benadryl	Liquid			Pepto Children's Chewable	Tablets
Benadryl Allergy & Cold	Caplets	Jevity	Liquid	Percy Medicine	Suspension
Benadryl Dye-Free Allergy	Liquigels	Kaopectate Cherry	Liquid	Polycose	Liquid, Powder
Benadryl Allergy Ultratab	Tablets	Kaopectate Peppermint	Liquid	Portagen	Powder
Benadryl Quick Dissolve Strips	Oral Films	Kaopectate Advanced Formula	Suspension	Prilosec OTC	Tablets
				Promote	Liquid
Benadryl Allergy Kapgels	Capsules	Kaopectate Vanilla	Liquid	Promote with Fiber	Liquid
Benadryl D Allergy Plus Sinus	Tablets	Konsyl	Powder	Pulmocare	Liquid
Benadryl Allergy Plus Sinus	Caplets	Konsyl Bladder Control	Capsules	RCF	Liquid
Benadryl Severe Allergy Plus Sinus Headache	Caplets	Lactaid	Tablets	Simply Sleep	Caplets
		Lactaid Fast Act	Caplets, Chewables	St. Joseph Adult Low Strength Aspirin	Tablets
Benadryl Children's Perfect Measure	Liquid	MCT Oil	Oil		
		Medi-Lyte	Tablets	Sucrets Children's	Lozenges
Benadryl Children's Allergy	Liquid	Metamucil	Capsules, Powder, Wafers	Sucrets Complete	Lozenges
Benadryl Children's Dye-Free Allergy	Liquid	Motrin Children's	Suspension	Sucrets Cough	Lozenges
		Motrin IB	Tablets	Sucrets Herbal	Lozenges
Benadryl-D Children's Allergy and Sinus	Liquid	Motrin Infant's	Drops	Sucrets Liquid	Liquid
		Motrin Junior Strength	Caplets, Tablets	Sucrets Maximum Strength	Lozenges
Caltrate 600	Tablets				
Caltrate 600 PLUS	Tablets	Mylanta Children's	Tablets	Sudafed	Tablets
Caltrate 600+D	Softchews	Mylanta Gas Maximum Strength	Softgels	Sudafed 12 Hour	Tablets
Caltrate 600+D Plus Minerals	Tablets, Chewables			Sudafed 24 Hour	Tablets
		Mylanta Maximum Strength	Liquid	Sudafed Children's	Liquid
Claritin-D 24	Tablets	Mylanta Regular Strength	Liquid	Sudafed Congestion	Tablets
Claritin-D Reditabs	Tablets (disintegrating)	Mylanta Supreme	Liquid	Sudafed OM Sinus Congestion Spray	Liquid
		Mylanta Ultimate Strength	Liquid, Tablets		
Colace	Capsules				

A315

LACTOSE- AND GALACTOSE-FREE DRUGS

TRADE NAME (OTC)	FORM	TRADE NAME (Rx)	FORM	TRADE NAME (Rx)	FORM
Sudafed PE Cold and Cough	Caplets	Apriso	Capsule	Kapidex	Capsules
Sudafed PE Sinus & Allergy	Tablets	Aromasin	Tablets	Keppra	Solution, Tablets
		Augmentin Chewable	Tablets	K-Lor	Powder
Sudafed PE Day and Night Cold	Caplets	Augmentin ES 600	Powder	K-Phos Neutral	Tablets
		Augmentin XR	Tablets	K-Phos Original Formula	Tablets
Sudafed PE Day and Night Congestion	Tablets	Augmentin	Suspension, Tablets	K-Tab	Tablets
		Axid	Solution	Lamisil	Tablets, Oral Granules
Sudafed PE Congestion	Tablets	Bactrim	Tablets	Lescol XL	Tablets
Sudafed PE Non-Drying Sinus	Caplets	Bactrim DS	Tablets	Lescol	Capsules
Sudafed PE Pressure and Pain	Caplets	Biaxin Granules	Suspension	Levaquin	Solution, Tablets
		Biaxin Filmtab	Tablets	Levothroid	Tablets
Sudafed PE Severe Cold Formula	Caplets	Calan SR	Tablets	Levoxyl	Tablets
		Cambia	Solution	Lexapro	Solution, Tablets
Sudafed PE Pressure & Pain	Caplets	Carafate	Suspension, Tablets	Librium	Capsules
Sudafed PE Triple Action	Caplets	Cardizem CD	Capsules	Lomotil	Tablets
Sudafed Sinus & Allergy	Tablets	Cardizem LA	Tablets	Lopid	Tablets
Sudafed Triple Action	Caplets	Ceftin	Suspension, Tablets	Lysteda	Tablets
Titralac	Tablets	Cefzil	Suspension, Tablets	Malarone Pediatric	Tablets
Titralac Plus	Tablets	Cipro XR	Tablets	Malarone	Tablets
Tums	Tablets	Cipro	Suspension, Tablets	Maxzide	Tablets
Tums E-X 750	Tablets	Citranatal RX	Tablets	Methylin ER	Tablets
Tums E-X Sugar Free	Tablets	Clinoril	Tablets	Micardis	Tablets
Tums Kids	Tablets	Coartem	Tablets	Micro-K	Capsules
Tums Quik Pak	Powder	Combivir	Tablets	Micronase	Tablets
Tums Smoothies	Tablets	Comtan	Tablets	Minipress	Capsules
Tums Ultra 1000	Tablets	Covera-HS	Tablets	Minocin	Capsules
Tylenol	Tablets	Creon	Capsules	Moxatag	Tablets
Tylenol Children's Plus Cold	Liquid	Cytotec	Tablets	Niaspan	Tablets
Tylenol Children's Plus Cold & Allergy	Liquid	Daypro	Tablets	Norpramin	Tablets
		Demerol	Tablets	Norvasc	Tablets
Tylenol Children's Plus Cold & Cough	Liquid	Depakene	Capsules, Solution	Omnicef	Capsules, Suspension
Tylenol Children's Plus Cold & Stuffy Nose	Liquid	Depakote Sprinkle	Capsules		
		Depakote	Tablets	Onsolis	Buccal film
Tylenol Children's Plus Cough & Runny Nose	Liquid	Detrol LA	Capsules	Pamelor	Capsules
		Detrol	Tablets	Pamine Forte	Tablets
Tylenol Children's Plus Cough & Sore Throat	Liquid	DiaBeta	Tablets	Patanase	Liquid
		Diovan HCT	Tablets	Paxil	Suspension, Tablets
Tylenol Children's Plus Flu	Liquid	Diovan	Tablets	Pepcid	Suspension, Tablets
Tylenol Children's Plus Multi-Symptom Cold	Suspension	E.E.S.	Suspension, Tablets	Percocet	Tablets
		Edluar	Tablets	Percodan	Tablets
Tylenol Infants'	Drops	Embeda	Capsules	Plaquenil	Tablets
Tylenol Meltaways Jr.	Tablets	Entereg	Capsules	Pletal	Tablets
Unisom SleepTabs	Gels, Melts, Tablets	Epivir	Tablets, Solution	PrandiMet	Tablets
		Epivir-HBV	Tablets, Solution	Prandin	Tablets
Unisom PM Pain SleepCaps	Caplets	Ery-Tab	Tablets	Precose	Tablets
Zantac 75	Tablets	Esgic-Plus	Capsules, Tablets	Prevacid	Capsules
Zantac 150 Cool Mint	Tablets	Exelon	Capsules, Solution	Prinivil	Tablets
Zantac Maximum Strength 150	Tablets	Exforge HCT	Tablets	Pristiq	Tablets
		Exforge	Tablets	Procardia XL	Tablets
TRADE NAME (Rx)	**FORM**	Fibricor (fenofibric acid)	Tablets	Procardia	Capsules
Actigall	Capsules	Fioricet with Codeine	Capsules	Promacta	Tablets
Advicor	Tablets	Fioricet	Tablets	Prometrium	Capsules
Aldactazide	Tablets	Flomax	Capsules	Protonix	Suspension, Tablets
Aldactone	Tablets	Gleevec	Tablets	Prozac	Capsules
Allegra Children's Oral	Suspension	Glucotrol XL	Tablets	Qualaquin	Capsules
Allegra	Suspension, Tablets	Glucovance	Tablets	Questran Light	Powder
Allegra-D 12 Hr, 24 Hr	Tablets	Glyset	Tablets	Questran	Powder
Altace	Capsules	GoLYTELY	Powder	Rapaflo	Capsules
Amicar	Solution, Tablets	Grifulvin V	Suspension, Tablets	Remeron SolTab	Tablets
Amnesteem	Capsules	Inderal LA	Capsules	Rifadin	Capsules
Antivert	Tablets	Isoptin SR	Tablets	Robaxin	Tablets
Aplenzin	Tablets	Kaletra	Solution, Tablets	Ryzolt	Tablets

TRADE NAME (Rx)	FORM	TRADE NAME (Rx)	FORM	TRADE NAME (Rx)	FORM
Sabril	Solution, Tablets	Treanda	Powder	Votrient	Tablets
Saphris	Tablets	Trental	Tablets	Welchol	Tablets, Suspension
Sarafem	Tablets	Treximet	Tablets	Wellbutrin SR	Tablets
Savella	Tablets	Trileptal	Suspension, Tablets	Wellbutrin XL	Tablets
Sectral	Capsules	Trilipix	Capsules	Wellbutrin	Tablets
Sinemet CR	Tablets	Trizivir	Tablets	Xenical	Capsules
Sinemet	Tablets	Twynsta	Tablets	Zantac	Efferdose Tablets, Syrup, Tablets
Soma	Tablets	Tyvaso	Liquid		
Stalevo	Tablets	Uniphyl	Tablets	Zarontin	Capsules, Solution
Stavzor	Capsules	Urex	Tablets	Zebeta	Tablets
Sucraid	Solution	Valcyte	Tablets, Solution	Zenpep	Capsules
Tamiflu	Capsules, Suspension	Valtrex	Caplets	Zestril	Tablets
		Valturna	Tablets	Ziac	Tablets
Tegretol/Tegretol-XR	Suspension, Tablets	Vibramycin Hyclate	Capsules, Suspension	Ziagen	Solution, Tablets
				Zipsor	Capsules
Tenoretic	Tablets	Vicodin ES	Tablets	Zofran	Solution, Tablets (disintegrating)
Tenormin	Tablets	Vicodin HP	Tablets		
Tessalon	Capsules	Vicodin	Tablets	Zoloft	Oral Concentrate, Tablets
Tiazac	Capsules	Vicoprofen	Tablets		
Ticlid	Tablets	Videx EC	Capsules, Delayed Release	Zonegran	Capsules
Tikosyn	Capsules			Zyban	Tablets
Tofranil-PM	Capsules	Vimpat	Tablets, Solution	Zyvox	Suspension, Tablets
Tofranil	Tablets	Visicol	Tablets		
Toprol-XL	Tablets	Vistaril	Capsules		

POISON ANTIDOTE CHART

WARNING: While every effort has been made to ensure the accuracy of this chart, it is not intended to serve as the sole source of information on antidotes. Guidelines may need to be adjusted based on factors such as anticipated usage in the hospital's local area, the nearest alternate sources of antidotes, and distance to tertiary care institutions. Contact your nearest regional poison control center (1-800-222-1222) for treatment information regarding any exposure, including indications for use of antidote therapy. Directions in this chart assume that all basic life support and decontamination measures have been initiated as needed.

ANTIDOTE	POISON/DRUG/TOXIN	SUGGESTED MINIMUM STOCK QUANTITY	RATIONALE/COMMENTS
N-Acetylcysteine [NAC] (Mucomyst®, Acetadote®)	Acetaminophen Carbon tetrachloride Other hepatotoxins	IV: 150 mL Acetadote PO: 8 x 30 mL of 20% NAC This would be enough to treat one 100 kg patient x 24 hours	Acetaminophen is the most common drug involved in intentional and unintentional poisonings. 600 mL (120 g) of the oral product provides enough to treat 3 adults for 24 h. Several vials may be stocked in the ED to provide a loading dose and the remaining vials in the pharmacy for the q 4 h maintenance doses. 150 mL (30 g) of IV product will treat 1 100 kg adult patient for an entire 21-hour IV protocol. Note: While controversial, IV NAC may be preferable in patients who have hepatic encephalopathy or are pregnant.
Amyl nitrite, sodium nitrite and sodium thiosulfate (Cyanide antidote kit)	Acetonitrile Acrylonitrile Bromates (thiosulfate only) Chlorates (thiosulfate only) Cyanide (e.g., HCN, KCN and NaCN) Cyanogen chloride Cyanogenic glycoside natural sources (e.g., apricot pits and peach pits) Hydrogen sulfide (nitrites only) Laetrile Mustard agents (thiosulfate only) Nitroprusside (thiosulfate only) Smoke inhalation (combustion of synthetic materials)	1 to 2 kits Each kit contains: 12x 0.3 mL amyl nitrite ampules 2 vials 3% sodium nitrite, 10 mL each 2 vials 25% sodium thiosulfate, 50 mL each	Stock 1 kit in the ED. Consider also stocking 1 kit in the pharmacy. Note: This kit has a short shelf life of 24 months. Stocking this kit may be unnecessary if an adequate supply of hydroxocobalamin HCl is available. Significant adverse reactions include methemoglobinemia and hypotension. For smoke inhalation victims, thiosulfate, without the use of nitrites, may be considered.
Antivenin, *Crotalidae* Polyvalent (Equine Origin)	Pit viper envenomation (e.g., rattlesnakes, cottonmouths, and copperheads)	None	As of March 31, 2007, this product is no longer available from the manufacturer. However, some supplies may still be available. See Antivenin, *Crotalidae* Polyvalent Immune Fab–Ovine in this chart.

(Continued)

This chart is adapted from material furnished by the Illinois Poison Center, a program of the Metropolitan Chicago Healthcare Council (MCHC).

POISON ANTIDOTE CHART

ANTIDOTE	POISON/DRUG/TOXIN	SUGGESTED MINIMUM STOCK QUANTITY	RATIONALE/COMMENTS
Antivenin, *Crotalidae* Polyvalent Fab–Ovine® (CroFab)	Pit viper envenomation (e.g., rattlesnakes, cottonmouths, and copperheads)	12-18 vials	Advised in geographic areas with endemic populations of copperhead, water moccasin, eastern massasauga, or timber rattlesnake. In low-risk areas, know nearest alternate source of antivenin. This product has a lower risk of hypersensitivity reaction than previously marketed equine product. Average dose in premarketing trials was 12 vials but more may be needed. 12 vials will cover 8 hours of treatment, while 18 vials will cover 24 hours of treatment. Stock in pharmacy. Store in refrigerator. Equine product is no longer available after March 31, 2007.
Antivenin, *Latrodectus mactans* (Black widow spider)	Black widow spider envenomation	0 to 1 vial	This product is only used for severe envenomations. Antivenin must be given in a critical care setting since it is an equine-derived product which may cause anaphylaxis. Stock in pharmacy. Product must be refrigerated at all times. Know the nearest source of antidote.
Atropine sulfate	Alpha₂ agonists (e.g., clonidine, guanabenz and guanfacine) Alzheimer drugs (e.g., donepezil, galantamine, rivastigmine, tacrine) Antimyesthenic agents (e.g., pyridostigmine) Bradyarrhythmia-producing agents (e.g., beta blockers, calcium channel blockers and digitalis glycosides) Cholinergic agonists (e.g., bethanechol) Muscarine-containing mushrooms (e.g., Clitocybe and Inocybe) Nerve agents (e.g., sarin, soman, tabun and VX) Organophosphate and carbamate insecticides	175 mg or greater Available in various formulations: 0.4 mg/mL (1 mL, 0.4 mg ampules) 0.4 mg/mL (20 mL, 8 mg vials) 0.1 mg/mL (10 mL, 1 mg ampules) Atropine Sulfate military-style auto-injectors: (Atropen®): 2mg/0.7 mL, 1 mg/0.7 mL, 0.5 mg/0.7 mL, 0.25 mg/0.3 mL Atropine Sulfate 2.1 mg/0.7 mL with Pralidoxime Chloride 600 mg/2 mL (DuoDote®)	The product should be immediately available in the ED. Some also may be stored in the pharmacy or other hospital sites, but should be easily mobilized if a severely poisoned patient needs treatment. Note: Product is necessary to be adequately prepared for WMD incidents; the suggested amount may not be sufficient for mass casualty events. Auto-injectors are available from Bound Tree Medical, Inc. Drug stocked in chempack containers is intended only for use in mass casualty events.
Botulinum antitoxin As of March 13, 2010, the only botulinum antitoxin available is HBAT (heptavalent types A-G). This product replaces bivalent antitoxins type AB and antitoxin type E. Baby Botulism Immune Globulin (BIG)	Food-borne botulism Wound botulism Botulism as a biological weapon Note: Heptavalent antitoxin not currently recommended for infant botulism	None. Product is stored at 9 CDC regional centers (including the Chicago Quarantine). To obtain antitoxin, hospitals must call the Illinois Department of Public Health which contacts the CDC in Atlanta. The CDC emergency operation center can be reached at 770-488-7100.	Antitoxin must be given in a critical care setting since it is an equine-derived product. Note: Product must be refrigerated at all times. Heptavalent antitoxin is stored in the CDC SNS. BabyBIG is available for infant botulism types A and B, through the Infant Botulism Treatment and Prevention Program, sponsored by the California Department of Public Health, telephone: 510-231-7600, http://www.infantbotulism.org/physician/obtain.php

(Continued)

ANTIDOTE	POISON/DRUG/TOXIN	SUGGESTED MINIMUM STOCK QUANTITY	RATIONALE/COMMENTS
Calcium disodium EDTA (Versenate®)	Lead Zinc salts (e.g., zinc chloride)	2x 5 mL amp (200 mg/mL)	One vial provides 1 day of therapy for a child. 2 to 4 g per 24 hours may be necessary in adult patients. Stock in pharmacy. Important note: Edetate disodium (Endrate®) is not the same as calcium disodium EDTA, and is used primarily as an IV chelator for emergent treatment of hypercalcemia, etc.
Calcium chloride and Calcium gluconate	Calcium channel blockers Fluoride salts (e.g., NaF) Hydrofluoric acid (HF) Hyperkalemia (not digoxin-induced) Hypermagnesemia	10% calcium chloride: 10x 10 mL vials 10% calcium gluconate: 30x 10 mL vials	Many ampules of calcium chloride may be necessary in life-threatening calcium channel blocker or HF poisoning. Stock in ED. More may be stocked in pharmacy. The chloride salt provides 3 x more calcium than the gluconate salt. Calcium chloride is very irritating and administration through a central line is preferable. Topical calcium gluconate or carbonate gels may be extemporaneously prepared by the pharmacy. Calgonate® (calcium gluconate 2.5% gel) is not FDA approved but is manufactured in an FDA-GMP approved facility and is distributed by Calgonate Corp in Port St. Lucie, Florida.
Deferoxamine mesylate (Desferal®)	Iron	12-36g (Available in 500 mg and 2g vials)	Quantity recommended supplies 8 to 24 hours of therapy for a 100 kg adult. Per package insert, the maximum daily dose is 6 g (12 vials). However, this dose may be exceeded in serious acute iron poisonings. Stock in pharmacy.
Digoxin immune Fab (Digibind®, DigiFab®)	Cardiac glycoside-containing plants (e.g., foxglove and oleander) Digitoxin Digoxin	15 vials Each vial (38 mg) neutralizes 0.5 mg of digoxin	An initial dose of 2-3 vials for chronic poisoning or 10 vials for acute poisoning may be given to a digoxin-poisoned patient in whom the digoxin level is unknown. More may be necessary in severe intoxications. 15 vials would effectively neutralize a steady-state digoxin level of 15 ng/mL in a 100 kg patient. Know nearest source of additional supply. Stock in ED or pharmacy.
Dimercaprol (BAL in oil)	Arsenic Copper Gold Lead Lewisite Mercury	2x 3 mL ampules (100 mg/mL)	This amount provides 2 doses of 3 to 5 mg/kg/dose given q 4 h to treat 1 seriously poisoned adult or provides enough to treat a 15 kg child for 24 h. Stock in pharmacy.
DMPS (2,3-dimercaptopropanol-sulfonic acid, Dimaval®, Unithiol)	Arsenic Bismuth Lead Mercury	None (Available as 50 mg/mL vials from McGuff Pharmacy)	DMPS is a water soluble analog of BAL. Unlike BAL, it does not have a potential risk of redistributing metals to the CNS. Also has a more favorable side effect profile, though further study is needed to fully elucidate advantages/disadvantages compared to other chelators.

(Continued)

ANTIDOTE	POISON/DRUG/TOXIN	SUGGESTED MINIMUM STOCK QUANTITY	RATIONALE/COMMENTS
Ethanol	Ethylene glycol Methanol	Consider stocking 180-360g in the form of 95% ethanol or equivalents. 10% alcohol in D_5W was discontinued in 2004; 5% alcohol in D_5W was discontinued in 2007. However, 10% alcohol can be prepared from dehydrated alcohol and D_5W. Consult PCC.	180 g provides loading and maintenance doses for a 100 kg adult for 8-24 h. More alcohol or fomepizole will be needed during dialysis or prolonged treatment. 95% or 40% alcohol diluted in juice may be given PO if IV alcohol is unavailable. Stock in pharmacy. Note: Ethanol is unnecessary if adequate amounts of fomepizole are stocked. See also fomepizole in this chart. May cause hypotension or metabolic abnormalities (e.g. hypoglycemia) esp. in pediatric patients.
Fat emulsion (Intralipid®, Liposyn II®, Liposyn III®)	Local anesthetics and possibly other cardiac toxins (e.g., bupropion, calcium channel blockers, cocaine, beta blockers, tricyclic antidepressants)	Quantity determined by institution. Available in 100 mL of 20% emulsion.	Fat emulsion is an experimental therapy showing promise in the reverse of cardiac toxicity induced by local anesthetics and other cardiac toxins. The evidence for the efficacy of fat emulsion therapy is solely based on animal studies and human case reports, and its safety has not yet been established. Consultation with a regional PCC toxicologist is advised. Initial dose: 1.5 mL/kg IV over 1 minute. Follow with infusion of 0.25 mL/kg/min over 30 minutes. Loading dose may be repeated once. Rate may be increased to 0.5 mL/kg/min for 60 minutes if blood pressure drops. Maximum total dose is 8 mL/kg. Consider storage in pharmacy, ED, and possibly surgical units.
Flumazenil (Romazicon®)	Benzodiazepines Zaleplon Zolpidem	Total 6-12 mg Available in 5 and 10 mL vials (0.1 mg/mL)	Due to risk of seizures, use with extreme caution, if at all, in poisoned patients. More may be stocked in the pharmacy for use in reversal of conscious sedation. Stock in ED, pharmacy, and any unit where procedural sedation is performed.
Folic acid and Folinic acid (Leucovorin)	Formaldehyde/Formic Acid Methanol Methotrexate, trimetrexate Pyrimethamine Trimethoprim	Folic acid: 3x 50 mg vials Folinic acid: 1x 50 mg vial	For adjunctive treatment of methanol-poisoned patients with an acidosis, give 50 mg folinic acid initially, then 50 mg of folic acid q 4 h for 6 doses. For methotrexate poisoned patients administer folinic acid only. Stock in pharmacy.
Fomepizole (Antizol®) 4-methylpyrazole (4-MP)	Ethylene glycol Methanol	1 to 2x 1.5 g vials Note: Available in a kit of 4x 1.5 g vials	One 1.5 g vial provides an initial dose of 15 mg/kg/12 h to an adult weighing up to 100 kg. Hospitals with critical care and hemodialysis capabilities should consider stocking 1 kit of 4 vials or more. More frequent dosing (i.e., every 4 h) is required if the patient is dialyzed. Note: Product has a 2-year

(Continued)

ANTIDOTE	POISON/DRUG/TOXIN	SUGGESTED MINIMUM STOCK QUANTITY	RATIONALE/COMMENTS
Fomepizole (Antizol®) 4-methylpyrazole (4-MP) *(continued)*			shelf life; however, the manufacturer offers a credit for unused, expired product. Ethanol is unnecessary if adequate supply of fomepizole is stocked. Fomepizole is preferred to ethanol because of ease of use, fewer adverse effects, simplicity of dosing, less need for close monitoring. Stock in pharmacy. Know where nearest alternate supply is located.
Glucagon HCl	Beta blockers Calcium channel blockers Hypoglycemia Hypoglycemic agents	50 to 90x 1 mg vials	This quantity provides 4 to 8 hours of maximum dosing, i.e., a 10 mg IV bolus dose followed by 10 mg/h. More may be necessary. Know where nearest alternate supply is located. Stock 30 mg in ED and remainder in pharmacy.
Hydroxocobalamin HCl (Cyanokit®)	Acetonitrile Acrylonitrile Cyanide (e.g., HCN, KCN and NaCN) Cyanogen chloride Cyanogenic glycoside natural sources (e.g., apricot pits and peach pits) Laetrile Nitroprusside Smoke inhalation (combustion of synthetic materials)	2 to 4 kits Each kit contains 2x 2.5 g vials Note: Diluent is not included in the kit.	Seriously poisoned cyanide patients may require 5 to 10 grams (1 or 2 kits). Stock 2 kits in ED. Consider also stocking 2 kits in the pharmacy. The product has a shelf-life of 30 months post-manufacture.
Hyperbaric oxygen (HBO)	Carbon monoxide and possibly the following: Carbon tetrachloride Cyanide Hydrogen sulfide Methemoglobinemia	Post the location and phone number of nearest HBO chamber in the ED.	Consult PPC to determine if HBO treatment is indicated.
Insulin and dextrose	Calcium channel blockers (diltiazem, nifedipine, verapamil) and possibly beta blockers	Quantity determined by institution. Humulin R is available as 100 units/mL in a 1.5 mL cartridge and 10 mL bottle. Dextrose 50% in water is available in 50 mL ampules and syringes. Dextrose 25% is available in 10 mL vials and syringes for pediatric use.	High dose insulin and dextrose therapy has reversed cardiovascular toxicity associated with calcium channel blocker overdose. Begin with 10 units to 1 unit/kg regular insulin IV bolus (with 1 amp D_{50}), then start a drip at 0.5 units/kg/h (consider addition of D_{10} drip with insulin drip) and titrate upward until hypotension improves. Stock in ED and pharmacy.
Methylene blue	Methemoglobin-inducing agents including: Aniline dyes Dapsone Dinitrophenol Local anesthetics (e.g., benzocaine) Metoclopramide Monomethylhydrazine-containing mushrooms (e.g., Gyromitra) Naphthalene Nitrates and nitrites Nitrobenzene Phenazopyridine	6x 10 mL ampules (10 mg/mL)	The usual dose is 1 to 2 mg/kg IV (0.1 to 0.2mL/kg). A second dose may be given in 1 hour. More may be necessary. 6 ampules provides 3 doses of 2 mg/kg for a 100 kg adult. Stock in pharmacy.

(Continued)

POISON ANTIDOTE CHART

ANTIDOTE	POISON/DRUG/TOXIN	SUGGESTED MINIMUM STOCK QUANTITY	RATIONALE/COMMENTS
Naloxone (Narcan®)	Alpha$_2$ agonists (e.g., clonidine, guanabenz and guanfacine) Unknown poisoning with mental status depression Opioids (e.g., codeine, diphenoxylate, fentanyl, heroin, meperidine, morphine and propoxyphene)	Naloxone: total 40 mg, any combination of 0.4 mg, 1 mg and 2 mg ampules	Stock 20 mg naloxone in the ED and 20 mg elsewhere in the institution. Note: Nalmefene (Revex), a longer-acting opioid antagonist, was discontinued by the manufacturer in July 2008.
Octreotide acetate (Sandostatin®)	Sulfonylurea hypoglycemic agents (e.g., glipizide, glyburide)	225 mcg Available in 1 mL ampules (0.05 mg/mL, 0.1 mg/mL, and 0.5 mg/mL) and 5 mL multidose vials (0.2 and 1 mg/mL).	Octreotide acetate blocks the release of insulin from pancreatic beta cells that along with IV dextrose can reverse sulfonylurea-induced hypoglycemia. The usual adult dose is 50 to 100 mcg IV or SC q 6 to 12 h. The usual pediatric dose is 1 to 1.5 mcg/kg IV or SC q 6 to 12 h. 225 mcg provides 4x 75 mcg adult doses. Stock in pharmacy.
D-Penicillamine (Cuprimine®)	Arsenic Copper Lead Mercury	None required as an antidote. Available in bottles of 100 capsules (125 mg or 250 mg/capsule)	D-Penicillamine is no longer considered the drug of choice for heavy metal poisonings. It may be stocked in the pharmacy for other indications such as Wilson's disease or rheumatoid arthritis.
Physostigmine salicylate (Antilirium®)	Anticholinergic alkaloid-containing plants (e.g., deadly nightshade and jimson weed) Antihistamines Atropine and other anticholinergic agents	2x 2 mL ampules (1 mg/mL)	Usual adult dose is 1 to 2 mg slow IV push. Note: Duration of effect is 30 to 60 min. Stock in ED or pharmacy.
Phytonadione (Vitamin K$_1$) (AquaMEPHYTON®, Mephyton®)	Indandione derivatives Long-acting anticoagulant rodenticides (e.g., brodifacoum and bromadiolone) Warfarin	100 mg injectable; 100 mg oral. Available as: 0.5 mL ampules (2 mg/mL) and 1 mL ampules (10 mg/mL) 5 mg tablets in packages of 10, 12, and 100	Patients who are poisoned by long-acting anticoagulant rodenticides may require 50 to 100 mg/day or more for weeks to months to maintain normal INRs. An oral suspension for pediatric patients may be extemporaneously prepared by the pharmacy. Stock in pharmacy.
Pralidoxime chloride (2-PAM) (Protopam®)	Organophospate insecticides (OPI) Nerve agents (e.g., sarin, soman, tabun and VX) And possibly: Antimyasthenic agents (e.g., pyridostigmine) Tacrine	18x 1 g vials. Also available as: Pralidoxime chloride military-style auto-injectors: 600 mg/2 mL Atropine Sulfate 2.1mg/0.7mL with Pralidoxime Chloride 600mg/2mL (DuoDote®)	18 g provides an adult dose of 750 mg/h for 24 h. More may be needed in severe poisoning. Health-care facilities located in agricultural areas where OPIs are used should maintain adequate supplies. Product is necessary to be adequately prepared for WMD incidents; the suggested amount may not be sufficient for mass casualty events. Auto-injectors are available from Bound Tree Medical, Inc. The drugs stocked in chempack containers is intended for use in mass casualty events only. Stock in ED or pharmacy.

(Continued)

ANTIDOTE	POISON/DRUG/TOXIN	SUGGESTED MINIMUM STOCK QUANTITY	RATIONALE/COMMENTS
Protamine sulfate	Heparin Low molecular weight heparins (e.g., enoxaparin, dalteparin, tinzaparin)	Variable, consider recommendation of hospital P&T Committee Available as 5 mL ampules (10 mg/mL) and 25 mL vials (250 mg/25 mL)	The usual dose is 1 to 1.5 mg for each 100 units of heparin. Stock in pharmacy in refrigerator. Preservative-free formulation does not require refrigeration.
Pyridoxine hydrochloride (Vitamin B$_6$)	Acrylamide Ethylene glycol Hydrazine Hydrazine MAOIs (isocarboxazid, phenelzine) Isoniazid (INH) Monomethylhydrazine-containing mushrooms (e.g., Gyromitra)	10 g (100 vials) Available as 1 mL vials (100 mg/mL)	Usual dose is 1 g pyridoxine HCl for each g of INH ingested. If amount ingested is unknown, give 5 g of pyridoxine. Repeat 5 g dose if seizures are uncontrolled. More may be necessary. Know nearest source of additional supply. For ethylene glycol, a dose of 100 mg/day may enhance the clearance of toxic metabolite. Stock in ED or pharmacy.
Silibinin (Legalon-SIL®)	Cyclopeptide-containing mushrooms (e.g., Amanita phalloides, Amanita verna, Amanita virosa, Galerina atumnalis, Lepiota josserandi, and others)	None. 350 mg/vial	Silibinin is a water-soluble preparation of silymarin; a flavolignone extracted from the milk thistle plant. It inhibits uptake of cyclopeptides in hepatocytes. These hepatotoxins are responsible for high morbidity and mortality following ingestion of these mushrooms. Silibinin is manufactured by Madaus, Inc. in Germany, and has been widely used in Europe since 1984. The initial adult loading dose consists of a 1 h infusion of 5 mg/kg followed by the recommended daily dosage of 20 mg/kg via continuous IV infusion. Product is now available in the U.S. under an open-treatment IND. Physicians can obtain the product free-of-charge by contacting the primary investigator at 866-520-4412.
Sodium bicarbonate	Chlorine gas Hyperkalemia Serum alkalinization: Agents producing a quinidine-like effect as noted by widened QRS complex on EKG (e.g., amantadine, carbamazepine, chloroquine, cocaine, diphenhydramine, flecainide, propafenone, propoxyphene, tricyclic antidepressants, quinidine and related agents) Urine alkalinization: Weakly acidic agents (e.g., chlorophenoxy herbicides, chlorpropamide, methotrexate, phenobarbital, and salicylates)	20 to 25x 50 mL vials of either 8.4% (50 mEq/50 mL) or 7.5% (44 mEq/50 mL) Consider stocking 4.2% (5 mEq/10 mL) for pediatric patients.	Stock 20 vials in ED and remainder in pharmacy Nebulized 2.5-5% sodium bicarbonate has been demonstrated in anecdotal case reports to provide symptomatic relief for chlorine gas inhalation.

(Continued)

ANTIDOTE	POISON/DRUG/TOXIN	SUGGESTED MINIMUM STOCK QUANTITY	RATIONALE/COMMENTS
Succimer (Chemet®) Dimercaptosuccinic acid (DMSA)	Arsenic Lead Lewisite Mercury	0 to 10 capsules Available in bottles of 100 capsules (100 mg/capsule)	Initial treatment of severely symptomatic heavy metal poisoning consists of parenterally administered chelators, e.g., BAL, Ca Na₂EDTA. Patients who markedly improve may eventually be started on oral DMSA. Asymptomatic or minimally symptomatic patients do not require parenteral therapy and are often treated as outpatients with an oral chelator. FDA approved only for pediatric lead poisoning, however it has shown efficacy for other heavy metal poisonings. 10 capsules represent an initial dose of 10 mg/kg in a 100 kg adult. Stock in pharmacy.

ADJUNCTIVE AGENTS

ADJUNCTIVE AGENT	POISON/DRUG/TOXIN	SUGGESTED MINIMUM STOCK QUANTITY	RATIONALE/COMMENTS
Benztropine mesylate (Cogentin®)	Medications causing a dystonic reaction or other EPS	Quantity determined by institution. Available in tablets of 0.5 mg, 1 mg, 2 mg (Bottles of 100 or 1,000) and in 2 mg/mL injectable ampules.	Maximum daily adult dose is 6 mg/d. Stock some in ED and some in pharmacy. See diphenhydramine also.
Bromocriptine mesylate (Parlodel®)	Medications causing NMS	Quantity determined by institution. Available in 2.5 mg tablets or 5 mg capsules (Bottles of 30 or 100).	Dose for NMS is 2.5 to 10 mg every 6 to 8 hours. Bromocriptine is a centrally acting dopamine agonist that reverses excessive dopamine blockade. Use with caution as this may worsen serotonin syndrome. Stock in pharmacy.
Centruroides Immune F(ab)₂ – Equine (Anascorp®)	Scorpion envenomation by *Centruroides sculpturatus*, the most venomous scorpion in the U.S. Note: It is found in southeastern California, Arizona, Nevada, southern Utah, and southwestern New Mexico.	None	This product is manufactured in Mexico by the Instituto Bioclon. In the U.S., it is marketed by Rare Disease Therapeutics, Inc. in Nashville, Tennessee. It is not FDA approved; however, it is available as an investigational new drug. Currently, the product is distributed to zoos and venom banks only. Usual dose: 1 to 3 vials.
L-Carnitine (Carnitor®)	Valproic acid	Quantity determined by institution. Available as 330 mg and 500 mg tablets, 250 mg and 300 mg capsules, 200 mg/mL IV solution and 100 mg/mL PO solution.	L-Carnitine may be considered in valproate intoxication associated with elevated serum ammonia levels and/or hepatotoxicity. Doses of 100 mg/kg/d up to 2 grams a day PO divided into 3 doses, or 150-500 mg/kg/d IV (maximum 3 grams daily) in 3 or 4 divided doses are recommended for a period of 3 to 4 days or until clinical improvement. Stock in pharmacy.
Cyproheptadine HCl (Periactin®)	Medications causing serotonin syndrome	Quantity determined by institution. Available in 4 mg tablets (Bottles of 100, 250, 500 and 1,000) and 2 mg/5 mL PO solution.	Cyproheptadine HCl is a nonspecific 5-HT antagonist that has been used in the treatment of serotonin syndrome. Adult dose is 4 to 8 mg PO repeated every 1 to 4 h until therapeutic effect is observed or maximum of 32 mg administered. Stock in pharmacy.

(Continued)

ADJUNCTIVE AGENT	POISON/DRUG/TOXIN	SUGGESTED MINIMUM STOCK QUANTITY	RATIONALE/COMMENTS
Dantrolene sodium (Dantrium®)	Medications causing NMS Medications causing malignant hyperthermia	Quantity determined by institution. Available in 25, 50 and 100 mg capsules (Bottles of 100 or 500) and injectable 20 mg/vial form.	The recommended dose for NMS is 1 mg/kg IV; may repeat as needed every 5 to 10 minutes for a maximum of 10 mg/kg. Dantrolene sodium inhibits calcium release from the sarcoplasmic reticulum of skeletal muscle and thereby reduces rigidity. Stock in pharmacy. Any hospital using inhalational anesthetics should strongly consider stocking dantrolene for treatment of malignant hyperthermia.
Diazepam (Valium®)	Chloroquine and related antimalarial drugs NMS Serotonin syndrome Severe agitation from any toxic exposure/overdose (e.g. cocaine, PCP, methamphetamine)	Quantity determined by institution. Available as 5 mg/mL injectables in 2mL Ampules, 2 mL disposable syringes, and 10 mL multidose vials. Diazepam military-style auto-injectors for nerve agent-induced seizures: 10 mg/2 mL.	Diazepam is used in conjunction with epinephrine for patients with chloroquine toxicity (seizures, dysrhythmias, hypotension) or if the amount ingested is more than 5 g. Intravenous loading dose of 2 mg/kg over 30 minutes. Maintenance dose of 1 to 2 mg/kg per day for 2 to 4 days. Diazepam and other benzodiazepines are also used in poisoned and nonpoisoned patients as an anticonvulsant, muscle relaxant, and antianxiety agent. They are usually the first-line therapy for drug-induced agitation, tachycardia, and hypertension. Benzodiazepines are a mainstay in the treatment of NMS and serotonin syndrome. Stock in ED and pharmacy. Adequate supply is necessary to be prepared for WMD incidents. Auto-injectors are available from Bound Tree Medical, Inc.
Diphenhydramine HCL (Benadryl®)	Medications causing a dystonic reaction or other EPS	Quantity determined by institution. Available in 25 and 50 mg capsules (Bottles of 30, 100 or 1,000). Also in oral liquid formulation of 12.5 mg/5mL (4 ounce bottle) and 50 mg/mL injectable syringes.	In addition to its use as an anticholinergic agent, diphenhydramine is a widely used antihistamine in the management of minor or severe allergic reactions. Stock in ED and pharmacy.
Glycopyrrolate Bromide (Robinul®)	OPIs Nerve agents	Quantity determined by institution. Available as 0.2 mg/mL in vials of 1 mL, 2 mL, 5 mL, and 20 mL.	The dose of glycopyrrolate for OPI poisoning is 0.01 to 0.02 mg/kg IV. Glycopyrrolate is a quarternary ammonium antimuscarinic agent which may assist in the control of hypersecretions caused by acetylcholinesterase inhibition. This agent produces less tachycardia and CNS effects than atropine. Stock in ED and pharmacy.

(Continued)

POISON ANTIDOTE CHART

ADJUNCTIVE AGENT	POISON/DRUG/TOXIN	SUGGESTED MINIMUM STOCK QUANTITY	RATIONALE/COMMENTS
Phentolamine mesylate (Regitine®)	Catecholamine extravasation Intradigital epinephrine injection	Quantity determined by institution. Available as a 5 mg/vial powder with 1 mL diluent.	Phentolamine is an alpha adrenergic antagonist which will reverse vasoconstriction and peripheral ischemia associated with extravasation of adrenergic agents. When phentolamine is not available, consider using subcutaneous terbutaline sulfate (Brethine®). Phentolamine also offers an additional option in the management of drug-induced hypertension. Stock in ED and pharmacy.
Sodium nitrite	Hydrogen sulfide (H₂S)	0 to 1 vial. Available as 3% sodium nitrite in 10 mL vial.	Nitrite therapy for H₂S poisoning is controversial. Seriously poisoned patients should receive nitrites within 1 hour of exposure. Sodium thiosulfate is not administered in H₂S poisoning. The product is available from Hope Pharmaceuticals in Scottsdale, Arizona. If the amyl nitrite/sodium nitrite/sodium thiosulfate CN antidote kits are stocked, additional sodium nitrite vials may not be necessary. Stock in pharmacy.
Sodium thiosulfate	Bromates Chlorates Mustard agents Nitroprusside Smoke inhalation	Quantity determined by institution. Available in 100 mg/mL, 10 mL vials and 250 mg/mL, 50 mL vials.	Sodium thiosulfate (without nitrites) has been advocated in the treatment of smoke inhalation related to CN exposure; however, it would not be necessary if hydroxocobalamin is available. Sodium thiosulfate may be used in conjunction with cisplatin to reduce toxicity of this chemotherapy agent. Sodium thiosulfate is found in the amyl nitrite/sodium nitrite/sodium thiosulfate CN antidote kits; however, additional vials may be stocked. Stock in pharmacy.
Thiamine	Ethanol Ethylene glycol	Quantity determined by institution. Available as 100 mg/mL in 2 mL vials.	Parenteral thiamine precedes IV dextrose in patients with chronic ethanol abuse. Thiamine 100 mg every 6 hours enhances clearance of toxic metabolites of ethylene glycol. Stock in ED and pharmacy.
AGENTS FOR RADIOLOGICAL EXPOSURES			
Calcium-diethylenetriamine pentaacetic acid (Ca-DTPA; Pentetate calcium trisodium injection) Zinc-diethylene-triamine pentaacetic acid (Zn-DTPA; Pentetate zinc trisodium injection)	Internal contamination with transuranium elements: americium, curium, plutonium	Quantity determined by institution. Supplied as 200 mg/mL, 5 mL ampules for IV or inhalation administration. The product is sponsored through Hameln Pharmaceuticals, GmbH, of Hameln, Germany. Distributed in the United States by Akorn, Inc.	1 ampule provides the usual adult dose of 1 g q 24 hours. More would be necessary in a mass casualty event. Ca-DTPA and Zn-DTPA are available through the SNS and REAC/TS, Oak Ridge, Tennessee, at 865-576-3131 (business hours) or 865-576-1005 (after hours).

(Continued)

ADJUNCTIVE AGENT	POISON/DRUG/TOXIN	SUGGESTED MINIMUM STOCK QUANTITY	RATIONALE/COMMENTS
Potassium Iodide, KI tablets (Iostat®, Thyrosafe®) KI liquid (Thyroshield®, SSKI®)	Prevents thyroid uptake of radioactive iodine (I-131)	Quantity determined by institution. Available in 130 mg and 65 mg tablets, and PO solutions: 65 mg/mL (30 mL bottle) and 1 g/mL (30 mL and 240 mL bottle).	One 130 mg tablet represents the initial daily adult dose. More would be necessary in a mass casualty event. KI tablets and oral solution are non-prescription. The Illinois Department of Nuclear Safety makes KI tablets available to healthcare facilities and the general public located near nuclear reactors.
Prussian blue, ferric hexacyanoferrate (Radiogardase®)	Radioactive cesium (Cs-137), radioactive thallium (Tl-201), and non-radioactive thallium	None recommended at the present time. Available in bottles of 30 capsules (500 mg/capsule).	The usual oral adult dose is 3 g, 3 times a day. The product is manufactured by Haupt Pharma Berlin GmbH for distribution by HEYL Chemisch-pharmazeutis-che Fabrik GmbH & Co. KG, Berlin, Germany, and is available in the U.S. from Heyltex Corporation. Prussian Blue is also available through the SNS and REAC/TS, Oak Ridge, Tennessee, at 865-576-3131 (business hours) or 865-576-1005 (after hours).

BAL=British anti-Lewisite; CDC=Centers for Disease Control and Prevention; CN=cyanide; ED=emergency department; EDTA=ethylenediaminete-traacetic acid; EPS=extrapyramidal symptom; FDA=Food and Drug Administration; HCl=hydrochloride; IV=intravenous; MAOI=monoamine oxidase inhibitor; NMS=neuroleptic malignant syndrome; OPI=organophosphate insecticide; P&T=pharmacy and therapeutics; PCC=poison control center; PO=oral; REAC/TS=radiation emergency assistance center/training site; SNS=Strategic National Stockpile; WMD=weapons of mass destruction

PRIMARY IMMUNODEFICIENCY DISORDER TREATMENT

DRUG (BRAND)	HOW SUPPLIED	IgA CONTENT	DOSAGE	MAXIMUM INFUSION RATE	SIDE EFFECTS	COMMENTS
IMMUNOGLOBULINS						
Immune globulin intravenous [human] (Carimune NF)	1, 3, 6 and 12 g vials, lyophilized powder	720 μg/mL	0.2 g/kg of body weight administered once monthly by intravenous infusion.	>2.5 mL/kg/hr	Increase in SrCr and BUN, flushing of face, tightness in chest, chills, fever, dizziness, nausea, diaphoresis, hypotension or HTN, arthralgia, myalgia, transient skin reactions (eg, rash, erythema, pruritus)	Do not shake excessively.
Immune globulin intravenous (human), dual inactivation plus nanofiltration (IGIV) (Flebogamma 5% DIF)	5% [10 mL, 50 mL, 100 mL, 200 mL, 400 mL]	Average: <3 μg/mL (Specification value: <50 μg/mL)	300 to 600 mg/kg body weight administered intravenously every 3 to 4 weeks.	6.0 mL/kg/hr	Increases in creatinine and BUN levels, bronchitis, cough, diarrhea, headache, nasal congestion, pyrexia, arthralgia, upper respiratory tract infection, wheezing	An in-line filter with a pore size of 15 to 20 microns is recommended for the infusion. Subjects over 65 y/o, the infusion rate should be limited to <0.06 mL/kg/min.
Immune globulin intravenous (human) [IGIV] solvent/detergent treated (Gammagard S/D)	5%, 10% Lyophilized	<2.2 μg/mL in a 5% solution	Approximately 300–600 mg/kg infused at 3 to 4 week intervals are commonly used.	5%: 4 mL/kg/hr 10%: 8 mL/kg/hr	Headache, local pain or irritation, chills, flushing, hypotension, N/V, rash, wheezing, fever, fatigue, backache, leg cramps, light-headedness, increased SrCr and BUN, renal dysfunction/failure	Must be at room temperature before administration.
Immune globulin intravenous (human) [IGIV] (Gammagard)	10% Liquid	37 μg/mL	Approximately 300–600 mg/kg infused at 3 to 4 week intervals are commonly used.	5 mL/kg/hr	Headache, fever, fatigue, N/V, chills, infusion-site events, dizziness, pain in extremity, diarrhea, cough, pruritus, pharyngeal pain	Must be at room temperature before administration.
Immune globulin intravenous (human) 5% (Gammaplex)	5% IgG (50 mg/mL) Liquid	Average: 4 μg/mL (Specification value: <10 μg/mL)	300–800 mg/kg every 3-4 weeks. Initial infusion rate: 0.5 mg/kg/min (0.01 mL/kg/min) for 15 min.	4.8 mL/kg/hr	Headache, fatigue, nausea, pyrexia, hypertension, myalgia, pain, vomiting	Use a separate infusion line, do not shake, promptly administer after piercing the cap.

(Continued)

DRUG (BRAND)	HOW SUPPLIED	IgA CONTENT	DOSAGE	MAXIMUM INFUSION RATE	SIDE EFFECTS	COMMENTS
IMMUNOGLOBULINS (Continued)						
Immune globulin intravenous (IGIV) & subcutaneous (IGSC) (human) (Gamunex-C)	1 g, 2.5 g, 5 g, 10 g, or 20 g single use bottles	46 µg/mL	IV route: 300 to 600 mg/kg body weight (3-6 mL/kg) administered every 3 to 4 weeks. SQ route: 1.37 x previous IGIV dose (in grams)/number of weeks between IGIV doses.	4.8 mL/kg/hr	IV route: headache, cough, injection-site reaction, nausea, pharyngitis, urticaria. SQ route: infusion-site reactions, headache, fatigue, arthralgia, pyrexia	SQ route: proper self-administration technique should be exemplified to patient or caregiver.
Immune globulin subcutaneous (human) [IGSC] (Hizentra)	0.2 g/mL (20%)	≤50 µg/mL	Initial dose = 1.53 x previous IGIV dose (in grams) / number of weeks between IGIV doses. Given SQ.	Up to 25 mL/hr/ injection site (50 mL/hr for all sites combined)	Swelling, redness, heat, pain, and itching at the injection site, headache, vomiting, pain, fatigue	Proper self-administration technique should be exemplified to patient or caregiver.
Immune globulin intravenous (human) [IGIV] (Octagam)	1.0 g, 2.5 g, 5 g or 10 g single use bottles	<100 µg/mL	300 to 600 mg/kg body weight administered intravenously every 3 to 4 weeks.	<4.2 mL/kg/hr	Nasal congestion, sinusitis, headache, cough, fever, sore throat, nausea, vomiting, diarrhea, URTI, fatigue, pain in limb	For patients judged at risk for developing renal dysfunction, reduce infusion time by infusing at a maximum rate less than 0.07 mL/kg/min.
Immune globulin intravenous [human] (Privigen)	Single-use 5, 10, and 20 g vials	≤25 µg/mL	200 to 800 mg/kg intravenously every 3 to 4 weeks.	4.8 mL/kg/hr	Headache, pain, nausea, fatigue, chills	For patients over 65 y/o at risk of renal insufficiency, infuse at a rate less than 2 mg/kg/min.
Immune globulin subcutaneous (human) (Vivaglobin)	16% (160 mg/mL) protein solution	<1700 µg/mL	Initial dose = 1.37 x previous IGIV dose (in grams)/number of weeks between IGIV doses. Weekly Dose: 100-200 mg/kg body weight. Given SQ.	20 mL/hr	Injection-site reactions, headache, gastrointestinal disorder, fever, nausea, sore throat, rash	Proper self-administration technique should be exemplified to patient or caregiver.

References: Information obtained from individual PI; Immune Deficiency Foundation

*Refer to the FDA-approved labeling for more information.

SUGAR-FREE PRODUCTS

The following is a selection of products by therapeutic category that contain no sugar. When recommending these products to diabetic patients, keep in mind that many may contain sorbitol, alcohol, or other sources of carbohydrates. This list is not all-inclusive and generics and alternate brands may be available. Check product labeling for a current listing of inactive ingredients.

Analgesics

Addaprin Tablets	Dover
Aminofen Tablets	Dover
Back Pain-Off Tablets ‡	Medique
I-Prin Tablets ‡	Medique
Medi-Seltzer Effervescent Tablets	Medique
Methadose Sugar Free Oral Concentrate	Covidien
Ms.-Aid Tablets ‡	Medique
Children's Silapap Liquid	Silarx

Antacids/Antiflatulants

Alcalak Chewable Tablets*† ‡ §	Medique
Diotame Chewable Tablets*† ‡ §	Medique
Pepto-Bismol Caplets † ‡	Procter & Gamble
Tums Extra Sugar Free Tablets* §	GlaxoSmithKline Consumer

Anti-asthmatic/Respiratory Agent

Jay-Phyl Syrup	JayMac

Antidiarrheal

Imogen Liquid	Pharm Generic

Blood Modifier/Iron Preparation

I.L.X. B-12 Elixir	Kenwood

Corticosteroid

Pediapred Solution* §	UCB

Cough/Cold/Allergy Preparations

Alacol DM Syrup	Ballay
Alacol Solution	Ballay
Aridex Solution	Gentex
Baltussin Solution	Ballay
Bromhist-DM Solution	Cypress
Bromhist Pediatric Solution	Cypress
Bromphenex DM Solution*† §	Breckenridge
Bromplex DM Solution*† §	Prasco
Broncotron Liquid	Seyer Pharmatec
Broncotron-D Suspension	Seyer Pharmatec
B-Tuss Liquid	Blansett
Carbaphen 12 Ped Suspension	Gil
Carbaphen 12 Suspension	Gil
Carbatuss-12 Suspension	GM
Carbetaplex Liquid* §	Breckenridge
Cetafen Cough & Cold Tablets ‡	Hart Health and Safety
Cetafen Cold Tablets ‡	Hart Health and Safety
Cheratussin DAC Liquid	Qualitest
Codal-DM Syrup	Cypress
Coldcough PD Syrup* §	Breckenridge
Coldcough Syrup* §	Breckenridge
Coldonyl Tablets	Medique
Corfen DM Solution	Cypress
Crantex Syrup	Breckenridge
De-Chlor DM Solution	Cypress
Despec Liquid	International Ethical
Despec-SF Liquid	International Ethical
Diabetic Tussin	Health Care Products
Diabetic Tussin DM Liquid §	Health Care Products
Diabetic Tussin Solution§	Health Care Products
Diphen Capsules ‡	Medique
Double Tussin DM Liquid	Reese
Dytan-CS Tablets	Hawthorn
Emagrin Forte Tablets	Medique
Gani-Tuss NR Liquid	Cypress
Genebronco-D Liquid	Pharm Generic
Genecof-HC Liquid	Pharm Generic
Genecof-XP Liquid	Pharm Generic
Genedel Syrup	Pharm Generic
Genedotuss-DM Liquid	Pharm Generic
Genelan Liquid	Pharm Generic
Genexpect DM Liquid	Pharm Generic
Genexpect SF Liquid	Pharm Generic
Gilphex TR Tablets	Gil
Giltuss Ped-C Solution§	Gil
Halotussin AC Liquid	Axiom
Halotussin DAC Solution	Axiom
Marcof Expectorant Syrup	Marnel
Metanx Tablets‡	Pamlab
Nalex DH Liquid	Blansett
Nalex A Liquid	Blansett
Neo DM Syrup*† §	Laser
Neotuss-D Liquid † §	A.G. Marin
Neotuss S/F Liquid † §	A.G. Marin
Phena-HC Solution	GM

* Contains sorbitol.
† May contain other sugar alcohols (eg, glycerol, isomalt, maltitol, mannitol, xylitol).
‡ May contain other sources of carbohydrates (eg, cellulose, lactose, maltodextrin, polydextrose, starch).
§ May contain natural or artificial flavors.

SUGAR-FREE PRODUCTS

Phena-S 12 Suspension	GM
Phena-S Liquid	GM
Poly Hist PD Solution	Poly
Rescon-DM Liquid* §	Capellon
Scot-Tussin Diabetes CF Liquid	Scot-Tussin
Scot-Tussin Expectorant Solution	Scot-Tussin
Scot-Tussin Senior Solution	Scot-Tussin
Siladryl Allergy Solution* §	Silarx
Siltussin DAS Liquid*† §	Silarx
Siltussin DM DAS Cough Formula Syrup*† §	Silarx
Siltussin SA Liquid*† §	Silarx
Children's Sudafed PE Cough & Cold Liquid*† §	McNeil Consumer
Children's Sudafed Nasal	McNeil Consumer
Sudatuss-SF Liquid	Pharm Generic
Supress DX Pediatric Drops † §	Kramer-Novis
Suttar-SF Syrup	Gil
Vazol Solution	Wraser
Z-Tuss DM Syrup † §	Magna

Fluoride Preparations

Fluor-A-Day Tablets*† §	Arbor
Fluor-A-Day Liquid	Arbor
Sensodyne with Fluoride Cool Gel*† ‡ §	GlaxoSmithKline Consumer
Sensodyne Tartar Control with Whitening † ‡ §	GlaxoSmithKline Consumer
Sensodyne w/Fluoride Toothpaste Original Flavor*† ‡ §	GlaxoSmithKline Consumer

Laxatives

Benefiber Powder	Novartis
Citrucel Powder ‡ §	GlaxoSmithKline Consumer
Colace Solution	Purdue Products
Fiber Choice Tablets* ‡ §	GlaxoSmithKline Consumer
Fibro-XL Capsules	Key
Konsyl Easy Mix Formula Powder ‡	Konsyl
Konsyl Orange Powder ‡ §	Konsyl
Konsyl Powder ‡	Konsyl
Metamucil Smooth Texture Powder ‡	Procter & Gamble
Reguloid Powder Regular Flavor ‡	Rugby
Reguloid Powder Orange Flavor ‡ §	Rugby

Mouth/Throat Preparations

Cepacol Dual Relief Sore Throat Spray † §	Combe
Cepacol Sore Throat + Coating Relief Lozenge † §	Combe
Cepacol Sore Throat Lozenges † §	Combe
Cheracol Sore Throat Spray †	Lee
Chloraseptic Spray*† §	Prestige
Diabetic Tussin Cough Drops † §	Health Care Products
Fisherman's Friend Sugar Free Mint Lozenges*	Physicians Total Care
Fresh N Free Liquid	Geritrex
Listerine Pocketpaks Film ‡ §	Johnson & Johnson
Luden's Sugar Free & Wild Cherry Throat Drops † §	McNeil Consumer
Medikoff Sugar Free Drops †	Medique
N'ice Lozenges* §	Heritage/Insight
Oragesic Solution* §	Parnell
Oragel Dry Mouth Moisturizing Gel*† ‡ §	Del
Orajel Dry Mouth Moisturizing Spray † ‡ §	Del
Sepasoothe Lozenges* ‡ §	Medique
Triaminic Sore Throat Spray*† §	Novartis

Vitamins/Minerals/Supplements

Adaptosode For Stress Liquid	HVS
Adaptosode R+R For Acute Stress Liquid	HVS
Alamag Tablets*† ‡ §	Medique
Alcalak Tablets*† ‡	Medique
Apetigen Elixir*†	Kramer-Novis
Apptrim Capsules	Physician Therapeutics
Apptrim-D Capsules	Physician Therapeutics
Bevitamel Tablets	Westlake
Biosode Liquid	HVS
Biotect Plus Caplet	Gil
Bugs Bunny Complete	Bayer
C&M Caps-375 Capsules	Key
Cal-Cee Tablets	Key
Calcet Plus Tablets	Mission Pharmacal
Calcimin-300 Tablets	Key
Cerefolin NAC Tablets	Pamlab
Chromacaps ‡	Key
Delta D3 Tablets ‡	Freeda Vitamins
Detoxosode Liquids	HVS

* Contains sorbitol.
† May contain other sugar alcohols (eg, glycerol, isomalt, maltitol, mannitol, xylitol).
‡ May contain other sources of carbohydrates (eg, cellulose, lactose, maltodextrin, polydextrose, starch).
§ May contain natural or artificial flavors.

DHEA Capsules	ADH Health Products
Diatx ZN Tablets ‡	Centrix
Diucaps Capsules	Legere
DL-Phen-500 Capsules	Key
Enterex Diabetic Liquid ‡	Victus
Evening Primose Oil Capsules †	Nature's Bounty
Ex-L Tablets Tablets ‡	Key
Extress Tablets	Key
Eyetamins Tablets ‡	Rexall Consumer
Fem-Cal Citrate Tablets ‡	Freeda Vitamins
Fem-Cal Tablets ‡	Freeda Vitamins
Fem-Cal Plus Tablets	Freeda Vitamins
Ferrocite Plus Tablets ‡	Breckenridge
Folacin-800 Tablets ‡	Key
Folbee Plus Tablets ‡	Breckenridge
Folbee Tablets ‡	Breckenridge
Folplex 2.2 Tablets ‡	Breckenridge
Foltx Tablets ‡	Pamlab
Gabadone Capsules	Physician Therapeutics
Gram-O-Leci Tablets*† ‡	Freeda Vitamins
Herbal Slim Complex Capsules	ADH Health Products
Hypertensa Capsules ‡	Physician Therapeutics
Lynae Calcium/Vitamin C Chewable Tablets	Boscogen
Lynae Chondroitin/ Glucosamine Capsules	Boscogen
Lynae Ginse-Cool Chewable Tablets	Boscogen
Mag-Ox 400 Tablets	Health Care Products
Mag-SR Tablets ‡	Cypress
Mag-SR Plus Calcium Tablets ‡	Cypress
Magimin Tablets ‡	Key
Magnacaps Capsules ‡	Key
Mangimin Tablets ‡	Key
Medi-Lyte Tablets ‡	Medique
Metanx Tablets ‡	Pamlab
Multi-Delyn with Iron Liquid †	Silarx
New Life Hair Tablets ‡	Rexall Consumer
Niferex Elixir* ‡ §	Ther-Rx
Nutrisure OTC Tablets	Westlake
Nutrivit Solution*† §	Llorens
Ob Complete Tablets	Vertical
O-Cal Fa Tablets ‡	Pharmics
Os-Cal 500 + D Tablets ‡	GlaxoSmithKline Consumer
Powervites Tablets ‡	Green Turtle Bay Vitamin

Prostaplex Herbal Complex Capsules	ADH Health Products
Protect Plus Liquid	Gil
Protect Plus Liquid NR Softgels	Gil
Pulmona Capsules	Physician Therapeutics
Quintabs-M Tablets ‡	Freeda Vitamins
Replace Capsules ‡	Key
Replace w/o Iron Capsules ‡	Key
Samolinic Softgels †	Key
Sea Omega 30 Softgels †	Rugby
Sea Omega 50 Softgels †	Rugby
Sentra AM Capsules	Physician Therapeutics
Sentra PM Capsules	Physician Therapeutics
Soy Care for Menopause Capsules	Inverness Medical
Span C Tablets ‡	Freeda Vitamins
Strovite Forte Syrup	Everett
Sunnie Tablets	Green Turtle Bay Vitamin
Sunvite Tablets † ‡	Rexall Naturalist
Super Dec B100 Tablets ‡	Freeda Vitamins
Super Quints B-50 Tablets ‡	Freeda Vitamins
Supervite Liquid	Seyer Pharmatec
Suplevit Liquid	Gil
Theramine Capsules	Physician Therapeutics
Triamin Tablets	Key
Triamino Tablets* ‡	Freeda Vitamins
Ultramino Powder	Freeda Vitamins
Uro-Mag Capsules ‡	Health Care Products
Vitafol Tablets † ‡	Everett
Vitamin C/Rose Hips Tablets	ADH Health Products
Xtramins Tablets	Key
Ze Plus Softgel	Everett
Miscellaneous	
Acidoll Capsules	Key
Alka-Gest Tablets	Key
Cafergot Tablets ‡	Sandoz
Cytra-2 Solution* §	Cypress
Cytra-K Solution* §	Cypress
Cytra-K Crystals	Cypress
Melatin Tablets ‡	Mason Vitamins
Namenda Solution*† §	Forest
Prosed/DS Tablets ‡	Ferring
Questran Light Powder ‡ §	Par

USE-IN-PREGNANCY RATINGS

The U.S. Food and Drug Administration's Use-in-Pregnancy rating system weighs the degree to which available information has ruled out risk to the fetus against the drug's potential benefit to the patient. Below is a listing of drugs (by generic name) for which ratings are available.

Contraindicated in pregnancy

Studies in animals or humans, or investigational or postmarketing reports, have demonstrated fetal risk, which clearly outweighs any possible benefit to the patient.

Acitretin
Ambrisentan
Amlodipine Besylate/Atovastatin
    Calcium
Anastrozole
Aspirin
Atorvastatin Calcium
Benzphetamine HCl
Bexarotene
Bicalutamide
Bosentan
Caffeine
Cetrorelix Acetate
Chenodiol
Cholecalciferol
Choriogonadotropin Alfa
Chorionic Gonadotropin
Clomiphene Citrate
Danazol
Degarelix
Desogestrel/Ethinyl Estradiol
Diclofenac Sodium
Dienogest/Estradiol Valerate
Dihydroergotamine Mesylate
Dronedarone
Dutasteride
Dutasteride/Tamsulosin
Ergotamine Tartrate
Ergotamine Tartrate/Caffeine
Estazolam
Estradiol
Estropipate
Ethinyl Estradiol/Drospirenone
Ethinyl Estradiol/Etonogestrel
Ethinyl Estradiol/Ferrous
    Fumarate/Norethindrone Acetate
Ethinyl Estradiol/Levonorgestrel
Ethinyl Estradiol/Norethindrone
    Acetate
Ethinyl Estradiol/Norgestimate
Ethinyl Estradiol/Norgetrel
Ethynodiol Diacetate
Ezetimibe/Simvastatin
Finasteride
Fluorouracil

Fluoxymesterone
Fluvastatin Sodium
Follitropin Alfa
Follitropin Beta
Ganirelix Acetate
Genistein Aglycone
Goserelin Acetate
Histrelin Acetate
Iodine I 131 Tositumomab
Isotretinoin
Leflunomide
Lenalidomide
Letrozole
Leuprolide Acetate
Lovastatin
Lovastatin/Niacin
Lutropin Alfa
Medroxyprogesterone Acetate
Megestrol Acetate
Menotropins
Meprobamate
Mequinol
Mestranol
Mestranol
Methotrexate Sodium
Methyltestosterone
Miglustat
Misoprostol
Nafarelin Acetate
Niacin
Niacin/Simvastatin
Norethindrone
Norethindrone Acetate
Oxandrolone
Peginterferon Alfa-2b
Pitavastatin
Pravastatin Sodium
Quazepam
Raloxifene HCl
Ribavirin
Rosuvastatin Calcium
Simvastatin
Tamsulosin HCl
Tazarotene
Temazepam
Tesamorelin
Testosterone
Testosterone Cypionate
Testosterone Enanthate
Thalidomide
Tositumomab
Tretinoin
Triazolam
Triptorelin Pamoate
Ulipristal Acetate
Urofollitropin

Warfarin Sodium
Zinc Bisglycinate

Positive evidence of risk

Investigational or postmarketing data show risk to the fetus. Nevertheless, potential benefits may outweigh the potential risk.

Aliskiren*
Aliskiren/Amlodipine/HCTZ*
Aliskiren/HCTZ*
Aliskiren/Valsartan*
Alitretinoin
Alprazolam
Altretamine
Amikacin Sulfate
Aminoglutethimide
Amiodarone HCl
Amlodipine
Amlodipine/Aliskiren*
Anthrax Vaccine Adsorbed
Arsenic Trioxide
Aspirin
Atenolol/HCTZ
Atenolol
Azacitidine
Azathioprine
Benazepril HCl/HCTZ*
Benazepril HCl*
Bendamustine HCl
Bismuth Subcitrate Potassium
Bismuth Subsalicylate
Bleomycin Sulfate
Bortezomib
Busulfan
Cabazitaxel
Candesartan Cilexetil*
Capecitabine
Captopril*
Captopril/HCTZ*
Carbamazepine
Carboplatin
Carmustine (BiCNU)
Celecoxib*
Chlorambucil
Chlorthalidone
Cisplatin
Cladribine
Clofarabine

---

* Category C or D depending on the trimester the drug is given.
HCTZ: Hydrochlorothiazide

Clonazepam
Cyclophosphamide
Cytarabine
Dactinomycin
Dasatinib
Daunorubicin HCl
Decitabine
Demeclocycline HCl
Dexrazoxane
Diazepam
Dipyridamole
Divalproex Sodium
Docetaxel
Doxorubicin HCl
Doxycycline Calcium
Doxycycline Hyclate
Doxycycline Monohydrate
Efavirenz/Emtricitabine/Tenofovir
   Disoproxil
Enalapril Maleate*
Enalapril Maleate/HCTZ*
Enalaprilat*
Epirubicin HCl
Eribulin Mesylate
Erlotinib
Ethotoin
Etoposide
Everolimus
Exemestane
Floxuridine
Fludarabine Phosphate
Fluorouracil
Flutamide
Fosphenytoin Sodium
Fulvestrant
Gefitinib
Gemcitabine HCl
Gentamicin Sulfate
Hydrochlorothiazide
Hydroxyurea
Ibritumomab Tiuxetan
Idarubicin HCl
Ifosfamide
Imatinib Mesylate
Irbesartan*
Irbesartan/HCTZ*
Irinotecan HCl
Ixabepilone
Lapatinib
Lithium Carbonate
Lomustine
Lorazepam
Losartan Potassium*
Losartan Potassium/HCTZ*
Mechlorethamine HCl
Megestrol Acetate
Melphalan
Mephobarbital
Mercaptopurine
Methimazole
Metronidazole
Midazolam HCl

Minocycline HCl
Moexipril HCl*
Moexipril HCl/HCTZ*
Mycophenolic Acid
Nelarabine
Neomycin Sulfate
Nicotine
Nilotinib
Oxaliplatin
Paclitaxel
Pamidronate Disodium
Paroxetine HCl
Pazopanib
Pemetrexed Disodium
Pentobarbital Sodium
Perindopril Erbumine
Phenytoin
Plerixafor
Polifeprosan 20 With Carmustine
Polymyxin B Sulfate
Potassium Iodide
Pralatrexate
Prednisolone Acetate
Prednisolone Sodium Phosphate
Procarbazine HCl
Propylthiouracil
Quinapril*
Quinapril/HCTZ*
Ramipril*
Romidepsin
Secobarbital Sodium
Small Pox Vaccine, Live
Sorafenib
Streptomycin Sulfate
Streptozocin
Sunitinib Malate
Tamoxifen Citrate
Telmisartan*
Telmisartan/HCTZ*
Temozolomide
Temsirolimus
Teniposide
Tetracycline HCl
Thioguanine
Tigecycline
Tobramycin
Topotecan
Toremifene Citrate
Trandolapril*
Trandolapril/HCTZ*
Triamcinolone Acetonide
Valproate Sodium
Valproic Acid
Valsartan*
Valsartan/HCTZ*
Valsartan/HCTZ/Amlodipine*
Valsartan/Amlodipine*
Vincristine Sulfate
Vinorelbine Tartrate
Voriconazole
Vorinostat
Zoledronic Acid

C

Risk cannot be ruled out

Human studies are lacking, and animal studies are either positive for risk or are lacking as well. However, potential benefits may outweigh the potential risk.

Abacavir Sulfate
Abacavir Sulfate/Lamivudine
Abacavir
   Sulfate/Lamivudine/Zidovudine
Abatacept
Abciximab
Absorbable Fibrin Sealant
Acamprosate Calcium
Acetaminophen
Acetaminophen/Butalbital/Caffeine
Acetaminophen/Codeine Phosphate
Acetaminophen/Hydrocodone
   Bitartrate
Acetaminophen/Oxycodone
Acetazolamide
Acyclovir
Adapalene
Adapalene/Benzoyl Peroxide
Adefovir Dipivoxil
Adenosine
Albendazole
Albumin (Human)
Albuterol
Alclometasone Dipropionate
Aldesleukin
Alemtuzumab
Alendronate Sodium
Alendronate Sodium/Cholecalciferol
Alfentanil HCl
Alglucerase
Allopurinol Sodium
Almotriptan Malate
Alpha1-Proteinase Inhibitor (Human)
Alprostadil
Alteplase
Amantadine HCl
Amcinonide
Amifostine
Aminocaproic Acid
Aminohippurate Sodium
Aminolevulinic Acid HCl
Aminosalicylic Acid
Amitriptyline HCl
Amlodipine Besylate
Amoxapine
Amphetamine Aspartate/
   Amphetamine Sulfate/
   Detroamphetamine Saccharate/
   Dextroamphetamine Sulfate
Anagrelide HCl
Anidulafungin

Anthralin
Antihemophilic Factor (Human)
Antihemophilic Factor (Recombinant)
Anti-Inhibitor Coagulant Complex
Antithrombin, Recombinant
Apomorphine HCl
Apraclonidine HCl
Arformoterol Tartrate
Aripiprazole
Armodafinil
Artemether/Lumefantrine
Articaine HCl
Asenapine
Asparaginase
Atomoxetine HCl
Atovaquone
Atovaquone/Proguanil HCl
Atracurium Besylate
Atropine Sulfate/Hyoscamine
  Sulfate/Scopolamine
Auranofin
Azelastine HCl
Baclofen
Bacitracin Zinc/Neomycin Sulfate/
  Polymyxin B Sulfate
BCG, Live (Intravesical)
Becaplermin
Beclomethasone Dipropionate
Belladonna
Bendroflumethiazide
Benzocaine
Benzoic Acid
Benzonatate
Benzoyl Peroxide
Bepotastine Besilate
Besifloxacin
Betamethasone Acetate
Betamethasone Dipropionate
Betamethasone Sodium Phosphate
Betamethasone Valerate
Betaxolol HCl
Bethanechol Chloride
Bevacizumab
Bimatoprost
Biperiden HCl
Bisacodyl/Polyethylene Gycol/
  Potassium Chloride/Sodium
  Bicarbonate/Sodium Chloride
Bisoprolol Fumarate
Black Widow Spider Antivenin
  (Equine)
Botulinum Toxin Type B
Brimonidine Tartrate
Brinzolamide
Bromfenac
Brompheniramine Maleate
Budesonide
Bumetanide
Bupivacaine HCl
Bupivacaine HCl/Epinephrine
  Bitartrate
Buprenorphine HCl

Bupropion HCl
Bupropion Hydrobromide
Butabarbital
Butalbital
Butenafine HCl
Butoconazole Nitrate
Butorphanol Tartrate
C1 Esterase Inhibitor (Human)
Caffeine Citrate
Calcipotriene
Calcitonin-Salmon
Calcitriol
Calcium Acetate
Calcium Chloride Dihydrate
Canakinumab
Capreomycin Sulfate
Carbachol
Carbetapentane Citrate
Carbidopa
Carbidopa/Levodopa
Carbidopa/Levodopa/Entacapone
Carbinoxamine Maleate
Carboprost Tromethamine
Carglumic Acid
Carisoprodol
Carisoprodol/Aspirin/Codeine
  Phosphate
Carisoprodol/Aspirin
Carisoprodol/Codeine
Carteolol HCl
Carvedilol
Caspofungin Acetate
Celecoxib*
Cetirizine HCl
Cetuximab
Cevimeline HCl
Chloral Hydrate
Chloroprocaine HCl
Chlorothiazide
Chloroxylenol
Chlorpheniramine Maleate/
  Pseudoephedrine HCl
Chlorpheniramine Polistirex/
  Hydrocodone Polistirex
Chlorpheniramine Tannate/
  Phenylephrine Tannate
Chlorpropamide
Cholestyramine
Ciclesonide
Cidofovir
Cilostazol
Cinacalcet
Ciprofloxacin
Ciprofloxacin/Dexamethasone
Citalopram Hydrobromide
Clarithromycin
Clarithromycin/Amoxicillin/
  Lanzoprazole
Clevidipine Butyrate
Clindamycin Phosphate
Clindamycin Phosphate/Benzoyl
  Peroxide Gel

Clocortolone Pivalate
Clomipramine HCl
Clonidine
Clotrimazole
Clotrimazole/Betamethasone
  Dipropionate
Coagulation Factor Ix (Human)
Coagulation Factor Viia, Recombinant
Coagulation Factor Viii Complex
  (Human)
Colchicine
Colistimethate Sodium
Colistin Sulfate
Conivaptan HCl
Corticorelin Ovine Triflutate
Cosyntropin
Crotalidae Polyvalent Immune Fab
  (Ovine)
Crotamiton
Cyclopentolate HCl
Cycloserine
Cyclosporine
Cysteamine Bitartrate
Cytomegalovirus Immune Globulin
Dabigatran Etexilate Mesylate
Dacarbazine
Daclizumab
Dalfampridine
Dantrolene Sodium
Dapsone
Darbepoetin Alfa
Darifenacin
Darunavir
Deferasirox
Deferoxamine Mesylate
Delavirdine Mesylate
Denosumab
Desloratadine
Desonide
Desoximetasone
Desvenlafaxine
Dexmedetomidine HCl
Dexrazoxane
Dextromethorphan Hydrobromide
Dextromethorphan Tannate
Diazoxide
Diclofenac Potassium*
Diclofenac Sodium
Diflorasone Diacetate
Diflunisal
Difluprednate
Digoxin
Digoxin Immune Fab (Ovine)
Diltiazem HCl
Dimethyl Sulfoxide
Dinoprostone
Diphenoxylate HCl
Diphtheria & Tetanus Toxoids
  Adsorbed (For Pediatric Use)
Diphtheria & Tetanus Toxoids And
  Acellular Pertussis Vaccine
  Adsorbed

---

* Category C or D depending on the trimester the drug is given.
HCTZ: Hydrochlorothiazide

Diphtheria Toxoid, Adsorbed
Disopyramide Phosphate
Dofetilide
Donepezil HCl
Dopamine HCl
Dorzolamide HCl
Doxazosin Mesylate
Doxepin HCl
Dronabinol
Drotrecogin Alfa (Activated)
Duloxetine HCl
Dyphylline
Ecallantide
Econazole Nitrate
Eculizumab
Edrophonium Chloride
Eflornithine HCl
Eletriptan Hydrobromide
Eltrombopag
Entecavir
Ephedrine Tannate
Epinastine HCl
Epinephrine
Epoetin Alfa
Eprosartan Mesylate*
Eprosartan Mesylate/HCTZ*
Ergocalciferol
Erythromycin
Escitalopram Oxalate
Esmolol HCl
Esomeprazole
Esomeprazole Magnesium/Naproxen*
Eszopiclone
Ethambutol HCl
Ethionamide
Etidronate Disodium
Etodolac
Etomidate
Everolimus
Exenatide
Ezetimibe
Febuxostat
Felbamate
Fenofibrate
Fenofibric Acid
Fenoprofen Calcium
Fentanyl
Fentanyl Citrate
Ferumoxides
Ferumoxytol
Fesoterodine Fumarate
Fexofenadine HCl
Fibrinogen (Human)
Filgrastim
Fingolimod
Flecainide Acetate
Fluconazole
Flucytosine
Fludeoxyglucose F-18
Fludrocortisone Acetate
Flumazenil
Flunisolide Hemihydrate

Fluocinolone Acetonide
Fluocinonide
Fluorescein Sodium
Fluorometholone
Fluoxetine HCl
Flurandrenolide
Flurbiprofen
Fluticasone Furoate
Fluticasone Propionate
Fluticasone Propionate/Salmeterol
Fluvoxamine Maleate
Fomepizole
Formoterol Fumarate
Formoterol Fumarate
    Dihydrate/Budesonide
Formoterol Fumarate
    Dihydrate/Mometasone Furoate
Fosamprenavir Calcium
Foscarnet Sodium
Fosinopril Sodium*
Fosinopril Sodium/HCTZ*
Frovatriptan Succinate
Furosemide
Gabapentin
Gadobenate Dimeglumine
Gadofosveset Trisodium
Gadopentetate Dimeglumine
Gadoxetate Disodium
Gallium Nitrate
Ganciclovir
Gatifloxacin
Gemfibrozil
Gemifloxacin Mesylate
Gentamicin Sulfate
Glimepiride
Glipizide
Globulin, Immune (Human)
Glutathione
Glyburide
Glycopyrrolate
Gold Sodium Thiomalate
Gramicidin
Guaifenesin
Haemophilus B Conjugate Vaccine
    (Meningococcal Protein
    Conjugate)
Haemophilus B Conjugate Vaccine
    (Tetanus Toxoid Conjugate)
Halcinonide
Halobetasol Propionate
Haloperidol Decanoate
Hemin
Heparin Sodium
Hepatitis A Vaccine, Inactivated
Hepatitis B Immune Globulin
    (Human)
Hepatitis B Vaccine, Recombinant
Hexachlorophene
Histidine
Homatropine Methylbromide
Hyaluronidase
Hydralazine HCl

Hydrochlorothiazide/Aldactone
Hydrocodone Bitartrate
Hydrocodone Polistirex
Hydrocortisone
Hydrocortisone Acetate
Hydrocortisone Sodium Succinate
Hydrocortisone Valerate
Hydromorphone HCl
Hydroquinone
Hydroxocobalamin
Hydroxyamphetamine Hydrobromide
Hydroxyethyl Starch
Hyoscyamine Hydrobromide
Hypericum Perforatum
Ibandronate Sodium
Ibuprofen/Hydrocodone
Ibuprofen/Oxycodone
Ibutilide Fumarate
Idursulfase
Iloperidone
Iloprost
Imiglucerase
Imipenem/Cilastatin
Imiquimod
Immune Globulin Intravenous
    (Human)
Incobotulinumtoxina
Indinavir Sulfate
Indomethacin
Influenza Virus Vaccine
Insulin Aspart Protamine, Human
Insulin Aspart, Human
Insulin Detemir (RDNA Origin)
Insulin Glargine (RDNA Origin)
Insulin Glulisine
Insulin, Human (RDNA Origin)
Interferon Alfa-2a, Recombinant
Interferon Beta-1b
Interferon Gamma-1b
Iobenguane I 123
Iodoquinol
Ipratropium Bromide
Ipratropium Bromide/Albuterol
Iron Dextran
Isocarboxazid
Isoflurane
Isoleucine
Isoniazid
Isosorbide Dinitrate
Isosorbide Mononitrate
Isradipine
Itraconazole
Ivermectin
Japanese Encephalitis Vaccine
    Inactivated
Ketoconazole
Ketoprofen
Ketorolac Tromethamine
Labetalol HCl
Lacosamide
Lamivudine
Lamotrigine

Lanreotide
Lansoprazole
Lanthanum Carbonate
Latanoprost
Leucovorin Calcium
Levalbuterol HCl
Levetiracetam
Levobunolol HCl
Levodopa
Levofloxacin
Levoleucovorin Calcium
Lincomycin HCl
Lindane
Linezolid
Liraglutide (RDNA Origin)
Lisdexamfetamine Dimesylate
Lopinavir/Ritonavir
Loteprednol Etabonate
Lubiprostone
Lymphocyte Immune Globulin, Anti-Thymocyte Globulin (Equine)
Mafenide Acetate
Measles Virus Vaccine, Live
Measles, Mumps & Rubella Virus Vaccine, Live
Measles, Mumps, Rubella And Varicella Virus Vaccine Live
Mebendazole
Mefenamic Acid
Mefloquine HCl
Meningococcal Polysaccharide Diphtheria Toxoid Conjugate Vaccine
Meningococcal Polysaccharide Vaccine
Meperidine HCl
Mepivacaine HCl
Mesalamine
Metaproterenol Sulfate
Metformin HCl
Methadone HCl
Methamphetamine HCl
Methenamine Mandelate/ Sodium Acid Phosphate
Methenamine Hippurate
Methionine
Methocarbamol
Methoxsalen
Methscopolamine Bromide
Methyl Aminolevulinate
Methyldopa
Methyldopate HCl
Methylergonovine Maleate
Methylphenidate
Methylprednisolone Acetate
Metipranolol
Metoprolol Succinate
Metoprolol Tartrate
Metyrapone
Metyrosine
Mexiletine HCl
Micafungin Sodium

Miconazole
Midodrine HCl
Milnacipran HCl
Milrinone Lactate
Minoxidil
Mirtazapine
Mitotane
Modafinil
Mometasone Furoate Monohydrate
Morphine Sulfate
Moxifloxacin HCl
Mumps Virus Vaccine, Live
Muromonab-CD3
Nabilone
Nabumetone
Nadolol
Naloxone HCl
Naltrexone HCl
Naphazoline HCl
Naproxen
Naratriptan HCl
Natalizumab
Natamycin
Nateglinide
Nebivolol
Nefazodone HCl
Neomycin Sulfate
Neostigmine Bromide
Nepafenac
Nesiritide
Niacin
Nicardipine HCl
Nifedipine
Nilutamide
Nimodipine
Nisoldipine
Nitisinone
Nitric Oxide
Nitroglycerin
Norepinephrine Bitartrate
Norfloxacin
Nystatin
Ofatumumab
Ofloxacin
Olanzapine
Olmesartan Medoxomil*
Olmesartan Medoxomil/HCTZ*
Olopatadine HCl
Olsalazine Sodium
Omega-3-Acid Ethyl Esters
Omeprazole
Oprelvekin
Orphenadrine Citrate
Oseltamivir Phosphate
Oxaprozin
Oxcarbazepine
Oxymorphone HCl
Palifermin
Paliperidone
Palivizumab
Pancrelipase
Pancuronium Bromide

Panitumumab
Paricalcitol
Pegademase Bovine
Pegaspargase
Pegfilgrastim
Peginterferon Alfa-2a
Peginterferon Alfa-2b
Pegloticase
Pemirolast Potassium
Penbutolol Sulfate
Pentazocine HCl
Pentoxifylline
Perflutren Protein-Type A
Phenazopyridine HCl
Phenobarbital
Phenoxybenzamine HCl
Phentermine HCl
Phentolamine Mesylate
Phenyl Salicylate
Phenylalanine
Phenylephrine HCl
Phenylpropanolamine HCl
Phosphoric Acid
Pilocarpine HCl
Pimecrolimus
Pimozide
Pioglitazone
Pioglitazone HCl/Metformin HCl
Pioglitazone/Glimepiride
Pirbuterol Acetate
Piroxicam
Pneumococcal Vaccine, Diphtheria Conjugate
Pneumococcal Vaccine, Polyvalent
Podofilox
Poglitazone/Metformin HCl
Polidocanol
Poliovirus Vaccine Inactivated
Porfimer Sodium
Posaconazole
Pralidoxime Chloride
Pramipexole DiHCl
Pramlintide Acetate
Pramoxine HCl
Prazosin HCl
Prednicarbate
Prednisolone Acetate
Pregabalin
Promethazine HCl
Propafenone HCl
Proparacaine HCl
Propranolol HCl
Protein C Concentrate (Human)
Pseudoephedrine HCl
Pyrazinamide
Pyridostigmine Bromide
Pyrilamine Tannate
Pyrimethamine
Quetiapine Fumarate
Quinidine Gluconate
Quinine Sulfate
Rabbit Antihymocyte Globulin

* Category C or D depending on the trimester the drug is given.
HCTZ: Hydrochlorothiazide

Rabies Immune Globulin (Human)
Rabies Vaccine
Raltegravir
Ramelteon
Ranibizumab
Ranolazine
Rasagiline Mesylate
Rasburicase
Regadenoson
Remifentanil HCl
Repaglinide
Reserpine
Reteplase
Retinyl Palmitate
Rho (D) Immune Globulin (Human)
Rifampin
Rifapentine
Rifaximin
Rilonacept
Riluzole
Rimantadine HCl
Rimexolone
Risedronate Sodium
Risperidone
Ritonavir
Rituximab
Rizatriptan Benzoate
Rocuronium Bromide
Romiplostim
Ropinirole HCl
Rosiglitazone
Rosiglitazone/Glimepiride
Rosiglitazone/Metformin HCl
Rotavirus Vaccine, Live, Oral, Pentavalent
Rubella Virus Vaccine, Live
Rufinamide
Sacrosidase
Salicylic Acid
Salmeterol Xinafoate
Salsalate
Sapropterin DiHCl
Sargramostim
Scopolamine Hydrobromide
Selegiline
Selenium Sulfide
Sertaconazole Nitrate
Sertraline HCl
Sevelamer Carbonate
Sevelamer HCl
Sibutramine HCl Monohydrate
Sirolimus
Smallpox Vaccine
Solifenacin Succinate
Somatropin
Spironolactone
Stavudine
Succinylcholine Chloride
Sufentanil Citrate
Sulconazole Nitrate
Sulfacetamide Sodium
Sulfamethoxazole/Trimethoprim
Sulfanilamide

Sulfisoxazole Acetyl
Sulindac
Sumatriptan
Tacrolimus
Tapentadol
Telavancin
Telithromycin
Tenecteplase
Terconazole
Teriparatide
Tetanus Immune Globulin (Human)
Tetanus Toxoid, Adsorbed
Tetrabenazine
Theophylline Anhydrous
Thiabendazole
Thonzonium Bromide
Threonine
Thrombin
Thyrotropin Alfa
Tiagabine HCl
Tiludronate Disodium
Timolol Hemihydrate
Timolol Maleate
Tinidazole
Tiotropium Bromide
Tipranavir
Tizanidine HCl
Tobramycin
Tobramycin/Dexamethasone
Tocilizumab
Tolazamide
Tolbutamide
Tolcapone
Tolmetin Sodium
Tolterodine Tartrate
Tolvaptan
Topiramate
Tramadol HCl
Travoprost
Trazodone HCl
Tretinoin
Triamcinolone Acetonide
Triamterene
Triamterene/HCTZ
Trifluridine
Trimethoprim HCl
Trimethoprim Sulfate
Trimipramine Maleate
Tropicamide
Trospium Chloride
Tuberculin Purified Protein Derivative, Diluted
Valganciclovir HCl
Valrubicin
Vancomycin HCl
Varenicline
Varicella Virus Vaccine, Live
Vecuronium Bromide
Venlafaxine HCl
Verapamil HCl
Verteporfin
Vigabatrin
Vilazodone HCl

Vitamin K1
Von Willebrand Factor (Human)
Yellow Fever Vaccine
Zaleplon
Zanamivir
Zeaxanthin
Ziconotide
Zidovudine
Zileuton
Zinc Oxide
Ziprasidone HCl
Zolmitriptan
Zolpidem Tartrate
Zonisamide
Zoster Vaccine Live

B

No evidence of risk in humans

Either animal findings show risk while human findings do not, or, if no adequate human studies have been done, animal findings are negative.

Aztreonam
Balsalazide Disodium
Basiliximab
Benzyl Alcohol
Bivalent Human Papillomavirus (Types 16, 18) Recombinant Vaccine
Bivalirudin
Brimonidine Tartrate
Bromocriptine Mesylate
Budesonide
Buspirone HCl
Cabergoline
Capsaicin
Cefaclor
Cefadroxil
Cefazolin Sodium
Cefdinir
Cefditoren Pivoxil
Cefepime HCl
Cefixime
Cefotaxime Sodium
Cefotetan Disodium
Cefpodoxime Proxetil
Cefprozil
Ceftaroline Fosamil
Ceftazidime
Ceftibuten Dihydrate
Ceftriaxone Sodium
Cefuroxime Sodium
Cephalexin
Certolizumab Pegol
Chlorhexidine Gluconate
Chlorthalidone
Ciclopirox

Cimetidine HCl
Cisatracurium Besylate
Clindamycin HCl
Clopidogrel Bisulfate
Clotrimazole
Clozapine
Colesevelam HCl
Collagenase Clostridium
   Histolyticum
Cromolyn Sodium
Cyclobenzaprine HCl
Cyproheptadine HCl
Dalfopristin
Dalteparin Sodium
Daptomycin
Desflurane
Desmopressin Acetate
Dexlansoprazole
Diclofenac Sodium
Dicloxacillin Sodium
Dicyclomine HCl
Didanosine
Diethylpropion HCl
Diphenhydramine HCl
Dipivefrin HCl
Dipyridamole
Dobutamine HCl
Dolasetron Mesylate
Doripenem
Dornase Alfa
Doxepin HCl
Doxercalciferol
Emedastine Difumarate
Emtricitabine
Enflurane
Enfuvirtide
Enoxaparin Sodium
Epinephrine
Eplerenone
Epoprostenol Sodium
Eptifibatide
Ertapenem
Erythromycin
Erythromycin Ethylsuccinate
Erythromycin Lactobionate
Erythromycin Stearate
Etanercept
Ethacrynate Sodium
Ethacrynic Acid
Etravirine
Famciclovir
Famotidine
Fenoldopam Mesylate
Flavoxate HCl
Fondaparinux Sodium
Fosaprepitant Dimeglumine
Fosfomycin Tromethamine
Fospropofol Disodium
Galantamine Hydrobromide
Glatiramer Acetate
Glucagon
Glyburide
Glycopyrrolate

Golimumab
Granisetron HCl
Guanfacine HCl
Hydrochlorothiazide
Hydrocortisone Acetate
Indapamide
Infliximab
Influenza Virus Vaccine
Insulin Aspart Protamine, Human
Insulin Aspart, Human
Insulin Aspart, Human Regular
Insulin Lispro Protamine, Human
Insulin Lispro, Human
Iopromide
Ipratropium Bromide
Iron Sucrose
Isosorbide Mononitrate
Japanese Encephalitis Vaccine
   Inactivated
Lactulose
Lansoprazole
Laronidase
Lepirudin
Levocarnitine
Levocetirizine DiHCl
Lidocaine HCl
Lodoxamide Tromethamine
Lurasidone HCl
Malathion
Maprotiline HCl
Maraviroc
Meclizine HCl
Memantine HCl
Meningococcal Oligosaccharide
   Diphtheria Crm197 Conjugate
   Vaccine
Mepenzolate Bromide
Meropenem
Mesalamine
Mesna
Metformin HCl
Methohexital Sodium
Methyclothiazide
Methyldopa
Methylnaltrexone Bromide
Metoclopramide
Metolazone
Metronidazole
Miglitol
Montelukast Sodium
Mupirocin
Nafcillin Sodium
Naftifine HCl
Nalbuphine HCl
Nedocromil Sodium
Nelfinavir Mesylate
Nevirapine
Nitazoxanide
Nitrofurantoin
Nitrofurantoin Macrocrystals
Nitrofurantoin Monohydrate
Nizatidine
Octreotide Acetate

Omalizumab
Ondansetron HCl
Orlistat
Oxiconazole Nitrate
Oxybutynin
Oxycodone HCl
Pancrelipase
Pantoprazole Sodium
Pegaptanib Sodium
Pegvisomant
Penciclovir
Penicillin G Benzathine
Penicillin G Potassium
Penicillin G Procaine
Pentosan Polysulfate Sodium
Permethrin
Phenazopyridine HCl
Phenobarbital
Pindolol
Piperacillin Sodium
Piperacillin Sodium/Tazobactam
   Sodium
Prasugrel
Praziquantel
Prilocaine
Progesterone
Propofol
Pseudoephedrine HCl
Quadrivalent Human Papillomavirus
   (Types 6, 11, 16, 18) Recombinant
   Vaccine
Quinupristin
Rabeprazole Sodium
Ranitidine HCl
Retapamulin
Rifabutin
Ritonavir
Rivastigmine Tartrate
Ropivacaine HCl
Saquinavir Mesylate
Saxagliptin
Sevoflurane
Sildenafil Citrate
Silodosin
Silver Sulfadiazine
Sitagliptin Phosphate
Sodium Fluoride
Sodium Oxybate
Somatropin (RDNA Origin)
Sotalol HCl
Spinosad
Sucralfate
Sulbactam Sodium
Sulfasalazine
Tadalafil
Tamsulosin HCl
Telbivudine
Tenofovir Disoproxil Fumarate
Terbinafine HCl
Terbutaline Sulfate
Tetracaine
Ticarcillin Disodium/Clavulanate
   Potassium

---

* Category C or D depending on the trimester the drug is given.
HCTZ: Hydrochlorothiazide

Ticlopidine HCl
Tinzaparin Sodium
Tirofiban HCl
Tobramycin
Torsemide
Tranexamic Acid
Trastuzumab
Treprostinil
Typhoid Vaccine Live Oral Ty21a
Ursodiol
Ustekinumab
Valacyclovir HCl
Vancomycin HCl

Vardenafil HCl
Velaglucerase Alfa
Zafirlukast

A

Controlled studies show no risk

Adequate, well-controlled studies in pregnant women have failed to demonstrate risk to the fetus.

Ferrous Sulfate
Folic Acid
Levothyroxine Sodium
Liothyronine Sodium

BRAND/GENERIC INDEX

Organized alphabetically, this index includes the brand and generic names of each drug in the Product Information section. Brand-name drug entries are capitalized; generic names are not. If more than one brand name is associated with a generic, each brand can be found under the generic entry.

THERAPEUTIC CLASS INDEX

Organized alphabetically, this index includes the therapeutic class of each drug in the Product Information section. Therapeutic class headings are based on information provided in the drug monographs. The drug entries listed under each bold therapeutic class are organized alphabetically by brand name or monograph title (shown in capitalized letters), followed by the generic name in parentheses.

ANTIMICROTUBULE AGENT

ANTIPROTOZOAL AGENT

ARB/CALCIUM CHANNEL BLOCKER (DIHYDROPYRIDINE)

ARB/CALCIUM CHANNEL BLOCKER (DIHYDROPYRIDINE)/THIAZIDE DIURETIC

ARGININE VASOPRESSIN ANTAGONIST

AROMATASE INACTIVATOR

ARTEMISININ-BASED COMBINATION THERAPY

ATYPICAL ANXIOLYTIC

AZOLE ANTIFUNGAL

B

BACTERIAL PROTEIN SYNTHESIS INHIBITOR

BARBITURATE

BARBITURATE/ANALGESIC

BENZISOXAZOLE DERIVATIVE

BENZODIAZEPINE

NOVACORT
(pramoxine HCl-hydrocortisone
acetate).........................827

CORTICOSTEROID/ANTI-INFECTIVE
ALCORTIN
(iodoquinol-hydrocortisone)............ 50

**CORTICOSTEROID/
AZOLE ANTIFUNGAL**
LOTRISONE
(betamethasone dipropionate-
clotrimazole)........................... 698

CORTICOSTEROID/BETA₂ AGONIST

CORTICOSTEROID/BETA$_2$ AGONIST
ADVAIR
(fluticasone propionate-salmeterol). 36
ADVAIR HFA ,
(fluticasone propionate-salmeterol). 38
DULERA
(mometasone furoate-formoterol
fumarate dihydrate) 398
SYMBICORT
(formoterol fumarate dihydrate-
budesonide) 1132

COX-2 INHIBITOR
CELEBREX
(celecoxib)..........................259

CYCLIC LIPOPEPTIDE
CUBICIN
(daptomycin).......................328

**CYCLIC POLYPEPTIDE
IMMUNOSUPPRESSANT**
NEORAL
(cyclosporine).......................797
SANDIMMUNE
(cyclosporine)......................1061

CYTOPROTECTIVE AGENT
FUSILEV
(levoleucovorin calcium) 537

D

DEBRIDING/HEALING AGENT
XIAFLEX
(collagenase clostridium
histolyticum)......................1326

DEPIGMENTATION AGENT
CLARIPEL
(hydroquinone).....................283
EPIQUIN MICRO
(hydroquinone).....................444

DIBENZAPINE DERIVATIVE
CLOZAPINE
(clozapine).........................292
FAZACLO
(clozapine).........................484
SAPHRIS
(asenapine)........................1064
SEROQUEL
(quetiapine fumarate)..................1077

SEROQUEL XR
(quetiapine fumarate)...................1079

DIBENZAZEPINE
TRILEPTAL
(oxcarbazepine)......................1214

DICARBAMATE ANTICONVULSANT
FELBATOL
(felbamate)........................ 486

**DIHYDROFOLIC ACID REDUCTASE
INHIBITOR**
FOLOTYN
(pralatrexate)..................... 518
METHOTREXATE
(methotrexate).....................739

**DIPEPTIDYL PEPTIDASE-4
INHIBITOR**
JANUVIA
(sitagliptin)...................... 618
ONGLYZA
(saxagliptin).......................855

**DIPEPTIDYL PEPTIDASE-4
INHIBITOR/BIGUANIDE**
JANUMET
(metformin HCl-sitagliptin)............. 617
KOMBIGLYZE XR
(metformin HCl-saxagliptin)...........638

**DIRECT ACTING SKELETAL
MUSCLE RELAXANT**
DANTRIUM
(dantrolene sodium)....................339
DANTRIUM IV
(dantrolene sodium) 340

DIRECT THROMBIN INHIBITOR
ARGATROBAN
(argatroban) 116

**DNA METHYLTRANSFERASE
INHIBITOR**
DACOGEN
(decitabine) 338

**DOPA-DECARBOXYLASE INHIBITOR/
DOPAMINE PRECURSOR**
PARCOPA
(levodopa-carbidopa) 885
SINEMET CR
(levodopa-carbidopa) 1088

**DOPA-DECARBOXYLASE
INHIBITOR/DOPAMINE PRECURSOR/
COMT INHIBITOR**
STALEVO
(entacapone-levodopa-carbidopa) 1108

**DOPAMINE ANTAGONIST/
PROKINETIC**
REGLAN
(metoclopramide HCl)..................1004

DOPAMINE RECEPTOR AGONIST
AMANTADINE
(amantadine HCl)............................ 69

F

NMDA RECEPTOR ANTAGONIST

NAMENDA
(memantine HCl)............................783

NUEDEXTA
(quinidine sulfate-dextrometho-
rphan hydrobromide) 836

NONBENZODIAZEPINE HYPNOTIC AGENT

LUNESTA
(eszopiclone) 705

NON-ERGOLINE DOPAMINE AGONIST

APOKYN
(apomorphine HCl)......................... 108

REQUIP
(ropinirole HCl) 1015

NON-ERGOT DOPAMINE AGONIST

MIRAPEX
(pramipexole dihydrochloride)........759

NON-HALOGENATED GLUCOCORTICOID

ALVESCO
(ciclesonide) 68

OMNARIS NASAL SPRAY
(ciclesonide) 851

NON-NARCOTIC ANTITUSSIVE

TESSALON
(benzonatate) 1169

NON-NUCLEOSIDE REVERSE TRANSCRIPTASE INHIBITOR

INTELENCE
(etravirine)...................................600

RESCRIPTOR
(delavirdine mesylate) 1016

SUSTIVA
(efavirenz) 1129

VIRAMUNE
(nevirapine) 1294

NON-NUCLEOSIDE REVERSE TRANSCRIPTASE INHIBITOR/ NUCLEOSIDE ANALOG COMBINATION

ATRIPLA
(tenofovir disoproxil fumarate-
emtricitabine-efavirenz) 138

NONSELECTIVE BETA-BLOCKER

BETAGAN
(levobunolol HCl) 187

BETIMOL
(timolol) 191

INDERAL LA
(propranolol HCl)...........................590

INNOPRAN XL
(propranolol HCl) 597

NADOLOL
(nadolol)......................................782

PINDOLOL
(pindolol) 913

PROPRANOLOL
(propranolol HCl)...........................967

TIMOLOL
(timolol maleate)..........................1183

TIMOPTIC
(timolol maleate)..........................1184

NONSELECTIVE BETA-BLOCKER/ ALPHA₁ BLOCKER

LABETALOL
(labetalol HCl) 644

TRANDATE
(labetalol HCl) 1199

NONSTEROIDAL ANTIANDROGEN

CASODEX
(bicalutamide) 242

NILANDRON
(nilutamide) 812

NONSTEROIDAL AROMATASE INHIBITOR

ARIMIDEX
(anastrozole)................................ 119

FEMARA
(letrozole) 488

NSAID

ACULAR
(ketorolac tromethamine).................26

ACULAR LS
(ketorolac tromethamine).................27

ANAPROX DS
(naproxen sodium)......................... 94

ANSAID
(flurbiprofen)................................101

BROMDAY
(bromfenac) 207

CALDOLOR
(ibuprofen) 222

CAMBIA
(diclofenac potassium) 223

CATAFLAM
(diclofenac potassium) 243

DAYPRO
(oxaprozin) 341

ETODOLAC
(etodolac).....................................464

FLECTOR
(diclofenac epolamine).................. 502

INDOMETHACIN
(indomethacin) 591

KETOROLAC
(ketorolac tromethamine)............... 634

MOBIC
(meloxicam)..................................765

MOTRIN
(ibuprofen)...................................770

NABUMETONE
(nabumetone) 781

NAPRELAN
(naproxen sodium).........................784

VISUAL IDENTIFICATION GUIDE*

ABILIFY
RX
(aripiprazole)
BRISTOL-MYERS SQUIBB/OTSUKA

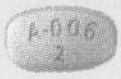

2 mg

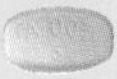

5 mg

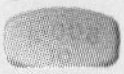

10 mg

15 mg

20 mg

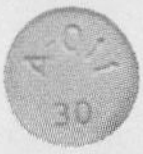

30 mg

Also available in Solution and IM Injection.

ABILIFY DISCMELT
RX
(aripiprazole)
BRISTOL-MYERS SQUIBB/OTSUKA

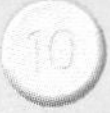

10 mg

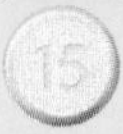

15 mg

Orally Disintegrating Tablets

ACTOS
RX
(pioglitazone HCl)
TAKEDA

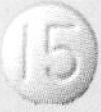

15 mg

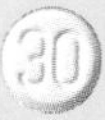

30 mg

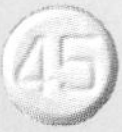

45 mg

ACTOPLUS MET XR
RX
(pioglitazone HCl/metformin HCl)
TAKEDA

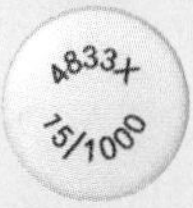

15 mg/1000 mg

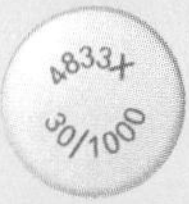

30 mg/1000 mg

Extended-Release Tablets

ADVICOR
RX
(niacin extended-release/lovastatin)
ABBOTT

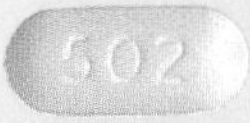

500 mg/20 mg

750 mg/20 mg

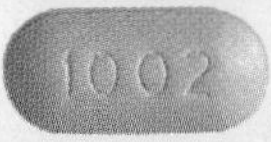

1000 mg/20 mg

1000 mg/40 mg

AFINITOR
RX
(everolimus)
NOVARTIS

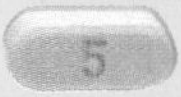

5 mg

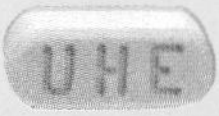

10 mg

Also available in 2.5 mg Tablet.

ALLEGRA
RX
(fexofenadine HCl)
sanofi-aventis

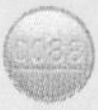

30 mg

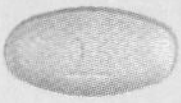

60 mg

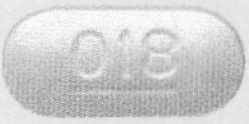

180 mg

ALLEGRA-D 12 HOUR
RX
(fexofenadine HCl/pseudoephedrine HCl)
sanofi-aventis

60 mg/120 mg

Extended-Release Tablets

ALLEGRA-D 24 HOUR
RX
(fexofenadine HCl/pseudoephedrine HCl)
sanofi-aventis

308
AV

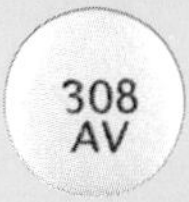

180 mg/240 mg

Extended-Release Tablets

AMBIEN
C-IV
(zolpidem tartrate)
sanofi-aventis

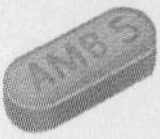

5 mg

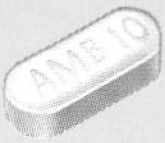

10 mg

*Other dosage forms and strengths may be available.

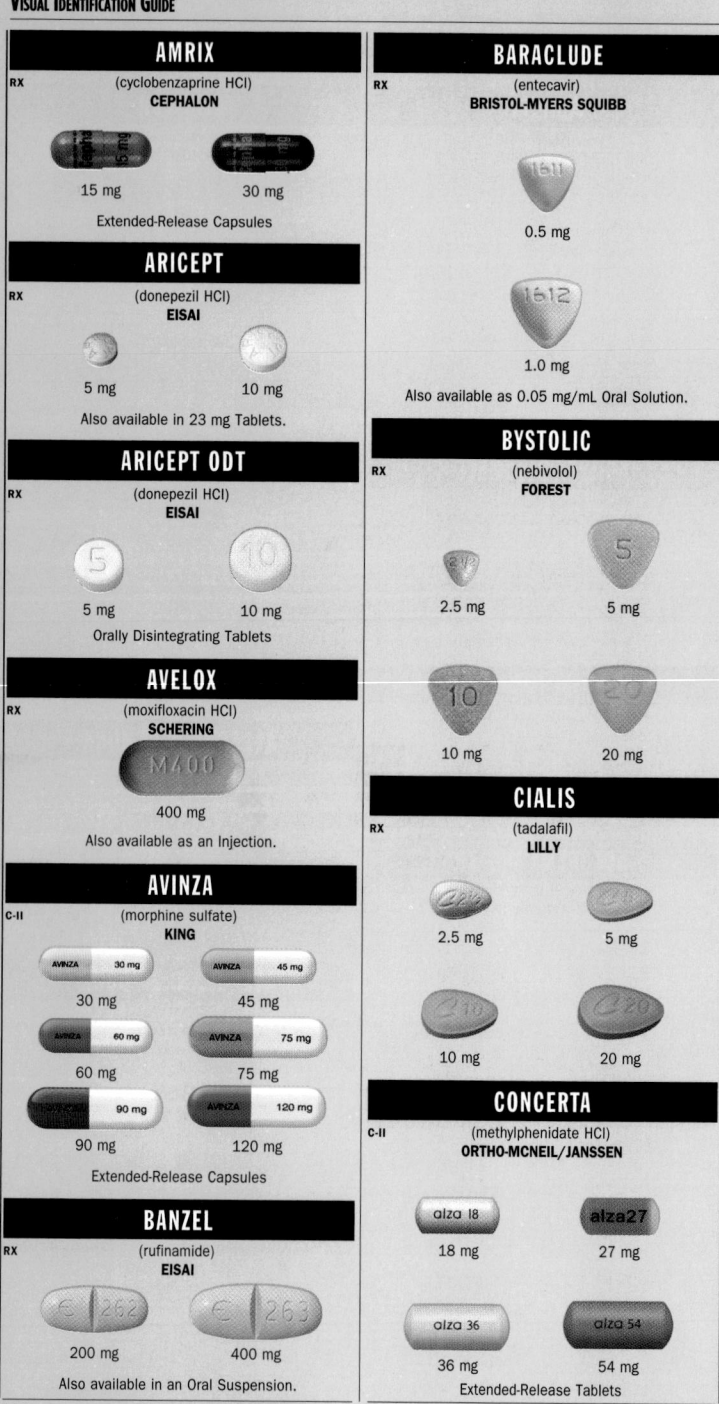

AMRIX

RX

(cyclobenzaprine HCl)
CEPHALON

15 mg   30 mg

Extended-Release Capsules

ARICEPT

RX

(donepezil HCl)
EISAI

5 mg   10 mg

Also available in 23 mg Tablets.

ARICEPT ODT

RX

(donepezil HCl)
EISAI

5 mg   10 mg

Orally Disintegrating Tablets

AVELOX

RX

(moxifloxacin HCl)
SCHERING

400 mg

Also available as an Injection.

AVINZA

C-II

(morphine sulfate)
KING

AVINZA 30 mg   AVINZA 45 mg

30 mg   45 mg

AVINZA 60 mg   AVINZA 75 mg

60 mg   75 mg

90 mg   AVINZA 120 mg

90 mg   120 mg

Extended-Release Capsules

BANZEL

RX

(rufinamide)
EISAI

262   263

200 mg   400 mg

Also available in an Oral Suspension.

BARACLUDE

RX

(entecavir)
BRISTOL-MYERS SQUIBB

1611

0.5 mg

1612

1.0 mg

Also available as 0.05 mg/mL Oral Solution.

BYSTOLIC

RX

(nebivolol)
FOREST

2 1/2   5

2.5 mg   5 mg

10   20

10 mg   20 mg

CIALIS

RX

(tadalafil)
LILLY

2.5 mg   5 mg

C10   C20

10 mg   20 mg

CONCERTA

C-II

(methylphenidate HCl)
ORTHO-MCNEIL/JANSSEN

alza 18   alza27

18 mg   27 mg

alza 36   alza 54

36 mg   54 mg

Extended-Release Tablets